TRATADO DE

Medicina Interna Veterinária

Doenças do **Cão** e do **Gato**

Volume 2

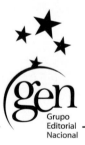

O GEN | Grupo Editorial Nacional – maior plataforma editorial brasileira no segmento científico, técnico e profissional – publica conteúdos nas áreas de ciências da saúde, exatas, humanas, jurídicas e sociais aplicadas, além de prover serviços direcionados à educação continuada e à preparação para concursos.

As editoras que integram o GEN, das mais respeitadas no mercado editorial, construíram catálogos inigualáveis, com obras decisivas para a formação acadêmica e o aperfeiçoamento de várias gerações de profissionais e estudantes, tendo se tornado sinônimo de qualidade e seriedade.

A missão do GEN e dos núcleos de conteúdo que o compõem é prover a melhor informação científica e distribuí-la de maneira flexível e conveniente, a preços justos, gerando benefícios e servindo a autores, docentes, livreiros, funcionários, colaboradores e acionistas.

Nosso comportamento ético incondicional e nossa responsabilidade social e ambiental são reforçados pela natureza educacional de nossa atividade e dão sustentabilidade ao crescimento contínuo e à rentabilidade do grupo.

TRATADO DE

Medicina Interna Veterinária

Doenças do **Cão** e do **Gato**

Volume 2

STEPHEN J. ETTINGER, DVM
DACVIM (Small Animal Internal Medicine and Cardiology)
FACC; FAHA; CCRP

EDWARD C. FELDMAN, DVM
DACVIM (Small Animal Internal Medicine)

ETIENNE CÔTÉ, DVM
DACVIM (Small Animal Internal Medicine and Cardiology)

Oitava edição

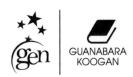

- Os autores deste livro e a editora empenharam seus melhores esforços para assegurar que as informações e os procedimentos apresentados no texto estejam em acordo com os padrões aceitos à época da publicação. Entretanto, tendo em conta a evolução das ciências, as atualizações legislativas, as mudanças regulamentares governamentais e o constante fluxo de novas informações sobre os temas que constam do livro, recomendamos enfaticamente que os leitores consultem sempre outras fontes fidedignas, de modo a se certificarem de que as informações contidas no texto estão corretas e de que não houve alterações nas recomendações ou na legislação regulamentadora.
- Data do fechamento do livro: 29/06/2022.
- Os autores e a editora se empenharam para citar adequadamente e dar o devido crédito a todos os detentores de direitos autorais de qualquer material utilizado neste livro, dispondo-se a possíveis acertos posteriores caso, inadvertida e involuntariamente, a identificação de algum deles tenha sido omitida.
- **Atendimento ao cliente:** (11) 5080-0751 | faleconosco@grupogen.com.br
- Traduzido de:

TEXTBOOK OF VETERINARY INTERNAL MEDICINE: DISEASES OF THE DOG AND THE CAT, EIGHTH EDITION
Copyright © 2017 by Elsevier, Inc. All rights reserved.
Previous editions copyrighted 2010, 2005, 2000, 1995, 1989, 1983, and 1975.

Christopher L. Mariani retains the copyright to his original videos.
Alexander M. Reiter retains the copyright to his original figures.
Angela E. Frimberger and Antony S. Moore retain copyright to their chapter.

Este livro foi produzido pela EDITORA GUANABARA KOOGAN LTDA., sob sua exclusiva responsabilidade. Profissionais da área da Saúde devem fundamentar-se em sua própria experiência e em seu conhecimento para avaliar quaisquer informações, métodos, substâncias ou experimentos descritos nesta publicação antes de empregá-los. O rápido avanço nas Ciências da Saúde requer que diagnósticos e posologias de fármacos, em especial, sejam confirmados em outras fontes confiáveis. Para todos os efeitos legais, a Elsevier, os autores, os editores ou colaboradores relacionados a esta obra não podem ser responsabilizados por qualquer dano ou prejuízo causado a pessoas físicas ou jurídicas em decorrência de produtos, recomendações, instruções ou aplicações de métodos, procedimentos ou ideias contidos neste livro.

This edition of *Textbook of Veterinary Internal Medicine: Diseases of the Dog and the Cat*, 8th Edition, by Stephen J. Ettinger, Edward C. Feldman and Etienne Côté, is published by arrangement with Elsevier Inc.
ISBN: 978-0-323-31211-0
Esta edição de *Textbook of Veterinary Internal Medicine: Diseases of the Dog and the Cat*, 8ª edição, de Stephen J. Ettinger, Edward C. Feldman e Etienne Côté, é publicada por acordo com a Elsevier Inc.

- Direitos exclusivos para a língua portuguesa
Copyright © 2022 by
EDITORA GUANABARA KOOGAN LTDA.
Uma editora integrante do GEN | Grupo Editorial Nacional
Travessa do Ouvidor, 11
Rio de Janeiro – RJ – CEP 20040-040
www.grupogen.com.br

- Reservados todos os direitos. É proibida a duplicação ou reprodução deste volume, no todo ou em parte, em quaisquer formas ou por quaisquer meios (eletrônico, mecânico, gravação, fotocópia, distribuição pela Internet ou outros), sem permissão, por escrito, da EDITORA GUANABARA KOOGAN LTDA.
- Capa: Bruno Sales
- Imagens da capa: iStock (© 1stGallery; © exopixel)
- Editoração eletrônica: Know-how Editorial
- Ficha catalográfica

CIP-BRASIL. Catalogação na Publicação
Sindicato Nacional dos Editores de Livros, RJ

E86
V.2

Ettinger, Stephen J.
Tratado de medicina interna veterinária : doenças do cão e do gato, volume 1 / Stephen J. Ettinger, Edward C. Feldman, Etienne Côté ; [tradução Aloysio Cerqueira ... et al.]]. - 8. ed. - Rio de Janeiro : Guanabara Koogan, 2022.
1.200 p. : il. ; 28 cm.

Tradução de: Textbook of veterinary internal medicine: diseases of the dog and the cat
Inclui bibliografia e índice
encarte colorido
ISBN 9788527736725

1. Medicina veterinária - Manuais, guias, etc. 2. Cães - Doenças. 3. Gatos - Doenças. I. Feldman, Edward C. II. Côté, Etienne. III. Cerqueira, Aloysio. IV. Título.

22-77951
CDD: 636.089
CDU: 636.09

Gabriela Faray Ferreira Lopes - Bibliotecária - CRB-7/6643

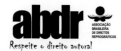

Aquele que estuda medicina sem livros navega em um mar inexplorado,
mas quem estuda medicina sem pacientes não vai para o mar.
Sir William Osler

Com amor, para minha esposa, Pat, e meus filhos,
Ricky, Robbie, Michael, Andrew e Nicole.
Vocês continuam sendo minha inspiração para tudo o que faço.
Steve Ettinger, Los Angeles, CA

Meu amor a Shawn, Rhonda, Shaina e Rowan,
que me deram tempo e apoio incondicional
para seguir meus sonhos.
Edward Feldman, Berkeley, CA

Para Jen e Hélène, com amor e gratidão.
Etienne Côté, Prince Edward Island, Canada

Revisão Técnica

Álan Gomes Pöppl (Capítulos 186 a 194, 266 a 270, 313 a 315, 317 a 320, 357 a 360)

Médico-veterinário. Residência em Clínica e Cirurgia de Pequenos Animais. Mestre em Ciências Biológicas: Fisiologia. Doutor em Ciências Veterinárias. Professor no Departamento de Medicina Animal da Faculdade de Veterinária da Universidade Federal do Rio Grande do Sul (UFRGS). Coordenador do Programa de Residência em Clínica Médica de Pequenos Animais do Hospital de Clínicas Veterinárias (HCV) da UFRGS. Coordenador do Serviço de Endocrinologia e Metabologia do HCV-UFRGS. Sócio Fundador e atual Diretor Científico da Associação Brasileira de Endocrinologia Veterinária (ABEV).

José Jurandir Fagliari (Capítulos 1 a 84, 91 a 103, 105 a 112, 115 a 119, 132 a 159, 178 a 185, 207 a 257, 280 a 300, 329 a 356)

Especialista em Patologia Clínica Veterinária e Mestre em Medicina Veterinária, área de concentração em Patologia Clínica Veterinária, pela Escola de Veterinária da Universidade Federal de Minas Gerais (UFMG). Doutor em Medicina Veterinária, área de concentração em Clínica: Fisiopatologia Médica, pela Faculdade de Medicina Veterinária e Zootecnia da Universidade

Estadual Paulista (Unesp), Campus de Botucatu. Pós-doutorado em Clínica e Patologia Clínica Veterinária no Department of Veterinary Pathobiology da University of Minnesota, EUA. Professor Titular da disciplina Semiologia Veterinária do Departamento de Clínica e Cirurgia Veterinária da Faculdade de Ciências Agrárias e Veterinárias da Unesp, Campus de Jaboticabal.

Thaís Rocha (Capítulos 85 a 90, 120 a 131, 160 a 177, 195 a 206, 258 a 265, 301 a 312, 316, 321)

Professora Titular de Semiologia e Clínica de Animais de Grande Porte na Universidade Vilha Velha (UVV/ES). Doutora em Clínica Médica Veterinária pela Faculdade de Ciências Agrárias e Veterinárias da Universidade Estadual Paulista (FCAV/Unesp), Jaboticabal. Mestre em Clínica Médica Veterinária pela FCAV/Unesp, Jaboticabal. Residência em Clínica Médica de Grandes Animais na FCAV/Unesp, Jaboticabal. Médica Veterinária pela Universidade Federal Rural do Rio de Janeiro (UFRRJ).

Vanessa Uemura da Fonseca (Capítulos 104, 113, 114, 271 a 279, 322 a 328)

Mestre em Ciências pela Faculdade de Medicina Veterinária e Zootecnia da Universidade de São Paulo (FMVZ-USP).

Tradução

Aloysio de Mello Figueiredo Cerqueira (Capítulos 271 a 279)

Angela Satie Nishikaku (Capítulo 8)

Douglas Futuro (Capítulos 136 a 150, 160 a 169)

Etiele Maldonado Gomes (Capítulos 6, 38 a 47, 170 a 194)

Felipe Gazza Romão (Capítulos 280 a 311, 321 a 360)

Flávia Thomaz Verechia Rodrigues (Capítulos 207 a 236)

Gabrielle Campos (Capítulos 7, 29 a 37, 151 a 156, 195 a 206)

Idilia Vanzellotti (Capítulos 1, 240 a 249)

Márcia Arêas Rédua (Capítulos 11, 250 a 270)

Mariângela Vidal Sampaio Fernandes (Capítulos 104 a 119)

Novaes Filho, L. F. (Capítulos 312 a 320)

Renata Scavone de Oliveira (Capítulos 3 e 4)

Roberta Martins Crivelaro (Capítulos 15 a 28, 65 a 91)

Roberto Thiesen (Capítulos 2, 5, 9, 10, 12 a 14, 48 a 64, 92 a 103, 120 a 135, 157 a 159, 237 a 239)

Editores

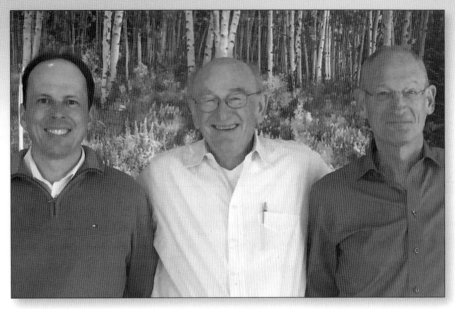

ETIENNE CÔTÉ STEPHEN J. ETTINGER EDWARD C. FELDMAN

Stephen J. Ettinger, DVM
DACVIM (Small Animal Internal Medicine and Cardiology)
FACC; FAHA; CCRP
Doctor Honoris Causa (University of Veterinary Medicine Bucharest)
VetCorp, Inc.
Los Angeles, California

Edward C. Feldman, DVM
DACVIM (Small Animal Internal Medicine)
Emeritus Professor of Small Animal Internal Medicine
University of California, Davis
Davis, California

Etienne Côté, DVM
DACVIM (Small Animal Internal Medicine and Cardiology)
Professor
3M National Teaching Fellow
Department of Companion Animals
Atlantic Veterinary College
University of Prince Edward Island
Charlottetown, PE, Canada

Material suplementar

Este livro conta com o seguinte material suplementar:

- Mais de 500 vídeos originais
- Referências bibliográficas

O acesso ao material suplementar é gratuito. Basta que o leitor se cadastre e faça seu *login* em nosso *site* (www.grupogen.com.br), clique no menu superior do lado direito e, após, em Ambiente de aprendizagem. Em seguida, clique no menu retrátil [≣] e insira o código (PIN) de acesso localizado na primeira capa interna deste livro.

O acesso ao material suplementar online fica disponível até seis meses após a edição do livro ser retirada do mercado.

Caso haja alguma mudança no sistema ou dificuldade de acesso, entre em contato conosco (gendigital@grupogen.com.br).

Consultores de seção

Agradecimentos especiais aos consultores de seção, que forneceram novas sugestões para os autores e tópicos para suas respectivas seções.

Os editores

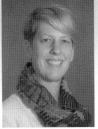

Vanessa R. Barrs, BVSc (Hons), PhD, MVetClinStud, FANZCVS (Feline Medicine), GradCertEd
Professor of Feline Medicine and Infectious Diseases, Faculty of Veterinary Science, School of Life and Environmental Sciences The University of Sydney, Sydney, NSW, Australia.
Seção 13, Doenças Infecciosas

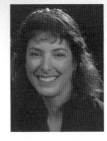

Lisa M. Freeman, DVM, PhD, DACVN
Professor, Department of Clinical Sciences, Cummings School of Veterinary Medicine, Tufts University, North Grafton, Massachusetts.
Seção 11, Considerações Dietéticas de Distúrbios Sistêmicos

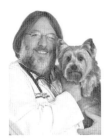

Joseph W. Bartges, DVM, PhD, DACVIM (Small Animal Internal Medicine), DACVN
Professor of Medicine and Nutrition, Department of Small Animal Medicine and Surgery, College of Veterinary Medicine The University of Georgia, Athens, Georgia.
Seção 24, Doenças do Trato Urinário Inferior

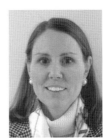

Ann E. Hohenhaus, DVM, DACVIM (Oncology and Small Animal Internal Medicine)
Staff Veterinarian, The Animal Medical Center, New York, New York.
Seção 12, Doenças Hematológicas e Imunológicas

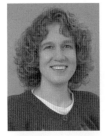

Leah A. Cohn, DVM, PhD, DACVIM, (Small Animal Internal Medicine)
Professor of Veterinary Medicine, Department of Veterinary Medicine and Surgery, Veterinary Health Center, University of Missouri, Columbia, Missouri.
Seção 15, Doença Respiratória

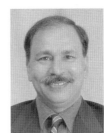

Safdar A. Khan, DVM, MS, PhD, DABVT
Senior Director of Toxicology Research, ASPCA Animal Poison Control Center, Adjunct Toxicology Instructor, College of Veterinary Medicine, University of Illinois, Urbana, Illinois.
Seção 8, Toxicologia

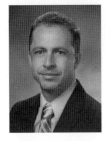

Ronaldo Casimiro da Costa, DMV, MSc, PhD, DACVIM (Neurology)
Professor and Service Head, Neurology and Neurosurgery, Veterinary Clinical Sciences The Ohio State University, Columbus, Ohio.
Seção 17, Doença Neurológica

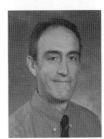

Mark G. Papich, DVM, MS, DACVCP
Professor of Clinical Pharmacology, College of Veterinary Medicine, North Carolina State University, Raleigh, North Carolina.
Seção 10, Considerações Terapêuticas em Medicina e Doença

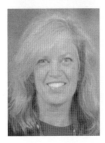

Autumn P. Davidson, DVM, MS, DACVIM (Small Animal Internal Medicine)
Clinical Professor, Veterinary Medical Teaching Hospital, School of Veterinary Medicine, University of California, Davis, California.
Seção 22, Doenças Reprodutivas

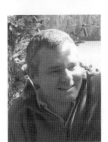

Jörg M. Steiner, med.vet., Dr.med. vet., PhD, DACVIM (Small Animal Internal Medicine), DECVIM-CA, AGAF
Professor and Director, Gastrointestinal Laboratory, Department of Small Animal Clinical Sciences, College of Veterinary Medicine and, Biomedical Sciences, Texas A&M University, College Station, Texas.
Seção 20, Doenças Pancreáticas

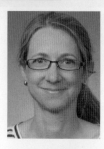

Jane E. Sykes, BVSc (Hons), PhD, DACVIM (Small Animal Internal Medicine)
Medicine & Epidemiology University of California, Davis, California.
Seção 13, Doenças Infecciosas

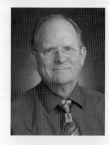

David Twedt, DVM, DACVIM (Small Animal Internal Medicine)
Professor, Department of Clinical Sciences, College of Veterinary Medicine and Biomedical Sciences, Colorado State University, Fort Collins, Colorado.
Seção 19, Doenças Hepatobiliares

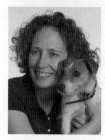

Harriet M. Syme, BSc, BVetMed, PhD, FHEA, DACVIM (Small Animal Internal Medicine), DECVIM, MRCVS
Professor of Small Animal Internal Medicine, Department of Clinical Sciences and Services, Royal Veterinary College, University of London, North Mymms, Hatfield, Hertfordshire, United Kingdom.
Seção 23, Doenças Renais

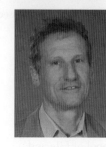

David M. Vail, DVM, MS, DACVIM (Oncology)
Professor and Barbara A. Suran Chair in Comparative Oncology, Department of Medical Sciences, School of Veterinary Medicine, University of Wisconsin-Madison, Madison, Wisconsin.
Seção 25, Câncer

Colaboradores

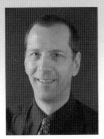

Anthony C.G. Abrams-Ogg, DVM, DVSc, DACVIM (Small Animal Internal Medicine)
Professor
Department of Clinical Studies
Ontario Veterinary College
University of Guelph
Guelph, Ontario, Canada

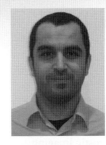

Suliman Al-Ghazlat, DVM, DACVIM (Small Animal Internal Medicine)
Small Animal Internist
Internal Medicine
BluePearl Veterinary Partners
New York, New York

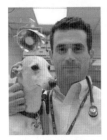

Mark J. Acierno, MBA, DVM, DACVIM (Small Animal Internal Medicine)
Professor
Department of Veterinary Clinical Science
Louisiana State University
Baton Rouge, Louisiana

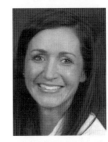

Erin Anderson, VMD, MSc, DACVIM (Cardiology)
Staff Cardiologist
Pittsburgh Veterinary Specialty and
    Emergency Center
Pittsburgh, Pennsylvania

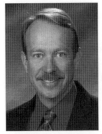

Larry G. Adams, DVM, PhD, DACVIM (Small Animal Internal Medicine)
Professor
Veterinary Clinical Sciences
Purdue University
West Lafayette, Indiana

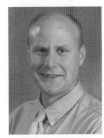

Todd M. Archer, DVM, MS, DACVIM (Small Animal Internal Medicine)
Assistant Professor and Service Chief,
    Small Animal Internal Medicine
Department of Clinical Sciences
Mississippi State University College of
    Veterinary Medicine
Mississippi State, Mississippi

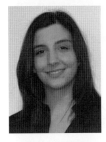

Maria Manuel Afonso, DVM, MScVet
PhD Candidate
Institute of Infection and Global Health
University of Liverpool, Leahurst Campus
Neston, Cheshire, United Kingdom

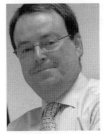

David John Argyle, BVMS, PhD, DECVIM-CA (Oncology), MRCVS
William Dick Professor of Veterinary
    Clinical Studies
Dean of Veterinary Medicine
Royal (Dick) School of Veterinary Studies
The University of Edinburgh Hospital for
    Small Animals
Edinburgh, Scotland, United Kingdom

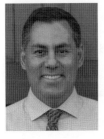

Ale Aguirre, DVM, DACVIM (Small Animal Internal Medicine)
Owner and Hospital Director
Internal Medicine and Interventional
    Radiology
Salt River Veterinary Specialists
Scottsdale, Arizona

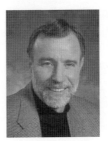

Clarke Atkins, DVM, DACVIM (Small Animal Internal Medicine and Cardiology)
Jane Lewis Seaks Distinguished Professor
    of Companion Animal Medicine,
    Emeritus
College of Veterinary Medicine
North Caroline State University
Raleigh, North Carolina

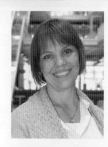

Eva Agneta Axnér, DVM, PhD, DECAR
Professor
Department of Clinical Sciences
Swedish University of Agricultural Sciences
Uppsala, Sweden

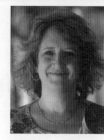

Ellen N. Behrend, VMD, PhD, DACVIM (Small Animal Internal Medicine)
Joezy Griffin Professor
Department of Clinical Sciences
Auburn University
Auburn, Alabama

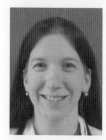

Kerry Smith Bailey, DVM, DACVIM (Neurology)
Staff Neurologist
Neurology
Oradell Animal Hospital
Ramsey, New Jersey

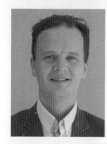

Niek J. Beijerink, DVM, PhD, DECVIM (Cardiology)
Senior Lecturer
School of Life and Environment Sciences,
  Faculty of Veterinary Science
University of Sydney
Sydney, NSW, Australia

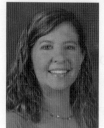

Elizabeth A. Ballegeer, BS, DVM, DACVR
Assistant Professor, Diagnostic Imaging
College of Veterinary Medicine
Michigan State University
East Lansing, Michigan;
IDEXX Telemedicine Consultants
Westbrook, Maine

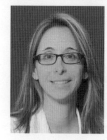

Marie-Claude Bélanger, DMV, MSc, DACVIM (Small Animal Internal Medicine)
Professor of Small Animal Internal
  Medicine and Cardiology
Clinical Sciences
University of Montreal
St-Hyacinthe, Quebec, Canada

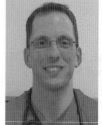

Matthew W. Beal, DVM, DACVECC
Professor
Emergency & Critical Care Medicine
Department of Small Animal Clinical
  Sciences
College of Veterinary Medicine
Michigan State University
East Lansing, Michigan

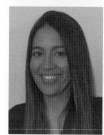

Elsa Beltran, Ldo Vet, DECVN, MRCVS
Lecturer in Veterinary Neurology and
  Neurosurgery
Department of Clinical Science and
  Services
The Royal Veterinary College, University
  of London
North Mymms, Hatfield, United Kingdom

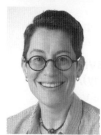

Julia A. Beatty, BSc (Hons), BVetMed, PhD, FANZCVSc (Feline Medicine)
Professor of Feline Medicine
Faculty of Veterinary Science
University of Sydney
Sydney, NSW, Australia

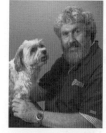

Peter Bennett, BVSc, FANZCVS, DACVIM (Oncology, Small Animal Internal Medicine)
Clinical Specialist in Oncology and Small
  Animal Medicine
Veterinary Teaching Hospital Sydney
University of Sydney
Sydney, NSW, Australia

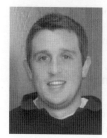

David P. Beehan, MVB (Hons), MS, DACT
Veterinary Inspector
Irish Department of Agriculture, Food and
  the Marine
Dublin, Ireland

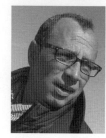

Emmanuel Bensignor, DVM, DECVD, DESV (Dermatology)
Dermatology
Clinique La Boulais
Rennes-Cesson, France;
Dermatology
Veterinary Clinic Paris 3
Paris, France;
Dermatology
Veterinary Hospital Atlantia
Nantes, France

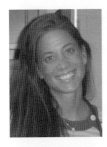

Allyson C. Berent, DVM, DACVIM (Small Animal Internal Medicine)
Staff Veterinarian, Interventional Radiology/Medicine
Director of Interventional Endoscopy
The Animal Medical Center
New York, New York

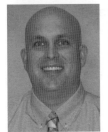

Darren Berger, DVM, DACVD
Assistant Professor of Dermatology
Veterinary Clinical Sciences
Iowa State University
Ames, Iowa

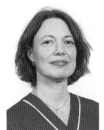

Annika Bergström, DVM, PhD, DECVS
Senior Lecturer
Department of Clinical Sciences
Faculty of Veterinary Medicine and Animal Sciences
Uppsala, Sweden

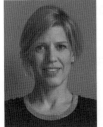

Alexa M.E. Bersenas, DVM, MS, DACVECC
Associate Professor
Department of Clinical Studies
Ontario Veterinary College, University of Guelph
Guelph, Ontario, Canada

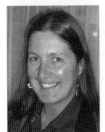

Sonya V. Bettenay, BVSc (Hons), DEd, FANZCVS, DECVD
Dermatologie Department
Fachklinik Haas & Link
Germering, Germany

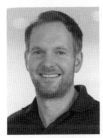

Nick Bexfield, BVetMed, PhD, DSAM, DECVIM-CA (Internal Medicine), FRSB, AFHEA, MRCVS
Clinical Associate Professor in Small Animal Medicine and Oncology
School of Veterinary Medicine and Science
University of Nottingham
Sutton Bonington, Leicestershire, United Kingdom

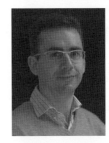

Frédéric Billen, DVM, MSc, PhD, DECVIM-CA (Internal Medicine)
Senior Lecturer in Internal Medicine of Companion Animals
Department of Clinical Sciences of Companion Animals and Equine
Faculty of Veterinary Medicine, University of Liege
Liege, Belgium

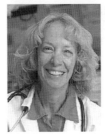

Barbara J. Biller, DVM, PhD, DACVIM (Oncology)
Associate Professor of Oncology
Clinical Sciences
Colorado State University
College of Veterinary Medicine and Biomedical Sciences
James L. Voss Veterinary Teaching Hospital
Flint Animal Cancer Center
Fort Collins, Colorado

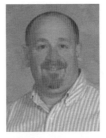

David S. Biller, DVM, DACVR
Professor
Department of Clinical Sciences
College of Veterinary Medicine
Kansas State University
Manhattan, Kansas

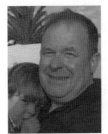

Vincent C. Biourge, DVM, PhD, DACVN, DECVCN
Health and Nutrition Scientific Director
R&D
Royal Canin
Aimargues, France

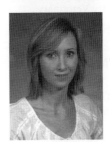

Petra Bizikova, MVDr, PhD, DECVD, DACVD
Assistant Professor of Dermatology
Department of Clinical Sciences
North Carolina State University
Raleigh, North Carolina

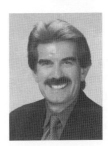

Byron L. Blagburn, MS, PhD
Distinguished University Professor
Department of Pathobiology
College of Veterinary Medicine
Auburn University
Auburn, Alabama

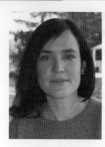
Shauna Blois, DVM, DVSc, DACVIM (Small Animal Internal Medicine)
Associate Professor
Clinical Sciences
Ontario Veterinary College, University of Guelph
Guelph, Ontario, Canada

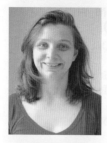
Amanda K. Boag, MA, VetMB, DECVECC, DACVECC, DACVIM (Small Animal Internal Medicine), FHEA, MRCVS
Clinical Director
Vets Now
Dunfermline, Fife, United Kingdom

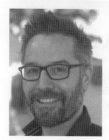
Manuel Boller, Dr.med.vet., MTR, DACVECC
Senior Lecturer, Veterinary Emergency and Critical Care
Faculty of Veterinary and Agricultural Sciences
University of Melbourne
Melbourne, Victoria, Australia;
Veterinary Emergency and Critical Care Service
UVet Werribee Hospital
Werribee, Victoria, Australia

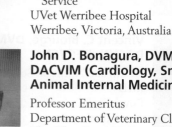
John D. Bonagura, DVM, MS, DACVIM (Cardiology, Small Animal Internal Medicine)
Professor Emeritus
Department of Veterinary Clinical Sciences
The Ohio State University
Attending Cardiologist
Cardiology and Interventional Medicine
The Ohio State University Veterinary Medical Center
Columbus, Ohio

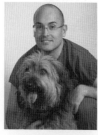
Juan F. Borrego, DVM, DACVIM (Oncology)
Head of the Oncology Department
Hospital Aúna Especialidades Veterinarias
Director
Instituto Veterinario de Oncología Comparada
Valencia, Spain

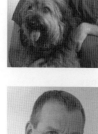
Adrian Boswood, MA, VetMB, DVC, DECVIM-CA (Cardiology), MRCVS
Professor of Veterinary Cardiology
Clinical Science and Services
The Royal Veterinary College
London, United Kingdom

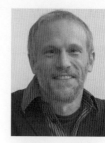
Søren Boysen, DVM, DACVECC
Professor
Veterinary Clinical and Diagnostic Sciences
University of Calgary, Faculty of Veterinary Medicine
Calgary, Alberta, Canada

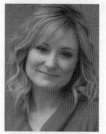
Christina Alanna Bradbury, DVM, MS, DACVIM (Small Animal Internal Medicine)
Staff Internist
Vista Veterinary Specialists
Sacramento, California

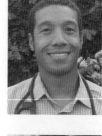
Allison Bradley, DVM, DACVIM (Small Animal Internal Medicine)
Small Animal Internal Medicine
VCA Veterinary Specialists of Northern Colorado
Loveland, Colorado

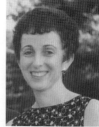
Fred C. Brewer, IV, DVM, DACVIM (Cardiology)
Owner
California Pet Cardiology
Long Beach, California

Marjory B. Brooks, DVM, DACVIM (Small Animal Internal Medicine)
Director, Comparative Coagulation Section
Population Medicine & Diagnostic Sciences
Animal Health Diagnostic Center, Cornell University
Ithaca, New York

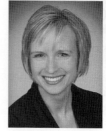
Ahna G. Brutlag, DVM, MS, DABT, DABVT
Associate Director of Veterinary Services & Senior Veterinary Toxicologist
Pet Poison Helpline & SafetyCall International, PLLC
Minneapolis, Minnesota;
Adjunct Assistant Professor
Department of Veterinary and Biomedical Sciences
College of Veterinary Medicine, University of Minnesota
St. Paul, Minnesota

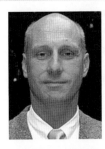

Steven C. Budsberg, DVM, MS, DACVS
Director of Clinical Research
Professor
Small Animal Medicine and Surgery
College of Veterinary Medicine, University of Georgia
Athens, Georgia

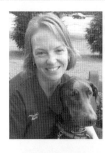

Amanda Callens, BS, LVT
Veterinary Technician
BluePearl Veterinary Partners Seattle
Seattle, Washington

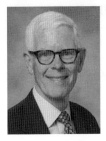

C.A. Tony Buffington, DVM, PhD, DACVN
Emeritus Professor
Veterinary Clinical Sciences
The Ohio State University
Columbus, Ohio

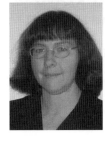

Karen L. Campbell, DVM, MS, DACVIM (Small Animal Internal Medicine), DACVD
Adjunct Clinical Professor and Dermatology Section Head
MU Veterinary Health Center at Wentzville
University of Missouri College of Veterinary Medicine
Columbia, Missouri;
Professor Emerita
Department of Veterinary Clinical Medicine
University of Illinois College of Veterinary Medicine
Urbana, Illinois

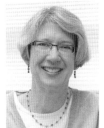

Shelley Burton, DVM, MSc, DACVP
Professor of Clinical Pathology
Department of Pathology and Microbiology
Atlantic Veterinary College, University of Prince Edward Island
Charlottetown, PE, Canada

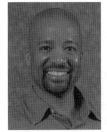

Stephan Anthony Carey, DVM, PhD, DACVIM (Small Animal Internal Medicine)
Assistant Professor
Department of Small Animal Clinical Sciences, College of Veterinary Medicine
Veterinary Medical Center
Michigan State University
East Lansing, Michigan

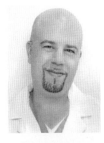

Christopher G. Byers, DVM, DACVECC, DACVIM (Small Animal Internal Medicine), CVJ
Medical Director
VCA Midwest Veterinary Specialists of Omaha
Omaha, Nebraska

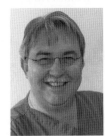

Didier-Noël Carlotti, Doct-Vét, DECVD (*in memoriam*)
Clinique Vétérinaire Aquivet, Parc d'Activités
Mermoz, Eysines
Bordeaux, France

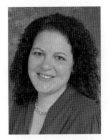

Julie K. Byron, DVM, MS, DACVIM (Small Animal Internal Medicine)
Associate Professor-Clinical
Veterinary Clinical Sciences
The Ohio State University
Columbus, Ohio

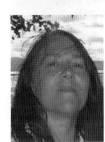

Margret L. Casal, Dr.med.vet., PhD, DECAR
Associate Professor of Medical Genetics
School of Veterinary Medicine
University of Pennsylvania
Philadelphia, Pennsylvania

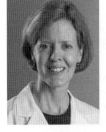

Mary Beth Callan, VMD, DACVIM (Small Animal Internal Medicine)
Professor of Medicine
Department of Clinical Studies
School of Veterinary Medicine
University of Pennsylvania
Philadelphia, Pennsylvania

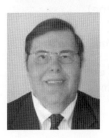

James L. Catalfamo, MS, PhD
Department of Population Medicine and Diagnostic Sciences
College of Veterinary Medicine
Cornell University
Ithaca, New York

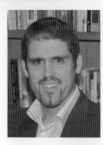

Nick John Cave, BVSc, MVSc, MANZCVS, PhD, DACVN
Senior Lecturer in Small Animal Medicine and Nutrition
Institute of Veterinary, Animal and Biomedical Sciences
Te Kunenga Ki Pūrehuroa
Massey University
Palmerston North, New Zealand

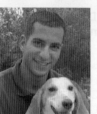

Serge Chalhoub, DVM, DACVIM (Small Animal Internal Medicine)
Instructor
Veterinary Clinical and Diagnostic Sciences
Faculty of Veterinary Medicine, University of Calgary
Calgary, Alberta, Canada

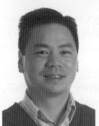

Daniel L. Chan, DVM, DACVECC, DECVECC, DACVN, FHEA, MRCVS
Professor of Emergency and Critical Care Medicine and Clinical Nutrition
Clinical Science and Services
The Royal Veterinary College, University of London
North Mymms, Hertfordshire, United Kingdom

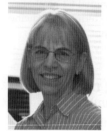

Marjorie Chandler, DVM, MS, MANZCVS, DACVN, DACVIM (Small Animal Internal Medicine), DECVIM-CA, MRCVS
Honorary Senior Lecturer in Small Animal Medicine and Clinical Nutrition
Internal Medicine
University of Edinburgh
Edinburgh, Scotland, United Kingdom;
Clinical Nutritionist
Clinical Nutrition
Vets Now Referrals
Glasgow, Scotland, United Kingdom

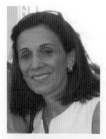

Valérie Chetboul, DVM, PhD, DECVIM-CA (Cardiology)
Professor of Cardiology
Alfort Cardiology Unit (UCA)
Centre Hospitalier Universitaire Vétérinaire d'Alfort (CHUVA)
Ecole Nationale Vétérinaire d'Alfort
Maisons-Alfort, France

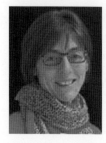

Cécile Clercx, DVM, PhD, DECVIM-CA (Internal Medicine)
Professor
Internal Medicine of Companion Animals
Department of Clinical Sciences of Companion Animals and Equids
CVU, Companion Animals Pôle
University of Liège
Liege, Belgium

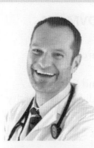

Craig A. Clifford, DVM, MS, DACVIM (Oncology)
Director of Clinical Studies
Oncology
Hope Veterinary Specialists
Malvern, Pennsylvania

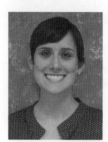

Martha G. Cline, DVM, DACVN
Clinical Veterinary Nutritionist
Department of Clinical Nutrition
Red Bank Veterinary Hospital
Tinton Falls, New Jersey

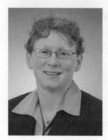

Joan R. Coates, BS, DVM, MS, DACVIM (Neurology)
Full Professor
Department of Veterinary Medicine and Surgery
Service Leader
Neurology and Neurosurgery Service
Veterinary Health Center (Small Animal Hospital), College of Veterinary Medicine
University of Missouri
Columbia, Missouri

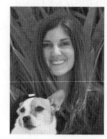

Sarah Cocker, DVM
Internal Medicine Resident
Internal Medicine
The Veterinary Specialty Hospital
San Diego, California

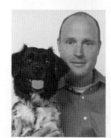

Ronald Jan Corbee, DVM, PhD, DECVCN
Assistant Professor
Clinical Sciences of Companion Animals
Utrecht University, Faculty of Veterinary Medicine
Utrecht, The Netherlands

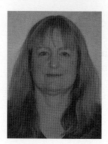

Susan Cox, RVT, VTS (Small Animal Internal Medicine)
Small Animal Internal Medicine Technician
Small Animal Internal Medicine Service
William R. Pritchard Veterinary Medical Teaching Hospital
University of California, Davis
Davis, California

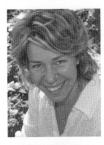

Sylvie Daminet, DVM, PhD, MSc, DECVIM-CA (Internal Medicine), DACVIM (Small Animal Internal Medicine)
Professor
Department of Companion Animals
Faculty of Veterinary Medicine
Ghent University
Merelbeke, Belgium

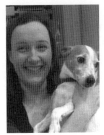

Lucy J. Davison, MA, VetMB, PhD, DSAM, DECVIM-CA (Internal Medicine), MRCVS
University Lecturer in Genetics and Small Animal Medicine
Department of Veterinary Medicine
The Queen's Veterinary School Hospital
University of Cambridge
Cambridge, United Kingdom;
Wellcome Trust Veterinary Postdoctoral Fellow
Wellcome Trust Centre for Human Genetics
University of Oxford
Oxford, United Kingdom

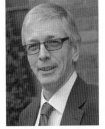

Michael J. Day, BSc, BVMs (Hons), PhD, DSc, DECVP, FASM, FRCPath, FRCVS
Professor of Veterinary Pathology
School of Veterinary Sciences
University of Bristol
Langford, North Somerset, United Kingdom

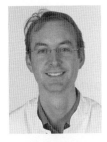

Jeffrey de Gier, DVM, PhD, DECAR-CA
Assistant Professor
Department of Clinical Sciences of Companion Animals
Faculty of Veterinary Medicine, Utrecht University
Utrecht, The Netherlands

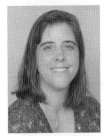

Armelle de Laforcade, DVM, DACVECC
Associate Professor
Department of Clinical Sciences
Tufts Cummings School of Veterinary Medicine
North Grafton, Massachusetts

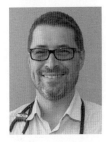

Louis-Philippe de Lorimier, DVM, DACVIM (Oncology)
Staff Medical Oncologist
Oncology Service
Centre Vétérinaire Rive-Sud
Brossard, Quebec, Canada

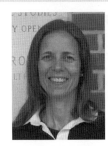

Luisa De Risio, DMV, MRCVS, PhD, DECVN, European and RCVS Recognized Veterinary Specialist in Neurology
Head of Neurology/Neurosurgery
Head of Research-Clinics
Neurology/Neurosurgery Service, Center for Small Animal Studies
Animal Health Trust
Newmarket, Suffolk, United Kingdom

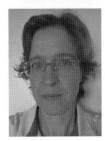

Hilde de Rooster, DVM, MVM, PhD, DECVS
Professor Doctor
Small Animal Medicine and Clinical Biology
Faculty of Veterinary Medicine, Ghent University
Merelbeke, Belgium

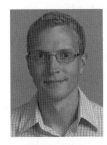

Jonathan D. Dear, DVM, DACVIM (Small Animal Internal Medicine)
Assistant Professor of Clinical Internal Medicine
Medicine & Epidemiology
University of California, Davis
Davis, California

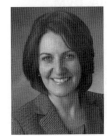

Camille DeClementi, VMD, DABT, DABVT
Adjunct Instructor
Department of Veterinary Biosciences
University of Illinois, College of Veterinary Medicine
Urbana, Illinois;
Senior Director
Animal Health Sciences
American Society for the Prevention of Animal Cruelty (ASPCA)
New York, New York

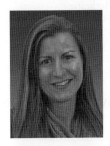

Amy E. DeClue, DVM, MS, DACVIM (Small Animal Internal Medicine)
Associate Professor
College of Veterinary Medicine
University of Missouri
Columbia, Missouri

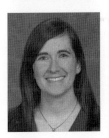

Andrea Dedeaux, DVM
Internal Medicine Resident
Department of Veterinary Clinical Sciences
Louisiana State University
Baton Rouge, Louisiana

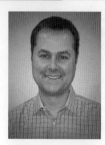

Sean J. Delaney, DVM, MS, DACVN
Founder
Balance IT, A DBA of DVM Consulting, Inc.
Davis, California

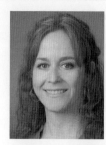

Katie Douthitt, RVT
Small Animal Clinic Medicine Services
Veterinary Medicine Teaching Hospital
University of California, Davis
Davis, California

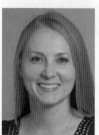

Ann-Marie Della Maggiore, DVM, DACVIM (Small Animal Internal Medicine)
Assistant Professor of Clinical Internal
   Medicine
School of Veterinary Medicine,
   Department of Medicine and
   Epidemiology
University of California, Davis
Davis, California

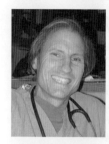

Kenneth J. Drobatz, DVM, MSCE, DACVIM (Small Animal Internal Medicine), DACVECC
Professor and Section Chief, Critical Care
School of Veterinary Medicine
Director, Emergency Services
Matthew J. Ryan Veterinary Hospital
University of Pennsylvania
Philadelphia, Pennsylvania

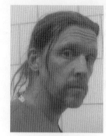

Curtis W. Dewey, DVM, MS, DACVIM (Neurology), DACVS
Associate Professor and Section Chief,
   Neurology/Neurosurgery
Department of Clinical Sciences
Cornell University
Ithaca, New York

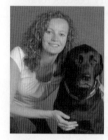

Marilyn E. Dunn, DMV, MVSc, DACVIM (Small Animal Internal Medicine)
Professor
Department of Clinical Sciences
University of Montreal
St-Hyacinthe, Quebec, Canada

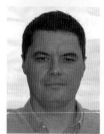

Ryan M. Dickinson, BA, DVM, DACVP
Assistant Professor
Department of Veterinary Pathology
Western College of Veterinary Medicine,
   University of Saskatchewan
Saskatoon, SK, Canada
*Cytology of the Skin and Subcutaneous
   Tissues*

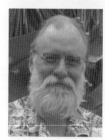

David A. Dzanis, DVM, PhD, DACVN
Chief Executive Officer
Regulatory Discretion, Inc.
Santa Clarita, California

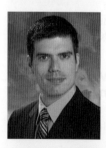

Pedro Paulo V.P. Diniz, DVM, PhD
Associate Professor of Small Animal
   Internal Medicine
College of Veterinary Medicine
Western University of Health Sciences
Pomona, California

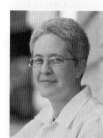

Melissa L. Edwards, DVM, DACVECC
Douglas, Alaska

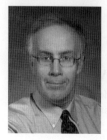

David C. Dorman, DVM, PhD
Professor of Toxicology
Department of Molecular Biomedical
   Sciences
North Carolina State University
Raleigh, North Carolina

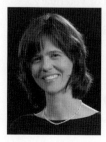

Laura Eirmann, DVM, DACVN
Clinical Nutritionist
Nutrition
Oradell Animal Hospital
Paramus, New Jersey;
Veterinary Communications Manager
Nestlé Purina PetCare
St. Louis, Missouri

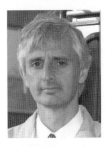

Gary C.W. England, BVetMed, PhD, DVetMed, DVR, DVRep, DECAR, DACT, FHEA, FRCVS
Foundation Dean & Professor of Comparative Veterinary Reproduction
School of Veterinary Medicine & Science
University of Nottingham
Loughborough, Leicestershire, United Kingdom

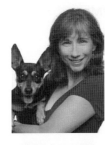

Deborah M. Fine-Ferreira, DVM, MS, DACVIM (Cardiology)
Cardiologist
Ali'i Veterinary Hospital
Kailua-Kona, Hawaii;
Cardiologist
Veterinary Emergency and Referral Center
Honolulu, Hawaii

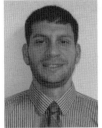

Steven Epstein, DVM, DACVECC
Assistant Professor of Clinical Small Animal Emergency and Critical Care
Department of Surgical and Radiological Sciences
University of California, Davis
Davis, California

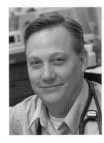

Daniel John Fletcher, PhD, DVM, DACVECC
Associate Professor of Emergency and Critical Care
Clinical Sciences
Cornell University College of Veterinary Medicine
Ithaca, New York

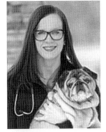

Chelsie Estey, MSc, DVM, DACVIM (Neurology)
Neurology/Neurosurgery Service
Upstate Veterinary Specialties
Latham, New York

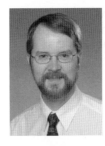

Peter Foley, MSc, DVM, DACVIM (Small Animal Internal Medicine)
Assistant Professor
Department of Companion Animals
Atlantic Veterinary College
University of Prince Edward Island
Charlottetown, PE, Canada

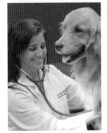

Amara H. Estrada, DVM, DACVIM (Cardiology)
Associate Professor and Associate Chair for Instruction
Department of Small Animal Clinical Sciences
Director of Teaching Academy
College of Veterinary Medicine
University of Florida
Gainesville, Florida

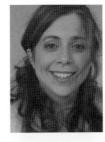

Yaiza Forcada, DVM, PhD, DECVIM-CA (Internal Medicine)
Lecturer in Small Animal Internal Medicine
Clinical Sciences and Services
The Royal Veterinary College
North Mymms, Hertfordshire, United Kingdom

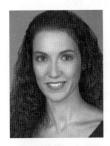

Amy Farcas, DVM, MS, DACVN
Owner, Veterinary Nutritionist
Veterinary Nutrition Care
San Carlos, California

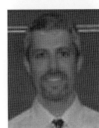

Marnin A. Forman, DVM, DACVIM (Small Animal Internal Medicine)
Head of Internal Medicine, Staff Internist
Internal Medicine
Cornell University Veterinary Specialists
Stamford, Connecticut

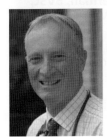

Luca Ferasin, DVM, PhD, CertVC, PGCert (HE), DECVIM-CA (Cardiology), GPCert (B&PS), MRCVS
European & RCVS Specialist in Cardiology
CVS Referrals
Cardiology
Lumbry Park Veterinary Specialists
Alton, Hampshire, United Kingdom
Coughing

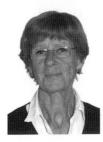

Catharina Linde Forsberg, DVM, PhD, DECAR
Professor Emeritus of Small Animal Reproduction
Department of Clinical Sciences,
Division of Reproduction
Swedish University of Agricultural Sciences
Private Company
Uppsala, Sweden

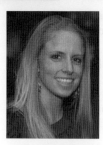

Amanda Foskett, DVM
Resident, Medical Oncology
The Oncology Service, LLC
Washington, DC

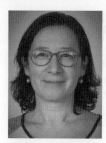

Sara Galac, DVM, PhD
Assistant Professor
Clinical Sciences of Companion Animals
Faculty of Veterinary Medicine, Utrecht
    University
Utrecht, The Netherlands

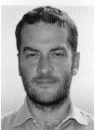

**Federico Fracassi, DVM, PhD,
DECVIM-CA (Internal Medicine)**
Professor
Department of Veterinary Medical
    Sciences
School of Agriculture and Veterinary
    Medicine
Bologna, Italy

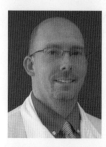

**Alex Gallagher, DVM, MS, DACVIM
(Small Animal Internal Medicine)**
Clinical Assistant Professor
Small Animal Clinical Sciences
University of Florida College of Veterinary
    Medicine
Gainesville, Florida

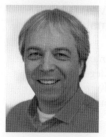

**Thierry Francey, DVM, DACVIM
(Small Animal Internal Medicine),
DECVIM-CA (Internal Medicine)**
Department of Clinical Veterinary
    Medicine
University of Bern
Bern, Switzerland

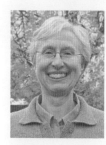

**Rosalind M. Gaskell, BVSc, PhD,
MRCVS**
Professor (Emeritus) and Honorary Fellow
School of Veterinary Science
University of Liverpool, Leahurst Campus
Neston, Cheshire, United Kingdom

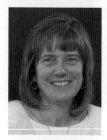

Diane Frank, DVM, DACVB
Professor (Behavioral Medicine)
Clinical Sciences
Université de Montréal
St-Hyacinthe, Quebec, Canada

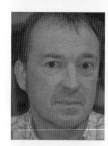

Olivier Gauthier, DVM, MSc, PhD
Professor of Small Animal Surgery and
    Dentistry
Small Animal Surgery
Oniris Nantes-Atlantic College of
    Veterinary Medicine, Food Science and
    Engineering
Nantes, France

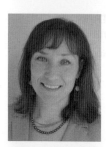

**Angela E. Frimberger, BS, VMD,
DACVIM (Oncology), MACVSc**
Director
Veterinary Oncology Consultants
Wauchope, NSW, Australia

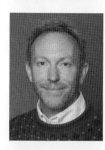

**James S. Gaynor, DVM, MS,
DACVAA, DAAPM**
Medical Director
Peak Performance Veterinary Group
Breckenridge, Colorado;
Medical Director
Animal Emergency Care Centers
Colorado Springs, Colorado

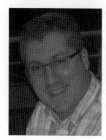

Jason W. Gagné, DVM, DACVN
Senior Manager, Veterinary Technical
    Marketing
Nestlé Purina PetCare
St. Louis, Missouri

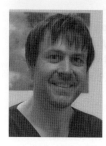

**Alexander James German, BVSc,
PhD, CertSAM, DECVIM-CA
(Internal Medicine), MRCVS**
Reader in Small Animal Medicine
Institute of Ageing and Chronic Disease
School of Veterinary Science
University of Liverpool
Neston, Merseyside, United Kingdom

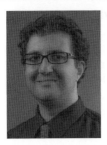

Alireza A. Gorgi, DVM, DACVIM (Neurology)
Department Head, Neurology/
 Neurosurgery
VCA West Coast Specialty & Emergency
 Animal Hospital
Fountain Valley, California;
Associate Clinical Professor
Western University of Health Sciences
 College of Veterinary Medicine
Pomona, California

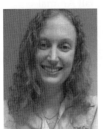

Susan A. Gottlieb, BVSc (Hons), BSc(vet), BAppSc, MANZCVS
Veterinarian
The Cat Clinic
Brisbane, Queensland, Australia

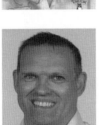

Peter A. Graham, BVMS, PhD, CertVR, DECVCP, MRCVS
Clinical Associate Professor
School of Veterinary Medicine and Science
University of Nottingham
Sutton Bonington, Leicestershire, United
 Kingdom

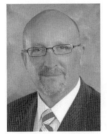

Thomas K. Graves, DVM, PhD, DACVIM (Small Animal Internal Medicine)
Dean and Professor
College of Veterinary Medicine
Midwestern University
Glendale, Arizona

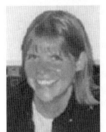

Amy M. Grooters, DVM, DACVIM (Small Animal Internal Medicine)
Professor
Companion Animal Medicine
Louisiana State University
Baton Rouge, Louisiana

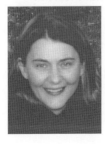

Sophie Alexandra Grundy, BVSc (Hons), MANZCVS, DACVIM (Small Animal Internal Medicine)
Internal Medicine Consultant
IDEXX Laboratories, Inc.
Westbrook, Maine

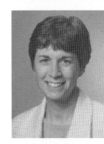

Lynn F. Guptill, DVM, PhD, DACVIM (Small Animal Internal Medicine)
Associate Professor
Department of Veterinary Clinical
 Services
Purdue University
West Lafayette, Indiana

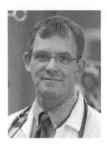

Tim B. Hackett, DVM, MS, DACVECC
Professor of Emergency and Critical Care
 Medicine
Department of Clinical Sciences
Colorado State University
Fort Collins, Colorado

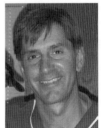

Jens Häggström, DVM, PhD, DECVIM-CA (Cardiology)
Professor
Department of Clinical Sciences
Faculty of Veterinary Medicine and
 Animal Science
The Swedish University of Agricultural
 Sciences
Uppsala, Sweden

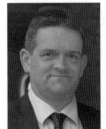

Edward James Hall, MA, VetMB, PhD
Professor of Small Animal Medicine
School of Veterinary Sciences
University of Bristol
Langford, Bristol, United Kingdom

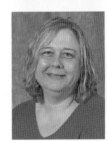

Meri F. Hall, RVT, LVT, CVT, LATG, VTS (Small Animal Internal Medicine)
Veterinary Technician
Internal Medicine
Veterinary Specialty Hospital
Palm Beach Gardens, Florida

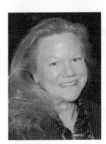

Cathleen A. Hanlon, VMD, PhD, DACVPM
Team Lead, Rabies; WHO Collaborating
 Center Head; OIE Expert (Retired)
Division of High Consequence Pathogens
 and Pathology
Centers for Disease Control and
 Prevention
Atlanta, Georgia

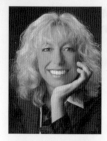

Katrin Hartmann, Dr.med.vet., Dr.habil., DECVIM-CA (Internal Medicine)
Professor
Head of Clinic of Small Animal Medicine
Director of Centre of Clinical Veterinary Medicine
Ludwig-Maximilian-Universitaet
Munich, Germany

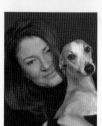

Camilla Heinze, DVM, RHD
Dyrlaege Camilla Heinze ApS
Karlslunde, Denmark

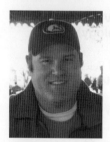

Eric J. Herrgesell, DVM, DACVR
Partner
Veterinary Medical Imaging
Sacramento, California

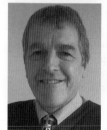

Michael E. Herrtage, MA, BVSc, DVSc, DVR, DVD, DSAM, DECVIM-CA (Internal Medicine), DECVDI, MRCVS
Professor of Small Animal Medicine
Department of Veterinary Medicine
University of Cambridge
Cambridge, Cambridgeshire, United Kingdom

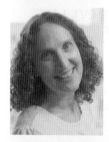

Rebecka S. Hess, DVM, DACVIM (Small Animal Internal Medicine)
Professor of Internal Medicine
Chief, Section of Medicine
Department of Clinical Studies, Philadelphia
School of Veterinary Medicine
University of Pennsylvania
Philadelphia, Pennsylvania

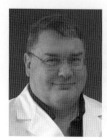

Richard C. Hill, MA, VetMB, PhD, DACVIM (Small Animal Internal Medicine), DACVN, MRCVS
Associate Professor
Department of Small Animal Clinical Sciences
University of Florida, College of Veterinary Medicine
Gainesville, Florida

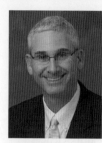

Daniel F. Hogan, DVM, DACVIM (Cardiology)
Professor, Cardiology
Veterinary Clinical Sciences
College of Veterinary Medicine, Purdue University
West Lafayette, Indiana

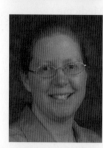

Kate Hopper, BVSc, PhD, DACVECC
Associate Professor of Small Animal Emergency & Critical Care
Veterinary Surgical and Radiological Sciences
University of California, Davis
Davis, California

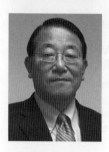

Takuo Ishida, DVM, PhD, DJCVP
Medical Director
Akasaka Animal Hospital
Minatoku, Tokyo, Japan;
President
Japanese Board of Veterinary Practitioners
Shibuyaku, Tokyo, Japan

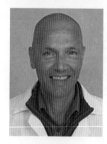

Nicholas Jeffery, BVSc, PhD, MSc, DECVN, DECVS, DSAS, FRCVS
Professor, Neurology and Neurosurgery
Veterinary Clinical Sciences
Texas A&M University
College Station, Texas

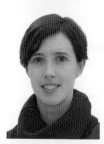

Rosanne Jepson, BVSc, MVetMed, PhD, DACVIM (Small Animal Internal Medicine), DECVIM-CA (Internal Medicine), FHEA, MRCVS
Lecturer in Small Animal Internal Medicine
Clinical Sciences and Services
Royal Veterinary College
London, United Kingdom

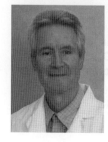

Albert Earl Jergens, DVM, PhD, DACVIM (Small Animal Internal Medicine)
Professor
Department of Veterinary Clinical Sciences
College of Veterinary Medicine
Iowa State University
Ames, Iowa

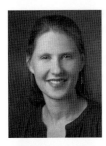

Jennifer L. Johns, DVM, PhD, DACVP (Clinical Pathology)
Assistant Professor
Comparative Medicine
Stanford University School of Medicine
Stanford, California

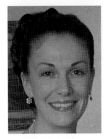

Andrea N. Johnston, DVM, DACVIM (Small Animal Internal Medicine)
Molecular Biology
University of Texas Southwestern Medical Center
Dallas, Texas

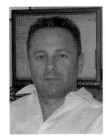

Ron Johnson, DVM, PhD, DACVCP
Associate Professor
Biomedical Sciences
University of Guelph
Guelph, Ontario, Canada

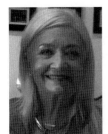

Dinah G. Jordan, BSPh, RPh, PharmD, DICVP
Chief of Pharmacy Services and Clinical Professor, Retired
College of Veterinary Medicine
Mississippi State University
Starkville, Mississippi

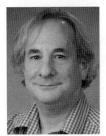

Philip H. Kass, DVM, MPVM, MS (Statistics), PhD (Epidemiology), DACVPM (Specialty in Epidemiology)
Professor of Analytic Epidemiology
Population Health and Reproduction, School of Veterinary Medicine
University of California, Davis
Davis, California

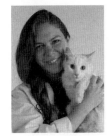

Eileen Kenney, DVM, DACVECC
Criticalist
Emergency/Critical Care
VCA West Los Angeles Animal Hospital
Los Angeles, California

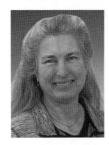

Marie E. Kerl, DVM, MPH, DACVIM (Small Animal Internal Medicine), DACVECC
Teaching Professor
Veterinary Medicine and Surgery
University of Missouri
Columbia, Missouri

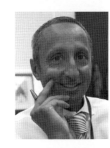

Chand Khanna, DVM, PhD, DACVIM (Oncology), DACVP (Hon)
Chief Science Officer
Ethos Veterinary Health
Woburn, Massachusetts;
The Oncology Service
President
Ethos Discovery
Washington, DC

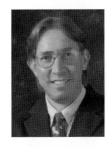

Peter P. Kintzer, DVM, DACVIM (Small Animal Internal Medicine)
Field Medical Specialist Manager
CAG Medical Organization
IDEXX Laboratories
Westbrook, Maine

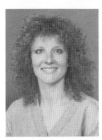

Karen Lynne Kline, DVM, MS, DACVIM (Neurology)
Staff Neurologist
Department of Neurology
VCA Veterinary Specialty Center of Seattle
Lynnwood, Washington

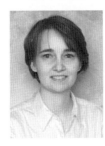

Amie Koenig, DVM, DACVIM (Small Animal Internal Medicine), DACVECC
Associate Professor of Emergency and Critical Care
Department of Small Animal Medicine and Surgery
College of Veterinary Medicine, University of Georgia
Athens, Georgia

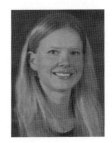

Amy M. Koenigshof, DVM, MS, DACVECC
Assistant Professor, Emergency and Critical Care Medicine
Small Animal Clinical Sciences
Michigan State University
East Lansing, Michigan

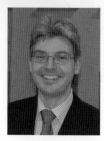

Hans S. Kooistra, DVM, PhD, DECVIM-CA (Internal Medicine)
Associate Professor
Department of Clinical Sciences of
 Companion Animals
University of Utrecht
Utrecht, The Netherlands

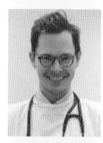

Peter Hendrik Kook, PD, Dr.med. vet., DACVIM (Small Animal Internal Medicine), DECVIM-CA (Internal Medicine)
Privatdozent
Clinic for Small Animal Internal Medicine
Vetsuisse Faculty, University of Zurich
Zurich, Switzerland

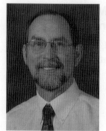

John M. Kruger, DVM, PhD, DACVIM (Small Animal Internal Medicine)
Professor, Internal Medicine
Small Animal Clinical Sciences
Michigan State University
East Lansing, Michigan

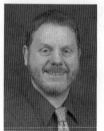

Butch KuKanich, DVM, PhD, DACVCP
Professor of Pharmacology
Department of Anatomy and Physiology
Kansas State University
Manhattan, Kansas

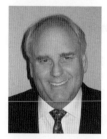

W. Douglas Kunz, MS, DVM
Medical Director
VCA Desert Animal Medical Hospital
Palm Springs, California

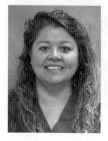

Michelle Anne Kutzler, DVM, PhD, DACT
Associate Professor of Companion Animal
 Industries
Animal and Rangeland Sciences
Oregon State University
Corvallis, Oregon

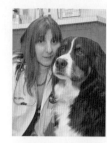

Mary Anna Labato, DVM, DACVIM (Small Animal Internal Medicine)
Clinical Professor
Section Head, Small Animal Medicine
Department of Clinical Sciences
Staff Veterinarian
Foster Hospital
Cummings School of Veterinary Medicine
Tufts University
North Grafton, Massachusetts

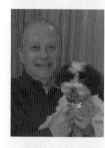

Gary Landsberg, DVM, DACVB, DECAWBM (Companion Animals)
Veterinary Behaviourist
North Toronto Veterinary Behavior
 Specialty Clinic
Thornhill, Ontario, Canada;
Vice President, Veterinary Affairs
CanCog Technologies
Toronto, Ontario, Canada

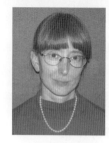

Cathy E. Langston, DVM, DACVIM (Small Animal Internal Medicine)
Associate Professor
Veterinary Clinical Sciences
College of Veterinary Medicine
The Ohio State University
Columbus, Ohio

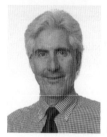

Michael R. Lappin, DVM, PhD, DACVIM (Small Animal Internal Medicine)
Professor
Department of Clinical Science
College of Veterinary Medicine and
 Biomedical Sciences
Colorado State University
Fort Collins, Colorado

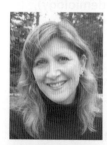

Jennifer Larsen, DVM, PhD, DACVN
Veterinary Medicine, Molecular
 Biosciences
School of Veterinary Medicine
University of California, Davis
Davis, California

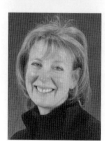

Martha Moon Larson, DVM, MS, DACVR
Professor
Department of Small Animal Clinical
 Sciences
Virginia-Maryland College of Veterinary
 Medicine
Virginia Polytechnic Institute and State
 University
Blacksburg, Virginia

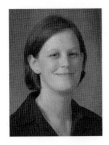

Patty Lathan, VMD, MS, DACVIM (Small Animal Internal Medicine)
Associate Professor, Small Animal Internal Medicine
Department of Clinical Sciences
Mississippi State University College of Veterinary Medicine
Mississippi State, Mississippi

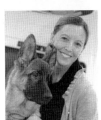

Jessica Lawrence, DVM, DACVIM (Oncology), DACVR (Radiation Oncology), MRCVS
Head of Oncology and Senior Lecturer in Oncology
Royal (Dick) School of Veterinary Studies
Easter Bush Campus, University of Edinburgh
Edinburgh, Scotland, United Kingdom;
Associate Professor of Radiation Oncology
Department of Veterinary Clinical Sciences
University of Minnesota, College of Veterinary Medicine
St. Paul, Minnesota

Justine A. Lee, DACVECC, DABT
VETgirl, LLC
St. Paul, Minnesota

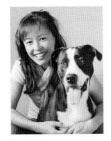

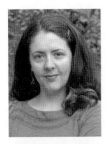

Tekla M. Lee-Fowler, DVM, MS, DACVIM (Small Animal Internal Medicine)
Assistant Professor
College of Veterinary Medicine
Auburn University
Auburn, Alabama

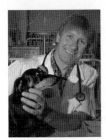

Andrew Lambert Leisewitz, BVSc, MMedVet(Med), PhD, DECVIM-CA (Internal Medicine)
Professor
Companion Animal Clinical Studies
University of Pretoria
Pretoria, Gauteng, South Africa

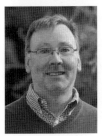

David Levine, PT, PhD, DPT, DABPTS (Orthopedics), CCRP, Cert. DN
Professor and Walter M. Cline Chair of Excellence in Physical Therapy
Physical Therapy
The University of Tennessee at Chattanooga
Chattanooga, Tennessee

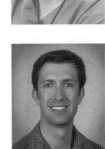

Julie K. Levy, DVM, PhD, DACVIM (Small Animal Internal Medicine)
Professor
Maddie's Shelter Medicine Program
College of Veterinary Medicine
University of Florida
Gainesville, Florida

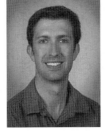

Jonathan Andrew Lidbury, BVMS, MRCVS, PhD, DACVIM (Small Animal Internal Medicine), DECVIM-CA (Internal Medicine)
Assistant Professor of Small Animal Internal Medicine
Gastrointestinal Laboratory Associate
Director of Clinical Services
Veterinary Small Animal Clinical Sciences
Texas A&M University
College Station, Texas

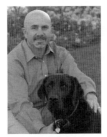

David Lipsitz, DVM, DACVIM (Neurology)
Staff Neurologist
Neurology
Veterinary Specialty Hospital of San Diego
San Diego, California

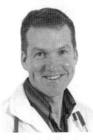

Julius M. Liptak, BVSc, MVetClinStud, FACVSc, DACVS, DECVS
Small Animal Surgeon and Surgical Oncologist
Alta Vista Animal Hospital
Ottawa, Ontario, Canada

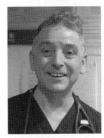

Christopher Little, BVMS, PhD, DVC, MRCVS
Veterinarian
Barton Veterinary Hospital
Canterbury, Kent, United Kingdom

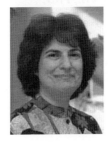

Meryl P. Littman, VMD, DACVIM (Small Animal Internal Medicine)
Professor of Medicine
Clinical Studies—Philadelphia
University of Pennsylvania School of Veterinary Medicine
Philadelphia, Pennsylvania

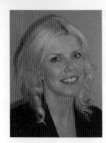
Ingrid Ljungvall, DVM, PhD
Associate Professor
Department of Clinical Sciences
Swedish University of Agricultural Sciences
Uppsala, Sweden

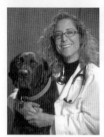
Cheryl London, DVM, PhD, DACVIM (Oncology)
Research Professor
Molecular Research Institute, Tufts Medical Center
Cummings School of Veterinary Medicine, Tufts University
Associate Faculty Professor
College of Veterinary Medicine
The Ohio State University
Columbus, Ohio

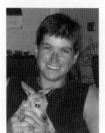
Cheryl Lopate, MS, DVM, DACT
Co-Owner and Clinical Veterinarian
Reproductive Revolutions
Aurora, Oregon;
Co-Owner and Clinical Veterinarian
Wilsonville Veterinary Clinic
Wilsonville, Oregon

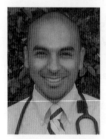
Julio López, DVM, DACVIM (Small Animal Internal Medicine)
Staff Internist
Studio City Animal Hospital
Los Angeles, California

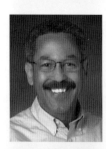
Jody P. Lulich, DVM, PhD, DACVIM (Small Animal Internal Medicine)
Professor
Minnesota Urolith Center
University of Minnesota
St. Paul, Minnesota

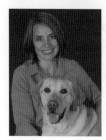
Kristin MacDonald, DVM, PhD, DACVIM (Cardiology)
Veterinary Cardiologist
VCA Animal Care Center of Sonoma
Rohnert Park, California

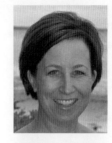
Valerie MacDonald, BSc, DVM, DACVIM (Oncology)
Associate Professor
Department of Small Animal Clinical Sciences
Western College of Veterinary Medicine, University of Saskatchewan
Saskatoon, SK, Canada

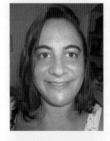
Lúcia Daniel Machado da Silva, DVM, PhD
Professor
Laboratory of Carnivores Reproduction
Veterinary Faculty
State University of Ceará
Fortaleza, Ceará, Brazil

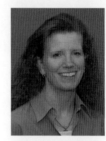
Catriona M. MacPhail, DVM, PhD, DACVS
Associate Professor, Small Animal Surgery
Department of Clinical Sciences
Small Animal Chief Medical Officer
Veterinary Teaching Hospital
Colorado State University
Fort Collins, Colorado

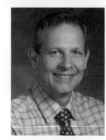
Denis J. Marcellin-Little, DEDV, DACVS, DECVS
Professor, Orthopedic Surgery
Department of Clinical Sciences
College of Veterinary Medicine, North Carolina State University
Raleigh, North Carolina

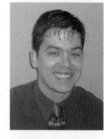
Christopher L. Mariani, DVM, PhD, DACVIM (Neurology)
Associate Professor of Neurology and Neurosurgery
Clinical Sciences
Director, Comparative Neuroimmunology and Neurooncology Laboratory
North Carolina State University
Raleigh, North Carolina

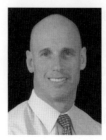
Stanley Leon Marks, BVSc, PhD, DACVIM (Small Animal Internal Medicine, Oncology), DACVN
Professor
Department of Medicine and Epidemiology
School of Veterinary Medicine
University of California, Davis
Davis, California

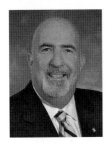

Steven L. Marks, BVSc, MS, MRCVS, DACVIM (Small Animal Internal Medicine)
Associate Dean and Director of Veterinary Medical Services
North Carolina State University
Raleigh, North Carolina

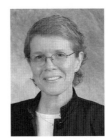

Margaret C. McEntee, DVM, DACVIM (Oncology), DACVR(RO)
Alexander de Lahunta Chair of Clinical Sciences, Professor of Oncology
Department of Clinical Sciences
College of Veterinary Medicine
Cornell University
Ithaca, New York

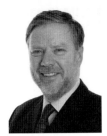

Mike Martin, MVB, DVC, MRCVS
Specialist Veterinary Cardiologist
Willows Referral Centre and Referral Service
Shirley, Solihull, West Midlands, United Kingdom

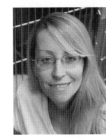

Maureen McMichael, DVM, DACVECC
Professor
Veterinary Clinical Medicine
University of Illinois
Urbana, Illinois

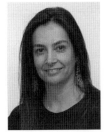

Ana Martins-Bessa, DVM, PhD
Professor
Department of Veterinary Sciences
Veterinary Teaching Hospital
University of Tras-os-Montes e Alto Douro, UTAD
Vila Real, Portugal

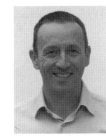

Carlos Melián, DVM, PhD
Director
Department of Veterinary Teaching Hospital
Universidad de Las Palmas de Gran Canaria
Clínica Veterinaria Atlántico
Las Palmas de Gran Canaria, Spain

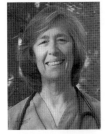

Karol A. Mathews, DVM, DVSc, DACVECC
Professor Emerita, Emergency & Critical Care Medicine
Department of Clinical Studies
Ontario Veterinary College
University of Guelph
Guelph, Ontario, Canada

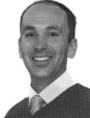

Richard John Mellanby, BSc, BVMS, PhD, DSAM, DECVIM-CA (Internal Medicine), MRCVS
Head of Small Animal Medicine
Royal (Dick) School of Veterinary Studies and The Roslin Institute
Hospital for Small Animals
The University of Edinburgh
Easter Bush Veterinary Centre
Midlothian, United Kingdom

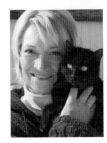

Glenna E. Mauldin, DVM, MS, DACVIM (Oncology), DACVN
Staff Veterinarian in Oncology and Nutrition
Cancer Centre for Animals
Western Veterinary Specialist and Emergency Centre
Clinical Instructor, Distributed Veterinary Learning Community
Faculty of Veterinary Medicine
University of Calgary
Calgary, Alberta, Canada

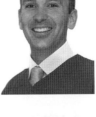

Linda Merrill, LVT, VTS (AIMVT-Small Animal Internal Medicine & AVTCP-Canine/Feline)
Executive Director
Academy of Internal Medicine for Veterinary Technicians
Seattle Veterinary Associates
Green Lake Animal Hospital
Seattle, Washington

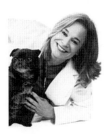

Elisa M. Mazzaferro, MS, DVM, PhD, DACVECC
Staff Criticalist
Cornell University Veterinary Specialists
Stamford, Connecticut

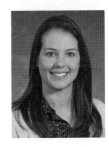

Kristen Messenger, DVM, DACVAA, DACVCP
Assistant Professor of Anesthesiology
Molecular Biomedical Science
North Carolina State University
College of Veterinary Medicine
Raleigh, North Carolina

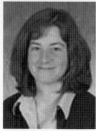

Kathryn M. Meurs, DVM, PhD, DACVIM (Cardiology)
Professor, Clinical Sciences
Associate Dean, Research and Graduate Studies
North Carolina State University
College of Veterinary Medicine
Raleigh, North Carolina

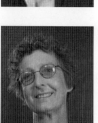

Kathryn E. Michel, DVM, MS, MSED, DACVN
Professor of Nutrition
Department of Clinical Studies
School of Veterinary Medicine
University of Pennsylvania
Philadelphia, Pennsylvania

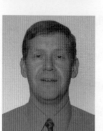

Darryl L. Millis, MS, DVM, DACVS, CCRP, DACVSMSR
Professor of Orthopedic Surgery
Small Animal Clinical Sciences
University of Tennessee College of Veterinary Medicine
Knoxville, Tennessee

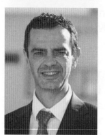

Luis Miguel Fonte Montenegro, Master's Degree
Clinical Director, Doctor Surgery
Hospital Veterinário Montenegro
Porto, Portugal

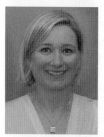

Carmel T. Mooney, MVB, MPhil, PhD, DECVIM-CA (Internal Medicine), MRCVS
Associate Professor
University Veterinary Hospital
University College Dublin
Belfield, Dublin, Ireland

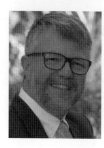

Antony S. Moore, BVSc, MVSc, DACVIM (Oncology)
Veterinary Oncology Consultants
Wauchope, NSW, Australia

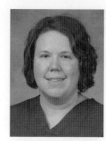

Sarah A. Moore, DVM, DACVIM (Neurology)
Associate Professor, Neurology and Neurosurgery
Department of Veterinary Clinical Sciences
The Ohio State University
Columbus, Ohio

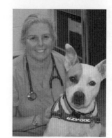

Lisa Moses, VMD, DACVIM (Small Animal Internal Medicine)
Pain Medicine Service
Angell Animal Medical Center
Fellow in Medical Ethics
Center for Bioethics
Harvard Medical School
Boston, Massachusetts

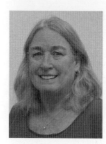

Jane D. Mount, MS, PhD
Research Fellow
Pathobiology
Auburn University
Auburn, Alabama

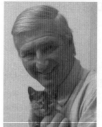

Ralf S. Mueller, Dr.med.vet., Dr.habil., DACVD, FANZCVSc, DECVD
Professor
Center of Clinical Veterinary Medicine
Clinic of Small Animal Medicine
Ludwig Maximilian University of Munich
Munich, Germany

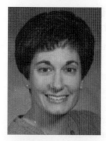

Karen R. Muñana, DVM, MS, DACVIM (Neurology)
Professor, Neurology
Department of Clinical Sciences
North Carolina State University
College of Veterinary Medicine
Raleigh, North Carolina

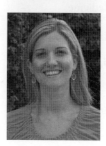

Laura A. Nafe, DVM, MS, DACVIM (Small Animal Internal Medicine)
Assistant Professor, Small Animal Internal Medicine
Veterinary Clinical Sciences
Oklahoma State University
Stillwater, Oklahoma

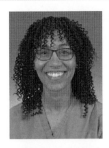

Thandeka Roseann Ngwenyama, DVM, DACVECC
Clinical Assistant Professor of Emergency
  and Critical Care
Veterinary Clinical Sciences
Washington State University
Pullman, Washington

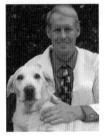

Brook A. Niemiec, DAVDC, DEVDC, Fellow AVD
Chief of Staff
Dentistry
Southern California Veterinarian
Dental Specialties & Oral Surgery
Founding Consultant, VetDentalRad. com
President, Practical Veterinary Publishing
Lead Instructor, San Diego Veterinary
  Dental Training Center
San Diego, California

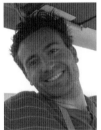

Stijn J.M. Niessen, DVM, PhD, DECVIM-CA (Internal Medicine), PGCVIM, PGCVetEd, FHEA, MRCVS
Senior Lecturer and Co-Head, Small
  Animal Internal Medicine
Clinical Science and Services
Director, Feline Diabetic Remission Clinic
Royal Veterinary College
London, United Kingdom;
Research Associate
Diabetes Research Group
Newcastle Medical School
Newcastle-upon-Tyne, Tyne and Wear,
  United Kingdom;
Consultant, Endocrinology
Veterinary Information Network
Davis, California

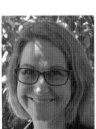

Carolyn R. O'Brien, BVSc, MVetClinStud, FANZCVS (Feline Medicine)
PhD Candidate
Faculty of Veterinary and Agricultural
  Sciences
University of Melbourne
Registered Specialist in Feline Medicine
Melbourne Cat Vets
Parkville, Victoria, Australia

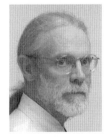

Dennis P. O'Brien, DVM, PhD, DACVIM (Neurology)
Chancellor's Chair in Comparative
  Neurology
Department of Veterinary Medicine &
  Surgery
University of Missouri
Neurology & Neurosurgery Service
Veterinary Health Center
Columbia, Missouri

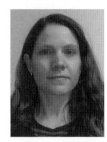

Mauria O'Brien, DVM, DACVECC
Clinical Associate Professor
Veterinary Clinical Medicine
University of Illinois
Urbana, Illinois

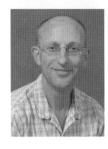

Robert T. O'Brien, DVM, MS, ACVR
Department of Veterinary Clinical
  Medicine
Director of Imaging, Epica Medical
  Innovations
Staff Radiologist, Oncura Partners
  Diagnostics, LLC
Nobleboro, Maine

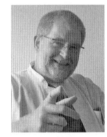

Gerhard Ulrich Oechtering, Dr.med. vet.habil., DECVAA
Professor
Small Animal Department—Ear, Nose and
  Throat Unit
University of Leipzig
Leipzig, Saxony, Germany

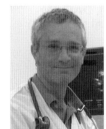

Dan G. Ohad, DVM, PhD, DACVIM (Cardiology), DECVIM-CA (Cardiology)
Clinical Senior Lecturer in Cardiology
Koret School of Veterinary Medicine
Robert H. Smith Faculty of Agriculture,
  Food and Environment
Hebrew University of Jerusalem
Rehovot, Israel

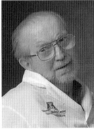

Carl A. Osborne, DVM, PhD, DACVIM
Veterinary Clinical Sciences Department
College of Veterinary Medicine
University of Minnesota
St. Paul, Minnesota

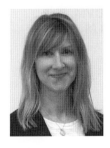

M. Lynne O'Sullivan, DVM, DVSc, DACVIM (Cardiology)
Associate Professor
Department of Clinical Studies
Ontario Veterinary College, University of
  Guelph
Guelph, Ontario, Canada

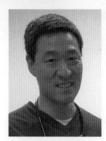
Mark A. Oyama, DVM, MSCE, DACVIM (Cardiology)
Professor and Chief, Section of Cardiology
Department of Clinical Studies
University of Pennsylvania
Philadelphia, Pennsylvania

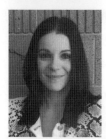
Caroline Page, BA, VetMB, DACVIM (Small Animal Internal Medicine)
Page Veterinary Consulting
Huntington Beach, California

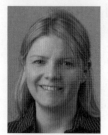
Carrie A. Palm, DVM, DACVIM (Small Animal Internal Medicine)
Assistant Professor
Medicine and Epidemiology
University of California, Davis
Davis, California

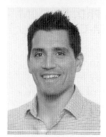
Douglas Palma, DVM, DACVIM (Small Animal Internal Medicine)
Staff Internist
Small Animal Internal Medicine
The Animal Medical Center
New York, New York

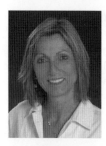
Manon Paradis, DVM, MVSc, DACVD
Professor of Dermatology
Department of Clinical Sciences
Faculté de Médecine Vétérinaire,
University of Montreal
St-Hyacinthe, Québec, Canada

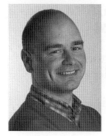
Dominique Peeters, DVM, PhD, DECVIM-CA (Internal Medicine)
Professor in Companion Animal Internal
  Medicine
Equine and Companion Animal Clinical
  Sciences
University of Liege
Liege, Belgium

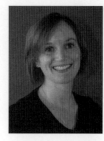
Sally C. Perea, DVM, MS, DACVN
Clinical Veterinary Nutritionist
Research and Development
Royal Canin, A Division of MARS, Inc.
Lewisburg, Ohio

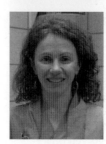
Dolores Pérez-Alenza, DVM, PhD
Professor
Animal Medicine and Surgery
Veterinary School, Complutense
University of Madrid
Head of Service
Small Animal Internal Medicine Service,
  Veterinary Teaching
Hospital Complutense
General Secretary, Board Member
AVEPA
Madrid, Spain

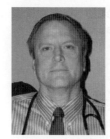
Michael Peterson, DVM, MS
Staff Veterinarian
Reid Veterinary Hospital
Albany, Oregon;
Associate Investigator
Viper Institute
University of Arizona
Tucson, Arizona

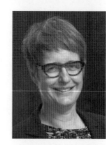
Christine Piek, DVM, PhD, DECVIM-CA (Internal Medicine)
Department of Clinical Sciences and
  Companion Animals
Faculty of Veterinary Medicine, Utrecht
  University
Utrecht, The Netherlands

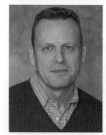
Simon R. Platt, BVM&S, MRCVS, DACVIM (Neurology), DECVN
Professor, Neurology and Neurosurgery
Small Animal Medicine and Surgery
College of Veterinary Medicine, University
  of Georgia
Athens, Georgia

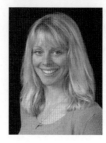
Rachel E. Pollard, DVM, PhD, DACVR
Department of Surgical and Radiological
  Sciences
School of Veterinary Medicine
University of California, Davis
Davis, California

Tratado de Medicina Interna Veterinária: Doenças do Cão e do Gato xxxiii

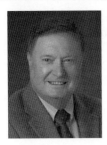

David James Polzin, DVM, PhD, DACVIM (Small Animal Internal Medicine)
Professor and Chief of Internal Medicine
Department of Veterinary Clinical Sciences
College of Veterinary Medicine
University of Minnesota
St. Paul, Minnesota

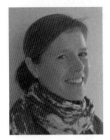

Nathalie Porters, DVM, MVM, PhD, DECVS
Professor Doctor
Small Animal Medicine and Clinical Biology
Faculty of Veterinary Medicine, Ghent University
Merelbeke, Belgium

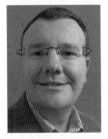

Simon Lawrence Priestnall, BSc (Hons), BVSc, PhD, PGCert(VetEd), FHEA, DACVP, FRCPath, MRCVS
Associate Professor of Veterinary Anatomic Pathology
Department of Pathology and Pathogen Biology
The Royal Veterinary College
Hatfield, Hertfordshire, United Kingdom

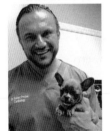

Robert Prošek, DVM, MS, DACVIM (Cardiology), DECVIM-CA (Cardiology)
Adjunct Professor of Cardiology
University of Florida
Gainesville, Florida;
President
Cardiopulmonary Medicine and Interventional Therapy
Florida Veterinary Cardiology
Miami, Florida

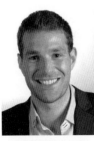

Yann Queau, DVM, DACVN
Research and Clinical Nutritionist
Research and Development Center
Royal Canin
Aimargues, France

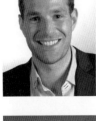

Oriana Raab, DVM, MVSc, DACVIM (Small Animal Internal Medicine)
Staff Internist
Internal Medicine
Tufts Veterinary Emergency Treatment and Specialties
Walpole, Massachusetts

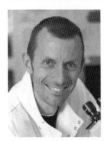

Alan Radford, BVSc, PhD, MRCVS
Reader in Infection Biology
Institute of Infection and Global Health
University of Liverpool
Neston, Cheshire, United Kingdom

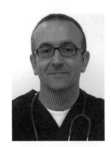

Juan José Ramos-Plá, DVM, PhD
Associate Professor
Medicine and Surgery
Cardenal Herrera CEU University
Clínica Veterinaria Vinaroz
Valencia, Spain

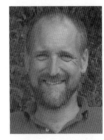

Ian K. Ramsey, BVSc, PhD, DSAM, DECVIM-CA (Internal Medicine), FHEA, MRCVS
Professor of Small Animal Medicine
University of Glasgow
Glasgow, Scotland, United Kingdom

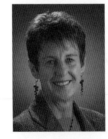

Jacquie Rand, BVSc (Hons), DVSc (Guelph), DACVIM (Internal Medicine)
Emeritus Professor
School of Veterinary Science
The University of Queensland
Executive Director and Chief Scientist
Australian Pet Welfare Foundation
Brisbane, Queensland, Australia

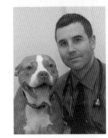

Kenneth M. Rassnick, DVM, DACVIM (Oncology)
Director, Oncology Consultation Service
Veterinary Medical Center of Central New York
Syracuse, New York;
Director, Oncology Consultation Service
Colonial Veterinary Hospital
Ithaca, New York

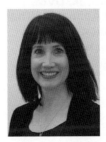

Carol R. Reinero, DVM, DACVIM (Small Animal Internal Medicine), PhD
Associate Professor
University of Missouri
Columbia, Missouri

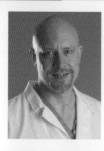

Alexander M. Reiter, Dipl. Tzt, Dr.med.vet., DAVDC, EVDC
Associate Professor of Dentistry and Oral Surgery
Department of Clinical Studies, Philadelphia
School of Veterinary Medicine, University of Pennsylvania
Philadelphia, Pennsylvania

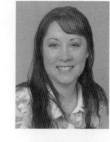

Elizabeth Rozanski, DVM, DACVIM (Small Animal Internal Medicine), DACVECC
Associate Professor of Critical Care
Cummings School of Veterinary Medicine
Tufts University
North Grafton, Massachusetts

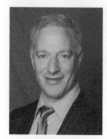

Keith Richter, DVM, MSEL, DACVIM (Small Animal Internal Medicine)
Chief Medical Officer
Ethos Veterinary Health
Staff Internist
Internal Medicine
Veterinary Specialty Hospital of San Diego
San Diego, California

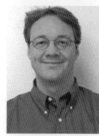

Craig G. Ruaux, BVSc, PhD, MACVSc, DACVIM (Small Animal Internal Medicine)
Associate Professor, Small Animal Medicine
Department of Clinical Sciences
Oregon State University
Corvallis, Oregon

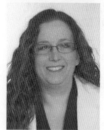

Teresa M. Rieser, VMD, DACVECC
Staff Criticalist
Department of Emergency and Critical Care
VCA West Los Angeles Animal Hospital
Los Angeles, California

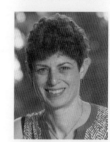

Clare Rusbridge, BVMS, PhD, DECVN, FRCVS
Chief of Neurology
Fitzpatrick Referrals
Eashing, Surrey, United Kingdom;
Reader in Veterinary Neurology
School of Veterinary Medicine
University of Surrey
Guildford, Surrey, United Kingdom

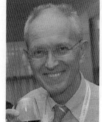

Stefano Romagnoli, DVM, MS, PhD, DECAR
Professor
Animal Medicine, Production and Health
University of Padova
Legnaro, Padova (Veneto), Italy

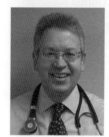

John E. Rush, DVM, MS, DACVIM (Cardiology), DACVECC
Tufts Cummings School of Veterinary Medicine
North Grafton, Massachusetts

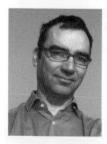

Dan Rosenberg, DVM, PhD
Internal Medicine Unit
MICEN VET
Créteil, France

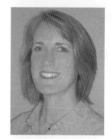

Helena Rylander, DVM, DACVIM (Neurology)
Clinical Associate Professor
Department of Medical Sciences
School of Veterinary Medicine
University of Wisconsin
Madison, Wisconsin

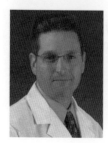

John Henry Rossmeisl, Jr., DVM, MS, DACVIM (Small Animal Internal Medicine and Neurology)
Professor, Neurology and Neurosurgery
Small Animal Clinical Sciences, VA-MD College of Veterinary Medicine
Virginia Tech
Blacksburg, Virginia

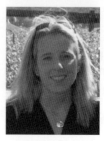

Veronique Sammut, DVM, MS, DACVIM (Neurology)
VCA West Los Angeles
Los Angeles, California

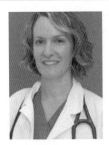

Kari Santoro Beer, DVM, DACVECC
Assistant Professor, Emergency and
 Critical Care Medicine
Department of Small Animal Clinical
 Sciences
Michigan State University
East Lansing, Michigan

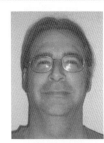

**Thomas Schermerhorn, VMD,
DACVIM (Small Animal Internal
Medicine)**
Professor
Department of Clinical Sciences
Kansas State University
Manhattan, Kansas

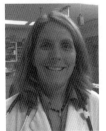

**Christine Savidge, DVM, DACVIM
(Small Animal Internal Medicine)**
Assistant Professor, Small Animal Internal
 Medicine
Department of Companion Animals
University of Prince Edward Island,
 Atlantic Veterinary College
Charlottetown, PE, Canada

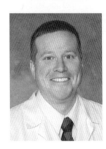

Chad W. Schmiedt, DVM, DACVS
Associate Professor
Department of Small Animal Medicine
 and Surgery
University of Georgia
Athens, Georgia

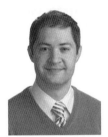

**Brian A. Scansen, DVM, MS,
DACVIM (Cardiology)**
Associate Professor
Clinical Sciences
Colorado State University
Fort Collins, Colorado

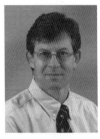

**Johan P. Schoeman, BVSc,
MMedVet, PhD, DSAM, DECVIM-CA
(Internal Medicine)**
Professor and Head of Department
Department of Companion Animal
 Clinical Studies
Faculty of Veterinary Science, University
 of Pretoria
Onderstepoort, Pretoria, South Africa

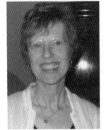

**Auke C. Schaefers-Okkens, DVM,
PhD, DECAR**
Department of Clinical Sciences of
 Companion Animals (retired)
Faculty of Veterinary Medicine, University
 of Utrecht
Utrecht, The Netherlands

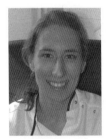

**Simone Schuller, Dr.med.vet.,
DECVIM-CA (Internal Medicine), PhD**
Professor
Department of Clinical Veterinary
 Medicine
Internal Medicine
Small Animal Hospital
Vetsuisse Faculty Bern
Bern, Switzerland

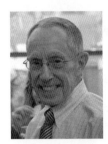

**Michael Schaer, DVM, DACVIM
(Small Animal Internal Medicine),
DCVECC**
Emeritus Professor
Adjunct Professor, Emergency and Critical
 Care Medicine
College of Veterinary Medicine
University of Florida
Gainesville, Florida

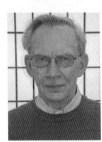

**Wayne Stanley Schwark, DVM,
MSc, PhD**
Emeritus Professor of Pharmacology
 Molecular Medicine
College of Veterinary Medicine, Cornell
 University
Ithaca, New York

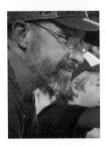

**Scott J. Schatzberg, DVM, PhD,
DACVIM (Neurology)**
Director of Neurology/Neurosurgery
The Animal Neurology and Imaging
 Center
Algodones, New Mexico

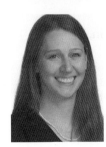

**Katherine F. Scollan, DVM, DACVIM
(Cardiology)**
Assistant Professor
College of Veterinary Medicine
Oregon State University
Corvallis, Oregon

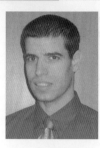

Gilad Segev, DVM, DECVIM-CA (Internal Medicine)
Senior Lecturer
Koret School of Veterinary Medicine
Hebrew University of Jerusalem
Rehovot, Israel

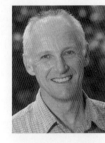

Kenneth W. Simpson, BVM&S, PhD, DACVIM (Small Animal Internal Medicine), DECVIM-CA (Internal Medicine)
College of Veterinary Medicine
Cornell University
Ithaca, New York

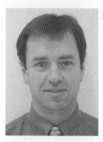

Rance K. Sellon, DVM, PhD, DACVIM (Small Animal Internal Medicine, Oncology)
Associate Professor
Department of Veterinary Clinical Sciences
College of Veterinary Medicine
Washington State University
Pullman, Washington

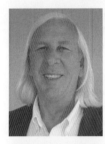

D. David Sisson, DVM, DACVIM (Cardiology)
Professor Emeritus
Veterinary Clinical Sciences
Oregon State University
Corvallis, Oregon

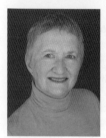

G. Diane Shelton, DVM, PhD, DACVIM (Small Animal Internal Medicine)
Professor
Department of Pathology, School of Medicine
Director, Comparative Neuromuscular Laboratory
University of California, San Diego
La Jolla, California

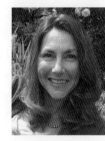

Barbara J. Skelly, MA, VetMB, PhD, CertSAM, DACVIM (Small Animal Internal Medicine), DECVIM-CA (Internal Medicine), MRCVS
University Senior Lecturer in Small Animal Medicine
Department of Veterinary Medicine
Queen's Veterinary School Hospital
University of Cambridge
Cambridge, Cambridgeshire, United Kingdom

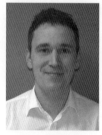

Robert E. Shiel, MVB, PhD, DECVIM-CA (Internal Medicine)
Lecturer
Small Animal Medicine Section, School of Veterinary Medicine
University College Dublin
Dublin, Ireland

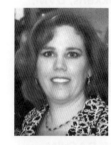

Stephanie A. Smith, DVM, MS
Research Assistant Professor
Department of Biochemistry, School of Molecular and Cellular Biology
Adjunct Clinical Assistant Professor
Department of Veterinary Clinical Medicine, College of Veterinary Medicine
University of Illinois
Urbana, Illinois

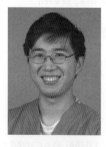

Andre C. Shih, DVM, DACVAA, DACVECC
Associate Professor
Large Animal Clinical Sciences
University of Florida College
Veterinary Medicine Anesthesia Service
Gainesville, Florida

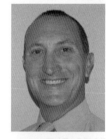

David Stephen Sobel, DVM, MRCVS
Director of Medicine
Metropolitan Veterinary Consultants
Hanover, New Hampshire; Clinical Consultant
Elands Veterinary Clinic
Dunton Green, Sevenoaks, United Kingdom

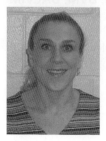

Deborah C. Silverstein, DVM, DACVECC
Associate Professor of Critical Care
University of Pennsylvania
Philadelphia, Pennsylvania

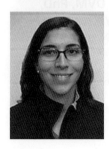

Maria M. Soltero-Rivera, DVM, DAVDC
Adjunct Assistant Professor
Dentistry and Oral Surgery
Penn Vet—Matthew J. Ryan Veterinary Hospital of the University of Pennsylvania
Philadelphia, Pennsylvania;
Veterinary Specialist
Dentistry and Oral Surgery
VCA San Francisco Veterinary Specialists
San Francisco, California

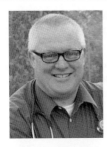
Dennis R. Spann, DVM, DACVIM (Small Animal Internal Medicine)
Staff Internist
Internal Medicine Department
Sacramento Area Veterinary Internal Medicine
Roseville, California

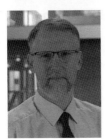
Thomas Spillmann, Dipl.med.vet, Dr.med.vet., DECVIM-CA (Internal Medicine)
Professor of Small Animal Internal Medicine
Department of Equine and Small Animal Medicine
Faculty of Veterinary Medicine, University of Helsinki
Helsinki, Finland

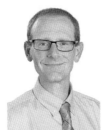
Timothy J. Stein, DVM, PhD, DACVIM (Oncology)
Medical Oncologist
Oncology
Austin Veterinary Emergency & Specialty Center
Austin, Texas

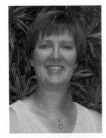
Rebecca L. Stepien, DVM, MS, DACVIM (Cardiology)
Clinical Professor of Cardiology
Department of Medical Sciences
School of Veterinary Medicine
University of Wisconsin—Madison
Madison, Wisconsin

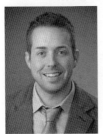
Joshua A. Stern, DVM, PhD, DACVIM (Cardiology)
Assistant Professor of Cardiology
Department of Medicine & Epidemiology
University of California, Davis
Davis, California

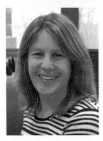
Tracy Stokol, BVSc, PhD, DACVP (Clinical Pathology)
Professor of Clinical Pathology
Department of Population Medicine and Diagnostic Sciences
College of Veterinary Medicine, Cornell University
Ithaca, New York

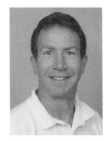
Michael Stone, DVM, DACVIM (Small Animal Internal Medicine)
Clinical Assistant Professor
Department of Clinical Studies
Cummings School of Veterinary Medicine at Tufts University
North Grafton, Massachusetts;
Traveling Ultrasonographer
Veterinary Internal Medicine Mobile Specialists
North Woodstock, Connecticut

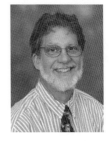
Joseph Taboada, DVM, DACVIM (Small Animal Internal Medicine)
Professor of Small Animal Internal Medicine and Associate Dean
School of Veterinary Medicine
Louisiana State University
Baton Rouge, Louisiana

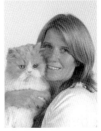
Séverine Tasker, BSc, BVSc (Hons), PhD, DSAM, DECVIM-CA (Internal Medicine), FHEA, MRCVS
Reader in Feline Medicine
The Feline Centre, Langford Veterinary Services
University of Bristol
Bristol, North Somerset, United Kingdom

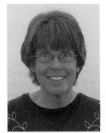
Susan M. Taylor, DVM, DACVIM (Small Animal Internal Medicine)
Professor
Small Animal Clinical Sciences
Staff Internist
Veterinary Teaching Hospital
Western College of Veterinary Medicine, University of Saskatchewan
Saskatoon, SK, Canada

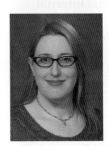
Karen M. Tefft, DVM, MVSc, DACVIM (Small Animal Internal Medicine)
Clinical Assistant Professor
Department of Clinical Sciences
North Carolina State University
Raleigh, North Carolina

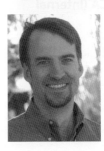
Douglas H. Thamm, VMD, DACVIM (Oncology)
Barbara Cox Anthony Professor of Oncology
Flint Animal Cancer Center,
Department of Clinical Sciences
Colorado State University
Fort Collins, Colorado

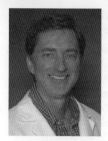

William B. Thomas, DVM, MS, DACVIM (Neurology)
Professor, Neurology and Neurosurgery
College of Veterinary Medicine
University of Tennessee
Knoxville, Tennessee

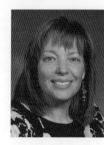

Shelly L. Vaden, DVM, PhD, DACVIM (Small Animal Internal Medicine)
Professor, Internal Medicine
College of Veterinary Medicine
North Carolina State University
Raleigh, North Carolina

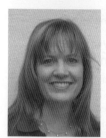

Melanie D. Thompson, DVM, MVSc, DACVIM (Small Animal Internal Medicine)
Internist
Small Animal Internal Medicine
Advanced Veterinary Care
Salt Lake City, Utah

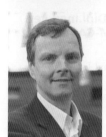

Thomas Wilhelm Vahlenkamp, Dr.med.vet., PhD
Institute of Virology
Center of Infectious Diseases
University of Leipzig
Leipzig, Germany

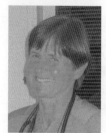

Anna Tidholm, DVM, PhD, DECVIM-CA (Cardiology)
Associate Professor
Albano Animal Hospital
Danderyd, Sweden

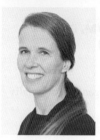

Alexandra van der Woerdt, DVM, MS, DACVO, DECVO
Staff Ophthalmologist
The Animal Medical Center
New York, New York

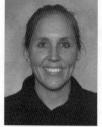

M. Katherine Tolbert, DVM, PhD, DACVIM (Small Animal Internal Medicine)
Assistant Professor
Small Animal Clinical Sciences
University of Tennessee
Knoxville, Tennessee

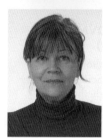

Astrid M. van Dongen, DVM, DRNVA
Assistant Professor
Department of Clinical Sciences of
  Companion Animals—Internal
Medicine/Nephrology
Faculty of Veterinary Medicine, Utrecht
  University
Utrecht, The Netherlands

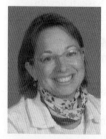

Lauren A. Trepanier, DVM, PhD, DACVIM (Small Animal Internal Medicine), DACVCP
Professor and Director of Clinical
  Research
Department of Medical Sciences
School of Veterinary Medicine,
University of Wisconsin—Madison
Madison, Wisconsin

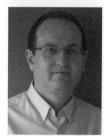

Lamberto Viadel Bau, DVM
Clínica Veterinaria Bau
Buñol, Valencia, Spain

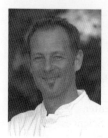

Stefan Unterer, Dr.med.vet., Dr. Habil., DECVIM-CA (Internal Medicine)
Oberarzt Innere Medizin
Leiter des Gastroenterologie-Service
Medizinische Kleintierklinik
Ludwig-Maximilians-Universität
Munich, Germany

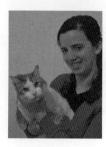

Cecilia Villaverde, BVSc, PhD, DACVN, DECVCN
Adjunct Professor
Ciència Animal i dels Aliments
Universitat Autònoma de Barcelona
Bellaterra, Spain

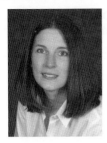

Lori S. Waddell, DVM, DACVECC
Clinical Professor of Critical Care
Department of Clinical Studies
School of Veterinary Medicine, University
of Pennsylvania
Philadelphia, Pennsylvania

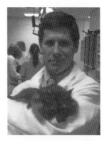

Craig B. Webb, PhD, DVM, DACVIM (Small Animal Internal Medicine)
Professor
Clinical Sciences Department
Head, Small Animal Medicine Section
Veterinary Teaching Hospital
Colorado State University
Fort Collins, Colorado

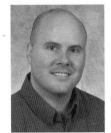

Joseph J. Wakshlag, DVM, PhD, DACVN, DACVSMR
Associate Professor
Clinical Sciences
Cornell University
Ithaca, New York

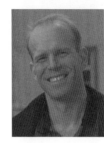

J. Scott Weese, DVM, DVSc, DACVIM
Professor
Pathobiology
Ontario Veterinary College
Guelph, Ontario, Canada

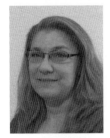

Valerie Walker, RVT
Small Animal Internal Medicine
  Technician
Small Animal Internal Medicine
University of California Veterinary
  Medical Teaching Hospital
Davis, California

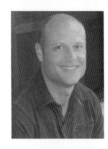

Chick Weisse, VMD, DACVS
Staff Veterinarian, Interventional
  Radiology/Surgery
Director of Interventional Radiology
The Animal Medical Center
New York, New York

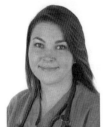

Julie Walter, BSc, DVM
Graduate Student
Companion Animals
Atlantic Veterinary College
Charlottetown, PE, Canada; Internal
  Medicine
Veterinary Emergency & Referral Hospital
Newmarket, Ontario, Canada

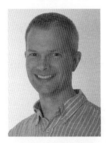

Nathaniel T. Whitley, BVMS, PhD, CertVC, DACVIM (Small Animal Internal Medicine), DECVIM-CA (Internal Medicine)
Head of Internal Medicine, Director
Department of Internal Medicine
Davies Veterinary Specialties
Higham Gobion, Hertfordshire, United
  Kingdom

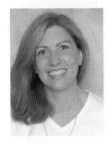

Cynthia R. Ward, VMD, PhD, DACVIM (Small Animal Internal Medicine)
Josiah Meigs Distinguished Teaching
  Professor
Small Animal Medicine and Surgery
University of Georgia College of
  Veterinary Medicine
Athens, Georgia

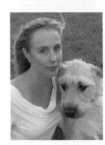

Joanna Whitney, BSc(vet), BVSc, MVetStud, FANZCVS
Lecturer in Small Animal Medicine
Faculty of Veterinary Science
University of Sydney
Sydney, NSW, Australia

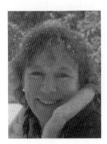

Penny J. Watson, MA, VetMD, CertVR, DSAM, DECVIM-CA (Internal Medicine), MRCVS
University Senior Lecturer in Small
  Animal Medicine
Department of Veterinary Medicine
University of Cambridge
Cambridge, United Kingdom

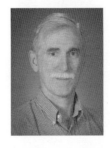

Michael D. Willard, DVM, MS, DACVIM (Small Animal Internal Medicine)
Professor
Department of Small Animal Clinical
  Services
Texas A&M University
College Station, Texas

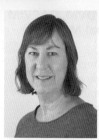

D. Colette Williams, PhD
Staff Research Associate
William R. Pritchard Veterinary
Medical Teaching Hospital
University of California, Davis
Davis, California

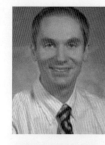

Michael W. Wood, DVM, PhD, DACVIM (Small Animal Internal Medicine)
Assistant Professor
Medical Sciences
University of Wisconsin—Madison
Madison, Wisconsin

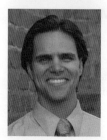

Justin G. Williams, DVM, DACVIM (Cardiology)
Staff Cardiologist
VCA San Francisco Veterinary Specialists
San Francisco, California

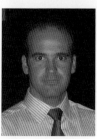

Panagiotis G. Xenoulis, DVM, Dr.med.vet., PhD
Assistant Professor of Small Animal
    Internal Medicine
Clinic of Medicine
Faculty of Veterinary Medicine, University
    of Thessaly
Karditsa, Greece;
Consultant in Internal Medicine
Section of Medicine
Animal Medicine Center of Athens
Athens, Greece

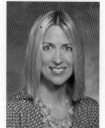

Laurel E. Williams, DVM, DACVIM (Oncology)
Adjunct Professor
Department of Clinical Sciences
College of Veterinary Medicine, North
    Carolina State University Oncologist
Veterinary Specialty Hospital of the
    Carolinas
Raleigh, North Carolina

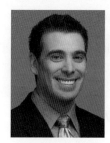

Brian M. Zanghi, PhD, MS
Research Scientist
Nestlé Research Center
Nestlé Purina PetCare
St. Louis, Missouri

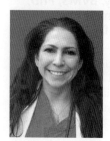

Sarah Elizabeth Winzelberg, VMD
Internal Medicine
Veterinary Emergency and Referral Group
Brooklyn, New York

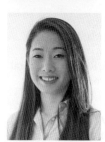

Bing Yun Zhu, BVCs (Hons I), DACVIM (Small Animal Internal Medicine)
Registered Specialist in Small Animal
    Internal Medicine
Internal Medicine
Small Animal Specialist Hospital
Ryde, NSW, Australia

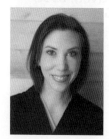

Angela L. Witzel, DVM, PhD, DACVN
Assistant Clinical Professor
Small Animal Clinical Sciences
The University of Tennessee
Knoxville, Tennessee

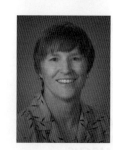

Debra L. Zoran, DVM, PhD, DACVIM (Small Animal Internal Medicine)
Professor and Operations Supervisor, Texas
    A&M VET
Department of Small Animal Clinical
    Sciences
College of Veterinary Medicine and
    Biomedical Sciences
Texas A&M University
College Station, Texas

Prefácio

Iniciamos o prefácio da sétima edição reconhecendo que já havíamos começado a trabalhar na oitava. Mal percebemos como ela iria evoluir, como o campo editorial mudaria e como as preferências de leitores juniores e seniores iriam desenvolver-se durante esse período relativamente breve. Quem teria imaginado, em 1975, quando publicamos a primeira edição, que se seguiriam pelo menos sete edições, que os números teriam cor, que haveria algoritmos em quase todos os capítulos, que mais de 500 vídeos estariam disponíveis ao clique de um *mouse* e que haveria 360 capítulos sucintos, mas completos, com a contribuição de mais de 300 autores? Um conteúdo mais abrangente sobre medicina interna foi compactado em dois volumes, o que não é significativamente diferente em tamanho em relação à primeira edição, de 1975. No entanto, pense nos avanços desde então! Esta edição é tão diferente das anteriores que é verdadeiramente única; afinal, atualmente todo livro didático é produzido tanto na versão impressa como na digital. O leitor pode escolher o formato preferido, e o recurso é compatível com *desktops/laptops*, *tablets* e *smartphones*.

Talvez a maior mudança tenha sido a participação de um terceiro coeditor para ajudar em todos os aspectos do desenvolvimento desta edição. Etienne Côté tem sido amigo, estagiário e, agora, um mentor. Ele realmente ajudou Ed e Steve com novas ideias, aprimorou o processo de edição e auxiliou na obtenção de novos contatos, trechos adicionais e orientação com informações de digitalização essenciais para o objetivo do livro. Agradecemos Etienne por seu tempo, sua experiência, sua diligência e seu interminável entusiasmo.

Esta oitava edição de *Tratado de Medicina Interna Veterinária: Doenças do Cão e do Gato* apresenta grandes mudanças. Nosso maior orgulho poderia ser os mais de 300 autores que concordaram em contribuir; ou talvez os mais de 20 países que eles chamam de lar; ou ainda as centenas de vídeos originais que tornam este livro vibrante. Poderia ser também a verdadeira competência dos autores, que se revela na capacidade de coletar o material mais importante, recente e relevante para o leitor, separando o que realmente importa e apresentando os assuntos claramente, sem floreio ou embelezamento. Como todos vão apreciar, é tudo isso e muito mais.

Anteriormente, o livro começava pela clínica médica, seguida por capítulos sobre doenças específicas de cada sistema do organismo. Embora isso não tenha mudado, enfatizamos a coesão e a profundidade do conteúdo das seções. Assim, convidamos o leitor a, em vez de apenas passar pelo sumário, examiná-lo cuidadosamente, a fim de perceber como é fácil pesquisar no livro e como os capítulos estão apresentados, de modo a imitar o processo de pensamento clínico do leitor praticante.

A obra é apresentada de maneira que reflita a medicina clínica veterinária; por isso, os primeiros capítulos contêm verdadeiros fundamentos do nosso trabalho profissional. As seções abordam também o diagnóstico diferencial entre as principais preocupações dos clientes e as razões para a busca de atendimento veterinário, como anormalidades no exame físico e clinicopatológicas. A última seção é totalmente nova e integra exames de laboratório com medicina clínica por meio de diagnósticos diferenciais detalhados e explicações da fisiologia de diferentes analitos. Há uma seção que inclui praticamente todos os procedimentos necessários para esclarecer ou confirmar um diagnóstico – técnicas que definem a medicina interna veterinária, desde a colocação do tubo de alimentação e a coleta de líquido cefalorraquidiano até a eletromiografia e a medicina hiperbárica. Outra nova seção consiste em capítulos sobre terapias intervencionistas, urológicas, cardiovasculares, gastrintestinais e outros procedimentos que estão na vanguarda da terapêutica de pequenos animais. Os capítulos específicos sobre doenças foram amplamente atualizados ou completamente reescritos. O livro termina com uma nova seção reconhecendo que as doenças nem sempre existem isoladamente. Essa seção de comorbidades identifica os pares de doenças que envolvem tratamento diametralmente oposto, requisitos e alguns casos complexos e especialmente desafiadores de medicina interna.

Todos os capítulos e seções foram configurados para facilitar a consulta. As referências cruzadas (que remetem o leitor de um capítulo para outro pertinente) foram implementadas pelos editores, com sua visão panorâmica de todo o livro. Isso não significa que o autor de um capítulo compartilhe do mesmo ponto de vista apresentado em um capítulo com referências cruzadas, mas auxilia o leitor a navegar rapidamente por informações relevantes e complementares entre si.

Bons vídeos transmitem, em poucos segundos, conteúdo que vários parágrafos levariam mais tempo para expressar, com menos eficácia. Esta edição tem uma biblioteca inteira de videoclipes originais de alta qualidade que incorporam a premissa de que "ver é crer". Todos foram cuidadosamente escolhidos pelos autores, adaptados para o aprendizado e incrementados com títulos e legendas que acreditamos fazer a medicina interna ganhar vida (conteúdo em inglês).

Cada capítulo termina com uma mensagem de direcionamento para as Referências Bibliográficas e/ou Leitura Sugerida, que estão *online* no Ambiente de Aprendizagem do *site* do Grupo GEN. No formato digital, as próprias referências já estão localizadas no final dos capítulos.

Por se tratar de uma produção mundial, envolvendo autores de mais de 20 nações, sabemos que diversos países e laboratórios utilizam os limites superior e inferior de maneira diferente ou mesmo em termos distintos para intervalos de referência. Preferimos que resultados laboratoriais típicos de qualquer condição sejam revistos de maneira geral, sugerindo que os valores podem estar acima, abaixo ou dentro da faixa de referência. Não é mais apropriado fornecer resultados específicos, uma vez que cada laboratório provavelmente usa diferentes ensaios e protocolos, que fazem com que cada faixa de referência seja específica ao laboratório em que o ensaio é realizado. Tal abordagem reflete nosso desejo de atender às necessidades dos leitores ao redor do mundo.

Tradicionalmente, inserimos fotos dos colaboradores da obra. Assim, o leitor pode reconhecer qualquer pessoa que tenha contribuído com um capítulo para o livro. É bom ver que nossos autores continuam entusiasmados em fazer parte desse esforço.

Não podemos agradecer-lhes o suficiente por cumprirem um cronograma tão curto e manterem seus capítulos atualizados, muitas vezes um mês antes do prazo final.

Escrever um capítulo com limite estrito de páginas provavelmente é uma das tarefas mais difíceis que se pode impor a um autor. Além disso, reunir material científico para um nível avançado exige conhecimento especial. Nosso objetivo é continuar atendendo às necessidades dos veterinários de hoje, bem como de estudantes, jovens graduados e profissionais da área que desejam um esforço enciclopédico em medicina de pequenos animais. Agradecemos também aos autores que contribuíram para edições anteriores e, assim, adicionaram um viés original às primeiras versões dos capítulos atuais.

Estamos orgulhosos de nosso esforço para incorporar excelentes colegas de tantos países. Este livro rapidamente tornou-se internacional, publicado em pelo menos cinco idiomas e lido na maior parte do mundo por veterinários e estudantes. É com honra, prazer e um distinto sentimento de orgulho que podemos oferecer ao leitor muitos dos melhores escritores veterinários e pesquisadores de todo o mundo. Em uma carta sobre seu capítulo, um dos colaboradores, Adrian Boswood, relatou algo que nos encorajou a continuar trabalhando. A carta dizia: "É uma honra poder contribuir para este livro. Ele tem uma fama que precede a minha carreira e, sem dúvida, também sobreviverá a ela!"

Obrigado a todos pelo apoio necessário em tão crucial processo de preparação. Nas edições anteriores, não tivemos editores de seção e decidimos continuar assim. No entanto, reconhecemos que há um número crescente de especialistas de destaque na profissão, embora não conheçamos todos. Assim, convidamos alguns de nossos amigos e colegas para ajudar com nomes de profissionais em potencial para escrever sobre suas áreas de especialização e revisar os títulos de capítulos propostos como representativos do campo. Somos muito gratos a esses colegas, que investiram tempo e esforço ao nos auxiliar nesse sentido. Em alguns casos, os autores são veterinários que conhecemos; em outros, foi oferecida uma extensa lista de novos nomes. Ficamos muito satisfeitos em convocá-los para contribuir. Sendo assim, agradecemos aos nossos consultores de seção pela ajuda, em especial aos Drs. Vanessa Barrs, Joe Bartges, Leah Cohn, Ronaldo da Costa, Autumn Davidson, Lisa Freeman, Ann Hohenhaus, Safdar Khan, Mark Papich, Jörg Steiner, Harriet Syme, Jane Sykes, David Twedt e David Vail.

Como sempre, a equipe da Elsevier foi muito prestativa ao elaborar esta nova edição. Tínhamos tantas ideias e tanto material novo para trabalhar, além de uma enorme lista de conteúdo em áudio e vídeo. Sozinhos, estávamos sobrecarregados. A execução de tudo isso não seria possível sem o apoio contínuo de Rhoda Howell, Jolynn Gower, Catherine Jackson, David Dipazo e, claro, Penny Rudolph. Muito obrigado pela paciência e presença contínua.

À nossas esposas e a nossos filhos, mais uma vez sentimos o esmagador desejo de lembrar o quanto são importantes para nós. Seu apoio, sua compaixão e sua vontade de compartilhar deste esforço significa muito. Nós amamos vocês!

Aos nossos colegas, que sempre foram tão solidários ao longo dos anos, obrigado por seus comentários construtivos, bem como por sua paixão pelo que tentamos fornecer. Suas calorosas boas-vindas, tanto em casa quanto aonde quer que viajemos, sempre foram uma verdadeira alegria para nós e nos fazem perceber o quanto todos nós estamos conectados neste mundo em expansão da medicina veterinária.

Steve Ettinger
Ed Feldman
Etienne Côté
Outubro de 2016

Sumário

VOLUME 1

SEÇÃO 1
Fundamentos Básicos da Medicina Veterinária

1 Histórico Clínico, *1*
Michael Schaer

2 Exame Físico, *4*
Stephen J. Ettinger, Edward C. Feldman e Etienne Côté

3 Genética Básica, *25*
Kathryn M. Meurs e Joshua A. Stern

4 Genômica Clínica, *27*
Kathryn M. Meurs e Joshua A. Stern

5 Medicina Veterinária Baseada em Evidências, *32*
Steven C. Budsberg

6 Estatística Biomédica: Tópicos Selecionados, *34*
Philip H. Kass

7 Eutanásia, *38*
W. Douglas Kunz e Stephen J. Ettinger

SEÇÃO 2
Diagnóstico Diferencial das Queixas Principais

GERAL

8 "O Animal Não Está Bem": Principal Queixa Inespecífica de Falha no Desenvolvimento, *43*
Stephen J. Ettinger, Edward C. Feldman e Etienne Côté

9 Diferenciação entre Alterações de Comportamento e Doenças Clínicas, *46*
Diane Frank

10 Manifestações Dermatológicas de Doenças Sistêmicas, *50*
Karen L. Campbell

11 Manifestações Oftálmicas da Doença Sistêmica, *54*
Alexandra van der Woerdt

12 Manifestações Neurológicas de Doenças Sistêmicas, *60*
Helena Rylander

13 Diferenciação entre Intoxicações e Doenças Não Tóxicas Agudas, *64*
Safdar A. Khan

14 Manifestações Ortopédicas de Doenças Sistêmicas, *70*
Bing Yun Zhu

15 Dor e Tumefação Articulares, *73*
Jonathan D. Dear

16 Ganho de Peso, *77*
Peter P. Kintzer

17 Distensão Abdominal, *79*
Julie Walter

18 Edema Periférico, *82*
Deborah M. Fine-Ferreira

19 Perda de Peso como Queixa Principal, *86*
Thomas Schermerhorn

20 Déficit de Crescimento, *89*
Hans S. Kooistra

21 Fraqueza, *92*
Fred C. Brewer IV

22 Inquietação, *95*
Michael D. Willard

23 Anorexia, *98*
Marnin A. Forman

24 Polifagia, *101*
Sylvie Daminet

25 Odores Corporais, *105*
Darren Berger

CARDIORRESPIRATÓRIO

26 Tosse, *108*
Luca Ferasin

27 Espirro e Secreção Nasal, *112*
Julio López

28 Taquipneia, Dispneia e Angústia Respiratória, *116*
M. Lynne O'Sullivan

29 Epistaxe e Hemoptise, *120*
Tim B. Hackett

30 Síncope, *124*
Mike Martin

NEUROLÓGICO

31 Distúrbios do Movimento, *128*
William B. Thomas

32 Tremores, *131*
Clare Rusbridge

33 Ataxia, Paresia e Paralisia, *135*
Ronaldo Casimiro da Costa

34 Estupor e Coma, *139*
Karen Lynne Kline

35 Convulsões, *143*
Karen R. Muñana

GASTRINTESTINAL

36 Ptialismo e Halitose, *147*
Camilla Heinze e Brook A. Niemiec

37 Engasgamento, *152*
Peter Hendrik Kook

38 Disfagia, *155*
Julio López

39 Vômito e Regurgitação, *159*
Alex Gallagher

40 Diarreia, *164*
Michael D. Willard

41 Melena e Hematoquezia, *167*
Karen M. Tefft

42 Constipação Intestinal, Tenesmo, Disquesia e Incontinência Fecal, *171*
Peter Foley

43 Flatulência, *175*
Alexander James German

UROGENITAL

44 Secreções Vulvar e Prepucial, *178*
Jeffrey de Gier e Auke C. Schaefers-Okkens

45 Poliúria e Polidipsia, *181*
Robert E. Shiel

46 Polaciúria, Estrangúria e Incontinência Urinária, *184*
Mary Anna Labato

47 Hematúria e Outras Condições que Causam Alteração na Cor da Urina, *189*
Thierry Francey

SEÇÃO 3

Diagnósticos Diferenciais para Anormalidades Detectadas no Exame Físico

48 Febre, *193*
Ian K. Ramsey e Séverine Tasker

49 Hipotermia, *201*
Justine A. Lee

50 Palidez, *203*
Dan G. Ohad

51 Hiperemia, *206*
Anthony C. G. Abrams-Ogg

52 Cianose, *208*
Anna Tidholm

53 Icterícia, *211*
Christina Alanna Bradbury

54 Petéquias e Equimoses, *214*
Shauna Blois

55 Sons Cardíacos Anormais e Sopros Cardíacos, *217*
Robert Prošek

56 Alterações de Pulso, *221*
Christopher Little

SEÇÃO 4

Diagnóstico Diferencial de Anormalidades Clinicopatológicas

57 Anemia e Eritrocitose, *225*
Tracy Stokol

58 Leucopenia e Leucocitose, *231*
Amy E. DeClue e Dennis R. Spann

59 Trombocitopenia e Trombocitose, *234*
Marjory B. Brooks

Tratado de Medicina Interna Veterinária: Doenças do Cão e do Gato

60 Hipoproteinemia e Hiperproteinemia, *239*
Shelley Burton

61 Hipoglicemia e Hiperglicemia, *242*
Yaiza Forcada

62 Creatinina e Nitrogênio Ureico Sanguíneo, *246*
Carrie A. Palm

63 Colesterol e Triglicerídeos, *248*
Panagiotis G. Xenoulis

64 Amilase e Lipase, *253*
Peter Hendrik Kook

65 Enzimas Hepáticas, *254*
Andrea N. Johnston

66 Creatinoquinase, *260*
Susan M. Taylor

67 Sódio e Cloro, *262*
Dan Rosenberg

68 Potássio e Magnésio, *267*
Ann-Marie Della Maggiore

69 Cálcio e Fósforo, *272*
Richard John Mellanby

70 Lactato, *276*
Kari Santoro Beer

71 Amônia, *278*
Allison Bradley

72 Exame de Urina, *280*
Peter A. Graham

73 Concentrações de Eletrólitos na Urina, *286*
Steven Epstein

74 Análise de Líquidos Corporais: Torácico,
Abdominal e Articular, *289*
Tracy Stokol

SEÇÃO 5
Técnicas

GERAL

75 Punção Venosa e Arterial, *297*
Linda Merrill

76 Cateterização da Veia Jugular e Mensuração
da Pressão Venosa Central, *299*
Meri F. Hall

77 Cateteres de Uso Intraósseo, *302*
Andre C. Shih

78 Taxa de Infusão Contínua, *304*
Steven L. Marks

79 Monitoramento da Glicemia em Amostra
de Sangue Obtida da Veia Auricular, *306*
Melanie D. Thompson

80 Tempo de Sangramento da Mucosa Bucal, *309*
Christine Savidge

81 Exame de Fezes, *311*
Byron L. Blagburn e Jane D. Mount

82 Técnicas para Colocação de Sonda por Via
Nasoesofágica e por Meio de Esofagostomia,
Gastrostomia e Jejunostomia, *319*
Stanley Leon Marks

83 Cuidados com o Equipamento de Endoscopia, *328*
Valerie Walker, Susan Cox e Katie Douthitt

84 Medicina Hiperbárica, *331*
Melissa L. Edwards

PELE

85 Otoscopia, Lavagem da Orelha e Miringotomia, *334*
David Stephen Sobel

86 Raspado, Aspiração por Agulha Fina e Biopsia
de Pele e Tecido Subcutâneo, *337*
Ralf S. Mueller e Sonya V. Bettenay

87 Citologia de Pele e Tecidos Subcutâneos, *340*
Ryan M. Dickinson

ABDOME

88 Ultrassonografia Abdominal, *343*
Rachel E. Pollard

89 Ultrassonografia Abdominal: Aspirações e
Biopsias, *346*
Eric J. Herrgesell

90 Abdominocentese e Lavagem Peritoneal
Diagnóstica, *348*
Oriana Raab

91 Laparoscopia, *350*
Keith Richter

PUNÇÕES E BIOPSIAS EM GERAL

92 Aspiração e Biopsia de Medula Óssea, *353*
Valerie MacDonald

93 Citologia de Órgãos Internos, *356*
Lamberto Viadel Bau

94 Artrocentese e Artroscopia, *359*
Jonathan D. Dear

95 Aspiração e Biopsia de Linfonodos, *361*
Takuo Ishida

96 Rinoscopia, Biopsia Nasal e Lavado Nasal, *364*
Caroline Page

RESPIRATÓRIAS E CARDIOVASCULARES

97 Terapia Respiratória e Inalatória, *367*
Laura A. Nafe

98 Oximetria de Pulso, *370*
Steven Epstein

99 Mensuração da Pressão Sanguínea, *372*
Rebecca L. Stepien

100 Colocação de Tubo Torácico, *377*
Tim B. Hackett

101 Lavado Transtraqueal e Broncoscopia, *379*
Tekla M. Lee-Fowler

102 Toracocentese/Pericardiocentese, *382*
Robert Prošek

103 Eletrocardiografia, *385*
Erin Anderson

104 Ecocardiografia, *388*
Marie-Claude Bélanger

RINS, VIAS URINÁRIAS, PRÓSTATA

105 Coleta de Urina, *406*
Amanda Callens e Joseph W. Bartges

106 Manuseio de Cateteres Urinários, *409*
Amanda Callens e Joseph W. Bartges

107 Desobstrução da Uretra, *411*
Jody P. Lulich e Carl A. Osborne

108 Cistoscopia e Uretroscopia, *415*
Julie K. Byron

109 Diálise Peritoneal, *418*
Alexa M. E. Bersenas

110 Terapia Renal Substitutiva Contínua/ Hemodiálise, *421*
Mark J. Acierno e Mary Anna Labato

111 Técnicas de Diagnóstico de Anormalidades da Próstata, *426*
Michelle Anne Kutzler

SISTEMA GASTRINTESTINAL

112 Intubação e Lavagem Gástrica, *430*
Deborah C. Silverstein

113 Endoscopia Gastrintestinal, *432*
M. Katherine Tolbert

114 Enemas e Desobstipação, *436*
Stefan Unterer

SISTEMA NERVOSO

115 Coleta e Exame do Líquido Cefalorraquidiano e Mielografia, *439*
John Henry Rossmeisl, Jr.

116 Biopsia de Músculos e Nervos, *442*
Kerry Smith Bailey

117 Eletromiografia e Velocidade de Condução Nervosa, *443*
David Lipsitz e D. Colette Williams

SISTEMA REPRODUTOR

118 Inseminação Artificial em Cadelas, *445*
Catharina Linde Forsberg

119 Vaginoscopia e Citologia Vaginal em Cadelas, *449*
Cheryl Lopate

SEÇÃO 6

Terapias Intervencionistas Minimamente Invasivas

120 Visão Geral Sobre a Medicina Intervencionista, *455*
Chick Weisse

121 Terapias Intervencionistas no Sistema Respiratório, *462*
Matthew W. Beal

122 Terapias Intervencionistas no Sistema Cardiovascular, *469*
Brian A. Scansen

123 Terapias Intervencionistas Gastrintestinais, *482*
Allyson C. Berent

124 Terapias Intervencionistas Urológicas, *489*
Marilyn E. Dunn e Allyson C. Berent

125 Terapias Intervencionistas Neoplásicas, *507*
Chick Weisse

SEÇÃO 7
Cuidados Intensivos

126 Fisiologia, Identificação e Manejo da Dor no Ambiente de Cuidados Intensivos, *513*
Lisa Moses

127 Choque, *522*
Teresa M. Rieser

128 Distúrbios Acidobásicos, Oximetria e Análise dos Gases Sanguíneos, *525*
Marie E. Kerl

129 Fluidoterapia com Cristaloides e Coloides, *530*
Christopher G. Byers

130 Transfusões Sanguíneas, Terapia com Hemocomponentes e Soluções Carreadoras de Oxigênio, *537*
Anthony C. G. Abrams-Ogg e Shauna Blois

131 Oxigenoterapia, *546*
Kate Hopper

132 Sepse e Síndrome da Resposta Inflamatória Sistêmica, *549*
Amy E. DeClue

133 Resposta Endócrina às Enfermidades Graves, *555*
Johan P. Schoeman

134 Insolação, *557*
Elisa M. Mazzaferro

135 Hemorragia, *561*
Armelle de Laforcade

136 Estado Epiléptico, *563*
Alireza A. Gorgi

137 Anafilaxia, *566*
Lori S. Waddell

138 Sedação e Anestesia em Pacientes em Unidade de Tratamento Intensivo, *569*
James S. Gaynor

139 Avaliação Inicial de Emergências Respiratórias, *573*
Carol R. Reinero

140 Parada e Reanimação Cardiopulmonares, *576*
Daniel John Fletcher e Manuel Boller

141 Emergências Cardíacas, *582*
Manuel Boller

142 Cetoacidose Diabética e Síndrome Hiperglicêmica Hiperosmolar, *587*
Mauria O'Brien

143 Abdome Agudo, *593*
Søren Boysen

144 Emergências Gastrintestinais, *599*
Amie Koenig

145 Emergências Hepáticas e Esplênicas, *603*
Amanda K. Boag

146 Emergências Reprodutivas, *606*
Luis Miguel Fonte Montenegro e Ana Martins-Bessa

147 Abordagem Geral do Paciente com Trauma, *612*
Kenneth J. Drobatz

148 Traumatismo Cranioencefálico, *615*
Eileen Kenney

149 Trauma Torácico, *618*
Elizabeth Rozanski

150 Traumatismo do Trato Urinário, *624*
Amy M. Koenigshof

SEÇÃO 8
Toxicologia

151 Descontaminação: Tratamento de Exposição a Toxinas, *627*
Camille DeClementi

152 Intoxicações Causadas por Produtos Químicos, *629*
Justine A. Lee

153 Intoxicação por Medicamentos que Necessitam de Receita e por Medicamentos de Venda Livre, *637*
Ahna G. Brutlag

154 Intoxicação por Drogas Utilizadas para Fins Recreativos, *643*
Safdar A. Khan

155 Intoxicações por Plantas, *647*
David C. Dorman

156 Mordidas e Picadas por Animais Peçonhentos (Zootoxicoses), *653*
Michael Peterson

SEÇÃO 9
Pressão Sanguínea

157 Fisiopatologia e Manifestações Clínicas da Hipertensão Sistêmica, *659*
Serge Chalhoub e Douglas Palma

158 Tratamento da Hipertensão Sistêmica, *666*
Dan G. Ohad

159 Hipotensão Sistêmica, *671*
Lori S. Waddell

SEÇÃO 10

Considerações Terapêuticas em Medicina e Doença

160 Princípios da Distribuição e Farmacocinética de Medicamentos, *677*
Butch KuKanich

161 Tratamento com Medicamentos Antibacterianos, *684*
Mark G. Papich

162 Terapia Antifúngica e Antiviral, *689*
Mark G. Papich

163 Terapia Antiparasitária, *693*
Byron L. Blagburn e Jane D. Mount

164 Terapia Anti-inflamatória, *696*
Shauna Blois e Karol A. Mathews

165 Terapia Imunossupressora, *701*
Todd M. Archer

166 Terapia Analgésica, *705*
Kristen Messenger

167 Antioxidantes, Nutracêuticos, Probióticos e Suplementos Nutricionais, *709*
Laura Eirmann

168 Medicamentos Manipulados, *712*
Ron Johnson e Dinah G. Jordan

169 Reações Adversas a Medicamentos, *716*
Wayne Stanley Schwark

SEÇÃO 11

Considerações Dietéticas de Distúrbios Sistêmicos

170 Avaliação Nutricional, *721*
Kathryn E. Michel

171 Nutrição Neonatal e Pediátrica, *724*
Cecilia Villaverde

172 Nutrição para Cães Adultos Saudáveis, *725*
Martha G. Cline

173 Manejo Nutricional do Cão Atleta, *728*
Joseph J. Wakshlag

174 Nutrição para o Gato Adulto Saudável, *730*
Jennifer Larsen

175 Nutrição de Cães e Gatos Geriátricos Saudáveis, *733*
Cecilia Villaverde

176 Obesidade, *736*
Juan José Ramos-Plá

177 Caquexia e Sarcopenia, *742*
Lisa M. Freeman

178 Manejo Nutricional das Doenças do Trato Gastrintestinal, *747*
Debra L. Zoran

179 Manejo Nutricional da Doença do Pâncreas Exócrino, *752*
Marjorie Chandler

180 Manejo Nutricional das Doenças Hepatobiliares, *754*
Craig G. Ruaux

181 Manejo Nutricional de Doenças Endócrinas e Metabólicas, *758*
Jennifer Larsen

182 Considerações Clínicas e Dietéticas em Casos de Hiperlipidemia, *762*
Richard C. Hill

183 Manejo Nutricional das Cardiopatias, *768*
Lisa M. Freeman e John E. Rush

184 Manejo Nutricional das Doenças Renais, *775*
Joseph W. Bartges

185 Controle Nutricional da Doença do Trato Urinário Inferior, *778*
Yann Queau e Vincent C. Biourge

186 Abordagem Nutricional de Afecções Dermatológicas, *781*
Manon Paradis

187 Distúrbios Esqueléticos Relacionados com a Nutrição, *783*
Ronald Jan Corbee

188 Abordagem Nutricional do Câncer, *788*
Glenna E. Mauldin

189 Nutrição em Cuidados Intensivos, *791*
Daniel L. Chan

190 Usos Nutricionais da Fibra, *796*
Amy Farcas

191 Reações Adversas aos Alimentos: Alergias *versus* Intolerância, *801*
Jason W. Gagné

192 Dietas Não Convencionais (Caseiras, Vegetarianas e Cruas), *806*
Sally C. Perea e Sean J. Delaney

193 Segurança Alimentar e Aspectos Regulatórios de Alimentos para Animais de Estimação, *811*
David A. Dzanis

194 Imunologia e Nutrição, *813*
Nick John Cave

SEÇÃO 12
Doenças Hematológicas e Imunológicas

195 Doenças Hematológicas e Imunológicas: Introdução e Terapia Medicamentosa, *819*
Suliman Al-Ghazlat e Ann E. Hohenhaus

196 Teste de Coagulação, *822*
Stephanie A. Smith e Maureen McMichael

197 Estados Hiper e Hipocoaguláveis, *827*
Shauna Blois

198 Anemias Hemolíticas Imunomediadas e Outras Anemias Regenerativas, *833*
Christine Piek

199 Anemias Não Regenerativas, *842*
Ann E. Hohenhaus e Sarah Elizabeth Winzelberg

200 Policitemia Primária e Eritrocitose, *848*
Ann E. Hohenhaus

201 Trombocitopenia Imunomediada, Doença de von Willebrand e Outros Distúrbios Plaquetários, *851*
Mary Beth Callan e James L. Catalfamo

202 Distúrbios Imunomediados e Não Neoplásicos em Leucócitos, *860*
Jennifer L. Johns

203 Poliartrite Imunomediada e Outras Poliartrites, *865*
Michael Stone

204 Doenças Dermatológicas Imunomediadas, *871*
Petra Bizikova

205 Lúpus Eritematoso Sistêmico, *877*
Michael Stone

206 Doenças Não Neoplásicas do Baço, *881*
David John Argyle e Robert T. O'Brien

SEÇÃO 13
Doenças Infecciosas

GERAL

207 Diagnóstico Laboratorial de Doenças Infecciosas, *893*
Michael R. Lappin

208 Vacinação de Animais de Companhia, *900*
Michael J. Day

209 Resistência Antimicrobiana, Vigilância e Infecções Nosocomiais, *906*
J. Scott Weese

210 Zoonoses, *909*
Michael R. Lappin

DOENÇAS BACTERIANAS

211 Doença de Lyme, *917*
Meryl P. Littman

212 Micobacteriose, Actinomicose e Nocardiose, *922*
Joanna Whitney e Carolyn R. O'Brien

213 Brucelose, *927*
David P. Beehan

214 Tétano e Botulismo, *930*
Simon R. Platt

215 Bartonelose em Cães, *935*
Pedro Paulo V. P. Diniz

216 Bartonelose em Gatos, *940*
Lynn F. Guptill

217 Leptospirose, *945*
Simone Schuller

218 Erliquiose, Anaplasmose, Febre Maculosa das Montanhas Rochosas e Neorriquetsiose, *950*
Jane E. Sykes

219 Micoplasmas Hemotrópicos, *957*
Séverine Tasker

220 Doenças Intestinais Bacterianas, *963*
Stanley Leon Marks

DOENÇAS CAUSADAS POR PROTOZOÁRIOS

221 Infecções por Protozoários, *968*
Michael R. Lappin

DOENÇAS VIRAIS

222 Infecção pelo Vírus da Imunodeficiência Felina, *977*
Julia A. Beatty

223 Infecção pelo Vírus da Leucemia Felina, *984*
Katrin Hartmann e Julie K. Levy

224 Infecções Causadas por Coronavírus (Cães e Gatos), Incluindo Peritonite Infecciosa Felina, *989*
Katrin Hartmann

225 Infecção por Parvovírus em Cães e Gatos, *997*
Andrew Lambert Leisewitz

226 Raiva, *1002*
Cathleen A. Hanlon

227 Doença Respiratória Infecciosa Canina, *1009*
Simon Lawrence Priestnall

228 Cinomose e Outras Infecções Virais em Cães, *1012*
Thomas Wilhelm Vahlenkamp

229 Infecções do Trato Respiratório Superior de Gatos, *1020*
Maria Manuel Afonso, Rosalind M. Gaskell e Alan Radford

230 Outras Infecções Virais em Gatos, *1023*
Maria Manuel Afonso, Rosalind M. Gaskell e Alan Radford

DOENÇAS FÚNGICAS

231 Criptococose, *1026*
Joseph Taboada

232 Coccidioidomicose, *1031*
Jane E. Sykes

233 Blastomicose e Histoplasmose, *1034*
Andrea Dedeaux e Joseph Taboada

234 Aspergilose em Cães, *1042*
Frédéric Billen e Dominique Peeters

235 Aspergilose em Gatos, *1046*
Vanessa R. Barrs

236 Infecções Fúngicas Diversas, *1051*
Amy M. Grooters

SEÇÃO 14
Doenças de Ouvido, Nariz e Garganta

237 Doenças do Ouvido, *1059*
Emmanuel Bensignor, Olivier Gauthier e Didier-Noël Carlotti

238 Doenças do Nariz, dos Seios Paranasais e da Nasofaringe, *1067*
Gerhard Ulrich Oechtering

239 Doenças da Laringe, *1085*
Catriona M. MacPhail

VOLUME 2

SEÇÃO 15
Doença Respiratória

240 Avaliação Clínica do Trato Respiratório, *1091*
Stephan Anthony Carey

241 Doenças da Traqueia e de Vias Respiratórias de Pequeno Calibre, *1102*
Cécile Clercx

242 Doenças do Parênquima Pulmonar, *1117*
Leah A. Cohn

243 Hipertensão Pulmonar e Tromboembolismo Pulmonar, *1141*
Justin G. Williams

244 Doenças do Espaço Pleural, *1146*
Elizabeth Rozanski

245 Doenças do Mediastino, da Parede Torácica e do Diafragma, *1153*
Martha Moon Larson e David S. Biller

SEÇÃO 16
Doença Cardiovascular

246 Fisiopatologia da Insuficiência Cardíaca, *1163*
Katherine F. Scollan e D. David Sisson

247 Insuficiência Cardíaca: Tratamento Clínico, *1173*
Adrian Boswood

248 Arritmias Cardíacas, *1186*
Etienne Côté e Stephen J. Ettinger

249 Marca-Passo Cardíaco, *1209*
Amara H. Estrada

250 Cardiopatias Congênitas, *1215*
Niek J. Beijerink, Mark A. Oyama e John D. Bonagura

251 Doenças Cardiovasculares no Início da Idade Adulta, *1256*
Ingrid Ljungvall e Jens Häggström

252 Cardiomiopatias: Cães, *1276*
Joshua A. Stern e Kathryn M. Meurs

253 Cardiomiopatias: Gatos, *1285*
Valérie Chetboul

254 Doenças do Pericárdio, *1312*
Kristin MacDonald

255 Dirofilariose Canina e Felina, *1323*
Clarke Atkins

256 Doença Arterial Tromboembólica, *1351*
Daniel F. Hogan

257 Doenças de Veias e Vasos Linfáticos, *1357*
Brian A. Scansen e John D. Bonagura

SEÇÃO 17
Doença Neurológica

258 Neurofisiologia, *1369*
Dennis P. O'Brien e Joan R. Coates

259 Exame Neurológico e Diagnóstico
Neuroanatômico, *1374*
Scott J. Schatzberg

260 Doenças do Cérebro: Anomalia, Degenerativa,
Metabólica, Neoplásica, Idiopática, Epiléptica
e Vascular, *1387*
Joan R. Coates e Dennis P. O'Brien

261 Doenças Cerebrais Inflamatórias, Infecciosas
e Multifocais, *1411*
Chelsie Estey e Curtis W. Dewey

262 Distúrbios do Sono, *1419*
Brian M. Zanghi

263 Disfunção Cognitiva em Cães e Gatos Idosos, *1422*
Gary Landsberg

264 Neuropatias Cranianas, *1426*
John Henry Rossmeisl, Jr.

265 Doença Vestibular, *1429*
Veronique Sammut

266 Doenças da Medula Espinal: Congênitas
(Desenvolvimento), Inflamatórias e
Degenerativas, *1437*
Ronaldo Casimiro da Costa e Simon R. Platt

267 Doenças da Medula Espinal: Traumáticas,
Vasculares e Doenças Neoplásicas, *1451*
Nicholas Jeffery

268 Neuropatias Periféricas, *1460*
Christopher L. Mariani

269 Distúrbios da Junção Neuromuscular, *1465*
Sarah A. Moore e Christopher L. Mariani

270 Transtornos Neurológicos Exclusivos
de Felinos, *1469*
Elsa Beltran e Luisa De Risio

SEÇÃO 18
Doença Gastrintestinal

271 Avaliação Laboratorial do Trato Gastrintestinal, *1475*
Jörg M. Steiner

272 Distúrbios Orais e das Glândulas Salivares, *1479*
Alexander M. Reiter e Maria M. Soltero-Rivera

273 Doenças da Faringe e do Esôfago, *1486*
Stanley Leon Marks

274 Interações Hospedeiro-Microbiota na Saúde
e Doença Gastrintestinal, *1500*
Albert Earl Jergens

275 Doenças do Estômago, *1504*
Kenneth W. Simpson

276 Doenças do Intestino Delgado, *1526*
Edward James Hall e Michael J. Day

277 Doenças do Intestino Grosso, *1575*
Edward James Hall

278 Doenças Anorretais, *1603*
Stefan Unterer

279 Peritonite, *1615*
Thandeka Roseann Ngwenyama e
Rance K. Sellon

SEÇÃO 19
Doenças Hepatobiliares

280 Avaliação Diagnóstica da Função Hepática, *1621*
Sarah Cocker e Keith Richter

281 Princípios Gerais do Tratamento de
Hepatopatias, *1632*
Jonathan Andrew Lidbury

282 Hepatopatias Inflamatórias/Infecciosas em
Cães, *1639*
Craig B. Webb

283 Hepatopatias Inflamatórias/Infecciosas em
Gatos, *1645*
Marnin A. Forman

284 Anomalias Vasculares Hepáticas, *1651*
Chick Weisse e Allyson C. Berent

285 Doenças Metabólicas Hepáticas, *1671*
Penny J. Watson

286 Doenças Hepatotóxicas, *1678*
Lauren A. Trepanier

287 Neoplasias Hepáticas, *1684*
Nick Bexfield

288 Doenças da Vesícula Biliar e do Sistema Biliar
Extra-hepático, *1688*
Ale Aguirre

SEÇÃO 20
Doenças Pancreáticas

289 Pancreatite: Etiologia e Fisiopatologia, *1695*
Thomas Spillmann

290 Pancreatite em Cães: Diagnóstico e
Tratamento, *1697*
Jörg M. Steiner

291 Pancreatite em Gatos: Diagnóstico e
Tratamento, *1702*
Craig G. Ruaux

292 Insuficiência Pancreática Exócrina, *1708*
Jörg M. Steiner

293 Neoplasia do Pâncreas Exócrino, *1712*
Peter Bennett

SEÇÃO 21
Doenças Endócrinas

294 Anormalidades Relativas ao Hormônio
de Crescimento em Gatos, *1715*
Stijn J. M. Niessen

295 Anormalidades Relativas ao Hormônio
de Crescimento em Cães, *1720*
Hans S. Kooistra

296 Diabetes Insípido, *1724*
Robert E. Shiel

297 Hiperparatireoidismo Primário, *1729*
Barbara J. Skelly

298 Hipoparatireoidismo, *1742*
Patty Lathan

299 Hipotireoidismo em Cães, *1745*
Carmel T. Mooney

300 Hipotireoidismo em Gatos, *1758*
Sylvie Daminet

301 Hipertireoidismo Felino, *1762*
Thomas K. Graves

302 Hipertireoidismo Canino, *1772*
Cynthia R. Ward

303 Tumores Secretores de Insulina, *1777*
Johan P. Schoeman

304 Diabetes Melito Canino, *1783*
Federico Fracassi

305 Diabetes Melito Felino, *1797*
Jacquie Rand e Susan A. Gottlieb

306 Hiperadrenocorticismo Canino, *1812*
Dolores Pérez-Alenza e Carlos Melián

307 Hiperadrenocorticismo Felino, *1828*
Ian K. Ramsey e Michael E. Herrtage

308 Tumores Adrenocorticais Não Secretores
de Cortisol e Incidentalomas, *1836*
Ellen N. Behrend

309 Hipoadrenocorticismo, *1842*
Rebecka S. Hess

310 Endocrinologia Gastrintestinal, *1851*
Thomas Schermerhorn

311 Feocromocitoma, *1856*
Sara Galac

SEÇÃO 22
Doenças Reprodutivas

312 Endocrinologia Reprodutiva e Manejo
Reprodutivo da Cadela, *1863*
Stefano Romagnoli e Cheryl Lopate

313 Efeito a Longo Prazo da Esterilização e da
Castração na Saúde de Cães e Gatos, *1879*
Hilde de Rooster e Nathalie Porters

314 Reprodução Felina Clínica, *1882*
Eva Agneta Axnér

315 Problemas na Gestação, no Parto e no Periparto
em Cães e Gatos, *1888*
Autumn P. Davidson

316 Piometra e Hiperplasia Endometrial
Cística, *1898*
Annika Bergström

317 Outras Causas Infecciosas de Infertilidade
e Subfertilidade em Cães e Gatos, *1903*
Sophie Alexandra Grundy

318 Exame de Saúde Reprodutiva e Distúrbios
de Reprodução em Cães Machos, *1906*
Gary C.W. England e
Lúcia Daniel Machado da Silva

319 Distúrbios Reprodutivos em Cães ou Cadelas Castrados, *1913*
Autumn P. Davidson

320 Cuidados dos Neonatos durante o Período Pós-Parto, *1921*
Margret L. Casal

SEÇÃO 23
Doenças Renais

321 Abordagem Clínica e Avaliação Laboratorial da Doença Renal, *1925*
Harriet M. Syme e Rosanne Jepson

322 Lesão Renal Aguda, *1939*
Cathy E. Langston

323 Transplante Renal, *1956*
Chad W. Schmiedt

324 Doença Renal Crônica, *1959*
David James Polzin

325 Glomerulopatias, *1981*
Shelly L. Vaden

326 Doenças Tubulares Renais, *1994*
Marie E. Kerl

327 Pielonefrite, *2000*
Astrid M. van Dongen

328 Doenças Renais Familiares e Congênitas de Gatos e Cães, *2003*
Gilad Segev

SEÇÃO 24
Doenças do Trato Urinário Inferior

329 Doenças de Ureter, *2009*
Larry G. Adams

330 Infecções do Trato Urinário Inferior, *2016*
Michael W. Wood

331 Urolitíase no Trato Urinário Inferior de Cães, *2021*
Jody P. Lulich e Carl A. Osborne

332 Urolitíase no Trato Urinário Inferior de Gatos, *2030*
Mary Anna Labato

333 Doenças Relacionadas com a Micção Anormal, *2035*
Julie K. Byron

334 Cistite Idiopática Felina, *2041*
C. A. Tony Buffington

335 Doenças da Uretra, *2045*
Joseph W. Bartges

336 Doenças Congênitas do Trato Urinário Inferior, *2053*
John M. Kruger, Joseph W. Bartges e Elizabeth A. Ballegeer

337 Doenças da Próstata, *2057*
Michelle Anne Kutzler

SEÇÃO 25
Câncer

338 Características/Origem do Câncer, *2063*
Chand Khanna e Amanda Foskett

339 Princípios e Práticas da Quimioterapia, *2066*
Angela E. Frimberger e Antony S. Moore

340 Princípios e Práticas de Radiologia Oncológica, *2073*
Jessica Lawrence

341 Imunoterapia no Tratamento de Câncer, *2079*
Barbara J. Biller

342 Terapia Molecular Dirigida, *2082*
Cheryl London

343 Complicações da Terapia Antineoplásica, *2085*
Louis-Philippe de Lorimier e Craig A. Clifford

344 Tumores Hematopoéticos, *2092*
David M. Vail

345 Tumores Cutâneos, *2106*
Kenneth M. Rassnick

346 Sarcomas de Tecidos Moles, *2111*
Margaret C. McEntee

347 Hemangiossarcoma, *2119*
Craig A. Clifford e Louis-Philippe de Lorimier

348 Tumores Ósseos e Articulares, *2128*
Julius M. Liptak

349 Mastocitose, *2140*
Douglas H. Thamm

350 Doenças Histiocíticas em Cães e Gatos, *2144*
Laurel E. Williams

351 Tumores do Trato Urogenital e da Glândula Mamária, *2147*
Juan F. Borrego

352 Síndromes Paraneoplásicas, *2155*
Timothy J. Stein

SEÇÃO 26

Doenças Musculoesqueléticas

353 Anormalidades Esqueléticas em Animais de Companhia, *2159*
Denis J. Marcellin-Little

354 Doenças Musculares, *2174*
G. Diane Shelton

355 Fisioterapia e Reabilitação, *2179*
David Levine e Darryl L. Millis

356 Dor Crônica: Fisiopatologia, Identificação e Procedimentos Gerais de Controle, *2187*
Lisa Moses

SEÇÃO 27

Comorbidades

357 Cardiopatia e Nefropatia, *2191*
Mark A. Oyama, Shelly L. Vaden e Clarke Atkins

358 Diabetes Melito e Doenças Responsivas a Corticosteroides, *2194*
Lucy J. Davison

359 Comorbidades Associadas à Obesidade, *2201*
Angela L. Witzel

360 Infecções e Imunossupressão Simultâneas, *2205*
Nathaniel T. Whitley

Índice Alfabético, *2213*

SEÇÃO 15
Doença Respiratória

CAPÍTULO 240

Avaliação Clínica do Trato Respiratório

Stephan Anthony Carey

INTRODUÇÃO

O objetivo de avaliar um cão ou gato com sinais respiratórios é obter um diagnóstico específico pelos meios menos invasivos. Primeiro, deve-se *verificar* se o histórico clínico (anamnese) e os sinais clínicos são compatíveis com doença ou disfunção respiratória. Em seguida, é importante *localizar* a disfunção em uma região específica ou mais no sistema respiratório. Verificada e localizada uma doença respiratória, usam-se os recursos disponíveis para *especificar* sua natureza exata e, em geral, recorre-se a meios mais invasivos (p. ex., amostragem para diagnóstico respiratório) e dispendiosos (p. ex., imagens avançadas, endoscopia).

HISTÓRICO CLÍNICO E RESENHA

Generalidades

A abordagem diagnóstica a um cão ou gato com sinais respiratórios começa na sala de exame. O conhecimento das condições específicas da raça e da idade do animal geralmente ajuda a agilizar o processo de localização. A mera resenha pode facilitar a priorização de uma lista de diagnóstico diferencial. Animais de estimação jovens, imunocomprometidos ou não vacinados são mais propensos a ter uma doença infecciosa. Distúrbios conhecidos ou suspeitos de terem etiologia hereditária ou genética em geral são específicos da raça (p. ex., fibrose pulmonar crônica em cães da raça West Highland White Terrier, malformação de laringe congênita em cães Norwich Terrier, asma em gatos das raças Siamês e Havana Brown).[1-3] A conformação também pode dar indícios a respeito da enfermidade. Por exemplo, cães de raças braquicefálicas costumam ter o palato mole espesso e alongado, narinas estenosadas, hipoplasia de traqueia ou outras características que contribuem para obstrução de via respiratória.[4,5] Cães dolicocefálicos parecem mais sujeitos a tumores nasais e aspergilose.[6,7]

Os clínicos devem esforçar-se para obter um histórico clínico completo e detalhado, incluindo alguma informação sobre quando o paciente esteve normal pela última vez. O entendimento de qualquer progressão, velocidade de alteração ou dos padrões quando ou onde os sinais clínicos foram notados pode ajudar. A prontidão em demonstrar um sinal clínico ao proprietário (p. ex., espirro reverso) também pode auxiliar a identificar a causa dos sintomas. Os proprietários devem ser estimulados a fazer vídeos de seus animais quando estão normais e ao

demonstrarem sinais de anormalidades. As perguntas devem visar não apenas a localizar a disfunção respiratória, mas também a verificar se o sistema respiratório é a fonte da disfunção (p. ex., tosse *vs.* náuseas em gatos). Pode ser preciso confirmar se os sinais clínicos antes atribuídos a outros sistemas orgânicos realmente são oriundos do trato respiratório (p. ex., vômito *versus* náuseas após a tosse, em cães).

Informações obtidas no histórico clínico sugestivas de doença respiratória

Espirro

Define-se espirro (ver Capítulo 27) como um reflexo expiratório involuntário protetor, após irritação da mucosa nasal, que pode ser difícil impedir. Durante um espirro, a cabeça em geral se move bruscamente para baixo. Isso pode ajudar os clientes a diferenciarem o espirro comum do espirro reverso (ver texto adiante). O espirro costuma ser uma resposta aguda à irritação e geralmente diminui ou cessa por completo nos casos de doença crônica ou progressiva, obstrução ou irritação da cavidade nasal.

Espirro reverso

É uma manifestação voluntária ou involuntária que envolve paroxismos ou uma série de esforços inspiratórios fortes e abruptos ("roncos"). O espirro reverso é uma resposta à obstrução ou irritação da nasofaringe. Quando o apresentam, os animais de estimação costumam caminhar ou parar, com o pescoço estendido, a cabeça inclinada para trás, os lábios repuxados também para trás e as narinas abertas (ver Capítulo 238). Esses esforços posturais alongam a nasofaringe e podem alargar ao máximo o meato nasofaríngeo. Os paroxismos podem durar segundos a alguns minutos e ocorrer à noite ou quando o animal está repousando e as narinas ficam mais estreitas. Embora não estejam tipicamente associados à dificuldade respiratória, os episódios podem ser bastante alarmantes.

Secreção nasal

Em geral, a secreção nasal (ver Capítulo 27) segue-se a um aumento das secreções líquidas da cavidade nasal, uma alteração nas propriedades viscoelásticas das secreções nasais, comprometimento da limpeza mucociliar nasal ou qualquer combinação dessas condições. Quando vista, a secreção nasal deve ser caracterizada em função de sua aparência e sua consistência (mucoide, serosa, hemorrágica etc.), informação que pode ajudar a localizar a fonte ou a razão do problema. É importante lembrar que nem sempre a secreção nasal pode ser óbvia. Gatos e alguns cães podem ficar tentando se limpar sem parar, para remover a secreção antes que o proprietário a veja. Em tais casos, o plano nasal pode apresentar ulceração ou hiperqueratose, e os pelos em torno dele se perdem devido à lambedura ou esfregação do nariz com as patas na tentativa de remover o incômodo. A limpeza mucociliar nasal normal da via respiratória também carreia as secreções da cavidade nasal para baixo, na direção do meato nasofaríngeo e da laringe, resultando em tosse iniciada em via respiratória superior. Secreção nasal franca nas narinas não será evidente até que a quantidade ou a característica das secreções ultrapasse a capacidade de limpeza mucociliar ou que o aparato de limpeza mucociliar tenha sido danificado ou comprometido o suficiente (p. ex., por infecções causadas por *Bordetella* [ver Capítulos 227 e 229], *Mycoplasma* ou vírus da parainfluenza [ver Capítulo 228], metaplasia escamosa [ver Capítulo 238]).[8,9] A secreção nasal também pode ser uma manifestação de doença não respiratória (p. ex., refluxo esofagofaríngeo).[10]

Respiração com a boca aberta/postural

Alterações posturais refletem tentativas de diminuir a resistência da via respiratória, por meio do aumento de seu diâmetro transverso.[11] Em cães, a respiração com a boca aberta é uma resposta comum à obstrução da via respiratória. Em gatos é rara, indicando que a capacidade de reserva ventilatória do sistema respiratório está próxima da exaustão. Quando o animal estende a cabeça e o pescoço, minimiza a curvatura da traqueia e da faringe. Abrir as narinas e a boca minimiza a resistência ao ar inspirado. Os animais também podem minimizar atividades estranhas (não respiratórias) e eliminar ações que exacerbam o estreitamento da via respiratória (deglutição, vocalização) (ver Capítulo 28).

Sons respiratórios audíveis

Ruídos respiratórios que são audíveis para os proprietários sem a ajuda de um estetoscópio devem-se quase sempre à obstrução de via respiratória e, em geral, têm origem no trato respiratório superior (cavidade nasal, nasofaringe, cavidade bucal, laringe, parte extratorácica da traqueia). Como o estresse e o tônus simpático associados a uma consulta clínica podem facilitar a abertura da via respiratória, é comum que os sons respiratórios observados no domicílio não sejam notados no consultório. Deve-se pedir aos proprietários que descrevam se os ruídos são contínuos (estridores) ou descontínuos (estertores), constantes (obstrução fixa) ou intermitentes (obstrução dinâmica ou episódica) e, se intermitentes, quais eventos desencadeiam o som (exercício, sono etc.). Pode ser útil o proprietário ter feito vídeos do animal apresentando os ruídos, tanto para caracterizar o som como para avaliar a postura do paciente durante o evento. Embora a determinação da fase da respiração durante a qual o ruído ocorre seja uma informação extremamente valiosa, pode ser difícil para os proprietários fazerem esse tipo de avaliação de maneira confiável.

Tosse

A tosse (ver Capítulo 26) é um mecanismo de defesa que protege as vias respiratórias inferiores, em geral desencadeado pela inalação de substâncias nocivas ou irritantes, ou pelo acúmulo de substâncias em qualquer parte da laringe ou da árvore traqueobrônquica. O som de uma tosse origina-se na laringe, como resultado da expulsão abrupta de ar intrapulmonar através da glote fechada. Cães e gatos com irritação ou estímulo oriundos de regiões diferentes da árvore traqueobrônquica podem exibir diferenças sutis na qualidade da tosse.

Diferenças nos sons da tosse podem ser úteis na localização e no tipo do estímulo. Por exemplo, a tosse que se origina em alvéolos ou vias respiratórias de pequeno calibre (broncopneumonia,

bronquite crônica) em geral é precedida de uma inspiração profunda. No início, os paroxismos podem ser brandos e tornam-se mais intensos à medida que as secreções traqueobrônquicas se direcionam às vias respiratórias centrais (de maior calibre). Essas tosses podem ser produtivas ou improdutivas e frequentemente são acompanhadas de náuseas, logo após, ou da deglutição das secreções. A tosse originária nas vias respiratórias centrais (traqueia, brônquios principais) em geral está associada a um som de "grasnar de ganso", à medida que o ar é expelido com força através de segmentos de vias respiratórias estenosadas ou colapsadas. Os paroxismos da tosse traqueal costumam ser "não progressivos". Na tosse traqueal, cada um soa como o som antecedente, desencadeia a subsequente e os episódios podem ser bastante prolongados (ver Capítulo 241). A tosse também pode ser induzida pelo estímulo da laringe, da traqueia e dos brônquios, pela drenagem pós-nasal de secreções nasais ou do conteúdo da cavidade bucal. Na tosse laríngea, o estímulo geralmente é abrupto e inesperado, causando laringospasmo reflexo. Isso impede a inspiração profunda antes do início da tosse e tipicamente resulta em uma tosse rápida, que pode ser fraca ou inefetiva, devido ao pequeno volume de ar expelido. Esses tipos de tosse também podem ser seguidos de esforços voluntários para limpar as vias respiratórias superiores (engasgos). Em termos técnicos, esse mecanismo é conhecido como *reflexo inspiratório*, em vez de reflexo de tosse, mas em geral é incluído nas descrições com outras formas de tosse.[12]

A tosse pode ser induzida por estenose da via respiratória, durante a expiração, como resultado de doença do espaço pleural (principalmente em cães, ver Capítulo 245), de cardiomegalia (cães, ver Capítulo 251) ou de estenose intrínseca da via respiratória secundária à doença dinâmica de via respiratória de pequeno calibre (bronquite crônica [cães e gatos], asma [gatos]; ver Capítulo 241), colapso de traqueia (principalmente cães) ou doenças pulmonares restritivas (ver Capítulo 242). Tipicamente, esses tipos de tosse são desencadeados por fluxo de corrente mais alto e podem ser notados nos estágios iniciais da doença apenas durante atividade física, mas podem tornar-se mais perceptíveis à medida que as reservas cardiopulmonares diminuem. A tosse "aferente" pode originar-se fora das vias respiratórias inferiores. Isso inclui o nariz, a nasofaringe, os seios paranasais, os canais auriculares, o diafragma e o pericárdio.[13] A participação exata de aferentes da tosse nesses locais não é inteiramente conhecido, porém sua presença sugere que locais extrapulmonares também podem ser causas importantes de tosse.

EXAME FÍSICO DO PACIENTE COM PROBLEMA RESPIRATÓRIO

Observações gerais

Os sinais respiratórios podem ser devidos inteiramente ou em parte à doença respiratória intrínseca. No entanto, tais sinais podem representar manifestações respiratórias de disfunção em outros sistemas (p. ex., gastrintestinal, sistema nervoso central [SNC], cardiovascular, hematológico, adrenal, tireóideo). Além disso, o estresse associado à doença não respiratória pode tornar evidente uma doença respiratória oculta, principalmente em gatos. Portanto, é sempre importante realizar um exame físico completo, se a estabilidade clínica do paciente permitir. O exame deve começar com a inspeção próxima do cão ou gato em repouso, se possível. No caso de pacientes estáveis, isso deve ocorrer enquanto se obtém o histórico clínico. Os pacientes podem ser retirados de suas caixas de transporte ou soltos de guias em uma sala de exame fechada, deixando-os livres para nela caminharem. Avaliam-se a frequência respiratória, o esforço para respirar, os sons pulmonares, o padrão respiratório e a postura do paciente. Se o animal estiver com dificuldade respiratória (ver

Capítulos 28 e 139), é importante, ainda, obter pelo menos uma avaliação superficial do padrão respiratório e da postura antes de manipulá-lo.

Padrões respiratórios

Normal

Durante a respiração normal, a parede torácica e a abdominal movem-se em conjunto durante a inspiração e a expiração. Esse movimento coordenado possibilita expansão pulmonar máxima, com esforço mínimo, durante a inspiração. A contração do diafragma, o relaxamento muscular passivo e a retração do pulmão por causa de sua elasticidade proporcionam a expiração.[14] As proporções normais entre tempo inspiratório e tempo expiratório são, aproximadamente, de 1:1 a 1:2. Alguns animais em repouso podem exibir uma pausa evidente no fim da expiração, durante a qual não são detectáveis movimentos da parede torácica ou abdominal. O aumento da carga de trabalho respiratório pode resultar em alteração do padrão respiratório. Essas alterações são respostas subconscientes, a fim de minimizar o trabalho respiratório. Elas variam em decorrência do tipo da carga respiratória (Figura 240.1).

Doenças pulmonares obstrutivas e restritivas

A *obstrução* da via respiratória causa aumento da resistência da via respiratória ou da pressão necessária para gerar um fluxo de ar. O aumento do esforço respiratório pode exacerbar o colapso dessa via respiratória e agravar a obstrução ao fluxo de ar. Obstruções extratorácicas (p. ex., tumor de laringe, paralisia laríngea, obstrução nasal ou nasofaríngea [ver Capítulo 238]) estão tipicamente associadas a um aumento no esforço e no ruído inspiratórios, enquanto obstruções intratorácicas (doença de via respiratória de pequeno calibre, tampão de muco, colapso da parte intratorácica da traqueia) estão associadas ao aumento do esforço e dos sons expiratórios. Uma estratégia compensatória comum em animais de estimação com obstrução de via respiratória é diminuir a velocidade do fluxo de ar para minimizar qualquer propensão ao colapso dessa via respiratória. Isso resulta em respiração profunda lenta, geralmente com prolongamento da fase inspiratória, nas obstruções extratorácicas (via respiratória superior), e da fase expiratória, nas obstruções intratorácicas.

A doença pulmonar *restritiva* resulta em diminuição da complacência pulmonar ou alteração no volume pulmonar associada a aumento da pressão na via respiratória envolvida. Animais de estimação com condições que causam padrão respiratório restritivo (broncopneumonia, fibrose pulmonar, doença do espaço pleural) requerem pressão mais elevada na via respiratória para a expansão total dos pulmões. Como o aumento da carga de trabalho está associado à expansão pulmonar, doenças pulmonares restritivas ou do espaço pleural podem ser compensadas pela diminuição do volume de ar corrente e aumento da frequência respiratória. O resultado é uma respiração rápida superficial.

Tanto as condições obstrutivas como as restritivas aumentam o trabalho respiratório. Com o tempo, esse aumento do esforço respiratório pode resultar em fadiga dos músculos respiratórios e um padrão respiratório *paradoxal*. À medida que os músculos respiratórios falham, a pressão intratorácica negativa gerada durante a inspiração tende a causar contração da parede torácica. A fadiga ou paralisia do diafragma pode ocasionar o recrutamento de músculos abdominais, causando expansão da parede abdominal durante a expiração. Esses movimentos das paredes torácica e abdominal são o oposto daqueles observados normalmente e

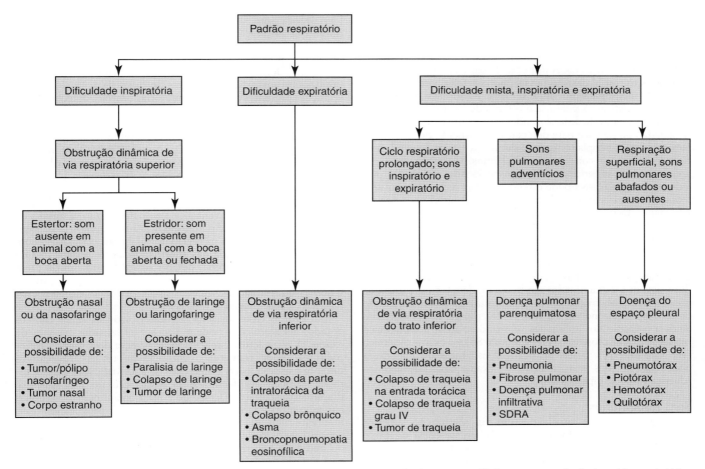

Figura 240.1 Algoritmo geral para avaliação de padrões respiratórios em cães e gatos. Esse algoritmo tem por objetivo nortear a avaliação de padrões respiratórios. Há exceções a essa abordagem algorítmica. *SDRA*, síndrome do desconforto respiratório agudo.

podem ser indicativos de disfunção respiratória grave ou crônica. Em cães e gatos com dispneia, a respiração paradoxal é fortemente relacionada à presença de doenças do espaço pleural (ver Capítulo 244).[15] A presença desse sinal clínico pode auxiliar na implementação do diagnóstico de emergência e dos procedimentos terapêuticos apropriados (ver Capítulo 139).

Postura

Animais de estimação com comprometimento respiratório significativo podem adotar uma postura que ajuda a maximizar a eficiência da respiração ou diminuir a resistência da via respiratória por aumentar o diâmetro transversal dessa via respiratória e facilitar a expansão da parede torácica. Quando o animal estende a cabeça e o pescoço, ocorre diminuição da redundância e da obstrução da faringe. A abertura das narinas abre a valva nasal (óstio interno). A respiração com a boca aberta desvia das resistências nasal e nasofaríngea e geralmente ocasiona perda significativa da reserva cardiopulmonar em gatos. Alguns animais podem sentar-se ou preferem permanecer em decúbito esternal com abdução dos cotovelos. Eles também podem minimizar a atividade extrapulmonar e eliminar ações que exacerbem a estenose da via respiratória (deglutição, vocalização).

Exame do sistema respiratório

Geral

O exame físico do sistema respiratório em geral confirma as informações obtidas na anamnese (histórico clínico) e os problemas observados, mas em alguns casos o histórico pode ser vago e não há sintomas respiratórios evidentes ou eles são discretos. O exame abrangente do sistema respiratório inclui a região nasal (focinho, cabeça, olhos, arcada dentária, palato duro, fluxo nasal de ar), a cavidade bucal, a palpação da laringe e da traqueia, a compressão torácica e auscultação do tórax e da entrada torácica. O exame da cavidade nasal geralmente envolve inspeção e palpação do focinho, da cabeça, dos olhos e do palato duro para avaliação da conformação e da simetria e para verificar se há defeitos nessas estruturas. A inspeção da parte externa das narinas e do aspecto rostral das vias nasais pode ser feita para verificação da cor da membrana mucosa e se há secreção nasal, bem como suas características. A patência e o fluxo de ar em cada cavidade nasal devem ser avaliados colocando-se na frente delas um pedaço de algodão ou de gaze para detectar o movimento de ar, ou uma lâmina de microscopia refrigerada durante a expiração nasal, verificando se ocorre condensação na lâmina. O palato duro e a arcada dentária superior devem ser inspecionados e palpados, pois a doença nasal invasiva pode estender-se para a cavidade bucal, e a doença dentária (p. ex., abscesso da raiz dentária) pode ocasionar manifestações nasais. A palpação e a retropulsão devem ser realizadas para avaliar a simetria. Tumores nasais invasivos ou rinite micótica destrutiva podem estender-se para a órbita. A cavidade bucal deve ser inspecionada para verificar a cor da membrana mucosa, o tempo de preenchimento capilar e o grau de hidratação. As tonsilas, a língua, a região sublingual e o palato duro devem ser examinados em busca de defeitos ou lesões que possam causar obstrução de via respiratória e para avaliar a função da faringe, verificando se há reflexo de engasgo. Estão indicados ainda a palpação dos linfonodos submandibulares e retrofaríngeo medial, o exame otoscópico (ver Capítulo 85) e o exame oftálmico (ver Capítulo 11). Sinais de doenças sistêmicas ou infecciosas podem ser notados primeiramente no exame nasal ou oftálmico (doença fúngica, hipertensão).

Sons respiratórios

As evidências de anormalidades em via respiratória superior incluem estertor, estridor e diminuição ou ausência de fluxo nasal de ar. Estertor é um som vibrante descontínuo de baixa intensidade que, em geral, se origina no meato nasofaríngeo e com frequência está associado à disfunção inspiratória, mas pode estar presente durante ambas as fases da respiração, inspiração e expiração. Como o meato nasofaríngeo tende a estreitar-se durante o repouso, o estertor pode ser mais evidente à noite. O estridor é um som inspiratório contínuo de alta intensidade, geralmente produzido como resultado de estenose da laringe ou da parte extratorácica da traqueia. Em contraste com o estertor, pode não haver ruído de estridor à respiração durante o repouso, mas pode ser exacerbado por fluxo de grande volume de ar (atividade física, respiração ofegante etc.). Anormalidades na via respiratória inferior podem causar sons adventícios (sibilos, crepitações), bem como alterações na característica do som broncovesicular normal. O fluxo inspiratório normal atinge velocidade máxima próximo ao fim da inspiração, e o fluxo expiratório normal o faz próximo do início da fase expiratória. Portanto, a auscultação torácica de fluxo de ar normal é tipicamente mais audível no fim da inspiração e no início da expiração. Sons broncovesiculares normais detectados à auscultação são gerados principalmente pelo fluxo laminar através das vias respiratórias centrais de maior calibre e que se infiltra nos alvéolos, no espaço pleural e na parede torácica. Alterações no volume (aumento ou diminuição) ou no padrão dos sons broncovesiculares podem ser indicadores precoces de doença respiratória, mesmo na ausência de sons pulmonares adventícios. Pode ocorrer uma detecção maior de sons broncovesiculares em decorrência de maior esforço respiratório, enquanto a diminuição nos sons broncovesiculares pode ser resultante de alterações estruturais no interstício pulmonar, nos alvéolos ou no espaço pleural.

Sons respiratórios adventícios indicam anormalidade. Sibilos (sons musicais contínuos, associados à estenose de via respiratória intratorácica), em geral, estão associados à disfunção expiratória. Sibilos de alta intensidade podem ser detectados quando há estreitamento das vias respiratórias inferiores ou de pequeno calibre, enquanto os de baixa intensidade podem indicar estreitamento de uma via respiratória de maior calibre. Crepitações ("estalidos", sons descontínuos de "estouros", mais audíveis durante a inspiração) representam um equilíbrio de pressão entre dois locais de uma via respiratória obstruída. Crepitações finas, tipicamente de origem alveolar ou bronquiolar, em geral são mais audíveis durante a inspiração. Crepitações sonoras úmidas costumam ser resultantes do fluxo de ar que atravessa secreções presentes em vias respiratórias centrais, detectadas por toda a inspiração ou durante a expiração.

Podem ocorrer diminuição ou ausência de sons respiratórios como resultado do acúmulo de ar ou líquido ou a presença de víscera no espaço pleural (ver Capítulos 28 e 244). Animais de estimação com doença no espaço pleural podem exibir um padrão respiratório superficial e rápido (restritivo). A localização da ausência de sons respiratórios deve dar indícios da natureza da anormalidade do espaço pleural. A ausência de sons respiratórios na região ventral é compatível com acúmulo de líquido (p. ex., sangue, pus, transudato, efusão quilosa). A ausência de sons respiratórios na região dorsal é mais compatível com pneumotórax. A maioria das anormalidades no espaço pleural de cães e gatos é bilateral, devido ao mediastino incompleto nessas espécies. No entanto, acúmulos de tecido (p. ex., mesotelioma) ou herniações viscerais podem resultar em sons assimétricos à auscultação.

Em muitos casos, os sons respiratórios ou os sinais clínicos notados no domicílio podem não ser observados na sala de exame. A espetacular capacidade de reserva do sistema cardiopulmonar pode requerer o emprego de testes provocativos durante o exame físico. A detecção de anormalidades cardiopulmonares pode ser facilitada pela indução de um "suspiro" durante a auscultação (fechando a boca do animal e obstruindo parcialmente as narinas por 4 a 5 respirações), provocando tosse mediante delicada palpação da traqueia ou submetendo o paciente à atividade física leve ou moderada. Registros em vídeo ou áudio de anormalidades observadas em casa e feitos pelo proprietário também podem ajudar os clínicos a verificarem e localizarem com acurácia a doença respiratória antes da realização de exames diagnósticos mais invasivos e dispendiosos.

TÉCNICAS DE DIAGNÓSTICO LABORATORIAL

Dados básicos iniciais: hemograma completo, perfil bioquímico sérico, exame de urina

A escolha de exames apropriados para entender e tratar melhor um animal de estimação com doença respiratória depende da resenha, da anamnese (histórico clínico), dos achados de exame físico, do diagnóstico diferencial e das opções ou limitações do proprietário. Os resultados dos dados básicos iniciais podem ajudar a diminuir ou priorizar causas prováveis dos sintomas, bem como facilitar a escolha de testes de diagnóstico mais avançados. No hemograma, a policitemia pode resultar de hipoxemia crônica e hipoxia tecidual. Leucocitose com neutrofilia é comum em animais de estimação com infecção da via respiratória (doença respiratória infecciosa canina, doença respiratória de trato superior felina); os animais com broncopneumonia podem apresentar leucocitose ou, na fase aguda, leucopenia. Eosinofilia periférica é comum em cães com broncopneumopatia e ocasionalmente é observada em animais de estimação com doença pulmonar parasitária, doenças fúngicas e em gatos com asma (ver Capítulo 241). Linfocitose em um animal de estimação jovem com doença respiratória e febre é compatível com infecção viral. Hipercalcemia em um paciente com sinais respiratórios pode ser sugestiva de neoplasia ou de doença fúngica.

Os dados básicos iniciais também possibilitam avaliação de doenças não respiratórias que podem interferir na função respiratória (p. ex., hiperadrenocorticismo, pancreatite, acidose metabólica grave) ou revelar doença respiratória. O acometimento sistêmico de um animal de estimação com dificuldade respiratória, que apresenta leucograma inflamatório e hipoalbuminemia, pode sugerir a presença de síndrome da dificuldade respiratória aguda (SDRA). Hipoalbuminemia grave pode acarretar efusão pleural e/ou ascite, com acúmulo de transudato naquelas cavidades. Isso pode causar aumento do esforço respiratório. Trombocitopenia, trombocitopatia, coagulopatia e hipertensão sistêmica podem resultar em hemorragia pulmonar, efusão hemorrágica ou epistaxe.

Exames sorológicos e outros testes de diagnóstico avançados

Testes sorológicos, pesquisa de antígeno na urina e nas fezes e reação em cadeia da polimerase (RCP) podem ser empregados em animais de estimação nos quais há suspeita de que os sintomas respiratórios são decorrências de causas infecciosas ou parasitárias. A ocorrência de doenças infecciosas (ver Capítulos 227 a 230) pode ser influenciada pela idade, pela região geográfica, por viagem, pelo estilo de vida (p. ex., gatos criados em ambiente externo *vs.* interno), pela presença de sintomas não respiratórios de comorbidades ou pelas condições sanitárias dos animais (p. ex., acometimento de vários filhotes de cães de uma mesma ninhada, diversos pacientes da mesma instituição ou abrigo, acometimento de um gato após a chegada de um filhote na residência). Infecções do trato respiratório recorrentes causadas por patógenos oportunistas são compatíveis com imunodeficiência. Por exemplo, o diagnóstico de criptococose nasal refratária ou recorrente em um gato pode requerer pesquisa dos vírus da leucemia e da imunodeficiência felina, enquanto rinite, traqueobronquite e pneumonia recorrentes em um cão jovem podem necessitar da pesquisa de discinesia ciliar primária ou deficiência hereditária de imunoglobulina.[16-18]

O método e o momento de coleta da amostra são fatores importantes a serem considerados quando se faz uma triagem para a detecção de causas infecciosas ou parasitárias da doença respiratória por meio de exames laboratoriais, em particular RCP (ver Capítulos 227, 229 e 234). As amostras coletadas para RCP devem ser obtidas mediante o uso de suabes com extremidade de poliéster, pois os resíduos presentes em suabes com ponta de algodão ou alginato de cálcio podem inibir o teste RCP para determinado patógeno ou para o seu genoma. A coleta de amostras superficiais de membranas mucosas pode ocasionar

---

Boxe 240.1 Fungos, vírus, bactérias e protozoários que comumente causam doença respiratória infecciosa em cães e gatos, detectáveis por meio de reação em cadeia da polimerase

Fungos
Blastomyces
Coccidioides
Cryptococcus
Histoplasma
Aspergillus
Pneumocystis

Vírus
Vírus da cinomose (em cães)
Adenovírus canino 2
Herpes-vírus canino
Vírus da parainfluenza canina 2
Coronavírus respiratório canino
Vírus da influenza canina (H3N2 e H3N8)
Vírus da influenza pandêmico (H1N1)
Pneumovírus canino
Herpes-vírus felino 1
Calicivírus felino

Bactérias
Bordetella bronchiseptica
Chlamydia felis
Mycoplasma cynos
Mycoplasma felis
Streptococcus equi subsp. zooepidemicus

Protozoários
Toxoplasma
Neospora
Acanthamoeba

---

resultados falsos negativos para patógenos virais (p. ex., coronavírus respiratório canino) ou para patógenos bacterianos facultativos (p. ex., *Mycoplasma cynos*). O desprendimento de patógenos pode cessar antes da resolução dos sinais clínicos (vírus da influenza canina). A realização de RCP após a excreção do microrganismo pode ocasionar resultado falso negativo. Em todos os casos, deve-se assegurar que o momento e o método de coleta da amostra sejam apropriados para os diagnósticos diferenciais considerados (Boxe 240.1).

DIAGNÓSTICO POR IMAGEM DO SISTEMA RESPIRATÓRIO

Considerações gerais

A investigação de suspeita de doença respiratória baseia-se muito no diagnóstico por imagem das vias respiratórias superiores (cavidade nasal, faringe, laringe, traqueia) e inferiores (brônquios, bronquíolos), do parênquima pulmonar (vasos sanguíneos, interstício, alvéolos) e de estruturas não pertencentes ao trato respiratório (coração, coluna vertebral, costelas, esterno, abdome etc.). A radiografia do tórax é o exame mais comum. Modalidades alternativas de imagem podem proporcionar níveis adicionais de detalhes e dimensões (tomografia computadorizada [TC] ou ressonância magnética [RM]); avaliação da função dinâmica da via respiratória em tempo real (fluoroscopia, ultrassonografia); ou indicação de função pulmonar regional (imagens obtidas em medicina nuclear). O diagnóstico por imagem deve ser completado antes de procedimentos mais invasivos (rinoscopia [ver Capítulos 96 e 238] e lavado broncoalveolar (LBA) [ver Capítulo 101]), para evitar hemorragia iatrogênica e dano de estruturas anatômicas que interferem nos exames de imagens.

SEÇÃO 15 • Doença Respiratória

Radiografia do trato respiratório superior

Introdução

Em termos anatômicos, as vias respiratórias superiores estendem-se da extremidade do nariz até a entrada do tórax. Em animais, a investigação de sinais clínicos e sons respiratórios suspeitos de estar localizados nas vias respiratórias superiores baseia-se fortemente em imagens dessas vias (cavidade nasal, faringe e laringe; ver Capítulos 238 e 239) e de estruturas não pertencentes ao trato respiratório (crânio, arcada dentária, órbitas ósseas, linfonodos, glândulas salivares). Como boa parte dessa região fica nos limites do crânio (cavidade nasal, nasofaringe) ou é circundada por estruturas de tecido mole sobrepostas (laringe, parte cervical da traqueia), podem ser necessárias técnicas avançadas de imagem para a confirmação de anormalidades. O posicionamento do paciente é fundamental, devendo-se evitar artefatos que provoquem movimento. Portanto, a melhor maneira para a obtenção de imagens das vias respiratórias superiores é sob sedação profunda ou anestesia geral.

Regiões nasal e facial

Radiografias nasais podem ser úteis para a localização e a caracterização de doença intranasal (ver Capítulo 238). Entretanto, radiografias nasais e dos seios nasais raramente detectam uma causa específica de doença (uma exceção seria um corpo estranho radiopaco). Os benefícios de radiografias nasais incluem a possibilidade de detectar assimetria, osteólise e opacidade de tecido mole na cavidade nasal e nas estruturas adjacentes. É possível obter radiografias nasais de alta qualidade com custo mínimo e sem equipamento especializado. Elas devem incluir um mínimo de duas imagens ortogonais. As imagens consideradas como padrão são: dorsoventral, ventrodorsal com a boca aberta (radiografia oclusal) e lateral. Imagens especiais (imagem oblíqua lateral, imagem "linha do horizonte") podem ser extremamente úteis para detectar acometimento do seio frontal e da bulha auditiva. Radiografias dentárias podem fornecer informação detalhada sobre o acometimento da arcada dentária maxilar e das raízes dentárias na patogenia da doença nasal. Contudo, as radiografias nasais não têm sensibilidade nem possibilitam o nível de detalhes obtidos na TC ou na RM. A complexidade do crânio de cães e gatos pode dificultar a detecção de lesões nasais iniciais ou discretas. Embora não seja um desafio técnico, o posicionamento do paciente tem extrema importância, porque um mau posicionamento resulta em imagens de pouco valor ou pode induzir a erro de diagnóstico.

Faringe, laringe e parte cervical da traqueia (ver Capítulos 238, 239 e 241)

A radiografia da parte lateral do crânio ou do pescoço em geral é adequada quando os sinais respiratórios estão localizados nessas áreas (p. ex., estridor, engasgo, tosse improdutiva, alteração ou perda da voz). A área específica de interesse deve estar centralizada na imagem, para minimizar o grau de paralaxe na visualização de estruturas pares simétricas (p. ex., bulhas auditivas, cartilagens aritenoides); o posicionamento é crítico na avaliação de tais radiografias, pois até mesmo a mais leve obliquidade pode dificultar a interpretação da imagem. Imagens centralizadas sobre a laringe são mais úteis para a avaliação de estridor laríngeo, enquanto aquelas centralizadas sobre a região mesocervical são preferíveis na avaliação de suspeita de colapso da parte cervical da traqueia. A investigação da suspeita de colapso na parte cervical ou na entrada torácica da traqueia também deve incluir imagens obtidas durante as fases inspiratória e expiratória, a fim de documentar colapso dinâmico (quando não se dispõe de fluoroscopia ou traqueoscopia).

Radiografia do tórax

Técnica e posicionamento

Radiografias do tórax para avaliação geral, com pelo menos duas imagens ortogonais (uma lateral e uma ventrodorsal ou dorsoventral) podem ajudar a localizar anormalidades na via respiratória inferior, no parênquima ou no espaço pleural. Exames que incluem ambas as imagens, lateral e ortogonal, são os ideais. Nas imagens laterais, os lobos pulmonares dependentes tendem a se colapsar, devido à compressão causada pelo coração e pelo diafragma, bem como ao menor movimento da parede torácica durante o ciclo respiratório.[19] Há casos esporádicos em que as imagens ventrodorsais (p. ex., doença do lobo acessório) e dorsoventrais (p. ex., aumento dos vasos sanguíneos pulmonares do lobo caudal) podem ser indicadas. O posicionamento e a técnica são particularmente importantes para a avaliação e a interpretação de estruturas intratorácicas (pulmões, coração, conteúdo mediastínico) e extratorácicas (costelas, coluna vertebral, estérnebras). Quaisquer dessas estruturas podem contribuir para a ocorrência de sinais clínicos de uma anormalidade respiratória. Deve-se ter cuidado para assegurar que as partes craniais dos membros sejam puxadas para a frente, de modo a evitar superposição da parte cranial do tórax em projeções laterais. A colimação das imagens deve incluir todos os campos pulmonares, a parte cranial do abdome e a entrada do tórax. As estruturas torácicas apresentam movimentação inerente em razão do movimento respiratório e do ciclo cardíaco, de maneira que o tempo de exposição das imagens torácicas deve ser o mais curto possível, enquanto há contraste adequado.

Classificação de anormalidades radiográficas dos pulmões

Os padrões radiográficos de pulmões anormais são: intersticial, brônquico e/ou alveolar (ver Capítulo 242). Os padrões pulmonares intersticiais são classificados, ainda, como não estruturados ou estruturados (nodulares). Padrões intersticiais não estruturados têm um aumento generalizado na opacidade de fundo do parênquima pulmonar e menor distinção dos vasos sanguíneos pulmonares. As causas comuns de padrão intersticial difuso incluem pneumonia viral ou hematogênica, edema pulmonar (cardiogênico e não cardiogênico), infiltração neoplásica (p. ex., linfoma pulmonar) e pneumonite secundária a doença sistêmica (p. ex., pneumonite urêmica). Os padrões intersticiais não estruturados podem ser artefatos ocasionados por técnica radiográfica inapropriada, hipoventilação ou uma variante do padrão normal em um paciente obeso.[20] Padrões intersticiais estruturados ou nodulares são vistos como nódulos de tecido mole discretos ou coalescentes nos campos pulmonares. Lesões nodulares > 2 cm, no parênquima pulmonar, em geral são denominadas "massas pulmonares". As lesões nodulares podem ser solitárias ou múltiplas, bem como sólidas ou cavitárias. O tamanho, a aparência e o número de lesões nodulares intersticiais podem ajudar a reduzir a lista de diagnósticos diferenciais (Tabela 240.1).

Tabela 240.1 Causas de nódulos e massas pulmonares intersticiais.

ACHADO	CAUSA	PREVALÊNCIA
Nódulos sólidos múltiplos	Metástase	Comum
	Micose	Incomum
	Êmbolos sépticos	Rara
Massa sólida solitária	Tumor primário	Comum
	Abscesso	Rara
Nódulos cavitários múltiplos	Metástase	Rara
	Parasitária	Rara
	Bolhas pulmonares	Incomum
Massa cavitária solitária	Tumor primário	Comum
	Abscesso	Rara
	Bolha pulmonar	Incomum

De Thrall DE: The canine and feline lung. In: Thrall DE, editor. *Textbook of veterinary diagnostic radiology*, 6 ed., St. Louis, 2013, Elsevier, p. 608-631.

Padrões pulmonares alveolares. Ocorre um padrão pulmonar alveolar quando o ar presente nos alvéolos é substituído por tecido mole ou líquido, resultando em aumento generalizado da opacidade pulmonar. Edema pulmonar, hemorragia e exsudatos inflamatórios ou neoplásicos são líquidos que podem substituir o ar alveolar, resultando em um padrão alveolar. A atelectasia, ou perda do ar alveolar com resultante colapso alveolar, também pode causar um padrão alveolar, que em geral também resulta em desvio do mediastino em direção ao local de atelectasia. Raramente, tumores sólidos podem resultar em um padrão alveolar, seja por substituição do ar alveolar ou por obstrução brônquica, que resulta em atelectasia. As características radiográficas do padrão alveolar incluem a presença de broncograma aéreo (sinal radiográfico de brônquio contendo ar), sinal lobar e silhueta de tecido mole (ou limite pouco claro) entre o pulmão acometido e o diafragma, o coração ou os vasos sanguíneos. As causas comuns de um padrão alveolar são broncopneumonia, edema pulmonar (cardiogênico ou não cardiogênico), hemorragia e atelectasia. Diagnósticos diferenciais menos comuns, mas importantes, para um padrão alveolar, identificam doença inflamatória grave de via respiratória (p. ex., broncopneumopatia eosinofílica), tromboembolia pulmonar e neoplasia (ver Capítulo 242).

Padrões pulmonares brônquicos. Ocorre um padrão pulmonar brônquico quando as paredes dos brônquios ficam espessadas ou o espaço peribrônquico imediato apresenta infiltrado de células ou muco. Em termos radiográficos, os brônquios aparecem como anéis com densidade de tecido mole e opacidade de ar no centro ("em forma de roscas") ou linhas paralelas radiopacas ("em forma de trilhos de trem"). Além do espessamento da parede brônquica, outras consequências da doença de brônquios podem alterar as imagens de radiografias do tórax, como bronquiectasia, atelectasia do lobo pulmonar cranial ou médio e campos pulmonares radiotranslúcidos, devido ao aprisionamento de ar e à hiperinsuflação. As causas comuns de padrão radiográfico brônquico em cães e gatos são doença alérgica de via respiratória (asma felina, broncopneumopatia eosinofílica canina), bronquite/pneumonite parasitária e bronquite crônica (ver Capítulo 241). A aparência ou a distribuição radiográfica de condições similares podem diferir entre as espécies; por exemplo, a aparência radiográfica clássica de insuficiência cardíaca congestiva esquerda em cães é um padrão intersticial peri-hilar ou alveolar, enquanto a mesma condição em gatos pode ocasionar uma distribuição pulmonar mais difusa; em geral, cães com broncopneumonia têm um padrão alveolar craniodistal, enquanto gatos costumam apresentar padrões alveolares multifocais ou difusos, assimétricos (ver Capítulo 242).

Efusão pleural

O acúmulo de líquido (sangue, quilo, exsudato inflamatório ou neoplásico, transudato, transudato modificado) no espaço pleural pode impedir a expansão pulmonar, ocasionando dificuldade respiratória, hipoxemia decorrente de hipoventilação e angústia respiratória. Os sintomas podem ser graves se o volume de líquido for grande ou quando ocorrer súbito acúmulo de líquido. A presença de líquido pleural de relevância clínica pode ser detectada por meio de radiografias de rotina, considerando que é necessário haver cerca de 100 mℓ de líquido no espaço pleural de um cão de porte médio para que tal anormalidade seja vista nas radiografias.[21] Volumes menores ou acúmulos localizados podem requerer outras modalidades de imagem (TC, ultrassom) para facilitar a detecção. Os sinais radiográficos indicativos de líquido pleural livre incluem o surgimento de linhas pleurais de fissura entre os lobos pulmonares, o afastamento dos lobos pulmonares da parede torácica, o arredondamento das bordas de lobos pulmonares dependentes e o ofuscamento das silhuetas diafragmática e cardíaca (ver Capítulo 244).

Pneumotórax

Ar ou outros gases no espaço pleural (pneumotórax) podem causar angústia respiratória e disfunção graves. O ar pode acumular-se no espaço pleural em decorrência de ruptura pulmonar, de alguma anormalidade no mediastino ou de difusão através da parede torácica. A aparência radiográfica mais comum de pneumotórax é o afastamento dos lobos pulmonares da parede torácica nas imagens laterais.[22] O pneumotórax também causa colapso pulmonar secundário ou atelectasia, resultando em aumento aparente da opacidade pulmonar. O colapso dos lobos pulmonares dependentes, em imagens laterais, possibilita que o coração desça para o hemitórax correspondente, o que resulta em uma linha de separação entre o coração e o esterno ("coração flutuante"). Pode ser necessário remover o líquido ou o ar da pleura, mediante toracocentese, antes da obtenção de imagens diagnósticas, para a estabilização do paciente (ver Capítulo 102), o que também pode melhorar o exame dos pulmões, do coração, do diafragma e do mediastino (ver Capítulos 244 e 245).

Tomografia computadorizada

Disponibilidade e uso em doenças nasais

Antigamente, para fazer uma TC em animais de estimação, era necessário anestesia geral, mas com os aparelhos mais recentes, com 32 ou 64 fileiras de detectores, pode-se obter uma série completa de imagens em alguns segundos. Atualmente, a TC pode ser realizada sem anestesia, em animais de estimação gravemente enfermos ou clinicamente instáveis.[23,24] Evitar o uso de anestesia permite avaliar a posição anatômica de estruturas das vias respiratórias superiores sem a interferência do tubo endotraqueal utilizado para a administração do anestésico.[25] A TC fornece uma imagem tridimensional (3D) detalhada da cavidade nasal, da nasofaringe e dos seios nasais. Devido às suas maiores sensibilidade e capacidade de resolução, a TC é considerada o exame de escolha para avaliar doença nasal (ver Capítulo 238). As imagens da TC são excelentes para a detecção de lesões nasais iniciais e para a determinação da extensão de um processo invasivo (p. ex., extensão para a lâmina cribriforme, acometimento orbitário). Embora a rinoscopia e a radiografia nasal não sejam exames sensíveis para distinguir rinite não infecciosa de neoplasia e/ou rinite micótica, a TC fornece detalhes úteis que podem sugerir uma dessas anormalidades. A TC é particularmente sensível para a detecção de alterações nas estruturas ósseas e cartilaginosas associadas à cavidade nasal. O uso exclusivo de TC não proporciona melhor distinção de estruturas de tecido mole *versus* líquido do que as radiografias nasais. No entanto, o uso de TC com contraste IV para evidenciação de estruturas vasculares e dos tecidos perfundidos pode ajudar a delinear as margens de tumores nasais invasivos e a distinguir acúmulo de líquido ou muco *versus* estruturas de tecido mole. É possível usar medições e reconstruções 3D de imagens de TC para orientar biopsias nasais subsequentes, bem como para o planejamento de procedimentos cirúrgicos e protocolos de radioterapia.

Tomografia computadorizada do tórax

Uma das principais vantagens da TC do tórax é a boa capacidade para detectar e localizar lesões discretas no pulmão, mediastino e na parede torácica que possam contribuir para a ocorrência de sintomas respiratórios. As mesmas cinco opacidades radiográficas (de gás, gordura, tecido mole, mineral e metal) detectadas em radiografias são usadas nas interpretações das imagens obtidas em TC. Contudo, a TC fornece melhor contraste entre opacidades adjacentes (p. ex., entre pulmões cheios de ar e vias respiratórias ou parede torácica) e tem maior sensibilidade para alterações na densidade em determinada opacidade. Para detectar nódulos pulmonares, a TC é mais sensível (detecta nódulos muito pequenos, como de 1 mm) do que a radiografia (detecta nódulos de 7 a 9 mm).[26,27] Tais fatores fazem da TC do tórax o exame preferido para a avaliação pulmonar quando o estadiamento das anormalidades pode alterar as recomendações para o tratamento. Embora os achados da TC não possam confirmar um diagnóstico, se específicos podem ter forte relação com algumas anormalidades. Em pessoas, foi estabelecido um conjunto de critérios relativos à TC para um diagnóstico "razoavelmente acurado" de fibrose pulmonar idiopática (FPI), com menor necessidade de biopsia pulmonar.[28] Similarmente, os achados de opacidade parecida com "vidro moído", faixas parenquimatosas, aspecto de favos de mel, espessamento peribroncovascular intersticial e bronquiectasia de tração, com distribuição predominantemente subpleural dessas lesões, são compatíveis com fibrose pulmonar idiopática canina (ver Capítulo 242). A gravidade desses achados na TC pode ter estreita relação com anormalidades pulmonares funcionais e a gravidade da doença.[29,30]

A natureza 3D da TC e a possibilidade de obter imagens de partes delgadas de estruturas respiratórias também contribuem para facilitar a localização e melhorar a resolução de vias respiratórias inferiores e de alvéolos. Esse nível de detalhe torna a TC útil não apenas para a detecção de anormalidades respiratórias, mas também para a quantificação de lesões morfológicas pulmonares. Medições do calibre de vias respiratórias e da espessura da parede brônquica com relação às artérias pulmonares adjacentes podem ser empregadas para a quantificação de alterações da parede brônquica na bronquite crônica e na bronquiectasia.[31,32] Imagens da TC em camadas delgadas de vias respiratórias pulmonares podem ser reformatadas em imagens broncoscópicas virtuais usadas para orientar a broncoscopia ou intervenções cirúrgicas.[33] A localização 3D de lesões pulmonares também facilita a coleta de aspirados percutâneos com agulha fina orientados pela TC, bem como biopsia com agulha de lesões da parede torácica, pleura e pulmão, em cães e gatos (ver Capítulos 93, 96 e 101).[34]

Ressonância magnética

A RM mostra melhor resolução de estruturas de tecido mole do que a radiografia ou a TC. É superior às radiografias na detecção de lesões discretas de tecido mole, incluindo neoplasias em fase inicial e granulomas fúngicos, e pode ser usada para a distinção imediata entre estruturas de tecido mole e acúmulo de líquido ou muco.[35,36] A RM é similar à TC na avaliação de doença nasal crônica e neoplasia nasal,[37] e pode ser útil na diferenciação de tipos diferentes de tumores nasais.[35] Uma limitação da RM é que, em comparação com a TC, é relativamente insensível para a detecção de alterações ósseas ou cartilaginosas na parte do crânio que circunda a cavidade nasal. Devido às limitações técnicas e práticas, a RM não é muito adequada para a obtenção de imagens pulmonares. A maioria das sequências da RM é afetada pela movimentação do paciente, de modo que, em regiões com movimento inerente, isto é, o sistema respiratório inferior, a RM padrão não é adequada. Gás emite muito pouco sinal à RM, de maneira que regiões preenchidas com gás, como os pulmões, tendem a resultar em imagens de baixa qualidade em comparação com a TC.[19] Outras limitações, como o custo e a necessidade de instalações especializadas, são semelhantes às da TC.

Fluoroscopia

Possibilita a visualização em tempo real de estruturas dinâmicas do trato respiratório superior e inferior, em repouso, quando o paciente manifesta um sinal clínico (p. ex., tosse), durante ou imediatamente após possíveis eventos desencadeantes (p. ex., deglutição, movimentação). Podem ser feitos exames fluoroscópicos das vias respiratórias superiores durante a ingestão de alimento ou líquido misturado com contraste (exame da deglutição) nos casos em que a transferência de ingesta por meio da faringe pode desencadear sintomas respiratórios. Os exemplos são refluxo nasofaríngeo em animais de estimação com espirros pós-prandiais ou refluxo esofagofaríngeo e aspiração como causa de broncopneumonia recorrente (ver Capítulo 238). A fluoroscopia é mais útil para detectar doença traqueal e brônquica dinâmica e é mais sensível que radiografias inspiratórias e expiratórias para a detecção de colapso dinâmico da traqueia, da carina e de brônquios lobares. É ainda mais acurada para a estimativa da magnitude e a localização de colapso de via respiratória.[38] Com a fluoroscopia durante a respiração normal, é possível avaliar se há colapso traqueal e/ou brônquico secundário à traqueobroncomalacia, bem como durante uma tosse induzida (Vídeo 240.1). Episódios de tosse podem ser provocados mediante a palpação leve da parte cervical da traqueia. Se não houver facilidade para provocar a tosse, então se pode aumentar transitoriamente a pressão intratorácica e cobrir brevemente a boca e o nariz do animal durante a expiração. A fluoroscopia também permite verificar se há cardiomegalia ou movimento cardíaco como causa de colapso de via respiratória intratorácica.[39] Podem ser colocados extensores traqueais sob orientação fluoroscópica e usar a fluoroscopia como procedimento de acompanhamento para monitorar a função desse extensor (ver Capítulo 121).

Ultrassonografia

Como quase todas as ondas geradas se refletem em interfaces de tecido mole/ar e osso/ar, a US tem utilidade limitada na avaliação de massas murais ou intraluminais das vias respiratórias superiores. A US do trato respiratório superior pode ajudar a identificar massas extraluminais em torno ou comprimindo a via respiratória. A US pode ser útil para determinar tanto a origem (p. ex., tireóidea, laríngea, em linfonodo) quanto a natureza (p. ex., preenchida com líquido, sólida) de lesões em forma de massa em torno da via respiratória superior. A US também foi avaliada como um recurso diagnóstico para paralisia de laringe e colapso de traqueia.[40,41] A US é sensível para a documentação de anormalidades morfológicas compatíveis com colapso de traqueia e paralisia de laringe, mas não é sensível para a documentação da presença de comorbidades (p. ex., colapso de laringe, colapso de brônquio) que precisa ser feita antes de procedimentos terapêuticos. Portanto, a US é um dos vários recursos que podem ser usados para obter informação a fim de determinar a causa de uma condição respiratória. Pode ser usada para identificar e caracterizar anormalidades da parede torácica e pleural que podem interferir na função respiratória, incluindo líquido ou massa pleural na parede torácica ou no espaço pleural (ver Capítulo 244). A US pode ser útil para identificar e caracterizar lesões pulmonares periféricas, como massas pulmonares, consolidação pulmonar, atelectasia e abscessos. O uso concomitante de US pode facilitar a coleta de aspirados com agulha fina de líquido ou lesões sólidas em forma de massas e orientar biopsias percutâneas de lesões pulmonares periféricas, pleurais ou da parede torácica (ver Capítulos 238 e 239).[42]

Medicina nuclear

A cintilografia nuclear é realizada mediante a administração de um radionucleotídio (em geral, o tecnécio 99m [Tc^{99m}]) marcado em um agente farmacêutico e que detecta a redução da radioatividade. O radionucliotídio e seu agente farmacêutico são selecionados de modo a assegurar sua liberação na região de interesse. A principal vantagem da imagem nuclear é a capacidade de proporcionar avaliações regionais da função pulmonar que não são possíveis nas modalidades de imagem mais convencionais. Os radionucleotídios podem ser administrados por via IV, para avaliar a perfusão pulmonar regional, ou por meio de nebulização, para avaliar a ventilação pulmonar. Podem ser realizadas cintilografias da perfusão em animais de estimação nos quais se suspeita de doença pulmonar tromboembólica (DPTE; ver Capítulo 243). A cintilografia vascular pulmonar é mais sensível e específica para a detecção e a localização de DPTE do que a angiografia.[43] No entanto, a natureza problemática da cintilografia e a necessidade de isolamento de pacientes em condições clínicas potencialmente graves fazem com que a angiografia seletiva seja usada mais comumente no diagnóstico de DPTE. A combinação de ventilação e cintilografia de perfusão (cintilografia V/Q) possibilita o cálculo das razões de ventilação de perfusão regional, que pode ser usada para localizar áreas de V/Q baixa, sem doença pulmonar difusa. A cintilografia V/Q pode dar informação importante sobre a função pulmonar regional antes de procedimentos intervencionistas, como biopsia pulmonar ou lobectomia pulmonar, bem como sobre a resposta ao tratamento. A deposição intratraqueal ou intranasal de Tc[99m] também foi usada na avaliação do transporte mucociliar, em cães e gatos.[44-46] A principal limitação das imagens nucleares é a baixa resolução espacial, de modo que os aspectos funcionais dessas imagens, em geral, são combinados com outras modalidades de imagem (p. ex., TC), quando se planeja alguma intervenção ou monitoramento da resposta ao tratamento da doença respiratória.

EXAME ENDOSCÓPICO DO TRATO RESPIRATÓRIO

Ver Capítulos 83, 96, 101 e 238.

COLETA DE AMOSTRAS PARA O DIAGNÓSTICO DE DOENÇAS DO TRATO RESPIRATÓRIO

Introdução

Em cães e gatos com doença respiratória, os achados de exame físico, as informações obtidas na anamnese e os resultados de exames laboratoriais e de imagens radiográficas costumam ser inespecíficos. Além disso, é difícil realizar testes da função pulmonar em cães e gatos. Portanto, a coleta de amostras de líquido ou tecido diretamente do trato respiratório, para cultura, citologia e/ou exame histológico pode ser muito útil (ver Capítulo 93). As amostras podem ser obtidas das vias respiratórias nasais por meio de suabe, escova, lavagem e biopsia. Faz-se LBA, endotraqueal e transtraqueal para colher amostras das vias respiratórias inferiores, embora se disponha de uma variedade de técnicas endoscópicas, cirúrgicas e toracoscópicas para a coleta de amostras de tecido do trato respiratório inferior (ver Capítulos 96, 101, 102, 244 e 245).

Coleta de amostras de vias respiratórias nasais (ver Capítulo 238)

Suabe e escova nasal

O uso de suabe nasal é uma técnica minimamente invasiva que geralmente não possibilita um diagnóstico acurado ou específico.[52] Em muitas circunstâncias, as células colhidas representam inflamação superficial secundária e microrganismos saprófitas que colonizam as vias respiratórias e não representam uma infecção verdadeira.[53,54] Por essas razões, a cultura de suabe nasal raramente é indicada e a sua utilidade limita-se ao diagnóstico citológico de algumas doenças específicas (p. ex., criptococose nasal em gatos)[52,55] ou para realização de RCP para a detecção de patógenos respiratórios. O suabe nasal é mais usado quando há suspeita de um diagnóstico específico. A técnica de escovação pode produzir células situadas mais profundamente na membrana mucosa nasal do que as colhidas por meio de suabe nasal e pode ser mais útil para a distinção entre doenças inflamatórias e neoplásicas.[56] Entretanto, na escovação nasal, é possível obter resultados tanto falsos negativos quanto falsos positivos na identificação de doenças nasais neoplásicas. As indicações para a escovação nasal são similares àquelas mencionadas para suabe nasal (ver Capítulo 96).

Hidropulsão salina

Na hidropulsão salina, faz-se lavagem com solução fisiológica sob alta pressão, a fim de obter amostras de tecido fragmentado de massas ou lesões localizadas no interior das vias respiratórias nasais e também pode proporcionar benefício terapêutico em alguns animais de estimação por eliminar secreções nasais acumuladas ou diminuir o volume de lesões expansivas (ver Capítulo 96).[57] Quando bem-sucedida, a hidropulsão salina pode fornecer amostras de tecido adequadas para histologia, o que aumenta a probabilidade de obter um diagnóstico acurado.

Devido à sensibilidade das vias respiratórias e dos seios nasais a maior risco de aspiração, os procedimentos de lavagem nasal devem ser realizados sempre com os pacientes anestesiados, com a utilização de um tubo endotraqueal com manguito.

Biopsia nasal

Amostras de biopsia nasal podem ser obtidas por meio de técnicas menos invasivas do que a cirurgia (ver Capítulo 96). Em termos específicos, a biopsia nasal por meio de uso de pinça é relativamente fácil. Biopsias nasais podem ser colhidas com orientação de um rinoscópio, da TC ou às cegas. O alto rendimento diagnóstico desse método se deve ao procedimento invasivo utilizado. É preciso tomar precauções específicas para diminuir o risco de complicações. A biopsia nasal é realizada sob anestesia geral, para a coleta de várias amostras e assegurar o bem-estar do paciente. Amostras colhidas via biopsia nasal podem ser ideais para o exame em microscopia óptica e para cultura microbiológica. As biopsias nasais também podem ser uma fonte de cílios móveis para o diagnóstico de discinesia ciliar, via microscopia eletrônica de transmissão. Deve-se avaliar a condição de coagulação de todos os animais de estimação, antes da biopsia nasal, pois pode ocorrer sangramento, às vezes intenso (ver Capítulos 80, 99 e 196).

Coleta de amostras para o diagnóstico de doenças de vias respiratórias inferiores

Lavado broncoalveolar

O LBA, realizado sob anestesia geral com ou sem orientação broncoscópica, possibilita a obtenção de amostras dos alvéolos, de vias respiratórias distais de pequeno calibre e do interstício para citologia e/ou cultura microbiológica (ver Capítulos 93 e 101).[52,58,59] O LBA é obtido com a introdução da extremidade de um broncoscópio em uma via respiratória distal de pequeno calibre e a instilação do líquido de lavagem; em seguida, retira-se o máximo possível desse líquido. Para obter um LBA sem o uso de broncoscópio, utiliza-se um tubo endotraqueal esterilizado para a intubação do animal, a fim de evitar, o máximo possível, a contaminação orofaríngea.[60] Em gatos e cães de pequeno porte, usa-se um cateter estéril de polipropileno ou de borracha vermelha French calibre 7 a 10 (Figura 240.2). O comprimento do cateter deve corresponder pelo menos a distância entre a extremidade do nariz até a última costela; mantém-se a técnica asséptica, ele avança pelo lúmen do tubo endotraqueal até encontrar resistência ocasionada pela via respiratória de pequeno calibre. Pode ser necessário um adaptador estéril para conectar firmemente o cateter a uma seringa.

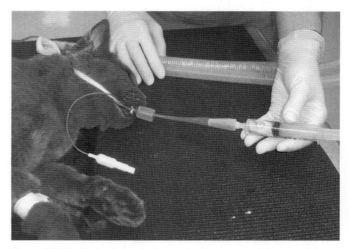

Figura 240.2 Técnica de lavado broncoalveolar, sem uso de broncoscópio, em gato. (Cortesia de Christine Venema, DVM, DACVIM.)

Em cães de grande porte, é possível instilar 1 a 2 mℓ de solução morna para o lavado (solução fisiológica 0,9% não bacteriostática)/kg de peso corporal (PC)[58] e, em cães menores e gatos, 2 a 4 mℓ/kg PC, por vez. Pode ser usado volume fixo de 10 a 25 mℓ. Cada volume de líquido deve ser acompanhado da introdução de 5 mℓ de ar, para garantir que todo o líquido instilado passe por toda a extensão do cateter. A dose de solução do lavado e o volume de ar são infundidos no broncoscópio ou cateter, por meio de uma seringa adaptada e, em seguida, aspirados imediatamente do cateter com a mesma seringa. Como alternativa, pode-se usar aspiração mecânica para aspirar uma amostra de líquido em um recipiente esterilizado próprio para isso.[59] Em cães e gatos, é esperada a recuperação de cerca de 40 a 60% do volume instilado,[61] mas já foram recuperados até 80% em gatos.[62] É recomendável colher amostras de pelo menos dois locais, inclusive em pacientes com doença difusa, pois a citologia do LBA pode variar em áreas diferentes do pulmão.[63] As amostras de líquido colhidas podem ser submetidas a exame citológico, cultura para microrganismos aeróbicos e anaeróbicos em geral, *Mycoplasma* e fungos.[52,64,65] As amostras de LBA também podem ser submetidas ao teste RCP para patógenos respiratórios. Hipoxemia decorrente do desequilíbrio entre ventilação e perfusão é a complicação mais comum do procedimento de obtenção de LBA e pode ser grave.[66,67] O fornecimento de oxigênio suplementar após o LBA em geral é suficiente para resolver a hipoxemia induzida pelo procedimento, mesmo em animais de estimação gravemente enfermos (ver Capítulo 131).

Lavado traqueal

Indicações. Geralmente, usa-se o lavado traqueal (ver Capítulo 101) para colher amostras de líquido de vias respiratórias proximais de grande calibre[52,68] em animais de estimação com tosse produtiva, pois tais amostras podem mostrar evidência de doença de via respiratória do trato respiratório inferior. Como a maior parte do líquido instilado não alcança a interface de trocas gasosas, é improvável que ocorra hipoxemia grave durante ou após esse procedimento. Faz-se lavado endotraqueal (LET) ou transtraqueal (LTT). O primeiro requer intubação e anestesia geral; portanto, pode ser uma opção mais apropriada para animais de estimação que não toleram a contenção necessária para LTT.

Lavado endotraqueal. A técnica e as diretrizes para o processamento das amostras obtidas são similares às mencionadas para LBA. Os animais de estimação são anesteiados e intubados com um tubo endotraqueal esterilizado. Introduz-se uma sonda de alimentação de borracha vermelha ou um cateter de polipropileno até a altura do quarto espaço intercostal, localização próxima à bifurcação da traqueia intratorácica (carina). Recomenda-se um volume de 0,5 a 5 mℓ de solução fisiológica 0,9%, não bacteriostática/kg PC, por vez. Igual volume pode ser instilado até três vezes e aspirado até que se obtenha uma amostra adequada. As amostras podem ser submetidas a exame citológico, cultura microbiológica, teste imunológico e RCP. São raras as complicações associadas ao LET. Agravamento transitório da condição respiratória, exacerbação da tosse e broncoespasmo podem ser notados durante e após o procedimento, embora sejam tipicamente brandos e de fácil reversão.[68]

Lavado transtraqueal. As amostras do LET e do lavado transtraqueal (LTT) são similares, mas o último é realizado em pacientes despertos ou levemente sedados,[52,59,68,69] o que evita a preocupação com a contaminação orofaríngea, que pode ocorrer no caso do LET.[70] O LTT restringe-se a cães com peso > 15 kg, que possam ser contidos, e é contraindicado para pacientes com anormalidades hemostáticas ou pioderma cervical ventral.[69] O LTT tem utilidade limitada na avaliação de animais de estimação com doença intersticial ou alveolar, porque pouco líquido alcança a parte distal do pulmão. Em geral, o animal é contido em decúbito esternal ou em posição sentada com o nariz direcionado dorsalmente. Faz-se tricotomia e preparação asséptica de uma área de pele em torno da laringe e da parte proximal da traqueia.

Em cães de médio porte, pode-se introduzir um cateter através do ligamento cricotireóideo. Em cães grandes, a agulha pode ser introduzida na linha média ventral da parte cervical da traqueia, entre dois anéis traqueais.[68,70] A introdução da agulha através do ligamento cricotireóideo evita o risco de penetração em ambas as paredes traqueais em cães de médio porte. Faz-se a aplicação intradérmica e SC de anestésico local (2 a 5 mg de lidocaína 2%/kg PC) no local em que se pretende introduzir a agulha e, em seguida, faz-se incisão da pele com lâmina de bisturi nº 11, nesse local, para facilitar a passagem de uma agulha estéril calibre 14 através do ligamento cricotireóideo. Alguns clínicos deslocam especificamente a pele para cima/cranialmente antes da introdução da agulha na pele e na traqueia, de modo que a agulha não deixa uma fístula após sua retirada. Antes de introduzir um cateter de borracha vermelha French calibre 3,5 ou um cateter de polipropileno através da agulha (Figura 240.3), deve-se marcar no cateter a distância desde o local de introdução pretendido até a altura da quarta costela, de modo a estimar a distância até a carina. Assim que a agulha estiver no lugar, o cateter é inserido através dela e avançado para o lúmen da traqueia até a distância previamente estabelecida. As recomendações para o volume de lavado varia de 0,5 a 5 mℓ/kg PC, por vez, como mencionado para o LET. Em geral, o volume da amostra do lavado traqueal é menor do que o obtido no LBA, mas pode ser suficiente para o exame citológico, cultura microbiológica e/ou RCP. Após a remoção do cateter e da agulha da traqueia, o local é recoberto com uma compressa de gaze estéril não aderente e uma bandagem leve, para evitar extravasamento de ar pelo local de introdução da agulha. As amostras de LTT devem ser manipuladas, preparadas e examinadas conforme recomendado para LET ou LBA.

As complicações associadas ao LTT são discretas, autolimitantes, incomuns e incluem enfisema SC, devido ao extravasamento de ar no local da introdução da agulha, hemorragia, arritmia cardíaca, hemoptise e laceração traqueal, que leva a pneumomediastino e, raramente, pneumotórax. A condição respiratória pode se agravar durante ou após o procedimento, como resultado da obstrução de via respiratória em decorrência de hemorragia ou hematoma, mas isso é incomum. Também é possível observar exacerbação da tosse após o procedimento. Pode ocorrer infecção no trajeto da agulha se houver uma falha significante na assepsia.

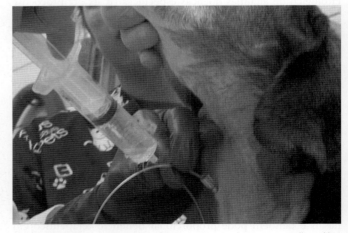

Figura 240.3 Lavado transtraqueal em um cão. Introduz-se uma agulha calibre 14 na traqueia, através do ligamento cricotireóideo, e, em seguida, introduz-se um cateter de polipropileno calibre 3,5 na traqueia, através da agulha, para instilação e recuperação do líquido do lavado. (Cortesia de Christine Venema, DVM, DACVIM.)

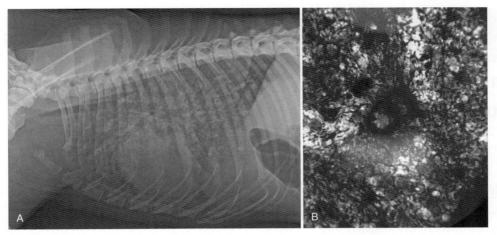

Figura 240.4 A. Radiografia lateral esquerda do tórax de um cão que apresentava febre e dificuldade respiratória. **B.** Citologia de aspirado transtorácico obtido com agulha fina do pulmão mostrado em (**A**), incluindo um brotamento de fungo de parede espessa e base ampla, compatível com *Blastomyces*. (Cortesia de Valerie Chadwick, DVM.) (*A figura B encontra-se reproduzida em cores no Encarte.*)

Coleta de amostra para citologia por meio de escovação transtraqueal e uso de agulha

Amostras endobrônquicas das vias respiratórias traqueal e brônquicas podem ser colhidas com orientação do broncoscópio, usando escova para citologia e agulha de aspiração transbronquial. Agulhas endobrônquicas e escovas para citologia permitem a obtenção de amostras de lesões focais de vias respiratórias. A amostragem endobrônquica de lesões focais da membrana mucosa é mais sensível para detectar inflamação de via respiratória do que o LBA, mas a sensibilidade de ambos os procedimentos é semelhante na detecção de alterações epiteliais.[61] A escovação endobronquial é segura e bem tolerada em cães, mas aumentam o tempo de anestesia e o custo do procedimento. Não há muitos relatos de complicações da aspiração endobrônquica com agulha em cães ou gatos. As descritas em pessoas são pneumotórax, hemorragia de via respiratória e pneumomediastino.[71]

Aspirado transtorácico com agulha e biopsia

Aspirado com agulha fina e amostra de pulmão obtida por meio de biopsia com agulha podem ser obtidos por via percutânea de animais de estimação com doença intersticial difusa ou naqueles com lesões pulmonares periféricas em forma de massas (Figura 240.4). A orientação com fluoroscópio, ultrassonografia e TC é útil para maximizar o rendimento e a acurácia da amostra para o diagnóstico, além de minimizar o risco de complicações.[72,73] As contraindicações à amostragem transtorácica incluem tendência a sangramento, lesões císticas ou bolhosas, pneumotórax, hipertensão pulmonar, dificuldade respiratória ou instabilidade do quadro clínico. Complicações potenciais da amostragem transtorácica podem ser sangramento, pneumotórax, contaminação do trajeto da agulha por células neoplásicas e morte.[74]

Biopsia pulmonar por meio de cirurgia e toracoscopia

Nos casos em que biopsias com agulha ou endobronquial podem não ser adequadas para confirmar o diagnóstico, é possível obter amostras maiores por meio de biopsia feita por cirurgia ou toracoscopia. A abordagem cirúrgica intercostal ou a esternotomia mediana, consideradas como padrão, proporcionam boa visualização do pulmão e acesso para a coleta de amostra grande por meio de biopsia. Nos casos de doença pulmonar periférica ou difusa, relata-se que uma abordagem por meio de um orifício mínimo ou minitoracotomia foi efetiva no sentido de propiciar o diagnóstico de doença pulmonar intersticial em cães e gatos, minimizando o tempo cirúrgico e o dano tecidual.[75]

A toracoscopia é uma técnica minimamente invasiva que permite a avaliação diagnóstica dos pulmões e do espaço pleural através de uma série de portais com 5 a 10 mm de diâmetro, em vez de uma única incisão grande, o que minimiza o dano tecidual e reduz o tempo de recuperação.[76] A cirurgia por meio de toracoscopia auxiliada por vídeo (VATS, do inglês *videoassisted thoracoscopic surgery*) proporciona melhor visualização das superfícies pleurais, dos pulmões, de estruturas mediastínicas e da parede torácica, comparativamente à toracotomia aberta, indicada para biopsia ou remoção de massas pulmonares ou de mediastino, massas pleurais, amostragem de líquido pleural e pericárdico, biopsia ou remoção de linfonodos traqueobrônquicos e na investigação de pneumotórax espontâneo.[76] Em um estudo, verificou-se que a VATS é comparável à toracotomia aberta, em termos de resultado cirúrgico e diagnóstico em cães submetidos à lobectomia pulmonar.[77]

OXIMETRIA DE PULSO E HEMOGASOMETRIA ARTERIAL

Ver Capítulos 75, 98 e 128.

REFERÊNCIAS BIBLIOGRÁFICAS

As referências bibliográficas deste capítulo se encontram online no Ambiente de Aprendizagem.

CAPÍTULO 241

Doenças da Traqueia e de Vias Respiratórias de Pequeno Calibre

Cécile Clercx

DOENÇAS DA TRAQUEIA

A maioria das anormalidades da traqueia pode envolver tanto o segmento intratorácico quanto o extratorácico. Traqueíte refere-se à inflamação do revestimento epitelial da traqueia. A resposta inflamatória pode ser de origem infecciosa ou não infecciosa.

As doenças não infecciosas da traqueia (que ocasionam inflamação da mucosa traqueal) são comuns e incluem flacidez da membrana traqueal dorsal, colapso de traqueia, lesão/laceração da traqueia, estenose pós-traumática, corpo estranho, tumor intratraqueal, inalação de fumaça, latidos prolongados (cães) e avulsão traqueal (gatos).

As anormalidades da traqueia também podem ser decorrências de doenças extratraqueais, como aumento extremo do coração, aumento do mediastino (tumor de linfonodo ou timoma, ou megaesôfago [Figura 241.1]), ou mesmo massas parenquimatosas, que podem causar desvio da traqueia, com possíveis efeitos na forma ou no lúmen do órgão (Figura 241.2) e subsequente obstrução e/ou inflamação. Doença alérgica de via respiratória inferior também pode ocasionar traqueíte secundária.

Em gatos, é mais provável que a traqueíte esteja associada à doença respiratória infecciosa felina (ver Capítulo 229). A traqueíte em gatos nem sempre induz tosse significativa, como acontece em cães.

Colapso de traqueia (cães)

Introdução

O colapso de traqueia (traqueia colapsada) é um distúrbio muito comum, que se caracteriza por achatamento dorsoventral dos anéis traqueais e flacidez da membrana traqueal dorsal. Vias respiratórias com malacia (ou colapso bronquial) em geral podem estar associadas a colapso de traqueia, e isso interfere negativamente no tratamento e no prognóstico. O som de "grasnar de ganso" da tosse é característico (Vídeo 241.1).

Etiologia e fisiopatologia

A causa de colapso de traqueia primário é complexa e mais corretamente considerada multifatorial. O desenvolvimento da doença clínica requer tanto uma anormalidade primária da cartilagem, que resulta em fraqueza intrínseca dos anéis traqueais, quanto fatores secundários capazes de iniciar a progressão para o estágio sintomático. O amolecimento de anéis cartilaginosos parece ser decorrência de uma redução no conteúdo de glicosaminoglicano e sulfato de condroitina, que provoca uma diminuição da capacidade de manter a rigidez funcional, isto é, fraqueza e achatamento dos anéis traqueais.[1,2] Fatores desencadeantes potenciais incluem obesidade, cardiomegalia, inalação de substâncias irritantes e alergênios, doença periodontal, infecções respiratórias e intubação endotraqueal recente.[3] As alterações dinâmicas do colapso de traqueia podem se limitar às regiões cervical e/ou torácica da traqueia e, frequentemente, são mais evidentes na junção cervicotorácica. O segmento cervical da traqueia se colapsa durante a inspiração, e o segmento torácico se colapsa durante a expiração, devido às pressões desenvolvidas durante o ciclo respiratório (Figura 241.3). O achatamento dorsoventral dos anéis traqueais cartilaginosos causa estiramento da membrana traqueal dorsal, que fica inflamada e pêndula, podendo prolapsar para o lúmen da traqueia, o que reduz ainda mais o diâmetro luminal, à medida que a pressão extraluminal exceda a intraluminal.[4] No interior do tórax, durante a inspiração, a

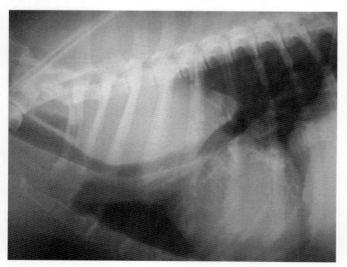

Figura 241.1 Radiografia lateral do tórax de um cão mestiço, de meia-idade, mostrando uma grande massa no mediastino, que causa deslocamento/desvio da traqueia.

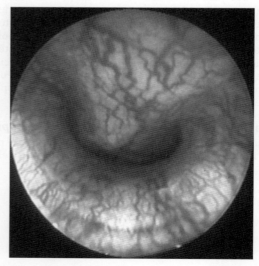

Figura 241.2 Endoscopia da traqueia em um cão com dificuldade respiratória grave e membranas mucosas cianóticas. Note a redução extrema e a forma modificada do lúmen traqueal, causadas por uma enorme massa no mediastino.

membrana dorsal redundante é aspirada pela pressão intratorácica negativa ou sujeita a ela durante a inspiração e pode aumentar excessivamente o lúmen traqueal, conforme se observa nas radiografias laterais (ver Figura 241.3). Em cães com colapso traqueal, em geral nota-se broncomalacia concomitante e não parece estar relacionada com inflamação da via respiratória.[5] Em contrapartida, também pode ocorrer broncomalacia independentemente do colapso de traqueia.

Também parece que o colapso de traqueia pode ser secundário a outros distúrbios. No cão da raça West Highland White Terrier (WHWT) com fibrose pulmonar idiopática (FPI), é frequente notar colapso de traqueia, pelo menos nos casos avançados.[6] Como o colapso de traqueia não é descrito nessa raça, exceto no caso de FPI, é possível supor que seja induzido secundariamente, devido ao aumento das pressões exercidas pela falta de elasticidade/complacência do pulmão fibrosado (ver no Capítulo 242 uma descrição mais detalhada da FPI).

No colapso de traqueia clássico ou possivelmente secundário, quando os sinais clínicos são aparentes, a síndrome é perpetuada pelo ciclo de inflamação crônica da mucosa traqueal, que exacerba e, por sua vez, é exacerbada pela tosse.

Manifestação clínica

É comum observar colapso de traqueia primário em cães de meia-idade a idosos de raças miniaturas, *toys* e pequenas. As mais representadas incluem Yorkshire Terrier, Lulu da Pomerânia, Pug, Poodle, Maltês e Chihuahua.[3,5,7]

Os sinais clínicos incluem tosse crônica em todos os casos, respiração ofegante discreta a grave, intolerância ao exercício e graus variáveis de dispneia inspiratória e expiratória (dificuldade respiratória), bem como grau variável de cianose nos casos avançados. É comum um histórico de doença clínica crônica.

A tosse é áspera, em geral descrita como "som de buzina"/"rasnado de ganso", e precipitada por atividade física, excitação, pressão traqueal (como a causada quando se puxa uma guia) ou ao beber água. Essa tosse característica pode ser provocada facilmente mediante palpação da traqueia. Um paroxismo de tosse em geral termina com uma tentativa terminal de vômito. O colapso do segmento cervical da traqueia às vezes pode ser visto como um achatamento dos anéis traqueais à palpação cervical. Em alguns casos, a tosse não é audível como tal e os proprietários relatam apenas um som semelhante a "grasnado de ganso" ou "grunhido/rosnar de porco" (Vídeo 241.2). Nos casos graves, a excitação pode acarretar

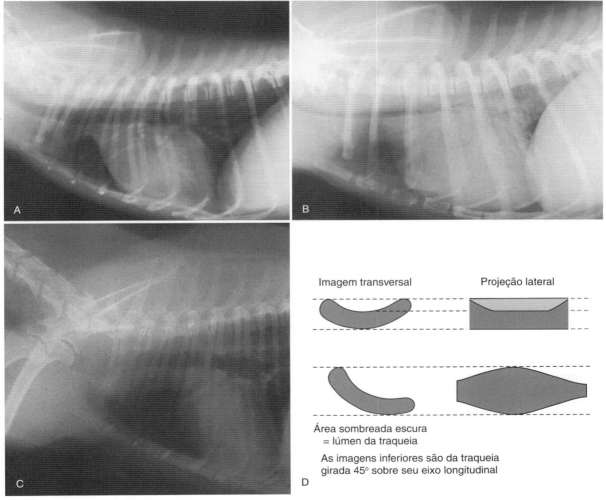

Figura 241.3 Radiografias torácicas laterais de um cão da raça Yorkshire Terrier durante (**A**) inspiração máxima e (**B**) expiração máxima. Note a alteração dramática no diâmetro traqueal que pode ocorrer durante o ciclo respiratório de animais com colapso de traqueia e como é importante obter imagens durante a inspiração e a expiração. Em casos graves como esse, o colapso expiratório não se limita ao segmento torácico da traqueia, mas estende-se também ao segmento cervical. **C.** Colapso de traqueia, observado na entrada torácica de um cão com rotação moderada da traqueia. Em decorrência da rotação, a traqueia parece mais larga que a colapsada, na imagem lateral. **D.** Diagrama do efeito da obliquidade nas radiografias de colapso traqueal cervical. O estreitamento do lúmen da traqueia é visível na radiografia lateral durante a inspiração (*parte superior, à direita*). No mesmo paciente, o colapso de traqueia é mascarado quando se obtém a mesma imagem com a traqueia girada sobre seu eixo longitudinal (*parte inferior, à direita*).

cianose e síncope (ver Capítulo 30), em decorrência da obstrução parcial ou completa da via respiratória, bradicardia mediada por estímulo vagal ou hipertensão pulmonar,[4] em especial quando há broncomalacia concomitante.

A auscultação sobre o trajeto da traqueia pode revelar sons estridentes tanto à inspiração como à expiração, o que precisa ser diferenciado de paralisia de laringe, relatada em cães com colapso de traqueia.[4] Durante a auscultação torácica, podem ser ouvidas crepitações à inspiração e à expiração em cães com colapso de via respiratória de pequeno calibre e/ou bronquite simultânea.

Recomenda-se auscultação cardíaca abrangente, pois um sopro cardíaco associado a regurgitação mitral pode ser ouvido; na verdade, doença mixomatosa/degenerativa da valva mitral é um achado comum em animais que apresentam colapso de traqueia, isto é, cães idosos de raças de pequeno porte. No entanto, o papel da cardiomegalia e especificamente do aumento do átrio esquerdo e a subsequente compressão e colapso da via respiratória ainda não foi esclarecido. Estudo recente revelou inflamação de via respiratória como a causa provável de tosse em cães que tinham aumento do átrio esquerdo e colapso de via respiratória.[8] Hepatomegalia é comum em cães com colapso de traqueia e pode ser reflexo de obesidade, embora tenha sido relatada disfunção hepática em cães com colapso traqueal.[9]

Diagnóstico diferencial

Os tipos de diagnósticos diferenciais incluem cardiopatia causada por valvulopatia mitral crônica, que pode ser uma doença concomitante, bronquite e/ou traqueíte crônicas, ambas possivelmente induzidas secundariamente pelo colapso de traqueia, e doenças crônicas do parênquima pulmonar (p. ex., FPI).

Diagnóstico

Suspeitas fortes do diagnóstico de colapso de traqueia baseiam-se na resenha, no histórico de tosse e nos achados ao exame físico.

Pode-se fazer uma avaliação diagnóstica adicional (radiografia, fluoroscopia, ecocardiografia, broncoscopia[10] e provas da função pulmonar[11]) para confirmar a extensão e a gravidade do colapso traqueal, com a finalidade de identificar doenças concomitantes (p. ex., broncomalacia, cardiomegalia, doença de via respiratória inferior) e quando é necessário obter medidas adequadas para avaliar as dimensões de um stent, no caso de se colocar um stent como um procedimento terapêutico (ver Capítulo 121).

O exame radiográfico de animais com traqueia colapsada pode ser feito com o animal em ambas as condições, imóvel e em movimento. Os exames radiográficos mais úteis incluem imagens laterais da entrada torácica, uma imagem tangencial (rostrocaudal) da entrada torácica (nessa projeção "skyline", a traqueia colapsada é vista como um formato oval, em "C" ou de lua crescente) e o exame fluoroscópico para mostrar os movimentos da membrana traqueal dorsal durante o ciclo respiratório.

Nas radiografias laterais, uma membrana traqueal dorsal redundante que se invagina no lúmen traqueal pode ser vista como uma opacidade de tecido mole ao longo do aspecto dorsal do lúmen traqueal cervical caudal, embora durante a inspiração ocasione aumento do diâmetro da traqueia. Essa condição pode ser vista em raças de pequeno e grande porte, como uma consequência de tosse e tem que ser diferenciada de superposição do esôfago. Portanto, são necessárias radiografias laterais obtidas durante as fases inspiratória e expiratória máximas do ciclo respiratório para demonstrar um colapso dinâmico. Na verdade, o colapso do segmento cervical da traqueia ocorre durante a inspiração, por causa da queda de pressão no lúmen da traqueia, enquanto o segmento torácico tende a colapsar durante a expiração, como consequência do aumento da pressão intratraqueal. Essas alterações dinâmicas são mais bem visualizadas em tempo real com o uso da imagem fluoroscópica intensificada.[7] Quando se compara a radiografia

com a fluoroscopia, supondo-se que a última seja obtida de modo correto, nota-se a evidência radiográfica de colapso em local incorreto em 44% dos cães e ela não é detectada em 8% dos cães submetidos apenas a radiografias.[7] Além disso, as medições radiográficas da traqueia de cães subestimam de maneira consistente o tamanho da traqueia; as mensurações com base em tomografia computadorizada (TC) são preferíveis para selecionar o tamanho do stent traqueal.[12]

Recentemente, identificou-se, em exame fluoroscópico, herniação do lobo pulmonar cervical (HLPC) ou protrusão do parênquima, além de entrada musculoesquelética do tórax, como um achado frequente em cães.[13] O colapso do segmento intratorácico da traqueia e dos brônquios principais (avaliado à fluoroscopia) foi fortemente associado à HLPC, em um estudo; embora uma membrana traqueal dorsal redundante em radiografias tenha sido associada à HLPC, o colapso do segmento extratorácico da traqueia não foi.[13]

A traqueoscopia, embora raramente necessária para confirmar o diagnóstico, revela desde uma diminuição do diâmetro dorsoventral, devido ao achatamento dos anéis cartilaginosos, com uma membrana dorsal pêndula, até um colapso grave que acarreta obstrução completa do lúmen traqueal (Figura 241.4). Portanto, a traqueobroncoscopia pode ser útil na determinação da gravidade do colapso de traqueia e, especialmente, de brônquio, bem como para avaliar doença concomitante de via respiratória (ver Capítulo 101). Na verdade, as radiografias subestimam sobremaneira a ocorrência de broncomalacia.[7] Portanto, a broncoscopia deve ser recomendada em todos os casos de suspeita de colapso de traqueia, antes da colocação de stent, pois a presença de broncomalacia grave e/ou doença de via respiratória inferior influencia muito o prognóstico após a colocação do stent (Vídeos 241.3 e 241.4).

Tratamento

Em animais com dificuldade respiratória acentuada, pode-se fornecer oxigênio (ver Capítulo 131); ademais, são necessários sedação e antitussígenos (ver Capítulo 138). Pode-se administrar butorfanol (0,05 a 0,2 mg/kg/4 a 6 h) ou acepromazina (0,01 a 0,1 mg/kg), por via SC, e succinato de prednisolona sódica (15 a 30 mg/kg IV), a fim de diminuir a inflamação aguda.

O tratamento a longo prazo visa principalmente minimizar os fatores potencialmente desencadeadores e a inflamação da mucosa traqueal.[3,4] No caso de animal obeso, a redução do peso é essencial (ver Capítulos 176 e 359). A mera perda de peso pode cessar os sinais clínicos. Da mesma forma, a substituição de coleiras duras pode ser efetiva. O afastamento do cão de produtos irritantes ao trato respiratório, como gases nocivos, fumaça e poeira, faz parte do senso comum e deve ser explicado com clareza ao proprietário. Também, é importante detectar e tratar outras doenças, inclusive doença crônica de via respiratória, doença cardíaca e hiperadrenocorticismo.

O tratamento a longo prazo consiste na administração de corticosteroides, em dose muito baixa (p. ex., 0,2 mg de prednisona/kg/24 h VO, durante 1 a 2 semanas, com intervalos de 3 meses) ou inalação (um "puff" de 120 mcg de fluticasona, a cada 12 h, usando máscara facial e espaçador; ver Capítulo 97), geralmente em combinação com um sedativo e um anti-histamínico. É preciso evitar sedação excessiva, pois o animal precisa se movimentar para evitar ganho de peso e estimular a limpeza da secreção traqueal. Medicamentos antitussígenos efetivos no controle da tosse incluem hidrocodona (0,22 mg/kg/12 h VO) e butorfanol (0,55 mg/kg/12 h VO). Também podem ser usados broncodilatadores (metilxantinas ou agonistas beta), sendo os seus benefícios atribuíveis à redução do espasmo em vias respiratórias de menor calibre, o que diminui a pressão intratorácica e, assim, a tendência de colapso de vias respiratórias de maior calibre, com melhora na limpeza mucociliar e redução da fadiga diafragmática.

Em cães cujo tratamento clínico falha, estão indicados anéis traqueais extraluminais para colapso do segmento cervical da

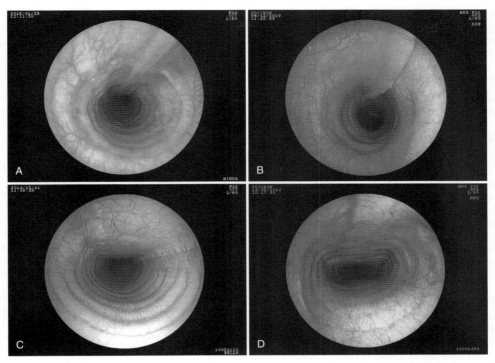

Figura 241.4 Endoscopia da traqueia de cães, mostrando traqueíte com prolapso e irritação da membrana dorsal **(A)**, hipoplasia de traqueia em um cão Buldogue Inglês **(B)** e diferentes graus de gravidade de colapso de traqueia, incluindo graus 1 **(C)** e 3 **(D)**.

traqueia, havendo relatos de resultados excelentes em cães tratados por cirurgiões habilidosos.[14] Se for diagnosticado colapso de traqueia e não for possível o tratamento clínico, o tratamento pode envolver a colocação de *stents* intraluminais autoexpansivos[15,16] (ver Capítulo 121).

Prognóstico
A maioria dos animais pode melhorar com um plano de tratamento individual, mas geralmente a doença é progressiva e o prognóstico a longo prazo é ruim, em especial quando há colapso irreversível de via respiratória.

Fístula traqueoesofágica ou broncoesofágica
É uma doença rara em cães. Os sinais clínicos incluem tosse crônica, infecções recorrentes do trato respiratório inferior e acúmulo de gás no trato gastrintestinal (GI) devido à passagem de ar da traqueia para o trato GI. A conexão entre a traqueia e o esôfago pode ser avaliada por meio de broncoscopia, radiografia contrastada, fluoroscopia ou TC.[17,18] Essa anormalidade é discutida em maiores detalhes no tópico adiante intitulado Doenças Brônquicas Primárias e no Capítulo 273.

Doenças de traqueia obstrutivas e/ou traumáticas

Etiologia
A obstrução parcial da traqueia pode ser causada pelo colapso de anéis traqueais, por estenose subsequente a lesões, corpos estranhos, neoplasias, granulomas, compressão externa, ou como uma complicação de traqueostomia.[19,20]

Lesões de traqueia. As lesões traqueais variam de pequenas lacerações a avulsões traqueais e podem ser causadas por traumatismo externo ou intraluminal. O traumatismo intraluminal é associado principalmente à intubação endotraqueal, enquanto o traumatismo externo é observado mais comumente como ocorrência secundária à briga de cães ou acidente automobilístico. Em gatos, um problema bastante relatado de traumatismo intraluminal diz respeito a estenose após necrose ou ruptura subsequente à insuflação excessiva do manguito do tubo endotraqueal.[21] Estenose após ruptura do segmento intratorácico da traqueia (ou brônquio) depois de traumatismo contuso no pescoço ou no tórax é uma causa relatada de traumatismo externo[22,23] (Vídeo 241.5). Tais problemas raramente são relatados em cães.

Corpos estranhos na traqueia. Em geral, quando corpos estranhos entram na traqueia, são pequenos o bastante para passar para um brônquio. Uma vez alojados em um brônquio, um corpo estranho típico causa broncopneumonia bacteriana, que responde a antibióticos, mas é recorrente. Quando os corpos estranhos são muito grandes, em geral se alojam na carina e causam obstrução de via respiratória, que tem o potencial de ser fatal (Figura 241.5). Os casos relatados de corpos estranhos em cães e gatos são raros, mas envolvem óleo mineral, pelos, projéteis, ossos, material vegetal e brinquedos.[19]

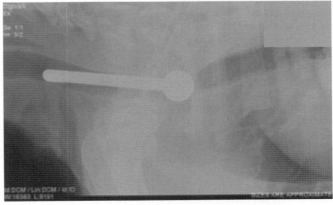

Figura 241.5 Imagem radiográfica lateral do tórax mostrando corpo estranho incomum, quase totalmente obstrutivo, na traqueia, obtida após a morte do paciente. O cão foi levado ao hospital como uma emergência, mas infelizmente morreu pouco antes de chegar. (Cortesia de G. Bolen.)

Tumores intratraqueais. São incomuns em cães e gatos. Em cães jovens, é possível a ocorrência de osteocondroma, enquanto cães e gatos idosos podem apresentar muitos outros tipos de neoplasias (p. ex., tumor de mastócito, carcinoma espinocelular, adenocarcinoma, osteossarcoma, plasmacitoma extramedular, leiomioma ou fibrossarcoma).[19,24-26]

Granulomas traqueais. Podem ser decorrências da colocação de *stent* intraluminal em cães com colapso de traqueia e resultar em grave redução do lúmen traqueal. O tratamento com corticosteroides VO ou mediante nebulização, na maioria dos casos resulta em diminuição do tamanho do granuloma (ver Capítulo 121).[15,27,28]

Granulomas parasitários. Também têm sido descritos. Em cães, há relatos de granulomas causados por vermes pulmonares (*Oslerus osleri*; *Filaroides osleri*) e, em gatos, foi descrita cuterebrose traqueal (ver diagnóstico diferencial para broncopneumopatia eosinofílica, adiante). Por meio de traqueoscopia, foram detectadas larvas de *Cuterebra* na traqueia ou na sua bifurcação para o lobo cranial. O tratamento efetivo consiste na remoção das larvas mediante traqueoscopia ou traqueotomia.[29]

Manifestação clínica

Lesões traqueais resultam, tipicamente, em enfisema subcutâneo nas regiões cervical e torácica, devido ao ar que escapa da traqueia para o tecido subcutâneo. É típico isso estar associado a estridor inspiratório em uma fase inspiratória prolongada, seguida de fase expiratória variável. Outros sinais clínicos incluem tosse, intolerância ao exercício, engasgo, desconforto durante exercício, febre, alteração no latido, cianose intermitente ou colapso e, em gatos, respiração com a boca aberta.[19,20] Além disso, pode ocorrer pneumomediastino, embora seja raro. Em estudo recente, a intubação endotraqueal e a ventilação com pressão positiva foram as causas mais comuns de pneumomediastino, seguidas de traumatismo e corpo estranho na traqueia.[30]

Após lesão por avulsão traqueal, acredita-se que o lúmen da via respiratória seja mantido pela adventícia traqueal intacta ou pelo espessamento do tecido mediastínico, o que leva ao desenvolvimento de uma pseudovia respiratória. Em seguida, ocorre estenose do lúmen em ambas as extremidades da lesão. Portanto, os sinais clínicos demoram a aparecer e devem-se à obstrução traqueal, como desconforto inspiratório e estridor traqueal.[22] No caso de corpo estranho na traqueia, os sinais clínicos apresentam início agudo.

Testes diagnósticos

O diagnóstico é confirmado por meio de radiografia do tórax (ver Figura 241.5) e traqueoscopia (Vídeo 241.6).

Tratamento

O tratamento cirúrgico de lesões traqueais consiste na ressecção das extremidades estenosadas da traqueia lesionada ou da parte da traqueia acometida por tumor e no reparo subsequente por anastomose, o prognóstico é bom.[22]

Traqueíte/traqueobronquite infecciosa

O complexo doença respiratória infecciosa canina (DRIC) também é conhecido como "tosse dos canis",[4,29,31-39] doença observada comumente em cães jovens, especialmente em canis comerciais. Em geral, essa doença contagiosa é autolimitada em cães, mas é possível notar uma ampla variedade de sintomas respiratórios. A etiologia e a fisiopatologia são discutidas em detalhes no Capítulo 227.

Resenha

Cães jovens são mais suscetíveis, em especial aqueles que vivem em ambiente com alta densidade populacional, pois os vírus e a bactéria *Bordetella* são altamente contagiosos. Apesar da ampla disponibilidade de vacinas contra *Bordetella*, a doença ainda é comum.

Manifestação clínica

Em geral, essa doença contagiosa é autolimitada em cães. Na infecção clássica, o único sinal clínico é tosse seca discreta. Pode haver secreção nasal, mas a infecção por *Bordetella* pode provocar tosse crônica, de cura mais difícil. Uma grande variedade de sintomas também pode ser verificada, desde doença branda até pneumonia grave que pode ser fatal, dependendo da gravidade da infecção e da presença de outros patógenos virais ou bacterianos, bem como do estado imune e da vacinação.[29,37]

Testes diagnósticos

O diagnóstico de bordetelose baseia-se na cultura bacteriana positiva ou, mais recentemente, na positividade na reação em cadeia da polimerase (PCR), na amostra do lavado broncoalveolar (LBA, ver Capítulos 101 e 240). Muitos laboratórios realizam PCR, mas não há estudo de avaliação da confiabilidade desse teste. *B. bronchiseptica (Bb)* foi isolada regularmente em cães que se mostravam sadios ao exame clínico, em culturas de amostras obtidas do trato respiratório superior e dos pulmões[38] e, mais recentemente, na PCR qualitativa em amostras de lavado broncoalveolar (LBA);[36] como a infecção e sua disseminação por aerossol pode persistir por semanas, ainda não está esclarecido como um resultado positivo da PCR deve ser interpretado no diagnóstico da doença, ou se pode ser considerado um achado acidental, ou indicativo de que o animal é um portador da infecção. A constatação de cocos pleomórficos ou cocobacilos aderidos aos cílios de células epiteliais é relatada como um achado citológico característico (Figura 241.6). Foi avaliada a acurácia diagnóstica da presença de *Bb* em preparações citológicas, como esfregaços de amostras de LBA ou de líquido obtido por meio de escovação brônquica centrifugadas,[34] juntamente com o valor diagnóstico respectivo da PCR quantitativa (PCRq) e de cultura bacteriana do LBA, no diagnóstico de infecção por *Bb* em cães. Em 24 cães jovens que apresentavam tosse dos canis, a cultura do LBA e a PCRq detectaram *Bb* em mais da metade e em 100% dos cães (com altos níveis CT), respectivamente.[34] Na maioria das amostras de LBA foram encontrados cocobacilos aderidos a células epiteliais ciliadas.[34]

Tratamento

É provável que não sejam necessários antibióticos em casos de traqueobronquite sem complicações (ver Capítulo 227). A vacinação não provou ter algum efeito positivo em cães com infecção ativa.[38] Em geral, o tratamento consiste em terapia antimicrobiana empírica; a doxiciclina (5 mg/kg/12 h VO) é o

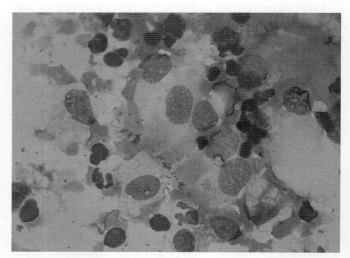

Figura 241.6 Preparação citológica (LBA, citospina) de um cão jovem infectado por *Bordetella bronchiseptica*: cocos pleomórficos ou cocobacilos aderidos aos cílios de células epiteliais são relatados como achados citológicos característicos.

CAPÍTULO 241 • Doenças da Traqueia e de Vias Respiratórias de Pequeno Calibre

antimicrobiano de escolha, devido à sua eficácia contra *Bb*, ao seu custo baixo e à facilidade de uso. Os cães que não respondem à administração oral ou parenteral de antibacterianos podem responder ao tratamento mediante nebulização. A aplicação tópica de antibacterianos não absorvíveis, na forma de aerossol, como a gentamicina, mostrou-se efetiva no sentido de reduzir a população de *Bb* na traqueia e nos brônquios de cães infectados (ver Capítulo 97).[4,39]

Em estudo recente de cães com tosse dos canis nos quais se confirmou a presença de *Bb*, a maioria deles foi tratada sem sucesso com vários antibióticos de uso oral, incluindo amoxicilina/ácido clavulânico, doxiciclina, marbofloxacino ou enrofloxacino, ao passo que o tratamento com gentamicina, mediante nebulização, por 3 semanas ou mais foi associado a melhora clínica significativa.[34]

DOENÇAS BRÔNQUICAS PRIMÁRIAS

Bronquite crônica em cães

Definição e considerações gerais

A bronquite crônica (BC) é uma doença incurável, de início insidioso, que se caracteriza por tosse, relacionada com alguma causa primária específica persistente, passível de identificação. É mais uma síndrome do que um diagnóstico definitivo.[40] Portanto, em cães, também é denominada bronquite crônica inespecífica/específica.

Em cães, considera-se bronquite crônica quando satisfaz 3 critérios diagnósticos: (1) tosse crônica (por pelo menos 2 meses); (2) evidência de hipersecreção mucosa ou excesso de muco; (3) exclusão de outras doenças cardiopulmonares crônicas (p. ex., insuficiência cardíaca congestiva, broncopneumonia infecciosa crônica, neoplasia pulmonar ou broncopneumopatia eosinofílica). No entanto, podem coexistir duas diferentes doenças (p. ex., insuficiência cardíaca congestiva e colapso de via respiratória), o que pode complicar o diagnóstico e o tratamento. Em seres humanos, a principal sequela funcional da bronquite crônica é a obstrução crônica de via respiratória, mencionada como doença pulmonar obstrutiva crônica (DPOC), com enfisema subsequente. Esse mecanismo parece ocorrer com menor frequência em cães, embora o diagnóstico de DPOC dependa da documentação de obstrução de via respiratória com base em testes de função pulmonar, que ainda não estão amplamente disponíveis em medicina veterinária. Cães com bronquite crônica grave de longa duração podem exibir bronquiectasia (dilatação e destruição de paredes dos brônquios) ou broncomalacia (colapso de via respiratória durante a expiração e tosse).

Etiologia, epidemiologia e fatores de risco

As causas primárias de bronquite crônica não são bem entendidas, razão pela qual também é denominada bronquite crônica inespecífica. A principal dificuldade é o fato de que a doença só é detectável em seus estágios avançados, pois tem início insidioso e progressão demorada. Portanto, a avaliação diagnóstica baseia-se na exclusão de todas as causas específicas potenciais, primárias ou secundárias, o que pode ser frustrante tanto para o clínico como para o proprietário. Na verdade, os achados clinicopatológicos típicos são variáveis e inconclusivos. A bronquite crônica inespecífica é diagnosticada principalmente em cães de raças de pequeno porte de meia-idade a idosos, mas também pode ocorrer em raças maiores. Muitos cães com bronquite crônica apresentam sobrepeso e doença periodontal, que parecem ser fatores de risco.

Em seres humanos, os fatores etiológicos mais importantes incluem tabagismo, ativo ou passivo, poluição atmosférica e infecção. É provável que os mesmos fatores sejam responsáveis pelo desenvolvimento de bronquite crônica em cães. Além disso, em cães, a infecção crônica ou prévia por *Bordetella bronchiseptica*,

pelo vírus da cinomose ou, ainda, por parasitas, ocasionando bronquite crônica eosinofílica, ou a presença de outras doenças, como colapso de traqueia ou cardiopatia crônica, são causas potenciais que levam ao desenvolvimento de bronquite crônica. Um estudo recente em que foram investigados fatores potenciais demográficos e históricos associados à tosse crônica não identificou a exposição ao tabagismo ambiental como um fator de risco.[41]

Em pessoas, o refluxo gastresofágico (RGE) geralmente é considerado uma das etiologias mais comuns de tosse crônica. Na verdade, as diretrizes para o tratamento da tosse publicadas por várias sociedades de pneumologistas em todo o mundo recomendam a avaliação e o tratamento de RGE como um componente integrante do algoritmo diagnóstico/terapêutico para a conduta nos casos de tosse crônica. Entretanto, falta provar se essa relação entre refluxo e tosse tem uma ligação causal,[42] embora atualmente seja sugerida na medicina canina que tal ligação não foi observada em larga escala em cães.

Fisiopatologia

A bronquite crônica resulta em alterações inflamatórias na mucosa brônquica, inclusive no aumento da produção de muco. O espessamento da parede do brônquio e, possivelmente, a broncomalacia progressiva contribuem para a obstrução da via respiratória e agravam ainda mais a inflamação, o que induz tosse, que, por sua vez, faz persistir a inflamação.

Manifestação clínica

Uma tosse persistente e sonora com paroxismos em geral seguidos, por fim, de ânsia de vômito, sem causa identificável, costuma ser a única queixa importante.

Diagnóstico

Deve-se excluir a tosse crônica relacionada a causas específicas, principalmente colapso de traqueia, fibrose pulmonar, broncopneumopatia eosinofílica, doença pulmonar parasitária, tumor de brônquio ou pulmão, primário ou secundário, e doença da valva mitral (ver Capítulos 26, 240 e 251).

São realizados testes diagnósticos para exclusão de outras causas de tosse crônica. Em geral, os resultados do hemograma completo são normais. Eosinofilia periférica tem interesse particular nos dados laboratoriais basais porque a eosinofilia circulante pode estar associada à eosinofilia pulmonar ou infecção parasitária. Outros exames laboratoriais que devem ser realizados incluem o teste para pesquisa de antígeno de dirofilária (ver Capítulo 255), exame de fezes para detecção de ovos e larvas de vermes pulmonares (ver Capítulo 81) e a avaliação da concentração circulante do pró-hormônio N-terminal (NT) do peptídio natriurético pró-cerebral (BNP), que se elevam na presença de aumento do átrio esquerdo/insuficiência cardíaca congestiva, bem como na hipertensão pulmonar (ver Capítulo 246). Teor elevado de NT-pró-BNP deve levar à avaliação adicional imediata por meio de ecocardiografia.[43]

As radiografias do tórax mostram espessamento da parede brônquica e/ou aumento generalizado da opacidade intersticial orientada para a via respiratória. Essas radiografias também são úteis para se excluírem outras condições que causam tosse, como insuficiência cardíaca congestiva, massa pulmonar, efusão pleural e doença pulmonar intersticial. A fluoroscopia é útil na avaliação de colapso de traqueia e de via respiratória de maior calibre. A ultrassonografia é útil quando se detecta uma lesão periférica isolada nas radiografias ou na presença de efusão pleural, mas não é útil na bronquite.

A tomografia computadorizada (TC), usada amplamente em pessoas com doenças das vias respiratórias, vem ganhando popularidade, também, na detecção de doença brônquica em cães. Em geral, a TC requer anestesia geral de curta duração, de modo que é comum combiná-la com avaliação da função da laringe, broncoscopia e coleta de amostras citológicas da via respiratória em cães com suspeita de bronquite crônica.

Os achados brônquicos são variáveis. Podem incluir superfície mucosa irregular, com perda do aspecto brilhante normal, adquirindo um aspecto granular e enrugado, bem como, às vezes, sinais de colapso de brônquio parcial. Contudo, foram relatados achados similares em cães idosos sadios, com algum grau de bronquiectasia[44] e, portanto, é preciso interpretar tais achados com cautela. A presença de quantidade excessiva de muco viscoso espesso nas vias respiratórias também é compatível com bronquite crônica.

A avaliação citológica do LBA tipicamente revela excesso de muco, possivelmente com hiperplasia de células epiteliais, aumento do número de neutrófilos, células globosas e macrófagos.[45] O exame de amostra obtida por escovação brônquica pode ser um indicador mais sensível de inflamação da via respiratória do que o exame citológico do LBA, pois mostra maiores porcentagens de leucócitos e neutrófilos.[46] Se uma amostra apresenta eosinofilia acentuada, deve-se considerar broncopneumopatia eosinofílica ou infecção parasitária (dirofilariose/angiostrogilose/infecção por *Crenosoma*), pois essas infecções são potencialmente emergentes em algumas regiões geográficas, especialmente na Europa.[47-50]

A ecocardiografia (ver Capítulo 104) ajuda a diagnosticar doença da valva mitral, que pode ocorrer concomitantemente nesses pacientes idosos e requer tratamento específico, bem como detectar aumento cardíaco direito e hipertensão arterial pulmonar, que podem ser secundários à doença traqueobrônquica crônica.

Tratamento e monitoramento

As alterações brônquicas não são prontamente reversíveis, quando o são. Portanto, o tratamento não cura a doença, mas o ideal é a prevenção ou redução da progressão da doença e a melhora dos sinais clínicos. A terapia baseia-se em uma avaliação da natureza e da gravidade dos problemas individuais do animal, confiando na responsabilidade do cliente.

Os objetivos do tratamento de cães com bronquite crônica incluem: evitar fatores que exacerbam a doença, diminuir a inflamação, limitar a tosse e melhorar a capacidade de atividade física.

Quaisquer poluentes ambientais devem ser eliminados. Os proprietários devem ser avisados para não fumar dentro de casa e limitar a exposição de cães a quaisquer irritantes presentes no ar, inclusive perfumes.

O controle do peso corporal é muito importante (ver Capítulos 176 e 359). A obesidade deve ser tratada de maneira intensiva, porque agrava bastante a tosse e limita a atividade. Além disso, a obesidade prejudica a função pulmonar e aumenta a resposta exagerada da via respiratória, mensurada por meio de pletismografia corporal total barométrica (PCTB) e do teste de caminhada por 6 min (TC6 M).[51,52] A perda de peso induz melhora significativa da função cardiopulmonar, avaliada pelo TC6 M, associada ao monitoramento da frequência cardíaca e da saturação sanguínea de oxigênio.[52] Em cães obesos com bronquite crônica, em geral nota-se melhora evidente dos sinais clínicos com a mera perda de peso, sem o uso de qualquer fármaco.

Nas atividades físicas, em vez de usar coleira, deve-se usar uma guia; episódios de latidos excessivos devem ser reduzidos com modificação apropriada do comportamento.

O controle de infecção bucal/periodontal e a higiene dentária são recomendados porque as bactérias da placa dentária podem ser inaladas, alcançar as vias respiratórias inferiores e se depositar nelas, em especial durante respiração ofegante.

Os glicocorticoides são a base do tratamento de bronquite crônica porque se supõe que reduzam a hipersecreção de muco e o espessamento da mucosa brônquica, o que diminui a tosse. Os glicocorticoides podem ser administrados por via oral ou mediante inalação. Prednisona é o glicocorticoide usado mais comumente, na dose inicial de 1 a 2 mg/kg/24 h VO, seguida da menor dose efetiva no controle dos sinais clínicos. A terapia em dias alternados é preferida por permitir a normalização do eixo hipotálamo-hipofisário e limitar os sinais clínicos associados ao uso de glicocorticoides exógenos.

Em pessoas, o uso de glicocorticoides inalantes tem sido bastante comum e cada vez mais em cães com bronquite crônica. Um estudo mostrou benefícios da terapia com fluticasona, liberada em uma câmara espaçadora e em máscara facial projetada especialmente para cães (p. ex., AeroDawg).[53] Tem relevância clínica o fato de que os glicocorticoides inalantes atuais são mais caros do que os de uso oral, embora o efeito poupador de esteroide sistêmico possa ser útil na melhora da qualidade de vida. Os broncodilatadores (agonistas beta-2, teofilina) são usados frequentemente, embora sua eficácia no tratamento de bronquite crônica não tenha sido bem esclarecida.

Os antibióticos são recomendados aos cães com exacerbação aguda da bronquite crônica e com suspeita razoável de infecção. A doxiciclina e os macrolídeos (azitromicina) são boas escolhas para cães com bronquite crônica devido a suas propriedades anti-inflamatórias, bem como por seus efeitos antimicrobianos.[40] As fluoroquinolonas também têm boa penetração tecidual, mas a sua administração concomitante à teofilina pode resultar em intoxicação por esta última (ver Capítulo 169).[54]

Os supressores da tosse são úteis para o conforto e o alívio tanto dos cães como dos proprietários, quando a tosse é estafante e refratária ao tratamento anti-inflamatório. Os supressores da tosse vendidos sem prescrição raramente são efetivos em cães; aqueles à base de narcóticos são mais efetivos. Em alguns países, as preparações de opioides de uso oral passaram a ter ampla disponibilidade. Nos países onde não se pode prescrever uma preparação de butorfanol de uso oral, algumas gotas da solução de uso injetável depositadas na língua podem ser efetivas, mas nem a dose necessária nem a relação dose-efeito foram estudadas (Tabela 241.1). Há relato de um estudo em pacientes humanos sobre a eficácia da gabapentina no controle da tosse relacionada à sensibilidade ao reflexo da tosse hiperativo em pessoas.[55]

Broncopneumopatia eosinofílica em cães

Etiologia e fisiopatologia

A broncopneumopatia eosinofílica (BPE) canina é uma doença que se caracteriza por infiltração eosinofílica no pulmão e na mucosa brônquica, considerada manifestação de hipersensibilidade imunológica. Embora a etiologia da BPE ainda seja desconhecida, a associação de infiltração eosinofílica e predominância de células T CD4+ favorece uma resposta imune Th2 dominante

Tabela 241.1	Supressores da tosse usados em cães com bronquite crônica.	
FÁRMACO	**DOSAGEM**	**COMENTÁRIO**
Opioides		
Butorfanol	0,25 a 1,1 mg/kg/ 8 a 12 h VO	Mais efetivo. Os efeitos colaterais potenciais incluem sedação excessiva. Pode ocorrer tolerância com o tempo
Hidrocodona	0,2 a 0,3 mg/kg/ 6 a 12 h VO	
Tramadol	2 a 5 mg/kg/ 8 a 12 h VO	
Não opioides		
Gabapentina	2 a 5 mg/kg/8 h VO	Eficácia não estabelecida
Metocarbamol	15 a 30 mg/kg/12 h VO	

VO, via oral. (Adaptada de Rozanski E: Canine chronic bronchitis. *Vet Clin North Am Small Anim Pract* 44:114, 2014.)

nas vias respiratórias inferiores.⁵⁶ Causas suspeitas e conhecidas de hipersensibilidade pulmonar em seres humanos e animais incluem fungos, mofos, fármacos, bactérias e parasitas. Todavia, em muitos casos, nenhuma causa primária é detectada. Ainda não foi esclarecida a participação de alergênios inalados na ocorrência de BPE. A BPE é diagnosticada principalmente em cães jovens. Cães das raças Husky Siberiano e Malamute são os mais predispostos à doença, mas muitas outras raças podem ser acometidas.

Manifestação clínica

Geralmente, por ocasião da consulta, a condição geral do paciente é boa, a menos que haja broncopneumonia bacteriana concomitante. Os sinais clínicos incluem principalmente tosse, engasgo e ânsia de vômito, notados em todos os casos. Nos casos agudos, engasgo e ânsia de vômito, às vezes, são as queixas principais, considerando até dispepsia no diagnóstico diferencial. Dispneia é um sinal muito frequente. Um sintoma menos comum é secreção nasal (≈ 50% dos cães acometidos).

Testes diagnósticos

Os elementos diagnósticos para BPE incluem fatores relacionados à resenha e ao histórico clínico (raça, idade jovem, resposta prévia a corticosteroides), sinais clínicos, achados radiográficos e broncoscópicos, eosinofilia, infiltração eosinofílica tecidual notada em exames citológicos e histopatológicos, resposta ao tratamento apropriado e exclusão de outras anormalidades. O achado radiográfico mais comum é um padrão broncointersticial misto, moderado a grave (Figura 241.7). Na TC, os achados associados à BPE são variáveis e heterogêneos e incluem espessamento moderado a marcante da parede brônquica, formação de tampão no lúmen brônquico por restos de muco, bronquiectasia, nódulos pulmonares e linfadenopatia.⁵⁷ A broncoscopia (ver Capítulo 101) pode revelar achados macroscópicos típicos, que incluem a presença de muco amarelo-esverdeado abundante ou material mucopurulento, espessamento marcante da mucosa com uma superfície irregular ou polipoide e, em alguns casos, obstrução parcial da via respiratória durante a expiração. Eosinofilia no sangue periférico é um achado frequente (≈ 60% dos casos). O exame citológico da amostra de LBA ou de escovação da via respiratória mostra intensa eosinofilia; frequentemente, mais de 50% das células inflamatórias são eosinófilos. Na maioria dos casos, também é possível notar infiltração eosinofílica na mucosa brônquica, em amostra obtida por meio de biopsia. No LBA de cães com BPE, tem-se verificado teor elevado do pró-peptídio aminoterminal do pró-colágeno do tipo III (PIIINP), uma proteína usada como marcador da síntese de colágeno do tipo III, possivelmente devido a alterações fibrosantes secundárias.⁵⁸

Diagnóstico diferencial

Vários parasitas, como *Strongyloides* spp., *Ascaris* spp., *Toxocara canis* e *Ancylostoma* spp., podem causar pneumonia eosinofílica em seres humanos e, provavelmente, em cães; os sintomas respiratórios são apenas discretos e, em geral, predominam os sintomas gastrintestinais (GI).

No cão, a dirofilariose subclínica causada por *Dirofilaria immitis* pode ocasionar pneumonite eosinofílica. A migração de larvas de *Angiostrongylus vasorum* através do parênquima pulmonar também pode resultar em pneumonia eosinofílica em cães (Vídeo 241.7). A infecção por esse nematódeo (também denominada dirofilariose francesa) é uma doença emergente, com aumento de relatos na distribuição e na prevalência no Reino Unido, na Europa, na África do Sul e na província de Newfoundland (Canadá). A faixa de expansão geográfica pode estar relacionada à influência do clima na distribuição do parasita. O verme infecta cães e raposas, e se dissemina a partir da ingestão dos hospedeiros intermediários, incluindo lesmas e caramujos. Os principais sinais clínicos incluem sintomas respiratórios, anormalidades hemorrágicas e sinais neurológicos,⁵⁹ de gravidade muito variável; a progressão da doença em geral é crônica e branda. No entanto, é necessário o diagnóstico precoce e correto, pois a estrongilose pode ser fatal, se não tratada. Nos casos acompanhados de sinais clínicos respiratórios e em regiões endêmicas, as alterações radiográficas pulmonares, exclusivamente, podem ser sugestivas do diagnóstico e incluem alterações broncointersticiais ou alveolointersticiais moderadas a graves em áreas periféricas e/ou caudodorsais (Figura 241.8). Outros parasitas broncopulmonares, como *Capillaria aerophila*, *Oslerus osleri*, *Filaroides hirthi*, *Crenosoma vulpis* (Vídeo 241.8) e *Paragonimus kellicotti*, também estão implicados na migração de eosinófilos para as vias respiratórias (*O. osleri*) ou ao pulmão (outros parasitas), em cães, e podem parecer BPE. Uma maior prevalência de doença brônquica causada pela infecção por *Crenosoma vulpis* também está se tornando evidente na Europa continental.⁶⁰

Por essas razões, é indispensável a triagem para doenças parasitárias mediante exame do LBA ou exames de fezes seriados

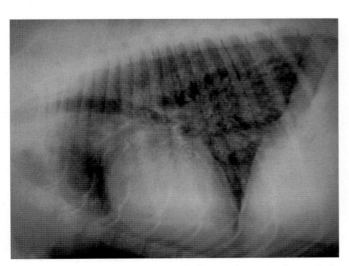

Figura 241.7 Radiografia lateral esquerda do tórax de um cão da raça Husky com 3 anos que apresentava BPE, mostrando padrão broncointersticial marcante, com infiltração brônquica. (Cortesia de G. Bolen.)

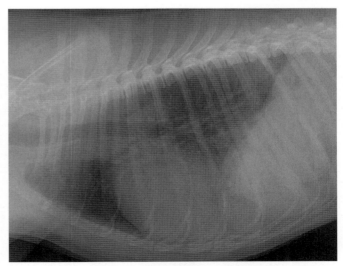

Figura 241.8 Radiografia lateral esquerda do tórax de um cão com angiostrongilose. Nota-se um padrão broncointersticial generalizado, com um padrão alveolar marcante na periferia dos lobos pulmonares caudais (note broncogramas aéreos). Uma linha de fissura pleural entre os lobos cranial e caudal esquerdos e discreto afastamento do lobo pulmonar da parede torácica são compatíveis com efusão pleural branda. As artérias e veias pulmonares estão dilatadas.

(Figura 241.9; ver Capítulo 81). É possível a detecção clínica de um antígeno liberado por vermes adultos da espécie *A. vasorum* em uma amostra de plasma (Angio Detect, IDEXX Laboratories),[61] ou esse antígeno pode ser detectado por PCR, em amostra de LBA.[50] Em áreas endêmicas, aconselha-se, com veemência, a realização de um teste com antígeno de dirofilária para excluir a possibilidade de dirofilariose subclínica. Entretanto, como alternativa, é possível usar anti-helmínticos apropriados para tratar o animal contra parasitas potenciais.[47]

Tratamento

A resposta à terapia com corticosteroide geralmente é muito boa, mas a cessação completa dos sinais clínicos nem sempre é conseguida. Inicia-se a administração de prednisolona na dosagem de 1 mg/kg/12 h VO, durante 1 semana, seguida da mesma dose, em dias alternados, por mais 1 semana e, então, a cada 24 horas, também em dias alternados, por mais 1 semana; a partir daí faz-se a diminuição gradual da dose até se obter a dose de manutenção. Como o tratamento oral prolongado com corticosteroide infelizmente pode desencadear efeitos colaterais sistêmicos bem conhecidos (*i. e.*, hiperadrenocorticismo iatrogênico) e seu uso pode ser contraindicado em cães com outros problemas de saúde concomitantes, como diabetes melito, obesidade ou cardiopatia (ver Capítulo 358), o tratamento alternativo com esteroides inalantes (TEI) tem sido empregado cada vez mais, nos últimos anos, tanto em medicina humana como em veterinária, com as supostas vantagens de ocasionar alta concentração do fármaco nos lúmens das vias respiratórias e baixa absorção sistêmica e, assim, reduzir potencialmente os efeitos secundários deletérios. A terapia com corticosteroide inalante é bem tolerada, resulta em melhora dos sinais clínicos e reduz os efeitos colaterais, possibilitando, ainda, a redução da dose oral de esteroide em animais que dependem do uso desse tipo de fármaco.[53,62] Entretanto, parece que o tratamento prolongado da BPE com o TEI, exclusivamente, não possibilita o controle total da doença em todos os cães acometidos e manutenção do TEI por longo período pode inibir o eixo hipófise-adrenal (EHA).[62] Outros fármacos com efeito imunomodulador foram propostos, mas até o momento não se dispõe dos resultados de ensaios clínicos.

Prognóstico

É frequente a ocorrência de recidiva após semanas a meses após a cessação da administração do fármaco, embora alguns cães possam continuar sem sinais clínicos depois disso.

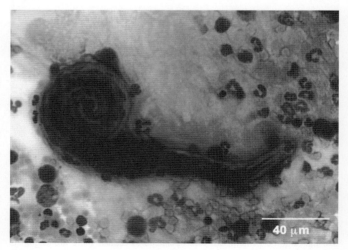

Figura 241.9 Exame citológico de esfregaço de LBA, após centrifugação, corado pelo método de May-Grunwald-Giemsa (MGG), no qual foi identificada uma larva L1 de *Angiostrongylus*.

Discinesia ciliar primária

Manifestação

Anteriormente conhecida como síndrome dos cílios imóveis, a discinesia ciliar primária (DCP) resulta de um grupo heterogêneo de doenças hereditárias que comprometem a motilidade ciliar. Tais alterações estão associadas principalmente a anormalidades ultraestruturais e causam infecção bacteriana recorrente das vias respiratórias superiores e inferiores. Nos cães acometidos, como acontece em seres humanos, a inefetividade e a incoordenação da função ciliar resultam em falha na limpeza do muco das vias respiratórias, o que, por sua vez, acarreta a formação crônica de tampão de muco e inflamação das cavidades nasais e das vias respiratórias. A disfunção dos monocílios do nodo embrionário também pode ocasionar assimetria aleatória do lado esquerdo do corpo e a transposição dos órgãos torácicos e/ou abdominais em 50% dos casos.[63] Isso é conhecido como síndrome de Kartagener, a qual representa uma tríade de sintomas que incluem bronquiectasia, transposição total de vísceras do lado esquerdo para o direito (*situs inversus*) e rinossinusite crônica. Essa síndrome foi relatada em seres humanos e em cães com DCP. Em cães, a DCP é uma doença rara que, ainda assim, foi relatada em mais de 19 raças.[64-68]

Etiologia

Atualmente, as mutações que causam DCP foram identificadas em mais de 20 genes humanos.[68] Cada gene causador pode estar associado a defeitos ciliares ultraestruturais particulares e esses 20 genes humanos explicam apenas 50% dos casos de DCP humana. Em geral, os casos em cães têm como foco um indivíduo de uma raça específica, mas às vezes ninhadas são acometidas ou casos diferentes podem segregar-se na mesma raça.[65,66,68] Essa doença genética geralmente é autossômica recessiva. Em cães, foi identificada uma mutação recente em um novo gene causador (*CCDC39*), em animais da raça Old English Sheepdog.[67] Essa nova mutação está dispersa mundialmente e é responsável pela DCP nessa raça. Foi desenvolvido um novo teste genético que está disponível em ampla escala para avaliação pré-acasalamento de cães dessa raça, mas ainda não em outras raças.

Manifestação clínica

Como consequência do comprometimento da limpeza mucociliar, os sinais clínicos consistem em anormalidades respiratórias crônicas causadas por rinossinusite, bronquite, broncopneumonia e bronquiectasia. Embora os sintomas respiratórios geralmente sejam as queixas que levam o paciente à consulta, podem ocorrer outros sinais clínicos relacionados à disfunção em outros tecidos que apresentam epitélio ciliado ou microtúbulos, como otite média, infertilidade em fêmeas, astenoteratoespermia em machos, hidrocefalia e fibrose renal ou dilatação de túbulos renais. Tipicamente, os sintomas surgem em um cão jovem de raça pura vacinado; contudo, alguns cães permanecem assintomáticos até vários meses a vários anos. Achados clínicos marcantes, isto é, secreção nasal bilateral recorrente e episódios repetidos de bronquite ou broncopneumonia, desde o nascimento, devem alertar o clínico para incluir DCP no diagnóstico diferencial.

Diagnóstico

A detecção de achados clínicos marcantes, em combinação com *situs inversus*, é muito sugestivo da doença. A maioria das outras causas possíveis deve ser excluída por um exame físico completo, bem como pelos testes complementares disponíveis atualmente. A confirmação de DCP requer a análise funcional e ultraestrutural dos cílios, tanto *in vivo* como *in vitro*. Para a análise funcional *in vitro* dos cílios em cães sob suspeita de terem

DCP, utiliza-se a cintilografia como um procedimento diagnóstico para avaliar a limpeza mucociliar. Na análise funcional *in vivo* dos cílios, os pacientes mostram consistentemente um movimento ciliar descoordenado ou discinético.

Cílios móveis são compostos por um microtúbulo de sustentação principal, o axonema, que consiste em nove pares de microtúbulos circundando um par central. Os braços de dineína, internos e externos, estendem-se a partir de cada dupla de microtúbulos externos e geram a força necessária para a motilidade do cílio, por meio de um mecanismo dependente de ATP. Em geral, a dismotilidade ou imobilidade ciliar está associada a defeitos ultraestruturais dos cílios, tais como ausência total ou parcial dos braços externos de dineína (BEDs) e/ou dos braços internos de dineína (BIDs), defeitos das projeções radiais ou de ligações de nexina e desorganização geral do axonema com transposição microtubular.[69] A microscopia eletrônica de transmissão pode revelar anormalidades ultraestruturais específicas (Figura 241.10), embora geralmente seja difícil fazer a distinção entre DCP e defeitos ciliares secundários causados por outra doença primária, com base apenas nos achados ultraestruturais. Portanto, uma técnica de cultura ciliar, a ciliogênese, mostrou-se capaz de distinguir de maneira definitiva etiologias primárias de secundárias.[64] Desenvolveu-se um teste TaqMan com sensibilidade e especificidade excelentes para a avaliação da prevalência da mutação em cães da raça Old English Sheepdog. O alelo com mutação foi encontrado em cães dessa raça, tanto na Europa como nos EUA, sugerindo uma distribuição mundial.[68] Esse teste genético também possibilitou o início de um programa de acasalamento que detecta portadores assintomáticos e previne o nascimento de indivíduos acometidos.

Diagnóstico diferencial

Outras causas de infecção bacteriana recorrente das vias respiratórias superiores (nos casos iniciais) e inferiores devem ser investigadas, como a presença de imunodeficiência, bactérias resistentes ou corpo estranho no brônquio. Em cães da raça Wolfhound Irlandês, foi descrita uma síndrome de rinite/broncopneumonia, caracterizada por rinorreia mucoide ou mucopurulenta transitória ou persistente, tosse e dispneia, em idade precoce; mesmo assim, a DCP ainda não foi identificada formalmente como a causa da doença.[70]

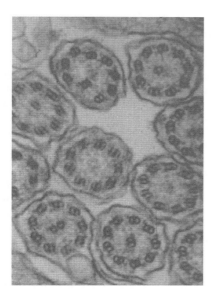

Figura 241.10 Microscopia eletrônica de transmissão mostrando anormalidades ultraestruturais primárias específicas, responsáveis por um defeito ciliar primário (ausência do par central, com transposição ocasional de um par periférico).

Tratamento

Embora a DCP não seja uma doença curável, frequentemente pode ser tratada por alguns anos (ver Capítulos 97 e 242). Um fator fundamental para o tratamento efetivo é o monitoramento adequado de microrganismos infectantes e o uso criterioso de antibióticos ao longo do tempo. Além disso, a hidratação sistêmica e local adequada, juntamente com tapotagem diária apropriada e exercício vigoroso, ajuda a eliminar o muco das vias respiratórias.

Prognóstico

Assim que o diagnóstico for estabelecido, o prognóstico em médio e longo prazos é ruim porque, apesar do tratamento adequado, em geral a doença progride com o tempo e a resposta ao tratamento é menos efetiva.

Fístula broncoesofágica

Define-se fístula broncoesofágica[17,29] como uma comunicação entre o esôfago e um ou mais brônquios. A maioria dos casos observados é secundária à ingestão e penetração de corpo estranho, em cães jovens ou de meia-idade (muito incomumente em gatos). Os sinais clínicos envolvem os tratos respiratório e GI, com estertores ruidosos, depressão, febre e perda de apetite. Também pode ocorrer efusão pleural, além de pneumonia localizada.

Em geral, o diagnóstico baseia-se em imagens de radiografias simples, com evidência de pneumonia, corpo estranho no esôfago, distensão do esôfago causada por gás e possível presença de efusão pleural. No hemograma completo, espera-se aumento do número de leucócitos, com desvio à esquerda. A melhor maneira de confirmar o diagnóstico é a obtenção de radiografias do tórax após a administração oral de pequeno volume de uma suspensão de bário. O exame endoscópico pode dar uma visão direta, porém se considera mais provável que a radiografia seja mais útil no diagnóstico. A correção bem-sucedida da fístula é mais provável mediante cirurgia torácica para corrigir o defeito, lavagem da área afetada e, muito provavelmente, lobectomia para remover os tecidos infectados. Se o distúrbio for identificado precocemente e tratado de maneira apropriada, o prognóstico em termos de recuperação pode ser bom. As complicações decorrentes da estenose esofágica podem ser um problema, principalmente quando há demora na detecção e no início do tratamento.

Mineralização brônquica, broncolitíase[29]

Raramente se constata mineralização brônquica, que pode ser secundária a qualquer doença crônica, inflamatória ou infecciosa. Na verdade, na mineralização brônquica pode não haver qualquer evidência clínica de disfunção. Em gatos normais, as glândulas mucosas peribrônquicas podem sofrer mineralização, vistas como opacidades multifocais mineralizadas.[71]

DOENÇAS BRÔNQUICAS SECUNDÁRIAS

Bronquiectasia

Introdução

Define-se bronquiectasia como uma dilatação anormal permanente e deformidade de vias respiratórias subsegmentares, resultantes de inflamação crônica de via respiratória que danifica os componentes elásticos dos brônquios, acarretando assim destruição da parede brônquica e comprometimento da limpeza de secreções respiratórias.[72] Considera-se uma entidade nosológica única, embora várias condições congênitas ou adquiridas que originam um ciclo de infecção e inflamação crônicas de via respiratória possam resultar em alterações bronquiectásicas.

Etiologia e fisiopatologia

Em seres humanos, a bronquiectasia pode ser classificada como bronquiectasia relacionada à fibrose cística (FC) e não relacionada à FC. A FC é uma doença hereditária causada por uma mutação no gene da proteína reguladora da condutância transmembrana na fibrose cística (CFTR, do inglês *cistic fibrosis transmembrane conductance regulator*). A formação de tampão de muco viscoso resulta em infecção e inflamação, ocasionando destruição da parede da via respiratória e bronquiectasia. Indivíduos com FC podem ser diagnosticados antes do nascimento por meio de testes genéticos ou um teste feito em amostra de suor no início da infância. Em nenhuma espécie animal não humana se detectou mutação de ocorrência natural no gene CFTR, que causa fibrose cística. Um estudo realizado em cães revelou que as mutações de ocorrência natural no CFTR são relativamente comuns em cães domésticos, mas não detectou uma taxa de expressão mais alta de mutações no CFTR em cães com bronquiectasia.[73] Portanto, é provável que a bronquiectasia em cães e gatos se deva principalmente à bronquiectasia não induzida por FC. Tanto em seres humanos como em cães, as etiologias da bronquiectasia, além de FC, incluem DCP, acompanhada ou não da síndrome de Kartagener. Ainda não foi esclarecido se ocorrem DCP e síndrome de Kartagener em gatos; caso ocorram, são extremamente raras. Em cães e gatos, a bronquiectasia focal se deve mais frequentemente à aspiração de corpo estranho e/ou obstrução de brônquio.[4,74]

Em geral, ocorre bronquiectasia difusa subsequente a doenças adquiridas,[4,41,76] incluindo lesão por aspiração ou inalação, broncopneumonia infecciosa crônica (inclusive a de origem parasitária), infecção crônica por *B. bronchiseptica* ou *Pneumocystis carinii* em cães com imunodeficiência, broncopneumopatia eosinofílica, bronquite crônica e, potencialmente, aspergilose broncopulmonar alérgica (uma causa rara de bronquiectasia cavitária localizada).[76] Em gatos, a inflamação brônquica crônica é sugerida como a causa mais comum de bronquiectasia, especialmente bronquite crônica, neoplasia e broncopneumonia,[77] e foi descrita em um caso de doença pulmonar fibrosante difusa.[78] As vias respiratórias acometidas em geral estão parcialmente obstruídas por exsudato purulento ou viscoso, pois a dilatação interfere muito na limpeza normal da via respiratória.

A disfunção na limpeza mucociliar, por sua vez, possibilita o acúmulo de muco, exsudato e microrganismos, e a infecção secundária estimula uma resposta inflamatória do hospedeiro, criando um círculo vicioso de dano adicional à parede da via respiratória e predisposição a infecções broncopulmonares recorrentes (Figura 241.11).

Resenha, histórico clínico e manifestação clínica

Em cães, parece haver predisposição racial à doença, pois a bronquiectasia é mais prevalente em algumas raças, como Cocker Spaniel Americano, Poodle Miniatura, Husky Siberiano e English Springer Spaniel.[74] Além disso, a maioria dos cães com bronquiectasia tem 7 anos ou mais.[74] É provável que os sinais clínicos reflitam uma doença primária e, em geral, incluem tosse (mais comum), engasgo, taquipneia, dispneia e, ocasionalmente, febre.[74] Pode-se detectar bronquiectasia por meio de radiografia torácica, tomografia computadorizada de alta resolução (TCAR) ou broncoscopia (Vídeos 241.9 e 241.10). As características radiográficas e broncoscópicas em cães foram descritas.[74,75] A broncoscopia não é considerada padrão-ouro, mas é extremamente útil no reconhecimento ou na visualização de lesões bronquiectásicas e, o mais importante, possibilita a coleta de amostras para identificação e tratamento potencial de possíveis doenças primárias (ver Capítulo 101). O exame broncoscópico detecta tampões mucopurulentos nas vias respiratórias dilatadas e revestimentos hiperêmicos enrugados nas paredes brônquicas.

Em pessoas, a radiografia de tórax simples não é considerada uma técnica muito sensível para a avaliação de alterações bronquiectásicas, tampouco se usa broncografia com essa finalidade. A TCAR foi descrita como o melhor procedimento não invasivo para o diagnóstico de bronquiectasia. Na TC, os principais achados em pessoas com bronquiectasia incluem dilatação anormal dos brônquios, ausência de redução do calibre dos brônquios periféricos e detecção de vias respiratórias distintas em 1 cm da superfície pleural. Os achados secundários incluem espessamento da parede brônquica, tampão de muco no lúmen brônquico e aprisionamento de ar periférico, constatado pela menor densidade pulmonar nas regiões acometidas.[79] O critério de uso mais utilizado para quantificar a dilatação brônquica anormal na TC é uma razão broncoarterial (BA; a razão do diâmetro do lúmen brônquico em corte transversal em relação ao diâmetro da artéria pulmonar a ele associada) > 1.[79] Em cães, estudo recente revelou que animais sadios podem ter uma razão BA de até 2.[80] Em um estudo retrospectivo realizado em cães com bronquiectasia diagnosticada por meio de broncoscopia e/ou histopatologia, as características mais comuns de bronquiectasia na TC foram dilatação, ausência de redução do diâmetro periférico da via respiratória e consolidação lobar.[80]

Em um grande número de cães com BPE, a TC revelou bronquiectasia em 60% deles.[57]

Como há carência de estudos correlacionando TC com achados broncoscópicos de bronquiectasia em cães, a sensibilidade do diagnóstico broncoscópico de bronquiectasia é questionável. Mostrou-se que a idade influencia os achados broncoscópicos em cães saudáveis da raça Beagle: a bronquiectasia foi descrita como um achado endoscópico normal em cães Beagle idosos e tal achado não parece estar associado ao aumento de neutrófilos no LBA.[44] Tais diferenças relacionadas à idade devem ser consideradas ao interpretar a presença de bronquiectasia em cães idosos com doença respiratória.

Cultura microbiológica e teste de sensibilidade (antibiograma) de amostra de LBA para bactérias aeróbicas e anaeróbicas são recomendados porque é provável que sejam úteis para orientar o tratamento do paciente. As bactérias frequentemente isoladas de pessoas com bronquiectasia incluem *Pseudomonas aeruginosa*, *Haemophilus influenzae*, *Staphylococcus aureus* e algumas outras.[81] Em cães, não se pode tirar qualquer conclusão a respeito da frequência de distribuição de bactérias em pacientes com bronquiectasia.[74]

O exame citológico de LBA tipicamente indica neutrofilia, eosinofilia, se de natureza alérgica ou parasitária, e metaplasia escamosa de células epiteliais. O teste PCR em amostra de LBA pode ser útil para identificar *Bordetella* spp., *Mycoplasma* spp. ou *Aspergillus* spp., pois a aspergilose broncopulmonar alérgica pode ser uma causa de bronquiectasia cavitária localizada,[76] como descrita em pessoas.

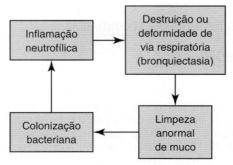

Figura 241.11 Hipótese do círculo vicioso na bronquiectasia. A resposta inflamatória mediada pelo hospedeiro diante do material estranho ou bactérias na via respiratória causa dano tecidual, resultando em bronquiectasia, que contribui para o comprometimento da limpeza de muco e a colonização bacteriana adicional.

CAPÍTULO 241 • Doenças da Traqueia e de Vias Respiratórias de Pequeno Calibre

Tratamento

O objetivo da terapia de bronquiectasia é o controle dos sinais clínicos e o tratamento ou prevenção de infecções bacterianas. Em medicina humana, a abordagem terapêutica inclui limpeza da via respiratória, para reduzir a infecção e a inflamação crônicas, e o tratamento dos casos que se agravam. Terapias inalantes são a base do tratamento (ver Capítulo 97). Em combinação com antibióticos administrados diretamente na via respiratória, são utilizados fármacos mucoativos, inclusive agentes mucolíticos e hiperosmolares, para melhorar a limpeza mucociliar e reduzir a infecção e a inflamação. Os antibióticos, em especial os inalantes, reduzem o agravamento da doença e a inflamação por diminuir a população de bactérias. Os macrolídeos reduzem a frequência de exacerbação e são a pedra fundamental da terapia anti-inflamatória na bronquiectasia.[82] Os antibióticos macrolídeos têm propriedades anti-inflamatórias e imunomoduladoras (sem supressão do sistema imune), além de atividade antibacteriana. São usados amplamente no tratamento da bronquiectasia em seres humanos.[82,83] A vantagem de usar macrolídeos, em vez de glicocorticoides, para tratar a inflamação é a imunomodulação sem imunossupressão. Não há estudo que tenha investigado os riscos e benefícios do uso prolongado de macrolídeos em cães. No momento, não há dados definitivos que sustentem o uso rotineiro de glicocorticoides, mesmo os inalantes, a menos que o paciente apresente asma ou BPE, simultaneamente.

Prognóstico

É fundamental o tratamento da doença primária para tentar reduzir a progressão da destruição de paredes brônquicas. Apesar das anormalidades clínicas substanciais, cães com bronquiectasia podem sobreviver por anos.[74] Pacientes com bronquiectasia focal são exceções, porque a ressecção cirúrgica do lobo pulmonar afetado pode ser curativa.

Broncomalacia

Considerações gerais e etiologia

A broncomalacia (BM) se caracteriza por fraqueza das paredes dos brônquios principais ou de menor calibre, que ocasiona colapso da parede brônquica. Em medicina veterinária, a broncomalacia tem sido diagnosticada cada vez mais.[5,84-86] A etiologia não foi esclarecida. Com base no exame endoscópico, a BM pode ser classificada como estática, dinâmica, ou ambas.[86] Enquanto a BM estática é comum em cães braquicefálicos,[85] a BM dinâmica (Vídeo 241.11) ocorre com maior frequência em associação ao colapso da traqueia e denomina-se traqueobroncomalacia. Na verdade, em uma população de 115 cães levados à consulta para avaliação de doença respiratória e examinados por meio de broncoscopia, documentou-se traqueobroncomalacia em 50% desses cães; constatou-se colapso de traqueia em 21% e broncomalacia em 47%.[5] Isso mostra que a BM dinâmica também pode ocorrer como uma doença clínica isolada, associada a infecção e/ou inflamação brônquica,[84] ou não. Em muitos casos, realmente não foi possível confirmar a participação da inflamação de via respiratória na ocorrência de BM.[5,87] Além disso, recentemente investigou-se a participação da cardiomegalia na ocorrência dessa anormalidade, mas não se conseguiu identificar associação alguma entre o aumento do átrio esquerdo e o colapso de via respiratória.[9]

Manifestação clínica

Como a BM costuma estar associada ao colapso da traqueia, os cães das raças Poodle e Yorkshire Terrier, em especial quando obesos ou com sobrepeso, são acometidos mais comumente.[5,84] Muitos cães braquicefálicos apresentam BM estática.[85] Todavia, outras raças podem ser acometidas, especialmente indivíduos idosos.

Os sinais clínicos incluem tosse crônica, sibilos, dispneia intermitente ou contínua, dificuldade para eliminar as secreções e, possivelmente, sinais de bronquite recorrente e pneumonia. À auscultação pulmonar, podem ser ouvidas crepitações pulmonares.[84] Como as radiografias parecem pouco sensíveis para detectar colapso de via respiratória, a documentação de BM requer broncoscopia (ver Capítulo 101).[5] Os tipos estático e dinâmico de BM podem coexistir, particularmente em cães de grande porte, com hipertensão pulmonar, padrão radiográfico brônquico e nodulações ao exame endoscópico.[86]

Diagnóstico

A broncoscopia pode revelar que ambos os pulmões estão acometidos; em cerca de metade dos casos, a doença parece afetar predominantemente o pulmão esquerdo.[84] O exame do LBA e a realização de biopsia da mucosa brônquica são procedimentos indispensáveis e podem revelar evidência de bronquite infecciosa em cerca de metade dos cães acometidos.

Tratamento e prognóstico

O tratamento é de suporte e inespecífico, devendo basear-se nos achados clínicos em cada caso. Até o momento, não há estudo que tenha investigado como os cães com BM respondem ao tratamento; ademais, não há disponibilidade de informação detalhada sobre o prognóstico.

DOENÇA DE VIA RESPIRATÓRIA INFERIOR EM GATOS

Em gatos, a tosse é um sinal clínico infrequente, ao contrário do que se observa em cães. Além disso, em gatos, a tosse é um tanto específica de doença traqueobrônquica, porque a de origem cardíaca é rara. Doença de via respiratória inferior de gatos (DVRIG) é uma designação que abrange todas as doenças brônquicas, incluindo inflamatórias e não inflamatórias, sendo as inflamatórias muito mais comuns.

A doença brônquica inflamatória de gatos (asma ou bronquite felina) caracteriza-se por inflamação das vias respiratórias inferiores sem uma causa óbvia identificável. É reconhecida clinicamente por várias combinações de tosse, sibilos, intolerância ao exercício e dificuldade respiratória, atribuíveis à obstrução de via respiratória causada por inflamação brônquica.

Muitos termos confusos são encontrados na literatura, como bronquite crônica, bronquite alérgica, bronquite eosinofílica e asma brônquica. Ainda é um desafio distinguir bronquite asmática da não asmática. Ainda é incerto se a asma felina e a bronquite crônica nessa espécie são de fato doenças diferentes ou duas facetas da mesma doença.[88] De acordo com alguns autores, a asma felina e a bronquite crônica atualmente devem ser consideradas duas doenças distintas.[89] Foram descritas diferenças na etiologia, nos achados radiográficos do tórax, nas porcentagens de eosinófilos/neutrófilos alveolares e na resposta aos testes de resposta das vias respiratórias (TRVR), nesse sentido, mas não há um teste discriminatório indiscutível.[106,118,145] A classificação baseia-se nas porcentagens de eosinófilos e neutrófilos no LBA. Vários estudos relataram as quantidades dos tipos celulares no LBA obtido de gatos,[94] mas não foram estabelecidas faixas de valores de referência específicas. Consequentemente, os limites dos valores de eosinófilos e neutrófilos para definir asma e bronquite crônica são definidos de maneira arbitrária.[105,106]

Devido a essa falta de consenso a respeito da definição exata de asma felina, a maioria dos estudos publicados falha em distinguir asma felina espontânea da bronquite crônica felina. Apesar de excelentes revisões publicadas recentemente,[96] é difícil obter informação separadamente sobre ambas as doenças. Portanto, as informações mencionadas nesta seção se referem mais à doença brônquica inflamatória felina.

Obteve-se um grande volume de informações interessantes com o estudo de modelos de asma felina, que representam um avanço relevante no estudo dessa doença, possibilitando tanto pesquisas farmacológicas quanto imunológicas. Entretanto, embora tenham sido obtidos resultados interessantes e promissores (ver detalhes na excelente revisão de Reinero[90]), é preciso muita cautela antes que os resultados de pesquisa possam ser colocados em prática. São necessários testes clínicos para explorar melhor o valor potencial das medicações inalantes propostas, da imunoterapia ou de outros tratamentos em pacientes felinos com doença brônquica inflamatória. Além disso, é necessário distinguir doença brônquica inflamatória felina de doenças não inflamatórias crônicas de vias respiratórias inferiores (p. ex., bronquite infecciosa ou crônica causada por várias infecções parasitárias), em razão de diferenças na patogenia, no tratamento e no prognóstico.[96]

Doença brônquica inflamatória felina

Patogenia e fisiopatologia

De acordo com Reinero,[90] a asma e a bronquite crônica em gatos devem ser consideradas duas síndromes distintas. Acredita-se que a bronquite crônica seja secundária a uma agressão que causou dano permanente da via respiratória, ocasionando muitos achados clinicopatológicos semelhantes aos da asma. Também se acredita que a asma seja alérgica, embora ainda não esteja claro se é possível diferenciar uma forma alérgica de uma doença crônica de outra etiologia. Em seres humanos, a asma é mediada por uma resposta alérgica após exposição a alergênios inalados. Isso induz a estimulação de uma resposta de linfócitos T auxiliar 2, levando à secreção de uma série de citocinas que direcionam a resposta imune, responsável pelas alterações patológicas nas vias respiratórias. Os detalhes da imunopatogenia da asma alérgica e evidências que confirmem a existência de asma alérgica em gatos foram revistos.[90] Na asma humana, os sinais clínicos estão relacionados com 3 fatores principais: (1) inflamação reversível da via respiratória e (2) obstrução/limitação do fluxo de ar, devido à (3) resposta inflamatória exagerada da via respiratória, além de hipertrofia do músculo liso, produção excessiva e acúmulo de muco (hipertrofia de glândulas mucosas), bem como edema da parede do brônquio.[91] Tais alterações às vezes são reversíveis. Contudo, a inflamação crônica pode ocasionar obstrução grave de via respiratória inferior, que causa hiperinsuflação pulmonar, pois os gatos não são capazes de eliminar completamente o ar de vias respiratórias estenosadas, o que resulta em aprisionamento de ar. A hiperinsuflação pulmonar pode provocar alteração permanente, evidenciada pelo remodelamento progressivo da via respiratória, inclusive com bronquiectasia, fibrose e/ou enfisema.

Resenha e sinais clínicos

Gatos jovens e de meia-idade são acometidos com mais frequência. Não há relato de predisposição evidente por gênero ou sexo,[88,92-95] embora fêmeas de meia-idade (2 a 8 anos)[4] e possivelmente gatos Siameses[92,95] pareçam ser mais acometidos. Os sinais clínicos consistem em tosse e aumento do esforço respiratório, cuja gravidade pode variar.[90,96] Em geral, os sinais clínicos são crônicos ou lentamente progressivos. Em alguns gatos, os sintomas passam despercebidos pelo proprietário por muito tempo. Em outros, as queixas incluem vômitos ou tentativas de expelir tricobezoares (bolas de pelos), o que pode desviar erroneamente a atenção quanto à conduta clínica para um exame e/ou tratamento de anormalidade gastrintestinal (GI). Pacientes com acometimento leve podem ter apenas episódios ocasionais e breves de tosse, intercalados por longos períodos sem sinais clínicos, enquanto nos casos moderados ou graves a tosse ocorre diariamente e os gatos podem ter qualidade de vida comprometida, com desconforto respiratório. Gatos com exacerbações graves ("crise asmática" ou "estado asmático") podem chegar ao veterinário com uma crise aguda, respirando com a boca aberta e apresentando dispneia e cianose. Pode ocorrer exacerbação associada à exposição a alergênios ou irritantes potenciais, como aerossóis em *spray*, fumaça de cigarro ou poeira ambiental, ou ainda após estresse associado à ida ao veterinário.

Diagnóstico

Em gatos com crise asmática, é contraindicada a manipulação excessiva do paciente. A auscultação, quando possível, pode revelar abafamento dos sons cardíacos, devido à hiperinsuflação pulmonar extrema. Inicialmente, o paciente deve ser estabilizado, o mais cedo possível (ver Capítulos 131 e 139). Em casos menos graves, os achados ao exame físico são variáveis; o exame físico pode ser normal em repouso ou indicar reflexo traqueal positivo e/ou presença de taquipneia ou dispneia obstrutiva expiratória. A auscultação pode não indicar achado notável algum ou revelar sibilos durante a fase expiratória ou, mais raramente, crepitações. A função cardíaca não está prejudicada, a menos que o gato tenha cardiopatia concomitante. Nesse estágio, são necessários testes adicionais, porque as doenças que podem simular achados clinicopatológicos de asma precisam ser excluídas.

Exames de imagem. O padrão radiográfico clássico em gatos com doença brônquica inflamatória consiste em evidência de espessamento da parede brônquica (em forma de roscas ou de trilhos de trem) ou um padrão broncointersticial; aprisionamento de ar também pode ser evidente (aumento do brilho e aplanamento do diafragma) e alguns gatos apresentam evidência de atelectasia no lobo pulmonar medial direito.[95,97] Em muitos casos, os achados radiográficos não são específicos o bastante para confirmar o diagnóstico e, em alguns gatos, tais achados estão dentro dos limites normais. A TC do tórax pode detectar anormalidades como espessamento da parede brônquica, padrão alveolar difuso e bronquiectasia,[98] bem como lesões que não são vistas em radiografias simples. Em gatos, a TC pode ser realizada usando-se uma câmara de plástico (a Vet-Mousetrap), que possibilita a obtenção de imagens sem necessidade de contenção química,[99] o que é muito benéfico em gatos incapazes de tolerar estresse. Estão em andamento estudos para determinar o impacto dessa abordagem promissora e refinada na bronquite felina.[100]

Hematimetria. Aproximadamente 20% (17 a 46%, dependendo do estudo) dos gatos acometidos apresentam eosinofilia em amostra de sangue periférico,[92,93,95,101] que não está relacionada com o grau de eosinofilia notado na via respiratória. Pode-se observar um leucograma de estresse, e nota-se hiperglobulinemia inespecífica em 14 a 50% dos casos.[102] Pode-se fazer um teste para pesquisa de anticorpo/antígeno de dirofilária, se as manifestações clínicas forem compatíveis com doença respiratória associada à dirofilariose (ver Capítulo 255).

Exame de fezes. Recomenda-se exame de fezes (ver Capítulo 81) como parte da pesquisa diagnóstica, na tentativa de excluir/detectar uma causa parasitária da infiltração eosinofílica, como infecção por *Aelurostrongylus abstrusus* (usando-se o teste de Baermann) ou *Toxocara cati* (por teste de flotação fecal).

Broncoscopia e exame do LBA. Em gatos, a broncoscopia é considerada menos segura do que em cães, principalmente devido ao pequeno calibre das vias respiratórias e à capacidade de resposta relativamente maior da via respiratória do gato.[103] Além disso, quando o gato apresenta dispneia, o procedimento torna-se mais perigoso, porque os riscos da anestesia aumentam e as complicações durante o procedimento ou a recuperação podem ser mais graves e potencialmente fatais. Os achados broncoscópicos não são altamente específicos e podem incluir quantidade moderada a grande de material mucoide ou viscoso, com ou sem hiperemia da via respiratória (ver Vídeo 241.11).

O exame citológico de amostras de lavado broncoalveolar (LBA) ou de lavado endotraqueal (LET) (ver Capítulo 101), em geral, fornece evidência de inflamação da via respiratória, com aumento do número de eosinófilos e/ou neutrófilos. Embora possa haver predomínio de eosinófilos nas amostras obtidas de vias respiratórias de gatos saudáveis, constatou-se relação entre o número de eosinófilos e neutrófilos no LBA e a gravidade da doença, em gatos com doença espontânea[94] ou induzida experimentalmente.[104] Sem dúvida, a doença asmática felina caracteriza-se principalmente pelo predomínio de eosinófilos no LBA, mas até o momento não há um meio incontestável capaz de distinguir o que é normal ou anormal, com base nas porcentagens de células no LBA. De acordo com alguns autores, em condições inflamatórias a infiltração pode ser considerada predominantemente eosinofílica quando preenche os seguintes critérios: mais de 20% de eosinófilos e porcentagem de neutrófilos dentro dos limites de referência, ou mais de 50% de neutrófilos; a infiltração pode ser considerada predominantemente neutrofílica quando o LBA contém mais de 7% de neutrófilos, e a porcentagem de eosinófilos situa-se nos limites de referência, ou mais de 50% de eosinófilos; finalmente, a inflamação é considerada mista quando há aumento concomitante nas porcentagens ou no número absoluto tanto de eosinófilos como de neutrófilos.[105] Em contrapartida, muitos estudos mencionam que a infiltração eosinofílica está relacionada com a presença de mais de 17% de eosinófilos, enquanto a bronquite crônica está relacionada com mais de 7% de neutrófilos no LBA, sendo que gatos com mais de 17% de eosinófilos e mais de 7% de neutrófilos são considerados asmáticos.[106] Tais definições são menos úteis quando o gato foi tratado previamente com glicocorticoides, que diminuem a contagem de eosinófilos. Estudo recente confirmou que nas vias respiratórias de gatos saudáveis pode-se esperar uma porcentagem de eosinófilos < 5% no LBA e que há uma boa correlação entre os achados (em particular a quantidade relativa de eosinófilos) no LBA e no tecido, na asma felina.[107]

Amostras de LBA e LET podem ser submetidas à cultura microbiológica ou PCR, para bactérias, micoplasmas e parasitas. A infecção por *Mycoplasma* pode causar infecção do trato respiratório inferior em gatos[88,108,109] e pode estar associada à ocorrência de doença brônquica felina;[88,109] as infecções por *Aelurostrongylus abstrusus* e *Troglostrongylus* spp. podem causar quadro clínico similar.[110] Espécies de *Mycoplasma* também podem ser detectadas no LBA de gatos doentes sem sintomas respiratórios e podem ser microrganismos comensais do trato respiratório inferior de gatos.[109]

Vários biomarcadores inflamatórios (como citocinas envolvidas na resposta alérgica, por exemplo, interleucina 4, interferona-gama e fator de necrose tumoral alfa) foram mensurados no LBA de gatos com doença brônquica felina, na tentativa de distinguir asma de bronquite crônica, mas o estudo não constatou qualquer diferença, comparativamente com gatos normais do grupo controle.[106] Mostrou-se que há diferença na concentração de endotelina 1 (ET-1) no LBA de gatos normais e de gatos com asma induzida experimentalmente; portanto, a concentração de ET-1 no LBA pode ser um biomarcador diagnóstico potencial para asma.[111] Biomarcadores potenciais também podem ser avaliados por um método não invasivo de coleta, obtendo-se amostra do ar exalado condensado,[112] e o peróxido de hidrogênio foi sugerido com um possível biomarcador não invasivo para monitorar a inflamação de via respiratória inferior, em teste de desafio com alergênio em gatos sensibilizados para *Ascaris suum* (AS).[113]

Testes de função pulmonar. Uma característica clínica importante da asma é a limitação do fluxo de ar, que é reversível, pelo menos em parte, com o uso de broncodilatador. Em medicina humana, os testes de função pulmonar são empregados comumente no diagnóstico e no monitoramento da resposta de pacientes com asma ou bronquite crônica. Em gatos, a espirometria é inadequada, porque requer a colaboração do paciente para a expiração forçada do ar através de um aparato bucal. Entretanto, foram desenvolvidos alguns testes não invasivos, como alça de fluxo-volume corrente (FVc), em que se utiliza máscara facial bem ajustada,[94,101] pletismografia de sangue total barométrica (PSTB)[104,114] ou uma combinação de FVc e PSTB[115] e curvas de fluxo-volume com o uso de uma técnica de compressão torácica[116,117] em gatos sadios e/ou naqueles com asma induzida experimentalmente. O FVc pode ser utilizado para estimar os parâmetros funcionais basais, bem como a resposta inflamatória exagerada da via respiratória, em geral quantificada calculando-se a concentração de uma substância broncoconstritora que induz aumento de 300% na pausa basal melhorada (Penh, do inglês *enhanced pause*).

FVc e PSTB foram usados em séries de casos clínicos,[101,107,115,118,119] juntamente com o teste de resposta da via respiratória com o uso de carbacol,[118,119] 5amp[120] ou metacolina[121] como teste de broncoprovocação.

Durante o teste FVc, a presença de limitação do fluxo de ar é afetada pela extensão geral da infiltração de granulócitos, enquanto a maioria dos testes PSTB possibilita evidência confirmatória de correlação entre a inflamação eosinofílica da via respiratória e as mensurações pletismográficas de broncoconstrição e da capacidade de resposta da via respiratória. A última sugere que a PSTB associada ao teste de capacidade de resposta da via respiratória pode ser um novo método para identificar gatos com doença inflamatória de via respiratória inferior e, possivelmente, para monitorar a progressão da doença ou a resposta ao tratamento.

Em gatos anestesiados, recentemente se provou que a mecânica pulmonar induzida por ventilação é útil.[121]

Diagnóstico diferencial

A lista de diagnósticos diferenciais para doença brônquica inflamatória felina inclui, principalmente, doença brônquica felina de origem não inflamatória (ver texto adiante) e doença do parênquima pulmonar (ver Capítulo 242), inclusive pneumonia/broncopneumonia infecciosa (p. ex., causadas por bactérias, vírus, parasitas ou protozoários),[5,105,122] que são raras, mas provavelmente subdiagnosticadas; corpo estranho em via respiratória; neoplasia; efusão pleural de várias etiologias (ver Capítulo 244); e doenças mais raras, como fibrose pulmonar felina[123,124] e a pneumonia lipídica endógena.[125]

Em gatos, as doenças brônquicas de origem inflamatória incluem:

- Doenças pulmonares parasitárias, incluindo infecção por *Aelurostrongylus abstrusus, Troglostrongylus brevior,*[126] *Eucoleus aerophilus* (antigamente denominado *Capillaria aerophila*),[127] *Dirofilaria immitis* e *Wolbachia*[128] (em regiões endêmicas), que podem resultar em achados clínicos similares, como inflamação eosinofílica de via respiratória. Não é fácil excluir com certeza essas doenças, porque o teste de sensibilidade não é infalível; portanto, recomenda-se o tratamento empírico, curativo ou preventivo, com fármacos efetivos (em regiões endêmicas)[128a]
- Infecção por *Toxocara cati* (ver Capítulos 81 e 276)
- Infecção bacteriana/por *Mycoplasma*[109,129,130] (ver Capítulos 227 e 242)
- Origem neoplásica (ver Capítulos 244, 344 e 346).

Controle/tratamento e monitoramento

Angústia respiratória aguda. Em gatos com angústia respiratória aguda grave deve-se minimizar o estresse e providenciar um ambiente rico em oxigênio (ver Capítulos 131 e 139). Deve-se realizar imediatamente o tratamento parenteral com broncodilatador (p. ex., o agonista beta-2 terbutalina, 0,01 mg/kg IV IM ou SC) ou corticosteroide de ação rápida (p. ex., dexametasona, 0,25 a 0,5 mg/kg IV ou IM).[4] O tratamento inalatório com broncodilatador também pode ser instituído, desde que uma quantidade mínima do fármaco possa alcançar os brônquios (o que é incerto em um animal com dificuldade respiratória grave). Esses tratamentos visam aliviar rapidamente, pelo menos em parte, a broncoconstrição. Quando o gato não responde à terapia, é preciso considerar a possibilidade de pneumotórax espontâneo e realizar toracocentese de emergência como procedimento para salvar-lhe a vida (ver Capítulos 102,[149] e 244). Na verdade, mostrou-se que a asma é a causa mais comum de pneumotórax espontâneo em gatos (4/16 casos, 25%).[131] Nesse estudo, os quatro gatos com pneumotórax espontâneo associado à asma sobreviveram à crise inicial de pneumotórax espontâneo, a ponto de terem tido alta do tratamento clínico.

Tratamento de longa duração. A maioria dos estudos retrospectivos em gatos com doenças de via respiratória inferior documentou resposta benéfica ao tratamento oral ou parenteral com glicocorticoides e/ou broncodilatadores.[92-94] A terapia clássica para doença brônquica crônica consiste na administração oral prolongada de corticosteroide (p. ex., 1 a 2 mg de prednisolona/kg/12 h VO, por 1 a 2 semanas, seguida de diminuição gradual da dose), que continua sendo um tratamento compatível, confiável e efetivo até o momento.[132] Sugeriu-se que a administração oral de propentofilina, um derivado da metilxantina com ação broncodilatadora, aos gatos com doença brônquica, além de uma dose baixa de prednisolona, pode ser mais efetiva que o tratamento exclusivo com prednisolona.[133]

Atualmente, há poucos parâmetros de mensuração práticos para avaliar/monitorar a resposta ao tratamento. Portanto, na prática, o monitoramento do tratamento em geral baseia-se principalmente na melhora dos sinais clínicos. A eosinofilia de via respiratória e a resposta exagerada da via respiratória são consideradas típicas da doença e seriam parâmetros interessantes a serem monitorados durante o tratamento.

Estudo recente avaliou a correlação entre a resolução dos sinais clínicos em gatos com doença de via respiratória que receberam glicocorticoides VO e a resolução da inflamação com base nos achados citológicos do LBA.[134] Dez gatos com doença brônquica inflamatória receberam glicocorticoide VO (dosagem média de prednisolona: 1,8 ± 0,2 mg/kg/dia) durante pelo menos 3 semanas. Todos apresentaram resolução dos sinais clínicos, mas em 7/10 gatos apresentaram achados inflamatórios citológicos persistentes no LBA, apesar da resolução dos sinais clínicos. Tal estudo mostra com clareza que as recomendações atuais para diminuir gradativamente a dose, com base na resolução dos sinais clínicos, são inadequadas e o ajuste apropriado da dose do tratamento oral deve basear-se nos resultados do exame citológico do LBA.

PSTB e o teste da alça de fluxo-volume pseudocorrente são meios não invasivos de avaliação da função pulmonar em gatos conscientes que estejam respirando espontaneamente; também se provou que ambos são úteis para monitorar a resposta ao tratamento tanto em modelos experimentais como em casos de ocorrência natural.[118-120,135]

O uso de medicações inalantes com auxílio de máscara facial e câmara apropriada, descrito pela primeira vez por Padrid,[136] está se tornando comum (ver Capítulo 97). Medicações inalantes têm a vantagem de propiciar alta concentração do fármaco nos lúmens das vias respiratórias, ao mesmo tempo que minimizam os efeitos colaterais. Corticosteroides inalantes (p. ex., propionato de fluticasona), utilizados essencialmente como terapia de uso prolongado, e broncodilatadores (p. ex., albuterol), usados como paliativos para os sintomas de uma exacerbação aguda, são os mais empregados e o foram pela primeira vez em modelos experimentais.[138-140] A resposta de pacientes felinos à terapia por nebulização foi avaliada em vários estudos. Um deles mostrou que a administração de budesonida por meio de inalação, na dose de 400 µg a cada 12 horas, poderia ser suspensa em 20 gatos, enquanto naqueles que ainda a estavam recebendo notou-se melhora dos sinais clínicos, bem como no índice de resposta da via respiratória mensurado pelo teste PSTB.[119] O mesmo estudo mostrou que, embora não tivessem sido observados efeitos colaterais induzidos pelo corticosteroide, em 3 de 15 casos detectou-se supressão do eixo hipotálamo-hipófise-adrenal. Em outro estudo, gatos foram tratados com propionato de fluticasona, por inalação (Flixotide, GlaxoSmithKline, 2 "puffs", 250 mcg/"puff", a cada 12 horas).[118] Apesar da melhora significativa nos escores clínicos – e, em alguns gatos, da resolução aparente dos sinais clínicos –, os valores do PSTB não indicaram diferença significativa na primeira avaliação, uma evidência a mais de que a resolução dos sinais clínicos pode preceder o restabelecimento da função normal da via respiratória. Não parece que isso se deva à dosagem insuficiente de fluticasona nebulizada. Na verdade, em um estudo com modelo de asma felina, uma dose de 44 µg, 2 vezes/dia, teve efeito idêntico ao de uma dose de 220 µg de fluticasona, por inalação, 2 vezes/dia;[141] esses achados sugerem que essa dose baixa deve ser avaliada no tratamento de gatos com doença brônquica inflamatória de ocorrência natural. Como a administração oral de prednisolona, exclusivamente, é capaz de resolver a reação asmática de fase tardia,[139] pode-se instituir uma combinação de medicações de uso oral e de inalação à base de glicocorticoide, seguida apenas de administração por inalação no período de acompanhamento.

Os broncodilatadores, como albuterol inalante (também denominado salbutamol), são muito úteis para aliviar os sinais clínicos rapidamente, porém, como falham no controle da inflamação da via respiratória, não devem ser usados sozinhos (como monoterapia). Eles devem ainda ser usados com cautela, por causa dos efeitos adversos possíveis, incluindo taquicardia, estimulação do sistema nervoso central, tremores e hipopotassemia. Além disso, a administração diária prolongada de albuterol racêmico foi associada à exacerbação da gravidade da inflamação de via respiratória em modelos experimentais de asma felina.[142]

Terapias adicionais

A perda de peso deve ser estimulada no caso de gatos obesos (ver Capítulo 176). Em estudo recente, foram comparadas algumas variáveis (índices) de função pulmonar entre gatos obesos e não obesos, com base no teste PSTB.[143] Embora a obesidade não esteja associada a um aumento significativo no índice de broncoconstrição, conforme relatado previamente em seres humanos e cães, confirmou-se um comprometimento significativo da função pulmonar, sugerindo que a perda de peso deve ser estimulada em gatos obesos com doença de via respiratória inferior (DVRI).

Não se comprovou que a nebulização com solução fisiológica e o uso de agentes mucolíticos ou fitoterápicos (VO ou por meio de nebulização) sejam benéficos, devendo ser usados com muita cautela. Em gatos, todas as substâncias nebulizadas têm o potencial de desencadear uma reação broncoespástica e/ou estresse ocasional extra, o que interfere negativamente no quadro clínico de um gato com DVRI. Em gatos com asma induzida experimentalmente, a nebulização endotraqueal com N-acetilcisteína, um fármaco com propriedades mucolíticas e antioxidantes, aumentou a resistência da via respiratória e causou outras reações adversas,[144] não sendo, portanto, recomendada.

Prognóstico

A doença brônquica felina está associada à morbidade considerável e, até mesmo, morte de gatos. Embora na maioria dos gatos se obtenha um bom controle com o tratamento VO ou mediante nebulização, ou ambas, em geral eles requerem tratamento vitalício. É importante ressaltar que a inflamação de via respiratória não diagnosticada pode ocasionar remodelamento irreversível, resultando na redução da função pulmonar.

Nos casos crônicos, quando o remodelamento já ocorreu, o alívio dos sinais clínicos pode ser um desafio e levar à eutanásia.

Contribuição de modelos experimentais de asma felina no desenvolvimento de possíveis tratamentos no futuro

O desenvolvimento e a implementação de modelos de asma felina contribuíram muito para o entendimento dos mecanismos fisiopatológicos e o diagnóstico, além de facilitarem a pesquisa de novos tratamentos. Na verdade, ao combinarem imagens estruturais/morfológicas (TC do tórax) e testes funcionais, os modelos propiciaram a possibilidade de acompanhamento seriado e padronizado de características clínicas, da função pulmonar, da inflamação e da imunologia da via respiratória. Foram descritos dois diferentes modelos de asma felina, com base na sensibilização artificial ao *Ascaris suum*[104,145] ou ao alergênio do capim Bermuda/alergênio do ácaro da poeira doméstica.[146] Investigou-se ou está sendo investigado em modelos experimentais de asma um grande número de novas terapias que podem ser efetivas ou ajudar a reverter os eventos imunes, na asma. Na verdade, a quantidade de dados gerados por uma equipe que usa o modelo de asma felina é fabulosa, fornecendo resultados experimentais interessantes e às vezes muito promissores (ver detalhes nas revisões de Reinero[89] e Trzil[96]). As novas abordagens terapêuticas avaliadas em modelos que utilizam gatos incluem nutracêuticos (ácidos graxos poli-insaturados ômega 3 mais luteolina),[147] diferentes broncodilatadores,[139,148] peptídio salivar imunomodulador feG-COOH,[149] antagonistas do leucotrieno,[150] fármacos antisserotoninérgicos,[151] doxiciclina,[139] imunoterapia rápida (*rush*),[152-154] lidocaína inalante,[155] masitinibe, um inibidor da tirosinoquinase,[121] e avaliação a longo prazo da terapia com célula-tronco mesenquimal.[100]

No entanto, embora essas pesquisas em modelos experimentais sejam muito úteis, elas não refletem necessariamente a situação em pacientes felinos com doença de ocorrência natural. Portanto, essas novas estratégias terapêuticas, testadas em contextos experimentais, ainda não podem ser recomendadas na rotina clínica.

REFERÊNCIAS BIBLIOGRÁFICAS

As referências bibliográficas deste capítulo se encontram online no Ambiente de Aprendizagem.

CAPÍTULO 242

Doenças do Parênquima Pulmonar

Leah A. Cohn

A estrutura do parênquima pulmonar possibilita a função primária de troca de gases no pulmão, órgão constituído por milhões de espaços de ar alveolares, cada um banhado por uma rede densa de capilares. Tecidos intersticiais de sustentação delgados e rendilhados ficam interpostos entre o revestimento epitelial dos alvéolos e o endotélio vascular circundante. Os tecidos intersticiais contêm arteríolas e vênulas pulmonares de calibres ligeiramente maiores. A doença parenquimatosa inclui doenças em alvéolos, na microvasculatura pulmonar ou nos tecidos intersticiais, excluindo as doenças de vias respiratórias de maior calibre (ver Capítulo 241), dos vasos pulmonares (ver Capítulo 243) e do espaço pleural (ver Capítulo 244).

MANIFESTAÇÕES DE DOENÇA DO PARÊNQUIMA PULMONAR

Cães e gatos com doença do parênquima pulmonar apresentam uma variedade de sinais clínicos relacionados com a disfunção respiratória ou doença sistêmica. Em geral, os sinais clínicos e as anormalidades notados ao exame físico, em animais com doença pulmonar, são semelhantes aos observados naqueles com doença de via respiratória, de mediastino ou do espaço pleural. Além disso, doenças não respiratórias (p. ex., doença neuromuscular, anemia, acidose) podem causar sintomas que simulam doença respiratória. As manifestações respiratórias comuns de doença do parênquima pulmonar consistem em tosse, intolerância ao exercício, taquipneia, respiração muito ofegante e maior esforço respiratório ou dificuldade respiratória. Com maior frequência, a dificuldade respiratória causada por doença do parênquima pulmonar resulta em esforço misto, inspiratório e expiratório, em contraste com o esforço predominantemente inspiratório observado em animais com obstrução de via respiratória superior (ver Capítulo 28) ou doença do espaço pleural (ver Capítulo 244), ou com o esforço expiratório observado em animais com doença de via respiratória inferior/brônquios (ver Capítulo 241). Algumas doenças do interstício pulmonar que limitam a complacência dos pulmões constituem exceções a essa regra geral, porque estão associadas a um esforço predominantemente inspiratório. Manifestações menos comuns de doença do parênquima pulmonar incluem hemoptise, colapso ou síncope e cianose. Também é possível que animais com comprometimento respiratório acentuado demonstrem evidência clínica mínima de doença respiratória. Isso é especialmente verdadeiro em gatos, espécie em que o primeiro sinal de doença do parênquima pulmonar acentuada pode ser morte súbita.[1-5]

O exame físico de animais com doença pulmonar pode não revelar achados notáveis ou identificar doença sistêmica ou torácica importante. Perda de peso, febre, linfadenopatia e edema na parte distal dos membros decorrentes de osteopatia hipertrófica são algumas das muitas manifestações sistêmicas potenciais de doenças pulmonares. Anormalidades na frequência respiratória ou esforço respiratório, cianose, aumento ou diminuição dos sons pulmonares broncovesiculares e/ou adventícios (*i. e.*, crepitações e sibilos) à auscultação são todos sugestivos de doença de via respiratória, do espaço torácico ou do pulmão (Figura 242.1). O exame do paciente com doença respiratória é descrito em detalhe nos Capítulos 2, 28 e 240. Qualquer animal que apresente dificuldade respiratória acentuada deve receber suplementação de oxigênio durante a avaliação (ver Capítulos 131 e 139).

AVALIAÇÃO DIAGNÓSTICA DE DOENÇA DO PARÊNQUIMA PULMONAR

Oxigenação

Em geral, a avaliação da oxigenação é útil em animais com suspeita de doença do parênquima pulmonar, embora doenças não parenquimatosas também possam causar hipoxemia. O reconhecimento visual de cianose confirma a presença de

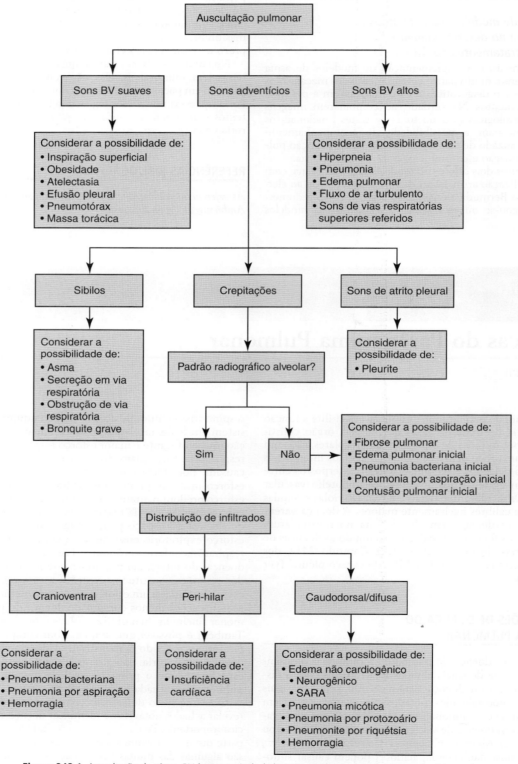

Figura 242.1 Auscultação do tórax. *BV*, broncovesicular(es); *SARA*, síndrome da angústia respiratória aguda.

CAPÍTULO 242 • Doenças do Parênquima Pulmonar

hipoxemia, mas não é um procedimento sensível, é subjetivo e não é útil em animais anêmicos. Os melhores testes de oxigenação são oximetria de pulso (ver Capítulo 98) e hemogasometria arterial (ver Capítulo 128). A última pode ser usada para a tomada de decisões quanto à necessidade de oxigênio suplementar ou de ventilação mecânica e para monitorar a resposta ao tratamento. Além disso, a Pa_{CO_2} e cálculos simples dos gradientes alveolar-arteriais podem ser usados para ajudar a determinar o mecanismo mais provável da hipoxemia.

Testes de triagem

As modalidades diagnósticas empregadas em cães e gatos com doença pulmonar variam de simples a complexas, de não invasivas a invasivas e de pouco a muito onerosas. Testes de triagem da condição clínica, como hemograma completo (HC), perfil bioquímico sérico e exame de urina, raramente esclarecem a ocorrência específica dos sintomas pulmonares, porém às vezes dão indícios de uma doença primária. Os resultados desses exames também são relevantes para o planejamento da anestesia necessária para a realização de muitas das técnicas diagnósticas respiratórias mais específicas. Ocasionalmente, testes como flotação fecal, sedimentação fecal de Baermann ou pesquisa de antígeno de dirofilária levam ao diagnóstico definitivo de doença pulmonar. Em algumas doenças infecciosas com manifestações pulmonares, um teste sorológico específico ou a reação em cadeia da polimerase (PCR) confirmam a suspeita clínica. Dispõe-se de testes sanguíneos simples para ajudar a distinção entre animais com sinais respiratórios devidos à doença cardíaca e aqueles com doença respiratória primária.

Peptídios natriuréticos

São um grupo de hormônios relacionados que interferem na homeostasia circulatória.[6] Muitos têm sido usados como biomarcadores de doença cardiovascular. O principal é o peptídio natriurético do tipo B (BNP; isto é, peptídio natriurético cerebral, do inglês *brain natriuretic peptide*), que induz natriurese, aumento da taxa de filtração glomerular, vasodilatação e inibe o sistema renina-angiotensina-aldosterona em animais com aumento do volume de líquido extracelular.[6] A concentração circulante de BNP aumenta em animais com sobrecarga de volume, hipertensão pulmonar e, em especial, disfunção cardíaca e insuficiência cardíaca (ver Capítulo 246). O peptídio é sintetizado como um pré-pró-hormônio e processado rapidamente em um pró-hormônio, que então sofre clivagem, originando o BNP ativo e o fragmento inativo NT-pró-BNP, este último com meia-vida mais longa que o hormônio ativo, daí a conveniência de sua estimativa diagnóstica. Como em geral é difícil estabelecer rapidamente se a dificuldade respiratória se deve à doença primária respiratória ou à cardiopatia e o tratamento de tais condições é bastante diferente, pode ser útil fazer um teste simples, seguro e rápido para distingui-las. Em cães com insuficiência cardíaca congestiva, foram detectadas concentrações circulantes médias de BNP mais altas que em cães normais ou naqueles com causas respiratórias de tosse ou dificuldade respiratória.[7,8] No entanto, o BNP também se apresentava elevado em cães com causas não cardíacas de tosse e cardiopatia concomitante.[7] Similarmente, foram avaliados testes ELISA para NT-pró-BNP em cães e gatos com causas cardíacas e não cardíacas de tosse ou dificuldade respiratória. Em animais de estimação com doença cardíaca foram constatadas concentrações mais elevadas de NT-pró-BNP do que naqueles com doença respiratória.[9-13] Em gatos, pode-se mensurar o teor de NT-pró-BNP no líquido pleural, para distinguir efusões de origem cardíaca daquelas de origem não cardíaca.[14] Diferentemente do que acontece em seres humanos, a idade e o gênero não parecem influenciar a concentração do peptídio natriurético;[7,12] entretanto, a concentração de NT-pró-BNP aumenta, juntamente com a elevação da concentração de creatinina, o que é um problema ao se fazer o teste em animais com azotemia.[12] Embora esses testes possam ser relativamente úteis na avaliação de animais de estimação com dispneia aguda, atualmente devem ser considerados testes auxiliares que não substituem exames mais apropriados, como os exames de imagem.[9,10,13,15]

Exames de imagem diagnósticos

Ajudam a excluir doença de via respiratória, de mediastino ou do espaço pleural como causa de sintomas respiratórios e fornecem importantes informações sobre doença do parênquima pulmonar. Em animais com doença pulmonar, as radiografias de tórax talvez sejam o exame diagnóstico isolado mais importante (depois da anamnese e do exame físico). A presença, a localização e a intensidade de padrões radiográficos anormais propiciam uma riqueza de informações que orientam o diagnóstico diferencial e o planejamento diagnóstico (Boxe 242.1). Ocasionalmente, ocorre doença pulmonar suficiente para causar sinais respiratórios, na ausência de alteração radiográfica no parênquima pulmonar. Por exemplo, as alterações radiográficas podem surgir após o desenvolvimento agudo de sintomas respiratórios em animais com pneumonia por aspiração, síndrome da angústia respiratória aguda (SARA) ou tromboembolismo pulmonar. Contudo, quando as imagens torácicas não mostram anormalidades em animais com sinais respiratórios das vias inferiores, deve-se considerar, adicionalmente, a possibilidade de anormalidade que pode simular doença respiratória, como anemia, dor, acidose ou distúrbios do sistema nervoso.

Boxe 242.1 Diagnóstico diferencial associado a padrões radiográficos comuns

Infiltrado alveolar
Pneumonia (bacteriana, parasitária, por protozoário, viral, por aspiração, intersticial)
Edema (cardiogênico ou não cardiogênico)
Hemorragia/contusão
Neoplasia pulmonar primária
Neoplasia metastática
Atelectasia
Tromboembolismo pulmonar
Afogamento
Inalação de fumaça

Infiltrado bronquiolar
Asma felina
Bronquite crônica
Bronquite eosinofílica
Aprisionamento peribronquiolar (p. ex., edema, inflamação)
Calcificação brônquica

Padrão intersticial
Alteração por envelhecimento (*i. e.*, "pulmão do cão idoso") (NE)
Fibrose pulmonar (NE)
Linfoma (NE)
Neoplasia pulmonar primária (E > NE)
Metástase pulmonar (E > NE)
Pneumonia/granuloma fúngicos (E > NE)
Pneumonia eosinofílica (E > NE)
Reação por corpo estranho (E > NE)
Hematoma (E ou NE)
Abscesso (E)
Cisto (E)

Padrão vascular
Dirofilariose
Doença tromboembólica
Hipertensão pulmonar
Insuficiência cardíaca congestiva

E ou *NE*, padrão estruturado ou não estruturado; *E*, padrão pulmonar intersticial estruturado; *NE*, padrão pulmonar intersticial não estruturado. Qualquer doença que cause um padrão alveolar pode iniciar com um padrão intersticial não estruturado que progressivamente se torna mais grave.

Tomografia computadorizada (TC) e ultrassonografia são usadas com menor frequência do que as radiografias torácicas simples para a obtenção de imagens dos pulmões de animais de estimação. TC tem vantagens sobre a radiografia de tórax padrão, incluindo maior sensibilidade para a detecção de pequenas lesões, como metástases, uma imagem tridimensional mais real da cavidade torácica e seu conteúdo, minimização de artefatos cumulativos e possibilidade de se observarem as imagens nos planos axial, coronal ou sagital.[16,17] Até recentemente, era necessária anestesia ou sedação profunda para fazer uma TC, o que limitava sua utilidade como exame de triagem. A combinação de aparelhos mais modernos com a aquisição mais rápida de imagens e a disponibilidade de dispositivos de contenção (p. ex., VetMousetrap, Urbana-Champaign, IL) fáceis de usar em gatos ou cães de pequeno porte com dispneia superaram algumas dessas limitações (Vídeo 242.1).[18] Apesar disso, para a obtenção das melhores imagens torácicas, a anestesia ainda é necessária e o ideal é que seja com ventilação controlada.[19] Como as ondas sonoras não produzem boas imagens quando atravessam espaços de ar, a ultrassonografia não é uma modalidade particularmente útil para a avaliação do parênquima pulmonar, sendo, às vezes, um procedimento auxiliar na avaliação de tecido pulmonar consolidado ou da patência vascular, e pode ser usada para orientar a obtenção de aspirados de massas torácicas com agulha.[20,21]

Exames invasivos

Em geral, são necessários exames invasivos para o diagnóstico de doença do parênquima pulmonar. Os de uso mais comum incluem lavado transtraqueal ou endotraqueal, broncoalveolar (LBA, com ou sem orientação broncoscópica; ver Capítulo 101), aspiração com agulha fina (AAF) de lesões pulmonares e biopsia pulmonar (ver Capítulo 240). Infelizmente, parece que a cultura de suabes simples de regiões profundas da boca/faringe não é um substituto aceitável para o lavado traqueal ou alveolar em cães com pneumonia bacteriana.[22] O lavado traqueal é um meio minimamente invasivo e relativamente seguro para a coleta de amostras de líquido de via respiratória, para cultura microbiológica e exame citológico. Como são colhidas mais amostras de grandes vias respiratórias que do parênquima, o lavado traqueal é particularmente útil para doença pulmonar acompanhada de tosse produtiva (p. ex., pneumonia bacteriana). O LBA propicia amostras diagnósticas de partes intrapulmonares mais profundas e, portanto, é útil em animais sem tosse produtiva. A broncoscopia pode orientar a coleta de LBA, de modo que sejam obtidas amostras de um local específico dos pulmões.[23] Na presença de doença difusa, o LBA pode ser colhido de maneira "cega", sem considerar o local de coleta nos pulmões.[24] Embora a AAF do parênquima pulmonar seja invasiva, não é onerosa e é relativamente segura. Na presença de massa focal ou lesão consolidada, a AAF é altamente produtiva. Todavia, a sensibilidade diminui quando a doença pulmonar é difusa.[20,25,26] A biopsia pulmonar é mais invasiva que o lavado de via respiratória ou o aspirado pulmonar; contudo, propicia maiores informações. A biopsia é indicada para a avaliação de animais com doença pulmonar progressiva ou grave, quando técnicas menos invasivas falham em esclarecer o diagnóstico. A biopsia é indispensável para demonstrar definitivamente a presença de muitas doenças do interstício pulmonar. Por exemplo, não se pode identificar fibrose pulmonar de maneira definitiva de outra maneira, a não ser por meio do exame histológico do tecido pulmonar.[1] A biopsia pulmonar pode ser feita mediante toracoscopia, uma abordagem "key-hole" (requer técnica e instrumentação especializada para a remoção máxima de tecido, com o mínimo de manipulação tecidual), ou toracotomia.[27]

DOENÇAS PULMONARES ESPECÍFICAS

Doença pulmonar parasitária

A doença pulmonar parasitária é causada tanto por vermes pulmonares como não pulmonares. Alguns vermes intestinais, em especial *Toxocara* (nematódeo) e *Ancylostoma* (anciléstomo),

migram para o pulmão antes que a forma adulta alcance o seu destino final, o intestino. Em geral, a migração pulmonar causa doença discreta e alguns (quando muito) sintomas respiratórios. No entanto, a migração maciça de larvas pode resultar em dano inflamatório tanto direto como indireto ao pulmão, causando pneumonia verminótica. Tais infecções profundas ocorrem tipicamente em filhotes de cães, que podem apresentar tosse e taquipneia. Geralmente não se faz um hemograma completo em cães muito jovens com tosse, mas é previsível que haja eosinofilia. O resultado do teste de flotação fecal pode ser negativo, porque a migração de larvas ocorre antes que as larvas maduras tenham alcançado o intestino. O tratamento empírico é razoável, caso se suspeite de migração pulmonar como a causa da tosse. Deve-se administrar um anti-helmíntico (pamoato de pirantel, na dose de 5 mg/kg VO), com intervalo de pelo menos 2 semanas. Felizmente, a maioria dos animais não precisa de tratamento adicional. Um esquema de curta duração, com uma dose anti-inflamatória de glicocorticoide, pode amenizar a tosse intensa, mas não deve ser usado antes da exclusão de outras causas de pneumonia infecciosa.

Em contraste com os vermes intestinais que migram através dos pulmões no trajeto para seu destino final, o destino dos vermes pulmonares é o trato respiratório.[28,29] Vários tipos de vermes pulmonares têm relevância em cães e gatos. Esses parasitas podem se instalar principalmente no parênquima pulmonar, nas vias respiratórias ou em ambos. A doença pulmonar parasitária pode ser confundida facilmente com outras condições, como broncopneumonia, pneumonia eosinofílica, asma, granulomatose pulmonar ou até mesmo com neoplasia pulmonar. Infelizmente, a excreção fecal intermitente de ovos ou larvas dos parasitas, após expectoração, significa que o exame de fezes é um método diagnóstico insensível. Por essa razão, costumam ser feitas tentativas terapêuticas quando se suspeita de vermes pulmonares. Em geral, usa-se alta dose de fembendazol (50 mg/kg/24 h VO, por 10 a 14 dias) ou ivermectina,[28] mas esta última deve ser usada com cautela em cães da raça Colly e outras raças que apresentam alta prevalência da mutação MDR-1 (ABCB1).[30] Embora o albendazol seja efetivo contra vermes pulmonares, tem maior potencial tóxico à medula óssea do que o fembendazol.[31-33]

Parasitas de parênquima pulmonar

Paragonimus kellicotti. Esse trematódeo pulmonar pode infectar cães e gatos. Encontrado em todo o mundo, nos EUA os trematódeos pulmonares são praticamente endêmicos na região dos Grandes Lagos, no centro-oeste e no sul do país. Como acontece com a maioria dos parasitas pulmonares, há um hospedeiro intermediário envolvido na transmissão. Animais de estimação se infectam após a ingestão de lagostim. O parasita migra do intestino para o peritônio, através do diafragma, e então para o espaço pleural. Logo em seguida, os trematódeos imaturos invadem os tecidos subpleurais, onde causam inflamação eosinofílica e neutrofílica.[34,35] Em geral, os parasitas formam bolhas e cistos no parênquima pulmonar. Os trematódeos maduros têm acesso aos bronquíolos através de uma série de "túneis" comunicantes, o que possibilita que os ovos sejam mobilizados pela tosse e deglutidos, antes da excreção nas fezes.

Os animais infectados com *P. kellicotti* costumam estar bem, mas podem apresentar tosse ou mesmo dificuldade respiratória.[36,37] A ruptura de lesões cavitárias pode ocasionar hemoptise ou pneumotórax.[36] Em geral, suspeita-se do diagnóstico quando animais com sintomas respiratórios têm eosinofilia concomitante ou achados radiográficos anormais.[38] Embora as lesões radiográficas não sejam detectadas de maneira uniforme, podem incluir algumas lesões nodulares ou císticas, ou bolhas, acometendo em especial os lobos pulmonares caudais direitos.[34,38-40] TC seriada de cães com infecção experimental detectou, inicialmente, efusão pleural e uma aparência subpleural de vidro moído, juntamente com opacidades lineares. Após 1 mês, foram observados nódulos peribrônquicos persistentes, dilatação brônquica e alterações cavitárias.[41] Podem ser detectados ovos em amostras do lavado de via respiratória ou nas fezes.[34] Para a detecção de ovos de parasitas prefere-se técnica de sedimentação fecal a outros métodos de exame de fezes.

Além do fembendazol, também se usa praziquantel (25 mg/kg/8 h VO, por 3 dias), com sucesso, no tratamento de infecção por *P. kellicotti*.[38,39,42] Deve-se avaliar a eficácia do tratamento com a realização de exames de fezes seriados, na busca de ovos.[39] O pneumotórax que resulta em dificuldade respiratória requer tratamento específico (*i. e.*, toracocentese; ver Capítulos 100, 102 e 139).

Filaroides. As espécies desse gênero são parasitas pulmonares relativamente incomuns de cães. Os nematódeos adultos das espécies *Filaroides hirthi* e *Filaroides milksi* (também conhecidos como *Andersonstrongylus milksi*) residem nos espaços alveolares e nos bronquíolos terminais; não é necessário fazer a diferenciação desses parasitas muito semelhantes.[43,44] As espécies desse gênero são reconhecidas com frequência como endêmicas em colônias de cães de pesquisa.[45-51] O parasita, ovovivíparo, é transmitido diretamente por via fecal-oral, o que permite a transmissão de uma fêmea infectada para sua ninhada ou entre filhotes infectados para os não infectados. A infecção repetida (autoinfecção) do hospedeiro com larvas, antes que elas deixem o hospedeiro, também é possível e aumenta o risco de "superinfecção".[52-57] Cães podem permanecer sadios enquanto parasitados ou desenvolver doença grave ou até mesmo fatal. A doença grave é particularmente provável em cães jovens de raças de pequeno porte, bem como naqueles com imunossupressão ou com superinfecção.[43,44,56,58,59]

Os sinais clínicos, quando ocorrem, podem incluir tosse e dificuldade respiratória. Infiltrados difusos broncointersticiais e alveolares resultam de inflamação granulomatosa em reação aos vermes mortos ou que estejam morrendo.[43,55,56,60] Usa-se o teste de flotação fecal, após centrifugação com sulfato de zinco, para identificar as larvas, mas sua sensibilidade é baixa devido à excreção intermitente (uma característica comum da maioria das infecções por vermes pulmonares). A detecção de ovos e/ou larvas no lavado obtido de via respiratória é um método alternativo de diagnóstico. Tem-se empregado uma variedade de tratamentos anti-helmínticos, mas os mais frequentemente utilizados são fembendazol (25 a 50 mg/kg/24 h VO, por 10 a 14 dias) ou ivermectina (0,4 a 1 mg/kg IV ou SC, para cães que não tenham a mutação MDR-1).[28,44,51] A resposta inflamatória aos vermes mortos pode agravar o quadro clínico após o tratamento, complicação que pode ser amenizada com um tratamento de curta duração com corticosteroide em dose anti-inflamatória (p. ex., predniso(lo)na, 0,5 a 1 mg/kg/24 h VO por 3 a 7 dias).[44,61]

Parasitas de vias respiratórias

Aelurostrongylus abstrusus. Verme pulmonar comum em gatos, cosmopolita; nos EUA, é mais comum nos estados do sul.[62,63] Embora a maioria dos gatos infectados permaneça bem, a infecção pode resultar em sinais clínicos que simulam doença broncopulmonar felina. Os vermes maduros se alojam nos bronquíolos; a inflamação dessas pequenas vias respiratórias pode resultar em tosse, sibilos e/ou dificuldade respiratória. As radiografias do tórax de gatos parasitados podem não apresentar nada notável ou mostrar um padrão nodular intersticial difuso e/ou peribronquiolar, ou ainda, às vezes, um padrão alveolar.[64] Em regiões endêmicas, deve-se considerar a infecção por *A. abstrusus* como um diagnóstico diferencial importante para a "asma" felina, em especial no caso de gatos expostos a ambientes externos, mais propensos a ingerir o molusco hospedeiro intermediário do parasita. O diagnóstico baseia-se na detecção de larvas em amostras de lavado de via respiratória ou em fezes, pelo método de sedimentação de Baermann.[28,63,65] Foi desenvolvido um teste PCR específico e muito sensível, utilizando-se amostras de fezes

ou material de suabe obtido da faringe, mas ainda não está disponível no comércio.[66] O tratamento pode ser com fembendazol (25 a 50 mg/kg/24 h VO, por 10 a 14 dias), ivermectina (300 a 400 mcg/kg SC) ou selemectina (6 mg/kg, em aplicação tópica).[29,63] Doses anti-inflamatórias de glicocorticoides inalantes ou de uso oral podem ser úteis durante o tratamento, bem como broncodilatadores para gatos com maior esforço respiratório.

Crenosoma vulpis. Nematódeo de via respiratória que pode infectar cães, mas não gatos.[28,67] Ocorre infecção indireta após a ingestão de moluscos que atuam como hospedeiros intermediários. A infecção é relatada mais frequentemente no nordeste dos EUA e na costa atlântica do Canadá, mas também ocorre na Europa. O parasita torna-se maduro (adulto) nas vias respiratórias, onde produz ovos contendo larvas que podem ser expelidos do trato respiratório durante a tosse e, então, deglutidos. A maioria dos cães infectados por *C. vulpis* permanece saudável, mas podem ocorrer sintomas de anormalidade de vias respiratórias inferiores (p. ex., tosse) e, às vezes, superiores (p. ex., secreção nasal). Chega-se ao diagnóstico mediante o reconhecimento dos parasitas imaturos no lavado de via respiratória ou no teste de sedimentação fecal de Baermann ou, ainda, utilizando testes de flutuação em amostras com sulfato de zinco, e centrifugação. O tratamento com fembendazol (50 mg/kg/24 h VO, por 3 dias), ivermectina ou milbemicina oxima (0,5 mg/kg VO, em dose única) pode ser efetivo.[68-70]

Oslerus osleri. Também conhecido como *Filaroides osleri*, esse parasita tem morfologia similar à de *F. hirthi* e *F. milksi* e, como acontece com tais patógenos, é transmitido diretamente, sem necessidade de hospedeiro intermediário. O principal local de alojamento de *O. osleri* maduro é a parte distal da traqueia e os brônquios mais proximais, onde formam nódulos granulomatosos na mucosa.[28,71] Em geral subclínica, a infecção pode resultar em tosse ou, menos comumente, intolerância ao exercício ou dificuldade respiratória, devido a obstrução da via respiratória ou pneumotórax. Como o nódulo que contém o parasita pode interferir nas defesas físicas do trato respiratório (p. ex., a camada mucociliar), há possibilidade de ocorrer infecção bacteriana secundária. É possível confirmar a infecção parasitária mediante a detecção de nódulos contendo o verme, em teste de flotação fecal, com sulfato de zinco, após a centrifugação da amostra ou mediante broncoscopia.

Eucoleus aerophilus. Também conhecido como *Capillaria aerophila*, esse nematódeo parasita do trato respiratório é cosmopolita e infecta a mucosa das vias respiratórias de cães e gatos, alojando-se na mucosa traqueal e brônquica, o que às vezes resulta em bronquite eosinofílica.[28,72] Embora a maioria das infecções permaneça subclínica, pode ocorrer tosse crônica ou mesmo desconforto respiratório ocasional. Ao contrário da maioria das infecções por vermes pulmonares, a melhor maneira de estabelecer o diagnóstico por meio de exame de fezes é o emprego de teste de flotação de rotina, não com a técnica de Baermann. O exame citológico do lavado de via respiratória pode ajudar na identificação dos ovos característicos, bioperculados, semelhantes aos do tricurídeo intestinal *Trichuris vulpis*.

Troglostrongylus spp. Esses nematódeos metastrongiloides foram reconhecidos recentemente infectando felinos domésticos e silvestres.[29,73] Embora algumas espécies infectem os seios nasais ou a traqueia, outras (em especial *T. brevior*) se alojam nos brônquios e bronquíolos do hospedeiro definitivo. Relatados principalmente em gatos, na Europa e África, esses parasitas são maiores do que *A. abstrusus* e causam maior patogenicidade, inclusive infecção fatal.[73,74] Embora seja possível identificar as larvas em amostras de fezes frescas, é difícil distingui-las daquelas de outros metastrongiloides.[73] Foi desenvolvido um teste PCR dúplex capaz de detectar e distinguir *T. brevior* e *A. abstrusus*, mas ainda não está disponível no comércio.[75]

Outros parasitas pulmonares relevantes

Dirofilaria immitis. É responsável pela dirofilariose, uma causa importante de doença pulmonar e cardíaca em regiões de clima temperado, em todo o mundo. Embora a infecção tenha sido bem descrita em cães há muitas décadas, apenas recentemente soube-se da ocorrência da infecção por dirofilária em gatos.[76-80] A interação do hospedeiro com o parasita, as consequências clínicas, o diagnóstico e o tratamento da doença causada por *D. immitis* diferem muito em cães e gatos, mas dispõe-se com facilidade de medidas profiláticas eficazes para ambas as espécies. No Capítulo 255 há mais detalhes sobre essa infecção.

Angiostrongylus vasorum. A infecção por esse parasita metastrongilídeo de canídeos foi relatada na Europa, na Ásia e na África, bem como na forma de um foco endêmico na província de Newfoundland, no Canadá.[70,81-83] Foi denominada "dirofilariose francesa" porque, como ocorre com os parasitas maduros de *D. immitis*, os de *A. vasorum* também se alojam na artéria pulmonar, na parte direita do coração e nas arteríolas pulmonares. Os cães se infectam após ingerir os hospedeiros intermediários (*i. e.*, moluscos) ou paratênicos (p. ex., rãs); larvas em estágio L3 são liberadas no intestino do cão antes de seguir seu caminho para os vasos sanguíneos pulmonares, onde eclodem. As larvas L1 então migram pelos alvéolos. Após alcançarem as vias respiratórias, podem ser excretadas com a tosse e deglutidas.

Os cães infectados podem parecer saudáveis ou ter uma variedade de sinais clínicos. As síndromes predominantes associadas à infecção são doença respiratória relacionada com a resposta inflamatória ao parasita e a síndrome de diátase hemorrágica.[83] A causa do sangramento não é bem entendida, mas pode ser que esteja relacionada com uma coagulopatia consumptiva desencadeada pelo parasita, e o sangramento pode ocorrer sem sinais respiratórios.[84,85] Sintomas neurológicos foram relatados em cães infectados, como consequência de hemorragia no sistema nervoso central.[86,87] Ocasionalmente, são relatadas hipertensão pulmonar grave, *cor pulmonale* e síncope resultantes, bem como pneumotórax espontâneo.[88-91] Embora a doença cardiopulmonar relacionada com a arterite pulmonar trombótica possa ser grave, os achados mais comuns são tosse crônica e debilitação generalizada. Diferentemente do que ocorre na dirofilariose causada por *D. immitis*, não são observadas alterações vasculares nas imagens torácicas. Em vez disso, relata-se alguma combinação dos padrões brônquico, intersticial e/ou pulmonar-alveolar periférico, sendo mais bem vista na TC do tórax (Figura 242.2).[92,93] Os achados laboratoriais associados à infecção podem incluir anemia, eosinofilia, trombocitopenia, anormalidades do tempo de coagulação e, em geral, hipercalcemia.[84,94-97]

O diagnóstico e o tratamento apropriados geralmente estão associados a um bom prognóstico, em termos de recuperação.[83] Como no caso de muitos parasitas pulmonares, o exame de fezes pela técnica de Baermann é o padrão para o diagnóstico e os parasitas também podem ser detectados no lavado de via respiratória.[98] Mais recentemente, foram descritos testes sorológicos e moleculares sensíveis e específicos para a detecção do parasita.[81,98,99] O fármaco de escolha para o tratamento da infecção por *A. vasorum* é o fembendazol (25 a 50 mg/kg/24 h VO, por 10 a 20 dias), embora tenham sido descritos outros tratamentos efetivos (p. ex., ivermectina [duas doses de 0,2 mg/kg SC, com intervalo de 1 semana], milbemicina oxima [0,5 mg/kg VO, com intervalos de 1 semana, por 4 semanas], solução de imidacloprida 10%/moxidectina 2,5%, em aplicação *spot-on*, levamisol).[70,81,100] O tratamento com espinosade e milbemicina oxima pode ser feito como um esquema profilático mensal.[101] Apesar da recuperação da maioria dos cães após tratamento, têm sido observadas reações que consistem em dispneia, ascite e morte súbita.[102]

Pneumonia bacteriana

Abrange um amplo espectro da doença, desde infecção aguda a crônica, uni ou multilobar e infecção subclínica a fatal. Há múltiplas vias potenciais de exposição pulmonar a bactérias potencialmente patogênicas. As bactérias podem ser inaladas ou aspiradas e se alojam nos pulmões, podem alcançá-los por propagação direta a partir do espaço pleural ou de estruturas intratorácicas ou podem chegar aos pulmões pela circulação sanguínea. A maioria das bactérias que causam pneumonia é representada por patógenos secundários, oportunistas, que causam doença apenas quando alguma condição favorece a sua multiplicação (*i. e.*, imunossupressão, aspiração). Em geral, a pneumonia bacteriana resulta de infecções microbianas mistas; microrganismos anaeróbios obrigatórios podem representar até 25% dos patógenos envolvidos.[103-106] As bactérias mais comumente implicadas são patógenos entéricos (p. ex., *Escherichia coli*, *Klebsiella*), *Pasteurella* spp., estafilococos coagulase-positiva, estreptococos, *Mycoplasma* spp. e *Bordetella bronchiseptica* (Tabela 242.1).[5,65,103-111] Pneumonia bacteriana é incomum em animais de estimação adultos sadios, em especial gatos. Com exceção de infecções causadas por patógenos respiratórios bacterianos primários (p. ex., *Bordetella bronchiseptica*), a

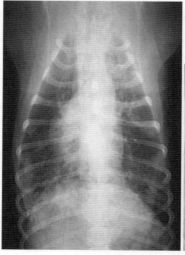
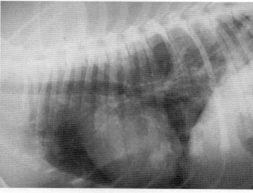

Figura 242.2 Radiografias de tórax obtidas de um cão com infecção por *Angiostrongylus vasorum*. Nota-se um padrão alveolar difuso em todos os lobos pulmonares, mais grave na parte periférica do lobo pulmonar caudal direito, da parte caudal do segmento cranial do lobo pulmonar esquerdo e por todo o lobo pulmonar caudal esquerdo. Também há espessamento peribrônquico discreto em todos os lobos pulmonares. Tanto a silhueta cardíaca como os vasos sanguíneos pulmonares não apresentam nada notável. (Cortesia da Dra. Harriet Syme, Royal Veterinary College.)

maioria dos animais com pneumonia bacteriana apresenta algum comprometimento clínico. O diagnóstico de pneumonia bacteriana deve levar imediatamente o clínico a buscar uma causa predisponente.

Manifestação

Cães desenvolvem pneumonia bacteriana com maior frequência do que gatos.[5,23,104,112,113] Muitos animais de estimação com pneumonia bacteriana têm um fator predisponente para a infecção, incluindo extremos de faixa etária, debilidade, comprometimento imunológico ou doença respiratória preexistente (Boxe 242.2).[107,112,114-119] Ocasionalmente, a pneumonia bacteriana é acompanhada apenas de sinais clínicos ou anormalidades mínimos ao exame físico, em especial quando se limita a uma região, envolvendo um único lobo pulmonar. Comumente, os sinais clínicos consistem em tosse (em geral branda e produtiva), secreção nasal, intolerância ao exercício ou dificuldade respiratória. Anorexia e letargia também são comuns. A febre, no máximo, é inconsistente; normotermia não exclui a possibilidade de pneumonia bacteriana. É possível notar perda da condição corporal, taquipneia, aumento (ou diminuição, quando há consolidação pulmonar) dos sons broncovesiculares, crepitações inspiratórias, arritmia sinusal e cianose.

Avaliação diagnóstica

Os testes de triagem diagnóstica para animais sob suspeita de pneumonia bacteriana incluem radiografias de tórax, hemograma completo e hemogasometria arterial ou oximetria de pulso. O ideal é solicitar, também, perfil bioquímico sérico e exames de urina e fezes, porque propiciam informações valiosas a respeito da saúde geral do animal e, às vezes, indícios como a presença de doença sistêmica que pode predispor à pneumonia. Neutrofilia (com ou sem desvio à esquerda), linfopenia e anemia discreta são achados inconsistentes, mas comuns no hemograma. Hipoxemia é comum, mas depende da gravidade do comprometimento da função pulmonar.[105,120] A aparência radiográfica clássica da pneumonia bacteriana é um padrão pulmonar alveolar, com distribuição predominantemente ventral.[112,121,122] Às vezes, apenas um único lobo pulmonar é envolvido (em particular após inalação ou aspiração de corpo estranho). O acometimento dorsocaudal pode predominar após exposição bacteriana hematogênica; no caso de pneumonia grave, todos os campos pulmonares podem estar envolvidos. Na pneumonia de menor gravidade ou no estágio inicial da doença, só é possível detectar um padrão intersticial. Ocasionalmente, complicações, como abscedação, efusão pleural e pneumotórax, são detectadas simultaneamente.[121]

O diagnóstico específico de pneumonia bacteriana é confirmado pela constatação de sepse pulmonar. O lavado de via respiratória fornece material para exame citológico, cultura microbiológica e teste de sensibilidade bacteriana (antibiograma). Em estudo recente do Ryan Veterinary Hospital da Universidade da Pensilvânia, verificou-se que a escolha empírica do antimicrobiano para o tratamento da pneumonia foi imprópria para os patógenos identificados na cultura bacteriológica e no antibiograma em 26% dos cães estudados.[106] Ainda mais preocupante, no caso de cães que tinham recebido antimicrobianos durante as 4 semanas prévias por alguma razão, foi a resistência ao antimicrobiano escolhido de maneira empírica em 64,7% dos cães com pneumonia adquirida na comunidade, ressaltando a importância de obter amostras para cultura e antibiograma antes de iniciar o tratamento.[106]

É provável que a duração do tratamento seja longa; a cultura microbiológica e o teste de sensibilidade bacteriana possibilitam a escolha dos antimicrobianos mais seguros, econômicos e que visem ao alvo corretamente. No entanto, após a obtenção da amostra, não se deve suspender a administração dos antimicrobianos à espera dos resultados do antibiograma. É preciso reconhecer que a terapia antimicrobiana prévia, a manipulação incorreta das amostras ou a infecção por microrganismos exigentes podem resultar em cultura negativa, mesmo na vigência de pneumonia bacteriana.[108,123,123a] Como em geral a pneumonia bacteriana resulta em tosse produtiva, o lavado de vias respiratórias de grande calibre (p. ex., transtraqueal ou transoral) pode ser seguro, de baixo custo e útil (ver Capítulos 101 e 240).[103] A amostra do LBA também pode ser usada para citologia e cultura microbiológica.[107,108] Na pneumonia bacteriana grave, naquela causada por corpo estranho ou na pneumonia por aspiração ou quando há áreas de consolidação pulmonar, deve-se solicitar cultura para microrganismos anaeróbicos, além da cultura de aeróbicos de rotina.[112,124] Como algumas espécies de *Mycoplasma* podem ser patógenos bacterianos primários das vias respiratórias, mas sua cultura é difícil pelos métodos de rotina, pode-se realizar também um teste PCR específico para *Mycoplasma*.[113,125] As vias respiratórias não são estéreis mesmo

---

Tabela 242.1 Patógenos bacterianos que causam infecção de trato respiratório inferior/pneumonia comumente isolados.

GÊNEROS E ESPÉCIES DE BACTÉRIAS	ISOLADOS EM CÃES[104-106,108,109]	ISOLADOS EM GATOS[5,65,110,111]
Escherichia coli	132	7
Pasteurella spp.	104	22
Bordetella bronchiseptica	105	15
Streptococcus spp.	149	12
Staphylococcus spp. coagulase +	101	1
Klebsiella spp.	45	
Enterococcus spp.	15	1
Pseudomomas aeruginosa	66	3
Mycoplasma spp.	95	34

Boxe 242.2 Fatores que predispõem à pneumonia bacteriana

Debilidade
Decúbito prolongado
Imunossupressão sistêmica
  Medicamentosa (p. ex., corticosteroides, quimioterapia)
  Infecciosa (p. ex., vírus da leucemia felina, vírus da imunodeficiência felina)
  Causada por doenças endócrinas (p. ex., hiperadrenocorticismo, diabetes melito)
Imunodeficiência
  Extremos de faixa etária
  Imunodeficiência congênita (p. ex., síndromes relacionadas com a raça, imunodeficiência combinada grave, defeitos fagocitários)
Anormalidades na defesa do trato respiratório
  Discinesia ciliar primária
  Deficiência de IgA
Dano ao epitélio respiratório
  Inalação de fumaça
  Afogamento
  Infecção viral, parasitária, por protozoário ou fúngica
  Neoplasia
  Síndrome da angústia respiratória aguda
Aspiração (ver Boxe 242.5, mais adiante)
Infecção de pleura/mediastino/via respiratória
Lesão penetrante no tórax
Obstrução de via respiratória (funcional ou estrutural)
Bronquiectasia
Sepse/bacteriemia

em pacientes saudáveis, sendo possível a associação de doença respiratória não infecciosa e infecção bacteriana secundária. Portanto, o diagnóstico de pneumonia bacteriana deve se basear na integração de todos os achados clínicos e radiográficos, de preferência em conjunto com a constatação citológica de inflamação neutrofílica de via respiratória e de bactérias intracelulares, além de cultura bacteriana positiva.

Tratamento

A pneumonia bacteriana deve ser tratada com antimicrobianos.[106,124] O tratamento empírico inicial pode ser ajustado depois, com base nos resultados da cultura bacteriana e do teste de sensibilidade (antibiograma). A terapia inicial pode ser baseada, em parte, na morfologia citológica e nas características de coloração dos microrganismos isolados na amostra do lavado de via respiratória.[107,109] Em animais gravemente acometidos ou instáveis, o tratamento inicial deve incluir antimicrobianos efetivos contra bactérias gram-positivas, gram-negativas, aeróbicas e anaeróbicas. Mais frequentemente, tal abordagem envolve terapia combinada, administrada por via parenteral (Boxe 242.3); a autora, em geral, inicia com uma combinação de ampicilina e enrofloxacino, embora a recomendação recente da International Society of Companion Animal Infecctious Disease (Iscaid) seja uma combinação inicial de fluoroquinolona com ampicilina ou clindamicina.[124] Animais com doença branda a moderada podem ser tratados inicialmente com antimicrobiano de menor espectro, administrado por via oral (ver Boxe 242.3). Embora muitos antimicrobianos (incluindo antibacterianos betalactâmicos) não atravessem prontamente a barreira hematobrônquica da via respiratória, isso é pouco preocupante com relação à pneumonia, que é uma infecção do tecido parenquimatoso e não de via respiratória. Embora a administração de antimicrobianos por meio de aerossóis possa ser benéfica (sem comprovação) no tratamento de alguns animais com pneumonia bacteriana, esse procedimento só deve ser realizado como terapia adjuvante e nunca em substituição aos antimicrobianos administrados por via sistêmica.[123,126] Em termos históricos na medicina veterinária, a duração recomendada do tratamento

---

Boxe 242.3 Escolhas empíricas de antimicrobianos para o tratamento inicial de pneumonia bacteriana

Doença grave, instável
Monoterapia
  Meropeném ou imipeném-cilastatina ou ticarcilina
Terapia combinada
  Betalactâmico (p. ex., ampicilina, amoxicilina/clavulanato, cefalosporina de segunda ou terceira geração) ou clindamicina
  E
  Fluoroquinolona (p. ex., enrofloxacino, marbofloxacino ou orbifloxacina)
  OU
  Aminoglicosídeo (p. ex., amicacina, gentamicina)

Doença moderada, estável
Monoterapia
  Amoxicilina/clavulanato ou trimetoprima-sulfonamida
Terapia combinada
  Betalactâmico E fluoroquinolona
  OU
  Clindamicina E fluoroquinolona

Doença branda, estável
Monoterapia
  Amoxicilina/clavulanato ou fluoroquinolona ou trimetoprima-sulfonamida

Nota: a escolha empírica inicial do antimicrobiano deve ser ajustada com base nos resultados da cultura microbiológica e do teste de sensibilidade bacteriana (antibiograma). Quanto mais grave a doença em seu início, mais importante que o tratamento proporcione cobertura de amplo espectro.

---

antimicrobiano era de 1 semana após a resolução radiográfica, tipicamente um mínimo de 3 a 4 semanas. Isso é um excesso extremo em comparação com a duração do tratamento recomendado para pneumonia em seres humanos[127,128] e provavelmente mais longo que o necessário em animais de estimação. Diretrizes da Iscaid recém-elaboradas para infecções respiratórias sugerem a reavaliação dos animais 10 a 14 dias após o início do tratamento, com emprego de tratamento antimicrobiano estendido, alterado ou suspenso com base na resposta clínica.[124]

Cães com pneumonia bacteriana grave, em geral, apresentam hipoxemia.[120] O ideal é mensurar a Pa_{O_2} mediante hemogasometria arterial (ver Capítulo 128), mas pode-se mensurar a Sp_{O_2}, com razoável correlação (ver Capítulo 98). Para animais com hipoxemia aguda, deve-se providenciar suplementação de oxigênio quando a Pa_{O_2} estiver < 80 mmHg ou a Sp_{O_2} < 94%. Os meios mais práticos de fornecimento de oxigênio incluem o uso de cânula nasal ou tenda de oxigênio (ver Capítulo 131). O oxigênio deve ser umidificado antes de seu fornecimento, para evitar ressecamento das vias respiratórias e consequente comprometimento da limpeza mucociliar. Hipoxemia persistente ou esforço respiratório acentuado contínuo, mesmo com suplementação de oxigênio, indicam a necessidade de ventilação mecânica. Infelizmente, o prognóstico em termos da recuperação de cães e gatos com doença respiratória primária que exige ventilação mecânica é ruim.[129] Em parte, isso pode estar relacionado com a presença de mais patógenos resistentes aos antimicrobianos em pacientes com insuficiência respiratória em decorrência de pneumonia.[130]

Para animais com pneumonia bacteriana grave indica-se terapia com reposição de líquido (ver Capítulo 129). Desidratação é comum em animais fracos, deprimidos, com anorexia, febre e taquipneia. Além dos efeitos sistêmicos da hipovolemia, a desidratação compromete a defesa mucociliar do trato respiratório. Nas vias respiratórias, o muco atua aprisionando bactérias e material particulado inalado. Os cílios epiteliais respiratórios impulsionam partículas aprisionadas craniais à orofaringe, que podem ser expelidas com a tosse ou deglutidos.[131] O revestimento de muco é constituído de duas camadas – uma camada aquosa, através da qual os cílios se movem, e uma camada de gel sobrejacente, que aprisiona os materiais particulados. Se a camada aquosa se desidrata, os cílios ficam aprisionados na camada de gel, inibindo a atividade do revestimento mucociliar. Devem ser administradas soluções cristaloides em taxa que mantenha a hidratação. O tratamento agressivo com excesso de líquido pode acarretar edema pulmonar iatrogênico e agravar o comprometimento respiratório. A nebulização com solução fisiológica estéril pode fluidificar o muco e tornar a função mucociliar mais efetiva, embora o benefício não esteja documentado em animais de estimação. A nebulização com solução fisiológica 3 a 4 vezes/dia parece melhorar a respiração em muitos animais com pneumonia.

Em animais com pneumonia bacteriana ocorre estímulo à tosse, sendo contraindicado o uso de supressores da tosse. Tapotagem (*i. e.*, fisioterapia torácica) é uma técnica simples de percussão torácica que ajuda na mobilização de secreções das vias respiratórias e estimula a tosse (Figura 242.3). Embora não haja documentação de que seja particularmente efetiva em seres humanos adultos com pneumonia, foi útil em outras situações, como na pneumonia associada à fibrose cística.[132] Segundo a autora, não há estudos que documentem a eficácia da técnica em cães e gatos. A tapotagem deve seguir-se à nebulização com solução fisiológica, quando ambas são usadas. Os animais devem ser estimulados a se movimentar, e aqueles em decúbito devem ser reposicionados com frequência para ajudar na mobilização de secreções respiratórias.

Em animais com pneumonia, o tratamento adicional consiste no uso de broncodilatadores, mucolíticos, cuidados nutricionais e de suporte. Broncodilatadores não são usados de forma rotineira no tratamento da pneumonia bacteriana. A inalação de albuterol ou broncodilatadores à base de metilxantina (p. ex., teofilina) é

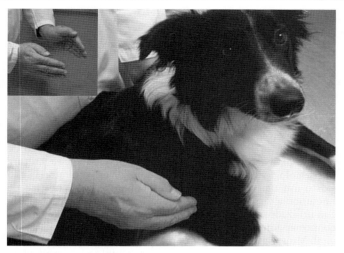

Figura 242.3 A percussão torácica (i. e., tapotagem) pode ajudar a mobilizar secreções das vias respiratórias. Usam-se as mãos em concha para fazer a percussão de cada lado do tórax do animal (com um pouco mais de força que a utilizada para aplaudir) repetidas vezes. A nebulização com solução fisiológica antes da tapotagem pode melhorar ainda mais a mobilização das secreções.

indicada aos animais que continuam com hipoxemia, mesmo após o fornecimento de oxigênio suplementar, quando há broncoconstrição concomitante (especialmente provável em gatos) ou antes da administração do fármaco inalante. A pneumonia bacteriana pode resultar na produção de quantidades abundantes de muco espesso e viscoso. Em termos teóricos, a liquefação do muco pode resultar em uma limpeza mucociliar mais efetiva. A simples manutenção da hidratação sistêmica e a umidificação das vias respiratórias costumam ser adequadas, mas às vezes há quem defenda o uso de mucolíticos. A N-acetilcisteína (NAC) diminui a viscosidade ao romper as pontes de dissulfeto de mucina, mas infelizmente a nebulização com NAC causa broncoconstrição.[133] A administração oral de NAC não foi investigada em animais de estimação com pneumonia de ocorrência natural, mas em outras espécies mostrou ter pelo menos alguma utilidade no tratamento tanto de doenças infecciosas como das não infecciosas de vias respiratórias acompanhadas de secreção excessiva de muco.[134-136] A autora usou NAC oral (disponível em lojas de alimentos naturais) em animais com acúmulo excessivo de muco devido à pneumonia, em dosagem de 125 mg a 600 mg VO, em intervalos de 8 a 12 horas, aparentemente com bom efeito. Animais com pneumonia podem ter relutância para comer, por isso é indispensável o cuidado com o suporte nutricional.

Ocasionalmente, indica-se lobectomia pulmonar como tratamento, quando a pneumonia não se resolve com o tratamento antimicrobiano apropriado.[137-139] Infecção residual em um único lobo pode estar relacionada com um problema físico primário, como corpo estranho no brônquio, abscesso ou tumor. Em tais casos, a remoção do lobo pode resultar em cura. Ocasionalmente, a falha em responder ao tratamento antimicrobiano apropriado se deve a um diagnóstico incorreto. Qualquer tecido pulmonar removido cirurgicamente deve ser submetido à cultura tecidual e exame histopatológico.

Patógenos bacterianos que causam pneumonia bacteriana

Bordetella bronchiseptica

É um patógeno respiratório primário. Basicamente, ele cria sua própria oportunidade para causar infecção mediante a secreção de endotoxinas que resulta em disfunção do movimento mucociliar.[140,141] A bordetelose é contagiosa; cães e gatos são suscetíveis, mas a doença é mais comum em cães.[142,143] Em geral, a infecção resulta em traqueobronquite, mas pode causar pneumonia grave em animais imunocomprometidos ou jovens. Em um estudo retrospectivo de pneumonia adquirida na comunidade, em cães com menos de 1 ano de idade, esse microrganismo foi responsável por quase metade de todos os casos.[105] Pode ser difícil eliminar tais infecções, apesar do uso de antimicrobianos aos quais B. bronchiseptica tenha suscetibilidade demonstrada in vitro. Diagnosticou-se pneumonia em filhotes de cães infectados com Bordetella tratados com amoxicilina ou amoxicilina-clavulanato, mesmo com a documentação in vitro da sensibilidade do microrganismo.[105] A adição de nebulização de aminoglicosídeos aos antimicrobianos sistêmicos foi proposta, mas não há documentação de eficácia no tratamento da pneumonia causada por Bordetella. O uso de antimicrobianos inalantes nunca deve substituir a administração sistêmica de antimicrobianos no tratamento de pneumonia. Para mais informações, consulte o Capítulo 97.

Streptococcus equi subespécie zooepidemicus

Pode causar pneumonia hemorrágica necrosante em cães e recentemente reconheceu-se que também infecta gatos.[144-146] Ao contrário de outras causas de doença respiratória infecciosa canina contagiosa, a doença pode tornar-se potencialmente fatal.[147-150] O patógeno é particularmente propenso a causar pneumonia hemorrágica grave e até mesmo fatal em cães de canis, inclusive naqueles criados em abrigos e colônias de animais de pesquisa. Como em outros tipos de pneumonia bacteriana, pode-se usar o lavado de via respiratória para identificar a infecção e orientar o tratamento antimicrobiano apropriado. Cães que morrem subitamente ou com evidência de pneumonia, no contexto de um canil, devem ser submetidos à necropsia e cultura bacteriana para confirmar a infecção.

Mycoplasma

As espécies de Mycoplasma, microrganismos exigentes, que não possuem parede celular, incluem microrganismos patogênicos (p. ex., M. pneumoniae, em seres humanos, M. hyopneumoniae em suínos) e comensais. Até 15 espécies diferentes foram isoladas de cães e muitas também de gatos.[151] Entretanto, como são difíceis a multiplicação desses microrganismos e a determinação da espécie, sua participação exata na doença respiratória de cães e gatos não está bem definida.

Também as espécies desse gênero são encontradas comumente nas vias respiratórias superiores e, ocasionalmente, nas vias inferiores de cães e gatos sadios.[152-154] A inoculação experimental de alguns micoplasmas causa pneumonia; a pneumonia de ocorrência natural em cães e gatos algumas vezes foi atribuída a Mycoplasma spp. (em especial M. cynos).[153,155-161] Contudo, em um estudo realizado com 93 cães com pneumonia bacteriana causada especificamente por micoplasmas, foram isoladas espécies de micoplasmas em apenas 7 cães como a única bactéria; em 58 cães, havia também bactérias de outros gêneros.[104] Isso, combinado com um desfecho clínico favorável mesmo quando o tratamento antimicrobiano não foi direcionado a micoplasmas, sugere que as bactérias desse gênero são principalmente oportunistas. Apesar disso, podem contribuir para a morbidade quando presentes como coinfecção com outros patógenos respiratórios.[151,157]

É preciso solicitar teste PCR ou cultura especial para identificar Mycoplasma spp. Em comparação com a cultura, a identificação de micoplasmas por PCR em amostras do trato respiratório resultou em sensibilidade de detecção de 81,8%, com especificidade de 78,9%.[125] Em geral, Mycoplasma spp. é sensível aos antimicrobianos macrolídeos, tetraciclinas, cloranfenicol e fluoroquinolonas, mas não aos que interferem na síntese da parede celular (p. ex., betalactâmicos), estrutura que esse gênero não possui.

Pneumonia causada por micobactérias

Gatos e cães ocasionalmente são diagnosticados com pneumonia causada por micobactérias. Tanto as infecções micobacterianas do tipo tuberculose (p. ex., causadas por Mycobacterium tuberculosis,

SEÇÃO 15 • Doença Respiratória

Mycobacterium bovis, Mycobacterium microti) quanto as não tuberculosas (p. ex., complexo *Mycobacterium avium, Mycobacterium fortuitum*) causam pneumonia em animais de estimação.[162-174] Pode ocorrer pneumonia como manifestação primária da infecção por micobactérias ou como um componente da infecção disseminada. Em geral, a pneumonia causada por micobactérias é granulomatosa, e as imagens radiográficas podem mostrar linfadenomegalia e efusão pleural, além de infiltrados intersticiais e alveolares. Padrões alveolares mistos são comuns, frequentemente incluem brônquicos, alveolares, intersticiais nodulares estruturados ou componentes intersticiais não estruturados.[174] Os microrganismos são encontrados em pequeno número, quando o são, em amostras obtidas de LBA ou em AAF, ou de aspirado de linfonodos. Como não absorvem os corantes utilizados na rotina, essas inclusões ácido-resistentes se apresentam como bastonetes de coloração negativa ("vazios") no exame citológico de rotina.[169,170,175] Cultura microbiológica e PCR são usadas para confirmar a presença de espécies de micobactérias em cães e gatos, mas aquelas semelhantes às causadoras de tuberculose apresentam crescimento notoriamente lento.[169,170,176,177] *M. tuberculosis* é primariamente um patógeno humano; quando identificado em cães, a doença é considerada uma zoonose reversa.[170,178] Em tais casos, deve-se entrar em contato com a secretaria de saúde local, e os proprietários de cães infectados devem ser instruídos a entrar em contato com um médico. As implicações de saúde pública, ao se tentar tratar infecções causadas por micobactérias do tipo daquelas causadoras de tuberculose, precisam ser muito bem consideradas. Tanto as infecções micobacterianas do tipo da tuberculose como as não tuberculosas requerem protocolos de tratamento de longa duração, com múltiplos fármacos, para obter seu controle. Para mais informações sobre infecções causadas por micobactérias, consulte o Capítulo 212.

Pneumonia causada por Yersinia pestis (peste bubônica)

Clínicos do centro-oeste e do extremo oeste dos EUA, em especial dos estados do Novo México e do Colorado, precisam considerar a peste bubônica como um diagnóstico diferencial, em qualquer gato com pneumonia. Embora a infecção seja relativamente rara, sua importância está associada ao seu potencial zoonótico. Cães são resistentes à peste bubônica e raramente desenvolvem sinais respiratórios (embora a transmissão zoonótica por cães também tenha sido relatada).[179,180] Já em gatos domésticos, a taxa de mortalidade da peste bubônica é próxima a 50% e a doença pode disseminar-se para seres humanos por contato ou inalação de gotículas de aerossóis.[181-183] Roedores (p. ex., cão-da-pradaria e esquilos) são os reservatórios naturais do cocobacilo gram-negativo *Yersinia pestis*. Gatos podem infectar-se por ingestão de roedores, ou coelhos infectados, ou pela picada de pulgas infectadas. Mais comumente, gatos que ingerem roedores infectados desenvolvem inicialmente linfadenite supurativa (adenite) nos linfonodos submandibulares e cervicais.[181] Essa forma bubônica pode progredir para uma forma septicêmica ou pneumônica secundária. Seres humanos podem desenvolver peste pneumônica primária após a inalação de gotículas infectadas oriundas da tosse de gatos. Sem tratamento, a peste pneumônica é fatal. Em regiões endêmicas, qualquer gato com pneumonia deve ficar em isolamento rigoroso e ser manuseado com extrema cautela. O exame citológico do exsudato ou do aspirado de linfonodos tipicamente revela bastonetes gram-negativos bipolares, em forma de alfinete de segurança. Nos EUA, deve-se entrar em contato com o Center for Disease Control and Prevention se houver suspeita da doença; a confirmação baseia-se na pesquisa de anticorpo fluorescente, em cultura microbiológica ou no título crescente de anticorpo. Com o diagnóstico ainda pendente, os gatos devem ser tratados com antipulgas e antimicrobianos imediatamente. Aminoglicosídeos, fluoroquinolonas, cloranfenicol e tetraciclinas são usados no tratamento da infecção por *Y. pestis*.

Pneumonia viral

Ao contrário da infecção respiratória bacteriana, a doença viral é causada predominantemente por patógenos primários e, em geral, é contagiosa. Alguns patógenos virais que causam pneumonia visam especificamente o trato respiratório (p. ex., vírus da influenza), enquanto outros vírus são polissistêmicos (p. ex., vírus da cinomose e vírus da peritonite infecciosa felina). As infecções virais consideradas como causas potenciais de pneumonia estão listadas no Boxe 242.4. As vacinas efetivas minimizam a morbidade associada a muitas causas potenciais de pneumonia viral. Embora seja fácil confirmar o diagnóstico de pneumonia bacteriana por meio de exame citológico e cultura microbiológica de rotina, do lavado de via respiratória, não existe um único teste simples que confirme o diagnóstico de pneumonia viral. Em geral, a infecção é meramente presuntiva. São utilizados exames sorológicos e PCR de alvo específico para confirmar a infecção mais frequentemente do que o isolamento viral. Muitos vírus que causam pneumonia são patógenos envolvidos na ocorrência de doença respiratória infecciosa contagiosa canina (*i. e.*, DRICC; ver Capítulo 227) ou causam, também, infecções do trato respiratório superior de gatos (ver Capítulo 229).[184,185] Vários laboratórios realizam testes PCR para muitos desses patógenos.

Em muitos aspectos, a pneumonia bacteriana e a pneumonia viral são semelhantes. Na verdade, muitas mortes associadas à pneumonia viral se devem a infecções bacterianas oportunistas. Uma vez que há poucas terapias antivirais específicas e pouca evidência que sustente o uso dessas medicações caras, quando existem, o tratamento da pneumonia viral, em grande parte, envolve o tratamento de suporte. Cães com suspeita de pneumonia viral devem ser isolados por causa da natureza contagiosa dessa infecção. Nos Capítulos 227 a 230 há informações adicionais sobre vírus relevantes para a saúde respiratória de cães e gatos.

Vírus influenza

Até recentemente, não se acreditava que o vírus influenza infectasse cães ou gatos. Em 2004, constatou-se que um surto de doença respiratória em um canil de cães da raça Greyhound foi causado pelo vírus influenza H3N8.[186,187] Desde então, vários outros vírus influenza do tipo A foram reconhecidos como causadores de infecção cruzada esporádica ou experimental em cães e gatos.[188-191] A maioria não resultou em transmissão mantida na espécie em que a infecção foi diagnosticada. Todavia, como o vírus influenza H3N8, o H3N2 desenvolveu capacidade de se disseminar entre cães, resultando em epidemias na Ásia e nos EUA.[188,192] Os vírus influenza são vírus RNA sujeitos a mutações, que podem ser espontâneas ou ocorrer quando um hospedeiro é infectado simultaneamente por dois vírus que se misturam entre si.[188,190,193] Aparentemente, o vírus canino H3N8 originou-se a partir de um vírus influenza equino, enquanto o H3N2 parece

---

Boxe 242.4 Vírus responsáveis pela ocorrência de pneumonia infecciosa de cães e gatos

Influenza aviária (rara)
Vírus da cinomose
Herpes-vírus canino
Hepatite infecciosa canina
Influenza canina (H3N8 e H3N2)
Vírus da parainfluenza canina
Coronavírus respiratório canino
Calicivírus felino
Herpes-vírus felino
Peritonite infecciosa felina/coronavírus

Nota: o vírus da leucemia felina e o vírus da imunodeficiência felina ocasionam imunossupressão e pneumonia infecciosa secundária, mas não causam, diretamente, pneumonia viral.

CAPÍTULO 242 • Doenças do Parênquima Pulmonar — 1127

ter origem aviária. Ambos são altamente contagiosos aos cães. Sabe-se menos sobre a infecção em cães infectados pelo H3N2 do que pelo H3N8. Início agudo de tosse, febre e letargia são sintomas típicos na infecção por ambos os vírus. A taxa de morbidade é elevada, mas a morte do animal é incomum. Quando ocorrem mortes, em geral estão relacionadas com pneumonia bacteriana oportunista. O H3N8 não parece ser zoonótico, mas a possibilidade de múltiplos eventos reagrupados significa que os veterinários precisam estar atentos a essa possibilidade.[192,194] Embora se disponha de fármacos anti-influenza específicos no comércio (fosfato de oseltamivir [Tamiflu]), seu uso não é estimulado. Esses fármacos de alto custo não foram avaliados na influenza canina. Mesmo quando usados de acordo com as prescrições da bula indicadas para influenza humana, eles devem ser administrados até 48 horas após o início da doença e resultam em apenas mínima redução na duração e gravidade da infecção. Dispõe-se de vacinas com vírus inativados contra influenza canina causada por H3N8 ou H3N2. Atualmente, a proteção contra influenza canina requer a administração de cada tipo específico de vacina, pois não há uma vacina com ambos os vírus.

A influenza é reconhecida com menor frequência em gatos do que em cães, mas os gatos são suscetíveis à infecção natural e experimental por vários tipos de vírus influenza A.[195-197] Gatos foram infectados com o vírus influenza H5N1 aviário patogênico após a ingestão de aves de granja infectadas e por transmissão direta de um gato para outro; a doença resultante, em geral, foi potencialmente fatal.[197-201] Os veterinários devem ficar atentos à possível infecção por vírus influenza em animais de estimação, tanto por causa da doença resultante no animal examinado como devido ao risco de contágio a outros animais de estimação e à infecção zoonótica por contato com humanos.[196,200]

Pneumonia causada por protozoário

A pneumonia causada por protozoário não é comum em cães ou gatos. Entre os protozoários patógenos que causam pneumonia, o *Toxoplasma* é o encontrado com maior frequência. Gatos são os hospedeiros intermediários de *Toxoplasma gondii* e, em geral, infectam-se sem manifestar doença clínica.[202] Quando ocorre doença, pode envolver o trato gastrintestinal, o sistema nervoso central, as vísceras abdominais, o coração, os olhos ou o trato respiratório. As manifestações respiratórias de pneumonia intersticial, agudas ou lentamente progressivas, estão entre as mais comuns.[203,204] Os resultados dos exames laboratoriais de rotina variam de acordo com o órgão acometido. A constatação sorológica de IgM específica confirma doença ativa, mas ocorrem resultados tanto falsos positivos quanto falsos negativos.[205] Ocasionalmente, são identificados taquizoítos de *T. gondii* em lavado de via respiratória de animais com pneumonia.[204,206,207] Espera-se uma resposta terapêutica rápida com o uso de sulfonamidas potencializadas ou clindamicina, mas a recorrência da infecção é possível. Mais informação sobre *T. gondii* pode ser encontrada no Capítulo 221.

Pneumonia micótica

Uma variedade de fungos sistêmicos (em especial *Blastomyces dermatitidis*, *Histoplasma capsulatum* e *Coccidioides immitis*) pode causar pneumonia micótica em cães e gatos.[208-210] Doença do trato respiratório inferior de progressão lenta pode ser a manifestação primária, mas também são comuns manifestações extratorácicas, inclusive perda de peso e linfadenopatia. As alterações radiográficas associadas à pneumonia micótica variam muito e, em geral, consistem em padrão pulmonar intersticial nodular ou nodular miliar e linfadenopatia hilar. O tratamento é dispendioso e potencialmente tóxico; portanto, é importante um diagnóstico definitivo em vez de presuntivo. Como as infecções intersticiais micóticas não resultam em esfoliação precoce de elementos fúngicos nas vias respiratórias, o lavado de via respiratória não é uma técnica sensível para a detecção dessas estruturas. Em geral, o diagnóstico é confirmado a partir de amostras obtidas de outros locais (p. ex., aspirado de linfonodos, "imprint" de lesões cutâneas). Recentemente, foram disponibilizados exames de urina para detecção de fungos relativamente sensíveis e específicos como auxiliares de diagnóstico e monitoramento do tratamento de pneumonia micótica.[211-213] Veja mais detalhes nos Capítulos 162 e 231 a 236.

O *Pneumocystis carinii* (também conhecido como *Pneumocystis jerovici*) foi classificado originalmente como um protozoário, mas atualmente é considerado um fungo. Embora esse microrganismo saprófita de ampla distribuição não seja altamente virulento, em hospedeiros imunocomprometidos de muitas espécies pode resultar em morbidade relevante, com alta taxa de mortalidade devido à pneumonia. A infecção foi descrita em vários cães de raças de pequeno porte com possível imunossupressão, mas é muitíssimo mais comum em cães das raças Dachshund Miniatura e Cavalier King Charles Spaniel.[214-220] Foi sugerida uma única imunodeficiência em cada raça (imunodeficiência variável comum em cães Dachshund e Lulu da Pomerânia; deficiência de IgG em cães Cavalier).[216,220,221] A maioria dos cães infectados é jovem e levada ao veterinário devido a sinais de doença de trato respiratório inferior progressiva. Embora não haja sinais físicos, radiográficos ou laboratoriais exclusivos, a ausência de febre, apesar de pneumonia grave, é um indício desse tipo de infecção.[221] O diagnóstico é difícil porque os patógenos não são isolados com facilidade no lavado de via respiratória, por isso pode ser necessário colorações especiais, como a coloração de metenamina de prata de Grocott-Gromori, para visualizar o microrganismo, quando presente.[222] Sulfonamidas potencializadas parecem ser o tratamento mais efetivo quando administradas no estágio inicial da doença. Embora a pneumonia causada por *Pneumocystis* seja importante em pessoas com imunossupressão (p. ex., durante infecção pelo HIV), acredita-se que os cães não abriguem a mesma cepa; portanto, o risco zoonótico deve ser baixo.[223]

Pneumonia por aspiração

Pneumonite e pneumonia por aspiração resultam da inalação de materiais que entram no trato respiratório inferior. O material aspirado, em geral, consiste em conteúdo estomacal com ou sem material particulado sólido. Pode ocorrer aspiração iatrogênica como resultado de alimentação forçada, administração oral de substâncias como bário ou óleo mineral, ou indução inapropriada de êmese após intoxicações orais (p. ex., com destilados de petróleo) (ver Capítulo 151). Dependendo do volume do material aspirado e das propriedades físicas do material (p. ex., pH, tonicidade, contaminação bacteriana, volume e tamanho do material particulado), o resultado pode variar de alteração mínima a edema pulmonar fulminante, necrose e hemorragia. Substâncias químicas irritantes (inclusive ácido gástrico) resultam em pneumonite, embora a aspiração de volume maior de um líquido menos agressivo possa resultar em um evento "catastrófico". A aspiração de soluções utilizadas para limpeza do intestino que contenham polietilenoglicol pode ser especialmente prejudicial, pois essas substâncias levam o líquido intersticial para os pulmões.[224,225] A aspiração de material particulado de tamanho grande pode resultar em obstrução aguda de via respiratória. Devido à baixa carga bacteriana do conteúdo gástrico, a infecção raramente é um componente inicial importante da aspiração. No entanto, o dano ao trato respiratório causado por ácido ou outras substâncias irritantes predispõe à infecção bacteriana secundária. Ocorre lesão por aspiração em etapas, que começa com uma resposta aguda da via respiratória, seguida de inflamação pulmonar e, em geral, culmina com infecção bacteriana oportunista.

Uma variedade de condições pode predispor os animais à aspiração (Boxe 242.5) e muitas envolvem animais hospitalizados em razão de diversas causas. Deve-se suspeitar de aspiração indesejada em qualquer animal hospitalizado com recorrência de sintomas do trato respiratório inferior. Embora a anestesia geral constitua um risco à aspiração, em um estudo

Boxe 242.5 Condições que predispõem à aspiração

Comprometimento da proteção consciente das vias respiratórias (p. ex., anestesia geral, sedação profunda, convulsões, coma)

Comprometimento da proteção inconsciente das vias respiratórias (p. ex., paralisia da laringe, alteração cirúrgica da anatomia da laringe [aprisionada], miastenia gravis)

Deglutição comprometida (p. ex., acalasia, déficit do V nervo craniano, raiva)

Regurgitação (p. ex., megaesôfago, distúrbio da motilidade, divertículo esofágico)

Hiperdistensão gástrica (p. ex., alimentação excessiva, íleo adinâmico, obstrução gastrintestinal)

Vômitos (p. ex., doença gastrintestinal primária, doença pancreática, uremia, doença hepática)

Alimentação forçada ou administração oral de medicamentos

---

multicêntrico recente constatou-se que a incidência de pneumonia por aspiração após anestesia foi de apenas 0,17%; foram detectados vários fatores que aumentam o risco de aspiração.[226] Em estudos retrospectivos realizados com 88 ou 120 cães com pneumonia por aspiração, pouco mais da metade estava febril (31 e 43%, respectivamente).[227,228] Respiração ofegante ou taquipneia foram achados comuns, porém inconsistentes. A maioria apresentava tosse e sons pulmonares adventícios ásperos/altos, ou diminuídos, à auscultação.[227,228] Leucocitose, com ou sem desvio à esquerda, foi um achado comum, mas inconsistente.[227,228] A aparência radiográfica clássica de pneumonia por aspiração é um infiltrado alveolar difuso ou focal (Figura 242.4), mas 25% dos cães acometidos, em um estudo retrospectivo, mostravam um padrão predominantemente intersticial.[227] Na aspiração, as alterações radiográficas podem ser tardias porque só ocorre acúmulo de líquido após lesão pulmonar química. A imagem lateral esquerda tem importância especial para melhorar o reconhecimento de um padrão alveolar no lobo pulmonar médio direito, cuja silhueta fica em grande parte sobreposta à sombra cardíaca. Como a aspiração de líquido depende da gravidade, os lobos pulmonares acometidos mais comumente são o médio direito, o cranial direito e a parte caudal do cranial esquerdo; no entanto, o lobo acometido depende da posição do animal no momento da aspiração.[227-229] Em um estudo, o prognóstico foi desfavorável em animais com envolvimento de mais de um lobo, e mais de um terço de todos os cães apresentou evidência radiográfica de acometimento de 2 ou mais lobos pulmonares.[228] Pode-se usar o lavado de via respiratória com fins diagnósticos quando não há uma história clara de aspiração nem qualquer predisposição conhecida para ela. Espera-se inflamação neutrofílica e é possível identificar macrófagos carregados com lipídios ou fragmentos particulados (p. ex., restos de alimentos). Em seres humanos, mensura-se a concentração de pepsina para confirmar a ocorrência de aspiração.[230] Infecções polimicrobianas e anaeróbicas são comuns, porém são complicações tardias da aspiração.

O tratamento da aspiração é, em grande parte, de suporte. Quando possível, deve-se fazer o máximo esforço para prevenir aspiração, preferivelmente corrigindo os fatores predisponentes (ver Boxe 242.5). Os animais devem estar em jejum antes da anestesia, usando-se manguito endotraqueal insuflado quando apropriado. No caso de animais conscientes com regurgitação ou vômitos frequentes, ou quando a proteção da via respiratória está comprometida, deve-se minimizar a ingestão oral. Alimentar animais de estimação com megaesôfago em recipientes colocados em lugares altos e mantê-los com a parte anterior do corpo elevada após a alimentação são práticas comuns, mas a eficácia dessas técnicas no sentido de prevenir aspiração é desconhecida. No caso de animais com regurgitação frequente devido a megaesôfago, a colocação de um tubo de gastrostomia pode facilitar a alimentação, ao mesmo tempo que minimiza o risco de aspiração (ver Capítulo 82). A administração de antagonistas do receptor de H2 ou de inibidores da bomba de prótons aumenta o pH do conteúdo gástrico e pode diminuir a lesão pulmonar química decorrente da aspiração, mas também pode aumentar o conteúdo gástrico de bactérias.[231] Fármacos procinéticos, como a metoclopramida, promovem o esvaziamento gástrico e comprimem o esfíncter esofágico inferior, o que pode diminuir o risco de aspiração de conteúdo gástrico.[232-234] Infelizmente, não houve diminuição da morbidade nem da mortalidade em seres humanos que receberam fármacos procinéticos ou antiácidos. Quando a aspiração é testemunhada (p. ex., durante anestesia), pode-se tentar a limpeza física das vias respiratórias. Também se empregou a lavagem terapêutica de vias respiratórias para retirar delas substâncias irritantes, após um evento de aspiração conhecido.[235] Após a constatação de aspiração, devem ser obtidas radiografias de tórax simples, além de monitorar a oxigenação. Se ocorrer dispneia pós-aspiração, o uso de broncodilatador pode amenizar o broncospasmo agudo. Deve-se fornecer oxigênio suplementar, conforme necessário (ver Capítulo 131); no entanto, a suplementação de oxigênio muito agressiva pode agravar a lesão pulmonar oxidativa associada à pneumonite química. A infecção bacteriana secundária pode requerer tratamento com antimicrobianos apropriados. O prognóstico quanto à recuperação, em geral, é bom, mas não pode ser previsto apenas com base na gravidade das alterações radiográficas.[236]

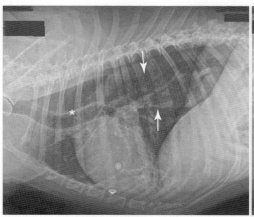
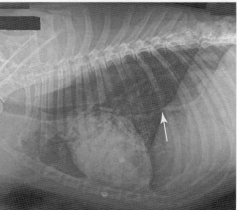
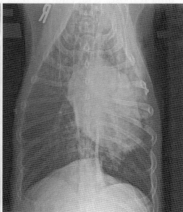

Figura 242.4 Radiografias ventrodorsal e laterais direita e esquerda de um cão mestiço castrado de 7 anos e histórico de megaesôfago, com início recente de aumento do esforço respiratório. O megaesôfago é evidente (*setas*; a margem dorsal visível da traqueia [*asterisco*] sugere realce de luz contra um esôfago cheio de ar) e um padrão alveolar compatível com pneumonia por aspiração é mais bem observado na parte média direita e na caudal dos lobos pulmonares craniais esquerdos. A sombra cardíaca foi desviada para o hemitórax esquerdo.

Edema pulmonar

Não é uma doença, e sim consequência de alguma. Como resultado do aumento da pressão hidrostática, diminuição da pressão oncótica, comprometimento da drenagem linfática ou aumento da permeabilidade vascular (ver Capítulo 18), o líquido se acumula no interstício e em seguida nos alvéolos a uma velocidade maior do que aquela com que pode ser reabsorvido. O acúmulo de líquido no espaço alveolar acarreta desequilíbrio da ventilação com relação à perfusão e hipoxemia. Felizmente, os pulmões são relativamente resistentes à formação de edema em comparação com outros tecidos.

O edema pulmonar é descrito como "cardiogênico" ou "não cardiogênico". A diferenciação é crucial, porque as condições são tratadas de maneiras diferentes. O edema cardiogênico, que se deve ao aumento da pressão hidrostática venosa pulmonar decorrente de insuficiência cardíaca do lado esquerdo, é tratado com diurético, redução da pós-carga e qualquer terapia específica que vise à causa da insuficiência cardíaca congestiva. O edema pulmonar cardiogênico e seu tratamento são discutidos em detalhes nos Capítulos 246 e 247. Nesta seção, são discutidas as causas não cardiogênicas de edema pulmonar.

É importante ter um conhecimento básico do movimento microvascular de líquido no pulmão.[237] Em animais saudáveis, quantidades diminutas de líquido e solutos extravasam pelas fendas entre as células endoteliais dos capilares e alcançam o espaço intersticial. Junções de oclusão, entre as células epiteliais dos alvéolos, impedem a entrada de líquido nos alvéolos. Em vez disso, o líquido intersticial se direciona ao espaço peribroncovascular, onde é removido pelos linfáticos e retorna à circulação. A equação de Starling, para a filtração através de uma membrana semipermeável, descreve os fatores que determinam a quantidade de extravasamento vascular (ver Capítulo 18). Na insuficiência cardíaca congestiva ou na sobrecarga de volume intravascular, o aumento da pressão hidrostática microvascular acarreta aumento também na filtração de líquido transvascular e edema pulmonar. Como a permeabilidade do endotélio capilar não se altera, esse líquido do edema contém pouca proteína. Em contrapartida, a maioria dos casos de edema pulmonar não cardiogênico ocorre quando a permeabilidade vascular aumenta em decorrência de lesão pulmonar direta ou indireta. Diferentemente do edema cardiogênico, o líquido do edema não cardiogênico contém concentração relativamente alta de proteína. O líquido com alto teor de proteína modifica o gradiente de pressão oncótica, o que altera ainda mais o fluxo de líquido. Tanto no edema cardiogênico como no não cardiogênico, o acúmulo de líquido alveolar, combinado com a diminuição da complacência pulmonar e a compressão de via respiratória, resultantes do edema, atuam em conjunto com esses fatores para aumentar a resistência vascular pulmonar. Hipoxemia é a consequência do desequilíbrio entre a ventilação e a perfusão, resultante de cada um desses fatores. A remoção espontânea do líquido alveolar depende do transporte ativo de sódio e cloreto, a partir da superfície luminal através das células epiteliais e da membrana basolateral. A direção do movimento da água segue passivamente a do sal. Como a remoção de líquido requer transporte ativo de sal através do epitélio, a lesão às células epiteliais não apenas leva à formação de edema, como impede a capacidade pulmonar de resolver o edema. Como resultado desses mecanismos de causa e resolução, o edema pulmonar não cardiogênico é mais refratário ao tratamento do que o cardiogênico.

Há uma ampla variedade de causas potenciais de edema pulmonar não cardiogênico (Boxe 242.6). A hipoalbuminemia grave (< 1,5 g/dℓ) está relacionada com a diminuição da pressão osmótica coloidal vascular. Embora a hipoalbuminemia possa contribuir na formação de edema pulmonar, os vasos linfáticos pulmonares são muito eficientes na remoção do líquido do espaço intersticial. Portanto, animais com pressão oncótica baixa são muito mais propensos a chegar ao veterinário com ascite, edema periférico ou mesmo efusão pleural do que com edema pulmonar.[238] Apesar disso, a hipoalbuminemia potencializa o edema pulmonar devido à alteração na permeabilidade vascular ou à administração excessiva de soluções cristaloides.[239] De maneira similar, embora a drenagem linfática seja importante para o equilíbrio intersticial normal de líquido, é mais provável que o comprometimento dela (p. ex., por causa de granuloma ou neoplasia, linfangite) resulte em efusão quilosa, do que em edema pulmonar. Choque elétrico ou lesão aguda ao sistema nervoso central podem levar a uma forma neurogênica particular de edema pulmonar não cardiogênico. Embora o mecanismo que causa o edema neurogênico não esteja completamente entendido, aventa-se a hipótese de que tanto a vasoconstrição pulmonar intensa (e o aumento resultante da pressão hidrostática pulmonar) quanto a resposta inflamatória aumentam a permeabilidade dos capilares pulmonares.[240] Mais comumente, o edema não cardiogênico está relacionado com a lesão (direta ou indireta) do epitélio pulmonar. Inflamação pulmonar e edema agudos ocasionados por uma variedade de lesões iniciais, resultando em comprometimento respiratório, podem ser denominados síndrome da angústia respiratória aguda (SARA).[241,242] Pode haver lesões pulmonares diretas (p. ex., pneumonia, aspiração, inalação de fumaça) ou indiretas (p. ex., pancreatite, uremia, sepse, traumatismo importante).[243,244] As definições em pesquisas veterinárias mais recentes relacionadas com essa síndrome foram elaboradas em 2007 e não estão mais alinhadas com as mais recentes definições elaboradas para uso em medicina humana.[241] Um painel de consenso desenvolveu um conjunto de definições relacionadas com a SARA em seres humanos, conhecido como "Definição de Berlim".[245] Nesse novo sistema de nomenclatura, a designação "lesão pulmonar aguda" foi abolida; a própria SARA atualmente é classificada como discreta, moderada ou grave, e foram desenvolvidos critérios diagnósticos específicos para ela. De acordo com tais critérios, a SARA é definida com um tempo característico de início (dentro de 1 semana do evento desencadeador ou início/agravamento de sintomas respiratórios), achados em radiografia ou TC do tórax (opacidades bilaterais, além das esperadas nas efusões, atelectasia ou lesões/massas expansivas) e origem não cardiogênica (exclusão de cardiopatia de gravidade suficiente para causar edema pulmonar cardiogênico).[245] A SARA é classificada como discreta (Pa_{O_2}/Fi_{O_2} = 200 a 300 mmHg, com pressão expiratória final positiva [PEFP] ≥ 5 cm H_2O), moderada (Pa_{O_2}/Fi_{O_2} = 100 a 200 mmHg, com PEFP ≥ 5 cm H_2O) ou grave (Pa_{O_2}/Fi_{O_2} = < 100 mmHg, com PEFP ≥ 5 cm H_2O), e essas categorias de gravidade têm valor preditivo quanto ao prognóstico de lesão pulmonar em seres humanos.[244,245] É muito provável que a medicina veterinária siga a humana e reveja as definições relacionadas com a SARA.

Boxe 242.6 Fatores predisponentes ao desenvolvimento de edema pulmonar não cardiogênico

Edema pulmonar neurogênico (p. ex., convulsões, eletrocussão, traumatismo craniano)

Edema pulmonar obstrutivo (p. ex., estrangulamento, paralisia de laringe, reexpansão pulmonar)

Doença sistêmica que predispõe à síndrome da angústia respiratória aguda (p. ex., sepse, choque, pancreatite grave, babesiose, intoxicação por paraquat, torção gástrica/esplênica/mesentérica, enterite viral, uremia)

Lesão pulmonar direta (p. ex., pneumonia por aspiração, pneumonia bacteriana, torção de lobo pulmonar, inalação de fumaça, pneumonite parasitária, contusão pulmonar, hiperóxia)

Hipoalbuminemia grave (p. ex., nefropatia com perda de proteína, linfangiectasia, insuficiência hepática)

Comprometimento da drenagem linfática (p. ex., linfangite, neoplasia linfática)

Causas diversas (p. ex., vasculite, afogamento, altitude elevada, embolia aérea, feocromocitoma)

Manifestação clínica

Qualquer que seja a causa, a manifestação clínica em animais com edema pulmonar não cardiogênico é similar. Os sinais clínicos podem surgir rapidamente ou demorar até 72 horas após a lesão desencadeante do edema. A gravidade dos sintomas depende da magnitude da lesão pulmonar e da quantidade de líquido acumulado; os sinais iniciais consistem em intolerância ao exercício e taquipneia. Uma tosse úmida pode produzir uma secreção espumosa. É possível observar dificuldade respiratória e ortopneia, e os animais podem apresentar cianose e/ou hemoptise. Esperam-se sons broncovesiculares ásperos e à auscultação notam-se crepitações durante a inspiração e/ou no fim da expiração. Ocasionalmente, quando o edema é grave, ocorre abafamento dos sons pulmonares. Em geral, animais com edema cardiogênico apresentam sopro cardíaco audível ou disritmia, mas esses achados também podem ser constatados em animais com edema não cardiogênico; portanto, sua *ausência* é fortemente sugestiva de uma anormalidade não cardiogênica, mas a presença de sopro ou arritmia é inespecífica. Taquicardia sinusal é comum em animais com edema cardiogênico, enquanto o estímulo vagal associado à doença pulmonar geralmente causa arritmia sinusal respiratória. Outras anormalidades notadas no exame físico podem estar relacionadas com uma anormalidade primária (p. ex., febre, dor).

Avaliação diagnóstica

Como os animais com edema pulmonar estão fragilizados, é preciso prosseguir com a investigação diagnóstica após estabilização clínica (ver tratamento adiante). As anormalidades no hemograma, no perfil bioquímico sérico e no exame de urina dependem quase inteiramente da doença primária. Da mesma forma, as alterações radiográficas variam dependendo da anormalidade primária e da magnitude do edema. Um padrão radiográfico intersticial não estruturado e/ou peribrônquico que progride com gravidade do edema gera um padrão alveolar; infiltrados difusos são comuns na SARA. Em geral, os campos pulmonares caudodorsais são os acometidos mais gravemente; porém, dependendo da fonte da lesão pulmonar, a localização predominante pode ser em qualquer local (p. ex., edema associado à aspiração de material particulado é mais grave nos lobos acometidos). Cardiomegalia (em especial o aumento do átrio esquerdo) ou congestão venosa pulmonar são mais sugestivas de edema cardiogênico do que de não cardiogênico. Hipoxemia é esperada, e tipicamente o gradiente alveolar-arterial de oxigênio encontra-se aumentado devido ao desequilíbrio entre ventilação e perfusão (ver Capítulo 128).

Tratamento

O tratamento do edema pulmonar não cardiogênico deve incluir medidas para tratar a doença primária. Em certos casos, pode ser impossível corrigir a causa desencadeante (p. ex., eletrocussão) ou fazer isso pode levar tempo (p. ex., pancreatite). O tratamento deve ser direcionado à hipoxemia. Quando a dificuldade respiratória é aparente, ou se a Pa_{O_2} for < 80 mmHg ou a Sp_{O_2} < 94% (ver Capítulo 98), deve-se fornecer oxigênio suplementar da maneira menos estressante possível (ver Capítulo 131). Como os animais com hipoxemia em geral estão estressados, o uso criterioso de sedativos (p. ex., sulfato de morfina ou acepromazina IV) pode estar indicado. É preciso cautela, porque os sedativos podem deprimir a respiração. Deve-se deixar que animais com dificuldade respiratória se posicionem como queiram para ficar mais confortáveis; porém, se estiverem em decúbito, devem ser mantidos em posição esternal ou colocados com o pulmão acometido mais gravemente na posição dependente. Animais com SARA geralmente têm comprometimento respiratório crítico; se a estabilização não for possível com medidas menos invasivas, intubação e suporte ventilatório podem ser necessários. Se o tratamento inicial for incapaz de manter a $Sp_{O_2} \geq 90\%$, a $Pa_{O_2} > 60$ mmHg e a Pa_{CO_2}

< 60 mmHg, deve-se providenciar ventilação com pressão positiva (VPP), que também pode ser indicada para aliviar o esforço respiratório persistente, que pode resultar em fadiga dos músculos respiratórios.

A administração de diurético é mais efetiva na resolução do edema cardiogênico ou daquele associado à sobrecarga de volume intravascular do que do edema não cardiogênico. O edema pulmonar neurogênico se deve ao aumento da pressão hidrostática e à alteração na permeabilidade vascular. Portanto, diuréticos como a furosemida podem ter algum benefício nessa condição. Em geral, o edema pulmonar neurogênico se resolve sem tratamento específico, supondo-se que as funções neurológica e respiratória possam ser preservadas por 48 a 72 horas após a lesão desencadeante.[240] A administração de bloqueadores alfa-adrenérgicos e de dobutamina foi sugerida como benéfica no tratamento de edema pulmonar neurogênico. Fármacos que resultam em vasodilatação cerebral devem ser evitados. O edema não cardiogênico resultante de hipoalbuminenia, ou exacerbado por tal condição, pode ser tratado com solução coloide. A transfusão de plasma para recuperar a pressão osmótica coloidal é impraticável, devido ao grande volume necessário e ao alto custo da transfusão de grande volume de plasma.[246] Em vez disso, em animais com edema pulmonar resultante de diminuição da pressão oncótica (ver Capítulo 130), deve-se realizar transfusão de albumina ou de soluções coloides sintéticas. Lamentavelmente, a administração de coloides sintéticos ou a transfusão de xenoalbumina podem causar reações adversas.[247-249] Como complicação adicional da administração de coloide, qualquer aumento na permeabilidade vascular pode ocasionar extravasamento de coloide para o espaço alveolar. Isso, por sua vez, pode agravar o edema. É preciso considerar o equilíbrio entre essas limitações e os benefícios do tratamento em cada caso.

O tratamento clínico da SARA, como o da síndrome da resposta inflamatória sistêmica (SRIS; ver Capítulo 132), que em geral acompanha a SARA, é complexo. No tratamento da SARA, usa-se uma variedade de fármacos que inibem a inflamação, alteram a produção de citocinas ou enzimas, ou atuam de diversas maneiras, com sucesso variável (em geral mínimo).[242,250] A administração intravenosa de líquido pode ser necessária para o tratamento apropriado da anormalidade primária (p. ex., uremia), mas precisa ser criteriosa, a fim de evitar o agravamento do edema devido ao aumento da pressão hidrostática.[251] Em contrapartida, em animais bem hidratados, pode-se induzir redução da pressão hidrostática pela administração de furosemida, que também pode causar broncodilatação e melhorar o fluxo linfático, mas não terá os efeitos marcantes observados quando há resolução do edema pulmonar cardiogênico. Embora, na verdade, a ventilação mecânica possa exacerbar as alterações pulmonares funcionais e estruturais, em geral é necessária no tratamento de seres humanos com SARA.[244] Provavelmente o mesmo se aplica aos animais.[252-254] O tratamento da SARA depende, em grande parte, do fornecimento de oxigênio e do tratamento da doença primária, enquanto se dá tempo para que os pulmões se recuperem por si mesmos.[244]

Câncer pulmonar

No pulmão, ocorrem neoplasia respiratória primária e metástases de cânceres não respiratórios. É importante diferenciar tumores pulmonares primários menos comuns de uma variedade de neoplasias metastáticas mais comuns, porque o diagnóstico, o tratamento e o prognóstico de tumores pulmonares primários diferem daqueles do câncer metastático. Animais com câncer pulmonar podem ser levados ao veterinário por causa de tosse, hemoptise, respiração ofegante ou outros sinais de disfunção respiratória. Em geral, os cânceres pulmonares são identificados em radiografias de animais sem sinais respiratórios durante a avaliação de sinais inespecíficos, como perda de peso ou neoplasia extratorácica. Ocasionalmente, animais com tumores pulmonares são trazidos para investigação de condições paraneoplásicas, como osteopatia hipertrófica ou polineuropatia.

Câncer pulmonar metastático e especial

Normalmente, o leito vascular pulmonar recebe todo o seu sangue do ventrículo direito, durante cada ciclo cardíaco. O sangue passa através de numerosos leitos capilares de pequeno diâmetro, bem oxigenados, o que faz do pulmão um local ideal para metástase. A hipótese "semeadura-solo" descreve o desprendimento de células tumorais, como sementes, que só podem germinar em solo (tecido) adequado.[255] Além da mecânica simples, o pulmão pode ser o alvo específico de certos tumores como local preferencial de metástase. A metástase do câncer é complexa; as células cancerosas precisam se desprender do tumor primário, ter acesso a vasos sanguíneos ou linfáticos para serem levadas a locais distantes, migrar a partir dos vasos para os tecidos, aderir a eles e, então, crescer no novo local (ver Capítulo 338).[255] Praticamente todas as neoplasias podem ocasionar metástase nos pulmões, porém algumas particularmente propensas a isso incluem melanoma bucal e do leito ungueal, carcinoma de tireoide, osteossarcoma, hemangiossarcoma e carcinoma de mama.

Manifestação clínica e avaliação diagnóstica. Em geral, os animais com câncer pulmonar metastático manifestam poucos sintomas respiratórios, mesmo com uma grande massa tumoral. A metástase pulmonar costuma ser detectada durante triagem por meio de radiografias do tórax. A triagem radiográfica para metástase deve incluir uma combinação de imagens obtidas em decúbito, nas posições dorsal, ventral, lateral direita e lateral esquerda, porque a atelectasia discreta que ocorre no pulmão acometido pode dificultar a detecção do tumor. A aparência radiográfica de câncer metastático varia muito, tipicamente com poucos a muitos nódulos intersticiais de tamanho variável, distribuídos por todo o pulmão (Figura 242.5). No entanto, a metástase pode surgir como nódulo solitário, padrão pulmonar intersticial ou alveolar, intersticial miliar ou até cistos múltiplos (Figura 242.6).[257-260] Mesmo com o posicionamento apropriado, o artefato de técnica pode dificultar a detecção de tumores com menos de 8 a 9 mm de diâmetro.[17] Embora se tenha postulado que a exibição inversa de radiografias digitais de tórax melhore a capacidade de detecção de nódulos pulmonares, isso não foi corroborado em um pequeno estudo recente.[261] A TC do tórax é o meio mais sensível de obtenção de imagens de tumores pequenos, mas a necessidade de anestesia ou sedação, equipamento e recursos financeiros impede que a TC seja um exame de triagem de rotina.[17,256,260,262] Como não há aparência radiográfica patognomônica de metástase pulmonar, os animais não devem ser diagnosticados com base apenas em radiografias do tórax quando um tumor primário não foi identificado de maneira definitiva. Em vez disso, a natureza neoplásica da doença pulmonar deve ser confirmada ou refutada por meio de técnicas de aspirado ou lavado de vias respiratórias ou de biopsia (ver Capítulo 240).

Tratamento. Infelizmente, o tratamento de câncer pulmonar metastático raras vezes tem benefício a longo prazo. O tratamento com tirosinoquinase pode ter eficácia limitada.[263] Nos casos em que há apenas um ou poucos nódulos pulmonares, a ressecção cirúrgica via toracoscopia ou toracotomia (com ou sem quimioterapia adjuvante) pode ser uma opção.[264,266] Particularmente, a metastesectomia pode ser útil nos casos em que ocorrem metástases bem depois do tratamento do tumor primário.[267] Foram descritas terapias inalatórias com quimioterápicos, moléculas imunológicas (i. e., interleucina 2 lipossômica) e terapia gênica resultando na produção de moléculas imunogênicas para o tratamento da neoplasia pulmonar primária e também da lesão metastática.[268-273] Tal tratamento ainda não está bem estabelecido nem disponível com facilidade para animais de estimação.

Linfoma pulmonar

O linfoma pode se instalar nos pulmões de cães e gatos, juntamente com órgãos linfoides e sólidos ou, raramente, sem massa tumoral adicional. Nas radiografias do tórax, observam-se padrões infiltrativos intersticiais, alveolares e mistos nos pulmões, com ou sem linfadenopatia no hilo e no mediastino concomitante. Quando a presença de linfoma é confirmada em outros tecidos e não há outras causas desencadeantes (p. ex., cardiopatia avançada), os infiltrados pulmonares vistos em radiografias podem ser atribuídos, de maneira presuntiva, ao linfoma. A técnica de AAF, o exame do LBA e biopsia pulmonar podem ser usados para confirmar a existência de um linfoma pulmonar solitário. No Capítulo 344, há uma discussão mais completa sobre linfoma e seu tratamento.

Granulomatose linfomatoide pulmonar

A granulomatose linfomatoide (GL) é um câncer linfoproliferativo raro no qual as células linfoides atípicas se infiltram em torno de vasos sanguíneos e os destroem. Em seres humanos, é considerada um precursor de baixo grau do linfoma de linfócito T. A imunofenotipagem de vários tumores de cães mostrou a presença de marcadores de linfócito T e, às vezes, marcadores de linfócito B.[274,275] Embora o acometimento pulmonar seja relatado com maior frequência, outros locais podem estar envolvidos, inclusive linfonodos, órgãos abdominais e derme. Cães de qualquer idade e gênero podem ser acometidos, mas há poucos relatos de casos em gatos.[274-281] Em vários cães acometidos, foi documentada leucocitose com eosinofilia e/ou basofilia, mas

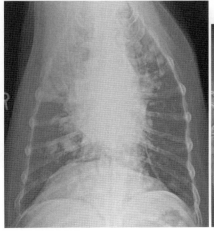
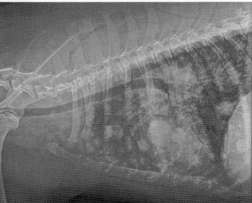

Figura 242.5 Radiografias lateral e ventrodorsal mostram a imagem estereotípica de metástase pulmonar. Nódulos múltiplos, amplamente distribuídos e de tamanhos variáveis, podem ser vistos em todos os campos pulmonares.

alguns desses animais tinham infecção parasitária concomitante. As radiografias de tórax mostram, tipicamente, massas pulmonares e/ou consolidação lobar. Infiltrados intersticiais e alveolares também são comuns, bem como linfadenopatia traqueobrônquica. Embora os resultados do AAF ou do lavado de via respiratória possam ser sugestivos de linfoma, a biopsia pulmonar é necessária para definir o diagnóstico, porque a relação particular entre o infiltrado granulomatoso linfoide e a vasculite define a doença. O emprego de exames menos invasivos é para, em grande parte, excluir causas mais comuns de consolidação pulmonar. Animais com hipoxemia podem precisar de cuidados de suporte, mas o tratamento definitivo baseia-se na quimioterapia.

Os protocolos usados no tratamento são idênticos aos empregados para tratar o linfoma (ver Capítulo 344). Em geral, o tratamento resulta em remissão duradoura, porém pode haver recorrência do acometimento pulmonar ou desenvolvimento de linfoma em outros sistemas orgânicos, meses a anos após o sucesso aparente do tratamento.

Histiocitose maligna

A histiocitose maligna (sarcoma histiocítico disseminado) é uma das várias doenças histiocíticas mais comuns em cães do que em gatos (ver Capítulo 350). A doença foi reconhecida pela primeira vez em cães da raça Pastor-de-Berna, nos quais se suspeita de uma

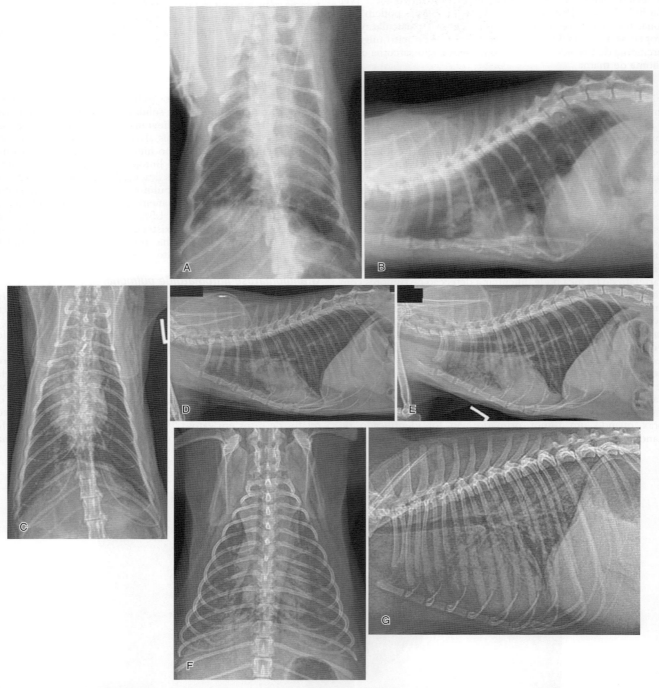

Figura 242.6 A aparência radiográfica de metástase pulmonar é muito variável. **A** e **B**. Múltiplas lesões císticas são vistas nas imagens lateral e dorsoventral desse gato com carcinoma espinocelular metastático. **C** a **E**. Nota-se um nódulo solitário dorsal à bifurcação da traqueia, na imagem lateral direita, notando-se padrões alveolares e intersticiais nessa gata com carcinoma de mama metastático. **F** e **G**. Note o padrão intersticial difuso a alveolar nesse cão com linfoma disseminado.

CAPÍTULO 242 • Doenças do Parênquima Pulmonar

base genética com um modo de herança poligênico.[282,283] Outras raças com alta predisposição entre aquelas diagnosticadas com essa condição são Retriever de Pelo Curto, Golden Retriever e Rottweiler. Como acontece no linfoma, a histiocitose maligna pode acometer qualquer combinação de órgãos, incluindo medula óssea, sistema nervoso central, vísceras abdominais e pulmões.[283,284] Células histiocíticas atípicas (uma linhagem de células mononucleares) acumulam-se nos órgãos acometidos, resultando em disfunção. A manifestação clínica, em geral, envolve sintomas inespecíficos, como letargia e anorexia; tosse e/ou dispneia são comuns.[284-287] Quando há acometimento pulmonar, as radiografias podem mostrar linfadenopatia torácica (linfonodos traqueobrônquicos e esternais, em especial), nódulos pulmonares (geralmente grandes e, com maior frequência, no lobo pulmonar medial direito) ou infiltrado intersticial e, algumas vezes, efusão pleural.[288] À TC, a maioria das massas é discreta a moderadamente acentuada e heterogênea, com margens pouco definidas e broncocêntricas.[288] O diagnóstico, em geral, baseia-se no exame histopatológico do tecido envolvido ou em achados clínicos sugestivos e características confirmatórias no exame citológico da medula óssea. Até o momento, a maioria dos protocolos quimioterápicos, em grande parte, não foi efetiva, e o prognóstico continua sendo reservado a grave.

Recentemente, outra doença pulmonar histiocítica, a histiocitose de células de Langerhans pulmonar felina, foi descrita em sete gatos,[283,289] todos adultos idosos com insuficiência respiratória progressiva. As radiografias mostraram um padrão broncointersticial difuso, com opacidades miliares a nodulares; todos foram diagnosticados durante a necropsia.

Câncer pulmonar primário

É incomum em cães e ainda menos comum em gatos. Foi proposta uma relação entre o acúmulo de poeira inalada (i. e., antracose) e cânceres pulmonares primários, mas não se confirmou uma relação definitiva com a convivência de animais de estimação com fumantes ou criados em ambiente urbano.[290,291] Quando ocorrem tumores pulmonares primários em animais de estimação, em geral são malignos. Os adenocarcinomas predominam, e a maioria dos outros tumores é classificada morfologicamente como carcinoma, carcinoma espinocelular ou carcinoma anaplásico.[292-297] Tumores pulmonares mesenquimais primários são extremamente raros.

Manifestação clínica. Na medicina de pequenos animais, a maioria dos tumores pulmonares primários é detectada em animais idosos. Metade dos cães com neoplasia pulmonar primária é levada à consulta para avaliação de tosse improdutiva crônica.[291,294,295,298] Embora também possa haver outros sintomas respiratórios, até um terço dos cães com tumores pulmonares primários não exibe sinais respiratórios clínicos.[294,295,298] Similarmente, gatos com tumores pulmonares primários geralmente não apresentam sintomas respiratórios. Apenas 20 a 40% dos gatos com tumores pulmonares primários exibem dispneia.[292,299] Tosse, taquipneia, cianose e hemoptise são ocorrências ocasionais em cães ou gatos. Os animais acometidos, de ambas as espécies, podem ser levados ao veterinário devido à perda de peso, letargia e diminuição do apetite, com ou sem sintomas respiratórios concomitantes. Pacientes com neoplasia pulmonar primária também são levados ao veterinário para avaliação de claudicação devido à osteopatia paraneoplásica ou, no caso de gatos, metástase de neoplasia pulmonar nas falanges (síndrome pulmonar-digital).[291,300] Outros problemas constatados na consulta veterinária podem incluir edema de cabeça e pescoço, ascite resultante da obstrução do fluxo de veias ou linfáticos causada pelo tumor, vômitos e diarreia. Às vezes, efusão pleural ou pneumotórax espontâneo acarretam dificuldade respiratória súbita.

Avaliação diagnóstica. Embora praticamente todos os padrões radiográficos sejam possíveis em animais com câncer pulmonar primário, em geral são observadas massas parenquimatosas raras ou solitárias.[293,299,301,302] Tumores nodulares solitários,

que não os histiocíticos, são detectados mais frequentemente nos lobos pulmonares caudais (Figura 242.7).[293,299] À TC, os tumores pulmonares primários costumam ser massas barocêntricas bem circunscritas, com broncogramas aéreos internos; até 25% desses tumores progrediram para metástase no momento do diagnóstico.[301] Como acontece na metástase pulmonar, o padrão radiográfico não pode ser considerado patognomônico, e o diagnóstico diferencial de nódulos pulmonares solitários ou multifocais precisa ser considerado (Boxe 242.7).

É preciso confirmar o diagnóstico pelo exame microscópico de células para satisfazer os critérios de malignidade. Amostras obtidas de LBA ou lavado traqueal (ver Capítulo 101) ajudam a excluir doença não neoplásica e raramente contêm células com morfologia neoplásica. A localização radiográfica de nódulos pode ser usada para nortear a introdução da agulha utilizada para AAF; ademais, podem ser obtidos aspirados com orientação fluoroscópica ou de TC.[16,26] Massas sólidas não aeradas localizadas próximo à margem pulmonar são viáveis para aspiração com agulha orientada por ultrassom, mas há risco, mínimo, de semeadura celular no trajeto da agulha.[303,304] Só se deve recorrer à biopsia percutânea orientada por exame de imagem devido ao risco de complicações (i. e., pneumotórax, hemotórax).[26] Embora se tenha encontrado uma boa correlação entre o diagnóstico obtido por AAF e por biopsia percutânea, é menos provável que os resultados do AAF forneçam um diagnóstico conclusivo.[25,26] Outras técnicas de biopsia pulmonar consistem em toracoscopia, biopsia "key-hole" e toracotomia parcial ou total.[305-307] Dependendo do tamanho e da localização do tumor, essas técnicas também possibilitam a extirpação completa do tumor pulmonar.

Como a ocorrência de metástase influencia muito o prognóstico, deve-se tentar fazer o estadiamento do tumor antes da lobectomia pulmonar. São necessários esforços razoáveis para detectar tumores distantes, porque os nódulos pulmonares solitários podem ser tanto metastáticos quanto tumores primários. Recomenda-se um exame físico completo (incluindo próstata, glândulas mamárias e ossos longos), bem como radiografias de abdome e imagens ultrassonográficas. O ideal é fazer TC do tórax antes de qualquer intervenção cirúrgica planejada, a fim de identificar pequenas massas em outros lobos pulmonares que possam passar despercebidas. Em cães, os tumores pulmonares primários aparecem tipicamente nas radiografias como uma massa solitária bem circunscrita na periferia de um lobo pulmonar caudal, mas até um terço desse tipo de neoplasia acomete múltiplos lobos.[292,293,295,301] Além disso, a TC melhora a capacidade de detectar acometimento de linfonodos traqueobrônquicos, o que influencia o prognóstico.[297,301]

Tratamento. A extirpação é o tratamento de escolha para tumores pulmonares primários restritos a um lobo. Como o envolvimento de linfonodos tem um impacto negativo no prognóstico, até mesmo linfonodos de tamanho normal devem ser submetidos a exame histológico.[296-298] Os achados prognósticos favoráveis incluem remoção completa do tumor, presença de um único tumor sem metástase, ausência de sinais clínicos relativos a um tumor pulmonar, baixo grau histológico ou tumor mais bem diferenciado, localização periférica do tumor e ausência de efusão pleural.[292,294,296,298,299,308] O tempo de sobrevida pós-operatória varia muito, mas pode ser até de 2 anos. Não se dispõe de grandes relatos sobre radiação tradicional ou quimioterapia no tratamento de tumores pulmonares primários em cães e gatos. O dano a estruturas intratorácicas e o movimento constante do alvo devido à respiração limitam o uso da radioterapia tradicional no tratamento dos tumores pulmonares, mas a radioterapia com intensidade modulada pode ser um tratamento efetivo, com poucos efeitos adversos.[309] A vinorelbina, um inibidor de mitose que atinge concentrações pulmonares mais altas do que outros alcaloides da vinca, foi usada com algum sucesso no tratamento de dois cães com carcinoma broncoalveolar.[310,311] Também aventou-se a possibilidade de o piroxicam, um antiinflamatório não esteroide que possui efeitos antitumorais, ser útil no tratamento de carcinoma pulmonar.[312] A quimioterapia

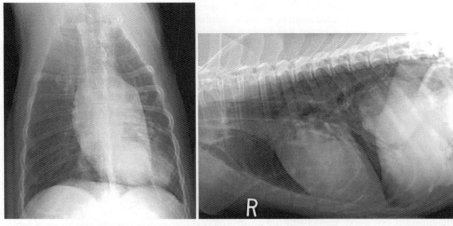

Figura 242.7 O carcinoma pulmonar primário em cães costuma surgir como um nódulo solitário nos lobos pulmonares caudais, conforme visto nas imagens lateral e ventrodorsal desse cão com uma massa solitária visível nas radiografias do lobo pulmonar caudal esquerdo.

Boxe 242.7 Diagnósticos diferenciais de nódulos pulmonares solitários ou multifocais

- Malformação arteriovenosa
- Atelectasia
- Pneumonia eosinofílica (também denominada infiltrado pulmonar com eosinofilia, broncopneumopatia eosinofílica, granuloma eosinofílico)
- Vesículas cheias de líquido
- Pneumonia focal
- Bronquiectasia focal com preenchimento de muco
- Granuloma fúngico
- Granuloma causado por corpo estranho
- Hematoma
- Neoplasia pulmonar metastática
- Impactação mucoide
- Granuloma parasitário
- Neoplasia pulmonar primária (em geral carcinoma)
- Abscesso pulmonar
- Cistos pulmonares
- Parasitas pulmonares
- Tromboembolismo pulmonar
- Tuberculose

intracavitária foi utilizada ocasionalmente, com bom resultado, em cães com efusão pleural maligna, carcinomatose, sarcomatose ou mesotelioma.[313,314] Vários relatos documentam a utilidade potencial da quimioterapia inalatória ou da administração, por inalação, de modificadores da resposta biológica, no tratamento do câncer pulmonar primário ou metastático.[268-273]

Doença pulmonar intersticial

As doenças pulmonares intersticiais (DPIs) representam um grupo heterogêneo de doenças não infecciosas e não malignas do trato respiratório, que podem ser diagnosticadas de maneira definitiva apenas com o exame histopatológico do tecido pulmonar.[315] As alterações teciduais situam-se no espaço entre a membrana basal das células epiteliais dos alvéolos e das células epiteliais dos capilares (i. e., o interstício pulmonar), além dos vasos sanguíneos e linfáticos adjacentes. Essas doenças relativamente raras caracterizam-se por inflamação, fibrose e/ou acúmulos anormais de proteína ou lipídio que restringem o volume pulmonar efetivo e diminuem a complacência pulmonar. Embora o diagnóstico de DPI esteja aumentando, elas continuam mal caracterizadas e, provavelmente, são subdiagnosticadas em cães e gatos.

Como seria esperado em um grupo heterogêneo de doenças, as causas de DPI são muitas. Inalação de substâncias tóxicas, alergênios e produtos irritantes (p. ex., fibras minerais) podem causar inflamação do epitélio alveolar e subsequente reação, ocasionando DPI. O dano tecidual também pode resultar da exposição sistêmica a fármacos ou toxinas, ou de reações de hipersensibilidade. Infelizmente, muitas DPIs continuam sendo idiopáticas. Várias DPIs foram reconhecidas em cães e gatos, incluindo pneumonia eosinofílica, fibrose pulmonar idiopática (FPI), pneumonite intersticial linfocítica (PIL), bronquiolite obliterante com pneumonia organizada (BOPO), pneumonia lipídica endógena, proteinose pulmonar alveolar, silicose e asbestose.[1,2,316-329] A maioria das DPIs é descrita como relatos de caso isolado ou um pequeno número de casos.

Pneumonia eosinofílica

Foram usados muitos nomes para descrever as doenças eosinofílicas dos bronquíolos terminais, alvéolos e vasos sanguíneos em cães e gatos (ver Capítulo 241). Denominada também, de maneira variável, de pneumonia eosinofílica, infiltrado pulmonar com eosinofilia/eosinófilos (IPE), broncopneumopatia eosinofílica, hipersensibilidade pulmonar, pneumonia granulomatosa eosinofílica, granulomatose pulmonar eosinofílica, síndrome hipereosinofílica e pneumonite eosinofílica, há pouca concordância sobre a classificação dos distúrbios pulmonares eosinofílicos.[327,330-336] Em seres humanos, a pneumonia eosinofílica pode ser classificada de maneira ampla, de origem determinada ou não determinada e aguda ou crônica. A pneumonia eosinofílica de origem determinada pode ser causada por parasitas, fungos ou outros microrganismos infecciosos, pela administração de fármacos ou pela exposição a toxinas.[337] Em seres humanos, a pneumonia eosinofílica (PE) de origem não determinada é subdividida em doença sistêmica com acometimento pulmonar (i. e., síndrome hipereosinofílica, SHE) ou pneumonia eosinofílica isolada.

Embora a doença de via respiratória eosinofílica reativa (i. e., asma) seja mais comum em gatos, a PE de origem não determinada é mais comum em cães. A pneumonia eosinofílica acomete mais frequentemente fêmeas do que machos.[338] Foi relatada predisposição à doença em cães das raças Husky Siberiano, Malamute do Alasca e Rottweiler, mas cães de qualquer raça podem ser acometidos.[336,338,339] A evolução clínica da doença pode ser aguda ou crônica. Tosse é o achado clínico mais consistente, mas às vezes são detectados engasgo, ânsia de vômito, esforço respiratório e sintomas não respiratórios, como perda de peso (em particular associados à infecção sistêmica, neoplasia ou SHE). Um padrão broncointersticial difuso é notado mais comumente em cães com PE, mas também se detecta padrão alveolar (Figura 242.8). É fácil confundir infiltrado denso com neoplasia pulmonar (Figura 242.9). A PE é uma das doenças mais comuns associadas à bronquiectasia,

CAPÍTULO 242 • Doenças do Parênquima Pulmonar 1135

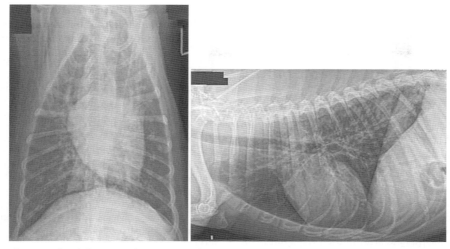

Figura 242.8 Imagem lateral e ventrodorsal de um cão da raça Rottweiler, macho, não castrado, com 1 ano de idade e pneumonia eosinofílica. Note o padrão broncointersticial grave em todos os lobos pulmonares; múltiplas linhas de fissura pleural são mais bem identificadas na imagem ventrodorsal. São vistos infiltrados alveolares em manchas focais na altura do ápice cardíaco.

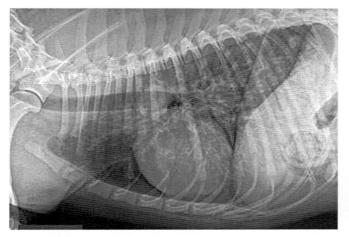

Figura 242.9 Imagem lateral esquerda do tórax de um cão mestiço com 3 anos que apresentava pneumonia eosinofílica. Note o padrão broncointersticial acentuado. Infiltrados pulmonares densos podem ser facilmente confundidos com neoplasia pulmonar.

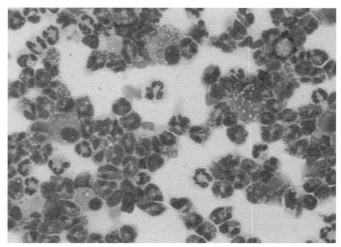

Figura 242.10 Fotomicrografia do lavado broncoalveolar de cão da raça Rottweiler, macho, não castrado, com 1 ano de idade, com pneumonia eosinofílica (aumento de 500×). As radiografias mostram padrão broncointersticial difuso, com infiltrado alveolar também difuso (ver Figura 242.8). A amostra altamente celular obtida do lavado broncoalveolar contém 90 a 95% de eosinófilos, com menor número de macrófagos alveolares. Não foram detectados microrganismos, tampouco células neoplásicas. (Cortesia da Dra. Linda Berent, University of Missouri.) (*Esta figura se encontra reproduzida em cores no Encarte.*)

em cães.[339] Embora se identifique eosinofilia periférica em aproximadamente 50 a 60% dos cães acometidos, a ausência de eosinofilia não exclui a possibilidade de PE. O exame de amostra de LBA de cães com PE indica aumento da celularidade (> 200 a 400 células/µℓ) com aumento acentuado na porcentagem de eosinófilos (Figura 242.10). Deve-se examinar com cuidado a amostra do lavado broncoalveolar de cães com suspeita de PE, em busca de células neoplásicas (p. ex., mastócitos, linfoma), elementos fúngicos ou parasitas pulmonares, e fazer cultura microbiológica. Em cães com lavado de via respiratória eosinofílico, deve-se excluir a possibilidade de infecção parasitária mediante exames de fezes seriados (*i. e.*, teste de flotação em amostra centrifugada, com sulfato de zinco e teste de sedimentação de Baermann) e/ou vermifugação, bem como pesquisa do antígeno de dirofilária.

Após a exclusão de causas infecciosas primárias, neoplásicas ou medicamentosas, o tratamento da PE idiopática baseia-se principalmente em um protocolo com doses decrescentes de corticosteroides (p. ex., predniso(lo)na, com dose inicial de 1 a 2 mg/kg/24 h). O prognóstico em termos de recuperação varia de razoável a excelente, a menos que haja bronquiectasia grave.[327,331,336,338,339] O prognóstico de cães com acometimento pulmonar isolado é melhor do que o daqueles com infiltrados em outros órgãos (*i. e.*, SHE).

Pneumonia lipídica

Resulta de uma resposta inflamatória ao acúmulo de glóbulos de lipídios nos espaços aéreos alveolares.[2,325] A pneumonia lipídica exógena segue-se à aspiração de lipídio – por exemplo, após a aspiração de óleo mineral – ou de produtos à base de petróleo usados no tratamento de constipação intestinal ou de tricobezoar.[340-342] A pneumonia lipídica endógena (PLEn) não está associada à aspiração. Embora incomum, a PLEn tem sido relatada em uma variedade de espécies animais, incluindo gatos e cães.[2,3,323,325,329,343] A lesão de pneumócitos associada à doença pulmonar obstrutiva, incluindo doenças relacionadas com a neoplasia pulmonar, foi associada à PLEn.[343,344] A lesão de pneumócitos acarreta degeneração celular, com liberação de colesterol e produção excessiva de surfactante com alto teor de colesterol.[2] Os lipídios então são fagocitados por macrófagos pulmonares; esses macrófagos espumosos acumulam-se nos alvéolos. O lipídio endógeno também está envolvido na patogenia de algumas pneumonias infecciosas, como a pneumonia micobacteriana atípica em gatos.[167] Em outras circunstâncias, não se consegue detectar qualquer anormalidade pulmonar primária associada à PLEn.[345]

A pneumonia lipídica endógena é tão rara que não é possível fazer afirmações sobre os dados de resenha típicos. Em uma série de 24 gatos com PLEn, diagnosticada durante a necropsia, as idades variaram de 1 a 15 anos, com média etária de 8,4 anos.[2] Gatos foram levados ao veterinário devido a uma variedade de sintomas inespecíficos, incluindo letargia, anorexia e perda de peso. Apenas 16 dos 24 animais apresentavam sinais respiratórios, como dispneia (11/24; 46%) ou tosse (8/24; 33%). Não se detectou lipemia em qualquer um desses gatos. As anormalidades radiográficas foram variáveis e inespecíficas. Como os animais com PLEn, em geral, têm outra doença pulmonar (p. ex., dirofilariose, neoplasia, infecção bacteriana), não é possível determinar quais lesões estão relacionadas com a PLEn e quais com a doença concomitante.[2,325,346] O LBA de animais com PLEn pode ser normal, sugestivo de doença respiratória simultânea ou conter macrófagos espumosos preenchidos por lipídios.[345] Na maioria das vezes, usa-se a necropsia para obter o diagnóstico de PLEn em pacientes veterinários, significando que há pouca informação sobre opções de tratamento potenciais ou sobre o prognóstico.[2,247,251,325,329] Quando se detecta uma doença pulmonar específica concomitante em animais com PLEn, deve-se tratar aquela doença diretamente. Em seres humanos, há relatos de que a PLEn idiopática responde ao tratamento com corticosteroides.[346a]

Fibrose pulmonar idiopática

A fibrose pulmonar pode ocorrer como uma reação à lesão pulmonar ou como uma doença primária de etiologia desconhecida (i. e., FPI).[347] FPI foi diagnosticada em cães e gatos. Na última espécie, a condição compartilha os aspectos histológicos da pneumonia intersticial habitual (PIH), que caracteriza a FPI em seres humanos.[348] Tais características incluem fibrose intersticial, proliferação de fibroblastos e miofibroblastos, aumento dos espaços de ar revestidos por epitélio proeminente (conhecidos como semelhantes a "favo de mel") e alterações inflamatórias relativamente brandas. Os pulmões são acometidos de maneira heterogênea, com áreas normais entremeadas com tecido doente. As lesões da FPI em cães possuem algumas características histopatológicas da PIH, mais do que a de outro tipo comum de pneumonia intersticial humana conhecida como "pneumonia intersticial inespecífica".[316,320,349,350]

Manifestação clínica. Predisposições raciais estão bem descritas para a FPI de cães, mas não de gatos, sendo os cães das raças West Highland White e Stafordshire Bull Terrier os mais predispostos. Em cães Terrier, a FPI acomete predominantemente indivíduos idosos (média etária de 8 anos) e se manifesta inicialmente com tosse e intolerância ao exercício. Em seguida, com a progressão da doença, nota-se dificuldade respiratória.[317,318,320,351-354] Ao contrário de cães, gatos de qualquer idade e gênero podem ser acometidos por FPI. Como os gatos conseguem ocultar sinais clínicos de doença pulmonar, eles podem se apresentar à consulta com o que parece ser um quadro de angústia respiratória de início muito agudo ou até mesmo morte súbita, em vez de tosse ou aumento insidioso do esforço respiratório.[1,354] É comum identificar sons pulmonares adventícios em animais com FPI. Especialmente em cães, auscultam-se crepitações inspiratórias proeminentes em todos os campos pulmonares. Um sopro cardíaco sistólico devido à regurgitação da tricúspide pode ser notado, em particular nos cães que apresentam hipertensão pulmonar/cor pulmonale. Cianose é um achado comum em cães (mas não em gatos) com FPI, na doença em estágio terminal. Não há alterações específicas nos exames de sangue ou de urina de rotina sugestivas de FPI, mas, no estágio final da doença, a hipoxemia pode resultar em policitemia e/ou aumento da atividade sérica de fosfatase alcalina.[350] Os achados radiográficos em gatos com FPI variam muito e incluem padrões bronquiolar, intersticial e alveolar; como essa doença costuma ser acompanhada de neoplasia pulmonar, é possível detectar nódulos pulmonares em gatos acometidos.[1,354,355] Em cães, o infiltrado broncointersticial é o padrão radiográfico pulmonar mais comumente constatado, porém essa anormalidade não é um sinal sensível, tampouco específico, da doença.

A percepção de crepitações inspiratórias sonoras, na ausência de um padrão pulmonar alveolar, pode ser importante indício da presença de FPI em cães.[315,350,351] Usa-se TC de alta resolução para confirmar o diagnóstico de FPI, na ausência de exame histológico, em seres humanos e, do mesmo modo, em cães.[350,356,357] Os poucos relatos de TC do tórax de gatos com FPI descrevem aumento focal da atenuação de tecido mole, massas teciduais e áreas de consolidação.[354] Pode-se usar ecocardiografia para excluir a possibilidade de insuficiência cardíaca congestiva como causa dos sinais clínicos, se não for identificada lesão cardíaca grave o suficiente para explicar os sintomas do paciente; uma cardiopatia primária pode coexistir independentemente na mesma população de pacientes, como aqueles acometidos com FPI e, em tais casos, pode ser um desafio determinar se a responsável pelos sinais clínicos é a doença pulmonar ou a cardiopatia (e assim encaminhar o paciente para um especialista em medicina interna e um cardiologista). Pode-se usar a mensuração da velocidade da regurgitação tricúspide para fazer uma estimativa da pressão na artéria pulmonar, medida útil porque a hipertensão pulmonar frequentemente está associada à FPI em cães e pode responder ao tratamento clínico (ver Capítulo 243).[350,358] Títulos sorológicos, broncoscopia, LBA e testes diagnósticos semelhantes ajudam a excluir outras doenças respiratórias, além da FPI. Foram investigados vários biomarcadores potenciais para FPI em cães, mas nenhum achado possibilitou a confirmação do diagnóstico.[351,359-365] Nenhuma técnica, além do exame histológico do tecido pulmonar, é útil para confirmar o diagnóstico de FPI e, mesmo quando a fibrose pulmonar é diagnosticada por biopsia, o diagnóstico de FPI depende da exclusão de causas conhecidas de lesão pulmonar que podem resultar em fibrose secundária.

Tratamento e prognóstico. Geralmente, o prognóstico a longo prazo para FPI é desfavorável; no entanto, cães com hipertensão pulmonar que respondem bem ao tratamento e/ou cães cujos proprietários estão satisfeitos com animais de estimação mais calmos podem viver um bom tempo e com qualidade de vida similar a de animais com a mesma idade. A maioria dos gatos dos relatos sobreviveu apenas dias a semanas.[1] Em cães, a doença progride mais lentamente, com sobrevida média, desde o início dos sintomas, de 32 meses ou menos.[351,353] Embora não haja teste terapêutico controlado para FPI em cães ou gatos, em seres humanos o uso de glicocorticoides, agentes citotóxicos e N-acetilcisteína não melhorou a sobrevida ou a qualidade de vida. Muito recentemente, o uso do inibidor da tirosinoquinase, nintedanibe, ou do antifibrótico pirfenidona, por via oral, mostrou alguma eficácia no tratamento de seres humanos com FPI, mas nenhum desses medicamentos foi testado em animais de estimação, e o seu uso é impraticável devido ao alto custo.[366,367] Como a tosse pode ser um componente proeminente da doença em cães, a supressão farmacológica da tosse grave pode melhorar a qualidade de vida do cão e de seu dono. A hipertensão pulmonar pode ser uma complicação grave da FPI, que pode ser beneficiada por tratamento direto. O controle farmacológico adequado da hipertensão pulmonar, sem causar hipotensão sistêmica, pode ser difícil. Mostrou-se que o tratamento com inibidores da fosfodiesterase 5 (p. ex., sildenafila, 1 mg/kg/8 h VO; tadalafila) reduz significativamente os sinais clínicos em cães com hipertensão pulmonar de ocorrência natural.[368-371]

Lesão pulmonar física

A lesão física aos pulmões pode ser mínima ou profunda, não sintomática ou fatal, dependendo de sua gravidade. Os meios mais comuns de lesão incluem traumatismo torácico contuso,

CAPÍTULO 242 • Doenças do Parênquima Pulmonar

afogamento e inalação de fumaça. Tais condições raramente implicam dificuldade no diagnóstico, porque as informações do histórico clínico e os ferimentos concomitantes costumam indicar a causa de lesão aparente.

Traumatismo torácico

Lesões decorrentes de acidentes automobilísticos e ferimentos provocados por briga são as causas mais comuns de traumatismo torácico em pequenos animais (ver Capítulo 149). Qualquer que seja a causa específica, o traumatismo pode resultar em lesão concomitante séria, incluindo hemorragia e choque. O exame completo do paciente é indispensável, não apenas porque lesões adicionais influenciam diretamente o resultado do tratamento, mas porque a descoberta de lesão simultânea grave (p. ex., lesão de medula espinal, ruptura da bexiga) pode interferir sobremaneira na duração do tratamento, no prognóstico e na decisão do proprietário de arcar com os custos do tratamento (ver Capítulo 147). O traumatismo pode resultar em ruptura de via respiratória (ver Capítulos 139 e 141), fratura de costela, contusão torácica, hérnia diafragmática (ver Capítulo 245), pneumotórax (ver Capítulos 102 e 244) e/ou contusão pulmonar; qualquer uma dessas condições pode resultar em taquipneia e angústia respiratória.

A contusão pulmonar resulta de hemorragia no interstício pulmonar e nos alvéolos. Ocasionalmente, a contusão ocorre mais como resultado da coagulopatia do que do traumatismo torácico. Nota-se angústia respiratória em decorrência do desequilíbrio entre ventilação e perfusão, devido à hemorragia em grande número de alvéolos. A lesão pulmonar por esmagadura, de via respiratória ou da parede torácica, bem como a dor costumam agravar a angústia respiratória. Embora crepitações e/ou sons vesiculares diminuídos possam ser ouvidos, sua presença não confirma contusão e sua ausência não exclui tal possibilidade. Hemoptise (ver Capítulo 29) é incomum após traumatismo torácico, mas sugere a presença de hemorragia pulmonar.[372] As radiografias de tórax são vitais para a avaliação de estruturas pulmonares (p. ex., costelas, diafragma, espaço pleural) e do parênquima pulmonar. A hemorragia intrapulmonar pode ser evidente como um padrão radiográfico pulmonar intersticial ou alveolar, ou como uma combinação de ambos. As alterações radiográficas no parênquima pulmonar, em geral, surgem até 24 horas após a lesão. Portanto, as radiografias obtidas após a lesão podem subestimar a gravidade da lesão pulmonar. O monitoramento eletrocardiográfico pode mostrar complexos ventriculares prematuros devido à miocardite traumática após traumatismo torácico relevante (ver Capítulos 141 e 248).

Animais que chegam à consulta com taquipneia ou angústia respiratória, após traumatismo torácico, devem receber suplementação imediata de oxigênio durante todos os procedimentos diagnósticos (ver Capítulos 131 e 149). Em muitos animais com contusão pulmonar, o quadro é brando a moderado e responde bem ao oxigênio suplementar e aos cuidados de suporte. Entretanto, quando a hipoxemia e/ou a dispneia persistem, apesar da suplementação de oxigênio, há necessidade de intubação e ventilação mecânica (de preferência com pressão ventilatória positiva).[373]

O tratamento específico da contusão pulmonar traumática não é possível; o tratamento da lesão traumática concomitante e suas complicações (p. ex., choque, hipovolemia) é vital. Em animais com contusão decorrente de ferimentos causados por mordida, a exploração cirúrgica da ferida e da cavidade torácica pode melhorar o desfecho.[374] Quando as contusões pulmonares se devem mais à coagulopatia do que ao traumatismo, indica-se o tratamento da coagulopatia. Como a intoxicação por rodenticida é a causa não traumática mais provável de hemorragia pulmonar, recomenda-se a administração de plasma fresco, plasma fresco congelado ou sangue total fresco e vitamina K, se o tempo de protrombina estiver prolongado em animais com contusão pulmonar (ver Capítulo 152). Antimicrobianos não estão indicados para contusão pulmonar na ausência de outras indicações para essa terapia (p. ex., traumatismo penetrante).

Embora a terapia com líquido possa ser um procedimento vital do tratamento de animais com traumatismo, deve ser monitorada com cuidado, para evitar edema pulmonar e agravamento da função pulmonar.[251] Complicações como lesões pulmonares cavitárias ou abscedação ocorrem raramente e a maioria dos animais que sobrevive às primeiras horas a 1 dia após a contusão pulmonar se recupera por completo da lesão pulmonar. O prognóstico piora quando o comprometimento pulmonar é suficiente para necessitar de ventilação mecânica, sendo pior em animais de menor porte do que naqueles de porte maior.[373]

Afogamento

Ocorre afogamento quando a submersão ou imersão em líquido causa um comprometimento respiratório primário.[375,376] Todo afogamento (fatal ou não) envolve aspiração de líquido. Embora a literatura antiga se referisse a laringospasmo durante ou após a submersão como "afogamento seco", agora se acredita que esse fenômeno seja muito raro e descrito de maneira imprópria como afogamento.[375,377] A fisiopatologia do afogamento difere um pouco quando a aspiração é de água doce, hipotônica, ou água salgada, hipertônica. Independentemente de diferenças mínimas nos volumes vasculares sistêmico e pulmonar e nas alterações eletrolíticas, as consequências imediatas mais importantes de cada tipo de afogamento estão relacionadas com a hipoxemia.[376,378,379] Alvéolos preenchidos com líquido, diluição e disfunção da substância surfactante, propiciando colapso alveolar e desvio vascular intrapulmonar, resultam em desequilíbrio na relação ventilação-perfusão e subsequente hipoxemia. A complacência pulmonar diminuída e a inflamação pulmonar, que resulta em edema pulmonar não cardiogênico devido à SARA, contribuem ainda mais para a hipoxemia, a qual acarreta acidose láctica; ademais, a hipercapnia decorrente do comprometimento pulmonar pode resultar em acidose respiratória e metabólica. A lesão pulmonar pode ser agravada pela aspiração de substâncias químicas ou bactérias contidas na água.[379] Raramente, ocorre infecção sistêmica invasiva, fúngica ou bacteriana, após o afogamento.[379-382]

O afogamento é mais comum em cães que em gatos, provavelmente porque gatos são menos propensos a entrar na água do que cães.[383] Como os cães em geral são bons nadadores, ocorre afogamento ou quase afogamento quando algo impede que saiam da água (p. ex., natação em piscina com declive íngreme e sem degraus, queda em um lago recoberto por gelo, corrente de água forte), quando alguma doença impede o reflexo de proteção das vias respiratórias apropriado (paralisia de laringe, estrangulamento), ou quando perdem a consciência enquanto estão nadando (p. ex., no caso de convulsão).[383] Uma proporção maior do que a esperada de cães que chega para cuidados veterinários após afogamento é jovem (tem menos de 4 meses de vida). Tipicamente, as vítimas de afogamento chegam para cuidados após serem resgatadas da água. As manifestações comuns por ocasião da consulta incluem parada respiratória, angústia respiratória, tosse, alteração do estado mental ou perda da consciência. Em geral, são detectados choque circulatório (ver Capítulo 127) e hipotermia (ver Capítulo 49) simultaneamente. A auscultação torácica pode revelar abafamento de sons broncovesiculares ou uma combinação de crepitações e sibilos. A oxigenação e o equilíbrio acidobásico devem ser avaliados, de preferência por meio de hemogasometria arterial (ver Capítulos 75 e 128). As radiografias mostram, tipicamente, padrão intersticial a alveolar difuso; porém, nos casos de contusão pulmonar, as alterações radiográficas podem subestimar a gravidade da lesão pulmonar porque em geral progridem após o resgate, devido ao desenvolvimento de SARA. A aparência radiográfica de "broncogramas de areia" (material radiopaco nas vias respiratórias) indica prognóstico ruim. Outros indicadores de prognóstico desfavorável incluem a necessidade de reanimação cardiopulmonar ou ventilação mecânica e acidose com pH sanguíneo < 7. O nível de consciência por ocasião da consulta não foi associado ao desfecho, em uma revisão retrospectiva de afogamento em água doce com recuperação total, mesmo no caso de animais que chegam em coma.[383] Deve-se administrar oxigênio suplementar imediatamente (ver Capítulo 131). Em geral, a hipoxemia persiste, mesmo com o fornecimento de oxigênio suplementar. Deve-se recorrer à ventilação mecânica, de preferência com pressão positiva contínua na via respiratória ou pressão expiratória final positiva, se o animal não conseguir manter a $Pa_{O_2} > 60$ mmHg, com uma $Fi_{O_2} > 50\%$.[129,379] Até mesmo animais que mantêm a normoxemia após o resgate podem desenvolver SARA e, portanto, devem ser observados por, no mínimo, 24 horas. Animais com hipotermia devem ser aquecidos, e o choque deve ser tratado imediatamente. Na vigência de lesão pulmonar, pode ser difícil manter o equilíbrio entre a administração de líquido para tratar o choque e a hiperidratação. Recomenda-se monitoramento hemodinâmico contínuo; também pode ser necessário suporte inotrópico. Desequilíbrios eletrolíticos e acidose graves (pH < 7,1) podem requerer tratamento. Apesar do alto risco de pneumonia bacteriana após o afogamento, não se comprovou que o uso profilático de antibiótico reduz o risco em seres humanos ou animais.[129,379,382-384] Se depois surgir evidência de pneumonia bacteriana, o exame citológico do lavado de via respiratória e a cultura microbiológica devem orientar a escolha do antimicrobiano. Corticosteroides não estão indicados, pois não melhoram a oxigenação nem aumentam a sobrevida.[379,385] Embora ainda não testado clinicamente, um estudo recente mostrou que a pentoxifilina (um inibidor inespecífico da fosfodiesterase), administrada em taxa de infusão contínua após o afogamento em água doce, reduziu a lesão pulmonar subsequente à SARA.[386]

Inalação de fumaça

Apesar da frequência com que ocorrem incêndios domésticos, a informação sobre lesão causada pela inalação de fumaça em animais de estimação é escassa.[387-392] Nem sempre a inalação de fumaça segue-se à exposição ao fogo, mas, quando ocorre, em geral resulta em lesão grave do trato respiratório. Obstrução de via respiratória do trato superior relacionada com broncospasmo e edema da laringe podem resultar de lesão térmica e química; tipicamente, tal lesão é máxima nas primeiras 24 horas.[390] A inalação de fuligem e gases nocivos liberados pela combustão de componentes domésticos (p. ex., cianeto de hidrogênio, amônia, aldeído, acroleína), inflamação de vias respiratórias e espaços de ar, mediadores inflamatórios sistêmicos, inativação da substância surfactante, broncoconstrição reflexa, atelectasia, edema de via respiratória e SARA contribuem para a ocorrência de lesão pulmonar nesse contexto.[388,390-393] A exposição a monóxido de carbono e cianeto compromete ainda mais a liberação de oxigênio e sua utilização pelos tecidos. A esfoliação de células epiteliais mortas e a fuligem podem resultar em obstrução tardia de via respiratória inferior, até mesmo dias após o evento, significando que o comprometimento respiratório decorrente da inalação de fumaça permanece dinâmico por até 1 semana após o evento desencadeante. Como uma preocupação a mais, o comprometimento dos mecanismos de defesa locais e sistêmicos predispõe de maneira acentuada à pneumonia bacteriana secundária.

Animais resgatados de incêndios podem ser levados ao veterinário aparentemente saudáveis ou com lesão grave. Os achados clínicos comuns consistem em tosse e engasgo, mucosas hiperêmicas, taquipneia, aumento do esforço respiratório, sons pulmonares broncovesiculares ou adventícios ásperos, som de via respiratória superior, secreção nasal, queimaduras ou lacerações.[388,391,392] Além disso, podem ser notadas anormalidades neurológicas (p. ex., ataxia, estupor), em decorrência da hipoxia do SNC, ou tais anormalidades podem ocorrer dias depois, devido a leucoencefalomalacia.[254,394,395] O ideal é mensurar a oxigenação por meio de hemogasometria arterial (ver Capítulos 75 e 128). Como em geral esses pacientes recebem oxigênio suplementar, a avaliação da razão $Pa_{O_2}:Fi_{O_2}$ é mais útil do que a simples verificação da Pa_{O_2}; uma razão < 300 significa comprometimento respiratório acentuado. Apenas o oxigênio dissolvido é mensurado por hemogasometria arterial, de modo que é preciso lembrar que a hipoxia tecidual pode ser marcante em animais com intoxicação por monóxido de carbono, apesar de Pa_{O_2} normal. Embora o

monóxido de carbono interfira na saturação de oxigênio na hemoglobina, a oximetria de pulso não possibilita distinguir oxiemoglobina de carboxiemoglobina. Portanto, a oximetria pode superestimar a capacidade de transporte sanguíneo de oxigênio, nos casos de intoxicação por monóxido de carbono.[396] Pode-se usar outro oxímetro para mensurar a concentração de carboxiemoglobina, se disponível. Nas radiografias do tórax, os cães frequentemente apresentam um padrão pulmonar alveolar, enquanto os padrões intersticial e alveolar foram constatados igualmente em gatos expostos à fumaça.[388,392]

Deve-se fornecer oxigênio suplementar pelo menos até se completar a avaliação inicial; a administração de oxigênio suplementar (iniciada de preferência no momento do resgate) pode resultar em melhora clínica rápida (ver Capítulo 131).[388] O oxigênio suplementar é útil para o tratamento da hipoxemia e também facilita a excreção pulmonar de monóxido de carbono. A utilidade da terapia com oxigênio hiperbárico continua controversa e sua disponibilidade é limitada para a maioria dos veterinários (ver Capítulo 84).[391,397] Hipoxemia persistente, mesmo com o fornecimento de oxigênio suplementar, pode necessitar de ventilação mecânica. Ocasionalmente, o edema de via respiratória superior requer intubação ou traqueostomia. Sem dúvida, a terapia com solução cristaloide é necessária para animais com queimaduras ou em choque. A terapia agressiva com líquido pode contribuir para a ocorrência de edema respiratório e, assim, requer monitoramento cuidadoso tanto da dose de líquido quanto da resposta do paciente.[389,391] O uso de coloides e solução fisiológica hipertônica em seres humanos com queimaduras (que podem acompanhar a inalação de fumaça) é discutível e deve ser decidido com cautela.[391] O uso profilático de antimicrobiano não se mostrou benéfico em seres humanos, mas não foi avaliado em animais de estimação com lesão causada por inalação de fumaça.[388,392,396] Embora algumas preparações de corticosteroides tenham sido benéficas em alguns modelos de inalação de fumaça em roedores, elas não foram efetivas em um estudo clínico no qual se usou um modelo canino; ademais, o seu uso de rotina também não se mostrou efetivo em seres humanos com lesão causada pela inalação de fumaça.[396,397a] Outras terapias, algumas vezes empregadas para tratar animais que inalaram fumaça, incluem broncodilatadores, nebulização com solução fisiológica e tapotagem, lubrificantes oculares, além do tratamento de queimaduras concomitantes (inclusive com uso de analgésico). Como a SARA pode desenvolver-se e agravar-se após a exposição inicial à fumaça, sugere-se o monitoramento nas primeiras 24 horas, mesmo quando o animal parece bem. Melhora na função respiratória no primeiro dia após o resgate é um indicador de prognóstico bastante positivo.[388,392] A deterioração da função respiratória após o primeiro dia de hospitalização, a presença de queimaduras concomitantes e a necessidade de ventilação mecânica são indicações de prognóstico ruim.

Miscelânea de doenças pulmonares

Atelectasia

Atelectasia pulmonar é simplesmente um pulmão não insuflado ou subinsuflado. Pode-se usar o termo para descrever pulmão de recém-nascido que ainda não se insuflou, aquele em colapso em decorrência de compressão mecânica (incluindo aquela associada ao decúbito), áreas de colapso alveolar resultante de preenchimento alveolar ou de colapso alveolar resultante de obstrução de via respiratória com reabsorção de ar aprisionado. A atelectasia não é uma doença primária, e sim uma consequência de doença.

Lesões pulmonares cavitárias

Essas lesões podem variar em tamanho, forma, espessura da parede, quantidade, localização e conteúdo. Há uma ampla variedade de causas potenciais de lesões pulmonares císticas ou cavitárias (Boxe 242.8).[398] Algumas causas específicas são comentadas a seguir.

Boxe 242.8 Causas potenciais de lesões pulmonares cavitárias ou císticas[41, 121, 258, 259, 341, 342, 403, 413, 441, 442]

Abscesso (parcialmente cheio de ar)
Bronquiectasia
Bolhas
Cistos congênitos
Doença hidática (rara)
Fibrose idiopática com aparência de favo de mel
Neoplasia metastática
Granuloma micótico (p. ex., causado por *Aspergillus*)
Parasitas (em especial *Paragonimus*)
Pneumatocele
Pneumonia causada por *Pneumocystis carinii*
Lesão após aspiração
Neoplasia pulmonar primária (p. ex., carcinoma broncogênico)
Infarto pulmonar
Cistos traumáticos

Abscessos. Abscesso pulmonar é um diagnóstico incomum em cães e gatos. Um abscesso pode ser preenchido predominantemente por ar ou ter uma aparência radiográfica nodular de tecido mole, devido ao acúmulo de líquido; uma linha de líquido pode ser visível quando há tanto ar quanto líquido, especificamente nas imagens obtidas com feixe de radiação horizontal. Tipicamente, ocorrem abscessos em áreas pulmonares que apresentam outras doenças (p. ex., focos de pneumonia, bronquiectasia); possuem parede espessa ou cápsula com borda interna irregular.[399,400] Em seres humanos, é provável que a formação de abscesso pulmonar seja uma sequela de pneumonia por aspiração, com infecção bacteriana secundária, ou quando há obstrução de vias respiratórias distais, como consequência de malignidade, inflamação, material estranho ou tampão de muco espesso.[401] Podem ser identificados sintomas respiratórios ou de infecção sistêmica em cães com abscesso pulmonar, semelhantes àqueles que podem ser evidências de osteopatia hipertrófica.[399,400,402-405] Quando apenas um lobo pulmonar é acometido, a extirpação cirúrgica é preferível ao tratamento exclusivo com antimicrobiano. A parte do pulmão extirpada pode ser submetida à cultura microbiológica e exame histológico. Às vezes, identifica-se uma causa primária de abscedação, como material estranho ou neoplasia.[137,406] A lobectomia cirúrgica também minimiza o risco de pneumotórax e piotórax, como consequência da ruptura do abscesso.[405] Quando a cirurgia não é possível, a terapia antimicrobiana é orientada pelos resultados da cultura microbiológica e do teste de sensibilidade bacteriana (antibiograma), mas a obtenção de uma amostra implica possíveis riscos: a ruptura do abscesso durante a aspiração com agulha pode ocasionar enfisema ou pneumotórax, enquanto o lavado de via respiratória pode resultar em ruptura de um abscesso repleto de ar.

Vesículas, bolhas e enfisema pulmonares. Bolhas são bolsas de ar presentes no parênquima pulmonar; elas resultam da destruição de paredes alveolares com a confluência de alvéolos adjacentes e não são revestidas por epitélio, como acontece nos cistos pulmonares. As bolhas foram classificadas em vários subtipos, dependendo do tamanho e de sua conexão com o tecido pulmonar circundante. As bolhas podem ser grandes ou pequenas e se instalar próximo da superfície pulmonar ou, profundamente, no parênquima.[407] As bolhas pulmonares são acúmulos de ar formados quando o ar que extravasou do pulmão fica aprisionado no interior da pleura visceral; as bolhas sempre são encontradas na superfície pulmonar.[407] *Enfisema bolhoso* é uma expressão usada para descrever a presença de bolhas.[408] A formação de bolhas é muito frequentemente idiopática, mas pode resultar de dano pulmonar devido a doenças parasitárias, neoplásicas, infecciosas ou outras morbidades em cães ou gatos. As bolhas podem estar relacionadas com doença congênita, inclusive com displasia broncopulmonar.[409-411] Bolhas idiopáticas ocorrem predominantemente em cães de meia-idade sadios, de tórax proeminente ou de raças de grande porte; em geral são detectadas em consequência de ruptura, seguida de pneumotórax espontâneo,[407,408,412] e podem ser vistas em radiografias como um achado acidental em cães ou gatos com doença pulmonar primária.[41,259,413,414] Infelizmente, a radiografia do tórax não é um método sensível (< 5 a 50% de detecção) na visualização de diversas bolhas.[407,408,412,415,416] A TC melhora a detecção (até 75%), mas ainda é limitada.[408,412] Assim que ocorre pneumotórax significativo, sempre que possível recomenda-se a lobectomia pulmonar parcial para remover o tecido pulmonar acometido.[407,408,415,416] No Capítulo 244 há mais informações sobre pneumotórax espontâneo.

Enfisema é qualquer condição pulmonar marcada por distensão e, por fim, ruptura de alvéolos, com consequente perda da elasticidade e da função pulmonares. Em seres humanos, o enfisema é detectado mais comumente simultâneo a doença pulmonar obstrutiva crônica (DPOC) e em geral é uma consequência da exposição a longo prazo ao tabagismo ou à poluição.[417] Essa forma de enfisema é extremamente rara em animais de estimação. No entanto, foi relatado enfisema lobar em vários cães jovens.[410,418-424] Ao contrário do enfisema de seres humanos adultos, o enfisema lobar congênito é uma condição de cães lactentes e jovens, em que o lobo pulmonar se apresenta hiperexpandido. Essa anormalidade pode ser idiopática ou resultar de obstrução, defeito ou compressão do brônquio.[418,424] O lobo enfisematoso aumentado causa compressão dos lobos normais, e o aumento da pressão alveolar no lobo acometido resulta em enfisema progressivo, com o desenvolvimento de bolhas e/ou vesículas.[420] Em geral, os achados radiográficos consistem em hiperinsuflação pulmonar com os vasos sanguíneos pulmonares estendendo-se para a margem do lobo, desvio do mediastino contralateral, deslocamento caudal do diafragma (uni ou bilateral), aumento da cavidade torácica, atelectasia de lobos não acometidos e, possivelmente, pneumotórax.[410,418,419,421,422,424,425] A comparação de radiografias obtidas durante a inspiração e a expiração pode ser útil, porque o pulmão enfisematoso não se esvazia durante a expiração. A remoção cirúrgica bem-sucedida do pulmão acometido foi relatada.[411,418,419,422,424]

Torção de lobo pulmonar

É incomum em cães e gatos.[426-430] Em geral, o lobo sofre rotação em relação ao eixo longitudinal, resultando em oclusão do brônquio e dos vasos sanguíneos do hilo.[429,431] Como a artéria pulmonar muscular continua a possibilitar a passagem de pequenas quantidades de sangue, enquanto a veia pulmonar de parede fina se colapsa completamente, o lobo acometido apresenta congestão e consolidação. Por fim, o líquido deixa a superfície do lobo e alcança o espaço pleural, resultando em efusão. Embora a torção resulte em efusão pleural, a efusão também pode predispor à torção. É possível que ocorra torção espontânea ou ela esteja associada à presença de neoplasia ou traumatismo torácico.

Manifestação clínica. Embora possa ocorrer torção em qualquer raça de cães, os das raças Afghan Hound e Pug são mais predispostos.[427,428,432-436] A maioria dos cães acometidos é jovem ou de meia-idade.[427,428] As queixas mais comuns são letargia, anorexia e aumento do esforço e da frequência respiratória, embora alguns animais apresentem alguns sintomas respiratórios.[436] Tosse, hemoptise e colapso também podem ser queixas iniciais. Anormalidades físicas comuns incluem febre, abafamento de sons pulmonares broncovesiculares e das bulhas cardíacas. Às vezes, é possível identificar cianose, taquicardia, tempo de preenchimento capilar prolongado e pulso fraco ou limitado.

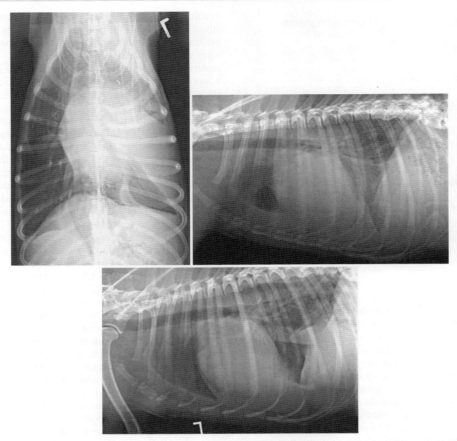

Figura 242.11 Radiografias de tórax, lateral e ventrodorsal, de um cão da raça Golden Retriever macho, castrado, de 4 anos, com torção do lobo pulmonar cranial esquerdo, mostrando consolidação do lobo.

Avaliação diagnóstica. Neutrofilia em sangue periférico (com ou sem desvio à esquerda) é comum. Em geral, as radiografias de tórax revelam efusão pleural; em caso afirmativo, devem ser repetidas após toracocentese (ver Capítulo 102), a fim de facilitar o reconhecimento de consolidação pulmonar (Figura 242.11). O posicionamento anormal do brônquio é identificado de forma inconsistente e é possível ver um brônquio proximal estenosado.[427,429,437] Quando detectado, um padrão gasoso vesicular (pequenas bolhas dispersas) no lobo acometido é fortemente sugestivo de torção.[429,437] Para a detecção de torção de lobo pulmonar, a TC torácica (com ou sem "broncoscopia virtual" reconstruída) é mais sensível e específica do que as radiografias.[429] Pode-se usar ultrassonografia quando há suspeita de torção de lobo pulmonar.[20,427,428,437] Ainda que raramente seja necessária, a broncoscopia (ver Capítulo 101) pode confirmar essa anormalidade.[438] O exame da efusão pleural geralmente revela um transudato sanguinolento modificado com grande quantidade de neutrófilos e linfócitos, mas ocorre efusão quilosa em alguns cães e gatos acometidos.[427,430] Em geral, são detectadas efusões quilosas em cães da raça Afghan Hound, com e sem torção de lobo pulmonar, o que especialmente nessa raça é difícil saber se a efusão causa torção, ou se a torção acarreta efusão, ou se ocorrem ambas.[427,432,433,439,440] Células mesoteliais reativas são identificadas frequentemente, mas raras vezes indicam mesotelioma. A cultura bacteriana da efusão ou de tecido pulmonar de 26 cães com torção de lobo pulmonar foi positiva em 8 cães (*Pseudomonas* spp., *E. coli*, *Enterococcus* spp., *Proteus* spp., *Staphylococcus* spp., *Enterobacter* spp. e *Serratia* spp.).[42]

Tratamento. Uma vez diagnosticada a torção de lobo pulmonar, a remoção do lobo acometido é o único tratamento apropriado. A torção pode ocorrer em qualquer lobo e em mais de um. De 58 cães avaliados em 3 séries de casos, constatou-se torção no lobo cranial esquerdo (n = 37), no lobo cranial médio (n = 34), no lobo cranial direito (n = 11), no lobo caudal direito (n = 2) e no lobo caudal esquerdo (n = 1).[427,428,437] Aproximadamente 60% dos cães se recuperam completamente após a cirurgia, talvez com melhor prognóstico naqueles da raça Pug.[427,428] Há relatos de taxas de morbidade tardia relevantes, incluindo pneumotórax, efusão quilosa e torção de lobos pulmonares adicionais em uma proporção pequena de cães que sobrevivem à cirurgia.[427,435]

Tromboembolismo pulmonar

É uma oclusão de vasos sanguíneos pulmonares para as partes aeradas do pulmão, que resulta em desequilíbrio na relação ventilação-perfusão e hipoxemia subsequente. Ver detalhes no Capítulo 243.

REFERÊNCIAS BIBLIOGRÁFICAS

As referências bibliográficas deste capítulo se encontram online no Ambiente de Aprendizagem.

CAPÍTULO 243

Hipertensão Pulmonar e Tromboembolismo Pulmonar

Justin G. Williams

HIPERTENSÃO PULMONAR

A hipertensão pulmonar (HP) pode ser definida como uma pressão sistólica na artéria pulmonar > 30 mmHg e/ou diastólica > 19 mmHg, conforme estimada por medições ecocardiográficas dos gradientes de regurgitação tricúspide ou pulmonar.[1-5] A pressão arterial pulmonar média normal é de 14 mmHg.[6] Um melhor entendimento das etiologias, dos sintomas e tratamentos da HP levou a melhor qualidade de vida e maior taxa de sobrevivência.

Fisiologia pulmonar e fisiopatologia

O leito vascular pulmonar é um sistema com pressão e resistência baixas e capacitância alta. O sangue flui do ventrículo direito (VD), através da artéria pulmonar (AP), por uma rede de artérias, capilares e veias, de paredes finas, antes de retornar ao átrio esquerdo, pelas veias pulmonares. A pressão na artéria pulmonar (PAP) é determinada pelo débito cardíaco do VD (ou fluxo sanguíneo pulmonar), pela resistência vascular pulmonar (RVP) e pela pressão na veia pulmonar. Ocorre hipertensão pulmonar quando há um desequilíbrio entre os fatores que controlam a vasoconstrição e a vasodilatação da artéria pulmonar, a ativação de plaquetas e a proliferação de células de músculo liso.

Os indutores de vasoconstrição pulmonar incluem hipoxia alveolar, endotelina 1 e serotonina. É provável que a vasoconstrição induzida pela hipoxia seja uma resposta fisiológica que resulta em desvio do sangue desoxigenado para áreas mais bem ventiladas do pulmão. Embora isso possa ser benéfico em uma situação aguda, em condições crônicas pode acarretar HP. A endotelina 1 (ET-1) é um peptídio liberado pelo endotélio vascular em resposta a alterações no fluxo sanguíneo, no estiramento vascular e na concentração de trombina. A ET-1 causa vasoconstrição, estimula o crescimento de músculo liso, aumenta a síntese de colágeno, promove remodelamento vascular e está aumentada em pessoas com HP.[7-9] Em cães ocorre elevação no teor de ET-1 em doenças associadas à HP, como dirofilariose[10] e cardiopatia esquerda adquirida.[11]

A prostaciclina e o tromboxano A_2 são ácidos araquidônicos metabólitos de células vasculares da AP com efeitos inibidores do tônus vascular da AP. A prostaciclina é um vasodilatador potente, que inibe a ativação plaquetária e tem propriedades antiproliferativas.[7] Em contrapartida, o tromboxano A_2 é um vasoconstritor e agonista plaquetário. Em pessoas com HP, o tromboxano A_2 predomina, resultando em vasoconstrição da AP, trombose e proliferação celular.[12] O fator de crescimento derivado de plaquetas (FCDP, ou PGDF em inglês) induz a proliferação e a migração de células do músculo liso da AP. A expressão do FCDP e de seu receptor está aumentada em pessoas com HP idiopática.[13,14]

O óxido nítrico (ON, ou NO em inglês) é um vasodilatador, inibidor da ativação plaquetária e inibidor da proliferação do músculo liso vascular. É sintetizado a partir de L-arginina e oxigênio por enzimas sintases ON, no endotélio da AP. Uma vez formado, o ON ativa o monofosfato cíclico de guanosina (GMPc), que causa vasodilatação pulmonar. Essa vasodilatação é limitada pela inativação do GMPc pela isoenzima fosfodiesterase 5 (PDE5).[7]

Classificação da hipertensão pulmonar

A hipertensão pulmonar pode ser classificada simplesmente com base na localização anatômica, como *pré* ou *pós-capilar*, ou como um sistema de cinco grupos baseado na doença primária. Desenvolvido para pessoas, esse sistema de grupos foi adaptado para etiologias veterinárias (Boxe 243.1). Os cinco grupos de HP são: hipertensão arterial pulmonar devido à doença vascular arteriolar (Grupo I), hipertensão venosa pulmonar devido à cardiopatia esquerda (Grupo II), hipertensão pulmonar causada por doença pulmonar crônica e/ou hipoxia (Grupo III), hipertensão pulmonar tromboembólica crônica (Grupo IV) e hipertensão pulmonar idiopática ou multifatorial (Grupo V).[15]

Boxe 243.1 Classificação da hipertensão pulmonar[1-5,15,17-19,21,30-33,35-37,39-50,53,60,62,71,89-96]

I. Hipertensão arterial pulmonar (HAP) devido à doença vascular pulmonar arteriolar
- Doença vascular pulmonar parasitária
  - *Angiostrongylus vasorum* (dirofilária francesa)
  - *Dirofilaria immitis* (dirofilariose)
- *Shunts* (desvios) sistêmico-pulmonares congênitos
  - Defeito do septo atrial (DSA)
  - Persistência do ducto arterioso (PDA)
  - Defeito do septo ventricular (DSV)
- Vasculite/arterite necrosante
- Idiopática.

II. Hipertensão pulmonar com cardiopatia esquerda (hipertensão venosa pulmonar)
- Doença da valva mitral
- Doença do miocárdio
- Miscelânea de cardiopatia esquerda.

III. Hipertensão pulmonar com doença pulmonar/hipoxemia
- Doença pulmonar obstrutiva crônica
- Doença da altitude elevada
- Fibrose pulmonar intersticial
- Neoplasia
- Vasoconstrição reativa da artéria pulmonar (decorrente de edema pulmonar e hipoxemia)
- Doença traqueobrônquica.

IV. Hipertensão pulmonar devido à doença trombótica e/ou embólica
- Tromboembolismo
  - Cardiopatia
  - Tratamento com corticosteroide
  - Coagulação intravascular disseminada
  - Endocardite (valva pulmonar/tricúspide)
  - Hiperadrenocorticismo
  - Anemia hemolítica imunomediada
  - Uso de cateter venoso de demora
  - Neoplasia
  - Pancreatite
  - Doença com perda de proteína (nefropatia ou enteropatia)
  - Sepse
  - Cirurgia
  - Traumatismo
- *Dirofilaria immitis* (dirofilariose).

V. Miscelânea
- Lesões compressivas em forma de massa tecidual (neoplasia, granuloma).

A HP do Grupo I inclui hipertensão arterial pulmonar (HAP) causada por doença vascular arteriolar pulmonar. Esse grupo inclui desvios sistêmico-pulmonares congênitos e dirofilariose (*Dirofilaria immitis*). Esta última condição causa HP em razão do dano vascular, resultando em lesões decorrentes de hipertrofia medial e proliferação e fibrose da camada íntima do vaso sanguíneo (ver Capítulo 255).[16] *Angiostrongylus vasorum*, também conhecido como dirofilária francesa, está associado a HAP em cães (ver Capítulo 241).[17,21] Os desvios cardíacos sistêmico-pulmonares apresentam baixa resistência pulmonar e alto fluxo, causando tensão no revestimento endotelial da artéria pulmonar, ocasionando HP.[22] A síndrome de Eisenmenger envolve grandes defeitos intra ou extracardíacos que surgem como *shunts* da esquerda para a direita, mas por fim acarretam aumento significativo da RVP e reversão do fluxo do desvio ou o torna bidirecional.[15,23]

Em pessoas, o Grupo I também inclui HP genética ou familiar.[15] Polimorfismos da PDE5 foram associados a respostas variáveis ao sildenafila e ao ON, bem como progressão da HP, em pessoas.[24-26] Em cães, um polimorfismo de PDE5 está associado à baixa expressão de GMPc.[27] Embora isso sugira possível predisposição à HP, um estudo realizado em cães infectados por *A. vasorum* não revelou diferença na frequência do polimorfismo em paciente com e sem HP.[17]

A HP do Grupo II envolve hipertensão venosa pulmonar (HVP) decorrente de cardiopatia esquerda, como doença degenerativa da valva mitral (DDVM), miocardiopatia dilatada ou qualquer cardiopatia que acomete o lado esquerdo do coração, seja atrial ou ventricular. A cardiopatia esquerda pode resultar em HP pela combinação de alta pressão no átrio esquerdo e HVP, bem como vasoconstrição arterial pulmonar reativa. Esses efeitos cardiovasculares são decorrentes de hipoxemia aguda ou crônica, menor disponibilidade de ON, alta expressão de endotelina 1 e dessensibilização aos peptídios natriuréticos.[28,29] As anormalidades do Grupo II foram sugeridas como as causas mais comuns de HP em cães, pois a DDVM pode ser a causa de HP em 30 a 74% dos casos de HP de ocorrência natural.[1-4,30-32]

A HP do Grupo III é secundária à doença pulmonar ou hipoxemia crônica. Em cães, a HP do Grupo III está associada à fibrose pulmonar, pneumonia, doença traqueobrônquica e neoplasia.[4,5] Até 40% dos cães da raça West Highland White Terrier com doença pulmonar intersticial crônica têm algum grau de HP.[5]

A HP do Grupo IV inclui hipertensão pulmonar causada por doença trombótica ou embólica. A dirofilariose é incluída novamente porque pode causar HP por embolização pelos vermes e obstrução direta do lúmen da artéria pulmonar.

A HP do Grupo V é um agrupamento de doenças idiopáticas ou com causas multifatoriais, que inclui doenças mieloproliferativas (como policitemia vera primária), doenças granulomatosas, anemia hemolítica imunomediada crônica e obstrução por tumor.[15,33]

A evidência de hipertensão pulmonar felina é limitada a relatos de casos. Ela foi associada a tromboembolismo pulmonar,[34-36] persistência de ducto arterioso com *shunt* da direita para a esquerda,[37] dirofilariose,[38,39] obstrução crônica de via respiratória superior[40] e infecção por *Aelurostrongylus abstrusus* (verme pulmonar felino).[41] Relata-se o tratamento de um gato com síndrome de Eisenmenger e defeito de septo atrial com sildenafila, por 10 meses.[41a]

Resenha

A maioria dos pacientes caninos com HP é de raças de pequeno porte e de meia-idade ou idoso, o que coincide com os dados de resenha de causas predisponentes, como doença degenerativa da valva mitral e doença pulmonar crônica.[2,4,42-46] Cães de raças Terrier podem ser mais sujeitos à anormalidade devido a sua predisposição a doenças pulmonares crônicas, como fibrose pulmonar intersticial.[5,42,47]

Sinais clínicos e exame físico

Como a HP compromete o transporte de oxigênio e diminui o débito cardíaco, na maioria dos casos os clientes observam intolerância ao exercício, tosse (ver Capítulo 26), dispneia (ver Capítulo 28) e síncope (ver Capítulo 30), em cães com HP.[3,4,32] Os pacientes também podem manifestar sinais clínicos específicos da doença primária. O exame físico pode revelar sons pulmonares anormais, cianose (ver Capítulo 52) e/ou ascite (ver Capítulo 17).[2-4,42] Em geral, a auscultação respiratória revela crepitações pulmonares, sibilos e sons respiratórios ásperos ou exacerbados.[4,32,42,48,49] Sopros do lado esquerdo ou direito do coração são auscultados na maioria dos cães com HP.[2,32,43,50] Pode-se notar uma segunda bulha cardíaca (B2) anormalmente alta ou o desdobramento dessa bulha (ver Capítulo 55). Os sinais clínicos constatados ao exame físico de HP felina incluem dispneia, congestão da veia jugular e sopro sistólico no lado direito do coração.[34-37,40,41]

Diagnóstico

A ecocardiografia (ECO) é o principal meio para diagnosticar HP em medicina veterinária. Embora o cateterismo cardíaco direito e a medição direta da pressão na AP sejam o padrão em medicina humana,[51,52] seu uso em pacientes veterinários costuma ser inviável pelo custo, pela pouca disponibilidade e pela necessidade de anestesia de um paciente geralmente instável.

O ecodoppler é um método não invasivo de mensuração da pressão na AP, em animais conscientes. A velocidade máxima de fluxo regurgitante na regurgitação tricúspide (RT) ou na insuficiência pulmonar (IP) pode levar ao diagnóstico de HP (Figura 243.1 A). Na ausência de estenose pulmonar, a velocidade da regurgitação possibilita estimar a pressão na AP usando a equação de Bernoulli modificada (gradiente de pressão = 4 × [velocidade máxima]^2). No entanto, a acurácia da pressão obtida depende da habilidade do profissional, da magnitude da RT e da tolerância do paciente ao exame, bem como de fatores fisiológicos, como a função sistólica do VD. Uma velocidade máxima da RT > 2,8 m/s (gradiente de pressão máxima da RT > 31 mmHg) ou uma velocidade máxima de IP > 2,2 m/s (gradiente de pressão máxima na IP > 19 mmHg) sugere fortemente HP.[2,4,5] Pode-se classificar a HP como branda (31 a 50 mmHg), moderada (51 a 75 mmHg) e grave (> 75 mmHg).[2,5,49,53,54] Se conhecida, a pressão do átrio direito, juntamente com o gradiente de pressão da RT, teoricamente possibilita uma predição mais acurada da pressão pulmonar sistólica. A pressão do átrio direito (AD) foi estimada por meio de ECO como sendo 5 mmHg em cães que não apresentavam aumento do VD, 10 mmHg se o VD estiver aumentado, mas sem insuficiência cardíaca direita, e 15 mmHg quando há sinais clínicos de insuficiência cardíaca direita.[30,32,55] Na HP, as medições ecocardiográficas e as invasivas diretas têm uma relação moderada, porém com ampla variabilidade.[55] Em um estudo de HP embólica aguda experimental em cães anestesiados, a ECO teve uma tendência a superestimar as medições diretas da HP; todavia, foram constatadas tanto subestimativa quanto superestimativa.[55]

Na ausência de RT ou IP, outros achados de ECO podem ser úteis para se diagnosticar HP. A ECO bidimensional pode revelar hipertrofia concêntrica ou excêntrica do VD, aumento do AE, achatamento septal e, potencialmente, disfunção sistólica do VD causada por HP moderada ou grave (Figura 243.1 B e C; Vídeo 243.1).[2,4,5,53,56,57]

Os perfis do fluxo na valva pulmonar, em exame Doppler espectral, potencialmente ajudam no diagnóstico e na classificação da gravidade da HP (Figura 243.1 D).[2,4,5,31,32,45,49] Outras medições de ECO que confirmam o diagnóstico de HP em cães incluem excursão sistólica plana anular tricúspide (ESPAT),[56] intervalos do tempo sistólico do ventrículo direito,[5,49] imagem Doppler do tecido direito (ITD),[31,58] razão artéria pulmonar: artéria aorta,[31] índice de Tei de desempenho miocárdico[31,32,58] e o índice de distensão da artéria pulmonar direita (DAPD).[59]

CAPÍTULO 243 • Hipertensão Pulmonar e Tromboembolismo Pulmonar

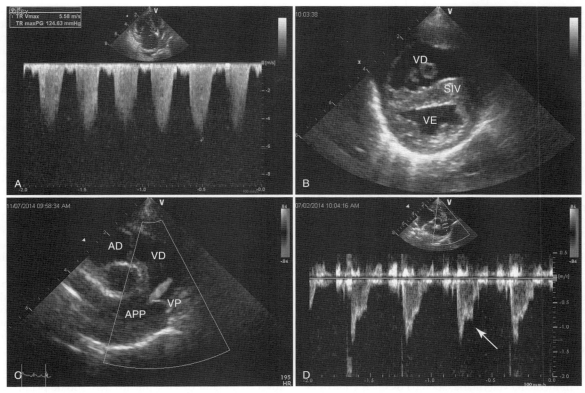

Figura 243.1 Imagens ecocardiográficas de um cão com hipertensão pulmonar grave. **A.** Onda Doppler contínua de interrogação de regurgitação tricúspide (RT) de uma projeção paraesternal esquerda modificada das quatro câmaras. A velocidade da RT é de 5,58 m/s e o gradiente é de 124,63 mmHg, valores calculados a partir da equação de Bernoulli modificada (gradiente de pressão = 4 × velocidade^2). Na ausência de estenose pulmonar e alta pressão do átrio direito, o gradiente de RT representa a pressão sistólica na artéria pulmonar. **B.** Achatamento do septo interventricular e hipertrofia da parede livre e dilatação da câmara ventricular direita. **C.** Projeção do eixo curto paraesternal direito, na base do coração. A imagem mostra marcante dilatação da artéria pulmonar principal e insuficiência pulmonar branda. **D.** Doppler espectral através da valva pulmonar, a partir de projeção do eixo curto paraesternal direito. Nota-se pico inicial e diminuição da velocidade, com ligeira reversão do fluxo no fim da sístole (*seta*). Esse perfil de velocidade na artéria pulmonar é do tipo III e confirma o diagnóstico de hipertensão pulmonar grave. *AD*, átrio direito; *APP*, artéria pulmonar principal; *SIV*, septo interventricular; *VD*, ventrículo direito; *VE*, ventrículo esquerdo; *VP*, valva pulmonar. (*Esta figura se encontra reproduzida em cores no Encarte.*)

Embora não sejam específicas para HP, as radiografias podem mostrar imagens que confirmam HP. Com base na causa primária da HP, o aumento do coração direito, a dilatação da artéria pulmonar e/ou infiltrados pulmonares podem ser evidentes (Figura 243.2). Em um estudo retrospectivo de pacientes com DDVM (< 15 kg) constatou-se que um eixo curto na escala cardíaca vertebral > 5,2 vértebras (v) e um comprimento de contato esternal > 3,3 v apresentou acurácia preditiva de 85,9%, na detecção de HP.[54]

Biomarcadores, como o peptídio natriurético do tipo NT-pró-B (NT-pró-BNP) ou troponinas cardíacas, podem ser úteis no diagnóstico de HP. O NT-pró-BNP é um peptídio liberado pelo miocárdio ventricular em resposta a tensão ou estiramento. Tradicionalmente, o NT-pró-BNP é usado como teste de triagem para detectar doença cardíaca, bem como na diferenciação entre doenças cardíacas e respiratórias.[60,61] Entretanto, o NT-pró-BNP pode estar elevado em cães com HP pré ou pós-capilar.[45,60,62] Cães com doença respiratória e HP (*i. e.*, do Grupo III) apresentam maior concentração sérica média de NT-pró-BNP em comparação com aqueles com doença respiratória, porém sem HP.[60,62] Além disso, pode haver correlação entre o NT-pró-BNP e o gradiente máximo de RT.[62] Contudo, o NT-pró-BNP não é específico o suficiente para distinguir cães com DDVM e aqueles com DDVM e HP.[54] Em termos gerais, a elevação de NT-pró-BNP aumenta a suspeita de HP, mas não é possível diferenciar HP e cardiopatia primária.

A concentração cardíaca de troponina I (cTnI) é uma medida de lesão miocárdica. Cães com HP pré e pós-capilar apresentaram aumento significativo de cTnI em comparação

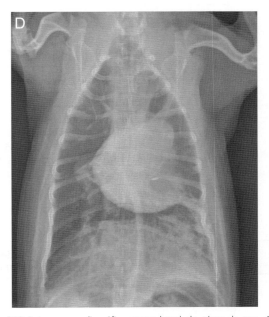

Figura 243.2 Imagem radiográfica ventrodorsal do tórax de um cão com hipertensão pulmonar grave e história de 1 ano de intolerância ao exercício, aumento do esforço expiratório, respiração ofegante progressiva e episódios de síncope. Note a grave dilatação da artéria pulmonar principal e da artéria pulmonar do lobo caudal direito, com infiltrados pulmonares no campo pulmonar caudal esquerdo.

com cães normais.[30] Todavia, a cTnI não foi diferente entre cães com doença respiratória e HP e aqueles com doença respiratória sem HP.[62]

Tratamento

A hipertensão pulmonar se instala a partir de um grupo heterogêneo de doenças, com vários subgrupos. Em consequência, o tratamento deve ser direcionado à causa primária (ver seções sobre Tratamento nos Capítulos 241, 242, 247 e 255), bem como à redução direta da HP para melhorar a qualidade de vida. Outrora designada "reino da quase morte",[63] em medicina humana, a HP pode ser tratada com diversos medicamentos. Antagonistas da endotelina (i. e., bosentana, ambrisentana, macitentano) e análogos da prostaciclina (i. e., beraprosta, epoprostenol, iloprost) têm custo proibitivo e, em geral, sua administração deve ser por via subcutânea contínua ou por meio de inalação, o que limita muito sua aplicação em pacientes veterinários. O valor dos antagonistas da endotelina ou análogos da prostaciclina ainda não foi confirmado em cães com HP; no entanto, é comum prescrever inibidores do tipo V da fosfodiesterase (PDE5-I).

Medicamentos à base de PDE5-I, como sildenafila (Viagra), tadalafila (Cialis) e vardenafila (Levitra), causam vasodilatação por aumentarem a concentração vascular pulmonar de GMPc. Subsequentemente, esse aumento resulta em elevação da concentração de ON endógeno.[2,3,64] Além de melhorar diretamente a HP, por meio da vasodilatação da AP, os medicamentos com PDE5-I reduzem o remodelamento cardíaco, a apoptose, a fibrose, a hipertrofia ventricular e melhoram a função cardíaca esquerda em pessoas.[64] O sildenafila é uma PDE5-I de curta ação, que, em medicina veterinária, abranda os sinais clínicos de HP e melhora a qualidade de vida.[2,3,46] Notou-se uma redução mensurável no gradiente de pressão da RT em alguns estudos,[3,46] mas não em outros.[2] Apesar disso, pesquisas mostram melhora clínica em cães que recebem sildenafila, independentemente de qualquer alteração na HP diagnosticada. O sildenafila é bem tolerado por cães na dose de 1 a 2 mg/kg VO, em intervalos de 8 a 12 h.[2,3,46] Embora não haja consenso quanto ao uso de sildenafila em cães, a Figura 243.3 mostra um processo de tomada de decisão potencial para o tratamento de HP nos Grupos II e III. O sildenafila tem sido usado de maneira empírica em gatos; inclusive há um relato de caso de um gato com HP decorrente da persistência de ducto arterioso (PDA), com desvio do fluxo da esquerda para a direita.[65] Não foram publicados ensaios clínicos em gatos.

O tadalafila é um inibidor da PDE5 de ação prolongada. Há um único estudo de caso publicado referente a um cão com HP idiopática tratado com tadalafila (1 mg/kg/48 h),[66] no qual notou-se redução da PAP e melhora dos sinais clínicos. Mostrou-se que o uso de tadalafila, oral e injetável, reduz a HP induzida experimentalmente em cães.[67] O vardenafila, outro PDE5-I de ação prolongada, ainda não foi avaliado no tratamento de HP em cães.

O pimobendana é um inibidor da fosfodiesterase 3 (PDE3) e sensibilizador ao cálcio. Seu emprego no tratamento da HVP (HP do Grupo II) em cães com DDVM reduziu a concentração NT-pró-BNP. Além disso, melhorou a qualidade de vida a curto prazo, mantendo uma baixa HVP a longo prazo.[45]

Considerando que ocorre trombose in situ e aumento da síntese de tromboxano A_2 em pessoas com HP idiopática, tem-se usado ácido acetilsalicílico (ácido acetilsalicílico) ou clopidogrel.[68] Alguns clínicos veterinários usam terapia antiplaquetária em cães com HP idiopática, mas sua indicação e efetividade são desconhecidas.

Estão surgindo terapias mais modernas na medicina humana, algumas já avaliadas em cães. O imatinibe (Gleevec) inibe a ativação do fator de crescimento derivado de plaquetas (FCDP, ou PDGF em inglês) e também inibe o receptor dele. Seis cães com insuficiência cardíaca congestiva e HP decorrentes de DDVM ou dirofilariose foram tratados com imatinibe, na dose de 3 mg/kg/24 h VO, por 30 dias, e mostraram melhora na velocidade máxima da RT, no tamanho do átrio esquerdo e na concentração plasmática do peptídio natriurético atrial.[69]

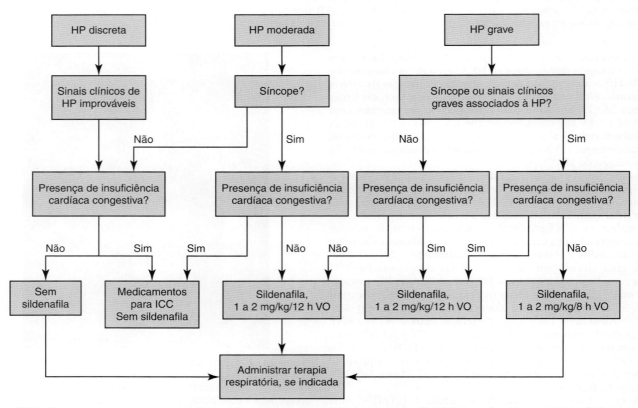

Figura 243.3 Abordagem para o tratamento de cães com hipertensão pulmonar (HP) dos grupos II e III. HP, hipertensão pulmonar; ICC, insuficiência cardíaca congestiva; VO, via oral.

Prognóstico

Em cães, o prognóstico para HP é bastante variável e costuma depender da causa primária. O prognóstico de HP grave é desfavorável. Antes da disponibilidade do sildenafila, em cães a HP estava associada a apenas alguns dias de sobrevivência após o diagnóstico.[4] Com o surgimento desse fármaco, a sobrevivência publicada aumentou para 91 dias,[3] com alguns pacientes sobrevivendo quase 2 anos.[2,3] Não há indicadores prognósticos bem definidos em medicina veterinária. Em pessoas, a gravidade dos sintomas induzidos pela HP e a obtenção dos objetivos do tratamento (melhora na função do VD, no teor de NT-pró-BNP. e na distância de caminhada durante 6 minutos) são os melhores indicadores de prognóstico de maior sobrevida.[70]

TROMBOEMBOLISMO PULMONAR

Etiologia/fisiopatologia

Tromboembolismo pulmonar (TEP) é a obstrução parcial ou completa da AP ou de seus ramos por trombos secundários a outras doenças. As enfermidades associadas à doença tromboembólica estão listadas no Boxe 243.1, Grupo IV. A patogenia do TEP baseia-se no dano endotelial, na estase do fluxo sanguíneo e em estados de hipercoagulação (ver Capítulo 197).[71] O TEP resulta em hipoxemia, broncoconstrição, desequilíbrio na relação ventilação-perfusão e hiperventilação. As complicações hemodinâmicas associadas ao TEP dependem da extensão da oclusão do vaso sanguíneo pulmonar e de disfunções cardíaca e pulmonar preexistentes. Com o tempo, surgem mais complicações, como atelectasia, edema pulmonar e efusão pleural.

Sinais clínicos e diagnóstico

Os sinais clínicos de TEP são altamente variáveis e inespecíficos. Os mais comuns são dispneia, taquipneia e letargia.[71-74]

É difícil estabelecer o diagnóstico *ante mortem* de TEP em medicina veterinária, devido à falta de um teste diagnóstico padrão viável e disponível. Radiografias do tórax estão indicadas, porém os achados em geral são inespecíficos, variando de infiltrados pulmonares focais a achados radiográficos normais.[73,75] Anormalidades na hemogasometria arterial podem aumentar o índice de suspeita, mas não são específicas o bastante para confirmar a presença de TEP. As alterações mais comuns na hemogasometria arterial associadas ao TEP consistem em hipoxemia, hipocapnia e aumento do gradiente de tensão alveolar-arterial de oxigênio (ver Capítulos 75 e 128).[71,73] Como o TEP é uma sequela de outra doença, uma pesquisa diagnóstica ampla, incluindo hemograma completo, perfil bioquímico sérico, exame de urina e teste para dirofilariose, pode detectar fatores predisponentes. Em geral, suspeita-se de TEP em pacientes nos quais não se consegue confirmar uma doença cardiopulmonar e, sabidamente, são predispostos à trombose. A tromboelastografia (TEG) possibilita uma avaliação global da coagulação e da fibrinólise, tendo o potencial de identificar condições de hipercoagulação e aumentar a suspeita de TEP (ver Capítulo 196).[71,75] Infelizmente, raras vezes se consegue a confirmação *ante mortem* de TEP em medicina veterinária.

Em pessoas, são usadas tomografia computadorizada (TC), angiografia pulmonar seletiva e cintilografia de ventilação e perfusão com uso de radionucleotídios para a triagem e confirmação de doença tromboembólica.[51,71] É difícil realizar angiografia seletiva em pacientes veterinários instáveis, considerando a necessidade de anestesia geral. Entretanto, um pequeno estudo prospectivo realizado em cães mostrou que a TC do tórax com injeção simultânea de um *bolus* de contraste (*i. e.*, angio-TC pulmonar) foi possível sob sedação, em pacientes com sintomas respiratórios, sendo útil para confirmar ou refutar a presença de TEP.[75]

Como a disponibilidade da angio-TC e a habilidade necessária em seu manejo são limitadas, tem-se recorrido aos exames de sangue mais amplamente disponíveis, como a mensuração de D-Dímeros, que são subprodutos da degradação da fibrina ocasionada pela plasmina e refletem a fibrinólise (ver Capítulo 196). Embora o D-Dímero não seja específico do TEP, em concentração normal ou baixa é altamente sensível para excluir a presença de TEP agudo em cães[76-80] e deve ser mensurado 1 a 2 horas após o surgimento de suspeita de TEP, pois sua concentração se eleva rapidamente e pode retornar ao valor basal em 24 a 48 horas.[81]

Tratamento

O objetivo principal do tratamento é limitar o crescimento do trombo e prevenir sua recorrência.[71] O tratamento antiplaquetário com anticoagulantes e trombolíticos tem sido empregado, mas não há uma abordagem ou consenso sobre tratamento com base em evidência. A terapia trombolítica com estreptoquinase, uroquinase ou ativador do plasminogênio tecidual é particularmente controversa; ademais, não há testes clínicos que avaliem seu uso no TEP veterinário. Foi descrita a infusão local de trombolíticos em um trombo, orientada por cateter, a qual pode resultar em risco menor de complicações hemorrágicas sistêmicas.[82,83] Sugeriu-se o uso de heparina não fracionada (injeção SC de 100 a 300 UI/kg, em intervalos de 6 a 8 h, ajustando a dose de modo a manter o tempo de tromboplastina parcial ativado [TTPa] em 1,5 a 2 vezes o valor basal)[84,85] ou de heparina de baixo peso molecular (dalteparina, na dose de 100 a 150 UI/kg/8 h, em cães,[84] e de 100 a 180 UI/kg a cada 8 a 24 h, em gatos[84,86]) como tratamento hospitalar inicial. Cuidados de suporte, incluindo o fornecimento de oxigênio (ver Capítulo 131), uso criterioso de soluções IV (ver Capítulo 129), sildenafila e broncodilatadores, são benéficos (ver Capítulo 139).[71] O tratamento efetivo de TEP agudo deve ser simultâneo à terapia antiplaquetária ou anticoagulante a longo prazo. O ácido acetilsalicílico é útil na prevenção de trombo na anemia hemolítica imunomediada e na nefropatia acompanhada de perda de proteína.[71,85] As doses de ácido acetilsalicílico comumente usadas são 0,5 mg/kg/24 h VO, em cães, e 5 a 81 mg/dose VO, a cada 3 dias, em gatos.[71,84,85,87] O clopidogrel também costuma ser usado nas doses sugeridas, de 2 a 3 mg/kg/24 h VO, em cães, e 18 a 75 mg/dose VO, a cada 24 horas, em gatos.[85,88]

REFERÊNCIAS BIBLIOGRÁFICAS

As referências bibliográficas deste capítulo se encontram online no Ambiente de Aprendizagem.

CAPÍTULO 244

Doenças do Espaço Pleural

Elizabeth Rozanski

ANATOMIA

O espaço pleural é definido como a área ou o espaço entre os pulmões e a parede torácica. Normalmente, não há estruturas de tecido mole ou ar livre nesse espaço. Uma quantidade muito pequena (1 a 5 mℓ) de líquido, que não é detectável em radiografias ou na ultrassonografia, pode estar presente na cavidade torácica. A cavidade pleural é revestida pelas pleuras visceral e parietal, que recobrem os pulmões e a parede torácica, respectivamente. Em pequenos animais, os dois hemitóraces são separados de maneira incompleta, o que geralmente resulta em troca de efusão pleural entre o lado direito e o esquerdo. Na efusão de longa duração, aderências fibrosas podem resultar na presença de doença unilateral, mas, como regra geral em cães e gatos, o mediastino é incompleto. Como acontece em todo o corpo, o movimento de líquido reflete as forças de Starling, bem como a permeabilidade tecidual e a drenagem linfática.[1] Em animais com efusão de longa duração, a taxa de drenagem linfática pode estar aumentada.

FISIOLOGIA

A função pulmonar normal depende de oxigenação e ventilação adequadas que, por sua vez, dependem da mecânica pulmonar e da facilidade de expansão pulmonar. A pressão intratorácica normal é subatmosférica, com uma média de – 5 cm de H_2O (– 3,7 mmHg). A pressão intratorácica negativa, juntamente com o surfactante pulmonar, mantém os pulmões insuflados, o que diminui o esforço respiratório.

A efusão pleural interfere na função pulmonar, restringindo a capacidade pulmonar total (CPT) e diminuindo a capacidade funcional residual (CFR). Nos casos avançados, há exacerbação do desequilíbrio da relação ventilação-perfusão e, se não tratada, a efusão pleural grave resultará em redução do débito cardíaco e, por fim, em parada cardíaca.[2] Esse fenômeno é mais comum no pneumotórax, em que a tensão pode surgir rapidamente, em contraste com as efusões pleurais, que tendem a desenvolver-se mais lentamente.

À medida que a efusão pleural se forma, há colapso gradual do parênquima pulmonar, bem como *aumento* na pressão intratorácica. Na presença de uma efusão acentuada, a pressão intrapleural será positiva. Embora geralmente se presuma que a remoção da efusão pleural isolada resultará em melhora imediata da função pulmonar, nem sempre é o caso. Em pessoas, são reconhecidas duas diferentes categorias de pulmão não recrutável com efusão pleural. A primeira denomina-se *pulmão aprisionado*, distúrbio que se desenvolve associado a inflamação ou neoplasia ativa na pleura.[3] Fibrina imatura e inflamação sobrejacente impedem a reexpansão e contribuem para a falha no recrutamento pulmonar após toracocentese. Nas efusões de longa duração, ocorrem espessamento e constrição da pleura visceral e espessamento da pleura parietal, o que pode levar ao desenvolvimento do *pulmão aprisionado*, ou muito constrito pela pleura visceral sobrejacente, sem poder se reexpandir adequadamente, mesmo na presença de pressão intratorácica negativa.[3] É provável que o pulmão aprisionado seja mais comum em pacientes veterinários, pois a maioria das efusões está associada à inflamação mais ativa. No entanto, o pulmão não recrutável foi muito menos avaliado em cães e gatos que em pessoas, mas poderia estar associado particularmente ao desenvolvimento de pneumotórax associado à toracocentese (ver adiante).

EXAME FÍSICO

Os sinais clínicos de doença no espaço pleural podem incluir taquipneia, ortopneia ou dificuldade respiratória evidente, tipicamente com respiração rápida/superficial, considerada a manifestação mais comum (Vídeo 244.1). Alguns animais apresentam esforço abdominal acentuado. Os achados ao exame físico podem incluir angústia respiratória, ação de músculos acessórios durante a respiração e abafamento de bulhas cardíacas/sons pulmonares (pneumotórax ou efusão pleural); ocasionalmente, os sons pulmonares podem parecer normais. Às vezes, é possível detectar macicez ventral à percussão do tórax em pacientes com efusão pleural. Outros achados clínicos podem refletir a doença primária (p. ex., som cardíaco de galope, lesão intratorácica em forma de massa, febre e traumatismo). A detecção de anormalidade no espaço pleural deve ser considerada um sinal clínico importante, mas não um diagnóstico definitivo. Em geral, o prognóstico de um paciente com efusão pleural é reservado, embora muitos casos respondam bem ao tratamento, pelo menos a curto prazo.

AVALIAÇÃO DIAGNÓSTICA INICIAL

O diagnóstico de efusão pleural ou pneumotórax pode ser feito por meio de toracocentese ou exames de imagens. A radiografia tem sido classicamente a técnica de imagem mais comum para a detecção de ambos os distúrbios, mas a ultrassonografia está sendo usada em maior escala nas emergências e na rotina clínica geral (Figura 244.1), especialmente para a detecção de efusão pleural, e cada vez mais para a detecção de pneumotórax (ver adiante). A tomografia computadorizada e a ressonância magnética

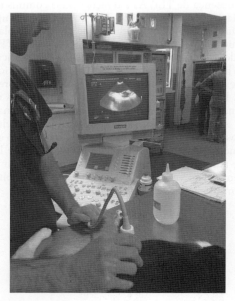

Figura 244.1 A triagem ultrassonográfica pode detectar efusão pleural como um espaço hipoecoico ou anecoico. Embora sejam necessárias habilidades ultrassonográficas avançadas para a identificação específica de muitas doenças, a maioria dos clínicos pode adquiri-las com relativa rapidez, suficiente para detectar líquido.

também podem mostrar efusões pleurais e pneumotórax, mas são usadas menos comumente como modalidades de imagens no diagnóstico inicial (Figura 244.2).

Os sinais radiográficos de efusão pleural incluem diminuição de detalhes ("ausência de brancos"), bordas pulmonares ventrais recortadas, linhas de fissura entre os lobos pulmonares e uma silhueta cardíaca obscurecida. Uma imagem radiográfica dorsoventral (DV) é útil para confirmar a presença de efusão pleural, com estresse mínimo ao paciente. Se disponíveis, radiografias com feixe horizontal também são muito úteis.[4] Efusões pleurais crônicas podem resultar em aparência radiográfica de bordas pulmonares "arredondadas", indicando fibrose pleural. À ultrassonografia, a efusão pleural é detectada como uma área livre de ecos, que aparece negra.[5,6]

Toracocentese

O tratamento de doença do espaço pleural objetiva tanto melhorar a função respiratória, ao remover líquido/ar, quanto identificar a causa primária. A toracocentese (ver Capítulo 102) é realizada após tricotomia e preparação asséptica de uma área entre a sétima e a nona costelas, próximo à junção costocondral (Vídeo 244.2 A e B). Ocasionalmente, o local pode ser mais ventral ou mais dorsal, com base na suspeita de líquido ou ar, respectivamente. O animal deve ser contido com cuidado, em decúbito esternal ou em estação. Tipicamente, em gatos e cães de pequeno porte, usam-se um cateter "butterfly" (com abas que parecem asas de borboleta), registro (torneira) e seringa de 5 a 30 mℓ. Em gatos maiores e na maioria dos cães, é necessária uma agulha mais longa. Em cães nos quais se espera a obtenção de um volume grande (> 1 ℓ) de efusão, pode-se recorrer a um cateter IV e aspiração, para a remoção mais rápida da efusão, em geral com menos estresse para o paciente e potencialmente menor risco de pneumotórax iatrogênico.

É recomendada técnica asséptica e pode-se fornecer oxigênio suplementar (ver Capítulo 131). Pode-se realizar um bloqueio anestésico local (lidocaína 2% e bicarbonato 8,4%, na proporção 9:1) ou ligeira sedação. No caso de pacientes que não cooperam, se resistirem por causa do temperamento ou da angústia respiratória, pode ser necessária anestesia ou sedação profunda (ver Capítulo 138), porém a equipe clínica deve estar preparada para a intubação e ventilação do paciente, se necessário, pois a sedação diminui o impulso respiratório. Percebe-se um som semelhante a "pop" quando a ponta da agulha penetra na cavidade pleural, embora isso possa ser mais difícil de notar por clínicos principiantes. Os volumes de líquido e ar obtidos devem ser registrados; em geral, é necessário retirar 5 a 30 mℓ para a mecânica ventilatória melhorar, mas uma quantidade menor pode ser útil para fins diagnósticos. Como o mediastino costuma ser incompleto, o hemitórax escolhido como o local de punção (i. e., lado direito ou esquerdo) é menos importante. Deve-se remover o máximo de efusão possível. A presença de fibrina ou efusão floculada pode dificultar a toracocentese. Se ela não for bem-sucedida, deve-se confirmar de novo a presença de efusão, de preferência com ultrassonografia. Se houver líquido, pode ser preciso usar uma agulha mais longa para alcançar o espaço pleural ou tentar a punção em outro local.

São incomuns complicações decorrentes de toracocentese, mas podem ocorrer. A mais relevante é o pneumotórax iatrogênico, que pode ser consequência de dano à pleura visceral e ao parênquima pulmonar, espessados/fibrosados, ou diminuição acentuada na pressão intratorácica, que resultam em lacerações espontâneas no pulmão ou na pleura e criação subsequente de uma fístula pulmonar-pleural. O pneumotórax iatrogênico de pequeno volume pode resolver-se sem tratamento, mas nos casos de extravasamentos grandes ou ativos pode ser necessária a colocação de um tubo de toracostomia ou até mesmo a realização de cirurgia. Outras complicações potenciais incluem hemorragia, se ocorrer punção inadvertida de um vaso de grande calibre ou do coração, ou extravasamento subcutâneo de efusão pleural infectada.

Tubos de toracostomia

Podem ser necessários tubos de toracostomia (tubos torácicos; ver Capítulo 100) para o tratamento de efusão pleural ou pneumotórax, em casos de ar ou efusão em grande volume que recorrem rapidamente, ou de efusão infecciosa, ou no pós-operatório. Cateteres de borracha vermelha podem ser usados como tubos torácicos, porém é mais comum a colocação de cateter com trocarte ou estilete, ou de cateter de pequeno calibre (p. ex., Mila International). Unidades de aspiração contínua podem ser utilizadas para ajudar na remoção de líquido ou ar e são mais usadas em casos de pneumotórax persistente do que nas efusões pleurais. No pneumotórax, como o acúmulo de ar pode ser bastante rápido, podem ser necessários tubos torácicos para facilitar a remoção de ar em tempo hábil. Em animais com traumatismo, pneumotórax ininterrupto ou sua recorrência após toracocentese, deve-se fazer a colocação imediata de um tubo de toracostomia. Como na efusão pleural, há uma variedade de opções para a escolha do tubo. Unidades de aspiração contínua podem ser úteis para prevenir novo acúmulo de ar, bem como promover a cicatrização do parênquima danificado.

Análise da efusão

Deve ser feita para ajudar a caracterizar as efusões pleurais (ver Capítulo 74). A aparência macroscópica da efusão pode ser purulenta, quilosa (leitosa), hemorrágica, serosa ou serossanguinolenta, ou ictérica. A maioria das efusões é serosa ou serossanguinolenta. A efusão pleural associada a piotórax pode ter odor desagradável (devido à presença de bactérias aeróbicas), bem como aparência macroscópica purulenta (Figura 244.3). O líquido deve ser caracterizado como transudato, transudato modificado ou exsudato, com base no conteúdo de proteína e na contagem celular (Tabela 244.1). Depois de avaliar a aparência macroscópica, a mensuração do teor de proteína e a contagem celular, o exame citológico da efusão geralmente é muito útil para obter o diagnóstico definitivo. Outros achados citológicos incluem a presença de células neoplásicas (carcinoma, linfoma), pequenos linfócitos, neutrófilos, bactérias, eritrócitos, macrófagos e células mesoteliais. Em casos raros, podem ser observados outros tipos celulares, como células de melanoma (Figura 244.4). Nas efusões de longa duração, as células mesoteliais podem assumir aparências citológicas bizarras, que podem dificultar a distinção de células neoplásicas.

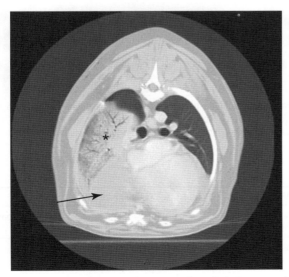

Figura 244.2 Imagem de tomografia computadorizada (TC) reconstruída de um cão com mesotelioma, que causou efusão pleural e subsequente torção pulmonar. A torção do lobo pulmonar é reconhecida pelo padrão vesicular no lobo (*asterisco*), enquanto o líquido é cinza (*seta*).

A avaliação bioquímica da efusão pleural é útil em alguns casos. Na medicina humana, os critérios de Light são amplamente aplicados à efusão pleural e recentemente foram descritos em gatos.[7] Em suma, os critérios de Light avaliam a razão entre o conteúdo de proteína da efusão e a concentração sérica de proteína, bem como a atividade da enzima lactato desidrogenase (LDH); em exsudatos, a razão é mais alta (> 0,5), bem como a atividade sérica de LDH.[8] Em pessoas, a análise bioquímica da efusão pleural é feita mais comumente do que em cães e gatos. O perfil bioquímico da efusão pleural consiste na mensuração do pH e das concentrações de glicose, amilase, creatinina ou BUN, colesterol, triglicerídios e uma variedade de outras substâncias. Em pessoas, a concentração de amilase no líquido pleural foi usada para confirmar perfuração esofágica, por exemplo, mas cães e gatos não produzem saliva com amilase.[9] O exame bioquímico da efusão pleural em cães e gatos é limitado. Baixo teor de glicose não está associado de maneira consistente à efusão pleural séptica, como é na efusão abdominal séptica.

A concentração de NT-pró-BNP na efusão pleural é alta em gatos com insuficiência cardíaca congestiva (ICC).[10] Concentração de NT-pró-BNP no líquido pleural > 323,3 pmol/mℓ foi associada a 100% de sensibilidade e 94% de especificidade, na diferenciação de efusão pleural cardiogênica da não cardiogênica, em uma série de casos em felinos.[10] Mais estudos sobre o perfil bioquímico da efusão pleural podem acrescentar informação útil à avaliação individual dos casos.

Cultura bacteriana e teste de sensibilidade (antibiograma) são indispensáveis nos casos em que se suspeita de infecção ou na efusão neutrofílica. A repetição da toracocentese pode predispor o paciente à infecção iatrogênica. A cultura bacteriana é empregada com maior frequência para avaliar se há microrganismos aeróbicos, embora geralmente o piotórax se deva às infecções anaeróbicas. Pode ser difícil a cultura de bactérias anaeróbicas, razão pela qual os dados sobre sua sensibilidade são limitados para serem obtidos. Microrganismos mais exigentes podem requerer meios de cultura especiais e um laboratório de microbiologia especializado. Infecção viral pode resultar em efusão pleural.[11] PCR também é um teste muito útil na identificação de microrganismos infecciosos, podendo ser solicitado, em especial, no caso de infecções atípicas.[12]

Outros exames diagnósticos

Em pacientes com efusão pleural, outros exames diagnósticos devem ser solicitados de acordo com os dados da resenha, os achados de exame físico e os resultados das análises da efusão. Os exames laboratoriais de rotina, incluindo hemograma completo, perfil bioquímico sérico e exame de urina, são aconselháveis para verificar se há uma doença sistêmica. Provas de função da tireoide, em gatos (ver Capítulo 301), e pesquisa de dirofilária em áreas endêmicas (ver Capítulo 255) também são recomendadas.

Radiografias do tórax após a remoção da efusão pleural geralmente são úteis para verificar se há ou não lesões em forma de massas, hérnia diafragmática ou aumento da silhueta cardíaca. A ecocardiografia é essencial na busca de evidência de cardiopatia direita ou efusão pericárdica. O exame ultrassonográfico do tórax pode ser útil para identificar e realizar biopsia de lesões

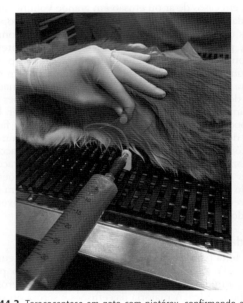

Figura 244.3 Toracocentese em gato com piotórax, confirmando a existência de material purulento.

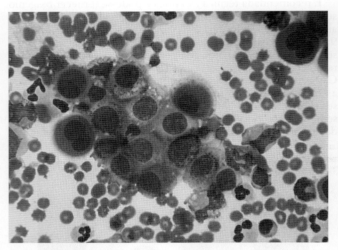

Figura 244.4 Células de melanoma metastático na efusão pleural de cão idoso mestiço da raça Border Collie. (Fotomicrografia por cortesia de Joyce Knoll, VMD, PhD, DAVCP.) (*Esta figura se encontra reproduzida em cores no Encarte.*)

Tabela 244.1 Características da efusão pleural.

	PROTEÍNA TOTAL	CELULARIDADE	TIPOS CELULARES	EXEMPLOS DE DOENÇA
Transudato	< 2,5 g/dℓ	< 2.500 células/µℓ	Neutrófilos não degenerados, macrófagos, células mesoteliais	Hipoalbuminemia (p. ex., enteropatia com perda de proteína)
Transudato modificado	2,5 a 7 g/dℓ	1.000 a 7.000 células/µℓ	Neutrófilos não degenerados, macrófagos, células mesoteliais, células neoplásicas, linfócitos	Insuficiência cardíaca congestiva (ICC), neoplasia, quilo
Exsudato	> 7 g/dℓ	> 7.000 células/µℓ	Diversos	Piotórax

Transudatos modificados são as causas mais comuns de efusão. A causa primária da efusão é o fator preditivo mais importante do prognóstico a longo prazo do paciente com efusão pleural.

expansivas (massas) e avaliar a integridade do diafragma. A tomografia computadorizada também é útil para detectar a causa da efusão.

Toracotomia ou toracostomia exploratória podem ser empregadas para uma avaliação mais completa da cavidade torácica, em especial quando há pneumotórax recorrente ou intratável, e para realização de biopsia, se indicada.

TIPOS DE EFUSÕES (VER CAPÍTULO 74)

Transudato puro

Esse tipo de efusão geralmente se desenvolve em animais de estimação hospitalizados ou naqueles com doenças crônicas acompanhadas de perda de proteína. No exame macroscópico, o líquido se assemelha à água e a celularidade é baixa. Cães da raça Yorkshire Terrier com linfangiectasia parecem mais propensos a desenvolver efusão pleural. O tratamento consiste em toracocentese (ver Capítulo 102), possivelmente tratamento de suporte com solução coloide (p. ex., plasma ou coloide sintético; ver Capítulo 129), diuréticos e terapia específica para a doença primária.

Transudato modificado

Este tipo de efusão é o mais comum em cães e gatos. As causas mais frequentes são as doenças mencionadas a seguir.

Insuficiência cardíaca congestiva

A insuficiência cardíaca direita pode resultar em acúmulo substancial de líquido pleural (ver Capítulos 246 e 247). A ICC é uma causa comum de efusão pleural em gatos. Pode desenvolver-se insuficiência cardíaca direita associada a doenças vasculares crônicas, ou certas malformações congênitas (p. ex., displasia da valva tricúspide). O exame físico mostra tipicamente outros sinais compatíveis com insuficiência cardíaca, como bulhas cardíacas anormais, taquicardia e/ou congestão de veia jugular. Gookin e Atkins relataram em um estudo, em um pequeno número de gatos, que qualquer efusão pleural de volume moderado a grande ($\geq$ 17 a 22 mℓ/kg) aumenta a pressão venosa central (PVC) em média 4,5 cm de H_2O (variação de 0 a 7 cm de H_2O), induzindo a um diagnóstico errôneo de efusão pleural como sendo cardiogênico.[13] O diagnóstico de insuficiência cardíaca baseia-se na demonstração ecocardiográfica de uma lesão cardíaca grave o suficiente para causar ICC. A elevação da concentração sérica[14] ou plasmática[6,14] de NT-pró-BNP também confirmam o diagnóstico de ICC. A adição recente de um teste SNAP confirmatório para NT-pró-BNP, em gatos, melhorou a disponibilidade em tempo real desse teste (IDEXX Laboratories, Westbrook, ME). Os achados citológicos na efusão pleural associados à ICC consistem em inflamação branda, embora alguns animais, em particular gatos, tenham efusão quilosa. O tratamento de efusão pleural associada à ICC é individualizado e o ideal é que se baseie na avaliação de um cardiologista veterinário; inclui, tipicamente, o uso de diurético, pimobendana e inibidores da enzima conversora de angiotensina. O tratamento clínico é mais útil para retardar o retorno da efusão pleural do que para a sua eliminação; portanto, recomenda-se toracocentese inicial para remoção da maior quantidade possível de líquido com segurança (ver Capítulo 102).

Doença pericárdica

A efusão pericárdica pode resultar no desenvolvimento de efusão pleural e ascite devido ao tamponamento cardíaco (ver Capítulo 254). A efusão pleural associada ao tamponamento cardíaco costuma se resolver após pericardiocentese (ver Capítulo 102). A presença de ascite com efusão pericárdica sugere uma progressão mais crônica e foi associada a um prognóstico melhor do que o tamponamento cardíaco agudo sem ascite secundária.[14] A pericardite constritiva também pode estar associada ao desenvolvimento de efusão pleural.

Malignidade

Neoplasia é uma causa comum de efusão pleural. Algumas neoplasias esfoliam facilmente (linfoma, alguns carcinomas), enquanto outras não apresentam critérios citológicos de malignidade. Conforme dito antes, efusões de longa duração podem estar associadas à presença de células mesoteliais reativas, o que pode dificultar a distinção de mesotelioma. A ausência de critérios citológicos para malignidade *não* exclui neoplasia da lista de diagnósticos diferenciais. O tratamento de efusões neoplásicas pode incluir toracocentese periódica, terapia intracavitária (p. ex., cisplatina, bleomicina, carboplatina) ou desvio do líquido neoplásico. Em animais com massas pulmonares que possam estar associadas à efusão maligna, a toracotomia e a ressecção da massa raramente são benéficas, podendo se constatar taxas de morbidade ou até mesmo de mortalidade significativas.

Exsudato

Infeccioso

As efusões pleurais podem ser de origem infecciosa. Os animais acometidos geralmente apresentam sinais sistêmicos de sepse (letargia, febre, leucocitose ou leucopenia; ver Capítulo 132). A avaliação citológica de efusões infecciosas mostra neutrófilos degenerados e, possivelmente, bactérias intra e extracelulares. As infecções podem ser aeróbicas ou anaeróbicas; as últimas podem produzir exsudatos de odor desagradável, sendo preciso tomar precauções para não expor pessoas aos agentes infecciosos por meio de inalação. Em gatos, ferimentos causados por mordeduras são considerados a fonte mais comum de infecção, enquanto em cães, além desses ferimentos, corpos estranhos penetrantes (farpas de madeira e espinhos de plantas) frequentemente são os responsáveis. Ocasionalmente, as efusões pleurais são secundárias à pneumonia bacteriana (*i. e.*, efusões parapneumônicas), mas são bastante raras em cães e gatos, em comparação com pessoas e equinos. Outras causas infecciosas menos comuns de efusão pleural são as infecções causadas por *Bartonella* spp., *Mycoplasma* spp. e vírus.

O tratamento de piotórax envolve drenagem (em geral, com auxílio de tubo de toracostomia; ver Capítulo 100) e uso de antibióticos com base na cultura microbiológica e no teste de sensibilidade (antibiograma). É possível que alguns animais precisem de intervenção cirúrgica para ressecção e drenagem de tecidos acometidos. O prognóstico de piotórax costuma ser bom, desde que o quadro clínico do animal de estimação não seja grave. O piotórax é uma das poucas efusões pleurais que pode ser curada.

A *peritonite infecciosa felina* (PIF) pode causar efusão pleural (ver Capítulo 224). Em geral, os gatos acometidos são jovens e apresentam concentração plasmática de globulina total elevada, bem como alto teor de proteína na efusão pleural (geralmente > 6 g/dℓ). No exame citológico, notam-se macrófagos reativos e neutrófilos, mas em pequena quantidade. Até o momento, não há tratamento efetivo para a PIF.

Hemorragia

Hemotórax pode ser decorrência de intoxicação por rodenticida anticoagulante (p. ex., brodifacoum; ver Capítulo 152), traumatismo, neoplasia ou torção de lobo pulmonar.[15] No hemotórax, por definição, o volume globular (hematócrito) da efusão pleural corresponde a um valor > 20% ou > 50% daquele verificado no sangue periférico do paciente. Os sinais clínicos de hemotórax refletem mais comumente hipovolemia do que a presença de efusão pleural. Em cães com anemia e efusão pleural, é prudente verificar o estado da coagulação antes da toracocentese, a fim de excluir a possibilidade de coagulopatia. O tratamento do hemotórax depende da causa primária e pode incluir transfusão de plasma, uso de vitamina K, cirurgia ou repouso. Tumores de costelas podem resultar em hemotórax, sendo necessária a ressecção para controlar a hemorragia. Pode-se deixar que o hemotórax traumático ou tóxico, de pequeno volume, que não comprometem a ventilação e cuja causa primária é controlada, sejam reabsorvidos espontaneamente.

Quilotórax

A efusão quilosa tem aparência branco-leitosa ou rosada e, no exame citológico, nota-se grande quantidade de pequenos linfócitos. Há muitas causas potenciais de efusão quilosa, sendo as doenças idiopáticas responsáveis por cerca de 50% dos casos. A avaliação de um paciente com efusão quilosa inclui a busca cuidadosa por uma causa primária, como doença cardíaca, trombo ou massa na veia cava cranial, dirofilariose ou neoplasia. Há relato de quilotórax pós-cirúrgico.[16] A efusão quilosa idiopática está associada à dilatação dos vasos linfáticos (linfangiectasia), mas o mecanismo permanece indefinido. O diagnóstico se baseia na detecção de alta concentração de triglicerídio no líquido pleural, comparativamente ao soro sanguíneo. Se for encontrada uma causa específica, o tratamento pode ser direcionado a ela. Na efusão idiopática, o tratamento pode consistir em toracocentese periódica (ver Capítulo 102) ou intervenção cirúrgica. Diversas técnicas cirúrgicas foram propostas como tratamento paliativo da efusão quilosa, mas nenhuma se mostrou efetiva na rotina clínica, com taxa de cura em torno de 50 a 70%. O melhor resultado cirúrgico parece estar associado a um cirurgião meticuloso e experiente.

Idiopático

Em alguns cães e gatos, apesar de todo o esforço concentrado, nenhuma causa de efusão pleural foi identificada. Nesses casos, o tratamento objetiva amenizar os sinais clínicos. Caso haja suspeita de doença imunomediada, antes de iniciar o tratamento imunossupressor, é fundamental a busca por infecções atípicas.

Miscelânea

Uma variedade de causas pode estar associada ao desenvolvimento de efusão pleural intermitente, incluindo torção de lobo pulmonar (ver Figura 244.2), pancreatite, doenças imunomediadas, hérnia diafragmática crônica, tromboembolismo pulmonar, lesões causadas por armas de fogo[17] ou cirurgias abdominais ou torácicas recentes. Gatos parecem especialmente predispostos ao desenvolvimento de efusão pleural no pós-operatório.

EFUSÕES CRÔNICAS

Podem ocorrer efusões pleurais crônicas secundárias a uma ampla variedade de doenças, mas são vistas mais comumente nas efusões idiopáticas, quilotórax, algumas cardiopatias congênitas e no mesotelioma. O tempo de sobrevivência com efusões crônicas depende da doença primária, bem como das características do paciente e do seu responsável. Alguns cães com efusões crônicas podem ser tratados durante meses a anos por meio de toracocentese intermitente, especialmente quando sua qualidade de vida for boa nos demais aspectos, a formação de aderências for limitada e o proprietário tiver condições emocionais e financeiras para arcar com os custos de uma doença crônica. É importante lembrar que animais com efusões crônicas são muito mais propensos a desenvolver pneumotórax após toracocentese, e o líquido da efusão pode ser infeccioso (piotórax).

Pneumotórax também é uma complicação iatrogênica comum da toracocentese em animais com efusão pleural crônica, quando a efusão resulta em espessamento da pleura e, possivelmente, aprisionamento pulmonar. Nesse contexto, o pneumotórax pode ser uma complicação devastadora, pois a cicatrização espontânea da pleura é improvável. Pode-se colocar um dreno pleural (Figura 244.5) para possibilitar a realização de toracocentese sem risco de laceração acidental da pleura.[18] Em cães de maior porte, o tamanho (20 G) da agulha de Hubber pode resultar em demora na drenagem da efusão. Além disso, nesse caso pode ocorrer infecção iatrogênica, principalmente se a drenagem for realizada por leigos, não treinados da maneira apropriada. Também foi descrita a omentalização como tratamento de efusão crônica.[19]

MENSURAÇÃO DA PRESSÃO PLEURAL

A mensuração da pressão pleural é muito útil na unidade de tratamento intensivo e no setor de emergência, podendo ser considerada indispensável na avaliação de respostas fisiológicas a uma enfermidade ou lesão grave. Em geral, a manometria pleural é recomendada às pessoas com efusão pleural e pode ser feita com facilidade em animais.[20] Pode-se monitorar a pressão pleural durante a toracocentese para drenar efusão pleural ou pneumotórax, ou continuamente se tiver sido colocado um tubo de toracostomia.

A manometria pleural foi projetada para monitorar a cavidade pleural em busca de sinais de pulmão não recrutável, condição evidenciada por grande decréscimo na pressão intrapleural que, posteriormente, poderia ocasionar dor ou pneumotórax espontâneo (PE). O pneumotórax iatrogênico é de interesse particular porque, na medicina veterinária, está associado à laceração acidental do pulmão. O conceito de pulmão não recrutável é convincente, pois aumentos maiores (p. ex., mais negativos) na pressão pleural também podem estar associados a PE, causado por laceração da pleura visceral em resposta à pressão acentuadamente negativa. Uma avaliação piloto de manometria pleural em nosso hospital, realizada pela médica veterinária Kendra LaFaunci, mostrou achados significativos, conforme ilustrado a seguir (Figura 244.6).

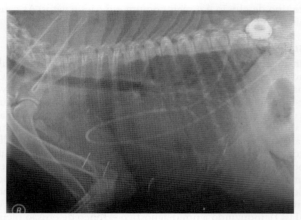

Figura 244.5 Radiografia do tórax de cão com efusão pleural crônica de causa desconhecida. Nota-se um dreno pleural.

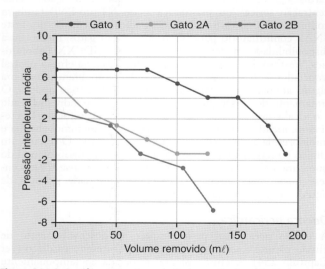

Figura 244.6 O gráfico representa a redução da pressão pleural devido à remoção da efusão pleural. A curva para o Gato 2B mostra leituras de pressão pleural quando se realizou toracocentese pela segunda vez. Desenvolveu-se uma pressão mais negativa associada ao mesmo volume de efusão removido; subsequentemente, esse gato desenvolveu pneumotórax, muito provavelmente causado por pulmão não recrutável. (*Esta figura se encontra reproduzida em cores no Encarte.*)

É interessante notar que o Gato 2B desenvolveu pneumotórax iatrogênico após toracocentese, potencialmente associado ao aprisionamento pulmonar, e pressão intratorácica substancialmente negativa. Além disso, o uso da manometria pleural também nos capacita a detectar se a agulha ou o cateter ainda está posicionado no espaço pleural após o movimento para reposicionar o paciente ou o término aparente do procedimento, o que em animais talvez seja a maior utilidade que obtemos.

RESUMO SOBRE EFUSÃO PLEURAL

A efusão pleural (Boxe 244.1) é uma anormalidade clínica, mas não um diagnóstico definitivo. Diversas condições podem resultar em efusão pleural; é mais provável que o tratamento seja efetivo, se for específico para a causa desencadeante. Pode ser necessária uma pesquisa diagnóstica abrangente para obter uma definição; em alguns casos, a etiologia permanece controversa.

PNEUMOTÓRAX

Define-se pneumotórax como a presença de ar livre no espaço pleural. Pode ser classificado como traumático, espontâneo ou iatrogênico, bem como aberto ou fechado[21] (Boxe 244.2). O *pneumotórax por tensão* é um tipo grave o suficiente para comprometer o débito cardíaco e, se não for prontamente esvaziado, resulta na morte do paciente. O pneumotórax por tensão pode ser decorrência de qualquer tipo de pneumotórax, embora quase sempre seja do tipo fechado (Figura 244.7).

Pneumotórax traumático

O pneumotórax traumático resulta de lesão ao tórax. É classificado como *aberto*, quando uma ferida aberta conecta o espaço pleural com o ar ambiente, e *fechado*, quando o extravasamento de ar é oriundo de tecido pulmonar danificado. Suspeita-se que a causa mais comum de pneumotórax em cães seja um traumatismo. Os ferimentos traumáticos podem ser contusos (p. ex., o impacto de uma batida de carro) ou penetrantes (p. ex., ferimentos causados por mordedura). O tratamento do pneumotórax traumático depende da gravidade dos sinais clínicos, com recomendação principal de tratar o paciente, não das anormalidades radiográficas.

Como em geral os animais com pneumotórax traumático têm, simultaneamente, contusão pulmonar ou fratura de costela, pode ser um desafio determinar a contribuição do pneumotórax na ocorrência de angústia respiratória. Se houver dúvida durante o exame clínico, é aconselhável toracocentese diagnóstica (ver Capítulo 102), para não perder a oportunidade de tratar uma condição clínica "tratável".

A detecção de pneumotórax traumático pode ser feita mediante toracocentese diagnóstica, ultrassonografia ou radiografias do tórax. Uma toracocentese diagnóstica negativa pode ser verdadeiramente negativa ou refletir o uso de agulha/cateter de comprimento inadequado ou a formação de bolsa de ar. Pode-se recorrer à avaliação ultrassonográfica (T-FAST), com foco no tórax, como teste diagnóstico padrão para pneumotórax (ver Capítulo 149), mas o clínico deve estar ciente de que pode ser mais difícil, para o menos experiente, identificar pneumotórax do que efusão pleural no exame ultrassonográfico.

O tratamento do pneumotórax traumático depende da gravidade e do mecanismo de desenvolvimento do pneumotórax (traumatismo contuso *versus* ferimento penetrante). A maioria dos casos de pneumotórax traumático se resolve rapidamente (1 a 4 dias) com cuidados de suporte e raramente requer cirurgia para controlar o extravasamento de ar. O prognóstico de pneumotórax traumático contuso é bom, sendo necessário apenas 1 dia de hospitalização, na maioria dos casos. É importante um exame completo do paciente na busca de outros ferimentos, porque pode haver lesões, como fraturas de coluna vertebral, que podem comprometer a cura e o prognóstico do paciente.

Em geral, ferimentos torácicos penetrantes requerem exploração cirúrgica, pois aqueles causados por mordeduras podem levar pelos e outros contaminantes à cavidade torácica. Em termos específicos, nos ferimentos por mordedura, o clínico deve lembrar que o local da perfuração causada pelo ferimento pode estar distante (vários centímetros) de onde ocorreu a penetração no tórax. Em cães de raças de pequeno porte (p. ex., Yorkshire Terrier) agarrados e sacudidos por cães maiores, é muito raro um ferimento por mordedura no tórax não penetrar realmente na cavidade torácica. Pequenas lesões na parede torácica (fraturas de costela ou laceração intercostal) podem ser detectadas como um movimento paradoxal da parede torácica ou palpada como uma depressão (ver Capítulo 149). Tórax instável, definido como a presença de duas ou mais fraturas em

---

Boxe 244.1 Resumo sobre efusão pleural

1. A detecção de efusão pleural deve levar a uma pesquisa abrangente da causa primária.
2. Muitos casos de efusão pleural podem ser tratados de maneira paliativa, com sucesso; todavia, a cura real é improvável, exceto nos casos de infecção, traumatismo ou intoxicação.
3. Durante a toracocentese pode ocorrer extravasamento de ar iatrogênico, em particular nas efusões crônicas.
4. Em cada toracocentese a avaliação citológica é indispensável, mesmo no caso de "agressores repetidos".

Boxe 244.2 Resumo sobre pneumotórax

1. O pneumotórax pode ser traumático, espontâneo ou iatrogênico.
2. Pode ser necessário o uso de tubo de toracostomia quando há grande volume de ar (ver Capítulo 100).
3. O pneumotórax causado por traumatismo contuso deve resolver-se com cuidados de suporte.
4. O pneumotórax causado por traumatismo penetrante pode necessitar de cirurgia, a fim de prevenir a ocorrência de infecção e reparar tecidos desvitalizados.
5. Em cães, o pneumotórax espontâneo (PE) deve levar à exploração cirúrgica.
6. Em gatos, o PE deve ser tratado individualmente.
7. O pneumotórax iatrogênico deve ser tratado de acordo o caso em questão.

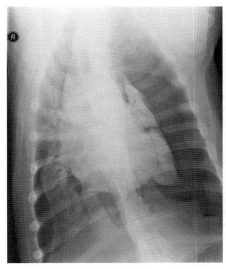

Figura 244.7 Radiografia do tórax de cão com pneumotórax por tensão.

duas ou mais costelas adjacentes, também pode ocorrer simultaneamente a traumatismo contuso ou penetrante. Embora se possa considerar a estabilização cirúrgica nos casos de ferimentos penetrantes, no traumatismo contuso o repouso e o alívio da dor devem ser procedimentos suficientes para possibilitar a cicatrização tecidual e normalização da mecânica pulmonar.

Pneumotórax espontâneo

É o que ocorre de forma atraumática, denominado primário quando não há doença pulmonar primária, e secundário se for decorrente de anormalidade pulmonar primária. É mais comum em cães do que em gatos; a ruptura de bolhas pulmonares resulta em PE primário. Cães de raças de grande porte parecem ser acometidos mais comumente. Os sinais clínicos refletem um padrão respiratório restritivo e consistem em inquietação, angústia respiratória e taquipneia. Deve-se perguntar aos proprietários de cães em que se suspeita de PE se algum traumatismo seria uma causa possível, porque em cães o PE é considerado uma doença cirúrgica, que requer intervenção e ressecção cirúrgicas imediatas do tecido pulmonar acometido, estando assim associado a um prognóstico melhor, ao passo que o pneumotórax decorrente de traumatismo contuso costuma ser tratado de maneira conservadora.[22] O diagnóstico diferencial pré-operatório inclui a obtenção de radiografias torácicas em três projeções, além de exames laboratoriais básicos. Podem ser realizados outros exames, a critério do clínico. Em geral, realiza-se exploração cirúrgica por meio de esternotomia mediana, que possibilita o exame de ambos os hemitóraces. Em alguns casos, apesar do procedimento cirúrgico aberto, é difícil detectar a causa do extravasamento de ar. Em tais casos, pode ser útil, ao explorar o tórax, providenciar ventilação com pressão positiva (p. ex., insuflando os pulmões a uma pressão de 15 a 20 cm de H_2O), enquanto se preenche o tórax com solução fisiológica estéril; isso faz com que os pulmões fiquem submersos e permite que o cirurgião veja as bolhas indicativas de extravasamento de ar. Em gatos, o PE primário é muito raro.

O PE secundário ocorre sem traumatismo, deve-se a uma doença pulmonar preexistente. Essa anormalidade foi relatada em cães, secundária a neoplasia, tromboembolismo pulmonar e, raramente, pneumonia. Em gatos, acredita-se que a causa mais provável seja asma/doença de via respiratória inferior ou dirofilariose. Pacientes com pequeno volume de ar podem ser tratados de maneira conservadora (tratamento clínico); no entanto, quando há grande volume de ar ou quando o pneumotórax está associado a uma lesão em forma de massa, o tratamento deve ser cirúrgico. Em geral, se tratado, o prognóstico de PE é bom, exceto quando há lesões neoplásicas.

Pneumotórax iatrogênico

É aquele que se instala durante o tratamento do paciente. As causas mais comuns são toracocentese em um animal de estimação com efusão crônica e fornecimento de ventilação com pressão positiva intermitente, com alta pressão inspiratória.

O tratamento de pneumotórax iatrogênico pode ser difícil, pois a efusão crônica preexistente pode ser uma causa de contraindicação de toracotomia ou aumentar o risco associado à intervenção cirúrgica. A remoção de pequeno volume de ar (5 a 20 ml) durante a toracocentese requer monitoramento cuidadoso do paciente, ao passo que a remoção de volumes maiores requer intervenções mais urgentes. Recomendou-se um "remendo sanguíneo" (*blood patch*) para o tratamento de um extravasamento de ar ativo.[23] Os principais benefícios desse procedimento são a facilidade de realizá-lo e a disponibilidade imediata de sangue do próprio paciente; recentemente foi descrito em uma população de oito cães, com resultados bastante promissores.[24] A complicação mais comum desse recurso em pessoas é infecção, embora também seja possível a ocorrência de pneumotórax por tensão devido à presença de um coágulo sanguíneo no tubo de toracostomia. Em geral, são colhidos 50 ml de sangue total, sem anticoagulante, e introduzidos no tórax com auxílio de um tubo de toracostomia. Está em andamento investigação adicional sobre esse procedimento em cães e gatos.

OUTRAS DOENÇAS DO ESPAÇO PLEURAL

Outras doenças também podem acometer o espaço pleural e resultar em angústia respiratória. Tais condições são abordadas com mais detalhes em outros capítulos (ver Capítulos 139, 149, 240, 245 e 273). É sensato avaliar se essas doenças podem estar envolvidas no quadro de angústia respiratória do paciente. Tais condições incluem massas na parede torácica, hérnia diafragmática, massas no mediastino e tumor ou corpo estranho no esôfago. As massas na parede torácica podem ser oriundas das costelas e as causas mais comuns são osteossarcoma, condrossarcoma e fibrossarcoma (ver Capítulo 245). Essas massas tumorais podem estar associadas a hemotórax grave e sua visualização pode ser difícil em imagens radiográficas, quando há grande volume de efusão.[15] Em tumores de baixo grau, a ressecção cirúrgica pode ser paliativa e até curativa. Tomografia computadorizada (Figura 244.8) pode ser muito útil para ajudar a elucidar a extensão dessas massas.

Hérnias diafragmáticas (HD; ver Capítulo 245) estão associadas mais comumente a traumatismo contuso e podem ser detectadas pela perda da continuidade do diafragma ou pela presença de conteúdo abdominal na cavidade torácica. Embora seja fácil detectar algumas HD em imagens do tórax de rotina, em alguns casos a documentação da lesão pode ser mais desafiadora. Pode-se recorrer a ultrassonografia, tomografia computadorizada ou, raramente, cirurgia exploradora, como métodos auxiliares na confirmação do diagnóstico. A correção cirúrgica deve ser imediata e emergencial, se o paciente apresentar instabilidade clínica ou herniação do estômago na cavidade torácica.

Lesões em forma de massas no mediastino (ver Capítulos 245 e 344) costumam resultar em angústia respiratória, devido ao desenvolvimento de efusão pleural. Todavia, massas muito grandes (p. ex., alguns timomas) podem resultar em compressão de estruturas intratorácicas; ademais, a miastenia gravis concomitante pode resultar em fraqueza neuromuscular e subsequente angústia respiratória.

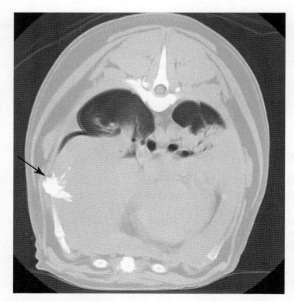

Figura 244.8 Imagem obtida em tomografia computadorizada (TC) de um cão com uma grande lesão em forma de massa (*seta*), na costela; o paciente chegou à consulta com baixo débito cardíaco (pulso fraco) e alta concentração de creatinina (5 mg/dℓ; 440 mmol/ℓ).

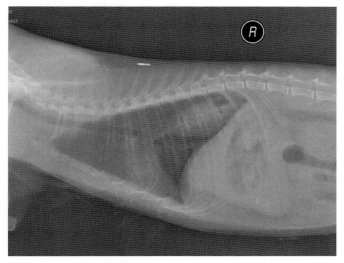

Figura 244.9 Radiografia lateral do tórax de gato com angústia respiratória grave, mostrando diversos corpos estranhos no esôfago (elásticos de prender cabelos).

A doença esofágica (ver Capítulo 273) geralmente resulta em regurgitação e dificuldade de deglutição, mas em alguns casos (Figura 244.9) ocasiona angústia respiratória evidente. A perfuração do esôfago também pode resultar em efusão pleural.

RESUMO

A doença do espaço pleural pode ser classificada como efusão, pneumotórax ou lesão que ocupa espaço (expansiva). A detecção imediata de doença do espaço pleural é vital em termos diagnósticos, porque um componente importante do tratamento é a resolução da causa primária. Muitas causas de efusão pleural estão associadas à doença crônica e podem necessitar de tratamento de longa duração, enquanto o pneumotórax pode ser tratado com mais sucesso. Lesões em forma de massas (HD) podem ser curáveis ou submetidas a tratamento paliativo apropriado.

REFERÊNCIAS BIBLIOGRÁFICAS

As referências bibliográficas deste capítulo se encontram online no Ambiente de Aprendizagem.

CAPÍTULO 245

Doenças do Mediastino, da Parede Torácica e do Diafragma

Martha Moon Larson e David S. Biller

MEDIASTINO

Anatomia

O mediastino é um espaço verdadeiro criado pelas reflexões pleurais e situa-se entre as cavidades pleurais direita e esquerda.[1,2] Está localizado primordialmente na linha média do tórax, embora se desvie um pouco para a esquerda, de modo a acomodar a extensão dos lobos pulmonares cranial direito e acessório. O mediastino contém e circunda o coração, a traqueia, o esôfago, o timo, os linfonodos torácicos, o ducto torácico, o nervo vago, a artéria aorta, as veias cavas cranial e caudal, bem como todos os outros vasos sanguíneos que entram ou saem do coração. O espaço mediastínico estende-se dorsalmente, do músculo longo ventral do pescoço até a coluna torácica, e ventralmente até o esterno, bem como da entrada do tórax até o diafragma. Não é um espaço fechado e se comunica com os tecidos moles cervicais através da entrada torácica e com o espaço retroperitoneal via hiato aórtico. Portanto, uma doença em qualquer desses compartimentos pode disseminar-se e comunicar-se. Por exemplo, o enfisema subcutâneo em tecidos moles cervicais pode estender-se para o mediastino, criando um pneumomediastino, e daí para o espaço retroperitoneal. O mediastino está separado do espaço pleural, mas fenestrações mediastínicas possibilitam que ar e líquido pleurais se comuniquem entre as cavidades torácicas. O mediastino é dividido em 5 compartimentos: cranioventral, craniodorsal, médio, caudoventral e caudodorsal.

Três conjuntos de linfonodos estão localizados no mediastino, mas geralmente não são visualizados, a menos que apresentem aumento de volume.[3-5] Os linfonodos mediastínicos craniais estão localizados ao longo da veia cava cranial, ventrais à traqueia e craniais ao coração. Seu número varia e eles recebem vasos linfáticos aferentes da traqueia, do esôfago, do pericárdio e da pleura, bem como de músculos do pescoço, do tórax e do abdome, da escápula, das seis últimas vértebras cervicais, das vértebras torácicas, das costelas, da tireoide, do timo e do mediastino. Os linfonodos traqueobrônquicos (hilares) são pares, com um par localizado na bifurcação dos brônquios principais (carina), pouco dorsais ao átrio esquerdo. A sua localização é um pouco mais cranial no gato em comparação com o cão. Outros linfonodos traqueobrônquicos estão localizados laterais à carina. Esses linfonodos recebem vasos linfáticos aferentes dos pulmões e brônquios. Os linfonodos esternais situam-se ao longo da parte ventral do mediastino cranial, um pouco dorsais à segunda e à terceira esternebras. Em gatos, os linfonodos esternais estão localizados um pouco mais caudalmente no esterno, em comparação com aqueles dos cães. Os linfonodos esternais recebem vasos linfáticos aferentes do diafragma, do pericárdio, das paredes torácicas ventral e abdominal, bem como da cavidade peritoneal.

Avaliação diagnóstica

O mediastino não é facilmente acessível ao exame físico, devido à sua localização intratorácica, e não há exames de sangue específicos para doença do mediastino. Ao exame físico, quando a parte cranial do tórax não for complacente durante leve palpação, pode-se suspeitar de uma grande massa na parte cranial do mediastino, particularmente em gatos. A ausência de sons respiratórios normais à auscultação também pode sugerir uma lesão em forma de massa; pneumotórax é um diagnóstico diferencial importante. A obtenção de imagens do mediastino (em radiologia, ultrassonografia [US], tomografia computadorizada [TC], ressonância magnética [RM] ou medicina nuclear) é essencial para uma avaliação não invasiva.

Radiografia simples

O mediastino é visto como uma opacidade de tecido mole apenas na parte cranial do tórax, ventral à traqueia. Essa opacidade se deve ao encobrimento das bordas de várias estruturas mediastínicas, inclusive esôfago, veia cava cranial, artéria subclávia esquerda, tronco braquiocefálico e linfonodos mediastínicos craniais. Tais estruturas são vistas individualmente apenas quando há ar no mediastino, atuando como um contraste negativo. Na imagem ventrodorsal (VD) ou dorsoventral (DV), o mediastino fica superposto à coluna vertebral, não devendo ter mais que o dobro da espessura dela, embora depósitos de gordura nele possam causar espessamento não patológico. O espessamento devido à gordura deve resultar em bordas retas lisas. Em animais jovens, o timo pode ser visualizado com uma estrutura opaca triangular de tecido mole, em forma de vela náutica, na parte cranioventral do mediastino, pouco à esquerda da linha média, e cranial ao coração.

A radiografia simples é ideal na primeira etapa de avaliação da presença de doença do mediastino, porque possibilita a avaliação do tamanho, da forma, da opacidade e dos locais de anormalidades. Em geral, as lesões de mediastino consistem em desvio do mediastino, pneumomediastino e aumento do tamanho e/ou da opacidade do mediastino (massa mediastínica).

Ocorre desvio do mediastino quando há diminuição do volume de um ou mais lobos pulmonares em um lado. O mediastino se desvia em direção ao lado afetado para compensar a perda de volume. O coração é o maior órgão contido no mediastino e um desvio para um dos lados (na imagem VD ou DV, em posição apropriada) é indicativo de desvio do mediastino. O diafragma do lado acometido também pode sofrer um desvio cranial para compensar. Como alternativa, o mediastino se desvia na direção do hemitórax normal, quando o lado oposto apresenta um aumento de volume secundário à efusão pleural unilateral de grande volume ou a uma grande massa pulmonar.

O aumento de tamanho do mediastino pode ser causado por tumor (massa tecidual) de mediastino, aumento de volume do esôfago ou presença de líquido no mediastino. Nas radiografias, tais condições são vistas como aumento difuso ou focal do mediastino. O aumento difuso de tecido mole pode ser causado por acúmulo de líquido secundário à inflamação ou hemorragia. O aumento focal geralmente se deve a uma lesão em forma de massa. Massas teciduais na parte cranial do mediastino são mais comuns e, se forem grandes o bastante, podem resultar em encobrimento da borda cranial do coração, elevação da traqueia e deslocamento caudal da carina (normalmente localizada no sexto espaço intercostal) e do coração. Nas imagens VD/DV nota-se aumento da parte cranial do mediastino. Massas mediastínicas de volume médio devem-se, mais comumente, a aumento de volume de linfonodos hilares, que criam um efeito de massa (expansivo) na base do coração, com desvio ventral da carina e dos brônquios principais (na imagem lateral) e desvio lateral dos brônquios principais (na imagem DV/VD). Massas na parte caudal do mediastino podem ser decorrências de abscesso, granuloma, tumor ou doença esofágica.

Ultrassonografia

A utilidade da ultrassonografia da cavidade torácica se limita à visualização do mediastino normal, pois o ar presente nos lobos pulmonares adjacentes impede a transmissão de ondas sonoras. No entanto, a avaliação sonográfica pode dar informação útil em animais com efusão pleural (que cria uma janela para o mediastino) ou com doença mediastínica.[6-9] A ultrassonografia possibilita a visualização de massas na parte mais cranial do mediastino.

Pode ser necessário colocar o transdutor em uma posição paraesternal cranial ou usar o coração como uma janela acústica para fazer uma avaliação adequada de massas teciduais menores. A ultrassonografia é especialmente útil para definir a arquitetura interna de massas sólidas ou císticas e mostrar a localização de estruturas vasculares em relação à massa. Embora a aparência ultrassonográfica de uma massa não seja específica da origem exata do tecido, ela pode ser usada para direcionar a introdução da agulha para obter aspirado com agulha fina (AAF) ou biopsia do núcleo do tecido.[10] A ultrassonografia transesofágica possibilita visualização excelente da base do coração, dos vasos sanguíneos das partes mais craniais do mediastino, da artéria aorta descendente e de parte da veia ázigos (ver Capítulo 104).[11-13] Essa modalidade elimina as dificuldades de obtenção de imagens em caso de obesidade, janelas intercostais de baixa qualidade e interferência do ar pulmonar.

Tomografia computadorizada

A tomografia computadorizada do tórax fornece informação mais detalhada sobre a presença, a localização e a extensão de doença. Ela possibilita melhor discriminação de contraste do que as radiografias simples, permitindo a distinção entre estruturas sólidas, gordurosas ou císticas.[14] O formato da imagem em corte transversal elimina o problema da sobreposição anatômica. A capacidade de reconstrução de planos múltiplos é uma vantagem a mais. A exacerbação do contraste após administração intravenosa de um composto iodado possibilita informações adicionais quanto à perfusão de tecidos moles e anomalias vasculares.[14-19] Em especial na presença de efusão pleural, a TC do tórax é superior às radiografias torácicas para localizar lesões em forma de massas no mediastino, determinar seu caráter (cístico *versus* sólido) e a extensão da doença, inclusive invasão vascular regional, informação fundamental para definir a possibilidade de ressecção cirúrgica de qualquer massa. A angiografia por tomografia computadorizada é necessária para avaliar, com maior confiança, se houve invasão vascular. Para controlar os movimentos respiratórios, geralmente é necessário anestesia geral para TC do tórax.

Avaliação diagnóstica adicional

Pode-se realizar cintilografia da tireoide com o uso de tecnécio-99m ou iodo-131, para identificar tecido tireoideano ectópico ou metastático funcional no mediastino.[20,21]

DOENÇAS DO MEDIASTINO

Pneumomediastino

É o acúmulo anormal de ar no mediastino, podendo ser causado por uma variedade de mecanismos.[22-25] A ruptura da traqueia pode provocar extravasamento de ar para o mediastino, tendo sido relatada em caso de traumatismo cervical, ventilação mecânica, aspiração transtraqueal, traqueostomia, intubação traqueal e hiperinsuflação ou colocação de cateter venoso central (ver Capítulo 241).[23,26] Anestesia geral com intubação endotraqueal e ventilação com pressão positiva (possibilidade de barotrauma e ruptura de traqueia), seguida de traumatismo e corpo estranho na traqueia, foram relatadas como as causas mais comuns de pneumomediastino em gatos.[25,27] Similar ao traumatismo traqueal, a ruptura de esôfago ou faringe pode resultar em pneumomediastino.[28,29] O enfisema subcutâneo de qualquer localização pode alcançar o mediastino por meio de tecidos moles cervicais e entrada torácica. Traumatismo ou hiperdistensão pulmonar e ruptura de alvéolos podem resultar em ar alveolar livre que se propaga ao longo do interstício pulmonar e da bainha broncovascular para o espaço mediastínico (efeito Macklin).[30] Isso pode ocorrer de forma completamente diferente do traumatismo pulmonar que resulta em pneumotórax. Lesão pulmonar grave ou doença respiratória preexistente podem ocasionar ruptura brônquica ou alveolar e subsequente pneumomediastino.[31,32] Menos comumente, pode penetrar ar no mediastino proveniente do acúmulo de gás no espaço retroperitoneal. Em alguns casos, a causa do pneumomediastino é desconhecida (pneumomediastino espontâneo).[24,25]

A presença de ar no mediastino exacerba o contraste de detalhes, possibilitando a visualização radiográfica de estruturas mediastínicas individuais (mais bem vistas em imagens laterais), incluindo veia cava cranial, tronco braquiocefálico e artéria subclávia esquerda, esôfago e veia ázigos (Figura 245.1). A visualização da parede da traqueia é exacerbada devido à presença de ar intra e extraluminal. O ar presente no mediastino pode comunicar-se com o espaço retroperitoneal, através do hiato aórtico, resultando em pneumorretroperitônio. Não ocorre pneumomediastino secundário a pneumotórax. Entretanto, um caso grave de pneumomediastino pode causar pneumotórax secundário.

Embora o pneumomediastino possa ocasionar alterações radiográficas marcantes, tipicamente não induz angústia respiratória, a menos que haja doença pleural ou pulmonar concomitante. Se o pneumomediastino progride para pneumotórax, em geral se observam taquipneia e dispneia (ver Capítulo 244). Animais com pneumomediastino associado à ruptura de esôfago manifestam sintomas associados à doença esofágica, como regurgitação, dor e disfagia (ver Capítulo 273). O ar aprisionado no mediastino não requer tratamento e se resolve espontaneamente em 2 semanas se não houver fonte de extravasamento de ar ativa.

Mediastinite

Os sinais clínicos associados a mediastinite consistem em taquipneia (provavelmente relacionada à dor torácica), dispneia, tosse, edema de cabeça e/ou pescoço e regurgitação. Podem ocorrer alterações na vocalização secundárias ao acometimento do nervo laríngeo recorrente. O exame físico pode revelar edema de cabeça e/ou pescoço, febre e abafamento dos sons pulmonares se também houver pneumotórax ou efusão pleural.

A inflamação mediastínica se manifesta radiograficamente como aumento focal ou difuso do mediastino. Espessamento da pleura mediastínica, ar e líquido no mediastino, aumento de linfonodos mediastínicos e lesões em forma de massas no mediastino foram relatados em TC.[33,34] Essas alterações podem resultar de perfuração de esôfago ou traqueia, infecção do tecido mole cervical profundo, que se estendem ao longo dos planos fasciais até o mediastino, ou extensão de infecção a partir do pericárdio, do parênquima pulmonar ou do espaço pleural.[35] Espinhos de gramíneas intratorácicos migratórios foram relatados como uma causa de mediastinite.[33] A mediastinite granulomatosa crônica pode ser causada por fungos, como *Histoplasma* ou *Cryptococcus* spp., ou bactérias, como *Actinomyces* ou *Nocardia* spp.[36,37] Foi documentada mediastinite secundária à espirocercose em cães.[38,39] A abscedação do mediastino pode resultar da progressão de doenças infecciosas crônicas ou neoplásicas no mediastino.[35] Abscessos e granulomas no mediastino costumam aparecer nas radiografias como massas mediastínicas e, portanto, podem ser confundidos com neoplasia.

O tratamento consiste na resolução da doença primária. A perfuração de esôfago pode necessitar de ressecção cirúrgica e/ou drenagem, juntamente com terapia antimicrobiana apropriada e cuidados de suporte.[35,37,39] A mediastinite, sem lesão expansiva (massa), pode responder à terapia antimicrobiana e cuidados de suporte exclusivamente.

Hemorragia no mediastino

Em geral, a hemorragia no mediastino se deve a traumatismo ou coagulopatia.[40-42] Os sinais clínicos associados à hemorragia no mediastino estão relacionados aos efeitos da perda de sangue aguda. Pode ocorrer dispneia, se a hemorragia de mediastino progredir para hemotórax ou a traqueia for comprimida pela hemorragia em torno dela. Os sinais radiográficos consistem em aumento do mediastino com opacidade de tecido mole, tanto nas imagens laterais quanto nas VD/DV. O diâmetro da traqueia pode estar estreitado devido à compressão, ou pode ocorrer espessamento da parede por causa da hemorragia submucosa (Figura 245.2).[41] O tratamento tem por objetivo a resolução da causa primária, como o uso de plasma e vitamina K no caso de intoxicação por rodenticida anticoagulante, juntamente com cuidados de suporte (ver Capítulo 152). A hemorragia de mediastino discreta geralmente não requer tratamento específico.

Massas mediastínicas

Em geral, as lesões em forma de massas no mediastino são classificadas de acordo com a sua localização (Tabela 245.1).

Tabela 245.1	Diagnóstico diferencial de lesões acompanhadas de aumento focal do mediastino.
REGIÃO	**DOENÇAS**
Cranioventral	Linfadenopatia; abscesso; massa no timo; tireoide ectópica; hematoma; granuloma; obesidade; massa vascular (artéria aorta, veia cava cranial); massa, corpo estranho ou dilatação de esôfago; massa na traqueia
Craniodorsal	Massa, corpo estranho ou dilatação de esôfago; massa na base do coração; tumor neurogênico; massa paraespinal ou espinal; hematoma; linfadenopatia; estenose aórtica; persistência do ducto arterioso; abscesso; massa na traqueia
Peri-hilar	Linfadenopatia; aumento do átrio esquerdo; massa, corpo estranho ou dilatação de esôfago; massa na artéria pulmonar principal (dilatação pós-estenose); massa na base do coração ou no átrio direito; massa espinal ou paraespinal
Caudodorsal	Massa, corpo estranho ou dilatação de esôfago; hérnia de hiato; hérnia ou massa diafragmática; espirocercose; massa espinal ou paraespinal; aneurisma aórtico; intussuscepção gastresofágica
Caudoventral	Hérnia diafragmática; hérnia diafragmática peritônio-pericárdica; abscesso; granuloma; hematoma

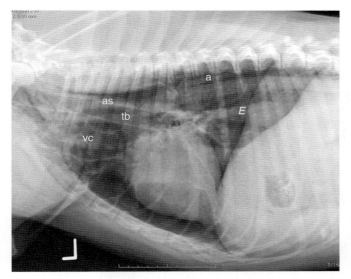

Figura 245.1 Pneumomediastino. Radiografia lateral do tórax de um cão mestiço com 6 anos de idade, levado à consulta após ter sido atropelado por um carro. O ar livre no mediastino delimita estruturas anatômicas que não são vistas normalmente, inclusive veia cava cranial (vc), esôfago (E), paredes interna e externa da traqueia, tronco braquicefálico (tb), artéria subclávia esquerda (as) e veia ázigos (a).

Cistos no mediastino

Os cistos benignos na parte cranial do mediastino podem originar-se de estruturas anatômicas diferentes (cisto paratireóideo, cisto tireoglosso, cisto tímico branquial e cisto pleural) e são mais comumente detectados em gatos idosos.[43,44] Em termos radiográficos, eles se apresentam como massas focais de tecido mole localizadas na parte cranioventral do mediastino, geralmente mais caudais do que outras massas mediastínicas (Figura 245.3). Pode-se realizar ultrassonografia ou TC para visualizar o conteúdo líquido e diferenciá-lo de lesões sólidas em forma de massas. Ao exame ultrassonográfico, os cistos de mediastino são ovoides/bilobados, de parede delgada, contêm líquido anecoico e, em geral, são acompanhados por exacerbação distal. Neoplasias sólidas, abscessos ou granulomas podem conter componentes

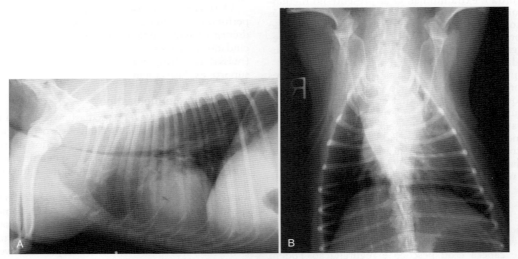

Figura 245.2 Hemorragia no mediastino. Imagens radiográficas lateral (**A**) e DV (**B**) do tórax de um cão com 5 anos que apresentava hemorragia no mediastino devido à intoxicação por rodenticida. Note a compressão da traqueia em decorrência da hemorragia de mediastino em torno dela (*imagem lateral*) e aumento do mediastino (*imagem DV*).

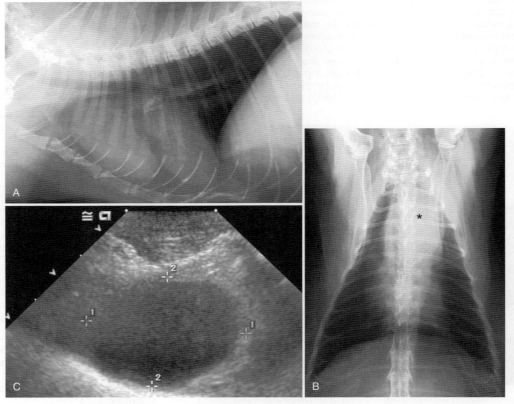

Figura 245.3 Cisto de mediastino. Imagens radiográficas lateral (**A**) e VD (**B**) do tórax de um gato com 6 anos levado à consulta para avaliação de vômitos. Há uma massa de tecido mole com borda bem definida na parte cranial do mediastino, um pouco cranial ao coração. Nota-se aumento do mediastino na imagem VD (*asterisco*). **C.** Imagem de ultrassonografia de massa na parte cranial do mediastino do mesmo gato. A massa é anecoica e está preenchida com líquido, achado compatível com cisto de mediastino benigno.

císticos e precisam ser diferenciados de um cisto simples. A aspiração com agulha fina orientada por ultrassom é o teste diagnóstico de escolha. O líquido aspirado é tipicamente transparente, incolor e com celularidade mínima. Em geral, os cistos de mediastino são achados acidentais que não ocasionam sinais clínicos, a menos que sejam grandes o bastante para comprimir estruturas adjacentes, como a traqueia.

Linfadenopatia no mediastino

O aumento de linfonodos mediastínicos é causado por uma variedade de doenças. O aumento de linfonodos hilares (traqueobrônquicos) mais comumente é secundário a linfoma ou pneumonia fúngica (histoplasmose, blastomicose, coccidioidomicose)[45] (Figura 245.4). Outras causas incluem sarcoma histiocítico, adenocarcinoma metastático (hepatocelular, da glândula anal, pancreático), micobacterioses, broncopneumopatia eosinofílica, granulomatose pulmonar eosinofílica e granulomatose linfomatoide.[45-55] Não parece haver relação entre o tamanho dos linfonodos traqueobrônquicos e o tipo de doença. Os linfonodos mediastínicos craniais recebem vasos linfáticos aferentes da cabeça e do pescoço (ver seção sobre Anatomia, mencionada anteriormente) e podem aumentar de tamanho quando há doenças nessas áreas. É provável que o linfoma seja a causa mais comum de aumento visível. É possível identificar linfadenopatia esternal em imagens radiográficas, pois os linfonodos esternais estão relativamente isolados de outras estruturas de tecido mole, o que torna seu aumento mais visível. Como esses linfonodos recebem drenagem aferente da cavidade peritoneal, o seu aumento deve levar à investigação imediata de doença abdominal.

Neoplasia de mediastino

Os tumores mediastínicos podem originar-se de qualquer estrutura do mediastino (linfonodos, timo, grandes vasos, traqueia, esôfago ou tecido ectópico tireóideo ou paratireóideo) ou pela disseminação de lesões neoplásicas de tecidos adjacentes.[56-59] As neoplasias de mediastino também podem ser lesões metastáticas ou componentes de um processo neoplásico multicêntrico.[59-61] Foram documentados tumores benignos.[62]

Em geral, os sinais clínicos associados a tumores de mediastino são causados por compressão ou invasão de estruturas, como grandes vasos sanguíneos, ducto torácico, esôfago e traqueia, ou devido à efusão pleural associada. Os sintomas consistem em tosse, dispneia, disfagia, regurgitação e edema da cabeça, do pescoço e/ou das partes inferiores dos membros. Os sinais clínicos causados pelo aprisionamento de nervo periférico são menos comuns e incluem paralisia de laringe, alterações na vocalização ou síndrome de Horner. Os sintomas associados à doença multicêntrica podem refletir outros locais de acometimento neoplásico ou estar relacionados com síndromes paraneoplásicas e consistem em anorexia, perda de peso, regurgitação, vômitos, diarreia e poliúria/polidipsia.

O linfoma de mediastino origina-se de um linfonodo ou de tecido do timo presente na parte cranial do mediastino (Figura 245.5 e Vídeo 245.1); é mais comum em gatos do que em cães,[56,58] tipicamente em gatos jovens (2 a 4 anos), em geral positivos para o vírus da leucemia felina.[56,58,61] Geralmente, o linfoma de mediastino está associado à efusão pleural, que pode prejudicar a visualização radiográfica do tumor de mediastino. O diagnóstico de linfoma mediastínico em geral pode ser confirmado pela detecção de linfócitos neoplásicos em amostra de líquido pleural ou em amostra obtida diretamente da neoplasia mediastínica por meio de aspiração com agulha fina (ver Capítulo 74). Em cães, o linfoma de mediastino pode estar associado à hipercalcemia.[62,63]

Os quimiodectomas, que costumam ser tumores aórticos ou do corpo carotídeo, são detectados com maior frequência como massas na base do coração (ver Capítulo 254) (Figura 245.6).

Outras massas neoplásicas no mediastino menos comuns incluem carcinoma ectópico da tireoide, carcinoma neuroendócrino e carcinoma anaplásico.[59] Não se pode determinar o tipo de tumor da massa mediastínica somente com base nos achados radiográficos. Contudo, é fundamental obter tal informação, porque o tratamento recomendado para tumor na parte cranial do mediastino, que não seja linfoma, é a ressecção cirúrgica. A tomografia computadorizada é de ajuda inestimável para uma avaliação mais detalhada da localização da massa, de sua morfologia, do envolvimento de vasos adjacentes e a identificação de metástases pulmonares.[64]

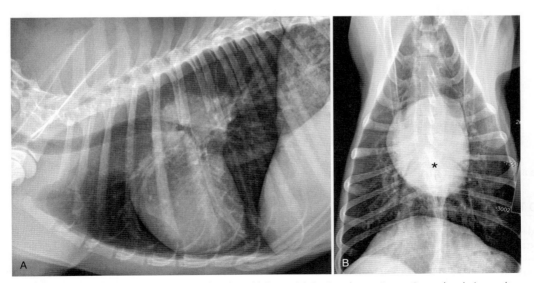

Figura 245.4 Linfadenopatia traqueobrônquica. Imagens radiográficas lateral (**A**) e VD (**B**) do tórax de um cão com 3 anos levado à consulta por apresentar tosse. Os linfonodos traqueobrônquicos estão aumentados e ocasionam um efeito de massa na região um pouco dorsal à carina, resultando em desvio ventral das partes caudais dos brônquios principais (imagem lateral). Na imagem VD, os linfonodos traqueobrônquicos aumentados (*asterisco*) causam uma opacidade maior sobre a base do coração e desvio lateral das partes caudais dos brônquios principais.

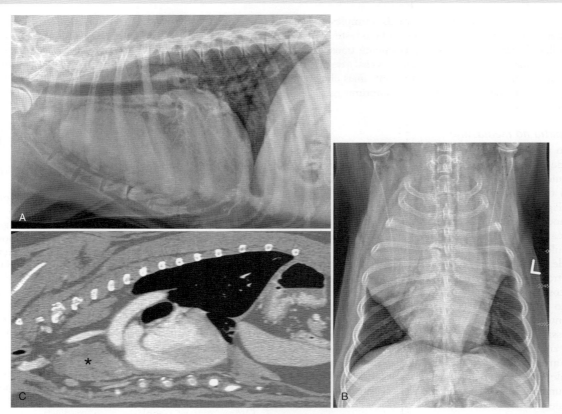

Figura 245.5 Linfoma de mediastino. Imagens radiográficas lateral (**A**) e VD (**B**) e imagem sagital reformatada obtida em TC (**C**) do tórax de um cão com 7 anos, para avaliação de letargia. Há uma grande massa na parte cranial do mediastino. Na imagem lateral, nota-se deslocamento dorsal da traqueia e há sobreposição da borda do órgão com a borda cranial do coração. Na imagem VD, nota-se que a massa está centralizada e cranial ao coração, mas se estende bilateralmente. A imagem da TC mostra a massa na parte cranial do mediastino (*asterisco*). O linfoma foi diagnosticado em amostra obtida por aspiração com agulha fina orientada por ultrassom e subsequentemente removido por cirurgia.

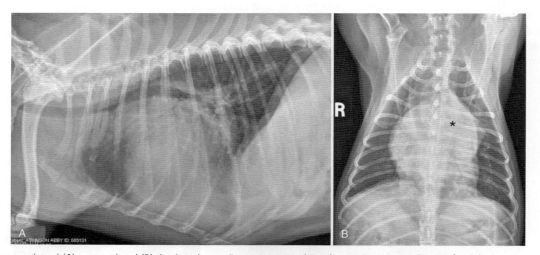

Figura 245.6 Imagens lateral (**A**) e ventrodorsal (**B**) do tórax de um cão com tumor na base do coração. Nota-se elevação focal da traqueia, na imagem lateral, e efeito de massa na margem cranial esquerda do coração, na imagem VD (*asterisco*).

DOENÇAS DO TIMO

O timo estende-se da entrada torácica até a quinta costela, no cão, e até a sexta costela, no gato. Dorsalmente, situa-se próximo aos nervos frênicos e aos lobos pulmonares craniais. A involução do timo em pequenos animais ocorre simultaneamente ao início da maturidade sexual e à perda dos dentes decíduos.[65] O timo atrofia, sendo substituído gradualmente por tecido conjuntivo e gordura, mas suas partes remanescentes persistem até uma idade avançada.[65]

Hemorragia no timo

Uma doença incomum, que consiste em hemorragia espontânea no timo, foi descrita em cães e em um gato.[56,66,67] Embora não seja uniformemente fatal, a maioria dos animais em que essa síndrome foi documentada morreu. A maioria dos animais acometidos tinha menos de 2 anos; portanto, parece que o problema está associado à involução do timo. Os sinais clínicos consistem em letargia, sinais de dor torácica, aumento do esforço respiratório e dispneia. Os achados de exame físico são atribuídos à perda de sangue/hipovolemia aguda e efusão pleural. Os sinais clínicos incluem mucosas pálidas, tempo de preenchimento capilar prolongado, taquicardia, taquipneia e abafamento dos sons pulmonares. As radiografias do tórax mostram uma massa no mediastino (hemorragia, hematoma), em geral associada à efusão pleural. O tratamento é de suporte e envolve a manutenção do volume intravascular (ver Capítulo 129), transfusão sanguínea (ver Capítulo 130) e toracocentese, conforme necessário (ver Capítulo 102).

Timoma

Os timomas são tumores bem reconhecidos em cães e gatos, surgem das células epiteliais do timo e podem ser benignos ou malignos.[56,57,61,68-71] Essa avaliação parece basear-se mais no grau de invasão tecidual e na possibilidade de ressecção do que nas características histopatológicas.[57] A malignidade está associada à capacidade de invasão tecidual, infiltração vascular e presença de metástases locais ou distantes. Em termos radiográficos, o timoma é visualizado como uma opacidade de tecido mole na região cranioventral ou, ocasionalmente, craniolateral do tórax (no mediastino). É possível notar desvio ou compressão da traqueia, efusão pleural ou, em alguns casos, megaesôfago e evidência de pneumonia por aspiração. À ultrassonografia, os timomas podem se apresentar como massas sólidas, císticas ou ambas. O exame citológico de amostras obtidas por AAF revela um número variável de linfócitos maduros, o que dificulta a diferenciação citológica entre timoma e linfoma mediastínico. Também é frequente identificar mastócitos em amostras citológicas obtidas de timomas. Para o diagnóstico definitivo, é necessária biopsia percutânea cirúrgica ou orientada por ultrassom. Síndromes paraneoplásicas são comuns em casos de timoma, em cães e gatos,[68,72] notadamente a miastenia gravis (ver Capítulo 269) que, em geral, está associada a megaesôfago (ver Capítulo 273) em cães com timoma (Figura 245.7).[68] Ver também Capítulo 352. A ressecção cirúrgica é o tratamento de escolha para timoma, mas há relatos de recorrência e metástase.

PAREDE TORÁCICA E DIAFRAGMA

Anatomia da parede torácica

O esterno e as costelas circundam e protegem a parte lateral e ventral do tórax. É normal constatar 13 pares de costelas e 8 esternebras. Todavia, são comuns anormalidades congênitas nesses números, em geral sem relevância clínica. O último par de costelas (o 13º) pode ser menor do que o normal ou nem estar presente. As esternebras podem estar fundidas ou em menor número. As lesões que acometem essas estruturas são mais bem avaliadas em radiografias ou TC do tórax.

Doenças de costelas

É comum notar fraturas de costelas associadas a traumatismo, devendo-se avaliar com cuidado as imagens do tórax obtidas após um acidente traumático. Nota-se tórax instável quando há fratura de pelo menos 2 costelas consecutivas, dorsal e ventralmente, resultando em um segmento de parede independente, que apresenta movimento respiratório paradoxal, movendo-se para dentro durante a inspiração e para fora durante a expiração. A falha mecânica secundária à angústia respiratória crônica/tosse pode resultar em fraturas não traumáticas de costelas em gatos com doença respiratória crônica.[73-74] Em geral, há envolvimento da parte média das costelas mais caudais (9ª a 13ª).

Os tumores de costela, mais comumente osteossarcoma e condrossarcoma, podem ocasionar uma lesão extrapleural em forma de massa (massa de base ampla que surge na periferia da pleura parietal, originando uma borda convexa de frente para os pulmões) e podem resultar em efusão pleural secundária (Figura 245.8). As costelas devem ser avaliadas com cuidado em pacientes com efusão pleural de etiologia desconhecida. A tomografia computadorizada é uma modalidade de imagem excelente para uma avaliação mais detalhada das costelas e do espaço pleural nesses casos.

Doenças do esterno

Pectus excavatum (ou "peito escavado") é uma deformidade do esterno e das cartilagens costais associadas, que se caracteriza por desvio dorsal das esternebras (geralmente as caudais) e compressão dorsal a ventral do tórax (Figura 245.9).[75-78] É mais comumente um defeito congênito, mas essa anormalidade foi descrita como uma condição secundária à resistência de via respiratória crônica, com aumento do esforço respiratório.[75] Os sinais clínicos dependem da gravidade da deformidade e são secundários à compressão do coração e dos pulmões. Embora alguns pacientes não tenham sinais clínicos, outros exibem intolerância ao exercício, taquipneia, cianose, angústia respiratória e sopro cardíaco, que pode ser funcional, secundário a mal posicionamento do coração ou devido a defeito cardíaco congênito concomitante ao peito escavado. Os sinais clínicos podem ser progressivos e, em alguns casos, potencialmente fatais. Um desvio dorsal discreto a grave das esternebras caudais, com desvio também da silhueta cardíaca são as alterações radiográficas mais comuns. O tratamento depende da gravidade da deformidade e dos sintomas associados, variando de conservador a reparo cirúrgico.

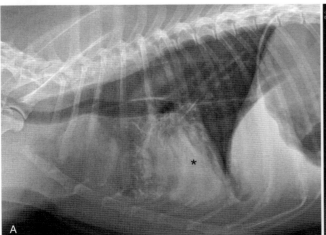
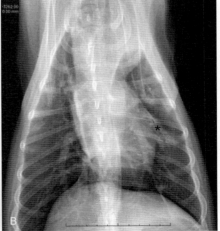

Figura 245.7 Imagens radiográficas lateral (**A**) e ventrodorsal (**B**) do tórax de um cão com 13 anos, com timoma e miastenia gravis. Nota-se uma massa na parte cranial do mediastino, juntamente com megaesôfago. Há um padrão pulmonar alveolar, compatível com pneumonia por aspiração, no subsegmento cranial do lobo pulmonar cranial esquerdo (*asterisco*).

Diafragma

Anatomia

O diafragma é a divisão musculotendinosa entre as cavidades torácica e abdominal.[79] A porção muscular é composta da parte lombar, inserida ao aspecto ventral da terceira e da quarta vértebras lombares (formando os pilares esquerdo e direito), da parte costal, que se insere desde a 8ª até a 13ª costela, e a parte esternal, inserida à cartilagem xifoide do esterno.

Hérnia diafragmática (traumática)

A doença mais comum do diafragma é a ruptura traumática, em geral secundária a traumatismo causado por acidente automobilístico ou queda. Com a ruptura, quantidades variáveis de vísceras abdominais são deslocadas em direção cranial ao diafragma; no gato, o órgão herniado mais frequentemente é o fígado, seguido de intestino delgado, estômago, omento, baço, pâncreas e intestino grosso.[80] Uma ordem similar de herniação de órgãos foi relatada em cães (fígado, intestino delgado, estômago, baço e omento).[81,82] Os sinais clínicos de hérnia diafragmática aguda estão relacionados, com maior frequência, com comprometimento respiratório e consistem em dispneia, tosse, intolerância ao exercício ou letargia. Nas radiografias do tórax, os órgãos herniados podem ser visualizados craniais ao diafragma, em especial quando preenchidos por gás, como estômago ou intestinos (Figura 245.10). Pode ser difícil distinguir o fígado ou o baço (órgãos sólidos) deslocados por efusão

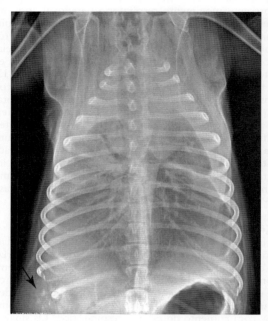

Figura 245.8 Condrossarcoma em costela. Imagem radiográfica dorsoventral do tórax de um cão com 10 anos, levado à consulta por apresentar angústia respiratória. Notam-se efusão pleural e uma lesão osteolítica na 12ª costela do lado direito do tórax (*seta*). Foi diagnosticado condrossarcoma.

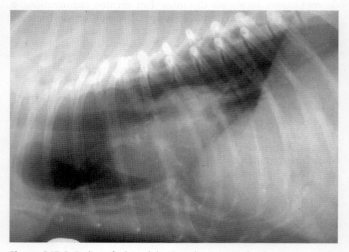

Figura 245.9 Radiografia lateral do tórax de cão portador de peito escavado. Note o desvio dorsal da parte caudal do esterno.

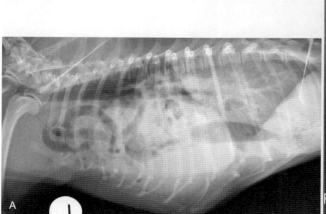
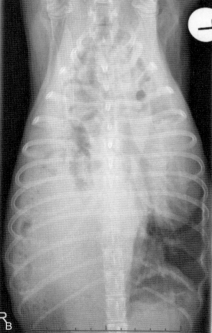

Figura 245.10 Imagens radiográficas lateral (**A**) e ventrodorsal (**B**) do tórax de um cão com hérnia diafragmática. É fácil visualizar múltiplas alças de intestino delgado preenchidas com gás, craniais ao diafragma, em ambas as imagens. Nota-se, também, herniação do fígado.

CAPÍTULO 245 • Doenças do Mediastino, da Parede Torácica e do Diafragma

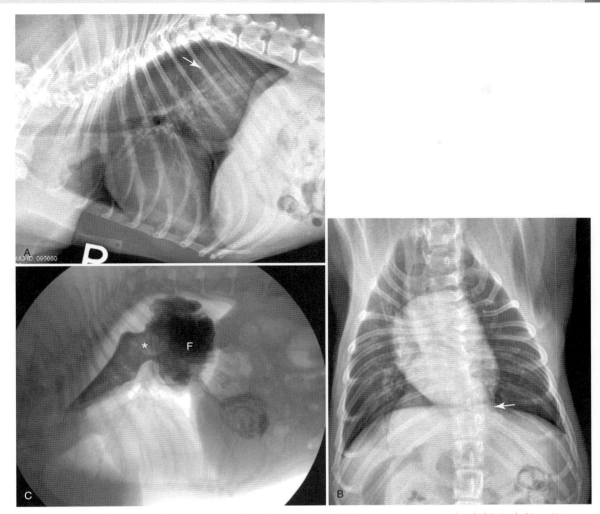

Figura 245.11 Imagens radiográficas lateral (**A**) e ventrodorsal (**B**) do tórax de um cão Buldogue com 4 anos, portador de hérnia de hiato. Nota-se opacidade de tecido mole pouco definida nas imagens lateral e ventrodorsal (*seta*), que representa a hérnia. Uma imagem fluoroscópica lateral (**C**) obtida após administração de bário, como contraste, mostra o deslocamento cranial da junção gastresofágica (*asterisco*) e da parte fúndica do estômago (*F*).

pleural ou consolidação pulmonar. É possível notar o deslocamento cranial de órgãos abdominais ou a ausência de visualização em sua localização normal. Ocasionalmente, as vísceras herniadas têm uma aparência focal, simulando uma massa pulmonar.[83] Em geral há efusão pleural, especialmente nas hérnias diafragmáticas crônicas.[82] Nem todas as hérnias diafragmáticas são reconhecidas imediatamente, talvez devido aos sinais clínicos mínimos, às alterações radiográficas pouco definidas ou ao desconhecimento de um acidente traumático. Os sinais clínicos de hérnias crônicas podem ser inespecíficos e incluem anorexia, letargia, vômitos ou perda de peso. Nem todos os pacientes manifestam sintomas respiratórios. Ultrassonografia e TC são úteis como modalidades de diagnóstico auxiliares na detecção de vísceras abdominais craniais ao diafragma, em especial quando a efusão pleural impede sua visualização em imagens radiográficas do tórax.

Hérnia diafragmática peritônio-pericárdica

A hérnia diafragmática peritônio-pericárdica (HDPP) será discutida juntamente com as doenças pericárdicas, no Capítulo 254.

Hérnia de hiato

As hérnias de hiato (Figura 245.11) são discutidas juntamente com as anormalidades do esôfago, no Capítulo 273.

REFERÊNCIAS BIBLIOGRÁFICAS

As referências bibliográficas deste capítulo se encontram online no Ambiente de Aprendizagem.

SEÇÃO 16
Doença Cardiovascular

CAPÍTULO 246

Fisiopatologia da Insuficiência Cardíaca

Katherine F. Scollan e D. David Sisson

O coração apresenta duas funções mecânicas fundamentais, essenciais para o funcionamento do sistema circulatório. Uma é ejetar sangue em volume suficiente para a artéria aorta e artérias pulmonares, de modo a suprir as necessidades de perfusão dos tecidos que participam do metabolismo. A outra função essencial do coração é receber sangue dos sistemas venosos pulmonar e sistêmico, de maneira a possibilitar a drenagem adequada dos leitos capilares pulmonares e sistêmicos, bem como manter uma distribuição apropriada do compartimento de sangue circulante. A pressão arterial média na árvore arterial sistêmica é cerca de 90 a 100 mmHg, em cães e gatos sadios, assegurando a distribuição adequada de sangue para os diversos leitos vasculares desse circuito de alta resistência. A pressão arterial média no circuito pulmonar, de baixa resistência, situa-se em torno de 20 mmHg.

Pode-se definir insuficiência cardíaca como o estado fisiopatológico em que o coração tem sua capacidade de ejetar ou receber sangue comprometida, o que acaba se tornando grave o bastante a ponto de superar os mecanismos compensatórios do sistema cardiovascular.[1] Define-se doença cardíaca como a presença de qualquer achado cardíaco fora dos limites aceitos de normalidade, incluindo sopro cardíaco, ritmo cardíaco anormal no eletrocardiograma (ECG) ou redução da contratilidade notada no ecocardiograma. A presença de cardiopatia identificável não implica, de maneira inerente, a existência de insuficiência cardíaca ou que ela vá se manifestar como um problema clínico. Há insuficiência cardíaca quando a função cardíaca anormal resulta em retenção de sódio e água, bem como em elevação das pressões venosa e capilar (*insuficiência cardíaca congestiva ou insuficiência retrógrada*) ou débito cardíaco inadequado (*insuficiência cardíaca de baixo débito ou insuficiência anterógrada*).

A insuficiência cardíaca pode resultar de comprometimento funcional do miocárdio, das valvas cardíacas ou do pericárdio, ou ainda ser uma consequência do aumento da resistência à ejeção. Define-se insuficiência miocárdica como uma diminuição na contratilidade cardíaca, não é sinônimo de insuficiência cardíaca. Embora a insuficiência miocárdica seja comum em pacientes com insuficiência cardíaca, alguns têm insuficiência cardíaca mesmo com a função miocárdica preservada. Exemplos relevantes são pacientes que apresentam tromboembolismo pulmonar grave, insuficiência valvular aguda ou tamponamento cardíaco. O clínico deve ter em mente que a função circulatória normal depende da integridade funcional geral do coração, do leito vascular e do sangue, juntamente com sua massa regular de células sanguíneas circulantes.[2] Com o comprometimento sério de qualquer um dos componentes desse sistema integrado, surgem sinais de insuficiência circulatória. Portanto, embora todos os pacientes com insuficiência cardíaca manifestem sintomas de insuficiência circulatória, o inverso não é necessariamente verdadeiro.

PATOGENIA

A insuficiência cardíaca é uma doença progressiva que começa com uma agressão ou um evento inicial que altera a função dos miócitos ou do miocárdio. Na prática clínica, é útil classificar os pacientes com insuficiência cardíaca conforme as consequências funcionais principais ou mais evidentes de sua doença primária (Boxe 246.1). De acordo com isso, alguns pacientes desenvolvem sinais de insuficiência cardíaca primariamente como uma consequência do comprometimento do enchimento cardíaco em decorrência de doenças pericárdicas restritivas, estenose mitral ou tricúspide, coração triatrial (ou *cor tritriatum*) ou doenças do miocárdio primárias que reduzem a complacência ventricular, incluindo miocardiopatia hipertrófica e restritiva. Os pacientes que desenvolvem insuficiência cardíaca a partir dessas doenças, em geral, são descritos de maneira apropriada como portadores de *insuficiência cardíaca diastólica* devido ao efeito primário da redução do enchimento diastólico. O conceito de complacência ventricular é mais bem explicado por meio de um gráfico que mostra a relação telediastólica do ventrículo, entre pressão e volume, como a curva que define a complacência em qualquer nível determinado de carga (Figura 246.1).[3] A distensibilidade tem uma relação estreita com a complacência e se refere à pressão necessária para encher o ventrículo com um volume específico. Dado o mesmo volume telediastólico, a pressão telediastólica será maior se o ventrículo estiver mais rígido (menos distensível e menos complacente) do que o normal.

Em outros pacientes, a insuficiência cardíaca se deve ao aumento acentuado na pós-carga, que impede a ejeção ventricular, incluindo estenose aórtica ou pulmonar, tromboembolismo pulmonar agudo e hipertensão sistêmica ou pulmonar crônica. A pós-carga representa a soma de todas essas forças que se opõem à ejeção de sangue do ventrículo para a circulação e, em geral, é expressa como a tensão sistólica ou o grau de estiramento da parede dos ventrículos durante o período de ejeção.[4]

Boxe 246.1 Classificação funcional da insuficiência cardíaca

Insuficiência cardíaca resultante de impedimento do enchimento cardíaco
Doença pericárdica
Efusão pericárdica com tamponamento
Pericardite constritiva

Obstrução ao fluxo de entrada valvular
Estenose da valva atrioventricular
Outras obstruções anatômicas
 Coração triatrial (*cor tritriatum*)
 Neoplasias, granulomas

Doença miocárdica intrínseca com comprometimento da função diastólica
Miocardiopatia hipertrófica
Miocardiopatia restritiva

Insuficiência cardíaca resultante de aumento da resistência à ejeção
Aumento da resistência à ejeção de sangue (pós-carga)
Obstrução discreta ao fluxo de saída
 Estenose pulmonar e aórtica (subvalvular)
 Miocardiopatia *obstrutiva* hipertrófica
Tromboembolismo em vasos de grande calibre
Hipertensão pulmonar

Insuficiência cardíaca resultante de comprometimento da ejeção ou de sobrecarga de volume
Doenças miocárdicas primárias e secundárias com comprometimento da função sistólica
Miocardiopatia dilatada
Doenças do miocárdio isquêmicas, infecciosas, nutricionais e tóxicas

Fluxo sanguíneo mal direcionado que resulta em sobrecarga de volume
Insuficiência valvular
Desvios da esquerda para a direita, fístulas arteriovenosas

Estados crônicos de alto débito
Tireotoxicose, anemia crônica

Insuficiência cardíaca resultante de arritmias e anormalidades de condução
Taquiarritmias sustentadas
Taquicardia supraventricular
Fibrilação atrial

Bradiarritmias crônicas
Bloqueio cardíaco completo

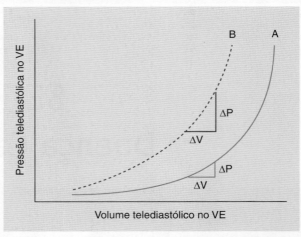

Figura 246.1 Complacência ventricular é a recíproca de rigidez, determinada pelo volume e pela geometria da câmara, bem como pela espessura e pelas características do tecido que constituem suas paredes. O gráfico mostra a relação entre pressão telediastólica ventricular e volume do ventrículo em um indivíduo sadio (**A**) e em um paciente com complacência ventricular reduzida (**B**), definida como o grau de inclinação da relação pressão-volume diastólica. Em qualquer volume, pacientes com a complacência ventricular reduzida terão pressão telediastólica mais elevada em comparação com um indivíduo saudável. *VE*, ventrículo esquerdo.

A pós-carga é determinada principalmente pela resistência vascular periférica (sistêmica; RVS), pelas propriedades físicas (complacência) da árvore arterial e pelo volume de sangue no ventrículo no início da sístole.

A sobrecarga de volume, seja resultante de um desvio da esquerda para a direita, seja de insuficiência valvular, é uma causa comum de insuficiência cardíaca, sempre que o desempenho ventricular sistólico é prejudicado pela influência combinada do fluxo sanguíneo mal direcionado e de um declínio progressivo na contratilidade miocárdica. Em contrapartida, pacientes com insuficiência miocárdica primária, inclusive miocardiopatias dilatada e isquêmica, desenvolvem sobrecarga de volume secundária devido à menor contratilidade e à alteração da geometria da câmara. Como as funções diastólica e sistólica são inter-relacionadas, ambas tendem a ficar comprometidas simultaneamente em animais com diversas doenças cardíacas. Sem dúvida, clinicamente é útil distinguir esses pacientes com redução na função de bombeamento sistólico daqueles com comprometimento da função diastólica, com função sistólica normal ou quase normal.

Arritmias cardíacas e anormalidades de condução podem ter efeitos adversos na função sistólica ou diastólica, dependendo do tipo e da duração da disritmia (ver Capítulo 248). Em algumas situações clínicas, pode ser bastante difícil determinar se uma arritmia específica é a causa do déficit funcional observado ou uma complicação de cardiopatia preexistente. Pacientes com anemia crônica grave, fístulas arteriovenosas ou hipertireoidismo podem apresentar sinais de insuficiência cardíaca, mesmo que seu débito cardíaco se iguale ou seja superior ao de animais normais, o que se denomina *insuficiência cardíaca de alto débito*.[5] Em tais circunstâncias, o débito cardíaco após o início de insuficiência cardíaca é sempre inferior àquele anterior ao início dessa insuficiência, indicando que o coração não pode mais suprir a maior necessidade de fluxo sanguíneo imposta pela doença primária.

Qualquer que seja a anormalidade desencadeante, muitos pacientes com cardiopatia permanecem assintomáticos por algum tempo, provavelmente devido à ativação de vários mecanismos compensatórios. Por fim, a ativação sustentada desses mecanismos compensatórios, neuro-hormonais e de citocinas, acarreta alterações em órgãos terminais e remodelamento cardíaco, ocasionando, assim, a progressão da insuficiência cardíaca.[2]

PROGRESSÃO DE DOENÇA CARDÍACA PARA INSUFICIÊNCIA CARDÍACA

Alterações neuro-hormonais

Há evidência sugestiva de que o desenvolvimento de insuficiência cardíaca se deve à hiperexpressão de substâncias biologicamente ativas capazes de ocasionar efeitos deletérios ao coração e à circulação sanguínea.[6] Foram bem documentadas as respostas neuroendócrinas à insuficiência cardíaca em desenvolvimento em pacientes humanos, nos quais há um aumento evidente da atividade do sistema nervoso adrenérgico, ativação do sistema renina-angiotensina-aldosterona (SRAA), hiperexpressão de peptídios natriuréticos atriais e cerebrais, aumento da síntese e liberação de adrenomedulina, endotelina e arginina vasopressina (AVP), além da expressão amplificada de numerosas citocinas pró-inflamatórias, como o fator de necrose tumoral alfa, a interleucina-1 e a interleucina-6.[7] Mais recentemente, estudos realizados em cães e gatos com cardiopatia indicaram respostas neuroendócrinas qualitativamente semelhantes.[8] O entendimento desses sistemas complexos é vital para compreender a patogenia da insuficiência cardíaca e das estratégias de tratamento racionais recentes. Com base na hipótese neuroendócrina de que a progressão da insuficiência cardíaca é uma consequência da excessiva ação de algumas respostas neuroendócrinas mal adaptativas, como a do sistema adrenérgico e do SRAA, muitas pesquisas foram direcionadas às estratégias terapêuticas que impeçam ou modifiquem de alguma forma essas respostas. A familiaridade com os mediadores dessas respostas adaptativas ajuda o clínico experiente a perceber que as concentrações plasmáticas de certos neuro-hormônios, como o NT-pró-BNP, são capazes de servir como biomarcadores valiosos, que podem ser usados para estabelecer um diagnóstico mais acurado de insuficiência cardíaca.

Ativação do sistema nervoso simpático

No início da progressão da insuficiência cardíaca, os aumentos da frequência cardíaca e da contratilidade, por meio da ativação do sistema nervoso simpático (SNS), são os mecanismos compensatórios predominantes no controle do desempenho cardíaco em declínio.[2] Os determinantes primários do volume sistólico e do débito cardíaco incluem a pré-carga, a pós-carga, a frequência cardíaca, a contratilidade miocárdica e o sincronismo ventricular. Em geral, o débito cardíaco em repouso é restabelecido a um nível quase normal em pacientes com insuficiência cardíaca, por meio de um aumento moderado da frequência cardíaca. A ativação simpática aumenta a frequência cardíaca ao interferir na taxa de despolarização do nodo sinoatrial (SA). A estimulação de receptores beta-adrenérgicos aumenta a frequência de estímulo das células do nodo SA, aumentando a corrente lenta de entrada de cálcio, I_{CaL}. Além disso, a ativação do SNS desvia a curva de ativação da corrente de entrada do marca-passo, I_f, para voltagens mais positivas, via estimulação dependente de G_s da adenilil ciclase. O efeito exato da frequência cardíaca no débito cardíaco tem imensa relevância clínica. O débito cardíaco aumenta linearmente com a frequência cardíaca até certo valor limiar; depois disso o intervalo diastólico encurtado causa redução no volume sistólico que impede a inclinação dessa curva (Figura 246.2).[9] Com frequência cardíaca muito rápida, o volume sistólico diminui à medida que o débito cardíaco começa a declinar. É digno de nota o fato de que o volume sistólico começa a declinar em uma frequência cardíaca baixa e em extensão maior em pacientes com insuficiência cardíaca do que em indivíduos normais. Isso impõe uma limitação muito real nessa resposta adaptativa e contribui para o desempenho sofrível de pacientes com insuficiência cardíaca quando tentam realizar exercícios.

A contratilidade do miocárdio, a força de contração intrínseca do miocárdio que não depende das condições de carga, aumenta com o estímulo nervoso adrenérgico, a ação das catecolaminas circulantes, a frequência cardíaca e, até certo ponto, o volume pós-carga. Nos estágios iniciais de insuficiência miocárdica, o declínio da contratilidade é impedido pela ativação adrenérgica. Mediante a ação da proteína estimuladora G_s, o estímulo beta-adrenérgico ativa a adenilil ciclase e a síntese de AMP cíclico (cAMP) que, então, ativa a proteinoquinase A (PKA).[10,11] A PKA induz a fosforilação de várias proteínas-chave (como os canais de cálcio do tipo L, a rianodina, o fosfolambano e a SERCA2), que facilitam o transporte de cálcio através do sarcolema, aumentam a liberação de cálcio pelo retículo sarcoplasmático (RS) induzida pelo próprio cálcio e a recaptação de cálcio pelo RS.[10,11] Ademais, a proteinoquinase A aumenta a atividade de uma variedade de outras proteínas que elevam a frequência cardíaca e a força de contração dos miofilamentos (troponina I e proteína C ligadora de miosina).

Em pacientes com insuficiência cardíaca, a constrição venosa adrenérgica resulta em aumento imediato do retorno venoso (volume pré-carga). O aumento do volume pré-carga induz uma contração cardíaca mais forçada e um aumento correspondente no volume sistólico, como descrito pela lei de Frank-Starling do coração (Figura 246.3). O aumento do estiramento sistólico de fibras miocárdicas aumenta a sensibilidade dos elementos contráteis ao cálcio do citosol, mecanismo às vezes mencionado como *ativação dependente do comprimento*.[12]

A ativação do SNS propicia um mecanismo de manutenção do desempenho cardíaco, a curto prazo, embora a exposição crônica a alta concentração de norepinefrina (NE) prejudique a sua ação de adaptação. O desempenho miocárdico em pacientes com reservas contráteis diminuídas pode ser impactado negativamente pela separação resultante entre pós-carga e contratilidade. Essa consequência também é exagerada em pacientes com insuficiência cardíaca crônica, nos quais a infrarregulação e o desacoplamento dos receptores cardíacos beta-1 diminuem ainda mais a resposta contrátil. A depleção da reserva de norepinefrina do miocárdio também aumenta o desequilíbrio porque

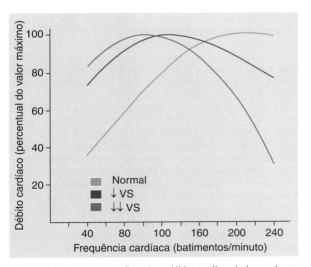

Figura 246.2 Em cães com cardiopatia, o débito cardíaco é alcançado em uma frequência cardíaca mais baixa que em cães saudáveis. Quando a função ventricular está comprometida, frequências cardíacas excessivas acarretam declínio substancial no volume sistólico (VS) e redução no débito cardíaco. Deve-se ressaltar que é muito difícil determinar a frequência cardíaca ideal para cada paciente. (*Esta figura se encontra reproduzida em cores no Encarte.*)

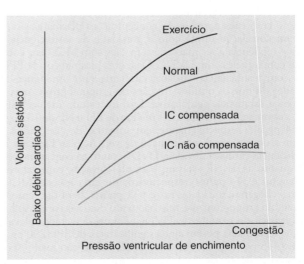

Figura 246.3 Em indivíduos normais, o volume sistólico ventricular aumenta à medida que aumenta a pressão de enchimento ventricular, o que é exacerbado pelo exercício, quando o aumento da contratilidade e a redução do volume pós-carga aumentam o mecanismo de Frank-Starling. Em pacientes com insuficiência cardíaca (IC), o mecanismo de Frank-Starling está comprometido pela combinação de redução da contratilidade, aumento da pós-carga e, em alguns pacientes, redução da função ventricular. (*Esta figura se encontra reproduzida em cores no Encarte.*)

torna o coração muito dependente das concentrações circulantes de catecolaminas. O processo de infrarregulação deve-se à redução da transcrição de RNAm e esse mecanismo está bem estabelecido para o receptor beta-1.[6,13] Por meio de um mecanismo diferente, o aumento da expressão miocárdica da quinase do receptor beta (BARK) facilita o desacoplamento dos receptores cardíacos beta-1 e beta-2 das proteínas G, pela ação da arrestina beta, reduzindo assim a produção subsequente de AMP cíclico.[14] A consequência dessas alterações é um menor aumento da frequência cardíaca e da contratilidade do miocárdio em resposta ao estímulo adrenérgico.

A medular da adrenal sintetiza e armazena NE e epinefrina (EPI), liberando-as na circulação em resposta ao estresse agudo. Ao contrário da glândula adrenal, os nervos periféricos não têm a enzima feniletanolamina N-metiltransferase e não sintetizam nem liberam epinefrina. Portanto, a NE, não a epinefrina, desempenha um papel central como um neurotransmissor e é liberada constantemente das terminações nervosas simpáticas terminais. Apesar da recaptação e da inativação da maior parte de NE liberada dessa maneira, uma pequena parte extravasa para o sangue circulante, de modo que a concentração plasmática de NE, em repouso, pode ser um parâmetro útil de atividade do sistema nervoso simpático. As concentrações plasmáticas de NE em pacientes humanos com insuficiência cardíaca congestiva (ICC) têm relação com a gravidade da insuficiência cardíaca e uma relação inversa com a taxa de sobrevivência.[15] Além disso, concentrações elevadas de NE em pacientes humanos tratados para ICC estão relacionadas com um declínio na condição clínica.[16] É importante saber que as concentrações plasmáticas de catecolaminas aumentam em muitas circunstâncias além de insuficiência cardíaca, inclusive estresse emocional e atividade física, o que enfatiza a baixa especificidade de tais mensurações. Por essas razões, a interpretação da concentração plasmática de catecolaminas, exclusivamente, sempre será difícil.

A estimativa da atividade adrenérgica em cães e gatos, em um contexto clínico, é um desafio e há grandes variações dos teores plasmáticos dessas catecolaminas, até mesmo em pacientes apropriadamente classificados de acordo com a gravidade da cardiopatia primária. Ware e colaboradores[17] foram os primeiros pesquisadores a relatar concentrações plasmáticas de NE muito elevadas em um pequeno número de cães com insuficiência cardíaca de ocorrência natural decorrente de miocardiopatia dilatada (MCD) e doença valvar degenerativa crônica (DVDC) em comparação com cães normais. As concentrações plasmáticas de NE tiveram correlação direta com a gravidade da insuficiência cardíaca e tendência a ser mais altas em cães com MCD em comparação com aqueles com DVDC. Os teores plasmáticos de EPI em cães com insuficiência cardíaca também eram um pouco mais elevados do que os obtidos em cães do grupo-controle, mas sem diferença estatística significativa. Em um estudo maior,[18] Sisson *et al.* constataram concentrações médias de EPI e NE de 133 pg/ml e 254 pg/ml, respectivamente, em amostras de cães sadios não errantes, obtidas mediante punção da veia jugular. Em cães com insuficiência cardíaca devida a DVDC, tanto as concentrações de EPI quanto as de NE estavam bastante elevadas, com valores de 314 pg/ml e 314 pg/ml, respectivamente; em cães com MCD, os valores chegaram a 211 pg/ml e 631 pg/ml, bem diferentes dos animais do grupo-controle, mas não tanto dos cães com insuficiência cardíaca decorrente de DVDC. Foram detectadas elevações menos acentuadas, porém ainda significativas, de EPI (290 pg/ml) e NE (445 pg/ml), em cães com DVDC que não manifestavam sintomas evidentes de insuficiência cardíaca congestiva. Em gatos com insuficiência cardíaca congestiva ou tromboembolismo sistêmico decorrente de miocardiopatia hipertrófica restritiva, constatamos concentrações plasmáticas de EPI e NE acima de 2.000 pg/ml e 2.500 pg/ml, em comparação com 250 pg/ml e 1.000 pg/ml, respectivamente, em gatos sadios cujas amostras foram obtidas mediante punção jugular.[19] Em gatos sadios relaxados, com cateteres colocados previamente na veia jugular, verificamos concentrações plasmáticas de EPI e NE de 221 pg/ml e 424 pg/ml,

respectivamente. Em gatos com miocardiopatia restritiva que não apresentavam insuficiência cardíaca, notamos concentrações plasmáticas de EPI e NE acima de 1.500 pg/ml e 1.700 pg/ml, respectivamente. Esses resultados indicam de maneira convincente que a atividade do sistema nervoso simpático aumenta em cães e gatos com cardiopatia de ocorrência natural, à semelhança do que acontece em pacientes humanos.[16,20]

Ativação do sistema renina-angiotensina-aldosterona

Na insuficiência cardíaca, a redução do débito cardíaco e a ativação do SNS ativam o SRAA. Na IC, os componentes do SRAA são ativados posteriormente ao SNS. Os principais estímulos para a liberação de renina pelas células justaglomerulares renais incluem diminuição da perfusão renal efetiva, redução da reabsorção de sódio nos túbulos renais e estímulo beta-adrenérgico.[21,22] Não é surpresa que dietas com baixo teor de sódio, desidratação, perda sanguínea e exercício vigoroso estimulam a liberação de renina pelo sistema justaglomerular. A principal ação da renina é acelerar a conversão do grande pré-hormônio angiotensinogênio no decapeptídio angiotensina I que, em seguida, é transformado em octapeptídio angiotensina II (AT II) pela enzima conversora de angiotensina (ECA). O angiotensinogênio é uma glicoproteína globular sintetizada no fígado e liberada no plasma sanguíneo, que atua como local de armazenamento primário.[21] A angiotensina II inibe a síntese de renina, sendo um exemplo do mecanismo clássico de inibição por retroalimentação (*feedback*).

Quando descoberto pela primeira vez, acreditava-se que o SRAA atuava quase exclusivamente nos limites do leito vascular. Atualmente, sabe-se que a maioria da ECA, no organismo, encontra-se nos tecidos, com menos de 10% na circulação.[23] Além disso, todos os vários componentes do SRAA podem ser encontrados em diversos tecidos, inclusive cérebro, miocárdio, vasos sanguíneos, glândulas adrenais e rins, de modo que muitos pesquisadores acreditam que o SRAA é ativado em um estágio mais precoce da insuficiência cardíaca do que os componentes circulantes.[24] É provável que a participação do SRAA tecidual varie em circunstâncias diferentes e de acordo com a natureza da doença primária. A angiotensina II, oriunda de cardiomiócitos e fibroblastos, tem uma participação particularmente importante no desenvolvimento de certos tipos de remodelamento patológico, atuando via G_q e pela ativação de proteínas quinases (MAPKs) por diversos mitógenos. A ECA é uma dipeptidil carboxipeptidase que atua na clivagem de dipeptídios terminais do fragmento C terminal dos peptídios que servem como substrato. A seletividade da ECA é tal que ela faz a clivagem de qualquer peptídio substrato, R1-R2-R3-OH, onde R1 é um L-aminoácido protegido, R2 é qualquer L-aminoácido, exceto prolina, e R3 é qualquer L-aminoácido com terminal carboxi livre. Portanto, a ECA transforma angiotensina I em angiotensina II ativa; ademais, inativa a bradicinina, um potente vasodilatador. A conversão de angiotensina I em angiotensina II pode ser realizada por outras enzimas além, da ECA, incluindo catepsina G, elastase, ativador do plasminogênio tecidual, quimase e a enzima geradora de AII sensível à quimostatina (CAGE).[25,26] A importância dessas vias alternativas depende da espécie, com vários relatos sugerindo que a quimase tecidual é mais ativa que a ECA no miocárdio e na matriz extracelular de cães e gatos.[26,27] As ações sequenciais da aminopeptidase e da ECA na angiotensina I originam angiotensina III, um 7-aminoácido peptídico (heptapeptídio) com ações similares às da angiotensina II, porém é menos potente.[25,28]

As ações fisiológicas da AT II foram bastante pesquisadas e todos os seus efeitos fisiológicos importantes parecem ser mediados por receptores AT_1, presentes em quantidade abundante nos vasos sanguíneos, rins, fígado, coração, hipófise e glândulas adrenais.[21,28] A meia-vida da AT II circulante é da ordem de 1 a 2 minutos, porque ela é rapidamente hidrolisada em fragmentos peptídicos inativos por angiotensinases circulantes. Além de sua ação como um vasoconstritor potente, a AT II promove retenção de sódio e água por ação direta nos túbulos renais e indiretamente ao estimular a síntese de aldosterona e sua liberação pelas glândulas adrenais. A angiotensina II e a aldosterona são fundamentais na regulação do equilíbrio de sódio e água e na manutenção da pressão vascular quando o volume sanguíneo diminui em razão de hemorragia ou privação de sal e água. Espécies de oxigênio reativo (EOR), geradas como consequência do aumento da expressão de AT II e de aldosterona, são fundamentais para o desenvolvimento de hipertrofia miocárdica e dos mecanismos de remodelamento vascular e ventricular prejudiciais, observados em pacientes com insuficiência cardíaca crônica.[25,29,30]

Os principais estímulos para a síntese e liberação de aldosterona incluem AT II, alta concentração plasmática de potássio e corticotropina (ACTH) (ver Capítulo 308). Outros mensageiros, incluindo as catecolaminas plasmáticas, a endotelina I e a AVP, também são conhecidos como promotores da síntese e liberação de aldosterona nos tecidos e no sangue.[25,30] Tradicionalmente, os principais efeitos fisiológicos da aldosterona são atribuídos a sua ação nos rins, que é a conservação de sódio. Nesse sentido, a aldosterona atua nas células epiteliais dos ductos coletores distais, onde se difunde ao citoplasma e se liga a receptores citoplasmáticos de mineralocorticoides (RM).[21,25,30] Após sua entrada no núcleo, os RM ativados induzem uma cascata de eventos que, por fim, aumenta a absorção de íons sódio e excreção de potássio. A síntese de aldosterona não se limita à glândula adrenal, e a distribuição dos receptores de mineralocorticoide é mais ampla do que se pensava. Em pacientes com insuficiência cardíaca, a aldosterona contribui para a disfunção de barorreceptores, facilitando a atividade do sistema nervoso simpático e diminuindo as ações do sistema nervoso parassimpático. A aldosterona também contribui para vasoconstrição generalizada via estimulação da atividade do sistema nervoso simpático mediada pelos receptores de mineralocorticoide, por inibir a captação e degradação de NE na periferia e por meio de outros mecanismos complexos que contribuem para a disfunção de células endoteliais.[21,29,31] A participação emergente da aldosterona como mediador de inflamação, fibrose e outros processos biológicos, como estresse oxidativo, envolvidos no remodelamento patológico dos vasos sanguíneos, nos rins e no coração, é de interesse particular.[29-31] A síntese de citocina induzida pela aldosterona é um componente importante desses processos de remodelamento. Muitos dos avanços no tratamento de insuficiência cardíaca e de hipertensão sistêmica obtidos nos últimos anos resultaram do uso de compostos que impedem a síntese de AT II por meio da inibição da ECA, que bloqueiam a interação da angiotensina II com receptores AT_1 (ARB), ou que inibem as ações da aldosterona.

Foram detectadas elevações substanciais da atividade plasmática da renina e dos teores séricos de aldosterona em cães com insuficiência cardíaca congestiva franca decorrente de regurgitação mitral (RM) e miocardiopatia dilatada (MCD), bem como em gatos com miocardiopatia hipertrófica ou restritiva (MCH ou MCR). A ativação do SRAA é particularmente exacerbada em cães e gatos com miocardiopatia adquirida quando se usa furosemida para aliviar os sintomas de congestão sanguínea. Há alguma discordância quanto ao papel do SRAA em pacientes com doença cardíaca menos grave. Vários pesquisadores notaram que a atividade da renina e a concentração de aldosterona, no plasma, estão na faixa normal ou apenas discretamente elevadas em cães e gatos com cardiopatia, antes do início evidente de insuficiência cardíaca.[32,33] Também é importante ressaltar que a atividade da renina e a concentração de aldosterona no plasma nem sempre estão elevadas em pacientes com insuficiência cardíaca franca.[34,35] Como os efeitos fisiológicos da ativação do SRAA incluem expansão de volume e vasoconstrição, ambos atuando para diminuir a produção de renina, a atividade desse sistema tende a ser física e com dissimulação de sua ativação. Portanto, embora haja unanimidade a respeito da ativação do SRAA em cães e gatos com insuficiência cardíaca congestiva franca, há incerteza quanto ao ponto exato de sua suprarregulação em pacientes com cardiopatia menos grave.

ALTERAÇÕES NEURO-HORMONAIS DA FUNÇÃO RENAL

Na insuficiência cardíaca, vários mecanismos resultam em retenção renal de sódio e água.[36] Apesar da expansão geral de volume, no contexto de insuficiência cardíaca, o débito cardíaco inadequado resulta em redução do volume de sangue arterial efetivo. Isso é percebido pelos barorreceptores arteriais, levando à ativação sustentada do SNS e do SRAA. A redução da perfusão renal e o aumento da vasoconstrição renal mediada pelo sistema nervoso simpático causam redução do fluxo sanguíneo renal e aumento da retenção de sódio e água. A angiotensina II induz aumento da sede e estimula a liberação de aldosterona e AVP (hormônio antidiurético [ADH]), ambas ocasionando maior retenção de água. Além disso, a norepinefrina aumenta a atividade do SRAA e estimula a síntese e liberação de ADH. O abrandamento da resposta renal aos peptídios natriuréticos exacerba o desequilíbrio dos mecanismos de competição, de vasodilatação/natriurese para vasoconstrição/retenção de sódio.[37] As consequências dessas alterações consistem em diminuição e redistribuição do fluxo sanguíneo renal, redução concomitante na excreção de sódio e elevação dos teores plasmáticos de AVP, com retenção de água livre de soluto. A retenção continuada de sódio e água na vigência de insuficiência cardíaca acaba por ocasionar aumento excessivo da pressão venosa e desenvolvimento de edema e efusão.

Peptídios natriuréticos

Os peptídios natriuréticos atrial e cerebral (tipo B), PNA e PNB, liberados pelo coração, e o tipo C, presente principalmente nos vasos sanguíneos, desempenham papéis reguladores importantes na circulação sanguínea e proporcionam equilíbrio aos agentes vasoconstritores e aqueles que ocasionam retenção de sódio. Em seres humanos, gatos e cães sadios, é provável que as formas circulantes de PNB e PNA sejam oriundas principalmente do átrio, onde são armazenados como moléculas precursoras, pró-PNA e pró-PNB, em grânulos ligados à membrana, para posterior liberação.[38-41] O terceiro peptídio natriurético, tipo C ou PNC, está presente principalmente no endotélio vascular. Em animais e seres humanos sadios, os teores circulantes de PNC são muito inferiores aos de PNA e PNB, sugerindo que eles atuam de maneira parácrina, induzindo relaxamento local do músculo liso vascular e inibindo o remodelamento vascular. Aumentos súbitos nas concentrações plasmáticas de PNA e PNB se devem à sua liberação dos grânulos atriais, onde são armazenados, principalmente pelo estímulo do estiramento atrial. Em pacientes com cardiopatia ocorrem aumentos sustentados de PNA e PNB circulantes, em razão da maior expressão de RNAm em diferentes locais do coração.[42] Em pacientes com doença miocárdica, as concentrações plasmáticas de PNB aumentam de maneira muito acentuada e, em geral, superam os teores de PNA, pois o principal local de produção de PNB deixa de ser os átrios e passa a ser os ventrículos.[43,44] Em gatos com miocardiopatia hipertrófica, há aumentos acentuados na expressão de PNB tanto nos átrios como nos ventrículos.[45] Outros pesquisadores, estudando cães com insuficiência cardíaca experimental induzida por marca-passo, relataram que a expressão ventricular de PNB permanece mais modesta e os átrios continuam sendo a fonte predominante da maioria do PNB circulante.[46]

As ações fisiológicas do PNA e do PNB geralmente se opõem às do SRAA.[47,48] Os peptídios natriuréticos atrial e os peptídios tipo B atuam via receptor do peptídio natriurético tipo A, RPN-A, para induzir natriurese e diurese por inibição do transporte tubular de sódio no ducto coletor da medular interna do rim. Esse mesmo tipo de receptor atua como mediador do relaxamento vascular de arteríolas sistêmicas e pulmonares, diminuindo assim a resistência vascular sistêmica e pulmonar. Outra ação do PNA e do PNB mediada pelo RPN-A é a inibição direta da liberação de renina pelo rim e de aldosterona pelo córtex adrenal. Um segundo receptor, o RPN-B, responde ao PNA e ao PNB, mas de preferência atua como mediador da vasodilatação causada pelo PNC produzido no local. O receptor de PNC (RPN-C) atua eliminando o PNA e o PNB da circulação. O PNA e o PNB também são eliminados pela ação de uma endopeptidase neutra ligada à membrana, que causa sua clivagem, originando fragmentos peptídicos inativos. A endopeptidase neutra e o RPN-C mostram maior afinidade pelo PNA do que pelo PNB, o que explica a meia-vida mais longa do PNB.[47-49] Acredita-se que os fragmentos N-terminais de pró-PNA e pró-PNB sejam removidos mais lentamente da circulação do que os do C-terminal porque a depuração desses peptídios é mais dependente da excreção renal. Como resultado, os teores plasmáticos de NT-pró-PNA e NT-pró-PNB são mais elevados do que o de C-terminal e não são tão lábeis como o do último. Ambos os fragmentos N-terminal dos peptídios são indicadores sensíveis de doença cardíaca em seres humanos e seus teores tendem a se relacionar bem com a gravidade de qualquer cardiopatia primária.[50,51]

As mensurações das concentrações plasmáticas de peptídios natriuréticos, em especial do PNB, são úteis para a diferenciação de pacientes humanos com dispneia decorrente de insuficiência cardíaca daqueles com doença pulmonar ou outras anormalidades.[51-55] As concentrações médias de PNB em pacientes humanos com cardiopatia das classes III e IV NYHA foram 8 a 10 vezes maiores do que o valor constatado em indivíduos sem insuficiência cardíaca.[56] Em estudos relatados recentemente, em gatos com doença miocárdica, as mensurações dos teores plasmáticos de PNB pareceram ter valor diagnóstico similar.[57,58] Os teores plasmáticos de PNB, com elevação superior a 10 vezes, distinguiram melhor os gatos com insuficiência cardíaca daqueles do grupo-controle do que as concentrações plasmáticas de PNA, que estavam aumentadas 4 a 5 vezes. O valor diagnóstico dos teores plasmáticos de PNB não parecem tão promissores em cães, nos quais a magnitude da alteração é menos acentuada do que a observada em gatos e seres humanos,[59,60] embora alguns estudos tenham mostrado que os níveis de PNB podem propiciar a diferenciação entre causas cardíacas e não cardíacas de angústia respiratória.[61-63] O desenvolvimento recente de um teste rápido para NT-pró-PNB em plasma de gatos deve proporcionar várias vantagens para o uso do PNB como um biomarcador cardíaco em gatos, inclusive com disponibilidade de resultados no domicílio, em 10 minutos.[64]

Arginina vasopressina/hormônio antidiurético

Na literatura veterinária, a AVP, em geral mencionada como ADH, é um composto não peptídio, com o aminoácido arginina na posição 8 (ver Capítulo 296).[65,66] A sequência de aminoácidos do peptídio maduro é altamente conservada na maioria dos mamíferos e idêntica em seres humanos, cães e gatos.[67] A pró-vasopressina, derivada da pré-pró-vasopressina, é sintetizada em neurônios cujos corpos celulares estão localizados no hipotálamo. Subsequentemente, a pró-vasopressina é processada no peptídio formado, vasopressina, em vesículas que são transportadas ao longo do axônio, para a neuroipófise, onde se tornam grânulos secretores contendo o peptídio ativo, nas terminações nervosas.[65] Os estímulos para a liberação de vasopressina pela neuroipófise, para a circulação sanguínea, incluem aumento da osmolalidade plasmática e hipovolemia. Quando o volume plasmático está reduzido, receptores de estiramento nos átrios e nas veias grandes diminuem sua frequência de descargas, estimulando a liberação de AVP.[65] A estimulação simpática e a AT II também estimulam a liberação de AVP. Após sua liberação, a vasopressina reage com receptores V1A, nos vasos sanguíneos e no coração, mediando ações vasoconstritoras e inotrópicas, e com receptores V2, no rim, estimulando a reabsorção de água.[66,68] Este último efeito ocorre via regulação da quantidade de canais de água aquaporina 2 inseridos na membrana luminal de células dos ductos coletores renais.[66,68] Receptores de barorreceptor V2 respondem a elevado teor plasmático de AVP, aumentando os reflexos barorreceptores, que diminuem a frequência cardíaca para manter a pressão arterial na faixa normal.

Em cães com insuficiência cardíaca induzida por marca-passo com frequência rápida, o teor plasmático de AVP se eleva antes do desenvolvimento de sintomas de congestão vascular em associação à ativação do SRAA. Aumentos acentuados são observados com o início de sintomas de congestão. Elevada concentração plasmática de AVP é detectada em alguns pacientes humanos com ICC, em particular naqueles com insuficiência cardíaca grave e hiponatremia por diluição.[66,69] O paradoxo de aumento da liberação de AVP ante a redução da osmolalidade plasmática e alta pressão de enchimento pode ser decorrência da sinalização de barorreceptor causada pela baixa pressão arterial.[70] Qualquer que seja o mecanismo, constatou-se que o receptor seletivo V2 ou os antagonistas combinados V1A/V2 normalizam a concentração plasmática de sódio e aliviam os sintomas de congestão nos pacientes assim acometidos.[66,71,72] Esses agentes às vezes são mencionados como aquaréticos, porque induzem a excreção de água sem alterar a excreção urinária de sódio ou potássio. O conivaptana, um bloqueador que combina V1A/V2, mostrou-se efetivo em cães com insuficiência cardíaca induzida experimentalmente e em pacientes humanos com ICC sintomática grave.[73,74] O tolvaptana é um antagonista do receptor V2 de vasopressina mais seletivo e ativo por via oral, que também está sendo avaliado em testes clínicos.[75] Foram documentados teores circulantes aumentados de AVP em cães com miocardiopatia dilatada[76,77] e doença valvar degenerativa crônica,[77] mas ainda não há tal relato em gatos.

ALTERAÇÕES NEURO-HORMONAIS DOS VASOS SANGUÍNEOS PERIFÉRICOS

A circulação sistêmica requer pressão relativamente alta e a manutenção da pressão sanguínea sistêmica é uma prioridade fisiológica obrigatória em todos os pacientes com insuficiência cardíaca. Isso envolve a ação tanto do sistema nervoso autônomo quanto de mediadores autorreguladores locais. Quando o débito cardíaco diminui, o fluxo sanguíneo sistêmico é direcionado preferencialmente para alguns centros vitais, por uma variedade de respostas de adaptação, aumentando o tônus dos vasos de resistência que suprem regiões menos vitais. Em pacientes com insuficiência cardíaca, o sistema nervoso adrenérgico tem uma participação predominante no redirecionamento do fluxo sanguíneo para centros vitais (cérebro e coração), sendo responsável por muito do aumento observado na resistência vascular periférica.[6] Outras influências que alteram as propriedades funcionais e estruturais da parede vascular incluem infrarregulação do tônus parassimpático, suprarregulação do SRAA, aumento da expressão e da liberação de endotelina e AVP e alterações no mecanismo de autorregulação do fluxo sanguíneo para leitos vasculares específicos.

Norepinefrina, angiotensina II, endotelina e AVP induzem vasoconstrição via receptores específicos da membrana do músculo liso ligados à proteína G, Gq, ativando a fosfolipase C e o trifosfato de inositol (IP3), que sinalizam o sistema.[78] O sistema IP3 regula a liberação de íons cálcio via receptor de IP3 (um canal de liberação de cálcio), no retículo sarcoplasmático das células do músculo liso, estimulando a vasoconstrição mediada pelo cálcio. Com a sinalização crônica do IP3, o diacilglicerol ativa a proteinoquinase C (PKC), iniciando uma cascata de sinais intercelulares que iniciam a hipertrofia e replicação do músculo liso, bem como uma pletora de alterações associadas na matriz extracelular (remodelamento vascular).[79] A baixa atividade do ramo parassimpático do sistema nervoso autônomo contribui para a vasoconstrição generalizada, com a remoção de seu efeito vasodilatador. Os receptores parassimpáticos muscarínicos, estimulados pela acetilcolina, ativam a guanilil ciclase, originando GMP cíclico, que inibe a entrada de cálcio na célula e diminui a concentração intercelular de cálcio. Na insuficiência cardíaca, o aumento da atividade simpática e dos vasoconstritores circulantes mantêm a pressão arterial e também aumenta o retorno venoso e o enchimento cardíaco via vasoconstrição periférica.

Infelizmente, o aumento do volume pós-carga associado estimula o remodelamento cardíaco e contribui ainda mais para a disfunção cardíaca.

Endotelina

O tônus vascular é modulado por vasodilatadores derivados do endotélio, óxido nítrico e prostaciclina, e pelas ações complexas do potente peptídio vasoconstritor derivado do endotélio, endotelina.[80] Três peptídios relacionados – endotelina-1, endotelina-2 e endotelina-3 – compreendem a família das endotelinas.[81] As endotelinas circulantes são derivadas de peptídios maiores produzidos por células do endotélio vascular (miócitos e uma variedade de outras células) em uma sequência de etapas análogas à descrita para os peptídios natriuréticos.[81-83] Portanto, a pré-pró-endotelina origina a pró-endotelina biologicamente inativa, também denominada grande endotelina, que subsequentemente é clivada no N-terminal pela enzima de conversão endotelial (ECE) para originar o peptídio maduro ativo, a endotelina-1 (ET-1). A expressão do RNAm da endotelina-1 e a produção de ET-1 são estimuladas por hipoxia e fatores mecânicos, incluindo estiramento e baixa tensão de cisalhamento; por substâncias vasoativas, como AT II, AVP, NE e bradicinina; e por fatores do crescimento e citocinas, incluindo o fator de transformação do crescimento beta, o fator de necrose tumoral alfa e a interleucina-1.[82,83]

A endotelina-1 atua por meio de dois receptores, ETA e ETB, para exercer efeitos biológicos que mantêm o tônus vascular normal.[82-85] A vasoconstrição de músculo liso, o aumento da contratilidade miocárdica e a secreção de aldosterona são os efeitos mais proeminentes mediados pelo estímulo do receptor ETA. Estimulação crônica de receptores ETA e teor persistentemente elevado de ET-1 causam proliferação e hipertrofia do músculo liso vascular e hipertrofia do miocárdio. Na insuficiência cardíaca, além de seus efeitos vasoconstritores diretos, a ET-1 inibe a ação do inibidor endógeno do ON sintase, dimetilarginina assimétrica (ADMA), e seu efeito pode ser inibido por antagonistas do receptor de ETA.[83] A vasodilatação, mediada pelo aumento na produção de ON e secreção de aldosterona, resulta em estímulo dos receptores de ETB na célula endotelial, propiciando uma maneira discreta e complexa de equilibrar o tônus vascular. Por sua vez, o aumento na concentração de ON inibe a síntese de ET-1, um exemplo de mecanismo de retroalimentação (feedback) negativa. Após injeção intravenosa de ET-1, inicialmente a pressão sanguínea diminui transitoriamente e em seguida aumenta, refletindo a ação desses dois subtipos de receptor. As interações da endotelina e do SRAA são complexas, mas a consequência final é a supressão da síntese de renina e o estímulo da secreção de aldosterona.[86] As estratégias terapêuticas baseadas no bloqueio dos receptores de ET e na inibição da enzima conversora de endotelina não resultaram em benefícios clínicos convincentes.

Em pessoas e animais saudáveis, a maior parte da ET-1 circulante é oriunda dos vasos sanguíneos e sua concentração é muito baixa, refletindo sua participação parácrina na manutenção do tônus vascular normal. Acredita-se que a produção de ET-1 pelo miocárdio contribua para o aumento de sua concentração plasmática observado em seres humanos, cães e gatos com insuficiência cardíaca. É digno de nota o fato de que a magnitude da elevação de ET-1 na insuficiência cardíaca não é tão marcante como a observada para os peptídios natriuréticos. A concentração plasmática de ET-1 mais que duplica em cães com ICC decorrente de DVDC ou MCD e aumenta mais de três vezes em gatos com miocardiopatia e ICC ou tromboembolismo sistêmico.[84,85] Elevações significativas, porém modestas, são observadas em cães e gatos com doença menos grave. Em um estudo de cães levados à consulta por apresentarem dispneia, o teor plasmático de ET-1 foi menos acurado que o de NT-pró-PNA na distinção de cães com ICC daqueles com dispneia por outras causas.[87] A concentração de ET-1 também está consistentemente elevada em pacientes com hipertensão pulmonar e algumas formas de doença renal, mas é interessante que isso não acontece em pacientes com hipertensão sistêmica.[88,89]

Óxido nítrico e adrenomedulina

O óxido nítrico, produzido nas células endoteliais a partir de L-arginina, pela ação da óxido nítrico sintase endotelial (eNOS), difunde-se nas células do músculo liso e contribui para a vasodilatação por meio de diversos mecanismos.[90] O óxido nítrico aumenta o teor intercelular de GMPc nas células do músculo liso vascular ao ativar a guanilato ciclase solúvel e ativar diretamente os canais de potássio, ocasionando hiperpolarização celular e vasodilatação. Em pacientes com insuficiência cardíaca, o comprometimento funcional das células endoteliais causa redução da síntese de ON, contribuindo ainda mais para a vasoconstrição excessiva.[91]

A adrenomodulina (ADM) é um peptídio composto de 52 aminoácidos, com efeito natriurético e potente ação vasodilatadora, com propriedades inotrópicas positivas, tendo sido detectada em uma variedade de tecidos, inclusive medular da adrenal, coração, pulmões e rins.[92,93] Os teores plasmáticos de ADM se elevam em pacientes humanos com insuficiência cardíaca e em cães com insuficiência cardíaca experimental induzida por marca-passo. Estudos recentes indicam que a AT II estimula a produção e secreção de ADM pelos miócitos cardíacos e fibroblastos, e a inibição da ECA pode inibir essa resposta. Portanto, a ADM parece ter efeitos endócrinos, autócrinos e parácrinos.[93] É interessante ressaltar que a ADM atua como um marcador de hipertrofia ventricular; sua função é atenuar a hipertrofia do miocárdio e a produção de colágeno. Deu-se pouca atenção à adrenomodulina em cães e gatos com cardiopatia de ocorrência natural. É provável que isso mude, porque cada vez mais aumenta o interesse na ADM como um possível agente terapêutico.

CITOCINAS E INTEGRINAS SINALIZADORAS

As citocinas, mais corretamente denominadas de fatores reguladores de proteína, são glicoproteínas ou pequenas proteínas sinalizadoras hidrossolúveis sintetizadas por uma ampla variedade de tipos celulares usados extensamente na comunicação intercelular.[94] As citocinas apresentam uma combinação de ações endócrinas, parácrinas e autócrinas, via receptores ligados à membrana, que suprem e causam infrarregulação da expressão de grupos de genes e seus fatores de transcrição, atuando como potentes modificadores da síntese de proteínas. Aumento da produção e alta concentração plasmática de citocinas pró-inflamatórias, incluindo interleucina-1, interleucina-6 e fator de necrose tumoral alfa (TNF-α), foram constatados em pacientes humanos com insuficiência cardíaca crônica e são considerados importantes indicadores de prognóstico desfavorável.[95] A elevação da concentração de TNF-α induz apoptose.[96] Infelizmente, os resultados de testes clínicos com agentes que bloqueiam as ações do TNF-α em pacientes humanos foram desapontadores.[97]

REMODELAMENTO CARDÍACO

Anormalidades circulatórias crônicas e danos patológicos no coração ocasionam alterações anatômicas e morfológicas no órgão, conhecidas, em termos gerais, como remodelamento cardíaco. Embora as respostas neuro-hormonais mal adaptadas à insuficiência cardíaca expliquem parte de sua natureza progressiva, o remodelamento cardíaco compromete ainda mais e, em geral, exacerba a disfunção cardíaca. O remodelamento cardíaco não interfere apenas no tamanho dos miócitos cardíacos, ele envolve também o volume de componentes do miócito e de não miócitos, a anatomia e a biologia dos miócitos cardíacos, bem como a geometria das câmaras cardíacas.

Alterações nos miócitos e não miócitos

A hipertrofia cardíaca, ou seja, o aumento de tamanho dos miócitos, é o fundamento da resposta de remodelamento, devido à capacidade extremamente limitada do coração para acrescentar novos cardiomiócitos. Quando o coração está sadio, os cardiomiócitos ocupam cerca de três quartos do volume do órgão e compreendem cerca de um terço do número total de células.[98] Essas células musculares estão embebidas em uma matriz extracelular rica em colágeno, produzida por um grande número de fibroblastos, e ambos os componentes são nutridos por uma rede extensa de vasos coronarianos revestidos por células endoteliais e ricamente dotados de células musculares lisas. Constituintes não celulares da matriz extracelular incluem, principalmente, colágeno dos tipos I e III, uma mistura rica em proteoglicanos e uma grande variedade de peptídios sinalizadores e proteases extracelulares.[99] O colágeno intersticial está organizado de um modo complexo, atua de modo a conectar e formar um feixe de miofibras em uma rede sofisticada que facilita a função primária do colágeno, que é a transmissão de força. O colágeno do endomísio circunda cada miócito, originando os suportes de colágeno que se conectam com os capilares e miócitos vizinhos. Fibras de colágeno do perimísio formam uma rede complexa de colágeno que circunda grupos de miócitos e une grupos de miócitos adjacentes entre si. O colágeno do epimísio forma uma bainha que abrange muitos feixes musculares e está conectado ao perimísio por filamentos fortes, semelhantes a tendões.[100] A partir dessa perspectiva, o coração pode ser visto como um material composto reforçado com fibra de colágeno, cuja função é sustentar os cardiomiócitos que atuam durante o enchimento diastólico e a ejeção sistólica. Como o interstício e o miocárdio estão conectados como um emaranhado, as alterações que ocorrem em um alteram as respostas biológicas e os mecanismos de remodelamento do outro.

Em seres humanos, o peso do coração pode diminuir até 25 a 30% durante repouso prolongado em cama ou na ausência de gravidade e aumentar até o extremo de 50 a 60% durante exercício extenuante.[101] Tensão mecânica, fatores de crescimento e estímulos neuro-hormonais atuam em conjunto para estimular mecanismos sinalizadores parácrinos e autócrinos fundamentais para esses processos fisiológicos de remodelamento. A reorganização do interstício é coordenada de maneira apropriada com o crescimento simétrico de células miocárdicas, e essas alterações são reversíveis assim que o desafio fisiológico é resolvido, como na hipertrofia cardíaca induzida por exercício ou pela gestação. O remodelamento reverso ocorre por meio da desativação de vias sinalizadoras pró-crescimento e ativação de outras vias sinalizadoras que desestruturam os componentes de adaptação do coração hipertrofiado. A quantidade de miócitos no coração maduro diminui com a idade, e os miócitos restantes precisam, por necessidade, remodelar-se à medida que assumem uma porcentagem maior da carga hemodinâmica.

O remodelamento cardíaco patológico compartilha muitos dos mecanismos de adaptação e das vias sinalizadoras do remodelamento fisiológico, mas o resultado final, em geral, é irreversível – redução do desempenho sistólico ou diastólico e, por fim, descompensação cardíaca. Há 40 anos, Meerson e colaboradores[102] identificaram três fases da resposta hipertrófica: (1) um estágio inicial em que a hipertrofia se desenvolve em resposta ao aumento da tensão da parede ventricular, (2) um estágio compensado em que a tensão da parede se normalizou pela resposta hipertrófica e (3) uma fase de exaustão, que se caracteriza pela morte de cardiomiócitos, desenvolvimento de fibrose miocárdica, dilatação ventricular e redução do débito cardíaco. Os mecanismos de remodelamento compensatório e adaptativo se alteram quando a tensão hemodinâmica é prolongada ou excessiva, os padrões fisiológicos de ativação neuro-hormonal são modificados excessivamente (SRAA, NE, ET-1) e o remodelamento vascular influencia a perfusão miocárdica.

A lei de Laplace enfatiza que qualquer aumento no tamanho da câmara cardíaca deve ser acompanhado de aumento proporcional na espessura da parede para manter a tensão normal da parede. A lei estabelece:

Tensão da parede = pressão × raio/2 × espessura da parede

Essa relação justifica as alterações observadas na arquitetura cardíaca quando uma carga hemodinâmica anormal crônica é imposta ao coração (Figura 246.4). Por esse motivo, a sobrecarga de pressão é compensada (a tensão da parede é normalizada) pelo aumento na espessura da parede, com poucas alterações, ou nenhuma, no tamanho da câmara cardíaca. Apesar dessa compensação, o trabalho total do coração submetido à sobrecarga de pressão aumenta, em relação ao normal, impondo necessidade persistente de maior produção de energia e liberação de oxigênio. A sobrecarga de volume, por sua vez, caracteriza-se por uma câmara cardíaca aumentada e um aumento apenas modesto na espessura da parede, suficiente para normalizar a tensão da parede. Assim, a sobrecarga de trabalho é redistribuída apropriadamente aos cardiomiócitos, o volume sistólico anterógrado é normalizado e a capacidade funcional do paciente, pelo menos teoricamente, é normalizada. O trabalho total do coração submetido à sobrecarga de volume aumenta, em relação ao coração normal, porém muito menos do que se observa no coração com sobrecarga de volume.[10]

Aumentos abruptos da tensão da parede durante a sístole, como acontece na estenose aórtica induzida experimentalmente, ocasionam elevação brusca no volume telessistólico do VE e diminuição concomitante do volume sistólico. Durante essa fase, o tamanho e a quantidade de mitocôndrias aumentam para suprir a maior demanda de energia.[103,104] Com o tempo, o miocárdio responde à sobrecarga de pressão mediante o processo de *hipertrofia concêntrica*, em que os sarcômeros se replicam de forma paralela (lado a lado), tornando as fibras musculares mais espessas, o que aumenta a espessura da parede do ventrículo esquerdo e do septo. O raio do ventrículo fica inalterado e pode até diminuir um pouco, graças à invasão da câmara pela parede ventricular espessada. Dessa forma, a tensão da parede durante a sístole é normalizada e o paciente manifesta pouco ou nenhum comprometimento funcional. Os fibroblastos do interstício também são submetidos ao aumento da carga de pressão e à elevação nos teores do fator de transformação do crescimento beta-1 gerado no local, da AT II e da aldosterona. Eles respondem a esses estímulos por meio de proliferação e aumento da síntese e deposição de colágeno, mediados pelo menos em parte pela baixa expressão da molécula de adaptação

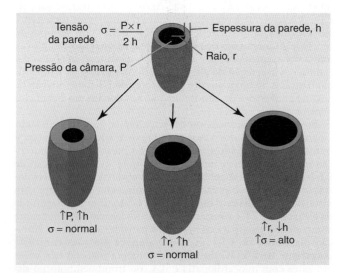

Figura 246.4 O coração responde a desafios hemodinâmicos de maneira previsível, de acordo com a equação de Laplace (já mencionada no texto). Em resposta à sobrecarga de pressão crônica, a espessura da parede ventricular aumenta para normalizar a tensão da parede (*à esquerda*). O diâmetro da câmara e a espessura da parede aumentam proporcionalmente durante o treinamento atlético e a gestação, para manter normal a tensão da parede (*no centro*). Em pacientes com insuficiência cardíaca decorrente de miocardiopatia dilatada, a tensão da parede aumenta, pois as dimensões da câmara aumentam de maneira desproporcional à espessura da parede (*à direita*).

DOC-2, nos fibroblastos ativados. No interstício, a quebra do colágeno é reduzida por causa da maior expressão do inibidor tecidual da metaloproteinase-1 (TIMP-1) e da correspondente redução da atividade das metaloproteinases da matriz, MMP-1 e MMP-9.[105]

Quando a agressão desencadeante é branda, ocorre compensação cardíaca a longo prazo, com comprometimento funcional mínimo, evidenciado pela longa sobrevida de cães com obstrução leve a moderada do fluxo sanguíneo. No entanto, quando a sobrecarga de pressão é grave o suficiente, a função miocárdica fica comprometida. A densidade capilar e a perfusão miocárdica não mantêm a regularidade proporcional a grandes aumentos na espessura da parede, e a hipoxia miocárdica crônica resulta em morte prematura de células miocárdicas e fibrose mais extensa do miocárdio. Não surpreende que a consequência mais comum da estenose aórtica subvalvar grave em cães seja a morte súbita decorrente de arritmia ventricular, presumivelmente como resultado da isquemia miocárdica e de suas sequelas. Em alguns pacientes, a hipertrofia concêntrica grave e a fibrose miocárdica induzida pela isquemia comprometem a complacência ventricular, ocasionando insuficiência cardíaca diastólica. Às vezes, ocorre falha global da bomba sistólica como consequência de mecanismos de remodelamento terminais que culminam em alongamento da fibra miocárdica, lise miofibrilar e morte de cardiomiócitos. Durante a fase de exaustão, a taxa de quebra do colágeno excede a de síntese, e o ventrículo hipertrofiado começa a se dilatar e progredir para insuficiência.

A resposta do coração à sobrecarga de volume difere substancialmente da observada na sobrecarga de pressão. As causas comuns de sobrecarga de volume incluem insuficiência valvular e lesões decorrentes de desvio (shunt) da esquerda para a direita, como acontece na persistência do ducto arterioso e no defeito do septo ventricular. A sobrecarga de volume simples se caracteriza por aumento da tensão da parede durante a diástole, ao qual os cardiomiócitos respondem replicando novos sarcômeros em série (terminação com terminação). O ventrículo se torna mais esférico e o diâmetro da câmara aumenta em um processo conhecido como hipertrofia excêntrica. A espessura da parede aumenta apenas modestamente para manter uma proporção normal com a do rádio, normalizando, assim, a tensão da parede. O modelo clinicamente relevante mais próximo de sobrecarga de volume é a regurgitação mitral, em que a carga adicional de volume é ejetada em um reservatório de baixa pressão, o átrio esquerdo. Outras formas de sobrecarga de volume, como acontece na insuficiência da valva aórtica e na persistência do ducto arterioso, são exemplos de sobrecarga de volume e pressão combinada, em que um volume adicional de sangue é ejetado em um reservatório de alta pressão, a artéria aorta. Ao examinar os mecanismos de sobrecarga de volume, é importante dar mais atenção à regurgitação mitral do que a outras anormalidades nas quais a adaptação cardíaca representa uma combinação de sobrecarga de volume e pressão.

Em comparação com a sobrecarga de pressão, a sobrecarga de volume induz um aumento relativamente modesto no peso do coração e na síntese de proteínas.[106] É interessante o fato de que o aumento de peso do coração secundário à regurgitação mitral resulta principalmente de uma baixa taxa de degradação de proteína. Tal observação reforça o conceito de que os sinais moderadores da sobrecarga de volume são diferentes daqueles que ocasionam sobrecarga de pressão e é preciso que haja uma diferença correspondente no padrão de ativação gênica. Os miócitos do coração com sobrecarga de volume são alongados em relação aos normais ou aos de coração com sobrecarga de pressão.[107] Presume-se que as diferenças na sinalização mecanorreceptora sejam amplamente responsáveis pelas diferenças no remodelamento, na sobrecarga de pressão e sobrecarga de volume, na medida em que é comum notar aumento dos teores de norepinefrina, cardiotrofina 1 e AT II na patogenia de ambas as formas de hipertrofia. Apesar disso, a ação integrada dessas vias sinalizadoras ainda é pouco entendida e pode ser que outros fatores, desconhecidos no momento, sejam responsáveis por algumas das diferenças observadas. A matriz extracelular apresenta alterações marcantes no coração de cães com regurgitação mitral induzida experimentalmente.[108,109] Tal alteração se caracteriza por perda de colágeno e ausência da estrutura elaborada dos cardiomiócitos com colágeno. A síntese de colágeno nos fibroblastos cardíacos se reduz substancialmente em cães com regurgitação mitral, juntamente com a redução na síntese de proteína nos sarcômeros. A taxa de degradação de colágeno aumenta devido à maior atividade de MMP-1 e MMP-9, em termos absolutos e relativos, com teores inibidores teciduais de MMP. Em cães com regurgitação mitral, ocorre aumento da quantidade de mastócitos no interstício.[108] Além disso, a expressão tecidual do fator de transformação do crescimento beta-1 diminui, juntamente com a infrarregulação dos genes da estrutura da matriz celular controlados por esse fator. Tais alterações são mais evidentes no início da sobrecarga de volume e tendem a se normalizar durante a fase compensada, voltando a se reativar apenas nos estágios finais da doença.

Os mecanismos de remodelamento na doença miocárdica isquêmica e na miocardiopatia dilatada diferem em termos qualitativos e quantitativos dos descritos para os casos de sobrecarga de pressão ou de volume. Na fase compensada da miocardiopatia isquêmica, as respostas de adaptação são mais semelhantes às observadas na sobrecarga de pressão devido à ação prolongada das potentes respostas neuroendócrinas de adaptação. No entanto, na fase descompensada, os cardiomiócitos começam a se alongar, a matriz de colágeno começa a se desintegrar e a câmara cardíaca se dilata, indicando anormalidade na sinalização intercelular. O coração de cães com miocardiopatia dilatada (MCD) também apresenta um padrão de remodelamento misto, mas o fenótipo de hipertrofia excêntrica predomina.

Alterações na biologia do miócito

Além da hipertrofia do miocárdio, a insuficiência cardíaca também resulta em alterações estruturais e funcionais nos componentes do acoplamento excitação-contração, nas proteínas contráteis e reguladoras, no citoesqueleto, nos mediadores de sinalização de apoptose e no metabolismo de energia.[110,111] O ciclo do cálcio é anormal na maioria dos pacientes com insuficiência cardíaca, e essa alteração contribui sobremaneira para a disfunção sistólica e diastólica.[112,113] É importante ressaltar que a quantidade de cálcio armazenada no retículo sarcoplasmático diminui em pacientes com insuficiência cardíaca. Essa redução foi associada a (1) diminuição do teor de SERCA ou da atividade da SERCA ATPase, (2) aumento da remoção do cálcio intercelular pelo intercambiador de sódio e cálcio, (3) alterações na liberação de cálcio via receptor de rianodina.[112,114] Como consequência, o início do pico transitório de cálcio nos cardiomiócitos funcionais é retardado, e o tempo de retorno ao nível basal é prolongado.[115] O aumento da atividade do intercambiador de sódio e cálcio compensa, até certo ponto, a menor recaptação via SERCA; porém, por fim, a taxa de remoção de Ca^{++} durante a diástole é reduzida.[116] Tais alterações no metabolismo do cálcio predispõem os cardiomiócitos a pós-despolarizações precoces e tardias, o que aumenta o risco de arritmias ventriculares graves e de morte súbita.

Ademais, a contratilidade do miocárdio é prejudicada pela redução da atividade da ATPase miofibrilar, que ocorre juntamente com alteração no padrão de fosforilação da troponina I, que resulta de aumento da PKC e redução dos processos mediados pela PKA.[117] Isoformas diferentes de proteínas contráteis e proteínas reguladoras associadas também podem contribuir para a diminuição da contratilidade, dependendo da espécie e da causa primária de insuficiência cardíaca.[118] Tais alterações têm relação com a expressão reduzida de isoformas adultas e o aumento da expressão de isoformas que se expressaram durante o desenvolvimento embrionário e, às vezes, é mencionado como programa genético fetal.[119,120] As vias e os mecanismos que regulam a expressão gênica, a transcrição de proteínas, a hipertrofia do miocárdio, bem como necrose e apoptose, são complexos, com inter-relação considerável entre si. Em parte, são mediados pela ativação de Gq ligada ao receptor adrenérgico alfa da fosfolipase C, translocação e ativação subsequentes de PKC e ativação da quinase extracelular relacionada com a sinalização, ERK1/2.[121] A quinase extracelular relacionada com a sinalização 1/2 é uma das quatro vias conhecidas da proteinoquinase ativada por mitógeno (MAPK) que atuam no coração e regulam a transcrição de proteínas e a expressão gênica.[13] Há envolvimento de vias MAPK adicionais, incluindo as proteínas quinases N-terminal c-Jun (JNK) e a via p38, envolvidas na diferenciação e na apoptose celular, bem como outros mecanismos celulares que modificam a expressão gênica, como a via do fator nuclear calcineurina de células T ativadas (NFAT) e o sistema sinalizador fosfoinositídeo 3-quinase/Akt/glicogênio sintase quinase-3 (PI3/Akt/GSK-3-beta).[122] Essa é uma supersimplificação compreensível e imperdoável dos mecanismos que comandam respostas diferentes a estímulos diferentes e, para obter maiores detalhes, o leitor interessado deve consultar diversas revisões excelentes sobre esses mecanismos complexos.[120,123]

Antes do início da insuficiência cardíaca, os cardiomiócitos que realizam trabalho externo adicional geram mais energia e reciclam mais cálcio do que as células que não realizam tais atividades. Quanto mais energia é produzida, mais calor é produzido, e a célula sofre maior estresse oxidativo. Como resultado, também é preciso destinar mais energia para a manutenção e o reparo dessas células. Portanto, não surpreende que uma das primeiras respostas de células sobrecarregadas seja aumentar o número de mitocôndrias para suprir a necessidade de energia.[104] Também é preciso energia adicional para a construção e manutenção das vias usadas para armazenar e distribuir energia. Por fim, esses mecanismos de adaptação se esgotam, resultando em anormalidades do ciclo do cálcio, disfunção sistólica e diastólica e morte celular. Em pacientes com insuficiência cardíaca, ocorre modificação na utilização de substrato, de ácidos graxos para carboidratos, e menor produção aeróbica de ATP.[124] A quantidade de ATP nos cardiomiócitos deficientes não se altera, mas as taxas de uso e de reposição de ATP diminuem à medida que a capacidade de produção de ATP das mitocôndrias fica limitada.[125] A insuficiência cardíaca se caracteriza por teores decrescentes de creatinofosfoquinase no citosol e nas mitocôndrias, além de diminuição da razão correspondente de fosfato de creatina/ATP. Tal alteração foi constatada em corações explantados de pacientes humanos com insuficiência cardíaca em estágio terminal, em cães com regurgitação mitral induzida experimentalmente e em cães com MCD de ocorrência espontânea.[126,127] O'Brien e colaboradores[128] verificaram redução do conteúdo de RNAm e da atividade enzimática de marcadores do ciclo do cálcio, glicólise e fosforilação oxidativa em cães com MCD. Mais recentemente, Oyama e Chittur[129] relataram menor expressão de genes envolvidos na glicólise e na fosforilação oxidativa. Lopes e colaboradores[130,131] relataram padrões similares de alteração na produção de energia refletidos nos perfis de expressão de proteína de mitocôndrias de cães com miocardiopatia induzida por marca-passo e naquela de ocorrência natural.

Essas alterações funcionais se refletem em alterações estruturais das mitocôndrias, que ficam menores e em maior quantidade.[104] Tais alterações são acompanhadas por modificações e ruptura das cristas mitocondriais internas. Nesse contexto, também ocorre alteração na arquitetura de outros constituintes celulares, com dissolução dos miofilamentos e desorganização de elementos do citoesqueleto. Isquemia é uma causa mais que óbvia da menor produção de energia e tem importância fundamental em pacientes humanos com aterosclerose. A isquemia regional, associada ao remodelamento vascular, é uma causa provável de alteração da produção de energia e morte celular em alguns de nossos pacientes, de maneira mais notável em gatos com miocardiopatia hipertrófica e cães com estenose subaórtica, em que o remodelamento de arteríolas coronarianas intramiocárdicas costuma ser bastante acentuado. É comum a associação dessas lesões vasculares com a formação de cicatrizes miocárdicas focais completamente desprovidas de miócitos funcionais.

SINAIS CLÍNICOS DE INSUFICIÊNCIA CARDÍACA

Por fim, os mecanismos ativados para compensar uma cardiopatia, inclusive as alterações neuro-hormonais e o remodelamento cardíaco, iniciam um ciclo vicioso de retenção inapropriada de sódio e água e diminuição da função cardíaca. A maioria dos pacientes, mas nem todos, com insuficiência cardíaca desenvolve congestão sanguínea sistêmica ou pulmonar, classificada como ICC direita ou esquerda, respectivamente. Essa classificação não é totalmente inclusiva, pois alguns pacientes apresentam tanto congestão sistêmica quanto pulmonar e, às vezes, não apresentam sinais de congestão quando a insuficiência cardíaca se desenvolve subitamente e o volume plasmático está normal ou diminuído.

Pacientes com insuficiência cardíaca são distinguidos mais claramente de indivíduos sadios por sua capacidade limitada de aumentar o débito cardíaco em resposta ao exercício. Na verdade, a maioria dos protocolos clínicos que classificam a gravidade da insuficiência cardíaca se baseia na resposta ao exercício. Na maioria dos pacientes com insuficiência cardíaca, a redução do débito cardíaco em repouso é apenas modesta, devido às respostas de mecanismos de adaptação que atuam aumentando a pré-carga, a frequência cardíaca e a contratilidade. O débito cardíaco em repouso só apresenta redução acentuada quando a insuficiência cardíaca é grave.

Na maioria dos animais com insuficiência cardíaca, desenvolve-se congestão pulmonar ou sistêmica como consequência da elevação excessiva da pressão venosa causada pelos efeitos combinados de aumento do volume plasmático (retenção de sódio e água) e diminuição da capacitância venosa (venoconstrição). Com o comprometimento funcional do lado esquerdo do coração, a pressão venosa pulmonar aumenta, resultando em edema pulmonar e sintomas de angústia respiratória (Figura 246.5 A). É possível notar sintomas de congestão, como tosse ou angústia respiratória, quando a pressão capilar pulmonar em cunha (PCPC) média ultrapassa 25 mmHg (normal < 10 mmHg). Com o comprometimento do lado direito do coração, a pressão venosa sistêmica aumenta, resultando em hepatomegalia e ascite, que em geral ficam evidentes quando a pressão venosa central excede 15 mmHg (normal < 5 mmHg) (Figura 246.5 B). Pacientes com insuficiência cardíaca de desenvolvimento gradual são mais tolerantes à elevação da pressão de enchimento cardíaco devido às alterações adaptativas na capacidade do fluxo linfático.[132] Em pacientes com insuficiência cardíaca, em geral, a pressão de enchimento é monitorada para determinar se o paciente está respondendo da maneira apropriada aos diversos procedimentos terapêuticos. Essa prática prudente só é útil se a atenção estiver voltada para a variável apropriada. Um erro comum na rotina clínica é mensurar a pressão venosa central (PVC) para orientar a administração de líquido em pacientes com comprometimento da função do coração esquerdo. A capacitância das veias esplâncnicas, por onde passa 70% do sangue circulante, é muito maior do que a da circulação pulmonar, além de serem complementadas por uma rede extensa de vasos linfáticos sistêmicos. Como resultado, a pressão se eleva lentamente nos leitos vasculares sistêmicos, quando o volume sanguíneo aumenta, e as manifestações de congestão no coração direito tendem a se desenvolver gradativamente. Como a capacitância das veias pulmonares é baixa, alterações relativamente pequenas no volume sanguíneo, ou em sua distribuição, podem causar um aumento rápido na pressão venosa pulmonar e edema pulmonar. Aumentos súbitos no tônus simpático (medo, ansiedade, exercício) causam constrição das veias esplâncnicas, desviando o volume de sangue circulante do reservatório venoso sistêmico para a circulação pulmonar. Isso pode desencadear um início súbito de edema pulmonar em pacientes propensos à insuficiência cardíaca esquerda.

As circulações pulmonar e sistêmica atuam em conjunto e, assim, como consequência direta, são interdependentes. A disfunção de um desses circuitos necessariamente influencia a função do outro. Por isso, um aumento na pressão do átrio esquerdo, como ocorre na regurgitação mitral, resulta em aumento correspondente na pressão da artéria pulmonar e no trabalho executado pelo coração direito. Na maioria das

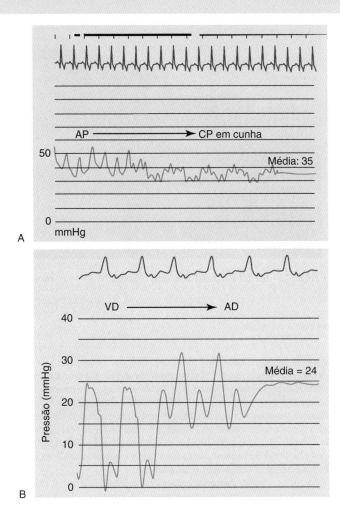

Figura 246.5 É possível que se desenvolva congestão pulmonar quando a pressão capilar pulmonar (*CP*) em cunha média excede 25 mmHg, conforme mostrado nesse cão com miocardiopatia dilatada (**A**). É possível que se desenvolva congestão sistêmica quando a pressão média do átrio direito excede 15 mmHg, como mostrado nesse cão com estenose da valva tricúspide (**B**). *AD*, átrio direito; *AP*, artéria pulmonar; *VD*, ventrículo direito.

circunstâncias, esse aumento de pressão é bastante modesto, mas uma vasoconstrição pulmonar grave pode ser induzida quando a saturação de oxigênio do sangue é reduzida devido à congestão pulmonar, resultando em hipertensão pulmonar debilitante e insuficiência cardíaca direita. O leito vascular pulmonar de gatos é mais reativo à hipoxemia do que o de cães e, como resultado, os gatos podem ser mais propensos ao desenvolvimento de hipertensão pulmonar grave como consequência de insuficiência cardíaca esquerda.[133] A relação complexa entre as circulações sistêmica e pulmonar também é evidenciada pelo padrão de congestão que se desenvolve quando há insuficiência de ambos os ventrículos simultaneamente. A efusão pleural, incomum na insuficiência cardíaca direita ou esquerda isolada, desenvolve-se frequentemente quando as pressões venosas sistêmica e pulmonar se elevam simultaneamente.[134] Em tal circunstância, ocorre acúmulo de líquido no espaço pleural porque a drenagem linfática, oriunda de ambos os sistemas circulatórios, não pode superar a rapidez de formação do líquido pleural.

RESUMO

A evolução do tratamento da insuficiência cardíaca (ver Capítulo 247) é paralela à evolução de nosso entendimento sobre a fisiopatologia dessa síndrome clínica complexa. A ênfase nos mecanismos de congestão e retenção de líquido levou ao desenvolvimento de diuréticos efetivos. O foco nas alterações hemodinâmicas na insuficiência cardíaca e nos mecanismos de redução da contratilidade cardíaca levou ao desenvolvimento de fármacos inotrópicos positivos e vasodilatadores. O reconhecimento das alterações neuro-hormonais reativas na insuficiência cardíaca serviu de base para o tratamento com inibidores da ECA, antagonistas da aldosterona e betabloqueadores. O entendimento dos mecanismos fundamentais envolvidos na excitação e na contração, na produção e na utilização de energia, bem como no remodelamento cardiovascular, sem dúvida, levou a uma variedade de novas abordagens terapêuticas e estratégias preventivas.

REFERÊNCIAS BIBLIOGRÁFICAS

As referências bibliográficas deste capítulo se encontram online no Ambiente de Aprendizagem.

CAPÍTULO 247

Insuficiência Cardíaca: Tratamento Clínico

Adrian Boswood

INTRODUÇÃO

Veterinários frequentemente se deparam com pacientes com insuficiência cardíaca que precisam de tratamento apropriado para o alívio dos sintomas e melhorar a qualidade de vida. O tratamento mais efetivo desses pacientes é obtido quando o clínico faz uma abordagem sistemática e tem conhecimento dos tipos de sinais clínicos que o paciente apresenta e dos mecanismos fisiopatológicos primários provavelmente envolvidos na manifestação dos sintomas em questão. Nem todos os pacientes com cardiopatia detectável ao exame clínico exibem sinais clínicos de insuficiência cardíaca; muitas doenças comuns apresentam fase pré-clínica ("assintomáticas") demorada durante a qual não se constata qualquer sinal clínico. Em pacientes idosos com cardiopatia é comum a presença de comorbidades; portanto, nem todos os sintomas manifestados pelos pacientes com cardiopatia se devem à insuficiência cardíaca, caso a tenham.

O QUE É INSUFICIÊNCIA CARDÍACA?

Pode-se dizer que há insuficiência cardíaca quando, como uma consequência de alguma anormalidade do coração, os pacientes manifestam sinais clínicos devido à incapacidade de manter um débito cardíaco suficiente para suprir suas necessidades metabólicas, com pressão de enchimento cardíaco normal (ver Capítulo 246). Portanto, os pacientes podem manifestar sinais de débito cardíaco inadequado, com pressão de enchimento anormal (insuficiência anterógrada); podem apresentar sinais clínicos como consequência de elevada pressão de enchimento cardíaco, porém com débito cardíaco normal (insuficiência retrógrada ou congestiva); ou, como costuma ser o caso em pacientes com manifestação clínica de emergência, podem ter sintomas causados por elevada pressão de enchimento cardíaco e, ao mesmo tempo, manifestar sinais clínicos associados a débito cardíaco inadequado. Os sinais clínicos típicos de débito cardíaco inapropriado consistem em intolerância ao exercício, síncope (ver Capítulo 30), palidez, extremidades frias e sinais de hipotensão (ver Capítulo 159), como letargia e depressão. Os sinais indicativos de que um paciente tem elevada pressão de enchimento cardíaco costumam ser decorrências de congestão da circulação venosa e incluem taquipneia e dispneia decorrentes de congestão e edema pulmonares (ver Capítulo 28); distensão abdominal devido à ascite (ver Capítulo 17); e taquipneia e dispneia decorrentes de efusão pleural (ver Capítulo 244). Ocasionalmente, o aumento da pressão de enchimento cardíaco pode ser indicada pelo desenvolvimento de edema subcutâneo (ver Capítulo 18), mas essa é uma apresentação rara em pacientes caninos e felinos.

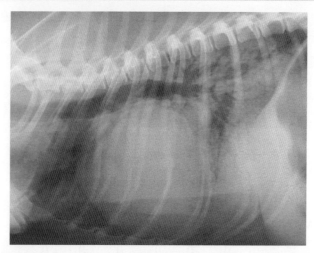

Figura 247.1 Insuficiência cardíaca esquerda em um cão. Esta imagem radiográfica lateral do tórax mostra alguns dos achados radiográficos clássicos associados à insuficiência cardíaca congestiva esquerda. Há aumento marcante da silhueta cardíaca, com opacificação difusa do parênquima pulmonar, compatível com edema pulmonar.

COMO DECIDIR DE MANEIRA DEFINITIVA QUE HÁ INSUFICIÊNCIA CARDÍACA?

Para confirmar que um paciente tem insuficiência cardíaca, é preciso estabelecer duas coisas: primeiro, que *o paciente tem evidência de cardiopatia*; segundo, que *ele está manifestando sinais clínicos em consequência da cardiopatia*.

Se um paciente apresenta sinais clínicos sugestivos apenas de cardiopatia, como sopro ou arritmia, mas não exibe quaisquer sinais clínicos resultantes daquela doença, então não há (ainda) insuficiência cardíaca. O tratamento de pacientes com cardiopatia adquirida que ainda não tenham sinais de insuficiência cardíaca é polêmico; as evidências contra e a favor do tratamento durante a fase pré-clínica de diferentes cardiopatias são discutidas em capítulos específicos (ver Capítulos 251 a 253).

Um fator que causa confusão e em geral complica o diagnóstico de insuficiência cardíaca é que os pacientes podem ter evidência clínica de cardiopatia e exibir sinais clínicos, porém causados por alguma outra doença concomitante. Por exemplo, cães com cardiopatia podem ter intolerância ao exercício devido a osteoartrite concomitante ou dispneia decorrente de paralisia de laringe. Portanto, para concluir que um paciente tem insuficiência cardíaca, é preciso estabelecer que ele tem cardiopatia *de gravidade suficiente para ser a causa provável dos sintomas e evidência de que tais sintomas têm relação direta com a cardiopatia do paciente*. Portanto, o diagnóstico de insuficiência cardíaca costuma ser feito com base na combinação de: histórico de sinais clínicos que apontam para insuficiência cardíaca, achados de exame físico indicativos de doença cardíaca e resultados de testes diagnósticos auxiliares que ajudam a estabelecer que os sinais observados são uma consequência da doença cardíaca do paciente.

Em paciente que chega à consulta com aumento da frequência e do esforço respiratórios (ver Vídeo 252.6), o teste diagnóstico mais útil para estabelecer se aqueles sintomas são de origem cardíaca ou não, em geral, é a radiografia do tórax. Considera-se que a detecção de anormalidades na forma e no tamanho da silhueta cardíaca, juntamente com achados compatíveis com insuficiência cardíaca, como congestão venosa pulmonar e um padrão alveolar, é indiscutível para estabelecer o diagnóstico de insuficiência cardíaca. A Figura 247.1 mostra uma imagem radiográfica lateral do tórax que exibe achados característicos em um cão com insuficiência cardíaca congestiva esquerda secundária à doença valvular degenerativa. A interpretação de radiografias do tórax pode ser mais difícil quando a silhueta cardíaca é encoberta pela presença de efusão pleural. Nesses casos, a detecção de aumento substancial do átrio no exame ecocardiográfico pode ajudar a incluir (ou, na ausência, excluir) a cardiopatia como a causa da efusão (ver Capítulo 104). Em pacientes que chegam à consulta com ascite como uma possível manifestação de insuficiência cardíaca direita, a evidência que confirma uma causa cardiovascular da ascite é a detecção de congestão venosa hepática na ultrassonografia abdominal e/ou evidência de cardiopatia direita substancial ou efusão pericárdica na ecocardiografia. Na Tabela 247.1, são mostrados exemplos de achados característicos obtidos à anamnese, ao exame físico e resultados de exames de imagem que sustentam o diagnóstico.

As mensurações das concentrações de biomarcadores cardíacos circulantes, como o fragmento N-terminal do peptídio natriurético tipo B (NT-pró-PNB), podem ajudar a estabelecer uma causa cardíaca para os sinais clínicos observados (ver Capítulo 246). Diversos estudos realizados em cães e gatos mostraram que os pacientes com sintomas que poderiam ser decorrências de insuficiência cardíaca congestiva (p. ex., dispneia) e apresentavam alta concentração circulante de NT-pró-PNB são mais propensos a ter uma causa cardíaca para tais sintomas; ou seja, a probabilidade de que os sinais clínicos do paciente se devam à insuficiência cardíaca aumenta de maneira considerável quando ele apresenta elevada concentração circulante de NT-pró-PNB.[1] Estudo recente também mostrou que alta concentração de NT-pró-PNB em amostra de efusão pleural de gatos ajuda a diferenciar aqueles cuja causa da efusão é cardíaca daqueles de etiologia não cardíaca.[2]

Assim que o clínico tenha convicção de que os sintomas do paciente são consequências de insuficiência cardíaca, ele deve avaliar qual é a melhor maneira de tratar esses sintomas. Em alguns pacientes atendidos como casos de emergência, com sinais clínicos potencialmente fatais, às vezes não é possível realizar exames diagnósticos auxiliares sem risco aos pacientes. Em tais circunstâncias, o clínico pode ter que tratar o paciente com base na doença primária mais provável e deixar para depois os exames diagnósticos apropriados, quando o paciente estiver mais estável e houver maior probabilidade de que vá tolerar esses procedimentos.

TRATAMENTO DA INSUFICIÊNCIA CARDÍACA

Há quatro etapas importantes no tratamento de pacientes com cardiopatia que causa insuficiência cardíaca:
1. Diagnóstico correto da doença primária.
2. Estadiamento da gravidade da doença.
3. Aplicação da abordagem "medicina baseada em evidência" (ver Capítulo 5).

CAPÍTULO 247 • Insuficiência Cardíaca: Tratamento Clínico

Tabela 247.1 Informações obtidas na anamnese, no exame físico e em exames diagnósticos auxiliares compatíveis com insuficiência cardíaca.

INFORMAÇÕES OBTIDAS NA ANAMNESE COMPATÍVEIS COM INSUFICIÊNCIA CARDÍACA	ACHADOS AO EXAME FÍSICO INDICATIVOS DE *CARDIOPATIA*	ACHADOS AO EXAME FÍSICO QUE PODEM INDICAR *INSUFICIÊNCIA CARDÍACA*	RESULTADOS DE EXAMES DIAGNÓSTICOS AUXILIARES QUE CONFIRMAM A CARDIOPATIA COMO CAUSA DOS ACHADOS AO EXAME FÍSICO
Taquipneia, dispneia e/ou angústia respiratória Intolerância ao exercício Cianose Apatia e depressão Fraqueza e letargia Inapetência	Sopro cardíaco Arritmia cardíaca Som de galope audível	Aumento da frequência e do esforço respiratórios, com ou sem crepitações pulmonares audíveis Aumento da frequência e do esforço respiratórios com abafamento central à auscultação ou percussão Distensão abdominal com uma onda de líquido palpável, em particular se acompanhada por congestão de veia jugular e/ou refluxo hepatojugular Palidez e extremidades frias	Imagem radiográfica do tórax com evidência de cardiomegalia, com congestão venosa pulmonar, e de um padrão alveolar/intersticial no parênquima pulmonar Imagem radiográfica do tórax com evidência de efusão pleural e de silhueta cardíaca anormal (se visível) Confirmação ultrassonográfica de efusão pleural com evidência de aumento atrial Evidência de congestão venosa hepática na ultrassonografia abdominal ou de cardiopatia direita significativa ou efusão pericárdica na ecocardiografia Hipotensão não atribuível a outra causa

Para estabelecer que os sintomas manifestados pelo paciente são causados por insuficiência cardíaca, com confiança razoável, ele deve ter um histórico clínico compatível com insuficiência cardíaca, anormalidades ao exame físico sugestivas de cardiopatia e insuficiência cardíaca, além de resultados de exames diagnósticos auxiliares que confirmem a cardiopatia. Quanto ao diagnóstico diferencial de alguns dos sinais clínicos aqui mencionados, o leitor deve consultar os Capítulos 26 a 30.

4. Na ausência de uma "melhor evidência", tomar uma decisão informada e racional, com base nos achados clínicos, a respeito do tipo de terapia que será mais efetiva.

O ideal é seguir essas etapas em todos os pacientes com sinais clínicos de insuficiência cardíaca; porém, em alguns casos, em particular naqueles com manifestação aguda e sinais clínicos graves, pode ser necessário primeiro estabilizar o paciente, antes de realizar as etapas 1 a 3. Os achados diagnósticos característicos de cada condição que podem resultar em insuficiência cardíaca são apresentados em detalhes nos Capítulos 250 a 255, assim como a terapia mais apropriada baseada em evidência para o tratamento de doenças específicas em estágios específicos. Portanto, no restante deste capítulo, vamos considerar os seguintes pontos: como escolher a terapia mais efetiva para um paciente com insuficiência cardíaca e quais achados clínicos orientam nossas opções de tratamento?

Quase todos os pacientes veterinários com sinais de insuficiência cardíaca necessitam de tratamento clínico para a resolução dos sinais clínicos. No entanto, há algumas exceções a essa condição geral – de maneira mais notável no caso de pacientes com efusão pericárdica (ver Capítulos 102 e 254). Em alguns pacientes, o tratamento clínico é a única intervenção necessária, enquanto em outros o tratamento clínico pode ser parte de um protocolo que inclui outras intervenções, como toracocentese (ver Capítulo 102) e fornecimento de oxigênio suplementar (ver Capítulo 131).

Alguns pacientes podem ter desenvolvido insuficiência cardíaca secundária a uma doença passível de tratamento cirúrgico, como persistência de ducto arterioso. Em pacientes como esses, pode-se aproveitar o tratamento clínico para estabilizá-los antes de instituir um tratamento mais definitivo.

JUSTIFICATIVA FISIOPATOLÓGICA PARA A ADMINISTRAÇÃO DE MEDICAMENTOS

Pacientes que chegam à consulta com sinais de insuficiência cardíaca apresentam anormalidades que consistem em uma ou mais das seguintes condições:

- Anormalidades do volume pré-carga
  - Pode-se pensar na pré-carga como a tensão da parede cardíaca no fim da diástole. Isso é determinado predominantemente pela pressão com que o sangue retorna ao coração, vindo da circulação venosa (embora também haja influência do tamanho do ventrículo). Muitos dos mecanismos de adaptação estimulados em pacientes com cardiopatia ocasionam retenção de líquido. Isso causa um aumento de volume de sangue na circulação venosa e, portanto, no volume pré-carga. A pré-carga é excessiva em pacientes que exibem sinais de congestão, sendo alterada principalmente por fármacos que reduzem o volume de líquido circulante (**diuréticos**) e dilatam as veias (**venodilatadores**)

- Anormalidades do volume pós-carga
  - Pode-se pensar na pós-carga como a força que resiste à contração do miocárdio. O principal determinante do volume pós-carga (na ausência de obstrução do fluxo de saída ventricular) é a resistência do leito vascular no qual o ventrículo está ejetando sangue, isto é, a resistência vascular sistêmica, no caso do ventrículo esquerdo, e a resistência vascular pulmonar, no caso do ventrículo direito. A resposta fisiopatológica à cardiopatia caracteriza-se pela estimulação de vários mecanismos que aumentam o volume pós-carga, incluindo o sistema nervoso simpático e o sistema renina-angiotensina-aldosterona (SRAA). O aumento da pós-carga inibe a ejeção ventricular, tende a reduzir o débito cardíaco, aumenta o trabalho do miocárdio e pode resultar em sinais de má perfusão. Os **vasodilatadores** são fármacos que reduzem a resistência vascular sistêmica ou pulmonar e podem ser usados para alterar o volume pós-carga

- Anormalidades da contratilidade do miocárdio
  - A contratilidade do miocárdio é um dos principais determinantes do débito cardíaco. Em muitos pacientes com sinais de insuficiência cardíaca há comprometimento primário ou secundário da contratilidade, embora seja difícil quantificá-lo, podendo haver sinais primários de débito cardíaco inadequado. **Fármacos inotrópicos positivos** ocasionam aumento da contratilidade

- Anormalidades do enchimento cardíaco
  - Para que haja um enchimento adequado das câmaras cardíacas, é preciso que o coração tenha tempo suficiente para isso e o miocárdio tenha elasticidade o bastante para possibilitar a entrada do retorno venoso adequado aos ventrículos durante a diástole. Doenças que tornam o miocárdio excessivamente rígido prejudicam o relaxamento (a lusitropia) ou não dão ao coração tempo ou espaço suficientes para se encher, podendo comprometer o seu enchimento. Isso requer um aumento no volume da pré-carga para manter um débito cardíaco adequado ou ocorre redução desse

débito cardíaco. Vários tipos de fármacos podem influenciar direta ou indiretamente a capacidade de enchimento do coração. Os fármacos que influenciam diretamente a capacidade de relaxamento do miocárdio são conhecidos como lusitrópicos, e incluem agentes simpaticomiméticos e bloqueadores dos canais de cálcio. Indiretamente, pode haver melhora no enchimento modificando-se a frequência e o ritmo cardíacos, de modo que haja mais tempo para o relaxamento ventricular e o enchimento efetivo

- Anormalidades da frequência e do ritmo cardíacos
  - Pacientes com sinais de insuficiência cardíaca frequentemente têm alterações na frequência e no ritmo cardíacos. É comum notar taquicardia em muitos pacientes com insuficiência cardíaca – a ponto de se esperar uma taquicardia sinusal discreta a moderada em muitos deles; todavia, algumas anormalidades do ritmo cardíaco causam comprometimento da função cardíaca suficiente para resultarem no desenvolvimento de insuficiência cardíaca (p. ex., bloqueio atrioventricular de terceiro grau ou miocardiopatia mediada por taquicardia) ou contribuírem para o agravamento dos sintomas de insuficiência cardíaca em pacientes com cardiopatia preexistente. Pacientes com bradicardia apresentam redução do débito cardíaco devido à diminuição da frequência cardíaca. Pacientes com taquicardia acentuada apresentam redução do débito cardíaco devido ao tempo insuficiente para o enchimento ventricular e, em alguns casos, à perda do padrão coordenado normal de contração ventricular (dissincronia ventricular).

Como em pacientes com sintomas de insuficiência cardíaca é provável a presença de algumas ou todas as anormalidades fisiopatológicas supracitadas, é fácil entender que fármacos que influenciam esses fatores provavelmente sejam os mais efetivos no tratamento de pacientes com insuficiência cardíaca. Portanto, podemos classificar os fármacos usados no tratamento da insuficiência cardíaca como aqueles que diminuem o volume pré-carga, reduzem o volume pós-carga, melhoram a função sistólica, o enchimento cardíaco ou otimizam a frequência e o ritmo cardíacos.

FÁRMACOS USADOS NO TRATAMENTO DE INSUFICIÊNCIA CARDÍACA

Fármacos que diminuem o volume pré-carga

Indicações para redução do volume pré-carga

Os sinais clínicos mais prováveis em um paciente com volume pré-carga excessivo são aqueles associados à congestão sanguínea. A pré-carga excessiva está associada ao aumento da pressão de enchimento ventricular, da pressão atrial e da pressão venosa, bem como congestão dos leitos vasculares que drenam o lado acometido do coração. Portanto, é provável que um paciente que requer redução do volume pré-carga tenha um ou mais dos seguintes sintomas: edema pulmonar, efusão pleural ou ascite.

Os dois tipos mais efetivos de fármaco na redução do volume pré-carga são diuréticos e venodilatadores. Os diuréticos reduzem o volume de líquido circulante do paciente e, assim, diminui a pressão de enchimento venoso (Figura 247.2 A a C). Os venodilatadores reduzem a pressão nas veias por aumentar o seu diâmetro (Figura 247.2 D).

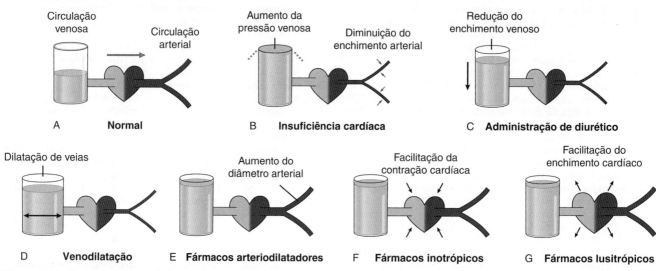

Figura 247.2 Consequências da insuficiência cardíaca e efeitos de seu tratamento na distribuição de líquido na circulação. **A.** Neste painel, são mostrados os constituintes básicos do sistema cardiovascular **normal**. O cilindro orientado verticalmente à esquerda indica a circulação venosa. O nível de sangue nesse cilindro reflete a pressão na circulação venosa. O coração está no meio do desenho e à sua direita está a circulação arterial, indicada pelos ramos dos cilindros. O diâmetro e o tamanho dessas "artérias" indicam a adequação do enchimento da circulação arterial. A seta verde, no alto da figura, indica a direção do fluxo na circulação, a partir da circulação venosa, através do coração, para a circulação arterial. **B.** Ilustra a consequência da **insuficiência cardíaca**. A retenção de líquido aumentou o enchimento do reservatório venoso, elevando a pressão venosa. Por fim, a pressão aumenta a tal ponto que o líquido começa a extravasar da circulação venosa para outros tecidos ou cavidades corporais, ocasionando insuficiência "congestiva" ou "retrógrada". O enchimento da circulação arterial é insuficiente porque o débito cardíaco reduzido acarreta insuficiência "de débito" ou "anterógrada". **C.** Ilustra o efeito da **administração de diurético**: redução do volume de líquido circulante. Isso culmina em redução do enchimento venoso, diminuição da pressão na circulação venosa, com valor inferior àquele que causa extravasamento de líquido; portanto, alivia os sinais de congestão. A administração de diurético, exclusivamente, não influencia o débito cardíaco; portanto, o enchimento arterial não se altera. **D.** Ilustra o efeito da **venodilatação**. A dilatação de veias reduz a pressão na circulação venosa, sem alterar o volume de líquido circulante. Isso se deve à maior capacidade das veias de manterem o volume de líquido presente, o que reduz a pressão na circulação venosa, para valor inferior àquele que ocasiona extravasamento de líquido. Portanto, o efeito primário é minimizar os sintomas de congestão, e o efeito no enchimento arterial será, no máximo, neutro. **E.** Ilustra o efeito da administração de **fármacos dilatadores arteriolares**. A diminuição da resistência à ejeção do sangue do ventrículo melhora a distribuição de sangue para a circulação arterial; portanto, o enchimento arterial melhora, embora isso possa ser acompanhado de prejuízo à redução da pressão sanguínea. Ademais, pode ajudar a reduzir a pressão na circulação venosa, ao possibilitar que o coração mantenha algum débito com um volume pré-carga menor. **F.** Ilustra o efeito de **fármacos inotrópicos**. Se a força de contração aumenta, o coração é capaz de manter um débito cardíaco maior, melhorando o enchimento arterial. O coração também pode ser capaz de alcançar esse débito com pressão de enchimento menor, ocasionando redução na pressão venosa e melhora nos sintomas de congestão. **G.** Ilustra o efeito de **fármacos lusitrópicos**. A melhora na capacidade de enchimento do coração durante a diástole propicia manutenção do débito cardíaco com pressão venosa de enchimento mais baixa. Portanto, pode haver redução da pressão venosa e/ou melhora do débito cardíaco e do enchimento arterial. (*Esta figura se encontra reproduzida, em cores, no Encarte.*)

Diuréticos

Por uma boa razão, os diuréticos são os medicamentos usados com maior frequência em pacientes com insuficiência cardíaca congestiva. Todos os diuréticos usados no tratamento de pacientes com insuficiência cardíaca têm um mecanismo de ação que resulta em aumento da excreção de sódio pelo paciente. Se a excreção de sódio aumenta (desde que não haja um aumento correspondente no consumo), ocorre redução no volume de líquido do compartimento extracelular do paciente, que resulta em menor volume de líquido circulante e redução do volume pré-carga. É provável que a redução do volume pré-carga resulte em rápida melhora dos sinais clínicos do paciente, se forem consequências de pressão de enchimento cardíaco excessiva.

Há várias classes de diuréticos que aumentam a excreção de sódio, por diferentes mecanismos, no néfron (Figura 247.3 e Tabela 247.2). A potência relativa de um diurético pode ser expressa pela extensão com que ele aumenta a fração de excreção de sódio – a proporção de sódio filtrado no glomérulo que é excretado na urina (ver Capítulo 73). De acordo com isso, a classe de diuréticos mais potente é a dos diuréticos de alça.

Três dos diuréticos usados mais frequentemente são furosemida, espironolactona e torsemida. Os diuréticos tiazidas também são usados, mas em geral combinados com diuréticos de alça, para controlar sintomas de congestão em pacientes com sinais mais avançados de insuficiência cardíaca.

A **furosemida** deve ser considerada o tratamento de primeira linha para qualquer paciente que requer tratamento clínico para alívio de sinais clínicos causados por congestão. Isso inclui pacientes que apresentam dispneia decorrente de edema pulmonar e efusão pleural, embora no último caso seja provável que o paciente também venha a se beneficiar de toracocentese (ver Capítulo 102). Pacientes com ascite ou (raramente) edema subcutâneo devido à cardiopatia também necessitam da indução da diurese para o alívio dos sinais clínicos. Se um paciente apresenta ascite marcante, a ponto de causar comprometimento respiratório, pode-se indicar abdominocentese (ver Capítulo 90) para propiciar alívio rápido dos sinais clínicos, mas ainda assim é necessário tratamento com diurético para prevenir novo desenvolvimento de efusão abdominal. A furosemida pode ser administrada por diversas vias, incluindo via oral, injeção de *bolus* e infusão em taxa constante.[3] Pacientes que não foram tratados previamente com o diurético são propensos a ter diurese intensa quando o fármaco é administrado pela primeira vez. Os que foram submetidos a tratamento de longa duração com furosemida podem se tornar refratários ao fármaco, tendem a apresentar diurese menos intensa e, para obter o controle dos sinais clínicos, podem necessitar de doses maiores de furosemida ou administração adicional de tipos diferentes de diurético que atuem em locais diferentes do néfron. Em cães refratários à ação da furosemida, parece que a administração de torsemida pode resultar em diurese melhor, com resolução sustentada dos sinais clínicos refratários, em alguns casos.[4,5] As doses orais iniciais de furosemida administradas a cães ou gatos devem variar de 1 a 2 mg/kg/12 horas, podendo ser aumentada para até 4 mg/kg, 3 vezes/dia (total de 12 mg/kg/dia). Se os pacientes estiverem recebendo quase a dose máxima de furosemida e os sinais de congestão se mostrarem refratários ao tratamento, provavelmente será mais benéfico usar também um segundo diurético, como espironolactona, tiazida ou torsemida, em vez de aumentar a dose de furosemida. Nos casos em que os pacientes aparentemente são refratários ao tratamento diurético no domicílio, é importante verificar se o medicamento está sendo administrado da maneira apropriada. Isso pode exigir um certo tato ao abordar a questão com os proprietários do animal quanto ao entendimento do esquema prescrito e à obediência a ele. Também é bom obter um histórico alimentar detalhado para determinar se um consumo alto de sódio é, em parte, responsável pela resistência constatada à terapia diurética (ver Capítulo 183).

A **espironolactona** é um diurético poupador de potássio que atua inibindo os receptores de aldosterona. Os benefícios demonstrados em pacientes humanos com insuficiência cardíaca[6] implicam uma ação independente do efeito diurético do agente. Portanto, o medicamento em questão deve ser considerado em escala mais ampla como um antagonista do receptor de aldosterona. A evidência de sua efetividade no tratamento de cães com doença valvular adquirida[7] levou à sua administração frequente aos cães com insuficiência cardíaca. Embora

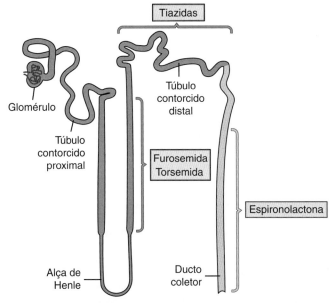

Figura 247.3 Locais de ação dos diuréticos comumente usados no néfron. A furosemida e a torsemida são diuréticos de alça, e seu principal local de ação é o ramo ascendente da alça de Henle. Os diuréticos tiazidas atuam predominantemente no túbulo contorcido distal. A espironolactona atua no ducto coletor. A administração de combinações de diuréticos com ação em mais de um local do néfron é conhecida como "bloqueio sequencial do néfron", que pode levar a intensa diurese.

Tabela 247.2 Classes de diuréticos, locais de ação, mecanismos de ação e potências relativas.

CLASSE DE DIURÉTICO	EXEMPLOS	PRINCIPAL MECANISMO DE AÇÃO	LOCAL DE AÇÃO NO NÉFRON	POTÊNCIA RELATIVA EXPRESSA COMO A EXCREÇÃO FRACIONADA MÁXIMA DE SÓDIO QUE PODE SER OBTIDA[15]
"Diurético de alça"	Furosemida Torsemida	Bloqueio do cotransportador de $Na^+/K^+/2Cl^-$	Alça de Henle	Até 25%
Tiazida	Hidroclorotiazida	Bloqueio de transportadores Na^+/Cl^-	Túbulo distal e segmento conector	Até 5%
Poupador de potássio	Espironolactona	Bloqueio de receptores da aldosterona	Túbulo coletor cortical	Até 2%

SEÇÃO 16 • Doença Cardiovascular

seja utilizado por seu efeito diurético, e outros efeitos hipotéticos, em gatos com cardiopatia e insuficiência cardíaca, um estudo que envolveu um pequeno número de animais sugeriu que o desenvolvimento de reações cutâneas adversas ao fármaco pode ser uma preocupação.[8] É possível que isso tenha limitado a frequência com que é administrado aos animais dessa espécie.

Em cães, mostrou-se que a dose efetiva de espironolactona é de 2 mg/kg/24 h por via oral.[9] Em contraste com a furosemida, há pouca evidência de que se consiga um controle melhor dos sinais clínicos com doses maiores ou com a administração mais frequente.

A espironolactona não tem efeito natriurético suficiente para ser usada como diurético único em pacientes que precisam de tratamento clínico para os sintomas de congestão. Portanto, é melhor considerá-la um agente para ser administrado junto a outros diuréticos, em particular os diuréticos de alça, para potencializar seu efeito. O outro argumento para sua administração é que se acredita que os benefícios associados à sua administração vão além dos efeitos diuréticos. Acredita-se que o bloqueio do receptor de aldosterona seja benéfico devido aos efeitos prejudiciais do bloqueio da aldosterona nos vasos sanguíneos e no remodelamento cardíaco.

A **torsemida** (torasemida) é um diurético de alça similar à furosemida que tem sido usado como medicamento de salvação em pacientes que são refratários a altas dosagens de furosemida durante tratamento crônico de insuficiência cardíaca. Há várias vantagens teóricas na administração de torsemida, incluindo uma probabilidade menor de pacientes ficarem refratários à sua administração[10] e também possíveis efeitos antialdosterona,[11] além dos efeitos na alça de Henle. Em pacientes com sinais refratários de insuficiência congestiva, a torsemida substitui a furosemida no esquema de tratamento, cessando o uso de furosemida. Essa substituição pode ser feita abruptamente, com a primeira dose de torsemida administrada quando a dose seguinte seria administrada. O método de administração recomendado é iniciar o tratamento com uma dose diária total de torsemida (fracionada em duas doses, com intervalo aproximado de 12 horas) que corresponde a cerca de um décimo da dose diária total de furosemida que o paciente estava recebendo[5] (Boxe 247.1).

Os **diuréticos tiazídicos** representam outra classe de diuréticos bastante usados em pacientes humanos, em particular naqueles com hipertensão sistêmica. Também têm sido usados em cães com insuficiência cardíaca, especialmente naqueles com sinais de congestão, refratários à furosemida e à espironolactona. As tiazidas atuam predominantemente inibindo a recaptação de sódio no túbulo contorcido distal; portanto, quando usadas com um diurético de alça e um poupador de potássio, tal combinação provoca um "bloqueio sequencial no néfron", sendo possível induzir maior diurese pela inibição da reabsorção de sódio em vários locais do néfron (ver Figura 247.3). A hidroclorotiazida é um diurético tiazídico que pode ser usado nessa situação.

Boxe 247.1 Exemplo de conversão de dosagem de furosemida para torsemida

Cão de 11 kg recebendo 40 mg de furosemida 3 vezes/dia, com evidência de ascite refratária ao tratamento atual. Qual dosagem de torsemida deve substituir o tratamento atual com furosemida?
- A dose total diária atual de furosemida é 120 mg/dia (= 10,9 mg/kg/dia)
- Portanto, a dose total diária de torsemida deve ser 120 mg/10 (i. e., 12 mg/dia)
- Essa dosagem total deve ser administrada em duas doses iguais, com intervalo aproximado de 12 horas
- Portanto, a dose de torsemida deve ser de 6 mg/12 h por via oral.

Complicações do tratamento diurético

Embora amplamente usado e em geral bem tolerado, há numerosas complicações e efeitos colaterais possíveis decorrentes da administração de diuréticos que exigem monitoramento cuidadoso dos pacientes que estejam sob tratamento de longa duração. Os "efeitos colaterais" mais óbvios dos diuréticos, da perspectiva do proprietário do animal, são polidipsia e poliúria causadas por eles. Os proprietários devem ser avisados, sempre, que esses efeitos do tratamento do animal são esperados.

Todas as complicações mais comumente observadas são consequências diretas dos mecanismos de ação desses fármacos e da adaptação do paciente à sua administração. Elas incluem depleção de volume e redução do débito cardíaco, além de anormalidades eletrolíticas.

Depleção de volume e redução do débito cardíaco. O efeito pretendido com a administração de diuréticos é reduzir de maneira apropriada o volume de líquido circulante do paciente. O objetivo é uma redução suficiente para aliviar os sinais de congestão, ao mesmo tempo que permita ao paciente manter perfusão adequada. Se, como consequência do tratamento, houver uma redução excessiva do volume de líquido circulante, ou se o paciente tiver uma dependência especial de uma alta pressão de enchimento ventricular para manter um débito cardíaco adequado (o que é particularmente provável em pacientes com insuficiência cardíaca predominantemente diastólica, como gatos com miocardiopatia hipertrófica), então pode ocorrer redução do débito cardíaco e consequente comprometimento da perfusão, após a diurese. Isso pode manifestar-se de diversas maneiras, inclusive com hipotensão ou azotemia. Se o paciente manifestar esses sinais após a indução de diurese, pode ser necessário realizar um ou ambos os procedimentos:
- Reduzir a intensidade do tratamento com diurético
- Instituir um esquema de tratamento de insuficiência cardíaca mais equilibrado, que controle a diminuição do débito cardíaco por outros meios, como, por exemplo, vasodilatação ou administração de fármacos inotrópicos.

Uma preocupação errônea comum é que os pacientes com esses sinais estejam "desidratados", portanto seriam beneficiados com a administração intravenosa de líquidos. A insuficiência cardíaca – conforme explicado anteriormente – é um problema de distribuição imprópria de líquido. Em um paciente com o coração normal, é provável que a administração de líquido na circulação venosa melhore o débito cardíaco, portanto, os sinais de baixo débito cardíaco e má perfusão. Em um paciente com insuficiência cardíaca, em particular naquele com sinais de congestão, já existe mais líquido que o suficiente na circulação venosa; o problema é que o coração é incapaz de transferir adequadamente aquele líquido para a circulação arterial. É provável que o acréscimo de mais líquido na circulação venosa agrave os sinais de congestão, sendo improvável que melhore a condição clínica do paciente.[12] Recentemente, foi demonstrado em pacientes humanos que a fluidoterapia intravenosa durante um episódio de insuficiência cardíaca descompensada aguda piora em vez de melhorar o resultado. Em geral, a terapia com líquido intravenoso está contraindicada em pacientes com sinais de insuficiência cardíaca congestiva.

Anormalidades eletrolíticas. Também são complicações comuns do tratamento com diurético. A resposta fisiológica normal ao aumento de sódio e à perda de água é a estimulação de mecanismos homeostáticos que tentam reter com mais vigor o sódio e a água. O SRAA é o mecanismo predominante entre eles. Menos comumente – embora de maneira significativa – a liberação de vasopressina às vezes também é estimulada por uma queda acentuada na pressão sanguínea, secundária à cardiopatia ou ao tratamento com diurético. Um dos efeitos da estimulação desses mecanismos homeostáticos é a alteração no controle de eletrólitos. A maior atividade da aldosterona tende a favorecer a retenção de sódio e a perda de potássio na parte distal do néfron. Isso leva a uma das consequências mais comumente observadas na administração de diuréticos de alça: hipopotassemia. É menos provável observar hipopotassemia em pacientes que estiverem recebendo tratamentos concomitantes que tendem a se contrapor ao SRAA.[13] O uso mais disseminado de inibidores da enzima conversora de angiotensina (IECA; ver adiante) e espironolactona, além de diuréticos de alça, mostra que agora a hipopotassemia é vista com menor frequência. A situação em que é mais provável detectá-la é durante a estabilização clínica emergencial de pacientes propensos a receber altas doses de furosemida e outros agentes que ainda não foram administrados.

Quando ocorre hipotensão substancial como consequência de cardiopatia grave ou tratamento vigoroso com diuréticos, a liberação de vasopressina pode ser estimulada. A vasopressina atua como mediadora na retenção renal de água livre. A retenção de água livre acarreta expansão do volume de líquido circulante, porém com redução na concentração de sódio. Portanto, uma cardiopatia grave avançada e o tratamento vigoroso com diurético podem ser associados ao desenvolvimento de hiponatremia.[13] Em estudos feitos com seres humanos, a presença de hiponatremia em pacientes com insuficiência cardíaca está associada a um prognóstico desfavorável.[14]

Depois de alguns dias de administração de diurético, o paciente se adapta fisiologicamente ao aumento do sódio e à perda de água e alcança um estado estável mediante o qual a maior perda de sódio fica equilibrada pela retenção de sódio mais vigorosa.[15] Nesse novo estado estável, o consumo de sódio é igual à perda de sódio, mas crucialmente esse novo estado estável é alcançado após uma redução no volume de líquido circulante do paciente. Após 10 a 14 dias de tratamento diurético, o paciente fica em um novo equilíbrio, mas com um volume menor de líquido circulante. Esse volume circulante menor é mantido, e os sinais de congestão continuam sob controle, enquanto o paciente estiver recebendo (e responder) a mesma dosagem de diurético, o consumo de sódio for consistente e a cardiopatia não se agravar de forma significativa. O período durante o qual esse novo equilíbrio se desenvolve é aquele em que o paciente está mais propenso a desenvolver complicações do tratamento diurético; portanto, é mais provável que ocorram sinais de depleção excessiva de volume e anormalidades eletrolíticas nos 10 a 14 dias após o início ou a modificação de um esquema diurético.

Ante a frequência com que ocorrem anormalidades da homeostasia de volume, da perfusão e das concentrações sanguíneas de eletrólitos em pacientes que estão recebendo diuréticos, é uma boa prática avaliar os indicadores de função renal e as concentrações sanguíneas de eletrólitos antes e depois do início de alguma modificação substancial no tratamento diurético. Verificar novamente as concentrações séricas de ureia, creatinina, sódio, potássio e cloreto 10 a 14 dias após o início ou a alteração de um esquema diurético permite a detecção precoce de anormalidades e fazer os ajustes necessários no tratamento.

No caso de pacientes hospitalizados com insuficiência cardíaca aguda que estejam recebendo terapia intensiva para insuficiência cardíaca e sendo feitos ajustes frequentes da dosagem, é prudente verificar regularmente as concentrações séricas de eletrólitos e indicadores da função renal: o ideal é pelo menos uma vez a cada período de 24 horas e mais frequentemente em pacientes que estejam tendo complicações.

Venodilatadores

São agentes que dilatam as veias da circulação sistêmica. Muitos vasodilatadores atuam tanto em veias como nas artérias e são descritos como vasodilatadores mistos ou "balanceados" (que serão discutidos adiante, ao se abordar a redução da pós-carga). Alguns vasodilatadores atuam predominantemente nas veias, portanto reduzem principalmente a pré-carga. Ao dilatar as veias, esses agentes aumentam o volume dos vasos de capacitância da circulação, diminuindo a pressão no interior das veias,

reduzindo a pressão em que o sangue retorna ao coração. Isso diminui a pressão hidrostática nas veias e nos capilares que drenam nelas – tendendo assim a reduzir os sintomas de congestão manifestados pelo paciente (ver Figura 247.2 D). Como os dois determinantes principais da pressão hidrostática venosa são o volume de líquido nas veias e até que ponto elas podem dilatar-se, é possível entender como os venodilatadores tendem a atuar de maneira complementar aos diuréticos na redução da pré-carga. Os diuréticos reduzem o volume de sangue nas veias, e os venodilatadores aumentam a capacidade venosa de manter aquele volume de sangue em pressão relativamente baixa. A classe de vasodilatadores que atuam predominantemente nas veias é a do nitrato, e o agente dessa classe administrado com maior frequência a pacientes veterinários é a nitroglicerina (trinitrato de glicerol). Alguns vasodilatadores à base de nitrato, em particular o nitroprussiato, influenciam a pós-carga e a pré-carga e serão discutidos adiante, juntamente com os vasodilatadores mistos (ou balanceados).

Os venodilatadores tendem a ser administrados em situações nas quais é necessária uma redução aguda da pré-carga, isto é, no tratamento de pacientes com sinais graves de congestão que precisam de tratamento de emergência. A nitroglicerina costuma ser administrada como um unguento cutâneo que requer absorção percutânea para ser efetivo. O método de administração e o desenvolvimento rápido de taquifilaxia (tolerância e perda rápida da eficácia) limitam o uso da nitroglicerina a períodos curtos em pacientes hospitalizados.

Há alguma evidência de efeitos favoráveis dos vasodilatadores à base de nitrato em pacientes humanos, em casos agudos, mas essa evidência é relativamente fraca e não indica superioridade dos nitratos em relação a outros métodos de controle dos sinais clínicos.[16] Não foram realizados estudos controlados a longo prazo desses agentes em pacientes veterinários. Estudos em cães normais anestesiados mostraram que o volume esplênico – portanto, por inferência, a capacitância vascular de volume – aumenta em resposta à administração transdérmica de nitroglicerina.[17] Em contraste, em outro estudo verificou-se que a administração oral do vasodilatador à base de dinitrato de isossorbida não interferiu na redistribuição do volume sanguíneo entre as cavidades corporais,[18] implicando que esse composto de nitrato pode não ser um vasodilatador efetivo em cães.

Fármacos que diminuem o volume pós-carga

A insuficiência cardíaca surge pela estimulação crônica de vários mecanismos homeostáticos que respondem a uma queda percebida na pressão da circulação arterial (ver Capítulo 246). Muitos dos sistemas estimulados na insuficiência cardíaca – inclusive o sistema nervoso simpático, o SRAA e o sistema vasopressina – resultam em aumento da resistência vascular sistêmica. Isso representa um esforço para restabelecer a pressão sanguínea para um valor mais próximo ao normal. Embora benéfica como uma resposta aguda à redução na pressão sanguínea, a vasoconstrição crônica é prejudicial à função cardíaca. O aumento da resistência vascular influencia o débito cardíaco ou requer aumento do trabalho cardíaco para manter um débito cardíaco adequado. O aumento do trabalho cardíaco aumenta o consumo de oxigênio pelo miocárdico e, se o aumento do trabalho cardíaco for crônico, haverá maior deterioração da função cardíaca, exacerbando o comprometimento do coração, já com insuficiência. No paciente com regurgitação mitral, a vasoconstrição arterial sistêmica resiste à ejeção de sangue do ventrículo esquerdo para a artéria aorta e pode favorecer o fluxo retrógrado do sangue, através da valva com insuficiência, para o átrio esquerdo. A via pela qual o sangue deixa o ventrículo esquerdo na presença de regurgitação mitral é determinada pela resistência relativa à ejeção para a artéria aorta ou o retorno para o átrio esquerdo. A redução na resistência à ejeção para a aorta (devido à resistência vascular sistêmica reduzida) tende a favorecer o sangue que deixa o ventrículo por essa via e reduzir a magnitude do jato regurgitante. Se a resistência à ejeção estiver reduzida, também é possível que um débito cardíaco similar seja mantido com uma pré-carga ventricular mais baixa – portanto, agentes que reduzem a resistência vascular sistêmica podem causar, indiretamente, redução do volume pré-carga.

É fácil entender as vantagens hipotéticas dos vasodilatadores: eles devem melhorar o débito cardíaco ou, como alternativa, manter o mesmo débito cardíaco, mas com trabalho miocárdico reduzido (ver Figura 247.2 E).

Foi estabelecida evidência clínica clara das vantagens dos vasodilatadores em vários estudos inovadores realizados em pacientes humanos com insuficiência cardíaca, incluindo o estudo V-HeFT[19] e o CONSENSUS,[20] que demonstraram aumento da sobrevida de pacientes com insuficiência cardíaca tratados com vasodilatadores.

Há várias classes de fármacos que são administrados a pacientes com insuficiência cardíaca e atuam total ou parcialmente por meio de um efeito vasodilatador; tais fármacos incluem nitrato, IECA, pimobendana e bloqueadores do canal de cálcio. Outras classes de vasodilatadores são usadas há tempo em cães, como a hidralazina[21] e o prazosina, mas seu uso diminuiu porque a evidência que apoia o uso de outros agentes foi mais forte.

Uma desvantagem potencial da administração de vasodilatador é que a redução na resistência vascular em um paciente com função cardíaca já comprometida pode acarretar queda da pressão sanguínea, resultando em sintomas de hipotensão, como síncope, fraqueza e hipoperfusão. Pacientes com algumas cardiopatias primárias podem ser capazes de aumentar seu débito cardíaco após redução da pós-carga em consequência do tipo de cardiopatia que apresentam e, portanto, ficar sob maior risco de apresentar tais complicações. Pacientes sob risco particular dessa complicação são aqueles com obstrução à ejeção do fluxo sanguíneo e com doenças que causam predominantemente disfunção diastólica, como a miocardiopatia hipertrófica em gatos. Apesar dessas preocupações, justificáveis, a grande variedade de benefícios, além da simples redução na resistência ventricular, associados à administração de agentes como IECA, significa que, na prática, muitas vezes eles são administrados a pacientes com tais doenças primárias. Nesses casos, é preciso maior cautela em seu uso, bem como monitoramento cuidadoso.

Nitroprussiato

É um vasodilatador do grupo nitrato que tem ação rápida, administrado por via intravenosa. Tem um efeito misto (balanceado), ou seja, pode reduzir o volume da pré-carga mediante venodilatação e também o da pós-carga por meio de dilatação arterial. Tem ação rápida, com efeitos potentes, e requer administração cuidadosa por meio de taxa de infusão contínua. Em uma unidade de tratamento intensivo, onde a pressão sanguínea pode ser monitorada com cuidado (ver Capítulo 99), pode ser um procedimento auxiliar muito útil a outros tratamentos, na assistência emergencial a um paciente que precisa de redução intensiva dos volumes da pré-carga e da pós-carga. É improvável que a administração de nitroprussiato no contexto de cuidados primários seja praticável. É difícil administrar nitroprussiato porque ele precisa ser protegido da luz durante a infusão. Como ocorre com relação à nitroglicerina, conforme já mencionado, os pacientes se tornam rapidamente refratários ao nitroprussiato, o que limita seu valor em tratamento de longa duração. Também é metabolizado em cianeto, o que limita o seu uso cumulativo.

Inibidores da enzima conversora de angiotensina

Como uma classe, os IECA são agentes mais comumente usados no tratamento de pacientes veterinários com insuficiência cardíaca. Há numerosos agentes com efeitos farmacodinâmicos similares; tais agentes incluem *enalapril, benazepril, ramipril, imidapril,* entre outros. A efetividade dos IECA no tratamento de cães com insuficiência cardíaca foi estabelecida em numerosos estudos na década de 1990.[22,23] Desde então, esses fármacos

se tornaram, com boa razão, parte padrão da terapia de longa duração na maioria dos pacientes com insuficiência cardíaca. A evidência de sua efetividade em gatos com insuficiência cardíaca está menos bem estabelecida. Resultados de um estudo preliminar sugeriram que os IECA eram superiores aos betabloqueadores no tratamento de insuficiência cardíaca secundária à miocardiopatia em gatos.[24] Devido a seus benefícios teóricos (maiores do que provados na prática), também são usados frequentemente como um componente fundamental da terapia em gatos com insuficiência cardíaca.

Mediante a inibição da enzima conversora de angiotensina, os IECA tendem tanto a causar vasodilatação quanto a inibição da retenção de líquido (ver Capítulo 246). Sua interferência nessa via é particularmente benéfica em pacientes que também tenham recebido diuréticos. Conforme descrito anteriormente, a administração de diurético acarreta perda de sódio e estimulação do SRAA. É vantajoso inibir a via pela qual o paciente tenta contornar os efeitos da perda de sódio pela diurese. Esse efeito complementar desses dois medicamentos costuma ser usado como argumento para a sua administração simultânea como rotina. Em geral, os IECA são administrados à maioria dos pacientes com insuficiência cardíaca que requerem diurese prolongada, a menos que haja alguma contraindicação à sua administração. Na prática, isso significa que a maioria dos cães e gatos sob terapia para insuficiência cardíaca vai receber um IECA. As dosagens de alguns desses agentes estão no Boxe 247.2.

Os IECA não são vasodilatadores particularmente potentes e é mais provável que seus benefícios estejam associados à administração prolongada do que de curta duração. Por essa razão, são mais propensos a fazer parte de um protocolo de tratamento prolongado do que um medicamento a ser administrado no contexto de insuficiência cardíaca aguda.

Houve muita controvérsia quanto aos IECA terem ou não efeito benéfico na cardiopatia pré-clínica. Dois estudos prospectivos controlados por placebo em cães com doença crônica da valva mitral[25,26] falharam em demonstrar de maneira conclusiva um prolongamento do tempo para o início de insuficiência cardíaca congestiva. Um estudo retrospectivo em cães com miocardiopatia dilatada[27] sugeriu que o benazepril poderia estar associado a um desfecho melhor, mas ainda não foi realizado um estudo prospectivo controlado por placebo desses medicamentos no estágio pré-clínico dessa doença. Atualmente, nenhuma evidência conclusiva confirma seu uso no estágio pré-clínico de doença miocárdica felina.

A melhor evidência, e a opinião da maioria dos especialistas, corrobora o uso de IECA na maioria dos pacientes com sinais de insuficiência cardíaca que requerem administração de diurético por tempo prolongado.

Pimobendana

O pimobendana é descrito como um "inodilatador": um agente com efeitos inotrópicos e vasodilatadores. É impossível separar esses dois efeitos; portanto, fica um tanto artificial considerar o fármaco como um "inotrópico" ou um "vasodilatador" aqui; entretanto, no tópico sobre os inotrópicos, adiante, há uma descrição mais detalhada do mecanismo de ação e das indicações para esse fármaco.

Bloqueadores do canal de cálcio

Como uma classe de medicamento, os bloqueadores do canal de cálcio têm numerosos e variados efeitos eletrofisiológicos cardíacos e vasculares. O bloqueador do canal de cálcio administrado em escala mais ampla a pacientes veterinários, por seu efeito vasodilatador, é o *anlodipino*, usado mais frequentemente como um agente anti-hipertensivo em gatos com hipertensão sistêmica (ver Capítulo 158); no entanto, seus potentes efeitos como um arteriodilatador levaram alguns veterinários a defender seu uso como vasodilatador em cães com insuficiência cardíaca. Pode ter benefício particular quando a insuficiência cardíaca é secundária à doença da valva mitral, pelas razões já

CAPÍTULO 247 • Insuficiência Cardíaca: Tratamento Clínico

Boxe 247.2 Fármacos comumente administrados no tratamento de insuficiência cardíaca em cães e gatos, com a justificativa para sua administração e o mecanismo de ação

Redução do volume da pré-carga
Diuréticos
- Furosemida
  - Oral: 1 a 4 mg/kg/8 a 12 h
  - IV: no tratamento emergencial: 1 a 4 mg/kg, na forma de *bolus*; repetir a dose em intervalos de 4 horas (ou menos, se os sintomas forem graves), até a melhora dos sinais clínicos
  - TIC IV: 0,5 a 1 mg/kg/h, até a melhora dos sinais clínicos
  - Se possível, deve-se evitar dose diária total > 12 mg/kg. A falha de um paciente em mostrar melhora após múltiplas doses intravenosas ou após TIC por mais de 4 h deve levar à reavaliação do diagnóstico e à modificação do esquema de tratamento
- Espironolactona
  - Oral: 2 mg/kg/24 h
- Torsemida
  - Calcular a dosagem com base na dose de furosemida que será substituída (ver Boxe 247.1)
- Hidroclorotiazida
  - Oral: 0,5 a 4 mg/kg/12 a 24 h. Usar a menor dose indicada, quando em combinação com outros diuréticos.

Venodilatadores
- Nitroglicerina
  - Administrada como unguento percutâneo
  - 2,5 cm de unguento transdérmico a 2% para 10 kg de peso corporal.

Redução do volume da pós-carga
Vasodilatadores
- Enalapril
  - Oral: 0,5 mg/kg/12 a 24 h
- Benazepril
  - Oral: 0,25 a 0,5 mg/kg/24 h
- Ramipril
  - Oral: 0,125 mg/kg/24 h

- Imidapril
  - Oral: 0,25 mg/kg/24 h
- Anlodipino
  - Para tratamento de insuficiência cardíaca em cães
  - Oral: 0,05 a 0,1 mg/kg/24 h
- Nitroprussiato
  - TIC IV: 1 a 5 mcg/kg/min
  - Iniciar com dose baixa, ajustar a dose e monitorar a pressão sanguínea.

Redução do volume da pós-carga no ventrículo direito
Vasodilatador pulmonar
- Sildenafila
  - Oral: relatadas amplas faixas de dosagem, de 0,25 mg/kg/12 h a 2 mg/kg/8 h
  - Iniciar lentamente e aumentar gradualmente.

Melhora do enchimento cardíaco
Agentes lusitrópicos
- Diltiazem
  - Oral: 10 mg/gato/8 h
  - Também são usadas várias preparações de liberação lenta, mas a farmacocinética destas está menos bem estabelecida.

Melhora da contratilidade cardíaca
Agentes inotrópicos
- Dobutamina
  - TIC IV: iniciar com a menor dose da faixa de dosagem indicada. Ajustar a dose até obter o efeito desejado, monitorando sinais de intoxicação, especialmente arritmias
  - Cão: 2 a 15 mcg/kg/min
  - Gato: 1 a 5 mcg/kg/min
- Pimobendana
  - Cão
  - Oral: 0,1 a 0,3 mg/kg/h (foram usadas dosagens similares em gatos)
  - IV: injeção na forma de *bolus* (disponível na Europa): 0,15 mg/kg.

IV, intravenoso(a); *TIC*, taxa de infusão contínua.

---

comentadas. Estudos experimentais mostraram redução na pressão do átrio esquerdo em cães com regurgitação mitral associada à administração de anlodipino, o que sugere uma justificativa fisiopatológica para sua administração a cães com insuficiência cardíaca secundária a essa condição;[28] contudo, ainda não foi publicado um estudo prospectivo sobre o efeito desse fármaco nos desfechos clínicos significativos em cães (ou gatos) com insuficiência cardíaca.

Portanto, a administração de anlodipino pode ser indicada a cães com insuficiência cardíaca, em particular quando secundária à regurgitação mitral, mas provavelmente deve ser considerada um vasodilatador de segunda ou terceira linha a pacientes que já estejam recebendo pimobendana e IECA e tenham sinais de insuficiência cardíaca refratária apesar de tal tratamento.

O *diltiazem* também é um bloqueador do canal de cálcio cujo uso tem sido defendido para cães e gatos com insuficiência cardíaca. Em cães, é bastante usado como antiarrítmico e em gatos como possível lusitropo positivo, sendo seus efeitos discutidos adiante e no Capítulo 248.

Vasodilatadores pulmonares

Os vasodilatadores que acabamos de descrever atuam de forma predominante ou exclusiva nas artérias sistêmicas. Alguns deles atuam principalmente, ou em parte, na circulação pulmonar. Em pacientes com insuficiência cardíaca congestiva direita, pode haver melhora dos sinais clínicos pela redução da resistência vascular pulmonar. Isso pode melhorar o débito sanguíneo do lado direito do coração (portanto, resultar em melhora geral do débito cardíaco) e também resultar em redução da pressão venosa sistêmica, graças à transferência mais efetiva de sangue das veias sistêmicas para as artérias pulmonares. É mais provável que a vasodilatação pulmonar melhore os sinais clínicos de um paciente quando forem, pelo menos em parte, consequências do aumento da resistência vascular pulmonar, isto é, em que o paciente tem hipertensão como causa primária ou uma complicação secundária da cardiopatia.

O *sildenafila* é um inibidor da fosfodiesterase V bastante usado com o objetivo de reduzir a resistência vascular pulmonar e melhorar os sinais clínicos em pacientes com sinais de cardiopatia secundária ao aumento da resistência vascular pulmonar (ver Capítulo 243). Foram publicadas séries de casos descrevendo melhora nos sinais clínicos associados à administração desse medicamento em cães.[29,30] Um estudo prospectivo cruzado cego sugeriu que o sildenafila, quando administrado a cães com insuficiência cardíaca e hipertensão arterial pulmonar secundária à doença degenerativa da valva mitral, ocasiona redução da pressão da artéria pulmonar e melhora a tolerância ao exercício e a qualidade de vida.[31] É mais provável que esse fármaco seja indicado aos pacientes com insuficiência cardíaca causada por doença vascular pulmonar parasitária ou doença pulmonar crônica. Sua administração também é indicada para cães em estágio terminal de doença mixomatosa da valva mitral, em que pode surgir insuficiência cardíaca do lado direito do coração secundária ao desenvolvimento de hipertensão pulmonar (ver Capítulo 251).

O pimobendana também tem propriedades vasodilatadoras pulmonares, além de seus efeitos vasodilatadores sistêmicos;

SEÇÃO 16 • Doença Cardiovascular

portanto, pode ser efetivo no controle dos sinais clínicos de insuficiência cardíaca direita em cães com doença da valva mitral em estágio mais avançado.

Há relatos ocasionais da administração de antagonistas do receptor de endotelina (p. ex., *bosentana*) a cães com hipertensão pulmonar, mas até o momento a evidência disponível de sua efetividade é insuficiente para que sejam recomendados. Seu custo também é proibitivo.

Fármacos que facilitam a função inotrópica

Um dos principais determinantes do débito cardíaco de um paciente é a contratilidade do miocárdio. Se ela for favorecida por meios fisiológicos ou farmacológicos, então obtém-se um aumento do débito cardíaco, com o mesmo enchimento cardíaco (pré-carga) ou o mesmo débito cardíaco pode ser conseguido com pressão de enchimento cardíaco mais baixa. Portanto, os fármacos que facilitam a contratilidade miocárdica têm a capacidade de aumentar o débito cardíaco ou diminuir indiretamente a pré-carga, permitindo que os pacientes mantenham um débito cardíaco similar com pressão de enchimento mais baixa (ver Figura 247.2 F).

A contratilidade do miocárdio costuma estar comprometida em pacientes com insuficiência cardíaca. O comprometimento da contratilidade pode ser a anormalidade primária que leva um paciente a ter insuficiência cardíaca, por exemplo, em pacientes com miocardiopatia dilatada, ou pode ser secundária a alterações crônicas na carga imposta ao coração por outras condições, como cardiopatia valvular ou hipertensão. A facilitação da contratilidade cardíaca melhora os sinais clínicos de muitos pacientes com insuficiência cardíaca. Aqueles com sinais de insuficiência anterógrada têm maior probabilidade de se beneficiar com a melhora do débito cardíaco. A redução indireta da pré-carga também pode melhorar os sinais clínicos de congestão.

Os inotrópicos podem ser administrados a pacientes hospitalizados com início agudo de insuficiência cardíaca (ou um paciente com deterioração aguda de uma insuficiência cardíaca crônica) ou administrados por tempo prolongado aos pacientes tratados em casa. O medicamento inotrópico mais comumente administrado aos pacientes com insuficiência cardíaca aguda é a *dobutamina*. O fármaco com propriedades inotrópicas mais comumente administrado por longo tempo é o *pimobendana*. Outros medicamentos com efeitos inotrópicos usados no tratamento de pacientes caninos incluem digoxina e milrinona. O primeiro ainda é administrado frequentemente aos cães, mas principalmente devido a seus efeitos parassimpaticomiméticos em cães com arritmia supraventricular (ver Capítulo 248). O último, um inibidor da fosfodiesterase, não é usado comumente.

Dobutamina

A dobutamina é um agente simpaticomimético que atua principalmente por meio de estimulação de receptores beta-1. Portanto, melhora a força de contração miocárdica e a frequência com que o miocárdio se relaxa, isto é, efeitos inotrópico e lusitrópico, respectivamente. Só pode ser administrada por via intravenosa, em taxa de infusão contínua. Isso significa que só pode ser administrada a pacientes hospitalizados. Há uma relação muito estreita entre a dose e a resposta, sendo mais provável que doses maiores estejam associadas a efeitos colaterais, como indução de arritmia. Por essa razão, é um medicamento administrado com maior segurança em uma unidade de cuidados intensivos, em que é possível assegurar dose apropriada e o monitoramento cuidadoso.

É mais provável que a dobutamina seja indicada aos pacientes com sinais agudos de insuficiência cardíaca complicada por hipotensão ou insuficiência primária da contratilidade do miocárdio (i. e., miocardiopatia dilatada). Também é útil como um fármaco de "resgate" no tratamento de pacientes com uma crise aguda que já estejam recebendo tratamento prolongado para insuficiência cardíaca congestiva de qualquer causa como, por exemplo, cães com doença da valva mitral e sinais de insuficiência cardíaca refratária à medicação oral.

Devido às restrições impostas ao uso de dobutamina pelo método de administração, é inevitável que seja administrada por curto período de tempo – no máximo alguns dias –, portanto, deve ser considerada como uma ponte na adoção de um protocolo de tratamento efetivo de longa duração.

Pimobendana

É um fármaco amplamente usado, com propriedades inotrópicas e vasodilatadoras decorrentes da inibição da fosfodiesterase e da sensibilização ao cálcio. Como esses efeitos são inseparáveis, é impossível determinar quais efeitos do pimobendana são decorrentes de qual mecanismo e, em termos mais amplos, provavelmente é mais útil referir-se ao fármaco como um "inodilatador". Devido aos efeitos supracitados, esses efeitos inodilatadores melhoram o débito cardíaco por meio da redução da resistência vascular sistêmica; ademais, melhora a contratilidade do miocárdio. Argumenta-se que esses efeitos combinados superam algumas das desvantagens dos agentes inotrópicos puros, possibilitando a melhora do débito cardíaco sem aumento substancial do trabalho miocárdico, devido à redução simultânea da pós-carga.

Esses efeitos hipotéticos do pimobendana são confirmados por uma enorme quantidade de resultados de ensaios clínicos prospectivos aleatórios, demonstrando melhores efeitos em cães com insuficiência cardíaca secundária tanto a doenças do miocárdio quanto das válvulas cardíacas.[32-34] Embora estritamente fora do âmbito de um capítulo sobre tratamento de insuficiência cardíaca, também há evidência mais recente sugestiva de benefício potencial do pimobendana por retardar o início dos sinais clínicos de insuficiência cardíaca em cães com miocardiopatia dilatada[35] e naqueles com doença degenerativa pré-clínica da valva mitral.[35a]

O pimobendana é indicado para administração de longa duração a todos os cães com insuficiência cardíaca secundária à doença degenerativa da valva mitral ou à miocardiopatia dilatada, as duas causas mais comuns de insuficiência cardíaca adquirida em cães. Embora a evidência de benefício de sua administração a pacientes caninos com insuficiência cardíaca secundária a outras causas seja menos evidente, esse medicamento pode ser indicado para a maioria dos pacientes caninos, a menos que o tratamento clínico não seja apropriado (p. ex., em cães com efusão pericárdica, causando tamponamento cardíaco) ou se sua administração for contraindicada (p. ex., em cães com obstrução do fluxo de sangue que sai do ventrículo).

Em geral, o pimobendana é administrado por via oral, mas na Europa há uma preparação de uso intravenoso para administração em condições emergenciais.

Os benefícios do pimobendana em gatos com insuficiência cardíaca parecem intuitivamente menos óbvios à luz dos tipos de doenças que levam mais comumente à insuficiência cardíaca nessa espécie. É mais difícil formular uma justificativa fisiopatológica para os benefícios de um inodilatador em pacientes com miocardiopatia hipertrófica, pois a doença primária não é uma daquelas que acreditamos estar associada ao comprometimento da contratilidade. Apesar disso, várias séries de casos[36,37] e um estudo de caso-controle[38] demonstraram que o pimobendana é tolerado, e provavelmente seguro, e pode estar associado a resultados melhores em gatos com insuficiência cardíaca, mesmo naqueles em que a doença primária é miocardiopatia hipertrófica. Portanto, pode-se considerar que o pimobendana é indicado para alguns gatos com insuficiência cardíaca. Em geral, é administrado aos gatos, juntamente com um IECA e um diurético. É indicado particularmente àqueles com sintomas de baixo débito cardíaco, simultâneos a sinais de congestão e àqueles já refratários à combinação mais convencional de diurético e IECA.

Fármacos que inibem a função inotrópica

Betabloqueadores

Alguns pacientes com cardiopatia podem ter sinais clínicos desencadeados por aumento da estimulação simpática, que aumenta a contratilidade e a frequência cardíacas. Acredita-se que esse seja particularmente o caso em gatos com miocardiopatia hipertrófica obstrutiva, em que o aumento da contratilidade pode estar associado ao agravamento da obstrução ao fluxo de saída de sangue; o aumento da frequência cardíaca pode prejudicar ainda mais o enchimento ventricular diastólico já comprometido. Portanto, argumentou-se que a administração de fármacos que reduzem a contratilidade e a frequência cardíacas pode ser benéfica a esses pacientes – em particular os fármacos que inibem o aumento da contratilidade associado à estimulação simpática. Por muitos anos, cardiologistas defenderam o uso de betabloqueadores, como o *atenolol*, no tratamento de gatos com miocardiopatia hipertrófica, em particular aqueles com evidência de obstrução dinâmica do fluxo de saída do sangue do ventrículo. Mais recentemente, estudos sugeriram possível efeito prejudicial dos betabloqueadores na recuperação de gatos com insuficiência cardíaca secundária à doença miocárdica[24] e um efeito neutro do atenolol no prognóstico de gatos com doença miocárdica pré-clínica.[39] Como resultado, atualmente o uso de betabloqueadores em gatos com doença do miocárdio não é mais indicado.

Foram realizados estudos para avaliar o efeito de betabloqueadores em cães com miocardiopatia dilatada[40] e doença da valva mitral.[41,42] A justificativa para esses estudos baseou-se na extrapolação de resultados clínicos favoráveis associados à administração de betabloqueadores a pacientes humanos com insuficiência cardíaca. Nenhum desses estudos demonstrou melhora evidente do quadro clínico de pacientes que receberam esses fármacos, nem melhora clínica relevante, como sobrevivência. Atualmente, há evidência insuficiente em defesa de sua administração a cães com cardiopatia pré-clínica e alguma evidência sugestiva de que sua administração a cães com evidência clínica evidente de insuficiência cardíaca é contraindicada.

A única indicação restante, sem controvérsia, para a administração de betabloqueadores a cães e gatos com insuficiência cardíaca deve-se a seus efeitos na frequência e no ritmo cardíacos em pacientes nos quais a arritmia esteja contribuindo para os sinais clínicos (ver Capítulo 248).

Aumento do enchimento cardíaco

Para manter um débito cardíaco normal, com pressão de enchimento intracardíaco normal, o coração precisa ser capaz de se encher normalmente entre as contrações. Para tanto, o relaxamento do miocárdio deve ser normal e o miocárdio ser complacente. O enchimento cardíaco pode ser prejudicado de diversas maneiras: o tempo de enchimento cardíaco pode ser inadequado se a frequência cardíaca for excessiva, o miocárdio pode estar muito rígido devido à fibrose ou hipertrofia e os mecanismos fisiológicos normais que reduzem a tensão da parede no início da diástole (principalmente os que acarretam redução da concentração intercelular de cálcio) podem estar prejudicados.

A terapia para insuficiência cardíaca pode influenciar direta ou indiretamente o enchimento cardíaco. Indiretamente, as intervenções que reduzem o tônus simpático e melhoram a oxigenação resultam em redução da frequência cardíaca e melhora da função diastólica. Fármacos que melhoram diretamente o relaxamento miocárdico são denominados agentes "lusitrópicos" (ver Figura 247.2 G). Parte da principal justificativa para a administração de diltiazem aos gatos com miocardiopatia hipertrófica baseou-se em um efeito lusitrópico positivo do fármaco. Foi mostrada apenas pouca evidência de benefício da administração de diltiazem aos gatos com miocardiopatia hipertrófica[43] e na literatura especializada não há evidência da superioridade do diltiazem comparativamente a outros métodos de tratamento, como o uso de IECA. Assim, atualmente o tratamento da miocardiopatia hipertrófica felina com diltiazem não é mais defendido por muitos clínicos.

Otimização da frequência e do ritmo cardíacos

Pacientes com insuficiência cardíaca geralmente têm anormalidades da frequência e do ritmo cardíacos. O débito cardíaco é o produto da frequência cardíaca e do volume sistólico. Bradiarritmias comprometem o débito cardíaco devido à redução da frequência cardíaca. Taquiarritmias comprometem o débito cardíaco devido a uma redução no volume sistólico, o qual está reduzido com frequências cardíacas altas por causa do tempo disponível reduzido para o enchimento cardíaco durante a diástole. Algumas taquiarritmias também causam perda da sincronia atrioventricular e/ou anormalidades da sequência de ativação do miocárdio ventricular; ambas podem comprometer ainda mais o volume sistólico.

Pacientes com sinais de insuficiência cardíaca atribuíveis diretamente à arritmia cardíaca, como aqueles com taquicardia supraventricular persistente rápida ou aqueles com bradiarritmias, como bloqueio atrioventricular de terceiro grau, têm uma melhora substancial com o controle da arritmia. Em pacientes cujos sintomas de insuficiência cardíaca são exacerbados por arritmia concomitante, embora possa não ser a causa primária dos sintomas, o tratamento apropriado de tal arritmia também deve ser um objetivo específico do tratamento geral, com outras tentativas de controlar os sinais de congestão e baixo débito (ver Capítulos 248 e 249).

É provável que o restabelecimento de uma frequência cardíaca mais próximo ao normal, seja redução, seja aumento da frequência de modo apropriado, melhore o débito cardíaco. Entretanto, não se deve esquecer que muitos pacientes com insuficiência cardíaca têm frequência cardíaca moderadamente elevada e taquicardia sinusal. Nesses pacientes, pode ser apropriado, durante um episódio agudo de insuficiência cardíaca, ter uma frequência cardíaca acima da esperada em um cão normal. A redução da frequência cardíaca nesses pacientes deve ser alcançada por meio de um controle melhor dos sinais de insuficiência cardíaca, e não pela administração direta de agentes cronotrópicos negativos (redutores da frequência cardíaca), como os betabloqueadores. Também é provável que o restabelecimento da ativação atrial e ventricular sincrônica, após a cessação de arritmia ventricular, melhore o débito quando tal arritmia estiver presente.

MONITORAMENTO E AJUSTE DA TERAPIA PARA INSUFICIÊNCIA CARDÍACA

Os dois propósitos principais do monitoramento de pacientes submetidos ao tratamento de insuficiência cardíaca são: estabelecer se as metas iniciais do tratamento foram alcançadas e se surgiram reações adversas à administração do tratamento (Figura 247.4).

As complicações do tratamento com diurético – especificamente, sua detecção e seu controle – foram discutidas na seção sobre diuréticos.

O sucesso da terapia é indicado pela resolução dos sinais clínicos e/ou achados diagnósticos que necessitaram da instituição do tratamento. Se um paciente precisou de tratamento devido à presença de efusão pleural que acarreta dispneia, então o tratamento bem-sucedido seria indicado pela resolução da efusão pleural e restabelecimento de frequência e esforço respiratórios mais próximo aos normais. De maneira similar, se a principal indicação para o tratamento foi dispneia, confirmada em radiografia como secundária a edema pulmonar, o tratamento bem-sucedido seria indicado pelo restabelecimento da frequência e do esforço respiratórios normais, juntamente com a resolução radiográfica do edema pulmonar.

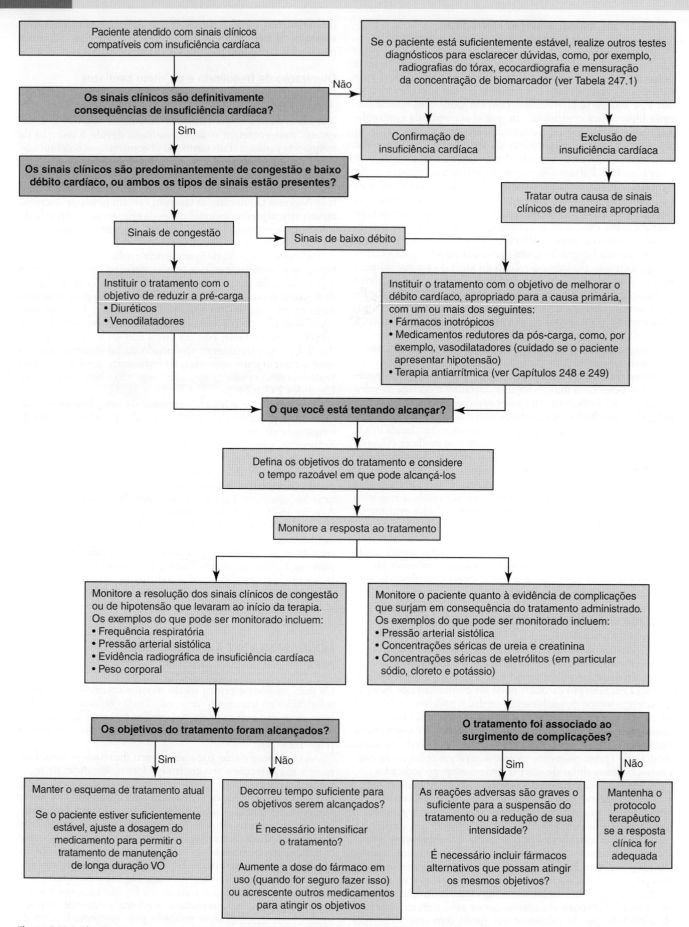

Figura 247.4 Algoritmo que indica algumas das principais etapas do tratamento de pacientes com insuficiência cardíaca. Os quadros em destaque e o texto em negrito indicam questões importantes que um clínico deve esclarecer para fazer escolhas mais apropriadas de tratamento e monitoramento.

Em um paciente hospitalizado para o tratamento inicial de insuficiência cardíaca congestiva, o ideal é que a eficácia terapêutica resulte em melhora da frequência e do esforço respiratórios nas primeiras horas após o início do tratamento. Em geral, a resolução do edema pulmonar detectável em radiografia demora mais que a observada nos sinais clínicos, podendo ser mais demorada, às vezes 24 a 48 horas. Se os indícios clínicos de insuficiência cardíaca congestiva, como a frequência respiratória, não melhoram, não é o bastante para a solicitação de nova radiografia do paciente, a menos que haja dúvida sobre o diagnóstico inicial de edema pulmonar cardiogênico e estejam sendo procuradas explicações alternativas para os sintomas manifestados pelo paciente. Portanto, em geral, o propósito de repetir radiografias é confirmar e documentar melhora nos sinais de insuficiência cardíaca em um paciente que já esteja mostrando evidência de melhora.

Em pacientes com sinais clínicos de má perfusão, é provável que a resolução daqueles sinais indique o sucesso do tratamento. Se um paciente chega para consulta com hipotensão, então a melhora na pressão sanguínea é um indício de resposta favorável ao tratamento. Extremidades com temperatura normal em um paciente é evidência de melhora na perfusão. Em pacientes com cardiopatia e que chegam à consulta com azotemia pré-renal, a melhora da perfusão pode resultar em melhora da azotemia.

Monitoramento da frequência respiratória em repouso

Um dos meios mais efetivos de monitoramento prolongado do sucesso na resolução de sinais clínicos de insuficiência cardíaca congestiva parece ser a estimativa da frequência respiratória em repouso, obtida pelo proprietário do animal no domicílio. Um estudo mostrou que, em cães submetidos ao tratamento para insuficiência cardíaca, uma frequência respiratória em repouso < 40 movimentos respiratórios por minuto foi altamente preditiva de que a insuficiência cardíaca do paciente está sob controle adequado.[44] Valores similares também são válidos para orientar a adequação do controle da insuficiência cardíaca em gatos. Um estudo mostrou que gatos normais e aqueles com cardiopatia subclínica raramente têm frequência respiratória superior a 30 movimentos respiratórios por minuto.[45]

A maioria dos proprietários consegue mensurar a frequência respiratória de seus animais de estimação, há uma variedade de aplicativos disponíveis para aparelhos telefônicos celulares que facilitam isso. É possível fornecer aos proprietários, ou eles mesmos podem estabelecer, parâmetros de frequência respiratória que representem um bom controle da insuficiência cardíaca, bem como valores que seriam motivo de preocupação. Após um período de monitoramento, os proprietários podem ter uma boa ideia da variação normal da frequência respiratória de seu animal. Eles podem, então, alertar o veterinário se a frequência respiratória de seu animal aumentar. Alguns proprietários podem até receber instruções sobre como ajustar a dosagem de diurético que seu animal recebe de acordo com a frequência respiratória; tal abordagem é particularmente útil no caso de pacientes instáveis que precisam de ajustes frequentes na terapia da insuficiência cardíaca, ou pacientes felinos que fiquem muito estressados quando vão a um hospital veterinário.

Ajuste da terapia domiciliar de longa duração

É possível aumentar ou diminuir a intensidade do tratamento de insuficiência cardíaca de um paciente. Em geral, um controle precário dos sinais de insuficiência cardíaca indica a necessidade de intensificar o tratamento. Embora a maioria dos pacientes responda bem à terapia para insuficiência cardíaca, em quase todos os casos os sinais clínicos de insuficiência cardíaca voltam a surgir após um período variável. No estudo QUEST, do American College of Veterinary Internal Medicine (ACVIM), que monitorou uma população de cães com doença degenerativa da valva mitral em estágio C, foi comum a necessidade de ajuste da terapia para insuficiência cardíaca e na maioria dos cães em que foi feito o ajuste nos três primeiros meses do tratamento foi preciso modificá-lo.[46]

A natureza da alteração necessária no tratamento costuma ser indicada pelo tipo de sinais clínicos do paciente naquele momento. O ajuste feito com maior frequência é a intensificação do tratamento diurético, devido ao ressurgimento de sinais de congestão (p. ex., taquipneia ou dispneia). Nos casos em que isso acontece, as dosagens de furosemida podem ser aumentadas até que os sinais clínicos do paciente sejam refratários ao tratamento, mesmo com dose de até 4 mg/kg/8 horas por via oral. Conforme discutido anteriormente, em geral isso requer a administração de vários diuréticos ou a substituição da furosemida por torsemida.

Ocasionalmente, após um longo período de estabilidade clínica, é possível reduzir a dose do diurético de um paciente. Isso pode ser feito mediante uma redução gradativa na dose administrada. Sempre que se modifica a dosagem de diurético ou a frequência de sua administração, deve-se monitorar o paciente para verificar se ocorre alteração na frequência respiratória. Se ela permanece estável, mesmo com a redução da dose de diurético, então pode-se tentar nova redução até se obter a menor dose efetiva no controle adequado dos sinais clínicos.

Se um paciente novamente apresenta sinais clínicos de baixo débito cardíaco, então pode ser necessário intensificar a terapia visando à melhora do débito cardíaco. Dependendo da natureza da doença primária do paciente, isso pode exigir modificação da dosagem de fármacos que já estão sendo administrados (como a otimização da dose de pimobendana) ou melhorar o controle da arritmia do paciente.

RESULTADO DO TRATAMENTO DA INSUFICIÊNCIA CARDÍACA

A maioria dos pacientes caninos e felinos pode ter muitos meses, em alguns casos mais de 1 ano, de boa qualidade de vida como resultado do sucesso do tratamento farmacológico de seu quadro clínico. Infelizmente, o desfecho mais comum para um paciente após o desenvolvimento de sinais de insuficiência cardíaca é a morte decorrente da cardiopatia, apesar do tratamento. Estudos realizados em cães[32,47] e gatos[48] com cardiopatia e insuficiência cardíaca mostraram que a maioria dos pacientes com insuficiência cardíaca morre no decorrer de 1 ano após o diagnóstico. No caso de cães com miocardiopatia dilatada, o tempo médio de sobrevida é inferior a 6 meses.[47]

Um objetivo realista e louvável da terapia é o alívio dos sinais clínicos do paciente, bem como prolongar sua vida, desde que ela tenha uma boa qualidade. Também deve ser responsabilidade do veterinário alertar o proprietário do paciente sobre a possibilidade da morte do animal e do tempo realista em que isso provavelmente vai ocorrer. Embora no início possa ser difícil e estressante para os proprietários ouvirem esse prognóstico, muitos sentem-se mais bem preparados para a morte de seu animal quando ela ocorrer.

Por fim, apesar da instituição do melhor tratamento, os pacientes sucumbem à cardiopatia. Priorizar o bem-estar do paciente durante o fim de sua vida também é muito importante nessa fase da doença.

REFERÊNCIAS BIBLIOGRÁFICAS

As referências bibliográficas deste capítulo se encontram online no Ambiente de Aprendizagem.

CAPÍTULO 248

Arritmias Cardíacas

Etienne Côté e Stephen J. Ettinger

Bem depois de sua invenção há mais de cem anos, o eletrocardiograma (ECG) continua sendo o exame diagnóstico de escolha para a avaliação clínica de pacientes com arritmia cardíaca.[1-5] Ele também é muito útil no monitoramento de pacientes com anormalidades sistêmicas, incluindo distúrbios eletrolíticos e hipoxemia. Além disso, anormalidades nas dimensões de vários componentes do ECG podem servir como um guia aproximado para a avaliação de cardiopatia estrutural. No entanto, esses critérios morfológicos do ECG raramente se baseiam em estudos controlados que indicam a especificidade e a sensibilidade; ademais, não foram estabelecidos parâmetros abrangentes do ECG para cães e gatos de acordo com a raça, a constituição corporal, a idade e o sexo. Um coração anormal pode ter um ECG normal e vice-versa. Portanto, o ECG, como acontece com o hemograma, nem sempre é um indicador absoluto de normalidade ou doença, sendo essencial a definição de padrões de traçados seriados ou informação clínica adicional para entender o verdadeiro significado do ECG na maioria dos pacientes. Os aspectos técnicos da eletrocardiografia e os intervalos de referência foram apresentados no Capítulo 103.

SISTEMA DE CONDUÇÃO CARDÍACA E ELETROCARDIOGRAFIA

Cada componente do traçado do ECG reflete um evento elétrico que está ocorrendo em uma parte específica do coração.[1,2,5] A sequência de eventos elétricos segue vias anatômicas específicas no coração e, na saúde, faz isso de maneira precisa e consistente, o que foi sujeito a revisão recente e perspicaz.[6]

O início do batimento cardíaco normal ocorre no nodo sinoatrial (SA), que está localizado nos tecidos subepicárdicos da crista terminal do átrio direito (AD) dorsolateral, na junção da veia cava cranial com o átrio direito e diretamente adjacente à crista terminal,[7,8] sendo perfundido pela artéria do nodo SA, um ramo da artéria coronária direita,[9] tendo extensa circulação colateral. No cão, o batimento cardíaco se origina na região mediana ou cranial do nodo,[10] exceto quando há alto tônus parassimpático, condição na qual as partes mais ventrais do nodo e os tecidos extranodais adjacentes são os locais de origem do batimento.[11] Essa alteração no local de formação do impulso explica a variação na morfologia da onda P às vezes observada no ECG de cães (e raramente de gatos) durante alterações no tônus autônomo, denominado *marca-passo errante*.

Por que o coração continua a bater? Nas células do marca-passo do nodo SA, o início do batimento cardíaco envolve vários desvios iônicos, em especial a corrente interna transportadora, predominantemente, de sódio (mas também de potássio), I_f.[6,12-14] Essa "corrente estranha" é assim denominada por causa de suas características incomuns de ser ativada por hiperpolarização, em vez de despolarização (o canal de entrada do nucleotídio cíclico, HCN4, ativado por hiperpolarização, é o que dá origem a I_f). Essa ativação inicia o processo de despolarização espontânea; uma redução nas correntes repolarizantes de potássio, I_{Kr} e I_{Ks}, dependente do tempo, o efeito da troca transmembrana de cálcio citosólico derivado do retículo sarcoplasmático por sódio extracelular e a liberação do cálcio local (citosólico)[12] também são importantes na elevação do potencial da membrana da célula nodal de SA para um valor menos negativo entre os batimentos cardíacos. Esse processo de despolarização diastólica espontânea, ou fase 4, é uma característica marcante de uma célula de marca-passo normal. O aumento resultante no potencial de membrana celular supera o limiar, ponto em que uma combinação de correntes transitórias (I_{Ca-T}, tipo T) e de longa duração (I_{Ca-L}, tipo L) de entrada de cálcio causa despolarização da célula. A despolarização termina quando as correntes repolarizantes de potássio, incluindo as correntes transitória de saída, retificadora tardia rápida e retificadora tardia lenta (I_{to}, I_{K-r} e I_{K-s}, respectivamente), são ativadas, extraindo íons potássio da célula. Em termos gerais, toda essa panóplia de correntes despolarizantes e repolarizantes, que são os eventos-chave da iniciação do batimento cardíaco, foi agrupada recentemente, juntas, com o "cronômetro" da membrana do nodo SA e o paradigma do "cronômetro" do cálcio (Figura 248.1).[6,12]

O impulso assim formado se propaga do nodo SA através de ambos os átrios, originando a onda P no ECG (Figura 248.2). Em termos específicos, parte do impulso que se propaga a partir do nodo SA segue ao longo de três conjuntos de fibras especializadas nos átrios, denominadas *vias ou tratos internodais*, que consistem no par de vias ventrais (anteriores), que leva atividade elétrica diretamente ao nodo atrioventricular (AV), e na via dorsal (posterior), denominada feixe de Bachmann, responsável pela ativação do átrio esquerdo.[15,16] Todas as três convergem ao nodo AV, no assoalho do AD.[7,17] Portanto, o movimento de saída de atividade elétrica do nodo SA desencadeia a contração muscular dos átrios e leva uma sequência de atividade elétrica transmitida aos ventrículos.

No nodo AV, o impulso que despolariza o coração é retardado propositalmente, devido à baixa quantidade de junções em hiato entre as células, o que torna lenta a condução intercelular.[9] Esse retardo é um processo normal e, na verdade, a falha do impulso em fazer uma pausa no nodo AV é uma anormalidade denominada pré-excitação (ver Síndromes de Macrorreentradas, adiante). O propósito desse retardo é otimizar o enchimento ventricular, possibilitando que os átrios finalizem sua contração. O período de quiescência elétrica negativa durante o qual o impulso passa lentamente através do nodo AV se reflete no ECG como um segmento plano entre a onda P e o complexo QRS, o segmento PR; em termos de nomenclatura, o *intervalo* PR consiste no segmento PR mais a onda P (ver adiante). Além de transmitir impulsos dos átrios para os ventrículos, o nodo AV sadio atua como um moderador, impedindo a passagem de impulsos atriais indesejáveis e a atividade dos ventrículos, como acontece quando esses impulsos são prematuros ou excessivos (p. ex., na fibrilação atrial [FibA]). Tal característica depende do período refratário das células do nodo AV e varia entre os indivíduos, e no mesmo indivíduo, dependendo de estímulos autonômicos. Em indivíduos normais, as fibras de condução unidirecional do complexo nodo AV-feixe de His fazem a única conexão elétrica entre os átrios e ventrículos.

Às vezes, considera-se que o nodo AV tem três componentes: as regiões atrionodal (AN), nodal (N) e nodal-feixe de His (NH) em sentido proximal (mais distante dos ventrículos) para distal (mais próximo aos ventrículos), respectivamente.[18] Essa divisão se baseia na demonstração experimental de diferenças no potencial de ação das três regiões e tem significado clínico limitado.

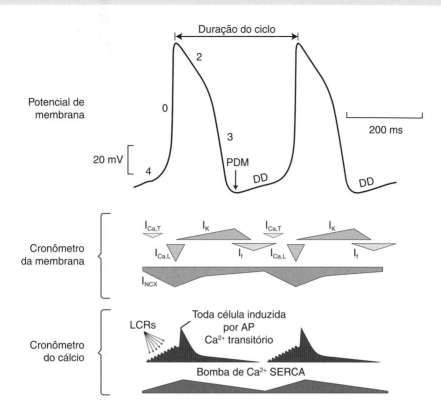

Figura 248.1 Componentes dos "cronômetros" da membrana e do cálcio, responsáveis pela despolarização do nodo sinoatrial. *DD*, despolarização diastólica; I_{Ca-L}, corrente de Ca^{2+} do tipo L dependente da voltagem; I_{Ca-T}, corrente de Ca^{2+} do tipo T dependente da voltagem; I_f, corrente "estranha"; I_K, corrente de potássio retificadora tardia; I_{NCX}, corrente de troca de sódio por cálcio; *LCR*, liberação local de Ca^{2+}; *PDM*, potencial diastólico máximo; *SERCA*, ATPase do retículo sarcoendoplasmático. (Reproduzida, com autorização, de Monfredi O, Maltsev VA e Lakatta EG. Modern concepts concerning the origin of the heartbeat. *Physiology [Bethesda]* 28:74-92, 2013.)

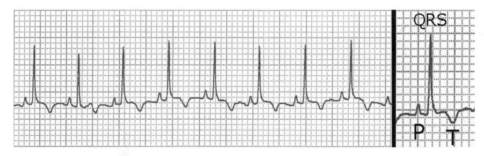

Figura 248.2 Ritmo sinusal normal do gato. Há uma onda P para cada complexo QRS, em intervalo PR fixo, e a morfologia da onda P e do complexo QRS não se altera. As ondas R são ligeiramente mais altas que o normal, aspecto compatível com hipertrofia de ventrículo esquerdo, nesse gato com miocardiopatia hipertrófica (onda R alta; 1 mV; faixa de referência para gatos: < 0,9 mV). A frequência cardíaca é de 155 bpm. Derivação II, 25 mm/s, 1 cm = 1 mV.

Importante é a automaticidade da região N, uma capacidade para formar impulsos espontaneamente muito parecida com a maneira que o nodo SA normalmente faz, porém em uma frequência menor. Assim, em geral o nodo AV é superado (e tem sua capacidade de marca-passo suprimida) durante o ritmo sinusal normal por impulsos sinusais normais, que passam através das células do marca-passo latentes no nodo AV – e as reajustam – antes que ocorra despolarização. Esse mecanismo normal impede a competição entre o nodo AV e o nodo SA como o marca-passo natural do coração. A região N do nodo AV ainda pode atuar como marca-passo do coração se os impulsos sinusais não chegam até ela – um mecanismo à prova de falhas que só é ativado quando há necessidade; é denominado *mecanismo de escape*, ou *ritmo de escape*. Em termos específicos, um ritmo de escape originário da região N é denominado *ritmo de escape juncional*, ressaltando que se origina da junção AV e não do sistema His-Purkinje nos ventrículos. Como a região N situa-se no centro do nodo AV, pode-se notar que o bloqueio AV (como o causado por fibrose do nodo AV) que afeta a região proximal (AN) possibilita o surgimento de um ritmo de escape juncional, enquanto no bloqueio AV, que ocorre na região N ou NH, há perda da possibilidade de tal ritmo e, geralmente, em vez disso ocorre ativação de um mecanismo de escape His-Purkinje/ventricular mais lento.

Tendo cruzado o nodo AV, o impulso elétrico de um batimento cardíaco normal segue rápida e uniformemente através dos ventrículos, via sistema His-Purkinje.[9,16] Essa rede de fibras condutoras assegura que o impulso seja levado rapidamente e distribuído de maneira uniforme, de modo que os ventrículos despolarizam e, então, se contraem de modo sincronizado.[19] As fibras surgem como um fio grosso, o feixe de His, que recebe a transmissão do nodo AV, alcança, através do coxim endocárdico, os ventrículos. O feixe de His logo se divide em ramos direito e esquerdo (RDF e REF), dirigidos para os seus respectivos ventrículos; o ramo esquerdo, por sua vez, divide-se em anterior esquerdo, posterior esquerdo e fascículos septais com forma e padrão de arborização altamente variáveis.[16] A relevância clínica dessa divisão em feixes tem relação com interrupções da condução elétrica através dos feixes, que podem ocorrer em várias condições patológicas e, ocasionalmente, em animais normais (ver Bloqueio de Ramos do Feixe de His, adiante). Em termos gerais, a despolarização dos ventrículos é aparente no ECG como o complexo QRS. Quando os ventrículos acabam de se despolarizar por completo, uma sequência de repolarização faz com que as células miocárdicas retornem ao seu estado de repouso. A sequência de repolarização, que acompanha a esteira da sequência de despolarização, é vista como a onda T no ECG.

A repolarização dos ventrículos ocorre de maneira transmural: miócitos do epicárdio se repolarizam primeiro, criando a parte ascendente da onda T. A amplitude da onda T é limitada pelo início da repolarização dos miócitos do endocárdio que, então, contribui para a parte descendente da onda T. A repolarização se completa quando a última população de miócitos ventriculares mesomurais, denominados células M ("mesomiocárdicas"), é repolarizada.[20] Alterações nesse mecanismo complexo podem ser patológicas, ocasionando alterações como onda "J" ou onda O, de Osborn, em pacientes com hipotermia, ou variantes normais, como a onda T de cães sadios, que pode ser positiva ou negativa. Deve-se ressaltar que os átrios também se repolarizam, mas a quantidade de atividade elétrica envolvida nesse processo, em geral, é direcionada a uma orientação que registra uma deflexão trivial, se houver alguma; na maioria das derivações do ECG, caso a deflexão ocorra, pode ser rotineiramente mascarada pelo complexo QRS subsequente.[21,22] Alterações graves na repolarização atrial podem ser observadas ocasionalmente como uma onda T atrial, ou onda T$_a$, e essas deflexões muito pequenas podem ser mais aparentes na presença de bloqueio AV, quando a pós-onda P do ECG não sofre restrições de um complexo QRS consequente.[21,22]

A frequência cardíaca é constantemente influenciada por estímulos autonômicos. Um cão de porte médio sem controle autonômico do batimento cardíaco tem uma frequência cardíaca intrínseca de 142 bpm, conforme demonstrado pelo antagonismo parassimpático e simpático simultâneo, em vez de uma frequência cardíaca em repouso normal de, aproximadamente, 100 bpm.[23] Estudos Holter confirmam a grande variabilidade a cada momento de estímulos autonômicos ao coração: em um ciclo de 24 horas, a frequência cardíaca varia de 55 a 243 bpm, em cães da raça Beagle[24] sadios, e de 77 a 282 em gatos sadios.[25,26]

Manipulações diagnósticas com eletrocardiografia

Manobra vagal

O aumento artificial do tônus vagal de um paciente tem valor diagnóstico e terapêutico potencial. Em termos diagnósticos, a redução da frequência cardíaca e o aumento da refratariedade do nodo AV mediante a realização de manobras vagais podem reduzir uma taquicardia marcante, possibilitando que algumas de suas características sejam mais aparentes, o que facilita o diagnóstico com base no ECG (Figura 248.3). Em termos terapêuticos, o aumento do tônus vagal, que interrompe circuitos de macrorreentrada, às vezes pode pôr fim em arritmias como a taquicardia de nodo AV reentrante e a taquicardia AV ortodrômica recíproca (ver Síndromes de Pré-excitação/Macrorreentrantes, adiante).

A massagem do seio carotídeo é um tipo de manobra vagal e envolve a simples aplicação de pressão digital leve, mantida pelo clínico, sobre um ou ambos os seios carotídeos do paciente, localizados imediatamente caudais ao aspecto dorsal da laringe (às vezes o ponto onde se provoca o reflexo do engasgo), por 5 a 10 segundos, enquanto o traçado do ECG é registrado. O paciente deve tolerar tal manobra; sinais de desconforto, aflição ou uma alteração acentuada na frequência cardíaca exigem a cessação imediata da manobra. Como cães e gatos muito raramente apresentam aterosclerose na artéria carótida, é improvável que a preocupação com consequências tromboembólicas da massagem do seio carotídeo, mencionadas na cardiologia humana, seja relevante na prática com pequenos animais. A pressão ocular, sobre as pálpebras fechadas, é outra forma de manobra vagal, que consiste na aplicação de pressão digital firme, porém leve e controlada, em ambos os globos oculares, com as pálpebras fechadas. A distância de retropulsão dos globos depende do formato da órbita e, subjetivamente, a força da pressão aplicada é a melhor referência, não devendo exceder a pressão digital que se faria em uma uva madura sem rompê-la. A pressão ocular é contraindicada em pacientes com problemas oculares. Parece haver variação interindividual na resposta às manobras vagais; alguns indivíduos manifestam um efeito mais marcante durante a massagem do seio carotídeo e outros à pressão ocular. Outro método simples de provocar uma resposta vagal sem infligir pressão sobre uma parte do corpo consiste em imergir a face do paciente ou a parte distal de um membro em um recipiente contendo água gelada, por um curto período.[27] Em cães ou gatos despertos, em geral, isso ocasiona, rapidamente, diminuição da frequência cardíaca sinusal mediada pelo nervo vago.

Teste de resposta à atropina

Pode-se administrar 0,04 mg de sulfato de atropina/kg IV como recurso diagnóstico para avaliar bradicardia.[3] Isso permite diferenciar bradicardias fisiológicas que são puramente de origem vagal (a atropina aumenta a frequência cardíaca) de bradicardias patológicas causadas por distúrbios intrínsecos da formação ou da condução do impulso (a atropina não tem efeito). A resposta ocorre dentro de segundos a minutos (até 15 minutos) após a injeção.[3] Uma resposta positiva à atropina não é um bom previsor de efeito benéfico de fármacos vagolíticos orais, como a hiosciamina ou a propantelina, em cães com bloqueio AV,[28] mas está associada a um efeito benéfico do tratamento clínico de disfunção do nodo sinusal (síndrome do nodo sinusal doente, SNSD).[28a]

ANORMALIDADES DO RITMO CARDÍACO

Os termos "disritmia" e "arritmia" são usados como sinônimos, embora seja preferível "arritmia".[29] Para avaliação e tratamento de pacientes com arritmias cardíacas, um esquema de classificação útil e prático é o que inclui as arritmias em três grupos: (1) anormalidades na formação do impulso (excitabilidade cardíaca), (2) anormalidades na transmissão do impulso (condução cardíaca) e (3) anormalidades complexas que envolvem tanto excitação quanto

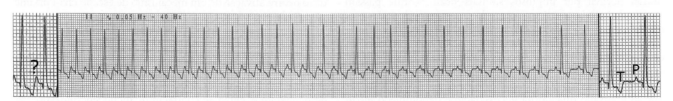

Figura 248.3 Manobra vagal em um cão adulto da raça Cairn Terrier. Inicialmente, nota-se uma taquicardia monomórfica. Não é possível identificar de maneira definitiva a deflexão entre dois complexos QRS como uma onda bifásica, ondas T e P sobrepostas ou ondas T e de *flutter* (*detalhe à esquerda*, "*?*"). A massagem do seio carotídeo começou 5 segundos antes; no fim do traçado, ondas P e T estão nitidamente separadas (*detalhe à direita*), possibilitando o diagnóstico de taquicardia sinusal. Derivação II, 25 mm/s, 1 cm/mV.

condução do estímulo. Alguns distúrbios do ritmo se enquadram mal em qualquer categoria. Algumas anormalidades da excitabilidade cardíaca são secundárias a anormalidades da condução (p. ex., ritmos de escape juncionais ou ventriculares). As anormalidades são apresentadas neste capítulo de acordo com o seu local anatômico de origem (i. e., atrial, juncional ou ventricular).

As anormalidades da excitação podem causar funcionamento excessivo ou inadequado do coração ou de suas partes. O aumento da excitabilidade acarreta extrassístoles, se for intermitente, e taquicardia, se mantido. Ectopia é o termo que descreve a produção espontânea de impulsos em qualquer local do coração, exceto o nodo SA. A diminuição da excitabilidade substitui a formação do impulso com quiescência elétrica, resultando em bradicardia ou assistolia.

As anormalidades da condução dentro do coração denominam-se *bloqueios*. Sua classificação depende da localização anatômica do bloqueio e de sua extensão ou magnitude (ver adiante). Pode ocorrer bloqueio no nodo SA (raramente detectado), no nodo AV ou em ramos do feixe de His (bloqueio de ramo do feixe de His, BRF).

Por fim, os distúrbios que combinam anormalidades da excitabilidade e da condução também têm relevância clínica. É comum notar influências das concentrações séricas de eletrólitos no ritmo cardíaco, que podem ocasionar anormalidades de excitação, condução ou ambas. Na pré-excitação e nas síndromes de macrorreentrada, vias acessórias de condução desviam parte da via de condução AV normal. A disfunção do nodo sinusal, também conhecida como *síndrome do seio doente* (SSD), em geral consiste em períodos de bradicardia e taquicardia causados por disfunção do nodo SA e de tecidos de condução supraventriculares e ventriculares.

Impacto clínico das anormalidades no ritmo cardíaco

As anormalidades do ritmo cardíaco mencionadas têm importância clínica variável. Seu impacto clínico varia de incômodo (algumas são variações benignas do ritmo normal) a gravemente prejudicial (potencialmente fatal). Em gatos, as extrassístoles ventriculares, a pré-dissociação e a dissociação AV isorrítmica foram associadas à miocardiopatia. Em cães, anormalidades da excitabilidade, em especial extrassístoles e FibA, são mais comuns que aquelas da condução, sendo a maioria destas últimas bloqueios AV.[1,2,30]

O impacto da arritmia cardíaca no paciente – as consequências hemodinâmicas – depende, no mínimo, de oito fatores: (1) frequência ventricular, (2) duração do ritmo anormal, (3) relação temporal entre os átrios e os ventrículos, (4) sequência de ativação ventricular, (5) função inerente do miocárdio e das valvas, (6) irregularidade da duração do ciclo, (7) terapia medicamentosa e (8) influências extracardíacas.[1-3] Por fim, a soma desses fatores – não o que aparece no ECG – determina o impacto da arritmia no paciente. Por exemplo, é essa a razão pela qual alguns animais com taquicardia ventricular (TV) parecem francamente normais, enquanto outros estão moribundos.

Identificação de anormalidades do ritmo cardíaco

Atualmente, a maior parte da eletrocardiografia clínica em medicina veterinária baseia-se em ECG de derivação única, realizado em pacientes hospitalizados. ECG com múltiplas derivações fornece um nível adicional de informações que, às vezes, é indispensável (ver Figura 248.13, mais adiante).

As anormalidades do ritmo cardíaco são identificadas no ECG, realizando-se um exame metódico de cinco pontos. Primeiro, uma avaliação rápida da esquerda para a direita em todo o traçado do ECG dá uma ideia geral da frequência e do ritmo cardíacos, proporcionando, assim, uma orientação diagnóstica. Essa etapa revela se há um único ritmo ou vários (Todos são complexos QRS com a mesma morfologia? Os intervalos R-R, ou *intervalos de acoplamento*, são os mesmos ou há variação? No último caso, a variação ocorre de maneira previsível?). A avaliação breve da frequência cardíaca (lenta, normal ou rápida) e se o ritmo é regular ou irregular (intervalos R-R iguais ou variáveis, respectivamente) leva à detecção de complexos prematuros ou tardios.

Em segundo lugar, os intervalos R-R são avaliados em partes representativas de todo o traçado do ECG. No contexto clínico, em gatos, a variabilidade no intervalo R-R normalmente não é vista, sendo considerada patológica.[31] Em cães, é normal haver uma variação cíclica (i. e., rítmica, padronizada, "regularmente irregular") do intervalo R-R, arritmia sinusal respiratória (Figura 248.4). Intervalos R-R sem padrão, "irregularmente irregulares" são sempre anormais, em ambas as espécies.

Terceiro, o exame de complexos QRS individuais consiste em determinar se são de base estreita ou larga. Em geral, QRS de base estreita indica despolarização ventricular normal (i. e., de origem supraventricular) (ver Figuras 248.2 a 248.4), enquanto QRS de base larga indica despolarização assincrônica dos ventrículos direito e esquerdo, que pode ser devido à origem ventricular da despolarização, ao BRF ou à pré-excitação/macrorreentrada (ver adiante). Como a repolarização ocorre imediatamente após a despolarização, um complexo QRS de forma anormal também deve ter uma onda T de formato anormal ou diferente. Se a onda T for normal, deve-se considerar a possibilidade de artefato, em vez de QRS verdadeiramente anormal, como a explicação para uma deflexão larga, bizarra.

Em quarto lugar, o exame das ondas P (presentes, ausentes; positivas, negativas) informa sobre a despolarização dos átrios. O exame do intervalo P-R: (1) determina se há uma onda P para cada complexo QRS e um QRS para cada onda P (para avaliar a sincronia AV); e (2) avalia a condução no nodo AV, confirmada por uma duração constante do intervalo P-R.

Por fim, são identificados o ritmo cardíaco básico primário e quaisquer ritmos adicionais ou secundários que se sobreponham. Normalmente, há uma onda P para cada complexo QRS (uma despolarização atrial para cada despolarização ventricular). As anormalidades que causam mais de uma onda P para cada complexo QRS incluem bloqueios AV de segundo e terceiro graus; as anormalidades que produzem complexos QRS sem ondas P incluem arritmias ventriculares, FibA e parada atrial.

Anormalidades da excitabilidade

Uma subdivisão importante envolve a classificação ampla de anormalidades da excitabilidade como sendo distúrbios da excitabilidade supraventricular,[32,33] incluindo TS, complexos atriais prematuros (CAP), taquicardias ventriculares, *flutter* atrial e FibA; ou como distúrbios da excitabilidade ventricular, que incluem extrassístoles ventriculares (CVP, CPV), TV, *torsade de pointes* (TdP),

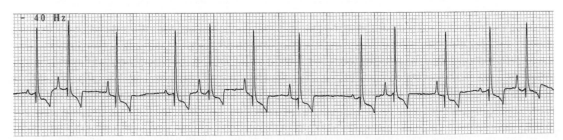

Figura 248.4 Arritmia sinusal respiratória e marca-passo errante em um cão. Derivação II, 25 mm/s, 1 cm = 1 mV.

flutter ventricular e FV. A classificação apropriada tem importância clínica: os fatores desencadeantes de arritmias nesses dois subgrupos, em geral, são específicos do subgrupo, e o tratamento antiarrítmico de ambos também costuma ser diferente.

Anormalidades e alterações da excitabilidade sinusal

Tais arritmias são variações do ritmo sinusal, estando associadas mais comumente a estímulos autonômicos normais ou excessivos.

Arritmia sinusal respiratória (normal). Mesmo no contexto hospitalar, o equilíbrio entre os estímulos simpáticos e os parassimpáticos ao coração, em geral, oscila a favor do sistema parassimpático na maioria dos cães em repouso.[23] Na clínica veterinária, essa característica contrasta com a média no gato. A predominância vagal no cão ocasiona duas características particulares do ritmo sinusal no ECG desses animais: arritmia sinusal respiratória (ASR) e marca-passo errante (MPE).

A ASR resulta de efeitos vagais e hemodinâmicos que ocorrem dentro do tórax durante cada ciclo respiratório (ver Figura 248.4). Em cães, é um mecanismo fisiológico normal que não requer tratamento. O resultado é uma correlação entre a frequência cardíaca e a respiratória, com lentidão da primeira durante a expiração e aumento do número de batimentos cardíacos durante a inspiração. A natureza cíclica repetitiva dessa arritmia é sua característica marcante. A ASR é notada pela primeira vez no filhote de cão, após 4 semanas de idade;[1] em geral, desaparece quando a frequência cardíaca excede 150 bpm, em qualquer idade (porque o tônus simpático supera o parassimpático na maioria das situações que acarretam essa frequência cardíaca rápida)[1,2] e pode ser exacerbada quando há dispneia grave (pneumotórax, fibrose pulmonar, enfisema, obstrução de via respiratória superior) devido a alterações marcantes na pressão intratorácica.[1] Em gatos, comumente ocorre arritmia sinusal respiratória durante o sono[34] e no ambiente doméstico em geral,[25] mas é provável que o estímulo adrenérgico causado pelo ambiente clínico explique sua raridade no contexto hospitalar. Em cães, a presença de ASR pode ser um indicador diagnóstico útil na rotina clínica, como na tosse em um cão adulto de raça de pequeno a médio porte. É comum que esses cães apresentem cardiopatia decorrente de doença de valva mitral mixomatosa/degenerativa (DVMD; durante a auscultação constata-se um sopro típico) e doença respiratória primária, como bronquite crônica asséptica. Pode ser difícil definir se a insuficiência cardíaca congestiva (ICC) ou um problema respiratório é o responsável pelos sintomas respiratórios do animal, daí a necessidade de tratamento imediato e prolongado; ademais, o prognóstico depende de saber qual doença predomina. A presença de ASR torna a DVMD descompensada a única causa improvável dos sintomas respiratórios porque o edema pulmonar cardiogênico da ICC quase que invariavelmente está associado ao aumento do tônus simpático e perda da ASR.

O tratamento efetivo da ICC pode levar ao reaparecimento de ASR em um paciente previamente com taquicardia sinusal ou outra taquicardia supraventricular, em particular se o tratamento incluir digoxina. O retorno da ASR deve-se à redução do tônus simpático associada à resolução da ICC; um benefício adicional do uso de digitálicos, ainda que teórico na clínica veterinária, é a reativação de barorreceptores, que de outra forma permanecem sob infrarregulação ("exaustos") pelo estímulo simpático que acompanha a ICC.

Arritmia sinusal ventriculofásica. É uma ocorrência incomum que consiste em alteração no intervalo P-P em pacientes com bloqueio AV de segundo ou terceiro grau.[35,36] Em termos específicos, o intervalo que sustenta o complexo QRS é mais curto que durante o bloqueio (ver Figura 248.22, mais adiante). Como o ritmo sinusal deve ser constante durante o bloqueio AV, essa variação cíclica repetitiva do intervalo P-P é incomum e pode ser explicada pelo aumento na perfusão arterial do nodo SA após a contração ventricular ou o estímulo do reflexo de Bainbridge com o enchimento atrial. O achado de arritmia sinusal ventriculofásica não tem importância clínica, além de não ser confundida com arritmia atrial.

Marca-passo errante. O MPE é uma ocorrência fisiológica normal em cães, não associada a doenças e não requer tratamento (ver Figura 248.4). Conforme discutido anteriormente, em cães, a origem da despolarização cardíaca não é fixa, podendo ser no AD ou mesmo entre o nodo SA e o nodo AV. No ECG, o resultado é uma alteração na amplitude da onda P, com intervalo P-R constante e complexos QRS que indicam uma aparência supraventricular normal. Em geral, essa variabilidade na onda P é cíclica e costuma estar associada a ASR (ver Figura 235.3, no Capítulo 235). Nessa situação, a amplitude da onda P aumenta com o aumento da frequência cardíaca (durante a inspiração) e diminui com a diminuição da frequência cardíaca (durante a expiração), às vezes a ponto de desaparecer (onda P isoelétrica) ou, raramente, negatividade da onda P nas derivações II, III e aVF.[1,2] No ECG, o diagnóstico diferencial de MPE inclui anormalidades morfológicas (p. ex., P pulmonar) e extrassístoles supraventriculares. Em alguns indivíduos com tônus vagal acentuado em repouso (p. ex., cães braquicefálicos), pode ser difícil diferenciar ASR ou MPE exagerado, porém normais em arritmia patológica, como CAP (extrassístoles supraventriculares). Tanto CAP quanto a combinação de MPE e ASR produzem onda P de morfologia diferente, intervalo R-R mais curto e complexos QRS de morfologia normal. A diferenciação baseia-se no grau de prematuridade (não devem ocorrer MP e ASR tão prematuramente, pois produzem uma onda P dentro da onda T precedente), na frequência cardíaca (não ocorrem MP e ASR em uma frequência acima de 150 bpm), na morfologia da onda P (como descrito antes, a ASR produz ondas P, que são mais altas, não mais curtas, quando a frequência cardíaca é mais rápida, enquanto no caso de CAP a onda P pode ser mais alta ou mais curta do que a onda P normal) e na aparência de uma série, ou "paroxismo", de batimentos cardíacos acoplados estreitamente entre si (o que corresponde a múltiplas extrassístoles supraventriculares [i. e., taquicardia supraventricular], não ASR). Se nenhuma dessas características for aparente, pode-se usar um monitor Holter para avaliar um grande número de batimentos cardíacos.

Bradicardia sinusal. A bradicardia sinusal (BS) é um ritmo sinusal em que a frequência cardíaca é anormalmente baixa (Figura 248.5). Há uma razão de 1:1 de complexos QRS e ondas

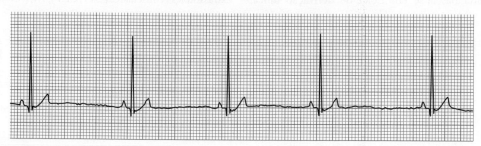

Figura 248.5 Bradicardia sinusal em um cão sadio calmo. A frequência cardíaca é de 45 bpm. Em geral, a bradicardia sinusal é atribuída a um tônus vagal alto, o que explica a ligeira variação no intervalo R-R (arritmia sinusal respiratória). Derivação II, 25 mm/s, 1 cm = mV.

P de aparência normal, com um intervalo P-R constante. Embora haja algumas variações normais aproximadas de frequência cardíaca para cães e gatos (p. ex., 70 a 160 bpm para cães, e 140 a 220 bpm para gatos; ver Capítulo 103), o conceito de bradicardia varia de acordo com a espécie, a idade, a raça e, em especial, o ambiente; cães mais velhos ou braquicefálicos tendem a ter frequência cardíaca mais lenta que a média; ademais, tanto os cães quanto os gatos apresentam frequências cardíacas normais que podem ser bastante influenciadas por estímulos ambientais.

Em geral, a BS indica a predominância fisiológica (p. ex., indivíduo braquicefálico, atlético, sono) ou predominância patológica do sistema parassimpático (p. ex., intoxicação sistêmica). Um teste auxiliar de diagnóstico é a resposta à injeção intravenosa de atropina (ver discussão anterior), que deve converter a BS fisiológica em ritmo sinusal normal ou taquicardia sinusal.[37] Como conceito geral, bradicardias graves ligadas diretamente a sinais clínicos francos (síncope, mal-estar, convulsões) requerem tratamento específico com fármacos ou implantação de marcapasso, e a BS quase nunca é a causa de tais manifestações clínicas. Pode ocorrer BS como manifestação cardíaca de asfixia (p. ex., paroxismo, obstrução de via respiratória superior devido a corpo estranho, neoplasia, pólipo nasofaríngeo ou palato mole alongado; válvula de escape [*pop-off*] fechada em um paciente intubado) e, em tal situação, o tratamento da BS com atropina (p. ex., 0,04 mg/kg IV) ou epinefrina em dose baixa (p. ex., 0,01 mg/kg IV) pode ser apropriado, se não for possível aliviar imediatamente a obstrução de via respiratória ou, se isso for conseguido, falhar no sentido de elevação imediata da frequência cardíaca. Em praticamente todas as circunstâncias, a BS é o efeito, não a causa, de um problema do paciente. Hipotermia, um plano anestésico excessivamente profundo e tônus vagal alto de qualquer origem (gastrintestinal [GI], respiratória, neurológica, oftálmica) são causas comuns de BS, e o tratamento da bradicardia consiste principalmente em tratar primeiro a causa primária. Talvez a única exceção seja a ocorrência de BS como parte da disfunção do nodo sinusal/SNSD, em que a BS pode ser uma bradicardia patológica primária, caso tipicamente acompanhado de bloqueio AV e/ou extrassístoles (ver disfunção do nodo sinusal/SNSD, adiante). Por fim, uma situação potencialmente perigosa é a transição instantânea de taquicardia para BS (ou outra bradicardia [p. ex., ritmo de escape ventricular]; ver ritmo de escape ventricular) em um paciente debilitado, instável e geralmente inconsciente. Tal alteração brusca pode prenunciar uma parada cardíaca próxima e deve ser considerada, com avaliação imediata do paciente em busca de causas primárias e preparação para reanimação cardiopulmonar (ver Capítulos 140 e 141).[38]

Taquicardia sinusal. A taquicardia sinusal (TS) é um ritmo sinusal que ocorre em uma frequência elevada (Figura 248.6). A ampla variação da frequência cardíaca em repouso, em cães e gatos normais, dificulta o ponto de corte para ritmo sinusal normal (RSN) e TS. Em cães, a TS é definida como uma frequência cardíaca superior a 160 bpm, mas de origem nodal (*i. e.*, complexos P-QRS-T de formato e sequência normais). Pode ser difícil diagnosticar essa arritmia no ECG quando a frequência cardíaca está extremamente elevada, fazendo com que ocorra sobreposição das ondas T e P. Uma manobra vagal, que reduza temporariamente a frequência cardíaca, separa as ondas P e T e esclarece que a taquicardia é de origem sinusal (ver Figura 248.3).

As causas de TS são diversas e em todas elas há predominância de estímulos simpáticos, em relação aos parassimpáticos. A TS é quase invariavelmente um resultado, não a causa, de problemas em um paciente. Portanto, é possível esperar que se resolva (retorne ao RSN) quando o distúrbio causador, como hipovolemia, ICC, anemia ou dor, receber o tratamento adequado. A supressão deliberada da TS na tentativa de restabelecer uma frequência cardíaca mais próximo do normal, especialmente em um paciente com doença aguda, pode ser (e tem sido) catastrófica, porque em muitas circunstâncias a TS é uma resposta compensatória. Nesses casos, a supressão da TS mediante o uso de betabloqueadores ou bloqueadores do canal de cálcio reduz um componente essencial do débito cardíaco adequado (frequência cardíaca) e pode causar hipotensão, colapso circulatório e parada cardíaca. Portanto, o tratamento da TS consiste em identificar a causa primária e tratá-la de maneira apropriada.

Um aspecto importante do tratamento cardiovascular é a prevenção de TS em pacientes com cardiopatia estrutural.[14,39] A justificativa é intuitiva: a taquicardia aumenta o consumo de oxigênio pelo miocárdio e também reduz a duração da diástole, a parte do ciclo cardíaco durante a qual ocorre a maioria da perfusão coronariana do miocárdio. Portanto, a taquicardia poderia forçar o coração a fazer mais com menos, o que pode ser especialmente prejudicial em pacientes com cardiopatia. Para evitar tal situação, a taquicardia pode ser limitada em cães e gatos com doença cardíaca mediante uma conduta relativa ao estilo de vida: substituição de períodos de corrida intensa em cães sem a guia por caminhadas mais leves com a guia, ou evitar perseguições a gatos e brincadeiras intensas. Mesmo assim, a experiência em seres humanos com cardiopatia indica que a prevenção de taquicardia por meios farmacológicos pode aumentar a sobrevida.[39] Na doença cardíaca pré-clínica (compensada, "assintomática") em pequenos animais, como uma abordagem terapêutica, envolveu o uso de betabloqueadores, bloqueadores do canal de cálcio e bloqueadores de corrente "estranha ou bizarra" de Na^+/K^+. No entanto, nenhum deles provou prolongar a sobrevida. O atenolol pode ser administrado com segurança a gatos com miocardiopatia hipertrófica subclínica (inaparente) (ver Capítulo 253)[40] e a cães com estenose subaórtica subclínica (inaparente) (ver Capítulo 250);[41] não se observou diferença no resultado entre animais tratados e animais do grupo-controle, não tratados, tampouco um benefício uniforme.

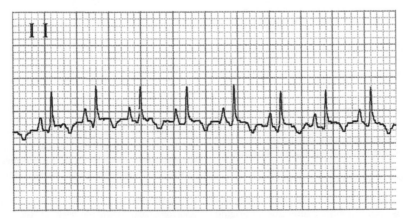

Figura 248.6 Taquicardia sinusal em um gato com miocardiopatia. A frequência cardíaca é de 210 bpm. Derivação II, 25 mm/s, 1 cm = 1 mV.

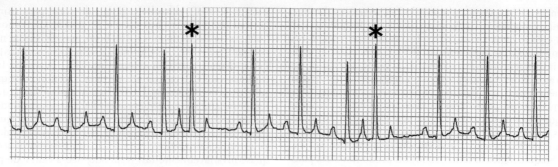

Figura 248.7 Complexos atriais prematuros (CAP) em um cão de 3 anos da raça Newfoundland; a arritmia foi um achado acidental. Note o ritmo sinusal normal, interrompido duas vezes por batimentos que apresentam complexos QRS com morfologia similar à dos complexos QRS sinusais (i. e., CAP [asteriscos]). Há superposição da onda P prematura no alto da onda T sinusal precedente; isso pode ser inferido notando-se o intervalo PR dos batimentos sinusais e contando de volta ao local esperado para a onda P de cada CAP. Ambos os CAP são seguidos de normalização, com pausa (ver Figura 248.8). Derivação II, 25 mm/s, 1 cm = 1 mV.

Cães com DVMD[42] ou com miocardiopatia dilatada[43] tratados com carvedilol não tiveram resultados melhores do que os do grupo-controle. É importante ressaltar que apenas um desses estudos foi prospectivo,[43] significando que a baixa força de evidência de estudos retrospectivos deixa um espaço para avaliação adicional da modulação da frequência cardíaca com o uso de betabloqueadores ou outros fármacos[44] em cães e gatos com doença cardíaca.

Anormalidades da excitabilidade atrial

São ocorrências comuns, em especial no cão. Na verdade, em cães com as formas mais comuns de cardiopatia (DVMD, miocardiopatia, muitas malformações congênitas), a distensão atrial acarreta alterações patológicas no tecido atrial que podem gerar estímulos atriais ectópicos. Tais alterações foram verificadas com o envelhecimento natural.[44a,44b]

Complexos atriais prematuros. Os CAP (sinonímia: contrações atriais prematuras, complexos ou contrações prematuras atriais [CPA], despolarizações atriais prematuras ou extrassístoles, batimentos supraventriculares [ou atriais] prematuros) são despolarizações prematuras que se originam em um foco atrial ectópico (Figura 248.7).

A identificação de CAP baseia-se em uma combinação das duas primeiras características mencionadas a seguir e, em geral, de todas as cinco: (1) prematuridade da sequência P-QRS-T; (2) complexos QRS que tenham uma aparência supraventricular, quando são estreitos e de forma comparável à dos QRS sinusais (incomumente, pode haver ausência de complexos QRS ou eles estarem ampliados em casos de CAP excepcionalmente precoces e, portanto, ocorrem durante o período refratário total e parcial, respectivamente); (3) uma onda P de amplitude diferente daquela das ondas P sinusais, incluindo negativas, bifásicas ou positivas, mas sempre precedendo o complexo QRS; (4) um intervalo P-R que pode ser ligeiramente diferente do sinusal, mais curto ou mais longo;[2] (5) uma pausa pós-sistólica que na maioria das vezes não é compensatória (Figura 248.8).

A patogenia dos CAP está relacionada mais comumente com uma lesão cardíaca (atrial) estrutural. A distensão do átrio é a causa principal desses focos ectópicos, mas tumores atriais (hemangiossarcomas), hipertireoidismo em gatos, intoxicação por digitálicos e outros distúrbios sistêmicos também são causas reconhecidas.[3,5]

As repercussões clínicas dos CAP são mínimas, exceto em casos de múltiplos surtos repetidos (ver Taquicardias Supraventriculares, adiante), e o principal interesse em identificar CAP em um ECG é levantar a suspeita de doença atrial. Portanto, o tratamento de CAP visa, em primeiro lugar, corrigir a causa primária, em vez de recorrer a fármacos antiarrítmicos.

Taquicardias atriais. As taquicardias supraventriculares são definidas em termos amplos como qualquer uma que se origine do nodo SA, do miocárdio atrial, do nodo/junção AV ou de veias que chegam aos átrios.[45] Em termos específicos, incluem taquicardia sinusal, de reentrada do nodo sinusal, atrial automática, de reentrada intra-atrial, *flutter* atrial, fibrilação atrial, de reentrada nodal AV (TRNAV), atrioventricular recíproca ortodrômica (TAVRO) e juncional automática.[46] A taquicardia sinusal foi discutida (anteriormente), e o *flutter* e a fibrilação atriais são discutidos separadamente (ver adiante), bem como a TRNAV e a

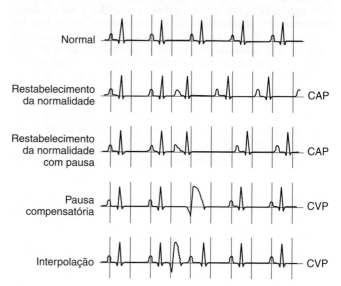

Figura 248.8 Representação esquemática do ritmo sinusal normal (RSN) e de complexos prematuros. **Normal**: a frequência cardíaca permanece constante e os intervalos de P a P e de R a R não se alteram. **Restabelecimento da normalidade**: um complexo atrial prematuro (*CAP*; batimento 3) restabelece o ritmo sinusal normal, de maneira que o período a partir do início da onda P prematura até a próxima onda P normal é exatamente igual a um intervalo P-P. **Restabelecimento da normalidade, com pausa**: o CAP (batimento 3) é seguido de uma pausa maior do que um intervalo P-P, porém menos de dois intervalos P-P. Tanto o restabelecimento da normalidade quanto o restabelecimento com pausa são exemplos de pausas não compensatórias (o ritmo do nodo SA é afetado pelo batimento prematuro, que altera a capacidade do nodo SA de proporcionar um batimento "compensatório" em tempo normal após o batimento prematuro). **Pausa compensatória**: o complexo ventricular prematuro (*CVP*; batimento 3) é seguido de uma pausa compensatória, ou seja, o período desde a onda P normal no batimento que precede o CVP até a onda P normal do batimento após o CVP é exatamente igual a dois intervalos P-P. Durante o CVP, a onda P sinusal ocorre no tempo, mas não é conduzida através do nodo atrioventricular (AV) para os ventrículos, que estão em um estado refratário devido ao CVP. **Interpolação**: ocorre um CVP (batimento 3) entre dois complexos sinusais normais, sem alterar o ritmo sinusal normal. Pode-se inferir a ausência de condução do CVP no nodo AV: a presença de CVP comumente retarda a transmissão nodal AV do próximo batimento, que se manifesta como prolongamento do intervalo P-R no batimento que segue o CVP inserido. Tal característica é útil para a diferenciação entre CVP e artefato de movimento.

TAVRO, ambas formas de arritmias de macrorreentrada (ver Síndromes de Macrorreentrada, adiante). As demais arritmias, em geral, são agrupadas na ampla categoria de "taquicardias atriais". Essa simplificação é exagerada para o paciente ocasional cuja taquicardia pode ser curada com ablação por meio de cateter de radiofrequência[47] e, na verdade, o ECG de 12 derivações fornece dois indícios importantes para a localização do foco ectópico em cães, como acontece em seres humanos.[48] Ainda, esse reagrupamento de taquicardia de reentrada do nodo sinusal, taquicardia atrial automática, taquicardia intra-atrial de reentrada e taquicardia juncional em uma categoria básica denominada taquicardias atriais é adequado para propósitos práticos, na maioria dos contextos de clínica veterinária. Taquicardia atrial pode ser definida como uma série de três ou mais CAP consecutivos que ocorrem em uma frequência maior do que o ritmo sinusal (Figura 248.9).

As taquicardias atriais podem ser intermitentes ou contínuas, e os impulsos podem ser transmitidos aos ventrículos ou pode ocorrer bloqueio AV fisiológico, como um mecanismo protetor, se a frequência dos impulsos atriais for alta o suficiente, e o nodo AV do paciente for apropriadamente discriminador. O mecanismo das taquicardias atriais pode envolver microrreentrada (p. ex., taquicardia reentrante do nodo sinusal, taquicardia reentrante intra-atrial) ou automaticidade espontânea de um foco atrial ectópico (p. ex., taquicardia atrial automática, taquicardia juncional automática).[32,46] Em geral, a identificação de taquicardias atriais intermitentes é direta: o ECG mostra uma "explosão" de CAP (Figura 248.9). No entanto, pode ser difícil estabelecer o diagnóstico de taquicardia atrial sustentada, porque as ondas P podem não ser claramente evidentes, pois elas ficam ocultas no complexo QRS prévio ou na onda T. Portanto, a diferenciação entre taquicardia atrial sustentada e taquicardia ventricular "alta" (i. e., que se origina próximo ao nodo AV) pode ser auxiliada pela exteriorização da onda P, o que pode ser obtido com uma manobra vagal (ver discussão anterior) e redução subsequente da taquicardia ou mesmo pela captura sinusal (i. e., restabelecimento do ritmo sinusal) (ver Figura 248.3).

A curto prazo, o mesmo objetivo pode ser alcançado farmacologicamente usando doses graduadas de um medicamento por via intravenosa. O tratamento intravenoso é reservado a cães ou gatos com taquicardia atrial muito rápida (p. ex., frequência cardíaca mantida > 200/min em cães e > 260/mim em gatos). As opções de tratamento incluem diltiazem (0,05 a 0,1 mg/kg, na forma de *bolus*, em aplicação intravenosa lenta, repetido até obter o efeito desejado ou até a dose máxima cumulativa de 0,25 a 0,35 mg/kg),[46,49] propranolol (0,02 mg/kg IV, quando necessário, tipicamente a cada 2 a 10 min; em um caso, há relato de 3 doses ao longo de 2 h),[27] esmolol (25 mcg/kg/min IV TIC,[50] com relatos até de 100 a 500 mcg/kg/min IV TIC[51] ou na forma de *bolus* de 500 mcg/kg IV em 1 min[46]), edrofônio (0,05 a 0,1 mg/kg IV; tenha disponíveis atropina e tubo endotraqueal),[52] ou fenilefrina (0,004 a 0,01 mg/kg IV).[52] Esses tratamentos requerem que o paciente tenha função sistólica e diastólica normal e nenhuma evidência de ICC, o que poderia tornar as dosagens mencionadas perigosas (hemodinamicamente comprometedoras). Em termos subjetivos, a injeção intravenosa de adenosina, usada com esse propósito, parece ser muito menos efetiva em cães que em seres humanos,[46] provavelmente, pelo menos em parte, devido à ocorrência rara de TRNAV em cães em comparação com pessoas.[53] O tratamento oral em longo prazo será discutido a seguir.

As causas de taquicardias atriais são as mesmas listadas para CAP (ver discussão anterior). Notou-se incidência significativamente mais alta de taquicardias atriais associadas à idade: em um estudo com cães monitorados por 1 semana após pneumonectomia, 7 de 8 cães que tinham 8 ou mais anos de idade desenvolveram episódios de taquicardia atrial, em comparação com nenhum de 7 cães com menos de 4 anos de idade submetidos ao mesmo procedimento.[54] Dois achados importantes foram que cães idosos tiveram um aumento progressivo na frequência cardíaca sinusal, começando 15 minutos antes do início de taquicardia atrial, e cães idosos tiveram evidências de fibrose e inflamação atrial, ocorrência que os mais jovens não apresentaram.[54]

O impacto clínico da taquicardia atrial depende de sua duração, da frequência e de lesões cardíacas subjacentes. No caso de taquicardias atriais rápidas, o bloqueio AV intermitente pode limitar a frequência ventricular, possibilitando melhor enchimento diastólico e menor impacto clínico. Quando a taquicardia atrial induz uma frequência cardíaca persistentemente elevada (e/ou síncope), conforme descrito anteriormente, o tratamento é necessário para evitar complicações a longo prazo, como miocardiopatia mediada por taquicardia.[49,55] Esse tratamento VO, é iniciado com a dose da faixa indicada e só após a resolução de quaisquer sinais de ICC (p. ex., eliminação de edema pulmonar com o uso de diuréticos). As opções de tratamento incluem um betabloqueador (p. ex., 0,3 a 1,5 mg de atenolol/kg/12 h VO ou 0,2 a 04 mg de metoprolol/kg/12 h VO ou 0,2 a 0,3 mg de carvedilol/kg/12 h VO), um bloqueador do canal de cálcio (p. ex., diltiazem regular [não de liberação lenta], na dose de 0,8 a 1,5 mg/kg/8 h VO),[49] digoxina (0,005 mg/kg/12 h VO) ou uma combinação desses medicamentos, se a monoterapia não for efetiva. Pode-se aumentar gradativamente a dose até obter o efeito desejado, o que requer monitoramento Holter para alcançar a frequência cardíaca ótima (seja mediante a indução de bloqueio AV em um nível que resulte em frequência ventricular apropriada, seja suprimindo a taquicardia atrial até um grau em que o ritmo dominante seja o RSN). Em geral, a taquicardia atrial precede o desenvolvimento de FibA, provavelmente em grande parte devido a uma causa patológica comum (aumento atrial e fibrose intersticial).[56] O tratamento da doença primária é uma parte essencial do tratamento dessas arritmias.

***Flutter* atrial.** Classicamente, o *flutter* atrial se caracteriza por uma série rápida e regular de despolarizações atriais, sem uma fase de repouso entre elas (Figura 248.10 e Vídeo 248.1).[32,46] As características do ECG, de acordo com o tempo, são: (1) ondas rítmicas rápidas de atividade elétrica atrial conhecidas como *ondas de flutter (F)*, em geral ocorrendo a uma frequência muito alta (280 a 400/min); (2) ausência de retorno das ondas F ao nível basal, conferindo uma aparência basal em "dentes de serra";

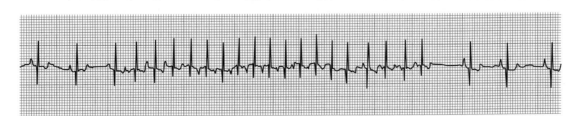

Figura 248.9 Taquicardia atrial. Uma "explosão" de batimentos cardíacos prematuros (rápidos) é visto no meio do traçado. Os complexos QRS permanecem do mesmo formato, como os sinusais, o que indica uma origem supraventricular. Durante muito tempo da taquicardia, as ondas P e T não são vistas com clareza; no entanto, como a forma dos complexos QRS está inalterada, a maioria das ondas T deve ter a mesma forma. Portanto, as deflexões negativas entre complexos QRS (meio do traçado) precisam ter uma superposição de ondas T normais e ondas P muito diferentes, intensamente negativas, indicando um foco atrial ectópico como origem da taquicardia. Nesse cão idoso da raça Golden Retriever não havia sinais clínicos, nem durante a consulta, nem durante o acompanhamento clínico; um ecocardiograma nada revelou de notável. Derivação II, 25 mm/s, 1 cm = 1 mV.

(3) complexos QRS de aparência supraventricular normal; (4) intervalo R-R variável, irregularmente irregular, caso ocorra bloqueio de alguns estímulos atriais, como costuma acontecer.

Ocorre *flutter* atrial como resultado da propagação do estímulo através de um circuito de macrorreentrada, ou seja, condução elétrica que se autoperpetua e ocorre ao longo de uma alça fechada preexistente de tecido de rápida condução no átrio direito.[32,46] Às vezes, a cessação do *flutter* atrial é espontânea; mais frequentemente, há necessidade de tratamento quando a maior parte ou todas as ondas do *flutter* se deve à frequência cardíaca resultante muito elevada (em cães, há risco de miocardiopatia mediada por taquicardia se uma frequência cardíaca > 240/min persiste continuamente por mais de 3 semanas).[49]

O diagnóstico de *flutter* atrial pode ser muito desafiador quando cada onda de *flutter* se propaga através do nodo AV para os ventrículos. A taxa de propagação 1:1 deixa as ondas F ocultas nos complexos QRS ou ondas T precedentes, dificultando o diagnóstico e, em geral, requerendo uma manobra vagal para induzir bloqueio AV transitório e revelar as ondas F (ver texto anterior). A avaliação eletrofisiológica intracardíaca em cães com taquicardia atrial mostrou que as características clássicas de *flutter* atrial nem sempre são aparentes no ECG de superfície.[57] Tal percepção é importante quando estão sendo consideradas terapias minimamente invasivas como uma forma de cura da taquicardia atrial. Entretanto, todas as opções de tratamento farmacológico para *flutter* atrial são as mesmas mencionadas para fibrilação atrial (ver adiante). Consegue-se abolir permanentemente o *flutter* atrial interrompendo-se o circuito do *flutter* por meio do emprego de cateter de radiofrequência.[57,58]

Fibrilação atrial. A fibrilação atrial (FibA) é uma arritmia comum e importante, que representa 14% de todas as arritmias de cães; em casos de miocardiopatia dilatada em cães, a taxa de prevalência é de 50%; pode ocasionar alterações hemodinâmicas de relevância clínica, que requerem tratamento específico.[32,59,60] Na população humana, estima-se uma prevalência de FibA de até 2%,[60] mas não há uma estatística similar em medicina veterinária. A FibA se caracteriza por desorganização elétrica completa no nível atrial, levando a uma série caótica e rápida de despolarizações atriais (400 a 1.200 por minuto) (Figuras 248.11 a 248.14).[61]

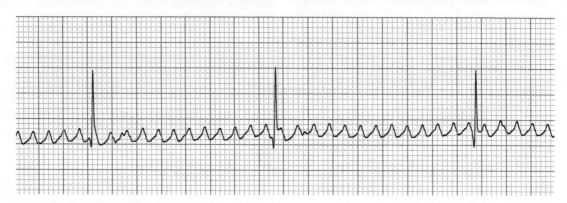

Figura 248.10 *Flutter* atrial. Notam-se despolarizações atriais de maneira distinta e organizada (ondas F), sem retorno ao nível basal entre cada uma, em um cão da raça Cocker Spaniel com 10 anos de idade. Isso produz a característica linha basal em dente de serra do *flutter* atrial. Nesse cão, a frequência cardíaca resultante é baixa (aproximadamente 40 bpm), que é incomum no *flutter* atrial e sugere doença de nodo AV concomitante. Derivação II, 25 mm/s, 1 cm = 1 mV.

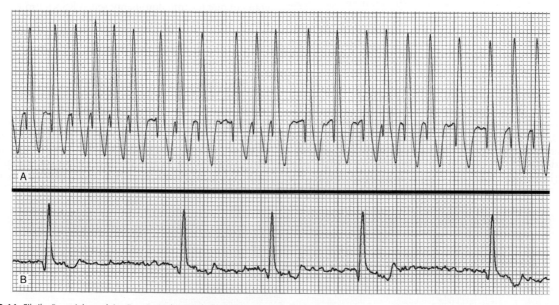

Figura 248.11 Fibrilação atrial em dois cães. **A.** Mal controlada. **B.** Bem controlada. Ambos os traçados mostram os aspectos característicos da fibrilação atrial: intervalo R-R irregularmente irregular, ausência de ondas P e um nível basal ondulante distinto (ondas F). Esses aspectos são mais claros no cão do painel **B**, porque o ECG em questão foi obtido quando o paciente permanecia estável. A frequência cardíaca (de resposta ventricular) é de 115 bpm. O aumento gradativo da dose de diltiazem com digoxina possibilitou esse resultado. No painel **A**, a frequência cardíaca é de 240 bpm. O cão do painel **A** teve o ECG obtido na consulta inicial, e tais frequências rápidas de resposta ventricular tornam a irregularidade do ritmo muito menos óbvia na fibrilação atrial. O painel **A** também mostra bloqueio de ramo do feixe esquerdo (duração do QRS = 0,08 s, com QRS positivo na derivação II), compatível com miocardiopatia dilatada primária do cão. **A.** Derivação II, 25 mm/s, 1 cm = 1 mV. **B.** Derivação II, 50 mm/s, 1 cm = 1 mV.

Em contraste com o *flutter* atrial, os estímulos de fibrilação na FibA aparecem no ECG como deflexões muito pequenas de formas altamente variáveis – essencialmente aleatórias – que não podem ser identificadas como atividade elétrica atrial organizada. O nodo AV atua como um "porteiro" em relação a essa atividade elétrica caótica, permitindo que apenas as despolarizações elétricas com intensidade, cronometragem e orientação ótimas passem através dos ventrículos e, assim, até certo ponto, controlam a frequência ventricular.

As três características da FibA no ECG são: (1) complexos QRS que parecem supraventriculares (estreitos, para cima e de amplitude ligeiramente variável na derivação II, a menos que haja aberração ventricular/BRF); (2) um ritmo irregularmente irregular, significando um intervalo R-R variável, com frequência ventricular que pode ser baixa, normal ou, mais comumente, alta, quando não tratada; (3) ausência de ondas P visíveis (substituídas por uma ondulação distinta da linha isoelétrica, denominada *ondas F*) (ver Figuras 248.11 e 248.12, e Vídeo 248.2). Durante a diástole, o enchimento ventricular é otimizado pela contração atrial, que pode ser responsável por 30% do enchimento total do ventrículo. Portanto, sua ausência pode reduzir o volume ventricular para níveis subótimos, originando sinais clínicos francos durante picos de atividade cardíaca, como acontece em atividade física intensa. Além disso, a frequência ventricular geral rápida, comumente resultante de FibA, pode limitar o enchimento diastólico quando há tempo insuficiente durante a diástole, antes que os ventrículos sejam estimulados a despolarizar novamente. Por essas razões, algumas contrações intermitentes podem ser inefetivas, podendo ocorrer um ou mais batimento(s) cardíaco(s) durante a auscultação, sem um pulso arterial palpável (*i. e.*, déficit de pulso). A FibA é uma das poucas arritmias de que se pode suspeitar, durante na auscultação e palpação, no exame físico, com base na irregularidade caótica do ritmo cardíaco à auscultação e à palpação do tórax, juntamente com déficit de pulso. No entanto, TV polimórfica, taquicardias atriais e frequentes CVP ou CAP devem ser incluídas no diagnóstico diferencial desse achado ao exame físico (ver adiante).

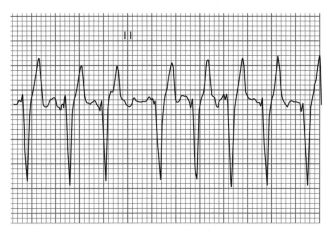

Figura 248.12 Fibrilação atrial com bloqueio de ramo do feixe direito em um cão. Esse tipo de arritmia ventricular se diferencia por apresentar intervalo R-R irregular e demora na resposta à manobra vagal. Derivação II, 25 mm/s, 1 cm = 1 mV.

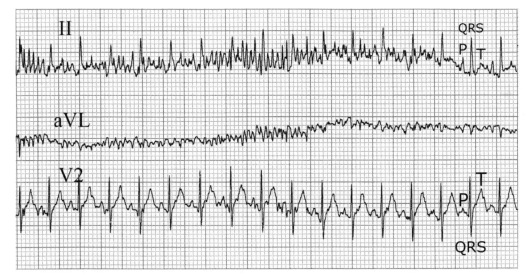

Figura 248.13 Artefato simulando fibrilação atrial em um gato, causado por tremedeira. Registro simultâneo das derivações II, aVL e V2. Nas derivações II e aVL, o extenso artefato de movimento confere ao nível basal uma aparência ondulante grosseira. O ritmo é sinusal normal, evidente, com maior clareza quando o animal para de tremer (3 últimos batimentos cardíacos) e em todo o traçado na derivação V2. Esse ECG mostra a vantagem de se registrarem múltiplas derivações simultaneamente porque, em geral, o artefato pode afetar uma ou mais derivações, mas não todas. 25 mm/s, 1 cm = 1 mV.

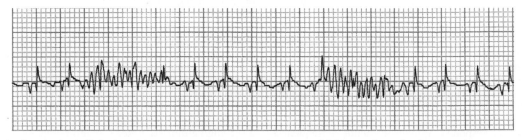

Figura 248.14 Artefato simulando fibrilação atrial em um gato, devido ao ato de ronronar. O início, o meio e o fim desse traçado mostram taquicardia sinusal. Entre eles, dois momentos de artefato pelo ato de ronronar do gato produzem uma ondulação grosseira do nível basal. Derivação I, 25 mm/s, 2 cm = 1 mV.

Um achado diagnóstico incomum no ECG, porém importante, é a combinação de FibA e BRF (ver Figura 248.12), que produz complexos QRS de base larga e, portanto, pode simular TV, mas sem ondas P que indiquem, de maneira conclusiva, uma dissociação (TV) ou associação (BRF) AV. Em tal situação, pode-se fazer uma manobra vagal (ver texto anterior), cujo efeito no nodo AV pode reduzir a frequência ventricular quando há FibA + bloqueio de ramo do feixe direito (BRFD), mas não na TV. Além disso, a TV monomórfica sustentada, em geral, caracteriza-se por intervalos R-R regulares, o que não acontece na FibA concomitante ao BRF.

Em cães, a FibA ocorre com maior frequência associada à cardiopatia primária, que ocasiona aumento do átrio.[62] Contudo, também ocorre FibA em indivíduos com coração normal, em termos estruturais ("FibA solitária"), associada à anestesia (em especial com opiáceos),[63] hipotireoidismo, pericardiocentese rápida de grande volume de líquido, doença GI e sobrecarga de volume que causa estiramento atrial, se o coração em questão apresentar massa de miocárdio atrial suficiente para perpetuar a fibrilação (i. e., cães de raças de porte médio a grande).[62] Em cães de raças gigantes, é comum detectar FibA solitária,[62,64,65] cujo prognóstico é melhor do que o da FibA associada a lesões cardíacas estruturais, talvez porque também esteja associada a uma frequência ventricular mais lenta (média de 120 bpm), em comparação com a FibA em cães com doença cardíaca estrutural subclínica (frequência cardíaca média: 155 bpm) ou cardiopatia estrutural e ICC (frequência cardíaca média: 203 bpm).[64] Ainda não se determinou se nos pacientes com FibA e coração normal, em termos estruturais, que progridem para miocardiopatia dilatada, isso acontece devido à sua arritmia ou, em contrapartida, a FibA é apenas o prenúncio arrítmico de uma doença que envolve, de maneira inerente, a dilatação subsequente da câmara cardíaca e disfunção sistólica.

Em gatos, a FibA é menos comum que em cães e quase sempre está associada a cardiopatia estrutural que causa aumento do átrio.[66] Em gatos, a FibA é um achado acidental em 20 a 25% dos casos e não confere, necessariamente, um prognóstico mais grave que o da doença cardíaca primária: mais da metade dos gatos diagnosticados com FibA vive 6 meses ou mais (6 a 12 meses: 21%; 1 ano ou mais: 33%).[66,67]

Em geral, a FibA é uma arritmia permanente e persistente; pode ser paroxística no cão[68,69] e muito rara em gatos. A FibA paroxística costuma ser de curta duração e se resolve espontaneamente em menos de 4 dias, se forem eliminados os estímulos que causam aumento do tônus vagal (p. ex., distúrbios GI, uso de opiáceos). Em alguns cães com átrios estruturalmente normais e em quase todos com aumento atrial grave, a FibA paroxística progride para persistente (permanente).

O início da FibA tem implicações prognósticas em cães de porte médio a grande com DVMD e ICC, sendo provável que outros grupos de doenças também. Aqueles com FibA vivem, em média, 142 dias (variação de 9 a 478 dias), após o início da ICC, em comparação com aqueles sem FibA (média: 234 dias; variação de 13 a 879 dias).[70] É possível que essa diferença se deva aos efeitos deletérios causados pela FibA, ou à ação da FibA como um marcador de DVMD mais avançado ou mais rapidamente progressivo.

Na maioria dos casos de FibA, o tratamento tem dois objetivos: (1) tratar a cardiopatia primária e (2) maximizar o débito cardíaco ao controlar (reduzir) a frequência de condução do estímulo através do nodo AV, se necessário (ver Figura 248.11). Na clínica de pequenos animais, a frequência ventricular ideal varia para cada paciente, dependendo de muitos fatores, inclusive a presença ou ausência de ICC e do peso corporal. Uma diretriz substanciada sugere que o tratamento deva visar uma frequência ventricular em cães com FibA que pesem 20 a 25 kg de, aproximadamente, 130 a 145 bpm.[71] Uma abordagem prática usada pelos autores deste capítulo é visar a uma frequência ventricular de resposta que corresponda, aproximadamente, à frequência sinusal esperada em condições ambientais (localização física, estado de despertar etc.) no momento do registro de ECG/Holter.

O ideal é usar o monitoramento Holter para avaliar o nível basal e, depois, novamente para verificar a resposta ao tratamento, pois a influência da variabilidade autonômica é muito substancial em cada paciente, e até no mesmo paciente, em ambientes diferentes. Em termos específicos, o ECG realizado em pacientes hospitalizados tem superestimado a frequência ventricular de resposta em cães com FibA, em média, 26 bpm (variação de 3 a 48 bpm), em comparação com o monitoramento Holter.[72] Para medir a frequência cardíaca na fibrilação atrial, a auscultação também é apenas subótima: em um estudo, o nível de acurácia da auscultação comparado ao ECG variou de 64% a um valor tão baixo como 12% em estudantes de veterinária e alguns veterinários.[73]

O tratamento da fibrilação atrial pode envolver a conversão para RSN (controle do ritmo) ou aceitar que a FibA persistirá e ter como foco a otimização da frequência ventricular/cardíaca resultante, se for muito rápida (controle da frequência).[60,74-76] A última abordagem foi validada para seres humanos;[60,74,77] é a estratégia de tratamento mais usada nos casos de FibA em cães e gatos. Os medicamentos de escolha são o diltiazem de liberação lenta (3 mg/kg/12 h VO) e digoxina (0,005 mg/kg/12 h VO), administrados simultaneamente.[78] É preciso ajustar a dose exata para obter uma frequência ventricular (frequência cardíaca) de resposta ótima, conforme descrito anteriormente; em geral, os ajustes de dose envolvem alteração na dose de diltiazem, mantendo fixa a da digoxina, a menos que haja sinais de intoxicação pela última (letargia, inapetência, vômitos, diarreia), o que levaria à diminuição da dose dela. A duração do tratamento costuma ser indefinida, a menos que ocorra conversão espontânea para RSN. Em cães com FibA, a combinação de digoxina e diltiazem controla melhor a frequência cardíaca (média: 126 bpm, em vez de 194 bpm pré-tratamento), em comparação com o uso apenas de digoxina (164 bpm) ou de diltiazem (158 bpm).[78] Os betabloqueadores, notadamente o atenolol, foram menos efetivos na redução da frequência ventricular de cães com FA, em comparação com a combinação digoxina + diltiazem.[70] O controle adequado da frequência cardíaca é importante porque está associado à sobrevida mais longa: em estudo realizado com cães de raças de médio e grande portes com DVMD e ICC, a associação de digoxina e diltiazem resultou em frequência cardíaca média de 144 bpm e tempo médio de sobrevida de 130 dias, em comparação com um tempo médio de sobrevida de 35 dias (e frequência cardíaca média de 180 bpm) com o uso apenas de diltiazem.[70] O tratamento inicial com baixa dose para começar a reduzir a frequência ventricular de resposta é feito simultaneamente ao início da administração de diuréticos, em pacientes com FibA de início agudo; aumenta-se a dose do medicamento de modo gradativo para conseguir o controle da frequência cardíaca com maior precisão, assim que ocorre a resolução dos sinais clínicos de ICC do paciente com o tratamento com diuréticos e o paciente estiver estável (alerta e se alimentando).

Em cães com FibA, a melhora da tecnologia da desfibrilação renovou o interesse na conversão elétrica da FibA em RSN.[79-82] Em um estudo, obteve-se a conversão de 36 de 39 cães (92,3%) por meio de desfibrilação bifásica, com duração média de RSN de 120 dias, daí em diante (pós-tratamento com cardioversão: 12 a 15 mg de amiodarona/kg/12 h VO, por 2 semanas, seguida de 5 a 7 mg/kg/24 h VO; monitoramento hematológico e do perfil bioquímico sérico a cada 6 meses).[79] FibA de início recente e ausência de cardiopatia estrutural foram associadas à manutenção mais duradoura do RSN.[80] A eficácia e a segurança da ranolazina, na dose de 22 mg/kg/12 h VO, acrescentada à amiodarona e iniciada após a cardioversão bem-sucedida de FA, estão sendo pesquisadas em cães com fibrilação atrial de ocorrência natural (Dra. Janice Bright, comunicação pessoal, 2016). Obteve-se a conversão farmacológica de FibA aguda em cães após aplicação intravenosa de amiodarona (infusão IV de 0,33 a 0,5 mg/kg/min até obter o efeito desejado; dose cumulativa de 3,78 a 8,3 mg/kg para a conversão de FibA em RSN, em 2 casos relatados),[83] procainamida (administração por via intravenosa lenta de *bolus* de 14,3 mg/kg; conversão para RSN 12 minutos após finalizar a dose, em 1 caso)[84] ou lidocaína (para FibA associada a tônus vagal alto [p. ex., paralisia de laringe, administração de opiáceos]: injeção IV única de *bolus* de 2 mg/kg; se não efetiva, pode-se repetir a dose uma vez; espera-se a conversão após 20 a 90 segundos).[85,86] Em um modelo experimental, a ranolazina (*bolus* IV de 3,2 mg/kg, seguido de 0,17 mg/kg/min) resolveu a FibA de 3 para 4 episódios (75%), em cães; a segurança e a eficácia em pacientes clínicos veterinários são desconhecidas.[87] Em termos gerais, atualmente o tratamento da maioria dos cães com FibA envolve o uso de medicamentos para o controle da frequência ventricular.

Dissociação atrial. A ocorrência de dois ritmos atriais organizados, porém independentes, um deles passando pelo nodo AV normalmente e desencadeando atividade ventricular, enquanto o outro está constantemente confinado aos átrios, é conhecida como *dissociação atrial*. Esse achado incidental incomum, aparentemente benigno, caracteriza-se, no ECG, por duas populações de ondas P, uma delas (em geral as maiores) acompanhada de maneira consistente por complexos QRS, e a outra exibindo bloqueio de saída – as ondas P menores (denominadas *ondas P'*) não ativam os ventrículos. A aparência resultante no ECG é uma superposição de ritmo sinusal normal e ritmo atrial independente, que pode ou não ser influenciado por estímulos autonômicos (alterando os intervalos P-P e/ou R-R). Não há ligação patológica conhecida entre a dissociação atrial e qualquer outra anormalidade cardíaca, e não é necessário tratamento ou intervenção alguma.[88,89]

Anormalidades da excitabilidade ventricular

As anormalidades da excitabilidade ventricular são importantes porque envolvem o principal elemento da bomba cardíaca, portanto podem ter repercussões hemodinâmicas e clínicas graves. Entretanto, é preciso reconhecer que as arritmias ventriculares têm muitos mecanismos e causas diversas (em especial não cardíacas), de modo que dependem mais da gravidade, do tratamento e do prognóstico que dos resultados do ECG.

Extrassístoles ventriculares ou complexos ventriculares prematuros. As extrassístoles ventriculares (sinonímia: contrações prematuras, batimentos ou despolarizações ventriculares prematuros [CVP, BVP, DVP, ectopia ventricular) são despolarizações prematuras geradas por um foco ectópico localizado no tecido ventricular.[1-5] Essas arritmias são os distúrbios patológicos do ritmo mais comuns em cães e gatos.[59,90] As principais características no ECG são intervalo R-R curto (*i. e.*, prematuridade) e complexo QRS de base larga, com morfologia (forma) diferente do complexo QRS sinusal normal. A maioria das extrassístoles ventriculares tem um complexo QRS de base larga de aparência frequentemente bizarra (> 0,07 segundo, em cães), sem onda P associada, e uma onda T associada diferente (em geral muito grande) (Figura 248.15).

Em geral, os CVP isolados são seguidos de uma pausa compensatória (ver Figura 248.8), mas podem ser interpolados. A alternância 1:1 entre batimentos sinusais e CVP é conhecida como bigeminismo ventricular; múltiplos de dois CVP são considerados um par; três ou mais CVP em um traçado constituem taquicardia ventricular (TV; ver a seguir).

Com a finalidade de identificar uma causa primária e instituir o tratamento correto, é importante diferenciar extrassístoles ventriculares de outras causas importantes de alteração da morfologia do QRS: (1) alterações decorrentes de cardiomegalia e desvio do eixo; (2) distúrbios da condução intraventricular em ramos do feixe (ver Figuras 248.24 e 248.25, mais adiante); (3) movimento abrupto ou outro artefato (ver Figura 248.19, mais adiante); (4) complexos QRS de base larga, mas não prematuros, de batimentos ventriculares de escape (ver Figura 248.23, mais adiante); (5) alterações na morfologia do QRS causadas por hiperpotassemia grave. Essas cinco causas de QRS de base larga não são arritmias ventriculares, não envolvem um foco patológico no ventrículo, portanto não são tratadas com fármacos antiarrítmicos (Figura 248.16).

As causas de extrassístoles ventriculares incluem praticamente todas as anormalidades cardíacas ou sistêmicas, sendo as mais comuns, no primeiro caso, doenças cardíacas primárias, como miocardiopatia,[91-93] cardiopatia valvular, cardiopatia congênita e endocardite[94], bem como anormalidades sistêmicas, como hipopotassemia, anemia, hipoxemia, traumatismo contuso,[95] síndrome vólvulo-dilatação gástrica,[96,97] massas abdominais (comumente esplênicas ou hepáticas),[98-100] intoxicação e acidose. Cães normais costumam ter até 24 CVP diários, registrados em estudos com Holter.[24,101] Em gatos, as extrassístoles ventriculares estão associadas predominantemente à doença de miocárdio. Em um estudo retrospectivo com 106 gatos com extrassístoles ventriculares, o ECG foi anormal em uma proporção significativamente maior de gatos com extrassístoles ventriculares (102 de 106; 96%), em comparação com um grupo equivalente de cães com extrassístoles ventriculares (95 de 138; 69%; $p < 0,001$), sugerindo que as extrassístoles ventriculares coexistem mais frequentemente com cardiopatia estrutural em gatos que em cães.[93] Os aspectos mais desafiadores, ao lidar com extrassístoles ventriculares, continuam sendo a avaliação de sua gravidade e da necessidade de tratamento. As abordagens e opções de tratamento são discutidas adiante (ver o tópico Taquicardia ventricular).

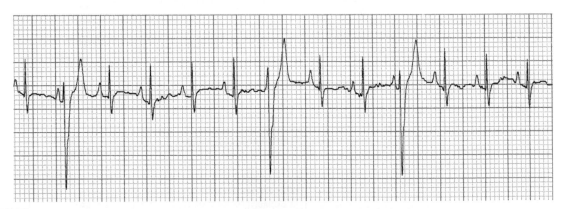

Figura 248.15 Complexos ventriculares prematuros (CVP) em Gato Doméstico de Pelo Curto de 10 anos de idade com miocardiopatia. O ritmo é sinusal normal, com 3 CVP monomórficos (com o mesmo formato) aparentes, como deflexões largas, bizarras e prematuras. Note que a função atrial não está alterada: as ondas P ainda são aparentes, mas não são responsáveis pelos complexos QRS de base larga bizarros, porque o intervalo P-R entre as ondas P e os CVP é muito curto para ser consistente com o tempo de trânsito AV nodal, conforme mostrado no intervalo P-R dos batimentos sinusais. Ou seja, os CVP são, por definição, despolarizações prematuras que precedem a sequência normal nodo SA/átrios/nodo AV/ventrículos. Os CVP não alteram a função do nodo SA; portanto, a pausa que acompanha cada um é compensatória (ver Figura 248.8). Derivação II, 25 mm/s, 2 cm = 1 mV.

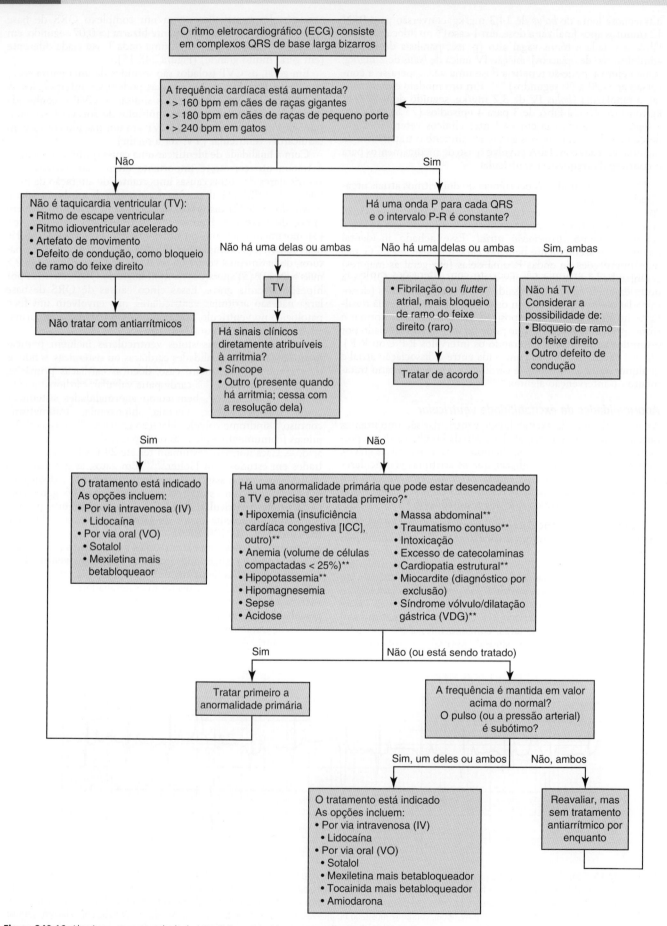

Figura 248.16 Algoritmo para a tomada de decisão clínica para pacientes com arritmias ventriculares. *Praticamente qualquer problema clínico, se grave o bastante, pode causar arritmia ventricular. **Mais comum.

Duas doenças cardíacas específicas de cães são quase exclusivamente arritmogênicas: causam CVP e TV, bem como costumam apresentar manifestações clínicas evidentes de arritmia aguda (mal-estar, síncope, convulsões hipóxicas/anóxicas ou morte súbita) como a anormalidade principal. A primeira, miocardiopatia ventricular direita arritmogênica (MVDA, arritmia ventricular familiar de cães da raça Boxer, miocardiopatia de cães da raça Boxer, displasia de VD arritmogênica), causa extrassístoles ventriculares e TV, descrita no Capítulo 252. A segunda é a morte cardíaca súbita hereditária de cães da raça Pastor-Alemão. Tal anormalidade pode se apresentar como um estado latente ou causar sinais clínicos evidentes.[102,103] A doença ocorre raramente, mas tem distribuição internacional e afetou várias gerações.[102] A anormalidade predominante é TV paroxística rápida. Cães com essa doença, em geral, desenvolvem sinais clínicos em idade precoce, que consistem em síncope e alta prevalência de morte súbita. Portanto, a doença causa manifestações clínicas principalmente em filhotes de cães ou cães adultos jovens (idade média: aproximadamente 1 ano; faixa etária média: 4 a 30 meses). Como regra, a arritmia não coexiste com alterações cardíacas estruturais, esperando-se que os resultados de radiografias do tórax e da ecocardiografia sejam normais nos cães acometidos. Um defeito na repolarização do miocárdio parece ser a causa da arritmia.[104] Embora os tratamentos que limitam a bradicardia (p. ex., fármacos vagolíticos, marca-passo ventricular) reduzam a ocorrência da arritmia, atualmente não há tratamento definitivo para essa anormalidade. Mais comumente, os cães acometidos que sobrevivem ao primeiro ano de vida se desenvolvem, apesar da doença, e levam vida normal daí em diante.

Ritmo idioventricular acelerado (RIVA). É um ritmo ventricular de frequência intermediária. No ECG, tem as mesmas características da TV, exceto a frequência, que é ligeiramente mais baixa que na TV. Portanto, em termos clínicos, o RIVA é considerado um subconjunto mais lento de TV e, na verdade, recebeu primeiro a denominação lógica, porém oximorônica, de "TV lenta". No ECG, observam-se dissociação AV, complexos QRS de base larga bizarros e possíveis batimentos de captura e de fusão, como notados na TV. Todavia, em um cão típico de porte médio, por definição, a frequência do RIVA situa-se entre 70 e 160 bpm, o que o coloca entre os ritmos idioventriculares (i. e., de escape; menos de 70 bpm) e TV verdadeira, em termos de frequência. As causas de RIVA são similares às de extrassístoles ventriculares, mas a frequência ventricular mais baixa compromete menos o tempo de enchimento ventricular diastólico; assim, em geral, o RIVA é bem tolerado.[105] Portanto, o tratamento é voltado para a causa primária; as medicações antiarrítmicas não são utilizadas, a menos que o tratamento da causa primária não seja efetivo na resolução da arritmia e o aumento da frequência cardíaca a ponto de satisfazer os critérios para TV.

Taquicardia ventricular (TV). É uma série de três ou mais extrassístoles ventriculares que ocorrem em uma alta frequência (Figura 248.17 e Vídeo 248.3). Pode ser contínua (sustentada) ou intermitente (paroxística). As causas são as mesmas listadas para extrassístoles ventriculares (CVP; ver discussão anterior). As manifestações clínicas são frequentes (fraqueza, síncope, convulsões hipóxicas/anóxicas), mas sua ocorrência depende diretamente das consequências hemodinâmicas do ritmo cardíaco. Uma TV cada vez mais rápida, por exemplo, ultrapassa um limiar de frequência ventricular além do qual um número maior de batimentos não representa maior débito cardíaco. Esse "ponto de retorno diminuído", que varia de acordo com as variáveis mencionadas anteriormente, acontece porque o tempo de enchimento diastólico fica mais comprometido em frequências cardíacas mais altas. Portanto, a TV muito rápida, como qualquer outra taquicardia muito rápida, pode desencadear sinais clínicos evidentes de redução do débito cardíaco.

A identificação de TV é mais fácil quando ela é intermitente. A aparência típica é a de uma ou várias séries de complexos QRS de base larga (> 0,07 s no cão, > 0,04 s no gato), não lembra complexos QRS sinusais, está associada a ondas T gigantes de aparência distinta, não está relacionada a ondas P e pode incluir batimento de captura (o primeiro complexo P-QRS sinusal normal após paroxismo de TV) e batimentos de fusão (complexos QRS com morfologia intermediária, entre a dos sinusais e a dos ectópicos, devido à colisão elétrica intraventricular entre um batimento sinusal normal e um CVP); os dois últimos são diagnósticos de TV. Na TV, há ondas P (os átrios despolarizam, mas o estímulo é bloqueado no nodo AV, ou logo após, porque o ritmo mais rápido [TV] predomina nos ventrículos), mas em geral são sobrepostos por complexos QRS de base larga bizarros e ondas T. Dessa forma, a presença de ondas P em intervalos regulares, mas não fixos, associadas a complexos QRS é compatível com TV (Figura 248.17) – os átrios não "foram informados" da presença de TV. O diagnóstico baseado no ECG pode ser mais desafiador quando a TV é contínua, em particular se for de origem septal ou no VD; portanto, causa complexos QRS de base um tanto estreita que podem lembrar os complexos supraventriculares. Complexos QRS de base larga causados por outros fatores (ver discussão anterior sobre extrassístoles ventriculares) não devem ser confundidos com TV.

O tratamento de TV começa com a confirmação do diagnóstico no ECG (i. e., exclusão de outras causas de complexos QRS de base larga bizarros) e a identificação e o tratamento da causa primária. Devido ao risco de pró-arritmia de qualquer tratamento antiarrítmico e à falta de evidência de que a resolução da TV reduz significativamente o risco de morte em cães ou gatos acometidos, a eliminação dos fatores desencadeantes de TV deve ser considerada a primeira e mais definitiva forma de tratamento.[106] Quando não é possível eliminar a causa, a presença ou ausência de sinais clínicos evidentes causados pela TV (em especial síncope ou pré-síncope – falha episódica e desorientação, sem perda da consciência) justifica o tratamento antiarrítmico. Na ausência de tais sinais, os fármacos antiarrítmicos devem ser administrados se a TV for hemodinamicamente grave; por sua vez, isso em geral depende da frequência cardíaca (frequência ventricular) induzida pela TV. Uma abordagem por etapas e as dosagens e aplicações dos fármacos são mostradas na forma de algoritmo na Figura 248.16.

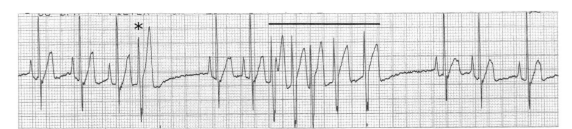

Figura 248.17 Taquicardia ventricular em um filhote de cão com 5 meses de idade, imediatamente após toracotomia e ligadura de ducto arterioso persistente. O ritmo sinusal normal e a arritmia sinusal respiratória são interrompidos por um complexo ventricular prematuro (*asterisco*) e em seguida uma série de 5 CVP monomórficos (com o mesmo formato), isto é, uma sequência de taquicardia ventricular. A arritmia se resolveu com o tratamento dos fatores desencadeantes (ver Figura 248.16). 25 mm/s, 1 cm = 1 mV.

Flutter ventricular. É um estágio muito rápido, em geral pré-fibrilatório, da TV. A percepção desse ritmo no ECG é a de uma série de ondas sinusoides altas, em intervalos curtos e idênticos, de modo que é impossível distinguir os complexos QRS das ondas T (Figura 248.18). Esse estágio intermediário, entre a TV e o FV, é raro, breve e melhora (reduz a TV, com ou sem conversão para RSN) ou progride para FV e parada cardíaca. É preciso diferenciar de artefato de movimento. O artefato que simula *flutter* ventricular mostra também evidência de atividade ventricular coordenada (complexos QRS normais dentro dos "impostores" do *flutter*) à inspeção próxima (Figura 248.19). O *flutter* ventricular é considerado uma arritmia ventricular grave e requer correção imediata das causas predisponentes (iniciando com a injeção IV de 2 mg de lidocaína/kg, na forma de *bolus*) e, possivelmente, desfibrilação elétrica (ver Capítulos 140 e 141).

Fibrilação ventricular (FibV). É um padrão desorganizado crônico terminal (fatal) de despolarizações ventriculares, que envolve dessincronização total da atividade elétrica ventricular. Em termos hemodinâmicos, acarreta colapso e parada circulatórios. Portanto, é um estado pré-agônico que leva à morte em questão de segundos a minutos. Na verdade, os ritmos cardíacos que definem parada cardíaca são FibV, assistolia e atividade elétrica sem pulso (notadamente TV sem pulso), não apenas assistolia.[107] A aparência da FibV no ECG consiste em ondas erráticas, sem um padrão, com morfologia, amplitude e frequência variáveis (Figura 248.20).

Por definição, a causa primária é uma anormalidade grave, como traumatismo miocárdico, anoxia, distúrbio eletrolítico grave e estados avançados de choque. Se o ECG indica suspeita de FibV, é preciso excluir imediatamente a possibilidade de artefato; a má conexão elétrica entre o paciente e as derivações do ECG pode simular uma FibV. A confirmação rápida de FibV consiste em: (1) aplicar álcool isopropílico na interface da pele com a derivação do ECG, para melhorar a condutividade (ajuda a excluir artefato); (2) avaliar a presença de arritmia em múltiplas derivações, não apenas na II; (3) sentir o pulso arterial (qualquer pulso palpável exclui FibV) e (4) notar se o paciente está inconsciente, porque a FibV é incompatível com perfusão cerebral adequada. A FibV, geralmente, é precedida, e portanto facilitada, por extrassístoles ventriculares (o que possivelmente representa a sobreposição da onda R à onda T), de modo que é possível que uma TV sustentada seja um *flutter* ventricular.[2] Infelizmente, o tratamento de CVP/TV com antiarrítmicos não reduz, de maneira confiável, o risco de FibV,[106] em vez disso, a causa primária e outros fatores desencadeantes, que podem ser arritmogênicos (hipopotassemia, anemia etc.), devem ser verificados e tratados devidamente. Quando o ritmo alcança valor de FibV, o tratamento (reanimação cardiopulmonar), embora não compensador, deve ser instituído imediatamente e em geral envolve desfibrilação elétrica, se disponível (ver Capítulos 140 e 141). A prevenção de FibV inicial ou sua recorrência pode ser obtida mediante o implante cirúrgico de um cardioversor-desfibrilador. Essa forma de terapia, bem mais efetiva e segura do que os medicamentos antiarrítmicos em pacientes humanos, vem ganhando interesse na medicina veterinária.[108,109]

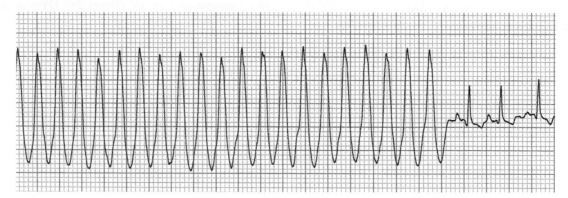

Figura 248.18 Taquicardia ventricular muito rápida, ou *flutter* ventricular, em um cão com miocardiopatia do ventrículo direito arritmogênica. A frequência cardíaca é de 320 bpm. Não são vistos complexos QRS e ondas T distinguíveis até os três últimos batimentos cardíacos, quando ocorre conversão do ritmo para taquicardia sinusal, na frequência de 180 bpm. Pode-se esperar que uma taquicardia rápida reduza acentuadamente o enchimento diastólico dos ventrículos, diminuindo o débito cardíaco e, em geral, ocasionando sinais clínicos, como síncope ou morte súbita (ver Vídeo 248.3). 25 mm/s, 1 cm = 1 mV.

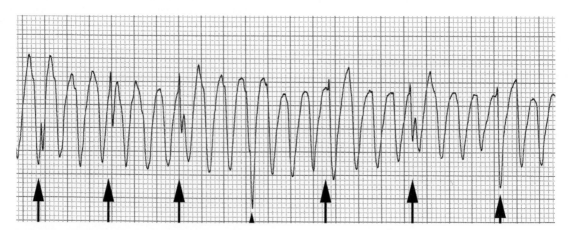

Figura 248.19 Artefato simulando taquicardia ventricular (TV), *flutter* ventricular ou hiperpotassemia grave. Essa é a aparência do ECG de respiração ofegante vigorosa, especialmente proeminente, em derivações precordiais como essa. O ritmo é sinusal normal. A inspeção próxima mostra ascensões positivas, estreitas e espaçadas (setas), que representam os complexos QRS sinusais normais emergindo através do artefato. Isso não seria visto na TV verdadeira, no *flutter* ventricular real ou na hiperpotassemia. Derivação V2, 25 mm/s, 1 cm = 1 mV.

Torsade de pointes **(TdP).** É uma arritmia ventricular que surge do prolongamento do intervalo Q-T.[110,111] A rotação dos picos dos complexos QRS no eixo horizontal do ECG deve-se à geometria sempre em mutação do circuito de reentrada, que oscila nos ventrículos. O diagnóstico de TdP baseia-se nos seguintes critérios: (1) o ritmo imediatamente anterior ao início da TdP é lento e o intervalo Q-T é prolongado (> 0,25 s no cão); (2) o início de TdP envolve uma extrassístole ventricular com sobreposição da onda R sobre a onda T (p. ex., ocorre despolarização [onda R] durante a fase vulnerável da onda T); (3) o ritmo ventricular rápido (> 180 bpm) que se segue aos complexos QRS é mais regular do que o verificado na FibV, mas sua amplitude e sua polaridade se alteram continuamente.

A duração total de um paroxismo de TdP que se resolve espontaneamente, em geral, é muito breve (5 a 10 segundos), mas pode persistir por mais tempo; em tais circunstâncias, pode progredir de maneira letal para FibV. TdP não é comumente detectada em cães; contudo, pode ser causada por qualquer anormalidade que prolongue o intervalo Q-T:[111] síndrome do intervalo Q-T longo congênita (em cães da raça Dálmata), hipopotassemia, hipocalcemia e dose excessiva ou intoxicação por antiarrítmicos, em particular da classe 1A, como a quinidina. O tratamento é altamente específico e requer a descontinuação de todos os antiarrítmicos e a administração intravenosa de sulfato de magnésio (administração por via intravenosa lenta de *bolus* de 20 a 60 mg/kg).[111]

Parassístole ventricular ("dois batimentos cardíacos como se fossem um"). É uma arritmia complexa que resulta da atividade concorrente e independente de dois marca-passos, um supraventricular normal e o outro em um local protegido em um ventrículo.[112] Por definição, a parassístole tem: (1) um foco ventricular com automaticidade anormal independente e uma frequência maior do que um foco de escape e (2) bloqueio unidirecional (entrada) que serve de escudo para esse foco de despolarizações sinusais. Na maioria das vezes, a parassístole é benigna, não requer tratamento antiarrítmico e costuma ser refratária a tal tratamento.

Dissociação atrioventricular isorrítmica (DAVI). É uma anormalidade do ritmo cardíaco na qual os átrios e ventrículos são comandados por marca-passos independentes, com frequências iguais ou quase iguais. Foi detectada em um grupo de 11 cães da raça Labrador Retriever, possivelmente relacionada com taquicardia juncional focal.[113] Os autores deste capítulo a têm observado com frequência mais desproporcional em cães da raça Samoieda, geralmente como um achado incidental (Figura 248.21). O achado característico no ECG consiste na presença de onda P no complexo QRS e até mesmo o precede (DAVI com sincronização do tipo I). Isso pode ocorrer periodicamente, com frequências atrial e ventricular idênticas ("enforcamento"), dando a aparência de sincronia AV.[113] Não se sabe se as implicações clínicas da DAVI são prejudiciais: não há associação comprovada com cardiopatia progressiva e, no momento, a DAVI é considerada um achado eletrocardiográfico casual.

Anormalidades da condução

As anormalidades que surgem de falhas na condução elétrica intracardíaca são denominadas, de maneira simples, como *bloqueios*, agrupados de acordo com critérios anatômicos e funcionais. Os primeiros se classificam de acordo com sua localização física: bloqueios SA, AV, BRF e fasciculares. Os critérios funcionais caracterizam os bloqueios de acordo com sua gravidade. Os de primeiro grau geram um retardo na condução; os de segundo grau causam bloqueio total, porém intermitente; e os de terceiro grau causam bloqueio total sustentado.

Bloqueio atrioventricular

Em um coração saudável, o nodo AV cumpre uma função importante de "porteiro", que ocasiona um atraso normal após cada batimento sinusal, possibilitando que os átrios finalizem a contração. O nodo AV também impede que estímulos atriais excessivos alcancem os ventrículos, nas taquicardias supraventriculares (ver texto anterior sobre fibrilação atrial). Essa função de filtro elétrico normal e vital ajuda a manter uma frequência

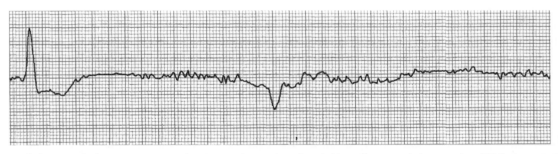

Figura 248.20 Fibrilação ventricular em um gato com síncope causada por miocardiopatia hipertrófica grave. Após o complexo QRS final, os ventrículos entram em fibrilação, produzindo uma ondulação fina na linha basal e nenhuma atividade sincronizada, ventricular ou atrial. O ritmo indica parada cardíaca e requer desfibrilação elétrica ou manutenção de reanimação no caso de morte humana. Um artefato de movimento externo explica a deflexão mais larga no meio do traçado. 25 mm/s, 1 cm = 1 mV.

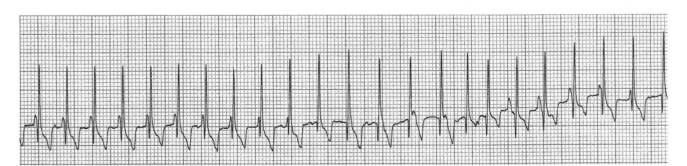

Figura 248.21 Dissociação atrioventricular isorrítmica em um cão da raça Samoieda. As ondas P e os complexos QRS estão estreitamente associados, mas o desvio de ondas P para dentro e para fora de complexos QRS indica ausência de sincronismo atrioventricular. Os marcos dessa arritmia são: complexo QRS de aparência supraventricular (de base estreita, positivo na derivação II) e frequências atrial e ventricular similares, mas não exatamente iguais. 25 mm/s, 1 cm = 1 mV.

cardíaca mais próximo do normal, quando ocorrem taquicardias supraventriculares, e esse efeito pode ser facilitado, se necessário, com o uso de medicamentos dromotrópicos negativos (retardam a condução no nodo AV), conforme descrito anteriormente, no tratamento de FibA. Contudo, a função do nodo AV pode ser excessiva ou extrema, dificultando a passagem de estímulos sinusais normais. A falha na condução AV normal, a partir dos átrios para os ventrículos, denomina-se *bloqueio AV* e sua relevância clínica depende das características descritas a seguir.

Bloqueio AV de primeiro grau. É simplesmente um retardo na condução AV, mais lenta que o normal; porém, cada estímulo consegue passar pelo nodo. Pode ser permanente ou transitório e ser decorrência de uma lesão estrutural ou ser meramente funcional. No ECG, o diagnóstico baseia-se na constatação de complexos QRS sinusais de aparência normal e intervalos P-R prolongados. Não há manifestação clínica; o bloqueio AV de primeiro grau é apenas um achado no ECG que não acarreta sinais clínicos evidentes, tampouco requer tratamento, devendo levar o clínico a ficar atento para causas possíveis de alto tônus vagal que, em geral, são fisiológicas e ocasionalmente podem ser tóxicas (p. ex., intoxicação causada por glicosídeos digitálicos). O bloqueio AV de primeiro grau não progride para bloqueio de segundo ou terceiro graus, exceto nos casos de intoxicação medicamentosa.

Bloqueio AV de segundo grau. Consiste na interrupção total (porém transitória) da condução AV. Portanto, há uma onda P para cada complexo QRS, mas não há um complexo QRS para cada onda P. Há dois subtipos importantes de bloqueio AV de segundo grau.[28] O primeiro, Mobitz do tipo I, caracteriza-se por um prolongamento progressivo do intervalo P-R até que, por fim, uma onda P é bloqueada (onda P sem complexo QRS), condição conhecida como *fenômeno de Wenckebach*. Em termos anatômicos, o bloqueio AV de segundo grau Mobitz do tipo I se origina na parte superior do nodo AV e diz-se que tem um bom prognóstico, pois está estreitamente relacionado ao bloqueio AV de primeiro grau e quase nunca causa sinais clínicos (Figura 248.22).

Em contraste, no segundo subtipo, bloqueio AV de segundo grau Mobitz tipo II, notam-se intervalos P-R perfeitamente regulares, até que uma ou mais ondas P seja(m) bloqueada(s) (Figura 248.22). Tal bloqueio surge do feixe AV e diz-se que seu prognóstico é mais reservado a ruim, pois lembra mais um bloqueio AV de terceiro grau. Entretanto, não há evidência objetiva que corrobore essa extrapolação da gravidade dos bloqueios Mobitz tipos I e II constatada na cardiologia humana para pacientes veterinários. No bloqueio AV de segundo grau Mobitz tipo II "simples", ocorre mais condução do que bloqueio de ondas P, enquanto no bloqueio AV de segundo grau Mobitz tipo II "avançado" ou "de alto grau" (como na Figura 248.22), ocorre o contrário. A presença ou ausência de sinais clínicos parece estar relacionada com a frequência ventricular. Em termos específicos, cães com bloqueio AV de segundo grau Mobitz tipo II têm uma expectativa de vida não diferente de cães com bloqueio AV de terceiro grau, e a implantação de marca-passo melhora de maneira significativa a sobrevida em ambos os grupos, independentemente da presença ou ausência de sinais clínicos associados à bradicardia.[28]

Portanto, os bloqueios AV de segundo grau Mobitz tipo I e tipo II simples raramente acarretam manifestações clínicas, como intolerância ao exercício, enquanto o bloqueio Mobitz tipo II mais avançado, por bloquear mais estímulos no nodo AV e resultar em frequência ventricular mais baixa, comumente ocasiona sinais clínicos semelhantes aos do bloqueio AV de terceiro grau: fraqueza, letargia, síncope e convulsões hipóxico-anóxicas de Stoke-Adams (convulsões verdadeiras causadas por hipoperfusão cerebral crítica induzida por bradicardia),[114] mesmo com exercício mínimo. A presença de tais sinais clínicos

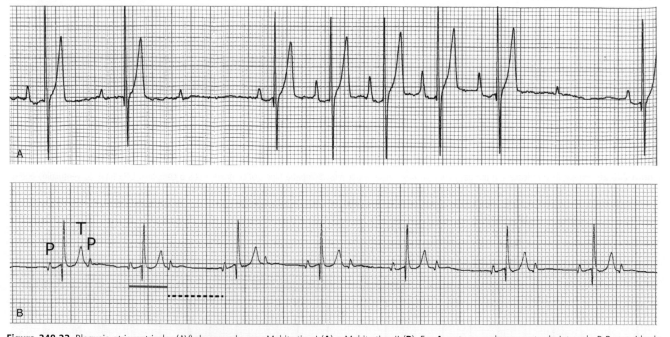

Figura 248.22 Bloqueio atrioventricular (AV) de segundo grau Mobitz tipo I (**A**) e Mobitz tipo II (**B**). Em **A**, nota-se prolongamento do intervalo P-R, seguido de bloqueio AV; então, o ritmo sinusal normal se restabelece, com intervalo P-R normal, até que ocorram, novamente, prolongamento de P-R e bloqueio. Essa condição é considerada uma variante fisiológica não prejudicial (*i. e.*, manifestação de alto tônus vagal). A alteração na onda P alta reflete um marca-passo errante (ver Figura 248.4), outra manifestação de alto tônus vagal. Em **B**, o estímulo atrial é bloqueado, sem prolongamento do intervalo P-R precedente. Em termos específicos, é um bloqueio 2:1; há duas ondas P para cada onda conduzida. As causas incluem etiologias farmacológicas (p. ex., agonistas alfa-2), fisiológicas (menos comumente) e patológicas (p. ex., fibrose do nodo AV). A frequência ventricular resultante é de 70 bpm. Dependendo da progressão – em especial para 3:1, 4:1 ou níveis mais altos de bloqueio – e da presença de sinais clínicos, tais pacientes podem precisar da implantação de marca-passo. Note que a arritmia sinusal ventriculofásica é um achado casual: em vez de um intervalo P-P constante em todo o traçado, o intervalo P-P ao lado dos complexos QRS (*linha contínua*) é mais curto que aquele verificado durante o bloqueio (*linha tracejada*). Derivação II, 25 mm/s, 1 cm = 1 mV.

e a frequência ventricular são os determinantes principais de o paciente precisar ou não de tratamento (implantação de marca-passo, ver Capítulo 249).

Bloqueio AV de terceiro grau. É o bloqueio AV total, com interrupção sustentada da condução AV. Os ventrículos despolarizam de acordo com um ritmo independente, lento e irregular, denominado *ritmo de escape* (juncional ou ventricular; ver a seguir) (Figura 248.23 e Vídeo 248.4). É importante reconhecer a atuação salva-vidas do ritmo de escape ventricular, porque ele previne assistolia. Portanto, ainda que os complexos QRS de escape ventricular sejam de base larga e bizarros, o tratamento antiarrítmico está absolutamente contraindicado.

No bloqueio AV de terceiro grau, não há comunicação elétrica entre os átrios e ventrículos (dissociação AV completa). Portanto, o diagnóstico ao ECG baseia-se na ausência total de condução da onda P (as ondas P ocorrem em intervalo P-R constante, mas não são seguidas imediatamente e de maneira consistente por complexos QRS; não há repetição do intervalo P-R) e no ritmo ventricular lento, regular (intervalo R-R constante), e os complexos QRS em geral têm morfologia uniforme, porém são bizarros e apresentam base ampla. É comum os bloqueios AV de terceiro grau causarem intolerância acentuada ao exercício, fraqueza e síncope. Ainda assim, é possível encontrar animais idosos, não muito ativos por natureza, com bloqueio AV de terceiro grau e "assintomáticos"; a implantação de marca-passo pode revelar de maneira retrospectiva a extensão e a duração dos sinais clínicos, quando o paciente exibe uma melhora substancial na tolerância ao exercício e vigor, no domicílio, no pós-operatório. Em gatos, especialmente, pode haver bloqueio de terceiro grau com um ritmo de escape ventricular apenas minimamente inferior ao ritmo cardíaco sinusal normal no domicílio (p. ex., 110 a 140 bpm) e o bloqueio ser um achado casual (Figura 248.23).[3,5,115]

As causas de bloqueios AV são diversas. Os de primeiro grau e segundo graus Mobitz tipo I em geral são funcionais (alto tônus vagal de indivíduos sadios; efeitos dromotrópicos negativos de digitálicos, antiarrítmicos ou sedativos estimulantes alfa-2); portanto, são variantes fisiológicas normais ou se resolvem com a interrupção da administração do fármaco. Raramente, pode haver cardiopatia com dilatação atrial e lesões no nodo AV como causa de um bloqueio AV de primeiro ou de segundo grau Mobitz tipo I. Os bloqueios AV de segundo grau Mobitz tipo II e os de terceiro grau às vezes são funcionais (hiperpotassemia, intoxicação por digitálicos, agonistas do receptor alfa-2, como a dexmedetomidina), porém mais comumente estão associados a uma lesão estrutural, seja inflamatória (endocardite, miocardite de Lyme, miocardite traumática) ou degenerativa (ruptura física do nodo AV, que acontece em decorrência de miocardiopatia, endocardiose ou fibrose).[116-118] Em cães, o bloqueio AV de terceiro grau em geral é considerado irreversível, mas mostrou-se que se resolveu espontaneamente ao RSN em 7% dos casos e reverteu para bloqueio AVF em 5% dos casos.[119]

O tratamento de bloqueio AV visa à causa primária, sempre que possível. No bloqueio AV de segundo grau Mobitz tipo II ou de terceiro grau, a resposta a fármacos parassimpaticolíticos ou simpatomiméticos tende a ser ineficaz porque esses agentes não revertem o processo mórbido do nodo AV, nem costumam impedir o bloqueio AV até um nível que tenha significado clínico.[28] A implantação de um marca-passo (ver Capítulo 249 e Vídeo 248.4) é mais efetiva e resulta em uma sobrevida bem

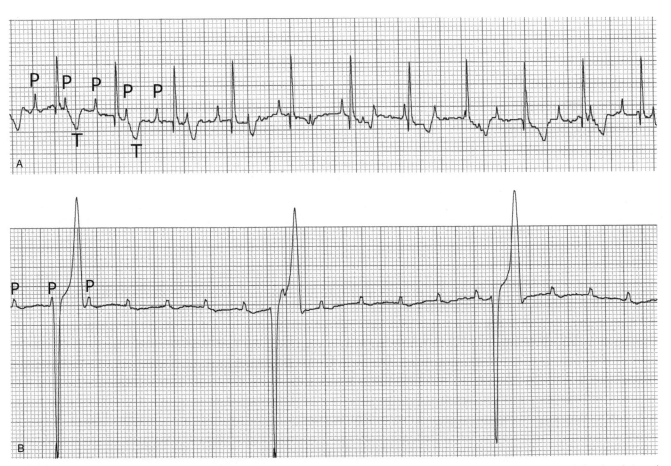

Figura 248.23 Bloqueio atrioventricular (AV) de terceiro grau em um gato (**A**) e um cão (**B**). Em ambas as circunstâncias, os átrios e ventrículos despolarizam de forma independente. Nos dois traçados, os intervalos P-P e R-R (ritmo de escape) também são constantes. A principal diferença está no ritmo de escape ventricular. Como em geral se observa em gatos com bloqueio AV de terceiro grau, o ritmo ventricular é rápido para um ritmo de escape (**A**. 120 bpm), enquanto em cães costuma ser muito mais lento (**B**. 30 bpm). Ambos os traçados: derivação II, 25 mm/s, 1 cm = 1 mV.

mais longa: a taxa de sobrevida de 1 ano para cães com bloqueio AV de alto grau, segundo ou terceiro, que recebem marca-passo é de 80 a 85%, em comparação com 50 a 55% para aqueles que não recebem marca-passo, e a de 2 anos é de 70 a 75% *versus* 30 a 35%, respectivamente.[28]

É importante ressaltar que a decisão de implantar um marca-passo pode ser um dilema aos proprietários que questionam se o cão idoso está chegando ao fim de sua vida natural porque ele "tem mostrado sinais de envelhecimento". Tais proprietários devem entender que esses sinais, em geral, foram as manifestações progressivas da bradicardia, não do envelhecimento, e a implantação do marca-passo – não sendo uma panaceia – pode resultar em uma qualidade de vida que os proprietários não viam em seus cães havia meses ou anos. Portanto, comorbidades (p. ex., doença renal crônica), sinais inespecíficos e idade avançada, embora relevantes para o paciente, devem ser vistos como situações em que a implantação de um marca-passo poderia ajudar, não como razões para ignorar o procedimento.

Gatos com bloqueio AV de terceiro grau apresentam características distintas de importância clínica. Muitos deles (11% de 18; 61%, em uma série de casos)[115] têm cardiopatias estruturais subjacentes, como miocardiopatia, que não serão revertidas com a implantação de um marca-passo. As frequências ventriculares de escape se aproximam do RSN (80 a 140, com média de 120 bpm, em uma série de casos),[115] de modo que o bloqueio AV de terceiro grau pode ser um achado casual em gatos. A sobrevida sem marca-passo pode ser surpreendentemente longa (em média, 386 dias; variação: 1 a 2.013 dias, em uma série de casos),[115] quaisquer que sejam os sintomas presentes.

Bloqueios de ramos do feixe

Os bloqueios de ramos do feixe (BRF) são retardos ou interrupções da condução que envolvem um ou mais ramos ventriculares do feixe de His. Os bloqueios podem ser funcionais (interrupções transitórias decorrentes de despolarização que ocorre durante o período refratário) ou estruturais (interrupções permanentes causadas por uma anormalidade física). O diagnóstico de BRF no ECG baseia-se no formato anormal dos complexos QRS, que se apresentam com base mais larga devido à dessincronização dos dois ventrículos. Não podem ser considerados arritmias porque não alteram o ritmo do batimento cardíaco; portanto, o diagnóstico ao ECG é estabelecido como "ritmo" (p. ex., sinusal normal "com bloqueio de ramo [direito ou esquerdo] do feixe" (ou "padrão de BRF"). A duração dos complexos QRS é > 0,07 s em cães com BRF (> 0,04 s em gatos com BRF) e a polaridade é positiva na derivação II, no caso de BRF esquerdo, e negativa na mesma derivação, no BRF direito[111] (Figuras 248.24 e 248.25).

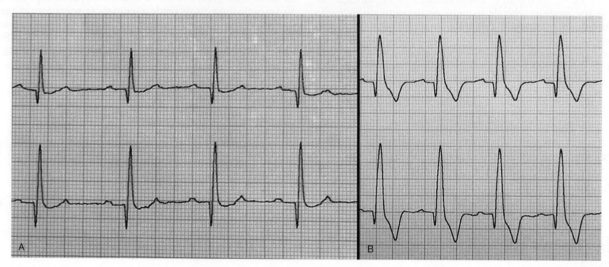

Figura 248.24 Ritmo sinusal normal sem **(A)** e com **(B)** bloqueio de ramo do feixe esquerdo. A principal diferença está na largura dos complexos QRS (0,09 s no painel **B**), que excede a variação normal para cães (até 0,06 s). O painel **A** foi obtido antes do tratamento com doxorrubicina para a neoplasia desse cão. O painel B foi obtido após dose cumulativa por toda a vida, de 150 mg/m², quantidade que às vezes pode estar associada à cardiotoxicose. Ambos os traçados: derivações I e II, 25 mm/s, 1 cm = 1 mV. (Cortesia da Dra. Glenna Mauldin, Animal Cancer Centre, Western Veterinary Specialist and Emergency Centre, Calgary, AB, Canadá.)

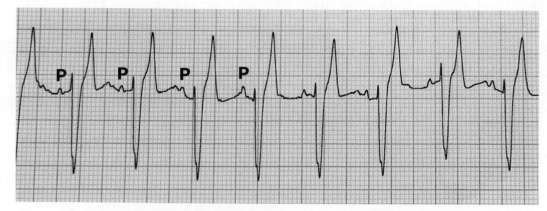

Figura 248.25 Ritmo sinusal normal com bloqueio do ramo direito do feixe (BRDF) em um cão com avaliação cardiovascular normal. Em cães, um BRDF detectado de maneira casual é considerado uma variante normal, sem consequências clinicamente relevantes. Os complexos QRS de base ampla e bizarros podem ser mal interpretados como CVP, se a associação entre a onda P e cada complexo QRS, em intervalo P-R constante, passar despercebida. Derivação II, 25 mm/s, 1 cm = 1 mV. (Cortesia da Dra. Glenna Mauldin, Animal Cancer Centre, Western Veterinary Specialist and Emergency Centre, Calgary, AB, Canadá.)

Caso ocorra BRF durante um ritmo sinusal, o diagnóstico no ECG é direto porque, além da aparência muito anormal dos complexos QRS, a sequência P-QRS-T é normal em todo o traçado do ECG. Ocorre uma onda P antes de cada QRS, e o intervalo P-R é constante e normal. Ainda assim, é preciso cuidado para identificar corretamente o ritmo como sinusal normal e evitar o diagnóstico errôneo de TV, com base apenas nos complexos QRS largos e bizarros. Se ocorrer bloqueio concomitantemente a um ritmo não sinusal, como na FibA, pode ser um desafio maior estabelecer o diagnóstico de BRF (ver Figura 248.12). Um BRF simultâneo a FibA simula extrassístoles ventriculares ou TV, o que pode interferir nas decisões terapêuticas (ver discussão anterior sobre fibrilação atrial). Gatos com cardiopatia (em especial miocardiopatia) são descritos classicamente como propensos a desenvolver bloqueio em um subtipo de REF denominado *fascículo anterior esquerdo* (FAE).[5] Essa observação eletrocardiográfica é confirmada pelo achado histológico em 63 corações de gatos com miocardiopatia em que 54 feixes esquerdos (86%) mostraram degeneração, fibrose, metaplasia óssea e outras lesões, em comparação com 20 feixes diretos (32%).[121] O bloqueio do FAE produz uma onda R alta na derivação I e na aVL e uma onda S profunda nas derivações II, III e aVF, portanto, um desvio do eixo esquerdo.[122]

As causas de BRF são muitas, porque os BRF podem ser decorrentes de uma variedade de alterações patológicas, incluindo hipertrofia concêntrica (como se observa na miocardiopatia hipertrófica),[121] dilatação (como se vê na miocardiopatia dilatada) e inflamação (endocardite, miocardite traumática). No cão, em geral, o bloqueio do ramo direito do feixe (RDF) é completamente normal, não necessariamente um achado preocupante no ECG. Em contrapartida, o BRFE quase sempre está associado ao aumento do ventrículo esquerdo (ver Figura 248.24). Manifestações clínicas isoladas de BRFs geralmente não ocorrem.[120,122] Esses distúrbios, portanto, não justificam tratamento específico além do problema subjacente, se houver. A importância de reconhecer o BRF está no fato de que o BRFE pode ser o primeiro indicador de cardiopatia primária que, em si, requer diagnóstico adicional e tratamento, além da possibilidade de ser interpretado erroneamente – o que não deve acontecer – como arritmias ventriculares.

Parada atrial (silêncio atrial)

É uma anormalidade do ritmo que se caracteriza pala ausência total de despolarização atrial (Figura 248.26). Os três diagnósticos diferenciais para parada atrial são: (1) hiperpotassemia moderada a acentuada ($K^+ > 7,5$ mEq/ℓ; ver discussão adiante), (2) miopatia atrial e (3) artefato no ECG (ondas P muito pequenas, ou isoelétricas, o que impede que sejam vistas da maneira apropriada). Embora a hiperpotassemia seja a causa mais comum de parada atrial (e a única reversível), pode ocorrer parada atrial devido a estiramento atrial acentuado,[123] como

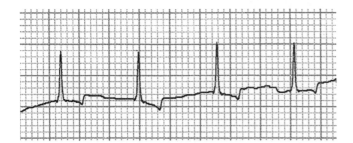

Figura 248.26 Parada atrial em um cão de 10 anos de idade da raça Labrador Retriever. Não se constata onda P nessa derivação, nem elas estavam presentes em qualquer outra derivação. O ritmo é regular, em frequência de 120 bpm. A causa mais provável é hiperpotassemia, que pode ser potencialmente fatal, mas foi excluída ao se detectar uma concentração sérica de potássio normal nesse cão. Portanto, por exclusão, o diagnóstico é miopatia atrial. Derivação II, 25 mm/s, 1 cm = 1 mV.

acontece particularmente em gatos com várias formas de miocardiopatia, ou hipoplasia do parênquima atrial, como se observa em associação com uma forma distrófica de neuromiopatia, em particular em cães da raça Springer Spaniel. Qualquer que seja a causa, a aparência no ECG é de um ritmo regular (intervalo R-R constante), em geral com complexos QRS com aparência supraventricular e frequência normal ou baixa, mas sem onda P detectável em qualquer derivação do ECG. A diferenciação entre as duas causas principais desse ritmo apenas no ECG é difícil, sendo indispensável a mensuração imediata da concentração sérica de potássio.

Dissociação eletromecânica

Em termos estritos, a dissociação eletromecânica (DEM) não é uma anormalidade do ritmo cardíaco. A DEM se refere à falha de conversão de um ritmo elétrico em forças mecânicas de sístole e diástole.[124,125] Portanto, o ECG pode mostrar praticamente qualquer ritmo; o diagnóstico se baseia na combinação de um paciente em colapso hemodinâmico com um ECG que mostra qualquer ritmo, porém com assistolia. Em geral, o pulso arterial é pouco perceptível ou ausente, o paciente costuma estar inconsciente e a DEM mais comumente é uma pré-parada ou uma condição terminal. O tratamento requer a correção das causas primárias, se possível, e em seguida visa aumentar a circulação para melhorar a perfusão do miocárdio (ver Capítulos 140 e 141). Como geralmente a DEM indica hipoxia miocárdica intensa, o prognóstico é ruim, qualquer que seja o tratamento.

Distúrbios complexos que envolvem anormalidades da excitabilidade e da condução

Efeitos cardíacos de anormalidades sistêmicas do potássio e do cálcio

Como a atividade cardíaca depende fundamentalmente dos movimentos dos íons através da membrana, concentrações sistêmicas patologicamente altas ou baixas de potássio e cálcio podem ocasionar distúrbios na função cardíaca, com efeitos importantes no ritmo do coração.

Hipopotassemia. A mensuração da concentração sérica de potássio é mais acurada se realizada em amostra de sangue obtida em tubo contendo heparina de lítio (tampa verde). Tubo com tampa roxa contém EDTA tripotássico, que dá ao teste um resultado falsamente elevado, incompatível com a vida, e tubo com tampa vermelha possibilita coagulação, processo que, durante a ativação e a agregação de plaquetas, libera potássio e pode causar pequena elevação de potássio, porém de relevância clínica significativa.

A concentração sérica baixa de potássio tem dois efeitos principais nos cardiomiócitos. Primeiro, torna o potencial de repouso da membrana cada vez mais negativo (Figura 248.27),[126,127] o que diminui a excitabilidade dos miócitos. Tal efeito se deve à maior diferença entre as concentrações inter e extracelular de potássio, na hipopotassemia, em comparação com a normocalemia (hiperpolarização); nos cardiomiócitos, em geral, é brando e transitório. Em segundo lugar, a hipopotassemia prolonga a repolarização, aumentando a duração do potencial de ação.[126,127] A repolarização do miócito depende, principalmente, da atividade das correntes de potássio, de maneira notável os canais retificadores tardios $I_{k,r}$ e $I_{k,s}$. Na vigência de hipopotassemia, essas correntes atuam mais lentamente. Esse prolongamento da repolarização prolonga o período normalmente muito breve de repolarização durante o qual o potencial de membrana diastólico se aproxima do potencial limiar. Portanto, o prolongamento da repolarização induzido pela hipopotassemia abre uma "janela" de maior excitabilidade durante a qual pode ocorrer atividade ectópica espontânea (como extrassístoles atriais ou ventriculares), dependendo do limiar alcançado após o período refratário absoluto por uma célula em repolarização lenta. Em termos clínicos, o segundo efeito (arritmogênico) predomina sobre o primeiro (supressivo) e o efeito cardiovascular

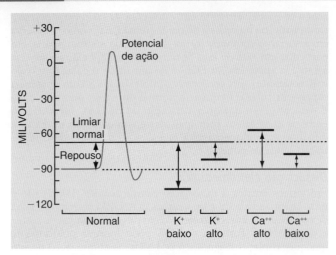

Figura 248.27 Efeitos de concentrações anormais de cálcio e potássio nas características da membrana celular em tecidos excitáveis. A concentração de potássio no líquido extracelular influencia o potencial de repouso, enquanto a concentração de cálcio no líquido extracelular interfere no potencial limiar. Igualmente ou mais importantes, embora não mostrados aqui, são os efeitos dessas anormalidades na repolarização. (Reproduzida, com autorização, de Leaf A, Cotran R: *Renal pathophysiology*, New York, 1976, Oxford University Press, p. 116.)

dominante de uma concentração sérica de potássio < 3,5 mEq/ℓ em cães e gatos é um risco maior de despolarizações espontâneas, notavelmente extrassístoles ventriculares (CVP). Outras manifestações de hipopotassemia no ECG podem incluir evidência de repolarização anormal prolongada na forma de ondas U, prolongamento do intervalo Q-T e dissociação AV.[128]

Como os antiarrítmicos da classe I (p. ex., lidocaína, mexiletina, quinidina) atuam nos canais de sódio, que requerem concentração sérica normal de potássio para funcionar, a hipopotassemia também é importante causa de refratariedade a tais fármacos: um paciente cujos CVP sejam causados por hipopotassemia em geral retornam ao ritmo sinusal normal apenas com suplementação de potássio, enquanto é improvável que o tratamento com lidocaína durante hipopotassemia altere a arritmia ventricular, podendo, ainda, causar intoxicação por lidocaína (distúrbios neurológicos, como convulsões), se a dose for administrada repetidas vezes, por não haver conversão para o ritmo sinusal. Essa observação importante tem implicações bastante diversas em pacientes com hipopotassemia por diluição (p. ex., paciente com a síndrome vólvulo-dilatação gástrica que recebe grande volume de líquido para reanimação) ou doença metabólica com perda de potássio (p. ex., doença renal crônica), quando ocorre CVP/TV e surge a questão: "Quando devo tratar essa arritmia com antiarrítmico?". Uma etapa inicial importante no sentido de responder a tal pergunta deve ser assegurar sempre que haja normocalemia, antes de iniciar o uso de antiarrítmico. A taxa de segurança máxima de infusão IV de cloreto de potássio é 0,5 mEq/kg/h (ver Capítulo 68).

Hiperpotassemia. Concentração sérica ligeiramente elevada de potássio (5,6 a 6,5 mEq/ℓ) está associada a maior permeabilidade da membrana celular ao potássio, durante a repolarização. Tal efeito na repolarização predomina sobre aquele que interfere na despolarização, mostrado na Figura 248.27; a hiperpotassemia discreta foi descrita como uma condição que estabiliza o ritmo cardíaco. Portanto, a hiperpotassemia em cães pode refletir-se no ECG como repolarização ventricular mais rápida (i. e., intervalo Q-T mais curto que o normal e onda T anormalmente estreita, em geral com picos ou na forma de "tenda").[126,127,129,129a] É um erro comum, porém grave, pensar que essa onda T representa sempre hiperpotassemia: em uma série de casos que abrangeu 205 cães com hipoadrenocorticismo, muitos apresentavam hipopotassemia, mas apenas 15% deles tinham ondas T em forma de "tenda" (altas, estreitas).[130] Similarmente, dentre 37 cães ou gatos com hiperpotassemia de ocorrência natural, apenas 2 (5%) tiveram ondas T altas,[131] e ambos apresentavam hiperpotassemia maior do que o esperado ante esse achado no ECG ([K⁺] sérica = 7 a 9,99 mEq/ℓ). O inverso também pode ocorrer: muitos cães sadios podem ter parâmetros de onda T que excedem a variação normal. Portanto, anormalidades da amplitude da onda T são parâmetros carentes de sensibilidade e especificidade e, particularmente nos casos de hipoadrenocorticismo, devem ser considerados "um grão de sal no oceano".

Pode ocorrer bradicardia sinusal (33% dos cães com hiperpotassemia e hipoadrenocorticismo), porque a hiperpotassemia diminui a atividade do marca-passo do tecido normal. Em termos específicos, diminui a inclinação da fase 4 da despolarização diastólica,[126] que reduz a frequência cardíaca. No entanto, também é comum a coexistência de hiperpotassemia de ocorrência natural com anormalidades no equilíbrio acidobásico ou alteração nas concentrações séricas de outros eletrólitos, dor, medo, sepse, hipovolemia e outros distúrbios, todos com tendência a causar o oposto – taquicardia sinusal. A observação rotineira de que muitos gatos e cães com hiperpotassemia, mesmo aquela grave, têm frequências cardíacas elevadas torna sua interpretação não confiável como inferência da concentração de potássio [K⁺] no soro sanguíneo de um paciente.[131,132]

Aumentos discretos a moderados na concentração sérica de potássio (6,6 a 7,5 mEq/ℓ) podem começar a interferir na velocidade de transmissão de uma célula para outra nos ventrículos. Em cães com hiperpotassemia decorrente de hipoadrenocorticismo, são observados complexos QRS largos em 32% dos casos.[130] Foi relatada uma diminuição na amplitude da onda R em 47% desses cães.

A hiperpotassemia moderada a grave (7 a > 8,5 mEq/ℓ) pode causar prolongamento do intervalo P-R (45%) ou ausência simultânea de ondas P (47% de um total de 92% de cães com hiperpotassemia e hipoadrenocorticismo), provavelmente os achados em ECG mais característicos de hiperpotassemia.[130] Os átrios são mais sensíveis à hiperpotassemia que os ventrículos e, neles, o miocárdio é mais sensível aos efeitos da hiperpotassemia que os tratos internodais. O resultado da hiperpotassemia grave é um *ritmo sinoventricular*, assim denominado porque o batimento cardíaco se origina no nodo SA, como de hábito, cruza os átrios através dos tratos internodais (mas o estímulo não se propaga para fora – sem ativação atrial, sem ondas P) e, em seguida, passa pelo nodo AV e o sistema His-Purkinje na sequência habitual. A aparência no ECG é a de um ritmo regular, com complexos QRS normais ou ligeiramente mais largos e ausência de ondas P em todas as derivações.

Concentração sérica de potássio muito alta (> 8,5 mEq/ℓ) pode ser fatal. São tantos os outros fatores que influenciam o ritmo cardíaco desses pacientes com doença gravíssima, que é impossível estabelecer um ponto de corte exato, em termos de letalidade, para a concentração sérica de potássio isoladamente. No caso de alta concentração, os complexos QRS e a onda T são ainda mais largos, podendo misturar-se em uma espécie de sino ondulado de ritmo pouco funcional ou até mesmo não funcional, ou um ritmo de escape do tipo ventricular em uma frequência muito baixa (ambos, provavelmente, ritmos pré-agônicos). Se não for corrigida imediatamente, a hiperpotassemia crítica que resultou nessas alterações gravíssimas no ECG pode causar parada cardíaca (fibrilação ventricular, ritmo de escape com dissociação eletromecânica) em questão de minutos (ver Capítulos 140 e 141).

Hipocalcemia. A baixa concentração sérica de cálcio induz efeitos cardíacos modestos e, em geral, clinicamente irrelevantes; em vez disso, no quadro clínico há predomínio dos efeitos sobre os músculos esqueléticos. A alteração da concentração sérica de cálcio afeta mais o limiar do potencial de ação dos miócitos do que o potencial de membrana em repouso (ver Figura 248.27).

A hipocalcemia diminui o limiar, facilitando a despolarização. A manifestação clínica consiste em discretas fasciculações dos músculos esqueléticos que progridem para tremores generalizados se concentração de cálcio não for normalizada. Tal efeito é mínimo nos cardiomiócitos. A hipocalcemia também prolonga a fase inicial da repolarização ventricular, podendo manifestar-se como um prolongamento do intervalo Q-T no ECG.[126]

Esses efeitos ajudam a explicar por que a administração intravenosa de cálcio é considerada "cardioprotetora" na hiperpotassemia grave, ainda que não possam alterar a concentração circulante de potássio. A hiperpotassemia aumenta o potencial de repouso da membrana (ver Figura 248.27) e, ao proporcionar cálcio adicional, eleva o limiar de despolarização, restabelecendo um gradiente iônico mais normal através da membrana celular. Considerando que 75% dos gatos com obstrução de uretra apresentam, simultaneamente, hipocalcemia discreta, moderada ou grave,[133] a administração por via intravenosa de gliconato de cálcio (infusão intravenosa lenta de 50 mg/kg, em um período de 10 a 30 minutos, até obter o efeito desejado) é um tratamento de primeira linha lógico para a hiperpotassemia nesses pacientes.

Ao administrar cálcio IV (sempre como infusão lenta e com monitoramento do ECG), às vezes os parâmetros do ECG atribuídos à hipercalcemia podem ser usados como marcadores de infusão excessivamente rápida. Uma redução súbita da frequência cardíaca, encurtamento do intervalo Q-T ou o aparecimento de extrassístoles ventriculares são justificativas para interromper a infusão e voltar a fazê-la depois, se necessário. Nesse caso, como ocorre na hiperpotassemia, o ECG é particularmente útil porque seus registros são obtidos por ocasião da admissão, possibilitando determinar se os parâmetros do paciente se modificam durante o tratamento em comparação com os valores basais.

Hipercalcemia. Similarmente, em geral, a hipercalcemia é mais preocupante devido aos seus efeitos extracardíacos que por qualquer alteração no ritmo cardíaco. A hipercalcemia grave aumenta o limiar do cardiomiócito, o que pode dificultar a despolarização. Ela também encurta a repolarização ventricular inicial, tornando mais curto o intervalo Q-T.[126,134] Tais consequências da hipercalcemia grave são preocupações secundárias em comparação com a desmineralização distrófica dos rins e de outros tecidos moles, por exemplo.

Síndromes de pré-excitação e macrorreentrada

Na pré-excitação, o estímulo normal originário do nodo SA é dividido no fim da despolarização atrial; parte dele segue normalmente através do nodo AV e parte segue, simultaneamente, através de um segmento anormal de fibras de condução rápida que liga os átrios e os ventrículos (a *via acessória* ou *ramo do circuito de reentrada*), desviando assim do nodo AV. O resultado é a ativação imediata, prematura e parcial dos ventrículos através do trato de desvio, sem o benefício de uma pausa no nodo AV, isto é, pré-excitação. Com uma exceção importante (ver adiante), o efeito desse padrão anormal de ativação é mínimo, porque ocorre perda apenas parcial da contribuição atrial ao enchimento do ventrículo. O ECG mostra que o retardo normal através do nodo AV foi antecipado pela condução através do ramo do circuito de reentrada (um segmento pequeno, ou nenhum, separa a onda P do complexo QRS) e aquela condução através do ramo do circuito de reentrada causa ativação sincrônica dos ventrículos (a condução pelo ramo do circuito de reentrada e pelo nodo AV normal acaba por compartilhar a ativação dos ventrículos), o que resulta em um entalhe no complexo QRS. O tamanho e a localização do entalhe no complexo QRS, a *onda delta*, dependem da distância que separa o ramo do circuito de reeentrada e o nodo AV no coração do indivíduo (Figura 248.28). Em geral, esses ramos do circuito são únicos, mas podem ser múltiplos, e a maioria se origina no átrio direito, não no esquerdo, em cães,[135] o que os torna mais acessíveis à ablação por meio de radiofrequência.

Em circunstâncias habituais, a pré-excitação é um achado casual subclínico. Todavia, em indivíduos com ela, uma despolarização prematura pode iniciar um ciclo de macrorreentrada capaz de ocasionar taquicardia extremamente súbita e persistente. Embora os ramos do circuito de reentrada conduzam estímulos rapidamente, seu período refratário costuma ser mais longo que o do nodo AV. Portanto, o momento de despolarização supraventricular prematura pode falhar no sentido de conduzir o estímulo através do nodo AV, despolarizando normalmente os ventrículos. À medida que o estímulo completa a despolarização dos ventrículos, o ramo do circuito de reentrada causa repolarização, sendo capaz de conduzir o estímulo. Em geral, os ramos do circuito de reentrada podem conduzir estímulos em outra

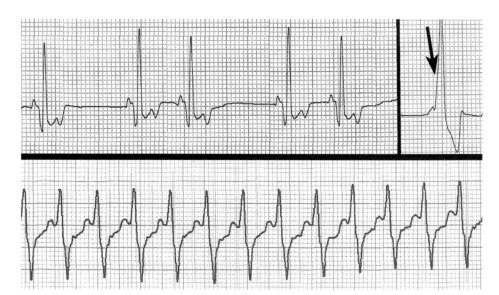

Figura 248.28 Pré-excitação e macrorreentrada. O intervalo P-R é anormalmente curto nesse cão da raça Golden Retriever adulto (*traçado superior*). Também se nota uma onda delta, mais bem observada na derivação V2 (*detalhe* do traçado superior, que mostra com maior clareza o encurtamento do intervalo P-R). O diagnóstico é arritmia sinusal respiratória, com evidência de pré-excitação ventricular. A frequência cardíaca é de 90 bpm. Derivação II, 25 mm/s, 1 cm = 1 mV. O mesmo cão foi hospitalizado devido ao início súbito de taquicardia grave, detectada pelo proprietário (*traçado inferior*). O traçado mostra uma taquicardia monomórfica de complexo largo, com frequência cardíaca de 330 bpm. Juntamente com o achado de pré-excitação no ECG basal, o diagnóstico mais provável é taquicardia com macrorreentrada. O intervalo P-R curto durante a taquicardia é incomum na síndrome de Wolff-Parkinson-White (taquicardia atrioventricular reentrante ortodrômica). Derivação precordial modificada (monitoramento em cuidado intensivo), 50 mm/s, 1 cm = 1 mV.

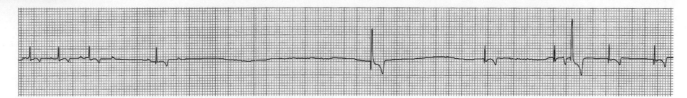

Figura 248.29 Disfunção do nodo sinusal (síndrome do seio sinusal doente) em um cão. O ritmo sinusal normal (3 batimentos) é seguido de bloqueio atrioventricular (AV) de segundo grau (Mobitz tipo II); batimento sinusal, outra condição do bloqueio AV de segundo grau Mobitz tipo II; e um período de assistolia que dura 3,5 s. A assistolia termina com um batimento de escape ventricular largo e de aparência bizarra, seguido de assistolia por 2 s, um batimento de escape juncional, um complexo ventricular prematuro (CVP) e dois batimentos de escape juncionais. Essa mistura de ritmos bradicárdicos e taquicardia (CVP), altamente variada, é característica de disfunção do nodo sinusal. Derivação II, 25 mm/s, 1 cm = 1 mV.

direção, de modo que a condução do estímulo ventricular é retrógrada, através do ramo do circuito de reentrada para os átrios, em seguida novamente através do nodo AV em direção normal e, de novo, através do ramo do circuito de reentrada, iniciando um ramo sem fim. Esse tipo de ciclo que se autoperpetua é um circuito macrorreentrante e pode provocar taquicardia AV reentrante potencialmente muito rápida e clinicamente evidente (desconforto aparente, sintomas gastrintestinais, intolerância ao exercício, letargia, síncope),[53] denominada *ortodrômica* (TAVRO, em que o estímulo segue em direção normal, "normógrada", através do nodo AV), a principal forma de macrorreentrada ventriculoatrial que se manifesta clinicamente, ou *síndrome de Wolff-Parkinson-White*, no cão.[32,46,53,136] Cães com essa síndrome podem ter frequências cardíacas notáveis, > 300 bpm. O tratamento inicial pode envolver manobras vagais que, ao reduzirem a condução AV (*i. e.*, ação dromotrópica negativa), interrompem o ciclo de reentrada (ver Figura 248.3). O tratamento mais efetivo consiste no uso IV de diltiazem ou esmolol, conforme descrito anteriormente para as taquicardias atriais.

Disfunção do nodo sinusal/síndrome do seio sinusal doente

A disfunção do nodo sinusal (síndrome do seio sinusal doente [SSSD], síndrome de bradicardia-taquicardia) é uma arritmia cardíaca bem reconhecida, que consiste na segunda indicação mais frequente para implantação de marca-passo em cães (após bloqueio AV).[28a,137-139] Envolve um distúrbio complexo dos tecidos de condução cardíaca, que acarreta anormalidades simultâneas na atividade sinusal (BS e parada sinusal), distúrbios da condução AV (bloqueios AV de primeiro e segundo graus) e distúrbios na excitabilidade supraventricular e ventricular (Figura 248.29). Portanto, a anormalidade não é um problema que envolve apenas o nodo SA, como a denominação SSSD sugere, mas sim uma doença que interfere na função do marca-passo cardíaco e nos tecidos de condução em todos os níveis.

A causa de SSSD é desconhecida. Algumas pessoas portadoras dessa síndrome possuem autoanticorpos direcionados ao tecido do nodo SA ou a receptores colinérgicos,[140,141] e tais mecanismos suscitam investigações na medicina veterinária porque poderiam explicar a panóplia de arritmias notadas em cães com esse distúrbio. Alguns aspectos epidemiológicos se destacam nos casos relatados na literatura veterinária. A doença é diagnosticada quase exclusivamente em cães, e a predileção racial estereotípica por fêmeas da raça Schnauzer Miniatura não é exclusiva. Muitas outras raças representam uma proporção cada vez maior de pacientes com essa síndrome, sendo dignas de nota as raças Cocker Spaniel[137,138] e West Highland White Terrier,[137,142] além de cães mestiços.[28a] É provável que o espectro da doença descrita como SSSD compreenda mais de um distúrbio distinto que pesquisas futuras possibilitarão classificar em anormalidades distintas.

A síndrome costuma surgir em adultos de meia-idade ou mais tardiamente (6 a 10 anos), e a associação com MVDA é comum, mas não obrigatória. Em termos histopatológicos, a depleção de células do nodo SA é vista como substituição fibrosa/fibrogordurosa, que causa impedimento de comunicação entre o nodo AV e o miocárdio atrial.[143] Em geral, o diagnóstico no ECG requer a obtenção de vários traçados, longos o bastante (de 2 a 3 min) para a demonstração convincente de algum ou todos os aspectos da SSSD:BS (em geral, com bloqueio AV de primeiro ou segundo grau), pausas sinusais prolongadas com batimentos de escape variáveis e episódios de taquicardia supraventricular ou extrassístoles ventriculares de várias frequências (Figura 248.29). Em alguns casos, ocorre apenas BS. Como essas manifestações são intermitentes, o diagnóstico só costuma ser estabelecido com a obtenção de um ECG durante um episódio de síncope, tropeço ou ataxia (quase síncope), que são as manifestações clínicas evidentes mais comuns dessa arritmia. O ECG ambulatorial, especialmente o registro de um evento cardíaco, é ideal para estabelecer o diagnóstico de SSSD quando o ECG de um paciente hospitalizado não ajuda (ver Capítulo 103). Tal procedimento mostrou que os episódios ocorrem mais durante a bradicardia do que a taquicardia. Uma resposta ao teste com atropina (ver texto anterior) pode confirmar a capacidade de o coração responder ao tratamento vagolítico, e recentemente tal fato mostrou ser uma resposta a longo prazo aos fármacos vagolíticos, em muitos cães acometidos.[28a] Tais medicamentos (p. ex., 0,5 a 3 mg de propantelina/kg/8 h VO,[142] ou 0,005 mg de hiosciamina/kg/8 h VO,[144] ou 10 mg de aminofilina/teofilina/kg/8 h VO)[145] podem melhorar a condição, reduzindo o impacto de episódios de bradicardia e pausas; de acordo com uma pesquisa retrospectiva recente, 54% dos cães com disfunção do nodo sinusal foram controlados com tratamento farmacológico.[28a] Quando os episódios são recorrentes, geralmente o tratamento definitivo requer a implantação de um marca-passo (ver Capítulo 249).

REFERÊNCIAS BIBLIOGRÁFICAS

As referências bibliográficas deste capítulo se encontram online no Ambiente de Aprendizagem.

CAPÍTULO 249

Marca-Passo Cardíaco

Amara H. Estrada

INDICAÇÕES PARA IMPLANTAÇÃO DE MARCA-PASSO

Bradicardia, como causa de sinais clínicos evidentes, continua sendo a principal indicação para a implantação de marca-passo em cães e gatos. Estão estabelecidos esquemas de classificação para marca-passo em pessoas com as categorias de "geralmente indicado", "pode ser indicado" e "não indicado", orientando as decisões de tratamento. Na medicina veterinária, as indicações são similares e o marca-passo cardíaco é implantado mais comumente em cães com bloqueio atrioventricular (AV) completo (de terceiro grau) ou disfunção do nodo sinusal (DNS) (Figura 249.1). Menos comumente são implantados marca-passos em pacientes veterinários com parada atrial persistente (não associada à hiperpotassemia) e bloqueio AV de segundo grau de alto nível.

Bloqueio atrioventricular

Cães com bloqueio AV (ver Capítulo 248) de segundo grau, de alto nível, ou bloqueio AV completo quase sempre devem ser considerados candidatos à implantação de marca-passo permanente (ver Capítulo 30). Até mesmo frequência de ritmo de escape > 50 bpm (bpm) é capaz de diminuir com o tempo. Gatos diferem em termos de frequência de ritmo de escape quando desenvolvem bloqueio AV, apresentando, tipicamente, um ritmo de escape ventricular mais rápido (90 a 120 bpm), de modo que não costumam precisar de marca-passo. Ocasionalmente, gatos com miocardiopatia desenvolvem bradicardia com ritmo de escape lento o bastante para precisar de marca-passo a fim de não apresentar insuficiência cardíaca congestiva ou, se a atividade física for afetada, melhorar a qualidade de vida.

Disfunção do nodo sinusal ("síndrome do seio doente"; ver Capítulo 248)

Pacientes com DNS que esteja causando sintomas evidentes, como síncope, são, definitivamente, candidatos a implantação de marca-passo (ver Capítulo 30). Pacientes com achados no ECG compatíveis com DNS, mas cujos proprietários acham que não estão manifestando sinais clínicos, representam um dilema. Muitos desses pacientes são idosos e os sinais clínicos podem existir, porém são confundidos com "lentidão causada pela idade avançada". O grau de bradicardia em que se deve considerar a implantação de um marca-passo é motivo de controvérsia, mesmo na medicina humana, devendo-se considerar cada paciente individualmente. Na opinião da autora, frequência sinusal consistentemente < 50 bpm durante períodos em que o animal está alerta/desperto é indicação para a implantação de marca-passo. Além disso, pausas sinusais > 3 segundos, em estado alerta/desperto, também devem ser consideradas anormais e indicações para uso de marca-passo, se o paciente tiver sinais de intolerância ao exercício ou letargia. Pausas que ocorrem durante o sono (em geral detectadas durante monitoramento Holter ou telemetria, em pacientes hospitalizados) são menos preocupantes. Alguns cães com DNS exibem uma resposta excessiva ao tônus vagal acentuado, provavelmente porque há um componente autônomo que contribui para o processo mórbido. A administração de um fármaco anticolinérgico, como a atropina, pode induzir uma frequência sinusal mais alta e a eliminação de pausas sinusais, mas isso não significa que a DNS seja benigna e, nesses casos, a implantação de marca-passo ainda deve ser considerada, em especial se houver sinais clínicos que poderiam ser atribuídos à bradicardia.

Parada atrial

A parada atrial persistente é uma arritmia incomum associada à miocardite atrial, que impossibilita a despolarização dos átrios a partir do estímulo iniciado no nodo sinusal. Embora o nodo sinusal continue a disparar estímulo, não é efetivo na despolarização dos átrios e na propagação ao nodo AV. No ECG, não há onda P e, em geral, há um ritmo de escape juncional ou ventricular. A implantação de marca-passo está indicada nessa doença, pois o aumento da frequência cardíaca pode amenizar os sinais clínicos de intolerância ao exercício ou síncope e ajudar no tratamento de insuficiência cardíaca congestiva, se presente. O prognóstico após a implantação de um marca-passo depende da gravidade ou da presença de doença miocárdica subjacente e geralmente não é tão favorável como o uso de marca-passo na DNS ou no bloqueio AV. A parada atrial temporária causada por hiperpotassemia é discutida em mais detalhes nos Capítulos 248 e 309, não sendo uma indicação para a implantação de marca-passo permanente.

Indicações menos comuns de implantação de marca-passo

Ainda há controvérsia a respeito da implantação de marca-passo cardíaco na *síncope vasovagal* (ver Capítulo 30), quando o tratamento clínico falha. Em ensaios clínicos feitos com seres humanos,[1,2] mostrou-se que a síncope vasovagal foi abolida ou impedida com o uso de marca-passo de câmara dupla e, mesmo que ocorra síncope, o marca-passo pode prolongar a consciência de modo a evitar lesão. Atualmente estão sendo investigados novos algoritmos para implantação de marca-passo em um ensaio clínico específico para pessoas com síncope vasovagal. A inclusão nesse ensaio clínico está completa e o estudo está em andamento.[3]

No momento, o uso de marca-passo em *taquiarritmias* em medicina veterinária não é comum. Entretanto, taquiarritmias supraventriculares crônicas (como fibrilação atrial, arritmias atriais de reentrada, taquicardia atrial) refratárias ao tratamento clínico tornaram-se uma indicação para a implantação de marca-passo em pessoas. Têm sido usadas várias técnicas, incluindo a denominada *ablate and pace* para fibrilação atrial crônica, na qual se faz a ablação do nodo AV por meio de radiofrequência e implanta-se um marca-passo no ventrículo para controlar a frequência cardíaca. Outra abordagem tem sido destinada à prevenção de fibrilação atrial em pacientes com taquiarritmias atriais refratárias, envolvendo marca-passo sincrônico biatrial.[4-6] Mostrou-se que esse marca-passo atrial de "duplo sítio" diminui os episódios de fibrilação atrial paroxística e *flutter*.[7] Além dessas técnicas alternativas de implantação de marca-passo, foram incluídos algoritmos para colocação de marca-passos na tentativa de diminuir o número de complexos atriais prematuros e manter um ritmo atrial consistente. Outra indicação comum para a implantação de um marca-passo permanente em pessoas é a taquicardia ventricular refratária, em especial no caso de distúrbios como a síndrome do QT longo, considerada resultante, em alta prevalência, de morte súbita devido à progressão da taquicardia ventricular para fibrilação ventricular. Muitos ensaios identificaram um benefício nítido no uso de marca-passos de câmara dupla/desfibriladores intracardíacos (DIC) em comparação com o tratamento clínico, exclusivamente, na

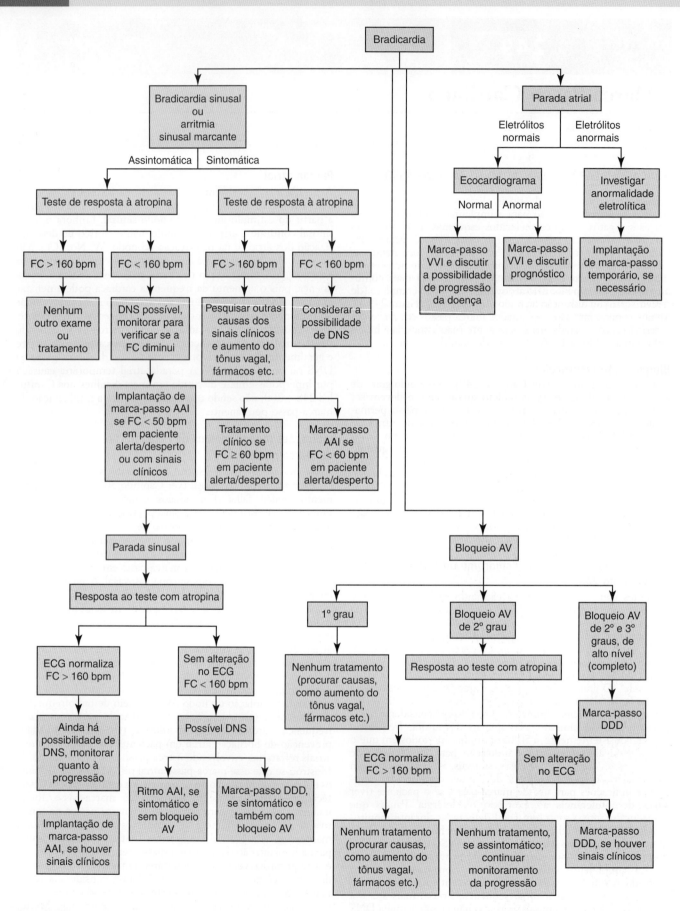

Figura 249.1 Esquema para a tomada de decisão terapêutica em pacientes com bradicardia. *AAI*, ritmo atrial, detecção de sinal atrial, inibido; *AV*, atrioventricular; *DDD*, ritmo de câmara dupla, detecção de câmara dupla, inibido; *DNS*, doença do nodo sinusal; *ECG*, eletrocardiograma; *FC*, frequência cardíaca; *VVI*, ritmo ventricular, detecção de sinal ventricular, inibido.

prevenção de morte súbita.[8-11] Atualmente há vários relatos na literatura veterinária sobre o uso bem-sucedido do tratamento com o emprego de DIC.[12-14]

Há mais de 25 anos, o marca-passo de câmara dupla foi indicado como um tratamento específico para pacientes com *miocardiopatia hipertrófica obstrutiva*, na ausência de anormalidade no sistema de condução. A hipótese era que, mediante o encurtamento do intervalo AV a fim de prevenir a condução normal através do nodo AV, seria possível assegurar um marca-passo no ventricular direito apical (VDA) "puro". Com essa abordagem, haveria então a contração tardia da parte basal do septo interventricular, com resultante redução ou eliminação do impedimento do fluxo sanguíneo de saída.[15-18] Atualmente não se utiliza essa abordagem por não ser efetiva[19,20] e pela preocupação com os efeitos negativos a longo prazo do marca-passo VDA.

Terapia de ressincronização cardíaca (TRC) é a terminologia aplicada ao restabelecimento da contração sincrônica entre a parede do ventrículo esquerdo (VE) livre e o septo ventricular por um marca-passo simultâneo, ou quase simultâneo, ao ventrículo direito apical e à parede livre do VE (marca-passo BiV). Atualmente esse tipo de marca-passo é um tratamento aceito e efetivo, considerando a relação custo/benefício em pacientes humanos com insuficiência cardíaca avançada, comprometimento da função do VE e complexo QRS largo.[21] Essa terapia agora também é uma opção realista para pacientes com insuficiência cardíaca leve e pode acabar substituindo o marca-passo VDA como um meio mais fisiológico de ritmo cardíaco. Por enquanto, os dispositivos são caros e obtidos para pacientes veterinários apenas por meio de doação; ademais, sua implantação e a programação subsequente requerem prática considerável do clínico para que sejam eficientes.[22]

TIPOS DE MARCA-PASSO E SUA HEMODINÂMICA

Identificada uma indicação para implantação de marca-passo, deve-se escolher o tipo mais apropriado para o paciente em questão. Os fatores a serem considerados incluem: (1) o débito subjacente do ritmo, (2) a condição física geral do paciente e quaisquer problemas clínicos associados, (3) capacidade de exercício/atividade do paciente, (4) resposta cronotrópica a exercício/excitação e (5) efeito do marca-passo na morbidade e mortalidade a longo prazo.

Nomenclatura dos marca-passos

A nomenclatura dos marca-passos é designada por numerais romanos de I a V. A posição I refere-se à(s) câmara(s) onde são implantados: A = átrio; V = ventricular; D = câmara dupla, ou seja, átrio e ventrículo. A posição II refere-se à(s) câmara(s) onde ocorre a detecção. As opções de letras são as mesmas da primeira posição. A designação O refere-se à ausência de detecção (portanto, refere-se a um ritmo fixo, assincrônico). A posição III refere-se à resposta do dispositivo aos eventos detectados. Um *I* representa o modo inibido, significando que, quando um evento é detectado, o dispositivo será inibido de continuar agindo; essa é a forma de detecção mais comum. *T* indica o desencadeamento de uma resposta. Quando um marca-passo detecta um evento e é programado nesse modo, ele vai disparar o dispositivo para liberar um estímulo de ritmo. *D* significa que as respostas *T* e *I* podem ocorrer. Em caso de marca-passo de câmara única, o evento detectado e o estímulo disparado ocorrem dentro da mesma câmara, de modo que essa função nunca é usada no marca-passo de câmara única. Contudo, no uso de marca-passo de câmara dupla, um evento detectado no átrio inibe o estímulo atrial e desencadeia a liberação de um estímulo ventricular com intervalo AV tardio programado para ser similar ao de um intervalo PR normal. A posição IV indica a programação e velocidade de modulação. Na prática, *R* é o único indicador comumente usado nessa posição e indica que o marca-passo inclui um sensor para modular a velocidade, independentemente da atividade cardíaca intrínseca. A posição V é usada para indicar se não há atividade rítmica em múltiplos locais sem câmara cardíaca (*O*), um ou ambos os átrios (*A*), um ou ambos os ventrículos (*V*) ou qualquer combinação de átrios e ventrículos (*D*). Por exemplo, para descrever um paciente com marca-passo de câmara dupla adaptado com estimulação biventricular, o código seria DDDRBiV.

Marca-passo de câmara única

Em termos práticos, basicamente há apenas dois tipos de marca-passo de câmara única: VVI e AAI, sendo o primeiro o mais comum em medicina veterinária.[23] A modulação da velocidade é uma opção em ambos os tipos de marca-passo (VVIR ou AAIR).

Marca-passo ventricular inibido (VVI)

É implantado no ventrículo e capaz de moderar o ritmo apenas no ventrículo (V na primeira posição do código do marca-passo), detectando apenas no ventrículo (V na segunda posição) e, se um batimento ventricular nativo for detectado, o disparo do marca-passo é inibido (I na terceira posição) (Figura 249.2). Embora esse marca-passo proteja o paciente de bradicardias letais, sua ação é bastante limitada, porque não restabelece nem mantém a sincronia AV e, em comparação com o VVIR, não induz resposta em paciente com incompetência cronotrópica, ou seja, no paciente em que a frequência cardíaca sinusal espontânea não aumenta em resposta a uma demanda fisiológica. Além disso, alguns pacientes com marca-passo VVI apresentam início ou agravamento de sinais clínicos durante a atividade ventricular. Os efeitos hemodinâmicos adversos associados a um marca-passo funcionando normalmente são conhecidos como "síndrome do marca-passo", expressão usada com referência às consequências hemodinâmicas e eletrofisiológicas adversas do marca-passo ventricular. Sinais neurológicos ou aqueles sugestivos de baixo débito cardíaco ou insuficiência cardíaca congestiva são os sinais clínicos indicativos da síndrome do marca-passo. Em um estudo realizado em pacientes humanos com marca-passos de câmara dupla (DDD) distribuídos aleatoriamente para implantação de DDD ou VVI, constatou-se que a síndrome

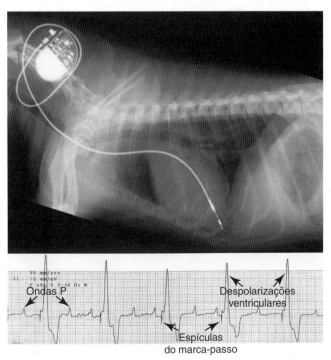

Figura 249.2 Radiografia cervical e lateral do tórax e ECG de um paciente com bloqueio cardíaco completo no qual foi implantado um marca-passo VVI transvenoso permanente. Note a dissociação entre as ondas P e os complexos QRS. Cada complexo QRS é precedido de uma espícula gerada pelo marca-passo e transmitida através da derivação no ápice do ventrículo direito.

do marca-passo estava presente em 83% dos pacientes submetidos à implantação de marca-passo VVI.[24] Os conceitos-chave identificados como causas da síndrome do marca-passo incluíram: (1) sequenciamento impróprio das contrações atriais e ventriculares e (2) impossibilidade de modulação da velocidade fisiológica. Tais efeitos podem ser subjacentes à síndrome do marca-passo observada em cães também.

Marca-passo atrial inibido (AAI)

O marca-passo atrial de câmara única é indicado apenas aos pacientes em que a bradiarritmia é um mecanismo sinusal e o bloqueio AV não é um problema. Nessa situação, é colocada uma derivação apenas no átrio (no apêndice atrial direito ou no septo atrial). A marcação do ritmo só ocorre no átrio (A, na primeira posição do código do marca-passo), se não houver atividade nativa detectada no átrio (A, na segunda posição), em um limite inferior específico programado ou abaixo dele. Se for detectado batimento atrial/sinusal nativo no átrio, então o marca-passo é inibido, impedido de disparar (I, na terceira posição). Esse marca-passo é apropriado para pacientes com DNS e condução AV normal (Figura 249.3). A desvantagem óbvia do marca-passo AAI é a falta de suporte ventricular que deve ocorrer no bloqueio AV. Se o paciente com DNS for avaliado com cuidado em busca de doença do nodo AV no momento da implantação do marca-passo, a ocorrência de doença nodal AV *clinicamente relevante* no futuro será rara.[25] A avaliação da função do nodo AV antes do uso de um sistema AAI deve incluir ritmo nodal incremental no momento da implantação do marca-passo. O critério usado pela instituição da autora é: o paciente deve ser capaz de condução no nodo AV 1:1 até a frequência de 120 bpm, enquanto estiver anestesiado. Se ocorrer bloqueio AV, com frequência mais baixa, são utilizados sistemas de marca-passo de câmara dupla. O benefício do marca-passo AAI em um paciente com DNS não se resume à manutenção da sincronia AV, mas também à manutenção do padrão normal de ativação no coração (via o nodo AV). Além disso, a condução retrógrada de estímulos através do nodo AV é comum em cães com marca-passo ventricular, em geral resultando em condução retrógrada e eco dos batimentos. Portanto, é importante que, quando se usa um marca-passo VVI em cães com DNS, ele seja programado em uma frequência baixa e só funcione como um *backup* em períodos de bradicardia, para reter o máximo possível da condução no nodo AV.

Marca-passo de câmara dupla

A manutenção do sincronismo AV (ritmo fisiológico) oferece benefícios substanciais à hemodinâmica e à mortalidade dos pacientes. Por essa razão, o ritmo fisiológico para bloqueio AV precisa envolver um sistema que "substitua" a capacidade do nodo AV de conduzir despolarizações atriais para o miocárdio ventricular. Atualmente os sistemas mais usados de marca-passo de câmara dupla são VDD, DDD ou DDDR com comutação de modo (discutida adiante).

Marca-passo atrial sincrônico (VDD)

Esse modo só funciona no ventrículo (V, na primeira posição do código do marca-passo), é sentido em ambas as câmaras (D, na segunda posição) e pode responder inibindo o débito ventricular, se a atividade ventricular intrínseca for sentida, ou desencadeando uma resposta ventricular, quando uma atividade atrial é sentida (D, na terceira posição). Esse modo de marca-passo é denominado atrial sincrônico, pois ele "rastreia" ondas P (sinusais) nativas. Esse modo possibilita a manutenção do sincronismo AV e a frequência ventricular é modulada pelo tônus autônomo inerente do paciente, pois é determinado pela própria frequência sinusal do paciente. Se houver uma pausa sinusal e nenhum evento atrial for sentido, o marca-passo será capaz de escape com um evento ventricular ritmado na frequência mais baixa programada. Ou seja, o marca-passo exibirá atividade VVI na ausência de um evento atrial sentido. O marca-passo VDD é apropriado para o paciente com função normal do nodo sinusal e anormalidade na condução do nodo AV. Esse marca-passo atrial sincrônico ventricular inibido (VDD) utiliza uma derivação que inclui um eletrodo colocado no ventrículo direito e um eletrodo atrial flutuante na parte intra-atrial da derivação ventricular para sentir as ondas P propagadas através do sangue. Essas ondas P nativas são sentidas pelo marca-passo e, então, seguindo um retardo AV programado apropriadamente, o sistema libera um estímulo ventricular (Figura 249.4). O ajuste da distância entre o eletrodo atrial flutuante e a extremidade ventricular do marca-passo em geral impede seu uso em cães de pequeno porte.

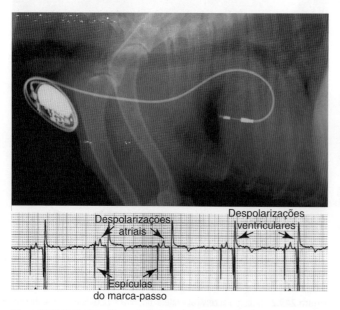

Figura 249.3 Radiografia cervical e lateral do tórax e ECG de um paciente com DNS no qual foi implantado um marca-passo AAI transvenoso permanente. Cada onda P é precedida de uma espícula gerada pelo marca-passo pela derivação no apêndice auricular direito.

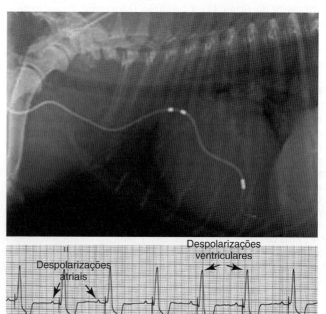

Figura 249.4 Radiografia cervical e lateral do tórax e ECG de um paciente com bloqueio cardíaco completo, no qual foi implantado um marca-passo VDD transvenoso permanente. Note o eletrodo atrial flutuante no átrio direito. Esse eletrodo detecta as ondas P nativas geradas pelo nodo sinusal, e uma espícula ventricular é, então, liberada pela derivação posicionada no ápice do ventrículo direito para causar despolarização ventricular.

Marca-passo de câmara dupla e sensibilidade com inibição e rastreamento

Conhecido como "marca-passo totalmente automático", o marca-passo de câmara dupla e sensibilidade com inibição e rastreamento (DDD) é capaz de sentir e dar o ritmo ao átrio e ao ventrículo. Esse tipo de marca-passo é apropriado aos pacientes com DNS que também apresentam bloqueio AV, ou aos pacientes com bloqueio AV de segundo grau completo ou de nível alto. Como é capaz de exercer funções duplas, em ambas as câmaras, a função normal do DDD pode aparecer no eletrocardiograma como (1) ritmo sinusal normal, (2) ritmo apenas atrial, (3) ritmo AV sequencial ou (4) ritmo atrial sincrônico.

Antigamente, considerava-se que a implantação dos sistemas de marca-passo de câmara dupla, em particular aqueles com duas derivações, era mais difícil e demorada, além de exigir uma programação mais complexa. Portanto, presumia-se que a implantação de marca-passos de câmara dupla teria taxas mais altas de complicações, tanto no início como a longo prazo. Recentemente, dados publicados mostraram que, embora a implantação de múltiplas derivações (Figura 249.5) prolongue o tempo de anestesia e do procedimento, os cães não apresentam incidência maior de complicações em curto ou longo prazos.[26]

IMPLANTAÇÃO DE MARCA-PASSO TRANSVENOSO

Marca-passo transvenoso temporário (provisório)

Para pacientes com bradiarritmias, o meio mais seguro para implantar um marca-passo permanente é após a implementação de algum método de marca-passo temporário (Vídeo 249.1). Isso possibilita que haja uma frequência cardíaca normal, o paciente esteja mais estável e o procedimento cirúrgico seja menos apressado durante a implantação do marca-passo permanente. O marca-passo temporário pode ser implantado por via transvenosa, transtorácica ou transesofágica, com cada técnica tendo seus prós e contras.[27-32]

Implantação de marca-passo permanente

O procedimento é mostrado no Vídeo 249.1; em outros textos também há descrições detalhadas do procedimento de implantação.[33] A maioria dos marca-passos permanentes é implantada por via transvenosa, através da veia jugular. As exceções são os pacientes em que há deslocamentos repetidos das derivações, aqueles com risco de hipercoagulação ou, para alguns clínicos, gatos e cães de raça de pequeno porte, em que é desejável a implantação epicárdica. Há relatos de obstrução da veia cava cranial[34], seguida de quilotórax[35], com a implantação transvenosa e, assim, a maioria dos cardiologistas prefere uma derivação epicárdica no ápice do ventrículo esquerdo por meio de abordagem abdominal/transdiafragmática em gatos e cães com menos de 2,2 kg que necessitam de marca-passo. No entanto, há derivações de pequeno diâmetro (4,1 French, Medtronic SelectSecure Model 3830), que podem servir para pacientes pequenos, mas a experiência veterinária com esse modelo de derivação é mínima.[36]

PROGRAMAÇÃO DO MARCA-PASSO

Os marca-passos podem ser programados e avaliados de maneira não invasiva, para ajuste e sintonia fina dos parâmetros do ritmo cardíaco. A programação e a consulta de marca-passos ocorrem, tipicamente, no período pós-operatório imediato (24 horas) e, em seguida, em 4 a 6 semanas, 3 e 6 meses e, daí em diante, anualmente, para avaliação de sua função e da carga da bateria. Os programadores de marca-passo não são intercambiáveis e um marca-passo específico vai requerer um certo programador. Os programadores podem ser emprestados para uso ou doados para instituições veterinárias por fabricantes de marca-passo. Alguns representantes de vendas locais também visitam uma instituição específica para reavaliações dos pacientes. Uma descrição detalhada da programação de marca-passo está além do âmbito deste texto, mas alguns parâmetros mais críticos merecem ser mencionados.

Programação da amplitude do pulso e da amplitude da voltagem

Há dois aspectos da liberação de energia que podem ser programados: a *voltagem*, ou amplitude do impulso, e a *amplitude do pulso*, ou até que ponto essa voltagem é aplicada ao miocárdio. A combinação delas representa a energia liberada no miocárdio. A liberação precisa ser alta o suficiente para induzir a despolarização e permitir uma margem adequada de segurança do ritmo, mas também deve ser programada com o intuito de maximizar a longevidade do marca-passo. Para determinar os ajustes apropriados, primeiro a amplitude do pulso é mantida constante e a voltagem é diminuída gradualmente até que uma perda de captura seja vista no ECG. O oposto é realizado em seguida; a tensão é mantida constante e a largura de pulso é gradualmente reduzida. É gerada uma curva de duração de apoio, que possibilita a determinação de valores apropriados para garantir uma adequada margem de segurança. Em geral, os valores limiares são ajustados considerando o dobro da amplitude de voltagem ou o triplo da amplitude do pulso. Quanto menor a liberação de energia, mais tempo a bateria vai durar. Alguns marca-passos determinam automaticamente os parâmetros de liberação, enquanto outros monitoram continuamente o limiar de captura (condição denominada conduta de captura) e ajustam automaticamente a liberação diária de energia. Os limiares para o ajuste do ritmo não são estáticos e podem mudar

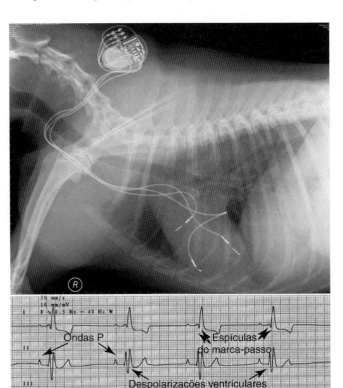

Figura 249.5 Radiografia cervical e lateral do tórax e ECG de um paciente no qual foi implantado um sistema CRT. Há uma derivação no apêndice auricular direito, uma no seio coronário e abaixo de uma veia coronária lateral, para marcar o ritmo da parede ventricular esquerda livre, além de uma terceira derivação em uma posição apical do ventrículo direito padrão.

rapidamente no decorrer do dia, o que justifica a programação com margem de segurança. É provável que o tempo cause a alteração mais importante no limiar. Em geral, uma derivação tem seu limiar mais baixo no momento da implantação. Em um período de 2 a 6 semanas, o limiar aumenta para seu nível mais alto ("amadurece") e em seguida se reduz para um limiar por longo tempo que costuma se estabilizar em aproximadamente duas ou três vezes o nível crítico.

Programação da frequência

A programação adaptativa da frequência pode ser feita em todos os marca-passos fabricados atualmente, na maioria dos modos de ritmo (p. ex., AAIR, VVIR, DDDR). Uma frequência programável típica é de 30 a 180 bpm, no caso de alguns marca-passos capazes de ser tão rápidos quanto 220 bpm. Os sensores que detectam movimento físico e ventilação minuto permitem que os pacientes tenham frequências mais lentas quando estão dormindo ou em repouso e mais altas quando estão se exercitando. A diminuição da frequência cardíaca quando não é necessária uma frequência mais alta também prolonga o tempo de uso da bateria do marca-passo. Algoritmos de ritmo são incluídos para "comunicar" ao marca-passo quando aumentar e diminuir a velocidade de estímulo. Embora esses algoritmos funcionem muito bem para as pessoas e a confiabilidade a longo prazo seja excelente, não se sabe se funcionam tão bem em pacientes veterinários, em especial aqueles que ficam ofegantes ou se arranham frequentemente!

Sensibilidade

Sensibilidade é a capacidade de o marca-passo reconhecer a atividade intrínseca do coração. Ela é vital para um marca-passo, porque permite que seu computador interno responda à atividade do próprio coração, o que significa inibir o ritmo quando necessário; ademais, o marca-passo não vai competir com ou interferir no próprio ritmo cardíaco do paciente. Em cães com bloqueio cardíaco completo e um marca-passo de câmara dupla, a sensibilidade é importante para rastrear ondas P nativas e liberar um estímulo ventricular em resposta. Em cães com DNS, é importante que o sistema reconheça batimentos normais e só entre em ação quando necessário. Todos os pacientes com marca-passo apresentam, potencialmente, arritmias, como complexos atriais ou ventriculares prematuros (CAP ou CVP), que precisam ser detectadas pelo marca-passo para assegurar que não ocorram durante o período vulnerável na onda T.

Os dois principais desafios à sensibilidade são *hipersensibilidade* (i. e., percepção de eventos que, na verdade, não existem ou não deveriam ser sentidos), como artefato de movimento, e *hipossensibilidade*, que se refere à ausência de sensibilidade a eventos que deveriam ser percebidos. Em geral, no ECG a hipersensibilidade se apresenta como pausas indevidamente longas entre espículas do marca-passo e podem ser detectadas de maneira definitiva, observando um canal marcador de programação. Ocorre *hipossensibilidade* quando há um evento intrínseco (onda P ou complexo QRS) que o marca-passo deveria ter detectado, mas passou despercebido. Na hipossensibilidade, o ECG mostra a atividade intrínseca seguida, com muita proximidade, de uma espícula do marca-passo.

A sensibilidade é um parâmetro programável, medido em milivolts (mV). Embora de início possa parecer contraintuitivo, o aumento da sensibilidade (tornando o dispositivo mais sensível) significa diminuição no ajuste de mV, enquanto a diminuição da sensibilidade significa aumento no ajuste do mV.

Período refratário

É um período breve em que a função de sensibilidade do marca-passo é desligada ou ignorada após a percepção de um sinal QRS ou a ocorrência de uma espícula causada pelo marca-passo. É programado para o intervalo QT do paciente, obtido no ECG de superfície. A vantagem de um período refratário é que ele não permite que o marca-passo perceba a onda T do complexo QRS

precedente ou o pós-potencial do marca-passo, que corresponde à atividade elétrica residual que ocorre após um batimento rítmico. A desvantagem é que podem não ser percebidos CVP ou CAP precoces. É possível prolongar o período refratário para eliminar sensibilidade imprópria de um sinal de QRS, onda T ou pós-potencial. Também pode ser encurtado para possibilitar que CVP ou CAP frequentes sejam percebidos e, assim, reduzir o risco de determinar o ritmo na onda T do batimento prematuro.

Características especiais

A tecnologia do marca-passo evoluiu a tal ponto que é impossível incluir uma discussão de todas as características especiais disponíveis no capítulo de um livro. Empresas diferentes usam terminologias distintas e a programação pode ser um pouco variada em cada tipo de marca-passo. Ao trabalhar com marca-passos, é aconselhável ter os manuais do dispositivo à mão, para consulta, ou utilizar materiais de treinamento dos diversos fabricantes. Técnicos regionais ou contatos de suporte técnico também podem ser úteis para a programação e a interpretação de gráficos de resolução de problemas durante as avaliações.

COMPLICAÇÕES DECORRENTES DO USO DE MARCA-PASSO

Relata-se que as complicações após a implantação de marca-passo têm relação direta com a experiência do profissional na medicina veterinária e humana.[37-39] O desenvolvimento de seroma é uma ocorrência relativamente comum, mas pode ser tratado com facilidade aplicando-se um envoltório no pescoço com ligeira pressão. Alguns cardiologistas também tratam empiricamente com antibióticos para diminuir o risco de infecção. É importante ressaltar que não se faz a drenagem do líquido que circunda o gerador com agulha e seringa, devido ao risco de introdução de bactérias no local e também de danificar as derivações e o gerador dentro da bolsa.

É provável que a trombose da veia jugular, parcial ou subclínica, seja comum após a colocação de derivação transvenosa, mas não costuma causar sinais clínicos. Às vezes, também se observa aderência ou formação de trombo na derivação, em ecocardiogramas de reavaliação, sem que o proprietário tenha notado sinais clínicos. Na experiência da autora, esses tipos de trombos não costumam se desalojar ou crescer muito com o tempo. Entretanto, é aconselhável tratar os pacientes com agentes antitrombóticos, como ácido acetilsalicílico ou clopidogrel, em dose baixa, se um trombo for detectado.

Perfuração de átrio ou ventrículo é uma ocorrência possível, embora rara.[36,37] Tamponamento cardíaco é o resultado mais grave da perfuração, mas é comum não haver sinais clínicos. Na verdade, os únicos sinais de perfuração podem ser aumento do limiar de estímulo, alteração no padrão de despolarização no ECG de superfície ou contração diafragmática a cada estímulo.

A complicação mais comum, em especial no período pós-operatório imediato, é o deslocamento ou mau posicionamento da derivação, causando perda de captura, vista no ECG como espículas do marca-passo não acompanhadas de captura elétrica da câmara apropriada. Para minimizar o risco dessa complicação, é importante que os pacientes fiquem em repouso e sejam impedidos de correr ou saltar após a implantação. Na instituição da autora, induz-se sedação antes da recuperação da anestesia e na alta hospitalar os proprietários são instruídos a manter o paciente quieto e com atividade apenas restrita por guia nas primeiras 6 semanas. Depois desse período, os pacientes podem voltar à atividade normal.

Se necessário, as arritmias que ocorrem como resultado da inflamação e da irritação associadas à colocação de derivação podem ser tratadas com segurança com agentes antiarrítmicos (ver Capítulo 248); elas se resolvem poucos dias após a implantação.

Às vezes, os cães manifestam contração do pescoço ou do diafragma a cada estímulo do marca-passo ("contração do marca-passo"; Vídeo 249.2). Em geral, isso se deve à corrente de alta voltagem ou à estimulação do nervo frênico e pode ser evitada reduzindo-se a voltagem da corrente. Os marca-passos doados por fabricantes, em geral, têm gravado no verso um aviso de que não são para uso humano. Isso, às vezes, pode causar extravasamento de voltagem em torno do gerador, razão pela qual devem ser implantados com o lado gravado para baixo, na tentativa de evitar contração do músculo sobrejacente.

Os geradores de pulso manufaturados duram, em média, 10 a 12 anos. A maioria dos geradores implantados em medicina veterinária não foi usada antes, mas a duração da bateria no implante é variável e pode ser avaliada usando um programador antes da implantação. Várias alterações na programação podem aumentar ou diminuir a vida útil do gerador de pulso. Quando a bateria de um gerador está prestes a descarregar, aparece um aviso conhecido em inglês como *end of life* (EOL, fim da vida útil) ou *elective replacement indicator* (ERI, indicador de substituição eletiva). Mais comumente, isso é percebido pela diminuição gradual na frequência do ritmo, dando assim bastante tempo para que se substitua o gerador antes que ele falhe.

Infecções

Em medicina veterinária, a prevalência relatada de infecção após implantação de marca-passo é de 5 a 10%,[40] muito maior do que em medicina humana, em que essa taxa é < 2%.[41,42] A atenção cuidadosa aos detalhes cirúrgicos e um procedimento asséptico têm extrema importância para evitar infecção no local de implantação do marca-passo. Na instituição da autora, a implantação é adiada (se possível) quando há sinais de infecção cutânea relevante ou de infecção do trato urinário, razão pela qual o exame de urina com urocultura e teste de sensibilidade (antibiograma) fazem parte da rotina, antes da implantação. O uso profilático de antibióticos antes da implantação e no período pós-operatório imediato continua sendo motivo de controvérsia, mas também é rotineiro.[43] A maioria dos estudos em seres humanos não mostra qualquer diferença significativa na taxa de infecção entre pacientes que receberam ou não profilaxia com antibióticos. O tratamento ideal de um marca-passo infectado (Figura 249.6) é a

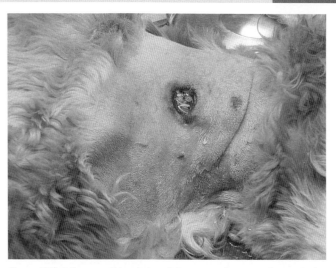

Figura 249.6 Imagem clínica da lateral do pescoço de um cão da raça Cocker Spaniel que apresenta infecção no local de implantação do marca-passo. Nota-se uma úlcera cutânea que acomete todas as camadas de pele e a protrusão do gerador do marca-passo na superfície. (Cortesia dos Drs. Etienne Coté e Nancy Laste, Angell Animal Medical Center.)

remoção de todo o sistema (derivação e gerador), se possível, terapia com antibiótico apropriado a longo prazo (de acordo com os resultados da urocultura e do teste de sensibilidade) e reimplantação do sistema de marca-passo no lado oposto do pescoço, se o adiamento não for viável.[44] O tratamento exclusivamente com antibiótico raramente é capaz de erradicar a infecção.[40-42]

REFERÊNCIAS BIBLIOGRÁFICAS

As referências bibliográficas deste capítulo se encontram online no Ambiente de Aprendizagem.

CAPÍTULO 250

Cardiopatias Congênitas

Niek J. Beijerink, Mark A. Oyama e John D. Bonagura

INTRODUÇÃO

O termo *cardiopatia congênita* (CC) engloba um grande número de anormalidades morfológicas e funcionais do coração e dos vasos sanguíneos contíguos presentes no momento do nascimento. Essas malformações geralmente surgem de alguma alteração ou interrupção do desenvolvimento embrionário do coração, causada por fatores genéticos ou ambientais. A gravidade da CC pode variar de trivial a risco de vida, e os sinais clínicos podem se manifestar a qualquer momento desde o período neonatal – antes do primeiro exame veterinário – até relativamente tarde na vida. Embora alguns tipos de CC sejam bem tolerados, consequências funcionais graves podem ocorrer, incluindo insuficiência cardíaca congestiva (ICC), hipoxemia, arritmia cardíaca ou morte súbita. Este capítulo fornece uma visão geral da CC em cães e gatos, bem como princípios de diagnóstico e controle dos defeitos comumente encontrados.

O leitor também é referido ao Capítulo 122 para uma descrição das técnicas intervencionistas usadas para corrigir defeitos cardíacos congênitos, ao Capítulo 257, que aborda algumas formas de anomalias vasculares venosas, e ao Capítulo 273, para considerações adicionais sobre o diagnóstico e tratamento da obstrução de esôfago causada por malformações do anel vascular.

Na maioria dos casos, o tratamento bem-sucedido da CC começa com o reconhecimento imediato de um distúrbio cardíaco pelo veterinário da família, seguido de encaminhamento para o cardiologista, a fim de uma avaliação mais detalhada. Na maioria das situações, um diagnóstico definitivo de CC pode ser obtido de forma não invasiva, após exame ecocardiográfico completo. No entanto, a definição precisa de algumas formas complexas de CC – assim como de certas malformações vasculares – pode exigir técnicas de imagem avançadas, conforme discutido mais adiante. O prognóstico para qualquer CC está relacionado com o tipo e a gravidade da malformação primária.

Algumas formas de CC não requerem tratamento e têm um prognóstico favorável. Outros defeitos são passíveis de terapia definitiva ou alguma forma de tratamento paliativo.

Etiologia

As malformações cardíacas congênitas podem ser causadas por fatores genéticos ou ambientais e, na maioria dos casos, um único agente causador não pode ser conclusivamente identificado. A interação de fatores toxicológicos, nutricionais, infecciosos e genéticos dificulta a determinação de uma única causa definitiva. A observação de que certos defeitos congênitos se apresentam em uma espécie ou raça predisponente[1-4] sugere fortemente uma base hereditária em muitos casos (Tabela 250.1). Essa hipótese tem sido demonstrada para diversos defeitos específicos em algumas raças de cães.[1,5-12] Vários estudos indicam uma simples base mendeliana de transmissão, dando suporte ao conceito de que fatores genéticos identificáveis contribuem para o desenvolvimento embrionário do coração e se relacionam com tipos específicos de CC. Outros genes podem ter efeitos aditivos ou efeitos modificadores e produzir um fenótipo discreto, uma vez que uma característica mendeliana tenha sido herdada, incluindo a variabilidade na penetração daquela característica.[13-17]

A complexidade e incerteza em torno da forma exata de herança de muitos defeitos cardíacos dificultam o aconselhamento aos proprietários que querem usar alguns cães como reprodutores. Embora os cardiologistas frequentemente tentem identificar CC em animais reprodutores durante a triagem clínica, esses esforços são prejudicados pela sensibilidade e especificidade limitadas dos testes diagnósticos disponíveis. Certamente, um exame físico normal não significa normalidade genética. Além disso, muitos sopros cardíacos discretos são difíceis de se interpretar,[18-20] e as triagens ecocardiográficas geralmente produzem resultados equivocados na ausência de critérios padrão-ouro, verdadeiros, para o diagnóstico de doença leve. Mesmo com uma atenção cuidadosa ao pedigree e os resultados dos testes de acasalamento, pode ser muito difícil inferir a prevalência geral de um defeito específico em uma população grande. O progresso nesse sentido depende do desenvolvimento de testes genéticos de baixo custo que possam detectar a presença de mutações genéticas responsáveis por malformações específicas.

A situação em gatos é ainda mais complicada e não há estudos genéticos detalhados em gatos com CC. Várias possíveis predisposições raciais têm sido relatadas, como displasia da valva tricúspide (DVT) e comunicação interatrial (CIA) em gatos da raça Chartreux,[21,22] e relatos mais antigos relacionam fibroelastose endocárdica e estenose mitral supravalvar em gatos Siameses. Outras predisposições de raça, em gatos, estão listadas a seguir como defeitos específicos.

Prevalência

Em levantamentos de cães, da década de 1960, conduzidos por Patterson e Detweiler,[23,24] a prevalência de CC em cães era de aproximadamente 0,56% dos casos hospitalares. Estudos subsequentes indicaram uma prevalência geral de CC em cães entre 0,46 e 0,85% das internações hospitalares; Buchanan relatou uma prevalência de aproximadamente 0,68%, considerando todos os cães examinados na Universidade da Pensilvânia.[25] A maioria dos estudos foi realizada em hospitais universitários, e essas pesquisas provavelmente englobam um número significativo de casos encaminhados para avaliação cardíaca. Em contraste, em um estudo recentemente publicado de uma população de cães de abrigos, Schrope reportou uma prevalência comparativamente menor de CC de 0,13% em 76.301 cães mestiços (rastreados por veterinários de abrigos e subsequentemente avaliados por um cardiologista).[26]

Apesar dessas diferenças de prevalência, as malformações cardíacas mais comuns em cães permaneceram praticamente inalteradas nos últimos 50 anos.[2-4,24-27]

Tabela 250.1	Predisposição das raças de cães para cardiopatias congênitas.

RAÇAS	DEFEITOS
Basset Hound	EP
Beagle	EP
Bichon Frisé	PDA
Boxer	ESA, EP, DSA
Boykin Spaniel	EP
Buldogue Inglês	EP, DSV, ToF
Bull Terrier	DVM, EA
Chihuahua	PDA, EP
Chow Chow	EP, CTD
Cocker Spaniel	PDA, EP
Collie	PDA
Doberman Pinscher	DSA
Dogue Alemão	DVT, DVM, ESA
German Shorthaired Pointer	ESA, DVM
Golden Retriever	ESA, DVT, DVM
Keeshond	ToF, PDA
Labrador Retriever	DVT, PDA, EP
Maltês	PDA
Mastiff	EP, DVM
Newfoundland	ESA, DVM, EP
Pastor-Alemão	ESA, PDA, DVT, DVM
Pomeranian	PDA
Poodle	PDA
Raças Terrier	EP
Rottweiler	ESA
Samoieda	EP, ESA, DSA
Schnauzer	EP
Shetland Sheepdog	PDA
Springer Spaniel Inglês	PDA, DSV
Weimaraner	DVT, HDPP
Welsh Corgi	PDA
West Highland/White Terrier	EP, DSV
Yorkshire Terrier	PDA

CTD, cor triatriatum dexter; DSA, defeito do septo atrial; DSV, defeito do septo ventricular; DVM, displasia da valva mitral; DVT, displasia da valva tricúspide; EA, estenose aórtica; EP, estenose pulmonar; ESA, estenose subaórtica; HDPP, hérnia diafragmática peritônio-pericárdica; PDA, persistência do ducto arterioso; ToF, tetralogia de Fallot.

Persistência do ducto arterioso (PDA), estenose subaórtica (ESA) e estenose pulmonar (EP) são as cardiopatias congênitas mais comuns na maioria dos inquéritos. Nos estudos de Patterson e Detweiler,[23,24] as frequências relatadas de diagnósticos foram de aproximadamente 28% para PDA, 20% para estenose da valva pulmonar (EP), 14% para ESA/estenose aórtica (EA), 8% para persistência de arco aórtico direito, 7% para defeito do septo ventricular (DSV) e menos de 5% para tetralogia de Fallot (ToF), persistência de veia cava cranial esquerda e defeito do septo atrial (DSA). O relatório de Buchanan,[25] que incluiu informações sobre prevalência obtidas de um banco de dados norte-americano de mais de 1.300 casos, indicou que a PDA foi mais frequentemente relatada (31,7%), seguida de ESA (22,1%) e EP com 18,3% dos casos. Entretanto, no estudo supracitado de CC em cães mestiços, as malformações mais comuns foram EP (31% dos casos de CC), PDA (17%), ESA (15%) e DSV (14%).[26] Estudos europeus indicaram uma prevalência maior de ESA e EP, comparativamente à PDA, com um maior estudo retrospectivo de 976 cães relatando uma prevalência de aproximadamente 32% para EP, 27% para estenose valvular ESA/EA e 21% para PDA. A mudança de popularidade de algumas raças de cães ao longo do tempo certamente influencia a prevalência regional de determinado defeito. Por exemplo, o número de cães das raças Golden Retriever, Labrador Retriever e Bull Terrier provavelmente aumentou o diagnóstico de ESA, DVT e displasia de valva mitral (DVM),[28] respectivamente. Scansen *et al.*[29] tabularam 4.694 malformações relatadas na literatura e calcularam a distribuição relativa de defeitos específicos. Conforme mostrado na Tabela 250.2, PDA, ESA/EA e EP são as malformações cardíacas gerais mais comuns em cães.

Tabela 250.2	Cardiopatias congênitas: dados de estudos combinados.	
DEFEITO	**NÚMERO**	**PORCENTAGEM**
Cães[1,3,4,25,28,167,341,345]		
Persistência do ducto arterioso (PDA)	1.207	25,7
Estenose subaórtica (ESA)	1.102	23,5
Estenose da valva pulmonar (EP)	1.039	22,1
Defeito do septo ventricular (DSV)	413	8,8
Displasia da valva tricúspide (DVT)	216	4,6
Displasia da valva mitral (DVM)	204	4,3
Outros defeitos	160	3,4
Persistência do arco aórtico direito ou outra anomalia do anel vascular (PAAD)	155	3,3
Tetralogia de Fallot (ToF)	110	2,3
Defeito do septo atrial (DSA)	89	1,9
Total	4.694	100
Gatos[28,33-35,344]		
Defeito do septo ventricular (DSV)	80	18,4
Persistência do ducto arterioso (PDA)	49	11,3
Displasia da valva tricúspide (DVT)	47	10,8
Displasia da valva mitral (DVM)	44	10,1
Defeito do septo atrioventricular (DSAV)	42	9,7
Estenose aórtica (EA)	31	7,1
Tetralogia de Fallot (ToF)	30	6,9
Defeito do septo atrial (DSA)	26	6,0
Persistência do arco aórtico direito (PAAD)	23	5,3
Fibroelastose endocárdica (FEE)	21	4,8
Estenose pulmonar (EP)	17	3,9
Outras malformações	11	2,5
Ventrículo direito de dupla saída (VDDS)	7	1,6
Cor triatriatum sinister	7	1,6
Total	435	100

Reproduzida de Scansen BA, Cober RE e Bonagura JD: Cardiopatia congênita. In: Bonagura JD, Twedt DC, editors: *Kirk's current veterinary therapy XV*, 15 ed., St. Louis, 2014, Elsevier/Saunders, p. 756-761.

Diversas pesquisas sobre CC em gatos foram relatadas.[30-36] A maior parte proveniente de centros urbanos, os quais incluem o Animal Medical Center (Nova York) e o Angell Memorial Animal Hospital (Boston). A prevalência mundial de CC em gatos é incerta. Os dois maiores levantamentos indicaram prevalência de 0,02 a 0,1% em internações hospitalares, e 1,95 a 2,9% em necropsias, conforme publicações de Harpster e Zook e por Liu *et al.*[32-34] Em um estudo de necropsia menor, 3,5% dos 368 filhotes de gatos foram diagnosticados com CC.[31] O estudo de uma população de 57.025 gatos mestiços de abrigos relatou uma prevalência global de 0,14%.[26]

Em termos de malformações cardíacas específicas em gatos, há diferenças notáveis entre as pesquisas, que podem representar diferenças de metodologia de amostragem ou diferenças geográficas reais.[37] Scansen *et al.*[29] tabularam os resultados dos maiores levantamentos (ver Tabela 250.2). Os defeitos mais comumente diagnosticados nesses levantamentos foram DSV (18,4%), PDA (11,3%), DVT (10,8%), DVM (10,1%), defeito do septo atrioventricular (DSAV) (9,7%) e EA (7,1%). Algumas pesquisas mostraram uma predisposição maior em machos. Em um estudo retrospectivo de gatos mestiços de abrigos,[26] DSV foi mais comum (21%), com ESA e EA valvar associadas respondendo por 17% dos diagnósticos de CC. Obstruções em toda a extensão do fluxo de saída do ventrículo direito (OSVD) também foram relativamente comuns nessa população.

Classificação

Embora vários esquemas tenham sido concebidos para classificar a CC, o padrão na pediatria humana hoje é uma análise segmentar sequencial que modela o coração como três segmentos maiores: átrios, ventrículos e grandes artérias. As relações entre esses segmentos – atrioventricular e ventriculoarterial – também são importantes para a classificação. Na análise segmentar, os átrios e ventrículos não são definidos por suas conexões venosas, arteriais ou outras, mas sim por sua morfologia. A posição (*situs*) de cada átrio também é relevante para o sistema de classificação. Essa abordagem é especialmente atraente para CC complexa, e o leitor interessado pode consultar os escritos de Richard Van Praagh e Robert Anderson,[38,39] os dois autores principais (embora às vezes opostos) que redefiniram a anatomia da CC. Recentemente foi publicado um exemplo desse esquema aplicado a gatos.[37]

Esquemas organizacionais mais antigos e mais simples ainda são relevantes para a medicina veterinária, e estes incluem a classificação de lesões como anomalias das valvas cardíacas, obstruções ao fluxo de saída ventricular e defeitos que possibilitam desvios (*shunts*) de sangue da esquerda para a direita, da direita para esquerda ou bidirecional. Outros tipos de malformações podem envolver a posição, ou *situs*, do coração (como ocorre na ectopia *cordis* e *situs inversus*);[37] defeitos ou cistos no pericárdio (ver Capítulo 254) e uma série de anomalias vasculares envolvendo ou conectando-se ao coração (ver Capítulo 257).

Abordagem clínica

Na obtenção do histórico clínico, é importante observar a espécie e a raça, já que muitas doenças congênitas têm uma base genética suspeita ou comprovada, e a maioria das malformações cardíacas em cães mostra predisposição de determinadas raças (ver Tabela 250.1). Sempre que possível, os registros de saúde dos pais e de irmãos devem ser revisados. O diagnóstico clínico de CC geralmente se baseia não nos sinais clínicos, mas na detecção de um sopro cardíaco durante um exame de rotina ou clínico de saúde. A maioria dos animais jovens com CC é assintomática, quando examinada pela primeira vez. Mesmo os cães e gatos com defeitos hemodinâmicos graves, regurgitantes, obstrutivos ou *shunts* (desvios) parecem ser completamente normais para muitos proprietários, especialmente nos primeiros 6 a 12 meses de idade. O clínico não deve necessariamente concluir, a partir de um histórico não digno de nota, que o defeito subjacente é discreto. Uma boa regra geral é que, quando um cão

SEÇÃO 16 • Doença Cardiovascular

ou gato com CC não exibe sinais clínicos de doença cardíaca, o paciente está em alto risco de morte, a menos que alguma terapia possa ser instituída com relativa rapidez.

Não há histórico característico ou sinais clínicos específicos de CC. Quando sinais respiratórios, como taquipneia, são atribuídos a doença cardíaca, a possibilidade de CC deve ser ao menos considerada, especialmente em animais mais jovens. Os autores avaliaram muitos pacientes, nos quais os sinais clínicos de CC se manifestaram durante a meia-idade ou mesmo mais tarde. Às vezes, uma arritmia, como taquicardia ventricular ou fibrilação atrial, sobrevém e ocasiona síncope ou insuficiência cardíaca crônica (ICC). Os sinais clínicos de CC relevante podem incluir intolerância ao exercício, colapso por esforço ou síncope, morte súbita ou sinais clínicos de ICC. Os gatos, ocasionalmente, apresentam tromboembolismo arterial, especialmente quando há dilatação do átrio esquerdo secundária à obstrução na passagem da valva mitral.[40]

Exame físico

Sopro cardíaco é uma característica marcante da CC (ver Capítulo 55); no entanto, um número significativo de sopros não é detectado na rotina clínica. Respiração ofegante e ronronar não tratáveis, ritmo cardíaco acelerado, rotação cardíaca e áreas auscultatórias muito próximas, típicas em filhotes de cães e gatos, representam desafios à auscultação. Além disso, a ausência de ruído na auscultação do lado esquerdo, na base cardíaca craniodorsal (para PDA) e na área da valva tricúspide (regurgitação tricúspide) são erros bastante comuns no exame. Sopros suaves são comuns em filhotes de cães e gatos, e na maioria dos casos é de origem funcional benigna (sopro funcional).[18,20,41-43] Infelizmente, durante a auscultação, não há achados específicos que distingam um sopro funcional daquele associado a CC leve. O sopro sistólico, que é suave, breve e musical ou vibratório, é mais provável que represente um sopro funcional (inocente), mas essas características não são absolutas. Mesmo os sopros intermitentes podem estar associados a malformações, como DVM com obstrução dinâmica da via de saída do ventrículo esquerdo (OSVE). O diagnóstico de ESA e EA de grau trivial a leve é especialmente problemático em cães, principalmente em raças propensas a essas doenças. Simplesmente não há padrão-ouro para o diagnóstico de condições clinicamente irrelevantes, porém, potencialmente hereditárias (ver adiante). Em contrapartida, um sopro sistólico de intensidade moderada a alta ou um sopro com intensidade palpável é indicativo de CC em um animal jovem. Estes devem ser prontamente investigados por meio de ecocardiografia Doppler,[20] lembrando que a intensidade de um sopro pode, mas não necessariamente, correlacionar-se com a gravidade da lesão. As características típicas dos sopros cardíacos associados aos defeitos congênitos mais comuns são discutidas no capítulo que abordam malformações específicas.

A maioria dos filhotes de cães e gatos saudáveis, com sopro de intensidade fraca ou suave – especialmente aqueles que não se destinam à reprodução –, pode ser razoavelmente acompanhada por meio de exame físico repetitivo durante o período sequencial de vacinação. As razões fisiológicas para sopros, como febre, infecções e anemia,[43] devem ser excluídas. A intensidade de muitos sopros funcionais diminui durante o período de vacinação, mas os sopros que aumentam em intensidade ou duração, especialmente em cães de raças de porte maior, propensos a ESA ou a DVT, devem ser avaliados por meio do exame ecocardiográfico. O exame deve ser indicado a um cliente, para seu animal de estimação, quando o sopro suave persistir. A detecção precoce de CC possibilita estabelecer o tratamento definitivo, quando aplicável (ver Capítulo 122). Aceitando o fato de que a maioria das pessoas desenvolve rapidamente um vínculo com seus animais de estimação, a detecção precoce de CC é valiosa para o proprietário que está disposto a aceitar a substituição de um animal de estimação saudável por um que possui malformação cardíaca.

A intensidade e a duração do sopro correlacionam-se com a gravidade de algumas lesões, especialmente com ESA e EP. Em contrapartida, um sopro pode ser discreto em alguns casos de CC grave. Em teoria, um grande DSV pode ser acompanhado apenas por um sopro suave devido ao equilíbrio da pressão ventricular, mas praticamente, na maioria dos casos, há pelo menos um sopro moderadamente alto, a menos que haja hipertensão pulmonar concomitante. No cenário de hipertensão pulmonar grave, como no PDA reverso, pode não haver sopro, e apenas um som cardíaco timpânico ou desdobrado é detectado. A eritrocitose secundária ao *shunt* de direita para esquerda também reduz a probabilidade de turbulência que acompanha os sopros. O sopro associado à displasia de válvula AV grave pode ser de baixa intensidade, especialmente na estenose de valva AV.

Os achados de exame físico auxiliares são, às vezes, úteis no diagnóstico diferencial e na avaliação clínica. A palpação de uma elevação ventricular (um impulso apical proeminente indicando aumento do ventrículo) ou a excitação precordial (indicando o ponto de intensidade máximo de um sopro cardíaco de alta intensidade) pode ser útil no que diz respeito à lesão subjacente. Pulsos arterial e venoso também podem oferecer uma visão sobre a anormalidade primária; no entanto, a frequência cardíaca rápida e o pequeno tamanho de muitos pacientes diminuem a sensibilidade do diagnóstico com base no exame físico, especialmente para clínicos inexperientes. Pulso arterial hipercinético (pulso em martelo d'água) é característico de lesões que provocam esvaziamento diastólico anormal do fluxo sanguíneo aórtico e baixa pressão arterial diastólica; as causas clássicas de tais condições são PDA e regurgitação aórtica grave. Pulsos arterial hipocinético ou tardiamente aumentado são típicos de OSVE de intensidade moderada a grave (p. ex., ESA) ou de defeitos graves acompanhados por baixo débito do ventrículo esquerdo (VE). Pulso venoso jugular proeminente ou congestão da veia jugular é indicativo de anormalidade do lado direito do coração, como acontece no DVT ou na EP.

A presença de cianose em um animal jovem, especialmente na ausência de dispneia ou doença pulmonar evidente, deve fazer pensar fortemente na possibilidade de malformação cardíaca e "cardiopatia cianótica" (ver Capítulo 52). O termo "cardiopatia congênita cianótica" é usado para categorizar esses defeitos congênitos que ocasionam mistura de sangue venoso e arterial, como na ToF. O *shunt* da direita para a esquerda refere-se a situações em que o sangue dessaturado flui para as artérias sistêmicas, permitindo a mistura de sangue dessaturado com sangue oxigenado, levando à hipoxemia. Isso pode ocorrer como resultado de defeitos, como a transposição dos grandes vasos ou uma combinação de um defeito comunicante, conectando os dois lados da circulação sanguínea, e algum mecanismo que eleva a pressão do lado direito, como acontece na ToF. *Shunt* reverso foi observado em casos de PDA, "janela" aorticopulmonar, DSV, DSA e EP ou DVT com patência do forame oval. Nota-se cianose evidente quando a pressão arterial parcial de oxigênio diminui para menos de $\approx$ 45 mmHg e o teor de hemoglobina arterial dessaturada atinge 5 g/dℓ. Cianose diferencial é típica de PDA reversa (ver a seguir).

Fisiologia do shunt da direita para a esquerda

O termo síndrome de Eisenmenger (fisiologia) é utilizado para descrever as circunstâncias em que a resistência vascular pulmonar aumentada causa reversão de um *shunt* da esquerda para a direita e causa cardiopatia cianótica.[44-46] Os fatores primários envolvidos na ocorrência da síndrome de Eisenmenger não estão completamente compreendidos, mas provavelmente estão relacionados a tensões de cisalhamento causadas pelas taxas de fluxo na vascularização pulmonar e nas alterações proliferativas na parede do vaso.[44,46-49] A síndrome de Eisenmenger geralmente se desenvolve rapidamente em cães e quase sempre antes dos 6 meses de idade. Em gatos, o desenvolvimento da doença vascular pulmonar pode ser mais gradual. Espessamento da camada íntima da artéria pulmonar, hipertrofia medial e lesões plexiformes em cães e gatos com fisiologia de Eisenmenger são semelhantes aos do homem, como descrito por Edwards e Heath e modificado por Roberts.[50] Em alguns casos, um componente do aumento de resistência vascular pulmonar está relacionado à vasoconstrição arterial. Esses pacientes podem responder clinicamente aos inibidores da fosfodiesterase V, como o sildenafila, que atuam como vasodilatadores pulmonares. Entretanto, as lesões plexiformes são geralmente consideradas irreversíveis. O fechamento cirúrgico do *shunt* força o ventrículo direito (VD) a trabalhar contra uma enorme resistência pulmonar, podendo ocasionar insuficiência do VD, colapso circulatório e morte.

Respostas sistêmicas à hipoxemia arterial incluem aumento da quantidade de hemácias, na tentativa de melhorar a disponibilidade de oxigênio. A hipoxia do tecido renal estimula a liberação de eritropoetina, que induz eritrocitose secundária. À medida que o valor do hematócrito (Ht) aumenta, a maior viscosidade do sangue predispõe os pacientes a trombose e complicações microvasculares.[44,47] Essa síndrome de hiperviscosidade, que tipicamente ocorre quando o valor do Ht excede 68%, é a principal causa de morbidade e mortalidade em animais com ICC, o que é raro. As manifestações clínicas dessa condição consistem em fraqueza; deficiências hemostáticas; disfunção renal; alterações metabólicas, como acidose; deficiência de ferro, eventos cerebrovasculares; síncope e convulsões.[51-54]

A direção do fluxo sanguíneo no *shunt* depende da resistência relativa dos mecanismos sistêmicos e da circulação pulmonar. O exercício promove vasodilatação arteriolar sistêmica e diminui a resistência sistêmica, aumentando, assim, a magnitude do *shunt* da direita para a esquerda. Nos casos de hipertrofia do VD e de DSV, a taquicardia ou o tônus simpático elevado pode aumentar a magnitude do *shunt* da direita para a esquerda por exacerbar a obstrução infundibular dinâmica e do aumento da resistência à ejeção do VD.[55] O bloqueio induzido por fármacos beta-adrenérgicos não específicos às vezes é utilizado para dessensibilizar ou prevenir essa ocorrência, particularmente em pacientes com ToF.[53,56] Betabloqueadores também tendem a limitar a atividade física, sendo outra explicação para sua eficácia em alguns pacientes. Anemia, absoluta ou relativa, reduz a relação entre resistência sistêmica e resistência pulmonar quando a resistência é estável.[52] Por esse mecanismo, a flebotomia excessivamente zelosa pode aumentar a gravidade da hipoxemia arterial, uma vez que diminui a capacidade de transporte de oxigênio pelo sangue.

O *shunt* da direita para a esquerda leva a aumentos compensatórios no fluxo sanguíneo sistêmico que nutre o pulmão, via artérias brônquicas. Esses vasos sistêmicos colaterais são facilmente reconhecidos na angiografia. Embora incomum, é possível que esses vasos se rompam, levando à hemoptise. Embolia paradoxal é outra complicação potencial do *shunt* da direita para a esquerda. Normalmente, os vasos sanguíneos pulmonares filtram os êmbolos venosos sistêmicos antes que eles atinjam o lado esquerdo da circulação. No *shunt* reverso, deve-se considerar a possibilidade de um êmbolo venoso atingir o sistema coronariano, cerebral ou outras artérias, particularmente quando se utiliza cateter. Por esse mecanismo, um trombo, microrganismos infecciosos ou o ar podem ter acesso a órgão vitais. Animais com doença cardíaca cianótica às vezes manifestam reações adversas (particularmente bradicardia) a sedativos e tranquilizantes.

Testes diagnósticos

A investigação diagnóstica no paciente com suspeita de CC atualmente se baseia na ecocardiografia com Doppler. Exames adicionais, incluindo radiografia, eletrocardiografia e exames clínico-laboratoriais podem ser úteis, porém raramente são definitivos em termos de diagnóstico. Exames de imagem avançados, como tomografia computadorizada (TC) com contraste (angiotomografia) ou angiografia por ressonância magnética são mais úteis no diagnóstico de CC complexa e anomalias vasculares. Cateterismo cardíaco com angiografia[30,57-60] é ainda o método de diagnóstico padrão-ouro, porém raramente é realizado, exceto durante terapias administradas via cateter (ver Capítulo 122).

Radiografias torácicas devem ser obtidas em todos os casos em que sinais respiratórios são encontrados. Além de mostrar a ICC, as radiografias também podem ajudar a verificar o estágio de gravidade da doença, especialmente em casos de sobrecarga de volume, causados por malformação da valva AV ou *shunt* da direita para a esquerda.[61-64] Os principais achados incluem identificação do aumento das câmaras específicas, dilatação dos grandes vasos e circulação pulmonar. Contudo, a hipertrofia concêntrica é subestimada em exame radiográfico e só pode ser detectada por meio da elevação do ápice (para o VD) ou pelo leve alongamento cardíaco (para o VE). A dilatação da artéria pulmonar principal é sugestiva de SP, *shunt* da esquerda para a direita ou de hipertensão pulmonar. A dilatação da artéria aorta é observada em casos de ESA, aortopatias[65] e PDA. O aumento da vascularização pulmonar é compatível com *shunt* da esquerda para a direita, enquanto indicadores de insuficiência vascular são frequentemente vistos em *shunt* da direita para a esquerda ou na hipertensão pulmonar.

Na ausência de arritmia cardíaca, na era da ecocardiografia Doppler, a utilidade do eletrocardiograma de múltiplas derivações (ECG; ver Capítulo 103) é menor. O resultado normal no ECG não exclui o diagnóstico de CC. Mesmo assim, o ECG pode frequentemente detectar anormalidades de condução ou aumento de volume moderado a grave de átrios ou ventrículos, que podem ser sugestivos de um ou mais distúrbios específicos.[66,67] Como exemplos, maior voltagem do segmento QRS nas derivações precordiais caudal e esquerda é típico de PDA; o *shunt* do eixo direito é comum na EP moderada a grave; e desdobramento de complexos QRS são relatados no DVT.[68] O achado frequente de um eixo frontal craniano frequentemente minimiza o valor das derivações padrão dos membros em gatos. O importante é que a principal indicação para um ECG na CC é a detecção de arritmias ou evidências de isquemia do miocárdio, que podem indicar uma forma mais complicada de CC. Um eletrocardiograma (Holter) ambulatorial pode ser útil para detectar arritmias induzidas por exercício ou isquemia que necessite de tratamento imediato. Deve-se ressaltar que algumas anormalidades do ritmo cardíaco devem ser considerados como uma forma de CC, em particular de vias acessórias associadas a pré-excitação ventricular e taquicardias supraventriculares reentrantes (ver Capítulo 248). Estas têm sido observadas em cães da raça Labrador Retriever com DVT.

Além do hematócrito (ou volume globular), os testes laboratoriais de rotina são de pouca utilidade, exceto em casos complicados por ICC, tromboembolismo ou outras comorbidades. A hipoxemia pode ser verificada por oximetria de pulso ou hemogasometria arterial, mas esses testes raramente são necessários.

Ecocardiografia

Estudos de ecocardiografia com Doppler (ver Capítulo 104) suplantaram amplamente o uso de cateterismo cardíaco e angiografia no diagnóstico e na avaliação da maioria das lesões cardíacas congênitas. Esse teste diagnóstico é descrito em detalhe no Capítulo 104 e em muitos exemplos e referências no presente capítulo.[69-85] Ecocardiografia com contraste salino às vezes é realizada para identificar desvios (*shunt*) da direita para a esquerda, especialmente através do forame oval patente (FOP), DSA ou DSV.

Os principais resultados do estudo ecocardiográfico na CC podem ser resumidos da seguinte forma: (1) identificação da morfologia das lesões, como os defeitos do septo, PDA, malformações valvares, e obstruções do fluxo sanguíneo por meio de uso de imagens 2D e 3D; (2) caracterização das respostas secundárias, como dilatação de câmaras cardíacas e grandes vasos, e detecção de hipertrofia do miocárdio por meio de estudos de imagens 2D, 3D e modo M; (3) detecção de fluxo sanguíneo anormal, como *shunts* e disfunção valvular, utilizando-se Doppler colorido e espectral; (4) quantificação da função ventricular sistólica e diastólica, usando múltiplas modalidades; (5) avaliação das pressões, fluxos e resistências, usando principalmente o método Doppler. Essas avaliações detalhadas geralmente requerem um profissional treinado nessa área, porque muitas avaliações precisam ser modificadas durante o exame, com base em achados recentes. Ecocardiografia transesofágica também é muito importante em CC, não apenas para o diagnóstico de algumas anormalidades, mas também para orientação durante o procedimento de cateterização.[86] Ecocardiografia epicárdica também é usada durante os chamados procedimentos híbridos – aqueles que associam técnicas cirúrgicas a técnicas em que se utilizam cateteres – para orientação de dispositivos colocados de forma transmural, através da parede atrial ou ventricular.

Ambos os aspectos da ecocardiografia, qualitativos (interpretação subjetiva) e quantitativos, são relevantes para o diagnóstico e avaliação de CC. Devido a diferenças no tamanho do corpo e do crescimento, pode ser difícil quantificar o tamanho do coração com base na raça ou no peso corporal. Isso pode ser um desafio, porém os profissionais mais experientes podem, de forma subjetiva, prever o aumento moderado ou o grave das câmaras cardíacas em casos de CC. Aspectos importantes dessa modalidade, como a equação de Bernoulli modificada, são apresentados em detalhes no Capítulo 104 e são ilustrados com exemplos no presente capítulo.

Cateterismo cardíaco

O cateterismo cardíaco é um procedimento hemodinâmico e angiográfico invasivo realizado para fim diagnóstico ou terapêutico. A maioria dos procedimentos de cateterismo envolve mensuração hemodinâmica – principalmente pressões intracardíaca e intravascular (Figura 250.1) – com angiografia e alguma forma de intervenção com uso de cateter. Devido aos efeitos anestésicos, mensurações hemodinâmicas, especialmente pressão sanguínea e débito cardíaco, são marcadamente deprimidos em comparação ao estado acordado ou levemente sedado, e não correspondem às mensurações obtidas em Doppler, a menos que sejam realizadas sob as mesmas condições.[75] Atualmente, o cateterismo cardíaco é reservado principalmente a procedimentos destinados ao reparo ou tratamento paliativo da CC. Exemplos específicos incluem valvuloplastia por cateter-balão para EP, colocação de dispositivo de oclusão para fechamento de PDA ou de DSA, e em estudos eletrofisiológicos utilizados para identificar e, em seguida, fazer ablação de uma via elétrica acessória. Princípios e exemplos de procedimentos de cateterização são discutidos mais detalhadamente no Capítulo 122.

PERSISTÊNCIA DO DUCTO ARTERIOSO

O ducto arterioso desenvolve-se a partir do sexto arco aórtico esquerdo embrionário. Essa estrutura fetal vital desvia o sangue não oxigenado da artéria pulmonar, por meio da artéria aorta descendente, para a placenta, onde o sangue é oxigenado, desviando assim a maior parte do fluxo sanguíneo do VD para longe do pulmão do feto, não funcional. Após o parto e início da respiração, a resistência vascular pulmonar diminui, o fluxo no ducto reverte e o aumento resultante na tensão de oxigênio arterial inibe a liberação local de prostaglandina. Esses processos levam à constrição do músculo liso da parede vascular e ao fechamento funcional do ducto arterioso. O ducto pode permanecer patente em filhotes com menos de 4 dias de idade, mas geralmente se fecha de maneira segura em 7 a 10 dias após o nascimento.[2,87,88] A PDA, além do período neonatal imediato, é denominada PDA e é o primeiro ou segundo defeito cardíaco congênito mais comumente diagnosticado em cães, dependendo da pesquisa. Gatos também são acometidos, mas com muito menos frequência que cães.

Patogênese

A falha do fechamento do ducto em cães e gatos ocasiona distintas anormalidades histológicas na parede do ducto. A parede do ducto, no feto saudável, apresenta um padrão de ramificação circunferencial frouxa do músculo liso, em todo o seu comprimento. Já em raças de filhotes que possuem alta probabilidade de apresentar PDA, diversas porções da parede do ducto são constituídas apenas por fibras elásticas. O aumento da prevalência de PDA em muitas raças (ver Tabela 250.1) indica que fatores genéticos provavelmente estão envolvidos na patogênese. Uma linhagem de cães da raça Poodle, com hereditariedade para PDA, tem sido extensivamente investigada, e um padrão poligênico de herança tem sido sugerido.[89] O aumento da probabilidade genética para a PDA resulta em "extensão da estrutura da parede não contrátil da artéria aorta para um segmento crescente do ducto arterioso, prejudicando progressivamente sua capacidade de fechamento fisiológico".[2] No homem, foram identificadas anormalidades nos genes que interferem na remodelação das células musculares lisas vasculares da parte média do ducto, a suposta causa de PDA.[90] É provável que defeitos genéticos semelhantes possam interferir no músculo liso vascular de cães com PDA.

Em sua forma mais branda, subclínica, o ducto se fecha completamente na extremidade da artéria pulmonar e forma-se uma bolsa de fundo cego em forma de funil na parte ventral da artéria aorta, conhecida como *ductus diverticulum*. Esse tipo de PDA, caracterizado por fechamento incompleto do ducto (a *forma branda* da doença), só pode ser diagnosticado por meio de angiografia ou necropsia, mas indica que o cão é portador da carga genética que causa esse defeito.[2,89] O diagnóstico ecocardiográfico de *ductus diverticulum* não foi relatado em cães ou outros animais. O aumento da probabilidade do envolvimento genético resulta em ducto cônico, em forma de funil, que persiste após o período pós-natal imediato, possibilitando um fluxo de sangue da artéria aorta para a artéria pulmonar, onde a pressão intravascular é mais baixa (Figura 250.2 A e B). Essa é a forma mais comum de PDA observada em cães.[91] A forma mais grave, porém relativamente não muito comum, é o ducto cilíndrico, não cônico, com persistente hipertensão pulmonar pós-natal (reação ou síndrome de Eisenmenger) e *shunt* bidirecional ou *shunt* da direita para a esquerda (Figura 250.2 C e D). PDA pode ser detectado também em animais com formas complexas de CC. Para informações adicionais sobre a morfologia e patogênese da PDA, o leitor pode consultar diversas revisões excelentes sobre o assunto.[92,94]

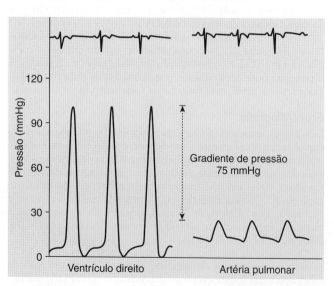

Figura 250.1 Traçado da pressão intracardíaca de cão mestiço de 1 ano, obtido durante o cateterismo do coração direito e artéria pulmonar (AP). As pressões de PA estão normais. Há um gradiente de pressão sistólica de 75 mmHg entre o VD e a AP, indicando a presença de uma obstrução ao fluxo do ventrículo direito (nesse caso, estenose da valva pulmonar [EP]). Há também um pequeno gradiente de pressão diastólica entre a AP e o VD, causado pelo fechamento diastólico da valva pulmonar, um achado normal. O ECG exibe uma onda S profunda, que é frequentemente encontrada em animais com EP e hipertrofia secundária do VD.

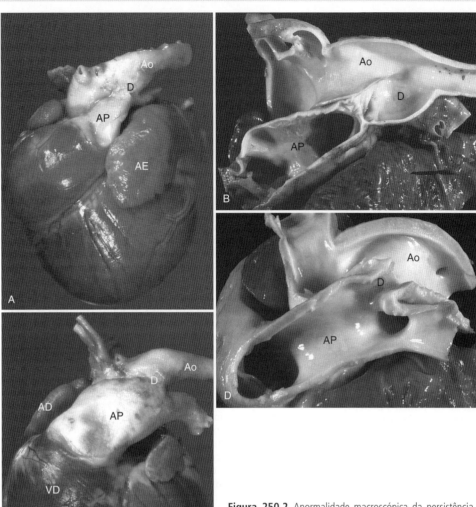

Figura 250.2 Anormalidade macroscópica da persistência do ducto arterioso (PDA). **A.** Visão do lado esquerdo do coração de um cão da raça Pastor-Australiano de 9 semanas de vida, com PDA com *shunt* da esquerda para a direita, mostrando a localização anatômica do ducto (*D*), entre a artéria aorta descendente (*Ao*) e a artéria pulmonar principal (*AP*). A aurícula esquerda (*AE*) está aumentada. **B.** Visão da direita para a esquerda de corte do PDA em um cão. O ducto apresenta forma de funil, com estreitamento na direção da extremidade da AP. **C.** Visão do lado esquerdo do coração de um cão com PDA e *shunt* da direita para a esquerda. Note o aumento do ventrículo direito (*VD*) e da aurícula direita (*AD*). A artéria pulmonar (*AP*) está aumentada. **D.** Visão de corte de um PDA, com *shunt* da direita para a esquerda, em um cão. Note a forma cilíndrica do ducto (*D*) e o fato de que a localização anatômica do ducto é distal aos ramos aórticos que suprem a porção cranial do corpo.

Fisiopatologia

A direção do fluxo sanguíneo na PDA é determinada pelas resistências relativas dos leitos vasculares pulmonar e sistêmico e, na grande maioria dos casos, segue da esquerda para a direita (ou seja, da artéria aorta para a artéria pulmonar). A extensão do *shunt* é determinada pelo gradiente de pressão relativo entre a circulação sistêmica e circulação pulmonar, bem como pelo grau de resistência no PDA. Na maioria das vezes, a região limítrofe situa-se na altura do óstio pulmonar, onde o ducto é mais estreito. Na PDA, o fluxo sanguíneo gera uma sobrecarga na circulação pulmonar, onde o sangue é desviado da artéria aorta para a artéria pulmonar. O aumento do volume de ejeção do VE, em consequência de um aumento do retorno venoso pulmonar e do volume diastólico final, associado com a hipertrofia excêntrica, contribui para um aumento da pressão sistólica na artéria aorta. Na diástole, o rápido escoamento do sangue da artéria aorta para a artéria pulmonar, de baixa pressão, via PDA, gera uma redução na pressão diastólica da aorta. A diferença de pressão resultante, entre as pressões arteriais sistólica e diastólica, gera o pulso arterial hipercinético (pulso em martelo d'água), detectado em cães com *shunts* consideráveis (ver Capítulo 56). Uma vez que o sangue passa continuamente pelo PDA durante a sístole e a diástole, surge um sopro contínuo que é tipicamente mais alto, próximo ao momento da segunda bulha cardíaca (ver Capítulo 55). Todas as estruturas vasculares envolvidas no transporte do sangue desviado aumentam, de modo a acomodar o volume extra, com dilatação da artéria aorta proximal, da artéria pulmonar principal e dos vasos sanguíneos pulmonares. A dilatação do átrio esquerdo (AE) e a hipertrofia excêntrica do VE desenvolvem-se em proporção ao volume de fluxo, ao longo do *shunt*. Esse mecanismo possibilita a compensação do volume, nessa condição de sobrecarga, por um período variável de tempo; contudo, se o *shunt* for grande, a insuficiência do miocárdio (cardiomiopatia por sobrecarga de volume) se desenvolve com a elevação progressiva da pressão diastólica final do VE e do evidente edema pulmonar. Como o *shunt* da esquerda para a direita ocorre em grandes vasos, o VD e a AD não são diretamente expostos ao sangue desviado, e essas estruturas permanecem normais, a menos que hipertensão pulmonar se desenvolva.

Em uma pequena porcentagem de casos de PDA em cães, o lúmen da PDA permanece amplo, sem estreitar-se no óstio pulmonar. A ausência de resistência do orifício do ducto possibilita que a pressão aórtica seja transmitida à circulação pulmonar sem resistência e, portanto, impedindo o declínio pós-natal normal da resistência vascular pulmonar. Nessa circunstância, as pressões das artérias aorta e pulmonar se equilibram, e o VD permanece com hipertrofia concêntrica após o nascimento, e pode ocorrer reversão do fluxo através do *shunt*. Em uma colônia de cães Patterson, esse padrão de hipertensão pulmonar de *shunt* reverso (direita para esquerda) desenvolveu-se nas primeiras semanas de vida.[89] Essas observações corroboram a manifestação clínica usual da maioria dos cães diagnosticados com PDA (reversa), geralmente sem histórico de sopro contínuo e nenhuma evidência de aumento do VE nos primeiros anos de vida. A maioria dos cães com PDA reversa exibe uma diminuição do fluxo sanguíneo pulmonar, VE normalmente é pequeno e hipertrofia concêntrica do VD acentuada. Em raras ocasiões, cães com PDA com *shunt* da esquerda para a direita de grau moderado a alto manifestam aumento repentino da resistência pulmonar devido à vasculite pulmonar necrosante. Da mesma forma, é raro detectar a gradual reversão da direção do *shunt*, normalmente com vários meses a vários anos de idade, após histórico de ICC do lado esquerdo.[49] Um aumento substancial do VE residual é evidente nas radiografias do tórax e no ecocardiograma. O fluxo sanguíneo pulmonar é reduzido, mas a hipertrofia do VD é menos marcante do que nos cães em que ocorre reversão da direção do *shunt* em idade precoce. A patogênese exata da hipertensão pulmonar não é completamente compreendida, mas as descrições anatômicas da vascularização pulmonar são semelhantes nos homens e animais. As alterações histológicas em pequenas artérias pulmonares consistem em hipertrofia da camada média, espessamento da camada íntima e redução da dimensão do lúmen vascular e desenvolvimento de lesões plexiformes na parede dos vasos.[49,50,95] A maioria dessas alterações é considerada irreversível, impossibilitando a correção cirúrgica da PDA reversa, exceto, possivelmente, em casos raros, quando a pressão arterial pulmonar se mantém subsistêmica, condição observada em gatos com PDA e menos frequentemente em cães.[96]

Achados clínicos

A PDA é o único defeito cardíaco congênito em que há predisposição sexual para as fêmeas (2,49/1.000, em fêmeas, e 1,45/1.000, em machos).[1] Muitas predisposições por raça para PDA foram relatadas (ver Tabela 250.1). Filhotes de cães e gatos gravemente comprometidos podem desenvolver baixa estatura, baixo escore corporal ou taquipneia, devido à ICC do lado esquerdo, e é provável que alguns filhotes venham a óbito devido à insuficiência cardíaca antes da primeira consulta pelo veterinário, o que normalmente ocorre entre 6 e 8 semanas de vida. A maioria dos filhotes é assintomática, com desenvolvimento físico normal no momento do diagnóstico.

Persistência do ducto arterioso com shunt da esquerda para a direita

Um exame físico completo geralmente é suficiente para sugerir o diagnóstico inicial. Na maioria das vezes, o pulso arterial é hipercinético. As membranas mucosas são rosadas, a menos que haja ICC grave do lado esquerdo. O estímulo precordial é frequentemente exagerado e abrange uma área maior da parede torácica do que é normal, devido ao aumento do VE. Um batimento é comumente palpado na região craniodorsal axilar esquerda, e um sopro contínuo clássico é ouvido melhor neste local (Figura 250.3 e ver Capítulo 55). O ponto de intensidade máxima do sopro está localizado sobre a artéria pulmonar principal, na base do coração esquerdo, na região craniodorsal e pode irradiar-se cranialmente até a entrada torácica e à base cardíaca direita, onde é quase sempre mais suave.[89,97,98] Frequentemente, apenas um sopro sistólico é audível sobre a área da valva mitral. Esse sopro pode resultar da radiação da porção mais alta do sopro contínuo da base do coração ou pode ser oriundo da regurgitação mitral secundária, que se desenvolveu em consequência da

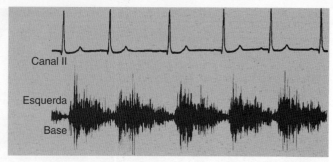

Figura 250.3 Fonocardiograma registrado na base do coração esquerdo de um cão com persistência do ducto arterioso (PDA) e *shunt* da esquerda para a direita. A derivação II do ECG é registrada simultaneamente para monitorar o ritmo (a sístole mecânica ventricular consiste em, aproximadamente, o período desde a metade do complexo QRS até o fim da onda T; o restante do tempo é diástole). O sopro gravado é contínuo, aumentando de intensidade durante a sístole, com pico próximo ao fim da sístole, e diminuindo de intensidade durante a diástole.

grande dilatação do VE. Em gatos, o sopro contínuo da PDA pode ser mais bem audível na região um pouco mais caudoventral do que em cães acometidos, e o sopro é frequentemente confundido com um "longo" sopro sistólico, especialmente se a hipertensão pulmonar estiver em desenvolvimento. Outros diagnósticos diferenciais para essa condição de um sopro contínuo como característica incluem desvio aortopulmonar, fístula arteriovenosa coronariana, ruptura de aneurisma do seio de Valsalva, janela aorticopulmonar, artéria coronária esquerda anômala e desvios arteriovenosos, embora sejam relativamente raros em comparação com a prevalência de PDA.[99-102]

Radiografias torácicas mostram aumento do tamanho do coração esquerdo e sobrecarga na circulação pulmonar, proporcionalmente à magnitude do *shunt* da esquerda para a direita (Figura 250.4). Na projeção dorsoventral, o arco aórtico, a aurícula esquerda e a artéria pulmonar principal podem ser anormalmente proeminentes. O achado radiográfico mais específico é o aparecimento de uma protuberância aórtica ("tumefação do ducto"), que é causada pelo estreitamento abrupto da artéria aorta descendente, somente na porção caudal até a origem do ducto, dilatação de aneurisma da artéria aorta e/ou o próprio ducto (Figura 250.4). O aumento moderado a grave do VE às vezes faz com que o ápice cardíaco se desloque para a direita (comum em gatos). Edema pulmonar surge após o início da ICC.

Quando o ritmo é normal, o ECG contribui pouco para a definição do diagnóstico. É possível constatar indicações de aumento do VE (aumento das ondas Q e R nas derivações II, III, aVF e precordiais esquerdas, V2 e V4) e aumento do AE (ondas P alargadas). Arritmia é a principal indicação para o registro de um ECG, e em cães com PDA de longa duração, fibrilação atrial, assim como complexos supraventriculares e ventriculares prematuros podem se desenvolver (ver Capítulo 248).

O diagnóstico de PDA pode ser confirmado pelo completo estudo ecocardiográfico com Doppler em quase todos os casos. A ecocardiografia em modo 2D e M demonstra hipertrofia excêntrica do VE e dilatação do AE, da artéria aorta ascendente e da artéria pulmonar (Figura 250.5 A e Vídeos 250.1 e 250.2). Função ventricular sistólica reduzida pode ser observada, e é sugerida por achados de redução do encurtamento da fração, aumento do ponto E de separação septal e/ou aumento do volume sistólico final do VE. O ducto pode ser visualizado e seu tamanho estimado a partir de imagem paraesternal craniana esquerda (Figura 250.5 B e Vídeo 250.3).[103] O exame Doppler da artéria pulmonar principal mostra fluxo contínuo de alta velocidade direcionado para a valva pulmonar (Figura 250.5 C e Vídeo 250.4). No caso típico, a velocidade máxima desse jato é de pelo menos 4,5 a 5 m/s e ocorre no fim da sístole (Figura 250.5 D). Outros achados ecocardiográficos comuns

CAPÍTULO 250 • Cardiopatias Congênitas   1223

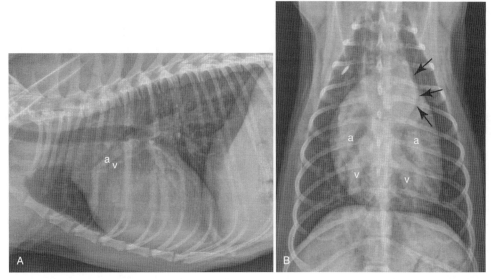

Figura 250.4 Radiografias do tórax de cão portador de PDA com *shunt* da esquerda para a direita. **A.** Projeção lateral mostra aumento do AE e aumento das veias (*v*) e artérias pulmonares craniais (*a*) **B.** Projeção dorsoventral mostra cardiomegalia moderada, protuberância característica na artéria aorta descendente (*setas*) e dilatação da artéria pulmonar principal. Os vasos sanguíneos pulmonares são proeminentes.

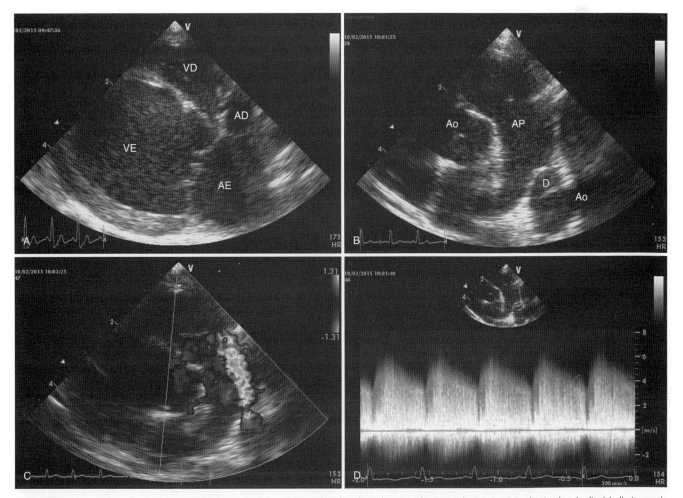

Figura 250.5 Ecocardiografia de cão com persistência do ducto arterioso (PDA) e *shunt* da esquerda para a direita. **A.** Visão do eixo longitudinal à direita revela dilatação excêntrica de ventrículo esquerdo (*VE*) e átrio esquerdo (*AE*). O ventrículo direito (*VD*) e o átrio direito (*AD*) são normais. **B.** Visão do canal (*D*) em imagem a partir da base do coração esquerdo. O ducto típico, com *shunt* da esquerda para a direita, é mais largo na extremidade aórtica (*Ao*) e se estreita próximo à artéria pulmonar principal (*AP*). **C.** Imagem de Doppler colorido de fluxo aplicada à imagem ecocardiográfica, em **B**, mostrando fluxo sanguíneo turbulento da esquerda para a direita, através do ducto. **D.** traçado de Doppler de onda contínua do jato da PDA obtido a partir da base do coração esquerdo mostrando fluxo contínuo e velocidade máxima em torno de 6 m/s. (*As figuras C e D encontram-se reproduzidas em cores no Encarte.*)

incluem aumento discreto da velocidade do fluxo expiratório (1,8 a 2,3 m/s, mas às vezes maior) e aumento secundário e leve da velocidade do fluxo mitral (Vídeo 250.5), insuficiência das valvas aórtica e pulmonar, embora em alguns cães possa ser detectada regurgitação mitral moderada a grave. Em cães com PDA, os defeitos cardíacos associados são incomuns; no entanto, ainda vale a pena excluir, por meio de um exame ecocardiográfico cuidadosamente realizado, a presença de defeitos congênitos concomitantes, como EP. Devido ao aumento do volume de ejeção e da velocidade do fluxo ao longo da OSVE, o diagnóstico de ESA/EA leve pode ser difícil de ser encontrado no cenário de ESA aberta, sua gravidade pode não ser evidente até que o ducto esteja fechado. Em animais que desenvolvem hipertensão pulmonar, hipertrofia concêntrica do ventrículo direito também pode estar presente, juntamente com acentuada dilatação da AP. Técnicas de ecocardiografia transesofágica também têm sido descritas e podem fornecer uma visualização aprimorada da anatomia do ducto.[86,104] Cateterismo e angiocardiografia cardíacos geralmente não são necessários para confirmar o diagnóstico de PDA (Vídeo 250.6) e não são recomendados, a menos que a avaliação ecocardiográfica Doppler seja ambígua ou malformações congênitas adicionais sejam suspeitas.

Persistência do ducto arterioso com hipertensão pulmonar e shunt *da direita para a esquerda*

A alta resistência vascular pulmonar, causando *shunt* da direita para a esquerda através da PDA, define a síndrome clínica comumente referida como "PDA reversa".[49,51,89,95,105-109] O *shunt* da direita para a esquerda é observado em uma minoria muito pequena de cães com PDA, mas a prevalência desse fenômeno é provavelmente subestimada e pode ser aumentada em cães que vivem em altitudes superiores a 1.500 metros acima do nível do mar. Os sinais clínicos são geralmente evidentes durante o primeiro ano de vida, mas muitos proprietários não reconhecem os sinais clínicos em seus animais de estimação durante os primeiros 6 a 12 meses de vida, e alguns animais não são diagnosticados até 3 a 4 anos de idade ou ainda mais tarde. Os sinais relatados incluem: fadiga por esforço, fraqueza de membros pélvicos, respiração superficial, hiperpneia, cianose diferencial e, raramente, convulsões. O exame clínico é bem diferente das PDA mais comuns de *shunt* da esquerda para a direita. O fluxo que passa da direta para a esquerda na PDA exibe pouca turbulência e o exame físico revela ausência de sopro cardíaco ou somente sopro sistólico na base esquerda do coração. O achado mais comum na auscultação é a exacerbação e o desdobramento da segunda bulha cardíaca. Cianose diferencial (cianose das membranas mucosas caudais, com membranas mucosas craniais róseas) pode ser observada, porém o reconhecimento pode exigir a avaliação após o exercício. A cianose diferencial é causada pela localização da PDA, que desvia o fluxo sanguíneo da direita para a esquerda, da artéria pulmonar para a artéria aorta descendente (ver Figura 250.2 C e D), mas poupa os ramos proximais da artéria aorta desta região e, então, fornece a demanda normal de oxigênio para a parte cranial do corpo. A perfusão dos rins com sangue com baixa oxigenação estimula a produção de eritropoetina e eritrocitose secundária, bem como hiperviscosidade sanguínea com o aumento gradativo do hematócrito (Ht) até um valor de 65% ou mais.[51] A eritrocitose pode ocorrer durante o primeiro ano de vida, mas muitas vezes não se agrava até os 18 a 24 meses de idade.

O ECG de cães com PDA reversa praticamente sempre revela evidências de hipertrofia do VD (desvio do eixo à direita, aumento da amplitude da onda S nas derivações I, II, III e precordiais esquerdas, V2 e V4). As radiografias do tórax indicam aumento do coração direito, dilatação da artéria pulmonar principal, uma visível "tumefação doo ducto" e aparência variável das artérias lobares e periféricas. A ecocardiografia mostra hipertrofia concêntrica do VD e dilatação da artéria pulmonar principal (Figura 250.6). Em alguns casos, um ducto largo e cilíndrico

pode ser visualizado (Figura 250.6). Hipertensão pulmonar pode ser verificada em alguns casos por meio do Doppler, averiguando-se os jatos de insuficiência tricúspide ou de insuficiência pulmonar (Figura 250.6). Ecocardiografia com contraste, cintilografia nuclear, oximetria e angiografia podem ser usadas para mostrar a presença de *shunt* da direita para a esquerda, caso o exame Doppler não comprove o diagnóstico com segurança. A ecocardiografia com contraste (ver Capítulo 104) é realizada por meio de injeção de solução salina agitada, com ar, na veia cefálica ou safena, opacificando, assim, o coração direito, a artéria pulmonar e a artéria aorta descendente (mais bem observado por imagem da artéria aorta abdominal dorsal até a bexiga). O cateterismo cardíaco pode mostrar hipertensão da artéria pulmonar, com equilíbrio entre as pressões sistólicas de VD e VE e da valva aórtica; a oximetria mostra diminuição da saturação de oxigênio distal à entrada da PDA na artéria aorta descendente; a angiografia do VD mostra hipertrofia do VD e geralmente delineia uma PDA ampla que parece ser uma continuidade distal da artéria aorta descendente (Figura 250.7). A morfologia das artérias pulmonares lobares podem parecer normais na angiografia, particularmente durante o primeiro ano de vida, ou podem apresentar aumento da tortuosidade. Injeções de contraste na artéria aorta ou no VE muitas vezes possibilitam a visualização de uma circulação colateral broncoesofágica extensa (Figura 250.7).

História natural

Filhotes de cães e gatos com PDA não são frequentemente comprometidos clinicamente por seu defeito no momento do diagnóstico. No entanto, se não há correção, a PDA tipicamente leva a complicações relacionadas ao *shunt* crônico da esquerda para a direita (ou seja, cardiomegalia do lado esquerdo, regurgitação da valva mitral, arritmias, ICC do lado esquerdo e morte). A progressão natural da PDA não tratada em pequenos animais tem um único estudo de uma série de 100 casos, em que o defeito não foi ocluído em 14 cães portadores da anomalia; 64% destes 14 cães morreram dentro de 1 ano após o exame.[110] Embora esses números sejam relativamente baixos, eles indicam claramente a necessidade de colocação de um dispositivo de fechamento do ducto ou sua correção cirúrgica para a maioria dos casos de PDA. A dissecação da artéria pulmonar é uma potencial complicação, recentemente reconhecida de casos de PDA não corrigida, em cães. Cães em idade mais avançada tem maior risco de apresentar essa complicação do que um cão jovem, típico, diagnosticado com PDA.[111] Em gatos, a literatura sobre a história natural da PDA é escassa. Gatos podem desenvolver hipertensão pulmonar significativa devido a *shunt* da esquerda para a direita, com mais frequência que os cães.[109,112-114] É importante ressaltar que a hipertensão pulmonar causada por PDA pode se desenvolver mais lentamente e cessar com intervenção imediata.[113,114] Quando persistente, a hipertensão pulmonar no recém-nascido leva a um quadro de *shunt* reverso, sinais clínicos resultantes de hipoxemia, eritrocitose, hiperviscosidade sanguínea e arritmias cardíacas. A ICC quase nunca se desenvolve, mas a morte súbita e as complicações inerentes à hiperviscosidade sanguínea são comuns. Cães e gatos com formas mais brandas de PDA geralmente sobrevivem até a idade adulta e podem viver além dos 10 anos de idade.[115,116]

Conduta clínica

A correção de PDA não complicada é considerada curativa. Além disso, o fechamento da PDA resulta em imediata diminuição da sobrecarga de volume do lado esquerdo, reversão da hipertrofia excêntrica do VE gradual ao longo do tempo[117] e um excelente prognóstico.[118] A correção pode não ser justificada em animais de estimação mais velhos se o fluxo sanguíneo no *shunt* for pequeno e a cardiomegalia for mínima ou ausente.

Geralmente, o fechamento da PDA é um procedimento eletivo que deve ser agendado imediatamente após a definição

CAPÍTULO 250 • Cardiopatias Congênitas 1225

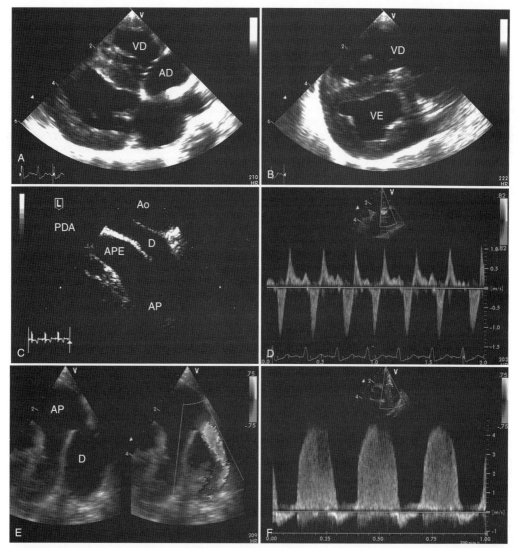

Figura 250.6 Ecocardiograma de paciente com persistência do ducto arterioso (PDA) e *shunt* da direita para a esquerda. **A.** A imagem do eixo longitudinal direito de um cão Esquimó Americano mostra aumento de ventrículo direito (*VD*) e átrio direito (*AD*). **B.** A imagem do eixo direito, curto, mostra aumento do VD e flacidez do septo interventricular em direção ao ventrículo esquerdo (*VE*). Esse achado é altamente sugestivo de sobrecarga de pressão do VD. **C.** Ecocardiograma transesofágico de cão com PDA e *shunt* da direita para a esquerda. O ducto (*D*) liga a artéria aorta (*Ao*) à artéria pulmonar (*AP*); é largo e cilíndrico. Tanto a AP quanto a artéria pulmonar esquerda (*APE*) estão aumentadas. **D.** O exame Doppler de onda contínua do cão de **A** mostra o fluxo bidirecional através do ducto. O fluxo da direita para a esquerda (*abaixo da linha basal*) ocorre durante a sístole, enquanto o fluxo da esquerda para a direita (*acima da linha basal*) ocorre durante a diástole. **E.** Exame Doppler bidimensional e colorido de fluxo, simultâneo do cão de **A**. Pode-se notar o fluxo da AP da direita para a esquerda, no grande ducto (*D*). **F.** Exame Doppler de onda contínua do cão de **A**, com insuficiência pulmonar. A velocidade máxima da insuficiência é de 4,5 m/s, indicando uma pressão diastólica na artéria pulmonar de, aproximadamente, 80 mmHg. Esse achado é compatível com o diagnóstico de hipertensão arterial pulmonar e presença de *shunt* da direita para a esquerda. (*As figuras D a F encontram-se reproduzidas em cores no Encarte.*)

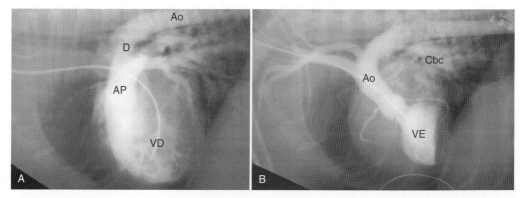

Figura 250.7 Diagnóstico angiográfico da persistência do ducto arterioso (PDA) com *shunt* da direita para a esquerda em um cão. **A.** A injeção de ventrículo direito (*VD*) opacifica o VD, a artéria pulmonar (*AP*), o ducto (*D*) e a artéria aorta descendente (*Ao*). Note que as artérias sistêmicas da porção craniana do cão não são opacificadas. **B.** Uma injeção no ventrículo esquerdo (*VE*) do mesmo cão opacifica o VE, a artéria aorta (*Ao*) e a circulação broncoesofágica colateral (*Cbc*) proeminente.

do diagnóstico e na idade mais precoce possível, de modo a evitar que a condição progrida de forma aguda. Se o paciente apresentar ICC com insuficiência miocárdica do VE, ele deve ser estabilizado por um curto período de tempo com medicamentos para ICC (furosemida, pimobendana, inibidores da ECA) antes de realizar anestesia. O tratamento medicamentoso de ICC geralmente continua durante vários meses após a reparação do defeito congênito nesses animais. Em alguns casos de fibrilação atrial, pode-se realizar eletrocardioversão no momento do fechamento do ducto ou em um momento posterior; no entanto, o tratamento medicamentoso prolongado (digoxina e diltiazem, com ou sem betabloqueador; ver Capítulo 248) pode ser necessário.

O fechamento da PDA reversa (com *shunt* da direita para a esquerda) é geralmente contraindicado devido às evidências baseadas em casos de desfechos desfavoráveis. O fechamento da PDA com *shunt* da esquerda para a direita e hipertensão pulmonar concomitante de gravidade variável foi relatado como bem-sucedido em ambos, cães[96] e gatos.[113,114] O tratamento com inibidores da prostaglandina não é efetivo em cães e gatos, muito provavelmente por causa da ausência de músculo liso na parede do ducto. Alguns cães têm demonstrado ser beneficiados pelo tratamento clínico com citrato de sildenafila (1 a 3 mg/kg/8 a 12 h via oral), e isso deve ser tentado durante pelo menos 3 a 4 semanas, para avaliar a resposta clínica.

A PDA típica pode ser cirurgicamente ligada ou fechada por meio de transcateterização usando espirais trombogênicas ou um oclusor, como o Amplatz Canine Duct Occluder (ACDO). Recentes abordagens de transcateterização representam o avanço mais importante no tratamento de PDA nas últimas duas décadas e atualmente são amplamente utilizadas. Esses procedimentos de cateterização intervencionista para PDA são discutidos no Capítulo 122. Apesar dos importantes avanços nas técnicas de transcateterização, a técnica de ligadura cirúrgica por meio de toracotomia esquerda continua sendo um método muito bem-sucedido para a oclusão da PDA e não deve ser vista como uma abordagem de importância inferior. A definição do tratamento apropriado depende da morfologia do ducto, do tamanho do paciente, da experiência do profissional e da preferência do proprietário. Algumas vantagens da oclusão de PDA por meio de cateterização, em relação à toracotomia e ligadura cirúrgica, incluem menor morbidade, menor tempo de internação e recuperação mais rápida. Em um grande estudo retrospectivo, comparando a ligadura cirúrgica e a oclusão com espirais via transcateterização, no tratamento da PDA, a ligadura cirúrgica foi associada a um elevado risco de complicações importantes, enquanto a técnica de oclusão transcateterização, usando espirais, foi associada a uma menor taxa de sucesso inicial ao tratamento, atribuída à incapacidade de estabilização da espiral, migração da espiral e fluxo residual significativo após a colocação apropriada da espiral.[119] Na era atual do ACDO, é difícil saber como comparar os métodos via transcateterização e os cirúrgicos, sem um estudo prospectivo adequado. Existem algumas desvantagens das abordagens que envolvem cateterização, incluindo: necessidade de fluoroscopia e exposição à radiação; necessidade de equipamentos especiais para cateterização e treinamento de operadores; incapacidade de fechar com segurança lesões cilíndricas que não apresentam estreitamente morfológico; e, em algumas situações, duração mais longa do procedimento (considerando que cirurgiões altamente experientes podem realizar o fechamento em menos de 40 minutos). A incapacidade atual da colocação de um ACDO em pacientes muito pequenos (< 2 a 2,5 kg) pode ser superada pela disponibilidade de um ACDO baixo.[120] À luz desses pontos, a maior vantagem da técnica de ligação cirúrgica é que ela pode ser realizada em animais com todos os tipos de morfologias de ductos e pesos corporais e, portanto, é método de escolha para cães e gatos muito pequenos, bem como animais com morfologia de ducto tipo III (sem estreitamento). A recuperação geralmente é rápida, com controle simultâneo da dor. As complicações do reparo cirúrgico da PDA em cães incluem:

hemorragia intraoperatória (11 a 15% dos casos), infecção, pneumotórax, arritmias cardíacas, parada cardíaca e insuficiência cardíaca. Taxas de mortalidade perioperatória entre 0 e 5,6% têm sido relatadas.[98,119,121]

Após o fechamento do ducto, a maioria dos cães se recupera sem complicações. Embora, de forma geral, o tamanho cardíaco diminua após a cirurgia, em muitos cães o aumento do tamanho do coração, do lado esquerdo, persiste.[122-125] Apesar de não haver sopro cardíaco contínuo e a recuperação clínica ser muito boa, o exame pós-operatório com Doppler pode indicar um discreto *shunt* residual.[98,126] Um sopro sistólico apical esquerdo, geralmente causado por regurgitação mitral secundária residual, é frequentemente perceptível por um período variável, após a ligadura do ducto.[97] Há relato de recanalização do ducto após a cirurgia, porém é incomum, ocorrendo em menos de 2% dos casos e mais comumente está associada à infecção.[92] Febre pós-operatória e infiltrados pulmonares podem indicar infecção no local da cirurgia e pneumonia hematogênica.[127]

Animais com PDA reversa têm doença pulmonar obstrutiva irreversível. A morbidade e mortalidade são geralmente o resultado de complicações relacionadas à eritrocitose e hipoxemia crônica, em vez de ICC. O tratamento desses pacientes consiste na restrição do exercício, na prevenção do estresse, na prevenção da desidratação e na manutenção do hematócrito entre 58 e 65% por meio de flebotomia periódica.[94] Conforme mencionado anteriormente, o tratamento com citrato de sildenafila também pode abrandar os sinais clínicos. O controle a longo prazo por essas técnicas é possível.[128] A flebotomia deve ser realizada com cautela para evitar fraqueza ou colapso, e o volume intravascular pode ser sustentado durante a flebotomia pela administração de solução cristaloide. Foram realizadas tentativas para reduzir o volume de hemácias em casos de PDA reversa por meio de terapia medicamentosa (p. ex., hidroxiureia), podendo ser uma alternativa a flebotomias repetidas.[129] A restrição à atividade física é geralmente recomendada, uma vez que a vasodilatação sistêmica induzida pelo exercício aumenta o grau de *shunt* da direita para a esquerda e predispõe à paresia ou colapso, bem como cianose, do membro pélvico. O fechamento da PDA reversa é fortemente contraindicado, já que invariavelmente ocasiona insuficiência cardíaca direita aguda no pós-operatório imediato ou no fim da cirurgia.

DEFEITOS DOS SEPTOS ATRIAL E VENTRICULAR

Durante o desenvolvimento embrionário cardíaco, os átrios e ventrículos atuam como uma câmara única. Subsequentemente, forma-se o coração normal com quatro câmaras, por meio do crescimento de septos cardíacos e valvas atrioventriculares (AV). Os átrios são separados por uma parede formada principalmente por dois septos: o septo primário, que se forma primeiro, e o septo secundário, que se desenvolve à direita do septo primário. O forame oval, uma passagem semelhante a uma fenda, que persiste entre esses septos, permite o *shunt* do fluxo sanguíneo da direita para a esquerda no átrio do feto, mas se fecha funcional e anatomicamente no recém-nascido assim que os pulmões se expandem e a pressão da AP aumenta. A maior parte do septo ventricular se forma pelo crescimento interno das paredes ventriculares. A área de confluência AV, incluindo o septo superior do ventrículo, o septo do átrio inferior e as valvas AV, é formada principalmente pelo crescimento e pela diferenciação dos coxins endocárdicos. As valvas AV normalmente se inserem em diferentes níveis do septo ventricular; a valva tricúspide se conecta em posição ligeiramente apical à valva mitral. O ramo resultante, definido como septo AV, forma essencialmente um septo atrial à direita e um septo ventricular à esquerda.[130]

Defeitos no desenvolvimento embrionário do septo ventricular, do septo atrial primário ou secundário, ou nos coxins endocárdicos, podem resultar em comunicação interventricular ou

DSV e/ou CIA ou DAS, respectivamente, juntamente com malformações nas valvas AV. Defeitos de septo congênitos são comuns em cães e gatos; manifestam-se como lesões isoladas ou componentes de lesões mais complexas, como defeito de septo AV completo (DSAV) e ToF.[22]

Patogênese dos defeitos de septo

Exceto o DSV em cães da raça Keeshond, uma alteração comprovadamente genética, com as chamadas malformações conotruncais,[11] não há dado sobre a(s) causa(s) de defeitos septais espontâneos em cães ou gatos. Os DSA são geralmente classificados com base na região anatômica da malformação. Os defeitos no forame oval ou próximo a ele são mais comuns e são denominados defeitos secundários do óstio (ou septo) (Figura 250.8). Os defeitos do septo atrial inferior são chamados de defeitos primários do óstio e podem ocorrer isoladamente ou como um componente do DSAV, parcial ou total. O raro defeito de septo atrial do tipo seio venoso é mais encontrado na região dorsocranial à fossa oval, próximo à entrada da veia cava cranial[131] e muitas vezes envolve a entrada de uma veia pulmonar no AD.

Uma vez que os coxins endocárdicos são amplamente responsáveis pela partição do septo atrial inferior, os defeitos na região imediatamente adjacente às valvas AV (septo primário) têm sido denominados "defeitos do coxim endocárdico", embora este termo seja menos usado atualmente. Um defeito nesse local também pode envolver o desenvolvimento anômalo das valvas AV. Estes podem variar de uma fissura no folheto septal da valva mitral até um folheto septal AV comum que atravessa os dois lados do coração. O DSAV total (defeito do coxim endocárdico) consiste em um amplo DSA inferior, um DSV de entrada (ventral ao folheto da valva tricúspide septal) e uma valva AV comum (passagem) que possui uma fenda no folheto mitral septal. As terminologias mais antigas para essas malformações graves incluem: defeito do ducto AV comum, pois desde a sua formação embrionária não ocorre partição da área do ducto AV e existe uma comunicação entre as quatro câmaras cardíacas. DSAV parcial ou total é mais comumente detectado em gatos[132,133] e pode causar ICC esquerda ou bilateral. Entretanto, o DSAV é comparativamente raro em cães.[134,135] Forame oval patente (FOP) não é um verdadeiro DSA, visto que o septo atrial se forma normalmente, mas as paredes que delimitam o forame são separadas. Na maioria das vezes, um FOP é devido a condições que aumentam a pressão da AD; todavia, dilatação grave do AE também pode levar à persistência do forame oval. O FOP normalmente alcança significado clínico quando ocorre *shunt* da direita para a esquerda, como pode acontecer na EP grave[136] ou DVT.

A maioria dos DSV está localizada no interior ou adjacente à porção membranosa do septo ventricular superior, logo abaixo da valva aórtica e cranial ao folículo tricúspide septal (Figura 250.9 A).[137] Estes são chamados de defeitos "membranosos", "perimembranosos" e "paramembranosos" por diferentes autores, e defeito "infracristal" na literatura antiga. Aneurisma de septo ventricular membranoso com ou sem um pequeno DSV perimembranoso patente também foi relatado em exame ecocardiográfico em cães e gatos.[138]

O típico DSV membranoso, quando visto do lado esquerdo do septo ventricular, localiza-se logo abaixo da valva aórtica, mais frequentemente centralizado entre a cúspide coronária direita e a cúspide não coronariana. No lado direito do septo, a abertura é frequentemente definida por sua posição em relação à crista supraventricular, à crista muscular que separa os fluxos de entrada e saída do sangue. Os defeitos membranosos são subcristais (infracristais), enquanto os defeitos subarteriais são localizados em uma posição supracristal, logo abaixo da valva pulmonar. Defeitos membranosos grandes podem obliterar a crista e estes são frequentemente associados a defeitos adicionais, tais como ToF (Figura 250.9 B).

A porção direita da raiz da artéria aorta, que inclui a cúspide coronária direita e a cúspide não coronária, pode ser deslocada para a direita (dextroposicionada), de modo que a artéria aorta atravesse o defeito, criando um "desalinhamento", o DSV. Desvios da raiz da aorta, na região cranial extrema e à direita, são observados na síndrome ToF – atresia pulmonar –, ventrículo direito de dupla saída. No entanto, a geometria alterada da raiz da artéria aorta que acompanha muitos casos de DSV pode resultar em substancial regurgitação na valva aórtica sem que haja essas graves malformações. Defeitos no septo ventricular muscular são raros em cães e gatos e podem ser localizados dorsalmente ou no ápice. Casos de DSV de entrada foram mencionados anteriormente sob DSAV.

Fisiopatologia

O *shunt* através de pequenos defeitos (resistentes ou restritivos) depende principalmente do tamanho do defeito e da diferença de pressão entre as duas câmaras, enquanto o *shunt* através de grandes defeitos (não resistentes) depende principalmente das resistências relativas nos sistemas vasculares sistêmico e pulmonar.[137,139-141] Na ausência de outras anormalidades, a pressão cardíaca no lado esquerdo excede as do lado direito e a direção do *shunt* é da esquerda para a direita. Nos desvios da esquerda para a direita, as câmaras cardíacas envolvidas no circuito do *shunt* aumentam para acomodar o excesso de volume sanguíneo e a

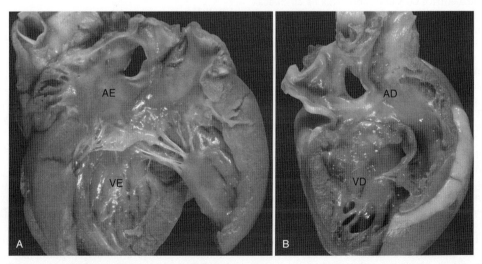

Figura 250.8 Anormalidade macroscópica do defeito do septo atrial (DSA) secundário em um cão. Vista do lado esquerdo (**A**) e do lado direito (**B**) mostrando a localização do DSA na região do septo atrial médio, onde deveria haver o forame oval.

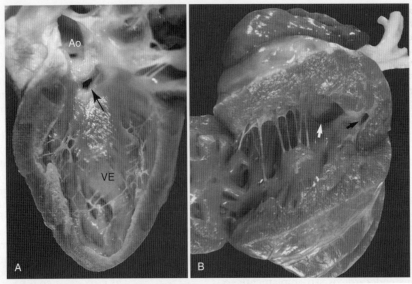

Figura 250.9 Anormalidade macroscópica do defeito de septo ventricular (DSV). **A.** Pequeno VSD resistente (seta) em um gato jovem, visto a partir do ventrículo esquerdo (VE). O DSV pode ser notado logo abaixo da artéria aorta (Ao). Uma rede fina de bandas moderadoras excessivas/falsos tendões é um achado não relacionado. **B.** Grande DSV não resistente em um cão jovem com ToF, visto a partir do ventrículo direito (VD). O grande defeito (seta branca) está localizado cranialmente ao aparato da valva tricúspide. O VD é acentuadamente espesso e um estreito anel subvalvular fibroso de EP subvalvular está presente (seta preta).

vascularização pulmonar torna-se sobrecarregada. Por fim, *shunt* da esquerda para a direita de grande volume pode resultar em insuficiência do miocárdio, elevando a pressão de enchimento cardíaco e desenvolvimento de ICC evidente. O *shunt* da direita para a esquerda se deve a defeito septal quando a pressão no lado direito do coração se eleva devido a EP, displasia da tricúspide (DSA) ou hipertensão pulmonar. As consequências do *shunt* reverso incluem cianose por hipoxemia arterial, eritrocitose, hiperviscosidade sanguínea e morte súbita (ver Fisiologia do *shunt* da direita para a esquerda, mencionada em texto anterior).

Defeito do septo atrial

O fluxo que passa através do DSA ocorre principalmente durante a diástole ventricular. A diferença de pressão através do DSA é baixa e a direção e magnitude do *shunt* são determinadas principalmente pelo tamanho do defeito e pela resistência diastólica em relação ao fluxo em cada ventrículo. Normalmente, o VD é mais complacente do que o VE e oferece pouca resistência ao enchimento cardíaco, fazendo com que o sangue desvie preferencialmente do AE para o AD e VD. O resultado é a dilatação do AD, hipertrofia excêntrica do VD e sobrecarga na circulação pulmonar. Na cateterização cardíaca, a saturação de oxigênio no coração direito e nas artérias pulmonares aumenta. O AE recebe o sangue desviado, mas a maior parte do aumento do retorno venoso pulmonar é desviado imediatamente para o AD, resultando em dilatação mínima do AE. Se um aumento considerável do AE for observado em um animal com um DSA, um DSAV com regurgitação mitral deve ser suspeitado.

O fluxo através do DSA geralmente não gera um sopro cardíaco audível, porque o gradiente de pressão e a velocidade do fluxo são baixos. Quando o sangue desviado se junta ao sangue que chega pela veia cava, o volume e a velocidade do fluxo que passa pelo coração direito aumentam, resultando em um sopro devido à estenose pulmonar (comumente) ou estenose de tricúspide (incomum). O fechamento tardio da valva pulmonar (e o fechamento precoce da valva aórtica) causa desdobramento da segunda bulha cardíaca.[139,142] Uma vez que a sobrecarga de volume afeta o VD e não o VE, grandes desvios culminam no desenvolvimento de insuficiência cardíaca direita ou lesão vascular pulmonar com sinais clínicos relacionados à hipertensão pulmonar e *shunt* da direita para a esquerda.

Defeito do septo ventricular

O fluxo através de um DSV ocorre principalmente durante a sístole ventricular. Na ausência de outros defeitos cardiovasculares, a pressão sistólica máxima do VE é cerca de cinco vezes maior que a do VD, e a direção do fluxo é do VE para o VD. A magnitude do *shunt* da esquerda para a direita em pequenos defeitos (restritivos) é determinada principalmente pelo diâmetro do defeito e pela diferença (gradiente) de pressão sistólica entre os ventrículos. A máxima diferença de pressão através do defeito pode ser estimada de forma não invasiva por meio de ecocardiografia com Doppler (ver Capítulo 104). No defeito restritivo com pressão relativamente normal no VD e no VE (aproximadamente 20 a 25 mmHg e 100 a 120 mmHg, respectivamente) espera-se uma velocidade máxima do fluxo através do defeito > 4,5 m/s, correspondendo a um gradiente de pressão > 80 mmHg. Esse fluxo de alta velocidade origina um sopro sistólico proeminente. Se a velocidade máxima for menor que a prevista, a pressão sistólica do VD provavelmente aumentará, por causa ou da presença de EP ou do aumento da pressão arterial pulmonar, que pode resultar de alto fluxo pulmonar, insuficiência cardíaca esquerda ou aumento da resistência vascular.

Quando um pequeno DSV está localizado no alto do septo membranoso, o sangue é ejetado do VE diretamente em direção à via de saída do ventrículo direito (VSVD) e à artéria pulmonar principal; o coração direito tem apenas uma sobrecarga moderada de volume, e o aumento do coração direito é mínimo. O aumento do coração direito é mais evidente quando o DSV é grande ou está localizado na porção muscular do septo interventricular (SIV). Nessas condições de um DSV membranoso ou subarterial, a cateterização cardíaca mostra saturação de oxigênio na VSVD e na artéria pulmonar maior do que o mensurado no AD ou ápice do VD. Os *shunts* grandes (razão fluxo pulmonar: fluxo sistêmico > 3:1) podem sobrecarregar o coração esquerdo a ponto de aumentar a pressão diastólica ventricular e causar sintomas de ICC esquerda. No DSV muito grande e não resistente, ambos os ventrículos apresentam pressão semelhante e os dois ventrículos se comportam como uma câmara de bombeamento comum. A menos que uma valva pulmonar estenosada proteja a circulação pulmonar, o desenvolvimento de ICC ou hipertensão pulmonar é inevitável. No caso de ambos, DSV com pequeno e grande desalinhamento, pode ocorrer regurgitação aórtica devido ao prolapso da cúspide da valva aórtica direita durante a diástole. Isso pode aumentar a tensão na parede do VE e predispor à ICC.

Achados clínicos

Defeito do septo atrial

As predisposições de raças de cães à ocorrência de DSA são apresentadas na Tabela 250.1. Em gatos com DSA, um estudo constatou elevada prevalência em gatos Domésticos de Pelo Curto e nas raças Persa e Chartreux.[22] Os achados clínicos de um típico DSA com *shunt* da esquerda para a direita incluem sopro suave de grau 2 a 3/6, sopro de ejeção sistólica na base do coração esquerdo e desdobramento da segunda bulha cardíaca (Figura 250.10).[22,143] O sopro é muitas vezes mal interpretado como oriundo de EP leve ou como um sopro inocente. Pode ocorrer sopro diastólico de baixa frequência no lado direito, na estenose tricúspide, mas isso é geralmente inaudível, especialmente em pacientes de menor porte. A cianose está ausente, a menos que exista um defeito adicional, como EP ou DVT,[144] ou exista complicação de hipertensão pulmonar, que é infrequente, para causar *shunt* da direita para a esquerda.[22] Sintomas de ICC do lado direito podem estar presentes em cães ou gatos com grandes defeitos.

As principais alterações estruturais cardíacas causadas pelo DSA incluem: aumento de volume do AD e hipertrofia excêntrica do VD. O ECG pode indicar aumento do VD (desvio do eixo direito, aumento da profundidade da onda S nas derivações I, II, III), mas também são observadas anormalidades da condução intraventricular, especialmente no defeito de óstio primário ou no DSAV.[2,133] Este último também pode exibir desvio esquerdo-cranial no eixo frontal. Radiografias torácicas mostram aumento do coração direito, artéria pulmonar principal e hipervascularização pulmonar proporcional à magnitude do *shunt* (Figura 250.11). O AE está apenas discretamente aumentado, a menos que exista concomitante regurgitação mitral decorrente de malformação da valva mitral ou de DSAV. A ecocardiografia 2D possibilita a obtenção de imagens diretas do DSA,[22] mas a detecção falso-positiva de DSA é comum devido a artefatos de imagem causados pela direção do feixe e da espessura delgada de algumas porções do septo interatrial normal. A detecção do *shunt* transatrial por meio de Doppler é mais confiável e tipicamente mostra fluxo diastólico laminar ou moderadamente turbulento através do DSA (Figura 250.12 e Vídeo 250.7), e aumento da velocidade na VSVD e das artérias pulmonares. Os estudos com Doppler também são úteis para mostrar anormalidades associadas, como regurgitação mitral ou outros defeitos.[145] Um erro muito comum é confundir o retorno venoso normal da veia cava caudal com o *shunt* atrial da esquerda para a direita, pois em imagem paraesternal do eixo longo este fluxo passa ao longo do septo atrial. Além disso, em imagens do eixo curto, o septo atrial pode ser encurtado, confundindo a localização de um DSA secundário de um DSA primário. A ecocardiografia com contraste é útil (ver Capítulo 104), particularmente quando o defeito é grande ou quando a elevada pressão do coração causa fluxo reverso através do defeito. O cateterismo cardíaco de animais com DSA pode ser útil para avaliar a magnitude e a direção do *shunt* e a resistência vascular pulmonar. No caso de *shunt* da esquerda para a direita, a oximetria mensurada em amostras de sangue obtidas da veia cava, do AD e do

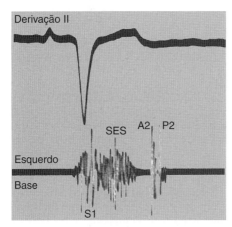

Figura 250.10 Fonocardiograma gravado na base do coração esquerdo de um cão com defeito do septo atrial (DSA) primário. Na derivação II, o eletrocardiograma (ECG) mostra um complexo QRS ligeiramente prolongado, negativo, que é indicativo de anormalidade de condução do ventrículo direito (VD) (bloqueio parcial ou incompleto do ramo direito). O fonocardiograma mostra um sopro de ejeção sistólico (*SES*) que termina bem antes da segunda bulha cardíaca, com amplo desdobramento da primeira bulha cardíaca (*S1*); *A2*, componente aórtico da segunda bulha cardíaca; *P2*, componente pulmonar da segunda bulha cardíaca.

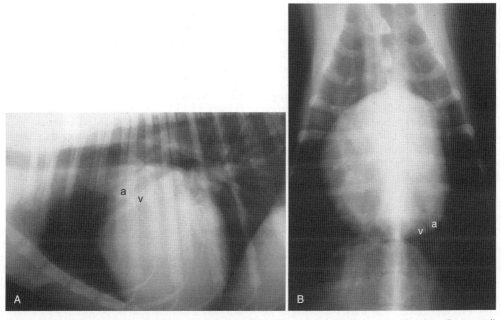

Figura 250.11 Radiografias laterais (**A**) e dorsoventrais (**B**) de cão da raça Poodle padrão com defeito de septo atrial (DSA). A silhueta cardíaca está aumentada, com destaque para átrio direito (AD), ventrículo direito (VD) e artérias pulmonares (*a*) e veias (*v*).

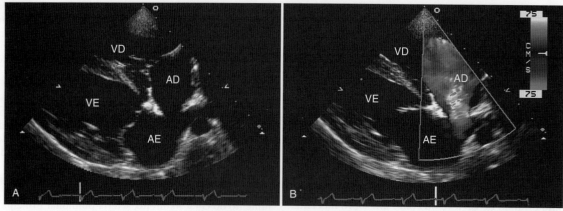

Figura 250.12 Ecocardiograma de comunicação interatrial secundária (ou defeito do septo atrial [DAS]) em um cão. **A.** A imagem do eixo longitudinal direito mostra ausência de um segmento do septo atrial entre os átrios direito (*AD*) e esquerdo (*AE*). O AD e o ventrículo direito (*VD*) estão moderadamente aumentados. **B.** Exame Doppler em cores indica fluxo da esquerda para a direita, de baixa velocidade, através do DSA. (*A figura B encontra-se reproduzida em cores no Encarte.*)

VD indica aumento da saturação de oxigênio entre a veia cava e o átrio e/ou ventrículo, e a magnitude do *shunt* sistêmico pulmonar pode ser estimada. A pressão venosa central e a pressão diastólica estão elevadas quando ICC está presente ou iminente. Aumento do fluxo sistólico na valva pulmonar pode ocasionar EP "relativa", identificada por um discreto gradiente de pressão sistólica (5 a 15 mmHg) entre o VD e a artéria pulmonar.[142] O fluxo sanguíneo no DSA pode ser avaliado por meio de angiocardiografia. O cateter, quando introduzido pela veia femoral, pode facilmente passar pelo AD através do DSA ou do FOP para o AE, a fim de realizar exame com contraste para a visualização do *shunt* da esquerda para a direita durante a fase de estudo. Alternativamente, a injeção de contraste na artéria pulmonar irá delinear defeitos de *shunt* da esquerda para a direita durante a fase do lado esquerdo do estudo. Após o retorno venoso pulmonar, o septo atrial geralmente pode ser visto entre o AE e a artéria aorta, em imagem lateral. A passagem do contraste do AE para o AD e a veia cava confirmam a presença do defeito. Quando há suspeita de um defeito de coxim endocárdico mais extenso, pode-se realizar uma injeção de contraste no VE para evidenciar DSV, regurgitação mitral e, ocasionalmente, o *shunt* do ventrículo esquerdo para o átrio direito através do DSA.

Defeito do septo ventricular

As predisposições de raças de cães para DSV estão indicadas na Tabela 250.1. O DSV é uma das anomalias congênitas mais frequentes em gatos,[36] e nenhuma predisposição por raça foi relatada, embora a experiência clínica sugira que esta anormalidade é relativamente comum em gatos da raça Maine Coon. Diferentemente, algumas raças de cães, incluindo Springer Spaniel Inglês, West Highland White Terrier e Lakeland Terrier, têm sido relatadas como sendo predispostas a DSV. As características clínicas do DSV dependem da magnitude do *shunt* e da presença de complicações ou de outros defeitos. Os animais com um pequeno DSV membranoso típico são assintomáticos e apresentam um sopro holossistólico áspero auscultado melhor na região precordial medial a cranial ventral, do lado direito.[137,146,147] Em casos raros de DSV subarterial, o defeito se abre logo abaixo da valva pulmonar, e o sopro sistólico é auscultado na base do coração, no lado esquerdo. Pode ocorrer desdobramento da segunda bulha cardíaca, mas muitas vezes não é detectada devido à sobreposição do sopro com a segunda bulha cardíaca. Se a deformidade da raiz da artéria aorta causar regurgitação aórtica significativa, um sopro cardíaco diastólico do tipo decrescente pode ser evidente sobre a área de saída do fluxo sanguíneo no VE. Isso resulta em uma combinação de sopros sistólico e diastólico que podem ser facilmente confundidos com PDA. A regurgitação aórtica também pode fluir para dentro do VD e ocasionar um sopro diastólico, auscultado melhor no hemitórax direito. Sopro sistólico na região das valvas AV também pode ser detectado se um DSV for parte de um DSAV total.

Os achados do ECG em animais com DSV são variáveis. No caso de *shunt* da esquerda para a direita de intensidade moderada ou alta, muitas vezes há indícios de aumento do AE ou VE, mas também podem ocorrer anormalidades de condução no VD. As derivações do plano frontal podem mostrar uma anormalidade sutil na ativação do septo ventricular precoce, caracterizada por uma onda Q larga ou que contém entalhe de alta frequência.[148] Desvio do eixo direito e um complexo QRS estreito em um cão com DSV geralmente indicam hipertrofia do VD e uma lesão mais complexa, como DSV com EP ou hipertensão pulmonar. Radiografias de tórax são muito úteis na avaliação da magnitude do DSV com *shunt* da esquerda para a direita. O grau de hipervascularização pulmonar e aumento de AE e VE são proporcionais à magnitude do *shunt* (Figura 250.13).[61] As artérias pulmonares principal, lobar e periférica são geralmente proeminentes. Em animais com pequenos defeitos, as radiografias torácicas podem parecer totalmente normais. Nos grandes defeitos, o VD também pode aumentar. A constatação de um grande segmento da artéria pulmonar, baixa perfusão pulmonar e escassa vascularização pulmonar periférica sugerem a possibilidade de EP ou hipertensão pulmonar e *shunt* da direita para a esquerda.

Na ecocardiografia, observam-se aumentos do AE e do VE em graus variáveis. No DSV moderados a grande, aumento do coração direito também pode estar presente. A ecocardiografia bidimensional do hemitórax direito é mais utilizada para detectar DSV membranoso, localizado logo abaixo da valva aórtica (Figura 250.14 A) e adjacente à borda cranioventral do folheto tricúspide septal. O raro DSV subarterial é mais bem detectado em imagens do eixo curto, na altura da artéria aorta, que inclui a entrada de fluxo sanguíneo no VD e a saída do sangue do VD para a artéria pulmonar. Visualizações fora do ângulo são frequentemente necessárias. A imagem de quatro câmeras apicais, à esquerda, é melhor para visualizar DSAV. Como regra geral, quando o diâmetro máximo do DSV é < 40% do diâmetro da raiz da artéria aorta, a lesão tende a ser restritiva e frequentemente bem tolerada, desde que não tenha regurgitação aórtica. Aneurismas pequenos de tecido semelhante a tecido membranoso podem ser, ocasionalmente, visualizados em forma de proeminência saindo do VD, nas bordas do DSV.[138] Como acontece no DSA, o exame Doppler do DSV deve ser realizado para confirmar a presença de *shunt*, e o Doppler colorido é particularmente útil para a identificação de pequenas lesões. Para um defeito perimembranoso, um fluxo de sangue se movendo em direção ao transdutor pode ser observado na imagem do eixo longo ou curto,

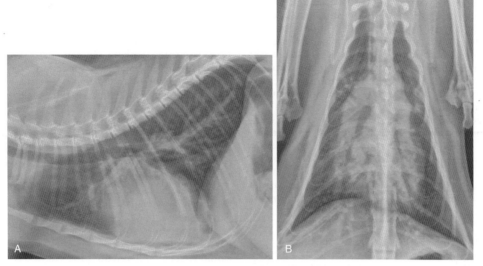

Figura 250.13 Radiografias torácica lateral (**A**) e dorsoventral (**B**) de gato com grande defeito do septo ventricular (DSV), ou comunicação interventricular (CIV), com *shunt* da esquerda para a direita. A silhueta cardíaca está aumentada e há arredondamento da borda cranial do coração, na imagem lateral. As artérias e veias pulmonares estão aumentadas na imagem dorsoventral.

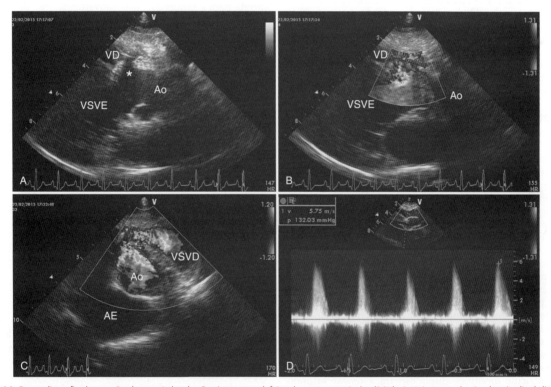

Figura 250.14 Ecocardiografia de um cão da raça Labrador Retriever com defeito de septo ventricular (DSV). **A.** A imagem do eixo longitudinal direito mostra o DSV (*asterisco*) localizado entre a via de saída do ventrículo esquerdo (*VSVE*) e a artéria aorta (*Ao*) e a abertura para o ventrículo direito (*VD*). Note a proximidade do DSV à raiz do Ao e à origem da valva aórtica. **B.** O estudo de Doppler de fluxo de cor de eixo longitudinal à direita revela *shunt* sistólico da esquerda para a direita através do VSD no VD. **C.** O exame Doppler com fluxo colorido do eixo curto paraesternal direito revela *shunt* sistólico da esquerda para a direita, através do DSV para a via de saída do ventrículo direito (*VSVD*). **D.** Registro do Doppler Espectral de todo o DSV, mostrando fluxo turbulento de alta velocidade, da esquerda para a direita, durante a sístole (complexo QRS para onda T). (*Esta figura se encontra reproduzida em cores no Encarte.*)

do lado direito (ver Figura 250.14 B e C e Vídeos 250.8 e 250.9). Exames Doppler espectral de onda contínua (CW) são úteis para quantificar o fluxo de alta velocidade através de pequeno DSV restritivo, conforme mencionado anteriormente (ver Figura 250.14 D). Quanto maior o DSV, menor a diferença de pressão entre os ventrículos e menor a velocidade do fluxo sanguíneo no DSV. Portanto, a velocidade máxima do fluxo sanguíneo no DSV, no Doppler CW, também pode ser usada para ajudar a definir o tamanho do defeito. A região da valva aórtica também deve ser observada quanto à regurgitação aórtica. A ecocardiografia com contraste também pode ser usada para identificar o fluxo no defeito, mas geralmente não é necessária se cuidadosos exames ecocardiográficos Doppler e bidimensional tiverem sido realizados.

Hoje o cateterismo cardíaco raramente é realizado para diagnosticar DSV. No entanto, se um paciente é considerado candidato cirúrgico, o cateterismo permite delinear ainda melhor o defeito anatômico e estimar o grau de *shunt*.[146] Além disso, métodos baseados em cateterização agora estão disponíveis para a oclusão de alguns DSV (ver Capítulo 122). Na cateterização, as amostras obtidas para oximetria mostram um "aumento" no conteúdo de oxigênio entre o AD e a artéria pulmonar, e as pressões intracardíaca e da artéria pulmonar geralmente são normais em cães e gatos com DSV pequeno. A pressão no VD frequentemente encontra-se elevada, 5 a 15 mmHg acima da pressão na artéria pulmonar. Aumentos mais marcantes na pressão sistólica do VD indicam hipertensão pulmonar ou EP concomitante, e a elevação da pressão ventricular diastólica final e pressão venosa central indica iminência de ICC. O *shunt* bidirecional ou o *shunt* da direita para a esquerda é observado quando a pressão sistólica do VD atinge e excede a pressão sistólica do VE. Alterações anatômicas das valvas semilunares ou dos grandes vasos, especialmente da raiz da artéria aorta, são mais bem visualizadas após a injeção de contraste na artéria aorta proximal, que também é o local preferido para determinar a presença e gravidade da regurgitação aórtica.

Defeito do septo atrioventricular

Um defeito parcial, com DSA primário e função da valva AV relativamente normal, deve comportar-se como um DSA isolado. Quando o DSA inclui uma importante malformação da valva AV, pode haver regurgitação valvular substancial, incluindo regurgitação mitral, regurgitação tricúspide e regurgitação mitral ao AD, através do DSA. A aparência ecocardiográfica clássica de um DSAV total inclui DSA, DSV de entrada e um folheto valvular AV "flutuante", que serve a ambos os ventrículos. Os desfechos podem incluir sinais clínicos de ICC ou de hipertensão arterial devido a doença pulmonar vascular secundária. Alguns desses detalhes foram descritos em outra publicação.[132] Uma manifestação particular do DSAV é o denominado átrio direito com dupla saída (ver a seguir).

História natural

As taxas de morbidade e mortalidade associadas a DSA e DSV dependem do tamanho e da localização do defeito, bem como da magnitude e direção do fluxo sanguíneo no *shunt* e da presença de lesões adicionais. O fechamento espontâneo de pequenos DSV geralmente ocorre em crianças, mas isso é aparentemente uma ocorrência incomum em gatos e cães.[149] Animais com defeitos pequenos não complicados que resultam apenas em *shunt* discreto geralmente levam uma vida normal, sem sinais clínicos aparentes. *Shunts* maiores, que causam cardiomegalia de intensidade moderada a grave, podem levar à ICC intratável, muito embora seja bem provável que a maioria dos pacientes com essas anormalidades venha a óbito quando a resistência vascular pulmonar diminui, sem que o animal nunca tenha sido examinado por um veterinário. A regurgitação aórtica de intensidade moderada a grave é uma complicação incomum do DSV e apresenta um risco muito substancial de insuficiência cardíaca esquerda e diminuição de sobrevida, embora possa levar mais de 5 anos para que a ICC venha a ocorrer. Quando o DSV está associado a obstrução do fluxo de saída do VD – devido à presença de ventrículo direito de dupla câmara, estenose infundibular ou obstrução próxima à valva –, o *shunt* da direita para a esquerda pode levar a sinais semelhantes aos da ToF. Muitas vezes, é difícil prever o desfecho em animais muito jovens com DSV, até que eles se aproximem do tamanho de um animal adulto, aos 6 a 12 meses de idade. Gatos com DSAV grave frequentemente desenvolvem ICC biventricular e cardiomegalia relevantes. Alguns irão sucumbir bem cedo, com idade < 2 anos, enquanto outros sobrevivem por muito mais tempo.[132] Animais que desenvolvem hipertensão pulmonar (síndrome de Eisenmenger) têm um prognóstico reservado a curto prazo e prognóstico muito reservado que progride para ruim a longo prazo, embora a sobrevivência além dos 7 anos seja possível.

Conduta clínica

Tratamento medicamentoso, cirurgia e tratamentos por meio de cateterização são possíveis, mas raramente necessários para pequeno DSA ou DSV isolado. Pacientes com ICC (unilateral ou biventricular) devem ser tratados como qualquer outro paciente com sobrecarga de volume cardíaco, com o uso de furosemida, inibidor da enzima conversora da angiotensina (ECA), espironolactona e pimobendana (ver Capítulo 247). Esses pacientes também são candidatos a um reparo paliativo ou definitivo, embora esses procedimentos não sejam amplamente disponíveis para pacientes veterinários.

O fechamento do orifício do defeito de septo é o tratamento definitivo para todos os defeitos dos septos atrial e ventricular. A correção cirúrgica pela abertura do coração é raramente tentada em animais devido à necessidade de circulação extracorpórea ou outras técnicas para induzir parada e perfusão do coração.[135,142,150-156] O tratamento cirúrgico paliativo de um DSV grande pode ser realizado sem *bypass*, por meio da colocação de uma faixa constritiva ao redor da artéria pulmonar principal. Essa técnica cria uma estenose pulmonar (EP) supravalvar e aumenta a pressão sistólica do VD, reduzindo a magnitude do *shunt* da esquerda para a direita.[157] Esse procedimento é recomendado para cães e gatos que apresentem sinais de cardiomegalia rapidamente progressiva e ICC evidente ou iminente. Uma faixa constritiva excessivamente agressiva deve ser evitada, porque muitas vezes é desnecessária e, se for muito apertada, ela pode provocar sobrecarga de pressão, insuficiência cardíaca direita aguda ou, em animais sobreviventes, *shunt* da direita para a esquerda. Alternativamente, vasodilatadores arteriais sistêmicos podem ser administrados para reduzir a resistência vascular sistêmica e a magnitude do *shunt* à esquerda.[158] Fechamento bem-sucedido de ambos, DSA[159,160] e DSV[161-164] podem ser realizados usando dispositivos de oclusão percutânea desenvolvidos na última década (ver Capítulo 122). Procedimentos híbridos, envolvendo toracotomia e colocação transmural cardíaca de dispositivo orientada por ultrassom, também foram relatados.[165,166] Conforme mencionado para PDA reversa, a correção cirúrgica de animais com síndrome de Eisenmenger não deve ser tentada. Atividade física restrita é provavelmente a estratégia mais prudente e eficaz em tais casos. O tratamento com citrato de sildenafil também pode abrandar os sinais clínicos. Flebotomia periódica pode ser útil em alguns pacientes que desenvolvem eritrocitose extrema. Recomenda-se a manutenção de um volume globular, ou hematócrito, de 58 a 65%.

DISPLASIA VALVAR

Regurgitação das valvas pulmonar e aórtica

Regurgitação pulmonar

A regurgitação pulmonar irrelevante é um achado comum em cães e gatos de todas as idades;[167] a regurgitação pulmonar (RP) congênita primária é uma anormalidade incomum decorrente do desenvolvimento anormal dos folhetos valvares ou da dilatação do anel da artéria pulmonar anômala.[168] A RP causa sobrecarga de volume e hipertrofia excêntrica no VD. Os ramos principal e proximal das artérias pulmonares direita e esquerda se dilatam para acomodar o aumento concomitante do volume sistólico do VD. A RP isolada é frequentemente bem tolerada. A RP congênita tem maior probabilidade de causar ICC, se a resistência vascular pulmonar aumentar subsequentemente como resultado de doença pulmonar parenquimatosa ou vascular grave, ou em casos em que a valva tricúspide também está comprometida. RP irrelevante é frequentemente observada em cães com PDA, presumivelmente por dilatação da artéria pulmonar principal. A maioria dos cães com EP tem insuficiência valvular moderada, mas, por vezes, observa-se RP grave concomitante. Geralmente, diferentes graus de gravidade de RP ocorrem como consequência de cirurgia ou de dilatação por balão para aliviar estenose pulmonar (EP). RP pode ser consequência de qualquer anormalidade que ocasione hipertensão pulmonar.

As características clínicas da RP incluem sopro sistólico variável (causado pelo aumento do fluxo de saída ou por outra lesão) e sopro diastólico, mais bem audível na base do coração esquerdo. Este sopro tipo "to-and-fro" não deve ser confundido com o sopro contínuo notado na PDA. O ECG de cães com RP congênita pode ser normal ou refletir o aumento do VD. Radiografias torácicas em casos graves de RP isolada geralmente mostram dilatação da artéria pulmonar principal e do VD, dando a impressão errônea de EP. A injeção de contraste na artéria pulmonar principal, utilizando um cateter de pequeno diâmetro, comprova a insuficiência valvar. A lenta excreção do contraste do VD, que se apresenta dilatado e com paredes finas, também confirmam o diagnóstico de RP. A ecocardiografia com Doppler colorido pode mostrar, de modo distinto, essas mesmas características de uma forma não invasiva e permite a visualização dos folhetos rudimentares ou disformes da valva (ver Capítulo 104). Portanto, o exame Doppler também auxilia na detecção de hipertensão pulmonar. Quando a velocidade do fluxo pulmonar regurgitante ultrapassa 2 m/s, a hipertensão pulmonar é possivelmente a provável causa da dilatação arterial e da insuficiência valvar. O tratamento de RP congênita não foi descrito em animais de companhia. Em cães com ICC, o tratamento medicamentoso convencional, que utiliza diuréticos, inibidores da ECA e pimobendana, é uma abordagem paliativa razoável (ver Capítulo 247).

Regurgitação aórtica

A regurgitação aórtica congênita isolada (RA, insuficiência aórtica) é uma anormalidade rara. É ocasionalmente detectada em cães jovens ou mais velhos com dilatação idiopática da artéria aorta (ectasia do anel aórtico). RA de grau leve a moderado também foi relatada em cães com valva aórtica bicúspide[169] ou quadricúspide[170,171] (Figura 250.15 A e B e Vídeos 250.10 a 250.12). Devido ao crescente uso da ecocardiografia com Doppler, a RA tem sido reconhecida com frequência crescente como uma complicação de outras malformações cardíacas.[172,173] A RA geralmente é acompanhada de estenose aórtica grave (EAS) e tem sido observada no DSV, na ToF e após o procedimento de dilatação de EA/EAS com cateter com balão. Os mecanismos prováveis para a ocorrência de insuficiência da valva aórtica nessas condições têm sido revisados.[173] Assim como na RP congênita, o sopro resultante da RA pode ser tanto sistólico quanto diastólico (tipo "to-and-fro") e é mais bem auscultado no hemitórax esquerdo. Todavia, muitos cães com RA não apresentam sopro audível. Em contraste, quando a RA é audível, a incompetência valvar é geralmente grave. O diagnóstico de RA clinicamente relevante é sustentado pela palpação de um pulso arterial hipercinético, resultante da combinação de maior volume sistólico e menor pressão diastólica, devido ao retorno do sangue da valva aórtica para o VE durante a diástole.

A hipertrofia excêntrica à mista do VE desenvolve-se proporcionalmente à gravidade da insuficiência. A RA grave geralmente resulta em ICC esquerda. O registro da RA e a estimativa de sua gravidade requer angiocardiografia ou, de uma forma mais prática, ecocardiograma com Doppler. O reparo definitivo requer cirurgia cardíaca e troca da valva. O uso de vasodilatadores arteriais pode reduzir o volume regurgitante e retardar o início da ICC, mas com risco de reduzir a perfusão coronariana. O tratamento com diuréticos, inibidores da ECA e pimobendana é indicado se a ICC estiver presente (ver Capítulo 247).

DISPLASIA DE VALVA ATRIOVENTRICULAR

Malformações congênitas das valvas mitral e tricúspide são relatadas em gatos e cães. Em gatos, a displasia da valva mitral (DVM) é uma das anomalias congênitas mais comuns descritas. As consequências dessa malformação abrangem (1) regurgitação em valva mitral ou tricúspide (mais comum); (2) obstrução do fluxo sanguíneo (i. e., estenose da valva mitral ou tricúspide); e (3) obstrução dinâmica da via de saída do ventrículo esquerdo VSVE devido ao deslocamento sistólico inadequado da valva mitral para dentro da VSVE. Obstrução fixa da VSVE também foi descrita em caso de malformação mitral.[174] A fisiopatologia e evolução clínica da regurgitação mitral congênita são similares às descritas na doença valvular degenerativa adquirida no cão (ver Capítulo 251). A anomalia de Ebstein é um defeito congênito relatado em cães relacionado à DVT, em que as origens dos folhetos da valva tricúspide são deslocadas em direção apical para dentro do VD.[21,175,176] Pode ou não estar associada à displasia de folhetos.

O movimento anterior sistólico (MAS) do aparato da valva mitral e a obstrução dinâmica da VSVE em gatos e cães foi considerado por muito tempo apenas uma manifestação de cardiomiopatia hipertrófica (ver Capítulos 252 e 253), talvez causada primariamente por alterações morfológicas no aparato da valva mitral em alguns animais. Quando a anormalidade primária é a displasia valvar, a hipertrofia concêntrica do VE geralmente regride se a obstrução for resolvida com tratamento (drogas bloqueadoras dos receptores beta).[177-179]

Patogênese

Relata-se que a DVT tem uma base genética em algumas das raças mais comumente atingidas;[9,10,180] em cães da raça Labrador Retriever uma mutação autossômica dominante com penetrância incompleta foi mapeada no cromossomo 9.[10] Um amplo espectro de anormalidades morfológicas congênitas das valvas mitral e tricúspide tem sido descrito, que abrange folhetos valvares encurtados, enrolados, entalhados e espessados; separação incompleta dos componentes da valva da parede ventricular ou

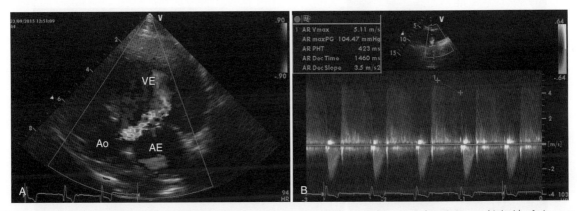

Figura 250.15 Ecocardiografia de um cão da raça Samoieda com regurgitação aórtica (RA) associada a uma valva aórtica quadricúspide. **A.** Imagem de exame com Doppler colorido de 5 câmaras apicais mostra fluxo diastólico da artéria aorta para o ventrículo esquerdo (VE). **B.** Registro em Doppler espectral do fluxo de insuficiência aórtica mostra fluxo diastólico, velocidade máxima de 5,11 m/s e tempo médio de pressão (TMP) de 423 ms. (Esta figura se encontra reproduzida em cores no Encarte.)

do septo (falha de separação em lâminas); alongamento, encurtamento, fusão e espessamento das cordas tendíneas; inserção direta da borda da valva no músculo papilar; e atrofia, hipertrofia, fusão e mau posicionamento dos músculos papilares e das cordas tendíneas.[175,181-185] A consequência usual dessas alterações é a insuficiência valvar. Exemplos de displasia das valvas mitral e tricúspide são mostrados nas Figuras 250.16 e 250.17. Alguns cães e gatos com DVM ou tricúspide apresentam, simultaneamente, FOP ou DSA, resultando em *shunt* da esquerda para a direita ou da direita para a esquerda.

Fisiopatologia

A anormalidade fisiopatológica fundamental das malformações de valva AV é a insuficiência que ocasiona sobrecarga de volume e se manifesta como dilatação atrial e hipertrofia excêntrica do ventrículo afetado. Alguns cães e gatos têm sobrevivido por 8 anos ou mais com anormalidade de valva AV relativamente grave, porém mais frequentemente a ICC se desenvolve mais cedo, especialmente no caso de doença mitral. O desenvolvimento de fibrilação atrial é especialmente desestabilizante para pacientes com essas lesões. Em alguns casos de DVT, cianose é observada como consequência do *shunt* da direita para a esquerda, no FOP ou no DSA. Estenose grave de valva AV limita a função do coração direito e, dessa forma, hipotensão, síncope ou colapso, após esforço físico, podem ser observados. A taquicardia abrevia a diástole e aumenta ainda mais o gradiente diastólico transvalvar, explicando-se, assim, a intolerância ao exercício. Hipertensão pulmonar e ICC do lado direito frequentemente se desenvolvem secundariamente à estenose mitral grave como consequência de elevações crônicas na pressão do AE; isso é mais comum em gatos. Como resultado, alguns pacientes inicialmente apresentando sinais de ICC do lado esquerdo, devido à estenose mitral, podem ser novamente levados à consulta meses depois com sintomas de ICC do lado direito. Como já mencionado, cães e gatos com displasia de valva AV são predispostos à fibrilação atrial, bem como à taquicardia supraventricular paroxística ou sustentada (ver Capítulo 248); sua ocorrência geralmente resulta em agravamento súbito do quadro clínico.

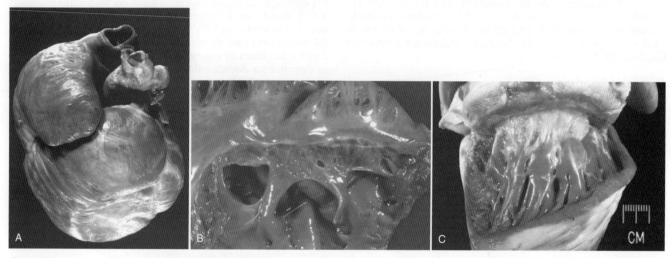

Figura 250.16 Anormalidade macroscópica da displasia da valva tricúspide (DVT). **A.** Imagem cranial do coração de um paciente com AR grave, aumento auricular e do ventrículo direito (VD) causado por DVT. **B.** Valva tricúspide de um cão da raça Labrador de 2 anos de idade com DVT grave. As bordas dos folhetos da valva se inserem diretamente nos músculos papilares; são evidentes a ausência e o encurtamento das cordas tendíneas. Há dilatação do AD e do VD. **C.** Deformidade tipo cortina da valva tricúspide de um cão da raça Samoieda de 2 anos de idade com DVT e estenose de tricúspide. A valva tricúspide encontra-se espessa e opaca. Existem múltiplos músculos papilares grandes e fundidos com cordas tendíneas curtas.

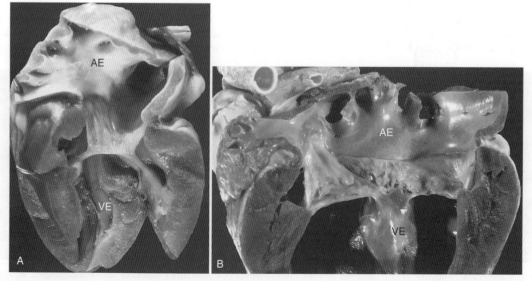

Figura 250.17 Anormalidade macroscópica da displasia da valva mitral (DVM). **A.** Amostra de um gato com DVM mostra um folheto da valva mitral espesso e opaco, inserção direta do músculo papilar à borda do folheto e aumento do AE. **B.** Amostra de um cão com DVM mostrando ligamentos cordiformes curtos do músculo papilar do ventrículo esquerdo (*VE*) até a borda do folheto, um folheto de valva mitral espessado e nodular e aumento acentuado do átrio esquerdo (*AE*).

Achados clínicos

A alta prevalência de DVM e DVT em várias raças (ver Tabela 250.1) sugere que fatores genéticos provavelmente estejam envolvidos na patogênese. A estenose da valva mitral, em particular, é comum em cães da raça Bull Terrier, nos quais a estenose ocorre frequentemente em associação com estenose da valva aórtica.[186] Gatos de todas as raças e cães Dogue Alemão, Pastor-Alemão, Bull Terrier, Golden Retriever, Newfoundland, Dálmata e Mastiff são predispostos à DVM.[182,187,188] Embora a DVT tenha sido descrita em gatos, parece ocorrer mais comumente em cães machos de grande porte, especialmente da raça Labrador Retriever.[189]

Cães e gatos com displasia valvular podem parecer clinicamente bem. Os sinais clínicos resultam de fadiga ao esforço, ICC do lado direito, do lado esquerdo ou biventricular, hipertensão pulmonar ou *shunt* da direita para a esquerda. Hemoptise pode ocorrer na estenose mitral. A principal característica da insuficiência valvar é um sopro holossistólico mais audível na área da valva afetada. Um ruído de galope alto também pode ser detectado.[187] Um sopro diastólico brando tardio e um "estalido" de abertura são às vezes auscultados em cães ou gatos com estenose valvular, mas esse achado geralmente está ausente ou não é percebido. Em casos de DVT, a intensidade do sopro nem sempre pode refletir a gravidade da doença. Em casos graves, um sopro pode ser muito discreto ou ausente, pois a valva não oferece resistência ao fluxo sanguíneo regurgitante. Congestão e pulsação da veia jugular são achados comuns na DVT; hepatomegalia e ascite estão presentes em cães que se apresentam com ICC do lado direito. Animais com ICC do lado direito geralmente apresentam baixo escore de condição corporal.

Desdobramentos dos complexos QRS (p. ex., Rr, RR, rR, rr) são achados distintos e comuns no ECG de cães e gatos com DVT (Figura 250.18).[68] Padrões de ampliação do coração direito também podem ser constatados. Ondas P altas ou largas são observadas em todos os tipos de displasia valvar, mas os padrões de aumento ventricular se limitam principalmente aos animais com fisiologia regurgitante e não são observados na estenose valvar isolada, exceto quando a hipertensão pulmonar se desenvolve secundária à estenose mitral. Arritmias atriais, incluindo complexos atriais prematuros, taquicardia atrial e fibrilação atrial são frequentemente registradas (Figura 250.18). O padrão de aumento da câmara nas radiografias de tórax geralmente reflete o envolvimento da valva afetada e as consequências fisiológicas resultantes (Figura 250.19). Nos casos de DVT, o grau de cardiomegalia é muitas vezes impressionante e pode assemelhar-se à aparência arredondada verificada no derrame pericárdico. A possibilidade de estenose valvar deve ser considerada sempre que o átrio estiver marcadamente dilatado, sem aumento do ventrículo ipsilateral.

O diagnóstico definitivo de malformação da valva AV requer ecocardiograma (ver Capítulo 104). Anormalidades de localização, forma, movimento ou fixação do aparelho valvar são facilmente observadas nesse exame (Figura 250.20 e Vídeos 250.13 e 250.14). Na insuficiência valvar, pode ocorrer sobrecarga de volume nos respectivos átrios e ventrículos; exames Doppler mostram fluxos regurgitantes fluindo do ventrículo para o átrio através da valva comprometida (Vídeo 250.15). Na estenose de valva isolada, o ventrículo parece pequeno e o átrio aumentado, e o espessamento dos folhetos valvares pode ser observado como um "domo" dentro do ventrículo, no início da diástole; exame Doppler colorido em caso de estenose AV mostra um fluxo de alta velocidade (geralmente > 2,0 m/s) adentrando o VE ou o VD no início da diástole, bem como um tempo médio de pressão prolongado, conforme determinado pela mensuração da extensão do declive E-F anormalmente raso. Na DVM e na obstrução dinâmica da VSVE, podem ser observados graus variáveis de hipertrofia concêntrica do VE (Figura 250.20 A) e fluxo turbulento de alta velocidade no interior da VSVE acompanhado de um fluxo de insuficiência mitral posterolateral.

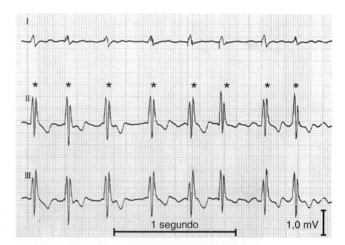

Figura 250.18 Eletrocardiograma (ECG) de três derivações obtido em um cão da raça Labrador Retriever de 1 ano de idade com displasia da valva tricúspide (DVT), mostrando desdobramento da morfologia de QRS (*asteriscos*) e fibrilação atrial em uma frequência ventricular de 200 despolarizações por minuto. Sensibilidade 10 mm/mV em velocidade do papel de 50 mm/seg.

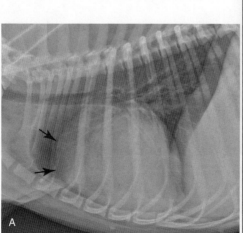 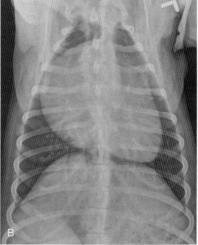

Figura 250.19 Radiografias torácicas lateral (**A**) e dorsoventral (**B**) de cão com displasia da valva tricúspide. O aumento do átrio direito (AD) e do ventrículo direito (VD) é visto em ambas as imagens. A imagem lateral mostra uma protuberância na cintura cranial (*setas*), provavelmente causada pelo aumento do átrio direito.

O exame da VSVE por meio de Doppler de onda contínua exibirá, em tais casos, um gradiente de pressão dinâmico e lábil secundário ao movimento anterior sistólico (MAS) da valva mitral (Figura 250.20 B). A DVT é identificada pelo deslocamento apical acentuado das inserções da valva tricúspide (Figura 250.20 C e D). Na anomalia de Ebstein, no homem, observa-se deslocamento apical com atrialização da parte proximal do VD. Entretanto, o diagnóstico de deslocamento apical deve ser feito com cautela, pois os pontos de inserção normais das valvas tricúspides são ligeiramente mais apicais do que o ponto normal de inserção da valva mitral; a razão para o deslocamento apical é especificamente uma falha da valva em separar em lâminas a parede do miocárdio. A melhor maneira de confirmar a anomalia de Ebstein é a cateterização cardíaca, em que um eletrograma ventricular é registrado juntamente com um traçado da pressão atrial dentro da câmara supravalvar.

Embora a ecocardiografia seja diagnóstica, também podem ser realizados cateterismo cardíaco e angiografia, especialmente se alguma intervenção for planejada. Gradientes de pressão diastólica (estenose valvar) e vários graus de ventricularização de formas de ondas atriais (na insuficiência valvar grave) podem ser registrados. A visualização angiográfica da insuficiência valvar é facilitada pela injeção ventricular de contraste, enquanto a estenose valvar é mais bem visualizada após injeção atrial que, no caso de estenose de mitral, frequentemente requer punção transeptal.

História natural

As taxas de morbidade e mortalidade associadas à displasia mitral ou tricúspide dependem da forma e da gravidade da disfunção valvar e da presença de lesões adicionais. Animais com pequena insuficiência geralmente têm uma vida normal, sem desenvolver sinais clínicos aparentes. Grande insuficiência e/ou estenose valvar grave, que causam cardiomegalia moderada a grave, levam frequentemente a arritmia atrial e ICC intratável. No entanto, essas consequências são variáveis, e a sobrevivência até 6 ou 8 anos de idade não é incomum, especialmente no caso de DVT.

Conduta clínica

Reparo da valva afetada tem sido realizado e a substituição cirúrgica da valva AV displásica tem sido realizada com sucesso em cães com displasia de mitral[190-192] ou tricúspide.[193] *Bypass* cardíaco é necessário para esses procedimentos raramente realizados. Valvuloplastia com balão foi descrita em cães com estenose mitral[194,195] e tricúspide[196,197], sendo mais discutida no Capítulo 122. O tratamento medicamentoso é instituído assim que a insuficiência cardíaca se instala; o tratamento de ICC causada por insuficiência valvar extensa consiste no uso de diuréticos, inibidores da ECA e pimobendana (ver Capítulo 247). O valor de qualquer terapia "preventiva" é desconhecido. Em cães com DVT e insuficiência cardíaca refratária, deve-se instituir paracentese periódica, embora a terapia medicamentosa concomitante seja frequentemente necessária (ver Capítulos 90 e 102). Como a taquicardia é pouco tolerada pelos pacientes com estenose de valva AV, todo esforço deve ser feito para evitar o estresse e restringir a atividade física. A administração de betabloqueadores, bloqueadores de canais de cálcio e/ou digoxina é útil, em alguns casos, para o controle da fibrilação atrial ou de outras taquiarritmias supraventriculares (ver Capítulo 248). Animais com obstrução significativa da VSVE secundária ao movimento anterior sistólico (MAS) da valva mitral, independentemente da presença ou ausência de sinais clínicos,

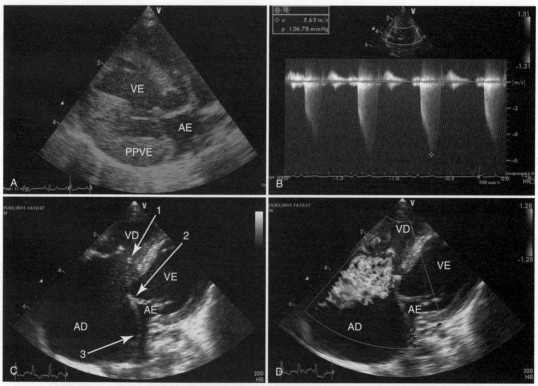

Figura 250.20 Ecocardiografia de displasia valvar mitral (DVM) e displasia da valva tricúspide (DVT). **A.** Imagem do eixo direito de cão da raça Lulu-da-Pomerânia de 6 meses de idade com DVM. Os folhetos da valva mitral estão marcadamente espessados e as cordas tendíneas estão encurtadas. O ventrículo esquerdo (*VE*), especialmente a parede posterior do VE (*PPVE*), apresenta hipertrofia concêntrica. **B.** Exame Doppler de onda contínua do mesmo cão mostra obstrução dinâmica da VSVE. O cursor está alinhado ao longo de um sinal sistólico cuja velocidade aumenta abruptamente no momento do movimento sistólico anterior da valva mitral. **C.** Imagem apical esquerda de um cão com displasia da valva tricúspide. A origem da valva tricúspide é deslocada em direção apical e o lobo septal é fundido ao septo interventricular (*1*). A origem do folheto da valva mitral (*2*) é mostrada para comparação. O septo atrial está acentuadamente marcante à esquerda (*3*). **D.** Exame com Doppler colorido do fluxo apical esquerdo de um cão com regurgitação de tricúspide grave causada por DVT. (*As figuras B e D encontram-se reproduzidas em cores no Encarte.*)

são comumente tratados com betabloqueadores (como o atenolol), com relato de ser efetivo para aliviar a obstrução dinâmica da VSVE.[177-179] Alguns pacientes toleram defeitos graves surpreendentemente bem por muitos anos. Em outros casos, há uma rápida progressão para insuficiência cardíaca e morte.

OBSTRUÇÕES DO FLUXO VENTRICULAR

Estenose pulmonar

A estenose pulmonar (EP) é o terceiro defeito cardíaco congênito mais comum em cães (ver Tabela 250.2);[3,167] ocasionalmente é detectada em gatos.[198-202] EP ocorre na maioria dos casos como um defeito cardíaco isolado, mas também é frequentemente acompanhado de anomalias cardíacas adicionais, como DVT. Obstruções congênitas da via de saída do coração direito podem se desenvolver nas regiões subvalvular e supravalvar, mas a malformação primária da valva pulmonar (displasia) é o defeito mais frequentemente observado em cães. Patterson *et al.* estudaram a hereditariedade e a patologia da displasia da valva pulmonar em cães da raça Beagle, e inicialmente sugeriram um modo poligênico de transmissão desse defeito.[203] Contudo, esses estudos de procriação não excluíram a possibilidade de um mecanismo de gene único de penetrância variável. O padrão de herança da EP não foi pesquisado em outras raças de cães predispostas, tampouco em gatos.

Patologia

As lesões valvares consistem em graus variados de espessamento valvar, fusão dos folhetos e hipoplasia dos componentes do anel valvar. Enquanto alguns cães apresentam uma valva fina em forma de domo, com um orifício central (Figura 250.21), muitos cães têm lesões mais complicadas que se assemelham à EP atípica em crianças.[47,203,204] Os folhetos valvares são geralmente espessados, deformados ou fundidos (Figura 250.21). Além do espessamento e da fusão comissural, as bordas distais dos folhetos podem estar presas à parede da artéria pulmonar, mimetizando uma obstrução supravalvar. O anel da valva pulmonar é hipoplásico em alguns cães, estreitando-se ainda mais a área disponível para a ejeção do VD. As anormalidades histológicas incluem espessamento da camada esponjosa da valva e presença de fileiras de células fusiformes em uma densa rede de colágeno. Acredita-se que essas modificações ocorrem devido à superprodução de elementos valvares normais ou por uma falha na conversão do tecido primordial embrionário da valva, semelhante a um coxim. Alguns cães com displasia valvar também apresentam um anel fibroso logo abaixo dos folhetos valvares, que acompanham as alterações valvares. Em outros cães e gatos[198] a lesão obstrutiva ocorre na região infundibular da VSVD. Ocasionalmente, a VSVD é separada do corpo (região do influxo) do VD por uma crista fibromuscular bem desenvolvida, resultando em uma anomalia denominada ventrículo direito duplo ou com dupla câmara ou estenose infundibular primária.[205,206] A distinção entre EP infundibular e ventrículo direito com dupla câmara nem sempre é clara, especialmente em gatos.[198] A EP supravalvar é incomum e, na experiência dos autores, é mais observada em cães da raça Schnauzer gigantes. A EP subvalvar foi associada ao desenvolvimento anômalo das artérias coronárias, especialmente em cães das raças Buldogue Inglês e Boxer.[207,208] Nessa condição, a circulação coronariana é derivada de um único óstio localizado no seio de Valsalva aórtico direito, e ambas as artérias coronárias, esquerda e direita, ramificam-se a partir de uma única grande artéria coronária (Figura 250.22).

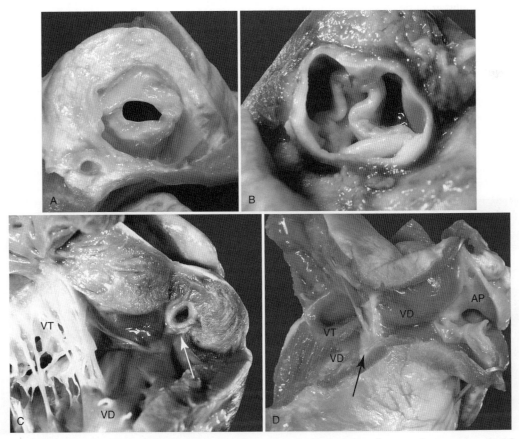

Figura 250.21 Amostras de anormalidades de cães com estenose pulmonar (EP). **A.** Os folhetos da valva pulmonar estão espessados e fundidos, com um orifício central; eles são semelhantes à valva em formato de domo, verificada em crianças com EP. **B.** Cúspides valvares muito espessas (displásicas) de um cão com EP. **C.** Anel fibroso na EP subvalvular (*seta*). **D.** Anel fibroso (*seta*) na área infundibular do ventrículo direito (*VD*), vários centímetros abaixo da valva pulmonar e da artéria pulmonar (*AP*). *VT*, valva tricúspide.

A partir desse local, a artéria coronária esquerda anômala circunda a VSVD, logo abaixo da valva pulmonar. Se essa lesão contribui para o componente subvalvular dessa malformação ou é simplesmente uma comorbidade ainda não está esclarecido, uma vez que já foi observada em cães da raça Buldogue sem EP. Independentemente disso, é clinicamente relevante porque a valvuloplastia efetiva com balão, na lesão subvalvular, foi associada à morte súbita (Figura 250.22).

O aumento da resistência à ejeção sistólica ocasiona hipertrofia concêntrica do VD, que provavelmente se inicia no útero e se desenvolve proporcionalmente à maior ou menor gravidade, dependendo do grau de obstrução do defeito. Embora essa resposta compensatória ocorra para normalizar a tensão da parede do miocárdio, ela pode comprometer a função diastólica do VD, bem como o suprimento e consumo de oxigênio no miocárdio. Em alguns cães com EP, a hipertrofia secundária da região infundibular da VSVD contribui principalmente para a obstrução do fluxo dinâmico de saída, particularmente evidente durante atividade física ou estresse. A presença desse mecanismo adicional de obstrução pode comprometer a resposta clínica à valvotomia cirúrgica ou à valvuloplastia com balão. Outros defeitos cardíacos podem interferir na fisiologia e alterar a manifestação clínica e o prognóstico de pacientes com EP. Por exemplo, EP e DVT podem ser uma associação particularmente prejudicial. Uma vez que o volume da regurgitação de tricúspide está diretamente relacionado ao tamanho do orifício regurgitante (gravidade da displasia) e da pressão do VD (gravidade do EP), a insuficiência de tricúspide grave tende a se desenvolver em cães acometidos, ocasionando insuficiência cardíaca direita intratável. Fibrilação atrial também pode desestabilizar o paciente com EP.

Um exame ultrassonográfico minucioso, na maioria das vezes usando ecocardiografia com contraste, revela conexões patentes entre os lados direito e esquerdo do coração, as quais ocorrem em uma porcentagem substancial de cães com EP; alguns cães com EP grave desenvolvem cianose devido ao *shunt* da direita para a esquerda, verificado em casos de DSA, FOP ou DSV. Alguns desses defeitos e suas consequências são discutidos mais detalhadamente na seção que aborda ToF.

Fisiopatologia
A obstrução ao fluxo de saída do VD aumenta a resistência à ejeção, causando aumento proporcional na pressão sistólica ventricular. A hipertrofia concêntrica do VD se desenvolve na tentativa de normalizar a tensão da parede ventricular. Durante a sístole, ocorre aumento da velocidade do sangue ejetado do VD, ao atravessar o orifício com obstruído. A velocidade do fluxo de sangue aumenta e torna-se turbulenta na região distal à obstrução. Uma dilatação pós-estenose se desenvolve na artéria pulmonar principal à medida que o fluxo de sangue turbulento desacelera e gasta parte de sua energia cinética contra a parede do vaso.

A hipertrofia concêntrica reduz a complacência diastólica do VD, prejudica o enchimento ventricular e frequentemente ocasiona aumento da pressão no AD. A regurgitação da tricúspide decorrente de dilatação ventricular progressiva, displasia valvar ou uma combinação dessas anormalidades pode contribuir para uma maior elevação da pressão atrial. À medida que a pressão do AD se aproxima de 15 mmHg, dilatação jugular, ascite, derrame pleural e outros sintomas de ICC direita se desenvolvem. Presume-se que a síncope secundária à hipotensão transitória seja decorrente da redução do débito cardíaco (secundária a bradicardia ou agravamento de uma obstrução infundibular dinâmica) e da combinação com vasodilatação arteriolar periférica (especialmente em caso de atividade física ou sua previsão). O estímulo dos mecanorreceptores do VD com sobrecarga de pressão também pode desencadear bradicardia reflexa e vasodilatação. Fluxo sanguíneo coronariano direito reduzido já foi documentado em alguns cães com EP e pode contribuir para a ocorrência de síncope devido a arritmias, intolerância ao exercício e insuficiência miocárdica. Em raras ocasiões, a hipertrofia septal grave e a diminuição do tamanho do VE causada por EP resultam em obstrução dinâmica do fluxo de saída do VE.[209]

Achados clínicos
Estenose pulmonar (EP) é comum em algumas raças de cães, como Beagle, Samoieda, Chihuahua, Buldogue Inglês, Schnauzer Miniatura, Cocker Spaniel, Boykin Spaniel, Labrador Retriever, Mastiff, Chow Chow, Newfoundland, Basset Hound e outras raças Terrier e Spaniel (ver Tabela 250.1).[25,105,108,210] Cães da raça Doberman Pinscher Miniatura também parecem predispostos à EP. A maioria dos cães com EP é assintomática durante o primeiro ano de vida, quando a doença geralmente é diagnosticada após a detecção de sopro cardíaco. Aproximadamente 35% dos cães com doença grave manifestam sinais clínicos, que podem incluir fadiga por esforço, síncope ou ascite.[211] Sintomas de ICC direita, como ascite, são mais frequentemente relatados em cães mais velhos.[204] Em gatos com EP grave, dispneia por esforço e letargia podem estar presentes.[199] A cianose pode ser notada quando a EP é complicada pelo *shunt* da direita para a esquerda, em função da presença concomitante de FOP, DSA ou DSV.

O achado de exame físico mais evidente na EP é um sopro de ejeção sistólica, mais audível na base do coração esquerdo, que, muitas vezes, se irradia dorsalmente. Em alguns casos, o sopro é auscultado na parte cranial do hemitórax direito.

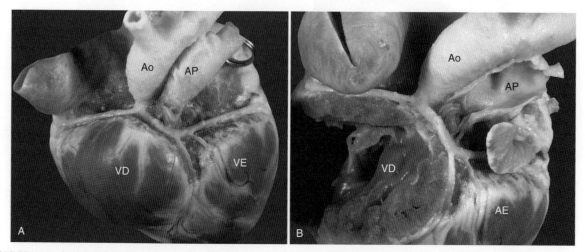

Figura 250.22 Anomalia da artéria coronária vista em alguns cães da raça Buldogue Inglês com estenose pulmonar. **A.** Notam-se ramificações das artérias coronárias esquerda e direita a partir de uma única artéria coronária grande que se origina no seio de Valsalva aórtico direito. A partir desse local, a artéria coronária esquerda circunda a VSVD, logo abaixo da valva pulmonar. **B.** As paredes anteriores da artéria pulmonar e o ventrículo direito (*VD*) foram removidos para mostrar o anel hipoplásico, a diminuta artéria pulmonar proximal (*AP*) e os folhetos da valva pulmonar espessados e agrupados. *Ao*, artéria aorta.

Em cães com insuficiência da valva pulmonar grave concomitante, o sopro de ejeção sistólica é acompanhado de discreto sopro diastólico do tipo decrescendo, mais bem auscultado na região imediatamente ventral à valva pulmonar. Um clique de ejeção sistólica é detectado com menor frequência, o que supostamente indica uma valva fundida, porém móvel. Um sopro holossistólico de regurgitação tricúspide pode ser audível no hemitórax direito. Pulso jugular de grande amplitude pode ser decorrência de uma grande onda causada pela contração atrial no VD rígido ou por ondas "cv", indicando regurgitação tricúspide significativa. Dilatação jugular e pulso jugular proeminente são evidentes na maioria dos cães com insuficiência cardíaca direita e ascite. Em geral, o pulso arterial periférico é normal.

Evidências de aumento do VD geralmente estão presentes no ECG, a menos que a lesão seja muito branda.[66,212,213] Desvio do eixo para a direita e ondas S profundas nas derivações I, II, III, aVF e precordiais esquerdas inferiores (V2, V4) são indicadores comuns de aumento do coração direito (Figura 250.23).

Radiografias de tórax mostram, tipicamente, um coração direito proeminente e dilatação pós-estenose da artéria pulmonar principal (Figura 250.24).[61,105,204,214] Essas alterações geralmente são mais evidentes na imagem dorsoventral. Achados adicionais e mais variáveis incluem dilatação da artéria pulmonar esquerda proximal, menor extensão do leito vascular pulmonar e dilatação da veia cava caudal.

A ecocardiografia é o método mais comumente utilizado para confirmar o diagnóstico de EP. O modo M e imagem 2D tipicamente mostram hipertrofia concêntrica do VD, aumento da proeminência dos músculos papilares, deformidade no(s) local(is) da(s) obstrução(ões), estreitamento da VSVD, graus variáveis de aumento do AD e dilatação pós-estenose da artéria pulmonar principal (Figura 250.25).[76,215] Das quatro valvas cardíacas, a valva pulmonar geralmente é a mais difícil de se visualizar com clareza no ecocardiograma transtorácico. Assim, pode ser impossível visualizar o local exato e a natureza da obstrução em alguns cães, sem modalidades adicionais de imagem, como ecocardiografia transesofágica. Muitas vezes, é particularmente difícil detectar uma discreta obstrução subvalvular próximo à valva pulmonar. Os folhetos da valva pulmonar se apresentam tipicamente espessados, frequentemente fundidos e parecem projetar-se sobre a artéria pulmonar durante a sístole (Figura 250.25). As bordas distais dos folhetos podem parecer parcialmente presas à parede da artéria pulmonar, criando um aspecto de ampulheta, em relação aos seios. Isso, por si, não é uma estenose supravalvular, mas indica um componente da valva displásica estenosada. Comparando a obstrução supravalvar isolada com outras valvas pulmonares normais, a obstrução supravalvar isolada é considerada rara. Quando presente, a hipoplasia do anel da valva pulmonar pode obscurecer ainda mais a anatomia valvar e confundir o tratamento. A ecocardiografia com Doppler colorido é útil para estabelecer a localização anatômica da obstrução, uma vez que uma região de aceleração do fluxo muda para um fluxo turbulento de alta velocidade que, geralmente, pode ser visto emergindo apenas distalmente ao orifício obstruído (Figura 250.25). A inspeção cuidadosa da anatomia da artéria coronária, especialmente à medida que esses vasos surgem dos seios aórticos, pode ajudar a identificar casos de anomalias das artérias coronárias. Isso é particularmente importante na EP subvalvular em cães das raças Boxer e Buldogue Inglês (Figura 250.26). Insuficiência de valva pulmonar leve a moderada também é constatada em muitos cães com EP.

Para quantificar com precisão a gravidade da obstrução, deve-se registrar a velocidade máxima do jato de fluxo sanguíneo em um traçado Doppler espectral, obtido com o feixe Doppler de onda contínua, em alinhamento paralelo à direção do fluxo (ver Figura 250.25 e Capítulo 104). Como regra geral, os gradientes

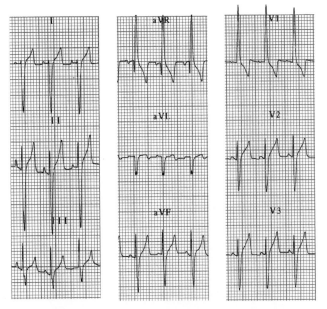

Figura 250.23 Eletrocardiograma (ECG) de um cão com estenose pulmonar mostrando um padrão típico de aumento do ventrículo direito (VD). O eixo elétrico médio é deslocado para a direita (−130°), e há ondas S proeminentes nas derivações I, II, aVF, V2 e V3 (V4).

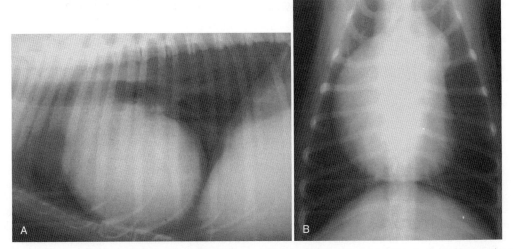

Figura 250.24 Radiografias torácicas lateral (**A**) e dorsoventral (**B**) de cão com estenose pulmonar. Há arredondamento da borda esternal e uma protuberância na cintura cardíaca cranial na imagem lateral. Notam-se aumento do coração direito e uma protuberância no segmento da artéria pulmonar (AP) principal na imagem dorsoventral. Os vasos pulmonares estão diminuídos, mesmo na ausência de *shunt* da direita para a esquerda.

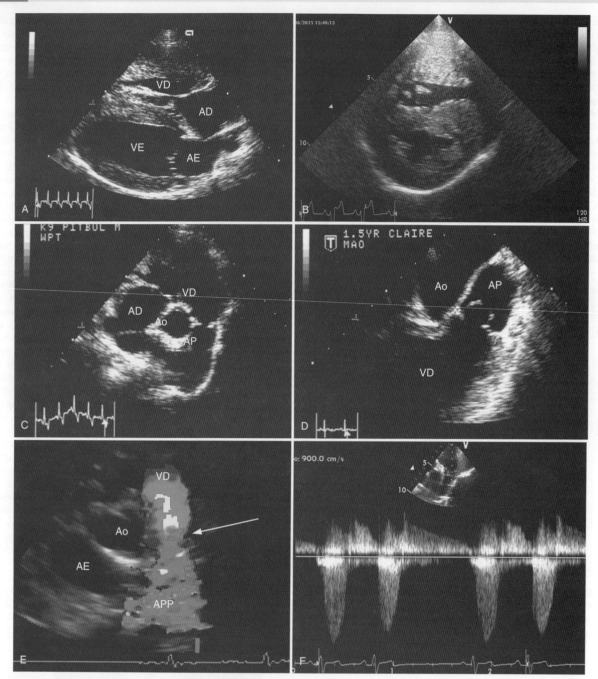

Figura 250.25 Ecocardiografia de estenose pulmonar. **A.** Imagem do eixo longitudinal direito de um cão revela hipertrofia concêntrica grave do ventrículo direito (*VD*). O átrio direito (*AD*) está dilatado. **B.** Imagem do eixo curto direito de um cão mostra flacidez do septo interventricular e hipertrofia concêntrica do VD causada por sobrecarga de pressão. **C.** Imagem do eixo curto direito da base do coração de um cão com estenose pulmonar (EP) mostra espessamento da valva pulmonar. Há uma dilatação pós-estenose da artéria pulmonar (*AP*). **D.** Ultrassonografia transesofágica de um cão jovem da raça Rottweiler com EP. Os folhetos da valva pulmonar podem ser vistos na forma de domo na AP durante a sístole. **E.** Exame do fluxo sanguíneo em Doppler colorido em um cão mostra alta velocidade e fluxo de sangue turbulento saindo do VD através da estenose (*seta*) e na artéria pulmonar principal (*APP*). **F.** Traçado de Doppler de onda contínua, obtido em imagem similar a **E**, mostra um fluxo sistólico de alta velocidade (5 m/s) através da lesão obstrutiva. A presença de insuficiência pulmonar também é notada durante a diástole. *Ao*, artéria aorta. (*A figura E encontra-se reproduzida em cores no Encarte.*)

derivados do Doppler são 40 a 50% maiores do que o gradiente medido durante o cateterismo cardíaco, em um cão, principalmente devido à anestesia geral necessária para o procedimento.[216] Além disso, estudos hemodinâmicos tipicamente indicam a gravidade da obstrução como um gradiente de pressão pico a pico, e essas medidas são quase sempre menores do que o gradiente instantâneo do pico de pressão calculado a partir das mensurações do Doppler da velocidade do pico de fluxo.[75] A subestimação do gradiente no paciente acordado é geralmente causada por um ângulo de incidência excessivo entre o feixe do ultrassom e o padrão do fluxo patológico. A superestimação pode ser mais comum e deve-se a registros espectrais que se sobrepõem durante a transmissão por ultrassom e são superconduzidas durante a fase de recepção. A pressão sistólica do VD pode ser estimada subtraindo-se a pressão sistólica da AP normal (20 a 25 mmHg) do gradiente de pressão, uma vez que a pressão da AP é invariavelmente normal em casos de EP isolada. Em cães com estenose dinâmica (infundibular) e fixa (valvar), o exame do fluxo de saída e da artéria pulmonar com Doppler pode originar um traçado que exibe a relação temporal e a velocidade entre os dois componentes da estenose. A avaliação do lado direito do coração com Doppler também pode detectar qualquer insuficiência da valva tricúspide

CAPÍTULO 250 • Cardiopatias Congênitas   1241

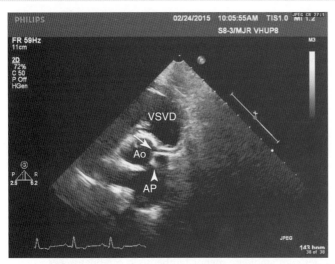

Figura 250.26 Ecocardiografia de um cão da raça Buldogue com estenose pulmonar (EP) subvalvar associada à anormalidade da artéria coronária. A imagem do eixo curto direito mostra uma artéria coronária aberrante (*seta*) que se origina da artéria aorta (*Ao*) e se estende ao longo da região subvalvular da via de saída do ventrículo direito (*VSVD*), logo abaixo da valva pulmonar (*ponta de seta*). A artéria pulmonar (*AP*) principal apresenta dilatação pós-estenose.

coexistente, e a pressão sistólica do VD também pode ser estimada usando a relação de Bernoulli e assumindo que a pressão do AD é de 0 a 5 mmHg (em cães sem ICC). Essa abordagem possibilita o controle de qualidade da estimativa obtida a partir do sinal da via de saída de fluxo do VD. A mensuração da velocidade desse jato regurgitante é particularmente útil para avaliar a gravidade da obstrução associada à EP, quando não é possível obter um alinhamento adequado com o fluxo através da via de saída.

A angiocardiografia é frequentemente realizada pouco antes da valvuloplastia com balão (Vídeo 250.16) ou para esclarecer a anatomia do coração direito antes da cirurgia (ver Capítulo 122). Tal exame mostra claramente a localização anatômica da(s) obstrução(ões), o grau de hipertrofia do VD, a presença de regurgitação tricúspide e a dilatação pós-estenose da artéria pulmonar. As características angiográficas da estenose valvar consistem em qualquer combinação das seguintes anormalidades: estreitamento na base imediata dos seios da valva; seios valvares assimétricos; hipoplasia do anel ou seio valvular; espessamento dos folhetos de valvas individuais que ocasiona defeito de enchimento cardíaco; estreitamento da coluna de contraste, com jato de contraste central ou assimétrico através de um orifício da valva estreito; valva em forma de domo durante a sístole (indicando fusão das comissuras); ou limitação do movimento do folheto supravalvar (Figura 250.27).[203,204] A obstrução muscular dinâmica do infundíbulo do VD é frequentemente vista em cães com EP (Figura 250.28). O termo ventrículo direito de dupla câmara é aplicado quando o VD é dividido em uma região de baixa pressão (o infundíbulo) e uma região de alta pressão (o ápice e a porção de entrada do VD) por uma crista muscular ou fibromuscular profunda, no infundíbulo (Figura 250.29). Alguma confusão pode ocorrer entre esta lesão e a EP subvalvar que não se localiza imediatamente adjacente aos folhetos valvares. A angiografia do ventrículo esquerdo ou a arteriografia coronariana devem ser realizadas quando houver suspeita de anormalidades no coração esquerdo ou na circulação coronariana. Tais exames devem ser realizados sempre que se faz cirurgia ou valvuloplastia com balão em um cão da raça Buldogue Inglês ou Boxer. Mesmo em raças com menor risco de anomalias coronarianas, a levofase (retorno do contraste ao lado esquerdo do coração após passar pelo pulmão) completa do ventriculograma direito pode ser útil na detecção de artérias coronárias direita e esquerda discretas. O aumento da artéria coronária direita é um achado esperado em todos os cães com EP e hipertrofia do VD bem desenvolvida.

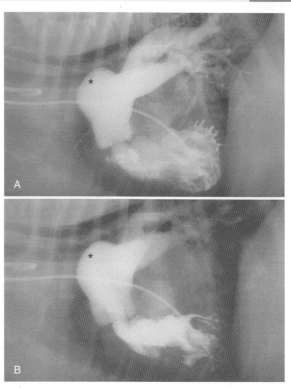

Figura 250.27 Imagens diastólica (**A**) e sistólica (**B**) de angiograma do ventrículo direito (VD) de um cão com estenose pulmonar. Note o fluxo estreito de contraste que passa pelo orifício pulmonar. A dilatação pós-estenose (*asteriscos*) da artéria pulmonar é visível em ambas as imagens, assim como a hipertrofia da parede do VD e dos músculos papilares.

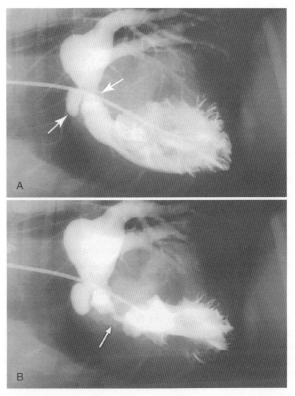

Figura 250.28 Angiocardiograma do ventrículo direito de um cão com estenose pulmonar grave. **A.** A comparação das imagens diastólica (**A**) e sistólica (**B**) mostra obstrução total da via de saída causada pela contração vigorosa do infundíbulo hipertrofiado (*seta* em **B**). Compare com a Figura 250.27. Note, também, a deformidade dos seios da valva pulmonar (*setas* em **A**).

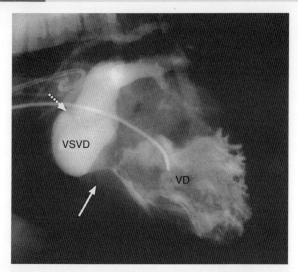

Figura 250.29 Angiocardiograma do ventrículo direito (*VD*) de um cão da raça Rottweiler com uma forma incomum de EP muscular subvalvar. Alguns profissionais se referem a essa lesão como "ventrículo direito de dupla câmara", para distingui-la do colapso dinâmico do infundíbulo hipertrofiado (ver Figura 250.28). Outros usam o termo apenas quando a lesão é mais profunda dentro do VD, e alguns evitam completamente o termo. A seta de traço contínuo mostra a lesão obstrutiva muscular na via de saída do ventrículo direito (*VSVD*). A seta tracejada indica a localização da valva pulmonar.

A confirmação hemodinâmica da obstrução da via de saída do fluxo é realizada medindo-se o gradiente de pressão sistólica ao longo da lesão (ver Figura 250.1). A gravidade da obstrução é geralmente definida como a diferença entre os picos de pressão sistólica medida acima e abaixo da obstrução (gradiente de pressão pico a pico). Como o gradiente registrado varia com a taxa de fluxo ao longo da obstrução, essa medida é muito influenciada pela contração do miocárdio e pelo protocolo anestésico utilizado. Apesar dessas limitações, o gradiente de pressão sistólica tem sido utilizado para incluir os pacientes com EP nas categorias leve (< 50 mmHg), moderada (50 a 80 mmHg) ou grave (> 80 mmHg).[204,217,218] Uma abordagem mais precisa requer a medição do débito cardíaco e o cálculo da área funcional do orifício estenosado (ver Capítulo 104). Outros achados potenciais no cateterismo incluem uma enorme onda "a" no AD, enorme onda "c-v" na regurgitação tricúspide grave, ou aumento da pressão diastólica final no VD devido à contração vigorosa do AD, ou desenvolvimento de insuficiência do VD.

História natural

Critérios confiáveis para estabelecer um prognóstico preciso não foram desenvolvidos para cães e gatos com EP. A experiência clínica indica que a maioria dos cães com EP leve ou moderada (gradiente < 80 mmHg, obtido no Doppler) geralmente tem uma vida normal, ou quase normal, especialmente se não houver sinais clínicos evidentes.[219] Essa generalização não inclui os cães com outros defeitos complicadores. O problema da DVT concomitante e sua relação com o desenvolvimento de insuficiência cardíaca já foi discutido. Embora o gradiente de pressão sistólica nem sempre seja preditivo do desfecho clínico, parece haver uma correlação geral entre o gradiente de pressão e a sobrevida. Cães com gradiente VD-AP > 125 mmHg, obtido no Doppler, frequentemente desenvolvem regurgitação tricúspide secundária, insuficiência cardíaca, síncope de esforço ou arritmia cardíaca grave (p. ex., fibrilação atrial). Quando há DSA, FOP ou DSV concomitante à EP, existe a possibilidade de *shunt* da direita para a esquerda. Se esse *shunt* for pronunciado, as consequências incluem hipoxemia arterial, eritrocitose e debilitação grave. Morte súbita ocorre em alguns cães com EP grave, mas essa ocorrência é incomum.

Conduta clínica

Pacientes com EP simples e assintomática, com gravidade leve ou moderada, geralmente não necessitam de tratamento. Exames ecocardiográficos seriados podem ser realizados para monitorar o grau de hipertrofia ventricular, o desenvolvimento de estenose infundibular secundária e a ocorrência de regurgitação tricúspide. A restrição de exercício geralmente é desnecessária. Alguns cães desenvolvem obstrução mais grave ao longo do tempo. Cães com doença grave ou sintomática são candidatos à cirurgia ou valvuloplastia por balão (ver Capítulo 122). Não foram realizados estudos prospectivos que investiguem o efeito da valvuloplastia por balão na sobrevida. Dados de estudos retrospectivos sugerem que a valvuloplastia por balão em cães com doença grave está associada à redução do risco de morte relacionada ao coração.[219-221] O gradiente de pressão exato que justifica a intervenção não pode ser afirmado com certeza. Cães com gradiente obtido em Doppler acima de 100 a 125 mmHg devem ser considerados candidatos à valvuloplastia por balão ou à cirurgia. Cães com gradiente menor também são candidatos a esses procedimentos se forem sintomáticos ou se apresentarem regurgitação de tricúspide. A intervenção em idade jovem deve ser encorajada, já que o desenvolvimento de ICC evidente reduz substancialmente a chance de um resultado bem-sucedido, independentemente do método de reparo ou método paliativo usado. Devido à alta probabilidade de hereditariedade, até mesmo os cães levemente comprometidos não devem ser utilizados como reprodutores.

O objetivo da intervenção em cães com EP grave consiste em abolir o gradiente de pressão sistólica ou reduzi-lo a um valor baixo e proporcionar alívio sintomático em cães que manifestam sinais clínicos. Por muitos anos, a cirurgia foi a única opção disponível para o tratamento de EP, e várias técnicas cirúrgicas têm sido defendidas, incluindo a dilatação da valva, o enxerto valvar ou a colocação de um conduto ligando o VD à artéria pulmonar.[217,218,222-228] A técnica de enxerto valvar aberta, apesar de difícil de realização, é um método particularmente versátil e econômico para o tratamento de cães com EP, particularmente quando há uma considerável obstrução subvalvar.[226-228] Esta técnica é bem adequada para o tratamento de alguns defeitos não passíveis de valvuloplastia por balão (p. ex., cães com obstrução muscular da VSVD, ventrículo direito de dupla câmara ou hipoplasia grave do anel da valva pulmonar). A técnica de enxerto valvar não deve ser realizada em cães com EP subvalvular associada à artéria coronária anômala, pois o corte da artéria resultará em morte.

A valvuloplastia percutânea por meio de cateter com balão é uma alternativa preferencial à cirurgia e deve ser recomendada para cães com EP valvar. Esse procedimento de cateterismo intervencionista para EP é discutido no Capítulo 122. A redução bem-sucedida do gradiente obstrutivo em 50% ou mais foi relatada em 75 a 80% dos cães tratados com essa técnica.[211,221,229,230] Uma análise retrospectiva de 40 cães submetidos à valvuloplastia por balão indicou uma redução de 53% na taxa de mortalidade em comparação com 41 cães que não realizaram o procedimento.[220] Cães com hipoplasia do anel da valva pulmonar ou desenvolvimento anômalo das artérias coronárias e EP subvalvular apresentam risco potencial de complicações graves da valvuloplastia por balão, incluindo avulsão da artéria coronária ou ruptura do anel da valva pulmonar.[231] Valvuloplastia por balão conservadora utilizando balão de tamanho 0,6 a 1 vez o diâmetro do anel valvar pulmonar foi relatada em um pequeno número de casos, com resultados variáveis.[232]

Estenose aórtica

A estenose aórtica subvalvar (EAS) é a malformação cardíaca congênita mais comum em cães de raças de grande porte.[4,172,173,233-242] A maioria dos casos de EAS ocorre em consequência de uma saliência ou anel de tecido fibroso fixo localizado na VSVE, logo abaixo da valva aórtica. A EAS é uma anormalidade problemática por várias razões. É muito difícil diagnosticar em cães levemente acometidos e é difícil tratar quando é grave. A EAS dinâmica também tem sido detectada com frequência crescente em cães e gatos com uma variedade de distúrbios cardíacos, incluindo EAS fixa, DVM, cardiomiopatia hipertrófica e outras condições que causam hipertrofia do septo interventricular e redução do tamanho do VE (ou seja, EP, ToF).[243] Cães da raça Bull Terrier são predispostos à estenose da valva aórtica, na qual os folhetos são espessos e o anel da valva aórtica é levemente hipoplásico. Cães da raça Boxer normais também apresentam diâmetro do anel aórtico menor que o de outras raças de cães, e isso confunde o diagnóstico da doença branda nessa raça.[244] EA discreta causada por uma valva bicúspide ocorre em raras ocasiões.[169] EA fixa foi descrita em um pequeno número de gatos,[32-34,245] incluindo um caso de estenose supravalvar.[246]

Patologia e patogênese

A estenose aórtica subvalvar (EAS) foi pesquisada extensivamente em cães da raça Newfoundland. Estudos de reprodução nessa e em outras raças estabeleceram uma base genética para a perpetuação da EAS.[2,247-249] Uma anomalia autossômica dominante no gene PICALM foi associada à ocorrência de EAS em cães dessa raça,[12] embora esses dados possam necessitar de validação adicional.[250] Um modo de herança autossômica recessiva é relatado em cães da raça Dogue de Bordeaux.[180] Assim, é provável que a EAS no cão possa ser resultante de diferentes anormalidades genéticas. Os estudos de colônia de reprodutores, de Pyle e Patterson, indicam ainda que a obstrução talvez ainda não esteja presente ao nascimento, mas se desenvolve durante as primeiras 4 a 8 semanas de vida.[2,235-237,247] Essa progressão tem uma significância particular em relação à identificação de sopros cardíacos em filhotes de raças reconhecidamente propensas a EAS. Trabalhos recentes em cães da raça Golden Retriever sugeriram que uma aortopatia ou estreitamento anormal do ângulo septo-aórtico pode ter participação no desenvolvimento ou progressão da EAS em cães, uma condição anteriormente relatada em crianças.[251]

As lesões de EAS em cães da raça Newfoundland têm sido descritas em estudos *post-mortem* como: leve (grau 1), que consiste em "pequenos nódulos esbranquiçados, levemente elevados na superfície do endocárdio do septo ventricular, logo abaixo da valva aórtica"; moderada (grau 2), que consiste em uma "crista estreita esbranquiçada espessa no endocárdio", estendendo-se, em parte, na SSVE; e grave (grau 3), que consiste em "uma faixa fibrosa, crista ou anel que circunda completamente a VSVE, logo abaixo da valva aórtica".[2,247] Esse anel é proeminente, acima do endocárdio, e estende-se até – e talvez envolva – a região cranioventral do folheto da valva mitral e a base da valva aórtica (Figura 250.30). O anel estenosante consiste em fibras reticulares dispostas de maneira frouxa, substância fundamental de mucopolissacarídeo e fibras elásticas. Feixes discretos de colágeno, e até de cartilagem, são encontrados em lesões avançadas.[247] O cateterismo cardíaco de cães com lesões de grau 1 não foi capaz de detectar com segurança a lesão visível após a morte, enquanto as lesões de grau 2 frequentemente estavam associadas a sopro cardíaco brando e gradiente de pressão sistólica mínimo. Conforme evidenciado por esses estudos e discutido a seguir, a detecção clínica de EAS discreta frequentemente é bastante difícil, e o aconselhamento genético pode estar repleto de erros. Diversas anormalidades cardíacas podem estar associadas a EAS, mais notavelmente DVM, PDA e uma série de anormalidades do arco aórtico. As lesões valvares observadas em cães da raça Bull Terrier, incluindo degeneração mixomatosa e metaplasia cartilaginosa dos folhetos valvares, assemelham-se à estenose valvar calcificada em humanos.[252] A maioria dos cães com EAS exibe algum grau de dilatação da artéria aorta distal. Essa dilatação pós-estenose pode variar de simples a grave e pode se estender até os vasos do arco. O grau de dilatação pós-estenose é frequentemente maior nas obstruções graves, mas essa relação é bastante variável.

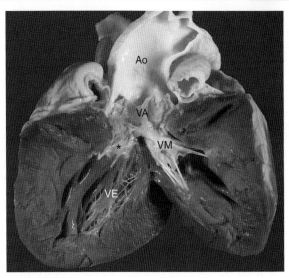

Figura 250.30 Anormalidade macroscópica da estenose subaórtica. A imagem da via de saída do ventrículo esquerdo (*VE*) no cão mostra a presença de um anel circunferencial de tecido fibroso pouco abaixo da valva aórtica (*VA*). Uma crista espessa de tecido fibroso é vista logo abaixo da valva aórtica e se estende até o septo ventricular (*asterisco*). Nota-se marcante espessamento das paredes ventriculares. Há espessamento da valva mitral (*VM*) anterior e cordas tendíneas associadas à direita da lesão. Nota-se dilatação pós-estenose da porção proximal da artéria aorta (*Ao*).

Em alguns cães acometidos, os achados patológicos divergem da descrição clássica. O folheto anterior da valva mitral é espesso, diferentemente da placa septal da fibrose endocárdica, em que o folheto mitral colide com o septo interventricular (SIV) devido à obstrução dinâmica.[253] Em vez de um anel fibroso, o septo apresenta hipertrofia uniforme ou uma crista fibromuscular ampla que surge da base do septo interventricular e se projeta para a VSVE. Músculos papilares malformados, mal posicionados ou desalinhados, cordas tendinosas espessadas e folhetos mitrais alongados ou deformados contribuem para o desenvolvimento da obstrução.[254] Malformação da valva mitral também está associada à EAS em gatos, embora a anormalidade seja relativamente rara nessa espécie.[245,255] Em alguns gatos, têm-se observado obstruções semelhantes a túneis relativamente longas.

Hipertrofia concêntrica do VE se desenvolve em cães com EAS fixa ou dinâmica, mais ou menos proporcional à gravidade da obstrução ao fluxo de saída, muito embora a correlação entre a espessura da parede e a magnitude do gradiente medido seja frequentemente inconsistente.[77] Anormalidades estruturais e funcionais do VE[78] e da circulação coronariana estão bem documentadas em cães com EAS.[235,237] O fluxo coronariano anormal também tem sido mensurado em artérias extramurais maiores, com diminuição do fluxo diastólico basal e reversão do fluxo coronariano durante a sístole.[105,237] Áreas focais de infarto e fibrose do miocárdio são comumente observadas nos músculos papilares e no subendocárdio de cães com EAS grave, muitas vezes com a presença de artérias coronárias intramurais anormais. As alterações histológicas das artérias coronárias intramurais nesses locais consistem em proliferação de tecido conjuntivo na camada íntima e no músculo liso e degeneração da camada medial. Essas alterações estão presumivelmente relacionadas à alta tensão da parede encontrada nessa condição patológica, e sua gênese pode estar relacionada à síntese de angiotensina II ou de outros mediadores bioquímicos de hipertrofia e remodelamento.[256-258] Além disso, essas lesões arteriais podem ser importantes na ocorrência de arritmias ventriculares malignas e morte súbita.

Fisiopatologia

A obstrução da via de saída do fluxo sanguíneo do VE provoca aumento da pressão sistólica e hipertrofia concêntrica do VE.

Consequentemente à obstrução fixa, a taxa de ejeção do VE sofre um retardo, causando um pulso arterial diminuído e tardio (pulso anacrótico). A alta velocidade e a turbulência do fluxo ao longo da área estenosada produzem um sopro de ejeção sistólica e contribuem para a dilatação pós-estenose, geralmente envolvendo a artéria aorta ascendente, o arco aórtico e a artéria braquiocefálica. A hipertrofia do átrio esquerdo se desenvolve como consequência do relaxamento prejudicado e da redução da complacência do VE hipertrofiado. Regurgitação aórtica leve está comumente presente, presumivelmente devido ao espessamento dos folhetos valvares ou à dilatação da artéria aorta ascendente. Danos ao endotélio da valva aórtica (lesões causadas pelo jato de sangue) predispõem os cães com EAS à endocardite infecciosa.[259,260] Cães com EAS grave podem desenvolver ICC esquerda devido à insuficiência miocárdica, disfunção diastólica, regurgitação mitral, fibrilação atrial ou uma combinação dessas anormalidades. Mais frequentemente, relata-se síncope por esforço ou morte súbita, presumivelmente como consequência de isquemia do miocárdio e desenvolvimento de arritmia ventricular maligna. Coerente com esse achado é que o ECG de esforço pode revelar depressão importante e instável do segmento ST. Em alguns cães, o colapso por esforço pode ser causado por hipotensão precipitada pelo aumento da pressão do VE induzido por exercício, ativação de mecanorreceptores ventriculares e bradicardia ou vasodilatação inapropriada.[261]

Achados clínicos

A EAS congênita é comum em muitas raças de cães (ver Tabela 250.1), especialmente Newfoundland, Boxer, Rottweiler, Golden Retriever e Pastor-Alemão.[167,262] EA valvar é comum apenas em cães da raça Bull Terrier. Os achados clínicos da EAS variam com a gravidade da obstrução e a presença de defeitos cardíacos concomitantes. Os achados clínicos em filhotes com EAS de grau leve são frequentemente discretos e facilmente negligenciados. Os cães assintomáticos têm um sopro de ejeção suave a moderadamente intenso que pode ser facilmente confundido com um sopro cardíaco fraco ou funcional.[263] A análise mais detalhada da frequência ou da turbulência dos sopros suaves pode fornecer informações sobre quais sopros estão associados à doença leve.[264,265] Na medida em que as lesões da EAS podem se desenvolver durante o período pós-natal, o sopro pode tornar-se cada vez mais proeminente durante os primeiros 6 meses de vida. Em cães de raças de rápido crescimento, como Newfoundland, a classificação da gravidade do EAS em um filhote deve ser reservada, até que o cão tenha atingido idade próxima a de adulto, porque a progressão, de leve a grave, foi observada durante esse período.[247,251,266] Cães gravemente acometidos podem apresentar fadiga por esforço, síncope ou ICC esquerda, mas a grande maioria dos cães é assintomática. Em cães com doença grave, uma observação comum do proprietário é que o cão acometido é menor do que os seus irmãos de ninhada saudáveis. A morte súbita, sem sinais premonitórios, é comum em cães severamente acometidos de 1 a 3 anos de idade.[260]

O diagnóstico de EAS grave não é difícil, pois o sopro sistólico geralmente se torna mais alto e, posteriormente, culmina em sopro holossistólico, quando a obstrução é mais grave.[267] Na EAS grave, o sopro geralmente é mais audível na base do lado esquerdo do coração, reconhecendo que, em alguns cães, o sopro sistólico é igualmente alto ou mais alto na base cardíaca direita, presumivelmente devido à irradiação na artéria aorta ascendente. O sopro da EA geralmente irradia-se para as artérias carótidas e pode ser auscultado na região cervical ventral. Frequentemente, o sopro se propaga para o ápice e pode ser confundido com regurgitação mitral. De fato, uma grande porcentagem de cães com EAS também apresenta regurgitação mitral, mas esses sopros geralmente são difíceis de serem diferenciados, devido ao seu tempo similar e à sobreposição de áreas de intensidade máxima. Apesar da ocorrência frequente de regurgitação aórtica detectada em ecocardiografia com Doppler, um sopro diastólico suave secundário à insuficiência da valva aórtica raramente é detectado. Em outras anormalidades físicas detectadas em cães moderada a severamente acometidos, notam-se pulso arterial diminuído e tardio e um impulso precordial proeminente do VE devido à hipertrofia do VE.

O ECG é frequentemente normal, mas pode, em casos graves, indicar hipertrofia do VE (aumento da amplitude da onda R nas derivações II, III, aVF, V2, V4). Depressão do segmento ST e alterações da onda T sugerem anormalidades de repolarização secundárias ou isquemia do miocárdio; o último é especialmente provável quando as alterações do segmento ST são desencadeadas por exercício ou ocorrem juntamente com ectopia ventricular (Figura 250.31). Em comparação com o ECG em repouso, o ECG com registros por um período de 24 horas (Holter) é o método mais sensível de detecção de arritmia ventricular intermitente ou induzida por exercício e alterações no segmento ST. A gravidade das arritmias assim detectadas corresponde frequentemente à gravidade da doença.[268]

As radiografias de tórax podem ser normais ou indicar hipertrofia do VE.[61,105,214] A dilatação pós-estenose da artéria aorta ascendente horizontalmente inclinada causa perda da cintura cranial na imagem lateral e alargamento do mediastino na imagem dorsoventral em casos graves (Figura 250.32). O aumento discreto do AE é comum em cães com EAS moderada ou grave, mas o aumento acentuado do AE sugere regurgitação mitral simultânea, insuficiência do VE ou *shunt* da esquerda para a direita concomitante. Embora desnecessária para o diagnóstico, a angiocardiografia é útil para delinear o local e a geometria da obstrução, que geralmente é mais evidente na porção ventral do fluxo, quando visto em imagem lateral (Figura 250.33 e Vídeo 250.17). Outros achados angiográficos incluem dilatação pós-estenose da artéria aorta ascendente, aumento da artéria coronária esquerda e seus ramos extramurais, pequena cavidade do VE e hipertrofia dos músculos papilares e da parede do VE. Injeção supravalvular da artéria aorta pode ser realizada para detectar insuficiência da valva aórtica, mas a ecocardiografia com Doppler é uma técnica mais sensível. Registros hemodinâmicos documentam a presença e a gravidade do gradiente de pressão sistólica através da obstrução (Figura 250.34). Esses registros também são úteis para detectar elevação da pressão diastólica final do VE e ICC iminente.[105,269] O gradiente de pressão registrado em cães com EAS é deprimido pela anestesia

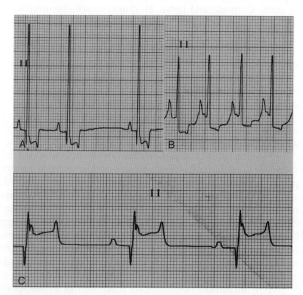

Figura 250.31 Eletrocardiograma (ECG) mostrando depressão (**A** e **B**) e elevação (**C**) do segmento ST em três cães com EAS grave, sugestivas de isquemia de miocárdio. Sensibilidade, 10 mm/mV. **A.** Traçado de um cão da raça Golden Retriever de 1 ano de idade, a 25 mm/s. **B.** Esse cão da raça Terra-Nova (Newfoundland) de 6 meses de idade apresentou colapso e morreu repentinamente 1 hora após a realização do ECG, a 25 mm/s. **C.** Traçado de um cão da raça Golden Retriever de 1 ano de idade, a 50 mm/s.

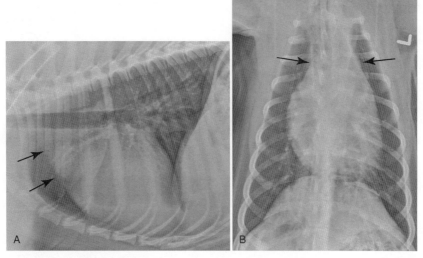

Figura 250.32 Radiografias lateral (**A**) e dorsoventral (**B**) de um cão jovem com estenose subaórtica. A protuberância proeminente na cintura cranial, na imagem lateral (*setas*), e o alargamento do mediastino cranial, na imagem dorsoventral (*setas*), são compatíveis com dilatação pós-estenose da artéria aorta ascendente.

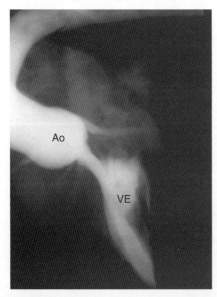

Figura 250.33 Angiograma de um cão com EAS. A injeção do ventrículo esquerdo (*VE*) causa opacificação do VE e da artéria aorta (*Ao*). Um estreitamento da coluna de contraste semelhante a um túnel é visto na via de saída do fluxo do VE. Também se nota uma artéria coronária circunflexa esquerda proeminente.

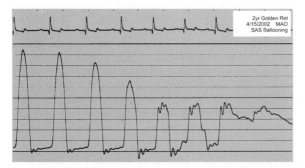

Figura 250.34 Pressões intracardíaca e na valva aórtica obtidas por meio de cateterismo cardíaco de um cão da raça Golden Retriever de 2 anos, com estenose subaórtica. O cateter é retirado do ventrículo esquerdo (VE; *esquerda*) pela via de saída do ventrículo esquerdo (VSVE; *centro*) e artéria aorta ascendente (*direita*). Um gradiente de pressão sistólica de 100 mmHg é mostrado entre o VE e a VSVE, indicando a localização subvalvar da obstrução (artefato de movimento do cateter sobreposto à via de saída do fluxo e registros da valva aórtica).

geral em aproximadamente 40 a 50%, comparativamente ao medido em pacientes não anestesiados, como resultado da diminuição do fluxo sanguíneo (volume sistólico).[270]

A EAS de intensidade moderada a grave é facilmente detectada na ecocardiografia 2D e Doppler (ver Capítulo 104). Os achados típicos consistem em hipertrofia concêntrica do VE, lesão subvalvar obstrutiva, área reduzida do orifício do VE e dilatação pós-estenose da artéria aorta (Figura 250.35).[71,76,201,215,239] Em cães da raça Golden Retriever, um ângulo mais agudo entre a artéria aorta ascendente e o septo interventricular (SIV) (ângulo aórtico-septal) tem sido associado a um aumento da velocidade do fluxo de saída do VE no desenvolvimento de EAS (Figura 250.36).[251] Os músculos papilares e a superfície endocárdica do miocárdio ventricular frequentemente aparecem hiperecoicos na doença grave, presumivelmente como resultado de isquemia miocárdica e substituição por fibrose ou calcificação. Alterações estruturais na valva mitral podem frequentemente ser apreciadas e o movimento anormal da valva mitral (movimento sistólico anterior, MSA) é evidente nos casos em que há DVM e obstrução dinâmica coexistentes.[253] O exame com Doppler espectral da VSVE é usado para avaliar a gravidade da doença, medindo a velocidade máxima do fluxo na VSVE.[271] Tais medidas mostram excelente correlação com mensurações invasivas (Figura 250.35).[75] As mensurações de Doppler podem ser feitas a partir de uma variedade de janelas de imagens subcostais, embora as velocidades obtidas em posição subcostal geralmente exibam valores mais altos.[272] Enquanto o gradiente de pressão estimado pelo Doppler, entre 80 e 100 mmHg (com velocidade máxima do fluxo variando de 4,5 a 5 m/s), é usado para detectar obstrução moderada da VSVE e velocidades mais altas usadas para detectar obstruções graves, essas designações são um tanto arbitrárias. O gradiente de pressão obtido no Doppler é influenciado pela quantidade de fluxo (volume sistólico) que atravessa o orifício obstruído e pode superestimar a gravidade da obstrução em caso de débito cardíaco elevado (p. ex., em cães estressados ou excitados, ou portadores de PDA), ou subestimar a gravidade se o fluxo for subnormal (p. ex., em cães sob anestesia ou com insuficiência de miocárdio concomitante). Nesses casos, a indexação do gradiente ao volume sistólico ou alguma medida relacionada ou a simples medida da área do orifício bidimensional pode fornecer uma estimativa melhor da gravidade da doença.[77,201,273] Registros de Doppler colorido de fluxo são importantes para detectar e estimar a gravidade da insuficiência da valva aórtica ou mitral coexistente, embora a concentração apenas na área do fluxo possa resultar em superestimação da gravidade.[202]

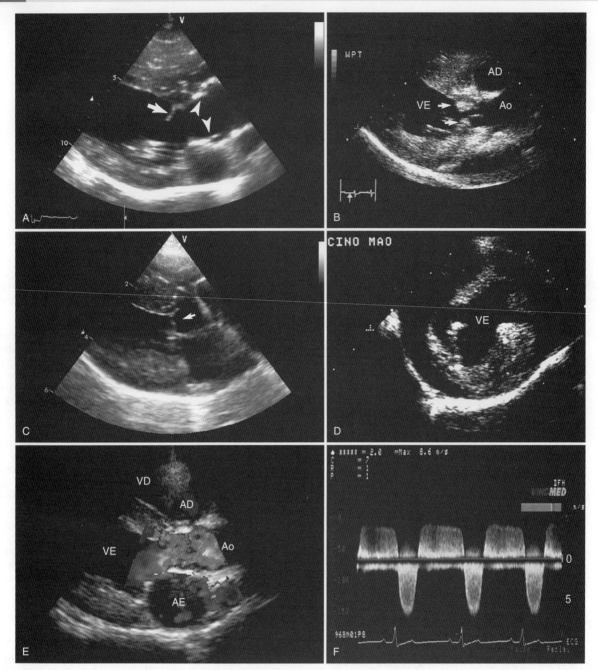

Figura 250.35 Ecocardiografia de estenose subaórtica (ESA). **A** a **C**. Imagens do eixo longitudinal direito mostram os vários tipos morfológicos de obstrução da via de saída do ventrículo esquerdo (VE) em cães com ESA. **A**. ESA membranosa discreta em um cão da raça Rottweiler de 5 anos de idade. Uma borda delgada de tecido membranoso se estende a partir do septo interventricular. Não se observa hipertrofia concêntrica significativa do VE. Os folhetos da valva aórtica aberta são indicados pelas setas. **B**. ESA grave semelhante a um túnel em um cão da raça Golden Retriever de 4 anos de idade. Duas cristas de tecido hiperecoico estão presentes na base da valva aórtica (setas). O VE está hipertrofiado, com superfície endocárdica hiperecogênica. **C**. ESA dinâmica em um cão da raça Poodle. O movimento anterior sistólico da valva mitral é visto projetando-se na via de saída do ventrículo esquerdo (seta). O VE apresenta hipertrofia concêntrica. A velocidade do fluxo sanguíneo ao longo da obstrução era superior a 5,5 m/s, indicando um grau grave de sobrecarga de pressão no VE. **D**. A imagem do eixo curto direito de um cão mestiço de 3 meses mostra hipertrofia concêntrica do VE e acentuada hiperecogenicidade do tecido subendocárdico e dos músculos papilares. Acredita-se que esse achado represente áreas de isquemia miocárdica e substituição por fibrose. **E**. O exame Doppler colorido do eixo longitudinal direito de um cão com ESA revela alta velocidade e fluxo sanguíneo turbulento na VSVE e artéria aorta (Ao). **F**. O traçado do Doppler de onda contínua, em imagem apical esquerda, em um cão com ESA grave mostra velocidade sistólica máxima de 6,5 m/s, indicando um gradiente de pressão de 169 mmHg através da obstrução. A presença de insuficiência aórtica também é detectada. (A figura E encontra-se reproduzida em cores no Encarte.)

A detecção *antemortem* das formas mais brandas de EAS por meio de auscultação, angiografia ou ecocardiografia muitas vezes não é possível e a velocidade de saída exata na qual o diagnóstico de EA torna-se sensível e específico é controversa e indefinida em qualquer exame padrão-ouro. Cães com anormalidades discretas (ou seja, lesão de grau 1, conforme descrito anteriormente) escapam à detecção até mesmo pelos clínicos mais experientes. Mesmo em cães com lesão de grau 2, a distinção de cães normais somente com base na velocidade de fluxo do VE é problemática. Há relato de um limite superior para a velocidade aórtica em cães normais, mas não está bem estabelecido para diferentes raças e condições de exame.[274] A velocidade média máxima da onda pulsada aórtica, no laboratório dos autores, para cães saudáveis sem qualquer sopro cardíaco é de 1,7 m/s, e este valor é semelhante aos valores relatados em um estudo de cães saudáveis sem sopro cardíaco em que a velocidade máxima na

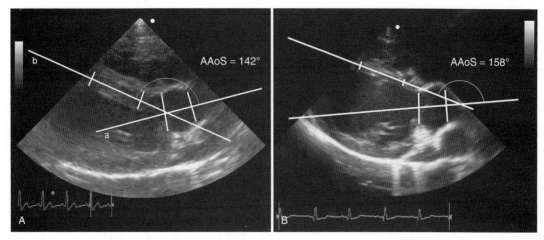

Figura 250.36 A. Medição do ângulo aórtico-septal em um filhote de cão da raça Golden Retriever que desenvolveu ESA quando adulto jovem. O ângulo é formado pelo longo eixo da aorta ascendente e o plano do septo interventricular (SIV). O eixo da linha média da raiz da aorta é obtido dividindo a raiz da artéria aorta no local do anel e acima da junção sinotubular (linha a). O eixo da linha média do SIV é obtido dividindo o septo nas extremidades dos folhetos da valva mitral, 2 cm em direção apical a partir desse ponto (linha b). AAoS = 142°. **B.** Medição do ângulo aórtico-septal em um filhote de cão da raça Golden Retriever normal. AAoS = 158°. *AAoS*, ângulo aórtico-septal; *ESA*, estenose subaórtica. (De Belanger MC, Cote E, Beauchamp G: Association between aortoseptal angle in Golden Retriever puppies and subaortic stenosis in adulthood. *J Vet Intern Med* 28:1498-1503, 2014.)

VSVE foi < 1,8 m/s, quando medida a partir do ápice esquerdo (limite superior do intervalo de confiança de 95%).[275] As velocidades registradas no exame Doppler de onda contínua em posição subcostal são minimamente mais rápidas, mas geralmente < 2 m/s em cães sem sopro cardíaco. No entanto, a velocidade de ejeção da VSVE acima desse valor é frequentemente registrada em cães com sopro de ejeção brando, mas sem evidência de obstrução discreta do fluxo de saída no ecocardiograma 2D (bidimensional). Tais velocidades são especialmente comuns em raças caracterizadas por dimensões da via de saída do fluxo levemente diminuídas (cães das raças Boxer e Bull Terrier). Um diagnóstico de EAS leve é mais seguro, uma vez que a velocidade máxima média é superior a 2,3 a 2,4 m/s e é associada a outros achados, particularmente: anormalidade de fluxo no Doppler de onda pulsada; lesão anatômica constatada em imagem bidimensional; regurgitação aórtica holodiastólica; e velocidade de fluxo acelerada abruptamente em uma pequena região da VSVE. Alguns pesquisadores consideram, no exame ecocardiográfico, uma área de saída de fluxo do ventrículo esquerdo, em relação à superfície corporal, < 1,46 cm/m² ou um ângulo aórtico-septal < 145°, como indicadores de EAS leve ou AES em desenvolvimento, em filhotes de cães da raça Golden Retriever.[201,251] A impossibilidade de detectar com segurança a EAS leve é uma grande fonte de frustração, quando se tenta fornecer conselho genético aos proprietários, que estão interessados em reduzir a incidência da doença.

História natural

EAS grave é uma condição desanimadora, já que muitos cães portadores dessa doença morrem prematuramente. Em uma pesquisa retrospectiva de 96 cães com EAS, constatou-se que 21 morreram repentinamente, na maioria das vezes nos primeiros 3 anos de vida.[260] Onze cães desenvolveram endocardite e/ou ICC, e 32 cães manifestaram intolerância ao exercício ou síncope. Cães com hipertrofia ventricular mínima, obstrução leve do fluxo ventricular e gradiente de pressão máxima do Doppler < 50 mmHg são mais propensos a ter uma vida normal, enquanto cães com gradiente de pressão > 125 a 130 mmHg têm grande probabilidade de desenvolver complicações sérias ou terem morte súbita.[276] Fatores complicadores que contribuem para um resultado adverso incluem: disfunção diastólica e sistólica progressiva do VE, regurgitação mitral, regurgitação aórtica, endocardite da valva aórtica e fibrilação atrial.[266,277,278] Morte súbita é mais provável de ocorrer durante ou logo após uma atividade intensa.

Conduta clínica

Cães com EAS de intensidade leve não são tratados, além da administração de antibióticos profiláticos, durante períodos previstos para bacteriemia, tais como durante procedimentos odontológicos, cirurgia ou sempre que houver suspeita de uma doença infecciosa concomitante. Essa prática permanece comum, apesar do fato de que a eficácia dos antibióticos profiláticos para reduzir o risco de endocardite infecciosa em cães com EAS não foi definitivamente estabelecida.[278] Diversas opções de tratamento podem ser consideradas no tratamento de cães com EAS de intensidade moderada a grave, mas a maioria dos tratamentos tem valor incerto. A ressecção aberta da lesão obstrutiva durante circulação extracorpórea oferece claramente a melhor oportunidade de reduzir substancial e permanentemente o gradiente de pressão sistólica;[279,280] no entanto, um procedimento bem-sucedido não parece alterar substancialmente a prevalência de morte súbita.[280] Outros procedimentos cirúrgicos empregados para dilatar ou controlar a obstrução falharam em alcançar uma redução sustentada do gradiente de pressão sistólica ou, então, acarretaram um risco inaceitável de complicações.[281,282] Além disso, esses procedimentos terapêuticos geralmente apresentam disponibilidade limitada e são proibitivamente caros para serem considerados opções terapêuticas de rotina.

Dilatação da EAS por balão foi tentada em cães, como alternativa à cirurgia ou ao tratamento com medicamentos ao longo da vida. Em média, a dilatação por balão, com uso de cateter, é capaz de reduzir a gravidade da obstrução da EAS em cães, em 50%[283]; entretanto, esse benefício a curto prazo é atenuado em alguns (e talvez na maioria) dos cães ao longo do tempo,[271] e a valvuloplastia por balão não aumentou a sobrevida, comparativamente ao tratamento com atenolol.[284] O uso de balões de "corte" que fazem incisão ou laceram a lesão de estenose, seguido de dilatação com balão de alta pressão foi descrito (ver Capítulo 122), mas, se esse procedimento produz resultados superiores em relação à dilatação por balão tradicional, isso até agora é desconhecido.[285] A dilatação da EAS por balão é mais desafiadora do que a valvuloplastia por balão, comparativamente à estenose pulmonar (EP). As complicações dessa técnica, com risco à vida, incluem arritmia fatal, desenvolvimento de endocardite da valva aórtica, ruptura do anel aórtico e avulsão da artéria braquiocefálica durante a retirada do balão. Além disso, a impossibilidade de ressecção cirúrgica para prevenir morte súbita sugere que o tratamento efetivo requer mais do que a redução do gradiente de pressão.

Os autores recomendam evitar atividade física intensa e prolongada, reconhecendo que, em cães jovens e muitas vezes saudáveis, essa recomendação, mesmo conservadora, nem sempre é prática. Com base em evidências clínicas e patológicas de isquemia miocárdica, os autores também administram bloqueadores de receptores beta-adrenérgicos aos cães com gradiente de pressão elevado ou com histórico de síncope. Os betabloqueadores (como o atenolol) reduzem a frequência cardíaca máxima, diminuem o consumo de oxigênio pelo miocárdio e aumentam o tempo para o fluxo diastólico da artéria coronária, oferecendo, assim, um benefício protetor teórico ao miocárdio contra a isquemia e contra o desenvolvimento de arritmia. Além disso, cães que recebem altas doses de betabloqueadores parecem menos dispostos (ou são menos capazes) para praticar atividades físicas intensas e prolongadas. Apesar dessas vantagens teóricas, um estudo retrospectivo não encontrou benefício do atenolol na sobrevida de cães com EAS (Figura 250.37).[276] Em teoria, o uso de bloqueadores de canais de cálcio ou inibidores da enzima conversora de angiotensina (ECA) também pode ser útil no tratamento de cães com ESA; entretanto, nenhum desses procedimentos terapêuticos foi avaliado em testes clínicos controlados com placebo.

TETRALOGIA DE FALLOT

As características anatômicas que definem a teratologia de Fallot (ToF) são: obstrução da via de saída do ventrículo direito devido à obstrução infundibular secundária à hipertrofia do VD, DSV perimembrano tipicamente grande e artéria aorta posicionada à direita (aorta dextro) (Figura 250.38). Na ToF, a valva pulmonar é frequentemente hipoplásica e pode contribuir para a obstrução da VSVD, além de, ou em vez de, EP puramente valvar. A fisiopatologia e os achados clínicos de EP valvar concomitante ao DSV isolado são semelhantes os da ToF; no entanto, não há desalinhamento do septo infundibular, a artéria aorta é normalmente posicionada e não ocorre estreitamento do infundíbulo do VD.[286] Em crianças, a atresia pulmonar é considerada uma variante extrema da ToF.

Patogênese

ToF tem sido extensivamente estudada em colônias de reprodutores de cães da raça Keeshond; provavelmente a etiologia seja oligogênica.[11] A patogênese dessa malformação provavelmente está relacionada ao desvio ventrocranial do septo de passagem do ventrículo.[287] Em medicina veterinária, persiste o termo "defeito de septo cardíaco conotruncal". Independentemente da terminologia, tem sido identificado o espectro de lesões, que variam de subclínica a clinicamente complicadas.[6,288-291] Patterson et al. classificaram os defeitos cardíacos conotruncais da seguinte forma: grau 1 – malformações subclínicas envolvendo persistência da linha de fusão do cone septal, aneurisma do septo ventricular e ausência do músculo papilar do cone; grau 2 – EP ou DSV, além das lesões de grau 1; grau 3 – ToF: EP, DSV e dextroposição da artéria aorta (com hipertrofia secundária do VD).[6] Anormalidades adicionais encontradas em alguns cães incluem dilatação e tortuosidade da artéria aorta ascendente, atresia pulmonar, hipoplasia da crista supraventricular e anomalias do arco aórtico. Com base em extensos estudos reprodutivos e análises genéticas sofisticadas, os defeitos conotruncais mostraram ser uma característica hereditária autossômica recessiva de expressão variável.[8]

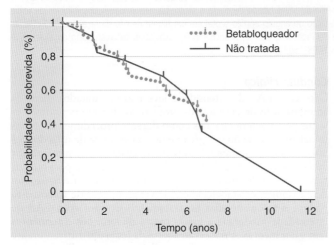

Figura 250.37 Curva de sobrevida de Cox ajustada de mortes relacionadas ao coração, em cães com EAS grave tratados com betabloqueador (n = 27), comparativamente a animais não tratados (n = 23). Não se constatou diferença significativa na sobrevida entre os grupos (P = 0,97). (De Eason BD, Fine DM, Leeder D, et al.: Influence of beta blockers on survival in dogs with severe subaortic stenosis. *J Vet Intern Med* 28:857-862, 2014.)

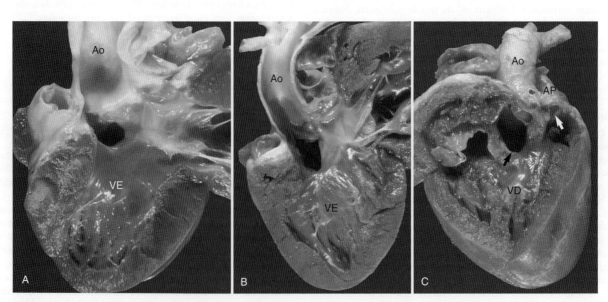

Figura 250.38 Anormalidade macroscópica da tetralogia de Fallot (ToF). **A. B.** As imagens laterais à esquerda de dois cães com ToF mostram uma grande comunicação interventricular (defeito do septo ventricular; DSV) não restritiva localizada entre a artéria aorta (*Ao*) e o ventrículo esquerdo (*VE*). Note a proximidade da raiz da artéria aorta e a possibilidade de prolapso de um folheto da valva aórtica no DSV. **C.** Imagem lateral direita do cão mencionado em **B** mostra grande DSV (*seta preta*), EP (*seta branca*) e hipertrofia do ventrículo direito (*VD*). *AP*, artéria pulmonar.

Fisiopatologia

Os componentes predominantes da ToF são obstrução da VSVD subvalvar grave e DSV. Em consequência da obstrução da via de saída do fluxo e da pressão sistólica elevada do VD, o sangue com dessaturação de oxigênio desvia-se do coração direito, através do defeito septal, e se mistura com o sangue oxigenado proveniente do VE.[292,293] O fluxo sanguíneo na artéria pulmonar e o retorno venoso pulmonar ficam reduzidos, e o AE e o VE se tornam pequenos e subdesenvolvidos. A adição de sangue dessaturado de oxigênio do VD ao lado sistêmico da circulação causa hipoxemia arterial, diminuição da saturação de oxigênio na hemoglobina, cianose e eritrocitose secundária. A circulação colateral sistêmica para o pulmão aumenta através do sistema arterial bronquial. Esses vasos fornecem sangue aos capilares do parênquima pulmonar, direta ou indiretamente, por meio de anastomose com a artéria pulmonar. Assim, uma grande parte desse sangue pode participar na troca gasosa pulmonar. Outros aspectos da fisiopatologia clínica já foram descritos anteriormente.

Achados clínicos

A ToF é comum nas raças de cães Keeshond, Buldogue Inglês e em algumas famílias de outras raças.[167] Também foi diagnostica em gatos.[108] As queixas e os sinais clínicos constatados durante a consulta são aqueles descritos anteriormente para cardiopatia cianótica. Na maioria dos casos de ToF, o sopro cardíaco se deve ao fluxo sanguíneo turbulento, de alta velocidade, através da VSVD obstruída.[286] Exercício ou excitação podem induzir ou agravar a cianose periférica, exacerbando o *shunt* da direita para a esquerda. A radiografia geralmente revela coração pequeno ou de tamanho normal e VD com bordas arredondadas (Figura 250.39). A artéria pulmonar principal não se mostra aumentada nas radiografias, ao contrário do que geralmente ocorre na EP, em que o septo ventricular se encontra íntegro. A vasculatura pulmonar apresenta-se diminuída e o átrio esquerdo pode ser pequeno devido ao menor retorno venoso. O ECG tipicamente exibe sinais de aumento do coração direito, incluindo desvio do eixo direito, embora em alguns gatos possam ser vistos vetores direcionados à esquerda ou em direção cranial.[294] Os achados ecocardiográficos incluem hipertrofia do VD, aumento das dimensões da câmara do VD, redução das dimensões do AE e do VE, grande derrame perimembranoso no orifício de saída do DSV e obstrução do fluxo do VD (Figura 250.40). Pode ser realizada ecocardiografia com contraste salino ou angiografia, a fim de documentar o *shunt* da direita para a esquerda, na saída do fluxo ventricular.[76,295] Em exame Doppler, o *shunt* geralmente é bidirecional, mas predominantemente da direita para a esquerda e de baixa velocidade devido ao baixo gradiente de pressão nos ventrículos.

O cateterismo cardíaco mostra o equilíbrio das pressões sistólicas do VE e do VD, semelhantes à obstrução da VSVD e a um grande DSV não restritivo (não resistente).[291] A oximetria de amostras de sangue revela que há decréscimo do fluxo de saída do VE e o sangue da artéria aorta apresenta relativa dessaturação de oxigênio. A angiocardiografia revela características morfológicas e consequências funcionais da malformação, incluindo: hipertrofia do VD; estreitamento do infundíbulo do VD; EP (tipicamente de uma valva pulmonar hipoplásica); dilatação pós-estenose mínima da artéria pulmonar; variados graus de hipoplasia da artéria pulmonar; grande DSV perimembranoso; VE pequeno, deslocado dorsalmente; aumento da artéria aorta, posicionada cranioventralmente e à direita; e circulação brônquica proeminente (Figura 250.41).[6,288-291] O *shunt* bidirecional através do DSV é comum. Nos casos de atresia pulmonar, o fluxo sanguíneo pulmonar é derivado do ducto arterioso, das artérias brônquicas ou colaterais sistêmicas. O cateterismo cardíaco é raramente necessário para o diagnóstico, mas, se for realizado, deve-se utilizar tratamento anticoagulante (p. ex., heparina), a fim de prevenir a ocorrência de embolismo sistêmico durante e logo após o procedimento.

Conduta clínica

A história natural e os tempos de sobrevivência de cães e gatos com ToF não são bem caracterizados. Como acontece com outras doenças cardíacas cianóticas, a ToF pode ser tolerada por anos, desde que o fluxo sanguíneo pulmonar seja mantido e a hiperviscosidade seja controlada.[128] A maioria dos animais portadores dessa doença apresenta capacidade de atividade física bastante limitada. A morte súbita é comum devido às consequências combinadas da hipoxemia, hiperviscosidade ou arritmia cardíaca. Diferentemente da EP com septo ventricular íntegro, a ICC é uma ocorrência incomum na ToF.

As opções de tratamento para animais com ToF incluem abordagens médicas e cirúrgicas. A correção definitiva do defeito (fechamento do DSV e remoção ou controle da estenose) pode ser feita sob circulação extracorpórea, mas esse tipo de cirurgia raramente é realizada em animais.[296,297] Como regra geral, a estenose não deve ser completamente aliviada se o DSV não puder ser fechado porque a perda da pressão do VD resulta em *shunt* acentuado da esquerda para a direita, com subsequente ICC esquerda.[291,298] Alguns cães foram tratados por meio da colocação cuidadosa de um balão na VSVD, a fim de aumentar

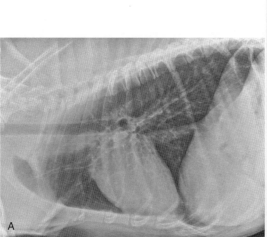
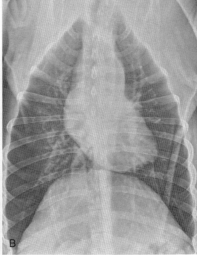

Figura 250.39 Radiografias lateral (**A**) e dorsoventral (**B**) de cão com tetralogia de Fallot. O aumento do coração direito é sugerido pelo arredondamento da borda esternal, na imagem lateral, e o aspecto de D invertido na imagem dorsoventral. A artéria pulmonar principal e os vasos pulmonares periféricos estão diminuídos.

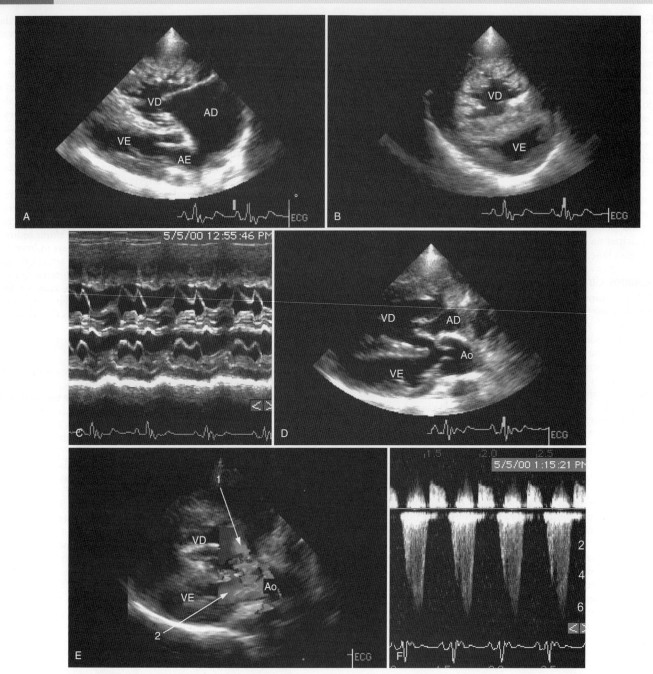

Figura 250.40 Ecocardiograma de um filhote de cão da raça Keeshond com tetralogia de Fallot. **A.** A imagem do eixo longitudinal direito mostra grave hipertrofia concêntrica do ventrículo direito (*VD*) e aumento do átrio direito (*AD*). **B.** A imagem do eixo curto direito mostra grave hipertrofia concêntrica do VD, flacidez do septo interventricular, um pequeno ventrículo esquerdo (*VE*) subpreenchido e hiperecogenicidade do subendocárdio do VD. **C.** O ecocardiograma em modo M mostra aumento do VD em comparação com o VE. As valvas tricúspide e mitral são vistas movendo-se no centro de seus respectivos ventrículos. Parece haver um movimento septal paradoxal em direção ao VD, durante a sístole. **D.** A imagem do eixo longitudinal direito mostra o DSV e o deslocamento à direita (dextroposição) da artéria aorta (*Ao*) e de sua raiz. **E.** O exame Doppler de fluxo colorido de uma imagem semelhante à mostrada em D revela um *shunt* da direita para a esquerda, do sangue do VD (*1*), através do DSV, e a mistura do sangue do VE (*2*), na Ao. **F.** O exame Doppler de onda contínua a partir da base do coração esquerdo, através da valva pulmonar, indica a presença de fluxo sanguíneo de alta velocidade causado pela estenose pulmonar (EP). (*A figura E encontra-se reproduzida em cores no Encarte.*)

o fluxo sanguíneo pulmonar. Como alternativa à correção definitiva, o tratamento paliativo cirúrgico por meio da criação de uma derivação sistêmico-pulmonar pode ser bastante gratificante.[291,299-301] Algumas variantes do *shunt* subclávio para a artéria pulmonar (Blalock-Thomas-Taussig) têm sido criadas com maior frequência em cães e gatos. Alguns cirurgiões preferem usar um enxerto, em vez de rebaixar a artéria subclávia. Ao criar um *shunt* da esquerda para a direita distal ao defeito cianótico, a perfusão pulmonar aumenta e há uma contribuição maior de sangue oxigenado para a circulação sistêmica.

O tamanho do *shunt* acessório deve ser controlado, de modo a evitar sobrecarga do pequeno VE e subsequente edema pulmonar. Não há relato do tempo em que esses *shunts* permanecem patentes em pacientes veterinários, mas um de nós, autores, acompanhou um cão com uma derivação de Blalock-Thomas-Taussig que permaneceu patente por mais de uma década. Outra opção, se o ducto arterioso ainda estiver presente, é o implante de um *stent* conduzido por um cateter, como o indicado para PDA, a fim de manter ou aumentar o fluxo sanguíneo pulmonar.

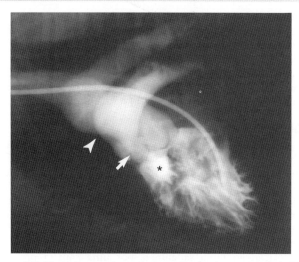

Figura 250.41 Angiograma de um cão da raça Keeshond com tetralogia de Fallot. A injeção no ventrículo direito (VD) opacifica o VD, a artéria pulmonar e a artéria aorta. O contraste pode ser visto no local suspeito de DSV (*asterisco*). A coluna de contraste se estreita na via de saída do ventrículo direito e na região da valva pulmonar (*seta*). Há uma grande dilatação pós-estenose da artéria pulmonar principal (*ponta de seta*). Pode-se notar uma artéria aorta larga, posicionada à direita.

A manutenção da hidratação é importante. A flebotomia periódica, realizada para manter o hematócrito entre 62 e 68%, produz um resultado satisfatório em muitos casos.[128] A retirada excessiva de sangue deve ser evitada, e o volume sanguíneo retirado deve ser substituído por líquidos cristaloides para manter o débito cardíaco e o suprimento de oxigênio nos tecidos.[52] Algumas crianças com ToF se beneficiam de betabloqueadores não específicos, com propranolol, para reduzir a contração hiperdinâmica do VD, que pode aumentar a obstrução ao fluxo de saída; no entanto, estudos controlados sobre a eficácia clínica desse tratamento em animais são escassos.[53,56] Hipoxemia grave deve ser tratada submetendo o paciente a repouso em gaiola e fornecimento de oxigênio, solução IV e bicarbonato de sódio (caso a acidose metabólica seja evidente). O tratamento com agentes vasoconstritores, como a fenilefrina, também pode ajudar a reduzir o fluxo no *shunt* da direita para a esquerda em uma situação de emergência. Medicamentos com propriedades vasodilatadoras sistêmicas marcantes, incluindo a acetilpromazina, devem ser evitados.

OUTRAS CAUSAS DE CARDIOPATIA CONGÊNITA CIANÓTICA

Atresia valvar

A atresia pulmonar com DSV é a forma mais grave de ToF (Figura 250.42). Todo o sangue ejetado do coração direito é desviado do lado direito do coração para o lado esquerdo, através de um grande DSV, e para a artéria aorta dilatada. A valva tricúspide é geralmente normal. O termo "pseudotronco arterioso" foi usado para descrever esse defeito. Difere-se de um verdadeiro "tronco arterioso" porque as artérias pulmonares não se originam do tronco e, na necropsia, a dissecção cuidadosa revela uma valva pulmonar não perfurada e a conexão do tronco pulmonar vestigial às artérias pulmonares esquerda e direita. Ocasionalmente, nota-se atresia de ambas as valvas, pulmonar e tricúspide (Figura 250.42). O VD é pequeno ou hipoplásico e o sangue que retorna às artérias radiculares passa por um FOP ou um DSA e ocorre cianose. Os pulmões são supridos através de um PDA ou de uma extensa circulação colateral broncoesofágica.

A atresia da valva aórtica, com hipoplasia do coração esquerdo, é uma forma rara de cardiopatia cianótica em cães. Geralmente não há perfuração do orifício aórtico e a artéria aorta ascendente apresenta hipoplasia; a valva mitral apresenta, na maioria das vezes, atresia ou hipoplasia. Na ausência de DSV, o VE é muito pequeno; quando há DSV, o VE é mais desenvolvido. O coração direito fornece toda a circulação pulmonar e sistêmica, resultando em cianose marcante e, na maioria dos casos, morte precoce.

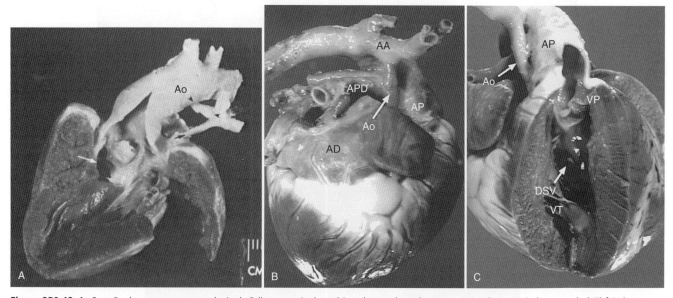

Figura 250.42 A. Coração de um gato com tetralogia de Fallot e atresia da artéria pulmonar (pseudotronco arterioso). O ventrículo esquerdo (VE) foi aberto para expor o grande *DSV* (*seta branca*), a artéria pulmonar hipoplásica (pequena seta preta) e a artéria aorta (*Ao*) dilatada. O fluxo pulmonar era através do ducto arterioso, cuja origem e terminação são mostradas pelas *setas*. Apesar da patência das artérias pulmonares lobulares, quase nenhum sangue foi encontrado na artéria pulmonar direita (*APD*). **B.** Coração de um cão que apresentava cianose grave desde o nascimento. Há hipoplasia da artéria aorta proximal; a abertura da valva aórtica não pôde ser identificada (atresia da valva aórtica). Uma grande artéria pulmonar (*AP*) origina os ramos pulmonares direito e esquerdo, e um grande segmento ductal patente conecta-se ao arco aórtico (*AA*), suprindo os vasos braquiocefálicos, a artéria aorta descendente e a artéria aorta hipoplásica. **C.** Mesmo cão mencionado em **B**. Note a hipertrofia acentuada do ventrículo direito aberto, bem como o defeito do septo ventricular (*DSV*), que recebeu sangue do coração esquerdo subdesenvolvido. *AD*, átrio direito; *VP*, valva pulmonar; *VT*, valva tricúspide.

Dupla via de saída do ventrículo direito

A dupla via de saída do ventrículo direito (DVSVD) consiste em um grupo heterogêneo de malformações em que ambos os grandes vasos saem do VD. Isso foi relatado em cães e gatos (Figura 250.43).[302,303] O DSV propicia ao VE uma via de saída para os grandes vasos. Dependendo da localização do DSV em relação à origem dos grandes vasos, a DVSVD pode se manifestar com sobrecarga da circulação pulmonar ou como uma forma de cardiopatia cianótica. Anormalidades concomitantes, como EP, hipertensão pulmonar e coarctação da artéria aorta, também podem contribuir para a manifestação de sinais clínicos. Tentou-se a correção cirúrgica dessa anormalidade em cães.

Transposição das grandes artérias

Na transposição das grandes artérias (TGA), a artéria aorta origina-se do VD e do tronco pulmonar do VE.[47,304] No caso complexo fatal, coexistem duas circulações independentes e as artérias sistêmicas nunca recebem sangue oxigenado. A sobrevivência de um animal com TGA depende da presença (ou desenvolvimento) de *shunts* entre as duas circulações, de modo a possibilitar a mistura do sangue para evitar hipoxemia fatal. Esses defeitos são complexos, geralmente letais e, muito provavelmente, subdiagnosticados em animais, em relação às crianças, uma vez que a maioria dos animais provavelmente morre sem diagnóstico em uma idade muito jovem.

Defeitos cardíacos variados

A possibilidade de variações no *situs* cardíaco, quanto a anormalidades nas conexões venoatrial, atrioventricular e ventriculoarterial e a malformações de câmaras cardíacas, septos e valvas, é imensa.[38,39] Está além do escopo deste capítulo discutir o espectro de todas as malformações cardíacas potenciais ou relatadas em animais. Deve-se ressaltar que a ectopia cardíaca é extremamente rara em gatos e cães em comparação com sua ocorrência em bovinos. Mais frequentemente encontradas são as anomalias congênitas do esterno. Algumas ocorrem com alguns defeitos cardíacos congênitos, inclusive hérnia diafragmática peritônio-pericárdica (HDPP) (ver Capítulo 254).

Malformações atriais

Os defeitos cardíacos congênitos que afetam os átrios incluem as formas de DSA mencionadas anteriormente, bem como os defeitos mais complexos. Estas últimas malformações incluem: *cor triatriatum* sinistra (CTS), *cor triatriatum dexter* (CTD), anel mitral supravalvar e dupla via de saída do átrio direito. Como implícito no nome, *cor triatriatum* refere-se a uma divisão do átrio esquerdo (sinistro) ou direito (dexter) em duas câmaras, criando "três átrios". A *cor triatriatum* é caracterizada, em relação ao fluxo sanguíneo, por uma câmara proximal (geralmente caudal), em continuidade com o retorno venoso, e uma câmara distal, em continuidade com a valva atrioventricular. A membrana intra-atrial obstrui o retorno venoso da câmara proximal, levando à congestão venosa posterior no lado acometido do coração. O particionamento do AE parece ser bastante raro em medicina veterinária, sendo mais frequentemente observado em gatos, enquanto CTD (ver a seguir) é aparentemente mais comum em cães. No caso de CTS, o átrio esquerdo está localizado distal à membrana que causa obstrução. Um diagnóstico diferencial importante para CTS é a estenose mitral supravalvar ou o anel supramitral. Esta é uma forma de estenose mitral caracterizada por uma membrana obstrutiva entre a valva mitral e o AE.[40,305] O átrio esquerdo é

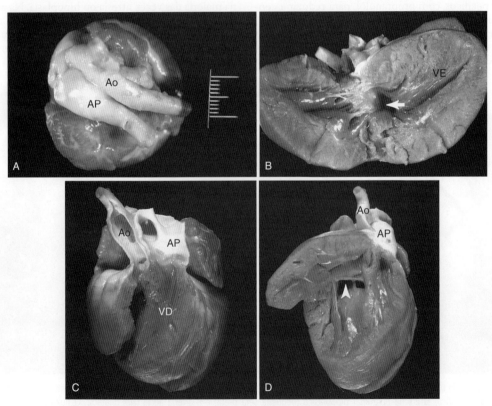

Figura 250.43 Dupla via de saída do ventrículo direito (DVSVD) em um Gato Doméstico de Pelo Curto com 6 meses de idade. **A.** Imagem dorsal do coração mostra o posicionamento lado a lado da artéria aorta (*Ao*) e da artéria pulmonar (*AP*) na borda direita cranial do coração. **B.** Imagem do DSV (*seta*) do lado do ventrículo esquerdo (*VE*). Note a ausência de DVSVD e artéria aorta se originando do VE e a descontinuidade entre o aparato da valva mitral e a artéria aorta ausente. **C.** Imagem do aspecto cranial direito mostra a origem da Ao e da PA no ventrículo direito (*VD*). A abertura do DSV no VD está abaixo da crista supraventricular e não é facilmente vista nessa imagem. **D.** Imagem do lado direito do septo interventricular mostra o local do DSV (*ponta de seta*), próximo à origem da artéria aorta (dupla via de saída do ventrículo direito, com envolvimento aórtico). (Cortesia do Dr. Richard Kienle.)

incorporado na câmara proximal de alta pressão do AE e a valva mitral pode estar normal ou malformada. Ambas as obstruções de retorno venoso pulmonar são mais frequentemente relatadas em gatos e ocasionam sinais clínicos de congestão pulmonar. As opções terapêuticas são limitadas, mas um procedimento híbrido bem-sucedido (cateter cirúrgico) foi relatado.[306] O diagnóstico diferencial de obstrução do retorno venoso pulmonar também deve incluir a condição denominada dupla via de saída do átrio direito. Essa malformação é caracterizada por um *shunt* extremo à esquerda do septo atrial ventral, com inserção da membrana dorsolateral à valva mitral. O retorno venoso pulmonar alcança o AE e atravessa um DSA primitivo para chegar ao AD, que se conecta a ambas as valvas atrioventriculares. Existem variações desse defeito que pode levar a sinais clínicos de congestão venosa pulmonar ou à dessaturação de oxigênio e sinais de cardiopatia cianótica.[307]

Das malformações atriais complexas, a CTD é mais frequentemente relatada e parece ocorrer principalmente em cães.[308-316] Essa condição envolve uma obstrução intra-atrial que impede o retorno venoso da veia cava caudal e do seio coronariano. A parte distal (cranial) do AD inclui a aurícula direita, que recebe o retorno venoso cranial normalmente. Esse defeito pode desenvolver-se isoladamente ou como parte de uma hipoplasia ou obstrução mais geral no coração direito. Estenose de tricúspide, valvar ou supravalvar,[316] hipoplasia do VD e EP foram, todas, observadas em cães com CTD. O caso típico de CTD isolado ocasiona obstrução venosa pós-hepática, sendo a manifestação clínica mais comum a ascite. O grau de obstrução do fluxo varia e, presumivelmente, pode se agravar com o tempo, pois alguns casos se manifestam após 2 anos de idade. Na maioria dos casos, o sangue da veia cava normalmente drena para dentro da câmara cranial e pelo orifício da tricúspide. A ausência de sopro cardíaco pode levar a um diagnóstico errôneo de doença hepática ou intra-abdominal. A ecocardiografia tem valor diagnóstico. Intervenções cirúrgicas e aquelas que utilizam cateter foram empregadas para monitorar efetivamente a CTD em cães.

Malformações ventriculares

Além do DSV e do ventrículo direito de dupla câmara, discutidos anteriormente, existem vários distúrbios relativamente raros dos ventrículos relatados em cães e gatos. A quase ausência de miocárdio do VD, substituído por tecido fibroso e gordura (semelhante à doença de Uhl, no homem), foi relatada em gatos e talvez em um cão.[317-319] Essa anormalidade deve ser considerada no diagnóstico diferencial de insuficiência e dilatação do VD.

A fibroelastose endocárdica (FEE) tem sido relatada em cães e gatos[3,320,321] e acreditava-se ser familiar em algumas linhagens de gatos Birmaneses e Siameses. Atualmente, é um diagnóstico raro e deve ser diferenciado do espessamento endocárdico secundário associado à dilatação crônica do VE. Como algumas das características gerais e clínicas da doença são semelhantes às da deficiência de taurina em gatos, aventa-se a possibilidade de que alguns dos casos relatados anteriormente em gatos tenham sido cardiomiopatia dilatada com FEE secundária. Os achados anatômicos macroscópicos de FEE primária incluem dilatação do VE e do AE, com espessamento grave do endocárdio, caracterizado macroscopicamente por espessamento branco-opaco difuso da superfície luminal (Figura 250.44). Obstrução ou anormalidades na drenagem linfática do miocárdio é uma causa sugerida. Os cães acometidos também podem ter espessamento dos folhetos da valva mitral. Em gatos, as lesões histológicas bem reconhecidas são espessamento fibroelástico hepatocelular difuso, espessamento fibroelástico do endocárdio com finas camadas de colágeno e fibras elásticas aleatoriamente organizadas. O edema do endocárdio, com dilatação dos vasos linfáticos, é proeminente e não há evidência de inflamação ou necrose do miocárdio. As características clínicas da FEE consistem em desenvolvimento inicial de insuficiência cardíaca esquerda ou biventricular, geralmente antes dos 6 meses de idade. Regurgitação mitral pode ser detectada. A dilatação do ventrículo esquerdo e do átrio esquerdo é evidente nas radiografias, no ECG e no ecocardiograma. Os diagnósticos diferenciais, clínicos e de necropsia, incluem DVM, EA/ESA, cardiomiopatia dilatada restritiva e miocardite com FEE secundária. Os animais acometidos são subdesenvolvidos. O tratamento medicamentoso da ICC (ver Capítulo 247) pode prolongar a vida, mas a recuperação é improvável.

ANOMALIAS VASCULARES

As anomalias vasculares, de artérias e veias podem ser classificadas, com base em sua localização no sistema vascular, como sistêmica, pulmonar ou coronariana. Várias malformações vasculares foram relatadas, das quais a PDA é a mais importante e já foi discutida anteriormente. Distúrbios vasculares periféricos,

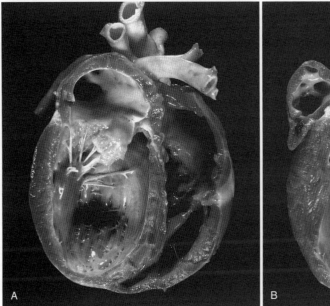
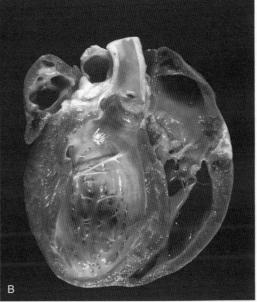

Figura 250.44 Anormalidades macroscópicas de um gato com fibrose endomiocárdica. As imagens do corte distante da via de entrada do fluxo do ventrículo esquerdo (VE) (**A**) e a VSVE (**B**) mostram fibrose difusa da superfície endomiocárdica, tanto do átrio quanto do ventrículo.

incluindo anormalidade da drenagem venosa abdominal e hepática e fístulas arteriovenosas, são discutidos nos Capítulos 284 e 257, respectivamente.

Anomalias arteriais

Malformações do tronco fetal incluem tronco arterioso persistente e defeito do septo aorticopulmonar ("janela"). A persistência do tronco arterioso comum é causada por falha na septação do tronco arterioso fetal e caracterizada por um grande DSV, pela existência de um único grande vaso saindo do coração; ademais, é classificada em função de sua origem e do número de ramos da artéria pulmonar que se originam no tronco. Há raros relatos dessa anomalia em cães e gatos,[322-325] e os sinais clínicos dependem, em grande parte, se o fluxo sanguíneo pulmonar está aumentado (p. ex., *shunt* da esquerda para a direita) ou se está restrito (caso em que, é provável que haja cianose). O defeito do septo aorticopulmonar é causado pela falha do tronco arterioso em se diferenciar completamente, originando uma abertura comum entre a artéria aorta e a artéria pulmonar, além de *shunt* entre os lados esquerdo e direito da circulação.[100] Enquanto uma condição clínica semelhante à PDA pode desenvolver-se, em outros casos instala-se hipertensão pulmonar somente durante o primeiro ano de vida e os sinais clínicos são similares àqueles de cães que desenvolvem síndrome de Eisenmenger juntamente com outros defeitos. A conduta clínica é semelhante àquela da PDA reversa. A cirurgia é difícil sem circulação extracorpórea e não deve ser tentada se a resistência vascular pulmonar estiver marcadamente elevada.

Pode haver desenvolvimento anômalo das artérias coronárias, mas raramente causa doença clínica documentada, com exceção dos casos de óstio único na coronária direita com passagem pré-pulmonar do ramo esquerdo da artéria coronária. Isso é mais comum em cães da raça Buldogue Inglês e foi discutido anteriormente no texto sobre EP. Entretanto, malformações coronárias também podem ser observadas na ausência de EP em alguns cães (inclusive em Buldogue Inglês); ademais, outras anormalidades coronárias são relatadas em cães com EP valvar. Por exemplo, óstio único na artéria coronária esquerda foi relatado em cães Buldogue Inglês com EP valvar.[326] Há raros relatos de *shunt* envolvendo conexões das artérias coronárias com as artérias pulmonares ou com o coração.[327,328] Os autores observaram outras malformações coronarianas durante a angiografia, incluindo fístulas e conexões anormais de vasos coronarianos a outras artérias sistêmicas.

Anormalidades aórticas são frequentemente associadas a ESA evidente. Conforme mencionado anteriormente, essas dilatações ou aneurismas aórticos podem ocorrer na ausência de ESA e podem representar aortopatias em algumas raças acometidas, incluindo cães das raças Rottweiler, Golden Retriever e Leonberger.[65] A coarctação da artéria aorta, um estreitamento semelhante a uma bolsa, próximo ao ducto arterioso, e exemplos mais extremos de obstrução aórtica, como hipoplasia tubular ou interrupção da aorta, são raramente observados em cães e gatos (dois casos são relatados em cães da raça Buldogue Inglês).[329,330]

Em medicina veterinária, as anomalias do anel vascular referem-se a malformações que aprisionam o esôfago, ocasionando regurgitação em animais recém-desmamados. A persistência do arco aórtico direito (PAAD), ao contrário do quarto arco aórtico esquerdo, é a mais comumente relatada. Anomalias do anel vascular incluem essa malformação comum, além de outras anomalias do anel, total ou parcial. Essas incluem compressão esofágica por artérias subclávias retroesofágicas, arco aórtico duplo ou arco aórtico esquerdo com deslocamento do ligamento arterioso para a direita.[4,25,29,37,331-334] Tais anormalidades são relativamente comuns em cães da raça Pastor-Alemão e foram detectadas em muitas outras raças de cães, incluindo Setter Irlandês, Dogue Alemão e Pinscher Alemão. Anomalias do anel vascular são menos comuns em gatos, mas foram observadas.[37,102,331,334] Ocasionalmente, outros defeitos cardíacos estão presentes, inclusive PDA e persistência da veia cava cranial esquerda (Figura 250.45). O diagnóstico de arco aórtico direito persistente geralmente pode ser obtido a partir do histórico clínico e mediante exame radiográfico, em imagem dorsoventral ou ventrodorsal, que mostra um desvio à esquerda da traqueia na base do coração.[335] Lesões mais complexas requerem tomografia computadorizada, ressonância magnética ou angiografia padrão. Essas anormalidades são descritas mais detalhadamente no Capítulo 273 e nas referências.[29,37]

Anormalidades das artérias pulmonares podem ser observadas sob várias condições. Atresia ou hipoplasia unilateral de artéria pulmonar foi reconhecida em gatos. A dissecção da artéria pulmonar é relatada como uma complicação da PDA em cães.[111] Um diagnóstico negligenciado é o de malformações vasculares arteriais sistêmico-pulmonares.[102,336,337] Essas malformações arteriovenosas são tipicamente múltiplas e podem conectar a artéria aorta, a artéria braquiocefálica ou outras artérias sistêmicas ao sistema arterial pulmonar. O resultado é uma sobrecarga de volume no lado esquerdo do coração. Sopros cardíacos geralmente são difíceis de ser detectados, mas podem incluir sopros contínuos, relacionados a *shunts*, ou sopros sistólicos, devido à regurgitação funcional da valva mitral devido à dilatação do VE e ao aumento do fluxo sanguíneo aórtico. O diagnóstico pode ser realizado por meio de imagem obtida em Doppler colorido da artéria pulmonar e com base na ausência de detecção de um ducto arterioso típico. Angiografia por tomografia computadorizada (TC) ou angiografia com contraste são técnicas diagnósticas. A conduta clínica pode incluir intervenção cirúrgica ou oclusão da malformação vascular com mola; entretanto, o clínico deve suspeitar sempre de múltiplos desvios e a possibilidade de abertura de novas malformações arteriovenosas com o fechamento de outras.

Anomalias venosas

Anomalias venosas, especialmente aquelas não relacionadas ao coração, são discutidas mais detalhadamente no Capítulo 257. Malformações venosas raramente causam problemas cardíacos em pequenos animais. O retorno venoso pulmonar anômalo, total ou parcial, tem sido raramente relatado e se comporta funcionalmente como um *shunt* da esquerda para a direita em

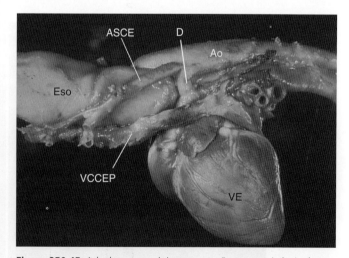

Figura 250.45 Achados macroscópicos em um cão com persistência do arco aórtico direito, PCA (*D*), origem anômala da artéria subclávia esquerda (*ASCE*) e veia cava cranial esquerda persistente (*VCCEP*). A imagem do lado esquerdo do coração, dos grandes vasos e do esôfago (*Eso*) mostra aprisionamento e dilatação cranial do esôfago (*Eso*) pelo anel vascular. A origem da artéria subclávia esquerda é deslocada distalmente de sua localização habitual, dorsal ao esôfago. A VCCEP pode ser vista lateralmente, ao lado do esôfago e base do coração esquerdo, e ao redor da cintura caudal do coração. *Ao*, artéria aorta.

nível atrial. Isso é mais comumente associado a um DSA tipo seio venoso, com drenagem venosa anômala parcial no átrio direito através do DSA. Anormalidades da drenagem venosa abdominal, como ducto venoso patente, podem induzir à encefalopatia hepática (ver Capítulo 284).

Uma anormalidade venosa relativamente comum, de relevância clínica, constatada durante cirurgia torácica ou cateterismo cardíaco, é a persistência da veia cava cranial esquerda (Figura 250.46).[70,338-340] Esta estrutura, normalmente presente no feto como parte do sistema venoso esquerdo principal, pode persistir e drenar para o seio coronário embrionariamente relacionado na face caudal do AD. O diagnóstico é direto na maioria dos casos e pode ser feito usando ecocardiografia 2D, através da detecção de um seio coronariano dilatado próximo ao sulco atrioventricular. O diagnóstico pode ser confirmado por contraste (salina), ecocardiograma, angiografia por TC ou angiografia contrastada (ver Capítulo 104). A persistência da veia cava cranial esquerda pode interferir na exposição cirúrgica, particularmente durante o tratamento cirúrgico da persistência do quarto arco aórtico direito, ou interferir na cateterização cardíaca, mas não tem relevância funcional conhecida (Figura 250.47). Tal como acontece na persistência do quarto arco aórtico direito, essa anomalia vascular é comum em cães da raça Pastor-Alemão; também foi relatada em outras raças de cães, bem como em gatos. A partição desse vaso geralmente não apresenta nenhum problema clínico, desde que a veia cava cranial direita normal também esteja presente (Figura 250.47).

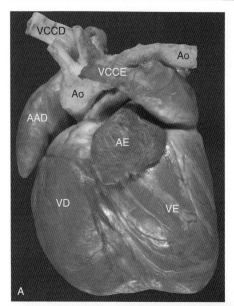

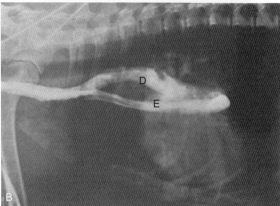

Figura 250.47 A. Exemplos de veia cava cranial esquerda persistente (VCCEP) em um cão. Note que a VCCEP envolve a cintura caudal do coração; é diferente da veia cava cranial direita (*VCCD*), anatomicamente correta. **B.** Angiograma não seletivo de um cão. O contraste é injetado nas veias jugulares direita e esquerda. A veia cava cranial direita normal (*D*) é evidente, assim como a VCCEP (*E*). Note que a VCCEP envolve a parte caudal do coração e entra na porção caudal do AD. *AAD*, apêndice auricular direito; *AE*, aurícula esquerda; *Ao*, artéria aorta.

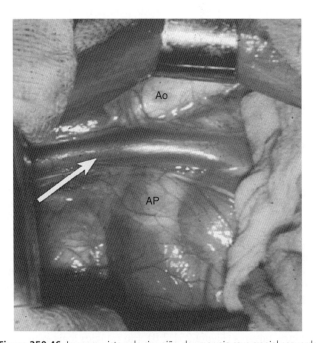

Figura 250.46 Imagem, vista pelo cirurgião, de uma veia cava cranial esquerda persistente (*seta*). Essa anomalia venosa é frequentemente encontrada durante a abordagem de PDA. Não há consequência hemodinâmica decorrente dessa anomalia. *Ao*, artéria aorta; *AP*, artéria pulmonar.

AGRADECIMENTOS

Os autores agradecem as contribuições de David Sisson, William Thomas e Peter Darke para a elaboração deste capítulo.

REFERÊNCIAS BIBLIOGRÁFICAS

As referências bibliográficas deste capítulo se encontram online no Ambiente de Aprendizagem.

CAPÍTULO 251

Doenças Cardiovasculares no Início da Idade Adulta

Ingrid Ljungvall e Jens Häggström

DOENÇA MIXOMATOSA DA VALVA MITRAL

A doença mixomatosa da valva mitral (DMVM) é caracterizada por uma degeneração mixomatosa lenta e progressiva do aparato da valva mitral e subsequente dilatação do átrio esquerdo (AE) e do ventrículo esquerdo (VE).[1-4] Embora a degeneração mixomatosa acometa mais comumente a valva mitral, qualquer uma das quatro valvas intracardíacas podem ser acometidas. No entanto, as valvas pulmonar e aórtica (valvas semilunares) raramente desenvolvem lesões degenerativas marcantes.[2,3,5] Diversos nomes têm sido atribuídos a essa anormalidade, como doença da valva mitral crônica, doença degenerativa da valva mitral, doença da valva mitral, endocardiose e, mais recentemente, doença mixomatosa da valva mitral. O termo "mixomatosa" descreve a característica histológica dessa anormalidade e exclui a maioria, se não todas, das outras formas de doença da valva mitral, porém a DMVM não necessariamente exclui o envolvimento de outras valvas. Assim, a denominação DMVM define com precisão e sucintamente o fenótipo patológico dessa condição.

Ocorrência

DMVM é a doença cardíaca mais prevalente em cães e estima-se que seja responsável por 75 a 80% das doenças cardíacas nessa espécie.[1,6-9] A DMVM é diagnosticada em todas as raças, mas a maior prevalência é observada em raças de cães de pequeno e médio portes, como Cavalier King Charles Spaniel (CKCS), Dachshund, Poodle Miniatura e Yorkshire Terrier.[8-13] Os cães acometidos não apresentam sinais de anormalidades valvares ao nascimento, mas desenvolvem DMVM mais tarde. A prevalência aumenta com a idade e é, em uma determinada idade, maior em machos.[1,2,6,7,9,12] A prevalência de DMVM em gatos sem doença primária do miocárdio é desconhecida, mas parece ser baixa. Alterações similares da valva mitral também são descritas no homem, em equinos e suínos.[14-16]

Herança e reprodução

A etiologia da DMVM não foi esclarecida, mas há muito tempo a hereditariedade é suspeita de ter um papel importante, devido à estreita associação dessa doença com algumas raças de cães de pequeno a médio porte. Estudos de famílias de cães das raças CKCS e Dachshund indicam evidências de que fatores genéticos têm importante participação na etiologia.[17-19] Esses estudos sugerem que a doença tem herança poligênica, isto é, múltiplos genes influenciam a característica, e um certo limiar deve ser alcançado antes que a DMVM se desenvolva.[17,18] O modo poligênico de herança significa que o acasalamento de um pai e uma mãe com início precoce de DMVM dará origem a uma prole que, em média, manifestará início precoce de DMVM (e ICC). O acasalamento de cães com início tardio da doença dará origem a descendentes que manifestarão a doença na velhice, ou nunca. Os machos apresentam um limiar mais baixo do que as fêmeas, o que significa que os machos desenvolverão a doença em uma idade mais jovem do que as fêmeas, em uma família de cães em que os descendentes, em média, possuem o mesmo genótipo. Dois *loci*, localizados nos cromossomos 13 e 14, mostraram estar associados ao início precoce de DMVM em cães da raça CKCS.[20] Esse achado provavelmente será precursor de mutações causais no futuro e tal descoberta aumentará sobremaneira o conhecimento dos mecanismos de ocorrência da doença, e poderá levar a testes genéticos, que ainda não estão disponíveis. A importância dos fatores genéticos implica que outros fatores, como nível de atividade física, grau de obesidade e dieta, tenham menor influência no desenvolvimento da doença. Programas de acasalamento de cães das raças CKCS e Dachshund, destinados a reduzir a prevalência de DMVM, foram lançados na Europa, na América do Norte e em outros lugares. Na ausência de testes genéticos confiáveis, esses programas de melhoramento utilizam a auscultação, para detectar sopro cardíaco, e/ou ecocardiograma, para detectar e quantificar a degeneração da valva mitral e/ou a regurgitação mitral (RM). Nesses programas, cães de uma idade específica que apresentam algum grau de sopro cardíaco ou achados ecocardiográficos compatíveis com DMVM não podem ser utilizados como reprodutores. Alguns programas, em parte, também se baseiam em avaliações da prevalência de DMVM nos pais. O limite de idade para potenciais cães e pais reprodutores é muito importante: o limite de idade deve ser aquele em que os cães com um início precoce de DMVM devem ser excluídos como reprodutores, mas não deve ser muito alta porque isso pode reduzir a população de reprodutores a um número baixo inaceitável.[21] Uma avaliação recente de um cruzamento mostrou redução na prevalência de sopro cardíaco e na gravidade das lesões da valva mitral avaliada em exame ecocardiográfico.[22]

Patologia

O aspecto macroscópico da degeneração mixomatosa depende de qual estágio da doença a valva é examinada; em casos de degeneração mixomatosa leve, os achados macroscópicos podem ser negligenciados, se não forem minuciosamente investigados.

As alterações começam na área de aposição dos folhetos valvares e são geralmente mais evidentes nos locais de inserção das cordas tendíneas. As bordas livres dos folhetos, que normalmente são delgadas, translúcidas e macias, tornam-se espessas e irregulares, com áreas de protuberância, em forma de balão, em direção à lateral do AE (Figura 251.1).[1-3,23,24] As cordas tendíneas, em si, também podem ser acometidas pela degeneração mixomatosa.[3,13,23] Com a progressão da doença, as protuberâncias se agravam e as lesões se espalham para outras partes dos folhetos valvares (Figura 251.2 B). Em estágios mais avançados, a fibrose pode causar espessamento acentuado e contração dos folhetos e das cordas tendíneas. As cordas tendíneas podem se romper, o que leva a uma borda livre, sem conexão. Podem ser observadas lesões no endocárdio atrial (fibrose) opostas ao orifício mitral (ou seja, "lesões de jato"). Em casos graves, é possível constatar vários graus de ruptura atrial, como lacerações endomiocárdicas, ruptura de músculos pectíneos do apêndice atrial, comunicação interatrial adquirida (defeito do septo atril) e hemopericárdio (ver Capítulo 254).[2,25]

Os achados histopatológicos nos folhetos valvares incluem degeneração mixomatosa (Figura 251.2 A e B), que se referem a um enfraquecimento e alteração patológica característica na organização do tecido conjuntivo, no qual o componente esponjoso é extraordinariamente proeminente, e as fibras de colágeno se apresentam desorganizadas na camada fibrosa (Figura 251.2 C a F).[26,27] É comum verificar aumento da quantidade de mucopolissacarídeos e glicosaminoglicanos nas valvas acometidas.[3,27,28]

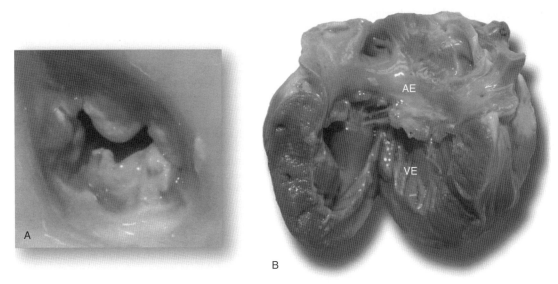

Figura 251.1 Exemplos de lesões *post mortem* de um cão que apresentava doença mixomatosa da valva mitral (DMVM) vista do átrio (**A**) e em imagem lateral (**B**), com o átrio esquerdo (*AE*) e o ventrículo esquerdo (*VE*) abertos. Os folhetos da valva mitral estão espessados e contraídos, com nódulos arredondados nas bordas livres e com áreas proeminentes/prolapsadas em direção à lateral do átrio esquerdo. Rompimento de cordas tendíneas, particularmente daquelas de menor ordem, é um achado comum. A lesão de jato, notada na parede atrial, é resultado do fluxo regurgitante de alta velocidade do sangue do VE, atingindo a parede atrial.

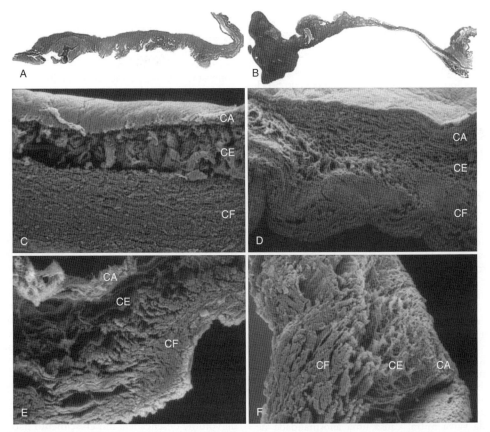

Figura 251.2 Cortes histológicos obtidos de um cão com doença mixomatosa da valva mitral (DMVM) branda (**A**) e grave (**B**). Microscopicamente, nota-se deposição marcante de glicosaminoglicanos (GAG) corados por ácido (cor azul, em reação do ácido periódico-*Schiff* [PAS]/coloração com azul de alcian) nas camadas esponjosa e fibrosa dos folhetos. Imagens obtidas em micrografia de varredura eletrônica de uma célula anormalmente macerada da valva mitral de cão, ao nível da zona intermediária (**C** a **F**). As imagens mostram o dano ao folheto valvar que ocorre quando a doença progride em diferentes graus Whitney (as micrografias C a F correspondem aos graus Whitney 1 a 4).[5] Ocorrem perda e deformidade da estrutura em camadas com o avanço da doença e redução simultânea da densidade de colágeno nas três camadas. *CA*, camada atrial; *CE*, camada esponjosa; *CF*, camada fibrosa. (A e B, Cortesia de Lisbeth Höier Olsen, Universidade de Copenhague, Dinamarca. C-F, De Han RI, Impoco G, Culshaw G *et al*.: Cell maceration scanning electron microscopy and computer-derived porosity measurements in assessment of connective tissue microstructure changes in the canine myxomatous mitral valve. *Vet J* 197:502-505, 2013. Publicado com permissão do editor.) (*As figuras A e B encontram-se reproduzidas em cores no Encarte.*)

Os achados característicos nas células endoteliais que cobrem a superfície da valva incluem pleomorfismo e lesão no revestimento celular. O dano endotelial, que é mais comumente evidente próximo às bordas dos folhetos valvares, pode causar perda local de células endoteliais, expondo assim a matriz subendotelial e as membranas basais subjacentes.[23]

Os achados histopatológicos nas câmaras cardíacas esquerdas incluem mudanças na composição e na estrutura da matriz extracelular (MEC) e dos miócitos, porém as bases celulares e moleculares que fundamentam essas mudanças permanecem pouco compreendidas. Tanto a fibrose miocárdica como a arteriosclerose intramiocárdica, especialmente nos músculos papilares, foram descritas em cães com DMVM em estágios avançados.[29,30]

Patogênese

Pouco se sabe sobre a patogênese do espessamento progressivo e da degeneração dos folhetos valvares. Provavelmente, um ou mais fatores desencadeantes primários aumentam o risco da doença em cães predispostos, pois nem todos os cães desenvolvem degeneração mixomatosa da valva atrioventricular.

O fato de o endotélio estar danificado ou até mesmo ausente em áreas doentes, provavelmente desempenha um papel importante para a progressão da doença, uma vez que[23,24,31] as células endoteliais são conhecidas por se comunicarem extensivamente com as células subendoteliais (p. ex., células intersticiais valvares, CIVs). O dano endotelial induz a liberação de peptídios vasoativos, como a endotelina-1, que está potencialmente envolvida na transformação das células CIVs subendoteliais a partir de um fenótipo predominantemente fibroblástico em fenótipos mais ativos de miofibroblastos e células musculares lisas.[23,26,32] A transformação de CIV também foi sugerida como sendo iniciada pela serotonina (5-HT),[33-35] e as concentrações séricas de 5-HT mostraram ser mais altas em cães da raça CKCS, comparados a algumas outras raças de cães,[33,36] e também aumento da valva mitral e do tecido miocárdico do ventrículo esquerdo (VE) em cães que apresentavam DMVM.[37] Da mesma forma, a expressão de receptores de 5-HT e moléculas de sinalização de matriz extracelular estão alteradas em folhetos mitrais acometidos pela doença.[34,38,39] Enzimas proteolíticas, como as metaloproteinases da matriz (MPMs), também podem estar envolvidas nos processos degenerativos, levando à organização atípica dos componentes do tecido conjuntivo.[38,40-42]

Fisiopatologia

Regurgitação mitral causada por doença mixomatosa da valva mitral

A deformidade da arquitetura valvar e das correspondentes cordas tendíneas levam ao deslocamento dos folhetos da valva mitral durante a sístole atrial (ou seja, prolapso da valva mitral)[43] e coaptação anormal dos folhetos da valva mitral durante a sístole ventricular. Assim, uma parte do volume sistólico, ou volume sistólico de ejeção, do VE retorna ao AE. O alongamento e a possibilidade de ruptura das estruturas das cordas tendíneas aumentam a regurgitação mitral (RM) por causarem prolapso total ou parcial (valva fluvial) dos folhetos para o interior do AE.[13]

O volume da RM foi descrito como dependente da área do orifício da valva mitral e do gradiente de pressão sistólico entre o AE e o VE,[44,45] ressaltando que este último é influenciado pela pressão intra-atrial, pela função do ventrículo esquerdo, bem como pela pressão arterial sistêmica. A degeneração mixomatosa do aparato da valva mitral causa uma anormalidade de aposição dos folhetos e, portanto, é uma causa primária de RM, enquanto a dilatação do lado esquerdo do coração exacerba a anormalidade da aposição da valva, levando à RM secundária.[2,46] Consequentemente, a regurgitação gera regurgitação. Geralmente, cães com DMVM têm um jato de RM dirigido lateralmente, presumivelmente, porque o folheto anterior é mais longo e tem uma mobilidade maior do que o folheto posterior (conforme descrito em cães e no homem);[46,47] portanto, é mais provável que ocorra prolapso do que quando se trata do folheto

posterior. No entanto, a orientação espacial do jato não é constante, particularmente em casos leves de RM, provavelmente devido a alterações na forma e orientação da área do orifício mitral durante a contração do VE.[48]

A RM primária de menor grau não induz qualquer alteração aparente nos índices de tamanho ou função cardíaca. O volume sistólico (ou volume sistólico de ejeção) cardíaco é mantido e o pequeno volume regurgitante é facilmente aceito pelo átrio esquerdo (AE). Com a progressão das lesões valvares, a parte regurgitante do volume total do débito cardíaco do ventrículo esquerdo (VE) aumenta, mas vários mecanismos compensatórios cardíacos e não cardíacos (p. ex., renais, neuro-humorais e vasculares) contribuem para manter o volume de ejeção sistólico.[49] A expansão do átrio esquerdo (AE) atenua o aumento de volume da RM e, assim, possibilita que a pressão intra-atrial permaneça comparativamente baixa, e o sangue pode ser ejetado facilmente para o AE durante a sístole ventricular, mesmo em cães com DMVM grave. Relata-se que mais de 75% do total do volume sistólico do VE é ejetado no AE durante a sístole em cães com DMVM grave.[50] A gravidade da dilatação do lado esquerdo do coração está associada à gravidade da RM, sugerindo que o volume da RM é o principal fator determinante do grau de dilatação do lado esquerdo do coração.[50,51]

O caminho extra (para o AE) do volume sistólico, ou volume de ejeção sistólico, reduz a pós-carga do VE (a resistência ao esvaziamento do VE), enquanto o aumento da carga de volume ocasiona aumento da pré-carga.[52] A ejeção retrógrada do volume sistólico do VE começa no início da sístole, levando a um curto período de contração isovolumétrica (definido como o intervalo entre o fechamento das valvas atrioventriculares e a abertura das valvas semilunares).[53,54] O AE tem uma importante função ao possibilitar que o volume regurgitante seja acolhido pela cavidade atrial e isso previne a hipertensão no leito vascular pulmonar.[55] O aumento da pressão do AE resulta em edema e congestão venosa pulmonar. O efeito do volume regurgitante na pressão e no volume do AE e, consequentemente, na pressão capilar pulmonar depende do tamanho do AE e da complacência da parede desse átrio. Consequentemente, a complacência do AE é determinada pela taxa de aumento do volume regurgitante, que é determinado pela taxa de progressão da DMVM e pela remodelação em resposta à sobrecarga de volume. Nos casos de DMVM de progressão lenta, há frequentemente um aumento drástico do AE; edema e congestão pulmonar se desenvolvem tardiamente. O edema também é retardado pelo desenvolvimento de uma drenagem linfática mais efetiva do interstício pulmonar na congestão pulmonar crônica.[56] Nos casos de RM com aumento agudo, como acontece na ruptura de cordas tendíneas de primeira ordem, ou de várias cordas tendíneas, o AE é incapaz de se adaptar, o que resulta em aumento rápido do AE e da pressão capilar pulmonar e, consequentemente, rápido desenvolvimento de congestão e edema pulmonar.

A transmissão reversa passiva do aumento da pressão de enchimento do VE para os capilares pulmonares pode, ainda, levar ao desenvolvimento de hipertensão pulmonar, e os cães com RM mais grave, e, portanto, com maior pressão no AE, têm risco maior de desenvolver hipertensão pulmonar.[57]

O VE compensa a perda do volume de ejeção sistólico aumentando o volume diastólico final e, para acomodar o aumento da pressão de enchimento (pré-carga), várias respostas compensatórias atuam no VE (ver Capítulo 246). A sobrecarga de volume desencadeia um crescimento não natural – denominado hipertrofia excêntrica, caracterizada pelo aumento da câmara cardíaca, porém mantendo a sua espessura relativa da parede. Isso é suficiente para normalizar a pressão no VE com sobrecarga de volume e manter um volume de ejeção adequado.[58-60] Tem sido sugerido também que a hipertrofia do miocárdio é estimulada pelo aumento da ativação neuro-hormonal, tal como o aumento da síntese de angiotensina II (AII),[61] embora os níveis circulantes de AII pareçam comparativamente inalterados durante a progressão de DMVM branda para ICC.[62]

No entanto, é bem provável que o miocárdio do cão seja capaz de realizar síntese local (no coração) de AII, em resposta à tensão hemodinâmica da parede da câmara cardíaca; ademais, há relato de que a enzima conversora de angiotensina (ECA), a quimase e a catepsina D são capazes de induzir a produção de AII no tecido cardíaco de cão com sobrecarga de volume.[61,63]

Embora ocorra aumento das dimensões dos eixos longo e curto em resposta à sobrecarga de volume crônica, a dimensão do eixo curto aumenta mais, o que leva a uma alteração morfológica do VE, de elíptico para uma forma mais globular.[64] O aumento do tamanho global do VE pode possibilitar a adaptação do miocárdio à tensão anormal da parede regional. Uma forma mais globular do VE pode contribuir para um aumento adicional na sobrecarga de volume por estímulo secundário da RM devido à desconfiguração da geometria anular normal da valva mitral.[49]

Os mecanismos compensatórios, como dilatação e hipertrofia do VE e aumento da atividade do sistema neuro-hormonal, inicialmente são considerados benéficos, por promover o suporte hemodinâmico necessário para manter um débito cardíaco suficiente, apesar da RM. No entanto, com a progressão da doença, esses mecanismos agravam a insuficiência cardíaca, devido à lesão do miócito e ao acúmulo de fibras de colágeno (i. e., fibrose miocárdica).[49,60]

O remodelamento cardíaco causado por sobrecarga de volume crônica em cães com DMVM, por sua vez, interfere na função mecânica do coração. O aumento da pré-carga aumenta a força de contração, de acordo com o mecanismo de Frank-Starling.[65] Dependendo da gravidade da RM, essas alterações ocasionam contração normal a hiperdinâmica do VE (hipercinesia), mesmo na presença de disfunção miocárdica intrínseca. Embora a função sistólica do miocárdio diminua com a progressão da doença, o processo de remodelação permite que o VE retenha uma função de bombeamento cardíaco relativamente bem preservada, mesmo em casos de DMVM avançada.[49,66] No entanto, devido à sobrecarga de volume crônica e ao fato de que a hipertrofia, enquanto necessária, é um remodelamento patológico, a contratilidade cardíaca diminui lentamente, mas de forma progressiva e inexorável, mesmo em cães clinicamente compensados.[67-69] Sugere-se que um aumento no grau de fibrose miocárdica influencia o mecanismo de Frank Starling, em cães com insuficiência cardíaca[65] e, dessa forma, impede uma transdução ótima de força contrátil gerada pelos miócitos durante a sístole. No entanto, o aumento do volume sanguíneo pulmonar, e não a diminuição do volume sistólico ejetado, mostrou ser a principal causa de função cardiopulmonar anormal em cães com DMVM.[51] Esse achado corrobora a observação clínica de que cães com MR grave manifestam mais comumente congestão e edema pulmonar (que provocam sintomas respiratórios) do que sinais clínicos causados pela redução do débito cardíaco direto (letargia, fraqueza, intolerância ao exercício).[70]

Regurgitação da tricúspide causada por doença mixomatosa da valva

A regurgitação tricúspide (RT) é um achado acidental comum em cães e gatos.[71] A RT comumente ocorre concomitantemente à degeneração mixomatosa da valva mitral, como consequência de alterações valvares primárias e/ou secundárias à hipertensão pulmonar, devido à degeneração mixomatosa do lado esquerdo. As alterações degenerativas do aparato da valva tricúspide são idênticas àquelas constatadas quando a valva mitral é afetada (ver seção Patologia).[72]

A degeneração mixomatosa da valva tricúspide comumente ocasiona RT de grau leve a moderado. A regurgitação tricúspide, na ausência de obstrução concomitante da valva pulmonar ou de hipertensão da artéria pulmonar, é comparativamente bem tolerada.[73] No entanto, como o ventrículo direito (VD) é projetado para se contrair contra uma artéria de baixa pressão, ele fica vulnerável a aumentos de pressão. Assim, responde mal ao aumento do trabalho; mesmo aumentos agudos relativamente pequenos de pressão da artéria pulmonar causam redução acentuada do volume

sistólico do VD.[74] Portanto, RT é relevante quando há hipertensão pulmonar. Além da dilatação do VD, ocorre aumento do átrio direito (AD), que exacerba a dilatação do anel da valva tricúspide e a RT. O aumento do AD pode resultar em taquiarritmias atriais, como fibrilação atrial e taquicardia supraventricular. Como consequência do aumento da pressão do AD, podem se desenvolver ascite, derrame pleural (especialmente em gatos), derrame pericárdico, hepatomegalia e esplenomegalia.

Sinais clínicos

DMVM branda a moderada (estágios A e B do American College of Veterinary Internal Medicine [ACVIM]) geralmente não está associada a nenhum sinal de doença. A maioria dos cães com DMVM não manifesta sinais clínicos; no máximo, apresenta sopro, embora possa se perceber intolerância ao exercício. Tosse é uma queixa comum em casos de DMVM. Embora esse sintoma não seja específico de doenças cardíacas, deve merecer uma avaliação adicional (ver Capítulo 26). Cães com compressão do tronco bronquial principal esquerdo, porém sem congestão ou edema pulmonar, podem ter crises de tosse a qualquer momento do dia, especialmente durante atividade física ou excitação. Caso contrário, os cães com DMVM branda a moderada não manifestam sinais clínicos de doença cardíaca.

Os primeiros sinais clínicos de ICC descompensada (Grau C do ACVIM) são geralmente leves, mas podem ser agravados em dias ou, às vezes, semanas (ver Capítulo 246). Uma vez que esses sinais são vagos e não específicos para ICC descompensada, o desafio para o diagnóstico diferencial de DMVM não é, comumente, estabelecer se a doença está ou não presente, mas se a DMVM é ou não responsável pelos sinais clínicos. Os sintomas estão relacionados com a presença e o grau de um ou vários dos seguintes eventos fisiopatológicos, listados em ordem de importância relativa: (1) aumento do AE e da pressão venosa pulmonar, podendo resultar em angústia respiratória e tosse devido a edema pulmonar e compressão do brônquio; (2) redução do fluxo de ejeção sistólica do VE ou VD, o que pode resultar em fraqueza e redução da resistência; (3) aumento do AD e da pressão venosa sistêmica, que pode resultar em derrame pleural e ascite; e (4) descompensação aguda devido à ruptura de cordas tendíneas, ruptura de átrio ou fibrilação ventricular, o que pode causar morte súbita.

Taquipneia e dispneia estão presentes quando há congestão e edema pulmonar.[75] A tosse também é comumente observada e, no caso de DMVM em estágio avançado, a tosse pode ser causada pela pressão do AE no brônquio principal esquerdo, por congestão e edema pulmonar ou, mais comumente, uma combinação dessas anormalidades.[76] Os cães com ICC descompensada costumam ficar ansiosos e inquietos durante a noite e geralmente preferem se posicionar em decúbito esternal. Sons respiratórios anormais, como sibilos, podem ser audíveis. Cães com ICC descompensada são frequentemente inativos e têm diferentes graus de inapetência. Pode se desenvolver caquexia cardíaca, embora a perda de peso corporal possa ser mascarada pela retenção concomitante de líquido e por edema.

Alguns cães com DMVM manifestam síncope (ver Capítulo 30). A síncope pode estar associada à taquiarritmia, mas o caráter desses eventos muitas vezes se assemelha à síncope vasovagal.[77-79] A frequência da síncope varia de episódios ocasionais a vários episódios por dia. Outras causas de síncope incluem desmaio, causado por tosse, que pode ocorrer em associação com paroxismos de tosse ou atividade física na presença de hipertensão pulmonar (ver Capítulo 243).[76]

A RT isolada, na ausência de hipertensão pulmonar, raramente resulta em sinais clínicos da doença.[72,76,80] Evidências de menor tolerância a exercício, fraqueza ou síncope são notadas principalmente em casos de hipertensão pulmonar, que se desenvolve como consequência de RM grave de longa duração ou taquiarritmia. É comum que esses animais apresentem sintomas de ICC direita e podem apresentar angústia respiratória devido ao derrame pleural; distensão abdominal causada por ascite, hepatomegalia ou esplenomegalia; ou sinais gastrintestinais, como diarreia, vômito e anorexia.

Embora a degeneração mixomatosa seja, às vezes, evidente no exame *post mortem* em uma ou ambas as valvas semilunares,[72,76,80] a degeneração mixomatosa dessas valvas raramente resulta em regurgitação relevante associada a sinais clínicos.

Exame físico

Um clique mesossistólico pode ser constatado no estágio inicial da DMVM (Áudio 251.5).[81,82] todavia, um sopro cardíaco sistólico é o achado clínico mais evidente durante a auscultação cardíaca em cães acometidos por DMVM (Figura 251.3). No entanto, a ausência de um sopro audível não elimina a possibilidade de regurgitação discreta.[83] O som começa como um sopro sistólico suave, com ponto de intensidade máxima no local sobre a valva mitral, no lado esquerdo do tórax, e pode ser intermitente (Áudio 251.1).[84,85] Nos estágios iniciais da DMVM, o sopro muitas vezes pode ser aumentado por manobras físicas, como uma corrida curta.[81] A presença de sopro cardíaco suave em um cão de raça pequena com DMVM é indicativo de que a gravidade da doença é leve e é improvável que haja ICC.[85] Com a progressão da doença, desenvolve-se um sopro "mais "grave", mais intenso e de maior duração (holossistólico) (Áudios 251.2 e 151.3, Figura 251.3).[21,82,83,86,87] Os sopros moderados a graves irradiam-se para outro ponto de intensidade máxima nos lados esquerdo e direito do tórax; sopros cardíacos altos também são acompanhados de pulso palpável no hemitórax esquerdo (área cardíaca apical; ver Capítulo 55). Cães que apresentam frêmito precordial raramente manifestam grau moderado da doença e têm maior risco de desenvolver ICC e/ou hipertensão pulmonar.[85] Sopros musicais de alta intensidade são menos frequentes e não refletem, necessariamente, a gravidade da DMVM (Áudio 251.4).[82] RT fisiológica irrelevante é comum em cães; geralmente essa regurgitação não é audível à auscultação. Já a RT patológica pode ser caracterizada por um sopro sistólico de intensidade variável, com ponto de intensidade máxima sobre a área tricúspide.

A sobreposição da primeira bulha cardíaca (S1) ao sopro vigoroso pode dar uma impressão de aumento da intensidade de S1, quando avaliado subjetivamente mediante auscultação cardíaca. No entanto, a análise avançada do sinal tem mostrado que a intensidade de S1 permanece inalterada comparativamente com o aumento da gravidade da RM.[83] A intensidade sonora de S2 diminui à medida que aumenta a gravidade da doença (ver Figura 251.3).[83,86] Considera-se que a intensidade de S2 depende principalmente do grau de alteração do gradiente de pressão na valva aórtica no momento do fechamento da valva;[88] um menor volume de ejeção sistólica[51] pode explicar a razão da diminuição da intensidade de S2 à medida que aumenta a gravidade da DMVM. Um terceiro som cardíaco de baixa intensidade pode estar presente, mas a detecção desse som frequentemente é difícil na auscultação padrão.[82,86,87] A presença de um som claramente audível (ruído de galope) é um forte indicador de insuficiência miocárdica.[82]

Em cães com DMVM, sem sinais de ICC, espera-se que os sons pulmonares e a frequência respiratória em repouso sejam normais.[75] Já em cães com DMVM mais grave, que manifestam sinais de ICC, os sons pulmonares são geralmente mais evidentes, podendo ser detectados crepitações, estalidos e sons subcrepitantes, mais bem audíveis no fim da inspiração. Sons anormais semelhantes são comuns em cães com doenças em vias respiratórias de pequeno calibre;[89] caso ocorram simultaneamente, pode ser um desafio diagnóstico determinar a causa dos sinais clínicos. No caso de congestão e edema pulmonar, espera-se aumento da frequência respiratória em repouso ou durante o sono (i. e., > 30 movimentos respiratórios/min).[75,90]

As membranas mucosas geralmente são normais, mesmo em cães com ICC, mas ocasionalmente podem ser cianóticas ou acinzentadas em casos avançados de ICC. Pulso fraco pode ser notado na ICC. Pulsos fracos e variáveis, com déficits, também podem ser observados em casos de anormalidades de ritmo (ver Capítulo 248). Se ocorrer tamponamento devido à hemorragia pericárdica causada por ruptura do AE, o pulso femoral será fraco e poderá notar-se dilatação da veia jugular (ver Capítulo 254).

Ascite na DMVM isolada é incomum, mas DMVM progressiva geralmente tende a envolver o lado direito do coração como consequência de hipertensão pulmonar e/ou degeneração mixomatosa avançada da valva tricúspide, ou devido ao desenvolvimento de taquiarritmia. Nesses cães, é possível notar sintomas de ICC direita, tal como distensão venosa, com sinais de hepatomegalia e/ou esplenomegalia e pulso jugular, além de ascite. Os sons cardíacos podem ser abafados pelo derrame pleural.

Achados eletrocardiográficos

A maioria das anormalidades do ECG associadas à DMVM é resultante de exacerbação de um ECG normal. Na DMVM, os achados eletrocardiográficos variam de traçados normais até anormalidades marcantes na frequência, ritmo ou configuração dos complexos. Com exceção da possibilidade de documentação e classificação de alguma arritmia, o ECG tem uso limitado no diagnóstico ou tratamento de DMVM.

A arritmia sinusal geralmente é preservada no estágio inicial da DMVM (ver Capítulo 248). Em cães com ICC, taquicardia sinusal e ausência de arritmia sinusal são achados comuns. Batimentos supraventriculares prematuros são comumente vistos em cães com DMVM,[79,91] mas esse achado tem pouca relevância hemodinâmica na maioria dos cães. Fibrilação atrial, taquicardia paroxística supraventricular, dissociação atrioventricular, batimentos ventriculares prematuros e taquicardia ventricular são menos comuns. Essas arritmias são mais frequentemente constatadas em casos avançados e, portanto, muitas vezes indicam um prognóstico ruim.

O ECG é um indicador que carece de sensibilidade no diagnóstico de aumento cardíaco e não detecta ICC (ver Capítulos 103 e 248). O eixo elétrico médio no plano frontal muitas vezes permanece na faixa de normalidade durante a progressão da doença. Nos casos de aumento significativo do AE, pode

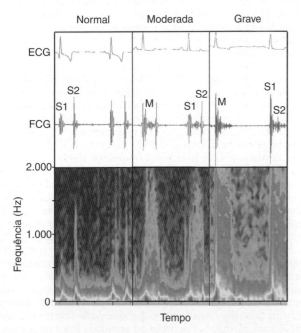

Figura 251.3 Fonocardiogramas (*FCG*) em cães com diferentes estágios da doença mixomatosa da valva mitral (*DMVM*). O registro é exibido em dois modos, obtidos simultaneamente: O modo superior exibe os traçados eletrocardiográficos (*ECG*, derivação II) e fonocardiográficos (*FCG*) sincrônicos; e o modo inferior mostra um gráfico de frequência de tempo em que diferentes frequências são exibidas de acordo com a intensidade, sendo as frequências de alta intensidade as vermelhas e as de baixa intensidade as em azul. Nota-se sopro holossistólico (*M*) nos fonocardiogramas dos cães com doença discreta a moderada e doença grave. Note que os componentes de frequência do sopro se alteram com a gravidade da doença. *S1*, primeira bulha cardíaca; *S2*, segunda bulha cardíaca. (*Esta figura se encontra reproduzida em cores no Encarte.*)

haver prolongamento da onda P. Em casos de aumento significativo do VE, pode haver prolongamento do complexo QRS e aumento da amplitude da onda R na derivação II.[92]

Na RT relevante, com hipertensão pulmonar, as alterações no ECG podem incluir evidências de aumento do AD (onda P alta), um padrão de aumento do VD e desvio do eixo elétrico médio à direita.[92] No entanto, mesmo em casos graves de RT e hipertensão pulmonar secundária à DMVM, esses sinais podem não ser evidentes devido às alterações concomitantes no lado esquerdo do coração. Nesses casos, o registro eletrocardiográfico só pode mostrar evidências de envolvimento do lado esquerdo.[72,76]

Achados radiográficos

Câmaras cardíacas do lado esquerdo. A radiografia é importante porque possibilita avaliar as consequências hemodinâmicas da DMVM (tamanho global do coração, presença de congestão e edema pulmonar). Além disso, a radiografia ajuda a excluir outras causas possíveis dos sinais clínicos. Em cães com DMVM, estruturas importantes a serem avaliadas são o AE, o VE, o tronco principal dos brônquios, os vasos pulmonares e o campo pulmonar. Cães com DMVM branda geralmente têm coração de tamanho normal, campos pulmonares normais e marcações vasculares normais.

O aumento do AE é uma das características radiográficas mais precoce e compatível de DMVM. O AE e o VE continuam a aumentar com a progressão da doença. O aumento da cavidade cardíaca, avaliado pelo escore cardíaco vertebral (ECV), tem sido caracterizado por uma fase lenta de progressão gradual da DMVM até cerca de 6 a 12 meses antes do início da ICC, quando a velocidade de alteração do aumento torna-se rápida.[93] Na imagem radiográfica lateral, os sinais de dilatação do VE e do AE incluem elevação da porção dorsal da região caudal da traqueia e da carina, deslocamento dorsal do brônquio principal esquerdo e proeminência visível do AE, fazendo com que a borda caudal do coração pareça reta ou com protuberância dorsocaudal (Figura 251.4 B). Na imagem dorsoventral (ou ventrodorsal), o apêndice do AE aumentado pode ser visto como uma protuberância na parte cranial esquerda da borda cardíaca (entre as posições de 2 e 3 horas). A borda do VE aumentada aparece arredondada e pode haver um deslocamento do ápice cardíaco para a esquerda ou para a direita.

Durante a progressão da DMVM, sinais radiográficos de congestão e edema pulmonar podem se desenvolver (Figura 251.4 C). Congestão e edema pulmonar são mais prováveis de estarem presentes em um cão com aumento relevante do coração (indicando DMVM avançada) do que em um cão com tamanho cardíaco normal ou levemente aumentado. Todavia, o grau de aumento cardíaco está pouco relacionado à gravidade da congestão e edema pulmonar. A dilatação da veia pulmonar, quando presente, é uma indicação precoce de congestão pulmonar; o diâmetro das veias é maior do que o das artérias pulmonares correspondentes e muitas vezes tornam-se tortuosas (especialmente em gatos). Entretanto, a dilatação venosa não é um achado consistente, mesmo em cães com edema pulmonar, e em alguns cães o delineamento da veia dilatada é indistinto, pois o edema intersticial prejudica, parcialmente, a visibilidade dos vasos pulmonares. Em cães, o edema pulmonar é frequentemente detectado na região peri-hilar e nas partes dorsais dos lobos pulmonares caudais, às vezes mais proeminentes no lado direito; porém, o edema agudo pode envolver os lóbulos cranianos. Em gatos, a localização do edema pulmonar cardiogênico não é tão previsível quanto nos cães com DMVM. Geralmente tem um aspecto mal definido e irregular.

Os achados pulmonares podem ser inconclusivos, já que as alterações radiográficas iniciais de edema pulmonar intersticial e do padrão bronquial se assemelham ao aspecto radiográfico da doença crônica de vias respiratórias, e a tendência é superestimar o diagnóstico de edema pulmonar quando se avaliam radiografias de cães com sinais de aumento cardíaco.

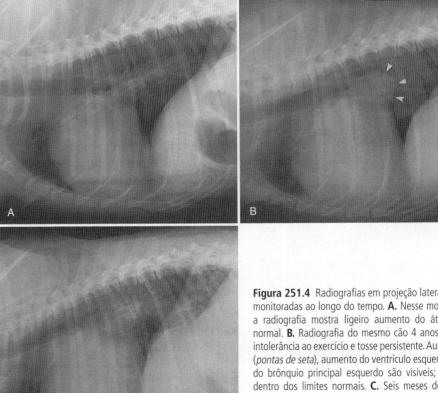

Figura 251.4 Radiografias em projeção lateral esquerda de um cão com DMVM monitoradas ao longo do tempo. **A.** Nesse momento o cão estava assintomático; a radiografia mostra ligeiro aumento do átrio esquerdo e perfusão vascular normal. **B.** Radiografia do mesmo cão 4 anos depois. O cão havia desenvolvido intolerância ao exercício e tosse persistente. Aumento acentuado do átrio esquerdo (*pontas de seta*), aumento do ventrículo esquerdo, elevação e discreta compressão do brônquio principal esquerdo são visíveis; já as marcações vasculares estão dentro dos limites normais. **C.** Seis meses depois, o cão também desenvolveu dispneia e havia apresentado episódios de síncopes. Além dos achados verificados na radiografia anterior (**B**), notam-se uma compressão mais evidente do brônquio principal esquerdo e evidência de congestão pulmonar e edema intersticial. (Cortesia de Kerstin Hansson, Uppsala, Suécia.)

Câmaras cardíacas do lado direito. Aumentos brandos do AD e do VD geralmente não estão associados a sinais radiográficos detectáveis. Sinais de aumento moderado a grave do AD, em imagem lateral, incluem proeminência do AD em direção craniodorsal. Isso faz com que a borda cranial do coração pareça reta, em vez de convexa, e eleva a traqueia à medida que ela percorre dorsalmente o AD. Além da elevação da traqueia e dilatação da veia cava caudal, os sinais de aumento do VD incluem o aumento do contato com o osso esterno e o abaulamento da borda direita do coração. Na imagem dorsoventral (ou ventrodorsal), o AD aumentado pode ser visto como uma protuberância na parte cranial direita da borda cardíaca (na posição de 9 a 12 horas). A borda do VD dilatado aparece arredondada e, se severamente aumentado, pode ter aparência de uma letra "D" invertida. Ocorre deslocamento do ápice cardíaco para a esquerda. Podem ser observados sinais de ICC direita, incluindo efusão pleural, efusão abdominal, hepatomegalia e esplenomegalia. Se há insuficiência biventricular, o tamanho cardíaco global aumenta e sinais de ICC esquerda e direita podem estar presentes.

Achados ecocardiográficos (ver Capítulo 104)

Valva mitral e câmaras cardíacas do lado esquerdo. A ecocardiografia é útil na obtenção do diagnóstico de DMVM e, posteriormente, para monitorar a doença. Embora algumas variáveis ecocardiográficas tenham sido sugeridas como úteis para predizer a presença de ICC,[94] nenhuma delas se mostrou mais precisa e sensível que outros parâmetros clínicos, como a frequência respiratória. A ecocardiografia bidimensional possibilita avaliar a anatomia da valva mitral e identificar o espessamento e a protrusão sistólica do folheto (prolapso da valva mitral) de um ou de ambos os folhetos no lado atrial do anel mitral (Figura 251.5 B). Foi relatado que a ecocardiografia tridimensional em tempo real (3DTR) transtorácica fornece uma avaliação mais precisa, extensa, não invasiva *in vivo* da anatomia valvar em pacientes cardíacos humanos (Vídeo 251.16 e Figura 251.5 C e D);[95] o seu uso potencial em pacientes caninos está atualmente sob avaliação. O prolapso da valva mitral é uma indicação precoce de DMVM e pode estar presente em cães com ou sem RM (Vídeos 251.1 a 251.4).[96,97] A presença e a gravidade da protrusão dos folhetos valvares podem ser avaliadas na imagem do eixo longo paraesternal direito, e relata-se que há boa correlação entre o seu grau de deslocamento e a gravidade da RM.[18,97,98] As alterações patológicas macroscópicas dos dois folhetos (anterior e posterior) são, frequentemente, igualmente graves no exame *post mortem*, porém as alterações degenerativas comumente são mais proeminentes no folheto anterior, na imagem do eixo longo paraesternal direito, no

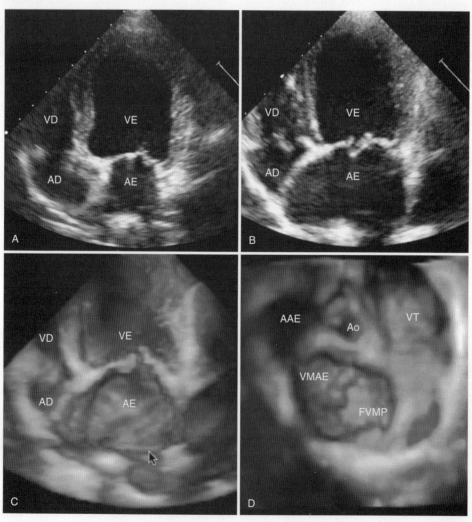

Figura 251.5 Ecocardiogramas de um cão normal (**A**) e de um cão com DMVM grave (**B** a **D**). A imagem de quatro câmaras apical esquerda, obtida em ecocardiograma bidimensional, durante a sístole, do cão com DMVM grave (**B**) mostra prolapso bilateral dos folhetos da valva mitral, prolapso do folheto da valva tricúspide e dilatação do AE e do VE. Imagem obtida na mesma projeção, em ecocardiograma tridimensional (3D) do mesmo cão, no fim da diástole (**C**), e imagem da valva mitral oposta, obtida em ecocardiograma 3D, do lado atrial (**D**) durante a sístole. O prolapso é evidente em vários locais em ambos os folhetos. *AAE*, apêndice atrial esquerdo; *AD*, átrio direito; *AE*, átrio esquerdo; *Ao*, artéria aorta; *FVMP*, folículo da valva mitral posterior; *VD*, ventrículo direito; *VE*, ventrículo esquerdo; *VMAE*, valva mitral anterior esquerda; *VT*, valva tricúspide.

ecocardiograma.[99] Com a progressão, as alterações degenerativas tornam-se mais evidentes (Vídeos 251.5 a 251.16) e os folhetos valvares geralmente têm aparência semelhante à clava, com maior espessamento na ponta (ver Figura 251.5 B e C). Pode-se detectar o espessamento de cordas tendíneas ou uma eversão da borda valvar (Vídeo 251.17 e Figura 251.5 B e C).[100,101] Relata-se a presença de eversão valvar quando a borda de um folheto ou, em casos graves, todo o folheto move-se em direção ao AE no momento da sístole, e isso indica ruptura de uma ou mais cordas tendíneas que, ocasionalmente, pode ser detectada no AE ou no VE.[100,102]

O AE é uma importante estrutura que deve ser avaliada em cães com DMVM, pois o seu tamanho reflete a gravidade da doença.[50] Embora o AE possa ser examinado a partir de diversas imagens, a de preferência é a imagem do eixo curto paraesternal direito, com a raiz da artéria aorta, o corpo do AE e a aurícula visíveis. A informação mais útil dessa imagem é o tamanho do AE, porque pode ser comparado com o tamanho da raiz da aorta, que é relativamente constante em determinado tamanho de cão. Em cães com DMVM, o diâmetro do corpo do AE pode ser consideravelmente maior que o do apêndice do AE.[103] Nos estágios iniciais de DMVM, com discreto grau de RM, os sinais de aumento do AE não são vistos no exame ecocardiográfico. Com a progressão da DMVM, a dimensão do AE aumentada, os cães com ICC frequentemente apresentam proporção entre o aumento do AE e a raiz da aorta (AE/Ao) de 2 ou mais.[104] A ecocardiografia 3D em tempo real (3DTR) possibilita estimar o volume do AE com maior precisão, e o potencial da avaliação do provável volume do AE por meio de 3DTR foi recentemente realizada em cães com DMVM.[105] No entanto, uma restrição à técnica 3DTR é a demora, em comparação com o exame ecocardiográfico tradicional; ademais, atualmente não há disponibilidade de uma faixa de referência normal para o volume do AE.

As dimensões anatômicas, o volume e a função do VE podem ser avaliados subjetivamente ou por meio de várias técnicas ecocardiográficas quantitativas. As avaliações clínicas ecocardiográficas tradicionais do VE baseiam-se em estimativas de dimensão de imagens unidimensionais (modo M) e/ou bidimensionais (2D). No entanto, o tamanho do VE também pode ser avaliado por meio de estimativas de volume com base em 2D (método do disco modificado de Simpson) ou técnicas de imagem 3D (Figura 251.6 A).[106] A possibilidade de avaliação do volume do VE tem sido mostrada em cães com DMVM,[64,107] mas os valores de referência normais para o volume do VE está disponível atualmente apenas para algumas raças. O tamanho normal do VE, ou apenas um VE discretamente aumentado, é observado em cães com DMVM branda. Com a progressão da doença, a dimensão e o volume do eixo curto diastólico final do VE aumentam, enquanto as medidas sistólicas finais não aumentam na mesma proporção.[64,93] A taxa de alteração aumenta e é maior quando os cães apresentam iminência de ICC (Figura 251.6 B e C).[93] A espessura da parede do VE está geralmente dentro dos limites normais. O aumento do tamanho do VE associado a uma espessura de parede normal indica sobrecarga de volume e hipertrofia excêntrica.

Alterações na morfologia do VE, acompanhadas de dilatação do VE, podem ser avaliadas por meio de um índice de esfericidade, tanto em imagens ecocardiográficas 2D quanto em 3D.[64] A ecocardiografia 3DTR fornece o índice de esfericidade, que pode ser obtido dividindo-se o volume diastólico final pelo

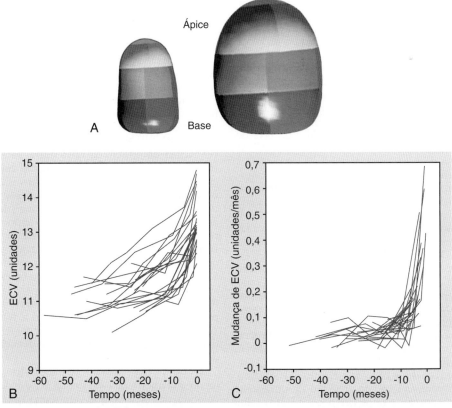

Figura 251.6 A. Moldes do ventrículo esquerdo (VE) obtidos a partir do conjunto de dados 3D de um cão saudável (à esquerda) e de um cão com DMVM grave (à direita). O molde do VE é automaticamente dividido em 17 segmentos. O volume do VE está claramente aumentado no cão doente; sua morfologia se altera de uma forma elíptica para uma forma mais globular (aumento da esfericidade) em resposta à sobrecarga de volume crescente. Demarcações radiográficas dos escores cardíacos vertebrais (ECV) (**B**) e taxa de variação do ECV (**C**) em função do tempo, em cães no estágio ACVIM B, progredindo para ICC (momento 0). Durante a progressão da DMVM, o tamanho do coração é caracterizado por um aumento lento até cerca de 6 a 12 meses antes do início da ICC; após esse período a taxa de alteração aumenta à medida que os cães progridem para ICC. (**B** e **C**, de Lord P, Hansson K, Kvart C et al.: Rate of change of heart size before congestive heart failure in dogs with mitral regurgitation. *J Small Anim Pract* 51:210-218, 2010. Publicado com permissão do editor.)

volume de uma esfera; este índice mostrou-se um preditor precoce e mais acurado do remodelamento cardíaco, comparativamente a outras variáveis ecocardiográficas, no homem.[108] O índice de esfericidade geralmente não é incluído no protocolo ecocardiográfico de rotina quando se avalia o remodelamento do VE em cães com DMVM, mas esse índice pode ser útil para a avaliação da progressão do remodelamento do VE em cães.[64]

Embora a função sistólica do miocárdio diminua com a progressão da DMVM, o processo de remodelação permite que o VE mantenha sua função de bombeamento cardíaco relativamente bem preservada, mesmo nos casos de DMVM avançada.[51,66] A identificação de disfunção sistólica por meio de modalidades ecocardiográficas é um desafio em cães com DMVM.[109] Muitos dos índices ecocardiográficos comumente usados para avaliar a função sistólica, como os índices da fase de ejeção (p. ex., encurtamento fracional do VE, fração de ejeção e velocidade média do encurtamento circunferencial) são, além de dependentes da contratilidade intrínseca, também influenciados pela carga hemodinâmica e pelo tônus simpático; portanto, possivelmente mascaram significativamente a disfunção miocárdica em cães com RM.[109] Em cães com DMVM branda, os valores dos índices da fase de ejeção são frequentemente normais; esses valores podem estar acima do normal em cães com DMVM moderada a grave. Portanto, no cenário de DMVM moderada ou grave, um encurtamento fracional normal comumente indica redução da contratilidade do miocárdio. A avaliação da dimensão ou do volume sistólico final do VE tem sido sugerida para refletir melhor a disfunção sistólica na presença de RM.[66,110] A dimensão ou volume final sistólico aumenta à medida que a função sistólica diminui, apesar do aumento do volume retrógrado do VE no AE de baixa resistência.[66] Porém, se a função contrátil do VE estiver preservada, o VE totalmente compensado diminuirá para uma dimensão sistólica final quase normal.[109] Os índices de volume sistólico final aumentam em cães com DMVM mais grave, indicando disfunção sistólica.[64,110] As técnicas de imagem mais recentemente introduzidas, como imagem Doppler de tecido (IDT) e técnica de rastreamento de pequenas alterações, foram consideradas comparativamente independentes das condições de carga cardíaca; entretanto, estudos sugerem que essas técnicas são influenciadas por condições de carga cardíaca e pela atividade do tônus simpático em maior extensão do que o anteriormente esperado. Semelhante ao encurtamento fracional, os valores de tensão e da taxa de deformação do VE parecem estar aumentados na DMVM moderada a grave, mas os valores podem diminuir (retornar aos valores constatados em cães normais) em estágios mais avançados, indicando insuficiência miocárdica.[111] Isso pode limitar o valor informativo adicional obtido com essa técnica, comparado ao uso de índices de volume sistólico final em cães com DMVM.

Regurgitações valvares podem ser detectadas e quantificadas no exame Doppler espectral e Doppler de fluxo colorido (Figura 251.7 A).[81] O ideal é que o fluxo regurgitante esteja alinhado com o feixe de ultrassom e isso é mais frequentemente alcançado na imagem de quatro câmaras apical esquerda. Como a direção do fluxo depende da direção da regurgitação, que, por sua vez, depende da morfologia do fluxo, outras imagens também podem propiciar um bom alinhamento.

A ecocardiografia com Doppler de fluxo colorido confirma a presença de um jato regurgitante, e o tamanho do jato pode ser comparado com o tamanho do AE (ver Vídeos 251.2, 251.4, 251.6, 251.8, 251.11, 251.13 e 251.15, e Capítulo 104). Essa medida depende das configurações do aparelho de ultrassom, sendo semiquantitativa em cães e gatos. Um pequeno jato exclui a presença de RM moderada a grave, mas muitas vezes é difícil distinguir claramente entre regurgitação moderada e grave com base nas informações do tamanho do jato. Pequenos jatos próximos à valva mitral não devem ser supervalorizados em cães sem qualquer outra anormalidade valvar, já que regurgitações irrelevantes podem frequentemente ser detectadas em cães normais.

O exame Doppler espectral fornece informações sobre a velocidade do jato regurgitante e os traçados do tempo de velocidade podem ajudar a estimar o volume regurgitante (ver Capítulo 104). O gradiente de pressão sistólica transmitral pode ser estimado pelo cálculo do pico do gradiente de RM usando a equação simplificada de Bernoulli: gradiente de pressão máximo de RM = 4 × (velocidade de RM).[2] Normalmente, cães com DMVM sem insuficiência miocárdica significativa têm uma velocidade do jato regurgitante de 5 a 6 m/s.[80] No entanto, a velocidade pode estar aumentada em indivíduos com hipertensão arterial sistêmica e diminuída em indivíduos com hipotensão, com aumento significativo da pressão no AE e/ou com insuficiência miocárdica. Assim sendo, a velocidade do jato regurgitante é tipicamente inferior a 5 m/s em cães com ICC fulminante aguda.

A fração regurgitante é a porcentagem do volume sistólico total do VE que retorna à câmara do AE. As medições da fração regurgitante em cães com RM moderada a grave indicam que o miocárdio desses animais pode ejetar mais de 75% do volume total de ejeção sistólico no AE.[50] Existem várias maneiras para estimar o volume e a fração regurgitante. O volume de ejeção da RM pode ser estimado indiretamente usando o método volumétrico pelo cálculo da diferença entre o volume sanguíneo de ejeção total menos o volume sanguíneo de ejeção na artéria aorta. O volume de ejeção sistólico total pode ser estimado usando o método biplanar da soma dos discos (método de Simpson modificado) do volume do VE, e o volume de ejeção sistólico pode ser estimado multiplicando a área transversal aórtica pela integral tempo-velocidade obtida no traçado do Doppler espectral do fluxo aórtico (ver Capítulo 104). Alternativamente, o volume de ejeção sistólico total pode ser estimado multiplicando-se a área transversal do anel da valva mitral, obtida em modo bidimensional, com a integral tempo-velocidade obtida a partir do traçado de Doppler espectral do fluxo diastólico através da valva. Ambos os métodos envolvem múltiplas medições, cada uma com seus próprios erros, o que significa que elas apenas fornecem estimativas do volume regurgitante. A fração regurgitante é calculada dividindo o volume sistólico regurgitante pelo volume de ejeção sistólico total do VE.

A fração regurgitante também pode ser quantificada pelo método da convergência de fluxo colorido na área da superfície de isovelocidade proximal (PISA) em cães com RM (Figura 251.7 B).[50,112] Na RM, o fluxo sanguíneo converge para o lado ventricular do orifício da valva mitral antes de passar pelo orifício regurgitante; no ecocardiograma com Doppler colorido essa área é caracterizada como um hemisfério. Pode-se calcular o volume sistólico regurgitante com base nos valores do raio desse hemisfério, da velocidade "aliasing", da velocidade máxima do jato regurgitante e da integral do tempo-velocidade do fluxo regurgitante (os dois últimos são obtidos a partir de medidas do Doppler espectral). A fração regurgitante é obtida dividindo-se o volume regurgitante pela soma do volume de ejeção sistólico e do volume regurgitante. Embora esse método tenha vantagens significativas em comparação com outros métodos de medição da fração regurgitante, ele possui várias limitações práticas e pode não ser prontamente aplicável a todos os casos de RM. Além disso, nenhum dos métodos Doppler mostrou ser indicador mais confiável da gravidade da doença do que o tamanho do AE em cães e gatos com RM.

Outro método mais direto para avaliar a gravidade da RM é medir o diâmetro da *vena contracta* no ecocardiograma de fluxo colorido, um método que vem sendo aplicado em cães.[101,113] A *vena contracta* é definida como a região de fluxo central mais estreita de um jato que passa pelo orifício de uma valva regurgitante, ou logo abaixo, onde a velocidade do sangue é maior (Figura 251.7 B).[114] Na RM ou na RT, a *vena contracta* é em geral medida no ecocardiograma bidimensional colorido como o diâmetro na visão esquerda de quatro câmaras apicais, mas a ecocardiografia 3D com fluxo colorido pode mostrar medidas

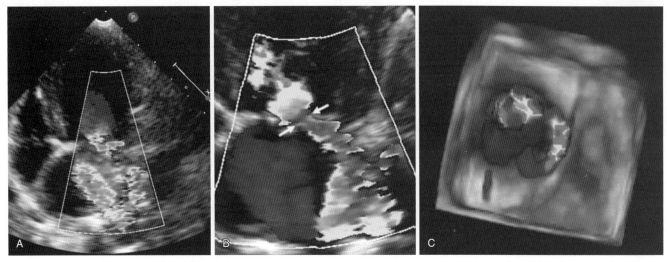

Figura 251.7 A. Imagem de quatro câmaras apical esquerda, obtida em ecocardiograma bidimensional com mapeamento de fluxo colorido, de cão com DMVM grave. Há evidências de regurgitação mitral moderada a grave. A velocidade do sangue aumenta no lado ventricular, em direção ao orifício regurgitante da valva, e há um jato direcionado lateralmente e um fluxo turbulento no átrio esquerdo. A gravidade da regurgitação mitral pode ser avaliada relacionando-se a área do jato com a área do átrio esquerdo, ou utilizando o raio do hemicírculo criado quando o fluxo sanguíneo converge para o lado ventricular, antes de passar pelo orifício regurgitante (método da área de superfície de isovelocidade proximal [PISA]; ver texto para detalhes), ou como ilustrado em um ecocardiograma com Doppler colorido em (**B**), medindo o diâmetro da contração da veia, que é a região de fluxo central mais estreita de um jato que ocorre em, ou apenas, a jusante do orifício da valva regurgitante (*setas*). A área da *vena contracta*, que é aproximadamente a mesma da regurgitação efetiva, pode ser avaliada por meio de ecocardiografia com Doppler 3D colorido, como ilustrado em **C**, onde a valva mitral é inspecionada do lado atrial e a regurgitação mitral é evidente em dois locais. (*Esta figura se encontra reproduzida em cores no Encarte.*)

da área da *vena contracta*, o que pode fornecer uma estimativa mais precisa do orifício regurgitante efetivo. De fato, a área da *vena contracta* na MR ou na TR não é um círculo; é mais esférica devido à ocorrência de regurgitação ao longo da linha de coaptação (ver Figura 251.7 C). Independentemente de o diâmetro ou a área da *vena contracta* serem medidos, o método mostrou boa concordância com o grau angiocardiográfico de RM e o volume regurgitante no homem.[114]

O Doppler espectral também pode ser usado para avaliar o fluxo transmitral durante a diástole. MR significativa é geralmente associada a maior velocidade de enchimento diastólico como consequência do aumento do fluxo diastólico transmitral.[115] Além disso, a função ventricular diastólica anormal, como consequência da grave sobrecarga de volume, pode ser detectada. É importante cronometrar os eventos ao avaliar o fluxo transmitral para distinguir regurgitação sistólica e fluxo diastólico, a fim de evitar diagnóstico falso positivo de RM clinicamente relevante. A regurgitação diastólica é comum em casos de bradicardia (e bloqueio AV de segundo grau) ou arritmias; provavelmente indica pequenos gradientes de pressão reversa durante o enchimento cardíaco.[116]

Valva tricúspide e câmaras cardíacas do lado direito. O aspecto ecocardiográfico da valva tricúspide que apresenta degeneração mixomatosa é semelhante, no modo bidimensional, às lesões mixomatosas da valva mitral, já descritas. Com o uso do Doppler com fluxo colorido, a RT pode ser detectada e semiquantificada. O AD, no entanto, não é tão facilmente acessível quanto o AE devido à sua posição anatômica; ademais, na RT a direção dos jatos não é consistente. A hipertensão pulmonar é uma complicação comum em cães com DMVM, e a ecocardiografia é a técnica veterinária não invasiva padrão para o diagnóstico da doença (ver Capítulo 243).[57] O Doppler espectral pode ser usado para estimar o volume sistólico do VD e detectar hipertensão pulmonar pela estimativa da pressão sistólica do VD e das pressões arteriais sistólica e diastólica pulmonares.[80] O gradiente de pressão entre o AD e o VD pode ser calculado com base na velocidade do pico do jato regurgitante e na equação de Bernoulli modificada, conforme descrito anteriormente.[57,117] A pressão sistólica do VD é obtida pela adição de uma estimativa da pressão do AD ao gradiente de pressão calculado na valva AV. E esse gradiente de pressão é arbitrariamente considerado como sendo 5 mmHg, na ausência de dilatação do AD; 10 mmHg na presença de dilatação do AD, mas nenhum sinal de ICC direita; e 15 mmHg em cães com ICC direita.[117]

Da mesma forma, podem ser usados o pico de velocidade da regurgitação da valva pulmonar e uma estimativa da pressão diastólica do VD para predizer a pressão diastólica da artéria pulmonar.[118]

Pode-se diagnosticar hipertensão pulmonar quando o pico de velocidade da RT for > 3 m/s, correspondendo a um gradiente de pico de RT > 36 mmHg.[57] A ausência de sinais de RT no ecocardiograma não exclui a possibilidade de hipertensão pulmonar em cães com DMVM. Os achados ecocardiográficos adicionais que indicam hipertensão pulmonar incluem sinais de hipertrofia e dilatação do VD, dilatação da artéria pulmonar e movimento paradoxal ou flacidez do septo interventricular.[57]

Significância e progressão

A doença mixomatosa da valva mitral, comparada a muitas outras doenças de cães, é considerada de alta morbidade e mortalidade nas raças acometidas, e a doença foi relatada como responsável por 75% dos casos de ICC em cães,[70] uma proporção consideravelmente maior em raças acometidas.[12,21,119] A progressão da doença varia entre os indivíduos, mas os cães acometidos geralmente podem compensar a RM por um longo período de tempo. A progressão da DMVM desde a detecção de um sopro cardíaco suave até a doença terminal é, muitas vezes, uma questão de anos, em cães de pequeno porte, mas alguns cães de grande porte parecem ser menos tolerantes à DMVM: nesses cães, a doença tem uma progressão mais drástica, com sinais clínicos mais graves do que em cães de pequeno porte.[120] É importante realizar o estadiamento da gravidade da doença para a avaliação de risco, a fim de tomar decisões terapêuticas e estabelecer o prognóstico. Em 2009, foi publicada uma recomendação do ACVIM, recomendando o estadiamento da DMVM em cães, em quatro grupos de pacientes: do estágio A ao D (Tabela 251.1).[121]

SEÇÃO 16 • Doença Cardiovascular

Tabela 251.1 Recomendação do American College of Veterinary Internal Medicine (ACVIM) quanto ao estadiamento da DMVM, em cães, em quatro classes (A a D).[121]

ESTÁGIO A	ESTÁGIO B		ESTÁGIO C	ESTÁGIO D
Cães com risco de desenvolver cardiopatia, mas que no momento não apresentam anormalidades cardíacas funcionais detectáveis (p. ex., cães da raça Cavalier King Charles Spaniel, sem sopro cardíaco)	Cães sem sinais clínicos, mas que apresentam clique sistólico (fase inicial) e/ou sopro sistólico		Cães com sinais clínicos anteriores ou atuais de ICC causada por cardiopatia estrutural. A gravidade dos sinais clínicos da ICC varia de leve a grave, sendo que a ICC grave requer terapia agressiva, que seria reservada para pacientes com doença refratária (ver Estágio D)	Cães com doença terminal que apresentam sinais clínicos de insuficiência cardíaca causada por regurgitação de valva AV refratária à terapia padrão de ICC. Esses pacientes necessitam de estratégias terapêuticas avançadas ou especializadas para se manterem clinicamente confortáveis com a doença
	B1	**B2**		
	Cães levados à consulta com evidência de RM branda (sopro cardíaco e sinais ecocardiográficos de regurgitação de valva AV), porém sem sinais de cardiomegalia	Cães assintomáticos que apresentam regurgitação de valva AV hemodinamicamente significativa evidenciada por achados radiográficos ou ecocardiográficos de cardiomegalia		

Embora exista risco de desenvolvimento futuro de ICC, muitos cães acometidos nunca desenvolvem sinais clínicos da doença durante a vida toda.[87,99,121,122] Os fatores de risco para progressão de DMVM, de branda para grave, incluem idade, sexo, raça, gravidade da lesão valvar, gravidade da RM, dilatação do VE e do AE, frequência cardíaca, concentrações circulantes do peptídio natriurético N-terminal tipo pró-B (NT-pró-BNP) e da troponina I cardíaca específica (cTnI), arritmias e síncope.[4,21,70,87,98,99,101,123-128]

Diagnóstico diferencial

Regurgitação mitral

Embora a causa comum de RM seja a degeneração mixomatosa, outras causas de RM são dignas de nota: cardiomiopatia dilatada e outras doenças miocárdicas; endocardite bacteriana da valva mitral; ou cardiopatia congênita previamente desconhecida, como displasia da valva mitral ou persistência do ducto arterioso (PDA). No entanto, as informações da resenha, os sinais clínicos e os achados de exame físico significantes são frequentemente tão característicos que sugerem fortemente a presença de DMVM. No estágio inicial de DMVM, é possível constatar discreto sopro cardíaco no início da sístole, que pode ser confundido com sopro fisiológico ou com sopros causados por cardiopatias congênitas, como discreta estenose aórtica ou pulmonar leve. No entanto, os cães com sopro fisiológico ou com sopro decorrente de estenose aórtica ou pulmonar geralmente são jovens e a intensidade máxima do sopro é constatada na área da base do coração, enquanto os cães com DMVM branda geralmente são mais velhos e a intensidade máxima do sopro é detectada na área da valva mitral. Todavia, a idade de início da DMVM é variável e um exame ecocardiográfico deve ser sempre realizado para confirmar o diagnóstico. Para fins de exclusão de cardiomiopatia dilatada e cardiomiopatia hipertrófica, também é necessário exame ecocardiográfico.

O aspecto ecocardiográfico da valva mitral comprometida por endocardite pode ser muito semelhante ao espessamento nodular de folhetos valvares, característico de degeneração mixomatosa. Entretanto, lesões de endocardite podem ser mais ecogênicas e mais isoladas. Além disso, pacientes com endocardite bacteriana geralmente têm histórico de febre, artrite, doença sistêmica, sopro cardíaco desenvolvido recentemente e sinais clínicos que podem indicar doença tromboembólica,[129] enquanto cães com DMVM frequentemente apresentam sopro cardíaco durante anos e não apresentam febre ou outros sintomas de doença sistêmica.

Regurgitação tricúspide

A RT (regurgitação tricúspide) secundária ou funcional pode ocorrer como consequência da dilatação do VD em todas as condições associadas a aumento adquirido na pressão do VD. Estas incluem dirofilariose, tromboembolismo pulmonar, hipertensão pulmonar secundária à doença cardíaca esquerda e hipertensão pulmonar idiopática. Além disso, a RT ocorre como consequência secundária à cardiomiopatia biventricular ou dilatada e à estenose pulmonar congênita. É incomum a valva tricúspide ser afetada por endocardite infecciosa ou ruptura de cordas tendíneas.[72,80] A regurgitação tricúspide pode ser observada em gatos com cardiomiopatia e hipertireoidismo.[130]

Sinais clínicos não específicos

Embora a DMVM possa ser prontamente diagnosticada em um paciente com sinais clínicos, o verdadeiro desafio diagnóstico consiste em determinar se a ICC descompensada é a causa primária dos sinais clínicos existentes. A maioria dos cães com DMVM é de idade avançada, de pequeno a médio porte, e muitos desses cães realizam menos atividades físicas diárias. Assim, a intolerância ao exercício pode ser difícil de se identificar. Além disso, os sinais clínicos da ICC esquerda, como tosse, dispneia e taquipneia, podem ser causados por várias condições, tais como doença de vias respiratórias de pequeno calibre (ver Capítulo 241), instabilidade traqueal (ver Capítulo 241), fibrose pulmonar (ver Capítulo 242), neoplasia (ver Capítulo 242), dirofilariose (ver Capítulo 255) e pneumonia (ver Capítulo 242). Muitos desses diagnósticos diferenciais podem ser excluídos por meio de diferentes testes clínicos, particularmente radiografia, mas em alguns casos os resultados podem ser inconclusivos. Isso inclui a mensuração de peptídios natriuréticos, que podem auxiliar na distinção entre DMVD leve e grave, e na diferenciação entre dispneia ocasionada por doença respiratória primária e dispneia causada por ICC.[131,132] Os cães podem apresentar uma combinação de DMVM relevante e doença respiratória primária, e nesse cenário o valor adicional da mensuração de peptídios natriuréticos é limitado. Nesses casos inconclusivos, um teste terapêutico com diurético por 48 a 72 horas, seguido de avaliação da frequência respiratória (a frequência respiratória é, então, comparada com os valores anteriores ao início do uso do diurético), e radiografias em série podem ajudar a identificar a causa primária.

Conduta

De forma ideal, a terapia de DMVM deveria deter a progressão da degeneração valvar ou melhorar a função valvar. Atualmente, não se conhece tratamento capaz de inibir ou prevenir a degeneração valvular, embora o reparo cirúrgico ou a troca da valva melhore a função valvar. Séries de casos com desfechos comparativamente bons foram relatados após correção cirúrgica da valva mitral,[133] porém esse procedimento está disponível apenas em poucos locais no mundo e, portanto, sua realização não é técnica, econômica ou eticamente possível para a maioria dos pacientes caninos e felinos. Portanto, no caso de DMVM, a conduta clínica tem como objetivo principal melhorar a qualidade de vida, prolongando a fase pré-clínica (assintomática), melhorando os sinais clínicos e aumentando a sobrevida. Isso geralmente implica que o tratamento deve ser ajustado às condições do paciente, do proprietário e do clínico, e geralmente envolve tratamento concomitante com dois ou mais medicamentos, logo que haja evidência de sinais de ICC. O tratamento de DMVM será discutido em quatro grupos de pacientes: (1) cães sem sinais de ICC (Estágio B do ACVIM); (2) cães com sintomas brandos a moderados de ICC (Estágio C do ACVIM); (3) cães com ICC recorrente (Estágio C ou D do ACVIM); e (4) cães com ICC grave e com risco à vida (fulminante) (Estágio C ou D do ACVIM).[121] Possíveis complicações serão discutidas separadamente. É incomum tratar casos de DMVM isolada em gatos e, portanto, os detalhes das dosagens de medicamentos para gatos não estão incluídos nesta seção.

Cães sem sintomas de ICC (Estágio B do ACVIM)

Cães em Estágio B do ACVIM representam um grupo relativamente heterogêneo de cães, variando de pacientes com apenas RM branda e tamanho cardíaco normal (Estágio B1 do ACVIM) a cães com RM grave e dilatação relevante do AE e do VE (Estágio B2 do ACVIM). Esse dilema leva a questões sobre quando iniciar o tratamento e se a terapia antes do início da ICC descompensada é benéfica, ineficaz ou prejudicial. Os inibidores da ECA são frequentemente prescritos para cães com DMVM, antes do início da ICC, mesmo para os animais em Estágio B1 do ACVIM. Atualmente, no entanto, não existem provas de que o tratamento com inibidores da ECA tenha um efeito preventivo no desenvolvimento e na progressão de sinais clínicos de ICC, ou melhore a sobrevida de cães com DMVM em Estágio B do ACVIM. Foram realizadas duas amplas pesquisas multicêntricas controladas com placebo, o Scandinavian Veterinary Enalapril Prevention (SVEP) e o Veterinary Enalapril Trial to Prove Reduction in Onset of Heart Failure (VETPROOF),[87,122] a fim de avaliar o efeito da monoterapia com enalapril, um inibidor da ECA, na progressão dos sinais clínicos de DMVM assintomática em cães. Em ambas, não se constatou diferença significativa entre os animais que receberam placebo e aqueles tratados, desde o início da terapia até a confirmação de ICC,[87,122] independentemente de os cães estarem no Estágio B1 ou B2 do ACVIM.[87] Na RM experimental, os antagonistas de receptores beta mostraram ter alguns efeitos benéficos, melhorando a condição hemodinâmica e a contratilidade do miocárdio.[134] Existem, no entanto, muito poucos estudos sobre o efeito dos antagonistas de receptores beta na ocorrência natural de DMVM,[135,136] e atualmente não há evidência conclusiva de que esses medicamentos tenham um efeito preventivo na DMVM assintomática. Na verdade, um amplo estudo clínico prospectivo controlado com placebo, incluindo cães com DMVM em Estágio B do ACVIM, foi finalizado prematuramente devido à carência de eficácia. Sabe-se que os vasodilatadores arteriais, como o anlodipino, são benéficos na DMVM em Estágio B2, porque a redução da impedância aórtica pode, teoricamente, reduzir a RM. O anlodipino foi avaliado na dose de 0,57 mg/kg, por via oral, administrado em intervalos de 12 horas em cães.[137] A documentação clínica do uso de anlodipino é escassa; no entanto, esse medicamento foi avaliado em um estudo ecocardiográfico não cego de cães com DMVM, no qual se constatou melhora significativa no volume sistólico regurgitante e na área do orifício regurgitante, bem como

redução da pressão arterial (10%).[138] O inodilatador pimobendana (uma combinação de sensibilizador de cálcio com inibidor da fosfodiesterase III) tem, além de sua ação inotrópica, efeito vasodilatador arterial em cães.[139,140] Demonstrou-se que o pimobendana reduz o tamanho cardíaco em cães com DMVM, tanto em curto quanto a longo prazo,[141,142] efeito que potencialmente poderia retardar o aparecimento de sintomas de ICC no Estágio B2 do ACVIM em cães. Realizou-se o estudo Evaluation of Pimobendana in dogs with Cardiomegaly Caused by Preclinical Mitral Valve Disease (EPIC), uma ampla pesquisa multicêntrica prospectiva controlada com placebo que incluiu cães com DMVM em Estágio B2 do ACVIM, a fim de comparar a eficácia do pimobendana com o placebo na prevenção do aparecimento de sintomas de ICC. Em 2015, o estudo foi encerrado prematuramente porque uma análise preliminar concluiu que havia evidências claras do benefício da administração de pimobendana no retardo de desenvolvimento de ICC esquerda, ou de morte presumivelmente de origem cardíaca. A análise preliminar não levantou qualquer preocupação com a segurança da administração de pimobendana. Os resultados completos e finais do estudo EPIC ainda não estavam disponíveis no momento da redação deste capítulo.

A progressão da doença pode ser monitorada em intervalos regulares de 3 a 12 meses, se houver cardiomegalia. Casos mais brandos não requerem monitoramento frequente (ver Significância e Progressão). Proprietários de cães com DMVM assintomática devem ser instruídos sobre os sinais de desenvolvimento de ICC e, no caso de reprodutores, sobre o fato de que a doença é significativamente influenciada por fatores genéticos. Os proprietários devem ser instruídos a aferir a frequência respiratória durante o sono/repouso, no domicílio, e serem informados que uma frequência respiratória recorrente > 30 movimentos respiratórios/minuto é anormal e merece uma investigação mais minuciosa, pois ela pode ser uma indicação de ICC.[75]

Atualmente, há poucas informações com base em evidências sobre os efeitos da atividade física e da dieta na progressão da DMVM em cães. Cães com DMVM branda não precisam ser submetidos à restrição dietética ou de exercício; em nossa experiência, observamos que cães com DMVM assintomática avançada geralmente toleram longas caminhadas em seu próprio ritmo, têm melhor qualidade de vida com esse tipo de atividade física e seu desempenho é melhor quando se evita a obesidade. No entanto, do ponto de vista fisiopatológico, deve-se evitar exercício extenuante ou dieta com alto teor de sódio, em cães com DMVM em Estágio B2 avançado, pois isso pode ocasionar edema pulmonar.

Cães com sintomas brandos a moderados de ICC (estágio C do ACVIM)

O estágio em que um paciente começa a manifestar sinais clínicos de DMVM (ou seja, desenvolveu ICC descompensada) é o fim de um processo que começou muito antes, com o início da regurgitação da valva. Considerando a fisiopatologia da DMVM, os objetivos do tratamento são: (1) reduzir a pressão venosa para aliviar o edema e a efusão; (2) manter o débito cardíaco adequado, a fim de evitar a ocorrência de fraqueza, letargia e azotemia pré-renal; (3) reduzir a carga cardíaca e a regurgitação valvar; e (4) proteger o coração dos efeitos negativos, a longo prazo, dos efeitos neuro-hormonais.

Cães com edema pulmonar brando a moderado geralmente podem ser submetidos a tratamento ambulatorial e regularmente examinados. Pacientes com edema pulmonar moderado a grave podem necessitar de cuidados intensivos, inclusive repouso em gaiola apropriada e, às vezes, suplementação de oxigênio (ver Capítulos 131 e 141). A base fundamental do tratamento de ICC é o uso de diurético, mais frequentemente a furosemida, bem como outros medicamentos com diferentes modos de ação, adicionados à terapia diurética (ver Capítulo 247). Uma combinação medicamentosa comumente usada nesse cenário inclui terapia tripla, com um diurético de alça (furosemida ou torsemida), pimobendana e um inibidor da ECA. Espironolactona e/ou digoxina também são usadas frequentemente.

A dosagem de furosemida deve ser preferencialmente baseada nos sinais clínicos, e não nos achados radiográficos. Um paciente pode respirar com facilidade, mesmo na presença de sinais radiográficos de edema intersticial, ou vice-versa. O curso usual do tratamento de um paciente com ICC branda a moderada é o tratamento intensivo inicial com furosemida (2 a 4 mg/kg/8 a 12 h IV, IM, SC), por 2 a 3 dias, seguido de redução da dose de diurético para uma dose de manutenção, como 1 a 2 mg/kg VO, em intervalos de 12 a 48 horas, ou menos. Casos mais graves de ICC podem necessitar de doses maiores. É importante usar uma dose adequada de diurético que alivie os sinais clínicos, mas evitar dose de manutenção desnecessariamente alta. O uso excessivo de diurético pode levar a fraqueza, hipotensão, síncope, agravamento da azotemia pré-renal e desequilíbrios acidobásicos e eletrolíticos. Dessa forma, deve-se utilizar, sempre, a menor dose possível de diurético, capaz de manter o cão livre de sinais clínicos de ICC. O proprietário deve ser informado sobre a necessidade de contato regular com o veterinário para uma estratégia de tratamento otimizada e individualizada para o cão. Muitas vezes, o proprietário pode ser instruído a alterar a dose, dentro de uma faixa de dose fixa, de acordo com a necessidade do cão. A torsemida é uma alternativa à furosemida. É também um diurético de alça, mas com maior duração de ação, menor suscetibilidade à resistência a diurético e propriedades adjuvantes de antagonista da aldosterona, em comparação com a furosemida.[143] A dose de torsemida recomendada é de 1/10 da dose de furosemida.[143]

Vários estudos clínicos indicam que o pimobendana é indicado como tratamento de primeira linha em cães com ICC causada por DMVM. De fato, atualmente o pimobendana é aprovado para uso veterinário em cães com CMD ou DMVM em muitos países, na dosagem de 0,25 mg/kg/12 horas VO. Há disponibilidade de dados de dois estudos clínicos multicêntricos controlados (Veterinary Study for the Confirmation of Pimobendana in Canine Endocardiosis [VetSCOPE] e Quality of life and Extension of Survival Time [QUEST])[124,144] e de um estudo clínico em um único centro[145], sobre a eficácia do pimobendana em cães com ICC causada por DMVM. Os resultados mostraram que os cães com ICC causada por DMVM que receberam pimobendana como adjuvante na terapia diurética apresentaram sintomas menos graves de ICC e sobrevida mais longa (como indicado por um tempo maior desde o início da terapia até um desfecho envolvendo morte/eutanásia em razão de problema cardíaco ou falha de tratamento), comparativamente àqueles que receberam inibidor da ECA e diuréticos.[124,144,145] De fato, no estudo QUEST mostrou-se que a terapia com pimobendana prolongou a sobrevida (medida como o tempo desde o início da terapia até o parâmetro de avaliação final) em 91%, e uma redução geral de 32% para atingir o primeiro parâmetro de avaliação, comparado com o grupo-controle positivo (benazepril).[124] Os tempos médios de sobrevida foram de 267 dias no grupo tratado com pimobendana, e 140 dias no grupo que recebeu benazepril, e a diferença máxima entre os dois tratamentos (> 20% de diferença na redução do risco) foi constatada, aproximadamente, aos 150 a 330 dias, indicando que o efeito benéfico de pimobendana não ocorreu apenas no início do estudo.[124,144]

O benefício do pimobendana na recuperação de cães com DMVM é provavelmente mediado pela combinação de vasodilatação e aumento da contratilidade, que reduzem a RM por diminuir o tamanho do VE e do anel da valva mitral, pelo aumento do volume de ejeção sistólico. De fato, estudos clínicos relatam redução no tamanho cardíaco em cães tratados com pimobendana em comparação com o grupo-controle positivo.[141,142,144] Os resultados dos testes clínicos com pimobendana

indicam que o risco de esse fármaco ocasionar aumento da RM (devido ao aumento do gradiente de pressão sistólica através da valva mitral) ou de causar ruptura de cordas tendíneas é comparativamente pequeno. Outros efeitos benéficos do pimobendana no tratamento de cães com DMVM em Estágio C do ACVIM incluem redução na frequência cardíaca e no tempo de trânsito pulmonar,[142] e menor tendência de retenção de água livre em comparação com o grupo-controle positivo.[141]

Os inibidores da ECA são indicados em combinação com diuréticos na DMVM avançada e com ICC, porque cães submetidos a testes clínicos controlados com placebo e com inibidor da ECA manifestaram sinais clínicos da doença menos graves, melhor tolerância ao exercício[146,147] e sobrevida mais longa do que os cães que não receberam inibidor da ECA.[148,149] No entanto, atualmente não se sabe se a combinação de pimobendana e inibidor da ECA confere um melhor resultado, em comparação com o uso exclusivo de pimobendana, quando qualquer um é adicionado à terapia diurética em curso. A dose do inibidor da ECA (p. ex., enalapril, benazepril, lisinopril, ramipril e imidapril) é geralmente fixa e depende do inibidor específico da ECA utilizado. Na faixa de dose recomendada para uso em cães e gatos, os efeitos vasodilatadores dos medicamentos não são proeminentes e os efeitos colaterais associados à hipotensão, como desmaio e síncope, são raros.[87,122,146,147,150] Uma razão para isso pode ser que os efeitos de curta duração dos inibidores da ECA na circulação dependam da atividade do sistema renina-angiotensina-aldosterona (SRAA) antes da administração do medicamento: quanto maior a ação, maior o efeito do fármaco.[151] Na combinação com diuréticos, como a furosemida, os inibidores da ECA têm um efeito sinérgico na ação do diurético, neutralizando o estímulo reflexo do SRAA, que ocorre na terapia diurética. Assim, os inibidores da ECA diminuem a tendência de retenção de líquido e neutralizam a vasoconstrição periférica e outros efeitos negativos no coração.

A espironolactona, que é antagonista da aldosterona e um diurético poupador de potássio, atualmente tem o seu uso aprovado na União Europeia como tratamento adjuvante à outra terapia de ICC em curso em cães com DMVM. Essa aprovação foi baseada em testes clínicos para registro do fármaco, que mostraram que a espironolactona, quando adicionada a outra terapia de ICC, reduziu o risco de atingir o parâmetro de avaliação primária do estudo, que consistia em morte cardíaca relacionada, eutanásia ou agravamento da ICC.[152] Isso sugere que pode ser mais vantajoso iniciar a terapia com espironolactona no estágio inicial da doença do que iniciá-la previamente (ver ICC recorrente). Esse estudo também mostrou que o tratamento de cães com espironolactona é comparativamente seguro e o risco de hiperpotassemia é baixo.

O uso de digoxina no tratamento de cães com DMVM é controverso. Existe uma carência geral de evidências científicas que apoiem o uso da digoxina. Alguns cardiologistas, no entanto, iniciam o tratamento com digoxina assim que surgem sinais clínicos de ICC. A digoxina é um inotrópico positivo fraco em comparação com o pimobendana, mas é útil para reduzir a taquicardia reflexa, normalizando a atividade dos barorreceptores e reduzindo a atividade simpática central.[153] Assim, a digoxina pode ser útil para reduzir a taquicardia sinusal, ou para tratar taquicardia supraventricular, como fibrilação atrial, e para abolir ou limitar a frequência dos episódios de síncope (ver texto anterior).

A conduta clínica de cães com ICC branda a moderada após o início do tratamento é variável. Contatos regulares com o proprietário, por telefone ou e-mail, devem ser mantidos quando o cão é submetido a tratamento ambulatorial, a fim de monitorar o resultado terapêutico e estabelecer uma dose de manutenção adequada de diurético. O paciente deve ser submetido a novo exame após 1 a 2 semanas de tratamento e, posteriormente, a cada 3 a 6 meses. Casos mais graves podem necessitar de monitoramento mais frequente da doença. O proprietário deve ser instruído a aferir a frequência respiratória durante o sono, várias vezes (de preferência deve ser < 30/min); também deve ser informado sobre a ocorrência de possíveis complicações no futuro. Em regiões de clima sazonal, pode ser útil um novo exame do cão antes que ocorra elevação da temperatura, recomendando ao proprietário que evite submeter o animal a alta temperatura ambiente, se possível. O uso de dietas com baixo teor de sódio como terapia complementar em pacientes com ICC é controverso. Atualmente, não há estudos clínicos de que tal procedimento seja benéfico no tratamento de ICC em cães e gatos. No entanto, cães com DMVM sintomática devem evitar ingestão excessiva de sódio. Cães que se mantêm estáveis com o tratamento da insuficiência cardíaca geralmente toleram caminhadas, em seu próprio ritmo, mas exercícios extenuantes devem ser evitados.

Cães com ICC recorrente (estágios C ou D do ACVIM; ver Capítulo 247)

A dose de manutenção do diurético (furosemida) em um paciente com DMVM geralmente deve ser gradualmente aumentada ao longo de semanas ou anos, a fim de evitar recidiva dos sinais clínicos de ICC. Frequentemente, as razões para o aumento da dose incluem dispneia recorrente causada por edema pulmonar ou, menos comumente, desenvolvimento de ascite. Ascite grave, que compromete a respiração, pode necessitar de abdominocentese (ver Capítulo 90). No entanto, muitos casos de DMVM com ascite menos grave respondem a doses crescentes de diurético. Mesmo em casos que requerem abdominocentese, a dose de diurético deve ser aumentada, pois ocorre recidiva de ascite sem uma mudança na medicação após a retirada do líquido peritoneal. Quando a dose de furosemida atingir um valor de, aproximadamente, 4 a 5 mg/kg/8 a 12 horas, por via oral, pode-se substituir a furosemida pela torsemida. Além disso, o bloqueio sequencial do néfron deve ser obtido pela adição de outro diurético. O medicamento de escolha é a espironolactona (1 a 3 mg/kg/12 a 24 h, por via oral) (ver texto anterior sobre ICC discreta a moderada). No entanto, pode-se utilizar um diurético tiazida, como a hidroclorotiazida (2 a 4 mg/kg/12 h, por via oral) ou trianereno (1 a 2 mg/kg/12 h, por via oral) ou amilorida (0,1 a 0,3 mg/kg/24 h, por via oral). Os estudos sobre trianereno e amilorida em medicina veterinária são limitados. Como o tratamento com furosemida precede e é usado concomitantemente com esses medicamentos, o risco de hiperpotassemia é baixo, mesmo quando são adicionados a um paciente que no momento é tratado com um inibidor da ECA. O risco de induzir azotemia pré-renal, hipotensão e desequilíbrio acidobásico e eletrolítico aumenta com a intensidade do tratamento diurético. No entanto, o clínico geralmente deve reconhecer que em algum grau tais distúrbios podem ocorrer ao tratar um paciente com ICC e, embora eles possam ocorrer, raramente resultam em problemas clínicos.

Cães com ICC grave e risco à vida (fulminante) (estágio C ou D do ACVIM)

As causas de ICC aguda grave geralmente incluem subtratamento de ICC existente, ruptura de corda tendínea importante, desenvolvimento de fibrilação atrial ou atividade física intensa, tal como perseguir pássaros ou gatos, na presença de DMVV relevante. Pacientes com ICC grave apresentam evidência radiográfica de edema intersticial e/ou alveolar grave e sinais clínicos importantes de ICC em repouso. Frequentemente manifestam dispneia e taquipneia graves e apresentam frequência respiratória na faixa de 40 a 90 movimentos/minuto. Durante a tosse podem expectorar espuma branca ou rósea, que é parte do líquido do edema. Esses cães necessitam de hospitalização imediata e tratamento agressivo. É importante não estressar os cães

com ICC grave ou fulminante, pois o estresse pode levar à morte. Uma sedação leve, para acalmar o cão, pode ser indicada em pacientes que se debatem para respirar (ver Capítulo 138). Um sedativo comumente usado nesse cenário é o butorfanol (0,25 mg/kg IM, IV, repetindo a dose após 30 a 60 minutos) ou a combinação de buprenorfina (0,0075 a 0,01 mg/kg IM) e acepromazina (0,01 a 0,03 mg/kg IV, IM ou SC). Além disso, radiografias de tórax e outros procedimentos diagnósticos podem ter que esperar até que o cão se torne clinicamente estabilizado com o tratamento com furosemida. Cães com dispneia relevante se beneficiam da administração intravenosa de furosemida, na dose de 1 a 4 mg/kg IV, em intervalos de 2 a 6 horas ou mais (ver Capítulo 141).[121,154] A furosemida pode ser administrada por via intramuscular, caso não seja impossível a colocação de um cateter intravenoso. A dose exata de furosemida depende não apenas da gravidade dos sinais clínicos, mas também do fato de o cão já estar ou não em tratamento oral com esse diurético. Caso a resposta inicial à administração de um *bolus* de furosemida não seja efetiva para melhorar a dispneia e a frequência respiratória após mais de 2 horas, a furosemida pode ser administrada na forma de taxa de infusão contínua (TIC), na dose de 1 mg/kg/h IV, após o tratamento com o *bolus* inicial.[121,154] Pode-se realizar tratamento com pimobendana, administrado como dose única IV de 0,15 mg/kg e continuado após 12 horas, por via oral, na dose de 0,25 a 0,3 mg/kg/12 horas, ou apenas por via oral.[121] A documentação clínica da eficácia do pimobendana na ICC aguda grave é limitada, mas nesse caso o seu uso é indicado devido a seu efeito hemodinâmico[155,156] em estudos experimentais (modelo de estimulação) em cães[157] e em experiência clínica.

Oxigenoterapia é sempre benéfica em pacientes com hipoxemia e pode ser administrada preferencialmente usando uma gaiola de oxigênio, desde que a temperatura na gaiola possa ser controlada (ver Capítulo 131). A insuflação nasal ou uma máscara facial também podem ser usadas, desde que o animal as aceite sem dificuldades.

Para os pacientes gravemente enfermos, pode-se administrar um vasodilatador arterial e/ou um venodilatador, a fim de reduzir a pós-carga e estabilizar a ICC (ver Capítulo 247). Os agentes vasodilatadores mais comumente usados nesse caso são pomadas venodilatadoras à base de nitroglicerina (4 a 12 mg/12 horas, uso tópico), que atuam aliviando a carga do coração e vasodilatadores arteriais, tal como anlodipino ou hidralazina, por via oral, ou nitroprussiato por via intravenosa, a fim de reduzir o volume pós-carga. A dose de vasodilatador arterial pode necessitar de ajustes em cães que já estejam em uso de inibidor da ECA. Mostrou-se que a administração de 0,1 mg de anlodipino/kg/24 h reduziu a pressão do AE, em cães com RM experimental,[158] bem como a gravidade da RM em cães com DMVM.[138] A hidralazina tem sido usada em pacientes com DMVM, em dose inicial de 0,5 a 2 mg/kg/12 h VO, mas deve ser usada com cautela devido a possíveis reações adversas. Ademais, o intervalo entre as doses deve ser aumentado de administração diária para semanal, com dose de manutenção apropriada de 1 a 2 mg/kg/12 h, por via oral, ou até que desenvolva hipotensão, detectada por medições da pressão arterial ou por sinais clínicos. Taquicardia reflexa pode se desenvolver em resposta à hipotensão, e problemas gastrintestinais às vezes são observados. Em cães considerados muito doentes para esperar pelos efeitos da administração oral do medicamento na redução da pós-carga ou para o suporte inotrópico (p. ex., pimobendana com ou sem hidralazina ou anlodipino), nitroprussiato (para redução da pós-carga em caso de edema pulmonar potencialmente fatal) ou dobutamina (para suporte inotrópico do paciente hipotenso) devem ser administrados por meio de TIC IV (ver Capítulo 141). Ambos os fármacos podem ser administrados na dose de 0,5 a 1 mcg/kg/minuto, com aumento gradual a cada 15 a 30 minutos, até a dose máxima de aproximadamente 10 mcg/kg/min. Esses fármacos, isoladamente ou em combinação, podem ser utilizados por 12 a 48 horas, para melhorar a condição hemodinâmica e controlar o edema pulmonar cardiogênico refratário. Recomenda-se o monitoramento contínuo do paciente por meio de eletrocardiografia e mensuração da pressão arterial, a fim de minimizar os riscos potenciais dessa terapia (ver Capítulos 99 e 103).

Pacientes com ICC grave ou fulminante necessitam de monitoramento inicial frequente da frequência respiratória, pois esse parâmetro reflete a resposta clínica ao tratamento com furosemida. A diminuição significativa da frequência respiratória nas primeiras horas indica uma terapia bem-sucedida, enquanto a ausência de alterações indica que é necessário aumentar a dose de furosemida ou sua administração deve ser mais frequente. Assim que ocorre redução da frequência respiratória, a dose de furosemida pode ser reduzida de acordo com a condição do cão e o julgamento clínico. Achados laboratoriais anormais, como azotemia pré-renal, desequilíbrio eletrolítico e desidratação, são comuns após altas doses de furosemida. Mais uma vez, essas anormalidades raramente são um problema clínico e os valores dos exames laboratoriais tendem à normalidade com a melhora clínica e quando o cão volta a se alimentar e beber água. A desidratação geralmente não é grave, mesmo após o tratamento intensivo com furosemida, e a reidratação intravenosa deve ser realizada lentamente e com cautela nos casos em que é necessária, pois o volume excessivo de líquido administrado pode ocasionar edema pulmonar.

Do ponto de vista ético, a eutanásia também deve ser considerada em cães em ICC grave ou fulminante, se o cão já recebe altas doses de diuréticos e outras terapias de insuficiência cardíaca, devido ao mau prognóstico a longo prazo, ao maior risco de ausência de resposta à intensificação adicional do tratamento da ICC e/ou à maior probabilidade de efeitos colaterais adversos.

Prognóstico após o início de ICC

Algumas variáveis clínicas fornecem informações prognósticas após o início da ICC em cães com DMVM. Tem se demonstrado que o tipo de terapia adjuvante influencia a sobrevivência (aumento da sobrevida constatada em cães tratados com pimobendana e os inibidores da ECA enalapril e benazepril).[124,148,149] Além disso, o tempo de sobrevida esperado diminui com doses de manutenção mais elevadas de furosemida, com maior intolerância ao exercício, gravidade do prolapso da valva mitral, aumento do tamanho cardíaco e gravidade da RM (escore VHS [vertebral heart size], tamanho do AE [AE/AO], dimensão do VE no fim da diástole, velocidade da onda E diastólica), piora da função sistólica (aumento da dimensão do VE no fim da sístole) e diminuição da concentração sérica de creatinina (indicando caquexia cardíaca em desenvolvimento).[4,101,124,148] Existem algumas evidências de que a raça também afeta as respostas clínicas após o início da ICC, mas os resultados atualmente não são conclusivos. Por fim, o desenvolvimento de uma complicação (ver a seguir) pode estar associado a um pior desfecho clínico.

Complicações associadas à doença mixomatosa da valva mitral

Tosse devido à compressão do brônquio principal esquerdo. O aumento grave do AE pode induzir tosse, mesmo na ausência de congestão e edema pulmonar, devido à compressão do brônquio principal esquerdo, que pode ser detectada na imagem radiográfica em projeção lateral. No entanto, a tosse devido a outros problemas respiratórios, como instabilidade traqueal, também é comumente observada em raças frequentemente acometidas por DMVM. A gravidade da tosse pode variar de alguns episódios por dia à tosse constante. Tosse branda ocasional não requer medicação diária devido ao esforço de dar medicação e possíveis efeitos colaterais adversos. Além disso, há pouca evidência disponível sobre o efeito dos tipos de medicamentos disponíveis para aliviar ou reduzir a tosse. No caso de tosse

relevante, provavelmente causada pela compressão do brônquio principal esquerdo, a terapia visa suprimir o reflexo da tosse ou reduzir a influência da causa primária da compressão, ou seja, o aumento do AE. A administração de supressores de tosse, como bitartrato de hidrocodona (2,5 a 10 mg/cão, via oral, em intervalos de 6 a 12 h), butorfanol (0,55 a 1,1 mg/kg, via oral, a cada 6 a 12 h), ou dextrometorfano (0,5 a 2 mg/kg, via oral, a cada 6 a 8 h), pode aliviar a tosse em alguns casos. Cães com evidência de instabilidade traqueal concomitante ou doença crônica de vias respiratórias de pequeno calibre podem melhorar com a administração de broncodilatador ou glicocorticoide por um breve período. Diversos derivados da xantina, como aminofilina (8 a 11 mg/kg, via oral, a cada 6 a 8 h), teofilina (ação prolongada), na dose de 20mg/kg, via oral, a cada 12 h, e oxitrifilina (ação prolongada), na dose de 25 a 30 mg/kg, via oral, a cada 12 h, são broncodilatadores comumente utilizados, embora a eficácia desses fármacos seja consideravelmente variável entre os indivíduos. Os agonistas do receptor beta-2, como a terbutalina e o salbutamol, devem ser usados com cautela em cães com DMVM, pois esses medicamentos podem causar elevações indesejáveis na contratilidade e frequência cardíaca, devido ao estímulo do receptor beta-2 do miocárdio.

Teoricamente, a tosse devida à compressão do brônquio principal esquerdo poderia melhorar com a redução do tamanho do AE e do VE. Isso pode ser conseguido reduzindo-se a RM e/ou a pressão venosa pulmonar. O benefício clínico real de tais tratamentos na gravidade da tosse é desconhecido atualmente. Medicamentos com potencial para reduzir a RM, diminuindo a pós-carga, incluem os vasodilatadores arteriais anlodipino e hidralazina e, em menor extensão, inibidores da ECA (ver texto anterior sobre ICC grave e com risco à vida [fulminante] [Estágio C ou D do ACVIM]). Além disso, relata-se que o inodilator pimobendana reduz o tamanho do coração em cães com DMVM, tanto em curto como em longo prazo.[141,142] A monoterapia diurética pode ser utilizada para diminuir a RM, reduzindo o volume sanguíneo e, assim, o tamanho do VE. No entanto, os diuréticos ativam o sistema renina-angiotensina-aldosterona (SRAA)[159] e a longo prazo podem causar distúrbios eletrolíticos. Assim, diuréticos devem ser reservados aos pacientes com sintomas de congestão e edema pulmonar ou àqueles em que supressores de tosse, glicocorticoides e vasodilatadores não aliviaram os sinais clínicos mais graves da tosse.

ICC direita devido à hipertensão pulmonar. Muitos pacientes com histórico de DMVM crônica desenvolvem ICC direita. Presume-se que essa condição se desenvolva como consequência de RT crônica concomitante, atribuível à degeneração mixomatosa, ou ao desenvolvimento de hipertensão pulmonar, ou uma combinação de ambas (Figura 251.8). Na DMVM, acredita-se que a hipertensão pulmonar se desenvolva secundariamente ao aumento persistente do AE e da pressão venosa pulmonar, mas a doença crônica concomitante das vias respiratórias também pode ser um fator contribuinte. Indivíduos com hipertensão pulmonar são sensíveis ao exercício, com sinais de fraqueza ou colapso, mesmo em atividades físicas leves. O exame físico pode revelar evidências de ICC direita, como ascite, derrame pleural, congestão hepática e esplênica e distensão das veias jugulares, com pulsações anormais. A presença e o grau de hipertensão pulmonar podem ser indiretamente quantificados por meio de ecocardiografia com Doppler (ver Capítulos 104 e 243). Recentemente mostrou-se que um gradiente de pressão > 55 mmHg é um indicador preditor negativo independentemente do desfecho da doença.[57]

O tratamento de cães com hipertensão pulmonar pode ser difícil. O objetivo da terapia é eliminar os fatores contribuintes e restringir a atividade física. A suplementação de oxigênio é indicada em casos de colapso agudo (ver Capítulo 131). Como a pressão venosa pulmonar persistentemente aumentada é, em grande parte, responsável pela ocorrência da doença, a terapia deve ser direcionada como se fosse para DMVM com congestão

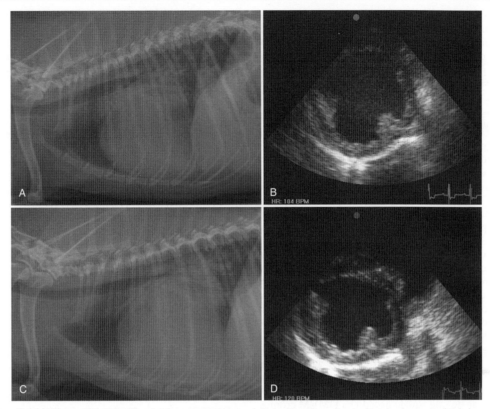

Figura 251.8 Radiografias laterais esquerdas (**A** e **C**) e do eixo curto paraesternal direito (**B** e **D**), no fim da diástole, de um cão (10 kg) com doença mixomatosa da valva mitral (DMVM) grave e aumento cardíaco grave, mostrando desenvolvimento de hipertensão pulmonar. O cão desenvolvera ICC, mas estabilizou-se com a terapia de insuficiência cardíaca, quando as imagens **A** e **B** foram obtidas. As imagens **C** e **D** foram obtidas 1 ano depois, quando o cão manifestava intolerância ao exercício mais marcante e evidência de ICC direita. Nessa fase, o tamanho radiográfico do coração tinha aumentado, de VHS (*vertebral heart scale*) de 13,8, em **A**, para 15, em C, mas o diâmetro diastólico final do ventrículo esquerdo diminuiu de 5,5 cm, em **B**, para 4 cm, em **D**, e o ventrículo esquerdo estava mais afastado do transdutor devido ao aumento do ventrículo direito. Também se nota evidência de flacidez do septo e o gradiente de pressão sistólica da regurgitação tricúspide era de 64 mmHg.

pulmonar (ver Conduta Clínica). Além disso, comumente utiliza-se sildenafila, um vasodilatador arterial pulmonar,[160,161] na dose de 0,5 a 2 mg/kg em intervalos de 8 a 24 h (em alguns casos pode ser necessária dose de 2 a 3 mg/kg/12 h VO). Uma série de casos de tratamento com sildenafila em cães, publicados, está disponível, nos quais muitos dos cães incluídos apresentavam hipertensão pulmonar devido à DMVM crônica grave.[160,161] Uma grande desvantagem desse fármaco é que ele é relativamente caro. Uma alternativa menos dispendiosa que o uso de sildenafila no tratamento de hipertensão pulmonar, nesse contexto, é o pimobendana. Em cães experimentais, constatou-se que esse fármaco diminui a pressão arterial pulmonar, devido à supressão da fosfodiesterase III;[139] em outro estudo cruzado de curta duração em cães com DMVM, também se relatou diminuição da pressão arterial pulmonar.[162] Assim, cães com DMVM e ICC crônica que desenvolvem hipertensão pulmonar provavelmente podem se beneficiar dessa terapia, se ainda não a receberam. Também pode ser indicado tratamento com broncodilatador, além de metilxantinas e agonistas seletivos de beta-2, porém estes últimos devem ser usados com cautela em cães com DMVM. Pode ser necessário um tratamento diurético agressivo para resolver a ascite, se presente. A drenagem física do líquido abdominal também propicia alívio temporário da ascite, dando aos medicamentos prescritos tempo adicional para fazerem efeito (ver Capítulo 90).

Desenvolvimento de arritmias que ocasionam episódios de síncope e/ou exacerbação aguda dos sintomas de ICC. Com a progressão da DMVM, não é incomum que ocorram episódios de síncope (ver Sinais Clínicos e Capítulo 30). Em cães com DMVM com episódios de síncope, é importante verificar se o paciente realmente está desmaiando ou se apresenta doença neurológica ou outra enfermidade. Além disso, é importante excluir a presença de ICC, hipertensão pulmonar ou bradiarritmias, como bloqueio AV de terceiro grau ou taquiarritmia sustentada, assim como fibrilação atrial. O aumento do AE predispõe à ocorrência de batimentos supraventriculares prematuros, fibrilação atrial e taquicardia supraventricular (ver Capítulo 248).[91] Embora as taquiarritmias ventriculares ocorram em cães com DMVM, geralmente em estágio avançado da doença, a taquiarritmia supraventricular intermitente é muito mais comum.[79,91] Tipicamente, o ECG de 24 horas (Holter) mostra episódios de ritmo supraventricular rápido imediatamente seguido de bradicardia, durante a qual o cão desmaia.[79,91] Cães que desenvolvem fibrilação atrial sustentada ou taquicardia supraventricular frequentemente têm um histórico prévio de DMVM, com início agudo de edema pulmonar. Além de outros achados característicos de DMVM; nesses casos, nota-se alteração do ritmo cardíaco. O objetivo do tratamento é aliviar o edema pulmonar, conforme descrito anteriormente, e reduzir a frequência cardíaca a um valor aceitável, para melhorar o débito cardíaco. Diltiazem e/ou digoxina são os medicamentos de escolha para os cães com taquicardia supraventricular.

O tratamento de cães com episódios de síncope, descrito anteriormente, ou fibrilação atrial sustentada/taquicardia supraventricular geralmente inclui a administração de digoxina (na dose de 0,22 mg/m² ou menos, via oral, a cada 12 h), a fim de controlar a taquiarritmia supraventricular. Caso isso não controle a frequência e a duração da taquicardia intermitente (e episódios de síncope) ou, em caso de fibrilação atrial com alta frequência ventricular, pode-se adicionar diltiazem (na dose de 0,5 a 2 mg/kg/8 h, via oral) ou um antagonista do receptor beta-1, como atenolol (0,25 a 2 mg/kg, via oral, a cada 12 a 24 h) ou metoprolol (0,5 a 1 mg/kg, via oral, em intervalos de 8 a 12 h). Ver Capítulo 248. Deve-se ressaltar que os indivíduos com DMVM geralmente são sensíveis a fármacos inotrópicos negativos, como os antagonistas dos receptores beta, que devem ser evitados em cães com ICC aguda. Portanto, esses medicamentos devem ser iniciados na menor dose possível, com aumentos gradativos e monitoramento cuidadoso. Nos casos de ICC, outro objetivo da terapia é aliviar o edema pulmonar, conforme descrito anteriormente no item sobre tratamento.

Exacerbação aguda da congestão e edema pulmonar devido à ruptura de cordas tendíneas. Pode-se suspeitar de ruptura de cordas tendíneas em todos os cães que apresentam DMVM, com desenvolvimento agudo de congestão e edema pulmonar (ver Vídeo 251.17); é uma ocorrência rara em gatos. As rupturas mais importantes envolvem as cordas tendíneas de primeira ordem (mais importantes) que estão conectadas ao folheto septal; em geral, esses pacientes morrem rapidamente devido à sobrecarga de volume aguda e ao edema pulmonar fulminante. A ruptura de cordas tendíneas menos importantes e, às vezes, de primeira ordem conectadas no lobo da parede livre podem resultar em sinais clínicos menos relevantes ou em nenhum sinal clínico.[100] A ruptura de cordas tendíneas importantes causa aumento agudo da RM e os achados clínicos podem diferir daqueles verificados na RM crônica. Devido ao aumento agudo da RM, pode haver um aumento acentuado do AE e da pressão venosa pulmonar, ocasionando edema pulmonar agudo, hipertensão pulmonar e insuficiência cardíaca direita.[55,67] O exame físico desses pacientes frequentemente revela um sopro cardíaco de menor intensidade do que aquele notado na DMVM crônica; nessa condição, é mais provável que haja um ritmo de galope S_3 (ver Capítulo 55) e distensão das veias jugulares, com pulsações, do que na DMVM crônica. Os achados radiográficos e ecocardiográficos quanto ao tamanho do coração são variáveis, dependendo de quanto a DMVM progrediu antes da ruptura das cordas tendíneas. A ecocardiografia com Doppler mostra RM grave, na imagem bidimensional (2D) pode-se notar um segmento flexível do folheto da valva mitral. As radiografias do tórax mostram um padrão intersticial e alveolar muito evidente, com dilatação das veias pulmonares. Esses pacientes necessitam de cuidados intensivos para estabilizar o quadro clínico e, posteriormente, terapia de manutenção para DMVM (consulte a seção Tratamento e o Capítulo 141). Desde que não haja ruptura de corda tendínea de primeira ordem, conectada ao folheto septal, muitos animais com essa cardiopatia podem ser mantidos com o auxílio de medicação apropriada.

Ruptura do átrio esquerdo e tamponamento cardíaco. Como consequência da dilatação na DMVM, o AE apresenta parede delgada e mais vulnerável ao aumento de pressão. A laceração do endocárdio é um achado frequente após a morte em cães com histórico de DMVM crônica (Vídeo 251.18).[72] O significado desse achado é que a lesão pode progredir para ruptura do AE, com desenvolvimento súbito de hemopericárdio, tamponamento cardíaco e morte súbita (Vídeo 251.19). Na maioria dos casos de ruptura atrial e tamponamento cardíaco ocorre morte súbita. Muitas vezes há histórico de trauma, excitação ou atividade física, que precede ruptura atrial e morte súbita. Em cães que sobreviveram ao evento inicial, podem ser notados sinais clínicos de tamponamento cardíaco associados a sintomas de DMVM. O desenvolvimento agudo de ascite, colapso ou intolerância ao exercício acentuada é uma condição prevista. O exame físico pode revelar sinais de derrame pericárdico (ver Capítulo 254). Para o diagnóstico definitivo, é necessária a realização de ecocardiografia, a fim de detectar a presença de efusão pericárdica relevante em associação com DMVM; todavia, no exame ecocardiográfico geralmente é difícil detectar a laceração. O tratamento da ruptura atrial com hemopericárdio e tamponamento cardíaco é geralmente em vão. Indica-se pericardiocentese imediata (ver Capítulo 102), com remoção do líquido pericárdico para aliviar o tamponamento, sem remover um volume tão elevado a ponto de causar hemorragia adicional. Se a hemorragia persistir após a pericardiocentese, a última opção é a realização de toracotomia de emergência, com pericardiectomia e fechamento da lesão; contudo, o prognóstico desse procedimento é muito reservado.

ENDOCARDITE INFECCIOSA

A endocardite infecciosa (EI) é uma doença acompanhada de risco à vida, causada por microrganismos que colonizam o endocárdio, geralmente resultando em lesões proliferativas ou erosivas da valva e outras estruturas cardíacas e, consequentemente, regurgitação da valva (Figura 251.9 A). A vegetação valvar pode causar tromboembolismo ou infecções metastáticas envolvendo múltiplos órgãos e ocasionando uma grande variedade de sinais clínicos, o que dificulta o diagnóstico.

Ocorrência

Em cães submetidos à necropsia, relata-se prevalência de endocardite infecciosa de 0,09 a 6,6%.[163] A avaliação dos dados de cães encaminhados para um hospital de ensino veterinário indica que a EI é uma condição clínica comparativamente rara, com prevalências que variam de 0,04 a 0,13%.[164,165] No entanto, dada a dificuldade para diagnosticar a doença, os sinais clínicos inespecíficos e a proporção comparativamente baixa de cães submetidos à necropsia, é provável que a real ocorrência seja consideravelmente maior. Raças de médio a grande porte, principalmente cães de raças puras, de meia-idade, têm maior risco de desenvolver endocardite.[166,167] A prevalência em gatos, com base na experiência clínica, é considerada 7 a 10 vezes menor do que em cães.[165,168,169] Animais com cardiopatia congênita têm baixa incidência de EI,[129] mas há relato de associação de EI com estenose subaórtica[170] e PDA.[171] Não se constatou qualquer relação entre EI e DMVM, em cães, mesmo após procedimentos odontológicos e em outras causas de bacteriemia.[129]

Etiologia e patogênese

A bacteriemia transitória ou persistente é um pré-requisito para o desenvolvimento de EI. A origem da bacteriemia pode ser uma infecção ativa localizada em algum local do corpo. Em alguns casos de EI não se consegue detectar clinicamente a origem da infecção.[172,173] Possível via para as bactérias atingirem e infectarem o endocárdio é o contato direto dos microrganismos com a superfície endotelial através da corrente sanguínea ou de capilares valvares (vasculite).[174] A maioria das bactérias requer fatores predisponentes para causar EI, como depressão do sistema imunológico ou lesão ao tecido endotelial,[129] por vezes associada a depósitos de complexos fibrina-plaquetas, para aderir à valva e causar EI.[175] Proteínas da matriz extracelular, tromboplastina e fator tecidual desencadeiam a coagulação. Ocorre ativação de fatores de coagulação no endotélio lesionado e de mediadores inflamatórios. O processo inflamatório, juntamente com as enzimas liberadas pelas bactérias, contribui para a degradação do tecido valvar.

Um grande número de bactérias foi identificado em cães com bacteriemia[176] (ver a seção sobre hemocultura a seguir), algumas sabidamente causadoras de EI.[172,173] Na verdade, os microrganismos que comumente causam EI são aqueles com maior capacidade de aderência à valva lesionada, incluindo *Staphylococcus* e *Streptococcus* spp. Bactérias como *Staphylococcus aureus* e *Bartonella* podem penetrar nas células endoteliais e outras células, e assim se protegerem do sistema imunológico. Além disso, as bactérias também são protegidas do sistema imunológico e de substâncias antibióticas por se incorporar ao coágulo.

As consequências da EI dependem de vários fatores: virulência do microrganismo infeccioso; local da infecção; grau de lesão valvar; influência da vegetação microbiana na função valvar;

CAPÍTULO 251 • Doenças Cardiovasculares no Início da Idade Adulta

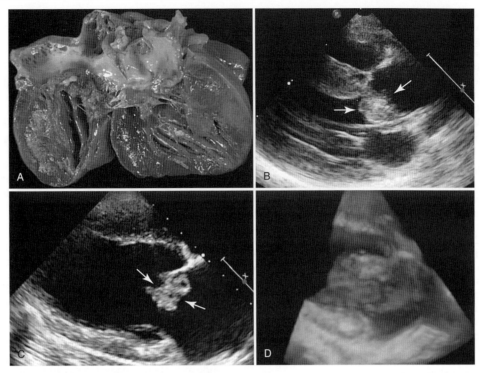

Figura 251.9 Endocardite infecciosa. **A.** Vegetação na valva mitral. Ecocardiograma bidimensional em um gato com endocardite infecciosa na valva aórtica (*setas*) vista no eixo longo paraesternal direito (**B**). Endocardite infecciosa na valva mitral (*setas*) vista no eixo longo paraesternal direito (**C**). Ecocardiograma 3D do mesmo cão de (**C**), mas a imagem é ligeiramente rotacionada para possibilitar a inspeção da valva mitral, no lado atrial (**D**). Note o tamanho da massa ecogênica de formato irregular presa ao folheto septal da valva mitral. (Cortesia Páll S. Leifsson, Universidade de Copenhague, Dinamarca.)

produção de exotoxinas ou endotoxinas; interação com o sistema imunológico, com formação de imunocomplexos; e desenvolvimento de tromboembolismo e infecções metastáticas. A bacteriemia por microrganismos gram-negativos frequentemente resulta em manifestações clínicas hiperagudas ou agudas, enquanto a bacteriemia por bactérias gram-positivas geralmente resulta em doença subaguda ou crônica. A necrose e a destruição do estroma valvar e/ou das cordas tendíneas ocorrem rapidamente na EI hiperaguda ou aguda, causando insuficiência valvar e insuficiência cardíaca. A deposição de imunocomplexos em diferentes órgãos pode causar glomerulonefrite, miosite ou poliartrite.[177] Complicações tromboembólicas como causas de sinais clínicos foram relatadas em aproximadamente 30 a 40% dos cães com EI[129,167] e os pulmões parecem ser o local mais comum de instalação de êmbolos, seguidos dos rins e da parte distal da artéria aorta.[129]

Patologia

A vegetação microbiana associada à EI afeta principalmente o lado esquerdo do coração, com maior prevalência de lesões na valva mitral, comparativamente à valva aórtica.[129,167] Pode haver envolvimento mural do endocárdio, com ou sem lesões valvulares concomitantes;[129] todavia, o envolvimento do lado direito do coração é incomum.[129] Os achados patológicos são variáveis e dependem da virulência do microrganismo infeccioso, do tempo de infecção e da resposta imune. A vegetação microbiana intracardíaca consiste em diferentes camadas de fibrina, plaquetas, bactérias, hemácias e leucócitos, frequentemente coberta por um endotélio intacto. As bactérias podem continuar a crescer apesar da terapia com antibiótico, devido a sua localização profunda na vegetação e à lenta atividade metabólica.[175]

Histórico e sinais clínicos

O diagnóstico de EI pode ser facilmente negligenciado, pois o histórico clínico e os sintomas não são específicos e pode não haver fatores predisponentes que levem à suspeita de EI.

Os fatores predisponentes que, em combinação com os sinais clínicos, devem levar à suspeita de EI são: terapia com drogas imunossupressoras, como corticosteroides,[129,166] cirurgia não bucal dentro de 3 meses, trauma em superfície mucosa do trato bucal ou genital e infecção nessas regiões do corpo, uso de cateter de demora, feridas infectadas, abscessos ou pioderma.[129,178]

Os sinais clínicos são variáveis e ocorrem em diferentes combinações. Claudicação tem sido descrita como a queixa mais frequente em cães com EI, seguida de sintomas inespecíficos, como letargia, anorexia, anormalidades respiratórias, fraqueza, febre (frequentemente recorrente), perda de peso e distúrbios gastrintestinais.[166,167] Rigidez e dor em articulações ou músculos podem ser causadas por reações imunomediadas; a dor abdominal pode ser causada por infarto renal ou esplênico secundário, embolização séptica ou formação de abscesso. Se a doença causar lesão valvular grave, podem ocorrer sinais de ICC e síncope devido a arritmias. Arritmias, principalmente ventriculares, foram relatadas em 62% dos cães com EI na valva aórtica.[172,173]

Exame físico

A maioria dos sinais clínicos carece de especificidade para EI. No entanto, febre, sopro cardíaco (particularmente se recentemente instalado) e claudicação são considerados sintomas clássicos.[129] A febre é relatada em 50 a 90% dos cães com EI.[166,167] A ausência de febre é relatada como mais comum em casos com envolvimento da valva aórtica,[167,172] um achado que pode ser atribuído à infecção por *Bartonella*. Relata-se que as infecções por *Bartonella* são frequentemente mais afebris,[167] mas esse achado também pode ser atribuído ao tratamento já iniciado com antibióticos. Como a insuficiência aórtica grave é incomum em cães, a detecção de sopro diastólico, e pulso periférico associado, deve levantar a suspeita de EI na valva aórtica. O sopro sistólico pode ser decorrência da destruição da valva mitral, resultando em regurgitação mitral (RM), ou por vegetações que causam obstrução do fluxo sanguíneo na valva aórtica, levando à estenose valvar.[166] Deve-se ressaltar o relato de que 26% dos cães com EI não apresentam sopros audíveis (Áudio 251.6).[166] Claudicação

SEÇÃO 16 • Doença Cardiovascular

também é um sintoma inconsistente na EI; em um estudo constatou-se incidência de 34%.[163] É possível constatar vários outros sinais ao exame físico, dependendo de quais órgãos são acometidos por imunocomplexos circulantes ou embolização séptica. Os achados possíveis são reações de dor em músculos ou abdome (baço, intestinos ou rins), extremidades frias, cianose e necrose cutânea causada por embolização grave, além de uma variedade de distúrbios neurológicos se o sistema nervoso central for acometido.

Testes diagnósticos

Achados ecocardiográficos

A ecocardiografia melhora significativamente as possibilidades de diagnóstico e monitoramento de animais com EI.[178] Vegetações valvares podem ser detectadas usando ecocardiografia 2D. As vegetações valvares são vistas como estruturas hiperecoicas (Vídeos 251.20 e 251.21; ver Figura 251.9 B a D), muitas vezes irregularmente delineadas, e com frequência se movem independentemente da valva. Algumas dessas lesões menores podem ser muito difíceis de se distinguir das lesões mixomatosas. Lesões erosivas podem ser mais difíceis de se identificar no ecocardiograma, mas a presença de regurgitação aórtica moderada a grave, detectada no ecocardiograma de fluxo colorido, deve levantar a suspeita de EI na valva aórtica. Outras causas associadas à regurgitação aórtica incluem estenose valvar ou subvalvar congênita, lesões mixomatosas (geralmente apenas regurgitação aórtica branda), hipertensão sistêmica grave e valva aórtica quadricúspide (uma malformação congênita muito incomum). A valva aórtica precisa ser vista de vários planos para ajudar a excluir os diagnósticos diferenciais e detectar a lesão erosiva. A regurgitação mitral ou aórtica pode ser detectada por meio de ecocardiografia Doppler de onda contínua ou com fluxo colorido. A gravidade da regurgitação aórtica pode ser avaliada em imagem da câmara apical esquerda, seja pela avaliação da inclinação do traçado do fluxo regurgitante no Doppler de onda contínua (inclinação mais acentuada indica insuficiência mais grave), seja pela avaliação do tamanho do jato regurgitante no ecocardiograma com fluxo colorido, que fornece uma estimativa semiquantitativa. A avaliação da gravidade da RM está descrita em outra parte deste capítulo e no Capítulo 104. Da mesma forma, as dilatações secundárias do AE e do VE podem ser detectadas por meio de ecocardiografia em modo 2D, 3D ou M, conforme descrito anteriormente. Em casos em que há forte suspeita clínica de EI, mas nenhuma lesão valvar é detectada no ecocardiograma transtorácico, pode-se realizar ecocardiografia transesofágica para se obter uma avaliação mais detalhada das valvas aórtica e mitral.

Achados eletrocardiográficos

Arritmia é relatada em 50 a 75% dos cães com EI.[166,167,172] Batimentos ventriculares prematuros e taquiarritmias ventriculares são as arritmias mais comumente encontradas, mas geralmente não são fatais. Desvio do segmento ST pode ser sugestivo de hipoxia no miocárdio e indicar embolia na artéria coronariana ou isquemia de miocárdio de outras etiologias.[92] Evidências de aumento da câmara cardíaca podem ser vistas na EI crônica. No entanto, todas as anormalidades do ECG mencionadas são inespecíficas.

Achados radiográficos

O exame radiográfico geralmente não adiciona nenhuma informação específica para o diagnóstico de EI. Na EI crônica com insuficiência mitral ou aórtica, pode-se detectar aumento do lado esquerdo do coração. Relata-se que aproximadamente 50% dos cães com EI apresentam ICC, indicada pela presença de infiltrados pulmonares peri-hilares e caudodorsais, sem diferença entre aqueles com EI da valva mitral ou da valva aórtica.[164,167] Surpreendentemente, não se constatou aumento

significativo do AE em uma proporção comparativamente grande dos cães com ICC, presumivelmente indicando um início agudo de regurgitação grave da valva e ICC.[164,176]

Hemocultura

A hemocultura positiva é essencial para estabelecer o diagnóstico de EI e para a escolha do tratamento antimicrobiano apropriado. Infelizmente, relata-se que 60 a 70% das hemoculturas realizadas em cães com EI são negativas.[164,172] A alta proporção de cães submetidos à terapia antimicrobiana antes do momento da obtenção da amostra de sangue para cultura microbiológica contribui, presumivelmente, para a ausência de crescimento bacteriano.[164] Outras causas de hemocultura negativa incluem infecções crônicas "encapsuladas", endocardite não infecciosa (contendo apenas plaquetas e fibrina na vegetação) ou falha de crescimento dos microrganismos da amostra. Algumas bactérias podem crescer lentamente e as amostras não devem ser consideradas definitivamente negativas antes de 10 dias de incubação (Bartonella requer incubação por até 4 semanas). Em 90% das hemoculturas, nota-se resultado positivo dentro de 72 horas após a incubação.[179] O teste PCR pode ser utilizado para amplificar e detectar ácido nucleico bacteriano no sangue e, assim, aumentar potencialmente a probabilidade de detectar bacteriemia. No entanto, parece que esse teste não é mais sensível do que a hemocultura, na detecção de bacteriemia em cães com suspeita de endocardite.[180] O risco de cultura negativa diminui quando a coleta e o manuseio das amostras são adequados.[175] O tempo para a amostragem provavelmente não é crítico, mas é crítico para evitar a contaminação da amostra. A técnica para obtenção de amostras de forma asséptica e anaeróbica é importante, sendo descrita em detalhes a seguir. Em caso de hemocultura positiva, é importante avaliar se o microrganismo é compatível com o diagnóstico de EI. Microrganismos que sabidamente causam EI em cães são: Staphylococcus spp. (S. aureus, S. intermedius, S. coagulase-positivo e S. coagulase-negativo), Streptococcus spp. (S. canis, S. bovis e estreptococo beta-hemolítico), Bartonella spp., Escherichia coli, Pseudomonas aeruginosa, Corynebacterium spp. e Erysipelothrix rhusiopathiae.[164,172,177] Bartonella vinsonii e proteobactérias relacionadas (B. henselae, B. clarridgeiae, B. washoensis) foram reconhecidas como causas potenciais de endocardite em cães.[164] Em um estudo envolvendo cães da Califórnia, Bartonella spp. foi a causa de EI em 28% dos casos, bem como em 45% dos casos de EI com hemocultura negativa.[164] Bartonella também é uma causa potencial de EI em gatos.[169] Estudos epidemiológicos sugerem que carrapatos e pulgas podem ser vetores de Bartonella. De fato, é comum notar sororreatividade concomitante para Ehrlichia canis, Anaplasma phagocytophilum e Rickettsia rickettsii, em cães com EI causada por Bartonella spp.[164] (ver Capítulos 215 e 216).

Realização de hemocultura. O ideal é que o laboratório de referência seja contatado para informação em relação ao tipo de frasco preferido, antes da obtenção da amostra de sangue. Para evitar contaminação da amostra, deve-se adotar técnica asséptica rigorosa. Devem ser coletadas, assepticamente, três ou quatro amostras de 5 a 10 mℓ de sangue (a chance de uma hemocultura positiva aumenta com o aumento do volume de sangue) de diferentes locais, com pelo menos 30 minutos a 1 hora de intervalo. As amostras devem ser submetidas às culturas aeróbica e anaeróbica. Os tubos para lise-centrifugação podem melhorar o resultado do teste diagnóstico. A obtenção de amostra de sangue por meio de cateter de demora deve ser evitada, mas tal procedimento pode ser utilizado como última opção. Para a cultura de Bartonella spp., faz-se o congelamento de 2 mℓ de sangue obtido assepticamente em tubo com EDTA, em temperatura de −70°C, até o momento da cultura.[173] As amostras são cultivadas em um meio de cultura especial para Bartonella e incubadas por até 4 semanas (ver Capítulos 215 e 216).

Outros achados laboratoriais

Anemia regenerativa discreta é constatada em 50 a 60% dos casos de EI.[129,166,167,172] A anemia sugere inflamação crônica e, geralmente, é do tipo normocítica e normocrômica. Nota-se leucocitose em cerca de 80% dos cães com EI, geralmente devido à neutrofilia (desvio à esquerda) e monocitose. Outros achados que podem ser encontrados incluem aumento da concentração de nitrogênio ureico sanguíneo (BUN) ou da concentração de creatinina no sangue, devido à embolização, infecção metastática, ICC ou doença imunomediada. Aumento da atividade sérica de fosfatase alcalina e hipoalbuminemia provavelmente são causados por endotoxinas circulantes e redução da função hepática.[163,178] A concentração sanguínea de glicose pode estar diminuída e testes sorológicos para doenças imunomediadas, como o teste de Coombs, podem ser positivos.[178] O exame de urina pode indicar hemoglobinúria, hematúria, piúria, bacteriúria e/ou proteinúria. Sempre deve-se realizar urocultura (preferencialmente realizada em amostra de urina obtida por cistocentese) em cães com suspeita de EI, na tentativa de isolar o microrganismo infectante.

Diagnóstico

Como os sinais clínicos da EI costumam resultar de complicações, em vez de refletir a infecção intracardíaca, o diagnóstico pode ser facilmente negligenciado. Embora em muitos cães possa haver suspeita de EI, o diagnóstico definitivo de EI requer exame histopatológico, o que não é possível no cão vivo. O diagnóstico de EI é frequentemente estabelecido pela identificação de critérios maiores e menores para EI. Foi proposto um sistema de pontuação, adaptado dos critérios de Duke modificados, para EI em pessoas,[181] para estabelecer um possível diagnóstico clínico de EI em cães (Tabela 251.2).[173]

Tratamento

O objetivo do tratamento é erradicar o microrganismo infeccioso e tratar todas as complicações secundárias. O resultado bem-sucedido da terapia baseia-se no diagnóstico precoce e no tratamento imediato agressivo. Devem-se realizar hemocultura (ver seção anterior) e teste de sensibilidade a antibióticos (antibiograma). Nos casos em que se suspeita que *Bartonella* seja a causa da EI, recomenda-se a coleta de uma amostra de sangue para exame sorológico. Enquanto se aguardam os resultados da cultura microbiológica e do teste de sensibilidade antimicrobiana (antibiograma), deve-se iniciar o tratamento intravenoso com um antibiótico bactericida de amplo espectro (p. ex., betalactâmicos [como a timentina, que é uma combinação de ticarcilina e clavulanato], na dose de 50 mg/kg/6 h IV ou imipeném, na dose de 10 mg/kg/8 h IV).[173] O aminoglicosídeo amicacina, na dose de 20 mg/kg/24 h, pode ser combinado com um dos antibióticos betalactâmicos supramencionados, a fim de obter um espectro de ação mais amplo.[173] Para cães com suspeita de EI causada por *Bartonella* o tratamento inicial é semelhante. Os aminoglicosídeos são potencialmente nefrotóxicos e seu uso é recomendado apenas por tempo limitado. Os pacientes tratados com aminoglicosídeo IV devem ser mantidos com administração intravenosa de líquido. A terapia concomitante com furosemida é contraindicada porque pode exacerbar a nefrotoxicidade. Isso limita o uso de aminoglicosídeos em cães com EI e ICC. Uma alternativa aos aminoglicosídeos é a enrofloxacina, quando há suspeita de EI causada por microrganismo gram-negativo, mas a resistência das diferentes bactérias a esse antibiótico parece ser variável em diferentes regiões geográficas. Um padrão de resistência relevante em determinada região geográfica pode limitar o uso de enrofloxacina como um antibiótico de primeira linha. A escolha do antibiótico depende também do local da infecção, pois sua distribuição e difusão nos órgãos são diferentes. A fonte primária da infecção deve ser detectada e tratada tão agressivamente quanto possível (p. ex., por meio de drenagem ou desbridamento cirúrgico).[182] É importante identificar possíveis problemas secundários, como ICC ou lesão renal, que podem influenciar a escolha do antibiótico, ou podem necessitar de terapia específica, ou, às vezes, indicam um prognóstico pior. Cães em ICC e/ou com arritmia requerem tratamento, como discutido anteriormente e nos Capítulos 247 e 248. Quando os resultados da hemocultura estiverem disponíveis, devem-se escolher os antibióticos apropriados e o tratamento IV agressivo deve ser continuado por 1 a 2 semanas, enquanto o paciente é rigorosamente monitorado, em particular no que diz respeito à função renal. Se o resultado da cultura for negativo, a decisão de continuar com o tratamento com antibiótico deve se basear na melhora clínica. Dependendo do resultado inicial do tratamento, a administração subcutânea pode substituir o tratamento IV após 1 a 2 semanas e, posteriormente, indica-se administração oral. A duração do tratamento deve ser de, pelo menos, 6 semanas com o antibiótico efetivo. Em pacientes com hemocultura positiva, recomenda-se realizar nova hemocultura 1 a 2 semanas após o início do tratamento com antibiótico e 1 a 2 semanas após o término do tratamento. Recomenda-se repetir exames ecocardiográficos, hemogramas e exames de urina durante e após antibioticoterapia, para monitorar a eficácia terapêutica e identificar possíveis complicações. Cães diagnosticados com EI causada por *Bartonella* podem ser monitorados repetindo-se

---

Tabela 251.2 Critérios sugeridos para o diagnóstico de endocardite infecciosa em cães.

CRITÉRIOS PRINCIPAIS (MAIORES)	CRITÉRIOS SECUNDÁRIOS (MENORES)	DIAGNÓSTICO
Ecocardiograma positivo: Lesão vegetativa ou erosiva, ou abscesso	**Febre**	**Definido**
	Cão de médio a grande porte (> 15 kg)	Histopatologia da valva
Insuficiência valvar recente: insuficiência	**Estenose subaórtica**	2 critérios principais
aórtica > discreta, sem estenose subaórtica	**Doença tromboembólica**	1 critério principal e 2 critérios secundários
ou ectasia do anel aórtico	**Doença imunomediada: glomerulonefrite,**	**Possível**
Hemocultura positiva: ≥ 2 hemoculturas	**poliartrite**	1 critério principal e 1 critério secundário
positivas, ou ≥ 3 se há contaminante	**Hemocultura positiva não satisfaz os**	3 critérios secundários
comum de pele	**principais critérios listados nesta tabela***	**Rejeitado**
	Sorologia para *Bartonella* ≥ 1: 1024	Outra doença diagnosticada
		Resolução de regurgitação ou anormalidade valvar dentro de 4 dias após o tratamento
		Sem evidência patológica de endocardite no exame pós-morte

*Ainda não aceito oficialmente como critério em medicina veterinária. Os critérios veterinários são modificados a partir dos critérios de Duke modificados, usados em medicina humana para o diagnóstico de endocardite.[181,184] (Adaptada de MacDonald KA: Infective endocarditis. In: Bonagura JD, Twedt D, editors: *Kirk's current veterinary therapy XV*, Philadelphia, 2015, WB Saunders, p. 786.)

o exame sorológico 1 mês após o início da antibioticoterapia.[173] Um título significativamente reduzido é indicativo de tratamento efetivo; um título aumentado sugere tratamento ineficaz e indica que é necessária a substituição do antibiótico (ver Capítulos 215 e 216).

Prognóstico

Fatores que podem indicar mau prognóstico incluem: diagnóstico tardio e retardo no início do tratamento, envolvimento da valva aórtica,[184] vegetação microbiana na valva,[183] infecção por *Bartonella* (causa, mais comumente, EI na valva aórtica),[176] infecção por bactérias gram-negativas, complicações cardíacas ou renais que não respondem ao tratamento, embolização séptica ou infecção metastática, trombocitopenia,[167] elevação da atividade sérica de fosfatase alcalina e hipoalbuminemia (relata-se taxa de mortalidade de 70%, se detectada em pacientes com EI),[163] tratamento concomitante com corticosteroides, independentemente de os antibióticos serem administrados simultaneamente,[167] tratamento com antibióticos bacteriostáticos ou interrupção prematura da antibioticoterapia. Fatores relatados como indicadores de prognóstico mais favorável incluem: envolvimento apenas da valva mitral (em um estudo, relatou-se tempo médio de sobrevida de 476 dias),[164] infecção por bactérias gram-positivas, infecção oriundas da pele, abscesso, celulite ou feridas.[178]

Prevenção

Pode-se indicar o uso profilático de antibióticos 1 a 2 horas antes e 6 horas depois de procedimentos cardíacos, quando há suspeita de que o fluxo sanguíneo turbulento tenha lesionado o endotélio (p. ex., nos casos de estenose aórtica, PDA ou DSV). Nesses casos, o tratamento precoce de todas as infecções é importante para evitar a instalação de bacteriemia e reduzir o risco de EI. A amoxicilina pode ser a primeira escolha, mas outros antibióticos, como a clindamicina, também podem ser utilizados, dependendo do sistema orgânico envolvido e do local da infecção.[175] Finalmente, é muito raro que cães com DMVM desenvolvam EI como consequência de procedimentos odontológicos, o que indica que o tratamento profilático desses cães é desnecessário.[129]

REFERÊNCIAS BIBLIOGRÁFICAS

As referências bibliográficas deste capítulo se encontram online no Ambiente de Aprendizagem.

CAPÍTULO 252

Cardiomiopatias: Cães

Joshua A. Stern e Kathryn M. Meurs

A cardiomiopatia (ou miocardiopatia) canina é uma das formas mais comuns de doença cardíaca adquirida em cães.[1] A forma mais comum de doença do miocárdio em cães é a cardiomiopatia dilatada; porém, cardiomiopatia arritmogênica ventricular direita, miocardiopatia hipertrófica e miocardite, entre outras, também são relatadas.

CARDIOMIOPATIA DILATADA EM CÃES

A cardiomiopatia dilatada (CMD) é uma doença do miocárdio caracterizada por aumento do coração e comprometimento da função sistólica de um ou ambos os ventrículos (Figura 252.1). Disfunção diastólica também pode ser observada.[2] O maior conhecimento da etiologia da doença em ambos, homem e cão, conduziu ao desenvolvimento da teoria de que CMD é o resultado final de uma variedade de insultos ao miocárdio, incluindo aqueles ocasionados por fatores virais, nutricionais, tóxicos e genéticos.[3] No homem, a doença tem demonstrado ser familiar em pelo menos 30 a 50% dos casos, e mutações causais foram identificadas em mais de 40 genes.[4,5] A etiologia permanece indeterminada e em muitos casos a doença é considerada idiopática.

Embora a CMD canina seja descrita como uma doença, tem-se observado uma variação significativa quanto à queixa relatada durante a consulta, a avaliação clínica e a taxa de progressão da enfermidade, dependendo da raça do cão e da causa primária.[6-12]

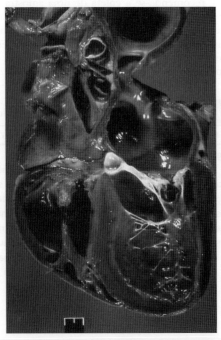

Figura 252.1 Coração de um cão da raça Doberman Pinscher com cardiomiopatia dilatada. Macroscopicamente, nota-se dilatação do ventrículo esquerdo e do átrio esquerdo. (Cortesia do Dr. Bruce Keene.)

Geralmente a CMD é uma doença de cães de raças de grande e médio portes. Algumas raças são claramente super-representadas, particularmente em regiões geográficas específicas. Publicações de resultados de pesquisas na América do Norte mostraram maior incidência da doença em cães das raças Doberman Pinscher, Wolfhound Irlandês, Dogue Alemão e Cocker Spaniel.[13,14] Já publicações europeias sugerem maior incidência em cães das raças Airedale Terrier, Doberman Pinscher, Newfoundland e Cocker Spaniel Inglês.[15] As diferenças de prevalência da raça entre as populações de cães podem sugerir uma influência de fatores genéticos no desenvolvimento de CMD, mas é mais provável que tais diferenças estejam relacionadas com fortes influências genéticas em algumas raças de cães populares em determinadas regiões. Essa estratificação populacional é vista quando estudos genéticos da mesma doença em uma única raça identificam resultados regionalmente específicos. Até o momento, foram relatadas duas mutações genéticas associados ao desenvolvimento de CMD em cães, que são detalhadas nas seções específicas da raça, a seguir.[16,17]

Manifestação clínica

A cardiomiopatia dilatada é uma doença que acomete animais adultos, com exceção de cães das raças Cão de Água Português e Manchester Toy Terrier, nos quais a doença é mais frequentemente diagnosticada antes de 1 ano de idade.[12,18]

Parece haver dois estágios da CMD: um estágio "assintomático", referido como subclínico ou oculto, que pode ser detectado durante um exame de triagem minucioso, e um estágio em que há sinais clínicos referido como doença evidente. Os sinais clínicos podem incluir tosse, dispneia, taquipneia, síncope, intolerância ao exercício e, ocasionalmente, ascite.

Exame físico

Pode-se auscultar sopro sistólico suave compatível com regurgitação da valva mitral e/ou um som de galope (S_3) na região apical esquerda (ver Capítulo 55). É possível constatar taquiarritmia de origem ventricular ou auricular. Em alguns casos, estes podem ser os primeiros sinais da forma oculta da doença e não devem ser negligenciados. Como a valvopatia primária é relativamente incomum em cães de raças de grande porte (ver Capítulo 251) e a detecção de CMD antes do desenvolvimento de insuficiência cardíaca congestiva (ICC) pode ser benéfica para o tratamento a longo prazo da doença, a identificação de um novo sopro, som de galope ou taquiarritmia em raças suspeitas pode justificar um exame cardíaco completo. Apesar de a CMD canina ser predominantemente uma doença de ventrículo esquerdo, com frequência, notam-se envolvimento biventricular e insuficiência cardíaca, com dilatação da veia jugular e ascite, particularmente em cães de raças gigantes.

Exame diagnóstico

Eletrocardiografia

Diversos cães com CMD têm eletrocardiograma normal, porém pode-se observar um padrão indicativo de aumento do átrio e/ou ventrículo (ver Capítulo 103). Além disso, é comum a ocorrência de taquiarritmia, particularmente fibrilação atrial e/ou taquiarritmia ventricular (ver Capítulo 248). Taquicardia sinusal pode ser observada, particularmente em casos de insuficiência cardíaca congestiva (ICC).

Radiografia

Cardiomiopatia dilatada (CMD) é uma doença progressiva do miocárdio. Se a CMD for diagnosticada no estágio inicial, os achados radiográficos podem ser discretos. Portanto, dependendo do estágio da doença, as radiografias do tórax podem apresentar padrão normal ou indicar aumento de volume do átrio e do ventrículo (tipicamente do lado esquerdo), com ou sem dilatação venosa e edema pulmonar. Em alguns casos, pode-se notar aumento de volume de ambos os átrios e ventrículos, particularmente na doença mais avançada acompanhada de taquiarritmia.

Ecocardiografia

A ecocardiografia é o exame de escolha para diagnosticar CMD em cães e também é um exame importante para diagnosticar doença oculta (ver Capítulo 104). Achados ecocardiográficos em paciente com doença avançada incluem: aumento de volume do átrio esquerdo e, às vezes, do ventrículo direito, quantificado por mensurações em ecocardiograma em modo M e bidimensional (Figura 252.2 e Vídeo 252.2). As medidas devem ser comparadas com os valores normais para raça ou tamanho (área de superfície corporal) específico do cão. Em alguns casos, a espessura da parede ventricular pode parecer delgada durante a diástole, mas geralmente, quando é mensurada, está na faixa de normalidade, uma vez que a CMD é caracterizada por hipertrofia excêntrica. Um importante parâmetro para o diagnóstico é a disfunção sistólica do ventrículo esquerdo concomitante, baseada na diminuição da fração de encurtamento (FEn, %), da fração de ejeção (FE, %) ou na área da fração de encurtamento e no aumento do volume sistólico final. Muitos cães podem também apresentar disfunção diastólica, determinada pela avaliação do fluxo transmitral, Doppler tecidual e fluxo venoso pulmonar.[2] A ecocardiografia com Doppler pode ser usada para documentar um jato central de regurgitação mitral que pode estar associado à dilatação do ventrículo. O diagnóstico diferencial de CMD é a doença da valva atrioventricular (AV) grave (ver Capítulo 251), uma vez que nesse caso ocasionalmente podem-se observar dilatação ventricular e disfunção sistólica graves. Para a diferenciação entre CMD e doença da valva AV, pode ser útil levar em consideração a raça do cão, uma vez que cães de raça de grande porte raramente desenvolvem doença valvar primária significativa. Além disso, a CMD é sustentada em casos em que não há o típico espessamento da valva AV associado com a degeneração clássica da valva AV. Uma exceção a isso pode ser o cão da raça Cocker Spaniel, uma raça com alta incidência de doença valvar primária e também alto risco de CMD.

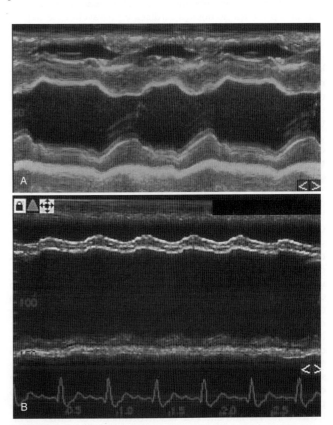

Figura 252.2 A. Ecocardiograma em modo M do ventrículo esquerdo de um cão normal mostrando função sistólica adequada. **B.** Ecocardiograma em modo M de um cão da raça Dogue Alemão com dilatação do ventrículo esquerdo, com função sistólica acentuadamente diminuída.

Infelizmente, o diagnóstico do estágio oculto da CMD é muito mais difícil. Em alguns casos, a dilatação do ventrículo precede o desenvolvimento de disfunção sistólica e é um indicador precoce de CMD.[20] Todavia, este nem sempre é o caso, e a disfunção sistólica pode preceder a dilatação. Anualmente, recomenda-se a realização de ecocardiografia bidimensional e ecocardiografia em modo M em cães adultos de raças predispostas a CMD ou casos em que são detectados sinais precoces (sopro cardíaco, som de galope, taquiarritmia). Exames adicionais sugeridos para obtenção de informações adicionais na avaliação de casos limítrofes da doença incluem mensuração do movimento do anel da valva mitral, índice de esfericidade, separação septal do ponto E, intervalos de tempo sistólicos, avaliação funcional de disco pelo método de Simpson, índice de desempenhos sistólico e diastólico e ecocardiografia sob estresse.[21-25] Uma vez que a idade de reprodução desejável pode preceder a idade de início da DCM, o diagnóstico precoce da doença é de suma importância na redução da prevalência dessa doença na população de cães.

Biomarcadores

Biomarcadores cardíacos são substâncias biológicas que induzem estresse cardíaco e lesão de miócitos (ver Capítulo 246).[26] O peptídio natriurético atrial (PNA), o peptídio natriurético tipo B (PNB) e a troponina I (TnI-c) são biomarcadores importantes na avaliação da doença cardíaca no cão.[21-31]

Relata-se que a concentração do peptídio natriurético atrial, um peptídio liberado em resposta ao aumento da pressão e do estiramento do átrio, eleva-se significativamente tanto na cardiomiopatia dilatada oculta (ou subclínica) quanto na cardiomiopatia dilatada clinicamente evidente, em cães da raça Doberman Pinscher.[28] Todavia, em outro estudo de cães de diversas raças com CMD notou-se que o PNA não era específico ou sensível o suficiente para ser utilizado como teste de triagem de CMD em estágio subclínico.[27] A capacidade do PNA para indicar a presença de doença cardíaca é provavelmente dependente do estágio da doença, permanecendo em níveis normais em casos iniciais da doença.

A troponina cardíaca I (TnI-c) também é um marcador de lesão de miocárdio. Constatou-se elevação da concentração plasmática de TnI-c em cães da raça Doberman Pinscher com CMD clinicamente evidente.[29] Teor elevado de troponina cardíaca I também foi observado em cães com CMD; portanto, a concentração de TnI-c não parece ter sensibilidade e especificidade como marcador de CMD em estágio inicial nesse grupo de cães.[27] Ensaios de alta sensibilidade para TnI-c recentemente tornaram-se disponíveis, muito embora sua utilidade na avaliação de CMD subclínica ainda não tenha sido relatada.

O peptídio natriurético tipo B (PNB) e o fragmento N-terminal pró-PNB (NT-pró-PNB) resultam da clivagem do pró-hormônio PNB, que é sintetizado nos miócitos (ver Capítulo 246). O pró-hormônio PNB é liberado quando os ventrículos apresentam dilatação, hipertrofia ou são submetidos a uma maior tensão na parede; após sua clivagem, ele resulta em dois polipeptídios.[26] Altos teores de PNB foram constatados em cães com insuficiência cardíaca congestiva (ICC), podendo ser usado como teste auxiliar de diagnóstico ou para excluir o diagnóstico de insuficiência cardíaca em cães que apresentam tosse ou dispneia.[30] Em estudo recente mensurou-se a concentração de NT-pró-PNB em cães com cardiomiopatia dilatada e verificou-se que o teor de NT-pró-PNB era significativamente mais elevado em cães com ICC.[31] O teste de triagem de PNB foi bastante sensível, mesmo em cães com CMD subclínica. Relata-se que os cães da raça Doberman Pinscher apresentam concentração plasmática elevada de NT-pró-PNB quando acometidos com CMD e até 1,5 ano antes do desenvolvimento de CMD.[32] Portanto, parece que o PNB pode ser o biomarcador mais útil tanto para o diagnóstico de CMD subclínica quanto para o diagnóstico de estágios mais avançados da doença, embora estudos adicionais sejam necessários para confirmar essas evidências.

Patologia

A patologia macroscópica da CMD tipicamente mostra dilatação dos átrios e ventrículos esquerdos e direitos, embora em alguns casos o lado esquerdo seja mais acometido que o direito.[33-35] Hipertrofia miocárdica excêntrica também é evidenciada pelo aumento da proporção coração/peso corporal.

Os achados histopatológicos podem variar e geralmente não são específicos. Achados comuns podem incluir ondulações atenuadas de miofibras, fibrose, vacuolização de miócitos, necrose e, em alguns casos, infiltração gordurosa.[33,35]

Etiologia

O termo *cardiomiopatia* pode ser usado para definir doenças do miocárdio causadas por uma variedade de fatores, incluindo fatores genéticos, virais e nutricionais, entre outros (ver Capítulo 253).[3] Em muitos casos da doença em cães, a causa é desconhecida. É evidente que diversas raças parecem ser mais predispostas; algumas raças parecem manifestar uma doença com características particulares, sugerindo que essas particularidades da doença são características de determinada raça. Uma forma familiar de CMD confirmada em várias raças é suspeita em outras raças.[9,17,18,36,37] Ocasionalmente, raças atípicas de cães desenvolvem DCM. A etiologia da doença nesses casos é desconhecida, e fatores externos que podem causar lesão de miocárdio, incluindo microrganismos infecciosos ou desequilíbrios nutricionais, devem ser considerados.[38-44]

Cardiomiopatia dilatada específica da raça

Cocker Spaniel. A cardiomiopatia dilatada foi relatada em cães Cocker Spaniel Americano e Cocker Spaniel Inglês.[1,6,45] Há relato de associação entre o desenvolvimento de CMD e baixa concentração plasmática de taurina em alguns cães Cocker Spaniel.[6] Em cães da raça Cocker Spaniel Americano com baixa concentração de taurina que receberam suplementação com taurina e L-carnitina, constatou-se aumento da porcentagem da função sistólica (FS%), bem como diminuição dos diâmetros diastólico e sistólico finais do ventrículo esquerdo, ao longo de 4 meses, embora sem retorno da função normal do miocárdio.[46] Esse estudo sugeriu que pelo menos alguns cães da raça Cocker Spaniel Americano com CMD podem se beneficiar da suplementação com taurina e talvez com L-carnitina.

Os teores de taurina podem ser mensurados em amostras de sangue ou de plasma, embora a concentração sanguínea seja menos afetada pela manipulação da amostra e por alimentação recente, comparada à concentração plasmática. Em cães da raça Cocker Spaniel Americano com CMD deve-se mensurar o teor sanguíneo ou plasmático de taurina e devem ser tratados com 500 mg de taurina e 1 grama de L-carnitina, por via oral, a cada 12 horas.[46] Quando necessário, deve-se administrar tratamento adicional para terapia de outras complicações da doença, incluindo insuficiência cardíaca congestiva e arritmias. Em muitos casos, as medicações de suporte cardiovascular podem ser gradualmente descontinuadas após o aumento da fração de encurtamento do ventrículo esquerdo de pelo menos 20% (geralmente após 3 a 4 meses de suplementação). Se possível, a suplementação com taurina e L-carnitina deve ser continuada por toda a vida.

Em alguns cães da raça Cocker Spaniel com CMD não se detecta deficiência de taurina. Nesses casos, geralmente o prognóstico é pior.

Cães da raça Cocker Spaniel Inglês também manifestam uma forma de CMD, porém sem relação com o teor de taurina ou de carnitina. Muitos cães reportados pertenciam ao mesmo canil, o que pode sugerir o envolvimento de um componente hereditário.[47,48] Foram observadas, frequentemente, evidências de aumento marcante do ventrículo esquerdo no eletrocardiograma, com amplitude da onda R > 3,0 mV na derivação II.[45] Alguns dos cães reportados morreram repentinamente, mas muitos tiveram um curso de doença prolongado, razoavelmente assintomático, ou longa sobrevida (anos), quando submetidos ao tratamento médico.[47]

Dálmata. Cães da raça Dálmata são ocasionalmente diagnosticados com CMD, todavia não tão comumente quanto em algumas outras raças, como Doberman Pinscher, Dogue Alemão e Irish Wolfhound.[1] Cães machos da raça Dálmata parecem mais predispostos à CMD, muito embora grandes estudos não tenham sido realizados.[7] Em todos os cães a doença surgiu na idade adulta, com sintomas compatíveis de insuficiência cardíaca esquerda (tosse, dispneia) ou síncope. Nenhum dos cães teve evidência de insuficiência cardíaca biventricular. A eletrocardiografia frequentemente indicou ritmo sinusal ou taquicardia sinusal com ectopia ventricular ocasional. Fibrilação atrial não foi observada em nenhum dos cães. A sobrevida variou de 1,5 mês a 30 meses; a realização de eutanásia se deveu à ICC refratária. Nenhum dos cães manifestou morte súbita. Curiosamente, a maioria (8/9) dos cães relatados foi alimentada com dieta com baixo teor de proteína por toda a vida ou parte de sua vida, para prevenção ou tratamento de urólitos de urato. A dieta com baixo teor proteico pode ter resultado em desequilíbrio e possível desenvolvimento de cardiomiopatia dilatada; no entanto, nos cães examinados não se constatou evidência de deficiência de L-carnitina ou de taurina. A causa e as consequências dessas dietas no desenvolvimento de CMD não são conhecidas; contudo, em cães da raça Dálmata que desenvolvem CMD e são alimentados com uma dieta com baixo conteúdo de proteínas, essa dieta deve ser substituída por uma dieta mais bem balanceada, se possível.

Ocasionalmente, cães da raça Dálmata desenvolvem doença de valva AV adquirida, de modo que isso deve ser considerado como um diagnóstico diferencial importante (ver Capítulo 251).

Doberman Pinscher. É uma das raças de cães mais comumente relatada com diagnóstico de CMD na América do Norte.[8,14,49,50] É uma doença que surge na idade adulta e resulta no desenvolvimento de insuficiência esquerda e/ou biventricular, muitas vezes com fibrilação atrial ou morte súbita.[51] O estágio subclínico (oculto) pode ser caracterizado por complexos ventriculares prematuros infrequentes, discreta dilatação ventricular e/ou disfunção sistólica.[51] A função diastólica é frequentemente preservada.[2] O estágio clínico é frequentemente caracterizado por fibrilação atrial, complexos ventriculares prematuros e insuficiência cardíaca congestiva. No início, muitos cães acometidos apresentam sintomas de taquiarritmia ventricular, incluindo síncope e, às vezes, morte súbita devido à cardiomiopatia.[52,53] Embora a síncope esteja frequentemente associada à presença de taquiarritmia ventricular, também há relato de bradicardia associada à fraqueza e síncope episódica em cães Doberman Pinscher com cardiomiopatia.[53] Portanto, deve-se tentar determinar a causa dos episódios de síncope com auxílio de Holter ou monitoramento dos eventos antes do início do tratamento.

No exame patológico de coração de cães da raça Doberman Pinscher acometidos, identificou-se uma série de achados inespecíficos. Dilatação moderada à grave das quatro câmaras cardíacas foi frequentemente observada, embora nas câmaras do lado esquerdo a dilatação tenha se mostrado mais grave do que nas do lado direito do coração. A relação entre o peso do coração e o peso corporal geralmente estava aumentada ($11,5 \pm 2,4$ g/kg; normal = $6,6 \pm 0,3$ g/kg, $p < 0,001$).[53b] As lesões histológicas foram caracterizadas por marcante degeneração e atrofia de miofibras, substituição do tecido miocárdico por espessas bandas de fibras de colágeno, fibrose intersticial, agregados de gordura, miocitólise multifocal e necrose miocárdica.

Em cães da raça Doberman Pinscher a cardiomiopatia dilatada parece ser hereditária. Um modo autossômico dominante de herança foi caracterizado pelo aparecimento da doença em múltiplas gerações, com igual representação de gênero e evidência de transmissão macho-macho[36] (Figura 252.3). Em cães da raça Doberman Pinscher Americano, identificou-se uma mutação *splice-site* no gene da enzima piruvato desidrogenase quinase 4 (PDK4), associada à ocorrência de CMD. Há disponibilidade de um teste de mutação, que pode ser utilizado para auxiliar na tomada de decisão quanto ao acasalamento. Essa mutação apresenta penetrância incompleta, o que significa que nem todos os cães com a mutação desenvolverão a doença e a expressão da doença é variável.[16] Estudos em andamento na Europa têm como objetivo identificar uma segunda mutação em cães da raça Doberman Pinscher, já que o gene da enzima PDK4 não parece ser a única causa de CMD em cães Doberman, nos EUA, e não foi associado ao estudo de coorte europeu de CMD em cães Doberman; além disso, uma região cromossômica diferente de interesse foi identificada pela análise de associação do genoma inteiro em cães europeus.[54,55]

A evidência de que a doença é de origem hereditária e a sugestão de que uma intervenção precoce pode aumentar a sobrevida têm levado a um significante interesse em rastrear cães assintomáticos com sinais ocultos da doença. Acredita-se que a realização anual de ecocardiografia e eletrocardiografia ambulatorial (monitoramento com *Holter*) são os melhores indicadores preditivos de CMD em estágio inicial.[50,56] Acredita-se que os critérios indicadores de doença subclínica (oculta) incluam exame ecocardiográfico, constatando-se diâmetro diastólico final do ventrículo esquerdo maior que 4,6 cm e diâmetro sistólico final do ventrículo esquerdo maior que 3,8 cm, mesmo na ausência de disfunção sistólica.[22] Esses números baseiam-se em cães de porte médio com CMD e pode ter menor valor em cães muito grandes (Vídeos 252.1 e 252.3). O monitoramento anual com Holter também tem sido recomendado aos cães Doberman Pinscher que possam desenvolver arritmia ventricular antes que

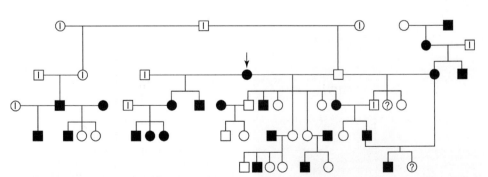

Figura 252.3 Pedigree de uma família de cães da raça Doberman Pinscher com cardiomiopatia dilatada, com um modo autossômico dominante de herança. O probando (indivíduo diagnosticado pela primeira vez com a doença genética na família) é indicado por uma seta. Círculos representam fêmeas; quadrados representam machos. Símbolos em preto representam animais afetados; a letra I, no símbolo, representa cães considerados indefinidos; símbolos brancos representam animais não afetados; um ponto de interrogação no símbolo representa animais não disponíveis para avaliação. (De Meurs KM, PR Fox, Norgard M et al.: A prospective genetic evaluation of familial dilated cardiomyopathy in the Doberman pinscher. *J Vet Intern Med* 21:1016-1020, 2007.)

ocorram dilatação ventricular e disfunção sistólica (Figura 252.4). Cães da raça Doberman Pinscher adultos que apresentam mais de 50 complexos ventriculares prematuros (CVP) no período de 24 horas ou com sequência de dois ou três CVP são propensos ao desenvolvimento de CMD.[56] A mensuração de PNB ou de NT-pró-PNB circulante também pode ser útil na detecção precoce da doença.[27,32] O teste genético para verificação da mutação de PDK4 associada pode auxiliar no desenvolvimento de protocolos de triagem.[16] Os proprietários devem ser informados de que essa doença surge na idade adulta, com variabilidade na idade de início e, assim, os testes de triagem devem ser realizados anualmente.

Dogue Alemão (Grande Dinamarquês). A cardiomiopatia dilatada (CMD) em cães da raça Grande Dinamarquês parece ser uma doença de origem familiar.[9] Em um estudo constatou-se que os machos são mais suscetíveis à CMD, sugerindo uma herança genética ligada ao cromossomo X, pelo menos em algumas famílias.[9] Se isso for verdadeiro, filhos de fêmeas afetadas têm maior risco de desenvolver a doença; filhas de pais acometidos podem ser portadoras subclínicas da doença. Os cães da raça Grande Dinamarquês acometidos apresentam, mais comumente, perda de peso e/ou tosse. Sopro cardíaco do lado esquerdo do coração, som de galope e ascite foram frequentemente observados. No eletrocardiograma, os achados mais comuns incluem fibrilação atrial, com complexo ventricular prematuro. Em alguns casos, nota-se fibrilação atrial antes de qualquer outra evidência de doença do miocárdio (aumento da câmara cardíaca ou disfunção sistólica). Portanto, cães com fibrilação atrial devem ser cuidadosamente avaliados quanto à possibilidade de CMD em estágio inicial e submetidos à avaliação anual para monitorar possível desenvolvimento da doença.

Wolfhound Irlandês. Em cães da raça Wolfhound Irlandês a cardiomiopatia dilatada (CMD) parece ser uma característica familiar.[37,57] O modo de herança é autossômico recessivo, com alelos específicos do sexo. Cães machos podem ser mais sujeitos à CMD.[10] Como acontece em cães da raça Grande Dinamarquês, a fibrilação atrial frequentemente precede o desenvolvimento de sopro cardíaco, sinais clínicos e ICC. Nota-se fibrilação atrial na maioria dos cães Wolfhound Irlandês no momento em que a CMD se desenvolve.[10,58] A progressão da doença não está bem entendida, mas parece ser lenta, com desenvolvimento de fibrilação atrial precedendo o desenvolvimento de ICC por um período médio de 24 meses.[10] Foram relatadas outras anormalidades ocasionais no eletrocardiograma, incluindo: complexos ventriculares prematuros e bloqueio fascicular anterior esquerdo.

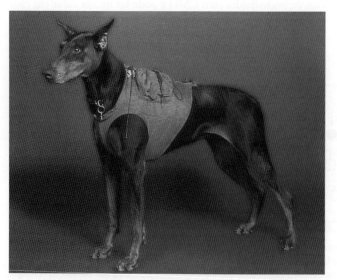

Figura 252.4 Cão da raça Doberman Pinscher adulto com um monitor Holter utilizado na triagem de cardiomiopatia dilatada subclínica (oculta).

Alguns cães da raça Wolfhound Irlandês acometidos apresentaram morte súbita, porém mais comumente foram submetidos à eutanásia devido à insuficiência cardíaca, mais comumente biventricular, e, às vezes, com quilotórax.[58,59] Há relatos ocasionais de baixo teor de taurina no sangue total em cães Wolfhound Irlandês; todavia, nesta raça não foi possível estabelecer uma clara relação entre o teor de taurina e a ocorrência de CMD.[60]

Newfoundland. Em cães da raça Newfoundland há relatos de surgimento de CMD em idade adulta, sem predisposição de gênero[11,23] A manifestação clínica incluía: dispneia, tosse, inapetência e ascite, com insuficiência cardíaca esquerda ou biventricular. Curiosamente, sopro cardíaco foi audível, por meio de auscultação, em apenas uma porcentagem muito pequena dos cães (4/37).[11] A anormalidade elétrica mais comum foi fibrilação atrial; contudo, constatou-se também complexo ventricular prematuro isolado.

Cão d'Água Português. Uma forma juvenil de CMD familiar foi relatada em Cão d'Água Português e acredita-se que seja uma doença herdada como uma característica autossômica recessiva ligada a uma região do cromossomo 8.[12,61] Filhotes de pais aparentemente não acometidos normalmente morriam com 2 a 32 semanas de idade, devido a colapso e morte súbita, sem quaisquer sintomas precedentes ou ao desenvolvimento de insuficiência cardíaca congestiva.[61]

Schnauzer Padrão. Há relato de CMD familiar em cães da raça Schnauzer Padrão; recentemente, constataram-se deleção e mutação *frame-shift* (também conhecida como mutação por erro de enquadramento) no gene da proteína *motif* 20 (uma sequência de nucleotídios ou aminoácidos padrão, diversificada, supostamente de relevância biológica) ligada ao RNA (RBM20). Esta mutação é herdada como uma característica autossômica recessiva. Embora atualmente não haja relato clínico desta doença e da mutação nesta raça, há disponibilidade de teste de mutação genética que pode ser usado para orientar a tomada de decisão quanto ao acasalamento.[17]

Manchester Terrier Toy. Uma forma de CMD familiar juvenil de rápida progressão foi relatada na raça Manchester Terrier Toy; é clinicamente semelhante à CMD verificada no Cão d'Água Português. A prevalência da doença é maior em cães com menos de 1 ano de idade; em geral, esses animais morrem repentinamente, sem sintomas evidentes de insuficiência cardíaca congestiva.[18]

Cardiomiopatia nutricional

Cardiomiopatia relacionada à taurina. O desenvolvimento de cardiomiopatia dilatada (CMD) devido à baixa concentração de taurina é muito menos comum no cão que no gato, uma vez que cães têm uma capacidade muito maior de sintetizar taurina que gatos. Todavia, conforme mencionado anteriormente, uma correlação entre anormalidades nos teores de taurina e L-carnitina e CMD foi previamente descrita em cães da raça Cocker Spaniel.[6,46] Atualmente existem relatos adicionais do desenvolvimento de CMD no cão, em que baixa concentração sanguínea ou plasmática de taurina foi documentada.[43,44] Os cães eram todos adultos no momento do início da doença e eram raças de grande porte. Um fator comum observado em diversos cães que desenvolveram CMD foi o baixo teor de taurina na dieta com ração seca destinada aos cães, tendo como ingredientes principais farinha de carne de cordeiro e/ou arroz.[44] Aventou-se a possibilidade de que produtos como farelo de arroz ou arroz integral podem resultar em diminuição do teor de taurina em alguns cães. Todavia, existe também relato de uma família de cães da raça Golden Retriever aparentemente com deficiência de taurina hereditária e cardiomiopatia dilatada. Em um estudo isolado sobre a concentração plasmática de taurina em cães com doença cardíaca, constatou-se que 4 de 6 cães Golden Retriever com CMD apresentavam baixo teor de taurina.[43] Esses achados sugerem que em algumas raças pode haver algumas variações no metabolismo da taurina que podem resultar no desenvolvimento de CMD.

Concentração sanguínea de taurina inferior a 150 nmol/mℓ ou concentração plasmática menor que 40 nmol/mℓ é indicativa de deficiência de taurina. Se houver suspeita de deficiência de taurina, a suplementação com taurina deve ser iniciada enquanto se aguarda o resultado da mensuração de seu teor sanguíneo ou plasmático. As dosagens publicadas para suplementação de taurina parecem variar ligeiramente, embora 1.000 mg/dia (via oral, em dose única ou fracionada) parece ser uma recomendação apropriada.[43,44] Ademais, devem ser fornecidos medicamentos para a disfunção cardíaca, conforme necessário, incluindo fármaco inotrópico, como pimobendana, e tratamento da insuficiência cardíaca, se necessário (ver Capítulo 247). Cães com deficiência de taurina e cardiomiopatia dilatada parecem responder de forma bastante rápida à suplementação; melhora nos resultados de exames, como ecocardiografia, deve ser observada dentro de 3 a 6 meses. O ideal é reavaliar a concentração sanguínea de taurina em intervalos de 1 a 2 meses, a fim de confirmar o aumento de sua concentração no sangue.[43]

Tratamento

Tratamento do cão com cardiomiopatia dilatada

O tratamento ideal para cardiomiopatia dilatada deveria ser diretamente direcionado à causa primária da lesão ao miocárdio. Infelizmente, na maioria dos casos, a causa primária não é conhecida e o tratamento deve ser direcionado às anormalidades cardíacas, por exemplo, disfunção sistólica, insuficiência cardíaca (ver Capítulo 247) ou arritmias (ver Capítulo 248).

Tratamento do cão com cardiomiopatia dilatada subclínica (oculta)

Existem poucos estudos que avaliaram o benefício do tratamento medicamentoso em cães diagnosticados no estágio subclínico (oculto) da doença; todavia, é provável que essa escassez de informação seja minimizada com a crescente possibilidade de diagnóstico precoce da doença. A administração de inibidores da enzima conversora da angiotensina (ECA) tem algum benefício em cão com dilatação ventricular inicial, com ou sem disfunção sistólica específica. O uso de inibidores da ECA em cães da raça Doberman Pinscher com dilatação ventricular foi associado a um período mais prolongado para o início de insuficiência cardíaca congestiva (ICC).[19] Muito embora este estudo seja retrospectivo, limitado à avaliação de cães Doberman Pinscher, o uso de inibidores da ECA em outras raças de cães com CMD subclínica deve ser levado em consideração.

O efeito cardioprotetor da administração de betabloqueadores em cães em estágio subclínico de CMD ainda está sendo avaliado. Constatou-se que a inclusão de baixa dose de betabloqueador no tratamento de pacientes com CMD e insuficiência cardíaca estável, no homem, reduziu tanto a taxa de mortalidade quanto a de morbidade.[63] No entanto, muitos pacientes humanos com CMD podem não tolerar o uso de betabloqueadores, mesmo em dose muito baixa, e rapidamente desenvolvem descompensação cardíaca. Um estudo prospectivo controlado com placebo em cães avaliou o efeito do betabloqueador carvedilol, administrado durante 3 meses, em dose gradualmente crescente, e não detectou diferença entre os animais tratados com o betabloqueador e aqueles que receberam placebo, quanto ao tamanho ou função do ventrículo esquerdo no exame ecocardiográfico, à ativação neuro-hormonal, ao tamanho do coração em exame radiográfico, à frequência cardíaca ou à percepção de melhora na qualidade de vida pelo proprietário.[64] É possível que um efeito melhor poderia ser obtido se a medicação fosse administrada por um longo período ou em dose maior. No geral, o uso de betabloqueadores em paciente canino com CMD ainda não foi bem estudado e ainda não há uma opinião consensual sobre o uso desses medicamentos em cães.

Os betabloqueadores podem ser utilizados nos pacientes com doença subclínica, porém esses pacientes devem ser cuidadosamente monitorados e os betabloqueadores não devem ser administrados se houver evidência de insuficiência cardíaca até que o paciente esteja clinicamente muito bem estabilizado. Deve-se ressaltar que o uso de betabloqueadores em cães com CMD requer muita cautela, com aumento de dose após um período de 2 semanas, e monitoramento cuidadoso de frequência cardíaca, pressão arterial e sinais clínicos.

O pimobendana, um inodilatador que sensibiliza o cálcio e inibe a ação da fosfodiesterase, é amplamente utilizado no tratamento de insuficiência cardíaca congestiva em cães (ver Capítulo 247).[65] O estudo multicêntrico PROTECT, duplo-cego e controlado com placebo, constatou um claro benefício do pimobendana durante a fase subclínica da doença em cães da raça Doberman Pinscher. O tempo médio de surgimento de insuficiência cardíaca congestiva ou morte súbita cardíaca foi significativamente prolongado (718 dias *versus* 441 dias) em cães Doberman com CMD subclínica que receberam dose padrão de pimobendana 2 vezes/dia.[66] Embora esse estudo tenha sido limitado à avaliação de pacientes da raça Doberman Pinscher, o uso de pimobendana em outras raças de cães com CMD subclínica deve ser considerado.

Tratamento do cão com cardiomiopatia dilatada e insuficiência cardíaca congestiva

Cães com CMD e insuficiência cardíaca se beneficiam do uso de medicamento inotrópico. O ideal é a administração de pimobendana, um inibidor das enzimas fosfodiesterase III e V com propriedades sensibilizadoras de cálcio, que apresenta efeito inotrópico positivo, assim como vasodilatador (inodilatador).[65] Notou-se que o pimobendana induz vasodilatação equilibrada e efeito inotrópico positivo, aumentando a sobrevida (média de 130 dias, no grupo tratado, *versus* a média de 14 dias, no grupo que recebeu placebo), em um estudo com pacientes da raça Doberman Pinscher com CMD que receberam a dose de aproximadamente 0,25 mg/kg/12 h, por via oral.[62,65] (Vídeo 252.6).

Outros medicamentos para insuficiência cardíaca, tais como inibidores de ECA e diuréticos, devem ser utilizados, quando necessários (ver Capítulo 247). Tratamento não específico incluindo suplementação nutricional com componentes como taurina deve ser considerado em cães com suspeita de baixo teor desse aminoácido, até que se prove o contrário.[67] A pacientes caquéticos pode-se recomendar a suplementação com ácidos graxos (ver Capítulos 177 e 183). Pode-se recomendar o tratamento de arritmias supraventriculares ou ventriculares indefinidas (ver Capítulo 248). Digoxina e/ou diltiazem são frequentemente utilizados no tratamento auxiliar de fibrilação atrial e insuficiência cardíaca congestiva.

Tratamento do cão com arritmia ventricular

Existe pouco consenso de quando e como se tratam arritmias ventriculares no cão com CMD. Taquicardia ventricular rápida, arritmias ventriculares complexas ou a combinação de arritmia ventricular, dilatação ventricular e disfunção sistólica parecem estar associadas a um risco maior de morte súbita causada por doença cardíaca e terem indicação para tratamento, mas isso ainda não foi bem estudado. Além disso, alguns cães morrem repentinamente sem ter nenhuma dessas arritmias documentadas. Caso se faça opção pelo tratamento, pode-se utilizar um dos vários antiarrítmicos ventriculares (ver Capítulo 248). Sotalol, uma combinação de betabloqueador e bloqueador de canal de potássio, pode ser benéfico em alguns casos, porém deve ser usado com um pouco mais de cautela (baixa dose) caso exista disfunção sistólica. A mexiletina, na dose de 5 a 6 mg/kg, via oral, em intervalos de 8 horas, pode ser muito efetiva para diminuição da arritmia. Em um número pequeno de pacientes pode provocar náuseas, mas tal ocorrência pode ser significativamente reduzida se for administrada simultaneamente a, pelo menos, uma pequena refeição; por isso, nunca deve ser administrada com o animal em jejum. Avaliou-se o uso de amiodarona em cães da raça Doberman Pinscher com arritmia ventricular, na dose de 10 mg/kg, via oral, a cada 12 h, durante 5 dias, seguida de 5 mg/kg/24 h. Foi sugerida a avaliação mensal cuidadosa da concentração sérica do fármaco, do hemograma completo (constatou-se neutropenia) e da atividade sérica das enzimas hepáticas.[51] Embora os objetivos do tratamento incluam a diminuição do número de complexos ventriculares prematuros, a melhora dos sinais clínicos e a redução do risco de morte súbita, ainda não há estudo quanto à eficácia de qualquer antiarrítmico para atingir esses objetivos.

Prognóstico para o cão com cardiomiopatia dilatada

O prognóstico de cardiomiopatia dilatada (CMD) em cães depende da causa primária, que geralmente não é conhecida. Todavia, na população de cães com CMD, foram identificados alguns preditores negativos de sobrevivência, incluindo idade ao início dos sinais clínicos, efusão pleural, edema pulmonar, ascite, fibrilação atrial, índice do volume sistólico, fração de ejeção e um padrão restritivo de fluxo transmitral.[68,69]

CARDIOMIOPATIA DO VENTRÍCULO DIREITO ARRITMOGÊNICA EM CÃES DA RAÇA BOXER

Desde o início da década de 1980, o termo cardiomiopatia do Boxer tem sido usado para descrever cães adultos da raça Boxer que apresentam arritmia ventricular e, por vezes, síncope.[70] Estudos recentes demonstraram que essa doença tem muitas semelhanças com uma doença no homem chamada cardiomiopatia do ventrículo direito arritmogênica (CVDA). As semelhanças entre elas incluem a manifestação clínica, a etiologia e uma histopatologia particular que consiste em um infiltrado gorduroso fibroso na parede livre do ventrículo direito[71] (Figura 252.5). A doença é mais comumente caracterizada por arritmia ventricular, síncope e morte súbita. Todavia, em um pequeno número de pacientes constatam-se disfunção sistólica e dilatação ventricular.

A CVDA é uma doença de origem familiar, em cães da raça Boxer; parece ser herdada como uma característica autossômica dominante.[72] Infelizmente, a doença também parece apresentar penetrância genética variável e os cães acometidos podem manifestar diferentes quadros clínicos, desde assintomático até síncope, morte súbita e disfunção sistólica com ICC. Constatou-se uma mutação por deleção no gene da estriatina, associada ao desenvolvimento de CVDA em cães da raça Boxer. Esta mutação é herdada como um padrão autossômico dominante com penetrância incompleta. É importante ressaltar que os cães homozigotos mutantes exibem formas mais graves de CVDA, incluindo maior número de arritmias ventriculares, morte súbita e uma forma rara de doença cardíaca estrutural, variante dessa condição, denominada CVDA tipo III.[73,74]

Diagnóstico

A queixa mais comum é a de síncope (ver Capítulo 30). Episódios de síncope podem estar associados a períodos de exercício ou excitação, mas nem sempre são. Alguns cães apresentam intolerância ao exercício ou letargia, outros morrem repentinamente sem nunca desenvolverem sintomas. Raramente (aproximadamente 10% dos cães são acometidos), o cão pode apresentar sinais de insuficiência cardíaca esquerda ou biventricular.

Na maioria dos cães da raça Boxer acometidos, os achados de exame físico são completamente normais. No entanto, pode-se constatar taquiarritmia durante a auscultação. Um pequeno número de pacientes apresenta dilatação ventricular e disfunção sistólica, condição denominada CVDA tipo III; pode-se auscultar sopro sistólico e/ou som cardíaco de galope (S3) no ápice esquerdo. Raramente, notam-se sinais de insuficiência cardíaca direita (ascite e dilatação de veia jugular). Ademais, em cães da raça Boxer verifica-se alta incidência de sopro sistólico basilar esquerdo. Esse sopro pode estar associado à estenose aórtica ou pode ser fisiológico. Muitos cães da raça Boxer com CVDA apresentam esse tipo de sopro, além de arritmia; no entanto, o sopro sistólico basilar esquerdo não é uma indicação de CVDA em cães Boxer.

Biomarcadores parecem ser de valor variável no diagnóstico de CVDA em cães da raça Boxer. Tem-se constatado elevação significativa da troponina cardíaca I (TnI-c) em cães Boxer com CVDA, correlacionada com o número e o grau do complexo ventricular prematuro (CVP) ou com a complexidade da arritmia[75] (Figura 252.6). No entanto, alguns cães acometidos

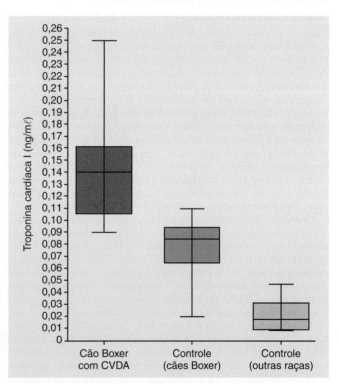

Figura 252.6 Diagrama de caixa das concentrações séricas de troponina cardíaca I de cães da raça Boxer com cardiomiopatia do ventrículo direito arritmogênica (CVDA) (n = 10), cães da raça Boxer controle (10) e cães de outras raças-controle (10). Nota-se elevação significativa no teor de troponina I em cães Boxer com CVDA. Linhas horizontais no interior das caixas representam valores médios. Cada caixa representa intervalos de confiança de 95%. As barras nas extremidades dos valores representam as faixas de variação. (De Baumwart RD, Orvalho J, Meurs KM: Evaluation of serum cardiac troponin I concentration in Boxers with arrhythmogenic right ventricular cardiomyopathy. Am J Vet Res 68:524-528, 2007.)

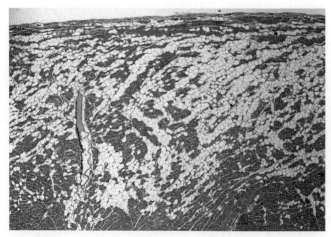

Figura 252.5 Achados histopatológicos na parede do ventrículo direito de cão da raça Boxer com CVDA, notando-se vacuolização multifocal de miócitos, perda de miócitos e infiltração gordurosa significativa. Aumento de 20×; coloração hematoxilina-eosina. (*Esta figura se encontra reproduzida em cores no Encarte.*)

apresentavam teor mais baixo de TnI-c, semelhante ao de cães Boxer normais. Portanto, embora a mensuração do teor de TnI-c possa fornecer informações auxiliares para um cão com suspeita de CVDA, são necessários estudos adicionais antes que o teste seja validado como um teste de triagem. A mensuração da concentração do peptídeo natriurético tipo B em grupos semelhantes de cães da raça Boxer não indicou diferença entre os cães acometidos, comparativamente a cães Boxer normais e não acometidos; portanto, o PNB não parece ser um indicador útil da doença.[76]

Um eletrocardiograma de 2 a 5 minutos (ver Capítulo 103) é frequentemente normal em cães Boxer acometidos; todavia, complexos ventriculares prematuros podem estar presentes isoladamente, em pares e na taquicardia ventricular paroxística (Figura 252.7). Os complexos ventriculares prematuros normalmente têm morfologia de bloqueio de ramo esquerdo, nas derivações I, II, III e aVF, compatível com arritmia de origem no ventrículo direito.[77] Em alguns casos, as arritmias ventriculares que causam síncope podem não ser observadas no eletrocardiograma, portanto um monitoramento com Holter, durante 24 horas, deve ser realizado para avaliar essas arritmias.

A interpretação dos resultados do Holter pode, às vezes, ser um desafio porque não há critérios confiáveis rigorosos para esse diagnóstico. No entanto, uma vez que é incomum para um cão normal ter qualquer CVP em um período de 24 horas, a observação de > 100 CVP, ou de pares, trios ou séries de taquicardia ventricular é anormal e pode ter valor diagnóstico em um cão com sinal clínico.[78] Os complexos supraventriculares prematuros também podem ser observados, particularmente em cães da raça Boxer com dilatação ventricular e disfunção sistólica.

As radiografias torácicas estão geralmente dentro dos limites normais. Entretanto, no pequeno número de casos com dilatação do ventrículo esquerdo e disfunção sistólica (CVDA tipo III), pode-se notar cardiomegalia generalizada, com edema pulmonar e/ou derrame pleural (Vídeo 252.5).

A ecocardiografia é uma parte importante da avaliação porque dilatação ventricular e disfunção sistólica podem ocorrer, mas na maioria dos casos os cães acometidos têm tamanho das câmaras cardíacas e função sistólica normais. Em alguns casos, o exame cuidadoso possibilita a detecção do aumento do ventrículo direito (Vídeo 252.4).

A etiologia familiar da CVDA despertou maior interesse na triagem de cães, antes de selecioná-los como reprodutores. Há disponibilidade de teste de mutação genética para o gene da estriatina, que pode ser usado para orientar a tomada de decisão na seleção de reprodutores e recomendação de esquemas de reavaliação.[73,74] No entanto, uma vez identificado o cão Boxer como positivo para CVDA, sem a mutação no gene da estriatina, é prudente a triagem clínica continuada quando há pelo menos uma outra causa de CVDA.

Como na maioria das vezes a CVDA se apresenta mais como uma anormalidade elétrica do que uma disfunção miocárdica, os esforços de triagem devem ser baseados no monitoramento anual com Holter e ecocardiografia. Infelizmente, não há critérios claros para o diagnóstico de CVDA subclínica. Todavia, os cães sintomáticos, que mostram sinais clínicos (síncope, insuficiência cardíaca) ou evidência de taquicardia ventricular no exame Holter não devem ser utilizados como reprodutores. Além disso, é provável que os cães com mais de 100 CVP com morfologia de bloqueio do ramo esquerdo, no período de 24 horas, sejam altamente suspeitos de serem acometidos. Porém, nem todos os cães acometidos desenvolvem sinais clínicos e muitos podem ter vida normal. É provável que existam múltiplos fatores que influenciam o desenvolvimento de sinais clínicos da doença em cães. Para ajudar a diminuir o risco de erro, introduzindo ou excluindo um cão de um programa de acasalamento, os proprietários devem ser encorajados a realizar teste de triagem anual em seus animais, em vez de dar uma ênfase significativa em um único resultado do exame Holter. Como a doença surge na idade adulta e tem sido notado aumento de CVP com o avanço da idade nos animais acometidos, não é possível garantir que um animal não acometido aos 2 anos de idade não permaneça sem a doença até o fim da vida. Além disso, um animal de 2 anos de idade com algumas centenas de CVP pode ter mais, menos ou o mesmo número de CVP no ano seguinte. Até que não haja maior compreensão quanto à hereditariedade e progressão da doença, deve-se ter cuidado ao aconselhar os criadores a excluir cães de programas de acasalamento. O excesso de zelo na exclusão de animais com base no resultado de um único exame Holter pode ter um impacto negativo significativo na raça.

Tratamento

Se uma arritmia for detectada no exame de rotina em um cão assintomático, um exame Holter deve ser realizado para avaliar a frequência e complexidade da arritmia. Embora não exista uma estreita relação entre o desenvolvimento de sinais clínicos e o número de CVP, o tratamento geralmente é iniciado quando se notam > 1.000 CVP/24 horas, taquicardia ventricular ou evidência de sobreposição da onda R na onda T. Pode-se realizar intervenção terapêutica precoce em cães da raça Boxer sabidamente homozigotos e positivos para a mutação no gene da estriatina, uma vez que já foi mostrado que eles manifestam a forma mais grave doença.[74] Os proprietários devem ser avisados de que os medicamentos utilizados no tratamento de arritmia ventricular podem causar efeitos pró-arrítmicos e não se sabe se esse tratamento reduz o risco de morte súbita. Até o momento, não há evidência de que o tratamento altere significativamente o desfecho da doença nos cães. Contudo, tem-se demonstrado que o tratamento diminui o número de complexos ventriculares prematuros, bem como os episódios de síncope.[79]

O tratamento geralmente é iniciado em cães com síncope e arritmia ventricular. Existem duas opções para o tratamento que são bem toleradas e têm mostrado diminuir o número e a complexidade de CVP: o sotalol, na dose de 1,5 a 3,5 mg/kg/12 h, via oral, ou a mexiletina, na dose de 5 a 6 mg/kg/8 h, via oral.[79] Em alguns casos, a combinação de sotalol e mexiletina, nas dosagens acima mencionadas, é indicada para um ótimo controle da arritmia. É provável que exista uma variação individual para a resposta ao fármaco e, se uma baixa resposta é observada com um ou o outro medicamento, ou a combinação dos dois,

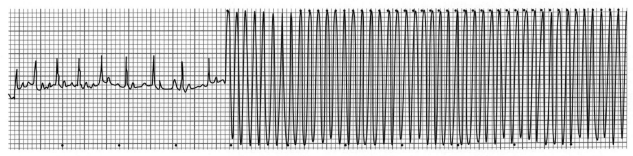

Figura 252.7 Eletrocardiograma de um cão da raça Boxer com cardiomiopatia do ventrículo direito arritmogênica (CVDA) e síncope. Nota-se um ritmo sinusal, com início súbito de taquicardia ventricular.

pode revelar-se mais efetiva. O ideal é que o monitor Holter seja colocado antes do início da terapia e repetido 2 a 3 semanas após, para monitorar o efeito da medicação. Existe significativa variação no número de CVP, no dia a dia, mas um efeito terapêutico é provável que exista se ocorrer ao menos uma redução de 85% no número de CVP após o início do tratamento.[80]

Em um estudo, foram administrados óleos de peixe (780 mg de ácido eicosapentaenoico [EPA] e 497 mg de ácido docosahexaenoico [DHA], por via oral, por dia) durante 6 semanas; notou-se redução do número de CVP, mas não em uma taxa acima daquela considerada como uma variação cotidiana. Assim, os antiarrítmicos continuam sendo indicados como tratamento, às vezes simultaneamente à suplementação com óleo de peixe.[81]

Se a ecocardiografia indicar disfunção sistólica e dilatação ventricular, pode-se recomendar o tratamento para CMD (pimobendana, inibidores da ECA, diuréticos). Adicionalmente, pode-se indicar suplementação com L-carnitina, na dose de 50 mg/kg, por via oral, a cada 8 a 12 horas, uma vez que um pequeno número de cães da raça Boxer manifestou melhora na função sistólica e no prognóstico após essa suplementação.[41]

Prognóstico

Cães com CVDA estão sempre em risco de morte súbita. No entanto, muitos pacientes podem viver anos quando tratados com antiarrítmico, sem sinais clínicos; todavia, eventualmente alguns podem desenvolver dilatação ventricular e disfunção sistólica. O prognóstico de cães Boxer que não apresentam disfunção sistólica e dilatação ventricular é comparável ao de cães dessa raça que não apresentam CVDA, com uma idade média de sobrevivência de 11 anos.[82]

MIOCARDITE

Miocardite é uma forma de doença do miocárdio caracterizada por necrose ou degeneração e inflamação do miocárdio. Uma variedade de agentes físicos, químicos e infecciosos podem lesionar o tecido miocárdico e provocar uma resposta inflamatória, que pode resultar em dilatação da câmara cardíaca e disfunção miocárdica, semelhante à observada na CMD e uma variedade de taquiarritmias e bradiarritmias.[83,84] Com frequência, nota-se elevação do teor plasmático de troponina cardíaca I (TnI-c), sugerindo lesão no miocárdio. Nos cães, microrganismos como protozoários e vírus são mais comumente relatados.

A doença de Chagas, causada pelo protozoário *Trypanosoma cruzi*, é comum em cães, particularmente na região sul da América do Norte. Três estágios de infecção têm sido descritos: agudo, latente e crônico. O estágio agudo é caracterizado por linfadenopatia generalizada, membranas mucosas pálidas, aumento do tempo de preenchimento capilar e hepatoesplenomegalia.[85] Este estágio está associado a uma série de anormalidades eletrocardiográficas, incluindo taquicardia sinusal, prolongamento do intervalo PR, diminuição da amplitude da onda R, desvios dos eixos e anormalidades da condução.[86] Pode ocorrer morte súbita. Cães que sobrevivem ao estágio agudo podem entrar em um período latente durante o qual os sinais clínicos parecem regredir.[86] A fase crônica da doença de Chagas está associada a sinais de disfunção cardíaca progressiva do lado direito, ascite, efusão pleural, hepatomegalia e distensão venosa jugular. Há relatos ocasionais de taquicardia ventricular.[86] Em um estudo, constatou-se que quase a metade dos cães diagnosticados histopatologicamente com miocardite por Chagas, na necropsia, manifestou morte súbita e 50% desses cães morreram com menos de 1 ano de idade.[84] O diagnóstico da doença de Chagas é mais frequentemente realizado por meio de sorologia e, às vezes, a forma aguda pode ser diagnosticada pela constatação da forma tripomastigota circulante em esfregaço sanguíneo espesso. Em geral, o tratamento da doença de Chagas é paliativo, direcionado aos sinais clínicos, uma vez que a destruição da forma intracelular do parasita pode resultar em exacerbação

grave da resposta inflamatória do hospedeiro. Todavia, existe um trabalho preliminar em cães sugerindo que um inibidor da cisteína-protease pode ser muito efetivo na redução da gravidade dos sintomas cardíacos da doença.[81]

Leishmania é um protozoário endêmico em certas regiões geográficas, inclusive a bacia do Mediterrâneo (ver Capítulo 221).[87] Acredita-se que os sinais clínicos da miocardite associada a *Leishmania* é resultante da ação direta do parasita no miocárdio, assim como da inflamação intensa em resposta ao parasita. Arritmias cardíacas, incluindo bloqueio AV de primeiro grau, têm sido observadas, e ambas, a epicardite e a miocardite, têm sido identificadas na necropsia. Outros protozoários parasitas, incluindo *Neospora caninum* e *Toxoplasma gondii*, foram associados ao desenvolvimento de miocardite.[88-90]

A miocardite causada por parvovírus é uma forma incomum da doença (ver também Capítulo 225). Pode se manifestar como doença hiperaguda, em filhotes com 3 a 8 semanas de idade. Esses filhotes apresentam dispneia aguda compatível com insuficiência cardíaca esquerda e morrem dentro de horas.[39] Na necropsia, nota-se aumento de volume do coração, com necrose de fibras musculares multifocal, infiltrado de células mononucleares e corpúsculos de inclusão intranucleares no miocárdio.[39,91] Uma outra forma da doença afeta cães jovens (geralmente com menos de 1 ano de idade), com manifestação clínica semelhante à CMD.[39,40]

O vírus do Nilo Ocidental raramente infecta os cães, e os sinais clínicos, muitas vezes vagos, incluem letargia, inapetência, sinais neurológicos, arritmia e febre.[92,93] Tem-se observado miocardite linfocítica neutrofílica grave e vasculite com hemorragia focal extensa e mionecrose. O diagnóstico pode ser confirmado de diversas maneiras, incluindo exame imuno-histoquímico, reação em cadeia da polimerase via transcriptase reversa (RT-PCR), isolamento do vírus e sorologia.[92]

Há relato de miocardite fúngica causada por *Blastomyces*, embora isso não pareça ser uma forma comum dessa infecção fúngica (ver Capítulo 233).[94] Três cães foram levados à consulta com sinais de síncope, um por morte súbita e três diagnosticados recentemente com sopro cardíaco. Achados cardíacos incluíam taquicardia sinusal; um cão apresentava prolongamento do segmento ST, e outro, bloqueio AV de terceiro grau. Dois cães tinham compressão cardíaca causada por granuloma extracardíaco, enquanto os demais tinham envolvimento miocárdico, epicárdico, pericárdico ou valvular. Embora haja relato de apenas um pequeno número de casos, geralmente os cães com blastomicose e envolvimento cardíaco têm um prognóstico ruim.

Raramente, microrganismos infecciosos, como as bactérias *Bacillus piliformis* e *Citrobacter koseri* e a espiroqueta *Borrelia burgdorferi*, têm sido consideradas como causas de miocardite.[95,96]

Miocardite atrial

Há relato de uma forma de miocardite limitada aos átrios.[97-99] Arritmias atriais inexplicadas, incluindo fibrilação atrial, foram associadas à inflamação ou presença de microrganismos infecciosos nos átrios. Miocardite multifocal em ambos os átrios foi observada durante a necropsia de um paciente com fibrilação atrial.[97] Assistolia intermitente com síncope foi observada em um cão que possuía linfócitos, macrófagos e neutrófilos em todo o átrio direito e, em menor quantidade, no átrio esquerdo.[98] Um caso de miocardite atrial foi associado a um diagnóstico concomitante de polimiosite.[99] O cão apresentava aumento significativo do átrio direito, complexos atriais prematuros e elevação no teor de troponina. No exame histopatológico identificou-se infiltração linfocítica no átrio direito.

CARDIOMIOPATIA HIPERTRÓFICA

A cardiomiopatia hipertrófica é uma doença miocárdica primária, caracterizada por hipertrofia concêntrica do septo interventricular e da parede livre do ventrículo esquerdo (ver Capítulo 253). A cardiomiopatia hipertrófica e a variante cardiomiopatia hipertrófica obstrutiva são formas raras de doença do miocárdio em cães (Vídeo 252.7). Parece haver diferenças significativas entre a doença verificada em cães e aquela mais comumente observada em gatos e no homem, no que diz respeito à etiologia e aos achados patológicos.[100,101] Há relatos de uma forma de cardiomiopatia hipertrófica obstrutiva de herança genética em cães da raça Pointer, mas na maioria dos casos parece ser esporádica.[100-103] Em função da relativa infrequência de cardiomiopatia hipertrófica e cardiomiopatia hipertrófica obstrutiva em cães, os pacientes suspeitos devem ser cuidadosamente avaliados quanto a outras causas de hipertrofia concêntrica do ventrículo esquerdo, inclusive a causa muito mais comum de obstrução do fluxo de saída do ventrículo esquerdo, em casos de estenose subvalvar e estenose da valva aorta.

HIPOTIREOIDISMO

Em alguns cães com hipotireoidismo têm sido observados redução na porcentagem da fração de encurtamento e aumento das dimensões do ventrículo esquerdo; todavia, os valores tiveram sobreposição significativa com os valores de cães normais.[104] Assim, embora a avaliação dos parâmetros da função da tireoide possa ser considerada em cães que apresentem alterações ecocardiográficas menores, além de outros sinais de hipotiroidismo, essa anormalidade não deve ser considerada como uma causa comum de disfunção miocárdica, tampouco de dilatação ventricular.[105] Apesar das muitas pesquisas sobre hipotireoidismo em cães da raça Doberman Pinscher, um estudo recente não identificou a influência do hipotireoidismo na etiologia ou na progressão da CMD nessa raça.[106]

INFARTO DO MIOCÁRDIO

Infarto agudo do miocárdio é uma forma rara de doença em cães e parece ser mais comumente associada à doença sistêmica ou doença cardíaca concomitante que causa tromboembolismo. Essas condições podem incluir: endocardite, neoplasia, doença renal, anemia hemolítica imunomediada e doença pancreática. Em cães que manifestam infarto raramente se constata aterosclerose, ao contrário do homem, que tem uma alta incidência de infarto associado à aterosclerose.[107]

REFERÊNCIAS BIBLIOGRÁFICAS

As referências bibliográficas deste capítulo se encontram online no Ambiente de Aprendizagem.

CAPÍTULO 253

Cardiomiopatias: Gatos

Valérie Chetboul

INTRODUÇÃO: CLASSIFICAÇÃO (CONSIDERAÇÕES NOSOLÓGICAS) E PREVALÊNCIA

As doenças do miocárdio (cardiomiopatias ou miocardiopatias) referem-se a um amplo espectro heterogêneo de doenças do músculo cardíaco e são, de longe, as doenças cardíacas mais comuns em gatos.[1-5] Ao longo das últimas 4 décadas, várias classificações de miocardiopatias em humanos for propostas e modificadas, devido ao aumento do conhecimento de suas várias causas primárias, das bases moleculares e genéticas e das características fisiopatológicas complexas, bem como devido à constatação de novas classificações patológicas.[6-14] Em 1980, a Organização Mundial da Saúde (OMS) definiu cardiomiopatias como *"doenças do músculo cardíaco de causa desconhecida"*, que foram diferenciadas das doenças específicas do músculo cardíaco (de causa conhecida).[6] Em 1995, uma nova classificação da OMS redefiniu as miocardiopatias como *"doenças do miocárdio associadas à disfunção cardíaca"* e acrescentou à lista duas doenças do miocárdio recentemente reconhecidas,[7] isto é, cardiomiopatia do ventrículo direito arritmogênica (CVDA) e cardiomiopatia restritiva (CMR), ambas descritas vários anos depois em gatos.[15-17] As cardiomiopatias foram classificadas em 5 grupos, de acordo com a sua fisiopatologia dominante, ou seja, cardiomiopatia dilatada (CMD), cardiomiopatia hipertrófica (CMH), CMR, CVDA e cardiomiopatias não classificadas (CMNC), que incluem os casos que não se enquadram nos 4 outros fenótipos.[7] Um grupo adicional nomeado "cardiomiopatias específicas" também foi reconhecido, e incluem doenças do miocárdio associadas a doenças cardíacas ou anormalidades sistêmicas (p. ex.,

doenças isquêmicas, valvares, hipertensivas, inflamatórias, cardiomiopatias metabólicas e tóxicas e anormalidades do miocárdio associadas a doenças do sistema neuromuscular ou do sistema geral). Em 2006, o comitê de especialistas da American Heart Association (AHA) [Associação Americana do Coração (AAC)] definiu cardiomiopatias como *"um grupo heterogêneo de doenças do coração associadas à disfunção mecânica e/ou elétrica que geralmente (mas não invariavelmente) é acompanhada de hipertrofia ou aumento de volume ventricular inapropriado ocasionadas por uma variedade de causas que frequentemente são genéticas".*[8] Em 2006, após discussão dos especialistas da AAC, houve consenso quanto à exclusão, dessa definição, de todas as doenças do miocárdio secundárias a outras anormalidades e propôs uma nova classificação das cardiomiopatias em dois grandes grupos (cardiomiopatia primária e cardiomiopatia secundária), com base no envolvimento predominante dos órgãos: cardiomiopatias primárias (genéticas, não genéticas e mistas), as únicas ou predominantemente restritas ao miocárdio, e cardiomiopatias secundárias, que acometem o miocárdico secundariamente a numerosos efeitos sistêmicos ou anormalidades de múltiplos órgãos.[8] Em 2008, a European Society of Cardiology Working Group on Myocardial and Pericardial Diseases (Sociedade Europeia do Grupo de Estudo de Doenças do Miocárdio e do Pericárdio) propôs uma atualização da classificação das cardiomiopatias com base, principalmente, nos 5 fenótipos da classificação da OMS de 1995 (*i. e.*, CMH, CMD, CVDA, CMR e CMNC), que foram subdivididos em formas familiares/genéticas e formas não familiares/não genéticas.[11] Todavia, ainda há controvérsia quanto à abordagem nosológica das cardiomiopatias,[18,19] de forma que uma determinada etiologia pode estar associada a um espectro de fenótipos miocárdicos e fenótipos morfológicos e funcionais e se sobrepor, e até mesmo progredir ao longo do tempo, enquanto o nosso conhecimento sobre a etiologia das cardiomiopatias previamente denominadas idiopáticas continua a evoluir. A fim de evitar confusão e ser mais claro para o leitor, este capítulo sobre cardiomiopatia em gatos vai se referir mais ao sistema de classificação "combinado" mencionado a seguir, por ser mais adequado e prático em cardiologia de gatos. Conforme a classificação proposta pela AAC, em 2006,[8] as cardiomiopatias vão ser referidas como doenças do músculo cardíaco não secundárias a outras doenças cardiovasculares, e cardiomiopatias primárias vão ser diferenciadas das cardiomiopatias secundárias de origens sistêmicas. As cardiomiopatias primárias vão ser subdivididas nos 5 fenótipos da OMS, de 1995, (Figura 253.1).[7] As cardiomiopatias primárias são as doenças cardíacas mais comuns em gatos e, portanto, constituem a parte central deste capítulo. Em um estudo com 287 gatos cardiopatas, a CMH foi a doença cardíaca mais comumente diagnosticada (68%), enquanto as anomalias congênitas representaram apenas 12% dos casos avaliados.[20] Da mesma forma, em um artigo sobre CMH, CMR e cardiomiopatias secundárias, a CMH representou 53% dos casos, enquanto 15% eram CMR e 32% eram cardiomiopatias secundárias, respectivamente.[21] Em outro estudo sobre cardiomiopatias primárias,[22]

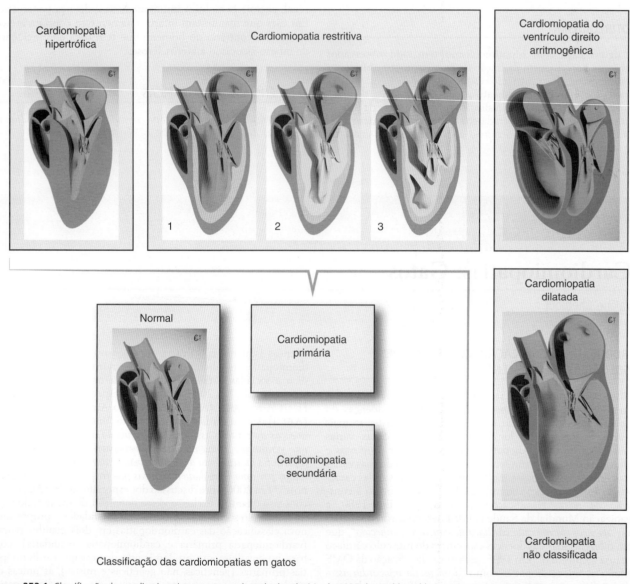

Figura 253.1 Classificação das cardiomiopatias em gatos, adaptada do relatório de 1995 da World Health Organization/International Society and Federation of Cardiology Task Force (Organização Mundial da Saúde/Sociedade Internacional e Federação de Força-Tarefa de Cardiologia) quanto à definição e classificação das cardiomiopatias.[7] As cardiomiopatias primárias incluem cardiomiopatia hipertrófica, cardiomiopatia restritiva (CMR), cardiomiopatia dilatada, cardiomiopatia do ventrículo direito arritmogênica e cardiomiopatia não classificada (que inclui casos que não se encaixam em nenhum outro grupo). A cardiomiopatia hipertrófica consiste em hipertrofia do ventrículo esquerdo (ou esquerdo e direito). A cardiomiopatia restritiva é caracterizada por enchimento limitado e redução do volume diastólico de qualquer um dos ventrículos (principalmente do ventrículo esquerdo), ou de ambos, com função sistólica normal ou próximo do normal e espessamento da parede ventricular. Duas formas básicas de CMR foram identificadas em gatos,[16] isto é, CMR miocárdica (a mais comum, n° 1) e CMR endomiocárdica (também conhecida como fibrose endomiocárdica), com cicatrização difusa que reduz a função do ventrículo esquerdo (n° 2) ou com cicatrização em ponte exuberante ligando o septo interventricular à parede livre do ventrículo esquerdo (n° 3). A cardiomiopatia dilatada é caracterizada pelo comprometimento da dilatação e contração do ventrículo esquerdo, ou de ambos os ventrículos. Por fim, a cardiomiopatia do ventrículo direito arritmogênica consiste em substituição fibrogordurosa progressiva do miocárdio do ventrículo direito, aumento global do lado direito do coração (e também potencial envolvimento do ventrículo esquerdo). (Ilustrações: execução e concepção pela Dra. Charlotte Taton e pela Profa. Valérie Chetboul.)

a CMH foi também, de longe, a doença mais comum (58%), seguida de CMR (21%), CMD (10%) e CMNC (10%), sem nenhum relato de CVDA (a cardiomiopatia primária mais rara em gatos).[1,20] No artigo mencionado, um gato apresentava alterações ecocardiográficas compatíveis com cardiomiopatia associada à presença de feixe de tendões musculares que conectam o septo à parede livre do ventrículo. Esses feixes de tendões musculares (*moderator band*), também denominados de falsos tendões, no ventrículo esquerdo (VE), são estruturas de grau de estiramento variável verificadas na cavidade do VE, conectadas ao septo interventricular (SIV), à parede livre do VE (PLVE) e/ou aos músculos papilares do VE e ápice.[23-25] Esses tendões são constituídos de quantidades variáveis de fibras de Purkinje, fibras de colágeno, tecido conjuntivo fibroso e miocárdico, tecido adiposo e vasos sanguíneos, recobertos pelo endotélio.[23-27] Como acontece no homem,[23-25,28] os falsos tendões são comumente achados ecocardiográficos acidentais em gatos, sem consequência na morfologia e função cardíaca (Figura 253.2 A e B).[29,30] No entanto, de forma semelhante ao homem,[23] há relato de redes excessivas desses tendões no VE de gatos, com vários efeitos deletérios secundários, como disfunção miocárdica do VE e remodelamento do VE, arritmias, insuficiência cardíaca congestiva (ICC) e tromboembolismo arterial (TEA), levando potencialmente à morte, mesmo em filhotes (Figura 253.2 C e D e Vídeos 253.1 e 253.2).[1,26,27] Como os feixes de tendões no VE são de origem congênita, o termo "cardiomiopatia ocasionada por feixes de tendões (*moderator band*) é comumente utilizado para definir esse estado de doença e não se encaixa na definição de cardiomiopatias estabelecida pela AAC.[8] No entanto, a prevalência de falsos tendões na via de saída do ventrículo esquerdo (VSVE) é maior em gatos com CMH obstrutiva (CMHO; também denominada cardiomiopatia obstrutiva hipertrófica ou CMOH), em comparação com gatos saudáveis e em gatos com CMH não obstrutiva, o que sugere possível participação dos falsos tendões na patogênese da obstrução dinâmica da VSVE (OVSVE; Figura 253.2 E).[29]

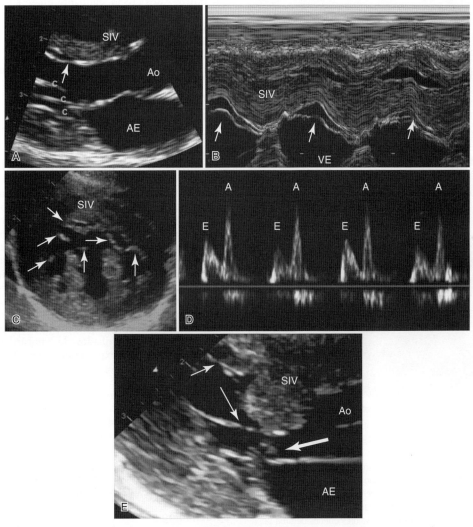

Figura 253.2 Falsos tendões (*moderator bands*) e cardiomiopatia hipertrófica em gato (ecocardiografia). **A** e **B**. Falsos tendões geralmente aparecem como estruturas lineares ecoicas delgadas (*setas*), mais tensos na diástole e mais relaxados na sístole, encontrados incidentalmente aqui ao longo do septo interventricular (*SIV*), em um gato saudável, no ecocardiograma bidimensional (imagem paraesternal direita de 5 câmaras, em **A**) e no ecocardiograma modo M (**B**). Em **C** e **D**, imagem transventricular do eixo curto mostrando uma rede excessiva de falsos tendões (*setas*) em um gato da raça Belga de 8 meses de idade (**C**), resultando em alteração diastólica, confirmada por meio de Doppler de onda pulsada através da avaliação da velocidade do fluxo mitral (**D**). Há um padrão de relaxamento prejudicado caracterizado por uma proporção entre a onda de enchimento inicial (*E*) e a onda de enchimento tardia (*A*) < 1 (E:A = 0,66), associada a tempo de desaceleração de E prolongado (> 100 ms) de (132 ms).[66] **E**. Imagem paraesternal da câmara direita, obtida no fim da sístole, de um gato com cardiomiopatia hipertrófica obstrutiva grave. O SIV se projeta para a via de saída do ventrículo esquerdo. Note a presença de falsos tendões (*setas finas*), inclusive um conectado ao SIV subaórtico, bem como o movimento sistólico anterior da valva mitral (*seta grande*); ambos contribuem para o agravamento da obstrução da via de saída do ventrículo esquerdo. *AE*, átrio esquerdo; *Ao*, artéria aorta; *c*, cordas tendíneas; *VE*, ventrículo esquerdo.

CARDIOMIOPATIA HIPERTRÓFICA

A cardiomiopatia hipertrófica é caracterizada fenotipicamente pelo aumento da massa cardíaca devido à hipertrofia do VE, não dilatado, na ausência de uma causa óbvia de hipertrofia do ventrículo esquerdo (HVE), tal como sobrecarga de pressão (p. ex., hipertensão arterial sistêmica) ou estímulo hormonal (p. ex., hipertireoidismo).[1,31]

Padrões, patologia macroscópica e histopatologia do ventrículo esquerdo com hipertrofia

Como acontece no homem, a CMH em gatos é caracterizada por fenótipos de variabilidade acentuada, incluindo HVE concêntrica discreta a grave, difusa ou segmentar (Figuras 253.3 e 253.4).[31-34] Na maioria dos gatos com CMH (até dois terços), a HVE é difusa, envolvendo partes ou ambos, o septo interventricular (SIV) e a parede livre do ventrículo esquerdo (PLVE), com hipertrofia dos músculos papilares do ventrículo esquerdo e, consequentemente, redução da cavidade do VE (Vídeo 253.3).[31,34] A HVE difusa pode ser simétrica ou assimétrica, com espessamento predominante do SIV ou da PLVE. Em cerca de um terço dos casos, a HVE está restrita a um único segmento, geralmente o SIV basal e, com menos frequência, ao ápice.[31,34] Em alguns casos, ocorre protrusão do SIV basal espesso para a VSVE, resultando em forma leve a grave de OVSVE, definindo assim as formas de CMHO (Vídeos 253.4 a 253.6). A combinação marcante de HVE e hipertrofia dos músculos papilares pode resultar em obstrução sistólica da cavidade médio-ventricular, associada à presença de placas de contato endocárdicas.[2,35] Embora raro, também pode ocorrer infarto do miocárdio devido a PLVE (Vídeo 253.12).[31] Tal variação de padrões geométricos também é revelada no ecocardiograma bidimensional (2D) e no ecocardiograma modo M (ver Capítulo 104), com variações entre as raças.[36,37] Em um estudo, constatou-se que gatos das raças Persa e Chartreux apresentavam prevalência significativamente maior de CMHO (44%) do que outros gatos (18%), enquanto quase a metade dos gatos da raça Maine Coon apresentavam HVE simétrica difusa (Figura 253.4).[37]

Nos casos de HVE discreta a moderada, o átrio esquerdo (AE) geralmente é normal.[2] A HVE grave é frequentemente associada a aumento leve a grave do AE (Figura 253.3 e Vídeos 253.7 e 256.2).[31] A hipertrofia do ventrículo direito (VD) também pode estar presente, associada ou não à hipertrofia do átrio direito (AD).

Histopatologia

Como no homem,[33] as características histológicas da CMH de gatos incluem vários graus de desarranjos de fibras do miocárdio do VE (menos comumente do miocárdio do VD), associados a arteriosclerose de grau leve a grave em artérias coronárias intramurais, fibrosamento intersticial no miocárdio e substituição por fibrose (Figura 253.5).[2,31,32,34] Em um relato, foram identificadas células musculares cardíacas desorganizadas no SIV de 30% dos gatos com CMH. A desorganizada arquitetura do PLVE foi menos comum (14%) e sistematicamente associada à desorganização do SIV.[32] Tais diferenças histológicas impactam a função miocárdica diastólica regional, como observado em imagens Doppler tecidual (IDT).[38,39] Em ambos, no homem e nos gatos, a desorganização das fibras do miocárdio também pode ser observada em casos de espessamento não graves, mesmo em segmentos não hipertrofiados do miocárdio do VE[2] que, do ponto de vista prático, explica por que nas IDT pode-se detectar disfunção miocárdica regional em segmentos miocárdicos aparentemente normais de gatos com CMH (Figura 253.6).[38] Na CMHO, pode-se observar uma placa de contato fibrosa da VSVE na superfície do SIV devido à aposição sistólica dos folhetos da valva mitral ao SIV. Maior deposição de colágeno miocárdico, associada a infiltrados de neutrófilos e linfócitos, também foi constatada no miocárdio de gatos com CMH pré-clínica, sugerindo possível contribuição de um processo inflamatório precoce à fibrose miocárdica (p. ex., [envolvendo] citocinas inflamatórias), fato que requer estudos adicionais.[40]

Epidemiologia

Em grandes populações de gatos com CMH, os machos são super-representados (70 a 79%), com predominância de gatos Domésticos de Pelo Curto (Shorthair) (65 a 70%), seguido de gatos Domésticos de Pelo Longo (Longhair) (9 a 22%) e gatos da raça Persa (3 a 12%).[37,41,42] Outras raças comumente relatadas variam de acordo com estudos (British Shorthair, Chartreux, Himalaia, Maine Coon, Sphynx, Ragdoll).[37,41-43] Gatos Birmaneses, Siameses, Pelo Curto Orientais e Abissínios são menos comumente acometidos[1,37,41,42] No momento do diagnóstico, a maioria dos gatos com CMH apresenta, em média, 5 a 7 anos.

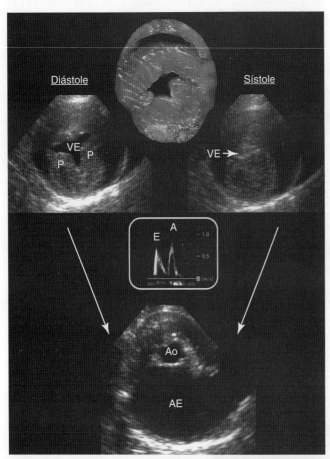

Figura 253.3 Miocardiopatia hipertrófica: relações macroscópicas entre imagens obtidas em ecocardiograma e em Doppler de um gato com hipertrofia do ventrículo esquerdo difusa simétrica. Ambas as imagens, do corte transversal da amostra e do eixo curto paraesternal direito (topo da figura), mostram grave hipertrofia do ventrículo esquerdo (VE), resultando em redução do lúmen do VE e consequente aumento acentuado do átrio esquerdo (AE), observado na região paraesternal direita da imagem transaórtica (parte inferior da figura; razão AE:artéria aorta (Ao) no fim da diástole de 3,7; valores obtidos de uma população de 100 gatos saudáveis: 0,5 a 1,2).[78] Note o desaparecimento da cavidade do VE no fim da sístole. O exame Doppler de onda pulsátil transmitral em imagem de 4 câmaras apicais esquerdas (imagem central) revela comprometimento do padrão de relaxamento do VE caracterizado por uma razão E:A invertida (< 1) (velocidades máxima do fluxo transmitral diastólico inicial [E] e tardio [A], respectivamente), confirmando, ambas, a redução inicial no enchimento do VE devido ao relaxamento prejudicado e à maior contribuição do AE no enchimento do VE (com contração do AE).[66] Ao, artéria aorta; P, músculos papilares do VE. (Cortesia do Prof. Jean-Jacques Fontaine, Departamento de Patologia da Escola Nacional de Veterinária de Alfort, França.)

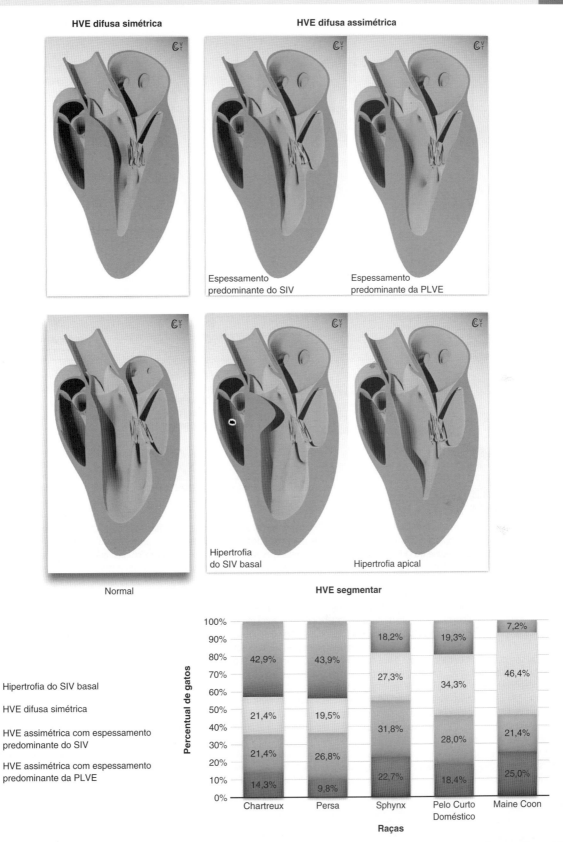

Figura 253.4 Variabilidade fenotípica das cardiomiopatias hipertróficas de gatos. A cardiomiopatia hipertrófica de gatos é caracterizada por vários padrões geométricos do ventrículo esquerdo (VE), incluindo hipertrofia do ventrículo esquerdo (HVE) difusa assimétrica e simétrica com espessamento predominante do septo interventricular (SIV) ou com espessamento da parede livre do VE (PLVE), e HVE segmentar (p. ex., hipertrofia de SIV apical ou subáortico). A hipertrofia subaórtica do SIV pode ser isolada ou associada a padrões geométricos difusos do VE. A hipertrofia dos músculos papilares do VE está frequentemente presente. Todas essas formas podem levar ao aumento do átrio esquerdo e a congestão das veias pulmonares, como mostrado aqui. Abaixo: histogramas representando a distribuição dos padrões geométricos do VE por raças avaliados por ecocardiografia em uma população de 344 gatos com cardiomiopatia hipertrófica, incluindo 239 Domésticos de Pelo Curto, 41 Persas, 22 Sphynx, 28 Maine Coon e 14 Chartreux (valores nas barras representam a porcentagem de gatos).[37] (Ilustrações: execução e concepção pela Dra. Charlotte Taton e Profa. Valérie Chetboul.) (*Esta figura se encontra reproduzida em cores no Encarte.*)

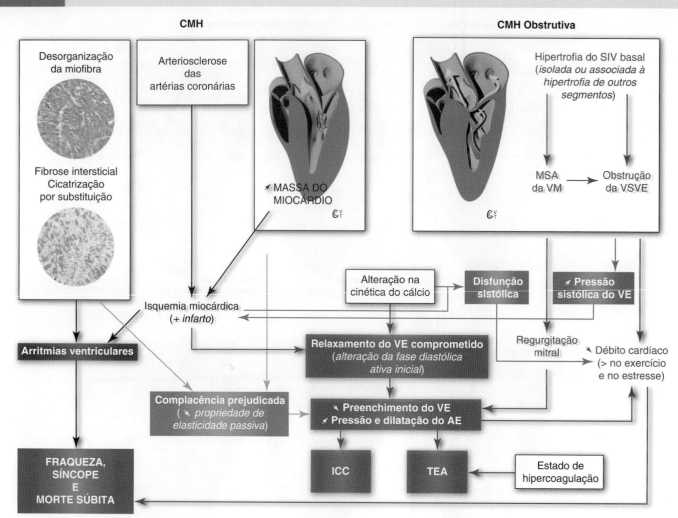

Figura 253.5 Principais consequências fisiopatológicas da cardiomiopatia hipertrófica (*CMH*) em gatos: disfunção miocárdica, arritmias e obstrução da via de saída do ventrículo esquerdo. (1) A disfunção diastólica refere-se tipicamente a anormalidades do relaxamento miocárdico ativo e da complacência passiva, ocasionando enchimento anormal do ventrículo esquerdo (*VE*), com diminuição do volume diastólico final ou volume diastólico final adequado apenas à custa do aumento da pressão de enchimento.[66] Na CMH, ocorre alteração no relaxamento e na complacência, mas há predomínio de anormalidades de relaxamento, que ocorrem precocemente, comprometendo a rápida fase inicial de enchimento do VE. A taxa e o volume de enchimento inicial do VE diminuem, resultando em aumento compensatório da contribuição da contração do átrio esquerdo (*AE*) para o enchimento do VE, associado principalmente à elevação da pressão do AE no fim da diástole.[66] A redução da complacência do VE, resultante de vários fatores (a própria hipertrofia do VE, fibrose intersticial, cicatrização por substituição e células miocárdicas desorganizadas), também contribui para aumento da pressão diastólica do VE e aumento subsequente da pressão do AE. A pressão no AE se agrava com a progressão da doença, que, por sua vez, ocasiona dilatação do AE e, por fim, é transmitida de volta ao sistema vascular pulmonar provocando congestão venosa e insuficiência cardíaca congestiva (*ICC*). A dilatação do átrio esquerdo também predispõe à estase sanguínea e ao tromboembolismo arterial (*TEA*), especialmente no caso de hipercoagulação sistêmica, bem evidenciada em gatos com CMH, mesmo sem ICC e TEA concomitantes.[70,71] (2) Embora não seja predominante, a disfunção sistólica resultante de isquemia do miocárdio, alteração da cinética do cálcio, aumento do tecido conectivo da matriz e assincronia miocárdica regional, pode contribuir para diminuição do débito cardíaco, particularmente nos estágios finais da doença e/ou no caso de CMH obstrutiva.[38,39,72] (3) Lesões histopatológicas associadas à CMH também representam um substrato eletricamente instável para taquiarritmias ventriculares reentrantes, responsáveis por fraqueza, síncope e morte súbita. (4) Na forma obstrutiva de CMH, a obstrução da via de saída do ventrículo esquerdo (*VSVE*) dinâmica pode ocasionar alto gradiente de pressão intraventricular sistólico (até mesmo > 100 mmHg), com várias consequências deletérias, incluindo diminuição do débito cardíaco e agravamento da hipertrofia e isquemia do miocárdio (pelo aumento da tensão na parede do miocárdio e demanda de oxigênio). Nessas formas particulares de CMH, a obstrução subaórtica resulta de ambos, protrusão do septo interventricular (*SIV*) basal espessado para a VSVE e movimento da valva mitral (*MSA*), caracterizado por contato discreto ou tardio do SIV (ver Figura 253.8). Em pacientes humanos com cardiomiopatia hipertrófica obstrutiva, quanto maior a duração do contato mitral-SIV, maior a gravidade da obstrução da VSVE.[33,73] A presença de MSA também pode resultar em perda da coaptação dos folhetos mitrais, levando à regurgitação mitral dirigida, que potencialmente contribui para o aumento da pressão do AE.[33,73] *VM*, valva mitral. (Cortesia da Dra. Charlotte Taton e da Profa. Valérie Chetboul. Histopatologia: cortesia do Prof. Jean-Jacques Fontaine, Departamento de Patologia, Escola Nacional de Veterinária de Alfort, França.) (*Esta figura se encontra reproduzida em cores no Encarte.*)

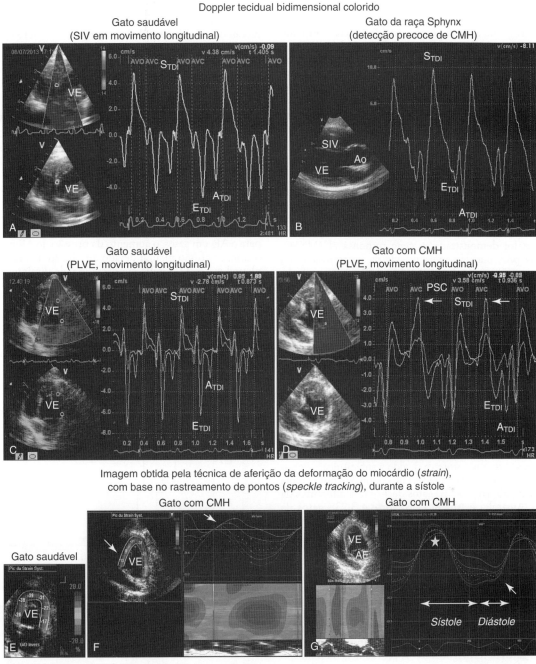

Figura 253.6 Disfunção miocárdica associada à cardiomiopatia hipertrófica (*CMH*), em gatos, observada em imagens de Doppler tecidual bidimensional colorido (*IDT*, **A** a **D**) e imagem de rastreamento de pontos (**E** a **G**). **A** a **D** mostram perfis de velocidade miocárdica longitudinal do septo interventricular (*SIV*, **A** e **B**) e a parede livre do ventrículo esquerdo (*PLVE*, **C** e **D**), em imagem no eixo longitudinal paraesternal esquerdo. S_{IDT}, E_{IDT} e A_{IDT} são picos de velocidade miocárdica registrados durante a sístole, no início da diástole e no fim da diástole, respectivamente. **A** e **B**. Comparativamente ao gato saudável (**A**), o perfil de velocidade registrado na base do SIV, no gato da raça Sphynx (**B**), mostra uma alteração diastólica típica; ou seja, uma inversão na proporção E_{IDT}:A_{IDT} (E_{IDT}: A_{IDT} < 1), apesar da ausência de hipertrofia do miocárdio no ecocardiograma bidimensional modo M (como mostrado na imagem paraesternal direita de cinco câmaras). Seis meses depois, esse gato desenvolveu hipertrofia moderada do SIV subaórtico, seguida de CMH obstrutiva difusa assimétrica. *Ao*, artéria aorta; *AVO*, abertura da valva aórtica; *AVC*, fechamento da valva aórtica; *SIV*, septo interventricular; *VE*, ventrículo esquerdo. **C** e **D**. Comparativamente ao gato saudável (**C**), os perfis de velocidade longitudinal registrados simultaneamente na base e no ápice da PLVE (*curvas amarela e verde*, respectivamente), o gato com CMH (**D**) mostra vários sinais de disfunção diastólica regional: (1) inversão na proporção E_{IDT}:A_{IDT} na base e (2) presença de ondas de contração pós-sistólica (CPS, *setas amarelas*), após as ondas S_{IDT} (e após AVC) e maior que a última, principalmente na base. Esse movimento marcante da onda de contração sistólica (*CPS*), confirmado na técnica de aferição da deformação do miocárdio (dados não mostrados), retarda os dois eventos diastólicos subsequentes (ondas E_{IDT} e A_{IDT}). **E** a **G**. Vários registros em ecocardiografia utilizando a técnica de aferição da deformação longitudinal do miocárdio (*strain*) baseada no rastreamento de pontos (*speckle tracking*), durante a sístole, usando ecocardiografia de rastreamento salpicada, visão paraesternal esquerda das quatro câmaras. *Strain* indica a deformação de um segmento do miocárdio ao longo do tempo, sendo expressa como a porcentagem de alteração de sua dimensão original. Nesses três exemplos, a deformação longitudinal sistólica foi registrada em seis segmentos do miocárdio do ventrículo esquerdo (*VE*), em 3 SIV e 3 PLVE. **E**. No gato saudável, todos os segmentos apresentam encurtamento sistólico regional. A *strain* sistólica é, portanto, negativa e codificada de forma homogênea em vermelho (há sobreposição dos valores de pico sobrepostos na imagem bidimensional colorida). **F**. No gato com hipertrofia segmentar do SIV, os segmentos septais afetados sofrem um alongamento anormal no início da sístole (*seta*) e são, portanto, codificados em azul (painel esquerdo). O painel da direita mostra as seis *strains* longitudinais do VE *versus* a curva de tempo, confirmando uma *strain* positiva anormal para esses dois segmentos do SIV (*seta*). **G**. No gato com CMH difusa, note a presença de CPS (*seta amarela*), durante a fase diastólica. Note também que todos os segmentos do miocárdio sofrem um alongamento anormal no início da sístole (*estrela amarela*). (*Esta figura se encontra reproduzida em cores no Encarte.*)

Contudo, em 3 relatos abrangendo 127 a 344 gatos com CMH[37,41,42] notaram-se amplas faixas etárias – 0,5 a 19, 0,2 a 18,3 e 0,2 a 16,7 anos, bem como variações raciais. Em um relato, o diagnóstico da doença em gatos das raças Maine Coon e Sphynx foi mais frequente nos mais jovens, comparativamente a outras faixas etárias (Figura 253.7 A).[37] Ademais, em outro artigo relata-se que os gatos da raça Ragdoll eram ainda mais jovens (2,5 anos de idade, com variação de 0,5 a 4,5 anos), em comparação àqueles de outras faixas etárias (5 anos de idade, com variação de 0,2 a 16,7 anos).[42]

Bases genéticas: relação entre genótipo e fenótipo

Cardiomiopatia hipertrófica no homem

No homem a CMH é uma doença de origem familiar em pelo menos 50 a 60% dos casos, sendo a herança autossômica dominante a mais comumente identificada.[44,45] Cardiomiopatia hipertrófica foi a primeira doença cardíaca humana na qual uma causa genética foi demonstrada; o gene responsável (MYH7, codificador da proteína da cadeia pesada da betamiosina) foi identificado em 1990.[46] No momento da redação deste capítulo, haviam sido identificadas mais de 1.400 mutações associadas à CMH, sendo a maioria os genes que codificam proteínas do miofilamento ou discos Z dos sarcômeros.[44,45]

Cardiomiopatia hipertrófica em gatos da raça Maine Coon

Em 2005, foi identificada uma mutação no gene sarcomérico da proteína C de ligação à miosina cardíaca (MyBPC3), herdada como herança autossômica dominante, em gatos da raça Maine Coon.[47] Esse foi o primeiro relato que demonstrou uma mutação espontânea causadora de CMH em uma espécie não humana.[47] Foi demonstrado que o gene MyBPC3 pode sofrer mutação no exon 3, e uma única alteração no par de bases (guanina em citosina) altera a estrutura proteica devido à substituição de um aminoácido essencial (*i. e.*, alanina [A] no códon 31) por prolina (P).[47] Em um estudo (n = 3.310 gatos de 17 raças diferentes da Ásia, Europa, Austrália e América do Norte e 3.238 gatos da raça Maine Coon), esta última foi a raça responsável por 100% de todos os gatos positivos para a mutação MyBPC3-A31 P.[48] Em um artigo europeu (n = 3.757 gatos de 17 raças diferentes, incluindo 2.744 gatos da raça Maine Coon), a mutação só foi detectada em gatos Maine Coon e em um gato British Longhair.[49] Assim, a substituição MyBPC3-A31 P (mutação) parece ser específica de gatos da raça Maine Coon, embora eventos marginais potenciais possam ocorrer.[48,49] A prevalência da mutação nessa raça é alta, variando de 31% (Ásia, América do Norte) a 42% (Europa) e 46% (Austrália), com predomínio acentuado (até 92%) em gatos heterozigotos.[48-50] A prevalência do fenótipo da CMH varia de 7 a 10%, aumenta com a idade e é fortemente dependente do estado genético (Figura 253.7 B).[49,50] A mutação MyBPC3-A31 P está associada a maior risco de CMH e o risco é muito maior em gatos homozigotos, com penetrância incompleta em gatos heterozigotos, pelo menos em meia-idade (risco relativo = 9,9 e 35,5, respectivamente).[49,50] Em um estudo constatou-se que mais de 80% dos gatos heterozigotos permaneciam saudáveis pelo menos até os 4 anos de idade.[50] Em contraste, alguns gatos da raça Maine Coon homozigotos podem desenvolver CMH, sugerindo o envolvimento de outras causas ou mutações.[39,50,51]

Cardiomiopatia hipertrófica em outras raças de gatos

Uma segunda mutação por substituição em MyBPC3 associada à CMH foi identificada em gatos da raça Ragdoll.[52] Essa mutação MyBPC3 R820W também é caracterizada por uma única substituição de par de bases (citosina por timina, no códon 820), com troca secundária de um aminoácido (arginina por triptofano).[52] Em uma pesquisa com 236 gatos da raça Ragdoll, a prevalência da mutação foi de 34%, com predomínio marcante da condição heterozigota (85%).[53] Formas de CMH familiar também foram relatadas ou sugeridas em várias outras raças, incluindo British Shorthair,[42] Sphynx,[54,55] Norwegian Forest,[56] além de gatos sem raça definida.[57,58] Na raça Sphynx detectou-se um padrão de herança autossômico dominante, com penetrância incompleta.[55]

Consequências fisiopatológicas

Arritmias ventriculares, disfunção miocárdica e OVSVE dinâmica são as principais consequências fisiopatológicas da CMH (ver Figura 253.5). A disfunção diastólica, considerada o principal mecanismo que explica o desenvolvimento de ICC,[33,34,59-62] ocorre no início do curso da CMH, mesmo antes da detecção de remodelação da câmara cardíaca, confirmada em imagem Doppler tecidual (IDT) (ver Figura 253.6).[33,38,39,61-66] Ocasiona aumento progressivo da pressão no AE, com DAE secundária e ICC (edema pulmonar). Como as veias pleurais viscerais drenam para o AE, em gatos, o aumento da pressão do AE pode, também, ocasionar efusão pleural devido à redução da drenagem venosa pleural visceral.[67] Como confirmado pela diminuição da velocidade sanguínea no apêndice do AE,[68] a estase sanguínea é outra

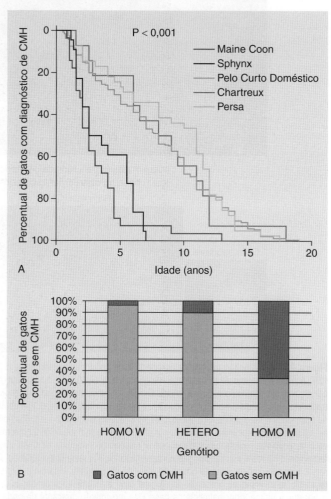

Figura 253.7 Cardiomiopatia hipertrófica (*CMH*) felina e raças específicas. **A.** Idade no momento do diagnóstico de CMH em uma população de 344 gatos com a doença, incluindo 239 gatos da raça Doméstico de Pelo Curto, 41 Persas, 22 Sphynx, 28 Maine Coon e 14 Chartreux. As curvas de Kaplan-Meier mostram as porcentagens de gatos com diagnóstico de CMH, de acordo com a idade.[37] **B.** Distribuição da população de gatos da raça Maine Coon (n = 96) de acordo com o genótipo (*Homo W, Hetero, Homo M*) e o fenótipo (presença ou ausência de CMH).[39] Grupo HOMO W: gatos selvagens homozigotos (*i. e.*, sem a mutação MyBPC3-A31 P). Grupos HETERO e HOMO M: gatos mutantes heterozigotos e homozigotos, respectivamente. (*Esta figura se encontra reproduzida em cores no Encarte.*)

complicação comum da DAE, predispondo à formação de trombo e tromboembolismo arterial (TEA) (ver Capítulo 256 e Vídeos 253.10 e 253.11).[69-71] A disfunção sistólica regional e, mais esporadicamente, a disfunção global, de várias causas, também podem estar presentes (ver Figura 253.6).[38,39,72] Por fim, um movimento anormal da valva mitral (movimento sistólico anterior, MSA; Figuras 253.5 e 253.8) contribui para ambos, OVSVE com diminuição do débito cardíaco e regurgitação da valva mitral, frequentemente relatada em gatos com CMH (29 a 67%).[29,34,41,42,60,62,73] O comprimento do folheto da valva mitral anterior e a prevalência de falsos tendões na VSVE são maiores em gatos com CMHO do que em gatos com CMH não obstrutiva (41% versus 22%), sugerindo possível participação dessas anormalidades na OVSVE (ver Figura 253.2).[29]

Apresentação clínica no diagnóstico

Sinais clínicos

Muitos gatos com CMH não apresentam sinais clínicos no momento do diagnóstico (33 a 77%).[37,41,42,60,74] Esses gatos são geralmente encaminhados por causa de uma ausculta cardíaca anormal detectada no exame de rotina, para fins de triagem antes do acasalamento, ou para avaliação cardiovascular antes de procedimentos anestésicos. A maioria dos gatos com CMH sintomática (70 a 80%) mostra sinais clínicos de ICC (*i. e.*, principalmente taquipneia e dispneia relacionadas a edema pulmonar e/ou derrame pleural, relatados em 18 a 46% dos gatos com CMH no momento da consulta; ver Vídeos 253.8 e 253.9).[37,41,42,74] Em gatos, tosse é mais raramente relatada do que em cães.[1]

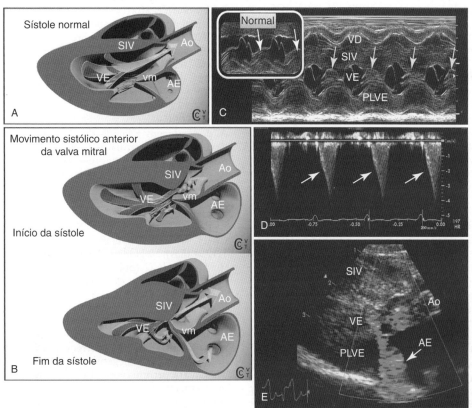

Figura 253.8 Movimento sistólico anterior (MSA) da valva mitral e cardiomiopatia hipertrófica obstrutiva: patogênese (**A** e **B**) e características de imagem (**C** a **E**). **A** e **B.** Em gatos normais (**A**) a valva mitral não se projeta para a via de saída do ventrículo esquerdo (VSVE) durante a sístole. A cardiomiopatia hipertrófica obstrutiva (CMHO) é caracterizada por obstrução dinâmica da VSVE, resultante da hipertrofia do septo interventricular (*SIV*) basal e/ou MSA da valva mitral, que é um movimento anormal da valva mitral para a VSVE durante a sístole (**B**), com um contato sistólico mediano a tardio entre a valva mitral e o SIV. A natureza das forças sistólicas hidrodinâmicas responsáveis pelo MSA da valva mitral tem sido discutida.[29,33,73] O mecanismo de Venturi, no qual o fluxo de alta velocidade flui para a via de saída do ventrículo esquerdo e suspende a valva mitral em direção ao SIV, foi a primeira proposta, mas estudos ecocardiográficos e com Doppler mais recentes em humanos com CMHO suportam a hipótese de que o arrasto, a força impulsionadora do fluxo, é a força hidrodinâmica dominante que se inicia com o MSA da valva mitral, como mostrado na figura.[73] No caso de CMHO o fluxo sistólico do VE é capaz de empurrar a parte inferior de ambos os folhetos da valva em direção ao SIV, devido à maior anormalidade no "ângulo de ataque" entre a direção do fluxo e os folhetos da valva mitral, no início da sístole. Esse aumento do ângulo de ataque resulta de dois mecanismos associados: (1) alterações locais na direção do fluxo intra-VE (aproximando-se da valva mitral) devido à protuberância do SIV; (2) protuberância dos folhetos da valva mitral (com o local de coaptação da valva mitral mais próximo ao SIV do que o normal) devido à hipertrofia dos músculos papilares, contribuindo também para maior mobilidade de cordas tendíneas.[73] Como mostrado na figura, a protrusão sistólica das cordas tendíneas na VSVE, seja isolada (14%), seja associada ao MSA da valva mitral (45%), é relatada em 59% dos casos de CMHO (*versus* 16 e 56% em gatos saudáveis e gatos com CMH não obstrutiva, respectivamente).[29] **C.** Traçado em modo M obtido de um gato com CMHO mostrando marcante MSA da valva mitral, caracterizado por um prolongado contato sistólico (*setas amarelas*) entre o folheto da valva mitral anterior e o SIV espessado, o que não é notado em um gato saudável (*painel superior esquerdo, setas brancas*). **D.** Registro de Doppler de onda contínua em um gato com CMHO e MSA da valva mitral, mostrando aumento da velocidade sistólica aórtica máxima (4 m/s; valor máximo normal de 1,9 m/s)[78] e perfil de fluxo máximo tardio, caracterizado por uma forma típica de onda côncava assimétrica, devido à aceleração súbita do fluxo no meio da sístole (*setas*). Isso confirma a obstrução dinâmica da VSVE. Usando a equação de Bernoulli modificada, o correspondente gradiente de pressão é de 64 mmHg, indicando obstrução moderada da VSVE. **E.** Mesmo gato mencionado na Figura **C**. O Doppler de fluxo colorido mostra imagem paraesternal direita com cinco câmaras, confirmando um jato sistólico turbulento duplo, incluindo um fluxo de ejeção para o interior da VSVE anormalmente estenosada e um jato de regurgitação mitral para o AE dilatado. Como comumente observado no MAS da valva mitral, e também ilustrado na Figura **B** (*figura inferior*), o jato de regurgitação mitral, que se origina do ponto de contato da valva mitral com o SIV, segue o vértice da valva mitral posterior e a direção dos folhetos (*seta*) e, em seguida, atinge a parte posterior da parede do AE. *AE,* átrio esquerdo; *Ao,* artéria aorta; *PLVE,* parede livre do ventrículo esquerdo; *VD,* ventrículo direito; *VE,* ventrículo esquerdo; *vm,* valva mitral. (Ilustrações: execução e concepção pela Dra. Charlotte Taton e Profa. Valérie Chetboul.) (*Esta figura se encontra reproduzida em cores no Encarte.*)

Ascite relacionada à ICC do lado direito também é rara.[37] Anorexia e letargia são comuns em gatos com ICC e podem preceder o aparecimento de ICC em 24 a 72 horas. Um evento antecedente que pode precipitar a descompensação é relatado em 14 a 50% dos casos, 7 a 15 dias antes do início da ICC (p. ex., terapia intravenosa [IV] com fluidos, anestesia recente, cirurgia, administração de corticosteroides e trauma).[37,41] O segundo sinal clínico mais relatado é relacionado a TEA, detectado em 4 a 17% dos gatos com CMH durante o diagnóstico, com ou sem ICC concomitante, caracterizado principalmente por paresia aguda bilateral e dolorosa dos membros pélvicos e, com menor frequência, paresia anterior (ver Capítulo 256).[37,41,42,60] Outros sinais clínicos incluem síncope e fraqueza, observadas em 1 a 6% dos gatos com CMH, por ocasião do diagnóstico.[37,41,60] Por fim, respiração com a boca aberta e dispneia, apesar da ausência de sinais radiográficos e ecocardiográficos de ICC, são relatadas em gatos com CMH.[42] Uma possível explicação é que esses gatos apresentam dor peitoral semelhante à angina, como aqueles relatados no homem com CMH.[42]

Auscultação cardíaca

A auscultação ou ausculta cardíaca é anormal na maioria dos gatos com CMH (78 a 92%).[37,41,42] As anormalidades mais comuns são sopros sistólicos (64 a 89% dos gatos com CMH), mais bem audíveis na região sobre o ápice esquerdo ou na parte cranial do esterno, resultantes da regurgitação mitral e da OVSVE, respectivamente (ver Capítulo 55).[37,41] Esses sopros são frequentemente dinâmicos (ou seja, de grau variável, aumentando com a frequência cardíaca) e encontrados mais comumente em gatos assintomáticos (89 a 92%) que em gatos sintomáticos (77%).[37,42] Isso pode ser explicado pelo fato de que os sopros cardíacos são as principais razões pelas quais os clínicos encaminham animais assintomáticos para ecocardiografia. Ritmo de galope e arritmias são detectados em até 33% e em 6 a 10% dos gatos com CMH, respectivamente.[37,41,42] Ao contrário dos sopros cardíacos, ambos são incomuns em gatos com CMH subclínica (< 10% e ≤ 5%, respectivamente), provavelmente porque esses sinais clínicos sejam reflexos de lesões graves no miocárdio.[37,42]

Achados eletrocardiográficos

Várias alterações eletrocardiográficas morfológicas inespecíficas (ECG; ver Capítulo 103) estão associadas a CMH em gatos, resultantes da HVE (amplitude do QRS > 0,9 mV) e DAE (duração da onda P > 0,04 segundos; intervalo PR > 0,09 segundos).[1,75] Os últimos índices do ECG relacionados à onda P têm baixa sensibilidade (12 a 60%), porém alta especificidade (81 a 100%) para predizer DAE em gatos com cardiomiopatia.[75] Um desvio do eixo esquerdo sugestivo de bloqueio fascicular anterior esquerdo é relatado em 11 a 33% dos gatos com CMH, mais frequentemente naqueles que apresentam outras cardiomiopatias.[1] Arritmias também são frequentemente diagnosticadas (em cerca de um terço dos gatos com CM, em um relato, com predomínio de complexos ventriculares prematuros: 65%; ver Capítulo 248).[60,76] Doenças do miocárdio, predominantemente CMH, são as causas mais comuns de arritmias ventriculares em gatos.[77] Outros relatos de arritmias incluem complexos supraventriculares prematuros, bloqueio atrioventricular ou dissociação atrioventricular (1%) e fibrilação atrial (0,5%).[1,37,60] Uso de Holter por 24 horas, que é mais sensível que o "ECG realizado na clínica" para detecção de arritmia, mostrou que gatos com CMH assintomática tiveram arritmias ventriculares e supraventriculares mais complexas e frequentes do que gatos normais, embora tenham apresentado frequências cardíacas semelhantes.[76] Todos os gatos assintomáticos exibiram arritmias ventriculares, sendo que 82% deles apresentavam arritmias complexas *versus* 20% dos gatos normais, e 87% tinham arritmias supraventriculares, com 23% deles exibindo complexidade *versus*, respectivamente, 60 e 13% dos gatos normais.[76]

De qualquer forma, tais arritmias estão associadas a um maior risco de morte súbita cardíaca ou a um menor tempo de vida, sendo necessária investigação adicional.

Curso clínico e prognóstico

O tempo de sobrevivência de gatos com CMH é altamente variável. Alguns vivem por anos, até mesmo têm uma expectativa de vida normal, e morrem por causa não cardíaca, enquanto outros morrem vários dias após o diagnóstico ou mesmo morrem subitamente antes que um diagnóstico *ante mortem* para CMH possa ser estabelecido. Por exemplo, uma média geral do tempo de sobrevivência de 709 dias, com uma ampla variação (2 a 4.418 dias), foi relatada em gatos com CMH que sobreviveram > 24 horas.[41] Esse tempo de sobrevida altamente variável também foi demonstrado em um outro estudo (1.276 dias, 0 a 3.617 dias).[42] Mortes cardíacas relacionadas à CMH incluem principalmente morte espontânea ou eutanásia, no caso de TEA ou ICC (cada uma delas representando cerca de 33 a 50% das mortes cardíacas), além de morte súbita (10 a 25% de todas as mortes relacionadas à CMH).[37,41,60] Foram identificados vários fatores de risco clínicos, raciais, genéticos e de exames de imagem associados à morte cardíaca.[37,41,42,53,60]

Sinais clínicos

A porcentagem relatada de gatos com CMH que morreram devido a causas cardíacas varia de 37 a 81%, dependendo da proporção de gatos que apresentavam sinais clínicos no momento do diagnóstico.[21,37,41,42,60] O tempo de sobrevida relatado é maior para gatos assintomáticos do que para gatos sintomáticos, dependendo muito dos sinais clínicos manifestados; todavia, com grande expectativa de intervalos de vida para cada categoria de estado clínico.[37,41,42,74] No artigo de Rush *et al.*, gatos com CMH subclínica tiveram uma sobrevida maior (mediana = 1.129 dias), seguidos de gatos que apresentaram síncope (654 dias), ICC (563 dias) e tromboembolismo atrial (TEA) (184 dias).[41] Payne *et al.* também constataram que gatos sem ICC (> 3.617 dias) sobreviveram mais tempo que aqueles com ICC (194 dias),[42] e Trehiou-Sechi *et al.* relataram que 80% dos gatos assintomáticos no momento do diagnóstico morreram devido a causas não cardíacas, enquanto 80% dos gatos sintomáticos morreram em decorrência de doença cardíaca.[37] Outros preditores clínicos negativos de morte cardíaca incluem idade, presença de arritmia com ritmo de galope e arritmia no momento do diagnóstico.[60]

Raça

Gatos da raça Ragdoll têm o tempo de sobrevivência mais curto do que outros gatos (sobrevida média de 19 dias *versus* 1.297 dias, respectivamente).[42] Em um estudo sem a inclusão da raça Ragdoll, a idade no primeiro evento cardíaco (ICC, TEA, síncope, morte súbita) foi menor em gatos da raça Maine Coon (idade média de 2,5 anos) do que em gatos de outras raças (7 anos), com a metade dos óbitos sendo de gatos da raça Maine Coon e atribuídos a causas cardíacas, enquanto a maioria (> 75%) das mortes de gatos das raças Chartreux e Persa foi atribuída a causas não cardíacas.[37]

Genética

Gatos da raça Ragdoll homozigotos para a mutação MyBPC3 R820W têm maior probabilidade de virem a óbito por causas cardíacas e têm um tempo mais curto para a morte cardíaca do que heterozigotos e gatos de raça selvagem (idade mediana na morte cardíaca de 5,7 anos *versus* > 16,7 anos e > 15,2 anos, respectivamente).[53]

Variáveis detectadas em exames de imagem

O aumento do átrio esquerdo, avaliado usando vários métodos,[66,78] está fortemente associado negativamente com o tempo de sobrevida em ambos os tipos de CMH, subclínica e clínica.[21,41,42,60,62] A sobrevida mediana de gatos com CMH com AE de tamanho normal (> 3.617 dias) é, portanto, maior que a dos gatos com HCM e DAE (229 dias).[42] Outros preditores de maior risco de morte devido à doença cardíaca nos exames de imagem incluem HVE grave (≥ 9 mm), diminuição da função sistólica (fração de encurtamento [FS%] ≤ 30%), diminuição da função do AE (avaliado por AE-FS%), aumento do VD, hipocinesia da parede regional, ecocontraste espontâneo/trombo, ou ambos, e padrão de enchimento diastólico restritivo.[21,41,42,60,79]

CARDIOMIOPATIA RESTRITIVA

Definição: lesões patológicas

Cardiomiopatia restritiva no homem

A CMR no homem é uma doença muscular cardíaca incomum caracterizada principalmente por disfunção no preenchimento ventricular devido à maior rigidez do miocárdio (ou menor complacência ventricular) de um ventrículo (principalmente VE), ou ambos, com função sistólica normal ou quase normal e espessamento da parede.[7,80-83] A complacência ventricular reduzida restringe o preenchimento ventricular (por isso o termo "restritivo") e resulta em aumento secundário da pressão de enchimento ventricular no fim da diástole, ocasionando aumento acentuado do AE ou aumento de ambos os átrios. Nos estágios iniciais, a função sistólica global é normal, porém, à medida que a doença progride, geralmente nota-se alteração da função sistólica.[11,83] No homem, a CMR na verdade representa um grupo heterogêneo de anormalidades cardíacas subdivididas em CMR primária e CMR secundária.[11,82,83] As causas de CMR secundária são várias, incluindo doenças infiltrativas (p. ex., amiloidose, sarcoidose, doença de Gaucher e doença de Hurler) e doenças de armazenamento (p. ex., hemocromatose, doença de armazenamento de glicogênio e doença de Fabry). CMR secundária, especialmente fibrose endomiocárdica, também é relatada na síndrome hipereosinofílica como uma complicação iatrogênica (radiação, drogas).[80,83] A CMR primária no homem é caracterizada por fibrose localizada ou intersticial difusa com possível fibrose nos nodos sinusal e atrioventricular, resultando em bloqueio atrioventricular.[80] A fibrose do endomiocárdio é uma forma específica de CMR primária, caracterizada por fibrose acentuada do endocárdio, além de fibrose miocárdica.[84,85] De forma semelhante à CMH, as formas familiares de CMR primária são relatadas como sendo a maioria causada por genes que codificam proteínas do sarcômero ou do disco-Z (p. ex., genes da troponina cardíaca e MYH7).[86-88] Interessante que, além dessas semelhanças genéticas, os fenótipos "sobrepostos" ou "cruzados" de CMR e CMH têm sido observados em famílias com mutações nos genes de sarcômeros, sugerindo que alguns casos de CMR podem ser considerados fenótipos de CMH "minimamente hipertrófica".[83]

Cardiomiopatia restritiva em gatos

"CMR miocárdica" e "CMR com fibrose endomiocárdica" semelhantes às formas de CMR primária no homem foram constatadas em gatos,[1,16,17,89] porém, com maior frequência em gatos em comparação ao homem[17], uma vez que a CMR é atualmente a segunda mais comum cardiomiopatia primária felina (Figura 253.9).[22] Até o momento da redação deste capítulo, nenhuma mutação causal para qualquer gato com CMR foi identificada. No entanto, e curiosamente, Fox et al. relataram que as características histopatológicas da CMH de gatos (p. ex., desarranjo de miócitos, arteríolas coronárias intramurais anormais, cicatrizes por substituição tecidual irregular) são constatadas na maioria dos gatos com CMR, sugerindo que a CMR de gatos pode ser a expressão fenotípica das mutações em sarcômeros.[17] A característica típica da fibrose endomiocárdica felina é a grave cicatriz endomiocárdica que comumente aparece

como uma lesão "tubular" distinta ligando o SIV e a PLVE, que pode resultar em estenose intracavitária média a apical (Figura 253.9 B).[16] A forma menos comum de fibrose endomiocárdica felina é caracterizada por cicatriz endomiocárdica difusa, resultando em redução ou obliteração da cavidade do VE (Figura 253.9 A). Em ambos os casos, o espessamento endocárdico pode envolver as câmaras atriais e o VD (raramente), e está associado com fibrose miocárdica intersticial, graus variados de hipertrofia de miócito e necrose, arteriosclerose coronária intramural e infiltrados inflamatórios.[16] Tais infiltrados inflamatórios também são descritos na forma felina de "CMR miocárdica", sugerindo possível participação de infecção viral e/ou de lesões mediadas por imunossupressão.[90] Em um artigo, pneumonia intersticial foi encontrada em > 25% dos gatos com CMR e uma questão levantada pelos autores era se o mesmo agente ou doença poderia afetar o coração e os pulmões.[89]

Epidemiologia: apresentação clínica no diagnóstico

No artigo de Fox et al., relata-se que, no momento do diagnóstico, 35 gatos com CMR tinham idade média de 10 ± 4 anos, variando de 1,5 a 17,1 anos.[17] Da mesma forma, em um estudo retrospectivo realizado na Alfort Cardiology Unit (UAC) em 112 gatos com CMR (2000-2011), a idade desses animais por ocasião do diagnóstico era 10 ± 4,8 anos (variando de 0,1 a 18,9 anos); apenas 10% dos animais apresentavam > 12 anos. Em uma série de casos de 22 gatos com CMR, constatou-se que a maioria era fêmea (73%).[22] Porém, na publicação de Fox et al.[17] a maioria dos animais era macho (71%), já na população de gatos examinados pela UAC a distribuição da doença foi semelhante em machos (52%) e fêmeas (48%). Nos três estudos, diferentes raças foram acometidas (p. ex., Birmanês, Siamês, Persa, Birman, Maine Coon), com predominância (59 a 78%) de gatos da raça de Pelo Curto (Shorthair), mas sem relato de ligação familiar.

Quase todos os gatos com CMR apresentam sinais clínicos no momento do diagnóstico, predominantemente relacionado à ICC.[17,21,22] Em um artigo sobre 35 gatos com CMR, verificou-se que 91% apresentavam ICC, 6% letargia e 3% síncope e paresia transitória.[17] Da mesma forma, a maioria dos 112 gatos com CMR (94/112, 84%) recrutados na UAC era sintomática por ocasião do diagnóstico, com 76% apresentando pelo menos 2 sinais clínicos. Os gatos restantes (16%) foram encaminhados para ecocardiografia devido à presença de sopros cardíacos ou arritmias, detectados durante a ausculta cardíaca de rotina. Os sinais clínicos mais comuns detectados em 94 animais sintomáticos foram dispneia (76%), seguida de sinais inespecíficos, como letargia, fraqueza, hipotermia, anorexia (56%), ascite (17%) e paresia/paralisia relacionada a TEA (10%). A dispneia foi associada à efusão pleural, na maioria dos gatos (71%), e ao edema pulmonar, no restante dos animais. Em gatos com CMR, constataram-se sopro cardíaco (sopro sistólico apical esquerdo, em 90% dos casos) e ritmo de galope, em 66 e 31%, respectivamente (ver Capítulo 55).

Achados eletrocardiográficos

Várias arritmias são comumente associadas a CMR, em gatos, com predomínio de complexos ventriculares prematuros (23 a 29%) e taquicardia supraventricular (9 a 23%) (ver Capítulos 103 e 248).[17,22] Fibrilação atrial é muito menos comum. Seis dos 112 gatos diagnosticados com CMR na UAC apresentavam fibrilação atrial (5%) e todos apresentavam DAE grave (razão AE:Ao = 2,5 ± 0,7).

Curso clínico e prognóstico

O prognóstico global da CMR no homem é ruim, e a maioria dos pacientes necessita de transplante cardíaco.[91] O prognóstico da CMR em gatos, da mesma forma, é ruim, com a maioria dos animais morrendo de causas cardíacas (60 a 86%).[17,21,22] Em 16 e 14 gatos com CMR relatou-se sobrevida média de 132 e

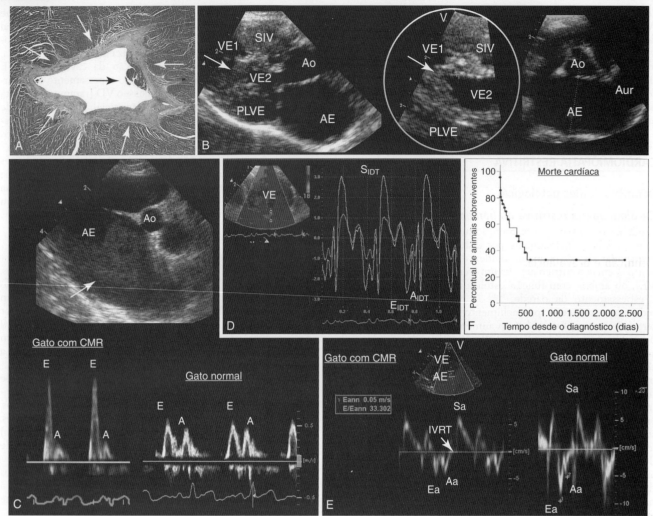

Figura 253.9 Achados representativos em gatos com cardiomiopatia restritiva (*CMR*, formas "miocárdica" e "endomiocárdica"). **A.** Imagem transversal panorâmica do ventrículo esquerdo mostrando uma cicatriz endocárdica circunferencial difusa grave no ventrículo esquerdo (*setas brancas*) de um gato com fibrose endomiocárdica que teve morte súbita. Nota-se, também, um trombo mural (*seta preta*). (Coloração Hematoxilina-Eosina-Saffron). **B.** Ecocardiogramas bidimensionais obtidos de um gato com fibrose endomiocárdica. Esquerda: a imagem paraesternal direita de cinco câmaras mostra uma grande cicatriz em ponte heterogênea (*seta*) conectando o septo interventricular (*SIV*) e a parede livre do ventrículo esquerdo (*PLVE*) e, assim, dividindo a cavidade do ventrículo esquerdo em duas partes, apical (*VE1*) e basal (*VE2*), com dilatação secundária do átrio esquerdo (*AE*), comparativamente à artéria aorta (*Ao*). *Centro*: imagem ampliada da cicatriz em ponte (*seta*), com áreas hiperecoicas focais (fibrose). *Direita*: imagem transaórtica paraesternal direita do eixo curto mostrando acentuado aumento auricular (*Aur*) e aumento do AE (razão AE no fim da diástole:Ao = 2,2; valores obtidos de uma população de 100 gatos saudáveis: 0,5 a 1,2).[78] **C.** Características de ecocardiografia e Doppler de um gato com CMR. *Figura do topo*: o aumento marcante do AE (razão AE no fim da diástole:Ao = 3,7) contém ecos semelhantes à fumaça (*seta*), indicativos de estase sanguínea. *Figuras embaixo*: quando comparado com um gato normal (*à direita*), o exame Doppler de onda pulsada transmitral do gato com CMR (*à esquerda*) obtido em imagem apical esquerda de 4 câmaras revela um padrão de enchimento restritivo típico caracterizado por uma razão aumentada (> 2)[66] entre as velocidades de pico do fluxo no início (onda E, m/s) e no fim (onda A, m/s) da diástole, resultante do aumento da pressão do AE e da redução da complacência ventricular, com elevação secundária da pressão diastólica do VE (ou seja, E:A = 4,6 *vs* 1,4 [0,65:0,45] para um gato normal). A diminuição da função do AE pode, também, contribuir para uma menor amplitude da onda A. O gato com CMR também apresenta um curto período de desaceleração da onda E por causa da rápida equalização das pressões do AE e do VE após o enchimento diastólico inicial (30 ms *versus* 92 ms para um gato normal; valores obtidos em 41 gatos sadios: 54 a 192 ms).[17] **D.** Disfunção diastólica radial diagnosticada em um gato com CMR, por meio de imagem de Doppler tecidual (*IDT*; imagem paraesternal direita do eixo curto) colorida bidimensional. Os perfis da velocidade radial são registrados simultaneamente em dois segmentos da PLVE, ou seja, subendocárdio (*amarelo*) e subepicárdio (*verde*). A disfunção diastólica é caracterizada por ondas diastólicas baixas, especialmente no subendocárdio (ou seja, onda E_{IDT} subendocárdica de 2,6 cm/s; valores normais registrados em uma população de 100 gatos saudáveis: 5,7 ± 1,5 cm/s [3,5 a 10,8]).[78] **E.** Registro de IDT de onda pulsada do anel mitral lateral de um gato com CMR (*à esquerda*) mostrando acentuada redução das velocidades diastólicas (Ea e Aa, cm/s), refletindo uma velocidade diminuída do movimento diastólico longitudinal, em comparação com o gato normal (*à direita*, mesmo animal que em **C**). O pico da velocidade anular no início da diástole (*Ea*) é de apenas 5 cm/s (*versus* 9,8 cm/s para o gato normal; valores normais > 6 cm/s).[66] Além disso, no gato doente, a razão entre a onda E mitral (1,66 m/s, valor não mostrado) e Ea é alta (33 *versus* 0,65:0,098 = 6,6 para o gato normal; valores normais < 12).[66] Por combinar o pico da onda E mitral (principalmente determinado pela pressão de preenchimento do VE e relaxamento) com Ea (que depende principalmente do relaxamento), a razão E:Ea é um índice que reflete a pressão de preenchimento do VE (à medida que o efeito do relaxamento em E é minimizado)[66], embora não existam estudos prospectivos envolvendo o uso dessa proporção em gatos com CMR. A*a* e S*a* correspondem aos picos das velocidades anulares no fim da diástole e na sístole, respectivamente. **F.** Curva de Kaplan-Meier ilustra o tempo até a morte cardíaca após o diagnóstico inicial de CMR na Unidade de Cardiologia de Alfort em 73 gatos que foram acompanhados e sobreviveram por mais de 24 horas após o exame inicial. O tempo médio de sobrevida foi de 364 dias (variando de 2 a 525 dias). A_{IDT}, pico da velocidade miocárdica no fim da diástole; E_{IDT}, pico da velocidade miocárdica no início da diástole; S_{IDT}, pico da velocidade miocárdica durante a sístole; VE, ventrículo esquerdo. (**A.** Cortesia do Prof. Jean-Jacques Fontaine, do Departamento de Patologia da Escola Nacional de Veterinária de Alfort, França; **F.** Cortesia do Prof. R Tissier, INSERM U955 e Unidade de Farmacologia-Toxicologia da Escola Nacional Veterinária de Alfort, França.) (*Esta figura se encontra reproduzida em cores no Encarte.*)

273 dias.[21,22] Morte espontânea ou eutanásia devido à ICC refratária (associada a TEA em > 25% dos casos) e morte súbita foram relatadas em 51 e 9% dos 35 gatos, respectivamente, com sobrevida mediana de 3,4 meses (0,1 a 52).[17] De forma similar, 47 de 87 gatos da população da UAC acompanhados evoluíram para óbito durante o período do estudo, ou seja, 14 (30%) de causas não cardíacas e 33 (70%) de causas cardíacas (incluindo 9% de morte súbita), sendo que um terço dos óbitos foi decorrente de morte súbita nas primeiras 24 horas após o diagnóstico (morte espontânea ou eutanásia devido à ICC aguda). Excluindo os gatos que sobreviveram menos de 24 horas (n = 14, incluindo 11 que morreram repentinamente), o tempo médio de sobrevida foi de 364 dias (2 a 525 dias), considerando morte cardíaca (ver Figura 253.9 F).

CARDIOMIOPATIA DILATADA

Definição e prevalência

Cardiomiopatia dilatada, uma cardiomiopatia primária caracterizada por dilatação do VE com disfunção sistólica (Figura 253.10 e Vídeo 253.15),[8,83] foi anteriormente reconhecida como a segunda doença cardíaca de gatos mais comum.[1] Todavia, Pion et al. demonstraram, em 1987, que a maioria dos casos de CMD em gatos não era realmente "primária", mas sim relacionada à deficiência de taurina e que ela pode ser reversível e evitada com a suplementação oral de taurina.[92-100] Assim, desde então, os alimentos comerciais destinados aos gatos têm sido suplementados com taurina (Boxe 253.1). Outras causas fenotípicas de CMD, tais como taquicardia sustentada, são relatadas também.[101] A prevalência do que se pensava inicialmente ser insuficiência miocárdica primária diminuiu significativamente e atualmente a CMD representa apenas 5 a 10% das cardiomiopatias primárias.[20,22] Um grande número de causas genéticas de CMD foram reconhecidas no homem, sendo a maioria relacionada aos genes que codificam proteínas do sarcômero, do disco-Z ou do citoesqueleto.[83] Uma mutação no gene que codifica uma proteína mitocondrial (PDK4) está similarmente associada ao desenvolvimento de CMD em cães da raça Doberman Pinscher.[102] Porém, até o momento da redação deste capítulo, nenhuma mutação foi identificada como causa de CMD em gatos, embora um envolvimento genético com padrão complexo de herança tenha sido evidenciado em uma grande colônia de gatos Domésticos de Pelo Curto (raça Shorthair).[103]

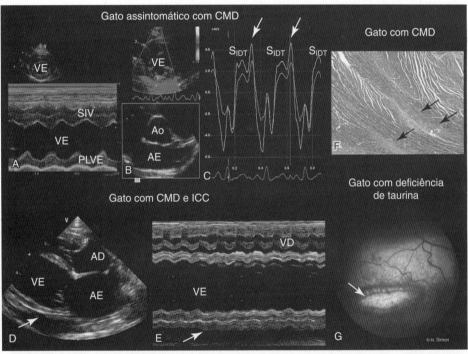

Figura 253.10 Achados representativos em gatos com cardiomiopatia dilatada primária (*CMD*, **A** a **F**) e insuficiência miocárdica induzida por deficiência de taurina (**G**). **A** e **B**. Ecocardiogramas modo M (**A**) e bidimensional (**B**) de um gato da raça Maine Coon assintomático, com CMD, encaminhado para exame ecocardiográfico antes do acasalamento. A insuficiência miocárdica é confirmada por uma diminuição moderada na fração de encurtamento (27%; valores obtidos de uma população de 100 gatos saudáveis: 33 a 66%).[78] O átrio esquerdo (*AE*) se mantém normal (no fim da diástole, razão AE:Ao = 1; valores obtidos de uma população de 100 gatos saudáveis: 0,5 a 1,2).[78] **C**. Mesmo gato de **A** e **B**. Perfis de velocidade miocárdica radial da parede livre do ventrículo esquerdo (*PLVE*) obtidos em imagem paraesternal do eixo curto direito usando Doppler bidimensional tecidual colorido. Os registros simultâneos das velocidades miocárdicas em um segmento subendocárdio (*amarelo*) e subepicárdio (*verde*) mostram que o subendocárdio se move mais rapidamente do que o subepicárdio durante a sístole e também durante a diástole, definindo, assim, os gradientes de velocidade sistólica e diastólica radial do miocárdio. No entanto, o gradiente sistólico médio situa-se no limite inferior de normalidade (0,9 cm/s; valores obtidos em uma população de 100 gatos sadios: 2,2 ± 0,7 cm/s).[78] Também são vistas ondas de contração pós-sistólicas (*setas*), após as ondas IDT e maiores do que as últimas (particularmente subendocárdica). Ondas de contração pós-sistólicas radiais, definidas como contrações miocárdicas radiais tardias anormais, durante a fase diastólica inicial (em vez de ocorrer durante a fase sistólica), não foram observados em uma população de 100 gatos saudáveis.[78] Picos de velocidades miocárdicas registradas durante a sístole (*IDT*). **D** e **E**. Ecocardiogramas obtidos de um gato com CMD e derrame pleural (*setas*) relacionados à insuficiência cardíaca congestiva. Nota-se dilatação das quatro câmaras cardíacas na imagem paraesternal direita das quatro câmaras (**D**). Função insuficiente do VE é confirmada pelo baixo valor da fração de encurtamento (15%) e hipocinesia do SIV e da PLVE no ecocardiograma modo M. **F**. Bandas largas de fibrose (*setas*) substituindo as fibras do miocárdio, devido à fibrose intersticial difusa, em um gato com DCM que morreu repentinamente (Coloração Hematoxilina-Eosina-Saffron, ×25). **G**. Fundo do olho direito de um gato com degeneração central da retina relacionada à deficiência de taurina. Note a típica lesão elipsoide e hiper-reflexiva (*seta*), com borda pigmentada, na área central (i. e., lateral ao disco óptico). *AD*, átrio direito; *Ao*, artéria aorta; *PLVE*, parede livre do ventrículo esquerdo; *SIV*, septo interventricular; *VD*, ventrículo direito; *VE*, ventrículo esquerdo. (**F**. Cortesia da Dra. Nathalie Cordonnier, Pathology Department, National Veterinary School of Alfort, França; **G**. Cortesia do Dr. Marc Simon, Paris, França.) (*Esta figura se encontra reproduzida em cores no Encarte.*)

Boxe 253.1 Caso particular de insuficiência do miocárdio induzida por deficiência de taurina; exemplo de cardiomiopatia secundária nutricional

A taurina (ou ácido 2-aminoetanossulfônico) é um ácido sulfônico que foi primeiramente identificado na bile de touros (daí o nome, da palavra latina *taurus*, que significa touro).[151,152] A taurina é amplamente distribuída nos tecidos animais, com maiores concentrações no coração, na retina, nos músculos esqueléticos e no sistema nervoso central.[151-153] Tem muitas ações biológicas diferentes, incluindo conjugação de ácidos biliares, manutenção das funções da retina e do miocárdio normais e desenvolvimento e manutenção das funções do sistema nervoso e dos músculos esqueléticos.[96,151-155]

Por que ocorre deficiência de taurina em gatos?

Os gatos podem sintetizar uma quantidade limitada de taurina, a partir da cisteína, devido à baixa concentração tecidual de cisteína-ácido sulfínico descarboxilase, uma enzima essencial para sua síntese.[96,156] Além disso, mesmo quando a dieta de taurina é restrita, os gatos usam taurina exclusivamente para a conjugação dos ácidos biliares, mais do que a via alternativa de conjugação com glicina.[157] A perda de taurina nas fezes, na forma de ácidos biliares, juntamente com a baixa capacidade de síntese, predispõem os gatos à deficiência de taurina, particularmente quando a ingestão dietética desse aminoácido é limitada.[96,157,158] Devido às várias funções da taurina, sua deficiência resulta em uma ampla gama de alterações clínicas, que podem ser prevenidas e/ou revertidas com o fornecimento de teor adequado de taurina na dieta. Elas incluem degeneração central da retina, anormalidades reprodutivas (p. ex., infertilidade, aumento da incidência de reabsorções fetais e abortos, baixo peso ao nascer), comprometimento da função imunológica e insuficiência do miocárdio, como foi constatado por Pion *et al.* em 1987 (ver Vídeos 253.17, 253.18 e 253.19).[92,96,153,156] No entanto, nem todos os gatos com deficiência de taurina desenvolvem insuficiência miocárdica sintomática (cerca de 25%), sugerindo a participação de outros fatores ainda não determinados.[96]

Problemas diagnósticos em relação à insuficiência do miocárdio induzida por deficiência de taurina

A suplementação rotineira de dietas comerciais com taurina destinadas aos gatos levou a uma diminuição dramática na prevalência de insuficiência do miocárdio induzida por deficiência de taurina, condição atualmente raramente diagnosticada em gatos, exceto em determinadas condições, como, por exemplo, o uso de dietas vegetarianas e veganas (ver Vídeos 253.17, 253.18 e 253.19).[4,96] No entanto, é muito provável que um pequeno número de casos continue a ser resultado de alimentos comerciais destinados aos gatos contendo quantidade inadequada de taurina.[96,159] Portanto, o diagnóstico de deficiência de taurina em gatos com o fenótipo ecocardiográfico de CMD baseia-se principalmente no histórico simultâneo de baixa concentração de taurina no plasma e/ou sangue total e evidência de deficiência sistêmica de taurina (p. ex., degeneração central da retina; Figura 253.10 G).[95,96] A concentração de taurina no plasma e no sangue total não é afetada pela idade ou pelo peso dos gatos,[160] e o melhor método clínico para avaliar o teor de taurina em gatos é a determinação e interpretação de ambas as concentrações de taurina, no plasma e no sangue total,[155] sendo o teor de taurina no sangue total menos sujeito a alteração do

que o do plasma durante o período pós-prandial ou após jejum alimentar.[95] Em geral, as concentrações normais de taurina no plasma e no sangue total são > 60 e > 200 nmol/mℓ, respectivamente, e há risco de insuficiência do miocárdio induzida por deficiência de taurina quando esses valores são < 30 e < 100 nmol/mℓ, respectivamente.[96] No entanto, jejum de 24 horas resulta em baixa concentração plasmática de taurina, levando a pensar em deficiência de taurina. Inversamente, a deficiência de taurina induzida pela dieta pode ser diagnosticada erroneamente em alguns gatos com insuficiência do miocárdio, como (1) pode ser difícil detectar dieta deficiente em taurina, pois a biodisponibilidade desse aminoácido pode diminuir com o processamento pelo calor (durante o envasamento do alimento), depleção de potássio, acidificação e teor de arroz integral ou farelo de arroz,[100,161,162] (2) resultado falso negativo (i. e., concentração normal de taurina) pode ser constatado em várias situações (coleta de amostra de sangue pós-prandial, TEA recente ou alteração na dieta), e (3) a degeneração central da retina é inconsistentemente verificada em gatos com insuficiência do miocárdio induzida por deficiência de taurina (em cerca de um terço dos animais); ademais, não fornece prova de deficiência atual de taurina (pois também pode indicar deficiência anterior do aminoácido).[92,94-96] A avaliação da resposta à suplementação de taurina pode, portanto, ser um método indireto auxiliar adicional na detecção de deficiência de taurina em gatos com fenótipo CMD e a todos eles recomenda-se a suplementação de taurina, independentemente dos valores da concentração de taurina.[93,96,105]

Suplementação de taurina, outros tratamentos e prognóstico

A terapia de insuficiência miocárdica induzida por deficiência de taurina inclui suplementação desse aminoácido (250 mg/12 h VO), juntamente com o tratamento de ICC (p. ex., diuréticos e inibidores da ECA; ver parágrafo no tratamento). Hipotermia e TEA estão associados a maior risco de morte prematura, que ocorre no primeiro mês em mais de um terço dos gatos.[93] No entanto, quase todos os gatos que sobrevivem mais de 1 mês manifestam evidente melhora clínica e ecocardiográfica. A melhora clínica, incluindo o comportamento e o apetite do gato, geralmente é observada dentro de 2 semanas e, na maioria dos pacientes, a evidência de melhora progressiva do ecocardiograma (em primeiro lugar, a diminuição do diâmetro sistólico e o aumento da porcentagem da FEn sistólica) é relatada 3 a 9 semanas após o início da suplementação de taurina.[93,98] O tratamento de ICC pode ser progressivamente descontinuado quando os sinais de insuficiência cardíaca regridem; a suplementação de taurina também pode ser interrompida assim que os valores ecocardiográficos normalizarem (geralmente dentro de 4 meses), desde que seja assegurada a ingestão adequada de taurina junto ao alimento, que deve ser confirmada por monitoramentos periódicos das concentrações plasmáticas e/ou de sangue total de taurina.[96] Embora a maioria dos gatos se recupere completamente da doença miocárdica, outros podem manifestar insuficiência miocárdica discreta persistente (FEn entre 25 e 30%), apesar da suplementação de taurina.[96] No entanto, esses animais são geralmente assintomáticos e não requerem terapia específica, exceto taurina.[96]

Consequências fisiopatológicas

Como no homem e nos cães,[83,104] a CMD felina é caracterizada por lesões degenerativas no miocárdio do VE ou de ambos os ventrículos, com vários graus de fibrose, miocitólise, arteriosclerose coronariana e alguns infiltrados inflamatórios.[1,90] Essas lesões são responsáveis pela diminuição da função sistólica, dilatação sistólica secundária e, posteriormente, dilatação diastólica dos ventrículos acometidos. A dilatação das cavidades ventriculares comumente resulta em dilatação do anel valvar atrioventricular correspondente e insuficiência valvar secundária, contribuindo potencialmente para a dilatação atrial com subsequente ICC e aumento do risco de TEA.[22,105] Em um relato, insuficiência valvular foi evidenciada em 69% de 32 gatos com

CMD, com as valvas mitral e tricúspide concomitantemente afetadas na metade dos casos e contraste ecogênico espontâneo no AE em 9% dos casos.[105]

Epidemiologia: manifestação clínica no momento do diagnóstico

Em uma série de casos de 11 gatos com CMD, a maior proporção da doença foi relatada em fêmeas (73%) com média de idade de 9,1 anos (intervalo 2 a 15,5 anos), enquanto uma proporção maior de machos (dois terços) de idade semelhante (10 anos, intervalo: 3 a 16 anos) foi relatada em 32 gatos com CMD, sem qualquer predisposição racial.[22,105] A maioria dos gatos com CMD apresentava sinais clínicos de ICC no momento do diagnóstico,[22,105] predominantemente dispneia resultante de derrame pleural e/ou edema pulmonar (diagnosticado em 69 e 34% dos casos, respectivamente)[105] e ascite (6 casos em uma série de 11 gatos com CMD).[22] Há relato de sinais de hipotensão sistêmica (p. ex., fraqueza) (55%),[22] bem como TEA (9%) e colapso (3%).[105] Ademais, em gatos a CMD pode ser diagnosticada incidentalmente em animais assintomáticos (ver Figura 253.10 A a C), indicando a evidência de uma fase subclínica da doença; contudo, atualmente isso não é tão bem caracterizado como em cães com CMD.[104] Anormalidades cardíacas na ausculta são detectadas na maioria dos gatos com CMD (97%), incluindo ritmo de galope (72%), sopro sistólico (34%), abafamento de sons cardíacos (3%) e arritmias (28%).[105]

Achados eletrocardiográficos

A maioria dos traçados de ECG de gatos com CMD é anormal (8/11 dos gatos com CMD, em duas séries de casos) (ver Capítulo 103).[20,22] Alterações morfológicas não específicas do ECG resultantes do aumento da câmara cardíaca são comumente encontradas.[20,22] Várias arritmias também são frequentemente diagnosticadas, predominantemente complexos ventriculares prematuros e taquicardia supraventricular (ver Capítulo 248).[105] A fibrilação atrial é muito menos comum (apenas 1 de 11 gatos com CMD em uma série de casos).[20]

Curso clínico e prognóstico

Entre os gatos com cardiomiopatia, aqueles diagnosticados com CDM têm um dos menores tempos de sobrevivência. A média de sobrevivência de 11 dias foi relatada em uma série de casos de 11 gatos com CMD.[22] Similarmente, um artigo recente relata tempo de sobrevivência dos gatos com CMD mais curto, apesar da inclusão de terapia com inotrópicos (pimobendana) ao tratamento padrão (furosemida, taurina, inibidor da ECA e/ou digoxina) (ou seja, 49 dias [1 a > 502 dias] *versus* 12 dias [1 a 244 dias] em gatos que receberam apenas tratamento padrão). Na maioria dos casos a morte foi devida à eutanásia por ICC refratária (42%) ou TEA (19%); e uma alta proporção de morte súbita também foi relatada (36%; ver Figura 253.10 F).[105] Ambas, hipotermia no momento da consulta e FEn < 20%, foram associadas à redução no tempo de sobrevivência.[105]

CARDIOMIOPATIA ARRITMOGÊNICA DO VENTRÍCULO DIREITO

Definições: comparação dos conhecimentos no homem e em pequenos animais

Seres humanos

A cardiomiopatia arritmogênica do ventrículo direito (CAVD) é, predominantemente, uma cardiomiopatia genética rara que afeta primariamente o VD, sendo patologicamente caracterizada pela substituição fibrogordurosa de miócitos do VD, levando à disfunção e insuficiência do VD, taquiarritmias ventriculares e maior risco de morte.[106-116] No estágio inicial da doença, as mudanças estruturais do miocárdio são discretas e limitadas a áreas localizadas no VD.[110,112] Em estágio mais tardio, as lesões fibrogordurosas no miocárdio do VD tornam-se difusas, com possibilidade de envolvimento do VE.[112] Além da forma "dominante direita clássica" da doença, duas outras formas menos comuns são relatadas: uma forma biventricular e outra forma dominante esquerda caracterizada pelo envolvimento inicial do VE, enquanto o VD permanece preservado.[112,114] Devido a esses subtipos, biventricular e dominante esquerdo, o termo CAVD não reflete estritamente as lesões miocárdicas reais, explicando por que o termo "cardiomiopatia arritmogênica ventricular" tem sido proposto.[111] Curiosamente, a CAVD foi descrita pela primeira vez por cardiologistas franceses, em 1978,[106] e o termo "displasia CAV" inicialmente foi escolhido para nomear a doença, pois se pensava que as lesões de miocárdio resultavam de

anomalias embriológicas.[106-108] Atualmente, a CAVD é conhecida como uma doença cardíaca adquirida ocasionada por mutação em genes que codificam proteínas do disco intercalado, principalmente proteínas do desmossomo (p. ex., placoglobina, desmoplaquina, desmocolina-2, placofilina-2 e desmogleína-2), em mais de 60% dos pacientes.[109,110,112] O desmossomo cardíaco desempenha vários papéis importantes: suporta a estabilidade estrutural do miocárdio, mantém a estabilidade e condutividade elétrica adequada através da regulação de junções comunicantes e homeostase do cálcio, e regula a transcrição de genes envolvidos na adipogênese e apoptose.[110] A CAVD geneticamente determinada quebra a integridade do desmossomo, resultando no desprendimento do miócito, apoptose e necrose, com infiltração inflamatória (como um processo reativo à morte cardíaca), e subsequente substituição por tecido fibrogorduroso (presume-se que represente um processo de "reparação" do miocárdio).[110,112] Essas lesões resultam em atrofia da parede do miocárdio do VD, com dilatação e hipocinesia secundária do VD, levando potencialmente à regurgitação da tricúspide, aumento do AD e ICC do lado direito. O comprometimento da integridade do desmossomo também ocasiona arritmias ventriculares em estágios iniciais da doença, devido à alteração e instabilidade elétrica no acoplamento elétrico do miócito.[112,115] A inflamação miocárdica associada ao CAVD também pode representar doenças imunes ou infecciosas. A predisposição de pacientes humanos com CAVD à miocardite viral ou bacteriana tem sido sugerida, e a miocardite é conhecida por mimetizar potencialmente lesões de CAVD. No entanto, a relação entre miocardite e CAVD ainda não foi esclarecida.[112,116]

Pequenos animais

Há relato de CAVD espontâneo em cães;[117-124] é uma doença familiar na raça Boxer (uma característica autossômica dominante de penetrância incompleta relacionada à idade; ver Capítulo 252), frequentemente associada à deleção no gene da estriatina, no cromossomo 17.[120,121] A estriatina está localizada na região do disco intercalado de cardiomiócitos e colocalizada com outras proteínas do desmossomo envolvidas na patogênese de CAVD no homem.[109,110,112] No gato, a CAVD recentemente foi reconhecida como cardiomiopatia, contabilizando < 5% de todas as cardiopatias (Figura 253.11).[1,20,125] Uma série de 12 casos de CAVD felino foi amplamente descrita em 2000.[15] Desde então, alguns casos esporádicos têm sido relatados.[126-128] No momento da elaboração deste texto, ao contrário da CAVD no homem e no cão, nenhuma transmissão genética foi identificada em associação com CAVD em gatos, o que permanece, portanto, de origem incerta. Na série de 12 gatos com CAVD[15] as lesões morfológicas foram semelhantes às descritas no homem, incluindo adelgaçamento difuso (7/12) ou segmentar (5/12) da parede do VD, aneurismas do VD de importância variada e dilatação do AD em 6/12 e 7/12 gatos respectivamente (ver Vídeo 253.16). As lesões histológicas também foram similares à CAVD no homem, incluindo atrofia acentuada do miocárdio do VD, com substituição fibrosa ou fibrogordurosa (9/12) e gordurosa (3/12) em todos os gatos, apoptose e miocardite focal ou multifocal em 9/12 e 10/12 gatos, respectivamente. Como descrito no homem e em cães,[112,117] lesões semelhantes foram observadas no VE da maioria dos gatos (10/12), inclusive com relato de envolvimento mais grave do VE.[127]

Epidemiologia: apresentação clínica no momento do diagnóstico

No momento do diagnóstico a maioria dos gatos com CAVD é de meia-idade (média de idade = 7,3 anos),[15] embora a faixa etária seja mais ampla (1 a 20 anos).[15,126,127] Não há relato de predisposição de raça ou sexo. O aspecto familiar da doença foi mencionado, porém não foi demonstrado.[125] Por ocasião da consulta, a maioria dos gatos com CAVD apresenta sinais clínicos de ICC do lado direito (ver Figura 253.11).[15,126,127] A síncope relacionada a taquiarritmias ventriculares é o sinal clínico menos

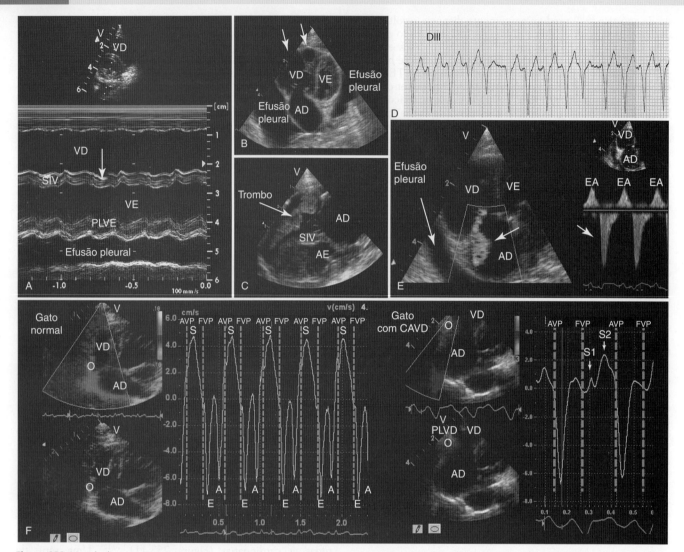

Figura 253.11 Achados representativos no eletrocardiograma, na ecocardiografia e em imagem Doppler tecidual em 4 gatos com cardiomiopatia arritmogênica do ventrículo direito (CAVD). **A.** Ecocardiograma em modo M confirmando uma grave dilatação do ventrículo direito (VD) com movimento paradoxal (seta) do septo interventricular (SIV). Note, também, a presença de efusão pleural como sinal de insuficiência cardíaca congestiva. **B.** Ecocardiograma bidimensional obtido de outro gato com CAVD (imagem apical esquerda) mostrando grave dilatação aneurismática do VD (setas), associada ao aumento do átrio direito (AD) e também efusão pleural **C.** Ecocardiograma bidimensional obtido de um terceiro gato com CAVD (imagem paraesternal direita das quatro câmaras) mostrando dilatação grave de ambas as câmaras cardíacas, com um trombo volumoso na cavidade do VD. **D.** Fibrilação atrial com configuração de bloqueio do ramo direito em um gato com CAVD grave (mesmo animal que em A). Derivação III, velocidade do papel = 25 mm/s, 2 cm = 1 mV. **E.** Insuficiência da valva tricúspide (setas) documentada em modo Doppler de fluxo colorido (à esquerda) e de onda contínua (à direita). Imagem de 4 câmaras em um quarto gato com CAVD em posição apical esquerda. Nenhum sopro cardíaco pode ser auscultado em razão do abafamento de sons cardíacos, devido à presença de efusão pleural. Note a dilatação acentuada das câmaras cardíacas direitas. **F.** Grave disfunção sistólica do miocárdio direito avaliada em modo Doppler bidimensional colorido em um gato com CAVD (à direita, mesmo animal que em B), comparativamente a um gato normal (à esquerda). No gato doente, o registro de velocidades longitudinais em um segmento basal da parede livre do ventrículo direito (PLVD) mostra uma onda sistólica dupla anormal (S1 e S2), com um pico de onda sistólica diminuído e retardado (S2) no fim da sístole, em vez de no meio da sístole (S) como no gato normal. AE, átrio esquerdo; AVP, abertura da valva pulmonar; EA, ondas diastólicas da tricúspide fundidas no início da diástole (E) e no fim da diástole (A); FVP, fechamento da valva pulmonar; PLVE, parede livre do ventrículo esquerdo; S, E e A, picos de velocidade da parede miocárdica direita durante a sístole, no início e no fim da diástole, respectivamente; VE, ventrículo esquerdo. (As figuras E e F encontram-se reproduzidas em cores no Encarte.)

comum.[15,125] Como no homem e em cães, os gatos com CAVD podem permanecer assintomáticos por um período variável de tempo. A doença pode, assim, ser diagnosticada em gatos aparentemente saudáveis encaminhados para ecocardiografia, principalmente em razão da ausculta cardíaca anormal (sopro cardíaco e/ou arritmias).[125,128] Sopro cardíaco sistólico apical direito suave, com regurgitação da valva tricúspide, é detectado na maioria dos gatos com CAVD (8/12 gatos na série de animais avaliados por Fox e colaboradores).[15,125] Arritmias também podem ser detectadas. No entanto, pode haver abafamento de sons cardíacos em caso de derrame pericárdico ou pleural.[125,126] Sintomas gerais inespecíficos (p. ex., letargia, anorexia) também são relatados em gatos com CAVD, mesmo naqueles sem evidência de ICC.[15,125]

Achados eletrocardiográficos

À semelhança do relatado no homem e em cães, os gatos com CAVD exibem grande variedade de alterações no ECG, incluindo complexos ventriculares prematuros/taquicardia de origem no VD e VE (particularmente com envolvimento do VE), fibrilação atrial, taquicardia supraventricular, bloqueio do ramo direito e bloqueios atrioventriculares de primeiro e terceiro graus (ver Figura 253.11 D e Capítulo 248).[15,125,126]

Curso clínico e prognóstico

Embora os gatos com CAVD possam permanecer assintomáticos por um período desconhecido, o prognóstico de CAVD manifesta é geralmente ruim. A maioria dos gatos com ICC relacionada à

CAVD morre alguns dias ou semanas após o diagnóstico inicial devido a causas cardíacas (morte espontânea ou eutanásia por agravamento do quadro clínico ou de ICC e/ou TEA que não responde ao tratamento).[15,126,127] No artigo de Fox et al., 6 dos 12 gatos com CAVD morreram em razão de ICC 2 dias a 4 meses após o início dos sinais clínicos (mediana = 1 mês).[15]

CARDIOMIOPATIAS NÃO CLASSIFICADAS

Este grupo de cardiomiopatias inclui as cardiopatias que não se enquadram em outras classificações (CMH, CMR, CMD e CAVD).[7] Em outras palavras, a cardiomiopatia não classificada (CMNC) não se caracteriza como uma única doença do miocárdio distinta, porém, em vez disso, engloba cardiomiopatias primárias incomuns cujas alterações ecocardiográficas não correspondem às características típicas dos quatro tipos de cardiomiopatias bem definidas anteriormente. Em gatos, o exame ecocardiográfico revela mais frequentemente uma miscelânea de alterações, incluindo HVE segmentar, hipocinesia regional e uma grande dilatação do átrio esquerdo (DAE).[4] No homem, a CMNC primária também inclui outras formas de cardiomiopatias (p. ex., não compactação do miocárdio).[11,129] Embora a patogênese seja pouco clara, ao menos algumas CMNC poderiam representar outras formas específicas ou estágios de outras cardiomiopatias, particularmente CMH, resultante de áreas mais ou menos extensas de isquemia e/ou infarto do miocárdio (secundário à arteriosclerose na artéria coronária, redução do fluxo sanguíneo coronariano devido ao aumento da pressão de enchimento do VE, constrição coronária funcional, densidade capilar inadequada relacionada ao aumento de massa miocárdica e/ou tromboembolismo vascular coronariano).[130-133] O acompanhamento de pacientes humanos e gatos com CMH tem evidenciado um estágio de CMH "dilatada" caracterizada por dilatação do VE, adelgaçamento relativo das paredes do miocárdio do VE, diminuição difusa ou regional da contratilidade e, geralmente, DAE grave.[131-134] Além da participação da isquemia e/ou infarto do miocárdio, apoptose e mutações genéticas têm sido evocadas para explicar essa evolução de CMH fenotípica no homem.[135,136] Essas formas particulares de CMH também são caracterizadas por cicatrizes multifocais no miocárdio, com grandes regiões de fibrose por reposição que podem mimetizar lesões de CMR.[133] Portanto, o diagnóstico de CMNC deve ser estabelecido com cautela e a hipótese de evolução de outra cardiomiopatia primária, em particular CMH ou CMR, deve ser primeiramente descartada. No entanto, pode ser difícil estabelecer o diagnóstico diferencial na ausência de exames ecocardiográficos sequenciais prévios. Em um estudo, a CMNC representou apenas 10% das 106 cardiomiopatias primárias.[22] Os gatos mais acometidos foram fêmeas adultas, com média de idade de 8,8 ± 4,8 (0,8 a 15 anos) e mais da metade com sinais de ICC. Surpreendentemente, um maior tempo de sobrevida foi observado em gatos com CMH (925 dias), em comparação com CMH (492 dias), CMR (132 dias) e CMD (11 dias).

CARDIOMIOPATIAS SECUNDÁRIAS

O diagnóstico definitivo de qualquer cardiomiopatia primária deve ser estabelecido após a exclusão de cardiomiopatias secundárias e outras doenças cardíacas caracterizadas por fenótipos ecocardiográficos similares. Embora às vezes difícil, o diagnóstico diferencial deve incluir, por exemplo, hipertireoidismo, particularmente em gatos idosos,[137-140] tumor infiltrativo (linfoma) ou miocardite, distrofia muscular,[141,142] acromegalia[143,144] cardiomiopatia induzida por esteroides[145] e causas cardiovasculares de HVE (p. ex., estenose aórtica e hipertensão arterial sistêmica)[146-149] nos casos do fenótipo CMH,[150] assim como deficiência de taurina (ver Boxe 253.1),[92-99,151-162] intoxicação por fármacos (p. ex., doxorrubicina) ou taquiarritmia sustentada em casos do fenótipo CMD.[4,92-99,101]

ABORDAGEM DIAGNÓSTICA DE CARDIOMIOPATIAS PRIMÁRIAS EM GATOS

Radiografia torácica

Cardiomegalia

Cardiomegalia é a anormalidade radiográfica mais comum associada às cardiomiopatias em gatos (Figura 253.12).[41,163-165] Como nos cães, o escore cardíaco vertebral (ECV) pode ser usado para avaliar e comparar, objetivamente, o tamanho do coração em radiografias sequenciais, com valores normais de 7,5 ± 0,3 vértebras (v) em radiografias em projeção lateral, com muito pouca variação entre raças (diferentemente do que ocorre em cães), e geralmente aceitam-se limites superiores ≤ 8,1 e 9 vértebras nas imagens lateral e dorsoventral ou ventrodorsal, respectivamente.[165-167] Porém, as radiografias de tórax apresentam algumas limitações diagnósticas. Gatos assintomáticos com CMH e com HVE discreta a moderada e sem DAE não apresentam alteração radiográfica, e como nos cães, edema pulmonar ou efusão pleural podem prejudicar a visualização das margens da silhueta cardíaca, impedindo a avaliação precisa do tamanho e da forma do coração. Guglielmini et al. demonstraram que o ECV é relativamente específico, mas não sensível para prever o aumento do coração em gatos.[165] Por exemplo, considerando um ponto de corte do ECV > 8,2 vértebras, em imagem lateral, a especificidade para predizer qualquer grau de DAE foi de 92%, mas o grau de sensibilidade variou de 63 a 78%, em gatos com DAE discreta e grave, respectivamente. Considerando o mesmo critério (ponto de corte), a especificidade para distinguir gatos com cardiopatia do lado esquerdo daqueles gatos saudáveis foi de 100%, mas a sensibilidade foi de apenas 52%.[165] Porém, o ECV continua sendo um procedimento auxiliar útil para diferenciar causas cardíacas de não cardíacas de dificuldade respiratória, em situações de emergência, quando a ecocardiografia não está imediatamente disponível ou tecnicamente alcançável: em casos de dispneia aguda, um ECV > 9,3 vértebras, em radiografias laterais, é altamente específico para doença cardíaca primária.[168]

Forma do coração

Até recentemente,[169,170] a forma típica do "coração dos namorados", avaliada em imagens dorsoventral ou ventrodorsal (Figura 253.12 D), era relacionada à dilatação biatrial e relativamente específica para CMH de gatos.[1,164] No entanto, uma forte correlação positiva entre o tamanho do AE e a gravidade da forma típica do "coração dos namorados" foi recentemente demonstrada, sem qualquer efeito do tamanho do AD neste último, exceto quando concomitante com DAE grave.[170] Da mesma maneira, em um relato recente, da maioria (83%) dos gatos com cardiomiopatia que apresentavam coração com forma de "coração dos namorados", somente 32% tinham CMH (CMR e CMNC representavam 17 e 34% dos casos restantes; Figura 253.12 H), com aumento biatrial confirmado em somente um terço dos gatos.[169] Em dois relatos, 10 a 19% dos gatos com coração em "forma de namorados" foram diagnosticados com outras condições que não eram miocardiopatias (p. ex., cardiopatia congênita e sobrecarga de volume), e até 7% não demonstraram nenhuma anormalidade ecocardiográfica.[169,170] O coração em "forma de coração de namorados", portanto, não deve mais ser considerado como uma característica específica da CMH em gatos. Nem isso prediz a presença de dilatação biatrial como causa primária de DAE isolado.[169,170] No caso particular de CAVD, radiografias torácicas mostram tipicamente aumento da silhueta cardíaca relacionada à dilatação do VD e do AD, frequentemente associada à dilatação da veia cava caudal (Figura 253.12 I e J).[1,15,125] O aumento global do coração também pode ser visto em casos de derrame pericárdico e/ou dilatação das cavidades cardíacas esquerdas.

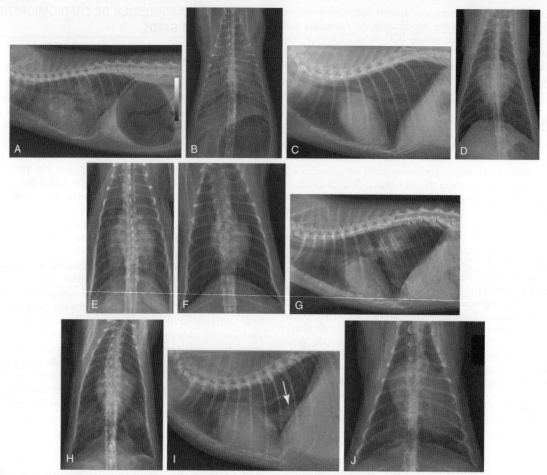

Figura 253.12 Radiografias torácicas representativas obtidas de gatos que apresentavam vários tipos de cardiomiopatia, por exemplo, cardiomiopatia hipertrófica (**A** a **F**), cardiomiopatia restritiva (**G** e **H**) e cardiomiopatia arritmogênica do ventrículo direito (**I** e **J**). **A** e **B**. Imagens lateral direita e dorsoventral mostram cardiomegalia grave, com escore cardíaco vertebral (ECV) de 8,9 na imagem lateral e um coração "em forma de coração dos namorados" (NR: termo comumente utilizado em radiologia veterinária para descrever uma silhueta cardíaca com aumento focal do coração na base do coração de gatos) na imagem dorsoventral. O exame ecocardiográfico confirmou um átrio esquerdo severamente aumentado, sem dilatação do átrio direito. Note o padrão pulmonar alveolar com distribuição simétrica, principalmente cranioventral e caudoventral. Uma grave distensão gasosa do estômago secundária à angústia respiratória também é vista. **C** e **D**. As imagens lateral direita e ventrodorsal mostram cardiomegalia grave (ECV = 9,4 na imagem lateral) e "coração dos namorados" na imagem ventrodorsal. O exame ecocardiográfico confirmou o grande aumento do átrio esquerdo (razão átrio esquerdo:aorta, no fim da diástole = 2,2; valor máximo normal = 1,2),[78] sem aumento do átrio direito. O edema pulmonar é aqui caracterizado por um padrão pulmonar intersticial desestruturado uniforme difuso. **E**. Essa imagem dorsoventral obtida de um gato da raça Maine Coon com cardiomiopatia hipertrófica mostra um aumento acentuado dos vasos pulmonares em comparação com a espessura da nona costela onde se cruzam. Note a largura grandemente aumentada da silhueta cardíaca (> 2/3 daquele da caixa torácica), sem constatação de coração em forma de "coração dos namorados". O edema pulmonar cardiogênico é caracterizado por um padrão pulmonar intersticial desestruturado difuso marcante. **F**. Mesmo gato que em **E**. A imagem ventrodorsal, obtida no dia seguinte ao tratamento com furosemida, mostra regressão do edema pulmonar, diminuição do tamanho da silhueta cardíaca, mas com persistente dilatação dos vasos pulmonares. **G** e **H**. Essas imagens lateral direita e ventrodorsal obtidas de um gato com cardiomiopatia restritiva mostram cardiomegalia grave (ECV de 9,2 na imagem lateral) e coração em forma de "coração dos namorados" na imagem ventrodorsal. Na ecocardiografia, foi documentado aumento marcante apenas do átrio esquerdo (razão átrio esquerdo no fim da diástole: aorta = 1,7). Note também manchas alveolares multifocais nos campos pulmonares cranioventral e caudodorsal compatíveis com edema pulmonar. Não há distribuição peri-hilar, como visto no cão. **I** e **J**. Essas imagens lateral direita e ventrodorsal obtidas de um gato com cardiomiopatia arritmogênica do ventrículo direito mostram um contato aumentado entre a silhueta cardíaca e o esterno e um desvio cardíaco à esquerda compatível com cardiomegalia do lado direito, com ECV de 9. Uma dilatação acentuada da veia cava caudal (*seta*) é também vista (duas vezes a altura da artéria aorta torácica). Note, também, a presença de duas manchas alveolares nos lobos pulmonares caudais. No diagnóstico diferencial deve-se considerar edema pulmonar ou tromboembolismo pulmonar. (Cortesia Dr. Pascaline Pey, Departamento de Diagnóstico por Imagem, Escola Nacional de Veterinária de Alfort, França.)

Sinais de insuficiência cardíaca congestiva

Como em cães, os sinais radiográficos de ICC incluem dilatação vascular, edema pulmonar e/ou derrame pleural. Em gatos com CAVD descompensada, as radiografias torácicas geralmente mostram efusão pleural, enquanto o edema é mais comumente diagnosticado que o derrame pleural em gatos com CMH descompensada (66% *versus* 34%; ver Figura 253.12 A a E).[41] Ao contrário do que acontece em cães, a distribuição peri-hilar a caudodorsal do edema pulmonar cardiogênico não predomina em gatos. O edema pulmonar relacionado à ICC, em vez disso, é caracterizado por maior opacidade, com uma gama de padrões mistos de distribuição variável. Em um estudo com 23 gatos com ICC, notou-se que a distribuição difusa (uniforme ou não uniforme) foi a mais comum, e todos os gatos tiveram evidência de um padrão intersticial reticular ou granular.[171] Padrões intersticiais difusos podem ser semelhante àqueles associados à bronquite crônica (ver Figura 253.12 C e D), o qual pode ser confundido. Uma distribuição ventral também é comum (ver Figura 253.12 A), mimetizando a opacidade pulmonar relacionada à broncopneumonia e levando, portanto, a outro risco de erro de diagnóstico.[171]

Exame ecocardiográfico e Doppler (Tabela 253.1 e Capítulo 104)

Ecocardiografia bidimensional e ecocardiografia em modo M

Ecocardiografias bidimensional e em modo M combinadas ao exame Doppler (Vídeos 253.3 a 253.19) são os procedimentos não invasivos mais precisos na identificação de cardiomiopatias e avaliação dos fenótipos do miocárdio (CMH, CMR, CMD ou CMNC). Contudo, os seguintes princípios básicos devem ser considerados para limitar o risco de erros no diagnóstico:

1. Se tecnicamente possível, exames ecocardiográficos completos devem sempre ser executados. Por exemplo, a CMH é caracterizada por um grande espectro de padrões de HVE de gravidade variáveis. Múltiplas visualizações de imagens 2D (imagens do eixo longo e do eixo curto, da base para o ápice) são, portanto, necessárias para confirmar a HVE e avaliar com precisão a sua distribuição e sua gravidade. A presença de contraste de eco espontâneo, mais especificamente no AE e em seu apêndice, deve ser também sistematicamente e exaustivamente determinada em gatos com alto risco para TEA (ver Vídeos 253.9 a 253.11 e 253.13).

2. A depleção de volume pode induzir a várias alterações, por exemplo, espessuras do SIV e da PLVE, diminuição dos diâmetros do VE com possível obliteração da cavidade no fim da sístole e levando potencialmente a um diagnóstico errôneo de CMH.[172] Em contrapartida, a administração de soluções IV pode aumentar o diâmetro do VE durante a diástole, a FEn (%) ou a proporção AE:Ao acima dos limites normais, mesmo com a detecção de sopros cardíacos sistólicos. Assim, o estado de hidratação e o tratamento diurético em curso devem sempre ser levados em consideração ao se interpretar as mensurações ecocardiográficas em gatos.

3. A influência da experiência do profissional na variabilidade de mensurações ecocardiográficas em gatos foi demonstrada, com maior variabilidade para profissionais menos experientes e há uma tendência frequente destes em superestimar a espessura da parede do miocárdio (até 2 mm), com risco subsequente de "superdiagnosticar" CMH, razão pela qual os profissionais devem estar atentos.[173]

4. Foram demonstrados efeitos de raça e de peso corporal em algumas mensurações ecocardiográficas (p. ex., diâmetro do VE no fim da diástole, espessura da PLVE e do SIV).[55,78] Por exemplo, o valor de corte no fim da diástole comumente utilizado para definir HVE é ≥ 6 mm, mas valores de corte mais baixos (p. ex., 5 mm e 5,5 mm) devem ser usados em gatos da raça Sphynx[5] com pesos < 4 kg e ≥ 4 kg, respectivamente.[55]

5. A mensuração do átrio esquerdo é de grande importância, uma vez que a DAE é considerada como a expressão estrutural de cronicidade e gravidade da disfunção diastólica em gatos com CMH e CMR, com alto valor prognóstico.[34,42,60,62,66] Orientações sobre uma técnica ideal para estimativa do tamanho do AE em gatos atualmente não estão disponíveis.[66] Alguns cardiologistas medem o diâmetro do AE, paralelo ao plano da valva mitral, a partir da camada média do septo atrial até a interface sangue-tecido da parede posterior do AE; um diâmetro < 16 mm é considerado normal na maioria dos gatos, sendo utilizados valores de 16 mm a < 20 mm, 20 mm a < 25 mm e > 25 mm para classificar DAE como discreta, moderada e grave, respectivamente.[66] A razão AE:Ao também é comumente usada para avaliar a DAE (ver Figura 253.9 B). No laboratório do autor, a razão AE:Ao é preferencialmente medida no fim da diástole (quando o tamanho do AE é menor) em imagens 2D do eixo curto, por ser altamente reprodutível, sem efeito de peso corporal, raça ou de gênero, e provavelmente reflete mais precisamente a pressão do VE no fim da diástole do que a mensuração da pressão no início da sístole (valor normal = 0,5 a 1,2).[66,78,173] Ao medir o AE no fim da sístole ou no início da diástole (primeira imagem diastólica em que o fechamento da valva aórtica é evidente), uma razão AE:Ao > 1,5 é compatível

com DAE (ecocardiografia 2D e em modo M, respectivamente).[174] No entanto, uma avaliação sistemática subjetiva do tamanho do AE comparada a outras estruturas (artéria aorta, septo interatrial) é recomendada.[66]

Doppler de onda pulsada

O Doppler de onda pulsada fornece medidas amostrais da função diastólica do VE (p. ex., velocidade do fluxo mitral, tempo de desaceleração do fluxo transmitral [E], tempo de relaxamento isovolumétrico), as quais são comumente usadas em gatos com CMH e CMR, juntamente com a velocidade no anel mitral avaliadas em IDT de onda pulsada (ver Figura 253.9),[66,175] porque a velocidade inicial no anel mitral (Ea) e a relação E:Ea são consideradas mensurações amostrais do relaxamento do VE e da pressão de enchimento (ver Tabela 253.1).[66] Por fim, **Doppler de onda contínua e de fluxo colorido** são usados para avaliar OVSVE e regurgitações em valvas atrioventriculares (ver Tabela 253.1 e Figura 253.8).

Imagem de Doppler tecidual para avaliação dos movimentos do miocárdio

A imagem do Doppler tecidual (IDT) (ver Tabela 253.1) quantifica as velocidades do miocárdio em tempo real e oferece uma análise sensível e quantitativa da função miocárdica regional.[176,177] Vários estudos demonstraram a capacidade do exame IDT 2D colorido para analisar a função do miocárdio do VE em gatos saudáveis acordados[78,178,179] e em gatos com CMH acordados.[38,39] Outros modos de IDT (modo onda pulsada e modo M colorido) também podem ser utilizados, embora a velocidade e as mensurações se limitem a um único segmento ou linha, respectivamente, o que diminui a capacidade técnica diagnóstica.[63,64,72,180] Outra desvantagem do IDT com onda pulsada é a impossibilidade de modificação de posição e tamanho da região de interesse do miocárdio com pós-processamento.

Movimentos diastólicos radiais e longitudinais da PLVE e do SIV avaliados pelo IDT 2D colorido são igualmente alterados em gatos com CMH (Vídeos 253.20 e 253.21) e em gatos com HVE devido à hipertensão arterial sistêmica.[38] A disfunção sistólica regional longitudinal é um componente adicional de alteração miocárdica associada a CMH caracterizada por diminuição nas velocidades e gradientes do miocárdio, assim como da pressão sistólica do miocárdio, em IDT, apesar da FEn (%) permanecer normal ou aumentada.[38,181] O mais importante é que o modo IDT 2D colorido mostrou-se mais sensível do que a ecocardiografia convencional na detecção de disfunção regional do miocárdio em ambas, na CMH de gatos e no modelo de CMH de gatos antes da ocorrência ou na ausência de hipertrofia do miocárdio evidente.[38,39,65,142] No entanto, é importante enfatizar que, para otimizar as capacidades do IDT para detectar disfunção miocárdica precoce, o IDT 2D colorido deve ser preferido pelas razões acima mencionadas. Gatos não devem ser sedados, e o uso da soma de velocidades do início e do fim da diástole deve ser evitado. Conforme realizado no laboratório do autor, o manuseio de um animal tranquilo em um ambiente relaxante, com mínima contenção para a realização de ultrassonografia, com o gato de pé, é altamente recomendado para reduzir o estresse e, assim, evitar a fusão de ondas diastólicas em cerca de 90% dos gatos.[66,78] A técnica IDT também é comumente usada para diferenciar pericardite de CMR no homem.[182] Todavia, atualmente não há dados sobre IDT na CMR de gatos.

Imagem de ressonância magnética do coração

A imagem de ressonância magnética do coração (IRMc) surgiu como uma ferramenta poderosa em pacientes humanos com cardiomiopatias, fornecendo dados sobre volume e função cardíacas e sobre a caracterização tecidual (fibrose e infiltração gordurosa).[183] IRMc tem sido usada em gatos da raça Maine Coon com CMH moderada a grave, porém nenhuma diferença nos índices de IRMc da função diastólica foi encontrada entre gatos controle e gatos com CMH, enquanto pela utilização da técnica de IDT pôde se detectar disfunção diastólica em todos os gatos com CMH.[184-186]

Tabela 253.1 — Critérios diagnósticos ecocardiográficos das quatro principais cardiomiopatias (ver Figuras 253.3, 253.6 e 253.8 a 253.11).*

	CARDIOMIOPATIA HIPERTRÓFICA	CARDIOMIOPATIA RESTRITIVA	CARDIOMIOPATIA DILATADA	CAVD
Ecocardiografia (2D e modo M) — Características mais comuns e formas específicas	• Hipertrofia do VE concêntrica difusa ou segmentada, simétrica ou assimétrica, com PLVE e/ou SIV no fim da diástole ≥ 6 mm+ • Hipertrofia dos músculos papilares • Possível obliteração da cavidade do VE no fim da sístole • Normal para aumento da função sistólica • Dilatação do AE • CMHO: forma específica, com hipertrofia do SIV subaórtico e MSA da valva mitral e/ou das cordas tendíneas, resultando em obstrução dinâmica da PLVE	• Dilatação marcante do AE ou dilatação biatrial • Espessuras normais da PLVE e do SIV (ou nos limites superiores de normalidade) • FEn (%) normal (ou no intervalo de referência) • Áreas hiperecoicas focais ou difusas no miocárdio e fibrose no endocárdio • FEM: forma específica, com ponte cicatricial entre a PLVE e o SIV e/ou espessamento circunferencial difuso hiperecoico do endocárdio, com redução da cavidade do VE	• Aumento do diâmetro do VE durante a diástole e a sístole (≥ 12 mm)[1] • Diminuição da % da FEn (< 30%)[1] • Adelgaçamento da PLVE, do SIV e/ou dos músculos papilares • Aumento, em modo M, da valva mitral, do ponto E à separação septal (> 4 mm) • Dilatação do AE	• Dilatações marcantes do AD e do VD • Movimento paradoxal do SIV • Adelgaçamento difuso ou segmentar da PMVD com hipocinesia, acinesia e/ou discinesia • Trabéculas anormais na PMVD (com predomínio no ápice) • Aneurismas no VD focais e grandes (predominantes no ápice e na região subtricúspide)
Outros achados potenciais	• Hipertrofia da PMVD • Dilatação do AD • Infarto do miocárdio (parede do miocárdio delgada e acinética)	• Discreta redução da função sistólica durante a progressão da doença • Hipertrofia leve a moderada do VE, em caso de fibrose grave do miocárdio	• Dilatação do AD e do VD	• Dilatação discreta do AE e do VE
Doppler de onda pulsada — Influxo mitral	Padrão de relaxamento: razão E:A invertida (< 1), prolongamento de E DT‡ e do TRIV (> 60 ms)§,||	Padrão restritivo: aumento da razão E:A (> 2), com aumento da onda E e diminuição da onda A, encurtamento de E DT‡ e do TRIV (< 34 ms)§,||	Padrões variáveis dependendo da pressão de preenchimento e condições de carga do VE. Padrão restritivo possível nas fases finais da doença, com alta pressão no AE	
Influxo na veia pulmonar	Padrão de fluxo dominante sistólico, com uma proeminente onda AR (e razão Adur:ARdur > 1, se a pressão de enchimento do VE permanece normal)	D reversa (padrão de fluxo diastólico dominante) com uma onda AR pequena ou ausente (e razão Adur:ARdur < 1), preditiva de contração ruim do AE		

Imagem de Doppler tecidual (IDT) com onda pulsada do anel mitral	Pequenas ondas diastólicas (com Ea < 6 cm/s), porém com razão onda E mitral:Ea normal (< 12), se as pressões de enchimento ainda não se elevaram (se elevada, E:Ea ≥ 12)[66] Ea / Aa	Pequenas ondas diastólicas,[66] ou seja, Ea < 6 cm/s, com razão Ea:Aa invertida (< 1) ou normal (> 1), associadas a razão E:Ea > 12 Aa / Ea		
Doppler com fluxo colorido	• Regurgitação mitral • CMHO: 2 jatos sistólicos turbulentos (jato de ejeção com inversão do sinal [aliasing] na OVSVE e jato aliasing de regurgitação mitral em direção posterior)	• Regurgitação mitral • *FEM com ponte de cicatrização*: obstrução no meio da cavidade do VE durante a sístole	Regurgitação de tricúspide e/ou mitral discreta a moderada devido à dilatação do anel correspondente	Regurgitação discreta a moderada na tricúspide
Doppler com onda contínua	• HCMO: perfis de picos tardios do fluxo ventricular (onda de forma assimétrica côncava típica) e altas velocidades de regurgitação mitral • Sinais de hipertensão arterial pulmonar no Doppler	• Sinais de hipertensão arterial pulmonar no Doppler • *FEM com ponte de cicatrização*: aumento de velocidade do fluxo sanguíneo no meio da cavidade do VE	Sinais de hipertensão arterial pulmonar no Doppler	Aumento moderado a grave da velocidade de regurgitação tricúspide devido ao aumento da pressão no VD
Doppler IDT 2D colorido dos movimentos radial e longitudinal do miocárdio	• Os primeiros sinais de disfunção diastólica (podem surgir antes da hipertrofia do VE): razão E_{IDT} longitudinal inversa:A_{IDT} (< 1),[38,39] com ondas CPS (> 50% dos casos) na PLVE e no SIV, e prolongamento longitudinal regional do TRIV em IDT; disfunção diastólica inicial do SIV em alguns gatos, por exemplo, aqueles da raça Maine Coon[39] • Estágios posteriores: razão E_{IDT} radial inversa:A_{IDT} (< 1)[38,39] • Diminuição do S_{IDT} (principalmente para os movimentos longitudinais da PLVE e do SIV)[38,39]	• Pequenas ondas radiais e longitudinais diastólicas da PLVE e do SIV (E_{IDT} e A_{IDT})[¶] • Pequenas S_{IDT} radiais e longitudinais nas formas graves da doença[¶]	• Redução da GVM sistólica radial principalmente devido à diminuição de S_{IDT} subendocárdico; ondas CPS radiais e/ou longitudinais de dissincronia regional do miocárdio[¶] • Diminuição do S_{IDT} longitudinal na PLVE e no SIV[¶] • Menos comumente: inversão da razão E_{IDT}: A_{IDT} radial e/ou longitudinal[¶]	Retardado, baixo (geralmente < 3 cm/s) e/ou S_{IDT} bifásico para o movimento longitudinal da PMVD na base[¶], com ou sem inversão da razão E_{IDT}:A_{IDT} (< 1) da PMVD, na base[¶]

*Outras características de imagem ultrassonográfica incluem sinais de insuficiência cardíaca congestiva (p. ex., efusões pleural e pericárdica, dilatação da veia cava caudal e ascite) e contraste de eco espontâneo ou trombo em câmaras atriais dilatadas. O diagnóstico definitivo de cardiomiopatia primária nunca deve ser baseado apenas nesses critérios de imagem. Cardiomiopatias secundárias caracterizadas pelo mesmo fenótipo sempre devem ser excluídas primeiro. [†]Valores de corte mais baixos devem ser usados de acordo com o peso corporal e as raças.[55,78] Ver texto com explicação. [‡]Vários intervalos de referência de E DT foram relatados (na maioria das vezes < 100 ms, mas variando de 45 a 192 ms, tornando assim essa variável menos confiável na tomada de decisão clínica).[17,66] [§]Os valores inferior e superior do intervalo de referência para TRIV avaliados em 100 gatos sadios acordados de várias raças foi de 34 ms e 56 ms, respectivamente,[78] com um valor de corte mínimo para TRIV (28 ms) na raça Sphynx.[55] O limite superior de TRIV de 60 ms é frequentemente utilizado na prática.[66] [‖] Nos estágios finais da cardiomiopatia hipertrófica, um padrão restritivo (razão E:A > 2, com encurtamento de E DT e TRIV) precedido por um padrão "pseudonormal" pode ser observado, enquanto nos estágios iniciais da cardiomiopatia restritiva pode-se notar um padrão de fluxo mitral de relaxamento anormal (razão E:A < 1, com E DT prolongada e TRIV). [¶]Dados não publicados (Unidade de Cardiologia de Alfort). 2D, bidimensional; A, velocidade máxima do fluxo transmitral no fim da diástole; Aa, velocidade máxima do movimento anular mitral no fim da diástole avaliada em IDT de onda pulsada; AD, átrio direito; Adur, duração da onda A mitral; AE, átrio esquerdo; AR, velocidade máxima do fluxo na veia pulmonar reverso durante a contração atrial; ARdur, duração da onda AR; AIDT, velocidade máxima no miocárdio avaliada em IDT colorida 2D no fim da diástole; CMHO, cardiomiopatia hipertrófica obstrutiva; D, pico de velocidade do fluxo diastólico na veia pulmonar; E, velocidade máxima do fluxo transmitral na diástole; Ea, pico de velocidade do movimento anular mitral no início da diástole, avaliado em IDT com onda pulsada; E DT, tempo de desaceleração da onda E mitral; EIDT, pico de velocidade no miocárdio avaliado em IDT 2D colorida no início da diástole; ES, fim da sístole; FEM, forma endomiocárdica de cardiomiopatia restritiva; FEn (S%), fração de encurtamento do ventrículo esquerdo; GVM, gradientes de velocidade no miocárdio avaliados em IDT colorida 2D e definidos como diferenças entre as velocidades no subendocárdio e no subepicárdio (GVM radial) ou entre as velocidades basal e apical (GVM longitudinal); MSA, movimento sistólico anterior; PLVE, parede livre do ventrículo esquerdo; PMVD, parede do miocárdio do ventrículo direito (livre); PSC, contração pós-sistólica; S, velocidade máxima do fluxo na veia pulmonar durante a sístole; SIDT, pico de velocidade no miocárdio avaliado em IDT colorida 2D durante a sístole; SIV, septo interventricular; TRIV, tempo de relaxamento isovolumétrico; VD, ventrículo direito; VE, ventrículo esquerdo; VSVE, via de saída do ventrículo esquerdo.

Outros procedimentos de diagnóstico (testes genéticos para cardiomiopatia hipertrófica e biomarcadores)

Testes genéticos

Testes genéticos (amostras de sangue ou *swab* bucal) estão disponíveis para identificação de mutações nos genes MyBP-C3-A31 P e MyBPC3 R820W em gatos das raças Maine Coon e Ragdoll, respectivamente, os quais são úteis para a definição de programas de acasalamento e para determinar o risco de um gato desenvolver CMH e vir a óbito por causa da doença.

Biomarcadores (ver Capítulo 246)[187-197]

As mensurações de troponinas cardíacas I e T (cTnI e cTnT) no soro/plasma são altamente sensíveis e são indicadores específicos de lesão aguda em células do miocárdio e devem ser pesquisadas em casos com suspeita ecocardiográfica de infarto, uma complicação rara da CMH.[31,133] Em gatos, a CMH está associada à elevação de cTnI e cTnT, verificando-se maior porcentagem de cTnI em gatos com lesão do miocárdio (67%) do que cTnT (28%).[188-190] Ambas são também preditores de óbito, mas com baixa sensibilidade e especificidade, e sem correlação entre alterações em suas concentrações e a espessura do VE ao longo do tempo.[188] A concentração de cTnI é maior em gatos com dispneia relacionada à ICC do que em gatos com dispneia não cardíaca, mas com marcante sobreposição entre as duas troponinas.[191] Entretanto, o teor plasmático do fragmento N-terminal do peptídio natriurético pró-B (NT-pró-BNP), o qual aumenta principalmente na resposta à tensão da parede do miocárdio, distingue ICC de doenças respiratórias em gatos com sintomas respiratórios com, aproximadamente, 90% de precisão diagnóstica e seu uso, além dos testes diagnósticos convencionais, aumenta significativamente a precisão do diagnóstico diferencial definido pelo clínico geral.[194,195] O NT-pró-BNP também discrimina de maneira confiável gatos normais de gatos com cardiomiopatia subclínica (especificidade e sensibilidade de 100 e 70,8%, respectivamente, para um valor de corte > 99 pmol/ℓ, com correlação positiva entre NT-pró-BNP e a espessura do VE ou a razão AE:Ao).[196,197]

TRATAMENTO DAS CARDIOPATIAS PRIMÁRIAS DE GATOS

Tratamento clínico das cardiomiopatias de gatos: tentativa de abordagem baseada em evidências

Tanto a medicina humana como a medicina veterinária se fundamentam em evidências atuais,[198-201] e a classificação da importância dessas evidências após avaliação crítica da literatura é fundamental.[202-205] Diferentes sistemas foram desenvolvidos para estratificar as evidências em medicina humana.[206] Como poucos ensaios clínicos são relatados em gatos com cardiopatia, a classificação simplificada de 3 níveis da força de evidência parece mais adequado nesta espécie:[207] **nível 1** (ou seja, melhor evidência), fundamenta-se em dados de pelo menos um ensaio clínico prospectivo aleatório controlado (ECPAC); **nível 2**, fundamenta-se em dados de pelo menos um ensaio clínico bem elaborado, não aleatório, estudos analíticos de coorte ou casos controlados, estudos usando modelos de laboratório ou simulações aceitáveis para a espécie em estudo, ou resultados dramáticos em experimentos não controlados; **e nível 3**, com base em opiniões de autoridades respeitadas por sua experiência clínica, estudos descritivos (relatos de casos, séries de casos), estudos em outras espécies, justificativa fisiopatológica ou relatórios de comitês de especialistas. A classificação AHA/American College of Cardiology (ACC), utilizada como consenso no diagnóstico de doença valvular crônica, em cães, talvez também possa ser aplicada a cardiopatias de gatos para esclarecer as diferentes situações terapêuticas:[208,209] **estágio A** corresponde aos gatos com risco de desenvolver cardiopatia, mas sem doença cardíaca

estrutural atual detectável (não se indica tratamento, pois não há doença); **o estágio B** inclui gatos com doença cardíaca estrutural, mas nunca desenvolveram sinais clínicos em decorrência da doença; **o estágio C** refere-se a gatos com sinais clínicos prévios ou atuais discretos a moderados (p. ex., dispneia devido à ICC) relacionados a doença cardíaca estrutural; e finalmente **o estágio D** aplica-se a gatos com sinais clínicos graves devido à doença cardíaca terminal.

Tratamento clínico de cardiomiopatia hipertrófica de gatos (estágios B a D; Tabela 253.2)

Objetivos terapêuticos: principais classes de fármacos

O objetivo geral nos estágios C e D é aliviar os sinais clínicos ou prevenir sua recorrência, a fim de melhorar a qualidade de vida e a sobrevivência do paciente. De forma ideal, o objetivo terapêutico específico deveria ser diminuir as lesões miocárdicas (remodelação e isquemia) e contrabalancear os principais eventos fisiopatológicos (disfunção diastólica e OVSVD dinâmica), a fim de melhorar o preenchimento do VE e aumentar o débito cardíaco. Betabloqueadores, ivabradina, bloqueadores de canais de cálcio, inibidores da ECA e espironolactona podem ser indicados para essa finalidade. Os efeitos potencialmente benéficos dos betabloqueadores na CMH são principalmente atribuíveis aos seus efeitos inotrópicos e cronotrópicos negativos, com subsequente prolongamento da fase diastólica e redução da OVSVD, respectivamente, ambos resultantes da redução da demanda de oxigênio pelo miocárdio (*i. e.*, redução da isquemia), associado a propriedades antiarrítmicas.[210-212] O atenolol, um betabloqueador seletivo, geralmente é preferível aos fármacos não seletivos (p. ex., propranolol) devido ao menor risco de broncospasmo.[5] O efeito potencialmente benéfico da ivabradina se deve ao seu efeito cronotrópico negativo pela inibição da corrente I_f no nó sinoatrial (ver Capítulo 248).[213,214] A ivabradina melhora a função diastólica em gatos saudáveis (nível de evidência 1),[61] mas o seu benefício em gatos com CMH necessita de avaliação adicional. As justificativas para o uso de bloqueadores do canal de cálcio incluem efeitos cronotrópicos e inotrópicos negativos, melhora direta do relaxamento do VE, vasodilatação coronariana e propriedades antiarrítmicas.[210,215-219] Devido aos seus potentes efeitos vasodilatadores, os bloqueadores do canal de cálcio di-hidropiridínicos (p. ex., anlodipino) podem ser prejudiciais nos casos de CMHO no homem[210] e também devem ser evitados na CMHO de gatos (nível de evidência 3). O diltiazem (um bloqueador do canal de cálcio benzotiazepínico) é mais comumente utilizado em gatos do que os bloqueadores do canal de cálcio fenilalquilaminas (Verapamil), porque os seus efeitos inotrópicos negativos e vasodilatadores são menos potentes.[1,5,218,219] Por fim, há vários dados de evidência nível 3 para o uso de antagonistas do sistema renina-angiotensina-aldosterona (SRAA) (p. ex., inibidores da ECA e espironolactona) no tratamento de CMH em gatos. Angiotensina II e aldosterona podem induzir hipertrofia e fibrose do miocárdio *in vitro* e *in vivo*, e em modelos animais de HVE, a espironolactona e bloqueadores da angiotensina II podem reverter essas lesões e melhorar a função diastólica, com efeito vasodilatador adicional aos inibidores da ECA.[220-226]

Estágio B

Gatos com CMH assintomática podem viver anos e a maioria (80%) vem a óbito por causas não cardíacas.[37,41,42] Assim como no homem, a terapia profilática para prevenir ou retardar o aparecimento de sinais clínicos permanece um assunto em discussão. De acordo com o ACC/CCE (Clinical Expert Consensus) sobre CMH humana, alguns casos em risco particularmente alto de morte súbita devem receber tratamento médico nesse estágio.[210] Se esse documento for aplicado aos gatos (nível de evidência 3), seria prudente que fosse de forma semelhante aos critérios adotados no homem, considerando os gatos no estágio B de CMH como pacientes em "categoria de risco", que poderiam requerer tratamento clínico (p. ex., gatos da raça Maine Coon ou Ragdoll mutante homozigoto, gatos com taquiarritmias ventriculares, OVSVD ou HVE grave, e gatos com DAE [um fator de risco de morte cardíaca e TEA,[21,41,42,60] mesmo no estágio B[62]]). Porém, atualmente não há dados que fundamentem o benefício do tratamento clínico ou funcional desse tipo de doença. Um estudo prospectivo, observacional, de coorte clínica aberto não demonstrou efeito do atenolol na sobrevida de 5 anos de gatos com CMH em estágio B (nível de evidência 1).[62] O atenolol também não reduziu a concentração dos biomarcadores em 6 gatos da raça Maine Coon com CMH em estágio B, sugerindo assim uma falta de efeito benéfico sobre a isquemia do miocárdio e a morte de miócito (nível de evidência 2).[227] E, finalmente, o atenolol diminuiu a função do AE e a velocidade do fluxo na aurícula esquerda de gatos saudáveis, que são dois fatores de risco conhecidos para DAE e TEA, levantando a questão do potencial efeito deletério se usado em gatos com CMH.[61] Portanto, se a opção por tratamento for escolhida em vez de "uma espera vigilante", muitos dos clínicos atualmente são a favor dos bloqueadores de canais de cálcio ou de antagonistas do SRAA (principalmente os inibidores da ECA), em vez do atenolol em gatos com CMH em estágio B, exceto nos casos de OVSVD grave e/ou taquiarritmia ventricular. Porém, nenhum benefício na sobrevivência ou nos sinais clínicos foi evidenciado para nenhuma dessas classes terapêuticas, e seus efeitos na função diastólica permanecem obscuros. Um estudo prospectivo aleatório duplo-cego em gatos com CMH em estágio B (nível de evidência 1) revelou aumento da razão onda E mitral:onda A no grupo tratado com benazepril, mas não naquele que recebeu diltiazem, porém sem qualquer diferença entre os dois no fim do estudo.[228] Ramipril ou espironolactona não melhoraram a função diastólica de gatos da raça Maine Coon com CMH em estágio B avaliados por IDT de onda pulsada híbrida em uma localização não miocárdica (com base na Ea, para alguns gatos, e pela soma de Ea e a velocidade anular tardia em outros).[186,229] Estudos adicionais são, portanto, necessários para avaliar com precisão o efeito dos antagonistas do sistema renina-angiotensina-aldosterona (SRAA) na função do miocárdio na CMH subclínica, utilizando vários índices diastólicos não híbridos, a partir de diferentes técnicas de imagem (Doppler convencional combinado com IDT de onda pulsada, bem como IDT 2D colorido, aplicado em vários segmentos do miocárdio), em gatos de várias raças. Em um relato, dermatite facial ulcerativa foi encontrada em 31% dos gatos cerca de 2,5 meses após iniciar tratamento com espironolactona (2 mg/kg/12 h, via oral).[229] Essa reação cutânea adversa (nível de evidência 1),[229] reversível após descontinuação do fármaco, sugere que devem ser usadas baixas doses de espironolactona em gatos (≤ 2 mg/kg/24 h, via oral, nível de evidência 3). Gatos com DAE ou gatos com contraste de eco espontâneo também se beneficiam da terapia antiplaquetária, embora sua eficácia profilática nesse estágio ainda não tenha sido demonstrada.

Estágio C
O fármaco de primeira linha para controlar os sinais de ICC é a furosemida (diurético de alça).[230,231] Na ICC aguda, a terapia hospitalar tipicamente inclui administração parenteral de furosemida, oxigênio (ver Capítulo 131), sedação para minimizar o estresse (p. ex., butorfanol; ver Capítulo 138), toracocentese em gatos com efusão pleural grave (ver Capítulo 102) e repouso em gaiola (nível de evidência 3).[231] Como a furosemida tem efeitos deletérios potenciais na perfusão renal e nas concentrações de eletrólitos, a dose inicial de emergência deve ser reduzida assim que os sinais de ICC melhorem, com a reavaliação dos parâmetros renais e dos eletrólitos (Na, K) na primeira semana de alta nos pacientes ambulatoriais.[231] Uma vez iniciada,

a furosemida é mantida na menor dose efetiva, diariamente, pelo resto da vida do gato (a cada 8 a 24 horas) ou em intervalos de 2 a 3 dias em casos muito raros de ICC relacionada a episódios de estresse. Os fármacos antiplaquetários também são prescritos devido ao risco de tromboembolismo arterial (TEA) (ver Capítulo 256). Um tratamento "específico" (mais comumente os inibidores da ECA)[232] é geralmente adicionado à furosemida, embora os efeitos benéficos na sobrevida a longo prazo justifiquem uma investigação mais aprofundada. Como mostrado com o enalapril,[233] a terapia com diltiazem em gatos com CMH em estágio C foi associada a melhora dos sinais clínicos e diversas variáveis de imagem (p. ex., tempo de relaxamento isovolumétrico), com 94% dos pacientes sobrevivendo após 6 meses, em um grupo de estudo prospectivo controlado sem placebo (nível de evidência 2).[218] Em estudo prospectivo não cego e sem placebo, a adição de benazepril para prolongar a ação do diltiazem foi bem tolerado, com alguns efeitos benéficos nos sinais clínicos e na HVE (nível de evidência 2), mas não no tempo de sobrevida.[234] Por fim, os resultados preliminares de um estudo multicentro sobre insuficiência cardíaca crônica em gatos (nível de evidência 1), em pacientes com ICC tratados com furosemida (incluindo 80% de gatos com CMH), mostraram que a taxa de sobrevida foi maior naqueles que receberam enalapril (sobrevida média = 920 dias), semelhante a de gatos tratados com diltiazem (227 dias) ou placebo (235 dias), e menor no grupo que recebeu atenolol (72 dias).[235] Todavia, as diferenças entre os grupos de tratamento não foram estatisticamente significativas, em parte devido ao número pequeno de gatos/grupo (comunicação pessoal do Dr. Philip Fox).

Estágio D
Em casos de efusão pleural refratária ao tratamento clínico, é necessária pleurocentese periódica (ver Capítulo 102). Espironolactona também pode ser usada (nível de evidência 3). Em alguns casos graves, a dose diária de furosemida pode ser bastante aumentada (p. ex., dose diária cumulativa de 6 a 12 mg/kg ou ainda mais para alguns autores) se os gatos continuarem a comer e beber (nível de evidência 3), embora a desidratação e a azotemia sejam comuns nessa posologia; os inibidores da ECA devem ser usados concomitantemente com muita cautela.[232,236] Outro diurético (hidroclorotiazida) pode ser cuidadosamente adicionado à furosemida (nível de evidência 3).[232] Por fim, o pimobendana, um potente inodilatador licenciado para o tratamento de cães com ICC, pode ser prescrito aos gatos com ICC refratária e/ou àqueles cujo exame ecocardiográfico indica disfunção sistólica do VE e insuficiência renal, em doses semelhantes às usadas em cães (nível de evidência 2), embora dados de ensaios clínicos prospectivos aleatórios controlados (ECPAC) ainda estejam faltando no momento da redação deste capítulo.[231,237-240] Pimobendana não é recomendado em casos de CMHO devido à sua ação inotrópica positiva e, potencialmente, ao agravamento da OVSVD e subsequente hipotensão sistêmica, como já relatado (nível de evidência 3).[239] Em função do efeito potencial de remodelação cardíaca do pimobendana mostrado em outras espécies (nível de evidência 3 para gatos),[241-243] recomenda-se o acompanhamento dos gatos com CMH tratados, com ecocardiograma, ao longo do tratamento.

Outras cardiomiopatias primárias
Nenhum ensaio clínico prospectivo aleatório controlado (ECPAC) foi especificamente realizado em gatos com CMR. O tratamento de gatos com CMR e CMH é, portanto, semelhante, já que ambas as doenças são fisiopatologicamente caracterizadas por disfunção diastólica e subsequente ICC (nível de evidência 3).

Devido às limitações em relação à identificação de gatos com insuficiência miocárdica induzida por deficiência de taurina, a suplementação de taurina é recomendada a todos os gatos com fenótipo CMD ecocardiográfico (nível de evidência 1), independentemente

FÁRMACOS		AÇÃO FARMACOLÓGICA DE INTERESSE	VIAS RELATADAS E DOSAGENS	INDICAÇÕES	CONTRAINDICAÇÕES	POTENCIAIS EFEITOS ADVERSOS	RECOMENDAÇÕES – COMENTÁRIOS
Antagonista da aldosterona	Espironolactona	Antagonista seletivo do receptor da aldosterona; assim, é um diurético poupador de potássio, com potencial de redução da remodelação e hipertrofia do coração	≤ 2 mg/kg/24 h VO ou 0,5 a 1 mg/kg/ 12 h VO	ICC refratária à terapia padrão	Hiperpotassemia	Dermatite facial ulcerativa relatada na dose de 2 mg/kg/12 h	Monitorar a função renal e as concentrações sanguíneas de eletrólitos
Fármacos usados como antiarrítmicos	Digoxina	Propriedades antiarrítmicas com discreta ação inotrópica positiva	0,007 mg/kg VO, a cada 24 h cada 2 d ou 0,03 mg/gato cada 24 h cada dia (gatos > 4 kg) ou cada 2 d (gatos < 4 kg)	• Taquiarritmias supraventricu-lares, inclusive fibrilação atrial • Insuficiência miocárdica (p. ex., CMD)	Taquiarritmias ventriculares	• Anorexia • Vômitos • Arritmias (arritmias ventriculares bradicardia, bloqueio AV) • Maior toxicidade no caso de hipopotassemia	• Concentrações estáveis atingidas em cerca de 8 a 10 dias, mas a meia-vida é variável • Avaliar a concentração sérica 8 h após administração de 8 a 10 dias de tratamento • Variação terapêutica = 0,7 a 2 ng/mℓ • Evitar o uso em gatos com insuficiência renal
	Esmolol	Betabloqueador de ação curta	50 a 200 mcg/kg/min IV, em TIC, ou 50 mcg a 200 mcg (até 500 mcg)/kg/ min IV, na forma de bolus, a cada 5 min	Tratamento agudo de taquiarritmias supraventriculares e ventriculares refratárias à lidocaína	• Hipotensão • Insuficiência do miocárdio grave	• Arritmias (bradicardia e bloqueio AV) • Hipotensão sistêmica • Efeito inotrópico negativo	Comece com a dosagem mais baixa em casos de insuficiência do miocárdio (confirmada em ecocardiografia)
	Ivabradina	Inibidor seletivo da corrente (I_f) no nó sinusal (efeitos cronotrópicos negativos)	0,3 mg/kg/12 h VO	CM com taquicardia sinusal	Bradicardia		
	Lidocaína	Antiarrítmico classe Ib	10 a 30 mcg/kg/min IV, em TIC, ou 0,2 a 0,75 mg/kg, na forma de bolus, lentamente (ao longo de 5 min); repetir apenas 1 a 2 vezes	Tratamento emergencial inicial de taquiarritmias ventriculares	• Hipotensão • Insuficiência do miocárdio grave	• Arritmias (bradicardia e bloqueio AV) • Tóxico para o SNC (p. ex., espasmos musculares e convulsões controladas com diazepam)	• Use com cautela por causa do risco de convulsões • Comece com a dose mais baixa, em casos de insuficiência do miocárdio (confirmada em ecocardiografia) • Monitorar a concentração sérica de potássio (a hiperpotassemia exacerba os seus efeitos eletrofisiológicos enquanto a hipocalcemia os diminui)

		Mecanismo de ação	Dose	Indicação	Contraindicações	Efeitos adversos	Comentários
	Sotalol	Betabloqueador com propriedades antiarrítmicas classe III	10 mg/gato/12 h VO ou 2 mg/kg/12 h VO	Tratamento oral crônico de taquiarritmias ventriculares	• Hipotensão • Insuficiência do miocárdio grave	• Bradicardia • Hipotensão sistêmica • Efeito inotrópico negativo • Anorexia • Fraqueza, depressão	• Diminua a dosagem em caso de doença renal concomitante • Comece com a dose mais baixa em caso de insuficiência do miocárdio (confirmada em ecocardiografia), bem como em gatos com ICC • Monitore a função do miocárdio (ecocardiografia)
Fármacos antiplaquetários	*Ácido acetilsalicílico*	Anti-inflamatório não esteroide que inibe a agregação plaquetária	5 a 81 mg/gato VO, a cada 3 d ou 5 mg/gato a 5 mg/kg a cada 3 d, administrada com alimento	Prevenção de TEA: • DAE discreta a moderada e/ou eco de contraste espontâneo em exame ecocardiográfico • Histórico de TEA	• Desidratação • Hipotensão • Sintomas gastrintestinais • Distúrbios hemorrágicos	• Anorexia, náuseas, vômito, hematêmese (risco de ulceração gastrintestinal) • Sangramento (maior risco em caso de altas doses ou quando combinada com outro fármaco anticoagulante)	• Menor risco de efeitos adversos na dose mais baixa • Efeito profilático de TEA inferior ao do clopidogrel em gatos que sobreviveram a evento anterior de TEA (ver Capítulo 256)[245] • Pode ser usada (com cautela) em associação com clopidogrel ou heparina (ver Capítulo 256)
	Clopidogrel	Derivado da tienopiridina (inibe a agregação plaquetária induzida pela adenosina difosfato (ADP))	18,75 mg/gato/24 h VO		• Sintomas gastrintestinais • Distúrbios hemorrágicos	• Anorexia, náuseas, vômito, diarreia	Pode ser usado (com cautela) em associação com dose baixa de ácido acetilsalicílico (5 mg/gato a cada 3 d) ou com heparina (ver Capítulo 256)
Inibidores da ECA	*Benazepril*	• Inibe o SRAA; portanto, tem ação vasodilatadora venosa e arterial (reduz a pré-carga e a pós-carga ventricular e diminui a isquemia do miocárdio), diminui a retenção de água e Na, potencial redução da remodelação e hipertrofia do coração • Efeito renal protetor	0,25 a 0,5 mg/kg VO, a cada 12 h a 24 h	• ICC em associação com furosemida • Remodelação do miocárdio associada com CMH e CMR	• Desidratação • Lesão renal aguda/oligúria/anúria • Hipotensão	Fármacos geralmente seguros, mas com possíveis efeitos colaterais: • Hipotensão (particularmente no caso do CMHO e grave insuficiência do miocárdio) • Insuficiência pré-renal, no caso de desidratação e/ou altas doses de furosemida	• Monitorar a hidratação; monitorar a pressão sanguínea, particularmente em casos de OHCM e insuficiência do miocárdio (nesses casos, comece com 1/4 a ½ da dose); se houver hipotensão, fracione a dose em 2 administrações/dia • Monitorar a função renal e as concentrações sanguíneas de eletrólitos • Imidapril: forma líquida licenciada para cães; prática para uso em alguns gatos, com boa tolerância à dosagem muito alta[246] • Descontinuar a administração do fármaco se houver desidratação e/ou anorexia e/ou lesão renal aguda
	Enalapril		0,25 a 0,5 mg/kg VO, a cada 12 a 24 h a cada dia ou a cada 2 dias				
	Imidapril		0,25 a 0,5 mg/kg/24 h VO (aumentar a dose se administrado com alimento)				
	Ramipril		0,25 a 0,5 mg/kg/24 h VO				

Continua

Tabela 253.2 Fármacos mais comumente utilizados no tratamento de gatos com cardiomiopatia.* (*Continuação*)

FÁRMACOS		AÇÃO FARMACOLÓGICA DE INTERESSE	VIAS RELATADAS E DOSAGENS	INDICAÇÕES	CONTRAINDICAÇÕES	POTENCIAIS EFEITOS ADVERSOS	RECOMENDAÇÕES – COMENTÁRIOS
Betabloqueador (outros que não sejam esmolol e sotalol; veja acima)	*Atenolol*	Betabloqueador (com atividade antagonista beta-1 relativamente seletiva): • Melhora a função diastólica devido a sua ação inotrópica negativa (resultando também em melhora da OVSVE) e efeitos cronotrópicos • Propriedades antiarrítmicas (taquiarritmias supraven-triculares e ventriculares)	6,25 a 12,5 mg/gato VO, a cada 12 a 24 h	Principalmente indicado aos gatos com CMHO em estágio B ou com CMH em estágio B com taquiarritmias ventriculares	Insuficiência grave do miocárdio	Arritmias (bradicardia, bloqueio AV) • Hipotensão • Fraqueza • Depressão	• Não deve ser iniciado em gatos com ICC • Realizar ecocardiografia antes da prescrição para confirmar a ausência de diminuição da função sistólica • Começar com a menor dosagem • Diminuir gradualmente a dose ao descontinuar o tratamento
Bloqueador de canais de cálcio	*Diltiazem*	• Melhora a função diastólica devido aos seus efeitos inotrópicos e cronotrópicos negativos e à dilatação de artérias coronárias • Melhora diretamente o relaxamento • Propriedades antiarrítmicas	1 a 3 mg/kg/8 h VO Para tratamento de emergência de arritmias supraven-triculares: 0,1 a 0,2 mg/kg IV, na forma de *bolus*, seguida de 2 a 6 mcg/kg/min IV	• Disfunção diastólica (CMH, CMR) • Arritmias supraventricu-lares	• Bradicardia • Bloqueio AV • Hipotensão • Hepatite • Insuficiência miocárdica (p. ex., CMD)	Geralmente bem tolerado, porém com dosagens altas ocorre: • Hipotensão • Anorexia, letargia em caso de maiores dosagens no início do tratamento • Reações cutâneas raras e sintomas GI (constipação intestinal, vômito, anorexia) • Bradicardia • Bloqueio AV	• Ecocardiografia antes da prescrição para confirmar a ausência de diminuição da função sistólica • Formulação de libertação prolongada (não licenciada para gatos), prática para uso nesta espécie: 5 a 10 mg/gato/12 h VO
Diuréticos	*Furosemida*	Ação diurética muito eficiente (diurético de alça)	Emergência: 1 a 4 mg/kg IV/IM/SC, ajustada de acordo com FR (dose máxima: 8 mg/kg/dia) Tratamento crônico: em geral 0,5 a 2 mg/kg VO, a cada 8 a 24 h	ICC (tratamento de primeira linha)	Cardiomiopatia em estágio B, com cavidades atriais normais	• Hipopotassemia • Hipocalcemia • Hiponatremia • Azotemia • Hipotensão • Letargia • Desidratação • Alcalose metabólica	• Estabeleça a menor dose efetiva • Absorção oral reduzida no estágio avançado de ICC (substituir a dose oral por injeção subcutânea) • Monitorar a hidratação e as concentrações sanguíneas de eletrólitos
	Hidroclorotiazida	Efeito diurético	1 a 2 mg/kg VO, a cada 12 a 24 h	ICC refratária a furosemida	O mesmo mencionado para furosemida	O mesmo mencionado para furosemida	O mesmo mencionado para furosemida

Inotrópicos	Dobutamina	Agonista adrenérgico (propriedades inotrópicas positivas)	1 a 5 mcg/kg/min TIC	Tratamento agudo de insuficiência miocárdica	Taquiarritmias ventriculares graves	• Taquiarritmias • Convulsões • Hipopotassemia (com uso prolongado) • Maior demanda cardíaca de oxigênio	Use com cuidado (monitorar a pressão sanguínea [ver Capítulo 99] e o ECG [ver Capítulo 103])
	Pimobendana	Inodilatador (sensibilizador de cálcio e inibidor de PDE III)	0,1 a 0,25 mg/kg/12 h VO; administrar 1 h antes da refeição	• CMD • Disfunção sistólica como complicação de qualquer outro tipo de CM, exceto CMHO • ICC refratária ao tratamento padrão	CMHO	• Agitação • Hipotensão, no caso de CMHO	Ecocardiografia antes da prescrição para excluir a possibilidade de OVSVE e confirmar insuficiência do miocárdio
Fármacos sedativos/ analgésicos	Butorfanol	Opioide sintético misto, agonista de receptor Kappa e antagonista de receptor Mu	0,1 a 0,4 mg/kg IV lenta ou IM (repetir, se necessário, a cada 1 a 4 h)	Reduz o estresse (ICC aguda)	Animais deprimidos	• Letargia • Depressão	
Taurina		Ácido 2-aminoetanossulfônico (ácido sulfônico)	250 mg/gato/12 h VO	• Insuficiência miocárdica por deficiência de taurina • CMD • Disfunção sistólica como complicação de qualquer outro tipo de CM			Em caso de insuficiência miocárdica por deficiência de taurina: melhora clínica em 1 a 2 semanas, achados ecocardiográficos melhoram dentro de 3 a 9 semanas (reduza e cesse o tratamento padrão de ICC assim que ocorrer resolução dos sintomas de ICC)

*Para tratamento de tromboembolismo arterial (ver Capítulo 256). *AV*, bloqueio atrioventricular; *CAVD*, cardiomiopatia arritmogênica do ventrículo direito; *CM*, cardiomiopatia; *CMD*, cardiomiopatia dilatada; *CMH*, cardiomiopatia hipertrófica; *CMHO*, CMH obstrutiva; *CMR*, cardiomiopatia restritiva; *DAE*, dilatação do átrio esquerdo; *ECA*, enzima conversora de angiotensina; *FR*, frequência respiratória; *GI*, gastrintestinal; *ICC*, insuficiência cardíaca congestiva; *IM*, via intramuscular; *IV*, via intravenosa; *OVSVE*, obstrução da via de saída do ventrículo esquerdo; *PDE*, fosfodiesterase; *SC*, via subcutânea; *SRAA*, sistema renina-angiotensina-aldosterona; *TEA*, tromboembolismo arterial; *TIC*, taxa de infusão constante; *VO*, via oral; *q 2 d*, a cada 2 dias; *q 3 d*, a cada 3 dias.

da concentração de taurina no sangue/plasma (ver Boxe 253.1).[92,93,96,105] A terapia com inotrópico positivo também é indicada; contudo, deve-se evitar o uso de fármacos com ação inotrópica negativa (p. ex., diltiazem, atenolol). A digoxina é um agente inotrópico fraco e, portanto, é prescrita principalmente por suas propriedades antiarrítmicas (em casos de taquicardia supraventricular).[244] O pimobendana é, portanto, preferido para o tratamento de gatos com CMD. Adicionado à terapia padrão (furosemida, taurina, inibidor da ECA, com ou sem digoxina), o pimobendana aumenta o tempo de sobrevida de gatos com CMD que não respondem ao tratamento com taurina, embora o prognóstico permaneça ruim (tempo de sobrevida média = 49 dias, nível de evidência 2).[105]

O tratamento de gatos com CAVD é semelhante ao da CMD (nível de evidência 3). A terapia antiplaquetária é geralmente prescrita devido ao risco de TEA relacionado ao aumento acentuado do AD. Casos refratários de taquicardia ventricular sintomática podem ser tratados com lidocaína IV ou esmolol IV. Sotalol pode ser prescrito para tratamento oral de longa duração, mas o seu efeito inotrópico negativo pode ser problemático.[125,219]

O tratamento de gatos com CMNC tem como objetivo controlar a ICC, se presente, e também se fundamenta no fenótipo miocárdico predominante (i. e., tratamento clínico de disfunção diastólica ou sistólica predominante, sendo semelhante ao de CMH ou CMD, respectivamente [nível de evidência 3]).

AGRADECIMENTOS

A autora é grata a toda a equipe de Cardiologia da Unidade Alfort, mais especificamente, Dra. Vassiliki Gouni, Dra. Cécile Damoiseaux, Dra. Charlotte Misbach, Dra. Emilie Trehiou Sechi e Prof. Jean-Louis Pouchelon. E também ao Prof. Renaud Tissier (INSERM U955 e Farmacologia-Toxicologia Unidade, Escola Nacional Veterinária de Alfort), Dr. Philip Fox (Centro Médico Animal, NYC, EUA), Prof. Jean-Jacques Fontaine e Dra. Nathalie Cordonnier (Departamento de Patologia, Escola Nacional de Veterinária de Alfort,) Dr. Marc Simon (Paris), Dr. Pascaline Pey (Departamento de Diagnóstico por Imagem, Escola Nacional Veterinária de Alfort), Dr. Patrick Verwaerde (Escola Nacional Veterinária de Toulouse), Sra. Diana Warwick e Dra. Charlotte Taton (ilustradora) por sua preciosa ajuda na compilação este capítulo. A autora também gostaria de agradecer sinceramente aos Drs. Stephen Ettinger e Etienne Côté por sua confiança e grande honra em pedir-lhe para contribuir para a 8ª edição do livro texto de *Veterinária em Medicina Interna*.

REFERÊNCIAS BIBLIOGRÁFICAS

As referências bibliográficas deste capítulo se encontram online no Ambiente de Aprendizagem.

CAPÍTULO 254

Doenças do Pericárdio

Kristin MacDonald

INTRODUÇÃO

Efusão pericárdica é a anormalidade pericárdica mais comum em cães e gatos. Quando causa tamponamento cardíaco, é uma causa comum de insuficiência cardíaca congestiva do lado direito em cães; no entanto, o tratamento é muito diferente da maioria das outras causas de insuficiência cardíaca direita. A efusão pericárdica é uma anormalidade multifatorial, incluindo causas infecciosas, inflamatórias e neoplásicas, com um amplo espectro de prognósticos que variam de bom até a morte.[2] Defeitos congênitos, incluindo hérnia diafragmática peritônio-pericárdica (HDPP), defeitos ou cistos pericárdicos, são menos comumente diagnosticados em cães e gatos. Pericardite constritiva é uma doença do pericárdio adquirida, incomum em cães e extremamente rara em gatos.

ANATOMIA E FISIOLOGIA DO PERICÁRDIO

O pericárdio é formado por duas membranas: uma membrana externa fibrosa, a membrana parietal, e uma membrana interna serosa, a membrana visceral, que forma o epicárdio. A base do pericárdio fibroso é continuada por grandes artérias e veias que adentram o coração e se misturam com a adventícia desses vasos. O ápice do pericárdio fibroso segue para a parte ventral do diafragma como o ligamento frênico-pericárdico ou reflexão mediastinal caudomedial.[7-9] As membranas parietal e visceral se unem na base cardíaca, e o espaço ao redor do coração entre as duas membranas é a cavidade pericárdica. Um pequeno volume de líquido (0,3 a 1 mℓ) normalmente está presente na cavidade pericárdica e serve para diminuir o atrito entre as duas membranas.

A membrana parietal é composta de células mesoteliais e tecido conjuntivo, incluindo fibras colágenas compactadas em uma orientação multicamada, intercaladas com fibras de elastina menos abundantes. Essa estrutura fornece propriedades fibroelásticas, para que seja facilmente distensível em baixo volume, porém menos distensível com grande volume de líquido pericárdico. Quando ocorre aumento crônico do volume pericárdico, o pericárdio alonga-se para suportar o volume intrapericárdico e, dessa maneira, torna-se mais distensível, parte complacente da curva volume-pressão. A pressão intrapericárdica é normalmente subatmosférica durante a maior parte do ciclo cardíaco (com a menor pressão durante a ejeção ventricular), semelhante ao que acontece com a pressão intrapleural. O pericárdio visceral é composto de células mesoteliais que se sobrepõem ao tecido conjuntivo e à elastina.

Embora o pericárdio tenha diversas funções para o coração, não é um requisito vital para manter as condições cardiovasculares normais, e a remoção cirúrgica ou agenesia congênita dessa estrutura não está associada a efeitos deletérios. As funções do pericárdio de restringir a excessiva dilatação cardíaca protege o coração de infecções e formação de aderências com os tecidos adjacentes, mantém o coração em uma posição fixa na cavidade torácica, regula a inter-relação entre o volume sistólico dos dois ventrículos e evita a regurgitação na valva tricúspide quando pressão ventricular se eleva durante a diástole. O efeito lubrificante do líquido pericárdico permite ao coração mover-se facilmente no saco pericárdico durante a sístole e a diástole.[10]

ANORMALIDADES CONGÊNITAS DO PERICÁRDIO

Hérnia diafragmática peritônio-pericárdica

HDPP é um defeito congênito que causa comunicação entre as cavidades pericárdica e peritoneal, possibilitando que órgãos abdominais entrem no espaço pericárdico, mantendo o espaço pleural intacto. A HDPP se forma quando há alterações no desenvolvimento embrionário da parte ventral do diafragma devido à fusão anormal do septo transverso com as pregas pleuroperitoneais.[3] Os órgãos mais comumente encontrados na hérnia são fígado e vesícula biliar, seguidos de intestino delgado, omento, baço e estômago.[4-6] A HDPP é uma anormalidade incomum, com prevalência variando de 0,02 a 0,15%, em cães, e 0,05 a 0,59% em gatos.[5-7] Gatos de pelos de tamanho médio ou longo são mais predispostos à HDPP (24/31 gatos em um estudo) e as raças predispostas incluem Maine Coon (prevalência de 12,9%), Himalaia (2,2%), gatos Domésticos de Pelo Longo (2,2%) e Persa (1%).[6] Os cães da raça Weimaraner também são predispostos.[5,6]

Sinais clínicos

Os sinais clínicos de HDPP variam dependendo dos órgãos ou tecidos contidos na hérnia. Aproximadamente metade dos cães e gatos de uma série de casos não apresentavam sinais clínicos e a HDPP foi um achado incidental.[5] Em animais sintomáticos, predominam sinais clínicos referentes aos sistemas respiratório e gastrintestinal (GI): taquipneia, angústia respiratória, vômito e anorexia são comuns. Outros possíveis sintomas são letargia, perda de peso, diarreia, intolerância ao exercício e tosse.

Diagnóstico

As anormalidades no exame físico em cães e gatos acometidos frequentemente incluem abafamento de sons cardíacos, ausência ou deslocamento do batimento apical, abafamento de sons pulmonares, taquipneia e baixo escore corporal. Outras alterações menos comuns são presença de sopro cardíaco, febre, borborigmo torácico, abdome vazio à palpação ou abdome cheio e doloroso à palpação.[5,6,10] Anormalidades associadas comumente em cães incluem malformações esternais (cartilagem xifoide incompleta); *pectus excavatum* (ou peito escavado); esternebra ausente (deformada ou fundida), hérnias abdominais cranioventrais e outras cardiopatias congênitas (estenose pulmonar e defeito do septo ventricular). Anormalidades associadas em gatos são menos comuns e geralmente limitam-se a malformações esternais e hérnias abdominais cranioventrais.

As radiografias de tórax geralmente são diagnósticas para HDPP (Figura 254.1).[5,10] Anormalidades compatíveis com HDPP incluem aumento da silhueta cardíaca e perda da distinção entre

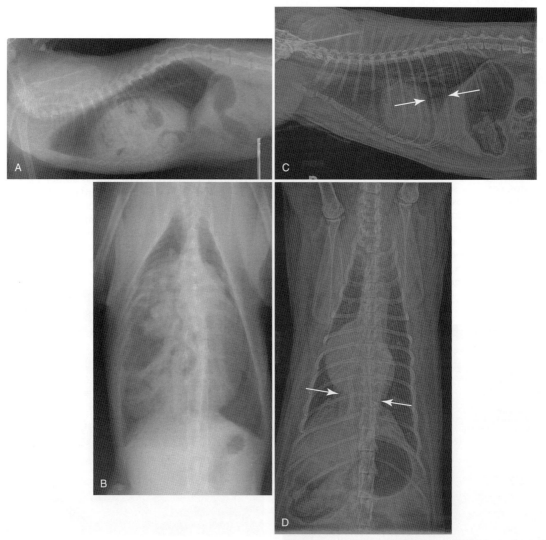

Figura 254.1 Radiografias torácicas lateral (**A**) e dorsoventral (**B**) de um gato com uma grande hérnia diafragmática peritônio-pericárdica (HDPP). A silhueta cardíaca está grandemente aumentada e o espaço pericárdico contém estruturas de diferentes opacidades e alças intestinais cheias de gás. A maior parte do conteúdo abdominal, incluindo o fígado e o intestino delgado, está deslocada para dentro do saco pericárdico. Radiografias lateral (**C**) e dorsoventral (**D**) de outro gato com HDPP. Embora as anormalidades sejam menos evidentes, a imagem lateral mostra claramente a persistência do retalho mesotelial remanescente dorsal (*setas*).

o coração e o diafragma, com opacidade devido à sobreposição de tecidos moles. A silhueta cardíaca geralmente contém alças intestinais cheias de gás, bem como estruturas de diferentes radiopacidades (ver Figura 254.1). A silhueta hepática pode ser pequena ou ausente, no abdome cranial, causando desvio cranial no eixo gástrico. Vários outros órgãos (intestino delgado, baço) podem estar ausentes do abdome. Nos gatos, um retalho mesotelial peritônio-pericárdico dorsal remanescente, que representa a borda dorsal da hérnia, pode ser visto em imagem visão lateral como uma opacidade curvilínea entre a silhueta cardíaca e o diafragma, na região ventral da veia cava caudal ou sobreposto a ela.[4-6] A obtenção de radiografias torácicas padrão e ecocardiografia eliminaram a necessidade de execução de série de radiografias do trato gastrintestinal (GI) superior, com contraste de bário, para o diagnóstico de HDPP.

O ecocardiograma é um exame confirmatório do diagnóstico de HDPP, no qual os órgãos abdominais (mais comumente o fígado) podem ser visualizados adjacentes ao coração no espaço pericárdico (Figura 254.2; Vídeo 254.1). Um importante diagnóstico diferencial é a consolidação (hepatização) do lobo pulmonar acessório; os achados radiográficos torácicos ajudam a diferenciar essa lesão e a HDPP. Discreta efusão pericárdica pode ser notada, porém efusão grave e tamponamento cardíaco são incomuns. O eletrocardiograma pode ser normal ou mostrar complexos de baixa voltagem e direção anormal do eixo elétrico principal. Os resultados do hemograma completo e do perfil bioquímico sérico geralmente são pouco notáveis; as anormalidades mais comuns incluem elevação da atividade sérica de alanina aminotransferase em cães (n = 10/26 cães) e aumento da concentração sérica de cálcio em gatos (9/29).[6]

Tratamento

Recomenda-se correção cirúrgica da HDPP em animais que apresentam sinais clínicos (Figura 254.3). A presença de sinais clínicos ou de intestino delgado no espaço pericárdico foi significativamente associada a tratamento cirúrgico em um grupo de 34 cães e gatos com HDPP. O prognóstico, após cirurgia bem-sucedida, é excelente, com taxa de mortalidade pós-operatória de 5 a 14%.[6,10] Complicações intraoperatórias ocorreram em 38% dos 37 gatos, em uma série de casos, e complicações pós-operatórias dentro de 3 dias após a cirurgia e entre 3 dias e 6 meses foram verificadas em 78 e 41% dos gatos, respectivamente, sendo a maioria discreta.[10] Notou-se resolução dos sinais clínicos em 75 a 85% dos pacientes submetidos ao procedimento cirúrgico; porém, estudo de uma série casos reportou não haver diferença na sobrevida, a longo prazo, entre animais submetidos a tratamento cirúrgico e não cirúrgico.[5,10] Aderências entre os órgãos herniados e o pericárdio podem complicar ou impedir a redução da HDPP em animais idosos. Consequentemente, no caso de animais idosos, em que a HDPP é um achado incidental, pode ser mais prudente recomendar a observação contínua, em vez do procedimento cirúrgico.

Cistos pericárdicos

Cistos pericárdicos são raros em cães e não foram relatados em gatos. No homem, os cistos pericárdicos podem surgir de anomalias do desenvolvimento do pericárdio, componentes linfáticos, cistos brônquicos e teratomas. Em cães, os cistos pericárdicos se assemelham a hematomas císticos. Uma vez que são vistos principalmente em cães jovens, isso sugere uma anomalia congênita ou de desenvolvimento. Anormalidades patológicas características incluem encapsulamento de cistos no tecido adiposo, com extensa hemorragia e necrose, ou organização de hematomas císticos. Em alguns casos, o cisto intrapericárdico benigno está associado a uma pequena HDPP. Em outros casos, o cisto é fixado por um pedículo ao ápice do pericárdio; o pedículo é resultado da herniação pré-natal do omento ou da gordura falciforme do peritônio no pericárdio e subsequente fechamento da HDPP. A obstrução vascular do tecido herniado e os traumas repetitivos ocasionados pelo batimento do coração resulta em formação de cisto.[19,20] Cistos intrapericárdicos causam tamponamento cardíaco por compressão cardíaca direta e associada à efusão pericárdica em alguns casos. O tratamento envolve a remoção cirúrgica do cisto e seu pedículo associado, pericardectomia e herniorrafia nos casos com HDPP.

Defeitos do pericárdio

Defeitos do pericárdio são raros em cães e não foram relatados em gatos. Eles podem ser congênitos ou adquiridos secundários a traumas e variam de formação parcial a ausência total do pericárdio.[11] Os defeitos dos lados esquerdo e direito parecem ser igualmente representados, com base na revisão de literatura de 15 cães (lado esquerdo, n = 7; lado direito, n = 6; lado esquerdo e direito, n = 1; e ausência de pericárdio, n = 1).[11-14] Até recentemente, a maioria dos casos eram achados acidentais durante a necropsia ou durante cirurgia torácica realizada para correção de causas não relacionadas ao defeito. Herniação com encarceramento da aurícula esquerda ou direita pode ocasionar graves consequências clínicas, de colapso ou síncope.[13,14]

O achado diagnóstico mais comum nos defeitos do pericárdio é uma forma incomum da silhueta cardíaca nas radiografias torácicas, devido a uma protuberância anormal da aurícula esquerda ou direita. Essa protuberância pode ser confundida

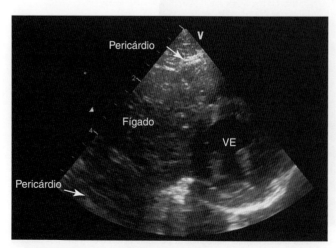

Figura 254.2 Ecocardiograma de um gato com hérnia diafragmática peritônio-pericárdica (HDPP). O fígado encontra-se no espaço pericárdico e toca o coração. A parte ventromedial do diafragma é incompleta. VE, ventrículo esquerdo.

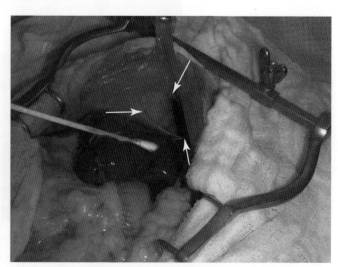

Figura 254.3 Correção cirúrgica de hérnia diafragmática peritônio-pericárdica (HDPP) em um gato; a parte cranial está localizada no *canto superior direito*. Uma HDPP grande está presente (*setas*), vista por laparotomia, após a retração dos lobos hepáticos do espaço pericárdico para a cavidade abdominal.

com tumor cardíaco ou dilatação atrial secundária à doença de valva atrioventricular (AV). É necessário o exame ecocardiográfico para distinguir a causa da silhueta cardíaca anormal; esse exame pode mostrar desproporção da dilatação da aurícula em comparação com o átrio e possível constrição do átrio/aurícula por um orifício fibrosado, semelhante a um anel, do defeito do pericárdio. O tratamento dos defeitos do pericárdio em animais sintomáticos inclui reparo do pericárdio, se o defeito for pequeno, ou pericardectomia, no caso de defeitos maiores.

DOENÇAS ADQUIRIDAS DO PERICÁRDIO

Efusão pericárdica

A efusão pericárdica é a anormalidade pericárdica mais comum em cães e gatos e, em geral, é uma doença cardíaca adquirida bastante comum em cães. A prevalência tem sido relatada em 0,43% (1 cão/233 casos) dos cães examinados em um hospital veterinário de referência e responde por aproximadamente 7% dos cães com sinais clínicos de cardiopatia.[1] É um distúrbio multifatorial, com um amplo espectro de prognóstico, que varia de bom a ruim, dependendo da causa.[2] As causas mais comuns de efusão pericárdica em cães são hemangiossarcoma (HSA; ver Capítulo 347), pericardite idiopática, mesotelioma e quimiodectoma.[3-5] A determinação da causa da efusão pericárdica fornece informações valiosas sobre o tratamento adequado, progressão clínica e prognóstico.

Fisiopatologia

A efusão pericárdica aumenta a pressão intrapericárdica, que é transmitida igualmente para todas as câmaras cardíacas durante a sístole e a diástole. No entanto, as paredes mais delgadas do coração direito, mais adaptáveis, suportam a tensão do aumento da pressão intrapericárdica, e isso ocasiona tamponamento cardíaco. O tamponamento cardíaco é definido como o comprometimento do preenchimento ventricular devido ao acúmulo de líquido no espaço pericárdico, levando à redução do volume sistólico e do débito cardíaco. O tamponamento cardíaco tem diferentes características fisiopatológicas baseadas na taxa de aumento da pressão intrapericárdica, classificado em tamponamento cardíaco agudo e tamponamento cardíaco crônico.

No tamponamento cardíaco agudo, o rápido acúmulo de efusão pericárdica leva a um rápido aumento da pressão intrapericárdica, em volume tão baixo quanto 50 a 150 mℓ (para um cão de 20 kg).[15] Se líquido adicional acumular-se cronicamente, ocorrerá estiramento do pericárdio para acomodar várias centenas de mililitros de líquido, sem aumento clinicamente relevante da pressão intrapericárdica (Figura 254.4).[16] O colapso do átrio e do ventrículo direito aumenta a pressão diastólica dessas duas câmaras cardíacas. O colapso do coração direito durante a diástole reduz o preenchimento e o volume sistólico do ventrículo direito, reduzindo, assim, o retorno venoso ao coração esquerdo. O volume sistólico do ventrículo esquerdo diminui (notado como redução do diâmetro do VE durante a diástole no exame ecocardiográfico), o qual diminui o débito cardíaco e causa hipotensão arterial e choque cardiogênico. O colapso diastólico do átrio direito e das câmaras ventriculares ocorre no início desse processo, quando o débito cardíaco diminui em aproximadamente 20% e antes da redução na pressão arterial.[17] Em um modelo experimental de tamponamento cardíaco agudo em cães, a pressão arterial média foi mantida até que o volume intrapericárdico aumentou para aproximadamente 100 mℓ e a pressão intrapericárdica era de aproximadamente 10 mmHg. A função sistólica do ventrículo esquerdo é mantida no tamponamento cardíaco agudo e não é a causa da hipotensão arterial; mais propriamente, a diminuição do preenchimento do ventrículo esquerdo durante a diástole é a causa do baixo débito cardíaco.[18] O aumento da atividade simpática em resposta à hipotensão arterial no tamponamento cardíaco é controlado de

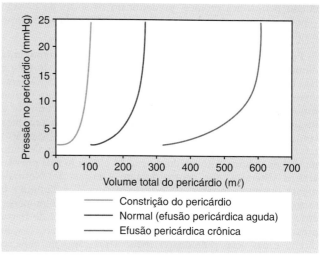

Figura 254.4 Efeitos da efusão pericárdica aguda, efusão pericárdica crônica e pericardite constritiva na pressão intrapericárdica. A pressão intrapericárdica aumenta sobremaneira com apenas 50 a 150 mℓ de efusão no quadro agudo. Na efusão crônica, ocorre acúmulo lento e por tempo prolongado de grande volume de efusão pericárdica, a curva volume-pressão é deslocada para a direita devido ao estiramento e à hipertrofia do pericárdio para acomodar o grande volume de líquido, sem aumento acentuado da pressão. Em contrapartida, na pericardite constritiva, a curva volume-pressão é deslocada para a esquerda devido à rigidez do pericárdio, sem complacência, que opera em uma curva íngreme de aumento dramático de pressão no pericárdio em pequenos aumentos de volume pericárdico. (Utilizada, com autorização, de Kittleson MD, Kienle RD: *Medicina cardiovascular em pequenos animais*, St. Louis, 1998, Mosby, Capítulo 25, p. 414.)

forma diferenciada: com base em um modelo de tamponamento cardíaco experimental em cães, notou-se aumento da atividade simpática no coração, na glândula adrenal e no fígado, mas diminuiu nos rins, reduzindo o débito urinário na tentativa de manter o volume sanguíneo.[19]

O tamponamento cardíaco crônico manifesta-se como uma elevação da pressão diastólica no coração direito e insuficiência cardíaca congestiva do lado direito do coração. Embora todas as câmaras cardíacas sejam submetidas ao mesmo aumento da pressão intrapericárdica, a elevação da pressão diastólica necessária para causar extravasamento de capilares sistêmicos é muito menor (10 a 15 mmHg) do que nos capilares pulmonares (25 a 30 mmHg), então a insuficiência cardíaca direita é vista, em vez de uma combinação de insuficiência cardíaca esquerda e direita. O acúmulo prolongado e lento da efusão pericárdica causa estiramento do pericárdio para acomodar normalmente centenas de mililitros de líquido, sem aumento clinicamente significativo da pressão (ver Figura 254.4). Os mecanismos precisos da expansão pericárdica são incertos e podem incluir desprendimento das camadas de colágeno seguido de estiramento das fibras de colágeno onduladas, ou possivelmente proliferação de fibroblastos com deposição de novo tecido conjuntivo.[20] Com base nas propriedades viscoelásticas do pericárdio, o seu estiramento inicial causa alisamento dos feixes de colágenos ondulados com estiramento concomitante das fibras de elastina; contudo, quando há estiramento adicional, essas estruturas não se distendem devido à falta de elasticidade das fibras de colágeno retas.

No tamponamento cardíaco ocorre ativação neuro-hormonal em resposta à diminuição do débito cardíaco. Isso inclui ativação do sistema nervoso simpático e do sistema renina-angiotensina-aldosterona, na tentativa de aumentar o débito cardíaco. Entretanto, diferentemente de outras formas de cardiopatia acompanhadas de elevada pressão de preenchimento diastólica, no tamponamento cardíaco não há aumento da concentração do peptídio natriurético atrial, o que limita a natriurese e sustenta a sobrecarga de volume e pressão venosa elevada.[21,56,57] Consequentemente, na efusão pericárdica crônica, predominam os sinais de pressão venosa sistêmica elevada e manifesta-se principalmente como insuficiência cardíaca congestiva do lado direito.

Pulso paradoxal. Pulso paradoxal é definido como uma diminuição da pressão arterial sistólica > 10 mmHg durante a fase inspiratória da respiração normal (Figura 254.5).[22] O paradoxo descrito por Adolf Kussmaul, em 1873, era um "pulso simultaneamente fraco e irregular que desaparecia durante a inspiração e retornava após a expiração", apesar da presença contínua do impulso cardíaco durante as duas fases respiratórias.[22] Pulso paradoxal é uma exacerbação do pequeno declínio normal do volume sistólico do ventrículo esquerdo e da pressão arterial sistêmica, que ocorre durante a inspiração. Normalmente, durante a inspiração, a pressão intratorácica diminui e o sangue flui preferencialmente para veia cava, veias pulmonares, átrio direito e ventrículo direito, que são estruturas de baixa pressão altamente complacentes. O sangue contido no coração direito e nas veias pulmonares reduz a pré-carga no coração esquerdo e, consequentemente, reduz o volume sistólico do ventrículo esquerdo. No homem, o volume sistólico do ventrículo esquerdo normalmente diminui, em média, 7% durante a inspiração e isso está associado a uma queda de 3% na pressão do sangue arterial durante a sístole. O volume sistólico do ventrículo direito, em contrapartida, aumenta durante a inspiração devido ao aumento do preenchimento do lado direito.

Na presença de efusão pericárdica as alterações recíproca e fásica com a respiração no preenchimento dos ventrículos direito e esquerdo e no débito cardíaco são exageradas. A expansão externa dos ventrículos é limitada na presença de efusão pericárdica e qualquer aumento de volume de um ventrículo pode ocorrer apenas à custa do outro, um processo conhecido como interdependência ventricular. Assim, quanto maior o preenchimento do ventrículo direito durante a inspiração, maior será a pressão no saco pericárdico, empurrando o septo interventricular para o lado esquerdo, e ambos reduzem o tamanho da câmara do ventrículo esquerdo, diminuindo o preenchimento do ventrículo esquerdo. Essa interação entre os ventrículos se sobrepõe à diminuição normal do débito cardíaco do ventrículo esquerdo que ocorre durante a inspiração, ocasionando o pulso paradoxal. No contexto clínico veterinário, a detecção do pulso paradoxo pode ser um desafio, especialmente quando a pressão intratorácica se altera rapidamente, como ocorre na respiração ofegante.

Etiologia

A efusão pericárdica é causada por uma variedade de anormalidades, incluindo causas neoplásicas, infecciosas, metabólicas, tóxicas, cardiovasculares, traumáticas e idiopáticas.[23-26] Em uma série de 107 cães com efusão pericárdica, as seguintes etiologias foram identificadas: HSA (33,6%; n = 36/107), pericardite idiopática (19,6%; n = 21/107), mesotelioma (14,0%; n = 15/107), quimiodectoma (8,4%; n = 9/107), adenocarcinoma de glândula tireoide (5,6%; n = 6/107), pericardite infecciosa (4,7%; n = 5/107), linfoma (2,8%; n = 3/107), sarcoma (1,8%; n = 2/107), bem como carcinomatose, ruptura do átrio esquerdo secundária à grave insuficiência da valva mitral, corpo estranho estéril e granuloma (cada um 0,9%, com n = 1/107).[23]

Neoplasia. A doença neoplásica é a causa mais comum de efusão pericárdica em cães. Em uma série de casos com 107 cães com efusão pericárdica, notou-se que 71% dos casos eram decorrentes de doença neoplásica.[23] HSA é a causa neoplásica mais comum de efusão pericárdica, com predominância no átrio direito (88% das neoplasias do átrio direito eram HSA;[23] Figura 254.6) e raramente ocorre na base do coração (13% dos tumores de base do coração eram HSA[23]).

As neoplasias de base do coração são caracterizadas por uma massa em crescimento no corpo aórtico da artéria aorta ascendente (Figura 254.7) e são causadas por uma variedade de etiologias neoplásicas, incluindo tumores neuroendócrinos (tumores de células quimiorreceptoras, tais como tumor do corpo aórtico, quemodectoma, paraganglioma não cromafina; 9/23 [39,1%]), adenocarcinoma da glândula tireoide (6/23 [26,1%]), mesotelioma (5/23 [21,7%]) e HSA (3/23 [13%]).[23] O mesotelioma causa uma propagação neoplásica das superfícies serosas do pericárdio, frequentemente pleura, sem causar tumor cardíaco ou pericárdico discreto, embora massas discretas possam ser vistas no caso de mesotelioma na base do coração e, raramente, no átrio direito. Outras causas neoplásicas menos comuns de efusão pericárdica são linfoma e sarcomas (p. ex., rabdomiossarcoma, não diferenciado, fibrossarcoma).[23]

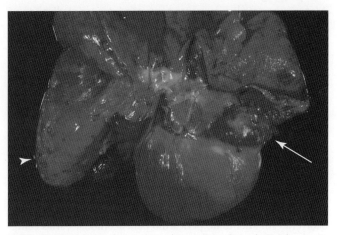

Figura 254.6 Amostra macroscópica do coração e dos pulmões de um cão com hemangiossarcoma (HSA) no átrio direito e metástase pulmonar. O átrio direito e a aurícula direita estão infiltradas por múltiplos tumores hemorrágicos nodulares (*seta*), uma característica de HSA do coração. Há muitos nódulos pequenos metastáticos em todo o parênquima pulmonar (*ponta de seta*), que não eram visíveis nas radiografias torácicas.

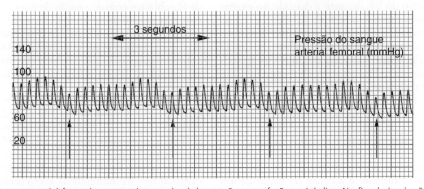

Figura 254.5 Pressão do sangue arterial femoral mostra pulso paradoxal de um cão com efusão pericárdica. No fim da inspiração (*setas verticais*), a pressão arterial sistólica diminui em mais de 10 mmHg e a pressão do pulso diminui.

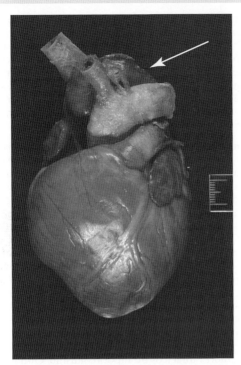

Figura 254.7 Amostra macroscópica do coração de um cão com neoplasia na base do coração. Nota-se uma grande massa, bem definida e lisa (seta), aderida à parte medial da artéria aorta, que é característica de tumor na base do coração.

Metástase de tumores cardíacos é comum e parece igualmente comum nas diferentes etiologias neoplásicas: HSA (67,9%; n = 19/28), mesotelioma (55,6%; n = 5/9]), adenocarcinoma da glândula tireoide (50%; n = 2/3) e quemodectoma (66,7%; n = 4/6).[23] HSA esplênico concomitante ocorre em aproximadamente 30% dos cães com HSA cardíaco, considerando os dados de 2 diferentes séries de casos.[23,27] Os pulmões são os locais mais comuns de metástase para o grupo combinado de todas as etiologias neoplásicas (30,5%; n = 18/59). Em cães com HSA cardíaco, os locais mais comuns de metástase são os pulmões (42,8%; n =12/28), baço (28,6%; n = 8/28), fígado (28,6%; n = 8/28) e rins (14,3%; n = 28/28).[23] Os locais mais comuns de metástase em cães com mesotelioma são os linfonodos intratorácicos (66,7%; n = 6/9), pulmões (22%; n = 2/9) e pleura (22%; n = 2/9).[23] Em cães com tumores neuroendócrinos, 50% dos animais (n = 3/6) apresentaram metástases nos pulmões, seguido do baço (16,7%; n = 1/6) e fígado (16,7%; n = 1/6).[23] O local mais comum de metástase em cães com adenocarcinoma da glândula tireoide é o pericárdio (66,7%; n= 2/3), seguido dos pulmões (33,3%; n = 1/3), da cavidade peritoneal (33.3%; n = 1/3 cães) e do miocárdio (33.3%; n = 1/3).[23]

Pericardite idiopática. Após o hemangiossarcoma (HSA), a pericardite idiopática (hemorrágica) é a segunda causa mais comum de efusão pericárdica em cães (causa em 20 a 75% dos casos).[23,28,29] Na verdade, a causa de pericardite idiopática é desconhecida, mas postula-se que a inflamação pericárdica secundária à doença viral ou imunomediada seja a causa. A inflação causada pela infiltração de células mononucleares e fibrose parece ter como alvo os vasos sanguíneos e linfáticos do pericárdio.[30] Vasos sanguíneos do pericárdio danificados são as prováveis fontes de hemorragia e efusão pericárdica. A efusão normalmente se acumula lentamente, ocasionando uma manifestação clínica comum de tamponamento cardíaco crônico. Esse processo pode se resolver espontaneamente após a pericardiocentese em aproximadamente metade dos casos; o restante dos casos apresenta efusão pericárdica recorrente em poucos dias ou alguns anos e requer pericardectomia subtotal. Pericardite constritiva é uma possível sequela crônica da pericardite idiopática.

Pericardite infecciosa. Pericardite infecciosa é uma causa incomum de efusão pericárdica em cães e foi relatada em apenas 4,7% de 107 cães com efusão pericárdica.[23] Um sítio comum da infecção é a migração de graveto (3/5 cães, naquela série de casos) ou outros corpos estranhos penetrantes intrapericárdicos. A efusão pericárdica tipicamente tem aspecto floculento e macroscopicamente supurativo, diferente da típica efusão hemorrágica escura de outras causas e do líquido pericárdico. O exame de amostras desses líquidos distingue pericardite infecciosa de outras causas de efusão pericárdica (ver a seguir). As bactérias e os fungos relatados com maior frequência são: *Bacteroides* spp., *Actinomyces* spp., *Streptococcus canis*, *Pasteurella* spp., *Peptostreptococcus* spp. e *Coccidioides immitis*.

Causas cardiovasculares. Uma causa menos comum de efusão pericárdica é a ruptura do átrio esquerdo em cães com grave insuficiência mitral causada por doença mixomatosa da valva mitral. Lacerações do endocárdio podem ocorrer em cães com dilatação e grave elevação da pressão do átrio esquerdo, acompanhadas de lesões por jato de alta velocidade oriundo de regurgitação mitral, atingindo a parede do átrio esquerdo. O cenário clínico é de tamponamento cardíaco agudo, fraqueza, choque cardiogênico e frequentemente morte aguda. Cães de raça de pequeno porte com grave degeneração da valva mitral são os mais predispostos à laceração do átrio esquerdo; cães das raças Shetland Sheepdog, Poodle macho, Dachshund e Cocker Spaniel parecem ser mais predispostos à ruptura do átrio esquerdo.[31,32]

Efusão pericárdica é frequentemente detectada em cães e gatos com insuficiência cardíaca congestiva, mas raramente em quantidade suficiente (e essencialmente nunca com pressão intrapericárdica suficientemente alta) para causar comprometimento hemodinâmico significativo.

Metabólicas e tóxicas. Causas metabólicas e tóxicas de efusão pericárdica são raras. Elas incluem efusão pericárdica secundária à uremia e efusão pericárdica devido a alto teor de colesterol associado ao hipotireoidismo.[33] Distúrbios de coagulação, levando à efusão pericárdica, ocasionalmente ocorrem na intoxicação por rodenticida anticoagulante e secundária à coagulação intravascular disseminada, intoxicação por varfarina e outras coagulopatias.[4,34] Embora os distúrbios hemorrágicos sejam uma causa incomum de efusão pericárdica, é necessária a avaliação da condição de coagulação (tempo de coagulação sanguínea, contagem de plaquetas) antes da pericardiocentese.

Histórico do paciente e características clínicas

Existem duas situações clínicas em pacientes com efusão pericárdica que causam sinais clínicos evidentes: tamponamento cardíaco agudo e tamponamento cardíaco crônico. Pacientes com tamponamento cardíaco agudo normalmente manifestam rápido início de fraqueza ou colapso, necessitando de atendimento clínico de emergência, com breve histórico prévio de anormalidades. Pacientes com tamponamento cardíaco crônico frequentemente apresentam vago histórico de inapetência, letargia, intolerância ao exercício, distensão abdominal progressiva e anormalidades respiratórias, como taquipneia ou dispneia.

Cães machos, de raças de médio a grande porte, principalmente Golden Retriever, são super-representados no grupo de cães que desenvolvem efusão pericárdica. Porém, cães de qualquer tamanho, sexo ou raça podem desenvolver efusão pericárdica. Como esperado, cães com tumor no coração são tipicamente mais idosos (idade média: 9,7 anos) do que cães sem tumor (idade média: 7,9 anos).[23] Cães das raças Buldogue Inglês, Boxer e Boston Terrier de meia-idade ou mais velhos são predispostos a tumores neuroendócrinos (quemodectomas) na base do coração, mas esses tumores também ocorrem em raças não braquicefálicas. Hiperplasia crônica induzida por hipoxia e neoplasia de quimiorreceptores podem explicar a predisposição de cães braquicefálicos a tumores do corpo aórtico.[35]

Anormalidades no exame físico

Abafamento de sons cardíacos, pulso fraco, taquicardia e mucosas pálidas são as principais anormalidades físicas verificadas no tamponamento cardíaco agudo. Além do abafamento dos sons cardíacos, com ou sem sons pulmonares, sinais de insuficiência cardíaca direita, como dilatação das veias jugulares ou pulsação jugular, teste de refluxo hepatojugular positivo, hepatomegalia e ascite com teste de balotamento indicando acúmulo de líquido (ver Capítulo 17) são anormalidades típicas em animais com tamponamento cardíaco crônico. Em uma série de casos que envolveu 107 cães com efusão pericárdica, constatou-se que 67 (62,6%) apresentavam evidências de insuficiência cardíaca direita.[23] Mais da metade dos cães com insuficiência cardíaca direita (36/107 [33,6%]) apresentavam efusão pleural e ascite concomitantes, enquanto poucos pacientes tiveram ascite isoladamente (17/107 cães [15,9%]) ou efusão pleural (14/107 cães [13%]).[23] Em relação à presença de efusão bicavitária, efusão pleural ou ascite, não houve diferença entre cães com causas neoplásicas ou não neoplásicas.[23] Arritmias cardíacas podem ser auscultadas em alguns casos, sendo a mais comum taquicardia sinusal devido ao choque cardiogênico. Sopro sistólico apical esquerdo pode estar presente em cães com ruptura do átrio esquerdo; é tipicamente de menor intensidade em comparação com exames prévios. Pulso paradoxal, no entanto, é incomum (10 a 20% dos casos) e pode ser identificado em cães com tamponamento cardíaco e padrão respiratório lento e regular (i. e., não ofegante).

Diagnóstico

O ecocardiograma é o teste essencial para diagnosticar efusão pericárdica e ajudar a diferenciar as etiologias de efusão pericárdica. Radiografias e eletrocardiogramas não são exames sensíveis, tampouco inespecíficos, mas podem aumentar a suspeita de doença pericárdica em alguns casos.

Radiografias do tórax. Embora as radiografias do tórax por excelência mostrem alterações radiográficas de cardiomegalia globoide, com margens cardíacas nítidas, e sejam clássicas para efusão pericárdica (Figura 254.8), a realidade é que as radiografias não são exames sensíveis, tampouco específicos para o diagnóstico de efusão pericárdica. De fato, a sensibilidade e a especificidade dos achados radiográficos em que a aparência da silhueta cardíaca era globoide foram de apenas 41,9 e 40%, respectivamente, para o diagnóstico de tamponamento cardíaco e efusão pericárdica em 50 cães de uma série e na realidade estava presente em aproximadamente metade dos 107 cães em outro estudo.[23,36] A cardiomegalia, definida como *vertebral heart size* (VHS; tamanho do coração em relação à unidade de vértebra torácica) > 10,7, também não foi um parâmetro sensível (sensibilidade = 77,6%), tampouco específico (especificidade = 47,8%), para o diagnóstico de tamponamento cardíaco, provavelmente devido aos acúmulos rápidos de pequenos volumes de efusão pericárdica no tamponamento agudo.[36] Hipoperfusão pulmonar e diminuição do tamanho da veia cava caudal são comuns em cães com choque cardiogênico devido ao tamponamento cardíaco agudo. Inversamente, dilatação da veia cava caudal, perda de detalhe abdominal e efusão pleural podem ser observadas com tamponamento cardíaco mais crônico e geralmente são acompanhadas de cardiomegalia globoide mais clássica. A detecção de tumor cardíaco em radiografias (Figura 254.8) não é um achado sensível, porém é específico (100% em um estudo); foi identificada em 10 dos 63 cães com tumores cardíacos.[23] Metástases pulmonares comumente ocorrem (Figura 254.8), mas as radiografias têm uma baixa taxa de detecção, de apenas 1/3 dos casos, sendo as metástases pulmonares confirmadas durante a necropsia ou toracotomia.[23]

Imagem tomográfica. A realização de tomografia computadorizada com múltiplos detectores aumenta a sensibilidade do diagnóstico na detecção de metástases pulmonares em comparação com as radiografias, mas não aumenta o valor diagnóstico de detecção de tumores cardíacos em comparação com o ecocardiograma transtorácico.[37] Da mesma forma, a imagem de ressonância magnética (RM) cardíaca não aumenta o valor diagnóstico para a detecção de tumores cardíacos em cães com efusão pericárdica em comparação com a ecocardiografia, mas pode fornecer informação descritiva sobre a extensão da doença, localização e características do tumor, se realizada por especialistas com extenso treinamento adicional em ressonância magnética do coração.[38]

Eletrocardiografia. Indica-se eletrocardiograma para qualquer paciente com arritmia cardíaca detectada durante o exame físico, mas não é um teste de diagnóstico preciso para efusão pericárdica (ver Capítulo 103). As anormalidades estão presentes de forma variável, e em uma série de 107 cães notou-se, em ordem de ocorrência: alternância elétrica (30/107 cães [28%]), taquicardia sinusal (30/107 cães [28%]), atenuação da voltagem de QRS (onda R < 1 mV) (26 cães [24,3%]) e arritmia ventricular (14/107 cães [13,1%]).[23] Alternância elétrica é a variação na amplitude QRS entre os batimentos cardíacos causada pela oscilação do coração para a frente e para trás na presença de um grande volume de efusão pericárdica; é bastante específica para efusão pericárdica em cães (Figura 254.9). A atenuação da voltagem de QRS se deve à efusão pericárdica, que isola o sinal elétrico transmitido à superfície corporal; também pode ocorrer em casos de efusão pleural, obesidade, grandes tumores torácicos ou hipotireoidismo. Outras anormalidades eletrocardiográficas menos comuns em cães com efusão pericárdica são: taquicardia supraventricular (3/107 cães [2,8%]), complexos atriais prematuros (2/107 cães [1,9%]), fibrilação atrial (2/107 cães [1,9%]) e alterações no segmento ST (2/107 cães [1,9%]).[23]

Ecocardiografia. O ecocardiograma é um exame essencial não apenas para confirmar o diagnóstico de efusão pericárdica em uma varredura de triagem; contudo, o uso de varredura de nível superior fornece informações adicionais sobre possível etiologia da efusão, bem como se há necessidade de pericardiocentese e se existe alguma cardiopatia estrutural ou funcional (ver Capítulo 104). A sensibilidade e a especificidade da ecocardiografia na detecção de tumor cardíaco são 82 e 100%, respectivamente, quando realizada por um cardiologista; esses valores são similares, independentemente de o tumor cardíaco situar-se no átrio direito (82 e 99%, respectivamente) ou na base do coração (74 e 98%, respectivamente).[23] A repetição do exame ecocardiográfico dentro de semanas a meses aumenta a sensibilidade (88%) para a detecção de neoplasias cardíacas.[23]

A efusão pericárdica é vista como um espaço anecoico ao redor do coração no espaço pericárdico. O pericárdio é visto em posição externa ao líquido anecoico, e é frequentemente realçado pela presença simultânea de efusão pleural. Juntamente com aos achados característicos do exame físico, o diagnóstico ecocardiográfico do tamponamento cardíaco é importante para ajudar a definir as estratégias de tratamento e o momento da pericardiocentese. Um volume de líquido pericárdico relativamente baixo pode causar tamponamento agudo, se ocorrer muito rapidamente, como pode ser observado no caso de hemorragia aguda causada por HSA. Entretanto, nos casos de acúmulo lento de efusão pericárdica, pode haver um volume extremamente grande de efusão pericárdica que, por fim, causa tamponamento crônico e insuficiência cardíaca direita. A evidência ecocardiográfica de tamponamento cardíaco inclui compressão diastólica do átrio direito, com curvatura côncava da parede para dentro da câmara atrial direita e, muitas vezes, compressão ou colapso do ventrículo direito, visto como uma curvatura interna da parede livre do ventrículo direito ou obliteração da câmara ventricular direita no tamponamento grave (Vídeo 254.2). Nota-se sobrecarga do ventrículo esquerdo, com tamanho da câmara reduzido, especialmente em casos de tamponamento cardíaco agudo. O tamponamento crônico, frequentemente, também causa dilatação venosa hepática, hepatomegalia

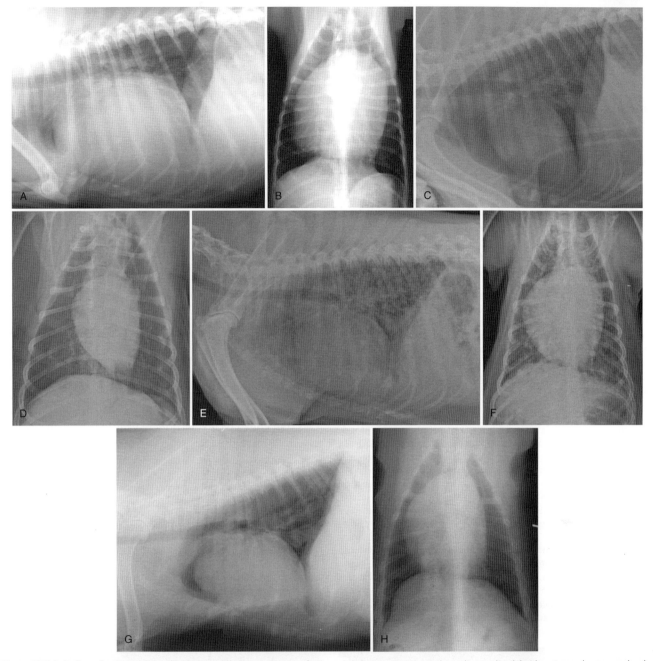

Figura 254.8 Radiografias lateral (**A**) e dorsoventral (**B**) de um cão com efusão pericárdica grave, mostrando cardiomegalia globoide extrema, bem como bordas cardíacas enrugadas, que confirmam o diagnóstico de efusão pericárdica. Há perda de detalhe abdominal, sugestiva de ascite. As radiografias obtidas após a pericardiocentese mostram silhueta cardíaca normal (**C** e **D**). Radiografias de outro cão com efusão pericárdica mostram cardiomegalia globoide discreta, devido ao tamponamento pericárdico agudo e à presença de um padrão pulmonar nodular compatível com metástases pulmonares (**E** e **F**); ver o ecocardiograma no Vídeo 254.4. Radiografias de um cão com um grande tumor na base do coração (**G** e **H**) mostram uma protuberância na cintura cardíaca cranial, na base do coração, na imagem lateral, com alterações menos evidentes na imagem DV, e cardiomegalia globoide discreta.

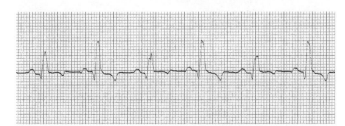

Figura 254.9 Alternâncias elétricas no eletrocardiograma de um cão com efusão pericárdica grave. Há uma variação na amplitude do segmento QRS entre os batimentos cardíacos devido à oscilação do coração na efusão pericárdica, bem como atenuação dos complexos QRS (< 1 mV). 50 mm/seg; 1 cm = 1 mV.

generalizada, ascite e efusão pleural. Pulso paradoxal pode ser diagnosticado por meio de ecocardiografia, usando-se Doppler com onda pulsada, verificando-se a velocidade do fluxo sanguíneo aórtico; conforme descrito anteriormente, ocorrem redução cíclica na velocidade do fluxo sanguíneo aórtico durante a inspiração e aumento da velocidade durante a expiração (e o inverso para as velocidades do fluxo sanguíneo pulmonar).

É necessário um exame cuidadoso de todas as câmaras, com foco particular na base do coração e no átrio/aurícula direita, para avaliar a presença de neoplasias cardíacas. Tipicamente, os tumores são classificados como neoplasias de base do coração, de átrio/aurícula direita ou outro. A razão dessa classificação é que há predisposição dos tipos de tumores para uma localização anatômica no coração e há um diferente comportamento biológico para cada uma das diferentes causas neoplásicas. Por exemplo, em uma série de casos constatou-se que 88% dos tumores do átrio direito eram HSA, enquanto na base do coração há maior propensão para tumores neuroendócrinos (40%) ou adenocarcinoma da tireoide (25%).[23] Apesar da generalização das predisposições tumorais pelo átrio direito e base do coração, há uma sobreposição de etiologias de tumores para cada local. Por exemplo, os tumores do átrio direito, além do HSA, incluem os seguintes (cada um respondendo por 2,5% dos casos): tumor neuroendócrino, adenocarcinoma de tireoide, mesotelioma, linfoma e sarcoma.[23] Da mesma forma, tumores da base do coração que não sejam neuroendócrinos ou adenocarcinoma da tireoide incluem mesotelioma (20%) e HSA (15%).[23]

As características ecocardiográficas teciduais do átrio ou aurícula direita com HSA consistem em uma massa irregular e heterogênea que se move simultaneamente à câmara e apresentam espaços cavitários ou intratumorais hipoecoicos compatíveis com hemorragia. A neoplasia pode estar localizada na aurícula direita, que deve ser visualizada em imagem do eixo longitudinal paraesternal cranial esquerdo (Figura 254.10; Vídeos 254.3 e 254.4) ou, mais comumente, pode se estender ao longo da parede do átrio direito e/ou sulco atrioventricular direito (Vídeos 254.3 e 254.5). Às vezes, há tumor no átrio direito e na base do coração, simultaneamente, provavelmente devido à disseminação da neoplasia primária, mas raramente de duas causas neoplásicas diferentes. Às vezes, os tumores do átrio direito penetram no lado direito do lúmen atrial e podem obstruir o retorno venoso ao átrio direito ou prejudicar o preenchimento do ventrículo direito (ver Vídeos 254.3 e 254.5; ver Capítulo 122).

Tumores na base do coração, que são tumores neuroendócrinos, geralmente são massas homogêneas encapsuladas que se desenvolvem a partir da artéria aorta ascendente, adjacente, porém separadas do átrio esquerdo ou do átrio direito (Figura 254.11; Vídeo 254.6). Como as neoplasias da base do coração compreendem uma variedade de etiologias, as características ecocardiográficas também podem variar. Alguns tumores da base cardíaca são pequenos e frequentemente não são detectáveis, a menos que a artéria aorta ascendente seja cuidadosamente examinada em imagem da via de saída do ventrículo esquerdo, no eixo longitudinal paraesternal direito, bem como em imagens do eixo curto, ao longo da base do coração. Outras neoplasias da base do coração podem ser tão grandes que é difícil determinar o local de origem. Em alguns casos, os tumores grandes na base cardíaca podem comprimir externamente a via de saída do ventrículo direito ou a artéria pulmonar. Às vezes, as neoplasias da base do coração não causam efusão pericárdica e são diagnosticadas incidentalmente com base na suspeita de uma massa na base do coração em radiografias ou durante o exame de um sopro cardíaco.

A presença de efusão pericárdica facilita muito a detecção de neoplasias intrapericárdicas, especialmente HSA cardíaco e tumores da base do coração, pois o líquido origina uma área anecoica ao redor do átrio e aurícula direita, bem como da artéria aorta ascendente. Consequentemente, se a condição clínica permitir, o procedimento de pericardiocentese deve ser postergado até que o exame ecocardiográfico seja concluído. Todavia, em cães com tamponamento cardíaco e colapso cardiovascular, a pericardiocentese não deve ser adiada, pois é um procedimento que salva a vida do paciente.

Efusão pericárdica secundária à ruptura do átrio esquerdo é acompanhada de evidência ecocardiográfica de doença mixomatosa da valva mitral e grave dilatação do átrio esquerdo (ver Capítulo 251). Um trombo hiperecoico alongado geralmente é visto estendendo-se da superfície epicárdica do átrio esquerdo para dentro do espaço pericárdico (Vídeo 254.7).

Em casos em que nenhuma massa é visualizada, os principais diagnósticos diferenciais incluem pericardite idiopática, mesotelioma, pericardite infecciosa ou um tumor muito pequeno ou muito distante para ser visto na imagem ecocardiográfica. No ecocardiograma é impossível distinguir pericardite idiopática e mesotelioma. O diagnóstico requer exame histopatológico e imuno-histoquímico do pericárdio para ajudar a diferenciar essas duas doenças em cães com efusão pericárdica recorrente submetidos à pericardectomia. Às vezes, o diagnóstico definitivo de mesotelioma é impossível, mas a suspeita é aumentada em cães com efusão pleural recorrente dentro de 4 a 6 meses após serem submetidos à pericardectomia subtotal.

Exame do líquido pericárdico. O exame do líquido pericárdico, com exame citológico, é inespecífico,[39] e o líquido geralmente é classificado como hemorrágico. No entanto, o exame do líquido continua sendo uma etapa essencial no diagnóstico de pericardite infecciosa e algumas causas neoplásicas, como o linfoma. O líquido pericárdico pode ser classificado como hemorrágico (40/47 [85%]), inflamatório supurativo (6/47 [12,7%]), inflamatório piogranulomatoso (4/47 [8,5%]), transudato modificado (2/47 [4,2%]) ou quilo (1/47 [2,1%]). A citologia pericárdica foi considerada não diagnóstica em 87 a 92,3% dos cães, mas foi capaz de identificar uma etiologia neoplásica específica em 4,6% de 250 cães (n = 7 neoplasias de células redondas, n = 3 células epitelioides atípicas, n = 1 neoplasia hematógena)

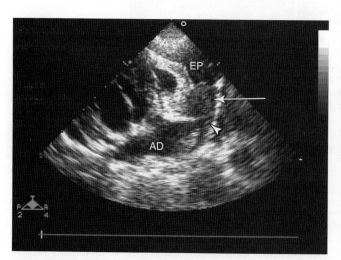

Figura 254.10 Ecocardiograma de um cão com neoplasia no átrio direito. Essa imagem do eixo longitudinal paraesternal cranial esquerdo mostra uma massa heterogênea e malhada na aurícula direita (seta), assim como efusão pericárdica (EP). A ponta de seta indica a aurícula direita. AD, átrio direito.

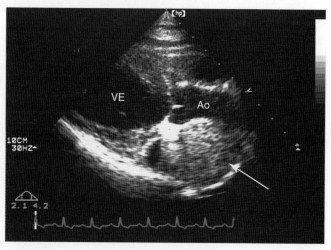

Figura 254.11 Ecocardiograma de um cão com neoplasia na base do coração. Essa imagem paraesternal do eixo longitudinal mostra uma massa bem definida e homogênea (seta) aderida à artéria aorta ascendente, característica de um tumor na base cardíaca. Ao, artéria aorta; VE, ventrículo esquerdo.

e todos os casos de pericardite infecciosa (n = 8; 3,1%).[23,40] Portanto, apesar do baixo valor diagnóstico, é essencial enviar amostra de líquido pericárdico para análise. Reatividade mesotelial foi detectada em 25 de 47 (53,2%) cães e normalmente não é útil para diferenciar pericardite idiopática do mesotelioma. Uma vez que as células mesoteliais hiper-reativas podem ser inadvertidamente classificadas erroneamente como mesotelioma, o diagnóstico de mesotelioma é feito por meio de exame histopatológico do pericárdio, após pericardectomia ou durante a necropsia. Entre os tumores do coração, o linfoma cardíaco é diferente, porque o exame citológico do líquido pericárdico define o diagnóstico em muitos casos (11/12 cães [88%] em uma série de casos) e essa neoplasia talvez seja passível de quimioterapia combinada.[35,38,55] A cultura microbiológica da efusão pericárdica para pesquisa de microrganismos aeróbicos e anaeróbicos deve ser realizada em casos de evidência macroscópica de líquido claro floculento e/ou quando o líquido é classificado como exsudato líquido. Indica-se o teste sorológico para C. immitis em cães com efusão pericárdica inflamatória que vivem em áreas endêmicas (ver Capítulo 232). O pH do líquido pericárdico apresenta uma grande sobreposição entre etiologias neoplásicas e não neoplásicas, e sua mensuração não é considerada confiável.[41,42] A mensuração da concentração sérica de troponina cardíaca I (cTn-I) mostrou resultados diferentes em diferentes estudos. A concentração sérica de cTn-I é significativamente mais elevada em cães com efusão pericárdica do que em cães normais, mas alguns resultados indicam um teor mais alto em cães com HSA em comparação com cães que tinham outros tumores ou outras doenças não neoplásicas; todavia, outros resultados não mostram essa diferença.[43-45]

Tratamento

Em pacientes com tamponamento cardíaco e comprometimento hemodinâmico, pericardiocentese e reanimação rápida com a administração de solução intravenosa salvam a vida imediatamente (ver Capítulo 102). O momento da pericardiocentese depende da gravidade do comprometimento cardiovascular e não deve ser adiada caso haja choque cardiogênico. Em pacientes estáveis, a pericardiocentese deve ser postergada, caso seja possível realizar um ecocardiograma de alto nível e, então, a seguir faz-se a pericardiocentese. Abdominocentese (ver Capítulo 90), com ou sem toracocentese (ver Capítulo 102), pode ser um procedimento paliativo em pacientes com tamponamento cardíaco crônico e ascite ou efusão pleural, respectivamente.

Aproximadamente 50% dos casos de pericardite idiopática são acompanhados de efusão pericárdica recorrente, sendo necessária a pericardectomia subtotal. Nos casos de efusão pericárdica recorrente, sem um tumor detectável, é necessário pericardectomia subtotal e exame histopatológico do pericárdio (frequentemente com emprego de corantes imuno-histoquímicos especiais), a fim de diferenciar pericardite idiopática de mesotelioma. A pericardectomia subtotal é curativa para pericardite idiopática: cães com pericardite idiopática submetidos à pericardectomia subtotal nunca atingiram um tempo médio de sobrevivência durante um período de 3 anos de estudo (obtiveram 100% de sobrevida), mas em cães com pericardite idiopática submetidos à janela pericárdica por meio de toracoscopia foi muito pior, com um intervalo livre da doença de 11,6 meses e tempo médio de sobrevida de 13,1 meses.[46]

Durante a toracotomia, pela aparência geral das superfícies serosas anormais da pleura e do pericárdio, pode-se clinicamente suspeitar da presença de mesotelioma, o qual requer a realização de biopsia de pleura e linfonodos. O tempo médio de sobrevida dos pacientes com mesotelioma submetidos à pericardectomia subtotal foi de 10,3 meses e não foi significativamente diferente daqueles submetidos à janela pericárdica por meio de toracoscopia (tempo de sobrevida médio de 8,6 meses). Infusões intracavitárias de carboplatina têm sido utilizadas para o tratamento de mesotelioma, porém com publicação de escassos relatos clínicos por especialistas. Um relato de caso documentou que um cão que estava livre da doença havia 27 meses, após o tratamento com carboplatina intratorácica e administração intravenosa de doxorrubicina.[47] Outro relato de caso documentou dois cães com mesotelioma peritoneal tratados com carboplatina intracavitária e piroxicam diário, com sobrevida de 8 meses e > 3 anos, respectivamente.[47,48]

A pericardectomia parcial é indicada para cães com tumores na base do coração, pois alivia o tamponamento cardíaco e está associada ao prolongamento significativo na sobrevida (sobrevida média de 730 dias após pericardectomia versus 42 dias sem pericardectomia).[49] Nesse estudo de 24 cães com tumores no corpo aórtico, apenas a pericardectomia se mostrou efetiva em aumentar a sobrevida e não outros tratamentos, inclusive quimioterapia.[49] Um segundo estudo mostrou resultados semelhantes.[50] Outros tratamentos adicionais não foram avaliados quanto à eficácia. Tratamento com radioterapia conformacional tridimensional foi realizado em um cão com quemodectoma confirmado em exame histopatológico: notou-se > 50% de redução do volume do tumor 25 meses após a terapia e o cão ainda estava vivo 42 meses depois do tratamento (após ter sido submetido à pericardectomia devido à efusão pericárdica recorrente).[51]

A realização de pericardectomia em cães com suspeita de HSA é controversa, a menos que seja associada à ressecção do tumor, que raramente é possível. Em um estudo, a pericardectomia parcial ou subtotal em cães com todas as causas neoplásicas combinadas resultou em taxas de sobrevida frustrantes, de 2,7 e 3,8 meses, respectivamente.[46] Em cães com HSA na aurícula direita apenas, a cirurgia de ressecção é uma opção viável, seguida de quimioterapia, porém os resultados ainda permanecem abaixo do esperado. Em um pequeno estudo de 23 cães com HSA no átrio direito ou com HSA na aurícula direita ressecado cirurgicamente, a quimioterapia aumentou a sobrevida (sobrevida média com quimioterapia e cirurgia de 175 dias versus 42 dias apenas com cirurgia).[52] Um estudo retrospectivo avaliando 64 cães com pressuposto HSA (i. e., tumores no átrio/aurícula direita com aparência heterogênea característica) tratados com doxorrubicina, comparativamente a 76 cães sem o tratamento com doxorrubicina, mostrou sobrevida mais longa após o tratamento (116 dias versus 12 dias, respectivamente); ademais, os cães do grupo tratado com doxorrubicina foram submetidos a maior número de pericardiocenteses e os proprietários estavam mais motivados a continuar a terapia do que aqueles do grupo não tratado.[53] Apenas 14% dos cães tratados com doxorrubicina tiveram probabilidade de sobrevida > 6 meses. Nenhum grupo foi submetido à pericardectomia ou ressecção do tumor. Ademais, a presença de metástase não interferiu na sobrevida, mas o volume do tumor e a trombocitopenia foram indicadores de prognóstico ruim. Por fim, um estudo retrospectivo de cães não submetidos à ressecção cirúrgica de HSA cardíaco, tratados com doxorrubicina com ou sem outros quimioterápicos, relatou um sobrevida média de 139,5 dias (intervalo de 2 a 302 dias), porém nenhum grupo-controle foi avaliado para fins comparativos.[54] Na experiência do autor, hemorragia aguda recorrente e tamponamento cardíaco são comuns em cães com HSA cardíaco e geralmente é letal antes que o animal sucumba à doença metastática.

O linfoma cardíaco é classificado como estágio V, subestágio b. Cães com linfoma em estágio III ou superior e sinais clínicos (subestágio b) têm um prognóstico ruim para remissão do tumor e sobrevivência. Em um estudo retrospectivo de 12 cães com linfoma cardíaco e efusão pericárdica tratados com várias combinações de pericardiocentese, pericardectomia e quimioterapia, a sobrevida média foi de 41 dias. No entanto, três dos cães ainda permaneciam vivos 328 dias após o diagnóstico inicial, sugerindo que o prognóstico de linfoma cardíaco nem sempre é ruim.[55]

Pericardectomia subtotal, drenagem torácica pós-operatória e terapia antimicrobiana de longa duração (pelo menos 6 meses) é o tratamento de escolha para pericardite infecciosa. O prognóstico de cães submetidos à pericardectomia que recebem tratamento prolongado com antibiótico é bom.[56] Em cães com infecção causada por C. immitis (ver Capítulo 232) pode ser necessário tratamento prolongado com antifúngico, durante muitos meses a anos.

PERICARDITE CONSTRITIVA

Pericardite constritiva ocorre quando o pericárdio parietal, pericárdio visceral, ou ambos desenvolvem fibrose, com ou sem fusão das camadas parietal e visceral. Esse processo diminui a complacência e, possivelmente, o volume intrapericárdico (Figura 254.12). O pericárdio fibrosado contrai as câmaras cardíacas e aumenta a pressão atrial e a pressão ventricular diastólica. Um pequeno volume de líquido pericárdico às vezes está presente em uma anormalidade conhecida como pericardite efusivo-constritiva, de modo que qualquer pequeno aumento de volume de efusão pericárdica ocasiona aumento marcante da pressão intrapericárdica. A consequência fisiopatológica da restrição pericárdica é semelhante àquela do tamponamento cardíaco crônico. Ascite é uma característica consistente e a dilatação da veia jugular é comum.[57] Pulso paradoxal é um achado incomum na pericardite constritiva, provavelmente porque o pericárdio rígido não transmite as variações respiratórias da pressão intratorácica ao coração, como acontece no caso de um pericárdio estruturalmente normal. As causas de pericardite constritiva não são claras, mas relatos de casos citam as seguintes etiologias: pericardite idiopática prévia, pericardite infecciosa (especialmente quando a infecção é causada por *C. immitis*), corpo estranho intrapericárdico, metaplasia óssea do pericárdio ou doença idiopática.[57-59] Cães de raças de grande e médio portes são mais comumente acometidos.

Diferentemente do que acontece em outras formas de doença do pericárdio, a ecocardiografia não é suficiente para fornecer um diagnóstico e detecta efusão pericárdica mínima, ou nenhuma, e não mostra colapso do ventrículo e átrio direitos; no entanto, geralmente há evidências de dilatação venosa hepática e ascite.

O diagnóstico de pericardite constritiva requer cateterização do coração direito. A constrição pericárdica não limita o preenchimento diastólico inicial ativo, mas limita o preenchimento no meio da diástole, quando a dilatação cardíaca é restrita pelo pericárdio enrijecido. Isso resulta em pressão em forma de onda "de mergulho e de platô" característica (o sinal de raiz quadrada) quando se mensura a pressão diastólica do ventrículo direito durante o cateterismo cardíaco (ver Figura 254.12). A parte "de mergulho" do traçado da pressão representa o preenchimento diastólico inicial rápido exacerbado do coração operando em baixo volume, não limitado pela restrição pericárdica. O platô ocorre assim que o volume da câmara cardíaca se expande até que seja limitada pela constrição do pericárdio, o que ocasiona um rápido aumento na pressão de preenchimento na metade e no fim da diástole e cessação do preenchimento diastólico, o qual pode ser mais evidente durante a infusão IV rápida de solução salina. Nota-se, também, o traçado da pressão diastólica do átrio direito em forma de W ou M, característico, na pericardite constritiva, onde há acentuado preenchimento no início da diástole após a sístole ventricular (Y descendente) e rápida diminuição da pressão do AD após a sístole (X descendente) (ver Figura 254.12).

O tratamento de pericardite constritiva requer pericardectomia subtotal e, se possível, remoção do pericárdio constritivo do miocárdio subjacente (Figura 254.13). O prognóstico, em geral, depende se a anormalidade está limitada ao pericárdio parietal (melhor prognóstico) ou se estende-se ao pericárdio visceral, o qual pode se aderir à superfície epicárdica (prognóstico ruim). Em uma série de casos de 13 cães, 8 apresentavam constrição pericárdica parietal, 5 tinham constrição pericárdica visceral e pericardectomia parietal, tais procedimentos conseguiram aliviar a síndrome em 6 de 10 cães.[57] A mortalidade perioperatória foi a mais frequente devido a tromboembolismo nesses casos. Em casos em que a pericardite constritiva seja uma complicação em função de infecção sistêmica por *C. immitis*, é necessária a terapia antifúngica a longo prazo adjunta. Em um

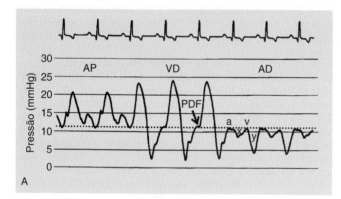

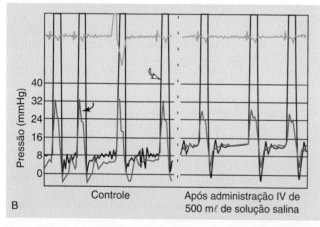

Figura 254.12 Anormalidades hemodinâmicas associadas à pericardite constritiva. **A.** Elevação e equilíbrio da pressão diastólica final (*PDF*) na artéria pulmonar (*AP*), ventrículo direito (*VD*) e átrio direito (*AD*). A pressão do átrio direito, em forma de onda, apresenta um padrão em forma de M devido ao reduzido X descendente e proeminente Y descendente. **B.** Registros simultâneos das pressões do ventrículo esquerdo (*seta vazada*) e do ventrículo direito (*seta sólida*) antes e depois da administração de solução salina. Sob condições controladas, as pressões em forma de onda mostram ligeiras elevações nas pressões diastólicas finais. Nota-se evidência de fisiologia constritiva patognomônica após infusão IV rápida de 500 mℓ de solução salina, resultando em elevação e equilíbrio da pressão diastólica dos ventrículos esquerdo e direito e surgimento do padrão de preenchimento diastólico de mergulho e platô. (De Sisson D, Thomas WP: Pericardial diseases and cardiac tumors. In: Fox PR et al., editors: *Textbook of canine and feline cardiology*, 2 ed., Philadelphia, 1999, Saunders, p. 697-698.)

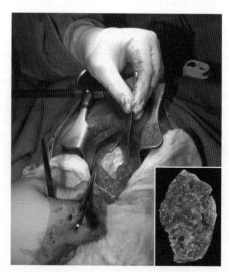

Figura 254.13 Pericardectomia subtotal em um cão com pericardite constritiva. O pericárdio encontra-se acentuadamente espessado, irregular, constritivo e fibrosado. Embora a superfície epicárdica estivesse pálida, não havia constrição do pericárdio visceral; realizou-se pericardectomia parietal subtotal. *Detalhe*: amostra macroscópica do pericárdio espessado obtida durante a ressecção.

estudo retrospectivo de 17 cães com pericardite constritiva de *C. immitis*, a mortalidade perioperatória foi alta (23,5%). Porém, a cirurgia foi bem-sucedida no alívio de sinais clínicos em alguns cães por > 2 anos.[58]

EFUSÃO PERICÁRDICA EM GATOS

A efusão pericárdica é o tipo de anormalidade pericárdica mais comum em gatos; está presente em aproximadamente 6% dos casos de cardiologia nessa espécie.[60] A maioria dos casos é discreta; não é causada por doença pericárdica, mas pela elevação da pressão intracardíaca de preenchimento, secundária à insuficiência cardíaca congestiva (44 a 75% dos casos de efusão pericárdica em gatos), pelo mesmo mecanismo fisiopatológico verificado na efusão pleural, na insuficiência cardíaca.[60,61] Ao contrário dos cães, os gatos raramente desenvolvem efusão pericárdica suficientemente grave para causar tamponamento cardíaco ou sinais clínicos, ou requerem pericardiocentese.[61,62] Depois de insuficiência cardíaca congestiva, neoplasia é a segunda causa mais comum de efusão pericárdica em gatos (19% de 83 casos, incluindo linfoma, adenocarcinoma, timoma e mesotelioma).[61] A neoplasia cardíaca é uma causa rara de efusão pericárdica em gatos, e os artigos mencionam quemodectoma e rabdomiossarcoma. A pericardite também é rara em gatos, detectada somente em 3 de 83 gatos nessa série de casos.[61] Da mesma forma, a pericardite infecciosa é rara em gatos, e as causas de infecção relatadas são *E. coli, Staphylococcus aureus, Enterococcus* e *Actinomyces*. Outras causas incomuns incluem: HDPP, peritonite infecciosa felina, hipoalbuminemia, infecção e inflamação sistêmicas e coagulação intravascular disseminada.

É necessária a pericardiocentese (ver Capítulo 102) em gatos com evidência ecocardiográfica de tamponamento cardíaco. O líquido pericárdico geralmente tem aspecto macroscópico semelhante à efusão pleural e, diferentemente dos cães, raramente é hemorrágico. Devem ser enviadas amostras da efusão para avaliação citológica e citológica com ou sem cultura microbiana, para elucidação de causas infecciosas, neoplásicas ou inflamatórias.

REFERÊNCIAS BIBLIOGRÁFICAS

As referências bibliográficas deste capítulo se encontram online no Ambiente de Aprendizagem.

CAPÍTULO 255

Dirofilariose Canina e Felina

Clarke Atkins

DIROFILARIOSE CANINA

A dirofilariose (infecção por verme do coração, dirofilaríase, dirofilariose), causada por *Dirofilaria immitis*, acomete principalmente os membros da família Canidae. A dirofilariose é uma doença amplamente disseminada, diagnosticada nas regiões temperadas do norte e do sul, nos trópicos e nos subtrópicos. Essas infecções são reconhecidas na maioria dos EUA, embora a distribuição seja mais favorável no sudeste e no vale do rio Mississippi (Figura 255.1). Em algumas áreas endêmicas dos EUA, a taxa de infecção se aproxima de 45% e em algumas regiões tropicais hiperendêmicas praticamente todos os cães são infectados. A dirofilariose geralmente não é frequente no Canadá, mas existem áreas endêmicas preocupantes no sul de Ontário. Uma pesquisa de veterinários realizada em 2001 indicou que havia 240.000 casos diagnosticados nos EUA, mas estimativas realistas consideram prevalência > 1.000.000 de casos.[1]

As espécies sabidamente infectadas por *D. immitis* incluem cães domésticos, lobos, raposas, coiotes, gatos domésticos, furões, ratos almiscarados, leões-marinhos, gatos não domésticos, quatis e homem. As espécies de maior interesse na prática veterinária são cães e gatos domésticos. Uma vez que as consequências do tratamento e do prognóstico diferem entre essas duas espécies, aspectos clínicos da dirofilariose canina e felina (verme do coração) são discutidos separadamente.

Quando a infecção por dirofilária é grave ou prolongada, pode resultar na condição patológica conhecida como dirofilariose. E isso pode variar desde um quadro assintomático (apenas com lesões radiográficas) a lesões graves com risco à vida, doença arterial pulmonar crônica e doenças pulmonar e cardíaca.

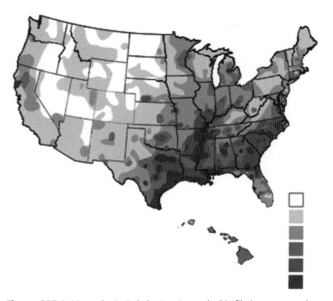

Figura 255.1 Mapa da Sociedade Americana de Dirofilariose mostrando a prevalência relativa da infecção nos EUA em 2013. Dados baseados em pesquisas da prática clínica. (Cortesia da Sociedade Americana de Dirofilariose.) (*Esta figura se encontra reproduzida em cores no Encarte.*)

Na dirofilariose crônica, também podem ocorrer glomerulonefrite, anemia e trombocitopenia. Ademais, a dirofilariose grave pode ocasionar efeitos multissistêmicos com apresentações agudas e fulminantes, como síndrome da veia cava (SVC) e coagulação intravascular disseminada (CID).

CICLO DE VIDA

D. immitis é transmitida por mais de 70 espécies de mosquitos, embora os vetores importantes do mosquito provavelmente sejam inferiores a 15. O conhecimento do complexo ciclo de vida de *D. immitis* é imperativo para médicos-veterinários que atuam em áreas endêmicas de dirofilariose (Figura 255.2). A terminologia para os estágios larvais pode ser confusa. O termo *L5* (último estágio ou quinto estágio larval) não é mais utilizado. A nomenclatura foi atualizada porque, embora muito menor do que um adulto maduro, esse estágio não sofre nova mudança; então, não é um estágio larval. A terminologia preferida para esse estágio pré-cardíaco é estágio imaturo 5 ([S5], adulto imaturo ou jovem). Para os fins deste capítulo, os termos *L5, estágio 5, jovem, adulto jovem, adulto imaturo* e *adulto maduro* são usados para descrever o estágio final de desenvolvimento da dirofilária. Além disso, o termo *L1* (1º estágio larval) refere-se ao 1º estágio larval após a ingestão pela fêmea do mosquito, enquanto antes disso, no hospedeiro, essas dirofilárias são denominadas microfilárias.

As dirofilárias adultas se instalam nas artérias pulmonares e, em menor quantidade, no ventrículo direito (nas grandes infecções). Após o acasalamento, as microfilárias (Mf; larvas de primeiro estágio), geradas por dirofilárias adultas maduras (S5 maduras), são liberadas na circulação sanguínea. Essas Mf são ingeridas por fêmeas de mosquitos durante o repasto sanguíneo e sofrem duas mudas (L1 em L2 e L2 em L3) ao longo de um período de 8 a 17 dias. É importante ressaltar que esse processo depende da temperatura; em épocas do ano em que não há dias suficientes com temperatura ambiente adequada, a muda no mosquito não ocorre durante a vida da fêmea do mosquito e, assim, não ocorre transmissão.[2,3] As mudas larvais e a maturação também dependem da presença de uma bactéria simbiótica intracelular, *Wolbachia pipientis*.[4] A L3 resultante é infectante e transmitida pelo mosquito ao se alimentar no hospedeiro original ou em outro hospedeiro, muito frequentemente um cão macho. Outra muda para L4 ocorre nos tecidos subcutâneo e adiposo e no músculo esquelético logo após a infecção (1 a 12 dias), com uma muda final para S5 (adulto imaturo) em 2 a 3 meses (50 a 68 dias) após a infecção.

Esse adulto imaturo (1 a 2 cm de comprimento) rapidamente alcança o sistema vascular e migra para o coração e para os pulmões, onde acontecem a maturação final (os machos adultos maduros medem 15 a 18 cm, e as fêmeas 25 a 30 cm) e o acasalamento. Sob condições ideais, o ciclo de vida leva de 184 a 210 dias. O cão hospedeiro torna-se microfilarêmico em 6 meses, mas tipicamente entre 7 e 9 meses após a infecção. As microfilárias, presentes em quantidade variável em cães infectados, apresentam ambas, periodicidade sazonal e periodicidade diurna, com maior número no sangue periférico durante a noite e durante o verão. Sabe-se que os vermes adultos vivem de 5 a 7 anos em cães, e as Mf vivem até 30 meses. Dillon enfatizou que a instalação de dirofilariose inicia-se com a muda do parasita para o estágio S5 (2 a 3 meses após a infecção), momento em que esses vermes adultos imaturos alcançam o sistema vascular, iniciando a doença vascular e possivelmente a doença pulmonar, com eosinofilia, infiltrados eosinofílicos e sintomas de doenças respiratórias.[5] É importante ressaltar que isso antecede a capacidade de o profissional diagnosticar a infecção por dirofilária.

FISIOPATOLOGIA

O termo "verme do coração" é impróprio porque o parasita adulto, em sua grande maioria, na verdade se instala no sistema arterial pulmonar, e o dano primário à saúde do hospedeiro é uma manifestação da lesão de artérias pulmonares e do pulmão. A gravidade das lesões e, portanto, as consequências clínicas

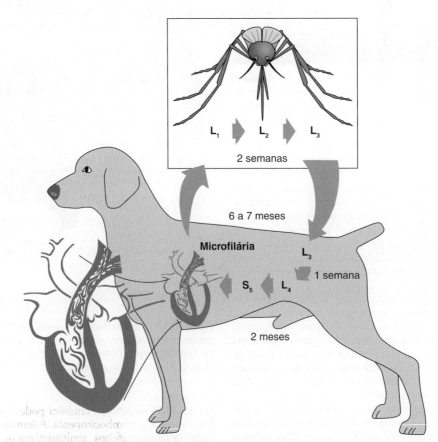

Figura 255.2 Ciclo de vida de *Dirofilaria immitis* no cão. L1-L4 = estágios larvais 1 a 4; *Mf*, microfilária; *S5*, 5º estágio ou adulto imaturo. (De Atkins CE: Heartworm disease. In: Allen DG, editor: *Small animal medicine*, Philadelphia, 1991, JB Lippincott, p. 341-363.)

estão relacionadas ao número relativo de vermes (variando de 1 a mais de 250), à duração da infecção e à interação hospedeiro-parasita. Os vermes adultos maduros e imaturos se instalam principalmente na árvore vascular pulmonar caudal, migrando ocasionalmente para as artérias pulmonares principais, o coração direito e as grandes artérias e veias em altas infecções.

A obstrução de vasos pulmonares por vermes vivos tem pouca relevância clínica, a menos que a carga parasitária seja alta ou o paciente seja pequeno. O principal efeito nas artérias pulmonares é ocasionado por proliferação de vilosidades miointestinais, inflamação, hipertensão pulmonar (HTP) induzidas pelo parasita (substâncias tóxicas, resposta imune e trauma físico) (ver Capítulo 243), bem como pelo dano à integridade vascular e fibrose. Isso pode complicar-se pela obstrução e vasoconstrição causada pela presença de vermes vivos,[6] por tromboembolismo de verme mortos e produtos da dirofilária.[7] As lesões pulmonares vasculares começam a se desenvolver alguns dias após a chegada dos vermes (3 meses após a infecção), com lesão e descamação endotelial, proliferação de vilosidades e ativação e quimiotaxia de leucócitos e plaquetas. A migração de tais células e a liberação de fatores tróficos induzem à proliferação e migração de células do músculo liso, com acúmulo de colágeno e fibrose. Lesões proliferativas acabam por invadir e até ocluir o lúmen vascular. Edema endotelial com alteração de junções intracelulares aumenta a permeabilidade dos vasos pulmonares. Parasitas que morreram naturalmente ou foram mortos provocam uma reação ainda mais grave, com trombose, inflamação granulomatosa e inflamação de vilosidades rugosa. No geral, ocorre aumento de tamanho das artérias pulmonares, com paredes espessas e tortuosas, e superfícies endoteliais rugosas. Essas anormalidades são, pelo menos parcialmente, reversíveis.[7]

Embora seja aceita a regra de que a atividade física exacerba os sintomas de tromboembolismo, na dirofilariose, a sua participação no desenvolvimento da doença vascular pulmonar e de HTP é menos clara. White Rawlings[8] não conseguiu mostrar o efeito de 2,5 meses de exercício controlado em esteira na HTP de cães com alta infestação. Dillon[9] relatou HTP mais grave em cães discreta e moderadamente infectados do que em animais altamente infectados, porém em cães não submetidos a exercício. A observação clínica sugere que os cães criados ao ar livre, principalmente cães de caça, apresentam lesões e HTP mais graves, possivelmente relacionadas à atividade física, mas o aumento da exposição e a carga parasitária também devem ser considerados.

As artérias pulmonares lesionadas se apresentam trombóticas, espessadas, dilatadas, tortuosas, não complacentes e funcionalmente incompetentes; assim, resistem ao recrutamento durante o aumento de demanda e, portanto, a tolerância ao exercício diminui. Vasos dos lóbulos pulmonares caudais são acometidos mais gravemente. A vasoconstrição pulmonar resulta, secundariamente, na liberação de substâncias vasoativas provavelmente liberadas por dirofilária, assim como de endotelina-1 produzida em excesso pelas células do endotélio vascular[10] e de substâncias vasoconstritoras, como serotonina, difosfato de adenosina (ADP) e tromboxano A_2, produzidas por plaquetas ativadas. Além disso, a hipoxia (induzida pelo descompasso do mecanismo de ventilação-perfusão pulmonar, secundário ao tromboembolismo pulmonar [TEP; ver Capítulo 243], pneumonia eosinofílica e consolidação pulmonar, ou a combinação das três) contribui ainda mais para a vasoconstrição. As consequências disso são HTP, aumento da pós-carga do ventrículo direito e comprometimento do débito cardíaco.[9-11] A HTP é exacerbada pelo exercício ou por outras condições que aumentam o débito cardíaco. O coração direito, que é uma bomba de volume eficiente, mas não suporta sobrecarga de pressão, inicialmente tenta se compensar pela hipertrofia excêntrica (dilatação e espessamento da parede ventricular); nas infecções graves ocorre descompensação (insuficiência cardíaca direita). Além disso, tensões hemodinâmicas, alterações geométricas e remodelação cardíaca podem contribuir para a insuficiência secundária da valva tricúspide e,

portanto, complicar ou propiciar descompensação cardíaca. Ocorre comprometimento adicional com o advento de arritmia cardíaca (ver Capítulo 248). Infarto pulmonar é incomum por causa da extensa circulação colateral existente no pulmão e devido à natureza gradativa da oclusão vascular. Porém, em função do aumento da permeabilidade vascular pulmonar, pode se desenvolver edema perivascular. Contudo, juntamente com o infiltrado inflamatório, esse acúmulo de líquido pode ser radiograficamente evidente como um aumento da densidade intersticial e até alveolar, aparentemente de mínima relevância clínica e certamente não indica insuficiência cardíaca esquerda (em outras palavras, não é edema pulmonar cardiogênico e, portanto, não se indica tratamento com furosemida).

O TEP espontâneo ou após o uso de medicamento adulticida e morte de parasitas pode precipitar ou agravar os sinais clínicos, ocasionando ou agravando a HTP, a insuficiência cardíaca direita ou, em casos raros, o infarto pulmonar. Parasitas mortos e desintegrados agravam a lesão vascular e exacerbam a coagulação. O fluxo sanguíneo pulmonar é comprometido e pode ocorrer consolidação dos lobos pulmonares acometidos. Com a morte súbita e maciça dos parasitas, esse dano pode ser grande, principalmente se associado a exercícios. A exacerbação pelo exercício provavelmente reflete o aumento do fluxo de sangue na artéria pulmonar e o escape de mediadores inflamatórios para o parênquima pulmonar pelas artérias pulmonares gravemente danificadas e permeáveis (ver Figura 255.12, mais adiante). Dillon sugeriu que a lesão pulmonar é semelhante à observada na síndrome de angústia respiratória aguda (SARA; ver Capítulo 242).[9]

Lesões pulmonares parenquimatosas também são resultantes de outros mecanismos além da consolidação pulmonar póstromboembólica. Pneumonia eosinofílica é mais frequentemente relatada na dirofilariose subclínica verdadeira, na qual a destruição imunomediada de microfilárias na microcirculação do pulmão provoca amicrofilaremia. Essa síndrome ocorre quando as Mf revestidas de anticorpos são aprisionadas na circulação pulmonar, induzindo uma reação inflamatória (pneumonia eosinofílica).[12] Uma forma mais grave, porém rara, de doença de parênquima pulmonar, denominada doença *pulmonar eosinofílica granulomatosa*, foi associada à dirofilariose. A causa exata e a patogênese não são conhecidas, mas são consideradas semelhantes às da pneumonia eosinofílica que ocorre na dirofilariose.[13] Postula-se que as Mf retidas nos pulmões são envolvidas por neutrófilos e eosinófilos e, por fim, originam granulomas associados à linfadenopatia brônquica.

Na dirofilariose, os complexos antígeno-anticorpo formados em resposta aos antígenos podem causar glomerulonefrite em cães com dirofilariose (ver Capítulo 325).[14] Isso resulta em proteinúria (albuminúria), raramente associada à insuficiência renal.

As dirofilárias também podem provocar doença quando ocorre migração errática. Esse fenômeno incomum tem sido associado a manifestações neuromusculares e oculares uma vez que tem sido descrita a presença do parasita em tecidos como músculo, cérebro, medula espinal e câmara anterior do olho. Além disso, foi observada trombose arterial sistêmica causada por S5 quando ocorre migração errática dos parasitas para a bifurcação aórtica ou mais distalmente para as artérias digitais (ver Capítulo 256).[15] Os parasitas adultos também podem "migrar" passivamente em sentido retrógrado da artéria pulmonar para o coração direito e para a veia cava, provocando a síndrome da veia cava (SVC), uma gravíssima complicação, descrita mais adiante.[16]

Recentemente foi reconhecido como importante o fato de que a bactéria *W. pipientis* se instala em parasitas filarídeos, inclusive *D. immitis*. Fato importantíssimo é que essas bactérias vivem em relação simbiótica com os parasitas filarídeos, sendo necessárias para a muda de fase larval no mosquito e no cão hospedeiro (L3-L4, L4-S5). A exata participação de *Wolbachia* na patogênese da dirofilariose não está bem esclarecido, mas foram identificadas proteínas de *Wolbachia* (proteínas de

SEÇÃO 16 • Doença Cardiovascular

superfície *Wolbachia* – PSW) no glomérulo e pulmão de cães infectados por dirofilária.[17,18] Além disso, as proteínas produzidas pela bactéria contribuem para a reação inflamatória do hospedeiro para a morte do parasita.

SINAIS CLÍNICOS

Os sinais clínicos de dilofilariose crônica dependem da gravidade e duração da infecção e, na maioria dos casos crônicos, refletem os efeitos do parasita nas artérias pulmonares e nos pulmões e, de forma secundária, no coração. É importante ressaltar que a grande maioria dos cães infectados por dirofilária é assintomática. O histórico dos cães acometidos inclui invariavelmente perda de peso, menor tolerância ao exercício, letargia, condição física ruim, tosse, dispneia, síncope e distensão abdominal (ascite). O exame físico (ver Capítulo 2) pode revelar evidências de perda de peso, desdobramento da segunda bulha cardíaca (13%), sopro cardíaco do lado direito devido à insuficiência de tricúspide (13%) e ritmo de galope cardíaco (ver Capítulo 55).[19] Se há insuficiência cardíaca direita, a distensão e o pulso da veia jugular são acompanhados de hepatoesplenomegalia e ascite. Na dirofilariose crônica, arritmias cardíacas e anormalidades de condução são incomuns (< 10%). Em casos de manifestações pulmonares parenquimatosas causadas por dirofilariose podem ser observadas tosse e crepitações pulmonares, com granulomatose (uma ocorrência rara). Além disso, também há relato de abafamento de sons pulmonares, dispneia e cianose. Quando ocorre TEP maciça (ver Capítulo 243) podem ser constatados, adicionalmente, sintomas de dispneia, febre e hemoptise.

DIAGNÓSTICO

Detecção de microfilária

O ideal é que seja obtido o diagnóstico precoce em exame de rotina, antes do aparecimento de sinais clínicos (*i. e.*, dirofilariose). Cães de áreas nas quais a dirofilariose é endêmica devem ser submetidos a teste anual para diagnóstico de dirofilariose, principalmente se não recebem medicação preventiva de dirofilariose. No passado, o diagnóstico era mais comumente realizado pela identificação microscópica de Mf em esfregaço sanguíneo direto de sangue obtido abaixo da camada de leucócitos, em um tubo de micro-hematócrito, usando-se o teste de Knott modificado ou a filtração em Millipore. A precisão desses testes, utilizados como triagem de rotina e no diagnóstico de suspeita de infecção por dirofilária, foi aprimorada por diversos testes. O teste de Knott modificado e a filtração em Millipore são mais sensíveis porque concentram as microfilárias, aumentando a chance de diagnóstico. A técnica de esfregaço direto possibilita o exame do movimento das larvas, ajudando na distinção entre *D. immitis* e *Dipetalonema reconditum* (atualmente denominado *Acanthocheilonema reconditum*); outros critérios de diagnóstico úteis estão incluídos na Tabela 255.1. Essa distinção é importante porque a presença deste último parasita não requer terapia onerosa e terapia à base de arsênico potencialmente

prejudicial, como no caso de *D. immitis*. Nenhum desses testes possibilita a exclusão definitiva de infecção por dirofilária por causa do risco de infecções amicrofilarêmicas (relatadas em 5 a 67% dos casos, sendo que 10 a 20% geralmente são confirmados)[20] e a possível ocorrência de resultado falso negativo, principalmente quando há pequena quantidade de microfilárias, coleta de pequeno volume de sangue ou se utiliza esfregaço sanguíneo direto. Não há boa correlação entre a quantidade de Mf circulantes no sangue periférico e o número de parasitas adultos e, portanto, não pode ser usada para determinar a gravidade da infecção. Na maioria das clínicas, o teste para detecção de microfilária tem sido amplamente substituído por testes de imunodiagnóstico para antígeno (*i. e.*, ensaio imunoenzimático [ELISA], imunoensaio de fluxo lateral e técnica de imunomigração rápida; Tabela 255.2). O teste modificado de Knott, o teste de filtragem em Millipore ou o esfregaço direto com sague fresco sempre devem ser realizados em cães positivos em testes de pesquisa de antígenos, a fim de determinar a condição da microfilariose. As razões para isso incluem saber se há grande quantidade de parasitas, o que possibilita o pré-tratamento ou tempo de observação programado após a primeira dose do tratamento com lactona macrocíclica (LM). Em segundo lugar, se há preocupação quanto à resistência do parasita à lactona macrocíclica, que pode ser facilitada quando esses fármacos são administrados em cães microfilarêmicos positivos para dirofilariose. Alguns veterinários optam por combinar os testes de pesquisa de antígeno e de microfilaremia. Essa prática é mais útil em cães que não recebem tratamento preventivo (o uso de LM normalmente torna o cão amicrofilarêmico). É geralmente aceitável que 1% dos cães infectados positivos para microfilária e negativos para o antígeno[20] podem ser subestimados, com base em novas informações sobre o complexo antígeno-anticorpo na infecção por dirofilária.[21-23]

Testes imunodiagnósticos para pesquisa de antígenos

Em cães que não recebem lactona macrocíclica (LM) como terapia preventiva, a prevalência de infecções amicrofilarêmicas é geralmente de 10 a 20%.[24] Isso pode ser observado em infecções pré-patentes (jovens), em infecções por parasitas de um único sexo (machos ou fêmeas, exclusivamente), com destruição imunomediada de microfilárias e com amicrofilaremia induzida por fármaco. Cães tratados preventivamente com LM são tipicamente amicrofilarêmicos. Portanto, os testes imunodiagnósticos são atualmente usados regularmente para triagem e em casos de suspeita de infecção por dirofilária. Esses testes são populares por causa de sua alta sensibilidade, especificidade e facilidade de execução (Tabela 255.2).[25-28] A limitação desses testes é que detectam exclusivamente antígeno de fêmeas de parasitas adultas e, portanto, produzem resultados negativos nos primeiros 6 meses (5 a 8 meses) de infecção, nas infecções causadas exclusivamente por machos e em infecções com baixa carga parasitária de fêmeas. De fato, em um estudo comparativo da acurácia de três kits de testes comerciais na detecção de carga parasitária baixa (≤ 4 fêmeas do parasita), constatou-se que nas infecções adquiridas naturalmente a sensibilidade geral (mediana

Tabela 255.1	Características para diferenciação de *Dipetalonema reconditum* e *Dirofilaria immitis*.			
	QUANTIDADE NO SANGUE	**MOVIMENTO**	**MORFOLOGIA**	**COMPRIMENTO (TESTE DE KNOTT MODIFICADO)**
D. reconditum	Geralmente pouca	Progressivo	Corpo curvado Cabeça romba Cauda curvada ou em forma de "gancho para abotoar"	263 μ (250 a 288 μ)
D. immitis	Geralmente muita	Estacionário	Corpo e cauda retos Cabeça em forma cônica	308 μ (295 a 325 μ)

Tabela 255.2 Testes de *kits* comerciais para pesquisa de antígeno e anticorpo para diagnóstico de dirofilariose em cães e gatos.[a]

FABRICANTE	PRODUTO	FORMATO	TESTE	AMOSTRA	ESPÉCIE	TEMPO	ETAPAS
Heska	Solo Step CH	M	IFL	P, S, ST	Canina	10 (ST), 5 (S, P)	1
Heska	Solo Step CH Batch Test Strips	M	IFL	P, S	Canina	5	1
Heska	Solo Step FH (anticorpo)	M	IFL	P, S,	Felina	5	1
IDEXX	PetCheck Heartworm Antigen PF	MP	E	P, S, ST	Canina e felina	20	9 ou 10
IDEXX	SNAP Heartworm Antigen Kit	M	E	P, S, ST	Canina	8	4
IDEXX	SNAP 3Dx, 4Dx	M	E	P, S, ST	Canina	8	4
IDEXX	SNAP Feline Heartworm Antigen Kit	M	E	P, S, ST	Felina	10	4
IDEXX	SNAP Feline Triple Antigen Kit	M	E	P, S, ST	Felina	10	4
Synbiotics	Witness HW	M	IMR	P, S, ST	Canina e felina	10	2
Synbiotics	DiroCHEK	MP	E	P, S	Canina e felina	15	4

[a]Testes listados em ordem alfabética pelo fabricante. *E*, ELISA; *IFL*, imunoensaio de fluxo lateral; *IMR*, imunomigração rápida; *M*, membrana; *MP*, micropoço; *P*, plasma; *S*, soro; *ST*, sangue total.

de três kits de teste) foi 79% e a especificidade mediana foi 97%.[29] A sensibilidade foi relativamente baixa (64%) para infecções com apenas uma fêmea parasita, mas melhorou com o aumento da carga parasitária de fêmeas parasitas (mediana de 85, 88 e 89% para duas, três e quatro fêmeas de parasitas, respectivamente). Obviamente, com carga parasitária mais alta, notou-se maior sensibilidade. Apesar do excelente resultado na detecção de pequena carga parasitária, ocorrem resultados falsos negativos (Figura 255.3).[29]

Alguns testes ELISA para pesquisa de antígeno são elaborados para prever quantitativamente a carga parasitária, com base na concentração do antígeno. O teste ELISA semiquantitativo (SNAP Canine Heartworm PF) foi elaborado para prever com sucesso a carga antigênica e, portanto, aproximar-se da carga parasitária. Rawlings *et al.*[30] demonstraram que isso pode ser útil para prever complicações tromboembólicas, em cães com maior carga parasitária que são mais propensos a sofrer essas complicações após o tratamento com fármaco adulticida. Essa aplicação é mais útil, no entanto, em casos de baixa concentração de antígeno (sugerindo baixa carga parasitária) porque altas concentrações do antígeno podem ser reconhecidas quando todos ou a maioria dos parasitas estão mortos, liberando uma grande quantidade de antígeno na circulação. A tecnologia ELISA também permite a determinação da eficácia da terapia adulticida. A concentração de antígeno ELISA normalmente diminui para níveis indetectáveis em 8 a 12 semanas após a terapia adulticida bem-sucedida; assim, um teste positivo que persiste por mais de 12 semanas após o tratamento é sugestivo de infecção persistente.[31] Porém, testes antigênicos podem permanecer positivos por períodos mais longos, e este autor não assume que seja falha na terapia adulticida, a menos que o teste antigênico seja positivo por > 6 meses após terapia adulticida, e não defende o uso do teste de rotina antes de 8 a 12 meses após o tratamento.

A American Heartworm Society (AHS) agora prefere o termo "antígeno não detectado" em vez do termo "negativo" quando se refere a resultados de teste de antígeno que não são positivos. Isso para enfatizar o fato de que testes negativos não descartam a possibilidade de infecção por parasitas imaturos, pequenos ou exclusivamente por machos do parasita.

Como previamente sugerido, a terapia com LM com ivermectina, milbemicina oxima, moxidectina ou selamectina elimina Mf dentro de 6 a 8 meses.[31-36] Além disso, a embriose pode ser permanente. Assim, o uso exclusivo de esfregaço sanguíneo direto, teste de Knott modificado ou teste em filtro Millipore (ou seja, testes para pesquisa de microfilária) em cães que recebem tratamento preventivo para dirofilariose com LM é inapropriado, embora esses métodos certamente sejam

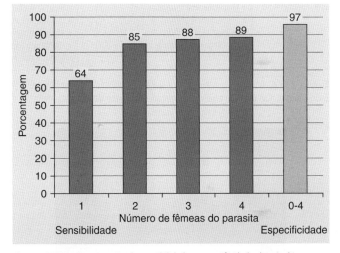

Figura 255.3 Comparação de sensibilidade e especificidade de três *kits* comerciais para teste de dirofilariose em amostras de soro de cães sabidamente infectados com baixa carga parasitária (zero a quatro fêmeas adultas de dirofilária). As barras mais escuras representam a sensibilidade mediana para os três testes para soro de cães com um, dois, três e quatro fêmeas de dirofilária adultas. A barra mais clara representa especificidade mediana para os três testes para soro de cães infectados com zero a quatro fêmeas adultas de dirofilária. (De Atkins CE: Comparison of results of three commercial heartworm antigen tests in dogs with low heartworm burdens. *J Am Vet Med Assoc* 222:1221-1223, 2003.)

suplementares. A única modalidade de teste rotineiramente efetiva em cães que recebem tratamento preventivo mensal é o teste para pesquisa de antígeno. Uma abordagem geral sobre o diagnóstico de infecção por dirofilária é mostrada na Figura 255.4.

Radiografia

Embora as imagens radiográficas não sejam um teste de triagem efetivo para dirofilariose, a radiografia torácica é um excelente método para detectar dirofilária, determinar sua gravidade, avaliar o parênquima pulmonar e suas alterações e definir os diagnósticos diferenciais. Anormalidades radiográficas, que se desenvolvem relativamente cedo no curso da doença, estão presentes em aproximadamente 85% dos casos. De acordo com o estudo de 200 cães infectados por dirofilária, realizado por Losonsky *et al.*,[37] as características radiográficas (Figura 255.5) incluem: aumento do ventrículo direito (60%), aumento da proeminência do principal segmento da artéria pulmonar (70%),

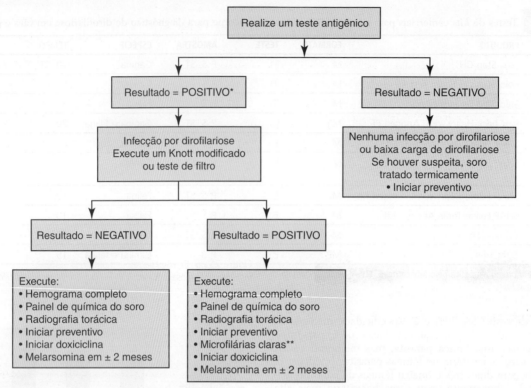

Figura 255.4 Abordagem esquemática para o diagnóstico de dirofilariose em cães. *O ideal é que o teste positivo seja confirmado. **O paciente deve ser observado quanto a reação adversa ou pré-tratado conforme descrito no texto.

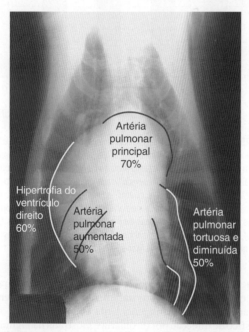

Figura 255.5 Frequência relativa de achados cardiovasculares radiográficos na dirofilariose. (De Losonsky JM, Thrall DE, Lewis RE: Thoracic radiographic abnormalities in 200 dogs with heartworm infestation. *Vet Radiol* 24:120-123, 1983.)

aumento do tamanho e da densidade das artérias pulmonares (50%), tortuosidade e diminuição da artéria pulmonar (50%). Se há insuficiência cardíaca, podem ser evidentes aumento da veia cava caudal, do fígado e do baço, bem como derrame pleural, ascite ou ambos. Thrall e Calvert[38] sugeriram que efusão pleural é incomum na dirofilariose, demonstrando que um acentuado aumento da artéria pulmonar lobar cranial foi o indicador mais sensível de dirofilariose associada à insuficiência cardíaca do que o aumento da veia cava caudal.

Radiografias torácicas obtidas na projeção ventrodorsal são preferíveis para avaliação da silhueta cardíaca e geralmente minimizam o estresse ao paciente. Todavia, a projeção dorsoventral é superior para a avaliação dos vasos pulmonares lobares caudais, que são considerados anormais caso sejam maiores do que o diâmetro da nona costela na intersecção entre a costela e a artéria (Figuras 255.5 e 255.6). A artéria pulmonar cranial é mais bem avaliada na projeção lateral e normalmente não deve ser maior que a veia que a acompanha ou o terço proximal da quarta costela (Figura 255.7).

O parênquima pulmonar pode ser bem avaliado por meio de radiografia. Em casos de pneumonite, os achados incluem uma mistura de densidade intersticial a alveolar, que é mais grave nos lobos pulmonares caudais (Figura 255.8). Na granulomatose pulmonar nodular eosinofílica, o processo inflamatório é organizado em nódulos intersticiais associados à linfadenopatia brônquica e, ocasionalmente, efusão pleural. Em casos de TEP, os achados radiográficos de coalescência de infiltrados alveolares e intersticiais, particularmente nos lobos pulmonares caudais, refletem inflamação e aumento da permeabilidade vascular pulmonar, descritos anteriormente (ver Figura 255.13). A consolidação pulmonar pode acompanhar uma embolização maciça, infarto ou ambos.

Eletrocardiografia

Em casos de dirofilariose, a eletrocardiografia é útil na detecção de arritmias, mas geralmente não é sensível na detecção de aumento da câmara cardíaca, quando comparada à radiografia e ao ecocardiograma. Se a radiografia não sugere dirofilariose, é improvável que o eletrocardiograma (ECG) seja útil no caso de ausência de arritmias. Com exceção da síndrome da veia cava e da insuficiência cardíaca, arritmias são raras (2 a 4%).[39,40] Todavia, a descoberta de um padrão de aumento do ventrículo direito (ver Capítulo 248) é uma evidência para a sustentação do diagnóstico de dirofilariose. Lombard e Ackerman[39] constataram anormalidades no ECG em 38 a 62% dos cães com dirofilariose, com alterações ecocardiográficas moderadas e graves, já Calvert e Rawlings[41] encontraram apenas um percentual de 6% dos 276 cães com dirofilarose que apresentavam alterações no ECG

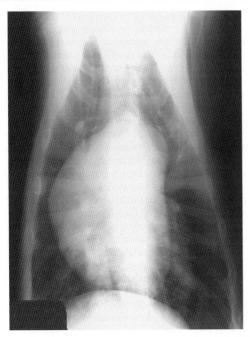

Figura 255.6 Radiografia torácica obtida em projeção dorsoventral de um cão com dirofilariose crônica. O leitor deve notar aumento da artéria pulmonar principal, aumento do ventrículo direito e artérias pulmonares lobares caudais tortuosas e aumentadas (ver Figura 255.5 com o diagrama de anormalidades radiográficas).

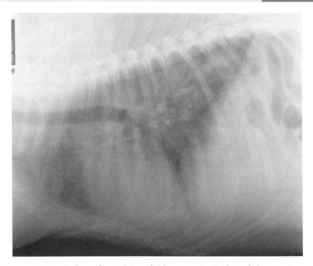

Figura 255.8 Radiografia torácica obtida em projeção lateral de um cão com tosse e dirofilariose crônica. O infiltrado alveolar intersticial difuso é grave e indica pneumonite eosinofílica. As alterações em artérias cardíacas e pulmonares são menos graves do que as mostradas nas Figuras 255.6, 255.7 e 255.13.

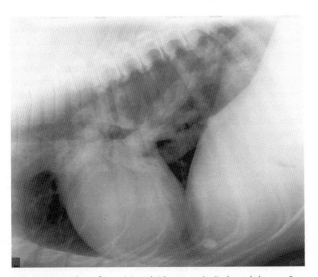

Figura 255.7 Radiografia torácica obtida em projeção lateral de um cão com dirofilariose crônica. O leitor deve notar o aumento do ventrículo direito (evidente no ápice; foi afastado do esterno), da artéria pulmonar apical e infiltrado intersticial nos lobos pulmonares caudais.

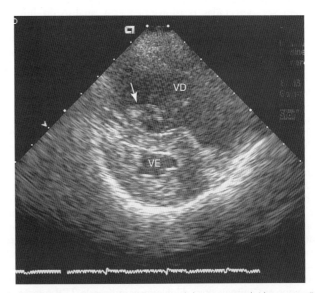

Figura 255.9 Ecocardiograma bidimensional do eixo curto obtido em um cão com dirofilariose crônica. O leitor deve notar o aumento do lúmen do ventrículo direito (*VD*) e do músculo papilar ventricular (*seta*). O septo é achatado e se curva em direção ao pequeno ventrículo esquerdo (*VE*). O eletrocardiograma, na parte inferior da figura, mostra que essa é uma imagem diastólica.

sugestivas de aumento do ventrículo direito. Esses pesquisadores[41] também constataram que os parâmetros do ECG mais sensíveis para detecção de dirofilária são as ondas SII mais profundas que 0,8 mv, eixo elétrico médio maior que 103° e mais que três parâmetros de ECG para aumento do coração direito. O último achado do ECG (mais de três critérios) é considerado o mais preciso. Na dilofilariose a ocorrência de P-pulmonale (ondas P altas, indicativas de aumento atrial) é incomum.

Ecocardiografia

O ecocardiograma é relativamente sensível na detecção de aumento do coração direito porque a dimensão diastólica final do ventrículo direito, o septo e a espessura da parede livre do ventrículo direito estão aumentados (Figura 255.9). Lombard relatou movimento septal anormal (paradoxal) em 4 de 10 cães com dirofilariose.[42] A proporção das dimensões internas do ventrículo esquerdo em relação ao ventrículo direito é uma estimativa útil; em cães com dirofilariose notou-se valor médio de 0,7, sendo menor que o valor normal de 3 a 4. Em alguns casos, o ecocardiograma bidimensional pode ser usado para mostrar parasitas na artéria pulmonar (ver Figura 255.21). Embora parasitas cardíacos possam ser ocasionalmente observados no ventrículo direito, esse método não é sensível, exceto em cães com síndrome da veia cava ou carga parasitária muito elevada, uma vez que os parasitas raramente se instalam nesse local.[42]

Patologia clínica

Os exames hematológicos e o perfil bioquímico sérico, apesar de uso limitado no diagnóstico de dilofilariose, são frequentemente úteis no fornecimento de evidências de suporte e na avaliação de anormalidades clínicas concomitantes que podem ou não estar relacionadas à dirofilariose. Calvert e Rawlings[41] relataram que cães com dirofilariose, no estado da Geórgia (EUA), geralmente apresentam anemia não regenerativa de baixo grau (presente em 10% dos cães com infecção discreta a moderada e em até 60% dos cães com infecção grave), neutrofilia (20 a 80% dos casos), eosinofilia ($\approx$ 85% dos casos) e basofilia ($\approx$ 60% dos casos). Trombocitopenia, que pode ser observada na dirofilariose crônica na síndrome da veia cava e na coagulação intravascular disseminada (CID), é mais comum 1 a 2 semanas após o tratamento com arsênico. Na dirofilariose grave, especialmente se há insuficiência cardíaca, as atividades das enzimas hepáticas podem estar aumentadas (10% dos casos) e ocasionalmente ocorre hiperbilirrubinemia. A azotemia é observada em apenas 5% dos casos e sua origem pode ser pré-renal, quando há desidratação ou insuficiência cardíaca ou devido à glomerulonefrite secundária. Em 10 a 30% dos casos nota-se albuminúria. Se a doença glomerular for grave, a hipoproteinemia (hipoalbuminemia) pode agravar o quadro clínico. Não é surpreendente que os achados clinicopatológicos sejam mais graves nos casos mais graves de dirofilariose.

A avaliação citológica do lavado traqueobrônquico (ver Capítulo 101) às vezes é útil, particularmente no cão com pneumonia e tosse, com dirofilariose subclínica e evidência radiográfica mínima de dirofilariose. O exame microscópico revela evidência de infiltrado eosinofílico. Em cães com microfilaremia, as Mf podem ser detectadas ocasionalmente. A análise do líquido abdominal, no caso de insuficiência cardíaca congestiva (ICC), normalmente revela a presença de transudato modificado. Cães com dirofilariose e insuficiência cardíaca direita apresentam pressão venosa central (PVC; ver Capítulo 76) que varia de 12 a mais de 20 cm H_2O; todavia, podem desenvolver ascite em PVC mais baixa, se houver hipoalbuminemia.

Apenas recentemente o uso de biomarcadores tem sido avaliado expressivamente em casos de dirofilariose. Venco et al.[43] relataram aumento na concentração sérica de proteína C reativa (PCR), que se liga a células mortas e estão para morrer, em resposta ao aumento das concentrações plasmáticas de citocinas. A concentração sérica de PCR de cães com e sem dirofilariose foi maior em pacientes doentes do que em animais do grupo-controle e havia correlação com o grau de lesão na artéria pulmonar e TEP. A esperança é que este biomarcador, que aumenta e diminui rapidamente com a ocorrência e resolução da doença, respectivamente, possa ser útil no estadiamento da dirofilariose e, portanto, possibilitando o monitoramento do tratamento, avaliando os resultados terapêuticos. Carreton et al. mostraram que o D-Dímero, a troponina cardíaca I e a mioglobina encontram-se anormalmente elevados em animais com dilofilariose, indicando TEP e lesão ao miocárdio, respectivamente.[41,44,45] Ao mesmo tempo que os resultados desses estudos preliminares são encorajadores, uso clínico apropriado de biomarcadores no diagnóstico e avaliação de dirofilariose necessita de estudo mais aprofundado.

CONDUTA CLÍNICA

A conduta clínica da dirofilariose é complexa por causa do ciclo de vida complexo do parasita, da acentuada variabilidade das manifestações clínicas e da gravidade da dirofilariose, dos métodos de profilaxia, das considerações sobre o uso de fármacos adulticidas e microfilaricidas, da toxicidade relativa e das complicações associadas à terapia com medicamento adulticida. Por esses motivos, o diagnóstico, a prevenção e o tratamento de dirofilariose continuam sendo um desafio.

Prevenção de dirofilariose

A prevenção de dirofilariose em animais de companhia é o objetivo óbvio e atingível do clínico veterinário. A falha na prevenção resulta da falta de conhecimento ou do mau entendimento por parte dos proprietários dos animais quanto à presença ou potencial gravidade da infecção causada por dirofilária, da falta de complacência do proprietário ou de orientações inadequadas do

veterinário quanto às medidas preventivas.[1,46-48] Estudos sobre a complacência do proprietário revelaram que aproximadamente 55% dos tutores de cães assistidos por veterinários compram medicamento preventivo para dirofilariose, mas os medicamentos utilizados são suficientes apenas para atender às necessidades de aproximadamente 56% desses cães. De forma que a proporção de cães da população que recebem cuidados adequados para profilaxia de dirofilariose é inferior a um terço dos animais.[47] Se forem levadas em consideração as doses compradas, mas não administradas, e cães que nunca foram levados a um veterinário, a porcentagem de cães cai drasticamente. Este último ponto foi enfatizado na Carolina do Norte, em 1999, quando o furacão Floyd causou extensas inundações e transtornos na região mais pobre do estado. Dos cães resgatados das enchentes, 67% apresentavam dirofilariose (comunicação pessoal do Dr. Kelli Ferris, da Universidade do Estado da Carolina do Norte [UECN], 2003). Além disso, as evidências sugerem que os profissionais veterinários estão deixando a desejar quanto à orientação dos proprietários. Uma pesquisa com clientes veterinários que compram LM como fármaco preventivo revelou que 38% não sabiam que o espectro de ação do medicamento prescrito era mais amplo do que aquele necessário apenas para prevenir a infecção por dirofilária.[49] Outro estudo que utilizou "atores-clientes" com animais de companhia para avaliar a participação de veterinários na falta de complacência do proprietário constatou que apenas 60% dos tutores de cães e $\approx$ 25% dos tutores de gatos foram alertados quanto ao risco de infecção por dirofilária, possíveis problemas relativos à doença e sobre os medicamentos, durante a visita agendada.[50]

Antibióticos derivados de lactonas macrocíclicas

A introdução da ivermectina, uma lactona macrocíclica (LM), em 1987, foi seguida pelo desenvolvimento e disponibilização de milbemicina oxima, selamectina e moxidectina. As LMs incluem avermectinas (ivermectina, doramectina, eprinomectina e selamectina) e milbemicinas (milbemicina oxima e moxidectina) e são oriundas de microrganismos do solo pertencentes ao gênero *Streptomyces*. Essa classe de fármacos possibilitou à medicina veterinária resultados altamente eficazes na prevenção de dirofilariose em várias formulações, combinações de medicamentos, espectros de ação e vias de administração. Esses medicamentos, uma vez que interrompem o desenvolvimento larval do estágio tecidual (L3 e L4) durante os primeiros 2 meses após a infecção, apresentam ampla janela temporal de eficácia e são administrados por via oral ou tópica, mensalmente, ou ainda por via injetável em intervalo de 6 ou 12 meses (o produto de 12 meses não está disponível nos EUA); sendo assim, o seu uso é muito prático. Além disso, esses produtos provocam reações menos graves do que os anteriormente utilizados, à base de dietilcarbamazina,[51] quando administrado acidentalmente em cães com microfilaremia. As LMs também propiciam, variavelmente, um efeito residual ("período de carência", "eficácia retroativa" ou "segurança líquida") em caso de lapso inadvertido de administração, sendo pelo menos parcialmente efetivas com intervalos de tratamento de até 2 a 3 meses, quando administradas continuamente pelos 12 meses seguintes.[52] Adicionalmente, as LMs atuam como microfilaricidas[28,52-54] e algumas têm ação adulticida, se usadas continuamente por um longo período.[54-57] É importante ressaltar que, no momento da redação deste capítulo, as dirofilárias apresentavam resistência a essa classe de fármacos (todas as moléculas e formulações) e efeito residual e presença sistêmica contínua de LM,[58] portanto, embora propiciem importantes vantagens que compensam falhas de compra, administração ou absorção, *não devem ser confiáveis*. Independentemente se as LMs são administradas sem interrupção (ou seja, todos os meses ou a cada 6 meses, dependendo do produto), essas vantagens se acumulam.

Ivermectina. A ivermectina, uma LM derivada da avermectina B_1, obtida de *Streptomyces* spp., é efetiva contra endoparasitas e ectoparasitas; é comercializada como um produto preventivo da infecção por dirofilária, administrada uma vez por mês. Também

CAPÍTULO 255 • Dirofilariose Canina e Felina

é comercializada em combinação com pamoato de pirantel (ancilóstomos e nematoides) e com pamoato de pirantel e praziquantel (ancilostomídeos, nematódeos e tênias), para melhorar a eficácia na prevenção contra helmintos intestinais (Tabela 255.3). Essas combinações de produtos são seguras em filhotes a partir de 6 semanas de vida. As LMs propiciam uma ampla janela de eficácia, além de alguma proteção quando ocorrem lapsos na terapia (período de carência). O uso de ivermectina é efetivo como profilático em casos de lapsos de até 2 meses. Em infecções experimentais a proteção é estendida, com administração contínua de 12 meses após a exposição, com lapsos de 3 meses (98% de eficácia) e de 4 meses (95% de eficácia).[52] Conforme afirmado anteriormente, a ivermectina é microfilaricida em dose preventiva (6 a 12 mcg/kg/mês), resultando em declínio gradual na quantidade de microfilárias. Apesar dessa destruição gradual de microfilárias, podem ocorrer reações adversas (diarreia transitória), geralmente discretas, se administrada em cães com microfilaremia.[52] Indivíduos portadores do gene de mutação ABCB1 (gene aka, resistente a multidrogas 1 [MDR-1] e de glicoproteína P1 [PGP-1]) (na maioria das vezes, mas não exclusivamente, na raças Collie, Shetland Sheepdog e outras raças de pastoreio) são suscetíveis à intoxicação por ivermectina (e a outras LM), em alta dose e em dose não indicada na bula (uso "extralabel"), que podem causar sintomas neurológicos.[59] Isso normalmente ocorre com o uso de preparados concentrados para animais, com sinais clínicos constatados em dose superior a 16 vezes a dose recomendada.[36] Por esse motivo, apenas as preparações formuladas para uso em animais de companhia devem ser administradas aos cães. Quando usada adequadamente, a ivermectina é muito efetiva na prevenção de infecção por dirofilária. Além disso, foram demonstradas propriedades adulticidas quando usada continuamente por 16 meses[55] e ser 95% eficaz na administração contínua por 30 meses[56] (consulte Controvérsias). Essa propriedade adulticida é exacerbada pela combinação com doxiciclina, por um período de 30 dias de tratamento. Ivermectina e doxiciclina parecem apresentar ação cinética, de várias maneiras, em relação à infecção por dirofilária (consulte Tratamento anti-*Wolbachia*).

Milbemicina oxima. A milbemicina oxima é um membro não macrolídeo de uma família de antibióticos milbemicinas (LM) oriunda de uma espécie diferente de *Streptomyces*. Na dose de 0,5 a 1 mg/kg, é efetiva na cessação do desenvolvimento de larvas em estágios L3 e L4, nas primeiras 6 semanas. Pode, portanto, ser administrada em intervalos mensais com um efeito residual de 2 meses quando ocorre atraso inadvertido na aplicação das doses. Com 12 meses contínuos de tratamentos após exposição ao parasita, esse efeito residual pode ser estendido em 3 meses (97% de eficácia), diminuindo para 41% com lapsos de 4 meses.[52] Na dose preventiva, a milbemicina oxima é um parasiticida de amplo espectro, sendo também efetiva contra alguns ancilóstomos, nematódeos e tricuris (ver Tabela 255.3), e pode ser iniciada em filhotes jovens com 2 meses de vida. Em cães com microfilaremia,

a milbemicina oxima pode causar reações adversas porque em dose preventiva é um excelente microfilaricida.[32,33] Raramente podem ser observadas reações adversas semelhantes às observadas com o uso de dose microfilaricida de ivermectina em cães que recebem dose preventiva de milbemicina oxima.[33] Com base no fato de que nas bulas das LM comercializadas os alertas referentes à morte de Mf e às reações são muito semelhantes, a importância dessas ocorrências tem sido questionada.[35] Como dose microfilaricida, podem ser administradas ivermectina (50 mcg/kg), difenidramina (2 mg/kg, IM) e dexametasona (0,25 mg/kg IV) antes da milbemicina oxima, a fim de eliminar a possibilidade de reações adversas em cães positivos para microfilária, particularmente aqueles com grande quantidade de microfilárias. Na dose preventiva, a milbemicina oxima, assim como outras LMs, é segura para uso em cães com mutação no gene ABCB1. Com o uso apropriado, a milbemicina oxima é altamente efetiva na profilaxia de dirofilariose. Atualmente, a milbemicina oxima está disponível em formulações como agente único e em combinação com lufenuron ou espinosade, para aumentar o seu espectro de ação, adicionando um efeito ectoparasiticida (ver Tabela 255.3).

Moxidectina. A moxidectina foi originalmente comercializada para prevenção de dirofilariose, por via oral, com estreito espectro de ação (dirofilária e ancilóstomo). Mostrou-se segura e efetiva na dose de 3 µg/kg, via oral, administrada mensalmente até 2 meses após a infecção.[60,61] A moxidectina de uso oral (atualmente não é comercializada nos EUA, mas sim em formulação de uso tópico aprovada pelo Federal Drug Administration – Center for Veterinary Medicine [FDA-CVM]) apresenta ação microfilaricida gradual nessa dose e não provocou reações adversas em cães com baixa infestação por microfilárias tratados com dose profilática.[53] Na dose de 15 mcg/kg, relata-se redução de 98% na quantidade de microfilárias 2 meses após o tratamento. O uso de moxidectina é seguro em cães da raça Collie e em outras raças com mutação no gene ABCB1,[62] mas não pode ser administrada por via oral a cães com menos de 6 meses de idade ou em gatos.

Uma formulação lipossômica de moxidectina de uso parenteral, de estreito espectro de ação (dirofilária e ancilóstomos), que propicia melhor complacência do tutor do animal, oferece proteção de 6 meses após uma injeção subcutânea. Com 12 meses (duas injeções) de tratamento contínuo, a moxidectina injetável é 97% efetiva na prevenção de infecção após um lapso de 4 meses de terapia preventiva, mas, surpreendentemente, parece ter ação adulticida limitada.[61] Não deve ser administrada a cães com < 6 meses de idade ou em gatos de qualquer idade.

Mais recentemente, a moxidectina (2,5% para cães e 1% para gatos) foi combinada com a imidacloprida (10%) e comercializada como um produto de uso tópico de amplo espectro (ver Tabela 255.3).[63,64] O produto combinado induz concentrações altas e sustentadas de moxidectina no organismo e aumentou a ação endoparasitária e a eficácia ectoparasitária. É um fármaco seguro, tem excelente efeito residual e é altamente

---

Tabela 255.3 Espectro de ação das lactonas macrocíclicas no cão.

FÁRMACO	D/MF	NEMATOIDES	ANCILÓSTOMO	TRICURIS/TÊNIAS	CARRAPATO	PULGA	ÁCARO
Iver/Pirantel	+	+	+				
Iver/PP/Prazi	+	+	+	Te			
Milbe-Lufen	+	+	+	Tr		+	
Milbe-Espino	+	+	+	Tr		+	
Milbemicina	+	+	+				
Moxi-injetável	+						
Moxi-Imida	+/+	+	+	Tr		+	
Selamectina	+		*		+	+	+

*Na bula da selamectina há indicação para ancilóstomos no Canadá. *D*, dirofilária; *Iver*, ivermectina; *Mf*, microfilária; *Milbe-lufen*, milbemicina-lufenuron; *Milbe-espino*, milbemicina-espinosade; *Moxi-imida*, moxidectina-imidacloprida; *Moxi-injetável*, injeção de moxidectina; *PP*, pamoato de pirantel; *Prazi*, praziquantel; *Te*, tênias; *Tr*, tricuris.

efetivo na prevenção de dirofilariose quando administrado mensalmente na dose aproximada de 2,5 a 6,8 mg de moxidectina/kg, para cães (1 a 2,5 mg/kg para gatos). Na dose recomendada, também é eficaz na prevenção e eliminação de pulgas; tratamento e controle de ancilóstomos, nematódeos e tricuris; bem como na eliminação de dirofilária, microfilária e sarna sarcóptica. Dois banhos, imediatos até 90 minutos após a aplicação, não altera a eficácia do produto. A segurança foi demonstrada com o uso de doses tópicas três e cinco vezes maiores do que a dose recomendada, em cães da raça Collie sensíveis à ivermectina. Esse produto pode ser administrado a filhotes de cães com 7 semanas de idade e de gatos com 9 semanas de idade.

Selamectina. É uma LM semissintética. É a única em que uma só molécula fornece amplo espectro de proteção com uso tópico uma vez por mês (ver Tabela 255.3). Em cães e gatos, sua eficácia no tratamento de dirofilariose é semelhante à de outras LMs.[66] Na dose de 6 a 12 mg/kg, com uso tópico, esse produto preventivo é efetivo contra dirofilária, pulgas e ovos de pulgas, ácaros de sarna sarcóptica, carrapatos e ácaros da orelha.[46] Banho e natação, até 2 horas após a aplicação, não alteram a eficácia do fármaco. A segurança foi demonstrada com o uso de dose tópica dez vezes maior que a dose recomendada, com administração oral de dose única e, em cães da raça Collie sensíveis à ivermectina, na dose em geral recomendada e em dose cinco vezes maior que a dose recomendada durante 3 meses.[67] Como acontece com outras LM, a selamectina tem um efeito residual de pelo menos 2 meses, e após 12 meses de tratamento contínuo apresenta 99% de proteção após 3 meses de profilaxia.[66,68] A selamectina tem ação microfilaricida lenta, semelhante a outras LMs.[68] A selamectina pode ser administrada em filhotes de cães a partir de 6 semanas de vida. A administração crônica e contínua de selamectina tem ação adulticida, embora nenhum dado publicado indique que seja tão eficaz nesse aspecto quanto a ivermectina.

Eprinomectina. É uma amino-avermectina derivada da avermectina B1 (uma fração oleandrose terminal modificada denominada 4(OO)-epiacetilamino-4(OO)-desoxiavermectina B1), foi originalmente utilizada como um agente tópico altamente efetivo contra parasitas internos e externos de bovinos. Esta LM também é formulada em uma combinação farmacêutica para gatos[69] com excelente biodisponibilidade, distribuição e ação sistêmica após aplicação tópica.[70] Após aplicação tópica, a concentração plasmática média máxima da eprinomectina foi constatada 24 horas após a administração, na maioria dos gatos, com biodisponibilidade média de 31%. A meia-vida terminal média é de 114 horas, devido à absorção lenta, em comparação com a meia-vida de eliminação média rápida de 23 horas, após administração intravenosa.[70] A combinação do produto (BROADLINE; fipronil, (S)-metopreno, eprinomectina e praziquantel) foi aprovada na Europa para o tratamento/prevenção de infecção por *D. immitis*, *Aelurostrongylus*, tênias, ancilóstomos, *T. cati* e pulgas. Diversos estudos mostraram que o uso tópico desse produto é efetivo e seguro, bem como preventivo, para dirofilariose, na dose mínima pretendida de 0,5 mg/kg, mensalmente.[70]

Em resumo, a classe de fármacos LM propicia uma maneira prática, efetiva e segura para profilaxia de dirofilariose, com variáveis espectros e modos de administração (ver Tabela 255.3). Todas são seguras em cães da raça Collie e outras raças que apresentam mutação no gene ABCB1, quando utilizadas como indicadas, em doses preventivas. Todas têm ação microfilaricida, embora apenas a formulação tópica de moxidectina imidaclopirida seja aprovada pela FDA-CVM para tal finalidade; acredita-se ela torna as fêmeas do parasita estéreis. Portanto, o teste de microfilária, para diagnóstico de infecção por dirofilária, não pode ser usado com segurança em cães que receberam esse produto. A profilaxia deve ser iniciada o mais tardar 6 a 8 semanas de idade, em áreas endêmicas, ou o mais breve possível, conforme as condições climáticas o exigirem.[27,71] Embora mais segura que a dietilcarbamazina (o medicamento preventivo original de uso diário, eventualmente, é substituído por LM) em cães com microfilaremia, há um risco variável quando se administra LM a esses cães. Antes da primeira dose, todos os cães

com mais de 6 meses de idade e em risco de infecção devem ser testados (teste antigênico, seguido de teste para pesquisa de microfilária, se o teste antigênico for positivo; ou, de forma ideal, em todos os casos), com um segundo teste após 7 a 8 meses.

É importante ter conhecimento do efeito residual dessa classe de medicamentos porque ele é uma vantagem dessas moléculas, mas não deve ser considerado no protocolo de rotina preventiva. Apesar da ação protetora verificada em condições experimentais durante pelo menos 8 semanas após a exposição, as LMs devem ser administradas *exatamente* como indicado pelo fabricante. As lactonas macrocíclicas (LMs) podem, no entanto, ser usadas para "resgatar" cães que tiveram falha na administração preventiva.[27,71] Se falhas acidentais ocorreram há mais de 6 a 8 semanas (dependendo do local e da época do ano), o tratamento preventivo deve ser restabelecido com a dose recomendada e mantido por pelo menos 12 dias consecutivos para obter novamente os benefícios da ação adulticida.[36] No caso de falha na administração preventiva durante um período de exposição conhecido, deve-se realizar um teste para pesquisa de antígeno de dirofilária 7 a 8 meses após a última exposição possível, caso tenha ocorrido infecção.

Tanto o AHS (*https://www.heartwormsociety.org*) quanto o Companion Animal Parasite Council ([CAPC], *www.CAPCvet. org*) recomendam prevenção ao longo de 1 ano, independentemente da localização geográfica.[72] Esse ponto de vista permanece controverso, pois sabe-se que os parasitas não são transmitidos durante todo o ano, exceto em alguns locais no extremo sul dos EUA. Como muitos veterinários e tutores de animais do norte dos EUA ainda usam abordagem sazonal para a profilaxia de dirofilariose, a AHS recomenda a prevenção inicial de dirofilariose com uso de LM dentro de 1 mês antes da temporada de transmissão[36] e continuação de 1 mês além da estação de transmissão.[27,71] Este autor recomenda a prevenção por 1 ano, pelo menos, abaixo da linha de Mason-Dixon, na América do Norte (consulte Controvérsias [adendo na edição eletrônica em ExpertConsult.com]).

Na última década, a preocupação com a resistência das dirofilárias às LMs veio à tona (ver Controvérsias [adendo na edição eletrônica em ExpertConsult.com]). Embora isso seja importante, a classe dos fármacos LMs ainda é amplamente efetiva na prevenção de infecção por dirofilária, e o uso desses produtos deve ser continuado.

Agentes bloqueadores: repelentes inseticidas

A permetrina é um piretroide de terceira geração que elimina rapidamente várias espécies de insetos. Esse produto atualmente está disponível para administração oral na forma de pelo menos 2 repelentes úteis no controle de mosquitos e, portanto, de vermes. Foi demonstrado que um deles atua como repelente durante 1 mês, além de eliminar três vetores de dirofilária (*A. aegypti*, *A. albopictus* e *C. pipiens*).[73] Foi demonstrado que o segundo pode repelir e matar mosquitos *A. aegypti* liberados para se alimentar em cães infectados com a cepa JYD-34 de *D. immitis*.[74] A alimentação em cães não tratados, do grupo-controle, propiciou taxa de ingurgitamento de ≈ 80 a 95%, com 95% dos mosquitos abrigando L1. No entanto, apenas 2% dos mosquitos tornaram-se ingurgitados em cães tratados, 28 dias após a aplicação do produto. A implicação desses estudos é que a aplicação mensal de permetrina pode repelir e matar mosquitos, impedindo efetivamente a transferência de dirofilárias para e de mosquitos, reduzindo também o desconforto causado por picadas de mosquitos e a população local de mosquitos. Essa abordagem também é efetiva para proteger contra dirofilárias resistente aos fármacos LM e se mostra promissora como procedimento auxiliar efetivo às medidas preventivas atuais.

Tratamento de parasitas com produtos adulticidas

Melarsomina

Na maioria dos casos de dirofilariose, é imperativo livrar o paciente do parasita causador. A tiacetarsamida (Caparsolato), há décadas é o único medicamento aprovado para esse propósito, mas não é mais comercializado, embora existam alguns estoques. Foi substituído pela melarsomina (Imiticida), um arsênico orgânico, superior em segurança e eficácia à tiacetarsamida.[75,76] Em um estudo com 382 cães infectados por *D. immitis* tratados com melarsomina, verificou-se que nenhum caso necessitou de descontinuação da terapia devido à intoxicação hepatorrenal (em comparação com os 15 a 30% dos animais tratados com tiacetarsamida); não ocorreu caso algum de TEP grave.[77]

A melarsomina tem um tempo de retenção médio cinco vezes maior que a tiacetarsamida, e seus metabólitos permanecem livres no plasma (dos quais os parasitas se alimentam).[75,76] Por isso, tem eficácia superior. Após administração de duas doses (de 2,5 mg/kg/24 h, IM) a eficácia se aproxima de 90%; obtém-se eficácia de 99% com a repetição do tratamento com duas doses após 4 meses ou com o fracionamento da dose, tema discutido mais adiante. É importante ressaltar que a morte de 90% dos parasitas não indica que 90% dos cães tratados ficam livres da infecção. As estimativas são de que apenas 70% cães se livram da infecção com o protocolo de 2 injeções, embora ocorra redução marcante de sua carga parasitária.[76]

Apesar da maior segurança desse produto, reações adversas ainda são encontradas.[19,24,78,80] Na verdade, o sucesso farmacológico da terapia adulticida, por definição, inclui eventos tromboembólicos. O clínico pode minimizar a gravidade dessa complicação restringindo a atividade física após a administração de melarsomina. Talvez a principal vantagem da droga seja a possibilidade de dosagem flexível ("doses fracionadas" – 1 injeção, seguida, de 2 injeções, com intervalo de não menos de 30 dias, e estas 2 injeções administradas com intervalo de 24 horas), possibilitando eliminação inicial segura de 50% dos parasitas, seguida de injeções subsequentes para atingir 100% de eficácia. Estudos têm mostrado que pacientes tratados com o protocolo de doses fracionadas têm maior soroconversão à condição de antígeno-negativo do que pacientes previamente tratados com Caparsolato ou com o protocolo posológico padrão da melarsomina.[81,82]

Pode-se utilizar protocolo de doses fracionadas em indivíduos gravemente infectados ou naqueles em que se prevê a ocorrência de tromboembolismo pulmonar (TEP) (Tabela 255.4). Inicialmente, esse procedimento (uma injeção IM de 2,5 mg/kg) possibilita a eliminação de apenas metade da carga parasitária e, portanto, diminuindo o risco de complicações embólicas. Essa dose única é seguida de um protocolo de duas doses em 1 mês, se as condições clínicas permitirem; o autor esperou até 3 meses quando houve adversidade significativa após a primeira injeção. Embora o fabricante recomende esse protocolo para cães gravemente infectados, o autor o utiliza em todos os casos, a menos que exista restrição financeira ou preocupação quanto à intoxicação por arsênico (p. ex., doença renal ou hepática grave preexistente; Figura 255.10).[78] As desvantagens do protocolo de doses fracionadas incluem despesa adicional, aumento da administração total de arsênico e necessidade de restrição de atividade física por 2 meses.

Tabela 255.4 Recomendações do fabricante para o uso de di-hidrocloreto de melarsomina, com base na condição do paciente.

CLASSE 1	CLASSE 2	CLASSE 3	CLASSE 4
Dirofilariose (assintomática, sem lesões radiográficas)	Dirofilariose sintomática (sintomas discretos a moderados)	Dirofilariose sintomática (sintomas graves)	Síndrome da veia cava
Duas doses de melarsomina com intervalo de 24 h (2,5 mg/kg IM)	Duas doses de melarsomina com intervalo de 24 h (2,5 mg/kg IM)	Uma dose de melarsomina (2,5 mg/kg IM), seguida de 2 injeções com intervalo de 24 h, depois de, aproximadamente, 1 mês	A melarsomina não é indicada para casos agudos

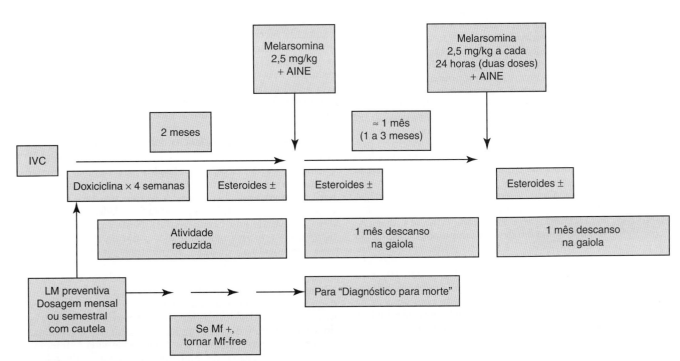

Figura 255.10 Abordagem para o tratamento de dirofilariose em cães. *AINE*, anti-inflamatório não esteroide; *D*, dirofilariose; *IVC*, infecção do coração por verme; *LM*, lactona macrocíclica como medicamento preventivo; *Mf*, microfilária. (Adaptada de Atkins CE, Miller M: Is there a better way to administer heartworm adulticidal therapy? *Vet Med* 98:310-317, 2003.)

Em 55 cães com dirofilariose grave assim tratados, verificou-se que em 96% dos casos o resultado foi bom ou muito bom, com mais de 98% de animais negativos para pesquisa de antígeno 90 dias após o tratamento.[77] Desses 55 cães gravemente infectados, 31% apresentaram TEP, mas nenhum morreu. Os sintomas mais comuns foram febre, tosse e anorexia 5 a 7 dias após o tratamento. Esses sinais clínicos estavam associados a opacidades radiográficas causadas por lesões perivasculares discretas no lobo pulmonar caudal que desapareceram espontaneamente ou após terapia com corticosteroides. Um pequeno estudo recente mostrou evidência de redução de biomarcadores de lesão pulmonar e cardíaca, utilizando protocolo de doses fracionadas, quando comparado ao protocolo padrão de 2 doses.[82] Além disso, o protocolo de doses fracionadas propiciou melhor resolução da proteinúria.

Sabe-se agora que a administração mensal de doxiciclina e ivermectina, 1 mês antes da administração de melarsomina, reduz a gravidade das lesões pulmonares em cães com dirofilariose, além de outros benefícios (ver Doxiciclina).[83]

No momento do diagnóstico (geralmente com teste de pesquisa de antígeno positivo para dirofilariose), é preenchido um banco de dados mínimo. Isso inclui teste de pesquisa de microfilária, hemograma completo, perfil bioquímico sérico, exame de urina e radiografia torácica. Se há suspeita de doença hepática com base nos achados clínicos e laboratoriais, a mensuração da concentração sérica de ácidos biliares pode ser útil para avaliar a função hepática. Nesse momento, deve ser prescrito o uso preventivo de LM (ver Figura 255.10).[78] Essa abordagem, que tem sido adotada pela AHS,[84] é utilizada para prevenir novas infecções, reduzir ou eliminar microfilárias (o tratamento crônico protege o próprio cão ou outros cães e gatos) e eliminar L4 em desenvolvimento (ainda não suscetível à terapia adulticida). Atualmente, em razão das preocupações quanto à resistência do parasita às lactonas macrocíclicas (LMs) as microfilárias devem ser eliminadas mais rapidamente do que fazem as doses de agentes preventivos. As microfilárias podem ser eliminadas mais rapidamente, embora nem sempre completamente, com imidaclorprida-moxidectina, doxiciclina + ivermectina, milbemicina oxima ou alta dose de ivermectina (50 µg/kg; não recomendada). A adição de doxiciclina a esse protocolo propicia inúmeras vantagens, discutidas a seguir. Em cães com microfilaremia, a primeira dose de LM é administrada no hospital ou no domicílio, sob observação; assim, uma reação adversa pode ser detectada e tratada imediatamente. Podem-se administrar corticosteroides, com ou sem anti-histamínico (0,25 mg de dexametasona/kg IV e 2 mg de difenidramina/kg IM; ou 1 mg de prednisolona/kg VO, 1 h antes e ± 6 h após a administração da primeira dose preventiva) para reduzir o risco de reação adversa em pacientes com alta microfilaremia. É importante ressaltar que reações adversas ao uso de dose preventiva de LM são incomuns, mas deve-se ter cautela, particularmente com a milbemicina oxima.

Dependendo da época do ano, tradicionalmente tem-se permitido um atraso, ou lapso, de até 2 a 3 meses antes da administração da terapia adulticida.[78] Embora o início da administração de LM previna infecção adicional, esse atraso permite a maturação larval até a idade adulta, garantindo que o único estágio do ciclo de vida é o parasita adulto, estágio vulnerável ao tratamento com melarsomina. Isso é mais importante se o diagnóstico é obtido durante ou no fim de uma temporada de exposição aos mosquitos. Se o diagnóstico é feito na primavera ou no fim do inverno, quando as larvas infectantes já tenham amadurecido, a terapia adulticida pode ser iniciada (ver Figura 255.10). Essa janela para possível escape larval de dirofilária também praticamente se fecha aos 30 dias de pré-tratamento com doxiciclina (98 a 100% de taxa de morte de larvas, se administrada durante os primeiros 60 dias pós-infecção, e 70%, se administrada 65 a 94 dias após a infecção; veja Doxiciclina).[85]

Protocolo de tratamento com fármaco adulticida

Aproximadamente 60 dias após o diagnóstico, incluindo 30 dias de tratamento com doxiciclina (10 mg/kg/12 h VO), 2 doses mensais ou 1 injeção de LM, inicia-se a terapia adulticida. O segundo mês de espera é opcional, mas, embora não haja dados de suporte, é lógico que, ao matar *Wolbachia* e eliminar a dirofilária, pensa-se que 30 dias extras diminuem ainda mais a biomassa dos vermes e a possibilidade de liberação potencial de proteínas, após a sua morte.

Na clínica do autor, administra-se um anti-inflamatório não esteroide (AINE) na manhã anterior à injeção, sendo continuado por um total de 4 a 5 dias, na maioria dos casos. A primeira injeção de melarsomina (2,5 mg/kg) é administrada por via intramuscular profunda, na musculatura lombar (como indicado na bula) e anota-se o local da injeção. Antes da injeção, troca-se a agulha e toma-se o cuidado de injetar profundamente no músculo e em nenhum outro lugar. Na clínica do autor alguns profissionais empregam sedação e preparação cirúrgica do local da injeção. Toma-se cuidado para garantir que o cão não se mova durante a injeção e realiza-se isso apoiando os membros pélvicos para evitar que o animal se sente/caia, com risco potencial de errar o local da injeção. Os pacientes são geralmente, mas não necessariamente, hospitalizados por um dia. A necessidade de restrição à atividade física por 1 mês é *fortemente enfatizada* e induz-se sedação, se necessário. Os tutores também são orientados quanto à ocorrência de reações adversas (febre, inflamação local, prostração, inapetência, tosse, dispneia, colapso), para ligarem se tiverem dúvidas e retornar para um segundo tratamento com duas injeções em aproximadamente 1 mês.

Se ocorrer reação sistêmica grave, a segunda etapa do tratamento adulticida é adiado ou ocasionalmente até cancelado. Normalmente, no entanto, mesmo com reações graves, todo o protocolo de tratamento é concluído dentro de 2 a 3 meses (ver Figura 255.10). Após um período mínimo de 1 mês, repete-se a injeção de melarsomina, novamente com registro do local da injeção. Se uma reação local significativa é observada após a primeira injeção, subsequentemente administra-se dexametasona ou AINE, por via oral, para minimizar a dor no local da injeção. No dia seguinte (aproximadamente 24 horas após a primeira injeção) repete-se o procedimento ao administrar a injeção de melarsomina na região lombar oposta. As orientações ao cliente são semelhantes àquelas previamente mencionadas, com ênfase à necessidade de rigorosa restrição à atividade física por 1 mês. O teste antigênico deve ser repetido 8 a 12 meses após a segunda série de injeções; um resultado positivo é indicativo de eficácia adulticida incompleta. Ressalta-se que, apesar da comprovada eficácia da melarsomina, nem todos os vermes morrem em todos os pacientes. Tipicamente, a carga parasitária é marcadamente reduzida, mas se restam apenas algumas fêmeas adultas, uma a três vivas, pode ocorrer teste antigênico positivo. Se a terapia adulticida deve ou não ser repetida, nessas condições, depende de cada caso, de acordo com a opinião dos proprietários.

Uso de lactonas macrocíclicas como adulticidas

Atualmente sabe-se que algumas LMs têm ação adulticida.[54-56] Quando esses fármacos são utilizados para eliminar dirofilárias adultas em um cão, os termos *morte suave* e *morte lenta* são usados para descrever essa abordagem. A ivermectina tem sido muito estudada e é a mais utilizada para essa finalidade, que geralmente deve ser evitada (ver Controvérsias). Neste capítulo, os termos *morte suave* e *morte lenta* são usados como sinônimos.

A ivermectina, quando administrada mensalmente por 31 meses consecutivos, tem 95% de eficácia adulticida, em infecções causadas por *D. immitis*.[56] A selamectina, quando administrada continuamente por 18 meses, eliminou aproximadamente 40% dos parasitas transplantados.[54] O tratamento mensal com imidaclorprida-moxidectina associado à terapia com doxiciclina por 30 dias (10 mg/kg/12 h) é efetivo na eliminação de infecções experimentais aos 5 meses de vida.[57] Injeção de liberação prolongada de milbemicina oxima e moxidectina parece ter eficácia adulticida mínima.[55,61] Embora possa haver uma regra para essa estratégia terapêutica em casos em que restrições ou problemas médicos concomitantes impeçam o tratamento com melarsomina, a recomendação atual é que as LMs não sejam utilizadas como o principal fármaco adulticida (ver Controvérsias).

Restrição à atividade física

O repouso em área restrita do canil é um aspecto importante no tratamento de dirofilariose após terapia adulticida, após ETP ou durante a terapia de insuficiência cardíaca. Isso geralmente pode ser melhor, ou apenas alcançado na clínica veterinária. Se restrições financeiras impedirem isso, canil ou permanência no banheiro ou na garagem da casa, com ou sem tranquilidade, e permitindo apenas caminhadas leves na coleira são soluções alternativas úteis. Mesmo assim, alguns proprietários não restringem ou não podem restringir a atividade física, resultando em piora ou complicações tromboembólicas. Na opinião do autor, a falha em restringir a atividade física após o tratamento com fármaco adulticida é a principal causa de complicação tromboembólica grave.

TRATAMENTO CIRÚRGICO

Sasaki, Kitagawa e Ishihara[86] descreveram um método de remoção mecânica dos parasitas usando uma pinça tipo jacaré flexível (Figura 255.11 e Vídeo 255.1). Esse método foi efetivo em 90% de 36 cães com dirofilariose discreta ou grave. Apenas dois dos cães gravemente afetados (n = 9) morreram de doença cardíaca e insuficiência renal 90 dias após o procedimento. Esses dados sugerem que, em mãos habilidosas, a técnica é segura. Estudos subsequentes de Morini et al.[87] demonstraram resultados superiores quando comparados com o tratamento com melarsomina, com menor ocorrência de TEP e SC. É importante ressaltar que a maioria dos cães tratados cirurgicamente requer administração subsequente de melarsomina para a cura. As vantagens dessa técnica incluem menor risco de complicações medicamentosas (terapia subsequente seria administração de fármaco adulticida em um cão assintomático, usando apenas 2 doses) e ausência relativa de complicações tromboembólicas. As desvantagens incluem a necessidade de anestesia geral, necessidade de habilidade do cirurgião, aparelho para fluoroscopia, risco de intercorrências anestésicas ou cirúrgicas e erradicação incompleta dos parasitas. No entanto, continua sendo uma alternativa possível para o tratamento de pacientes de alto risco.

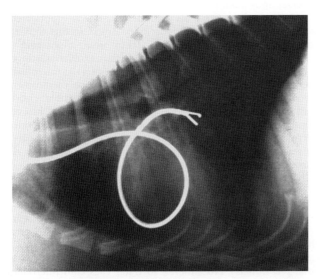

Figura 255.11 Retirada de dirofilária com auxílio de uma pinça do tipo jacaré flexível. (De Sasaki Y, Kitagawa H, Ishihara K: Clinical and pathological effects of heartworm removal from the pulmonary arteries using flexible alligator forceps. In: Otto GF, editor: *Proceedings of American Heartworm Symposium 1989*, Batavia, IL,1990, American Heartworm Society, p. 45.)

TERAPIA DE SUPORTE

Corticosteroides

Os efeitos anti-inflamatórios e imunossupressores inerentes aos corticosteroides são úteis para o tratamento de alguns casos de dirofilariose. A prednisona, esteroide mais frequentemente preconizado, reduz a arterite pulmonar, mas na realidade agrava a proliferação vascular notada na dilofilariose, diminui o fluxo arterial pulmonar e reduz a eficácia da tiacetarsamida (não existem dados que relatam esse efeito da melarsomina). Por essa razão, os corticosteroides são indicados no tratamento de dilofilariose apenas em razão das complicações pulmonares parenquimatosas (pneumonia eosinofílica, granuloma eosinofílico e tromboembolismo pulmonar [TEP]), para tratar ou prevenir reações adversas aos fármacos microfilaricidas, e possivelmente para minimizar a reação tecidual à melarsomina. No caso de pneumonia, administra-se prednisona (1 mg/kg/dia), por via oral, durante 3 a 5 dias; o tratamento é descontinuado ou a dose ajustada conforme necessário.[12,24] A resposta é geralmente favorável. A prednisona também tem sido recomendada, juntamente com repouso no canil, para o tratamento de TEP, na dose de 1 a 2 mg/kg/dia, via oral, até que a melhora radiográfica e clínica seja notada.[24] Devido à possibilidade de retenção de líquido induzida por esteroides, essa terapia deve ser usada com cautela no caso de insuficiência cardíaca. Além disso, é necessário cuidado, porque estudos anteriores mostraram que a terapia com corticosteroide reduziu o fluxo sanguíneo pulmonar e agravou a doença da túnica íntima vascular, em um modelo de infecção por dirofilária;[88] ademais, os corticosteroides também são procoagulantes.[24] Conforme mencionado para terapia com fármacos adulticidas (discutido anteriormente) e microfilaricidas (discutido a seguir), os corticosteroides podem ser utilizados para minimizar possíveis reações adversas à melarsomina e às lactonas macrocíticas (LMs) em razão da morte súbita de Mf.

Ácido acetilsalicílico

Os fármacos antitrombóticos têm recebido muita atenção no tratamento de dirofilariose[88-92] e o tema recentemente foi revisto.[93] Benefícios potenciais incluem redução da gravidade das lesões vasculares, redução de HP e da vasoconstrição da artéria pulmonar induzida por tromboxano, e menor ocorrência de TEP após o tratamento com adulticida.[90] O ácido acetilsalicílico foi efetivo em diminuir a lesão vascular causada por fragmentos de parasitas mortos,[90] reduzindo a extensão e a gravidade da proliferação da camada íntima muscular dos vasos sanguíneos causada por parasitas vivos implantados[91] e na melhora da doença do parênquima pulmonar e da proliferação da camada íntima em cães com vermes implantados e tratados com tiacetarsamida.[88] Estudos mais recentes, no entanto, obtiveram resultados polêmicos. Quatro cães submetidos à implantação de dirofilária e tratados com fármaco adulticida e ácido acetilsalicílico não apresentaram melhora nas lesões angiográficas pulmonares, e os cães tratados apresentaram tortuosidade vascular mais grave do que os cães do grupo-controle e aqueles que receberam heparina.[89] Boudreau et al.[92] constataram que a dose de ácido acetilsalicílico necessária para diminuir a reatividade plaquetária em pelo menos 50% foi aumentada em quase 70%, no caso de dirofilariose (implantação experimental), e em quase 200%, no caso de tromboembolismo pulmonar (implantação experimental de parasita morto). Não se verificou diferença significativa na gravidade de lesões vasculares pulmonares em pacientes tratados com ácido acetilsalicílico, comparativamente aos cães do grupo-controle. Por esse motivo, a AHS não recomenda tratamento antitrombótico de rotina em caso de dirofilariose.[28] Calvert et al.,[24] no entanto, utilizaram com sucesso a combinação de ácido acetilsalicílico e confinamento rigoroso em gaiola com terapia adulticida para dirofilariose grave. Se usado, o ácido acetilsalicílico (5 a 7 mg/kg) é administrado por via oral, diariamente, começando 1 a 3 semanas antes e continuando por 4 a 6 semanas após a administração do fármaco adulticida. No caso de tratamento prolongado com ácido acetilsalicílico, deve-se monitorar periodicamente o volume globular (VG), ou hematócrito, e a concentração sérica de proteína total. Deve-se evitar o uso ou descontinuar o tratamento com ácido acetilsalicílico em caso de terapia corticosteroide concomitante, hemorragia gastrintestinal (melena ou diminuição do VG), êmese persistente, trombocitopenia (< 50.000 plaquetas/$\mu\ell$) e hemoptise.[24] O clopidogrel (Plavix) não foi avaliado na dirofilariose.

Terapia com heparina

Doses baixas de heparina de cálcio foram avaliadas em cães com dirofilariose e demonstrou reduzir as reações adversas associadas à tiacetarsamida em cães com sinais clínicos graves, inclusive insuficiência cardíaca.[94] Nesse estudo, a heparina de cálcio, na dose de 50 a 100 UI/kg SC, a cada 8 a 12 h, por 1 a 2 semanas antes e 3 a 6 semanas após a terapia com fármaco adulticida, reduziu as complicações tromboembólicas e aumentou a sobrevida, em comparação com o ácido acetilsalicílico e o indobufeno. Os cães de ambos os grupos também receberam 1 mg de prednisona/kg/dia. Ressalta-se que esse tratamento não foi avaliado com a terapia adulticida com melarsomina. Calvert et al.[24] recomendam heparina sódica (50 a 70 UI/kg) em cães com trombocitopenia e/ou coagulação intravascular disseminada (CID), com uso contínuo até que a contagem de plaquetas seja superior a 150.000 células/$\mu\ell$ por pelo menos 7 dias e possivelmente por semanas.

Doxiciclina

Wolbachia pipientis, detectada pela primeira vez na década de 1920 em mosquitos, é agora conhecida como um microrganismo endossimbiôntico em filarídeos e em outros parasitas, inclusive D. immitis. É essencial para desenvolvimento, reprodução, infecciosidade, bem-estar e sobrevivência de filarídeos. Kramer e Genchi publicaram uma excelente revisão sobre a relação entre Wolbachia e D. immitis.[18] Com o conhecimento relativamente recente de que Wolbachia pode contribuir na patogênese da infecção por dirofilária e das reações adversas à morte de parasitas espontânea e induzida farmacologicamente, há métodos de eliminação de Wolbachia em estudo.[17,18,57,83,85,95-100] Embora a doxiciclina seja muito benéfica no tratamento e na prevenção de dirofilariose, parece que em tais condições a ivermectina e a doxiciclina parecem atuar sinergicamente. Em infecções experimentais (transplante de verme adulto na jugular) constatou-se que um protocolo terapêutico complexo com ivermectina (semanalmente, em dose preventiva [ou seja, quatro vezes a dose típica]) e doxiciclina (10 mg/kg/dia, em protocolo terapêutico interrompido por 14 de 36 semanas), durante 36 semanas, reduziu/eliminou Wolbachia em casos de dirofilariose, provocou involução uterina do parasita, eliminou microfilárias em 8 semanas, reduziu a ocorrência de TEP após terapia com melarsomina e reduziu a infestação por dirofilária com ivermectina, em protocolo de morte suave, comparado com aquele de até 78% de cães do grupo-controle após 9 meses de tratamento.[17,18,83,96-98] Deve-se reconhecer que esse protocolo terapêutico é preliminar, prova de conceito, não indicado em bula e impraticável. No entanto, parece ser um tratamento de eliminação de Wolbachia possível, com uso de doxiciclina ou outros medicamentos na dirofilariose. Também não houve perda da característica protetora de TEP no estudo com ivermectina administrada mensalmente na dose recomendada e no tratamento com doxiciclina durante 30 dias. Um protocolo mais prático, empregando dose preventiva de ivermectina 2 vezes/semana, durante 6 meses, combinada com doxiciclina (10 mg/kg/dia), por 30 dias, acelerou o processo de morte lenta das dirofilárias em 73% dos cães infectados experimentalmente, convertendo-os em animais negativos ao teste antigênico por até 300 dias após a infecção.[100] Além disso, monoterapia com dose de 10 mg de

doxiciclina/kg/12 h mostrou-se efetiva na eliminação de estágios larvais em desenvolvimento nos tecidos, conforme mencionado anteriormente.[85,99] A terapia com a combinação de doxiciclina e ivermectina torna todos os estágios do hospedeiro "livres de Wolbachia" e as subsequentes L3 transmitidas por mosquitos não são infectantes.[97,99] Também demonstrou-se que a doxiciclina, como monoterapia na dose de 10 mg/kg/12 h, por 30 dias, provocou efeitos negativos na dirofilária, em todas as fases de desenvolvimento.[97,99] Isso é particularmente importante porque interrompe o ciclo de transmissão da dirofilária, reduzindo/eliminando as subsequentes infecções do hospedeiro tratado, diminuindo assim as chances de a resistência do parasita ser propagada ao hospedeiro seguinte. Os dados ora disponíveis indicam que a doxiciclina ou outros fármacos que impedem o desenvolvimento de Wolbachia são indicados a todos os cães com dirofilariose.

Terapia microfilaricida

Apesar do fato de que antes de 2014 não havia fármaco algum aprovado pela FDA-CVM para a eliminação de microfilária, foi instituída a terapia microfilaricida tradicional 3 a 6 semanas após a administração do fármaco adulticida.[24,36] As lactonas macrocíclicas (LMs) oferecem uma solução segura e efetiva como alternativa ao levamisol e à ditiazanina usados anteriormente. As microfilárias são rapidamente eliminadas com o uso de ivermectina na dose de 50 mcg/kg (aproximadamente oito vezes a dose preventiva) ou milbemicina oxima na dose de 0,5 mg/kg (dose preventiva), embora isso não seja indicado na bula (uso "extralabel"). Reações adversas, provavelmente relacionadas à quantidade de microfilárias e à taxa de eliminação dos parasitas, foram observadas em 6% dos 126 cães tratados com ivermectina, na dose microfilaricida.[101] Sinais de reações adversas incluíram choque, depressão, hipotermia e vômito. Todos os cães se recuperaram com fluidoterapia e tratamento com corticosteroide (2 a 4 mg de dexametasona/kg, IV), dentro de 12 horas. Uma fatalidade, no entanto, foi observada 4 dias após a terapia microfilaricida. Achados e frequências semelhantes, porém menos graves, foram relatados após o uso de dose preventiva de milbemicina oxima.[33] Cães tratados devem ser hospitalizados e cuidadosamente observados durante o dia. Cães com peso inferior a 16 kg, contendo mais de 10.000 microfilárias por mililitro de sangue, são mais predispostos a reações adversas.[101] Podem ser administradas difenidramina (2 mg/kg, IM) e dexametasona (0,25 mg/kg, IV) a fim de prevenir a ocorrência de reações adversas após a administração de dose microfilaricida de LM.

Uma taxa de morte mais lenta de microfilária é obtida com ivermectina, selamectina e imidacloprida-moxidectina tópica na dose preventiva.[31,32,53,54,65,66,101,102] Tanto uma abordagem de morte rápida quanto de morte lenta das microfilárias atinge o objetivo do paciente, ou seja, livrar-se da maioria das microfilárias e esterilização da fêmea de dirofilária. O único medicamento aprovado pela FDA-CVM reconhecido como microfilaricida é a imidacloprida-moxidectina.[102] A combinação de doxiciclina com ivermectina (ou, possivelmente, outro LM) também elimina microfilárias, prontamente e com segurança. Atualmente não há necessidade ou razão para usar a formulação de ivermectina destinada a bovinos para eliminar microfilárias em cães.

Este autor adota uma abordagem alternativa (ver Figuras 255.6 e 255.10), iniciando a administração de LM e doxiciclina no momento do diagnóstico, geralmente dias a semanas antes da terapia adulticida.[78] Essa abordagem é mais simples, mais segura e induz proteção imediata contra dirofilariose. Existe pouca chance de reações adversas com o uso de microfilaricidas de ação mais lenta (ivermectina, moxidectina ou selamectina, em doses preventivas). No entanto, ao tratar cães com microfilaremia, o proprietário deve ser avisado dessa possibilidade e aconselhado a administrar o medicamento (1) em 1 dia em que esteja em casa, (2) no hospital ou (3) após pré-tratamento, conforme descrito a seguir. Embora o uso de milbemicina oxima de forma preventiva pareça causar raras reações adversas, a primeira dose é administrada no hospital e/ou pode ser precedida da administração de dexametasona e difenidramina, quando se detecta grande quantidade de microfilárias (ver Terapia adulticida).

COMPLICAÇÕES E SÍNDROMES ESPECÍFICAS

Dirofilariose assintomática

A maioria dos cães com dirofilariose é assintomática, embora muitos apresentem infecção pelo parasita (lesões radiográficas e patológicas). O tratamento, conforme descrito anteriormente, consiste no uso de melarsomina, no protocolo de dose fracionada, juntamente com a dose preventiva de LM. Cães assintomáticos podem, no entanto, tornar-se sintomáticos após a terapia adulticida devido a TEP e lesão pulmonar (conforme descrito em outra parte deste capítulo). O risco de TEP pode ser previsto de maneira imperfeita por semiquantificação da carga parasitária, usando alguns testes antigênicos, e pela gravidade das lesões radiográficas.[30] Claramente, um cão com lesões radiográficas graves não tolera bem as complicações tromboembólicas, mas nem todos os cães com sinais radiográficos apresentam alta carga parasitária. Por exemplo, um cão com lesões radiográficas moderadas a graves e antigenemia alta pode não estar em alto risco de TEP após o uso de fármaco adulticida porque é possível que os parasitas tenham morrido, fato que explica tanto a antigenemia (liberação de antígenos por parasitas mortos) quanto as anormalidades radiográficas (dirofilariose crônica). Essa conclusão pode também ser válida em cães com lesões radiográficas graves e antigenemia negativa ou baixa (presumindo-se que a maioria ou todos os parasitas tenham morrido e liberado antígenos). Alternativamente, a evidência antigênica de alta carga parasitária em um cão com sinais radiográficos mínimos ainda pode indicar uma reação grave após o uso de melarsomina, porque os achados são compatíveis com grande quantidade de parasitas, porém sem a depauperação natural dos parasitas (ou seja, uma infecção relativamente recente, com doença mínima). Sem dúvida, uma baixa carga parasitária e lesões radiográficas mínimas sugerem menor risco de reação adversa ao fármaco adulticida.

É importante ressaltar que, em cada situação, algumas suposições estão envolvidas e devem ser tomadas precauções. Quando o risco de TEP é grande, às vezes administra-se uma dose de 5 a 7 mg de prednisona/kg/dia VO, por 10 a 14 dias, inicialmente no diagnóstico, e após cada dose de melarsomina ou clopidogrel (18,75 mg/kg/dia VO; não há dados disponíveis para dirofilária).

Alguns profissionais recomendam o uso de corticosteroide ou mesmo heparina.[24] Restrição ao exercício forçado é o mais importante. Os tutores devem ser orientados quanto ao risco de sinais sugestivos de ETP e da importância de assistência veterinária imediata em caso reação adversa.

Glomerulonefrite

A maioria dos cães com dirofilariose crônica apresenta glomerulonefrite, que pode ser grave (Figura 255.12 e Capítulo 325).[14] Portanto, quando um cão apresenta doença glomerular, deve-se considerar dirofilariose no diagnóstico diferencial. Embora se considere que geralmente as lesões glomerulares sejam provocadas por dirofilária, dificilmente a dirofilariose causa insuficiência renal; há um dilema terapêutico quando um cão chega à consulta com proteinúria, azotemia e dirofilariose. A lógica sugere que a terapia adulticida é indicada porque a dirofilariose contribui para a ocorrência de doença glomerular, mas também traz riscos. A abordagem adotada por este autor é manter o paciente hospitalizado e administrar líquido (2 a 3 mℓ de solução de Ringer com lactato/kg/h; ver Capítulo 129), por via intravenosa, por 48 horas (começando 12 horas antes da primeira dose de melarsomina em protocolo de dose fracionada). O paciente é então liberado e indica-se uma consulta para

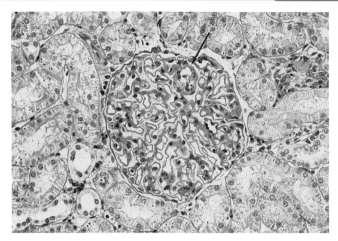

Figura 255.12 Lâmina corada com hematoxilina e eosina (H&E); corte histológico de 3 mícrons de um cão com dirofilariose crônica e resultante glomerulonefrite membranoproliferativa. Nota-se espessamento das paredes capilares e aumento generalizado da celularidade. Note um capilar com parede espessa com microfilária em seu lúmen (seta). (Cortesia do Dr. Greg Grauer.)

reavaliação depois de 48 horas para mensuração das concentrações de nitrogênio ureico e de creatinina no sangue. A segunda e a terceira injeções são previamente agendadas para 1 a 3 meses, com a tomada de decisão sobre o tratamento baseada na idade, no estado clínico geral, na função renal e na resposta do paciente à terapia adulticida inicial.

Pneumonia eosinofílica

Relata-se que a pneumonia eosinofílica acomete 14% dos cães com dirofilariose; o seu desenvolvimento é relativamente precoce no curso da doença.[12,24] Na verdade, a patogênese provavelmente envolve uma reação imunológica à morte da microfilária nos capilares pulmonares. Os sinais clínicos incluem tosse e, algumas vezes, dispneia, além de outros sintomas típicos da dirofilariose, como perda de peso e intolerância ao exercício. Os achados específicos no exame físico podem ser ausentes ou incluir dispneia e crepitações pulmonares audíveis em casos mais graves. Os achados radiográficos incluem aqueles típicos de dirofilariose, com infiltrado intersticial a alveolar, geralmente mais grave nos lobos pulmonares caudais (ver Figura 255.8). No sangue periférico e em amostras de lavado de vias respiratórias podem ser encontrados eosinófilos e basófilos em excesso.

O tratamento com corticoide (prednisona ou prednisolona, na dose de 1 a 2 mg/kg/dia VO) resulta em atenuação rápida dos sinais clínicos, com melhora radiográfica em menos de 1 semana. O fármaco pode então ser descontinuado após 3 a 5 dias, caso ocorra melhora dos sinais clínicos. Apesar de a terapia microfilaricida geralmente não ser indicada porque as infecções são frequentemente subclínicas, a profilaxia com LM é indicada para evitar mais infecções. A terapia adulticida pode ser empregada após a melhora clínica.

Granulomatose eosinofílica

A granulomatose eosinofílica pulmonar, uma manifestação mais grave, porém rara, responde menos favoravelmente. Essa síndrome é caracterizada por um processo inflamatório nodular mais organizado associado à linfadenopatia brônquica e, ocasionalmente, efusão pleural. Na granulomatose pulmonar, tosse, respiração ofegante e crepitações pulmonares são frequentemente audíveis. Em casos muito graves, pode ocorrer abafamento dos sons pulmonares associado à dispneia e cianose. O tratamento com prednisona, com o dobro da dose geralmente usada na pneumonia, induz remissão parcial ou completa dos sintomas em 1 a 2 semanas. O prognóstico permanece reservado porque é comum a recidiva da doença dentro de várias semanas. A prednisona pode ser combinada com ciclofosfamida ou azatioprina na tentativa de aumentar a ação imunossupressora (ver Capítulo 165). Essa última combinação parece para ser a mais efetiva. A terapia com fármaco adulticida deve ser postergada até que ocorra a remissão dos sinais clínicos. Como o prognóstico quanto à eficácia do tratamento clínico é reservado, tem-se recomendado a extirpação cirúrgica das lesões lobares.[103]

Embolia pulmonar

Trombose espontânea ou tromboembolismo pulmonar (TEP) associado à morte e/ou ao processo de morte dos parasitas (a principal complicação da dirofilariose) pode precipitar ou agravar os sinais clínicos, provocar ou agravar hipertensão pulmonar (HTP), insuficiência cardíaca direita ou, em casos raros, hemoptise e infarto pulmonar (ver Capítulo 243). Morte súbita pode ser resultado de insuficiência respiratória fulminante, exsanguinação ou DIC (ver Capítulo 197), ou podem ser inexplicáveis e repentinas (arritmia ou embolia pulmonar grave). A manifestação mais comum, no entanto, é um início repentino de letargia, anorexia e tosse 7 a 10 dias após a terapia adulticida, frequentemente após exercício leve. No exame físico é possível constatar dispneia, febre, palidez de membranas mucosas e sons pulmonares anormais (crepitações).

As radiografias torácicas (Figura 255.13) revelam infiltrados pulmonares significantes, mais graves nos lobos pulmonares caudais. A gravidade, em comparação com as radiografias pré-tratamento, é tipicamente dramática. O infiltrado, geralmente alveolar, é mais grave nos lobos caudais e, ocasionalmente, notam-se áreas de consolidação pulmonar. As anormalidades laboratoriais variam de acordo com a gravidade dos sinais clínicos, mas podem incluir leucocitose com desvio à esquerda, monocitose, eosinofilia e trombocitopenia. O grau de trombocitopenia pode fornecer informações prognósticas.

O tratamento clínico da doença pulmonar tromboembólica é, em grande parte, empírico e não há consenso geral. Normalmente concorda-se que o confinamento rigoroso no canil, o fornecimento de oxigênio em cuba de oxigênio ou por meio de insuflação nasal (50 a 100 mℓ/kg/min; ver Capítulo 131) e a administração de prednisona (1 mg/kg/dia, por 3 a 7 dias) são indicados nos casos mais graves.[19,24,104] Alguns profissionais recomendam cuidadosa terapia com líquidos (ver Síndrome da veia cava) para maximizar a perfusão tecidual e prevenir desidratação.[104] Alguns clínicos indicam o uso de heparina (75 UI/kg SC 3 vezes/dia até a normalização da contagem plaquetária [5 a 7 dias]) e de ácido acetilsalicílico (5 a 7 mg/kg/dia),[41] mas tal procedimento é controverso.[5,88-93]

Outras estratégias terapêuticas podem incluir o uso de supressores da tosse, antibióticos (se a febre não ceder) e, embora especulativos nesse momento, vasodilatadores (anlodipino, sildenafila, hidralazina, diltiazem; ver a discussão sobre insuficiência cardíaca a seguir e, com mais detalhes, no Capítulo 247).[105,106] Se a terapia vasodilatadora for empregada, será preciso monitorar a pressão arterial por causa da hipotensão (ver Capítulo 159), que é um efeito colateral potencial. A melhora clínica pode ser rápida, com possível alta hospitalar após vários dias de tratamento. Para cães menos severamente comprometidos, o uso de prednisona e o confinamento domiciliar são frequentemente suficientes.

Insuficiência cardíaca congestiva

A insuficiência cardíaca direita resulta do aumento do volume sanguíneo pós-carga do ventrículo direito (secundário à doença crônica da artéria pulmonar e ao tromboembolismo resultante de HTP; ver Capítulo 246). Quando grave e crônica, a HTP pode ocasionar insuficiência da valva tricúspide e insuficiência cardíaca direita. Os sintomas de congestão sanguínea (ascite) são agravados pela hipoproteinemia (Figura 255.14). Calvert sugeriu que até 50% dos cães com grave complicação vascular pulmonar causada por dilofilariose desenvolvem insuficiência cardíaca.[24] Os sinais clínicos (Figura 255.14) incluem, variavelmente, perda de peso, intolerância ao exercício, membranas mucosas acinzentadas com tempo de preenchimento capilar prolongado, ascite, dispneia, distensão jugular venosa e pulsação (Vídeo 255.2), arritmias com déficit de pulso e sons pulmonares adventícios (crepitações e possivelmente chiado). A dispneia pode ser causada por infiltrado pulmonar eosinófilo (IPE) ou ETP, mas *não* por edema pulmonar cardiogênico, distensão abdominal ou derrame pleural.

A terapia com fármaco adulticida deve ser postergada até que se constate melhora clínica. O tratamento envolve dieta e intervenções farmacológicas e de procedimentos. Os objetivos específicos incluem abrandamento dos sintomas de congestão vascular (diuréticos, restrição de sódio e paracentese), de hipertensão pulmonar (HTP) (terapia vasodilatadora, de preferência com sildenafila e/ou pimobendana; ver Capítulo 243), melhora do débito cardíaco (reduzindo o volume pós-carga e melhorando a função sistólica pelo uso de terapia inotrópica [pimobendana]) e minimizando a resposta neuro-humoral à diminuição

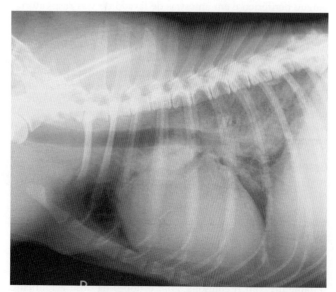

Figura 255.13 Radiografia torácica lateral obtida de um cão com dirofilariose crônica após tratamento com fármaco adulticida. Note aumento do ventrículo direito e da artéria pulmonar apical parcialmente ofuscado pelos infiltrados pulmonar, intersticial e alveolar, mais grave nos lobos pulmonares caudais.

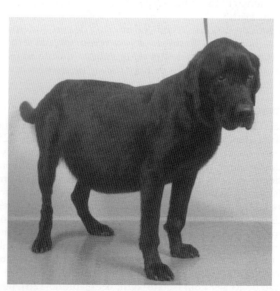

Figura 255.14 Cão de raça Labrador Retriever, macho, adulto, com insuficiência cardíaca congestiva devido à dirofilariose. Note distensão abdominal (ascite) e caquexia cardíaca.

do débito cardíaco (sistema renina-angiotensina-aldosterona (SRAA) e sistema nervoso simpático, com uso de inibidores da enzima conversora de angiotensina [ECA] e bloqueadores de receptores de mineralocorticoides [espironolactona]).

A restrição moderada de sal é lógica e provavelmente útil para diminuir a necessidade de diuréticos. Para conseguir isso, o autor escolhe uma dieta destinada a pacientes idosos ou a pacientes com insuficiência cardíaca precoce. Diuréticos podem ser úteis na prevenção de recidiva de ascite, mas normalmente não são capazes de mobilizar efetivamente grande acúmulo de líquido. Isso então requer paracentese abdominal e/ou torácica, periodicamente, quando há desconforto aparente (ver Capítulo 102). A furosemida é normalmente usada na dose de 2 a 6 mg/kg/dia, dependendo da gravidade e da resposta do paciente. Diuréticos adicionais, que propiciam um efeito suplementar atuando em diferentes partes do néfron, incluem espironolactona (2 mg/kg/dia, via oral) e hidroclorotiazida (1 a 2 mg/kg VO, a cada 12 a 48 h). A torsemida, um diurético de alça mais potente, pode ser utilizado para substituir a furosemida em 10% de sua dose atual (ver Capítulo 247).[107]

Os inibidores da ECA (p. ex., enalapril, benazepril, lisinopril, ramipril), por atuarem no SRAA, podem ser utilizados como vasodilatadores mistos no remodelamento da doença obstrutiva cardíaca e na redução da retenção de líquido, particularmente em casos de ascite refratária. O vasodilatador arterial, hidralazina, conforme demonstrado por Lombard,[105] melhora o débito cardíaco em um pequeno número de cães com dilofilariose e insuficiência cardíaca. Também foi demonstrado reduzir a pressão na artéria pulmonar e a resistência vascular, o trabalho do ventrículo direito e a pressão aórtica, sem alterar o débito cardíaco ou a frequência cardíaca de cães com dirofilariose experimental grave (porém, sem insuficiência cardíaca).[106]

A experiência clínica sugere que, em ordem de preferência, pimobendana, sildenafila, hidralazina, anlodipino e diltiazem podem ser úteis nesse cenário. Estudos adicionais são necessários. Na insuficiência cardíaca, a primeira escolha do autor é a combinação de pimobendana (0,25 mg/kg/12 h VO) e sildenafila (0,5 a 1 mg/kg VO, a cada 8 a 12 h). Se o custo for um fator limitante na escolha do medicamento, poderá ser feita a substituição por 0,5 a 2 mg de hidralazina/kg/12 h, via oral, 0,1 a 0,25 mg de anlodipino/kg/24 h, via oral, ou 0,5 a 1,5 mg de diltiazem/kg/8 h VO ou uma formulação de ação prolongada com ajuste da dose para 2 a 4 mg/kg VO, a cada 12 a 24 h. O risco de hipotensão com essas terapias deve ser considerado, e a pressão arterial monitorada. Na prática clínica do autor, o inodilatador pimobendana é empregado nessas circunstâncias, exclusivamente ou com sildenafila, para propiciar vasodilatação arterial e suporte inotrópico para reduzir o risco de hipotensão.

Devido ao risco de toxicidade e vasoconstrição pulmonar associado ao uso de digoxina, esta não é rotineiramente utilizada pelo autor no tratamento de insuficiência cardíaca decorrente de dirofilariose. No entanto, a digoxina combinada com o diltiazem pode ser útil no controle de fibrilação atrial, por controlar a taxa de resposta ventricular.

O ácido acetilsalicílico ou o clopidogrel, teoricamente úteis por sua capacidade de abrandar algumas lesões vasculares pulmonares e a vasoconstrição induzida por plaquetas, podem ser usados nas doses de 5 e 2 a 3 mg/kg/dia VO, respectivamente. A restrição rigorosa ao exercício com duração indefinida é fortemente recomendada.

Frequentemente, a insuficiência cardíaca se instala após terapia com fármaco adulticida, mas, se estiver presente antes da terapia adulticida, a questão difícil de responder será quando (ou se) deve administrar melarsomina. Se ocorrer boa resposta clínica ao tratamento da insuficiência cardíaca, a terapia adulticida poderá ser administrada em 4 a 12 semanas, conforme as condições permitirem. A melarsomina é geralmente evitada em caso de insuficiência cardíaca refratária, com base em uma abordagem de morte lenta (ivermectina e tratamento com doxiciclina por 30 dias).

Síndrome da veia cava

A síndrome da veia cava (SVC) é uma variante relativamente incomum, porém uma variante ou complicação grave da dilofilariose. A maioria dos estudos mostrou acentuada predisposição sexual, 75 a 90% dos cães com SVC são machos. É caracterizada por alta carga parasitária (geralmente > 60, com a maioria dos parasitas instalada no átrio direito e na veia cava); o prognóstico é ruim.[26] Estudos realizados no laboratório do autor indicam que a migração retrógrada das dirofilárias adultas para a veia cava e o átrio direito, 5 a 17 meses após a infecção, causa obstrução parcial do fluxo sanguíneo do lado direito do coração, pela interferência no aparelho valvar, ocasionando insuficiência da valva tricúspide (resultando em sopro sistólico, pulso jugular e aumento da PVC).[108] Cães acometidos também apresentam hipertensão pulmonar (HTP) preexistente induzida por dirofilariose, o que aumenta acentuadamente os efeitos hemodinâmicos adversos da insuficiência tricúspide. Esses efeitos combinados reduzem substancialmente a pré-carga do ventrículo esquerdo e, portanto, o débito cardíaco. Arritmias cardíacas podem comprometer a função cardíaca (Figura 255.15).

Essa constelação de eventos precipita um início repentino de sinais clínicos, incluindo anemia hemolítica (ver Capítulo 198) causada pelo dano às hemácias (He) à medida que passam através de uma rede de parasitas que ocupam o átrio direito e a veia cava, bem como através de filamentos de fibrina nos capilares, no caso de CID. Hemólise intravascular, acidose metabólica e comprometimento da função hepática com prejuízo à remoção de procoagulantes circulantes contribuem para o desenvolvimento de CID. O efeito desse dano traumático ao éritron é exacerbado pelo aumento da fragilidade das hemácias, devido a alterações da membrana eritrocitária em cães com dirofilariose. Hemoglobinemia, hemoglobinúria e disfunção hepática e renal também são observadas em muitos cães. A causa da disfunção hepatorrenal não está clara, mas provavelmente resulta da combinação de efeitos da congestão passiva, perfusão diminuída e efeitos deletérios dos produtos da hemólise. Sem tratamento, a morte frequentemente ocorre dentro de 24 a 72 horas, devido ao choque cardiogênico, complicado pela anemia, alterações decorrentes de acidose metabólica e CID. Um início repentino de anorexia, depressão, fraqueza e, ocasionalmente, tosse é acompanhado na maioria dos cães por dispneia e hemoglobinúria. A hemoglobinúria é considerada um sinal patognomônico dessa síndrome. O exame físico revela palidez de membranas mucosas, tempo de preenchimento capilar prolongado, pulso fraco, distensão e pulso jugular, hepatoesplenomegalia e dispneia. A ausculta torácica pode indicar sons pulmonares adventícios; sopro cardíaco sistólico devido à insuficiência da valva tricúspide (87% dos casos); som evidente de desdobramento da segunda bulha (67%); e ruído de galope cardíaco (20%) (ver Capítulo 55). Outros achados relatados incluem ascite (29%), icterícia (19%) e hemoptise (6%). A temperatura corporal varia de subnormal a levemente elevada.[18]

Hemoglobinemia e microfilaremia estão presentes em 85% dos cães que apresentam SVC.[26] Anemia regenerativa moderada (com valor médio do hematócrito de 28%) caracterizada pela presença de reticulócitos, hemácias nucleadas e aumento do volume corpuscular médio (VCM) é vista na maioria dos casos. Essa anemia, do tipo macrocítica normocrômica, tem sido associada à presença de hemácias-alvo, esquistócitos, acantócitos e esferócitos. Há relato de leucocitose (contagem média de leucócitos de, aproximadamente, 20.000 células/µℓ) com desvio à esquerda, neutrofilia e eosinofilia. Cães que desenvolvem CID (ver Capítulo 197) caracterizam-se pela presença de trombocitopenia e hipofibrinogenemia, bem como prolongamento do tempo de protrombina (TP) de estágio único, tempo de tromboplastina parcial (TTP), tempo de coagulação ativado (TCA) e alta concentração de produtos da degradação de fibrina. A análise bioquímica do soro sanguíneo normalmente revela aumento de enzimas hepáticas, bilirrubina e indicadores da função renal. O exame de urina revela altas concentrações de

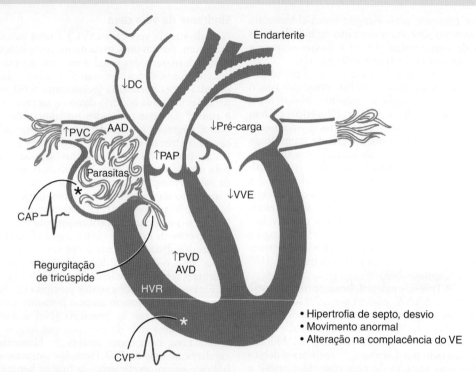

Figura 255.15 Esquema demonstrativo da patogênese da disfunção cardíaca síndrome da veia cava (SVC) causada por dirofilariose. A SVC complica a dirofilariose crônica quando ocorre migração retrógrada do parasita à artéria pulmonar, com a maioria dos parasitas instalando-se na veia cava e no átrio direito. A função da valva tricúspide é comprometida, resultando em insuficiência valvular. A regurgitação da valva tricúspide é sobreposta à hipertensão pulmonar. A pré-carga do ventrículo esquerdo diminui. Ocorre insuficiência cardíaca congestiva de baixo débito. O desvio do septo para a esquerda e a movimentação septal anormal à direita contribuem para a menor pré-carga do ventrículo esquerdo. A obstrução do fluxo do ventrículo direito em decorrência da presença de dirofilárias e arritmia cardíaca pode contribuir ainda mais para a disfunção cardíaca, mas provavelmente são fatores menos importantes. *AAD*, aumento do átrio direito; *AVD*, aumento do ventrículo direito; *CAP*, complexo atrial prematuro; *CVP*, complexo ventricular prematuro; setas, aumentada(o) ou diminuída; *DC*, débito cardíaco; *HVR*, hipertrofia do ventrículo direito; *PAP*, pressão na artéria pulmonar; *PVC*, pressão venosa central; *PVD*, pressão no ventrículo direito; *VVE*, volume do ventrículo esquerdo. (De Atkins CE: Pathophysiology of heartworm caval syndrome: recent advances. In: Otto GF, editor: *Proceedings of American Heartworm Symposium* 1989, Batavia, IL, 1990, American Heartworm Society, p. 27-31.)

bilirrubina e proteínas em 50% dos casos e, mais frequentemente, hemoglobinúria. A PVC é alta em 80 a 90% dos casos (média de 11,4 cm de H_2O; normal, < 5 cm H_2O; ver Capítulo 76). Anormalidades eletrocardiográficas incluem taquicardia sinusal em 33% dos casos e complexos atriais e ventriculares prematuros em 28 e 6% dos casos, respectivamente (ver Capítulo 248). O eixo elétrico médio cardíaco tende a girar para a direita (em média, + 129°), com um padrão S1,2,3 evidente em 38% dos casos. A profundidade da onda S em CV6 LU (V_4), indicador mais confiável de aumento do ventrículo direito (> 0,8 mv), está presente em 56% dos casos. A radiografia torácica revela sinais graves de dirofilariose, com cardiomegalia, aumento da artéria pulmonar principal, aumento da vascularização pulmonar e tortuosidade da artéria pulmonar, em ordem de frequência decrescente (ver Figuras 255.5 a 255.7). No ecocardiograma nota-se presença maciça de parasitas evidente no átrio direito com movimentação para o ventrículo direito durante a diástole (Vídeo 255.3). Esse achado no ecocardiograma bidimensional em modo M é patognomônico de SVC em um cenário clínico apropriado (Figura 255.16). Nota-se aumento do lúmen do ventrículo direito e diminuição do tamanho do ventrículo esquerdo, sugerindo HTP acompanhada de redução do preenchimento do ventrículo esquerdo. O movimento septal paradoxal, causado por alta pressão do ventrículo direito, é comumente observado. Não há evidência ecocardiográfica de disfunção do ventrículo esquerdo. No cateterismo cardíaco verifica-se hipertensão pulmonar, ventricular e do átrio direito, com débito cardíaco reduzido.

O prognóstico é ruim, a menos que a causa da síndrome – presença de dirofilárias no átrio direito e na veia cava – seja removida. Mesmo com esse procedimento, a taxa de mortalidade pode se aproximar de 40% ou mais. Em um estudo retrospectivo de 21 cães com SVC constatou-se morte perioperatória (6) ou falha na recuperação (1) em 33% dos animais.[109] Todos os 14 cães submetidos à remoção bem-sucedida de parasitas receberam alta hospitalar; 10 sobreviveram 18 meses ou mais.

A fluidoterapia (ver Capítulo 127) é necessária para aumentar o débito cardíaco e a perfusão tecidual, prevenir ou ajudar a reverter a CID, prevenir nefropatia por hemoglobinúria e auxiliar na correção da acidose metabólica. O excesso de líquido, no entanto, pode agravar ou precipitar sintomas de ICC. Na clínica do autor, introduz-se um cateter na veia jugular esquerda (ver Capítulo 76) e institui-se fluidoterapia intravenosa com solução de dextrose 5% ou metade de solução fisiológica e metade de dextrose 2,5%. O cateter não deve atingir a veia cava cranial porque isso interfere na embolectomia dos parasitas. Um cateter cefálico pode substituir o cateter de jugular, porém um tanto quanto inconveniente, mas não possibilita o monitoramento da PVC. A taxa de infusão intravenosa de líquido depende da condição clínica do animal. Uma recomendação útil é fazer a infusão o mais rápido possível (até 1 volume cardiovascular durante a primeira hora) sem elevar a PVC ou sem elevá-la acima de 10 cm H_2O se a pressão estiver normal ou quase normal desde o início. A terapia inicial (ver Capítulos 127 e 129) deve ser agressiva (10 a 20 mℓ/kg na primeira hora) se o choque for acompanhado de PVC normal (< 5 cm H_2O) e deve ser reduzida para aproximadamente 1 a 2 mℓ/kg/h se a PVC for de 10 a 20 cm H_2O. A transfusão de sangue total não é indicada na maioria dos casos porque a anemia geralmente não é grave e os fatores de coagulação transfundidos podem agravar a CID. O uso de bicarbonato de sódio não é indicado, a menos

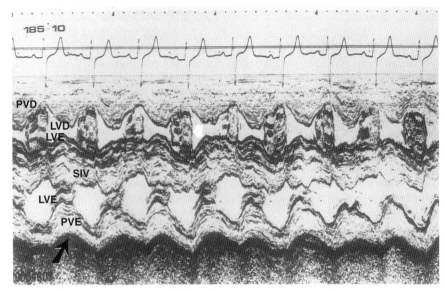

Figura 255.16 Ecocardiograma em modo M de um cão com síndrome da veia cava de início recente mostra espessamento das paredes dos septos ventricular direito e intraventricular, hipertrofia excêntrica do ventrículo direito e diminuição do ventrículo esquerdo. Uma massa ecogênica (*seta vazada*) de dirofilárias pode ser vista deslocando-se para o ventrículo direito em cada diástole. O movimento septal paradoxal é evidente. A *seta sólida* indica o pericárdio. *LVD*, lúmen do ventrículo direito; *LVE*, lúmen do ventrículo esquerdo; *PVD*, parede do ventrículo direito; *PVE*, parede posterior do ventrículo esquerdo; *SIV*, septo intraventricular. (De Atkins CE: Heartworm caval syndrome. *Semin Vet Med Surg* 2:64-71, 1987.)

que a acidose metabólica seja grave (pH 7,15 a 7,20). Podem ser administrados antibióticos de amplo espectro e ácido acetilsalicílico (5 mg/kg/dia). O tratamento para CID é descrito em outra parte deste livro (ver Capítulo 197).

Jackson desenvolveu uma técnica para remoção cirúrgica dos parasitas da veia cava e do átrio direito.[110] Esse procedimento deve ser realizado o mais breve possível no curso da terapia, quando viável. A sedação pode não ser necessária no paciente moribundo; nesse caso, o procedimento pode ser realizado apenas com anestesia local. Para facilitar o procedimento e manter a técnica asséptica, a anestesia geral é pode ser empregada na clínica. O cão é contido ou posicionado em decúbito lateral esquerdo, após tricotomia e preparação cirúrgica. A veia jugular é isolada distalmente. Faz-se uma ligadura frouxa ao redor da porção cranial da veia até que se faça a sua incisão, após a qual a ligadura é realizada. Uma pinça tipo jacaré (20 a 40 cm, preferencialmente de diâmetro pequeno) é suavemente guiada veia abaixo enquanto ela é segura frouxamente entre o polegar e o indicador. A veia jugular pode ser temporariamente ocluída com fita umbilical. Se houver dificuldade na passagem da pinça, a manipulação suave do cão, por um assistente, para estender ainda mais o pescoço ajuda na passagem da pinça após a entrada no tórax; pode ser necessário direcionar medialmente a pinça na base do coração. Uma vez introduzida a pinça, ela é aberta e ligeiramente avançada, em seguida fechada, e os parasitas são removidos. Um a quatro vermes são geralmente removidos de cada vez. Esse processo é repetido até que cinco a seis tentativas sucessivas sejam infrutíferas. Um esforço deve ser feito para remover 35 a 50 parasitas. Cuidado deve ser tomado para não fragmentar o parasita durante a retirada. Após a remoção dos parasitas, a veia jugular é ligada distalmente e realiza-se sutura subcutânea e de pele de rotina. Outros cateteres, como cateter uretral com cesto conhecido como basket ou dormia, pinça em escova (*horsehair brush*), laço (*homemade snare*) e pinça tipo jacaré flexível também já foram utilizados para execução desse procedimento.[111] A orientação fluoroscópica, quando disponível, é útil nesse procedimento. A remoção bem-sucedida de parasitas está associada à redução na intensidade do sopro cardíaco e do pulso jugular, ausência de sombreamento na imagem obtida em exame ultrassonográfico, causado por dirofilária, rápida cessação de hemoglobinemia e hemoglobinúria e retorno das atividades séricas de enzimas a valores normais. Melhora imediata e latente da função cardíaca ocorre nas primeiras 24 horas. É importante ter em mente que a remoção dos parasitas não reduz adequadamente a pós-carga do ventrículo direito (HTP) e, portanto, a fluidoterapia deve ser monitorada cuidadosamente antes e depois da cirurgia para evitar precipitação ou agravamento da insuficiência cardíaca direita. E o repouso no canil deve ser reforçado por um período de tempo dependente do progresso do paciente.

Embolectomia de parasitas por meio da venostomia jugular frequentemente é bem-sucedida e consegue-se estabilizar o quadro clínico do animal, possibilitando que a terapia adulticida seja instituída para eliminar os parasitas remanescentes em um período de no mínimo 1 mês. Mensurações cuidadosas das concentrações de nitrogênio ureico sanguíneo (NUS) e de creatinina sérica e as atividades séricas de enzimas hepáticas devem preceder o fim do tratamento. Se ácido acetilsalicílico ou outra terapia anticoagulante for empregada, deve ser mantida por 3 a 4 semanas após a terapia adulticida. Melhoria substancial da anemia não deve ser esperada antes de 2 a 4 semanas depois da embolectomia dos parasitas. O tratamento preventivo com LM, como descrito anteriormente, é administrado no momento da alta hospitalar.

Migração errática

Embora nos cães as dirofilárias se instalem tipicamente nas artérias dos lobos pulmonares caudais, elas podem ser encontradas no ventrículo direito e raramente (ver Síndrome da veia cava) no átrio direito e na veia cava. Com muito menos frequência, larvas imaturas S5 migram de modo errático para outros locais, inclusive cérebro, medula espinal, espaço epidural, câmara anterior do olho, humor vítreo, tecido subcutâneo, escroto e cavidade peritoneal. Além do mais, os parasitas podem permanecer na circulação sanguínea sistêmica e provocar doença tromboembólica sistêmica.[15] O tratamento de migração parasitária errática (como, por exemplo, na cavidade peritoneal) pode não requerer nada ou pode necessitar de extirpação cirúrgica do parasita, terapia com fármaco adulticida e tratamento sintomático (p. ex., controle de crises convulsivas, em caso de migração cerebral). O método de remoção cirúrgica do parasita das artérias ilíaca interna e femoral já foi descrito.[15]

PROGNÓSTICO

O prognóstico de dirofilariose assintomática geralmente é bom e, embora o prognóstico de dirofilariose grave seja reservado, uma grande porcentagem desses casos pode ser tratada com sucesso.[112] Uma vez que a crise inicial tenha passado e a terapia adulticida tenha sido bem-sucedida, as resoluções das manifestações subjacentes da dirofilariose crônica então se iniciam. O prognóstico é mais reservado em casos graves de CID, SVC, embolia pulmonar maciça, granulomatose eosinofílica, doença arterial pulmonar grave e insuficiência cardíaca. Após a terapia adulticida, as lesões da camada íntima dos vasos sanguíneos regridem rapidamente, embora não completamente, dependendo da gravidade.[113-115] A melhora é percebida 4 semanas após o tratamento da artéria pulmonar principal, com todas as artérias pulmonares submetidas a resolução acentuada dentro de 1 ano. Lesões radiográficas e arteriográficas da dirofilariose começam a se resolver dentro de 3 a 4 semanas, a HTP diminui em meses e pode estar normal 6 meses após a terapia adulticida. Alterações do parênquima pulmonar são mais graves nos 6 meses após a terapia adulticida e posteriormente começam a diminuir em gravidade, com resolução acentuada nos próximos 2 a 3 meses. A persistência dessas lesões é sugestiva de infecção ativa. A terapia com corticosteroide acelera a resolução dessas lesões. Da mesma forma, doença renal irreversível é incomum, com lesões glomerulares resolvendo-se dentro de meses após o tratamento bem-sucedido com fármaco adulticida. Os sintomas de insuficiência cardíaca também são reversíveis com terapia sintomática, repouso em gaiola e eliminação efetiva da infecção.

DIROFILARIOSE FELINA

CICLO DE VIDA

O ciclo de vida de *D. immitis* é semelhante em gatos e cães (ver Figura 255.2). A infecção difere nos gatos, pois estes geralmente não são o alvo preferido de alimentação dos mosquitos; para ser um vetor efetivo para os gatos, o mosquito tem que ter se alimentado primeiro em um canídeo, já que, como hospedeiros não naturais, os gatos são inerentemente resistentes à infecção por dirofilária. Infecções em gatos, portanto, tendem a ser relativamente pouco frequentes e brandas. Além disso, no gato o ciclo de vida do parasita é mais longo, de modo que o período de patência (observado em < 20% dos gatos) é de até 7 a 8 meses após a infecção. Por fim, o gato está sujeito a doenças vasculares pulmonares e doenças pulmonares, mesmo sem a manifestação clínica da infecção.

Essa condição, conhecida como dirofilariose associada à doença respiratória (DADR; em inglês HARD),[152,153] tem causado confusão na nomenclatura relativa à infecção por dirofilária *versus* exposição à dirofilária. Na maioria das doenças infecciosas e parasitárias, a presença de anticorpos sem uma infecção estabelecida (ou seja, madura) é denominada "exposição", que significa que o hospedeiro foi exposto e eliminou a infecção ou foi (ou está) infectado. Porém, na infecção por dirofilária, uma vez que se constata teste de anticorpo positivo quando as larvas de dirofilária se instalam no hospedeiro e realizam duas mudas e, assim, com o potencial de causar doença, alguns pesquisadores consideram tal condição como "infecção", *mesmo que não ocorra infecção*, antes da maturação dos parasitas. Nesta seção deste capítulo, o autor utiliza o termo "infecção por dirofilária madura" para a infecção causada por dirofilárias adultas, ou maduras (ou dirofilariose, que é a infecção por dirofilária madura, com lesões patológicas identificáveis) e se refere a essas infecções, que são finalmente eliminadas, como "infecções imaturas", para gatos, ou "exposição" quando se refere a populações, sabendo-se que cerca de 50% desses gatos podem desenvolver doença pulmonar devido à exposição à DADR.[152,153]

FISIOPATOLOGIA

O gato doméstico, embora seja um hospedeiro atípico, pode ser parasitado por *D. immitis* e como resultado desenvolver dirofilariose. As manifestações clínicas da doença são diferentes e frequentemente mais graves nesta espécie, mas, se considerarmos apenas infecções causadas por parasitas maduros, a taxa de infecção corresponde a apenas 5 a 20% da verificada em cães.[154] A infecção experimental no gato é mais difícil de se estabelecer do que no cão, com menos de 25% de L3 atingindo a idade adulta.[155] Essa resistência também se reflete em infecções naturais, nas quais em felinos com carga parasitária de dirofilariose é quase sempre inferior a 10 e, normalmente, de 1 a 4 dirofilárias.[154] Outros indicadores inerentes de resistência dos gatos à dirofilária são período reduzido de latência, alta frequência de amicrofilaremia, pequena quantidade de microfilárias e menor tempo de vida dos vermes adultos (em geral pensa-se ser de 2 a 3 anos, com novas evidências sugerindo que pode demorar mais tempo em infecções naturais – até 4 anos).[156] Todavia, estudos demonstraram que a prevalência de infecção por dirofilária madura pode ser tão alta como 14% em gatos de abrigo.[154] Um estudo realizado em gatos bem cuidados no Texas e na Carolina do Norte revelou a presença de infecção de dirofilária madura em 9 de 100 gatos com sintomas cardiorrespiratórios.[157] Além disso, o teste de anticorpos mostrou que 26% desses gatos tinham sido "expostos" à infecção por dirofilária.[157] Estudos recentes não conseguiram fundamentar a hipótese de que os machos são mais sujeitos à infecção natural por dirofilária, embora, em infecções experimentais de gatos machos, a carga parasitária seja maior.[157,159] A migração errática de vermes foi sugerida como uma ocorrência mais frequente em gatos do que em cães.

Novamente, é importante esclarecer a distinção entre infecção por dirofilária madura (presença de parasitas adultos na artéria pulmonar ou em outro local) e infecções eliminadas ("exposição" sem parasita adulto, maduro). A morte de adultos imaturos (S5 imaturo ou juvenil, adultos imaturos ou juvenis, ou juvenis) pode causar lesões pulmonares e vasculares pulmonares em gatos, antes da maturação dos parasitas. De forma exclusiva, a doença se desenvolve *mesmo em gatos que resistem à infecção madura*, e os sinais clínicos e a doença antecedem a capacidade dos clínicos em diagnosticar a doença por meios convencionais. Estudos demonstraram que lesões pulmonares anatômicas e radiográficas se desenvolvem em gatos infectados experimentalmente,[152,153,160] e ocorrem lesões vasculares pulmonares em gatos naturalmente infectados[151] em que a maturação de parasitas adultos imaturos *não* ocorre. Além disso, em infecções experimentais eliminadas com o uso de medicamentos antes da maturação da dirofilária, constatou-se recentemente a ocorrência não apenas de lesões arteriais proliferativas e pulmonares inflamatórias, mas também de doença inflamatória proliferativa nos bronquíolos e no parênquima pulmonar.[152,153] Presumivelmente, esses achados estão associados aos sintomas de doenças respiratórias, frequentemente observados em gatos sem infecção por dirofilária madura, e foram chamadas de DADR.[152,153] Esses estudos importantes mostraram que gatos "expostos" (infectados sem ocorrência de maturação total do parasita) à dirofilária desenvolvem lesões respiratórias e sinais clínicos de dirofilariose. Esses achados são importantes, pois não apenas demonstram que a infecção por dirofilária é geralmente eliminada e normalmente causa sinais clínicos semelhantes à asma, mas muito mais gatos desenvolvem sinais clínicos de dirofilariose do que se acreditava anteriormente. Isso porque 38 a 74% dos gatos com infecção por dirofilária madura desenvolvem quadro clínico estimado em 50% daqueles que eliminam a infecção (ou seja, DADR estimada em 5 a 10 vezes mais comum do que as infecções maduras).[156,160] Essa distinção também é importante a fim de comunicação com o tutor(a), já que o gato com DADR provavelmente vai recuperar-se, enquanto o gato com infecção por dirofilária madura pode morrer em função da doença.

A exata importância clínica da DADR, no entanto, é difícil de ser mensurada porque é um diagnóstico de exclusão, e a suspeita inerente de veterinários para a infecção por dirofilária felina é baixa. Assim, é provável que uma grande porcentagem de casos não seja reconhecida. Além disso, no modelo experimental foi utilizada carga infectante muito alta (100 L3 por gato), muito maior do que um gato poderia adquirir naturalmente. Portanto, é difícil transferir diretamente nosso conhecimento de DADR experimental para o gato naturalmente infectado.

A resposta da artéria pulmonar aos parasitas adultos, maduros, é mais grave em gatos do que em cães (devido, em parte, à presença de macrófagos intravasculares pulmonares [PIM][162], embora a HTP tenha sido pouco frequentemente relatada. Dillon[5] demonstrou um aumento pulmonar dentro de 1 semana após o transplante de parasitas adultos, sugerindo uma interação hospedeiro-parasita intensa. Isso foi confirmado pelo exame *post mortem*, que revelou endarterite grave com hiperplasia da camada íntima das vilosidades.[158] Tal resposta da camada íntima muscular e de eosinófilos provoca estreitamento e tortuosidade de vasos sanguíneos pulmonares, trombose e possivelmente HTP (Figura 255.17).[163,164] Maia *et al.* demonstraram inflamação arterial pulmonar difusa e hipertrofia, lesões bronquiolares e intensa pneumonia intersticial, em 6 semanas após a introdução de 2 parasitas adultos na veia jugular.[164] A hiperplasia de pneumócitos tipo II foi evidente em microscopia eletrônica de varredura, indicando dano ao parênquima pulmonar. Como a ramificação da artéria pulmonar de gatos é menor que a dos cães e possui menor circulação colateral, a embolização, mesmo de pequeno número de parasitas, provoca resultados desastrosos, com infarto e até óbito. Embora incomum, a ocorrência de *cor pulmonale* e insuficiência cardíaca direita pode estar associada à dirofilariose crônica felina, e é manifestada por efusão pleural (hidrotórax ou quilotórax), ascite, ou ambos.

Na dirofilariose, o pulmão, em si, também sofre dano, com infiltrado eosinofílico no parênquima pulmonar (pneumonite) e nas artérias pulmonares (Figura 255.18). Os vasos pulmonares podem extravasar plasma, provocando edema pulmonar (e, possivelmente, síndrome da angústia respiratória aguda). Além disso, ocorre proliferação de células tipo II induzida por PIM. Essa combinação de danos ao sistema respiratório altera a difusão de O_2, ocasionando hipoxemia.[162] Adicionalmente, os achados radiográficos sugerem aprisionamento de ar, compatível com broncoconstrição.[158,160]

A real importância da broncoconstrição nesse processo é pouco conhecida. Estudos experimentais levaram a diferentes conclusões, concentraram-se em ambos os aspectos, a infecção por dirofilária e a DADR, usando experimentos com infecções por dirofilárias maduras e imaturas, testes de antígeno de *Wolbachia* positivo e negativo, infecções naturais, dirofilárias obtidas de cães tratados com doxiciclina e de cães que não receberam doxiciclina e infusões de homogenato de dirofilárias.[166-170] Embora uma revisão aprofundada desses manuscritos não seja possível, os resultados de destaque estão resumidos a seguir.

Apesar do aumento da espessura da parede bronquiolar em gatos acometidos por dirofilariose, uma resposta hiper-reativa do músculo liso bronquiolar não parece ser o mecanismo primário dos sinais clínicos do trato respiratório. A reconhecida resposta atenuada das vias respiratórias ao isoproterenol pode indicar refratariedade ao relaxamento bronquiolar induzido por catecolamina em gatos com dirofilariose.[165] Possivelmente, resultados contraditórios têm sido obtidos usando pletismografia para avaliação da função das vias respiratórias em gatos sintomáticos com evidência sorológica de infecção por dirofilária. E houve diferenças significativas em vários indicadores *in vivo* de broncoconstrição entre gatos com dirofilariose e aqueles normais, do grupo-controle.[166] Estudos subsequentes, usando pletismografia para comparar proteína específica de *Wolbachia* (PSW) positiva em gatos negativos, demonstraram anormalidades significativas nos índices de broncoconstrição e anticorpos positivos em gatos sintomáticos.[167] Isso indica a possibilidade de participação de *Wolbachia*, ou mais provavelmente de suas proteínas, na patogênese da broncoconstrição em gatos com dirofilariose. Em contrapartida, um estudo com gatos normais que receberam, por 18 dias, homogenato de dirofilária por via intravenosa não demonstrou diferença nas lesões pulmonares ou nos indicadores de broncoconstrição, não importando se o parasita utilizado tinha sido coletado de cães tratados com doxiciclina ou em cães não tratados.[168] Esse estudo também revelou que a infusão de homogenato causou proliferação intersticial e peribrônquica de músculo liso e miofibrócitos, aparentemente causada por uma substância humoral, pois as lesões não foram claramente relacionadas aos locais nos quais as dirofilárias são normalmente encontradas.

Mediadores inflamatórios (eicosanoides) parecem contribuir para as lesões associadas à dirofilariose. Morchon *et al.* demonstraram que gatos naturalmente infectados apresentavam concentrações séricas significativamente maiores de prostaglandina E_2 (PGE_2), tromboxano B_2 (TXB_2) e leucotrieno B_4 (LTB_4) do que gatos não infectados.[170] Em gatos infectados experimentalmente, acompanhados sequencialmente por 180 dias, a concentração de PGE_2 aumentou significativamente durante os primeiros 60 dias pós-infecção, diminuindo progressivamente até o 180º dia pós-infecção, enquanto os teores de TXB_2 e LTB_4 aumentaram progressivamente, atingindo valores máximos

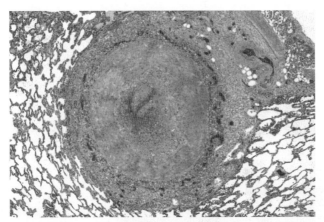

Figura 255.17 Coloração com H&E mostrando grande artéria pulmonar com obstrução do lúmen devido a grave hipertrofia e hiperplasia do músculo liso medial, fibrose das camadas subíntima e íntima, endarterite e, possivelmente, trombose. Note pneumonia intersticial periarterial (provavelmente eosinofílica). (*Esta figura se encontra reproduzida em cores no Encarte*.)

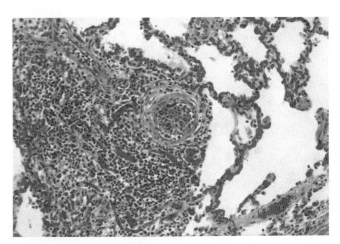

Figura 255.18 Artéria pulmonar pequena do gato visto na Figura 255.17 mostra hipertrofia medial leve. Note o alongado manguito perivascular de células inflamatórias ao redor do vaso, que representa um infiltrado eosinofílico. (*Esta figura se encontra reproduzida em cores no Encarte*.)

180 dias após a infecção. Isso sugere que a PGE_2 pode estar relacionada à morte de parasita S5 imaturo (DADR), enquanto TXB_2 e LTB_4 podem estar envolvidos na reação à dirofilária adulta ou madura.

O resultado final desse dano multifacetado é a diminuição da função pulmonar, hipoxemia, dispneia, tosse e até morte. A morte súbita em gatos com dirofilariose pode envolver uma reação anafilática a parasitas prestes a morrer, com ou sem DADR.[171] Parece improvável que seja devido ao antígeno PSW.[169]

SINAIS CLÍNICOS

As manifestações clínicas da dirofilariose em gatos podem ser hiperagudas,[171] agudas ou crônicas.[157,158,173-175] No entanto, em um estudo retrospectivo, constatou-se que 28% dos gatos com infecção causada por dirofilária madura, atendidos em um centro de referência, foram levados à consulta em razão de sintomas não relacionados à dirofilariose.[174] Além disso, dados mais recentes e prospectivamente obtidos de dois estudos italianos com 77 gatos atendidos em clínica geral revelaram que apenas 58% dos gatos assintomáticos desenvolveram sinais clínicos de dirofilariose, com um terço de casos fatais.[156,161]

A manifestação aguda ou hiperaguda geralmente é causada pela morte do parasita e/ou embolização ou migração errática, e os sinais clínicos variavelmente incluem salivação, taquicardia, choque, dispneia, hemoptise, vômito e diarreia, síncope, demência, ataxia, andar em círculo, inclinação e rotação da cabeça, cegueira, convulsões e morte. O exame *post mortem* muitas vezes revela infarto pulmonar, com congestão e edema. Mais comumente, o início dos sintomas é menos agudo (forma crônica). Relatos de achados históricos de dirofilariose felina crônica incluem anorexia, perda de peso, letargia, intolerância ao exercício, sinais de insuficiência cardíaca direita (efusão pleural é incomum), tosse, dispneia e vômito. O autor e seus colaboradores constataram que dispneia e tosse são sintomas relativamente frequentes e, quando presentes, devem levar à suspeita de dirofilariose, em áreas endêmicas.[174] Quilotórax, pneumotórax e SVC também foram reconhecidos como manifestações incomuns de dirofilariose felina.

Em um relato de 50 casos de infecção natural por dirofilária em gatos na Carolina do Norte, os sinais clínicos mais comumente relatados foram relacionados ao sistema respiratório (32 gatos; 64%); com dispneia (24 gatos; 48%) foi o sintoma de maior frequência, seguido de tosse (19 gatos; 38%) e respiração ofegante (Figura 255.19).[174] Vômito foi relatado em 17 gatos (38%) e em 8 (16%) foi observado com frequência. Verificou-se que 5 (10%) gatos com dirofilariose exibiram vômitos sem sinais respiratórios concomitantes, e vômito foi notado em 7 gatos (14%) por ocasião da consulta. Sintomas neurológicos (incluindo colapso ou síncope [10%]) foram relatados em 7 gatos (14%). Cinco (10%) dos gatos estavam mortos no momento da consulta. Sopros cardíacos foram raramente observados em gatos que não tinham doença cardíaca concomitante, independentemente da infecção por dirofilária. Um gato manifestava insuficiência cardíaca, mas era portador de cardiomiopatia hipertrófica concomitante. A dirofilariose foi considerada um achado acidental em 14 gatos desse estudo (28%). É digno de nota que em uma região hiperendêmica da Itália estudos sobre infecção natural por dirofilária em gatos assintomáticos apresentaram cura espontânea em aproximadamente 80% dos gatos infectados.[156,161]

O exame físico geralmente é pouco relevante, embora possam ser observados sopro, ritmo de galope ou sons pulmonares diminuídos ou adventícios (ou uma combinação desses achados) (ver Capítulo 55). Adicionalmente, os gatos podem ser magros, dispneicos, ou ambos. Quando há insuficiência cardíaca, raramente são detectadas dilatação da veia jugular, dispneia e ascite.

DIAGNÓSTICO

O diagnóstico de dirofilariose em gatos apresenta uma abordagem única e um conjunto de questões problemáticas.[5] Primeiro, os sinais clínicos geralmente estão ausentes e, quando presentes, são bem diferentes daqueles verificados em cães. Além do mais, a incidência geral de dirofilariose em gatos é baixa, então a suspeita clínica é baixa; a eosinofilia é transitória ou ausente; os resultados de testes imunológicos são frequentemente falsos negativos; achados eletrocardiográficos são mínimos; sinais radiográficos são inconsistentes e podem ser transitórios; e a maioria dos gatos apresenta amicrofilaremia. Por fim, o clínico deve ter em mente que gatos com teste antigênico positivo quase sempre apresentam infecção por dirofilária madura, e os gatos com teste de anticorpo positivo (teste de antígeno negativo) normalmente não têm infecção por dirofilária. Contudo, aproximadamente 50% dos gatos positivos para anticorpos e negativos para antígenos desenvolvem lesões pulmonares devido à DADR. O diagnóstico de DADR é feito por exclusão e requer um alto índice de suspeita (Tabela 255.5).

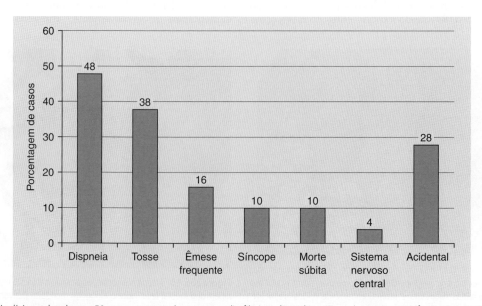

Figura 255.19 Sinais clínicos relatados em 50 gatos comprovadamente com dirofilariose. (De Atkins CE *et al.*: Heartworm infection in cats: 50 cases [1985-1997]. *J Am Vet Med Assoc* 217:355-358, 2000.)

CAPÍTULO 255 • Dirofilariose Canina e Felina

Tabela 255.5 Comparação de doenças respiratórias associadas à dirofilariose (DADR) causadas por morte de dirofilária (adultas imaturas) nos vasos sanguíneos pulmonares e por dirofilariose felina causada por dirofilária adulta madura.

PARÂMETRO	DADR	DIROFILARIOSE CRÔNICA
Início dos sinais clínicos depois da infecção	cerca de 3 meses	> 7 meses
Etiologia	Instalação e morte de formas imaturas de dirofilária na artéria pulmonar	Resposta cardíaca e parenquimatosa e vascular pulmonar à presença, morte e deterioração de vermes adultos
Sinais clínicos	Dispneia, tosse, respiração ofegante	Dispneia, tosse, hemoptise, colapso, vômito, sinais neurológicos, insuficiência cardíaca, morte súbita
Resultados de testes sorológicos		
Antígeno	Negativo	Positivo ou negativo
Anticorpo	Frequentemente +	Frequentemente +
Microfilaremia	Ausente	Ocasionalmente presente
Achados radiográficos	Padrão broncointersticial	Padrão broncointersticial variável, aumento da artéria pulmonar e hiperinsuflação do pulmão; menos comumente, derrame pleural ou consolidação pulmonar
Achados ecocardiográficos	Normal (sem dirofilária discernível)	Dirofilária(s) frequentemente encontrada(s) na artéria pulmonar, no átrio direito ou no ventrículo direito; possível hipertensão pulmonar

De Lee ACY, Atkins CE: Understanding feline heartworm infection: disease, diagnosis, and treatment. *Top Companion Anim Med* 25:224-230, 2010.

Não existem razões médicas convincentes para a triagem de gatos com dirofilariose antes da administração preventiva de lactona macrocíclica (LM), porque o risco de reações adversas associadas à morte por presença de microfilária é pequeno (gatos não apresentam microfilaremia ou têm um pequeno número de microfilárias ou as reações adversas são mínimas com o uso preventivo de LM). No entanto, a triagem possibilita ao clínico alertar aos tutores de animais que os seus gatos foram expostos (teste de anticorpo positivo) à dirofilária, para que eles possam optar pela busca da confirmação do diagnóstico de infecção por dirofilária madura. Também minimiza as dificuldades de relações públicas, caso o gato desenvolva dirofilariose, enquanto submetido à medicação preventiva. Adicionalmente, a triagem de rotina permite que o clínico entenda o risco de ocorrência de dirofilariose em sua área de atuação. A abordagem do autor para a triagem de rotina de dirofilariose em gatos difere um pouco desta, quando há suspeita de infecção (Figura 255.20).

Os métodos de imunodiagnóstico (ver Tabela 255.2) não são apropriados aos gatos devido à baixa carga parasitária e, portanto, à carga antigênica.[175] Em um estudo utilizando teste ELISA para pesquisa de antígeno em amostras de soro sanguíneo de gatos infectados experimentalmente, verificou-se soropositividade em 36 a 93% de 31 gatos, que continham 1 a 7 fêmeas de dirofilária, com maior sensibilidade quando havia alta carga de fêmeas do parasita.[176] Gatos com apenas um parasita ou apenas parasitas machos não foram detectados como positivos. Portanto, testes falsos negativos ocorrem com frequência, dependendo do teste utilizado, da maturidade do parasita, do gênero e da carga parasitária. No entanto, a especificidade de todos os testes foi de, praticamente, 100%. É importante ter em mente que os sinais de infecção podem ser observados antes da presença de antígeno detectável (oriundo de fêmeas adultas). McCall *et al.*[177] relataram que, em infecções naturais, o teste antigênico detecta menos que 50% dos casos comprovados, enquanto Snyder *et al.*[178] apresentaram dados diferentes (de infecções naturais nas quais o sangue obtido de até 2 horas após a eutanásia) que mostram que o teste antigênico é mais sensível (74%) do que anteriormente relatado. Como os testes para pesquisa de antígeno continuam a melhorar, sua sensibilidade exata é um pouco ofuscada, mas é estimada em 50 a 75%, nas infecções naturais causadas por dirofilária adulta ou madura.

Os testes para pesquisa de antígeno não detectam gatos com DRAD, mas os testes de anticorpos são rotineiramente positivos nesses gatos (ver Tabela 255.5).[175] Um teste para pesquisa de antígeno (IDEXX's SNAP Feline Heartworm Antigen Test) tem sido comercializado para uso em gatos e faz parte da plataforma SNAP de testes para doenças infecciosas de gatos. É uma adaptação do teste realizado em cães, com relato de aumento da sensibilidade em 15% em relação aos testes de antigênicos convencionais.

Embora menos específico para infecções por dirofilária madura, os testes para pesquisa de anticorpos para dirofilariose são úteis na detecção de dirofilariose felina, mesmo quando os testes antigênicos são negativos. Em um estudo sobre dirofilariose em 257 gatos com teste de anticorpo positivo, verificou-se que apenas 13,1% dos animais apresentavam teste antigênico positivo.[179] O teste para pesquisa de anticorpo também serve como marcador de exposição e risco de dirofilariose (mesmo que o gato nunca desenvolva infecção por dirofilária madura) e possibilidade de DRAD. Um teste para pesquisa de anticorpos para dirofilariose felina para utilização em clínica também está disponível (HESKA: Solo Step FH). É importante ressaltar que se estima que a metade dos gatos com teste de anticorpo positivo e de antígeno negativo tem manifestações *post mortem* de dirofilariose e, nesses gatos, a condição de anticorpo positivo pode diminuir com o tempo. Muitas vezes, o teste para pesquisa de anticorpo é usado em associação com o teste antigênico; esses testes estão disponíveis nos formatos *cage-side* e *send-off*.

Recentemente, a utilização de teste para pesquisa de antígeno de *Wolbachia* (proteína específica de *Wolbachia* – PSW) e de PCR para pesquisa do DNA de *Wolbachia* mostrou-se promissora no diagnóstico de dirofilariose em gatos.[180,181] Foi demonstrado que o tratamento térmico do soro sanguíneo pode aumentar a sensibilidade do teste antigênico.[22] Em 6 gatos com infecção experimental testados, notou-se que 4 apresentavam resultado falso negativo em testes comerciais para pesquisa do antígeno e o tratamento térmico do soro a 39,44°C por 10 minutos tornou o soro positivo em 5 de 6 gatos. Isso pode ser um estímulo necessário para possibilitar, definitivamente, o diagnóstico de dirofilariose em gatos, mas é improvável que detecte todas as infecções causadas por parasitas machos.

Radiografias de tórax são úteis no diagnóstico de dirofilariose (ou de outras doenças que mimetizam dirofilariose). Porém, gatos assintomáticos raramente apresentam lesões radiográficas, portanto essa modalidade de diagnóstico não é ideal para fins de triagem.[161,182] O critério radiográfico mais sensível (artéria

1346   SEÇÃO 16 • Doença Cardiovascular

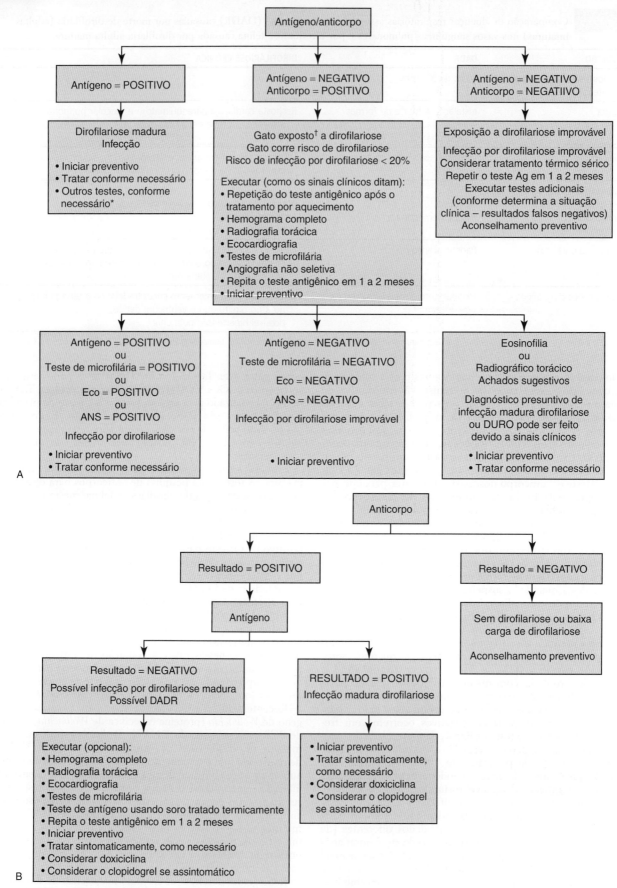

Figura 255.20 A. Algoritmo da abordagem utilizada pelo autor no diagnóstico de dirofilariose em gatos com suspeita da infecção. **B.** Algoritmo da abordagem do autor para triagem de gatos com dirofilariose. *Radiografias de tórax e exames de sangue; †*exposição* significa que o gato foi exposto e permitido o desenvolvimento ao estágio L4, mas pode ou não ter permitido a maturação do parasita. Alguns clínicos preferem considerar esse gato como *infectado*, já que a infecção provavelmente foi eliminada no estágio de S5 imaturo e pode manifestar sinais clínicos. *ANS*, angiografia não seletiva; *DADR*, doença respiratória associada à dirofilariose.

pulmonar caudal esquerda 1,6 vez maior que a nona costela, no nono espaço intercostal, na projeção ventrodorsal) foi detectado apenas em 53% dos casos. Portanto, embora a maioria dos gatos com sinais clínicos tenha alguma anormalidade radiográfica, os achados não são específicos para dirofilariose. Adicionalmente, um estudo realizado por Selcer et al.[160] demonstrou que os achados radiográficos frequentemente eram transitórios, e as anormalidades radiográficas que foram encontradas em gatos que resistiram à maturação da dirofilária e foram negativos no exame *post mortem*, provavelmente, apresentavam o que mais tarde ficou conhecido como DRAD. Os achados radiográficos incluem aumento de artérias pulmonares caudais (Figura 255.21) e frequentemente bordas do parênquima pulmonar mal definidas com alterações que incluem infiltrados focais ou difusos (intersticial, broncointersticial ou mesmo alveolar), densidade perivascular e ocasionalmente atelectasia (Figuras 255.22 e 255.23). Hiperinsuflação pulmonar também pode ser evidente, e os erros de diagnóstico da doença brônquica felina podem ser facilmente cometidos (ver Figuras 255.21 A e 255.22 A). A angiografia pulmonar também é utilizada para demonstrar corpos estranhos lineares radiolucentes intravasculares e aumento, tortuosidade e ofuscação das artérias pulmonares (Figura 255.24).

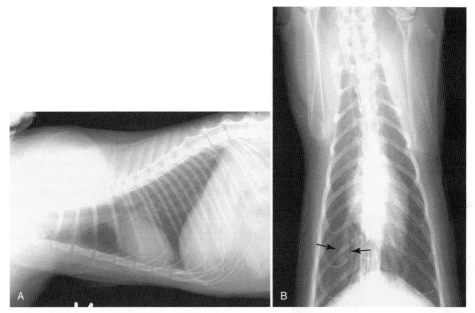

Figura 255.21 A. Radiografia lateral do tórax de um gato com dirofilariose. Nota-se um bom padrão intersticial nos lobos caudais do pulmão e o tórax com certo grau de hiperinsuflação. Esse padrão radiográfico é parecido e, portanto, confundido com o da doença brônquica felina. **B.** Radiografia dorsoventral do tórax do mesmo gato mostrado em **A**. Novamente, as alterações não são marcantes, mas a artéria pulmonar do lobo caudal direito está aumentada (> 1,6 vez maior que a nona costela, no nono espaço intercostal; *setas*). Pode-se notar tortuosidade da artéria pulmonar contralateral.

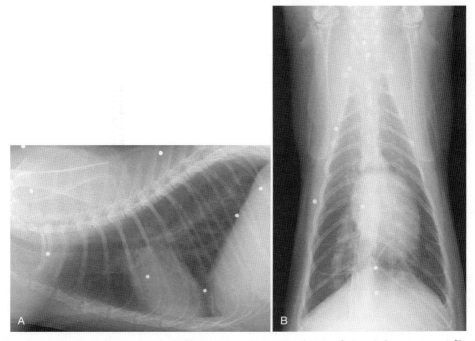

Figura 255.22 A. Radiografia lateral do tórax de um gato com dirofilariose e tosse. Note o tórax hiperinsuflado, o diafragma reto e o infiltrado intersticial pulmonar moderado. O ventrículo direito está moderadamente aumentado. **B.** Radiografia dorsoventral do tórax do mesmo gato mostrado em **A**. O infiltrado pulmonar é mais facilmente observado nessa imagem do lobo pulmonar caudal direito. Note o aumento da artéria pulmonar do lobo caudal direito.

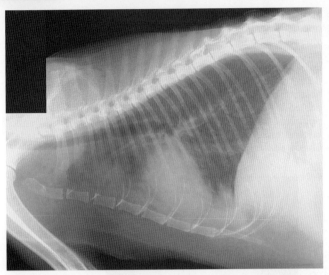

Figura 255.23 Radiografia lateral do tórax de um gato com quadro grave de dificuldade respiratória e dirofilariose. Note o infiltrado alveolar na região ventral do pulmão e infiltrado intersticial menos grave mais dorsalmente nos lobos pulmonares caudais. Essa doença pulmonar grave provavelmente se deve à morte de dirofilária e pode representar a síndrome da angústia respiratória aguda.

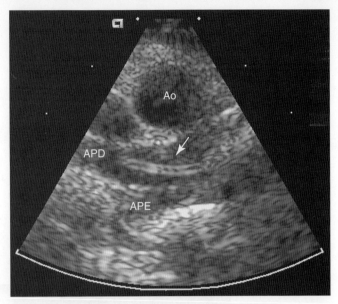

Figura 255.25 Ecocardiograma bidimensional de eixo curto de um gato de 18 anos de idade, macho, castrado, com câncer e sopro cardíaco assintomático. É possível notar uma dirofilária adulta, identificada por duas linhas paralelas ecodensas, na artéria pulmonar direita (seta). Ao, artéria aorta; APD, artéria pulmonar direita; APE, artéria pulmonar esquerda.

TRATAMENTO E PREVENÇÃO

Surge a pergunta se a profilaxia de dirofilariose é justificada para gatos uma vez que eles não são o hospedeiro natural e a incidência nessa espécie é baixa. Achados de necropsia em gatos com dirofilariose no Sudeste mostraram prevalência de infecção causada por dirofilária madura de 2,5 a 14%, com mediana de aproximadamente 5% (Figura 255.26).[154] Ao considerar a questão da instituição de tratamento profilático, vale ressaltar que essa prevalência se aproxima ou até supera a das infecções pelo vírus da leucemia felina (FeLV) e pelo vírus da imunodeficiência felina (FIV). Uma pesquisa de anticorpos nacional, em 1998, em mais de 2.000 gatos claramente assintomáticos revelou prevalência de exposição ao redor de 12% (Figura 255.27)[185] e sugeriu ser de 16%,[186] embora outras estimativas tenham sido menores (1 a 8%).[187] Considera-se que uma taxa de 12% de animais anticorpo-positivos indica taxa de prevalência de infecção causada por dirofilária madura de 1 a 2% e de 5 a 6% para DRAD; assim, em todo o país estima-se uma taxa de morbidade DRAD (doença respiratória associada à dirofilariose) em gatos em torno de 6 a 8%. Também é digno de nota que, com base nas informações dos tutores, quase um terço dos gatos diagnosticados com dirofilariose na UECN eram mantidos apenas em ambiente fechado.[174] Por fim, as consequências da dirofilariose felina são potencialmente terríveis, sem soluções terapêuticas claras. Portanto, o autor recomenda o tratamento preventivo de gatos criados em áreas endêmicas – onde os cães são submetidos à terapia preventiva.

Cinco endoparasiticidas e ectoparasiticidas de amplo espectro aprovados pela FDA-CVM são (ou serão) comercializados para uso em gatos nos EUA (Tabela 255.6). A ivermectina é disponibilizada em formulação mastigável, a milbemicina oxima como comprimido aromatizado e a selamectina, moxidectina/imidacloprida e eprinomectina/fipronil/praziquantel são disponibilizados para uso tópico. Os espectros de ação e as formulações desses produtos são variáveis; portanto, na maioria dos casos, as necessidades individuais dos clientes são facilmente atendidas.

Como a grande maioria dos gatos não apresenta microfilaremia, a terapia microfilaricida é desnecessária nessa espécie. O uso de medicamentos adulticidas arsenicais é problemático. A tiacetarsamida (caparsolato de sódio), se disponível, apresenta

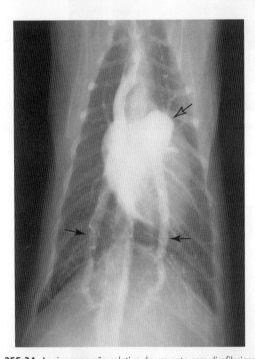

Figura 255.24 Angiograma não seletivo de um gato com dirofilariose. Note o aumento da artéria pulmonar principal (seta vazada) e aumento, tortuosidade e obscurecimento de artérias pulmonares caudais (setas sólidas). O exame cuidadoso revela radiolucências lineares na artéria pulmonar caudal direita. (Cortesia da Dra. Kathy Spaulding. De Atkins CE: Heartworm disease. In: Allen DG, editor: *Small animal medicine*, Philadelphia, 1991, JB Lippincott, p. 341-363.)

Na experiência do autor, a sensibilidade de ecocardiograma é maior em gatos do que em cães.[157,183,184] Normalmente, uma linha dupla de ecodensidade é evidente na artéria pulmonar principal, em um de seus ramos, no ventrículo direito ou, ocasionalmente, na junção atrioventricular direita (AV) (Figura 255.25 e Vídeo 255.4). Atkins et al.[157] visualizaram dirofilária por meio de ecocardiografia em 78% de 9 casos clínicos; Selcer et al.[160] encontraram casos de infecção experimental em 16 animais.

CAPÍTULO 255 • Dirofilariose Canina e Felina   1349

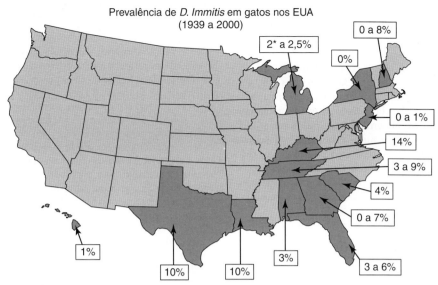

Figura 255.26 Prevalência de dirofilariose em estudos de achados de necropsia em gatos de abrigo. Nos estados sombreados os estudos foram concluídos. Em um estudo em Michigan verificou-se prevalência de 2%; foi realizado estudo antigênico. *Esse número representa testes antigênicos positivos e não positivos baseados em achados de necropsia, como todos os outros. (Adaptada de Ryan WG, Newcomb KM: Prevalence of feline heartworm disease – a global review. In: Soll MD, Knight DH, editors: *Proceedings of the 1995 American Heartworm Symposium,* Batavia, IL, 1996, American Heartworm Society.)

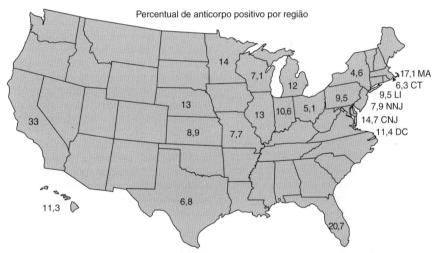

Figura 255.27 Prevalência (%) de exposição à dirofilariose (teste positivo para anticorpos) em mais de 2.000 gatos claramente assintomáticos em 19 estados (21 regiões). *CNJ,* Central New Jersey; *LI,* Long Island, Nova York; *NNJ,* Norte de Nova Jersey. (Adaptada de Miller MW, Atkins CE, Stemme K et al.: Prevalence of exposure to *Dirofilaria immitis* in cats from multiple areas of the United States. In: Soll MD, Knight DH, editors: *Proceedings of the 1998 American Heartworm Symposium,* Batavia, IL, 1998, p. 161-166.)

Tabela 255.6 Fármacos utilizados na prevenção de dirofilariose disponíveis nos EUA e respectivos espectros de ação.

FÁRMACO	DIROFILÁRIA	ANCILÓSTOMOS	NEMATOIDES	TÊNIAS CESTÓDIOS	PULGAS E OVOS	CARRAPATOS	SARCOPTES	ÁCARO DE ORELHA
Ivermectina mastigável (Hartguard para gatos)	+	+						
Milbemicinaoxima (comprimido aromatizado) Interceptor	+	+		+				
Selamectina (tópico) Revolution	+	+		+	+/+			+
Moxidectina/Imidaclorida (tópico) Advantage Multi	+	+		+	+/-			+
Eprinomectina/Fipronil/ Praziquantel* (tópico) BROADLINE	+	+		+	+			

*Atualmente não comercializado nos EUA; as indicações da bula são para a Europa e na bula prevista para a União Europeia também inclui *Aelurostrongylus abstrusus.*

riscos, mesmo em gatos em condições normais. Turner et al. relataram óbito decorrente de edema pulmonar e insuficiência respiratória em 3 dos 14 gatos normais tratados com tiacetarsamida (duas doses de 2,2 mg/kg, com intervalo de 24 horas).[188] Dillon et al.[189] não confirmaram essa reação pulmonar aguda em 12 gatos normais que receberam esse fármaco, mas um gato morreu após a última injeção. Mais importante ainda, uma significativa, mas não quantificada, porcentagem de gatos com dirofilariose desenvolve tromboembolismo pulmonar (TEP) após terapia adulticida.[172-174] Isso surge vários dias a 1 semana após o tratamento e geralmente é fatal. Em 50 gatos com dirofilariose atendidos na UECN, 11 receberam tiacetarsamida. O resultado desse estudo mostrou que não houve diferença significativa na sobrevida de animais tratados com tiacetarsamida e aqueles submetidos a tratamento sintomático.[174]

Em gatos, os dados sobre o uso de melarsomina no tratamento de infecção experimental por dirofilária (parasitas transplantados) são limitados e contraditórios. Embora haja um relato resumido de que uma injeção (2,5 mg de melarsomina/kg; metade da dose recomendada para cães) em gatos infectados experimentalmente sem que dados de mortalidade fosse relacionado ao tratamento, a carga parasitária pós-tratamento não foi significativamente diferente daquela verificada em gatos do grupo-controle não tratados.[190] Diarreia e sopro cardíaco foram frequentemente observados nos gatos tratados. Em outro relato que utilizou o protocolo padrão para cães (duas doses de 2,5 mg/kg, com intervalo de 24 horas) ou de dose fracionada (uma injeção, seguida de duas injeções, com intervalo de 24 horas, em 1 mês), os resultados foram mais favoráveis.[191] O tratamento com protocolo padrão de dose única e com o protocolo de dose fracionada resultou em redução de 79 e 86% da carga parasitária, respectivamente, e não ocorreram reações adversas. Embora promissores, esses dados não publicados precisam ser interpretados com cautela, pois os parasitas transplantados eram imaturos (< 8 meses e mais suscetíveis) e nos gatos do grupo-controle a taxa de mortalidade de vermes foi 53% (a média da carga parasitária foi reduzida em 53% pelo ato de transplante). Adicionalmente, a experiência clínica em gatos naturalmente infectados tem sido geralmente desfavorável, com taxa de mortalidade inaceitável. Por causa desse risco inerente, a falta de um benefício claro e a curta expectativa de vida dos parasitas nesta espécie, o autor não recomenda terapia adulticida em gatos.

A remoção cirúrgica das dirofilárias tem sido bem-sucedida e é atraente porque minimiza o risco de tromboembolismo. A taxa de mortalidade relatada na única série de casos publicada foi, infelizmente, inaceitável (dois de cinco gatos).[192] Recentemente tivemos sucesso em gatos com dirofilariose associada à insuficiência cardíaca, utilizando um cateter com cesto de nitinol para a remoção dos parasitas pela veia jugular.[193] Mesmo com suas vantagens, essa abordagem ainda é impraticável na grande maioria dos casos. Gatos com dirofilariose devem ser submetidos a tratamento preventivo com corticosteroide (1 a 2 mg de prednisolona/kg, via SC, em intervalos de 8 a 48 horas), de curta duração e terapia mensal para o controle dos sintomas respiratórios. Se os sinais clínicos reaparecerem, pode-se administrar terapia com esteroide em dias alternados (na menor dose para o controle dos sintomas) e pode ser continuado indefinidamente. Para emergências embólicas podem ser usados oxigênio, corticosteroides (1 mg de dexametasona/kg IV ou IM ou 50 a 100 mg de succinato de prednisolona sódica/gato IV) e broncodilatadores (6,6 mg de aminofilina/kg/12 h IM, 15 a 20 mg de teofilina de liberação prolongada/kg/24 h VO ou 0,01 mg de terbutalina/kg SC). O uso de broncodilatadores é justificável porque alguns deles, como as xantinas (aminofilina e teofilina) melhoram a função dos músculos das vias respiratórias em fadiga. Além disso, o achado de hiperinsuflação em campos pulmonares pode indicar broncoconstrição, uma condição na qual a broncodilatação seria indicada. Mesmo assim, este autor não utiliza rotineiramente broncodilatadores em casos de dirofilariose felina.

O uso de ácido acetilsalicílico tem sido questionado porque as alterações vasculares associadas ao consumo de plaquetas que ocorre na dirofilariose aumentam sua taxa de rotatividade e diminuíram efetivamente os efeitos antitrombóticos do fármaco. Relata-se que a dose convencional de ácido acetilsalicílico não preveniu lesões vasculares causadas por infecção experimental por dirofilária detectadas por angiografia.[194] A dose de ácido acetilsalicílico necessária para causar benefício histológico, mesmo que limitado, aproxima-se da dose tóxica. Como os estudos citados foram baseados em estimativas de sensibilidade relativamente baixas da função plaquetária e da doença pulmonar arterial (possivelmente não detectando benefícios sutis),

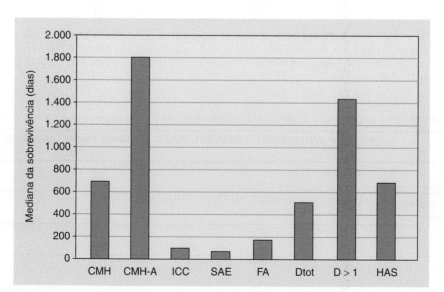

Figura 255.28 Sobrevida média verificada em quatro relatos anteriores de gatos com diversas doenças cardiovasculares. A sobrevida média mostrada de 5 anos foi, na verdade, superior a 5 anos. CMH, cardiomiopatia hipertrófica; CMH-A,* cardiomiopatia hipertrófica assintomática; D > 1, dirofilariose com sobrevida além de 1 dia; Dtot, todos os casos de dirofilariose; FA, fibrilação atrial; HAS, hipertensão arterial sanguínea; ICC, cardiomiopatia hipertrófica com insuficiência cardíaca; SAE, cardiomiopatia hipertrófica com embolia sistêmica. (De Atkins CE, Côté E, DeFrancesco TC et al.: Prognosis in feline heartworm infection: comparison to other cardiovascular disease. In: Seward LR, Knight DH, editors: Proceedings of American Heartworm Society: 2001, Batavia, IL, 2003, American Heartworm Society, p. 41-44.)

porque as opções terapêuticas são limitadas e porque na dose de 40 a 80 mg/72 h VO o ácido acetilsalicílico geralmente não é tóxico, é barato e prático, o autor continua defendendo o uso de ácido acetilsalicílico para gatos com infecção por dirofilária. No entanto, o ácido acetilsalicílico não deve ser prescrito simultaneamente ao tratamento com corticosteroide. Dados recentes sobre tromboembolismo arterial mostram que o clopidogrel é um medicamento antiplaquetário melhor que o ácido acetilsalicílico, em gatos e em pessoas.[195] Embora o clopidogrel (18,75 mg/gato/24 h) não tenha sido estudado na dirofilariose felina, parece a melhor opção para gatos com infecção por dirofilária do que o ácido acetilsalicílico, embora mais dispendioso. O tratamento de outros sinais clínicos de dilofilariose em gatos é amplamente sintomático.

PROGNÓSTICO

No estudo anteriormente mencionado sobre 50 gatos com infecção natural por dirofilária, ao menos 12 animais morreram por outras causas que não a infecção por dirofilária. Destes, 7 e outros 2 gatos que sobreviveram foram considerados sobreviventes de dirofilariose (viveram > 1.000 dias).[174] A mediana da sobrevida de todos os gatos acometidos por dirofilariose, que sobreviveram além da confirmação do diagnóstico, foi de 1.460 dias (4 anos; com intervalo de 2 a 4.015 dias), enquanto a mediana da sobrevida de todos os gatos (n = 48, com acompanhamento adequado) foi de 540 dias (1,5 ano; com intervalo de 0 a 4.015 dias). A sobrevida de 11 gatos tratados com caparsolato de sódio (média de 1.669 dias) não foi significativamente diferente daquela de 30 gatos tratados com fármaco adulticida (média de 1.107 dias). Da mesma forma, variáveis como idade (< 3 anos de idade), presença de dispneia, tosse, positividade no teste de ELISA para antígeno de dirofilária, detecção ecocardiográfica de parasitas e sexo do gato parecem não influenciar a sobrevivência.[174] Dados recentes mencionados indicam que aproximadamente 40% de 75% dos gatos infectados podem ser assintomáticos e 80% desses gatos podem progredir para cura espontânea.[156,161] Isso é interpretado como evidência de que a infecção por dirofilária em gatos é provavelmente muito mais comum do que atualmente se imagina e os efeitos adversos podem ser menos graves do que se acredita. O efeito da infecção por dirofilária na sobrevivência foi comparável ao de outras doenças cardiovasculares (Figura 255.28).[196]

REFERÊNCIAS BIBLIOGRÁFICAS

As referências bibliográficas deste capítulo se encontram online no Ambiente de Aprendizagem.

CAPÍTULO 256

Doença Arterial Tromboembólica

Daniel F. Hogan

FUNDAMENTAÇÃO

O tromboembolismo arterial (TEA) é definido como infarto de um ou mais leitos arteriais por material embólico, geralmente oriundo de um trombo em um local distante do infarto no leito arterial. É importante diferenciar o TEA da trombose arterial por várias razões. Primeiro, a lesão primária geralmente é muito diferente; a superfície endotelial do vaso infartado é normal nos casos de TEA, enquanto as anormalidades no endotélio vascular e/ou parede vascular são características de trombose arterial. Segundo, o TEA geralmente está associado a fluxo estagnado ou estase sanguínea, enquanto a trombose arterial está associada a um fluxo de alto cisalhamento em um vaso sanguíneo com lúmen diminuído. Terceiro, o TEA ocorre comumente em pacientes veterinários, enquanto a trombose arterial verdadeira é extremamente rara.

Em alguns casos, o local do trombo inicial é conhecido ou confiável. No embolismo cardiogênico (EC), os trombos são mais comumente encontrados no interior do átrio ou aurícula esquerdos dilatados. O coração também é a origem de êmbolos, que se desenvolvem no caso de endocardite (ver Capítulo 251). No entanto, muitas vezes a origem do trombo não pode ser determinada, e esta inclui condições como neoplasia e nefropatia acompanhadas de perda de proteínas. Alguns profissionais sugerem que trombos venosos profundos são fontes de material embólico, mas isso não explicaria a localização arterial do êmbolo na ausência de uma anormalidade cardiovascular, como desvio (*shunt*) da direita para a esquerda. A *embolia paradoxal*, que é um acidente vascular cerebral tromboembólico arterial resultante de trombose venosa profunda, ocorre no homem e geralmente está associada a uma comunicação interatrial, como a persistência do forame oval, que possibilita a passagem do êmbolo da circulação venosa para a arterial. Isso foi relatado em medicina veterinária[1] e poderia ocorrer muito mais nas espécies de animais domésticos, como um estudo recente que sugere que os defeitos do septo atrial são muito mais comuns no cão do que originalmente se suspeitava.[2] A neoplasia pulmonar é a única doença em que a trombose em veia pulmonar poderia gerar um êmbolo capaz de alcançar a circulação arterial sistêmica.

PATOGÊNESE

No paciente saudável normal, há um equilíbrio entre a formação de trombos e a sua dissolução. Esse delicado equilíbrio possibilita o reparo contínuo da lesão endotelial, enquanto impede o desenvolvimento descontrolado de trombos. A hemostasia primária começa com a exposição do colágeno subendotelial e é caracterizada pela aderência de plaquetas ao tecido subendotelial local. Em seguida, ocorre ativação e agregação plaquetária, com liberação de agentes com propriedades de pró-agregação e vasoconstrição. Essas substâncias, em conjunto com os fatores circulantes no plasma, iniciam a cascata de coagulação, resultando em hemostasia secundária. À medida que ocorre a formação do tampão hemostático e a cicatrização endotelial, mecanismos profibrinolíticos são ativados para cessar o desenvolvimento de tampão hemostático, prevenindo a formação excessiva de trombos. A trombose patológica ocorre quando há desequilíbrio entre a formação de trombos e a fibrinólise, em favor do primeiro.

Classicamente, o desenvolvimento de trombose patológica tem sido descrito com base na tríade de Virchow: lesão endotelial, estase sanguínea e hipercoagulação. A lesão endotelial pode ser decorrência da dilatação do átrio esquerdo em gato com cardiomiopatia hipertrófica, de lesão de válvula aórtica em cão com estenose subaórtica ou de invasão tumoral à árvore arterial. Já a estase sanguínea pode estar associada à dilatação de câmaras cardíacas (Vídeo 256.1) ou fluxo sanguíneo restrito de crescimento tumoral. A presença de uma condição de hipercoagulação é muito mais difícil de ser identificada especificamente, principalmente em animais domésticos. Em humanos, condições de hipercoagulação conhecidas incluem anormalidades hereditárias dos fatores procoagulantes IIa (trombina), Va e VIIIa, e nas proteínas antitrombóticas antitrombina (AT), proteína C e proteína S.[3-7] Outras condições de hipercoagulação foram associadas à hipersensibilidade de plaquetas e ao aumento dos teores de homocisteína, lipoproteína (a), inibidor do ativador do plasminogênio (PAI-1) e do inibidor da fibrinólise ativada pela trombina (IFAT). Em cães e gatos, a trombose clínica foi associada ao aumento da hipersensibilidade plaquetária, diminuição das atividades de AT e de proteína C e aumentos dos fatores II, V, VII, VIII, IX, X, XII e de fibrinogênio.[8-14] Parece prudente considerar o desenvolvimento de doenças trombóticas a partir do conceito de risco cumulativo, em que cada componente da tríade de Virchow pode contribuir para um maior risco de trombose.

A composição inicial do trombo patológico consiste em grande quantidade de plaquetas, mas progressivamente se torna mais rica em fibras, à medida que aumenta o tamanho do trombo. Conforme o trombo amadurece, ele se torna lamelar, em que porções superficiais podem se romper, formando êmbolos que ocasionam infarto de leitos arteriais distantes. A gravidade do infarto depende do tamanho e da estabilidade do êmbolo, pois a obstrução ocorre quando o tamanho do êmbolo excede consideravelmente o diâmetro do vaso sanguíneo.

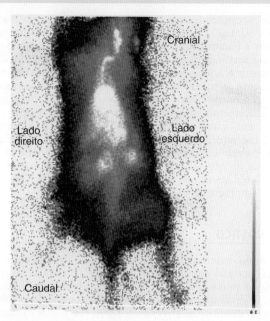

Figura 256.1 Varredura de perfusão nuclear em gato com tromboembolismo arterial (TEA) assimétrico usando ^{99m}Tc não ligado. Nota-se redução marcante na perfusão do membro pélvico direito e abaixo do joelho do membro pélvico esquerdo. (*Esta figura se encontra reproduzida em cores no Encarte.*)

SINAIS CLÍNICOS

Os sinais clínicos atribuíveis ao ATE dependem da gravidade do infarto e localização do leito vascular infartado. A gravidade dos sinais clínicos é inversamente proporcional ao volume do fluxo sanguíneo arterial. Muitos órgãos possuem uma rede de vasos colaterais que podem suprir o fluxo sanguíneo à área irrigada pela artéria principal obstruída; no entanto, essas redes se desenvolvem mais plenamente quando a perda de fluxo sanguíneo é gradual; ademais, existem fortes evidências de que o infarto agudo causado por TEA está associado ao comprometimento no desenvolvimento dessas redes de vasos colaterais.[15,16]

O infarto renal tem sido associado a sinais de dor renal e insuficiência renal aguda, enquanto o infarto mesentérico pode resultar em evidências de dor abdominal, vômito e diarreia. O infarto esplênico pode estar associado a letargia, anorexia, vômitos e diarreia.[17] Déficits neurológicos importantes e convulsões foram associados a infarto cerebral, bem como a morte súbita em casos graves.[1]

Embora os infartos cerebral, renal e esplâncnico ocorram ocasionalmente, o infarto da trifurcação aórtica é responsável pela maioria dos casos de TEA em cães e gatos.[18] O infarto da trifurcação aórtica (o clássico êmbolo em sela) resulta em perda de fluxo sanguíneo para os membros pélvicos e causa neuromiopatia isquêmica (NMI) (Figura 256.1). Os sinais clínicos de NMI incluem paresia ou paralisia dos membros pélvicos, com ausência segmentar de reflexos, músculos dos membros pélvicos rígidos e doloridos, membros frios e sem pulso, e leitos vasculares das unhas cianóticos (Vídeo 256.2). As alterações podem ser bilaterais, simétricas ou assimétricas, ou unilaterais, dependendo do grau de obstrução arterial e do desenvolvimento de vasos colaterais. O início dos sinais clínicos é agudo e podem se agravar, mas geralmente permanecem estáveis ou melhoram dentro de alguns dias a 3 semanas. O principal fator contribuinte para o desenvolvimento de NMI parece ser a liberação de substâncias vasoativas pelas plaquetas ativadas, reduzindo o fluxo colateral em torno do local da obstrução. Doenças semelhantes foram diagnosticadas em pessoas que sofreram acidente vascular cerebral trombótico, embolia cardiogênica, acidente vascular cerebral tromboembólico cardiogênico e embolia pulmonar.[19-22] Na obstrução aórtica experimental, verificou-se que o fluxo sanguíneo em gatos é mantido por uma extensa circulação colateral no sistema vertebral e nos músculos epaxiais (Vídeo 256.3).[15,16,23] No entanto, ocorre perda dessa circulação colateral em graus variados com a presença de trombo no segmento da artéria aorta e sinais clínicos evidentes de NMI. A serotonina liberada pelas plaquetas ativadas parece ser pelo menos um fator importante para essa ocorrência. Modelos de pesquisa mostraram que a presença de serotonina em um segmento de artéria aorta isolada resulta em ausência de rede vascular colateral e sinais evidentes de NMI, enquanto o pré-tratamento com agonistas serotoninérgicos previnem essas alterações.[16,24]

O infarto da artéria subclávia direita é o segundo local mais comum de TEA em gatos com doença cardíaca subjacente. Os sinais clínicos associados ao infarto nesse local são essencialmente idênticos aos do infarto da trifurcação aórtica, embora os sintomas estejam restritos ao membro torácico direito.[25]

Além dos sinais clínicos associados ao infarto do leito vascular, é possível notar sinais clínicos adicionais relacionados à doença primária. Estes podem incluir febre, depressão e dispneia na sepse; depressão, taquipneia e palidez na anemia hemolítica imunomediada (AHIM); depressão e ascite ou edema periférico na síndrome nefrótica; taquipneia, fraqueza e poliúria/polidipsia no hiperadrenocorticismo; dispneia e sopro cardíaco ou ruído de galope na doença cardíaca primária. Em gatos com embolia cardiogênica, constatou-se insuficiência cardíaca congestiva (ICC) concomitante em 44 a 66% dos casos.[18,26,27]

TRATAMENTO

Os elementos-chave para o tratamento emergencial do TEA incluem prevenção da formação continuada de trombos associada à embolia, melhora do fluxo sanguíneo ao órgão infartado, controle da dor com tratamento clínico apropriado de acordo com anormalidades clínicas e cuidados de suporte.

Redução da formação de trombos

A **heparina não fracionada (HNF)** consiste em um grupo heterogêneo de moléculas com peso molecular médio de ≈ 15.000 dáltons (Da) (variando de 3.000 a 30.000 Da). Devido à variabilidade do tamanho das moléculas, pode ocorrer variação nas propriedades farmacocinéticas e anticoagulantes. As moléculas de heparina contêm uma sequência de pentassacarídeos que se ligam à AT, facilitando a inibição de IIa, Xa, IXa e XIIa. Também ocorre inibição da ativação dos fatores V e VIII, catalisados pela trombina. A heparina não fracionada também tem ação antiplaquetária em pessoas normais, inibindo a agregação plaquetária induzida por trombina e se ligando e inibindo o fator de von Willebrand (FVW). O efeito adverso mais comum da terapia com heparina no homem é hemorragia, já que até 10% de pacientes podem desenvolver trombocitopenia induzida por heparina. Não há estudos objetivos sobre a avaliação do risco de hemorragia em cães e gatos tratados com heparina, embora certamente já haja relato a respeito. No conhecimento do autor, não há relato clínico de trombocitopenia induzida por heparina em cães ou gatos. O ideal é a obtenção de parâmetros que possibilitem avaliar o padrão de sangramento, incluindo contagem de plaquetas, tempo de protrombina (TP), tempo de tromboplastina parcial ativada (TTPa) e, se possível, tromboelastografia (TEG) antes da terapia com heparina (ver Capítulo 196). Isso determinaria a função de coagulação básica e identificaria anormalidades hemorrágicas, como coagulação intravascular disseminada (CID), que podem estar associadas à TEA ou suas causas primárias. Em cães e gatos, a dose apropriada de heparina tem-se mostrado muito variável e a dose necessária pode mudar com o tempo devido à diminuição do teor de AT na circulação sanguínea.[28-30a] Os protocolos terapêuticos razoáveis consistem em doses iniciais de 250 a 375 UI/kg IV seguida de 150 a 250 UI/kg SC, a cada 6 a 8 h, para gatos, e 200 a 300 UI/kg IV seguida de 200 a 250 UI/kg SC, a cada 6 a 8 h, para cães. Historicamente, têm sido utilizadas mensurações seriadas de TTPa para monitorar a terapia com heparina no limite de 1,5 a 2 vezes o valor basal, e esse teste está prontamente disponível.[29] No entanto, um estudo em gatos sugere que a TTPa não se correlaciona bem com a concentração plasmática de HNF.[28] Portanto, pode-se realizar o monitoramento anti-Xa, embora as pesquisas não tenham avaliado se há inibição efetiva do crescimento do trombo.[31]

O tamanho das **heparinas de baixo peso molecular (HBPM)** é menor que o das HNF e poderiam ser usadas em substituição às HNF. O custo desses medicamentos é muito superior ao das HNF (aproximadamente $3 a $5/dose), mas em pessoas podem ser administrados por via SC, a cada 12 h, no tratamento emergencial de anormalidades trombóticas. Dalteparina e enoxaparina têm sido usadas em cães e gatos, nas doses de 100 UI/kg SC, a cada 24 a 12 h, e 1 a 1,5 mg/kg SC, em intervalos de 24 a 12 h, respectivamente.[32,33] Todavia, não há testes clínicos avaliando a inibição do crescimento do trombo com o uso desses produtos em medicina veterinária, de forma que, no momento, a dose exata e a resposta clínica são desconhecidas.

Aumento do fluxo sanguíneo

Fluxo arterial – terapia trombolítica

No infarto, o principal objetivo é restabelecer o fluxo arterial nos órgãos infartados. Isso requer a remoção do trombo, seja por meio de embolectomia, seja por dissolução com fármacos trombolíticos. Fármacos trombolíticos têm sido utilizados em cães e gatos para dissolver o trombo e restabelecer o fluxo arterial.[34-39] O ideal é que os fármacos sejam administrados o mais breve possível após a ocorrência do evento embólico, mas a dissolução efetiva tem sido observada até 18 h após os sinais clínicos iniciais.[34] Efeitos adversos graves podem estar associados à terapia trombolítica; portanto, cuidado deve ser tomado ao se utilizar esses fármacos. A súbita retomada do fluxo arterial aos órgãos infartados pode resultar em rápido desenvolvimento de hiperpotassemia, com risco à vida do paciente e acidose metabólica grave. Essa condição é denominada *lesão por reperfusão*, cuja ocorrência é mais provável no infarto aórtico terminal. A frequência de lesão de reperfusão após terapia trombolítica em gatos com embolia cardiogênica (EC) é de 40 a 70%.[34-36] A lesão por reperfusão é a causa mais comum de morte em gatos em tratamento farmacológico trombolítico, com taxa de sobrevivência relatada de 0 a 43%.[34-36] Devido a possíveis efeitos adversos e ao custo, a terapia trombolítica não deve ser usada em todos os casos de TEA. Todavia, a terapia trombolítica deve ser fortemente considerada em casos de infarto cerebral, infarto esplâncnico ou infarto renal para o restabelecimento do fluxo arterial, que é da maior importância.

Estreptoquinase (EQ). Combina-se com o plasminogênio para formar um complexo ativador que transforma o plasminogênio em plasmina, uma enzima proteolítica. O plasminogênio degrada fibrina, fibrinogênio, plasminogênio, fatores de coagulação e EQ. O complexo EQ-plasminogênio converte plasminogênio circulante e o ligado à fibrina e, portanto, é considerado um ativador inespecífico da plasmina. A estreptoquinase é produzida por estreptococos e pode induzir estimulação antigênica, especialmente após repetidas doses. Esses anticorpos anti-EQ também podem reduzir a eficácia do fármaco. Em cães e gatos, a estreptoquinase é tipicamente administrada na dose de 90.000 UI IV, ao longo de 1 h, seguida de infusão de 45.000 UI/hora, por até 12 h. Em um estudo, constatou-se que os oito gatos tratados apresentaram, durante a fase de manutenção, angústia respiratória e morreram repentinamente.[36] Em um segundo estudo, notou-se que, em aproximadamente 50% de 46 gatos com EC, ocorreu retorno do pulso femoral dentro de 24 h após o início do tratamento como EQ;[35] a função motora retornou em 30% dos pacientes, a maioria (80%) em 24 h. Gatos com infarto em um único membro melhoraram sobremaneira; 100% recuperaram o pulso e em 80% houve retorno da função motora. Verificou-se sangramento espontâneo VO, retal ou no local de introdução do cateter em 24% dos gatos e lesão por reperfusão em aproximadamente 40% dos gatos. A hemorragia foi grave o suficiente para requerer transfusão sanguínea em 27% dos gatos; apenas 18% sobreviveram à terapia com EQ. A taxa de sobrevivência total foi de 33% durante a hospitalização. Há um artigo publicado sobre o tratamento com EQ em três cães com TEA.[37] A resolução parcial do trombo foi observada em um cão, enquanto outros 2 tiveram resolução completa após 1 a 3 doses de EQ. Todos os três pacientes apresentaram resolução parcial ou completa dos sinais clínicos com apenas pequeno sangramento, que foi resolvido com a descontinuação da infusão de EQ. Não ocorreu lesão por reperfusão em qualquer um dos cães. A estreptoquinase não está mais disponível nos EUA, embora haja uma disponibilidade limitada em um pequeno número de outros países.

Uroquinase (UQ). Sua atividade é semelhante à da estreptoquinase, mas é considerada mais específica para a fibrina devido às características físicas do composto. As preparações comerciais consistem em ambas, fração de alto peso molecular (APM) e fração de baixo peso molecular (BPM). No mercado há disponibilidade muito maior de produtos com APM, as quais são rápida e continuamente convertidas na forma BPM na circulação sanguínea. A fração APM tem maior afinidade com a forma lisina-plasminogênio do plasminogênio, que se acumula preferencialmente em trombos. Isso confere alguma especificidade da fibrina à UK. A uroquinase foi administrada, por via IV, a gatos e cães com TEA, na dose de carregamento de 4.400 UI/kg, ao longo de 10 min, seguida de 4.400 UI/kg/h, por 12 h.[38,39] Dos 12 gatos tratados, 56% recuperaram a função motora, enquanto em apenas 27% notou-se retorno do pulso. Não foi observado sangramento, mas evidência de lesão por reperfusão foi observada em 25% dos gatos tratados. No geral, 5/12 (42%) sobreviveram ao tratamento.[38] No Reino Unido, a experiência clínica foi muito menos satisfatória em cães, com taxa de mortalidade de 100% em cães tratados.[39] A uroquinase não está mais disponível nos EUA.

Ativador do plasminogênio tecidual (AP-t). É o principal ativador da plasmina *in vivo*; no entanto, ele não se liga prontamente ao plasminogênio circulante. Ambos, o plasminogênio e o AP-t, têm alta afinidade pela fibrina, com estreita relação no interior dos trombos, resultando em conversão fibrinoespecífica do plasminogênio em plasmina. Contudo, a especificidade da fibrina é relativa e, quando o AP-t é administrado em altas doses, podem ocorrer uma condição proteolítica sistêmica e hemorragia.[40]

Há pouquíssima experiência clínica com o uso de AP-t recombinante humano em cães e gatos com TEA espontâneo.[34,41,42] O fármaco tem sido administrado por via intravenosa, tanto na forma de infusão IV contínua em gatos (0,25 a 1 mg/kg/h, na dose total de 1 a 10 mg/kg/h) quanto na forma de terapia de *bolus* múltiplos em cães (1 mg/kg IV). Em dois cães com TEA tratados, um apresentou retorno gradual do pulso arterial femoral[43] após a administração de múltiplos *bolus* de AP-t, enquanto o outro cão não apresentou resposta.[41] Há relato de um teste clínico com terapia com AP-t em seis gatos com EC.[34] As complicações incluíram discreta hemorragia no local de introdução do cateter (50%), febre (33%) e lesão por reperfusão (33%). A taxa de sobrevivência emergencial foi de 50%, sendo as mortes atribuídas a lesão por reperfusão e choque cardiogênico. Dos gatos que sobreviveram, 100% apresentavam infarto de ambos os membros. A perfusão foi restabelecida em 36 h e a função motora retornou em 48 h em 100% dos gatos sobreviventes. O ativador do plasminogênio tecidual atualmente é o único fármaco trombolítico aprovado para uso humano nos EUA.

Melhora do fluxo colateral

Se a dissolução do êmbolo não for bem-sucedida ou não foi tentada, pode-se tentar aumentar a perfusão ao órgão infartado pelo aumento do fluxo por meio da rede de vasos sanguíneos colaterais. O uso de vasodilatadores, como a acepromazina, geralmente não é efetiva, pode resultar em hipotensão clínica e, posteriormente, redução da perfusão sanguínea. Os produtos liberados das plaquetas, serotonina e tromboxano, foram considerados como potenciais responsáveis pela perda do fluxo colateral associado ao infarto da artéria aorta. Portanto, fármacos antiplaquetários podem ajudar a melhorar o fluxo colateral, reduzindo a concentração de substâncias vasoativas liberadas pelas plaquetas. Em gatos, relata-se que o ácido acetilsalicílico reduziu a quantidade de tromboxano liberado pelas plaquetas ativadas e melhorou o fluxo colateral em um modelo experimental de infarto aórtico, mas foi utilizada dose de ácido acetilsalicílico muito alta (associada a intoxicação em casos clínicos).[44] Tem-se demonstrado que o clopidogrel reduz a liberação de serotonina das plaquetas ativadas em gatos, enquanto estudos em outras espécies demonstraram menor produção de tromboxano.[45,46] Há também evidências de que o clopidogrel atua como vasomodulador *ex vivo* (reduz a vasoconstrição) em ratos, coelhos e cães[47,48] e com ação semelhante em gatos *in vivo* utilizados em pesquisa, incluindo abrandamento significativo dos sinais clínicos.[49] Enquanto a ação antitrombótica máxima do clopidogrel é obtida 72 h após a administração diária de 2 a 4 mg/kg VO, em cães e gatos,[45,50] uma dose oral de aproximadamente 10 mg/kg administrada a cães resultou em ação antitrombótica semelhante após 90 min, sem efeitos adversos.[50] Adicionalmente, a administração diária de 75 mg VO, para gatos (≈ 15 mg/kg) foi bem tolerada e não tem sido associada a efeitos adversos. Portanto, embora não haja dados objetivos para sustentar esta afirmação, a administração emergencial de clopidogrel em casos de TEA pode ser útil e melhorar o fluxo colateral sem causar efeitos adversos.

Controle da dor

O TEA pode resultar em dor intensa, e o controle dessa dor é um aspecto criticamente importante do tratamento emergencial de TEA (ver Capítulo 126). Fármacos narcóticos são mais comumente utilizados, com resultado muito bom. Butorfanol (0,1 a 0,4 mg/kg SC IM IV, a cada 1 a 4 h; cães e gatos), hidromorfona (0,08 a 0,3 mg/kg SC IM IV, a cada 2 a 6 h; cães e gatos), buprenorfina (0,005 a 0,02 mg/kg SC IM IV, a cada 6 a 12 h; cães e gatos) ou oximorfona (0,05 a 0,2 mg/kg SC IM IV, a cada 1 a 3 h; cães e gatos) têm sido amplamente utilizados e parecem fornecer boa analgesia com poucos efeitos adversos. Em casos de condições graves ou refratárias, fentanila (4 a 10 mcg/kg na forma de *bolus* IV seguido de 4 a 10 mcg/kg/h IV; cães e gatos). Injeções devem ser aplicadas em local cranial ao diafragma para assegurar boa absorção.

SOBREVIDA

As taxas de sobrevivência relatadas para EC inicial em gatos são notavelmente semelhantes, seja com tratamento conservador (35 a 39%),[18,26,27] seja com terapia trombolítica (33%).[35] Gatos com infarto em um único membro pélvico apresentam melhora mais evidente (68 a 93%)[18,26,27,35] do que gatos com infarto bilateral em membros pélvicos (15 a 36%), independentemente da terapia utilizada.[18,26,27,35] A taxa de pacientes não sobreviventes varia de 61 a 67%, com taxa de mortalidade natural (28 a 40%) semelhante à taxa de eutanásia (25 a 35%).[18,26,27,35] A não sobrevivência tem sido significativamente associada à hipotermia,[18,35] baixa frequência cardíaca[18] e ausência de função motora.[18] A sobrevida mediana relatada a longo prazo, após o evento inicial de CE, variou de 51 a 345 dias.[18,26,27,35,51,52]

PREVENÇÃO

A prevenção primária de TEA é o tratamento que reduz o risco do primeiro evento tromboembólico em um animal com risco de TEA. Embora a prevenção primária seja o ideal e um objetivo lógico, existe uma compreensão insuficiente do risco trombótico em nossos pacientes. Sabemos que algumas condições primárias estão associadas a TEA, mas não podemos prever com precisão quais os animais realmente desenvolverão TEA. O melhor conjunto de evidências está associado a EC em gatos. Os gatos com aumento do átrio esquerdo ou evidência de disfunção sistólica parecem mais sujeitos a TEA.[52] Padrões similares foram detectados no homem. Esses achados combinados com a experiência clínica levaram à recomendação de que a terapia antitrombótica profilática deve ser considerada em gatos com mensurações ecocardiográficas do diâmetro do átrio esquerdo no fim da sístole > 1,7 cm, ou proporção átrio esquerdo-artéria aorta (AE/Ao) > 2.[53] A terapia antitrombótica profilática também é indicada em gatos com contraste espontâneo no átrio esquerdo no ecocardiograma (ver vídeo 256.1).[53]

Em medicina veterinária, a **prevenção secundária** recebeu mais atenção; é definida como a prevenção de novo caso de TEA em um animal com histórico prévio de TEA. Novamente, o maior conjunto de evidências em medicina veterinária está relacionado a EC em gatos. As taxas de recidivas relatadas em estudos retrospectivos não controlados em gatos tratados com algum antitrombótico variaram de 17 a 75%,[18,26,27,34,35] com taxa de recidiva em 1 ano de 25 a 50%.[27,35] Recentemente, o primeiro estudo prospectivo publicado avaliou a prevenção secundária de EC em gatos.[54] TEA Felino – Clopidogrel *versus* Ácido acetilsalicílico (FAT-CAT, do inglês *Feline Arterial Thromboembolism – Clopidogrel versus Aspirin trial*) foi um estudo multicentro duplo-cego aleatório com grupo-controle positivo, que avaliou 75 gatos depois que sobreviveram a um evento de EC. A dose de 18,75 mg de clopidogrel/gato/24 h VO, reduziu significativamente a probabilidade de recidiva de EC, em comparação com o ácido acetilsalicílico, e propiciou maior tempo médio para a ocorrência de recidiva (443 dias *versus* 192 dias). O uso de clopidogrel também foi associado à redução significativa da proporção entre o ponto final composto de recidiva de EC ou morte cardíaca e o tempo médio mais longo para a ocorrência do evento (346 dias *versus* 128 dias).

Fármacos antitrombóticos

Devido ao seu efeito direto na formação do trombo, o uso de fármacos antitrombóticos tornou-se o principal procedimento para prevenção primária e secundária de TEA em cães e gatos. No entanto, deve-se ressaltar que o objetivo da prevenção total de recidivas de eventos embólicos em animais com doenças crônicas, como doença cardíaca ou síndrome nefrótica, provavelmente não é realista. O objetivo deve ser postergar a ocorrência do próximo evento de TEA ou abrandar os sinais clínicos associados ao evento.

Fármacos antiplaquetários

Esses fármacos inibem algumas etapas da aderência, agregação ou reação de liberação plaquetária e interferem na formação do trombo inicial, rico em plaquetas, no local da lesão endotelial. Alguns desses fármacos também apresentam alguma ação vasomoduladora por interferir na ação de substâncias vasoativas, como serotonina e tromboxano.

Ácido acetilsalicílico. É o fármaco antiplaquetário disponível mais utilizado e estudado atualmente. Provoca acetilação irreversível da ciclo-oxigenase plaquetária, impedindo a formação de tromboxano A2, que possui potentes propriedades pró-agregadoras e vasoconstritoras. O ácido acetilsalicílico é considerado um antiplaquetário moderado de ação indireta que inibe a agregação plaquetária secundária, mas não a primária. O ácido acetilsalicílico tem ação semelhante na ciclo-oxigenase endotelial, reduzindo a produção de prostaciclina, uma substância com propriedades antiagregantes e vasodilatadoras. No entanto, as células endoteliais são capazes de superar essa inibição, ao contrário das plaquetas; assim, as propriedades antitrombóticas predominam no cenário clínico. Os efeitos farmacológicos, analgésicos e antiplaquetários do ácido acetilsalicílico foram avaliados em cães e gatos.[55-58] As taxas de recidivas em estudos retrospectivos variaram de 17 a 75%.[18,26,27,34] Os efeitos adversos são tipicamente gastrintestinais (GI; por exemplo, anorexia, vômito) e foram relatados em até 22% dos gatos tratados.[18] Um estudo que avaliou um protocolo com baixa dose de ácido acetilsalicílico não detectou diferença significativa nas taxas de recidivas, em comparação com o uso da dose padrão de ácido acetilsalicílico, porém houve menor taxa de eventos gastrintestinais adversos.[18] No estudo FAT-CAT notou-se apenas um caso de efeitos GI adversos causado pelo ácido acetilsalicílico, embora outro gato tenha morrido em decorrência de um evento de EC recorrente, no qual foi observada uma grande úlcera gástrica durante a necropsia.[54] O protocolo de estudo FAT-CAT exigia que os medicamentos do estudo fossem administrados na forma de cápsula gelatinosa, e isso pode ter resultado em menor irritação gástrica.

Há pouquíssima evidência clínica publicada sobre o uso de ácido acetilsalicílico na prevenção de trombose em cães. Um estudo relatou maior sobrevida em cães com anemia hemolítica imunomediada (AHIM) tratados com dose baixa de ácido acetilsalicílico, além de terapia imunossupressora.[59] Além disso, há um estudo retrospectivo sobre o tratamento de trombose em cães no qual se verificou que 3/9 (33%) pacientes apresentaram melhora ou resolução do trombo.[59a] Há relato de que cães saudáveis que receberam ácido acetilsalicílico desenvolveram lesões endoscópicas gastroduodenais moderadas, inclusive erosão e hemorragia submucosa, embora em dose consideravelmente maior que a dose utilizada clinicamente.[60] Nesse estudo, êmese foi observada em aproximadamente 7% dos cães durante o período de tratamento sem evidência de diarreia.

Clopidogrel. Clopidogrel é uma tienopiridina de segunda geração com ação antagônica específica e irreversível no receptor ADP 2Y12 da membrana plaquetária. Inibe a agregação plaquetária primária e secundária em resposta a múltiplos agonistas. Esses efeitos são mais potentes do que os induzidos pelo ácido acetilsalicílico. A alteração conformacional do complexo glicoproteína IIb/IIIa induzida pelo ADP também é inibida, o que reduz a ligação do fibrinogênio e do fator de von Willebrand.[61] Também prejudica a reação de liberação plaquetária, diminuindo a liberação de agentes pró-agregadores e vasoconstritores, como serotonina e ADP.[46] Efeitos vasomoduladores também foram verificados in vitro e in vivo.[48,49] O composto original não tem ação antiplaquetária; deve sofrer biotransformação hepática para formar um metabólito ativo. Ao contrário do ácido acetilsalicílico, o clopidogrel não está associado à ulceração gastroduodenal. Em gatos normais que receberam 18,75 mg/gato/24 h VO, constatou-se ação antiplaquetária máxima 3 dias após a administração do medicamento e cessou dentro de 7 dias após a descontinuação do medicamento;[45] resultados semelhantes foram observados em cães tratados com 1 a 3 mg/kg/24 h VO.[50,62] A estimulação do sistema enzimático hepático P450 em cães resulta em ação antiplaquetária, em doses mais baixas, presumivelmente devido à maior biotransformação do composto original. Nenhum efeito adverso foi observado durante o estudo, mas há relatos de êmeses esporádicas em gatos que recebem clopidogrel clinicamente, o que pode ser atribuído ao sabor extremamente amargo do fármaco. Em relação à tromboprofilaxia, um pequeno estudo comparou a sobrevida de 90 dias em cães com AHIM tratados com clopidogrel e/ou ácido acetilsalicílico em dose baixa.[63] A maioria dos cães desses grupos sobreviveu nos primeiros 90 dias, com número muito pequeno de casos clínicos suspeitos de trombose e nenhum animal apresentou complicações hemorrágicas. A agregação plaquetária não foi monitorada com nenhum dos fármacos; portanto, não se sabe se havia real efeito da farmacodinâmica do ácido acetilsalicílico ou do clopidogrel. Nos gatos, o clopidogrel está associado a probabilidade significativamente reduzida de EC recidivante em comparação com o ácido acetilsalicílico em gatos (ver ácido acetilsalicílico, já mencionada). Até o momento, em cães ou gatos, não há relatos de casos de agranulocitose ou púrpura trombocitopênica trombótica (PTT), efeitos adversos possíveis em pessoas em tratamento com clopidogrel.

Fármacos anticoagulantes

Este grupo de fármacos inibe a cascata de coagulação, interferindo na formação de um ou mais fatores de coagulação ativos. Alguns desses medicamentos também possuem ação antiplaquetária menor.

Varfarina. A varfarina inibe a formação dos fatores de coagulação dependentes de vitamina K, ou seja, fatores II, VII, IX e X, bem como as proteínas anticoagulantes C e S. Em humanos, após a administração de varfarina, o conteúdo circulante de proteína C diminui antes da redução dos fatores de coagulação, resultando teoricamente em uma condição de hipercoagulação que dura de 4 a 6 dias. Por esse motivo, normalmente a heparina não fracionada (HNF) é administrada durante esse período. A varfarina é indicada em muitas doenças de humanos com risco de TEA, inclusive fibrilação atrial e prótese de valva cardíaca. Numerosos estudos têm demonstrado a eficácia da varfarina como procedimentos primário e secundário da prevenção de EC com fibrilação atrial, mesmo quando são empregados protocolos de anticoagulação de menor intensidade. Em humanos, hemorragia é a complicação mais comum.[64] A varfarina apresenta diversas interações com outros medicamentos que podem aumentar ou diminuir o efeito anticoagulante. No homem, a terapia com varfarina é ajustada por meio do monitoramento de um parâmetro normalizado para diferentes reagentes de tromboplastina em diferentes laboratórios, a razão normalizada internacional (INR, do inglês International Normalized Ratio). Em humanos, recomenda-se intensidade de anticoagulação média (valor de INR 2 a 3) para a maioria das condições.

Estudos farmacocinéticos e farmacodinâmicos em cães e gatos[65,66] demonstraram que a absorção de varfarina após administração oral é rápida. Ocorre recirculação êntero-hepática, o que poderia contribuir para o conhecido intervalo de resposta anticoagulante variável intraindividual.[66] A varfarina não é distribuída uniformemente por todo o comprimido e recomenda-se que seja triturado e preparado por um farmacêutico, em vez de fracionado. É necessário um monitoramento cuidadoso e os tutores devem estar cientes disso antes de iniciar a terapia, pois requer dedicação e gastos por parte do proprietário. Foi recomendado que ajustes na dose de varfarina devem ser feitos alterando-se a dose semanal total e não a dose diária, em resposta ao monitoramento do INR.[67] Enquanto não definido, o valor de INR de 2 a 3 é considerado um indicador de anticoagulação adequado para cães e gatos. Não há testes clínicos objetivos que avaliem a eficácia da varfarina na prevenção de eventos trombóticos para cães e gatos. Em estudos retrospectivos, as taxas de recidivas de EC publicadas para gatos tratados com varfarina variaram de 42 a 53%, com tempo médio estimado de sobrevivência de 210 a 471 dias.[26,35] Hemorragia (ambas, maior e menor) é a complicação mais comum observada em 13 a 20% dos gatos; relata-se hemorragia fatal em até 13% dos gatos.[26,33,35]

Heparinas de baixo peso molecular. O tamanho das heparinas de baixo peso molecular (HBPM) é menor (4.000 a 5.000 dáltons), comparativamente à heparina não fracionada (HNF), mas elas mantêm a sequência de pentassacarídeos que se liga à AT, inibindo o fator Xa, com redução marcante da inibição de IIa. A menor atividade anti-IIa se traduz em ação irrelevante na aPTT e na tromboelastografia (TEG), na terapia com HBPM.[68] Por esse motivo, o monitoramento do tratamento da HBPM é realizado com base na mensuração da atividade anti-Xa.[69,70] Em pessoas com trombose ativa, a terapia com enoxaparina pode induzir ação anti-Xa máxima de 0,6 a 1 UI/mℓ em 4 h e há correlação desse valor com a redução de eventos trombóticos.[69,71] Em humanos, não é comumente aceita a faixa terapêutica da atividade anti-Xa na terapia tromboprofilática com HBPM 1 vez/dia, embora em humanos haja relato de atividade máxima média (em 4 h) de 0,42 UI/mℓ e mediana da atividade mínima (em 24 h) de 0,03 UI/mℓ (variação de 0 a 0,188 UI/mℓ).[72] No homem o efeito adverso mais comum do uso de HBPM é hemorragia menor (5 a 27%) ou maior (0 a 6,5%), semelhante ao que acontece com o uso de HNF.

Em gatos saudáveis,[32,68] relata-se que a dalteparina e a enoxaparina propiciaram resultados semelhantes: atividade anti-Xa máxima em 4 h, a qual diminui para valor abaixo do limite de detecção em 8 h.[32,68] Esses resultados podem sugerir a necessidade de um curto intervalo entre as doses; no entanto, conforme mencionado anteriormente, em humanos a atividade anti-Xa máxima não deve ser mantida durante todo o intervalo entre as doses. De fato, em um modelo de estase venosa modificado, em gatos saudáveis, a enoxaparina (1 mg/kg/12 h SC) resultou em 100% de inibição no desenvolvimento de trombo em 4 h e 91,4% de inibição em 12 h após sua administração. Notou-se fraca correlação entre a ação antitrombótica da enoxaparina e a atividade anti-Xa; no entanto, também não havia atividade anti-Xa mensurável 12 h após a administração do medicamento.[73] Na opinião do autor, a enoxaparina possui efeito antitrombótico no protocolo terapêutico atualmente relatado de 1 mg/kg SC, a cada12 a 24 h, e a atividade anti-Xa máxima precisa obter correlação com a redução de eventos trombóticos em testes clínicos, antes que se possa recomendar a administração de protocolos mais precisos.

Em estudo semelhante com enoxaparina em cães, utilizou-se modelo farmacocinético para avaliar se a atividade anti-Xa era mantida durante todo o intervalo entre doses.[75] Como esse não é o objetivo da terapia com HBPM, pode-se seguir a recomendação da dose atual de 1 mg/kg SC, a cada 12 a 24 h, até que os testes clínicos forneçam informações precisas de dosagem.

Um estudo retrospectivo que comparou o uso de dalteparina e de varfarina na prevenção de recidiva de EC em gatos mostrou semelhantes taxas de recidiva e tempo médio de sobrevida entre os grupos de animais.[33] Nenhum dos gatos tratados com dalteparina manifestou complicações hemorrágicas e notou-se sangramento pouco frequente com a terapia com dalteparina em outro estudo em gatos.[74]

Anticoagulantes mais recentes. Recentemente, foram desenvolvidos novos medicamentos anticoagulantes para comercialização e uso humano, com excelente eficácia; geralmente não requerem monitoramento e o risco de hemorragia é relativamente baixo. O primeiro fármaco que desafiou o domínio clínico da varfarina foi a dabigatrana, um inibidor direto da trombina, cuja ação não era inferior a da varfarina na prevenção de EC associada à fibrilação atrial.[76] Não há estudo publicado conhecido sobre o uso clínico de dabigatrana em cães ou gatos.

Uma classe maior de fármacos consiste em inibidores de Xa. Como sugere o nome, esses medicamentos inibem o fator Xa diretamente ou por meio da potencialização da antitrombina. Também foi demonstrado que sua ação não é inferior à da varfarina na prevenção de EC associada à fibrilação atrial.[77,78] O efeito adverso mais comum é hemorragia, com frequência semelhante à verificada com o uso de HBPM. Até o momento esses medicamentos não foram criticamente avaliados em cães ou gatos, mas os dados farmacológicos básicos estão se acumulando. O fondaparinux é um inibidor sintético do fator Xa que potencializa a ação da antitrombina. Em um pequeno número de gatos saudáveis, constatou-se que o fondaparinux (0,06 mg/kg/12 h SC) induziu atividade anti-Xa que se aproxima dos níveis terapêuticos em humanos.[79] Atualmente, o custo desse protocolo é maior do que o da HBPM, e como não se espera uma resposta clínica superior, o fondaparinux não pode ser fortemente incentivado para uso clínico. Rivaroxabana e apixabana são inibidores diretos de Xa de uso oral aprovados para uso em humanos. Ambos os fármacos apresentam efeito dose-dependente *in vitro* em ensaios de coagulação em gatos.[80,81] Além disso, o apixabana foi usado experimentalmente em cães na prevenção de trombose associada à implantação de valva cardíaca.[82]

É provável que a classe de fármacos inibidores do fator Xa tenha grande impacto na profilaxia clínica nos próximos 5 a 10 anos. É uma opção terapêutica que pode ser administrada por via oral, não requer monitoramento, tem baixo risco de hemorragia, é eficaz em termos de custo e melhoraria sobremaneira o tratamento clínico de cães e gatos em risco de trombose.

REFERÊNCIAS BIBLIOGRÁFICAS

As referências bibliográficas deste capítulo se encontram online no Ambiente de Aprendizagem.

CAPÍTULO 257

Doenças de Veias e Vasos Linfáticos

Brian A. Scansen e John D. Bonagura

Sinais clínicos resultantes de doenças do sistema venoso periférico ou de vasos linfáticos são raramente constatados na prática veterinária. Todavia, doenças desses vasos devem ser considerados no diagnóstico diferencial de cães ou gatos com edema de extremidades (inclusive cabeça e pescoço), em pacientes com efusão cavitária ou em casos inexplicáveis de edema (ver Capítulo 18). Comprometimentos da microcirculação que alteram a pressão hidrostática ou oncótica venosa aumentam a permeabilidade vascular ou linfática, ou que impedem a drenagem venosa ou linfática podem justificar tais sinais clínicos. Essas anormalidades podem ser primárias, incluindo anomalias do desenvolvimento ou síndromes herdadas, ou secundárias à compressão, inflamação ou infiltração de veias ou vasos linfáticos. Este capítulo resume brevemente a fisiologia sistêmica de veias e de vasos linfáticos, técnicas de exame de imagem para avaliação desses leitos vasculares e, por fim, considera condições selecionadas associadas a anomalias sistêmicas de veias ou vasos linfáticos (Boxe 257.1).

FISIOLOGIA DOS FLUXOS LINFÁTICO E VENOSO SISTÊMICOS

As veias sistêmicas atuam como reservatório complacente de baixa pressão para o volume intravascular, com aproximadamente 60% do volume de sangue contido dentro dos vasos.[1] O retorno venoso sistêmico é controlado por várias forças. Estas incluem pressões intravasculares positivas retrógradas (*vis a tergo*) e as pressões intracardíacas mais negativas anterógradas (*vis afronte*) da coluna de sangue venoso; as forças laterais (*vis a latere*), especialmente de contração e relaxamento alternados do músculos esqueléticos; força da gravidade e postura; resistência vascular modulada pelo sistema autônomo, hormônios e mediadores vasoativos locais; e alterações nas pressões intratorácicas operantes durante ambas, ventilação espontânea e ventilação mecânica. No estado saudável essas forças direcionam o sangue sistêmico de volta ao átrio direito, com auxílio de

Boxe 257.1 Anormalidades venosas e linfáticas

Doenças de veias
Flebectasia
Varicose
Flebite e tromboflebite
Trombose venosa
Malformações venosas

Doenças de vasos linfáticos
Linfangite
Linfedema
Linfangiectasia
Hipoplasia, aplasia e hiperplasia linfática
Linfangioma, linfocistos
Linfangiossarcoma

Tumores de vasos sanguíneos periféricos
Angioma, hemangioma, hemangiossarcoma

válvulas venosas unidirecionais que impedem o retorno sanguíneo.[2] Disfunção ou insuficiência de veias sistêmicas, causada por anormalidade nas válvulas venosas, disfunção das bombas musculares, refluxo venoso, dilatação venosa, trombose venosa ou obstrução do fluxo venoso, é ocorrência comum em pessoas.[2] Condições similares em pequenos animais raramente são reconhecidas, embora condições trombóticas ocorram, particularmente quando se utiliza cateter venoso central de longa permanência. Insuficiência venosa e obstrução do fluxo sanguíneo também podem ser secundárias à compressão extraluminal ou estreitamento intraluminal, flebite e trombose.

O sistema linfático desempenha um papel crítico na regulação do volume de líquidos cavitários corporais e do volume de líquido intersticial. Os vasos do sistema linfático também auxiliam na remoção de material inorgânico do tecido subcutâneo e na modulação da absorção de gordura no trato gastrintestinal, contribuindo para o transporte de antígenos e para a vigilância imunológica.[3] Além disso, o sistema linfático é a via metastática preferida para muitos tipos de câncer. Essa diversidade de funções destaca o papel central desempenhado pelo sistema linfático em ambas, na saúde e na doença.

Os vasos linfáticos são oriundos do interstício, na forma de capilares revestidos por endotélio especializados no transporte de líquido, solutos e partículas macromoleculares de volta ao sistema venoso. Líquidos, proteínas, células e partículas macromoleculares do espaço intersticial adentram os vasos linfáticos iniciais, que consistem em uma série de pequenos capilares linfáticos de fundo cego nos tecidos. A linfa, então, flui por um sistema de vasos linfáticos, cujos diâmetros aumentam progressivamente. À medida que a linfa flui para a circulação central, ela passa por pelo menos um linfonodo antes de ser depositada em troncos linfáticos maiores.[4] Os troncos profundos se unem para formar dois vasos linfáticos principais: o ducto linfático torácico e o ducto linfático direito. O ducto torácico drena a maior parte do líquido do corpo e faz retornar o líquido linfático (linfa) para o sistema venoso, na veia braquicefálica ou na veia subclávia esquerda. O ducto linfático direito drena o lado direito da cabeça, o pescoço e o membro torácico direito.

Os vasos linfáticos contêm muitas junções entre as células endoteliais individuais, que estão conectadas ao redor da matriz extracelular formada por fibras reticulares e colágeno. Estas junções se abrem quando a pressão hidrostática do tecido se eleva e os filamentos de ancoragem se estiram, possibilitando a transferência de líquido para dentro do vaso.[5] À medida que o líquido é removido do interstício, as fibras de conexão se contraem e as junções entre as células endoteliais se fecham. A abertura e o fechamento dessas junções permitem atuar como valvas de entrada, impedindo o refluxo da linfa ao interstício. Os vasos maiores do sistema linfático têm progressivamente menos junções abertas, paredes musculares maiores e frequentes valvas intralinfáticas que também impedem o refluxo da linfa. A ação da contração muscular externa, juntamente com a contratilidade intrínseca dos vasos linfáticos, auxilia no movimento da linfa através do sistema linfático e de linfonodos. Enquanto estiver no linfonodo, a linfa está em contato com a circulação sanguínea e aproximadamente metade do líquido é drenado antes de deixar os ductos linfáticos maiores.[4] Além de sua função de transporte, o sistema linfático desempenha um papel importante na resposta imunológica a microrganismos infecciosos e células neoplásicas.[3] Os componentes celulares, em particular os linfócitos, são indispensáveis para reações imunológicas e produção de anticorpos.[3,5]

TÉCNICAS USADAS PARA AVALIAR DOENÇAS VENOSAS E LINFÁTICAS

Angiografia

A angiografia é o teste diagnóstico tradicionalmente utilizado para avaliar doenças vasculares periféricas devido à sua capacidade de caracterizar e permitir a visualização da anatomia vascular normal e anormal. O resultado diagnóstico requer atenção cuidadosa a três elementos importantes: escolha do contraste radiopaco, técnica para distribuição vascular do contraste e alta qualidade da imagem radiográfica.

Conforme discutido no Capítulo 122, as partículas à base de iodo são utilizadas de forma singular como agentes de contraste no sistema vascular. Atualmente, uma segunda geração (iohexol, iopamidol) e uma terceira geração (iodixanol) de agentes de contraste são administradas devido ao melhor perfil de segurança do que o dos agentes de primeira geração. Os fatores a serem considerados ao selecionar um agente de contraste incluem segurança do paciente, qualidade da imagem e custo. Para animais com insuficiência renal, a administração de agentes de contraste deve seguir um protocolo conservador e diurese com administração concomitante de líquido.

A realização de venografia é muito mais fácil do que a linfangiografia e geralmente é menos desafiadora do que a angiografia arterial devido ao acesso vascular mais fácil e à pressão mais baixa no sistema venoso. Um cateter intravenoso de pequeno calibre pode ser introduzido em uma veia superficial, distal ao local suspeito da lesão vascular e injeta-se o contraste. As imagens são obtidas durante e após a injeção, a fim de avaliar a anatomia e a taxa de depuração venosa. A venografia pode ser usada para detectar trombos venosos ou invasão vascular por neoplasia (ambas aparecem como defeitos de preenchimento vascular), estenose venosa (Figura 257.1 e Vídeo 257.1) ou obstrução venosa total. Em imagens fluoroscópicas, pode-se avaliar a insuficiência venosa. A presença de vasos sanguíneos colaterais abundantes sugere obstrução crônica.

A linfangiografia facilita a avaliação regional do sistema linfático. A técnica da linfangiografia indireta depende do agente de contraste infundido no tecido, para ser seletivamente absorvido e transportado através do sistema de vasos linfáticos.[6] A linfangiografia direta é mais desafiadora (a menos que haja linfangiectasia), mas fornece resultados superiores, quando executada com sucesso (Vídeo 257.2). A canulação linfática seletiva requer incisão asséptica na região linfática de interesse (observação: a identificação de linfangiectasia pode ser facilitada pela injeção subcutânea de corante vital [por exemplo, corante azul de Evans 3% ou azul patente 11%] nos vasos venosos plantares ou ingestão de refeição rica em gorduras, para os vasos linfáticos intestinais). O vaso linfático, então, é canulado com uma agulha de calibre 27 ou 30 G ou com cânula linfática especial.[6] Um meio de contraste solúvel à base de iodo, conforme mencionado anteriormente, é então lentamente injetado no vaso. Como os contrastes solúveis aquosos rapidamente difundem-se através das paredes dos tecidos linfáticos adjacentes, os detalhes radiográficos ficam obscuros, a menos que radiografias sejam obtidas logo após a injeção do contraste. Alternativamente, são utilizados agentes de contraste contendo iodo oleoso (p. ex., lipiodol), reduzindo o extravasamento de contraste dos vasos linfáticos. Os contrastes oleosos são retidos nos vasos linfáticos e linfonodos ao longo das vias de drenagem; em humanos, alguns relatos sugerem que a linfangiografia com esse agente pode até ser curativa para extravasamento quiloso.[7] Durante a linfangiografia, pode-se notar permeabilidade dos vasos linfáticos, além do tamanho dos linfonodos regionais. Doença metastática nos linfonodos ou granulomas aparecem como defeitos de preenchimento no linfonodo repleto de contraste. Linfangiografia também pode ser realizada para identificar o local do extravasamento ou a localização do ducto torácico em pequenos animais com derrame quiloso.[8-10]

Diagnóstico ultrassonográfico

A ultrassonografia é uma técnica direta e não invasiva de avaliação de anormalidades venosas, patência e função.[11,12] O ultrassom pode auxiliar no diagnóstico de trombose venosa, aneurisma, doença vascular traumática e compressão de estruturas vasculares no local do processo patológico (Figura 257.2). Métodos especiais de ultrassonografia têm sido utilizados em pessoas para obter imagem da entrada venosa do ducto torácico, mas esse método ainda não foi relatado em cães e gatos.

A ultrassonografia duplex consiste na obtenção de imagem bidimensional em escala de cinza, simultaneamente ao Doppler pulsado e Doppler de fluxo colorido.[12,13] A presença de trombo, corpo estranho, compressão e anatomia vascular anormal pode ser detectada na imagem bidimensional.[13] A sobreposição das imagens obtidas no Doppler de fluxo colorido à imagem bidimensional pode facilitar a definição da anatomia e a detecção de turbulência associada a malformação vascular e lesões estenosantes.[11] A falha em comprimir uma veia aplicando-se pressão com o transdutor do ultrassom sobre a veia é indicativo de

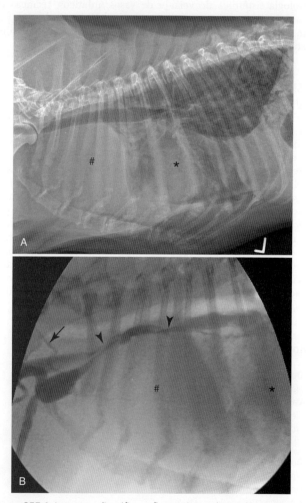

Figura 257.1 Imagens radiográficas e fluoroscópicas de cão da raça Labrador Retriever de 10 anos de idade com timoma. Uma grande massa de tecido mole (#) está presente cranialmente ao coração (asterisco) na radiografia lateral do tórax, como mostra a imagem **A**, com pouca efusão pleural aparente. Venografia não seletiva via cateter cefálico é mostrada na imagem **B**, revelando estreitamento e compressão extraluminal da uma veia cava cranial (pontas de seta) e desenvolvimento de varicosidades venosas colaterais (seta).

CAPÍTULO 257 • Doenças de Veias e Vasos Linfáticos

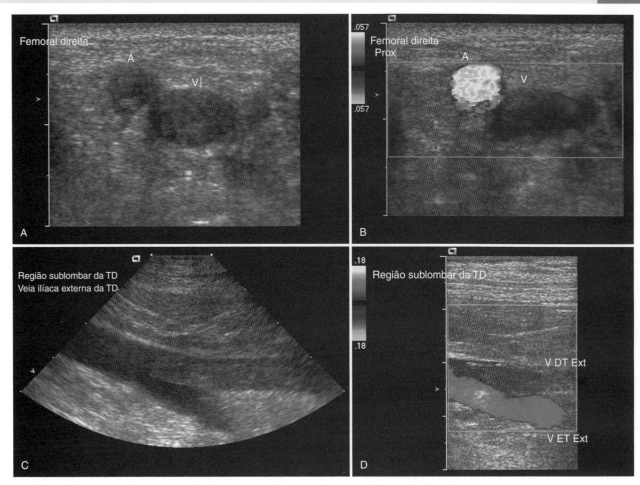

Figura 257.2 Imagens obtidas em ultrassonografia e Doppler colorido das artérias e veias ilíacas e femorais de um cão mestiço de 9 anos de idade com peritonite séptica e coagulação intravascular disseminada. A imagem de corte transversal em **A** mostra que o lúmen da veia (V) femoral direita (TD) é preenchido com um trombo hiperecoico não compressível, enquanto **B** mostra Doppler de fluxo colorido na artéria (A) femoral proximal (Prox) normal, mas fluxo quase ausente na veia (V). **C** e **D**. Imagens sagitais das veias ilíacas externas (Ext), com trombo hiperecoico e obstrução do fluxo na veia ilíaca externa direita (V DT Ext), comparado ao lúmen patente e fluxo na veia ilíaca externa esquerda (V ET Ext). (As figuras B e D encontram-se reproduzidas em cores no Encarte.)

trombose parcial ou total.[13] A avaliação ultrassonográfica da duração do fluxo venoso reverso após a manobra de Valsalva ou a compressão e o relaxamento do músculo da panturrilha são testes diagnósticos para insuficiência venosa em humanos, mas sua realização é um desafio, se não impossível, em animais.[14]

Linfocintilografia

A linfocintilografia consiste na injeção de um marcador radioativo, monitorado por uma câmera gama. Embora comumente empregado em medicina humana para avaliação da drenagem linfática e estadiamento oncológico,[15] não é rotineiramente utilizado em medicina veterinária. A linfocintilografia para avaliação da drenagem linfática das glândulas mamárias de cães já foi descrita.[16]

Imagens transversais

Atualmente é possível obter imagem tridimensional de estruturas vasculares por meio de angiografia por tomografia computadorizada (ATC) ou de angiografia por ressonância magnética (ARM). Ambas, ATC (Figura 257.3) e ARM (Figura 257.4), foram empregadas na avaliação de estruturas vasculares em animais.[17-19] O benefício de imagens transversais, como aquelas obtidas em ATC ou ARM, é que elas substituem o cateterismo central seletivo, pois esses procedimentos requerem apenas acesso venoso periférico. A maior parte da literatura publicada sobre essas técnicas visou avaliar o delineamento anatômico de desvios portossistêmicos,[17,20,21] embora possam ser utilizadas para a avaliação de qualquer outra estrutura vascular. Recomenda-se o bloqueio respiratório ou fazer com que o animal prenda a respiração, ou mantê-lo em apneia durante o período do exame, a fim de evitar movimentos durante a realização do exame, principalmente quando se faz avaliação das veias abdominais ou torácicas; isso pode não ser necessário para ATC dos vasos dos membros.

Além de impedir ou prender a respiração, o método de processamento e visualização das imagens obtidas durante ATC ou ARM pode melhorar sobremaneira as informações obtidas no exame. Visualizadores que propiciam projeções de intensidade máxima (PIM), projeções de intensidade mínima e volume tridimensional, com capacidade de arquivar imagens, podem facilitar a interpretação da imagem, particularmente em estudos vasculares. A PIM é uma técnica na qual há visualização de imagens em que o programa de computador cria uma única imagem projetando o *voxel* (menor unidade em espessura na imagem tomográfica) como um valor de atenuação máxima em uma série de imagens, ou placa, em uma imagem bidimensional. Quando as séries de imagens são processadas dessa maneira, todo o curso do vaso e sua relação com as estruturas circundantes podem ser mais claramente observados. A imagem tridimensional do volume de um ATC permite que a relação espacial completa da vasculatura seja realizada e pode melhorar muito a cirurgia ou o planejamento da intervenção.

Exclusivamente na ARM, as técnicas de imagem estão disponíveis para a clara visualização do sangue, em imagem, sem necessidade de administração de contraste (Figura 257.4). Os agentes

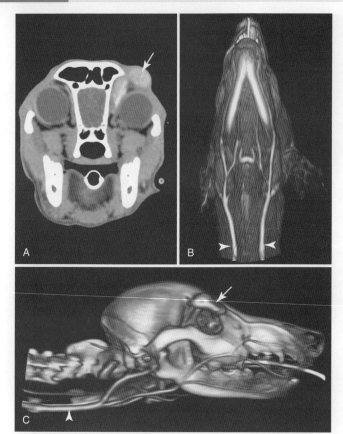

Figura 257.3 Angiotomografia realizada com tomografia computadorizada de uma variz venosa acima do olho direito de um cão da raça Dachshund de 6 meses de idade. Aplicou-se contraste iodado por meio de injeção intravenosa periférica, realizando-se varredura cronometrada até a chegada do contraste à lesão de interesse. Nesse caso, a imagem transversal mostrada em **A** é uma imagem axial da cabeça, com grande estrutura venosa (*seta*) acima e medial à órbita direita. As reconstruções tridimensionais nas projeções ventral (**B**) e lateral (**C**) mostram sobreposição da anatomia das estruturas venosas e musculoesqueléticas à veia jugular externa, indicada por pontas de seta e uma variz indicada pela *seta*. (*Esta figura se encontra reproduzida em cores no Encarte.*)

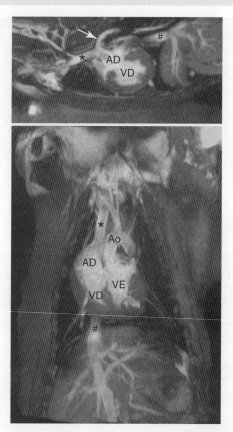

Figura 257.4 Angiografia por ressonância magnética (ARM) do coração e dos grandes vasos de um cão da raça Scottish Terrier, macho, com 2 anos de idade, com estenose da valva pulmonar. A ARM sem contraste, com imagens de sangue claras, realça a anatomia venosa e arterial, possibilitando a visualização das veias cavas cranial (*asterisco*) e caudal (*#*), veia ázigos (*seta*), átrio direito (*AD*), ventrículo direito (*VD*), ventrículo esquerdo (*VE*) e arco aórtico (*Ao*).

de contraste ainda podem ser utilizados e são preferidos em alguns estudos (como varredura de perfusão), mas podem não ser necessários para o delineamento anatômico de vasos sanguíneos.

A linfangiografia por tomografia computadorizada é comumente empregada em pessoas para avaliar estruturas linfáticas e tem sido aplicada para obtenção de imagem em cães (Figura 257.5), particularmente para avaliação da anatomia do ducto torácico antes de cirurgia para quilotórax idiopático (Vídeo 257.3).[9,22,23] A melhor detecção de ramos linfáticos e subtração digital da sobreposição de estruturas anatômicas são dois benefícios notados na linfangiografia por TC, em relação à linfangiografia radiográfica em cães.[9] Atualmente realiza-se linfangiografia por ressonância magnética em humanos,[24,25] como estudo preliminar, sugerindo utilidade similar em medicina veterinária.

DOENÇAS DE VEIAS

As doenças do sistema venoso raramente resultam em morbidade em pequenos animais, embora a presença de trauma, tromboembolismo, edema, inflamação local, invasão tumoral e doenças sépticas comumente acomete as veias. Muitas dessas condições, no entanto, não são reconhecidas. Doenças venosas incluem lesões traumáticas, flebites superficial e profunda, trombose (tromboflebite), embolização causada por cateter, aneurismas, síndromes de compressão venosa e varizes.

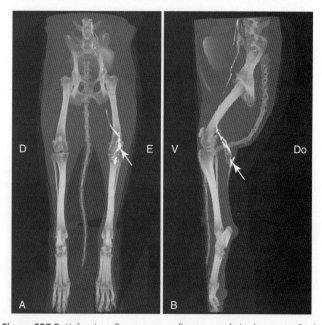

Figura 257.5 Linfangiografia por tomografia computadorizada em um cão da raça Irish Wolfhound de 6 anos de idade com linfedema no membro pélvico esquerdo. Imagens em projeção tridimensional de intensidade máxima dos membros posteriores e da pelve em perspectiva dorsal (**A**) e sagital (**B**) realçam drenagem linfática normal no membro posterior esquerdo, após injeção de contraste iodado, no linfonodo poplíteo esquerdo (*seta*). Note o discreto edema de tecidos moles no membro distal esquerdo, compatível com linfedema de etiologia desconhecida. *D*, direito; *Do*, dorsal; *E*, esquerdo; *V*, ventral.

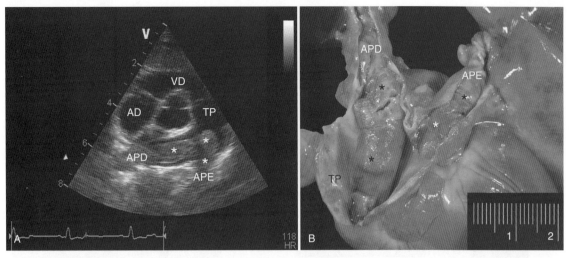

Figura 257.6 Grande trombo pulmonar em um cão da raça Cavalier King Charles Spaniel de 6 anos de idade. **A.** O ecocardiograma destaca um grande trombo hiperecoico (*asterisco*) que obstruiu as artérias pulmonares direita (*APD*) e esquerda (*APE*) e estendeu-se para o tronco pulmonar (*TP*). **B.** Imagem de necropsia do mesmo cão, revelando trombo organizado (*asterisco*) em todo o TP e ramos das artérias pulmonares. *AD*, átrio direito; *VD*, ventrículo direito.

Os trombos venosos se formam na circulação venosa quando há baixo fluxo sanguíneo e são compostos de fibrina e eritrócitos. Considera-se que os trombos venosos se desenvolvem secundariamente aos componentes clássicos da tríade de Virchow: estase de fluxo, lesão endotelial e condição de hipercoagulação.[26] Trombose venosa causa menos anormalidades clínicas evidentes do que a trombose arterial e, consequentemente, muitas vezes não é detectada. A trombose venosa profunda é um importante fator de risco para embolia pulmonar no homem, mas não é considerada um fator de risco de tromboembolismo pulmonar em animais. O tromboembolismo pulmonar (TEP) é uma doença comum e muitas vezes com complicações com risco à vida do paciente associadas a diversas doenças sistêmicas e metabólicas. Um trombo formado nas veias periféricas, veia cava e/ou no lado direito do coração pode causar embolia na artéria pulmonar. O desenvolvimento de TEP pode ocorrer em vários casos de doença protrombótica, inclusive síndrome nefrótica, hiperadrenocorticismo, anemia hemolítica imunomediada, trombocitose, doença cardíaca, sepse, coagulação intravascular disseminada, dirofilariose e neoplasia.[27-35] A deficiência de antitrombina (AT) pode estar envolvida na trombogênese, em várias dessas doenças, alterando a química intravascular do sangue e aumentando o risco de trombose. Na anemia hemolítica imunomediada, por exemplo, a hemólise libera substâncias trombogênicas.[34] A trombina e outros fatores de coagulação são inibidos pela AT, de tal forma que mesmo uma leve redução na concentração de AT pode resultar em trombose ou tromboembolismo. A presença de múltiplos distúrbios concomitantes em animais com tromboembolismo é comum. Por exemplo, 47% dos gatos submetidos à necropsia e confirmados com TEP apresentavam várias anormalidades predisponentes.[36] Também podem ocorrer grandes trombos pulmonares *in situ*, relatados principalmente em cães da raça Cavalier King Charles Spaniel[37] (Figura 257.6) e em cães ou gatos com dirofilariose (ver Capítulo 255). O tromboembolismo pulmonar é discutido em detalhes no Capítulo 243.

Varicose venosa, uma condição que consiste em tortuosidade e dilatação de veias, é rara em cães e gatos (Figura 257.7). Quando detectadas, as varizes venosas podem ser acompanhadas de fístulas arteriovenosas[38] ou se desenvolver como consequência de obstrução venosa crônica (ver Figura 257.1). Uma revisão recente classificou quatro vias de fluxo venoso colateral na obstrução da veia cava caudal em cães.[39] A flebectasia cutânea é uma lesão benigna às vezes erroneamente chamada telangiectasia. É relatada quase exclusivamente em cães com síndrome de Cushing espontânea ou iatrogênica (ver Capítulo 306).[40] A flebectasia é uma dilatação, extensão ou reduplicação anormal das veias ou de capilares ou uma combinação dessas alterações.

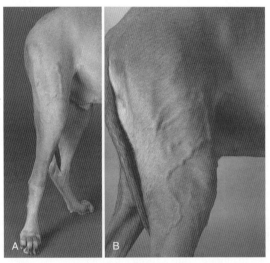

Figura 257.7 Veias varicosas em um cão da raça Mastiff, macho, de 4 anos de idade, com histórico de trombocitopenia imunomediada, edema e tumefação do membro pélvico direito e suspeita de trombose venosa profunda. Note veias superficiais dilatadas e tortuosas que se desenvolveram para propiciar drenagem colateral como visto nas imagens cranial (**A**) e lateral (**B**).

A perfuração venosa ou trauma contuso nas veias geralmente é bem tolerada porque a rápida coagulação resulta em oclusão venosa e impede hemorragias graves. Quando há ampla oclusão venosa, o edema e a cianose resultantes são geralmente temporários, razão da circulação colateral. Se todas as veias de drenagem da região forem comprometidas, podem surgir edema e necrose acentuados. Trauma contuso tem sido associado à obstrução da veia cava ou torção da veia cava caudal intratorácica e ascite subsequente.[41-43]

As malformações venosas são achados acidentais frequentes e podem se manifestar como duplicação, interrupção, transposição ou conexão anômala; a persistência da veia cava cranial esquerda é digna de atenção.[44] Em cães e gatos normalmente a veia cava cranial situa-se no lado direito. Quando a veia embriológica cardeal anterior esquerda não regride nessas espécies, ocorre persistência da veia cranial esquerda (ver Capítulo 250). A veia cava cranial esquerda pode ocorrer individualmente ou, mais frequentemente, notam-se ambas, veias cavas craniais esquerda e direita (Figura 257.8; ver também Figuras 250.45 e 250.46, no Capítulo 250). Buchanan descreveu dois tipos de

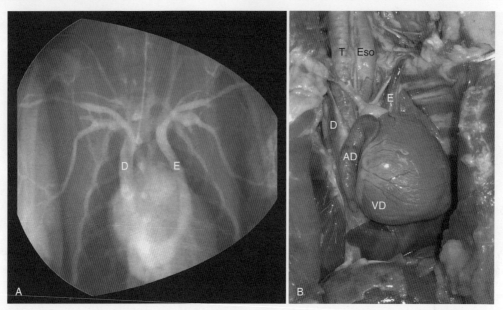

Figura 257.8 Imagens de uma cadela mestiça de 7 anos de idade com persistência de veia cava cranial esquerda e estenose da valva pulmonar. **A.** Veias cavas craniais bilaterais separadas e veia cava cranial direita normal (*D*) e veia cava cranial esquerda persistente (*E*); note a entrada da veia cava cranial esquerda persistente no seio coronariano, na face caudal do átrio direito. **B.** Imagem de necropsia do mesmo animal com as duas veias cavas aparentes. *AD*, átrio direito; *Eso*, esôfago; *VD*, ventrículo direito; *T*, traqueia.

veia cava cranial esquerda persistente no cão: completa e incompleta.[45] A veia cava cranial esquerda se conecta na face caudoventral do átrio direito, na região do seio coronariano, em contraste com a entrada da veia cava cranial direita na face cranial do coração. A persistência da veia cava cranial esquerda geralmente não causa problema clínico ao animal, embora um relato de caso de veia cava cranial persistente incompleta em um cão da raça Brittany Spaniel tenha sugerido a possibilidade de essa estrutura causar megaesôfago, se houver atresia parcial.[46] Anomalias venosas de transposição são comuns em animais, como, por exemplo, persistência do arco aórtico direito. Pode haver relatos de implantação de marca-passo e extração de dirofilariose através de uma veia cava cranial esquerda persistente,[47,48] embora essa abordagem cirúrgica seja tecnicamente mais desafiadora do que a técnica padrão.

Anomalias venosas adicionais têm sido relatadas. Notavelmente, ausência unilateral da veia jugular externa esquerda já foi descrita no gato[49] e o autor já observou ausência de veia jugular externa direita em dois cães da raça Buldogue Inglês.[50] A veia ázigos esquerda está presente em algumas espécies, mas é tipicamente ausente em cães e gatos. Se presente, é remanescente do sistema supracardinal esquerdo, que também adentra o seio coronário. Há relatos ocasionais de casos de veia ázigos esquerda como única fonte de retorno venoso caudal, se concomitante com interrupção da veia cava caudal.[51,52] Numerosas anormalidades da veia cava caudal têm sido relatadas em animais.[18,53-63] A veia cava caudal pode exibir duplicação, transposição para a esquerda ou interrupção com continuação com a veia ázigos; essas malformações estão às vezes associadas a desvio (*shunt*) portossistêmico (ver Capítulo 284). A maioria dessas malformações não causa sinais clínicos (a menos que concomitantes com *shunt*/desvio portocaval), mas podem ser detectadas durante exploração cirúrgica ou exame de diagnóstico por imagem e, portanto, devem ser levadas em consideração. As malformações venosas ou hemangiomas venosos podem ser considerados como crescimentos vasculares benignos que podem se desenvolver localmente ou podem se disseminar, consistindo em um espectro de anormalidades anatomicamente classificadas como malformações capilares, linfáticas, venosas ou arteriovenosas.[64,65] A literatura veterinária ainda não definiu completamente um esquema de classificação ou nomenclatura padronizada para essas lesões em animais, embora uma revisão histopatológica de tumores vasculares tenha sugerido uma classificação semelhante a de humanos.[66] As malformações arteriovenosas são discutidas com mais detalhes no Capítulo 284.

Dilatação cística das veias também pode ocorrer; dilatação venosa ou aneurisma geralmente permitem apenas fluxo sanguíneo de baixa velocidade e as pequenas lesões são assintomáticas. A expansão da lesão pode ocorrer, especialmente após trauma. Trombose pode resultar de fluxo sanguíneo lento e consequente sensibilidade e tumefação localizadas. Lesões maiores em áreas dependentes podem aumentar, causando dilatação vascular relevante, com risco potencial de alterações na cor da pele, ulceração dérmica e hemorragia. As áreas afetadas se apresentam como locais com hipertermia, moles e com massa compressível. Não se constata pulso arterial ou ruído devido ao baixo fluxo sanguíneo. A dor pode ser decorrência da pressão exercida nos tecidos e nervos profundos. O diagnóstico se baseia no histórico clínico, nos achados de exame físico e na ultrassonografia. Pode ser necessária venografia ou imagem transversal, como ATC ou ARM, para definir a lesão, particularmente no caso de aneurisma intra-abdominal.[67] A terapia sintomática com o uso de bandagens compressivas suaves às vezes é útil no controle emergencial. A excisão cirúrgica dos vasos afetados é ocasionalmente necessária, mas a ressecção completa é difícil e a recidiva da lesão no local é comum.

Aneurisma venoso raramente é reconhecido em medicina veterinária. Há relatos de aneurismas na veia jugular externa, veia linguofacial e veias maxilares, assim como na veia cava cranial.[68-70] Nesses casos, as lesões foram consideradas anomalias vasculares congênitas, não associadas a um processo obstrutivo ou traumático. O autor já detectou aneurisma na veia caudal em associação à interrupção da veia cava caudal e continuação da veia ázigos em um cão (Figura 257.9). Quinze casos de aneurismas venosos portais foram descritos em uma revisão de angiografia por tomografia computadorizada (ATC) em mais de 3 mil cães; nenhum dos cães desse estudo mostrou sinais clínicos, embora trombose venosa portal no local de um aneurisma tenha sido descrita em um caso.[67]

Embolização de fragmentos de cateter intravascular é uma complicação ocasional do uso de cateter intravenoso.[71-73] No homem, complicações relacionadas à embolização por cateter incluem perfuração da parede cardíaca, endocardite, embolia pulmonar e arritmias cardíacas graves.[74,75] Portanto, geralmente é considerado prudente remover os fragmentos de cateter. A remoção

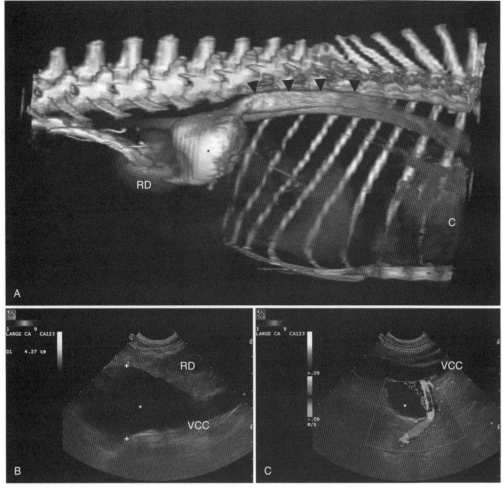

Figura 257.9 Imagens obtidas de um cão da raça Greyhound, macho, de 10 anos de idade, com interrupção da veia cava caudal pré-hepática, continuação da veia ázigos e grande aneurisma na veia cava (*asterisco*). **A.** Reconstrução tridimensional sagital de uma angiotomografia computadorizada mostrando grande dilatação do aneurisma na veia cava caudal e continuação por toda a veia ázigos (*pontas de seta*). **B** e **C.** Imagens de ultrassonografia em escala de cinza (**B**) e em Doppler colorido (**C**) do aneurisma, que mede cerca de 4,3 cm de diâmetro. *C*, coração; *RD*, rim direito; *VCC*, veia cava caudal. (*Esta figura se encontra reproduzida em cores no Encarte.*)

não cirúrgica e transvenosa de fragmentos de cateter usando cateter de laço, pinça e cateter em cesta foi descrita em animais.[72,73] Sempre que possível devem ser tomadas medidas para evitar situações que predispõem à fragmentação do cateter, inclusive contenção inadequada durante a colocação do cateter, retirada do cateter por meio de sua agulha de colocação durante o reposicionamento, falha na fixação adequada do cateter ao paciente, corte inadvertido do cateter durante a substituição da bandagem e uso de cateter cardíaco reesterilizados, porém danificados.

Flebite pode ocorrer a partir de um processo inflamatório local estendendo-se para veias ou pode originar-se de uma lesão na camada íntima da veia. As causas comuns de lesões à camada íntima das veias são injeção perivenosa ou intravenosa de fármacos irritantes, infusão de grande quantidade de líquido e manutenção do cateter por longo período. A flebite relacionada à infusão ocorre por três causas: (1) química (lesão à veia causada por fármacos irritantes), (2) física (traumatismo na camada íntima provocado por cateter, agulha, hipertonicidade ou problemas particulares do líquido infundido) e (3) microbianos (líquido, pele ou extremidade do cateter contaminados). Ambas, tromboflebite estéril ou tromboflebite séptica, podem ocorrer como consequência. A tromboflebite é tipicamente localizada e é caracterizada por dor, edema e exsudação (Figura 257.10). Pacientes com doenças graves ou sistema imunológico comprometido, no entanto, podem desenvolver sepse, pneumonia tromboembólica ou endocardite.

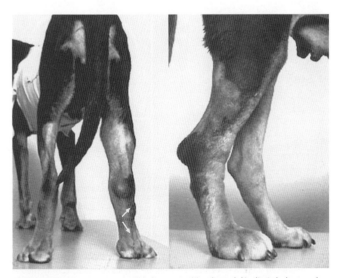

Figura 257.10 Imagens caudal (*à esquerda*) e lateral (*à direita*) do membro pélvico direito de um cão jovem com edema grave causado por tromboflebite. O problema se desenvolveu após a colocação de cateter na veia safena. O membro está marcadamente edemaciado e há extravasamento do edema (*setas*) através de uma pequena úlcera cutânea. A trombose venosa impede a drenagem venosa e aumenta a formação de líquido linfático.

A flebite é uma das causas principais de dano à camada íntima das veias, levando à trombose venosa. A trombose, geralmente, tem pouca consequência local se ocorrer em vasos pequenos. Porém, o êmbolo pode ser carreado para o pulmão e causar tromboembolismo pulmonar (TEP). Na maioria dos animais, os coágulos sanguíneos transportados para o pulmão são rapidamente fragmentados e não causam complicações. Todavia, quando há doença inflamatória, desidratação ou insuficiência circulatória, a formação de trombos pode continuar nos vasos pulmonares e levar à oclusão vascular, dispneia, dor e morte.[31] Na tromboflebite infecciosa, êmbolos bacterianos podem ser carreados para os pulmões e causar pneumonia tromboembólica. Trombose venosa espontânea é rara, embora trombose do sistema venoso portal, inclusive nas veias esplênicas, seja ocasionalmente diagnosticada em cães (Figura 257.11).[76] Na maioria dos casos, doenças hepáticas primárias ou condições associadas à condição protrombótica (nefropatia com perda de proteínas, anemia hemolítica imunomediada ou hiperadrenocorticismo) ou compressão (torção esplênica) são identificadas.[76] Os sinais clínicos incluem ascite, dor abdominal, desvio (*shunt*) portossistêmico adquirido e choque hipovolêmico.[76]

Nos casos de oclusão venosa, os sinais clínicos dependem da localização anatômica, extensão e duração da obstrução. A obstrução aguda de veias centrais, veias sistêmicas profundas, causa edema, cianose, desconforto e dilatação venosa distal ao local da obstrução. Obstrução da veia cava cranial causa edema no pescoço, na cabeça, nos membros torácicos e nas porções dependentes da parte cranial do tórax (Figura 257.12; ver Capítulo 18). A efusão pleural geralmente resulta de lesão obstrutiva em veia central. As causas comuns de obstrução da veia cava cranial incluem tumores no mediastino cranial, cateter venoso central de uso prolongado e eletrodos de marca-passo transvenoso.[77-85] Em animais com ascite e edema subcutâneo também há relato de sinais clínicos resultantes de torção, compressão, obstrução neoplásica ou trombose da veia cava caudal intratorácica (Figura 257.13).[41,86-89] As obstruções do sistema venoso intra-abdominal ou do sistema venoso pélvico causam edema em membros pélvicos e escroto. Os sinais clínicos dependem da quantidade de vasos sanguíneos colaterais e da capacidade dos vasos linfáticos regionais em drenar o líquido intersticial e seroso da cavidade. Além da trombose, causas de obstrução venosa incluem neoplasias malignas invasivas e compressão venosa causada por abscessos, hematomas, tumores e linfadenopatia. Vários tumores tendem a invadir a veia, entre eles quimiodectomas, tumores adrenais, como feocromocitoma e hemangiossarcomas (Figura 257.14). A angiografia pode indicar lesão oclusiva ou compressiva, ou evidenciar aumento da circulação colateral (ver Figura 257.1). O exame ultrassonográfico é útil para detectar massas ou anormalidades de fluxo; ATC ou ARM pode definir a anatomia tridimensional da obstrução e avaliar as causas extraluminais (Figura 257.14). O prognóstico e a terapia da obstrução venosa dependem da doença primária. Estes temas são discutidos em vários capítulos deste livro.

DOENÇAS DE VASOS LINFÁTICOS PERIFÉRICOS

As anormalidades linfáticas podem ser aquelas de órgãos internos, como linfangiectasia intestinal, e os distúrbios linfáticos

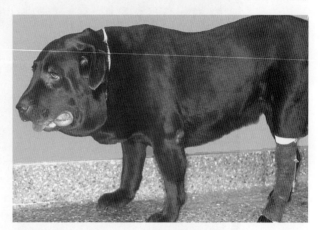

Figura 257.12 Síndrome da veia cava cranial em um cão, causada por tumor de mediastino e compressão da veia cava cranial. Nota-se edema periférico intenso na extremidade cranial.

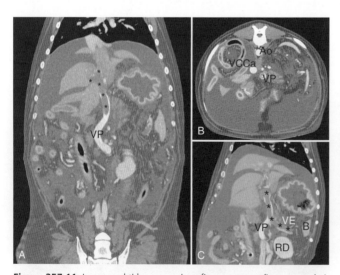

Figura 257.11 Imagens obtidas em angiografia por tomografia computadorizada de um cão da raça Doberman Pinscher de 2 anos de idade, com trombose das veias esplênica e porta. Reconstruções de projeção de intensidade máxima dorsal (**A**), transversal (**B**) e fora do eixo (**C**) mostram uma estrutura hipoatenuante compatível com trombo (*asterisco*) no lúmen da veia esplênica que se estende para o tronco portal e ramos intra-hepáticos. Ascite moderada também é aparente. *Ao*, aorta; *B*, baço; *RD*, rim direito; *VCCa*, veia cava caudal; *VE*, veia esplênica; *VP*, veia porta.

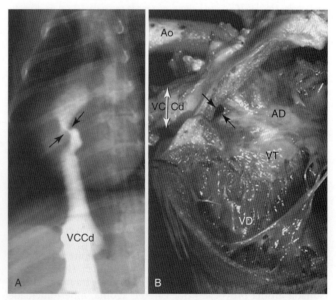

Figura 257.13 Estenose adquirida (fibrose) da veia cava caudal em um cão idoso. **A.** Angiograma da veia cava caudal (*VCCd*), verificando-se estreitamento marcante da coluna do corante (*setas*) na conexão da veia com o átrio direito caudal. **B.** Imagem *post mortem* do coração obtida em perspectiva lateral direita. As paredes do átrio e do ventrículo direito foram retraídas para mostrar a estenose do lúmen da veia cava (pequenas setas). Compare essa abertura com o diâmetro da veia cava caudal (à esquerda, seta dupla vertical). São mostrados: ventrículo direito (*VD*), valva tricúspide (*VT*), átrio direito (*AD*) e artéria aorta descendente (*Ao*).

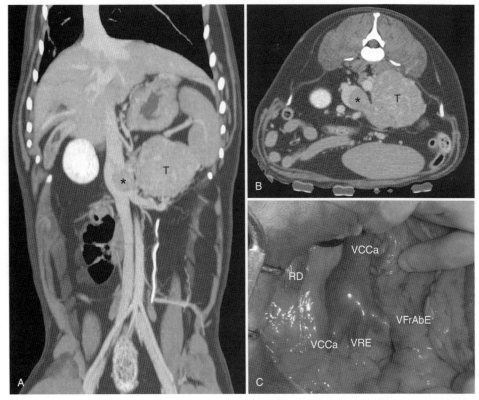

Figura 257.14 Imagens de um cão mestiço com 11 anos de idade com feocromocitoma adrenal esquerdo. O tumor (*T*) invadiu a veia frenicoabdominal e pode-se notar que o trombo tumoral (*asterisco*) se estende para o lúmen da veia cava caudal. A exposição cirúrgica do mesmo cão é vista em **C**, destacando a anatomia da veia cava caudal (*VCCa*), veia renal esquerda (*VRE*), veia frenicoabdominal esquerda (*VFrAbE*) e rim direito (*RD*). O tumor e o rim esquerdo não são visíveis, obscurecidos pelo omento. (Imagem cirúrgica; cortesia de Kathleen Ham, DACVS.)

periféricos. Diversas doenças linfáticas, incluindo linfedema, linfangiectasia intestinal, quilotórax, linfadenite, linfocistos, linfoma, linfangioma e linfangiossarcoma, foram reconhecidas em animais. Os tipos e as causas das doenças de vasos linfáticos periféricos estão resumidos no Boxe 257.2.

Boxe 257.2 Causas de doenças de vasos linfáticos periféricos

Linfangite, linfedema, linfadenite, linfadenopatia
  Infeção
  Neoplasia
  Hiperplasia reativa
  Granuloma
Linfedema
  Primário – anormalidade de desenvolvimento de vaso linfático
    Hipoplasia
    Aplasia
    Linfangectasia
    Hiperplasia
  Secundário – anormalidades adquiridas de vaso linfático
    Excisão cirúrgica do vaso linfático ou do linfonodo
    Linfangiopatia pós-traumática
    Invasão neoplásica
    Compressão extrínseca de vasos linfáticos ou tecidos
    Linfadenite obstrutiva aguda
    Linfadenite esclerosante crônica/linfangite
    Atrofia linfática com fibrose intersticial
    Terapia por radiação
  Linfocistos
Higroma cístico, linfocele, pseudocisto
Linfangiomas
Linfangiossarcomas

Doenças inflamatórias de vasos linfáticos (linfangite e linfadenite)

Linfangite e linfadenite geralmente são secundárias à inflamação local, particularmente envolvendo a pele, as membranas mucosas e os tecidos subcutâneos. A linfangite também pode resultar de infecções bacterianas e fúngicas, doença neoplásica ou doença inflamatória. Os vasos linfáticos podem ser acometidos e ocluídos, à medida que drenam agentes inflamatórios e seus subprodutos dos espaços teciduais. Nos linfonodos (ou gânglios linfáticos), os microrganismos são fagocitados e inativados ou mortos por mecanismos humorais e celulares. Durante esse processo, os linfonodos podem sofrer obstrução, aumentar de volume e se apresentarem quentes e dolorosos. Os membros afetados podem apresentar edema local, que pode resultar em claudicação. Pirexia, anorexia e depressão são sintomas comuns; é possível notar leucocitose no caso de linfangite aguda grave.

A linfangite pode se tornar crônica quando associada à lesão granulomatosa ou estática, como corpo estranho, ou à inflamação aguda tratada sem sucesso. A linfangite tem sido associada à coccidioidomicose cutânea em cães e gatos, nos casos de linfadenite intestinal secundária a feridas por mordida, esporotricose e linfangite lipogranulomatosa crônica na enteropatia crônica acompanhada de perda de proteínas (ver Capítulo 276).[90-94] A persistência de edema inflamatório nas infecções cutâneas resulta na proliferação de células mesenquimais que, por sua vez, pode causar espessamento irreversível de pele e de tecido subcutâneo. O prognóstico é variável, dependendo da causa e, em geral, mais favorável se o tratamento for precoce. A terapia consiste em umidificação, calor, compressas ou banhos locais, que reduzem o edema e favorecem a drenagem. O tratamento agressivo com antibiótico, local e sistêmico, geralmente propicia a recuperação dos animais com febre e anorexia. A cultura microbiológica, o teste de sensibilidade bacteriana (antibiograma) e o exame citológico dos linfonodos regionais devem ser realizados em casos de linfangite aguda que não respondem ao tratamento e de linfangite crônica. Exames com uso de contraste e exploração cirúrgica podem ser indicados quando há fístula ou abscesso, ou suspeita de corpo estranho.

Linfedema

Ocorre acúmulo de líquido patológico no interstício quando a taxa de filtração microvascular excede a drenagem linfática.[3] O conceito das forças de Starling envolve a interação entre a pressão oncótica e a pressão hidrostática, associada à permeabilidade vascular, que aciona a filtração microvascular.[5] No leito microvascular, existe uma rede de movimento do líquido ultrafiltrado para o interstício de tal forma que, no caso de fluxo linfático inadequado ou prejudicado, o ultrafiltrado se acumula, levando ao linfedema. Linfedema, especificamente, refere-se ao acúmulo de líquido no espaço intersticial resultante da drenagem linfática anormal.[4] Esse termo não deve ser usado para outras formas de edema, como o edema relacionado à obstrução venosa ou ao edema generalizado relacionado à hipoproteinemia. O líquido rico em proteínas do linfedema (2 a 5 g/dℓ) causa um gradiente osmótico elevado e exacerba o acúmulo de líquido.[95] Numerosos esquemas de classificação foram utilizados para categorizar o linfedema. As categorias etiológicas de linfedema comumente usadas incluem sobrecarga de líquido, inadequação da coleta de linfa nos capilares linfáticos, contratilidade linfática anormal, vasos linfáticos insuficientes, obstrução de linfonodo e defeitos dos ductos linfáticos principais.

Tradicionalmente, um esforço clínico é realizado para diferenciar linfedema primário de secundário. Linfedema primário refere-se a uma anormalidade dos vasos linfáticos ou linfonodos. Linfedema secundário refere-se a doença nos vasos linfáticos ou linfonodos devido a um processo patológico diferente. Linfedema secundário pode ocorrer como resultado de neoplasia, cirurgia, trauma, parasitas, terapia por radiação ou infecção, sendo mais comum que o linfedema primário. Distinguir entre linfedema primário e secundário é frequentemente difícil. Uma doença que envolve um linfonodo pode resultar em fibrose e obstrução, com desenvolvimento secundário de edema.

Linfedema primário

Linfedema primário pode resultar de três anormalidades morfológicas e funcionais principais, incluindo (1) anormalidades de grandes vasos, como aplasia ou hipoplasia do ducto torácico e da cisterna do quilo, (2) aplasia de vasos linfáticos periféricos ou incompetência valvar congênita e (3) fibrose do linfonodo ou deficiência no tamanho e quantidade de linfonodos.[96]

Linfedema causado por aplasia, hipoplasia ou displasia de vasos linfáticos proximais ou linfonodos ocorre com maior frequência nos membros pélvicos de cães jovens (Figura 257.15). O edema pode ser transitório, observado apenas durante o período juvenil, ou permanente. Casos leves são restritos aos membros pélvicos, enquanto casos graves podem progredir para edema em todo o corpo.[97-101] Embora a condição seja frequentemente bilateral, um membro é geralmente mais edemaciado que o outro. Vários casos de suspeita congênita de linfedema foram relatados, embora quase todos representem relatos de casos únicos de décadas atrás.[100-102] Uma série de cães com linfedema primário de origem familiar foi descrita e os estudos dessa família sugeriram uma associação autossômica dominante hereditária, com gravidade variável de sintomas e alta taxa de mortalidade nos cães severamente acometidos.[97,103] As raças de cães relatadas incluem: Buldogue, Poodle, Old English Sheepdog e Labrador Retriever, embora não esteja claro se essas raças são as de maior risco.

O histórico clínico pode esclarecer se há tumefação crônica dos membros desde o nascimento ou se o edema surgiu mais tarde. O edema apresenta magnitude variável; não é quente nem frio (ver Vídeo 18.1, no Capítulo 18). O edema geralmente não é acompanhado de claudicação ou dor, a menos que ocorra grande aumento ou celulite. O crescimento e a atividade são geralmente normais, mas o repouso e a massagem dos membros não reduzem a gravidade do edema. Os linfonodos regionais, normalmente, são proeminentes em filhotes em fase de crescimento, e às vezes são difíceis de se identificar. Em geral, ocorrem alterações pouco evidentes na concentração plasmática de proteína total, no traçado eletroforético de proteínas séricas, no hemograma e no perfil bioquímico sanguíneo. O diagnóstico de linfedema primário é baseado no histórico clínico (idade ao início da anormalidade, progressão da doença, membros afetados e distribuição do edema) e nos sinais clínicos. Cirurgia prévia, trauma ou infecções anteriores devem também ser considerados. Pode ser necessária linfangiografia radiográfica para confirmar o diagnóstico em casos brandos; ademais, esse exame auxilia na determinação da morfologia de sistemas linfáticos anômalos (Figura 257.16).

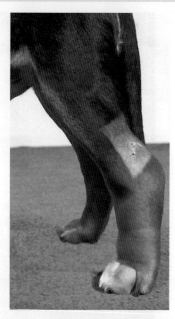

Figura 257.15 Edema acentuado não doloroso no membro pélvico esquerdo de um cão jovem com displasia linfática congênita.

O prognóstico para a resolução do linfedema congênito é reservado e depende da etiologia. Alguns cães que desenvolvem edema de membros pélvicos durante o período neonatal melhoram espontaneamente. Cães com edema grave de membros e tronco têm maior probabilidade de sucumbir nas primeiras semanas após o nascimento.[97,98] A dilatação crônica dos vasos linfáticos leva à disfunção de válvula linfática permanente. Subprodutos metabólicos acumulados levam à deposição de colágeno e fibrose. Complicações como abrasões e infecções recorrentes frequentemente se desenvolvem. Cães com linfedema primário não devem ser usados como reprodutores; conforme mencionado anteriormente, testes de acasalamento de cães com linfedema apoiam a hipótese de doença hereditária autossômica dominante de expressão variável.[97]

Linfedema secundário

Linfedema persistente ocorre somente após destruição ou bloqueio de um número considerável dos principais vasos linfáticos ou de vários linfonodos sequenciais e seus linfáticos aferentes ou eferentes.[95] Os fatores que podem retardar ou impedir a formação de edema incluem abertura do reencaminhamento do fluxo linfático através das anastomoses linfáticas e vias perilinfáticas de drenagem linfática e aumento da captação de líquido do sistema venoso. Linfedema secundário está frequentemente relacionado a uma combinação de obstrução de veias e vasos linfáticos.[104] A inibição do retorno venoso inibe o fluxo linfático por alterar as forças de Starling, exacerbando o acúmulo de líquido nos tecidos. Isso sobrecarrega os capilares linfáticos e resulta no acúmulo de líquido no espaço intersticial.[95] Os vasos linfáticos distais podem ficar mais distendidos, causando perda de competência valvular e estagnação do fluxo linfático,

CAPÍTULO 257 • Doenças de Veias e Vasos Linfáticos 1367

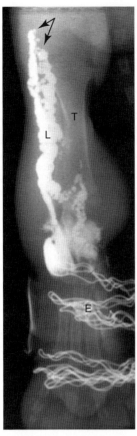

Figura 257.16 Linfangiograma de um cão jovem com displasia de vasos linfáticos. Após a canulação de um vaso linfático distal, o meio de contraste foi infundido no sistema linfático. Note a dilatação e tortuosidade dos canais linfáticos (*L*) que terminam em fundo cego, na articulação do joelho (*setas*). *E*, esponjas cirúrgicas radiopacas; *T*, tíbia.

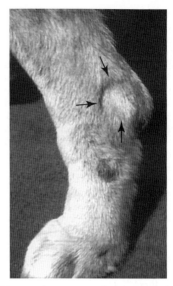

Figura 257.17 Edema cutâneo em um cão com neoplasia lombar caudal. O edema foi causado pela obstrução do retorno venoso dos membros pélvicos ou pela obstrução da drenagem linfática. O líquido edematoso do tecido foi deformado por pressão digital leve, resultando em afundamento visível do tecido subcutâneo do membro pélvico (*setas*).

insuficiência mural e acúmulo adicional de líquido proteináceo nos tecidos subcutâneos. Outras etiologias comuns incluem: terapia pós-traumática, pós-radiação ou interrupção pós-cirúrgica de linfáticos; excisão de linfonodos; bloqueio de linfonodos e vasos linfáticos por compressão ou invasão neoplásica.[105-108] Linfedema resultante de neoplasia local é geralmente um sinal de propagação amplamente disseminada de uma doença de alto grau de malignidade e invasiva.

Os sinais clínicos associados ao linfedema secundário variam dependendo da causa primária e da resposta sistêmica, bem como da sobreposição de sinais clínicos de obstrução venosa sistêmica. Portanto, o exame físico e o exame de imagem apropriado devem avaliar os dois sistemas orgânicos. O linfedema pode estar localizado na periferia de uma extremidade (Figura 257.17) ou se estender no sentido proximal aos tecidos subcutâneos.[105] A localização e a gravidade da obstrução determinam a extensão do edema. Por exemplo, obstrução sublombar ou intrapélvica causa edema bilateral dos membros pélvicos e edema de coxas e genitália externa. Tumores de mediastino e trombose da veia cava cranial provocam edema bilateral dos membros torácicos e dos tecidos da parte ventral do tórax, pescoço e cabeça. O clínico deve palpar todos os linfonodos cuidadosamente para observar aumento de volume e sensibilidade. No edema bilateral dos membros pélvicos, é importante realizar palpação retal ou abdominal para avaliar os linfonodos sublombares. Próstata, região anal, glândulas mamárias e área vaginal devem ser cuidadosamente inspecionadas quanto à presença de neoplasias, as quais podem causar doença obstrutiva intrapélvica. Deve-se suspeitar de tumor intrapélvico em todos os cães com edema dos membros pélvicos e sinais vagos de dor sublombar, desconforto durante a deambulação ou dificuldade para defecar ou urinar. Dependendo do tipo e da extensão da doença sistêmica primária, o edema de membros pode ser a única anormalidade detectável ou pode ser acompanhado de febre, anorexia e perda de peso. Os achados clinicopatológicos dependem da doença primária.

O diagnóstico de linfedema baseia-se amplamente nos achados do histórico clínico e do exame físico; é facilitado pela realização de exame de imagem e exclusão da possibilidade de obstrução venosa. Exames radiográficos devem ser realizados em áreas suspeitas, as quais frequentemente incluem a pelve ou a parte cranial do tórax. Em um número substancial de casos, podem ser detectadas massas de tecidos moles ou lesões ósseas destrutivas. Ocasionalmente, a detecção de efusão pleural subclínica em caso de edema periférico sugere doença linfática mais generalizada. A ultrassonografia pode fornecer informações sobre tumores de tecidos moles e rapidamente identifica linfonodos aumentados e outras estruturas, tanto periféricas quanto intra-abdominais. Deve-se realizar exame duplex scan, conforme descrito anteriormente, para excluir a possibilidade de trombo e/ou obstrução venosa. Linfangiografia, linfocintilografia, venografia ou ATC podem ser indicadas para avaliar a anatomia e integridade do lúmen das veias e dos vasos linfáticos, caso o diagnóstico permaneça incerto. Linfangiografia era tradicionalmente utilizada para o diagnóstico definitivo de doenças linfáticas. Em alguns casos, os vasos linfáticos são hipoplásicos por todo o seu trajeto. Se aplásicos, não é possível encontrar vasos linfáticos apropriados para canulação e injeção de radiocontraste. Falha em delinear um linfonodo após linfografia não é prova absoluta de sua ausência.[6] A linfangiografia característica do linfedema primário consiste em aplasia de linfonodos e pequenos vasos linfáticos que terminam em fundo cego ou fazem anastomose com vasos colaterais ao derredor (em vez de dentro) dos locais onde os linfonodos seriam normalmente encontrados.

Para cães com edema restrito a um dos membros, os diagnósticos diferenciais incluem inflamação, trauma, obstrução vascular, hemorragia, celulite, flebite e fístula arteriovenosa (AV) (ver Capítulo 18). Considerações diagnósticas para cães com edema envolvendo ambos os membros torácicos incluem: trombose, compressão ou invasão da veia cava cranial por um tumor do mediastino. Neste último, o edema geralmente envolve as regiões da cabeça e do pescoço, assim como os membros. Causas apenas de edema bilateral dos membros pélvicos incluem obstrução de linfonodos sublombares por infiltração neoplásica, insuficiência cardíaca congestiva do lado direito e efusão pericárdica, aceitando o fato de que em alguns cães nenhuma causa é identificada. Na experiência dos autores, cães da raça Irish Wolfhound parecem mais predispostos a linfedema idiopático (ver Figura 257.5). Se os quatro membros estiverem envolvidos, os diagnósticos diferenciais devem incluir hipoproteinemia, insuficiência cardíaca congestiva, insuficiência renal, hipertensão portal ou neoplasia linfática (linfangiossarcoma). Conforme mencionado anteriormente, a estreita associação entre as estruturas linfáticas e venosas pode dificultar a distinguir entre obstrução linfática e venosa, e ambas podem ocorrer ao mesmo tempo. Ulceração, dermatite, cianose, varizes chorosas ou necrose gordurosa são sinais de obstrução em vez de estase linfática.

A terapia geralmente não é bem-sucedida, a menos que o edema tenha como causa primária a elevação da pressão venosa (diferentemente do linfedema verdadeiro). Nos estágios iniciais do linfedema, o tratamento clínico é direcionado à manutenção do conforto do animal e à redução do edema. Doenças infecciosas requerem terapia antimicrobiana de longa duração. Algumas doenças neoplásicas podem se beneficiar de quimioterapia ou radioterapia. Aplicação de bandagem compressiva (comparável à compressão por meias em pessoas) por longo tempo e fisioterapia podem facilitar o fluxo linfático e reduzir o acúmulo de linfa no subcutâneo (ver Capítulo 355).[109] Cuidados locais tópicos com a pele e terapia antibiótica intermitente são úteis na redução da celulite secundária. Com exceção de casos isolados, os tratamentos farmacológicos geralmente não são efetivos. As benzopironas (p. ex., a rutina) são um grupo de fármacos recomendados para reduzir o linfedema com alto conteúdo de proteína, estimulando os macrófagos, promovendo proteólise e aumentando a absorção de fragmentos proteicos, embora não haja comprovação de sua eficácia no tratamento de linfedema.[110,111] A administração prolongada de diurético é contraindicada, uma vez que a redução do líquido intersticial concentra proteínas no espaço intersticial residual, que pode causar lesão tecidual.[6] As opções cirúrgicas podem incluir (1) procedimentos para facilitar a drenagem linfática dos membros (linfangioplastia, procedimentos de ponte, desvios, transposição omental) e (2) procedimentos para extirpação do tecido anormal. A excisão cirúrgica do tecido subcutâneo edematoso deve ser estadiada para diminuir a desvascularização.[6] A administração, a curto prazo, de fármacos anti-inflamatórios, colocação de bandagem e fisioterapia pode ser útil em casos de trauma ou no período pós-cirúrgico de linfedema.

Linfangioma, linfangiossarcoma

Os linfangiomas são tumores benignos de vasos linfáticos de pequeno calibre e acredita-se que se desenvolvem quando os sacos linfáticos primitivos falham em estabelecer comunicação venosa.[112] Em uma pesquisa de 5 anos, com avaliação de 221 tumores vasculares de cães, constatou-se que apenas um caso de linfangioma foi definitivamente identificado, sugerindo que essa neoplasia é rara.[66] Os linfangiomas podem ser classificados em três categorias, com base em sua característica histológica: (1) linfangioma capilar, composto de uma rede de vasos linfáticos do tamanho dos capilares, (2) linfangiomas cavernosos, compostos de vasos linfáticos dilatados que se infiltram no tecido circundante e (3) higromas císticos (tumores císticos uniloculares ou multiloculares revestidos por uma única camada de endotélio sustentada por estroma de tecido conjuntivo, contendo um líquido proteináceo cor de palha [com 1,3 a 4,5 g de proteína/dℓ]).[113] As lesões se apresentam como grandes tumores flutuantes no tecido subcutâneo, em fáscias, no mediastino, no tecido hepático, nos linfonodos e no espaço retroperitoneal.[114-117] Linfangiomas também foram diagnosticados em extremidades corporais, coxins metacarpianos, nasofaringe, axila, regiões inguinal e mamária, espaço retroperitoneal e pele em cães.[112,118-120] Os sinais clínicos estão relacionados ao tamanho, à localização e extensão do linfangioma. Os linfangiomas podem exercer pressão sobre as estruturas circundantes e podem interferir na função muscular, respiração (compressão da traqueia), micção ou função intestinal. A linfa pode extravasar para a superfície cutânea através de uma ou várias fístulas. Os diagnósticos diferenciais incluem outras massas que ocupam espaço, como

abscessos, linfonodos aumentados, neoplasias e cistos congênitos de origem não linfogênica. O prognóstico pode ser bom após excisão cirúrgica apropriada, marsupialização ou radioterapia.[121] O risco de recidiva é alto devido à incapacidade inerente de identificação dos limites distintos do tumor.

O linfangiossarcoma se origina em células endoteliais linfáticas.[122] É um tumor maligno raro em cães e gatos, embora seja frequentemente relatado secundário a linfedema crônico em humanos.[123-125] O diagnóstico microscópico de tecido corado com hematoxilina e eosina pode ser difícil, já que as características da neoplasia se assemelham às do hemangiossarcoma. Artigos sugerem que a distinção entre hemangiossarcoma e linfangiossarcoma pode se basear na ausência de eritrócitos nos espaços vasculares do linfangiossarcoma.[122] A marcação por meio de exames imuno-histoquímicos mais recentes parece caracterizar melhor essas neoplasias.[66,122] A predisposição por raça ou sexo ainda não foi estabelecida, mas raças de médio a grande porte podem ser mais suscetíveis, e tanto animais jovens quanto idosos são acometidos.[107,122,126-131] É comum a ocorrência de metástase em cães e gatos; estima-se que é verificada em um terço a metade dos casos no momento do diagnóstico.[122,129,132] Os sinais clínicos incluem edema em extremidades, região inguinal, axila, cabeça e pescoço.

Em um relato de 12 gatos com linfangiossarcoma, constatou-se que 9 apresentavam tumores subcutâneos não circunscritos de rápido crescimento e os demais com tumor no tórax ou abdome.[129] Em todos os gatos acometidos, o tumor era invasivo e não foi possível a ressecção cirúrgica total da lesão.[129] As queixas por ocasião da consulta foram semelhantes àquela de uma série de 12 cães com linfangiossarcoma, em que 10 apresentavam edema de pescoço, parte ventral do abdome ou membros, quase todos com extravasamento de secreção serossanguinolenta no tecido sobrejacente.[122] Foram relatados derrames quilosos associados (pleural, abdominal e subcutâneo).[133-135] Linfangiossarcoma pulmonar foi diagnosticado em um cão que apresentava efusão torácica quilosa.[136] O exame citológico da massa tumoral ou da tumefação não é esclarecedor; a maioria dos laudos citológicos relata inflamação discreta sem sinais de malignidade.[122] O diagnóstico é confirmado pela obtenção de uma amostra por meio de biopsia. Histologicamente, os tumores linfáticos de origem endotelial são caracterizados por proliferação de células endoteliais neoplásicas. Têm-se utilizado corantes como marcadores imunocitoquímicos, como o gene homeobox 1 associado ao domínio próspero para confirmar o diagnóstico da neoplasia em cães e gatos.[122,137,138] O prognóstico de linfangiossarcoma é de reservado a ruim, com altas taxas de recidiva local e metástase. Nos primeiros artigos publicados, a maioria dos animais era submetida à eutanásia ou morria devido a linfedema grave, efusão pleural ou metástases distantes. Em um relato de caso, documentou-se ausência de recidiva e de metástase por um período de 9 meses após a ressecção do tumor e tratamento com doxorrubicina.[139] Na série de 12 cães,[122] várias estratégias de tratamento foram empregadas incluindo excisão cirúrgica incompleta em 5 cães, com sobrevida média de 513 dias; quimioterapia exclusiva, com sobrevida de 182 dias; e tratamento exclusivo com prednisona em 1 cão, com sobrevida de 90 dias. A combinação das terapias (cirurgia, quimioterapia, com ou sem radioterapia) propiciou sobrevida de 574 dias em um cão e de 248 dias em outro. A sobrevida média dos três cães não tratados foi de 368 dias.[122] Atualmente não se conhece o tratamento ideal para linfangiossarcoma em cães e gatos.

AGRADECIMENTOS

Os autores agradecem contribuições anteriores para este capítulo de Philip R. Fox e Jean-Paul Petrie.

REFERÊNCIAS BIBLIOGRÁFICAS

As referências bibliográficas deste capítulo se encontram online no Ambiente de Aprendizagem.

SEÇÃO 17
Doença Neurológica

CAPÍTULO 258

Neurofisiologia

Dennis P. O'Brien e Joan R. Coates

A unidade básica do sistema nervoso é constituída de membranas estimuláveis. A capacidade de transmitir o estímulo (potencial de ação) para outros neurônios começa com o potencial de repouso da membrana, uma bateria recarregável que alimenta o processo. A condutância flutuante dos canais de Na^+ e K^+ voltagem-dependentes ao longo do axônio transmite o estímulo adiante em forma de potencial de ação. Essa transmissão é facilitada pela bainha de mielina, que funciona como um isolante e permite uma transmissão rápida dos impulsos elétricos ao longo do axônio neuronal de forma saltatória. O potencial de ação se encerra na terminação nervosa (sinapse), com a abertura dos canais Ca^{++} voltagem-dependentes, os quais acionam uma cascata de proteínas sinápticas, acoplam-se no terminal sináptico de membrana e liberam neurotransmissores. Esses neurotransmissores se ligam ao receptor pós-sináptico e, posteriormente, sua ação é finalizada por proteínas específicas de recaptação ou inativação enzimática. Os neurotransmissores podem agir a curto ou longo prazo em neurônios pós-sinápticos, tornando-os mais ou menos suscetíveis a propagação do impulso. Os potenciais excitatórios ou inibitórios se somam no cone axonal, onde a "decisão" para interromper qualquer sinal adicional ou iniciar novamente o processo com um novo potencial de ação é tomada. Esse processo básico de transmissão e inibição neuronal ocorre na anatomia complexa do sistema nervoso a fim de produzir atenção, percepção, motivação e ação.

MEMBRANAS EXCITÁVEIS: POTENCIAL DE REPOUSO DE MEMBRANA E CANAIS IÔNICOS

Em repouso, uma célula nervosa como o neurônio possui uma carga elétrica que pode ser medida através de sua membrana celular, sendo o meio intracelular de membrana relativamente negativo em relação ao meio extracelular (potencial de repouso da membrana). Esse potencial de repouso da membrana é criado pelo transporte ativo de íons ao longo da membrana, resultando em concentrações diferentes de íons nos meios intra e extracelular. As moléculas de ATPases de Na^+ e K^+ utilizam energia do ATP para bombear 3 íons de Na^+ para fora da célula em troca de 2 íons de K^+. Esse mecanismo cria um gradiente de concentração de sódio Na+ muito maior no meio extracelular e uma concentração de potássio K^+ muito maior no meio intracelular. Dessa forma, um gradiente elétrico é estabelecido também, uma vez que um

íon a mais de Na^+ é bombeado para o meio extracelular, enquanto os íons de K^+ são bombeados para o meio intracelular. Ânions com carga negativa, tais como as proteínas e os aminoácidos, não podem se difundir através das membranas; portanto, mantêm a carga negativa no interior da membrana. Essa diferença de potencial em neurônios é de –65 a –70 mV. Em processos patológicos como a hipoglicemia, ocorre prejuízo na capacidade de neurônios fornecerem ATP suficiente para o bombeamento de Na^+/K^+ ATPase intra e extracelular. A célula não consegue manter seu potencial da membrana em repouso; por isso, seu estado decai para um estado mais despolarizado, o que pode desencadear convulsões ou evolução para um estado de coma.

A permeabilidade da membrana a um íon é determinada pelo estado dos canais da membrana, que são seletivamente permeáveis a diferentes tipos de íons. O grau e a direção do fluxo são dependentes dos gradientes de concentração e da carga da membrana. Quando, por exemplo, um canal K^+ se abre, o íon difunde a favor do gradiente de concentração: no caso do K^+, do meio intracelular para o meio extracelular. O equilíbrio dessa força iônica, portanto, é a diferença entre as cargas elétricas. Os ânions carregados negativamente no meio extracelular atraem os elementos de cargas positivamente carregadas, como o K^+, gerando a difusão oposta para o meio extracelular (Figura 258.1).

Potencial de equilíbrio para potássio (E_k)

$$E_k = 61\ mV\ Dentro\ \frac{[K^+]\ fora}{[K^+]\ dentro} = 61\ Dentro\ \frac{5}{150} = -90\ mV$$

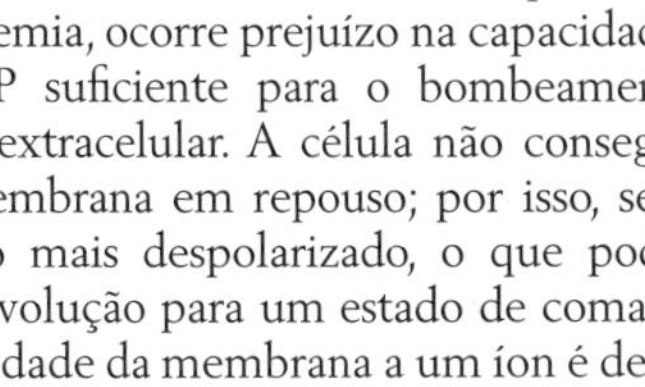

Figura 258.1 A maior concentração de K^+ dentro da célula propicia a difusão para fora da célula. Essas forças são opostas pela carga negativa dentro da membrana, o que atrai positivamente o K^+ com carga. A tensão da membrana onde essas duas forças estão em equilíbrio é o potencial de equilíbrio (E_k), calculado pela equação de Nernst. Assim, quando a membrana está em –90 mV, não há difusão de K^+. (De O'Brien, D.P. Vet Med 8415: *Advanced Veterinary Neurology*, http://bblearn.missouri.edu, 2015. Usada com permissão.)

A diferença de voltagem elétrica através da membrana axonal onde a difusão não ocorre e essas forças estão em equilíbrio é chamada de potencial de equilíbrio (E_k). Esse estado de equilíbrio depende da diferença de concentração de difusão ($[K^+]_{fora}/[K^+]_{dentro}$) e é calculada pela multiplicação do log desse quociente por uma constante (a equação de Nernst).

O mecanismo de abertura e fechamento dos canais iônicos é regulado por uma membrana de voltagem ou por um neurotransmissor, ligado a um receptor que está acoplado a um canal iônico. Quando o canal está aberto, o íon que é permeável à difusão difunde-se até que o equilíbrio potencial seja atingido. Se um canal de K^+ se abre, o K^+ difunde-se para o meio extracelular a favor do gradiente de concentração menor, até o interior da célula atingir o equilíbrio potencial de –90 mV, e quando as forças de voltagem e de difusão estão em equilíbrio. Portanto, torna a célula mais negativa (hiperpolarizada). Em contrapartida, a concentração de Na^+ no meio extracelular é muito maior que a concentração Na^+ no meio intracelular, favorecendo o gradiente eletrolítico de difusão para o meio intracelular. A célula é altamente impermeável ao Na^+ durante o potencial de repouso celular, mas, quando um canal de sódio se abre, o Na^+ difunde-se para o meio intracelular até que o potencial de equilíbrio seja atingido em 59 mV, despolarizando a célula. Outro íon que é importante para o potencial de repouso celular é o Cl^-. O Cl^- tem seu próprio mecanismo de transporte ativo, que cria um gradiente de concentração de Cl^- no meio extracelular muito maior do que no meio intracelular, com E_{Cl} de –70 mV.

O gradiente de concentração e a permeabilidade em repouso da membrana neuronal para esses íons diferentes contribuem para o potencial da membrana em repouso. A equação de Goldman, Hodgkin e Katz prevê o potencial da membrana da célula com base no equilíbrio dessas duas variáveis. Em repouso, as concentrações de Na^+ e de Cl^- são maiores no meio celular comparadas com as do seu interior, e o oposto acontece para a concentração K^+. A permeabilidade de repouso para o K^+ (P_k) aumenta à medida que numerosos canais de "vazamento" são abertos naquela determinada voltagem. A permeabilidade de repouso para P_{Cl} é maior, uma vez que vários canais estão abertos (vazando). O somatório de todos esses fatores dá origem ao potencial de membrana em repouso de cerca de –65 mV para neurônios.

As patologias de canais são doenças que afetam a função do canal iônico e alteram a excitabilidade da membrana neuronal. Gatos com crises convulsivas parciais complexas possuem anticorpos contra canais de voltagem regulados por potássio. Cães com mutação nos genes que codificam uma porção desse complexo canal de potássio têm epilepsia juvenil familiar benigna.[1,2] Essas doenças alteraram a P_k e, portanto, alteraram a excitabilidade da membrana celular, predispondo a atividade neuronal excessiva e a convulsões.

TRANSMISSÃO DE ESTIMULAÇÃO: O POTENCIAL DE AÇÃO

Quando um neurônio despolariza além do seu limiar (–55 mV), os canais Na^+ voltagem-dependentes no axônio se abrem, iniciando um potencial de ação que transmite o estímulo para outros neurônios (Figura 258.2 A). A quantidade de Na^+ que se difunde para o meio intracelular através de um canal permeável é expressa em condutância (g_{Na}). À medida que o Na^+ se difunde para o meio intracelular, a membrana celular se despolariza até que o equilíbrio potencial para Na^+ (E_{Na}) igual a 59 mV seja atingido. Os canais Na^+ têm um mecanismo secundário de bloqueio, por inativação dos canais, que ocorre com o fechamento do canal por um breve período de tempo, impedindo maior difusão de sódio pelo poro do canal (Figura 258.2 B). Canais voltagem-dependentes de K^+ abrem-se em resposta à despolarização produzida por g_{Na}. O K^+ nesse momento se difunde através desses canais iônicos em direção ao seu potencial de equilíbrio de –90 mV. Uma vez que esse valor fica abaixo do

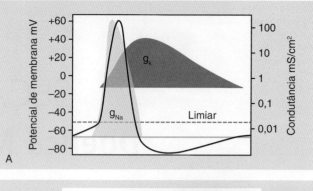

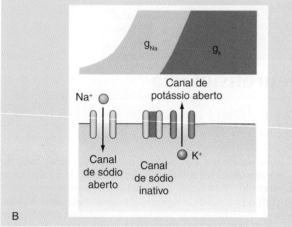

Figura 258.2 A. O potencial de ação (*linha preta*) é gerado por mudanças na condutância de Na^+ (g_{Na} em *cinza-claro*) e K^+ (g_K em *cinza-escuro*). Quando a célula despolariza além de um limiar de –55 mV, os canais de Na^+ se abrem (**B**) e o Na^+ se difunde para dentro da célula até atingir o potencial de equilíbrio de 59 mV. Canais de Na^+ se inativam, impedindo qualquer difusão adicional desse íon. Canais de voltagem de K^+ se abrem com despolarização, permitindo a difusão do K^+ para fora da célula até que seu potencial de equilíbrio de –90 mV seja alcançado. (Utilizada, com autorização, de O'Brien, D.P. Vet Med 8415: *Advanced Veterinary Neurology*, http://bblearn.missouri.edu, 2015.)

potencial de repouso normal da membrana de –65 mV, ocorre uma pós-hiperpolarização da membrana até que a condutância de repouso normal traga a voltagem de volta ao potencial de repouso. Fármacos antiepilépticos, como a fenitoína, melhoram a inativação de canais de sódio, tornando-os menos suscetíveis a transmitir a propagação de um potencial de ação.[3] Toxinas como as piretrinas bloqueiam o canal de inativação de sódio, aumentando a formação do potencial de ação e causando tremores e convulsões (ver Capítulo 152).[4]

Dois fatores influenciam a velocidade com que o potencial de ação se propaga pelo axônio: o diâmetro axonal e a bainha de mielina. Com o aumento do diâmetro do axônio, eleva-se o número de íons disponíveis para as correntes de fluxo iônico (*i.e.*, diminui a resistência do fluxo iônico). Ao mesmo tempo, entretanto, ocorre o aumento da área de superfície, onde a diferença de carga entre o meio intracelular e o extracelular é armazenada (*i.e.*, aumenta-se a capacitância de resistência ao fluxo iônico). Se uma camada isolante de mielina é colocada no axônio, a capacidade de armazenamento de carga da membrana diminui (*i.e.*, diminui-se a capacitância) nessa área de isolamento sem afetar a resistência do fluxo iônico dentro do axônio, permitindo assim que o fluxo iônico passe entre áreas não mielinizadas (nódulo de Ranvier) de forma saltatória. Doenças desmielinizantes, como polirradiculoneurite (ver Capítulo 268), aumentam a capacitância da membrana axonal; portanto, diminuem a velocidade de condução e potencialmente bloqueiam a propagação do potencial de ação.

COMUNICAÇÃO NEURONAL: SINAPSE

Os neurônios se comunicam através de sinapses. Enquanto algumas sinapses permitem um fluxo direto de íons entre os neurônios (sinapses elétricas ou junções comunicantes), a maioria das sinapses utiliza sinais químicos via neurotransmissores. Os neurotransmissores são armazenados em vesículas estocadas no terminal nervoso. Quando o potencial de ação despolariza a terminação nervosa, canais de cálcio voltagem-dependentes se abrem, permitindo a entrada de íons Ca^{++} para o interior da célula. O Ca^{++} ativa uma série de proteínas de vesículas sinápticas que se ancoram na vesícula na membrana pré-sináptica, onde elas se fundem com a membrana celular, liberando o neurotransmissor dentro da fenda sináptica. A toxina botulínica se liga a uma dessas vesículas proteicas, impedindo a liberação de acetilcolina na junção neuromuscular (ver Capítulo 214).[5]

O neurotransmissor difunde-se pela fenda sináptica e liga-se a um receptor na superfície da membrana pós-sináptica. O receptor pós-sináptico pode ser outro neurônio, um músculo ou outro efetor como uma célula endócrina. Os receptores podem ser divididos em receptores inotrópicos, regulados por canais iônicos, e receptores metabotrópicos, regulados por meio de mensageiros secundários. Os efeitos dos neurotransmissores cessam por difusão através da sinapse neuronal, por degradação enzimática ou por um mecanismo de recaptação ativa.

Os receptores ionotrópicos clássicos têm subunidades compostas de domínios de membrana que formam um poro central, que é permeável seletivamente a determinados íons. Diversas moléculas estruturais são importantes para a junção das regiões pré e pós-sinápticas, assim como para a ancoragem de canais iônicos e de proteínas, de receptores, e de vários mensageiros secundários de membrana nas regiões sinápticas. Quando o neurotransmissor se liga a um sítio da região de ligação extracelular da célula ligante, ocorre uma alteração na conformação e na permeabilidade do poro da célula ligante. As três famílias dos receptores ionotrópicos são (1) acetilcolina nicotínico (ACh), ácido gama-aminobutírico (GABA) e glicina, (2) glutamato e (3) receptores ATP ou purina P2X.[6] Os efeitos sobre a célula pós-sináptica podem ser excitatórios ou inibitórios, dependendo do íon que se difunde pelo poro aberto.

Quando a ACh se liga ao receptor nicotínico, o poro se torna permeável a cátions.[6] No potencial de repouso da membrana (período refratário), o Na^+ é o íon que mais se difunde para o meio intracelular, despolarizando a membrana pós-sináptica. Quando se registra o potencial pós-sináptico de membrana na célula, essa despolarização aparece como um potencial pós-sináptico excitatório (PPSE) (Figura 258.3). Na fenda sináptica, a acetilcolinesterase degrada a ACh em colina e ácido acético, que são levados para dentro do terminal pré-sináptico e recaptados para ressintetizar ACh. Na miastenia gravis, autoanticorpos são direcionados contra a subunidade alfa 1 e bloqueiam parcialmente o receptor ACh na junção neuromuscular (ver Capítulo 269).[7] Esse processo dificulta a abertura do canal ACh e produz fadiga, que é a marca da doença. Os inibidores da acetilcolinesterase prolongam a interação da ACh com o receptor e revertem os sinais clínicos.

O GABA é o principal neurotransmissor inibitório. O receptor GABA-A e o receptor de glicina estreitamente relacionado têm uma estrutura molecular semelhante ao receptor ACh, mas o canal iônico é permeável apenas ao ânion Cl^-.[6] Quando o canal se abre, Cl^- pode difundir-se para o meio intracelular, criando um potencial pós-sináptico inibitório (PPSI) que hiperpolariza a célula (Figura 258.3). Uma vez que o potencial da membrana em repouso em muitos neurônios é próximo ao potencial de equilíbrio para o Cl^-, pode não ocorrer uma grande movimentação de íons Cl^- através da membrana quando o canal iônico se abre. Ainda assim, a abertura do canal diminui a probabilidade de a célula pós-sináptica alcançar seu limiar de ação para gerar um potencial de ação, já que qualquer despolarização desloca o equilíbrio de difusão de Cl^- para o meio intracelular. Fármacos antiepilépticos comumente usados, como o diazepam e o fenobarbital, ligam-se a sítios extracelulares no receptor GABA-A. Esses fármacos não abrem o canal iônico, mas alteram a cinética do canal, aumentando o tempo de abertura dos poros quando o GABA se liga ao seu receptor.[8]

A função do mais importante neurotransmissor excitatório no sistema nervoso central, o glutamato, é um pouco mais complicada.[6,9] Existem dois subtipos de receptores inotrópicos para o glutamato, os quais foram classificados de acordo com os primeiros fármacos utilizados neles pela primeira vez para diferenciá-los, o receptor AMPA (alfa-amino-3-hidroxi-5-metil-4-i-soxazolepropionato) e o receptor NMDA (N-metil D-aspartato), que são frequentemente encontrados em proximidade. O glutamato tem que se ligar a ambos os receptores para produzir um efeito. Quando se liga ao receptor AMPA, despolariza

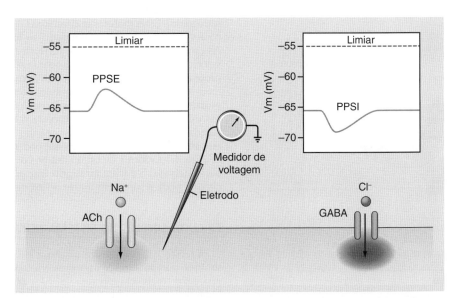

Figura 258.3 Quando o canal nicotínico de ACh se abre e o Na^+ se difunde para dentro da célula, um sublimiar de despolarização da membrana pode ser registrado como um potencial pós-sináptico excitatório (*PPSE*). Quando um neurotransmissor inibitório, como o ácido gama-amino butírico (*GABA*), liga-se ao seu receptor, o influxo de Cl^- polariza ainda mais a célula e é registrado como um potencial pós-sináptico inibitório (*PPSI*). (De O'Brien, D.P. Vet Med 8415: *Advanced Veterinary Neurology*, http://bblearn.missouri.edu, 2015. Usada com permissão.)

parcialmente a membrana celular, liberando um íon Mg^{++} que bloqueia o canal do receptor NMDA. Quando se liga ao receptor NMDA, pode possibilitar uma condutância adicional dos íons Na^+, que melhora o PPSE produzido por ativação do receptor AMPA. O canal NMDA também é permeável ao Ca^{++}. E o aumento do Ca^{++} intracelular pode acionar o sistema de segundo mensageiro que possui efeitos mais prolongados na sinapse, conforme discutido a seguir. A ativação excessiva do receptor NMDA e o acúmulo de Ca^{++} intracelular podem desencadear a morte celular, um processo chamado excitotoxicidade.[10]

A segunda classe de receptores de neurotransmissores, os receptores metabotrópicos, incluem os receptores muscarínicos da acetilcolina, receptores metabotrópicos do glutamato, receptores GABA-B e a maioria dos receptores de serotonina, assim como os receptores para norepinefrina, epinefrina, histamina, dopamina, neuropeptídios e endocanabinoides.[6,9] Esses receptores atuam através de sistemas de mensageiro secundário, como proteína G, e produzem influências mais prolongadas na função. Às vezes, esses sistemas afetam indiretamente a condutância do canal iônico e o mesmo neurotransmissor pode ter efeitos opostos, dependendo do receptor. Quando a ACh se liga ao receptor de ACh muscarínico M_2, a proteína G se liga ao GTP e dissocia uma subunidade, que então se liga à proteína G acoplada ao potássio retificador interno (GIRK). Esse mecanismo abre o canal iônico e permite que o K^+ se difunda para o meio extracelular, hiperpolarizando a membrana. Em contrapartida, a ativação do receptor M1 fecha o canal de K^+ tipo M, produzindo um PPSE prolongado.[9]

Os receptores metabotrópicos também podem promover mudanças a longo prazo na função sináptica. Por exemplo, o receptor glutamato metabotrópico mGluR1 é encontrado em alta concentração nas células de Purkinje do cerebelo. Quando o glutamato se liga a esse receptor, a proteína G é ativada e ativa uma série de outros mensageiros secundários para finalmente ativar uma proteinoquinase C (Figura 258.4). Esse mecanismo remove um fosfato do receptor AMPA, promovendo internalização e degradação do receptor. Isso torna a sinapse menos responsiva à estimulação excitatória glutamatérgica, um processo denominado depressão a longo prazo, que é uma parte essencial do processo de aprendizado e da memória. Cães da raça Coton Tulear com mutação no gene *mGluR1* (*GRM1*) não são capazes de fazer essas mudanças ao longo de seu desenvolvimento. Portanto, apresentam aprendizagem motora comprometida e ataxia cerebelar grave (Vídeo 258.1).[11] Outros neurotransmissores metabotrópicos produzirão potencialização da força sináptica a longo prazo.

Outra classe de neurotransmissores que funciona por meio de receptores metabotrópicos são as monoaminas, como dopamina ou serotonina. A dopamina e a adenosina agem por meio de receptores diferentes para intervir na atividade do AMP cíclico. A estimulação do receptor dopaminérgico D2 diminui os níveis de AMP cíclico e aumenta a excitabilidade celular. Já a estimulação do receptor de adenosina aumenta os níveis de AMP cíclico e diminui a excitabilidade celular. Fármacos como a cafeína bloqueiam os receptores de adenosina, deixando a atividade dopaminérgica sem inibição; portanto, aumentam a excitabilidade.[12]

A serotonina é um neurotransmissor importante na regulação de humor; a deficiência de atividade da serotonina é responsável pela depressão clínica. A atividade da serotonina no seu receptor pós-sináptico é cessada em função da recaptação de serotonina para o terminal pré-sináptico por um transportador serotoninérgico. Fármacos como a fluoxetina bloqueiam seletivamente os transportadores de serotonina com outros efeitos menores sobre outros transportadores monoaminérgicos correlacionados. Tais fármacos são usados para tratar ansiedade por separação e comportamentos compulsivos em cães.[13,14]

MANUTENÇÃO DO MAQUINÁRIO: TRANSPORTE AXONAL

Todas as proteínas são sintetizadas perto do núcleo e devem ser transportadas por meio do citoplasma para o local onde são necessárias. Os neurônios diferem de outras células, uma vez que as proteínas, vesículas e mitocôndrias precisam ser transportadas ao longo do eixo axonal, e em um animal como o cavalo o axônio neuronal pode ter metros de comprimento. Proteínas danificadas e outros subprodutos, então, têm que ser transportados de volta ao corpo celular para serem degradados e reciclados. Dessa forma, o sistema de transporte axonal teve que evoluir para a realização dessa tarefa. O percurso da via celular na qual a carga é transportada é composto por microtúbulos, que ficam dispostos ao longo do comprimento do axônio. Dois motores moleculares separados carregam a carga ao longo dos microtúbulos: as cinesinas, que realizam o transporte do corpo celular para as terminações nervosas (transporte anterógrado), e as dineínas, responsáveis pelo transporte da terminação nervosa de volta ao corpo celular (transporte retrógrado). Esses motores utilizam o ATP e passam por alterações conformacionais para "caminharem" ao longo dos microtúbulos. As cargas vesiculares movem-se de maneira consistente e em alta velocidade. Inicialmente pensava-se que as proteínas citosólicas, as proteínas citoesqueléticas e as proteínas mitocondriais moviam-se mais lentamente. Todavia, pesquisas recentes mostraram que as proteínas citosólicas, as proteínas musculoesqueléticas e as proteínas mitocondriais trafegam na mesma velocidade; porém, fazem paradas frequentes ao longo do caminho.[15] Toxinas ou mutações que atrapalham o transporte axonal podem resultar em acúmulo de material na forma de esferoides no corpo celular ou na terminação nervosa. E a falha no suprimento adequado da terminação nervosa pode resultar em morte de axônios mais longos.[16]

CIRCUITO SIMPLES NO SISTEMA NERVOSO

O processo básico de estimulação e inibição permite circuitos simples, que podem ser dispostos em camadas para produzir os processos mais complexos da função do sistema nervoso. Quando um único potencial de ação libera um neurotransmissor excitatório, o PPSE produzido normalmente não atinge o limiar para gerar outro potencial de ação no neurônio pós-sináptico. Os PPSEs oriundos de muitos potenciais de ação podem se somar para despolarizar a membrana pós-sináptica acima do

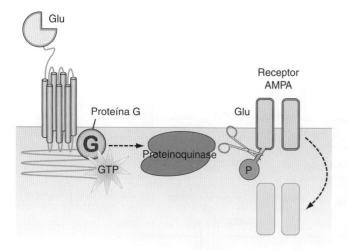

Figura 258.4 Ativação do receptor metabotrópico de glutamato mGluR1, que produz mudanças em longo prazo na função sináptica. Através de uma série de etapas intermediárias, a proteína G ativa uma proteinoquinase C (PKC), que remove o fosfato do receptor AMPA. Isso leva à internalização e degradação do receptor, enfraquecendo a força da sinapse. Essa depressão em longo prazo da função sináptica é um dos blocos de construção de plasticidade sináptica e do aprendizado. (De O'Brien, D.P. Vet Med 8415: *Advanced Veterinary Neurology*, http://bblearn.missouri.edu, 2015. Usada com permissão.)

limiar, processo denominado somação temporal. Alternativamente, axônios de neurônios pré-sinápticos múltiplos podem convergir para um único neurônio. Quando mais de um potencial de ação converge para um neurônio simultaneamente, os PPSEs também podem se somar para despolarizar o neurônio pós-sináptico acima do limiar, chamado de processo de somação espacial. Em contrapartida, um neurônio estimulado pode se ramificar e fazer sinapse com muitos neurônios pós-sinápticos. Tais circuitos divergentes permitem a propagação de um sinal por meio de múltiplos neurônios de segunda ordem.

Neurônios inibitórios normalmente funcionam como interneurônios no circuito neuronal para controlar a excitabilidade. Geralmente os neurônios inibitórios fazem sinapse próximo ao corpo celular do neurônio no qual podem bloquear a propagação do PPSE para o cone axonal, onde o potencial de ação é gerado. A célula de Renshaw na medula espinal é um exemplo de interneurônio inibitório. Um impulso excitatório para o neurônio motor também ativa a célula de Renshaw. A célula de Renshaw, então, inibe os neurônios motores adjacentes em um processo de inibição colateral. A toxina tetânica bloqueia a liberação de glicina, resultando em estimulação excessiva dos neurônios motores e o sinal clínico clássico da tetania (ver Capítulo 214).

A inibição também pode ser direcionada para o local de origem da estimulação. As células piramidais gigantes do córtex cerebral são neurônios glutaminérgicos excitatórios que enviam fibras de projeção longas ao córtex. Um ramo dessas sinapses axonais nos interneurônios GABAérgicos do córtex faz sinapse retrógrada com as células piramidais. E essa inibição de retorno ajuda a evitar o excesso de disparo das células piramidais; uma falha dessa inibição pode estar relacionada a alguma atividade convulsiva.[17]

PROCESSO SENSORIAL

A combinação de alguns desses circuitos simples ilustra como o sistema nervoso processa a informação (Figura 258.5). Um estímulo sensorial, como o toque ou a luz, ativará receptores imediatamente abaixo do estímulo com maior intensidade que os receptores localizados ao seu redor. Os receptores mais intensamente estimulados geram mais potenciais de ação, quando comparados aos receptores localizados perifericamente. A inervação divergente de cada um desses receptores inerva um certo número de células pós-sinápticas adjacentes. Os ramos dos axônios, tanto os receptores centrais altamente estimulados como os ramos dos axônios receptores periféricos menos estimulados, convergirão para o neurônio central de segunda ordem. A combinação da somação temporal e espacial garantirá que o neurônio de segunda ordem atinja o seu limiar de ativação para gerar um potencial de ação. Ramos desses axônios de neurônios de segunda ordem fazem sinapse com interneurônios inibitórios que se projetam em torno dos neurônios de segunda ordem (inibição lateral).

Embora esses neurônios recebam algum estímulo excitatório de entrada, essas estimulações de entrada são muito mais fracas e a inibição lateral evita que esses neurônios de segunda ordem atinjam o limiar de ação. Esse mecanismo tem como foco a estimulação central do estímulo e ao mesmo tempo a inibição dos neurônios adjacentes. Quando essa programação ao redor do centro se espalha ao longo de populações inteiras de circuitos sensoriais, ela pode ser usada para detectar margens e formas. Quando associada à duração e ao tempo de ativação de áreas adjacentes, o movimento é percebido.

FUNÇÃO COGNITIVA, ATENÇÃO E MOTIVAÇÃO

Nas áreas do córtex cerebral e nas áreas subcorticais, as informações sensoriais agem de acordo com o nível de estimulação, estado motivacional e experiências passadas do animal. A estimulação do cérebro é essencial para a consciência e atenção. Esse processo é em grande parte mediado por projeções para

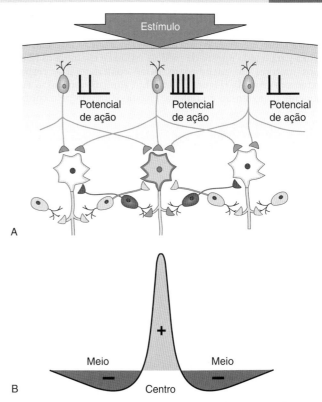

Figura 258.5 Nos sistemas sensoriais, quanto mais forte o estímulo em um receptor, maior o número de potenciais de ação (PA) gerados. Convergência de excitação forte e fraca de receptores adjacentes ativa neurônios de segunda ordem no centro do estímulo (**A**). A inibição lateral de neurônios de segunda ordem circundante cria um halo de inibição que foca a resposta a um grupo seleto de neurônios de segunda ordem (**B**). (De O'Brien, D.P. Vet Med 8415: *Advanced Veterinary Neurology*, http://bblearn.missouri.edu, 2015. Usada com permissão.)

o prosencéfalo, neurotransmissores monoaminérgicos (principalmente norepinefrina, dopamina, serotonina e histamina), neurônios colinérgicos do tronco cerebral e do prosencéfalo basal,[9] um sistema que às vezes é referido como sistema de ativação reticular. Lesões grandes dentro dessas vias de projeções podem produzir estupor e coma; já lesões mais seletivas podem afetar diferentes aspectos da atenção ou motivação sem perda de consciência.

CONTROLE MOTOR

Assim como no sistema sensorial, o entendimento da função do sistema motor começa com circuitos simples. Quando um músculo é estendido, os receptores no fuso muscular são estimulados. Os potenciais de ação gerados pelo estímulo trafegam pela medula espinal onde fazem sinapse diretamente com o neurônio motor que inerva esse músculo, produzindo uma contração muscular. Essa extensão ou reflexo miotático faz parte de um circuito projetado para regular comprimento e tensão muscular, mas também é uma ferramenta essencial do exame neurológico (ver Capítulo 259). O reflexo de retirada ou reflexo flexor, um reflexo importante no exame neurológico, possui um circuito mais complexo. Quando um animal pisa em um espinho ou o clínico pressiona a falange do membro (dedo do pé), neurônios aferentes periféricos relacionados com a dor farão sinapse com interneurônios dentro da medula espinal e se projetarão para o córtex cerebral, onde a dor será percebida. Porém, independentemente de qualquer percepção, o circuito reflexo será ativado e responderá para o membro. Os interneurônios excitatórios na medula espinal fazem sinapse com os neurônios motores para os músculos flexores do membro, afastando o membro do estímulo nocivo. Essa flexão repentina de um membro muda o peso para o membro contralateral. Para fornecer o suporte necessário para essa mudança, outro interneurônio cruza para o lado oposto da medula espinal e estimula os neurônios motores do membro extensor contralateral – resposta extensora cruzada (Figura 258.6). Em animais normais, o componente de extensão do reflexo cruzado é inibido pelo controle motor descendente; se o animal está em decúbito lateral, ocorrerá apenas o reflexo de retirada. Se esse controle descendente for abolido por uma lesão afetando os neurônios motores superiores, o reflexo de extensão cruzada é liberado da inibição e ocorre quando o reflexo de retirada for induzido. Levando essa interferência entre neurônios para outro nível, os geradores de padrões centrais podem gerar atividades rítmicas como ocorre em caminhadas. Alguns geradores de padrões são compostos por células que sofrem disparos espontâneos, mas padrões também podem ser gerados através de um sistema recíproco de inibição chamada meio-centro.[9] O sistema neuronal superior motor descendente facilita ou inibe esses geradores de padrões locais através de entradas neuromodulatórias para produzir ritmo na caminhada normal, que é posteriormente modificado no nível da medula espinal, dependendo do retorno sensorial. Se o controle normal desse processo pelo neurônio motor superior é perdido em razão de lesão na medula espinal, esses geradores de padrão espinal podem funcionar espontaneamente, resultando em "caminhada espinal" ou "andar espinal" (Vídeo 258.2).

Essa hierarquia de controle do movimento é contínua e central. A posição da cabeça e do pescoço influencia o tônus dos músculos extensores e flexores nos membros através dos reflexos tônicos do pescoço, preparando o corpo para o movimento com base na direção para a qual a cabeça e o pescoço estão dirigindo a atenção. Sinais modulatórios diferentes para geradores de padrão espinal produzem caminhadas diferentes. As áreas locomotoras do tronco cerebral que geram esses sinais modulatórios, por sua vez, são regidas pelo córtex e pelo sistema motor de núcleos basais. Esses sistemas são regulados por experiências passadas através de projeções monoaminérgicas que medeiam a motivação e o estímulo.

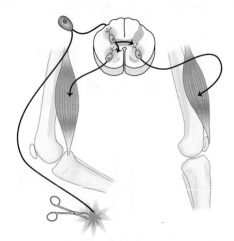

Figura 258.6 Um estímulo doloroso à pata provoca dois reflexos como resposta: retirada e extensão cruzada. Neurônios aferentes de dor fazem sinapse com um interneurônio que excita neurônios motores que inervam os músculos flexores do membro. Essa retirada é um reflexo independente de percepção consciente. Outras fibras nervosas interneuronais cruzam para o lado contralateral e fazem sinapse com as fibras musculares dos músculos extensores para suportar o aumento de peso deslocado para esse lado pela retirada. A extensão cruzada componente só é vista quando há perda de inibição dos reflexos do NMS. (De O'Brien, D.P. Vet Med 8415: *Advanced Veterinary Neurology*, http://bblearn.missouri.edu, 2015. Usada com permissão.)

REFERÊNCIAS BIBLIOGRÁFICAS

As referências bibliográficas deste capítulo se encontram online no Ambiente de Aprendizagem.

CAPÍTULO 259

Exame Neurológico e Diagnóstico Neuroanatômico

Scott J. Schatzberg

O *diagnóstico neuroanatômico* preciso permanece indispensável para a realização de um diagnóstico diferencial adequado, que permita ao clínico interpretar corretamente os testes neurodiagnósticos. Este capítulo tem como objetivo fornecer ao clínico informações de neuroanatomia funcional básica e habilitá-lo para realizar o exame clínico e obter um diagnóstico neuroanatômico preciso. O modelo do exame foi amplamente fundamentado nas recomendações de Lahunta.[1] Os videoclipes deste capítulo mostram os diversos componentes do exame neurológico e as anormalidades silenciosas associadas aos diagnósticos neuroanatômicos mais frequentes.

Os últimos 15 anos foram marcados pelo aumento drástico na disponibilidade de testes neurodiagnósticos avançados para pacientes veterinários, principalmente a imagem de ressonância magnética (RM), que tem aprimorado a capacidade de diagnosticar problemas complexos e distúrbios neurológicos indefinidos. A "desvantagem" de tais avanços é que os clínicos têm desenvolvido uma tendência natural de confiar fortemente (ou exclusivamente!) em testes avançados de imagem em pacientes com distúrbios neurológicos. Embora a RM e a tomografia computadorizada (TC) sejam sensíveis para a identificação de anormalidades do sistema nervoso central (SNC) e do sistema nervoso periférico (SNP), ambas as modalidades de imagem carecem de especificidade e podem ser enganosas quando interpretadas fora do contexto de diagnóstico neuroanatômico e do diagnóstico diferencial. Apesar da disponibilidade excepcional de imagens em corte transversal, a habilidade do clínico em prover diagnóstico, prognóstico e tratamento com sucesso para pacientes com doença neurológica permanece criticamente dependente do exame neurológico.

EXAME NEUROLÓGICO

O exame neurológico pode ser dividido em cinco partes, que incluem a avaliação do (1) sistema sensitivo e comportamento,

CAPÍTULO 259 • Exame Neurológico e Diagnóstico Neuroanatômico

(2) postura e marcha, (3) reações posturais, (4) massa muscular, tônus e reflexos espinais e sensibilidade cutânea e (5) nervos cranianos. A ordem de realização do exame neurológico não é tão importante, mas o clínico deve desenvolver uma abordagem consistente na rotina para avaliar cada cão ou gato.

Sistema sensitivo e comportamental

O tutor geralmente é a melhor pessoa para avaliar as mudanças de nível de consciência e comportamento de um animal de companhia, portanto deve ser questionado cuidadosamente. Exemplos de mudanças comportamentais incluem animais dóceis que se tornam agressivos (e vice-versa) ou animais que se esquecem de habilidades aprendidas. A busca de um histórico preciso pode ser crucial, uma vez que as mudanças comportamentais podem ser secundárias a lesões intracranianas que, de outra forma, não teriam impacto no exame neurológico (ver Capítulos 9 e 13).

O sistema sensitivo deve ser avaliado cuidadosamente em animais de companhia em decúbito. O decúbito pode estar associado a distúrbios do tronco encefálico, medula espinal cervical ou distúrbio neuromuscular difuso (DNM); das três localizações, apenas as lesões no tronco encefálico devem afetar o trato sensitivo. A alteração desse sistema normalmente decorre de um distúrbio no sistema ativador reticular ascendente (SARA) e/ou em componentes do sistema límbico do cérebro ou do tronco encefálico rostral (diencéfalo). Muitos termos têm sido utilizados para descrever mudanças no sistema sensitivo e/ou comportamental, incluindo depressão, letargia, falta de resposta, estupor, coma, ansiedade, desorientação, hiperatividade, histeria, propulsão e agressão (ver Capítulo 148).

Postura e marcha

Postura

O clínico deve avaliar a postura quando o animal de companhia estiver em posição quadrupedal e andando. Devem ser observadas a inclinação da cabeça (p. ex., doença vestibular), virada da cabeça ou do corpo (tronco encefálico rostral ou doença cerebral), posição do pescoço (baixa, em casos de doença medular espinal cervical ou doença neuromuscular difusa), ângulo do jarrete (plantígrado com neuropatias periféricas), evidência de tremor (doença neuromuscular) e posição da cauda (flácida, em casos de doença lombossacra). O clínico também deve reconhecer alterações específicas de postura da raça, como o tarso afundado em Pastores-Alemães.

Lesões intracranianas graves podem levar a duas posturas de opistótono: descerebrado ou descerebelado de rigidez. No *opistótono descerebrado*, a rigidez é caracterizada por um opistótono com extensão rígida do pescoço e de todos os quatro membros e está tipicamente associada a lesões no mesencéfalo ou cerebelo rostral. Já o *opistótono descerebelado de rigidez* resulta de lesões cerebelares graves e é caracterizado por um opistótono com rigidez extensora dos membros, mas com os quadris flexionados.

Pleurototótono refere-se ao desvio da cabeça e pescoço para um lado e pode estar presente em lesões do tronco encefálico médio a rostral ou lesões cerebrais.

Marcha

A força e a coordenação são os principais componentes da marcha a serem avaliados. A marcha deve ser observada em um local onde o animal de companhia possa se mover com ou sem a coleira (se possível) e sempre em uma superfície não escorregadia. O reconhecimento de padrões de anormalidades da marcha é um componente chave para o diagnóstico neuroanatômico.

Paresia. Paresia refere-se à deficiência na capacidade de suportar peso ou de gerar a marcha. Em pacientes neurológicos, a paresia pode resultar de uma lesão no sistema de neurônio motor inferior (NMI)/sistema neuromuscular, no sistema de neurônios motor superior (NMS) ou em ambos.

Animais com "paralisia de NMI" manifestam uma grande variação na capacidade de suportar peso. Os membros torácicos ou pélvicos (ou ainda ambos os membros, em casos de doença do NMI difusa) podem ser afetados. Um cão com DNM moderado pode ser tratado de forma ambulatorial e apresenta marcha curta e irregular (Vídeos 259.1 e 259.41), enquanto um paciente com DNM grave pode ser tetraplégico. Alguns animais de companhia com doença do NMI podem ter uma evolução ambulatorial, e a doença pode acometer ambos os membros pélvicos simultaneamente, mas também é possível ocorrer em distúrbios ortopédicos e da medula espinal.

Animais com "paresia de NMI" podem igualmente apresentar variação na habilidade de produzir a marcha. Dependendo da localização da lesão na medula espinal ou na região médio-caudal do tronco encefálico, os membros torácicos e/ou pélvicos podem ser afetados com sinais de NMS. Animais de companhia com apresentação de paresia ambulatória de NMS andam com marcha espástica longa que normalmente é acompanhada por ataxia *proprioceptiva generalizada* (PG; Vídeos 259.2 e 259.39). A ataxia PG ocorre porque a maior parte das principais vias dos NMS (reticuloespinal e trato rubroespinal) que funcionam para gerar a marcha é anatomicamente adjacente às vias PG (tratos espinocerebelar e a via proprioceptiva consciente). Lesões de medula espinal e de tronco encefálico médio-caudal perturbam as vias NMS descendentes e as vias PG ascendentes, resultando em graus variáveis de paresia e ataxia.

Alguns clínicos utilizam um esquema de classificação para ajudar no prognóstico e no monitoramento da resposta ao tratamento das lesões na medula espinal. Tais esquemas verificam a força e a propriocepção da marcha. A classificação em geral é uma escala de 0 a 5, mas é relativamente inconsistente; alguns esquemas utilizam a nota 0 como normal, enquanto outros, o contrário (p. ex., a nota 5 é normal). Se um esquema de classificação for utilizado, os clínicos devem qualificar a nota como descrição de força, propriocepção e nocicepção (em animais em decúbito) para evitar confusão. Para lesões medulares, o grau de disfunção foi classificado recentemente, usando a pontuação de Frankel modificada.[2,3]

- Grau 0: tetraplegia ou paraplegia sem nocicepção profunda
- Grau 1: tetraplegia ou paraplegia sem nocicepção superficial
- Grau 2: tetraplegia ou paraplegia com nocicepção
- Grau 3: tetraparesia ou paraparesia não ambulatória
- Grau 4: tetraparesia ou paraparesia ambulatória e ataxia PG
- Grau 5: apenas hiperestesia espinal ou sem disfunção.

Ataxia. Existem três formas clínicas de ataxia (incoordenação): (1) PG, (2) vestibular e (3) cerebelar.

A ataxia PG foi mencionada anteriormente em relação à paresia de NMS, uma vez que as duas em geral são simultâneas. Ela resulta da interrupção dos longos tratos ascendentes que estão localizados na medula espinal e transmitem a informação do grau de contração muscular dos membros, do tronco e do pescoço. Quando a informação PG não chega ao cérebro, resulta em incoordenação, que pode incluir cruzamento dos membros, afastamento ou arrastamento dos dígitos, apoio ou aterrissagem sobre o aspecto dorsal das patas e, às vezes, atraso na fase de voo da marcha. Associada aos sinais de NMS, a incoordenação produz uma marcha relativamente característica que reflete ambas as paresias de NMS e ataxia PG (ver Vídeos 259.2 e 259.39).

A *ataxia vestibular* resulta da perda de orientação da cabeça em relação aos olhos, pescoço, membros e tronco. Animais com doença vestibular podem perder o equilíbrio e ter tendência à andar sem direção, inclinar-se ou cair para um lado (Vídeo 259.3). A cabeça inclinada e o nistagmo anormal geralmente acompanham a ataxia (Vídeo 259.28). Animais de companhia com lesões vestibulares periféricas mantêm força e propriocepção normais, mas, em casos de lesão vestibular central, tetraparesia de NMS e déficits PG geralmente estão presentes (Vídeo 259.34).

A *ataxia cerebelar* é caracterizada por marcha hipermétrica com episódios repentinos de atividade motora (Vídeo 259.4). A hipermetria cerebelar pode ser diferenciada de uma marcha de NMS pela hiperflexão acentuada na fase de avanço do membro, porém essa diferenciação é desafiadora. Em razão da conexão estreita entre os sistemas cerebelar e vestibular, podem ser observados rotação de cabeça (*head tilt*), perda de equilíbrio e nistagmo anormal em lesões cerebelares (Vídeo 259.35).

Reações posturais

Após a observação da marcha, as reações posturais devem ser avaliadas para identificar déficits sutis de força e coordenação. A capacidade do animal de realizar reações posturais exige que todos os principais componentes sensoriais (PG) e motores (NMS e NMI) do SNC e do SNP estejam intactos. Embora muitos clínicos usem as reações posturais para avaliar a propriocepção consciente (PC), esse é um termo inadequado, pois todas as reações posturais dependem dos sistemas motor e proprioceptivo. Portanto, ao avaliar as reações posturais, ambos os tratos sensoriais consciente e inconsciente devem ser testados; deficiências nos dois componentes principais do PG não podem ser separadas na prática.[1]

O clínico deve ser cauteloso ao interpretar as reações de déficit postural, pois elas não têm valor para a localização da lesão quando realizadas sem o exame de outros componentes do sistema nervoso (Figura 259.1). Por exemplo, um cão ou gato em decúbito com DNM grave e difuso ou com lesão grave da medula espinal cervical pode ter um atraso (ou ausência) de reações posturais nos quatro membros. A avaliação minuciosa dos reflexos espinais, bem como da massa e do tônus muscular, é necessária para diferenciar entre essas duas localizações. Outro exemplo seria o de um paciente com déficit de reação postural unilateral que possui muitas localizações possíveis, incluindo lesão unilateral do prosencéfalo (cérebro e/ou tálamo), tronco encefálico ou medula espinal. Lesões prosencefálicas unilaterais em geral resultam em déficits de reação postural *contralateral* e marcha normal (e provavelmente acompanhada de déficit na resposta de ameaça contralateral, déficits sensoriais contralaterais e alterações sensoriais; Vídeo 259.33). Lesões do tronco encefálico unilateral (caudal) ou da medula espinal causam déficits de reação postural ipsilateral, e a presença de anormalidades no nervo craniano e/ou de alterações sensoriais pode ajudar na diferenciação entre as duas localizações e sugere disfunção do tronco encefálico.

Em pacientes em decúbito, o teste de reação postural pode ajudar a diferenciar entre tetraparesia do NMS e do NMI. Um cão com doença do NMI "isolado" que mantém alguma atividade voluntária de movimento deve ter reações posturais relativamente normais (se a maior parte do peso corporal é sustentada; ver Vídeo 259.41). Isso ocorre porque o sistema PG não é afetado pela doença do NMI isolado. Em contrapartida, um animal em decúbito com lesão do tronco encefálico ou da medula tem atraso ou ausência de reações posturais em todos os quatro membros.

As respostas do saltitar e do posicionamento são as reações posturais mais valiosas (Vídeos 259.5 a 259.7). Todavia, testes adicionais (p. ex., carrinho de mão e propulsão extensora) podem ser úteis quando essas respostas forem ambíguas.

Testes de reação postural

Saltitar. Seguro pelos membros pélvicos, o animal deve ser apoiado em um membro torácico enquanto o outro membro é mantido fora do chão. O animal deve ser movido lateralmente, e a força e a coordenação dos membros devem ser observadas, comparando os dois lados (ver Vídeo 259.5). O clínico deve observar o aspecto lateral do membro torácico testado, que deve se mover assim que o ombro for movimentado em sentido lateral sobre a pata. Qualquer atraso, irregularidade ou exagero na resposta é anormal. Pode ocorrer atraso no saltitar (simétrico ou assimétrico) em casos de disfunção motora (lesões do NMS ou do NMI) ou

sensorial (PG). Comumente, os sistemas de NMS e PG (p. ex., doenças do tronco encefálico e da medula espinal) são afetados simultaneamente e a resposta de saltitar anormal é um reflexo de ambos (p. ex., déficits de NMS/PG). Lesões no sistema PG ou cerebelo podem produzir respostas exageradas (ver Vídeo 259.6).

Respostas ao saltitar dos membros pélvicos devem ser avaliadas de forma similar. Enquanto se apoiam o tórax e os membros torácicos, um membro pélvico deve ser sustentado e o cão ou gato salta lateralmente no membro de apoio. Respostas de saltitar dos membros pélvicos devem ser comparadas entre si, e não à dos membros torácicos (ver Vídeo 259.6). Normalmente, as respostas ao saltitar dos membros pélvicos são mais espásticas, com uma amplitude de movimento um pouco maior que a dos membros torácicos.

Respostas de posicionamento da pata e de colocação tátil. Respostas de posicionamento avaliam se o cão ou gato corrige a posição da pata após ter sido flexionada, de forma que o peso seja suportado na superfície dorsal (ver Vídeo 259.7). Animais de companhia saudáveis rapidamente colocam a pata na posição anatômica normal. O teste de resposta de posicionamento da pata deve ser realizado nos membros torácicos e pélvicos individualmente. O clínico deve suportar a maior parte do peso do animal durante o teste. Embora alguns clínicos atribuam um atraso na resposta à diminuição da PC (p. ex., "déficit PC"), esse seria um erro de interpretação por três razões: (1) um animal com paresia grave com doença do NMI isolado (p. ex., miastenia *gravis*) pode ter atraso na resposta (ou mesmo estar ausente) ao teste de posicionamento da pata, apesar de não apresentar lesão no sistema de PC (p. ex., o cão pode estar fraco demais para retornar sua pata para a posição anatômica normal); (2) as respostas de posicionamento da pata *não* isolam as vias da PC de outras vias sensoriais aferentes (p. ex., tratos espinocerebelares) do SNP e SNC; por fim, (3) raramente (e inexplicavelmente!) alguns animais de companhia sem doenças neurológicas atrasam as respostas de posicionamento da pata.

Respostas de colocação táteis são tipicamente realizadas em gatos ou cães de pequeno porte. O animal deve ser apoiado no chão e seus membros torácicos devem ser trazidos para a borda de uma mesa, para que a superfície dorsal das patas entre em contato (Vídeo 259.8). O animal deve pisar rapidamente sobre a mesa com a posição anatômica correta da pata. O teste deve ser realizado nos membros torácicos simultaneamente e individualmente. Cobrir os olhos do animal pode ajudar, pois a ausência de visão pode compensar o senso de posicionamento quando o sistema PG estiver anormal.

Propulsão extensora. Embora esse teste seja realizado apenas ocasionalmente, pode ser útil em pacientes com sinais sutis dos membros pélvicos. O animal deve ser mantido fora do chão, apoiado caudalmente às escápulas e abaixado ao chão, permitindo estender os membros pélvicos a fim de suportar seu peso. Durante a movimentação do animal para frente e para trás, avalia-se a simetria, a força e a coordenação dos membros pélvicos (Vídeo 259.9).

Hemilocomoção. Essa reação postural não é realizada rotineiramente, mas pode ser útil em cães grandes. De um lado do corpo, os membros torácicos e pélvicos devem ser afastados no chão, e o cão então é forçado a andar para frente ou para o lado. Cães saudáveis pulam suavemente nos membros torácicos e pélvicos (Vídeo 259.10).

Carrinho de mão. Essa reação postural também é realizada raramente, mas pode ser útil em pacientes com déficits sutis nos membros torácicos. O animal deve ser apoiado sob o abdome, para que os membros pélvicos sejam mantidos fora do chão, e depois deve andar sobre os membros torácicos (Vídeo 259.11). Com essa postura, a visão é comprometida, e o animal depende muito da PG. Com a cabeça estendida na posição normal, cães e gatos devem andar com movimentos simétricos de ambos os membros torácicos e pélvicos. Pacientes com lesões graves podem apresentar a cabeça flexionada com o nariz orientado perto do chão para apoio.

CAPÍTULO 259 • Exame Neurológico e Diagnóstico Neuroanatômico

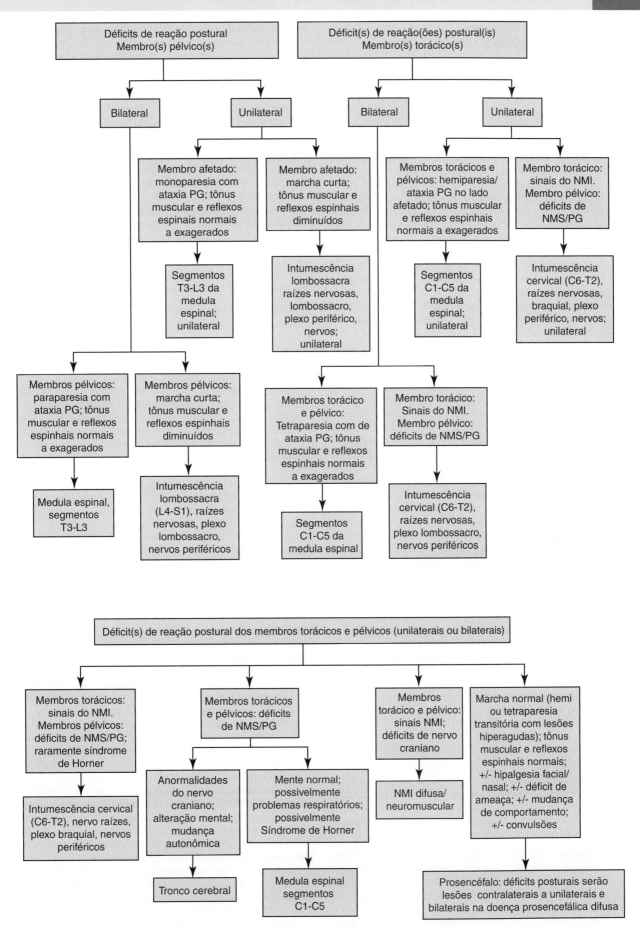

Figura 259.1 Fluxograma para o diagnóstico neuroanatômico associado a déficits de reação postural. *NMI*, neurônio motor inferior; *NMS*, neurônio motor superior; *PG*, proprioceptivo geral.

Massa muscular, tônus muscular, reflexo espinal e sensibilidade cutânea

A massa e o tônus musculares devem ser avaliados quando o animal estiver relaxado, preferencialmente em decúbito lateral. A resposta ao estímulo doloroso pode ser avaliada por último, para manter a cooperação.

Massa e tônus muscular

A cabeça e os músculos epaxiais da região do pescoço e toraco-lombar devem ser avaliados quanto à simetria e qualquer evidência de atrofia. Cada membro torácico e pélvico precisa ser observado da mesma forma, desde a região proximal até a região distal. O tônus muscular deve ser avaliado por sua amplitude de movimento passiva em cada membro. O grau de resistência é definido como normal, hipotônico ou hipertônico/espástico; este varia de leve à acentuado, sendo o grau acentuado ocasionalmente associado a um sinal de canivete (refere-se a tentativas feitas para flexionar o membro que de fato *aumentam* o grau de extensão do membro, até que ele ceda subitamente para flexão completa sem resistência).

A hipertonia ou espasticidade geralmente resulta de lesões em vias de NMS (embora também possa ser observada em distúrbios miotônicos; Vídeos 259.12 e 259.15). O NMS normalmente influencia a atividade do NMI para facilitar a atividade motora voluntária e manter o tônus muscular, dando suporte ao corpo contra a gravidade. Lesões que prejudicam as vias do NMS podem "liberar" a via inibitória do NMI, levando a hiperatividade do mecanismo facilitador (ver Capítulo 258).

Em contrapartida, a hipotonia está relacionada a doença neuromuscular/do NMI (Vídeo 259.13). A integridade funcional completa da "unidade de NMI" (corpo celular, raiz nervosa, nervo periférico, junção neuromuscular e músculo) é necessária para produzir contração das células musculares e manter efetivamente o tônus muscular. Quando a unidade de NMI está enferma, uma consequência é uma perda de tônus muscular. Na doença do NMI, a denervação também pode levar à degeneração das células musculares, e atrofia neurogênica pode ser percebida.

Cães tetraplégicos devem ser mantidos em posição quadrupedal, e o clínico precisa avaliar o tônus muscular e respostas voluntárias dos membros. Cães com doença da medula espinal cervical frequentemente apresentam hipertonia e membros hipertônicos, enquanto o tronco e os membros podem apresentar-se espásticos. Ocasionalmente, a hipertonia associada à doença cervical de medula espinal é tão intensa que o animal pode manter-se em posição quadrupedal, mesmo sem apoio. Em contrapartida, cães tetraplégicos com doença neuromuscular/do NMI difusa tipicamente são hipotônicos (ou atônicos) e entram em colapso quando o clínico tenta apoiá-los em uma posição ereta. É difícil diferenciar entre tetraplegia do NMS e do NMI, já que os diagnósticos diferenciais são acentuadamente diferentes, assim como os diagnósticos, o manejo e as recomendações de tratamento.

Reflexos espinais

Embora a maioria dos livros de neurologia descreva diversos reflexos tendinosos e musculares, muitos deles são de uso limitado, pois não estão presentes em todos os animais de pequeno porte em condições normais. Os reflexos mais confiáveis são os reflexos patelares e de retirada descritos a seguir. Outros reflexos espinais serão abordados sucintamente.

Reflexo patelar. O reflexo tendíneo mais confiável é o reflexo patelar, mediado pelo nervo femoral através dos segmentos da medula espinal L4-L7. Com o membro mantido em flexão parcial, o clínico deve obter o reflexo ao bater levemente no tendão patelar com um martelo plexor ou martelo pediátrico (Vídeo 259.14). Esse reflexo deve ser testado com o animal em decúbito lateral, tanto direito quanto esquerdo. Por motivos inexplicáveis, é comum o reflexo ser eliciado mais facilmente com o

membro adjacente ao solo. Vale ressaltar que um ou ambos os reflexos patelares podem estar ausentes em cães mais velhos sem outros sinais neurológicos.[4] As respostas são tipicamente classificadas como ausente (0), hiporreflexia (+1), normal (+2), hiper-reflexia (+3) ou clônica (+4). O reflexo ausente ou hiporreflexia ocorre quando há doença em uma parte do arco reflexo (mais comumente na unidade NMI). Hiper-reflexia ou clônus podem estar presentes em doenças do NMS (ver Vídeo 259.15).

Reflexos bicipital e tricipital. Nos membros torácicos, o reflexo do bíceps e do tríceps geralmente pode ser eliciado em animais de companhia que estão relaxados em decúbito lateral. O clínico deve colocar um dedo e bater levemente nas extremidades distais dos bíceps e nos músculos braquiais ao nível do cotovelo. A resposta normal é a leve flexão do cotovelo. O nervo musculocutâneo medeia o reflexo bicipital por meio dos segmentos C6-C8 da medula espinal. O reflexo do tríceps é provocado tocando levemente no tendão de inserção do músculo tríceps, proximal ao olécrano, o que causa uma leve extensão do cotovelo. O nervo radial medeia o reflexo tricipital através dos segmentos C7-T2 da medula espinal.

Reflexo de retirada/flexor – membros torácicos e pélvicos. O reflexo de retirada/flexor avalia a integridade do arco reflexo de retirada do membro torácico e do pélvico. Eles são eliciados aplicando pressão firme na base da unha com uma pinça manual ou uma hemostática (Vídeos 259.16 e 259.17). Uma resposta normal é a retirada imediata e forte do membro, com flexão completa de todas as articulações. Animais com redução do reflexo de retirada ocasionalmente estendem o membro ou chutam em resposta ao estímulo nocivo (Vídeos 259.18 e 259.19). No membro torácico, os nervos toracodorsal, axilar, musculocutâneo, mediano, ulnar e radial são responsáveis pela flexão do ombro, cotovelo, carpo e dígitos. Os nervos responsáveis por esse reflexo surgem dos segmentos da medula espinal C6-T2. A estimulação específica do nervo sensitivo depende da localização do estímulo nocivo. O nervo ulnar inerva a pele na superfície palmar da pata; o nervo radial inerva a superfície dorsal e as superfícies cranial e lateral do antebraço. Os nervos ulnar e musculocutâneos inervam as superfícies caudal e medial, respectivamente. É preciso ter cuidado para não interpretar excessivamente as zonas autônomas, pois há algumas áreas de sobreposição da inervação cutânea suprida por esses nervos e um grau de variação individual do paciente.

Deficiências no reflexo de retirada do membro torácico (Vídeos 259.18, 259.39, 259.41 e 259.42) sugerem lesão em C6-T2 (segmentos da medula espinal, raízes nervosas, plexo braquial, nervos periféricos) ou uma potencial lesão mais difusa no NMI/NMS (esta última seria acompanhada por redução dos reflexos nos membros pélvicos, tônus reduzido e outros sinais neuromusculares). Tem sido sugerido que cães com lesões na medula espinal em nível C1-C5 podem *erroneamente* responder em C6-T2, em função da resposta reduzida do reflexo de retirada, que pode estar presente nos membros torácicos.[5] Entretanto, a explicação para esse fenômeno não foi bem esclarecida.

No membro pélvico, o reflexo de retirada/flexor é mediado pelo nervo isquiático através dos segmentos L6-S1 da medula espinal. Lesões do componente motor do nervo isquiático (distal à pelve) podem resultar em hipotonia, atrofia e paralisia dos músculos do joelho (flexores), quadril (extensores), tarso e dígitos (ambos). Em caso de lesões isquiáticas, o reflexo de retirada/flexor do membro pélvico está reduzido ou ausente (ver Vídeo 259.19). Cães e gatos podem andar com paralisia do nervo isquiático, mas o tarso normalmente é "caído" ou mais próximo ao solo do que o normal no lado afetado (disfunção tibial) e a pata muitas vezes fica mal posicionada na superfície dorsal (disfunção fibular); no entanto, o membro pode suportar peso se o nervo femoral estiver intacto.

A superfície dorsal e plantar das patas do membro pélvico são inervadas pelos ramos sensoriais dos nervos fibular e tibial, respectivamente. O nervo safeno (ramo do femoral que adentra na medula espinal no nível de L4-L6) inerva o aspecto medial. Portanto, os animais com o nervo isquiático gravemente contundido em geral mantêm a sensibilidade no aspecto medial da pata. Se a superfície medial é estimulada em um animal com lesão isquiática isolada, ele flexiona o quadril, uma vez que a inervação do músculo iliopsoas está intacta, porém o calcanhar, o tarso e os dígitos *não* flexionam. Portanto, tanto a superfície medial quanto a lateral do membro pélvico devem ser testadas para o reflexo de retirada/flexor e para nocicepção (ver adiante).

Reflexo extensor cruzado. Animais com lesões das vias de NMI em decúbito podem apresentar reflexo extensor cruzado quando o reflexo de retirada é avaliado, ou seja, o reflexo pode ocorrer no membro oposto ao que está sendo testado. Embora tipicamente anormal e indicativo de doença NMI, cães normais às vezes apresentam reflexo extensor cruzado. A fim de evitar extensão voluntária do membro contralateral como resposta ao estímulo nocivo, o reflexo de retirada/flexor deve ser eliciado com um beliscamento leve enquanto o membro oposto é observado.

Reflexo perineal. O reflexo perineal é provocado por estimulação levemente dolorosa do ânus. O esfíncter anal e a cauda devem ser observados quanto a contração e flexão, respectivamente. O reflexo perineal é mediado por ramos dos segmentos sacral e caudal da medula espinal através do nervo pudendo.

Reflexo musculocutâneo. Esse reflexo é observado pela contração do músculo cutâneo do tronco em resposta à leve estimulação da pele dorsal. O estímulo pode ser eliciado na região torácica e grande parte da região lombar. Nervos espinais regionais segmentares carreiam impulsos sensoriais (Vídeo 259.20) na medula espinal, os quais são retransmitidos cranialmente à medula espinal até o segmento C8. Nesse local, ocorre uma sinapse com os NMI de *ambos* os nervos torácicos laterais, que inervam o tecido do músculo cutâneo do tronco. Esse reflexo pode exigir várias tentativas para ser provocado, e é raro que cães e gatos normais não o manifestem. O reflexo pode ser particularmente útil no diagnóstico do nível de uma lesão toracolombar transversal da medula espinal ou no monitoramento de uma lesão progressiva da medula espinal (p. ex., mielomalácia ascendente ou descendente). Normalmente, o reflexo é preservado por um a dois corpos vertebrais caudais ao nível da lesão da medula espinal.

Nocicepção (percepção da dor)

Em animais em decúbito, o clínico pode aplicar um estímulo nocivo a um dígito (Vídeo 259.21). Isso gera impulsos aferentes que entram na coluna vertebral via nervo periférico e fazem sinapses nos neurônios das raízes nervosas dorsais, localizadas nos tratos bilaterais no funículo lateral da medula espinal. Esses tratos ascendem à medula espinal, continuam através dela, da ponte e do mesencéfalo para núcleos específicos no tálamo e retransmitem a informação nociceptiva para áreas sensoriais somáticas do córtex cerebral. Uma resposta positiva é evidenciada por vocalização, virada da cabeça ou dilatação das pupilas, uma vez que os impulsos alcançam o tálamo ou cérebro.

Embora muitos esquemas de classificação para lesão medular diferenciem entre a percepção da dor superficial e a profunda, isso pode ser extremamente desafiador e em geral não é necessário. No entanto, é fundamental diferenciar entre a nocicepção e o componente do reflexo de retirada/flexor (ver anteriormente). *Animais com lesões transversais da medula espinal mantêm o reflexo flexor, o que não deve ser confundido com nocicepção intacta.*

Nervos cranianos

É importante desenvolver um método sistemático de avaliação dos nervos cranianos. Esse componente do exame neurológico é idealmente realizado com um cão ou gato cooperativo. Esta seção oferece uma abordagem gradual para avaliar os nervos cranianos quanto a: (1) visão e resposta pupilar à luz (RPL);

(2) fissura palpebral e simetria de terceira pálpebra; (3) posição e movimento do globo ocular; (4) função vestibular; (5) função facial e trigêmeo; e (6) função da língua e laringofaringe. Os sinais clínicos associados à disfunção de nervos cranianos são resumidos na Tabela 259.1.

Visão e respostas pupilares à luz (II, III, VII)

O teste de resposta à ameaça é o mais confiável para avaliar a visão em animais. É uma resposta aprendida, que pode não estar presente em cães e gatos filhotes com menos de 10 a 12 semanas (rastreamento de objeto em movimento pode ser útil nesses animais jovens). A resposta à ameaça requer nervo óptico, trato óptico (diencéfalo) e radiação óptica funcionais até a região do córtex occipital, bem como via eferente, que inclui os neurônios faciais. Embora o mecanismo exato seja desconhecido, um cerebelo funcional também é necessário para a resposta à ameaça.[1] A maioria das vias visuais caudais ao quiasma óptico é contralateral ao olho testado. Com um olho do animal coberto, o clínico deve fazer um gesto ameaçador para o olho aberto (com muita atenção para não tocar ou estimular o animal com correntes de ar! Vídeo 259.22).

Uma resposta normal de ameaça se manifesta com o fechamento palpebral completo, que depende da inervação do nervo facial no músculo orbicular do olho. Se a resposta de ameaça for ausente ou retardada, as pálpebras devem ser avaliadas quanto à sua capacidade de fechamento, realizando-se o teste de reflexo palpebral (Vídeo 259.23). Se houver paralisia facial, a retração do globo ocular, a elevação da terceira pálpebra e a retração da cabeça podem ajudar na avaliação da visão (Vídeo 259.29). Como alternativa, a capacidade do paciente de passar em uma pista com obstáculos pode ser avaliada.

Após o teste de resposta de ameaça, o clínico deve avaliar o tamanho da pupila e o RPL (Vídeo 259.24). As pupilas devem ser avaliadas em luz natural e em ambiente escuro quanto à simetria. Uma fonte de luz brilhante deve ser direcionada para cada olho individualmente (Vídeo 259.25). Animais normais têm uma rápida constrição da pupila na qual a luz é direcionada (RPL direta), e a pupila do olho oposto também deve contrair (RPL indireto ou consensual). A resposta indireta ocorre porque a maioria das fibras do nervo óptico cruza o quiasma óptico e novamente no nível do núcleo pré-tectal, com estimulação bilateral dos núcleos oculomotores parassimpáticos.

Além das lesões dos nervos óptico e oculomotor, existem várias possibilidades de localizações para déficits de RPL (Tabela 259.2). Se um RPL direto não for desencadeado em um olho, o clínico deve aproximar ao máximo a luz desse olho e movê-la para avaliar todos os aspectos do fundo do olho. Se não houver resposta, então o clínico deve balançar a luz para o olho responsivo, e a pupila não responsiva deve ser avaliada quanto à constrição. Se o resultado for não responsivo, então significa que ocorreu lesão do nervo óptico ou do ocular, e a contração pupilar ocorrerá quando a luz for direcionada para o olho contralateral (p. ex., RPL indireto positivo). Tais testes talvez tenham que ser repetidos várias vezes para diferenciar entre um problema no nervo ocular/nervo óptico e um no nervo oculomotor.

Fissura palpebral e simetria de terceira pálpebra (III, V, nervos simpáticos)

O clínico deve observar a pálpebra quanto a tamanho e simetria. O tamanho reduzido (ptose) pode ser causado por disfunção do nervo craniano III (oculomotor), com paresia secundária do músculo elevador palpebral superior, disfunção do nervo craniano V (mandibular, ramo do nervo trigêmeo) e atrofia secundária dos músculos mastigatórios (Vídeo 259.26) ou disfunção simpática com perda de tônus do musculo liso orbital. Tanto a atrofia dos músculos mastigatórios quanto a disfunção simpática podem resultar em elevação da terceira pálpebra.

SEÇÃO 17 • Doença Neurológica

Tabela 259.1 Função, teste e sinais clínicos associados à disfunção do nervo cranial.

NERVO CRANIAL	FUNÇÃO	TESTE	SINAIS CLÍNICOS DA DISFUNÇÃO
I NC Olfatório	Odor	Não testado rotineiramente	Anosmia; hiposmia
II NC Óptico	Visão; resposta à luz	Resposta à ameaça; RPL; desvio de obstáculo em curso; rastreamento de objetos em movimento	Cegueira; pupilas dilatadas ou não responsivas
III NC Oculomotor	Motor para os músculos extra-oculares; parassimpático à pupila	Nistagmo fisiológico; globo ocular em posição de repouso; respostas à luz pupilar	Estrabismo ventrolateral; ptose; pupila dilatada; RLP diminuídos a ausentes
IV NC Troclear	Motor para o músculo oblíquo dorsal	Posição do globo ocular em repouso (gato); exame de fundo de olho (cão)	Estrabismo dorsomedial (gato); lateral desvio da veia da retina (cão)
V NC Trigêmino	Motor para os músculos da mastigação (mandibular); sensorial para enfrentar (oftalmológico e maxilar)	Tom da mandíbula; massa muscular; sensação de mucosa facial, córnea e nasal	Atrofia muscular mastigatória; queixo caído se bilateral; diminuição/ausência facial/sensação nasal
VI NC Abducente	Motor para reto lateral e afastador bulbi	Nistagmo fisiológico; globo ocular na posição em repouso	Estrabismo medial
VII NC Facial	Motor para os músculos da expressão facial; glândulas parassimpáticas a lacrimais; língua sensorial (paladar) a rostral	Resposta à ameaça; reflexo palpebral; retração labial; movimento da orelha; teste de ruptura de Schirmer	Incapacidade de fechar a pálpebra, mover a orelha ou retrair o lábio; tetania hemifacial; desvio de filtro nasal (contralateral); olho seco
VIII NC Vestibulococlear	Saldo; audição	Postura do corpo e da cabeça; maneira de andar; movimento e posição do olho; audição	Inclinar a cabeça; ataxia vestibular; nistagmo; estrabismo posicional; surdez
IX NC Glossofaríngeo	Sensorial e motor da faringe	Reflexo de vômito; capacidade de engolir	Reflexo de vômito diminuído; disfagia
X NC Vago	Sensorial e motor da faringe, laringe e vísceras	Reflexo de vômito; reflexo oculocárdico	Reflexo de vômito diminuído; disfagia; paralisia da laringe; megaesôfago
XI NC Acessório	Motor para trapézio	Avaliação da massa muscular	Atrofia do trapézio
XII NC Hipoglosso	Músculos motores da língua	Músculos motores da língua	Atrofia da língua; incapacidade de retrair língua se bilateral

RPL, resposta pupilar à luz.

Tabela 259.2 Locais das lesões (apenas lesões do lado direito, como exemplo) e tamanho associado da pupila em repouso, respostas pupilares leves (RPLs) e respostas de ameaça.

TAMANHO DO FILHOTE DE RESTAURAÇÃO RPLS, AMEAÇA	II CN DIREITO (*NERVO ÓPTICO*)	III CN DIREITO (*NERVO OCULOMOTOR*)	LOCALIZAÇÃO DA LESÃO		
			RETROBULBAR DIREITO	TRATO ÓPTICO CERTO (*THALAMUS*)	CÓRTEX OCCIPITAL DIREITO
Pupila esquerda Tamanho de descanso	Tamanho normal	Tamanho normal	Tamanho normal	Tamanho normal	Tamanho normal
RPLs	Luz no olho esquerdo, ambas as pupilas contraem	Luz no olho esquerdo, apenas a pupila esquerda contrai	Luz no olho esquerdo, ambas as pupilas contraem	Luz no olho esquerdo, ambas as pupilas contraem	Luz no olho esquerdo, ambas as pupilas contraem
Ameaça esquerda	Positiva	Positiva	Positiva	Déficit grave	Déficit grave
Pupila esquerda Tamanho de descanso	Dilatação normal a parcial	Dilatação completa	Dilatação completa	Tamanho normal	Tamanho normal
RPLs	Luz no olho direito, nenhuma pupila contrai	Luz no olho direito, apenas a pupila esquerda contrai	Luz no olho direito, nem aluno contrai	Luz no olho direito, ambas as pupilas contraem	Luz no olho direito, ambas as pupilas contraem
Ameaça certa	Negativo	Positivo	Negativo	Déficit leve	Déficit leve

RPL, resposta pupilar à luz.

Posição e movimento dos olhos (III IV, VI, VIII)

Ao avaliar a cabeça, o clínico deve verificar se os olhos estão em uma posição central à órbita, que requer uma função normal dos componentes periféricos e centrais do sistema vestibular, dos nervos cranianos III (oculomotores) IV (troclear) e VI (abducente) e dos músculos extraoculares que eles inervam. O estrabismo ventrolateral está associado à disfunção do nervo oculomotor, enquanto o estrabismo medial está associado à disfunção do nervo abducente. Já a extorsão (estrabismo dorsolateral) do globo ocular está associada à disfunção do nervo troclear. Em gatos, a disfunção troclear causa rotação lateral do aspecto dorsal da pupila, mas não pode ser reconhecida no exame ocular externo em cães, uma vez que suas pupilas são redondas. Em cães, o exame de fundo de olho é necessário, pois mostra desvio lateral da veia da retina.

Função vestibular (VIII)

O nistagmo fisiológico (respostas oculocefálicas ou oculovestibulares) é avaliado com o movimento da cabeça de um lado para o outro em um plano horizontal (Vídeo 259.27). Isso estimula o nervo craniano VIII a transmitir impulsos para o tronco encefálico, para os núcleos vestibulares e fascículo longitudinal medial e, por fim, para os neurônios abducente e oculomotor, para a abdução e a adução do globo ocular, respectivamente.

Estrabismo e nistagmo são comumente associados a disfunção do sistema vestibular. O estrabismo posicional ventrolateral geralmente está associado a doença vestibular. Nistagmo é uma oscilação involuntária do globo ocular (Vídeo 259.28). O nistagmo de repouso ou espontâneo é contínuo e observado quando a cabeça está em qualquer posição, enquanto o nistagmo posicional é visto apenas quando a cabeça é mantida em certas posições e costuma ser observado em pacientes que possuem lesões no sistema vestibular. Ocasionalmente, o nistagmo posicional pode ser induzido em pacientes compensados, quando são colocados de costas e com a cabeça e o pescoço estendidos. A utilidade do nistagmo para a localização da lesão vestibular é revisada na seção "Diagnóstico neuroanatômico" deste capítulo.

Funções dos nervos facial e trigêmeo (V, VII)

O clínico deve avaliar o reflexo palpebral tocando suavemente os cantos medial e lateral do olho (ver Vídeos 259.23 e 259.29). A resposta normal é imediata e consiste no fechamento completo da fenda palpebral. Os ramos sensoriais do nervo trigêmeo (nervo oftálmico, medialmente; nervo maxilar, lateralmente) medeiam o braço aferente do reflexo palpebral, enquanto o ramo do nervo facial medeia o braço eferente motor. O clínico também deve avaliar a simetria facial; a queda do lábio ou da orelha (ver Vídeo 259.29) ou salivação unilateral sugere disfunção do nervo facial. Ocasionalmente, o filtro nasal será desviado para a frente, superestimando a musculatura facial em decorrência de tetania facial.

Para avaliação do ramo mandibular do nervo trigêmeo, o clínico deve observar os músculos temporal e masseter quanto a tamanho e simetria. Na disfunção mandibular unilateral (p. ex., neoplasia na bainha do nervo trigêmeo), nenhuma perda da função da mandíbula será vista, porém uma profunda atrofia muscular pode estar presente (ver Vídeo 259.26). Em casos de disfunção bilateral do nervo mandibular (p. ex., neurite idiopática do trigêmeo), o paciente pode ter a mandíbula decídua e saliva excessiva (Vídeo 259.30). A paralisia mandibular pode ser acompanhada de hipoalgesia facial, dependendo da extensão do envolvimento dos nervos sensoriais oftálmico e maxilar.

A função sensorial trigeminal é mais facilmente avaliada por teste de sensibilidade nasal. O clínico deve tocar suavemente o aspecto medial da mucosa nasal com a ponta de uma caneta ou uma pinça hemostática fechada (Vídeo 259.31). Pacientes normais afastam rapidamente a cabeça (pacientes estoicos ocasionalmente não reagem). Esse teste avalia duas vias neurais: primeiro, o ramo ipsilateral do nervo oftálmico, que inerva a mucosa nasal; segundo, as vias nociceptivas, que se projetam em direção ao tálamo contralateral e ao córtex somestésico cerebral. Portanto, a hipoalgesia nasal deve ser interpretada à luz do restante do exame neurológico. Ele pode indicar uma lesão do nervo trigêmeo *ipsilateral* ou uma lesão prosencefálica *contralateral* (ver Vídeo 259.33).

Função da língua e da laringofaringe (IX, X, XII)

O clínico pode usar o "reflexo de vômito" para avaliar simultaneamente os nervos cranianos glossofaríngeo, vago e hipoglosso. Ao abrir a boca do paciente, a língua deve ser primeiramente avaliada quanto à atrofia e à movimentação, a fim de averiguar a função da musculatura do hipoglosso. Dependendo da cooperação do paciente, o clínico pode então inserir um dedo através da cavidade oral na orofaringe e laringofaringe. O tônus muscular e o reflexo de vômito devem ser observados para avaliar os ramos faríngeos do glossofaríngeo e do nervo vago. A utilidade clínica desse teste é limitada, em razão da variabilidade nas respostas normais. Disfagia (ver Capítulos 38 e 273) é um indicador mais confiável de disfunção dos nervos IX e X.

DIAGNÓSTICO NEUROANATÔMICO

Após a realização do exame neurológico completo, o clínico deve tentar fazer o diagnóstico neuroanatômico de uma das cinco principais regiões do sistema nervoso: (1) prosencéfalo (cérebro e/ou tálamo); (2) tronco encefálico médio a caudal (mesencéfalo, medula e ponte); (3) cerebelo; (4) medula espinal; e (5) NMI/sistema neuromuscular. Sinais neurológicos associados a lesões em cada uma dessas regiões estão descritos nas Tabelas 259.3 a 259.6; os principais déficits neurológicos e os exames-padrão para cada região também são explicados.

O clínico inicialmente deve tentar conciliar todas as informações dos déficits neurológicos em uma única lesão. Se uma única lesão não puder explicar todos os sinais, é provável que o diagnóstico neuroanatômico seja multifocal ou difuso (ver mais adiante). Após localizar a lesão para uma das cinco regiões principais do SNC ou SNP, uma localização mais precisa deve ser determinada (p. ex., lado e segmentos anatômicos específicos afetados, como C1-C5 ou C6-T2). Como mencionado anteriormente, um diagnóstico neuroanatômico preciso fornece informações críticas para o estabelecimento de diagnósticos diferenciais e ajuda na seleção e interpretação de testes neurodiagnósticos.

Prosencéfalo

Embora comumente utilizado como termo embriológico para designar a área do cérebro composta pelo telencéfalo (hemisférios cerebrais) e pelo diencéfalo (epitálamo, tálamo e hipotálamo), essa grande região é uma chave para o diagnóstico neuroanatômico. Em razão da sobreposição dos sinais clínicos associados às doenças cerebral e talâmica, lesões que afetam essas duas áreas não podem ser diferenciadas de maneira confiável. Quando os sinais neurológicos sugerem doença cérebro-talâmica ("prosencéfalo"), o diagnóstico neuroanatômico de lesão prosencefálica é feito.

Animais com doença prosencefálica costumam ter histórico de convulsões generalizadas ou parciais e/ou comportamento anormal (ver Tabela 259.3). Alterações de comportamento típicas incluem depressão (decorrente de lesões no SARA), letargia, desorientação, perda do comportamento aprendido (treinamento), maior agressividade/docilidade, irritabilidade, histeria ou comportamento maníaco, pressão na cabeça, estimulação propulsiva e andar em círculos (Vídeo 259.32). Anormalidades no sistema autonômico e na função endócrina (sede, apetite, temperatura, eletrólitos e equilíbrio hídrico) e padrões de sono também podem estar presentes.

Tabela 259.3 Sinais neurológicos que podem estar associados à doenças do prosencéfalo.

TESTE NEUROLÓGICO	POSSÍVEIS ANORMALIDADES
Sensório/comportamento	Convulsões; comportamento anormal; atividade propulsiva; depressão ao coma
Postura/marcha	Virada da cabeça, marcha normal (a menos que seja lesão); circulação propulsiva (geralmente ipsilateral à lesão) ou estimulação; vagando sem rumo; pressionando a cabeça; distúrbios do movimento (raros)
Reações posturais	Déficits contralaterais
Massa/tônus muscular	Reflexos na coluna vertebral
Reflexos na coluna vertebral	Hipalgesia contralateral (geralmente facial/nasal)
Sensação cutânea	Hipalgesia contralateral (geralmente facial/nasal)
Nervos cranianos	Déficits de ameaça contralateral com RPL normal (radiação óptica e córtex occipital) ou anormal (quiasma óptico, tratos ópticos); facial; língua ou faringe fraqueza (rara)
Outros	Anormalidades na sede, apetite, termorregulação

RPL, resposta pupilar à luz.

Tabela 259.4 Sinais neurológicos que podem estar associados à doenças do tronco encefálico.

TESTE NEUROLÓGICO	POSSÍVEIS ANORMALIDADES
Sensório/comportamento	Depressão – coma
Postura/marcha	Tetraparesia NMS (ou tetraplegia) e déficits PGs; ataxia vestibular (pontina ou lesões medulares); opistótono (lesões no mesencéfalo)
Reações posturais	Déficits ipsilaterais (ponte e medula), déficits contralaterais (mesencéfalo rostral)
Massa/tônus muscular	Normal a aumentado (todos os quatro membros)
Reflexos na coluna vertebral	Normal a aumentado (todos os quatro membros)
Sensação cutânea	A hipalgesia do tronco e dos membros pode ser presente (raro)
Nervos cranianos	Anisocoria (III, simpático); queixo caído (V bilateral); atrofia dos músculos de mastigação (V); hipalgesia facial (V); inclinação da cabeça (VIII); nistagmo em repouso ou posicional (VIII); nistagmo fisiológico anormal (III, IV, VI, VIII); estrabismo de descanso ou posicional (III, IV, VI, VIII); paresia ou paralisia facial (VII); disfagia (IX, X); paresia ou paralisia da língua (XII)
Outros	Anormalidades respiratórias ou cardíacas

NMS, neurônio motor superior; *PG*, proprioceptivo geral.

Tabela 259.5 Sinais neurológicos que podem estar associados à doença cerebelar.

TESTE NEUROLÓGICO	POSSÍVEIS ANORMALIDADES
Sensório/comportamento	Não afetado
Postura/marcha	Tremor intencional de cabeça, pescoço ou olhos; opistótono e rigidez extensiva de todos os membros com quadris fledados (grave, rostral lesões); balanço truncal; inclinar a cabeça; marcha hipermétrica/espástica com força preservada; perda de equilíbrio
Reações posturais	Atrasadas e depois exageradas em todos os membros com doença difusa ou no membro ipsilateral com lesões unilaterais
Massa/tônus muscular	O tônus muscular pode ser exagerado
Reflexos na coluna vertebral	Normais ou exagerados
Sensação cutânea	Não afetada
Nervos cranianos	Ameaça de déficit (ipsilateral); anisocoria (rara)

CAPÍTULO 259 • Exame Neurológico e Diagnóstico Neuroanatômico

Tabela 259.6 Sinais torácicos e pélvicos dos membros associados a lesões na medula espinal.

LOCALIZAÇÃO DA LESÃO	MEMBROS TORÁCICOS	MEMBROS PÉLVICOS	LESÕES GRAVES
C1-C5	Paresia NMS; déficits de PG; reflexos de retirada normais* e tônus muscular	Paresia NMS; déficits de PG; reflexos espinais e tônus muscular normais a exagerados	Tetraplegia espástica; complicações do potencial respiratório; síndrome de Horner do NMS
C6-T2	Paresia do NMI (curto e agitado maneira de andar); reflexos de retirada e tônus muscular reduzidos	Paresia NMS; déficits de PG; andar com passos largos; reflexos da medula espinal e tônus muscular normais a exagerados	Paralisia flácida do NMI em membros torácicos; paraplegia espástica em membros pélvicos; complicações do potencial respiratório; síndrome de Horner (T1-T3)
T3-L3	Normal	Paresia NMS; déficits de PG; andar com passos largos; reflexos da medula espinal e tônus muscular normais a exagerados	Paraplegia espástica; Schiff-Sherrington pode ocorrer em membros torácicos; possíveis sinais paradoxais do NMI (choque espinal) nos membros pélvicos
L4-S3	Normal	Paresia NMI (marcha curta e agitada); déficits de PG (substância branca); reflexos patelares (L4-L6) ou de retirada (L6-S1) reduzidos	Paraplegia flácida em membros pélvicos, que podem incluir ânus e cauda flácidos com redução da sensação de ausência do períneo

*As lesões em C1-C5 podem estar associadas a reflexos reduzidos na retirada do membro torácico.[5] *NMI*, neurônio motor inferior; *NMS*, neurônio motor superior; *PG*, proprioceptivo geral.

Embora convulsões, alterações comportamentais e autonômicas/endócrinas suportem um diagnóstico neuroanatômico prosencefálico, essas anormalidades raramente ajudam a identificar o lado da lesão no cérebro ou tálamo. Animais com lesões prosencefálicas manifestam comumente déficits visuais, sensitivos (facial/nasal hipoalgesia) e reações posturais, todos contralaterais ao lado da lesão (ver Vídeo 259.33). Apesar de apresentarem déficits de reações posturais (um verdadeiro déficit de "PC"), animais com doença prosencefálica normalmente têm marcha normal (déficit de marcha pode estar presente em lesões agudas, como acidente vascular cerebral [AVC]). A marcha é normal em lesões prosencefálicas, já que os NMS responsáveis pela formação da marcha em espécies domésticas (tratos rubroespinal e reticuloespinal) são poupados, localizando-se mais caudalmente no mesencéfalo, na ponte e na medula.

Um fenômeno incomum conhecido como *síndrome da negligência* (heminegligência ou hemidesatenção) ocorre algumas vezes em lesões prosencefálicas unilaterais. Nessa síndrome, o animal "ignora" todas as informações sensoriais percebidas em seu ambiente que são contralaterais à lesão prosencefálica. O paciente pode andar em círculos propulsivamente ou comer somente um lado da tigela (ipsilateral para a lesão). A Tabela 259.3 resume os potenciais sinais clínicos associados à doença prosencefálica.

Tronco encefálico

O tronco encefálico é ventral aos dois hemisférios cerebrais e ao cerebelo. Embora anatomicamente o diencéfalo seja uma extensão rostral do tronco encefálico, ele é considerado parte da região prosencefálica (acima) em termos de localização. Um diagnóstico neuroanatômico do "tronco encefálico" é usado para denotar lesões que incluem o mesencéfalo, a ponte e a medula oblonga (bulbo). Funcionalmente, o tronco encefálico contém os núcleos dos pares de nervos cranianos, o centro de consciência (SARA), o centro respiratório, os neurônios motores descendentes e as vias sensoriais ascendentes. Portanto, anormalidades dos nervos cranianos, alterações comportamentais e perda de funções autonômicas, de força e de coordenação podem estar presentes em doenças do tronco encefálico (ver Tabela 259.4).

O tronco encefálico conecta os hemisférios cerebrais à medula espinal via neurônios sensoriais ascendente (PG) e via neurônios motores descendentes (NMS). Assim como nas lesões da medula espinal C1-C5, a tetraparesia da NMS (por

tetraplegia) e os déficits PG podem acompanhar doenças do tronco encefálico. Em razão da presença de núcleos vestibulares na ponte e na medula, ataxia vestibular pode estar presente e sobreposta à ataxia PG (ver Vídeo 259.34).

Dependendo da região do tronco encefálico afetada (médio a caudal), podem ocorrer disfunções dos nervos cranianos III a XII. O exame neurológico permite a avaliação de diversas funções motoras e sensoriais desses nervos (ver Tabelas 259.1 e 259.4). Lesões que afetam os nervos cranianos caudais ao tronco encefálico geralmente causam alterações posturais ipsilaterais e déficits de reações posturais, em razão do seu impacto no NMS e no sistema PG. A presença de anormalidades nos nervos cranianos e de reações posturais normais sugere neuropatia periférica (craniana); porém, a compressão precoce ou lenta do tronco encefálico não pode ser excluída. Se houver ambiguidade nos testes de reação postural, uma avaliação neurodiagnóstica deve ser considerada.

Doença vestibular

Inclinação da cabeça, ataxia vestibular, nistagmo e estrabismo são comumente observados em doença vestibular (ver Vídeos 259.28, 259.34 e 259.35), porém raramente ajudam o clínico a diferenciar entre a doença vestibular central e a periférica. A chave para essa diferenciação é a presença ou ausência de déficits de reações posturais. Em pacientes com lesões vestibulares que envolvem o tronco encefálico caudal, os déficits de reações posturais ipsilaterais estão presentes em razão do envolvimento das vias do NMS/PG (ver Vídeo 259.34) Em contrapartida, as reações posturais são normais com lesões vestibulares periféricas, já que não há envolvimento das vias do NMS/PG.

Lesões que afetam o nervo vestibular periférico resultam em inclinação da cabeça, ipsilateralmente à lesão (a orelha baixa está do lado da lesão); isso é menos previsível com lesões do tronco encefálico. Embora a maioria dos animais com doença vestibular central tenha inclinação ipsilateral de cabeça no lado da lesão, aqueles com lesões no tronco encefálico envolvendo o pedúnculo cerebelar caudal (ou lóbulo floculonodular do cerebelo) podem manifestar inclinação da cabeça contralateral – ou a chamada "inclinação paradoxal da cabeça" (ver Vídeo 259.35).

Nistagmo de repouso ou nistagmo posicional geralmente acompanha tanto a doença vestibular central quanto a periférica (ver Vídeo 259.28). A direção do nistagmo é definida pela fase rápida de deslocamento do globo ocular. O plano de rotação pode ser *rotatório*, *horizontal* ou *vertical*. Normalmente, o nistagmo vertical está associado a lesões vestibulares centrais (ver Vídeo 259.34), enquanto o rotatório ou horizontal pode estar presente com lesões centrais ou periféricas. Na lesão vestibular periférica, a fase rápida do nistagmo é oposta à lesão, o que não é confiável quando se refere a doença central, em que o nistagmo pode ser em qualquer direção. Além disso, a fase rápida do nistagmo ocasionalmente muda de direção em lesões no tronco encefálico.

Déficits adicionais de nervos cranianos geralmente acompanham distúrbios vestibulares. Os distúrbios do nervo facial são os mais comuns e podem ser observados na doença vestibular tanto *periférica* quanto *central*. Ocasionalmente, a síndrome de Horner acompanha lesões vestibulares periféricas, uma vez as fibras do sistema nervoso simpático passam pela orelha média a caminho da órbita. Raramente, a síndrome de Horner pode estar associada a uma lesão do tronco encefálico por envolvimento do NMS (*hipotalamotecto-tegumentar*); isso normalmente requer lesão grave do tronco encefálico e, em geral, o animal é tetraplégico, com mudanças marcantes do estado mental. A via sensitiva não é afetada por lesões vestibulares periféricas, enquanto animais com lesões vestibulares centrais podem estar apáticos a comatosos, dependendo do grau de envolvimento do SARA.

Cerebelo

A função do cerebelo é *regulatória*, e não precursora primária de atividade motora. Ele coordena movimentos em relação à postura do animal, proporcionando sinergia de atividade muscular. A doença cerebelar produz *dismetria* única, caracterizada por incapacidade de regular a taxa, a amplitude e a força de um movimento (ver Vídeo 259.4). Embora um cão ou gato com doença cerebelar possa estar incapacitado e não consiga permanecer em posição quadrupedal, movimentos voluntários devem ser provocados com força normal.

Animais ambulatórios com ataxia cerebelar em geral manifestam movimentos hipermétricos "explosivos" em todas as amplitudes de movimento. Normalmente, movimentos voluntários são atrasados no início, mas, uma vez iniciados, são exagerados. Na caminhada, os membros em geral têm levantamento excessivo e retornam forçosamente ao solo em cada passada. O tônus muscular normalmente é aumentado, e os reflexos espinais podem ser normais ou exagerados. Embora o PC não seja afetado na doença cerebelar, as reações posturais são tipicamente atrasadas e exageradas. Na extensão de cabeça, após a retirada de apoio repentino, um *fenômeno de ricochete* pode ocorrer, em que a cabeça cai excessivamente na direção ventral.

Em razão da conexão estreita com o sistema vestibular, a inclinação da cabeça (geralmente paradoxal) e outros sinais vestibulares podem acompanhar a doença cerebelar (ver Vídeo 259.35). Em geral, um leve *tremor de intenção* de cabeça, pescoço ou olhos está presente nas doenças cerebelares (Vídeo 259.37), mas isso não deve ser confundido com tremores generalizados de corpo inteiro associados com distúrbios difusos do SNC (Vídeo 259.38). Por fim, vale ressaltar que a doença cerebelar pode estar associada a déficit da resposta de ameaça ipsilateral (doença cerebelar difusa bilateral). Embora seja mais comum o cerebelo ser afetado difusamente (p. ex., hipoplasia cerebelar ou abiotrofia), em algumas ocasiões lesões cerebelares unilaterais ou focais (infarto ou neoplasia cerebelar) produzem sinais cerebelares ipsilaterais (Vídeos 259.35 e 259.36). A Tabela 259.5 resume os sinais clínicos potenciais associados à disfunção cerebelar.

Medula espinal

Um segmento da medula espinal é definido como uma porção da medula que dá origem a um par de nervos espinais. Existem 8 segmentos cervicais, 13 torácicos, 7 lombares, 3 sacrais e pelo menos 2 caudais em cães e gatos. Funcionalmente, a coluna vertebral pode ser dividida em quatro regiões neuroanatômicas: cervical (C1-C5), cervicotorácica (C6-T2), toracolombar (T3-L3) e lombossacra (L4-S3).

Os corpos celulares do NMI dos membros torácicos e pélvicos estão localizados dentro da substância cinzenta, na intumescência

ventral do segmento cervicotorácico (C6-T2) e lombossacro (L4-S3), respectivamente. As vias ascendentes (sensitivas) e descendentes (motoras) compreendem a substância branca da medula espinal e estão localizados mais superficialmente. Com raras exceções, as lesões de medula espinal resultam previsivelmente em perda sequencial ou geral da propriocepção, da função motora, da função da bexiga e da nocicepção. A recuperação da função geralmente ocorre na direção inversa.

Conforme discutido na seção de marcha e postura, lesões na medula espinal normalmente produzem uma combinação de déficits de NMS e PG nos membros, caudal ao nível da lesão (ver Vídeos 259.2 e 259.39). Se a lesão da medula espinal estiver na intumescência cervical ou lombar, produzirá sinais de NMI nos membros torácicos ou pélvicos correspondentes. Por outro lado, lesões na medula espinal também podem produzir uma combinação de sinais NMS e NMI nos membros torácicos ou pélvicos (ver Vídeo 259.39). Por exemplo, a herniação de disco no espaço intervertebral C6-C7 pode causar marcha com passos longos dos membros torácicos (sinal NMS), mas reflexos de retirada reduzidos do membro torácico (sinal NMI). Pacientes ambulatórios com lesões C6-T2 tipicamente apresentam uma marcha desconexa "bimotora", na qual os membros torácicos apresentam passos mais curtos e picados (sinal NMI) e membros pélvicos mais longos (sinal NMS) com ataxia PG[1] (Vídeo 259.40).

Estabelecer um diagnóstico neuroanatômico para um dos quatro segmentos da medula espinal normalmente é simples e fundamenta-se nas quatro combinações possíveis de sinais de normalidade, NMI e NMS, que podem estar presentes nos membros torácicos e pélvicos (Tabelas 259.7 a 259.10; ver Figura 259.1 e Tabela 259.6). No entanto, existem alguns cenários clínicos que podem criar confusão com a doença da medula espinal em T3-L3. Essas situações são consideradas a seguir.

As lesões da medula espinal toracolombar (T3-L3) tipicamente poupam os membros torácicos e causam uma combinação de sinais de NMS e de déficits PG nos membros pélvicos (ver Vídeo 259.2). Contudo, lesões agudas de T3-L3 podem produzir espasticidade acentuada nos referidos membros torácicos, como síndrome de *Schiff-Sherrington*, resultante da interrupção da ascensão de axônios inibitórios oriundos de interneurônios (células da borda), localizados na borda dorsolateral da substância cinzenta ventral dos segmentos medulares espinais L1-L7.[1] Os interneurônios ascendentes exercem efeito inibitório nos NMI da intumescência cervical, que pode ser perdida com lesões transversais em nível de T3-L3. O teste de reação postural diferencia entre uma lesão grave em C1-C5 e a síndrome de Schiff-Sherrington. Há retardo nas reações posturais no caso de a lesão ser em função do envolvimento das vias NMS e PG, mas são normais na síndrome de Schiff-Sherrington, apesar da presença de espasticidade.

Um segundo cenário clínico desafiador está associado a lesões agudas de T3-L3, que produzem sinais contrários do NMI (reflexos espinais reduzidos e hipotonia) nos membros pélvicos. Essa situação geralmente é acompanhada por síndrome Schiff-Sherrington, e os sinais de NMI nos membros pélvicos têm sido referidos como *choque espinal*. Pensa-se que essa condição pode ser secundária a uma desconexão transitória entre os NMS descendentes e os NMI da intumescência lombossacra.[6] Embora o choque espinal possa persistir por semanas no homem, geralmente é transitório (horas a dias) em cães e gatos.

Ocasionalmente, lesões de T3-L3 produzem sinais de NMI nos membros pélvicos que não são acompanhados por síndrome Schiff-Sherrington, sendo mais comum com mielopatia fibrocartilaginosas embólica (MFCE) e raramente com doença de disco.[7] Por horas, ou até dias, sinais contraditórios de NMI podem ser identificados nos membros pélvicos com tais lesões de T3-L3. A hipótese é que isso também represente uma variação do choque espinal.[6]

Uma terceira situação desafiadora está relacionada às lesões de L4-L7, que podem produzir sinais de NMI e ataxia PG, além dos sinais NMI previstos nos membros pélvicos. Isso pode resultar de lesões que afetam predominantemente a substância branca na coluna vertebral nesse nível.

CAPÍTULO 259 • Exame Neurológico e Diagnóstico Neuroanatômico

Tabela 259.7 Sinais neurológicos que podem estar associados à disfunção da medula espinal C1-C5.

TESTE NEUROLÓGICO	POSSÍVEIS ANORMALIDADES
Sensório/comportamento	Normal
Postura/marcha	Variável: varia de tetraparesia/ataxia PG de NMS a tetraplegia espástica
Reações posturais	Atraso para ausência nos quatro membros
Massa/tônus muscular	Massa muscular normal (atrofia leve devido a desuso em doenças crônicas), normal a tônus muscular exagerado nos quatro membros; possível bexiga NMS
Reflexos na coluna vertebral	Normal a aumentado nos quatro membros, refluxos de retirada ocasionalmente reduzidos em membros torácicos*
Sensação cutânea	Hipalgesia caudal a uma lesão focal (rara)
Nervos cranianos	Miose ipsilateral (rara devido à síndrome de Horner do NMS)
Outras	Uma lesão focal e grave entre esses segmentos pode resultar em morte devido a disfunção respiratória

*Lesões Ci-C5 podem estar associadas à retirada reduzida de membros torácicos.[5] *NMS*, neurônio motor superior; *PG*, proprioceptiva geral.

Tabela 259.8 Sinais neurológicos que podem estar associados à disfunção da medula espinal C6-T2.

TESTE NEUROLÓGICO	POSSÍVEIS ANORMALIDADES
Sensório/comportamento	Normal
Postura/marcha	Variável: marcha NMI em membros torácicos, NMS paresia/ataxia PG em membros pélvicos através de tetraplegia espástica
Reações posturais	Atraso para ausência nos quatro membros
Massa/tônus muscular	Atrofia neurogênica de membros torácicos (lesões crônicas); tônus reduzido nos membros torácicos; tom normal a exagerado nos membros da região pélvica; possível bexiga do NMS
Reflexos na coluna vertebral	Reflexos de retirada normais a reduzidos em membros torácicos; reflexos patelares e flexores de retirada normais a exagerados nos membros pélvicos
Sensação cutânea	Hipalgesia ou normal nos quatro membros ou hipalgesia apenas nos membros torácicos
Nervos cranianos	Síndrome de Horner ipsilateral (lesões T1-T3)
Outras	Uma lesão focal e grave entre esses segmentos pode resultar em morte devido a disfunção respiratória

NMI, neurônio motor inferior; *NMS*, neurônio motor superior; *PG*, proprioceptivo geral.

Tabela 259.9 Sinais neurológicos que podem estar associados à disfunção da medula espinal T3-L3.

TESTE NEUROLÓGICO	POSSÍVEIS ANORMALIDADES
Sensório/comportamento	Normal
Postura/marcha	Variável: NMS paresia/ataxia PG em pélvica membros através de paraplegia espástica
Reações posturais	Normal em membros torácicos; atrasado para ausente nos membros pélvicos
Massa/tônus muscular	Tom normal nos membros torácicos (exceto por espasticidade de Schiff-Sherrington na região torácica); tônus normal a exagerado em membros pélvicos; massa muscular normal, a menos que atrofia por desuso em membros pélvicos; possível bexiga do NMS
Reflexos na coluna vertebral	Reflexo de retirada normal em membros torácicos; patelar normal a exagerada e reflexos de abstinência nos membros pélvicos; "trunci" cutâneo pode se apresentar levemente caudal à lesão
Sensação cutânea	Normal em membros torácicos; hipalgesia, analgesia ou normal nos membros pélvicos
Nervos cranianos	Normal
Outras	Lesões L4-L7 da substância branca podem produzir sinais semelhantes

NMS, neurônio motor superior; *PG*, proprioceptivo geral.

Tabela 259.10 Sinais neurológicos que podem estar associados à disfunção da medula espinal L4-S3.

TESTE NEUROLÓGICO	POSSÍVEIS ANORMALIDADES
Sensório/comportamento	Normal
Postura/marcha	Variável: paraparesia acidificada e ataxia PG nos membros pélvicos devido a paraplegia flácida
Reações posturais	Atraso para ausência nos membros pélvicos
Massa/tônus muscular	Tom normal em membros torácicos; tom reduzido nos membros pélvicos, redução da massa muscular em membros pélvicos (crônicos); bexiga do NMS (raro) ou NMI
Reflexos na coluna vertebral	Hiporreflexia devido a arreflexia patelar (L4-L6), retirada (L7-S1) e reflexos perineais (S1-S3)
Sensação cutânea	Normal em membros torácicos; normal, hipalgesia ou analgesia em membros pélvicos, cauda, períneo, ânus (pênis)
Nervos cranianos	Normal
Outras	Lesões L4-L7 (substância branca) podem produzir sinais que imitam T3-L3

NMI, neurônio motor inferior; *NMS*, neurônio motor superior; *PG*, proprioceptivo geral.

SEÇÃO 17 • Doença Neurológica

Tabela 259.11 Anormalidades neurológicas associados à disfunção do neurônio motor inferior e disfunção neuromuscular.

TESTE NEUROLÓGICO	POSSÍVEIS ANORMALIDADES
Sensório/comportamento	Normal
Postura/marcha	Variável: paresia acidificada no(s) membro(s) afetado(s) através de paralisia flácida do(s) membro(s); exercício pode exacerbar a paresia
Reações posturais	Atraso para ausência no(s) membro(s) afetado(s); normal na doença NMI "pura" se o paciente mantém alguma função motora voluntária
Massa/tônus muscular	Tom diminuído do(s) membro(s) afetado(s); atrofia neurogênica pode ser grave; pseudo-hipertrofia em certas miopatias; possível bexiga NMI
Reflexos na coluna vertebral	Variável: hiporreflexia através de arreflexia de membro(s) afetado(s); reflexo perineal possivelmente reduzido (S1-S3)
Sensação cutânea	Normal na doença NMI "pura" (mas se um polineuropatia com sensibilidade pode estar presente hipalgesia)
Nervos cranianos	Variável: múltiplos nervos cranianos podem ser afetados
Outras	Paralisia laríngea, disfagia, megaesôfago comum com doença do NMI

NMI, neurônio motor inferior.

Sistema nervoso periférico

Neurônio motor inferior/sistema neuromuscular

A unidade do NMI consiste no corpo celular dentro da substância cinzenta ventral no SNC, da raiz nervosa ventral, do nervo periférico e do músculo. Doenças de qualquer componente dessa unidade produzem sinais do NMI. A força normal depende não apenas da função da unidade NMI, mas também da transmissão neuromuscular efetiva via acetilcolina (ACh), através da junção neuromuscular (JNM). Doenças que afetam a transmissão neuromuscular (p. ex., miastenia *gravis* ou paralisia por carrapatos), as chamadas juncionopatias, podem produzir sinais de NMI indistinguíveis de neuropatias e miopatias.

Como as DNM podem mimetizar umas às outras, o exame neurológico raramente confirma o componente exato do NMI que está comprometido. O clínico pode requisitar exames complementares (atividade de creatinoquinase sérica [ver Capítulo 66] e aspartato aminotransferase [ver Capítulo 65], teste de edrofônio, titulação de anticorpo receptor de acetilcolina [ver Capítulo 269], eletrodiagnóstico [ver Capítulo 117], biopsias de nervos e de músculos [ver o Capítulo 116]) para, posteriormente, localizar o problema no nervo, no músculo ou na JNM. A unidade do NMI pode ser afetada de forma difusa ou periférica, ou ainda nervos cranianos podem estar comprometidos. Quando déficits dos nervos cranianos (p. ex., paresia facial) estão presentes, eles devem ser interpretados com outros achados neurológicos para a diferenciação entre a doença neuromuscular e o distúrbio do tronco encefálico.

A fraqueza neuromuscular é caracterizada por flacidez e diminuição ou ausência de reflexos espinais. As reações posturais geralmente são normais na presença de DNM isolada (nenhum envolvimento de nervo sensorial; ver Vídeo 259.41); todavia, o paciente deve estar bem apoiado, já que pode haver falhas no teste postural, atribuídas à fraqueza muscular. Pacientes ambulatórios com DNM isoladas em geral têm marcha "curta e irregular", sem ataxia, uma vez que o PG não é afetado (ver Vídeos 259.1 e 259.41). Intolerância ao exercício pode ser a única anormalidade presente em alguns pacientes com DNM.

Uma exceção importante ao clássico padrão "curto e irregular" da doença neuromuscular é a marcha do membro pélvico associada à disfunção isquiática em cães e gatos com polineuropatias. Uma vez que a disfunção isquiática não afeta a sustentação de peso, a marcha pélvica não é curta. Apesar de ser um problema do NMI, há uma marcha exagerada do membro pélvico, na qual o animal inicia repetidamente a marcha de uma posição plantígrada (andar com os dedos dos pés e os metatarsos planos no chão) e "arremessa" seus membros pélvicos para frente (ver Vídeo 259.42). Isso não deve ser confundido com lesão em T3-L3 ou hipermetria cerebelar. A flexão do quadril é exagerada em razão da falta de contração antagônica dos músculos caudais da coxa. Pacientes com polineuropatias também podem ter atraso nas reações posturais, em razão do envolvimento das fibras do nervo sensitivo na neuropatia periférica.

Em algumas DNM (p. ex., polineuropatias), o envolvimento do nervo laríngeo recorrente pode levar a uma alteração ou perda de voz (disfonia) e aumento do ruído inspiratório (estridor). O desenvolvimento do megaesôfago em várias DNMs pode causar regurgitação, geralmente acompanhada de pneumonia aspirativa. Esses pacientes também correm o risco de hipoventilação, em razão do envolvimento dos músculos respiratórios. Finalmente, alterações na massa muscular podem variar de atrofia neurogênica grave (p. ex., avulsão do plexo braquial) a "pseudo-hipertrofia", que acompanha miopatias (distrofia muscular; Tabela 259.11).

Nervos periféricos sensoriais

As fibras aferentes dos nervos sensoriais são paralelas e trabalham junto ao NMI dentro dos nervos periféricos. Os axônios sensoriais têm o corpo celular na raiz dos gânglios dorsais ou nos gânglios homólogos dos nervos cranianos. Uma região cutânea inervada por fibras nervosas aferentes de um único nervo espinal ou nervo craniano é chamado de *dermátomo*. Doenças que afetam exclusivamente o sistema sensorial são raras (p. ex., neuropatias sensoriais e gangliorradiculoneurite) e são caracterizadas por déficits sensoriais variáveis, desde hipoalgesia até analgesia de várias regiões do corpo.

Localização multifocal e difusa no sistema nervoso central

Entre os muitos distúrbios neurológicos, os déficits neurológicos não podem ser explicados por uma única lesão. Por exemplo, um cão da raça Pug com meningoencefalite necrosante pode manifestar sinais de convulsões prosencefálicas e alterações vestibulares (inclinação da cabeça, ataxia vestibular). Nesse cenário, é feita a localização intracraniana multifocal.

Localizações multifocais não são análogas a distúrbios que afetam o SNC de forma difusa, em que a maior parte do eixo neuronal está afetado. O sinal neurológico mais comum associado a doença difusa do SNC é um tremor do corpo inteiro (ver Vídeo 259.38), que não deve ser confundido com os breves tremores de intenção da cabeça, do pescoço ou do torso, os quais podem estar presentes na doença cerebelar (ver Vídeo 259.37). A lista de diagnósticos diferenciais para uma localização difusa do SNC é relativamente estreita e inclui dismielinogênese, meningite difusa (síndrome do tremor idiopático, meningoencefalomielite granulomatosa disseminada, meningite infecciosa) e várias toxicoses (p. ex., bolores, algas e etilenoglicol).

REFERÊNCIAS BIBLIOGRÁFICAS

As referências bibliográficas deste capítulo se encontram online no Ambiente de Aprendizagem.

CAPÍTULO 260

Doenças do Cérebro: Anomalia, Degenerativa, Metabólica, Neoplásica, Idiopática, Epiléptica e Vascular

Joan R. Coates e Dennis P. O'Brien

"Todas as doenças mais agudas, mais poderosas e mais mortais e aquelas mais difíceis de serem compreendidas... caem sobre o cérebro."

Hipócrates

RESPOSTA CEREBRAL À LESÃO

Respostas gerais e seus resultados

O sistema nervoso tem relativamente poucas respostas a lesões, e a complexidade dos sinais neurológicos em resposta ao trauma depende da localização da lesão (Tabela 260.1). Como os neurônios são células excitáveis, uma resposta potencial a uma determinada doença é a descarga excessiva; o exemplo mais drástico seria uma atividade convulsiva. Se uma condição destrói os neurônios de um sistema, ele perde sua função. Por exemplo, a destruição de um núcleo do nervo craniano no tronco encefálico leva à paralisia dos músculos inervados por esse nervo. Se o sistema perde a via inibitória, então o sistema que não está mais inibido pode mostrar uma resposta exagerada. O exemplo clássico de tal desinibição são os reflexos exagerados vistos com a perda do neurônio motor superior (NMS). Ao lidar com funções cerebrais superiores, essas respostas podem ser complexas. Por exemplo, agressão paradoxal às vezes observada em cães que receberam benzodiazepínicos ou barbitúricos pode representar uma desinibição do comportamento agressivo. O sistema nervoso é especialmente sensível às mutações genéticas, uma vez que muitos genes são expressos apenas por breves períodos durante o desenvolvimento. Poucos neurônios são capazes de se reproduzirem após a maturidade, pois o processo de construção complexo e sistemático inicial não pode ser duplicado. Mutações que interferem na capacidade das células de responder aos insultos, como estresse oxidativo ou deficiências enzimáticas, podem levar a danos acumulativos e degeneração precoce ou tardia.

Pressão intracraniana aumentada

Além dos efeitos locais, o processo de doença no cérebro pode produzir efeitos generalizados secundários ao aumento da pressão intracraniana. Uma vez que a calvária é um globo ósseo, os três principais componentes dentro dele são cérebro, líquido cefalorraquidiano [LCR] e sangue, que estão confinados em um espaço fixo. De acordo com a doutrina Monro-Kellie, qualquer aumento em um desses componentes teria que ser acompanhado por uma diminuição em um dos outros dois. Um aumento gradual no volume de um dos componentes, como na hidrocefalia progressiva lenta, pode ser compensado, em certa extensão, por atrofia do tecido cerebral. Doença aguda não permite tempo suficiente para a atrofia compensatória, e mesmo a doença crônica (tumor cerebral) eventualmente excederá a capacidade de compensação, resultando em aumento da pressão intracraniana. Com o aumento da pressão intracraniana, sinais generalizados de doença prosencefálica se desenvolvem, mesmo se a causa inicial for um processo localizado, como a neoplasia. A pressão arterial sistêmica aumenta para manter perfusão cerebral, que pode causar aumento do reflexo no tônus vagal e diminuição das frequências respiratória e cardíaca (fenômeno de Cushing). Vômito também pode ocorrer.

O aumento contínuo da pressão intracraniana leva à herniação. O tecido cerebral pode tanto herniar lateralmente abaixo da foice cerebral quanto caudalmente abaixo do tentório, ou ainda através do forame magno.[1] A herniação tentorial leva à deterioração progressiva rostral-caudal do estado neurológico quando o mesencéfalo, a ponte e a terminação da medula são comprimidos. A compressão do tronco encefálico resulta em alterações pupilares, perturbação do NMS e das vias respiratórias. A progressão pode ser rápida ou evoluir lentamente ao longo de horas ou mesmo de dias. As herniações são mais frequentemente associadas a lesões no prosencéfalo, tais como neoplasia ou trauma. O aumento de pressão que surge

---

Tabela 260.1 Resumo dos mecanismos fisiopatológicos associados às categorias de doenças cerebrais.

DEGENERATIVA	ANOMALIA	METABÓLICA	NEOPLÁSICA	INFLAMATÓRIA	TRAUMA	TÓXICA	VASCULAR
Degeneração e perda neuronal específica (corpo celular, axônio) Axonopatia Mielinopatia Degeneração esponjosa Neuroinflamação Astrocitose Mutações genéticas que causam morte celular prematura, canalopatia etc.	Fatores genéticos e ambientais (vírus, toxinas) causando migração anormal ou perda, desenvolvimento neural, orientação e transporte axonal Destruição do tecido Hidrocefalia congênita	Fatores genéticos e ambientais Decorrente de doença sistêmica Perda de função enzimática, causando acúmulo de produtos de armazenamento (ver também Tóxica) Encefalomalacia	Destruição tecidual Compressão Edema vasogênico Obstrução de vaso Obstrução do LCR Neuroinflamação Astrocitose Disseminação ao longo do eixo neural ("metástase de descida")	Destruição tecidual Compressão Edema vasogênico e citotóxico Obstrução do LCR Mediadores inflamatórios causando comprometimento vascular, função neural e de condutância alterada, astrocitose	Lesão de tecido Compressão, concussão Hemorragia Lesão isquêmica Neuroinflamação	Depleção energética Desequilíbrio da excitação-inibição Toxicidade direta aos neurônios Lesão anóxica Desequilíbrio iônico Edema citotóxico Edema de mielina	Hemorragia causando compressão, vasoespasmo, produção de radicais livres Lesão isquêmica Obstrução vascular Obstrução do LCR Neuroinflamação

LCR, líquido cefalorraquidiano.

SEÇÃO 17 • Doença Neurológica

abaixo do tentório (p. ex., um tumor cerebelar) causa herniação do cerebelo através do forame magno, mimetizando os eventos terminais da herniação tentorial; porém, sem nenhum dos sinais anteriores.

Edema cerebral

Existem três tipos de edema cerebral (citotóxico, vasogênico, intersticial), e uma resposta comum aos insultos pode coexistir. O edema citotóxico é resultado do acúmulo de líquido nos neurônios. O esgotamento de energia ocorre em razão da falha da bomba de Na^+/K^+ ATPase dependente de ATP e outros canais iônicos que resultam na translocação de água do meio intracelular para extracelular. O edema citotóxico geralmente ocorre como resultado de isquemia ou de processos que alteram a membrana celular. O edema vasogênico resulta de perturbação física ou funcional do endotélio vascular, muitas vezes associado à barreira hematencefálica (BHE). O acúmulo de líquido é extracelular e geralmente distribuído na substância branca porque suas fibras neuronais mielinizadas são distribuídas difusamente dentro da matriz da glia e nos capilares. O edema intersticial frequentemente acompanha hidrocefalia obstrutiva, causando compartimentalização do LCR que cruza os revestimentos ependimários, criando edema cerebral intersticial extracelular e periventricular. Determinar o tipo de edema permite o tratamento mais adequado. Ambos os edemas citotóxico e intersticial são manejados pelo tratamento da causa subjacente, enquanto o edema vasogênico pode ser tratado com o uso de terapias com osmóticos e corticosteroides.

Além das doenças inflamatórias primárias do SNC, a neuroinflamação desempenha um papel importante na fisiopatologia de muitas condições cerebrais em animais.[2] A neuroinflamação é caracterizada por uma ampla gama de respostas imunológicas, diferindo da inflamação periférica principalmente em relação às células principais envolvidas, que são mais perceptivelmente os astrócitos e a micróglia.[3] A BHE (incluindo a barreira hematomedular) refere-se à proteção do fluxo de células e de macromoléculas da circulação sistêmica para o SNC.[4] Essa barreira seletivamente permeável é composta por células endoteliais, membranas basais e periócitos perivasculares vizinhos, células gliais (astrócitos, micróglia) e neurônios. Juntas, essas células moderam a intensidade de respostas da inflamação no SNC.[4-6] No entanto, embora o SNC tradicionalmente tenha sido considerado "imunologicamente privilegiado", dados atuais confirmam que o SNC é imunocompetente e interage ativamente com o sistema imunológico periférico.[7] A inflamação periférica pode desencadear uma resposta neuroinflamatória envolvendo o endotélio da BHE, glia e neurônios por meio de mediadores e citocinas.[2]

LOCALIZAÇÃO DA LESÃO

Um dos objetivos do exame neurológico é localizar a lesão em uma das quatro áreas cerebrais: (1) prosencéfalo (cérebro e diencéfalo), (2) mesencéfalo, (3) ponte e medula ou (4) cerebelo (Tabela 260.2). Embora mais de uma lesão possa ser localizada dentro de uma área, alocando corretamente a lesão em uma das divisões amplas é o suficiente para se ter uma lista razoável de diagnósticos diferenciais e um plano de diagnóstico (ver Capítulo 259 e Vídeo 260.1). Ao localizar a lesão, a primeira pergunta que o clínico deve responder é se os sinais refletem uma doença focal, difusa ou multifocal. Lesões focais são suspeitas se os sinais exibidos são fortemente lateralizados (p. ex., andar em círculos, convulsões de início focal, déficits de nervos cranianos unilaterais). Uma lesão focal é mais sugestiva em casos de neoplasia, doença vascular ou infecção localizada. Normalmente, processos degenerativos ou metabólicos ou insultos tóxicos devem afetar o cérebro de uma forma mais geral e não afetam preferencialmente um lado. Embora sinais simétricos da doença prosencefálica sugiram um processo difuso da patologia, eles não descartam uma doença focal. A doença focal pode produzir sinais difusos através de mecanismos como hidrocefalia obstrutiva, edema difuso e aumento da pressão intracraniana. Todo esforço deve ser feito para explicar os sinais clínicos com base em uma única lesão. Se uma única lesão não pode explicar todos os sinais, então deve-se suspeitar de uma doença multifocal. Por exemplo, uma lesão isolada não pode explicar um animal que tenha convulsões (córtex cerebral) e paralisia facial unilateral (medula ou nervo facial).

DIAGNÓSTICO DIFERENCIAL

Idade, sexo, raça

Uma vez localizada a lesão, uma lista de diagnósticos diferenciais pode ser feita e um plano de diagnóstico desenvolvido. A maioria das doenças em medicina veterinária é categorizada por sua apresentação e/ou alterações patológicas; porém, os sinais clínicos podem ser inespecíficos. Os sinais clínicos muitas vezes fornecem a primeira dica para o diagnóstico. Doenças congênitas e hereditárias são mais comuns em animais jovens de raça pura. As anomalias congênitas referem-se a qualquer malformação presente ao nascimento, incluindo ambas as condições genéticas e aquelas resultantes de influências externas durante a gestação, tais como toxinas, desnutrição ou infecção. Muitas doenças hereditárias neurológicas são congênitas, ou pelo menos aparentes em idade jovem, mas há exceções notáveis. Algumas doenças lisossomais de armazenamento requerem tempo para o acúmulo de subprodutos. Animais com ataxia cerebelar hereditária (abiotrofia) podem se apresentar normais

---

Tabela 260.2 Sinais clínicos associados à localização intracraniana.

SÍTIO DE LOCALIZAÇÃO	SINAIS CLÍNICOS
Cérebro	Convulsão, comportamento e nível de consciência anormais, marcha normal, marcha propulsiva, andar em círculos ipsilateral e desvio de cabeça (*head turn*), déficits de reação postural contralateral e déficits de resposta à ameaça e de sensibilidade facial contralaterais
Diencéfalo	Comportamento e nível de consciência anormais, andar em círculos para qualquer direção, marcha normal, déficits de reação postural, anorexia ou polifagia, disautorregulação da temperatura, anormalidades endócrinas, déficits visuais
Mesencéfalo	Nível de consciência anormal, andar em círculos e desvio de cabeça (*head turning*), déficits de reação postural, hemi ou tetraparesia, ataxia PG, déficits NC III
Tronco encefálico	Nível de consciência normal a anormal, inclinação da cabeça ipsilateral e andar em círculos, ataxia vestibular, déficits posturais ipsilaterais, hemi ou tetraparesia, déficits ipsilaterais de NC V-XII
Cerebelo	Nível de consciência normal, postura de base ampla, disfunção vestibular paradoxal, postura descerebelada, tremor de intenção, ataxia cerebelar, pode ser visto déficit de resposta à ameaça ipsilateral

NC, nervo cranial; *PG*, proprioceptiva geral.

CAPÍTULO 260 • Doenças do Cérebro: Anomalia, Degenerativa, Metabólica, Neoplásica, Idiopática... 1389

clínica e histologicamente por um tempo imprevisível até que os sinais clínicos sucedam com a morte dos neurônios de Purkinje. Finalmente, algumas condições (epilepsia idiopática ou lipofuscinose ceroide neuronal) não apresentam sinais no início ou mesmo até a idade adulta tardia. Já condições como infecção, trauma e intoxicação podem ocorrer a qualquer momento, e animais jovens têm maior probabilidade de serem afetados. Com o aumento da idade, neoplasias, encefalopatias metabólicas e doenças degenerativas tornam-se cada vez mais comuns.

Início, progressão e tipos de sinal

O início e a progressão dos sinais clínicos podem fornecer informações importantes na prioridade da lista de diagnóstico diferencial. As malformações congênitas estão presentes desde o nascimento e são relativamente estáticas. Todavia, condições como a hidrocefalia podem progredir com o tempo. Sinais clínicos de início agudo são mais prováveis em doenças vasculares, traumas, bem como na maior parte das intoxicações e doenças infecciosas/inflamatórias ou metabólicas. Sinais clínicos flutuantes (que melhoram e pioram) podem ser característicos na inflamação e nas doenças metabólicas. Algumas doenças infecciosas/inflamatórios, metabólicas, neoplásicas e degenerativas são crônicas e progressivas. O início do episódio é característico de epilepsia, alguns distúrbios associados a movimentos anormais e canalopatias.

Os resultados do exame neurológico podem sugerir o tipo do processo da doença (ver Capítulo 259). Algumas doenças terão predileção por regiões específicas do cérebro. Geralmente, sinais de lateralização (andar em círculo, hemiparesia ou déficit do nervo craniano unilateral) sugerem um processo de doença localizada, como infecção, doença vascular, neoplasia ou lesão traumática. Da mesma forma, convulsões com início focal sugerem lesão cortical localizada, muito embora a epilepsia idiopática possa produzir crises focais.[8,9] Dessas, doenças neoplásicas infecciosa/inflamatória, vasculares ou metastáticas seriam as com maior probabilidade de produzirem sinais multifocais. Insultos metabólicos ou tóxicos geralmente não causam sinais focais ou assimétricos. Uma vez que o córtex cerebral é a área do cérebro mais exigente metabolicamente, os sinais prosencefálicos tendem a predominar. Todavia, processos de doença localizada podem resultar em sinais de doença prosencefálica difusa em função do aumento da pressão intracraniana. O clínico deve suspeitar fortemente de doenças hereditárias em casos de animais jovens de raça pura com sinais de doença cerebral difusa simétrica quando as etiologias tóxica, metabólica e infecciosa de rotina foram descartadas. Tabelas publicadas de raça para doenças específicas podem ser consultadas.[10-12]

DIAGNÓSTICO E ABORDAGEM DA DOENÇA CEREBRAL

Avaliação laboratorial de rotina

Ao considerar a abordagem diagnóstica para doenças que afetam o cérebro (Figura 260.1), os clínicos devem considerar custo, disponibilidade de imagens, riscos e possibilidades promissoras. O valor do histórico completo e exame neurológico nunca devem ser subestimados (ver Capítulo 259). Mesmo se imagens avançadas revelam uma lesão nítida, se essa lesão não corresponde aos resultados do exame neurológico, seu significado preciso ser questionado. Os exames de patologia clínica de rotina podem fornecer informações criticamente importantes, e estão prontamente disponíveis, com boa relação custo-benefício e não são invasivos. Mesmo com uma doença aparentemente focal, revisar o banco de dados mínimo sobre qualquer animal doente é essencial. O hemograma completo (HC) pode sugerir etiologias infecciosas/inflamatórias, assim como pode prover indicações sobre outras causas. O perfil bioquímico sérico e a análise de urina serão essenciais para descartar deficiências de energia, distúrbios eletrolíticos ou acúmulo de toxinas endógenas.

Animais com sinais de doenças prosencefálicas difusas ou convulsões devem ter a função hepática avaliada por mensuração de ácidos biliares ou de tolerância à amônia (ver Capítulo 284). Se erros inatos de metabolismo são suspeitos, exames de urina para mensurar metabólitos anormais podem ser necessários. Exames para toxinas exógenas específicas como chumbo ou organofosforados podem ser indicados se houver sinais e o histórico for sugestivo de intoxicação (ver Capítulo 152). Triagem para todas as possíveis neurotoxinas não é viável. Uma vez que hipotireoidismo (ver Capítulo 299), hiperadrenocorticismo (ver Capítulo 306), tumores que secretam insulina (ver Capítulo 303) e outras condições endócrinas podem ser acompanhados de sinais neurológicos, o exame endócrino deve ser considerado se indicado por informações coletadas. Imagens torácicas e abdominais são importantes, particularmente em pacientes geriátricos, a fim de descartar doenças metastáticas e coexistentes.[13,14]

Imagem cerebral

Visão geral

A disponibilidade de tomografia computadorizada (TC) ou imagens de ressonância magnética (RM) para animais com doenças cerebrais revolucionou a neurologia. Embora dispendiosas, as informações obtidas geralmente justificam o investimento. As radiografias de crânio de rotina são de pouco valor no diagnóstico de doença cerebral, já que apenas o crânio pode ser avaliado sem estudos de contraste ou angiografia, e a sobreposição de estruturas torna a interpretação difícil. Imagens de ultrassom (US) do cérebro, embora úteis, são uma opção apenas quando uma fontanela aberta ou a craniotomia fornecem uma janela acústica. Imagens transversais com tomografia computadorizada ou ressonância magnética permitem a detecção de mudanças dentro do cérebro.[15,16] TC e RM produzem imagens que são orientadas por fatias, eliminando assim o efeito somatório associado à radiografia convencional. Ressonância magnética por varredura fornece melhor resolução de contraste dos tecidos nervosos, enquanto a TC fornece melhor resolução espacial e imagem rápida. Por meio de varreduras por TC, reconstrução de imagens do plano sagital e dorsal transversais causam resolução espacial inferior. As imagens multiplanares diretas adquiridas por ressonância magnética resultam em melhor resolução espacial de cada plano, embora as varreduras sejam mais demoradas. O menor tempo necessário para adquirir imagens de TC pode ser vantajoso em pacientes pós-trauma. A ressonância magnética não pode ser usada quando implantes de metal ou marca-passos cardíacos estão presentes. Às vezes até mesmo os microchips de identificação podem interferir nas varreduras de ressonância magnética.

Tomografia computadorizada

A tomografia computadorizada depende dos princípios tradicionais de radiografia. Um tom de cinza atribuído para um pixel pelo computador, normalizado para as características de absorção de água, é associado a um número denominado unidade Hounsfield (HU; Tabela 260.3). Apenas imagens transversais são adquiridas, embora reconstruções de computador possam gerar imagens em um plano sagital, plano dorsal ou em três dimensões. A tomografia computadorizada tem a vantagem de ser capaz de captar imagens ósseas, o que é útil na detecção de mineralização e de hemorragia. O sistema ventricular é prontamente apreciado na TC, mas finos detalhes anatômicos de lesões parenquimatosas frequentemente não são visíveis. Edema pode ser visível como uma densidade reduzida do parênquima, enquanto hemorragia ou calcificação produzem aumento da densidade. A resolução da TC é limitada pela atenuação de raios X pelo crânio. A densidade dos ossos petrosos na base do crânio limita a qualidade da imagem da TC ao *tentorium cerebelli*.

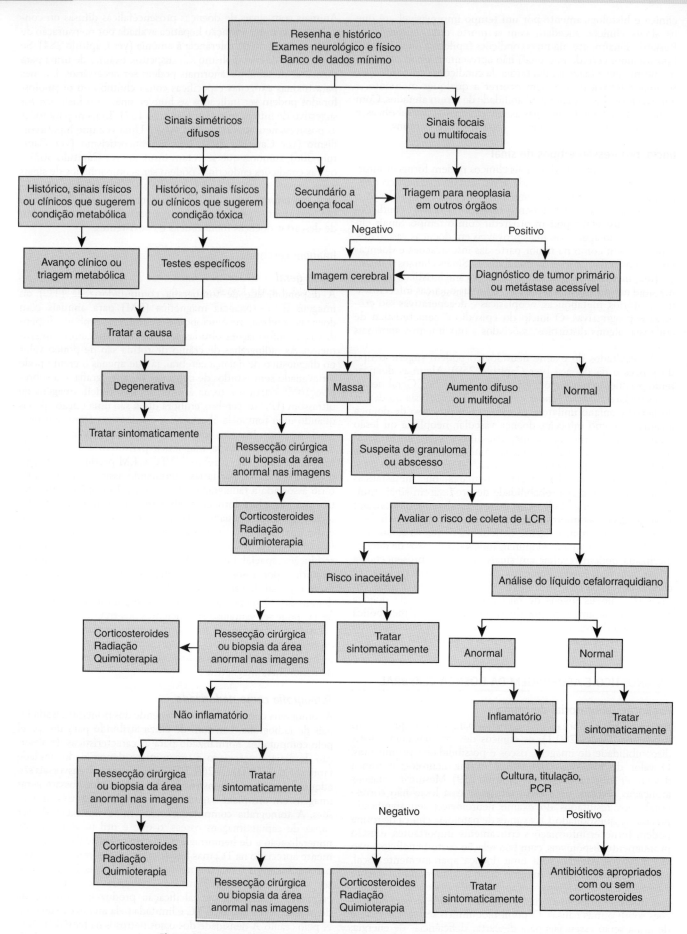

Figura 260.1 Acesso diagnóstico para a doença cerebral. *LCR*, líquido cefalorraquidiano.

CAPÍTULO 260 • Doenças do Cérebro: Anomalia, Degenerativa, Metabólica, Neoplásica, Idiopática...

Tabela 260.3 Unidades de Hounsfield para vários tecidos intracranianos.

TECIDOS	UNIDADES DE HOUNSFIELD
Ar	−1.000
Gordura	−50 a −100
Água	0
LCR	0 a 15
Cérebro	25 a 50
Hemorragia hiperaguda a aguda	60 a 100
Mineral e ósseo	100 a > 1.000
Metal (p. ex., contraste de iodo metálico)	Variável conforme a diluição, 100 a > 3.000

LCR, líquido cefalorraquidiano.

A atenuação dos raios X será semelhante aos raios gama usados na terapia de radiação, de forma que as imagens de TC podem ser usadas para calcular a dose de administração.

Imagem por ressonância magnética

A imagem por ressonância magnética orienta átomos de hidrogênio, com seus elétrons despareados, em alinhamento com base em suas propriedades magnéticas. Quando a energia – um pulso de radiofrequência – é aplicada, há mudanças no alinhamento dos átomos e, quando o pulso é removido, os átomos realinhados retornam à orientação anterior, enquanto liberam energia de volta ao meio ambiente. É essa liberação de energia que ajuda na formação das imagens. A taxa na qual a energia é liberada é baseada nas características inerentes do tecido. Duas constantes de tempo, denominadas T1 e T2, descrevem esse processo. Uma série de imagens, chamada sequência de pulso, pode ser adquirida com base "ponderada" nas propriedades T1 ou T2, referidas como imagens ponderadas em T1 (T1W) ou imagens ponderadas em T2 (T2W). As imagens resultantes são imagens em tons de cinza em que o grau de brilho relativo e é referida como intensidade (Tabela 260.4). Imagens T1W são caracterizadas por gordura brilhante e água escura enquanto as imagens T2W são caracterizadas por água clara e gordura escura. Edema é rapidamente aparente como sinais aumentados em imagens T2W. A densidade de prótons é uma sequência intermediária que caracteriza áreas com alta densidade de prótons (brilhante) e áreas com baixa densidade de prótons (escura). O contraste diminui entre os ventrículos e o cérebro, mas aumenta entre a substância cinzenta e substância branca, revelando detalhes anatômicos finos. Várias sequências foram desenvolvidas para suprimir o sinal em certos tecidos, por exemplo, LCR e gordura. A sequência atenuada inversa de recuperação de fluido (*fluid attenuated inversion recovery* [FLAIR]) suprime o sinal do fluido com pouca

ou nenhuma proteína (*i. e.*, LCR), ou seja, o que é hipointenso e permite o aumento da identificação de enfermidades (edema de tecido) e de lesões perto dos ventrículos. Sequências de recuperação de inversa de tau curta (*short-tau inversion recovery* – STIR) permitem a supressão da gordura. Gradiente eco da imagem T2W (GRE) (T2*) é usado para detectar artefatos de produtos sanguíneos que são formados na hemorragia.

Técnicas de ressonância magnética mais avançadas podem ser usadas para investigar distúrbios funcionais no SNC. RM de espectroscopia (EMR) avalia a química e o metabolismo do cérebro (conteúdo molecular de tecidos) que podem ser alterados em doença e fornecer produtos químicos marcadores para processos patológicos como em neoplasias e inflamação. Imagem ponderada por difusão (IPD) depende do movimento molecular ou difusão da água, alterada em muitos processos patológicos. Acompanhada pelo cálculo de coeficientes de difusão aparente (CCDA), a IPD pode auxiliar na identificação de problemas como edema citotóxico associado a infarto isquêmico. A imagem do tensor de difusão (ITD), também conhecida como rastreamento de fibra, avalia a direção de difusão (anisotropia) na substância branca importante para fornecer mais informações sobre a conectividade neuronal. A angiografia por RM (ARM) usa sequências de ecogradiente para detectar mudanças de sinal de fluxo sanguíneo (vasos) nos tecidos.

Descrição da lesão para imagem transversal

Para ambas, tanto a tomografia computadorizada (TC) quanto a ressonância magnética (RM), uma abordagem padrão é usada para caracterizar anomalias estruturais primárias e secundárias. Nas anomalias primárias, as descrições das lesões são baseadas em seu número (único ou múltiplo) e densidade/intensidade (hipodenso, hiperdenso, isodenso) (Tabela 260.5) em relação à área adjacente normal, à sua distribuição (homo ou heterogênea),

Tabela 260.4 Sequências comumente usadas em ressonância magnética para definir a intensidade do tecido* e indicações.

	T2W	FLAIR (T2W)	T1W	STIR	GRE (T2*)
Gordura	Hipo	Hiper	Hiper	Hipo	Hiper
LCR	Hiper	Hipo	Hipo	Hiper	Hiper
Edema	Hiper	Hiper	Hipo	Hiper	Hiper
Indicações para sequência selecionada	Permite distinção entre líquido e tecido; executada em todo estudo de IRM	Supressão (anulação) de líquido de baixa proteína (*i. e.*, LCR), permitindo a visualização de lesões periventriculares	Comparação de imagens pré e pós-contraste para avaliar suprimento do tecido vascular e interrupção da BHE	Permite a supressão de sinal hiperintenso da gordura	Mais sensível para detecção do sinal vazio na hemorragia, osso e mineralização

*Aparência da intensidade do tecido na sequência em comparação com o córtex cerebral (substância cinzenta). *BHE*, barreira hematencefálica; *FLAIR*, recuperação de inversão atenuada por fluido; *GRE*, gradiente eco; *STIR*, recuperação de inversão de tau curto.

SEÇÃO 17 • Doença Neurológica

Tabela 260.5 Patologias com densidade aumentada de tomografia computadorizada (TC) ou intensidade aumentada de ressonância magnética.

DENSIDADE DA TC	INTENSIDADE T1W	INTENSIDADE T2W
Proliferações ósseas	Gordura	LCR e outros fluidos
Tecido mineralizado	Estágio de metemoglobina em hemorragia	Edema
Hemorragia (hiperaguda, aguda)	Líquido mucinoso	Necrose
Lesão enriquecida com iodo	Necrose laminar cortical Lesão enriquecida com gadolínio	Desmielinização
Tecidos de alta densidade celular (fibrosa)	Melanina	Mudanças celulares (gliose, inflamação, neoplasia)
Objeto metálico	Deposição de ferro	

LCR, líquido cefalorraquidiano.

bordas, anatomia e localização em relação ao SNC (extra-axial, intra-axial) e meninges (intradural, extradural, intraparenquimatosa). Efeitos secundários na anatomia e ao redor também são descritos para incluir a extensão e o tipo de edema e efeito da massa, causando mudança nas estruturas da linha média, herniação de tecido ou distorção dos ventrículos. Alterações do fluxo de LCR podem causar edema periventricular, hidrocefalia obstrutiva ou ventriculomegalia e siringo-hidromielia.

Agentes de contraste podem ser empregados com TC ou com varreduras RM a fim de melhorar a resolução do tecido e ampliar a detecção de processos patológicos. As imagens podem ser obtidas imediatamente após o contraste IV para avaliar a vasculatura ou podem ser feitas após vários minutos para avaliação da absorção tecidual. Os agentes de contraste usados para TC são iodados e alteram a atenuação de raios X, enquanto os agentes de contraste usados para ressonância magnética são paramagnéticos e funcionam mudando as taxas de relaxamento dos prótons. As lesões são caracterizadas pelo grau e pela distribuição do realce do contraste. Após a administração por via intravenosa, a BHE normalmente excluiria tais agentes. A presença ou ausência de realce de contraste com doença do SNC depende do grau de ruptura da BHE ou presença de vasodilatação ou neovascularização e, como tal, é um achado inespecífico associado a muitas doenças do SNC.[17-19] A ruptura dessa barreira por neoplasia ou inflamação resulta em acúmulo de contraste e realce da lesão, aumentando assim a capacidade de identificar a(s) lesão(ões) primária(s).

Outras modalidades de imagem

A tomografia por emissão de pósitrons (PET, do inglês *positron emission tomography*) e a tomografia computadorizada de emissão de fóton único (*single photon emission computed tomography* [SPECT]) são técnicas de imagem funcional que permitem mensurações qualitativas e quantitativas do metabolismo tecidual e estão ganhando utilidade na medicina veterinária.[20] As maiores utilidades da técnica incluem definição de áreas metabolicamente ativas para biopsia *versus* lesões isquêmicas inativas. Imagens produzidas por PET são corregistradas com TC ou IRM para obtenção de relações anatômicas. Imagens de PET têm sido avaliadas em cérebros caninos normais e em cães com doença intracraniana.[21-24]

Biopsia cerebral

Embora imagem avançada forneça excelentes imagens do sistema nervoso, elas não podem fornecer diagnósticos definitivos para muitas doenças cerebrais que são fundamentadas na histologia. A biopsia cerebral *ante mortem* pode produzir um diagnóstico mais definitivo para orientar abordagens de tratamento; em contrapartida, tais procedimentos são dependentes da obtenção de material de biopsia de porções representativas da lesão. Técnicas de biopsia guiada por imagem diminuem a morbidade e aumentam a viabilidade. Sistemas estereotáxicos guiados por tomografia

computadorizada ou ressonância magnética, técnicas de mão livre que utilizam US, TC ou IRM e biopsia guiada por endoscopia têm sido desenvolvidas para biopsia cerebral em cães.[25-35] A eficácia do diagnóstico da biopsia de lesões cerebrais pode ser influenciada pelo tamanho da amostra e pela dificuldade em distinguir entre a lesão primária e alterações secundárias da lesão, tais como edema e necrose. A avaliação citológica intraoperatória de uma amostra de biopsia pode melhorar a precisão do diagnóstico.[36,37] Além das limitações em precisão do diagnóstico por biopsia, também existem riscos que não podem ser negligenciados; um estudo recente em cães com encefalite sugeriu que a taxa de mortalidade e morbidade é de 6 e 29%, respectivamente.[34] Neuronavegação moderna pode refinar ainda mais as técnicas de biopsia e diminuir a morbidade.[31,38,39] O uso combinado de marcadores externos rigidamente fixados para pontos de referência dentro e fora da calota craniana e instrumentos cirúrgicos rotulados fornecem informações em tempo real durante o procedimento de coleta de material.

Análise do líquido cefalorraquidiano

Uma vez que uma lesão em massa produz aumento da pressão intracraniana, o risco de complicações aumenta significativamente; portanto, exames de imagem devem preceder a coleta de LCR. O exame de LCR é mais útil para identificar doença inflamatória, mas pode fornecer outras informações (aumento da proteína em neoplasia). Em alguns casos, a análise do LCR pode ser diagnóstica. Na criptococose (ver Capítulo 231), por exemplo, os microrganismos podem ser vistos no exame. Mais comumente, a análise do LCR simplesmente confirma a inflamação ou a presença de doença. Testes adicionais são necessários para fazer um diagnóstico definitivo. A cultura do LCR tem baixo custo. A cultura microbiana de sangue ou urina podem ser consideradas em casos de suspeita de infecção bacteriana.

O LCR, soro ou ambos podem ser analisados para a presença de anticorpos em casos de doenças infecciosas, mais comumente *Neospora caninum*, *Toxoplasma gondii*, *Ehrlichia* spp., *Anaplasma* spp., *Rickettsia rickettsii* e *Coccidioides immitis*. A prevalência varia com a localização geográfica. A infecção por *Cryptococcus* spp. geralmente é detectada por teste de antígeno. Outros DNA ou RNA microbianos podem ser detectados pela reação em cadeia da polimerase altamente sensível e específica (PCR).[40-42] Os resultados devem ser interpretados com cuidado para evitar falsos positivos e controles negativos rigorosos devem ser avaliados em paralelo (ver Capítulo 207). Um resultado de PCR negativo pode indicar que níveis indetectáveis de ácido nucleico estão presentes, um agente pode estar no tecido neural, mas não está no LCR, ou o distúrbio pode ter sido desencadeado por um agente que não está mais presente.[41] Outras análises no LCR têm sido estudadas para doenças no SNC, mas carecem de especificidade quanto à doença. A composição de proteína do LCR pode ainda ser definida por técnicas semiquantitativas de eletroforese, e anormalidades têm sido relatadas como úteis na identificação de doenças

CAPÍTULO 260 • Doenças do Cérebro: Anomalia, Degenerativa, Metabólica, Neoplásica, Idiopática...

inflamatórias, neoplásicas e doenças degenerativas.[43-45] Citometria de fluxo e imunofenotipagem, usadas para identificar células mononucleares em distúrbios inflamatórios do LCR[46] e a identificação de linhagem de células neoplásicas, não são práticas por serem necessários grandes volumes (4 a 5 mℓ) de LCR, a menos que a contagem de células seja muito alta.

Eletroencefalograma, genoma, resposta à terapia e outros diagnósticos

O eletroencefalograma (EEG) é usado principalmente para confirmar a atividade epiléptica cerebral de pacientes com suspeita de convulsão. É particularmente útil no *status* epiléptico para confirmar que a atividade convulsiva cessou. A resposta auditiva evocada (RAE) no tronco encefálico é usada principalmente para avaliar a função coclear, mas intervalos das últimas ondas podem também avaliar a condução do tronco encefálico.[47,48] Os potenciais evocados somatossensorial e visual podem avaliar a função desses sistemas.

Avanços no estudo de genoma animal permitiram a identificação de mutações causadoras de doenças e desenvolvimento de testes de DNA para detectar alelos mutantes. Isso simplificou o diagnóstico de muitas doenças cerebrais hereditárias, a maioria nas quais em cães e gatos tem traços autossômicos recessivos ou são resultado de uma herança genética complexa. Traços dominantes podem ser eliminados de uma raça não reproduzindo animais afetados. Doenças familiares não são necessariamente genéticas, uma vez que famílias podem compartilhar a mesma dieta, ambiente, e exposição à infecção e assim por diante. A predileção da raça por uma determinada doença sugere uma contribuição genética, mas, novamente, outros fatores podem estar refletidos, como o uso típico de uma determinada raça ou administração de suplementos da moda. Em última análise, a natureza hereditária de alguns distúrbios é classificada no gene ou seu produto que é alterado. Muitos sites agora estão disponíveis para identificar os laboratórios que realizam esses testes. No entanto, o clínico deve ser capaz de selecionar o teste e interpretar os resultados adequadamente.[49-51] Isso requer uma compreensão da terminologia usada, dos tipos de testes genéticos disponíveis e da investigação das potenciais armadilhas do teste de DNA (ver Capítulo 4).

A resposta à terapia pode ser importante para o diagnóstico, principalmente quando fatores financeiros ou outros limitam a realização do teste. A terapia para a condição mais provável pode ser iniciada e a resposta ao tratamento monitorada. Por exemplo, uma grande melhora com o uso da tetraciclina poderia dar suporte ao seu uso na doença transmitida por carrapatos. Em contrapartida, ao mesmo tempo que o uso de corticosteroides desempenha um papel importante no tratamento de doença cerebral, o risco de efeitos adversos, incluindo a exacerbação de doenças infecciosas, precisa ser avaliado cuidadosamente. Uma grande melhora com o uso dos corticosteroides seria compatível com neoplasia ou doença inflamatória infecciosa/não infecciosa. A melhora da neoplasia costuma durar pouco, enquanto algumas doenças não inflamatórias e não infecciosas podem ser mantidas em remissão com o tratamento prolongado com corticosteroides. Também doenças infecciosas frequentemente podem responder muito bem ao uso corticosteroides, podem piorar apenas em casos nos quais antibioticoterapia apropriada não é instituída. A resposta a fármacos antiepilépticos (FAE) ajuda a confirmar um distúrbio convulsivo, mas não descarta uma causa subjacente às convulsões.

DOENÇAS ESPECÍFICAS DO CÉREBRO

O cérebro é o órgão mais exigente metabolicamente no corpo. Uma grande parte da energia do corpo é reservada para manter potenciais de membrana em repouso e a neurotransmissão. O sistema nervoso tem vias de metabolismo energético mais limitadas do que outros tecidos e, portanto, é mais sensível a

distúrbios de glicose ou suprimento de oxigênio. O cérebro também é sensível a toxinas exógenas ou endógenas, e centros superiores mais sensíveis a insultos metabólicos. Portanto, os sinais de doença prosencefálica são uma manifestação comum de doenças sistêmicas (ver Capítulo 12). Os distúrbios são descritos de acordo com o esquema de classificação DAMNEITV (d = degenerativo, a = anomalia, m = metabólico, n = neoplásico e nutricional, e = epilepsia idiopática, i = inflamatória, t = traumática, v = vascular). Enfermidades decorrentes de processos inflamatórios, que na sua maioria são multifocais e traumas de cabeça são discutidos nos Capítulos 148 e 261, respectivamente.

Doenças degenerativas cerebrais primárias

As doenças neurodegenerativas do cérebro têm curso progressivo e geralmente são diagnosticadas em animais bastante jovens ou geriátricos (ver Capítulo 263). As encefalomielopatias degenerativas podem ser seletivas, difusas ou multifocais, já que o neurônio ou mielina frequentemente envolvem o cérebro e a medula espinal. Sinais talamocorticais, do tronco encefálico, da medula espinal e/ou cerebelares podem ser predominantes. Os achados de ressonância magnética do cérebro podem mostrar lesões simétricas seletivas na substância cinzenta ou branca que podem ter distribuição regional ou difusa. Adicionalmente, achados de ressonância magnética de atrofia cerebral também podem ser regionais ou difusos. Todavia, um diagnóstico definitivo para muitos desses distúrbios é feito em biopsia ou necropsia. Teste de DNA pode ser útil. Atualmente, não há tratamento eficaz para a maioria das doenças neurodegenerativas. Descobertas genéticas permitiram melhor compreensão das vias subjacentes causadoras de doenças e podem fornecer estudos terapêuticos direcionados. Essas estratégias terapêuticas incluem terapia de transferência de genes somáticos, terapia de reposição de enzimas, transplante de células heterólogas e silenciamento de RNA. Elas são promissoras e testes clínicos em vários modelos de doenças em cães e gatos estão em andamento.

Anomalias cerebrais

Malformações congênitas do cérebro normalmente estão presentes desde o nascimento e não são progressivas. Algumas exceções, como coma hidrocefalia congênita, podem se manifestar mais tarde na vida com sinais progressivos O sistema nervoso se origina de uma placa na superfície dorsal do embrião, que se dobra para formar o tubo neural, começando na área torácica e se estendendo rostro-caudalmente. Defeitos genéticos e infecção no útero, intoxicação ou desnutrição podem causar falha do fechamento normal do tubo neural, normalmente observado no aspecto rostral ou extremidades caudais do sistema nervoso em desenvolvimento. Células da crista neural cranial são necessárias para dobrar o tubo e se tornar o mesênquima da face e base da calvária.[162] Defeitos de fechamento do tubo neural do cérebro podem variar em gravidade, e o mais grave é a anencefalia com completa falta de desenvolvimento do cérebro e nenhuma indução da formação da calvária.

Malformações graves são aparentes no exame físico e em imagens cerebrais.[163] O exame *post mortem* pode ser necessário para detectar deficiências mais sutis. Anomalias cerebrais podem acompanhar outros defeitos, como fenda palatina ou anomalias cardíacas. Para a maioria das malformações congênitas, o tratamento é sintomático e o prognóstico depende da gravidade da condição. O histórico e a sorologia podem ajudar a descartar etiologias tóxicas ou infecciosas tratáveis. Aconselhamentos genético, vacinal e nutricional podem ajudar a prevenir futuras ocorrências em criadouros.

Encefalopatia metabólica

Erros inatos do metabolismo

Erros inatos do metabolismo interferem na função em nível bioquímico ou levam à morte neuronal prematura. Frequentemente, os sinais se manifestam aumentando e diminuindo e encefalopatia difusa e simétrica em neonatos ou no animal jovem. Os primeiros e mais consistentes sinais anormais são debilidade e convulsão. Encefalopatia neonatal com convulsões (ENCC), por exemplo, é uma doença hereditária em cães Poodles Standard caracterizada por atraso no desenvolvimento com convulsões e morte antes do desmame com poucas informações bioquímicas ou histológicas sobre a causa. Uma mutação foi identificada em um importante fator de transcrição (ATF2), o que afeta a programação normal de desenvolvimento neuronal.[239] Outros sinais neurológicos variam com a distribuição regional das lesões e a gravidade do distúrbio metabólico. Algumas doenças mostram características bilaterais e sinal simétrico de mudanças na ressonância magnética do cérebro. A dieta pode influenciar na gravidade dos sinais.

Alguns erros inatos do metabolismo podem ser aparentes em testes de laboratório. As deficiências nas enzimas do ciclo da ureia aumentam as concentrações de amônia no sangue durante a cetonúria ou acidose, sem uma causa subjacente clara, como diabetes melito, que pode refletir em erros no metabolismo mitocondrial. Se há acúmulo anormal de um metabólito, esse produto às vezes pode ser detectado, como anormalidades no lactato sanguíneo e no piruvato em distúrbios mitocondriais. A identificação de concentrações anormais de certos metabólitos na urina pode ser um cuidado diagnóstico ideal, uma vez que os metabólitos podem ser excretados pelos rins em altas concentrações, e volumes de urina suficientes podem ser coletados para os testes, mesmo em neonatos. Testes simples de triagem de urina estão disponíveis para alguns erros inatos do metabolismo, mas a maioria requer testes em laboratórios especializados. Soro ou LCR podem ser testados para metabólitos que não são detectados na urina, enquanto outros testes medem atividades enzimáticas específicas.

Lesões simétricas bilaterais do SNC podem ser tanto manifestações de suscetibilidade seletiva de populações celulares a metabolismo alterado ou serem determinadas pela anatomia vascular (isquemia). Muitos erros inatos do metabolismo afetam outros órgãos avaliados mais rapidamente que o cérebro. Se nervos periféricos estão envolvidos, uma biopsia de nervo pode fornecer informações, por exemplo, a presença de macrófagos vacuolados em células globoides na leucodistrofia. Ocasionalmente, tais células vacuoladas podem ser visíveis em esfregaços de sangue de rotina ou análise de LCR. Como o músculo também tem uma alta demanda metabólica, as doenças que afetam o metabolismo energético podem mostrar mudanças na biopsia do músculo. No caso de hepatomegalia ou linfadenopatia acompanhar sinais neurológicos, uma biopsia de um desses órgãos mais acessíveis pode revelar produtos de armazenamento.[240,241]

Encefalopatia mitocondrial

Encefalopatia mitocondrial necrosante subaguda, conhecida como síndrome de Leigh ou síndrome semelhante à síndrome de Leigh no homem, consiste em defeitos na cadeia respiratória ou no metabolismo do piruvato da mitocôndria. As lesões são atribuídas à congestão vascular, causada por acidose láctica resultante na hipoxemia e necrose. Os sinais clínicos incluem ataxia, paresia, distúrbios do movimento, déficits cognitivos, nistagmo e convulsões. A encefalopatia mitocondrial tem sido reconhecida por ataxia proprioceptiva aguda, convulsões, mudanças de comportamento, cegueira central, tetraparesia e/ou deficiências da sensibilidade facial em cães da raça Husky do Alasca com idade inferior a 1 ano. Lesões cavitárias e espongiformes da substância cinzenta são observadas simetricamente no tálamo e *striatum*, na junção da substância cinzenta e branca do córtex cerebral, no tronco encefálico e no *vermis* cerebelar.[145-147] Essas lesões são claramente visíveis na ressonância magnética como hiperintensidade T2W.[147,242] Foi determinado que uma mutação no SLC19A3, que codifica uma proteína transportadora de tiamina, desempenha papel importante na encefalopatia no Husky do Alasca.[146,242] Encefalopatia necrosante subaguda

associada a defeitos combinados da cadeia respiratória também foi relatada em cães da raça Yorkshire Terriers e American Staffordshire Bull Terriers.[148,149,243]

Acidúrias orgânicas

Essas doenças são caracterizadas por ácidos orgânicos anormais decorrentes de erros em uma via metabólica. Embora relativamente poucas tenham sido descritas em medicina veterinária, elas são comuns na medicina humana e provavelmente ocorrem ocasionalmente em alguns cães de raça pura. A doença pode ser diagnosticada através da identificação de ácidos orgânicos na urina e existe a possibilidade de intervenção terapêutica, se a via deficiente puder ser contornada. Os níveis celulares do ácido malônico regulam o uso de carboidratos ou dos ácidos graxos como fontes de energia na alimentação *versus* a condição de jejum, respectivamente. Um cão da raça Maltês de uma família com acidúria malônica desenvolveu convulsões, estupor, hipoglicemia, acidose e cetonúria após um breve período de anorexia. A alimentação frequente com uma dieta rica em carboidratos e baixa em gordura eliminou a necessidade de contar com ácidos graxos como fonte de energia e melhorou os sinais clínicos.[244]

A cobalamina (vitamina B12) é um cofator necessário na conversão de metilmalonil CoA em succinil CoA, um passo significativo para entrada no ciclo de Krebs. A má absorção seletiva hereditária da cobalamina foi relatada em cães das raças Schnauzers Gigante, Beagle, Border Collie e Pastor-Australiano.[245-247] Mutações em ambos os genes *amnionless* (AMN) ou no gene cobulina (CUBN) podem ocasionar à síndrome de Imerslund-Grasbeck (IGS) ou a má absorção seletiva de cobalamina. Estudos genéticos em cães mostraram mutações em AMN em Schnauzers Gigantes e Pastores-Australianos e CUBN em Beagles e Border Collies.[248-251] Os sinais clínicos característicos incluem nível de consciência alterado, inapetência e convulsões associadas a hiperamonemia e discrasias sanguíneas. A identificação de alto nível de ácido metilmalônico (AMM) urinário e baixas concentrações de cobalamina séricas confirmam o diagnóstico. A disfunção do ciclo da ureia é uma consequência do acúmulo de AMM. Os sinais clínicos se resolvem com a administração parenteral de cianocobalamina. A deficiência de cobalamina tem sido associada a teores elevados de MMA urinário e sinais neurológicos em gatos, presumivelmente em razão de deficiência do fator intrínseco necessário para a absorção de vitamina B_{12} (cianocobalamina).[252] A doença gastrintestinal também pode interferir na absorção de cobalamina em gatos.[253,254] Gatos com doença gastrintestinal também podem desenvolver a acidose D-láctica, provavelmente em razão da produção excessiva da isoforma D por bactérias nos intestinos.[255] D-lactato não é detectado pela maioria dos ensaios de lactato de rotina, os quais são projetados para detectar a isoforma L produzida por mamíferos, mas é muito mais provável que produza encefalopatia.[256]

Concentrações aumentadas de ácidos metilmalônico e malônico, bem como outros metabólitos intermediários, foram encontrados na urina de um filhote de Labrador Retriever com 12 semanas de vida e sinais neurológicos progressivos. O filhote não era cetoacidótico ou hiperamonêmico, e os teores de cobalamina eram normais. Atrofia difusa do SNC foi encontrada na necropsia, mas nenhum defeito metabólico foi identificado.[257] Cães da raça Staffordshire Bull Terriers e Yorkshire Terriers com acidúria L-2-hidroxiglutárica hereditária desenvolvem convulsões, ataxia e comportamento alterado, geralmente entre 4 e 5 anos. Nas regiões do tronco encefálico, cerebelo, tálamo e substância cinzenta cerebral, a hiperintensidade difusa na ressonância magnética foi observada com T2W.[258] Os teores de ácido L-2-hidroxiglutárico estavam aumentados na urina, LCR e plasma de cães acometidos.[258,259] Mutações na desidrogenase (L2 HGDH) que metaboliza o ácido orgânico foram descritas nas raças Staffordshire Bull Terriers e Yorkshire Terriers.[259-261]

Doenças de armazenamento lisossomal

Definições. As doenças de armazenamento lisossomal são caracterizadas pelo acúmulo de subprodutos metabólicos dentro dos lisossomos, a organela celular responsável pela quebra do complexo de macromoléculas. Os lisossomos mantêm o pH ácido e substratos para o catabolismo que incluem esfingolipídios (um dos principais componentes da mielina), oligossacarídeos, mucopolissacarídeos, glicoproteínas e proteínas (Tabela 260.6). As doenças do armazenamento são causadas por deficiências enzimáticas importantes, resultando em uma falha da quebra de moléculas e no acúmulo de substrato. A maioria das síndromes é nomeada de acordo com o produto que é acumulado. As proteases são menos substrato-específicas, e as deficiências isoladas por protease são incomuns e menos prováveis de produzir problemas, embora a lipofuscinose ceroide possa ser um desses defeitos.[240,241,262,263] Alguns defeitos interferem na capacidade das células de utilizar uma enzima normal. Na doença das células I (mucolipidose) em gatos, por exemplo, parece ocorrer um distúrbio no tráfego de enzimas para o lisossomo, afetando várias enzimas.[264] Alguns substratos devem ser engolfados (endocitose) em uma organela de parede dupla, o autofagossomo, e posteriormente entregues ao lisossomo para degradação. Mutações em genes que interrompem esse processo (autofagia) recentemente foram associadas a doenças neurodegenerativas em cães. A ataxia cerebelar hereditária em cães das raças Setter Gordon e Pastor-Inglês e a doença neurodegenerativa em Lagotto Romagnolo caracterizada por ataxia cerebelar, mudanças de personalidade e vacuolização neuronal têm sido associadas a mutações nos genes autofágicos RAB24 e ATG4D, respectivamente.[133,265] Revisões recentes de doenças de armazenamento em animais estão disponíveis.[240,241,262,263,266,267] O acúmulo de produtos de armazenamento ocorre ao longo do tempo e o início dos sinais é retardado na maior parte das doenças de armazenamento, apesar da deficiência enzimática estar presente desde o nascimento. A idade de início dos sinais clínicos e a gravidade do processo podem depender da função enzimática residual e dos sistemas afetados, uma vez que algumas doenças de armazenamento afetam vários órgãos e outros afetam apenas o sistema nervoso. Ainda não foi esclarecido como o acúmulo dos produtos de armazenamento produz doenças neurológicas. Na leucodistrofia de células globoides, um dos produtos de armazenamento é claramente tóxico para as células da oligodendróglia. Em outros, a formação de esferoides pode estar relacionada à morte neuronal.[240,241,263,268]

Sinais. Sinais cerebelares de dismetria, ataxia do tronco e nistagmo geralmente são os primeiros sinais de doenças de armazenamento.[241] O cerebelo depende de condução rápida para retorno sensorial durante o movimento, e é bastante sensível a distúrbios que afetam a mielina ou o processamento de informações, e até mesmo deficiências sutis pode causar sinais. Déficits de aprendizagem ou demência mais profundas podem ser necessários em outras condições para atingir um limite para o aparecimento dos sinais, que muitas vezes progridem para fraqueza do neurônio motor superior (NMS), anormalidades comportamentais e convulsões.[241] Algumas doenças (p. ex., lipofuscinose ceroide neuronal) causam disfunções visuais e prosencefálicas antes que a disfunção cerebelar seja observada.[269] Nervos periféricos estão envolvidos em algumas condições, como leucodistrofia de células globoides, fucosidose, glicogenose tipo IV, manosidose e doença de Niemann-Pick.[98,270] Em algumas doenças de armazenamento lisossomal, sinais de envolvimento de outros órgãos podem ser visíveis. Podem-se observar anormalidades na retina ou formação de catarata (ver Capítulo 11). Anormalidades do tecido ósseo e conjuntivo frequentemente caracterizam-se por mucopolissacaridoses, mucolipidose e alfamanosidose, nas quais o exame radiográfico revela malformações ósseas dismórficas da coluna e/ou face. Aumento cardíaco, hepático, esplênico ou de linfonodos podem acompanhar os sinais neurológicos.

Diagnóstico. A distribuição multissistêmica de anomalias da doença de armazenamento lisossomal permite obter um diagnóstico de tecidos extraneurais. Vacúolos de armazenamento podem estar visíveis em células brancas do esfregaço de sangue periférico ou, na leucodistrofia de células globoides ou fucosidose, na análise do LCR. Biopsias ou aspirado de gânglios linfáticos (ver Capítulo 95), fígado (ver Capítulos 89 e 91), baço ou músculo (ver Capítulo 116) podem ser realizadas para revelar armazenamento de vacúolos. Em algumas doenças de armazenamento lisossomal, a imagem transversal de ressonância magnética pode mostrar várias hiperintensidades e atrofia cerebral.[241,267] A necropsia pode ser necessária para mostrar produtos de armazenamento acumulados quando apenas o sistema nervoso está envolvido. A microscopia eletrônica pode mostrar material de armazenamento contido nos lisossomos. Metabólitos anormais podem ser detectados na urina em alguns casos de doenças de armazenamento. O diagnóstico definitivo é baseado no teste para a mutação conhecida (ver Tabela 260.6) e/ou para a demonstração de atividade enzimática deficiente em tecidos afetados, por cultivo de leucócitos ou fibroblastos.

Lipofuscinose ceroide neuronal

Definições. A lipofuscinose ceroide neuronal (LCN), também conhecida como doença de Batten, é um subconjunto de doenças de armazenamento lisossomal na qual os produtos de armazenamento são proteínas com características de autofluorescência, semelhantes a pigmentos ceroides e lipofuscina, que se acumulam normalmente com o envelhecimento. Os produtos armazenados na LCN são subunidade c de ATP mitocondrial ou de proteínas ativadoras de esfingolipídios (saposinas A e D), em razão da deficiência das enzimas solúveis. As membranas proteicas estão localizadas no lisossomo, retículo endoplasmático, ou em proteínas associadas à vesícula sináptica.[271,272]

Sinais. Os sinais clínicos decorrentes de LCN incluem deficiências visuais (geralmente o primeiro sinal, especialmente na penumbra), declínio na cognição e nas funções motoras, convulsões, atrofia cerebral generalizada e morte no período de juventude à meia-idade. Mudanças de comportamento se tornam proeminentes com a progressão da doença e incluem timidez, hiperestesia, confusão, agressão não provocada, convulsões, bater de dentes, bruxismo e mioclonia. A ataxia proprioceptiva generalizada e ataxia cerebelar tendem a ser manifestações posteriores em muitas raças, embora sejam os sinais mais proeminentes em American Bulldogs com deficiência de catepsina D.[273,274]

Diagnóstico e tratamento. A atrofia cerebral generalizada pode ser observada em imagens transversais em estágios posteriores da doença, mas o diagnóstico definitivo requer o reconhecimento de material autofluorescente no cérebro ou outros tecidos. Mutações responsáveis por muitas das LCN em cães foram identificadas em testes DNA e estão disponíveis (ver Tabela 260.6). Mutações genéticas das LCN em cães incluem LCN1 (Dachshund), LCN2 (Dachshund de Pelo Longo), LCN4 (Staffordshire Terrier Americano), LCN5 (Border Collie, Golden Retriever), LCN6 (Pastor-Australiano), LCN7 (Cão de Crista Chinês), LCN8 (Setter Inglês, mix de Pastor-Australiano), LCN10 (Buldogue Americano), LCN12 (Terrier Tibetano).[274-285] Esses testes auxiliam na confirmação do diagnóstico e auxiliam os criadores de cães nos esforços para reduzir a incidência de LCN nas raças. Não existe terapêutica eficaz para as doenças do armazenamento. Terapia de genes, terapia com células-tronco e terapia de reposição enzimática são promissoras.[262,266,267] Terapia sintomática para controle das convulsões e dos fármacos que alteram o comportamento pode ajudar a melhorar alguns dos sinais.

Tabela 260.6 — Classificação de doenças de armazenamento lisossomal em caninos e felinos.

DOENÇA DE ARMAZENAMENTO (DOENÇA HUMANA)	DEFICIÊNCIA DE ENZIMA/PROTEÍNA (MUTAÇÃO GÊNICA)	ESPÉCIE – RAÇA	SINAIS CLÍNICOS
Glicoproteinoses Fucosidose	Alfa-L-fucosidase (*FUCA1*)	C – *Springer Spaniel Inglês*	Ataxia cerebelar, mudança comportamental, disfonia, disfagia, convulsões
Manosidose (alfamanosidose)	Alfa-D-manosidase (*MANB*)	F – PCD, PLD, *Persa*	Ataxia cerebelar, tremor, opacidade de córnea, anomalias esqueléticas, neuropatia
Doença de Lafora	Alfaglucosidase (*EPM2A*)	C – Beagle, Basset Hound, Poodle, *Dachshund Pelo de Arame*; F – PCD	Epilepsia mioclônica, apatia
Oligossacaridoses/glicogenoses GSD tipo 1 (Doença de von Gierke)	Glicose-6-fosfatase (*M121I*)	C – Silky Terrier, *Maltês*, outras raças Toy; F – PCD	Fraqueza, convulsões, estupor
GSD tipo 2 (Doença de Pompe)	Alfaglucosidase ácida (*GAA*)	C – Lapphund; F – PCD	Ataxia, fraqueza muscular
GSD tipo 3 (Doença de Cori)	Amilo-1,6-glucosidase (*AGL*)	C – Akita, Pastor-Alemão, *Retriever de Pelo Crespo* (IIIA)	Letargia, intolerância ao exercício, organomegalia
GSD tipo 4 (Doença de Andersen)	Enzima ramificadora de glicogênio (*GBE-1*)	F – *Gato Norueguês da Floresta*	Ataxia cerebelar, tremor muscular, organomegalia
GSD tipo 7 (Doença de Tarui)	Fosfofrutoquinase (*PFKM*)	C – *Springer Spaniel Inglês, Cocker Spaniels Americano, Whippets*, cães de raças mestiças, *Wachtelhund*	Intolerância ao exercício, rabdomiólise
Mucolipidose Mucolipidose II (Doença das células I)	N-acetilglucosamina 1-fosfotransferase (*GNPTA*)	F – *PCD*	Dismorfismo facial, da retina, apatia, ataxia
Esfingolipidoses GM1-gangliosidose tipo 1 (Doença de Norman-Landing)	Beta-D-galactosidase (*GLB1*)	C – Mestiços de Beagle, *Cão-d'Água Português*, Springer Spaniel Inglês, *Husky Siberiano, Shiba*; F – *PCD, Siamês, Korat*	Ataxia cerebelar, opacificação da córnea, tremor, convulsões, paralisia, dismorfismo esquelético facial
GM2-gangliosidose (Doença de Tay-Sachs) (variante B)	Beta-N-acetil hexosaminidase A (subunidade alfa) (*HEXA*)	C – Pointer Alemão de Pelo Curto; Chin Japonês	Ataxia cerebelar
GM2-gangliosidose (Doença de Sandhoff) (variante O)	Beta-N-acetil hexosaminidase B (subunidade beta) (*HEXB*)	C – Golden Retriever, *Poodles Toys*; F – PCD – Korat Japonês, Birmanês-Europeu	Ataxia cerebelar
GM2AB-gangliosidose (doença de Bernheimer-Seitelberger) (variante AB)	GM2 Proteína ativadora da deficiência (*GM2A*)	F – *PCD*	Ataxia cerebelar
Galactosialidose	Galactosialidose com alfaneuraminidase	C – Schipperke (5 anos)	Ataxia cerebelar
Glicocerebrosidose (Doença de Gaucher)	Beta-D-gluco cerebrosidase	C – Sydney Silky	Ataxia cerebelar
Leucodistrofia de células globoides (Doença de Krabbe)	Beta-D-galactosil ceramidase (*GALC*)	C – *West Highland White Terrier, Cairn Terrier, Beagle, Poodle*, Kelpie Australiano; Basset Hound, Tick Hound Azul, Lulu da Pomerânia, *Setter Irlandês*; F – PCD, PLD	Ataxia cerebelar, tremor, paraparesia, neuropatia

Continua

CAPÍTULO 260 • Doenças do Cérebro: Anomalia, Degenerativa, Metabólica, Neoplásica, Idiopática... — 1397

Tabela 260.6 Classificação de doenças de armazenamento lisossomal em caninos e felinos. (*Continuação*)

DOENÇA DE ARMAZENAMENTO (DOENÇA HUMANA)	DEFICIÊNCIA DE ENZIMA/PROTEÍNA (MUTAÇÃO GÊNICA)	ESPÉCIE – RAÇA	SINAIS CLÍNICOS
Leucodistrofia metacromática	Arilsulfatase A	F – PCD	Disfunção motora progressiva, convulsões, opistótono, neuropatia
Esfingomielinose (Doença de Niemann-Pick tipo A)	Esfingomielinase	C – Poodle Miniatura F – Balinês, Siamês	Ataxia cerebelar, tremor, paraparesia, neuropatia; biopsia
(Doença de Niemann-Pick tipo C)	Deficiência de esterificação de colesterol (*NPC1, NPC2*)	C – Boxer; F – *PCD*	C – Ataxia cerebelar, hepatomegalia, neuropatia; F – ataxia cerebelar
Mucopolissacaridoses MPS I (Síndrome de Hurler)	Alfa-L-iduronidase (*IDUA*)	C – *Plott Hound*, Rottweiler, raças mestiças; F – *PCD*	C – Retardo de crescimento, deformidade facial, claudicação, opacidade da córnea
MPS II	Iduronato-2-sulfato sulfatase	C – Labrador Retriever	Ataxia cerebelar, intolerância ao exercício, opacidade da córnea, dismorfismo facial
MPS II (A, B, E)	A: Heparina sulfamidase (*SGSH*) B: N-acetil-alfa-D-glucosaminidase (*NAGLU*) E: Arilsulfatase G (*ARSG*)	C – *Cão Huntaway* (IIIA), *Dachshund Pelo de Arame* (IIIA) *Schipperke* (IIIB) *Staffordshire Terrier Americano* (IIIE)	Ataxia cerebelar, tremor, degeneração da retina, opacidade da córnea
MPS VI (Doença de Maroteaux-Lamy)	N-acetilgalactosamina 4-sulfase (Arilsulfatase B) (*ARSB*)	C – Pinscher Miniatura, Schnauzer Miniatura, *Poodle Miniatura*, Welsh Corgi; F – *Gato Siamês*, PCD	Retardo de crescimento, deformidade facial, opacidade da córnea, proliferações espinais
MPS VII (Síndrome de Sly)	Beta-D-glucuronidase (*GUSB*)	C – mestiços F – *PCD*	C – Paraparesia, cardíaca; F – Retardo do crescimento, deformidade facial, opacidade da córnea, proliferações espinais
Lipofuscinoses neuronais ceroides (doença de Batten) LNC 1	Proteína palmitoil-tioesterase 1 (*PPT1*)	C – *Dachshund Miniatura*	Déficits visuais, ataxia cerebelar, comprometimento cognitivo, mioclonia, convulsão
LNC 2	Tripeptidil-peptidase (*TPP1*)	C – *Dachshund de Pelo Longo*	Idem
LNC 5	Proteína lisossomal solúvel LNC5 (*LNC5*)	C – *Border Collie; Golden Retriever*	Idem
LNC 6	Proteína transmembrana LNC6 (*LNC6*)	C – *Pastor-Australiano*	Idem
LNC 7	Principal superfamília de domínio facilitador MFSD8 (*MFSD8*)	C – *Cão de crista chinês*	Idem
LNC 8	Proteína transmembrana LNC8 (*LNC8*)	C – *Setter Inglês; mestiço de Pastor-Australiano*	Idem
LNC 10	Catepsina D (*CTSD*)	C – *Buldogue Americano*	Idem
LNC 12	ATPase tipo P (*ATP13A2*)	C – *Terrier Tibetano*	Idem
Outras	Mutação genética desconhecida	C – Pastor-Australiano, Chihuahua, Cocker Spaniel, Collie, Dachshund, Dálmata, Golden Retriever, Retriever Japonês, Labrador Retriever, Poodle Miniatura, Sheepdog da Planície Polonesa, Saluki, Spitz, Welsh Corgi; F – Gato Siamês, PCD Japonês, DSH Europeu	

Raças em itálico significam mutação genética descoberta. *C*, canino; *F*, felino; *GSD*, doença de armazenamento de glicogênio; *LNC*, lipofuscinose ceroide; *MPS*, mucopolissacaridose; *PCD*, Gato Doméstico de Pelo Curto; *PLD*, Gato Doméstico de Pelo Longo.

NEOPLASIA

Neoplasia intracraniana é uma condição comum em cães e gatos. Revisões evidenciam o diagnóstico, tratamento, exames de imagem e histologia.[17,286-290] Tumores no tecido cerebral são, de forma geral, classificados como primários ou secundários. Neoplasias intracranianas primárias (Tabela 260.7) incluem tumores neurais derivados da glia ou dos tecidos meníngeos, enquanto as neoplasias intracranianas secundárias são extraneurais e invadem localmente ou espalham-se para os tecidos neurais a partir de um sítio distante.

Tumores cerebrais primários

Tipos, metástases e incidências

Meningiomas compreendem cerca de 50% de incidência dos tumores cerebrais primários em cães, gliomas 30 a 40% e os tumores do plexo coroide são menos comuns (Tabela 260.8).[291-293] Os tumores cerebrais primários também incluem sarcoma histiocítico, tumores de células granulares, linfoma e tumores neuroectodérmicos primitivos (TNEP). Em gatos, os meningiomas representam cerca de 60% de todos os tipos de tumores com gliomas ocorrendo em uma frequência mais baixa.[294,295]

Raramente, neoplasias intracranianas primárias podem disseminar-se por todo o SNC por vias hematogênicas ou LCR ("metástase descendente"). Os tumores com probabilidade de disseminação extraneural incluem meningiomas, TNEPs, gliomas malignos, tumores histiocíticos e tumores do plexo coroide. Áreas estreitas do sistema ventricular são predispostas a hidrocefalia obstrutiva com seus sinais clínicos. Os meningiomas olfatórios de cães podem invadir o cérebro por meio da placa cribriforme.[296] Raramente, o meningioma pode fazer metástase para fora do SNC, para o pulmão ou para o pâncreas.[297,298] Tumores gliais raramente fazem metástase, a menos que ocorra o envolvimento ventricular. Ependimomas e os tumores do plexo coroide têm a possibilidade de implantarem-se ao longo das vias do LCR e enviam "sementes" que se alocam a distância no tecido da medula espinhal.[299-301] A incidência de tumores primários do SNC foi relatada como sendo de 14,5 em 100 mil cães (similar no homem) e 3,5 em 100 mil gatos.[302-304] A prevalência de neoplasia intracraniana em cães, com base em dados de necropsia, foi relatada como de 2 a 4,5% com prevalência de neoplasias primárias de 2,3% da população total (2,8% em cães > 1 ano) e neoplasias secundárias a 2,2% (2,6% em cães > 1 ano).[291]

Tabela 260.7 Neoplasias intracranianas primárias.

TIPO	EXEMPLOS HISTOLÓGICOS
Tumores de tecido neuroepitelial	
Tumores astrocíticos	Pilocítico, célula gigante subependimária, xantoastrocitoma pleomórfico, difuso (gemistocítico fibrilar, protoplasmático), anaplásico, gliobastoma, gliomatose cerebral
Tumores oligodendrogliais	Oligodendroglioma, oligoastrocitoma anaplásico
Tumores oligoastrocíticos	Oligoastrocitoma, oligoastrocitoma anaplásico
Tumores ependimários	Subependimoma, mixopapilar, ependimoma (celular, papilar, tanicítico de células claras), ependimoma anaplásico
Tumores do plexo coroide	Papiloma do plexo coroide, papiloma atípico do plexo coroide, carcinoma do plexo coroide
Outros tumores neuroepiteliais	Astroblastoma, glioma de coroide, glioma angiocêntrico
Tumores neuronais e neuronais-gliais mistos	Gangliocitoma displásico do cerebelo, astrocitoma infantil desmoplásico, tumor neuroepitelial disembrioplásico, gangliocitoma, ganglioglioma, ganglioglioma anaplásico, neurocitoma central, neurocitoma extraventricular, liponeurocitoma cerebelar, tumor glioneuronal papilar, tumor glioneuronal formador de roseta do 4º ventrículo, paraganglioma
Tumores da região pineal	Pineocitoma, tumor do parênquima pineal de diferenciação intermediária, pineoblastoma, tumor papilar da região pineal
Tumores embrionários	Meduloblastoma (meduloblastoma desmoplásico/nodular, meduloblastoma com extensa nodularidade, meduloblastoma anaplásico, meduloblastoma de células grandes), tumor neuroectodérmico primitivo do SNC (neuroblastoma do SNC, ganglioneuroblastoma do SNC, meduloepitelioma ependimoblastoma), tumor teratoide/rabdoide atípico
Tumores das meninges	
Tumores de células meningoteliais	Meningioma (meningotelial, fibroso, transicional, psamomático, angiomatoso, microcístico, secretor, linfoplasmocitário, metaplásico, cordoide, célula clara, atípico papilar, rabdoide, anaplásico)
Tumores mensenquimais	Lipoma, angiolipoma, hibernoma, lipossarcoma, tumor fibroso solitário, fibrossarcoma, histiocitoma fibroso maligno, leiomioma, leiomiossarcoma, rabdomioma, rabdomiossarcoma, condroma, condrossarcoma, osteoma, osteossarcoma, osteocondroma, hemangioma, epitelioide, hemangiopericitoma, hemangiopericitoma anaplásico, angiossarcoma, sarcoma de Kaposi, sarcoma de Ewing
Lesões melanocíticas primárias	Melanocitose difusa, melanocitoma, melanoma maligno, melanomatose meníngea
Outras neoplasias relacionadas às meninges	Hemangioblastoma
Linfoma e neoplasias hematopoéticas	Linfomas malignos, plasmocitoma, sarcoma granulocítico
Tumores de células germinativas	Germinoma, carcinoma embrionário, tumor do saco vitelino, coriocarcinoma, teratoma (maduro, imaturo, com transformação maligna), tumor de células germinativas misto
Tumores da região de Sellar	Craniofaringioma (adamantinomatoso, papilar), tumor de células granulares, pituicitoma, oncocitoma de células fusiformes da adeno-hipófise

SNC, sistema nervoso central. Adaptada do Sistema de Classificação da Organização Mundial da Saúde (OMS). De Louis DN, Ohgaki H, Wiestler OD et al.: The 2007 WHO Classification of tumors of the central nervous system. Acta Neuropathol 114: 97-109, 2007.

CAPÍTULO 260 • Doenças do Cérebro: Anomalia, Degenerativa, Metabólica, Neoplásica, Idiopática... 1399

Tabela 260.8 Recursos de imagem de ressonância magnética de tumores cerebrais caninos e felinos comuns.[17,288,289,301,305,334,337,338,343,344]

TIPO DE TUMOR	LOCALIZAÇÃO ANATÔMICA	CARACTERÍSTICAS* DO SINAL DE RM	APRIMORAMENTO POR CONTRASTE	MARGINAÇÃO DE TUMOR E EDEMA
Tumores de origem neuroepitelial (intra-axial)				
Astrocitoma Origem histológica: astrócitos	Rostrotentorial (frontal, periforme, lobos temporais); tálamo em grau superior; pode ocorrer infratentorial; contato ventricular, mas não invade	T1W-leve a moderado hipointenso; T2W-moderado hiperintenso	Variável; baixo grau – baixo a médio; alto grau – moderado a acentuado, não uniforme ou periférico (anel)	Margens distintas a não distintas; edema peritumoral variável; tumores de escore alto podem conter hemorragia; podem conter regiões císticas
Oligodendroglioma Origem histológica: oligodendrócito	Normalmente rostrotentorial (frontal, piriforme, lobos temporais); podem ter superfície e contato ventricular, metástase descendente	T1W-moderado hipointenso; T2W-hiperintenso, marcado quando mucinoso	Variável; grau baixo – leve a médio; alto grau – moderado a acentuado, não uniforme ou periférico (anel)	Margens distintas a não distintas, globular; tendem a ter menos edema peritumoral do que astrocitomas; tumores de alto grau podem conter hemorragia; podem conter regiões císticas
Gliomatose cerebral Origem histológica: a maioria astrocítica; oligodendroglial?	Lesões focais ou multifocais, espalhadas pela sustância branca, periventricular, lesões subpiais ou lesões meníngeas difusas; origem histológica como as oligodendrogliais ou as astrocíticas	T1W-iso a hipointenso; T2W-hiperintenso; não detecção	Minimamente ou não evidenciado; lesões meníngeas podem melhorar	Margens indistintas; edema peritumoral mínimo; não tem feito de massa
Meduloblastoma/tumor neuroectodérmico primitivo (TNEP) Origem histológica: Tumor neuronal embrionário	Meduloblastoma cerebelar; (TNEP)/lobos olfatórios/ frontoparietais	T1W-iso a hipointenso; T2W-hiperintenso; não detecção	Minimamente ou não heterogêneo; (TNEP) podem ter melhora acentuada	Margens distintas a não distintas
Ependimoma Origem histológica: células de revestimento ependimal do sistema ventricular	Comum nos ventrículos laterais, 3° e 4°; região suprasselar; menos comum do que os TPC	T1W-hipo a leve hiperintenso; T2W-moderado a hiperintenso	Variável; evidenciação heterogênea ausente a marcada	Normalmente depende da forma do ventrículo; edema peritumoral varia de ausente a mínimo; pode conter cistos ou hemorragia; causa ventriculomegalia
Tumor do plexo coroide (TPC) Origem histológica: epitélio do plexo coroide	Ventrículos laterais, 3ª e 4ª e aberturas laterais; a maioria ocorre no 4° ventrículo; metástase descendente	T1W – hipo, iso ou hiperintenso; T2W – hiperintenso; pode aparentar heterogêneo quando tem hemorragia		Normalmente depende da forma do ventrículo com invasão para dentro do tecido; edema peritumoral; pode conter cistos ou hemorragia; causa ventriculomegalia
Tumores de meninges (extra-axial)				
Meningioma (cães) Origem histológica: leptomeninges ou células formadoras de granulações aracnoides	Mais comum nas meninges dos bulbos olfatórios e lobos frontais e cerebral, convexidades (sulcos) cerebelar associadas com as regiões basilar, tentorial, falcine e suprasselar; pode penetrar a placa cribriforme	T1W – geralmente isointenso, heterogêneo; T2W – hiperintenso	Evidenciação normalmente acentuada, homogênea, pode ser heterogênea	Margens distintas, globoide, cauda dural, tipo placa, base ampla; edema peritumoral; cistos são comuns

Continua

Tabela 260.8 — Recursos de imagem de ressonância magnética de tumores cerebrais caninos e felinos comuns.[17,288,289,301,305,334,337,338,343,344] *(Continuação)*

TIPO DE TUMOR	LOCALIZAÇÃO ANATÔMICA	CARACTERÍSTICAS* DO SINAL DE RM	APRIMORAMENTO POR CONTRASTE	MARGINAÇÃO DE TUMOR E EDEMA
Meningioma (gatos) Origem histológica: leptomeninges ou células formando granulações aracnoides	Mais comum nas meninges da convexidade cerebral parietal comum, cerebelo; pode ser múltiplo	T1W-iso a hipointenso; T2W – hiperintenso; sinal vazio de ossificação em tumor e hiperostose de calvaria	Evidenciação acentuada, uniforme; pode ser heterogênea	Margens distintas com bordas suaves ou irregulares; edema peritumoral; cistos são comuns
Tumor de células granulares Origem histológica: desconhecido, origem meníngea é suspeita	Massa em forma de placa que se estende ao longo das meninges na convexidade cerebral e assoalho, falx, suprasselar	T1W moderado hiperintenso; T2W hiperintenso	Evidenciação acentuada, homogênea; envolvimento meníngeo	Irregular, mas com margens definidas, semelhantes a placas; edema peritumoral
Linfoma e tumores hematopoéticos				
Linfoma (primário ou metastático) Origem histológica: célula B ou T; Cão – células B, Gato – células B ou célula T	Intra ou extra-axial; suprasselar primário-rostrotentorial, frequentemente perto do ventrículo; metastático – frequentemente meninges com invasão do parênquima; focal ou multifocal	T1W-iso a hipointenso; T2W-isoa hiperintenso	Evidenciação variável; homo a heterogêneo evidenciação meníngea difusa	Margens indistintas; edema peritumoral mínimo a moderado
Sarcoma histiocítico Origem histológica: surge a partir de células intersticiais dendríticas das meninges	Normalmente extra-axial, mas pode ser intra-axial; restrito às meninges e plexo coroide próximo ao olfatório, convexidade cerebral, cerebelo; focal ou difuso	T1W-iso a hipointenso; T2W – iso a hipointenso, heterogêneo	Evidenciação moderada, homo a heterogênea; evidenciação suave a acentuada, evidenciação meníngea difusa	Margens indistintas a distintas, cauda dural, tipo placa; edema peritumoral leve a acentuado
Tumores da região selar Tumores hipofisários	A maioria surge da adeno-hipófise na região selar (> 10 mm)	T1W-isointenso; T2W-suave hiperintenso	Evidenciação acentuada e homogênea	Margens distintas; edema peritumoral leve a moderado quando grande; pode ser cístico ou hemorrágico
Tumores metastáticos Metástase	Geralmente lesões multifocais; interface substância cinzenta/branca cerebelar	Intensidade mista T1W; Intensidade mista T2W	Evidenciação com contraste variável; evidenciação periférica (borda)	Margens indistintas; edema peritumoral acentuado; alguns tumores (p. ex., hemangiossarcoma) têm hemorragia e cistos

*Em comparação com a substância cinzenta.

Idade, gênero, raça e fatores de risco

Tumores cerebrais primários geralmente afetam cães mais velhos, sem predileção por sexo e idade média de 9 anos (variação de 4 a 13 anos); 95% dos cães têm idade maior que 5 anos.[292,293] A idade média relatada para cães com meningiomas, gliomas (astrocitoma, oligodendroglioma) e tumores de plexo coroide é de 10 a 14 anos, 8 anos e 5 a 6 anos, respectivamente.[291,293,301,305] Tumores cerebrais primários, particularmente gliomas, podem ser vistos em cães mais jovens.[291,306] Os cães das raças Boxer, Boston Terrier, Golden Retriever, Buldogue Francês e Rat Terrier têm risco maior para neoplasia intracraniana primária.[291] Raças dolicocefálicas podem apresentar risco maior para meningiomas, enquanto raças braquicefálicas podem ter maior risco para gliomas.[291,293] Certas raças têm um nível significativo de risco para neoplasias intracranianas primárias específicas, incluindo Golden Retrievers, raças mestiças e Schnauzers Miniatura; Rat Terriers têm risco significativo para meningiomas; Spaniels Ingleses Toy, Boston Terriers, Buldogues Franceses, Boxers, Buldogues Ingleses e Bullmastiffs para gliomas; e Dálmatas e Setter Inglês para neoplasias do plexo coroide/ependimomas.[291] Cães que pesam mais que 15 kg aumentaram o risco de meningioma.[291] Doberman Pinschers e Cocker Spaniels têm diminuição significativa do risco de neoplasias intracranianas primárias.[291]

Gatos com tumores cerebrais são mais velhos, com idade média de aproximadamente 12 anos.[294] Em meningiomas felinos, gatos machos são mais acometidos do que as fêmeas.[294,307] A raça Doméstico de Pelo Curto é a raça mais comumente

CAPÍTULO 260 • Doenças do Cérebro: Anomalia, Degenerativa, Metabólica, Neoplásica, Idiopática...

identificada.[294] Fatores de risco definitivos para o desenvolvimento de tumores cerebrais são desconhecidos para cães e gatos. A genética pode ter um papel em algumas raças de cães, uma vez que meningiomas (como no homem) têm fenótipos semelhantes e podem compartilhar alterações genéticas semelhantes que levam à tumorigênese.[308] A forte associação de raça a tumores específicos, como os gliomas com raças braquicefálicas, pode fornecer uma oportunidade para diminuir a incidência por meio de reprodução seletiva.[291,309] Gatos jovens com mucopolissacaridose tipo 1 têm alta incidência de desenvolvimento de meningiomas, o que fornece indícios para suspeita de correlação com base genética.[310] Hormônios como o estrogênio e a progesterona podem influenciar a tumorogênese.[311,312] Superexpressão do fator de crescimento endotelial vascular (FCEV) parece ser comum em tumores cerebrais primários de cães e pode ser correlacionada com a malignidade do tumor.[313,314]

Tumores cerebrais secundários

Tipos

Neoplasias intracranianas secundárias podem ser seguidas por metástase no parênquima cerebral em um local primário distante ou por extensão direta nos tecidos adjacentes à neoplasia. É mais comum que os tumores nasais se espalhem por extensão direta através da placa cribriforme.[315-317] Os tipos de tumor que invadem por extensão direta incluem carcinoma ótico de células escamosas, tumores de hipófise, tumores da calvária (osteocondrossarcomas, condrossarcomas osteocondrossarcoma multilobular) e tumores de bainha de nervo (tumores do V nervo craniano). Metástase intracraniana geralmente ocorre por via hematogênica em cães, com embolização na junção da substância cinzenta-branca ou na "divisa" das distribuições da vasculatura intracraniana no córtex cerebral e do cerebelo.[13] A metástase leptomeníngea pode ocorrer quando as células tumorais adentram o espaço aracnoide de forma hematogênica por meio da leptomeninge e por veias diploicas ou pelo plexo coroide, ou ainda por propagação perineural ao longo dos nervos periféricos e dos nervos cranianos. Apesar de rara, uma infiltração difusa ou multifocal de leptomeninges com células do carcinoma pode causar carcinomatose meníngea.[299,318,319]

Cães

A neoplasia secundária é responsável por aproximadamente 50% de todos os tumores intracranianos em cães. Em dois grandes grupos de cães, hemangiossarcoma (29, 35%), tumores hipofisários (11,25%), linfoma (12,20%), carcinomas metastáticos (12,19%) neoplasias nasais por extensão (6%), melanoma maligno (3%) e sarcoma histiocítico (3%) foram os tumores intracranianos mais comuns.[13,291] Tumores da bainha do nervo (0,9%) e neoplasias de células redondas mal diferenciadas não foram tão comuns (0,48%).[291] As metástases afetam mais frequentemente o cérebro.[13,289] Os tumores hipofisários secundários podem consistir em linfomas, carcinomas, ou, menos frequentemente, sarcoma histiocítico ou melanoma.[13,320-322] A realização de exames de imagem para identificação de metástases intracranianas é responsável pelo aumento do conhecimento de alguns tipos de tumores. O uso de imagens tem levado a melhores regimes de tratamento para muitas condições, resultando em maior longevidade e mais tempo para ocorrência de metástase. A distribuição multifocal de tumores secundários cerebrais ocorre em apenas 30% e neoplasias não relacionadas concomitantes ocorrem em cerca de 18% dos cães.[13,293]

Gatos

A prevalência de neoplasias intracranianas secundárias em gatos representa cerca de 22% dos tumores cerebrais; os mais comuns são linfoma e tumores hipofisários.[294,295,303,323] Linfomas renais primários frequentemente se espalham para o SNC e as meninges podem ser um local para os linfomas.[324] A distribuição por via hematogênica (o adenocarcinoma pulmonar é o mais comum) e em gatos é observada em cerca de 6%.[294] Outros tipos de tumor secundários em gatos incluem adenocarcinoma, carcinoma de células escamosas, fibrossarcoma, histiocitoma fibroso maligno, sarcoma e hemangiossarcoma.[294]

Sinais clínicos

Os sinais clínicos refletem a localização do tumor intracraniano. Independentemente da origem do tecido, o foco da neoplasia intracraniana causa sinais típicos em cães em razão da compressão do tecido cerebral adjacente pela expansão da massa ou pelo edema peritumoral que compromete o fluxo sanguíneo ou por hidrocefalia obstrutiva. Tumores intracranianos podem causar edema vasogênico cerebral distribuído preferencialmente em espaço extracelular peritumoral da substância branca. À medida que a condição progride, os sinais clínicos podem evoluir e refletir em danos adicionais em razão do aumento da pressão intracraniana que causa mudanças no tecido nervoso intracraniano. Danos adicionais e sinais clínicos podem resultar da expansão do tumor em tecidos não neurais, como a cavidade nasal, periórbita ou a calvária circundante. Sinais neurológicos comuns observados em animais com tumores cerebrais incluem alteração do estado mental (p. ex., obnubilação, estupor, coma), convulsões, ataxia, andar em círculos e alterações comportamentais. Convulsão (45 a 51%) é mais comum; porém, andar em círculo (23%), ataxia (21%) e inclinação da cabeça (13%) ocorrem.[292,293] Cães com neoplasias intracranianas que apresentam maior risco de convulsões e com tumores que afetam o lobo frontal apresentam aumento acentuado da possibilidade de gadolínio e de hérnia subfalcina e subtentorial.[325] Neoplasia cerebral deve ser considerada uma doença diferencial quando o cão tem seu primeiro episódio de convulsão após os 4 anos de idade.[292]

Os sinais clínicos em gatos são semelhantes, mas muitas vezes são vagos ou inespecíficos, sendo a anorexia e a letargia os sinais mais comuns. Em 160 gatos, os sinais neurológicos mais comuns foram nível de consciência alterado (26%), andar em círculo (22,5%) e convulsões (22,5%).[294] Gatos com sinais neurológicos inespecíficos são comuns (21%).[294] Mudanças de comportamento foram observadas em 81% de 121 gatos com meningioma.[307]

Diagnósticos

Teste de linha basal. Quando existe suspeita de neoplasia intracraniana, o exame de neuroimagem é fundamental, mas, quando realizado isoladamente, pode priorizar apenas um diagnóstico diferencial. Hemograma, análise bioquímica e urinálise podem ser úteis para identificar distúrbios metabólicos, inflamatórios ou tóxicos subjacentes, que podem assemelhar-se às neoplasias intracranianas. Radiografias torácicas, abdominais e ultrassom abdominal (US) são ferramentas úteis para descartar doença metastática e comorbidades, que podem alterar os planos de tratamento.[326] Em um estudo retrospectivo de 177 cães com neoplasia intracraniana secundária, 76% tinham doenças metastáticas pulmonares no exame *post mortem* e 39% tinham evidência de doença metastática em radiografia de tórax.[13] O exame US do abdome deve ser incluído na avaliação de qualquer cão com sinais no SNC.[14]

Imagem em corte transversal. Imagens em corte transversal com ressonância magnética ou tomografia computadorizada geralmente são necessárias para a tentativa de realização de um diagnóstico provisório e para identificar a área para retirada de tecido. A biopsia requer equipamento especial ou cirurgia. Anormalidades na TC em neoplasia intracraniana consistem em distribuições multifocais ou focais, efeito de massa associado a edema, massa neoplásica e estrutura do ventrículo assimétrica. As lesões podem ser difíceis de detectar na TC se estiverem localizadas na fossa caudal em razão da interferência do ambiente circundante do osso temporal petroso ou à falta de realce de contraste. A TC é necessária para o planejamento da radiação, uma vez que a atenuação da radiação na estrutura óssea é usada para os cálculos.

Preferência pela realização de varreduras de ressonância magnética. A ressonância magnética é a técnica preferida para diagnóstico *ante mortem* de neoplasias intracranianas. A aquisição imagem em vários planos é especialmente útil para o planejamento cirúrgico. A ressonância magnética pode fornecer detalhes sobre o tamanho do tumor, margens, propriedades do tecido e localização anatômica. As varreduras por ressonância magnética podem identificar efeitos patológicos secundários (p. ex., edema, obstrução, hidrocefalia) causados pelo tumor.[17,289] Massas extra-axiais podem surgir de fora do cérebro (p. ex., meninges, calvária, ventrículos) e intra-axiais de dentro do parênquima cerebral. As características de ressonância magnética de neoplasias intracranianas são frequentemente usadas para priorizar o diagnóstico diferencial.[17-19,288,289,305,327] Padrões de ressonância magnética em massas meníngeas e ventriculares extra-axiais, lesões intensificadoras, moderadas ou não intensificadoras e multifocais intra-axiais foram descritas em cães. Cada um desses padrões pode fornecer recursos para a suspeita de um tipo específico de tumor (ver Tabela 260.8).[288]

Tumor cerebral primário na RM. A maioria das neoplasias cerebrais primárias com base em exames de ressonância magnética é isolada. Meningiomas, gliomas e tumores do plexo coroide podem ser multifocais.[293,305,311,328-332] Os tumores cerebrais são frequentemente hipo a isointensos na imagem T1W e hiperintensos na imagem T2W. O efeito de massa (deslocamento da linha média, distorção dos ventrículos e parênquima adjacente e hérnias cerebrais) pode ser identificado. O efeito de massa também pode ser causado por edema peritumoral, que tende a seguir a massa branca (corona radiata) e é evidente na hiperintensidade em imagens T2W e FLAIR. Edema difuso é relatado em 52% dos meningiomas caninos.[305] A maioria das massas meníngeas (p. ex., meningioma, sarcoma histiocítico, tumor de células granulares, carcinomatose meníngea, linfoma) tende a apresentar contato dural de base ampla e, às vezes, sinais de uma "cauda dural".[288,289,329,333,334] Uma borda distinta com o neuroparênquima ajuda a distinguir meningioma de meningioma extra-axial.[305] Contudo, granulomas menores e outras massas intradurais podem ter localizações semelhantes, cauda dural, contraste homogêneo e realce intenso, edema perilesional e hiperintensidade em T2.[293,305,323,329,335] Como massas intra-axiais, gliomas, incluindo oligodendroglioma e astrocitoma, variam amplamente em seu aspecto na ressonância magnética e podem ser confundidos com um êmbolo ou doença inflamatória.[289,336] As margens tumorais frequentemente aparecem indistintas na ressonância magnética.[337,338] Não há recursos na ressonância magnética que possam distinguir com segurança astrocitoma de oligodendroglioma.[338]

Muitos tumores cerebrais primários na ressonância magnética mostram realce pelo contraste após a administração de agentes de contraste à base de gadolínio.[13,17,19,288,289,293,301,305,323] O realce do contraste, margens bem definidas e forma regular são as principais características da neoplasia na ressonância magnética, quando comparadas a doenças inflamatórias ou vasculares.[19,339] O realce do contraste do anel periférico é um achado inespecífico compatível com necrose central, associada a doenças cerebrais neoplásicas e não neoplásicas.[17,288,289,340] Uma vez que as paquimeninges estão assentadas fora da BHE, a maioria dos tumores (p. ex., meningioma, sarcoma histiocítico, tumor de células granulares, carcinomatose meníngea, linfoma) e granulomas que surgem nessa área aumenta o contraste.[299,305,334,341-344] Das massas ventriculares, os tumores de plexo coroide tendem a se intensificar fortemente,[301] enquanto o realce de ependimomas é mais variável.[335,345] A característica do aumento do contraste de gliomas na ressonância magnética é o de uma massa difusa realçada, variável ou semelhante a um anel comparado em imagens T1W hipointenso a isointenso no pré-contraste.[288,293,337]

Esse tipo de aumento padrão pode se sobrepor às características de ressonância magnética do linfoma intra-axial e do granuloma.[19,293,294,335] Mais comumente, gliomas de baixo grau geralmente têm realce leve a nenhum realce, quando comparados a gliomas de alto grau.[337,338] Gliomas que são classificados como de alto grau na histopatologia tendem a ter realce moderado ou acentuado após administração contraste IV.[293,337,338,346] Todavia, contraste mínimo ou nenhum realce é uma característica de imagem da gliomatose cerebri.[347]

Tumor metastático na ressonância magnética. Os tumores metastáticos na ressonância magnética são geralmente lesões multifocais no parênquima cerebral ou meninges.[13,17,288] Múltiplas lesões de pequenas massas geralmente estão presentes, embora lesões isoladas possam ocorrer. Tumores cerebrais hematogênicos metastáticos na imagem de ressonância magnética aparecem como lesões ovoides a esféricas em interface entre as substâncias branca e cinzenta, enquanto é mais provável que a embolia ocorra em arteríolas corticais. Outras características de tumores metastáticos do SNC em ressonância magnética incluem múltiplas lesões hiperintensas em imagens T2W circunscritas por edema acentuado e variável aumento de contraste ou aumento periférico em imagens T1W pós-contraste.[13,17,288]

Outros recursos de imagem. Técnicas de ressonância magnética metabólica e fisiológica, combinadas com dados obtidos de ressonância magnética tradicional ou de tomografia computadorizada geralmente são mais usadas para identificação e monitoramento de neoplasias intracranianas e outras doenças do SNC.[286,348] Especificamente, tomografia por emissão de pósitrons (PET) usando 2-desoxi-2 [^{18}F] fluoro-D-glicose (FDG), que reflete o aumento do metabolismo da glicose em tumores cerebrais, vem sendo usada para definir as melhores áreas para biopsia.[23,24] Exame por imagem de difusão ponderada com base na imagem ADC e MRS tem sido descrito em tumores cerebrais de cães, mas não tem especificidade na determinação do tipo histológico de doença intracraniana.[349] Alterações metabólicas usando MRS têm sido usadas para diferenciar lesões neoplásicas inflamatórias de outras neoplásicas que têm N-acetilaspartato (NAA) mais baixa e altas concentrações de colina.[350]

Análise do líquido cefalorraquidiano. A análise do LCR pode ajudar no diagnóstico e exclusão de doença inflamatória evidente e pode ser benéfica como um teste de triagem (ver Capítulo 115).[351,352] Coleta de LCR deve ser evitada em razão do risco de herniação, quando há suspeita de aumento da pressão intracraniana e com base nos sinais clínicos e de imagem (desvio da foice do cérebro, compressão dos ventrículos ou das cisternas quadrigeminais e hidrocefalia obstrutiva). A concentração aumentada de proteína e uma contagem total de células nucleadas normal a um moderado aumento (dissociação albuminocitológica) são típicos em neoplasias intracranianas.[353-355] Tumores do plexo coroide estão associados às elevações mais marcantes no total de proteína do LCR, e em outras neoplasias, o LCR pode apresentar aumento do número de células brancas do sangue, proteína total aumentada, mas a citologia é geralmente pleocitose mista não específica.[293,353,354,356] Achados semelhantes são relatados em gatos.[294,357] Raramente, células neoplásicas podem ser encontradas no LCR em associação com neoplasias nas proximidades do sistema ventricular ou das meninges, tais como tumor no plexo coroide, linfoma, glioma, ependimoma, neurocitoma e sarcoma histiocítico.[293,301,333,358-361] A composição de proteína do LCR pode ser ainda definida por técnicas semiquantitativas com eletroforese, e anormalidades foram relatadas como úteis na identificação de doenças inflamatórias, neoplásicas e doenças degenerativas.[43,352] Estudos que definem biomarcadores para neoplasias em cérebro de cães (metaloproteinases de matriz de [MMP, do inglês *matrix metalloproteases*], ácido úrico, atividade fibrinolítica) para determinar a carga tumoral e o tipo de neoplasia têm limitações em relação à especificidade e sensibilidade.[362-365]

Biopsia cerebral e histopatologia. O desenvolvimento de técnicas de imagem melhoradas permite um maior grau de definição da lesão a partir de características anatômicas e patológicas. A biopsia cerebral é particularmente útil quando as lesões são pequenas, profundamente enraizadas ou em uma área cirurgicamente inacessível. A escolha do local para a biopsia depende da suspeita diagnóstica e da extensão da lesão. A heterogeneidade do tecido na imagem deve ser levada em consideração realizando-se a coleta de amostra adequada de diferentes áreas, incluindo a interface entre o tumor e áreas adjacentes ao cérebro. A coleta de áreas de amostra no local de necrose deve ser evitada, pois geralmente não compensa. As chances de diagnóstico são consideradas mais altas quando os alvos de biopsia incluem ambas as áreas sem contraste (necróticas) e com realce de contraste do tumor.[366] A biopsia tru-cut é considerada mais confiável do que a aspiração por agulha fina para determinar o tipo específico de tumor.[366] A avaliação citológica de preparações para esmagamento de tumor cerebral pode ser realizada minutos após a coleta da biopsia.[37] As chances de diagnóstico são geralmente > 90% para lesões neoplásicas.[286] Os primeiros estudos de biopsia cerebral relatam taxas de morbidade e mortalidade que variam de 7 a 27%.[25,28]

O diagnóstico definitivo de neoplasia intracraniana, o subtipo de tumor e a graduação são realizados por exame histológico do tecido.[52,53] A imuno-histoquímica tem sido usada para identificar com mais precisão o fenótipo celular, usando-se marcadores antigênicos específicos de células para classificar mais claramente as neoplasias intracranianas.[290] A caracterização molecular e genética da neoplasia está se tornando mais comum em neuropatologia e neuro-oncologia veterinária.[286,313,367,368]

Tratamento

Objetivos. Os objetivos para o tratamento de tumores cerebrais são a completa remoção de tumor ou redução de tamanho e o controle de efeitos (edema, aumento da pressão intracraniana).[286,287] As opções de tratamento dependem do tipo e da localização do tumor, início dos sinais clínicos, custos e morbidade/mortalidade associadas.[286,287] As diretrizes de tratamento para os tipos específicos de tumores cerebrais consistem em terapias paliativas e definitivas. Ressecção cirúrgica e radioterapia fracionada são os métodos definitivos mais comuns usados para tratar tumores cerebrais em caninos e felinos. Outros avanços terapêuticos contemporâneos para tumor cerebral em animais incluem radiocirurgia estereotáxica, entrega por convecção melhorada e imunoterapia.[287]

Terapia paliativa. A terapia paliativa consiste em controlar efeitos secundários causados por tumor e minimizar os sinais clínicos. Para animais com tumores cerebrais, a terapia paliativa tem focado no controle de edema vasogênico e controle das convulsões. O tratamento com corticosteroides neutraliza os efeitos secundários de edema peritumoral e da hidrocefalia obstrutiva e reduz a pressão intracraniana. Doses anti-inflamatórias de corticosteroides podem ser usadas e ajustadas de acordo com a resposta clínica. A osmoterapia – como o manitol – é útil para o controle do aumento agudo da pressão intracraniana.[369] O manitol é mais amplamente usado em uma solução a 25% administrada em bolus IV (0,5 a 2 g/kg). A furosemida (0,7 mg/kg IV) pode ter um efeito sinérgico na redução rápida do edema vasogênico.[370] Doses únicas têm efeito breve e pode ser necessário repeti-las. Os sinais clínicos de obstrução ventricular associada à obstrução ventricular por massa podem ser melhorados com o procedimento de desvio ventricular.[204] Terapia com fármacos antiepilépticos para convulsão aguda (p. ex., diazepam) e para o controle a manutenção é indicada para convulsões associadas a tumores.

Cirurgia. A cirurgia por si só pode ser curativa quando a ressecção completa é alcançada, mas muitas vezes é limitada pela anatomia e extensão da doença. A cirurgia pode alcançar citorredução, produzir um diagnóstico definitivo e fornecer informações de prognóstico para o planejamento de tratamento adjuvante. A craniectomia pode aliviar os sinais decorrentes do aumento secundário na pressão intracraniana.[371] Critérios para uma cirurgia bem-sucedida incluem: que a massa tumoral seja isolada, não invasiva, localizada perto da superfície do cérebro, no hemisfério cerebral, e que a remoção cause prejuízo neurológico mínimo. Cirurgia tem sido mais comum para meningioma prosencéfalico, porém, tem um prognóstico pior em cães do que em gatos, pois são mais invasivos e frequentemente atípicos em cães.[328,372-375] Cães com meningiomas excisados cirurgicamente têm sobrevida média de 7 meses, enquanto a média da sobrevivência em gatos é de cerca de 36 meses.[307,328,372,373] O tratamento cirúrgico incorporando aspiração ultrassônica e técnicas endoscópicas aumentou o acesso a tumores localizados nas regiões profundas do parênquima cerebral.[35,374] A eletroporação irreversível (IRE) é uma nova técnica de ablação de tecido não térmico que envolve eletrodos e entrega de pulsos elétricos.[376] O uso seguro e viável de IRE fornecido estereotaticamente com um sistema NanoKnife foi relatado para o tratamento de gliomas caninos.[377]

Radioterapia. A radioterapia tornou-se um pilar no manejo de tumores malignos e benignos do SNC em animais. A radioterapia pode ser administrada em vários tratamentos (radioterapia fracionada) ou em um único tratamento (radiocirurgia) (ver Capítulo 340).[286,287] A radioterapia fracionada é benéfica no tratamento de tumores cerebrais como terapia única ou como coadjuvante na ressecção cirúrgica.[328,378,379] Estudos investigando o diagnóstico presuntivo de tumores cerebrais em cães tratados com o uso da radioterapia fracionada relataram tempos médios de sobrevivência que variaram entre 5 e 24 meses.[378-383] Quando pesquisando a morte por causas não relacionadas ao tumor cerebral e usando a sobrevivência com base nas mortes atribuíveis à piora dos sinais neurológicos, o tempo médio de sobrevida global foi de 39 meses para radioterapia isolada em tumores cerebrais extra-axiais, intra-axiais e hipofisários combinados.[378] A radiação como única terapia produziu tempos médios de sobrevivência de 11,5 a 19 meses em cães com diagnóstico histológico de meningioma.[378,379]

Deterioração recorrente dos sinais neurológicos causada tanto pela recidiva da doença quanto de necrose geralmente é a causa do óbito ou é o motivo de eutanásia em cães com tumores cerebrais tratados com radiação.[328,378-380] O risco de necrose do SNC aumenta à medida que aumenta a dose de radiação.[384] Efeitos adversos agudos da radiação incluem edema cerebral ligado ao distúrbio da BHE, os quais podem resultar em desmielinização e respondem à terapia com corticosteroide.[385,386] Complicações tardias incluem necrose após radiação focal do SNC e lesões vasculares graves.[385] Como a tecnologia continua a evoluir, planos de tratamento desenvolvidos por meio de computador e métodos mais precisos para o posicionamento do paciente contribuíram para melhor homogeneidade da dose e redução da toxicidade para o tecido cerebral normal.[378,387-389] Radioterapia tridimensional conformada mostrou uma sobrevida média de 19 meses em cães tratados com meningioma; essa taxa foi aumentada para 30 meses ao obter-se informações sobre os pacientes que morreram de causas não relacionadas ao meningioma.[330] Em alguns centros veterinários, radiocirurgia estereotáxica (p. ex., acelerador linear, GammaKnife, CyberKnife) para tumores cerebrais tem sido usada para administrar uma única dose grande de radiação em um alvo definido. Radiocirurgia estereotáxica envolve o uso de radiação ionizante convergente para interceptar o alvo do tratamento. Uma única sessão de terapia aplica uma dose precisa e alta (> 10 gray) causando lesão vascular significativa e hipoxia ao tecido tumoral, poupando os tecidos normais adjacentes. Meningiomas têm sido os tumores mais comumente relatados tratados por radiocirurgia estereotáxica. O tempo médio de sobrevivência em cães é de 13,3 meses para todos os tumores cerebrais e para meningiomas.[390,391] Assim, apenas a radiocirurgia isoladamente tem se mostrado promissora no tratamento de tumores cerebrais em cães com menos efeitos adversos agudos do que a terapia por radiação convencional.

Quimioterapia. Quimioterápicos administrados sistemicamente para tratamento de tumores cerebrais em medicina veterinária foram inicialmente pragmáticos. A BHE é considerada um importante obstáculo ao uso de quimioterapia para tumores cerebrais, iatrogenicamente pode-se até mesmo cruzar-se a BHE por meio de administração de manitol antes da administração de agentes.[392] Hidroxiureia tem sido defendida como quimioterápico em cães com meningioma.[393] A citosina arabinosídeo intratecal e metotrexato foram avaliados com segurança a curto prazo em cães com doença do SNC, incluindo neoplasia.[394] Um estudo recente não conseguiu mostrar diferença na sobrevida média em cães com tumores cerebrais tratados com prednisona paliativa e FAEs em comparação com os animais que receberam terapia paliativa e lomustina.[395]

Novas terapias. O reconhecimento de tumores cerebrais caninos como um modelo de doença translacional criou oportunidades para novos métodos de tratamento.[286,287] A aplicação por convecção melhorada (ACM) contorna a BHE, resultando em altas concentrações intratumorais de fármacos com toxicidade mínima. A técnica envolve a entrega local direcionada de macromoléculas por fluxo em massa usando microinfusão de baixa pressão com cateteres projetados especificamente. Em cães com gliomas, ACM tem sido realizado como uma única modalidade terapêutica antes e depois da ressecção cirúrgica.[396] Uso da aplicação de nanopartículas de ACM de CPT-11 lipossomal e cetuximabe bioconjugado magnético de óxido de ferro mostraram ter eficácia em gliomas caninos.[397,398] Durante o ACM, as infusões podem ser monitoradas com IRM em tempo real e com uso de marcadores baseados em gadolínio.[287,399]

As imunoterapias em oncologia consistem no uso da resposta imune do hospedeiro para matar tumores (ver Capítulo 341). Na imunoterapia ativa, os pacientes são tratados com uma combinação de antígenos de tumor ou células apresentadoras de antígenos com um agente estimulador como uma citocina ou imunoadjuvante que muitas vezes são combinadas com outra terapia definitiva.[287] Essa imunoterapia combinada tem sido utilizada em cães com tumores cerebrais.[400,401] Nesses estudos, mostrou-se que vacinas induziram anticorpos sistêmica e localmente no sitio do tumor.

Prognóstico e sobrevida

Exceto para os meningiomas felinos e caninos, o prognóstico para outros tipos de tumor cerebral é bastante variável. O tempo de sobrevida para gliomas após o diagnóstico por imagem tende a ser curto, com uma média < 80 dias.[338] O prognóstico para cães com tumores cerebrais tratados com paliativos é ruim. Cães com tumores cerebrais diagnosticados definitivamente na necropsia obtiveram uma sobrevida média de 2 meses, após o diagnóstico por imagem do cérebro.[402] Tempos de sobrevivência mais longos podem ocorrer dependendo do tamanho, tipo e localização do tumor, da gravidade dos sinais clínicos e da decisão do tutor em prosseguir com a terapia. Tumores supratentoriais tendem a ter um tempo de sobrevivência mediano mais longo em comparação com os tumores infratentoriais.[402] Tumores cerebrais metastáticos têm duração média de 21 dias dos sinais clínicos até a morte.[13]

Conclusões prognósticas para terapias definitivas de tumores cerebrais em animais são limitadas pelo pequeno número de casos, desenho de estudo retrospectivo, falta de histopatologia diagnóstica definitiva e falta de critérios objetivos monitorados facilmente.[286,287] O tempo médio de sobrevivência para todos os tipos de tumor relatados em cães após a cirurgia isolada variam de 2 a 7 meses.[328,380] Normalmente nos primeiros 30 dias após a cirurgia, os animais com tumores infratentoriais não apresentam risco significativamente maior de mortalidade em comparação com aqueles animais com tumores supratentoriais.[403] A complicação perioperatória devastadora comum é a pneumonia por aspiração (ver Capítulo 242). Conforme descrito anteriormente em cães com tumores cerebrais, a cirurgia associada com a radioterapia resulta em maior tempo de sobrevivência. Em estudos anteriores, o tempo médio de sobrevivência em cães com meningiomas cerebrais tratados por excisão cirúrgica combinada e radioterapia foi entre 11 e 28 meses.[311,328,379,381] Uma vez que os gatos têm meningiomas que podem ser completamente removidos por cirurgia, seu prognóstico de sobrevida em geral é melhor do que o dos cães. Um estudo retrospectivo grande e recente de meningiomas após excisão cirúrgica relatou um tempo médio de sobrevivência de 37 meses (95% – intervalo de confiança de 28 a 54 meses).[307]

Os objetivos de caracterização molecular de tumores cerebrais caninos têm sido direcionados para a obtenção de informações sobre prognóstico. Expressão aberrante de genes específicos de tumor, receptores, citocinas e proteínas celulares têm sido identificados em tumores cerebrais caninos e felinos, incluindo receptores de progesterona, de antígeno nuclear de proliferação celular, de fator de crescimento vascular endotelial (FCVE) e de um marcador proliferativo Ki-67.[312,313,404-407] Receptores de progesterona foram identificados em meningiomas caninos e perda de receptores pode estar associada a maiores frações proliferativas tumorais, que podem afetar indiretamente o prognóstico.[311,312] Pode existir uma associação positiva entre o grau de malignidade e um fator angiogênico, FCVE[312,406] em meningiomas caninos, mas pode não ser correlacionado com a sobrevida.[405] Em cães, tumores com índice alto de fração proliferativa medido por técnicas imuno-histoquímicas para detectar o antígeno nuclear de proliferação celular foram associados a taxas de sobrevivência mais baixas.[311,408] O maior reconhecimento de epidemiologia, neuropatologia, biologia molecular e semelhanças genéticas entre os tumores do cérebro canino e humano continuarão a impulsionar o uso de tumores cerebrais caninos como modelos de doença translacional.[286,287,396,409]

EPILEPSIA IDIOPÁTICA

Declarações do consenso
Em 2014, a Força-Tarefa Internacional de Epilepsia Veterinária (IVETF) foi fundada e desenvolveu uma série de relatórios de consensos baseados em conhecimentos publicados sobre epilepsia.[410] Os relatórios de consenso focaram definição, classificação, terminologia, raças, diagnóstico, tratamento, medidas de resultados de ensaios terapêuticos, neuroimagem e neuropatologia.[410-417] Em 2015, uma Declaração de Consenso de Pequenos Animais da ACVIM foi estabelecida para focar o manejo da convulsão canina com fundamentação na literatura e *expertise* complementar clínica.[418] Ambas as declarações de consensos fornecem uma plataforma contínua e de futuras pesquisas de epilepsia em medicina veterinária que aprimoram nossa compreensão da epilepsia e do seu tratamento.[410,418]

Epilepsia primária e síndrome epiléptica
Definições
Convulsões epilépticas são definidas como sinais transitórios decorrentes da atividade neuronal anormal excessiva ou sincrônica no cérebro. Epilepsia refere-se a pelo menos duas crises não provocadas em um intervalo > 24 horas (ver Capítulo 35).[419,420] O termo idiopático significa uma doença de causa desconhecida, mas, para ser significativo, o termo deve definir claramente uma entidade.[421] No homem, muitas epilepsias anteriormente classificadas como "idiopáticas" foram associadas a mutações específicas. Isso levou à recomendação da International League Against Epilepsy (ILAE) para a mudança da classificação anterior de sistema idiopático, sintomático e criptogênico para termo

genético, estrutural/metabólico e desconhecido.[422] Todavia, até que a genética da epilepsia em animais seja mais bem definida, ainda há utilidade em usar o termo bem conhecido como epilepsia idiopática (EI) para animais de estimação, nos quais uma causa estrutural ou metabólica de convulsões ainda não tenha sido identificada.[411,423]

Incidência

A incidência de epilepsia por todas as causas em cães tem sido estimada em 0,62 a 0,75%, comparável ao índice estimado no homem (0,22 a 4,1%).[424-426] A maioria dos cães com epilepsia tem doença idiopática, enquanto apenas 0 a 22% dos gatos epilépticos têm doença idiopática.[427-430] Cães machos são mais comumente acometidos que cadelas em uma proporção de cerca de 1,4:1, enquanto, diferenças de gênero não foram encontradas em gatos.[424,425,430,431] A maioria dos cães epilépticos tem sua primeira convulsão entre 1 e 5 anos e são esses os mais propensos a serem diagnosticados como idiopáticos. Cerca de 1/3 de cães de 1 a 5 anos é diagnosticado com uma doença estrutural ou metabólica que causa convulsão. Cães de qualquer idade podem não ter uma causa identificada para sua convulsão.[431-435] Em um estudo, a idade média de início da doença epiléptica idiopática em gatos foi de 3,8 anos, enquanto gatos com epilepsia familiar tiveram sua primeira crise quando tinham < 1 ano.[430,436] Cães epilépticos têm maior probabilidade de serem diagnosticados como idiopáticos se o tempo entre a primeira e a segunda convulsão for > 4 semanas.[431] No início, as convulsões na EI podem ser generalizadas ou focais, mesmo quando se suspeita de causa genética.[8,9,431,437-441]

Causa

Existem fortes evidências de que a EI seja de origem genética em muitas raças de cães. A prevalência da epilepsia é significativamente maior em cães de raça pura do que em cães de raças mestiças.[442] Filhos de cães epilépticos têm uma chance significativamente maior de terem convulsões e uma idade mais precoce de início das crises epilépticas.[434] Estudos genéticos específicos em diversas raças mostram uma base genética com incidência de até 33% em algumas raças.[9,434,435,437-439,441,443-456] Quando calculada, a herdabilidade chega a 0,87, sugerindo um papel significativo da genética no risco de epilepsia. Em contrapartida, apenas uma família de gatos com epilepsia genética foi relatada.[436] Apesar dessa forte evidência de uma causa genética, a associação de variantes genéticas específicas para epilepsia na maioria das raças permaneceu não descrita.[457]

Mutações específicas têm sido identificadas em uma série de doenças em que as convulsões recorrentes são parte de uma síndrome mais ampla. Por exemplo, as epilepsias mioclônicas progressivas têm outros sinais neurológicos progressivos.[458] Em cães, as mutações genéticas têm sido identificadas no gene malin (EPM2b ou NHCLRC1) em Dachshunds com doença de Lafora e em vários genes lipofuscinoses ceroide dos neurônios associados a epilepsia mioclônica progressiva (genes TPP1 e PPT1 em Dachshunds) ou outra síndrome de convulsão (CLN5 em Border Collies, CLN8 em cães de apartação de gado, na raça Setter Inglês, e ATP13A2 em cães da raça Terriers Tibetanos) (ver Tabela 260.6).[278-283,459,460] Em todas essas doenças, outros sinais como ataxia, cegueira ou declínio cognitivo também estão presentes. Outros exemplos de síndrome epiléptica incluem mutações em canais iônicos, como o canal de potássio KCNJ10 na ataxia espinocerebelar com miocimia e convulsões em cães da raça Jack Russell Terrier[96] ou mutações em fatores de transcrição ATF2 em Poodles Standard neonatos com convulsões por encefalopatia.[239]

A única mutação associada a EI em cães está no gene LGI2 em cães da raça Lagotto Romagnolo com epilepsia focal remitente.[461] Variantes no gene ADAM23 foram associadas ao risco maior de convulsões em cães da raça Pastor-Belga.[462] Os genes LGI2 e ADAM23 fazem parte de um sistema pré-sináptico, complexo de canal de potássio controlado por voltagem e de anticorpos agonistas a esse complexo, que foram mostrados na epilepsia de lobo temporal em gatos.[463,464] Esses gatos mostram evidências de necrose do hipocampo, que os classificam com convulsões estruturais/metabólicas, mas ilustram que pode haver outras causas de EI, além das causas por predisposições genéticas.

Diagnóstico com os critérios da Força-Tarefa Internacional de Epilepsia Veterinária

Tradicionalmente, o diagnóstico clínico de EI é por exclusão, após o teste diagnóstico para causas de convulsões reativas e epilepsia estrutural. O IVETF estabeleceu um sistema de três níveis de critérios de confiança para o diagnóstico de epilepsia idiopática.[413] O nível de confiança I para o diagnóstico de EI é baseado no histórico de dois ou mais episódios epilépticos não provocados, ocorrendo com pelo menos com 24 horas de intervalo, observado pela primeira vez entre 6 meses e 6 anos, com exames físicos e neurológicos interictais normais, sem anormalidades significativas no exame de sangue básico e na urinálise. O nível de confiança II para o diagnóstico de EI é baseado em fatores do nível I mais aferição de ácidos biliares em jejum e pós-prandial, ressonância magnética do cérebro e análise do LCR. O nível de confiança III é fundamentado nos níveis I e II, além da identificação de anormalidades características da convulsão no EEG. Para o diagnóstico de EI, preconiza-se o uso de imagens avançadas e exames do LCR, porém esses exames não são essenciais para o diagnóstico. O IVETF recomenda a realização de ressonância magnética do cérebro e análise do LCR após exclusão de convulsões reativas em cães com um dos seguintes critérios: (1) idade no início da crise epiléptica < 6 meses ou > 6 anos; (2) anormalidades neurológicas interictais compatíveis com localização intracraniana; (3) estado epiléptico ou convulsão de *cluster*; (4) diagnóstico prévio de EI e resistência farmacológica a um único FAE titulado com a maior dose de tolerância.[413]

Exame de imagem e análise do LCR

A atividade epiléptica convulsiva, em si, pode causar alterações nos exames de ressonância magnética e no LCR. A histopatologia do cérebro de cães e gatos epilépticos pode revelar evidências de lesão neuronal e perda de áreas cerebrais suscetíveis, como lobos piriformes/temporais, giro cingulado, hipocampo e córtex cerebral.[465-468] Mudanças de sinal de ressonância magnética podem ser localizadas unilateral ou bilateralmente nessas áreas cerebrais suscetíveis e são caracterizadas por vários graus de hiperintensidade em T2W, imagens FLAIR e T1W pós-contraste.[467,469] Essas mudanças de sinal foram mostradas parcial ou completamente em imagens de ressonâncias magnéticas repetidas 10 a 16 semanas depois do controle da convulsão, indicando edema vasogênico ou citotóxico decorrente de atividade convulsiva.[467] Atrofia do hipocampo também pode ser um componente dos achados de ressonância magnética em cães e gatos com epilepsia crônica.[436,470] Se as alterações na ressonância magnética são compatíveis com crises associadas, o IVETF recomenda repetir a ressonância magnética 16 semanas após o controle da crise.[413] Anormalidades do LCR às vezes refletem pleocitose leve e pode ocorrer aumento da concentração de proteína como resultado de atividade convulsiva epiléptica.[471] Quanto maior o intervalo após a convulsão, menor contagem de células brancas sanguíneas no LCR.[471] Se houver anormalidades no LCR, doenças infecciosas devem ser desconsideradas; recomenda-se repetir a análise do LCR após um intervalo sem convulsões.[413]

Tratamento

Objetivos do tratamento. Os objetivos da terapia são diminuir a frequência, gravidade e duração das crises com poucos efeitos colaterais aceitáveis e nenhum efeito adverso, visto que a eliminação completa das convulsões é praticamente impossível em cães. O uso de fármacos antiepilépticos (FAE) tem sido a base da terapia para epilepsia em cães e gatos. No entanto, a falta de uniformidade e de diretrizes com fundamentação científica sobre o tratamento de FAE tem dificultado a tomada de decisão apropriada. Ao decidir sobre a terapia com FAE, os médicos devem seguir uma abordagem de tratamento levando em consideração: (1) o tempo de início do tratamento com FAE; (2) a seleção do FAE e a dose mais adequada; (3) o monitoramento do FAE e o ajuste do tratamento; (4) saber o momento de adicionar ou mudar o FAE; (5) promover a adesão do tutor.[414,472-475]

Início da terapia com fármacos antiepilépticos. A decisão de iniciar o tratamento com o FAE é fundamentada em uma série de fatores, incluindo etiologia, risco de recidiva, tipo de crise e tolerabilidade.[475] Os médicos-veterinários devem considerar também a saúde geral do animal, o estilo de vida do proprietário, as limitações financeiras e a capacidade de cumprir qualquer protocolo proposto.[472] Em humanos, não há benefício em iniciar a terapia com o FAE após uma única convulsão não provocada, mas há evidências para iniciar o controle de convulsão precoce após um segundo episódio.[476-478] Em cães, o monitoramento de convulsões a longo prazo é considerado mais bem-sucedido se a terapia com o FAE for iniciada logo após o início do episódio de convulsão, especialmente em cães com convulsões frequentes e em raças conhecidas por terem epilepsia grave.[437,438,479,480] Para resumir, IVETF e ACVIM recomendam o início do tratamento a longo prazo para animais com epilepsia quando qualquer um dos seguintes critérios estiver presente: (1) lesão estrutural identificável ou histórico prévio de doença cerebral ou lesão; (2) ocorrência de convulsões repetitivas agudas (estado epiléptico); (3) período interictal < 6 meses (*i. e.*, 2 ou mais convulsões dentro de um período de 6 meses); (4) períodos pós-ictais incomuns prolongados ou graves; (5) frequência de crises epilépticas e/ou duração aumentada e/ou a gravidade da convulsão ter piorado em três períodos interictais.[414,418]

Visão geral das opções médicas. Uma variedade de FAEs pode ser usada para o tratamento de cães e gatos epilépticos, mas não há diretrizes baseadas em evidências disponíveis para ajudar na escolha de um FAE de primeira linha para manejo a longo prazo do controle de convulsão em cães e gatos. A maioria das convulsões em cães com EI pode ser controlada com monoterapia. Após a primeira revisão sistemática em medicina veterinária para avaliar a eficácia do fármaco no tratamento de EI, a maioria dos dados é derivada de estudos retrospectivos e não padronizados.[481] Um estudo com metanálise de 3 ensaios com fármacos randomizados controlados em cães epilépticos revelou que 30% dos cães experimentaram redução de 50% ou mais nas convulsões com o uso de placebo, uma consideração ao avaliar estudos retrospectivos abertos, especialmente aqueles que envolvem um pequeno número de animais, pois os resultados relatados podem ser exagerados.[482] Em razão de questões éticas do estudo controle-placebo que são de relevância para cães epilépticos e seus tutores, há um consenso de que os ensaios clínicos de FAE para pacientes veterinários devem ser conduzidos de forma controlada, cega e randomizada, a fim de alcançar um alto nível de evidência e ajustar o efeito placebo.[415,481]

A princípio, é preferível a administração de um único FAE, pois isso evita interações medicamentosas, além de facilitar para o proprietário. Outros fatores a serem considerados ao escolher um FAE incluem o mecanismo de ação, a eficácia, os efeitos adversos, as potenciais interações medicamentosas, a frequência de administração com base nas propriedades farmacocinéticas e o custo.[472] O mecanismo de ação para muitos FAEs inclui aumento nos efeitos inibitórios dos canais de cloreto ativados por GABA, modulação da membrana associada aos canais de cátions (sódio e cálcio) e redução da neurotransmissão excitatória. O FAE mais comumente utilizado em medicina veterinária aumenta mecanicamente a inibição no cérebro.[475] Em geral,

os FAEs são iniciados com dose baixa e, em seguida, adaptados às necessidades individuais com base no controle de convulsões, nos efeitos adversos e nas concentrações séricas do fármaco. Uma série de FAEs com melhor tolerabilidade, menos efeitos colaterais e menos interações farmacológicas foi desenvolvida para tratar pessoas com epilepsia e muitos (p. ex., levetiracetam, zonisamida, gabapentina, pregabalina) foram utilizados em cães e gatos. Atualmente, esses medicamentos estão sendo usados como FAE de primeira linha ou como complemento no tratamento de cães com epilepsia refratária; no entanto, a eficácia para ambos os usos ainda precisa ser estabelecida. A Tabela 35.2 (ver Capítulo 35) lista os FAEs comumente usados com efeitos adversos relatados no tratamento de convulsões em cães e gatos. Outros estudos recentes mostram as propriedades e recomendações de uso de FAEs em cães e gatos.[414,418,472,475]

Até recentemente, fenobarbital (FB) e brometo de potássio (KBr) foram os únicos FAEs de primeira escolha para o tratamento a longo prazo de EI em cães, com base em seu histórico, disponibilidade e custo.[483-486] Pesquisas de revisão sobre a eficácia do FAE relataram um melhor nível de evidência com o uso de FB oral em comparação com KBr oral.[481] Em um estudo clínico randomizado em cães que tinham presumivelmente EI comparando FB a KBr como FAEs de primeira linha, mostrou-se que 85% dos cães tratados com FB tornaram-se livres de convulsões por 6 meses em comparação com 52% dos cães que receberam KBr, e ainda o FB foi mais bem tolerado.[486] Em 2013, a imepitoína foi aprovada na Europa como um FAE de primeira linha para cães com EI, com base em estudos clínicos randomizados que mostraram a eficácia do fármaco antiepiléptico, com alta tolerabilidade e segurança. A evidência para recomendar o uso de imepitoína como o único FAE em cães com crises epilépticas é boa.[481,487-489] Em um estudo controlado randomizado, a eficácia da imepitoína foi semelhante ao FB, com menos efeitos colaterais.[489] O painel do consenso ACVIM sugere forte recomendação e estabelece a eficácia do tratamento com FB e imepitoína como FAEs de primeira linha para cães com IE.[418]

Monitoramento terapêutico. Uma vez que a terapia com FAE é iniciada, é importante monitorar sistematicamente o controle das convulsões, efeitos sistêmicos dos fármacos e concentrações séricas, associados às metas de controle de convulsões com efeitos adversos mínimos.[472] O monitoramento da epilepsia depende da observação acurada do tutor quando se avalia a eficácia da terapia.[472] Os tutores devem ser instruídos a manter um livro de registro para documentar as ocorrências de convulsão e as mudanças da administração de medicamentos. Os objetivos do monitoramento das concentrações séricas incluem a determinação do nível de eficácia do fármaco após o início da terapia; se a falha do medicamento é decorrente de fatores farmacocinéticos (tolerância metabólica) ou fatores farmacodinâmicos (tolerância funcional) em relação a uma mudança de fármacos; se a falha do tratamento é decorrente de má adesão ou nível inadequado do fármaco; prevenção de ocorrência de efeitos tóxicos; e ajuda na individualização da terapia.[418] A mensuração das concentrações de fármacos ocorre após o estabelecimento de um estado de platô da concentração sanguínea com base em 5 meias-vidas de eliminação. O pico e os níveis mínimos são recomendados para fármacos com meia-vida curta de eliminação e quando as convulsões não são bem controladas.[490] Concentrações séricas de fármacos estão disponíveis para alguns medicamentos para determinar se o intervalo do alvo terapêutico foi atingido ou não. Uma queda de 20% ou mais na concentração sérica mínima frequentemente é um indicador de má conformidade da administração.[475] As concentrações terapêuticas séricas são baseadas em estudos que avaliam a concentração pela qual a maioria (população) dos cães com EI tem a convulsão controlada. Todavia, poucos FAEs (*i. e.*, FB, KBr) em medicina veterinária estabeleceram concentrações terapêuticas e ajustes de dose baseados no controle da convulsão, concentrações séricas do fármaco e efeitos adversos. É importante ter uma avaliação regular das concentrações séricas mesmo nos momentos em que as convulsões estão bem controladas, a fim de monitorar os teores tóxicos, especialmente para medicamentos com uma janela terapêutica estreita (*i. e.*, FB e KBr), para monitorar a concentração de flutuações no soro e ter conhecimento quando houver necessidade de fazer mudanças na terapia (ver Capítulo 35).

Combinação de terapias. Nem todos os pacientes epilépticos podem ser controlados com um único FAE, e tais pacientes podem exigir medicamentos complementares para controle das convulsões. Aproximadamente 30% de cães com EI requerem dois ou mais FAEs para controle das convulsões.[481,483,484] Além disso, cerca de 50% de todos os cães epilépticos são capazes de manter um estado livre de convulsões sem ter efeitos adversos da medicação.[491] Antes de iniciar um segundo fármaco, deve-se esperar um tempo para determinar os efeitos do primeiro medicamento e garantir que concentrações séricas adequadas foram alcançadas antes de assumir que houve falta de eficácia. Um fármaco não deve ser considerado ineficaz até que a dose máxima ou as concentrações séricas-alvo tenham sido alcançadas, ou até que efeitos adversos inaceitáveis tenham ocorrido.

Epilepsia refratária. O termo epiléptico refratário ou fármaco-resistente é utilizado na medicina veterinária para descrever uma condição em que um animal com epilepsia não consegue atingir o controle da convulsão ou sofre efeitos colaterais intoleráveis, apesar da utilização de terapia apropriada com FAEs convencionais.[473,474] Embora a resistência aos fármacos seja um problema sério para alguns cães com EI, é menos frequente em gatos. Fatores para EI refratária podem estar relacionados a três variáveis: doenças, medicamentos e a doenças cerebrais subjacentes,[475] como malformação cortical, lesão cerebral traumática anterior ou outro processo de doença ativo. Os mecanismos relacionados a medicamentos incluem tolerância metabólica ou funcional, conhecidos como resistência a fármacos, os quais têm duas teorias sobre a patogênese: a hipótese-alvo, que propõe alterações genéticas ou relacionadas a doenças em alvos celulares de FAEs, e a hipótese do transportador, que postula sobre o transporte alterado de fármacos através da BHE.[492,493] A tolerância metabólica ocorre quando o aumento da dose do medicamento não resulta em um aumento paralelo na concentração sérica do fármaco. Embora a genética da epilepsia canina e felina estejam se tornando mais bem compreendidas, questões relacionadas ao paciente podem se tornar mais relevantes, como as que dizem respeito à resposta ao tratamento.[412] Evidências para prever a farmacorresistência em cães são limitadas, embora a densidade de convulsões (várias convulsões em um curto período de tempo) seja um fator preditivo influente de farmacorresistência.[494]

Faltam critérios para a tomada de decisão sobre o início de um segundo ou terceiro FAE na medicina veterinária. Vários fatores deveriam ser considerados ao se decidir a respeito de um segundo FAE: selecionar um FAE com mecanismo de ação diferente, minimizando o uso de interações farmacológicas, limitando a toxicidade aditiva, determinando o risco *versus* o benefício da politerapia e os efeitos na qualidade de vida do animal de estimação e de seu tutor.[418] O painel de consenso ACVIM recomendou o uso de FB, KBr, levetiracetam, zonisamida e imepitoína (Europa), considerado para pacientes epilépticos resistentes a medicamentos.[418,473,485,495-499] O único estudo clínico publicado realizado com gatos com epilepsia refratária avaliou o uso de levetiracetam; 7/10 gatos tiveram uma avaliação favorável na resposta ao tratamento e toleraram bem o fármaco.[500]

Prognóstico

Com base em um consenso do IVETF, a condição livre de convulsão é o principal objetivo do tratamento e do manejo terapêutico da epilepsia canina e felina.[415] O termo livre de convulsão foi definido como o intervalo entre crises três vezes mais longo do que o intervalo pré-tratamento após no mínimo de 3 meses de tratamento. O sucesso terapêutico parcial foi definido como prevenção de convulsões ou prevenção do estado epiléptico, redução relevante da frequência de convulsões levando em consideração a frequência dos episódios de convulsão pré-tratamento e a redução da gravidade das crises.[415] A avaliação da eficácia do tratamento com FAEs foi realizada pela proporção de cães em estudo populacional que teve a frequência das convulsões reduzida. Quando mais de 50% de redução na frequência de convulsões foi usada como uma medida de resultado de redução, cerca de 2/3 dos cães alcançaram esse objetivo.[494] Fatores associados com a redução de convulsões incluíram fêmeas, castração, nenhum histórico de convulsões e idade avançada no início das convulsões. No homem, fatores associados com a permanência do estado de livre de convulsões incluem: ausência de lesão cerebral estrutural, epilepsia de curta duração, poucas convulsões antes do controle farmacológico e monoterapia com FAE.[478]

Cães e gatos com epilepsia podem experimentar convulsões epilépticas recorrentes debilitantes, que podem levar a alterações do comportamento, outros efeitos clínicos e redução da qualidade de vida.[501,502] Além disso, a qualidade de vida também é impactada para o tutor do paciente epiléptico.[503-505] Em um estudo realizado, 60% dos tutores relataram que a epilepsia de seu cão teve um impacto negativo em sua qualidade de vida.[501] Vários estudos mostraram expectativa de vida normal para cães com epilepsia idiopática, enquanto outros estudos mostraram uma redução de até 2 anos na expectativa de vida.[444,501,506,507] O tempo médio de sobrevivência de 1,5 ano para epilepsia canina após o diagnóstico foi relatado em um grande estudo de coorte de cães epilépticos.[424] Esse mesmo estudo descobriu que raças mantidas exclusivamente para companhia viveram um tempo maior após o diagnóstico, comparadas àqueles raças com dupla finalidade, como as raças caçadoras e de trabalho.[424] As raças com menor probabilidade de entrar em remissão ou ter > 50% em redução de convulsão foram Border Collie, Pastor-Alemão e Staffordshire Terrier.[494] Muitos animais de estimação são sacrificados em razão da gravidade das convulsões ou em função dos graves efeitos colaterais induzidos pelos fármacos.[485,501,508]

Os fatores de risco para a eutanásia incluem idade mais jovem de início das convulsões, alta frequência inicial, controle deficiente das convulsões e dos episódios de estado epiléptico.[437,479,506,507] Aproximadamente 40 a 60% dos cães com epilepsia têm um ou mais episódios de grupos de convulsões ou estado epiléptico e uma média de vida de 8 anos, quando comparados a 11 anos para aqueles com epilepsia e sem estado epiléptico.[428,507-510] Cães que tiveram grupos de convulsões são significativamente menos propensos a atingir remissão com qualquer tratamento com FAE.[494] Embora a expectativa de vida do animal de estimação não seja afetada, as chances de um epiléptico obter remissão completa sem necessidade de tratamento é baixa: 6 a 8% em cães[438,479,501] e 17% em gatos.[430] Assim, a epilepsia em animais de companhia geralmente requer terapia ao longo da vida e comprometimento do tutor. Um equilíbrio entre a qualidade de vida, e o sucesso terapêutico é muitas vezes a chave para o comprometimento do tutor com o tratamento do seu animal.[503]

Embora o tratamento com FAE deva ser considerado por toda a vida, a descontinuação de FAEs pode ser considerada em animais de estimação com remissão das crises. A decisão de diminuir gradualmente a dose do FAE deve ser de forma individual, mas a remissão da convulsão por pelo menos 1 a 2 anos é recomendada.[414,474] Existem poucas informações de recidiva de convulsão, e os tutores devem estar cientes de que convulsões podem ocorrer a qualquer momento. É aconselhável diminuir a dose de FAE em 20% ou menos em periodicidade mensal.[414] Apenas em caso de efeitos adversos com risco de vida, o FAE deve ser imediatamente interrompido. Nessa situação, o animal está sob observação atenta e um FAE que tenha um metabolismo diferente deve ser administrado simultaneamente em uma dose de ataque inicial.

DOENÇA VASCULAR CEREBRAL

Classificação

A alta demanda metabólica do tecido cerebral necessita de um fornecimento adequado de sangue. A redução do suprimento sanguíneo causa falta de oxigenação e/ou glicose, levando à isquemia neuronal e morte tecidual. A doença cerebrovascular é definida como qualquer anormalidade do cérebro resultante de um processo patológico que afeta seu fornecimento de sangue.[511] Doenças vasculares cerebrais podem ser resultantes de um fluxo excessivo de sangue através da vasculatura cerebral (hipertensão), ruptura da vasculatura (sangramento) ou redução de fluxo de sangue (infarto).[53,175] Acidente vascular encefálico (AVE), também conhecido como derrame, é a manifestação clínica da doença cerebrovascular, resultante de isquemia cerebral (acidente vascular encefálico isquêmico) e menos frequentemente de hemorragia cerebral (derrame hemorrágico).

Os sinais clínicos devem estar presentes por > 24 horas para serem considerados derrame.[512] Se os sinais de um AVE se resolverem dentro de 24 horas, o termo usado é ataque isquêmico transitório. Isquemia global refere-se à hipoxia/anoxia de todo o cérebro e morte simétrica bilateral em populações neuronais seletivamente vulneráveis (p. ex., córtex cerebral, hipocampo, córtex cerebelar, núcleos basais e tálamo).[53]

O infarto cerebral pode resultar de uma ruptura da vasculatura levando a um infarto hemorrágico ou pela oclusão vascular ocasionando pelo infarto isquêmico.[513] O trombo ou êmbolo causa uma oclusão focal, mas, com menor frequência, pode ser multifocal. Os infartos isquêmicos que têm hemorragia secundária são chamados infartos hemorrágicos; quando a hemorragia não está presente, os infartos são denominados infartos não hemorrágicos. De acordo com o tamanho do vaso, os infartos podem ser consequência de doença dos pequenos vasos, que dá origem a infartos lacunares, ou de doença de grandes vasos, que dá origem a um infarto territorial. Infartos territoriais tendem a ocorrer no cerebelo e no cérebro. AVEs não hemorrágicos traumáticos são decorrentes da ruptura de um vaso cerebral e desenvolvimento de um hematoma. A hemorragia pode ser localizada como intra-axial no parênquima cerebral ou extra-axial, tal como no espaço intraventricular, subdural ou subaracnoide e LCR.[514] A hemorragia subaracnoide pode produzir vasospasmo cerebral, uma constrição temporária de uma artéria intracraniana causando isquemia regional transitória. O vasospasmo é difícil de determinar clinicamente em animais, mas foi associado à hemorragia subaracnoide em cães.[515]

Fisiopatologia

Infarto isquêmico

O infarto é uma área comprometida no parênquima cerebral que é resultante da oclusão vascular focal, trombose ou embolia. Em relação ao tromboembolismo relacionado ao acidente vascular encefálico (AVE), a oclusão é decorrente de uma fonte embólica (séptica, parasitária, metastática, aterosclerótica) que trefegou de outro leito vascular ou do coração.[512,516] A área infartada do cérebro consiste em um núcleo isquêmico com perda permanente de fluxo sanguíneo e lesão neuronal irreversível circundada por uma penumbra, na qual o fluxo sanguíneo diminui, mas ainda há neurônios viáveis que estão em risco de lesão irreversível. A terapia é direcionada para a reversão desse processo patológico em 4 a 6 horas, mas a cascata de edema isquêmico vasogênico pode progredir dentro da penumbra e continuar por 24 a 48 horas.[512,516]

Os infartos isquêmicos não hemorrágicos são os mais comuns em AVEs reconhecidos em cães.[517,518] Sítios comuns para acidentes vasculares cerebrais isquêmicos em cães incluem cerebelo,

região estriatocapsular e tálamo.[517-521] Nenhuma causa *ante mortem* subjacente é detectada para cerca de 50% dos AVEs em cães.[522] Nenhum fator relacionado a idade ou sexo foi identificado, e a incidência é desconhecida.[512] Os cães da raça Cavalier King Charles Spaniel e Galgo parecem super-representados.[517,518,522] Os cães Galgos parecem mais predispostos ao AVE isquêmico do que todas as outras raças juntas, sendo a hipertensão um possível fator contribuinte.[523] Infartos cerebelares territoriais são mais prováveis em cães de raças pequenas, especialmente em animais da raça Cavalier King Charles Spaniel, já infartos lacunares talâmicos/ mesencéfalos ocorrem mais frequentemente em cães de raças de grande porte.[518,522] Cães Schnauzer Miniatura podem ter maior risco, possivelmente relacionado à hiperlipidemia.[524]

Várias etiologias foram associadas ao AVE isquêmico em cães e gatos, incluindo sepse, aterosclerose associada a hipotireoidismo primário, e cães Schnauzer Miniatura com hiperlipidemia primária, migração parasitária aberrante, doença tromboembólica e neoplasia.[512-529] Doenças que predispõem a acidente vascular encefálico isquêmico não hemorrágico incluem distúrbios metabólicos (hipotireoidismo, feocromocitoma, hipertensão) ou hipercoagulopatia (diabetes melito, hiperadrenocorticismo, doença renal, nefropatia com perda de proteína).[512-531] Infartos cerebrais hemorrágicos podem resultar em trombose venosa ou dano vascular com extravasamento de sangue quando a reperfusão ocorre no foco da isquemia.[53] Várias condições são subjacentes ao acidente vascular encefálico hemorrágico isquêmico, tais como coagulopatia, hipertensão, sepse, inflamação e metástase (hemangiossarcoma).[512,531,532]

Derrame hemorrágico

A hemorragia pode lesionar os tecidos vizinhos, interrompendo vias vitais, exercendo pressão local nas estruturas cerebrais adjacentes e causando isquemia dos tecidos ao redor. Os hematomas podem ser grandes o suficiente para aumentar a pressão intracraniana, causando deslocamento e herniação do tecido cerebral. A hemorragia intracraniana não traumática ocasiona ruptura de vasos sanguíneos ou distúrbios hemorrágicos, que podem ser primários ou secundários. Múltiplas hemorragias podem indicar distúrbio de sangramento, toxicidade, traumas ou tumores vasculares metastáticos.[53] A incidência de AVE hemorrágico em cães e gatos é desconhecida. Hemorragia intracraniana ocorre mais comumente secundária a traumatismo cranioencefálico.[514] Em um estudo com 75 cães com hemorragia intracraniana não traumática, foi relatado que as lesões eram intraparenquimatosas (n = 72), subdurais (n = 2) ou intraventricular (n = 1); desse grupo de cães, 33 animais apresentaram uma condição concomitante, incluindo infecção por *Angiostrongylus vasorum*, hipertensão, hemangiossarcoma metastático, doença renal crônica, hiperadrenocorticismo, linfoma intracraniano, meningioma meningotelial, sepse e hipotireoidismo.[533] Distúrbio de sangramento em associação com infecção por *A. vasorum* provavelmente predispõe a infecções com hemorragias intracranianas.[534] As condições simultâneas mais comumente associadas a lesões múltiplas < 5 mm (microssangramentos cerebrais) foram endocrinopatias e hipertensão.[533] Adenoma hipofisário, infarto ou hemorragia (apoplexia hipofisária) podem causar convulsões de início súbito, alterações de comportamento ou perda de visão.[535]

Pouco se sabe sobre gatos, mas AVEs hemorrágicos e acidentes vasculares isquêmicos foram relatados.[532] Encefalopatia isquêmica felina, uma síndrome de infarto cerebral, geralmente envolve a artéria cerebral média. Alguns casos foram associados à migração aberrante de larvas *Cuterebra* spp. para o cérebro.[528,536] Uma vez que nem todos têm lesões vasculares óbvias, vasospasmos podem ser o resultado de hemorragia na região do espaço subaracnóideo causado pela migração da larva ou resultado da toxina produzida por larvas.[196] Deve-se suspeitar de infartos hemorrágicos em gatos com doença hepática e sinais vestibulares centrais.[532]

Isquemia global

A isquemia cerebral global é um diagnóstico diferencial em cães e gatos com disfunção neurológica aguda após anestesia ou pós-reanimação cardiopulmonar.[537,538] O divisor de águas do infarto se desenvolve quando o fluxo sanguíneo cerebral é reduzido abaixo do ponto de compensação por mecanismos autorregulatórios cerebrais, causando disfunção cerebral bilateral generalizada. O uso da cetamina predispõe à isquemia, e as raças braquicefálicas também são predispostas a isquemia global.[537] O uso de abridores de boca em gatos foi associado como um provável fator de risco para o desenvolvimento de isquemia cerebral, perda auditiva e cegueira.[538] Se a boca for aberta ao máximo, o fluxo de sangue através das artérias maxilares é obstruído em alguns gatos.[539,540] Descobertas adicionais sugerem que deficiências de visão e audição podem não ser apenas os resultados da perfusão reduzida ao cérebro, mas também podem ser resultado da interrupção do fluxo de sangue diretamente para retina ou orelha interna.[539] Abridores de boca pequenos não foram associados a anormalidades em testes de função da retina ou angiografia por ressonância magnética e permanecem fornecendo uma abertura suficiente, minimizando os riscos de reduções no fluxo sanguíneo da artéria maxilar.[541]

Sinais clínicos

O início dos sinais neurológicos varia de superagudo a agudo e geralmente não são progressivos após 24 horas.[512] Os sinais comuns observados por tutores incluem alteração do estado mental, hemiparesia, convulsões e disfunção vestibular. Déficits neurológicos em cães com AVE geralmente têm localização anatômica focal e refletem o local e a extensão da lesão vascular.[512,517,521,522,531,542] O infarto de uma região específica do cérebro está associado aos sinais clínicos (i. e., prosencefálico, talâmico, mesencefálico, pontíneo, medular, cerebelar).[517,542] Em 38 cães com infartos cerebrais, as localizações envolvidas foram cérebro (29%), tálamo/mesencéfalo (21%), cerebelo (47%) e multifocais em 7%. O acidente vascular encefálico isquêmico em 27 cães envolveu a artéria cerebral média em 70% dos em cães.[542]

Disfunção motora e ataxia proprioceptiva geral foram relatadas em 78% dos animais, incluindo sinais de heminegligência sensorial e déficits motores contralaterais como consequência de infarto da artéria cerebral média. Um estudo relatou convulsões em 50% dos cães após acidente vascular encefálico isquêmico,[542] porém outro estudo relatou convulsão em apenas 1 cão. O início do AVE isquêmico geralmente varia de agudo a hiperagudo. Normalmente, a deterioração ocorre após o insulto, provavelmente em razão do edema, mas depois torna-se estável ou melhora após as primeiras 24 horas. No AVE hemorrágico, muitas vezes a área comprometida envolve mais de uma artéria, e os sinais secundários decorrem do aumento da pressão intracraniana. Se a hemorragia estiver associada ao efeito de massa, a deterioração pode resultar em formação de edema ou aumento do hematoma.

Diagnóstico

Inicialmente, outras doenças cerebrais agudas como as doenças metabólicas, neoplásicas, inflamatória e trauma devem ser considerados. Isso é importante para determinar a presença de distúrbios subjacentes extraneurais (Figura 260.2). Cães e gatos com doença isquêmica e AVE hemorrágico devem ser avaliados para doença hipertensiva, endócrina, renal, cardíaca e metastática.[522,530] Juntamente com o exame físico (ver Capítulo 2) e exame neurológico (ver Capítulo 259), exames da retina (ver Capítulo 11) devem ser considerados, mudanças podem revelar evidências de vasos tortuosos sugestivos de hipertensão (ver Capítulo 157) e hemorragia, que pode sugerir um distúrbio hemorrágico ou hipertensivo. O hemograma permite a identificação de índices hematimétricos anormais ou anomalias plaquetárias. O perfil bioquímico sérico e urinálise devem ser usados para avaliar a hipercoagulabilidade ou outra doença sistêmica subjacente. Teste de coagulação específico é recomendado (ver Capítulo 196). O monitoramento da pressão arterial seriado

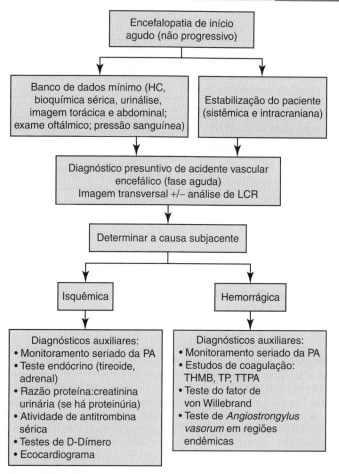

Figura 260.2 Algoritmo de abordagem diagnóstica para suspeita de acidente cerebrovascular. *HC*, hemograma completo; *LCR*, líquido cefalorraquidiano; *PA*, pressão arterial; *THMB*, tempo de hemorragia da mucosa bucal; *TP*, tempo de protrombina; *TTPA*, tempo de tromboplastina parcial ativada.

pode detectar hipertensão subjacente (ver Capítulo 99). A encefalopatia hipertensiva pode ser observada com quadros agudos (> 30 mmHg do nível de repouso) ou sustentados (> 180 mmHg) de aumento na pressão arterial sistólica (ver Capítulo 157).[543] Outros testes adjuvantes incluem exames de imagens torácica, abdominal e cardíaca, teste endócrino para doença adrenal (ver Capítulo 306) e da tireoide (ver Capítulo 299).

O diagnóstico definitivo de acidente vascular encefálico requer histologia por biopsia ou necropsia. Estudos de imagem são necessários para fazer uma estimativa diagnóstica, determinar a extensão da lesão e distinguir entre acidente vascular encefálico isquêmico e hemorrágico.[512,531] Além disso, reconhecer o infarto e/ou a hemorragia auxilia no manejo adequado do paciente. Imagens de TC frequentemente são normais durante a fase aguda da isquemia; assim, um diagnóstico definitivo depende de exclusão de outras doenças semelhantes. Os primeiros sinais de lesão isquêmica na TC incluem hipodensidade parenquimatosa, perda da distinção do aspecto acinzentado da substância branca, achatamento sutil de sulcos corticais e efeito de massa local oriundo do edema.[512,531] A ressonância magnética é considerada mais sensível que a TC para detectar lesões isquêmicas agudas.[513] Achados de imagem por RM característicos associados a infarto isquêmico incluem lesões em forma de cunha bem demarcadas com efeito de massa mínimo. A lesão intra-axial é hiperintensa nas sequências T2W e FLAIR e hipointensa em sequências T1W com realce mínimo.[336,513,517] A distribuição de lesões deve se correlacionar com sua perda do suprimento arterial regional fornecido.[336,517,518,542] Lesões de AVE crônicas tendem a contrastar um pouco melhor alguns dias após o início do processo,[517,518,531,544] o que pode ser confundido com neoplasia e inflamação.[19,336]

SEÇÃO 17 • Doença Neurológica

Tabela 260.9 Momento da hemorragia e descrição de ressonância magnética (RM)/tomografia computadorizada (TC).

	< 24 H	1 A 3 DIAS	> 3 DIAS	> 7 DIAS	> 1 MÊS
Estágio clínico	Hiperaguda	Agudo	Subagudo precoce	Subagudo a crônico	Crônico
Estado da hemoglobina (HB)	OxiHb	DeoxiHb	MetHb	MetHb	Hemossiderina e ferritina
Localização celular nos eritrócitos	Intra	Intra	Intra	Extra	
Intensidade do sinal T1W	Iso	Iso a hipo	Hiper	Hiper	Iso a hipo
Intensidade do sinal T2W/FLAIR	Ligeiramente hiper	Hipo	Hipo	Hiper	Hipo
T2* (GRE) Perda de intensidade do sinal (sinal vazio)	Presente (borda)	Presente	Presente	Presente	Presente
Densidade TC	Hiper	Hiper	Hiper	Iso	Iso a hipo

FLAIR, recuperação de inversão atenuada por fluido; *GRE*, gradiente seco.

Dificuldade para diferenciar lesões isquêmicas agudas de crônicas por meio de ressonância magnética podem ser superadas com técnicas funcionais de ressonância magnética. Imagem ponderada por difusão (DWI) complementa outras sequências convencionais de RM com sensibilidade para edemas citotóxicos, especialmente na isquemia inicial, e em sua avaliação de evolução temporal em isquemia aguda versus AVE crônico.[513,545] O contraste do tecido por DWI reflete o movimento browniano de moléculas de água. O infarto isquêmico hiperagudo (horas a 4 dias) aparece como hiperintenso na imagem por DWI que corresponde a hipointensidade em mapas de ADC, e é compatível com edema citotóxico e redução do movimento browniano das moléculas de água. Com o passar do tempo, o edema vasogênico desenvolve-se e, no DWI e mapeamento ADC correspondente, o sinal torna-se hiperintenso à medida que a difusão se torna maior em razão do aumento de volume de água extracelular. A angiografia por RM (ARM) pode ser útil para identificar oclusão vascular subjacente ou malformação.

O reconhecimento da hemorragia é importante no diagnóstico e manejo apropriado. Tomografia computadorizada é considerada altamente sensível para detecção de hemorragia aguda, que parece hiperdensa em razão da atenuação dos raios X pela porção globina da hemoglobina (Tabela 260.9). Ao longo de dias a semanas, hematomas eventualmente tornam-se isodensos com o aumento de contraste variável. Na ressonância magnética, lesões hemorrágicas agudas e subagudas frequentemente estão associadas a edema vasogênico circundante, que tem aparência de imagem hiperintensa em sequências T2W e FLAIR. Existem estágios distintos de aparências das lesões das hemorragias intracranianas na ressonância magnética em razão da quebra das células sanguíneas vermelhas em várias formas da hemoglobina, as quais criam diversos padrões de intensidades de sinal em sequências definidas (ver Tabela 260.9).[546-548] As sequências gradiente-eco (T2*) são recomendadas para visualização de hemorragia. A sequência T2*W aproveita a vantagem das propriedades magnéticas da hemossiderina, oxi, desoxi e metaemoglobina para identificar áreas de produtos sanguíneos, acúmulo e evolução temporal da hemorragia intracraniana. As propriedades paramagnéticas da desoxiemoglobina na hemorragia aguda causam um artefato de suscetibilidade na sequência T2*W, que é visualizado como um sinal vazio (escuro). Às vezes a sequência T2*W pode melhorar a distinção de microssangramentos (< 4 mm) que não são facilmente visualizados em uma sequência T2W.[549]

Tratamento

O manejo dos AVEs é predominantemente de suporte: controle de convulsões, da pressão intracraniana e tratamento de qualquer causa subjacente, como vasculite ou hipertensão.[512] Após um acidente vascular encefálico isquêmico, a recuperação geralmente ocorre dentro de várias semanas com cuidado de suporte. O tratamento inclui correção de anormalidades, minimizando os efeitos da cascata isquêmica e melhorando o fluxo sanguíneo

cerebral. Com base no desenvolvimento da penumbra em pacientes humanos com AVE, a "janela de oportunidade" para instituir essas terapias é dentro de 6 horas.[516]

Os princípios do tratamento agudo para AVE incluem monitoramento de parâmetros vitais (vias respiratórias, respiração, circulação), estabilização intracraniana e investigação das causas subjacentes. O foco da estabilização intracraniana de redução do edema cerebral, otimizando fluxo sanguíneo cerebral e, se indicado, remoção do espaço ocupado pelo hematoma. A perfusão cerebral é otimizada com o manejo da pressão arterial sistêmica e da pressão intracraniana elevada. No AVE hemorrágico, os benefícios provavelmente superam os riscos ao considerar a administração de um agente, como o manitol. O uso de agentes trombolíticos (i. e., o ativador tecidual de plasminogênio, estreptoquinase) durante o tratamento agudo é infrequente em razão do custo, e raramente coágulos sanguíneos estão associados a infarto em cães e gatos e existe falha na administração desses agentes dentro da janela temporal de 6 horas.[512,516] Embora não comprovado como sendo benéficos, a longo prazo antitrombóticos (p. ex., ácido acetilsalicílico) podem ser considerados na doença tromboembólica para reduzir o risco de outro infarto. O paciente deve ser monitorado seriamente a longo prazo para sinais de recidiva de AVE e sinais de progressão da doença subjacente.

Prognóstico

O prognóstico depende do tipo e da localização do AVE, da gravidade da disfunção neurológica, da ocorrência de deterioração ou complicações e da causa subjacente.[522] Estudos de sobrevivência de AVEs são difíceis, pois cães geralmente têm sinais neurológicos graves que levam os tutores a optar pela realização da eutanásia. No acidente vascular encefálico isquêmico, a maioria dos cães se recupera semanas após o início dos sinais.[517,518,522] Em um estudo com 20 cães com AVE isquêmico, o prognóstico era bom, caso eles sobrevivessem aos primeiros 30 dias pós-AVE, porém existiu o risco de recidiva.[550] A recidiva tem sido baseada em um episódio repetido da disfunção neurológica aguda.[522,542] Cães com uma condição médica concomitante que cause acidente vascular encefálico isquêmico tem sobrevida mais curta do que cães sem condição subjacente identificada.[522] Em um estudo de 75 cães com hemorragia intracraniana não traumática, 61% dos animais tiveram um resultado excelente a longo prazo.[533] Todavia, acidente vascular encefálico hemorrágico no cerebelo é associado a maior mortalidade.[518] A identificação de hipertensão em cães com doenças intracranianas hemorrágicas não traumáticas é um indicador de prognóstico ruim.[533] Em cães com hemorragia intracraniana e múltiplas lesões > 5 mm, A. vasorum (ver Capítulo 242) foi a única condição concomitante com um bom resultado.[533]

REFERÊNCIAS BIBLIOGRÁFICAS

As referências bibliográficas deste capítulo se encontram online no Ambiente de Aprendizagem.

CAPÍTULO 261

Doenças Cerebrais Inflamatórias, Infecciosas e Multifocais

Chelsie Estey e Curtis W. Dewey

Distúrbios cerebrais em que o exame neurológico revela envolvimento multifocal ou difuso são relativamente comuns na prática clínica. O envolvimento multifocal ou difuso do cérebro refere-se a evidências clínicas de que mais de uma divisão funcional do cérebro está acometida por um processo mórbido. Por exemplo, considera-se que um cão com disfunção prosencefálica e cerebelar apresenta envolvimento multifocal ou difuso do cérebro. Chamar uma localização neurológica de multifocal ou difusa é, de certa forma, uma questão semântica, mas *difusa* sugere uma forma mais generalizada e constelação simétrica de deficiências, enquanto *multifocal* conota um grupo mais assimétrico de anormalidades. São muitas as implicações da localização multifocal/difusa em um paciente com sinais, por exemplo, de encefalopatia, o tipo de distúrbio mais provável em tal neurolocalização. Em geral, distúrbios inflamatórios, metabólicos, neoplasia multifocal/metastática e toxinas são mais recorrentes na lista de diagnósticos diferenciais para cães e gatos com encefalopatia multifocal/difusa. No entanto, é importante notar que essas implicações às vezes são imprecisas. Pacientes com distúrbios metabólicos ou tóxicos que causam doenças cerebrais mais provavelmente manifestam déficits neurológicos simétricos (*i. e.*, encefalopatia difusa), porém isso não é absoluto.

O clínico deve estar ciente de que as lesões cerebrais focais podem levar a sinais multifocais de encefalopatia em razão de muitos mecanismos: (1) uma extensa massa que invade mais de uma região do cérebro; (2) edema em torno de uma massa focal, produzindo efeito de massa; (3) obstrução de fluxo normal do líquido cefalorraquidiano (LCR) por uma lesão cerebral, levando ao acúmulo de LCR ventricular (p. ex., hidrocefalia obstrutiva associada a uma lesão da fossa caudal); (4) lesões que afetam uma área do cérebro que tem influência sobre uma região separada do cérebro (p. ex., lobo floculonodular ou pedúnculo cerebelar caudal).

Este capítulo analisa as características clínicas mais evidentes dos distúrbios cerebrais multifocais/difusos mais comuns encontrados em cachorros e gatos. Distúrbios que comumente levam à disfunção cerebral multifocal/difusa são resumidos de acordo com o esquema DAMNIT (degenerativo, anomalia, metabólico, neoplásico, nutricional, inflamatório [não infeccioso], infeccioso, toxinas, trauma) no Boxe 261.1. Nem todos esses distúrbios serão discutidos em detalhes, e alguns não são discutidos, pois aparecem em outras partes deste livro. A ênfase é dada aos distúrbios cerebrais inflamatórios não infecciosos de cães em razão da sua ocorrência frequente na prática clínica e propensão para causar disfunção cerebral multifocal.

Boxe 261.1 Doenças que podem causar disfunção cerebral multifocal ou difusa

Degenerativa
Doença de armazenamento lisossomal* (ver Capítulo 260)
Síndrome de disfunção cognitiva (ver Capítulo 263)
Leucodistrofia/degeneração esponjosa (ver Capítulo 260)
Vacuolização neuronal e degeneração espinocerebelar de cães Rottweiler e Boxer

Anomalia
Síndrome de malformação occipital caudal (ver Capítulo 260)
Cisto aracnoide intracraniano
Hidrocefalia congênita (ver Capítulo 260)
Distúrbios de migração neuronal
Sobreposição atlanto-occipital
Síndrome de Dandy-Walker (ver Capítulo 260)

Metabólica
Encefalopatia hepática (ver Capítulos 281 e 284)
Encefalopatia hipoglicêmica (ver Capítulo 303)
Encefalopatia associada a eletrólitos
Encefalopatia relacionada ao sistema endócrino (p. ex., hipotireoidismo [ver Capítulo 299], hipertireoidismo [ver Capítulo 301])
Encefalopatia associada ao sistema renal (ver Capítulo 322)
Kernicterus
Encefalopatia mitocondrial
Acidúrias orgânicas

Neoplásica
Tumores cerebrais primários (ver Capítulo 260)
Tumores cerebrais metastáticos/multifocais (p. ex., linfoma; ver Capítulo 260)

Nutricional
Deficiência de tiamina (ver Capítulo 12)
Deficiência de cobalamina (Border Collies) (ver Capítulo 292)

Inflamatória, não infecciosa
Meningoencefalomielite granulomatosa
Encefalite necrosante
Meningoencefalite eosinofílica

Infecciosa
Bacteriana
Fúngica
Viral
Riquetsial
Protozoário
Verminose
Hidrocefalia com encefalite periventricular

Tóxicas
Brometalina (ver Capítulo 152)
Maconha (ver Capítulo 154)
Metaldeído (ver Capítulo 152)
Antidepressivos tricíclicos (ver Capítulo 153)
Brunfelsia (ver Capítulo 155)
Pista
Sobredose de metilxantina
Nicotina (ver Capítulo 155)
Intoxicação por sal (bolas de tinta; ver Capítulos 13 e 152)

Trauma (ver Capítulo 148)
Hemorragia intracraniana
Edema
Lesão intraxonal difusa

*Esses distúrbios também podem ser considerados de natureza metabólica.

DISTÚRBIOS CEREBRAIS INFLAMATÓRIOS E NÃO INFECCIOSOS

A terminologia associada a esses distúrbios pode ser confusa. Um conceito importante a lembrar é que esses termos são baseados em descrições histopatológicas, e não em etiologias conhecidas. Além disso, estimou-se que aproximadamente 1/3 de todos os distúrbios cerebrais inflamatórios caninos não chega a um diagnóstico específico. Os dois distúrbios mais comumente reconhecidos nessa categoria de doença são meningoencefalomielite granulomatosa (MEG) e encefalite necrosante (EN). A encefalite necrosante frequentemente é subdividida em duas formas: meningoencefalite necrosante (MEN) e leucoencefalite necrosante (LEN). Os autores encontraram vários pacientes com características de ambos, MEG e EN. Em razão desse fenômeno e da falta de causas identificáveis específicas para esses distúrbios, o "guarda-chuva" *meningoencefalite de etiologia desconhecida* (MED) tem sido sugerido.[1] Embora tal termo tenha alguma utilidade, características clínicas e resposta à terapia tendem a diferir entre os casos "clássicos" de MEG e EN. Por isso, os autores entendem que é importante considerá-las como entidades clínicas separadas quando é possível usar informações clínicas e/ou diagnósticas para ajudar a diferenciar entre os dois processos de doença.

Meningoencefalomielite granulomatosa

É uma doença inflamatória idiopática comum e enigmática do sistema nervoso central (SNC) em cães e é considerada extremamente rara em gatos. A MEG é diagnosticada definitivamente por meio de características histológicas, tipificadas por infiltrados perivasculares de células principalmente mononucleares (linfócitos, macrófagos e plasmócitos) no cérebro e/ou medula espinal. Os infiltrados celulares perivasculares característicos de MEG definem a síndrome da doença e são responsáveis pelos déficits neurológicos observados. A causa subjacente dessa doença continua a ser um mistério, mas acredita-se amplamente que a MEG seja um distúrbio autoimune, especificamente uma reação de hipersensibilidade do tipo retardado (mediada por células T). As lesões predominam na substância branca. Autoanticorpos direcionados contra astrócitos foram mostrados em casos de MEG, apoiando ainda mais a suspeita de que essa é uma doença cerebral autoimune. No entanto, não está claro se esses anticorpos antiastrócitos representam uma resposta imune primária ou secundária. Estudos recentes de reação em cadeia da polimerase (PCR) não conseguiram detectar o material genético viral em tecido cerebral de cães com MEG. Há três formas clínicas reconhecidas de MEG: focal, multifocal (disseminada) e ocular. A forma ocular é a menos comum. Na experiência dos autores, a MEG multifocal é a forma mais comum da doença.

A MEG pode afetar qualquer raça de cão de qualquer idade e sexo. Todavia, animais jovens a de meia-idade (idade média de 5 anos) e fêmeas de raças pequenas (p. ex., Poodle, Terrier) parecem ser predispostos. Convulsões, disfunção cerebelovestibular e hiperestesia cervical são características comuns de MEG multifocal. Pacientes com MEG ocasionalmente podem ficar febris após apresentação. Existem relatos de casos de MEG confirmados por biopsia em cães, mas a grande maioria foi diagnosticada na necropsia. Um diagnóstico presuntivo *ante mortem* de MEG é baseado na epidemiologia, no histórico e em sinais clínicos característicos, além de resultados de testes diagnósticos. A avaliação do LCR (ver Capítulo 115) geralmente fornece as informações mais importantes no diagnóstico *ante mortem* de MEG. Uma pleocitose principalmente mononuclear, com porcentagem variável de neutrófilos e teor elevado de proteína, é típica de MEG. Os resultados dos estudos de imagem são altamente variáveis em cães com MEG. Na maioria dos casos, porém, imagens de tomografia computadorizada/ressonância magnética (TC/RM) do cérebro em pacientes com MEG apresentam lesões isoladas ou múltiplas (mais comumente) (Figura 261.1), ou podem revelar áreas de realce de contraste com margens indistintas.

A terapia imunossupressora com glicocorticoides (p. ex., prednisona oral, 1 a 2 mg/kg a cada 12 horas; ver também Capítulo 165) há muito tempo é considerada o protocolo de tratamento padrão para MEG, apesar de uma alta taxa de falha clínica. A dose pode ser reduzida lentamente ao longo do tempo se o paciente apresentar resposta clínica ao tratamento. No entanto, os pacientes com MEG normalmente requerem terapia imunossupressora vitalícia. O prognóstico para MEG permanece reservado, mas melhorou drasticamente nos últimos anos em razão dos novos protocolos de tratamento da doença. Em um estudo, o tempo médio de sobrevivência de cães com MEG multifocal tratados com terapia com glicocorticoides foi de 8 dias.[2] Muitos fármacos imunossupressores alternativos foram avaliados como opções de tratamento adjuvante para pacientes com MEG. As três opções mais promissoras incluem procarbazina, citosina arabinosídeo e ciclosporina.[3-6] Tempos de sobrevivência superiores a 12 meses foram relatados para cada um desses três fármacos. Ademais, o uso desses medicamentos parece permitir diminuições sucessivas nas doses de glicocorticoides, minimizando efeitos adversos associados ao uso de esteroides. Procarbazina é um fármaco antineoplásico que atravessa a barreira hematencefálica (BHE) e tem alguma especificidade para células T. Acredita-se que os efeitos citotóxicos da procarbazina ocorram principalmente por meio da metilação das bases de DNA. Em um estudo de cães com diagnóstico presuntivo de MEG, o uso de procarbazina como adjuvante da prednisona foi associado a um tempo médio de sobrevida de 14 meses,

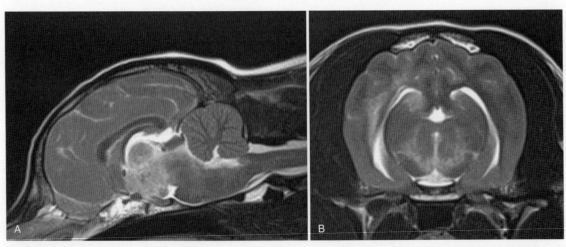

Figura 261.1 Imagens de ressonância magnética ponderadas em T2 sagital (**A**) e transversal (**B**) do cérebro de um cão mostram múltiplas lesões intensificadoras de contraste típicas de meningoencefalomielite granulomatosa.

independentemente da forma clínica de MEG (a maioria era multifocal). A dose utilizada pelos autores é de 25 mg/m^2, por via oral a cada 24 horas. A mielossupressão é o efeito adverso mais provável, embora gastrenterite hemorrágica também possa ocorrer. O hemograma deve ser verificado semanalmente durante o primeiro mês, depois, mensalmente, para monitorar a mielossupressão.[3] Citosina arabinosídeo é um nucleosídio sintético análogo que cruza a BHE. Esse medicamento se insere nas moléculas de DNA após a ativação enzimática, causando a terminação prematura da cadeia em células ativas mitoticamente. O protocolo usado para cães com MEG é uma taxa contínua de infusão IV (CRI, do inglês *continuous rate infusion*) (400 mg/m^2) administrada durante 24 horas. O CRI IV é a via de administração preferida dos autores, uma vez que o platô alcançado por essa via pode permitir uma exposição mais prolongada a citarabina em níveis citotóxicos no plasma.[7] A administração subcutânea de 50 mg/m^2 a cada 12 horas por 2 dias subsequentes é menos eficaz do que a CRI em razão da natureza específica do ciclo celular desse medicamento. A administração do medicamento deve ser repetida inicialmente a cada 3 semanas, com o intervalo estendendo-se gradualmente ao longo do tempo. O medicamento deve ser diluído 2:1 com solução salina estéril (para evitar a irritação do tecido) antes da injeção, e luvas devem ser usadas ao manusear a citosina arabinosídeo. Como a mielossupressão é um efeito adverso potencial desse fármaco, o hemograma deve ser verificado semanalmente no primeiro mês, e o hemograma e o perfil bioquímico sérico devem ser verificados antes de cada tratamento subsequente. A mielossupressão parece ser muito pouco frequente com esse protocolo. Em um artigo com 10 cães com encefalite não infecciosa de etiologia indeterminada, o tratamento com citosina arabinosídeo foi associado a um tempo de sobrevida médio de aproximadamente 1,5 ano. Em dois desses cães, um tratamento terciário (procarbazina, leflunomida) também foi administrado.[4] A ciclosporina (ciclosporina A) é um peptídio lipofílico que não cruza facilmente a BHE. Apesar disso, pensa-se que o fármaco pode ficar preso nas células endoteliais no SNC, e a natureza inflamatória da MEG pode permitir que mais ciclosporina atravesse a BHE do que ocorreria na ausência de inflamação. O modo de ação da ciclosporina é por meio do bloqueio da transcrição de genes em células T ativadas que levam à produção de citocinas inflamatórias. Houve vários relatórios clínicos do uso de ciclosporina no tratamento de MEG em cães; o fármaco parece ter sucesso, com média do tempo de sobrevivência de 2,5 anos em um relato de 10 cães.[5] Vários regimes terapêuticos têm sido sugeridos. Os autores usam 3 a 5 mg/kg por via oral a cada 12 horas. Efeitos adversos relatados atribuíveis ao uso de ciclosporina em cães incluem vômito, diarreia, anorexia, perda de peso, hiperplasia gengival, papilomatose, hipertricose e queda excessiva de pelos.[5]

Houve um relato que descreveu o uso de leflunomida, um análogo da pirimidina, para doença inflamatória cerebral não infecciosa em três cães. Os cães responderam favoravelmente à leflunomida e ainda estavam vivos mais de 12 meses após o início da terapia.[8] As doenças inflamatórias cerebrais específicas que afetaram esses cães não foram determinadas nesse relatório. Nos últimos anos, os autores têm combinado os três novos medicamentos para tratar pacientes suspeitos de MEG, mais comumente com uso de prednisona, ciclosporina e citosina arabinosídeo. Os resultados são preliminares, mas as respostas têm sido favoráveis, e os efeitos colaterais mínimos.

Encefalite necrosante

Essa subcategoria de doença inclui MEN e LEN. Assim como na MEG, suspeita-se que sejam doenças autoimunes. Ambos os distúrbios necrosantes são semelhantes, pois são caracterizados por múltiplas lesões necróticas não supurativas inflamatórias cavitárias do cérebro, que envolvem tanto a substância cinzenta quanto a branca (Figura 261.2). Na MEN, essas lesões são normalmente encontradas no cérebro, com envolvimento consistente das meninges. Cavitações cerebrais extensas com perda de demarcação entre substância cinzenta e branca são frequentemente encontradas em imagens de MEN. LEN exibe lesões semelhantes, que muitas vezes envolvem o tronco encefálico, além do cérebro, com envolvimento menos consistente das meninges e do córtex cerebral (i. e., principalmente a substância branca). Os primeiros relatos desses distúrbios em raças predispostas levaram aos termos *encefalite do Pug* ou *encefalite do Pug/Maltês* para MEN e *encefalite do Yorkshire Terrier* para LEN. Pug e Maltês são cães comumente acometidos por MEN, mas outras raças têm sido relatadas com esse distúrbio, incluindo Chihuahua, Shih Tzu, Pekingese, Papillion, Yorkshire Terrier, Coton de Tulear, Bruxelas Griffon e cães mestiços da raça Staffordshire Terrier.[9,10] A raça Yorkshire Terrier parece ser a raça mais acometida por LEN, mas essa doença também pode acometer outras raças de cães de pequeno porte, como o Buldogue Francês. É muito possível que MEN e LEN representem variantes do mesmo processo de doença. É esperado que mais raças sejam relatadas com EN idiopática. Os testes de PCR não conseguiram identificar o DNA viral associado a esses distúrbios. Tal como acontece com MEG, as lesões necróticas observadas na histopatologia cerebral são responsáveis pelos sinais clínicos e pela disfunção e definem a síndrome da doença.

A EN tende a ocorrer em cães jovens de raças pequenas, mas uma ampla faixa etária foi relatada. Os sinais clínicos (ver Capítulo 259) geralmente correspondem à distribuição das lesões cerebrais. Atividade convulsiva é frequente com EN, sendo muitas vezes a reclamação clínica primária. Cães Pug e Maltês com MEN têm idades variadas na apresentação da doença, entre

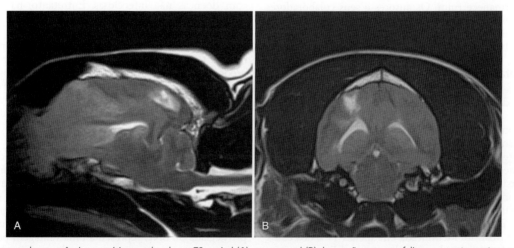

Figura 261.2 Imagens de ressonância magnética ponderada em T2 sagital (**A**) e transversal (**B**) de um cão com encefalite necrosante mostram uma região característica de necrose cerebral.

6 meses e 7 anos. O início e a progressão dos sinais clínicos da disfunção neurológica podem ser agudos (curso da doença de 2 semanas ou menos) ou crônicos (curso da doença de 4 a 6 meses). Sinais clínicos de disfunção do prosencéfalo (convulsões, andar em círculos, estado de apatia, déficits visuais com reflexo pupilar à luz normal, pressão de cabeça contra obstáculos etc.) predominam. Dor no pescoço é uma característica comum e pode ser causada por meningite e/ou doença do prosencéfalo. A idade de apresentação da doença em Yorkshire Terriers com LEN tem sido relatada entre 1 e 10 anos. Esses cães geralmente apresentam um quadro crônico e progressivo de agravamento da disfunção neurológica ao longo de vários meses. Além de sinais clínicos de disfunção do prosencéfalo e dor no pescoço, Yorkshire Terriers com LEN geralmente apresentam sinais clínicos de disfunção do tronco encefálico (p. ex., doença vestibular central). O diagnóstico definitivo de EN é baseado em lesões cerebrais histopatológicas características observadas na necropsia. Um diagnóstico presuntivo é baseado principalmente nos sinais clínicos, histórico e achados do exame neurológico. Os resultados dos exames de sangue são caracteristicamente normais. Os achados do LCR (ver Capítulo 115) na maioria das vezes são anormais; com maior frequência, é comum encontrar predominante ou exclusivamente pleocitose mononuclear com teores elevados de proteína. Em geral, as células mononucleares na MEN são principalmente linfocíticas, enquanto uma mistura de linfócitos e monócitos em geral é observada no LCR de pacientes com LEN. Achados de ressonância magnética e tomografia computadorizada foram descritos em vários casos de EN. Na ressonância magnética, as lesões são geralmente isointensas ou hipointensas em imagens ponderadas em T1, hiperintensas em imagens ponderadas em T2 e FLAIR com realce de contraste de maneira inconsistente e não uniforme. Dilatação assimétrica ventricular e áreas de hipointensidade no cérebro (correspondendo ao parênquima cerebral malácico), às vezes aparece contínua com os ventrículos laterais, são achados consistentes.

O tratamento de pacientes com suspeita de EN com glicocorticoides e fármacos anticonvulsivantes (se houver convulsões) deve ser tentado, mas muitas vezes tem pouco ou nenhum efeito clínico apreciável. O prognóstico para MEN varia de ruim a grave. A maioria dos cães morre ou é sacrificada em razão de disfunção neurológica progressiva dentro de 6 meses a partir do início dos déficits neurológicos. O mesmo protocolo de fármacos usados nos últimos anos para MEG tem sido sugerido para uso em casos de EN. Em razão do baixo número de casos em comparação com MEG, bem como da falta de distinção entre MEG e EN em alguns relatos, não está claro se esses fármacos são eficazes ou não para EN. Na experiência dos autores, procarbazina não parece ser tão eficaz em casos suspeitos de EN, em comparação com casos MEG. O prognóstico para esse grupo de doenças permanece ruim. Os autores e seus colaboradores obtiveram sucesso empírico no tratamento de muitos casos de pacientes suspeitos com MEN usando micofenolato de mofetila (ver Capítulo 165).

Meningoencefalite eosinofílica

A meningoencefalite eosinofílica (MEE) é uma causa incomum diagnosticada de doença intracraniana canina. É caracterizada principalmente por inflamação meníngea e quadro de pleocitose eosinofílica com contagem de eosinófilos superior a 10% no líquido cefalorraquidiano (LCR) em animais acometidos, independentemente de contagens circulantes de eosinófilos no sangue. Na medicina veterinária, MEE é frequentemente de natureza idiopática, embora MEE infecciosa possa ser causada por agentes comum *Cryptococcus neoformans* (ver Capítulo 231), *Neospora caninum* (ver Capítulo 221) e *Baylisascaris procyonis* (ver Capítulo 210). Em um estudo retrospectivo, uma causa infecciosa para MEE foi identificada em apenas 17% dos casos, enquanto 70% foram considerados idiopáticos.[11] Em contrapartida a outras encefalites caninas, como a meningoencefalite

granulomatosa, meningoencefalite necrosante e leucoencefalite, às quais os cães *toys* e de raças de pequeno porte são predispostos, a MEE idiopática é mais comumente diagnosticada em raças maiores. Especificamente, Rottweiler, Golden Retriever e Tervuren Belga parecem sobrerrepresentados para essa condição.[12-14] A ocorrência de MEE idiopática foi relatada apenas em uma parcela de cães de raças pequenas, incluindo Yorkshire Terrier, Beagle, Pug e Pinscher Miniatura. O diagnóstico pode ser feito com base nos achados clínicos, no aspecto na ressonância magnética e na análise do LCR com uma pleocitose eosinofílica (ver Capítulo 115). Uma grande variedade de aspectos de ressonância magnética é observada na MEE idiopática canina, incluindo varreduras normais.[11] Os mesmos protocolos de medicamentos usados para o tratamento de MEG e EN também têm sido usados com sucesso pelos autores.

Meningoencefalite não supurativa do Galgo

A meningoencefalite não supurativa dos Galgos é uma doença associada à raça, com distribuição de lesão única. Esse processo de doença afeta animais jovens da raça Galgo geralmente menores de 12 meses de idade. Assume-se a possibilidade de um fator de risco genético, uma vez que a doença foi mostrada em irmãos, e uma causa infecciosa ainda não foi identificada. Foi encontrada uma associação entre o haplótipo classe II de antígeno leucocitário e a meningoencefalite do cão Galgo.[15] Os sinais clínicos relatados são variados e incluem sinais prosencéfalicos (alteração do nível de consciência, mudanças de comportamento, cegueira) e sinais de tronco encefálico (inclinação de cabeça, andar em círculos, ataxia).[16] A ressonância magnética mostra anormalidades com predileção para as porções rostroventrais do cérebro, particularmente os lobos e bulbos olfatórios.[17] O exame histopatológico revela gliose grave e gemistocitose com infiltrado de células mononucleares perivasculares no núcleo caudato, na substância cinzenta cortical do cérebro e na sustância cinzenta periventricular em sua porção rostral do tronco encefálico. Lesões mais brandas também são encontradas na camada molecular do cerebelo, do tronco encefálico caudal e medula espinal cervical cranial.[18]

DOENÇAS INFECCIOSAS DO CÉREBRO

Infecções do cérebro podem resultar em disfunção neurológica produzindo efeito de massa (*i. e.*, abscesso organizado) ou liberação de toxinas e mediadores inflamatórios. Acredita-se que uma das principais causas dos déficits neurológicos sejam os fatores inflamatórios secundários em resposta induzida por microrganismos. Doenças infecciosas do cérebro são muito menos comumente encontradas em cães e gatos em comparação com doenças não infecciosas. Entretanto, há uma suposição dogmática de que esses distúrbios sejam raros, combinados à progressão clínica frequentemente rápida de tais doenças, o que pode colocar um paciente acometido em risco indevido de não receber terapia oportuna e apropriada. Essa é, obviamente, uma preocupação específica com as doenças infecciosas que podem responder a agentes antimicrobianos. Em alguns casos, descompressão cirúrgica ou remoção de abscesso cerebral ou de granuloma também podem ser indicadas em caráter de emergência.

Meningoencefalite bacteriana

As bactérias podem obter acesso ao cérebro por meio da via hematogênica ou por extensão da infecção de um foco vizinho (p. ex., extensão de otite interna). A BHE e a ausência de um sistema linfático no SNC ajudam a protegê-lo da invasão por microrganismos. Contudo, uma vez que um agente infeccioso tenha sucesso ao ultrapassar a BHE, a natureza imunologicamente privilegiada do SNC representa uma vantagem para o microrganismo invasor e um prejuízo para o hospedeiro. Microrganismos comumente implicados na meningoencefalite bacteriana canina e felina incluem espécies de *Staphylococcus* e *Streptococcus*, *Pasteurella multocida* (especialmente gatos), espécies de *Actinomyces* e *Nocardia*, bem como anaeróbios (p. ex., *Bacteroides*, *Peptostreptococcus*, *Fusobacterium* e *Eubacterium*). Em um relato de meningoencefalite bacteriana canina, os microrganismos causadores mais comuns foram *Escherichia coli*, espécies de *Streptococcus* e espécies de *Klebsiella*. As infecções gram-negativas foram as mais comuns, e as infecções por microrganismos múltiplos ou únicos foram igualmente prováveis.[19]

Cães e gatos de qualquer idade, raça ou sexo podem desenvolver meningoencefalite bacteriana, mas é mais comum em animais jovens do que em animais de meia-idade (p. ex., 1 a 7 anos). Sinais clínicos das disfunções neurológicas são frequentemente agudas e rapidamente progressivas. Febre e hiperestesia cervical são consideradas características clássicas da meningoencefalite bacteriana, mas podem não ser evidentes. Um diagnóstico provisório de meningoencefalite bacteriana é feito mediante dados do histórico e sinais clínicos, bem como resultados de exames laboratoriais. Uma resposta positiva aos antibióticos também apoia o diagnóstico. Os resultados do hemograma podem indicar uma resposta inflamatória sistêmica, mas nem sempre é o caso. Anormalidades em perfis de bioquímica sérica (p. ex., aumento da atividade de ALT e SAP, hipoglicemia, hiperglicemia) são aparentes na maioria dos casos. Imagens avançadas (TC, RM) podem ser úteis no diagnóstico de lesões de massa (Figura 261.3) ou hidrocefalia obstrutiva. As informações mais valiosas são obtidas por análise do LCR (ver Capítulo 115), que geralmente é anormal. Em casos agudos de meningoencefalite bacteriana, um padrão supurativo do LCR, frequentemente com neutrófilos degenerados e de aparência tóxica, é comum. Os teores de proteína também costumam ser elevados. A presença de bactérias intracelulares na amostra do LCR confirma o diagnóstico. Bactérias extracelulares podem representar agentes causadores, mas também podem ser contaminantes. Resultados positivos da cultura do LCR, sangue e/ou da urina também apoiam o diagnóstico de meningoencefalite bacteriana, mas muitas vezes são falsamente negativos (ver Capítulo 221).

O tratamento com antibiótico da meningoencefalite bacteriana de forma ideal deve ser baseado em resultados de cultura/sensibilidade do microrganismo causador. Uma vez que isso geralmente não pode ser obtido, a antibioticoterapia frequentemente baseia-se nos resultados da coloração de gram de microrganismos observados na análise do LCR ou no(s) patógeno(s) mais provável(is), caso os microrganismos não sejam observados. Antibióticos adequados para bactérias causadoras de meningoencefalite devem ser, de forma ideal, bactericidas, ter um baixo nível de ligação às proteínas e serem capazes de cruzar a BHE. A terapia intravenosa é recomendada por, pelo menos, 3 a 5 dias iniciais de terapia. Altas doses intravenosas de ampicilina (p. ex., 22 mg/kg a cada 6 horas) foram recomendadas como uma escolha terapêutica apropriada para a maioria dos casos de meningoencefalite bacteriana canina e felina. A ampicilina atravessa a BHE inflamada relativamente bem e é bactericida. Se uma infecção gram-negativa é suspeita ou confirmada, enrofloxacino (p. ex., 10 mg/kg IV, a cada 12 horas em cães) ou uma cefalosporina de terceira geração (p. ex., cefotaxima a 25 a 50 mg/kg IV a cada 8 horas) são boas escolhas terapêuticas. Metronidazol (10 mg/kg IV lentamente a cada 8 horas) é um excelente antibiótico de escolha para a maioria das infecções anaeróbicas. O metronidazol intravenoso deve ser administrado durante 30 a 40 minutos porque a infusão rápida pode causar hipotensão.

Em casos graves de meningoencefalite bacteriana, pode ser prudente instituir terapia antimicrobiana combinada enquanto se aguardam os resultados dos exames laboratoriais de LCR (coloração de gram, resultados de cultura). Com base nas informações sobre os agentes causais de meningoencefalite bacteriana canina, a inclusão de antibióticos com forte atividade contra bactérias gram-negativas é altamente recomendada. Uma vez que uma resposta positiva com antibioticoterapia intravenosa é alcançada, o paciente pode começar a receber terapia oral. Trimetoprima-sulfonamida (15 mg/kg, via oral a cada 12 horas) é de amplo espectro e bactericida, e penetra rapidamente na BHE, mesmo quando a BHE não está inflamada. Também estão disponíveis formulações orais de enrofloxacino e metronidazol. As recomendações para a duração da terapia antibiótica oral variam. A descontinuação da antibioticoterapia, de forma ideal, é baseada tanto nos sinais clínicos como nos resultados normais do LCR de acompanhamento. No entanto, as informações mencionadas anteriormente muitas vezes não estão disponíveis. A antibioticoterapia deve ser administrada durante 10 a 14 dias após a resolução dos sinais clínicos da doença. O uso de glicocorticoide em casos de infecção é teoricamente contraindicado, mas há evidências de que o uso transitório (máximo de 4 dias) de doses anti-inflamatórias de glicocorticoides melhora os resultados em pessoas com meningite bacteriana.[9] Essa terapia deve ser considerada para cães e gatos com esse distúrbio. Se as imagens de TC ou RM localizarem um abscesso acessível cirurgicamente, a intervenção cirúrgica poderá desempenhar um papel importante no tratamento da meningoencefalite bacteriana. Infelizmente, não há relatórios que descrevam grandes grupos de cães ou gatos que receberam tratamentos apropriados para meningoencefalite bacteriana confirmada.

A informação disponível escassa sugere um mau prognóstico. Em geral, as infecções bacterianas semelhantes no SNC de pessoas mostram que a chave para o tratamento bem-sucedido de cães e gatos com meningoencefalite bacteriana é um diagnóstico precoce e uma terapia rápida e agressiva.

Meningoencefalite fúngica

Existe uma grande variedade de microrganismos fúngicos que podem invadir o SNC, incluindo *Cryptococcus* (ver Capítulo 231), *Coccidioides* (ver Capítulo 232), *Blastomyces* (ver Capítulo 233), *Histoplasma* (ver Capítulo 233), *Aspergillus* (ver Capítulos 234 e 235) e as *feo-hifomicoses* (p. ex., *Cladosporium*; ver Capítulo 236). *Cryptococcus neoformans* é de longe o microrganismo fúngico mais comumente associado a meningoencefalite em cães e gatos. Meningoencefalite decorrente de coccidioidomicose foi relatada em 36 cães.[20] A doença fúngica é normalmente contraída por cães e gatos por meio de inalação de esporos de fungos. A infecção do SNC pode ocorrer via extensão local (p. ex., seio nasal/frontal) ou via hematógena. De forma semelhante à meningoencefalite bacteriana, cães e gatos com meningoencefalites fúngicas são frequentemente jovens à meia-idade. Embora os sinais clínicos de disfunção neurológica possam ter início agudo e progredir rapidamente, a meningoencefalite fúngica frequentemente é caracterizada por progressão lenta (semanas a meses) de

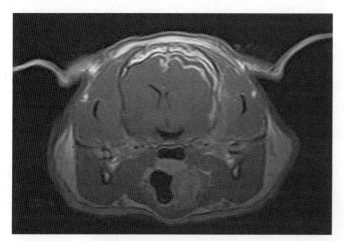

Figura 261.3 Imagem de ressonância magnética cerebral axial ponderada em T1 (com contraste) de um gato com abscesso cerebral. (Utilizada com permissão de Dewey CW: Encephalopathies: disorders of the brain. In Dewey CW, editor: *A practical guide to canine and feline neurology*, 2 ed., Hoboken, NJ, 2008, Wiley-Blackwell.)

disfunção neurológica, muitas vezes precedida por um período de doença inespecífica (p. ex., letargia, anorexia). Evidência clínica de infecção fúngica extraneural é comum em casos de meningoencefalite fúngica. Na criptococose, a infecção extraneural ao redor da região da cabeça (olhos, seios nasais e frontais) é mais provável. Em coccidioidomicose, a infecção inicial do sistema pulmonar é típica.

O diagnóstico da meningoencefalite fúngica é feito por identificação da presença do microrganismo fúngico no paciente que apresenta sinais de encefalopatia. O achado da presença do microrganismo fúngico em um sítio extraneural em um paciente com disfunção cerebral é uma forte evidência de meningoencefalite fúngica. É provável que a imagem cerebral (de preferência ressonância magnética) mostre lesões intra-axiais que intensificam fortemente o contraste (Figura 261.4). Esses granulomas fúngicos geralmente têm evidências de edema perilesional substancial. A identificação do microrganismo em uma amostra de LCR é a evidência mais forte para apoiar o diagnóstico, e é mais provável que isso ocorra com infecções por *Cryptococcus* do que com outras infecções fúngicas (ver Capítulo 115). Colorações especiais estão disponíveis para ajudar na identificação de fungos específicos em amostras de citologia. Infecções fúngicas do SNC geralmente causam pleocitose de células mistas com aumento do teor da proteína no exame do LCR. A natureza da pleocitose é altamente variável, mas geralmente inclui uma grande proporção de ambas as células mononucleares, bem como neutrófilos, típicos de doença granulomatosa. No relato de cães com coccidioidomicose intracraniana, pleocitose mononuclear foi a mais comumente mostrada, seguida de pleocitose por células mistas. Os eosinófilos também podem constituir uma grande proporção dos leucócitos no LCR em pacientes com meningoencefalite fúngica. O teste de LCR e/ou soro para anticorpos para antígenos fúngicos também podem ser realizados. Esses testes são muito confiáveis para infecções por *Cryptococcus*, *Coccidioides* e *Blastomyces*, menos fidedignos para infecções por *Aspergillus* e não confiáveis para infecções por *Histoplasma*. Esses testes não estão disponíveis para as feo-hifomicoses. Os vários fungos também podem ser cultivados a partir de líquidos corporais, usando meios de crescimento especiais; isso pode ser perigoso para a saúde humana no caso da blastomicose, coccidioidomicose e histoplasmose. As anormalidades do hemograma são variáveis e inespecíficas. Elementos fúngicos podem ser identificáveis em amostras de urina. O exame oftálmico pode mostrar evidências de doença inflamatória (p. ex., uveíte, coriorretinite; ver Capítulo 11). Lesões pulmonares podem ser identificáveis em alguns casos (p. ex., *Histoplasma Blastomyces, Coccidioides*) em radiografias torácicas. Gatos com suspeita ou confirmação de meningoencefalite fúngica devem ser testados para o vírus da leucemia felina (ver Capítulo 223) e o vírus da imunodeficiência felina (FIV; ver Capítulo 222).

O tratamento e prognóstico para meningoencefalite fúngica canina e felina são mal definidos. Embora medicamentos antifúngicos constituam a base do tratamento para esses casos, a remoção cirúrgica/citorredução de grandes granulomas intracranianos às vezes pode ser indicada. De forma semelhante à meningoencefalite bacteriana, dados que descrevem um grande número de cães e gatos com doença fúngica no SNC tratados com agentes antifúngicos de forma apropriada estão em falta. É provável que a meningoencefalite causada por *Aspergillus* ou feo-hifomicose seja fatal. Poucos fármacos antifúngicos são capazes de cruzar a BHE de forma eficaz, mesmo quando está inflamada. A flucitosina (5-fluorocitosina) e o fármaco triazol/fluconazol são dois antifúngicos que cruzam facilmente a BHE. Existem vários relatos de remissões ou curas em pacientes com criptococose do SNC tratados com combinações de medicamentos que incluíam flucitosina e/ou os fármacos triazólicos mais recentes (itraconazol e fluconazol). O uso de flucitosina isoladamente pode levar ao desenvolvimento de resistência ao medicamento. Em uma publicação na qual 36 cães estavam com coccidioidomicose intracraniana, 84% melhoraram, ou o caso foi resolvido com o uso de fluconazol.[20] Uma vez que os sinais clínicos da doença estejam controlados, a maioria dos pacientes com meningoencefalite fúngica necessita de terapia antifúngica a longo prazo (meses). Na experiência do autor, a terapia com fluconazol para casos de meningoencefalite fúngica pode precisar ser muito prolongada. No relato com 36 cães com meningoencefalite por coccidioidomicose, o tempo mínimo de tratamento foi de 1 ano.[20] A decisão do momento para interromper o tratamento antifúngico deve ser com base em sinais clínicos, resultados repetidos do LCR e títulos sorológicos ou do LCR para o microrganismo (se apropriado). Uma vez que o fluconazol penetra bem na BHE e o itraconazol não, o fluconazol é o agente antifúngico de escolha para o tratamento de infecção fúngica do SNC (5 mg/kg VO a cada 12 horas). A principal desvantagem do uso de fluconazol é o alto custo do medicamento. Embora controverso, pode ser benéfico administrar baixas doses de prednisona oral (p. ex., 0,5 mg/kg a cada 12 horas) no período inicial de tratamento (1 a 2 semanas), para combater o edema perilesional.

Meningoencefalite viral

As infecções virais mais frequentemente encontradas no cérebro em cães e gatos na prática clínica são o vírus da cinomose (paramixovírus; ver Capítulo 228) e vírus da peritonite infecciosa felina (PIF – coronavírus; ver Capítulo 224), respectivamente.

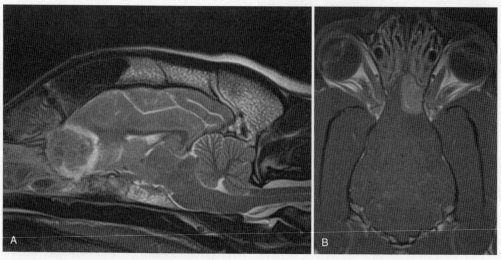

Figura 261.4 Imagens de ressonância magnética ponderada em T2 sagital (**A**) e ponderada em T1 dorsal pós-contraste (**B**) de um cão com granuloma criptocócico.

Outras causas menos comuns de meningoencefalites virais incluem vírus da raiva (cães e gatos; ver Capítulo 226), FIV (um lentivírus; ver Capítulo 222), herpes-vírus canino (ver Capítulo 228), parvovírus felino (vírus da panleucopenia; ver Capítulo 225), vírus da doença de Borna felina (BDV; ver Capítulo 270), pseudorraiva (cães e gatos, causada por um herpes-vírus suíno; ver Capítulo 228) e o vírus do Nilo Ocidental (flavivírus transmitido por mosquitos; ver Capítulo 228). O envolvimento do SNC raramente é relatado em associação com adenovírus canino (vírus da hepatite infecciosa canina), vírus da parainfluenza canina (também um paramixovírus) e parvovírus canino. Existem múltiplas vias de infecção viral, mas a inalação é a mais comum. A raiva é normalmente contraída por meio de feridas por mordida do animal infectado e pseudorraiva pela ingestão de carne de porco crua infectada. O FIV pode ser transmitido por feridas de mordida. Os vírus podem causar danos no parênquima cerebral por via direta (p. ex., citolítica) e indireta (p. ex., efeito imunomediado). Alguns vírus têm predileção por células neuronais e gliais e são denominados "neurotrópicos". Esses vírus incluem os agentes causadores de cinomose canina, raiva, pseudorraiva e doença de Borna felina.

Tal como acontece com outras doenças infecciosas do SNC, os animais acometidos frequentemente são jovens à meia-idade. Infecções virais do SNC normalmente têm um curso agudo a subagudo, mas pode ser hiperagudo (p. ex., pseudorraiva) ou insidioso (PIF) no início e na progressão. Os sinais clínicos de encefalopatia multifocal são comuns. Sinais extraneurais (p. ex., febre, doença oftálmica, doença respiratória) de infecções virais podem ou não estar presentes. Na meningoencefalite canina, histórico ou evidência clínica de doença gastrintestinal e/ou respiratória antes ou concomitante às disfunções neurológicas são achados clássicos que dão suporte ao diagnóstico. Hiperqueratose, ou "almofada dura", que afeta os coxins plantares e/ou o plano nasal, é outro achado clássico e ainda indicador incompatível com infecção por cinomose canina. Outras manifestações extraneurais de infecção pelo vírus da cinomose em cães incluem conjuntivite mucopurulenta, rinite mucopurulenta e coriorretinite (ver Capítulo 11). O envolvimento extraneural pode ser inexistente ou subclínico e, portanto, pode não ser estimado. Mioclonia (contração muscular rítmica e repetitiva), em um ou mais membros e/ou músculos da cabeça, é um achado clínico relativamente específico e comum na infecção canina por cinomose do SNC (ver Capítulo 31). Pensa-se que a mioclonia seja decorrente da atividade anormal do marca-passo nos neurônios danificados pelo vírus. "Mastigar chiclete" – movimentos rítmicos de mandíbula apresentados por alguns cães com cinomose – pode representar uma forma de mioclonia ou atividade convulsiva focal. A infecção do SNC por PIF (coronavírus) está frequentemente associada à forma não efusiva da doença. O histórico e os sinais clínicos de doença sistêmica (p. ex., febre, perda de peso) são comuns em gatos com meningoencefalite por coronavírus. A encefalopatia multifocal é comum, muitas vezes com disfunção no tronco encefálico e cerebelo.

Um histórico de vacinação ruim ou inexistente em uma situação aguda de encefalopatia em cão ou gato com possível exposição à vida selvagem ou a outros cães ou gatos não vacinados deve alertar o clínico a considerar o diagnóstico diferencial para raiva (ver Capítulo 226). As formas típicas de raiva "furiosa" e "paralítica" foram descritas. A forma furiosa é mais comum em gatos e é caracterizada por apreensão e agressão, sugerindo principalmente disfunção do prosencéfalo. A forma paralítica, encontrada com maior frequência em cães, é caracterizada por disfunção do neurônio motor inferior dos núcleos do tronco cerebral, levando a uma mandíbula caída (NC V), dificuldade para engolir e ptialismo concomitante (NCs IX a XI). Dificuldades respiratórias e anormalidades da marcha também podem estar presentes. Atividade convulsiva focal e/ou generalizada pode ocorrer com ambas as formas de raiva. Cães e gatos com raiva podem se apresentar com uma ampla variedade de

sinais clínicos e de disfunções neurológicas, e as formas anteriormente mencionadas da raiva devem ser observadas como um guia geral.

O diagnóstico de meningoencefalite viral geralmente é feito na necropsia. A identificação do vírus causador no parênquima cerebral é feita por meio de vários métodos (p. ex., visualização de corpúsculos de inclusão, imunocitoquímica, isolamento viral) e o aparecimento de padrões histológicos característicos (p. ex., piogranulomas em PIF, lesões desmielinizantes do tronco encefálico na cinomose) ajudam a confirmar o diagnóstico de uma encefalopatia induzida por vírus específico. No caso de um cão ou gato não vacinado que morreu ou foi sacrificado por causa de doença cerebral (de início recente) e teve exposição a pessoas (especialmente feridas por mordidas), exame do cérebro (p. ex., teste de anticorpo fluorescente direto) para raiva é obrigatório. O diagnóstico *ante mortem* de meningoencefalite viral muitas vezes é difícil de ser obtido e depende da combinação de achados históricos e clínicos característicos com diversos testes diagnósticos. Testes diagnósticos específicos e confiáveis para meningoencefalite viral estão em falta. Intuitivamente, a identificação da presença de um agente viral em um paciente que apresenta sinais encefalopáticos apontaria esse vírus como o fator causal. Todavia, a identificação de vírus ou antígenos virais em tecidos corporais ou fluidos geralmente não é bem-sucedida. O teste do anticorpo fluorescente indireto para cinomose canina, geralmente realizado por raspado de conjuntiva, esfregaço de capa leucocitária e/ou sedimento urinário, pode produzir muitos resultados falsos negativos e falsos positivos, por isso não é de grande valia no uso clínico. A identificação de anticorpos circulantes contra vários vírus no sangue e no LCR pode ser realizada. Uma vez que o paciente pode ter sido exposto natural ou intencionalmente (vacinação) ao vírus patógeno suspeito no passado, um título positivo de anticorpos séricos frequentemente tem pouco significado clínico. Da mesma forma, um paciente previamente imunizado para uma doença viral específica que mostra um título positivo no LCR para esse agente viral tem pouco significado clínico. Se a BHE é ultrapassada por qualquer motivo, os anticorpos séricos podem se mover passivamente através do LCR. A demonstração de um gradiente de títulos (*i. e.*, título para um anticorpo antiviral no LCR superior ao título sérico) é a evidência mais definitiva do vírus como agente causador da doença.

Mais recentemente foi descrito o uso de um teste de transcriptase reversa, reação da polimerase em cadeia (RT-PCR), para amplificar o vírus da cinomose canina, produtos de RNA específicos no soro e no LCR. Esse procedimento de PCR parece ser um teste *ante mortem* específico para infecção pelo vírus da cinomose canina. Os autores têm tido uma série de resultados positivos de RT-PCR para coronavírus do LCR obtidos de gatos com suspeita ou PIF neurológica comprovada. A sensibilidade e especificidade de RT-PCR para LCR em PIF neurológica são atualmente desconhecidas; é provável que esse teste seja sensível, mas não específico para PIF neurológica. Alguns testes básicos de laboratório podem fornecer evidências de suporte para infecções virais específicas, caso estejam anormais. Linfopenia pode ocorrer com infecções pelo vírus da cinomose canina (ver Capítulo 228), e a hiperglobulinemia é comum com infecções por PIF (ver Capítulo 224). O exame oftálmico pode fornecer evidências clínicas valiosas em algumas doenças (p. ex., lesões de retina hiper-reflexiva na cinomose canina; ver Capítulo 11).

Os valores do LCR costumam ser anormais na meningoencefalite viral. Cães imaturos com cinomose que afeta principalmente a substância cinzenta podem ter resultados normais do LCR. O resultado característico da análise da LCR em um paciente com doença viral do SNC consiste predominantemente em pleocitose mononuclear (linfocítica) com proteína elevada. A exceção a essa regra é o LCR do paciente com PIF. O coronavírus tende a induzir uma resposta imunológica intensa nessa doença, e o tipo de célula predominante na meningoencefalite por PIF geralmente é o neutrófilo, com números variáveis de linfócitos e macrófagos (uma resposta piogranulomatosa). Os títulos de IgG no LCR para coronavírus felino provavelmente não são úteis para o diagnóstico.

Imagens avançadas (TC/IRM) podem mostrar lesões no cérebro (p. ex., regiões de realce de contraste e focos inflamatórios) em alguns casos de meningoencefalite viral. Embora a imagem cerebral provavelmente não revele anormalidades características específicas na maioria dos casos, pode ser útil descartar outras doenças (p. ex., cistos intra-aracnóideos intracranianos em cães e gatos jovens). A hidrocefalia pode ser uma sequela comum da meningoencefalite por PIF, que pode ser observada em imagem de TC ou RM. Realce de contraste periventricular também foi descrito em imagens do cérebro na RM de gatos com meningoencefalite por PIF. Gatos com meningoencefalite por PIF confirmada podem ter imagens normais de RM do cérebro.

Não existem agentes antivirais eficazes disponíveis para meningoencefalite por vírus, e o prognóstico para essas doenças geralmente varia de ruim a grave para a sobrevida. Raiva e pseudorraiva progridem rápido e invariavelmente são fatais (com frequência em razão de falha respiratória) em 1 semana e 48 horas, após o início do quadro clínico, respectivamente. A PIF normalmente progride por várias semanas e também é invariavelmente fatal. Os cães com infecções do SNC por cinomose, em sua maioria, morrem ou são sacrificados em razão da disfunção neurológica progressiva. Entretanto, os sinais clínicos da doença podem permanecer estáticos ou melhorar em alguns cães, e a sobrevivência é possível com os devidos cuidados ambulatoriais. Doses anti-inflamatórias de prednisona frequentemente são prescritas para diminuir os efeitos secundários de infecção viral no tecido do SNC nesses casos. Encefalopatia associada a FIV parece ter um curso crônico sem progressão dos sinais clínicos em muitos casos.

Outras doenças infecciosas

Outros microrganismos infecciosos que podem levar à encefalopatia multifocal em cães e gatos incluem riquétsia (p. ex., erliquiose, febre maculosa das Montanhas Rochosas [FMMR] em cães; ver Capítulo 218), protozoário (p. ex., *Toxoplasma* em cães e gatos, *Neospora* em cães; ver Capítulo 221) e verminose (p. ex., *Cuterebra* em gatos). *Toxoplasma gondii* e *Neospora caninum* são protozoários conhecidos por ocasionalmente causarem meningoencefalite em cães. *Toxoplasma* também foi relatado como causador de meningoencefalite em gatos. Infecção experimental de gatos com *Neospora* pode causar meningoencefalite, mas nenhum caso de ocorrência natural foi relatado. Meningoencefalite canina e felina decorrente de um microrganismo que parece ser *Sarcocystis* também foi relatada.

Para infecções por riquetsioses e protozoários, o diagnóstico *ante mortem* é geralmente baseado em testes sorológicos para a presença do microrganismo agressor (i. e., aumento dos títulos de anticorpos), em conjunto com outras evidências de suporte (p. ex., trombocitopenia em um cão com infecção por FMMR). Infelizmente, o diagnóstico de meningoencefalite verminótica requer a identificação do parasita, o que muitas vezes não é possível. Imagem avançada (de preferência ressonância magnética) pode mostrar o aumento de contraste nas lesões cerebrais nessas infecções, e os resultados do LCR são provavelmente anormais. Distribuições variáveis de tipos de células foram relatadas em análises de LCR de pacientes com essa doença infecciosa.

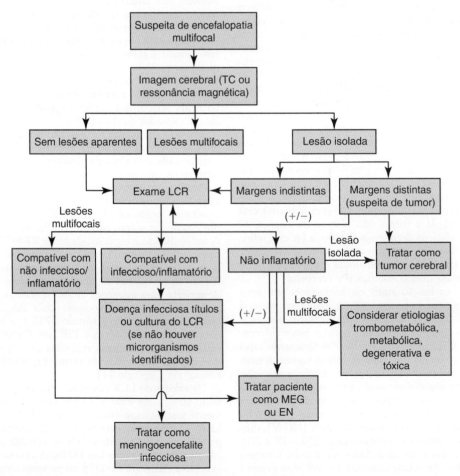

Figura 261.5 Algoritmo para suspeita de encefalopatia multifocal. *EN*, encefalite necrosante; *LCR*, líquido cefalorraquidiano; *MEG*, meningoencefalomielite granulomatosa; *RM*, imagem de ressonância magnética; *TC*, tomografia computadorizada.

Fármacos usados para tratar cães com meningoencefalite por riquetsiose incluem doxiciclina, cloranfenicol e enrofloxacino. Clindamicina ou sulfonamidas combinadas com trimetoprima ou pirimetamina são recomendadas para meningoencefalite protozoária. Em casos suspeitos de cuterebríase do SNC em gatos, o tratamento com ivermectina é recomendado. Esses gatos deveriam ser pré-tratados com difenidramina e glicocorticoides a fim de melhorar as reações alérgicas a larvas mortas e as que morrem na região intracraniana. Além disso, é recomendado tratar esses gatos por 2 semanas com antibióticos (p. ex., amoxicilina/ácido clavulânico) após o tratamento com ivermectina, para minimizar a probabilidade de meningoencefalite bacteriana secundária.

DISTÚRBIOS DEGENERATIVOS E ANOMALIAS DO CÉREBRO

Distúrbios cerebrais degenerativos (ver também Capítulo 260) que podem causar encefalopatia multifocal ou difusa são numerosos e incluem doenças de armazenamento lisossomal, encefalopatias mitocondriais e acidúrias orgânicas. Essas categorias de doenças degenerativas compreendem uma grande variedade de anormalidades genéticas (principalmente autossômicas recessivas), que têm em comum o acúmulo intracelular de um ou mais

produtos de uma via metabólica de degradação interrompida. O defeito metabólico é responsável pelo desenvolvimento de doença intracraniana, normalmente por meio de um acúmulo de subproduto(s) que leva à disfunção celular, presumivelmente decorrente do inchaço celular, um efeito tóxico do(s) material(is) acumulado(s), ou ambos. Em geral, o diagnóstico dessas doenças requer a identificação do defeito enzimático específico, do acúmulo ou armazenamento um produto e/ou um gene defeituoso responsável pela anormalidade. Atualmente, os tratamentos são limitados para esses distúrbios e o prognóstico é frequentemente reservado a ruim. Existem várias anomalias cerebrais que podem levar a sinais clínicos multifocais ou difusos de disfunção cerebral, que incluem síndrome de malformação occipital caudal (SMOC, também conhecida como malformação de *Chiari tipo I* e *hipoplasia óssea occipital*), cisto aracnoide intracraniano e hidrocefalia congênita. Esses distúrbios são mais bem diagnosticados em imagem de ressonância magnética e tratados com uma combinação de manejo cirúrgico e clínico (Figura 261.5).

REFERÊNCIAS BIBLIOGRÁFICAS

As referências bibliográficas deste capítulo se encontram online no Ambiente de Aprendizagem.

CAPÍTULO 262

Distúrbios do Sono

Brian M. Zanghi

O sono é um processo fisiológico complexo, determinado por um estado neurocomportamental ativo, mantido pelo sistema nervoso central (SNC). Em última análise, o sono desempenha um papel essencial na restauração das funções físicas e cognitivas e é indispensável para uma vida saudável. A ocorrência natural de distúrbios do sono é relativamente incomum em gatos e cães. Em todos os tipos de distúrbio, a condição pode variar de sutil a grave, mas também pode indicar outra doença neurológica subjacente. Ter alguma familiaridade tanto com o sono normal quanto o anormal ajuda no diagnóstico de anormalidades associadas ao sono.

SONO NORMAL

O sono não é um estado de repouso passivo, mas uma fisiologia dinâmica controlada por processos neurológicos muito ativos.[1] Os horários de pico da atividade locomotora "normal" ou sono em gatos e cães são influenciados pela frequência de alimentação,[2-4] idade,[2,3,5] habitação (interna e/ou externa)[6] e rotina do proprietário.[7,8] Além disso, a atividade durante a vigília e o descanso nos períodos de sono podem ser influenciados por muitos outros fatores, incluindo luz ambiente, temperatura, presença de outros animais e fome. Desse modo, considerar o ambiente doméstico, a idade e o padrão de alimentação do animal de companhia, além do horário do proprietário, ajuda a avaliar o padrão de sono normal de cada animal e os fatores que influenciam e, portanto, auxiliam na avaliação de um distúrbio intrínseco ou extrínseco do sono antes de conduzir uma avaliação diagnóstica mais completa.

A cronobiologia e as características do sono têm sido bem documentadas em humanos e roedores nas últimas décadas.[9-15] Além disso, existe uma compreensão das características normais de eletroencefalografia (EEG) mensurada durante o sono em cães[16-19] e em gatos.[20-23] O sono normal consiste nos estados de REM (em inglês *rapid eyes movements*, movimento rápido dos olhos) e não REM (ou sono de ondas lentas [SOL]), que todas as espécies de mamífero experimentam. O processo de sono começa com a transição para SOL, seguido pelo sono REM e um breve estado de vigília, antes de entrar novamente no ciclo e reiniciar o SOL.[16,18] Os estágios SOL e o sono REM são mais bem determinados por polissonografia (PSG), que permite a geração simultânea de dados de EEG, eletro-oculograma (EOG) e/ou eletromiografia (EMG), que são resumidos para gerar um hipnograma (Figura 262.1). Embora PSG seja considerado o padrão-ouro na determinação do estado de sono/vigília, é difícil conduzir esse exame em um cenário clínico normal por ser demorado, caro e requer a fixação de vários eletrodos, de maneira que evite o deslocamento. Como consequência, o PSG é amplamente limitado ao uso experimental e não é oferecido pelos clínicos.

As proporções relativas de diferentes estados de sono e vigília observados em cães alojados em canis são geralmente semelhantes em múltiplos estudos.[16-19] A vigília de cães adultos predomina durante o dia, compreendendo de 7 a 8 horas das 12 horas do dia (ciclo de luz),[19,24] em comparação a aproximadamente 5 horas durante a noite. Em contraste com os cães, gatos alojados com ciclos de luz/escuridão de 12 horas exibem comportamento noturno (42% do dia em estado de vigília/sonolência contra 53% durante a fase escura).[23]

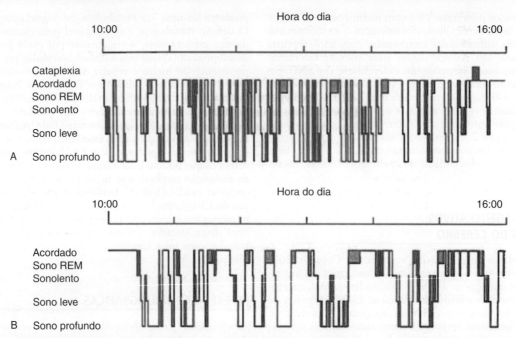

Figura 262.1 Hipnogramas de um Dobermann narcoléptico (**A**) e de Dobermann e saudável (controle) (**B**). As gravações foram realizadas por eletroencefalografia (EEG) cortical e músculo do pescoço. O monitoramento de eletromiografia (EMG) com eletrodos implantados cronicamente (Shelton e colegas de trabalho, 1995). O sono foi avaliado com base nos sinais de EEG e EMG e a cada período de 30 segundos foi classificado como vigília, sonolência, sono leve, sono profundo ou sono de movimento rápido dos olhos (*REM*) (ou cataplexia para o cão narcoléptico). (Utilizada, com autorização, de Tonokura M, Fujita K, Nishino S: Revisão da fisiopatologia e manejo clínico da narcolepsia em cães. *Vet Rec* 161: 375-380, 2007.)

ALTERAÇÕES GERIÁTRICAS NO SONO E RITMO CIRCADIANO

Como em humanos,[25,26] foram relatadas mudanças nos ritmos de sono/vigília mensurados por PSG em cães de acordo com a idade,[27] e os proprietários têm percebido que a atividade declina conforme o animal envelhece.[28-30] Cães idosos (com mais de 9 anos) podem ter atividade locomotora menor, sono diurno mais prolongado, diminuição do sono REM, sono fragmentado durante o dia (cochilos mais curtos, porém mais frequentes) e aumento da vigília PSG noturna.[3,27,31] No entanto, não foi definido se as interrupções do sono noturno relatadas por tutores estão relacionadas ao aumento da vigília PSG noturna ou se são sintomas de outra alteração comportamental/física relacionada à idade.

Mudanças de sono relacionadas à idade nas pessoas estão ligadas a alterações do ritmo circadiano[25,26,32,33] e a disfunção cognitivas, como em pacientes com Alzheimer, que têm significativamente mais sono diurno, sono noturno interrompido[34] e hiper e hipoatividade exageradas.[35,36] Cães com deficiência cognitiva[31] também experimentam um atraso no pico de atividade (mudança de ritmo circadiano), mas, na ausência de disfunção cognitiva, isso não parece ocorrer como consequência da idade avançada.[2] A relação entre idade avançada, padrões comportamentais de sono/atividade e comprometimento cognitivo tem sido inicialmente explorada apenas em cães.[31,37,38] Além disso, a hiperatividade relacionada a idade (9 a 15 anos) parece associada a uma progressão da disfunção de múltiplos domínios cognitivos,[31,37] e não apenas de um único domínio.[38] Caso seja grave, pode ser mais bem tratada por meio da abordagem do comprometimento cognitivo subjacente (ver Capítulo 263).

ABORDAGEM DIAGNÓSTICA

Os distúrbios do sono são primários ou secundários. *Distúrbios secundários do sono* podem resultar de encefalite por massas intracranianas, trauma, administração de fármacos ou outros processos mórbidos. Além de histórico completo e de exame físico e neurológico (ver Capítulo 2 e 259), um vídeo do tutor documentando o evento é inestimável – caso ocorra durante o sono –, uma vez que a maioria dos animais não vai relaxar o suficiente para dormir no consultório do veterinário. Informações sobre o início do evento após o sono, como duração e se o animal despertou, ajudam o clínico a determinar a possibilidade de um distúrbio do sono. Uma convulsão verdadeira deve ser descartada, uma vez que a maioria dos animais tem o início de ataques epilépticos durante o sono. Em contrapartida, um distúrbio do sono deve ser considerado caso um animal seja tratado por suspeita de epilepsia mas com resposta mínima ou nenhuma resposta a doses apropriadas de fármacos anticonvulsivantes.

Triagem sistemática com exames de sangue, radiografias do tórax e abdome e ultrassom abdominal descartam outras doenças. Anormalidades no exame neurológico devem aumentar a suspeita de doença primária do SNC, mas a imagem intracraniana com ressonância magnética (RM) e a análise do líquido cefalorraquidiano (LCR) são necessários para descartar doença cerebral estrutural ou doença infecciosa/inflamatória. Se uma doença intracraniana for identificada em um paciente com distúrbio do sono, a doença primária deve ser tratada, se possível, antes de qualquer tratamento específico do distúrbio do sono, pois o distúrbio pode ser secundário a uma doença cerebral subjacente.

DISTÚRBIO DE COMPORTAMENTO DO SONO REM

Durante o sono REM, a inibição normal dos neurônios motores faz a maioria dos músculos se tornar atônica. Existem exceções com atividade contrátil menor e/ou aleatória do diafragma, músculos intercostais e pequenos músculos distais da face, patas, laringe e cauda.[39-42] Essa atividade muscular localizada resulta em espasmos característicos dos olhos, rosto, laringe e patas, com menor contração coordenada às vezes levando a movimentos de "pedalagem" dos quatro membros (não em gatos),[39,41] representando um estado de "sonho". No transtorno do sono (TS) durante a fase REM, nenhuma atonia muscular está presente, e ocorre movimento coordenado significativo, que muitas vezes resulta em movimentos violentos dos membros,[39,41,43] mas também pode se apresentar na forma de mastigação e ranger de dentes, mordedura do ar ou da roupa de cama e atacar o dono ou outro cão.[43]

No homem, a suspeita diagnóstica de TS é baseada nos critérios clínicos e PSG,[44] que requer: (1) o PSG determinando o sono REM sem atonia; (2) o PSG documentando anormalidades durante o sono REM (aumento do tom da EMG e/ou contração excessiva física dos membros); e (3) a ausência de uma atividade epileptiforme no EEG durante o sono REM. Em razão da raridade de TS em medicina veterinária, há pouca necessidade do uso de PSG em casos com suspeita de TS. Portanto, o diagnóstico de TS na maioria das vezes se baseia em: (1) uma descrição dos sinais clínicos que são característicos de comportamentos do TS; e (2) a avaliação de vídeos dos eventos que ocorrem durante o sono.

Relatos fornecidos por tutores de animais de companhia revelam que, em 93% dos cães com TS (13 de 14 casos), os eventos não tiveram sucesso quando tratados com melatonina, gabapentina, diazepam, difenidramina, acepromazina, clonazepam ou fenobarbital.[41,43] Todavia, a dose e a frequência desses tratamentos não foram relatadas pelos tutores durante o estudo de revisão.[43] O brometo de potássio (44 mg/kg, 1 vez/dia) diminuiu a gravidade e a frequência de eventos de TS relatados por 78% dos tutores de cães (11 casos).[43] Além disso, a redução da gravidade do episódio de TS durante o sono noturno a longo prazo (6 meses) foi observada com o uso da clomipramina, começando na dose de 1 mg/kg VO, a cada 12 horas, e aumentando progressivamente para 4 mg/kg VO, a cada 12 horas por 12 semanas.[45]

DISTÚRBIOS RESPIRATÓRIOS DO SONO OU APNEIA DO SONO

A apneia do sono é um problema comum em humanos. As características dos distúrbios respiratórios do sono (DRS) incluem saturação de oxigênio arterial normal quando acordado, mas respiração desordenada e episódios de dessaturação de oxigênio durante o sono, particularmente no sono REM, com frequência causando o despertar. A hipersonolência, ou sonolência diurna excessiva, também está presente, provavelmente como resultado de uma interrupção contínua do sono. A conformação braquicefálica tem características anatômicas (estenose das narinas, palato mole alongado, traqueia hipoplásica), que aumentam a resistência das vias respiratórias superiores e podem causar padrão de obstrução respiratória (ver Capítulo 238). Clinicamente, a respiração de um cão braquicefálico pode ser exacerbada pela excitação ou esforço (aumento da passagem de ar) ou pelo relaxamento da região faríngea (anestesia, sedação, sono).

A raça Buldogue Inglês foi proposta como um modelo natural de DRS. Esse cão mostra dessaturação de oxigênio acentuada no sono REM, padrões de respiração paradoxais (movimentos torácicos e abdominais não sincronizados) e despertar durante eventos de apneia.[46,47] O Buldogue também adormece mais rápido do que cães-controle, sugerindo hipersonolência. Melhora clínica da hipersonolência em um cão foi observada após uma cirurgia das vias respiratórias superiores para aliviar o quadro clínico.[46] O Buldogue também foi usado para avaliar a eficácia de muitas terapias medicamentosas experimentais com serotoninérgicos.[48-50]

NARCOLEPSIA (NARCOLEPSIA-CATAPLEXIA)

A narcolepsia ocorre em animais e humanos e é uma doença crônica de distúrbio do sono de origem neurológica, caracterizada em cães por sonolência diurna excessiva e/ou ataque cataplexico pronunciado (perda repentina de tônus muscular). Por apresentarem características clínicas muito semelhantes ao homem com narcolepsia/cataplexia, cães acometidos passaram por muitas pesquisas para determinar a patologia subjacente, o que facilitou os critérios para o diagnóstico positivo de narcolepsia primária em animais e no homem.

Formas de narcolepsia primária e fisiopatologia

A narcolepsia canina primária existe na forma familiar ou esporádica e é estimada com prevalência muito baixa em cães (menos de 0,2%).[51] A forma esporádica é a mais comum, tendo sido observada em mais de 17 raças,[51,52] e seu início ocorre em uma ampla faixa de idades (7 semanas a 7 anos). Para família de cães acometidos, ela começa antes dos 6 meses de idade[53,54] e é resultado de uma mutação no gene do receptor-2 da hipocretina (*Hcrtr2*), hereditária através da genética mendeliana clássica. A etiologia de ambas as formas está associada a um déficit na neurotransmissão de hipocretina.[52,55]

Sinais clínicos de narcolepsia

O diagnóstico de narcolepsia em cães concentra-se principalmente na ocorrência de cataplexia, que pode se manifestar como uma leve perda de tônus muscular esquelético ou fraqueza muscular, provavelmente observada como colapso de ambos os membros pélvicos e acompanhada por queda do pescoço. Em condições moderadas, o cão pode parecer sonolento ou resistente à "sonolência", enquanto em formas mais grave os ataques podem levar a uma paralisia completa e colapso, durando de alguns segundos a minutos. Salivação excessiva e incontinência *não* são observados durante um ataque cataplético como nas convulsões. Como a narcolepsia é um distúrbio do sono, os cães que apresentam ataques catapléticos prolongados podem apresentar também características do sono REM. Após um ataque cataplético, os cães se levantam e retomam a atividade normal ou possivelmente entram em sono normal.

Diagnóstico

Para um diagnóstico adequado, é importante descartar ataques cataplépticos resultantes de outros distúrbios episódicos, como convulsões ou síncope.[56] Informações relatadas pelos tutores sobre ataques prévios e idade de início também ajudam a avaliar como e quando os ataques ocorrem.

Um ataque cataplético pode ser desencadeado por experiências emocionais positivas, como brincadeiras ou oferecimento da comida favorita. Assim, a cataplexia pode ser avaliada clinicamente usando o teste de cataplexia induzida por alimentos (FIAT).[57] Porém, se o cão estiver nervoso durante o exame, pode não exibir os ataques e, portanto, testes em casa com gravação de vídeo são benéficos. Videoclipes de ataques típicos de cataplexia e FIAT estão incluídos (Vídeos 262.1 e 262.2), assim como estão disponíveis *on-line* no site da Escola de Medicina de Stanford, Center for Narcolepsy, em *http://med.stanford.edu/psychiatry/narcolepsy* (2014).

Mensurar a concentração de peptídio hipocretina-1 (inferior a 80 pg/mℓ; normal = 250 a 350 pg/mℓ) no LCR é a ferramenta mais específica e sensível para diagnosticar a forma esporádica de narcolepsia.[55] Casos da forma familiar, que resulta de uma mutação no gene do receptor Hcrtr2, têm concentrações "normais" de hipocretina no LCR, o que, portanto, não exclui o diagnóstico de narcolepsia.[55]

Se houver suspeita de uma forma leve de narcolepsia/cataplexia, o desafio farmacológico pode ser útil para diagnosticar cães, além de ser bem tolerado. Tem-se estabelecido aumento da atividade colinérgica para desencadear o sono REM,[57] e inibidores centrais ativos da acetilcolinesterase (salicilato de fisostigmina; 0,025 a 0,1 mg/kg, via intravenosa) aumentam a frequência de ataques catapléticos em 15 minutos em cães narcolépticos, mas não têm efeito em cães não narcolépticos. Recomenda-se iniciar com a dose mais baixa, por causa de possíveis efeitos adversos de salivação e diarreia.

SEÇÃO 17 • Doença Neurológica

Tabela 262.1 Medicamentos anticatapléticos para o tratamento da narcolepsia em cães.

TIPO DE FÁRMACO	COMPOSTO	DOSAGEM DIÁRIA (MG/KG VIA ORAL)	MEIA-VIDA (HORAS)	EFEITOS COLATERAIS (CLASSIFICAÇÃO)	COMENTÁRIOS	REFERÊNCIAS
Antidepressivo tricíclico	Imipramina	1,5-3	5-30	Vômito, anorexia, letargia, diarreia, anticolinérgico, anti-histaminérgico	Deve-se tomar cuidado se o cão for epilético	57-59
	Clomipramina	3-6	15-60			57
	Desipramina	2-3 vezes ao dia	10-30			57, 61
Inibidor de recaptação serotonina/ noradrenalina	Venlafaxina	6-12	4*	Sem lado anticolinérgico efeitos		62
Antagonista alfa-2 adrenérgico	Ioimbina	0,045 duas vezes diariamente†	< 1	Convulsões, excitação, músculos tremor, ptialismo		61

*O metabólito ativo é O-desmetilvenlafaxina, que tem meia-vida de 11 horas. †Pode desenvolver-se tolerância e os sinais clínicos são moderadamente bem controlados com alteração do regime mensal entre ioimbina e desipramina.

Tratamento e prognóstico

O tratamento da narcolepsia em animais visa principalmente reduzir a frequência e a duração dos ataques catapléticos. A melhor forma de tratar cães com ataques catapléticos leves a moderados é evitar a causa precursora, limitando assim as brincadeiras ou comportamentos que desencadeiam os episódios. Em casas com vários cães, alimentar o cão narcoléptico em local ou horário diferente dos demais cães pode reduzir as ocorrências. Mostrou-se eficácia em reduzir (mas não curar) os episódios catapléticos uma mudança na rotina e a administração oral de vários medicamentos (Tabela 262.1). A ativação do sistema adrenérgico, que inibe a cataplexia, é a principal forma de tratamento.[57] Registrar a frequência dos ataques catapléticos e a hora do término de uma refeição quando ocorrem os ataques é útil para avaliar a eficácia do tratamento e a dose diária do fármaco.

A narcolepsia canina não é progressiva, nem ameaça a vida, mas requer cuidados adequados por parte do tutor ao longo da vida do animal. A qualidade de vida do cão pode ser mantida com o conhecimento do tutor sobre a doença, para que provisões possam ser feitas, tornando o ambiente melhor e mais seguro. O cuidado deve incluir o uso de vasilhas de comida inquebráveis e de água elevada (possivelmente ao nível do ombro) para prevenção de acidentes caso o animal sofra um ataque cataplético próximo a tigela ou enquanto bebe. Também é necessário restringir o acesso às escadas.

REFERÊNCIAS BIBLIOGRÁFICAS

As referências bibliográficas deste capítulo se encontram online no Ambiente de Aprendizagem.

CAPÍTULO 263

Disfunção Cognitiva em Cães e Gatos Idosos

Gary Landsberg

Muitas mudanças comportamentais em cães e gatos podem estar associadas à idade avançada, incluindo aparecimento ou aumento de medos, fobias e ansiedade, irritabilidade, agressividade, distúrbios repetitivos, despertar noturno, vocalização e sujeira na casa.[1,2] Tais sinais são consistentes com manifestações de doenças do envelhecimento cerebral. Entretanto, alguns desses comportamentos não estão relacionados ao envelhecimento patológico do cérebro, mas a condições médicas, incluindo outras doenças neurológicas, e os sinais podem ser decorrentes de distúrbios de comportamento primários resultantes de mudanças no ambiente doméstico. Além disso, animais de companhia idosos podem se estressar com mais facilidade e são menos capazes de se adaptar a mudanças, quando comparados a animais mais jovens. Portanto, para determinar se tais sinais clínicos estão relacionados a doenças do envelhecimento cerebral, as causas médicas e comportamentais devem ser primeiramente excluídas (ver Capítulo 9).

SINAIS CLÍNICOS

A síndrome de disfunção cognitiva (SDC) é um distúrbio neurodegenerativo de cães e gatos idosos caracterizado por mudanças comportamentais a partir de uma série de motivos. Acredita-se que tem origem cognitiva em associação ao desenvolvimento de padrões distintos de lesões cerebrais. A SDC não é uma consequência inevitável do envelhecimento em cães e gatos, e é provável que diferenças individuais sejam mais uma regra do que uma exceção. Alguns animais idosos apresentam apenas alterações comportamentais discretas, enquanto outros desenvolvem sinais graves ou múltiplos, que podem incluir declínio de consciência, resposta alterada a estímulos e deficiências de aprendizagem e de memória, o que pode atrapalhar o comportamento normal e reduzir drasticamente a qualidade de vida. Sinais clínicos de SDC em cães foram descritos na forma do acróstico DISUDA (*DISHA* em inglês), que se refere a

*D*esorientação, *I*nterações alteradas com o dono ou outros animais de companhia, alterações do ciclo do *S*ono-despertar, *U*rinar e *D*efecar em local não habitual e *A*tividade alterada (que pode ser aumentada, repetitiva ou reduzida).[1-4] Sinais adicionais podem incluir aumento da agitação e da ansiedade, alteração da capacidade de resposta a estímulos (ou seja, aumentada ou reduzida), interesse do apetite e/ou auto-higiene alterados (ou seja, aumentado ou reduzido) e habilidade diminuída para executar comandos ou tarefas treinadas previamente. Esse mesmo cenário se aplica a SDC em gatos, embora a prevalência de sinais individuais possa ser diferente.[5,6]

A detecção e intervenção precoce podem diminuir o declínio do quadro clínico, prevenir complicações, aumentar a longevidade e incrementar o bem-estar do animal. Os sinais de SDC muitas vezes não são relatados, porque os clínicos veterinários podem não solicitar as informações necessárias e os proprietários dos animais podem considerar os sinais comportamentais insignificantes ou não tratáveis.

A prevalência de SDC tem sido avaliada em uma série de pesquisas baseadas em questionários. Em um estudo, aproximadamente 48% dos tutores de 150 cães relataram que seus cães mais velhos (7 anos ou mais) exibiam pelo menos um sinal clínico de SDC. Porém, apenas 17% relataram esses sinais ao clínico (dados próprios, 1999, Pfizer Animal Health). Em outro estudo, 180 proprietários de cães idosos sem problemas clínicos identificáveis relataram pelo menos um sinal consistente com SDC em cães entre 11 e 12 anos (28%) e 15 a 16 anos (68%).[4] Prevalências de 22,5 e 5%[7] em cães de 10 a 12 anos e de 41% em cães maiores de 14 anos foram relatadas mais recentemente.[7,8] A prevalência geral descrita no último estudo foi de 14,2% (68 cães de um total de 479 cães estudados), enquanto o diagnóstico de SDC foi de apenas 1,9% (9 cães de 479) ou de 13% (9 dos 68 cães acometidos).[8] Ademais, SDC é uma doença progressiva, cuja prevalência e gravidade aumentam de acordo com o envelhecimento.[7,9] Em alguns estudos, fêmeas e machos castrados são mais acometidos do que machos e cães não castrados, respectivamente.[7,10] Porém, embora as fêmeas possam viver mais se forem castradas, uma vida útil longínqua não foi associada à castração em machos, exceto em raças gigantes, que são menos propensas a atingir uma idade na qual a SDC se tornaria uma preocupação clínica.[11,12] Em um estudo com 151 gatos acima dos 11 anos, 35% foram diagnosticados com SDC (28% de 95 gatos com idade entre 11 e 15 anos e 50% de 46 gatos com mais de 15 anos).[5,6]

A prevalência alta e o subdiagnóstico de SDC tornam essencial que clínicos veterinários e suas equipes informem aos proprietários sobre a importância de relatar os sinais clínicos de SDC para a identificação precoce da doença. Os clínicos devem ser proativos em perguntar aos donos se houve qualquer mudança no comportamento ou outros sinais que possam ser indicativos de SDC. Um questionário comportamental deve incluir perguntas que extraem informações sobre (a) desorientação ou confusão, (b) diminuição do interesse em interações sociais (p. ex., acariciar, brincar), (c) sono/despertar alterado à noite, (d) sujeira na casa, (e) atividades repetitivas, como andar de um lado para o outro ou em círculos, (f) diminuição na atividade ou apatia em relação a alimentação ou auto-higiene, (g) aumento da ansiedade ou irritabilidade, (h) resposta alterada a estímulos (visão, audição, olfato) e (i) diminuição da capacidade de resposta aos comandos aprendidos anteriormente.

ESTUDOS LABORATORIAIS

Questionários usados como ferramenta de base para identificar cães e gatos com SDC fornecem evidências de disfunção cerebral global, mas tendem a ser insensíveis a mudanças iniciais e sutis na aprendizagem e memória associadas ao envelhecimento cerebral patológico.[1,5,13] A disfunção cognitiva é avaliada com mais precisão com o uso de testes neuropsicológicos, projetados para fornecer medidas quantitativas da função cognitiva a partir de um aparelho padronizado (Toronto General Testing Apparatus; Figura 263.1). Esses testes são sistemáticos, padronizados e objetivos e fornecem uma medida quantitativa do declínio cognitivo relacionado à idade.[14-18] De fato, muito embora os sinais de SDC possam não ser reconhecidos até os 11 anos ou mais, os testes neuropsicológicos podem identificar deficiências de aprendizagem e memória em cães e gatos a partir dos 6 anos.[8,15,18,19] De forma similar, mudanças funcionais nos neurônios do núcleo caudado promovem deficiências no processamento de informação em gatos jovens de 6 anos.[19] Muitas funções cognitivas testadas com tarefas baseadas em experimentos laboratoriais provavelmente também contribuem para identificar os sinais clínicos que podem ser observados pelos donos dos animais.[20,21] Recentemente pesquisadores têm mostrado que essas tarefas podem ser usadas em um ambiente clínico para identificar déficits cognitivos em cães, embora esses testes laboratoriais em geral sejam muito longos e complexos para aplicar na rotina clínica.[22-25]

Estudos em laboratório usando uma série de testes neuropsicológicos motivados por recompensa possibilitam que vários domínios ou funções cognitivas possam ser avaliados independentemente em cães e gatos idosos.[18-26] Esses testes envolvem problemas de aprendizagem simples, como discriminação de tarefas, em que dois objetos de aparência diferente são apresentados ao animal e um deles está associado a recompensa em forma de alimento (Figura 263.1 e Vídeo 263.1). Cães e gatos em idade avançada podem aprender a solucionar esses problemas e talvez não difiram de animais jovens no tempo de aprendizagem.[17,27,28] Uma vez que cães e gatos aprendam a discriminar visualmente, o objeto de recompensa pode ser trocado, de forma que o objeto incorreto se torne agora o da recompensa. Isso é chamado de *aprendizagem reversa* – um tipo de habilidade cognitiva que depende da função intacta do córtex pré-frontal (ver Vídeo 263.1).[27,28] Cães e gatos idosos, quando comparados a animais jovens homólogos, são prejudicados em sua capacidade de selecionar o objeto incorreto anterior, o que sugere falta de habilidade de modificar comportamentos aprendidos.[17,26-28] Outras mudanças comportamentais que são provavelmente associadas à disfunção do córtex pré-frontal incluem: comportamentos estereotipados (como o andar compulsivo); alteração

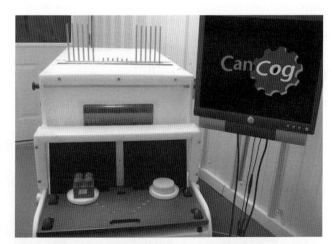

Figura 263.1 Aparelho de teste geral de Toronto (ATGT). Este aparelho e o *software* de computador são a versão felina do aparelho teste avaliação de tarefas de aprendizagem e memória. Na discriminação de tarefa, primeiro o gato aprende a deslocar um dos objetos (p. ex., o *círculo à direita*), colocando-o aleatoriamente em um dos locais, por ser recompensado por comida. Uma vez que o gato pode consistentemente deslocar o objeto correto para o alimento, este é então colocado sob o objeto oposto (*quadrado à esquerda*) até que o gato aprenda a deslocar o novo objeto consistentemente (tarefa de reversão). (Usada com autorização de CanCog Technologies.)

da personalidade, incluindo o aumento de medo, irritabilidade ou agressão; e incapacidade de inibir comportamentos aprendidos anteriormente (sujar a casa).

O processo de envelhecimento também pode afetar significativamente a memória. A memória espacial é mensurada pela capacidade dos cães de se lembrarem do local onde obtiveram uma recompensa alimentar escondida pela última vez, mas essa capacidade está comprometida em um subconjunto de animais idosos (Figura 263.2).[14-18,26,29,30] Funcionalmente, esse tipo de prejuízo da memória pode estar presente clinicamente em animais de companhia na forma de desorientação e delírio. Cães idosos também apresentam prejuízo em sua capacidade de reconhecer objetos vistos anteriormente,[14] assim como pessoas ou animais conhecidos. Em um estudo em laboratório avaliando o desempenho felino durante uma tarefa de teste de placa de buraco, o envelhecimento não afetou de forma significativa a aprendizagem espacial, porém os erros de memória aumentaram.[30]

Diferenças comportamentais relacionadas à idade também foram mostradas em testes de reatividade.[20,21,31] O teste de curiosidade, por exemplo, permite que os cães examinem e interajam com muitos brinquedos, a fim de avaliar sua reação e atenção aos objetos. Em um teste de 10 minutos, os cães jovens mostram um comportamento de exploração e contato mais significativo com os novos objetos do que os cães seniores, com o cão idoso com deficiência cognitiva mostrando o menor contato.[21] Além disso, os cães idosos com deficiência cognitiva mostraram maior locomoção que seus pares não deficientes da mesma idade, o que poderia estar ligado a um comportamento estereotipado ou errante.[21,31] Medidas de comportamento exploratório são mais aceitáveis em avaliação clínica, porque exigem breves sessões de teste e uma pequena área para realização, sugerindo que são mais úteis no ambiente clínico para animais idosos com SDC.[21,31]

BASES NEUROBIOLÓGICAS

Mudanças morfológicas gerais do envelhecimento do cérebro canino incluem diminuição da massa cerebral (particularmente no córtex frontal), aumento do volume ventricular e espessamento das meninges.[27,32] Mudanças adicionais podem incluir acúmulo de lipofuscina, surgimento de corpos apoptóticos, degeneração neuroaxonal, redução de neurônios e desmielinização.[32-34]

Cães idosos apresentam perda de neurônios no hipocampo – uma região do cérebro que desempenha papel importante para a memória.[35] É interessante prover aos cães idosos enriquecimento comportamental (caminhadas ao ar livre, interação social, brinquedos, treinamento cognitivo) para a manutenção desses neurônios.[35] Cães idosos também perdem sua capacidade de gerar novos neurônios no hipocampo (ou seja, neurogênese), o que está ligado à perda de aprendizagem e habilidade de memória.[36] Estudos de espectroscopia por ressonância magnética (RM) têm identificado uma relação da idade com o declínio de neurônios.[37]

Gatos idosos também apresentam atrofia cerebral, perda neuronal, alargamento dos sulcos, aumento de volume dos ventrículos laterais e diminuição de volume das substâncias cinzenta e branca, embora essa diminuição possa não ser tão marcante como nos cães.[6,19,38-40] Mudanças no lobo piriforme podem estar relacionadas com o declínio cognitivo, e uma redução nas células de Purkinje cerebelares pode estar associada ao processamento da informação e às deficiências motoras.[5,6,38,40]

Em nível bioquímico, várias mudanças foram relatadas no envelhecimento canino, incluindo redução na função colinérgica e lesão oxidativa; o envelhecimento felino está associado a atrofia acentuada do sistema colinérgico no *locus coeruleus*.[39-45] O papel da lesão oxidativa é suportado pela descoberta de que a dieta rica em antioxidantes e cofatores mitocondriais pode melhorar significativamente a função cognitiva em cães e gatos idosos.[18,46]

O acúmulo de beta amiloide (beta-A) no cérebro humano é uma das primeiras características patológicas para o desenvolvimento da doença de Alzheimer, e acredita-se que ele preceda a disfunção sináptica e perda neuronal, atrofia cerebral e os sintomas subsequentes.[47] A mudança de beta-A em cães é surpreendentemente semelhante às observadas em pacientes humanos com doença de Alzheimer em sua sequência de Peptídio, distribuição temporal e bioquímica,[48,49] e o comprometimento cognitivo em cães está correlacionado ao aumento e deposição beta-A (Figura 263.3).[35,50,51] Em contrapartida, gatos com mais de 10 anos mostram placas de beta-A mais difusas e predominantemente menos tipos de proteínas.[7,9,48,51-54] Há controvérsias entre os estudos sobre uma associação entre lesões SDC e beta-A em gatos.[51,53,54] Ao contrário de pacientes humanos com Alzheimer, nem os cães nem os gatos apresentam emaranhados neurofibrilares, embora a Tau hiperfosforilada seja relatada em ambas as espécies e possa representar um início da anormalidade.[53-56] Infartos ou mudanças cerebrovasculares e perivasculares, incluindo acúmulo de beta-A e micro-hemorragia periventricular, também podem causar alguns dos sinais clínicos associados à disfunção cognitiva em animais de estimação seniores.[2,6,27,32,34,48,50,51,53] (Figura 263.3). Beta-A vascular pode contribuir para hipoperfusão cerebral.[57]

OPÇÕES DE TRATAMENTO

Dieta, medicamentos ou suplementos podem ser eficazes para melhorar os sinais e retardar o progresso da SDC. Estudos em

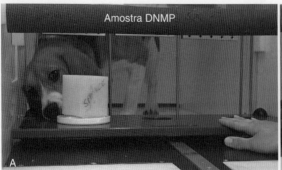
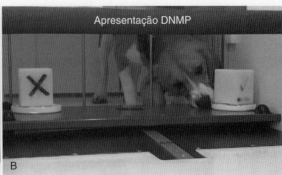

Figura 263.2 Teste com atrasado e não correspondência com a posição (DNMP) para memória espacial de curto prazo. **A.** A figura evidencia a fase da amostra do teste, com apenas um bloco apresentado com o alimento abaixo do objeto. Este é retirado, seguindo-se a fase de apresentação, durante a qual dois objetos idênticos são exibidos, com o objeto não correspondente cobrindo a comida. **B.** O alimento está localizado sob o novo objeto (*à direita*). A memória pode ser avaliada aumentando o atraso entre a retirada do objeto inicial (amostra) e a colocação de dois objetos (apresentação). (Usada com autorização da CanCog Technologies.)

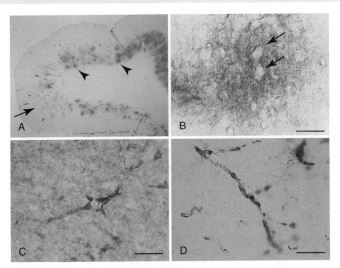

Figura 263.3 Lesões de beta-amiloide (beta-A) no cérebro de cão idoso (Border Collie de 15 anos). **A.** Beta-A se acumula extensivamente no córtex temporal como depósitos difusos (*pontas de seta*) ou na cerebrovasculatura (*seta*). **B.** Ampliação maior de uma placa beta-A difusa demonstra pequenas fibrilas se acumulando no espaço entre os neurônios (*setas*). **C.** Beta-A também podem ser observadas nas membranas dos neurônios. **D.** Vasos sanguíneos dentro do parênquima cerebral também podem acumular beta-A. Todas as seções imunocoradas com anticorpo anti-beta-A-1-42. As marcações em barras em B-D = 20 μ. (Tecido cerebral gentilmente cedido por Carolyn Wilki.)

cães têm mostrado que a estimulação mental na forma de treinamento, brincadeiras, exercícios e manipulação de brinquedos pode ajudar a manter a qualidade de vida, assim como a função cognitiva, mas são mais eficazes associados à nutrição apropriada.[58,59] Esse fato é consistente com estudos em humanos, que mostram que educação e exercícios cerebrais e físicos retardam o início da demência.

Atualmente, existe um fármaco na América do Norte, a selegilina, que foi aprovado para o tratamento de SDC em cães idosos. Cloridrato de selegilina é um inibidor seletivo reversível de monoamina oxidase B, que mostrou melhora significativa dos sinais de doença cognitiva em cães idosos.[60,61] No cérebro canino, a selegilina aumenta a concentração de 2-feniletilamina, um neuromodulador que aumenta a função da dopamina e das catecolaminas. Seus metabólitos l-anfetamina e l-metanfetamina podem aumentar a função cognitiva e melhorar o comportamento. Selegilina também pode contribuir para a diminuição de radicais livres no cérebro.

Propentofilina, um derivado da xantina, é licenciada na Europa e na Austrália para o tratamento, diminuindo a capacidade perceptiva, a letargia e o comportamento depressivo em cães idosos. A propentofilina pode aumentar o fluxo de sangue e inibir a agregação plaquetária e a formação de trombos. Todavia, não foi encontrado efeito sobre a atividade comportamental em testes laboratoriais realizados com cães Beagle idosos.[62]

Uma vez que cães idosos são particularmente suscetíveis aos efeitos dos fármacos anticolinérgicos, é prudente evitar medicamentos com efeitos anticolinérgicos em tais pacientes.[41] Na verdade, fármacos ou produtos naturais que melhoram a transmissão colinérgica podem ter benefícios potenciais para os sinais de SDC em cães e gatos, porém mais pesquisas são necessárias para encontrar fármacos e doses eficazes.[63]

Nenhum fármaco foi aprovado para o tratamento de SDC em gatos, embora tanto a selegilina quanto a propentofilina tenham sido relatadas como úteis.[1,5,6]

Outra estratégia terapêutica para disfunção cognitiva em cães, gatos e humanos são as dietas e os suplementos naturais que podem reduzir os fatores de risco que contribuem para o envelhecimento do cérebro e o declínio cognitivo. É provável que uma abordagem integrativa seja necessária para alcançar e manter a saúde do cérebro, como dietas suplementadas com ácidos graxos poli-insaturados, antioxidantes e cofatores mitocondriais.[64-66] Duas dietas veterinárias terapêuticas, desenvolvidas para o manejo de SDC e aplicadas durante um estudo, mostraram melhora da aprendizagem e memória em cães. A dieta da Hills *Pet Nutrition* (Canina b/d) é suplementada com ácidos graxos, antioxidantes (vitaminas C, betacaroteno, selênio, flavonoides, carotenoides), ácido alfa-lipóico-dl e carnitina-l para melhorar a função mitocondrial.[58,59,67] Quando a dieta foi combinada com enriquecimento ambiental, a melhora foi ainda maior.[58,59] Em um ensaio clínico, efeitos significativos foram obtidos apenas com a dieta.[68] A dieta da Nestlé Purina® (*Purina Pro Plan Bright Minds*) é suplementada com óleos botânicos contendo triglicerídeos de cadeia média para fornecer corpos cetônicos como fonte alternativa de energia para neurônios em envelhecimento.[69] O suplemento dietético da Nestlé Purina® (ainda não disponível comercialmente) com antioxidantes (vitaminas E, C e selênio), arginina, vitaminas B e óleo de peixe melhorou significativamente a aprendizagem e as tarefas de memória em gatos idosos de 5,5 a 8,7 anos.[18]

Baseados em estudos laboratoriais e/ou clínicos, diversos suplementos nutricionais também podem ser eficazes no manejo da SDC. *Senilife* (CEVA Saúde Animal) contém fosfatidilserina (um fosfolipídio de membrana), Gingko biloba, vitaminas E, B6 e resveratrol, e é indicado para cães e gatos, mas só foi avaliado em estudos com cães até o momento.[70,71] *Activait* (Vet Plus Ltd), que contém fosfatidilserina, ácidos graxos ômega-3, vitaminas E e C, carnitina-l, ácido alfalipoico, coenzima Q e selênio, foi avaliado em uma pesquisa clínica canina.[72] Um produto felino também está disponível com ácido alfalipoico removido. *S-adenosil-metionina* (Novifit, Virbac Animal Health) pode ajudar a manter a fluidez da membrana celular e a função do receptor, regular os níveis de neurotransmissores e aumentar a produção de glutationa.[73,74] *Apoaequorin* (Neutricks, Neutricks, LLC) é uma proteína encontrada em águas-vivas que tampona cálcio e que, em experimentos laboratoriais, melhorou a aprendizagem e atenção em cães.[75] A imunoterapia também tem sido avaliada em cães idosos, envolvendo a vacinação de animais idosos contra a proteína beta-A. Embora o estudo não tenha tido sucesso em reverter o déficits cognitivo, essa abordagem pode ser promissora para tratamentos futuros.[76]

REFERÊNCIAS BIBLIOGRÁFICAS

As referências bibliográficas deste capítulo se encontram online no Ambiente de Aprendizagem.

CAPÍTULO 264

Neuropatias Cranianas

John Henry Rossmeisl, Jr.

O termo *neuropatia craniana* refere-se a qualquer condição que cause disfunção de um nervo craniano (NC), em qualquer lugar ao longo de seu curso anatômico.[1] As neuropatias cranianas afetam mais frequentemente um único NC (mononeuropatia), mas podem envolver vários NC (polineuropatias) ou aparecer associadas a polineuropatias generalizadas.[2-5] É necessário um exame neurológico completo (ver Capítulo 259) para localizar corretamente o nível de disfunção do NC, com foco na identificação dos componentes centrais ou periféricos envolvidos, a fim de formular a lista de diagnósticos diferenciais e um plano de manejo adequado (Tabela 264.1).[1] Por exemplo, a identificação de deficiências envolvendo dois ou mais NC geralmente é indicativa de lesão em uma região anatômica na qual os nervos estão próximos um do outro, como no caso da síndrome de Horner (SH), em que a paresia facial e disfunção vestibular periférica são causadas por doenças da orelha média e interno.[6] As etiologias comuns de neuropatias cranianas incluem doenças degenerativas, idiopáticas, inflamatórias, metabólicas e neoplásicas.[1-6] Por convenção, uma neuropatia craniana idiopática é diagnosticada somente após a exclusão de doenças cujas causas estruturais e metabólicas têm propensão a comprometer o NC, o que pode ser um desafio quando se trata de um paciente vivo. As mononeuropatias idiopáticas afetam os nervos cranianos com mais frequência do que outros nervos periféricos, e várias dessas síndromes são autolimitantes.[2,3,5]

NERVO ÓPTICO (NC II) | NEURITE ÓPTICA

A neurite óptica é caracterizada por início agudo de perda de visão, frequentemente bilateral e associada a pupilas midriáticas e não responsivas (ver Capítulo 11).[7] Com frequência ocorrem mudanças visíveis no segmento posterior do olho, como edema no disco óptico (Figura 264.1), congestão vascular, hemorragia e neurorretinite peripapilar, embora o exame oftálmico possa apresentar-se normal em casos de doença retrobulbar.[7,8] Se o edema do disco óptico é visível, os diagnósticos diferenciais incluem papiledema ou edema do nervo óptico, possivelmente acompanhados de uveíte ou glaucoma. Essas condições em geral são diferenciadas com base nos achados do exame clínico geral.[7] O papiledema é um edema não inflamatório de disco, resultante de hipertensão intracraniana, que não causa perda aguda de visão.

As etiologias prováveis de neurite óptica incluem infecções (p. ex., cinomose viral canina, infecções por fungos e por protozoários) e causas imunomediadas (meningoencefalite granulomatosa) meningoencefalites e neoplasias (ver Figura 264.1), que podem infiltrar ou comprimir os nervos ou quiasma óptico (meningioma, glioma, tumores de hipófise).[7-10] Assim, exames de imagem de ressonância magnética (RM) cerebral (ver Capítulos 260 e 261), análise do líquido cefalorraquidiano (ver Capítulo 115) e ensaios sorológicos são recomendados para o diagnóstico em casos de neurite óptica.[8-10] O manejo da meningoencefalite é revisado no Capítulo 261.

Tabela 264.1 — Nervos cranianos: nomes, funções e manifestações da disfunção.

NÚMERO	NOME	PRINCIPAIS FUNÇÕES	SINAIS CLÍNICOS DE DOENÇA
I	Olfativo	Cheiro	Incapacidade de cheirar
II	Ótico	Visão	Cegueira
III	Oculomotor	Movimento do olho e constrição da pupila	Posição anormal dos olhos, tamanho da pupila ou reatividade da pupila à luz
IV	Troclear	Movimento do olho	Posição anormal dos olhos
V	Trigemino	Sensação para os olhos e rosto, movimento da mandíbula	Esfregar ou apalpar o rosto Perda de massa muscular na cabeça Mandíbula caída – flacidez, incapacidade de fechar a boca
VI	Abducente	Movimento do olho	Posição anormal dos olhos
VII	Facial	Movimento dos músculos faciais Gosto Produção de rasgo e saliva	Inclinação da orelha ou bochecha, desvio do nariz, sialorreia Olho seco
VIII	Vestibulococlear	Equilíbrio e audição	Posição anormal da cabeça, movimentos anormais dos olhos, vertigem Surdez
IX	Glossofaríngeo	Sensação e movimento dos músculos da garganta Gosto	Dificuldade de comer ou engolir
X	Vago	Movimento dos músculos da garganta	Perda de voz, tosse, regurgitação
XI	Acessório	Movimento dos músculos do pescoço e ombros	Difícil de apreciar em pequenos animais
XII	Hipoglosso	Movimento da língua	Desvio ou paralisia da língua, dificuldade para comer

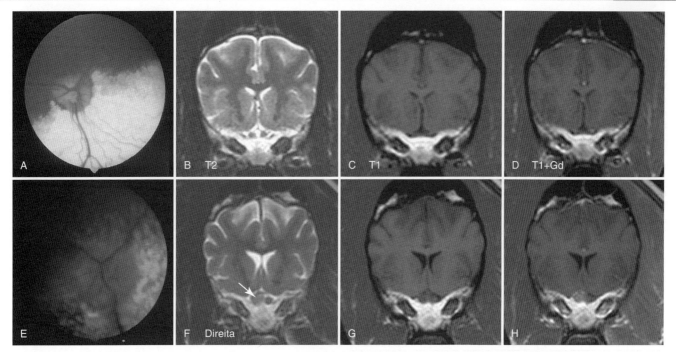

Figura 264.1 Morfologia do nervo óptico canino normal no exame fundoscópico (**A**), e em transversal ponderada em T2 (**B**), ponderada em T1 (**C**) e ponderada em T1 pós-contraste (**D**) ressonância magnética da região retrobulbar. Neurite óptica associada a evidências fundoscópicas de disco óptico edemaciado (**E**), causada por astrocitoma do nervo óptico, que aparece como alargamento unilateral do nervo óptico direito na ressonância magnética transversal (**F** [seta], **G** e **H**). (As figuras A e E encontram-se reproduzidas em cores no Encarte.)

A eletrorretinografia (ERG) é o exame de preferência para pacientes com neurite óptica. Em muitos cães, se nenhuma causa subjacente for identificada, presume-se que a neurite óptica é idiopática, e a terapia sistêmica com doses imunossupressoras de prednisona é realizada na tentativa de tratamento (ver Capítulo 165).[7] Já a síndrome degenerativa da retina adquirida súbita (SDRAS) é outra causa de cegueira aguda bilateral associada a pupilas midriáticas.[10,11] Porém, muitos cães com SDRAS apresentam reflexo pupilar à luz lento e incompleto, e o exame de fundo de olho é inicialmente normal; nesses casos, o ERG é debelado.[10,11] O prognóstico de neurite óptica para a completa recuperação visual varia entre reservado a ruim.[7]

NERVOS OCULOMOTOR (NC III), TROCLEAR (NC IV) E ABDUCENTE (NC VI)

Coletivamente, os nervos oculomotor (NC III), troclear (NC IV) e abducente (NC VI) inervam os músculos extraoculares. Juntamente aos sistemas vestibular e proprioceptivo, esses nervos são responsáveis pelo posicionamento do globo ocular e pela coordenação dos movimentos dos olhos.[12] A porção parassimpática do NC III é responsável pela constrição pupilar. Sinais clínicos de disfunção desses nervos ou de suas projeções vestibulares correlacionadas produzem estrabismo, nistagmo fisiológico anormal em função da oftalmoplegia externa, nistagmo patológico (caso a lesão envolva o sistema vestibular) e oftalmoplegia interna (ou seja, pupila midriática e fixa), se a lesão afetar a porção parassimpática do NC III.[12-14]

As síndromes de seio cavernoso (SSC) e de fissura orbital (SFO) são definidas pela disfunção clínica de dois ou mais dos nervos cranianos III IV e VI e pelos ramos oftálmicos ou maxilares do nervo trigêmeo (NC V).[13,14] Os axônios desses NC cursam em grande proximidade anatômica entre si ao longo no assoalho do crânio, em uma área adjacente ao seio cavernoso, antes de emergirem do crânio através da fissura orbital. Os sinais clínicos observados frequentemente na SSC e na SFO são oftalmoplegia externa e interna, sensibilidade reduzida da córnea, ceratite neurotrófica e ptose.[13,14] A diferenciação entre as síndromes requer demonstração do nível anatômico da lesão por meio de diagnóstico por imagem. As causas mais comuns são neoplasias primárias ou metastáticas, embora causas infecciosas já tenham sido relatadas, principalmente em gatos.[13,14]

NERVO TRIGÊMEO (NC V) | NEUROPATIA TRIGEMINAL

O nervo trigêmeo consiste em três ramos principais, responsáveis pela sensibilidade da cabeça (ou seja, nervo oftálmico, maxilar e mandibular) e pela função motora dos músculos de mastigação (ou seja, nervo mandibular).[1,2] As apresentações clínicas comuns de mononeuropatias trigeminais envolvem disfunção mandibular motora; casos de disfunção trigeminal sensorial isolada são raros.[15] Primeiramente, há um início agudo de uma paresia bilateral e flacidez dos nervos mandibulares, resultando em queda da mandíbula e incapacidade de fechar a boca (Vídeo 264.1).[2] Essa apresentação clínica pode ser consequência de distúrbios que afetam a função mecânica da mandíbula (p. ex., fratura da articulação temporomandibular ou avulsão), de doenças que desencadeiam dor associada ao movimento da mandíbula (miosite do músculo mastigatório, lesões de massa retrobulbar), de doenças inflamatórias (Neospora, Toxoplasma, Criptococos, raiva), de doenças idiopática ou neoplásica (neoplasia hematopoética, tumor de bainha do nervo [TBN]) e de lesões nervosas do NC V.[2,16-18] Animais com sinais clínicos limitados à queda aguda da mandíbula geralmente possuem doença nas porções periférica do NC V, pois uma lesão bilateral nos núcleos motores trigeminais pontíneos estariam correlacionadas a sinais clínicos adicionais e graves e a um quadro clínico grave de síndrome pontomedular, que muitas vezes engloba disfunção vestibular central, nível de consciência deprimida e/ou déficits no NC VI e no nervo facial (NC VII).[1]

Neurite idiopática do trigêmeo (NIT) é a causa mais comum de queda da mandíbula em cães (ver Vídeo 264.1). A doença prejudica principalmente a função motora do músculo mastigatório, embora déficits sensoriais do trigêmeo possam estar correlacionados à NIT em aproximadamente um terço dos cães e sejam observadas ocasionalmente paralisia do NC VII concomitante, atrofia muscular mastigatória ou SH.[2] O tratamento inclui cuidados de suporte com alimentação assistida (ver Capítulo 82). Cães acometidos geralmente se recuperam em 2 a 4 semanas. O exame de RM cerebral em animais com neuropatia trigeminal fornece o melhor método não invasivo para diferenciação das etiologias de neuropatia trigeminal. Na RM, nervos trigêmeos normais e anormais apresentam realce do contraste.[19] Em caso de NIT, o nervo é caracterizado por sinal e morfologia normais ou aparece difusamente aumentado e hiperintenso em T2.[20]

Outra apresentação da neuropatia trigeminal é o quadro de início agudo de atrofia unilateral, muitas vezes grave, dos músculos de mastigação ipsilateral ao nervo mandibular disfuncional. O TBN trigeminal é uma etiologia comum de atrofia unilateral neurogênica do músculo mastigatório (Figura 264.2).[20] Podem ser observadas também hipoalgesia ou parestesia facial, que se manifestam como fricção facial, coceira ou dor, além da SH. O TBN é invasivo localmente e lento para fazer metástase. As opções de tratamento englobam citorredução cirúrgica, radioterapia ou cuidados de suporte com glicocorticoides.[20,21] O prognóstico é reservado, embora uma média geral de sobrevida de 881 dias tenha sido relatada em 4 cães tratados com radiocirurgia estereotáxica para TBN trigeminal.[21]

NERVO FACIAL (NC VII) | NEUROPATIA/PARALISIA FACIAL

A paralisia facial é caracterizada por incapacidade aguda de fechamento da fissura palpebral, queda da orelha e do lábio e sialorreia no lado comprometido.[1] As causas da paralisia do nervo facial (NC VII) periférico incluem otite média interna, lesão cirúrgica iatrogênica (p. ex., osteotomia da bula), doença idiopática, doença metabólica (hipotireoidismo), neoplasias óticas, trauma e hipersensibilidade a sulfamida.[3,6,22,23] Em função da estreita relação anatômica entre os nervos vestibulococlear e facial, a medula espinal e o osso temporal petroso, sintomas vestibulares podem apresentar etiologias tanto do sistema nervoso periférico quanto do sistema nervoso central (p. ex., neoplasia, meningoencefalite) e etiologia da paralisia do NC VII.[6,24] A paresia facial também pode ser uma característica de neuropatias generalizadas ou de doenças neuromusculares, como polirradiculoneurite canina aguda, paralisia por doença de carrapatos e miastenia *gravis*.[25-27] A paralisia facial é relatada como de origem idiopática em 75% dos cães e 25% dos gatos com neuropatia facial.[3] Aproximadamente 60% dos casos de doença idiopática apresentam sinais unilaterais e 40% sinais bilaterais (Vídeo 264.2).[28] A paralisia facial idiopática está comumente associada a vários segmentos do NC VII realçados na RM.[28,29] É possível a recuperação espontânea de paralisia idiopática do NC VII. Em cães, o aumento de contraste do nervo na RM pode fornecer informações prognósticas. Um estudo indicou que é menos provável que a recuperação da função do NC VII ocorra ou seja prolongada em casos que mostram contraste do nervo na RM.[29] Os animais que se recuperam geralmente o fazem dentro de 3 a 8 semanas.[3,29]

NERVO VESTIBULOCOCLEAR (NC VIII)

O ramo vestibular do nervo vestibulococlear (NC VIII) participa da manutenção do equilíbrio e da postura, e distúrbios que afetam o sistema vestibular são revisados no Capítulo 265.[1,12] A disfunção do ramo da cóclea resulta em surdez, que pode ser classificada como condutiva (p. ex., otite externa/média) ou de origem neurossensorial.[30] A causa mais comum é neurossensorial congênita hereditária, associada a genes da coloração de pelagem branca, malhada e merle.[30,31] Em cães e gatos, a surdez neurossensorial adquirida pode ocorrer secundariamente à degeneração coclear, em função do envelhecimento (ou seja, presbiacusia) ou de tratamento com fármaco ototóxico (p. ex., aminoglicosídeos).[30] A surdez é diagnosticada via teste de resposta auditiva evocada de tronco encefálico.[30,31]

GLOSSOFARÍNGEO (NC IX), VAGO (NC X) E ACESSÓRIOS (NC XI) | DISFAGIA, MEGAESÔFAGO E PARALISIA LARÍNGEA

Os nervos glossofaríngeo (NC IX), vago (NC X) e acessório (NC XI) são importantes para a função da faringe, da laringe e do esôfago.[1] No paciente disfágico, é importante diferenciar problemas neurogênicos de preensão que interferem na disfunção da mandíbula (NC V), lábios (NC VII) e/ou língua (NC XII) de problemas de deglutição neurogênicos. Distúrbios de preensão e disfagia orofaríngea podem ser identificados com o exame físico, observando o animal comer, enquanto a caracterização e o diagnóstico de distúrbios da faringe, cricofaringe e/ou fase esofágica da deglutição frequentemente requerem exames diagnóstico de imagem, incluindo radiografia de contraste e videofluoroscopia (ver Capítulo 38).[32] A disfagia pode estar associada a sinais clínicos de engasgo e tosse após beber ou comer, acúmulo de saliva ou comida na faringe e reflexo de deglutição anormal. Doenças neurológicas que comumente causam disfagia incluem miopatias primárias (ver Capítulo 354), polineuropatias (ver Capítulo 268), distúrbios da junção

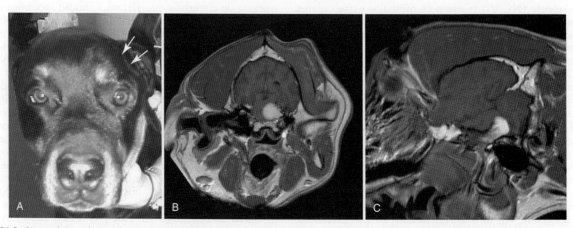

Figura 264.2 Características clínicas de ressonância magnética de tumor de bainha do nervo trigêmeo em um cão. **A.** Atrofia unilateral dos músculos temporal esquerdo (*setas*) e masseter, juntamente com síndrome de Horner parcial ipsilateral. Transversal (**B**) e parassagital esquerda (**C**) pós-contraste de ressonância magnética ponderada em T1 demonstrando massa extra-axial lobular, com realce de contraste envolvendo o nervo trigêmeo, resultando em compressão mesencefálica e perda de massa muscular (**B**; temporal esquerdo).

neuromuscular (p. ex., miastenia *gravis*, botulismo; ver Capítulo 269) e lesão caudal do tronco cerebral (encefalite e neoplasia; ver Capítulos 260 e 261).[25,27,33,34]

O esôfago é inervado pelo nervo vago e ramo interno do NC XI.[1] O megaesôfago é caracterizado por dilatação generalizada e peristaltismo anormal do esôfago (ver Capítulo 273).[35,36] A regurgitação é o principal sinal clínico observado, e pneumonia aspirativa secundária é comum (ver Capítulo 242). Megaesôfago é mais comum em cães do que em gatos e pode ser congênito ou adquirido, embora a maioria dos casos caninos seja adquirida e idiopática.[35] Apesar de o megaesôfago poder ser identificado rapidamente com radiografia torácica e histórico completo, métodos diagnósticos auxiliares são necessários para estabelecer a etiologia.[32] O megaesôfago adquirido pode ser causado por polineuropatias, polimiopatias, *Myasthenia gravis*, endocrinopatias (p. ex., hipoadrenocorticismo, hipotireoidismo) e intoxicações (chumbo, organofosforados, tálio); para um diagnóstico de megaesôfago idiopático, essas causas precisam ser descartadas.[25,27,32,33,35-40] O tratamento é direcionado à causa subjacente, se presente, e focado nos diversos tipos de procedimentos de alimentação assistida (p. ex., cadeira Bailey, tubo de gastrostomia). O prognóstico associado ao megaesôfago é altamente variável e depende da etiologia subjacente (ver Capítulo 273).[35-39]

A laringe é inervada por ramos do nervo vago.[1] O nervo laríngeo recorrente inerva os músculos abdutores da laringe. Lesões que afetam esse nervo podem resultar em disfonia, estridor inspiratório e agonia respiratória.[4] A paralisia laríngea congênita tem sido descrita em diversas raças, enquanto a[25,41,42] paralisia laríngea adquirida tem sido associada a doença metabólica (p. ex., hipotireoidismo), trauma no nervo laríngeo recorrente, neoplasia (carcinoma de células escamosas, carcinoma de tireoide), intoxicações (chumbo) e doença do tronco cerebral (neoplasia, encefalite).[25,42-44] Em cães mais velhos de raças grandes, a paralisia laríngea é frequentemente a manifestação clínica inicial de um quadro polineuropatia degenerativa progressiva (ver Capítulo 239).[4,25,42]

SÍNDROME DE HORNER

A SH é resultante de lesões que afetam qualquer porção dos três neurônios da via oculosimpática.[5,45] Os sinais clínicos consistem em miose, ptose, protrusão da terceira pálpebra e enoftalmia. Neurônios de primeira ordem (neurônio motor superior ou central) que se originam no tronco cerebral rostral trafegam pela medula espinal cervical, fazendo sinapse com os neurônios de segunda ordem (pré-ganglionar), que têm seu corpo celular nos segmentos espinais T1-T3. Axônios de neurônios de segunda ordem percorrem o tronco vagossimpático e fazem sinapse com neurônios de terceira ordem (pós-ganglionar) no gânglio craniocervical e então projetam-se para o olho e anexos.[5,46] O teste tópico de fenilefrina pode ajudar na localização da lesão ao longo dessas vias.[5] A observação de midríase por 20 minutos após a aplicação tópica de fenilefrina indica lesão pós-ganglionar, enquanto midríase após 20 minutos sugere lesão pré-ganglionar.[5] A SH pode ser causada por lesões degenerativas, inflamatórias, isquêmicas, metabólicas, neoplásicas ou traumáticas em qualquer local da via oculossimpática, embora na maioria dos casos nenhuma etiologia seja identificada, e a condição seja presumivelmente idiopática.[5,46] Entretanto, dados recentes indicam que a SH é idiopática e pós-ganglionar na maioria dos casos, o que contradiz os resultados de publicações anteriores[45,46] Golden Retrievers são predispostos a desenvolver SH idiopática.[45,46] Esta é principalmente uma questão estética, uma vez que a visão não é prejudicada, a menos que o problema seja bilateral, e a condição se resolve em muitos cães dentro de 3 a 4 meses.[45,46]

REFERÊNCIAS BIBLIOGRÁFICAS

As referências bibliográficas deste capítulo se encontram online no Ambiente de Aprendizagem.

CAPÍTULO 265

Doença Vestibular

Veronique Sammut

Inclinação da cabeça e nistagmo são manifestações clínicas de doenças vestibulares e problemas neurológicos comuns em pequenos animais, que podem ter apresentação clínica dramática. A disfunção vestibular pode se originar do sistema vestibular periférico ou central.

NEUROANATOMIA FUNCIONAL

O sistema vestibular é o sistema sensorial responsável por manter a postura, o equilíbrio e o tônus da cabeça e do corpo em relação às forças gravitacionais e ao movimento e está dividido em componentes periféricos e centrais (Figura 265.1). O sistema vestibular periférico está localizado principalmente na porção petrosa do osso temporal e inclui o labirinto e a porção vestibular do nervo vestibulococlear (nervo craniano [NC] VIII). O labirinto membranoso é composto por uma série de estruturas preenchidas com fluido, que consiste em três canais semicirculares, no utrículo e no sáculo, que são responsáveis pela função vestibular.

Os componentes vestibulares centrais incluem os quatro pares de núcleos vestibulares adjacentes à parede do quarto ventrículo, na parte dorsal da ponte e da medula, e o núcleo fastigial e lobo floculonodular do cerebelo. A partir do NC VIII, alguns axônios fazem sinapse em um dos núcleos vestibulares, enquanto outros sobem diretamente para o cerebelo através do pedúnculo cerebelar caudal. A maioria dos axônios dos núcleos vestibulares projeta-se para a medula espinal via trato vestibulospinal lateral ipsilateral, para influenciar o tônus extensor por facilitação nos músculos extensores ipsilaterais e inibição nos músculos flexores ipsilaterais e o fascículo dos músculos longitudinais mediais (FLM), que faz sinapse nos núcleos dos nervos oculomotor (NC III), troclear (NC IV) e abducente (NC VI), para ajustar os olhos em relação à posição e ao movimento da cabeça. Alguns axônios se projetam para o centro do vômito na formação reticular do bulbo (desempenhando um papel no enjoo do movimento), enquanto outros ascendem ao córtex cerebral (prosencéfalo) para percepção consciente da posição, por meio de uma retransmissão dos núcleos talâmicos. Por essa

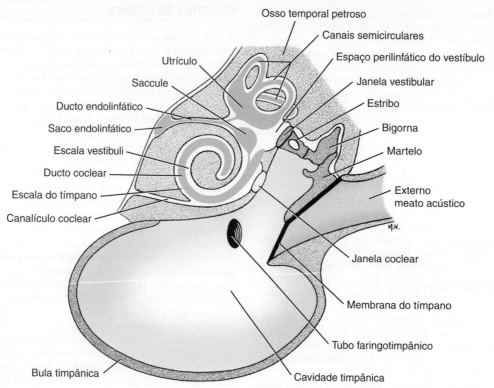

Figura 265.1 Seção transversal diagramática das orelhas média e interna do cão. (Adaptada de Evans H, de Lahunta A: *Guide to the dissection of the dog*, 8 ed., St. Louis, 2017, Saunders.)

razão, a doença vestibular às vezes pode ser vista com lesões talâmicas. O cerebelo tem função inibitória sobre os núcleos vestibulares, evitando o tônus extensor excessivo.

SINAIS CLÍNICOS

A lesão vestibular causa uma falta de facilitação dos músculos extensores de um dos lados, com o lado normal "empurrando" o corpo e a cabeça em direção ao lado anormal, levando ao desequilíbrio. Como a maioria dos processos de doença é unilateral ou assimétrica, geralmente são observadas perda de equilíbrio e inclinação da cabeça para um lado. No entanto, o envolvimento bilateral também é possível.

Inclinação de cabeça

A inclinação da cabeça é o sinal mais comum e consistente de um distúrbio vestibular unilateral ou assimétrico. É caracterizada por rotação da cabeça no plano mediano, deixando uma orelha mais baixa que a outra. É importante diferenciar a inclinação e a torção de cabeça ou torcicolo decorrente de uma lesão prosencefálica, na qual as orelhas e os olhos estão paralelos ao solo, mas o nariz está voltado para um dos lados do corpo. Pacientes com envolvimento vestibular bilateral podem não ter inclinação da cabeça, a menos que um lado seja mais afetado do que o outro, porém eles tendem a ter amplas excursões da cabeça de um lado para o outro. Com envolvimento cerebelar, a cabeça pode ser inclinada para o lado oposto ao da lesão (ver Síndrome paradoxal).

Ataxia vestibular

A ataxia vestibular é caracterizada por uma postura ampla e perda de equilíbrio do lado da lesão. A cabeça e o corpo podem oscilar, e o animal muitas vezes se inclina, cai ou mesmo rola para um lado. O animal pode andar em círculos (vestibular), que são tipicamente erráticos e de pequeno diâmetro (Vídeo 265.1). Isso deve ser diferenciado do andar em círculos compulsivo, secundário a uma lesão no prosencéfalo, na qual os círculos são tipicamente grandes, regulares e bem formados. A presença de paresia e/ou deficiências proprioceptivas gerais (PG) indicam lesão central que afeta as vias motoras descendentes e os tratos proprioceptivos ascendentes. No entanto, a avaliação inicial da PG pode ser difícil se o paciente estiver gravemente afetado. Com perturbação bilateral, o animal em geral fica em pé próximo no chão e pode perder o equilíbrio para ambos os lados.

Nistagmo

O nistagmo é um movimento rítmico e involuntário dos olhos. Pode ser igual para ambos os lados (nistagmo pendular) ou, mais comumente, ter uma fase rápida e uma lenta (nistagmo espasmódico), além de poder ainda ser caracterizado como fisiológico ou patológico e horizontal, vertical ou rotatório. Por convenção, a direção do nistagmo é descrita durante sua fase rápida. O nistagmo pendular não é um sinal de disfunção vestibular e é principalmente reconhecido em gatos da raça Siamês, Himalaia, Birmanês e cruzamentos delas.

Fisiológico

O nistagmo fisiológico é o movimento conjugado do olho que ocorre durante a movimentação da cabeça, a fim de estabilizar imagens na retina. Pode ser provocado em pacientes normais com movimento da cabeça de um lado para o outro (reflexo oculovestibular). Nas doenças vestibulares, o nistagmo fisiológico pode ser reduzido em ambos os olhos quando a cabeça está voltada para o lado da lesão. Em casos de envolvimento bilateral, o aspecto fisiológico (e patológico) do nistagmo pode estar completamente ausente, em razão da falta de ativação vestibular em ambos os lados.

Patológico

O nistagmo patológico é frequente, mas nem sempre está presente na doença vestibular. Pode ser espontâneo (quando a cabeça está na posição normal) ou posicional (visível apenas quando a cabeça é colocada em uma posição incomum; por exemplo, em extensão completa ou com o animal em decúbito dorsal). O nistagmo patológico é descrito pela orientação do plano em que os globos oculares estão se movendo (vertical, rotatório ou horizontal) e, por convenção, pela direção da fase rápida (esquerda ou direita; Vídeos 265.2 e 265.3). Com o distúrbio vestibular, os olhos tendem a "desviar" na direção da lesão (fase lenta) e redefinem rapidamente para sua posição original por meio de um reflexo do tronco encefálico (fase rápida). Isso faz a fase rápida do nistagmo ser oposta ao lado da lesão. O nistagmo espontâneo está frequentemente presente em lesões agudas e pode desaparecer dentro de alguns dias, em razão da compensação central. Por essa razão, e porque a presença de nistagmo patológico (seja espontâneo ou posicional) é sempre anormal e indicativa de doença vestibular, é importante tentar incitar o nistagmo posicional.

Na doença vestibular periférica, o nistagmo patológico pode ser horizontal ou rotatório, e a fase rápida é sempre para o lado oposto ao da lesão. Na doença central, o nistagmo patológico pode ser em qualquer plano (incluindo vertical) e mudar de direção com diferentes posições da cabeça, enquanto na fase rápida pode ser em direção à lesão. Portanto, a identificação de um nistagmo vertical ou com a fase rápida em direção à lesão é uma indicação de envolvimento central. Contudo, deve-se ter cuidado ao diagnosticar um paciente com base apenas no nistagmo vertical, uma vez que é fácil confundir com nistagmo com um ligeiro componente rotatório. Um estudo clínico comparativo também sugeriu que o número de batidas do nistagmo em repouso foi significativamente maior na doença periférica em comparação à central. Verificou-se que uma taxa de nistagmo em repouso de mais de 66 batimentos por minuto (bpm) foi muito específica (95%) e sensível (85%) para doença periférica.[2]

Estrabismo

Estrabismo vestibular é caracterizado por um desvio ventral do globo ocular do lado da lesão quando a cabeça está em extensão (estrabismo posicional). No entanto, o olho pode mover-se normalmente de um lado para o outro, porque não há paralisia de qualquer um dos músculos extraoculares. Esse tipo de estrabismo pode ser visto com uma lesão vestibular tanto periférica quanto central.

Déficits do nervo craniano

Embora não seja exatamente parte da síndrome vestibular, outros déficits de NC podem ser vistos junto aos sinais vestibulares. No tronco encefálico, o nervo facial (NC VII) está próximo ao nervo vestibulococlear (NC VIII) e se desloca perto da orelha interna. Por essa razão, a paralisia do NC VII pode ser observada com ambas as doenças periféricas e centrais. A inervação simpática do olho também passa perto da orelha interna, e a síndrome de Horner (SH) pode ocorrer em casos de doença periférica, mas raramente é vista em doenças centrais. Qualquer outro envolvimento de NC indica origem central da doença.

Náuseas e vômito

Náuseas e vômitos são frequentemente vistos com doenças vestibulares e podem estar relacionados ao enjoo ou ser resultado de um problema nas vias entre os núcleos vestibulares e o centro do vômito no tronco encefálico. Podem ser vistos também em doenças periféricas e centrais, embora o vômito possa ser mais comum com doenças periféricas.[1]

Mudança no nível de consciência

Pacientes com doença vestibular são frequentemente muito ansiosos e bastante desorientados pela falta de equilíbrio. No entanto, isso deve ser diferenciado de depressão central ou obnubilação, o que indica envolvimento do tronco encefálico.

Algum grau de depressão mental geralmente ocorre com doenças centrais, pois os núcleos vestibulares estão próximos ao sistema de ativação reticular ascendente (SARA), responsável pelo estado de alerta normal.

Síndrome paradoxal

O cerebelo é inibidor dos núcleos vestibulares ipsilaterais. Com a falta de inibição decorrente de uma lesão cerebelar, os núcleos vestibulares aparecem "hiper" desse lado, o que causa um excesso no tônus extensor do lado da lesão, que vai "empurrar" a cabeça e o corpo para o outro lado. O lado da lesão pode ser identificado pela presença de déficits concomitantes (déficit de PG ipsilateral, paresia, hipermetria ou déficits de NC).

A síndrome vestibular paradoxal pode ser vista com lesões no lobo floculonodular do cerebelo, no pedúnculo cerebelar caudal e nos núcleos vestibulares rostral e medial na medula.[3]

NEUROLOCALIZAÇÃO

O aspecto mais importante na avaliação de um paciente com vestibulopatia é localizar a lesão tanto no sistema vestibular periférico quanto no caso de origem central (Tabela 265.1). Um bom histórico, exame físico e exame neurológico cuidadosos e completos são essenciais (ver Capítulos 1, 2 e 259).

Para diagnosticar o envolvimento central, é necessária a identificação de déficits que não podem ser atribuídos aos componentes periféricos, como déficits de PG, paresia, estado mental alterado ou de NC (além do NC VII). A presença de nistagmo vertical sem componente rotatório ou de nistagmo com a fase rápida em direção à lesão também sugere envolvimento central.

A presença da SH sugere uma lesão na orelha média/interna. Embora possa parecer um processo simples de distinção entre doenças periférica e central, os sinais clínicos frequentemente se sobrepõem.

Tabela 265.1 Sinais clínicos associados a doenças centrais e periféricas.

SINAIS CLÍNICOS	PERIFÉRICO	CENTRAL
Nistagmo	Horizontal ou rotativo Fase rápida da lesão	Horizontal, giratório ou vertical Fase rápida ou em direção à lesão
Estrabismo posicional	Possível	Possível estrabismo real também possível (de NC III, IV, VI)
Déficit do nervo cranial (NC)	Possível estrabismo real também possível (de NC III, IV, VI)	Qualquer NC possível (principalmente NC V a XII)
Síndrome de Horner	Possível	Rara
Estado mental	Alerta, pode ser ansioso ou desorientado	Alterado Pode ser obtundido, estuporado, comatoso, e desorientado
Propriocepção geral/paresia	Não	Possível, geralmente ipsilateral
Hipermetria	Não	Possível se cerebelar lesão (ipsilateral)

PROCEDIMENTOS DE DIAGNÓSTICO

Para a avaliação das doenças vestibulares periféricas, os testes de diagnóstico devem incluir um exame otoscópico (idealmente sob sedação ou anestesia), imagens das bulas timpânicas com radiografias ou, idealmente, imagens avançadas (tomografia computadorizada [TC] ou ressonância magnética [RM]), miringotomia para citologia e cultura (ver Capítulos 33, 85 e 259) e avaliação da tireoide. A TC é mais sensível do que as radiografias, mesmo com otite média (84 e 75% de apuração, respectivamente), mas a RM tem sensibilidade ainda maior e pode detectar otite interna também.[53]

O diagnóstico de doenças centrais (Figura 265.2) muitas vezes requer imagem avançada do cérebro com TC ou RM, análise do líquido cefalorraquidiano (LCR) e títulos para doenças infecciosas. A RM é preferível à TC, porque fornece melhores detalhes de tecidos moles e porque o artefato de endurecimento ósseo na TC torna mais difícil a avaliação do componente vestibular na fossa caudal. A RM também permite a visualização de estruturas da orelha interna, assim como da LCR, meninges e parênquima cerebral (Figura 265.3).[4] Outros procedimentos de diagnóstico potencialmente úteis incluem um exame fúndico para avaliar as lesões de coriorretinite ou hemorragia retinal (ver Capítulo 11) e um teste de potencial auditivo evocado do tronco encefálico (BAER), que também avalia o componente do tronco encefálico da audição.

TRATAMENTO DE SUPORTE E COMPENSAÇÃO EM DOENÇAS VESTIBULARES

O sistema vestibular central possui um grande potencial de compensação, mesmo para sinais vestibulares extremamente graves. Pacientes com doença vestibular se beneficiam da terapia geral destinada a reduzir alguns sinais clínicos, como vômito e doença do movimento. Promover a atividade normal e fisioterapia igualmente acelera a recuperação na maioria dos casos. A correção dos déficits vestibulares pelo sistema nervoso central (SNC) requer que o paciente se mova a fim de fornecer o *feedback* somatossensorial necessário para compensação.

Antieméticos e fluidoterapia (ver Capítulos 39 e 129) podem ser necessários se o paciente estiver vomitando e/ou desidratado. Meclizina (12,5 a 25 mg, via oral, a cada 24 horas) tem propriedades antieméticas e antivertiginosas,[5] que provavelmente ajudam por meio da sua atividade anti-histamínica fraca, propriedades depressoras do SNC e efeitos anticolinérgicos. Maropitant (1 mg/kg, via subcutânea, a cada 24 horas ou 2 a 8 mg/kg, via oral, a cada 24 horas em cães e 1 mg/kg, via oral, a cada 24 horas em gatos) é um inibidor de neurocinina-1, que bloqueia a ação da substância P para a via final comum no centro emético do cérebro. Contudo, o maropitant não parece possuir qualquer efeito antivertiginoso, portanto a meclizina pode ser benéfica mesmo em conjunto com maropitant.

DOENÇAS VESTIBULARES PERIFÉRICAS

Otite interna/média

Otite interna/média (OIM) é uma causa comum de doença vestibular periférica em cães e gatos (Vídeo 265.4). O envolvimento do NC VII e a SH também estão com frequência presentes. A etiologia é mais comumente uma extensão da otite externa em cães, mas uma infecção ascendente da nasofaringe (via tuba auditiva) parece mais comum em gatos.[8] A propagação hematogênica também é possível. As bactérias mais encontradas são *Staphylococcus* spp., *Streptococcus* spp., *Pseudomonas* spp., *Proteus* spp. e a levedura *Malassezia pachydermatis*. O diagnóstico geralmente é feito por exame otoscópico, imagem das bulhas e miringotomia para cultura e sensibilidade. Todo o tímpano pode não ser visualizado com otoscopia padrão, e uma membrana timpânica intacta não exclui o diagnóstico de OIM. Se houver material na orelha média, as amostras devem ser obtidas, se possível, para citologia e cultura. As radiografias são normais em até 25 a 33% dos casos confirmados, enquanto os resultados de TC são falsamente negativos em cerca de 17%.[9,10]

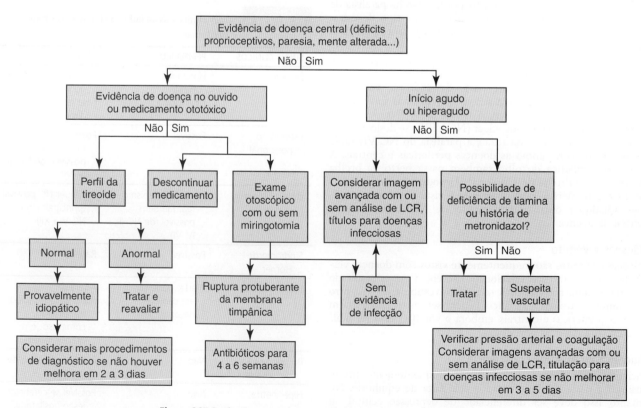

Figura 265.2 Algoritmo para doença vestibular. *LCR*, líquido cefalorraquidiano.

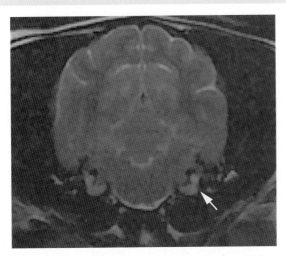

Figura 265.3 Ressonância magnética transversal ponderada em T2 imagem do cérebro de cão mostrando o fluido hiperintenso nas orelhas internas normais (seta).

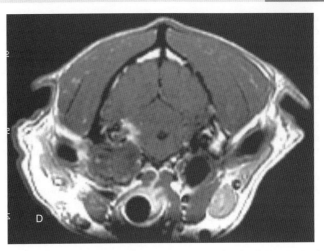

Figura 265.4 Imagem de ressonância magnética ponderada em T1 transversal mostrando cérebro de um cão ao nível da bula timpânica após a administração de gadolínio – DTPA. A bula certa é preenchida com material isointenso e há realce de contraste no tronco encefálico no mesmo nível. O diagnóstico de infecção de orelha média/interna foi confirmado em cirurgia.

Tratamento de OIM consiste em terapia antibiótica com base nos resultados da cultura e sensibilidade por um período mínimo de 4 a 6 semanas. Na ausência de cultura, deve ser escolhido um antibiótico eficaz contra a maioria dos microrganismos causadores comuns e com boa penetração óssea (p. ex., amoxicilina/clavulanato ou uma fluoroquinolona; ver Capítulos 161 e 162). Em alguns casos, uma osteotomia de bulha pode ser necessária para controlar a infecção ou confirmar o diagnóstico. O prognóstico é bom para a resolução da infecção.[12] No entanto, é possível que uma leve inclinação da cabeça e o dano ao NC VII sejam irreversíveis. Ocasionalmente, a infecção pode se estender para a cavidade craniana, causando uma meningoencefalite otogênica, empiema epidural ou um abscesso cerebral, que pode ser fatal (Figura 265.4).

O tratamento é agressivo e consiste em drenagem cirúrgica da cavidade timpânica com terapia antibiótica, mas o prognóstico é geralmente favorável.[6,11]

Pólipos nasofaríngeos

Os pólipos nasofaríngeos são crescimentos pedunculados resultantes de inflamação crônica (ver Capítulo 238). Em gatos, podem ser congênitos.[13] Eles se originam da tuba auditiva, nasofaringe ou forro da bula timpânica. Gatos jovens entre 1 e 5 anos são mais comumente afetados, mas isso pode ocorrer também em cães (Figura 265.5).[15] Além dos sinais de doença da orelha média/interna, são possíveis sinais de vias respiratórias superiores (espirros, estridor) ou faríngeos (engasgo, disfagia).

O tratamento envolve a remoção do pólipo, que pode ser feito por uma simples tração-avulsão, mas a recidiva é possível em 30 a 50% dos casos.[13,14] Quando há envolvimento da orelha média, uma osteotomia da bulha geralmente é necessária para evitar a recidiva. Um estudo retrospectivo recente de tração de pólipos transtimpânica perendoscópica em 37 gatos sugeriu uma resolução em 94% dos casos com menos complicações do que a osteotomia da bulha e tração simples (8 contra 57% a 81 e 43%, respectivamente).[54]

Doença vestibular idiopática

Essa é uma condição comum observada em gatos de todas as idades e em cães mais velhos – por isso às vezes é chamada de "doença vestibular do cão idoso" ou "doença vestibular geriátrica canina".[16,17] É caracterizada por um início agudo ou hiperagudo de sinais vestibulares periféricos. Sinais unilaterais são mais comuns, mas às vezes é observada doença bilateral, especialmente em gatos, que pode ser facilmente mal interpretada como um derrame ou uma convulsão. Os sinais vestibulares podem ser leves, mas em geral são bastante graves, na medida em que o paciente está gravemente incapacitado, tornando um exame

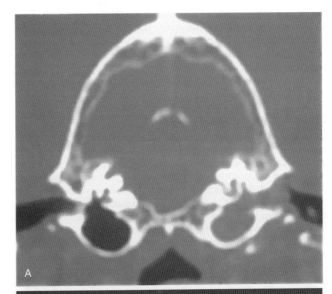

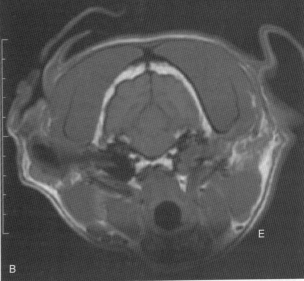

Figura 265.5 A. Imagem de tomografia computadorizada de cão com pólipo na orelha média esquerda. **B.** Imagem de ressonância magnética ponderada em T1 transversal do mesmo cão no mesmo nível.

neurológico completo difícil inicialmente. Náuseas e vômitos são comuns, bem como ansiedade, mas não há sinal de envolvimento central ou doença da orelha média (ou seja, sem paralisia ou SH). A etiologia é desconhecida, mas pode ser uma anormalidade no fluxo da endolinfa. Em gatos, a condição é mais comum no Nordeste dos EUA e no Canadá durante o verão e início do outono e pode ser causada pela migração de pequenas larvas de *Cuterebra* através do canal auditivo.[18] Uma apresentação semelhante é vista no Sudeste dos EUA em gatos que ingerem a cauda do lagarto-de-cauda-azul.[1,19] O diagnóstico é por exclusão, e a maioria dos pacientes melhora significativamente em 72 horas, embora a recuperação completa possa levar de 2 a 3 semanas. O tratamento é direcionado para náuseas e vômitos e é apenas de suporte. Apesar da apresentação frequentemente dramática, o prognóstico é muito bom, mas pequenos déficits residuais são possíveis. Tratamento direcionado para *Cuterebra* em gatos geralmente não é necessário, nem recomendado.

Hipotireoidismo
Doença vestibular secundária ao hipotireoidismo é reconhecida principalmente em cães de meia-idade a mais velhos (ver Capítulo 299).[20] Os sinais vestibulares são geralmente leves a moderados e podem ser unilaterais ou bilaterais, resultado de um déficit no metabolismo de energia com distúrbio no transporte axonal e possível desmielinização segmentar.[21] Pode haver envolvimento concomitante do nervo facial, e é possível que o paciente fique letárgico, o que torna difícil a diferenciação da doença central.[22] O diagnóstico definitivo é feito com teste de tireoide, e resolução ou melhora dos sinais clínicos é esperada dentro de 2 meses, com suplementação adequada de hormônio tireoidiano.

Ototoxicose e trauma iatrogênico
Uma lista de agentes ototóxicos foi compilada principalmente a partir de extrapolações da literatura humana ou relatos anedóticos, que incluem aminoglicosídeos, diuréticos de alça, clorexidina e cisplatina.[23,24] Entre esses, os aminoglicosídeos (sobretudo estreptomicina) e clorexidina são provavelmente os mais comuns. Em razão da ototoxicose potencial, esses fármacos nunca devem ser usados topicamente se a membrana timpânica não puder ser visualizada.

O trauma iatrogênico durante a limpeza do ouvido é provavelmente mais comum do que a ototoxicose verdadeira. A ruptura iatrogênica da membrana timpânica durante a limpeza do ouvido permite a entrada de material na bulha, o que pode levar a uma otite média inflamatória grave.[8,26] A paralisia do NC VII e/ou SH pode ser vista concomitantemente.

Outras

Congênitas
Doença vestibular unilateral congênita foi relatada em algumas raças de cães, incluindo Pastor-Alemão, Cocker Spaniel Inglês, Doberman e Fox Terrier de Pelo Liso, e em raças de gatos, incluindo Siamês, Birmanês e Tonkinês.[25,27-29] A doença congênita bilateral tem sido relatada em Akitas e Beagles.[25] A etiologia pode ser uma malformação ou degeneração das estruturas da orelha interna.

Os sinais clínicos são geralmente notados quando o animal começa pela primeira vez a deambular e incluem ataxia vestibular e inclinação da cabeça – a menos que a condição seja bilateral. O nistagmo patológico em geral não é uma característica da doença, mas alguns pacientes também têm audição prejudicada. Não há tratamento, mas os sinais vestibulares geralmente melhoram em razão da compensação.

Neoplasia
Tumores do canal auditivo ou orelha média não são comuns, mas, quando se desenvolvem, tendem a ser agressivos, especialmente em gatos. Eles incluem adenocarcinoma de glândula ceruminosa, carcinoma de células escamosas, fibrossarcoma, osteossarcoma ou condrossarcoma e linfoma (sobretudo em gatos). No geral, a maioria tende a apresentar um prognóstico muito reservado.

Em razão da proximidade entre o nervo trigêmeo (NC V) e o NC VIII, cães com tumor na bainha do NC V podem apresentar sinais vestibulares.

DOENÇAS VESTIBULARES CENTRAIS

Qualquer processo de doença que pode afetar o cérebro tem o potencial de causar uma síndrome vestibular. No entanto, algumas condições e doenças tendem a afetar preferencialmente os componentes vestibulares.

Doenças inflamatórias
Doenças inflamatórias do cérebro (encefalite), tanto infecciosas quanto não infecciosas, podem afetar qualquer parte do SNC e frequentemente produzem sinais multifocais. Elas são uma causa comum de distúrbio vestibular. Algumas doenças tendem a causar sinais vestibulares com mais frequência e são discutidas brevemente aqui, mas o Capítulo 261 traz uma discussão mais completa sobre doenças inflamatórias.

Doenças infecciosas
O vírus da cinomose canina comumente causa sinais cerebelares e vestibulares, que podem progredir para tetraparesia. Em cães mais velhos, sinais sistêmicos e mioclonia muitas vezes estão ausentes, tornando o diagnóstico difícil.[30,31] O diagnóstico pode ser feito por ensaio de imunofluorescência (IFA) de uma raspagem conjuntival ou por análise do LCR, mas isso em geral não traz informações importantes em casos crônicos. A análise de reação em cadeia da polimerase (PCR) de urina ou de LCR provou ser mais útil no diagnóstico *ante mortem* de cinomose do SNC.[30,32] Não há tratamento específico, e o prognóstico é reservado a desfavorável. No entanto, alguns cães podem se recuperar, embora deficiências neurológicas residuais sejam comuns (ver Capítulo 228).

Em gatos, os sinais vestibulares podem ser vistos com a infecção pelo vírus da peritonite infecciosa felina (PIF). Sinais neurológicos são relatados em um quarto a um terço dos gatos com a forma seca de PIF.[33] Gatos afetados geralmente têm menos de 3 anos e vivem em residências ou abrigos com vários animais. O vírus da PIF induz uma vasculite piogranulomatosa mediada por imunocomplexos. O diagnóstico *ante mortem* é difícil. O prognóstico é ruim, e a doença geralmente é fatal (ver Capítulo 224).

Febre maculosa das Montanhas Rochosas (FMMR) e erliquiose são relatadas como causas de sinais neurológicos em cerca de 40 e 20% dos casos, respectivamente, e a disfunção vestibular é uma manifestação comum, especialmente na FMMR.[7,34] A presença de achados laboratoriais típicos (trombocitopenia, anemia, leucocitose) deve levantar a suspeita dessas doenças, mesmo que não haja histórico de exposição a carrapatos.[31,35] Doenças fúngicas, em particular criptococose, podem levar à disfunção vestibular, enquanto doenças bacterianas são raras e resultam principalmente da extensão de doenças da orelha média. Infecção por *Toxoplasma gondii* em cães e gatos e *Neospora caninum* em cães também pode ser observada. Raiva tem sido relatada como causadora de sinais vestibulares rapidamente progressivos (ver Capítulos 226 e 231).[31,36-40]

Doenças não infecciosas
Doenças inflamatórias não infecciosas do cérebro também são chamadas de meningoencefalite de etiologia desconhecida (MOD) ou encefalite responsiva a esteroides (ver Capítulo 261).

Essas doenças afetam os cães, mas raramente os gatos. Entre as doenças não infecciosas estão a meningoencefalite granulomatosa (MEG) e algumas encefalites específicas de raças (p. ex., leucoencefalite necrosante do Yorkshire Terrier e encefalite necrosante de Pug), que carregam um prognóstico reservado a desfavorável. Os sinais clínicos podem ser agudos ou insidiosos e geralmente progressivos. O diagnóstico definitivo requer histopatologia (ver Capítulo 261), mas um diagnóstico presuntivo pode ser feito com base nos resultados de imagem avançada (TC ou, idealmente, RM), análise de LCR e títulos negativos para doenças infecciosas. O tratamento consiste em esteroides (p. ex., prednisona 1 a 2 mg/kg/dia, via oral) juntamente a outros fármacos imunossupressores (p. ex., citosina arabinosídeo, lomustina, procarbazina, ciclosporina) ou radioterapia. A maioria dos pacientes melhora com a terapia, mas recidivas são comuns. O prognóstico é reservado, mas extremamente variável e, se for aplicada terapia agressiva, considerado melhor do que o relatado antigamente.

Neoplasia

Tumores primários ou secundários podem afetar o tronco encefálico e cerebelo. Eles são uma causa comum de doença vestibular central. O tumor primário que afeta mais comumente os componentes vestibulares do SNC em cães é o meningioma, o tumor da bainha nervosa do NC V (afetando o tronco encefálico ou NC VIII por extensão) e o tumor do plexo coroide no quarto ventrículo. Em gatos, o meningioma e o linfoma são mais frequentemente diagnosticados. Sinais clínicos podem ser agudos ou insidiosos, e a condição geralmente é progressiva durante um período de semanas a meses (Vídeo 265.5). O diagnóstico requer imagens avançadas do cérebro (TC ou, idealmente, RM). A análise do LCR pode ser útil na tentativa de descartar doenças inflamatórias, mas raramente é diagnóstica de um processo tumoral (Figura 265.6). O tratamento pode ser paliativo com glicocorticosteroides ou direcionado ao processo tumoral (excisão cirúrgica, quimioterapia, radioterapia). O prognóstico geralmente é ruim. O Capítulo 260 discute com mais detalhes os tumores cerebrais.

Vascular

Um acidente vascular encefálico (AVE) ou derrame é caracterizado por um início repentino de sinais focais não progressivos de disfunção cerebral (ver Capítulo 260). Ocorre quando o sangue que flui para uma região do cérebro é obstruído por um infarto (trombo ou embolia), uma hemorragia ou um espasmo arterial, e pode resultar na morte do tecido cerebral. Anteriormente, acreditava-se que era incomum em cães e gatos, mas agora sua maior frequência é reconhecida com o uso de RM.[41,42] O local mais comum para AVE em cães é o cerebelo, em áreas irrigadas pela artéria cerebelar rostral.[42] A maioria dos AVE resulta de infartos não hemorrágicos, mas um componente hemorrágico é possível.[43] A etiologia não pode ser determinada em muitos casos.[45] No entanto, condições como insuficiência renal crônica ou hiperadrenocorticismo estão presentes em pouco mais de 50% dos pacientes. Gatos com infartos hemorrágicos muitas vezes têm uma patologia hepática e/ou nefrite. O diagnóstico é feito com o histórico (início de deficiências neurológicas hiperagudas e não progressivas) e achados de RM, que incluem uma lesão bem definida com demarcação nítida hiperintensa em imagens ponderadas em T2 e sequências de recuperação de inversão atenuada por fluido (FLAIR) com efeito de massa mínimo ou nenhum (Figura 265.7) e sem realce de contraste periférico, nem contraste mínimo. A sensibilidade e a especificidade da RM no diagnóstico de AVE são melhoradas com o uso de estudos funcionais mais recentes, como o de imagem de difusão ponderada, mas seu uso não está amplamente disponível na medicina veterinária.[42] Imagens de eco gradiente (T2* ou T2-GRE) são úteis para identificar infartos hemorrágicos, pois as hemorragias aparecem hipointensas nessa sequência, independentemente da idade da hemorragia.

A avaliação da coagulação pode ser útil no diagnóstico de infartos hemorrágicos. Tromboelastografia (TEG), que avalia a formação e a lise do coágulo, pode detectar um estado hipercoagulável. Infelizmente, esse teste tem disponibilidade atual muito limitada. Se um estado hipercoagulável for confirmado ou suspeito, o tratamento com clopidogrel (1 a 3 mg/kg, via oral, a cada 24 horas), um antagonista do receptor ADP, pode ajudar a reduzir a agregação plaquetária.

O tratamento é principalmente de suporte, e a atenção deve ser dada para garantir uma boa hidratação, pressão arterial e oxigenação (Vídeo 265.6). O prognóstico é muito bom, mas cães com doença concomitante têm sobrevida mais curta e

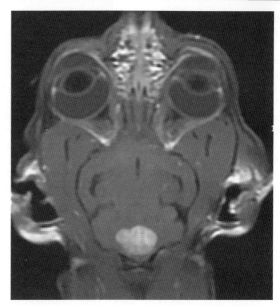

Figura 265.6 Imagem de ressonância magnética ponderada em T1 dorsal do cérebro de gato após a administração de gadolínio – DTPA. Há grande massa com realce difuso e marcante contraste no cerebelo. O diagnóstico presuntivo foi tumor encefálico primário. Todavia, *Cryptococcus* foram identificados em análise do líquido cefalorraquidiano, e o gato respondeu ao fluconazol.

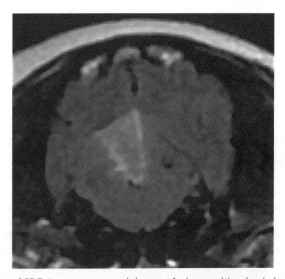

Figura 265.7 Imagem transversal de ressonância magnética do cérebro de um cão, recuperação inversa atenuada por fluido. Há uma lesão hiperintensa definida com demarcação nítida e sem massa no cerebelo, compatível com AVE (artéria cerebelar rostral).

aumento do risco de recidiva.[44] Um estudo retrospectivo de 23 cães com AVE isquêmico relatou uma taxa de mortalidade de 23% em 30 dias, mas uma sobrevida média de 505 dias.[55] Ocasionalmente, episódios de eventos neurológicos paroxísticos são vistos antes da apresentação (às vezes descrita como convulsão, por causa de sua curta duração) e podem representar ataques de isquemia transitória (AIT).[42] Os AIT são episódios de déficit neurológico focal breve secundário à embolia, constrição vascular ou espasmos que se resolvem dentro de 24 horas (na maioria dos casos, de minutos a algumas horas).[46] Em humanos, os AIT precedem o infarto cerebelar em 26 a 41% dos casos, mas são mal reconhecidos e entendidos na medicina veterinária.

Toxicose

A toxicidade do metronidazol em cães provoca sinais vestibulares centrais, de agudos a subagudos bilaterais, geralmente acompanhados por sinais cerebelares (tremores de intenção, hipermetria; Vídeo 265.7). Nistagmo vertical posicional em repouso é um achado comum. Anorexia e vômitos frequentemente precedem os sinais vestibulares. O mecanismo exato de toxicidade é desconhecido, mas metronidazol parece interagir com os receptores ácido gama-aminobutírico (GABA) no cerebelo e núcleos vestibulares. A toxicose é geralmente observada com a administração diária de mais de 60 mg/kg/dia durante 3 a 14 dias, mas foram relatados em cães que receberam apenas 33 mg/kg/dia.[47]

A recuperação geralmente ocorre em 1 a 2 semanas após a interrupção do metronidazol com cuidados de suporte. A adição de diazepam (0,5 mg/kg, intravenoso, seguido por 0,5 mg/kg, via oral, a cada 8 horas) para o tratamento acelera a recuperação em cerca de 1 a 3 dias, em razão de seu efeito sobre os receptores GABA.[47] Em gatos, a intoxicação por metronidazol tende a causar distúrbios no prosencéfalo (convulsões, cegueira, ataxia) em vez de sinais vestibulares.[48]

Outras

Deficiência de tiamina

Deficiência de tiamina (vitamina B_1) causa necrose bilateral e hemorragia nos núcleos suscetíveis do cérebro (ver Capítulo 12). Em gatos, os núcleos vestibular e ocular são frequentemente afetados, levando a sinais vestibulares e pupilas dilatadas e sem resposta, muitas vezes com ventroflexão profunda da cabeça e do pescoço. A deficiência de tiamina pode ocorrer em pacientes alimentados com uma dieta rica em tiaminase (peixe cru) ou comida enlatada submetida a calor excessivo (acima dos 100°C ou 212°F).[50] Dióxido de enxofre, usado como conservante, pode destruir a tiamina nos alimentos.

O diagnóstico é baseado no histórico, achados típicos de RM e teor sanguíneo de tiamina.[57] O tratamento consiste na administração de tiamina (12,5 a 50 mg por paciente por dia, intramuscular, subcutâneo ou via oral), e o prognóstico em geral é bom, se a doença for reconhecida e tratada rapidamente.

Anomalia

Algumas malformações e anomalias congênitas podem causar sinais vestibulares. Entre elas, a síndrome de malformação occipital caudal é provavelmente a mais comum, vista normalmente em Cavalier King Charles Spaniels, mas possível em outras raças pequenas. Um cisto aracnoide, especialmente na cisterna quadrigeminal, também pode causar deficiências cerebelares.

Trauma

Traumatismo craniano pode causar sinais vestibulares, em razão do envolvimento cerebelar e/ou do tronco encefálico. Se o tronco cerebral é afetado, obnubilação e até estupor ou coma são prováveis. O prognóstico para traumatismo craniano é bom para uma lesão cerebelar, mas muito reservado quando há envolvimento do tronco cerebral.

Doenças degenerativas

Doenças do armazenamento e degenerativas, abiotrofia e hipoplasia cerebelar, entre outras, podem causar sinais vestibulares. São geralmente progressivas, e o prognóstico é reservado a ruim.

Síndrome vestibular pós-anestésica em gatos

O autor e outros médicos-veterinários da província de Quebec (Canadá) relataram casos de síndrome vestibular aguda após anestesia em gatos jovens. Em um estudo retrospectivo, 18 casos foram avaliados ao longo de 4 anos.[51]

Nesse estudo, 90% dos gatos tinham entre 3 e 6 meses (destes, 72% tinham entre 3 e 4 meses). Os animais se recuperaram normalmente da anestesia sem deficiências observadas, e os sinais vestibulares apareceram 2 a 24 horas após a recuperação. A maioria estava alerta, embora salivação e náuseas fossem ocasionalmente relatadas. Nenhuma limpeza de ouvido foi realizada durante o procedimento. A recuperação demorou 48 h a 10 semanas, com a grande maioria de volta ao normal dentro de 1 semana. A causa da doença é desconhecida, e complicações anestésicas não foram relatadas em nenhum dos casos. Nem um único medicamento ou combinação de medicamentos ou técnica foi identificado como comum a todos os casos (Vídeo 265.9).

EPISÓDICO

Às vezes, uma perturbação vestibular episódica é observada, principalmente em cães (Vídeo 265.8). Os episódios podem durar alguns segundos a minutos e são caracterizados por inclinação da cabeça, perda de equilíbrio e nistagmo. Em alguns pacientes, os episódios parecem ser induzidos por excitação ou certas atividades e movimentos.

A etiologia desses "episódios vestibulares" é provavelmente variada. Alguns casos podem representar AIT, enquanto outros provavelmente são secundários à encefalopatia hipertensiva, o que deve incitar, portanto, avaliações seriadas de pressão arterial. A encefalopatia hipertensiva foi relatada com elevação aguda e sustentada da pressão arterial sistólica (ver Capítulos 99 e 157). Os sinais clínicos são frequentemente reversíveis, com normalização da pressão arterial.[56] No entanto, a etiologia permanece indeterminada em muitos casos, apesar de uma extensa avaliação diagnóstica. É possível que algumas convulsões possam estar presentes com os sinais vestibulares. Em humanos, epilepsia do lobo temporal pode causar tontura e vertigem.[52] Duas condições tendem a causar distúrbio vestibular episódico em humanos: vertigem posicional paroxística benigna (VPPB) e doença de Meniere.

Com a VPPB, os episódios geralmente são desencadeados por determinadas posições da cabeça. Eles duram alguns segundos, e a condição pode se resolver em alguns meses.[52] Embora essas condições não sejam relatadas em medicina veterinária, a síndrome vestibular episódica pode representar uma delas.

REFERÊNCIAS BIBLIOGRÁFICAS

As referências bibliográficas deste capítulo se encontram online no Ambiente de Aprendizagem.

CAPÍTULO 266

Doenças da Medula Espinal: Congênitas (Desenvolvimento), Inflamatórias e Degenerativas

Ronaldo Casimiro da Costa e Simon R. Platt

ESPONDILOMIELOPATIA CERVICAL

Etiologia e patogenia

A espondilomielopatia cervical (EMC) é a doença mais comum da coluna vertebral cervical em cães de raça grande e gigante. Quinze nomes diferentes têm sido usados para descrever esta doença (síndrome de wobbler, instabilidade vertebral cervical, síndrome da malformação-malarticulação cervical, entre outros), refletindo a compreensão limitada da patogênese da doença.[1-4]

A causa do EMC ainda não é clara. Fatores genéticos, congênitos, de conformação corporal e nutricionais têm sido propostos; contudo, tanto a conformação corporal quanto a nutrição não parecem ser significantes.[5,6] As evidências atuais apoiam a etiologia congênita com base genética, o que tem sido documentado em Dobermans como traço autossômico dominante com penetrância variável.[7]

Existem duas formas de EMC, que, apesar de algum grau de sobreposição, podem ser amplamente divididas em compressão óssea-associada e compressão disco-associada.[1,8,9] A *compressão disco-associada* em geral é observada em cães de meia-idade (principalmente Dobermans) e é causada por protrusão intervertebral de disco com ou sem hipertrofia do ligamento dorsal longitudinal ou ligamento flavo (Figura 266.1 A). Na grande maioria dos casos, são afetados os discos C5-6 e C6-7. A fisiopatologia da forma óssea é diferente, vista predominantemente em cães adultos jovens de raça gigante, sobretudo Dogue Alemão. Raças gigantes em geral têm compressão da medula espinal secundária à proliferação do arco vertebral (dorsalmente), processos articulares (dorsolateralmente) ou processos articulares e pedículos (lateralmente) (Figura 266.1 B). A causa da compressão parece ser uma combinação de malformação vertebral e mudanças osteoartrítico-osteoartróticas que afetam os processos articulares.[1]

Achados clínicos

Cães com EMC apresentam tipicamente uma longa história de deficiências de marcha crônicas e progressivas que afetam sobretudo os membros pélvicos. A principal anormalidade neurológica é a ataxia proprioceptiva, que leva a uma marcha "vacilante" (em inglês, *wobbler*, daí o nome "síndrome de wobbler"), além de graus variáveis de fraqueza que afetam os membros pélvicos ou todos os quatro membros. Uma vez que a maioria das lesões está localizada na região cervical caudal, muitos cães apresentam a chamada "marcha de dois motores", na qual a marcha do membro torácico pode parecer instável e apresenta passos curtos, enquanto a do membro pélvico é muitas vezes baseada na largura (abduzida), com um comprimento de passada mais longo e marcadamente descoordenado (Vídeo 266.1). Déficits de reação postural (déficits de posicionamento proprioceptivo) são geralmente observados, mas podem não ser evidentes em casos de história crônica, apesar da presença de ataxia proprioceptiva, reforçando assim a importância de uma avaliação cuidadosa da marcha (ver Capítulo 259). Os reflexos espinais dos membros torácicos geralmente revelam diminuição do reflexo extensor (retirada) com aumento de tônus ou tônus normal. Os reflexos dos membros pélvicos são normais a aumentados.

A palpação da coluna cervical pode revelar dor, porém a hiperestesia cervical não é uma característica proeminente dessa doença. Manipulações vigorosas da coluna cervical são desnecessárias e podem levar à descompensação neurológica grave.

Diagnóstico

O diagnóstico definitivo deve ser feito usando imagens avançadas (tomografia computadorizada [TC], ressonância magnética [RM]) ou mielografia. As radiografias de triagem não podem ser usadas como o único critério de diagnóstico, mas apenas como um teste de triagem para descartar outros diagnósticos diferenciais e para um diagnóstico presuntivo. Achados radiográficos observados na forma associada à discopatia são principalmente mudanças na forma do corpo vertebral, estreitamento do espaço do disco intervertebral e estenose do canal vertebral. Alterações osteoartríticas e escleróticas dos processos articulares são as marcas radiográficas em cães de raça gigante com compressões ósseas e podem ser observadas em projeções lateral e ventrodorsal.[10] A mielografia já não é o método de escolha para diagnosticar a EMC, mas pode ser usada se a TC e RM não estiverem disponíveis. A TC é um exame rápido que permite a visualização de cortes transversais da coluna cervical. Tem que ser combinada com a mielografia para identificar a localização exata da(s) lesão(ões) compressiva(s). Além disso, fornece uma visualização superior da direção e da gravidade da compressão da medula espinal, em comparação com a mielografia.[11] A RM é o exame padrão-ouro para avaliação diagnóstica e é comprovadamente superior à mielografia e complementar à TC.[12-14] A principal vantagem da RM é a detecção do sinal de alterações da medula espinal (observadas em aproximadamente 50% dos cães comprometidos), permitindo a identificação precisa do(s) local(is) em estado mais grave.[15]

Tratamento

Idealmente, a história natural de uma doença deve ser entendida de modo que as recomendações para o tratamento e prognóstico possam ser fundamentadas nesse conhecimento. Infelizmente, a história natural de EMC não está definida, porque parece que a doença progride com lentidão em muitos cães com ambas as formas de EMC.[4,16] As duas opções amplas de tratamento são clínico (conservador) ou cirúrgico. O tratamento conservador é uma opção viável para muitos cães, principalmente os de raça gigante, com múltiplas lesões compressivas afetando o aspecto lateral da medula espinal. Esta opção também pode ser apropriada para iniciar cães sob controle médico – em um primeiro momento, para avaliar a melhoria obtida com o tratamento e, depois, para dar aos proprietários a oportunidade de decidir sobre a cirurgia. A resposta ao manejo clínico pode ser usada para avaliar indiretamente o grau de reversibilidade das lesões da medula espinal, e o componente mais importante é a restrição de exercícios para minimizar o componente dinâmico da lesão.[1,17] Os cães podem passear na guia, mas de forma livre, e a atividade não supervisionada é fortemente desencorajada. Em vez disso, deve ser usado um arnês (peitoral) corporal em vez de coleira. Os corticosteroides parecem beneficiar os cães com EMC, e as dosagens anti-inflamatórias de prednisona são com

1438 SEÇÃO 17 • Doença Neurológica

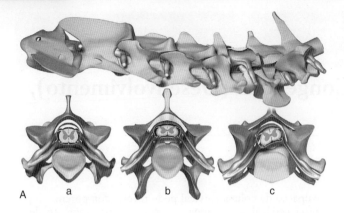

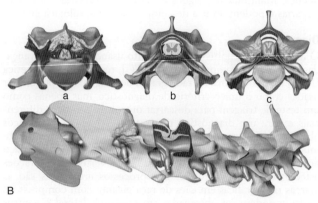

Figura 266.1 A. Espondilomielopatia cervical associada a discopatia. Superior: compressão da medula espinhal ventral e compressão da raiz nervosa em C5-6 causado pela protrusão do disco intervertebral. Dorsalmente, hipertrofia do ligamento flavum causa leve compressão da medula espinhal. *a*, seção transversal em nível do disco C4-5, região mostrando medula espinhal e canal vertebral normais. *b*, Compressão ventral na região C5-6 causada pela protrusão do disco intervertebral e hipertrofia do ligamento longitudinal dorsal e ligamento flavum (levando a leve compressão dorsal). *c*, protrusão assimétrica do disco intervertebral em C6-7 causando medula espinhal e compressão da raiz nervosa. **B.** Espondilomielopatia óssea cervical. *a*, compressão severa dorsolateral da medula espinhal em C2-3 causada por malformação óssea e alterações osteoartríticas. *b*, Região do disco C3-4 normal. *c*, compressão bilateral em C4-5 causada por osteoartrite mudanças e proliferação medial das facetas, resultando em estenose absoluta do canal vertebral e estenose do forame, que levam à compressão da medula espinhal e da raiz nervosa, respectivamente. Inferior: Compressão da medula espinhal dorsal em C3-4 causada por malformação da lâmina e hipertrofia do ligamento *flavum*. Mudanças osteoartríticas também são mostradas em C2-3. (De da Costa RC: Cervical espondilomielopatia [síndrome de wobbler] em cães. *Vet Clin North Am Small Anim Pract* 40 [5]: 881-913, 2010.)

frequência usadas (0,5 a 1 mg/kg, via oral, a cada 12 a 24 h), diminuindo progressivamente ao longo de 2 a 4 semanas. O mecanismo proposto de ação dos corticosteroides é a redução do edema vasogênico, proteção contra a toxicidade do glutamato e redução de apoptose de neurônios e oligodendroglia.[18-20] Axônios sobreviventes desmielinizados também podem remielinizar com o tratamento. Devido à possibilidade de complicações gastrintestinais, omeprazol ou famotidina são frequentemente usados em associação com corticoterapia. Por volta de 50% dos cães melhoram com o manejo.[16,21-23]

A cirurgia é em geral considerada como representante do tratamento de escolha para a maioria dos cães com EMC.[2,24] Uma vez que a maioria dos animais comprometidos tem compressão da medula espinal, descomprimi-la fornece, em teoria, o tratamento definitivo. É importante, porém, considerar vários fatores, por exemplo a gravidade de sinais neurológicos, tipo e gravidade da(s) lesão(ões) compressiva(s), resposta (ou sua ausência) ao manejo clínico, expectativas de curto e longo prazo do proprietário e presença de outros fatores concomitantes (doenças neurológicas, ortopédicas, sistêmicas ou cardíacas, como a cardiomiopatia dilatada que afetaria o resultado a longo prazo).

Esse é um dos tópicos mais polêmicos em relação à doença: 27 técnicas cirúrgicas têm sido propostas para tratar a EMC.[24,25] As técnicas podem ser divididas, de forma geral, em descompressão direta (p. ex., ventral fenda ou laminectomia dorsal), descompressão indireta (técnicas de distração com tampão de polimetilmetacrilato) e técnicas de preservação de movimento (substituição de disco).[24-28] Atualmente nenhuma técnica tem clara superioridade. Aproximadamente 70 a 80% dos cães melhoram com o tratamento cirúrgico, embora muitos se deteriorem em 2 a 3 anos após a cirurgia. Uma discussão extensa sobre opções cirúrgicas está além do escopo deste capítulo.

ESTENOSE LOMBOSSACRAL DEGENERATIVA

Etiologia e patogenia

A estenose lombossacral degenerativa é uma doença comum de cães adultos de raças grandes. Vários termos foram usados para descrevê-la, como síndrome da cauda equina, compressão da cauda equina, estenose ou doença lombossacral, instabilidade lombossacral e estenose lombossacral degenerativa.[29-31] Esses termos abrangem uma síndrome caracterizada por estenose (estreitamento) da região lombossacra, frequentemente causada por protrusão do disco intervertebral (Figura 266.2). A fisiopatologia básica envolve degeneração progressiva crônica do disco intervertebral, com subsequente protrusão do disco intervertebral L7-S1 no canal vertebral associada à proliferação dos tecidos moles ao redor da cauda equina, como hipertrofia do ligamento interarcuado (ligamento Flavo) e da cápsula articular e fibrose epidural.[29,32,33]

As causas específicas para a alta incidência desse processo degenerativo são desconhecidas. Uma base genética foi proposta recentemente em Pastores-Alemães.[34] Parece que a presença de vértebras transicionais ou osteocondrose sacral na junção lombossacral nessa raça, assim como em outras raças grandes, está associada ao desenvolvimento da estenose lombossacral degenerativa.[34-37] Pastores-Alemães também mostraram ter estenose do canal vertebral e um grau mais alto entre L7-S1 em comparação com outras raças.[34]

Achados clínicos

Os sinais refletem a compressão dos nervos espinais e dos nervos das raízes nervosas na região lombossacra. O principal sinal clínico é a dor lombossacral. Os pacientes apresentam uma história sugestiva de dor, como dificuldade ou relutância em sentar, pular e subir escadas e claudicação. Palpação cuidadosa

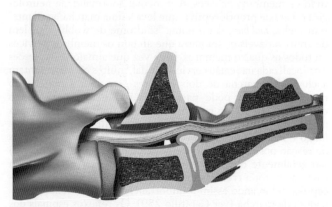

Figura 266.2 Ilustração esquemática da protrusão do disco intervertebral em L7-S1 comprimindo a cauda equina. (De Dewey CW, da Costa RC: *Guia prático de neurologia canina e felina*, 3 ed., Ames, IA, 2015, Wiley.)

CAPÍTULO 266 • Doenças da Medula Espinal: Congênitas (Desenvolvimento), Inflamatórias e Degenerativas

da área lombossacra (incluindo lordose da coluna caudal) enquanto a área lombossacra é pressionada, elevação da cauda ou palpação retal devem causar dor. É importante sempre realizar exame retal nesses cães, uma vez que neoplasias no canal pélvico podem estender-se dorsalmente, causando sinais de disfunção da cauda equina.[29]

O exame de marcha de cães comprometidos revela fraqueza do membro pélvico (sem ataxia proprioceptiva) e, muitas vezes, uma "rigidez" na forma de andar. Em alguns casos, o único sinal é claudicação uni ou bilateral, que pode ser mal interpretada como um sinal de doença ortopédica. Muitos cães grandes também têm doenças ortopédicas concomitantes, destacando a importância de uma boa avaliação neurológica (ver Capítulo 259) e palpação espinal. A maioria dos animais tem déficits em testes de posicionamento proprioceptivo dos membros pélvicos, com diminuição do reflexo flexor (principalmente flexão dificultosa do jarrete) e um reflexo patelar normal (às vezes, com "pseudo-hiper-reflexia"). Nos últimos estágios da doença, os pacientes podem apresentar incontinência urinária e/ou fecal.

Diagnóstico

O diagnóstico de estenose lombossacral degenerativa é baseado em sinalização (principalmente em cães de meia-idade a mais velhos de raças grandes), achados históricos e clínicos e resultados de exames de imagem da região lombossacra. O exame radiográfico deve sempre ser o teste inicial de imagem. Apesar de raramente ser diagnóstico por si só, o exame pode ser usado para descartar discopondilite, neoplasias espinais e lesões traumáticas. Descobertas radiográficas comuns são colapso do espaço do disco intervertebral, esclerose das placas vertebrais terminais, desalinhamento do sacro com a vértebra L7, estreitamento do forame craniano do sacro e espondilose.

Vários procedimentos foram propostos para diagnosticar definitivamente a estenose lombossacral degenerativa, mas está claro que a TC e a RM (sobretudo a RM) fornecem informações estruturais mais detalhadas sobre a cauda equina, incluindo sobre o forame intervertebral L7-S1 e as raízes nervosas L7.[32,38-43] É importante ter em mente que cães clinicamente normais (sobretudo cães mais velhos) podem ter compressão da região lombossacra sem sinais clínicos associados e que o grau de compressão da cauda equina visto na imagem não se correlaciona com a presença de doença ou com sua gravidade.[42,44] Esse é um dos desafios associados ao diagnóstico da estenose lombossacral degenerativa.[45]

Tratamento

O tratamento do paciente com estenose lombossacral degenerativa pode ser não cirúrgico ou cirúrgico. As decisões de tratamento são baseadas principalmente na gravidade dos sinais clínicos, na idade do paciente e na presença de doenças concomitantes (neurológicas e não neurológicas). A terapia não cirúrgica consiste inicialmente em repouso forçado por um algumas semanas, seguido por um período de caminhadas curtas regulares para manter a massa muscular. Além disso, medicamentos anti-inflamatórios (não esteroidais ou prednisona, mas não ambos; ver Capítulo 164), analgésicos (como gabapentina; ver Capítulos 126, 166 e 356) e redução do peso corporal (ver Capítulo 176) são recomendados.[29,33] O tratamento não cirúrgico (ou conservador) é uma opção inicial razoável, principalmente em pacientes idosos com doenças ortopédicas múltiplas ou sistêmicas. Um estudo retrospectivo recente avaliou o acompanhamento de curto e longo prazo de cães tratados clinicamente e encontrou um resultado bem-sucedido em 55% dos casos (17 de 31 cães).[46] O uso de esteroides no espaço epidural é uma abordagem terapêutica popular no ser humano para hérnias de disco comprimindo raízes nervosas lombar e lombossacral.[47] Um estudo retrospectivo avaliou o uso de injeções de esteroide peridural guiado por fluoroscopia e demostrou um resultado de melhora em 79% dos cães.[48]

O tratamento cirúrgico é o tratamento de escolha quando os sinais do paciente são graves ou refratários ao tratamento clínico. Em geral, a cirurgia consiste em uma laminectomia dorsal sobre o interespaço L7-S1, frequentemente associada à remoção de tecidos moles hipertrofiados. A extensão lateral da descompressão (facetectomia) pode ser necessária, dependendo da lesão. A estabilização também pode ser necessária em alguns casos. Em pacientes com estenose foraminal lateralizada, em oposição à estenose do canal vertebral, foraminotomia (alargamento cirúrgico do forame) pode precisar ser executado.[49] O prognóstico para a recuperação funcional desse distúrbio é, em geral, bom a excelente com intervenção cirúrgica. Os resultados de sucesso variam de 66,7 a 95% dos casos.[50-52] O tratamento cirúrgico é menos bem-sucedido em cães com incontinência fecal ou urinária, com um artigo indicando falha na resolução da incontinência em 55 a 87% de casos.[29,33,50-52]

CISTOS SINOVIAIS EXTRADURAIS

Etiologia e patogenia

Cistos sinoviais extradurais (CSE) ou cistos intraespinais extradurais são cistos decorrentes do tecido articular periarticular. Eles podem ser divididos em dois tipos: sinoviais e ganglionares. Os cistos sinoviais têm um revestimento sinovial contendo líquido, enquanto os cistos ganglionares possuem material mixoide sem revestimento específico. Essas são diferenças patológicas que podem de fato refletir estágios distintos da mesma doença.[53] Considerando que os dois tipos de cistos ocorrem em estreita proximidade com as articulações intervertebrais, o termo "cistos de justaposição" foi adotado para abranger ambos os cistos.[53]

A fisiopatologia não está bem estabelecida. Considera-se que a degeneração da articulação zigapofisário (alterações osteoartríticas) causa protrusão da membrana sinovial, por meio de defeitos da cápsula articular. A protrusão forma uma cavidade pararticular preenchida com fluido sinovial, que leva a compressões extradurais.[53,54] Outros mecanismos propostos são proliferação de células mesenquimais pluripotentes, degeneração mixoide com formação de cisto no tecido de colágeno e aumento na produção de ácido hialurônico por fibroblastos.[54] Alguns dos cães acometidos com cistos lombossacrais tinham vértebras transicionais, o que pode ser um fator de risco.[55]

Achados clínicos

Os sinais clínicos dos cistos sinoviais refletem sua localização na coluna vertebral, sendo os dois locais mais frequentes as regiões lombossacra e cervical. Os sinais clínicos de cistos cervicais são aqueles de uma mielopatia cervical com ataxia proprioceptiva e tetraparesia, enquanto claudicação de membro pélvico ou fraqueza, com ou sem dor à palpação, pode ser observada em cistos lombossacrais.[54,55]

Diagnóstico

A maioria dos relatos de cães com cistos sinoviais lombossacra/caudal lombares era de raças grandes, de meia-idade ou mais velhos (idade média de 8 anos).[53] Já os cistos sinoviais cervicais são relativamente comuns em associação com a forma óssea da EMC em cães jovens de raça gigante.[3,56,57] Dois estudos de RM indicam que eles ocorrem em 20% dos cães com EMC.[3,56,57]

O diagnóstico de cistos sinoviais é mais bem feito quando usada RM (Figura 266.3). No homem, é relatado que a RM tem uma sensibilidade de 90% para o diagnóstico de CSE, em comparação com 70% utilizando TC.[58] Tanto as janelas de tecido mole quanto as de osso devem ser usadas para aumentar a precisão da TC e detectar esses cistos. A RM em cães revela os cistos como massas extradurais bem circunscritas em um ou ambos os lados do canal vertebral. Eles são hiperintensos em imagens ponderadas em T2, com características variáveis

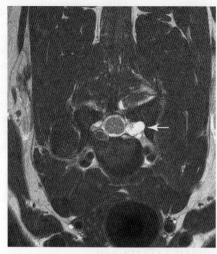

Figura 266.3 Cisto sinovial extradural em um Dogue Alemão com a forma óssea de espondilomielopatia cervical (seta).

em imagens ponderadas em T1.[55,56,59] As alterações radiográficas são inespecíficas e apenas indicam doença articular degenerativa nos locais comprometidos. As alterações mielográficas podem ser sugestivas, mas não são diagnósticas. Mudanças na projeção lateral são compressão(ões) extradural(s) dorsais e, na vista ventrodorsal, compressões axiais uni ou bilaterais.[54] O fluido cerebrospinal (LCR) tipicamente revela dissociação albuminocitológica, mas também pode ser observada pleocitose mononuclear leve.[53,54]

Tratamento

O tratamento desses cistos é tipicamente cirúrgico, muitas vezes feito ao mesmo tempo que a cirurgia descompressiva (laminectomia dorsal) para EMC ou estenose lombossacral degenerativa. No entanto, muitos desses cistos no homem são assintomáticos e, em muitos casos, podem ser descobertas por acidente.[60] O mesmo pode ser verdade para os cães; portanto, a tentativa de manejo clínico com restrição de atividade e anti-inflamatórios é recomendado no início. Todos os casos relatados de tratamento cirúrgico de cistos sinoviais tiveram resultados positivos.[53]

DIVERTÍCULO ARACNOIDE ESPINAL (CISTO)

Etiologia e patogenia

Divertículos aracnoides espinais são dilatações focais do espaço subaracnoide, que podem levar a uma mielopatia progressiva por compressão. Esses divertículos eram anteriormente chamados de cistos aracnoides, mas este era um nome impróprio, porque eles não são cavidades epiteliais revestidas fechadas.[53,61,62] Também são chamados de cistos intra-aracnóideos ou subaracnóideos, cistos meníngeos, cistos leptomeníngeos e pseudocistos.[63-65] Atualmente, parece que esses divertículos estão sendo reconhecidos com mais frequência, pelo uso generalizado da RM. No homem, estruturas semelhantes a cistos nas meninges foram classificadas em três tipos, sendo o tipo III (formas intradurais) a forma que melhor se ajusta aos divertículos encontrados em cães.[53,61]

A etiologia desses cistos não é totalmente compreendida. Um recente relatório indicou uma predisposição genética em Pugs.[62] Parece que uma etiologia congênita é provável nos casos observados em cães jovens. Outras causas propostas são a presença de doenças concomitantes: uma grande série de casos recentes indicou que 21,3% dos cães tinham doenças concomitantes nas proximidades dos divertículos (p. ex., doença de disco intervertebral, malformações vertebrais, mielite), o que pode ter influenciado seu desenvolvimento.[66]

Dois estudos recentes revisaram 215 casos de divertículos da aracnoide e revelaram que aproximadamente 55% deles ocorrem na região cervical, enquanto 45% são vistos na região toracolombar.[53,66] Os locais específicos mais comuns foram C2, C3 e T9 a T13. Raças grandes têm uma predileção por divertículos cervicais, enquanto raças pequenas têm tendência a ter divertículos toracolombares.[53,66] Aproximadamente 88% dos divertículos parecem estar localizados no aspecto dorsal da medula espinal; 8%, na região ventral; e o restante nas regiões laterais ou circunferenciais.

Achados clínicos

Os sinais clínicos refletem a localização da mielopatia. Esta doença é caracterizada principalmente por ataxia proprioceptiva com vários graus de tetraparesia ou paraparesia, sem dor espinal evidente. Alguns cães com divertículos cervicais apresentam sinais mais graves nos membros torácicos, sugerindo uma lesão intramedular. Uma característica comum é uma marcha espástica grave nos membros torácicos, dando a aparência de "pseudo-hipermetria".[67] A hiperpatia espinal não é um sinal proeminente, mas foi relatada em 18,9% dos cães em uma grande série de casos (embora uma boa proporção tivesse doenças concomitantes, tornando difícil saber a origem exata da dor).[66] As incontinências urinária e fecal foram relatadas em aproximadamente 8% dos cães, sobretudo nos pacientes com divertículos toracolombares.

Diagnóstico

Duas raças estão sobrerepresentadas: Rottweilers e Pugs. Os Buldogues Franceses também são predispostos a divertículos toracolombares. No geral, há uma clara predisposição em machos, sendo a proporção de macho e fêmea de 2:1 a 3:1 em grandes séries de casos. A idade média é de 2,5 anos, mas podem ser acometidos entre os 2,5 meses e os 13 anos. Pugs tendem a ser comprometidos em idade mais avançada (média de 59 meses).[53,66]

Mielografia, TC-mielografia ou RM são necessárias para diagnosticar esse distúrbio (Figura 266.4). A mielografia e a TC pós-mielografia demonstram esses divertículos como expansões em forma de lágrima, cheias de contraste no espaço subaracnoide.[53,63] Também podem revelar um bloqueio da coluna de contraste subaracnóidea sem preenchimento dos divertículos subaracnóideos. A RM é geralmente considerada a modalidade de imagem de escolha para avaliar esses divertículos, porque também permite a avaliação do parênquima da medula espinal e a detecção de comorbidades, como a siringo-hidromielia. É importante usar sequências de mielograma de RM (imagens ponderadas em T2) para facilitar a visualização do divertículo.[68] A análise do LCR é normal na maioria dos casos. Aproximadamente 20% dos cães mostram dissociação albuminocitológica e 10% podem mostrar pleocitose mononuclear leve.[53,63]

Tratamento

O manejo clínico (ou seja, terapia com glicocorticoides) pode ser tentado inicialmente. Em alguns casos, os sinais podem ser manejados por longos períodos, e a doença parece se estabilizar. Entretanto, o manejo cirúrgico é geralmente o tratamento de escolha. As técnicas cirúrgicas descritas envolvem fenestração com durotomia ou durectomia e marsupialização do divertículo. Nos casos em que a instabilidade vertebral pode estar presente, a estabilização é recomendada. Dos dados limitados disponíveis, o tratamento cirúrgico de cistos aracnoides espinais parece ter um bom prognóstico. Parece que 65 a 80% dos casos têm bons resultados.[53,65] Não está claro quantos cães têm recorrência, porque o acompanhamento dos casos notificados é variável, mas aparentemente pelo menos 10 a 20% dos casos apresentam recorrência dos sinais. Os fatores associados a um melhor resultado foram a idade (menos de 3 anos) e a duração dos sinais clínicos (menos de 4 meses).[65]

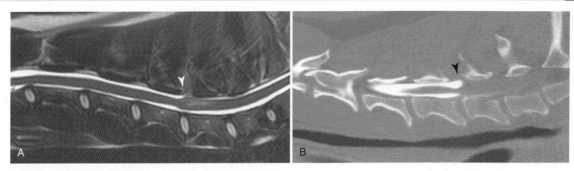

Figura 266.4 Imagens de um cão Rottweiler com um divertículo aracnoide cervical. **A.** Ressonância magnética (RM) sagital ponderada em T2. **B.** Imagem de mielograma de tomografia computadorizada (TC). Observe que o divertículo não tem a aparência típica de lágrima na ressonância magnética (*ponta de seta branca*). A mielografia por TC facilita a visualização (bloqueado da *ponta de seta* para frente) e confirmação. (De Dewey CW, da Costa RC: *Guia prático de neurologia canina e felina*, 3 ed., Ames, IA, 2015, Wiley.)

ESPONDILOSE DEFORMANTE

Etiologia e patogenia

A espondilose é um processo degenerativo muito comum da coluna vertebral, essencialmente sem significado clínico por si só.[69] É caracterizada pela formação de exostoses ou proliferações ósseas ao redor da região ventral (e às vezes lateral) das margens da placa terminal vertebral, que podem resultar em uma ponte óssea entre as vértebras adjacentes.[70] Essa é uma condição não inflamatória que se acredita estar associada a alterações degenerativas no anel fibroso dos discos intervertebrais em um esforço para estabilizar a região do disco. Osteófitos variam de pequenos esporos a pontes ósseas ao longo do espaço entre os discos vertebrais, deixando ao menos parte da superfície ventral do corpo vertebral não afetada. Um recente estudo retrospectivo em 2.041 cães encontrou espondilose em 367 animais (18,1%).[70] A espondilose comumente afeta as regiões torácica, lombar e lombossacra.

Achados clínicos

É muito tentador atribuir à espondilose sinais de doença da medula espinal, como paresia, paralisia ou ataxia proprioceptiva, mas tal associação nunca foi documentada (apesar da alta prevalência de espondilose). Um estudo sugeriu que a espondilose pode predispor os cães à doença do segmento adjacente, tornando-os suscetíveis ao desenvolvimento de protrusão do disco intervertebrais (tipo II) nos segmentos cranial ou caudal para os espaços de disco fundidos.[71] Assim, a presença de déficits deve indicar a possibilidade de doenças neurológicas concomitantes. O único sinal relatado para ocorrer em cães de trabalho é uma redução do nível de atividade, secundária à diminuição da flexibilidade da coluna vertebral.[70] A compressão da raiz do nervo (causando dor e claudicação) foi documentada em cães com hiperostose esquelética idiopática difusa. É possível (porém raro) que também ocorra em casos de espondilose com grave proliferação óssea lateralizada, causando estenose do forame intervertebral.[72]

Diagnóstico

A espondilose pode ser observada em animais adultos de vários tamanhos e idades, mas é mais proeminente em cães de meia-idade a mais velhos, de raças médias a gigantes. Boxers, Pastores-Alemães e Retrievers "Flat Coated" parecem ser os principais predispostos.[70,73] O diagnóstico é estabelecido com base na aparência radiográfica de osteófitos vertebrais oriundos da periferia da placa terminal, associados a placas terminais escleróticas, e na preservação da porção central dos corpos vertebrais.[70] É importante diferenciar espondilose de discopondilite e hiperostose esquelética idiopática disseminada (HEID). Como afirmado anteriormente, a espondilose por si só não causa sinais neurológicos; então, em pacientes com sinais neurológicos óbvios, um diagnóstico adicional e exames complementares com mielografia, TC, RM e LCR são recomendados para diagnosticar definitivamente a causa dos sinais (ver Capítulo 115).

Tratamento

A espondilose não tem significado clínico na grande maioria dos cães, e o tratamento não é necessário.[69] Nos casos em que seja documentado compressão da raiz nervosa, o tratamento com analgésicos, como gabapentina, ou descompressão cirúrgica das raízes nervosas pode ser necessário.[72]

HIPEROSTOSE ESQUELÉTICA IDIOPÁTICA DISSEMINADA

Etiologia e patogenia

A HEID é um distúrbio sistêmico caracterizado por proliferação fibrocartilaginosa, seguida de ossificação endocondral dentro dos tecidos moles do esqueleto axial e apendicular. A ossificação de HEID parece afetar uma área, em vez de estruturas anatômicas específicas. Em cães, é caracterizada principalmente pela formação de osso novo generalizado, que aparece como ossificação que flui ao longo dos aspectos ventral e lateral da coluna vertebral.[70] Inicialmente foi considerada uma condição rara, porém um artigo recente descreveu HEID em 78 cães (3,88% de 20.141 cães). Entre 78 desses cães, também tinham espondilose 53 (67,9%). As regiões vertebrais T6-T10 e a L2-L6 foram as localizações mais comuns para a HEID.[70]

Achados clínicos

Semelhante a espondilose, a HEID é tipicamente um achado radiográfico com pouco significado clínico. Pode causar rigidez espinal e desempenho limitado em cães de trabalho.[70] Dor na coluna pode ser vista, embora seja uma possibilidade bastante incomum. Tem sido demonstrada como uma causa de estenose foraminal, levando à dor e claudicação do membro pélvico (sinal de raiz nervosa).[72] Como a HEID pode predispor à doença do segmento adjacente, qualquer cão com claros déficits neurológicos devem ser investigados minuciosamente.[67]

Diagnóstico

A HEID é vista principalmente em cães mais velhos (idade média de 8 anos) e de raças grandes, com os Boxers sendo super-representados. A aparência radiográfica característica é ossificação "fluida", principalmente no aspecto ventrolateral da coluna vertebral, estendendo-se por pelo menos quatro vértebras contíguas (Figura 266.5).[70,74] A proliferação óssea não invade o canal vertebral e, portanto, não causa compressão da medula espinal ou deficiências neurológicas. Também pode haver ossificação dos ligamentos interespinhosos dorsalmente, que pode ser bastante extensa.[75,76] É importante diferenciar HEID de espondilose deformante.[70] Lesões de espondilose

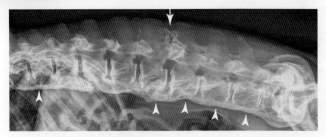

Figura 266.5 Radiografia lateral de um cão da raça Boxer mostrando HEID. Observe que a proliferação óssea envolve todo o aspecto da região ventral dos corpos vertebrais por mais de quatro corpos vertebrais contíguos (*pontas de seta*). A proliferação óssea também é vista no aspecto dorsal da coluna vertebral em L3-4 (*seta*).

geralmente poupam pelo menos parte das superfícies ventrais dos corpos vertebrais adjacentes, e isso é a diferença radiográfica mais importante em relação à HEID.

Um estudo de RM revelou que a intensidade do sinal das lesões ósseas proliferativas era de intensidade igual à do osso vertebral medular (em ambas as sequências ponderadas em T1 e T2). Em contraste, em cães com espondilose, o sinal dos osteófitos foi hipointenso em comparação com o sinal da medula óssea em ambas as imagens ponderadas em T1 e T2.[77]

Tratamento

Semelhante ao que acontece na espondilose, a grande maioria dos cães com HEID não apresenta sinais secundários à proliferação óssea da doença. Se a compressão da raiz do nervo for documentada como a fonte de dor, tratamento com analgésicos ou descompressão cirúrgica de raízes nervosas pode ser necessário.[72]

MIELOPATIA DEGENERATIVA

Etiologia e patogenia

A mielopatia degenerativa (MD) é uma doença degenerativa que afeta principalmente a medula espinal toracolombar de cães de porte médio a grande.[78,79] Também é chamada de radiculomielopatia degenerativa, devido ao envolvimento da raiz nervosa.[80]

Mecanismos imunológicos, inflamatórios, metabólicos, nutricionais, oxidativos, excitotóxicos e genéticos têm sido explorados como subjacentes à patogênese da MD.[79,81-87] Faltam evidências causais definitivas para a maioria desses mecanismos. Uma forma autossômica incomplete penetrante de herança genética foi proposta após a identificação de uma mutação genética na superóxido dismutase 1 (SOD1) em alguns cães acometidos.[85] Mielopatia familiar degenerativa foi relatada em Boxers e Rhodesian Ridgebacks.

A MD é uma axonopatia central primária restrita à medula espinal, que começa no segmento medular torácico e ascende/descende ao longo da medula espinal. A degeneração do axônio e da mielina da medula espinal ocorre em todos os funículos, mas principalmente na face dorsal dos funículos laterais e dorsais. Portanto, a descrição da lesão é mais bem denotada como uma degeneração segmentar do axônio e mielina associada, em vez de degeneração Walleriana.[88,89]

Achados clínicos

Os sinais clínicos são os de mielopatia toracolombar crônica (T3-L3) (Vídeo 266.2). Eles começam com ataxia proprioceptiva leve e paraparesia que progride lentamente, levando a paresia mais grave, até que o cão não seja capaz de deambular. Essa progressão geralmente leva de 6 a 12 meses em raças grandes.[78,79] A falta de hiperestesia espinal é uma característica típica e auxilia bastante no diagnóstico diferencial com outras mielopatias compressivas que ocorrem em cães mais velhos de raças grandes (como protrusão do disco intervertebral e neoplasia espinal). Os déficits proprioceptivos são comumente observados nos estágios iniciais da doença. Os reflexos espinais nos membros pélvicos são frequentemente normais a hiper-reflexivos. Reflexos patelares reduzidos a ausentes são encontrados em aproximadamente 10 a 15% dos pacientes, mas isso não indica necessariamente uma lesão do neurônio motor inferior; em vez disso, pode refletir um dano seletivo às raízes nervosas lombares dorsais (sensoriais). O tônus extensor desses cães está sempre aumentado na fase inicial da doença, sugerindo que a arreflexia patelar ou hiporreflexia seja sensorial, em vez de distúrbio do neurônio motor inferior. A doença implacavelmente progride e, se os cães forem mantidos vivos, envolve as regiões lombar e cervical da medula espinal, bem como o tronco encefálico, causando déficits do neurônio motor inferior, tetraparesia e, eventualmente, disfonia e disfagia.

Diagnóstico

Várias raças grandes podem ser mais afetadas com MD, mas os Pastores-Alemães e os Boxers são as mais comumente atingidas. A idade de início dos sinais neurológicos é geralmente 5 anos ou mais, com a idade média de 9 anos em cães de raças grandes. Em um estudo, a idade média para os cães Pembroke Welsh Corgis foi de 11,2 anos.[84] Parece haver uma maior prevalência em fêmeas Corgis (1,6:1), mas não em outras raças.[79]

O diagnóstico é baseado principalmente na exclusão de outras mielopatias. A imagem da coluna vertebral (mielograma, RM e TC) é geralmente normal, mas alguns cães podem ter protusão de disco intervertebral com leves elevações ósseas. O clínico deve então considerar a duração dos sinais, bem como os achados do exame neurológico para determinar o significado dessas lesões. A RM é a modalidade de imagem de escolha para garantir que todos os outros diferenciais sejam descartados, incluindo lesões intramedulares como neoplasias.[90] Pacientes com MD geralmente apresentam resultados normais de LCR ou níveis elevados de proteína com uma contagem normal de células.[84] Um teste de DNA baseado na mutação SOD1 está disponível comercialmente. Cães que são homozigotos para a mutação correm o risco de desenvolver MD e contribuem com um cromossomo que possui o alelo mutante para todos os seus filhos. Os heterozigotos são portadores de DM, mas improváveis de desenvolver DM clínico, ainda que possam transmitir um cromossomo com o alelo mutante para metade de sua prole.[78] Os corticosteroides podem ser usados para auxiliar no diagnóstico diferencial dessa doença. Eles geralmente levam à melhora em cães com mielopatias compressivas crônicas (como protrusão do disco intervertebral), mas não beneficiam cães com MD. Essa estratégia pode ser útil para convencer o tutor a buscar imagens avançadas.[67]

Tratamento

Nenhuma terapia farmacológica tem demonstrado alterar o curso da MD. A suplementação com vitaminas e a administração de glicocorticoides, ácido aminocaproico e N-acetilcisteína já foram usadas, mas nenhum desses medicamentos apresentou efeitos benéficos.[91] O único tratamento que demonstrou alterar o curso a longo prazo da doença é fisioterapia (ver Capítulo 355).[92] Em um estudo retrospectivo, cães com MD confirmada e suspeita fizeram fisioterapia controlada, incluindo caminhada, amplitude passiva de movimento dos membros pélvicos, massagem do membros pélvicos e músculos paravertebrais e hidroterapia. Cães que eram tratados com um regime de fisioterapia mais intenso tiveram um tempo médio de sobrevivência de 255 dias, em comparação com os que receberam um regime moderado (130 dias) ou nenhuma fisioterapia (55 dias).[92] O prognóstico a longo prazo é ruim, e a maioria dos cães são sacrificados devido a disfunção grave dos membros pélvicos dentro de 6 a 12 meses. No estudo de Pembroke Welsh Corgis, o tempo médio desde o diagnóstico até a morte foi de 1,25 anos.[93]

DOENÇA DO DISCO INTERVERTEBRAL

Etiologia e patogenia

Os discos intervertebrais são interpostos em cada espaço (exceto entre C1 e C2), unindo os corpos do vértebras adjacentes.[94,95] Cada disco intervertebral consiste em um anel fibroso laminado externo (*annulus fibrosus*) e um central, centro amorfo e gelatinoso (núcleo pulposo).[96] O núcleo pulposo é mesodérmico altamente hidratado remanescente da notocorda.[95] Raças condrodistróficas apresentam colagenização progressiva e calcificação no núcleo pulposo e anel fibroso interno em idade precoce.[95] O *annulus fibrosus* consiste em bandas de fibras paralelas que correm obliquamente de um corpo vertebral para o seguinte. Eles providenciam um meio para a transmissão de tensões e deformações que é exigida por todos os movimentos laterais e ascendentes.[96]

A degeneração ou doença do disco intervertebral (DDIV) leva a extrusão ou protrusão (ambas denominadas "herniação") do material do disco para o canal vertebral, resultando em sinais clínicos devido a compressão e/ou contusão da medula espinal.[94,97] A fisiopatologia resultante da lesão medula espinal, que foi bem descrita em outro lugar,[97] nem sempre explica o grau de disfunção neurológica associada.[98] A DDIV é classificada como Hansen tipo I e tipo II.[99] A DDIV tipo I é a herniação do núcleo pulposo através das fibras anulares e extrusão de material nuclear para dentro do canal vertebral. É tipicamente associada com degeneração condroide do disco, mas às vezes a extrusão de um núcleo pulposo hidratado pode ser responsável pela disfunção da medula espinal.[100,101] O disco é expulso através do anel dorsal, causando compressão ventral, ventrolateral ou circunferencial da medula espinal. A DDIV tipo I geralmente afeta raças condrodistróficas e tem um início agudo. No entanto, raças grandes não condrodistróficas, como Doberman Pinscher e Labrador Retriever, também podem ser comprometidas,[102] sobretudo após um trauma.[103] Malformações vertebrais congênitas resultam em degeneração precoce dos discos intervertebrais adjacentes,[104] embora doença discal clínica nesses locais possa não ser tão comum como em outras partes da coluna vertebral.[105] Costas compridas, miniaturização e excesso de peso também aumentam o risco de DDIV tipo I.[106] Hansen tipo II é uma protrusão anular causada pelo deslocamento do material nuclear central e está comumente associada à degeneração do disco fibroide. O anel fibroso lentamente se projeta para dentro do canal espinal, causando compressão da medula espinal. A compressão crônica pode levar a distúrbios isquêmicos focais e outras degenerações microvasculares da medula espinal. A DDIV tipo II geralmente ocorre nos pontos móveis da coluna vertebral e é mais comum em cães idosos, de raças não condrodistróficas. Não é incomum identificar vários espaços de disco comprometidos. A instabilidade espinal crônica pode ser uma predisposição subjacente à DDIV tipo II.

Doença de disco cervical

Achados clínicos

A maioria dos cães com doença do disco cervical, que é responsável por 14 a 25% dos distúrbios do disco intervertebral nesses animais,[107,108] têm extrusão de disco em vez de protrusão.[109] Animais de raças condrodistróficas e outras raças pequenas são de maior risco. Têm sido documentado que Dachshunds, Poodles Toys e Beagles representam a maioria dos casos,[110] porém raças grandes, como Labrador Retrievers, Dálmatas e Dobermans, podem ser acometidos com extrusões de disco cervical, representando até 24% de todos os casos.[94,109,111,112] Os cães mais acometidos têm entre 4 e 8 anos quando apresentam sinais clínicos, com idade média variando de 6,3 a 8,6 anos; é extremamente raro que cães com menos de 2 anos sejam afetados.[109-113] Machos e fêmeas são igualmente comprometidos.[110] Quando cães de raças grandes são comprometidos por doença do disco cervical aguda ou crônica, uma malformação concorrente subjacente e/ou instabilidade como parte de uma síndrome EMC deve ser sempre considerada (ver seção Espondilomielopatia cervical). A maioria dos casos de doença de disco cervical em cães condrodistrofoides ocorre na coluna cervical cranial, com 80% afetando os espaços C2-C4 e 44 a 59% afetando C2-C3 isoladamente.[107,108] No entanto, a maioria dos cães de raças grandes é comprometida no espaço do disco intervertebral C6-C7, e a maioria das protusões *versus* extrusões é localizada mais caudalmente.[109,113]

Aproximadamente 45% dos cães com extrusão de disco cervical têm início dos sinais de forma aguda, com 55% tendo um início mais lento, sejam de raças grandes ou não condrodistróficos.[109] O sinal clínico predominante é dor no pescoço, que pode ser observada em até 60% dos cães sem deficiências neurológicas e em quase 90% dos cães acometidos em geral.[109,114] A dor no pescoço, evidente pela postura do animal ou pela palpação da coluna e músculos do pescoço, podem ser extrema, incessante e refratária à medicação, o que é aparentemente menos provável em casos de extrusões do núcleo pulposo hidratado do que em outras doenças relacionadas ao disco.[101] O "sinal de raiz" do nervo é outro achado frequente na doença do disco cervical, com possibilidade de ser observada em 22 a 50% dos cães.[108,114] Os déficits neurológicos podem ser restritos a um membro torácico ou o animal pode apresentar hemiparesia, tetraparesia ou mesmo tetraplegia com hipoventilação. Tetraparesia ambulatória é observada em até 42% dos cães, e 11 a 22% exibem tetraparesia não ambulatória.[109,114,115] Tetraplegia é incomum e tem sido descrita em 2 a 7% dos casos.[109] Os déficits neurológicos são mais comum inclusive com lesões em C4-C5 a C6-C7, que pode refletir o maior grau de espaço no canal vertebral cranial em comparação com mais caudalmente.[116] A redução ou perda dos reflexos do membro torácico geralmente implicam uma lesão na medula espinal C6-T2; no entanto, 36% dos cães com redução ou ausência de reflexos dos membros têm, na verdade, uma lesão C1-C5 da medula espinal.[112]

Diagnóstico

Pesquisas radiográficas podem ajudar a descartar discopondilite, neoplasia e malformações anatômicas, que podem ser consideradas dependendo dos sinais clínicos.[117] Embora sinais radiográficos, como estreitamento do espaço do disco intervertebral e deslocamento dorsal do material do disco mineralizado, possam ser altamente sugestivos de extrusão de disco, mielografia, TC ou RM são essenciais para um diagnóstico definitivo.[117] A taxa geral de precisão para identificar corretamente o(s) local(ais) da extrusão do disco com radiografia é de 35%.[117] A análise do LCR deve ser considerada para descartar doença inflamatória (ver Capítulo 115). O desvio de contraste da coluna ventral é o achado mielográfico mais comum de doença do disco cervical; vistas oblíquas podem ajudar nas localizações lateralizadas ou foraminais.[118,119] Já a TC realizada após a mielografia pode fornecer informações mais detalhadas sobre a localização da lesão compressiva (Figura 266.6), particularmente para discos lateralizados e discos intradurais.[120,121] Por fim, a RM é o melhor método para avaliação da medula espinal cervical e fornece um método seguro e não invasivo para obter imagens de alta resolução (ver Figura 266.6).[122,123] Essa modalidade de imagem pode fornecer informações detalhadas sobre a estrutura dos discos intervertebrais e medula espinal e ajudar no prognóstico.[124,125]

Tratamento

O repouso rígido em gaiola por 4 a 6 semanas é o aspecto mais importante de uma abordagem conservadora na doença de disco cervical e pode ser seguido por exercícios incrementais restritos e graduais ao longo do próximo mês, usando um peitoral corporal em vez de uma coleira e uma guia. O período prolongado de descanso permite a resolução da inflamação e estabilização do disco rompido por fibrose, evitando herniação posterior.[94]

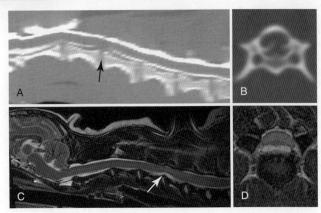

Figura 266.6 A. Tomografia computadorizada sagital reconstruída pós-mielografia da medula espinhal cervical de um cão com dor aguda no pescoço. A coluna ventral de contraste é afinada e desviada dorsalmente sobre o espaço do disco C3-C4 (seta) devido a uma extrusão do disco (Doença tipo I). **B.** A imagem transversal de TC-mielográfica em nível do espaço do disco C3-C4 confirma a compressão do cordão ventral. **C.** Imagem de ressonância magnética sagital ponderada em T2 da medula espinhal cervical de um cão com tetraparesia aguda. A compressão do cordão ventral pode ser identificada acima do espaço do disco C4-C5 devido a uma lesão hiperintensa (seta). **D.** Imagem de ressonância magnética transversal ponderada em T2 no espaço do disco C4-C5 confirma que o cordão está ventralmente comprimido por uma estrutura hiperintensa, que é compatível com extrusão agudo do núcleo pulposo hidratado.

O uso de medicamentos anti-inflamatórios, como corticosteroides ou analgésicos não esteroides, pode ser recomendado por alguns dias para acompanhar o repouso (ver Capítulo 164). Medicamentos analgésicos podem ser necessários em alguns cães além ou em vez de anti-inflamatórios (ver Capítulos 126, 166 e 356). O uso da acupuntura em cães com doença do disco cervical foi descrito e relatado como associado a uma recuperação inicial em 69% dos casos (ver Capítulo 356).[126] Relaxantes musculares, como o Diazepam e o Metocarbamol, são medicamentos adjuvantes úteis em cães com dor cervical relacionada à doença discal. Sinais de envolvimento da raiz nervosa, como assinatura da raiz nervosa ou hérnia foraminal identificada em imagens avançadas, podem ser tratados com Gabapentina (10 a 20 mg/kg VO a cada 8 h). Taxas de recorrência de 33 a 36% ou mais foram relatadas com abordagens conservadoras.[126-128] Um estudo avaliando 88 cães com manejo conservador presumivelmente com hérnia de disco intervertebral cervical encontrou um resultado de sucesso de 49% dos casos, enquanto 33% recorreram e 18% obtiveram falha terapêutica.[128] Duração mais crônica da doença e déficits neurológicos mais graves podem resultar em menos sucesso quando tratados de forma conservadora, como é o caso da doença de disco toracolombar.[128]

A decisão de tratar cirurgicamente é baseada em vários fatores. Os critérios pertinentes incluem gravidade neurológica, cronicidade (se os sinais representam recorrência), resposta a tratamento médico, saúde sistêmica do paciente e aspectos financeiros do tutor. Os pacientes sintomáticos podem ser divididos em três grupos: grupo I, primeiro episódio envolvendo somente dor cervical; grupo II, episódios repetidos de dor cervical apenas; e grupo III, dor no pescoço e deficiências neurológicas concomitantes.[94] O tratamento clínico muitas vezes pode ser recomendado para cães do grupo I. A descompressão cirúrgica é mais apropriada para o grupo II e é necessária para o grupo III.

Quando tratado apenas com descompressão da fenda ventral, a recuperação completa é observada em até 90% dos cães em 1 mês e 98% dos cães 12 meses após a cirurgia.[114] O acompanhamento a longo prazo (6 meses a 4 anos) após a descompressão da fenda ventral para protrusão de disco cervical caudal em cães de raças grandes revelou uma taxa de sucesso de apenas 66%, e concluiu-se que a dinâmica das lesões compressivas podem precisar de um procedimento de estabilização.[129] A taxa de recorrência após a cirurgia para doença de disco cervical tem sido sugerida para aproximadamente 5 a 10%, com uma média de tempo de recorrência de 91 dias para todos os cães.[109,127] Vários eventos adversos significativos foram relatados em até 10% de cães submetidos à cirurgia da fenda ventral, que incluem deterioração do estado neurológico, dificuldade respiratória, hemorragia intraoperatória e dor persistente.[130]

Doença de disco toracolombar

Achados clínicos

A DDIV Hansen tipo I ocorre mais comumente dentro da região toracolombar em raças condrodistróficas. A junção toracolombar (T12-T13 a L1-L2) é responsável pela maior incidência de todas as lesões de disco.[131] A incidência de DDIV toracolombar tem uma diminuição progressiva de T12-T13 caudalmente. O local mais comum para DDIV Hansen tipo I em raças grandes não condrodistróficas é o espaço intermediário entre L1 e L2;[102] todavia, Pastores-Alemães podem ser acometidos particularmente por discos entre T1-T5.[132,133] O início dos sinais neurológicos pode ser hiperagudo (antes de 1 hora), agudo (antes de 24 horas) ou gradual (depois de 24 horas). Cães se apresentando com extrusões de disco toracolombar hiperagudas ou agudas podem manifestar sinais clínicos de choque espinal ou posturas de Schiff-Sherrington.[131] Isso é indicativo de lesão da medula espinal aguda e grave, mas não determina o prognóstico. O grau de disfunção neurológica é variável e afeta o prognóstico. Os sinais clínicos variam de apenas hiperestesia de coluna vertebral até paraplegia com ou sem percepção de dor. A taxa de incidência de mielomalácia focal e ascendente/descendente tem sido relatada como bem alta (10%) em cães com DDIV toracolombar aguda e perda de nocicepção;[131,134,135] o risco de desenvolver esta condição pode ser superior em certas raças, como Buldogue Francês.[105] Disfunção neurológica grave também não é um cenário incomum com extrusões agudas do núcleo pulposo não compressiva (DDIV Hansen tipo III, extrusão de disco traumático, extrusão de disco de baixo volume e alta velocidade), onde o núcleo extrusor se espalha ao longo do espaço epidural e pode completamente circundar ou penetrar na dura-máter (Figura 266.7).[136,137] A extrusão intervertebral do disco clinicamente relevante foi relatada em gatos com menos de 5 anos, porém é mais comum em animais de meia-idade a mais velhos.[138,139] Sinais clínicos devido à doença de disco em gatos pode refletir uma mielopatia transversa dolorosa em qualquer região da medula espinal, mas a probabilidade de extrusão de disco clinicamente significativa parece ser maior na região toracolombar e lombar. O início do DDIV tipo I em gatos é geralmente agudo.[138]

Diagnóstico

O diagnóstico inicial de DDIV toracolombar é obtido a partir dos sinais clínicos, histórico e exame neurológico. A radiografia da coluna vertebral pode ajudar a determinar o diagnóstico e o local da extrusão do disco toracolombar se os sinais radiográficos estiverem bem definidos e consistentes com a localização neuroanatômica (ver Figura 266.7).[140,141] Estudos de cães cirurgicamente confirmados com DDIV toracolombar mostraram que, quando identificado o local da extrusão de disco, a radiografia prévia teve uma precisão de 68 a 72%, mas o percentual de precisão com mielografia foi maior:[131] a localização de lesão longitudinal por mielografia para DDIV toracolombar varia em precisão de 40 a 97%, mas geralmente está perto de 90%.[131] A TC ou a RM são usadas isoladamente ou como um adjuvante da mielografia para delinear a lateralização do material de disco extrusado e a extensão da lesão mais completas.[97] A TC isoladamente tem demonstrado ser mais precisa, mais rápida e com menos efeitos colaterais do que a mielografia na identificação do local principal de hérnia de disco.[142,143] Material de disco mineralizado e hemorragia aguda podem ser identificados no

CAPÍTULO 266 • Doenças da Medula Espinal: Congênitas (Desenvolvimento), Inflamatórias e Degenerativas

canal vertebral usando TC sem contraste. Material de disco extrusado de forma aguda normalmente é reconhecido como uma massa extradural hiperatenuante heterogênea comprimindo a medula espinal,[144,145] e material de disco extrusado cronicamente tem uma aparência hiperatenuante mais homogênea. A imagem de ressonância magnética (RM) fornece uma técnica mais sensível no reconhecimento da patologia da medula espinal (p. ex., edema, hemorragia e delineamento tridimensional da compressão da medula espinal), permitindo uma abordagem cirúrgica precisa e determinando a extensão de descompressão cirúrgica necessária (Figura 266.7).[146] A IRM é considerada o melhor método para reconhecimento precoce de *disco in situ*, com base na degeneração e diminuição de intensidade do sinal dentro do núcleo pulposo em imagens ponderadas em T2, e para determinar a localização e extensão do material do disco extrusado dentro do espaço peridural.[147,148] A IRM também demonstrou ser superior para a avaliação de DDIV recorrente.[149]

Tratamento

As indicações para o tratamento não cirúrgico de DDIV toracolombar incluem um primeiro incidente de apenas dor na coluna, paraparesia leve a moderada e restrições financeiras do tutor. Este último é o único motivo para o tratamento não cirúrgico de um paciente recumbente, que deve sempre ser considerado um candidato cirúrgico. Cães podem ser manejados com repouso absoluto em gaiolas por 4 a 6 semanas, associado com o alívio da dor pelo uso de anti-inflamatórios, opioides e relaxantes musculares (ver Capítulo 356). A acupuntura também tem sido defendida como um tratamento para o controle da dor. Os cães devem ser monitorados de perto quanto à deterioração do estado neurológico. Se a dor persistir ou o estado neurológico piorar, o manejo cirúrgico é recomendado. Estudos têm mostrado que as taxas de recuperação são mais baixas em cães não deambuladores e as de recorrência, mais altas após tratamento conservador em vez de cirúrgico. Taxas de sucesso com manejo conservador em cães ambulatórios com dor ou leve paresia variam de 82 a 100%.[131] Estudos retrospectivos mais recentes de cães tratados de forma conservadora com doença de disco toracolombar documentaram 30 a 50% taxas de recorrência em cães ambulatórios com estado minimamente comprometido.[131,150] A recorrência de dor em cães com DDIV na coluna toracolombar que são tratados de forma conservadora geralmente ocorre dentro de 6 meses a 1 ano a partir do início dos sinais clínicos. Indicações para tratamento cirúrgico de DDIV toracolombar incluem dor na coluna ou paresia não responsiva a terapia clínica, recorrência ou

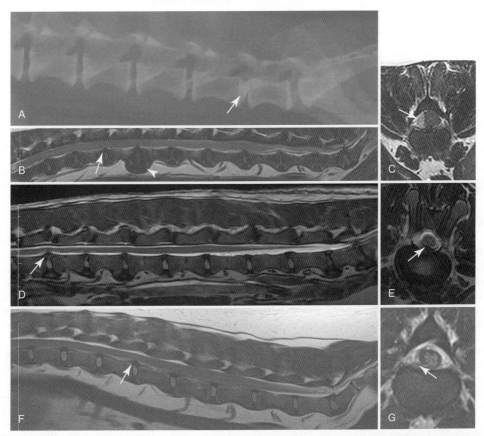

Figura 266.7 A. Radiografia lateral da coluna vertebral lombar de um cão apresentando paraparesia. O espaço do disco L6-L7 (*seta*) é reduzido em comparação com os espaços dos discos adjacentes. Além disso, o disco aparece calcificado *in situ* e há opacidade no forame intervertebral. Todas essas características são compatíveis com a extrusão do disco intervertebral neste local. **B.** Imagem de RM sagital ponderada em T2 da coluna vertebral toracolombar de um cão com dor nas costas de início agudo e paraparesia. Há espondilose em ponte do corpo vertebral ventral moderada em L1-L2 (*ponta de seta*). Além disso, há um leve desvio ventral da medula espinhal em T13-L1 (*seta*), que é não convincente de uma lesão que exigiria cirurgia. No entanto, a compressão de cordão lateral marcada pode ser observada neste local (*seta*) na ressonância magnética transversal ponderada em T2 (**C**), que foi devido a uma extrusão aguda de disco. **D.** Imagem de ressonância magnética sagital ponderada em T2 da coluna vertebral toracolombar de um cão de raça grande porte com paraparesia e ataxia moderada. O desvio do cordão ventral pode ser identificado em T12-T13 devido à protrusão anular compatível com lesão de disco do tipo II. O leve desvio do cordão pode ser observado na ressonância magnética ponderada em T2 transversal (**E**), devido à protrusão anular ventrolateral (*seta*). **F.** Imagem de ressonância magnética sagital ponderada em T2 de um cão de raça grande com paralisia aguda revela novamente uma lesão moderada ventral no cordão em L2-L3 (*seta*) que parece ser semelhante ao da Figura 266.2 D. No entanto, em imagens transversais ponderadas em T2 neste local (**G**), o sinal anormal está presente dentro o espaço epidural (*seta*) e o cordão parece heterogeneamente hiperintenso. A lesão de dentro o cordão foi devido a uma extrusão aguda de núcleo não compressiva, frequentemente associada a trauma.

progressão dos sinais, paraplegia com percepção de dor intacta e paraplegia sem percepção de dor por menos de 24 a 48 horas. Perda prolongada da percepção de dor (mais de 48 horas) tem um prognóstico ruim, e os tutores devem ser informados a respeito antes da cirurgia. A cirurgia inclui descompressão da coluna vertebral pela remoção do material do disco extrusado. As diferenças nas taxas de recuperação de cães não ambulatórios variam de acordo com a gravidade da disfunção neurológica (grau neurológico), intervalo de tempo desde os sinais clínicos iniciais até a cirurgia e velocidade de aparecimento dos sinais.[131] Em cães ambulatórios, um grau crescente de deficiências no pré-operatório está significativamente associado a tempos de recuperação mais longos.[151] Administração de corticosteroides ou alta dose de succinato de sódio de metilprednisolona parece não melhorar o resultado em cães submetidos a cirurgia para extrusão do disco intervertebral e tem sido associada a maior prevalência de complicações gastrintestinais e urinárias, aumento da permanência no hospital e despesas para o proprietário.[97,150] A percepção de dor é considerada o indicador prognóstico mais importante para uma recuperação funcional. Em geral, a maioria dos cães com percepção de dor intacta tem um prognóstico excelente, sobretudo se tratada cirurgicamente.[152] Cães com perda de percepção de dor por mais de 24 a 48 horas antes da cirurgia têm um prognóstico pior para o retorno da função. Um estudo com 87 cães com perda de percepção de dor profunda relatou que 58% dos animais recuperaram a percepção de dor profunda e a capacidade de andar.[134] Em geral, o prognóstico é ruim se a percepção de dor não retorna dentro de 2 a 4 semanas a partir do momento da cirurgia.[131,134,135] A recorrência de sinais clínicos após cirurgia descompressiva em cães com DDIV toracolombar é entidade clínica comum, com taxas de incidência relatadas de 2 a 42%.[131] O tempo de recorrência geralmente ocorre entre 1 mês e 2 anos após a cirurgia. Recorrência de sinais clínicos dentro de 1 mês após a cirurgia está provavelmente relacionada ao espaço de disco herniado original; recorrência posterior a mais de 1 mês é causada por uma hérnia de disco em um local distinto da extrusão inicial.[131]

INSTABILIDADE ATLANTOAXIAL

Etilogia e patogenia

A instabilidade da articulação atlantoaxial (AA) leva à compressão e concussão da medula espinal cervical, resultante do deslocamento das vértebras (subluxação) para o canal vertebral;[153] a subluxação atlantoaxial resulta de uma anormalidade no ligamento e/ou osso entre o atlas (primeira vértebra cervical) e o *axis* (segunda vértebra cervical). O *axis* tem uma projeção cranioventral em forma de pino, chamada de processo ou pino odontoide. O pino encontra-se dentro do forame vertebral do atlas, estabilizado ventralmente pelo ligamento transverso, o que impede seu movimento no canal espinal, mas ainda permite o movimento rotacional. O pino também é fixado ao forame magno pelo ligamento apical, e os côndilos occipitais, pelos ligamentos alares. Há também um ligamento atlantoaxial dorsal, articulando o arco dorsal do atlas e a coluna craniodorsal do eixo.

A subluxação atlantoaxial foi relatada pela primeira vez em cães em 1967.[154] Desde então, várias deformidades congênitas e de desenvolvimento da articulação AA foram documentadas como causadoras da instabilidade da coluna vertebral, predispondo à subluxação de AA, particularmente em cães jovens de raças pequenas.[155-158] As possíveis anomalias incluem displasia (34% dos cães), hipoplasia ou aplasia (46% dos cães), angulação dorsal e fratura do processo, bem como ausência do ligamento transverso.[155,156,159,160] Qualquer anormalidade no processo odontoide predispõe à instabilidade da junta AA, devido ao seu

papel importante na estabilidade normal desta articulação. Contudo, até aproximadamente 24% dos cães com subluxação AA têm um pino normal.[160]

Pequenas raças, incluindo Yorkshire Terriers, Chihuahuas, Poodles em miniatura, Pomeranians e Pekingese, são mais frequentemente comprometidas por anomalias congênitas e de desenvolvimento que predispõem à instabilidade AA e possível subluxação.[159,161,162] Isso ocorre principalmente porque as facetas ósseas são propensas a mau desenvolvimento em raças miniatura, graças a aberrações de fechamento da placa de crescimento fisário. No entanto, a subluxação atlantoaxial devido a anomalias vertebrais congênitas também foi relatada em cães de raças grandes.[163,164] Já a subluxação atlantoaxial devido a anomalias vertebrais congênitas em gatos é muito rara.[165-167] A subluxação traumática de AA pode ocorrer em qualquer raça e idade do cão. Ela resulta da sobreflexão forçada da cabeça, que pode romper os ligamentos ou causar uma fratura do pino ou arco dorsal do eixo.[159] Um impacto considerável pode ser necessário para causar tais lesões em uma articulação AA normal; muitas vezes, até mesmo luxações AA traumáticas estão associadas a um defeito congênito subjacente e instabilidade da articulação.[159,160]

Achados clínicos

Dor no pescoço é o sinal mais comum associado a subluxação AA, sendo observada na maioria dos cães com lesões traumáticas e em 30 a 60% dos cães com lesões congênitas.[59,160,162,168] Os déficits neurológicos associados (ver Capítulo 259) são determinados pelo grau de dano presente na medula espinal tanto após a concussão quanto na compressão residual. Os déficits neurológicos podem variar de anormalidades leves de reação postural (56%) a tetraplegia (10%); no geral, a disfunção da marcha foi relatada em até 94% dos cães.[160,168,169] Esses déficits podem ser assimétricos, além de parecerem piores tanto nos membros pélvicos quanto nos torácicos. Nos raros casos que se apresentam com tetraplegia, é possível progressão dos sinais clínicos para um estado de comprometimento respiratório clínico e até mesmo parada.[159]

Diagnóstico

A subluxação atlantoaxial pode ser diagnosticada a partir do estudo radiográfico da coluna cervical, embora deva ser tomado extremo cuidado ao restringir e mover cães nos quais a doença é suspeita. Em radiografias laterais, um espaço aumentado pode ser visto entre a lâmina dorsal do atlas e o processo espinhoso dorsal do *axis* (Figura 266.8).[153] Em casos graves, o desalinhamento dos corpos do atlas e do *axis* é claramente visível. A presença e o tamanho do processo odontoide podem ser avaliados mais precisamente em vistas ventrodorsais, assim como em radiografias oblíquas.[170] Estas visualizações são preferíveis, em vez da visualização com abertura de boca, que coloca o paciente em risco grave de trauma da medula espinal. Se não houver evidência de subluxação na vista lateral, o pescoço pode ser flexionado cuidadosamente para procurar por instabilidade (o espaço entre a lâmina dorsal do atlas e o processo espinhoso dorsal do eixo devem ser avaliados). É preferível fazer este procedimento com a fluoroscopia, para que o movimento possa ser monitorado, a fim de prevenir a subluxação iatrogênica acidental; isso pode fornecer um diagnóstico rápido em um cão consciente. A TC e a RM podem adicionar informações vitais, que ajudam na tomada de decisão em relação ao tratamento do paciente individual.[171-173] A TC é um possível auxílio na identificação de conformação do processo, presença de fratura de processo ou vertebral e colocação de implante cirúrgico.[171,173] A reconstrução por TC tridimensional da articulação AA consegue adicionar um nível extra de compreensão ao diagnóstico, o que pode auxiliar na decisão cirúrgica. A RM pode fornecer

CAPÍTULO 266 • Doenças da Medula Espinal: Congênitas (Desenvolvimento), Inflamatórias e Degenerativas 1447

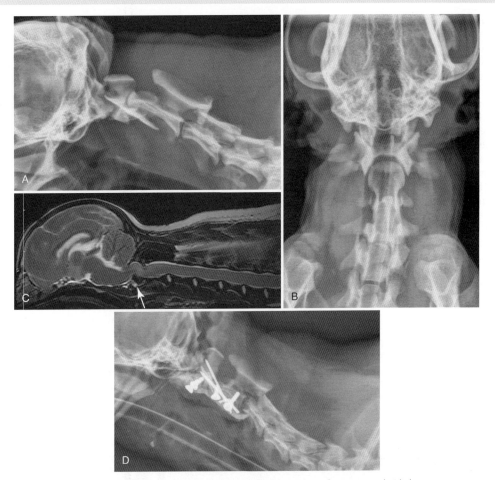

Figura 266.8 A. Imagem radiográfica lateral da coluna vertebral cervical de um Yorkshire Terrier de 11 meses de idade, que apresentou tetraparesia e dor no pescoço. Subluxação dorsal de C2 com em relação a C1 causa um aumento do espaço entre a lâmina dorsal de C1 e o arco dorsal de C2. **B.** Imagem radiográfica ventrodorsal da coluna vertebral cervical do cão da Figura 266.3 A. O espaço articular entre a primeira e a segunda vértebras cervicais está aumentado e não há evidências de uma fossa, um fator predisponente para a subluxação atlanto-axial. **C.** Imagem de ressonância magnética sagital ponderada em T2 da coluna vertebral cervical de um cão com subluxação atlantoaxial identifica a compressão da medula espinhal associada à lesão vertebral e um espaço articular atlanto-axial alargado (seta). **D.** A radiografia pós-operatória lateral de um cão com fixação cirúrgica da articulação atlantoaxial usando pinos transarticulares, parafusos do corpo vertebral e cimento de metilmetacrilato.

informações adicionais sobre patologia da medula espinal, como hemorragia ou edema e siringo-hidromielia, o que pode ser importante para o prognóstico (ver Figura 266.8).[173,174]

Tratamento

O objetivo do tratamento conservador é estabilizar a articulação AA enquanto as estruturas ligamentares cicatrizam.[161] O tratamento não cirúrgico de subluxação AA, incluindo confinamento estrito da gaiola por 6 semanas, analgesia e uma cinta cervical rígida, teve sucesso em alguns pacientes; no entanto, abordagens não cirúrgicas ou conservadoras são suscetíveis a recorrência ou aparecimento progressivo dos sinais clínicos.[161,175,176] A tala deve imobilizar a junção AA, e, assim, todo o envoltório deve passar por cima da cabeça cranialmente às orelhas e voltar ao nível do peito. Complicações associadas ao uso de tala e bandagem de pescoço incluem recorrência da doença, úlceras da córnea, migração do tala e consequentemente sua ineficácia, dermatite úmida e úlceras de decúbito, hipertermia, comprometimento respiratório (dispneia, aspiração), anorexia, otite externa e acúmulo de alimentos entre a tala e a mandíbula.[161] Um resultado bom a longo prazo foi documentado em 10 de 26 casos (38%) manejados de forma conservadora.[161,175,176] Cães que foram acometidos por menos de 30 dias eram significativamente mais propensos a ter um bom resultado a longo prazo quando tratados de forma conservadora, em comparação com cães acometidos por um período superior a 30 dias.[161] O objetivo do tratamento cirúrgico é de estabilizar a articulação AA, evitando assim mais danos à medula espinal (ver Figura 266.8). Embora a cirurgia seja designada para reduzir o componente compressivo da doença, ela não aborda nenhuma doença do parênquima subjacente, resultante da concussão associada à doença. A cirurgia deve ser considerada em todos os cães, pois tem o potencial de fusionar a articulação AA permanentemente e reduzir a chance de uma recorrência catastrófica. A taxa de mortalidade perioperatória associada à fixação de AA foi relatada entre 10 e 30%.[160,162] Fatores de risco que afetam o resultado cirúrgico em cães têm sido identificados.[160] A idade de início (antes dos 24 meses) foi significativamente associada a maiores chances de sucesso na primeira cirurgia e no resultado.[160] A duração (menos de 10 meses) e a gravidade dos sinais clínicos foi significativamente associada a maiores chances de um resultado bem-sucedido;[160] apesar do prognóstico reservado para cães com graves deficiências neurológicas, muitos pacientes que são incapazes de andar antes da cirurgia têm um bom resultado.[162] Se um procedimento dorsal ou ventral é realizado, não parece mudar as chances do resultado.[160]

MALFORMAÇÕES CONGÊNITAS DA MEDULA ESPINAL

Malformações congênitas incidentais das vértebras são descritas comumente em várias raças de cães, como o Buldogue, e ocasionalmente em gatos.[177-179] Os defeitos podem estar associados a anormalidades estruturais da medula espinal, que podem surgir durante o desenvolvimento embrionário ou fetal. As anormalidades de desenvolvimento embrionário afetam sobretudo a formação do corpos vertebrais (p. ex., vértebra borboleta e hemivértebra, causando predominantemente escoliose), enquanto as anomalias fetais são mais comumente defeitos de origem segmentar (p. ex., bloqueio de vértebras e defeitos centrais, que causam predominantemente cifose), mas podem ocorrer cruzamentos.[178] As pesquisas radiográficas muitas vezes detectam uma coluna vertebral anômala, mas imagens avançadas, como RM, são necessárias para avaliar a compressão da medula espinal associada ou doença (Figura 266.9). Um esquema de classificação radiográfica humana modificado tem sido proposto para auxiliar na descrição dessas anomalias,[180,181] enquanto o grau de curvatura espinal radiograficamente calculado tem sido associado à presença de deficiências neurológicas.[182,183] Reconstruções tomográficas tridimensionais podem ajudar com uma maior compreensão da anomalia vertebral presente no caso individual; já no homem, a TC serve para ajudar a classificar a anomalia subjacente (ver Figura 266.9).[178,184]

Vértebras de borboleta
Assim chamadas por causa de sua aparência ventrodorsal na radiografia, as vértebras de borboleta resultam da falha de formação do tubo ventral e nas porções centrais do corpo vertebral.[178,185] Essas anomalias são mais frequentemente vistas em raças braquicefálicas de cauda em parafuso e, embora sejam muitas vezes clinicamente insignificantes, podem resultar em desvio da coluna.[178]

Hemivértebras
Essas anomalias surgem devido à falha de uma metade sagital da vértebra no desenvolvimento, devido a uma possível ausência congênita de vascularização, que resulta em uma vértebra lateralmente encravada e com angulação escoliótica.[178] Elas são mais comumente descritas em Buldogues Franceses e Ingleses e em Boston Terriers, embora outras raças possam ser afetadas;[183] são consideradas hereditárias em Buldogues Ingleses, Yorkshire Terriers e Pastores-Alemães de Pelo Curto, como uma anormalidade autossômica recessiva.[186] A maioria das vértebras afetadas estão localizada entre T5-T9, mas as hemivértebras podem surgir em qualquer local.[183,187] Não estão associadas a grave estenose de canal; no entanto, compressão da medula espinal resulta em mais associação entre cifose e subluxação.[183] Além disso, no local da anomalia, não é incomum encontrar hérnia de disco concomitante e/ou divertículo aracnoide, ambos podendo ser responsáveis por sinais neurológicos. Embora as hemivértebras possam ser clinicamente insignificantes, quando associadas a sinais clínicos, estes são referentes à sua localização neuroanatômica e ocorrem em animais muito jovens ou tardiamente na idade adulta.[183,187] O realinhamento cirúrgico e a estabilização, em vez de apenas uma laminectomia dorsal, foram aconselhados em casos clínicos com o prognóstico variando de bom a reservado.[183,188]

Hipoplasia do centro
Hipoplasia ou aplasia do centro resulta em perda do corpo vertebral variável (uni ou bilaterais), resultando em um grau de escoliose.[178] O grau de desvio da coluna vertebral resultante está relacionado com a gravidade do defeito e o número de vértebras acometidas. A anomalia é considerada distinta da hemivértebra, embora potencialmente pareçam semelhantes na imagem

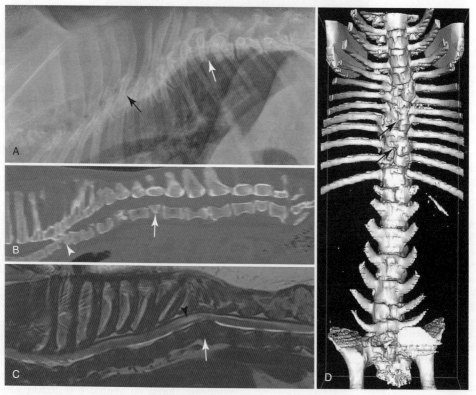

Figura 266.9 A. Imagem radiográfica lateral da coluna vertebral torácica cifoescoliótica em um Buldogue Francês de 7 meses de idade, devido às malformações vertebrais presentes. As anormalidades do corpo vertebral mais graves, compatíveis com hipoplasia central, podem ser observadas afetando T10 (seta branca) e T5 (seta preta). **B.** Imagem de tomografia computadorizada sagital da vértebra toracolombar coluna de um Buldogue Francês diferente torna mais fácil discernir a forma da coluna vertebral e inferir como eles podem estar afetando o canal vertebral. A anomalia afetando L1 (seta) não parece estar associada a estenose do canal. As anomalias que afetam a coluna vertebral cranial torácica (ponta de seta) está associada a uma estenose significativa. **C.** Imagem sagital ponderada de ressonância magnética da coluna vertebral toracolombar de um cão Pug demonstra o efeito que um corpo vertebral anômalo (seta) associada a estenose na medula espinhal causando compressão e siringe (ponta de seta preta) cranial à lesão. **D.** Imagem de tomografia computadorizada tridimensional reconstruída da coluna vertebral de um Buldogue Francês ajuda a identificar várias anomalias do corpo vertebral (setas).

CAPÍTULO 266 • Doenças da Medula Espinal: Congênitas (Desenvolvimento), Inflamatórias e Degenerativas

radiográfica e resultante das mesmas etiologias hipotéticas e nas mesmas raças de cauda enroscada. Embora esses defeitos estejam presentes ao nascimento, os sinais clínicos associados podem não ser aparentes até os 10 meses de idade,[189] quando podem surgir de forma aguda ou ter início crônico; sinais clínicos em um estágio posterior da vida são possivelmente associados a uma condição concorrente, como doença do disco.[178]

Vértebras bloqueadas
Esta anomalia resulta da fusão parcial ou total de duas vértebras em qualquer ponto. As vértebras bloqueadas podem estar associadas a angulação da coluna vertebral, subluxação atlantoaxial e/ou doença do disco.[158,190]

Aplasia da faceta articular
Anormalidades do processo articular ou faceta das vértebras podem resultar da disgenesia dos dois arcos neurais de ossificação central ou do desenvolvimento anormal de centros de ossificação secundários.[191] Frequentemente localizados entre T1-T9 e assintomáticos, a aplasia da faceta articular foi ocasionalmente relatada caudal a esta região e associada à estenose do canal vertebral.[191-193]

Vértebra transicional
Encontrada na junção entre duas divisões estruturais da coluna vertebral (p. ex., toracolombar e lombossacra), as vértebras transicionais são anomalias vertebrais congênitas que compartilham características de ambas as divisões. A anormalidade mais comum é a presença ou a ausência de uma costela ou processo transverso, frequentemente assintomática e descrita em cães e gatos.[178] Semelhante ao bloqueio de vértebras, essa anomalia pode estar associada à doença de disco, que foi bem descrita na junção lombossacral em Pastores-Alemães.[194-196]

MENINGOMIELITE

Meningomielite é definida como inflamação no parênquima da medula espinal e meninges circundantes. É relativamente incomum estar presente sem encefalite; uma revisão retrospectiva de 220 cães com doenças do sistema nervoso central (SNC) inflamatória revelou que apenas 41 animais tinham envolvimento focal na medula espinal.[197] O vírus da cinomose canina (ver Capítulo 228) e protozoários (ver Capítulo 221) têm sido a causa infecciosa mais comumente identificada, enquanto a meningitearterite responsiva a esteroides é a causa provável reconhecida com mais frequência em processo de doença inflamatória não infecciosa.[197] Rickettsiae, fungos, bactérias, helmintos e meningites de etiologia desconhecida (MED), como meningoencefalomielite granulomatosa, são outras causas relatadas de meningomielite em cães.[198-204] Todavia, em muitos casos, o processo da doença subjacente permanece indeterminado. Uma revisão com 28 cães acometidos com meningomielite revelou que MED era o diagnóstico mais comum e que cães de raças Hound e Toys com idade inferior ou igual a 3 anos tiveram 13 vezes mais chances de meningomielite em comparação com outras raças.[205]

Os sinais clínicos associados à meningomielite refletem a região do SNC envolvida e podem incluir hiperestesia paravertebral, ataxia proprioceptiva geral e paresia de membro ou paralisia. O diagnóstico definitivo de doença inflamatória do SNC requer histopatologia, mas pode ser presumido usando uma combinação de análise LCR (ver Capítulo 115), imagem avançada e teste de doenças infecciosas (ver Capítulo 207). O prognóstico pode ser especificado de acordo com o processo subjacente da doença e da gravidade dos sinais clínicos.[205] Para uma descrição mais detalhada de doenças inflamatórias do SNC, o leitor é referido ao Capítulo 261.

MENINGITE-ARTRITE RESPONSIVA A ESTEROIDES

Etiologia e patogenia
Suspeita-se de uma causa imunológica para a meningite-artrite responsiva a esteroides (MARE), resultando em uma vasculite, embora nenhum fator desencadeante específico tenha sido identificado.[206,207] Notavelmente, níveis aumentados de imunoglobulina A (IgA) no LCR e no soro, aumento na relação células B/células T no sangue e no LCR e níveis de interleucina (IL) 6 e IL-8 no LCR são considerados compatíveis com a estimulação do sistema imunológico.[208-210] Alta expressão de CD1 em células polimorfonucleares parece ser um fator importante na patogênese da MARE e pode estar envolvida na passagem intensificada de neutrófilos para dentro do espaço subaracnóideo, levando à meningite e aos sinais clínicos.[211] A metaloproteinase da matriz (MMP) 2 parece estar envolvida na invasão neutrofílica do espaço subaracnoide.[212] O envolvimento de tais marcadores moleculares fornecem um potencial alvo terapêutico. Com a progressão crônica das lesões, ruptura e hemorragia da vasculatura enfraquecida podem estar presentes, acompanhadas por leptomeninges espessadas com inflamação menos intensa.

Achados clínicos
A MARE, também denominada vasculite necrosante, síndrome de poliarterite juvenil, meningite/meningomielite responsiva a corticosteroides, meningite supurativa asséptica, panarterite e síndrome de dor, é relatada em Beagles, Bernesianos de Montanha, Boxers, Pastores-Alemães de Pelo Curto, Border Collies, Jack Russell Terriers, Weimaraners e Nova Scotia Duck Tolling Retrievers,[207,213,214] mas é observada e provavelmente ocorre em outras raças de médio a grande porte. Os cães acometidos são frequentemente adultos jovens (8 a 18 meses), mas podem ter qualquer idade; em geral apresentam febre e hiperestesia, com rigidez cervical e anorexia. Déficits neurológicos podem ser observados na forma crônica da doença e, raramente, disfunção motora grave pode resultar de sangramento espontâneo no espaço subaracnóideo.[213] Alguns cães (até 46%) com poliartrite imunomediada (ver Capítulo 203), especialmente Bernesianos de Montanha, Boxers e Akitas, podem apresentar sinais clínicos semelhantes aos dos cães com MARE e ter meningite concomitante (ver Capítulo 261).[215]

Diagnóstico
Uma neutrofilia periférica marcada com um desvio à esquerda pode ser vista no momento dos sinais clínicos. O LCR (ver Capítulo 115) muitas vezes revela uma intensa pleocitose neutrofílica e elevação de proteínas; contagens de célula superior a 100 células/$\mu\ell$ são comuns. Os neutrófilos são não degenerados, ao contrário da meningite bacteriana. Na maioria dos cães com doença aguda ou crônica, há elevações dos níveis de IgA no LCR e no soro, embora isso não seja específico para essa doença. As concentrações de IgA no LCR são significativamente maiores em cães com MARE quando comparadas com outras categorias de doenças, com exceção da doença inflamatória do SNC; portanto, são consideradas não específicas. A sensibilidade para concentrações de IgA no soro e no LCR foi de 91%, com uma especificidade de apenas 78% na avaliação de 311 cães com MARE.[216] A proteína C reativa (PCR) é a principal proteína de fase aguda (PFA) canina e demonstrou ser imediatamente responsiva tanto à inflamação quanto à sua resolução; outras PFA incluem amiloide-A sérica (SAA), haptoglobina e glicoproteína ácida alfa-1 (GAP). Foi demonstrado que a PCR no soro é significativamente maior em cães com MARE em comparação a cães com outras doenças neurológicas.[217] Resultados de um estudo recente com 9 cães acometidos por MARE demonstrou um aumento significativo de todas as PFA séricas acima das concentrações normais e que todas diminuíram (com exceção da haptoglobina) em resposta ao tratamento com corticosteroides.[218] A PCR sérica e a SAA também foram encontradas

consistentemente elevadas em todos os pacientes, exibindo sinais consistentes com uma recidiva durante o tratamento, porém com resultados normais de LCR e leucograma. No entanto, assim como a IgA, as elevações da PCR são consideradas inespecíficas e são elevadas na sepse; portanto, a PCR só pode ser usada como um teste de suporte diagnóstico.[219]

Tratamento

O prognóstico pode ser bom se os cães forem tratados precoce e agressivamente com doses imunossupressoras de corticosteroides (ver Capítulo 165), com até 80% dos casos seguindo para uma remissão a longo prazo.[220,221] Doenças infecciosas devem ser descartadas antes do tratamento ser iniciado. O tratamento é a longo prazo: foi relatado ser necessário mais de 2 anos em alguns cães; contudo, após esse tempo, os níveis séricos e de LCR de IgA permaneceram elevados em alguns cães, portanto, esses títulos não são considerados valiosos para o monitoramento da doença.[221] O controle da contagem de células no LCR em cães com essa condição é um indicador sensível de sucesso de tratamento. Em casos refratários ou em pacientes com efeitos colaterais relacionados a esteroides, terapia de imunomodulação alternativa deve ser considerada, como a azatioprina.

DISCOPONDILITE

Etiologia e patogenia

Discospondilite deve-se à infecção do disco intervertebral e placas terminais vertebrais adjacentes; se a infecção for confinada ao corpo vertebral, é chamada de osteomielite vertebral ou espondilite.[222] *Staphylococcus* spp. (*S. pseudintermedius* ou *S. aureus*) é o agente etiológico mais comum associado à discopondilite canina;[213] outros organismos menos comumente identificados incluem *Streptococcus* spp., *Escherichia coli*, *Actinomyces* spp. e *Brucella canis*, bem como *Aspergillus* spp. Cadelas jovens da raça Pastor-Alemão parecem ser predispostas à aspergilose (ver Capítulo 234),[223] enquanto os jovens Basset Hounds contraem discopondilite devido a tuberculose sistêmica (ver Capítulo 212).[224] A propagação hematógena de focos distantes de infecção (trato urogenital, pele, doença dentária), feridas penetrantes, cirurgia[225] ou migração de material vegetal podem causar infecção direta do espaço do disco ou vértebras, o que geralmente é observado em nível de L2-L4 na inserção da crura diafragmática. Os locais mais comumente comprometidos são L7-S1, coluna cervical caudal, médio-torácica e coluna toracolombar.[213] A infecção em geral é lentamente progressiva, mas pode resultar em sinais agudos devido a fraturas vertebrais patológicas secundárias e doença do disco intervertebral. Uma associação com empiema foi documentada em vários cães, o que pode representar uma extensão da doença e deve ser considerado na seleção dos testes de diagnóstico e/ou ao lidar com um caso refratário.[226-228]

Achados clínicos

Dor na coluna é o sinal clínico inicial mais comum nessa doença, mais frequentemente vista em cães machos grandes e intactos, jovens a meia-idade.[229] Com a proliferação de tecido inflamatório, a compressão do tecido neural pode levar a ataxia, paresia e, ocasionalmente, paralisia, dependendo do local da lesão. Aproximadamente 30% dos cães apresentam sinais de doença sistêmica, como febre e perda de peso.

Diagnóstico

As alterações hematológicas geralmente não estão presentes, a menos que haja condições concomitantes, como endocardite (ver Capítulo 251). A citologia da urina pode revelar agentes bacterianos ou fúngicos (ver Capítulo 72). As culturas de sangue e urina devem ser realizadas em todos os casos suspeitos, sendo positivas em até 75 e 50% dos casos, respectivamente (ver Capítulo 207).[213,222] De forma ideal, a cultura deve ser realizada antes do início da antibioticoterapia. A sorologia para brucelose também deve ser realizada, principalmente tendo em vista seu potencial zoonótico (ver Capítulo 213); ela tem sido relatada positiva em até 10% dos casos. O diagnóstico definitivo em geral é feito com radiografias da coluna (Figura 266.10), embora a alteração radiográfica possa não ser evidente nas primeiras 2 a 4 semanas de infecção. O local mais comumente comprometido é L7-S1, mas outros locais acometidos com frequência incluem vértebras cervicais caudais, vértebras craniais torácicas e junção toracolombar. Como esta pode ser uma doença multifocal, toda a coluna deve ser radiografada. A evidência radiográfica inclui estreitamento do espaço do disco acompanhado por irregularidade sutil de ambas as placas terminais, lise, proliferação óssea do osso vertebral adjacente e até mesmo fraturas. Radiografias também podem ser usadas para monitorar a resposta ao tratamento ou a progressão da doença,[230] embora a progressão clínica seja igualmente importante, pois a mudança radiográfica pode ficar em atraso em relação à melhora clínica. A mielografia costumava ser recomendada em pacientes com déficits neurológicos substanciais para descartar doença discal concomitante e subluxação que afetasse o sistema tecidual neural; todavia, isso deve ser reservado para quando nem TC, nem RM estão disponíveis. Um estudo de 27 cães com discopondilite descobriu que as radiografias com contraste revelaram compressão mediana da medula em apenas 5% dos cães que não estava relacionada com sinais clínicos ou resultados clínicos.[231] A TC pode identificar erosão sutil na placa terminal e edema dos tecidos moles paravertebrais mais rapidamente do que a radiografia. A TC pós-mielograma, assim como a RM, define com clareza a compressão dos tecidos neurais por tecidos infectados. Discospondilite parece ter aumento da intensidade do sinal em imagens ponderadas em T2 e diminuição da intensidade do sinal em imagens ponderadas em T1; alterações também são observadas em tecidos na região paravertebral em todos os casos.[232,233] Em um estudo, um aumento de contraste foi visto em placas terminais das vértebras acometidas em 15 de 17 (88%) pontos, assim como erosão da placa terminal na medula óssea com T2-hipointenso. A RM também pode destacar a inflamação nos músculos ao redor (ver Figura 266.10).

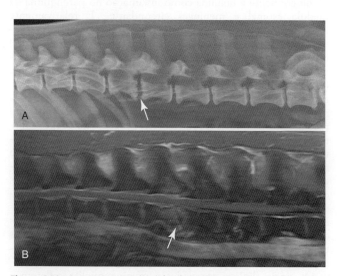

Figura 266.10 A. Imagem radiográfica lateral toracolombar coluna vertebral de um Golden Retriever adulto com dor nas costas devido a discopondilite em L2-L3. As placas terminais vertebrais associadas com o espaço do disco intervertebral L2-L3 (*seta*) são irregulares devido à lise e à proliferação óssea. **B.** Imagem sagital ponderada em T1 de ressonância magnética pós-contraste da coluna vertebral toracolombar representada na Figura 266.5 A, revela absorção de contraste (hiperintensidade) dentro do corpo vertebral e processo espinhoso dorsal de L1 e associado às placas terminais de L1 e L2 (*seta*). Tecido macio, proliferação e disseminação da infecção para o espaço epidural secundária à discopondilite está associada a um ligeiro estreitamento da medula espinal acima do espaço do disco.

Tratamento

O tratamento inicial da discopondilite consiste em antibióticos (amoxicilina ou cefalexina potenciada), repouso em gaiola e analgésicos. Os antibióticos intravenosos devem ser considerados se houver comprometimento neurológico grave ou se estiverem presentes sinais de sepse; caso contrário, antibióticos orais são aceitáveis. Por mais rápido que seja a melhora do paciente, a continuação dos antibióticos por 8 a 16 semanas é recomendada, embora um estudo avaliando 513 casos observou uma duração média de tratamento de 54 semanas.[213,222,229] A resolução dos sinais clínicos, como dor e febre, deve ser esperada dentro de 5 dias após o início da terapia; no entanto, a resolução neurológica completa pode levar de 2 a 3 meses. Deficiências residuais podem permanecer, mas a dor persistente indica doença ativa, e os pacientes devem ser tratados com um antibiótico adicional e considerados para mais diagnósticos, na medida em que uma infecção fúngica potencial ou lesão cirúrgica pode estar presente. Discospondilite associada a *Aspergillus* spp. tem sido tratada com Itraconazol (5 mg/kg de peso corporal, via oral, a cada 24 horas), e, embora não existam relatos de sucesso a longo prazo, acredita-se que a recorrência crônica e progressão sejam prováveis (ver Capítulo 234). O prognóstico para a doença é geralmente muito bom, a menos que a etiologia seja fúngica, existam múltiplas lesões, fratura vertebral ou subluxação ou haja endocardite; o potencial de recorrência deve ser considerado, especialmente se a brucelose foi diagnosticada ou uma condição imunossupressora estiver presente.

REFERÊNCIAS BIBLIOGRÁFICAS

As referências bibliográficas deste capítulo se encontram online no Ambiente de Aprendizagem.

CAPÍTULO 267

Doenças da Medula Espinal: Traumáticas, Vasculares e Doenças Neoplásicas

Nicholas Jeffery

MECANISMOS DE DISFUNÇÃO ESPINAL

Distúrbios traumáticos, vasculares e neoplásicos podem não parecer relacionados, mas cada um causa disfunções na medula espinal, principalmente por prejudicar o fluxo de sangue. Trauma de impacto agudo e interrupção vascular comprometem instantaneamente o fluxo sanguíneo, que dispara uma série de eventos secundários autodestrutivos dentro da medula espinal, formando um nítido contraste com a compressão lenta e progressiva dos vasos sanguíneos e a diminuição da circulação associada geralmente a lesões neoplásicas. Lesão por impacto pode causar poucos danos imediatos à medula espinal, como alguns axônios cortados e hemorragia focal, mas isso não pode ser usado para prever a gravidade de eventos destrutivos subsequentes.[1]

As consequências funcionais de lesões por impacto em geral surgem porque o trauma inicia uma cascata de reações moleculares, culminando em grave comprometimento da microcirculação, que, por sua vez, causa apoptose celular, necrose do tecido e dano progressivo ao longo de 3 a 7 dias.[2,3] A destruição transversal quase completa pode ocorrer, embora a extensão do dano esteja claramente relacionada com a gravidade da lesão inicial.[4,5] A extensão da lesão é mediada em grande parte por mediadores inflamatórios. A perda de circulação leva a consequências secundárias, causadas pela falta de oxigênio e de glicose. Em última análise, a despolarização dos neurônios e axônios permite o acúmulo de cálcio como segundo mensageiro-chave, que ativa muitas enzimas autodestrutivas, especialmente calpaínas, caspases e xantina oxidase.[2] Eventos semelhante são secundários a lesões vasculares primárias, mas comumente têm efeitos espaciais mais limitados, uma vez que os vasos afetados são em geral de diâmetro mais estreito e com menores regiões de distribuição. Eles também diferem no fato de que o trauma externo pode estar associado com a compressão prolongada. Por exemplo, fraturas vertebrais deslocadas podem comprometer ainda mais o fluxo sanguíneo.

Os mecanismos subjacentes à destruição do tecido associada à compressão crônica da medula espinal não são muito bem entendidos. Há evidências de microcirculação prejudicada.[6,7] As lesões neoplásicas geralmente causam compressão progressiva de medula espinal durante um período que persiste de semanas a meses. Inicialmente, o fluxo sanguíneo é suficiente para preservar a função adequada da medula espinal, mas, ao final, um "ponto de inflexão" é alcançado, no qual a compressão se torna muito grave para permitir compensação e progressão rápida dos sinais clínicos.

DIAGNÓSTICO DAS LESÕES DE MEDULA ESPINAL

Introdução

A abordagem inicial para doenças do sistema nervoso é usar o exame físico neurológico para tentar localizar o problema (ver Capítulo 259). Por meio dessas informações, pode-se então considerar as possíveis causas de uma lesão no local dentro do contexto da sinalização e do histórico. O início, a taxa e o grau de progressão ou regressão dos sinais clínicos são importantes. Essa abordagem é usada para localizar doenças traumáticas, vasculares ou neoplásicas da medula espinal. Crucialmente, tanto a doença traumática quanto a neoplásica podem estar associadas a dor na coluna sem evidência de deficiência neurológica. Nesses casos, uma observação cuidadosa e palpação suave podem ajudar a localizar a lesão, embora as observações possam ser enganosas em animais ansiosos ou estoicos. Às vezes, uma avaliação precisa pode ser auxiliada pela observação clínica durante um período de 24 horas ou mais.

Histórico

Ouvir atentamente e avaliar as observações do proprietário pode ser de extrema importância para desenvolver um "índice de suspeita" aos tipos de lesões específicas na medula espinal.

Informações de histórico e sinais clínicos são cruciais.[8] Em humanos, estima-se que por voltar de 80% dos diagnósticos são derivados apenas da história, embora o aspecto de espécie de "sinalização" seja um dado importante.[9]

Diagnóstico diferencial

Em geral, as lesões traumáticas podem ter poucos diagnósticos diferenciais. Os sinais clínicos em animais de estimação com lesões vasculares são geralmente muito óbvios.

Testes diagnósticos

A maioria das doenças traumáticas, vasculares e neoplásicas requerem imagem para confirmar a localização e sugerir uma etiologia, embora o diagnóstico preciso geralmente dependa do exame histológico. A doença inflamatória pode ser identificada usando a análise do líquido cefalorraquidiano (LCR), mas, por causa dos riscos (p. ex., hemorragia exacerbada e disseminação de células tumorais), raramente é um primeiro teste de diagnóstico razoável, e exames de imagens são com frequência necessários para auxiliar a interpretação dos resultados. Por exemplo, o aumento da proteína no LCR é um achado não específico comum, mas não invariável, associado à compressão da medula espinal.[10,11] Radiografia e tomografia computadorizada (TC) são excelentes modalidades para o diagnóstico de lesões que afetam vértebras, mas fornecem poucos detalhes da própria medula espinal. Imagens de ressonância magnética (RM) são preferíveis para diagnóstico de lesões da medula espinal e também podem ser usadas para detectar lesões ligamentares. As RM têm a desvantagem de fornecer detalhes ósseos relativamente ruins e poder ser dispendiosas e demoradas. As TC e RM podem ser consideradas complementares, mas, na medicina veterinária, uma delas é frequentemente selecionada, dependendo da lesão, se há suspeita de ser óssea ou de tecidos moles (afetando especialmente a medula espinal). Essa decisão em geral é feita tendo em mente a natureza da incitação da lesão (p. ex., trauma externo), a gravidade, a necessidade de diagnosticar para posterior intervenção cirúrgica e as evidências de dor (que tende a sugerir envolvimento esquelético). Animais com suspeita de uma lesão vascular são inicialmente avaliados com ressonância magnética (RM), porque essas lesões não são visíveis com o uso de outras modalidades de exames de imagens (Tabela 267.1).

Tratamento

Visão geral

As categorias de doenças neste capítulo têm etiologias e prognósticos extremamente variados. Por exemplo, lesões traumáticas podem requerer estabilização cirúrgica meticulosa (p. ex., fraturas-luxações instáveis; Figura 267.1), mas, às vezes, estratégias conservadoras (para fraturas estáveis, por exemplo) ou cuidados de suporte não específicos (para extrusão de disco hiperagudo), como repouso em gaiola, podem ser recomendados. Lesões vasculares primárias que causam danos na medula espinal geralmente não respondem à terapia no momento em que os animais acometidos são diagnosticados. Isso não implica um prognóstico desesperançoso, porque muitas lesões são incompletas, e tais animais recuperam sua função à medida que a inflamação é resolvida e as alterações plásticas ocorrem nos

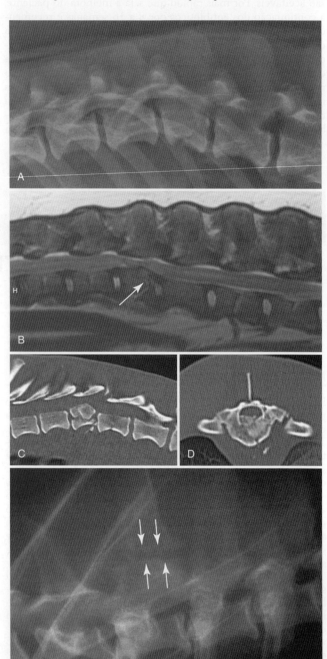

Figura 267.1 Fratura toracolombar-luxações vertebrais frequentemente causa instabilidade que ameaça a integridade da medula espinhal e em geral requer estabilização cirúrgica. **A.** Fratura do aspecto caudal da vértebra L1 claramente visível apenas com a radiografia. **B.** A ressonância magnética sagital ponderada em T2 também mostra a fratura (seta) e revela detalhes da lesão da medula espinhal. **C.** A tomografia computadorizada sagital reconstruída revela detalhes excelentes de uma fratura vertebral T13 em outro cachorro. **D.** Imagem de tomografia computadorizada (TC) transversal correspondente revela a extensão do comprometimento do canal vertebral associado a esta fratura de "explosão", provavelmente resultante de compressão ao longo do longo eixo da coluna vertebral. **E.** Fratura patológica de processo espinhoso da vértebra T1 (setas). Esta lesão não causa déficits neurológicos, mas foi associada a dor intensa.

| Tabela 267.1 | Capacidade das modalidades de imagem para detectar lesões da medula espinhal e da coluna vertebral. |

TIPO DE LESÃO	RADIOGRAFIA	TC	RM
Traumática			
Fratura-luxação	+	++	+
Extrusão de disco	–	±	++
Vascular (qualquer tipo)	–	–	++
Neoplásica			
Extradural	±	±	++
Intradural/extramedular	–	–	++
Intramedular	–	–	++

RM, ressonância magnética; TC, tomografia computadorizada.

CAPÍTULO 267 • Doenças da Medula Espinal: Traumáticas, Vasculares e Doenças Neoplásicas

circuitos.[12] Lesões neoplásicas também mostram extrema variabilidade no prognóstico; alguns casos são desesperadores com ou sem tratamento (p. ex., metástases disseminadas de hemangiossarcoma), enquanto em outros animais acometidos espera-se que vivam por vários anos (p. ex., mieloma múltiplo[13]).

Corticosteroides

O papel da corticoterapia em lesões traumáticas e vasculares da medula espinal é fonte de persistente controvérsia.[14] Por décadas, clínicos humanos e veterinários usaram corticosteroides, muitas vezes em altas doses, para reduzir as consequências funcionais e patológicas de insultos agudos na coluna vertebral. Apesar dos efeitos positivos dos corticosteroides que às vezes são relatados em pesquisas de laboratório, eles não têm sido replicados em estudos clínicos.[15] Publicações iniciais sobre o uso de succinato de metilprednisolona sódica em altas doses para lesão da medula espinal humana sugeriu benefício,[16] mas isso já foi contestado, e o consenso atual é que os corticosteroides não são úteis na melhora aguda de insultos da medula espinal.[17] Além disso, o uso de corticosteroides é prejudicial em traumatismo craniano, talvez porque reduza a massa muscular e seja imunossupressor.[18]

No entanto, os corticosteroides costumam ter um efeito de alívio dramático sobre os déficits neurológicos associados com compressão (prolongada) do sistema nervoso central (SNC), reduzindo a permeabilidade dos vasos sanguíneos e o edema circunjacente à lesão compressiva.[14] Embora isso possa ser útil na perspectiva do proprietário do animal, os esteroides podem obscurecer ambas as informações funcionais como informações de imagem. A administração indiscriminada de corticosteroides também pode expor o animal a um risco de efeitos colaterais desnecessários e prejudiciais, como imunossupressão.

DOENÇAS TRAUMÁTICAS

Sinalização e histórico

Nenhuma sinalização específica precisa estar associada com a lesão traumática, mas é bem sabido que animais jovens, especialmente machos, tendem a ser super-representados. O histórico pode ser de grande valor para levantar suspeitas por lesões traumáticas. Quase sempre há um início agudo de sinais clínicos, e, muitas vezes, o evento traumático foi testemunhado. Há poucas exceções, mas os animais que sustentam luxações de fratura vertebral em algumas ocasiões não exibem sinais neurológicos imediatamente após o incidente; com o tempo, as vértebras da região comprometida podem se deslocar, produzindo sinais de deterioração neurológica e dor. Isso parece ser particularmente prevalente em associação com lesões da região cervical superior, sobretudo da região atlanto-axial e L7/S1 (embora as lesões nesse nível não afetem a medula espinal). Apesar do trauma externo que ocasiona lesões espinais sintomáticas em geral grave, alguns animais desenvolvem sinais de lesão da medula espinal após o que havia sido considerado como trauma sem gravidade; por exemplo, cães com subluxação atlanto-axial congênita que desenvolvem sinais clínicos após trauma trivial, como bater a cabeça na parte inferior de móveis ao levantar da posição reclinada.

Apresentação e manejo imediato

O impacto veicular ou quedas de altura são as causas mais comuns de lesões traumáticas da coluna vertebral que causam deficiências neurológicas óbvias. No entanto, alguns animais de companhia têm apenas sinais de dor mal localizada. É importante ressaltar que alguns animais podem apresentar choque circulatório, de forma que o exame neurológico não seja imediatamente confiável em função da má perfusão do SNC, que pode causar deficiências neurológicas temporárias. Por este motivo, é imperativo reexaminar os animais afetados em

intervalos frequentes para determinar se o estado neurológico está mudando. Quando examinado pela primeira vez, pode ser tentador atender ferimentos marcantes primeiro, mas é importante priorizar o tratamento de acordo com o sistema ABC (vias respiratórias, respiração [breathing], circulação; ver Capítulo 147).[19] Por outro lado, é fundamental estar ciente da possibilidade de lesão neurológica, acima de tudo fratura-luxação. Isso é especialmente verdadeiro para animais que têm dor inespecífica, porque o manuseio descuidado pode levar a um prejuízo maior. É importante não mover os animais mais do que o absolutamente necessário se apresentados em decúbito após o trauma. Em muitas ocasiões, é sensato fazer radiografias da coluna vertebral em um estágio inicial, mesmo às vezes antes de um exame neurológico completo, de modo a identificar locais que possam estar em risco de lesão iatrogênica. Em animais em que uma única luxação de fratura na coluna vertebral foi identificada, é essencial considerar a possibilidade de outras lesões adicionais, que podem não estar produzindo sinais tão óbvios.[20] Portanto, é prudente obter com frequência radiografias ou, melhor ainda, imagens de TC de toda a coluna vertebral.

Testes diagnósticos

Para quase todos os animais de companhia que sofreram traumas, resultados de exames de imagem são decisores críticos. As radiografias torácicas são sempre indicadas por causa de pneumotórax (ver Capítulos 149 e 244) e hemorragia pulmonar (ver Capítulos 149 e 242), que são comuns. Radiografias simples da coluna vertebral são melhores como testes de "regra geral" do como testes de "exclusão", porque muitas lesões traumáticas, mesmo as que afetam as vértebras ou, de fato, o próprio canal vertebral, podem ser negligenciadas. A TC é indicada em animais com suspeita de lesão das estruturas esqueléticas, por exemplo aqueles que exibem forte dor na coluna apesar dos achados negativos na radiografia. No entanto, algumas lesões traumáticas podem não ser aparentes, apesar do uso da TC. Varreduras por RM são excelentes para detectar lesões traumáticas dentro da medula espinal, embora forneçam uma definição menos precisa de contornos ósseos.

Doenças específicas

Diagnóstico diferencial

As lesões traumáticas têm poucos diagnósticos diferenciais, principalmente se o trauma foi observado. O trauma também deve ser considerado como uma possível explicação para quaisquer sinais clínicos agudos de animal com indicativos de lesão medular. Os principais diagnósticos diferenciais são hérnia de disco intervertebral ou lesões vasculares da medula espinal. Embora teoricamente a doença inflamatória possa causar sinais clínicos agudos, não é comum que se desenvolva tão rapidamente como ocorre após o trauma. O trauma pode ser esquecido como uma possível causa, especialmente em animais com sinais agudos de letargia ou obtundação (que pode indicar dor).

Fratura-luxação vertebral

O resultado mais comumente observado de trauma externo é fratura ou luxação de vértebras.[21] A menos que tais lesões afetem o canal vertebral, elas não causam sinais clínicos indicativos de lesão da medula espinal (embora os nervos espinais possam ser afetados). Todos os pacientes exibem dor. Na maioria dos casos, a subluxação é causada por fratura parcial da vértebra, mas pode haver subluxações simples resultantes de lesão ligamentar isolada, mais especificamente na região cervical craniana (Figura 267.2). O tratamento de luxações de fraturas vertebrais depende muito da gravidade dos sinais do quadro clínico, de uma estimativa de "estabilidade" e da localização da lesão.[21] É fundamental determinar se a resposta de "dor profunda" está intacta, porque ela fornece informações de prognóstico mais precisas (ver Capítulo 259). É importante lembrar que os animais em choque circulatório podem ficar temporariamente amortecidos em resposta à dor.

As opções de tratamento para luxações de fratura da coluna vertebral podem variar muito. Por exemplo, animais deambulatórios exibindo déficits neurológicos leves nos membros pélvicos associados com fraturas estáveis das vértebras torácicas podem não exigir intervenção cirúrgica e se recuperam com restrição simples de exercício enquanto a lesão cicatriza. Em contradição, um animal com paraplegia (mas sensação de dor intacta) causada por uma fratura de um corpo vertebral lombar seria um bom candidato para estabilização cirúrgica. O tratamento das fraturas-luxações vertebrais é o assunto de muitas revisões na literatura.[21] A tomada de decisão pode ser auxiliada com a ideia de que a coluna vertebral é uma série de três planos sagitais que percorrem todo o seu comprimento. Se dois dos três planos são interrompidos pela lesão, então é sugestivo de instabilidade, fornecendo uma forte indicação para fixação interna. A magnitude da subluxação no local da lesão nem sempre é um bom guia ao prognóstico, porque a posição dos elementos esqueléticos durante a imagem pode não refletir adequadamente a extensão de movimento durante o processo de lesão.

Extrusão traumática de disco

Ocasionalmente, animais (sobretudo cães) que sofreram trauma externo na coluna vertebral ainda apresentam sinais de lesão medular grave sem nenhuma evidência óbvia de luxação de fratura vertebral. Em alguns, há estreitamento aparente do espaço do disco intervertebral. Por meio do uso da RM, é possível demonstrar que muitos desses pacientes têm espaços de discos colapsados associados com o escape e a extrusão de núcleo pulposo direcionados dorsalmente.[22,23] Quase sempre, essa extrusão de disco não é de um núcleo doente, como ocorre normalmente na hérnia de disco tipo I em cães condrodistróficos (ver Capítulo 266). Em vez disso, a fuga de um núcleo normal é feita por meio de um anel que foi rompido.[24] A extrusão forçada de um pequeno volume de núcleo cria uma lesão na medula espinal, devido a contusão que não causa uma compressão persistente (Figura 267.3). Os sinais clínicos são frequentemente lateralizados, porque a hérnia de disco se desvia para o lado do ligamento longitudinal dorsal na linha média. Os sinais podem ser semelhantes aos de embolia fibrocartilaginosa (EFC). Exame pós-morte de tais casos sugeriu que o núcleo extruído pode realmente passar algumas vezes pela substância da medula espinal.[25] A lesão resultante não pode ser vista em imagens que não sejam RM.

Trauma de microchip

Existem vários relatos de introdução inadvertida de microchips de identificação no canal da medula espinal.[25a] Os relatos sugerem que cães muito pequenos podem estar em risco elevado para esse tipo de lesão, que pode ocorrer imediatamente após a implantação ou se desenvolver após a migração dos microchips.[26,27]

Prognóstico

O prognóstico para as lesões traumáticas da medula espinal, é claro, depende da gravidade da lesão, mas, muitas vezes, ele é surpreendentemente bom. O melhor indicador de prognóstico disponível continua sendo a sensação de "dor profunda". Quando presente, a maioria dos animais recupera (eventualmente) capacidade locomotora suficiente para viver uma vida normal ou quase normal. Animais com lesões cervicais quase sempre retém a sensação de dor profunda – aqueles que não, em geral morrem de comprometimento respiratório.[28] A perda da sensação de dor profunda após trauma externo toracolombar é indicativa de um prognóstico extremamente cauteloso, na melhor das hipóteses.

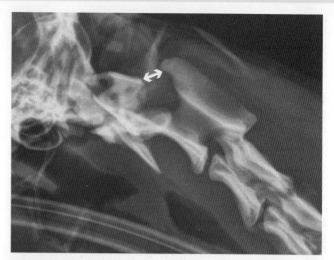

Figura 267.2 Radiografia lateral mostrando subluxação atlantoaxial em um Yorkshire Terrier jovem, resultante de laceração parcial ou alongamento dos ligamentos intervertebrais. Distância aumentada entre o arco do atlas e a ponta cranial do processo espinhoso do eixo (*seta dupla*). Este sinal deve ser interpretado com cautela porque também pode ser observado em certa medida em cães aparentemente normais.

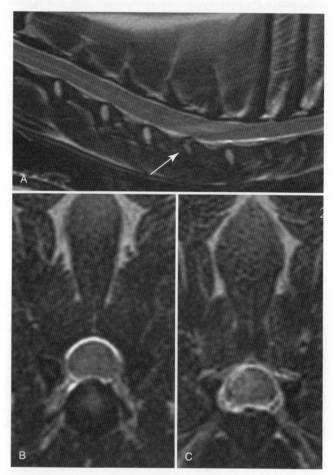

Figura 267.3 Imagens típicas de ressonância magnética (RM) de um cão que sofreu uma hérnia de disco intervertebral traumática associada a uma queda. **A.** Imagem ponderada em T2 sagital revela perda do normal hiperintensidade do núcleo do disco intervertebral entre as vértebras C6 e C7 (*seta*), além de hiperintensidade da medula espinhal imediatamente adjacente, sugestiva de edema. **B.** Transversal. A imagem ponderada em T2 na porção média da vértebra C6 ilustra intensidade normal do parênquima da medula espinal. **C.** Transversal. A imagem ponderada em T2 na porção média do corpo vertebral C7 revela hiperintensidade anormal dentro da medula espinal.

Poucos animais recuperam a locomoção de novo. Animais com lesão toracolombar e sensação de dor intacta em geral recuperam as funções extraordinariamente bem.

A recuperação após grave lesão traumática da medula espinal pode ser um processo longo – os animais frequentemente requerem pelo menos 10 dias antes de demonstrar *qualquer* mudança. A recuperação total pode levar 3 meses ou mais. Após grave lesão da medula espinal, uma "cicatriz" se desenvolve dentro da medula espinal, consistindo principalmente de um processo astrocítico e uma matriz secretora de proteoglicanos. Ambos podem inibir a regeneração axonal.[29] Cicatrização por fibroblastos também pode se desenvolver no espaço subaracnoide e prejudicar o fluxo de LCR. O resultado de tal cicatrização pode levar ao acúmulo de fluido dentro da medula espinal, mas, às vezes, é grave o suficiente para ser reconhecido como siringomielia (ver Capítulo 266). Essas lesões secundárias podem dar origem a síndromes de dor em pessoas que são incomumente reconhecidas em cães e gatos. Perda de continência fecal pode ocorrer (ver Capítulo 42).[30]

DOENÇAS VASCULARES

Introdução

Uma ampla gama de distúrbios circulatórios pode levar à disfunção da medula espinal, incluindo qualquer causa de redução da pressão arterial (ver Capítulo 159). Todavia, outros sinais clínicos são prováveis de predominar em certas condições suficientemente graves para causar tais distúrbios circulatórios sistêmicos (p. ex., insuficiência cardíaca). Sendo assim, pode ser prudente medir a pressão arterial em casos sem causa óbvia de disfunção da medula espinal (ver Capítulo 99). Sinais associados com trombose aórtica (ver Capítulos 256), doença dos nervos periféricos (ver Capítulo 268) ou doenças musculares (ver Capítulo 354) também podem ser consistentes com doença da medula espinal. A aferição da pressão sanguínea pode fornecer teste direto para incluir/excluir um diagnóstico diferencial.[31] Da mesma forma, doenças sistêmicas que afetam a coagulação do sangue (ver Capítulo 197), incluindo os estados hipercoaguláveis, como o hiperadrenocorticismo, e os hipocoaguláveis, como trombocitopenia, podem causar lesões na medula espinal e devem ser considerados durante o exame físico (ver Capítulo 196). A maioria dos animais de companhia com danos na medula espinal devido a uma lesão vascular tem doença regionalmente específica, que são discutidas a seguir.

Sinalização

Lesões vasculares na medula espinal são, em geral, mais comuns em animais de meia-idade a mais velhos. Embolização fibrocartilaginosa, especificamente, é mais comum no homem e em raças não condrodistróficas – talvez, o Schnauzer Miniatura esteja risco.[32] Em geral, a sinalização não é especialmente sugestiva desse tipo específico de lesão, e, de fato, infartos espinais foram documentados em animais relativamente jovens.[33]

Histórico

Lesões da medula espinal de origem vascular têm um efeito inicial instantâneo, durante o qual o animal pode apresentar sinais de dor. Com muita frequência, o animal está se exercitando e, de repente, grita ou apenas entra em colapso e já está neurologicamente prejudicado.[34] No momento em que o animal é examinado pelo veterinário, em geral não há nenhuma evidência de dor (mas cuidado com pacientes ansiosos e estoicos; ver Capítulo 126). Ao longo de vários dias subsequentes (se o animal não for visto por longo tempo), muitas vezes há uma regressão gradual dos sinais neurológicos. Animais com lesões vasculares da medula espinal não parecem ter dor quando examinados após algum tempo. O histórico, especialmente combinado com outras sinais típicos, pode ser tão característico de lesões vasculares que são quase patognomônicos.

Apresentação

As lesões vasculares da medula espinal com frequência têm uma apresentação típica altamente estereoscópica. A causa subjacente pode ser obstrução da vasculatura (trombose ou embolia), mas ruptura de um vaso sanguíneo (frequentemente anormal) é menos comum. Em ambos os casos, o vaso em geral é pequeno, e os sinais são quase sempre fortes e lateralizados. Portanto, a apresentação típica é um aparecimento de sinais neurológicos hiperagudo, que muitas vezes são altamente lateralizados (Vídeo 267.1). Porém, apresentações alternativas ocorrem; por exemplo, animais em que a artéria espinal ventral é comprometida mostram evidências de doença bilateral grave. A progressão típica após a apresentação imediata é de recuperação gradual da função perdida. A rapidez da recuperação depende da localização precisa e da gravidade da lesão. Animais com lesões que não afetam os neurônios motores inferiores (que se encontram dentro da medula espinal nos segmentos C5-T2 e L4-S3) normalmente se recuperam logo, caso a lesão seja insuficientemente grave para causar perda de sensação de dor profunda. Em certas ocasiões, o paciente com uma lesão vascular extremamente grave não sobrevive. Na necropsia, trombose grave ou disseminada é em geral identificada. Animais em que as regiões de neurônio motor inferior são afetadas estão especialmente em risco, por necessitar de um tempo de recuperação prolongado ou por um lapso na recuperação.

Diagnóstico diferencial

Os sinais típicos de lesões vasculares são altamente sugestivos da etiologia. No entanto, hérnia de disco intervertebral (ver Capítulo 266) e lesão traumática da medula espinal devem ser considerados. Cada diagnóstico diferencial requer varredura de RM para confirmar a etiologia.

Testes diagnósticos

A aparente falta de dor na coluna, somada à lateralização estereotípica, muitas vezes sugere fortemente uma origem vascular. Tal suspeita leva à IRM como a única modalidade de imagem que pode revelar doença dentro do parênquima da medula espinal. Outras modalidades de imagens não podem descartar esse diagnóstico. Apenas se houver dúvida sobre outros diagnósticos vale a pena usar outros exames.

Doenças específicas

Embolia fibrocartilaginosa

Esta condição é bem descrita na literatura veterinária e pode ocorrer em cães e gatos. A lesão incitante é uma oclusão do suprimento arterial da medula espinal pelo material condroide, que oblitera o lúmen do vaso. Isso causa o equivalente a um "acidente vascular encefálico" na medula espinal. A região dependente da medula espinal após o infarto torna-se de imediato desvitalizado e não funcional e, posteriormente, necrótico.[35] Nas horas após o insulto inicial, o edema pode se acumular ao redor do parênquima da medula espinal, levando a um moderado agravamento dos sinais clínicos, que podem ser visíveis ao proprietário e ao veterinário. A fonte do material condroide não é conhecida. Ele tem sido sugerido como derivado do disco intervertebral (núcleo) e, em seguida, finaliza dentro do suprimento arterial.[36] Todavia, não há explicações satisfatórias para sua eventual localização. Explicações alternativas incluem paredes dos vasos sanguíneos submetidos a metaplasia condroide com esse material, que finalmente descoloca-se e/ou aloja-se mais abaixo ou, talvez, induza a um trombo no local original.

A EFC é suspeita em animais que apresentam sinais clínicos típicos, com lesão observada na IRM, mas o diagnóstico definitivo só pode ser feito no exame *post mortem*. As lesões clássicas são pequenas, normalmente localizadas em um quadrante da medula espinal, que aparenta estar hiperintensa ou normal em varreduras ponderadas em T2 e iso ou hipointensa em varreduras ponderadas em T1.[37] No entanto, muitos cães com suspeita de exibir EFC apresentam grandes regiões de hiperintensidade em T2 e STIR em varreduras de IRM (Figura 267.4).[38] Uma vez que muitos se recuperam naturalmente, o diagnóstico não é definitivo e a natureza da lesão permanece especulativa. Por esse motivo às vezes é usado o termo *mielopatia isquêmica*: para refletir com mais exatidão a falta de um diagnóstico preciso.[39] Antes do acesso generalizado à IRM, a EFC era suspeita em uma maior proporção de casos. Com o uso da RM, alguns pacientes mostraram ter um dos vários tipos de hérnia de disco intervertebral hiperagudos (ver Figura 267.3 e Capítulo 266). A maioria dos cães suspeitos de EFC exibe sinais lateralizados leves a moderadamente graves, mas que mostram considerável melhora dentro de cerca de 48 horas. Outros, porém, podem ter deficiências funcionais devastadoras, cuja melhora espontânea não ocorre. É claro que apenas lesões definitivamente diagnosticadas são aqueles casos (incomuns) encontrados no exame *post mortem*; portanto, fornecendo uma visão possivelmente tendenciosa da natureza da doença. Os fatores de risco para a condição não foram estabelecidos, mas talvez seja prudente analisar o estado de coagulação dos animais acometidos (ver Capítulo 196).

O prognóstico depende da gravidade e da localização da lesão inicial. Em geral, os animais com lesões nas regiões T3-L3 ou C1-C5 da medula espinal têm um bom prognóstico se sua sensação de dor profunda for intacta (ver Capítulo 259). Animais que perderam a dor profunda ou com grandes lesões afetando as intumescências da medula espinal (ou seja, C6-T2 ou L4-S3) têm um prognóstico resguardado, uma vez que há menos espaço para respostas plásticas que melhoram os déficits funcionais, caso essas regiões da substância cinzenta tenham sido destruídas. Lesões que afetam a medula espinal sacral podem ser particularmente problemáticas, já que incontinências fecal e/ou urinária são comuns e difíceis de controlar a longo prazo. Nenhum tratamento é necessário, mas, semelhante ao prognóstico para lesões traumáticas, um período de até 3 meses ou mais deve ser dado para se observar a completa recuperação.

Ruptura do vaso sanguíneo/hematomielia

Um pequeno número de casos com hematoma dentro da substância da medula espinal foi relatado.[40] Muitos foram de animais jovens, e presume-se que o hematoma se desenvolveu devido à ruptura de um vaso anômalo. Na verdade, vasos anômalos foram descritos na medula espinal em alguns casos, apoiando essa teoria. Os fatores de risco para essa condição não são conhecidos, mas seria presumível que ela ocorra com mais frequência durante os períodos de aumento da pressão arterial sistêmica, embora isso não tenha sido documentado. Trauma não tem sido associado a essa condição. Embora se possa esperar que tais lesões ocorram de forma aguda, há evidências de que o sangramento se acumule ao longo de um período de várias semanas. A gravidade dos sinais clínicos varia consideravelmente. Os casos diagnosticados em definitivo tendem a ser bastante graves, mas isso pode refletir a necessidade implícita de diagnóstico em tais casos.

O diagnóstico dessa lesão intraparenquimatosa depende da IRM. O acúmulo de sangue na medula espinal sofre uma série de mudanças na característica da imagem ao longo do tempo, que pode ajudar na identificação da duração do processo. No entanto, as mudanças podem ser não confiáveis e variar consideravelmente, dependendo do campo de força magnética, precisão do tempo de aquisição de imagens e vários outros fatores.[41] Pequenos hematomas dentro da medula espinal com bastante frequência são suspeitos, mas, quando associados com sinais clínicos relativamente moderados que tenham se desenvolvido de forma aguda, os animais acometidos são frequentemente tratados de forma conservadora. Portanto, um diagnóstico definitivo não é alcançado, porque muitas vezes os animais se recuperam. Os casos gravemente afetados com grandes massas intraparenquimatosas requerem intervenção cirúrgica de emergência. Se não for verificado, o hematoma em expansão causa danos progressivos à medula espinal, o que pode levar a déficits clínicos irreversíveis. A intervenção cirúrgica tem como objetivo drenar o hematoma via incisão através da *pia matter* e partes superficiais do parênquima da medula espinal.[40] Vasos sanguíneos anômalos, se presentes, podem ser identificados e uma biopsia, realizada. O prognóstico para o tratamento cirúrgico depende principalmente da gravidade dos sinais clínicos.

Hematoma extradural

Os hematomas extradurais são comumente encontrados em associação com hérnias de disco agudas e ocasionalmente com distúrbios de hemostasia. Em casos raros, os cães são apresentados com sinais neurológicos progressivos agudos ou crônicos, associados com a dor, em que a causa subjacente é um hematoma

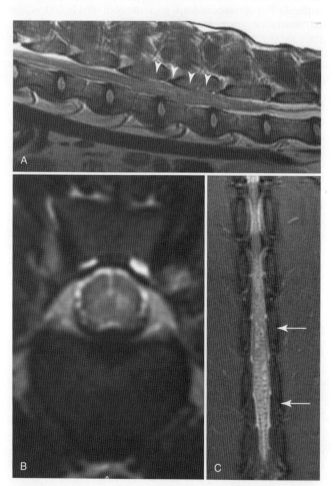

Figura 267.4 Imagens de ressonância magnética (RM) ilustrando características de suspeita de fibrocartilagem embolização. **A.** Imagem ponderada em T2 sagital médio ilustrando hiperintensidade parenquimatosa leve dentro das vértebras lombares caudais (*pontas de seta*). Observe o tamanho normal, forma e intensidade dos núcleos do disco intervertebral, indicando que o disco herniado não é uma causa provável. **B.** Imagem transversal ponderada em T2 no nível médio da lesão ilustrando hiperintensidade assimétrica da matéria cinzenta. **C.** Imagem STIR dorsal da região lombar caudal. Esta sequência de varredura é frequentemente sensível a lesões vasculares e revela hiperintensidade parenquimatosa irregular característica (*região entre as setas*).

idiopático.[42] A descompressão cirúrgica está associada com um prognóstico bom a excelente. É importante reconhecer que tal patologia é encontrada, porque a aparência de imagem também é consistente com neoplasia extradural, que tem um prognóstico muito pior.

Anomalias vasculares

As anomalias vasculares são frequentemente incriminadas no desenvolvimento de hemorragia intraparenquimatosa.[43] Elas também podem, às vezes, formar lesões em massa, que podem ser detectadas em exames de RM e ser candidatas para remoção cirurgia.[44]

Doença sistêmica associada a hemorragia e trombose na medula espinal

A hemorragia no parênquima da medula espinal também pode surgir de uma doença sistêmica que cause estados hipocoaguláveis. Distúrbios da coagulação do sangue, como hemofilia, são causas raras de lesões espinais em cães (ver Capítulo 197).[45] No entanto, existem vários distúrbios de coagulação que podem estar associados com disfunção espinal, incluindo doença da marca de von Wille e, raramente, trombocitopenia imunomediada (ver Capítulo 201).[46,47] Fragilidade vascular associada com inflamação (vasculite) também pode ser uma causa de hemorragia dentro ou ao redor da medula espinal. Causas reconhecidas em cães incluem infecção por *Angiostrongylus vasorum* (ver Capítulo 242) e leishmaniose (ver Capítulo 221).[48-50] Por outro lado, a vasculite também pode levar a lesões da medula espinal, causando trombose, em vez de hemorragia.[51]

LESÕES NEOPLÁSICAS

Sinalização

Lesões neoplásicas da medula espinal ou coluna vertebral estão associadas a determinadas raças. Cães grandes são mais suscetíveis a osteossarcoma, um tumor espinal comum.[52,53] Acredita-se que haja risco de hemangiossarcoma para Golden Retrievers nos EUA, outra neoplasia espinal comum.[52] A idade mais avançada (por volta dos 4 anos para cães gigantes) é um fator de risco reconhecido para qualquer condição neoplásica, embora cães mais jovens (frequentemente por volta dos 12 meses) são suscetíveis ao nefroblastoma, um tumor espinal intramedular.[54] A idade não deve ser usada como regra para doença neoplásica. O nefroblastoma pode ser mais comum em cães Pastores-Alemães, embora nem todos os estudos concordem com esta afirmação.[53-55] O linfoma é uma lesão medular comum em cães e gatos (ver Capítulo 344), sendo a principal causa de lesões na coluna vertebral em gatos adultos.[56] Lesões metastáticas da medula espinal ocorrem ocasionalmente,[7] então vale a pena considerar essa possibilidade durante o exame clínico, especialmente em animais caquéticos.

Histórico

Animais com doença neoplásica comumente têm uma doença de aparecimento capcioso de sinais clínicos, à medida que a lesão aumenta gradativamente. Contudo, alguns animais com tumores na medula espinal apresentam um início agudo de sinais clínicos, que pode surgir por meio de dois mecanismos principais: (1) desenvolvimento de fratura patológica, no qual há um progressivo enfraquecimento do osso até a fratura que causa imediata lesão espinal; e (2) lesão vascular aguda associada com embolização tumoral ou compressão e trombose associadas a pressão prolongada ou excessiva. Portanto, é importante considerar a possibilidade de tumor em qualquer cão que tenha evidência de disfunção da medula espinal, mesmo em caso de início agudo.

Apresentação

A maioria dos animais com neoplasias espinais tem um início lento de deficiências neurológicas progressivas e dor. No entanto, os sinais clínicos variam de acordo com a natureza do tumor. Neoplasia extradural é tipicamente dolorosa, provavelmente porque distorce as meninges ou os nervos da medula espinal, ou porque causa danos a elementos esqueléticos. Lesões dentro da dura-máter não são tipicamente associadas com sinais de dor até os estágios tardios, mas alguns dados recentes sobre lesões intramedulares sugerem que isso pode não ser acurado.[57]

A taxa de crescimento tumoral é altamente variável. Tumores semelhantes podem crescer de forma diferente, a depender do local na medula espinal, embora a progressão dos sinais possa ser enganosa, uma vez que as lesões podem se tornar muito grandes antes de qualquer sinal ser notado (Figura 267.5). Em geral, os sinais clínicos associados com lesões intradurais progridem lentamente, e alguns animais podem ter sinais clínicos por muitos meses ou até anos antes de sua apresentação clínica.[58] Por outro lado, os animais que têm sinais clínicos associados com lesões extradurais tipicamente mostram progressão rápida (dias a semanas).

Diagnóstico diferencial

A disfunção crônica progressiva da medula espinal é mais frequentemente associada com neoplasia ou hérnia de disco crônica (geralmente tipo II). Porém, há uma razoável amplitude de diagnósticos diferenciais possíveis, que inclui doenças inflamatória ou infecciosas, como discopondilite meningoenencefalomielite, cuja origem é desconhecida.[60] Em animais mais velhos, doenças degenerativas costumam ser consideradas em cães da raça Corgi e Pastor-Alemão,[61] principalmente a mielopatia degenerativa (ver Capítulo 266). Siringomielia congênita,[62] pós-traumática ou associada com a adesão (acúmulo de fluido no parênquima da medula espinal) podem produzir sinais clínicos semelhantes em alguns casos, especialmente em cães pequenos.[30] Além disso, existem muitas massas não neoplásicas ou anomalias que podem estar associadas com déficits progressivos graduais da medula espinal e com déficits neurais, como seio dermoide, calcâneo circunscrito, hematomas (descrito anteriormente), exostose cartilaginosa, lipoma, proliferação óssea associada a erros congênita do metabolismo e distúrbios mal classificados, como meningioangiomatose.[63-68] Esta ampla lista de diagnósticos diferenciais, incluindo muitas lesões benignas, envolve a necessidade do diagnóstico preciso para evitar suposições de prognóstico ruim. Para animais com disfunção aguda da medula espinal, o principal diagnóstico diferencial é a hérnia de disco aguda (mesmo em cães de raças grandes) e as lesões traumáticas e vasculares discutidas antes. Muitos, mas nem todos, os casos de lesão medular aguda associados com lesões neoplásicas exibem sinais de dor.

Testes diagnósticos

Como na maioria das condições do SNC, após localizar uma lesão, o próximo passo usual para o diagnóstico é a imagem da área afetada. Frequentemente, é útil começar com radiografias, já que uma proporção razoável de animais afetados tem lesões de elementos esqueléticos que possam ser identificadas (ver Figura 267.1). No entanto, é importante reconhecer que apenas uma proporção de neoplasias espinais causa perda óssea suficiente ou proliferação óssea possível de ser reconhecida em radiografias simples. Lesões dentro da dura-máter geralmente não alteram a densidade óssea, nem todas as neoplasias peridurais estão associadas com alterações ósseas. Portanto, a radiografia é um bom teste de "inclusão", mas ruim para a "exclusão". O próximo passo é geralmente uma varredura por IRM (ver Figura 267.5). A IRM é excelente para detectar lesões, independentemente da localização fora ou dentro do parênquima da medula espinal. A TC é limitada à detecção de lesões radiopacas ou daquelas que causam alterações na densidade óssea, embora isso possa ser extremamente útil para tipos específicos de lesões (Figura 267.6).

1458　SEÇÃO 17 • Doença Neurológica

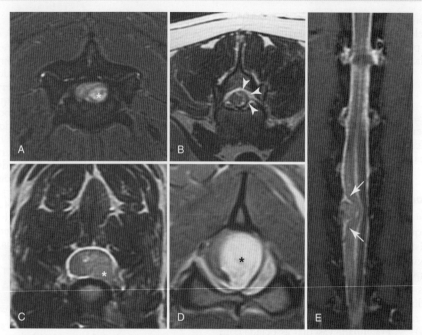

Figura 267.5 Imagens de ressonância magnética (RM) ponderadas em T2 de tumores da coluna vertebral. **A.** Tumor extradural (*asterisco*); medula espinal comprimida (histologia indicou fibrossarcoma). **B.** Tumor intradural-extramedular (meningioma) (*pontas de seta*). **C.** Tumor da bainha nervosa (intradural-extramedular para intramedular) (*asterisco*). **D.** Grande tumor extradural (*asterisco*) foi diagnosticado em um cão que deambulava no momento da apresentação clínica. **E.** Meningioma cervical ilustrando a aparência típica de um "tee de golfe" criado pelo LCR circundante (*setas*).

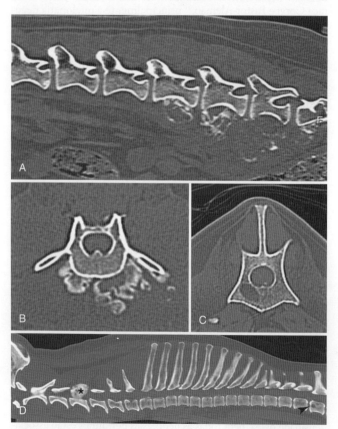

Figura 267.6 A tomografia computadorizada (TC) pode ser útil para definir lesões ósseas associados a tumores. **A.** Imagem sagital reconstruída ilustrando extensa proliferação óssea ao longo do aspecto ventral das vértebras lombares caudais, associadas a um tumor prostático metastático. **B.** Imagem transversal da mesma lesão. **C.** Imagem transversal que ilustra uma lesão lítica dentro do corpo vertebral L2 causada por mieloma múltiplo. **D.** Imagem de TC sagital reconstruída ilustrando uma lesão primária na vértebra C4 (*asterisco*) e suspeita de lesão metastática no corpo vertebral de L1 (*ponta de seta*).

Doenças específicas

Visão geral

A doença neoplásica da medula espinal é mais bem categorizada de acordo com a localização da lesão em relação às meninges ao redor da medula. Assim, a divisão clínica (e patológica) são extradurais, intradurais/extramedular e intramedular. Destas, as mais comuns são as extradurais, com os tipos intradural/extramedular sendo provavelmente o segundo tipo mais comum.[53,58,59]

Tumores extradurais

Essas lesões encontram-se dentro do espaço peridural, normalmente preenchido por gordura. De acordo com seu local de origem, neoplasias que surgem neste local geralmente são tumores ósseos ou vários tipos de sarcoma de tecidos moles, como osteossarcoma, hemangiosarcoma, fibrossarcoma, linfoma, lipossarcoma e mieloma múltiplo. Os raros tumores benignos que se encontram nesta localização incluem os lipomas.[66] Contudo, a maioria dos tumores epidurais são malignos e frequentemente causam danos ósseos secundários, levando ao enfraquecimento ósseo e, comumente, às fraturas patológicas. Muitos desses tipos de câncer (p. ex., hemangiossarcoma e osteossarcoma) já fizeram metástase no momento do diagnóstico, e é comum observar lesões metastáticas em outros locais do esqueleto ou nos pulmões (ver Figura 267.6). É importante ressaltar que muitos cães acometidos por neoplasia espinal extradural parecem sentir dor considerável, o que pode ajudar a suspeitar desse tipo de lesão *versus* outros tipos de tumores.

Tumores intradurais/extramedulares

Estas são lesões de tecido que revestem ou projetam-se através do espaço subaracnoide, como as meninges e raízes nervosas. Tanto os meningiomas quanto os tumores da bainha nervosa tendem a crescer lentamente, produzindo sinais clínicos durante meses a anos.[58] Os tumores da bainha nervosa parecem ser mais comuns na intumescência da medula espinal, embora isso também possa refletir a maior probabilidade de diagnóstico de lesões em locais que causem claudicação. Meningiomas podem ocorrer em qualquer local, mas parecem ser especialmente comuns no espaço C1/C2 em cães, com uma possível predisposição na raça Boxer. Embora os tumores da bainha nervosa e os meningiomas sejam em geral considerados como relativamente benignos na histologia, é típico invadir localmente o tecido normal, e pode ser difícil extirpá-los por completo. Alguns tumores de bainha nervosa parecem estar associados com síndromes neuropáticas de dor, incluindo depressão generalizada e alterações de comportamento.[58]

Tumores intramedulares

Esses tumores não são comuns.[57] Eles surgem de elementos do neurópilo, como células da glia (de vários tipos) e, raramente, neurônios. Os tipos comuns de tumor nesta categoria incluem astrocitoma e ependimoma, que podem variar consideravelmente em seu comportamento histológico: alguns são bem circunscritos por uma cápsula e podem ser extirpados, enquanto outros são altamente invasivos e agressivos. Normalmente, eles têm um crescimento lento e progressivo até vários meses. Nefroblastoma é um exemplo de neoplasia encontrada nesse compartimento, embora também possa cruzar para o espaço extramedular/intradural. Esse tumor parece se desenvolver perto da junção toracolombar de cães jovens como consequência de um erro durante a embriogênese, em que um pequeno número de células progenitoras renais são incorporadas ao tubo neural em desenvolvimento e, mais tarde, tornam-se neoplásicas.[55] Esse tipo de tumor geralmente tem um fenótipo histológico benigno, mas pode ser localmente invasivo.

Diagnóstico do tipo de tumor espinal

Tendo em mente a extrema variabilidade no comportamento do tumor e, portanto, o prognóstico, é altamente desejável um diagnóstico específico sem a realização de uma cirurgia aberta tradicional. A análise do LCR também pode ser útil ocasionalmente, na medida em que as células cancerosas podem se esfoliar no fluido e ser detectadas ou, alternativamente, o fluido pode revelar evidências de uma condição infecciosa (ver Capítulo 115).[69,70] A análise de sangue e/ou aspiração de medula óssea (ver Capítulo 92) pode ser útil em alguns casos, como aqueles com suspeita de mieloma múltiplo (ver Capítulo 344).[13] Da mesma forma, pode ser útil obter aspirados de linfonodos para identificar casos de linfoma multifocal ou aspirados de lesões pulmonares suspeitas de serem metástases. Se uma lesão em forma de massa foi identificada nas imagens, é possível obter amostras de biopsia de dentro ou fora do parênquima da medula espinal sem a realização de cirurgia aberta.[71,72] Ultrassonografia, fluoroscopia ou biopsias guiadas por TC podem ser obtidas usando agulhas, ferramenta tru-cut de biopsia e agulhas Jamshidi. Existem potenciais perigos óbvios e graves. Para lesões na medula espinal em si, pode ser possível colocar uma agulha na medula e obter biopsia por aspiração criteriosa.[71] Tais biopsias podem ser úteis para descartar outros diagnósticos diferenciais, como granulomas fúngicos ou lesões de massa benignas. Apesar da grande variedade de métodos, pode ser difícil diagnosticar o câncer percutâneo, a menos que

se esfolie facilmente. A maioria dos tumores espinais são suspeitos em imagem, mas não confirmados até que a histologia seja realizada. Massas extradurais não devem ser consideradas neoplásicas, porque os animais acometidos podem ser inadequadamente sacrificados.

Tratamento e prognóstico

As doenças neoplásicas que afetam a medula espinal têm uma ampla gama de tratamentos e prognósticos, dependendo da natureza da lesão. Por exemplo, os meningiomas muitas vezes podem ser cirurgicamente extirpados, embora com frequência cresçam de novo durante um período de meses a anos. Os tumores da bainha nervosa podem, teoricamente, ser extirpados na íntegra, mas, como muitas vezes estão perto da medula espinal e requerem grandes margens para a excisão total, isso raramente é alcançado quando estão dentro do canal vertebral. No entanto, o intervalo livre de doença a longo prazo (mais de 12 meses) pode ser obtido apenas por ressecção cirúrgica. Algumas outras lesões neoplásicas têm um prognóstico desesperançoso, como hemangiossarcoma que já obteve metástase. Outros têm um prognóstico intermediário e podem ocasionalmente responder à quimioterapia (p. ex., mieloma múltiplo).[13] Embora mielite induzida por radiação seja uma sequela potencialmente devastadora da radioterapia direta na medula espinal, um planejamento cuidadoso pode produzir resultados gratificantes.[73,74] A radioterapia é a opção mais notável para uma terapia adjuvante em casos que tenham recorrência de um tumor previamente excisado ou nos quais houve extirpação primária incompleta.[55]

Em geral, o prognóstico para a maioria dos tumores epidurais é ruim, principalmente porque são com frequência malignos e podem muito bem já terem feito metástase no momento do diagnóstico. A redução cirúrgica de volume pode fornecer alívio rápido e eficaz da compressão, que é frequentemente associado à rápida recuperação da perda da função. Infelizmente, os resultados, sobretudo para sarcomas, são com frequência de curta duração, com recorrência dos sinais clínicos dentro de algumas semanas a meses. Os tumores intradurais/extramedulares são passíveis de excisão cirúrgica, e esta é a principal modalidade de tratamento. O resultado pode ser bastante gratificante para meningiomas, porque frequentemente são de crescimento lento e os sinais clínicos podem ser aliviados por mais ou menos 12 meses. Em contradição, tumores da bainha nervosa tendem a ter um prognóstico pior por causa da dificuldade de remoção do tumor em sua totalidade. Os tumores intramedulares são frequentemente do tipo benigno e podem até ser encapsulados, o que significa que podem ser potencialmente extirpados. Isso, é claro, envolve a incisão do parênquima da medula espinal e o uso de técnicas de microdissecção, mas os resultados podem ser muito gratificantes,[55,75] embora a recorrência dos sinais clínicos tenha sido relatada em alguns dos casos (muito pequenos) relatados na literatura veterinária.

REFERÊNCIAS BIBLIOGRÁFICAS

As referências bibliográficas deste capítulo se encontram online no Ambiente de Aprendizagem.

CAPÍTULO 268

Neuropatias Periféricas

Christopher L. Mariani

O sistema nervoso periférico (SNP) inclui todos as estruturas nervosas fora do sistema nervoso central (SNC), ou seja, o cérebro e a medula espinal. O SNP é composto de fibras nervosas motoras que inervam o músculo esquelético, fibras nervosas sensoriais que são responsáveis pelo tato, dor e posição proprioceptiva a partir da pele, das articulações e dos músculos, fibras aferentes que carregam informações de sentido especial (p. ex., sistemas auditivo e vestibular) e fibras autonômicas que inervam as vísceras torácicas e abdominais, bem como outras estruturas (p. ex., glândulas salivares, íris e barorreceptores). O sistema autônomo é ainda dividido em sistemas simpático e parassimpático. Fibras nervosas periféricas podem surgir do corno ventral da medula espinal, saindo pela raiz ventral (fibras motoras e simpáticas); do gânglio da raiz dorsal adjacente a medula espinal, entrando na medula através da raiz dorsal (fibras sensoriais); ou do tronco cerebral ou gânglios adjacentes (fibras motoras e fibras parassimpáticas), entrando ou saindo nos nervos cranianos. Embora alguns nervos carreguem informações puramente motoras ou sensoriais, a maioria dos nervos é composta por uma combinação das duas fibras. Uma neuropatia se refere à doença do nervo periférico (nervos espinais ou cranianos; ver Capítulo 264), enquanto polineuropatias afetam vários nervos periféricos, muitas vezes de forma difusa.

SINAIS CLÍNICOS

Os distúrbios nervosos periféricos mais reconhecidos em medicina veterinária têm sua apresentação clínica dominada pela disfunção dos nervos motores, embora os sinais sensitivos e autonômicos sejam observados em algumas condições. Os sinais clínicos característicos incluem paresia, hipotonia, atrofia muscular, depressão ou ausência de reflexos espinais segmentares (Vídeo 268.1). A paresia pode envolver todos os membros ou se manifestar como paraparesia e, muitas vezes, resulta em uma marcha curta. Disfonia, disfagia, estridor inspiratório, megaesôfago e reflexos palpebrais e deglutição reduzidos ou ausentes podem ser observados, graças ao envolvimento dos nervos laríngeo recorrente, glossofaríngeo, vago e facial (ver Capítulo 259).[1-3] Distúrbios da junção neuromuscular (ver Capítulo 269) e dos músculos (ver Capítulo 354) podem resultar em muitos dos mesmos sinais, e pode ser difícil distingui-los de doença do nervo periférico fundamentando-se no exame clínico isolado. Os sinais de disfunção sensorial incluem ataxia, perda da capacidade de posicionamento proprioceptivo, redução ou ausência de reflexos espinais e parestesia ou anestesia, resultando potencialmente em automutilação. A disfunção autonômica pode resultar em vômito ou regurgitação, diarreia, íleo, retenção urinária, incontinência, lacrimejamento e salivação prejudicadas e disfunção pupilar. Esses distúrbios podem ser exibidos de forma aguda e progressiva ou com sinais episódicos, porém mais frequentemente se apresentam de forma crônica e com curso progressivo.

PLANO DIAGNÓSTICO

Um hemograma completo, uma avaliação da bioquímica sérica e uma urinálise são indicadas para identificar distúrbios metabólicos responsáveis por disfunção do nervo (p. ex., diabetes melito e hipotireoidismo) e doença por comorbidade e para avaliar a adequação de pacientes para anestesia geral. Testes metabólicos adicionais, incluindo avaliação da tireoide (ver Capítulos 299 a 302) e frutosamina sérica (ver Capítulos 304 e 305), também podem ser considerados. Creatinoquinase sérica (ver Capítulo 66), carnitina e piruvato pré e pós-exercício, lactato (ver Capítulo 70) e avaliação de gasometria (ver Capítulo 128) podem ser úteis para identificar certos distúrbios musculares. Exames de imagem das cavidades torácica e abdominal são frequentemente indicados para identificar doenças neoplásicas. Titulação sérica ou testes baseados em reação em cadeia da polimerase (PCR) para doenças infecciosas (ver Capítulo 207), como toxoplasmose ou neosporose (ver Capítulo 221), também podem ser apropriados.

O diagnóstico por imagem avançada (imagens de ressonância magnética [RM] ou tomografia computadorizada [TC]) é útil em alguns casos para demonstrar processos neoplásicos, inflamatórios e outras doenças que afetam nervos específicos ou raízes nervosas ou que apresentam lesões do SNC. No entanto, essas modalidades normalmente desempenham um papel maior na exclusão de outros distúrbios na lista de diagnóstico diferencial. Da mesma forma, a avaliação do líquido cefalorraquidiano (LCR; ver Capítulo 115) é mais útil para eliminar outros processos de doenças, mas ocasionalmente é anormal em distúrbios dos nervos periféricos que envolvam as raízes nervosas ou tanto o SNC quanto o SNP.

Os testes de diagnósticos mais úteis para doenças dos nervos periféricos são os eletrodiagnósticos (ver Capítulos 117) e a histopatologia de biopsias de músculos e nervos (ver Capítulo 116). O eletrodiagnóstico inclui eletromiografia (EMG), teste de condução de velocidades de nervo motor e sensorial (CVNM e CVNS, respectivamente), avaliação da onda F, potenciais do dorso do cordão, avaliação de reflexo H, estimulação magnética e resposta evocada auditiva de tronco encefálico (RETE).[4,5] Juntos, a EMG e a CVNM são úteis para confirmar a disfunção do sistema neuromuscular, para diferenciar a doença de nervo periférico da doença muscular e para distinguir a doença de desmielinização axonal. A avaliação da onda F permite a investigação do nervo proximal e das raízes nervosas ventrais, enquanto a CVNS e o teste do dorso do cordão avaliam os nervos sensoriais e o nervo das raízes dorsais. No entanto, os testes de eletrodiagnóstico raramente permitem o diagnóstico de uma etiologia específica. Exames histopatológicos de biopsias de músculos e nervos são úteis para confirmar e detectar mais anormalidades definidas com o teste eletrodiagnóstico e são mais propensos a identificar uma etiologia específica.[6,7] Os testes eletrofisiológicos e biopsia de músculos e nervos são descritos com mais detalhes em outros capítulos (ver Capítulos 116 e 117). Testes específicos para disfunção autonômica também podem ser úteis para identificar animais com envolvimento dessa parte do sistema nervoso.[8,9]

DISTÚRBIOS DEGENERATIVOS

Existem vários distúrbios neuropáticos degenerativos que afetam raças específicas de cães e gatos e, portanto, parecem ser hereditários por natureza. Esses distúrbios são bastante raros, e uma discussão detalhada está além do escopo deste capítulo. O leitor é encaminhado para análises mais abrangentes do tópico.[10-16]

DISTÚRBIOS METABÓLICOS

Diabetes melito

A neuropatia diabética é uma das causas mais comuns de disfunções do nervo periférico em pacientes humanos,[17] porém parece ocorrer com muito menos frequência na medicina veterinária. Os sinais clínicos são percebidos principalmente em gatos (ver Capítulo 305), enquanto evidências da doença raramente são reconhecidas em cães (ver Capítulo 304). A fisiopatologia da neuropatia diabética tem sido intensamente estudada, com uma série de teorias causais propostas.[18-20] Os sinais clínicos incluem paraparesia, progredindo em alguns casos para tetraparesia, ataxia de membro pélvico (ver Vídeo 305.2), dificuldade em salto, reações posturais e de reflexos espinais segmentares reduzidas e atrofia muscular distal.[12,18-24] Uma postura plantígrada é frequentemente observada em gatos (ver Vídeo 305.3). Embora mal reconhecida, a disfunção do nervo sensorial que resulta em parestesias, hiperestesia e irritabilidade provavelmente ocorre com alguma frequência nesse transtorno.[12,19,22,23,25] Sintomatologia de nervos cranianos e sinais autonômicos são comuns no homem, mas raramente são relatados em animais.[19,26] No entanto, a disfunção subclínica do nervo aparece com certa regularidade.[27-30]

O diagnóstico é fortemente suspeito quando há demonstração de hiperglicemia e glicosúria em um animal com sinais clínicos consistentes. A frutosamina sérica também pode ser de alguma utilidade, já que a neuropatia é mais comum em pacientes desregulados. O teste de eletrodiagnóstico pode revelar atividade dentro dos músculos acometidos e redução da condução de velocidade nervosa sensorial e motora, embora essas mudanças possam ser sutis e irregulares.[12,18,21,24,26,28] No entanto, anormalidades consistentes são detectáveis em CVNM, CVNS, onda F e avaliação do dorso do cordão, mesmo quando as anormalidades na EMG são sutis ou ausentes.[22] A evidência de bloqueio de condução foi igualmente notada em cães.[28] Juntos, esses achados sugerem que a desmielinização predomina sobre as mudanças axonais, o que é suportado em animais pela histopatologia de biopsias musculares e nervosas,[22,27,31] embora pelo menos um artigo documente a contribuição de lesão axonal no processo da doença.[23] Lesões microscópicas e evidências de anormalidades ultraestruturais perineurais e microvasculares também foram documentadas em cães e gatos diabéticos.[32,33]

A terapia é principalmente dirigida para o controle da causa subjacente do distúrbio diabético e a melhora do controle glicêmico que normalmente resulta no alívio ou resolução dos sinais clínicos.[18,20,21] Existem poucos relatos de terapia adicional em medicina veterinária. A acetil-L-carnitina tem múltiplos mecanismos de ação potencialmente benéficos e demonstrou eficácia em experimentos com modelos e pacientes humanos.[34] Ela tem sido usado em gatos com neuropatia diabética com sucesso anedótico.[35] O pesquisador notou uma melhora dramática dos sinais em alguns pacientes felinos após terapia antioxidante com vitamina E e N-acetilcisteína.

Hipotireoidismo

Sinais de disfunção neuromuscular têm sido frequentemente associados ao hipotireoidismo tanto em pacientes caninos quanto humanos (ver Capítulo 299).[18,20,36,37] A fisiopatologia subjacente dessa associação permanece mal caracterizada, mas potencialmente envolve os nervos periféricos e os músculos. Tendo como base estudos eletrofisiológicos, a deficiência do hormônio tireoidiano parece levar a danos axonais e desmielinização.[36-39] O acúmulo de glicosaminoglicanos e glicogênio dentro das células de Schwann pode ser responsável pela disfunção celular e pela resultante mudança desmielinizante. Também existem evidências experimentais de um papel do hormônio tireoidiano no conjunto de microtúbulos para o transporte axonal normal, que, quando prejudicado, pode resultar em axonopatias.[18] A atividade alterada de sódio-potássio ATPase, com transporte axonal prejudicado, é outro potencial mecanismo.[39-41] Em pacientes humanos, mononeuropatias (particularmente síndrome do túnel do carpo) são comuns, sendo atribuídas a depósitos de mucina nas estruturas dos tecidos moles, o que causa uma neuropatia compressiva.[42] Tem sido sugerido um processo semelhante como um possível responsável pela compressão de nervos cranianos em pacientes veterinários.[18]

Os animais podem apresentar paresia ou, em casos raros, claudicação envolvendo um único membro, dois membros ou todos os quatro membros.[41,43,44] Deficiências dos nervos cranianos, incluindo paresia facial, sinais vestibulares e disfunção do nervo trigêmeo, são com frequência reconhecidas, em geral unilaterais, e comumente afetam vários nervos (ver Capítulo 264).[18,45-48] Esses sinais podem ocorrer secundários a uma neuropatia ou, em outros casos, estar relacionados ao envolvimento do SNC.[49] Uma associação também foi feita entre hipotireoidismo, megaesôfago (ver Capítulo 273) e paralisia laríngea (ver Capítulo 239),[41,50] embora um papel causal seja tênue e ainda precise ser provado.[45,51-53] Há possibilidade de animais acometidos apresentarem sinais clínicos clássicos, como letargia, ganho de peso, alopecia e seborreia. Hemograma completo e perfil bioquímico sérico podem mostrar anemia não regenerativa leve, hipercolesterolemia ou nível elevado de creatinoquinase. O diagnóstico é confirmado pela demonstração de um nível reduzido de tiroxina sérica livre e total (T4) com elevado nível do hormônio estimulador da tireoide (ver Capítulo 299).[54] A análise de LCR pode mostrar um aumento da proteína sem pleocitose concomitante.[40,46] Testes eletrofisiológicos mostram potenciais de denervação na EMG, com reduções em CVNM e CVNS.[41,43,44] Os RETE também podem ser anormais.[41,46] A biopsia de músculo mostra atrofias de fibra tipo I e II, consistentes com mudança neuropática, ou uma atrofia seletiva de fibra do tipo II, sugestiva de uma miopatia. A biopsia do nervo pode mostrar alterações características mistas, tanto da degeneração axonal quanto da desmielinização.[12,15,41,43] Em muitos casos, o diagnóstico é parcialmente baseado na administração de levotiroxina e na demonstração da resposta clínica, que em geral começa dentro de vários dias e é concluído em 3 a 8 semanas.[45] Deficiências dos nervos cranianos, megaesôfago e paralisia laríngea podem ter menor probabilidade de melhorar.[18,41,45,50]

NEOPLASIAS

A disfunção do nervo periférico devido à neoplasia pode ser resultado de compressão do tecido nervoso devido a um tumor do nervo ou da bainha nervosa[55-57] do tecido neoplásico adjacente[58-62] ou pode ocorrer como um processo paraneoplástico. Tumores da bainha nervosa com frequência exibem características malignas, baseado na histopatologia e em sua tendência de ser localmente invasivos, crescendo proximamente acima dos nervos ou das raízes nervosas.[15,56,63-67] Essas neoplasias podem ocorrer em qualquer paciente de pequeno porte (Vídeo 268.2), embora sejam mais comuns em cães de raças grandes e sejam raros em gatos.[57,65,66,68] As neoplasias comumente surgem do plexo braquial. Claudicação e atrofia muscular são os sinais mais comuns e, muitas vezes, os únicos por longos períodos antes dos sinais clínicos adicionais, tais como paresia e déficits de reflexo ou de reações posturais.[56,57,65,66,69] O tumor pode eventualmente invadir a medula espinal, levando a ataxia, paresia e déficits de reação postural caudal à invasão. A dor pode ser provocada com a manipulação do membro ou com palpação da axila ou da região inguinal.[56] A síndrome de Horner pode estar presente com envolvimento da região caudal do plexo braquial.[56,69] Tumores da bainha do nervo trigêmeo são as neoplasias de nervos cranianos mais comuns e geralmente levam a atrofia muscular mastigatória unilateral.[70] Já tumores envolvendo outros nervos cranianos são vistos com menos frequência.[71,72]

O diagnóstico de tumores da bainha do nervo periférico pode ser desafiador. Ocasionalmente, uma massa é palpada na axila ou via retal.[73] A ressonância magnética (RM) ou TC podem permitir a visualização do tumor em muitos casos.[58,70,74-80] A ultrassonografia (US) também pode ser útil por facilitar a aspiração com agulha fina ou biopsia de lesões de massa identificáveis.[58,71,81-85] Já a EMG pode ser útil na demonstração de potenciais de denervação, dando suporte a um processo neuropático em pacientes com claudicação sem uma causa ortopédica óbvia.[56,65,73] A terapia definitiva para tumores de bainha nervo periférico consiste na remoção cirúrgica da neoplasia, que pode ser muito difícil. Embora tumores envolvendo porções de nervos periféricos distais possam ser completamente ressecáveis, a maioria dos tumores envolve o plexo braquial ou lombar e as raízes nervosas associadas a esses plexos.[77,86-89] A intervenção cirúrgica para esses tumores geralmente requer amputação do membro afetado, e a remoção definitiva pode requer laminectomia com secção das raízes nervosas o mais próximo possível da medula espinal. Apesar de ser uma terapia tão agressiva, muitos tumores recidivam, uma vez que possuem a tendência de crescer proximamente e invadir múltiplas raízes nervosas.[56,87]

A remoção cirúrgica de tumores da bainha do nervo trigêmeo foi relatada.[70] Outras neoplasias que possam envolver nervos periféricos incluem os sarcomas,[58,61] os carcinomas[60] e os tumores de células redondas.[59,80,90-94] Linfoma e outras neoplasias de células redondas podem envolver um único ou, em muitos casos, vários nervos ou raízes nervosas, levando a sinais focais ou multifocais.[80,90-93,95,96]

Neuropatia paraneoplásica

Uma polineuropatia associada ao câncer em um local remoto tem sido descrita em vários cães, mas em apenas um gato (ver Capítulo 352), e foi relatada com mais frequência com insulinoma (ver Capítulo 303),[97-104] embora uma variedade de outros tumores também tenha sido relacionada.[12,105-112] O mecanismo da doença é suspeito de ser primariamente imunomediado, devido ao antígeno mimetizador, em que o sistema imunológico gera uma resposta aos antígenos presentes dentro da neoplasia que são compartilhados com os nervos periféricos.[113,114] Em pacientes com insulinoma, hipoglicemia também tem sido sugerida como uma causa. Neuropatias sensoriais, motoras e autonômicas foram descritas no homem,[115] mas os sinais motores têm predomínio em artigos veterinários. Embora raramente relatadas, evidências eletrofisiológicas ou histológicas de disfunção de nervo periférico estão presentes em uma grande proporção de animais com câncer, e essa condição é provavelmente uma causa não reconhecida de fraqueza nos pacientes.[97,116,117] Um número substancial de autoanticorpos circulantes têm sido associados com neoplasias em humanos com polineuropatias paraneoplásicas, muitas vezes anterior ao diagnóstico por meios convencional.[113,114,118] Tais autoanticorpos ainda não foram identificados em pacientes veterinários. O diagnóstico consiste em documentar apropriadamente os sinais clínicos (p. ex., paresia, hiporreflexia e atrofia muscular), as alterações eletrofisiológicas e os resultados da biopsia de músculos e nervos no animal com uma neoplasia identificada, enquanto se elimina outras possíveis etiologias.

Uma melhora drástica ou resolução dos sinais clínicos foi documentada após a excisão cirúrgica ou outra terapia para câncer.[98,102,105,108,119,120] Como o mecanismo subjacente é uma provável terapia imunomoduladora, tem sido utilizado em pacientes humanos, incluindo corticosteroides plasmaférese, imunoglobulina intravenosa e outros fármacos imunossupressores. Essa terapia pode ser ineficaz em resolver os sinais neurológicos se a destruição neuronal tiver já ocorrido, embora estabilização dos sinais possa ser visto.[113,121] A terapia imunomoduladora é raramente relatada em pacientes veterinários, embora uma melhora drástica tenha sido documentada após a terapia com corticosteroides ser registrada em um cão com insulinoma.[98]

DISTÚRBIOS INFECCIOSOS E INFLAMATÓRIOS

Poliadiculoneurite por protozoários

A neosporose surgiu como um importante causa de doenças neuromusculares em cães (ver Capítulo 221).[122-124] O organismo protozoário responsável, *Neospora caninum*, foi identificado pela primeira vez em 1988, e a espécie canina foi confirmada como um hospedeiro definitivo em 1998.[125-129] Muitos casos de polirraduculoneurite protozoária anteriormente atribuídos a *Toxoplasma gondii* eram provavelmente causados por *N. caninum*.[123,124,130] Esses organismos podem ser distinguidos com imuno-histoquímica e, ocasionalmente, estudo cuidadoso da estrutura do cisto com microscopia de luz ou eletrônica.[122,131] Tanto *T. gondii* quanto *N. caninum* exibem uma predileção por tecido nervoso e podem invadir nervos periféricos, músculos e o SNC. Os sinais clínicos incluem paresia envolvendo um ou vários membros, atrofia e dor muscular, redução do tônus muscular, déficits de reação postural e redução ou ausência de reflexos espinais segmentares.[132,133] Sinais de nervos cranianos, como inclinação da cabeça, disfagia e paresia da língua, foram ocasionalmente relatados.[132] A apresentação clássica da infecção por *N. caninum* é paraparesia em cães jovens, que progressivamente leva a uma condição não ambulatória caracterizada por extensão rígida dos membros pélvicos associada a contraturas musculares.[122,134-136] Os pacientes são infectados por via transplacentária, e 25% ou mais desses filhotes podem apresentar sinais clínicos.[124,130,133,137] A ingestão de carne crua parece ser um risco fator para infecção por *T. gondii* e *N. caninum*.[124,133,138]

Testes sorológicos estão disponíveis para *T. gondii* e *N. caninum*, mas devem ser interpretados com cuidado, pois os animais expostos podem soroconverter e não apresentar sinais clínicos da doença.[122,138-141] Titulação pareada aguda, titulação convalescente e avaliação dos níveis de IgM (para *T. gondii*) talvez ajudem a distinguir pacientes infectados de animais meramente expostos,[133] embora títulos séricos para *N. caninum* raramente excedam 1:800 em cães não afetados clinicamente.[132,139] Testes de PCR tem sido desenvolvidos para esses organismos e agora estão disponíveis em vários laboratórios.[142-144] A EMG tipicamente mostra atividade espontânea nos músculos dos membros acometidos. A análise do LCR pode demostrar celularidade mista ou pleocitose não supurativa com elevação de proteína.[123,124] Biopsias de músculos e nervos com frequência mostram evidências de infiltrados celulares inflamatórios e, em alguns casos, organismos protozoários.[145]

A Clindamicina continua sendo o tratamento de escolha para infecção por *T. gondii* em cães e gatos, embora outros fármacos, incluindo Sulfonamidas, Pirimetamina, Doxiciclina e Minociclina, tenham alguma eficácia.[133] Para *N. caninum*, terapia com Clindamicina ou drogas Sulfonamidas potencializadas, com ou sem Pirimetamina, muitas vezes é eficaz e pode levar à resolução de sinais.[132,146,147] No entanto, alguns pacientes progridem com a terapia, e uma melhora significativa é bastante improvável se ocorrerem contraturas musculares.[136,148]

Polirradiculoneurite aguda

Polirradiculoneurite aguda pode ser observada em cães e gatos e causa uma tetraparesia flácida aguda ascendente (Vídeo 268.3). Os sinais clínicos em geral progridem rapidamente ao longo de vários dias, embora a progressão possa continuar por até 10 dias.[18,149-152] Os membros pélvicos geralmente são envolvidos primeiro, seguidos pelos membros torácicos, sendo que esses podem, em raros casos, estar primária ou exclusivamente envolvidos. Os casos graves evoluem e envolvem os nervos cranianos e a musculatura respiratória, levando à hipoventilação. Os reflexos espinais segmentares ficam de reduzidos a ausentes, mas a sensibilidade permanece intacta, e muitos animais parecem hiperestésicos. Esse distúrbio foi primeiramente reconhecido em cães por volta de 7 a 10 dias após contato com um guaxinim e foi originalmente denominado "paralisia de Coonhound". No entanto, sinais idênticos são vistos em animais sem exposição ao guaxinim, e, embora outras causas predisponentes, como vacinação ou infecção, possam ser identificadas, em muitos casos o gatilho é desconhecido.[151-153] As evidências sugerem fortemente que essa é uma doença imunomediada, similar à síndrome de Guillain-Barré (SGB) no homem, resultante de um antígeno dividido entre o estímulo incitante e o tecido do SNP.[18] Infiltrados celulares inflamatórios ocorrem dentro e ao redor dos nervos periféricos e particularmente envolvem a porção ventral das raízes nervosas.[18,149-151,154] Recentemente, anticorpos gangliosídeo anti-GM2 foram detectados em um subconjunto de cães com polirradiculoneurite.[155]

A suspeita diagnóstica é feita com base nas características clínicas dos sinais, no curso da doença e na história da possível causa desencadeadora. Os principais diagnósticos diferenciais são paralisia do carrapato, botulismo, envenenamento e miastenia *gravis* fulminante, que são todas doenças da junção neuromuscular (ver Capítulo 269). Os testes eletrofisiológicos podem ajudar a distinguir outras doenças de polirradiculoneurite aguda pelas causas anteriormente mencionadas (ver Capítulo 117). A atividade espontânea é observada no exame EMG, que pode ser detectável 1 a 2 dias após o início da doença.[156,157] Anormalidades em estudos de condução nervosa motora incluem amplitudes do potencial de ação muscular composto reduzido (PAMC) e dispersão temporal com latências PAMC prolongadas.[4,156] As velocidades de condução nervosa motora e sensorial são relativamente preservadas. A avaliação da onda F é particularmente sensível na detecção dessa condição, devido ao envolvimento das raízes nervosas ventrais, e revela latências de onda F aumentadas, razões F anormais ou ondas F completamente ausentes.[18,156] A análise de LCR coletado da cisterna lombar (ver Capítulo 115) pode revelar aumento da concentração de proteína sem pleocitose.[18] A terapia é principalmente de suporte, e a maioria dos animais se recupera caso haja tempo suficiente (Vídeo 268.4).[151,152] No entanto, o tempo de recuperação é variável e pode levar algumas semanas ou até 6 meses em casos raros.[18,158] Em pacientes com doenças respiratórias, o envolvimento muscular pode exigir ventilação mecânica.[159] Apesar da natureza imunomediada da doença, a terapia com corticosteroide não mostrou ser benéfica, piorando a atrofia muscular e predispondo os pacientes a infecções.[149] Um estudo recente sugeriu que a administração intravenosa de imunoglobulina humana pode encurtar o tempo de recuperação em cães com polirradiculoneurite aguda,[160] embora esta e outras terapias imunomoduladoras, como plasmaférese, requerem um estudo mais aprofundado em pacientes veterinários.

Neurite do plexo braquial
A neurite do plexo braquial é uma condição rara, com apenas alguns relatos na literatura veterinária.[88,161-165] Os sinais clínicos incluem claudicação, paresia, atrofia muscular, depressão de reflexos espinais segmentares e deficiência sensorial afetando exclusivamente os membros torácicos, normalmente com uma lesão bilateral, mas com distribuição assimétrica. A atividade espontânea é observada em EMG, enquanto a condução nervosa pode ser normal ou ligeiramente prolongada. A análise do LCR também pode ser normal ou demostrar uma moderada pleocitose linfocítica e elevação de proteínas.[164] No diagnóstico de imagem, particularmente a RM, podem aparecer nervos espessados e raízes nervosas sugestivas da condição, porém é possível que a histopatologia seja necessária para diferenciar de neurite

neoplásica por infiltração dos nervos.[15,88,164] Uma resposta aos glicocorticoides foi observada em alguns casos,[164,165] e remissões espontâneas, embora frequentemente demoradas, tem sido descritas.[15,158] A causa da síndrome é incerta, mas um mecanismo imunomediado é provável.

Polineuropatia inflamatória desmielinizante crônica
Neuropatias inflamatórias crônicas caracterizadas por desmielinização foram descritas em cães e gatos usando diversos termos, incluindo polineuropatia desmielinizante inflamatória crônica (PDIC), neuropatia recorrente crônica, neuropatia desmielinizante adquirida e polirradiculoneurite desmielinizante crônica.[14,18,158,166,167] Paralelos têm sido feitos com a doença humana, também denominada PDIC.[167,168] A etiologia subjacente é desconhecida, mas suspeita-se que seja imunomediada, com base nos infiltrados de células inflamatórias mononucleares endoneurais, na imunocoloração de anticorpo IgG de mielina, na ausência de agentes infecciosos detectáveis e em uma resposta positiva a administração de corticosteroides.[15,18,158,166] A desmielinização é o achado patológico predominante no exame de biopsia do nervo, com degeneração axonal observada menos frequentemente.[15,158] Infiltrados de células inflamatórias têm uma distribuição irregular e podem não ser apreciados em amostras de biopsia. As biopsias de músculo esquelético podem apresentar variação no tamanho da fibra, consistente com desnervação.[166,169,170] Os sinais clínicos costumam se desenvolver de forma insidiosa e progredir lentamente, em geral envolvendo primeiramente os membros pélvicos e depois os torácicos.[167] A monoparesia é a manifestação inicial menos frequente. Alguns pacientes apresentam um curso recidivo remitente,[167,169,170] e o início de sinais agudos também já foi descrito.[171] Os sinais clínicos consistem em vários graus de paresia, intolerância ao exercício, perda de massa muscular, redução dos reflexos espinais segmentares e, ocasionalmente, tremores musculares, claudicação, ventroflexão do pescoço, paralisia facial, disfonia, megaesôfago e paralisia laríngea (Vídeo 268.5).[15,167,169,170] A EMG pode ser normal ou mostrar atividade espontânea irregular, mas a CVNM é diminuída de forma consistente, muitas vezes com evidências do bloco de condução (ver Capítulo 117).[18,167,169,170] Muitos animais respondem à administração de corticosteroides em doses imunossupressores, embora seja uma resposta incompleta em alguns casos.[18,158,167,169] Regimes imunossupressores adicionais não foram bem estudados em pacientes veterinários, embora imunoglobulina intravenosa, plasmaférese, Azatioprina, Ciclofosfamida e outras drogas imunomoduladoras têm sido recomendadas para pacientes humanos.[168,172]

Poligangliorradiculoneurite sensorial
Uma neuropatia inflamatória que afeta preferencialmente os nervos sensoriais, as raízes nervosas e os gânglios da raiz dorsal foi descrita em várias raças de cães de 1,5 a 9 anos.[149,173-176] A causa subjacente da doença é desconhecida, embora etiologias infecciosas (virais), imunomediadas e tóxicas têm sido sugeridas.[173,176] Um envolvimento semelhante do nervo sensorial tem sido visto com algumas toxinas, incluindo mercúrio, doxorrubicina e a administração de grandes quantidades de piridoxina (vitamina B6).[158,177,178] Há infiltração de células mononuclear inflamatórias nas estruturas nervosas sensoriais e, ocasionalmente, nos gânglios autônomos por linfócitos, sobretudo os CD3+.[15,173-176] Os sinais clínicos consistem em ataxia, redução ou ausência da propriocepção e dos reflexos espinais segmentares (particularmente o reflexo patelar) e hipalgesia da face, tronco ou membros.[149] Disfagia, regurgitação, megaesôfago, anisocoria e automutilação foram relatadas em alguns casos.[149,173,175] Cursos clínicos agudo e crônico têm sido observados, e a condição é tipicamente progressiva. A massa, o tônus e a força muscular do membro são preservados, embora atrofia muscular mastigatória tenha sido relatada em alguns casos e seja atribuída a danos nas fibras motoras à medida que passam

SEÇÃO 17 • Doença Neurológica

através do gânglio trigêmeo.[15] A EMG e a CVNM são geralmente normais, embora o CVNS seja anormal e possa não ser registrada.[173] A análise do LCR é com frequência normal.[173] Alterações histológicas caracterizadas por degeneração axonal podem ser observadas com a biopsia do nervo, porém é necessário tomar cuidado para fazer a biopsia de um nervo sensitivo de função mista (p. ex., antebraquial cutâneo caudal ou nervo sural cutâneo caudal).[6,7,179] Infiltrados inflamatórios não podem ser observados, a menos que seja feita a biopsia de um gânglio da raiz dorsal. A biopsia muscular geralmente é normal. Como a doença é inflamatória e com suspeita de imunomediação, terapia imunossupressora com corticosteroides e outros medicamentos foi tentada, mas não foi relatado sucesso até a presente data.[158,173] Uma condição semelhante foi descrita em um gato jovem.[180]

DISTÚRBIOS TRAUMÁTICOS

Trauma nos nervos periféricos pode ocorrer secundário a uma variedade de eventos, incluindo trauma contuso, lesões por laceração (p. ex., mordidas de animais e feridas de faca), lesões por estiramento ou rasgamento (acidentes automobilísticos), compressão de fraturas, edema compartimentado de tecido e lesão iatrogênica (por injeção no local ou trauma cirúrgico). Diversas terminologias e sistemas de classificação foram desenvolvidas para descrever o grau de lesão do nervo com base na ruptura da bainha de mielina, axônio e tecido de suporte.[158,181] As lesões mais comuns são aquelas que envolvem o plexo braquial secundário a um acidente de veículo motor (Vídeo 268.6),[165,181] o nervo ciático secundário a trauma ou lesão iatrogênica[181-187] e os nervos caudais secundária a lesão por lesão de tração da cauda. A disfunção do nervo femoral[181,188-190] também tem sido cada vez mais reconhecida como secundária a trauma envolvendo o músculo ileopsoas em cães.[191-193]

Os principais sinais clínicos são vários graus de paresia e desuso do membro ou cauda, reações posturais e função de reflexo prejudicadas, dor na deambulação ou manipulação de membros e sensibilidade possivelmente prejudicada.[181,184,186] O diagnóstico geralmente é óbvio com base na história e no exame. No entanto, a avaliação da gravidade da lesão pode ser auxiliada por exame de EMG para documentar estudos de denervação ou por condução nervosa para documentar a presença ou ausência de condução no local afetado (ver Capítulo 117).[69,181,183,194-196] A US, TC ou RM podem ser úteis para a documentação de trauma de nervo ou músculo associado à lesão.[191-193,197,198] A terapia foca tipicamente nos cuidados de suporte e na reabilitação, incluindo alcance passivo de movimento, massagem e outros exercícios de fisioterapia, para ajudar manter a integridade muscular e articular enquanto a recuperação é aguardada (ver Capítulo 355). A remoção de fragmentos ósseos compressivos (se houver) ou implantes é indicada. Alguns animais podem traumatizar os membros devido ao arrastamento durante a deambulação ou por automutilação; portanto, cobrir o membro com uma bandagem ou "sapatinho" pode ajudar a evitar a complicação.[199] Outras intervenções potencialmente úteis incluem analgésicos e medicamentos para modular as parestesias (p. ex., Gabapentina ou Pregabalina) e órteses ou colchetes para suporte de membro.[199-203] Embora empregados em raras ocasiões, as técnicas para reconectar com cirurgia o nervo periférico parcial ou totalmente cortado e o uso de enxertos de nervos foram descritos em pequenos animais.[184,204-208] A recuperação depende da integridade das estruturas endoneurais, bem como a distância necessária para reinervar o tecido alvo, à medida que a regeneração axonal ocorre em uma taxa de aproximadamente 1 a 2 milímetros por dia.[181] A perda de sensibilidade no membro ou na cauda distal à lesão geralmente indica um prognóstico ruim; todavia, de forma ideal, 4 a 6 semanas devem ser esperadas para uma potencial recuperação. Em última análise, a amputação do membro ou da cauda muitas vezes é necessária.

DISTÚRBIOS TÓXICOS

Várias toxinas, produtos farmacêuticos e outros agentes foram relados como causas de neuropatias periféricas em pequenos animais, embora raramente sejam vistos e documentados. Tais substâncias incluem metais pesados (p. ex., mercúrio, tálio, chumbo), antibióticos (lasalocida, nitrofurantoína, salinomicina), pesticidas (organofosfatos), solventes orgânicos e produtos químicos (acrilamida, hexacarbonos), vitaminas (piridoxina) e fármacos antineoplásicos (vincristina, vimblastina, cisplatina).[15,18,120,177,178,209-218]

NEUROPATIAS AUTONÔMICAS

Disautonomia refere-se à disfunção generalizada do sistema nervoso autonômico e é observada em várias espécies em veterinária.[219-223] A discussão detalhada dessa condição está além do escopo deste capítulo, e os leitores interessados são encaminhados para análises mais abrangentes do tópico.[9,219,224,225] Disfunção autonômica também pode ocorrer como parte de um processo mais generalizado de neuropatia periférica, que foi bem documentada em pacientes humanos em uma variedade de condições, incluindo diabetes melito, polineuropatia paraneoplásica, SGB e neuropatias tóxicas.[115,226,227] Relatos de tal envolvimento autonômico são infrequentes na literatura veterinária, mas esse componente do processo da doença pode ser sub-reconhecido.[26,104,225,228] Lesões autonômicas seletivas têm sido relatadas em cães com ganglionite mioentérica apresentando diarreia ou megacólon,[229,230] um cão com pupilotonia e vários gatos com síndrome de Pourfour du Petit apresentando midríase unilateral.[231,232] Também são frequentemente observadas em animais com síndrome de Horner ou lesões no nervo oculomotor, devido a causas neoplásicas, inflamatórias, traumáticas ou idiopáticas.[233]

NEUROPATIAS IDIOPÁTICAS DIVERSAS

A doença denervante distal é uma polineuropatia canina idiopática com envolvimento principalmente axonal que afeta os nervos motores em uma distribuição distal e em geral melhora espontaneamente em 4 a 6 semanas.[158,234,235] Outras axonopatias com distribuição semelhante distal, mas com cursos crônicos e ininterruptos, também têm sido descritas e denominadas de polineuropatia simétrica distal ou degeneração axonal crônica.[18,158,236] Neuropatias idiopáticas que afetam os nervos trigêmeo, facial e vestibular são frequentemente reconhecidas.[47,158,237-241] Considerando que a disfunção dos nervos trigêmeo e vestibular são tipicamente autolimitantes na melhora espontânea, a paralisia do nervo facial com frequência não melhora e requer manejo a longo prazo. A paralisia idiopática laríngea que ocorre em cães mais velhos é provavelmente uma manifestação de uma neuropatia periférica mais generalizada, e o Labrador Retriever é super-representado em relatos dessa condição (ver Capítulo 239).[242-244]

REFERÊNCIAS BIBLIOGRÁFICAS

As referências bibliográficas deste capítulo se encontram online no Ambiente de Aprendizagem.

CAPÍTULO 269

Distúrbios da Junção Neuromuscular

Sarah A. Moore e Christopher L. Mariani

INTRODUÇÃO

Definição

A junção neuromuscular (JNM) é composta pelo terminal nervoso motor pré-sináptico, fenda sináptica e placa muscular terminal pós-sináptica (Figura 269.1). Ele fornece comunicação unidirecional entre o terminal do axônio do nervo motor e o músculo através do neurotransmissor acetilcolina (ACh). A JNM é um dos vários componentes da unidade motora, e pacientes com doença nesse local apresentam sinais clínicos consistentes com doença do neurônio motor inferior (NMI; ver Capítulo 268).

Função

Potenciais de ação originados dentro do corno ventral da medula espinal pelos neurônios motores são propagados para baixo, em direção aos nervos motores periféricos. Processos achatados de terminações dos nervos motores (o terminal pré-sináptico) formam um pequeno recuo em fibras no músculo esquelético, chamado de fenda sináptica. Uma porção alargada de membrana da fibra muscular adjacente à fenda sináptica constitui o terminal pós-sináptico. O terminal pré-sináptico contém um grande estoque de vesículas com ACh, que são liberadas na fenda sináptica em resposta à despolarização do terminal do nervo pré-sináptico. O íon do cálcio é um cofator importante nesse processo, pois facilita a fusão de vesículas de ACh para a membrana pré-sináptica e subsequente exocitose da ACh para a JNM. A ACh se difunde pela fenda sináptica para se ligar aos receptores ACh (AChR) na fase pós-sináptica da membrana muscular para resultar em contração da fibra muscular. A ação da ACh livre que persiste dentro da fenda sináptica é interrompida pela ação da enzima acetilcolinesterase (AChE; ver Figura 269.1). Em unidades motoras de funcionamento normal, há um excesso de ACh e AChR disponíveis. Os potenciais da membrana muscular produzidos pela despolarização do nervo também excedem em muito o necessário para a contração da fibra muscular. Isso é conhecido como fator de segurança da transmissão neuromuscular.

Sinais clínicos

Os distúrbios que afetam a JNM podem ser classificados como pré-sinápticos ou pós-sinápticos. Eles resultam da incapacidade de liberação da ACh no terminal pré-sináptico para a fenda sináptica, ou da incapacidade da membrana muscular pós-sináptica para responder à ACh. Qualquer um dos distúrbios resulta em transmissão neuromuscular prejudicada. Manifestações clínicas de deficiência na transmissão neuromuscular são normalmente simétricas na natureza e podem incluir tetraparesia aguda ou tetraplegia, tetraparesia crônica estática ou progressiva e fraqueza episódica que é exacerbada pela atividade. Animais com sinais clínicos referenciáveis para JNM têm paresia acompanhada por diminuição de tônus muscular (paresia flácida) e podem não ser capazes de segurar a cabeça erguida devido à fraqueza da musculatura cervical. Esses pacientes também podem ter reflexos espinais segmentares diminuídos, déficits dos nervos cranianos e sinais autonômicos, dependendo da doença e da gravidade. Pacientes com doença na JNM geralmente apresentam função sensorial e nível de consciência normais.

DOENÇAS PRÉ-SINÁPTICAS DA JUNÇÃO NEUROMUSCULAR

Paralisia do carrapato

A paralisia do carrapato é mais comumente associada à exposição a carrapatos *Dermacentor* sp. ou *Ixodes* sp.[1,2] Os sinais clínicos são resultado de uma neurotoxina produzida nas grandes glândulas salivares dos carrapatos fêmeas, que é liberada na circulação após o carrapato se fixar e se alimentar por vários dias. O mecanismo celular exato da neurotoxina salivar não está definido, mas parece interferir com a liberação de ACh no terminal do nervo pré-sináptico por meio de um mecanismo mediador de cálcio.[1,3,4] A paralisia do carrapato não causa alteração no hemograma completo (HC), nos testes bioquímicos séricos, no diagnóstico por imagem ou na avaliação do líquido cefalorraquidiano (LCR).[5] Os procedimentos de eletrodiagnóstico geralmente não são realizados. Os sinais clínicos ocorrem quando um carrapato ingurgitado se fixa na pele do animal e se resolvem quando o carrapato causador do problema é removido. O diagnóstico é presuntivo na maioria dos casos e é baseado na identificação e remoção de um carrapato ingurgitado (ver Vídeo 211.1, no Capítulo 211).

Na América do Norte, os carrapatos *Dermacentor* sp. são os mais comumente associados à paralisia do carrapato.[1] Os cães são acometidos com frequência, enquanto os gatos parecem resistentes. Os sinais clínicos começam entre 5 e 9 dias após a fixação do carrapato.[6] Os cães têm um quadro agudo, com paresia flácida ascendente de progressão rápida, que pode evoluir para tetraplegia durante 12 a 72 h. Os reflexos espinais

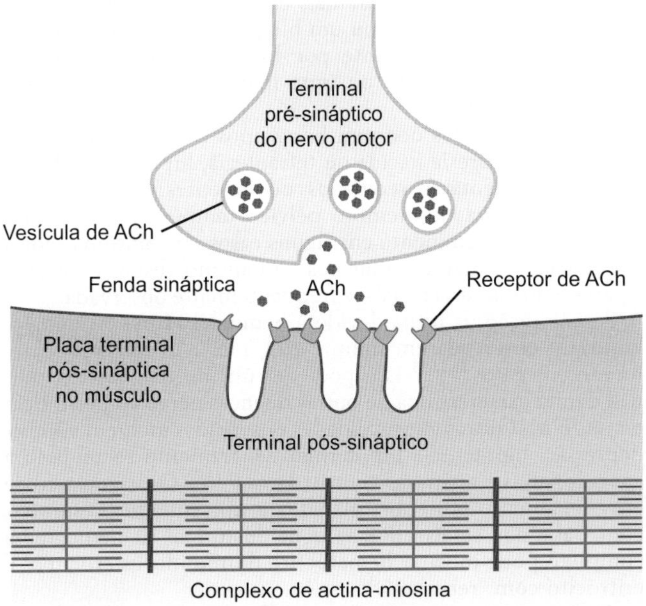

Figura 269.1 Representação esquemática do sistema da junção neuromuscular. *ACh*, acetilcolina. (Reproduzida com autorização da Universidade Estadual de Ohio.)

segmentares são desde severamente diminuídos a ausentes em todos os quatro membros, enquanto o tônus muscular é diminuído.[5,7-9] Deficiências em nervos cranianos são incomuns em cães da América do Norte, mas disfonia e leve fraqueza muscular facial e mastigatória são ocasionalmente observadas.[7] Anormalidades autonômicas, sensoriais e esfincterianas não ocorrem em cães com paralisia de carrapato americano. Em casos graves, paralisia respiratória pode exigir ventilação mecânica, mas é possível resultar em morte devido à hipoventilação. Remoção do carrapato causador do problema resulta em melhora dramática dos sinais, geralmente dentro de horas.

Na Austrália, a paralisia por carrapato é muito mais grave e é mais frequentemente causada por *Ixodes* sp. Tanto os gatos como os cães podem ser acometidos.[3,6-8] Semelhante à paralisia do carrapato americano, os animais com paralisia do carrapato australiano têm paresia flácida ascendente aguda e rapidamente progressiva, que pode evoluir para tetraplegia em horas. Disfunção autonômica, disfunção urinária e insuficiência cardíaca congestiva devido à disfunção diastólica podem ocorrer.[5,7,8,10] A dilatação pupilar é comum em gatos e muitas vezes observada em cães com a doença avançada.[6] Animais acometidos podem desenvolver edema pulmonar, pneumonia aspirativa e hipoventilação progressiva.[5,8,10] Deficiências de nervos cranianos unilaterais e síndrome de Horner também foram relatadas.[11] Diferente da paralisia de carrapato americano, animais de companhia com paralisia de carrapato australiano podem continuar a enfraquecer por vários dias após a remoção do carrapato.[12]

A remoção do carrapato, somada a cuidados de suporte, é o tratamento primário para paralisia por carrapatos americanos e australianos. Animais de companhia devem ser examinados cuidadosamente em busca de carrapatos, e pode ser necessária a realização da tosa. Examinar os canais auditivos, o períneo, a boca, as cavidades nasais e os espaços interdigitais também é importante. Se um carrapato não for encontrado, acaricidas tópicos podem ser aplicados. Na paralisia do carrapato australiano, fenoxibenzamina e a acepromazina podem ser usados para tratar os sinais autonômicos.[7,8,13] Os glicocorticoides não são usados rotineiramente para tratar a paralisia do carrapato, e a antibioticoterapia não ajuda.[7,9]

Botulismo

O botulismo é uma condição aguda difusa do neurônio motor inferior, resultante da exposição a neurotoxinas produzidas pela bactéria *Clostridium botulinum*, um anaeróbio gram-positivo onipresente no solo, na água e no trato gastrintestinal (GI) de mamíferos e peixes. A maioria dos animais de companhia desenvolve botulismo ao ingerir a neurotoxina botulínica pré-formada presente em carne estragada ou não cozida, embora raramente a toxina possa ser produzida *in vivo* após infecção do fígado ou GI. Este último é referido como toxinfecção. Oito tipos diferentes de toxinas botulínicas foram identificados, mas o mais comum em cães é a neurotoxina botulínica do tipo C (BoNT-C).[15-18] A ocorrência natural de botulismo é extremamente rara em gatos, mas foi relatada com BoNT-C.[19]

A toxina botulínica bloqueia a liberação de ACh no terminal pré-sináptico do músculo esquelético e a sinapse autonômica colinérgica por clivagem enzimática irreversível do receptor solúvel da proteína de ativação de fator sensível a N-etilmaleimida (RSPA).[6,15,20,21] A proteína RSPA é essencial para o "encaixe" das vesículas ACh sinápticas nas membranas présinápticas, permitindo a liberação de ACh na fenda sináptica. A liberação prejudicada causa um início agudo de tetraparesia progressiva acompanhada por sinais autonômicos, como íleo, taquicardia ou bradicardia, midríase e retenção urinária. Também são comuns deficiências de nervos cranianos, como megaesôfago e diminuição do reflexo palpebral e pupilar à luz.[15,16,22] A taxa de desenvolvimento e a gravidade dos sinais clínicos dependem da quantidade de toxina ingerida, com sinais ocorrendo dentro de horas até 6 dias após a ingestão dos alimentos contaminados.[8,10]

O diagnóstico de botulismo pode ser feito demonstrando BoNT-C no sangue, nas fezes, no conteúdo estomacal ou na fonte de alimento de um animal acometido. Historicamente, o padrão-ouro para o diagnóstico do botulismo era o teste de inoculação em camundongos: instilar uma amostra oriunda do paciente na cavidade peritoneal de um camundongo e observar o desenvolvimento dos sinais clínicos.[15,16] Na verdade, um diagnóstico clínico de botulismo é muitas vezes presuntivo com base no histórico e no exame clínico. O hemograma de rotina não mostra anormalidades. Os testes de eletrodiagnóstico podem confirmar envenenamento por botulismo ao demonstrar aumentos incrementais nos potenciais de ação composto do músculo (PACM) com estimulação em altas taxas.[18] Esse achado está presente em cerca de 60% dos humanos adultos com botulismo, mas não foi descrito em cães.[23]

O tratamento para o botulismo por natureza é principalmente de suporte. Os antibióticos geralmente não são indicados, mas podem ser considerados se a toxinfecção for uma possibilidade ou se outras indicações, como pneumonia aspirativa, estiverem presentes. Certos antibióticos, como aminoglicosídeos e ampicilina, podem potencializar o bloqueio neuromuscular, portanto devem ser evitados.[24] Embora a administração de antitoxina venha sendo recomendada, a maioria dos produtos disponíveis não contém anticorpos contra BoNT-C e, portanto, não são úteis para cães.[15,22] As antitoxinas não podem prender a toxina após ela entrar nos terminais nervosos, mas podem ser eficazes para prender a toxina circulante e cessar parcialmente a progressão da doença.[15,20] Se forem administradas, uma injeção de teste deve ser realizada, uma vez que esses produtos são de origem equina, e reações anafiláticas são possíveis (ver Capítulo 137).[20] A recuperação do botulismo ocorre espontaneamente ao longo de 1 a 4 semanas, e o prognóstico para a maioria os animais é excelente, se o suporte for dado de forma adequada.[8,15]

Envenenamento por cobras elapídeas (ver Capítulo 156)

As cobras elapídeas incluem o leste (*Micrurus fulvius*) e Texas (*Micrurus tener*) cobra-coral na América do Norte, a tigre (*Notechis scutatus*), a marrom (*Pseudonaja spp.*) e preta-de-barriga-vermelha (*Pseudechis porphyriacus*) na Austrália, e uma variedade em outros continentes, incluindo najas, kraits e mambas.[25-29] Ao contrário das cobras crotalídeas, as cobras elapídeas têm presas curtas, rígidas e imóveis, e pode não haver evidência de um ferimento de punção nos animais envenenados.[25] Dependendo da cobra, o veneno causa ou um bloqueio neuromuscular pós-sináptico não despolarizante por forte ligação ao AChR na membrana pós-sináptica, ou uma inibição pré-sináptica com liberação de ACh.[25,27,30]

Os sinais clínicos ocorrem horas após o envenenamento e incluem tetraparesia flácida ou tetraplegia, hipotonia, reflexos espinais segmentares reduzidos ou ausentes e hipoventilação.[25-32] A ataxia de membro pélvico também pode ser um sinal clínico proeminente em alguns casos.[33-35] Sintomatologia relacionada aos nervos cranianos – ptialismo, disfagia, disfonia e paresia ou paralisia facial – é frequentemente observada.[28,31,32] A descoloração da urina devido à hemoglobinúria ou mioglobinúria é observada em muitos cães, mas não tão frequentemente em gatos.[26,32,33] Isso pode ser útil no diagnóstico, pois não é uma característica de outras doenças nervosas periféricas ou da JNM. Outras anormalidades observadas incluem vômito, depressão, hipotensão, hipotermia, sangramento secundário a coagulopatias e arritmias ventriculares.[27,31-35] O diagnóstico de envenenamento por cobra elapídea é tipicamente presuntivo, com base nos sinais clínicos e no histórico. O hemograma completo pode mostrar hematócrito diminuído, esferocitose e eritrócito com "rebarbas".[32]

O tratamento é principalmente de suporte. O uso de um curativo compressivo no local do envenenamento pode ajudar a prevenir a circulação do veneno pelos vasos linfáticos.[27] A diurese fluida deve ser considerada se hemoglobinúria ou

CAPÍTULO 269 • Distúrbios da Junção Neuromuscular

miodobinúria estiverem presentes (ver Capítulo 129). A administração de soro antiofídico tem sido defendida e pode ser benéfica na prevenção ou redução da gravidade dos sinais clínicos.[25,26,29,33-36] Produtos de origem equina apresentam riscos de anafilaxia, e injeções-testes devem ser consideradas. Uma variedade de soro antiofídico está disponível na Austrália e outros países. Os suprimentos norte-americanos de soro antiofídicos para cobra-coral não estão mais sendo fabricados. No entanto, há uma proteção cruzada entre o soro antiofídico de cobra-tigre e o de cobra-coral-mexicana, e este produto é usado rotineiramente com bons resultados por alguns clínicos.[37-39] A maioria dos animais se recuperam totalmente dentro de 1 a 2 semanas depois de cuidados de suporte adequados.[29,31-33,39]

DOENÇAS PÓS-SINÁPTICAS DA JUNÇÃO NEUROMUSCULAR

Miastenia *gravis* adquirida

Patogênese e predisposição da raça

Miastenia *gravis* (MG) adquirida é uma doença autoimune caracterizada pela produção de autoanticorpos contra AChR nicotínico no terminal muscular pós-sináptico.[40-42] Esses autoanticorpos levam a destruição mediada pelo complemento do AChR, redução dos números de receptores funcionais e diminuição da capacidade do músculo de responder à ACh liberada na fenda sináptica.[43-47] O resultado é fraqueza do músculo esquelético, que geralmente é exacerbado pela atividade. Existe uma distribuição bimodal de idade para o desenvolvimento da MG adquirida: os cães geralmente têm menos de 4 ou mais de 9 anos.[44,48,49] Raças super-representadas incluem Akita, German Shorthaired Pointer, Chihuahua, Pastor-Alemão, Golden Retriever e Newfoundland.[6,50-52] A MG adquirida é menos comum em gatos, mas as predileções por Abissínio, Somali e outras raças puras são relatadas.[48,53,54] A MG adquirida pode se apresentar em uma de suas três formas, sendo a "generalizada" a mais, porém as formas "focal" e "grave fulminante" também são relatadas.[48]

Miastenia gravis generalizada

Pacientes com MG generalizada geralmente apresentam um exame neurológico normal em repouso (ver Capítulo 259). No entanto, demonstram fraqueza durante uma sessão de exercício ou atividade induzida, além de uma marcha agitada e comprometida, observada primeiramente nos membros pélvicos.[44] Se a atividade contínua for encorajada, o envolvimento do membro torácico se torna aparente. Alguns animais de companhia mostram um reflexo palpebral diminuído ou fatigável, embora não esteja consistentemente presente. Reflexos espinais segmentares são em geral normais. Os sinais de disfunção faríngea ou laríngea podem se manifestar como ptialismo (devido à dificuldade para engolir; ver Capítulo 36) e/ou disfonia e estão presentes de forma variável.[44,48] Cães com MG generalizada normalmente apresentam megaesôfago concomitante e história de regurgitação (ver Capítulos 39 e 273). Em gatos, o megaesôfago é menos frequente.[53] Ventroflexão do pescoço devido à fraqueza dos músculos cervicais é mais comum em gatos que em cães.[48,54-56]

Formas fulminantes e focais de miastenia gravis

Pacientes com MG fulminante apresentam fraqueza súbita, rápida e progressiva grave e difusa, que não melhora com o repouso. A condição dos pacientes progride rapidamente para tetraparesia não ambulatória e decúbito lateral.[6] Os reflexos espinais podem estar preservados ou diminuídos.[6] A regurgitação frequente de grandes volumes de líquido associada ao megaesôfago é típica, e a pneumonia aspirativa é comum (ver Capítulos 242 e 360).[40] Sinais adicionais incluem fraqueza dos músculos respiratórios e retenção de urina. Foi relatado que a

prevalência de miastenia fulminante é 16% em cães e 15% em gatos. Timoma foi associado com o desenvolvimento dessa forma da doença em ambas as espécies.[42,55,57-63]

A MG focal se apresenta como fraqueza de um grupo muscular isolado, mais comumente os músculos ocular, facial, esofágico, faríngeo ou laríngeo. Fraqueza generalizada não é observada em animais de companhia, e as queixas de apresentação típicas incluem regurgitação, disfagia, disfonia ou estrabismo.[44,49,64]

Condições associadas

Várias doenças foram associadas à MG em cães e gatos, incluindo timoma, hipotireoidismo, hipoadrenocorticismo, polimiosite e miosite mastigatória.[42,63,65,66] Em gatos com hipertireoidismo, uma associação entre MG adquirida e tratamento com metimazol foi relatada, resolvida com a descontinuação da medicação.[53,67,68]

Diagnóstico

Nenhuma mudança no hemograma completo ou na bioquímica sérica é patognomônica para MG. A evidência de inflamação é comum em animais de companhia com pneumonia aspirativa. Esses testes são valiosos na triagem de causas metabólicas de fraqueza neuromuscular (hipocalcemia, hipotireoidismo, hiperadrenocorticismo) e na avaliação de creatinina quinase como um indicador de polimiosite (ver Capítulo 66).[69] Radiografia ou TC torácicas devem ser obtidas para documentar a presença ou ausência de timoma e para rastrear pneumonia aspirativa secundária. Os estudos de contraste da deglutição podem ser usados para avaliar disfagia (ver Capítulo 273), mas são contraindicados em casos de megaesôfago e de regurgitação. A US abdominal também pode ser considerada para descartar causas paraneoplásicas de MG adquirida em pacientes idosos (ver Capítulo 88).[70-73]

O padrão-ouro para o diagnóstico de MG adquirida generalizada em pacientes veterinários é a demonstração de autoanticorpos anti-AChR no soro.[69,73,74] Embora ocorra alguma reatividade cruzada entre as espécies, os autoanticorpos contra o AChR são relativamente específicos para cada espécie. Por esse motivo, é fundamental o uso de um sistema de ensaio típico para cães e para gatos.[69] Níveis de anticorpos são altamente variáveis entre os pacientes e não se correlacionam bem com a gravidade dos sinais clínicos; no entanto, em determinados pacientes, uma diminuição nos níveis de anticorpos se correlaciona bem com a melhora dos sinais clínicos, que pode ser seguida pela avaliação da remissão da doença.[69] Foi sugerido que a medição de autoanticorpos anti-AChR específicos da espécie detectam aproximadamente 98% dos cães com MG adquirida generalizada,[69] mas os anticorpos são relatados em uma porcentagem menor de cães com MG focal. A titulação de anticorpos pode ser negativa no início do curso da doença e ser afetada pela administração de corticosteroides antes da mensuração.[75] Um novo teste é sugerido para pacientes em que qualquer cenário for suspeito. Um pequeno número de pacientes pode ter MG adquirida soronegativa verdadeira. Nesses casos, é possível confirmar o diagnóstico documentando decréscimos no CMAP em resposta à estimulação nervosa repetitiva e pela normalização da fraqueza muscular dos membros após a terapia com anticolinesterase.[75]

A administração do edrofônio anticolinesterásico de curta ação pode ser usada como diagnóstico para avaliar a melhora da força muscular, a marcha ou a capacidade de deglutir.[42] Esse fármaco inibe a AChE, permitindo que mais ACh permaneça na JNM e, assim, beneficiando a transmissão neuromuscular. Animais geralmente mostram melhora segundos após o recebimento do medicamento (Vídeo 269.1). O efeito dura vários minutos, seguido pelo retorno dos sinais clínicos. Deve-se notar que a melhora após a administração de edrofônio não é completamente específica para MG, portanto alguns animais com outras formas de fraqueza neuromuscular podem apresentar o mesmo resultado.[43,73,76] Além disso, nem todos os animais com MG melhoram com edrofônio.[43,73,77] A precipitação de uma crise colinérgica é possível por superestimulação de AChR, levando ao agravamento da fraqueza, salivação, tremores, vômito, bradicardia, broncoconstrição e dificuldade respiratória. Animais devem ser monitorados imediatamente após a administração de edrofônio. Atropina e equipamento para fornecer intubação e suporte respiratório devem estar disponíveis e prontos para uso, se necessário.

Tratamento em longo prazo

O tratamento em longo prazo para animais com MG adquirida almeja dois objetivos: (1) aumentar a quantidade de ACh disponível na fenda sináptica para neutralizar a deficiência de números de AChR e (2) reduzir os autoanticorpos anti-AChR. Fármacos anticolinesterásicos, como brometo de piridostigmina (oral) ou neostigmina (IM), são os pilares da terapia, atuando na inibição da AChE para que a ação da ACh seja mais longa dentro das fendas sinápticas.[8,42,78,79] Esses medicamentos devem ser cuidadosamente titulados para fazer efeito. A neostigmina é geralmente usada apenas em pacientes hospitalizados que são incapazes de tomar medicamentos via oral, como aqueles em crise aguda ou com regurgitação profunda e frequente. Ambos os medicamentos citados têm uma janela terapêutica estreita e significativa. Podem ocorrer efeitos colaterais graves, como bradicardia, hipersalivação, vômito, diarreia, cãibras musculares e fraqueza.[79] Isso pode ser problemático, pois os sinais clínicos associados à administração excessiva de drogas anticolinérgicas podem ser difíceis de distinguir dos sinais clínicos da MG não controlada.

Fármacos imunossupressores, como Ciclosporina, Micofenalato de Mofetila (MMF) e Azatioprina, também são frequentemente usados no tratamento de MG adquirida para reduzir os níveis de autoanticorpos circulantes, visando uma resposta do sistema imune adaptativo, enquanto poupa a imunidade inata e a função dos neutrófilos (ver Capítulo 165).[78,80-83] O MMF já foi o medicamento imunossupressor preferido para MG com base na experiência humana; no entanto, um estudo recente comparando Piridostigmina somada ao MMF e Piridostigmina sozinha não mostrou diferença no tempo de sobrevivência ou taxas de remissão.[83]

Os corticosteroides também podem ser eficazes no tratamento de MG (ver Capítulo 165), mas devem ser usados com cautela em pacientes com pneumonia aspirativa (ver Capítulo 242 e 360). Os corticosteroides conseguem potencializar a fraqueza muscular e exacerbar os sinais clínicos em alguns pacientes, e um aumento gradual na dosagem de esteroides é recomendado para ajudar a evitar esta complicação.[41,57,73,75,77,78] Outras estratégias para imunomodulação também podem ser empregadas em pacientes com MG, incluindo troca plasmática terapêutica e imunoglobulina IV (IVIG).[84-86] Nenhuma das técnicas foi avaliada exaustivamente em um grande número de cães com MG, embora existam algumas evidências para apoiar sua utilidade nesta e em outras doenças imunomediadas.[86-91] A longo prazo, foi relatada uma taxa de remissão espontânea de até 88% para cães com causas não paraneoplásicas de MG adquirida.[92]

Miastenia *gravis* congênita

A MG congênita presumível, ou síndrome miastênica, foi relatada em cães das raças Jack Russell Terrier, Smooth Fox Terrier, Springer Spaniel, Samoieda, Dachshund Miniatura de Pelo Liso, Gammel Dansk Hønsehund (GDH) e mestiços, além de gatos.[54,93-104] A deficiência de AChR é assumida na maioria raças e foi documentada em Jack Russell Terrier, Springer Spaniel e Dachshund em miniatura.[101,105] A doença muitas vezes afeta vários animais dentro da mesma ninhada e geralmente se torna evidente após 6 a 9 semanas de idade. A fraqueza generalizada

dos membros e músculos cervicais que pioram com a atividade é comum. Megaesôfago pode ou não estar presente.[98,101] Os cães da raça GDH são incomuns, porque a condição começa por volta dos 4 meses de idade e é relativamente insensível aos medicamentos bloqueadores da AChE.[102,106] Considera-se que esses cães tenham um defeito pré-sináptico na transmissão neuromuscular.[106,107] Uma herança de modo autossômico recessivo foi demonstrada em Smooth Fox Terrier, Jack Russell Terrier e GDH.[94,97,108] Um diagnóstico definitivo de MG congênita pode ser feito por meio da quantificação de AChR em uma biopsia muscular (ver Capítulo 116), embora esse teste não esteja prontamente disponível.[101,105] Piridostigmina ou neostigmina são os pilares da terapia e muitas vezes proporcionam melhora. No entanto, a resposta a longo prazo para a terapia é variável, e relatos na maioria das raças descrevem morte ou eutanásia devido à dificuldade de controle dos sinais clínicos.[98,99] Exceções são MG congênita em Dachshund Miniatura, que se resolveu espontaneamente aos 6 meses de idade, e GDH, que permanece estável com leve sinais clínicos.[101,102]

OUTROS

Colapso induzido pelo exercício do Labrador Retriever

Embora não seja uma doença da JNM, o colapso induzido por exercício do Labrador Retriever (CIE) causa fadiga e flacidez ou tetraparesia durante ou após atividades vigorosas. Os achados de exames são normais em repouso. Ataxia, fraqueza dos membros pélvicos e colapso se desenvolvem em associação com treinamento de campo intenso ou prolongado, caça ou brincadeiras vigorosas. Os sinais clínicos podem progredir para envolver os membros torácicos se o animal continuar com a atividade. A recuperação ocorre com o repouso, e a maioria dos cães são clinicamente normais dentro de 30 minutos; no entanto, episódios graves podem resultar em morte.[109-111] A condição é hereditária no Labrador, associada a uma mutação hereditária autossômica recessiva (Arg256 Leu) no gene que codifica a proteína dinamina 1 (DNM1).[109,110] A família de genes de dinamina codifica um grupo de enzimas que mantém a função da vesícula sináptica durante a neurotransmissão sustentada (p. ex., durante a atividade física intensa).[109,112] Especificamente, a DNM1 é expressa em membranas terminais sinápticas dentro do sistema nervoso central (SNC) e é importante na reciclagem de vesículas sinápticas durante a estimulação neurológica de alta frequência. Um fenótipo de colapso também é reconhecido em outras raças, mas a associação entre colapso e a mutação Arg256 Leu é variável.[112]

Cães com CIE associado a DNM1 (d-EIC) normalmente experimentam seu primeiro episódio de colapso antes dos 2 anos.[111] A perda do reflexo patelar é comum, e os cães mantêm um estado mental normal.[111,113] Hipertermia e lactato plasmático elevado frequentemente se desenvolvem durante um episódio, mas não são diferentes do que é observado em exercícios normais para cães.[113] As relações lactato/piruvato sérico são normais em cães com CIE tanto em repouso quanto durante o exercício, e biopsias musculares são normais.[113] Um teste genético para a mutação Arg256 Leu DNM1 está comercialmente disponível agora para auxiliar no diagnóstico. Embora não exista cura para a CIE, os cães acometidos têm um excelente prognóstico se eles se abstiverem de atividades físicas intensas conhecidas que desencadeiem os episódios.[113]

REFERÊNCIAS BIBLIOGRÁFICAS

As referências bibliográficas deste capítulo se encontram online no Ambiente de Aprendizagem.

CAPÍTULO 270

Transtornos Neurológicos Exclusivos de Felinos

Elsa Beltran e Luisa De Risio

DOENÇAS DO SISTEMA NERVOSO CENTRAL

Malformações congênitas

Panleucopenia felina

Hipoplasia cerebelar causada por infecção perinatal com o vírus da panleucopenia felina (VPF) é o distúrbio cerebelar difuso mais comum em gatos.[1] A exposição ao VPF durante as últimas 3 semanas de gestação ou as primeiras 3 semanas de vida podem induzir a destruição da divisão da camada externa germinativa e causar hipoplasia cerebelar granuloprival em filhotes de gatos (ver Capítulo 225).[2,3] Infecções fetais antes das últimas 3 semanas de gestação podem resultar em hidroencefalia.[4,5] A vacina VPF viva modificada durante a gravidez pode resultar em filhotes clinicamente acometidos.[5] Os sinais clínicos incluem ataxia cerebelar, tremor de intenção, déficits de resposta à ameaça e nistagmo (Vídeo 270.1) e geralmente permanecem estáveis ou mesmo melhoram ao longo do tempo, pois alguma compensação é possível. Não existem testes de diagnóstico específicos. Exames de imagem avançada, em particular imagem de ressonância magnética (IRM), podem revelar atrofia cerebelar. A análise do líquido cefalorraquidiano (LCR) em geral é normal. Não há tratamento, mas os gatos podem ter uma boa qualidade de vida quando seu ambiente é modificado para acomodar suas deficiências (consulte a Folha de Informações do Cliente online). A prevenção pode ser alcançada pela vacinação de fêmeas antes da prenhez.

Erros inatos do metabolismo

Poucos erros são relatados exclusivamente em gatos e normalmente também afetam o sistema nervoso periférico (PNS; Tabela 270.1).

Doença Prion

A *encefalopatia espongiforme felina* (EEF) é uma doença induzida por príons que afeta a família *Felidae*.[6-8] Estudos experimentais sugerem que a EEF é provocada pelo mesmo agente que causa a encefalopatia espongiforme bovina (EEB) e uma nova variante da doença de Creutzfeldt-Jakob no homem.[6,7] Acredita-se que gatos contraiam a doença ao ingerir alimentos contaminados com EEB. Até o momento, a EEF só foi relatada na Europa. Um estudo experimental recente demonstrou que a doença debilitante crônica (encefalopatia espongiforme transmissível de veado-mula, veado-de-cauda-branca, rena e alce) pode ser transmitida ao gato doméstico, levantando assim a questão de potencial transmissão cervídeo-felino.[9] A doença clínica se apresenta em gatos adultos e é caracterizada por sinais clínicos de doença crônica progressiva (de semanas a meses), incluindo anomalias de comportamento, ataxia, tremores musculares, hipersalivação, dilatação e pupilas sem resposta e hiperestesia. O diagnóstico é baseado na avaliação histopatológica do cérebro.[7,8,10-12] Não há tratamento atual, e a doença é progressiva e fatal.

Doenças inflamatórias do sistema nervoso central infecciosas e não infecciosas

Doenças virais do sistema nervoso central

Peritonite infecciosa felina.   A peritonite infecciosa felina (PIF) é a doença infecciosa do sistema nervoso central (SNC) mais comum em gatos.[13-15] Até 33% dos casos mostram sinais neurológicos, e todas as três formas (efusiva [úmida], não efusiva [seca] e mista) têm sido associadas ao envolvimento do SNC, sendo a forma não efusiva a mais comum (ver Capítulo 224).[14,16,17] A PIF em geral é observada em gatos de raça pura expostos a ambientes com vários gatos, normalmente com menos de 4 anos.[14,18-20] Os sinais neurológicos refletem a área de envolvimento do SNC, que muitas vezes inclui a fossa caudal (cerebelo, ponte e bulbo),[17,21] e podem apresentar-se isoladamente ou associados a sinais sistêmicos.[16,18,19] Lesões oftálmicas (irite, uveíte anterior e ceratite) foram relatadas em até 53% dos casos com PIF neurológica (ver Capítulo 11).[16,18,21] Os sinais neurológicos mais comuns são estado mental alterado, déficits de resposta à ameaça, síndrome vestibular, convulsões, ataxia e paresia (Vídeo 270.2).[16,18,21-25] As convulsões ocorrem em até 33% dos gatos com doenças neurológicas por PIF e têm sido associadas a um prognóstico ruim.[21,24] A PIF é a causa mais comum de mielopatia em gatos jovens com menos de 2 anos (Vídeo 270.3).[23] O diagnóstico geral para a avaliação da PIF está descrito no Capítulo 224. Atualmente, os testes de diagnóstico *ante mortem* para PIF neurológica visam excluir outras condições que possam causar uma apresentação clínica semelhante, mas não podem confirmar diretamente o diagnóstico. Achados de imagem avançada incluem hidrocefalia obstrutiva, dilatação ventricular e contraste periventricular, realce ependimal e meníngeo refletindo a natureza superficial e das lesões PIF ventricular no SNC (Figura 270.1).[15,18] No entanto, mais de 37% dos gatos com PIF neurológica confirmada histologicamente podem ter resultados normais de ressonância magnética (RM).[15] A coleta de LCR deve ser realizada após descartar a possibilidade de aumento de pressão intracraniano (PIC), idealmente por RM, porque a alta PIC pode aumentar a morbidade e mortalidade associadas a esse procedimento em gatos com PIF neurológica (ver Capítulo 115).[15,21,26] O máximo de achados comuns no LCR são concentração de proteína superior a 2 g/ℓ (mais de 200 mg/dℓ) e a contagem de células nucleadas acima de 100 células/mcℓ com uma pleocitose neutrofílica.[14,16,21,27] A concentração elevada de proteína no LCR pode aumentar a viscosidade e, portanto, o LCR pode não fluir adequadamente durante a coleta. Anticorpos de coronavírus têm pouco valor diagnóstico como títulos séricos negativos ou títulos inferiores a 1:400 e foram relatados em gatos com PIF neurológica.[14,18,21] Anticorpos de coronavírus CSF (IgG) não são necessariamente mais sensíveis do que os anticorpos séricos.[17] O uso de albumina quociente e índice de IgG não conseguiram identificar um padrão de proteína específico para PIF neurológica, indicando que o distúrbio de função de barreira sangue-LCR e síntese de IgG intratecal não é uma característica comum da PIF.[28] Uma reação em cadeia da polimerase reversa em tempo real fortemente positiva (RT-PCR) no LCR apoia o diagnóstico. No entanto, alguns gatos com PIF neurológica confirmada histologicamente têm RT-PCR negativa.[18] A imuno-histoquímica foi usada com sucesso em um gato para identificar macrófagos infectados com PIF no LCR; no entanto, outros estudos são necessários para avaliar sua sensibilidade e especificidade.[29] O diagnóstico definitivo requer uma combinação de exame macroscópico e histopatológico com a demonstração de antígeno viral em amostras pós-morte do SNC. Ainda não há cura

SEÇÃO 17 • Doença Neurológica

Tabela 270.1 Doenças neuromusculares e do sistema nervoso central herdadas específica do felino.

DOENÇAS, RAÇA(S) ACOMETIDA(S), IDADE DE INÍCIO E PADRÃO DE HERANÇA DE SEXO	SINAIS CLÍNICOS	TESTES DE DIAGNÓSTICO	TRATAMENTO E PROGNÓSTICO
Manosidose (deficiência de alfa-manosidase)[74-77] • Raças DSH, DLH, Persa • 7-15 meses • AR	Disfunção cerebelar progressiva, comportamento anormal, letargia, opacificação da córnea e lente	Teste genético	Sem tratamento Prognóstico ruim
Doença de armazenamento de glicogênio tipo IV[78,79] • Gato Noruguês da Floresta • 5 meses • AR	Tremores musculares generalizados e fraqueza que progride para tetraplegia (envolvimento do PNS e SNC)	Teste genético	Sem tratamento Prognóstico ruim Morte por volta de 12 meses
Doença de Niemann-Pick tipo A[80-82] • Gatos Siameses e Balineses • 2-5 meses, machos e fêmeas • AR	Tetraparesia progressiva, postura palmípede e plantígrada, reflexos espinhais diminuídos	EMG: atividade espontânea MNCV reduzido Ensaio enzimático em leucócitos e fibroblastos de cultura (reduzida atividade de esfingomielinase)	Sem tratamento Prognóstico pobre Morte em torno de 10 meses
Polimiopatia periódica hipocalêmica[83-85] • Raças Birmanês e parentesco do Birmanês • 2 meses a 2 anos, fêmeas e machos • AR	Início episódico e agudo de ventroflexão passiva do pescoço, mialgia, cabeça balançando, marcha rígida, fraqueza. Normal entre os episódios	Hipocalemia intermitente (< 3,0 mmol/ℓ) e CK elevada Teste genético disponível	Suplementação oral de potássio Pode melhorar com o tempo
Distrofia muscular associada a deficiência de alfa-distroglicano[86,87] • Gatos Sphynx e Devon Rex • 3-23 semanas, fêmeas e machos • AR	Incapacidade de pular, ventroflexão passiva do pescoço, dificuldade para engolir, dorsal protrusão das escápulas, marcha agachada, fadiga após curtos períodos de atividade	CK: valores leves a normais EMG: atividade espontânea leve RNS: mostra de 1-3 Hz resposta decremental Biópsia muscular	Sem tratamento Progressão lenta ou pode estabilizar Morte por aspiração/possível laringoespasmo
Polineuropatia associada a hipercilomicronemia[88,89] • DSH, DLH, Himalaia, Persa, Siamês • 4-8 semanas, fêmeas e machos • AR	Progressivo, focal/multifocal, mononeuropatia assimétrica devido a granulomas lipídicos comprimindo os nervos periféricos	Atividade LPL reduzida Mutação em LPL caracterizada	Dieta com baixo teor de gordura pode resolver a neuropatia periférica
Hiperoxalúria primária (L-glicérico acidúria)[90] • DSH • 5-9 meses, fêmeas e machos • Suspeita de AR	Início agudo, fraqueza, tetraparesia, diminuição dos reflexos da medula espinal, diminuição da nocicepção, e dor abdominal	Análise de urina (L-glicérico acidúria) Doença renal, uremia	Prognóstico ruim devido a lesão renal aguda e uremia
Polineuropatia axonal[91] • Gatos com raquetes de neve • 3-6 meses, machos • Suspeita de herança	Início insidioso, ligeiramente progressivo, pélvico, intermitente fraqueza dos membros com diminuição dos reflexos de retirada bilateralmente	EMG com atividade espontânea MNCV reduzido Biópsias de músculos e nervos	Tratamento de suporte Estabilização em 6-12 meses, com tendência para remissão
Distal central e axonopatia periférica[92] • Gatos da raça Birmanês • 10 semanas, fêmeas • Suspeita ser hereditário	Postura palmípede lentamente progressiva com adução dos jarretes. Marcha hipermétrica e paraparesia	EMG: atividade espontânea MNCV reduzido Biópsias de músculos e nervos	Tratamento de suporte Prognóstico desconhecido

AR, autossômico recessivo; *CK*, concentração sérica de creatina quinase; *DLH*, doméstico de pelo longo; *DSH*, doméstico de pelo curto; *EMG*, eletromiografia; *LPL*, lipase de lipoproteína; *MNCV*, velocidade de condução nervosa motora; *PNS*, sistema nervoso periférico; *RNS*, estimulação nervosa supramáxima repetitiva; *SNC*, sistema nervoso central.

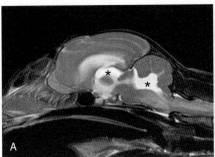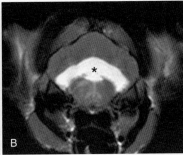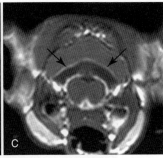

Figura 270.1 Gato doméstico com cinco meses com peritonite infecciosa felina neurológica. **A.** Imagem de ressonância magnética (RM) ponderada em T2 mediana. **B.** T2 transversal e (**C**) Imagens de RM pós-contraste ponderadas em T1 ao nível do 4º ventrículo mostrando dilatação severa do sistema ventricular (*asteriscos*) com realce periventricular marcado (*setas*) após administração de contraste.

nem prevenção confiável da PIF (ver Capítulo 224), e o prognóstico para gatos com PIF neurológica é ruim: o tempo médio de sobrevivência relatado em dois estudos foi de 6,5 dias (variando de 2 a 330 dias) e 21 dias (variando de 7 a 150 dias).[16,21]

Vírus da imunodeficiência felina. O vírus da imunodeficiência felina (FIV) é um retrovírus neurotrópico que causa a síndrome de imunodeficiência adquirida, que pode resultar em infecções oportunistas do SNC e neoplasias (linfoma). O FIV compartilha muitas características com o vírus da imunodeficiência humana (HIV) e tem sido usado como modelo animal para compreensão da neuropatogênese do HIV (ver Capítulo 222). No entanto, os sinais neurológicos (início insidioso e curso progressivo) em gatos infectados naturalmente são muito incomuns[30-32] e incluem comportamento anormal, seguido de espasmos faciais, ataxia, convulsões, distúrbios do sono e tremores de intenção.[32,33] Ligeiras elevações na contagem de células nucleadas (pleocitose mononuclear) e concentração de proteína total têm sido relatadas no LCR.[34] Em gatos infectados experimentalmente, a IRM mostrou atrofia cortical e dilatação ventricular leve, alterações na substância branca e aumento dos coeficientes de difusão aparente na substância branca, na substância cinzenta e nos núcleos basais.[35,36] Resultados positivos de testes sorológicos e PCR positivo em soro e LCR podem apoiar o diagnóstico. O tratamento é focado no gerenciamento de infecções oportunistas do SNC. O prognóstico é ruim; contudo, alguns gatos permanecem assintomáticos por muitos anos.[37]

Vírus da leucemia felina. O vírus da leucemia felina (FeLV) (ver Capítulo 223) tem sido associado com mielopatia degenerativa crônica em gatos adultos e geriátricos.[38] Não existe predileção de raça ou gênero, e o aparecimento de sinais clínicos é insidioso, com curso lentamente progressivo. Os sinais neurológicos incluem comportamento anormal, vocalização, hiperestesia e paraparesia que evolui para paraplegia com incontinência urinária.[38] A RM (cérebro e medula espinal) e a análise do LCR são normais. O resultado positivo de testes sorológicos e PCR positivo em soro e LCR podem apoiar o diagnóstico. Essa doença é incomum; portanto, outras doenças concomitantes devem ser consideradas para gatos infectados com FeLV com mielopatia. O prognóstico é ruim e o tratamento é de suporte.

Vírus da doença de Borna felina. A doença assombrosa dos felinos refere-se a uma meningoencefalomielite causada por um vírus de RNA de cadeia negativa, o vírus da doença de Borna (VDB). Tem sido relatada principalmente na Europa, mas também ocorre em outras partes do mundo, incluindo Ásia e Austrália.[39-43] Os prováveis reservatórios são pássaros e roedores; portanto, gatos adultos jovens de vida livre em áreas rurais correm maior risco.[44] Os sinais neurológicos mais comuns incluem marcha instável e "cambaleante" (ataxia) e déficits de reação postural, seguidos por comportamento anormal e ausência ou diminuição da resposta à ameaça.[44] Os achados de exames de imagens avançadas geralmente não apresentam alterações dignas de nota. O LCR pode ser anormal em 50 a 60% dos gatos infectados (pleocitose mononuclear com aumento da concentração de proteína total).[44] Títulos sorológicos e RT-PCR em tempo real em soro e LCR podem apoiar, mas não confirmam o diagnóstico.[44,45] A doença é progressiva, e, apesar do tratamento de suporte, a maioria dos gatos afetados morre ou é sacrificada durante o primeiro mês após o início de sinais clínicos.[44,46]

Doenças parasitárias do sistema nervoso central

Gurltia paralisante. Gurltia paralisante é um nematoide metastrongilídeo neurotrópico de gatos domésticos na América do Sul.[47-51] O ciclo de vida de *G. paralysans* é desconhecido. Vermes e ovos adultos podem ser encontrados na região toracolombar e parênquima medular lombossacral e veias leptomeníngas que causam meningomielite crônica e lentamente progressiva (gurltiose felina). Não há predileção por raça ou gênero, e gatos adultos jovens de áreas rurais ou periurbanas são geralmente acometidos. Os sinais clínicos incluem ataxia proprioceptiva de membros pélvicos, paraparesia, paraplegia, hiperestesia lombossacral, incontinência fecal ou urinária e/ou paralisia da cauda (Vídeo 270.4). A tomografia computadorizada mielográfica (TC-mielografia) e a RM mostram aumento difuso da medula espinal toracolombar e lombossacra.[48] A pleocitose mononuclear do LCR foi relatada em até 55% dos gatos afetados.[48] O diagnóstico presuntivo *ante mortem* de gurltiose felina é baseado em sinais neurológicos, fatores epidemiológicos e exclusão de outras causas de mielopatias felinas.[48-51] Nenhuma larva ou ovo de parasita foi encontrado no exame fecal. O diagnóstico definitivo é baseado na histopatologia por meio da detecção de *G. paralysans* adultos na medula espinal (Figura 270.2). Amostras PCR de soro e LCR estão sendo avaliadas como uma possível ferramenta de diagnóstico para infecção por *G. paralysans* em gatos domésticos.[52] Não há tratamento, e o prognóstico é ruim.

Distúrbios do sistema nervoso central de origem desconhecida

A *necrose felina hipocampal* (NFH) é um distúrbio convulsivo caracterizado por eventos epilépticos (convulsões generalizadas e/ou focais com envolvimento orofacial) e comportamento interictal anormal.[53-56] Não há predileção por raça ou gênero.[56-61] A idade de apresentação varia de 3 meses a 14 anos.[56-58,61,62] O início dos sinais clínicos é agudo, com uma rápida progressão. As crises tendem a se tornar recorrentes em alguns dias ou semanas após o início.[54,56] Dois grupos principais de NFH devem ser considerados: a NFH primária ou idiopática, que parece ser a causa direta das convulsões, e a NFH secundária, que aparece como consequência de atividade convulsiva devido a uma doença precipitante do prosencéfalo hipocampal ou extra-hipocampal (encefalite límbica autoimune do felino, neoplasia).[54,56,59,60,63] O diagnóstico definitivo é feito histopatologicamente; no entanto, os achados de RM podem confirmar lesões do hipocampo

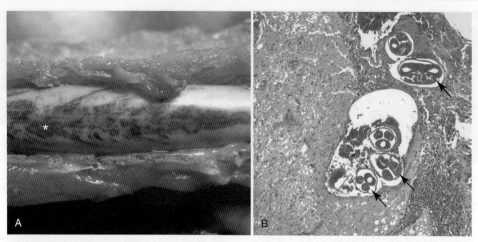

Figura 270.2 Lesões patológicas associadas à infecção por *Gurltia paralysans* em um gato adulto. **A.** Segmentos da medula espinal lombar mostrando congestão vascular marcada (*asterisco*). **B.** Seção histológica da medula espinhal mostrando seções do parasita dentro da vasculatura (*setas*) dentro do espaço subaracnóideo e parênquima medular. (Cortesia do Dr. Marcelo Gomez.)

(Figura 270.3).[56] O tratamento consiste em fármacos antiepilépticos. A medicação imunossupressora também tem sido recomendada em casos suspeitos de encefalite límbica autoimune.[56,61,63] O prognóstico geralmente é ruim, pois a maioria dos gatos torna-se resistente aos medicamentos antiepilépticos durante a fase aguda da doença; entretanto, se essa fase for superada, o resultado a longo prazo pode ser favorável.[54,57,60,61,63]

A *meningoencefalomielite linfo-histiocítica vagarosa progressiva* é caracterizada por um início tardio (média de 9 anos) e progressão lenta (média de 11 meses).[64] Não há predileção por raça ou gênero e todos os casos relatados ocorreram em gatos de vida livre (caçadores ativos que vivem no nordeste da Escócia). Sinais neurológicos incluem estado mental entorpecido ou desorientado, marcha espástica, postura da cauda rígida e estendida, reações posturais diminuídas ou ausentes em todos os quatro membros e resposta à ameaça diminuída a ausente bilateralmente (Vídeo 270.5). Exame de imagens avançadas pode mostrar atrofia cerebral. A análise do LCR foi normal em um gato testado. O diagnóstico definitivo é baseado na análise histopatológica do tecido cerebral.[64] Os possíveis agentes causais sugeridos incluem um gatilho imunogênico infeccioso ou ambiental. Não há tratamento, e o prognóstico é ruim.[64]

A *polioencefalomielite felina* é uma encefalomielite subaguda a crônica não supurativa, com predomínio de alterações patológicas na substância cinzenta, que acomete principalmente as medulas oblonga e espinal.[65,66] Achados patológicos são altamente sugestivos de um agente viral. Não há predileção de raça, gênero ou idade. A doença é considerada rara (prevalência de 1% em gatos com mielopatia).[23] Os sinais clínicos incluem ataxia, paresia e diminuição das reações posturais em todos os quatro membros.[65-68] O diagnóstico é baseado na análise histopatológica do tecido.[65,66,69] Não há tratamento, e o prognóstico pode ser favorável quando há sinais neurológicos leves e não progressivos.[67]

DOENÇAS DO SISTEMA NEUROMUSCULAR

Doenças neuromusculares hereditárias

As doenças neuromusculares hereditárias são raras, de progressão lenta e afetam predominantemente gatos jovens (ver Tabela 270.1).

Doenças neuromusculares adquiridas

Polineuropatia motora de origem desconhecida em gatos jovens

A polineuropatia motora recorrente ou progressiva tem sido relatada em gatos jovens de 3 a 44 meses de idade, principalmente gatos da raça Bengalis (mas qualquer raça ou gênero pode ser acometido).[70,71] Os sinais clínicos incluem fraqueza generalizada (recorrente ou progressiva), postura palmígrada e plantígrada, ventroflexão do pescoço e reflexos espinais reduzidos a ausentes.[70,71] O diagnóstico é baseado em testes de eletrodiagnóstico (ver Capítulo 117) e avaliação histopatológica de músculos e biopsias dos nervos. O tratamento é de suporte, e o prognóstico varia de excelente a ruim, o que destaca as possíveis etiologias diferentes.[70,71]

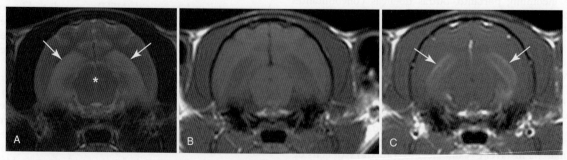

Figura 270.3 Gato Doméstico de Pelo Curto de quatro anos com necrose primária do hipocampo felino. **A.** Imagem de ressonância magnética (RM) ponderada em T2 transversal. **B.** Imagem ponderada em T1 e (**C**) pós-contraste ponderada em T1 (RM) ao nível do aqueduto mesencefálico (**A**, *asterisco*). É moderado hiperintensidade bilateral em imagens ponderadas em T2 (**A**, *setas*) e hipointensidade a normal da sustância cinzenta em imagens ponderadas em T1 da formação do hipocampo (**B**). Há aprimoramento marcado do hipocampo (**C**, *setas*) em imagens ponderadas em T1 após a administração de contraste.

DISTÚRBIOS PAROXÍSTICOS ESPECÍFICOS DE ORIGEM DESCONHECIDA

A *síndrome da dor orofacial felina* (*SDOF*) é um distúrbio de dor caracterizado por sinais comportamentais agudos de desconforto oral com ou sem mutilação da língua. É prevalente em gatos da raça Birmaneses; todavia, qualquer raça, sexo ou idade pode ser acometido.[72,73] A SDOF foi hipotetizada como análoga a neuralgia do trigêmeo no homem. Os sinais clínicos incluem eventos paroxísticos de início agudo de lambidas exageradas, movimentos de mastigação e patas na boca, geralmente confinadas a um lado da cavidade oral e lábios (Vídeo 270.6). Os eventos duram 5 minutos a 2 horas, e o gato normalmente pode se distrair disso. Os achados do exame neurológico são normais.

O diagnóstico baseia-se na exclusão de outras possíveis causas de dor oral ou disfunção do nervo trigêmeo. Lesões orais e estressores ambientais podem precipitar esses episódios. Alguns gatos conseguem ser resistentes aos analgésicos tradicionais, incluindo gabapentina.[73] Medicamentos antiepilépticos adjuvantes (fenobarbital) podem ajudar a controlar o efeito da alodinia, e o estresse ambiental devem ser limitado.[73] Ocasionalmente, é necessária terapia para toda a vida; contudo, remissão tem sido relatada em até 45% dos gatos acometidos.[73]

REFERÊNCIAS BIBLIOGRÁFICAS

As referências bibliográficas deste capítulo se encontram online no Ambiente de Aprendizagem.

SEÇÃO **18**
Doença Gastrintestinal

CAPÍTULO **271**

Avaliação Laboratorial do Trato Gastrintestinal

Jörg M. Steiner

INTRODUÇÃO

Sinais de doença no trato gastrintestinal são muito comuns em cães e gatos, mas o diagnóstico definitivo pode ser desafiador. Há uma ampla gama de testes laboratoriais que podem ajudar a avaliar os pacientes com suspeita de doença gastrintestinal. Dependendo dos sinais clínicos que o paciente apresenta (p. ex., perda de peso [ver Capítulo 19], vômito [ver Capítulo 39], diarreia [ver Capítulo 40]), uma abordagem sistemática específica deve ser adotada para incluir/excluir as várias causas possíveis. Independentemente dos sinais clínicos observados, os principais objetivos do clínico devem ser: (1) descartar de início as causas secundárias de sinais gastrintestinais; (2) descartar causas comuns de doenças gastrintestinais antes de considerar causas raras; (3) usar ferramentas de diagnóstico menos invasivas e mais acessíveis antes de optar por aquelas mais invasivas e caras.

A avaliação citológica de aspirados com agulha fina (ver Capítulo 89) ou impressões de tumor (ver Capítulo 93) e avaliação histopatológica de biopsias coletadas por endoscopia (ver Capítulo 113), laparoscopia (ver Capítulo 91) ou cirurgia também são modalidades de diagnóstico laboratorial importantes para se chegar a um diagnóstico definitivo e são discutidos na Seção 5.

AVALIAÇÃO LABORATORIAL DE ETIOLOGIAS ESPECÍFICAS

Miastenia *gravis*

O megaesôfago envolve a perda de motilidade do esôfago, que leva a um aumento do seu diâmetro, regurgitação e, em muitos casos, pneumonia aspirativa. Em vários pacientes, a causa subjacente do megaesôfago não pode ser determinada, mas alguns casos têm uma forma localizada de miastenia *gravis*, que pode ser diagnosticada pela demonstração de anticorpos contra receptores de acetilcolina no soro de cães afetados, um teste que é altamente sensível e específico para essa doença (ver Capítulo 269).[1]

Estratégias laboratoriais para o diagnóstico de enteropatógenos

Microrganismos do tipo Helicobacter

O real impacto patogênico de infecções por microrganismos do tipo *Helicobacter* em cães e gatos não é completamente compreendido. Muitos animais sadios apresentam evidências desses microrganismos no estômago.[2] No entanto, há cães e gatos que mostram sinais de gastrite crônica (ou seja, sinais clínicos de vômito) sem outra causa identificável e evidências de microrganismos do tipo *Helicobacter* no estômago e respondem à terapia tripla ou quádrupla indicada para o tratamento de infecções por *Helicobacter pylori* em humanos. A presença desses microrganismos na mucosa estomacal pode ser determinada usando colorações especiais (p. ex., coloração de Warthin-Starry), reação em cadeia da polimerase (PCR) ou hibridização fluorescente *in situ* (ver Capítulo 275).[3] O microrganismo também pode ser identificado indiretamente por um teste de urease em uma biopsia gástrica ou um com[13] C-ureia no sangue ou urina (apesar de este atualmente não estar mais disponível comercialmente para uso em cães ou gatos).[3,4]

Parvovirose

Na prática clínica, um ensaio de imunoabsorção enzimática (ELISA) *in house* que detecte o antígeno CPV-2 nas fezes é atualmente o teste usado com mais frequência para parvovirose em cães. Ele pode, no entanto, ser falso positivo em cães que foram recentemente vacinados.[5] O CPV-2 também pode ser diagnosticado por PCR, que é associado a uma maior sensibilidade, mas é menos indicado em pacientes com doença hiperaguda grave (ver Capítulo 225).[5]

Salmonella spp.

Cães e gatos podem ser portadores de *Salmonella* spp. por um longo período sem apresentar sinais clínicos (ver Capítulo 220).[6,7] No entanto, diarreia aguda ou crônica são possíveis positivos nas fezes. A identificação de *Salmonella* spp. é tradicionalmente por isolamento em meio de cultura seletivo e específico, seguido de teste de suscetibilidade. No entanto, em muitos pacientes, o organismo não é eliminado consistentemente nas fezes (ver Capítulos 40 e 220). Além disso, *Salmonella* spp. pode ser diagnosticada por uma cultura enriquecida seguida de PCR ou de PCR direto.

Campylobacter spp. patogênico

Embora haja diversas espécies de *Campylobacter* spp. que tenham sido identificadas no trato intestinal de cães e gatos, apenas um número limitado desses microrganismos, principalmente *C. jejuni* e *C. coli*, foi associado com diarreia (ver Capítulos 40 e 220).[8] Essas subespécies podem ser diagnosticadas por PCR.

Clostridioides difficile e Clostridium perfringens

Clostridioides difficile tem sido associado a diarreia em cães e gatos (ver Capítulo 220).[9-11] A virulência de C. *difficile* está associada com a presença de genes que codificam várias toxinas, mais notavelmente a toxina A (uma enterotoxina) e a toxina B (uma citotoxina), que podem ser detectadas por ELISA; entretanto, resultados positivos nem sempre se correlacionam com a doença.[9,11]

Clostridium perfringens também tem sido comumente associado a diarreia em cães e gatos. O principal fator de virulência é a enterotoxina de *Clostridium perfringens* (CPE), que induz danos à mucosa, aumenta a permeabilidade intestinal e reduz a absorção de água, levando à diarreia.[12] A coprocultura para C. *perfringens* tem pouco valor diagnóstico, visto que pode ser um microrganismo comensal e ser detectado em até 80% das amostras fecais.[9,11] Exame microscópico de esfregaços fecais e enumeração de endosporos fecais também não são úteis para o diagnóstico de diarreia associada a C. *perfringens*.[11,13] A recomendação recorrente é a detecção da enterotoxina de C. *perfringens* por ELISA, mas um resultado positivo não prova definitivamente uma relação causa-efeito.[12]

FISH para Escherichia coli aderente e invasiva

A colite histiocítica ulcerativa é uma forma grave de colite que tradicionalmente afeta os cães da raça Boxer, mas também pode ser vista em outras raças (ver Capítulos 40 e 277).[14] O diagnóstico é baseado em achados histopatológicos de colite ulcerativa histiocítica em uma amostra de biopsia do cólon e a detecção de um E. *coli* aderente e invasivo por hibridização fluorescente in situ.[14,15] Esse teste é baseado no uso de uma sonda genética dirigida contra uma região específica do DNA desse microrganismo, que foi marcado com fluorescência.[15] Evidenciar microrganismos marcados com fluorescência na mucosa do cólon confirma a presença do organismo e da doença (ver Capítulos 133 e 277).

Ferramentas laboratoriais para o diagnóstico de endoparasitas (ver Capítulo 81)

Esfregaço fecal

Um esfregaço fecal pode ser usado para identificar infecções por protozoários, mais comumente *Giardia lamblia* tanto em cães quanto em gatos e *Tritrichomonas foetus* em gatos. No entanto, a sensibilidade de um esfregaço fecal para o diagnóstico de qualquer infecção é geralmente baixa, e um resultado negativo não descarta uma infecção por protozoário.[16,17] Ocasionalmente, outras infecções parasitárias (p. ex., *Trichuris* spp.) podem ser detectadas por avaliação direta de um esfregaço fecal.

Flotação Fecal

A flotação fecal é uma ótima ferramenta para detecção de ampla variedade de ovos de helmintos e cistos de *Giardia* em cães e gatos. Há técnicas avançadas (i. e., flotação com centrifugação e flotação com sulfato de zinco) que aumentam sua sensibilidade.[18]

Imunofluorescência para Giardia e Cryptosporidium

A imunofluorescência é uma excelente técnica diagnóstica para a detecção de *Giardia* spp. e *Cryptosporidium* spp. tanto em cães como em gatos (ver Capítulos 210 e 211).[19,20] A imunofluorescência usa anticorpos marcados com fluorescência direcionados contra antígenos específicos destes protozoários para diferenciá-los de outros materiais de origem fecal (Figura 271.1).

ELISA para Giardia lamblia

Há testes de ELISA para a detecção de antígenos de *Giardia* em amostras fecais que se mostram altamente sensíveis, mas a especificidade é menor que a imunofluorescência, sobretudo em pacientes que foram recentemente tratados.[20,21]

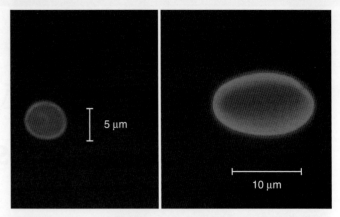

Figura 271.1 Ensaio de imunofluorescência (IFA) para *Cryptosporidium* spp. e *Giardia* spp. Um criptosporídeo pode ser visto à esquerda, enquanto a imagem à direita mostra um cisto de giárdia em uma amostra de um cão (ampliação × 1000). (Reimpressa do GI Lab Newsletter, Suchodolski, *Update on the diagnosis of enteropathogens*, p. 3, © 2012, com permissão do Laboratório Gastrintestinal.)

PCR para Tritrichomonas foetus

Tritrichomonas foetus é uma das causas de infecções por protozoários mais importantes em gatos. Em geral, T. *foetus* pode ser diagnosticado por esfregaço fecal, cultura (InPouch™ TF-Feline) ou PCR, mas somente esta última apresenta uma sensibilidade aceitável.[22,23] Muitos laboratórios oferecem testes de PCR para esse patógeno. No entanto, não há um padrão definido, pois alguns laboratórios usam a PCR em tempo real, enquanto outros fazem o mais tradicional *Nested* PCR. Portanto, o número mínimo de organismos detectáveis por grama de fezes pode variar dramaticamente entre laboratórios. Alguns gatos eliminam o organismo de forma intermitente, e uma lavagem do cólon pode oferecer maior sensibilidade.

PCR para Heterobilharzia americana

Heterobilharzia americana é um trematódeo que causa esquistossomose em cães e foi descrito principalmente em algumas áreas do Texas e Louisiana (EUA). O ovo do trematódeo pode ser identificado pela sedimentação com cloreto de sódio, que só é realizada em casos de solicitação especial. Um ensaio baseado em PCR para a detecção de DNA dos ovos desse microrganismo nas fezes está disponível e se mostrou mais sensível que a sedimentação.[24]

Ferramentas laboratoriais para avaliação da função e da doença intestinal

Concentração de folato sérico

O folato é uma vitamina B hidrossolúvel (vitamina B9), abundante na maioria dos alimentos comerciais para animais de companhia. No entanto, o folato na dieta é fornecido principalmente como folato poliglutamato, que não pode ser absorvido de imediato. No intestino delgado proximal, o folato poliglutamato é desconjugado pela folato desconjugase, e o folato monoglutamato resultante é absorvido por meio de transportadores específicos de folato no intestino delgado proximal (Figura 271.2 e Vídeo 271.1).[25,26] Em pacientes com doença proximal do intestino delgado, tanto a folato desconjugase quanto os carreadores de folato podem ser destruídos, levando à má absorção de folato em pacientes com doença grave. Se a condição for crônica, os estoques corporais de folato podem se esgotar e a concentração sérica do folato diminui. O mesmo é verdade em pacientes com doença difusa do intestino delgado quando a sua porção proximal estiver envolvida no processo da doença.[27,28] Muitas espécies bacterianas sintetizam folato, e acredita-se que um aumento no número de certas espécies bacterianas (ou seja, disbiose do intestino delgado) pode levar a aumentos significativos na concentração de folato sérico.[29]

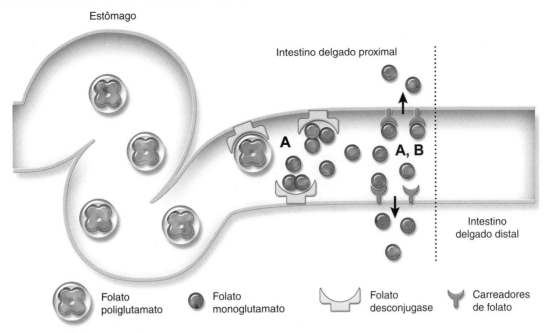

Figura 271.2 Absorção do folato. O folato da dieta entra no trato gastrintestinal predominantemente como poliglutamato. A folato desconjugase, uma enzima da região apical dos enterócitos do intestino delgado cranial, desconjuga o folato poliglutamato em folato monoglutamato. Carreadores específicos de folato nos enterócitos localizados no intestino delgado cranial permitem a absorção do monoglutamato. Tanto a desconjugase quanto as moléculas carreadoras estão localizadas apenas no intestino delgado cranial, não havendo absorção de folato no intestino delgado distal ou no cólon. (Reimpressa de *Clinical Techniques in Small Animal Practice*, 18(4): Suchodolski e Steiner, "Laboratory assessment of gastrintestinal function", p. 208, © 2003, com permissão da Elsevier.)

Concentração sérica de cobalamina

Cobalamina (vitamina B12) é uma vitamina hidrossolúvel abundante na maioria dos alimentos comerciais para animais de companhia, portanto deficiências dietéticas não são muito comuns. No entanto, os proprietários que alimentam seus animais exclusivamente com dietas vegetarianas ou veganas que não sejam enriquecidas com cobalamina podem causar, inadvertidamente, uma deficiência de cobalamina. A cobalamina da dieta está ligada a proteínas de origem animal em uma forma não absorvível. No estômago, as proteínas são digeridas por pepsina e HCl, liberando a cobalamina, que é imediatamente ligada à proteína R (uma proteína transportadora de cobalamina, sintetizada pela mucosa gástrica). No intestino delgado, a proteína R é digerida por proteases pancreáticas, e a cobalamina livre é ligada pelo fator intrínseco (Figura 271.3 e Vídeo 271.2).[30] Em cães e gatos, a maior quantidade de fator intrínseco é secretada pelo pâncreas exócrino.[31-33] Isso é diferente dos humanos, que secretam a maioria do fator intrínseco pela mucosa estomacal.[34] O fator intrínseco complexado/cobalamina é absorvido por receptores específicos no íleo (Figura 271.3 e Vídeo 271.2).[33] Uma doença do intestino delgado distal, se for grave, levará à destruição de receptores de cobalamina no íleo, resultando em má absorção da cobalamina, que acabará por levar ao esgotamento dos estoques corporais e consequente deficiência. A doença difusa do intestino delgado também pode causar má absorção se o íleo estiver envolvido no processo de doença.[29,35-39] Insuficiência pancreática exócrina comumente também leva à deficiência de cobalamina.[40,41] Finalmente, alguns pacientes com disbiose do intestino delgado têm uma diminuição da concentração sérica de cobalamina, porque algumas bactérias intestinais podem competir pela cobalamina disponível (ver Capítulo 277).[42]

Concentração fecal do inibidor da alfa₁-antitripsina

Muitos distúrbios gastrintestinais, se forem graves, podem estar associados com perda de proteína gastrintestinal. A alfa₁-antitripsina (alfa₁-AT) é sintetizada no fígado e inibe uma variedade de diferentes proteases.[43] Ela tem uma massa molecular de aproximadamente 60.000 Da, semelhante ao da albumina; portanto, quando a doença intestinal é grave o bastante para estar associada à perda gastrintestinal de albumina, a alfa₁-AT é perdida aproximadamente na mesma taxa (Figura 271.4).[44] Em contraste com a albumina, a alfa₁-AT não é hidrolisada por proteases digestivas e bacterianas no lúmen gastrintestinal,[44] portanto a concentração fecal de alfa₁-AT pode ser usada como uma estimativa para a perda de proteína gastrintestinal.[45,46] Clinicamente, a concentração fecal de alfa₁-AT deve ser avaliada em cães com hipoalbuminemia que não apresentem sinais clínicos de doença gastrintestinal e cuja perda de proteína extra gastrintestinal não pode ter a fonte identificada. Além disso, cães pertencentes a raças associadas com uma alta prevalência de enteropatia com perda de proteínas (p. ex., Lundehund, Wheaten Terrier e Yorkshire Terrier), sem quaisquer sinais clínicos de doença gastrintestinal, mas destinados a reprodução, devem ser testados.[45]

Concentração sérica de proteína C reativa

A proteína C reativa (pCr) é uma proteína de fase aguda que está recebendo crescente interesse pela avaliação de cães com uma variedade de doenças inflamatórias. Ela está aumentada em cães com doença inflamatória intestinal (DII) idiopática e mostrou se correlacionar bem com o índice de atividade da doença clínica.[47-49] Assim, a maior utilidade clínica da concentração sérica de pCr é monitorar a resposta ao tratamento em cães com DII, uma vez que uma dieta ou terapia médica eficaz estará associada com uma diminuição na concentração.[48] Uma variedade de ensaios para a medição de pCr no soro estão disponíveis, mas infelizmente nem todos eles fornecem resultados confiáveis.[50]

Teste de permeabilidade gastrintestinal

Uma importante propriedade da parede gastrintestinal é atuar como uma barreira contra a perda de proteínas plasmáticas e a absorção descontrolada de substâncias nocivas do lúmen gastrintestinal. Durante uma doença intestinal, a parede intestinal torna-se mais permeável, e o teste de permeabilidade gastrintestinal pode ser usado para avaliar a função de barreira.

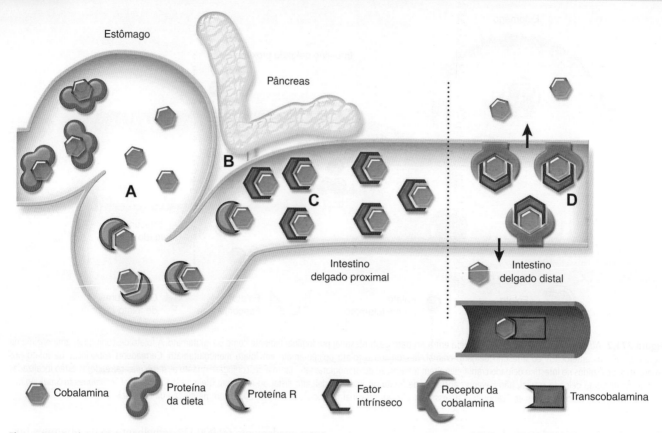

Figura 271.3 Absorção de cobalamina. A cobalamina da dieta liga-se às proteínas. No estômago, a pepsina e ácido clorídrico degradam a proteína, liberando a cobalamina (A). A cobalamina é imediatamente se ligada à proteína R, que é produzida pela mucosa gástrica. No duodeno, as proteases pancreáticas digerem a proteína R, liberando a cobalamina, que se liga ao fator intrínseco (B) no duodeno. Em cães e gatos, o fator intrínseco é produzido principalmente pelo pâncreas exócrino. A cobalamina permanece ligada ao fator intrínseco durante a passagem através do intestino delgado cranial (C). No intestino delgado distal, o complexo cobalamina/fator intrínseco é capturado por receptores específicos encontrados apenas em enterócitos no íleo (D) e os enterócitos processam o complexo fator intrínseco/cobalamina, liberando a cobalamina na circulação, onde um conjunto final de proteínas de ligação (transcobalaminas) complexam a vitamina e a carreiam para as células. (Reimpressa de *Clinical Techniques in Small Animal Practice*, 18(4): Suchodolski e Steiner, *Laboratory assessment of gastrintestinal function*, p. 207, © 2003, com permissão da Elsevier.)

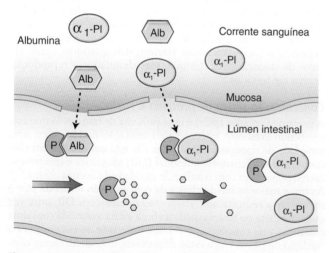

Figura 271.4 Alfa$_1$ antitripsina (alfa$_1$-AT). Em pacientes com integridade da mucosa alterada, proteínas plasmáticas podem ser perdidas no lúmen intestinal. Ao contrário da albumina, que é degradada por proteases digestivas e bacterianas, a alfa$_1$-AT é resistente a degradação proteolítica e possivelmente ao trânsito intestinal. Portanto, a alfa$_1$-AT pode ser quantificada nas fezes usando um imunoensaio. (Reproduzida de Clínicas Veterinárias da América do Norte: Práticas em Pequenos Animais, 41: Berghoff e Steiner, Testes laboratoriais para o diagnóstico e tratamento de enteropatias caninas e felinas crônicas, p. 321, © 2011, com permissão da Elsevier.)

Tradicionalmente, a captação e/ou absorção diferencial de açúcares simples, como lactulose, ramnose e/ou manitol, tem sido usada para avaliar a permeabilidade gastrintestinal.[51,52] No entanto, nenhum ensaio de rotina para a avaliação de rotina da permeabilidade gastrintestinal está disponível. Nos últimos anos, o iohexol tem sido explorado como um novo marcador, mas estudos adicionais são necessários antes que esse teste possa ser sugerido para uso na rotina.[53]

Concentrações séricas ou fecais de marcadores de inflamação

Vários marcadores para avaliar inflamações gastrintestinais foram recentemente descritos. A calprotectina e o S100A12 são marcadores para inflamação neutrofílica e se mostram aumentados tanto no soro quanto nas fezes de alguns cães com DII.[54,55] A metil-histamina é um marcador estável de degranulação de mastócitos, e foi descrito aumento da concentração fecal e sérica de metil-histamina em alguns cães com DII.[56] A tirosina bromada é um marcador da atividade dos eosinófilos, e concentrações séricas aumentadas foram descritas.[57] Mais pesquisas serão necessárias antes que a utilidade clínica desses marcadores possa ser definitivamente estabelecida, mas é uma especulação atrativa que, no futuro, seja possível avaliar os tipos específicos de células inflamatórias envolvidas em um paciente com suspeita de DII sem biopsias intestinais e determinar a abordagem terapêutica ideal baseada em um painel desses marcadores.

Endocrinologia gastrintestinal

O trato gastrintestinal é provavelmente o maior órgão endócrino do corpo, mas muito pouco se sabe sobre as doenças que o acometem, devido a um desequilíbrio de seus hormônios:[58] muitos não podem nem mesmo ser mensurados de forma confiável e outros mostram concentrações cíclicas complexas que tornam a interpretação de uma única mensuração muito difícil. Há ensaios validados para a mensuração de insulina e gastrina em cães e gatos e para a medição de CCK e motilina em cães. A dosagem da concentração sérica de gastrina demonstrou ser útil para o diagnóstico de gastrinoma, mas nenhum dos outros ensaios desempenham atualmente um papel na prática clínica diária.[59,60]

REFERÊNCIAS BIBLIOGRÁFICAS

As referências bibliográficas deste capítulo se encontram online no Ambiente de Aprendizagem.

CAPÍTULO 272

Distúrbios Orais e das Glândulas Salivares

Alexander M. Reiter e Maria M. Soltero-Rivera

Este capítulo fornece informações sobre a importância de se reconhecer achados anatômicos normais da cavidade oral frequentemente confundidos com lesões patológicas. Considerações perioperatórias são levantadas, e o uso criterioso de antimicrobianos é discutido. Distúrbios comuns da cavidade oral e das glândulas salivares são revisados, com foco no seu manejo não cirúrgico.

ESTRUTURAS NORMAIS FREQUENTEMENTE CONFUNDIDAS COM LESÕES PATOLÓGICAS

Não é incomum que dentistas e cirurgiões orais sejam consultados por causa da presença de um achado anatômico normal que pode parecer destoante e maior do que o esperado ou que apresenta coloração distinta em comparação com os tecidos circundantes (Figura 272.1).

A papila incisiva é uma eminência arredondada de mucosa do palato duro, situada na linha média caudal aos primeiros incisivos superiores. Ocasionalmente, pode ser mais ou menos pigmentada em comparação com a mucosa circundante e, desse modo, confundida com lesões patológicas.

A mucosa do palato duro mais rostral frequentemente aparece "inchada", como se estivesse sentada em uma almofada de ar. Quando um dedo pressiona essa mucosa, normalmente é suave, cedendo à pressão exercida, e o aparente inchaço retorna assim que o dedo é removido. Isso é normal e deve-se à presença de um plexo arterial fino e extenso resultante de profusa ramificação e de anastomose das principais artérias palatinas que recobrem as fissuras palatinas.

Cães e gatos têm quatro pares de glândulas salivares principais: parótida, zigomática, mandibular e sublingual. O tecido glandular também está difusamente presente na submucosa nos lábios, na língua, no palato mole e nas paredes da faringe. Gatos, mas não cães, têm uma pequena glândula situada na face lingual de cada primeiro dente molar inferior. Essa glândula do molar lingual aparece como uma protuberância da mucosa macia e não deve ser confundido com um inchaço anormal.

Gatos e cães têm dobras mucosas (frênulos) medianas muito discretas, que conectam os lábios superior e inferior às mandíbulas na linha média. Uma estrutura semelhante a um frênulo, muito mais forte e evidente, está situada imediatamente caudal a cada dente canino mandibular. Esse "frênulo" lateral do lábio às vezes pode ser mais pigmentado de um lado, causando preocupação quanto a presença de uma neoplasia.

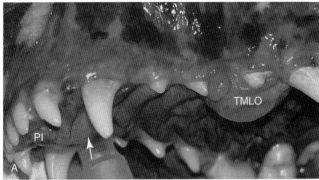

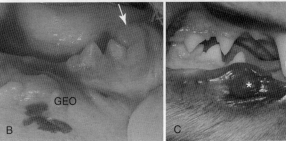

Figura 272.1 A. Estruturas normais muitas vezes mal interpretadas como lesões patológicas em cães e gatos incluem a papila incisiva (*PI*) e a mucosa rostral do palato duro "inchada" (*seta*). Esse cão foi diagnosticado com tumor multilobular ósseo (*TMLO*) em sua mandíbula superior esquerda. **B.** A glândula do molar lingual (*seta*) é uma pequena glândula salivar situada na face lingual do primeiro dente molar inferior de gatos; esse gato também foi diagnosticado com granuloma eosinofílico (*GEO*) na margem do lábio inferior. **C.** Uma estrutura semelhante a um frênulo (*asterisco*) está situada imediatamente caudal ao dente canino inferior em cães e gatos normais. (Copyright Alexander M. Reiter.) (*Esta figura se encontra reproduzida em cores no Encarte.*)

A pigmentação oral está mais comumente associada a melanina produzida por melanócitos. Embora essas células possam estar envolvidas no desenvolvimento de lesões pigmentadas na boca, a mucosa oral geralmente apresenta vários tipos de pigmentação normais. Pigmentações suspeitas de lesões de melanoma maligno inicial frequentemente apresentam discreto relevo, enquanto a pigmentação normal não altera a superfície da mucosa.

CONSIDERAÇÕES PERIOPERATIVAS

Abertura da boca

Há relatos de que a abertura prolongada e ampla da boca reduz o fluxo sanguíneo da artéria maxilar, potencialmente resultando em cegueira pós-anestesia temporária ou permanente e/ou outras deficiências neurológicas em gatos.[1] A colocação de abre-bocas e de suportes em cunha auxilia na visualização e permite o acesso a tecidos profundos na cavidade oral, na faringe e na laringe. Entretanto, a duração da abertura deve ser minimizada para reduzir o risco de tensão do músculo mastigatório e lesão das articulações temporomandibulares. Quanto maior for a abertura da boca de um gato, mais apertados o lábio e a bochecha se tornam e mais difícil será desviar esses tecidos para realizar procedimentos como limpeza ou extração dentária. A colocação de abre-bocas de plástico com 20 mm ou 30 mm de espessura entre os caninos superiores e inferiores permite uma abertura bucal adequada para esses procedimentos.[2] Surdez pós-anestésica foi relatada em cães e gatos após procedimentos de limpeza dentária e de orelha. Pacientes geriátricos podem ser mais propensos, e a função vestibular também pode ser comprometida. No entanto, muitos casos são temporários, em que os animais se recuperam.[3]

Insuflação do manguito do tubo endotraqueal

Em um gato adulto, uma vedação clinicamente hermética pode ser obtida pelo enchimento do *cuff* do tubo endotraqueal com $1,6 \pm 0,7$ mℓ de ar. A hiperinsuflação do manguito pode resultar em ruptura traqueal em gatos, o que tem sido relatado principalmente em associação com procedimentos odontológicos usando anestesia. Várias outras causas foram sugeridas, incluindo trauma iatrogênico de movimento do tubo endotraqueal durante as manipulações orais e a mudança de decúbito do paciente.[4] Os sinais clínicos associados a ruptura traqueal incluem evidência palpável de enfisema subcutâneo, tosse, engasgo, dispneia, anorexia e febre (ver Capítulo 241).

Manipulação oral e de estruturas adjacentes

Tamponamento faríngeo excessivo, manipulação da língua, elevação excessiva da mucosa alveolar nas faces linguais das mandíbulas e outras complicações iatrogênicas podem resultar em edema oral, o que agravaria o edema tecidual já existente em pacientes com inflamação ou trauma oral.[5] Quando grave o suficiente, a respiração pode ser comprometida durante recuperação de uma anestesia, e tais pacientes são capazes de se beneficiar com uma dose única de dexametasona (0,1 a 0,2 mg/kg IV) no final do procedimento. Também é possível enrolar a língua com uma esponja de gaze embebida em solução hipertônica antes da extubação. Se mostra adequado estar preparado para uma potencial necessidade de realização de traqueostomia de emergência. As compressas de gaze usadas para o tamponamento faríngeo devem ser contadas para a recuperação segura e completa no final do procedimento. Compressas pequenas de gaze podem se deslocar para dentro do esôfago. A garganta de cada paciente deve ser cuidadosamente inspecionada com a ajuda de um laringoscópio antes da extubação, para garantir que todo o material estranho tenha sido removido.

Extensão ventral excessiva da língua em um gato antes da intubação pode provocar a perfuração da mucosa sublingual ou da mucosa na parte inferior da língua por causa de dente canino mandibular muito pontiagudo. Proprietários de cães com doença periodontal grave devem ser avisados sobre aumento do risco de fratura mandibular, que pode ocorrer durante uma manipulação relativamente rotineira (ao abrir a boca para intubação, colocar um suporte de boca ou mordaça ou durante a extração de um dente). Isso enfatiza a importância da radiografia dentária pré-operatória, para determinar a saúde do osso da mandíbula.

Aplicar regularmente lubrificante ocular ou manter as pálpebras fechadas durante a anestesia ajuda a prevenir lesões na córnea.[6]

Hipo e hipertermia

A prevenção da hipotermia do paciente é de particular importância quando a água é usada para resfriar instrumentos dentários ou para enxaguar os debris da boca (ver Capítulo 49).[7] Por outro lado, a hipertermia também é uma preocupação, especialmente em gatos, quando são usados opiáceos como a hidromorfona, com ou sem anestesia inalatória, cetamina ou ambos.[8] Gatos com hipertermia pós-operatória costumam responder favoravelmente a administração de fluidos intravenosos, remoção de cobertores da gaiola, métodos mecânicos de resfriamento (como um ventilador), aplicação de compressas de gelo e fricção de álcool nos coxins (ver Capítulo 134).

Sangramento oral e hemostasia

Um sangramento oral grave pode ser decorrente de lesão de vasos sanguíneos maiores, discrasias hemorrágicas (p. ex., doença de von Willebrand), lesão lingual ou palatina, inflamação oral, trauma de tecidos moles, neoplasia oral ou fratura de mandíbula. A reposição de volume intravascular é realizada com cristaloides, coloides e/ou hemoderivados.[9] Um sangramento difuso da mucosa nasal (p. ex., após maxilectomia ou cirurgia do palato) pode ser interrompido por irrigação, com uma mistura de 0,25 mℓ de fenilefrina a 1% e 50 mℓ de lidocaína a 2% (0,05 a 0,1 mℓ/kg em gatos; 0,1 a 0,2 mℓ/kg em cães),[10] ligadura de vasos, cera óssea, selantes de fibrina e muitos outros.

Enfisema subcutâneo ou submucoso

O enfisema ocorre às vezes após o uso de equipamento movido a ar, com ar soprado ou spray de ar/água nos tecidos submucosos, particularmente após dissecção profunda de grandes retalhos mucoperiosteais. Na mandíbula, o enfisema geralmente é subcutâneo, pois o ar migra para o espaço intermandibular e, daí, para a região ventrolateral da face; um enfisema submucoso pode acontecer tanto na mandíbula superior quanto na inferior. Em geral, se resolve dentro de alguns dias, mas pode ser reduzido ou prevenido de forma eficaz com pressão digital suave, aplicada ao retalho suturado por alguns minutos, para eliminar as bolhas de ar e possibilitar uma vedação adesiva entre o tecido mole e o osso. Sopro ou pulverização de ar/água nas cavidades alveolares e no osso desnudado ou tecidos sangrando podem causar êmbolos aéreos e são fortemente desencorajados.[11]

Deiscência incisional

A deiscência de locais de cirurgia oral geralmente é resultado da tensão nas linhas de sutura. Outras causas incluem infecção ou necrose de ossos e/ou tecidos moles quando a cirurgia foi excessivamente traumática e/ou causou perda de suprimento vascular aos tecidos. Feridas orais podem ser tratadas por meio de nova sutura ou são deixadas para granular e epitelizar. Qualquer ferida oral que não esteja cicatrizando depois de 7 dias ou mais após a cirurgia deve ser biopsiada para descartar a possibilidade de neoplasia.

USO RACIONAL DE ANTIMICROBIANOS

A possível transferência de bactérias resistentes a antibióticos de gatos e cães para humanos foi recentemente reconhecida como uma potencial ameaça à saúde pública;[12,13] logo, drogas antimicrobianas devem ser usadas apropriadamente (ver Capítulo 209). Os antibióticos sistêmicos podem ter um espectro mais amplo de atividade do que os antibióticos tópicos e atingir todos os tecidos periodontais, mas só alcançam uma baixa concentração local. Antibióticos como amoxicilina-clavulanato (14 mg/kg PO 12/12 h), cloridrato de clindamicina (11 mg/kg PO 12/12 h) e, para osteomielite grave, metronidazol (30 mg/kg PO a cada 24 horas × 10 dias e 10 mg/kg PO a cada 24 horas × 20 dias, com desbridamento cirúrgico radical) são as drogas de escolha contra os patógenos periodontais isolados em cães.

A utilização de baixa dosagem de doxiciclina (1 a 2 mg/kg PO a cada 12 horas) considera mais sua ação anti-inflamatória do que antibacteriana. A aplicação local de gel de doxiciclina (8,5%) ou clindamicina (2%) em bolsas periodontais limpas mais profundas que 4 mm tem a vantagem de liberar uma concentração local elevada da droga e resulta em desfecho clínico favorável em cães.[14,15]

Uma bacteriemia temporária secundária a uma condição oral ocorre diariamente em pacientes com doença periodontal e tem sido descrita em cães e gatos durante e após a limpeza e a extração dentária. Geralmente é de curta duração em animais saudáveis, uma vez que as bactérias são eliminadas pelo sistema imunológico do hospedeiro, portanto a bacteriemia esperada não é uma indicação para o uso peri operatório de antibióticos sistêmicos em um paciente saudável. Infecção sistêmica como resultado de extração dentária mal realizada foi relatada apenas de modo observacional.[16] Antibióticos podem ser necessários em pacientes específicos, com condições preexistentes que podem piorar durante ou após o procedimento cirúrgico dentário ou oral (p. ex., hiperadrenocorticismo, diabetes melito, doença renal e hepática e pacientes em quimioterapia oncológica). A droga de escolha é ampicilina intravenosa (22 mg/kg, em procedimentos apenas na boca) ou cefazolina (20 mg/kg, quando a pele fora da boca está incluída na cirurgia), administrada na indução anestésica e repetida a cada 2 a 4 horas durante o procedimento. Além da bacteriemia em animais de companhia com doença periodontal, há um quadro crônico de liberação de mediadores inflamatórios, imunocomplexos e subprodutos da degradação bacteriana e celular no sangue e nos vasos linfáticos que pode produzir lesões de órgãos distantes de forma direta ou imunomediada. Os efeitos sistêmicos da doença periodontal são bem documentados em humanos (doenças cardíacas, acidente vascular cerebral, diabetes, doenças respiratórias, parto prematuro e bebês com baixo peso ao nascer) e têm sido cada vez mais investigados em cães e gatos.[17,18]

INFLAMAÇÃO ORAL

A maioria dos cães e gatos tem algum grau de doença periodontal. A gengivite é a inflamação da gengiva, enquanto a periodontite é a inflamação da gengiva, do ligamento periodontal, do osso alveolar e do cemento (Figura 272.2). Os patógenos periodontais na placa dentária causam a doença, mas a reação do hospedeiro às bactérias e suas toxinas também desempenha um papel na destruição tecidual durante o processo inflamatório (recessão gengival, perda de fixação, bolsa periodontal, reabsorção óssea alveolar, mobilidade e perda dentária). Os dentes afetados são escamados e polidos sob anestesia por um profissional, e existem várias opções de terapia e cirurgia (incluindo extração). O uso rotineiro de antibióticos para o tratamento da doença periodontal não é recomendado.

Úlceras de contato

Em cães, a inflamação além da doença periodontal tende a ser localizada na mucosa oral voltada para as superfícies dentais com placas. Tais lesões comumente são referidas como "úlceras em beijo" ou "úlceras de contato." Animais adultos jovens a meia-idade das raças Cocker Spaniel, Labrador Retriever, Poodle Standard, Terrier Escocês, Maltês e Dachshund às vezes apresentam osteomielite grave e celulite adjacente (ossos e raízes dentárias expostas, infectadas, inflamadas e necróticas, rodeadas por mucosa oral ulceronecrótica), que os tornam letárgicos, febris e sem apetite devido à dor oral. Alguns deles também têm otite externa, dermatite das pregas labiais e pododermatite. O tratamento envolve extração dentária parcial ou total, desbridamento tecidual, controle da dor, suporte nutricional e terapia anti-inflamatória, antisséptica e antimicrobiana.[19]

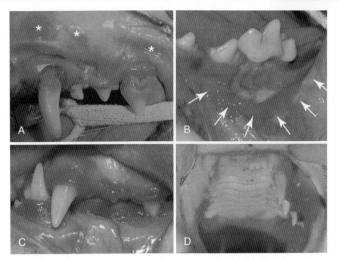

Figura 272.2 A. Cão com gengivite e periodontite mostrou também ulcerações na mucosa labial e bucal (*asteriscos*), que entram em contato com os dentes carregados de placa da mandíbula superior esquerda. **B.** Cão com osteomielite idiopática e osteonecrose do lado esquerdo da mandíbula circundada por mucosa oral ulceronecrótica (*setas*). **C.** Gato adolescente com gengivite hiperplásica juvenil. **D.** Gato adulto com estomatite; observe que os dentes do quadrante superior esquerdo já tinham sido extraídos, resultando na redução de inflamação daquele lado da boca. (Copyright Alexander M. Reiter.) (*Esta figura se encontra reproduzida em cores no Encarte.*)

Gengivite hiperplásica juvenil

A gengivite hiperplásica juvenil pode ser encontrada em gatos filhotes, adolescentes e adultos jovens que se apresentam com gengiva aumentada e inflamada (outras mucosas orais não são afetadas), principalmente em torno dos dentes maxilares e mandibulares pós-caninos. Certos medicamentos (p. ex., bloqueadores dos canais de cálcio e ciclosporinas) também podem causar hiperplasia gengival. Uma cuidadosa gengivectomia e a gengivoplastia devem ser realizadas (incluindo exame histológico de lesões suspeitas), seguidas por limpeza dentária profissional. Os proprietários são encorajados a realizar diariamente a escovação dentária com dentifrício contendo azitromicina (8,5%). A azitromicina já demonstrou reduzir a ocorrência de aumento da gengiva nos cães.[20]

Granuloma piogênico

O granuloma piogênico é uma lesão ulceroproliferativa benigna em gatos, resultando desde o quarto dente pré-molar, que traumatiza a gengiva e as mucosas alveolar e bucal adjacente, até um primeiro molar mandibular presente ou ausente. Excisão cirúrgica da massa e embotamento ou extração do dente ou dentes envolvidos são os tratamentos de escolha.[21]

Estomatite

A estomatite em gatos adultos geralmente se manifesta como inflamação do revestimento mucoso da cavidade oral caudal lateral às dobras do palatoglosso, estendendo-se rostralmente na gengiva, nas mucosas alveolar, bucal, labial e sublingual e, em algumas ocasiões, na superfície ventral e dorsal da língua. A etiologia não é clara, mas calicivírus felino (FCV) e herpes-vírus-1 felino (FHV-1) foram implicados (ver Capítulo 229).[22] História e sinais clínicos de estomatite incluem inapetência, perda de peso, secreções oral, nasal e ocular, linfadenopatia regional e sinais de dor oral. Em casos graves, os tecidos orais inflamados tornam-se proliferativos e ulcerados e sangram espontaneamente. Vários graus de doença periodontal e reabsorção dentária podem estar presentes. Um aumento na proteína total sérica geralmente é devido às concentrações elevadas de gamaglobulina. Uma amostra de biopsia deve ser obtida para descartar neoplasia ou outras causas de doenças de inflamação oral. É necessária uma abordagem de tratamento multimodal, usando uma combinação de terapias cirúrgicas e clínicas. A gestão da dor é imperativa (ver Capítulo 356). O controle da placa é conseguido com limpeza dentária profissional, terapia antimicrobiana tópica e sistêmica e extração dentária. A extração parcial e total ainda é o padrão-ouro para o tratamento da estomatite felina.[23] Os corticosteroides muitas vezes são necessários para diminuir a inflamação, reduzir a dor e estimular o apetite. Alguns gatos podem se beneficiar de aplicações periódicas subcutâneas ou intramusculares de acetato de metilprednisolona (Depo-Medrol; 4 mg/kg). Outros apresentam melhora com pomada de prednisolona (1 mg/kg por 0,1 mℓ a cada 12 a 24 horas), que é aplicada no pavilhão auricular. A ciclosporina (p. ex., Neoral) pode ser útil (começando em 2,5 mg/kg PO a cada 12 horas por 6 semanas antes de avaliar a eficácia; monitorar valores renais; níveis de ciclosporina no sangue total superiores a 300 ng/mℓ foram associados a uma melhora significativa de inflamação oral). Melhora clínica da estomatite também foi relatada com lactoferrina bovina (250 mg PO a cada 24 horas). Doxiciclina em baixa dosagem (1 mg/kg PO a cada 24 horas) e interferona ômega (5 MU diluídos e divididos, conforme necessário para injeção na submucosa de todas as áreas inflamadas; os 5 MU restantes são adicionados a 100 mℓ de solução salina e congelados em dez alíquotas de 10 mℓ; o proprietário dará 1 mℓ PO a cada 24 h por 100 dias; a fração de 10 mℓ em uso é refrigerada e as outras alíquotas são mantidas congeladas até serem necessárias) também foram sugeridos como opções de tratamento médico.[24] Cirurgia com *laser*, para remover o tecido proliferativo e inflamado da mucosa, pode ser usada como uma coadjuvante em pacientes com estomatite que não respondem a extrações e terapia médica.[25]

COMPLEXO GRANULOMA EOSINOFÍLICO

O complexo granuloma eosinofílico inclui várias condições da mucosa oral de cães e gatos e lábios e pele de apenas gatos que são caracterizadas por um infiltrado histopatológico eosinofílico.[26] As lesões são mais comuns em gatas adultas jovens e cães machos. As causas sugeridas incluem ectoparasitas e outros insetos, alergênios ambientais e hipersensibilidade alimentar. Os sinais clínicos dependem da localização da lesão, e incluem disfagia, ptialismo e inapetência. Em gatos, a condição se manifesta como nódulos (pontilhados com pequenas áreas densas, brancas ou amareladas) nas superfícies dorsal e lateral da língua, no palato duro e mole, nas dobras palatoglossais e no queixo ou como úlceras bem demarcadas (bordas em relevo em torno de uma superfície ulcerada) no lábio superior e filtro (ocasionalmente também no lábio inferior). Em cães, lesões ulceradas únicas ou múltiplas (frequentemente confluentes) podem estar presentes no palato mole e na mucosa lateral faríngea (normalmente em cães da raça Cavalier King Charles Spaniel), enquanto lesões em relevo, irregulares, ulceradas e com bordas bem demarcadas estão localizadas na língua lateral ou ventral (principalmente em cães das raças Husky Siberiano e Malamute do Alasca). Biopsia com avaliação histopatológica é uma garantia para descartar outros diagnósticos diferenciais (como carcinoma de células escamosas, linfoma e outras doenças de pele). Além de eliminar a causa subjacente, o tratamento de escolha é prednisona ou prednisolona (1 a 2 mg/kg PO a cada 12 horas inicialmente; em seguida, diminuir para a menor dose efetiva) ou injeções periódicas de acetato de metilprednisolona (4 mg/kg por vias subcutânea ou intramuscular). É possível também tentar moxicilina-clavulanato (14 mg/kg PO a cada 12 horas). A excisão cirúrgica das áreas afetadas raramente é recomendada. Lesões não tratadas podem resultar em grande perda de tecido mole (lábio superior) e em comunicação oronasal (palato duro).[26]

CONDIÇÕES AUTOIMUNES ORAIS

Doenças autoimunes que causam lesões cutâneas em cães e gatos também podem ocorrer nas áreas de junção mucocutânea ao redor da boca e na mucosa oral dentro da boca (lúpus eritematoso com autoprodução de anticorpos contra tecido e proteínas nucleares; ver Capítulos 204 e 205). Em certas ocasiões, eles estão totalmente contidos na cavidade oral, como acontece com o pênfigo vulgar e o penfigoide bolhoso, com autoprodução de anticorpos contra estruturas epiteliais escamosas específicas, ou o penfigoide de membrana mucosa, com autoprodução de anticorpos contra proteínas teciduais. Ao contrário do que acontece na estomatite em gatos e na ulceração de contato em cães, a mucosa do palato duro pode ser afetada. Uma biopsia da borda frontal da lesão quando uma bolha intacta não for encontrada pode ser suficiente. O armazenamento das amostras em solução de Michel é recomendado por alguns patologistas para preservar a antigenicidade do tecido à temperatura ambiente.[27]

As bolhas passam por diferentes estágios, desde a formação (vesícula) até a erosão e a ulceração. As vesículas são características, mas podem não estar mais presentes no momento do diagnóstico e serem substituídas por escamas, crostas, erosões e úlceras. A lesão no pênfigo vulgar é suprabasilar (fenda intercelular), com formação de acantócitos. A lesão no penfigoide bolhoso é subepidérmica, sem formação de acantócitos. Lamina 5 e 6, colágeno XVII e integrina alfa-6/beta-4 foram implicados como autoantígenos no penfigoide de membrana mucosa em cães, mas apenas laminina 5 foi reconhecida em gatos. As abordagens de tratamento são descritas nos Capítulos 204 e 205.

HIPERSENSIBILIDADE E CONDIÇÕES METABÓLICAS ORAIS

Eritema multiforme e necrólise epidérmica tóxica

O eritema multiforme pode ser mediado pela deposição de imunocomplexos nos capilares superficiais da pele e menos frequentemente da mucosa oral, como resultado de uma infecção ou exposição a drogas.[28,29] Necrólise epidérmica tóxica é caracterizada por uma necrose coagulativa de espessura total com mínima inflamação da derme;[30] é uma forma extrema de reação a medicamentos (ver Capítulo 169), com o animal deprimido, febril e inapetente. A causa subjacente deve ser preferencialmente eliminada (p. ex., cessação do uso de determinado medicamento). Anti-inflamatório e terapia imunossupressora ou imunomoduladora são instituídos junto aos cuidados de enfermagem.

A uremia resulta da retenção de resíduos urêmicos após rápido declínio da função renal[31] (ver Capítulo 322). Um forte odor de amônia está presente na respiração (ver Capítulo 36), e ulcerações orais ocorrem, especialmente nas mucosas labial e bucal, nas margens laterais da língua, no frênulo labial lateral e nas comissuras labiais. Vasculite urêmica e trombose podem levar à necrose e à descamação da mucosa. Em casos graves, resulta em descamação da ponta da língua. As lesões costumam ser dolorosas, contribuindo para a anorexia já observada em animais de companhia com doença renal. Qualquer condição que produza um estado de hipercoagulabilidade (p. ex., leptospirose e diabetes melito) pode levar à formação de trombos e subsequente descamação das áreas afetadas.[32] O tratamento é de suporte, até que a causa possa ser removida ou resolvida e inclui o manejo da dor (tal como buprenorfina 0,01 mg/kg a cada 8 a 12 horas por via intravenosa), contornando a alimentação oral com suplementação nutricional enteral ou parenteral (ver Capítulo 82) e uso de protetores gástricos (sucralfato 0,5 a 1 g PO a cada 4 a 6 h). Enxaguantes bucais tópicos, como uma mistura de difenidramina, sucralfato/alumínio, hidróxido de magnésio (Maalox, Novartis) e lidocaína, podem fornecer algum controle local da dor. O enxágue com clorexidina diluída (0,12%) ajuda a prevenir infecção secundária de áreas necróticas.[31]

CORPO ESTRANHO ORAL

A penetração de corpos estranhos pode provocar feridas profundas e contaminadas na área sublingual, na prega palatoglossal, no palato mole, na tonsila palatina, no piso da órbita ou na parede faríngea.[33] Eles também podem se alojar em todo o palato duro entre os dentes maxilares da bochecha (p. ex., pedaços de madeira), presos na mucosa oral (bardana e grama vulpino) ou presos na língua e atravessando o frênulo lingual (uma agulha com linha). Animais de estimação afetados apresentam halitose, diminuição do apetite e de ingestão de água, patadas na face, inchaço na região intermandibular ou região do pescoço, tratos sinusais, secreção de saliva com aspecto claro ou translúcido tingido de sangue, náuseas, e ânsia de vômito, engasgo ou vômito. Ultrassonografia (US), tomografia computadorizada (TC) e ressonância magnética (RM) são mais úteis do que radiografias para localizar um corpo estranho oculto.[9] O manejo requer exploração cirúrgica, remoção do corpo estranho, limpeza de feridas e, se apropriado, colocação de drenos e sutura. Amostragens para cultura são realizadas, e a antibioticoterapia empírica é instituída antes da disponibilidade de resultados de cultura e sensibilidade. Feridas intraorais frequentemente são fechadas para evitar o aprisionamento de alimentos, cabelos e outros debris. Se o ponto de entrada intraoral cicatrizou quando o paciente apresentou sinais clínicos, a abordagem cirúrgica é escolhida, com base em descobertas diagnósticas para determinar a rota mais direta e segura para a recuperação de corpos estranhos.[9]

QUEIMADURAS ORAIS (FIGURA 272.3)

Lesões elétricas geralmente ocorrem em animais jovens que mastigam cabos de energia.[24] Complicações com risco de vida estão relacionadas a edema pulmonar neurogênico ou inalação de fumaça (ver Capítulo 242). Os tecidos afetados em geral incluem lábios, bochechas, mucosa oral, língua e palato. Queimaduras mais extensas também afetam dentes e ossos. Se ocorreu edema pulmonar não cardiogênico, o paciente inicialmente é estabilizado, então tratado de forma conservadora (lavagem da ferida). Mais tarde, uma vez que o tecido necrótico esteja evidente, o desbridamento conservador pode ser iniciado. A necrose da língua pode fazer que um grande pedaço de tecido se desprenda. A necrose do palato pode causar um defeito oronasal. Queimaduras térmicas resultantes da exposição a itens quentes às vezes são vistas no plano nasal, lábios, mucosa labial, língua e palato. Os proprietários são aconselhados a não superaquecer os alimentos e líquidos quando tentam torná-los mais palatáveis para pacientes com inapetência. Queimaduras químicas por exposição a produtos de limpeza caseiros, compostos fenólicos, óleos essenciais, metal pesado (tálio) ou toxinas vegetais (p. ex., *Dieffenbachia* – "comigo-ninguém-pode") se apresentam como úlceras agudas cobertas por detritos necróticos. A terapia inicial para queimaduras térmicas e químicas é a lavagem com solução de Ringer com lactato, seguida por conduta conservativa. O pelo de um animal de companhia afetado deve ser limpo se houver suspeita de que contenha resíduos do agente responsável por uma queimadura química.[24]

MIOSITE DE MÚSCULOS MASTIGATÓRIOS

A miosite de músculos mastigatórios (MMM) é uma doença autoimune que afeta os músculos temporal, masseter e pterigoides medial e laterais em cães (ver Capítulo 354). Cães adultos jovens a meia-idade de raças de grande porte parecem ser afetados mais comumente.[34] Um estágio agudo (inchaço muscular doloroso/inflamação) normalmente dura 2 a 3 semanas, seguido por um estágio latente (animal com aparência saudável) e por um estágio crônico (atrofia muscular) ou uma etapa aguda recorrente. Cães com MMM aguda têm um histórico de diminuição de atividade, letargia, relutância em comer e sinais de dor ao bocejar ou ao abocanhar guloseimas e brinquedos, além de possivelmente apresentarem febre, linfadenopatia regional, inchaço dos músculos temporais e masseter (dolorosos à palpação) e exoftalmia. Cães com MMM crônicos em geral são ativos e alertas, mas mostram atrofia progressiva dos músculos mastigatórios e enoftalmia. O cão resiste à abertura da boca ou não consegue abri-la totalmente. O edema e atrofia muscular podem ser assimétricos.[34]

Os músculos temporal, masseter e pterigóideo medial e lateral possuem fibras 2 M que diferem do tipo comum de fibras 2C de outros músculos esqueléticos. Nessa doença, autoanticorpos visam o componente único de miosina das fibras do tipo 2 M, resultando em inflamação muscular, necrose e fagocitose. Um diagnóstico definitivo de MMM pode ser feito se os anticorpos contra fibras do tipo 2 M forem identificadas no soro e/ou complexos imunes detectados em amostras de músculos biopsiados.[35] Um título de anticorpos contra a fibra tipo 2 M de inferior a 1:100 é negativo, enquanto 1:100 é limítrofe e superior a 1:100 é positivo.

A TC ajuda a descartar a maioria dos diagnósticos diferenciais de MMM, permite aspiração guiada por agulha fina de músculos pterigoides cirurgicamente inacessíveis e mostra alterações de tamanho (maiores devido ao edema ou inflamação e menores devido a atrofia, necrose ou fibrose), atenuação do tecido pré-contraste (hipoatenuado devido ao edema) e aumento heterogêneo de contraste (devido à inflamação) nos músculos afetados e presença de linfadenopatia regional.[35]

As biopsias musculares são retiradas de áreas dos músculos temporais ou masseter que mostrem o aumento de contraste mais óbvio na TC. Uma amostra de tecido muscular de 0,5 a 1 cm de diâmetro é excisada, envolta em uma esponja de gaze seca ou minimamente umedecida e colocada em um recipiente à prova d'água (p. ex., um tubo de tampa vermelha de 10 mℓ; ver Capítulo 116). A amostra é mantida refrigerada e enviada ao laboratório dentro de 18 a 24 horas. Deve-se prestar atenção

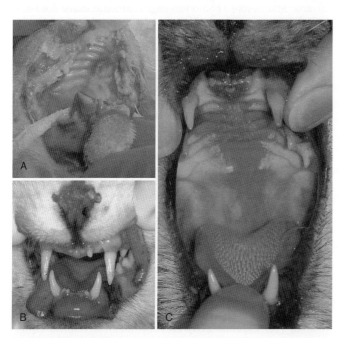

Figura 272.3 A. Gato com queimaduras por choque elétrico, que causaram necrose dos lábios, língua, palato e mucosa oral. **B.** Gato com queimaduras por calor no plano nasal, lábios e ponta e lados da língua, devido a alimento oferecido após aquecimento em forno micro-ondas. **C.** Gato com queimaduras por produtos químicos, que resultaram em erosões de início agudo da ponta e lados da língua e do palato. (Copyright Alexander M. Reiter.) (*Esta figura se encontra reproduzida em cores no Encarte.*)

especial ao fechamento completo da ferida, porque os corticosteroides atrasam a cicatrização do tecido conjuntivo[36] e eles não devem ser iniciados antes da coleta de sangue e amostragem muscular. Uma injeção de dexametasona (1 mg/kg IV, uma vez após a biopsia muscular) é útil na redução imediata da inflamação em cães com MMM aguda. O paciente recebe alta com indicação de prednisona (1 a 2 mg/kg PO a cada 12 horas), geralmente resultando em melhora rápida dos sinais clínicos (redução de dor e sinais de doença sistêmica, bem como visível melhora da abertura da boca, 1 a 2 dias após o início da terapia com corticosteroide). Após 2 a 3 semanas, a dosagem pode ser diminuída para 1 mg/kg PO a cada 24 horas por mais 3 a 4 semanas e então diminuída lentamente, até a menor dosagem eficaz possível em dias alternados durante um período de 8 a 12 meses. Cães incapazes de receber corticosteroides, sem resposta aos corticosteroides isoladamente ou mostrando efeitos colaterais inaceitáveis em resposta podem se beneficiar da administração de azatioprina (1 a 2 mg/kg PO a cada 24 horas). Os exames de acompanhamento devem ocorrer após 2 semanas e 1, 2, 6, 9 e 12 meses após o início da corticoterapia; depois, uma vez a cada 6 a 12 meses, com foco no peso corporal, grau de atrofia muscular, dor à palpação da cabeça e amplitude de abertura da boca (que é medida com uma régua entre as bordas incisais dos incisivos superiores e inferiores). Os testes periódicos de titulação de anticorpos são importantes antes de diminuir as dosagens de prednisona, particularmente quando a dosagem já é muito baixa (p. ex., 0,1 a 0,2 mg/kg PO a cada 48 horas). Em cães com recidivas, o tratamento deve ser reinstituído na dosagem máxima de prednisona e diminuir lentamente para a dosagem eficaz mais baixa possível em dias alternados.[34]

CONDIÇÕES DA GLÂNDULA SALIVAR

A *sialocele* (extravasamento de saliva para os espaços submucosos ou subcutâneos) requer tratamento cirúrgico, e o leitor é encorajado a consultar livros de cirurgia para obter informações sobre o diagnóstico e tratamento.[37,38]

A *sialadenite*, uma inflamação de uma glândula salivar, é vista em cães de meia-idade a mais velhos. A glândula salivar zigomática é mais comumente afetada, e o cão pode apresentar um edema doloroso na área orbital/retrobulbar com exoftalmia. Os sinais clínicos incluem mal-estar, inapetência, linfadenopatia, febre, sinais de dor na retropulsão do olho através da pálpebra fechada e ao abrir a boca, disfagia e secreção mucopurulenta na abertura do ducto na boca. O palato mole pode ter uma aparência assimétrica devido a uma glândula zigomática aumentada e inflamada. Sialolitos podem ser fatores contribuintes. A TC e a RM devem ser considerados para descartar os diagnósticos diferenciais. Aspiração por agulha fina e avaliação citológica da glândula salivar zigomática (através da mucosa oral) e dos nódulos linfáticos regionais (ver Capítulo 95), cultura bacteriana e teste de sensibilidade (se houver suspeita de infecção) e três projeções de radiografias torácicas (se houver suspeita de neoplasia) podem ser realizadas. Um diagnóstico definitivo de sialadenite requer uma biopsia incisional e avaliação histopatológica. É possível tentar drenagem intraoral para aliviar o acúmulo de fluido mucopurulento e pressão associada que causem desconforto. O tratamento médico inclui o controle da dor (se houver; ver Capítulos 126 e 356) e uso de antibióticos (com base na cultura e resultados de sensibilidade do aspirado de fluido/tecido), anti-inflamatórios não esteroides (AINEs) e doses anti-inflamatórias de corticosteroides (ver Capítulo 164).[39]

A *sialadenose* é um aumento não inflamatório de uma glândula salivar sem anormalidades citológicas ou histológicas óbvias. A *sialometaplasia necrosante* (com necrose ou infarto da glândula salivar) é um aumento doloroso de uma glândula salivar, com metaplasia escamosa dos ductos das glândulas e necrose isquêmica lobular. A sialadenose e a sialometaplasia necrosante ocorrem principalmente em cães de raças pequenas, de jovens adultos a meia-idade. O histórico e os sinais clínicos são menos graves na sialadenose (perda de peso, relutância ao exercício, fungar, estalar os lábios, secreção nasal, hipersalivação, inapetência, depressão, náuseas, ânsia de vômito e engolir em seco). Além desses sintomas, cães com sialometaplasia necrosante frequentemente mostram engasgo, regurgitação, vômito crônico, tosse, taquipneia, dispneia, espirro reverso e esforços respiratórios abdominais. Eles ficam sensíveis à palpação da região faríngea, mostram sinais de dor associados à abertura da boca e estão deprimidos, nauseados e anoréxicos. Um mecanismo patogenético neurogênico é suspeito de se correlacionar com anormalidades do nervo vago, e condições associadas com sialometaplasia necrosante incluem distúrbios esofágicos. O manejo da dor e estratégias diagnósticas e terapêuticas semelhantes à sialadenite devem ser realizadas. A administração de fenobarbital oral (1 a 2 mg/kg PO a cada 12 horas) resultou em intensa melhoria em alguns casos, fornecendo suporte para um mecanismo neurogênico.[39]

DISTÚRBIOS NÃO NEOPLÁSICOS DOS OSSOS DA MANDÍBULA

A *osteopatia craniomandibular* é caracterizada por proliferação de tecido ósseo bilateralmente no corpo da mandíbula, na articulação temporomandibular e na bula timpânica em raças de pequeno porte. Espessamentos da calvária, do tentório do cerebelo e das extremidades podem ser observados.[40] O cão pode mostrar sinais de dor, falta de vontade ou incapacidade de abrir totalmente a boca e relutância em comer. Hipertermia pode estar presente e sinais neurológicos ocasionalmente são vistos. O tratamento consiste em drogas anti-inflamatórias (AINEs ou corticosteroides; ver Capítulo 164), drogas analgésicas (ver Capítulos 126 e 356) e suporte nutricional (ver Capítulo 82).

A *hiperostose calvariana*, observada principalmente em cães jovens da raça Bulmastife, é caracterizada pela proliferação óssea irregular e progressiva e pelo espessamento da cortical óssea da calvária. Manifesta-se como um engrossamento suave dos ossos da calvária, tornando-o diferente do espessamento irregular visto na osteopatia craniomandibular. Os sinais clínicos incluem inchaço doloroso do crânio, exoftalmia, febre e linfadenopatia. Na maioria casos, é autolimitante.[41]

A *osteodistrofia fibrosa* resulta de uma condição congênita associada ao hiperparatireoidismo primário ou secundário nutricional/renal (ver Capítulo 297).[42] Há osteopenia generalizada com manifestação mais pronunciada nos ossos da mandíbula, causando mobilidade dentária, inchaço facial, maxilares espessos e "emborrachados" e mucosa oral ulcerada. As radiografias mostram diminuição difusa e marcada da densidade óssea, perda de estrutura óssea trabecular normal, bem como perda de lâmina dura. Os dentes em geral não parecem estar desmineralizados e raramente sofrem reabsorção. O prognóstico é muito ruim, exceto para casos de hiperparatireoidismo secundário nutricional, que pode ser tratado com uma dieta adequada.

TUMORES ORAIS BENIGNOS

Os *papilomas* são lesões esbranquiçadas semelhantes a uma couve-flor, induzidas por vírus nas membranas mucosas e junções mucocutâneas da boca em cães com menos de 1 ano de idade (ver Capítulo 228). Eles costumam se resolver espontaneamente em 1 a 3 meses, a menos que o paciente apresente imunocomprometimento; descartar linfoma é particularmente importante em cães mais velhos que apresentem papilomatose oral grave.

Fibromas odontogênicos periféricos são tumores odontogênicos mistos (comuns em cães e raros em gatos), localizados frequentemente na gengiva perto dos dentes incisivos, caninos ou pré-molares.[43] O fibroma do tipo ossificação (anteriormente denominado epúlide ossificante) é distinto do tipo fibromatoso (epúlide fibromatosa) pelo seu conteúdo com quantidades variáveis de osso ou tecido dentário duro dentro do tecido mole do tumor. Esses tumores são excisados juntamente à extração do dente envolvido e curetagem completa do alvéolo. A biopsia distinguirá esses tumores da hiperplasia gengival (Figura 272.4).

Ameloblastomas são tumores odontogênicos epiteliais. O ameloblastoma acantomatoso canino (anteriormente chamado epúlide acantomatoso) é um tumor invasivo local que causa lise óssea ao redor das raízes dos dentes e alterações císticas. Contudo, apesar desse comportamento localmente agressivo, não causa metástase, portanto é considerado benigno.[43] Externamente, em muitas ocasiões tem uma superfície áspera, semelhante a uma couve-flor, e às vezes se parece com um carcinoma de células escamosas. É mais comum na área dos dentes incisivos e caninos dos maxilares superior ou inferior e menos comum na área dos dentes carnassiais.

Odontomas não são verdadeiras neoplasias, mas sim um conglomerado de células desorganizadas de tecido normal. Esmalte, dentina, cemento e pequenas estruturas semelhantes a dentes podem compor a massa. Lesões com características semelhantes a dentes normais são considerados odontomas compostos, enquanto odontomas complexos tem um arranjo mais desorganizado.[44]

Outros tumores orais benignos que são menos comuns incluem cementoma, granuloma de células gigantes, tumor odontogênico indutivo felino, tumor odontogênico produtor de amiloide, tumor de células plasmáticas, osteoma e lipoma.

TUMORES ORAIS MALIGNOS

O *melanoma maligno* geralmente ocorre em cães mais velhos com pigmentação, mas é muito raro em gatos (ver Capítulo 345). O tumor é pigmentado ou não pigmentado (amelanótico), muitas vezes cresce com rapidez e invade o osso precocemente. A superfície do tumor em geral está ulcerada e com odor fétido, devido à necrose causada pela lesão que ultrapassa o limite de seu suprimento sanguíneo. As localizações típicas são gengiva, palato, superfície dorsal da língua e superfície mucosa e junções mucocutâneas dos lábios e bochechas. Metástases regionais e à distância são comuns no momento do diagnóstico.[45]

O *carcinoma de células escamosas* não tonsilar normalmente é um tumor de cães e gatos mais velhos, mas o carcinoma papilífero de células escamosas também pode ocorrer em cães adolescentes e jovens adultos. Os tumores, na maioria das vezes, são encontrados na gengiva como lesões proliferativas e ulceradas e, menos frequentemente, na mucosa dos lábios, bochechas, língua e área sublingual. A invasão óssea é comum em lesões gengivais. Se ocorrer no maxilar superior em gatos, o tumor pode ser menos protuberante, enquanto a invasão óssea é mais grave. O uso de coleiras antipulgas, a ingestão de atum enlatado e a exposição ambiental à fumaça do tabaco foram identificados como fatores de risco para carcinoma de células escamosas em gatos.[46] A metástase para os linfonodos regionais é comum, enquanto à distância pode ocorrer no final do processo da doença. Estudos recentes sugerem uma taxa de metástase para os linfonodos mandibulares superior a 30%.[47] O carcinoma de células escamosas tonsilar e lingual em cães é altamente metastático (ver Capítulo 345 para o tratamento e informações de prognóstico no carcinoma de células escamosas).

O *fibrossarcoma* é o segundo tumor maligno oral mais comum em gatos e o terceiro em cães. É um tumor altamente invasivo que tende a ocorrer em cães jovens adultos de raças grandes e cães de meia-idade de pequeno porte, afetando a gengiva, a mucosa do lábio/bochecha e o palato duro/mole. Muitas vezes, ele aparece como uma lesão ulcerada protuberante, mas, ocasionalmente, surge da superfície lateral do osso incisivo e da maxila, apresentando uma massa firme e lentamente crescente no focinho. Metástases regionais e à distância de fibrossarcomas são menos comuns em comparação com melanoma maligno e carcinoma de células escamosas. Os fibrossarcomas de baixo grau parecem ter histologia benigna, mas são biologicamente malignos[48] (ver Capítulo 348 para o tratamento e informações prognósticas sobre o fibrossarcoma).

O *osteossarcoma* afeta a mandíbula e, com menos frequência, o maxilar. Em várias ocasiões, manifesta-se como uma massa carnuda, ulcerativa ou necrótica, com extensa evidência radiográfica de invasão óssea (lise óssea em vez de proliferação de tecido duro). Metástases regionais e à distância parecem ser menos comuns do que para o osteossarcoma de membro.[49] O tumor multilobular ósseo é uma variante menos agressiva, manifestando-se como uma massa dura, bem circunscrita e não ulcerada na maxila, palato, ramo da mandíbula, arco zigomático e calvária. Parece radiograficamente como uma combinação de tecido mineralizado e não mineralizado (aparência de "bola de pipoca") (ver Capítulo 348 para tratamento e informações prognósticas sobre osteossarcoma).

Tumores da bainha de nervo periférico às vezes são diagnosticados incorretamente como fibrossarcoma. Eles tendem a crescer ao longo dos principais nervos da face (infraorbital, alveolar inferior, palatino principal), maxilar superior e inferior e palato (ver Capítulo 268).

Outras lesões malignas menos comuns incluem hemangiossarcoma, linfoma, tumor de mastócitos e tumores anaplásicos ou indiferenciados.

ABORDAGEM PARA AVALIAR MASSAS ORAIS

O sistema tumor-nódulo-metástase (TNM) auxilia na descrição da extensão clínica (estágio) da doença neoplásica por meio da avaliação do tumor primário, linfonodos regionais e locais distantes de possível metástase.[50] Três projeções de radiografia torácica (e ocasionalmente também um ultrassom abdominal, se houver razão para suspeitar de doença intra-abdominal) devem ser realizadas antes de colocar um paciente com tumor oral sob

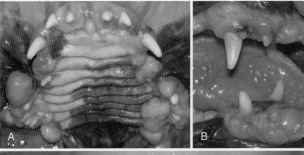
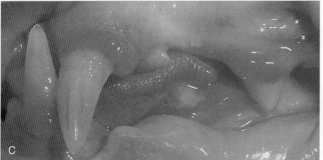

Figura 272.4 A. Cão com numerosos tumores odontogênicos periféricos. **B.** Hiperplasia gengival induzida por anlodipino em um cão. **C.** Hiperplasia gengival induzida por ciclosporina em um gato. (Copyright Alexander M. Reiter.) (*Esta figura se encontra reproduzida em cores no Encarte.*)

anestesia, particularmente quando há suspeita de lesão oral maligna. No entanto, lesões metastáticas com diâmetro inferior a 5 mm podem não ser visíveis nas radiografias. Por outro lado, a inclusão do tórax durante uma TC da cabeça (para avaliar o tumor primário) e pescoço (para avaliar os linfonodos) pode permitir a detecção de lesões metastáticas com menos de 2 mm de diâmetro.[51] O uso de radiografias dentárias convencionais ou digitais (em particular com filmes dentais de tamanho 4 ou placas de fósforo) é superior à radiografia médica padrão quanto à avaliação da qualidade e à extensão óssea de lesões dos maxilares superior e inferior.

Uma biopsia é preferencialmente obtida de uma área que pode ser incluída na ressecção definitiva. Áreas de tecido necrótico podem estar presentes em tumores de crescimento rápido, mas tal tecido não é útil no diagnóstico; o tecido viável deve ser incluído na amostra de biopsia. A amostragem citológica pode ser realizada no paciente acordado ou sedado. Técnicas de agulha fina são úteis para lesões que esfoliam bem, e a amostragem frequentemente é realizada com uma agulha 22G por meio de uma biopsia ou aspiração por agulha (ver Capítulos 93 e 95). A palpação dos nódulos linfáticos não é sensível nem específica para detectar metástases de linfonodos regionais.[52] Portanto, o exame citológico de biopsias de agulha de linfonodo e aspirados deve ser realizado, o que pode ser adequado para o diagnóstico de melanoma metastático e carcinoma de células escamosas, mas é menos satisfatório para outros tumores orais. Esfregaços de impressão e raspagens obtidos da superfície de um tumor epitelizado ou ulcerado não tem valor diagnóstico, apenas se obtido a partir do corte da superfície de um tumor excisado (ver Capítulos 86 e 87).

A amostragem histológica, mais precisa do que a citológica, requer uma anestesia geral e o exame microscópico de uma amostra fixada em formalina. Fórceps Rongeur são ideais para amostras de osso e lâminas de bisturi para amostras incisionais e excisionais de tecido mole. Instrumentação que danifique tecidos (p. ex., eletrocautério) não deve ser usada durante o procedimento de amostragem, para que o diagnóstico não seja obscurecido. Múltiplas amostras devem ser obtidas. A hemostasia é feita com pressão digital, e locais de biopsia de tumores invasores mais profundos são suturados. Para fixação adequada, a amostra é colocada em 10% de formalina tamponada, a 1 parte de tecido para 10 partes de fixador. Linfonodos parotídeos, mandibulares e retrofaríngeos medial e lateral devem ser de preferência avaliados histologicamente após a excisão (ver Capítulo 95). Uma biopsia negativa de linfonodo, no entanto, não exclui a possibilidade de metástases regionais, que podem ocorrer ao longo das vias perineurais ou vasculares, ou metástases para outros linfonodos menos acessíveis. Se os resultados citológicos ou histológicos não correspondem aos achados clínicos, um segundo espécime, maior e mais profundo, é obtido. Um retalho de mucosa pode ser levantado para acessar o tecido mais profundo e encontrar tumores que são cobertos por uma camada de tecido normal de espessura variável.

RESULTADO E CONCLUSÃO

A comunicação com o proprietário é extremamente importante antes de decidir por um procedimento cirúrgico oral. Em geral, os cuidados domiciliares no pós-operatório imediato, a higiene bucal a longo prazo em casa e a necessidade de reavaliações periódicas devem ser discutidos. Considerando essencial a anestesia geral para avaliar completamente quaisquer lesões dentais e orais e para realizar o tratamento conforme necessário, o risco de complicações perioperatórias também deve ser discutido. Além disso, algumas das doenças discutidas neste capítulo requerem tratamento médico para o resto da vida ou procedimentos cirúrgicos que podem levar a uma mudança na aparência estética ou funcionalidade do paciente.

O diagnóstico de um tumor oral maligno ou localmente agressivo deve levar a uma discussão aprofundada sobre seu comportamento biológico, a possibilidade de complicações intraoperatórias, a expectativa de qualidade de vida do animal, a expectativa de vida após o procedimento ou as possibilidade de a cirurgia não ser realizada e alternativas subsequentes de tratamento (como radioterapia, imunoterapia e quimioterapia).

A colaboração com oncologistas clínicos e radioterapeutas é útil para permitir que o veterinário e o proprietário tomem uma decisão consciente, que se adeque ao animal de companhia e sua família.

REFERÊNCIAS BIBLIOGRÁFICAS

As referências bibliográficas deste capítulo se encontram online no Ambiente de Aprendizagem.

CAPÍTULO 273

Doenças da Faringe e do Esôfago

Stanley Leon Marks

ANATOMIA E FUNÇÕES NORMAIS

A cavidade oral, a orofaringe e o esôfago podem ser pensados como uma série de câmaras de expansão e contração divididas por esfíncteres musculares. A propulsão do bolo alimentar através dessa parte do trato alimentar é o resultado da pressão positiva desenvolvida atrás dele e de um vácuo ou pressão negativa desenvolvida na sua frente. Qualquer perturbação nos elementos anatômicos, no funcionamento ou na coordenação desse sistema pode resultar na transferência anormal do bolo alimentar para o estômago, resultando em disfagia (dificuldade para engolir).

A disfagia é relativamente comum em cães, e a lista de possíveis causas é extensa (Boxe 273.1), mas não é tão frequente em gatos, com exceção de causas estruturais da disfagia orofaríngea (DOF) associada a tumores orais, úlceras e gengivoestomatite.

O mecanismo da deglutição é complexo, envolvendo 31 pares de músculos estriados e cinco nervos cranianos com núcleos no tronco encefálico (fibras sensoriais e motoras do trigêmeo; facial; glossofaríngeo e vago; e fibras motoras do hipoglosso), e o centro da deglutição na formação reticular do tronco encefálico. O reflexo normal da deglutição é um processo de quatro fases: preparatória oral, oral, faríngea e esofágica.[1] O esôfago transporta o bolo alimentar da faringe para o estômago. A camada externa de tecido conjuntivo frouxo do esôfago, chamada de adventícia, está presente na porção cervical, mas é amplamente substituída por serosa no tórax. Em cães, a musculatura do esôfago, do músculo cricofaríngeo à junção gastresofágica, é totalmente estriada. Em gatos, o músculo estriado é substituído por músculo liso em cerca de um terço do esôfago. A parede interna consiste em submucosa e mucosa, dividida pela muscular da mucosa fenestrada, mais proeminente no esôfago torácico. A submucosa contém vasos sanguíneos, nervos e glândulas, e a mucosa é composta de epitélio escamoso estratificado queratinizado. A inervação do músculo estriado do esôfago em cães e gatos é fornecida por neurônios eferentes viscerais especiais do núcleo ambíguo bilateral no bulbo. Axônios são transportados nos nervos vagos e distribuídos com os nervos faringoesofágico e laríngeo recorrente, e com os troncos vagais. As inervações do músculo liso em gatos provêm do núcleo ambíguo bilateral rostral via eferentes viscerais gerais e são distribuídos via ramos do nervo vago bilateral.

FASES DA DEGLUTIÇÃO

Fases oral preparatória, oral e faríngea

A *fase preparatória oral* é voluntária e começa quando o alimento ou o líquido entra na boca. A mastigação e lubrificação dos alimentos são marcas dessa fase, pois o bolo alimentar é modificado e preparado para a deglutição. Anormalidades estão associadas a doenças dentárias (ver Capítulo 272), xerostomia e fraqueza dos lábios (nervos cranianos V e VII), da língua (nervo craniano XII) e das bochechas (nervos cranianos V e VII) (ver Capítulo 264). A *fase oral* consiste nos eventos musculares responsáveis pelo movimento do bolo alimentar da língua para a faringe e é facilitada pelos movimentos musculares da língua, da mandíbula e do músculo hioide. A *fase faríngea* começa com o bolo alimentar alcançando as amígdalas, a elevação do palato mole para evitar que o bolo entre na nasofaringe, a elevação e o movimento para a frente da laringe e hioide, a retroflexão da epiglote e o fechamento das pregas vocais para impedir a entrada na laringe. Então, há contração sincronizada dos músculos constritores médio e inferior da faringe, juntamente ao relaxamento do músculo cricofaríngeo, que constitui grande parte do esfíncter esofágico superior (EES). Isso permite a passagem do bolo alimentar para o esôfago (Figura 273.1). A respiração é interrompida brevemente (momento de apneia).[2] A sincronia entre a constrição dos músculos da faringe e o relaxamento do músculo cricofaríngeo é essencial para permitir a passagem do bolo alimentar para o esôfago.

Anormalidades da fase faríngea incluem fraqueza faríngea devido a neuropatias ou miopatias, tumores ou corpos estranhos na faringe e obstrução do EES secundária à hipertrofia do músculo cricofaríngeo.

Apesar das inúmeras causas de DOF, os resultados fisiopatológico finais caem em uma de duas categorias interrelacionadas: (1) anormalidades da transferência de bolo ou (2) anormalidades de proteção das vias respiratórias. As anormalidades da transferência do bolo podem ser agrupadas posteriormente naquelas causadas por (a) falha da bomba orofaríngea (fraqueza

Boxe 273.1 Causas de disfagia orofaríngea e esofágica em cães

Sistema nervoso central (SNC)
Acidente vascular encefálico (AVE)
Tumor de tronco encefálico

Iatrogênica
Anti-histamínicos
Anticolinérgicos
Fenotiazinas
Quimioterapia
Pós-cirúrgico muscular ou neurogênico
Radiação
Ingestão de uma substância corrosiva
Antibióticos (clindamicina, doxiciclina)
Medicamentos anti-inflamatórios não esteroidais

Infecciosa/inflamatória
Esofagite
Botulismo
Tétano
Candidíase
Raiva
Abscesso
Infecção por calicivírus (gatos)
Infecção pelo vírus da rinotraqueíte (gatos)

Metabólica
Hiperadrenocorticismo
Hipoadrenocorticismo
Hipotireoidismo (não é uma causa importante em cães)
Miopatia associada à tireotoxicose (humanos)

Miopática/neuropática
Neuropatias periféricas
Miopatias inflamatórias (infecciosas, imunomediadas, pré-neoplásico)
Dermatomiosite
Distrofias musculares
Miastenia *gravis*
Megaesôfago

Estrutural
Neoplasia orofaríngea ou esofágica
Barra cricofaríngea
Teias esofágicas proximais
Tumores esofágicos
Estenose esofágica
Fístula esofágica
Divertículo esofágico
Anomalia de anel vascular
Corpo estranho
Anomalia congênita (fenda palatina, divertículo)
Hérnia de hiato
Refluxo gastresofágico
Intussuscepção gastresofágica

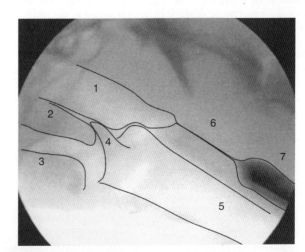

Figura 273.1 Visão fluoroscópica lateral normal da faringe em repouso. Observe que a radiopacidade é revertida nas imagens de fluoroscopia comparadas com imagens radiográficas convencionais (ou seja, o ar é branco, o osso é preto). *1*, nasofaringe; *2*, palato mole; *3*, base da língua; *4*, epiglote; *5*, traqueia; *6*, esfíncter esofágico superior (EES); *7*, esôfago proximal com bário no lúmen. (De Pollard RE, Marks SL, Davidson A et al.: *Quantitative videofluoroscopic evaluation of pharyngeal function in the dog. Vet Radiol Ultrasound* 41[5]:409-412, 2000.)

SEÇÃO 18 • Doença Gastrintestinal

faríngea); (b) assincronia orofaríngea e faringo-EES (neuropatias); e (c) obstrução do fluxo faríngeo (acalasia cricofaríngea, tumores da faringe, corpos estranhos).

Fase esofágica

A *fase esofágica* é involuntária, começando com o relaxamento do EES e o movimento do bolo alimentar no esôfago. O feedback sensorial provavelmente desempenha um papel importante na regulação da velocidade e na intensidade das ondas peristálticas, dependendo das características do bolo alimentar. O peristaltismo induzido pela deglutição é o peristaltismo primário. O peristaltismo secundário ocorre em resposta à distensão do lúmen esofágico por um bolo que falhou em ser impulsionado para o estômago. O relaxamento do EES antes das pressões propagadas permite que o alimento seja esvaziado no estômago, e, uma vez que o bolo alimentar passa, o EES se contrai para evitar o refluxo do conteúdo gástrico para o esôfago.

ABORDAGEM DIAGNÓSTICA

Sinais

O diagnóstico de doenças que afetam a fase orofaríngea da deglutição pode ser extremamente desafiador. Histórias de deglutição repetitiva, engasgo e náuseas associadas a refeições, regurgitação nasal nas refeições, tosse relacionada à deglutição, comida caindo da boca durante a deglutição e pneumonia recorrente devem causar suspeita de DOF (Figura 273.2). A DOF pode causar apneia transitória e síncope em alguns cães. Em contraste, os animais com disfagia esofágica são tipicamente mais fáceis de diagnosticar, embora alguns tenham doenças da faringe e do esôfago associadas. Os sinais típicos de disfagia esofágica incluem regurgitação (sólidos ou líquidos), odinofagia (dor ao engolir), tentativas repetidas de engolir e salivação excessiva. A regurgitação é o sinal mais consistente de doença esofágica e deve ser diferenciada dos sinais de DOF ou vômito. Doença faríngea ou esofágica pode ser parte de uma doença sistêmica em animais que manifesta apenas sinais de disfagia, ressaltando a importância de uma avaliação sistêmica abrangente. A avaliação de cães e gatos com sinais de disfagia faríngea ou esofágica inclui uma revisão dos sinais clínicos, história de medicação e questionário sobre qualquer anestesia recente (Boxe 273.2). Exames físicos (avaliação da pré-alimentação) e neurológicos e avaliação de exames laboratoriais são valiosos antes de observar a deglutição e usar estudos de imagem e avaliações endoscópicas.

Sinais clínicos

As causas de DOF em cães filhotes incluem fenda palatina, disfagia cricofaríngea, distrofia muscular e fraqueza faríngea. Raças com predisposição hereditária ou alta incidência de DOF

Boxe 273.2 Avaliação do animal disfágico com base no histórico

Idade de início?
Início repentino ou início gradual?
Disfagia durante ou entre as refeições?
Dificuldade com sólidos, líquidos ou ambos?
Disfagia intermitente ou progressiva?
Padrão temporal da disfagia (a disfagia orofaríngea ocorre segundos após a deglutição)
História de tosse?
História da administração de medicamentos?
História de disfonia?
Anestesia geral recente?
Histórico de odinofagia?

---

incluem o Golden Retriever (fraqueza da faringe),[3] Cocker e Springer Spaniels (disfagia cricofaríngea), Bouvier des Flandres e Cavalier King Charles Spaniel (distrofia muscular),[4] Boxer e Terra-nova (miopatia inflamatória). Cães de raças grandes são predispostos a distúrbios da musculatura mastigatória. Uma predisposição familiar para megaesôfago congênito foi sugerida nas raças Dogue Alemão, Pastor-Alemão, Labrador Retriever, Setter Irlandês, Shar-pei, Terra-nova, Schnauzer Miniatura e Fox Terrier.[5] O megaesôfago congênito é raro em gatos, embora os siameses sejam predispostos. Megaesôfago idiopático adquirido é mais comum em cães de raças grandes.

Exame físico e neurológico

O exame físico do animal disfágico inclui cuidadosa avaliação da orofaringe, usando sedação ou anestesia se necessárias, para ajudar a descartar doenças dentárias, corpos estranhos, fenda palatina, anormalidades glossais e tumores orofaríngeos. A faringe e o pescoço devem ser palpados cuidadosamente em busca de massas, assimetria ou dor, e o tórax, auscultado cuidadosamente por evidências de pneumonia aspirativa. A avaliação de nervos cranianos deve incluir avaliação da língua, do tônus da mandíbula e da habilidade para abduzir as cartilagens aritenoides com a inspiração. Exames físicos (ver Capítulo 2) e neurológicos (ver Capítulo 259) completos podem revelar evidências de um distúrbio neuromuscular generalizado: atrofia muscular, rigidez e reflexos espinais diminuídos ou ausentes. O reflexo de engasgo deve ser avaliado colocando um dedo na faringe; no entanto, a presença ou ausência desse reflexo não indica eficácia da deglutição faríngea, nem proteção deglutiva adequada das vias respiratórias.[6]

Observação da alimentação e ingestão de líquidos

A importância de observar cuidadosamente o animal disfágico enquanto come (ração e comida enlatada) e bebe não pode ser supervalorizada. As observações ajudam a localizar o problema, caso esteja na cavidade oral, na faringe ou no esôfago. Cães com uma fase oral anormal da deglutição em geral tem dificuldade com a preensão ou o transporte aboral do bolo alimentar para a base da língua, o que muitas vezes pode ser diagnosticado a partir da observação dos animais comendo. DOFs que afetam a fase faríngea da deglutição podem ser um desafio diagnóstico. Esses casos costumam apresentar sinais não específicos: engasgo, ânsia de vômito e múltiplas tentativas de deglutição antes que um bolo seja movido com sucesso para o esôfago proximal (Vídeo 273.1). Esses animais de companhia costumam ter um transporte anormal do bolo alimentar da orofaringe para a hipofaringe ou da hipofaringe para o esôfago proximal. A disfagia cricofaríngea, com sinais semelhantes aos observados nos distúrbios da faringe, causa transporte anormal do bolo alimentar através do EES. Cães com megaesôfago, estenoses esofágicas ou esofagite podem exibir evidências de odinofagia e regurgitação segundos a minutos após a ingestão do bolo alimentar.

Avaliação laboratorial

Testes laboratoriais abrangentes são justificados em animais com DOF e disfagia esofágica para fornecer um mínimo conjunto de dados neuromusculares. Os testes devem conter um hemograma completo, painel bioquímico sérico (incluindo concentrações de creatinina quinase [CK] e eletrólitos), urinálise, avaliação da função tireoidiana (ver Capítulo 299) e título de anticorpo antirreceptor da acetilcolina (AChR) para miastenia gravis adquirida (ver Capítulo 269). Concentrações de CK persistentemente elevadas (2.000 a 20.000 UI/ℓ) podem indicar miosite generalizada, enquanto aumento marcante de CK (superior a 20.000 UI/ℓ) são mais sugestivos de miopatia necrosante ou distrófica (ver Capítulo 354). Uma concentração normal de CK não exclui miopatia, particularmente quando focal (miosite do músculo mastigatório; ver Capítulo 272) ou crônica. A miastenia *gravis* adquirida é uma importante causa neuromuscular de

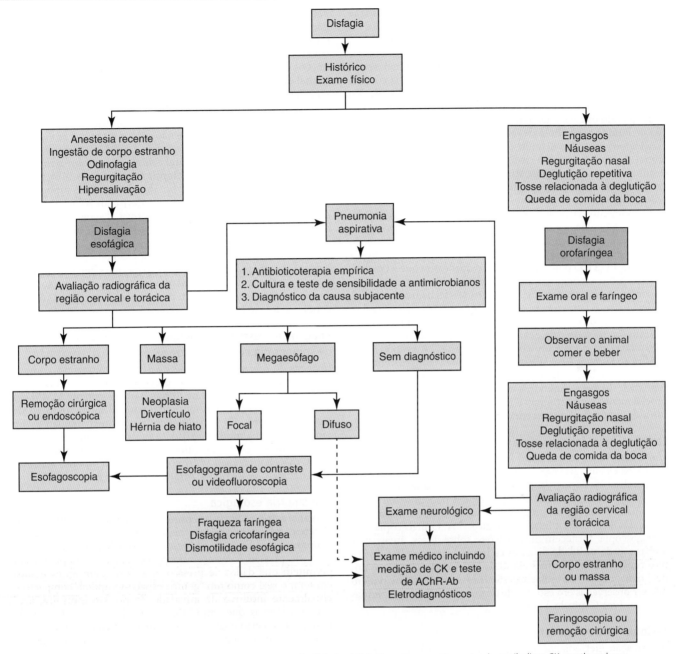

Figura 273.2 Algoritmo para ajudar a determinar a causa da disfagia. *AChR-Ab*, anticorpo antirreceptor da acetilcolina; *CK*, creatinoquinase.

DOF, provocando fraqueza de faringe e esôfago e/ou laringe sem fraqueza muscular clinicamente detectável nas extremidades. Fraqueza faríngea como o único sinal clínico de miastenia *gravis* foi descrita em 1% dos cães afetados.[7] O teste de AChR deve ser realizado em todos os animais de estimação com disfagia adquirida. O padrão-ouro para o diagnóstico da miastenia *gravis* adquirida continua sendo a demonstração de autoanticorpos séricos contra o receptor nativo AChR por radioimunoensaio de imunoprecipitação. Individualmente, os níveis de anticorpos AChR se correlacionam com a gravidade da doença, mas os níveis de anticorpos entre os pacientes são altamente variáveis e não se correlacionam bem com a gravidade. Esse teste não é útil para disfagia congênita em que uma base imunológica é improvável.

Radiografia cervical e torácica

A faringe de animais saudáveis é preenchida com ar e facilmente vista em radiografias. O tamanho do espaço preenchido de ar pode diminuir por causa de uma inflamação/edema, uma neoplasia ou um alongamento do palato mole e aumentar com disfunção da faringe ou do EES, doença respiratória crônica (inspiratória) ou megaesôfago grave crônico. O esôfago normal não é visível nas radiografias, exceto após aerofagia, devido a excitação, náuseas, dispneia ou anestesia.

Estudo videofluoroscópico da deglutição

A videofluoroscopia de contraste envolve imagens em tempo real do animal engolindo bário líquido ou ração embebida em bário e é um dos procedimentos mais importantes para avaliar a integridade funcional do reflexo da deglutição (ver Figuras 273.1 e 273.2). Os estudos fluoroscópicos da deglutição geralmente envolvem a avaliação de cinco deglutições de 5 a 10 mℓ de bário líquido (60% peso/volume), cinco deglutições de comida enlatada e cinco deglutições de ração embebida em bário. A videofluoroscopia é usada para determinar a sequência de eventos que compõem uma deglutição e para cronometrar esses eventos, comparando uns aos outros. O movimento de certas estruturas anatômicas pode ser medido a partir de um ponto fixo para avaliar melhor a função. Eventos de deglutição que ocorram fora da sequência, em momentos inadequados ou com redução do vigor podem causar morbidade significativa.

O posicionamento não é padronizado para a videofluoroscopia. Alterações na posição corporal (decúbito esternal *versus* lateral) não parecem afetar a medição da proporção da constrição faríngea ou o tempo de deglutição em cães saudáveis. No entanto, o trânsito esofágico cervical é significativamente retardado quando os cães estão em decúbito lateral.[8] Assim, a retenção de líquido ou de bolo de ração no esôfago cervical não seria considerada anormal quando cães doentes estão em decúbito lateral durante a imagem. Estudos de deglutição em cães em decúbito esternal são significativamente mais propensos a resultar na geração de ondas peristálticas primárias para bolo de ração e líquidos.

O momento da deglutição pode ser determinado facilmente quando o vídeo é visto quadro a quadro, com cada quadro representando 1/30 de segundo do sistema do Comitê Nacional do Sistema de Televisão (NTSC – sistema de televisão analógica usado nos EUA). O ponto de partida é o quadro em que a epiglote se fecha sobre a laringe. Os quadros são contados até a observação da contração faríngea máxima e da abertura e fechamento do EES. A deglutição é considerada completa quando a epiglote reabre geralmente após cinco ou seis quadros em cães saudáveis.[9] Foi descrito um método para quantificar a contratilidade faríngea em cães através de videofluoroscopia de contraste.[10] A proporção de constrição faríngea é calculada dividindo a área faríngea contraída ao máximo pela área faríngea em repouso. À medida que a contratilidade faríngea diminui, a relação se aproxima de 1.[10] Esse procedimento simples fornece informações importantes sobre a força da contração faríngea em cães disfágicos.

Laringoscopia, faringoscopia e esofagoscopia

Um exame laríngeo completo (ver Capítulo 239) é importante em todos os animais com DOF e disfagia esofágica para descartar paralisia da laringe associada a polineuropatia (ver Capítulo 268). Cães geriátricos de raças grandes podem desenvolver neuropatia generalizada progressiva com fraqueza faríngea associada, DOF e dismotilidade esofágica.[11] A faringoscopia e a esofagoscopia fornecem informações sobre essas áreas, mas ambas são de utilidade diagnóstica limitada para avaliar distúrbios funcionais em animais anestesiados. A esofagoscopia é útil para o diagnóstico de esofagite, estenoses esofágicas (que podem não ser observadas em estudos de deglutição de bário) e hérnias de hiato (ver Capítulo 113).

Teste de eletrodiagnóstico

A avaliação eletrodiagnóstica, incluindo a eletromiografia e a medição da velocidade de condução nervosa motora e sensorial, não fornece um diagnóstico específico na maioria dos casos, mas pode fornecer informações importantes quanto à gravidade, à distribuição e ao caráter de um processo de doença miopática ou neuropática e auxiliar na seleção do local anatômico ideal para uma biopsia (ver Capítulo 117). Os testes de eletrodiagnóstico devem incluir os músculos da faringe e a língua. O estado de saúde deve ser considerado, porque esses procedimentos são realizados sob anestesia geral.

Biopsias de músculos e nervos

Biopsias de músculos e nervos geralmente são essenciais para alcançar um diagnóstico específico (ver Capítulo 116). As biopsias musculares devem ser coletadas precocemente no decorrer de uma avaliação em animais com suspeita de doença neuromuscular, antes que a fibrose e a perda de fibras musculares se tornem extensas, mas após o resultado sérico negativo do título do anticorpo AChR ser obtido. Se o início dos sinais clínicos for recente e o título de anticorpos for de 0,3 a 0,6 nmoL/ℓ, um novo teste após 4 a 6 semanas pode ser de valor, pois um número significativo de cães com os primeiros sinais clínicos

pode ter títulos de anticorpos na "zona cinzenta" durante o teste inicial. Em cães com suspeita de doença miopática, biopsias musculares são geralmente obtidas de músculos grandes (o vasto lateral ou tríceps). Biopsias da faringe e dos músculos cricofaríngeos devem ser obtidas em cães com DOF.[12] O fino músculo frontal encontra-se diretamente sob a pele e é comum ser biopsiado em vez do músculo temporal em cães com suspeita de miosite muscular mastigatória (MMM; ver Capítulo 272). O músculo frontal não é afetado em uma MMM e, se biopsiado por engano, o diagnóstico pode não ser corretamente realizado.[12] Faça uma incisão e retraia o músculo frontal e a fáscia espessa, que se encontra abaixo do frontal e diretamente sobre o músculo temporal para expô-lo para a biopsia (ver Capítulo 116). Enrole os espécimes do músculo (0,5 × 0,5 × 1,0 cm) em esponjas de gaze umedecidas (não muito molhadas) com solução salina e coloque em um contêiner seco à prova d'água, mantendo-o refrigerado até o envio. Um segundo espécime de biopsia menor próximo a biopsia original deve ser colocado em formalina tamponada a 10%. Todos os espécimes são enviados em embalagens refrigeradas durante a noite, para que cheguem ao laboratório dentro de 24 a 36 horas após a coleta (ver Capítulo 354). As biopsias musculares devem permanecer frias para otimizar a condição dos espécimes.

Imagens de ressonância magnética e varreduras de tomografia computadorizada

Imagens de ressonância magnética (RM) e tomografia computadorizada (TC) de cabeça e pescoço têm sido usadas para diagnosticar miopatias inflamatórias, particularmente MMM em cães.[13] As imagens podem ser usadas para selecionar os locais de biopsia muscular. Os achados comuns incluem mudanças no tamanho (atrofia ou inchaço) de todos os músculos mastigatórios, exceto o digástrico, e aumento de contraste predominantemente não homogêneo visto nos músculos temporal, masseter e pterigoide.[13] A RM pode também detectar neoplasias.

Manometria esofágica

A manometria esofágica permite que a pressão no lúmen esofágico e esfíncteres sejam medidos para avaliar a atividade neuromuscular. Envolve alta resolução (HRM), com até 36 sensores de pressão.[14] Avanços no processamento computacional permitem que dados de pressão objetivos sejam apresentados em tempo real como um "gráfico espaço-temporal" compacto e visualmente intuitivo de atividade de pressão esofágica, avaliando as forças que impulsionam os alimentos e fluidos da faringe para o estômago. Esse teste diagnóstico pode ser empregado em cães totalmente acordados e fornece uma avaliação funcional sensível do EES, do esôfago e do EEI.[14]

Teste de pH/impedância esofágica

O teste de pH/impedância esofágico é usado para avaliar o refluxo ácido e não ácido em animais com suspeita de RGE troesofágico (RGE), esofagite inexplicada ou hérnias de hiato. Os clínicos têm várias opções ao selecionar as sondas de pH esofágico. O Sistema Bravo de Monitoramento de pH sem cateter (Sistema de Teste de Refluxo Bravo™) da Medtronic é o primeiro sistema sem cateter usado para medir o pH esofágico em pessoas com suspeita de RGE. Esse é um teste de pH esofágico revolucionário, pois permite que as pessoas mantenham sua dieta e atividades durante o mesmo. O sistema é uma alternativa ao tradicional cateter transnasal de pH, que pode causar desconforto e é facilmente deslocado em cachorros e gatos. A principal desvantagem do Sistema Bravo é que ele apenas registra o pH esofágico e não utiliza tecnologia de impedância que permitiria uma medição mais precisa de eventos de refluxo ácido e não ácido. O teste de pH esofágico tem sido utilizado em cães acordados e anestesiados em um esforço para identificar fatores de risco para RGE e/ou os efeitos de agentes procinéticos no RGE.[15,16]

DOENÇAS DA FARINGE

Faringite

Anatomia, causas e sinais

A faringe é dividida em três regiões: nasofaringe, orofaringe e laringofaringe. As manifestações clínicas de inflamações variam de acordo com sua localização e sua extensão, além da etiologia e do envolvimento de estruturas adjacentes. A inflamação faríngea pode ocorrer devido a corpos estranhos, massas obstrutivas (pólipos nasofaríngeos, linfoma, carcinoma de células escamosas), doença infecciosa, ingestão de substâncias cáusticas ou irritantes e como uma extensão da estomatite, rinite ou sinusite. As manifestações clínicas mais comuns incluem disfonia, ronco, engasgo, tosse, disfagia, hiporexia e hipersalivação. Amigdalite é frequentemente reconhecida em associação com faringite.

Diagnóstico e tratamento

Histórico e exame oral são em geral suficientes para confirmar o diagnóstico, embora um exame oral abrangente sob sedação ou rinoscopia com nasofaringoscopia retrógrada possa ser necessário em casos selecionados. A avaliação por meio de radiografias da região cervical pode ser pouco efetiva, a menos que um corpo estranho radiodenso ou uma faringite secundária a doença extrafaríngea esteja presente. A remoção ou o tratamento da causa primária é essencial. Analgésicos, enxágue/lavagem com antimicrobianos tópicos, antimicrobianos sistêmicos, hidratação e nutrição de suporte são importantes. Pólipos inflamatórios nasofaríngeos em gatos com bula timpânica normal podem ser removidos por avulsão por tração. É possível tratar a estenose nasofaríngea por dilatação por balão sob anestesia geral.

Fraqueza faríngea

Anatomia, causas e sinais

Uma falha de bombeamento orofaríngeo, chamada de fraqueza da faringe, é uma interrupção no transporte coordenado de alimento e água da orofaringe para a hipofaringe ou da hipofaringe para o esôfago. A fraqueza de faringe pode ocorrer secundária a anormalidades morfológicas (infecção, inflamação, trauma, neoplasia, obstrução do EES [acalasia cricofaríngea]) ou por causas funcionais (doença neuromuscular). Doenças neuromusculares específicas que devem ser consideradas incluem miastenia *gravis*, distrofia muscular, polimiosite, hipotireoidismo e neuropatia de nervo craniano. Os sinais clínicos geralmente incluem disfonia, engasgo, disfagia, tentativas repetidas de engolir um único bolo alimentar e tosse.

Diagnóstico e tratamento

Radiografias torácica e cervical devem ser obtidas em todos os cães antes de completar um estudo videofluoroscópico da deglutição. A fluoroscopia pode demonstrar ausência de contração aboral da faringe, transporte incompleto do bolo e refluxo nasofaríngeo ocasional de bário. Esse exame é fundamental para diferenciar a fraqueza de faringe da disfagia cricofaríngea. Uma avaliação sistêmica (nível de CK, título de anticorpo AChR, teste de hormônio da tireoide, eletrodiagnósticos) é um esforço necessário para descartar uma doença sistêmica, uma neuropatia ou uma miopatia subjacente (ver Figuras 273.2 e 273.3). A terapia da fraqueza de faringe secundária à doença neuromuscular subjacente é principalmente paliativa, sobretudo quando uma causa subjacente não pode ser identificada, e inclui suporte nutricional enteral, alterações na dieta e consistência da água e alimentação

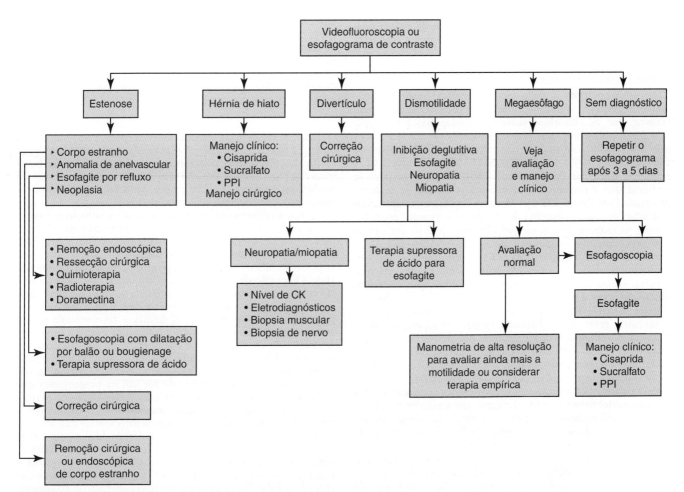

Figura 273.3 Algoritmo para auxiliar na determinação das considerações diagnósticas e terapêuticas para os achados videofluoroscópicos mais comuns em cães disfágicos. *CK*, creatinoquinase; *PPI*, inibidor da bomba de próton.

com elevação. Cães com miastenia *gravis* devem ser tratados com inibidores da acetilcolinesterase (p. ex., piridostigmina, 1 a 3 mg/kg PO a cada 8 a 12 horas). Glicocorticoides (p. ex., 1 a 2 mg/kg de prednisolona ou equivalente PO a cada 12 horas, com redução gradual ao longo de 10 a 12 semanas dependendo da resposta) ou ciclosporina (5 mg/kg PO a cada 12 a 24 horas por 10 a 12 semanas) são utilizados para gerenciar as polimiopatias inflamatórias (ver Capítulos 354 e 360), e a terapia de reposição tireoidiana deve ser tentada em animais com hipotireoidismo documentado (ver Capítulo 299).

DOENÇAS DO ESÔFAGO

Disfagia cricofaríngea

Definição e sinais clínicos

A disfagia cricofaríngea é um distúrbio neuromuscular congênito ou adquirido do EES, caracterizado por falha de seu relaxamento (acalasia) ou uma falta de coordenação entre seu relaxamento e a contração faríngea (assincronia). Os cães afetados têm transporte anormal do bolo alimentar da hipofaringe para a região proximal do esôfago. A assincronia cricofaríngea é essencialmente um "problema de bombeamento", onde os músculos fracos da faringe são incapazes de impulsionar o bolo alimentar através do EES. A etiologia de nenhuma condição é determinada, embora estudos preliminares deem suporte para uma neuropatia focal subjacente. Os animais afetados demonstram disfagia progressiva (geralmente pior quando bebem água) no momento do desmame ou logo após. Os sinais clínicos sinais são caracterizados por repetidas tentativas de engolir, engasgo, ânsia de vômito e regurgitação nasal (ver Vídeo 273.1). Os sinais clínicos de cães com acalasia são indistinguíveis da assincronia. O exame físico pode revelar evidências de pneumonia aspirativa (tosse, estertores úmidos à ausculta, febre).

Diagnóstico e tratamento

Cães com suspeita de disfagia cricofaríngea devem ser cuidadosamente avaliados antes de uma intervenção cirúrgica, para garantir que os distúrbios sistêmicos (miopatias [ver Capítulo 354], polineuropatias [ver Capítulo 259 e 268]) tenham sido descartados com titulação de anticorpos AChR e níveis de CK (ver Capítulo 66), eletromiografia (EMG; ver Capítulo 117) e biopsia muscular (ver Capítulo 116). Além disso, deve-se certificar que a pneumonia aspirativa seja tratada de maneira adequada (ver Figura 273.1).[17] Radiografias torácicas ajudam a descartar as causas estruturais da disfagia (corpo estranho, massa); no entanto, um estudo videofluoroscópico da deglutição é o procedimento diagnóstico de escolha (Vídeo 273.2). A maioria dos cães afetados com acalasia cricofaríngea tem um músculo cricofaríngeo espessado proeminente ("barra" cricofaríngea), visível na videofluoroscopia ou endoscopia, causando obstrução grave à propulsão do bolo alimentar através do EES (Figura 273.4). Radiografias estáticas de contraste podem demonstrar retenção de bário na faringe ou aspiração para a traqueia; no entanto, estudos estáticos não permitem a integridade funcional do EES ou a avaliação da contração coordenada da faringe e relaxamento do EES.

O tratamento definitivo para acalasia cricofaríngea envolve miotomia cirúrgica ou miectomia do músculo cricofaríngeo. Os músculos cricofaríngeos e tireofaríngeos são acessados pela linha média ventral padrão com 180° de rotação da laringe em seu eixo longitudinal ou por abordagem via lateral com rotação de 90° da laringe.[18] A miotomia cricofaríngea envolve a secção do músculo cricofaríngeo ao nível da mucosa faríngea. Uma miotomia cricofaríngea endoscópica fechada com *laser* de CO$_2$ vem sendo cada vez mais utilizada em pessoas e cães, com tempo de anestesia e morbidade reduzidos em comparação com a miotomia cricofaríngea transcervical mais tradicional.[19]

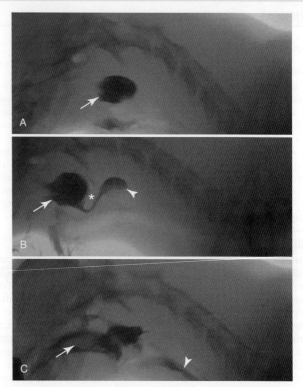

Figura 273.4 Estudo fluoroscópico da deglutição em um filhote fêmea castrada de 7 meses de idade da raça Dachshund miniatura com disfagia secundária grave à acalasia cricofaríngea. **A.** A faringe (*seta*) é preenchida com bário líquido. **B.** O músculo cricofaríngeo hipertrofiado ("barra" cricofaríngea) (*asterisco*) obstrui o movimento do bolo alimentar da faringe (*seta*) para o esôfago proximal (*ponta de seta*). Observe a coluna atenuada de bário sendo espremida através da abertura estreita do EES. **C.** O movimento retrógrado do bário líquido na orofaringe (*seta*) é causado pela obstrução do esfíncter esofágico proximal e subsequente aspiração de bário na traqueia (*ponta de seta*). (De Marks SL: Oropharyngeal dysphagia. In Bonagura JD, Twedt DC: *Kirk's current veterinary therapy XV*, St. Louis, 2014, Saunders.)

Existem evidências menos convincentes para miectomia cirúrgica em cães com assincronia cricofaríngea; no entanto, um relato descreveu uma miectomia cricofaríngea bilateral bem-sucedida para manejar um cão sem raça definida de 8 meses de idade com assincronia cricofaríngea, após falha inicial de uma miectomia cricofaríngea unilateral padrão.[20]

Um procedimento menos invasivo para a resolução temporária de acalasia cricofaríngea envolve a injeção de toxina botulínica no músculo cricofaríngeo.[21] A toxina botulínica A (BTA), uma neurotoxina sintetizada pelo bacilo *Clostridium botulinum*, atua nos terminais nervosos colinérgicos pré-sinápticos bloqueando a liberação de acetilcolina. De um modo dose-dependente, ela enfraquece a contração ao ser injetada no músculo alvo e tem sido usada com sucesso em pessoas e cães para o manejo temporário da acalasia esofágica. A toxina é reconstituída pouco antes da injeção com 0,9% de solução salina estéril a uma concentração de 25 unidades/mℓ e é injetada no músculo cricofaríngeo em 3 locais (10 unidades por local), usando uma agulha transbrônquica. A duração limitada do efeito da toxina botulínica (cerca de 3 a 4 meses) pode ser útil na triagem cães que conseguem se beneficiar de uma miectomia cirúrgica permanente, porque os animais que respondem favoravelmente à toxina devem também se beneficiar da miectomia cirúrgica. Um esforço para identificar a melhor consistência do alimento e água (adicionando espessantes alimentares comerciais, como o *Thick-It*) para esses cães pode ser útil. Alguns sucumbem a episódios repetidos de pneumonia aspirativa e desnutrição. A alimentação enteral via tubo PEG é um método viável alternativo; no entanto, podem ocorrer aspiração silenciosa e pneumonia, apesar do advento dos dispositivos de alimentação enteral.

Esofagite

Anatomia, causas e sinais clínicos

A esofagite é uma doença aguda ou distúrbio inflamatório crônico da mucosa esofágica que ocasionalmente envolve a submucosa subjacente e a muscular da mucosa. Existem diversas causas, incluindo ingestão de agentes cáusticos, vômito crônico, corpos estranhos esofágicos, tubos de alimentação nasoesofágicos ou de esofagostomia fragilizados e refluxo gastresofágico associado a anestesia geral ou hérnia de hiato. Doxiciclina e clindamicina administradas por via oral podem causar esofagite "induzida por medicação", particularmente em gatos.[22] Um refluxo gastesofágico durante a anestesia é precedido pelo desenvolvimento de uma estenose esofágica benigna em 46 a 65% dos casos e representa a causa mais comum de esofagite de alto grau e formação de estenose em cães.[23] O relaxamento do EEI é mediado por vias não adrenérgicas não colinérgicas e demonstrou ocorrer com a administração de pré-anestésico injetável e agentes anestésicos inalantes de utilização comum.[24,25] A exposição prolongada da mucosa esofágica a ácidos é uma causa importante de esofagite e uma possível formação de estenose, particularmente quando o pH é inferior a 4,0, já que o pH para a conversão proteolítica do pepsinogênio em pepsina está dentro da faixa do 1,5 e 3,5.[26] Além disso, a esofagite diminui o tônus do EEI, o que leva a mais refluxo e inflamação da mucosa. Distúrbios na motilidade do esôfago podem ocorrer como uma sequela de esofagite, independentemente da causa. Os sinais clínicos dependem da gravidade da inflamação, extensão do envolvimento esofágico e tipo de lesão. Animais com inflamação leve podem não exibir sinais clínicos, enquanto os com esofagite moderada a grave podem apresentar sinais de anorexia, disfagia, odinofagia, regurgitação e hipersalivação. A tosse pode ser observada com pneumonia aspirativa concomitante.

Diagnóstico e tratamento

Resultados de hemograma completo, de bioquímica sérica e de urinálise são geralmente normais, e o esôfago parece normal nas radiografias torácicas. A pneumonia aspirativa pode ser evidente nas áreas dependentes do pulmão. A dilatação esofágica segmentar ou difusa pode ser vista com inflamação grave da mucosa. A videofluoroscopia consegue confirmar uma superfície esofágica irregular, dismotilidade esofágica (Vídeo 273.3) ou formação de estenose (ver Figura 273.3). O diagnóstico definitivo da esofagite requer endoscopia e biopsia esofágica; no entanto, o diagnóstico presuntivo é frequentemente feito a partir da aparência da mucosa esofágica: eritema e superfície granular com áreas de ulceração e sangramento ativo (Figura 273.5). Uma esofagite leve pode aparecer normal no exame endoscópico; portanto, a biopsia da mucosa é necessária para confirmar o diagnóstico. As lesões são geralmente mais evidentes no esôfago distal e adjacente, além do EEI.

A esofagite discreta geralmente se resolve com tratamento mínimo, além de uma alimentação em refeições menores e mais frequentes, com restrição de gordura, para aumentar o esvaziamento gástrico e minimizar o RGE. Animais com esofagite moderada a grave ou aqueles exibindo sinais de disfagia, regurgitação, salivação ou anorexia devem ser tratados com supressores de ácido gástrico e procinéticos. Os benefícios dos inibidores da bomba de prótons (PPI), como o omeprazol em pessoas com RGE moderado a grave, são documentados, e vários estudos têm mostrado o efeito supressor de ácido superior dos PPI em comparação com os antagonistas do receptor H2 (famotidina, ranitidina).[27,28] Os PPI são administrados por via oral ou IV (1 a 1,5 mg/kg a cada 12 horas) e devem ser gradualmente reduzidos ao longo de 7 a 10 dias, se usados por mais de 2 semanas. O sucralfato, um medicamento que atua como barreira de difusão, pode ser administrado como uma suspensão (0,5 a 1 g PO, 3 vezes/dia) para o manejo da esofagite de refluxo. Ele se liga à mucosa erodida e fornece uma barreira eficaz de proteção contra os conteúdos do refluxo. Agentes procinéticos, tais como cisaprida (0,5 mg/kg PO a cada 8 a 12 horas) ou metoclopramida (0,2 a 0,4 mg/kg SC ou IV, como uma injeção em bolo a cada 8 horas, ou 1 a 2 mg/kg/24 horas em infusão contínua [CRI]), podem ser usados para aumentar a pressão EEI e melhorar o esvaziamento gástrico. A cisaprida é um procinético mais potente do que a metoclopramida e é mais eficaz na redução do RGE em cães.[14] Antibióticos de amplo espectro são recomendados para animais com pneumonia aspirativa (ver Capítulo 242). A duração da terapia diverge de acordo com a gravidade da esofagite e dos sinais clínicos, mas varia entre 5 e 7 dias (casos leves) e 2 a 3 semanas (esofagite moderada a grave). Uma combinação de cisaprida, sucralfato e omeprazol é eficaz para o tratamento de esofagite grave causada por vômito persistente, RGE ou trauma induzido por corpo estranho.

Estenose esofágica

Definição, anatomia e sinais clínicos

A estenose esofágica, um estreitamento anormal do lúmen esofágico, é mais comumente causada por RGE durante anestesia geral, lesão química por ingestão de substâncias, corpos estranhos esofágicos, cirurgia esofágica e lesões de massas intra ou extraluminais (neoplasia ou abscesso). Os gatos são particularmente suscetíveis a esofagite associada à doxiciclina e à clindamicina e estenose esofágica subsequente.[22] O RGE durante anestesia geral foi relatado como precedendo a estenose em até 65% dos casos. Os sinais clínicos são observados cerca de 7 a 8 dias após a anestesia.[29] A incidência de RGE em cães durante a anestesia varia de 16 a 55% e ocorre de modo secundário a uma diminuição na pressão do EEI induzida por uma variedade de agentes anestésicos, incluindo atropina, morfina, acepromazina, tiopentol, xilazina e isoflurano.[24,25] Danos à camada muscular da mucosa do esôfago estão associados à proliferação fibroblástica e contração, levando à formação da estenose. Os sinais clínicos (regurgitação progressiva e disfagia) estão relacionados com a gravidade e a extensão da estenose. Os primeiros sinais clínicos podem incluir um sutil "engolir em seco" por alguns dias, que é facilmente esquecido pelos tutores. Os sinais clínicos progressivos incluem disfagia, odinofagia, regurgitação, salivação, anorexia, tosse e perda de peso.

Diagnóstico e tratamento de dilatação

O diagnóstico de estenose esofágica é frequentemente sugerido pelo histórico e confirmado com radiografias de contraste usando bário líquido ou bário misturado com ração enlatada (esofagograma) ou via análise videofluoroscópica da deglutição (ver Figura 273.2). As radiografias de contraste são úteis para

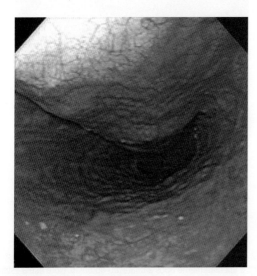

Figura 273.5 Esofagite grave caracterizada por eritema grave, ulceração e mucosa granular em Labrador Retriever de 3 anos secundária a refluxo gastresofágico durante anestesia procedimento.

determinar o número, a localização e a extensão das estenoses. A esofagoscopia é o procedimento de diagnóstico definitivo; é útil para diferenciar estenoses benignas de malignas e facilita a dilatação por balão (Figura 273.6). A dilatação mecânica da estenose é melhor realizada usando a dilatação com balão ou bougienage. A vantagem teórica da dilatação do balão (Figura 273.7) é que as forças aplicadas à estenose são radiais, em contraste com as forças longitudinais aplicadas com o instrumento rígido de bougienage. No entanto, uma série de casos retrospectivos em 20 cães e 8 gatos com estenoses esofágicas benignas submetidos a tratamento de bougienage sugeriu que este procedimento foi seguro e eficaz para a maioria dos pacientes, com desfechos semelhantes à dilatação por balão.[30] Dilatadores de balão estão disponíveis em vários diâmetros (até 20 mm) e comprimentos (3 a 8 cm) e são feitos de um material plástico rígido que pode suportar uma pressão relativamente alta (até 147 psi). Eles são fabricados para passar pelo canal de biopsia do endoscópio ou ao lado do endoscópio com o uso de um fio-guia, que passa através do canal do endoscópio (ou com imagens de fluoroscopia) e avança além da estenose no estômago ou no esôfago caudal. O escopo é removido à medida que o fio-guia prossegue pelo canal, deixando assim o fio-guia perto de sua posição original. O cateter balão é então passado sobre o fio-guia (com o balão desinflado), até que esteja posicionado dentro da estenose. A posição do balão é visualizada através do endoscópio ou por fluoroscopia. Um dispositivo inflador com manômetro é conectado no balão, e a pressão é lentamente aumentada até a especificada pelo fabricante. O balão é mantido inflado por 60 a 90 segundos e então esvaziado. Pressões sequencialmente crescentes são aplicadas para dilatar a estenose em incrementos de 1 a 2 mm, sem causar ruptura ou sangramento excessivos (Figura 273.8). O procedimento é repetido 3 a 5 dias mais tarde, em um esforço para dilatar ao máximo a estenose.

Triancinolona transendoscópica

A administração transendoscópica de triancinolona na submucosa do local da estenose, usando uma abordagem de quatro quadrantes antes do procedimento de dilatação por balão, tem sido associada a uma redução na taxa de formação de novas estenoses.[31,32] Aproximadamente 2,5 mg de triancinolona por quadrante é injetada com uma agulha de aspiração transbrônquica, que pode ser aplicada pelo canal de biopsia do endoscópio. O esteroide é geralmente usado nos dois ou três primeiros procedimentos de dilatação. Mitomicina C tópica (5 mg de mitomicina C embebida em uma esponja de gaze colocada endoscopicamente no local da estenose por aproximadamente 5 minutos, e o local lavado com 60 mℓ de água após remoção da esponja) também se mostrou benéfica para prevenir nova estenose.[33] A terapia médica contínua é garantida após a dilatação por balão usando os mesmos medicamentos e modificações alimentares como as discutidas para esofagite.

Stents intraluminais

Os *stents* intraluminais podem ser usados com animais em que a dilatação do balão falhou ou aqueles com estenoses recorrentes (ver Capítulo 123).[34] Há disponíveis *stents* revestidos ou não com polipropileno para evitar o crescimento de tecido dentro deles. Os materiais disponíveis incluem Nitinol (níquel e titânio), Elgiloy (cobalto, níquel e cromo), aço inoxidável, plástico de poliéster/silicone ou biodegradável (p. ex., PDS). A seleção é baseada na localização da estenose, no comprimento e na necessidade de sua remoção. Uma vez implantados, os *stents* devem ser ancorados no lugar ou migram rapidamente para o

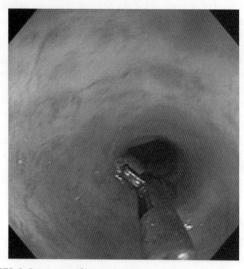

Figura 273.6 Estenose esofágica vista através do endoscópio antes da dilatação do balão. A distância entre as pontas das asas do fórceps de biopsia mede 5 mm e pode ser usada para medir o diâmetro da pequena estenose. (*Esta figura se encontra reproduzida, em cores, no Encarte.*)

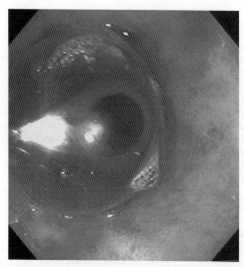

Figura 273.7 Dilatação por balão da estenose esofágica mostrada na Figura 273.6, utilizando um balão dilatador CRE que foi passou pelo lúmen da estenose antes da insuflação. (*Esta figura se encontra reproduzida, em cores, no Encarte.*)

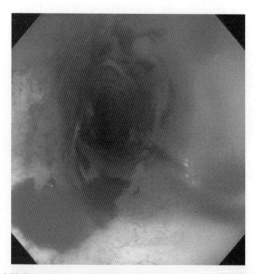

Figura 273.8 Aparência endoscópica da estenose esofágica mostrada na Figura 273.6 imediatamente após a dilatação do balão. Note que a estenose foi desfeita com sucesso, mas o sangramento secundário à ruptura da estenose na posição das 7 horas impediu uma maior dilatação durante o procedimento. (*Esta figura se encontra reproduzida em cores no Encarte.*)

estômago. Eles podem ser fixados usando um dispositivo de sutura (GI Stitch™, Pare Surgical), projetado para ser usado em um endoscópio de canal duplo.

Corpos estranhos esofágicos

Definição e sinais clínicos

Os corpos estranhos são uma causa comum de disfagia em cães, mas menos comuns em gatos. Os corpos estranhos esofágicos mais frequentes em cães são ossos, anzóis, agulhas e gravetos, enquanto brinquedos são mais costumeiros em gatos. Normalmente se alojam em pontos de distensão esofágica mínima: entrada torácica, base do coração ou no hiato diafragmático. Abrasão, ulceração e perfuração da mucosa podem ocorrer com objetos pontiagudos ou angulares que estão alojados intraluminalmente. A gravidade do dano esofágico e os sinais resultantes dependem do tamanho, da forma, das bordas e da duração da obstrução. Em alguns casos, o proprietário observa a ingestão. O início dos sinais clínicos está frequentemente relacionado ao grau de obstrução esofágica e tipo de corpo estranho ingerido. Animais com corpos estranhos menores com uma superfície lisa que causam obstrução incompleta podem ter sinais durante dias a semanas, enquanto a obstrução completa causa disfagia aguda, regurgitação, odinofagia, engasgo e salivação excessiva.

Diagnóstico e tratamento

O exame físico é variável, alternando de normal a halitose (necrose de tecido), febre e letargia. Corpos estranhos ósseos podem ocasionalmente ser palpados se estiverem alojados no esôfago cervical. O diagnóstico definitivo em geral requer radiografia. Corpos estranhos radiodensos podem ser detectados, mas a identificação de corpos estranhos radiolucentes requer um esofagograma. Radiografias são indispensáveis para a detecção de pneumonia aspirativa ou perfuração esofágica (pneumomediastino, enfisema ou mediastinite; Figura 273.9). Deve ser usado um agente de contraste positivo solúvel em água (ioexol, Gastrografin™ [diatrizoato]), em vez de sulfato de bário, se a perfuração esofágica for suspeita. A esofagoscopia pode ser realizada para confirmar o diagnóstico e avaliar o dano secundário à mucosa.

Os corpos estranhos esofágicos devem ser removidos prontamente, porque a retenção aumenta o risco de dano à mucosa esofágica, ulceração e perfuração. Corpos estranhos no esôfago proximal ou ossos grandes podem ser removidos com um sigmoidoscópio rígido, enquanto os mais distais além do alcance de um endoscópio rígido devem ser removidos usando um endoscópio flexível. Para uma remoção segura, uma pinça fórceps que passe pelo lúmen do endoscópio rígido é usada para apreender o corpo estranho e puxá-lo para dentro do endoscópio. Corpos estranhos esofágicos distais podem ser empurrados para o estômago para uma remoção por gastrotomia se não forem removidos pela boca. Corpos estranhos menores são mais bem removidos com um endoscópio flexível e cesta, pinça de biopsia ou pinça de recuperação a laço. Anzóis que ficam alojados no esôfago proximal ao medial podem ser desalojados com a extremidade distal de um endoscópio rígido, inserindo-a entre o eixo e a parte do gancho e empurrando aboralmente. Uma vez desalojado da mucosa, o gancho pode ser puxado para o lúmen do endoscópio rígido para uma remoção segura. Um endoscópio flexível pode ser usado para remover anzóis que estão alojados fora do alcance de um endoscópio rígido. Animais com necrose ou ulceração esofágica devem jejuar por 24 a 48 horas após a remoção do corpo estranho. Uma sonda de gastrostomia (ver Capítulo 82) pode ser inserida durante a remoção do corpo estranho em animais com esofagite grave ou necrose para contornar temporariamente o esôfago durante a alimentação. A terapia específica para esofagite deve incluir suspensões de sucralfato e inibidores da bomba de prótons por 7 a 10 dias após a remoção do corpo estranho. Antibióticos de amplo espectro são indicados em animais com ulceração grave ou pequenas perfurações. Uma esofagotomia é indicada caso a endoscopia falhe na remoção do corpo estranho; no entanto, é preferível tentar empurrá-lo para o estômago para a remoção por gastrotomia. A cirurgia também é indicada para reparar perfurações esofágicas maiores.

Anomalias do anel vascular
Ver Boxe 273.3.

Neoplasia esofágica
Ver Boxe 273.4.

Divertículos esofágicos
Ver Boxe 273.5.

Fístula esofágica
Ver Boxe 273.6.

Megaesôfago e hipomotilidade esofágica

Megaesôfago congênito

O megaesôfago, a causa mais comum de regurgitação em cães, é caracterizado por dilatação esofágica focal ou difusa e dismotilidade esofágica concomitante. Pode ser uma doença congênita ou adquirida. A forma adquirida é mais comum e pode ser idiopática ou secundária a uma doença reconhecida. O megaesôfago congênito idiopático é caracterizado por hipomotilidade e dilatação do esôfago, causando regurgitação e falta de crescimento em filhotes logo após o desmame. A predisposição familiar foi sugerida para as raças Setter Irlandês, Dogue Alemão, Pastor-Alemão, Labrador Retriever, Shar-pei, Terra-nova, Schnauzer Miniatura e Fox Terrier. O megaesôfago congênito em gatos é raro, mas os siameses podem ser predispostos. A patogênese da forma congênita é mal compreendida, mas possivelmente envolve um defeito na inervação vagal aferente do esôfago.[44,45]

Megaesôfago secundário adquirido

A causa subjacente do megaesôfago secundário adquirido (ASM) é desconhecida, mas um defeito na resposta neural aferente à distensão esofágica, semelhante ao megaesôfago congênito, é suspeita.[46] A miastenia *gravis* é responsável por 25 a 30% de ASM em cães[47,48] e pode envolver apenas o esôfago (miastenia *gravis* focal) ou, mais comumente, o esôfago e os músculos periféricos (ver Capítulo 269). O ASM também foi associado a miosite lúpica (ver Capítulo 205), polineuropatias (ver Capítulo 268), hipoadrenocorticismo (ver Capítulo 309), polimiopatias (ver

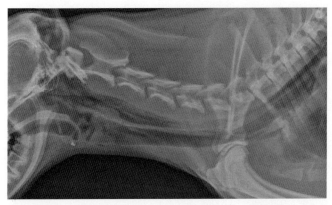

Figura 273.9 Projeções ortogonais do pescoço cervical realizadas em um cão da raça Border Collie de 9 meses, que foi observado brincando com uma vareta que ficou presa no seu esôfago. Um grande volume de gás livre (enfisema) é visto dorsalmente à faringe dissecando entre os planos retrofaríngeos, estendendo-se caudalmente na entrada torácica e no mediastino craniano (pneumomediastino). Nenhum corpo estranho radiográfico foi identificado durante o estudo, e uma avaliação endoscópica do esôfago foi recomendada.

SEÇÃO 18 • Doença Gastrintestinal

Boxe 273.3 Anormalidades do anel vascular

Definições e prevalência

As anomalias do anel vascular são malformações congênitas das principais artérias do coração; elas prendem o esôfago intratorácico e causam obstrução esofágica. O arco aórtico direito persistente (PRAA) é a anomalia mais comum em cães e gatos e ocorre quando o arco aórtico embrionário direito (em vez do quarto arco aórtico esquerdo) torna-se a aorta adulta funcional. Uma compressão circular do esôfago acomete a aorta à direita, o ligamento arterioso dorsolateralmente à esquerda, o tronco pulmonar à esquerda e a base do coração ventralmente. Essa anomalia é considerada um transtorno familiar com evidência de base hereditária em cães da raça Pastor-Alemão e Setter Irlandês.[35] Outras anomalias vasculares menos comuns incluem artérias subclávia direita ou esquerda persistentes, arco aórtico duplo, aorta dorsal direita persistente, arco aórtico esquerdo com ligamento arterioso direito e artérias intercostais aberrantes.

Sinais clínicos

Cães e gatos filhotes afetados geralmente apresentam regurgitação de alimentos sólidos no momento do desmame (ver Capítulo 39). É comum observar perda de peso com falha no desenvolvimento apesar de um bom apetite. A presença de tosse úmida, dispneia e febre sugerem pneumonia aspirativa (ver Capítulo 242). O exame físico muitas vezes revela um animal magro, atrofiado, mas que, de resto, parece normal. Ocasionalmente, um esôfago dilatado pode ser observado ou palpado na região cervical.

Diagnóstico

As anomalias do anel vascular devem ser diferenciadas de outras causas de regurgitação em animais jovens, como megaesôfago congênito, corpo estranho e estreitamento esofágico (ver Figura 273.3). Os sinais e um histórico compatível com regurgitação iniciada durante o desmame são altamente favoráveis a uma anomalia de anel vascular. Radiografias torácicas geralmente demonstram dilatação do corpo esofágico cranial à base do coração. Desvio focal para a esquerda da traqueia perto da borda cranial do coração em radiografias dorsoventral ou ventrodorsal é um sinal confiável de PRAA em cães jovens.[36] Um esofagograma pode ser realizado para confirmar a localização da obstrução esofágica e a gravidade da distensão do esôfago. A esofagoscopia (ver Capítulo 113) pode ajudar a diferenciar uma estenose intraluminal de uma compressão extraluminal. As estenoses aparecem como anéis fibrosos distintos intraluminais que permanecem estáticos quando vistos endoscopicamente, enquanto as pulsações rítmicas das principais artérias comprimindo o esôfago externamente são observadas com uma anomalia do anel vascular. Além disso, anomalias do anel vascular ocorrem na base do coração, enquanto estenoses intraluminais podem acometer qualquer segmento do corpo do esôfago e são mais comuns em animais adultos.

Tratamento

A terapia definitiva para PRAA é a ligadura cirúrgica e a transecção do ligamento arterioso por meio de uma abordagem intercostal esquerda. Durante a cirurgia, as áreas de fibrose periesofágica devem ser reduzidas, e o local estreitado precisa ser dilatado com um cateter balão de dilatação. Animais gravemente debilitados por desnutrição exigem suporte nutricional enteral por meio de alimentação por uma sonda de gastrostomia antes da cirurgia (ver Capítulo 82). Pneumonia aspirativa deve ser efetivamente tratada com antibióticos de amplo espectro (ver Capítulo 242). A melhora clínica significativa geralmente segue a cirurgia corretiva na maioria dos pacientes (mais de 90%); no entanto, hipomotilidade esofágica e regurgitação podem persistir, particularmente naqueles animais que têm um retardo na cirurgia. Animais afetados podem se beneficiar de alimentação elevada, conforme descrito para o megaesôfago idiopático. Infelizmente, não existem medicamentos para melhorar a motilidade do músculo estriado esofágico.

Boxe 273.4 Neoplasias esofágicas

Definições e prevalência

Os tumores do esôfago são relativamente raros, representando menos de 0,5% de todos os tipos de câncer em cães e gatos.[37] Os tumores podem ser esofágicos primários, de origem periesofágica ou metastáticos. O fibrossarcoma esofágico e o osteossarcoma são os tumores malignos mais comuns em cães e se desenvolvem como uma transformação maligna de granulomas esofágicos associada com infecção por *Spirocerca lupi*.[38,39] O carcinoma de células escamosas é o tumor esofágico primário mais comumente diagnosticado em gatos. Outros tumores esofágicos primários relatados com menos frequência no cão e no gato incluem leiomiomas e leiomiossarcomas, adenocarcinomas e carcinomas indiferenciados. Tumores periesofágicos provenientes de linfonodos regionais, tireoide, timo e base do coração causam invasão esofágica local, obstrução mecânica direta ou ambas. Lesões metastáticas (carcinomas de tireoide, pulmonar ou gástrico) comumente envolvem o esôfago, mas estão associados com menos frequência a sinais clínicos de doença esofágica.

Sinais clínicos

Os sinais clínicos se desenvolvem gradualmente e refletem uma obstrução esofágica progressiva. Os mais comuns incluem regurgitação, disfagia, odinofagia, ptialismo e perda de peso. Animais com doença metastática podem ter debilitação geral, anorexia e sinais de envolvimento pulmonar, como dispneia e tosse. O exame físico pode revelar emagrecimento, embora alguns tumores periesofágicos e esofágicos envolvendo o esôfago cervical sejam palpáveis.

Diagnóstico

As radiografias torácicas podem ser normais ou revelar dilatação esofágica variável, uma massa intraluminal ou evidência de uma lesão periesofágica deslocando o esôfago. Os pulmões devem ser avaliados para pneumonia aspirativa e metástases. Um esofagograma geralmente confirma a presença de uma massa intraluminal ou lesão obstrutiva. Uma esofagoscopia com biopsia da mucosa e citologia ou histopatologia esfoliativa são necessárias para o diagnóstico definitivo de uma neoplasia esofágica. Biopsias pequenas por pinça, obtidas por endoscopia, podem ser superficiais e não representativas do tumor, portanto uma técnica de mordida dupla deve ser realizada para maximizar a eficiência do diagnóstico.

Tratamento

Quimioterapia, ressecção cirúrgica e radioterapia representam as modalidades primárias para o tratamento da neoplasia maligna do esôfago; no entanto, a radioterapia pode ser complicada por lesões agudas ou crônicas nas estruturas mediastinais adjacentes, enquanto a ressecção cirúrgica é complicada por causa da exposição cirúrgica limitada, da tensão na anastomose e do risco de formação de estenose no pós-operatório. O linfoma pode ser tratado com quimioterapia (ver Capítulo 344). Neoplasias esofágicas benignas de crescimento lento (p. ex., leiomioma) geralmente têm um prognóstico favorável com a ressecção cirúrgica completa.[40] Os granulomas esofágicos associados a *Spirocerca lupi* podem ser tratados com doramectina, administrada na dosagem de 200 mcg/kg SC para três tratamentos, com intervalos de 14 dias,[38] ou 500 µg/kg de uma solução injetável administrada por via oral, 1 vez/dia durante 6 semanas. Esse regime é repetido por mais 6 semanas em cães que exibam qualquer evidência de formação de granuloma detectada via esofagoscopia.[39]

CAPÍTULO 273 • Doenças da Faringe e do Esôfago

Boxe 273.5 Divertículo esofágico

Definições e prevalência
Divertículos esofágicos são saculações circunscritas da parede do esôfago que afetam a sua motilidade. Divertículos congênitos ocorrem de forma secundária a anormalidades durante o desenvolvimento embriológico que permite a herniação da mucosa esofágica através de um defeito na muscular da mucosa. Os divertículos adquiridos são subdivididos em formas de pulsão ou tração. Os divertículos de pulsão se desenvolvem em associação com aumentos na pressão intraluminal secundária à obstrução (estenose ou corpo estranho) ou à motilidade alterada[41] se desenvolvem de modo secundário à obstrução de anomalias do anel vascular. Os divertículos de tração resultam da inflamação periesofágica e de fibrose. Aderências ao tecido adjacente (p. ex., pulmão, brônquio, linfonodo) distorcem o lúmen esofágico e criam saculações. O desenvolvimento de um abscesso devido à migração de um corpo estranho (p. ex., espigueta de grama) é uma causa comum de divertículos de tração no oeste dos EUA. O acúmulo de ingesta (impactação) dentro dos divertículos leva a esofagite, obstrução mecânica (observada com divertículos grandes) e dismotilidade esofágica.

Sinais clínicos
Os sinais clínicos dos divertículos esofágicos são semelhantes aos de muitos outros distúrbios esofágicos e incluem regurgitação, odinofagia e ânsia de vômito. Os divertículos podem ocasionalmente ser um achado incidental em animais sem sinais clínicos associados. O enfraquecimento da muscular da mucosa pode ocorrer em casos raros, resultando em perfuração do divertículo com vazamento de alimento e de líquido para o mediastino e em sinais de sepse e de dificuldade respiratória.

Diagnóstico
As radiografias torácicas podem revelar um tecido cheio de ar ou tecido mole com opacidade adjacente ou envolvendo o esôfago; no entanto, a radiografia de contraste é necessária para diferenciar um divertículo esofágico de uma massa na região periesofágica, mediastinal ou pulmonar. A esofagoscopia (ver Capítulo 113) confirma o diagnóstico, embora possa ser necessário aspirar alimentos e líquidos para visualizar o divertículo. Os divertículos não devem ser confundidos com a redundância esofágica normal, observada em animais jovens braquicefálicos das raças Buldogue e Shar-pei. Outros diferenciais para divertículos epifrênicos incluem hérnia de hiato e intussuscepção gastresofágica.

Tratamento
A diverticulectomia é a terapia preferida, particularmente para grandes divertículos que são uma causa contínua de impactação esofágica. Divertículos pequenos em pacientes subclínicos podem ser tolerados ou manejados com porções menores de alimentos de consistência líquida ou semilíquida, ofertados em uma alimentação vertical para minimizar a impactação da ingesta no divertículo. Divertículos de tração são frequentemente tratados com antibióticos de amplo espectro, enquanto os de pulsão são tratados por sua causa-base específica (estenose, corpo estranho, esofagite). A maioria dos casos justifica um prognóstico reservado, porque a cirurgia corretiva pode induzir a formação de estenose e a hipomotilidade segmentar pode persistir após a cirurgia.

Boxe 273.6 Fístula esofágica

Uma fístula esofágica é uma via de comunicação anormal entre o esôfago e as estruturas adjacentes. A maioria das fístulas esofágicas envolve os pulmões ou as estruturas das vias respiratórias (p. ex., fístulas esofagopulmonar, esofagotraqueal e esofagobrônquica; ver Capítulo 242). Fístulas congênitas e adquiridas têm sido descritas, embora ambas as formas sejam raras em cães e gatos.[42,43] As congênitas são incomuns e resultam da separação incompleta da árvore traqueobrônquica do trato digestivo, a partir da qual é formada durante o período de desenvolvimento embriológico. Cães da raça Cairn Terriers parecem ser predispostos. As fístulas esofágicas adquiridas são geralmente associadas com corpos estranhos esofágicos retidos, especialmente ossos e gravetos que causam perfuração esofágica e vazamento do conteúdo para os tecidos adjacentes. A cura leva ao desenvolvimento de um trato comunicante com contaminação das vias respiratórias, resultante do conteúdo esofágico. Outras causas menos comuns das fístulas esofágicas incluem trauma e neoplasia.

Sinais clínicos
Os sinais clínicos estão relacionados principalmente ao sistema respiratório e incluem tosse e dispneia. Tossir depois de beber é um sinal comum de apresentação. Regurgitação, disfagia, letargia, anorexia, febre e perda de peso são sinais mais raros de ser observados.

Diagnóstico
As radiografias torácicas geralmente revelam uma localização alveolar, brônquica, padrão pulmonar intersticial ou uma combinação deles. Os lobos caudal direito e médio do pulmão em cães e os lobos caudal esquerdo e acessórios em gatos são os mais comumente afetados.[42,43] Corpos estranhos radiopacos podem ser observados no esôfago; contudo, um esofagograma é necessário para o diagnóstico definitivo da comunicação da via respiratória esofágica. O uso de agentes de contraste iodados deve ser evitado, porque são hiperosmolares e quimicamente irritantes para o pulmão. Esofagoscopia ou broncoscopia são de valor limitado para confirmação de fístulas pequenas.

Tratamento
É necessária uma excisão cirúrgica da fístula, com o fechamento do defeito esofágico. A lobectomia do lobo pulmonar afetado pode ser necessária, como resultado de consolidação pulmonar ou material estranho contido dentro das vias respiratórias. A terapia pós-cirúrgica inclui repouso esofágico por 48 a 72 horas e administração de antibióticos de amplo espectro para combate de infecções com base em cultura e teste de suscetibilidade de amostras dos tecidos envolvidos. Um bom prognóstico é dado após uma cirurgia bem-sucedida, reservado em caso de complicações graves, como derrame pleural grave, pneumonia ou abscedação pulmonar.

Capítulo 354), disautonomia, envenenamento por chumbo e formas graves de esofagite. A disautonomia, uma neuropatia autonômica generalizada em que o megaesôfago e a hipomotilidade esofágica são achados consistentes, é reconhecida com mais frequência em gatos e atribuída a lesões degenerativas envolvendo gânglios autonômicos.[49] Outras causas de hipomotilidade esofágica segmentar ou difusa incluem corpos estranhos, estenose, anomalias do anel vascular e esofagite.

Sinais clínicos e diagnóstico
A regurgitação é o sinal clínico mais comumente associado ao megaesôfago. Existe uma considerável variabilidade na frequência e no tempo dos episódios de regurgitação após a ingestão da refeição. Filhotes com megaesôfago congênito geralmente começam a regurgitar quando desmamados para introdução de alimentos sólidos. Animais afetados podem sofrer de desnutrição e pneumonia aspirativa (ver Capítulo 242). Sinais adicionais dependem da causa subjacente do megaesôfago e incluem dores musculares e rigidez da marcha (polimiosite), fraqueza generalizada, intolerância ao exercício (doença neuromuscular) e sinais gastrintestinais (intoxicação por chumbo, hipoadrenocorticismo).

O megaesôfago deve ser suspeito em qualquer animal com uma história de regurgitação (ver Capítulo 39). Radiografias do pescoço e tórax são os exames diagnósticos de preferência para a maioria dos casos de megaesôfago (ver Figuras 273.2 e 273.10), embora, se as imagens forem ambíguas, a radiografia de contraste

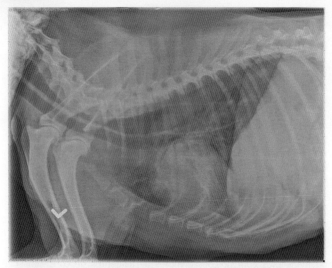

Figura 273.10 Radiografia torácica lateral direita de um cão da raça Braco Húngaro de 3 anos com história de regurgitação, ptialismo e disfonia há 3 semanas. O esôfago está difusamente distendido por gás e há infiltrados intersticiais a alveolares ventrais na região cranial esquerda e direita dos lobos pulmonares mediais, consistentes com pneumonia aspirativa. O cão foi diagnosticado com miastenia *gravis* focal; teve resolução completa do megaesôfago e sinais clínicos associados após a administração de piridostigmina.

(esofagograma) possa ser considerada para ajudar a excluir um megaesôfago por causa de corpo estranho ou para avaliar a motilidade esofágica. As radiografias podem revelar opacidades alveolares consistentes com pneumonia aspirativa. Hematologia de rotina, bioquímica sérica e urinálise devem ser realizadas para triagem para causas de ASM. Um título de anticorpo AChR para MG adquirida deve ser feito, mesmo na ausência de fraqueza muscular generalizada, porque MG pode causar megaesôfago focal. O teste deve ser repetido 4 a 8 semanas mais tarde em todos os cães com um título inicial na "zona cinzenta" (0,3 a 0,6 nmol/ℓ), particularmente quando o início do megaesôfago for considerado de natureza aguda. Um cortisol basal ou teste de estimulação com ACTH devem ser considerados para ajudar a descartar hipoadrenocorticismo. Procedimentos diagnósticos adicionais que devem ser baseados na apresentação de cada caso individual incluem esofagoscopia (ver Capítulo 113), eletromiografia, biopsia de músculos e nervos (ver Capítulo 116) e velocidade de condução nervosa (ver Capítulo 117). Uma associação clara com hipotireoidismo não foi comprovada, e uma baixa concentração de T4 total é mais consistente com a síndrome do eutireóideo doente (ver Capítulo 299).

Tratamento

Animais com ASM devem ser diferenciados daqueles com megaesôfago idiopático adquirido e ter seus transtornos subjacentes tratados. O tratamento do megaesôfago idiopático e das formas adquiridas que falham em responder à terapia clínica específica é de suporte e sintomático. O clínico deve recomendar refeições pequenas e frequentes, em uma posição elevada ou vertical (p. ex., cadeira de Bailey) para auxiliar a passagem da ingesta para o estômago. A consistência deve ser variada (líquida, carne enlatada ou ração) para determinar quais tipos de alimentos são mais bem tolerados. Em animais gravemente desnutridos ou que sofrem episódios repetidos de pneumonia aspirativa, deve ser colocada uma sonda de gastrostomia temporária ou permanente para suporte nutricional enteral (ver Capítulo 82). A alimentação através de uma sonda de gastrostomia reduz o risco de pneumonia aspirativa; no entanto, cães com megaesôfago ainda podem aspirar saliva ou refluxo de ingesta do estômago para o esôfago. Antibióticos de amplo espectro devem ser considerados na pneumonia aspirativa (ver Capítulo 242). Os clientes devem ser informados de que a pneumonia recorrente é um problema comum, necessitando de detecção e tratamento imediatos para o sucesso a longo prazo.

Atualmente, drogas procinéticas não têm benefício comprovado no manejo do megaesôfago idiopático em cães. Metoclopramida e cisaprida são agentes procinéticos de músculo liso que não têm efeito no músculo estriado esofágico e podem exacerbar os sinais clínicos. Cisaprida pode ser um agente procinético útil em gatos com distúrbios da motilidade esofágica distal, afetando o componente do músculo liso do esôfago felino.

Os animais afetados devem ser reavaliados em intervalos de 1 a 2 meses para monitorar a progressão da doença. Radiografias torácicas devem ser repetidas para avaliar a dilatação esofágica e pneumonia aspirativa. Alguns animais com megaesôfago congênito melhoram ao longo dos meses com cuidados de suporte diligentes.

O prognóstico do megaesôfago idiopático adquirido é em geral ruim. Esses animais normalmente sucumbem a episódios repetidos de pneumonia aspirativa ou são eutanasiados devido a irreversibilidade de sua doença. Animais com ASM podem responder à resolução da causa subjacente O prognóstico em cães com megaesôfago causado por MG adquirida é favorável, com aproximadamente 50% dos pacientes respondendo a terapia de suporte.[47]

Hérnia de hiato

Definições e prevalência

A hérnia de hiato é definida como qualquer protrusão de conteúdo abdominal (mais comumente uma porção do estômago) através do hiato esofágico do diafragma na cavidade torácica na presença de um ligamento frênico-esofágico intacto. São reconhecidos três tipos de hérnias de hiato em cães e gatos: o Tipo I é a hérnia de hiato de deslizamento, em que o segmento abdominal do esôfago e partes do estômago são deslocadas cranialmente através o hiato esofágico; o Tipo II é a hérnia de hiato paraesofágica, em que o segmento abdominal do esôfago e o esfíncter esofágico inferior permanecem em uma posição fixa, mas uma porção do estômago hernia para o mediastino ao longo do esôfago torácico.[50,51] Foi relatado um caso de hérnia de hiato esofágico do Tipo IV, em que o fígado, o estômago e o intestino delgado foram deslocados para o tórax.[52] A hérnia de hiato do Tipo I é a forma mais comum e pode ocorrer como lesão congênita ou adquirida em cães e gatos. Hérnias de hiato deslizantes congênitas foram documentadas em raças braquicefálicas: Shar-pei, Chow Chow, Buldogue Inglês, Buldogue Francês, Pug e Boston Terriers.[53] Os animais afetados desenvolvem sinais clínicos logo após o desmame. A hérnia de hiato adquirida pode ocorrer em qualquer cão ou gato e decorrer de aumentos repentinos na pressão intra-abdominal secundários a trauma (via dano aos nervos e músculos diafragmáticos, resultando em frouxidão hiatal) ou dificuldade respiratória (causada por aumento da pressão intratorácica negativa, observada com obstrução das vias respiratórias [paralisia laríngea]). Não obstante à causa, a hérnia de hiato reduz a pressão do EEI e leva a refluxo gastresofágico, esofagite e hipomotilidade esofágica segmentar ou difusa.

Sinais clínicos e diagnóstico

Os sinais clínicos mais comuns são regurgitação intermitente, vômito e hipersalivação, frequentemente precipitada por excitação ou exercício. O refluxo persistente do suco gástrico pode causar esofagite secundária com sinais de odinofagia. Dispneia e tosse podem ocorrer com hérnia grave ou pneumonia aspirativa. Radiografias torácicas devem ser obtidas em todos os cães com suspeita de hérnia de hiato e podem revelar uma opacidade dorsocaudal de tecidos moles intratorácicos, cheios de ar (Figura 273.11). Também podem ser observados graus variáveis de dilatação esofágica e opacidades alveolar, consistentes com pneumonia aspirativa. Radiografias são de sensibilidade relativamente baixa para o diagnóstico de hérnia de hiato, e é muito mais provável um procedimento dinâmico com bário (videofluoroscopia) identificar herniação intermitente do estômago, que pode permitir ainda a avaliação da motilidade esofágica (ver Vídeo 273.3 e as Figuras 273.3 e 273.12). Um estudo videofluoroscópico normal da deglutição não descarta uma hérnia de hiato, porque o problema ocorre de forma intermitente e pode não ser observado. É possível usar uma esofagoscopia para diagnosticar a hérnia de hiato por deslizamento, quando a separação aparente entre a junção escamocolunar e a impressão diafragmática, usando uma manobra em J, for maior que 2 cm.[54] A esofagoscopia é também usada para procurar evidências de esofagite. A manometria de alta resolução (HRM) é uma ferramenta não invasiva que pode ser usada para diagnosticar hérnias de hiato em pessoas e animais.

Tratamento

Uma hérnia de hiato por deslizamento nem sempre está associada com sinais clínicos, principalmente quando adquirida. O manejo clínico deve ser implementado em animais com sinais de RGE grave, esofagite e regurgitação antes da intervenção cirúrgica. Inibidores da bomba de prótons, como omeprazol, são supressores de ácido superiores em comparação com os antagonistas do receptor H2 e devem ser administrados com uma suspensão de sucralfato para proporcionar maior citoproteção da mucosa. Drogas que aumentam o tônus do EEI (cisaprida ou metoclopramida) podem ser administradas com PPI e sucralfato.

Animais em que os manejos clínicos não surtem efeito podem se beneficiar de cirurgia reconstrutiva, especialmente para hérnias de hiato congênitas grandes. A anatomia normal do hiato pode ser restaurada por aposição crural diafragmática, esofagopexia e técnicas de gastropexia fúndica esquerda com tubo.[40,42] É importante também considerar o tratamento cirúrgico para a síndrome braquicefálica em cães afetados de modo concomitante com hérnia de hiato, porque a obstrução das vias respiratórias superiores cria um aumento na pressão negativa intratorácica que pode agravar a hérnia. O prognóstico para a maioria dos cães após a correção cirúrgica é geralmente favorável, embora regurgitação persistente seja descrita nos animais com distúrbios de motilidade esofágica concomitantes.

Refluxo gastresofágico

Definição e sinais clínicos

O refluxo gastresofágico (RGE) está associado a refluxo de fluidos gástricos ou intestinais ou a ingesta para o esôfago, secundário à perda de integridade da barreira gastresofágica (Figura 273.13). As consequências do RGE incluem vários graus de esofagite resultante do prolongado contato da mucosa esofágica com ácido gástrico, pepsina, tripsina, sais biliares e bicarbonato duodenal. Apenas o ácido gástrico produz uma esofagite leve; no entanto, a combinação de ácido gástrico com pepsina ou tripsina pode causar esofagite grave. As causas mais comuns do RGE em cães e gatos incluem hérnia de hiato, redução da pressão do EEI induzida por anestesia geral, vômito crônico que causa um enfraquecimento do tônus do EEI e atonia gástrica causando GER. Os sinais clínicos são semelhantes aos da esofagite e podem incluir regurgitação, hipersalivação, odinofagia e anorexia. Animais que apresentam refluxo na boca podem estalar os lábios, ofegar ou "engolir a seco" imediatamente após esses episódios. O refluxo noturno ocorre mais comumente em pessoas e animais por causa de relaxamentos transitórios do EEI durante o sono e a perda do reflexo de deglutição.

Diagnóstico e tratamento

O diagnóstico de RGE é suspeitado a partir do histórico: respiração ofegante noturna, engolir a seco, estalar os lábios, anestesia geral recente e vômito crônico. A videofluoroscopia pode demonstrar RGE intermitente; no entanto, episódios intermitentes podem ser observados em animais com função esofágica normal.

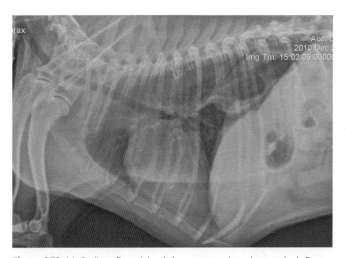

Figura 273.11 Radiografia torácica de levantamento lateral esquerdo de Boston Terrier de 5 anos com história crônica de regurgitação. O estômago é visto estendendo-se através do diafragma até o tórax craniodorsal na projeção lateral esquerda. Ele então retorna para um local mais normal em projeções subsequentes. Esses achados são altamente favoráveis a uma hérnia hiatal deslizante.

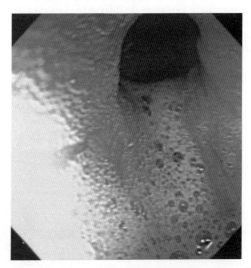

Figura 273.13 Esofagoscopia realizada em cão da raça Boston Terrier de 5 anos de idade com história crônica de regurgitação secundária a uma hérnia de hiato por deslizamento (Tipo I). O leitor deve notar a flacidez do esfíncter esofágico inferior e a evidência de refluxo gastresofágico. A mucosa esofágica na posição 9 a 11 horas depois parece eritematosa, secundária à esofagite. (*Esta figura se encontra reproduzida em cores no Encarte.*)

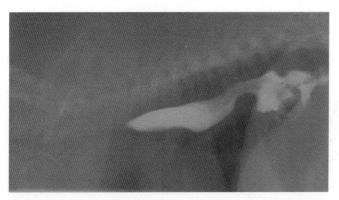

Figura 273.12 Estudo videofluoroscópico contrastado da deglutição em Boston Terrier de 5 anos com história crônica de regurgitação documentar, refluxo gastresofágico grave em associação com hérnia hiatal deslizante (Tipo I).

A esofagoscopia é um procedimento útil para documentar inflamação associada ao RGE. O teste de impedância/pH esofágico é útil para diagnosticar refluxos ácidos e não ácidos em pessoas e cães com suspeita de RGE e esofagite inexplicável ou hérnia de hiato (ver a seção Teste de pH/impedância esofágica).

A terapia medicamentosa visa a administração de supressores de ácido (inibidores da bomba de prótons), barreiras de difusão (sucralfato) e agentes procinéticos (cisaprida e metoclopramida). A cisaprida é um agente procinético superior à metoclopramida e tem sido prescrito em cães para aumentar o tônus do EEI e melhorar o esvaziamento gástrico. Os animais devem ser alimentados com uma dieta restrita em gordura, porque ela retarda o esvaziamento gástrico e pode reduzir a pressão do EEI. Em pessoas com RGE grave, a cirurgia antirrefluxo é comumente realizada por laparoscopia e visa reforçar e reparar a barreira defeituosa por meio da plicatura do fundo gástrico.[55] As terapias endoscópicas antirrefluxo vem sendo utilizadas em seres humanos, mas ensaios clínicos em cães ainda são necessários.

REFERÊNCIAS BIBLIOGRÁFICAS

As referências bibliográficas deste capítulo se encontram online no Ambiente de Aprendizagem.

CAPÍTULO 274

Interações Hospedeiro-Microbiota na Saúde e Doença Gastrintestinal

Albert Earl Jergens

INTRODUÇÃO

O trato gastrintestinal (GI) é colonizado por uma complexa comunidade de bactérias, arqueias, fungos, protozoários e vírus, que promove o desenvolvimento do sistema imunológico e contribui para a saúde do hospedeiro.[1,2] A carga microbiana total nos intestinos é estimada na faixa de 10^{12} a 10^{14} microrganismos, o que é aproximadamente 10 vezes o número de células do hospedeiro. O conjunto de microrganismos que habitam o intestino é conhecido como *microbiota intestinal*, e o conjunto dos seus genomas, como *microbioma intestinal*.

Essas bactérias exercem um efeito condicionador na homeostase intestinal, ao fornecer sinais regulatórios para o epitélio e influenciar nas respostas imunológicas da mucosa. Esse hábitat é separado do meio intestinal por uma única camada de células epiteliais e contém centenas de diferentes espécies. A escassez de bactérias no estômago e no intestino delgado proximal deve-se, respectivamente, às secreções ácidas, biliares e pancreáticas, que matam a maioria das bactérias ingeridas, e à atividade motora de propulsão, que impede a colonização bacteriana estável. No entanto, a densidade bacteriana aumenta dramaticamente no intestino delgado distal, enquanto no intestino grosso aumenta para 10^{11} a 10^{12} bactérias/g de conteúdo luminal. Uma grande proporção da massa fecal consiste em bactérias (cerca de 60% dos sólidos fecais).[3]

As principais funções da microbiota intestinal que contribuem para a manutenção da saúde do trato GI incluem: atividades metabólicas que produzem energia e nutrientes; importantes efeitos tróficos sobre epitélio intestinal e estrutura/função imunológica; e proteção do hospedeiro colonizado contra invasão por microrganismos patogênicos (Figura 274.1). A microbiota intestinal também pode ser um fator essencial em distúrbios patológicos específicos, incluindo doença inflamatória intestinal (DII), "supercrescimento bacteriano no intestino delgado" (SIBO) e causas infecciosas de gastrenterite. Além disso, pró e prebióticos, simbióticos e transplante de microbiota fecal (TMF) podem ter um papel na prevenção ou tratamento de algumas doenças gastrintestinais.

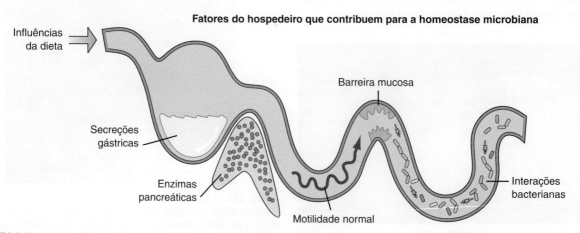

Figura 274.1 Mecanismos do hospedeiro que contribuem para a homeostase da mucosa. A composição da microbiota intestinal em animais saudáveis é influenciada por diversos fatores, incluindo secreções alimentares, motilidade gastrintestinal, integridade da barreira mucosa, tecido linfoide associado ao intestino e interações entre bactérias.

COMPOSIÇÃO DA MICROBIOTA EM ANIMAIS SAUDÁVEIS

A colonização do trato GI começa imediatamente após o nascimento e ocorre dentro de alguns dias. As bactérias comensais parecem ser adquiridas por colonização oportunista de espécies particulares, como resultado de encontros ambientais aleatórios. Essas bactérias de "primeira hora" podem modular a expressão de genes das células epiteliais no hospedeiro e criar um hábitat favorável para si mesmas ao mesmo tempo que evitam o crescimento de outras bactérias introduzidas posteriormente. Análises quantitativas recentes da microbiota fecal, independentes de cultura, mostraram que as bactérias anaeróbias superam as bactérias aeróbias por um fator de 100:1000.[1,2] Essas técnicas moleculares avaliam genes codificadores do RNA ribossômico 16S (rRNA), que são comuns a todas as bactérias, mas cujas sequências precisas variam entre as espécies, podendo ser usadas para identificação e classificação de bactérias. Exemplos dessa tecnologia incluem o desenvolvimento de sondas moleculares para microarranjos de DNA, sequenciamento genômico de alto rendimento (p. ex., plataforma Illumina®) para avaliação da quantidade e diversidade microbiana, técnicas de hibridização *in situ* fluorescente (FISH) para avaliar a distribuições espacial da microbiota da mucosa e chips de genes para identificar e enumerar espécies bacterianas específicas. Mais de 99% da microbiota intestinal humana é composta por bactérias divididas em 4 espécies: *Firmicutes, Bacteriodetes, Proteobacteria* e *Actinobacteria*.[1,2,4] Enquanto a composição da microbiota de um humano adulto parece ser relativamente estável ao longo do tempo, existe um grau notável de variação interindividual.

Parece óbvio que a composição da microbiota intestinal em cães e gatos saudáveis é claramente diferente. Usando cultura bacteriana tradicional, gatos saudáveis demonstraram ter muitas bactérias totais e anaeróbicas no intestino delgado proximal.[5,6] As bactérias anaeróbias mais comumente isoladas compreenderam os gêneros *Bacteroides, Clostridium, Eubacteria* e *Fusobacteria*, enquanto *Pasteurella* spp. foram as espécies anaeróbicas facultativas predominantes. Um estudo separado mostrou que a microbiota duodenal dos cães contém normalmente uma contagem bacteriana superior a 10^5 UFC/ml de suco duodenal; no entanto, contagens significativamente mais altas foram observadas em algumas raças e em cães sem sinais de doença do trato intestinal.[7,8] Estudos de sequenciamento de última geração do gene 16S rRNA definiram ainda mais os microbiomas canino e felino, que, em termos filogenéticos elevados, se assemelham ao microbioma humano e de outros mamíferos. Em média, 10 diferentes filos bacterianos foram identificados no intestino saudável de cães e gatos, com *Firmicutes, Bacteroidetes, Proteobacteria, Fusobacteria* e *Actinobacteria* compreendendo a maioria dos micróbios encontrada nas fezes.[9,10] Além do mais, estudos emergentes indicam que a ingestão alimentar atual também desempenha um papel importante, potencialmente ainda maior do que a genética do hospedeiro, na formação da ecologia microbiana intestinal.[11] A investigação dos metagenomas caninos e felinos (através de sequenciamento *shotgun* de DNA genômico) forneceu uma visão recente e valiosa sobre a capacidade funcional da microbiota (Figura 274.2).[12,13] Apesar das diferenças nas populações microbianas desses animais, sua capacidade funcional parece ser altamente conservada.

INTERAÇÕES FISIOLÓGICAS MICRORGANISMO-HOSPEDEIRO

Estudos comparativos de animais livres de microrganismos e colonizados convencionalmente forneceram informações importantes sobre o efeito da comunidade microbiana intestinal nos mecanismos fisiológicos do hospedeiro associados a doenças.

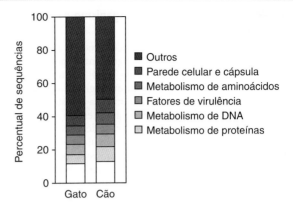

Figura 274.2 Proporções relativas das principais funções de genes microbianos em cães e gatos. Observe que a capacidade funcional da microbiota é bastante semelhante entre essas espécies de mamíferos, apesar da variação em suas populações microbianas. (De Honneffer JB, Minamoto Y, Suchodolski JS: *Microbiota alterations in acute and chronic gastrintestinal inflammation of cats and dogs.* World J Gastroenterol, 20(44):16489-16497, 2014.) (*Esta figura se encontra reproduzida em cores no Encarte.*)

Funções metabólicas

Uma das principais funções metabólicas da microbiota do cólon é a fermentação de resíduos alimentares não digeríveis em ácidos graxos de cadeia curta (AGCC), incluindo acetato, propionato e butirato.[14] Este último é consumido quase completamente pelo epitélio do cólon, onde serve como uma importante fonte de energia para os colonócitos. A diversidade de genes dentro da comunidade microbiana fornece as enzimas e as vias bioquímicas necessárias para esse fim e distintas dos recursos próprios do hospedeiro. Os resultados dessa complexa atividade metabólica são a recuperação de uma lesão metabólica e a disponibilidade de substratos absorvíveis para o hospedeiro, assim como o fornecimento de energia e nutrição para o crescimento e a proliferação das bactérias. Essas bactérias residentes podem neutralizar carcinógenos da dieta, sintetizar biotina, folato e vitamina K, metabolizar sais biliares e auxiliar na absorção de cálcio, magnésio e ferro.[15,16] A colonização aumenta a captação de glicose no intestino, enquanto camundongos livres de microrganismos requerem uma maior ingestão calórica para manter o peso corporal normal. Tem sido proposto que a microbiota intestinal de um indivíduo possui uma eficiência metabólica específica, e diferenças na composição microbiana podem regular o armazenamento de energia e predispor à obesidade em adultos.[17]

Efeitos tróficos e protetores ao epitélio

Bactérias entéricas conferem numerosos e diversos efeitos estruturais e protetores sobre o epitélio intestinal.[1,2] A expressão dos genes do hospedeiro induzida por bactérias influencia a absorção de nutrientes, o metabolismo, a angiogênese, a integridade da barreira mucosa e o desenvolvimento do sistema nervoso entérico. Os ligantes de bactérias residentes influenciam o desenvolvimento e a função normais da imunidade da mucosa.[18,19] Essas bactérias educam o sistema imunológico da mucosa e modulam o ajuste fino/regulação do repertório das células T e o perfil de citocinas das células T auxiliares tipo 1 (Th1)/Th2. Ao longo do epitélio, bactérias entéricas residentes formam uma barreira natural (biofilme) contra a colonização por microrganismos exógenos. A resistência à colonização por microrganismos patogênicos envolve vários mecanismos, incluindo o deslocamento, a competição por nutrientes e locais de ligação epitelial e a produção de substâncias antimicrobianas, como ácido láctico e bacteriocinas.[20] É digno de nota que a exposição de linhagens de células epiteliais do cólon com ligantes bacterianos aumenta a zônula de oclusão-1 (ZO-1) associada à integridade da barreira intestinal.[21]

Interação (*cross-talk*) entre microrganismo e hospedeiro na superfície mucosa

A manutenção da homeostase da mucosa requer a interpretação precisa do microambiente para distinguir entre bactérias comensais e microrganismos patogênicos. Uma perturbação nesses processos pode levar a respostas imunológicas inadequadas do hospedeiro e subsequente lesão da mucosa intestinal. A interação entre o tecido linfoide associado ao intestino e a microbiota na vida precoce parece ser crucial para o desenvolvimento adequado de complexos circuitos imunorreguladores da mucosa e sistêmicos. Vários tipos de células imunossensoriais amostram ativamente bactérias comensais, patógenos e outros antígenos luminais. Essas células incluem enterócitos de superfície, células M e células dendríticas (DC). Enterócitos de superfície são interconectados por junções oclusivas e cobertos por muco que promove exclusão de antígenos. Eles detectam sinais de perigo dentro do microambiente luminal e respondem secretando defensinas, quimiocinas e citocinas e induzindo a produção de IgA, que inicia e direciona as respostas imunes inatas e adaptativas.[1,22,23] As células M, células epiteliais especializadas que se sobrepõem aos folículos linfoides, amostram antígenos luminais e entregam seus produtos para as DC e outras células apresentadoras de antígeno. Células dendríticas fornecem vigilância imunológica adicional por meio de amostragem direta do conteúdo intestinal, inserindo ou estendendo os dendritos entre enterócitos superficiais.[24] Além disso, as DC podem ingerir e reter bactérias comensais vivas e transportá-las para linfonodos mesentéricos, onde podem ser produzidas localmente as respostas imunológicas a estas bactérias.[25] Assim, o acesso de bactérias comensais para o ambiente interno do hospedeiro é impedido.

RECONHECIMENTO DAS BACTÉRIAS NA MUCOSA

As células imunossensoriais devem reconhecer rapidamente os micróbios patogênicos no lúmen para iniciar uma resposta imune controlada, mas precisam manter a hiporresponsividade a bactérias comensais inofensivas (ou seja, tolerância oral). Esse processo discriminatório é amplamente mediado por dois grandes sistemas hospedeiros de receptores de reconhecimento padrão (PRR): a família de receptores semelhantes a Toll (TLR) e os receptores similares ao domínio de oligomerização ligante de nucleotídio (NOD1 e NOD2).[26] Os TLR compreendem uma classe de PRR transmembrana que desempenham um papel-chave no reconhecimento microbiano, na indução de genes antimicrobianos e no controle das respostas imunes adaptativas. Os NOD são uma família estruturalmente distinta de PRR intracelulares, que exercem atividade antimicrobiana e previnem a invasão de patógenos. Tanto TLR quanto NOD são amplamente expressos em vários tipos de células da mucosa do trato GI e participam da defesa do hospedeiro contra patógenos microbianos por meio de: (1) reconhecimento de moléculas-padrão presentes em patógenos; (2) expressão na interface com o "ambiente" do trato GI; (3) indução da secreção de citocinas e quimiocinas pró e anti-inflamatórias que se associam a imunidade adaptativa; e (4) indução de vias efetoras antimicrobianas.[23] Assim, os TLR expressos por células não epiteliais (p. ex., macrófagos e DC) e células epiteliais intestinais (p. ex., TLR4 para LPS e TLR5 para flagelina bacteriana) desempenham papéis funcionais importantes na sinalização de células epiteliais da defesa imune inata.[27]

Diferentes TLR reconhecem seletivamente diferentes PRR (ou seja, cada TLR liga "assinaturas moleculares" específicas de diferentes classes de microrganismos) e iniciam a sinalização através de vias conservadas, como as de transdução de sinal NFkB e proteínas quinases ativadas por mitógenos (MAPK).[4,26] Os efeitos envolvem a ativação transcricional de genes que codificam citocinas pró e anti-inflamatórias e quimiocinas, bem como a indução de moléculas coestimulatórias.[28] No intestino saudável, a sinalização TLR/NOD promove a defesa do hospedeiro e respostas de reparo de tecido, mantendo assim a mucosa em homeostase comensal. Essa resposta programada cria um gradiente quimiotático para a entrada de neutrófilos, monócitos e linfócitos T na mucosa, o que facilita a eliminação de patógenos invasores. Por outro lado, uma doença intestinal pode se desenvolver quando a homeostase comensal e/ou da mucosa está prejudicada devido a fatores genéticos específicos (p. ex., NOD2/mutação CARD15 na doença de Crohn) ou desencadeadores ambientais (p. ex., constituintes da dieta, infecção por patógenos, uso de drogas anti-inflamatórias não esteroidais).[4,26,29] Portanto, um erro no reconhecimento de bactérias e a intolerância da mucosa por meio de sinalização TLR/NOD aberrantes estimula respostas pró-inflamatórias exageradas, levando à inflamação crônica via produção de citocinas e quimiocinas em hospedeiros geneticamente suscetíveis.

DESEQUILÍBRIOS MICROBIANOS E DOENÇA ENTÉRICA

Doença inflamatória intestinal idiopática

A DII é um distúrbio intestinal crônico, imunologicamente mediado, resultante de complexas interações entre fatores ambientais e imunológicos em hospedeiros geneticamente suscetíveis (ver Capítulo 276).[30-32] Há evidências abundantes de que bactérias comensais estão envolvidas na patogênese da DII humana e em modelos animais experimentais de colite. A interação direta da microbiota comensal com a mucosa intestinal estimula a atividade inflamatória das lesões intestinais em humanos com DII.[4,30,33] Lesões intestinais também ocorrem em regiões anatômicas de maiores concentrações de bactérias luminais, como o cólon.[34] Flagelina derivada de bactérias comensais foi identificada como um antígeno dominante em humanos e cães, sugerindo que o reconhecimento de flagelina dependente de TLR5 desempenha um papel nas respostas imunológicas à microbiota comensal observada em DII.[35] Além disso, mutações de NOD2/CARD15 foram fortemente associadas com o desenvolvimento da doença de Crohn, implicando um papel da disfunção de PRR e da detecção bacteriana prejudicada na DII.[4,26,29]

Os modelos animais também sugerem que a microbiota residente seja um fator causal de DII. Em vários modelos de animais diferentes, a colite e a ativação imune não se desenvolvem na ausência de bactérias comensais.[1,2,4,30] Outros modelos também respondem à terapia antimicrobiana para a sua doença. Além disso, foi demonstrado que diferentes espécies bacterianas podem causar fenótipos diversos de doenças em um único hospedeiro e que outras espécies podem fornecer os estímulos dominantes para a expressão da doença.[36]

Os dados clínicos e de pesquisa indicam que a microbiota residente provavelmente desempenha um papel fundamental na condução do processo inflamatório de DII em animais de companhia. A participação das bactérias luminais é fortemente sugerida por observações da atenuação da doença clínica em gatos pelos níveis terapêuticos de metronidazol e em cães pela tilosina.[32,37] Em estudos separados, um aumento de macrófagos mieloides/histiócitos positivos para antígeno da lâmina própria,[38] regulação positiva da expressão da molécula de MHC de classe II epitelial[39] e aumento da reatividade de anticorpos para componentes da microbiota bacteriana indígena normal[40] foram associados com inflamação intestinal crônica de DII felina. Além disso, o número de *Enterobacteriaceae* associada com a mucosa mostrou correlação com as anormalidades na histologia duodenal, a regulação positiva de RNA mensageiro (mRNA) de citocinas da mucosa e o número de sinais clínicos em gatos com DII.[41] Em estudos separados, cães com DII mostraram comunidades microbianas duodenais distintas em comparação com cães saudáveis,[42] e TLR2, 4 e 9 responsivos a bactérias foram regulados positivamente na mucosa duodenal e na colônia inflamada de cães doentes.[43] Isso pode levar a um aumento da inflamação por meio da interação com bactérias comensais. Uma associação entre *E. coli* aderente/invasiva (AIEC) e colite granulomatosa (GC, anteriormente colite ulcerativa histiocítica) foi atualmente reconhecida, em que cães afetados respondem a terapia antimicrobiana com fluoroquinolona.[44] Estudos filogenéticos detalhados têm confirmado uma notável semelhança entre isolados AIEC obtidos de cães Boxer com GC e isolados AIEC derivados de tecidos ileais de humanos com doença de Crohn.[45]

Diarreia responsiva a antibióticos

Perturbações na microbiota intestinal e/ou respostas desreguladas do hospedeiro aos seus componentes podem causar sinais crônicos de diarreia e perda de peso (ver Capítulo 276). O SIBO canino tradicionalmente é definido com base no aumento do número de bactérias anaeróbias obrigatórias no suco duodenal, mas existem controvérsias sobre quais são as quantidades bacterianas normais.[46] Embora os limites numéricos de bactérias encontradas em cães assintomáticos possam variar (como mencionado anteriormente), há um consenso geral de que SIBO pode ocorrer de modo secundário à insuficiência pancreática exócrina, depuração prejudicada de bactérias (p. ex., obstrução intestinal, distúrbio de motilidade) ou lesão da mucosa (doença infiltrativa da mucosa).[47] Pouco se sabe sobre a etiologia do SIBO idiopático em cães, e o termo diarreia responsiva a antibióticos (DRA) foi proposto para enteropatias responsivas a antibióticos sem uma causa subjacente.[48,49]

O aumento do número de bactérias intestinais (ou seja, SIBO) poderia causar má absorção e diarreia por meio de: (1) competição por nutrientes – a ligação bacteriana da cobalamina que prejudica sua absorção intestinal; (2) metabolismo bacteriano de nutrientes em produtos secretores (p. ex., ácidos graxos hidroxilados, sais biliares desconjugados), que promovem as secreções do cólon; e (3) lesão bioquímica na mucosa intestinal, que diminui a sua atividade enzimática.[49] A DRA pode se desenvolver de modo secundário à alteração da função de barreira, à imunidade de mucosa aberrante ou às alterações qualitativas na microbiota entérica. Estudos mostram que cães com DRA podem ter deficiência seletiva de IgA (raça Pastor-Alemão) e aumento das células T CD4 + e dos plasmócitos produtores de IgA da mucosa, o que refletiria uma patogênese imunológica subjacente.[50] A microbiota presente na DRA em geral consiste em uma população mista de aeróbios e anaeróbios comensais que normalmente habitam o intestino.

Critérios de diagnóstico para diferenciar SIBO de DRA permanecem mal definidos. Avaliações diagnósticas completas para eliminar outras causas para sinais no trato GI devem ser realizadas. Devido às limitações da bacteriologia quantitativa tradicional, foram desenvolvidos testes indiretos para SIBO/DRA, como determinação da concentração de folato sérico, cobalamina e ácidos biliares não conjugados, mas eles não são confiáveis.[46,47] O teste diagnóstico atual de escolha para DRA idiopática é a remissão dos sinais clínicos após administração de antibiótico.

Gastrenterite infecciosa

Bactérias enteropatogênicas podem causar diarreia em cães e gatos jovens e adultos (ver Capítulo 220). As bactérias que são incriminadas por causar enterocolite com mais frequência incluem *Clostridium perfringens*, *Clostridioides difficile*, *Campylobacter* spp., patotipos de *E. coli* e *Salmonella* spp.[51] A verdadeira prevalência de diarreia mediada por bactérias é confundida pela presença de muitos desses microrganismos em animais sadios. No entanto, diarreia atribuída à perturbação na microbiota intestinal pode resultar da proliferação de microrganismos, produção de enterotoxinas e/ou invasão da mucosa. Informações sobre a patogênese da diarreia associada a *C. perfringens* são limitadas, mas o mecanismo provavelmente envolve cepas comensais enterotoxigênicas.[51] A administração de antimicrobianos antes da internação e a de drogas imunossupressoras durante a hospitalização foram fatores de risco para colonização por *C. difficile* em um estudo.[52] A infecção por *C. jejuni* é elevada em ambientes lotados e insalubres, e a produção de uma citotoxina e uma toxina termolábil promove inflamação da mucosa e secreção de fluidos, respectivamente. Muito ainda precisa ser aprendido sobre o papel da infecção por *Helicobacter* spp. na gastrite crônica canina e felina, mas estudos concluídos até o momento indicam que essa bactéria é altamente prevalente em cães e gatos saudáveis e doentes e que não existe uma relação simples entre infecção e doença.[53,54]

PROBIÓTICOS, PREBIÓTICOS E SIMBIÓTICOS

As bactérias podem ser usadas para melhorar a saúde do trato GI. *Probióticos* são microrganismos vivos que, após a ingestão em quantidade suficiente, promovem benefícios de saúde além daqueles inerentes à nutrição básica.[55] Lactobacilos e bifidobactérias têm sido os mais comumente usados, mas coquetéis multicepas (p. ex., VSL#3), *E. coli* Nissle 1917 e *Saccharomyces boulardii* (não bacteriano) também têm sido usados por seus efeitos probióticos.[56,57] Bactérias probióticas conferem benefícios mensuráveis ao hospedeiro, incluindo a capacidade de melhorar a função da barreira epitelial, modular o sistema imunológico da mucosa e alterar a microbiota intestinal (Figura 274.3). Os *prebióticos* são carboidratos não digeríveis da dieta – lactossacarose, fruto-oligossacarídeos (FOS), Psyllium, farelos – que estimulam o crescimento e o metabolismo de bactérias entéricas endógenas protetoras.[58] Os efeitos benéficos dos prebióticos também estão associados com a produção de SCFA, devido à fermentação por

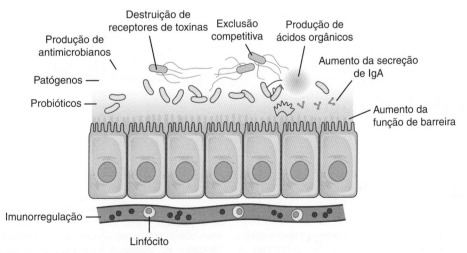

Figura 274.3 Mecanismos propostos de atividade probiótica. *IgA*, imunoglobulina A. (Adaptada de Ewaschuk JB, Dieleman LA: *Probiotics and prebiotics in chronic inflammatory bowel diseases.* World J Gastroenterol 12:5941-5950, 2006.)

SEÇÃO 18 • Doença Gastrintestinal

bactérias do cólon. *Simbióticos* são combinações de probióticos e prebióticos, uma modalidade terapêutica emergente. Evidências crescentes apoiam um papel terapêutico para probióticos, prebióticos e simbióticos em doenças gastrintestinais em humanos, incluindo diarreia infecciosa, infecção por *H. pylori*, síndrome do intestino irritável, deficiência de lactase e alguns tipos de DII.[1,2,59]

Estudos científicos investigaram os efeitos da suplementação alimentar com prebióticos na microbiota de cães e gatos saudáveis. Em um estudo, um suplemento de FOS a 0,75% de matéria seca produziu alterações qualitativas e quantitativos na microbiota fecal de gatos saudáveis.[60] Comparados com amostras de gatos alimentados com uma dieta basal, um aumento do número de lactobacilos e de *Bacteroides* spp. e uma diminuição do número de *E. coli* foram associados à dieta FOS. No entanto, o exame bacteriológico do suco duodenal desses mesmos gatos mostrou grande variação na composição da microbiota durante os períodos de amostragem, que não foram afetados pela suplementação de FOS.[61] Além disso, cães saudáveis da raça Beagle alimentados com uma dieta de 1% de FOS em um ensaio de 3 meses mostraram excreção fecal inconsistente de *Lactobacillus* spp. e *Bifidobacterium* spp.[62]

Existem poucos relatos sobre o uso de bactérias probióticas em cães e gatos. Estudos recentes *in vitro* confirmaram a capacidade de um coquetel probiótico liofilizado (p. ex., três cepas diferentes de *Lactobacillus* spp.) para modular a expressão de citocinas regulatórias *versus* pró-inflamatórias em cães com enteropatias crônicas.[63] No entanto, um ensaio clínico usando esse mesmo coquetel em cães com diarreia responsiva a alimentos falhou em induzir padrões consistentes da expressão de citocinas regulatórias (p. ex., efeito benéfico), apesar da clara melhoria clínica.[64] É relatado que um probiótico fabricado comercialmente (FortiFlora – *Enterococcus faecium* SF68, Nestlé Purina) tem benefício potencial no controle da diarreia e no aumento das respostas imunológicas em cães e gatos.[65] Mais recentemente, o probiótico humano VSL#3 mostrou aumentar a remissão clínica e reduzir a inflamação histopatológica em cães com IBD quando administrado continuamente por 8 semanas.[66]

TRANSPLANTE DE MICROBIOTA FECAL

O transplante de microbiota fecal (TMF) descreve "a infusão de uma suspensão fecal de um indivíduo saudável para o trato GI de um indivíduo com doença do cólon."[67] O fundamento lógico por trás do TMF inclui a reintrodução de uma comunidade microbiana completa e estável, destinada a reparar ou substituir a microbiota nativa alterada para corrigir um desequilíbrio subjacente. Supõe-se que a microbiota repara, erradica ou impede patógenos, que podem estar causando doenças específicas no trato GI, como a colite por infecção de *Clostridioides difficile*

Tabela 274.1 Considerações práticas para o transplante de microbiota fecal (TMF).

PARÂMETRO	CONSIDERAÇÃO
Seleção do doador	Raça – suscetível a doenças gastrintestinais? Histórico de vacinação Triagem diagnóstica para agentes infecciosos História recente de uso de antibióticos
Preparação do receptor	Papel da dieta? Realizar lavagem intestinal? Realizar teste com antibiótico antes?
Estocagem da amostra do doador	Fezes frescas *versus* congeladas
Tipo de diluente	Solução salina *versus* água *versus* leite
Volume de fezes requerido	Aproximadamente 60 g de fezes em 250 a 300 mℓ de diluente
Rota de administração	Nasogástrica/entérica *versus* colonoscopia

As diretrizes práticas para TMF estão em revisão, e seu estabelecimento para cães, gatos ou mesmo humanos ainda está em suspenso.

(CDI) em humanos.[67,68] Evidências recentes têm implicado a microbiota intestinal na patogênese de outros distúrbios que não afetam o trato GI em pacientes humanos, incluindo obesidade, diabetes melito, autismo, miastenia *gravis* e artrite reumatoide. Apenas dados clínicos muito esparsos descrevem o uso de FMT para tratar doenças GI crônicas em cães e gatos, incluindo CDI e DII idiopática. Diretrizes práticas formais para a realização do TMF estão sendo elaboradas, mas devem incluir: (1) as indicações clínicas para seu uso; (2) procedimentos adequados de triagem de doadores; (3) preparação do material fecal; e (4) possíveis vias de administração (Tabela 274.1).[67] A ligação entre a microbiota intestinal e a saúde do trato GI é reconhecida, e a manipulação fisiológica da microbiota intestinal representa uma excitante estratégia terapêutica para prevenção e tratamento da inflamação GI crônica.

REFERÊNCIAS BIBLIOGRÁFICAS

As referências bibliográficas deste capítulo se encontram online no Ambiente de Aprendizagem.

CAPÍTULO 275

Doenças do Estômago

Kenneth W. Simpson

ANATOMIA E FISIOLOGIA FUNCIONAL

Visão geral

A principal função do estômago é a de atuar como um reservatório que controla o tamanho e a taxa de passagem da ingesta para o intestino delgado. O estômago também inicia a digestão das proteínas e gorduras, e facilita a absorção de vitaminas e minerais.

Anatomicamente, o estômago é composto por quatro regiões: cárdia, fundo, corpo e antro (Figura 275.1). O fundo e o corpo se expandem para acomodar a ingesta. O antro é grosso e muscular e tritura os alimentos em partículas menores que são liberados no duodeno. O esfíncter esofágico posterior evita o refluxo da ingesta para o esôfago, e o esfíncter pilórico controla o efluxo para o duodeno.

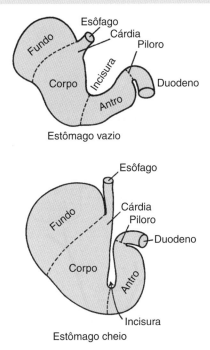

Figura 275.1 Anatomia gástrica do estômago vazio e cheio. (De Guilford WG, Strombeck DR: Gastric structure and function. In Guilford WG et al., editors: *Strombeck's small animal gastroenterology*, 3 ed., Philadelphia, 1996, Saunders, p 239.)

A parede gástrica tem três camadas: mucosa, muscular e serosa. A mucosa possui um epitélio superficial, glândulas gástricas e uma camada mais interna de músculo liso, com estrutura fina e função variável dependendo da região gástrica. A mucosa da cárdia e do piloro é mais fina e menos glandular do que no fundo e no corpo. A mucosa do corpo contém células mucosas do colo (pepsinogênio A, lipase gástrica), células parietais (ácido, pepsinogênio A, fator intrínseco) e células principais (pepsinogênio A; Figura 275.2).[1-3] Uma variedade de células neuroendócrinas envolvidas com a secreção de ácido gástrico são intercaladas entre as glândulas. As células predominantes são células do tipo enterocromafim e células produtoras de somatostatina no fundo com gastrina e células produtoras de somatostatina no antro. Pequenos agregados localizados de tecidos linfoides são observados na base das glândulas gástricas. Entrelaçada entre glândulas gástricas há uma rica rede de vasos sanguíneos, linfáticos e nervos. Abaixo da submucosa há duas camadas de músculos perpendiculares uns aos outros. A serosa é a camada mais externa.

Regulação da secreção de ácido

A secreção de ácido é regulada por uma variedade de substâncias neuroquímicas e estímulos neuro-humorais.[4,5] Peptídeos luminais, proteína digerida, acetilcolina e peptídeo liberador de gastrina estimulam a secreção de gastrina pelas células G e promovem a liberação de histamina por células do tipo enterocromafins (Figura 275.3). A liberação de histamina de mastócitos e a ligação de acetilcolina e gastrina às células parietais também contribuem para a secreção. A somatostatina, liberada em resposta aos níveis de pH gástrico abaixo de 3, diminui a secreção de gastrina, histamina e ácido.

A secreção de ácido não estimulada em cães e gatos é mínima (em cães, < 0,04 mmol/kg^{0,75}/h)[6] e a H$^+$/K$^+$-ATPase, "a bomba de ácido", está presente em tubulovesículas dentro do citoplasma de células parietais.[7] No estado estimulado, H$^+$/K$^+$-ATPase e transportadores de KCl são incorporados na membrana canalicular da célula parietal; íons de hidrogênio, derivados da ionização da água dentro das células parietais, são transportados para o interior do lúmen do estômago em troca de K pela H$^+$/K$^+$-ATPase. Transportadores de potássio e de cloreto na membrana canalicular

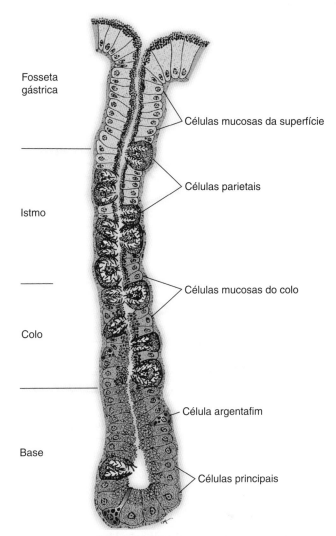

Figura 275.2 Aparência histológica da mucosa fúndica. (© Kenneth W. Simpson.)

permitem a transferência luminal de potássio e cloreto. O OH$^-$ se combina com o minúsculo CO$_2$, catalisado pela anidrase carbônica, para formar HCO$_3^-$, que se difunde no sangue (a "maré alcalina"). A estimulação resulta em um rápido aumento na secreção de íons de hidrogênio e fluidos, com o pH diminuindo rapidamente para cerca de 1. As concentrações de K$^+$ (10 a 20 mmol/ℓ) e Cl$^-$ (aproximadamente 120 a 160 mmol/ℓ) no suco gástrico são mais elevadas do que no plasma.

O estômago é protegido do ácido gástrico por uma unidade funcional conhecida como *barreira mucosa gástrica* (BMG).[8-10] A BMG compreende uma compacta camada de células epiteliais revestidas com uma camada de muco rica em bicarbonato e um abundante suprimento de sangue na mucosa que fornece bicarbonato, oxigênio e nutrientes. A produção local de prostaglandinas (PGE$_2$) é importante na modulação do fluxo sanguíneo, secreção de bicarbonato e renovação celular epitelial. Quando ocorre um dano, as células epiteliais migram rapidamente sobre a superfície mucosa lesionada, auxiliadas pela produção local de fatores de crescimento, como o fator de crescimento epidérmico (EGF, do inglês *epidermal growth fator*).

Motilidade gástrica

A motilidade gástrica normal é o resultado da interação organizada dos músculos lisos com estímulos neurais e hormonais. A taxa de esvaziamento gástrico é determinada pela diferença de pressão entre o estômago e o duodeno e a resistência do

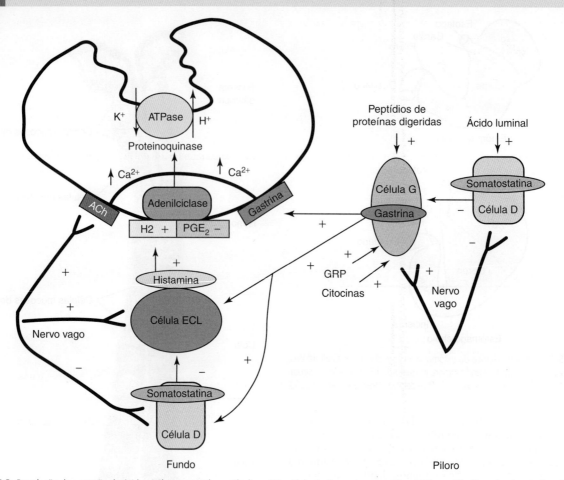

Figura 275.3 Regulação da secreção de ácido. *ACh*, receptor de acetilcolina; *ECL*, célula do tipo enterocromafim; *GRP*, peptídio liberador de gastrina; *H2*, receptor de histamina H2; *PGE*, receptor de prostaglandina E2. (Adaptada de Simpson KW: In DiBartola SP, editor: *Fluid, electrolyte, and acid-base disorders in small animal practice*, 4 ed., Philadelphia, 2012, Saunders.)

fluxo através do piloro. Os líquidos são liberados mais rapidamente do que os sólidos, e a taxa de liberação de líquidos aumenta com o volume. A taxa de liberação de sólidos depende da densidade calórica. Em cães, sólidos digestíveis de tamanho < 2 mm são esvaziados no duodeno. O esvaziamento gástrico é modulado via osmorreceptores e quimiorreceptores intestinais. Carboidratos, aminoácidos e, especialmente, gorduras retardam o esvaziamento gástrico. A liberação de colecistocinina (CCK) em resposta a ácidos graxos e aminoácidos, como o triptofano, é um fator que retarda o esvaziamento gástrico. Sólidos grandes e indigeríveis são liberados do estômago em jejum pela fase III do complexo motor migratório em resposta à liberação de motilina.

Digestão e assimilação de nutrientes

O estômago tem um papel limitado na digestão de proteínas, gorduras e micronutrientes. A pepsina, que digere proteínas, é secretada como pepsinogênio em resposta à acetilcolina e histamina em conjunto com o ácido gástrico. A lipase gástrica canina, que digere a gordura, é secretada em resposta à pentagastrina, histamina, prostaglandina E_2 e secretina, paralelamente à secreção de muco gástrico. Embora a pepsina seja ativa apenas em pH ácido, a lipase gástrica canina permanece ativa no intestino delgado e constitui até 30% da lipase total secretada em um período de 3 horas.[11] Embora a lipase gástrica e a pepsina não sejam essenciais para a assimilação de gordura e proteína da dieta, a entrada de peptídios e ácidos graxos no intestino delgado provavelmente ajuda a coordenar o esvaziamento gástrico e a secreção pancreática. O fator intrínseco, necessário para a absorção da cobalamina (vitamina B12), é produzido por células parietais e células na base das glândulas antrais em cães, mas não em gatos.[1,12] A importância da secreção do fator intrínseco gástrico é questionável, pois o pâncreas é o principal local de secreção tanto em cães quanto em gatos. A acidez gástrica também pode afetar a disponibilidade de minerais, como ferro e cálcio.

Microbiota gástrica

O conceito de um conteúdo gástrico estéril foi alterado quando a bactéria gástrica *Helicobacter pylori* foi isolada do estômago humano em 1983.[13] O estômago em cães e gatos também abriga um amplo espectro de espécies de *Helicobacter* grandes, espirais e tolerantes a ácidos e uma variedade de microrganismos aeróbios e anaeróbios que podem desempenhar um papel no desenvolvimento de gastrite ou mesmo câncer (ver Gastrite crônica). Uma microbiota mista de aeróbios e anaeróbios (aproximadamente 10^6 a 10^7 CFU/mℓ) é estabelecida logo após o nascimento em cães e a colonização por *Helicobacter* spp., que é provavelmente adquirida da mãe, e tem sido descrita logo às 6 semanas de idade.[14] *Helicobacter* spp. são adaptados para vida em um ambiente ácido e produzem urease que catalisa a formação de amônia a partir da ureia para tamponar a acidez gástrica. Outras espécies bacterianas cultivadas a partir do estômago canino (*Proteus*, *Streptococcus*, *Lactobacillus*) podem aumentar temporariamente após uma refeição ou após coprofagia.[15] A aplicação de métodos moleculares modernos para identificar bactérias demonstrou que a maioria das sequências no estômago de cães saudáveis da raça Beagle pertence a Proteobacteria (99,6%) com apenas alguns Firmicutes (0,3%). As Proteobacterias incluíram o gênero *Helicobacter* (98,6%) em biopsias gástricas, conforme análises com

CAPÍTULO 275 • Doenças do Estômago

prévias *in situ*.[15-18] A secreção de ácido e o esvaziamento gástrico provavelmente regulam grande parte dessa microbiota transitória, e bactérias podem proliferar em caso de hipossecreção de ácido gástrico devido à atrofia glandular ou inibição farmacológica. O pirossequenciamento de amplicons do gene *16S* rRNA (região V1-V3) revelou uma diminuição de *Helicobacter* spp. durante administração de omeprazol (mediana de 92% das sequências durante a administração em comparação com > 98% antes e depois da administração; P = 0,0336), o que foi acompanhado por maiores proporções de Firmicutes e Fusobacteria. Hibridização fluorescente *in situ* (FISH, *fluorescence* in situ *hybridization*) confirmou essa diminuição de *Helicobacter* gástrico (P < 0,0001) e mostrou um aumento no total de bactérias no duodeno (P = 0,0033) durante a administração de omeprazol.[15] Do ponto de vista do diagnóstico, é importante perceber que bactérias como *Proteus* spp. produzem urease, o que pode levar a um resultado de teste falso positivo para *Helicobacter* spp.

AVALIAÇÃO CLÍNICA DAS DOENÇAS DO ESTÔMAGO

Visão geral

A doença gástrica é geralmente o resultado de inflamação, ulceração, neoplasia ou obstrução. Manifesta-se clinicamente como vômito (ver Capítulo 39), hematêmese, melena (ver Capítulo 41), náuseas, ânsia de vômito, eructação, hipersalivação, distensão abdominal (ver Capítulo 17), dor abdominal ou perda de peso (ver Capítulo 19). A abordagem clínica pode ser simplificada considerando as doenças gástricas como um grupo de síndromes clínicas com base na combinação de etiologia, patologia e apresentação clínica (Tabela 275.1). Uma vez que um grande e variado grupo de doenças não gástricas pode causar sinais clínicos semelhantes, uma abordagem sistemática é essencial para determinar se uma doença gástrica primária é a causa. A abordagem de diagnóstico inicialmente se concentra no histórico e em achados físicos, com testes de patologia clínica e diagnóstico por imagem empregados em pacientes com envolvimento sistêmico ou sinais crônicos (Figura 275.4).

Sinais, histórico e exame físico

A idade e a raça podem ser úteis no diagnóstico de certas desordens gástricas. Cães jovens são mais propensos a ingerir corpos estranhos ou sofrer de obstrução de fluxo causada por *Pythium insidiosum*, enquanto o câncer gástrico é frequentemente encontrado em cães e gatos muito mais velhos. Dilatação volvulogástrica são geralmente encontrados em raças gigantes e cães com peito profundo, como Dogue Alemão e Setter Irlandês. Existem também predisposições reconhecidas em algumas raças caninas à gastropatia hipertrófica (Spaniel Perdigueiro de Drenthe, Basenji, Shih Tzu), gastrite atrófica (Norsk Lundehund) e câncer gástrico (p. ex., Pastor-Belga, Collie, Staffordshire Bull Terrier, Beagle e

Norsk Lundehund). O vômito é o principal sinal clínico de doença gástrica (ver Tabela 275.1), e um dos principais objetivos do histórico é distinguir o vômito da regurgitação (esforço abdominal ativo, presença de bile; ver Capítulo 39). Deve-se tentar obter informações sobre duração, frequência, conteúdo, cor, progressão e relação com a alimentação. Se o vômito não puder ser adequadamente diferenciado da regurgitação, é importante observar os episódios. Deve-se solicitar ao tutor que grave os episódios em casa. Se a regurgitação for apenas uma possibilidade, um vídeo será útil. Além disso, radiografias torácicas podem ser usadas para detectar dilatação ou obstrução esofágica.

Uma revisão completa do ambiente, incluindo se o animal vive dentro de casa ou ao ar livre, se é um domicílio com um único animal ou com diversos animais, se tem acesso a corpos estranhos, toxinas ou medicamentos, o estado de vacinação, os sistemas corporais (atitude, comportamento, presença de poliúria, polidipsia, perda de peso, diarreia, tosse, espirro, tolerância ao exercício), histórico médico anterior e exame físico ajudam a diferenciar causas de vômito não gástricas de gástricas. O exame físico é frequentemente normal em animais de estimação com doença gástrica primária. Distensão abdominal pode ser detectada em animais com dilatação gástrica/dilatação volvulogástrica (DG/DVG) ou retardo no esvaziamento gástrico. Perfusão anormal, estado de hidratação, temperatura, frequência respiratória, palidez da mucosa e dor abdominal, muitas vezes acompanham doenças como DG/DVG, obstrução do fluxo gástrico, ulceração e perfuração. Achados históricos e físicos devem ser integrados para determinar se o paciente está sistemicamente bem ou mal e se os sinais clínicos podem ser agudos, crônicos, discretos ou graves (ver Figura 275.4).

Vômito não produtivo, náuseas, ânsia de vômito e distensão abdominal em cães de peito profundo e de raças grandes são frequentemente associados com DG/DVG, que requer diagnóstico rápido e tratamento (ver Capítulos 143 e 144). A presença de sangue fresco ou digerido ("borra de café") no vômito, com ou sem melena, aumenta a possibilidade de úlceras gástricas ou erosões. Vômito de alimentos > 8 a 10 horas após a ingestão sugere retardo no esvaziamento gástrico, necessitando de discriminação entre obstrução do fluxo gástrico de propulsão gástrica defeituosa. A perda de peso é raramente associada a doença gástrica, mas pode acompanhar câncer, infecções fúngicas, obstrução do fluxo e gastropatias que podem fazer parte de um processo de doença mais generalizado, como gastroenteropatia em cães das raças Basenji e Norsk Lundehund. Se o vômito for agudo e o animal estiver sistematicamente bem, sem histórico ou "alertas vermelhos" físicos, testes diagnósticos adicionais são frequentemente adiados em favor da terapia sintomática. Se o animal está sistemicamente doente ou tem histórico significativo ou anormalidades físicas, a ênfase se volta para a identificação de condições que necessitem de intervenção cirúrgica, como dilatação gástrica e peritonite séptica, além de excluir causas não gastrintestinais de vômito antes de prosseguir para procedimentos mais especializados ou invasivos de diagnóstico destinados a detectar distúrbios gástricos e intestinais primários (Figura 275.4).

Exames laboratoriais

Os exames laboratoriais ajudam a diferenciar a doença gastrintestinal (GI) primária de doença não GI e para averiguar as consequências metabólicas da doença GI (ver Capítulo 39). Amostras de sangue e urina devem ser obtidas antes do tratamento. Em animais de estimação doentes, uma avaliação rápida do micro-hematócrito (M), proteínas plasmáticas totais (PPT), glicose e nitrogênio da ureia no sangue (NUS), gravidade específica, glicose, cetonas e proteína da urina, e as concentrações plasmáticas de sódio (Na) e potássio (K) ajudam a detectar doenças potencialmente fatais: por exemplo, insuficiência renal (azotemia, isostenúria; ver Capítulos 322 e 324) e hipoadrenocorticismo (ver Capítulo 309), e para orientar a terapia inicial enquanto se fazem testes mais definitivos.

Tabela 275.1 Doenças do estômago.

SÍNDROME CLÍNICA	CARACTERÍSTICAS PREDOMINANTES
Gastrite aguda	Início súbito de vômitos
Ulceração ou erosão	Vômitos, hematêmese, melena, ± anemia
Dilatação gástrica/vólvulo	Ânsia de vômito, distensão abdominal, taquicardia
Gastrite crônica	Vômito crônico de alimento ou bile
Esvaziamento gástrico retardado	Vômito agudo a crônico após mais de 8 a 10 h da alimentação
Neoplasia	Vômito crônico, perda de peso, ± anemia

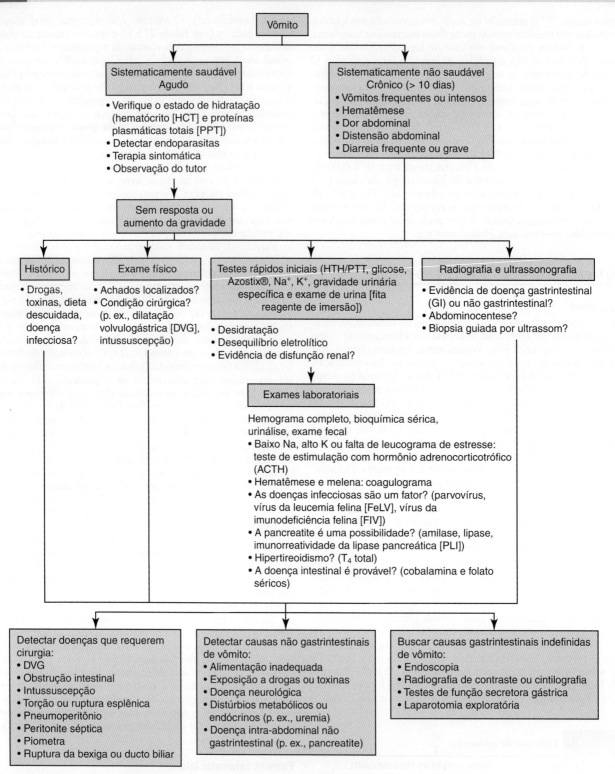

Figura 275.4 Abordagem diagnóstica do paciente com vômito. (© Kenneth W. Simpson.)

Anormalidades no hemograma completo (CBC) são infrequentes em doença gástrica primária. A hemoconcentração como uma consequência de desidratação ou choque frequentemente acompanha uma DVG, perfuração gástrica ou obstrução gástrica. A combinação de um nível de hematócrito superior a 55% e concentrações de proteína normais ou diminuídas é encontrada em cães com gastrenterite hemorrágica e foi associada à proliferação de *Clostridium* spp. e a elaboração da toxina necrosante, netF (ver Capítulo 276).[19,20]

Anemia, microcitose eritrocitária e trombocitose podem estar presentes em cães com sangramento gástrico crônico. Cães da raça Spaniel Perdigueiro de Drentse podem ter estomatocitose-gastrite hipertrófica familiar. Um pontilhado basofílico dos eritrócitos sugere toxicose por chumbo. Anormalidades bioquímicas na doença gástrica primária são geralmente restritas a alterações nos eletrólitos e equilíbrio ácido-base, aumentos pré-renais na creatinina e NUS, e ocasionalmente hipoproteinemia.

CAPÍTULO 275 • Doenças do Estômago

O vômito do conteúdo gástrico e intestinal geralmente envolve a perda de fluido contendo cloreto (Cl), K, Na e bicarbonato. A desidratação é variavelmente acompanhada por diminuições de Na, K e Cl.[21,22] A determinação do estado ácido-base avaliando o CO_2 total ou gasometria venosa permite o reconhecimento de acidose metabólica ou alcalose (ver Capítulo 128). Acidose metabólica é geralmente mais comum do que a alcalose metabólica em cães com doença GI.[21] Quando a via de saída gástrica ou o duodeno está obstruído, a perda de Cl pode exceder a de bicarbonato, com diminuição de Cl e K, e alcalose.[21-23] A alcalose metabólica é aumentada pela retenção de HCO_3^- devido ao volume e depleção de K e Cl.[24] O efeito final é a conservação do volume em detrimento do pH extracelular. A reabsorção renal de quase todo bicarbonato filtrado e a troca de sódio por hidrogênio no túbulo distal promovem um pH urinário ácido apesar de uma alcalemia extracelular ("acidúria paradoxal").[24,25] Alcalose metabólica em pacientes com sinais gastrointestinais não está invariavelmente associada a obstrução do fluxo de saída e também foi encontrada em cães com enterite por parvovírus e pancreatite aguda.[26] Doenças caracterizadas por hipersecreção ácida, como o gastrinoma, também podem estar associadas com alcalose metabólica e acidúria. A secreção ácida gástrica basal em dois cães com tumores produtores de gastrina (1,7 e 2,7 mmol/h/kg^{0,75} HCl) foi máxima no estado não estimulado.[21] Nesta situação, a hipocloremia, hipocalemia, alcalose e desidratação são provavelmente devido à hipersecreção de ácido gástrico e sua perda no vômito.[27] A gasometria de sangue venoso e osmolalidade do plasma são frequentemente determinadas em animais com suspeita de ingestão de etilenoglicol, com os achados de acidose metabólica e um gap osmolal alto (calculado pela subtração da osmolalidade calculado e medida) sugestivos de ingestão (ver Capítulo 152).

Um NUS elevado na ausência de creatinina elevada é compatível com sangramento gástrico. A albumina baixa pode ser detectada em cães das raças Basenji ou Lundehund com gastroenteropatia perdedora de proteínas, cães com pitiose e cães ou gatos com neoplasia. O aumento das concentrações de globulinas foi observado na gastroenteropatia em cães Basenji, infecção por *Pythium* e plasmocitoma gástrico. Elevações de creatinina, ureia, cálcio (Ca), K, glicose, enzimas hepáticas, bilirrubina, colesterol, triglicerídeos e globulina e diminuição de Na, Ca, ureia ou albumina frequentemente se associam a causas não gastrointestinais de vômito.

A urina deve ser avaliada quanto à gravidade específica, pH, glicose, cilindros, cristais e bactérias. A urinálise completa é importante, por exemplo, cilindros de leucócitos na urina podem ser a única evidência de que uma pielonefrite é a causa do vômito (ver Capítulo 72). O teste de coagulação é indicado em pacientes com melena ou hematêmese para detectar coagulopatias subjacentes e naqueles com abdome agudo para detectar coagulopatia intravascular disseminada (CID; ver Capítulo 196). Doenças infecciosas associadas a vômitos e diarreia requerem exame fecal para diagnóstico de *Giardia*, endoparasitas, *Salmonella* spp., *Campylobacter* spp., e parvovírus (ELISA) ou teste sorológico (vírus da leucemia felina [FeLV], vírus da imunodeficiência felina [FIV]). Testes adicionais para confirmar o hipoadrenocorticismo (estimulação de ACTH), disfunção hepática (ácidos biliares pré e pós-prandiais), hipertireoidismo (T4), pancreatite (ultrassom e vários testes [ver Capítulo 289-291]), e doença intestinal (cobalamina e folato séricos; ver Capítulo 276). Em cães com DGV, avaliação do lactato sérico (ver Capítulos 70 e 144) no momento da admissão e sua resposta à terapia pode ajudar a determinar o prognóstico e a necessidade de terapia agressiva.[28-30]

IMAGEM

Radiografia abdominal

As radiografias são o teste de escolha na avaliação inicial de doença gástrica, vômito ou dor abdominal. Radiografias fornecem informações sobre a posição gástrica e conteúdos que podem ajudar a identificar DG/DVG, corpos estranhos e obstrução de fluxo gástrico. Elas também permitem avaliar o tamanho e a forma do fígado, rins e baço, além de auxiliar na detecção de intussuscepção, peritonite, pneumoperitônio e alterações sugestivas de pancreatite. As radiografias de contraste podem fornecer mais informações quando as radiografias comuns são inconclusivas. No entanto, a combinação de ultrassonografia (US) e endoscopia é geralmente mais eficaz para detectar obstrução, distúrbios gastrintestinais inflamatórios e neoplásicos do que radiografias de contraste. O uso de radiografia de contraste é frequentemente limitado à investigação de retardo no esvaziamento gástrico associado a defeitos na propulsão ou distúrbios intestinais "funcionais".[31]

Ultrassonografia abdominal, estudos com contraste, fluoroscopia

US pode ser empregada para avaliar a espessura da parede gástrica, estratificação da parede e esvaziamento gástrico (ver Capítulo 88). US é menos precisa do que a endoscopia para a detecção de neoplasia gástrica, particularmente linfoma, mas pode aumentar a suspeita de lesões gástricas e facilitar a detecção de lesões não gástricas em animais de estimação com sinais de doença gastrintestinal.[32,33] Quando US e endoscopia não estão disponíveis, a distensão do estômago com ar (contraste negativo) pode revelar espessamento gástrico, massas ou corpos estranhos. Contraste positivo com o sulfato de bário pode fornecer mais informações e também é usado para avaliar a permeabilidade do fluxo gástrico. A combinação de fluoroscopia e contraste positivo é útil para avaliar a permeabilidade pilórica e o esvaziamento gástrico. Na ausência de endoscopia e US, a radiografia de contraste pode ser seguida de biopsia cirúrgica para obter um diagnóstico definitivo.

Endoscopia

A endoscopia (ver Capítulo 113) permite a visualização direta e biopsia do estômago e duodeno, e é o melhor método para diagnosticar inflamação gástrica primária, ulceração ou neoplasia, remoção de pequenos corpos estranhos e avaliação dos pacientes antes da quantificação do esvaziamento gástrico. Ela não fornece boas informações sobre lesões submucosas ou desordens funcionais. Com espessamento mural ou massas gástricas endoscópicas, as biopsias muitas vezes não são profundas o suficiente para obter o tecido-alvo, sendo necessária uma biopsia cirúrgica. Avanços recentes em imagem por endoscopia, como endomicroscopia confocal e cromoendoscopia, podem ajudar a distinguir uma inflamação crônica da neoplasia.[34] Os equipamentos, seus cuidados, suas técnicas e fotografias de uma ampla gama de lesões GI são apresentadas nos Capítulos 83 e 113.[35,36]

A necessidade de anestesia geral frequentemente impede o uso de endoscopia digestiva alta em animais de estimação instáveis com sinais de doença gástrica (p. ex., hematêmese). O advento da endoscopia sem fio por cápsula revolucionou a imagem não invasiva do trato GI superior humano. Estudos preliminares em cães mostram a sua utilidade para identificar lesões da mucosa no fundo gástrico, piloro e intestino delgado associado ao parasitismo ou sangramento gastrointestinal.[37-39]

Avaliação do esvaziamento gástrico

Procedimentos e ferramentas usadas para avaliar o esvaziamento gástrico incluem contraste de bário (líquido ou misturado com alimentos), poliesferas impregnadas de bário, cintilografia nuclear, testes respiratórios de ^{13}C-octanoato e ^{13}C-acetato e cápsulas de endoscopia e motilidade sem fio.[37,40-44] Testes de esvaziamento gástrico são frequentemente usados para confirmar a suspeita de retardo no esvaziamento gástrico em pacientes com radiografias normais ou duvidosas. Eles também são usados quando a obstrução do fluxo gástrico e causas óbvias de propulsão defeituosa foram descartadas antes e após o uso de drogas

SEÇÃO 18 • Doença Gastrintestinal

procinéticas. As limitações e os benefícios dessas abordagens são discutidos em Esvaziamento gástrico retardado e Distúrbios da motilidade.

Teste de secreção gástrica

O teste de secreção gástrica é realizado principalmente em pacientes com esofagite, ulceração gastrintestinal, hipertrofia da mucosa ou com grandes quantidades de fluido gástrico quando a hipersecreção de ácido é suspeita. Em sua forma mais simples, o pH gástrico e a gastrina sérica em jejum são medidos para determinar se a hipersecreção de ácido é provável (ver Capítulo 273). A terapia antissecretória deve ser interrompida por 48 horas antes do teste. As disfunções renal e hepática devem ser descartadas, pois qualquer uma das condições pode causar aumento nas concentrações circulantes de gastrina. A ampla faixa de pH gástrico em jejum, não estimulada em cães e gatos (pH 1 a 8), torna difíceis declarações definitivas sobre a produção de ácido. No entanto, a presença de um pH gástrico de < 3 com aumentos simultâneos nas concentrações de gastrina sérica exclui a possibilidade de acloridria ou tumor de mastócitos e aumenta a possibilidade de gastrinoma.[27] Cães com tumores de mastócitos e hipersecreção de ácido induzida por hiper-histaminemia têm baixas concentrações séricas de gastrina. Provavelmente cães com acloridria têm concentrações aumentadas de gastrina, mas um pH gástrico > 3.[45] A determinação da concentração sérica de gastrina após infusão IV de secretina ou Ca é usada para investigar a possibilidade da produção de gastrina exógena por tumores pancreáticos (gastrinomas; síndrome de Zollinger-Ellison; ver Capítulo 310). Foi relatado que cães da raça Basenji com gastroenteropatia e diarreia apresentaram maior liberação de gastrina em resposta à estimulação de secretina sem evidência de gastrinoma.[46] Teste provocativo da secreção de ácido gástrico com estimulação de pentagastrina ou bombesina pode ser realizado para detectar acloridria em pacientes com gastrite atrófica, ou gastrina sérica elevada e pH gástrico > 3, para determinar a provável contribuição da acloridria. A secreção de ácido estimulada por pentagastrina em cães atinge um pico de 28 mℓ/kg^{0,75}/h, 4,1 mmol de HCl/kg^{0,75}/h, 0,34 mmol K$^+$/kg^{0,75}/h e 0,09 Na$^+$ mmol/kg^{0,75}/h.[6] Sedação com oximorfona e acepromazina é uma alternativa à anestesia para estudos de secreção em cães.[28] Em gatos, a produção de ácido (média ± DP) em resposta à pentagastrina (8 mcg/kg/h) varia de pH 0,9 a 1,1, com taxas de secreção (valores medianos) de 1,2 mmol/15 min a 1,4 ± 0,5 mmol/15 min em gatos conscientes e 1,2 (0,6 a 2,7) mmol/kg^{0,75}/h em gatos anestesiados.[47] O desenvolvimento de sistemas telemétricos de pH podem facilitar a avaliação não invasiva do pH gástrico em cães com suspeita de hipo e hipersecreção de ácido gástrico.[48,49]

GASTRITE AGUDA

Definições

Gastrite aguda é o termo aplicado à síndrome marcada por vômito de início súbito, presumivelmente devido a uma lesão ou inflamação da mucosa estomacal (Boxe 275.1). Na maioria dos animais de estimação, a causa é inferida pelo histórico, como alimentação inadequada; o diagnóstico raramente é confirmado por biopsia, e o tratamento é sintomático e de suporte (ver Capítulo 39). Animais com gastrite aguda associada à intoxicação por drogas, ingestão de corpo estranho, ou distúrbios metabólicos frequentemente apresentam hematêmese, melena, diarreia concomitante ou outros sinais de doença sistêmica, exigindo uma abordagem de diagnóstico completa para determinar a causa e fornecer cuidados ideais. Existem poucas evidências para apoiar uma causa de infecções virais (parvovírus, cinomose, hepatite infecciosa canina) na gastrite aguda.

Boxe 275.1 Causas da gastrite aguda

Alimentação inadequada ou intolerância (não alérgica e alérgica)
Corpos estranhos (ossos, brinquedos, bolas de pelo)
Drogas e toxinas (medicamentos anti-inflamatórios não esteroides, corticosteroides, metais pesados, antibióticos, plantas, produtos de limpeza, alvejante)
Doença sistêmica (uremia, doença hepática, hipoadrenocorticismo)
Parasitas (*Ollulanus, Physaloptera* spp.)
Bactérias (toxinas bacterianas, *Helicobacter*)
Vírus

Achados clínicos e diagnóstico

Vômito de início súbito é o principal sinal clínico do quadro agudo da gastrite. Em alguns casos, é acompanhado de hematêmese ou melena e graus variáveis de doença sistêmica. O histórico pode revelar acesso ou ingestão de comida estragada, lixo, toxinas, medicamentos ou corpos estranhos. Os sinais de intoxicação podem ser evidentes, como icterícia e palidez na ingestão de zinco, salivação ou defecação na intoxicação por organofosforados ou ingestão de cogumelos, e salivação e ulceração oral na ingestão de produtos químicos. O diagnóstico da gastrite aguda é geralmente com base nesses achados clínicos e resposta ao tratamento sintomático. Um diagnóstico específico pode ser buscado se o animal tem acesso a objetos estranhos ou toxinas, está sistematicamente indisposto, ou tem hematêmese, melena ou vômito que não responde a terapia sintomática ou outros sinais de doença mais séria. Os testes laboratoriais na maioria dos animais com gastrite aguda primária refletem desidratação leve e muitas vezes não são realizados na ausência de suspeita de doença mais grave. Radiografias abdominais podem ser feitas para detectar objetos estranhos ou obstrução GI. Diagnósticos adicionais, como ultrassonografia e endoscopia, raramente são indicados; a maioria dos animais com gastrite simples responde à terapia sintomática.

Tratamento

Fluidoterapia

Fluidos administrados por via oral, em pequenas quantidades, mas de modo frequente, podem ser dados a animais de estimação que estão vomitando, com o volume aumentado à medida que o vômito diminui. Administrar soluções eletrolíticas SC isotônicas balanceadas pode ser suficiente para corrigir déficits leves de fluido (< 5%), mas é insuficiente para desidratação moderada a grave. Animais de estimação que requerem fluidos IV (ver Capítulo 129) devem passar por uma avaliação diagnóstica mais extensa.

Restrição e modificação da dieta

Quando o vômito é agudo, a ingestão oral é interrompida por pelo menos 24 horas. Pequenas quantidades de uma dieta líquida podem ser oferecidas, apesar do vômito, para manter a função de barreira GI e determinar se o vômito foi resolvido. Uma dieta branda caseira não picante, com restrição de gordura (p. ex., frango cozido e arroz, queijo *cottage* de baixo teor de gordura e arroz [1: 3]), ou uma dieta comercial à base de arroz com restrição de gordura podem então ser introduzidas, dando pouco e frequentemente com uma transição feita de volta para uma dieta normal ao longo de 1 semana ou mais.

Protetores/adsorventes

Subsalicilato de bismuto, caulim-pectina, carvão ativado e magnésio, alumínio e produtos que contêm bário são frequentemente administrados a animais de estimação com vômito agudo ou diarreia para ligar bactérias e suas toxinas, e para revestir a mucosa GI. Esses agentes são provavelmente mais seguros e mais eficazes do que antibióticos ou modificadores de motilidade na gastrenterite aguda. Subsalicilato de bismuto (Pepto-Bismol 1 ml/5 kg via oral a cada 8 h), subcitrato de bismuto, caulim-pectina (1 a 2 ml/kg via oral a cada 8 h) e sucralfato (0,25 a 1 g via oral a cada 8 h) são frequentemente empregados. Drogas redutoras de ácido, como antagonistas do receptor H2, podem ser administradas, mas geralmente são reservadas para aqueles com sinais de erosão gástrica ou ulceração (melena, hematêmese) ou gastrite persistente, conforme descrito a seguir. Em geral, os antieméticos não devem ser administrados a animais de estimação com gastrite aguda para evitar mascarar a resposta à terapia. Pacientes que continuam a vomitar requerem investigação adicional.

Prognóstico

O prognóstico para gastrite aguda não complicada é geralmente de recuperação completa.

EROSÃO GÁSTRICA E ULCERAÇÃO

Definições e causas

Erosões gástricas e úlceras estão associadas a uma série de distúrbios gástricos e não gástricos primários (Tabela 275.2). Os sinais clínicos variam em duração e gravidade, de agudo a crônico e de discreto a fatal. O mecanismo do dano gástrico subjacente pode ser amplamente atribuído a comprometimento do BMG (definido anteriormente) por meio de lesão direta, interferência com prostaglandinas gastroprotetoras (PGE_2), muco ou bicarbonato, diminuição do fluxo sanguíneo e hipersecreção de ácido gástrico. Talvez a causa mais previsível para erosão gástrica e ulceração seja o uso de um medicamento anti-inflamatório não esteroide (AINE) ou um glicocorticoide, seja isoladamente, seja em combinação com doença do disco intervertebral.[50] Os AINEs causam danos diretos à mucosa e podem interferir na síntese de prostaglandinas.[9] Flunixino meglumina, ácido acetilsalicílico e ibuprofeno causam erosões gástricas e úlceras em cães saudáveis (Figura 275.5).[51] A administração de agentes anti-inflamatórios também é considerada um risco significativo para perfuração gástrica em cães e gatos.[52,53] Doses altas de glicocorticoides isoladamente, como dexametasona e metilprednisolona, causam erosões gástricas, mas os mecanismos pelos quais induzem danos ainda não estão claros.[60] Ao contrário dos AINEs, seus efeitos não são amenizados por análogos da PGE_2.[61]

Para contornar a toxicose causada pela inibição das "prostaglandinas amigáveis" (PGE_2), drogas que bloqueiam preferencialmente a "ciclo-oxigenase indutível (COX-2)" foram desenvolvidos.

Tabela 275.2	Associação de ulceração e erosão gástricas com doenças específicas.
PROBLEMA GÁSTRICO	**DOENÇAS RELACIONADAS**
Metabólico/endócrino	Hipoadrenocorticismo, uremia, doença hepática, mastocitose, CID, hipergastrinemia e outros APUDomas
Inflamação	Gastrite
Neoplasia	Leiomioma, adenocarcinoma, linfoma
Induzido por drogas	Anti-inflamatórios não esteroides e esteroides
Hipotensão	Choque, sepse
Idiopático	Estresse, cirurgia da coluna vertebral, induzida por exercício (cães de trenó)

CID, coagulopatia intravascular disseminada.

Esses agentes COX-2 seletivos (p. ex., carprofeno, meloxicam, deracoxibe, etodolaco) são menos ulcerogênicos em cães.[54,55] No entanto, mesmo drogas seletivas de COX-2, como meloxicam e deracoxibe, são ulcerogênicas, especialmente em combinação com dexametasona ou outros AINEs, sendo associadas à perfuração gástrica, mas a sua segurança em animais de estimação doentes ainda não foi determinada.[51,56-59]

Hipersecreção de ácido gástrico em resposta à histamina liberada por mastócitos e gastrina de gastrinomas são causas claras de ulceração gastroduodenal e esofagite em cães e gatos. Uremia, insuficiência hepática, hipoadrenocorticismo e hipotensão são frequentemente propostas como fatores de risco para erosão gástrica ou ulceração, embora poucos detalhes tenham sido publicados sobre patogênese, frequência ou gravidade do dano gástrico nessas condições. Em um estudo recente de cães com doença renal crônica (DRC), a ulceração estava presente em apenas 1 de 28 cães. Os achados predominantes nesses cães foram edema de mucosa, vasculopatia e mineralização, que se correlacionaram com o grau de azotemia e do produto cálcio-fósforo.[62,63] Achados semelhantes também foram observados em gatos com DRC.[63] Cães de trenó na corrida "Iditarod" (Iditarod Sled Dog Race) no Alasca são propensos a desenvolver erosões gástricas e úlceras (ver Capítulo 173).[64,65] Esse achado é semelhante ao provocado por atividades físicas de humanos e equinos nos quais a patogênese não é compreendida, mas responde à supressão de ácido. Erosões e úlceras também são sequelas de gastrite e câncer gástrico, e são discutidos neste capítulo.

Achados clínicos

Vômito, hematêmese e melena podem estar presentes em pacientes com erosões gástricas ou úlceras. Mucosas pálidas, dor abdominal, fraqueza, inapetência, hipersalivação (potencialmente associada a esofagite como consequência da hipersecreção de ácido gástrico; ver Capítulo 273) e evidências de comprometimento circulatório podem estar adicionalmente presentes de maneira variável. O acesso a toxinas e medicamentos, particularmente AINEs, deve ser determinado. A avaliação visa identificar as consequências atuais e doenças associadas a erosões gástricas e úlceras (ver Tabela 275.2). O hemograma completo pode revelar anemia, que é inicialmente regenerativa, mas pode progredir e se tornar microcítica, hipocrômica e minimamente regenerativa. Quando acompanhados de trombocitose e diminuição da saturação de ferro ou ferritina sérica baixa, esses achados são característicos de sangramento crônico e deficiência de ferro (ver Capítulos 57, 198 e 199). Eosinofilia e falta de um leucograma de estresse em cães é compatível com hipoadrenocorticismo, alergia alimentar (ver Capítulo 186), gastrenterite eosinofílica, mastocitose (ver Capítulo 349) ou uma síndrome hipereosinofílica. Leucocitose neutrofílica e desvio à esquerda

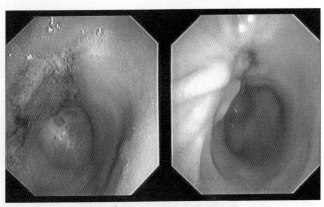

Figura 275.5 Ulceração gástrica causada pela ingestão de ibuprofeno antes e depois (1 semana) do tratamento com cimetidina e sucralfato. (© Kenneth W. Simpson.)

podem indicar inflamação ou possível perfuração gástrica. O exame de um esfregaço da capa leucocitária pode ajudar a detectar mastocitose.

Bioquímica e urinálise podem revelar achados compatíveis com desidratação (azotemia e hiperestenúria), doença renal (azotemia e isostenúria), doença hepática (aumento de enzimas hepáticas ou bilirrubina; diminuição do colesterol, albumina ou NUS) ou hipoadrenocorticismo (i. e., hiponatremia e/ou hiperpotassemia). Eles também identificarão anormalidades de eletrólitos e equilíbrio acidobásico associadas a vômitos e ulceração gastrintestinal. A presença de alcalose metabólica, hipocloremia, hipopotassemia e urina ácida é compatível com obstrução gastrintestinal superior (física ou funcional) ou um estado hipersecretor. Testes devem ser realizados para detectar anormalidades na hemostasia primária e secundária que podem estar associadas a sangramento gastrintestinal. As concentrações séricas de gastrina e histamina podem ser avaliadas quando a hipersecreção de ácido é suspeita como causa de ulceração.

Diagnóstico

Diagnóstico por imagem

Radiografias simples geralmente não são úteis no diagnóstico de erosões gástricas ou úlceras, mas podem ajudar a descartar outras causas de vômito, como corpos estranhos, peritonite e perfuração gástrica. Radiografias de contraste podem revelar defeitos de preenchimento, mas não permitem uma avaliação detalhada ou amostragem da mucosa. A ultrassonografia (ver Capítulo 88) pode ser usada para avaliar a parede gástrica quanto ao espessamento associado a úlceras ou massas e também ajuda a descartar causas não gástricas de vômito. As informações fornecidas por radiografia e ultrassom são complementares à avaliação endoscópica, o teste diagnóstico de escolha (Figura 275.6).

Endoscopia

A endoscopia permite a avaliação direta da mucosa estomacal e a coleta de amostras (ver Capítulo 113). Úlceras associadas a AINEs tendem a ser encontradas no antro e geralmente não são relacionadas a espessamento acentuado da mucosa ou a bordas irregulares (ver Figura 275.5). Isso contrasta com os tumores ulcerados que frequentemente têm bordas espessadas e mucosa circundante (Figura 275.7). As úlceras devem ser biopsiadas na periferia para evitar perfuração. As biópsias obtidas por endoscopia não são ideais para o diagnóstico de neoplasia gástrica infiltrativa, mas várias biópsias do mesmo local podem ser feitas para permitir a amostragem de tecido mais profundo. Uma aspiração com agulha fina guiada por endoscopia que emprega uma agulha e tubo no canal de biópsia também pode ser usada para amostrar lesões profundas. Mesmo com essa abordagem, o diagnóstico pode ser perdido e a biópsia cirúrgica pode ser necessária para um diagnóstico definitivo.

pH gástrico e gastrina sérica

A combinação erosão ou ulceração da mucosa, hipertrofia da mucosa antral, suco gástrico abundante e esofagite é altamente sugestiva de hipersecreção (Figura 275.7). É prudente medir o pH gástrico e a gastrina sérica em animais de estimação com erosão gástrica ou ulceração não associada a drogas ou tumores gástricos.

Cães com tumores de mastócitos e hipersecreção ácida induzida por hiper-histaminemia têm baixas concentrações de gastrina sérica.[27] A combinação de pH gástrico < 3 e aumento de gastrina sérica deve levar a investigação adicional para gastrinoma por teste de estimulação de secretina, US (fígado e pâncreas) e cintilografia com pentertreotídio (análogo da somatostatina).[27] A utilidade do monitoramento de pH baseado em cápsula e da endoscopia na detecção de hipersecreção de ácido gástrico e anormalidades mucosas associadas não foi determinada em ambiente clínico. A administração de omeprazol ou famotidina (ambos a 1 mg/kg via oral a cada 24 horas) para o controle da secreção de ácido de pode aumentar a gastrina sérica dentro de 3 a 7 dias, de 37,2 ng/ℓ a 71,3 ± 19 e 65,5 ± 39,52 ng/ℓ, respectivamente.[66] O aumento da gastrina sérica induzida por terapia antiácida a curto prazo é resolvido após uma suspensão em um período de 7 dias.[66,67] Omeprazol (1,1 mg/kg via oral a cada 12 horas por 15 dias) foi associado a um grande aumento na gastrina, de um valor de base mediana de 10 ng/ℓ (intervalo: 10 a 27) até uma mediana máxima de 379,5 ng/ℓ (intervalo: 49,9 a 566) no nono dia do tratamento. A gastrina sérica permaneceu significativamente aumentada acima dos valores de linha de base do sexto ao décimo quinto dia de tratamento, mas retornou aos valores pré-tratamento no prazo de 3 dias após a cessação.[67]

Tratamento

Visão geral

O tratamento de erosões e úlceras gástricas é dirigido à causa subjacente. Deve-se tratar de anormalidades em hidratação (ver Capítulo 129), perfusão, eletrólitos e/ou acidobásicas (ver Capítulo 128). A transfusão de sangue pode ser indicada (ver Capítulo 130). O suporte adicional do BMG é aprimorado através da proteção da mucosa, citoproteção e diminuição da secreção de ácido gástrico. Quando o vômito é persistente, antieméticos (ver Capítulo 39) podem ajudar a reduzir a perda de fluidos, o desconforto e o risco de esofagite (ver Capítulo 273).

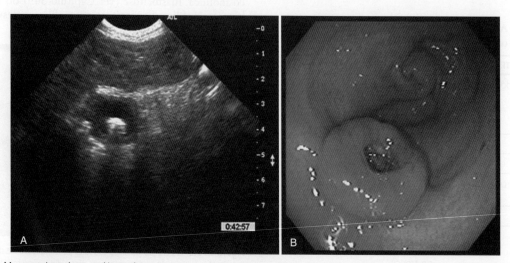

Figura 275.6 A. Massa projetando-se no lúmen do estômago de um cão apresentando vômito e hiperglobulinemia (IgA). **B.** A presença da massa é confirmada, permitindo o diagnóstico de plasmocitoma gástrico através de biopsia. (© Kenneth W. Simpson.)

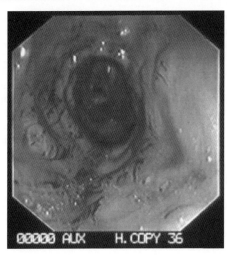

Figura 275.7 Erosão gástrica e hipertrofia da mucosa em cão com gastrinoma. (© Kenneth W. Simpson.) (*Esta figura se encontra reproduzida em cores no Encarte.*)

Fluidoterapia

A taxa de administração de fluidos (ver Capítulo 129) depende da presença ou ausência de choque (ver Capítulo 127), o grau de desidratação e a presença de doenças (p. ex., cardíaca ou renal), que predispõem à sobrecarga de volume. Pacientes com histórico de vômitos que estão levemente desidratados geralmente respondem a cristaloides (p. ex., LR ou NaCl 0,9%) a uma taxa que fornecerá os requisitos de manutenção bem como substituirá déficits e perdas em progresso. A depleção de potássio é muitas vezes uma consequência de vômitos prolongados ou anorexia, e a maioria dos fluidos de substituição poliônica contém apenas pequenas quantidades. Portanto, KCl é adicionado a fluidos parenterais com base nos níveis séricos. O monitoramento da pressão venosa central (ver Capítulo 76) e a avaliação da produção de urina (ver Capítulo 322) são necessários em pacientes com doença gastrintestinal grave, particularmente aqueles com complicações por perdas de fluido no terceiro espaço no intestino ou peritônio. Pacientes em choque requerem suporte mais agressivo (ver Capítulos 127, 129 e 144).

Redução da secreção de ácido

A inibição farmacológica da secreção de ácido (ver Figura 275.3) pode ser efetuada pelo bloqueio de receptores H2 (cimetidina, ranitidina, famotidina), gastrina (proglumida) e acetilcolina (atropina, pirenzipina) e pela inibição da adenilciclase (análogos de PGE) e H$^+$/K$^+$-ATPase (p. ex., omeprazol).[68] Análogos de somatostatina de ação prolongada, como a octreotida, diminuem diretamente a secreção de gastrina e ácido gástrico. Foi demonstrado que a diminuição da secreção de ácido gástrico com um antagonista de receptor H2 promoveu a cicatrização da mucosa em cães com uma variedade de úlceras e erosões induzidas experimentalmente (ver Figura 275.5). A famotidina é interessante, pois não inibe as enzimas P450 e pode ser administrada 1 vez/dia. A atividade procinética adicional da ranitidina ou nizatidina (mediada pela atividade anticolinesterásica) pode torná-las boas escolhas em casos de esvaziamento gástrico retardado associado à propulsão defeituosa.[40] Em pacientes com ulceração gástrica grave ou persistente e refratária a antagonistas H2, a inibição mais efetiva da secreção de ácido pode ser alcançada com um inibidor da H$^+$/K$^+$-ATPase, como o omeprazol (1 mg/kg via oral a cada 24 h [cães]). O omeprazol é o medicamento inicial de escolha em pacientes com hipersecreção ácida secundária a tumores de mastócitos e gastrinoma (síndrome de Zollinger-Ellison). O omeprazol demonstrou ter poucos efeitos colaterais a longo prazo em cães (0,7 a 1 mg/kg via oral a cada 24 horas), mas deve ser usado com cautela em animais de estimação com doença hepática e deve ser revisado para interações com drogas como a cisaprida. Em dosagens mais altas (1,1 mg/kg via oral a cada 12 horas), o omeprazol tem sido associado a hipergastrinemia e disbiose gástrica significativas.[67] Cães de trenó tratados com omeprazol para hemorragia gástrica associada ao exercício tiveram escores de gravidade gástrica significativamente reduzidos em comparação com o placebo. No entanto, a droga causou um aumento na frequência de diarreia (omeprazol 54%, placebo 21%).[64] Investigações adicionais são necessárias sobre o papel dessa droga para atletas com úlceras gástricas.[64] A combinação de omeprazol e a octreotida, um análogo da somatostatina de ação prolongada, reduziu efetivamente o vômito em um cão com gastrinoma (octreotida 2 a 20 µg/kg SC a cada 8 horas).[69] A octreotida também pode ser empregada para diminuir rapidamente a secreção de ácido gástrico em animais de estimação com úlceras grandes reveladas na endoscopia e tem sido usada para controlar o sangramento gástrico em humanos. Acetato de octreotida de liberação sustentada (5 mg/IM a cada 4 semanas) suprimiu transitoriamente a secreção de gastrina em um cão da raça Shiba Inu com gastrinoma.[70]

Fornecimento de proteção da mucosa

O misoprostol, análogo da PGE$_2$, protege contra erosões gástricas induzidas por AINEs em cães em dosagens que não inibem a secreção de ácido (3 a 5 µg/kg VO a cada 8 horas) e pode ser dado a cães tratados a longo prazo com AINEs para artrite.[71,72] O principal efeito colateral do misoprostol é a diarreia e não deve ser administrado a fêmeas grávidas. O complexo hidróxido de alumínio e sacarose sulfatada (sucralfato), protetor de mucosa, liga-se a áreas desnudadas de epitélio da mucosa, independentemente da causa subjacente e é útil para o tratamento de erosões gástricas, úlceras e esofagite. O sucralfato pode ser dado para pacientes que recebem antiácidos injetáveis, mas pode comprometer a absorção de outros medicamentos orais, e sua administração provavelmente é melhor quando separada destes por várias horas. Em contraste com a eficácia do misoprostol e antagonistas H2 na prevenção de erosões induzidas por AINEs, a administração profilática de várias combinações de misoprostol, cimetidina e omeprazol não demonstrou prevenir erosões gástricas em cães, com ou sem doença do disco intervertebral, recebendo altas doses de glicocorticoides.[60,73,74] No entanto, essas drogas podem acelerar a cura de suas lesões gástricas. O sucralfato é provavelmente a droga de escolha para o tratamento de ulceração gastrintestinal em animais de estimação que recebem altas dosagens de glicocorticoides, porque é eficaz independentemente se o ácido está causando ou retardando a cura.

Tumores de mastócitos (ver Capítulo 349) são também considerados separadamente, pois a ulceração gástrica é uma complicação frequente e grave. Acredita-se que os tumores de mastócitos causem vômito por meio dos efeitos centrais da histamina na zona de gatilho quimiorreceptora (ZGQ) e pelos efeitos periféricos da histamina sobre a secreção de ácido gástrico, com hiperacidez e ulceração resultantes. O tratamento da mastocitose com antagonistas H1 e H2 da histamina (p. ex., difenidramina e famotidina) deve reduzir os efeitos centrais e periféricos da histamina. Os corticosteroides são usados para diminuir a carga tumoral. Se a hipersecreção de ácido estiver presente ou for suspeita, isso é provavelmente mais bem gerenciado com inibidores da bomba de prótons (p. ex., omeprazol 1 mg/kg VO a cada 24 horas). Os análogos da somatostatina também podem ser úteis para controlar a hipersecreção refratária de ácido gástrico (p. ex., octreotida 2 a 20 µg/kg SC a cada 8 horas, ou acetato de octreotida 0,5 mg/kg a cada 4 semanas).[27,70]

Antieméticos

Os antieméticos (ver Capítulo 39) podem ser usados quando o vômito é grave e compromete o equilíbrio de fluidos e/ou eletrólitos ou causa desconforto.[68] Antieméticos comumente usados em cães incluem a metoclopramida, que antagoniza os receptores D2-dopaminérgicos e 5HT3-serotonérgicos e tem

SEÇÃO 18 • Doença Gastrintestinal

efeitos colinérgicos no músculo liso (1 mg/kg/q 24 h CRI IV); derivados de fenotiazina, como clorpromazina e proclorperazina, que são antagonistas de receptores adrenérgicos alfa-1 e alfa-2, H1 e H2-histaminérgicos e D2-dopaminérgicos no centro do vômito e ZGQ; ondansetrona (0,5 mg/kg IV), que antagoniza os receptores periféricos 5 HT3; e maropitant, que antagoniza os receptores da neurocinina-1 (1 mg/kg IV a cada 24 horas, ou 2 mg/kg PO a cada 24 horas, não mais de 5 dias). Uma comparação desses antieméticos indicou maior eficácia do maropitant e da ondansetrona para controlar o vômito periférico induzido por ipecacuanha do que metoclopramida ou clorpromazina e uma eficácia semelhante a maropitant, clorpromazina e metoclopramida para controlar o vômito mediado centralmente induzido pela apomorfina.[75] O maropitant foi associado à evidência histológica de hipoplasia da medula óssea em filhotes e não deve ser usado em cães < 8 semanas ou gatos < 16 semanas de idade. O maropitant a 1 mg/kg foi eficaz na prevenção do vômito induzido por movimento e por xilazina em gatos e reduziu o vômito (1,1 mg/kg PO diariamente por 2 semanas) em gatos com doença renal crônica.[76,77] Antagonistas não seletivos de receptores colinérgicos, como atropina, escopolamina, aminopentamida e isopropamida, são geralmente evitados, pois podem causar íleo paralítico, esvaziamento gástrico retardado e boca seca.

Antibióticos e analgésicos
Uma cobertura antibiótica profilática (p. ex., cefalosporinas, ampicilina) pode ser necessária para animais em choque com disfunção importante da barreira GI. Leucopenia, neutrofilia, febre e fezes com sangue são indicações adicionais para antibióticos profiláticos em animais com vômitos ou diarreia. As escolhas iniciais nessas situações incluem ampicilina ou uma cefalosporina (eficaz contra gram-positivas e algumas bactérias gram-negativas e anaeróbicas), que podem ser combinadas com um aminoglicosídeo (eficaz contra gram-negativas aeróbias) quando a sepse está presente e o estado de hidratação é adequado (ver Capítulo 161). A enrofloxacino é uma alternativa adequada para um aminoglicosídeo em pacientes esqueleticamente maduros com risco de nefrotoxicose provocada por uso de aminoglicosídeo. Pode ser fornecida analgesia usando opioides, como buprenorfina (0,0075 a 0,01 mg/kg IM). Estudos recentes indicam que o maropitant antiemético tem propriedades analgésicas durante a estimulação visceral laparoscópica, mas os efeitos analgésicos em outras situações permanecem por ser determinados.[78] A cirurgia pode ser necessária quando a causa da ulceração não está clara ou para ressecção de úlceras grandes que não cicatrizam ou as que estão prestes a perfurar. A perfuração pilórica foi associada a AINEs, e taxas de mortalidade (cerca de 64%) são similares à perfuração em outros locais no trato GI.[52]

DILATAÇÃO VOLVULOGÁSTRICA

Definições e patogênese
Dilatação gástrica (DG) e dilatação volvulogástrica (DVG) são caracterizadas pelo estômago dramaticamente distendido com ar (ver Capítulos 143 e 144). Com o vólvulo, o estômago gira em torno de seu eixo, movendo-se dorsalmente e à esquerda do fundo. Ambas, DG e DVG, causam obstrução da cava caudal e prejudicam o retorno venoso ao coração, resultando em choque hipovolêmico que pode ser agravado pela desvitalização da parede gástrica, torção ou avulsão esplênica, congestão das vísceras abdominais, choque endotóxico e CID.

Nenhuma causa única de DG ou DVG foi identificada. Cães de raças grandes e com peito profundo, como Akita, Bloodhound, Collie, Dogue Alemão, Setter Irlandês, Wolfhound Irlandês, Newfoundland, Rottweiler, São Bernardo, Poodle Padrão e Weimaraner, correm maior risco. A incidência cumulativa de DVG foi estimada em 6% para cães de raças grandes e gigantes. O risco ao longo da vida é influenciado pela raça, variando de 3,9% para Rottweiler a 39% em Dogue Alemão.[79] Em cães de raça grande e gigante, fatores significativamente associados a um risco aumentado de DGV incluem a idade, como de maior importância relativa no histórico de DGV, alimentação rápida, alimentação 1 vez/dia, uso de tigela elevada e aerofagia.[80,81] A personalidade do cão também pode ter um impacto, pois cães mais felizes têm uma incidência menor.[48] A esplenectomia anterior não parece aumentar o risco de DGV.[82] A análise do gás gástrico na DG/DGV tem sido interpretada para associar a aerofagia como a causa da distensão, com a dilatação explicada por uma incapacidade para eructar ou esvaziar o ar nos intestinos.[83] No entanto, um estudo recente descobriu que a composição de CO_2 variou de 13 a 20%, com um cão tendo uma concentração de H_2 de 29%.[84] Uma vez que o teor de CO_2 do ar atmosférico é inferior a 1%, esses resultados sugerem que a distensão gástrica gasosa em DGV não é o resultado de aerofagia.[84] Fontes prováveis de gás incluem a fermentação bacteriana da dieta, mas a dieta específica e fatores microbianos ainda precisam ser determinados.[84] Estudos em cães com DGV em recuperação de gastropexia sugerem que a atividade elétrica e o esvaziamento gástrico também podem estar relacionados ao desenvolvimento da DG.[85] A inter-relação do vólvulo e a distensão gástrica não está clara, embora o comprimento do ligamento hepatogástrico possa facilitar a torção.

Características do diagnóstico
Um histórico de náuseas, ânsia de vômito, salivação, distensão abdominal, fraqueza ou colapso aumenta a possibilidade de dilatação ou vólvulo, particularmente em cães de raças grandes e tórax profundo. Os achados físicos geralmente incluem distensão abdominal e timpanismo, taquicardia e palidez da mucosa. Hipotermia, depressão e coma podem ser observados quando o choque é grave. Arritmias cardíacas, como batimentos ventriculares prematuros ou taquicardia ventricular, podem ser detectados no exame ou podem se desenvolver até 72 h após a apresentação (ver Capítulos 127 e 144). A radiografia é geralmente realizada após suporte de fluido e descompressão e ajuda a distinguir dilatação simples de dilatação e vólvulo. Geralmente, são necessárias incidências reclinadas laterais direita e esquerda. A dilatação é associada à distensão de gás, e em uma posição lateral direita, o ar está presente no fundo (Figura 275.8). Com vólvulo, o piloro move-se dorsalmente e para a esquerda, e o estômago é compartimentalizado. Em uma radiografia lateral direita, o fundo é visualizado como um grande compartimento ventral com o piloro, menor e cheio de gás, localizado dorsalmente e separado do fundo por uma faixa de tecido mole, formando o sinal do "braço de Popeye" (Figura 275.9). A perda de contraste abdominal pode indicar ruptura gástrica ou sangramento de vasos esplênicos avulsionados, enquanto o contraste aumentado devido a pneumoperitônio sugere ruptura gástrica.

Achados de patologia clínica
As alterações hematológicas são frequentemente restritas a um aumento no hematócrito. Uma variedade de distúrbios acidobásicos e eletrolíticos foi observada em cães com DGV (ver Capítulo 128).[86,87] Acidose metabólica e hipopotassemia foram as anormalidades mais comuns em um estudo e ocorreram em 15 e 16 de 57 cães, respectivamente.[86] A acidose metabólica é provavelmente devido a hipoperfusão tecidual, metabolismo anaeróbio e acúmulo de ácido láctico (ver Capítulo 70).[86] Alcalose metabólica também pode ocorrer e estar relacionada ao sequestro de ácido gástrico ou vômito.[86] A medição do lactato plasmático no momento da admissão e sua resposta à terapia (> 43 a 50% de redução dentro de 12 horas é um bom achado) pode ajudar a determinar a presença de necrose gástrica, prognóstico e necessidade de terapia agressiva.[28-30] A acidose e a alcalose respiratória têm sido observadas de modo variável e

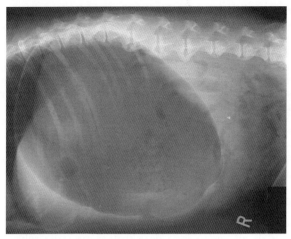

Figura 275.8 Radiografia de dilatação gástrica (lateral direita). O fundo está distendido com ar. (© Kenneth W. Simpson.)

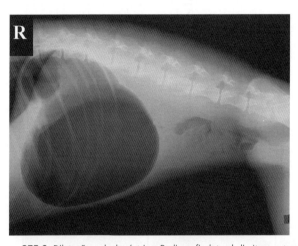

Figura 275.9 Dilatação volvulogástrica. Radiografia lateral direita mostrando compartimentação gástrica, com o piloro (dorsal) separado do fundo por um tecido de baixa densidade (© Kenneth W. Simpson.)

refletem hipoventilação ou hiperventilação, respectivamente. A natureza variável das anormalidades acidobásicas e de eletrólitos em cães com DGV indicam que a terapia com fluidos deve ser individualizada com base na gasometria e níveis de eletrólitos. O monitoramento e a correção de anormalidades do equilíbrio acidobásico são importantes, porque podem predispor a arritmias cardíacas e fraqueza muscular. Anormalidades de coagulação são geralmente compatíveis com CID (trombocitopenia, D-Dímero aumentado ou PDFs, ATIII reduzido, prolongamento do TTPa; ver Capítulo 196).

Tratamento

Fluidoterapia (ver Capítulo 127) e descompressão gástrica (ver Capítulo 112) são as abordagens mais importantes.

Suporte de fluidos

A fluidoterapia tradicionalmente consiste em doses de ataque de LR (60 a 90 mℓ/kg/h) administradas por meio de cateteres de grosso calibre nas veias cefálica ou jugular (ver Capítulos 127 e 129). Estudos experimentais comparando cristaloides (60 mℓ/kg, seguidos de NaCl 0,9% 20 mℓ/kg/h) com solução salina hipertônica (7% NaCl em 6% dextrana, 5 mℓ/kg, seguidos de NaCl 0,9% 20 mℓ/kg/h) em cães com choque induzido por DGV indicam que a solução salina hipertônica mantém melhor o desempenho miocárdico, maior frequência cardíaca e menor resistência vascular sistêmica.[88] A dose de reanimação de solução salina hipertônica foi administrada em 5 a 10 minutos *versus* uma hora para cristaloides. A fluidoterapia deve ser intensamente monitorada por medições frequentes da pressão arterial, frequência cardíaca, HT, PPT e oligúria. Potássio e bicarbonato são mais bem administrados com base na gasometria e medições de eletrólitos no sangue. Hipopotassemia é comum após a terapia com fluidos, e 30 a 40 mEq KCl/ℓ devem ser adicionados aos fluidos após a dose de choque inicial, ao mesmo tempo que garante que a taxa máxima de infusão de KCl de 0,5 mEq/kg/h não seja excedida (ver Capítulo 324).

Descompressão gástrica

A descompressão pode ser realizada por intubação orogástrica com um tubo estomacal bem lubrificado (ver Capítulo 112), ou um cateter de calibre 16 pode ser usado para trocarização do estômago (ver Capítulo 144). A descompressão oral também pode ser realizada após a trocarização. A descompressão deve ser mantida até a cirurgia. A sedação com butorfanol (0,5 mg/kg IV) ou oximorfona (0,1 mg/kg IV) e diazepam (0,1 mg/kg IV lento) pode ser necessária para passar um tubo estomacal.

Terapia adjuvante para choque endotóxico e lesão por reperfusão

A terapia adjuvante de lesões frequentemente inclui succinato sódico de prednisolona (10 mg/kg IV) ou fosfato sódico de dexametasona para o choque e antibióticos de amplo espectro, como uma cefalosporina em combinação com uma fluoroquinolona, para contornar a translocação bacteriana e a endotoxemia (ver Capítulo 127). Alguns clínicos defendem a flunixino meglumina para o choque endotóxico, mas o autor não. A administração de agentes para diminuir a peroxidação lipídica (U70046F) e quelação do ferro (desferroxamina) reduziu a mortalidade atribuída à lesão de reperfusão em cães com DGV experimental.[89,90] Esses agentes são mais bem administrados antes de ocorrer a reperfusão, isto é, antes de se desfazer uma torção.

Arritmias cardíacas

Arritmias cardíacas (p. ex., complexos ventriculares prematuros, taquicardia ventricular) são relativamente frequentes (cerca de 40% dos cães) e podem ou não contribuir para a mortalidade.[91-94] Arritmias podem se desenvolver até 72 horas após a apresentação e são consideradas uma consequência da anormalidade de eletrólitos, equilíbrio acidobásico e hemostáticas, bem como lesões de reperfusão (ver Capítulos 141 e 248). As arritmias devem ser tratadas se associadas à fraqueza, síncope ou frequência cardíaca > 150 bpm. As arritmias são gerenciadas com a correção dos distúrbios acidobásicos, eletrolíticos e hemostáticos subjacentes e a administração de lidocaína em *bolus* (1 a 2 mg/kg IV) ou continuamente (até 50 a 75 mcg/kg/min) e procainamida (10 mg/kg IM q 6 h e depois por via oral se eficaz) quando as arritmias são persistentes (ver Capítulos 141 e 248). É importante que as concentrações plasmáticas de K^+ e Mg^{2+} sejam normalizadas para permitir uma terapia antiarrítmica eficaz. Foi relatado que cães com DGV tratados na apresentação com lidocaína (2 mg/kg, *bolus* IV) seguido por taxa de infusão contínua (CRI) de 0,05 mg/kg/min IV por 24 h tiveram diminuição da frequência de arritmias, lesão renal aguda e duração da hospitalização.[95]

Cirurgia

Os objetivos da cirurgia são reposicionar o estômago e baço e realizar uma gastropexia para permitir descompressão a curto prazo e prevenir a recorrência. A cirurgia pode ser complicada por necrose gástrica, que requer gastrectomia parcial e avulsão ou torção do baço, que pode requerer ressecção ou remoção.

Prognóstico

As taxas de mortalidade para cães com DGV são de cerca de 10 a 15%.[93,94] Cães com necrose gástrica, ressecção gástrica, esplenectomia, arritmias cardíacas pré ou pós-operatórias e tempos mais longos da apresentação até a cirurgia têm maior taxa de mortalidade, atingindo > 30% em alguns estudos.[7,91,93,94] A dosagem de lactato plasmático na admissão (> 6 a 9 mmol/ℓ; ver Capítulo 70) e sua resposta à terapia (> 43 a 50% de redução dentro de 12 h é considerada um bom sinal) podem ajudar a determinar a presença de necrose gástrica, prognóstico e necessidade de terapia agressiva (ver Capítulos 127 e 144).[28-30]

Profilaxia

A taxa de recorrência de DG/DGV foi estimada em 11% em animais com mais de 3 anos em um estudo, com sobrevida mediana de 547 dias para cães que fizeram gastropexia versus 188 dias para cães que não fizeram.[58] Gastropexia profilática em cães das raças Dogue Alemão, Setter Irlandês, Rottweiler, Poodle Padrão e Weimaraner reduziram a mortalidade de apenas 2,2 vezes em Rottweiler para até 29,6 vezes em Dogue Alemão.[79] Dois estudos recentes que avaliaram o efeito da gastropexia incisional profilática mostraram que esta evitou completamente o DGV, com o DG relatado em 5 a 11% de 101 casos.[96,97]

GASTRITE CRÔNICA

Prevalência e definições

A gastrite é comum em cães, afeta 35% dos cães investigados com vômitos crônicos e 26 a 48% de cães assintomáticos.[98,99] A prevalência em gatos não foi determinada. O diagnóstico de gastrite crônica é baseado no exame histológico de biopsias gástricas e geralmente é subclassificado de acordo com as alterações histopatológicas e a etiologia.

Características histopatológicas da gastrite

A gastrite em cães e gatos é geralmente classificada de acordo com a natureza do infiltrado celular predominante (eosinofílico, linfocítico, plasmocítico, granulomatoso, folicular linfoide), a presença de anormalidades morfológicas (atrofia, hipertrofia, fibrose, edema, ulceração, metaplasia) e sua gravidade subjetiva (discreta, moderada, grave). Um esquema padronizado de graduação visual foi proposto por Happonen et al. e foi adaptado para patologistas (Figura 275.10).[99,100] A forma mais comum de gastrite em cães e gatos é a gastrite linfoplasmocítica superficial discreta a moderada com concomitante hiperplasia do folículo linfoide (Figura 275.11).[101] Gastrites eosinofílica, granulomatosa, atrófica e hiperplásica são menos comuns.

Etiologia

Visão geral da condição inflamatória

Apesar da alta prevalência de gastrite, uma causa subjacente raramente é identificada. Na ausência de doença sistêmica, ulcerogênica ou drogas irritantes, objetos estranhos gástricos, parasitas (Physaloptera e Ollulanus spp.) e, em casos raros, infecções fúngicas ou similares (Pythium insidiosum, Histoplasma spp.), a gastrite é geralmente atribuída a alergia ou intolerância alimentar, parasitismo oculto, uma reação a antígenos bacterianos ou patógenos desconhecidos. O tratamento é frequentemente empírico, mas pode servir para definir a causa da gastrite, como responsivo a dieta (ver Capítulo 178), antibiótico, esteroides ou parasitário.

Embora a base da resposta imunológica da gastrite em caninos e felinos seja desconhecida, estudos experimentais recentes em animais lançaram luz sobre o ambiente imunológico no trato GI para revelar uma interação complexa entre a microbiota de GI, o epitélio, células imunes efetoras (p. ex., linfócitos e macrófagos) e mediadores solúveis (p. ex., quimiocinas e citocinas).[100,102]

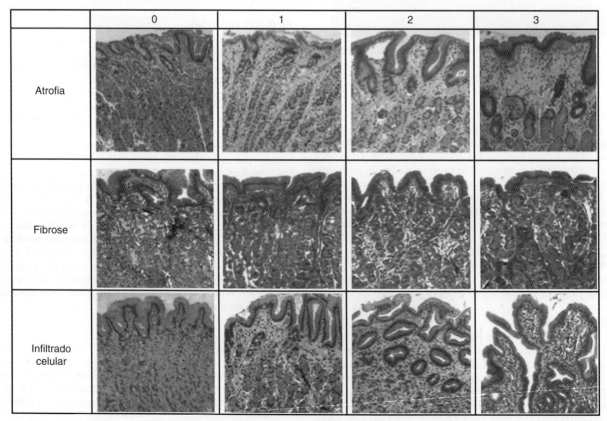

Figura 275.10 Esquema fotográfico padronizado para avaliação da atrofia gástrica, fibrose e infiltrados celulares em cães. (De Wiinberg B, Spohr A, Dietz HH et al.: Quantitative analysis of inflammatory and immune responses in dogs with gastritis and their relationship to Helicobacter spp. infection. J Vet Intern Med 19[1]:4-14, 2005.) (Esta figura se encontra reproduzida em cores no Encarte.)

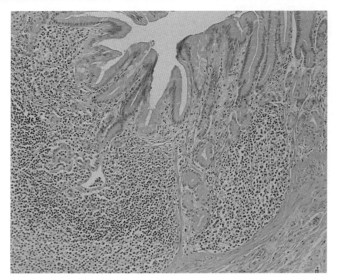

Figura 275.11 Hiperplasia do folículo linfoide e gastrite linfoplasmocítica em um gato com infecção por *Helicobacter felis*. (© Kenneth W. Simpson.)

Nos saudáveis, esse sistema evita inflamação ativa por exclusão de antígeno e tolerância imunológica induzida. O desenvolvimento da inflamação intestinal em camundongos sem as citocinas interleucina (IL) 10, fator de transformação do crescimento-beta (TGF-beta) ou IL-2 indicam sua importância central no controle da inflamação da mucosa. Em modelos murinos, a inflamação GI se desenvolve apenas na presença de microbiota intestinal indígena, levando à hipótese de que a inflamação espontânea da mucosa pode ser o resultado de uma perda de tolerância à microbiota GI indígena. O papel desses mecanismos em espécies exogâmicas, como o cão e o gato, ainda precisa ser determinado, mas claramente a perda de tolerância a antígenos bacterianos ou a dieta deve ser considerada.

O papel das células epiteliais na resposta inflamatória está sendo elucidado, com bactérias gram-negativas ou patogênicas induzindo a secreção de citocinas pró-inflamatórias (p. ex., IL-8, IL-1-beta) por células epiteliais, enquanto comensais ou bactérias, como *Enterococcus faecium* ou *Lactobacillus* spp., induzem a produção das citocinas imunomoduladoras TGF-beta ou IL-10.[63] As citocinas pró-inflamatórias produzidas por células epiteliais são moduladas pela produção de IL-10 a partir de macrófagos e potencialmente pelas próprias células epiteliais.[103] Nesse contexto, cães com gastrite linfoplasmocítica de etiologia indeterminada mostraram uma correlação entre a expressão da citocina imunomoduladora IL-10 e citocinas pró-inflamatórias (IFN-α, IL-1-beta, IL-8).[16] A expressão simultânea de mRNA de IL-10 e IFN-alfa também foi observada no intestino de cães da raça Beagle, nas células da lâmina própria e do epitélio intestinal, apesar da microbiota bacteriana luminal que era mais numerosa do que no grupo-controle de cães.[104] Portanto, é tentador visualizar um "ciclo homeostático" consistindo em estímulos pró-inflamatórios e respostas contrárias por imunomodulação e reparo, com um desequilíbrio em qualquer desses braços manifestando-se como uma gastrite.

Papel dos patógenos

A importância de patógenos desconhecidos no desenvolvimento de inflamação na mucosa é bem demonstrada pelo *H. pylori* gástrico, uma bactéria gram-negativa que infecta cronicamente mais da metade de todas as pessoas no mundo.[13] Essa infecção é caracterizada por infiltração de células polimorfonucleares e mononucleares e regulação positiva de citocinas pró-inflamatórias e da quimiocina IL-8 (CXCL8). As células T da mucosa em indivíduos infectados são direcionadas para a produção de interferona-gama (IFN-γ), em vez de IL-4 ou IL-5, indicando uma forte tendência em direção a uma resposta tipo Th1.[105,106] As respostas sustentadas à infecção, imunes e inflamatórias gástricas, parecem ser fundamentais para o desenvolvimento de úlceras pépticas e câncer gástrico em humanos.

Prevalência de Helicobacter

Há uma alta prevalência da infecção gástrica por *Helicobacter* spp.: de 67 a 100% dos cães de estimação sadios, 74 a 90% de cães apresentam vômitos, 100% de cães da raça Beagle (modelo animal de experimentação) e de 40 a 100% em gatos saudáveis e doentes.[107-109] Cães e gatos são colonizados por uma variedade de grandes microrganismos espirais (5 a 12 mícrons; Figura 275.12). Em gatos na Suíça, nos EUA e na Alemanha, *H. heilmannii* é a espécie predominante, e *H. bizzozeronii* e *H. felis* são muito menos frequentes. Gatos também podem ser colonizados por *H. pylori* (2 a 5 µ), mas a infecção foi limitada a uma colônia fechada de gatos usados em experimentação de laboratório.[110] Em cães da Finlândia, Suíça, EUA e Dinamarca, *H. bizzozeronii* e *H. salomonis* são as mais comuns, seguidas por *H. heilmannii* e *H. felis*; *H. bilis* e *Flexispira rappini* também foram descritas. Esses *Helicobacter* spp. gástricos são distintos dos *Helicobacter* spp. êntero-hepáticos que colonizam o intestino delgado distal e o cólon.[18] A tutoria de cães e gatos foi correlacionada com um risco aumentado de infecção por *H. heilmannii* em humanos.[111] Estudos recentes confirmam claramente que cães e gatos abrigam *H. heilmannii*, mas os subtipos de *H. heilmannii* presentes em cães e gatos, os tipos 2 e 4, são de menor importância em humanos (cerca de 15% dos casos), que são predominantemente colonizados por *H. heilmannii* tipo 1 – o *Helicobacter* spp. predominante em porcos.[17] A transmissão de uma variedade de *Helicobacter* spp. não *H. pylori*, incluindo *H. felis*, *H. salomonis*, *H. bizzozeronii*, de animais de estimação para o homem parece mais comum do que inicialmente se estimava.[112]

Tratamento associado a Helicobacter

O efeito da erradicação de *Helicobacter* spp. sobre a gastrite e sinais clínicos em humanos, a principal evidência que apoia o papel patogênico de *H. pylori*, não foi completamente investigado em cães ou gatos. Um ensaio de tratamento não controlado de cães e gatos com gastrite e infecção por *Helicobacter* spp. mostrou que os sinais clínicos em 57 de 63 cães e gatos responderam a uma combinação de metronidazol, amoxicilina e famotidina. Uma segunda endoscopia mostrou que 14 de 19 animais tiveram resolução da gastrite e nenhuma evidência de *Helicobacter* spp. em biopsias gástricas.[113] Um ensaio controlado de amoxicilina, metronidazol e bismuto ± famotidina em 24 cães encontrou uma diminuição semelhante no vômito (86,4%), mas apenas 43% de eliminação de *Helicobacter* em 6 meses.[114] Esse estudo também observou que a pontuação de avaliação de gastrite em cães que eram negativos para *Helicobacter* aos 6 meses diminuiu, enquanto nos cães positivos para *Helicobacter* aumentou. A razão para a taxa bem maior de recrudescência ou reinfecção aparente em cães e gatos do que em humanos (1 a 2% ao ano observado após o tratamento de *H. pylori*) ainda não foi determinada. Com informações limitadas de ensaios de erradicação, a maioria dos conhecimentos atuais sobre a patogenicidade do *Helicobacter* spp. para cães e gatos vem da avaliação de animais com e sem infecção, de sinais clínicos e de um pequeno número de infecções experimentais.

As espécies de *Helicobacter* de tamanho maior são encontradas em cães e gatos, não se ligam ao epitélio, mas colonizam a mucosa superficial e as glândulas mucosas e gástricas, particularmente do fundo e da cárdia, e podem ser observadas intracelularmente.[107,109] Degeneração das glândulas gástricas com vacuolização, picnose e necrose de células parietais é mais comum em animais infectados do que em animais não infectados. A inflamação é geralmente de natureza mononuclear e varia de discreta a moderada em gravidade. Hiperplasia linfoide

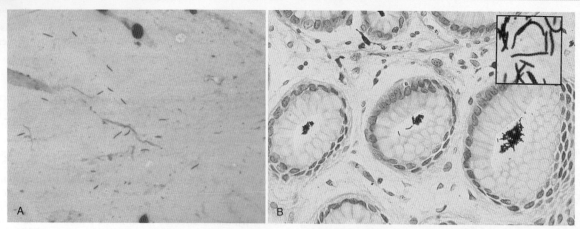

Figura 275.12 *Helicobacter* spp. visualizados em (**A**) esfregaço de impressão (coloração Diff-Quik) e (**B**) biopsia endoscópica (coloração de Steiner), com ampliação de um grupo de *Helicobacter* no canto superior direito. (© Kenneth W. Simpson.)

gástrica é comum e pode ser extensa em cães e gatos infectados com *Helicobacter* spp., particularmente quando biopsias gástricas de espessura total são avaliadas. Além dessa resposta imune gástrica local, uma resposta sistêmica caracterizada pelo aumento da circulação de IgG anti-*Helicobacter* foi detectada em soros de cães e gatos naturalmente infectados. Contudo, a gastrite observada em cães e gatos infectados com essas grandes bactérias espiraladas é geralmente menos grave do que a observada com *H. pylori* em humanos infectados. Úlceras gastrintestinais, neoplasia gástrica ou alterações na gastrina sérica ou na secreção de ácido não foram associadas à infecção por *Helicobacter* spp. em cães ou gatos.

Diferenças no padrão da doença entre humanos, cães e gatos podem ser atribuídas às diferenças na virulência do *Helicobacter* spp. infectante ou na resposta do hospedeiro. Estudos que abordam esse problema indicam que *H. pylori* evoca uma resposta pró-inflamatória de citocinas e celular mais grave em cães e gatos do que a infecção experimental ou natural por *Helicobacter* spp.[110,115]

A resposta inflamatória de mucosa limitada e a ausência de sinais clínicos na maioria dos cães e gatos infectados com *Helicobacter* spp., não *H. pylori*, apesar da estimulação antigênica significativa comprovada por soroconversão e hiperplasia de folículos linfoides, sugere que *Helicobacter* spp. é mais comensal do que patogênico. É interessante especular que é a perda de tolerância ao *Helicobacter* spp. gástrico, em vez da patogenicidade inata dessas bactérias, que explica o desenvolvimento de gastrite e sinais clínicos em alguns cães e gatos.

Achados clínicos

O principal sinal clínico de gastrite crônica é vômito de alimento ou bile. Apetite diminuído, perda de peso, melena ou hematêmese são encontrados de forma variável. A presença simultânea de doenças dermatológicas e os sinais GI aumentam a probabilidade de alergia alimentar.[116] Práticas dietéticas e acesso a toxinas, medicamentos e corpos estranhos devem ser cuidadosamente revisados. Os sinais são importantes, pois podem aumentar a probabilidade de que a gastrite crônica seja a causa do vômito. Hipertrofia da mucosa fúndica é frequentemente associada a uma enteropatia grave em cães da raça Basenji, com estomatocitose, anemia hemolítica, icterícia e polineuropatia em cães da raça Spaniel Perdigueiro de Drente.[117,118] A hipertrofia da mucosa pilórica é observada em cães pequenos braquicefálicos, como os da raça Lhasa Apso, associada à obstrução do escoamento gástrico (ver Esvaziamento gástrico retardado e desordens na motilidade, a seguir). A atrofia da mucosa gástrica que pode progredir para adenocarcinoma foi relatada em cães da raça Norsk Lundehund com gastroenteropatia e perda de proteínas.[119] Cães machos jovens de raças de grande porte nos estados do Golfo do México nos EUA podem ter gastrite granulomatosa causada por *Pythium* spp., com a infecção mais prevalente no outono, no inverno e na primavera.[120] O exame físico muitas vezes é normal. A distensão abdominal pode ser relacionada ao esvaziamento gástrico retardado causado por obstrução ou propulsão defeituosa. Massas abdominais, linfadenopatia, ou alterações oculares podem ser encontradas em cães com infeções fúngicas gástricas.

Diagnóstico

Análises laboratoriais

Um perfil bioquímico, hemograma completo, urinálise e T4 (para gatos > 5 anos de idade), deve ser realizado como uma triagem básica para causas metabólicas, endócrinas, infecciosas e outras causas não gastrintestinais de vômito, bem como para as alterações acidobásicas e eletrolíticas associadas a vômitos, obstrução do fluxo ou hipersecreção ácida. Os resultados dos testes costumam ser normais em animais de estimação com gastrite crônica. A eosinofilia pode levar à consideração de gastrite associada a hipersensibilidade alimentar, endoparasitas ou tumores de mastócitos. Hiperglobulinemia e hipoalbuminemia podem estar presentes em cães da raça Basenji com gastropatia ou enteropatia, ou em cães com pitiose gástrica. Pan-hipoproteinemia é uma característica da gastroenteropatia em cães da raça Norsk Lundehund, doença inflamatória intestinal (DII) generalizada moderada a grave, linfoma GI e histoplasmose GI. Testes mais específicos, como um teste de estimulação ACTH ou sorologia para *Pythium insidiosum*, são realizados com base nos resultados desses testes. A determinação de IgE específica para alimentos não demonstrou ser útil no diagnóstico de hipersensibilidade alimentar em cães ou gatos. A utilidade de testes não invasivos, como pepsinogênio sérico e permeabilidade gástrica à sacarose, usada para diagnosticar gastrite em humanos, não foi determinada em cães e gatos.

Imagem

Radiografias abdominais frequentemente são normais em cães e gatos com gastrite. Distensão gástrica ou esvaziamento gástrico retardado (alimentos retidos mais de 12 h após uma refeição) podem ser observados. Uma radiografia de contraste pode revelar úlceras ou espessamento das pregas gástricas ou da parede, mas tem sido amplamente substituída pela combinação de ultrassonografia (US) para detecção de anormalidades murais e endoscopia para observação e coleta de amostra da mucosa gástrica.[31]

Endoscopia

O exame endoscópico (ver Capítulo 113) permite a visualização de corpos estranhos, erosão, ulceração, hemorragia, espessamento das pregas, hiperplasia de folículos linfoides (evidente como marcas de pústulas na mucosa), aumento de muco ou líquido (claro ou com cor de bile) e aumento ou diminuição da friabilidade da mucosa (ver Capítulo 113). Nódulos de mucosa focais discretos ou multifocais podem ser observados com infecção por *Ollulanus* spp. A ficomicose gástrica pode estar associada a massas irregulares na saída do piloro e podem ser necessários testes sorológicos por ELISA, *Western blotting* e cultura de biopsias gástricas recentes. Parasitas como *Physaloptera* spp. podem ser observados como vermes de 1 a 4 cm de comprimento. Excesso de líquido com coloração de bile é sugestivo de gastrite associada a refluxo duodenogástrico, enquanto o excesso de líquido claro pode indicar hipersecreção de ácido gástrico. O fluido gástrico pode ser aspirado para citologia (*Helicobacter* spp., ovos ou larvas do parasita) e medição do pH. Esfregaços de impressão de biopsias gástricas são uma forma eficaz de identificar *Helicobacter* spp. (microrganismos espiralados de 5 a 12 µ) e são mais sensíveis do que o teste de urease de biopsia (*Helicobacter* spp. produzem urease; ver Figura 275.12 A). A gastrina sérica deve ser quantificada se erosões gástricas inexplicáveis, úlceras, acúmulo de líquido, ou hipertrofia da mucosa forem observados.

Gotejamento de antígenos e biopsia

O procedimento endoscópico de gotejamento de antígenos da dieta na mucosa gástrica para verificar a presença de alergia alimentar não foi útil em cães ou gatos: é altamente subjetivo, detecta apenas hipersensibilidade imediata e não se correlaciona com os resultados dos ensaios de eliminação da dieta.[116] O estômago deve ser biopsiado mesmo quando parece normal (geralmente três biopsias de cada região: piloro, fundo e cárdia). Pregas espessadas podem exigir várias biopsias, e uma biopsia de espessura total é frequentemente necessária para diferenciar gastrite de neoplasia ou infecção fúngica e diagnosticar hipertrofia submucosa ou muscular. Os resultados da US gástrica podem ajudar a prever essas possibilidades e complementar os achados endoscópicos (ver Figura 275.6).

As seções gástricas devem ser coradas com HE para avaliação de celularidade e arquitetura, e a coloração de Steiner modificada para bactérias espirais gástricas (ver Figura 275.12 B). Colorações especiais adicionais, como a metenamina de prata de Gomori, são indicadas, se inflamação piogranulomatosa estiver presente, para detectar fungos. O tricromo de Masson pode ser usado para destacar a fibrose gástrica, enquanto corante vermelho da Síria e azul de Alcian ajudam a revelar eosinófilos e mastócitos, respectivamente. A imunocitoquímica pode ser empregada para ajudar a distinguir o linfoma da gastrite linfocítica grave. A coloração de mucina é realizada em cães da raça Norsk Lundehund com atrofia gástrica mostrando uma presença anormal de células mucosas do colo e metaplasia pseudopilórica.[121]

Os achados da biopsia costumam ser usados para orientar o tratamento. Por exemplo, gastrite linfoplasmocítica discreta pode ser tratada com uma mudança na dieta, enquanto gastrite linfoplasmocítica moderada sem infecção por *Helicobacter* spp., que falha em responder à mudança na dieta, pode se beneficiar do tratamento com corticosteroides. Uma vez que a avaliação histológica das biopsias gástricas não são uniformes entre os patologistas, mesmo quando um esquema de pontuação padronizado é usado (ver Figura 275.10), um clínico prudente deve revisar cuidadosamente os cortes histológicos para entender a interpretação do patologista.[16] Mesmo com uma avaliação ideal, alterações histológicas semelhantes podem ser observadas em pacientes com diferentes etiologias subjacentes; desse modo, ensaios de tratamento bem estruturados muitas vezes formam a base de um diagnóstico etiológico.

Tratamento

O tratamento da gastrite inicialmente se concentra na detecção e no tratamento de distúrbios metabólicos subjacentes e na remoção de drogas, toxinas, corpos estranhos, parasitas e infecções fúngicas.

Gastrite parasitária

Ollulanus tricuspis

Ollulanus tricuspis é um verme microscópico (0,7 a 1 mm de comprimento, 0,04 mm de largura) que infecta o estômago de felinos. Sua transmissão predominante de gato para gato ocorre através da ingestão de vômito. Também pode sofrer autoinfecção interna, com cargas de vermes chegando a 11 mil por estômago. As anomalias da mucosa variam de nenhuma a hiperplasia de pregas e gastrite nodular (2 a 3 mm). Os achados histológicos incluem infiltrados linfoplasmocitários, hiperplasia folicular linfoide, fibrose e até 100 leucócitos globulares/campo (grande aumento). *Ollulanus* spp. não são detectados por exame fecal e requerem avaliação de suco gástrico, vômito ou seções histológicas para larvas ou vermes. Lavagem gástrica e êmese induzidas por xilazina foram descritas para auxiliar no diagnóstico. Tratamento com fenbendazol (10 mg/kg PO a cada 24 horas 2 d) pode ser eficaz.

Physaloptera spp.

Physaloptera spp. são vermes longos de cerca de 2 a 6 cm que são esporadicamente detectados no estômago de cães e gatos. *Physaloptera rara* é a mais comumente descrita e parece ser principalmente um parasita de coiotes. O diagnóstico é difícil, pois a carga de vermes costuma ser baixa, e os ovos são transparentes e difíceis de se ver na flotação com açúcar. O tratamento com pamoato de pirantel (5 mg/kg PO: cães, dose única; gatos, duas doses, com 14 dias de intervalo) pode ser eficaz. O controle da infecção pode ser difícil devido à ingestão de hospedeiros intermediários, como baratas e besouros, e hospedeiros paratênicos, como lagartos e ouriços. Dado o difícil diagnóstico de *Ollulanus* e *Physaloptera* spp., a terapia empírica com um anti-helmíntico, como fembendazol, pode ser necessária em cães e gatos com gastrite inexplicada.

Outros parasitas

Infecção gástrica com *Gnathostoma* spp. (gatos), *Spirocerca* spp. (cães) e *Aonchotheca* spp. (gatos) foi associada a nódulos gástricos, tratados por ressecção cirúrgica do tecido gástrico afetado.[122]

Pitiose gástrica

A presença de espessamento transmural na saída gástrica (Figura 275.13) e histologia que indica inflamação piogranulomatosa aumenta a possibilidade de infecção por fungos como *Pythium insidiosum* (ver Capítulo 236).[120] Uma coloração especial (metenamina de prata de Gomori), cultura, sorologia e PCR de tecidos infectados podem ser usadas para ajudar a confirmar o diagnóstico. O tratamento consiste em ressecção cirúrgica agressiva combinada com itraconazol (10 mg/kg PO a cada 24 horas) e terbinafina (5 a 10 mg/kg PO a cada 24 horas) por 2 a 3 meses após a cirurgia. Títulos ELISA de amostras de pré e pós-tratamento podem mostrar uma queda acentuada durante o tratamento bem-sucedido, e as drogas podem ser interrompidas. A terapia médica é mantida por mais 2 a 3 meses se os títulos permanecerem elevados. O prognóstico é pobre, pois < 25% dos animais afetados são curados apenas com medicamentos.[120,123]

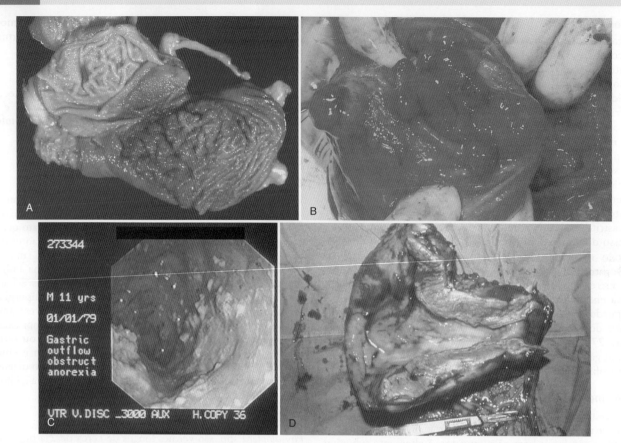

Figura 275.13 Aparência macroscópica de gastropatias hipertróficas. **A.** Hipertrofia fúndica difusa. **B.** Hipertrofia fúndica multifocal. **C.** Hipertrofia da mucosa antral (pilorogastropatia hiperplásica idiopática em um cão braquicefálico). **D.** Espessamento da saída do piloro devido a *Pythium* spp. (**A**, **B** e **D**, cortesia da Cornell University; **C**, cortesia da Ohio State University.) (© Kenneth W. Simpson.)

Gastrite associada a *Helicobacter*

A falta de definições sobre a patogenicidade de *Helicobacter* spp. no estômago faz com que os veterinários sejam confrontados com o dilema de tratar ou ignorar bactérias em espiral observadas em biopsias de pacientes com vômitos crônicos e gastrite. À luz de sua patogenicidade em humanos, furões, chitas e ratos, parece prudente que a erradicação de *Helicobacter* spp. gástrico seja tentada antes de iniciar o tratamento com agentes imunossupressores para controlar a gastrite. No entanto, isso deve ser decidido de modo individual. Por exemplo, no paciente com um infiltrado linfoplasmocítico do estômago e do intestino delgado com uma infecção por *Helicobacter* spp. concomitante, deve-se tratar a DII, *Helicobacter*, ou ambos?

O autor recomenda o tratamento apenas de pacientes sintomáticos em que tenham sido confirmadas por biopsia infecção por *Helicobacter* spp. e gastrite. Os protocolos de tratamento atuais são baseados naqueles considerados eficazes em humanos infectados por *H. pylori*. Um ensaio de tratamento não controlado de cães e gatos com gastrite e infecção por *Helicobacter* spp. mostrou que os sinais clínicos em 90% de 63 cães e gatos responderam ao tratamento com uma combinação de metronidazol, amoxicilina e famotidina, e 74% dos 19 animais submetidos a uma segunda endoscopia não tinham evidências de *Helicobacter* spp. em biopsias gástricas.[113] Um recente ensaio controlado com amoxicilina (15 mg/kg PO a cada 12 horas por 14 dias), metronidazol (10 mg/kg PO a cada 12 horas por 14 dias) e bismuto ± famotidina em 24 cães encontrou uma diminuição semelhante no vômito (86,4%) e redução dos escores de gastrite em cães que seram negativos poara *Helicobacter* após 6 meses. O uso de famotidina não melhorou a resolução dos sinais clínicos ou a erradicação do *Helicobacter*. Infelizmente, apenas 43% dos cães estavam isentos de *Helicobacter* após 6 meses,[114] o que ecoa os resultados de estudos em cães e gatos assintomáticos infectados com *Helicobacter*. As combinações de tratamento avaliadas nesses animais assintomáticos incluem (1) amoxicilina (20 mg/kg PO a cada 12 horas por 14 dias), metronidazol (20 mg/kg PO a cada 12 horas por 14 dias) e famotidina (0,5 mg/kg PO a cada 12 horas por 14 dias) em cães;[124] (2) claritromicina (30 mg PO a cada 12 horas por 4 dias), metronidazol (30 mg PO a cada 12 horas por 4 dias), ranitidina (10 mg PO a cada 12 horas por 4 dias) e bismuto (20 mg PO a cada 12 horas por 4 dias; protocolo CMRB) em gatos infectados com *H. heilmannii*;[125] e (3) azitromicina (30 mg PO a cada 24 horas por 4 dias), tinidazol (100 mg PO a cada 24 horas por 4 dias), ranitidina (20 mg PO a cada 24 horas por 4 dias) e bismuto (40 mg PO a cada 24 horas por 4 dias; protocolo ATRB) em gatos infectados por *H. heilmannii*.[125] A reavaliação do estado de infecção em 3 dias (cães) ou 10 dias (gatos) após o tratamento revelou 6 de 8 cães, 11 de 11 gatos tratados com o protocolo CMRB e 4 de 6 gatos tratados com o protocolo ATRB estavam livres de *Helicobacter* com base em histologia e teste de urease (cães) ou teste respiratório com ^{13}C-ureia (cães e gatos).[125,126] No entanto, aos 28 dias (cães) ou 42 dias (gatos) após completar a terapia antimicrobiana, 8 de 8 cães, 4 de 11 gatos que receberam o protocolo CMRB e 5 dos 6 gatos que receberam o protocolo ATRB foram infectados novamente. Um efeito transitório da terapia combinada (amoxicilina 20 mg/kg PO a cada 8 horas por 21 dias, metronidazol 20 mg/kg PO a cada 8 horas por 21 dias e omeprazol 0,7 mg PO a cada 24 horas por 21 dias) na colonização bacteriana também foi observado em 6 gatos com infecção por *H. pylori*.

Uma análise mais aprofundada de biopsias gástricas de cães e gatos infectados assintomáticos e gatos infectados por *H. pylori* usando PCR com *primers* específicos para *Helicobacter* revelaram a persistência de DNA de *Helicobacter* em biopsias gástricas que se mostraram negativas na histologia e no teste de urease.[127] Esses estudos sugerem que regimes de antibióticos eficazes contra *H. pylori* nos humanos podem apenas causar supressão transitória, em vez de erradicação de *Helicobacter* spp. em cães e gatos.

Um estudo recente que incluiu metronidazol (11 a 15 mg/kg PO a cada 12 horas), amoxicilina (22 mg/kg PO a cada 12 horas) e subsalicilato de bismuto (0,22 mℓ/kg PO a cada 8 horas) para 5 animais infectados com *Helicobacter* (3 cães e 2 gatos) por 21 dias demonstrou a resolução dos vômitos e a erradicação a longo prazo de *Helicobacter* (9 a 38 meses) em todos os animais.[128] O autor empregou a combinação de amoxicilina (20 mg/kg PO a cada 12 horas), claritromicina (7,5 mg/kg PO a cada 12 horas) e metronidazol (10 mg/kg PO a cada 12 horas) por 14 dias com sucesso em erradicar a infecção por *H. pylori* em gatos. Uma combinação semelhante de antibióticos acrescido de omeprazol suprimiu *Helicobacter* transitoriamente em 4/13 gatos de rua adultos assintomáticos.[127] Esses estudos sugerem que uma maior duração do tratamento (21 dias) ou o uso de antibióticos que podem erradicar o *Helicobacter* intracelular (claritromicina) podem melhorar a erradicação, mas estudos adicionais são necessários para traçar diretrizes claras sobre o tratamento de *Helicobacter* spp. gástrico em cães e gatos.

Gastrite crônica de causa desconhecida

Gastrite linfoplasmocítica de causa desconhecida é comum em cães e gatos e pode estar associada a infiltrados semelhantes nos intestinos.[101] Gatos com gastrite linfoplasmocítica e enterite também devem ser avaliados quanto à presença de doença pancreática e biliar concomitantes, relacionadas à "tríade felina".[129] O infiltrado celular varia amplamente em gravidade e pode ser acompanhado por atrofia da mucosa ou fibrose e menos comumente por hiperplasia. Pacientes com gastrite linfoplasmocítica discreta, gastrite sem hiperplasia folicular e evidência de *Helicobacter* spp. são inicialmente tratados com dieta. A dieta geralmente é restrita em antígenos aos quais o paciente foi exposto anteriormente, como uma dieta à base de cordeiro, se o paciente já tiver sido alimentado com frango, e carne bovina, ou que contenha proteínas hidrolisadas (geralmente frango ou soja) que podem ser menos alergênicas do que proteínas intactas. Muitas dessas dietas também são ricas em carboidratos e restritas em gordura, o que facilita o esvaziamento gástrico, e podem conter outras substâncias, como óleo de peixe (*Menhaden*, clupeiformes) ou antioxidantes que podem alterar a inflamação. A dieta de exclusão é oferecida exclusivamente por um período de cerca de 2 semanas e episódios de vômitos são gravados.[116] Se os sinais melhorarem, um desafio com a dieta original é necessário para confirmar o diagnóstico de hipersensibilidade alimentar. A introdução de um componente alimentar específico, tal como a carne bovina, à dieta de teste é necessária para confirmar a hipersensibilidade alimentar. Se o vômito não regredir, pode ser oferecida uma dieta diferente por mais 2 semanas, geralmente o limite de tolerância do proprietário, ou o paciente pode iniciar o tratamento com prednisolona (1 a 2 mg/kg/dia PO, diminuído para dias alternados, na mínima dosagem que mantém a remissão ao longo de 8 a 12 semanas).

Em pacientes com gastrite linfoplasmocítica moderada a grave que são livres de HLO, pode-se iniciar uma combinação de uma dieta de exclusão e prednisolona. Se os pacientes entrarem em remissão, eles serão mantidos na dieta de exclusão enquanto a prednisolona for reduzida e interrompida se possível. Antiácidos e protetores de mucosa são adicionados ao regime terapêutico se úlceras ou erosão forem detectadas na endoscopia ou se hematêmese ou melena forem observadas. Se a gastrite não responder à dieta, prednisolona e antiácidos, imunossupressão adicional pode ser indicada, mas isso nem sempre é necessário. As biopsias gástricas devem ser cuidadosamente

reavaliadas para evidência de linfoma. Em cães, a imunossupressão geralmente é aumentada com azatioprina (2 mg/kg PO a cada 24 horas por 5 dias, a seguir a cada 48 horas em dias alternados com prednisolona). O clorambucila é uma alternativa mais segura à azatioprina em gatos (PO) e tem sido empregado com sucesso no controle da DII e linfoma de células pequenas (ver a seguir). Agentes procinéticos, como metoclopramida, cisaprida e eritromicina, podem ser usados como medicamentos adicionais quando o esvaziamento gástrico retardado está presente. Eles são discutidos a seguir.

A gastrite eosinofílica difusa de etiologia indefinida é geralmente abordada de forma semelhante à gastrite linfoplasmocitária A presença de eosinofilia, alterações dermatológicas e infiltrados eosinofílicos podem ser ainda mais sugestivos de sensibilidade alimentar. Em gatos, deve ser determinado se faz parte de uma síndrome hipereosinofílica. Tratamento para parasitas ocultos, dietas teste e imunossupressão podem ser realizados conforme descrito anteriormente. Granulomas eosinofílicos focais podem ser associados a parasitas ou infecção fúngica que deveriam ser excluídos antes da imunossupressão com corticosteroides.

ESVAZIAMENTO GÁSTRICO RETARDADO E TRANSTORNOS DE MOTILIDADE

Definições

Distúrbios da motilidade gástrica podem interromper o armazenamento, a mistura dos alimentos e sua liberação para o duodeno.[40] A motilidade gástrica normal é o resultado da interação organizada do músculo liso e estímulos neurais e hormonais. O esvaziamento gástrico retardado é a manifestação mais comumente reconhecida de distúrbios da motilidade gástrica. Esvaziamento gástrico rápido e distúrbios de motilidade associados ao trânsito retrógrado da bile ou ingesta são menos bem definidos. O esvaziamento gástrico retardado é causado por obstrução do fluxo ou propulsão defeituosa (Boxe 275.2) e geralmente é suspeitado quando um animal de estimação vomita alimentos após pelo menos 8 e geralmente até 10 a 16 horas após uma refeição.

Boxe 275.2 Causas de esvaziamento gástrico retardado

Obstrução do fluxo
Estenose congênita
Corpo estranho
Hipertrofia da mucosa pilórica
Granuloma
Pólipos
Neoplasia
Massas extragástricas

Propulsão defeituosa
Desordens gástricas
Gastrite
Úlceras
Neoplasia
Gastrenterite
Peritonite
Pancreatite
Metabólica (hipopotassemia, hipocalcemia, hipoadrenocorticismo)
Inibição nervosa (trauma, dor, estresse)
Disautonomia
Dilatação volvulogástrica
Cirurgia
Medicamentos (anticolinérgicos, narcóticos)
Idiopática

Sinais, histórico e exame físico

O vômito de alimentos 8 a 10 horas após a sua ingestão é o sinal mais comum. O vômito pode ser em jato com estenose pilórica. Distensão abdominal, perda de peso, melena, desconforto abdominal, distensão, inchaço e anorexia estão variavelmente presentes. Os sinais e o histórico podem ser úteis para priorização de diagnósticos. O vômito observado no desmame aumenta a possibilidade de estenose pilórica. Acesso a corpos estranhos, ossos e medicamentos são de óbvia relevância para a obstrução do fluxo. Cães braquicefálicos, de meia-idade e de raças pequenas, como o Shih Tzu, parecem predispostos a uma síndrome de vômito secundária à obstrução do fluxo pilórico causada por hipertrofia da mucosa pilórica e/ou muscular.[136,137] Neoplasia gástrica é geralmente detectada em animais mais velhos com perda de peso, hematêmese e palidez. A pitiose gástrica (ver Capítulo 336) é mais prevalente em cães jovens de raças grandes nos estados do Golfo do México dos EUA. Cães de raça de grande porte e peito profundo são mais propensos a DVG que pode ter um problema subjacente com esvaziamento gástrico (ver DG/DVG anteriormente). Um exame físico completo é realizado para detectar as causas do vômito: corpos estranhos; massas ou espessamentos intestinais; causas não GI, incluindo tireoide (nódulos em gatos), fígado (icterícia, hepatomegalia) ou doença renal (anormal à palpação); e os efeitos sistêmicos do vômito, como desidratação e fraqueza.

Avaliação laboratorial

Hematologia, bioquímica sérica, urinálise, exame de fezes (parasitas [ver Capítulo 81], parvovírus [ver Capítulo 225]) e sorologia (FeLV; ver Capítulo 223) são empregados para detectar causas não GI de vômito ou esvaziamento gástrico retardado e para determinar as consequências do vômito. Os achados laboratoriais variam dependendo da gravidade do vômito, extensão da obstrução pilórica e a presença de distúrbios associados à perda de sangue ou inflamação. O hemograma completo costuma ser normal, mas a anemia pode acompanhar úlceras gástricas ou neoplasia. Hiperglobulinemia pode estar presente quando a obstrução do fluxo de saída é secundária a granuloma fúngico. A presença de hipocloremia, hipopotassemia e alcalose metabólica, com ou sem acidúria, aumenta a suspeita de uma obstrução gastrintestinal superior ou potencial hipersecreção de ácido gástrico.

Diagnóstico: imagens, endoscopia, teste de pH gástrico, técnicas cintilográficas

As radiografias são essenciais para diagnosticar a retenção de alimentos ou fluidos no estômago por mais de 8 h após uma refeição e para detectar distúrbios extragástricos, como peritonite (ver Capítulo 279). A US (ver Capítulo 88) pode detectar espessamento mural ou irregularidade do estômago sugestivo de neoplasia, granuloma, hipertrofia, um objeto estranho radiotransparente ou detectar causas não gástricas de esvaziamento retardado, por exemplo, pancreatite. Uma radiografia de contraste pode ser usada para detectar anormalidades murais e confirmar suspeita de obstrução gástrica quando as radiografias simples são inconclusivas (Figura 275.14).

Geralmente dá-se preferência à endoscopia (ver Capítulo 113), em vez de procedimentos radiográficos, para confirmação de obstrução pilórica ou de causas gástricas/duodenais de redução da propulsão (p. ex., úlceras, gastrite; ver Figura 275.13). O rendimento da endoscopia pode ser comprometido pela administração recente de bário; portanto, costuma ser realizada antes dos estudos radiográficos contrastados. A biopsia endoscópica é limitada à mucosa superficial e, com frequência, é necessária biopsia cirúrgica para se obter um diagnóstico definitivo de condições granulomatosas, neoplásicas ou hipertróficas. A determinação do pH gástrico e dos níveis séricos de gastrina pode ajudar a diferenciar a pilorogastropatia da hipertrofia associada a hipergastrinemia. Tumores pancreáticos produtores de polipeptídios também podem estar associados a hipertrofia de mucosa.

Procedimentos mais sofisticados podem ser usados para avaliar diretamente a motilidade e o esvaziamento gástricos e para otimizar a terapia pró-cinética.[40,41] Eles incluem contraste baritado (líquido ou misturado com os alimentos), poliesferas impregnadas com bário, ultrassonografia, cintilografia, testes de depuração respiratória com ^{13}C-octanoato e ^{13}C-acetato e cápsulas de motilidade *wireless*.[40-44,49]

Já existem vários procedimentos radiográficos contrastados; contudo, são comprometidos pela ampla variabilidade nos tempos de esvaziamento do bário na forma líquida e na forma misturada com os alimentos. A administração de poliesferas impregnadas com bário é um procedimento contrastado simplificado adequado à prática clínica rotineira. Exige menos radiografia do que a seriografia esôfago-estômago-duodeno (SEED), e o desempenho e a interpretação são padronizados. Sua utilidade em animais de estimação ainda precisa ser determinada. A ultrassonografia pode ser útil na detecção de anormalidades da

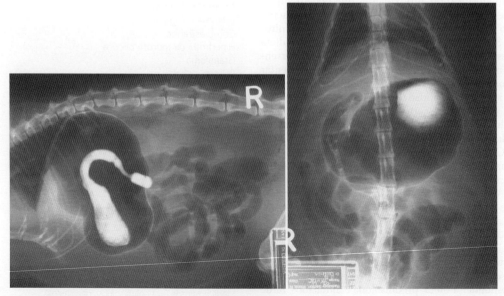

Figura 275.14 Dilatação gástrica marcada e retenção de bário líquido em um Gato Doméstico de Pelo Curto de 12 anos de idade. Biopsias gástricas de espessura total mostraram infiltração submucosa com neutrófilos e linfócitos. (Cortesia da Universidade Cornell. © Kenneth W. Simpson.)

parede gástrica e na mensuração da atividade contrátil, com mensuração padronizada de um índice de motilidade considerado comparável ao ^{13}C-octanoato.[138]

As técnicas cintilográficas eram, tradicionalmente, consideradas a maneira mais acurada de avaliar o esvaziamento gástrico, mas envolvem radioatividade e são realizadas apenas em centros especializados. Os testes com ^{13}C-octanoato e ^{13}C-acetato não radioativos foram avaliados em seres humanos e cães, e constatou-se que refletem o esvaziamento gástrico (os valores são maiores do que os da cintigrafia porque os substratos ^{13}C precisam ser absorvidos e metabolizados antes da liberação de ^{13}C). Recentemente, constatou-se que a telemetria *wireless* com cápsula possibilita mensuração acurada do esvaziamento gástrico, com coeficientes médios de variação (8%) semelhantes aos da cintigrafia (11%) e tempos de esvaziamento consideravelmente maiores do que os da cintigrafia.[43,44] A endoscopia *wireless* com cápsula possibilita a visualização simultânea do piloro e a determinação do tempo de esvaziamento gástrico.[37]

Tratamento

Conduta direta

O tratamento dos distúrbios de esvaziamento gástrico é direcionado à causa subjacente. Úlceras gástricas, erosões e inflamação devem ser investigadas e manejadas clinicamente, conforme descrito. Corpos estranhos devem ser removidos endoscópica ou cirurgicamente. Estenose pilórica, pólipos e gastropatia hipertrófica que não estão associadas à hipergastrinemia são tratados cirurgicamente. Quando gastropatia hipertrófica, úlceras ou erosões, ou excesso de suco gástrico são encontrados na endoscopia, antagonistas H2 podem ser administrados por via intravenosa durante o procedimento para tentar prevenir perfuração ou esofagite pós-operatória. Neoplasia, pólipos e granulomas podem exigir ressecção gástrica extensa e procedimentos Billroth.

Alterações de dieta

A modificação de dieta para facilitar o esvaziamento gástrico pode ser benéfica, independentemente da causa. Quantidades pequenas de dietas semilíquidas, com restrição de proteínas e gorduras oferecidas com intervalos frequentes podem facilitar o esvaziamento, como uma "dieta para doenças intestinais" misturada com água e igual volume de arroz cozido (ver Capítulo 178).

Medicamentos

Nenhum ensaio controlado em cães e gatos avaliou a eficácia de diferentes procinéticos em diferentes estados de doença, sendo o tratamento geralmente baseado na "melhor escolha/menor prejuízo". Quando uma real atividade procinética é necessária, a cisaprida e a eritromicina parecem ser as mais eficazes.[40] Os ensaios de tratamento com procinéticos devem ser provavelmente estruturados para um período entre 5 e 10 dias para determinar o seu benefício. Um diário de sinais clínicos e a avaliação objetiva do esvaziamento do estômago usando os testes descritos anteriormente, antes e depois da terapia, ajudam a otimizar o tratamento. Terapia combinada, como eritromicina e cisaprida, não é recomendada devido ao potencial para interações medicamentosas adversas (ver Capítulo 169). O prognóstico para pacientes com esvaziamento gástrico retardado depende da causa. Um distúrbio de motilidade caracterizado por refluxo duodenogástrico é considerado como suspeita da *síndrome do vômito bilioso*. Os cães afetados geralmente vomitam no início da manhã, e a remissão pode ser alcançada alimentando o animal à noite. Agentes procinéticos também podem ser empregados.

Em situações não obstrutivas, o esvaziamento gástrico pode ser aumentado, e o refluxo duodenogástrico, inibido por agentes procinéticos, como metoclopramida, cisaprida, eritromicina ou ranitidina.[40,68,139] A escolha do procinético depende se um efeito antiemético central é necessário, como a metoclopramida, ou um antiácido procinético combinado (ranitidina) é indicado, ou se o tratamento com um agente foi ineficaz ou causou efeitos adversos, como alterações comportamentais com a metoclopramida. Além de

sua atividade procinética no estômago e trato gastrintestinal superior, a metoclopramida (0,2 a 0,5 mg/kg PO SC a cada 8 horas) tem propriedades antieméticas centrais e é uma escolha inicial em pacientes com doenças metabólicas subjacentes associadas a vômitos e esvaziamento gástrico retardado. No entanto, a metoclopramida pode apenas facilitar o esvaziamento de líquidos e é menos eficaz na promoção organizada da motilidade gastroduodenal e intestinal do que a cisaprida. A cisaprida (0,1 a 0,5 mg/kg PO a cada 8 horas) não tem efeitos antieméticos centrais, geralmente é mais potente na promoção do esvaziamento gástrico de sólidos do que a metoclopramida, tem mais interações medicamentosas, e sua disponibilidade é limitada. A eritromicina (cão: 0,5 a 1 mg/kg PO a cada 8 horas, entre refeições) libera a motilina, atua nos receptores da motilina e imita a fase III do complexo mioelétrico migratório interdigestivo, promovendo o esvaziamento de sólidos. A nizatidina e a ranitidina (0,5 a 1 mg/kg PO a cada 8 horas) têm atividade procinética em cães de experimentação atribuídos a um efeito semelhante ao organofosfato.[140] O cloridrato de ranitidina (75 mg PO a cada 12 horas) foi recentemente observado não ter efeito sobre o tempo de esvaziamento gástrico avaliado por cápsula de motilidade sem fio.[43]

NEOPLASIA GÁSTRICA

Visão geral

Os tumores gástricos representam < 1% de todas as neoplasias caninas e felinas relatadas.[141] Tumores malignos são mais comuns do que os benignos e a maioria dos tipos de neoplasias gástricas foi relatada como de ocorrência mais frequente em machos, exceto os adenomas.[142] As neoplasias gástricas descritas são o leiomiossarcoma, linfoma (ver Capítulo 344), fibrossarcoma, sarcoma anaplásico raro e plasmocitoma extramedular gástrico (Tabela 275.4).

Tumores benignos

Os tumores benignos do estômago incluem leiomiomas e, menos frequentemente, pólipos adenomatosos. Leiomiomas gástricos caninos são vistos em cães velhos, idade mediana de 16 anos, com alguns identificados incidentalmente na necropsia ou vistos devido a sangramento gastrintestinal e anemia microcítica (Figura 275.15). Pólipos adenomatosos são raros em cães, mas foram relatados como elevados, sésseis ou crescimentos pedunculados únicos ou múltiplos no estômago, geralmente no antro pilórico terminal. Embora a maioria seja descoberta incidentalmente, também pode causar sinais de distúrbios GI com vômito (Figura 275.16). Em humanos, pólipos adenomatosos são

Tabela 275.4	Características da neoplasia gástrica em cães.		
TUMOR	**LOCALIZAÇÃO MAIS COMUM**	**IDADE MEDIANA (ANOS)**	**PREDISPOSIÇÃO DE RAÇA RELATADA**
Adenocarcinoma	Antro pilórico, curvatura menor	10	Pastor-Belga Collie de Pelo Longo, Staffordshire Bull Terrier Norsk Lundehund, Bouvier, Pastor-Belga Groenendael, Poodle Grande, Elkhound Norueguês
Leiomioma	Cárdia	16	Beagle
Leiomiossarcoma		7	Nenhuma
Linfoma	Difuso	10	Nenhuma

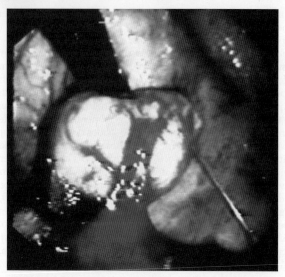

Figura 275.15 Leiomioma gástrico ulcerado na cárdia de um cão. (Cortesia da Ohio State University. © Kenneth W. Simpson.) (*Esta figura se encontra reproduzida em cores no Encarte.*)

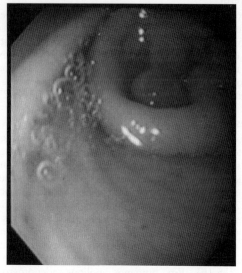

Figura 275.16 Pólipo adenomatoso na via de saída do piloro de um cachorro. (Cortesia da Universidade de Londres. © Kenneth W. Simpson.) (*Esta figura se encontra reproduzida em cores no Encarte.*)

geralmente considerados como possíveis lesões pré-malignas, e alterações consideradas focalmente malignas foram encontradas em cães. Neoplasia gastrintestinal benigna no gato ocorre em uma frequência muito inferior do que no cão, embora até 36% de todas as neoplasias GI sejam consideradas benignas.

Tumores malignos

Adenocarcinoma

O adenocarcinoma maligno é a neoplasia gástrica mais comum em cães, responsável por 47 a 72% de todas as doenças malignas gástricas caninas.[143-146] O adenocarcinoma gástrico é extremamente raro em gatos. A idade máxima dos cães com carcinomas gástricos foi relatada como sendo de 10 a 12 anos com faixa de 3 a 13 anos e idade média de 9 a 10 anos. Uma predisposição da raça para o carcinoma gástrico em Pastor-Belga, Collie de Pelo Longo e Staffordshire Bull Terriers foi sugerida, embora alguns estudos não mostrem predileções por raças. O Registro Norueguês de Câncer Canino indicou que Pastor-Belga Tervuren, Bouvier de Flandres, Groenendael, Collie, Poodle Grande e Elkhound Norueguês têm um risco significativamente maior de desenvolver carcinoma gástrico.[141] Os machos foram mais propensos a ser afetados do que as fêmeas. Gastrite atrófica em Lundehunds parece ser frequente, e atrofia gástrica e inflamação podem preceder a tumorigênese, como acontece em humanos.[134]

Os carcinomas gástricos de cães ocorrem mais comumente na curvatura menor e região pilórica como lesões anulares ou estenosantes, e metástases são frequentes com envolvimento dos linfonodos, pulmões e fígado (Figura 275.17). Os carcinomas podem ser divididos em três padrões morfológicos de distribuição: (1) lesões difusamente infiltrantes e não ulcerativas que envolvem a maior parte do estômago e são compatíveis com a aparência de "garrafa de couro" descrita em humanos; (2) localizado, placa elevada e espessada, geralmente contendo uma úlcera central elevada e escavada; e (3) lesão elevada, polipoide, séssil projetando-se no lúmen do estômago. Dois tipos histológicos de carcinoma gástrico foram descritos em humanos: (1) *difuso* e (2) *intestinal* ou *tubular*. O tipo difuso consiste em infiltrados aleatórios generalizados de células neoplásicas dispersas entre os elementos do estroma da parede gástrica. O tipo intestinal é caracterizado por uma estrutura tubular e glandular. O tipo difuso é mais comum em cães.

Linfoma

A neoplasia gastrintestinal mais comum em ambos, gatos e cães, é o linfoma. No linfoma canino originado na submucosa gástrica, o processo pode ser descrito como difuso ou nodular, com o infiltrado

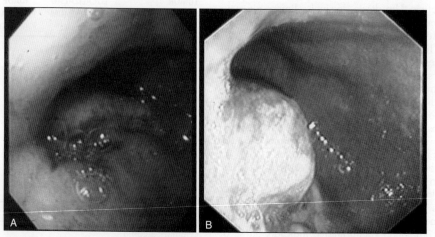

Figura 275.17 Aparência endoscópica de adenocarcinoma gástrico em um cão. **A.** Adenocarcinoma difuso. **B.** Adenocarcinoma focal. (Cortesia The Ohio State University. © Kenneth W. Simpson.) (*Esta figura se encontra reproduzida em cores no Encarte.*)

difuso sendo mais comum (Figura 275.18). O envolvimento do fígado, de linfonodos regionais, do intestino delgado e da medula óssea é comum. O linfoma gástrico felino não está associado à infecção por FeLV, sendo categorizado como linfoblástico ou de células grandes e linfocítico ou de células pequenas, sendo este último mais localizado no trato GI e apresenta um prognóstico muito melhor do que o linfoma de células grandes.[147,148] Em cães e gatos, uma inflamação linfoplasmocítica pode preceder ou coexistir com o linfoma gástrico. Foi sugerido que a inflamação linfoplasmocítica é uma mudança pré-linfomatosa no trato GI. O desenvolvimento de linfoma gástrico em resposta à estimulação antigênica crônica e inflamação é exemplificado pelo linfoma MALT gástrico em pessoas com gastrite associada a H. pylori.

Leiomiossarcoma

Os leiomiossarcomas são tumores de crescimento lento de origem em músculos lisos. A idade mediana dos cães afetados é > 10 anos. O leiomiossarcoma intestinal é mais comum em fêmeas, e uma predisposição foi relatada na raça Pastor-Alemão. No entanto, nem raça nem predisposição sexual foram relatadas para leiomiossarcoma gástrico.[149] Em um estudo, em grupo de cães com leiomiossarcoma no baço, estômago, intestino delgado e ceco, 79% não mostraram evidência de metástases na cirurgia e 64% sobreviveram por mais de 2 semanas.[149] A invasão da parede gástrica por leiomiossarcomas e linfomas é frequentemente difusa. Esses tumores podem causar ulceração semelhante a adenocarcinomas, ou podem aparecer como massas discretas. A sobrevida mediana desses cães foi de 10 meses (intervalo: 1 mês a 7 anos). Do grupo do estômago/intestino delgado, 29% eventualmente morreram de leiomiossarcoma. O leiomiossarcoma e leiomioma têm sido associados a hipoglicemia paraneoplásica e convulsões, provavelmente devido à produção de fatores de crescimento semelhantes a insulina (ver Capítulo 352).[150]

Achados clínicos

Os sinais clínicos mais comuns associados à neoplasia gástrica são vômito crônicos, perda de peso, anorexia, diarreia e hematêmese, melena ou palidez se houver ulceração. Alguns cães têm dor abdominal ou abdome distendido. Com o linfoma GI, o início dos sinais é frequentemente insidioso, gradualmente aumenta em gravidade e se torna refratário a tratamento sintomático.

Diagnóstico

As radiografias podem ser completamente normais ou podem sugerir espessamento focal da parede gástrica, uma massa abdominal, evidências de peritonite, esplenomegalia, hepatomegalia ou linfadenopatia. A perfuração gastrintestinal espontânea em gatos foi associada ao linfoma.[151] Uma US pode revelar espessamento mural ou irregularidades que podem indicar que as lesões podem ser mais de submucosa ou musculares do que superficiais. Linfadenopatia ou metástases regionais podem ser evidentes. US pode ser empregada para avaliar a espessura e estratificação da parede gástrica e o esvaziamento gástrico. A US é menos precisa do que a endoscopia para detecção de neoplasia gástrica, particularmente linfoma, mas pode aumentar a suspeita de uma lesão gástrica e facilitar a detecção de lesões não gástricas em animais de estimação com sinais de doença GI.[32,33]

A gastroscopia (ver Capítulo 113) é capaz de detectar com eficiência a maioria dos tumores gástricos e substituiu amplamente a radiografia de contraste. O linfoma é visto como espessamento das pregas com mucosa rosada ou branca, de forma difusa, suave ou "semelhante a paralelepípedos", podendo haver hemorragias petequiais ou equimóticas dispersas. Os carcinomas gástricos tendem a ser massas focais rosa-escuras a vermelhas que podem parecer ligeiramente pedunculados. Áreas roxas desbotadas a pretas indicam hemorragia, enquanto os focos amarelos a marrons geralmente representam úlceras necróticas. Algumas lesões são submucosas e pode-se ter a impressão de que algo está recuando o estômago, ou a parede parece menos distensível ou espessa. A endoscopia de cápsula sem fio pode facilitar a detecção não invasiva de neoplasias gástricas.

Várias amostras de biopsia devem ser coletadas de áreas suspeitas, e as massas devem ser biopsiadas várias vezes no mesmo lugar para se aprofundar no tecido, pois tumores gástricos podem ter áreas de necrose superficial, inflamação e ulceração que devem ser evitadas ao coletar biopsias. Focar na periferia ajuda a evitar a perfuração. As biopsias cirúrgicas devem ser tomadas onde a aparência endoscópica macroscópica não corresponde ao diagnóstico histológico, tal como uma grande massa gástrica focal com um resultado de biopsia endoscópica de gastrite linfoplasmocítica. Quando a endoscopia não está disponível, a radiografia de contraste pode ser útil, com características da neoplasia gástrica, incluindo espessamento da parede gástrica, defeitos de preenchimento e desarranjo do padrão normal das pregas, e esvaziamento gástrico retardado com retenção e acumulação irregular de bário. A cirurgia é então realizada para coletar amostras da área afetada.

Tratamento

Exceto pelo linfoma (ver Capítulo 344), a cirurgia é a forma mais comum de tratamento do câncer gástrico. A ressecção pode ser curativa se a área afetada for localizada, ou se o tumor for benigno. Se uma área extensa estiver envolvida, uma gastrectomia parcial ou antrectomia seguida por gastroduodenostomia (Billroth I) pode ser tentada. No entanto, muitos pacientes estão em um estágio avançado da doença, e as lesões são frequentemente extensas demais para serem ressecadas. O adenocarcinoma gástrico frequentemente causa metástases; logo, os gânglios linfáticos e o fígado devem ser inspecionados e biopsiados. Mesmo com a cirurgia, o prognóstico para neoplasia gástrica maligna é ruim, a maioria dos animais de estimação morre dentro de 6 meses, de recorrência ou doença metastática. O leiomiossarcoma é uma exceção e carrega um prognóstico bom a excelente se a massa for cirurgicamente ressecável. Mesmo que as metástases sejam evidentes na cirurgia, um resultado favorável pode ser alcançado, porque o tumor apresenta crescimento lento. A sobrevivência de cães com leiomiossarcoma no estômago, intestino delgado, pâncreas e ceco varia de 0 a 47 meses após a cirurgia, e a sobrevida média é de 12,5 meses.[149]

O linfoma GI tem um prognóstico ruim em cães.[152] Em gatos o prognóstico depende se o tumor é de alto ou baixo grau, epiteliotrófico ou transmural.[153] Linfomas de células T pequenas (tipicamente epiteliotróficos) alcançam remissão substancial quando tratados com clorambucila e prednisolona.[147,148] Linfomas de células grandes (B ou T) são tratados com uma combinação de quimioterapia cíclica e tem um prognóstico muito pior.

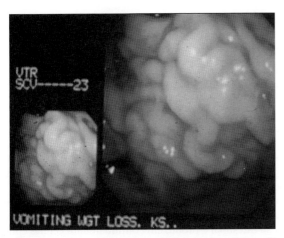

Figura 275.18 Espessamento de pregas gástricas devido ao linfoma. (Cortesia da Universidade de Londres. © Kenneth W. Simpson.)

REFERÊNCIAS BIBLIOGRÁFICAS

As referências bibliográficas deste capítulo se encontram online no Ambiente de Aprendizagem.

CAPÍTULO 276

Doenças do Intestino Delgado

Edward James Hall e Michael J. Day

As funções conflitantes do intestino delgado (ID), ou seja, digestão e absorção de nutrientes *versus* proteção do corpo de ameaças ambientais, o tornaram o maior e mais complexo órgão imunológico do corpo, bem como o principal órgão digestivo. Nas edições anteriores deste livro, o capítulo sobre doenças do ID inicialmente focava em doenças relacionadas a distúrbios de sua função digestiva e, posteriormente, em doenças associadas ao sistema imune de mucosas.[1,2] A última edição, então, destacou como o terceiro componente principal do ID, o *microbioma* (microbiota intestinal), interage com o sistema imune da mucosa, enquanto parte das funções integradas do órgão.[3] Agora está claro que o microbioma é importante não apenas para a saúde intestinal, mas também para a doença (ver Capítulo 274). A disbiose, por exemplo, é um distúrbio do microbioma normal e está envolvida na inflamação intestinal, podendo resultar até mesmo em carcinogênese e em morte,[4-7] o que levou ao surgimento de novas terapias, como probióticos, transplantes microbianos fecais e terapia com células-tronco para enteropatias crônicas.[8-13] O microbioma é ainda mais notável por reconhecidamente poder afetar todo o animal; o eixo intestino-cérebro envolve uma comunicação bidirecional, com evidências crescentes de que o microbioma pode afetar o comportamento e as funções cognitivas, um fenômeno que será, sem dúvida, explorado mais em edições futuras.[14-20] Entretanto, mesmo com a nossa melhor compreensão atual dos três elementos principais – mucosa, sistema imune de mucosa e microbioma –, o clínico já é mais capaz de compreender e tratar muitas doenças do ID.

O sinal cardinal dessas doenças é a diarreia, um aumento significativo na frequência, fluidez ou volume das fezes (ver Capítulo 40). No entanto, a diarreia pode ser uma manifestação de doença em outra parte do trato gastrintestinal (GI) ou em órgãos de outros sistemas (Boxe 276.1). Em contrapartida, a diarreia não está presente em todos os casos de doença do ID, e há diversos sinais de disfunção do ID, sendo alguns não especificados (Boxe 276.2).

ANATOMIA FUNCIONAL DO INTESTINO DELGADO

Estrutura normal[21-33]

O ID começa no piloro do estômago e termina na válvula ileocólica, sendo dividido arbitrariamente em três segmentos: o duodeno proximalmente, onde entram o ducto biliar comum e um ou mais ductos pancreáticos; o jejuno; e, finalmente, o íleo. O sangue é fornecido por ramos das artérias mesentéricas celíacas e craniais e é drenado para o fígado pela veia porta. Os vasos lácteos nas vilosidades drenam para os vasos linfáticos mesentéricos, que passam para a cisterna do quilo. A inervação autônoma do ID é pelos nervos vago e esplâncnicos.

O ID é, em essência, um tubo conectado ao ambiente externo pela boca e pelo ânus, com uma estrutura transversal básica de serosa, muscular (camadas musculares longitudinal externa e circular interna), submucosa e mucosa ao redor do lúmen. A camada mucosa interior é clinicamente a mais importante e é responsável pelas funções secretoras, absortivas e de barreira. Ela varia em espessura ao longo do ID, sendo mais fina distalmente, e compreende o epitélio e a lâmina própria (LP), que contém componentes

---

Boxe 276.1 Causas da diarreia

Doença gastrintestinal
- Doença GI difusa (p. ex., inflamação ou linfoma)
- Doença gástrica
  - Acloridria*
  - Síndromes de dumping*
- Doença intestinal
  - Relacionada à dieta (p. ex., intoxicação alimentar, gula, mudança súbita de dieta e toxinas)
  - Doença primária do intestino delgado
    - Dietética
    - Disbiose
    - Infecciosa
    - Inflamatória
    - Neoplástica
    - Tóxica
  - Doença primária do intestino grosso (ver Capítulo 277).

Doença não gastrintestinal
- Doença pancreática
  - Insuficiência pancreática exócrina‡
  - Pancreatite (aguda, crônica)
  - Carcinoma pancreático‡
  - APUDomas (gastrinoma causando síndrome Zollinger-Ellison)*
- Doença hepática
  - Insuficiência hepatocelular
  - Colestase intra-hepática e extra-hepática
- Doença endócrina
  - Hipoadrenocorticismo clássico‡ (ver Capítulo 309)
  - Hipoadrenocorticismo atípico‡ (ver Capítulo 309)
  - Hipertireoidismo† (ver Capítulo 301)
  - Hipotireoidismo‡ (ver Capítulo 299)
- Doença renal
  - Uremia (ver Capítulo 322)
  - Síndrome nefrótica‡ (ver Capítulo 325)
- Infecção polissistêmica (p. ex., cinomose, leptospirose e hepatite infecciosa canina em cães; PIF, FeLV e FIV em gatos)
- Diversos
  - Toxemias (p. ex., piometra e peritonite)
  - Hipertensão portal e insuficiência cardíaca direita
  - Doença autoimune
  - Neoplasia metastática
  - Várias toxinas e fármacos.

*Condições raras. ‡Raro apenas em gatos. †Raro apenas em cães. *APUD*, tumor de captação e descarboxilação do precursor de amina; *FeLV*, vírus da leucemia felina; *FIV*, vírus da imunodeficiência felina; *PIF*, peritonite infecciosa felina.

---

do sistema imune. A mucosa é modificada por dobras grosseiras e processos semelhantes a dedos – as vilosidades –, cobertos por uma camada epitelial de enterócitos e células caliciformes que aumentam sua área de superfície em centenas de vezes.

Uma vilosidade e suas criptas alimentadoras constituem a unidade funcional do ID. As células das criptas são o local de secreção intestinal e produzem continuamente células epiteliais indiferenciadas. A maioria se desenvolve como enterócitos à medida que migram da cripta para a ponta das vilosidades, onde,

Boxe 276.2 Sinais clínicos de doença do intestino delgado

Sinais cardinais
- Diarreia
  - Aumento na frequência, volume e consistência das fezes.

Outros sinais
- Vômito
- Perda de peso e deficiência/retardo de crescimento
- Hematêmese
- Melena
- Apetite alterado
  - Inapetência/disorexia
  - Anorexia
  - Polifagia
  - Coprofagia
  - Pica
- Desconforto abdominal, dor
- Distensão abdominal: ascite
- Edema periférico
- Borborigmos e flatulências
- Halitose
- Desidratação
- Polidipsia (compensatória)
- Choque.

em última análise, são eliminadas após aproximadamente 3 dias. Os enterócitos diferenciados realizam processos digestivos e absortivos por meio de enzimas digestivas e proteínas transportadoras expressas na membrana celular luminal (apical), uma membrana com microvilosidades (MMV) também chamada de "borda em escova", em razão de sua aparência microscópica.

Função normal[34-38]

A função do enterócito é voltada para a produção de proteínas da face apical, a fim de digerir, absorver e transferir nutrientes simples e água do lúmen para o sangue e os vasos linfáticos. A glutamina derivada dos alimentos é a principal fonte de energia dos enterócitos, o que explica o declínio na estrutura das vilosidades, barreira epitelial e funções imunológicas durante a fome.

Digestão[39,40]

Os principais constituintes da dieta devem ser hidrolisados em moléculas simples para ser transportados através da mucosa. Isso é amplamente alcançado dentro do ID pela emulsificação dos sais biliares e pela hidrólise enzimática luminal: o ID apenas fornece o ambiente ideal em termos de temperatura, de pH e de mistura com sais biliares e enzimas digestivas pancreáticas. Apenas a hidrólise terminal de carboidratos e proteínas é realizada por enzimas da MMV.

Absorção[41-52]

Açúcares simples, aminoácidos e oligopeptídeos são absorvidos por transporte ativo ou facilitado, enquanto as vitaminas lipossolúveis (A, D, E e K) e os produtos da digestão de gorduras são absorvidos por difusão passiva para os vasos lácteos. A endocitose de peptídios pelo ID de um adulto não apresenta significado nutricional, mas a absorção de anticorpos colostrais intactos é crucial em um neonatal.

A absorção de ácido fólico e vitamina B_{12} é complexa (Figura 276.1 A) e importante clinicamente, pois a má absorção pode ajudar a determinar o local e a gravidade da doença intestinal (Figura 276.1 B). O ácido fólico é absorvido no ID proximal, enquanto a cobalamina (vitamina B_{12}), ligada ao fator intrínseco, é absorvida no íleo. Cães e gatos têm menor capacidade de armazenar cobalamina em comparação aos humanos; gatos também carecem da proteína de ligação transcobalamina I e rapidamente perdem a cobalamina por meio da reciclagem enterohepática. Desse modo, a má absorção grave dessa vitamina pode esgotar os estoques em gatos dentro de 1 mês.

Motilidade[53-70]

As ondas lentas e as contrações segmentares e peristálticas do ID são geradas pela contração coordenada dos músculos lisos longitudinais e circulares, em resposta à atividade elétrica espontânea: células intersticiais de Cajal são as células marca-passo. A motilidade intestinal de cães em jejum é caracterizada por um ciclo de três fases, em que uma fase quiescente é seguida de uma atividade contrátil menor e por complexos mioelétricos (motores) migratórios (CMM), que eliminam o material não digerível. As ondas CMM de limpeza intestinal são induzidas pelo hormônio motilina e podem ser replicadas por baixas doses de eritromicina, que estimula o receptor da motilina. Contrações segmentares retardam o trânsito intestinal e garantem a mistura e a digestão dos nutrientes, enquanto o peristaltismo impulsiona a ingestão em sentido aboral. A duração e o padrão da atividade contrátil no estado de alimentação são determinados pela natureza da dieta, com gorduras não absorvidas e fibras prolongando a atividade.

Absorção e secreção de água e eletrólitos[71]

A fisiopatologia da diarreia é detalhada no Capítulo 40. A diarreia é o resultado de um desequilíbrio entre a quantidade de líquidos e de eletrólitos secretados e absorvidos. A absorção líquida ocorre quando o cão está saudável, mas os fluxos através do intestino são massivos (por volta de 2 ℓ por dia em um animal de 20 kg), e as perdas líquidas resultam em diarreia e desidratação graves. A absorção no cólon é importante, pois pode ajudar a compensar as perdas líquidas do ID, mas a diarreia ocorre se sua capacidade de reserva estiver sobrecarregada (ver Capítulo 277).

MICROBIOMA DO INTESTINO DELGADO[72-74]

Microbiota normal[75-114]

O microbioma compreende bactérias, protozoários, fungos e vírus e é uma parte integrante do ID saudável. Ele afeta muitos aspectos da função do ID – tamanho das vilosidades, renovação de enterócitos e de enzimas da MMV e motilidade –, e a presença de um microbioma estável é importante para o desenvolvimento e o equilíbrio contínuo do sistema imune da mucosa e sistêmico e para prevenção da colonização por patógenos. Na doença intestinal, a diversidade do componente bacteriano do microbioma é reduzida, e há uma mudança para espécies potencialmente prejudiciais, enquanto o componente viral (o viroma) é diversificado.

A microbiota bacteriana é o maior componente do microbioma e compreende uma mistura diversa de bactérias aeróbias, anaeróbias e anaeróbicas facultativas, com mais de duzentas espécies presentes no ID de qualquer animal. Muitos microrganismos no microbioma não são cultiváveis, mas técnicas moleculares de impressões digitais (do inglês *fingerprint*), usando sequenciamento do gene do rRNA 16S de alto rendimento, agora podem identificá-los. O microbioma saudável é relativamente resistente às mudanças ambientais, mas pode ser modificado, tanto positiva quanto negativamente, por mudanças na dieta, uso de antibióticos e até estilo de vida. Embora os efeitos da terapia com antibióticos na microbiota muitas vezes sejam clinicamente leves e autolimitantes, podem ocorrer mudanças persistentes no microbioma; portanto, o uso indiscriminado de antibióticos na diarreia é desaconselhável, especialmente porque também pode aumentar a resistência aos antibióticos. Salmonelose pós-antibiótica fatal foi registrada em gatos.

O número de bactérias aumenta do duodeno ao cólon: os fatores que mantêm esse gradiente aboral são a permeabilidade luminal, a motilidade, a disponibilidade de substrato, as secreções bacteriostáticas e bactericidas (ácido gástrico, bile e secreções das células caliciformes e pancreáticas) e uma válvula ileocólica intacta. Uma análise bacteriológica quantitativa, realizada em amostras de suco intestinal não diluído do ID proximal, revelou

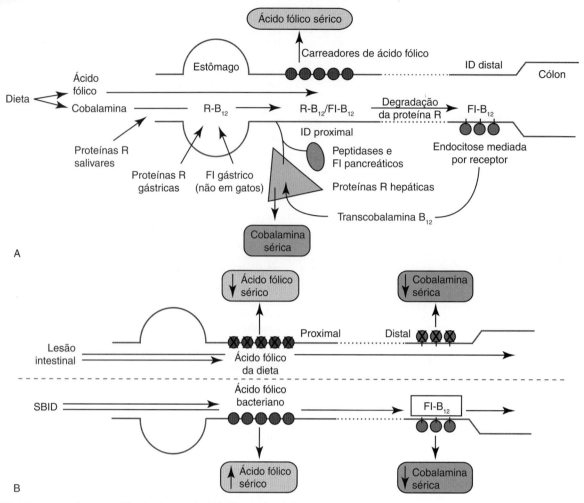

Figura 276.1 Representação esquemática da absorção de ácido fólico e da cobalamina. **A.** No intestino normal, o folato é absorvido no ID proximal por meio de difusão mediada por carreador. A cobalamina presente na dieta inicialmente é protegida da digestão pelas proteínas R e, em seguida, é absorvida no íleo por endocitose mediada por receptor, quando se liga ao fator intrínseco. **B.** No intestino doente, lesões proximais e distais da mucosa causam má absorção de folato e cobalamina, respectivamente. O ácido fólico e a cobalamina séricos reduzidos são marcadores de lesão do ID proximal e/ou distal. Classicamente, o supercrescimento bacteriano do intestino delgado (SBID) causa aumento da captação de ácido fólico, em razão da síntese e da diminuição da captação de cobalamina decorrente da incorporação bacteriana. No entanto, essas mudanças são pouco perceptíveis e não podem ser usadas para diagnóstico, pois não se correlacionam com a responsividade a antibióticos. *ID*, intestino delgado; *FI*, fator intrínseco.

contagens bacterianas em cães e gatos saudáveis que variavam de 10^2 a 10^8 unidades formadoras de colônias (UFC) de bactérias totais/mℓ. Esses números são consideravelmente superiores aos 10^5 UFC/mℓ ou menos relatados em humanos saudáveis e extrapolados incorretamente para cães no passado.

Interações bactéria-mucosa[115-133]

As interações entre as bactérias e a mucosa normalmente são mediadas por receptores de superfície epitelial que fazem parte do sistema imune inato. O epitélio usa receptores-padrão de reconhecimento (RPR, do inglês *pattern recognition receptors* [*PRR*]), para identificar elementos conservados da estrutura bacteriana (ver Capítulo 274). Originalmente referidos como "padrões moleculares associados a patógenos" (PAMP, do inglês *pathogen-associated molecular patterns*) expressos por microrganismos potencialmente patogênicos, a terminologia alternativa "padrões moleculares associados a microrganismos" (MAMP, do inglês *microbe-associated molecular patterns*) engloba o conceito de interação com microrganismos comensais normais, além de patógenos (Figura 276.2).

Os RPR de enterócitos incluem muitos receptores semelhantes a Toll (TLR, do inglês *Toll-like receptors*) e a domínios de oligomerização de nucleotídios (NOD, do inglês *nucleotide oligomerization domain-like receptors*), que podem ser expressos na superfície da membrana ou dentro de compartimentos citoplasmáticos. Exemplos dessas moléculas incluem: TLR2 e TLR4, que reconhecem lipopeptídeos e lipopolissacarídeos encontrados em bactérias gram-negativas, respectivamente; TLR5, que reconhece a proteína do flagelo bacteriano (flagelina); e NOD2, que reconhece o lipopolissacarídeo.

SISTEMA IMUNE GASTRINTESTINAL

A mucosa do ID tem uma função de barreira geral e deve permanecer "tolerante" a antígenos inofensivos, como bactérias comensais e alimentos, embora seja capaz de gerar uma resposta imune protetora também contra patógenos. A resposta-padrão do sistema imune do ID é de tolerância, que é expressa não apenas no trato intestinal; respostas de tolerância em outras superfícies mucosas e dentro do sistema imune podem ser induzidas a partir de interações no trato intestinal. Essas respostas conseguem ser conduzidas por subconjuntos específicos de células apresentadoras de antígenos (APC, do inglês *antigen-presenting cells*) tolerogênicas, que induzem células T reguladoras específicas do antígeno (Treg), que, por sua vez, mediam esses efeitos. Elementos específicos do microbioma parecem ser responsáveis por amplificar e manter a atividade Treg para prevenir doenças imunomediadas locais e sistêmicas.

CAPÍTULO 276 • Doenças do Intestino Delgado 1529

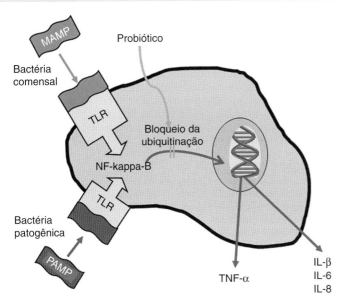

Figura 276.2 Reconhecimento de bactérias comensais e invasoras pelo tecido linfoide associado à mucosa. Receptores semelhantes a Toll (TLR) são encontrados em células endoteliais, monócitos, macrófagos e células dendríticas do tecido linfoide associado à mucosa intestinal (MALT, do inglês *microbe-associated molecular pattern*), bem como na superfície basolateral dos enterócitos. Os TLR reconhecem padrões moleculares associados a microrganismos (MAMP) expressos por todas as bactérias e estimulam, via sinalização intracelular, a produção do fator de transcrição nuclear NF-kappa-B. Quando a célula é exposta a um padrão molecular associado a patógeno (PAMP), o NF-kappa-B é ubiquitinado e pode então ativar a transcrição do mRNA, que codifica citocinas proinflamatórias, como o fator de necrose tumoral (TNF-α, do inglês *tumor necrosis factor*) e várias interleucinas (IL), desencadeando a cascata inflamatória. No entanto, quando estimulado por microrganismos comensais ou probióticos, a ubiquitinação de NF-kappa-B é bloqueada. O mecanismo de diferenciação dos comensais e dos patógenos ainda não foi totalmente compreendida.

Anatomia funcional do sistema imune de mucosa[134-138]

O tecido linfoide associado a mucosa (MALT, do inglês *mucosal associated lymphoid tissue*) ocorre em superfícies internas do corpo; no intestino, é denominado tecido linfoide associado ao intestino (GALT, do inglês *gut associated lymphoid tissue*) e consiste em locais indutíveis, que compreendem as placas de Peyer (PP), os folículos linfoides isolados e os linfonodos mesentéricos (LM), e os locais efetores, que compreendem a LP e o epitélio intestinal. No entanto, essa distinção não é absoluta, e as funções diferentes desses locais se sobrepõem. A LP consiste em uma matriz de tecido conjuntivo com um componente misto de células imunes, mas predominantemente linfoplasmocitário. Uma grande população de linfócitos intraepiteliais (LIE) também existe entre os enterócitos.

Células e moléculas do sistema imune de mucosa

Linfócitos[139-157]

Os linfócitos B estão presentes na região folicular das PP e dos LM. A LP é dotada de uma grande população de plasmócitos e é o estágio de diferenciação terminal de uma célula B ativada. Eles estão predominantemente localizados na LP pericriptal, e a maioria é voltada à produção de imunoglobulina (Ig) A. A maioria dos linfócitos T intestinais tem um receptor de células T (TCR, do inglês *T-cell receptor*) formado por uma cadeia alfa e beta e está localizada principalmente dentro da LP e dos tecidos linfoides organizados; alguns dos linfócitos são LIE. Também existe uma população de células T evolutivamente mais velha expressando um TCR composto por uma cadeia gama e delta, e esses, em grande parte, são LIE. Em razão da sua localização, essas células são consideradas uma defesa primitiva de primeira linha contra patógenos.

Os linfócitos T podem ser subdivididos adicionalmente com base na expressão de moléculas CD4 e CD8. As células T CD4 (células T "auxiliares" clássicas) reconhecem peptídios antigênicos apresentados por moléculas de classe II do complexo principal de histocompatibilidade (MHC II, do inglês *major histocompatibility complex*) em APC, enquanto as células T CD8 (geralmente células citotóxicas) são restritas ao MHC I. Na LP canina, as células T são mais numerosas nas regiões vilosas superiores e são principalmente do TCR alfabeta, fenótipo CD4. No entanto, na LP felina, as células T CD8 superam a população CD4. Existem vários subconjuntos funcionais da população T auxiliar (Th), que são descritos a seguir. Além disso, agora são reconhecidos vários subconjuntos de "células linfoides inatas", que têm morfologia linfoide, mas não carregam moléculas receptoras de linfócitos clássicas (ver a seguir). A maioria dos linfócitos da LP é altamente diferenciada, o que implica que eles recebem estimulação antigênica e mitogênica contínua, provavelmente do microbioma endógeno.

Células dendríticas[118,158-166]

As células dendríticas (CD) funcionam predominantemente como APC, podendo ser encontradas tanto em tecidos induzíveis (p. ex., PP) como tecidos efetores (LP). As CD foliculares armazenam antígenos para fornecer estimulação contínua às células B de memória. As CD também são proeminentes na LP da vilosidade, onde sua função principal é a "amostragem" de antígenos. Essas células muitas vezes estão localizadas imediatamente abaixo da camada de enterócitos e são capazes de estender os processos citoplasmáticos (dendritos) entre os enterócitos e dentro do lúmen intestinal para amostras de antígenos. Nos locais induzíveis, elas são responsáveis por gerar respostas imunes e induzir tolerância. Em roedores, as CD da LP responsáveis por cada um desses efeitos são definidas pela expressão da molécula CD103, de modo que aquelas que induzem respostas inflamatórias são CD103⁻ e aquelas que induzem tolerância mediada por Treg são CD103⁺.

Outras células do sistema imune[143,145,167-170]

Os macrófagos estão presentes na PP e na LP, e suas funções incluem fagocitose, apresentação de antígenos e imunorregulação. Eles secretam citocinas, quimiocinas e mediadores inflamatórios, incluindo o fator de necrose tumoral alfa (TNF-alfa), eicosanoides e leucotrienos. Os neutrófilos estão normalmente presentes em pequeno número, embora aumentem com a inflamação da mucosa. Mastócitos (MC) e eosinófilos podem ser encontrados na LP normal e produzir ativamente mediadores químicos de inflamação (p. ex., histamina, heparina, eicosanoides e citocinas). Os MC expressam o receptor de IgE de alta afinidade (Fc-epsilon-RI), que pode se ligar a IgE e causar sua degranulação e liberação de seus mediadores inflamatórios. Em cães, os eosinófilos são uma população proeminente na LP, especialmente nas criptas. Os eosinófilos podem ter papéis pró-inflamatórios, sobretudo em processos alérgicos, porque são uma fonte rica de mediadores pró-inflamatórios, citocinas e quimiocinas. Uma "conversa cruzada triangular" pode ocorrer entre os eosinófilos, os MC e os linfócitos T.

Enterócitos[167,171-174]

Os enterócitos têm funções importantes na imunidade. Em primeiro lugar, eles excluem antígenos. Em segundo, expressam TLR de superfície, que interagem com a microbiota entérica. Além disso, podem apresentar antígenos por meio da expressão de MHC II. O MHC II é expresso constitutivamente por enterócitos em cães, mas está ausente em enterócitos de gatos, embora seja regulada positivamente na inflamação. Por último, os enterócitos podem produzir mediadores inflamatórios, quimiocinas e citocinas.

Neurônios entéricos[175,176]

Os neurônios entéricos conseguem liberar neuropeptídeos imunoativos, incluindo a substância P, que pode causar inflamação neurogênica via receptores de neurocinina (NC). Na comunicação bidirecional, que também pode existir, a liberação de mediadores por células imunes (p. ex., mastócitos) consegue gerar reflexos dos axônios e, assim, modular a motilidade intestinal, a secreção e a absorção.

Citocinas[177-187]

Uma grande variedade de citocinas é produzida por células no ID. Essas moléculas podem ser agrupadas em tipos pró-inflamatórios, imunorreguladores e quimiocinéticos. Diferentes populações de linfócitos T CD4 têm padrões variados de secreção de citocinas e podem regular diferencialmente as respostas do sistema imunológico (humoral e mediada por células). *In vitro*, existem duas populações principais de linfócitos T CD4 +: as células T helper 1 (Th1) que produzem interleucina-2 (IL-2) e interferona gama (IFN-gama) e medeiam a imunidade celular, envolvendo a ativação de linfócitos T citotóxicos CD8 + e macrófagos, classicamente em resposta à infecção por patógenos intracelulares ou ao câncer; e os linfócitos T helper 2 (Th2), que produzem IL-4, IL-5, IL-6 e IL-13 e atuam para promover a ativação e a diferenciação de linfócitos B em células plasmáticas secretoras de anticorpos. Os linfócitos Th2 medeiam a "troca de classe de imunoglobulina" durante a ativação de linfócitos B, que, no ID, é principalmente para IgA ou IgG. As células Th17 são caracterizadas pela produção de IL-17 e atuam nas respostas inflamatórias, possuindo, inclusive, um papel fundamental na patogênese das enteropatias inflamatórias.

Entretanto, existem outras populações, que têm função de regulação negativa. Os linfócitos Th3 produtores de TGF-beta foram identificados como efetores de "tolerância oral" clássica, mas o linfócito Treg CD25 + Foxp3 + (produzindo IL-10 como uma citocina de assinatura) é a população "supressora" mais importante em termos de tolerância intestinal local ou sistêmica. Muitos outros tipos de células também produzem citocinas, e é o perfil local comum de citocinas que determina o tipo predominante de resposta imune.

Os papéis polarizados desses subconjuntos clássicos de linfócitos T são espelhados pelas atividades complementares das "células linfoides inatas" (CLI), identificadas recentemente. As CLI do grupo 1, que incluem as células *natural killer* (NK), têm uma produção de IFN-gama semelhante a dos linfócitos Th1. As CLI do grupo 2, por sua vez, produzem IL-5 e IL-13 de modo similar aos efeitos dos linfócitos Th2. Os CLI do Grupo 3 produzem IL-17 e IL-22 e podem ter um efeito pró-inflamatório (como para linfócitos Th17) ou, em algumas circunstâncias, ter um efeito protetor anti-inflamatório.

Homing dos linfócitos no tecido linfoide associado ao intestino[143,149,188-191]

Os linfócitos trafegam entre os locais induzíveis e efetores. As vias de *homing* são mediadas por interações entre leucócitos e células endoteliais, por meio da expressão diferencial de "receptores de *homing*" na superfície do leucócito interagindo com o adressinas vasculares endoteliais. A interação mais importante para os linfócitos da mucosa ocorre entre alfa$_4$/beta$_7$ no linfócito e na molécula de adesão celular adressina de mucosa-1 (MAdCAM-1, do inglês *mucosal addressin cell adhesion molecule-1*) na célula endotelial. Um fator final importante para o *homing* de linfócitos é a produção de quimiocinas e seus receptores. O conjunto de quimiocinas de certo tecido determina quais tipos de células T auxiliares e outros subconjuntos de células são recrutados do sangue circulante para o tecido.

Respostas imunológicas inatas do intestino delgado[192-194]

As defesas imunológicas inatas do ID têm sido amplamente descritas, e incluem fatores como movimentos peristálticos, presença do microbioma intestinal, camada de muco e barreira de enterócitos e a presença e função de células imunes inatas (p. ex., CD, macrófagos, granulócitos, CLI e LEI, que expressam gamadelta-TCR). Apesar de mal definido no cão e no gato, a produção de peptídios antimicrobianos relacionados à catelecidina (ou seja, defensinas) por enterócitos (e, particularmente, por células de Paneth das criptas) é de grande importância em outras espécies.

Respostas imunes adquiridas do tecido linfoide associado ao intestino

As respostas imunes adquiridas se desenvolvem após uma série de etapas envolvendo a captação de antígeno, a apresentação a linfócitos virgens, a coestimulação por linfócitos auxiliares, a proliferação e diferenciação clonal, o direcionamento para locais efetores e o desempenho das funções efetoras. Os mecanismos específicos envolvidos são descritos em detalhes em outro momento, mas algumas características particulares para o GALT são descritas neste capítulo.

Captação e apresentação de antígeno[161]

A captação de antígenos particulados ocorre através das células M localizadas dentro da cobertura epitelial das PP. As células M transferem antígenos luminais para as CD e macrófagos dentro desses tecidos linfoides. Essas APC processam e apresentam antígeno aos linfócitos no contexto das moléculas MHC II. Os antígenos solúveis podem ser absorvidos via enterócitos e apresentados às células T. A amostragem direta de antígenos luminais por CD foi descrita anteriormente.

Respostas de linfócitos T e B[181,195-198]

O papel de linfócitos Th1 e Th17 em respostas citotóxicas e inflamatórias na mucosa intestinal e dos linfócitos Treg na tolerância local e sistêmica foi discutido anteriormente.

Os linfócitos B reconhecem epítopos antigênicos conformacionais intactos por meio de seu receptor superficial de membrana (Ig; sinal 1) e requerem a "ajuda" dos linfócitos T na forma de interações moleculares intercelulares diretas (sinal 2) e o fornecimento de citocinas de Th2 atuando em um receptor de citocinas dos linfócitos B (sinal 3). A troca de classe de imunoglobulina do linfócito B permite a produção diferencial de anticorpos IgA, IgE ou IgG, em resposta a diferentes classes de antígenos. Após a troca de classe, os linfócitos B passam por uma expansão adicional e, em seguida, se deslocam para locais efetores, onde se diferenciam em plasmócitos.

A síntese de IgA predomina na mucosa intestinal saudável. Os plasmócitos na LP liberam moléculas de IgA dimérica, dois monômeros ligados pela cadeia de união (J). A IgA dimérica é capturada pelo receptor da imunoglobulina polimérica (RIgP), expresso na superfície basolateral dos enterócitos. O complexo de receptor e IgA passa pelo enterócito e é entregue por meio da MMV. Na superfície luminal, o RIgP é clivado para formar o componente secretor (CS), que permanece associado à pIgA, protegendo-a da degradação enzimática no lúmen intestinal. A principal função de IgA secretora (SIgA) é a exclusão imune, isto é, a ligação e neutralização do seu respectivo antígeno. Isso ajuda a manter a tolerância e protege a mucosa da invasão do antígeno. A deficiência de SIgA pode predispor a doenças intestinais.

As respostas aos parasitas envolvem a produção de IgE determinada por Th2, que se liga ao Fc-epsilon-RI nos mastócitos da mucosa. Quando os mastócitos são posteriormente expostos ao antígeno, ocorre sua degranulação, iniciando uma reação inflamatória local, o recrutamento de eosinófilos teciduais e o aumento das células caliciformes produtoras de muco. Esses muitos mecanismos efetores podem levar à morte das formas larvais dentro da mucosa ou à expulsão de parasitas luminais. Respostas de IgE inadequadas também podem ser geradas, fornecendo um mecanismo proposto para alergia alimentar por meio de uma resposta clássica de hipersensibilidade tipo I.

Tolerância da mucosa[199-203]

As descrições anteriores se relacionam às respostas imunológicas específicas a patógenos, mas tais respostas são a exceção, não a regra, e a resposta-padrão aos antígenos da mucosa é a tolerância, o que não é uma surpresa, dado que a maioria dos antígenos luminais é derivada de componentes inofensivos da dieta e da microbiota comensal. A geração de respostas imunes ativas a moléculas comuns seria um desperdício e potencialmente prejudicial, pois poderia levar a uma inflamação descontrolada. Apesar de os mecanismos pelos quais a tolerância da mucosa ocorre serem bem caracterizados, permanece não resolvida a questão fundamental do que leva à tolerância ou a uma resposta imune pelo GALT.

A tolerância da mucosa pode resultar tanto da anergia/deleção (apoptose) de células T específicas para o antígeno quanto da supressão ativa por células supressoras antígeno-específicas. As subpopulações de células T CD4 + alfa/beta que medeiam a supressão ativa produzem citocinas de regulação negativa (p. ex., TGF-β, IL-10 e IL-17) ou atingem seu efeito por meio de interações célula a célula (através, por exemplo, do CD25 e receptor de IL-2). No entanto, qualquer célula capaz de produzir perfis semelhantes de citocinas pode desempenhar um papel; portanto, a tolerância pode surgir dos efeitos de linfócitos T CD8 +, macrófagos, células do estroma e enterócitos. Além disso, uma vez que TGF-β e IL-10 também são importantes na produção de IgA, a geração de tolerância da mucosa provavelmente ocorre em paralelo às respostas específicas de IgA, o que ajuda a manter imune a tolerância por exclusão.

Consequências da ativação inadequada da imunidade no intestino delgado[124,132,204-226]

Em indivíduos saudáveis, o sistema imune intestinal é mantido em equilíbrio homeostático complexo com uma configuração tolerogênica dominante. Muitas das doenças discutidas neste capítulo surgem quando essa homeostase é perturbada por influências multifatoriais, inclusive fatores genéticos, disfunção de barreira e disbiose, levando à exposição inadequada a antígenos luminais, à indução da inflamação tecidual e à alteração no equilíbrio entre as células efetoras imunes e reguladoras na mucosa.

Se o desafio antigênico inadequado for contido, a mucosa entra em fase de reparo, e o ambiente de tolerância retorna ao normal. No entanto, se o perigo persistir, seja porque a barreira da mucosa permanece violada e/ou a agressão patogênica continua inalterada, seja em razão de uma anormalidade inerente no GALT, um estado de inflamação crônica se instala. A inflamação causa o aumento da expressão de moléculas de MHC II e a ativação de linfócitos e células endoteliais, alterando a expressão de adressinas vasculares. A expressão aumentada de MAdCAM-1 leva ao aumento do recrutamento de linfócitos específicos da mucosa, enquanto a expressão de outras adressinas (p. ex., E-selectina, P-selectina e adressina de nodo periférico) consegue levar ao recrutamento de um leque mais amplo de especificidades de imunócitos. Proteólise extracelular por metaloproteinases de matriz pode levar a mudanças na arquitetura. Em última análise, a inflamação crônica resulta em mudanças histopatológicas que provavelmente são semelhantes, independentemente da causa inicial. Além disso, foi levantada a hipótese de que a estimulação crônica de linfócitos em pacientes geneticamente predispostos poderia resultar na expansão de um clone maligno de linfócitos T e linfoma da mucosa.

MECANISMOS FISIOPATOLÓGICOS NA DOENÇA INTESTINAL

Uma série de mecanismos fisiopatológicos potenciais podem levar à disfunção do ID, e um ou mais dos mecanismos a seguir podem estar presentes em qualquer doença específica do ID.

Perturbação luminal[227-232]

A falta de enzimas pancreáticas na insuficiência pancreática exócrina (IPE; ver Capítulo 292), o aumento da destruição das enzimas por hipersecreção de ácido (p. ex., síndrome de Zollinger-Ellison; ver Capítulo 275) ou o crescimento excessivo de bactérias resulta em falha de digestão. A "disbiose" é um termo mais aceitável do que "crescimento excessivo" para descrever a perturbação do microbioma normal que pode ocorrer após infecção, uso de antibióticos, mudança repentina na dieta ou imunoincompetência/inflamação da mucosa subjacente. Algumas bactérias competem por nutrientes e produzem metabólitos (p. ex., sais biliares desconjugados e ácidos graxos hidroxilados), que podem estimular a secreção intestinal. A interrupção da circulação enterohepática normal e a falta de sais biliares resultam em má absorção de gorduras. A deficiência de sais biliares pode ser causada por disfunção hepática acentuada, obstrução do ducto biliar, desconjugação por bactérias ou doença ileal.

Doenças superfície apical da membrana[40,47,48,52,233-254]

As doenças primárias da superfície apical da membrana são alterações bioquímicas que ocorrem na ausência de lesões estruturais. A falta de uma enzima-chave digestiva leva à má digestão/absorção, diarreia osmótica e perda de peso. A deficiência de sacarase-isomaltase é reconhecida em humanos, mas ainda não foi descrita em cães ou gatos. A deficiência de lactase no ser humano pode ser uma falha congênita em expressar a enzima graças a uma mutação genética à regulação negativa da sua expressão em adultos. A deficiência congênita de lactase não foi relatada em cães e gatos, mas ocorre deficiência relativa, particularmente em gatos adultos, pois a expressão é reduzida após o desmame. A deficiência congênita de aminopeptidase N na MMV dos enterócitos foi descrita em cães, mas não tem significado clínico em razão da compensação por outras peptidases.

O mecanismo da deficiência de cobalamina, comumente visto em cães da raça Shar-pei com doença intestinal, não foi elucidado ainda, mas a deficiência na captação do fator intrínseco de cobalamina no íleo pode decorrer de uma mutação na molécula receptora, a cubilina. As mutações genéticas que causam má absorção seletiva da cobalamina, também conhecidas como síndrome de Imerslund-Gräsbeck, foram identificadas em cães das raças Pastor-Australiano, Beagle, Collie e Schnauzer Gigante. Todas as mutações resultam em deficiência de cobalamina com consequente acidúria metilmalônica e uma constelação de sinais clínicos, incluindo: inapetência, deficiência de crescimento, degeneração hepática, hepatoencefalopatia, neutropenia, anemia e/ou proteinúria. A diarreia pode ser uma característica, uma vez que dietas deficientes em cobalamina resultam em anormalidades histológicas e na disfunção do ID.

A ressecção cirúrgica do íleo (p. ex., em razão da intussuscepção ileocólica irredutível) e doença afetando o ID distal causam má absorção de sais biliares e cobalamina. Contudo, a deficiência congênita do transportador de sal biliar ileal relatada no ser humano – uma causa de diarreia grave – ainda não foi relatada em cães ou gatos.

Lesão da membrana de microvilosidades (apical)[255-260]

A MMV está obviamente lesionada quando danos histológicos das vilosidades estão evidentes, mas, mesmo sem alterações à microscopia óptica, pode ocorrer comprometimento maciço da função da mucosa. Esse dano é observado na infecção por *Escherichia coli* enteropatogênica, com goma de carragena ou com lectinas, que causam a perda de enzimas e transportadores da membrana apical, como também da área de superfície. O supercrescimento bacteriano está associado a lesões sutis, mas específicas à membrana, pois os anaeróbios são muito eficazes na degradação de glicoproteínas e liberação de enzimas da membrana.

Disfunção no enterócitos[261,262]

As lesões dos enterócitos por toxinas bacterianas, sem alteração histológica, ainda podem interferir com sua função, bem como causar perda subcelular de proteínas da membrana apical. Desnutrição e isquemia também prejudicam a função e aumentam a permeabilidade epitelial. A abetalipoproteinemia em humanos é uma falha do transporte transcelular de lipídios, resultando em acúmulo anormal de lipídios nos enterócitos, e, embora essa condição ainda não tenha sido relatada em cães e gatos, o fármaco dirlopatida, utilizado para perda de peso, atua bloqueando a proteína de transferência de triglicerídeo microssomal dentro dos enterócitos e, portanto, absorvendo gordura; a diarreia é um efeito adverso comum e previsível desse medicamento.

Ruptura da barreira epitelial[263-272]

A integridade epitelial é crucial para manter a tolerância oral e excluir patógenos. No modelo experimental de camundongo quimérico N-caderina dominante negativo, em que a integridade epitelial é interrompida em razão da falta de expressão normal de E-caderina nas junções oclusivas, a inflamação intestinal é restrita às regiões do intestino nas quais o gene mutante é expresso. Em outros animais-modelo, a desnutrição resulta tanto na atrofia das vilosidades quanto no aumento da absorção macromolecular transepitelial, na produção de mucina anormal e na secreção reduzida de IgA. As causas naturais da diminuição da função de barreira incluem fatores luminais agressivos e mediadores inflamatórios endógenos. A lesão na barreira pode levar à entrada de antígenos, às reações alérgicas e/ou inflamatórias subsequentes e até mesmo à translocação de bactérias para a circulação. Medicamentos anti-inflamatórios não esteroidais (AINE) danificam a barreira, aumentando a permeabilidade intestinal, mas a presença de fibras solúveis (p. ex., pectina) é protetora. A norepinefrina, que é naturalmente aumentada pelo estresse, altera a permeabilidade das junções oclusivas dos enterócitos, permitindo a invasão por *Campylobacter* e o recrutamento de neutrófilos pela indução de IL-8. A perda de líquido tecidual rico em proteínas na direção oposta também tem significado clínico, causando uma enteropatia com perda de proteínas (EPP).

Atrofia das vilosidades[270,273]

A atrofia das vilosidades causa perda de área de superfície intestinal e resulta em má absorção de gordura. Além disso, há limitação na taxa de captação de produtos de digestão de proteínas e de carboidratos mediada por transportadores, porque há um número finito de transportadores de nutrientes. A atrofia é causada pela diminuição da produção ou pelo aumento na taxa de perda dos enterócitos. Se esta ultrapassa o aumento da proliferação, resulta em atrofia das vilosidades; mas, se a causa inicial puder ser removida, a atrofia é completamente reversível. Por outro lado, uma taxa persistentemente elevada de perda de enterócitos pode resultar em aumento compensatório da taxa de proliferação de células da cripta, de modo a não diminuir a altura das vilosidades se a perda de células for correspondida pelo aumento da proliferação. No entanto, um efeito funcional significativo ainda ocorre, já que os enterócitos maduros são substituídos por enterócitos imaturos, de funcionalidade subótima.

Agentes infecciosos que lesionam os enterócitos podem infectar a extremidade da vilosidade (p. ex., rotavírus) ou o meio da vilosidade (coronavírus), causando perda de células e diarreia leve a moderada. Medicamentos citotóxicos (vincristina) e infecção por parvovírus, que causam parada na maturação e destruição da cripta, respectivamente, podem ser devastadores, causando colapso total das vilosidades e das criptas e diarreia grave. Supondo que algumas células-tronco sobrevivam ao ataque, a regeneração é possível, mas provavelmente levará vários dias.

Distúrbios na motilidade[274-282]

Alterações da motilidade intestinal como causa primária de disfunções no ID em cães e gatos são pouco caracterizadas. A síndrome do intestino irritável (SII) é um distúrbio funcional com mudanças principalmente na motilidade. Alterações de motilidade secundárias ocorrem com obstrução intestinal, pseudo-obstrução, íleo adinâmico ou enteropatias inflamatórias e infecciosas. Ondas rápidas de contrações podem ser causadas por isquemia no ID e por bactérias enterotoxigênicas. Na má absorção, os solutos não absorvidos retêm líquidos osmoticamente, causando distensão intestinal e hipermotilidade reflexa. O hipertireoidismo em gatos diminui o tempo de trânsito e causa diarreia.

Entretanto, a diarreia está realmente associada com a hipomotilidade intestinal ou íleo adinâmico na maioria dos casos. O íleo adinâmico é uma obstrução funcional transitória e reversível do intestino com muitas causas (Boxe 276.3). Em infecções virais entéricas, por exemplo, o íleo adinâmico é comum,

---

Boxe 276.3 Causas potenciais de íleo adinâmico

Funcional
- Cirurgia abdominal
- Isquemia
- Síndrome do intestino irritável (diarreia/constipação intestinal mistas).

Inflamatória
- Pancreatite
- Parvovírus
- Peritonite.

Metabólica
- Diabetes melito
- Endotoxemia
- Hipopotassemia
- Hipocalcemia/hipomagnesemia
- Uremia.

Neuromuscular
- Medicamentos anticolinérgicos e opioides
- Disautonomia
- Miopatia visceral
- Neuropatia visceral.

Física
- Obstrução intestinal
  - Corpo estranho
  - Intussuscepção
  - Massas – neoplasia, granuloma
  - Mecânica – torção, vólvulo, encarceramento, aderências
- Distensão excessiva por aerofagia.

---

promovendo mais diarreia, já que a estase permite a fermentação bacteriana. O íleo adinâmico pós-operatório é causado por uma combinação de inflamação induzida cirurgicamente e inibição simpática, potencialmente complicada por peritonite, administração de opioides ou ambas. A má absorção leva à presença de alimento não digerido no íleo e no cólon, inibindo a motilidade intestinal através de vias neuro-hormonais, e pode retardar o esvaziamento gástrico. Hipomotilidade e constipação intestinal são esperadas com hipotireoidismo, mas, ocasionalmente, é verificada diarreia responsiva a antibióticos.

Inflamação da mucosa[283-286]

A inflamação é uma resposta celular e vascular a uma série de causas incitantes, inclusive infecção, isquemia, trauma, toxinas, neoplasias e reações imunomediadas. De fato, qualquer coisa que rompa a barreira da mucosa pode desencadear uma inflamação e danos teciduais por meio da regulação positiva das metaloproteinases da matriz.

Modelos experimentais de inflamação GI em roedores geneticamente modificados permitiram uma melhor compreensão da patogênese da inflamação da mucosa e dos mecanismos que a acionam. Várias alterações do sistema imune da mucosa são capazes de levar a respostas inflamatórias crônicas histologicamente semelhantes e podem ser induzidas de três maneiras: através da alteração da microbiota endógena, através da interferência com a barreira mucosa ou através da desregulação do sistema imunológico da mucosa. Seja pela ruptura da barreira mucosa, seja pela desregulação do sistema imunológico, a presença de uma microbiota entérica é essencial para a expressão da inflamação. Isso sugere que indivíduos saudáveis são tolerantes à sua própria microbiota intestinal, mas pacientes com doença inflamatória intestinal (DII) idiopática têm a tolerância quebrada.

Hipersensibilidade[287,288]

A sensibilização de um paciente a um antígeno da dieta pode provocar uma reação alérgica mediada por IgE quando o animal

CAPÍTULO 276 • Doenças do Intestino Delgado

é exposto novamente a ele. A liberação de numerosos mediadores de mastócitos pode ter efeitos sistêmicos generalizados (como anafilaxia), efeitos remotos (prurido e urticária) ou apenas efeitos intestinais locais, induzindo mudanças rápidas na absorção e secreção, secreção de muco, permeabilidade epitelial e endotelial e motilidade intestinal.

Neoplasia

Tumores difusos que infiltram a mucosa, como o linfoma, causam disfunção no ID. As células malignas podem apenas obstruir o fluxo sanguíneo e linfático, mas a função dos enterócitos provavelmente pode ser prejudicada ou a mucosa pode apresentar atrofia das vilosidades ou ser ulcerada em razão da isquemia. Tumores isolados são possíveis causas de disfunção, provavelmente por meio dos efeitos da obstrução parcial, com estase da ingesta e supercrescimento bacteriano secundário. Mais tipicamente, os tumores sólidos estão associados a sinais como obstrução intestinal, sangramento e caquexia associada ao câncer. A peritonite pode ocorrer se a integridade da parede do intestino estiver comprometida. Os tumores cutâneos de mastócitos conseguem causar hipersecreção de ácido gástrico mediada por histamina, levando a ulceração gastroduodenal e até perfuração.

Falha na distribuição de nutrientes[289,290]

Após a absorção, os nutrientes são transportados pelo sangue e linfonodos, mas apenas doenças linfáticas intestinais são bem descritas em animais. A dilatação e disfunção linfática primária (linfangiectasia) que causa má absorção pode ser idiopática ou estar associada a linfangite. Linfangiectasia secundária é observada em qualquer condição que cause obstrução dos vasos linfáticos.

Anormalidades congênitas[291-302]

São relatadas estenose intestinal, atresia, não rotação e duplicações aleatórias de segmentos do ID e do intestino grosso (IG) em cães e gatos. Duplicações são lesões semelhantes a cistos que raramente causam sinais clínicos, a menos que sejam obstrutivas. Divertículos com terminação cega podem predispor a aprisionamento de corpo estranho, supercrescimento bacteriano, sangramento GI ou perfuração. Ductos vitelinos císticos podem ocorrer, com vazamento umbilical de conteúdo do ID, se houver um *ductus omphaloentericus* persistente. As fístulas arteriovenosas podem causar hemorragia do ID.

ASPECTOS CLÍNICOS DA DOENÇA DO INTESTINO DELGADO

Diarreia[303-305]

O sinal cardinal de disfunção do ID é a diarreia, que é um aumento significativo na frequência, na fluidez ou no volume das fezes, causado por aumento no teor de água e/ou sólidos nas fezes. No entanto, deve-se lembrar que doenças de outros órgãos também podem causar diarreia e que a ausência de diarreia reconhecível não exclui a possibilidade de doença do ID significativa; outros sinais são possíveis (ver Boxe 276.2).

A diarreia pode ser classificada de várias maneiras (Boxe 276.4), porém as categorias não são mutuamente exclusivas e permitem que o problema seja visto de diferentes perspectivas, facilitando a abordagem diagnóstica e a escolha do tratamento apropriado. Uma abordagem mecanicista ajuda a compreender o motivo do desenvolvimento de diarreia evidente. A maioria das doenças do ID tem um componente de diarreia osmótica, mas mecanismos mistos ocorrem mesmo em uma situação tão simples quanto a deficiência de lactase (Figura 276.3). A má absorção normalmente causa diarreia osmótica, mas a fermentação bacteriana de solutos não absorvidos pode complicar o quadro; o pH fecal muitas vezes é baixo graças à produção de

ácidos graxos voláteis e alguns produtos como ácidos graxos hidroxilados e ácidos biliares não conjugados, que causam secreção no cólon. Por esse motivo, sinais de diarreia do ID frequentemente acompanham uma doença prolongada. A diarreia por permeabilidade é decorrente de inflamação ou infiltração neoplásica, causando exsudação, e a diarreia secretora é causada por toxinas químicas ou bacterianas (Boxe 276.5).

Boxe 276.4 Esquemas de classificação para a diarreia

Anatômico
- Extraintestinal
- Do intestino delgado
- Do intestino grosso
- Difusa.

Causal
- Insuficiência pancreática exócrina, salmonelose, linfoma, entre outras.

Clínico
- Não fatal, leve, autolimitada
- Com perda de proteína
- Grave, potencialmente fatal
- Multissistêmica.

Etiológico
- Bacteriana
- Dietética
- Idiopática
- Neoplástica
- Parasitária
- Viral.

Mecanicista
- Dismotilidade
- Osmótica
- Secretora
- Permeabilidade (exsudativa)
- Mista.

Fisiopatológico
- Alérgica
- Bioquímica
- Infecciosa/inflamatória
- Neoplástica
- Vascular/linfática.

Temporal
- Aguda
- Crônica.

Boxe 276.5 Causas da diarreia secretora

- Enterotoxinas e endotoxinas bacterianas (p. ex., *Clostridium perfringens*, *Escherichia coli*, *Salmonella* spp.[a])
- Ácidos graxos hidroxilados da fermentação bacteriana
- Ácidos biliares não conjugados da fermentação bacteriana
- Infecção por *Giardia*
- Laxantes estimulantes (p. ex., óleo de rícino, dioctil sulfossuccinato de sódio, bisacodil)
- Glicosídeos cardíacos
- Neoplasias de captação e descarboxilação do precursor de amina (CDPA, excesso de polipeptídeos intestinais vasoativos, serotonina, prostaglandinas, substância P)
- Inflamação intestinal.

[a]N.T.: a diarreia secretora provocada por salmonela é, principalmente, consequência da inflamação decorrente do processo invasivo de mucosa relacionado com o patógeno.

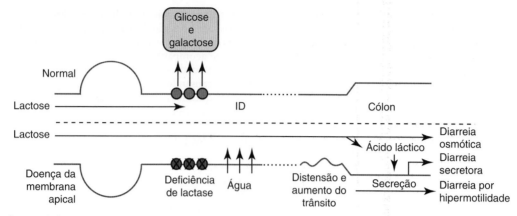

Figura 276.3 Deficiência de lactase. Representação esquemática dos mecanismos da diarreia causada pela deficiência de lactase. A ausência da enzima lactase na membrana apical leva a má digestão e má absorção, diarreia osmótica e trânsito mais rápido, em razão da distensão por água. A fermentação bacteriana de lactose não digerida em ácido láctico estimula a secreção do cólon.

Má absorção[306-309]

A deficiência na assimilação dos alimentos às vezes é classificada como uma falha primária de digestão (má digestão) ou uma falha primária de absorção (má absorção). No entanto, essa distinção é enganosa, pois a falta de absorção é uma consequência inevitável da falta de digestão. Prefere-se usar o termo "má absorção" para descrever a absorção defeituosa de um constituinte da dieta que resulta da interferência com o processamento digestivo e/ou absortivo dessa molécula. O local da anormalidade primária pode ser a região luminal, a mucosa ou as fases de transporte (Tabela 271.1). As manifestações clínicas da má absorção – ou seja, diarreia, perda de peso e alteração do apetite (polifagia, coprofagia, pica) – são, em grande parte, resultado da falta de absorção dos nutrientes e de sua perda nas fezes. Contudo, a capacidade de reserva do ID distal e cólon pode evitar a diarreia, mesmo com extensa má absorção e perda de peso. A polidipsia é uma manifestação incomum e peculiar do apetite excessivo: os animais muitas vezes são sistemicamente saudáveis e têm um apetite aumentado, mas perdem peso, a menos que uma neoplasia ou uma condição inflamatória grave esteja presente. Apenas quando o paciente estiver gravemente desnutrido ou desenvolver hipoproteinemia, ele parecerá doente.

Melena[310]

A melena é uma condição em que sangue escuro e oxidado está presente nas fezes, refletindo sangue engolido ou sangramento GI localizado ou generalizado proximal ao IG (Tabela 276.2; ver Capítulo 41). Estima-se que a perda de 350 a 500 mg/kg de hemoglobina no trato GI seja necessária para que a melena esteja visível. Como advertência, medicamentos com sulfato ferroso ou suspensões de bismuto (p. ex., Pepto-Bismol) também podem conferir cor escura às fezes. No hemograma, a presença de microcitose, principalmente com trombocitose, sugere deficiência de ferro secundária à perda crônica de sangue. No perfil bioquímico sérico, um aumento da proporção de ureia para creatinina no sangue (da digestão bacteriana do sangue) fornece evidências de suporte. Hipoproteinemia pode indicar perda de sangue ou EPP.

Enteropatia com perda de proteínas[289,290,311-315]

Quando a doença do ID é grave o suficiente para causar perda de proteína e, por consequência, o lúmen intestinal excede a síntese de proteínas plasmáticas, uma hipoproteinemia se desenvolve. Uma diarreia crônica associada a pan-hipoproteinemia geralmente requer biopsia intestinal para definir a causa da EPP (Tabela 276.3). Linfangiectasia alimentar, linfoma e DII são as três doenças subjacentes mais comuns, embora histoplasmose e pitiose devam ser consideradas em áreas endêmicas. Doenças não intestinais que causam ascite por meio de hipertensão portal em geral causam ascite antes da diarreia. A hipoproteinemia associada a doença GI é muito menos comum em gatos do que em cães e, quando ocorre, frequentemente está relacionada a linfoma GI; raramente resulta em ascite em gatos.

Os sinais clínicos associados à EPP incluem perda de peso, diarreia, vômito, edema periférico, ascite e derrame pleural. A perda de massa muscular é com frequência uma característica predominante, mas a diarreia não está invariavelmente presente, sobretudo na linfangiectasia e neoplasia intestinal focal, onde ela pode estar ausente. Os achados físicos podem incluir edema depressível, ascite, emagrecimento, intestinos espessados e melena. Tromboembolismo secundário à hipoproteinemia é uma característica de alguns casos de EPP, porque os pacientes afetados são hipercoaguláveis (ver Capítulo 197).

Borborigmos e flatulência[316]

Borborigmos são ruídos abdominais estrondosos causados pela propulsão de gás no estômago e através dos intestinos. O ar engolido e a fermentação bacteriana da ingesta são as principais causas de borborigmo e flatulência, resultando, muitas vezes, em um odor desagradável. Alimentar-se de uma dieta altamente digerível, com baixo teor de fibra (p. ex., queijo cottage e arroz em uma proporção 1:2), deixa pouco material no intestino para a fermentação bacteriana, e biscoitos de carvão podem beneficiar sintomaticamente em alguns casos. Se os borborigmos ou flatulência continuarem apesar da modificação da dieta ou adição de adsorventes, o animal pode ser excessivamente aerofágico ou ter má absorção, sobretudo se diarreia ou perda de peso também estiverem presentes. Investigações para uma doença do ID subjacente devem ser realizadas.

Perda de peso ou deficiência de crescimento

As causas gerais de perda de peso são a redução da ingestão de nutrientes, o aumento da perda de nutrientes ou o aumento do catabolismo (ver Capítulo 19). O histórico deve revelar se o tipo e a quantidade de dieta fornecida são adequados e se anorexia, disfagia ou vômito são causas potenciais. A perda de peso ou falta de crescimento acompanhada de diarreia muitas vezes é uma característica de má absorção, e a abordagem diagnóstica é a mesma da diarreia crônica. No entanto, a diarreia não acompanha invariavelmente a má absorção que causa perda de peso, pois a capacidade reserva de absorção do cólon pode remover o excesso de água das fezes.

CAPÍTULO 276 • Doenças do Intestino Delgado

Tabela 276.1 Mecanismos fisiopatológicos da má absorção.

MECANISMO	EXEMPLO
Fase luminal	
Dismotilidade	
Trânsito intestinal rápido	Hipertireoidismo
Hidrólise defeituosa do substrato	
Inativação enzimática	Hipersecreção gástrica
Falta de enzimas pancreáticas	Insuficiência pancreática exócrina
Liberação prejudicada de CCQ, secretina	Prejuízo da secreção pancreática decorrente de doença grave do ID
Má digestão de gorduras	
Secreção diminuída de sais biliares	Doença hepática colestática, obstrução biliar
Aumento da perda de sais biliares	Doença ileal
Desconjugação dos sais biliares	Supercrescimento bacteriano
Hidroxilação de ácidos graxos	Supercrescimento bacteriano
Má absorção da cobalamina	
Deficiência de fator intrínseco	Insuficiência pancreática exócrina
Deficiência no receptor da cobalamina	Deficiência hereditária seletiva de cobalamina (síndrome de Imerslund-Gräsbeck)
Competição por cobalamina	Supercrescimento bacteriano
Fase mucosa	
Deficiência enzimática da membrana apical	
Congênita	Trehalase congênita (gatos) Aminopeptidase N (cães da raça Beagle)
Adquirida	Deficiência relativa de lactase
Disfunções dos enterócitos	
Processamento deficiente dos enterócitos	Abetalipoproteinemia,* doença de inclusão das microvilosidades,* administração de dirlopatide
Redução na área de superfície	Atrofia das microvilosidades
Enterócitos imaturos	Aumento da renovação dos enterócitos
Inflamação da mucosa	Doença inflamatória intestinal
Fase de transporte	
Obstrução linfática	
Primária	Linfangiectasia
Secundária	Obstrução causada por neoplasia, infecção ou inflamação
Comprometimento vascular	
Vasculite	Infecção, imunomediada
Hipertensão portal	Hepatopatia, insuficiência cardíaca direita, tamponamento cardíaco

*Condição humana, ainda não relatada em cães ou gatos. *CCQ*, colecistoquinina; *ID*, intestino delgado.

Tabela 276.2 Causas de melena.

MECANISMO	FONTE
Doenças hemorrágicas	Trombocitopenia, trombocitopatia, deficiências fatoriais, CID
Deglutição de sangue	Oral, nasal, faríngea, esofágica ou pulmonar
Erosão/ulceração gastrointestinal	
Metabólica	Uremia, doença hepática
Inflamatória	Gastrite/úlcera, enterite, GH
Neoplásica	leiomioma, TEGI, adenocarcinoma, linfoma
Paraneoplásica	Mastocitose, hipergastrinemia (gastrinoma)
Vascular	Fístula AV, aneurisma, angiodisplasia
Isquemia	Choque hipovolêmico, hipoadrenocorticismo, trombose/infarto, reperfusão
Medicamentosa	Agentes anti-inflamatórios não esteroides e glicocorticoides
Objetos externos afiados	

AV, arteriovenosa; *CID*, coagulação intravascular disseminada; *GH*, gastrenterite hemorrágica; *TEGI*, tumor estromal gastrintestinal.

Tabela 276.3 Enteropatias com perda de proteínas.

CAUSAS	EXEMPLOS
Inflamação	Linfoplasmocítica, eosinofílica, granulomatosa
Linfangiectasia	Distúrbio linfático primário, hipertensão venosa (p. ex., insuficiência do coração direito, cirrose hepática)
Neoplasia	Linfoma
Infecção	Parvovirose, salmonelose, histoplasmose, ficomicose
Hemorragia gastrintestinal	GH, neoplasia, ulceração
Endoparasitas	*Giardia*, *Ancylostoma* spp.
Estrutural	Intussuscepção

GH, gastrenterite hemorrágica.

DIAGNÓSTICO DE DOENÇA DO INTESTINO DELGADO

Abordagem diagnóstica[317-322]

Diarreia

A maioria dos casos de diarreia é aguda, não fatal e autolimitante e requer apenas cuidados gerais de suporte, não um diagnóstico específico. No entanto, alguns casos precisam de diagnóstico e manejo, pois são potencialmente fatais e/ou infecciosos para outros animais, representando um risco zoonótico. Se hipovolemia ou desidratação clinicamente significativa estiver presente, os déficits de líquidos e eletrólitos devem ser abordados simultaneamente com o esforço de diagnóstico, mas a extensão das investigações necessárias é variável. Investigações são essenciais se a diarreia for hemorrágica, acompanhada por sinais sistêmicos, ou sem resposta a tratamento de suporte não específico. Por definição, a diarreia crônica não é autolimitante, e um diagnóstico etiológico geralmente é necessário para permitir o tratamento. Abordagens diagnósticas para diarreia aguda e crônica são discutidas no Capítulo 40 e descritas nas Figuras 276.4 e 276.5, respectivamente.

O objetivo da abordagem diagnóstica é eliminar doenças extraintestinais da lista de diferenciais e distinguir entre doença de ID e doença do IG (Tabela 276.4). O histórico (Boxe 276.6 e Capítulo 1), a suscetibilidade da raça e o exame físico (Tabela 276.5; ver Capítulo 2) são passos cruciais e, em alguns casos, suficientes para chegar a um diagnóstico. Um exame retal deve ser realizado para confirmar diarreia, identificar qualquer melena insuspeitada e obter amostras para exames citológicos retais e fecais.

As investigações preliminares também podem incluir coleta de dados básicos por meio de CBC, perfil bioquímico sérico, análise de urina e exame fecal. Elas podem identificar casos de hipoadrenocorticismo, mas uma proporção anormal de sódio para potássio sérico às vezes é observada na doença primária de ID, notavelmente na salmonelose e na tricuríase. O diagnóstico por imagem pode ser indicado, sobretudo se for suspeitada uma doença com a necessidade de intervenção cirúrgica pelo histórico e/ou achados do exame físico (ver "Distúrbios intestinais cirúrgicos", a seguir). Outras investigações em casos de doença diarreica crônica incluem exclusão de IPE, testes indiretos de função (p. ex., folato e cobalamina séricos), lesões intestinais (inibidor de alfa$_1$-protease [alfa$_1$-IP] fecal, calprotectina fecal) e, finalmente, inspeção direta do ID por endoscopia ou cirurgia com exame histológico de biopsias, mas estas raramente são necessários na doença aguda.

Melena[310,323-334]

A abordagem geral para melena é descartar diáteses hemorrágicas generalizadas, ingestão de sangue de outras lesões (p. ex., massas orais), toxicoses (AINE), e distúrbios metabólicos subjacentes (hipoadrenocorticismo) antes de buscar as causas GI primárias. A ultrassonografia (US) é particularmente útil para detectar massas GI e espessamento. A próxima etapa é a endoscopia para identificar sangramento. Uma enteroscopia e uma endoscopia de videocápsula podem ser usadas para localizar o sangramento mais distal, mas raramente são acessíveis. Se a fonte do sangramento GI ainda assim não for determinada, uma cintilografia ou angiografia com hemácias marcadas podem ser consideradas, mas, em última análise, a laparotomia exploratória pode ser indicada.

Enteropatia com perda de proteínas[289,290,312,314,335-338]

A identificação de uma EPP é baseada na descoberta de hipoalbuminemia. Normalmente, as concentrações séricas de albumina e globulina estão reduzidas em pacientes com EPP. No entanto, é uma exceção hiperglobulinemia com hipoalbuminemia, encontrada tanto na histoplasmose quanto na doença imunoproliferativa de ID da raça Basenji; ocasionalmente, também é localizada na DII grave e no linfoma alimentar. A EPP causadora de hipoalbuminemia substancial é rara em gatos, mas há raças de cães que parecem predispostas, como Basenji, Lundehund, Rottweiler, Wheaten Terrier de Pelo Macio, Yorkshire Terrier e Shar-pei. A raça levanta

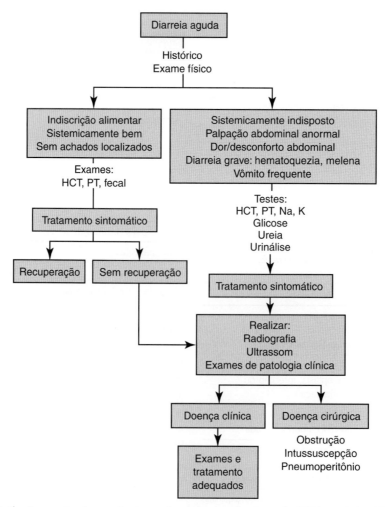

Figura 276.4 Algoritmo mostrando uma abordagem diagnóstica para diarreia aguda. *HCT*, hematócrito; *PT*, proteína total.

CAPÍTULO 276 • Doenças do Intestino Delgado

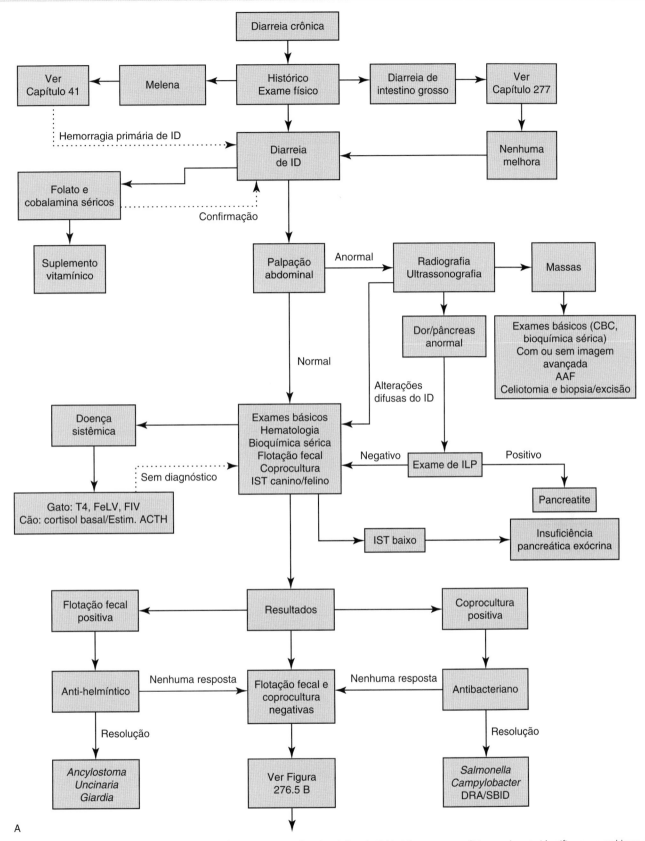

Figura 276.5 Algoritmos mostrando uma abordagem diagnóstica para diarreia crônica. **A.** O histórico e o exame físico geralmente identificam um problema de ID, mas a falha da terapia específica para um problema suspeito de IG também deve levar o clínico veterinário a considerar uma doença de ID. Concentrações séricas anormais de folato e cobalamina são uma indicação suplementar e conseguem prover mais evidências de doença ID. Um conjunto de dados básico pode fornecer evidências de doença sistêmica, levando à investigação de condições que não do ID, e em geral são indicados cortisol basal (ou teste de estimulação do ACTH) para cães e T4 sérico para gatos mais velhos. A palpação abdominal anormal é uma indicação para imagens abdominais, mas um hemograma e perfil do bioquímico sérico devem ser realizados antes de investigações mais invasivas. Imunorreatividade semelhante a tripsina (IST) provavelmente deve ser avaliada em todos os casos caninos que não apresentarem anormalidades na palpação abdominal, já que os sinais de insuficiência pancreática exócrina nem sempre são típicos e as concentrações séricas de folato/cobalamina podem estar alteradas. O exame fecal identifica parasitas GI e bactérias patogênicas, mas podem ser achados coincidentes.

Continua

1538 SEÇÃO 18 • Doença Gastrintestinal

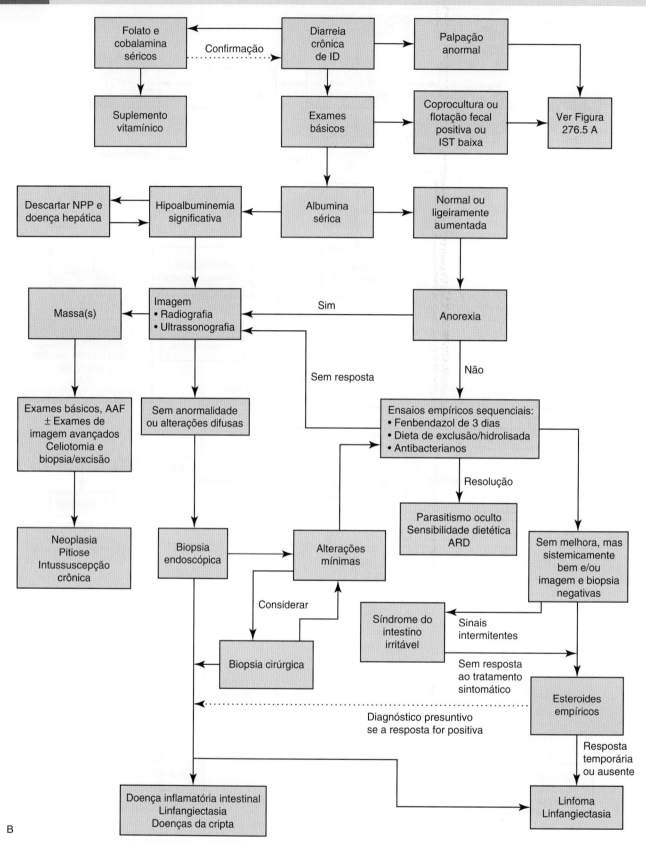

Figura 276.5. (Continuação) B. Investigações adicionais de casos com palpação abdominal normal dependem da concentração de albumina sérica e do apetite do paciente. Se a albumina não estiver substancialmente diminuída e se o paciente estiver bem sistemicamente e se alimentando, ensaios empíricos sequenciais com fenbendazol e uma dieta de exclusão ou hidrolisada e com antibacterianos, como o metronidazol, podem ser realizados antes de considerar a biopsia intestinal. Imagens e biopsia endoscópicas são indicadas se o paciente tiver evidências de enteropatia com perda de proteína ou estiver anoréxico. Se os resultados da biopsia forem normais, então pode ser considerada a biopsia cirúrgica ou devem ser iniciados os ensaios empíricos com glicocorticoides. *AAF*, aspirado com agulha fina; *CBC*, hemograma; *DRA*, diarreia responsiva a antibióticos; Estim. *ACTH*, teste de estimulação do hormônio adrenocorticotrófico; *FeLV*, vírus da leucemia felina; *FIV*, vírus da imunodeficiência felina; *ID*, intestino delgado; *ILP*, imunorreatividade da lipase pancreática; *IST*, imunorreatividade semelhante à tripsina; *NPP*, nefropatia com perda de proteína; *SBID*, supercrescimento bacteriano no intestino delgado.

Tabela 276.4 Sinais clínicos associados a doenças do intestino delgado e intestino grosso.

SINAIS	DOENÇA DE INTESTINO DELGADO	DOENÇA DE INTESTINO GROSSO
Fezes		
Volume de fezes	Grande	Pequeno
Muco	Raro	Comum
Sangue (se presente)	Melena	Sangue fresco
Gordura	Às vezes	Ausente
Cor	Variável	Normal
Alimentos não digeridos	Ocasionalmente	Ausentes
Defecação		
Tenesmo	Raro	Comum
Frequência	Duas a 3 vezes/dia	Mais de 3 vezes/dia
Urgência	Incomum	Comum
Outros sinais		
Vômito	Às vezes	Incomum
Gás	Às vezes	Ausente
Perda de peso	Comum	Rara

Tabela 276.5 Manifestações físicas em animais com sinais de distúrbio do intestino delgado.

MANIFESTAÇÕES	INTERPRETAÇÃO
Gerais	Descartar outra doença sistêmica
Orofaringe	
Membrana mucosa	Estado de hidratação, estado cardiovascular, anemia, icterícia
Língua	Corpo estranho linear
Região cervical	
Glândula tireoide	Nódulo na tireoide (hipertireoidismo)
Palpação abdominal	Efusões, massas, inchaço das alças intestinais, corpos estranhos, acúmulo anormal de alimento, dor associada, fezes, linfadenopatia, outras doenças sistêmicas
Ausculta abdominal	Íleo, borborigmo
Exame retal	
Digital	Massas, corpos estranhos, distúrbios hemostáticos, desidratação
Coleta de amostra de fezes	Análise laboratorial, identificação de melena
Raspagem da mucosa retal	Citologia
Exame cutâneo	
Pelagem em mau estado	Desnutrição
Prurido	Hipersensibilidade alimentar
Prurido facial	Hipersensibilidade alimentar
Prurido nos pés	Hipersensibilidade alimentar, infecção por *Uncinaria stenocephala* (migração larval)

Boxe 276.6 Informações do histórico úteis no diagnóstico de doenças do intestino delgado

Informação do paciente
- Idade
- Gênero
- Espécies e raça.

Histórico ambiental
- Interior *versus* exterior
- Vida livre
- Catador (*carniceiro*)
- Exposição a parasitas
- Contato com animais infectados
- Mudança recente de ambiente
- Área de doenças endêmicas.

Histórico médico
- Status de vacinação
- Status de vermifugação
- Cirurgia abdominal anterior
- Excisão prévia de tumor de mastócitos cutâneo
- Histórico de medicações.

Sinais clínicos
- Duração
- Frequência
- Gravidade
  - Apetite alterado
  - Presença de sangue
  - Perda de peso
- Progressão
  - Ordem de apresentação
  - Contínuo ou intermitente por natureza
  - Duração dos intervalos sem sinal
- Outros sinais (p. ex., vômito e ascite)
- Fatores que melhoram ou pioram os sinais (p. ex., tratamentos e dietas).

a suspeita em um cão hipoproteinêmico, mesmo que a diarreia esteja ausente, mas causas renais e hepáticas de hipoalbuminemia devem ser eliminadas pela dosagem de ácidos biliares séricos e perda de proteína urinária (ou seja, razão proteína:creatinina urinária), respectivamente, com a ressalva de que EPP e nefropatia com perda de proteína (NPP) simultâneas são observadas em Wheaten Terriers de Pelo Macio. Hipocolesterolemia e linfopenia são comuns na EPP, e hipocalcemia ionizada e hipomagnesemia podem ocorrer. Dosar o aumento do inibidor de alfa$_1$-IP fecal pode ser um teste sensível para EPP antes que uma hipoalbuminemia significativa se desenvolva.

As radiografias abdominais não são úteis para os pacientes com EPP e ascite, devido à perda de contraste na radiografia, mas a US pode revelar espessamento intestinal e/ou linfadenopatia mesentérica, bem como efusão abdominal. As radiografias torácicas podem mostrar derrame pleural, neoplasia metastática ou alterações consistentes com histoplasmose. Embora possam confirmar a presença de má absorção, os testes de função intestinal raramente fornecem um diagnóstico definitivo, mas a biopsia intestinal é mais útil. Uma vez que muitas causas intestinais de EPP são difusas, a endoscopia é a maneira mais segura para obter biopsias, porém a biopsia cirúrgica pode ser necessária para obter um diagnóstico definitivo do linfoma transmural e da linfangiectasia.

Exames laboratoriais

Exames básicos

As investigações preliminares incluem hemograma, perfil bioquímico sérico e urinálise.

Citologia retal

No final de um exame retal, esfrega-se o dedo enluvado em uma lâmina de microscópio e o esfregaço é corado. Embora o resultado frequentemente seja negativo ou, na melhor das hipóteses, mais representativo de uma doença de IG, um número elevado de neutrófilos pode ser sugestivo de etiologia bacteriana, indicando a necessidade de coprocultura. Elementos fúngicos também podem ser identificados. O teste é rápido e simples, mas em todos os casos são indicados testes confirmatórios.

Exames fecais

Os exames fecais são uma parte importante da investigação da doença de ID (ver Capítulo 81). Testes como a quantificação da excreção de gordura fecal são inadequados para a prática clínica, e a coprocultura às vezes tem valor questionável, mas a identificação de parasitas é importante.

Esfregaço direto

A coloração de esfregaços para grânulos de amido não digerido (iodo de Lugol), glóbulos de gordura (coloração de Sudan) e fibras musculares (coloração de Wright ou Diff Quik) pode indicar má absorção, mas os resultados são inespecíficos. A presença de elementos fúngicos e clostrídios esporulados é de significado incerto, mas a citologia retal pode ser útil para identificar inflamação neutrofílica associada. Montagens úmidas frescas não coradas podem ser usadas para observar trofozoítos móveis de protozoários. A produção de enterotoxina por *Clostridium perfringens* é uma causa potencial de diarreia; no entanto, a presença de muitos endosporos clostridiais (mais de 5 por campo em objetiva de imersão em óleo) em esfregaços corados com Diff-Quik não é mais considerada um indicador confiável, enquanto um ensaio fecal positivo para enterotoxina (ensaio imunoenzimático [ELISA] ou aglutinação passiva reversa de látex é mais provável de ser significativo.

Métodos de concentração fecal[339-345]

Os métodos de concentração fecal são muito efetivos para a detecção da maioria dos parasitas intestinais (Figura 276.6; ver Capítulo 81). O exame de três amostras fecais por flutuação com sulfato de zinco é recomendado para detectar oocistos de *Giardia*. Um esfregaço direto, a sedimentação ou a técnica de Baermann podem identificar larvas de *Strongyloides* spp.

Testes de antígenos[342,346-348]

Testes de coproantígenos em fezes podem ser usados para detectar infecções por cestódeos, trematódeos e nematódeos, mas os testes de antígenos são usados com maior frequência para detectar infecções por protozoários ou por vírus. Disponíveis comercialmente, os testes rápidos baseados em ELISA podem ser usados para detectar antígenos de *Giardia* (ver Capítulo 221) e parvovírus canino (ver Capítulo 225) nas fezes.

Imunofluorescência[348,349]

A marcação de esfregaços fecais com anticorpos imunofluorescentes é considerada um dos métodos mais sensíveis para detectar *Giardia* e *Cryptosporidium* (ver Capítulo 221).

Coprocultura de rotina[350,351]

A tentativa de cultivar todas as espécies bacterianas presentes em uma amostra fecal é de pouco valor, sobretudo porque a microbiota fecal não reflete necessariamente a do ID, e muitas

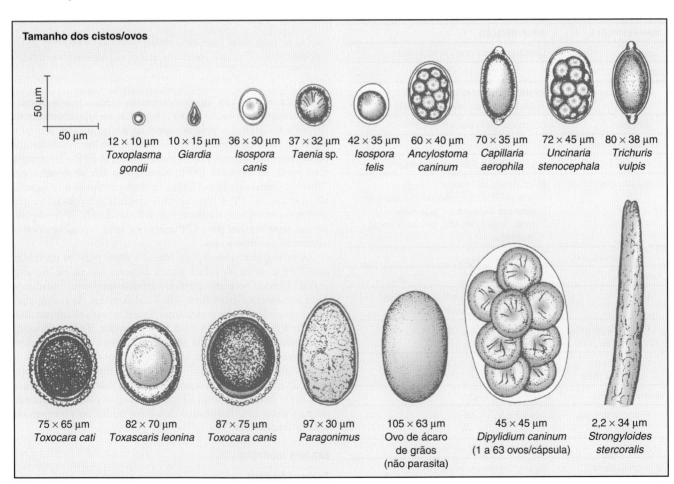

Figura 276.6 Flutuação fecal. Identificação de cistos de protozoários e ovos de parasitos que podem ser encontrados nas fezes de cães e gatos. (Cortesia de Hoechst-Roussel-Agri Vet Company, Somerville, Nova Jersey, EUA.)

espécies não são cultiváveis. No entanto, a identificação direcionada de patógenos potenciais pode ser útil. A coprocultura é indicada em animais com diarreia hemorrágica, febre, leucograma inflamatório ou neutrófilos na citologia retal. A identificação de *Salmonella* spp., *Campylobacter jejuni* e *Clostridioides difficile* é útil, embora seja importante interpretar um isolado positivo à luz do histórico clínico, pois esses microrganismos podem estar presentes nas fezes de animais clinicamente saudáveis. É possível cultivar as fezes para fungos, como *Histoplasma capsulatum*, mas o isolamento é difícil e lento.

Reação em cadeia da polimerase de material fecal[352-362]

Embora a reação em cadeia da polimerase (PCR, do inglês *polymerase chain reactions*) de material fecal possa ser difícil em razão da presença de inibidores da reação a partir do uso de iniciadores específicos e controles adequados, bactérias e parasitas podem ser identificados nas amostras fecais. A PCR é potencialmente mais sensível do que a cultura bacteriana, pois os microrganismos vivos não precisam estar presentes, além de ser possível identificar a espécie. No entanto, a PCR é mais frequentemente usada para classificar microrganismos após terem sido cultivados; *E. coli* pode ser cultivada a partir da maioria das amostras fecais, mas apenas certas cepas são patogênicas (ensaios de PCR são capazes de detectar genes associados a patogenicidade). A PCR é o método de escolha para o diagnóstico da infecção por *Tritrichomonas* em gatos (ver Capítulos 221 e 277).

Perfil molecular (molecular fingerprinting)[72,74,85,104,108,228,363,364]

Muitas bactérias intestinais não são cultiváveis *in vitro* e só podem ser identificadas por sequenciamento de genes do rRNA 16S bacteriano. Esse método é usado para observar o padrão da microbiota no líquido intestinal, nas biopsias e nas fezes de uma população e é de utilidade restrita para pacientes individuais.

Exame virológico[365-368]

A diarreia viral geralmente é aguda e autolimitante e não requer um diagnóstico positivo. A microscopia eletrônica pode ser usada para identificar partículas virais características, como rotavírus, coronavírus e parvovírus. Também estão disponíveis testes fecais de ELISA e PCR para parvovírus.

Sangue oculto[310,369-371]

Esse teste é usado para identificar sangramento intestinal de mucosa ulcerada e tumores, tanto benignos quanto malignos, antes que a melena seja vista; entretanto, o sangue oculto não ajuda a localizar a fonte. Infelizmente, a maioria dos ensaios testa de forma inespecífica para qualquer hemoglobina e, por ser muito sensível, reage a qualquer carne da dieta, bem como ao sangue do paciente. Portanto, a dieta deve excluir a carne ou ser hidrolisada por pelo menos 72 h para que um resultado positivo tenha algum significado. Os exames imunológicos são muito sensíveis e detectam hemoglobina em cães saudáveis.

Inibidor de alpha₁-protease[315,372-382]

Esse teste avalia a presença do inibidor de alfa₁-IP nas fezes. A alfa₁-IP é uma proteína sérica endógena que ocorre naturalmente e é resistente à degradação bacteriana no lúmen intestinal. Parece ter valor para o diagnóstico da EPP, pois correlaciona-se ao histórico de testes de excreção fecal de albumina radioativa marcada com ^{51}Cr (cromo). Aparentemente, ela é um marcador mais sensível para a detecção de doença precoce do que a medição da albumina sérica. Para melhorar a precisão do diagnóstico o ensaio ser válido, devem ser avaliadas três amostras fecais frescas, coletadas após a defecação voluntária, porque a abrasão da parede do cólon durante a evacuação digitalmente induzida é suficiente para elevar as concentrações fecais de alfa₁-IP.

Calprotectina fecal[383-389]

O ensaio da calprotectina fecal é um marcador comprovado de inflamação intestinal na DII humana, pois a molécula identificada é liberada com atividade da elastase de neutrófilos. Um ensaio específico para cães foi desenvolvido, e concentrações fecais aumentadas tendem a se correlacionar à inflamação intestinal e ao grau de alterações histológicas, mas não necessariamente aos sinais clínicos.

3-Bromotirosina e N-metil histamina[390-392]

A molécula de 3-bromotirosina (3-BrY) é um produto estável da peroxidase de eosinófilos, e sua concentração sérica serve como um marcador de ativação de eosinófilos. No entanto, estudos indicam que ela pode estar aumentada em qualquer forma de DII, e não apenas na enterite eosinofílica. As concentrações urinária e fecal de N-metil-histamina são marcadores fracos de ativação de mastócitos ou de atividade clínica da doença em cães com enteropatias crônicas.

Concentrações séricas de folato e cobalamina[52,234,237-239,242,377,393-410]

Os ensaios de concentrações séricas de folato e de cobalamina geralmente são realizados na mesma amostra de soro coletada para o teste de IST. Esse ensaio tem valor limitado no diagnóstico de doenças específicas do ID e não é recomendado para diagnosticar supercrescimento bacteriano. As concentrações subnormais de folato e cobalamina são marcadores primários de doença GI (ver Figura 276.2), mas também são indicadores da necessidade de suplementação. A hipercobalaminemia não tem significado em cães ou gatos com doença GI e pode ser decorrente da suplementação, mas tem sido associada a doenças hepáticas e neoplásicas em gatos.

Testes indiretos especiais[411-414]

Em casos de má absorção, a biopsia intestinal geralmente é necessária para obter um diagnóstico definitivo. No entanto, a IPE deve ser descartada antes da biopsia, porque os sinais de má absorção são inespecíficos e não permitem a diferenciação da causa. Assim, a medição da IST deve ser realizada em todos os casos (ver Capítulo 292). Também é sabido que metade das biopsias são consideradas normais pela microscopia óptica. Portanto, uma série de testes indiretos pode ser realizada, geralmente antes da biopsia, para avaliar lesões intestinais, permeabilidade alterada e disfunção, embora sua sensibilidade e especificidade limitem sua utilidade.

Testes de absorção intestinal[415-419]

Testes de função intestinal que avaliam a absorção mediada de vários substratos – como lactose, glicose, amido, triglicerídeos e vitamina A – não são mais realizados, em razão da falta de sensibilidade e especificidade. Até mesmo o teste da D-xilose foi abandonado, pois é muito pouco sensível em cães e não discriminatório em gatos. A absorção diferencial de dois açúcares – xilose/3-O-metil-D-glicose – elimina os efeitos não mucosos que prejudicam o teste de xilose, mas esse ensaio não entrou na prática de rotina.

Permeabilidade intestinal[266,416,420-449]

A permeabilidade intestinal é um índice de integridade da mucosa e é avaliada pela determinação da captação não mediada de marcadores não digeríveis e não metabolizáveis no plasma e/ou na urina. A sonda de permeabilidade com ácido etileno diamino tetra-acético marcado com ^{51}cromo (^{51}Cr-EDTA) foi usada em estudos originais, mas a segurança de seu uso é limitada por ser um emissor gama. O teste lactulose/ramnose tornou-se o teste-padrão de permeabilidade do ID. Recentemente, o iohexol tem se mostrado um marcador útil, porque é seguro e seu ensaio está disponível comercialmente. Na DII, há reduções na E-caderina e na alfacatenina, essenciais para a estrutura

SEÇÃO 18 • Doença Gastrintestinal

e a função das junções oclusivas. Consequentemente, a permeabilidade intestinal é aumentada pela atrofia das vilosidades, pelo dano epitelial ou por ambos. Os AINE também aumentam a permeabilidade intestinal

Testes para enteropatia com perda de proteínas[315,450,451]
Historicamente, a perda de proteína intestinal era detectada medindo a perda fecal de moléculas radiomarcadas, como albumina marcada com ^{51}Cr e ceruloplasmina marcada com ^{67}Cu. Contudo, esses testes são desagradáveis para o paciente e potencialmente perigosos; portanto, foram descartados, embora continuem a ser o padrão pelo qual outros testes, como alfa$_1$-IP fecal, são avaliados.

Testes de respiração[405,452-467]
Os testes de respiração são usados para avaliar o metabolismo bacteriano no trato GI. As bactérias sintetizam um gás, que é absorvido e excretado na respiração. Testes de hidrogênio respiratório têm sido usados mais amplamente, porque as células de mamíferos não podem produzir hidrogênio; portanto, qualquer detecção deve ser de origem bacteriana. Esses testes podem avaliar potencialmente a má absorção de carboidratos, a colonização bacteriana do ID e o tempo de trânsito orocecal, mas não são amplamente usados.

Sais biliares não conjugados[468-472]
A hipótese por trás do teste de ácidos biliares não conjugados séricos (ABNS) é de que algumas espécies de bactérias do ID podem desconjugar os ácidos biliares, que são então absorvidos passivamente pelo ID e não passam por reciclagem êntero-hepática. Portanto, em teoria, aumentos na atividade bacteriana no ID podem resultar em um aumento nos ABNS. Contudo, os resultados não se correlacionam com o diagnóstico – em parte porque há um aumento pós-prandial significativo nos ABNS em cães sadios –, e o teste não é mais recomendado.

Testes diversos de atividade bacteriana[460,472-479]
Vários testes foram planejados para detectar a atividade metabólica bacteriana intestinal e o supercrescimento bacteriano ou para avaliar o tempo de trânsito oro cecal. Entre eles estão o teste do nitroso-naftol, a excreção urinária de índico, o D-lactato sérico e a liberação bacteriana de sulfapiridina da sulfassalazina ou do ácido para-aminobenzoico (PABA) de um conjugado de sal biliar (PABA-UDCA). A avaliação dos gases voláteis emitidos pelas fezes pode fornecer um perfil característico de infecções específicas, porém nenhum desses testes é amplamente utilizado em animais de companhia.

Avaliação indireta da motilidade intestinal[458,460,479-491]
O tempo de trânsito intestinal pode ser avaliado diretamente por estudos de bário com e sem alimentos, US (incluindo Doppler de onda pulsada) e cintilografia. O registro da atividade mioelétrica *in vivo* não é praticado na rotina clínica, embora a pressão peristáltica possa ser medida com a cápsula SMART. As avaliações indiretas da motilidade intestinal incluem o hidrogênio respiratório após a administração de carboidratos e os marcadores visuais (corante vermelho carmim, óxido crômico) ou químicos (sulfassalazina, paracetamol, nitrofurantoína, PABA-UDCA) VO. Os resultados são variáveis, e, muitas vezes, as metodologias não se correlacionam bem. Muitos são tecnicamente difíceis, e a composição da dieta do teste e o estresse afetam as taxas de trânsito tanto quanto as doenças.

Diagnóstico por imagem[492-496]
Historicamente, a imagem do trato intestinal era limitada a radiografias simples e contrastadas, mas agora é complementada por US e endoscopia flexível. A cintilografia, a tomografia computadorizada (TC) e a ressonância magnética (RM) estão sendo mais adotadas, e a "endoscopia virtual" por TC helicoidal está se tornando disponível.

Radiografia simples[483,497-503]
Radiografias simples para avaliação são mais úteis na investigação de vômitos primários, diarreia associada a vômito, evidência de dor abdominal e anormalidades palpáveis. O rendimento do diagnóstico é melhorado se as duas incidências laterais forem obtidas, além da incidência ortogonal, embora uma única radiografia lateral possa ser suficiente se for combinada à US. Geralmente, o objetivo é a detecção de um distúrbio cirúrgico agudo (corpos estranhos, gás peritoneal livre, deslocamento intestinal, massas, obstruções), uma diminuição dos detalhes da serosa e um íleo.

Íleo é uma dilatação anormal de um segmento imóvel do intestino, e o diagnóstico diferencial depende se é localizado ou generalizado e se um acúmulo de gás ou líquido está presente (Boxe 276.7). A interpretação deve ser cautelosa se o paciente foi tratado com medicamentos que podem afetar o trato GI. Nem sempre as comparações do grau de dilatação intestinal com marcos ósseos para determinar se há obstrução são úteis, e a utilidade de radiografias simples na má absorção é mínima, especialmente se ascite estiver presente, já que todos os detalhes são obscurecidos por líquidos.

Radiografia de contraste
Desde a introdução da US abdominal e da endoscopia, os estudos radiográficos de contraste tiveram seu valor limitado na avaliação da doença de ID, mas permanecem úteis para a doença gastresofágica (ver Capítulo 273).

Exames de acompanhamento.[504-506] Estudos usando suspensões microfinas de bário podem identificar úlceras e detalhes irregulares da mucosa e confirmar a presença de corpos estranhos radioluscentes, mas são insensíveis para massas murais e obstruções parciais e raramente fornecem mais informações do que radiografias simples de boa qualidade. A administração de bário pode atrasar a endoscopia por pelo menos 24 horas. Se houver suspeita de perfuração, um contraste à base de iodo deve ser usado. A enteróclise (deposição de contraste diretamente no estômago ou no intestino por meio de intubação orogástrica ou orointestinal, para distensão ideal) fornece mais informações, mas é tecnicamente exigente e não é adotada. Embora os estudos de contraste permitam a avaliação da taxa de trânsito intestinal do agente de contraste, o resultado não é fisiológico e não se correlaciona intimamente com o movimento da ingesta avaliado pelo padrão-ouro da cintilografia. Além disso, a evidência de dismotilidade não fornece informações etiológicas.

Boxe 276.7 Diagnóstico diferencial do íleo adinâmico

Íleo gasoso
- Generalizado
  - Aerofagia
  - Enterite
  - Peritonite generalizada
  - Fármacos paralisantes de musculatura lisa (p. ex., atropina)
- Localizado
  - Interrupção do suprimento arterial mesentérico
  - Obstrução intestinal em estágio inicial
  - Peritonite localizada (p. ex., pancreatite).

Íleo com líquido
- Generalizado
  - Enterite
  - Neoplasia intestinal difusa
- Localizado
  - Corpo estranho
  - Intussuscepção ou outra obstrução mecânica (p. ex., encarceramento)
  - Tumor causando obstrução.

Esferas de polietileno impregnadas com bário[491,507-510]

As esferas de polietileno impregnadas com bário (EPIB) são marcadores radiopacos de fase sólida que fornecem informações sobre o esvaziamento gástrico, o trânsito intestinal e os distúrbios obstrutivos. Uma vez que o tempo de trânsito das EPIB é altamente variável, seu uso para estudos de trânsito é limitado, e elas são mais úteis na detecção de obstruções parciais.

Ultrassonografia[494,511-562]

O exame de US abdominal do ID é agora uma parte rotineira da investigação de doenças (ver Capítulos 88 e 89), embora sua utilidade diagnóstica na diarreia crônica tenha sido questionada. Um exame convencional pode detectar perda de camadas da parede do ID, ulceração, heterogeneidade e estriações da mucosa, evidências de fibrose, peristaltismo, íleo, conteúdo luminal e corpos estranhos, além de ser usado para medir a espessura da parede do ID. A US tem maior sensibilidade do que a radiografia e excelente especificidade para a detecção de lesões, com intussuscepções, massas, corpos estranhos radiopacos e radioluscentes, espessamento da parede intestinal e linfadenopatia em enteropatias crônicas inflamatórias, linfáticas e neoplásicas (Figura 276.7). Até mesmo as placas de Peyer e locais de cirurgia intestinal anterior podem ser identificados com um equipamento adequado e um operador experiente. O desenvolvimento da US endoscópica agora permite que a parede da mucosa e as vísceras adjacentes sejam examinadas com ainda mais detalhes.

Valores para a espessura normal da parede do ID são relatados para cães e gatos; a espessura diminui de 5 a 6 mm proximalmente para 4 a 5 mm distalmente, mas há variações de acordo com o tamanho do corpo, e paredes mais espessas são observadas em cães maiores. As intussuscepções em geral são reconhecidas como múltiplos anéis concêntricos no plano transversal e como um segmento espesso de múltiplas camadas no longitudinal. A alteração da aparência ultrassonográfica normal de cinco camadas (superfície da mucosa, mucosa, submucosa, muscular e serosa) é típica de neoplasia, enquanto o espessamento da parede também pode resultar de outros distúrbios infiltrativos e edema, embora a musculatura espessada tenha sido associada a linfoma em gatos. A heterogeneidade da mucosa é uma possível indicação de inflamação ou de abscesso de cripta. Estriações refletem dilatação linfática; a administração de óleo de milho antes do exame pode melhorar sua identificação, embora a especificidade do achado seja reduzida. A US de alta frequência pode diferenciar agregados linfoides da mucosa. A aspiração de massas ou paredes grosseiramente espessadas com agulha fina guiada por US para exame citológico é possível, e a biopsia por agulha é uma opção para lesões maiores.

Endoscopia[325,326,331,480,563-586]

A endoscopia permite a visualização da mucosa do ID e a coleta de várias amostras de tecido sem a necessidade de cirurgia invasiva, nem o risco de biopsia cirúrgica; complicações de bacteriemia ou perfuração são raras. Um equipamento endoscópico de ótima qualidade, a manutenção adequada e um operador experiente são mais importantes do que a manipulação farmacológica para conseguir uma intubação bem-sucedida do ID (ver Capítulos 83 e 113). O ID proximal é visualizado durante a gastroduodenoscopia (Vídeo 276.1), e o íleo pode ser amostrado passando o endoscópio de modo retrógrado através da válvula ileocólica durante uma colonoscopia. Portanto, apenas a porção média do jejuno não é examinada satisfatoriamente por endoscopia de rotina. No entanto, dado que a maioria dos casos de má absorção envolve doença difusa, essa limitação pode não ser significativa, embora a discordância entre os achados de biopsias duodenais e ileais pareadas signifique que o ideal é ambos os locais serem amostrados.

Atualmente, a endoscopia flexível é o método diagnóstico-padrão, com tecnologias emergentes que incluem endoscopia de cápsula, enteroscopia, endoscopia de balão duplo e endomicroscopia confocal. A enteroscopia usa um endoscópio muito mais longo e fino (com ou sem um guia) e/ou balões de avanço; ela permite o exame da maior parte do jejuno, assim como uma cápsula de videoendoscopia que passa da boca ao ânus e transmite imagens por telemetria. A cápsula SMART coleta dados fisiológicos (pH, pressão) por telemetria, mas sem imagens, enquanto a endomicroscopia confocal avalia a morfologia celular do ID e o potencial para detecção precoce de displasia epitelial e neoplasia.

Achados anormais no exame endoscópico macroscópico incluem granulação e friabilidade da mucosa, erosões e úlceras, alimentos retidos, lesões de massa e hiperemia/eritema (Figura 276.8). Um exsudato branco leitoso e/ou vasos linfáticos dilatados são sugestivos de linfangiectasia, e a presença de parasitas intraluminais pode ser diagnosticada em alguns casos (Vídeo 276.2), mas a identificação de nematoides geralmente é um achado acidental. Um sistema de pontuação endoscópica qualitativa simples para DII foi desenvolvido (Tabela 276.6). No entanto, nenhuma dessas características é patognomônica para doenças específicas, e os achados brutos frequentemente não se correlacionam com os resultados histopatológicos.

Suco duodenal[103,469,587-591]

O suco duodenal pode ser coletado durante a duodenoscopia, através de um tubo estéril de polietileno passado pelo canal de biopsia, ou por aspiração com agulha, através da parede intestinal na laparotomia. No entanto, pode ser difícil coletar amostra suficiente sem contaminação por sangue e tecido. A amostra pode ser examinada para trofozoítos de *Giardia*, embora isso não tenha se mostrado confiável no diagnóstico. Alternativamente, podem ser realizadas culturas quantitativas e qualitativas para microrganismos aeróbios e anaeróbios, consideradas o padrão-ouro para o diagnóstico de supercrescimento bacteriano, mas há grandes problemas de interpretação, e os resultados não ajudam na tomada de decisão para casos de doença GI. Portanto, a cultura bacteriana de rotina do suco duodenal não é recomendada.

Biopsia intestinal[565,577,592-608]

Na maioria dos casos de diarreia aguda, um diagnóstico de tecido não é necessário, e a biopsia intestinal raramente é realizada. No entanto, na diarreia crônica, um diagnóstico definitivo muitas vezes depende do exame histológico do tecido intestinal, ainda que haja grandes limitações. As amostras de biopsia são coletadas endoscópica ou cirurgicamente, ou seja, laparotomia ou laparoscopia.

Na laparotomia, biopsias de espessura total em geral são coletadas de pelo menos três locais: o duodeno, o jejuno e o íleo. No entanto, o risco de deiscência após a biopsia cirúrgica pode ser substancial, especialmente se o paciente estiver desnutrido e/ou hipoproteinêmico, se o tecido for neoplásico ou se o cirurgião for inexperiente. A administração de plasma reduz os efeitos oncóticos da hipoproteinemia, mas é apenas transitório e só vale a pena durante o período perioperatório, já que o suporte oncótico não ajuda na cicatrização de feridas.

O risco reduzido da biopsia endoscópica em comparação com a cirúrgica é equilibrado por uma série de desvantagens, e o tutor deve sempre ser avisado de que uma biopsia cirúrgica pode, em última instância, ser necessária para o diagnóstico definitivo. O duodeno e, se possível, o jejuno proximal são biopsiados rotineiramente, e as biopsias ileais podem ser obtidas por colonoscopia. Realizar biopsia endoscópica antes de um procedimento cirúrgico é a melhor conduta, a menos que haja evidências de que a doença está além do alcance do endoscópio. A opção cirúrgica é preferida se há qualquer possibilidade de existir doença extraintestinal ou lesões intestinais focais. O tamanho e a qualidade das biopsias endoscópicas dependem não apenas do equipamento disponível, mas também da pressão exercida pela pinça, que depende, em parte, de um operador experiente e do processamento das biopsias. As biopsias sempre ser feitas, mesmo na ausência de anormalidades graves, porque alterações microscópicas podem estar presentes. Várias amostras (6 ou mais) devem ser coletadas, porque o tamanho dos espécimes, os artefatos de esmagamento e a fragmentação podem dificultar a interpretação (Figura 276.9).

1544 SEÇÃO 18 • Doença Gastrintestinal

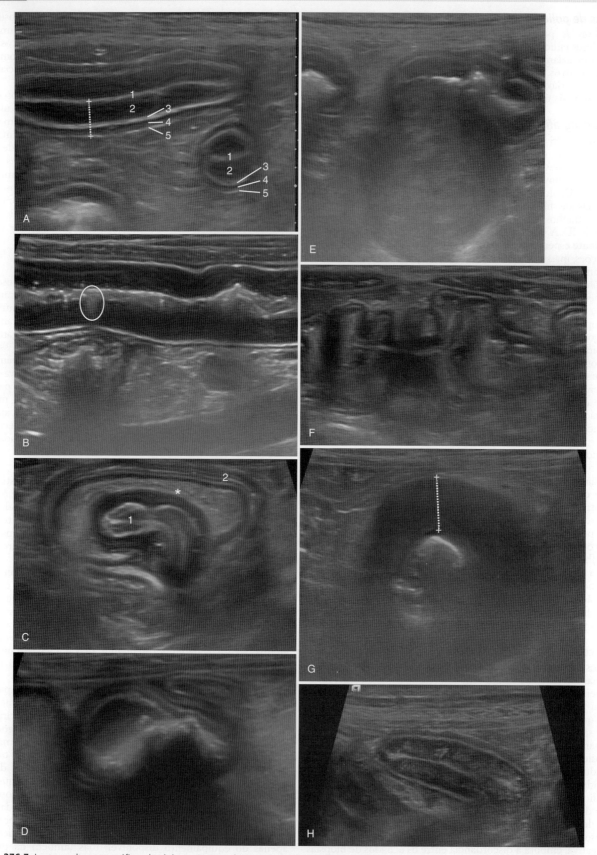

Figura 276.7 Imagens ultrassonográficas do abdome. **A.** Estratificação normal (lúmen [branco; *1*]; mucosa [preta; *2*]; submucosa [branca; *3*]; muscular [preto; *4*]; serosa [branca; *5*]) de alças do jejuno nas seções longitudinal e transversal em um cão. **B.** Seção longitudinal do duodeno canino com camadas normais e uma placa de Peyer atravessando a mucosa (*circulado*); note que o duodeno é mais reto e tem uma parede mais espessa que o jejuno. **C.** Uma intussuscepção com a estrutura clássica de parede dupla; o *intussusceptum* (*1*) é circundado por ingesta (*asterisco*) no *intussuscipiens* (*2*). **D.** Um corpo estranho intestinal com sombra acústica. **E.** Uma lesão em massa excêntrica, passível de aspirados com agulha fina ou biopsia *Tru-Cut*. **F.** Um corpo estranho linear com plicatura das alças intestinais. **G.** Parede intestinal espessada com perda de camadas causada por um linfoma. **H.** Manchas e estrias heterogêneas e hiperecoicas na mucosa de um cão com linfangiectasia (ver Figura 276.8 H). (Cortesia de Chris Warren-Smith, *Langford Veterinary Services.*)

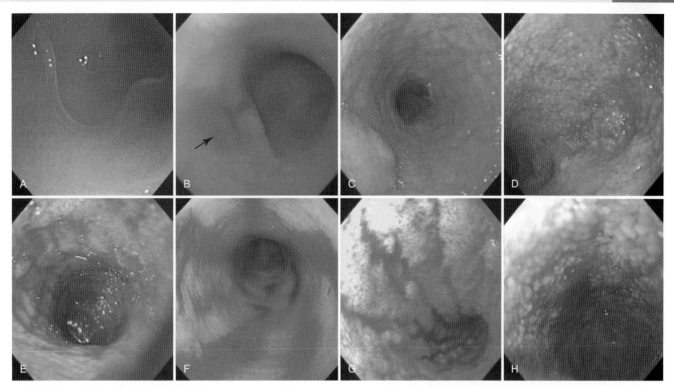

Figura 276.8 Exemplos de lesões duodenais endoscópicas. **A.** Achado incidental de um verme *Toxocara* isolado no duodeno de um gato. **B.** Úlcera duodenal proximal (*seta*) em um gato com enterite linfoplasmocitária apresentada devido à hematêmese. **C.** Doença inflamatória intestinal leve: enterite linfoplasmocitária; observe a irregularidade e a papila duodenal principal em aproximadamente 7 horas. **D.** Doença intestinal inflamatória grave: enterite linfoplasmocitária; observe a granulação marcante, envolvendo inclusive as placas de Peyer. **E.** Abscedação acentuada das criptas associada à enteropatia com perda de proteínas em um Chihuahua. **F.** Doença inflamatória intestinal: sangramento associado a enterite eosinofílica. **G.** Doença inflamatória intestinal grave: enterite eosinofílica. **H.** Linfangiectasia; observe os múltiplos lácteos dilatados contendo linfa branca. (**B.** Cortesia de Natasha Hetzel. **E.** Cortesia Jenny Reeve.) (*Esta figura se encontra reproduzida em cores no Encarte.*)

Tabela 276.6 Avaliação quantitativa do aspecto endoscópico da mucosa.

APARÊNCIA	PONTUAÇÃO	DESCRIÇÃO
Friabilidade	0	Ausente
	1	Sangramento leve ao toque
	2	Sangramento nítido ao toque
Granulação	0	Textura normal
	1	Textura aumentada
	2	Textura nitidamente aumentada
Erosões	0	Ausente
	1	Somente algumas erosões
	2	Erosões difusas
Dilatação linfática	0	Ausente
	1	Focos brancos – focais ou multifocais
	2	Focos brancos difusos

Escore máximo da enteroscopia = 8. Adaptada de Slovak JE, Wang C, Sun Y, et al. Development and validation of an endoscopic activity score for canine inflammatory bowel disease. *Vet J* 203:290-295, 2015.

Exame das biopsias[604,609-616]

Histopatologia. Embora a avaliação histopatológica de biopsias intestinais continue sendo o suposto padrão-ouro para o diagnóstico da doença intestinal, ela tem limitações marcantes. Vários espécimes de biopsia podem ser normais à microscopia ótica, o que sugere que muitas doenças têm um aspecto funcional, em vez de uma causa morfológica (Boxe 276.8) ou que problemas ocorreram na amostragem ou na interpretação. Muitas vezes, não há concordância entre histopatologistas, especialmente ao examinar biopsias endoscópicas, que necessitam de uma abordagem padronizada. Em um estudo, alguns histopatologistas fizeram o diagnóstico de linfoma após avaliarem tecidos de cães saudáveis, e houve apenas uma concordância razoável entre 5 patologistas independentes em cerca de metade das amostras examinadas.

Um esquema de pontuação histopatológica e critérios foram sugeridos pelo grupo de padronização GI da Associação Mundial de Veterinários de Pequenos Animais (AMVPA, do inglês *World Small Animal Veterinary Association*) como um meio de estabelecer a concordância. No entanto, os membros do grupo também mostraram que a experiência do endoscopista, a qualidade e o número de biopsias e a qualidade do processamento e coloração podem influenciar a confiabilidade da interpretação histológica. Como esperado, quanto melhor for a qualidade das biopsias, menos fragmentos são necessários para detectar com segurança mudanças arquitetônicas (ou seja, tamanho, profundidade e integridade); por outro lado, mais espécimes são necessários para identificar lesões mais profundas (criptas). As biopsias ileais são mais propensas a mostrar alterações histopatológicas do que as duodenais. Portanto, o clínico deve sempre interpretar os resultados da biopsia endoscópica com cautela à luz da apresentação clínica; resultados devem ser questionados se o diagnóstico do tecido não se enquadrar no quadro clínico ou se a resposta à terapia aparentemente apropriada for fraca. Em alguns casos, pode ser necessário repetir a biopsia (p. ex., por laparotomia exploratória).

Citologia.[617-620] Um exame citológico de preparações de esmagamento e esfregaço de biopsia endoscópica ou as escovações de mucosa são apenas adjuvantes ao exame histopatológico. Esfregaços de impressão mostram a melhor correlação entre os achados histológicos e são mais úteis para massas neoplásicas.

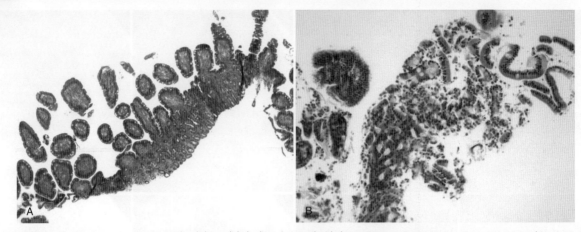

Figura 276.9 Biopsia endoscópica. **A.** Biopsia duodenal de qualidade diagnóstica; vilosidades e criptas estão presentes na amostra, mas a biopsia, normalmente, não é mais profunda do que a mucosa muscular. **B.** Biopsia endoscópica de má qualidade; o tecido está traumatizado e rompido; portanto, não é adequado para fazer um diagnóstico. (Reproduzida, com autorização, de Hall E, Williams D, Simpson J, editors: BSAVA Manual of Canine and Feline Gastroenterology, 2 ed., Quedgely, Gloucester, England, 2005, BSAVA Publications.)

Boxe 276.8 Causas de diarreia crônica cujos resultados de biopsias do intestino delgado podem ser normais*

- DRA, SBID
- Doença da membrana apical (p. ex., hipolactasia)
- Indiscrição alimentar
- Intolerância alimentar
- Esclerose intestinal (se as biopsias não forem de espessura total)
- Distúrbio de motilidade/síndrome do intestino irritável
- Doença da mucosa irregular não coletada
- Diarreia toxigênica/secretora
- Hipersensibilidade do tipo I ao alimento (se o cachorro passar fome antes da biopsia)
- IPE ou doença do cólon ou sistêmica não diagnosticada.

*A detecção de anormalidades histológicas depende do tamanho e da qualidade da biopsia, da qualidade do processamento e da experiência do patologista.
DRA, diarreia responsiva a antibióticos; IPE, insuficiência pancreática exócrina; SBID, supercrescimento bacteriano no intestino delgado.

Tabela 276.7 Causas da diarreia aguda.

CAUSAS	EXEMPLOS
Anatômica	Intussuscepção
Dietética	Hipersensibilidade (alergia), intolerância, dieta repentina mudança, intoxicação alimentar (má qualidade, alimentos/bacterianos)
Infecciosas	
Bacterianas	Salmonella, Campylobacter jejuni, Clostridium spp. (?) e Escherichia coli (?)
Parasitárias*	
Helmintos	Ancylostoma caninum, Trichuris vulpis
Protozoários	Coccidia, Giardia spp., Tritrichomonas foetus
Virais	
Leve	Adenovírus, coronavírus, norovírus, rotavírus
Grave	Podem ou não estar relacionadas ao FeLV/FIV
Metabólica	Hipoadrenocorticismo
Tóxica	Alimentos ou outras fontes
Pancreática	Pancreatite aguda

*Muitas vezes começam de forma aguda, mas tornam-se crônicas se não forem tratadas. FeLV, vírus da leucemia felina; FIV, vírus da imunodeficiência felina.

Exames alternativos.[144,621-635] Outros exames de biopsia disponíveis incluem: microscopia eletrônica; ensaio bioquímico de enzimas da membrana apical com fracionamento subcelular; caracterização imunocitoquímica de células B, T e seus subconjuntos (p. ex., células CD4 e CD8); expressão de MHC por imuno-histoquímica e citometria de fluxo; expressão de mRNA de citocinas; e avaliação da clonalidade das células T. Estas são, em grande parte, ferramentas de pesquisa. Hibridização fluorescente in situ (FISH) permite a identificação de microrganismos nos tecidos e seu arranjo espacial.

DOENÇA AGUDA DO INTESTINO DELGADO

Diagnóstico[320,636-639]

As potenciais causas de diarreia aguda estão listadas na Tabela 276.7; porém, se é buscado um diagnóstico definitivo ou é instituída uma terapia empírica de suporte, trata-se de um julgamento clínico e às vezes econômico. Pacientes que estão ativos, alertas e não desidratados podem não exigir mais investigação, porque os sinais geralmente são autolimitantes.

A abordagem diagnóstica da diarreia aguda é discutida no Capítulo 40 e resumida na Figura 276.4. Causas não intestinais, como pancreatite ou hipoadrenocorticismo, devem ser descartadas antes de focar no ID. A investigação adicional é indicada se o paciente estiver entorpecido ou deprimido, febril, desidratado, taquicárdico ou bradicárdico; se apresentar desconforto abdominal, melena, fezes mucoides com sangue ou vômitos frequentes; ou se tiver anormalidades físicas óbvias que localizam o problema no ID, como massas intestinais, espessamento e plicatura. O diagnóstico por imagem (Figura 276.10), uma biopsia não invasiva ou uma cirurgia podem definir a causa. As anormalidades sistêmicas também podem ser definidas a partir de um conjunto de exames básicos e outros testes ou na ausência de resposta do animal a uma terapia geral não específica.

Tratamento da diarreia aguda[640-644]

O manejo inicial da diarreia aguda é inespecífico, de suporte, e escolhido com base nos achados clínicos, especialmente a presença de desidratação, enquanto os resultados dos exames iniciais e adicionais estiverem pendentes. A administração de antieméticos é indicada se o paciente estiver vomitando e se obstrução intestinal tiver sido descartada. É importante que o paciente seja reavaliado regularmente para monitorar a resposta à terapia e detectar quaisquer novos sinais que causem preocupação.

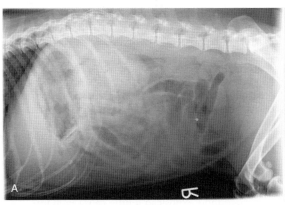 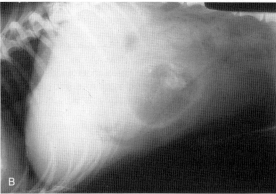

Figura 276.10 Radiografias abdominais laterais. **A.** Cão jovem sem raça definida com infecção por parvovírus mostrando evidência de íleo generalizado. **B.** Yorkshire Terrier de 10 anos com obstrução intestinal devido a um adenocarcinoma anular. Observe a alça intestinal dilatada proximal à massa e o sinal de cascalho (i. e., acúmulo de material próximo à massa).

Fluidoterapia[645-652]

Fluidoterapia oral e terapia de reposição eletrolítica podem ser suficientes se a diarreia aguda estiver associada a desidratação insignificante ou for apenas leve e se o vômito for raro ou ausente. São usadas soluções contendo glicose e eletrólitos – às vezes com adição de glicina, glutamina ou peptídios (p. ex., água de arroz) –, pois promovem a absorção osmótica de água (ver Capítulo 189). A inclusão da glutamina, um nutriente utilizado preferencialmente pelos enterócitos, pode promover a recuperação e diminuir a translocação bacteriana. No entanto, quando a diarreia é acompanhada por vômito ou desidratação significativa, devem ser administrados fluidos parenterais, a uma taxa que reponha os déficits, supra as necessidades de manutenção e compense as perdas contínuas (ver Capítulo 129). Pacientes com hipovolemia acentuada requerem suporte mais intensivo. Os antieméticos podem ser benéficos para reduzir a perda de líquidos e o desconforto do paciente, mas possivelmente mascararam sinais de obstrução intestinal. O tipo de líquido e a necessidade de suplementação de potássio são mais bem avaliados por meio de exames e hemogasometria. É melhor administrar líquidos parenterais IV; a via intraóssea pode ser usada se o acesso venoso não estiver disponível (ver Capítulo 77), mas a administração de fluidos SC é inadequada.

Dieta[644,648,649,653-658]

As recomendações atuais sobre o papel da dieta no tratamento da diarreia aguda são amplamente baseadas no bom senso, em evidências práticas e na extrapolação das diretrizes de manejo para o tratamento de humanos. A melhor conduta, em geral, consiste em suspender a alimentação por 24 a 48 horas, para "descansar" o intestino; em seguida, é oferecida uma dieta leve em porções pequenas e frequentes, por 3 a 5 dias, e, depois, a dieta original é gradualmente reintroduzida. As opções comuns de uma dieta leve e com restrição de gordura para cães são arroz e frango cozidos, peixe branco ou queijo cottage com baixo teor de gordura. Os gatos têm uma tolerância menor ao amido e podem se beneficiar de uma dieta com maior teor de proteína e gordura. Pouca atenção precisa ser dada à adequação nutricional geral de dietas leves preparadas em casa quando fornecidas por pouco tempo. Dietas GI veterinárias comerciais estão disponíveis e são mais convenientes.

O dogma do "repouso intestinal" para cães e gatos foi contestado por estudos que mostraram que alimentar bebês humanos durante a diarreia secretora e infecciosa promovia a recuperação e o fortalecimento da imunidade da mucosa. Existem algumas evidências em cães de que a alimentação acelera a recuperação da gastrenterite hemorrágica (GH). No entanto, a diarreia secretora em geral é menos comum em cães e gatos em comparação a bebês; o volume aumentado resultante da diarreia (embora em um período mais curto) pode ser cosmeticamente inaceitável e a presença de vômito pode impedir essa abordagem de qualquer maneira.

Teoricamente, qualquer doença intestinal predispõe o animal ao desenvolvimento de uma sensibilidade alimentar. Portanto, a alimentação com uma nova fonte de proteína durante esses períodos pode impedir o desenvolvimento de sensibilidade à dieta básica. Contudo, a evidência para esse conceito de alimentação com uma "proteína de sacrifício" é circunstancial.

Protetores e adsorventes[659,660]

Subsalicilato de bismuto, caulim, montmorilonita (uma forma refinada de argila esmectita ou caulim), pectina, carvão ativado, magnésio e produtos contendo alumínio e bário são frequentemente administrados durante a diarreia aguda para se ligar a bactérias e suas toxinas e proteger a mucosa intestinal. Eles também se ligam à água e podem ser antissecretores. A terapia não deve exceder 3 dias se não houver melhora.

Agentes modificadores da motilidade e da secreção[661-669]

Os anticolinérgicos e opiáceos ou opioides (loperamida, difenoxilato) costumam ser usados para o manejo inespecífico da diarreia aguda, mas os agentes anticolinérgicos podem potencializar o íleo adinâmico e não são recomendados. Acredita-se que os analgésicos opioides exerçam seus efeitos estimulando a motilidade segmentar, o que diminuiria o trânsito, mas na verdade eles diminuem a secreção intestinal e promovem a absorção. São indicados no manejo de suporte a curto prazo da diarreia aguda em cães e contraindicados em casos de obstrução ou de etiologia infecciosa. A loperamida pode ter efeitos colaterais no sistema nervoso central na raça Collie e outros cães com a mutação do gene de resistência a múltiplos fármacos (MDR-1). Fármacos antimuscarínicos, como a hioscina (butilescopolamina), geralmente não são recomendados, pois podem produzir um ID paralisado e não funcional, predispor à intussuscepção e causar intoxicação. No entanto, em casos leves de gastrenterite aguda, seu efeito antiespasmódico pode ajudar a aliviar a dor, como a de cólica.

Terapia antimicrobiana[670-675]

Os antimicrobianos são com frequência prescritos para diarreia aguda, mas são verdadeiramente indicados apenas para animais com infecção bacteriana ou protozoária confirmada no ID. O consenso atual é de que também são indicados quando há suspeita de quebra generalizada da integridade da barreira intestinal, a partir de evidências de diarreia hemorrágica quando, consequentemente, o paciente está sob risco de sepse. No entanto, não há benefício se o paciente não for bacterêmico nem apresentar sinais de sepse. Leucopenia, neutrofilia com desvio à esquerda, febre, presença de sangue nas fezes e choque são indicações potenciais para antibióticos profiláticos em animais com diarreia. As escolhas iniciais nessas situações incluem amoxicilina com clavulanato ou cefalosporina (eficaz contra bactérias gram-positivas, algumas gram-negativas e anaeróbias). Se houver suspeita de translocação sistêmica de bactérias entéricas, são indicados antimicrobianos eficazes contra microrganismos anaeróbicos (p. ex., metronidazol ou clindamicina) e aeróbios gram-negativos "difíceis" (um aminoglicosídeo ou uma fluoroquinolona). Os aminoglicosídeos potencialmente nefrotóxicos, como a gentamicina, não devem ser administrados até que o volume do paciente seja expandido. Mostrou-se que as quinolonas intravenosas alcançam concentrações terapêuticas no lúmen do intestino canino e podem ser eficazes contra enterococos e *E. coli*.

Prebióticos e probióticos (simbióticos)[10,676-729]

Prebióticos são substratos seletivos usados por um número limitado de espécies microbianas "benéficas", que, portanto, causam alterações na microbiota luminal. Os mais frequentemente usados são carboidratos não digeríveis (p. ex., a lactulose), inulina, fruto-oligossacarídeos (FOS) e mananoligossacarídeos (MOS) e imunomoduladores (lactoferrina). Seu uso combinado com probióticos, que receberá o nome de "simbiótico", é projetado para estimular o crescimento do microrganismo; os prebióticos também podem ter um efeito sobre o sistema imunológico.

Já os probióticos são definidos como "microrganismos vivos administrados por via oral que exercem benefícios para a saúde além dos da nutrição básica." No entanto, o que constitui a saúde entérica não está definido por completo, e não estão plenamente explicadas quais características da atividade probiótica são benéficas. Por exemplo, probióticos que aumentam a secreção de IgA podem indicar exclusão imunológica aprimorada, mas, inversamente, são indicativos de piora na função da barreira da mucosa.

Além das propriedades antagônicas diretas contra bactérias patogênicas, os probióticos modulam as respostas imunes da mucosa (p. ex., são capazes de induzir células Treg) e conseguem alterar a permeabilidade intestinal. Há evidências de que o efeito positivo dos probióticos é espécie-específico e está presente apenas enquanto o probiótico for administrado continuamente. É improvável que a prática tradicional de se alimentar com iogurte, como forma de repovoar o intestino com lactobacilos benéficos após um distúrbio GI agudo, ou o uso de antibióticos funcione, mas os probióticos estão agora disponíveis para uso em cães e gatos. Há evidências crescentes de alguma eficácia na diarreia aguda, e os probióticos são uma escolha terapêutica mais responsável do que a administração geral de antimicrobianos em casos de gastrenterite.

Etiologia da diarreia aguda[730-732]

Em muitos casos de doença primária do ID que causa diarreia aguda, um agente etiológico não é identificado. A falta de um diagnóstico definitivo é vista comumente em humanos com GH que sobrevivem e, embora academicamente insatisfatória, essa inespecificidade em cães e gatos não importa se o problema for resolvido, não se repetir e não representar riscos para terceiros. Muitos mecanismos etiológicos foram descritos.

Diarreia aguda induzida por dieta, medicamentos ou toxinas[320,733]

A diarreia aguda e autolimitada em cães está mais comumente associada a mudanças rápidas de dieta, indiscrição alimentar, intolerância à dieta, hipersensibilidade ou intoxicação alimentar. O histórico pode permitir que um diagnóstico fundamentado e presuntivo seja feito. No entanto, a causa exata raramente é determinada. A mudança repentina na dieta com bastante frequência causa diarreia – talvez por alterar o microbioma. Ingestão de medicamentos (p. ex., fármacos AINE ou antibacterianos) ou toxinas (inseticidas) também pode causar vômito e diarreia. O prognóstico geralmente é excelente, e uma investigação é necessária apenas se a diarreia não for resolvida ou a condição do paciente se deteriorar.

Gastrenterite hemorrágica[644,674,675,734-749]

Existem inúmeras causas potenciais de vômito com sangue e diarreia, mas gastrenterite hemorrágica (GH) é o nome dado a uma síndrome caracterizada por diarreia aguda hemorrágica acompanhada de hemoconcentração acentuada em cães. Essa condição foi recentemente renomeada para síndrome da diarreia hemorrágica aguda (SDHA), mas nem todos os casos relatados têm a hemoconcentração característica. A causa é desconhecida, mas a hipótese atual é de que seja uma consequência da produção de enterotoxina de *Clostridium perfringens*, embora isso tenha sido questionado. A disbiose está presente, mas não está claro se é uma causa ou um efeito. Além disso, a GH pode representar uma reação de hipersensibilidade tipo 1 relacionada à dieta, já que a recidiva é observada em alguns cães, sugerindo exposição a uma causa incitante.

Achados clínicos. Raças pequenas, sobretudo Schnauzer Miniatura, são afetadas com mais frequência, mas a GH pode atingir cães grandes também. Os pacientes apresentam diarreia aguda hemorrágica e fétida, às vezes precedida de vômito. A febre é incomum, mas o estado mental deprimido e o desconforto abdominal são comuns. O início pode ser agudo e estar associado a mudanças marcantes de líquidos no ID, levando a um choque hipovolêmico grave, mesmo antes de aparecerem sinais clássicos de desidratação (p. ex., aumento da tensão da pele; ver Capítulo 127).

Diagnóstico. A evidência direta de invasão clostridial já foi demonstrada em biopsias endoscópicas, mas raramente é obtida, já que esse exame normalmente não é indicado. Em vez disso, um diagnóstico presuntivo de GH é feito com base em achados clínicos associados a mais de 60% de hematócrito (Ht). A concentração de proteína total no soro com frequência é normal ou não tão alta quanto seria esperado em relação ao Ht, provavelmente em razão da perda de plasma intestinal. As radiografias podem mostrar evidência no íleo. A ausência de leucopenia e a hemoconcentração marcada ajuda a distinguir GH de infecção por parvovírus; contudo, precisam ser descartados pancreatite (ver Capítulo 290) e hipoadrenocorticismo (ver Capítulo 309).

Tratamento. Cristaloides intravenosos são essenciais (ver Capítulo 129), mas alguns pacientes tornam-se hipoproteinêmicos e então requerem plasma (ver Capítulo 130). Antibióticos parenterais são administrados muitas vezes em razão de uma possível infecção clostridial e do alto risco de sepse, mas esse procedimento pode não ser necessário e aumentar o risco relativo à resistência do microbioma (ver Capítulo 161). A melhora clínica em geral é observada dentro de algumas horas, embora a diarreia possa levar vários dias para desaparecer. Uma vez que o paciente esteja na fase de recuperação, uma terapia de suporte padrão para diarreia aguda pode ser encorajada. O prognóstico para a maioria dos animais é bom, embora a recidiva possa ocorrer, mas se a GH for complicada por hipoproteinemia grave ou sepse, o prognóstico é mais reservado.

Causas infecciosas e parasitárias[750-753]

Diarreia causada por agentes infecciosos e parasitários é considerada comum em animais jovens, imunologicamente *naives* (imaturos) ou imunocomprometidos e alojados em grande número ou em locais pouco higiênicos. Parvovírus (ver Capítulo 225), *Giardia* (ver Capítulo 221), *Tritrichomonas* (ver Capítulo 221), *Salmonella* spp. (Ver Capítulo 220), *Campylobacter* spp. (Ver Capítulo 220), ancilostomídeos e tricurídeos (ver a seguir) podem ser causas significativas de diarreia. A importância do coronavírus, *C. perfringens* e *E. coli* como causas de diarreia ainda não foi definida. Trematódeos são raros em cães e gatos e têm maior probabilidade de causar doença hepática, bem como portar *Neorickettsia* (envenenamento por salmão; ver Capítulo 218). Miíase intestinal é um problema muito raro.

Existe um potencial zoonótico para muitas dessas infecções, e boas precauções de higiene sempre devem ser adotadas.

Infecções específicas do ID são discutidas posteriormente. A maioria das enterites virais de cães e gatos causa diarreia aguda e geralmente autolimitada, embora casos graves em pacientes jovens ou imunocomprometidos possam ser fatais.

DOENÇA CRÔNICA DO INTESTINO DELGADO

Etiologias da diarreia crônica

Em muitos casos de doença primária do ID que causa diarreia crônica, uma inflamação da mucosa está presente, mas sem a identificação de um agente etiológico. Essa situação foi denominada "enteropatia crônica", uma vez que abrange doenças responsivas a dieta, antibióticos e esteroides. A doença responsiva a esteroides foi equiparada a DII idiopática, embora existam muitas variações histológicas (ou seja, linfoplasmocitária, eosinofílica, neutrofílica ou granulomatosa), sugerindo que mesmo a verdadeira DII não é uma única doença. As causas conhecidas de inflamação intestinal incluem parasitas (especialmente *Giardia*; ver Capítulo 221), infecção bacteriana (ver Capítulo 220) e alergia alimentar (ver a seguir); apenas a inflamação idiopática deve ser denominada DII. Outras causas primárias de diarreia crônica incluem linfangiectasia, linfoma e anormalidades estruturais (p. ex., intussuscepção crônica).

Caracterização[754-759]

Historicamente, as enteropatias crônicas têm sido definidas por sua aparência histológica. Esse critério fornece poucas informações quanto à sua etiologia, e, de fato, muitos casos não têm alterações histológicas evidentes. Então, mais recentemente, as enteropatias crônicas foram definidas por sua resposta a tratamentos empíricos testados em sequência. Doenças responsivas a alimentos, antibióticos e corticosteroides foram comparadas à sensibilidade dietética, doença bacteriana ou DII idiopática, respectivamente. Uma análise de risco-benefício da biopsia intestinal sugere que a busca de um diagnóstico histológico antes do tratamento parasiticida e do manejo da dieta e dos antibióticos pode não valer a pena se o paciente ainda estiver comendo e não houver evidência de EPP, especialmente se for um animal jovem. Os achados de inflamação intestinal ainda requerem ensaios empíricos a fim de chegar ao diagnóstico presuntivo, e a resposta ao tratamento e o prognóstico em gatos mais velhos é semelhante se eles tiverem DII ou linfoma alimentar.

Manejo de enteropatias inflamatórias crônicas[760]

Se um diagnóstico histológico específico for feito (p. ex., linfangiectasia ou linfoma), podem ser usados tratamentos específicos. No entanto, há inflamação intestinal sem causa identificável em muitas circunstâncias, em razão da falta de alterações histopatológicas específicas. Nesses casos, é apropriado realizar tratamentos empíricos sequenciais. É mais lógico e seguro tratar primeiro com parasiticidas para tentar identificar o parasitismo oculto, antes de seguir uma modificação na dieta, seguido pelo uso de antibacteriano e, finalmente, por uma tentativa de imunossupressão. Portanto, um tratamento de 3 dias de fenbendazol é a conduta mais adequada inicialmente, com o objetivo de identificar ou descartar giardíase e helmintíase (ver Capítulo 163).

Manejo dietético[103,591,654,655,761-778]

O manejo da dieta é uma modalidade muito importante no tratamento geral de enteropatias crônicas (ver Capítulo 178); a anorexia, por exemplo, tem efeitos adversos no sistema imunológico. A dieta ideal é altamente digerível, com restrições moderadas em gordura, sem lactose, sem glúten, não marcadamente hipertônica, nutricionalmente equilibrada e palatável. As dietas hidrolisadas são uma alternativa potencial (ver a seguir). Oferecer o necessário para uma nutrição diária em diversas refeições (geralmente entre duas e quatro) reduz a carga em um intestino comprometido. Comer com mais frequência é desnecessário,

porque o esvaziamento gástrico impõe uma alimentação natural por gotejamento do ID. A inclusão de fibra moderadamente fermentável (p. ex., *Psyllium*) é reconhecida por promover a saúde do cólon; a fibra solúvel também promove a saúde do ID, mas as fibras podem diminuir o trânsito intestinal e o excesso é contraindicado. Suplementos prebióticos, como FOS e MOS, alteram a microbiota, mas seu efeito na microbiota do ID é limitado.

Dietas de carne ou alimentos crus biologicamente apropriados (ACBA) estão em alta, e a prática indica o sucesso no tratamento de enteropatias crônicas. A preocupação, no entanto, é o da segurança microbiológica, pois essa alimentação pode estar contaminada com *Salmonella*, *Campylobacter* e *Toxoplasma*, nenhum dos quais é adequadamente destruído pelo congelamento (ver Capítulo 192).

Antibacterianos

Os antibacterianos são indicados para as condições específicas em que um patógeno bacteriano foi detectado durante o tratamento de DRA ou SBID secundário e outras enteropatias crônicas, como DII, em que a modulação da microbiota pode ser desejável. Tilosina, metronidazol ou oxitetraciclina são comumente usadas, mas quaisquer efeitos benéficos podem ir além de sua atividade antibacteriana, com potenciais efeitos sobre o sistema imune das mucosas (ver Capítulo 161).

Imunossupressão[779]

Os medicamentos imunossupressores são indicados quando há evidência de inflamação da mucosa e nenhuma causa subjacente foi encontrada. No entanto, dado o potencial para efeitos adversos, o diagnóstico deve ser revisto antes da instituição de tal terapia, especialmente se ela foi feita apenas com base na biopsia endoscópica, que é notoriamente não confiável. Os glicocorticoides são a escolha preferida para a imunossupressão, uma vez que são geralmente eficazes e têm o efeito colateral positivo de aumentar o apetite. No entanto, se tais esteroides são ineficazes ou os efeitos colaterais são inaceitáveis, então outros agentes não esteroides podem ser usados, como azatioprina, clorambucila, metotrexato, ciclosporina ou micofenolato (ver Capítulo 165).

Suplementação vitamínica[408,780-783]

Baixas concentrações séricas de folato e cobalamina podem ser encontrados em casos de má absorção causadora de diarreia crônica e são úteis para o diagnóstico. O significado clínico da redução do folato sérico é incerto, e o valor da suplementação não foi comprovado. No entanto, a hipocobalaminemia está associada a um prognóstico pior. Mudanças metabólicas significativas ocorrem com a deficiência de cobalamina e com o acúmulo de homocisteína e de ácido metilmalônico, que podem levar à hiperamonemia. A acidemia pode causar inapetência, fraqueza e piora da doença intestinal. A cobalamina, portanto, deve ser suplementada: injeções parenterais semanais são aplicadas por pelo menos 4 semanas e até as concentrações séricas estarem altas.

Probióticos[718,784]

A maioria dos relatos de uso de probióticos em animais diz respeito ao tratamento da diarreia aguda (ver também Capítulo 167). Um estudo indicou que um simbiótico produziu redução da diarreia crônica felina, mas há evidências de *Enterococcus faecium* SF68 eliminando infecções crônicas, como *Giardia* de cães.

Tratamentos adjuvantes[785-787]

Agentes procinéticos, como metoclopramida, cisaprida e mosaprida, podem melhorar o bem-estar e o apetite, superando a náuseas associada ao íleo. A mirtazapina é frequentemente administrada para melhorar o apetite, mas também tem efeito procinético. A loperamida e o difenoxilato diminuem o trânsito intestinal e a frequência da diarreia, mas são principalmente úteis como agentes cosméticos para reduzir a probabilidade de liberação inadequada da diarreia, assim como os adsorventes e as fibras oferecem tratamento geral inespecífico.

Tratamentos alternativos[788-797]

A aplicação de acupuntura tem sido relatada por estimular a motilidade do ID, e várias preparações de ervas (p. ex., agrimônia, araruta, mirtilo, camomila, olmo, casca, casca de nim e alteia [Althaea officinalis]) são recomendadas para o tratamento de enteropatias crônicas. Algumas se ligam à água, como o caulim, enquanto outras contêm moléculas que reduzem a secreção intestinal. No entanto, não há estudos cegos controlados com placebo para apoiar seu uso. A lactoferrina bovina foi proposta como uma forma de estimular o sistema imune inato, mas não há evidências que confirmem tal efeito. Além disso, os remédios homeopáticos não têm base científica. Beta-1,3/1,6-D-glucano, beta-hidroxibetametil-butirato e levamisol foram associados à redução da inflamação do ID em DII, com glucano sendo o mais eficaz e de início mais rápido. Enterovacinas genéricas e autógenas foram testadas, mas sem prova de eficácia até o momento da publicação deste livro.

Manejo de enteropatia com perda de proteínas

Suporte de coloide ou transfusão de plasma (ver Capítulo 130) podem ser indicados no período perioperatório durante a coleta de amostras de biopsia, mas são ineficazes na manutenção da pressão osmótica coloide a longo prazo. Diuréticos podem reduzir a ascite; a espironolactona é possivelmente mais segura (ou seja, poupadora de potássio e menos drástica) e, em última análise, mais eficaz do que a furosemida. Tratamentos específicos são discutidos posteriormente.

ENTERITES VIRAIS

Várias infecções virais em cães e gatos podem causar enterite enquanto um componente importante de suas síndromes clínicas. As seguintes infecções são abordadas em detalhes em seus respectivos capítulos: infecções por parvovírus canino[365-368,653,798-912] e felino/panleucopenia[807,913-926] (ver Capítulo 225), infecções por coronavírus caninos e felinos[802,927-955] (ver Capítulo 224), vírus da imunodeficiência felina[956,957] (FIV; ver Capítulo 222) e vírus da leucemia felina[958] (FeLV; ver Capítulo 223). Outros vírus de prevalência mais baixa também são causas potenciais de enterite.[959-977] Os rotavírus podem infectar cães e gatos, mas a infecção geralmente é tão transitória que nenhum sinal é reconhecido. Norovírus foi isolado de gatos e cães com enterite, e há evidências sorológicas de infecção generalizada. Um agente semelhante ao torovírus foi isolado das fezes de gatos afetados com uma síndrome de diarreia crônica característica e um prolapso da terceira pálpebra, mas não foi mostrada uma associação clara com sinais clínicos. O circovírus foi isolado de cães com diarreia e vasculite. Bocavírus é um pequeno vírus não envelopado com um genoma ssDNA linear e membro da família Parvoviridae. Cepas caninas de bocavírus (vírus diminutos de cães) foram incriminadas como causa de enterite em filhotes, e uma infecção fatal foi associada a uma nova cepa: bocavírus canino 2. Muitos outros novos vírus entéricos, como astrovírus (mamastrovírus 1 e 2), kobuvírus e sakobuvírus foram identificados, mas seu papel patogênico ainda precisa ser elucidado.

ENTERITES BACTERIANAS (VER CAPÍTULO 220)

Relevância do isolamento bacteriano[943,978-982]

Bactérias potencialmente enteroinvasivas, como Campylobacter jejuni, Salmonella spp. e E. coli, podem ser patogênicas em cães e gatos e estar associadas à diarreia aguda. A incidência de infecção é maior em animais jovens, em canis e em pacientes imunocomprometidos; além disso, a coinfecção é provavelmente comum. No entanto, esses microrganismos também podem ser isolados de animais saudáveis e daqueles com diarreia crônica; portanto, existe confusão sobre seu significado quando isolado. Embora esses microrganismos ainda apresentem um risco zoonótico, e medidas preventivas devam ser tomadas com animais de companhia de pacientes imunocomprometidos ou famílias com crianças pequenas (ver Capítulo 210), tentar erradicar os microrganismos com antibióticos quando o animal não mostra sinais clínicos pode ser inútil e desnecessário e até induzir um estado de portador.

Campylobacter spp.[263,980,983-1020]

Campylobacter (ver Capítulo 220) pode ser encontrada nas fezes de até 100% de cães e gatos saudáveis que tiveram diarreia em algum momento da vida; a bactéria adere às células epiteliais intestinais e, em condições adequadas, pode invadir e causar enterocolite ulcerativa. Campylobacter jejuni, C. coli, C. helveticus, C. lari e C. upsaliensis foram detectadas e identificadas por análise molecular do 16S RNA ribossômico. Em humanos, todas as espécies de Campylobacter são consideradas patogênicas, mas sua presença nas fezes de animais saudáveis levanta a dúvida sobre sua patogenicidade em cães e gatos. Comer carne de frango é um grande fator de risco para infecção; mostrou-se que a patogenicidade de C. jejuni em aves está relacionada à sua capacidade invasiva quando expostas a norepinefrina e durante o recrutamento de neutrófilos para um processo inflamatório. Estudos in vitro usando linhagens de células epiteliais mostraram a ativação de NF-kappa-B, a produção de quimiocina IL-8 e a capacidade de induzir migração de neutrófilos através da produção bacteriana de peptídios n-formil quimiotáticos.

Há evidências experimentais de que C. jejuni causa enterocolite em cães, mas parece ser mais patogênica quando há coinfecção viral. A infecção por C. coli foi associada à diarreia em gatos filhotes e enterite neutrofílica. É possível que o isolado mais comum de cães, C. upsaliensis, seja um comensal, porque estudos longitudinais mostraram que ele persiste em cães saudáveis. Assim, muitas infecções por Campylobacter são assintomáticas, com taxas de portador relatadas em cães e gatos saudáveis em 50% ou mais dos casos; animais de canil e mais jovens têm as taxas de isolamento mais altas. Os sinais clínicos dependem da quantidade e das espécies de Campylobacter que infectaram um animal e de suas condições, podendo variar amplamente de enterocolite branda a grave, com sinais clínicos de diarreia aquosa, mucoide ou hemorrágica acompanhada de vômito, tenesmo, febre, anorexia e desidratação grave. Animais mais jovens, com sistema imune menos desenvolvido e menor capacidade de concentração renal para resistir à desidratação são mais propensos a ser mais gravemente afetados.

Diagnóstico

A presença de bactérias delgadas em forma de asa de gaivota em um esfregaço fecal corado fornece um diagnóstico presuntivo. O microrganismo é frágil in vitro, e a cultura de amostras de fezes frescas ou PCR é recomendada para evitar falso-negativos. A identificação da espécie por testes bioquímicos dos microrganismos cultivados é incerta, e PCR é o teste preferido.

Tratamento[1021]

O tratamento é necessário dependendo da espécie de Campylobacter identificada, do estado de saúde do animal e da gravidade dos sinais clínicos, se presentes. Em animais saudáveis, a terapia antimicrobiana deve ser reservada para os casos em que pode haver contato com humanos imunocomprometidos, embora o risco zoonótico seja pequeno se as precauções normais de higiene forem tomadas (ver Capítulo 210). A eritromicina é um tratamento eficaz em cães e gatos (cães: 20 mg/kg VO, a cada 8 h; gatos: 10 mg/kg VO, a cada 8 h), reduzindo a eliminação em 48 h quando administrada em cães, mas pode causar vômitos. Tilosina e clindamicina são alternativas se uma terapia antimicrobiana for considerada necessária. A bactéria geralmente é sensível a fluoroquinolonas, mas é difícil justificar seu uso para eliminar um microrganismo que poderia ser um comensal ou apenas produzir sinais autolimitantes. Foi relatada resistência a antibióticos. Foram recomendadas várias culturas pós-tratamento para confirmar a erradicação de C. jejuni, mas, a menos que a identificação da espécie por PCR esteja disponível, esta pode não ser uma abordagem sensata.

Prognóstico
O prognóstico de recuperação geralmente é bom, mas a colonização persistente, sobretudo por C. upsaliensis, pode ocorrer.

Salmonella spp.[990,1022-1058]
Salmonella tem potencial zoonótico (ver Capítulos 210 e 220) e pode causar sinais clínicos significativos, embora sejam incomuns e ocorram com maior frequência em animais jovens, parasitados, em canis ou imunocomprometidos. O estado de portador subclínico é visto com maior frequência, e a bactéria foi isolada das fezes em até 30% de cães sadios e 18% dos gatos sadios. Taxas de isolamento de aproximadamente 2% são relatos comuns, a menos que o animal seja coprofágico ou ingira carne crua com regularidade (dietas ACBA). Foram relatadas taxas de contaminação por *Salmonella* através de dietas ACBA de até 20%. Pode ocorrer infecção humana por cães, gatos e seus alimentos.

Achados clínicos[1036,1059-1061]
Quatro cenários são possíveis depois de uma infecção: portador subclínico transitório, gastrenterite aguda, bacteriemia e endotoxemia (ou um estado portador). Se causar diarreia aguda, a infecção varia de leve a grave e com sangue, além de provocar anorexia, febre, dor abdominal e vômito. Invasão da mucosa e translocação podem resultar em sepse, endotoxemia, coagulação intravascular disseminada e morte em animais suscetíveis (ver Capítulo 132). O receptor para invasão é a proteína transmembrana reguladora de condutância da fibrose cística (CFTR), expressa por enterócitos, mas modulada por bactérias comensais. Gatos com infecção por *Salmonella* podem apresentar apenas sinais vagos (p. ex., febre, leucocitose e conjuntivite) e nenhum sinal GI. Uma doença diarreica sazonal, aguda e febril, conhecida como "febre dos pássaros canoros", foi relatada em gatos de países do Mediterrâneo após a ingestão de pássaros canoros em migração, portadores de S. Typhimurium.

Diagnóstico[318,321,354,1062]
O diagnóstico é baseado no isolamento de *Salmonella* nas fezes ou no sangue – em casos de pacientes com septicemia – por cultura em meio seletivo ou por PCR. As características clinicopatológicas são inespecíficas: hiperpotassemia e possível hiponatremia (pseudo-hipoadrenocorticismo).

Tratamento[1063]
O tratamento com antibióticos pode estimular bactérias resistentes e um estado de portador, por isso não é recomendado quando a *Salmonella* é isolada de animais saudáveis ou estáveis apenas com diarreia. Em animais com diarreia hemorrágica grave, depressão acentuada, choque, febre persistente ou sepse, antibióticos parenterais precisam ser administrados. A escolha do antibiótico deve ser orientada por testes de sensibilidade quando possíveis, mas as fluoroquinolonas parecem ser eficazes contra muitas estirpes de *Salmonella* spp. e são menos propensas a induzir um estado portador. A terapia deve ser administrada inicialmente por 10 dias, mas uma terapia prolongada pode ser necessária. Várias coproculturas devem ser feitas para garantir que a infecção tenha sido eliminada. No entanto, microrganismos invasores podem ser vistos em biopsias do ID por FISH, mesmo quando a coprocultura é negativa.

Prognóstico
Na maioria dos casos, o prognóstico para a diarreia associada a infecção por *Salmonella* é bom. Um prognóstico reservado deve ser considerado em pacientes com septicemia. Indicadores de prognóstico negativos incluem início hiperagudo, febre alta (acima dos 40°C), hipotermia, diarreia hemorrágica grave, desvio à esquerda degenerativo e hipoglicemia.

Clostridium spp.
C. perfringens foi associado a GH (SDHA; ver anteriormente e Capítulo 220). Esse microrganismo e *Clostridioides difficile* podem fazer parte da microbiota residente de cães, mas também podem causar sinais semelhantes aos da colite (ver Capítulo 277).

Escherichia coli[351,358,1057,1064-1080]
E. coli é uma possível causa importante de diarreia aguda, embora o microrganismo frequentemente faça parte de infecções mistas com outros patógenos, como parvovírus, enquanto algumas cepas podem causar diarreia crônica (ver Capítulo 220). Muitas estirpes de *E. coli* são comensais, mas, em outras, genes cromossômicos e/ou plasmídeos codificam para mecanismos de patogenicidade. *E. coli* enterotoxigênica (ETEC), enteropatogênica (EPEC; causadora da lesão A/E, do inglês *attaching and effacing*) e entero-hemorrágica (EHEC) podem causar diarreia tanto aguda quanto crônica. EHEC também têm sido associada à síndrome hemolítico-urêmica e à *E. coli* aderente e invasiva (AIEC) com colite granulomatosa (ver Capítulo 277).

ETEC causa doença do ID principalmente ao produzir toxinas termoestáveis (ST) e termolábeis (LT) que estimulam o excesso de secreção pelo ID, enquanto EHEC tem tropismo para o IG (ver Capítulo 277). EPEC, que causa a lesão A/E nos enterócitos da mucosa intestinal (Figura 276.11) através da expressão de intimina pelo gene *eae*, pode lesionar tanto o ID quanto o IG. Uma infecção fatal por EPEC foi relatada em gatos filhotes e em um gato adulto, cujas lesões A/E foram encontradas no íleo e no cólon. A morte de cães filhotes com infecção por EPEC parece ser mais comum, porém muitas vezes há uma infecção mista com cinomose, parvovírus e protozoários patogênicos, o que contribui para o agravamento do quadro clínico.

A identificação de cepas patogênicas requer testes específicos, como bioensaios para toxinas ou ensaios de PCR para detectar marcadores de patogenicidade, mas mesmo o isolamento de microrganismos carreadores de genes associados a patogenicidade não comprova a causa. Convencionalmente, o

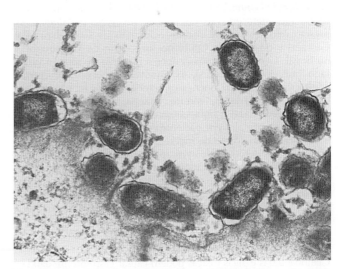

Figura 276.11 *Escherichia coli* enteropatogênica (EPEC). Micrografia eletrônica mostrando a lesão A/E (*attaching and effacing*) de EPEC na superfície luminal de um enterócito, causando lesão generalizada às microvilosidades. (Cortesia de R. J. Higgins e G. R. Pearson.)

SEÇÃO 18 • Doença Gastrintestinal

tratamento consiste em antibióticos apropriados; vacinação e imunoglobulinas orais são alternativas não comprovadas que, pelo menos, não influenciam na resistência antimicrobiana.

Microrganismos enteroaderentes[1081-1085]

Tal qual *E. coli*, microrganismos aderentes como *Streptococcus* spp. foram relatados enquanto causadores de diarreia crônica em cães, e *Enterococcus hirae* foi isolado de gatos filhotes.

Yersinia pseudotuberculosis[216,1086-1088]

Yersinia pseudotuberculosis pode ser ingerida quando gatos comem roedores ou pássaros contaminados. A bactéria infecta o trato GI, fígado e nódulos linfáticos, causando perda de peso acentuada, diarreia, anorexia, letargia, icterícia e linfadenopatia mesentérica. A suscetibilidade em humanos está relacionada à expressão das proteínas NOD. O tratamento pode ser tentado com oxitetraciclina ou sulfatrimetoprim, mas a doença em geral é progressiva e fatal. *Yersinia enterocolitica* é predominantemente um patógeno do IG (ver Capítulo 277).

Tuberculose[1089]

Em cães e gatos, *Mycobacterium* spp. causa infecções granulomatosas multissistêmicas, que ocasionalmente envolvem o trato GI (ver Capítulo 212). Gatos podem desenvolver infecção do ID com *M. bovis* pela ingestão de leite de vaca infectado, porém, mais comumente, têm infecções cutâneas ou pulmonares. Uma enterocolite granulomatosa com linfadenopatia mesentérica associada a infecção por *M. avium* foi relatada em cinco cães da raça Basset Hound.

Bactérias diversas[1090-1099]

Muitas bactérias GI podem ser patógenos oportunistas ou parte de uma infecção mista, mas, ocasionalmente, os sinais clínicos estão relacionados diretamente a um microrganismo específico. *Clostridium piliforme* (anteriormente *Bacillus piliformis*) causa a doença de Tyzzer, uma doença rara que provoca uma diarreia aguda e fatal em cachorros e gatos filhotes, para a qual nenhum tratamento eficaz foi descrito. *Providencia alcalifaciens* foi relatada como causa primária de enterite bacteriana em três cães. *Anaerobiospirillum* foi associado a ileocolite em gatos, mas as espiroquetas *Brachyspira pilosicoli*, embora patogênicas e zoonóticas, são mais propensas a causar colite (ver Capítulo 277).

Diarreia riquetsial (envenenamento por salmão; ver Capítulo 218)[1100-1112]

Neorickettsia helminthoeca e *Neorickettsia elokominica* são encontradas nas metacercárias do verme *Nanophyetus salmonicola*, presente no salmão nas regiões ocidentais da Cordilheira das Cascatas e do norte da Califórnia, no centro de Washington e no Brasil. Cerca de 1 semana após a ingestão de salmão infectado por cães (e coiotes), as riquétsias emergem do verme adulto e causam uma doença caracterizada por febre alta, gastrenterite hemorrágica, vômito, letargia, anorexia, polidipsia, secreção oculonasal e linfadenopatia periférica. A mortalidade é extremamente alta em pacientes não tratados. O diagnóstico é baseado no histórico de ingestão de peixe cru em uma área endêmica, na detecção de ovos operculados do verme em fezes e na presença de corpúsculos de inclusão intracitoplasmáticos em macrófagos de aspirados de linfonodos. Oxitetraciclina (7 mg/kg, intravenoso, a cada 8 h) é o tratamento de escolha e deve ser mantido por pelo menos 5 dias. O trematódeo vetor é erradicado com praziquantel.

Infecções por cianobactérias e algas[1113-1121]

Cianobactérias e algas tóxicas podem causar gastrenterite aguda e morte. Sua proliferação pode liberar uma anticolinesterase na água que induz vômito, diarreia, ataxia e morte rápida em cães que bebem a água contaminada. *Prototheca* spp. são algas aclorofiladas que causam a prototecose, uma infecção cutânea normalmente de gatos, mas que, em cães, pode envolver o intestino e o SNC. A doença disseminada fatal que afeta o ID tem sido relatada, mas a doença do IG é mais comum (ver Capítulo 277).

Infeções fúngicas

Patogenicidade[85,109,1122-1131]

Uma quantidade baixa de fungos é encontrada no microbioma intestinal normal em culturas convencionais de rotina, porém mais são identificados por técnicas moleculares. Eles geralmente não são considerados patogênicos. Um número maior de fungos pode ser encontrado na DII idiopática, mas não está claro se isso é a causa ou o efeito, embora um benefício empírico da administração de nistatina tenha sido relatado em casos intratáveis de diarreia, sugerindo um papel para fungos. A levedura *Cyniclomyces guttulatus* foi isolada de cães e gatos com diarreia crônica, mas é encontrada com mais frequência nas fezes de animais saudáveis e provavelmente não é significativa, a menos que esteja em grande número. No entanto, em circunstâncias apropriadas como a imunossupressão, os fungos podem invadir a mucosa intestinal e até mesmo se disseminar por todo o corpo. A aspergilose intestinal (ver Capítulos 234 e 235), a mucormicose (ver Capítulo 236) e a criptococose (ver Capítulo 231) são ocasionais, mas a incidência de infecções fúngicas varia em todo o mundo; alguns são onipresentes (p. ex., candidíase[840,1130,1132] e zigomicose;[1124,1160-1165] ver Capítulo 236) e outros são localizados de acordo com regiões geoclimáticas (p. ex., histoplasmose;[1166-1169] ver Capítulo 233). Infecção intestinal primária com oomiceto aquático *Pythium* spp. (pitiose; ver Capítulo 236) é de longe a ficomicose mais comum (ou seja, uma infecção com um fungo fracamente septado).[1133-1159] O envolvimento GI pode ser extenso e grave.

HELMINTOS

Importância[1170-1178]

A infestação por helmintos é comum em cães e gatos e atinge majoritariamente o ID; *Trichuris* são parasitas do IG (ver Capítulo 277). Algumas espécies são patogênicas, sobretudo quando presentes em grandes números; outras não são patogênicas, exceto em filhotes, mas podem predispor a novas doenças e algumas são zoonóticas. Tratamento anti-helmíntico regular, portanto, é importante para a saúde dos animais jovens (ver Capítulo 163) e a proteção dos seres humanos (ver Capítulo 210). Diversos anti-helmínticos estão disponíveis (p. ex., benzimidazóis [albendazol, fenbendazol, febantel, flubendazol, mebendazol, oxfendazol, tiabendazol], milbemicina oxima, moxidectina, niclosamida, piperazina, pirantel, selamectina), embora sua disponibilidade possa variar geograficamente.

Ascarídeos[996,1179-1211]

Os ascarídeos são onipresentes em cães e gatos, e muitos estudos mostraram variações geográficas na prevalência, que dependem da propriedade, do padrão econômico e das práticas de vermifugação. Normalmente, *Toxocara canis* é encontrado em cães e *Toxocara cati* (*T. mystax*) em gatos. *Toxascaris leonina* é menos comum tanto em cães quanto gatos. *Baylisascaris procyonis*, o ascarídeo de guaxinins, ocasionalmente infecta cães.

Epidemiologia[1208,1212-1221]

Cães e gatos adultos podem ser infectados por *Toxocara* spp. através da ingestão de ovos embrionados ou de hospedeiros paratênicos, como roedores. No entanto, os filhotes são os mais comumente infectados, porque a principal via de infecção é a transmissão transplacentária para *T. canis* e a transmamária para *T. canis* e *T. cati*. A migração juvenil de *T. canis* pode causar lesão hepática, pulmonar e ocasionalmente ocular. Os nematódeos adultos vivem no ID.

Achados clínicos[1222,1223]

Na maioria das vezes, os ascarídeos causam doença em animais jovens e sinais de infestação intensa são diarreia, perda de peso ou retardo no crescimento. Uma pelagem sem força e abdome distendido podem ser evidentes em filhotes. Obstrução intestinal e ruptura foram descritos em infestações graves.

Diagnóstico[341,342,345,1224]

Pode-se presumir que quase todos os filhotes tenham infecção por *T. canis*. O diagnóstico pode ser confirmado por exame de flutuação fecal (ver Figura 276.6 e Capítulo 81) e ocasionalmente por endoscopia (ver Figura 276.8 A).

Tratamento[1213,1225-1235]

Uma ampla gama de anti-helmínticos é eficaz contra os ascarídeos, e quaisquer reações adversas geralmente são leves ou não relatadas (ver Capítulo 163). O tratamento deve ser repetido em intervalos de 2 a 3 semanas.

Aspectos de saúde pública[1189,1221,1236-1246]

A infecção de humanos por *Toxocara* se dá pela ingestão de ovos, que não são embrionados e infectantes quando eliminados (ver Capítulo 210). A progressão para a fase L3 embrionada é necessária para a infecção, logo, fezes frescas não são um risco zoonótico, pois a embrionação leva de 2 a 7 semanas. Os seres humanos podem ser infectados por ingestão acidental de solo ou alimentos contaminados e por contato com ovos aderidos aos pelos do animal. *T. canis* representa um problema substancial de saúde pública, pois pode causar *larva migrans* visceral, ocular e neural, enquanto até 30% das pessoas são soropositivas, indicando exposição. As taxas de infecção e contaminação do solo variam muito de acordo com fatores socioeconômicos, geografia e clima, mas as crianças apresentam o maior risco em razão da geofagia e pica. O risco aumenta em três vezes se a pessoa é proprietária de um cão e cinco vezes se possuir mais de um.

Os animais jovens devem ser rotineiramente desparasitados com 2, 4, 6, 8, 12 e 16 semanas de idade e em um intervalo mínimo de 6 meses para proteger a população, mas há preocupação de que a falta de estimulação antigênica fornecida por endoparasitas afete a imunocompetência. *T. canis* pode ser controlado através das cadelas grávidas, pela administração seja de fenbendazol 50 mg/kg VO, a cada 24 h do dia 40 da gestação até 2 dias após o parto, seja de duas doses de moxidectina.

Strongyloides sp.[1179,1219,1247-1252]

Strongyloides tumefaciens é um parasita do IG (ver Capítulo 277), mas *S. stercoralis* é um pequeno nematódeo que pode causar enterite hemorrágica em filhotes jovens. Larvas infectantes são ingeridas, transmitidas através do leite da mãe ou da penetração pela pele, e, após a migração através do pulmão, amadurecem no ID. A avaliação fecal usando a técnica Baermann ou a demonstração de larvas móveis de primeiro estágio em esfregaços de frescos de fezes (ver Figura 276.6) ajuda a diferenciar as larvas de *Angiostrongylus*, *Oslerus* e ancilóstomos adultos. A infecção pode ser tratada com tiabendazol e possivelmente fenbendazol ou ivermectina (ver Capítulo 163).

Ancilostomídeos[1216,1253-1263]

Infecções por *Ancylostoma* spp. são mais comuns em regiões tropicais e subtropicais e tratam-se de zoonoses importantes, que causam *larva migrans* cutânea (ver Capítulo 210). Os ancilóstomos têm ciclo de vida direto, e a infecção pode ser adquirida no pré-natal, na lactação (não em gatos), na ingestão de larvas, na migração de larvas através da pele e na ingestão de um pequeno roedor hospedeiro paratênico.

Ancylostoma caninum é o ancilóstomo mais importante de cães e está associado a perda de sangue e enterite hemorrágica. *Ancylostoma braziliense* ocorre em cães no sul dos EUA e em gatos. *Ancylostoma tubaeforme* é o ancilóstomo mais comum em gatos, porém é mais raro e menos patogênico. *Uncinaria stenocephala* é a ancilostomíase de cães da Europa Ocidental, do norte dos EUA e do Canadá. A infecção é mais comumente relatada em canis, particularmente com a raça Galgo e muito raramente em gatos.

Achados clínicos

Diarreia, vômito, desidratação e crescimento deficiente são comuns em cães filhotes com infecção por *A. caninum*. Fraqueza e palidez refletem perda de sangue intensa, e a infecção pode causar anemia rápida e potencialmente fatal ou anemia crônica com deficiência de ferro. *U. stenocephala* não causa anemia, mas infestações graves podem estar associadas à diarreia. Penetração interdigital na pele e migração larval de *U. stenocephala* causa prurido podal.

Diagnóstico[341,342,357,1224,1264,1265]

O diagnóstico é feito por demonstração de ovos nas fezes (ver Figura 276.6 e Capítulo 81). Os ancilóstomos podem ser vistos na endoscopia (ver Vídeo 276.2), mas a infecção deve ser diagnosticada ou tratada empiricamente antes do procedimento.

Tratamento[1225,1264,1266-1269]

Para infecção por *Ancylostoma* em filhotes anêmicos, pamoato de pirantel foi sugerido como o tratamento de escolha, pois tem uma atuação muito rápida e é comparativamente seguro (ver Capítulo 163). Filhotes anêmicos podem necessitar de transfusão de sangue (ver Capítulo 130) e cuidados de suporte. Administração mensal de milbemicina ou ivermectina e pamoato de pirantel foi aprovada para a prevenção ou controle da ancilostomíase em cães.

Tênias[1225,1236,1270-1274]

Dipylidium caninum é a tênia mais comum que infecta cães e gatos nos EUA e na Europa, com pulgas como seus hospedeiros intermediários. Normalmente, não há sinais clínicos, exceto "grãos de arroz" móveis (proglotes), visíveis na área perineal ou nas fezes. Infestações pesadas de *D. caninum* raramente são associadas a diarreia, perda de peso e retardo de crescimento. O diagnóstico da infecção por *D. caninum* é confirmado pela demonstração de cápsulas ovígeras características, contidas em proglotes e obtidas da área perineal ou fezes (ver Figura 276.6).

Várias tênias são comuns em cães e gatos, tendo bovinos, ovinos, caprinos e leporídeos como os hospedeiros intermediários mais comuns. *Sensu stricto*, os cães são hospedeiros definitivos da pequena tênia *Echinococcus granulosus*; humanos e ovinos são hospedeiros intermediários. A infecção ocorre por meio da ingestão de carne crua infectada, e os cães pastores normalmente são contaminados por ingestão de carcaças de ovinos. A infecção por *E. granulosus* não é associada a sinais clínicos em cães, mas é uma zoonose importante, pois causa a hidatidose humana. *Echinococcus multilocularis* pode ser carreado por cães e é uma zoonose igualmente importante. *Mesocestódios* spp. é uma causa rara de doença intestinal (EPP), mas ocasionalmente provoca infecção intraperitoneal. O gato é o hospedeiro definitivo de *Spirometra* spp., que raramente causa sinais intestinais.

D. caninum, *Echinococcus* spp. e *Taenia* spp. são adequadamente controlados pela administração de rotina de praziquantel (alternativas incluem diclorofeno, epsiprantel ou niclosamida; ver Capítulo 163). O tratamento da infecção por *D. caninum* também envolve o controle adequado das pulgas.

PROTOZOÁRIOS

Os coccídeos geralmente são considerados patógenos menores que causam doenças em cães e gatos jovens ou imunossuprimidos, mas a infecção por *Giardia* pode ser clinicamente significativa. *Tritrichomonas fetus*, *Pentatrichomonas hominis*, *Balantidium coli* e *Entamoeba histolytica* são habitantes do cólon (ver Capítulo 277).

Isospora spp.[1275-1288]

Isospora spp. (sin. *Cystisospora*) são os coccídeos parasitas mais comuns de cães (*I. canis, I. ohioensis*) e gatos (*I. felis, I. rivolta*). A transmissão ocorre por ingestão de ovos ou hospedeiros paratênicos. Os esporozoítos são liberados no ID e entram nas células para começar o desenvolvimento. O período pré-patente varia de 4 a 11 dias, dependendo da espécie. A infecção por *Isospora* comumente não produz sinais clínicos. Cães e gatos filhotes mantidos em condições anti-higiênicas ou animais imunossuprimidos são capazes de desenvolver infestações pesadas, que podem estar associadas a diarreia em geral mucoide, mas às vezes com sangue. Agentes infecciosos concomitantes são comuns e, clinicamente, podem ser mais significativos.

Oocistos de *Isospora* são encontrados no exame direto de um esfregaço ou por flutuação. A infecção geralmente é autolimitante, mas sulfadimetoxina ou sulfatrimetoprim podem ser usados quando os sinais clínicos justificam o tratamento. Coccidiostáticos, como toltrazurila e diclazurila, são os preferidos, quando disponíveis (ver Capítulo 163). O prognóstico de recuperação é bom.

Cryptosporidium spp.[349,359,360,844,1287-1322]

A taxonomia desse gênero está mudando à medida que novas informações genéticas surgem, de modo que esses microrganismos já não são considerados intimamente relacionado aos coccídios. *Cryptosporidium parvum*, um patógeno clinicamente significativo em humanos e bezerros, agora é reconhecido como não sendo uma única espécie. Mais de 20 genótipos de C. *parvum* foram identificados, incluindo "espécies" de cães e de gatos, às vezes denominadas C. *canis* e C. *felis*, respectivamente (ver Capítulo 221). Os cães podem transmitir os genótipos de bovinos e murinos para humanos, mas genótipos específicos para cães e gatos são provavelmente zoonóticos apenas para humanos imunocomprometidos (ver Capítulo 210).

C. *parvum* é um parasita intracelular obrigatório, com transmissão fecal-oral. A infecção pode ser assintomática, mas tem sido associada à diarreia autolimitante em gatos e raramente em cães e à diarreia hemorrágica grave em animais imunocomprometidos e animais coinfectados. A infecção é mais comum em pacientes jovens, frequentemente com infecções parasitárias concomitantes, mas a prevalência varia com a região geográfica também. Gatos eliminam o microrganismo com maior frequência do que cães, e a excreção pode ser reativada pela administração de corticosteroide ou estresse cirúrgico.

Diagnóstico[347,349,359,1307,1315,1323-1325]

Oocistos de *Cryptosporidium* são extremamente pequenos (por volta de 1/10 do tamanho dos oocistos de *Isospora*) e devem ser identificados por flutuação fecal, microscopia de imersão, imunofluorescência direta, coloração ácido-resistente modificada de esfregaços fecais, ensaios imunoenzimáticos ou PCR. Os microrganismos podem ser reconhecidos em biopsias intestinais.

Tratamento[1291,1298,1326-1329]

A paromomicina foi relatada como eficaz contra *Cryptosporidium* em um gato. No entanto, a eficácia do medicamento é provavelmente fraca, e ele pode causar lesão renal aguda e uremia. Tilosina e azitromicina são opções, mas os efeitos positivos podem decorrer do tratamento de outros agentes infecciosos. A nitazoxanida parece ser tão eficaz quanto em humanos, mas, felizmente, a doença é em geral autolimitante em animais imunocompetentes e não necessita de nenhum tratamento específico.

Giardia sp.

Epidemiologia[361,990,1031,1032,1183,1190,1293,1301, 1314,1316,1319,1320,1330-1369]

Giardia sp., anteriormente denominada G. *lamblia*, pode infectar cães e gatos (ver Capítulo 221). Estudos epidemiológicos moleculares indicam que existem sete genótipos (A-G), mas os que infectam cães (C e D [*G. canis*]) e gatos (F [*G. felis*]) não são os tipicamente encontrados em infecções humanas (A [*G. duodenalis*] e B [*G. enterica*]). Por outro lado, gatos e cães podem abrigar o genótipo zoonótico A; o genótipo B foi encontrado em cães, mas não em gatos.

O parasita geralmente é transmitido pela via fecal-oral. Os oocistos ingeridos excisam no ID superior, e os trofozoítos se ligam à mucosa intestinal, do duodeno ao íleo. Após a multiplicação dos trofozoítos, os oocistos são eliminados nas fezes 1 a 2 semanas após a infecção.

Prevalência[356,1183,1199,1200,1203,1204,1209,1210,1219,1287,1321,1364,1370-1392]

A prevalência da infecção em estudos com cães depende da região geográfica, do método de diagnóstico e da idade e estado de saúde do animal, variando de menos de 2 a 100% em canis. Os casos de infecção em gatos são menos comuns.

Achados clínicos[1363,1393-1397]

A maioria das infecções é assintomática, mas os sinais podem variar de diarreia aguda leve e autolimitante a diarreia grave ou crônica do ID associada à perda de peso.

Diagnóstico[340,342-344,348,412,590,1307,1315,1382,1398-1406]

Giardia pode ser vista na superfície das biopsias intestinais, mas a sensibilidade é baixa, pois podem ser perdidas durante o processamento; o número de células caliciformes costuma aumentar. A infecção também pode ser diagnosticada pela demonstração de trofozoítos móveis no suco duodenal ou em um esfregaço fecal muito fresco. A identificação de oocistos nas fezes por flutuação com sulfato de zinco é preferível, mas a eliminação de oocistos ocorre de forma intermitente; portanto, três análises fecais em 5 dias são necessárias para uma sensibilidade de 95% (ver Capítulo 81). Antígeno de *Giardia* também pode ser detectado por meio de testes de ELISA fecal (teste SNAP *Giardia*, ProSpecT *Giardia* ensaio em microplaca), que tem 95% de especificidade, mas sensibilidade de aproximadamente 90% (ver Capítulo 221). Esse pode ser o método preferido de técnicos inexperientes, em comparação à flutuação com sulfato de zinco. IFA fecal e PCR também estão disponíveis.

Tratamento[714,718,1328,1332,1407-1428]

Metronidazol 25 mg/kg VO, a cada 12 h por 5 dias foi o medicamento mais comumente usado para tratar a infecção por *Giardia* em pequenos animais. Ronidazol pode ser usado, mas tem efeitos colaterais. Metronidazol elimina a infecção de *Giardia* em aproximadamente dois terços dos casos, mas pode causar efeitos colaterais neurológicos nessas doses altas, especialmente em gatos. A eficácia pode ser aumentada com a suplementação de metronidazol com silimarina. O fenbendazol (50 mg/kg VO, a cada 12 h por 3 a 5 dias) geralmente elimina a infecção por *Giardia* e pode ser combinado com o metronidazol para resolver os sinais clínicos e liberação de cistos. O albendazol não é recomendado, porque está associado a intoxicação da medula óssea. A eficácia do febantel (em um produto combinado com praziquantel e pirantel) é discutida, mas é provável que a nitazoxanida seja eficaz, e secnidazol só precisa ser administrado uma vez. A descontaminação dos pelos do paciente por banho e do ambiente por limpeza a vapor ou com compostos quaternários de amônio é recomendada para prevenir a reinfecção. Vacinas de *Giardia* não estão mais disponíveis, e a administração de probióticos não mostrou nenhum benefício para eliminar a infecção.

Prognóstico

O prognóstico geralmente é bom, mas alguns pacientes podem exigir vários tratamentos para eliminar a infecção, porque a reinfecção é um problema comum. A reativação de uma infecção latente pela administração de corticosteroides também foi relatada.

REAÇÕES ADVERSAS AOS ALIMENTOS

Uma reação adversa aos alimentos é uma resposta repetida e deletéria a um componente da dieta. Pode ser a manifestação de uma reação imunológica a um antígeno da dieta (*i. e.*, uma alergia alimentar verdadeira, também chamada de hibersensibilidade) ou uma reação não imunológica (ou seja, intolerância). Embora a alergia alimentar e a intolerância difiram em sua etiopatogênese, os sinais clínicos são semelhantes, e a abordagem no tratamento – exclusão do componente alimentar ofensivo – é a mesma. A intolerância alimentar pode estar associada a um único ingrediente de um alimento preparado, como lactose ou conservantes, que pode estar presente em alimentos imunologicamente não relacionados. Em contrapartida, a alergia confirmada a um alimento específico pode se estender a alimentos relacionados. Em humanos, a intolerância alimentar é diagnosticada com mais frequência do que a hipersensibilidade, mas sua verdadeira prevalência em pequenos animais é desconhecida.

Testes de exclusão de dieta são necessários para diagnosticar tanto a alergia quanto a intolerância alimentar, mas não as diferenciam.

Alergia alimentar/hipersensibilidade (ver Capítulos 10, 186 e 191)[287,288,1429-1437]

Uma doença cutânea pruriginosa é a manifestação mais comumente relatada de alergia alimentar, mas a verdadeira prevalência da doença intestinal é incerta, porque nenhum teste indireto fácil e confiável está disponível, e até mesmo uma resposta positiva a uma exclusão da dieta não é uma prova absoluta. Isso ocorre porque outras causas de sinais GI podem responder, por motivos não alérgicas, à manipulação da dieta (Boxe 276.9). O manejo da alergia alimentar é simples – oferecer qualquer alimento que não contenha o alergênio –, mas a dificuldade está no reconhecimento inicial de que a alergia alimentar está presente, e então na identificação do que deve ser excluído (ver Capítulo 186).

Mecanismos[1438-1454]

Hipóteses atuais de alergia alimentar propõem um mecanismo ou uma combinação destes que levam à quebra da tolerância oral: barreira mucosa inadequada, microbioma anormal, apresentação anormal de antígenos da dieta para o sistema imune da mucosa ou desregulação do sistema imune. Tais hipóteses poderiam explicar tanto a suscetibilidade genética à alergia e ao seu desenvolvimento após uma lesão GI primária que danifica a barreira da mucosa, quanto a enterite viral que pode danificar o sistema imune e a barreira mucosa. Em vez da tolerância, uma resposta imune ativa pode então ocorrer direcionada para antígenos presentes (*i. e.*, sensível a antígenos da dieta) e envolve muitos mecanismos, incluindo reações do tipo I (mediada por IgE, imediata), tipo III (mediada por imunocomplexos) e tipo IV (hipersensibilidade retardada). A modulação da resposta também depende da composição do microbioma. Uma associação recente entre a ingestão de determinado alimento e o aparecimento de sinais é sugestiva de uma reação do tipo I. Em reações mistas ou retardadas, a demora entre a ingestão de alimentos e o início dos sinais obscurece qualquer ligação causal, particularmente se a ingestão repetida causar doença crônica.

Sinais clínicos[1455-1460]

Sinais clínicos de alergia alimentar em geral envolvem a pele ou o trato GI (Boxe 276.10); sinais cutâneos e gastrintestinais podem ocorrer simultaneamente, mas são relatos raros. Sinais sistêmicos (anorexia, letargia) são registrados raramente, assim como urticária-angioedema e até mesmo anafilaxia (ver Capítulo 137). Sinais como comportamento anormal e asma são, em grande parte, observacionais, mas há relatos de que lambidas anormais de superfícies (p. ex., concreto) cessam com a introdução de uma dieta de exclusão (ver Capítulo 9). O principal sinal cutâneo de alergia alimentar é o prurido; outras lesões de pele, com exceção de complexos eosinofílicos em gatos, surgem por meio de autotrauma e pioderma secundário. Os sinais de doença GI alérgica a alimentos não são patognomônicos e incluem vômito, diarreia, dor abdominal, flatulência, borborigmos e perda de peso ou falha no crescimento.

Abordagem diagnóstica[443,525,759,1461-1464]

Após a investigação preliminar negativa (exames básicos e fecais, imagem) e um ensaio com fenbendazol, o diagnóstico da sensibilidade alimentar é feito a partir da resposta à manipulação da dieta. Embora a análise detalhada de biopsias intestinais de cães com doença responsiva a alimentos mostre uma tendência para o aumento de eosinófilos na mucosa, um ensaio de dieta

---

Boxe 276.10 Sinais clínicos reconhecidos como manifestações de alergia alimentar

Sinais sistêmicos
- Anorexia
- Letargia
- Linfadenopatia periférica (gatos)
- Urticária-angioedema
- Anafilaxia.

Sinais cutâneos
- Pápulas primárias
- Eritroderma
- Prurido e autotrauma
  - Pioderma secundário
  - Descamação
- Otite externa
- Dermatite miliar (gatos)
- Complexo de granuloma eosinofílico (gatos).

Sinais gastrintestinais
- Desconforto/dor abdominal ou "cólica"
- Vômito
- Hematêmese
- Diarreia
- Sinais semelhantes ao intestino delgado
- Sinais semelhantes a colite
- Apetite alterado
  - Lambidas em superfícies
  - Pica
  - Perda de peso e/ou retardo de crescimento.

Não comprovado
- Asma
- Mudanças comportamentais
- Claudicação.

Boxe 276.9 Condições que podem melhorar clinicamente em resposta à modificação da dieta

- Gastrite crônica
- Insuficiência pancreática exócrina
- Alergia alimentar
- Intolerância alimentar
- Distúrbios de esvaziamento gástrico
- Refluxo gastresofágico
- Doença inflamatória intestinal
- Linfangiectasia
- Dieta nutricionalmente inadequada
- Pancreatite
- Desvio portossistêmico
- Supercrescimento bacteriano no intestino delgado.

é recomendado, seja antes da biopsia intestinal em pacientes que se alimentam e não estão hipoproteinêmicos, seja após a biopsia que revela inflamação intestinal. Os sinais clínicos devem ser resolvidos com a exclusão do componente ofensivo da dieta e a reexposição à dieta original. Ainda faltam critérios objetivos para julgar tal resposta: monitorar as mudanças na permeabilidade intestinal ou os padrões de fluxo de sangue arterial mesentérico através da US Doppler não é específico o suficiente, e mesmo a repetição da biopsia não mostra necessariamente a resolução de qualquer alteração histológica, embora isso possa ser porque ela demore mais do que a melhora dos sinais clínicos. Uma resposta clínica positiva a uma dieta de exclusão pode ocorrer por acaso ou refletir uma alergia ou intolerância, cuja confirmação do diagnóstico requer um novo desafio, mas muitos tutores o recusam.

Testes sorológicos.[1465-1477] Foram feitas tentativas para desenvolver testes para alergia alimentar que evitem ensaios com dieta, mas, infelizmente, nenhum na medicina veterinária é confiável. IgE e/ou IgG sérica específica para antígenos alimentares pode ser dosada *in vitro*, mas uma avaliação crítica sugere que esses testes não são úteis, pois existem discrepâncias entre laboratórios e os resultados não se correlacionam com a resposta do paciente a um ensaio de dieta de exclusão. O teste cutâneo intradérmico e o teste de contato também não se mostraram confiáveis no diagnóstico de doença GI alérgica a alimentos. O teste gastroscópico de sensibilidade alimentar (TGSA), em que os antígenos da dieta são instilados diretamente na mucosa gástrica, teoricamente deveria dar resultados mais específicos em casos com sinais GI, porém a correlação entre o TGSA e o desafio clínico é fraca. A utilização da mucosa do cólon como superfície-teste (teste de provocação colonoscópica de alergênio [PCA]) poderia ser mais reprodutível, mas não foi amplamente adotada.

Teste de dieta de exclusão.[1478-1482] O princípio de uma dieta de exclusão (eliminação) é fornecer componentes aos quais o animal não foi prévia ou pelo menos recentemente exposto (ver Capítulo 186). Essa dieta deve ser a única fonte de nutrição durante o teste, e todas as guloseimas e suplementos devem ser evitados. A concordância total do tutor é essencial. Opções incluem dietas preparadas em casa, dietas de proteína de fonte única e dietas de proteína hidrolisada. As caseiras têm sido preferidas às comerciais, pois há relatos de recaída quando os pacientes são alimentados com uma dieta comercial equivalente, e análises de alimentos mostraram proteínas não declaradas em algumas comerciais. No entanto, muitos clínicos recomendam o uso inicial de uma dieta comercial, porque a conveniência auxilia na concordância do tutor ao teste.

Em dietas de proteína de fonte única, o alimento contém apenas uma fonte de proteína e uma fonte de carboidrato. Se for caseira, é improvável que seja nutricionalmente equilibrada, mas em geral não é algo importante para a curta duração do ensaio. No entanto, alimentos específicos para filhotes, embora convenientes, não são adequados para gatos, porque são relativamente deficientes em taurina e muitas vezes contêm cebola em pó, que pode causar anemia hemolítica por corpúsculo de Heinz. Cordeiro ou frango com arroz têm sido as escolhas-padrão, mas dada a maior diversidade de alimentos para animais de companhia, o paciente pode já ter sido exposto a essas opções, portanto elas nem sempre são apropriadas, e fontes mais alternativas tornaram-se um requisito. Uma alternativa para dietas preparadas em casa é o uso de uma dieta comercial de exclusão, e uma ampla variedade agora está disponível, contendo diferentes fontes de proteínas (p. ex., frango, soja, salmão, bagre, veado ou pato) e carboidratos (arroz, milho, tapioca ou batata).

Dietas de proteína hidrolisada,[763,1483-1491] que geralmente são baseadas em proteína de frango ou soja, são dietas de exclusão alternativas e estão amplamente disponíveis. A princípio, o processo hidrolítico divide proteínas em componentes cujo peso molecular estaria abaixo do esperado para ativar uma resposta do sistema imune. Para abolir completamente toda a antigenicidade, os peptídios precisam ter menos de 1 kD, mas nesse tamanho eles quase invariavelmente têm um gosto amargo; apenas dietas analergênicas, baseadas na proteína da pena e contendo somente peptídios menores que 1 kD, estão disponíveis. No tamanho alcançado na maioria das dietas hidrolisadas (7 a 10 kD), as proteínas ainda são potencialmente antigênicas, mas são muito pequenas para fazer ligações cruzadas com moléculas de IgE em mastócitos, e, desse modo, as reações do tipo I são abolidas; no entanto, as reações do tipo IV ainda são possíveis. Dietas hidrolisadas também são substancialmente mais caras de produzir do que as de exclusão padrões, e tanto a palatabilidade quanto a concordância do tutor podem ser problemáticas. No entanto, essas dietas atualmente são a maneira mais fácil de garantir a alimentação com novos antígenos, e essa abordagem tornou-se o método preferido de muitos clínicos. Estudos sugeriram seu efeito benéfico significativo, e elas parecem ter uma vantagem sobre a tradicional dieta de exclusão de fonte única de proteína. No entanto, a falta de resolução histológica após um ensaio bem-sucedido pode indicar que o paciente tinha na verdade uma DII idiopática, e a melhora clínica foi simplesmente decorrente da alimentação mais digerível.

Um protocolo padronizado para ensaios de dieta de exclusão não foi estabelecido, e a duração ideal não é conhecida.[1432] Três semanas foram escolhidas arbitrariamente, mas é preferível estender para 6 semanas, sobretudo se houve uma resposta apenas parcial. Na verdade, casos de doença de pele decorrente de alergia alimentar podem levar até 10 semanas para responder, provavelmente porque o antígeno translocado para a pele e armazenado nas células dendríticas precisa ser eliminado. A doença GI alérgica a alimentos com frequência responde mais rápido, de forma que, felizmente, é raro precisar empregar a dieta de exclusão por esse tempo, porque pode se tornar difícil manter a observação do paciente e/ou tutor. Os testes de desafio e provocação geralmente são conduzidos por até 14 dias, mas são concluídos mais cedo se os sinais se repetirem em 2 dias consecutivos.

1. Fase de exclusão. A dieta de exclusão é fornecida como única fonte de alimento por um mínimo de 3 semanas.
2. Fase de desafio. Uma vez que a remissão é alcançada, o animal deve ser desafiado com a dieta original para demonstrar recidiva e confirmar o diagnóstico. Alguns animais podem não recidivar, talvez porque a barreira mucosa tenha sido restaurada e outras reações são evitadas. No entanto, alguns tutores recusam o desafio, especialmente se houver probabilidade de recidiva da diarreia.
3. Fases de resgate e provocação. Após a recaída durante a fase de desafio, para tutores que desejarem, uma série de testes de provocação pode ser realizada para identificar o(s) alimento(s) ofensivo(s). A remissão é recuperada por "resgate" com a dieta de exclusão original, e alimentos individuais são então introduzidos sequencialmente. Se não houver recaída, o alimento é identificado como "seguro" e o próximo alimento é testado; se houver uma recaída, o resgate é repetido, e o alimento é identificado como "inseguro".
4. Fase de manutenção. Quando todos os alimentos ofensivos, ou pelo menos os suficientemente seguros, forem identificados para permitir a escolha de uma dieta regular, o animal é mantido com uma dieta-padrão segura. Após o teste de alimentação, a maioria dos animais pode ser mantida em uma das dietas disponíveis com antígenos limitados.

Tratamento[1492]

O tratamento é simples, uma vez que o diagnóstico tenha sido feito: evitar o alimento ofensivo impede a ocorrência de sinais. Dietas comerciais geralmente são mais adequadas como manutenção e são preferíveis às refeições preparadas em casa, pois são nutricionalmente equilibradas. Manter uma dieta hidrolisada é uma alternativa cara. Imunoterapia de peptídios é usada em humanos, mas ainda não está disponível para animais.

Intolerância alimentar[1433,1434]

A gula, o "hábito catador" (*scavenging*) e a intoxicação alimentar são ocorrências comuns que podem ser consideradas exemplos de intolerância alimentar, porém com tendência a ser incidentes isolados e agudos, enquanto as intolerâncias alimentares verdadeiras são repetíveis, ainda que possam ser previsíveis ou imprevisíveis. As intolerâncias previsíveis ocorrem em qualquer animal após a ingestão de um alimento contaminado, de uma toxina reconhecida ou de quantidades excessivas de alimentos. Já as intolerâncias alimentares imprevisíveis, embora repetíveis em um indivíduo suscetível, são reações idiossincráticas, cujas razões incluem diferenças, de base genética ou não, nas atividades de enzimas intestinais, permeabilidade intestinal, metabolismo pós-absorção, estabilidade dos mastócitos e microbioma.

Mecanismos

A maioria dos mecanismos sugeridos de intolerância alimentar é explorada de estudos em humanos e pode ou não ser válida para cães e gatos.

Intoxicação alimentar. A intoxicação alimentar é mais provável em cães que fazem catação e é causada por alimentos com toxinas, contaminados com microrganismos produtores de toxinas ou infectados por microrganismos que se multiplicam e, subsequentemente, causam sinais gastrintestinais agudos, como a campilobacteriose.

Intolerâncias farmacológicas. Essas intolerâncias são resultado da presença de compostos farmacologicamente ativos (p. ex., envenenamento por chocolate com metilxantinas). Em humanos, intolerâncias podem resultar de compostos de ocorrência natural (aminas vasoativas, glicosídeos cardíacos, alcaloides vegetais e alucinógenos e tremórgenos fúngicos) ou substâncias produzidas pelo metabolismo bacteriano intestinal.

Mecanismos pseudoalérgicos.[1493,1494] Essas reações adversas são mediadas por histamina, mas surgem de mecanismos não imunológicos. Uma alta concentração de histamina pode estar presente naturalmente em alguns alimentos, como atum, cavala e alguns alimentos comerciais para cães, ou em razão de contaminação, por exemplo de queijo ou peixe enlatado, com microrganismos produtores de histamina, como *Proteus* ou *Klebsiella*. Alguns alimentos, como crustáceos, morangos e alguns aditivos alimentares, como a tartrazina, podem causar liberação de histamina de mastócitos sem mediação de IgE. Esse mecanismo é bem documentado em humanos, mas não em pequenos animais.

Reações metabólicas.[40,252,1495] São pouco documentadas em pequenos animais. Má absorção de carboidratos e intolerância podem ser características de uma série de doenças intestinais, e a intolerância específica à lactose pode estar associada à sua deficiência. No desmame, as atividades da lactase diminuem, especialmente em gatos, e os animais podem se tornar intolerantes se alimentados com leite em excesso. Se um animal tem uma doença de ID subjacente, produtos lácteos devem ser evitados, porque a atividade da lactase é reduzida ainda mais. No entanto, alergia a proteína do leite bovino ou doença intestinal subclínica prévia também pode explicar as reações adversas ao leite.

Sinais clínicos[1496]

Os sinais clínicos de intolerância alimentar incluem vômito, diarreia e aparente desconforto abdominal. No entanto, prurido e até anafilaxia são possíveis se a liberação de histamina estiver envolvida. Problemas comportamentais (ver Capítulo 9) podem ser responsivos à dieta por meio de mecanismos não imunológicos.

Diagnóstico

O único meio confiável de diagnosticar a intolerância a alimentos é monitorando a resposta a um teste de dieta. Novamente, tais ensaios não definem o mecanismo patogênico exato envolvido. Os resultados dos testes sorológicos de alergia alimentar são irrelevantes.

Enteropatia sensível ao glúten[623,1497-1510]

A doença intestinal causada pelo glúten do trigo foi mostrada na raça Setter Irlandês. Os animais afetados normalmente são encaminhados para avaliação veterinária em razão do baixo ganho de peso e diarreia crônica intermitente após o desmame. No entanto, a idade do cão quando o glúten é introduzido e a quantidade afetam a expressão da doença, com alguns cães se tornando assintomáticos com o tempo.

A condição se assemelha à doença celíaca (sensibilidade ao glúten) em humanos, embora os sinais clínicos e a atrofia da mucosa sejam menos intensos. A doença celíaca mostra uma clara predisposição genética, assim como a enteropatia sensível ao glúten (ESG) é uma doença autossômica recessiva hereditária na raça Setter Irlandês. No entanto, ao contrário da doença celíaca humana, não há relação com os genes *DQA* e *DQB* do complexo principal histocompatibilidade, e a patogênese é diferente. A ESG pode afetar outras raças de cães, mas não foi relatada em gatos. A sensibilidade ao glúten foi sugerida em cães da raça Wheaten Terriers de Pelo Macio com EPP e nefropatia perdedora de proteínas.

Patogênese[430,1511-1524]

A patogênese da ESG no Setter Irlandês permanece caracterizada de forma incompleta. O glúten ingerido ou é diretamente tóxico para a mucosa intestinal ou induz uma reação imunológica adversa. Em contraste com a doença celíaca, onde há reatividade cruzada entre os peptídios do glúten e a transglutaminase tecidual, respostas de células T e imunoglobulina ao glúten ou aos antígenos da mucosa não são observados nesses animais. No entanto, o envolvimento do sistema imunológico é sugerido pelo aumento das células T CD4 + e diminuição das populações CD8 + na lâmina própria. Os sinais clínicos e alterações histológicas e bioquímicas são resolvidos com uma dieta sem glúten, e uma recaída ocorre quando dietas que contenham glúten são reintroduzidas. Uma permeabilidade anormal da mucosa precede o desenvolvimento da doença em cães afetados dessa raça, sugerindo que uma anormalidade na barreira mucosa poderia permitir a entrada anormal de peptídios do glúten.

Diagnóstico[1498,1502,1525]

As alterações histológicas mostram atrofia parcial das vilosidades e infiltração de linfócitos intraepiteliais, com um infiltrado variável na lâmina própria. A remissão dessas alterações e dos sinais clínicos ocorre quando uma dieta sem glúten é fornecida, e ocorre recaída no desafio do trigo e do glúten.

Tratamento

O sucesso do tratamento depende da exclusão de glúten da dieta. Alimentos patenteados sem glúten (ou seja, trigo, cevada ou centeio) são recomendados.

SUPERCRESCIMENTO BACTERIANO NO INTESTINO DELGADO E DIARREIA IDIOPÁTICA ANTIBIÓTICO-RESPONSIVA

Definições[255,469,1526-1538]

O supercrescimento bacteriano verdadeiro no intestino delgado (SBID) é definido por um aumento no número absoluto de bactérias na parte superior do ID durante um estado de jejum. A população bacteriana normal do ID é controlada por uma série de mecanismos, e o crescimento excessivo é a proliferação descontrolada dessas bactérias em vez de uma infecção específica. Na medicina humana, o SBID primário como causa de diarreia e a síndrome do intestino irritável permanecem controversos, mas é aceito que ocorram de modo secundário a distúrbios que interferem nos mecanismos normais de controle (Boxe 276.11). Historicamente, o termo "SBID *idiopático*" foi usado para descrever

SEÇÃO 18 • Doença Gastrintestinal

Boxe 276.11 Causas secundárias do supercrescimento bacteriano no intestino delgado

Estrutura anatômica anormal
- Alça cega (congênita ou induzida cirurgicamente)
- Ressecção cirúrgica da válvula ileocólica.

Acloridria
- Bloqueadores de ácido, especialmente inibidores da bomba de prótons
- Espontânea (gastrite atrófica).

Insuficiência pancreática exócrina
Distúrbio de motilidade
- Funcional
- Hipotireoidismo
- Pseudo-obstrução intestinal.

Doença da mucosa
- Giardíase crônica
- Sensibilidade alimentar
- Doença inflamatória intestinal (causa ou efeito?)
- Patógenos primários ocultos.

Obstrução intestinal parcial
- Intussuscepção crônica
- Estenose
- Tumor.

uma condição responsiva a antibióticos em cães de raças grandes, especialmente o Pastor-Alemão, mas nenhuma causa subjacente pôde ser encontrada, e o supercrescimento foi reivindicado como a causa provável. Uma resposta positiva a muitos antibióticos geralmente é observada, mas uma enteropatia responsiva apenas a tilosina foi relatada. Por outro lado, em razão das preocupações sobre a existência de um aumento verdadeiro no número de bactérias em casos idiopáticos caninos, o nome alternativo de diarreia responsiva a antibióticos (DRA) foi adotado, enquanto SBID é mais considerado como um sinal clínico ou um mecanismo patogênico secundário. Embora os gatos possam sofrer de SBID secundário, uma condição idiopática responsiva a antibióticos semelhante àquela vista em cães não foi documentada, mas a eficácia do metronidazol na DII leve às vezes é notada.

O limite máximo normal de bactérias duodenais (número de unidades formadoras de colônias cultivadas por mililitro [UFC/mℓ] de suco duodenal) em humanos é inferior a 10^5 UFC/mℓ de bactérias totais ou a 10^4 UFC/mℓ de bactérias anaeróbias. Esse número foi incorretamente extrapolado para cães, e estudos subsequentes mostraram que uma contagem total de 10^5 UFC/mℓ ou superior é comumente encontrada em cães assintomáticos. Portanto, embora um SBID verdadeiro possa ocorrer secundariamente a condições equivalentes às dos humanos, a premissa para definir uma doença idiopática e responsiva a antibióticos como SBID com base na linha de corte numérica original é falha. Neste capítulo, pacientes com uma causa subjacente documentada são diagnosticados com SIBO secundário, e o termo "DRA *idiopática*" é usado para condições idiopáticas responsivas a antibióticos.

Etiologia e patogênese[255,1539-1541]

Diarreia responsiva a antibióticos idiopática[255,760,1542-1562]

Existem muitas hipóteses quanto à causa da DRA idiopática. Originalmente, elas eram baseadas na crença de que um SBID verdadeiro estava presente. Mecanismos que permitem SBID verdadeiros, como motilidade anormal do ID, não foram comprovados em cães ou gatos. Acloridria secundária ao tratamento com omeprazol altera qualitativamente o microbioma em cães, mas não se correlaciona à doença. Hipóteses mais recentes focam nas interações hospedeiro-bactéria.

Outro mecanismo hipotético é a deficiência de IgA secretória (SIgA). Estudos que documentaram concentrações séricas baixas de IgA são irrelevantes, já que a secreção de SIgA na mucosa não reflete as concentrações séricas. Uma deficiência absoluta de IgA fecal associada a infecção por EPEC foi mostrada uma vez em cães da raça Pastor-Alemão, mas não foi reproduzida por outros pesquisadores. Além disso, uma deficiência secundária de SIgA poderia existir nessa raça, explicando a baixa produção de IgA por biopsias intestinais cultivadas *in vitro*, apesar do aumento do número de plasmócitos IgA + da mucosa. A causa da deficiência não é clara, mas um defeito complexo é provável, envolvendo anormalidades tanto na produção quanto na liberação de IgA do plasmócito ou na via de translocação de IgA através do epitélio durante a secreção. Nenhuma anormalidade na cadeia J ou na expressão de pIgR foi detectada. Os cães dessa raça possuem uma variante específica do gene IgHA e quatro mutações no código da região de dobradiça da cadeia pesada de IgA que podem afetar a eficácia da molécula ou sua suscetibilidade à proteólise. Ainda assim, todo Pastor-Alemão, independentemente do seu estado de saúde, é da mesma variante (C), e é provável que esse achado seja apenas um fenômeno específico da raça.

Cães com DRA têm aumento de células T CD4 + na lâmina própria e da expressão de certas citocinas, sugerindo uma desregulação imunológica. Hipermetilação de genes controladores da troca para IgA foi mostrada na DII e está associada à diminuição da expressão de IgA na mucosa e, talvez, uma perda de tolerância a bactérias endógenas. Alternativamente, um polimorfismo em TLR-5 (o receptor para flagelina bacteriana) é sugerido em cães da raça Pastor-Alemão com fístula perianal e DRA. Tal hipótese é apoiada pela resolução dos sinais clínicos e diminuição da expressão de citocinas, sem um declínio no número de bactérias, por meio de antibacterianos. O fato de os antibacterianos mais eficazes também serem aqueles com propriedades imunomoduladoras (p. ex., oxitetraciclina, metronidazol, tilosina) também pode apoiar essa hipótese. Além disso, há evidências práticas de que alguns Pastores-Alemães afetados por DRA na juventude desenvolveram DII mais tarde. Uma hipótese alternativa é que um patógeno não identificado esteja envolvido; candidatos incluem *Helicobacter* spp. intestinal ou *E. coli* enteropatogênica. A predisposição da raça Pastor-Alemão para DRA poderia então ser explicada por uma infecção no período perinatal e/ou suscetibilidade genética à infecção como resultado de polimorfismos do MHC II ou TLR.

Um aumento verdadeiro no número de bactérias no ID pode causar má absorção e diarreia por muitos mecanismos: competição por nutrientes, produção de nutrientes para criar produtos que provocam diarreia (p. ex., sais biliares desconjugados e ácidos graxos hidroxilados) e/ou dano direto a mucosa. No entanto, esses mecanismos podem não ser relevantes na DRA idiopática, porque não há aumento nos números, embora mudanças reversíveis na atividade enzimática da mucosa sejam observadas em cães que respondem a antibióticos.

Supercrescimento bacteriano do intestino delgado secundário[232,1563-1565]

SBID verdadeiro pode ocorrer de modo secundário a doenças que resultam em excesso de substrato no lúmen intestinal, doenças que afetam a depuração de bactérias ou distúrbios morfológicos ou funcionais da mucosa (ver Boxe 276.11).

Apresentação clínica

Diarreia idiopática responsiva a antibióticos

A DRA idiopática é mais comumente observada em cães jovens da raça Pastor-Alemão, embora casos tenham sido relatados em outras raças grandes, mas não em gatos. A microbiota presente é composta predominantemente de bactérias aeróbias ou anaeróbias, mas tende a ser uma população mista com estafilococos, estreptococos, coliformes, enterococos, corinebactérias e anaeróbios como bacteroides, fusobactérias e clostrídios. Essas bactérias geralmente são comensais encontradas na orofaringe, ID e IG. A cultura de bactérias fecais não pode ser correlacionada com a microbiota bacteriana do ID, nem ser usada para o diagnóstico dessa condição.

Os cães afetados apresentam com maior frequência sinais de diarreia crônica intermitente acompanhada de perda de peso e/ou crescimento retardado, muitas vezes associado à produção intestinal excessiva de gás, manifestada como borborigmos e flatulências. No entanto, vômito e sinais de colite são relatados, e, ocasionalmente, os cães têm crescimento retardado, mas não apresentam diarreia evidente. O apetite é variável; os cães mais afetados têm polifagia, pica e/ou coprofagia, mas alguns são anorexígenos, talvez em associação à deficiência adquirida de cobalamina. Uma resposta positiva para antibióticos é esperada, e a condição pode piorar se corticosteroides forem administrados. Os principais diagnósticos diferenciais são IPE e DII, ambos comuns na raça.

Supercrescimento bacteriano do intestino delgado secundário

SBID secundário pode ocorrer após muitas condições primárias (ver Boxe 276.11), mas os sinais clínicos relacionam-se de início com a condição subjacente. Quando SBID desenvolve-se secundário a uma obstrução parcial ou dismotilidade focal, o número de bactérias pode ser superior a 10^9 UFC/mℓ. No entanto, sinais de SBID secundário também podem ser vistos e são indistinguíveis dos de DRA idiopática, com predomínio da diarreia. Os sinais clínicos podem ser intermitentes, porque a diarreia regular pode eliminar temporariamente o crescimento excessivo. Usando o ponto de corte numérico histórico de 10^5 UFC/mℓ de bactérias totais, o SIBD secundário foi considerado comum em enteropatias crônicas. Na realidade, esses números são normais, e o SIBD secundário verdadeiro é incomum, com exceção de SBID secundário a IPE. Foi documentado um aumento no número de bactérias no ID em IPE induzida experimentalmente, mas diminuiu após tratamento com reposição enzimática. Portanto, em muitos casos, o SIBD propriamente dito não tem importância. No entanto, uma proporção de casos de ocorrência natural de IPE responde de forma subótima à suplementação de apenas enzima pancreática e pode exigir terapia antibiótica concomitante. Dado que a maioria dos cães afetados com IPE é da raça Pastor-Alemão, não está claro se esse é o resultado do SBID secundário ou de DRA idiopática concomitante.

Diagnóstico[588,1528,1532,1566,1567]

O diagnóstico de SBID e DRA é controverso. Em todos os casos, é fundamental que uma investigação completa seja conduzida para eliminar as causas de SBID secundário antes que o paciente seja tratado com antibacterianos. Distúrbios sistêmicos devem ser descartados com um conjunto de exames gerais, a IPE eliminada por ensaio de IST sérica (ver Capítulo 290) e um diagnóstico por imagem realizado para identificar obstruções intestinais parciais (ver Capítulo 88). Um exame fecal de patógenos parasitários e bacterianos conhecidos é obrigatório (ver Capítulo 81).

A cultura quantitativa de aeróbios e anaeróbios do suco duodenal foi o padrão-ouro para o diagnóstico de SBID, mas não é mais recomendado pelos motivos descritos anteriormente. Esse excesso de diagnóstico de SBID provavelmente explica por que ele foi relatado em 50% dos cães com doença intestinal crônica. Cultura de biopsias endoscópicas não mostrou ser útil.

Testes indiretos para SBID/DRA

Os testes indiretos incluem marcadores bioquímicos séricos e análise do hidrogênio respiratório.

Concentrações séricas de folato e cobalamina.[405,469,1568-1570] As bactérias podem sintetizar folato e evitar a absorção de cobalamina. Portanto, SBID está associado ao aumento da concentração sérica de folato, à diminuição da concentração de cobalamina ou a ambos, como visto em humanos com SBID secundário. No entanto, estudos têm mostrado que esses testes são de valor limitado no diagnóstico de DRA idiopática. O desempenho fraco pode estar relacionado a fatores da dieta, à presença de doenças concomitantes, ao uso de medicamentos que alteram as concentrações séricas de vitaminas ou apenas ao fato de o número de bactérias não necessariamente ter aumentado. Quaisquer alterações observadas de folato e cobalamina séricos na IPE podem refletir a disfunção pancreática em vez de SIBD secundário. Embora frequentemente sejam os únicos disponíveis para os profissionais, esses testes em geral não auxiliam no diagnóstico de DRA idiopática e não são recomendados.

Ácidos biliares não conjugados séricos.[469,470] Um estudo preliminar em cães sugeriu que a concentração dos ácidos biliares não conjugados séricos (ABNCS) aumentou no SBID em razão da desconjugação de sais biliares pelas bactérias. No entanto, estudos posteriores mostraram que as concentrações de ABNCS não eram sensíveis nem específicas para diagnóstico de DRA idiopática.

Outros testes bioquímicos.[473] Uma avaliação do aumento da quantidade de um produto bacteriano produzido naturalmente (p. ex., indican urinário, p-nitrosonaftol) ou após administração oral de uma substância de teste (sulfapiridina, PABA) poderia diagnosticar SBID, mas esses testes não são confiáveis.

Excreção de hidrogênio respiratório.[1571] A fermentação bacteriana no trato intestinal libera hidrogênio, que, após absorção sistêmica, é exalado e pode ser medido em amostras de ar expirado. Teoricamente, o SBID resultaria em uma elevada concentração de hidrogênio respiratório de repouso e/ou um pico inicial (ou dobrado) de excreção de hidrogênio após a ingestão de uma refeição de teste. No entanto, concentrações aumentadas de hidrogênio na respiração também podem ser vistas com má absorção de carboidratos ou tempo de trânsito orocecal diminuído, e a falta de especificidade fez o teste, em grande parte, ser abandonado.

Permeabilidade intestinal[1572-1574]

A permeabilidade intestinal pode ser anormal no SBID e melhorar após tratamento antibiótico. No entanto, tais achados não são patognomônicos para SIBO secundário nem DRA idiopática e não estão prontamente disponíveis na prática.

Ausência de alterações histológicas na biopsia intestinal

As biopsias na maioria das vezes são histologicamente normais ou mostram apenas anormalidades sutis na DRA. No entanto, tais achados não podem ser diagnósticos, porque outras condições produzem resultados semelhantes, e tais achados foram descritos como "enteropatias de alterações mínimas".

Resposta empírica aos antibióticos

O atual teste diagnóstico definitivo para DRA idiopática é, logicamente, a resposta à terapia empírica. No entanto, uma resposta clínica aos antibacterianos não é específica e, de fato, pode ser vista com DII, diarreia infecciosa e até mesmo uma série de doenças não entéricas, como anomalias portovasculares. Além disso, a resposta à terapia antibiótica não discrimina a DRA idiopática do SBID secundário, e a DRA é um diagnóstico válido apenas depois que investigações diagnósticas completas eliminaram outras causas possíveis.

Identificação de DRA idiopática[469]

Tanto testes diretos quanto indiretos preconizados para o diagnóstico de SBID idiopático são de valor limitado. Portanto, o único teste de diagnóstico disponível para DRA é a resposta a um tratamento antibacteriano. Contudo, tal processo de diagnóstico é apropriado somente após uma investigação completa que elimine todas as outras causas de responsividade a antibacterianos. Há quatro critérios sugeridos para um diagnóstico de DRA idiopática: (1) resposta clínica positiva ao teste com antibióticos; (2) recidiva dos sinais após a retirada dos antibióticos; (3) remissão na reintrodução de antibióticos; e (4) eliminação de outras causas com base nos resultados de outros testes de diagnóstico e avaliação histopatológica.

Identificação do supercrescimento bacteriano do intestino delgado secundário

Embora muitos testes estejam disponíveis para documentar o supercrescimento, na prática é mais importante identificar a causa subjacente.

Tratamento

Diarreia responsiva a antibióticos idiopática[75,102,107,1529-1531,1539,1545,1575-1579]

Antibacterianos. Nenhuma cura está disponível para DRA idiopática, mas os sinais podem ser controlados com antibióticos. Um antibacteriano de amplo espectro é indicado; escolhas adequadas incluem oxitetraciclina (10 a 20 mg/kg VO, a cada 8 h), metronidazol (10 a 15 mg/kg VO, a cada 12 h) e tilosina (20 mg/kg VO, a cada 8 a 12 h). A oxitetraciclina (OTC) é barata, mas não está disponível universalmente. Ela pode ser dada com os alimentos, porque a absorção sistêmica não é necessária, mas não pode ser usada antes da erupção dos dentes permanentes, pois causa manchas no esmalte. Alguns autores criticaram seu uso, porque está associado ao rápido desenvolvimento de resistência a antibióticos mediada por plasmídeo. No entanto, dada a eficácia a longo prazo na maioria dos casos, a OTC pode não agir por meio de suas propriedades antibacterianas, especialmente por não reduzir significativamente o número de bactérias no ID, mas fornecer pressão seletiva sobre a microbiota intestinal, colaborando para o estabelecimento de bactérias menos nocivas, da mesma forma que a tilosina mostrou aumentar os lactobacilos e enterococos fecais. Alternativamente, a OTC pode exercer efeitos imunomoduladores, que foram sugeridos para esse grupo de antibióticos e outros antibacterianos comumente usados para o tratamento da DRA, como o metronidazol e a tilosina. A OTC tem mostrado exercer um efeito sobre a atividade das enzimas da membrana apical dos enterócitos, mas não se sabe se por meio da inibição da atividade de bactérias.

Qualquer que seja o antibacteriano escolhido, um tratamento de 4 a 6 semanas é administrado inicialmente, embora o antibiótico possa ser trocado após 2 semanas se a resposta tiver sido abaixo do ideal. Em alguns casos, a interrupção prematura do tratamento pode levar à recaída, e uma terapia prolongada frequentemente é necessária. Em alguns animais, há uma recaída tardia, que ocorre vários meses após a interrupção dos antibióticos e requer cursos repetidos ou terapia prolongada. Muitas vezes a eficácia é mantida, apesar da redução na dose ou na frequência de administração: um antibacteriano, 1 vez/dia, pode manter o controle dos sinais, e tilosina a 5 mg/kg mostrou ser tão eficaz quanto o padrão de dose de 20 mg/kg. Os cães também conseguem "superar" o problema com a idade, como resultado da diminuição na ingestão calórica ou de um sistema imune maduro e desenvolvido da mucosa. Em função de preocupações de saúde pública com o uso prolongado de antibióticos, é apropriado interromper o tratamento periodicamente para determinar sua necessidade.

Tratamentos auxiliares.[79,103,591,773,775-777,1577,1580,1581] A manipulação da dieta pode ser um tratamento auxiliar útil tanto para DRA idiopática quanto para SBID secundário (ver Capítulo 178). Uma dieta altamente digerível e com baixo teor de gordura é desejada para reduzir o substrato disponível para uso bacteriano. A adição de FOS tem sido defendida para reduzir o número de bactérias no ID, embora a evidência da eficácia seja

conflitante, com o maior efeito visto na microbiota do cólon. O uso de probióticos não foi avaliado exaustivamente na DRA. Por fim, se ocorrerem baixas concentrações de cobalamina sérica, a terapia parenteral com cobalamina é justificada.

Supercrescimento bacteriano do intestino delgado secundário

Embora a terapia antibacteriana melhore os sinais clínicos, o tratamento adequado para as condições subjacentes é preferível. Para IPE, a suplementação de enzimas pancreáticas pode reduzir o número de bactérias, pois as proteases exógenas têm propriedades antibacterianas (ver Capítulo 290).

DOENÇA INFLAMATÓRIA INTESTINAL

Definição[754,757,760,1544,1582-1592]

Doença inflamatória intestinal (DII) é um termo coletivo que descreve distúrbios do trato GI caracterizados por sinais GI persistentes ou recorrentes e evidência histológica de inflamação intestinal. A doença tem pouca semelhança clínica ou histologicamente com a DII humana (doença de Crohn e colite ulcerativa), mas pode compartilhar a etiologia. No entanto, o uso indiscriminado do termo DII não é recomendado, pois várias doenças estão associadas à inflamação intestinal crônica (Boxe 276.12), ao passo que, por definição, a causa é idiopática. Variações na aparência histológica da inflamação sugerem que a DII idiopática não é uma única doença (Figura 276.12), e a nomenclatura reflete meramente a distribuição anatômica e o tipo celular predominante. A inflamação pode ser confinada ao ID ou é possível existir gastroenterocolite difusa. A enterite linfoplasmocitária (ELP) é o tipo histológico mais comumente relatado; enterite eosinofílica (EE) e gastrenterite eosinofílica (GEE) são menos comuns, e a enterite granulomatosa é rara. Infiltração neutrofílica subjacente é uma característica da DII humana precoce, e enterite neutrofílica às vezes é vista em gatos, mas raramente em cães.

Apresentação clínica[780,1592-1602]

A DII idiopática é uma causa comum de vômito crônico e diarreia em cães e gatos, mas sua verdadeira incidência é desconhecida. Na realidade, é provavelmente sobrediagnosticada em

---

Boxe 276.12 Causas da inflamação crônica do intestino delgado

Infecção crônica
- *Giardia* sp.
- *Histoplasma* sp.
- *Toxoplasma* sp.
- *Mycobacterium* sp.
- Prototecose
- Pitiose
- Bactérias patogênicas (*Campylobacter*, *Salmonella* spp., *E. coli* patogênica).

Alergia alimentar
Inflamação do intestino delgado associada a outras doenças gastrintestinais primárias
- Linfoma
- Linfangiectasia.

Causas idiopáticas
- Enterite linfoplasmocitária (ELP)
- Gastroenterocolite eosinofílica (GEE)
- Enterite granulomatosa (igual à enterite regional?)
- Enterite neutrofílica (possivelmente secundária a invasão bacteriana).

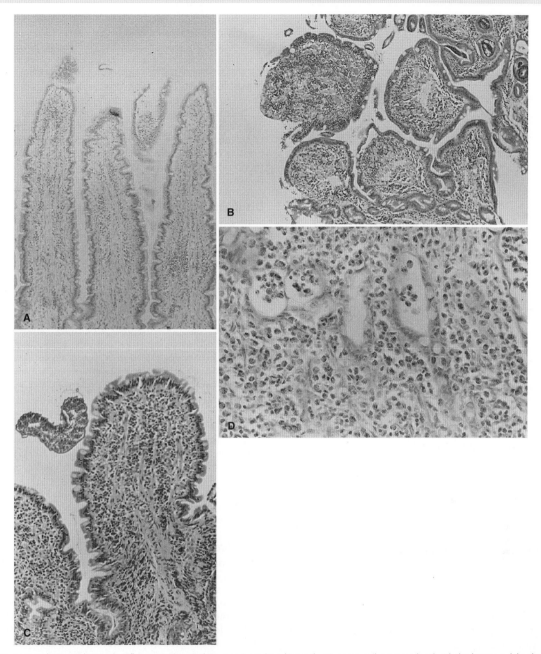

Figura 276.12 Aspecto histopatológico da inflamação intestinal. **A.** Aparência histológica de jejuno normal, mostrando vilosidades longas e delgadas e um número mínimo de células na lâmina própria. **B.** Enterite linfoplasmocitária (ELP) idiopática em um cão da raça Dachshund, mostrando vilosidades atrofiadas e um infiltrado linfoplasmocitário **C.** Inflamação intestinal linfoplasmocitária associada à infecção por *Strongyloides* (um parasita é visível na seção da superfície mucosa). **D.** Enterite eosinofílica (EE) em um cão da raça Pastor-Alemão, mostrando infiltração maciça da área da cripta com eosinófilos. (Cortesia de G. R. Pearson.)

razão da facilidade relativa de obtenção de biopsias endoscópicas e da dificuldade na interpretação de espécimes histopatológicos tão pequenos, além da falha em eliminar outras causas de inflamação da mucosa. Não ocorre predisposição de gênero, mas a DII parece se desenvolver mais comumente em cães e gatos de meia-idade, com sinais intermitentes, às vezes vistos em uma idade mais precoce. Embora a DII possa ocorrer potencialmente em qualquer animal, certas raça são reconhecidamente mais predispostas e têm padrões característicos da doença. Em gatos, uma associação chamada *triaditis* existe entre DI, colangite linfocítica e pancreatite crônica (ver Capítulo 283).

Vômito e diarreia são os sinais clínicos mais comuns na DII, mas um caso individual pode mostrar alguns ou todos os sinais listados no Boxe 276.13. Às vezes, um evento precipitante óbvio (p. ex., estresse, mudança na dieta, gastrenterite aguda) está presente no histórico, mas os sinais clínicos podem aumentar ou diminuir espontaneamente. A natureza dos sinais se correlaciona com a região afetada do trato GI: o vômito é mais comum se inflamação gástrica ou do ID superior estiver presente; em gatos, o vômito frequentemente é o sinal predominante de DII do ID; perda de peso está associada a doença do ID; e diarreia do tipo de IG pode ser o resultado de inflamação colônica primária ou ocorrer de modo secundário à diarreia prolongada do ID (ver Capítulo 277). A presença de sangue no vômito ou na diarreia geralmente está associada a doenças mais graves, particularmente EE e GEE. DII grave também está associada a perda de peso e ELP, com consequente hipoproteinemia e ascite. O apetite é variável; polifagia pode estar presente em face à perda de peso significativa, enquanto a anorexia normalmente ocorre com uma inflamação grave. O ato de comer grama pode crescer na DII, mas em geral é considerado um mecanismo para induzir o vômito em um animal nauseado. Uma inflamação mais leve pode não afetar o apetite, embora os sinais de dor pós-prandial possam ser significativos, mesmo sem outros sinais.

SEÇÃO 18 • Doença Gastrintestinal

Boxe 276.13 Sinais clínicos associados a doença intestinal inflamatória

- Vômito
  - Bile
  - Alimento
  - Com ou sem pelos em gatos
  - Com ou sem grama em cães
  - Sangue (hematêmese)
- Diarreia do tipo de intestino delgado
  - Grande volume
  - Aquosa
  - Melena
- Alças intestinais espessadas
- Diarreia de tipo de intestino grosso (ver Capítulo 277)
  - Hematoquezia
  - Fezes mucoides
  - Frequência e tenesmo
- Desconforto/dor abdominal
- Borborigmos e flatulências excessivos
- Perda de peso
- Apetite alterado
  - Polifagia
  - Diminuição do apetite/anorexia
  - Comer grama
- Hipoproteinemia
  - Ascite
  - Edema subcutâneo
  - Derrame pleural.

Etiologia e patogênese[125,149-151,183-186,204-207,225,266,282-285,434,1545,1603-1658]

A etiologia subjacente da DII de pequenos animais é desconhecida, mas comparações foram feitas com a DII humana. A esse respeito, a quebra da tolerância imunológica aos antígenos luminais (bactérias e componentes da dieta) é considerada crítica, talvez resultante da ruptura da barreira mucosa, desregulação do sistema imune ou distúrbios no microbioma, com regulação positiva de TLR. Fatores de crescimento intestinal (como o peptídio trifólio de células caliciformes), de crescimento e epidérmico podem ser regulados negativamente na DII, inibindo o reparo da mucosa.

Antígenos derivados da microbiota endógena são provavelmente importantes na patogênese da doença, e um papel potencial para fatores relacionados à dieta é sugerido graças ao benefício clínico da terapia dietética em alguns casos de DII. A enteropatia autoimune é uma condição rara em humanos, que se assemelha um pouco à ELP (i. e., achatamento das vilosidades, infiltrado de células mononucleares e abscessos de cripta). No entanto, não há evidências de autoimunidade em DII de pequenos animais.

Uma infecção não diagnosticada como causa da inflamação do ID permanece uma possibilidade alternativa, considerando a identificação recente de AIEC em colite granulomatosa de cães da raça Boxer, uma condição previamente considerada como uma manifestação de DII idiopática. A toxoplasmose foi associada à inflamação do ID (ver Capítulo 221), e uma análise de PCR identificou *Mycobacterium avium*, subespécie *paratuberculosis*, em cerca de 20% dos casos presumidos de DII idiopática (ver Capítulo 212). A presença de leveduras no ID e, em alguns casos de DII, de anticorpos anti-*Saccharomyces*, além de relatos práticos de melhora com nistatina oral, sugerem que as leveduras podem eventualmente estar envolvidas na DII.

Fatores genéticos provavelmente contribuem para a patogênese da DII, e, em humanos, as associações mais fortes são com genes do MHC humano (antígeno leucocitário humano [ALH]). Além disso, alguns pacientes humanos com doença de Crohn têm uma mutação no gene NOD2-CARD15. O produto desse gene detecta o lipopolissacarídeo bacteriano e consegue ativar o fator de transcrição pró-inflamatório NF-kappa-B. Essa associação poderia explicar o desenvolvimento de respostas imunes aberrantes a bactérias em certos indivíduos. Polimorfismos genéticos em genes NOD2 ou TLR foram mostrados em algumas raças de cães. Por exemplo, polimorfismos de nucleotídio único (*snps*) no exon 3 do gene NOD2 ocorrem na raça Pastor-Alemão com DII, mas não em outras raças; *snps* também são reconhecidos em genes que codificam TLR4 e TLR5 em cães afetados dessa raça. A regulação positiva de TLR foi mostrada em DII. Esse pode ser um epifenômeno associado à inflamação, mas poderia levar a uma hiper-responsividade de TLR a bactérias luminais.

Diagnóstico[609,1659-1661]

A biopsia intestinal é necessária para o diagnóstico de inflamação, mas o diagnóstico de DII idiopática deve ser limitado a casos em que é encontrada evidência histológica de inflamação sem uma causa subjacente óbvia. Todas as outras etiologias, incluindo infecciosas e responsivas à dieta e a antibacterianos, devem ser excluídas. Portanto, antes de realizar uma biopsia intestinal, são feitos avaliação laboratorial e diagnóstico por imagem. Esses testes não podem confirmar se a inflamação é idiopática, mas podem ajudar a eliminar causas da inflamação intestinal e doença intestinal por alterações anatômicas (p. ex., tumor, intussuscepção) ou doença extraintestinal (pancreatite). Além disso, ao determinar se uma doença intestinal focal ou difusa está presente, o clínico pode escolher o método mais adequado de biopsia intestinal.

Hemograma[1662]

Ocasionalmente, observa-se neutrofilia com ou sem desvio à esquerda. Uma eosinofilia poderia sugerir EE/GEE, mas não é patognomônica, nem invariavelmente presente. A anemia pode refletir inflamação crônica ou perda crônica de sangue. A trombocitopenia é observada em menos de 3% dos casos, mas a trombocitose geralmente é observada com sangramento gastrintestinal crônico.

Perfil bioquímico sérico[780]

Nenhuma alteração patognomônica é observada na DII, mas doenças de outros sistemas e órgãos devem ser reconhecidas e excluídas. Além disso, hipocolesterolemia sugestiva de má absorção, hipocalcemia e hipomagnesemia também podem ser encontradas. Hipoalbuminemia e hipoglobulinemia são características de ELP, e hipoalbuminemia correlaciona-se com um pior prognóstico. A inflamação intestinal em cães pode causar uma "hepatopatia reativa", com elevações discretas na atividade sérica das enzimas hepáticas. Em contrapartida, em razão da sua meia-vida mais curta em gatos, é mais provável que o aumento na atividade sérica das enzimas hepáticas nessa espécie seja resultado de uma doença hepática primária.

Exame fecal[374,384,1660]

Exames fecais são importantes para eliminar outras causas de inflamação da mucosa, como ancilóstomos e tricurídeos, *Giardia* e bactérias patogênicas (ver Capítulo 81). Dado o potencial para infecção oculta por *Giardia*, o tratamento empírico é recomendado em todos os casos (ver anteriormente). O aumento nas concentrações fecais de alfa$_1$-IP seria esperado na DII como marcador de perda de proteína intestinal, mesmo antes de a hipoproteinemia se desenvolver, e a concentração de calprotectina fecal deve estar aumentada se houver inflamação.

Concentrações séricas de vitaminas[50,234,395,401,402,780,783,1663-1665]

A hipovitaminose D pode ocorrer na DII e estar associada a hipocalcemia ionizada. A captação de folato e cobalamina são potencialmente reduzidos pela má absorção intestinal, portanto a inflamação do ID pode resultar em concentrações de folato sérico subnormal (inflamação proximal), cobalamina sérica subnormal (inflamação distal) ou ambos (inflamação difusa). O grau de hipocobalaminemia na DII se correlaciona ao grau de lesão histológica e um pior prognóstico. Embora não seja patognomônica para DII, a deficiência de cobalamina requer correção terapêutica, pois tem consequências metabólicas sistêmicas (ver Capítulo 292). As evidências práticas sugerem que gatos com DII e deficiência de cobalamina requerem suplementação parenteral para responder de forma otimizada à imunossupressão.

Diagnóstico por imagem[498,524-529,551,556,561,1666]

Informações a partir de imagens, juntamente a sinais específicos, permitem ao clínico escolher o método de biopsia mais adequado. Radiografias simples podem ser úteis para detectar doenças anatômicas do ID, mas em geral não são relevantes na DII, e estudos com contraste raramente acrescentam mais informações específicas. O exame ultrassonográfico pode documentar doença focal ou difusa e/ou se outros órgãos foram afetados, além de ser superior à radiografia para identificar doença de ID. Ele permite a avaliação da espessura da parede intestinal e pode documentar linfadenopatia mesentérica, enquanto a aspiração por agulha fina (AAF) guiada por US pode fornecer amostras para análise citológica (ver Capítulos 89 e 93). No entanto, o aumento da espessura da parede intestinal não é uma característica de todos os casos de DII idiopática canina e não é patognomônico. A heterogeneidade da mucosa é consistente com a inflamação ou abscedação da cripta, enquanto estrias são indicativas de dilatação de vasos linfáticos.

Biopsia intestinal[144,565,570,571,577,581,603,604,609-616,1544,1590,1596,1667-1672]

A biopsia intestinal é necessária para documentar a inflamação, o que é essencial para o diagnóstico de DII. A endoscopia é o método mais seguro para a biopsia, mas tem limitações: as amostras são superficiais e podem ser pequenas e esmagadas, enquanto a interpretação histopatológica está sujeita à disparidade entre patologistas, assim como sua aparência endoscópica grosseira. Um sistema de pontuação endoscópica foi publicado pelo *WSAVA GI Standardization Group* (Grupo de Padronização GI) para tentar obter confiabilidade na avaliação subjetiva do eritema, da irregularidade e da friabilidade da mucosa,[609] semelhante a um sistema padrão de graduação histológica para DII de ID e IG em cães e gatos. Essas diretrizes não são um sistema numérico para contagem de características e "pontuação" da inflamação intestinal, nem uma escala ponderada; em vez disso, são um modelo que permite comparações objetivas de achados individuais a um ponto de referência. Elas destinam-se a permitir estudos comparativos prospectivos para identificar quais mudanças são importantes na definição histológica da DII e, assim, compreender a correlação entre a gravidade clínica e a histológica. Um modelo simplificado avalia apenas atrofia de vilosidades, lesão epitelial, LIE, alterações de cripta e infiltrado na LP.

Biopsias endoscópicas (ver Capítulo 113) só podem ser coletadas do segmento proximal do ID, a menos que uma ileoscopia via intubação colônica também seja realizada. No entanto, as biopsias ileais parecem fornecer um diagnóstico melhor. Em alguns casos, a biopsia cirúrgica de espessura total é necessária, embora o procedimento seja mais invasivo e a deiscência possa ser problemática, especialmente se hipoproteinemia grave estiver presente. A laparotomia pode ser mais adequada para gatos, dada a tendência para envolvimento de vários órgãos (ou seja, *triaditis*). A avaliação histopatológica do material de biopsia permanece o padrão-ouro para o diagnóstico da inflamação intestinal, e o padrão de mudança histopatológica dita o tipo de DII presente. No entanto, são reconhecidas limitações na interpretação histopatológica de biopsias intestinais: a qualidade de amostras pode variar, a concordância entre os patologistas é fraca e a diferenciação entre amostras normais e ELP leves e entre ELP graves e linfoma pode ser difícil. Esquemas de graduação histológica foram sugeridos, e critérios padronizados foram produzidos e devem ser adotados. É importante ressaltar que a inflamação da mucosa em biopsias endoscópicas é descrita de forma ampla, enfatizando tanto as alterações morfológicas quanto o número de células inflamatórias na LP. Essa abordagem considera que o aumento da celularidade poderia ser meramente uma resposta reativa, equivalente ao aumento de um linfonodo de drenagem, e que evidências de lesão à mucosa também são necessárias para confirmar a inflamação.

Índices de atividade da doença inflamatória intestinal[524,780,1673-1678]

Índices de atividade clínica ajudam na quantificação da gravidade da DII e mostram alguma correlação com achados de ultrassom. Eles auxiliam os pesquisadores na avaliação da resposta ao tratamento e na comparação dos estudos, permitindo aos profissionais fazer um prognóstico comparado aos estudos publicados. O índice de atividade da DII canina (Tabela 276.8) se correlaciona à gravidade histológica e às concentrações séricas de proteínas de fase aguda, como a proteína C reativa. A avaliação de tendências na concentração de proteínas de fase aguda também pode ser útil no monitoramento da resposta ao tratamento. O índice de atividade clínica da enteropatia crônica canina é uma modificação que inclui a concentração sérica de albumina e a presença de ascite e prurido, mas ainda precisa ser avaliada de forma independente.

Outros métodos de diagnóstico[108,384,420,434,618-627,633,1603,1679-1692]

Dadas as limitações da histopatologia, outras modalidades diagnósticas podem ser necessárias. O exame citológico é provavelmente menos sensível ou específico, mas a imuno-histoquímica ou a citometria de fluxo podem ser usadas para analisar subconjuntos de células imunes, enquanto a RT-PCR permite medir a expressão de mRNA de citocinas. No entanto, essas técnicas são trabalhosas e fracamente padronizadas, sendo pouco provável que tenham ampla disponibilidade em um futuro próximo. A presença de anticorpos antineutrofílicos citoplasmáticos e perinucleares (pANCA), o aumento sérico de proteínas de fase aguda, as concentrações alteradas de hormônios GI, o aumento da permeabilidade intestinal e da concentração sérica de 3-BrY e a excreção fecal de calprotectina podem ser marcadores úteis de inflamação intestinal. A avaliação imuno-histoquímica de marcadores de células T e B e o teste de clonalidade do rearranjo do receptor de antígeno por PCR para distinguir linfoma de DII grave também são de valor potencial, mas o rearranjo clonal é igualmente observado em alguns pacientes com DII.

Tratamento[1631,1693-1696]

Independentemente do tipo histológico da DII, o tratamento em geral envolve uma combinação de modificações de dieta com agentes antibacterianos e/ou terapia imunossupressora. Informações objetivas da eficácia são limitadas, e a maioria das recomendações é com base na experiência clínica. Uma abordagem em fases da terapia é recomendada sempre que possível; tratamentos sequenciais com parasiticidas, dieta de exclusão e antibacterianos são testados para descartar causas conhecidas de inflamação antes de usar uma medicação imunossupressora. Casos leves com frequência respondem a uma mudança na dieta e/ou ao metronidazol, especialmente gatos. No entanto, em alguns casos, os sinais clínicos ou a inflamação da mucosa são tão graves que a intervenção precoce com imunossupressão é essencial. Se os sinais clínicos forem intermitentes, o tutor deve manter um diário para anotar sinais e atividades que possibilitem comparações mais objetivas.

Modificação da dieta[658,1485,1697-1701]

Uma dieta facilmente digerível que diminui a carga antigênica intestinal e a inflamação da mucosa é indicada para pacientes com DII (ver Capítulo 178). Tradicionalmente, são recomendadas

SEÇÃO 18 • Doença Gastrintestinal

Tabela 276.8 Índices para a avaliação objetiva da gravidade da doença na doença inflamatória intestinal.

CARACTERÍSTICA	IADIIC	PONTUAÇÃO	IACECC	PONTUAÇÃO	FCECAI	PONTUAÇÃO
Atitude/atividade	Normal	0	Normal	0	Normal	0
	Ligeira diminuição	1	Ligeira diminuição	1	Ligeira diminuição	1
	Diminuição moderada	2	Diminuição moderada	2	Diminuição moderada	2
	Diminuição intensa	3	Diminuição intensa	3	Diminuição intensa	3
Apetite	Normal	0	Normal	0	Normal	0
	Ligeira diminuição	1	Ligeira diminuição	1	Ligeira diminuição	1
	Diminuição moderada	2	Diminuição moderada	2	Diminuição moderada	2
	Diminuição intensa	3	Diminuição intensa	3	Diminuição intensa	3
Vômito	Nenhum	0	Nenhum	0	Nenhum	0
	Leve (uma vez/semana)	1	Leve (uma vez/semana)	1	Leve (uma vez/semana)	1
	Moderado	2	Moderado	2	Moderado	2
	(2 a 3/semana)	3	(2 a 3/semana)	3	(2 a 3/semana)	3
	Grave (> 3/semana)		Grave (> 3/semana)		Grave (> 3/semana)	
Consistência	Normal	0	Normal	0	Normal	0
das fezes	Um pouco mole,	1	Um pouco mole,	1	Um pouco mole,	1
	sangue fecal, muco	2	sangue fecal, muco	2	sangue fecal, muco	2
	ou ambos	3	ou ambos	3	ou ambos	3
	Fezes muito moles		Fezes muito moles		Fezes muito moles	
	Diarreia aquosa		Diarreia aquosa		Diarreia aquosa	
Frequência	Normal	0	Normal	0	Normal	0
das fezes	2 a 3/dia	1	2 a 3/dia	1	2 a 3/dia	1
	4 a 5/dia	2	4 a 5/dia	2	4 a 5/dia	2
	> 5 por dia	3	> 5 por dia	3	> 5 por dia	3
Perda de peso	Normal	0	Normal	0	Normal	0
(não	Leve (< 5%)	1	Leve (< 5%)	1	Leve (< 5%)	1
intencional)	Moderado (5 a 10%)	2	Moderado (5 a 10%)	2	Moderado (5 a 10%)	2
	Grave (> 10%)	3	Grave (> 10%)	3	Grave (> 10%)	3
Albumina sérica			> 2 g/ℓ	0		
			15 a 19,9 g/ℓ	1		
			12 a 14,9 g/ℓ	2		
			< 12 g/ℓ	3		
Lesão endoscópica					Não	0
					Sim	1
Proteína total					Normal	0
					Aumentada	1
ALT/ALP					Normal	0
					Aumentada	1
Fosfato					Normal	0
					Diminuído	1
Pontuação Final	Clinicamente insignificante	0 a 3	Clinicamente insignificante	0 a 3	Clinicamente insignificante	0 a 3
	DII leve	4 a 5	DII leve	4 a 5	DII leve	4 a 5
	DII moderado	6 a 8	DII moderado	6 a 8	DII moderado	6 a 8
	DII grave	≥ 9	DII grave	≥ 9	DII grave	≥ 9

Para converter a concentração de albumina sérica em mg/dℓ, divida o valor em g/ℓ por 10. *ALT/ALP*, alanina aminotransferase/fosfatase alcalina; *DII*, doença inflamatória intestinal; *IACECC*, índice de atividade clínica de enteropatia crônica canina; *IADIIC*, índice de atividade de doença inflamatória intestinal canina; *IAECF*, índice de atividade de enteropatia crônica felina.

dietas limitadas em antígenos com base em uma preparação altamente digerível de proteína de fonte única, eliminando a possibilidade de reação alimentar adversa como causa da inflamação GI. Tal ensaio de dieta de exclusão é recomendado em todos os casos em que não há um ELP e o paciente estiver comendo; a maioria dos tutores fica satisfeita em tentar isso primeiro, por estarem preocupados com os efeitos adversos da terapia medicamentosa.

O arroz bem cozido é a fonte preferida de carboidratos, em razão de sua alta digestibilidade, mas batata, amido de milho e tapioca também são opções por não conterem glúten. Restrição de gordura reduz os sinais clínicos associados à má absorção de gordura. A modificação da proporção de ácidos graxos $\Omega3{:}\Omega6$ pode igualmente modular a resposta inflamatória e ter algum benefício tanto no tratamento quanto na manutenção da remissão. A suplementação com folato e cobalamina é indicada caso as concentrações séricas estiverem abaixo do normal, embora ainda não esteja claro se a cobalamina deve ser suplementada via parenteral ou se a suplementação oral produz efeito fisiológico.

As dietas de exclusão também conseguem ajudar a resolver quaisquer sensibilidades secundárias aos componentes da dieta que possam ter surgido após a ruptura da barreira mucosa. Desse modo, após a inflamação ser resolvida, a dieta normal

CAPÍTULO 276 • Doenças do Intestino Delgado 1565

muitas vezes pode ser reintroduzida sem o risco de sensibilidade adquirida. Mais recentemente, dietas hidrolisadas têm sido usadas na DII com um suposto sucesso maior, mesmo em pacientes que falharam em um ensaio com uma dieta de exclusão limitada em antígenos. No entanto, a melhora histológica na celularidade da mucosa não foi aparente, apesar da resolução dos sinais clínicos. Mostrou-se regulação negativa de mRNA de algumas citocinas pró-inflamatórias. Portanto, a resposta a uma dieta hidrolisada poderia indicar: (1) a dieta hidrolisada simplesmente é tão digerível que mesmo um paciente com doença de ID pode assimilá-la; (2) a DII está em remissão ou mesmo curada, mas a melhora histológica na celularidade leva mais tempo do que a dos sinais clínicos. A última explicação talvez espelhe o que acontece com um linfonodo de drenagem após a eliminação da infecção primária.

Terapia antibacteriana[691,1702-1708]

O tratamento com antimicrobianos pode ser justificado na DII, em parte para tratar qualquer SBID secundário, em parte por causa da importância dos antígenos bacterianos na patogênese da DII. No entanto, o único estudo-controle não mostrou nenhum benefício em ministrar metronidazol com prednisolona. Fluoroquinolonas e metronidazol muitas vezes são usados em DII humana, e o metronidazol é o medicamento preferido para pequenos animais. A eficácia do metronidazol, especialmente na DII felina, pode não estar relacionada apenas à sua atividade antibacteriana, pois ela consegue exercer efeitos imunomoduladores na imunidade celular. Outros antibacterianos (p. ex., oxitetraciclina, tilosina) também podem ter efeitos imunomoduladores e alguma eficácia.

Medicamentos imunossupressores

A modalidade de tratamento mais importante na DII idiopática é a imunossupressão, embora deva ser usada apenas como último recurso (ver Capítulo 165). Na DII humana, glicocorticoides e tiopurinas (p. ex., azatioprina, 6-mercaptopurina) são usados mais amplamente.

Glicocorticoides.[1702,1709-1711] Em cães, os glicocorticoides são usados com mais frequência, sendo prednisona, prednisolona e metilprednisolona os medicamentos de escolha. A dexametasona talvez deva ser evitada, pois, em roedores, ela (e não a prednisolona) é deletéria para a atividade enzimática da borda em escova dos enterócitos. A budesonida é usada ocasionalmente, sendo mais comum para a DII felina.

Prednisolona/prednisona. Uma dose inicial de 1 a 2 mg/kg VO, a cada 12 h (ou seja, 2 a 4 mg/kg/dia) é indicada durante 2 a 4 semanas; na DII grave, é possível administrá-la via parenteral, pois a absorção oral pode ser fraca. A dose é então reduzida lentamente ao longo das semanas ou meses subsequentes, em geral a cada 3 a 4 semanas; o tempo e as quantidades exatas de reduções de dose são baseadas na resposta clínica *versus* a tolerabilidade dos efeitos colaterais, a conveniência do tamanho do comprimido e a disponibilidade de reexame. Em cães, sinais de hiperadrenocorticismo iatrogênico são comuns inicialmente, mas a maioria, exceto atrofia muscular, são transitórios e se resolvem conforme a dose é reduzida. Normalmente, a primeira redução é de 1 a 2 mg/kg a cada 12 h para 1 a 2 mg/kg a cada 24 h; cada redução subsequente em geral diminui a dose pela metade. Em alguns casos, a terapia pode ser completamente retirada ou pelo menos reduzida a uma dose baixa administrada a cada 48 horas.

Budesonida.[1712-1717] Esse é um corticosteroide revestido entericamente, ativo localmente, sendo 90% destruído durante sua primeira passagem pelo fígado. É usado para manter a remissão na doença de Crohn ileal humana com supressão hipotalâmica-hipofisária adrenal mínima. É uma alternativa interessante para gatos com DII e diabetes melito secundária a pancreatite crônica e é relativamente barata para gatos e cães pequenos. No entanto, a supressão adrenal foi documentada em cães, e uma hepatopatia por esteroide pode se desenvolver. Um estudo preliminar mostrou eficácia aparente em cães e gatos, mas outro mais recente não mostrou nenhum benefício sobre a prednisolona na DII canina em termos de remissão e taxas de efeitos adversos. Informações publicadas sobre o uso desse medicamento são limitadas, com intervalos de doses muito amplas sendo sugeridos, mas uma dose oral diária inicial de 1 mg para gatos e 1, 2 e 3 mg para cães pequenos, médios e grandes, respectivamente, são usadas com mais frequência.

Medicamentos citotóxicos[1693,1718-1728]

Se os sinais clínicos da DII recidivarem consistentemente quando a dose de corticosteroide for reduzida, medicamentos citotóxicos podem ser adicionados para fornecer um efeito poupador de esteroides. Em cães, a azatioprina (2 mg/kg VO, a cada 24 horas) é normalmente usada em combinação com prednisona ou prednisolona quando a resposta inicial à terapia é fraca ou quando os efeitos colaterais dos corticosteroides são pronunciados. No entanto, ela pode ter início de atividade retardado (até 3 semanas), e, dado seu potencial mielossupressor, o monitoramento regular do hemograma é necessário. A toxicose pode estar parcialmente relacionada à falta de tiopurina s-metiltransferase (TPMT) em alguns cães, enquanto a ausência completa de TPMT em gatos significa que apenas doses baixas de azatioprina são necessárias, e ela não é recomendada, a menos que a reformulação esteja disponível. O clorambucila (2 a 6 mg/m^2 VO, a cada 24 h até a remissão, seguido por redução gradual) com prednisolona provavelmente é uma escolha melhor para gatos. Da mesma forma, uma combinação clorambucila-prednisolona em cães tem se mostrado mais eficaz do que uma combinação prednisolona-azatioprina.

Outros medicamentos imunossupressores às vezes são usados. O metotrexato é eficaz no tratamento da doença de Crohn humana, mas não é amplamente utilizado em cães, pois muitas vezes causa diarreia. A ciclofosfamida tem poucas vantagens sobre a azatioprina e raramente é usada. A eficácia do micofenolato de mofetila na DII em pequenos animais é desconhecida, mas não é muito bem-sucedida como terapia única na DII humana. Por outro lado, a ciclosporina mostrou um efeito previsivelmente promissor, dado sua atividade específica para linfócitos T e eficácia em cães para tratamento da fístula perianal. Infelizmente, ela é cara, e estudos de DII em humanos mostraram eficácia variável e toxicidade. A resistência a esteroides se correlaciona à indução da expressão da glicoproteína P; embora seja esperado que isso também confira resistência à ciclosporina, foi relatada uma resposta adequada à ciclosporina em 11 de 14 cães com enteropatia resistente a esteroides.

Prebióticos e probióticos[686,688,694,703,1650,1706,1729-1736]

A modulação da microbiota entérica com probióticos ou prebióticos poderia ter benefícios em direcionar a patogênese da DII, pois ambos demonstraram reduzir a inflamação intestinal em modelos de camundongos com DII. Ensaios com probióticos controlados por placebo em pacientes humanos com DII mostraram resultados promissores, e os primeiros ensaios em cães e gatos indicaram modulação do sistema imune de mucosa e alguma eficácia clínica. Um maior efeito foi visto com as cepas Probiótico VSL#3,[a] porém mais probióticos espécie-específicos são necessários.

Novas terapias para doença inflamatória intestinal[8-13,690,1724,1737-1749]

Novas terapias medicamentosas são cada vez mais usadas em DII humana para atingir o processo de doença subjacente com mais precisão. Essas terapias incluem novos medicamentos imunossupressores, anticorpos monoclonais, citocinas e fatores de transcrição. Medicamentos que têm como alvo TNF-α (p. ex., talidomida, oxpentifilina) são usados na DII humana e podem

---

[a]N.T.: Na verdade, uma mistura de oito cepas de três espécies bacterianas distintas.

ser adequados para o tratamento de cães, em razão da importância dessa citocina na patogênese da doença. Terapia com anticorpo monoclonal anti-TNF-α é usada em casos graves de DII humana. No futuro, anticorpos monoclonais espécie-específicos poderão ser usados para tratar DII canina e felina, assim como o oclacitinibe (Apoquel) é usado na dermatite atópica.

O transplante de microbiota fecal (TMF) foi desenvolvido para tratar humanos com infecção por *Clostridioides difficile*, mas agora está sendo testado para o tratamento da doença de Crohn. Relatórios preliminares de sucesso no tratamento de DII canina por TMF estão surgindo. Foi relatada uma terapia com células-tronco bem-sucedida na enteropatia crônica felina, mas sem uma avaliação objetiva do sucesso. O transplante intestinal total foi realizado experimentalmente em suínos e humanos, mas não em cães ou gatos.

Resposta ao tratamento e prognóstico[317,780,1659,1677,1750-1758]

Há uma percepção de que o tratamento da DII idiopática canina com corticosteroides geralmente é bem-sucedido e a completa remissão é o resultado mais provável, porém essa noção não é suportada pela avaliação crítica da literatura: os relatos de respostas positivas a parasiticidas, terapia dietética ou antimicrobianos, por si só, sugerem que nunca houve um verdadeiro sucesso relatado para DII idiopática. Um resultado negativo em cães foi associado a doença mais grave (conforme avaliado clínica, endoscópica ou histologicamente) e com suspeita de doença pancreática concomitante indicada por alta imunorreatividade da lipase pancreática, hipocobalaminemia e hipoalbuminemia. A expressão de Glicoproteína P e a expressão diferencial de TLR-2 e TLR-4 também são preditivas de resposta ao tratamento. Não está claro se a correlação com hipoalbuminemia simplesmente reflete a gravidade da doença ou uma maior probabilidade de morte por doença tromboembólica, uma vez que a antitrombina (58 kDa) e a albumina (70 kDa) são moléculas de tamanho semelhante.

A resposta ao tratamento da DII felina parece melhor e mais frequente, com a remissão prolongada; o metronidazol como única terapia em casos mais brandos pode ter sucesso, e os gatos são mais resistentes aos efeitos metabólicos do uso crônico de corticosteroide. Sobrevivência prolongada também foi observada na terapia simples com prednisolona e clorambucila.

Um achado importante foi que a melhora clínica não é necessariamente acompanhada por melhora histológica, o que pode refletir a dificuldade em avaliar a inflamação intestinal histologicamente, mas essa discordância também é vista na doença de Crohn humana, em que a remissão histológica é mais lenta do que a remissão clínica. Alguns pacientes caninos apresentam inicialmente uma boa resposta, seguida por recaída refratária ao tratamento adicional, e uma taxa de eutanásia de 10 a 20%. A falha em manter a remissão pode indicar desenvolvimento da resistência aos corticosteroides por meio da expressão glicoproteína-P, um diagnóstico inicial equivocado de linfoma alimentar ou transformação da inflamação crônica em linfoma.

Enterite linfocítico-plasmocítica[1759-1767]

A enterite linfocítico-plasmocítica (ELP) é a manifestação histológica mais comum de inflamação intestinal, caracterizada por um infiltrado de linfócitos e células plasmáticas na mucosa, associada a alterações morfológicas (ver Figura 276.12). No entanto, existem muitas outras causas de infiltração linfoplasmocitária no ID (ver Boxe 276.13), incluindo enteropatógenos, outras bactérias e *Toxoplasma*. Todas essas causas subjacentes devem ser excluídas antes de um diagnóstico de ELP idiopática ser confirmado. A ELP é prevalente em vários cães com pedigree e gatos de raça pura, e em cães com frequência causa uma EPP. A ELP normalmente afeta animais mais velhos; é rara (mas não impossível) em indivíduos com menos de 2 anos.

Etiopatogênese[629,1524,1656,1768]

Alterações das populações de células imunes na ELP canina incluem aumentos de células T na lâmina própria (especialmente células CD4 +), células plasmáticas IgG+, macrófagos e granulócitos, variando de uma infiltração leve a grave. Diversas alterações inespecíficas na expressão dos genes de citocinas e de quimiocinas entre animais com DII e animais normais foram mostradas tanto pelos métodos de arranjo de genes como expressão de mRNA. Concentrações aumentadas de proteínas de fase aguda (p. ex., proteína C reativa), que normalizam após tratamento, indicam resposta inflamatória. Fibrose de mucosa pode ocorrer, especialmente em gatos. Existem mudanças na expressão de metaloproteinase na ELP, e a fibrose pode ser reconhecível por US.

Sinais clínicos[1762]

Sinais de ELP, incluindo diarreia crônica e perda de peso, não são patognomônicos. Vômito crônico pode ser o sinal predominante, especialmente em gatos.

Diagnóstico

A abordagem para o diagnóstico da ELP é o mesmo de qualquer enteropatia crônica, embora um diagnóstico definitivo dependa, em última análise, da descrição histopatológica do aumento do número de linfócitos e células plasmáticas em associação a mudanças morfológicas, mas nenhuma causa subjacente identificável (ver Capítulo 113). Atrofia completa ou parcial das vilosidades pode estar presente, com fusão de vilosidades e abscedação de criptas em casos graves. A distinção entre ELP grave e linfoma alimentar pode ser difícil, e diferenças podem existir entre biopsias endoscópicas e espécimes *post-mortem* do mesmo paciente. Essas discrepâncias são possíveis porque as duas condições podem estar presentes simultaneamente, já que inflamação intestinal crônica, em conclusão, pode resultar em transformação maligna, ou porque o linfoma de baixo grau pode não ter sido diagnosticado corretamente logo de início.

Tratamento e prognóstico

O tratamento e prognóstico para ELP é igual ao descrito anteriormente para DII idiopática.

Enterite eosinofílica[1172,1769-1772]

A enterite eosinofílica (EE) é relatada como a segunda forma mais comum de DII idiopática. Frequentemente também envolve o estômago (gastrenterite eosinofílica, GEE) e/ou o cólon. A doença difusa é mais comum, mas a EE segmentar foi relatada em cães e gatos, e a fibroplasia esclerosante eosinofílica felina pode ser uma variante da EE. Histologicamente, distúrbios morfológicos variáveis da mucosa (p. ex., atrofia de vilosidades) estão presentes, com um infiltrado misto de células inflamatórias onde os eosinófilos predominam. Tal como acontece com a ELP, os critérios de diagnóstico variam entre patologistas; alguns definem EE puramente com base no aumento subjetivo no número de eosinófilos na mucosa, enquanto outros aplicam critérios mais rígidos (eosinófilos devem predominar na LP). Outro critério é a presença de eosinófilos entre as células epiteliais das vilosidades e criptas, que sugere migração transepitelial. No entanto, o número de eosinófilos da mucosa pode variar acentuadamente em cães normais e, portanto, essa condição pode ser sobrediagnosticada. Assim como ocorre com outras formas de DII, um diagnóstico de EE idiopática deve ser feito apenas após outras causas de inflamação eosinofílica, como parasitismo e enteropatia responsiva a alimentos, terem sido eliminadas.

Sinais clínicos[1772-1775]

A EE pode ser vista em cães e gatos de qualquer raça e idade, embora seja mais comum em adultos jovens. As raças Boxer e Doberman podem ser predispostas, e um aumento da incidência no Pastor-Alemão foi sugerido. EE e GEE também podem ser associadas a distúrbios eosinofílicos sistêmicos em cães e gatos. Os sinais clínicos relatados, que dependem da área do trato GI envolvida, incluem vômito, diarreia de ID e diarreia de IG. Erosão/ulceração de mucosa e hemorragia podem ocorrer com

CAPÍTULO 276 • Doenças do Intestino Delgado 1567

maior frequência na EE do que em outras formas de DII (ver Figura 276.8 F e G); portanto, hematêmese, melena ou hematoquezia são possíveis. A EE grave tem sido associada à ELP e, raramente, à perfuração espontânea do trato GI.

Etiopatogênese[1172,1222,1256,1776-1778]
Um infiltrado eosinofílico na mucosa pode estar relacionado a sensibilidade dietética, endoparasitismo, larva migrans visceral ou ser idiopático. Uma infecção zoonótica por A. caninum foi associada a GEE em humanos. A infiltração de eosinófilos é provavelmente o resultado da produção local e sistêmica de citocinas e quimiocinas, como IL-5 e membros da família das eotaxinas. Esses mediadores podem ser produzidos pelo subconjunto Th2 das células T CD4 +. A infiltração de eosinófilos também é vista como um efeito paraneoplásico de tumores de mastócitos e, às vezes, de linfoma.

Diagnóstico[1779]
O diagnóstico da EE, em última análise, é feito pela avaliação histopatológica de biopsias intestinais (ver Capítulo 113) em conjunto à exclusão de parasitas e hipersensibilidade alimentar. A eosinofilia não está invariavelmente presente, nem é patognomônica para a EE, pois também pode ocorrer com parasitismo, hipoadrenocorticismo, doença alérgica cutânea ou respiratória, linfoma e neoplasia de mastócitos. Alças intestinais espessadas podem ser palpadas em alguns gatos afetados, o que é possível confirmar por US.

Tratamento
Dado que os infiltrados eosinofílicos da mucosa podem estar relacionados a doenças endoparasitárias, o tratamento empírico com fenbendazol sempre é aconselhável. Em seguida, um ensaio de dieta de exclusão deve ser feito para eliminar a possibilidade de sensibilidade à dieta antes de considerar uma terapia imunossupressora. O prognóstico na EE idiopática é reservado, mesmo com uma boa resposta inicial ao tratamento, porque a recidiva é comum.

Fibroplasia esclerosante eosinofílica felina[545,1161,1780-1785]
Essa variante histológica de DII provavelmente representa uma manifestação incomum de EE em gatos. A fibrose da parede intestinal felina pode ser induzida por inflamação crônica, pois também é relatada em ficomicose intestinal e tumores de mastócitos. A condição idiopática ocorre mais frequentemente em gatos de meia-idade e da raça Ragdoll. Vômito e diarreia são sinais clínicos comuns, e massas intestinais no duodeno e no íleo podem ser palpáveis. Histologicamente, observa-se um infiltrado de eosinófilos intercalado com fibroblastos e bandas de colágeno. Bactérias são encontradas dentro das lesões em cerca de metade dos casos, mas os relatos tendem a responder à prednisolona.

Enterite neutrofílica[634,1544,1786]
Embora os neutrófilos estejam presentes na mucosa intestinal normal e sejam as primeiras células a se infiltrar na mucosa de pacientes humanos com a doença de Crohn, a enterite neutrofílica é rara em cães e apenas ligeiramente mais comum em gatos quando a doença sai da remissão. Tradicionalmente, quando uma predominância de neutrófilos era encontrada na biopsia da mucosa intestinal, um tratamento empírico com antibióticos era recomendado primeiro em vez de imunossupressão, graças à preocupação com uma causa potencialmente infecciosa. Estudos recentes com o uso de FISH justificam essa abordagem, pois parece haver uma associação entre enterite neutrofílica e invasão por Campylobacter coli em gatos e com C. jejuni e Salmonella em cães.

Enterite granulomatosa[1787-1792]
Enterite granulomatosa é uma forma rara de DII do ID, caracterizada por infiltração da mucosa com macrófagos, resultando na formação de granulomas. A distribuição da inflamação pode ser irregular. Essa condição provavelmente é a mesma que "enterite regional", na qual granulomas ileais foram relatados. A colite granulomatosa está associada a AIEC (ver Capítulo 277). Em gatos, uma inflamação piogranulomatosa transmural foi associada à infecção pelo vírus da peritonite infecciosa felina (PIFV; ver Capítulo 224).

Enterite proliferativa[1793-1796]
Enterite proliferativa é caracterizada por hipertrofia segmentar da mucosa intestinal. Embora muitas espécies possam ser afetadas, a condição é mais comum em suínos e rara em cães. Há sugestões de uma etiologia infecciosa subjacente, e Lawsonia intracellularis foi implicada em alguns casos de DII canina. Outros agentes infecciosos com uma ligação proposta são Campylobacter spp. e Chlamydia.

Formas de doença inflamatória intestinal raça-específicas[1797]
A DII idiopática é observada em todos os cães, de raças puras e mestiços, mas certas raças podem ser super-representadas. Em algumas, como o Pastor-Alemão, em que tanto a ELP quanto a EE são comuns, a suposição ainda é de que elas sejam afetadas pelas mesmas condições que outras. De modo similar, gatos siameses são predispostos a ELP. Ainda que a mesma etiopatogenia da inflamação intestinal ocorra em todos os cães, pode haver disfunções imunológicas e genéticas subjacentes, relacionadas à raça, que aumentam o risco dessas doenças. No Pastor-Alemão, snps nos genes que codificam os TLR mostram polimorfismos, sugerindo uma base genética. Cães das raças Rottweiler, Yorkshire Terrier e Lundehund são predispostos a inflamação intestinal, mas geralmente está associada a vasos lácteos dilatados, e eles são classificados como tendo linfangiectasia primária. Outras raças de cães, no entanto, também são propensas a inflamação intestinal idiopática, mas características de sua condição sugerem que elas não têm a forma classicamente reconhecida de DII.

Enteropatia do cão Basenji[1666,1798-1805]
Uma forma grave de enteropatia, hereditária de ELP, é bem caracterizada em cães Basenji, embora o modo da herança não esteja claro. Tem sido comparado à doença imunoproliferativa do intestino delgado (DIID) em humanos, porque ambas envolvem inflamação intestinal intensa. No entanto, a DIID está associada a uma gamopatia (doença da cadeia pesada alfa) e uma predisposição ao linfoma, enquanto cães afetados com enteropatia costumam ter hiperglobulinemia, mas não doença de cadeia pesada alfa, embora possam estar predispostos a linfoma. As lesões intestinais são caracterizadas por aumentos de células T CD4+ e CD8+. Os sinais de diarreia crônica intratável e perda de peso são mais comuns e, geralmente, progressivos; perfuração intestinal espontânea pode ocorrer. Gastrite linfoplasmocítica, junto a hipergastrinemia e hiperplasia da mucosa, pode ser vista, além da enteropatia. ELP com hipoalbuminemia ocorre com frequência, embora a ascite seja menos comum. A abordagem para o diagnóstico é a mesma para DII idiopática e depende do exame histopatológico de espécimes de biopsia (ver Capítulo 113). Contudo, o tratamento geralmente é malsucedido, com a maioria cães morrendo poucos meses após o diagnóstico. Por outro lado, um tratamento combinado, precoce e intensivo com prednisolona, antibióticos e a modificação dietética alcançou remissão em alguns casos.

Enteropatia com perda de proteína familiar e nefropatia com perda de proteína em cães Wheaten Terrier de Pelo Liso[1504,1509,1679,1680,1754,1806-1810]
Uma síndrome clínica única para cães da raça Wheaten Terrier de Pelo Liso foi caracterizada. Os cães afetados apresentam sinais de ELP, de nefropatia perdedora de proteína (NPP) ou de ambos (ver Capítulo 325). Uma base genética é provável, já que uma análise de pedigree mostrou um ancestral macho comum, e mutações nos genes NPHS1 e KIRREL2 foram encontrados em cães com o NPP. A doença provavelmente é imunomediada, dada a presença de infiltração de células inflamatórias no ID.

Um papel potencial para a hipersensibilidade alimentar foi sugerido, pois os cães afetados mostraram reações adversas durante os testes provocativos de alimentos e as alterações nas concentrações de IgE fecal antígeno-específicas.

Os sinais de ELP tendem a se desenvolver em uma idade mais jovem do que os sinais de NPP e podem incluir vômito, diarreia, perda de peso e derrames pleurais e peritoneais. Ocasionalmente, doença tromboembólica pode ocorrer. As investigações laboratoriais preliminares, na maioria dos cães com ELP, mostram pan-hipoproteinemia e hipocolesterolemia. Em contrapartida, hipoalbuminemia (sem hipoglobulinemia), hipercolesterolemia, proteinúria e, finalmente, azotemia são vistas apenas se NPP se desenvolver. Um teste pANCA positivo pode ser preditivo da doença. A biopsia intestinal revela evidência de inflamação, achatamento das vilosidades e erosões epiteliais. O tratamento para ELP/NPP é semelhante ao descrito para DII idiopática, mas o prognóstico geralmente é pior.

Enterite linfoplasmocítica e deficiência de cobalamina em cão da raça Shar-pei[400,1811-1815]

Essa raça é reconhecida como predisposta a enterite linfoplasmocitária e, frequentemente, tem uma hipocobalaminemia grave associada. Suspeita-se de uma causa genética, mas essa hipótese não foi comprovada, e nenhuma ligação com a febre/amiloidose do Shar-pei foi demonstrada; na verdade, essa condição pode apenas representar uma DII.

Linfangiectasia

Definição e causa[290,336-338,1816-1839]

Linfangiectasia intestinal é caracterizada por dilatação marcada e disfunção dos vasos linfáticos intestinais. Há ruptura de vasos lácteos anormais e vazamento de linfa rica em proteínas das vilosidades para o lúmen intestinal, uma EPP que, em última instância, causa hipoproteinemia. A perda simultânea de linfócitos pode levar a imunodeficiência, e os cães afetados correm o risco de inflamação ou doença neoplásica; a raça Lundehund, que herdou essa forma da doença, tem predisposição a gastrite e carcinoma gástrico, por exemplo. A linfangiectasia pode ser um distúrbio primário ou desenvolver-se de modo secundário à obstrução linfática. A linfangiectasia primária geralmente é limitada ao intestino, embora possa ser parte de uma anormalidade do sistema linfático mais disseminada, envolvendo, por exemplo, um quilotórax. A linfangiectasia frequentemente é considerada congênita, ainda que os sinais clínicos, em geral, não estejam presentes desde o nascimento. A linfangiectasia não foi descrita em gatos.

Uma inflamação da mucosa e a linfangite lipogranulomatosa às vezes são relatadas em associação à linfangiectasia, e alguns autores consideram essa condição uma variante da DII idiopática. No entanto, as anormalidades linfáticas predominam e envolvem toda a espessura da parede intestinal, enquanto, na maioria dos casos da DII idiopática, apenas uma dilatação láctea leve é vista (Figura 276.13). Não está claro qual é o principal

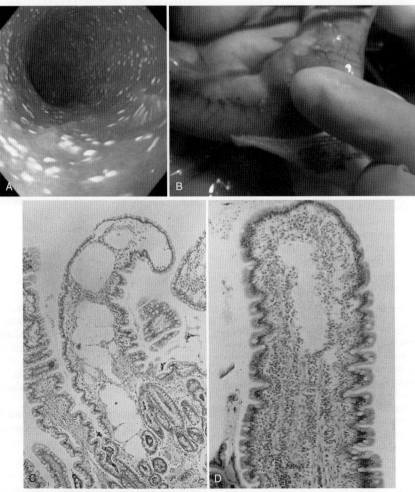

Figura 276.13 Linfangiectasia. **A.** Aparência endoscópica do duodeno de um cão com linfangiectasia, mostrando lácteos dilatados e cheios de gordura. Observe a natureza irregular das mudanças. **B.** Aspecto de linfangite lipogranulomatosa em cão com linfangiectasia à celiotomia. Observe as manchas brancas no lado mesentérico da serosa jejunal. **C.** Aparência histológica de uma biopsia jejunal de um cão da raça Jack Russell Terrier com enteropatia acompanhada de perda de proteína, em que lácteos marcadamente dilatados são consistentes com o diagnóstico de linfangiectasia. **D.** Aparência histológica de uma biopsia jejunal de um cão da raça Retriever com enterite linfoplasmocítica moderada e dilatação secundária leve dos lácteos. (**B.** Cortesia de Sophie Tyler.) (*As figuras A e B encontram-se reproduzidas em cores no Encarte.*)

evento: o vazamento de linfa pode causar inflamação e formação de granuloma ou a linfangite pode causar obstrução linfática. O desenvolvimento de linfangite lipogranulomatosa associada, sobreposta às anomalias congênitas, é uma possível razão para o início e a progressão tardios. A doença é mais comumente vista em raças pequenas de Terrier (p. ex., Yorkshire, Maltês), Rottweiler e o Lundehund norueguês.

A linfangiectasia secundária é causada por obstrução dos vasos linfáticos intestinais. As causas subjacentes incluem: (1) infiltração ou obstrução dos vasos linfáticos por inflamação, fibrose ou processo neoplásico; (2) possivelmente obstrução do ducto torácico; e (3) insuficiência cardíaca direita, decorrente de insuficiência cardíaca congestiva ou tamponamento cardíaco.

Histórico e sinais clínicos[1840-1847]

As manifestações clínicas da linfangiectasia são amplamente atribuíveis aos efeitos da perda entérica de linfa e à consequente hipoproteinemia. Outras funções intestinais permanecem intactas, e a hipoproteinemia pode até estar presente sem diarreia. Esteatorreia, perda profunda de peso, polifagia e diarreia são mais típicos, e vômitos, letargia e anorexia são vistos ocasionalmente. Os sinais podem ser insidiosos no início e ter um padrão intermitente ou flutuante. Ascite ou edema subcutâneo pode ocorrer secundariamente à hipoalbuminemia; o líquido ascítico em geral é um transudato puro, mas, se houver insuficiência cardíaca direita causando linfangiectasia secundária, um transudato modificado desenvolve-se por meio da hipertensão portal. Ascite quilosa é uma possibilidade se a cisterna do quilo estiver anormal ou se os vasos linfáticos abdominais estiverem obstruídos por neoplasia abdominal, como o feocromocitoma. A linfangiectasia foi associada à hepatopatia granulomatosa e, em cães da raça Lundehund, à gastrite e carcinoma gástrico.

Diagnóstico[338,550,556,1845-1851]

Dado que a linfa é rica em lipoproteínas e linfócitos, análises laboratoriais frequentemente mostram pan-hipoproteinemia, hipocolesterolemia e linfopenia decorrente do vazamento de linfa. Hipomagnesemia e hipocalcemia ionizada foram relatadas, sendo a última sugestiva de má absorção de vitamina D e cálcio, e a perda intestinal da proteína de ligação da vitamina D pode estar envolvida. É possível documentar ELP medindo as concentrações fecais de alfa$_1$-PI. Em cães da raça Lundehund afetados, alta excreção fecal de alfa$_1$-PI ocorre antes das alterações nas proteínas séricas.

Estrias hiperecoicas da mucosa são observadas nessa condição, mas a especificidade dessa mudança ultrassonográfica não é conhecida. Os achados gerais na endoscopia incluem a presença de exsudato branco leitoso e gotículas lipídicas brancas ou bolhas mucosas proeminentes, que provavelmente são o resultado da distensão da ponta das vilosidades com o quilo (ver Figuras 276.8 H e 276.12 A). As biopsias endoscópicas podem apoiar o diagnóstico, mas as de espessura total podem ser necessárias para fazer um diagnóstico definitivo. As biopsias endoscópicas podem ser muito superficiais, ou a doença é potencialmente irregular e não detectada. Na laparotomia exploratória, a maioria dos cães apresenta anormalidades macroscópicas, incluindo ID espessado, vasos linfáticos dilatados (no mesentério e serosa intestinal) e ocasionalmente aderências. Os linfonodos mesentéricos também podem estar aumentados, e massas nodulares branco-amareladas (1 a 3 mm de diâmetro) frequentemente são observadas dentro e ao redor dos vasos linfáticos mesentéricos e serosos (ver Figura 276.13 B). Esses nódulos são lipogranulomas, consistindo em acúmulos de macrófagos carregados de lipídios, e parecem resultar de extravasamento peri linfático do quilo ou estão associados a uma linfangite.

O diagnóstico definitivo de linfangiectasia depende de uma biopsia intestinal, e alguns patologistas acreditam que biopsias de espessura total também são necessárias para um diagnóstico confiável. No entanto, existem riscos envolvidos com a cirurgia exploratória em cães desnutridos e hipoproteinêmicos. Alterações

histopatológicas características incluem "dilatação em balão" dos linfáticos na mucosa e na submucosa. A linfangiectasia verdadeira deve ser distinguida da dilatação pós-prandial normal dos vasos lácteos e da dilatação do vaso lácteo secundário ocasionalmente observada com a DII (ver Figura 276.13 C e D).

Tratamento[1693,1852,1853]

A linfangiectasia secundária é manejada pelo tratamento específico de doença subjacente, como pericardiocentese ou pericardiectomia para tamponamento cardíaco (ver Capítulo 102). O objetivo do tratamento da linfangiectasia primária é diminuir a perda entérica de proteína e resolver a inflamação associada para interromper a diarreia, controlando qualquer edema ou efusões. A manipulação da dieta e glicocorticoides são os tratamentos mais importantes.

Doses anti-inflamatórias de glicocorticoides (prednisolona a 0,5 a 1 mg/kg VO, a cada 12 h, e, em seguida, reduzida) podem ser benéficas em alguns casos, especialmente se linfangite associada, lipogranulomas e/ou infiltrado linfocítico-plasmocítico estiverem presentes na LP. Infelizmente, nem todos os casos respondem a tal terapia. O uso de antimicrobianos (tilosina, metronidazol) não mostrou nenhum benefício nítido. Os diuréticos são indicados no tratamento das efusões, e combinações de diuréticos são preferidas (p. ex., furosemida e espironolactona).

A dieta ideal para casos de linfangiectasia é restrita em gordura, densa em calorias e altamente digerível, com afirmações de que pode ser curativa mesmo que a prednisolona seja ineficaz, contanto que seja instituída antes do desenvolvimento dos lipogranulomas. Dietas de redução de peso – ainda que com baixo teor de gordura – são inadequadas, pois os pacientes requerem uma dieta rica em energia; as gastrintestinais com restrição de gordura são preferidas. Anteriormente, a administração de triglicerídeos de cadeia média (TCM) era recomendada, porque pensava-se que esses lipídios eram absorvidos diretamente para o sangue portal. No entanto, essa teoria foi contestada, e o uso do óleo de TCM não é mais recomendado, pois não é muito palatável. A suplementação com vitaminas lipossolúveis é recomendada. O tratamento com ciclosporina pode ser eficaz, mas há confusão se tais casos são, na verdade, DII com dilatação linfática secundária ou linfangiectasia verdadeira.

A resposta ao tratamento é imprevisível, mas a suspensão dos sinais clínicos pode ser espontânea ou alcançada temporariamente com o tratamento, com remissões ocorrendo de meses a muitos anos. No entanto, o prognóstico geral a longo prazo é fraco, e os pacientes quase invariavelmente sucumbem, em última instância, por desnutrição grave, derrames incapacitantes e diarreia intratável

Doença da cripta[1854,1855]

As causas mais comuns de ELP são linfoma, DII e linfangiectasia. No entanto, existem relatos de ELP associada a lesões de cripta intestinal sem evidência de neoplasia, linfangiectasia ou inflamação substancial. Uma baixa frequência de abscedação de cripta é observada no tecido normal, já que várias criptas formam uma unidade cripta-vilosidade, mas um aumento no número de lesões de cripta foi associado a ELP. Biopsias endoscópicas superficiais podem não detectar essas lesões, porém biopsias mais profundas mostram abscedação (ver Figura 276.8 E) ou muitas criptas dilatadas cheias de muco, células epiteliais descamadas e/ou células inflamatórias. A etiologia subjacente não é conhecida. A resposta à terapia com antibacterianos e medicamentos imunossupressores é variável; alguns cães se deterioram repentinamente e podem morrer de doença tromboembólica.

NEOPLASIA DO INTESTINO DELGADO

Espectro da doença[1856-1865]

Linfoma, adenocarcinomas e tumores de mastócitos são os tumores gastrintestinais mais comuns em gatos, com predomínio do linfoma, enquanto os adenocarcinomas, os tumores de músculo liso e outros tumores de células estromais são mais comuns em cães. Fibrossarcoma intestinal (cães), hemangiossarcoma (gatos), Schwannoma, tumores neuroendócrinos, carcinoides e tumores plasmócitos são raros. Os sinais clínicos geralmente incluem perda de peso (se o tumor for maligno), anorexia, diarreia, melena, vômito, desconforto abdominal, efusão abdominal e anemia. Outras consequências mais raras de neoplasia intestinal incluem intussuscepção, perfuração intestinal e efeitos paraneoplásicos. A perda ultrassonográfica da estratificação de parede é altamente indicativa de um aumento de 50 vezes na probabilidade de neoplasia. Exames citológicos de AAF mostram apenas por volta de 70% de concordância com a avaliação histológica. O diagnóstico é baseado na detecção de uma massa ou alças intestinais espessadas na palpação abdominal e/ou em imagens, com o diagnóstico definitivo, em última análise, exigindo biopsia.

Linfoma intestinal[6,7,1866-1877]

O linfoma alimentar (LA) é caracterizado por infiltração da mucosa, submucosa e/ou epitelial por linfócitos neoplásicos, invadindo o intestino de forma difusa ou focal (Figura 276.14). A infiltração focal pode ser nodular, semelhante a uma placa ou circunferencial, mas distribuição difusa é mais comum. Formas focais podem causar obstrução, enquanto a infiltração difusa resulta em má absorção e frequentemente EPP em cães. Microscopicamente, as células neoplásicas podem infiltrar o epitélio (i. e., epiteliotrópicas) ou a lâmina própria, estendendo-se para as camadas musculares mais profundas e linfonodos mesentéricos. A maioria dos gatos afetados apresenta teste negativo para FeLV no momento do diagnóstico, e o LA tornou-se a forma mais comum de linfoma felino após o declínio da infecção por FeLV. O LA pode surgir por mutação em genes promotores e/ou supressores ou talvez por progressão do ELP. A estimulação antigênica crônica pode levar à seleção de um clone maligno e há evidências de suprarregulação de IL-6 em felinos com DII e LA. A estimulação antigênica crônica em pacientes geneticamente predispostos pode estimular a transformação e seleção de células T malignas e progressão para LA de baixo grau, como foi visto em humanos com linfomas gástricos de MALT associados a infecção por *Helicobacter*. O LA frequentemente está associado a mudanças na distribuição espacial do microbioma, embora este seja muito provavelmente um efeito, não a causa do LA. Uma discussão mais ampla de linfoma é apresentada no Capítulo 344.

Achados clínicos[1877-1890]

Cães de meia-idade ou mais velhos são mais comumente afetados por LA. Perda de peso, diarreia crônica e a inapetência progressiva são características comuns; vômito, hematêmese e melena também podem ser notados. Intestinos difusamente engrossados, massa abdominal, linfadenopatia mesentérica e evidências de dor são achados possíveis na palpação abdominal. Hepatoesplenomegalia concomitante e linfadenopatia generalizada são sugestivas de linfoma multicêntrico ou de uma forma alimentar envolvendo o fígado. Raramente há leucemia associada. Sinais decorrentes de hipoproteinemia podem se desenvolver se o LA difuso resultar em uma EPP. Sinais clínicos comuns em gatos são vômito (65%), diarreia (52%), perda de peso (46%) e massas palpáveis.

Complicações[1025,1891,1892]

Além dos problemas esperados de má absorção e EPP, o LA pode causar perfuração intestinal com consequente peritonite. O envolvimento de outros órgãos (baço, pâncreas) pode ocorrer. Infecção secundária por *Salmonella* e trombose arterial femoral foram relatadas.

Achados laboratoriais[50,1665,1771,1778,1893-1898]

A anemia, caracterizada como normocítica-normocrômica não regenerativa ou microcítica e hipocrômica, geralmente é o resultado de doença crônica ou de perda crônica de sangue, mas anemia secundária Coombs positiva às vezes ocorre. Neutrofilia pode ser evidente, e, ocasionalmente, hipereosinofilia paraneoplásica é encontrada. A maioria dos gatos afetados são FeLV negativos. Testes bioquímicos de rotina em cães com LA podem revelar pan-hipoproteinemia em animais com linfoma difuso causando EPP, embora LA de células B ocasionalmente cause hiperglobulinemia via gamopatia monoclonal. É incomum uma EPP causar hipoproteinemia acentuada no LA felino. As reduções nas concentrações séricas de folato ou cobalamina podem ser o resultado de má absorção, SBID secundário a obstrução intestinal ou consumo de ácido fólico pelas células tumorais. Uma hipovitaminose D pode ocorrer.

Diagnóstico por imagem[519,553,1880,1895,1899-1904]

A US pode mostrar espessamento difuso ou focal da parede intestinal, perda de estratificação da parede intestinal e linfadenopatia mesentérica (ver Capítulo 88); também facilita a AAF de lesões tumorais e de espessamento (ver Capítulo 89). Em gatos, o espessamento da muscular de mucosa é sugestiva de LA: uma proporção de muscular para submucosa superior a 1 é indicativa de segmento intestinal anormal, mas não é patognomônica, pois pode ser igualmente causada por obstrução por corpo estranho e enteropatias crônicas. A linfadenopatia mesentérica também não é discriminatória. Endoscopicamente,

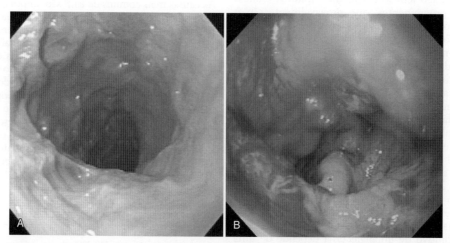

Figura 276.14 Linfoma alimentar. Imagem endoscópica do duodeno de (**A**) cão de 8 anos da raça Collie com mucosa muito irregular e protuberante e (**B**) cão da raça Retriever de 6 anos, mostrando protuberância da mucosa causada por infiltração difusa. A biopsia é necessária para confirmar a causa dessas alterações como linfoma. (**B**. Reimpressa, com autorização, de Lhermette P, Sobel D, editores: *BSAVA manual of canine and feline endoscopy and endosurgery*, Quedgely, Gloucester, England, 2008, BSAVA Publication.) (*Esta figura se encontra reproduzida em cores no Encarte*.)

anormalidades decorrentes de DII ou linfoma podem não ser distinguíveis visualmente de modo confiável, e biopsias devem sempre ser feitas para análise histopatológica (ver Figuras 276.7 G e 276.14).

Biopsia intestinal[517,577,604,605,610,617,1905]

Biopsia de espessura total é preferível a biopsias de pinça endoscópica, que pode perder a lesão ou simplesmente mostrar EPP adjacente. Isso está, em parte, relacionado ao tamanho e à profundidade limitados das biopsias endoscópicas, mas também reflete a tendência do LA de ser predominante mais distalmente no ID. Assim, as biopsias endoscópicas podem ser menos sensíveis do que as cirúrgicas, a menos que seja realizada uma ileoscopia. Biopsias de espessura total dão diagnóstico mais confiável quando os linfócitos neoplásicos podem ser visualizados infiltrando as camadas musculares intestinais. No entanto, a laparotomia exploratória é um procedimento arriscado, pois muitos pacientes estão gravemente debilitados e hipoproteinêmicos e, subjetivamente, a cura de qualquer incisão intestinal pode ser prejudicada pela infiltração neoplásica de tecido conjuntivo normal. Amostras para avaliação citológica podem ser coletadas na endoscopia por escova de citologia, preparação de esfregaço ou via percutânea AAF sob orientação de ultrassom, mas na maioria dos casos é necessária a biopsia intestinal. Uma biopsia percutânea, guiada por ultrassom, de ID espessado e linfonodos mesentéricos aumentados às vezes é possível.

Achados histológicos

Histopatologia de rotina.[1906-1911] Embora a avaliação histopatológica do material de biopsia seja o padrão-ouro para o diagnóstico do LA, a diferenciação de EPP grave pode ser difícil, especialmente em biopsias endoscópicas. Uma infiltração simultânea com eosinófilos pode ocorrer e causar diagnósticos incorretos, como um tumor de mastócitos. A fenotipagem adicional pode ser necessária para um diagnóstico definitivo e fornecer informação prognóstica.

Tipificação.[627,633,1682,1686,1906-1920] Imuno-histoquímica, citometria de fluxo e avaliação da clonalidade de células T por análise por PCR dos rearranjos dos genes do receptor das células T e B melhoram a precisão do diagnóstico (ver Capítulo 334). Essas técnicas moleculares permitem a classificação da linhagem de linfócitos e uma distinção mais precisa de linfoma da EPP. A imuno-histoquímica pode ajudar no diagnóstico se todos os linfócitos pertencerem a uma única linhagem. LA primários de células B e T foram relatados em proporções diferentes, e claramente a crença original de que todos os LA foram sempre de células B na origem está incorreta.

Estudos recentes mostraram que a incidência do LA felino parece estar aumentando. Clinicamente, três formas principais foram definidas, e todas afetam gatos mais velhos (10 a 13 anos), que são geralmente negativos para FeLV. LA de grau intermediário a alto frequentemente apresenta-se como uma massa intestinal focal (às vezes, com envolvimento extraintestinal). Esses são tumores de células T ou B, com um tempo médio de sobrevida de 7 a 10 meses após quimioterapia multiagente. LA de baixo grau apresenta-se como um espessamento intestinal difuso (às vezes, com uma massa intestinal e envolvimento de linfonodos mesentéricos). Esses são principalmente tumores de células T, com um tempo médio de sobrevida de 19 a 29 meses após a quimioterapia com prednisolona e clorambucila. Linfoma linfocítico granular grande apresenta-se como uma massa intestinal focal (às vezes, com envolvimento extra intestinal). Esses são principalmente tumores de células T (com expressão imuno-histoquímica da granzima B), cujo tempo médio de sobrevivência é de apenas 17 dias após quimioterapia multiagente. Os patologistas classificaram LA felinos usando terminologias alternativas baseadas na classificação humana da OMS como: (1) linfoma de células T da mucosa de tipo de células pequenas a intermediárias com envolvimento do epitélio e lâmina própria; (2) linfoma transmural de células T de células grandes que pode mostrar epiteliotropismo e, na maioria das vezes, é um linfoma linfocítico grande granular; e (3) linfoma transmural de grandes células B.

Tratamento e prognóstico[1884,1894,1903,1915,1921-1933]

Cães com LA alimentar difuso ocasionalmente respondem a quimioterapia de multiagentes (ver Capítulo 344), mas a maioria apresenta uma resposta ruim, e, naqueles que respondem, existe o risco de perfuração intestinal. A resposta pobre é diferente do linfoma multicêntrico canino ou linfoma restrito ao reto canino (ver Capítulo 277).

Em contrapartida, o prognóstico em gatos é mais favorável: alguns alcançam remissão prolongada. A linhagem celular parece ser importante para determinar a resposta ao tratamento e prognóstico: (1) linfoma de células T da mucosa de células pequenas a intermediárias tem um tempo longo de sobrevida, com média de 29 meses; (2) linfoma transmural de células T de células grandes tem um tempo médio de sobrevida curto de 1,5 meses; (3) linfoma transmural de células B tem um tempo médio de sobrevida de 3,5 meses. Há evidências de que o primeiro tipo (células pequenas) está aumentando em incidência e, felizmente, tem um prognóstico muito melhor do que linfomas de grau intermediário e alto. Foram relatadas boas respostas para quimioterapia combinada seja com protocolos multifármacos padrão, seja com um regime "apenas oral" (p. ex., prednisolona e clorambucila) para a forma de células pequenas. Este último tratamento é bem tolerado e pode ser particularmente aplicável aos casos em que a diferenciação entre LA de grau baixo e EPP é incerta; o tratamento também é aplicável a DII grave. A radioterapia abdominal tem sido usada como terapia de resgate.

Plasmocitoma extramedular[1934-1938]

São tumores raros no trato GI e ocorrem principalmente no estômago ou IG, sendo, às vezes, encontrados no ID. Eles podem estar associados a uma gamopatia monoclonal, mas essa também foi encontrada na gastroenterocolite plasmocítica.

Adenoma e adenocarcinoma intestinal[1857,1939-1954]

Em cães, tanto o adenoma quanto o adenocarcinoma são encontrados mais comumente no IG do que no ID; o oposto é verdadeiro em gatos.

No ID canino, o carcinoma tem predileção pelo duodeno, enquanto o jejuno e o íleo são mais comumente afetados em gatos. O adenocarcinoma é mais comum em cães mais velhos (idade média de 9 anos) e gatos (idade média de 11 anos). Os adenomas podem ser polipoides, enquanto os carcinomas são mais propensos a crescer como lesões estenóticas em placas ou anulares. O adenocarcinoma intestinal é mais comum do que o adenoma e mais frequente em gatos da raça Siamês, porém pólipos adenomatosos também são vistos no ID felino. Não há associação conhecida com infecção por retrovírus em gatos, e há expressão variável de p53 em cães.

Achados clínicos e diagnóstico[546,547,1862,1941,1950-1955]

Os adenocarcinomas são localmente infiltrativos e podem se estender à serosa e ao mesentério, levando a metástases nos linfonodos locais e/ou na cavidade peritoneal, bem como via hematógena. Consequentemente, os sinais clínicos estão relacionados à obstrução parcial ou peritonite quando ocorre perfuração ou carcinomatose intracelômica. A palpação abdominal consegue revelar espessamento focal do intestino. Melena e anemia podem estar presentes se ocorrer ulceração significativa; a anemia em geral é fortemente regenerativa, mas pode se tornar hipocrômica e microcítica em razão da deficiência de ferro. O diagnóstico por imagem consegue delinear uma lesão em massa, e AAF guiados por ultrassom podem ser úteis, embora o diagnóstico definitivo geralmente requeira biopsia percutânea (Tru-Cut) ou cirúrgica (ver Capítulo 89).

Tratamento e prognóstico[1945,1956-1962]

A ressecção cirúrgica é o tratamento de escolha. No entanto, o prognóstico em geral é grave, porque os tumores quase invariavelmente levam a metástases no momento do diagnóstico. Tempos de remissão após cirurgia de até 2 anos foram relatados, mas o tempo de sobrevida é frequentemente inferior a 6 meses. Para os cães, é relatado um tempo médio de sobrevida de 10 meses, com taxas de 40,5 e 33,1%, após 1 e 2 anos, respectivamente. O tempo de sobrevida é significativamente mais curto para cães com evidência histológica de metástase no momento da cirurgia (média de 3 meses) do que para cães sem (média de 15 meses). A propagação metastática comumente envolve linfonodos locais e do fígado, bem como carcinomatose, com metástases para os testículos, a pele e outros órgãos. A expressão "COX-2" foi documentada em cães, mas não em tumores epiteliais intestinais felinos, e é um potencial alvo terapêutico; quimioterapia adjuvante padrão não foi mostrada como efetiva.

Tumores de células musculares lisas do estroma[1963-1981]

Tumores de músculo liso do ID (leiomioma e leiomiossarcoma) são incomuns em cães mais velhos (idade média de 10 anos) e raros em gatos. O local anatômico em cães normalmente é o jejuno ou ceco, enquanto em gatos estão quase exclusivamente no ID. Os tumores frequentemente são nodulares na borda antimesentérica. A distinção histológica entre tumores benignos e malignos é difícil, mas a disseminação metastática do leiomiossarcoma para o fígado e linfonodos locais é incomum de qualquer maneira. Outro tumor dentro desse espectro é o tumor estromal GI (TEGI), que é histologicamente semelhante, mas surge das células intersticiais de Cajal.

A distinção de tumores de músculo liso de TEGI é pela expressão diferencial de moléculas de CD, como CD34 e c-KIT (CD 117) e marcadores de músculo liso (vimentina, desmina, alfa-actina de músculo liso [AML]) e neurogênicos (S100, enolase específica de neurônios [NSE] e sinaptofisina). Normalmente, tumores de músculo liso expressam AML, mas são negativos para o marcador c-KIT (CD117). A expressão não controlada de c-KIT, um receptor da tirosinoquinase, é um marcador importante de TEGI. Tumores que se assemelham a TEGI, mas não mostram nenhuma expressão de c-KIT, são classificados como TEGI-semelhantes.

Diagnóstico[1982-1990]

Sinais clínicos. A apresentação clínica pode variar e incluir vômito, diarreia, anorexia, poliúria, polidipsia, melena, colapso agudo e perda de peso. Muitos desses sinais são resultado dos efeitos locais do tumor (ou seja, obstrução, intussuscepção), do sangramento agudo ou da anemia por deficiência de ferro. No entanto, efeitos paraneoplásicos são relatados, especialmente hipoglicemia, como resultado da produção de um peptídio semelhante ao fator II de crescimento, parecido com a insulina. Outras síndromes paraneoplásicas associadas a leiomiossarcomas incluem eritrocitose, decorrente da elaboração de uma molécula semelhante a eritropoetina, e diabetes insípido nefrogênico (ver Capítulo 352).

Exames laboratoriais. Achados como eritrocitose ou hipoglicemia refletem as consequências de efeitos diretos ou paraneoplásicos, mas os resultados dos testes podem ser normais. A anemia por deficiência de ferro pode se desenvolver sem quaisquer sinais GI evidentes, em razão da perda crônica de sangue oculto.

Diagnóstico por imagem. Radiografias e especialmente ultrassom podem auxiliar na identificação de uma lesão de massa (ver Capítulo 88), enquanto a endoscopia digestiva alta pode confirmar a presença de uma lesão se estiver ao alcance e rompendo a mucosa (ver o Capítulo 113). No entanto, as biopsias por pinça costumam ser muito superficiais, e a laparotomia exploratória é a técnica de escolha tanto para o diagnóstico quanto para o tratamento.

Tratamento e prognóstico[1991,1992]

O tratamento de escolha é a excisão cirúrgica, e o prognóstico é excelente para leiomiomas. Leiomiossarcomas têm crescimento e metástase lentos; logo, se a ressecção cirúrgica for completa, o prognóstico é bom, com tempo médio de sobrevida de 21 meses. O prognóstico é afetado por características macroscópicas, histológicas e imuno-histoquímicas, como tamanho e localização do tumor, índice mitótico, pontuação AgNOR e rotulagem Ki67. Mesmo que a metástase seja evidente no momento da cirurgia, o prognóstico é razoável, com sobrevida prolongada relatada em alguns casos. Parece não haver diferenças no prognóstico para TEGI em comparação a tumores de músculo liso. Em humanos, o imatinibe, um inibidor da tirosinoquinase, prolonga a sobrevivência em TEGI irressecáveis; ensaios clínicos com masitinib e toceranib para TEGI em cães estão em andamento.

Tumores de captação e descarboxilação de precursores da amina[1993-1996]

Tumores neuroendócrinos funcionais, os chamados tumores de captação e descarboxilação de precursores da amina (APUDomas) – tumores de peptídio vasoativo intestinal (VIPomas), tumores de polipeptídeo pancreático (PPomas) –, ainda não foram adequadamente descritos em cães e gatos. Foi descrito um carcinoide funcional, com teores séricos aumentados de 5 HT.

Outras neoplasias gastrintestinais[1776,1781,1857-1861,1943,1952,1993,1994,1997-2012]

Tumores raros, como fibrossarcoma, osteossarcoma, Schwannoma e carcinoides não funcionais, tendem a ser focalmente invasivos e em geral causam sinais clínicos semelhantes aos do adenocarcinoma intestinal. Os tumores intestinais de mastócitos tendem a se comportar mais como LA, mas, em gatos, podem ser associados a uma reação fibrótica marcante e são descritos como tumores esclerosantes de mastócitos felinos (ver anteriormente). Sarcoma histiocítico pode infiltrar o ID e causar má absorção grave. Hemangioma do ID é muito raro, assim como hemangiossarcoma, mas este é mais comum em gatos, nos quais os sinais costumam estar relacionados à hemorragia e, ocasionalmente, à trombose mesentérica. O melanoma intestinal é muito raro. Pólipos hamartomatosos em cães e pólipos adenomatosos que afetam o ID em gatos de meia-idade podem causar vômito, hematêmese ou melena. No entanto, é possível ocorrer perda crônica de sangue oculto, e os animais podem apresentar anemia por deficiência de ferro. A ganglioneuromatose é uma proliferação benigna muito rara de gânglios e células gliais entéricas. Na maioria das espécies, ocorre entre as camadas submucosa e muscular, mas uma lesão da mucosa, ressecada com sucesso, foi relatada em um cão.

OUTRAS DOENÇAS DO INTESTINO DELGADO

Íleo adinâmico e pseudo-obstrução intestinal

Definição e apresentação clínica[63,274-278,483,484,2013-2036]

O íleo adinâmico é uma sequela comum de muitos problemas gastrintestinais primários – cirurgia abdominal, enterite parvoviral, pancreatite, peritonite, hipopotassemia – e disautonomia (ver Boxes 276.3 e 276.7). O íleo pós-operatório pode ocorrer após qualquer cirurgia abdominal graças a uma combinação de inflamação, aumento do efeito inibitório simpático no tônus e, frequentemente, o uso de analgésicos opioides. É de importância clínica, pois aumenta a morbidade e prolonga a hospitalização.

A disautonomia frequentemente mostra envolvimento de vários órgãos, afetando a função da pupila, da saliva e da bexiga, bem como motilidade gastresofágica e intestinal. Uma epidemia foi controlada em gatos do Reino Unido na década de 1980 (a chamada síndrome de Key-Gaskell), talvez em razão da retirada de um potencial componente alimentar tóxico não identificado. Entretanto, casos esporádicos ainda são vistos em todo o mundo em cães e gatos.

O termo "pseudo-obstrução intestinal" descreve uma condição em que os pacientes mostram evidências clínicas consistentes com uma obstrução, mas nenhuma causa mecânica é encontrada. A condição foi associada tanto às neuropatias viscerais quanto às miopatias em humanos, e tais causas podem ocorrer em pequenos animais. Existem muitos relatos na literatura de casos isolados em cães, mas poucos em gatos. A maioria dos casos está associada a leiomiosite idiopática e enteropatia esclerosante, com fibrose e um infiltrado de células mononucleares da túnica muscular. A deficiência de alfa-actina do músculo liso foi descrita em um gato de Bengala, e pseudo-obstrução intestinal felina também pode ser secundária ao linfoma intestinal.

Manejo[490,2022,2037-2048]

Após a possibilidade de obstrução mecânica ter sido eliminada, o manejo do íleo adinâmico e da pseudo-obstrução intestinal visa identificar qualquer causa subjacente e fornecer o tratamento específico. Terapia não específica para estimular a motilidade intestinal também é indicada. Os agentes procinéticos adequados incluem os agonistas do receptor 5-HT 4 cisaprida ou mosaprida, o antagonista dopaminérgico D2 metoclopramida, os inibidores da acetilcolinesterase (como a acotiamida) e medicamentos semelhantes à motilina (como a eritromicina). Em cães e gatos, a cisaprida parece ser o agente mais eficaz, mas não está mais disponível em muitos países graças à toxicose humana. Os antibacterianos também podem ser apropriados, dada a probabilidade de SBID secundário. A alimentação é benéfica para humanos, e é possível continuar o suporte nutricional indefinidamente, embora vômito e constipação intestinal ou diarreia em geral continuem. Infelizmente, a maioria dos casos de pseudo-obstrução idiopática relatada na literatura veterinária respondeu mal à terapia, e o prognóstico é grave; foi relatado apenas um caso que respondeu a doses imunossupressoras de corticosteroides combinadas com procinéticos.

Distúrbios intestinais cirúrgicos

Obstrução intestinal[499,501,503,523,2049-2094]

A obstrução intestinal pode ser o resultado de lesões extraluminais, intramurais ou intraluminais e classificada como aguda ou crônica, parcial ou completa e simples ou estrangulante. A maioria das obstruções intraluminais é causada por muitos objetos estranhos; os radiotransparentes (meias, caroços de pêssego, espigas de milho) podem ser os mais difíceis de identificar. As causas intramurais de obstrução incluem neoplasia, parasitas (raros), hematomas (que, acredita-se, ocorrem espontaneamente), granulomas (p. ex., PIF focal, ficomicose, pelos encravados) e estenoses (depois de compactação por corpo estranho ou cirurgia). As causas extraluminais incluem aprisionamento por hérnias, lacerações mesentéricas, aderências congênitas e adquiridas e intussuscepções.

A maioria dos casos de obstrução do ID pode ser identificada por meio de radiografias abdominais simples (ver Figura 276.10). Um intestino dilatado, com mais de 1,6 multiplicado pela altura do corpo de L5 em seu ponto mais estreito, tem sido considerado altamente preditivo de obstruções do ID, mas a validade de tal fórmula é debatida. Corpos estranhos lineares causam agrupamento do ID e um padrão característico de bolhas de gás em forma de vírgula. A US é útil na detecção de corpos estranhos radioluscentes, intussuscepções e obstruções intramurais, mas o acúmulo de gás intestinal pode obscurecer a lesão.

O prognóstico para a cura cirúrgica depende da causa da obstrução, da presença de perfuração e peritonite, da viabilidade do intestino remanescente e da gravidade de quaisquer anormalidades metabólicas associadas. A recuperação é auxiliada por um retorno rápido à nutrição enteral. O resultado provavelmente será favorável com corpos estranhos simples, mas é reservado para corpos estranhos lineares, pois é provável que haja várias perfurações, e é grave para animais com vólvulo ou neoplasia intestinal metastática. O paciente corre risco de desenvolver síndrome do intestino curto se uma parte extensa do ID precisar ser ressecado (ver a seguir).

Intussuscepção[1858,1997,2095-2138]

A causa extraluminal mais comum da obstrução é intussuscepção, e a intussuscepção ileocólica é a variante anatômica mais frequente. Em casos graves, o *intussusceptum* pode migrar através do *intussuscipiens* e sair pelo ânus, onde pode ser confundido como um prolapso retal. São relatadas intussuscepções retrógrada, médio-jejunal e dupla, enquanto as intussuscepções duodenogástricas são raras e podem causar vômito e choque, embora possam ser redutíveis por endoscopia (Figura 276.15). Animais mais jovens são mais propensos a desenvolver intussuscepções, especialmente após um caso de gastrenterite ou cirurgia intestinal, e os gatos da raça Maine Coon também podem ser predispostos. Existe risco aumentado após cirurgia renal experimental, toxicoses que afetam a motilidade intestinal, hipotireoidismo congênito e pós-parto. Neoplasia é a causa mais frequente em animais de meia-idade a mais velhos, com a massa tumoral atuando como um nicho para o dobramento interno do ID. Intussuscepções também foram associadas à lesão renal aguda decorrente de leptospirose.

O diagnóstico da intussuscepção é feito por meio de uma combinação do histórico, da palpação de uma massa abdominal "em forma de salsicha", da evidência radiográfica de uma massa e uma obstrução do ID e da demonstração ultrassonográfica de uma estrutura característica de parede dupla (ver Figura 276.7 C). Intussuscepções transitórias, clinicamente silenciosas, e reduções espontâneas após obstrução foram relatadas, mas a correção é necessária na maioria dos casos clinicamente afetados, o que pode envolver redução simples ou ressecção real da região afetada com anastomose ponta a ponta. A recidiva é um risco reconhecido e pode, em parte, estar relacionada a danos dos nervos entéricos da região. Um rápido retorno à alimentação e a normalização da motilidade intestinal são recomendados, em vez de paralisar o ID no pós-operatório com medicamentos antimuscarínicos. A enteroplicatura pode ser realizada para tentar prevenir a recidiva, mas acarreta riscos de perfuração, aprisionamento e estenose.

Estrangulamento intestinal[558,2066,2139-2146]

O estrangulamento pode ocorrer se as alças do intestino estão encarceradas em: hérnias umbilicais ou inguinais; uma hérnia interna, por meio de um defeito induzido cirurgicamente no

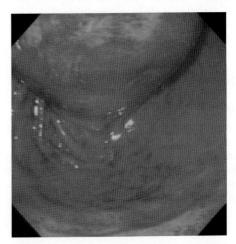

Figura 276.15 Intussuscepção duodeno-gástrica. Imagem endoscópica do intussuscepto do duodeno por meio do piloro no antro gástrico em um cão Pastor-Alemão encaminhado para avaliação de vômito. (*Esta figura se encontra reproduzida em cores no Encarte.*)

mesentério; rupturas ligamentares omentais, mesentéricas ou duodenocólicas; ou aprisionamento por aderências após fratura óssea púbica ou lipomas intra-abdominais. Além de causar obstrução, é provável que ocorra isquemia intestinal, com risco de lesão de reperfusão após a correção cirúrgica ou a perfuração se não for corrigida.

Vólvulo intestinal[2070,2110,2147-2156]

Nessa condição, os intestinos giram em torno do eixo mesentérico, comprometendo a artéria mesentérica cranial, e uma obstrução vascular completa consequente pode levar ao infarto. O achado radiográfico típico é a distensão de gás, marcante de grande parte do ID. A confirmação é feita na cirurgia, e a possibilidade de eutanásia na mesa de operação deve ser discutida com o tutor se a laparotomia revelar isquemia intestinal difusa e necrose. Os relatos são esporádicos e, felizmente, raros, porém o prognóstico é grave.

Perfuração intestinal[2068,2071,2157-2179]

Uma perfuração do ID levando a peritonite séptica é causada mais frequentemente por administração de AINE, pela ingestão de corpos estranhos lineares e de objetos afiados não digeríveis (p. ex., palitos de coquetel, agulhas) ou pela demora no diagnóstico de qualquer corpo estranho no ID. Perfuração por fragmentos ósseos pontiagudos raramente é relatada e pode não ser tão arriscada quanto o público foi levado a acreditar, pois os ossos são amolecidos e até dissolvidos no ácido gástrico. A ingestão de vários ímãs foi associada a perfuração, provavelmente em razão da necrose da parede intestinal entre dois objetos atraídos magneticamente. Avulsão traumática de um vaso mesentérico leva a isquemia e perfuração retardada do segmento intestinal relevante. Tumores e granulomas fúngicos podem provocar perfuração, e ilhas de mucosa gástrica heterotópica no ID também são propensas a ulceração ou mesmo perfuração.

Síndrome do intestino curto[2180-2191]

A síndrome do intestino curto (SIC) refere-se à situação em que uma grande porção do ID (mais de dois terços) está ausente, em razão de ressecção ou, raramente, de uma anomalia congênita. Casos de SIC felizmente são raros em gatos e cães, com a opção de eutanásia para casos graves, e muita informação sobre o manejo tem sido extrapolada da cirurgia GI humana.

Sinais clínicos. Os sinais clínicos (p. ex., diarreia) são resultado da porção funcional do ID insuficiente para assimilação de nutrientes e eletrólitos. Em alguns casos, a SIC ocorre temporariamente após ressecção, pois uma hiperplasia adaptativa no restante do intestino pode levar à melhora clínica subsequente. O grau de má absorção depende do comprimento do intestino ressecado; em cães, estudos experimentais sugerem que a remoção de até 85% do intestino pode ser tolerada. O local da ressecção é igualmente importante: a remoção da válvula ileocólica predispõe à colonização bacteriana ascendente. Ressecção massiva também precipita mudanças nos hormônios GI, levando a hipergastrinemia e aumento da secreção de ácido.

Diagnóstico. O diagnóstico da SIC geralmente é baseado em um histórico de ressecção intestinal com consequente diarreia e perda de peso. Se houver suspeita de lesão congênita, uma radiografia de contraste pode demonstrar o comprimento do ID encurtado.

Tratamento.[2192-2195] Após uma ressecção maciça, a terapia parenteral intensiva com fluidos (ver Capítulo 129) e a nutrição parenteral (ver Capítulo 189) devem ser adotadas. A alimentação oral é restrita, mas não totalmente retirada, porque a presença de alimentos, bile e secreções pancreáticas no intestino é um estímulo importante para adaptação intestinal. Uma dieta líquida isotônica, oligomérica e com restrição de gordura pode ser fornecida inicialmente, com transição gradual para uma dieta líquida polimérica e, em seguida, com restrição de gordura e fibra de fácil assimilação. Má absorção de gordura, vitaminas hidrossolúveis e minerais também pode ocorrer, e suplementação parenteral ou na dita pode ser necessária. A suplementação parenteral de cobalamina é essencial se o íleo for ressecado. Antagonistas do receptor H_2 ou inibidores da bomba de prótons podem ser usados no período pós-operatório para neutralizar uma possível hipergastrinemia. Agentes antimicrobianos podem ser necessários se a junção ileocecocólica foi ressecada ou se SBID secundário for suspeitado. Se a resposta à dieta e aos antibióticos for pobre, agentes antissecretores (loperamida, difenoxilato, octreotida) podem ser necessários. Uma resina de ligação de sais biliares (p. ex., colestiramina) pode ajudar a reduzir a secreção do cólon causada pelos sais biliares mal absorvidos após ressecção ileal; o ácido ursodesoxicólico foi descrito por melhorar a adaptação intestinal em um modelo cirúrgico felino.

Prognóstico.[1742] O prognóstico depende da quantidade de ID preservada e da resposta à terapia. Alguns animais sofrem notável hiperplasia adaptativa e podem retornar a uma dieta normal, enquanto outros nunca respondem adequadamente. Complicações da SIC humana incluem cálculos biliares, urólitos de oxalato e acidose d-láctica. Em casos refratários, uma modificação GI cirúrgica experimental para retardar o trânsito intestinal e aumentar a área de absorção foi descrita; reconstrução, regeneração ou transplante intestinal podem ser viáveis no futuro.

Síndrome do intestino irritável

Definição e diagnóstico[2196-2198]

A síndrome do intestino irritável (SII) é caracterizada por episódios recorrentes, geralmente agudos, de dor abdominal, borborigmos e diarreia que mais comumente causam sinais de disfunção no IG (ver Capítulo 277). A motilidade intestinal disfuncional pode ser de importância principal (Boxe 276.14), porque, na ausência de alterações morfológicas, um distúrbio funcional é considerado a causa desse problema enigmático.

Boxe 276.14 Causas potenciais da síndrome do intestino irritável

- Distúrbios primários de motilidade
- Transtornos psicossomáticos
- Intolerância alimentar não diagnosticada
- Doença inflamatória não diagnosticada
- Hiperalgesia visceral.

REFERÊNCIAS BIBLIOGRÁFICAS

As referências bibliográficas deste capítulo se encontram online no Ambiente de Aprendizagem.

CAPÍTULO 277

Doenças do Intestino Grosso

Edward James Hall

ESTRUTURA E FUNÇÕES NORMAIS

Em princípio, o intestino grosso (IG) de caninos e felinos são simples estruturas tubulares, compreendendo o cólon, um pequeno divertículo cecal e o reto. No entanto, ele desempenha um papel fundamental no controle da homeostase de fluidos, nas interações do hospedeiro com o microbioma intestinal e no armazenamento e evacuação regular de matéria fecal. Distúrbios do IG são comuns nesses animais, podendo causar diarreia ou constipação intestinal, além de, se houver ulceração, eliminação de sangue fresco (*hematoquezia*; ver Capítulo 41). É importante ressaltar que a maioria dos distúrbios do IG, embora quase sempre não seja fatal, pode ter um efeito significativo na qualidade da vida do paciente (QV). Crianças com doença crônica do IG têm baixa QV,[1] e o sofrimento causado a cães, gatos e seus tutores frequentemente é evidente na prática veterinária,[2] se bem que a QV não seja facilmente quantificada.

Estrutura

Anatomia macroscópica[3-8]

No que diz respeito à anatomia, o IG tubular continua a partir do intestino delgado distal (ID), começando no esfíncter ileocólico e terminando no ânus, sendo composto de três seções anatomicamente distintas: o ceco, o cólon, e o reto (Figura 277.1 A). A seção do cólon compreende três segmentos maldelineados – cólon ascendente, transverso e descendente –, demarcado por flexuras que não são muito pronunciadas, sobretudo em gatos, em que o cólon transverso é muito curto. O cólon é apoiado em um mesentério frouxo, o mesocólon, de modo que sua posição nas radiografias laterais pode estar no abdome dorsal ou médio.

A estrutura bruta do cólon é relativamente simples, sem faixas longitudinais de músculo (tênias), como visto no cólon humano, e em geral sem saculações (haustros). O diâmetro do lúmen do cólon é variável, dependendo do volume de gás e do conteúdo de fezes, mas quase sempre é o dobro do diâmetro do ID. Em média, o IG tem 60 a 75 cm de comprimento em cães (faixa de 25 a 90 cm), variando de 20 a 45 cm em gatos. Em ambos os animais, contribui com 20 a 25% do comprimento intestinal total (delgado e grosso).

Esfíncter ileocólico. A papila ileocólica pode ser visualizada durante a colonoscopia flexível. Em cães, ela aparece como uma protuberância elevada semelhante a um cogumelo (Figura 277.2 A), mas em gatos costuma ser bastante achatada e em forma de fenda. É um esfíncter pelo qual o conteúdo ileal líquido entra periodicamente. Adjacente a ele, fica o orifício cecocólico, que leva a um ceco com terminação cega.

Ceco. O ceco é um divertículo que surge do cólon proximal; o orifício ceco-cólica é separado da papila ileocólica e tem o próprio músculo esfíncter. Situa-se aproximadamente a meio caminho entre o flanco direito e o plano mediano, ventral ao duodeno no nível das 3ª e 4ª vértebras lombares, separadas pelo omento maior. O ceco canino varia de 8 a 30 cm de comprimento e é sigmoide, espiralando em direção ao fundo cego arredondado. De modo ventral, está ligado à borda antimesentérica do íleo. O ceco em gatos é menos torcido, mais curto (2 a 4 cm) e estreito, tornando difícil a intubação endoscópica.

Cólon proximal. O cólon corre de maneira cranial pela papila ileocólica como o cólon ascendente ou direito, que é o

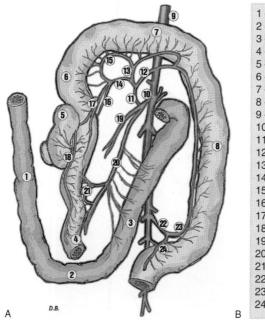
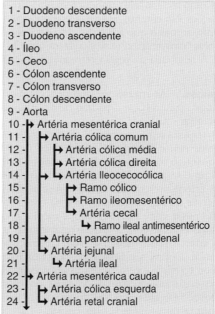

1 - Duodeno descendente
2 - Duodeno transverso
3 - Duodeno ascendente
4 - Íleo
5 - Ceco
6 - Cólon ascendente
7 - Cólon transverso
8 - Cólon descendente
9 - Aorta
10 - ↳ Artéria mesentérica cranial
11 - ↳ Artéria cólica comum
12 - ↳ Artéria cólica média
13 - ↳ Artéria cólica direita
14 - ↳ Artéria Ileocecocólica
15 - ↳ Ramo cólico
16 - ↳ Ramo ileomesentérico
17 - ↳ Artéria cecal
18 - ↳ Ramo ileal antimesentérico
19 - ↳ Artéria pancreaticoduodenal
20 - ↳ Artéria jejunal
21 - ↳ Artéria ileal
22 - ↳ Artéria mesentérica caudal
23 - ↳ Artéria cólica esquerda
24 - ↳ Artéria retal cranial

Figura 277.1 Anatomia funcional do intestino grosso canino. **A.** Arranjo anatômico do intestino grosso e seu suprimento de sangue. O duodeno é mostrado para fins de referência espacial. **B.** Representação esquemática das seções do intestino grosso e as divisões de seu fornecimento arterial de sangue. (Adaptada e redesenhada de Lecoindre P, Gaschen F, Monnet E, editores: *Canine and Feline Gastroenterology*, França, 2010, Wolters Kluwer.)

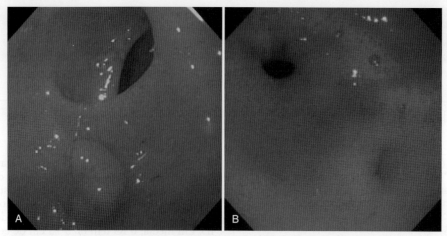

Figura 277.2 Junção ileocólica normal, conforme observada durante a colonoscopia flexível em: **A.** Cão: a papila ileocólica em forma de cogumelo é vista abaixo do orifício cecal. **B.** Gato: a papila ileocólica é muito mais plana, e o ceco, muito menor e mais curto do que nos cães. (*Esta figura se encontra reproduzida em cores no Encarte.*)

segmento colônico mais curto em cães. O apêndice cecal surge no cólon direito proximal, a não mais do que 1 cm da papila ileocólica. O cólon, então, gira na flexura cólica direita ou hepática para passar pelo corpo como o cólon transverso, adjacente à grande curvatura do estômago e do lobo pancreático esquerdo e cranial à raiz do mesentério. Os cólons direito e transverso, juntos, são funcionalmente considerados proximal.

Cólon distal. O cólon transverso gira de modo caudal no abdome cranial, na flexura cólica esquerda ou esplênica, tornando-se o esquerdo ou descendente, considerado o distal. O cólon esquerdo é o mais longo segmento e passa, de maneira causal, além da borda ventromedial do rim esquerdo e ventral à musculatura sublombar e dos linfonodos. Ao nível da borda pélvica, torna-se o reto.

Reto. O reto quase sempre está totalmente dentro do canal pélvico, iniciando onde a artéria retal cranial entra e terminando no canal anal. Tem 4 a 6 cm de comprimento e 3 a 4 cm de largura em cães de tamanho médio, sendo sua porção média ligeiramente mais larga, formando um bulbo rudimentar. Em geral, fica a meio caminho entre o sacro e o solo da pelve em radiografias laterais. Como o cólon, ele também tem uma superfície lisa sem indentações. No entanto, apenas a metade cranial é coberta por peritônio, ao passo que a distal é retroperitoneal. A mucosa forma dobras transversais que se suavizam quando o reto está distendido. A anatomia da região reto-anal é descrita no Capítulo 278.

Suprimento sanguíneo.[9] As artérias mesentéricas craniais e caudais fornecem sangue para o IG, e o padrão de distribuição é importante ao planejar qualquer ressecção cirúrgica (ver Figura 277.1 B). A artéria mesentérica cranial supre o ceco e o cólon ascendente pelos ramos ileocecocólico e cólico direito, respectivamente, enquanto o cólon transverso o faz por meio da artéria cólica medial, que se anastomosa com as artérias cólica direita e esquerda. A artéria mesentérica caudal supre a artéria cólica esquerda que corre de maneira cranial, ao longo do cólon esquerdo, para anastomosar com a artéria cólica média, e de modo caudal, para anastomosar com a artéria retal cranial. O reto é suprido pelas artérias retais medial e caudal, bem como pela artéria retal cranial. Destas, a última supre a maior parte do sangue para o cólon terminal e reto, devendo ser preservada durante qualquer ressecção colônica/retal. As veias do cólon terminam na veia porta, malgrado as veias do segmento retal retroperitoneal possam terminar na veia cava caudal.

Vasos linfáticos.[10-11] A linfa do cólon drena para linfonodos cólicos segmentais – direito, meio e esquerdo – associados às raízes das artérias mesentéricas craniais e caudais. O número de linfonodos varia de um a nove, com uma média de quatro. Isso é importante no planejamento cirúrgico de qualquer ressecção de IG, conquanto a drenagem colateral seja estabelecida rapidamente.

Inervação.[12-14] O nervo vago fornece inervação para o cólon proximal, enquanto os pélvicos suprem o cólon distal. Nervos simpáticos se originam dos gânglios paravertebrais e seguem as artérias mesentéricas e os nervos esplâncnicos lombares para o IG. Os intestinos também contêm um sistema nervoso intramural, localizado entre as camadas musculares longitudinais, circulares, e na submucosa. Fibras pré-ganglionares parassimpáticas e pós-ganglionares simpáticas fazem sinapse em corpos celulares e dendritos do sistema nervoso intrínseco. Vias de reflexo controlam o movimento da parede do cólon, secreção de água e eletrólitos, além do fluxo sanguíneo local.

Anatomia microscópica[7,8,15-37]

O IG se assemelha à estrutura do ID (ver Capítulo 276), compreendendo quatro camadas: mucosa, submucosa, muscular e serosa (Figura 277.3).

Mucosa. Em comparação com a estrutura microscópica do ID, o IG é uma superfície plana, sem vilosidades, e os colonócitos epiteliais expressam menos microvilosidades, mas existem muito mais células caliciformes secretoras de muco (Figura 277.4).

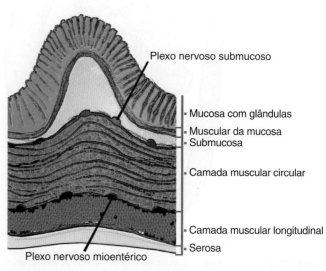

Figura 277.3 Microestrutura da parede do cólon, mostrando as quatro camadas e o plexo nervoso entérico.

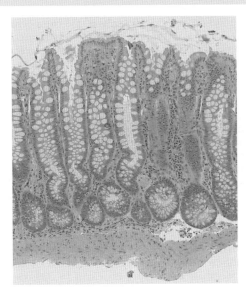

Figura 277.4 Aspecto histológico da mucosa do cólon. Observe a superfície plana com muco, criptas profundas e grande número de células caliciformes na mucosa, bem como a muscular da mucosa subjacente. (Cortesia de Michael Day, Universidade de Bristol.)

Epitélio. Várias criptas tubulares retas (≈ 500 μ de comprimento) estão presentes no cólon, estendendo-se por quase toda a espessura da mucosa. Elas apresentam células epiteliais, produtoras de muco e endócrinas. As células na base das criptas se dividem e proliferam continuamente, migrando para o topo do epitélio à medida que amadurecem. A renovação celular é mais lenta do que no ID – 4 a 7 dias, em comparação com 3 dias no ID –, porém é afetada pelo hormônio do crescimento (GH) com a expressão aumentada dos receptores de GH durante o reparo no cólon. À medida que os colonócitos migram para cima, diferenciam-se e amadurecem em células epiteliais, caliciformes ou endócrinas. Por fim, essas células sofrem apoptose e descamam para o lúmen.

A superfície plana de absorção é revestida por uma única camada de células colunares situadas em uma membrana basal e intercaladas com células caliciformes (10 a 25 células caliciformes para cada 100 epiteliais). As primeiras são importantes no IG, pois produzem muco que inibe a invasão bacteriana, além de lubrificar a passagem das fezes. As células endócrinas secretam somatostatina, polipeptídeo P, fatores de crescimento semelhantes à insulina e peptídios similares ao glucagon. Os linfócitos intraepiteliais consistem predominantemente no subtipo de células T CD8+.

Lâmina própria. Os linfócitos intraepiteliais do cólon migram da lâmina própria (LP), que contém os vários componentes do sistema imunológico da mucosa semelhante àqueles encontrados na LP do ID (ver Capítulo 276), em especial linfócitos e plasmócitos, com mastócitos, macrófagos, eosinófilos e neutrófilos presentes em menor número. Os linfócitos da LP do cólon são predominantemente células T CD4+, B secretoras de IgA e plasmáticas. A estrutura geral do sistema imunológico da mucosa e do tecido linfoide associado ao intestino (GALT) é descrita em mais detalhes nos Capítulos 274 e 276. Os outros elementos celulares do LP do cólon incluem fibroblastos e neurônios entéricos que interagem com as células do sistema imune e os colonócitos.

Muscular da mucosa. A camada mais interna da mucosa é separada da submucosa pela fina camada muscular da mucosa (*muscularis mucosae*).

Submucosa. A submucosa do cólon se assemelha à do ID: contém numerosos vasos sanguíneos e linfáticos, matriz extracelular densa bastante infiltrada por fibroblastos e células imunes, com fibras nervosas amielínicas e células dos gânglios que formam o plexo submucoso (de Meissner). As células intersticiais de Cajal estão localizadas na superfície submucosa do músculo liso circular e desempenham um papel duplo como células de marca-passo do músculo liso e mediadores da transmissão neuromuscular no cólon. A submucosa é dobrada, esticando-se e achatando-se quando o cólon é distendido com gás ou fezes.

Muscular. O músculo liso do cólon é composto por camadas musculares circulares internas e longitudinais externas, com o plexo mioentérico (de Auerbach) interposto.

Serosa. Essa camada é composta por células mesoteliais que cobrem as porções do IG encontradas na cavidade peritoneal. Sua secreção serosa lubrifica e reduz o atrito causado pelos movimentos intestinais.

Função

A interação da microbiota com as células do sistema imunológico do cólon é uma parte importante do sistema imunológico da mucosa (ver Capítulo 274). No entanto, as principais funções do cólon são absorção de água e eletrólitos na região proximal do cólon, para produzir fezes de consistência adequada, e seu armazenamento no cólon distal e reto, para permitir a evacuação em um momento apropriado por meio do processo coordenado de defecação.

O IG não é principalmente um órgão digestivo, porém a fermentação microbiana de material não digerido ocorre dentro dele, com uso pelos colonócitos dos ácidos graxos de cadeia curta (AGCC) produzidos. Curiosamente, também foi demonstrada a capacidade da mucosa do cólon canino em transportar aminoácidos e açúcares simples. Mas, exceto em neonatos, ao que tudo indica, ela não tem papel nutricional em comparação com a captação realizada pelo ID.[38] No entanto, pode fazer parte do mecanismo adaptativo visto na síndrome do intestino curto.

Absorção e secreção de água e eltrólitos[39-49]

O IG saudável tem uma grande capacidade de absorção e é capaz de absorver até 90% da água que entra no cólon para produzir fezes de consistência aceitável. De fato, ele tem alguma capacidade de reserva que pode absorver quantidades maiores se alguma diarreia do ID entrar no cólon, mas é sobrecarregado se volumes maiores de conteúdo ileal entrarem. Na doença do IG, o cólon tem uma capacidade reduzida, o que também leva à diarreia.

A água é absorvida por osmose passiva após a absorção de sódio, que ocorre sobretudo na região proximal do cólon. A absorção de sódio e a secreção de potássio para o lúmen do cólon também são moderadas pela aldosterona e por glicocorticoides, que estimulam a atividade da Bomba ATPase Na+/K+. A captação de sódio não está ligada à absorção de glicose no IG, e fluidos de reidratação oral contendo glicose não têm valor no tratamento da diarreia de origem colônica.

O potássio é absorvido por meio de um transportador de troca K+/H+, contudo pode ser secretado ativamente no cólon distal. Esses mecanismos complementam o controle da homeostase do potássio pelos rins. A absorção de cloreto segue o gradiente eletroquímico mantido pela absorção ativa de sódio e pela troca cloreto-bicarbonato. O pH do cólon é mais ácido do que o do ID, sendo mantido pela troca de sódio e potássio contra bicarbonato e cloreto – o bicarbonato também neutraliza os ácidos orgânicos produzidos pelas bactérias luminais.

Muco[50-55]

O muco do cólon é uma mistura de glicoproteínas ou mucinas de alto peso molecular produzidas por células caliciformes e epiteliais esfoliadas. A secreção de mucina depende da secreção de cloreto por meio do regulador transmembrana da fibrose cística (CFTR) e da exocitose. O muco não é produzido só como um lubrificante, facilitando a defecação, mas também para proteger a mucosa de danos. Patógenos e enterotoxinas podem se ligar ao muco antes de atingir o epitélio, atuando como uma barreira física. Entretanto, as células caliciformes também secretam moléculas antibacterianas e fatores de crescimento e reparo, como trifólio. Deficiências na camada de muco podem predispor ou potencializar a inflamação intestinal com aumento da quantidade de muco secretado na colite ou após estimulação parassimpática.

Motilidade[13]

A fim de realizar suas funções primárias de absorção de água e eletrólitos no cólon proximal e de armazenamento e controle da defecação no cólon distal e no reto, a motilidade do IG e sua coordenação pelo sistema nervoso entérico são complexas, mas cruciais. A falta congênita de gânglios entéricos em uma seção do cólon distal e reto de crianças causa a doença de Hirschsprung.[86] A seção afetada requer ressecção cirúrgica, mas a condição foi descrita apenas em um gato e nunca em cães.[87]

A habilidade inerente, espontânea e contrátil da musculatura lisa normal do cólon é influenciada pelo sistema nervoso entérico e por uma variedade de transmissores, como colecistocinina, neurotensina, somatostatina, serotonina e substância P, bem como acetilcolina e epinefrina/norepinefrina do sistema nervoso autônomo.

Há diferenças regionais nos padrões de motilidade colônica para facilitar as distintas funções do cólon proximal e distal. No primeiro, o tônus do músculo liso, junto com a atividade elétrica de ondas lentas, chamada contrações fásicas rítmicas (CFRs), permite a mistura de conteúdo e absorção de água. Essa função é aprimorada por contrações retrógradas gigantes (CRGs) iniciadas no cólon transverso e propagadas em direção ao ceco, causando antiperistalse. No segundo, explosões de pico e poderosas contrações migratórias gigantes (CMGs) impulsionam as fezes em direção ao reto e ajudam a expulsá-las.

O sistema nervoso simpático atua principalmente para restringir a progressão do conteúdo em direção ao reto, inibindo a atividade dos neurônios entéricos que controlam a motilidade por relaxar os músculos não esfincterianos e contrair os esfincteres. A ativação simpática também suprime a secreção de água e eletrólitos no lúmen do cólon. Desse modo, a atividade simpática atua para reduzir a necessidade de defecar, o que é apropriado durante uma situação de "lutar ou fugir".

O controle da defecação é discutido em detalhes no Capítulo 278. Em resumo, trata-se de um reflexo que pode ser moderado por processos conscientes para que, em condições de saúde, ocorra no momento e no lugar adequados. O reflexo de defecação pode ser desencadeado pela ingestão de uma refeição (reflexo gastrocólico), bem como pela distensão do cólon distal e reto. A estimulação causa contração do músculo reto do cólon e do reto, em geral começando com CMGs e relaxamento do esfincter anal, ao mesmo tempo que o paciente adota a postura necessária. A contração voluntária do esfincter anal pode inibir temporariamente a defecação, mas, em última análise, o desejo pode superar esse controle. No IG doente, o limite para o desejo de defecar é reduzido, e, assim, o animal quase sempre defeca após uma pequena quantidade de matéria fecal acumulada no reto, continuando a se esforçar de forma improdutiva (tenesmo fecal), como se ainda desejasse defecar mais, não obstante nenhum conteúdo retal permaneça para ser eliminado. Dificuldade ou dor ao defecar (disquezia) é um sinal de doença retoanal (ver Capítulos 42 e 278).

Microbioma colônico[43,88-106]

O microbioma colônico tem funções essenciais interagindo com o sistema imune da mucosa, fornecendo energia para utilização pelos colonócitos e sintetizando aminoácidos e vitaminas (ver Capítulo 274). O cólon abriga a maior concentração de bactérias no intestino, com até 10^{12} organismos por grama de fezes, representando $\approx 50\%$ da matéria seca fecal. Além das bactérias, fungos e alguns protozoários costumam estar presentes.

O conjunto de espécies bacterianas que compõem o microbioma individual de um animal saudável é relativamente estável, mas influenciado por idade, raça, localização geográfica, condições de habitação, coprofagia e dieta, sendo alterado em condições inflamatórias. Cada animal tem uma microbiota única, a despeito de apresentar microrganismos relacionados com a classe que ocupa um nicho ecológico específico no IG. Historicamente, a composição da microbiota colônica, com base na cultura de fezes de rotina, acredita-se ser composta sobretudo de bactérias anaeróbias, com gêneros como *Bifidobacterium*, *Bacteroides* e *Clostridium/Clostridioides* sendo predominantes e com menos bactérias anaeróbias facultativas ou aeróbias, como lactobacilos, enterobactérias e estreptococos em cães. Números iguais de bactérias aeróbias/anaeróbias facultativas e anaeróbias estritas foram encontrados nas fezes de gatos. No entanto, a maioria das bactérias no IG não pode ser cultivada *in vitro*, e até 70% podem representar espécies desconhecidas. Usando o sequenciamento do gene 16S rRNA de alta *performance*, é possível identificar quase todo o DNA bacteriano nas fezes. Fusobactérias são mais abundantes no cólon ($\approx 33\%$ de todos os clones identificados), seguido por Bacteroidales ($\approx 30\%$) e Clostridiales do *cluster* XIVa ($\approx 26\%$). Foi mostrado que a diversidade bacteriana no trato gastrintestinal (GI) aumenta em direção ao cólon em cães saudáveis e é reduzida pela administração de antibióticos.

A microbiota colônica metaboliza carboidratos, proteínas e lipídios nos AGCCs acetato, propionato e butirato, com subprodutos de hidrogênio, metano, compostos de sulfa e dióxido de carbono. Fibras fermentáveis que não são digeridas pelo ID são substratos importantes para as bactérias. Os AGCCs produzidos pelas bactérias são metabolizados pelos colonócitos e fornecem um importante suprimento de energia para o epitélio do IG. Eles também promovem a proliferação e a diferenciação de colonócitos, estimulam a absorção de água e eletrólitos e modificam a motilidade do cólon. Além disso, o butirato produzido por bactérias comensais pode induzir citocinas anti-inflamatórias, como a interleucina (IL)-10.

A microbiota bacteriana do cólon normal tem uma importante função na mediação da proteção contra bactérias patogênicas por meio de uma variedade de mecanismos, incluindo competição por substratos e por sítios de ligação. A inflamação intestinal crônica está ligada a alterações na composição da população bacteriana, e a alimentação com uma dieta livre de fibras mostrou induzir colite.

Vigilância imunológica[7,23,107-112]

O sistema imune da mucosa saudável no intestino evolui para ser tolerante a antígenos alimentares e microrganismos comensais, porém permanece capaz de responder rapidamente a microrganismos patogênicos. A anatomia funcional do GALT é descrita em detalhes nos Capítulos 274 e 276. No IG, ela consiste em sítios indutivos, incluindo folículos linfoides no cólon e no reto, além dos linfonodos colônicos e dos sítios efetores dentro da LP. As células denominadas microfenestradas (M) são abundantes no epitélio, recobrindo os folículos linfoides no IG que contêm células dendríticas (CDs). As CDs na LP têm o papel importante da amostragem contínua de antígenos do lúmen, estendendo dendritos entre as células epiteliais e, em seguida, ativando várias células imunes diferentes do sistema adaptativo (células T e B), conforme descrito no Capítulo 276. Além disso, as células epiteliais intestinais podem atuar como fagocíticas e apresentadoras de antígenos não profissionais, por meio de amostragem contínua de antígenos do lúmen intestinal e apresentação destes às células da LP, por meio da expressão do complexo principal de histocompatibilidade (MHC) II e da produção de citocinas que influenciarão as respostas imunes na LP.

O sistema imune inato, composto em particular de células epiteliais, macrófagos e CDs, parece determinar a resposta imune subsequente. Desregulação do equilíbrio entre tolerância e inflamação pode contribuir para o desenvolvimento da

CAPÍTULO 277 • Doenças do Intestino Grosso

doença. Células epiteliais intestinais constantemente também reconhecem microrganismos comensais por sua ligação com receptores semelhantes ao Toll (TLRs). Quando há microrganismos comensais e homeostase de um intestino normal, um equilíbrio entre subpopulações efetoras e reguladoras de células T é mantido por meio de um conjunto controlado de citocinas (ver Capítulo 276).

AVALIAÇÃO DIAGNÓSTICA

A investigação diagnóstica de doenças do cólon é orientada pelas informações obtidas no histórico e no exame físico, pela ausência de quaisquer sinais de doença sistêmica e pelo fato de a doença ser aguda, crônica, ou ter ocorrido antes, o que influencia na lista de diagnóstico diferencial (Boxe 277.1). Abordagens lógicas diagnósticas para diarreia do intestino grosso, hematoquezia e constipação intestinal são mostradas na Figura 277.5.

Histórico
Cães e gatos com doença de IG geralmente apresentam diarreia, constipação intestinal e/ou hematoquezia. As perguntas padrão incluem aquelas sobre dieta do animal, meio ambiente, histórico de viagens, vacinação, tratamentos parasiticidas, doenças simultâneas e quaisquer problemas de outros animais em contato. A perda de peso não é uma característica da doença de IG, exceto em condições neoplásicas avançadas ou quando o tutor tenta controlar a diarreia restringindo a ingestão de alimentos.

O tutor deve ser perguntando sobre a característica e a consistência fecal do animal, bem como sobre a frequência de defecação. Alguns dados do histórico, como presença de muco nas fezes (Figura 277.6), urgência, aumento da frequência, com ou sem hematoquezia, e tenesmo após defecação são típicos de diarreia de IG (Tabela 277.1). A hematoquezia indica ulceração do IG, e uma vez que o problema de sangramento generalizado seja descartado, são sugestivos de inflamação grave, ancilostomíase, tricuríase, intussuscepção ou neoplasia.

A constipação intestinal se refere à defecação reduzida ou ausente por vários dias a semanas. As sequelas incluem desidratação, perda

---

Boxe 277.1 Diagnósticos diferenciais a serem considerados em gatos com constipação intestinal crônica[50]

Disfunção neuromuscular
Músculo liso do cólon: megacólon idiopático, envelhecimento
Doença da medula espinal: doença lombossacral, síndrome da cauda equina, deformidades sacrais da medula espinal (gato da raça Manx [Manês])
Distúrbios do nervo hipogástrico ou pélvico: lesão traumática, malignidade, disautonomia
Neuropatia submucosa ou do plexo mioentérico: disautonomia, envelhecimento

Obstrução mecânica
Intraluminal: material estranho, neoplasia, divertículo retal, hérnia perineal, estenoses anorretais
Intramural: neoplasia
Extraluminal: fraturas pélvicas, neoplasia

Inflamação
Fístula perianal, proctite, abscesso do saco anal, corpos estranhos anorretais, feridas de mordida perianal

Metabólico e endócrino
Metabólico: desidratação, hipopotassemia, hipercalcemia
Endócrino: hipotireoidismo, obesidade, hiperparatireoidismo nutricional secundário

Ambiental e comportamental
Caixa de areia suja, inatividade, hospitalização, mudança de ambiente

---

de peso, dor abdominal e linfadenopatia mesentérica leve a moderada. Tenesmo também é visto na constipação intestinal, mas quase sempre nenhum material fecal é eliminado. No entanto, às vezes, o proprietário pode relatar que o animal produz algumas gotas de líquido fecal que podem ser confundidas com diarreia, à medida que as secreções passam pelas fezes impactadas. Fatores ambientais, como hospitalização, cama de gato suja e desidratação, podem predispor a constipação intestinal e ser determinadas durante a anamnese.

Esquemas de pontuação clínica como os Índices de Atividade de Doença Inflamatória Intestinal Canina e Felina (CIBDAI, FIBDAI), de Atividade de Enteropatia Crônica Clínica Canina (CCECAI) e de Atividade de Enteropatia Crônica Felina (FCEAI) foram publicados na tentativa de correlacionar sinais clínicos com os desfechos da doença.[113-115] Essa pontuação faz o monitoramento antes e depois do tratamento mais objetivo e permite comparações de gravidade clínica entre estudos (ver Capítulo 276). Cães jovens com escores de gravidade leve para colite mostraram responder bem às dietas de eliminação sozinhas e ter os melhores resultados.

Exame físico
O exame físico de rotina de cães e gatos com diarreia de IG pode não revelar anormalidades. Atenção deve ser dada a descobertas como pirexia (perfuração cecal ou colônica, infecção fúngica) ou uveíte (prototecose, linfoma, peritonite infecciosa felina). É necessária uma palpação abdominal cuidadosa para identificar dor abdominal (colite, neoplasia do cólon, perfuração), massas abdominais (neoplasia colônica, colite granulomatosa, intussuscepção cecocólica ou ileocólica), espessamento do ID (inflamação ou linfoma do ID concomitante), linfadenopatia mesentérica (colite, linfoma, doenças fúngicas disseminadas) e hepatoesplenomegalia (linfoma, doenças fúngicas disseminadas).

A constipação intestinal é o segundo sinal mais comum em pacientes com doença do cólon subjacente e geralmente é nítida na palpação abdominal ou no exame retal. Ainda que fatores ambientais possam predispor a constipação intestinal, deve-se enfatizar encontrar as causas-base, como massas abdominais (neoplasia, prostatomegalia), dor abdominal (corpos estranhos, perfuração do cólon), defecação dolorosa (furunculose anal/ fístulas perianais, abscesso do saco anal), neuropatia autonômica (disautonomia), paresia de membro posterior (lesões da medula espinal), fraturas pélvicas e hérnia perineal.

Em todos os casos de suspeita de doença de IG, um exame retal digital é obrigatório, ainda que possa exigir anestesia geral em gatos e cães muito pequenos. Lesões reto-anais, como anormalidades do saco anal, hérnia perineal, estenoses e pólipos retais e outras neoplasias retais, devem ser palpáveis, e doenças prostáticas podem ser avaliadas simultaneamente como causa da constipação intestinal (ver Capítulos 111 e 337). Irregularidades palpáveis da mucosa do cólon são sugestivas de infiltrações inflamatórias ou neoplásicas. No final do exame, a citologia retal pode ser realizada esfregando o dedo enluvado em uma lâmina de microscopia, submetendo-a à coloração com Diff-Quik ou corante de Wright. Uma amostra fecal também pode ser coletada, e uma diarreia ou hematoquezia prévia não reconhecida, identificada.

Investigação laboratorial[116,117]

Exames básicos
As análises laboratoriais de rotina que incluem hemograma completo, perfil de bioquímica sérica e urinálise são indicadas na maioria dos casos de doenças crônicas do cólon, mas podem ser desnecessárias na doença aguda leve. Não há alterações hematológicas ou bioquímicas patognomônicas em pacientes com doença do IG, porém resultados anormais podem fornecer pistas diagnósticas. Anormalidades associadas a sinais do cólon e seus diagnósticos diferenciais potenciais são listados na Tabela 277.2.

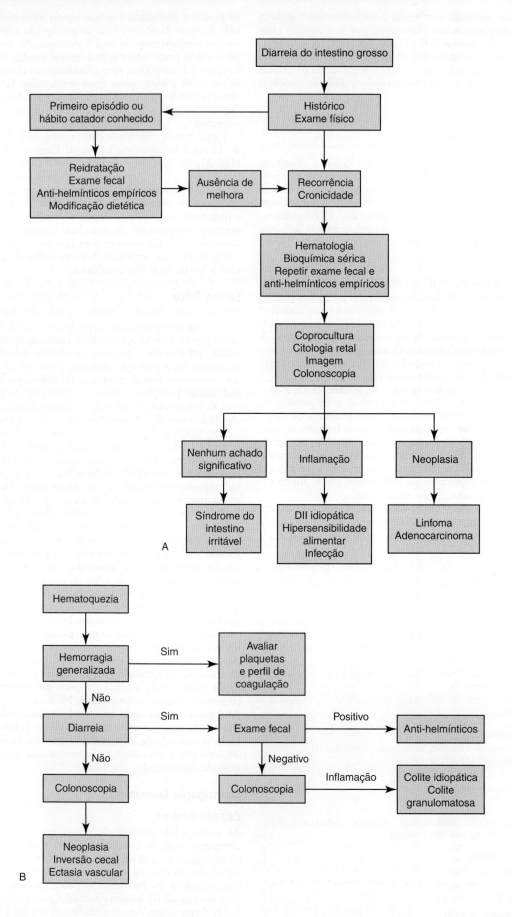

Figura 277.5 Algoritmos para uma abordagem diagnóstica de (**A**) diarreia do intestino grosso, (**B**) hematoquezia e (**C**) constipação intestinal. *DII*, doença inflamatória intestinal.

Continua

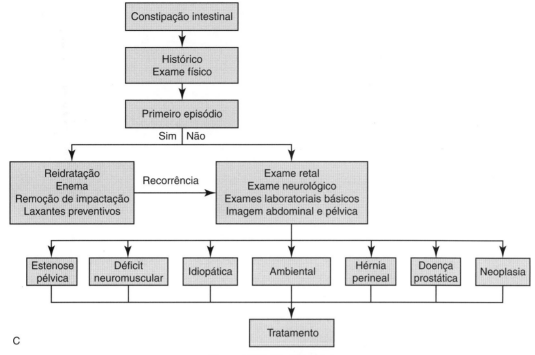

C

Figura 277.5 (*Continuação*)

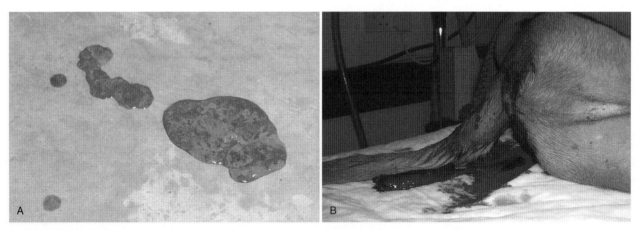

Figura 277.6 Hematoquezia. **A.** Material fecal de um cão com colite grave. Observe o sangue fresco e o muco, eliminados em múltiplos pequenos volumes, sugerindo aumento da frequência e tenesmo. **B.** Hematoquezia em um cão com colite grave. (*Esta figura se encontra reproduzida em cores no Encarte.*)

Tabela 277.1	Sinais clínicos associados à diarreia do intestino grosso.
SINAIS	**FREQUÊNCIA**
Perda de peso	Incomum
Vômito	Incomum
Flatulência	Incomum
Frequência de defecação	Aumento marcante
Volume fecal	Normal a leve diminuição
Urgência	Geralmente presente
Tenesmo	Geralmente presente
Muco nas fezes	Quase sempre presente
Hematoquezia	Quase sempre presente
Cor anormal das fezes (p. ex., verde)	Raro
Melena	Ausente
Esteatorreia	Ausente

Exames adicionais

Mesmo na ausência de sinais típicos de doença ID, concentrações séricas de cobalamina e folato devem ser avaliadas em animais com presumível doença do cólon (ver Capítulo 276). Baixos níveis de cobalamina sérica indicam doença que afeta o ID distal, mesmo quando a apresentação clínica é mais típica de colite – na verdade, uma diarreia persistente de ID pode ser a causa da inflamação do cólon. Biopsias ileais, obtidas por colonoscopia (ver Capítulo 113), são indicadas se a cobalamina sérica estiver anormal.

A extensão da inflamação pancreática também pode causar inflamação das regiões adjacentes do cólon e sinais de colite. Assim, a medição da imunorreatividade da lipase pancreática (PLI) pode ser indicada se houver qualquer suspeita de pancreatite (ver Capítulos 290 e 291). Da mesma forma, dependendo do índice de suspeita, os testes sorológicos para doenças fúngicas podem ser indicados (ver Capítulos 233 e 236).

Em gatos com colite crônica ou constipação intestinal, o teste do vírus da leucemia felina (FeLV; ver Capítulo 223) e FIV (ver Capítulo 222) devem ser realizados, e a tiroxina sérica, medida, se houver diarreia em gatos mais velhos (ver Capítulo 301).

Tabela 277.2	Anormalidades associadas à doença do cólon e suas causas potenciais.
ACHADO	**CAUSA POTENCIAL**
Anemia não regenerativa leve a moderada	Doença crônica
Anemia regenerativa (hipocrômica, microcítica, deficiência de ferro, se hemorragia crônica)	Perda de sangue • Ancilostomídeos e tricurídeos • Intussuscepção e inversão cecal • Colite • Neoplasia • Ectasia vascular
Leucocitose	• Inflamação • Infecção • Neoplasia
Eosinofilia	• Parasitismo • Hipoadrenocorticismo • Tumor de mastócitos • Síndrome hipereosinofílica • Paraneoplásico (linfoma, saco anal adenocarcinoma etc.)
Hipoalbuminemia	• Sangramento • Reação de fase aguda negativa • Enteropatia perdedora de proteína concomitante
Hiperglobulinemia	• Peritonite infecciosa felina • Inflamação intestinal • Neoplasia
Hipercalcemia	• Neoplasia • Granulomas fúngicos • Infecção por *Heterobilharzia*
Hipoglicemia	• Leiomiossarcoma • Tumor estromal GI (GIST) • Grande tumor abdominal
Hiponatremia e hiperpotassemia concorrente	• Hipoadrenocorticismo • Salmonelose • Infecção por *Trichuris*

Não há alterações laboratoriais patognomônicas em pacientes com doença do cólon, mas resultados anormais podem fornecer pistas diagnósticas.

Exame fecal[118-128]

Exame parasitológico fecal (ver Capítulo 81), como esfregaços diretos e flotação de sulfato de zinco, deve ser feito em todos os animais antes da colonoscopia, e a administração empírica de parasiticidas de amplo espectro também pode ser testada primeiro, sobretudo em áreas onde a infecção por *Trichuris* é endêmica. Embora seja principalmente um parasita de ID, *Giardia* também pode estar envolvida na colite e ser identificada não só por flotação fecal, mas por um teste imunocromatográfico (SNAP® teste) ou por coloração imunofluorescente (ver Capítulo 221).

Existem vários métodos para detectar infecção por *Tritrichomonas* em gatos.[129,130] A infecção pode ser identificada em uma amostra fecal fresca – uma gota de diarreia recente é misturada com uma de soro fisiológico quente em uma lâmina, coberta com uma lamínula e examinada com uma objetiva de microscópio de 40x. Trofozoítos com mobilidade progressiva podem ser observados, mas o teste é de baixa sensibilidade. Mais sensíveis são o sistema de cultura InPouch ou a reação em cadeia da polimerase (PCR), para a qual uma amostra diarreica é necessária, podendo ser obtida por uma lavagem alta do cólon. A contaminação da amostra com a caixa de areia do gato deve ser evitada, pois pode inibir a reação de PCR.

A coprocultura geralmente é realizada em cães e gatos com colite crônica.[119,131-136] A inflamação do cólon pode estar

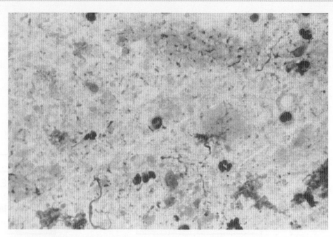

Figura 277.7 Citologia retal de um cão com colite aguda. Entre bactérias e detritos fecais, vários neutrófilos estão presentes, o que sugere colite bacteriana. (*Esta figura se encontra reproduzida em cores no Encarte.*)

associada à infecção por *Campylobacter* spp., *Clostridium perfringens*, *Clostridioides difficile*, *Salmonella* spp. e, possivelmente, *Yersinia* spp. No entanto, esses microrganismos também podem ser encontrados nas fezes de animais saudáveis, e as culturas positivas devem ser interpretadas à luz de outros achados clínicos, sendo a terapia experimental, por vezes, a mais efetiva para identificar essas infecções. PCRs para diversos desses microrganismos estão disponíveis, sendo mais sensíveis, já que não requerem microrganismos vivos, especialmente em relação a *Campylobacter* spp. que são bastante frágeis e que logo morrem em amostras *ex vivo*.

A cultura quantitativa de bactérias do cólon não é recomendada, uma vez que o número de espécies bacterianas cultiváveis no cólon abrange apenas cerca de 30% do microbioma total. Existem poucas informações disponíveis sobre anormalidades específicas do microbioma no cólon de cães e gatos com colite, mas é provável que a composição seja alterada especificamente para diferentes doenças, como foi demonstrado no caso de humanos com doença de Crohn ou câncer de cólon, além de gatos com doença inflamatória intestinal (DII).[137]

Citologia[138,139]

A citologia pode ser realizada após o exame retal digital, usando um dedo enluvado ou um aplicador com ponta de algodão para limpar o reto, ou escovas de citologia, por endoscopia, durante a colonoscopia. Em geral, bactérias e detritos predominam, mas às vezes os agentes causadores podem ser identificados, incluindo fungos, células neoplásicas ou inflamatórias, como linfócitos, eosinófilos ou neutrófilos (Figura 277.7).

Imagem

Radiografias simples lateral e ventrodorsal do abdome e da região pélvica podem ser úteis em pacientes com hematoquezia, disquezia ou suspeita de constipação intestinal, potencialmente identificando obstruções, megacólon, e confirmando a constipação intestinal. Elas são menos úteis em pacientes com diarreia de IG, nos quais a ultrassonografia pode ser mais eficiente.

Radiografia[140-144]

As radiografias podem identificar corpos estranhos radiopacos, impactação fecal e causas extraluminais de obstrução, como estenose do canal pélvico ou prostatomegalia. Massas discretas no cólon provavelmente só são detectadas se houver gás luminal para destacá-las, todavia a linfadenopatia sublombar pode dar uma pista para doença metastática.

Às vezes, pode ser difícil diferenciar entre ID cheio de gás, cólon, e, portanto, detectar uma obstrução do ID. Um colonograma de contraste negativo, insuflando com ar quando o cólon estiver vazio, pode ajudar a determinar qual estrutura na radiografia é o cólon, bem como destacar potenciais espessamentos e massas da parede do cólon (Figura 277.8). Assim, um pneumocolonograma pode ser útil, se bem que possa impedir a realização em sequência de uma ultrassonografia, haja vista que o gás interfere no ultrassom. A torção do cólon é rara, mas pode ser identificada em radiografia, por distensão gasosa e deslocamento do cólon dentro do abdômen.[145-149]

A pneumatose cólica, uma forma de pneumatose cística intestinal, é uma manifestação muito rara de doença do cólon em animais vivos, ainda que seja uma característica reconhecida em espécimes *post mortem* após a putrefação. O gás livre é visualizado na parede do cólon, abaixo da submucosa ou serosa. Pode ser associado à colite ou à neoplasia do cólon, assim como idiopático e de resolução espontânea.[150-155]

Radiografias de contraste positivo tiradas após um estudo de acompanhamento mostrarão bário no cólon, e as lesões podem ser ocasionalmente identificadas (Figura 277.9). Contudo, o preenchimento costuma ser incompleto, e um enema de bário é mais adequado para mostrar problemas como intussuscepção, inversão cecal e estenose. No entanto, enemas de bário, em especial estudos de duplo contraste,[144] raramente são realizados hoje em dia, a menos que a colonoscopia não esteja disponível. Estudos de contraste positivo são desagradáveis e sujeitos a artefatos, já que fezes retidas podem mimetizar um defeito de preenchimento causado por massa, como também o estreitamento normal do cólon na borda pélvica às vezes é mal-interpretado como estenose.

Um diagnóstico avançado por imagem do IG é possível,[156-159] e é especialmente útil para obter imagens do IG dentro do canal pélvico. "Endoscopia Virtual" usando Tomografia Computadorizada helicoidal foi desenvolvido em humanos para identificar pólipos e carcinomas do cólon, embora possa não ser tão sensível quanto a colonoscopia.

Ultrasonografia[143,160-169]

Por meio de um ultrassom abdominal, o íleo, a junção ileocecal, o ceco e o cólon ascendente, transverso e descendente podem ser potencialmente identificados (ver Capítulo 88). Uma abordagem perineal é indicada se as anormalidades forem suspeitas no IG intrapélvico.

Se distendido, um cólon normal deve ter três camadas e uma espessura ≤ 2 mm. Um cólon não distendido pode dar um aspecto de espessamento da parede, mas a presença de ar no lúmen pode dificultar a avaliação de todo o órgão. Na colite, muitas vezes não há achados radiográficos, ultrassonográficos ou apenas espessamento difuso da mucosa. Infiltração focal e massas intramurais são mais sugestivas de neoplasia de IG.

Colonoscopia[170]

A colonoscopia é indicada em pacientes com diarreia de IG e/ou hematoquezia e, às vezes, naqueles constipados após o IG ter sido esvaziado (ver Capítulo 113). Endoscópios rígidos ocos podem ser usados para visualizar o reto e o cólon descendente, entretanto a visão é limitada e o cólon proximal não pode ser examinado. A endoscopia flexível é o método de escolha para visualização de todo o cólon e obtenção de biopsias da mucosa. A ileoscopia concomitante é recomendada, a menos que uma lesão que explique todos os sinais clínicos seja encontrada no IG. A cirurgia para obter biopsias colônicas de espessura total não é recomendada por causa dos riscos de deiscência da ferida e peritonite séptica.

Preparação[171-175]

A colonoscopia bem-sucedida depende da adequada limpeza do cólon. Cães e gatos devem ficar em jejum de 36 a 48 horas antes do procedimento e, se forem usados vários enemas, com grandes volumes (cada 30 ml/kg), enemas altos são necessários para fornecer limpeza adequada. Apenas água quente é usada para os enemas, podendo ser introduzida com auxílio de um balde ou uma bomba de Higginson (ver Capítulo 114). Sabão ou laxantes, muito usados no manejo de pacientes constipados, devem ser evitados ao preparar o paciente para colonoscopia, pois podem induzir alterações na mucosa do cólon. Enemas de fosfato podem causar hiperfosfatemia fatal em gatos e cães pequenos.

A limpeza mais completa é produzida pela administração de uma solução de lavagem oral que é um potente laxante osmótico. Soluções de polietilenoglicol (PEG), tornadas isotônicas com adição de eletrólitos, são preferidas, como Colyte®, Golytely® e Klean-Prep®. Como essas soluções têm um sabor desagradável (gosto de sabão) ou aroma de frutas adicionado para palatabilidade humana, poucos pacientes caninos os bebem voluntariamente. Elas, portanto, devem ser administradas por tubo estomacal em cães ou por tubo nasoesofágico em gatos no dia anterior ao procedimento (ver Capítulo 112). A instilação nas vias respiratórias deve ser evitada, uma vez que foi registrada pneumonia fatal por inalação. Um grande volume (25 a 30 ml/kg PO 2 vezes e de preferência 3 vezes) deve ser fornecido com intervalo de aproximadamente 2 horas. Laxantes osmóticos orais de volume menor, como o fosfato de sódio, produzem uma limpeza menor e podem induzir cólicas abdominais e vômitos. Enemas de água morna são administrados no dia seguinte antes do procedimento ou enquanto o animal estiver sob anestesia, até o IG estar limpo.

Exame

Um exame colonoscópico completo inclui a visualização de todo o cólon até a junção ileocólica (Vídeo 277.1 e Capítulo 113). Sempre que possível, o ceco e o íleo também devem ser

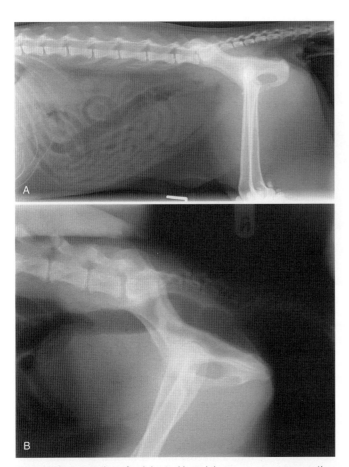

Figura 277.8 A. Radiografia abdominal lateral de um gato com pneumocólon, destacando o espessamento da parede dorsal do cólon para a bexiga urinária. (Cortesia de Virginie Barberet, Universidade de Bristol.) **B.** Radiografia abdominal lateral de um cão com um pólipo adenomatoso colônico na região pélvica. A massa foi visualizada por insuflação do cólon com ar antes de tirar a radiografia.

1584   SEÇÃO 18 • Doença Gastrintestinal

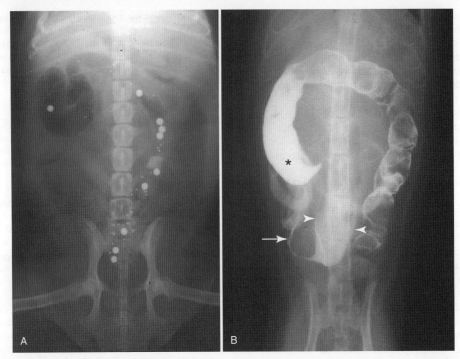

Figura 277.9 A. Radiografia abdominal ventrodorsal de um cão 24 horas após receber esferas de polietileno impregnadas com bário (BIPS) *per os*. Todos os BIPS atingiram o cólon, indicando que não há obstruções parciais impedindo sua passagem. Gás preenche o ceco enrolado e o cólon proximal; material fecal está presente no cólon distal. **B.** Radiografia abdominal ventrodorsal de um gato siamês 24 horas após a administração oral da suspensão de bário. O bário preenche o ceco pontiagudo e o cólon (*asterisco*), mas uma alça do intestino delgado dilatada (*pontas de seta*) é vista conectada ao cólon proximal por uma fina faixa de bário (*seta*). Esse sinal de "caroço de maçã" é consistente com uma massa ileal, e um carcinoma foi confirmado na cirurgia.

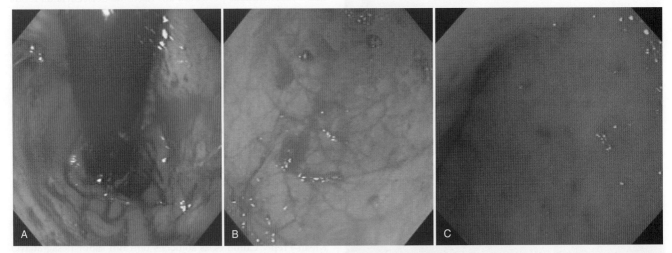

Figura 277.10 Endoscopia digestiva baixa em um cão da raça Weimaraner com hematoquezia causada por uma inversão cecal, conforme mostrado na Figura 277.16. Em ambas as imagens, a parede do intestino grosso está histologicamente normal, e a presença de sangue luminal se dá em razão do sangramento da inversão cecal mais proximal. **A.** Visão retroflexada do cólon distal e reto. **B.** Cólon transverso normal, mostrando vasos sanguíneos na submucosa. **C.** Múltiplos folículos linfoides visíveis na mucosa retal de um cão da raça Pastor-Alemão. (*Esta figura se encontra reproduzida em cores no Encarte.*)

examinados e biopsiados. O paciente é posicionado em decúbito lateral esquerdo, de modo a permitir a insuflação do cólon proximal. Após a sucção e a lavagem de qualquer material fecal remanescente, o endoscópio é avançado em torno das flexuras até que a papila ileocólica seja identificada. Em cães grandes, o endoscópio também pode ser retroflexado para permitir um melhor exame do reto (Figura 277.10 A), pois muitas vezes não consegue permanecer inflado durante a endoscopia flexível, já que o ar vaza pelo ânus, mesmo que um assistente tente mantê-lo fechado. Na verdade, a endoscopia rígida com um proctoscópio é um método melhor para examinar a mucosa retal.

A mucosa do cólon normal deve ser rosa, lisa e cintilante, com os vasos submucosos visíveis (Figura 277.10 B). A perda de visualização desses vasos sugere que a mucosa está infiltrada e espessada, mas são necessárias biopsias para confirmação. No reto, várias pequenas manchas escuras na mucosa são folículos linfoides (Figura 277.10 C).

As biopsias dos pacientes para o exame histológico devem ser coletadas de áreas alteradas, com aparência normal e de zona de transição. Se toda a mucosa parecer normal, seis a oito biopsias do cólon descendente, transverso e ascendente ainda devem ser coletadas. O número e a qualidade das biopsias feitas durante a endoscopia são cruciais para um diagnóstico histológico preciso. Além disso, usar a maior pinça possível (≥ 2,8 mm de diâmetro) e descartáveis pode auxiliar em biopsias endoscópicas de melhor qualidade.

Outras técnicas endoscópicas[176-178]

Além de ser usada para um diagnóstico histológico, a colonoscopia também pode ser empregada tanto para testes diagnósticos avançados quanto de modo terapêutico – por exemplo, polipectomia e dilatação de estenose –, conquanto estas sejam indicações raras em cães e gatos. Se a eletrocirurgia for realizada para remover pólipos, o cólon deve ser insuflado com dióxido de carbono, a fim de evitar uma mistura de gases potencialmente explosiva.

O teste de provocação de alergênio por colonoscopia (TPAC) foi desenvolvido para identificar antígenos associados à alergia ou à intolerância alimentar e tem sido usado com sucesso em cães, mas não em gatos.[179] De modo resumido, uma agulha de escleroterapia com bainha é avançada pelo colonoscópio, ao passo que soluções de antígeno, histamina (controle positivo) ou solução salina (controle negativo) são injetadas na mucosa do cólon, em torno da junção ileocólica, em um teste com tempo controlado. Uma reação positiva é um demarcado inchaço com edema e hiperemia no local da injeção, 1 a 2 minutos após a injeção do antígeno. Assim, essa reação pode ser avaliada diretamente na mucosa do cólon com mais facilidade do que um teste de gastroscopia para hipersensibilidade alimentar.[180,181] No entanto, falsos positivos e negativos são possíveis, e o TPAC parece não funcionar em gatos. Além disso, o teste TPAC só é útil se os sinais clínicos em cães alérgicos a alimentos forem causados por uma reação de hipersensibilidade imediata do tipo I. Portanto, ele raramente é utilizado, mesmo em centros de referência terciários.

DOENÇAS INFLAMATÓRIAS

A inflamação do IG quase sempre é difusa e denominada de colite, porém a de regiões específicas é identificada por nomes específicos, como tiflite (ceco), colite (cólon) e proctite (reto). A tiflite isolada foi observada em associação com impactação e formação de fecólitos.[182] Infecção por *Trichuris* é muito mais comum, apesar de estar mais associada à inflamação generalizada do IG. A colite é vista com mais frequência em cães, quando comparado com gatos, e pode ser aguda ou crônica.

Colite aguda[183-184]

A colite aguda é, por definição, de início súbito e geralmente autolimitada. A condição quase sempre é diagnosticada, com base nos sinais clínicos característicos de diarreia mucoide, hematoquezia causada por inflamação e aumento da frequência, bem como tenesmo oriundo da alteração da motilidade do cólon (ver Figura 277.6). Muitas vezes, a causa nunca é identificada, porém há muitas causas potenciais infecciosas (bactérias, protozoários, helmintos), como as descritas a seguir.

A colite aguda em cães, em geral, ocorre após indiscrição na dieta, embora a causa exata raramente seja identificada. A carragenina é um mucopolissacarídeo extraído de algas marinhas e adicionado a alguns alimentos para gatos, de modo a formar géis e um ingrediente de muitos alimentos humanos processados, tendo sido apontado como causa de colite aguda em cães que "roubam" comida de gatos. Ela pode danificar os colonócitos e tem sido associada à ulceração do cólon e à neoplasia em modelos de roedores. A colite traumática é causada pela ingestão inadequada de ossos, areia ou material pontiagudo indigestível dos chamados ossos, além de brinquedos de náilon.

O manejo da colite aguda é de suporte e inespecífico, pois a maioria dos casos é autolimitante. Interrupção temporária da alimentação e modificação na dieta (baixo teor de gordura, dietas altamente digeríveis) podem ser todo o necessário. Antidiarreicos à base de caulim podem ligar toxinas bacterianas e produzir fezes mais firmes. O difenoxilato ou a loperamida podem reduzir o tenesmo que o paciente e o tutor acham mais desconfortável. Antibióticos raramente são indicados, todavia o tratamento empírico com metronidazol muitas vezes é eficaz. O costume de usar sulfatrimetoprim para tratar a colite felizmente passou. Os relatos de tratamento bem-sucedido com metronidazol raramente são estudos controlados, e talvez probióticos ou um placebo sejam igualmente eficazes. A colite aguda que não responde à conduta terapêutica se torna crônica.

Colite crônica idiopática

Definição[185-191]

A doença inflamatória intestinal (DII) idiopática afeta o trato gastrintestinal de cães e gatos onde nenhuma causa para a inflamação pode ser identificada. Ela pode ser classificada com base na região do trato GI afetada e em critérios clínicos e histopatológicos. Em geral, é diagnosticada em animais com sinais GI crônicos (> 3 semanas de duração), incluindo anorexia, vômito, diarreia e perda de peso para o qual nenhuma outra causa conhecida pode ser identificada.

Se o cólon estiver envolvido na DII, o principal sinal é diarreia, normalmente com muco, hematoquezia, urgência, frequência e tenesmo. Os animais afetados não respondem ao tratamento sintomático com dieta, parasiticidas ou antibióticos.

Além desse processo de eliminação empírica, a avaliação histopatológica das biopsias intestinais permite a classificação com base no tipo de célula inflamatória que infiltra a mucosa (Figura 277.11). Tais células encontradas na mucosa do cólon incluem linfócitos e/ou plasmócitos (colite linfocítico-plasmocítica), eosinófilos (colite eosinofílica), neutrófilos (colite neutrofílica ou supurativa), macrófagos (colite granulomatosa) ou, mais frequentemente, uma combinação delas, mas com um tipo de célula predominante. Pouco se sabe por que o tipo de célula predominante difere na colite linfoplasmocitária e eosinofílica, porém se acredita, com pouca evidência, que a doença eosinofílica se deva mais ao resultado de uma reação imune a antígenos

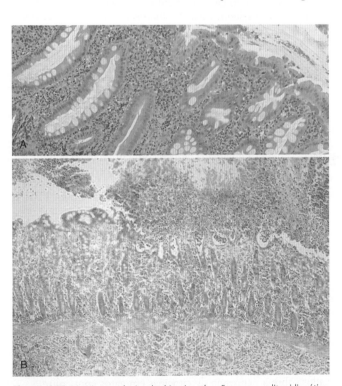

Figura 277.11 Histopatologia de biopsias de cães com colite idiopática. **A.** Colite linfoplasmocitária. Observe a separação das glândulas por uma população mista de células inflamatórias, em que as predominantes são linfócitos e células plasmáticas. **B.** Colite eosinofílica grave. A mucosa está ulcerada e infiltrada com grande número de eosinófilos que estão extravasando para o lúmen do cólon. (**A.** Cortesia de Michael Day, Universidade de Bristol. **B.** Cortesia de Geoff Pearson, Universidade de Bristol.) (*Esta figura se encontra reproduzida em cores no Encarte.*)

alimentares. Diferenças na resposta dos tipos histológicos ao tratamento também são pouco documentadas. A inflamação gastrintestinal neutrofílica é muitas vezes assumida como reflexo de uma causa bacteriana, e *Campylobacter* spp. são conhecidas por atrair neutrófilos. Dessa forma, antibióticos são geralmente prescritos antes da imunossupressão.

O processo inflamatório pode afetar todo o trato GI (gastro-enterocolite), porém pode envolver apenas o cólon (colite), quando a sugestão é que o prognóstico é melhor. A colite idiopática é discutida aqui, porém todo o espectro de DII é discutido em detalhes no Capítulo 276.

Fisiopatologia e mecanismos da doença[192-203]

Em humanos, a DII engloba dois distúrbios principais: a doença de Crohn, caracterizada por uma inflamação granulomatosa transmural ou piogranulomatosa, podendo ocorrer em qualquer parte do trato GI, embora em geral esteja centrada no íleo, e a colite ulcerativa (CU), restrita ao cólon e caracterizada por uma inflamação neutrofílica mais superficial, restrita à mucosa. A patogênese exata da DII em pequenos animais não foi elucidada, porém estudos em modelo murino de colite e em humanos levaram à hipótese atual de que se trata de uma perda de tolerância imunológica a bactérias luminais e/ou antígenos alimentares que levam a uma resposta inflamatória.

Pesquisas recentes realizadas em cães e gatos sugerem um processo patogenético molecular similar, potencialmente incluindo uma barreira mucosa defeituosa, um sistema imune anormal e mudanças no microbioma. Predisposições genéticas e mecanismos envolvidos na inflamação intestinal são discutidos em detalhe no Capítulo 276 e não são repetidos aqui, já que até o momento não há evidência de diferenças significativas entre DII no ID e no IG. Na verdade, a maioria das DII é difusa, envolvendo ambas as regiões, ou limitada ao ID. Na experiência do autor, a colite idiopática isolada é incomum. Relatos anteriores de colite podem não ter reconhecido o envolvimento do ID por causa da predominância de sinais semelhantes aos da colite e, portanto, não analisando biopsias do ID. No entanto, de que modo pode haver variações na distribuição regional da inflamação e se as formas associadas a ID e IG têm diferentes etiologias são questões ainda não respondidas.

Resposta imune.[204] Vários estudos com cães e gatos investigaram o processo inflamatório associado à colite. Os primeiros se concentraram na descrição dos tipos de células inflamatórias predominantes encontrados, e ambos os linfócitos T e B, bem como plasmócitos produtores de IgG, parecem aumentados na mucosa colônica inflamada de cães com DII. Mais recentemente, usando PCR quantitativo com transcriptase reversa (qRT-PCR), a expressão de mRNA de citocinas foi avaliada em biopsias da mucosa do cólon. Na DII humana, doença de Crohn (Th1 e Th17) e CU (Th2) mostram diferentes perfis de citocinas, mas os resultados relativos à natureza do padrão específico observado em cães com DII é conflitante. Em um estudo, o padrão predominante da expressão mRNA de citocinas em cães foi o de uma resposta imune Th1. Contudo, a precisão desses resultados foi questionada desde então. Por exemplo, o qRT-PCR, mais confiável, não mostrou diferença na expressão de mRNA de citocinas da mucosa duodenal em comparação com cães saudáveis e doentes. A expressão de mRNA de citocinas do cólon não foi investigada novamente usando qRT-PCR, portanto é prudente não sobrevalorizar os resultados do estudo inicial. As citocinas do tipo IL-17 podem ser importantes na DII canina e felina e não foram investigadas originalmente. Existem dados não publicados sobre a expressão de citocinas em gatos com colite.

Efeitos da inflamação na função do cólon.[205-207] Como descrito antes, as principais funções do cólon são a absorção de água e eletrólitos (cólon proximal), além do armazenamento de fezes (cólon distal). A inflamação do cólon pode interromper essas funções de várias maneiras. A colite pode diminuir a capacidade de absorção total da mucosa por meio da perda de colonócitos

funcionais, aumentar a permeabilidade e desequilibrar o transporte de sódio e cloreto. Além disso, a colite tem efeitos diretos na motilidade do cólon, diminuindo a motilidade não propulsiva, explicada por distúrbios nas células musculares lisas circulares do cólon, e aumentando as grandes contrações migratórias (GCMs), resultando em defecação e tenesmo frequentes. A inflamação pode prejudicar a mobilização de cálcio, alterar a expressão de moléculas de sinalização-chave de acoplamento de excitação e contração, inibir a sinalização muscarínica e aumentar a transcrição do fator nuclear *kappa* B (NF-*kappa* B), um passo importante para causar inflamação. Por fim, os distúrbios na absorção e na motilidade podem alterar a composição do microbioma comensal luminal que desempenha um papel importante na manutenção da função colônica, contribuindo para uma deterioração adicional.

Influência da dieta.[208] A alergia alimentar tem sido associada à inflamação intestinal, mas a resolução completa seria esperada em resposta a uma dieta de exclusão apropriada (ver Capítulos 178, 186 e 276). No entanto, os antígenos alimentares provavelmente não desempenham um papel direto na patogênese da DII humana, ainda que vários componentes da dieta possam exercer efeitos deletérios ou benéficos no microbioma e na mucosa intestinal, modificando o processo inflamatório da mucosa. Os efeitos dos antígenos da dieta na DII não foram estudados em detalhes em cães ou gatos, porém o tratamento dietético é visto como um componente integral da terapia. Uma grande proporção de cães e gatos com colite responde clinicamente à terapia dietética de maneira isolada, embora a resolução histológica quase sempre não ocorra.

Dietas hidrolisadas são reconhecidas como eficazes em muitos casos de DII que antes teriam sido tratados por imunossupressão. No entanto, as biopsias de acompanhamento costumam não mostrar resolução histológica, apesar da cessação dos sinais clínicos. Ainda não se sabe se isso reflete a necessidade de aguardar mais para que as alterações histológicas se resolvam ou se a dieta altamente digestível está apenas mascarando as deficiências funcionais de um intestino inflamado.

Exame clínico e histórico

Cães com todas as formas de DII tendem a ser de meia-idade – idade mediana de 6,5 anos, com uma ampla faixa etária –, enquanto em gatos com colite linfocítico-plasmocítica a idade média de início dos sinais clínicos é semelhante – média de 5,2 anos, faixa de 0,5 a 10 anos. Uma predisposição de certas raças de cães, como Pastor-Alemão e Shar-pei, é descrita e tem sido sugerida também para gatos de raça pura, mas sem influência do sexo em ambas as espécies.

Os sinais de colite crônica são caracterizados por diarreia de IG com defecação frequente de pequenos volumes de fezes amolecidas a aquosas, muitas vezes misturadas com muco e/ou sangue fresco. Urgência para defecar e tenesmo após a defecação costumam ser notados, contudo o vômito é menos frequente do que na DII de ID. Dor abdominal, perda de peso, anorexia e letargia podem ocorrer durante os episódios em animais gravemente afetados ou naqueles com envolvimento gástrico e/ou de ID.

Um sistema de pontuação clínica para classificar objetivamente a gravidade da doença em um animal de estimação com colite é recomendado para monitorar a resposta ao tratamento e realizar possíveis estudos comparativos.[113-115] Cães jovens com colite e pontuação de gravidade baixa demonstraram responder bem apenas com o controle na dieta e apresentam os melhores resultados.

Exame físico

A maioria dos cães e dos gatos com colite idiopática está em bom estado geral, exceto na doença grave, visto que seu estado nutricional permanece inalterado, a menos que o tutor promova restrição alimentar para tentar controlar a diarreia. Se não houver envolvimento de ID, a palpação abdominal muitas vezes é inconclusiva, conquanto deva ser realizada para descartar intussuscepção ou neoplasia afetando o cólon. O exame retal digital pode ser doloroso em razão da inflamação anal e retal associada à colite. Furunculose anal/fístula perianal (ver Capítulo 278) também é vista em associação com colite em cães da raça Pastor-Alemão.[209-212] O reto pode parecer vazio ou conter sangue, muco e/ou fezes diarreicas. Uma superfície irregular e anormal da parede retal pode ser perceptível na palpação do reto.

Investigação laboratorial

Os resultados da bioquímica sérica, do hemograma completo e do exame de urina, em geral, não são significativamente anormais em cães e gatos com colite idiopática. Isso pode ser diferente em animais com inflamação GI generalizada que inclua o ID, em que leucocitose com neutrofilia e desvio à esquerda, hipoproteinemia com hipoalbuminemia e hipoglobulinemia, e às vezes atividade de enzimas hepáticas leve a moderadamente aumentadas, podem estar presentes (ver Capítulo 276). A proteína C reativa (PCR) pode estar elevada, entretanto é um marcador não específico que aumenta em muitas doenças que causam inflamação, e os resultados em cães e gatos com DII grave são inconsistentes. A relevância clínica precisa de marcadores séricos de autoimunidade, como anticorpos anticitoplasma e perinucleares de neutrófilos (pANCA), e ainda precisa ser determinada em cães com DII.[213-219]

Um exame parasitológico (ver Capítulo 81) pode identificar a presença de parasitas como *Trichuris*, que causam colite. Mas, mesmo na ausência de uma identificação positiva, tratamento empírico com fembendazol (50 mg/kg PO diariamente, por 3 dias) é recomendado para eliminar a maioria dos helmintos e dos protozoários GI. Exame citológico de raspagem retal pode revelar *Histoplasma capsulatum* (ver Capítulo 233), neutrófilos – um sinal de inflamação (ver Figura 277.7) – ou aumento do número de bacilos gram-negativos curvos ou em "asa de gaivota", além de bastonetes gram-positivos, talvez indicativos de infecção por *Campylobacter* ou *Clostridium perfringens*, respectivamente, ainda que seja impreciso identificar espécies bacterianas com base na morfologia (ver Capítulo 220). Em geral, o diagnóstico por imagem com radiografias e ultrassonografia não é útil em gatos e cães com colite, a menos que haja massas ou lesões focais visíveis, ou se a doença se estender ao ID. O engrossamento da parede do cólon pode ser encontrado no exame de ultrassom abdominal, porém sua ausência é mais útil para descartar neoplasia.

Biopsia por endoscopia

Quando os resultados indicam a possibilidade de DII de IG, um diagnóstico definitivo é mais bem alcançado com a colonoscopia (Figura 277.12; ver Vídeo 277.1; ver Capítulo 113). Isso deve ser precedido por uma gastroduodenoscopia em animais com suspeita de envolvimento ID simultâneo. A colonoscopia flexível permite a visualização completa do IG, e muitas vezes é possível para realizar também a biopsia do íleo. O exame histopatológico permite que processos neoplásicos sejam excluídos e diferencia entre os vários tipos de inflamação do cólon.

A colite linfoplasmocitária é a forma histológica mais descrita, ao passo que a eosinofílica é menos comum (Figura 277.12). Por sua vez, a piogranulomatosa é incomum e está associada a massas proliferativas de vários milímetros a centímetros de tamanho visível durante a colonoscopia ou palpável pelo reto – os cães afetados têm graves sinais clínicos. A supurativa (neutrofílica) foi relatada como uma variante provável de DII em gatos e, muitas vezes, responde ao tratamento empírico da colite. Uma evidência emergente indica que isso pode se dar em razão de uma infecção bacteriana específica, já que microrganismos são vistos nos tecidos usando técnicas de hibridização fluorescente *in situ* (FISH, do inglês *Fluorescence in situ Hybridization*). Por fim, a colite granulomatosa (CG) é descrita em detalhes em uma seção separada, pois não é mais considerada parte da DII idiopática.

Infelizmente, não há concordância entre patologistas sobre a interpretação da avaliação de amostras de biopsia intestinal submetidas a exame histopatológico, porque, em última análise, é uma avaliação subjetiva e complicada por artefatos causados pela qualidade da amostra, pelo processamento e pelas técnicas de coloração. Um sistema de graduação histológica padronizado para DII de ID e IG em cães e gatos, com base em imagens e descrições escritas de alterações patológicas, foi publicado pelo grupo de padronização GI da Associação Mundial de Veterinários de Pequenos Animais (WSAVA, do inglês World Small Animal Veterinary Association).[220] Foi necessária uma abordagem ampla para descrever as alterações inflamatórias na mucosa das biopsias endoscópicas, enfatizando as mudanças arquitetônicas e o número de células inflamatórias na LP (Boxe 277.2). De maneira controversa, omitiu-se deliberadamente a avaliação do número de células caliciformes como um indicador de colite por causa de uma visão de que células que já tenham liberado seu conteúdo de mucina poderiam ser desconsideradas. Essa visão foi questionada, e esquemas futuro precisarão avaliar seu valor na identificação precisa da colite. No entanto, houve um mal-entendido geral quanto ao que as diretrizes WSAVA buscavam alcançar. Elas não são um sistema de pontuação numérica que adicionam pontos para cada característica, pela qual a inflamação

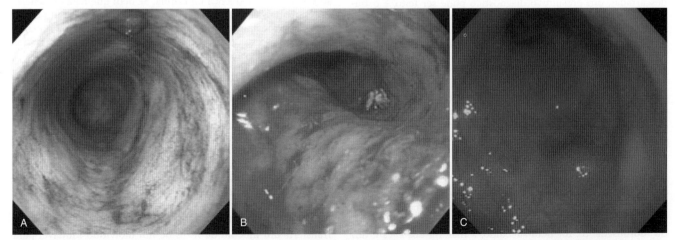

Figura 277.12 Imagens colonoscópicas de cães com diarreia do intestino grosso. Em resumo, a colite linfoplasmocitária, a colite eosinofílica e o linfoma podem parecer semelhantes, por isso devem ser coletadas biopsias por endoscopia. **A.** Cólon descendente de um Pastor-Alemão com colite linfoplasmacítica moderada. **B.** Cólon descendente e flexura cólica esquerda em um Labrador Negro com colite eosinofílica moderada. Os vasos submucosos são obscurecidos pela mucosa espessada e inflamada, que é irregular e ulcerada com sangramento espontâneo. **C.** Cólon terminal de um Husky Siberiano com linfoma alimentar nodular difuso. Áreas de mucosa normal mostrando vasos da submucosa são intercaladas com áreas espessadas, quase nodulares, de infiltração tumoral. (*Esta figura se encontra reproduzida em cores no Encarte.*)

Boxe 277.2 Sistema de pontuação histológica para um relatório objetivo da inflamação do cólon em cães e gatos

Recursos para avaliar e pontuar em normal, discreta moderado e grave

Características morfológicas
Lesão da superfície epitelial
Hiperplasia de cripta
Dilatação/distorção de cripta
Fibrose/atrofia

Inflamação
Linfócitos e plasmócitos da lâmina própria
Eosinófilos da lâmina própria
Neutrófilos da lâmina própria
Macrófagos da lâmina própria

Adaptado de Day MJ, Bilzer T, Mansell J et al.: Histopathological standards for the diagnosis of gastrintestinal inflammation in endoscopic biopsy samples from the dog and cat: a report from the World Small Animal Veterinary Association Gastrintestinal Standardization Group. J Comp Pathol 138(Suppl 1):S1-S43, 2008. Nota do autor: Os números das células caliciformes foram excluídos.

intestinal pode ser graduada. Trata-se apenas de um modelo para que todos possam ter confiança em que diferentes patologistas indicam a mesma coisa quando descrevem uma alteração como discreta/moderada/grave. Não é uma escala ponderada, portanto uma pontuação cumulativa pode ser irrelevante, pois ainda não se sabe quais características examinadas são as mais significantes. As diretrizes foram publicadas para permitir estudos comparativos prospectivos para analisar quais alterações são importantes na definição histológica da DII e, assim, entender a correlação entre gravidade clínica e histológica.

Tratamento e conduta

É importante saber se um paciente tem colite idiopática ou se há uma causa subjacente que faz parte de uma DII mais generalizada, pois os tratamentos diferem. Um paciente com sinais de colite, mas com anormalidades de concentrações séricas de folato e cobalamina, quase sempre também apresenta doença do ID. Portanto, idealmente, biopsias de ID, obtidas por endoscopia digestiva alta e ileoscopia, também devem ser coletadas, em vez de apenas proceder a uma biopsia colonoscópica quando há suspeita de colite.

Uma vez que as causas conhecidas de colite tenham sido descartadas, um presuntivo diagnóstico pode ser feito, e o tratamento empírico baseado em modificação da dieta e medicamentos com efeitos colaterais mínimos se inicia. De modo ideal, um diagnóstico preciso, com base no exame histológico das biopsias do cólon, deve ser realizado antes do uso de glicocorticoides, que podem ter efeitos colaterais e mascarar condições, caso testes adicionais de diagnóstico sejam necessários. No entanto, de maneira pragmática, a terapia empírica com glicocorticoides pode ser tentada se outros tratamentos falharem. Um diagnóstico histológico é obrigatório antes do uso de outras drogas imunossupressoras, haja vista que podem ter efeitos colaterais potencialmente permanentes e até fatais.

Manejo dietético[43,221-223]

As dietas recomendadas para animais de estimação com colite crônica incluem exclusão com base naquelas altamente digestíveis e de baixo resíduo, ou em uma nova dieta de proteína única ou hidrolisada. Se for bem-sucedido, a maioria dos cães e dos gatos com colite terá respondido a tal mudança em 2 semanas.

As fibras dietéticas insolúveis adicionais podem reduzir a digestibilidade dos nutrientes, mas também ter um efeito benéfico e sintomático na colite, em parte por meio da modificação da motilidade do cólon. Como alternativa, a Psyllium é uma fibra indigestível e solúvel derivada da semente de *Plantago*

ovata, muitas vezes recomendada no manejo da colite. Ela tem grande capacidade de retenção de água e forma géis com água, contribuindo para a melhora da consistência fecal. A Psyllium demonstrou ser eficaz no tratamento da colite idiopática crônica em cães quando adicionada a uma dieta altamente digerível. Uma dosagem diária inicial variando de meia colher de sopa para raças miniatura a três colheres para cães grandes é adicionada a cada refeição, sendo a dosagem ajustada para o efeito desejado.

A fibra fermentável é solúvel e resiste à digestão no ID, sendo metabolizada pelas bactérias do cólon. A adição de dela provou benefício adjuvante nos estudos clínicos de colite crônica canina e felina, muitas vezes adicionada a alimentos comerciais para animais de estimação. Exemplos incluem não só o Psyllium, mas também polpa de beterraba, fruto-oligossacarídeos (FOSs), inulina e mananoligossacarídeos (MOSs). As fibras fermentáveis são metabolizadas em AGCCs pelas bactérias do IG e fornecem uma fonte de energia para os colonócitos. Quando essa fibra está ausente da dieta, a estrutura do epitélio intestinal se torna anormal e pode ocorrer diarreia. Goma de acácia e alfaglucano butirogênico – um amido resistente sintetizado a partir de 1,4-alfa-D-glucanos com comprimentos de cadeia do polímero de 10 ± 35 unidades de glicose – são bons substratos para a produção de AGCCs, sendo muito encontrados em produtos combinados com probióticos, caulim e outros antidiarreicos. Além de fornecer uma fonte de energia para os colonócitos, os efeitos benéficos conhecidos das fibras fermentáveis incluem a proliferação de colonócitos por meio do aumento do fluxo sanguíneo para a mucosa do cólon e promoção da diferenciação de células epiteliais em colonócitos totalmente funcionais. Além disso, FOSs e MOSs são prebióticos e podem influenciar a composição do microbioma do IG. Em gatos, relatou-se aumento nas concentrações fecais no cólon de *Bacteroides* e *Lactobacillus* spp. e diminuição de *Escherichia coli* e *Clostridium perfringens*.

Probióticos[224-231]

Probióticos são microrganismos vivos benéficos para o trato GI do hospedeiro (ver Capítulo 167). Nenhum estudo clínico foi capaz de documentar efeitos positivos convincentes dos probióticos em cães e gatos com doenças gastrintestinais crônicas, embora experimentos *in vitro* e estudos em gastrenterite aguda canina e felina, bem como em pacientes humanos, indiquem benefícios potenciais. A bactéria probiótica *Enterococcus faecium* (SF68) foi administrada com segurança ao trato GI canino e aumentou o conteúdo de IgA fecal e as células B maduras circulantes em filhotes. Esse probiótico pode ser útil na prevenção ou no tratamento de doença GI canina. Se bem que haja evidências experimentais emergentes de que probióticos exercem um efeito sobre a permeabilidade intestinal e a resposta imune da mucosa, até que mais estudos provem a eficácia clínica, os veterinários devem ver as alegações do produto com algum ceticismo.

Terapias adjuvantes

O MPS Protect é um mucopolissacarídeo também encontrado em alguns produtos antidiarreicos combinados e que, teoricamente, aumenta a produção de muco protetor do cólon. Medicamentos herbais têm mostrado oferecer alguma proteção para danos por anti-inflamatórios não esteroides.[232,233] Existem dados derivados de tutores de que a homeopatia é eficaz em cerca de dois terços de cães com diarreia, mas nenhum estudo controlado prova qualquer benefício.[234]

Transplante fecal microbiano[235-240]

Transferir um inóculo de fezes de um indivíduo saudável para um paciente com doença gastrintestinal está se tornando um tratamento aceito para infecção por *Clostridioides difficile* resistente em pacientes humanos e tem sido aplicado na DII. O conceito foi extrapolado para o tratamento da DII canina, com relatos observacionais de sucesso até aqui. Como o material transplantado é dado em um enema de retenção, talvez seja mais adequado para tratar a colite. Contudo, até que mais estudos tenham sido feitos, não pode ser recomendado, em particular porque ainda é debatido como rastrear e escolher doadores saudáveis.

Terapia medicamentosa

A intervenção farmacológica (Tabela 277.3) é necessária se a terapia dietética e adjuvante (probiótico etc.) falhar no controle dos sinais clínicos ou, em casos graves, pode ser iniciada junto com a modificação da dieta.

Metronidazol[241-245]

Entre os antimicrobianos, o metronidazol é muito usado em cães e gatos com colite. Além de seus efeitos antimicrobianos contra bactérias anaeróbias obrigatórios, também é eficaz contra a *Giardia*, malgrado, em doses antibacterianas padrão (ou seja, 10 mg/kg), apenas suprima, e não elimine a infecção. Além disso, o metronidazol demonstrou ter efeitos imunomodulatórios e ser genotóxico para os linfócitos felinos, afetando várias etapas inatas e adaptativas da resposta imune. Ele é usado em cães e gatos com colite para modificar a microbiota intestinal, diminuindo os microrganismos anaeróbios e a inflamação. Apresenta gosto desagradável, sobretudo para gatos, contudo outros efeitos colaterais são bastante raros e incluem vômitos e diarreia. Hepatotoxicose e neurotoxicose ocorrem em dosagens mais altas.

Ácido 5-amino salicílico

O ácido 5-amino salicílico (5-AAS ou mesalazina) é um droga anti-inflamatória não esteroide eficaz no tratamento da CU em humanos. A molécula nativa é potencialmente nefrotóxica, se absorvida pelo ID, por isso só está disponível como uma preparação com revestimento entérico dissolvido pelo pH ácido cólon e como um enema de espuma.[a] A segurança da preparação do revestimento entérico não foi estabelecida em cães e gatos, por isso seu uso não é recomendado, enquanto as preparações de enema são improváveis de serem adequadas. Portanto, é administrado a cães e gatos como pró-drogas.

A sulfassalazina (Azuflin, Salazoprin) é uma pró-droga que consiste em 5-ASA ligado por uma ligação azo a sulfapiridina.[223,246,247] É administrada por via oral e atinge o ponto distal do ID e do cólon, inalterada. Lá, as bactérias quebram a ponte azo e liberam ambas as moléculas. A 5-ASA exerce efeitos inflamatórios diretamente na mucosa do cólon, inibindo a síntese de prostaglandina e leucotrieno. A sulfapiridina é, em essência, uma molécula transportadora, e acredita-se que não tenha efeito antes de ser absorvida e eliminada pelo metabolismo no fígado e na excreção urinária. O principal efeito adverso da sulfassalazina é a ceratoconjuntivite seca (CCS). Apesar de seu mecanismo de ação exato ser desconhecido, a sulfassalazina pode danificar as glândulas lacrimais. A detecção precoce com imediata descontinuação do tratamento é necessária para prevenir o início da CCS irreversível. Portanto, a produção de lágrimas deve ser medida em intervalos regulares em todos os cães que recebam sulfassalazina. Vômito pode ocorrer e ser prevenido se o medicamento for administrado com comida, mas a pancreatite aguda foi registrada como efeito colateral. Outras pró-drogas com o mesmo mecanismo de ação estão disponíveis.

A olsalazina (Dipentum) consiste em duas moléculas de 5-ASA ligadas por uma ponte azo. Como duas moléculas 5-ASA

---

[a]N.T.:Também disponível na forma de supositórios.

| **Tabela 277.3** | Terapia farmacológica da inflamação do intestino grosso. |

CATEGORIA DA DROGA E NOME	DOSAGEM RECOMENDADA	INDICAÇÃO
Antimicrobianos Enrofloxacino	5 mg/kg PO a cada 24 h (C), por 4 a 8 semanas; cultura e teste de sensibilidade para *Escherichia coli* recomendado antes de iniciar o tratamento	CG
Metronidazol	10 a 15 mg/kg PO a cada 12 h (C, G) a cada 8 h (C) Para benzoilmetronidazol, aumente a dosagem acima em aproximadamente 50%	Colite aguda e crônica
Drogas anti-inflamatórias Sulfassalazina	10 a 30 mg/kg PO a cada 8 h, por 4 a 6 semanas, dose total máxima de 1 g (C); 5-12,5 mg/kg PO a cada 8 h, por 2 a 4 semanas (G) Administre com alimento. Diminua lentamente em etapas de 10 a 14 dias para a cada 12 h; depois, metade da dose a cada 12 h; por fim, 1 vez/dia. Controle regularmente a produção de lágrimas	DII colônica refratária à dieta e metronidazol
Olsalazina	5 a 15 mg/kg PO a cada 8 h, por 4 a 6 semanas, dose total máxima de 1 g (C); 2,5 a 7,5 mg/kg PO a cada 8 h, por 2 a 4 semanas (G)	
Drogas imunossupressivas Prednisona (prednisolona)	1 a 2 mg/kg PO a cada 12 h, por 10 a 14 dias, depois diminuindo lentamente ao longo de várias semanas	DII colônica refratária a dieta e antibióticos
Azatioprina	Dose inicial: 2 mg/kg PO a cada 24 h (C), por 2 semanas; depois, 2 mg/kg dia sim, dia não, por 2 a 4 semanas; por fim, 1 mg/kg PO dia sim, dia não. Pode levar de 2 a 4 semanas para o efeito total.	DII colônica refratária a esteroides
Clorambucila	Gatos > 4 kg: 2 mg por gato PO em dias alternados, por 2 a 4 semanas; em seguida, diminuir para a menor dose eficaz (2 mg/kg por gato PO, a cada 3 a 4 dias) Gatos < 4 kg: iniciar com 2 mg/kg por gato PO, a cada 3 dias	DII felina refratária ou grave; combinada com prednisolona
Ciclosporina	5 mg/kg PO a cada 24 h (C), por 10 semanas	DII colônica refratária crônica refratária a esteroides

C, Cão; *G*, Gato; *CG*, colite granulomatosa; *DII*, doença inflamatória intestinal.

são liberadas para cada molécula de olsalazina administrada, a dosagem é de 50% da droga sulfassalazina. Esperava-se que isso eliminasse o risco de CCS, mas ela ainda foi relatada, embora mais raramente.

A balsalazida é outra pró-droga (4-aminobenzoil-beta-ala-nina-mesalamina) com 5-ASA ligado a um transportador inerte, porém sua segurança e eficácia em cães e gatos não foi demons-trada e não pode ser recomendada.

Glicocorticoides

Os glicocorticoides são usados como uma segunda linha de tratamento para cães com DII do cólon refratária a modificação dietética, metronidazol e sulfassalazina (ver Capítulos 164 e 165). Por causa dos efeitos colaterais, as dosagens de prednisona são reservadas a pacientes com colite confirmada e quando as causas subjacentes forem descartadas. Como os efeitos colaterais tendem a ser menos graves em gatos e eles podem não tolerar medicação 3 vezes/dia com sulfassalazina, sendo mais suscetí-veis à intoxicação por mesalamina, os glicocorticoides costu-mam ser uma opção de tratamento considerada antes em gatos do que em cães com colite. A budesonida, que é 90% metabo-lizada pela primeira passagem pelo fígado, é usada em alguns casos de DII, mas não há relatos de seu sucesso em casos isolados de colite idiopática.

Agentes citotóxicos

Agentes citotóxicos podem ser usados como poupadores este-roides para tratar todas as formas de DII, e não especificamente para colite idiopática (ver Capítulo 276). Graças a potenciais efeitos colaterais e considerações financeiras, eles devem ser reservados a animais com doença inflamatória colônica docu-mentada sem resposta a qualquer outro tratamento. O cloram-bucila tem sido usado com sucesso em cães e gatos com DII. A azatioprina foi recomendada para cães com DII refratária a doses imunossupressoras de corticosteroides, sendo raramente eficaz como agente único. Em vez disso, deve ser usada como terapia adjuvante, pois leva a uma significativa economia no uso de esteroides na DII canina, conquanto possa demorar várias semanas para alcançar a eficácia máxima. Doses de 2 mg/kg por via oral a cada 24 horas, em cães, e 0,3 mg/kg por via oral a cada 48 horas, em gatos, foram usadas com algum sucesso na DII. Por ser citotóxico, os comprimidos não devem ser quebrados. Assim, uma reformulação é necessária para produzir comprimidos de tamanho apropriado para gatos e cães pequenos.

Ciclosporina

A ciclosporina (Ciclosporina) reduz a produção de IL-2 em células T, tornando-as mais suscetíveis à apoptose (ver Capítulo 165). Sua eficácia na dosagem de 5 mg/kg PO a cada 24 horas, por 10 semanas, foi relatada em 9 de 14 cães com DII resistentes a esteroides, mas nenhum deles tinha só colite idiopática.[248-250]

Prognóstico

O prognóstico para DII do cólon depende da resposta ao trata-mento e da gravidade inicial da doença. Cães jovens que res-ponderam bem apenas com a terapia de eliminação de dieta tiveram um bom prognóstico, com a maioria em remissão em 1 ano. Cães mais velhos com doença grave e aqueles que precisam de esteroides para controlar os sinais clínicos apresentam um prognóstico muito mais reservado.[113]

COLITE GRANULOMATOSA[251-292]

Definição

Antes conhecida como colite ulcerativa histiocítica (CUH), a colite granulomatosa (CG) foi por muitos anos considerada uma forma de DII idiopática, mas hoje é associada a uma infecção intracelular por cepas de E. coli aderente e invasiva (AIEC). Ocorre com mais frequência em cães jovens da raça Boxer, mas vem sendo vista com frequência crescente em cães da raça Buldogue Francês, à medida que a raça ganha popularidade. Também foi descrita ocasionalmente em outras raças, como Mastiff, Malamute do Alasca e Buldogue Inglês, além de um gato. Desde que foi descrita, há 50 anos, a condição tem sido reconhecida mundialmente, ainda que hoje seja mais comum nos EUA e na Austrália, com raros relatos na Europa. A doença é restrita quase exclusivamente ao cólon, não obstante casos com envolvimento ID tenham sido observados e causem sinais graves de colite com diarreia mucoide, hematoquezia, urgência e tenesmo. A condição é caracterizada, de modo histopatológico, pela presença de macrófagos corados pelo ácido periódico de Schiff (PAS) subjacente a uma mucosa colônica ulcerada. Ten-tativas de tratar a condição com terapias usadas para colite idiopática, como metronidazol, sulfassalazina e glicocorticoides, falharam, e, historicamente, a gravidade da doença quase sempre leva à eutanásia do paciente.

Etiopatogênese

A causa da CG canina tem sido debatida por décadas, a despeito de sua ocorrência em grupos de animais e em alguns canis, além da presença do material PAS-positivo nos macrófagos, sugerir uma etiologia infecciosa. Estudos iniciais com microscopia ele-trônica demonstraram os chamados corpos residuais, que se assemelham a organismos semelhantes a bactérias em grânulos dentro de macrófagos PAS-positivos. Agentes infecciosos espe-cíficos, como micobactérias, micoplasmas, clamídias e riquétsias, foram todos propostos como causadores da CG. Tentativas de reproduzir a doença por infecção de cães com Mycoplasma spp. não tiveram sucesso. Em estudos de imuno-histoquímica, as lesões da CG são caracterizadas por aumento do número de células CD3-positivas, células plasmáticas produtoras de IgG e células MHC classe II positivas, que demonstram uma resposta inflamatória. De maneira alternativa, a restrição de raça marcada de GC, com a maioria dos cães afetados no primeiro relato de HUC em 1965 sendo rastreado até um único ancestral, sugere uma predisposição genética.

Mais recentemente, dois estudos independentes relataram ao mesmo tempo a remissão bem-sucedida e a provável cura após tratamento prolongado com enrofloxacino.[256,263] Doze casos foram descritos, cada um deles mostrando uma forte resposta ao tratamento com enrofloxacino (5 mg/kg PO a cada 24 h, por 4 a 8 semanas) ou um protocolo de combinação com enroflo-xacino, amoxicilina (20 mg/kg PO a cada 12 h) e metronidazol (10 a 15 mg/kg PO a cada 12 h). A resposta relatada à enroflo-xacino foi efetiva, com todos os cães respondendo dentro de 3 a 12 dias após o início da terapia e vários ficando livres da doença após um curso de terapia de 4 a 6 semanas. Alguns aparentemente necessitaram de tratamento por muito mais do que 6 semanas. Cinco foram biopsiados novamente quando estavam em remissão clínica após o término do tratamento com antibióticos. A melhora nas lesões histológicas foi evidente em todos, com desaparecimento de macrófagos PAS-positivos em três cães e uma redução acentuada no número de macrófagos nos outros dois.

O sucesso do tratamento com enrofloxacino em CG ressus-citou a questão de uma etiologia infecciosa. Usando FISH, um grande número de cocobacilos foi encontrado na mucosa do cólon em cães Boxer afetados com CG, mas não em tecidos normais na mucosa de cães com outros tipos de colite.[275,276,282] Estudos adicionais identificaram a bactéria como Escherichia coli localizada no compartimento intracelular dos macrófagos PAS-positivos. Elas, quando cocultivadas com células epiteliais e macrófagos, revelaram propriedades aderentes e invasivas espe-cíficas. Na verdade, a variante de E. coli associada com CG tem um fenótipo semelhante ao do comportamento adesivo e inva-sivo exibido por E. coli de infecções crônicas do trato urinário em mulheres e endometrite bovina.[293] E. coli semelhantes foram associadas à doença de Crohn em pessoas, que tem uma doença com aparência histológica semelhante. AIECs replicam nos fagolisossomos de macrófagos, provocando uma lesão granulomatosa, em vez de serem eliminadas. Essas descobertas apoiam a hipótese de que a genética desempenha um papel fundamental na infecção que causa a CG. Pessoas com doença de Crohn têm polimorfismos em certos receptores de reconhecimento de padrão (PRRs) do sistema imunológico inato, como NOD2 (receptor de domínio de oligomerização de ligação de nucleotídio 2), ligado a um defeito genético na imunidade inata com doença funcional.[294] Foi hipotetizado que defeitos semelhantes em PRRs podem estar presentes na CG como uma predisposição genética subjacente, graças à preponderância de casos em cães jovens da raça Boxer. A confirmação e a identificação de mutações em PRRs, como receptores *toll-like* (TLRs) ou NODs, em Boxers com CG, ainda não foram descritas. No entanto, um defeito na atividade de fagocitose de neutrófilos foi identificado e parece ser a razão mais provável pela qual a infecção AIEC não foi eliminada.

Avaliação do paciente

Histórico e exame físico

O início da doença geralmente ocorre antes dos 2 anos. Os sinais clínicos são aqueles de inflamação grave a crônica do IG e incluem diarreia, hematoquezia, aumento da frequência de defecação, tenesmo e presença de muco excessivo nas fezes. Achados de exame físico são normais em muitos cães com CG, mas perda de peso e inapetência podem ser observadas em casos graves. Sangue fresco e muco são encontrados no exame retal.

Diagnóstico

A abordagem diagnóstica para cães com CG é a mesma descrita para colite idiopática. Hemograma completo, bioquímica sérica e urinálise são necessários para excluir quaisquer doenças extraintestinais. Exame parasitológico de amostras fecais e coprocultura devem ser realizados (ver Capítulos 81 e 221). Um exame de ultrassom do abdome (ver Capítulo 88) pode revelar uma mucosa do cólon difusamente espessada. No entanto, em muitos cães, nenhuma anormalidade é detectada. Em geral, a colonoscopia revela locais de hemorragia e ulceração graves intercaladas com trechos de mucosa de aparência mais normal (Figura 277.13). As biopsias devem ser retiradas das úlceras, de mucosa normal e de zonas de transição.

As lesões iniciais podem consistir em um infiltrado inflamatório misto na LP, logo abaixo de um epitélio degenerativo.

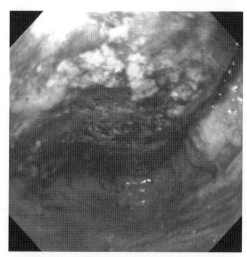

Figura 277.13 Colite granulomatosa. Visão endoscópica do cólon de um cão jovem da raça Boxer afetado, mostrando irregularidade grave, ulceração e hemorragia. (*Esta figura se encontra reproduzida em cores no Encarte.*)

Com o aumento da cronicidade e da gravidade, a ulceração piora, com perda generalizada da superfície epitelial e das células caliciformes. Abaixo, há infiltração grave da LP e da submucosa por neutrófilos, macrófagos, linfócitos, células plasmáticas e mastócitos, representando uma resposta inflamatória mista, talvez refletindo a invasão secundária por bactérias luminais. Acumulação de grandes macrófagos PAS-positivos costuma ser patognomônica para CG. Hibridização *in situ* fluorescente (FISH) feita em biopsias demonstra a presença de *E. coli* no tecido. A coloração com PAS e FISH continua a ser a melhor forma de confirmar o diagnóstico e distinguir CG de colite linfoplasmocitária idiopática, que é vista com mais frequência mesmo em cães da raça Boxer.

Tratamento e conduta

O prognóstico para CUH foi considerado grave quando a conduta consistia em várias combinações de gestão dietética e tratamento anti-inflamatório ou imunossupressor com sulfassalazina, prednisolona e azatioprina (ver anteriormente, na seção sobre colite crônica). Inevitavelmente, essas estratégias não tinham sucesso, e os cães mais afetados eram eutanasiados por serem refratários ao tratamento. O sucesso do tratamento com enrofloxacino reverteu o prognóstico e a cura é possível. No entanto, a resistência ao fármaco se desenvolveu, talvez em razão de seu uso inadequado em cães da raça Boxer com colite oriunda de outras causas, e algumas AIEC isoladas de CG são sensíveis apenas à amicacina.[274]

INFECÇÃO

Infecções gastrintestinais podem causar colite aguda ou crônica. Elas são comuns em cães e gatos, mas a maioria afeta o ID principal, sequencial ou simultaneamente a ID e IG. A gastroenterocolite aguda quase sempre começa com inapetência, vômito e diarreia do tipo ID antes de ocorrerem sinais de colite (hematoquezia, muco, urgência, tenesmo), ao que parece refletindo a passagem do agente infeccioso no trato GI. Agentes infecciosos que visam sobretudo o IG são descritos aqui.

Não há infecções virais que afetem apenas o IG, embora uma manifestação incomum de peritonite infecciosa felina (PIF) seja uma massa piogranulomatosa na região ileocecocólica, causando diarreia ou obstrução.[295-297] Informações sobre parvovírus, coronavírus entérico e outras doenças virais que causam uma infecção gastrintestinal generalizada podem ser encontradas nos Capítulos 224, 225, 228 e 276. Da mesma forma, uma série de causas bacterianas de gastroenterocolite são discutidas em mais detalhes no capítulo anterior e no Capítulo 220. Infecções específicas do IG são causadas principalmente por parasitos protozoários e metazoários que, ao que parece, ocupam um nicho ecológico que faz do IG seu local predileto de interação.

Bactérias[298-300,320]

Enteropatógenos, como *Campylobacter*, *Escherichia coli*, *Salmonella* e *Yersinia*, costumam infectar o ID, mas também podem causar colite. Aqui, novamente, a dificuldade é que o isolamento não prova a causa, pois esses organismos podem ser encontrados nas fezes de animais clinicamente saudáveis. Uma *E. coli* aderente e invasiva está associada à colite granulomatosa em cães da raça Boxer (ver anteriormente).

Anaerobiospirillum[301,302]

Um pequeno bacilo anaeróbio gram-negativo levemente espiralado, *Anaerobiospirillum* spp., pode ser isolado das fezes de cães e gatos. Existem, no entanto, relatos de casos agudos de ileocolite ulcerativa ou necrosante em gatos associada a esse organismo. Ela pode ser demonstrada nas criptas de biopsias coradas com colorações Giemsa ou Steiner, ou por PCR. Não há dados publicados sobre o tratamento.

Brachyspira pilosicoli[303-309]

Esse microrganismo é uma espiroqueta e causa a disenteria suína, podendo ser patogênica em cães. Infecção maciça com sinais de colite aguda foi descrita em cães mantidos em colônias com más condições de higiene.

Campylobacter spp[131,132,141,299,310-314]

Campylobacter são bacilos gram-negativos espiralados, móveis, muitas vezes encontrados nas fezes, inclusive de animais saudáveis. Ainda não se sabe se eles são patogênicos em cães e gatos (ver Capítulo 220). Eles costumam causar doenças do intestino delgado e são discutidos em detalhes no Capítulo 276. No entanto, existem relatos de Campylobacter causando enterocolite e colite isolada.

Clostridioides difficile[119,133,315-328]

Um bacilo gram-positivo anaeróbico formador de esporos C. difficile é um patógeno nosocomial significativo em humanos (ver Capítulos 210 e 220). C. difficile produz duas toxinas principais, A (uma enterotoxina) e B (uma citotoxina), que podem causar colite pseudomembranosa fatal em humanos hospitalizados que receberam antibióticos. No intestino humano, as toxinas causam perda de integridade epitelial e morte celular por meio da glicosilação e da inativação de guanosina trifosfatases, resultando na despolimerização da F-actina. Também causam inflamação ao estimular a produção de prostaglandinas e substância P, promovendo a degranulação de mastócitos. Seu efeito sobre o epitélio intestinal canino é desconhecido, e os dados sobre a colite pseudomembranosa em cães após terapia antibiótica não são claros. Na verdade, o isolamento do organismo em cães diarreicos é mais associado a sinais tanto do ID quanto do IG.

O organismo pode ser cultivado pelas fezes em até 40% de cães saudáveis e com diarreia, se bem que suas toxinas sejam mais encontradas em cães com diarreia. Também é relatada a presença de toxinas nas fezes de mais de 90% de cães neonatos sem sinais clínicos. Assim, é difícil provar uma relação causal entre enterotoxina e doença em cães, ainda que o organismo tenha sido incriminado como causa de infecção hospitalar e diarreia. Metronidazol (10 mg/kg PO a cada 8 a 12 h) é um tratamento eficaz, pois a resistência antibacteriana parece ser rara em isolados caninos.

Clostridium perfringens[320,321,328-345]

Esse bacilo gram-positivo anaeróbio formador de esporos causa toxinfecção alimentar em humanos e foi incriminado como causa de colite canina aguda e gastrenterite hemorrágica (GEH). No entanto, muitas vezes está presente no ID canino saudável, com taxas de isolamento descritas de até 80%. Pode produzir toxinas Tipo A, incluindo a toxina principal A e uma enterotoxina (enterotoxina de Clostridium perfringens [CPE]). Cepas de C. perfringens produtoras de toxinas do tipo A têm sido associadas a doenças agudas e, com frequência, enterocolite hemorrágica em cães, sobretudo em canis e em condições de hospedagem. A CPE pode estimular a secreção do intestino e iniciar apoptose, mas C. perfringens também pode carregar outros fatores de virulência, como a toxina beta$_2$.

Historicamente, a secreção de CPE foi associada à esporulação do microrganismo em condições ambientais adequadas, supostamente levando à diarreia. Isso era muitas vezes ligado ao estresse de hospitalização ou canil, ou a uma repentina mudança na dieta, talvez causando uma mudança no pH do cólon, com diarreia mucoide ocorrendo 1 a 5 dias após admissão e quase sempre respondendo ao metronidazol ou à adição de fibras na dieta. A observação de cinco microrganismos esporulados por campo de alto aumento em um esfregaço fecal era considerado diagnóstico. No entanto, foi demonstrado que a esporulação não se correlaciona com a produção de CPE e, uma vez que cerca de 15% dos cães saudáveis também podem abrigar C. perfringens produtor de CPE, sua patogenicidade não está confirmada.

O isolamento de C. perfringens por coprocultura é insuficiente para provar que ele é a causa da colite, mas imunoensaios estão disponíveis para detectar CPE nas fezes. O PCR também está disponível para a detecção do gene cpe. Todavia, o valor clínico de todos esses testes é questionável, pois o CPE é detectado com frequência semelhante em fezes de cães saudáveis.

C. perfringens é suscetível a metronidazol (8 a 15 mg/kg PO a cada 8 a 12 h), amoxicilina, eritromicina e tilosina, sendo comum resistência às tetraciclinas. O prognóstico é bom, e o tratamento de suporte com a adição de fibras na dieta ou probióticos às vezes é tão bem-sucedido quanto tratamento com antibióticos, levantando a dúvida sobre se eles são necessários.[341] Contudo, se a C. perfringens é uma causa de colite, ainda motivo de debate, conquanto evidências emergentes indiquem que causa GEH. Estudos recentes demonstram C. perfringens na mucosa intestinal de cães com GEH, mas não há associação com a produção de CPE.[330]

Escherichia coli[346-356]

E. coli é encontrada no trato GI de quase todos os cães e da maioria dos gatos, e é provável que seja um comensal a menos que carregue genes plasmidiais ou cromossômicos específicos que codificam para mecanismos patogênicos. Alguns isolados costumam causar sobretudo doença do ID, como E. coli enterotoxigênica (ETEC), que produz toxinas termoestáveis (STs) e termolábeis (LTs) que estimulam o aumento da secreção pelo ID (ver Capítulos 220 e 276). Outros podem causar danos tanto ao ID quando ao IG, como E. coli enteropatogênica (EPEC), que causa aderência íntima e "apagamento" das microvilosidades epiteliais intestinais (lesão "attaching and effacing" [A/E]) por meio, entre outros fatores, da interação da adesina intimina codificada pelo gene eae. Infecção fatal por EPEC foi relatada em um gato filhote e em um gato adulto nos quais lesões A/E foram encontradas no íleo e no cólon. Acredita-se que morte de cachorros filhotes com infecção por EPEC sejam mais comuns, porém muitas vezes há uma infecção mista e contribuição para o vírus da cinomose, parvovírus e protozoários patogênicos.

Alguns isolados de E. coli, como E. coli entero-hemorrágica (EHEC), tem um tropismo pelo IG. Malgrado, em geral, não sejam invasivos, as EHEC produzem as toxinas Shiga (Stx, também chamada de verocitotoxina [VT]), que matam os colonócitos por inibição da síntese de proteínas, levando a edema, hemorragia submucosa, arterite, trombose arteriolar no cólon e diarreia hemorrágica. Outras toxinas participam da patogênese, como os fatores citotóxicos necrosantes 1 e 2 (CNF 1 e 2). As taxas de isolamento variam até 15% em cães saudáveis e 5% em gatos saudáveis.

A EHEC do sorotipo O157: H7, um comensal no gado bovino, também produz as toxinas Stx e está associada à potencialmente fatal síndrome hemolítico-urêmica (SHU) em humanos. Embora o O157: H7 tenha sido isolada das fezes de cães saudáveis, não há evidências conclusivas de SHU na espécie, mesmo que possa ser produzida experimentalmente por inoculação IV de Stx. O organismo também foi associado à "podridão do Alabama", onde ocorrem lesões ulcerativas na pele e lesão renal aguda.[357] Outros sorotipos são isolados com mais frequência em taxas de até 25% em cães da raça Greyhound, provavelmente associados à alimentação com carne crua. E. coli produtoras de Stx são encontradas mais em gatos com diarreia do que em saudáveis.

Como a patogenicidade de qualquer E. coli depende de quais genes carrega, o simples isolamento pela cultura de rotina não tem sentido, e o PCR é necessário para identificar o gene ou os genes que codificam para patogenicidade. Mesmo assim, a identificação não necessariamente confirma a causalidade, uma vez que o organismo pode estar presente em animais saudáveis e a vacinação de cães contra E. coli é especulativa.

Helicobacter spp. entero-hepáticos[358]

Helicobacter spp. gástricos são bem conhecidos, não obstante seu potencial patogênico em cães e gatos ainda seja um debate.

CAPÍTULO 277 • Doenças do Intestino Grosso

Entretanto, helicobacteres êntero-hepáticos também foram identificados e possivelmente incriminados em colangite de felinos. Recentemente, foi identificada uma associação entre *Helicobacter* em criptas colônicas e muco superficial e a evidência histológica de colite em cães e gatos. Todavia, a falta de comprovação dos postulados de Koch significa que ainda não sabemos seu significado na etiologia da colite supostamente idiopática.

Salmonella *spp.*[356,359-388]

Salmonella spp., com mais frequência o sorotipo *S. Typhimurium* em cães e gatos, é um potencial risco zoonótico. Ela se liga a células epiteliais e M no ID e no IG, podendo causar enterocolite. A infecção, felizmente, é pouco frequente (< 2%), mas a taxa de isolamento fecal é semelhante em pacientes saudáveis e diarreicos, variando de 1 a 36% de todos os cães e de 1 a 18% dos gatos saudáveis. As taxas mais altas de isolamento relatadas quase sempre são associadas à ingestão de alimentos crus, mastigação de couro cru e carne malcozida. Mais informações sobre fisiopatologia, apresentação clínica, tratamento e prognóstico são discutidos nos Capítulos 220 e 276.

Yersinia enterocolitica[389-391]

Y. enterocolitica é um cocobacilo gram-negativo móvel, que pode ser isolado das fezes de cães e gatos clinicamente saudáveis. Também foi associado, com mais raridade, a desconforto abdominal e/ou diarreia com sangue. Em humanos, a infecção foi correlacionada com polimorfismos de/NOD2, uma molécula de reconhecimento de padrão bacteriano no sistema imunológico inato.[392]

Algas

Prototheca *spp.*[393-406]

Prototheca spp. são algas aclorofiladas que podem causar prototecose em cães, gatos e humanos. *Prototeca zopfii* costuma estar associada a GI e disseminada em cães jovens, ao passo que a *Prototheca wickerhamii* está mais associada a infecções cutâneas em cães e gatos. As algas vivem em lixo orgânico e alimentos, solo e água contaminados com esgoto, de modo que a imunidade celular prejudicada do hospedeiro parece desempenhar um papel na infecção e na disseminação de doenças. A infecção colônica primária é seguida por endosporulação e disseminação para outros tecidos.

A maioria dos cães com doença disseminada apresenta sinais de diarreia prolongada com sangue. Sinais oculares e neurológicos geralmente acompanham colite e cinomose, devendo ser incluídos na lista de diagnóstico diferencial, o qual se dá por citologia de raspado retal ou colônico e/ou por histologia dos tecidos afetados, mostrando os organismos encapsulados. A cultura dos tecidos afetados é prontamente realizada e permite a diferenciação de espécies. O tratamento da prototecose disseminada com combinações variadas de anfotericina B e itraconazol (ver Capítulo 162) foi tentado, mas apenas retarda a progressão, sendo o resultado final invariavelmente fatal.

Fungos

Infecções fúngicas sistêmicas, que podem infectar o trato gastrintestinal, ocorrem em certas áreas geográficas e são descritas em detalhes em outros capítulos. O *histoplasma* (ver Capítulo 233) costuma afetar o ID; o *Aspergillus* (ver Capítulos 234 e 235) pode causar infecção gastrintestinal em pacientes imunossuprimidos e foi observado durante terapia com ciclosporina; por fim, Oomycetes, como *Pythium insidiosum* e zigomicetos (ver Capítulo 236), podem infectar o trato GI (ficomicose).

Histoplasma capsulatum[407-409]

O *H. capsulatum* é um fungo um dimórfico cujo estágio micelial de vida livre cresce em clima quente, solo úmido e rico em nitrogênio, contaminado com excrementos de morcegos ou pássaros. Nos EUA, ocorre principalmente ao longo dos rios Ohio, Mississippi e Missouri. Os esporos de fungos são inalados e, em seguida, disseminados por macrófagos para o trato GI e outros órgãos. Suspeita-se que a infecção direta do trato GI após a ingestão, sem envolvimento pulmonar, também possa ocorrer. Reações inflamatórias granulomatosas com ulceração e perda de sangue ocorrem no trato GI e causam os sinais clínicos típicos.

O organismo causa diarreia crônica de ID em cães jovens e gatos, sendo os sinais comuns tenesmo, hematoquezia e muco nas fezes. Os cães também podem apresentar pirexia, anorexia, vômito e perda de peso. O ID pode ser afetado, com sinais de perda de peso e, às vezes, enteropatia perdedora de proteínas. A colonoscopia revela inflamação granulomatosa grave.

O *histoplasma* é diagnosticado de forma mais confiável dentro de macrófagos em esfregaços citológicos de raspados retais ou amostras de citologia de escova obtidas durante a colonoscopia. Como alternativa, aspirados de linfonodos ou amostras histológicas podem ser usados para o diagnóstico. Colorações para fungos, como PAS e metenamina de prata de Gomori, podem ajudar a demonstrar os organismos em tecidos fixados.

O tratamento de suporte com modificação da dieta, antimicrobianos, antidiarreicos e 5-aminossalicilatos pode fornecer algum alívio dos sintomas, mas o tratamento definitivo é com itraconazol a 10 mg/kg PO a cada 24 h, por 4 a 6 meses. O tratamento deve ser mantido por pelo menos 2 a 3 meses após a resolução dos sinais clínicos. O prognóstico parece favorável em cães e gatos.

Pythium insidiosum[410-412]

O *Pythium insidiosum* é um microrganismo aquático pertencente à classe Oomycetes e que causa a pitiose. Cães machos de raças grandes, usados como cães de caça, são mais afetados, pois o microrganismo vive em águas quentes pantanosas. As áreas endêmicas são a região da Costa do Golfo dos EUA, porém a doença foi diagnosticada no extremo norte da Virgínia e na Califórnia.[b]

O microrganismo tem predileção pela pele e/ou pelo GI trato. Quando este é afetado, a obstrução GI superior se dá com mais frequência em razão da infiltração grave da parede gastrintestinal. Às vezes, o cólon também é afetado, resultando em diarreia de IG. Mais informações sobre o diagnóstico e o tratamento podem ser encontradas nos Capítulos 236 e 276.

Protozoários

O trato GI hospeda uma série de microrganismos protozoários que fazem parte do microbioma normal, porém algumas espécies são consideradas enteropatogênicas (ver Capítulo 221). A maioria, como coccídios – *Cryptosporidium* e *Cystoisospora* (antes *Isospora*) e *Giardia* –, é considerada infecção de ID, mas alguns (*Tritrichomonas*) são claramente patógenos de IG. O significado de outros protozoários, como *Balantidium* e *Pentatrichomonas*, é incerto.

Balantidium coli[413-418]

Os hospedeiros primários desse parasita ciliado são suínos e primatas não humanos. A infecção é raramente relatada em cães e está associada ao acesso a suínos. O *Balantidium coli* supostamente causa colite ulcerosa em cães, com sinais clínicos típicos de diarreia de IG e extrapolando a infecção humana. Tratamento com tetraciclinas ou metronidazol costumam ser eficaz. No entanto, a coinfecção com *Trichuris vulpis* em casos relatados confunde o significado da presença do organismo, já que o tratamento da infecção dos helmintos por si só pode resolver os sinais.

---

[b]N.T.: No Brasil, casos de pitiose já forma descritos, e a região do Pantanal parece ser a de maior ocorrência, principalmente em equinos.

Entamoeba histolytica[419,420]

Em particular um parasita intestinal em humanos e primatas não humanos, a *Entamoeba histolytica* causa disenteria amebiana. Embora a amebíase seja geralmente uma doença leve em cães e gatos, e o microrganismo também possa ser encontrado em cães e gatos saudáveis, um relato descreve colite grave em um cão e em um gato. O microrganismo vive no cólon ou ligado à parede do cólon, raramente se disseminando para outros órgãos. Os raros casos descritos apresentaram sinais de diarreia aguda de ID, hematoquezia e tenesmo. A fonte de infecção em animais de estimação quase sempre é de origem humana, o que aumenta a importância das considerações de saúde pública, caso seja diagnosticado em um animal de estimação. O diagnóstico é mais bem feito por esfregaços fecais diretos. A erradicação é alcançada com metronidazol a 30 mg/kg PO a cada 12 h, por 3 semanas, sendo indicado o monitoramento para neurotoxicose.

Giardia intestinalis (lamblia)[421]

Infecção de cães e gatos que pode causar sinais clínicos sugestivos de colite, mas geralmente é considerada uma infecção SI. A maior concentração de organismos é encontrada no duodeno de cães e no íleo de gatos (ver Capítulos 221 e 276).

Pentatrichomonas hominis[422-428]

Este protozoário flagelado é geralmente considerado um comensal em cães e é mais importante porque pode ser confundido com *Giardia* em preparações fecais frescas. No entanto, existe alguma suspeita de que pode causar colite, especialmente em filhotes de gatos, embora infecções concomitantes geralmente compliquem o quadro. Na pior das hipóteses, só podem ser um patógeno oportunista.

Tritrichomonas foetus[129,130,423,425,426,429-451]

Esse protozoário é de importância emergente como causa de diarreia persistente em gatos. Ele coloniza principalmente o IG e causa colite crônica. Irritação anal e incontinência fecal também podem ser características da infecção. Embora seja sobretudo um enteropatógeno felino, foi relatado em cadelas reprodutoras na França, mas não foi encontrado em uma pesquisa com 215 cães filhotes.[424] O *Tritrichomonas foetus* é um protozoário flagelado semelhante em tamanho e forma a *Giardia*, todavia só existe na forma de trofozoíta. É um importante patógeno em bovinos, causando infertilidade e aborto, mas a transmissão venérea parece não ser importante em gatos, nos quais a transmissão ocorre diretamente pela via fecal-oral.

Apresentação clínica. Gatos de qualquer idade, raça ou sexo podem ser infectados, mas a infecção ocorre com mais frequência em animais jovens (< 1 ano), com *pedigree* em gatis lotados, centros de realocação ou famílias com vários felinos. A prevalência em gatos sintomáticos no Reino Unido foi estimada em 20% dos animais saudáveis, porém pode ser de até 31%. A infecção persistente é mais comum, e, embora os sinais possam se resolver espontaneamente, a infecção pode permanecer latente, fazendo os animais sofrerem recrudescência quando estressados. É, portanto, mais apropriado procurar o microrganismo em filhotes e em jovens com diarreia, em especial se houver um ambiente predisposto à infeção, bem como em gatos mais velhos com sinais de colite recorrente. Na verdade, a infecção de qualquer gato é possível e não deve ser considerada restrita apenas àqueles com *pedigree*. Além disso, os gatos que não respondem ao tratamento para uma infecção por *Giardia* devem ser testados em razão de um possível diagnóstico incorreto.

Oscilação na intensidade da diarreia de IG, com muco ou sangue fresco em fezes com odor fétido, é um sinal típico. Gatos infectados podem ter fezes semiformadas, exibindo incontinência fecal e um ânus edematoso e dolorido. Por outro lado, podem se apresentar saudáveis. Os sinais clínicos dependem da resposta imunológica do hospedeiro, da microbiota endógena, da patogenicidade da cepa do parasita e de coinfecções, como *Giardia*. Gatos infectados também devem ser testados para infecção por FeLV e FIV.

Diagnóstico. O microrganismo pode ser identificado por biopsia de cólon, mas é preferível fazer o diagnóstico da infecção de *T. fetus* por exame de fezes (ver Capítulo 81). Existem vários métodos disponíveis, porém nenhum é 100% sensível, e o uso de antibimicrobianos nos últimos 7 dias pode causar falso-negativos. A repetição do teste deve ser considerada quando houver um alto índice de suspeita e um resultado negativo. Resultados falso-negativos são mais prováveis se fezes formadas forem examinadas. A sensibilidade do teste pode ser melhorada quando se examinam apenas amostras diarreicas. As lavagens altas do cólon fornecem a melhor amostra, e as lavagens com solução salina são centrifugadas ou deixadas para sedimentar, sendo o sedimento submetido a exame.

Os métodos de diagnóstico incluem a identificação da mobilidade dos microrganismos em uma montagem úmida direta. Amostras muito frescas mantidas aquecidas devem ser usadas e examinadas em minutos. Mesmo assim, a sensibilidade é relatada apenas em 14% dos casos. A especificidade pode ser baixa se o microrganismo for diagnosticado incorretamente como *Giardia* spp. ou *Pentatrichomonas*. *Tritrichomonas fetus* têm uma motilidade progressiva característica, giratória e espasmódica, com uma membrana ondulante e três flagelos anteriores (ver Capítulo 207 e Vídeo 207.1), enquanto *Giardia* tem um movimento lento cambaleante.

O organismo pode ser cultivado usando um sistema de cultura comercial disponível (InPouch™ TF, Biomed Diagnostics), originalmente desenvolvido para o diagnóstico de infecção venérea bovina. Embora mais sensível do que o exame de esfregaço direto, o método é trabalhoso e o diagnóstico, potencialmente demorado, pois os resultados só podem ser considerados negativos quando não há crescimento após 12 dias.

A análise de PCR de fezes é relativamente rápida e é o método mais sensível de detecção de *T. fetus* – apenas 10 microrganismos por grama de fezes podem ser detectados. O PCR é baseado na região espaçadora transcrita interna conservada e o no gene rRNA 5,8S. De preferência, fezes frescas devem ser testadas. Mas, se houver uma demora entre a coleta e a chegada ao laboratório, elas podem ser mantidas refrigeradas por até 1 semana, conquanto isso diminua a sensibilidade. A PCR quantitativa permite a determinação do número de microrganismos presentes e pode ser usada para monitorar a resposta ao tratamento. Mais uma vez, a sensibilidade é melhorada por amostragem de diarreia ou lavagens do cólon, e as amostras não devem incluem resíduos da caixa de areia de gato, que podem conter inibidores da reação de PCR.

Tratamento. Apenas ronidazol (30 a 50 mg/kg PO a cada 12 h, por 2 semanas) demonstrou ser eficaz no tratamento de gatos com infecção por *T. fetus*. No entanto, efeitos colaterais neurológicos foram relatados, ainda que desapareçam após a interrupção da terapia, e os sinais clínicos podem se resolver sem tratamento em até 9 meses depois do início da diarreia. Recaídas são comuns e podem ser provocadas por mudança de dieta, tratamento médico, viagens e estresse. A doença tem um razoável prognóstico a longo prazo para resolução espontânea.

Helmintos

Heterobilharzia americana[452-460]

A esquistossomose em cães é causada por *Heterobilharzia americana*, um parasita hepático que produz diarreia aguda ou crônica do ID. Guaxinins são os hospedeiros reservatórios mais importantes, mas outros incluem camundongos, nutria ("ratão do banhado") e coelhos. A infecção canina é restrita ao sudeste e a áreas da Costa do Golfo dos EUA. O ciclo de vida de *H. americana* envolve pelo menos um hospedeiro intermediário, em geral caracóis. As cercárias provenientes do caracol penetram na pele do

CAPÍTULO 277 • Doenças do Intestino Grosso

cão e migram pelo pulmão e pelo fígado. Os parasitas amadurecem no fígado e põem ovos nas vênulas mesentéricas terminais. Os ovos, então, migram pela parede intestinal, liberando enzimas proteolíticas, e causam inflamação granulomatosa grave no local de penetração. Alguns ovos não chegam ao lúmen intestinal e podem se disseminar para fígado, pâncreas e pulmões, onde causam mais lesões granulomatosas que podem resultar em insuficiência hepática.

Os sinais clínicos incluem vômitos, diarreia do ID e hematoquezia. A bioquímica sérica pode revelar diminuição albumina e concentrações aumentadas de globulina. Um aumento das enzimas hepáticas quase sempre é observado. Além disso, os granulomas podem causar hipercalcemia. O diagnóstico é confirmado pela identificação dos ovos em esfregaços fecais diretos ou flotação salina, ou por biopsia de fígado ou intestinos. Um ELISA está disponível para infecções ocultas. Um protocolo de combinação de fenbendazol com praziquantel é uma terapia eficaz. O prognóstico é bom em casos agudos, mas de médio para ruim na doença prolongada que envolve o fígado, onde a cirrose está frequentemente presente.

Strongyloides tumefaciens[461,462]

Os *Strongyloides* spp. são parasitas incomuns em cães[c] e normalmente infectam o ID. *S. tumefaciens*, um verme filiforme, é uma infecção rara observada sobretudo na costa do Golfo dos EUA e em áreas tropicais. As larvas infecciosas penetram pela pele ou na mucosa oral/esofágica, alcançando os pulmões. Elas se dividem entre os alvéolos e são tossidas e engolidas. Os parasitas adultos são exclusivamente fêmeas partogenéticas que penetram e persistem na submucosa do cólon, em cavidades revestidas com epitélio com um poro luminal, causando nódulos visíveis por endoscopia e que podem coalescer para formar massas adenomatosas. Ovos embrionados ou larvas estão presentes nas fezes. Gatos infectados podem ser assintomáticos, contudo o parasita pode causar uma diarreia intratável em animais jovens. O tratamento com fembendazol (50 mg/kg PO a cada 24 h, por 5 dias) é eficaz, e o prognóstico é bom.

Trichuris spp.[463-470]

Infecção por tricurídeos é bastante comum em cães em regiões temperadas e subtropicais do mundo, podendo causar sinais agudos ou crônicos de diarreia de ID. Os cães infectados podem ser assintomáticos o ter fezes mucoides, hematoquezia e tenesmo. *T. vulpis* é um parasita comum em cães e outros canídeos, mas muito raro em gatos. *T. campanula* e *T. serrata*, esporadicamente, infectam gatos na Austrália, nas Índias Ocidentais e na Ásia. *T. vulpis* tem um ciclo de vida direto, sendo transmitido pela rota orofecal e tendo os ovos eclodindo no ID do hospedeiro, onde as larvas permanecem por 2 a 10 dias após penetrarem na mucosa. As larvas, então, emergem e migram para o cólon, onde se aderem à mucosa. Seus locais de predileção são o ceco e o cólon proximal, onde sua fina porção anterior penetra na mucosa, causando uma reação granulomatosa localizada, podendo até provocar uma inversão cecal. O período pré-patente é de 70 a 110 dias, e os vermes adultos vivem até 18 meses.

Os sinais clínicos dependem da natureza da resposta do sistema imune do hospedeiro, do seu nutricional, do seu ambiente e da presença de outros parasitas GI. Os sinais e o grau do sangramento aumentam com a gravidade da carga parasitária e podem incluir dor abdominal, vômito, inapetência e perda de peso, além dos sinais mais comuns de diarreia e hematoquezia. No perfil bioquímico, alguns cães podem mostrar evidências de hiperpotassemia e hiponatremia, simulando hipoadrenocorticismo, mas eles têm uma resposta normal à estimulação de ACTH. Eosinofilia e anemia podem

---

[c]N.T.: No Brasil, outras espécies, como *S. stercolaris*, parecem ser frequentes em cães.

estar presentes. O diagnóstico é feito pela identificação na flotação fecal dos ovos de paredes grossas, em forma de barril com dois tampões polares (ver Capítulo 81). No entanto, falso-negativos podem ocorrer quando os ovos são eliminados intermitentemente e o tratamento é empírico, apesar de um exame fecal negativo ser recomendado em áreas endêmicas antes da colonoscopia, a fim de investigar colite, a despeito de a extremidade posterior livre do verme ser vista na colonoscopia. Os parasiticidas mais usados e eficazes contra *T. vulpis* incluem fembendazol, pamoato de pirantel, febantel, moxidectina e milbemicina oxima (ver Capítulo 163). Graças a um longo período pré-patente (70 a 107 dias), o tratamento deve ser repetido em 3 semanas e, depois, em 3 meses. A reinfecção é provável em cães que vivem em ambientes contaminados, pois os ovos são bastante resistentes. A profilaxia da dirofilariose com milbemicina oxima pode ajudar a controlar a infecção.

HEMATOQUEZIA

Sangue fresco nas fezes é indicativo de sangramento do ID. Hematoquezia em associação com diarreia mucoide, urgência e tenesmo são mais sugestivos de colite (ver anteriormente), mas sangue sem diarreia e/ou com disquezia é mais indicativo de uma lesão focal com sangramento, assumindo que um problema de sangramento generalizado tenha sido descartado. A abordagem diagnóstica para hematoquezia é apresentada na Figura 277.5 B.

Neoplasia de intestino grosso[471]

Tumores do IG estão associados a sinais de ulceração da mucosa e/ou de obstrução, como hematoquezia, tenesmo e disquezia. Eles são mais comuns do que os do estômago e ID em cães, e a idade média dos cães afetados é de 7 a 11 anos, enquanto a dos com neoplasia IG é de 12,5 anos. A maioria dos tumores do cólon canino é maligno, com adenocarcinoma seguido por linfoma sendo os mais comuns. A maioria dos adenocarcinomas de IG se desenvolve no cólon descendente e no reto, sendo frequentes em cães das raças Pastor-Alemão, Collie e West Highland White Terrier. Leiomiossarcomas do IG são encontrados com mais frequência no ceco. Neoplasias benignas, como adenomas e leiomiomas, são muito menos comuns no IG do que tumores malignos em caninos, embora pólipos adenomatosos sejam relativamente comuns. No IG felino, o adenocarcinoma é mais comum (46%) do que o linfoma (41%), enquanto os tumores de mastócitos (9%) também são observados (ver Capítulo 349).

Adenocarcinoma colorretal[472-481]

Os adenocarcinomas intestinais caninos são mais encontrados na região distal do cólon e no reto, podendo causar obstrução mecânica, que leva à disquezia e à prisão de ventre, com esforço de defecação improdutivo. Tutores observadores podem reconhecer que seus cães estão eliminando fezes progressivamente deformadas que são espremidas pelo tumor à medida que o lúmen se estreita. A ulceração da superfície do tumor leva à hematoquezia, mesmo se a consistência fecal estiver normal, e sangue pode ser visto em listras na superfície das fezes. A diarreia é menos característica, a menos que a obstrução e a invasão do tumor causem inflamação, secreção de fluidos ou má absorção de água e sais. A invasão local do tumor ocorre em uma taxa relativamente lenta, com o adenocarcinoma colorretal canino e metástases para locais distantes sendo incomuns. A desvitalização e a necrose do tumor podem levar ao aparecimento espontâneo de perfuração e peritonite séptica. Cães podem se apresentar moribundos, com febre, letargia, anorexia, vômito, dor abdominal e colapso.

Os locais mais comuns de adenocarcinoma em gatos são o cólon descendente (39%) e a região ileocólica (28%), ainda que os adenocarcinomas exclusivamente ileais sejam mais comuns, com predisposição em gatos idosos da raça Siamês. Hematoquezia, em vez de obstrução e constipação intestinal, é o sinal mais provável em gatos, pois o tumor tende a ser proximal. Ao contrário dos cães, os tumores do cólon felino têm uma alta taxa (> 60%) de metástase, que está associada à diminuição do tempo de sobrevida.

Diagnóstico. Adenocarcinomas colorretais caninos são palpáveis em cerca de 70% dos casos. A estenose do lúmen retal encontrado no exame digital retal é sugestiva de neoplasia, já que estenoses benignas são muito raras. Lesões no cólon proximal e no ceco não são tão facilmente aparentes, conquanto mais de 50% de gatos com massas colônicas tenham uma massa palpável no abdome. Estudos radiográficos de contraste e ultrassonográficos têm sido usados com vários níveis de sucesso no diagnóstico de neoplasia colônica canina e felina. Lesões estenóticas anulares associadas a adenocarcinoma do cólon podem aparecer como dilatação do cólon proximal em radiografias. O material de contraste radiográfico delineia com mais precisão o estreitamento do lúmen no local do tumor, mas análise com contraste foi amplamente substituída pela ultrassonografia, que é útil na avaliação de lesões murais e linfadenopatia. A ultrassonografia foi relatada como efetiva na localização de cerca de 84% das neoplasias do cólon em felinos. TC não foi suficientemente avaliada para que uma comparação razoável seja feita com a ultrassonografia, porém é provável que seja mais sensível à medida que o gás luminal não interfere.

A colonoscopia flexível com biopsia da mucosa é o método preferido para o diagnóstico definitivo de adenocarcinoma do cólon (Figura 277.14, Vídeo 277.2; ver Capítulo 113). Anormalidades endoscópicas podem incluir massas, sangramento espontâneo, aumento da friabilidade, ulceração e estreitamento da circunferência luminal. Várias amostras de biopsia devem sempre ser obtidas de tecido doente, tecido saudável adjacente e da zona de transição entre essas áreas. O patologista tem uma chance muito melhor de diagnosticar e estadiar a doença por avaliar tecido não necrótico.

Tratamento. A modalidade de tratamento mais adequada depende da localização anatômica e da presença e da extensão das metástases. A excisão cirúrgica completa é o tratamento recomendado para adenocarcinomas focais, mas acesso a massas intrapélvicas pode exigir a abertura da pelve e um abaixamento endorretal, procedimento estética e funcionalmente insatisfatório. Cães com adenocarcinomas colorretais costumam ter um prognóstico ruim, com um tempo mediano de sobrevivência (TMS) de apenas 1,6 mês, ainda que em um estudo cães com ressecção da massa tumoral tenha sobrevivido, em média, 7 meses mais do que aqueles que fizeram apenas uma biopsia. A radioterapia tem sido usada de forma inconsistente como paliativo de adenocarcinomas recorrentes, mas peritonite pós-radiação e perfuração foram relatadas. A regulação positiva da ciclo-oxigenase 2 (COX-2) pode contribuir para as características de crescimento de alguns tumores. Desse modo, inibidores seletivos de COX-2, como piroxicam ou meloxicam, podem ser úteis, embora, em última análise, a eutanásia é indicada.

O adenocarcinoma do cólon felino é um tumor invasivo, altamente metastático, tratado com uma ampla cirurgia de excisão (colectomia subtotal) e quimioterapia sistêmica, com ou sem medicamentos anti-inflamatórios não esteroidais. Em um estudo retrospectivo, os resultados da colectomia subtotal e da carboplatina adjuvante em 18 gatos foram avaliados – o intervalo médio livre de doença foi de 251 dias (variação, 37 a 528 dias), e o TMS, de 269 (variação, 40 a 533 dias). Fatores prognósticos negativos incluíram metástases nodais e a distância – 178 contra 328 dias, e 200 contra 340 dias, respectivamente. Assim, a colectomia subtotal associada à carboplatina adjuvante é um tratamento seguro e potencialmente eficaz para gatos com adenocarcinoma do cólon, com um tempo de sobrevivência mais longo do que aqueles submetidos à ressecção tumoral apenas (TMS de 138 dias contra 68 dias).

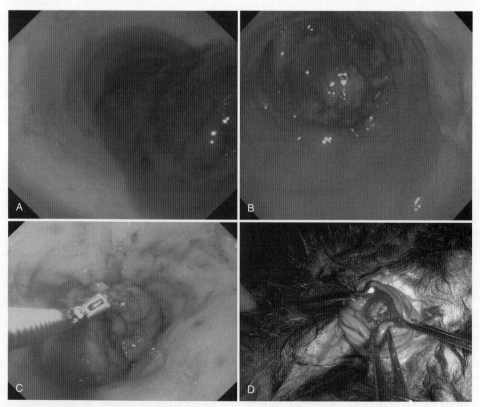

Figura 277.14 Adenocarcinoma colorretal. **A.** Grande coágulo de sangue encontrado na colonoscopia, cobrindo a massa vista em **B**. **B.** Vista colonoscópica de uma massa no cólon de um cão da raça Border Collie de 12 anos, após a remoção do coágulo sanguíneo. **C.** Biopsia endoscópica de um adenocarcinoma do cólon em um cão da raça West Highland White Terrier de 10 anos que apresentava episódios de constipação intestinal. **D.** Adenocarcinoma no reto de um gato de 12 anos visualizado por eversão progressiva gradual do reto usando uma pinça de tecido. (*Esta figura se encontra reproduzida em cores no Encarte.*)

Pólipo colorretal adenomatoso[157,162,177,178,482-494]

Pólipos benignos às vezes ocorrem no cólon terminal e reto de cães adultos e são reconhecidos pela passagem de sangue fresco e coágulos na superfície das fezes. Às vezes são confundidos com colite, e sua característica principal é não haver diarreia. Ocorre com frequência em cães da raça Dachshund Miniatura. E, na experiência do autor, as raças Cocker Spaniel e Pastor de Shetland também são predispostas. Uma polipose adenomatosa de ocorrência familiar é reconhecida em humanos. A transformação maligna de pólipos adenomatosos em carcinoma *in situ* e adenocarcinoma invasivo é uma ameaça real em humanos e foi demonstrada em cães, se bem que, na maioria dos casos, o pólipo permaneça benigno. O diagnóstico, em geral, pode ser feito à palpação retal, onde uma massa tumoral móvel com um pedúnculo pode ser sentida. No entanto, o tecido pode ser tão macio que é difícil reconhecer a massa tumoral em um cão consciente, mesmo com sangramento abundante. O exame retal deve, portanto, ser repetido assim que o animal estiver preparado e anestesiado para colonoscopia. Pode ser possível exteriorizar o pólipo pelo esfíncter anal se ele estiver no reto terminal, ou visualizá-lo com um espéculo anal ou proctoscópio. Além disso, ele pode passar despercebido por endoscopia flexível, pois a ponta do endoscópio pode ser inserida além da lesão antes de a visualização ser possível (Figura 277.15, Vídeo 277.3).

Às vezes, a manipulação retal digital dos pólipos resulta na sua remoção acidental, porém permanecendo o pedúnculo, o que faz o pólipo crescer novamente e a hematoquezia recomeçar. Da mesma forma, a remoção acima do ponto de fixação do pedúnculo pode permitir a recorrência. A eversão suave da mucosa retal com uma pinça Allis e a ressecção submucosa da base do pedúnculo do pólipo é curativa. Para pólipos no cólon distal e no reto proximal, a remoção por meio de um laço de polipectomia com um ressectoscópio foi relatada. De maneira alternativa, a ressecção via laparotomia é possível para pólipos do cólon. Pólipos múltiplos foram tratados com polipectomia e coagulação com plasma de argônio.

A histologia pode indicar um pólipo benigno ou inflamatório, um adenoma ou mesmo um carcinoma *in situ*. A pseudopolipose é uma condição muito rara em que vários nódulos são encontrados no cólon (Figura 277.15 D). Eles não são pólipos verdadeiros porque não têm pedúnculo. São tratados com glicocorticoides.

Linfoma alimentar[481,495-501]

O linfoma alimentar quase sempre é uma doença difusa que afeta o ID, com ou sem envolvimento do IG, e pode produzir uma variedade de sinais, incluindo anorexia, vômito, diarreia, melena, hematoquezia e perda de peso. Está emergindo como a forma mais comum de linfoma em gatos. Em cães, é potencialmente uma causa de enteropatia de perda de proteínas se envolver o ID, mas é rara em comparação com a doença multicêntrica. O linfoma retal em cães é um subgrupo da condição, em que a doença é restrita anatomicamente e responde bem à quimioterapia combinada. Todas as outras formas de linfoma alimentar canino respondem muito mal à quimioterapia ou a lise do tumor leva à perfuração intestinal e à peritonite séptica. A remissão é muito rara.

Aspiração por agulha fina transabdominal (ver Capítulo 89), citologia de fluidos peritoneais e citologia endoscópica esfoliativa podem ser úteis no diagnóstico do linfoma, mas a histologia pode ser necessária para um diagnóstico definitivo.

Os sinais clínicos comuns em gatos com linfoma alimentar são vômito (65%), diarreia (52%), perda de peso (46%) e massas palpáveis. A maioria dos gatos afetados é FeLV-negativo, e a maioria dos linfomas colônicos em gatos tem origem em células B. A quimioterapia combinada (prednisona, vincristina, ciclofosfamida) tem sido usado para tratar o linfoma do cólon.

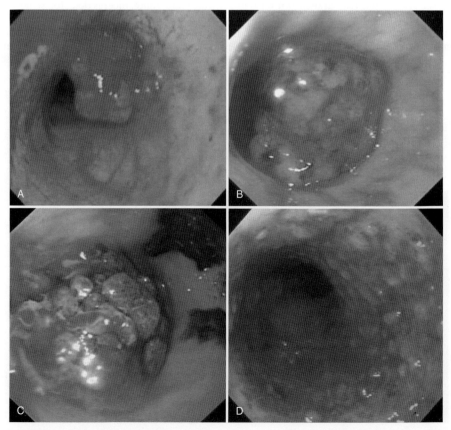

Figura 277.15 Visualizações endoscópicas de pólipos colorretais. **A.** Pólipo adenomatoso retal hemorrágico em um cão da raça Cocker Spaniel. **B.** Pólipo adenomatoso retal grande em um cão Pastor de Shetland, conforme visto no Vídeo 277.3. **C.** Pólipo adenomatoso do cólon em um cão. **D.** Pseudopolipose em um cão da raça Jack Russell Terrier. (*Esta figura se encontra reproduzida em cores no Encarte.*)

Outros tumores[483,502-520]

O leiomiossarcoma ocorre com mais frequência no ceco canino. Tumores do estroma GI (GIST), que surgem das células intersticiais de Cajal, são muito semelhantes clinicamente e antes não podiam ser diferenciados. De fato, 42% dos 50 tumores relatados como leiomiossarcoma foram caracterizados como GISTs por imuno-histoquímica, pela detecção da expressão de desmina, actina de músculo liso e marcadores c-kit (ver Capítulo 276). Tumores de músculo liso têm sido associados à hipoglicemia, fraqueza e atividade convulsiva, em razão da liberação de uma substância semelhante à insulina e da eritrocitose causada pela liberação de eritropoetina. O prognóstico para leiomiomas, em geral, é favorável.

Plasmacitoma extramedular é um tumor raro do trato GI, mas pode ocorrer no cólon e no reto. O plasmocitoma funcional secreta uma única classe de imunoglobulina, e os animais afetados podem desenvolver a síndrome de hiperviscosidade, como sangramento retinal e epistaxe. Os plasmocitomas podem ser tratados com quimioterapia adjuvante, como prednisona ou melfalana, após a excisão cirúrgica.

Uma variedade de outros tumores mesenquimais pode ocorrer no IG, como neurofibrossarcoma, fibrossarcoma, ganglioneuroma e hemangiossarcoma, sendo o último mais comum no trato gastrintestinal de gatos do que de cães.

Intussuscepção cecocólica (inversão cecal)[521-524]

A invaginação do ceco para o cólon é anormal e, inicialmente, pode ocorrer de forma intermitente. No entanto, em última análise, ficará preso pelo esfíncter no orifício ceco-cólico. O comprometimento da drenagem venosa leva a descamação da mucosa e sangramento intraluminal. A diarreia não é um achado consistente, mas sangue fresco e coágulos podem ser vistos parcialmente misturados com as fezes. Os cães podem mostrar sinais de desconforto abdominal e a intussuscepção pode ser palpável. A lesão pode ser visível com radiografia, com ou sem contraste de bário ou com ultrassonografia, porém um diagnóstico definitivo é feito por colonoscopia (Figura 277.16 A) quando uma protuberância com sangramento é vista adjacente à papila ileocólica.

Essa condição incomum é relatada exclusivamente em cães e considerada rara em gatos porque eles têm o ceco muito mais curto e menos móvel. A infecção por *Trichuris* é associada a predispor os cães a tal condição, todavia pode ser vista em cães após diarreia causada por outros fatores. O tratamento é feito pela tiflectomia (Figura 277.16 B).

Ectasia vascular colônica (angiodisplasia)[525-529]

Existem alguns relatos de casos de angiodisplasia no cólon ou no reto de cães jovens. A(s) lesão(ões) da ectasia vascular frequentemente sangram muito, levando à hematoquezia marcada, com os pacientes às vezes necessitando de transfusões. O diagnóstico é feito por colonoscopia quando áreas de coalescência e vasos sanguíneos tortuosos da mucosa são observados. Pode ser tratada com sucesso pela excisão cirúrgica da região afetada, entretanto pode ser um desafio detectar a lesão na cirurgia da superfície serosa, além de várias cirurgias poderem não ter sucesso. A ablação a *laser* e a eletrocoagulação também podem ser tentadas. Contudo, em alguns casos, a condição pode afetar grande parte do cólon, e, em vez de realizar colectomia subtotal, há relatos de manejo bem-sucedido com estrogênios.

Miopatia visceral e impactação cecal[530]

Um caso de impactação cecal associado à miopatia visceral e à pseudo-obstrução intestinal foi relatado (ver Capítulo 276).

Perfuração colônica[170,472,531-534]

Perfurações colorretais são raras, mas podem ser causadas por trauma (p. ex., fraturas pélvicas ou biopsia colônica muito vigorosa) e irradiação, ou por inserção de um termômetro ou outros objetos estranhos. Também podem ocorrer após ulceração neurogênica do cólon.

Ulceração neurogênica do cólon[535-537]

Muito raramente, úlceras do cólon se desenvolvem em pacientes com doenças agudas do disco intervertebral ou após cirurgia da coluna vertebral. Elas tendem a ocorrer no cólon proximal, em especial na flexura colônica esquerda. O mecanismo é malcompreendido e complicado, pois muitos desses pacientes também

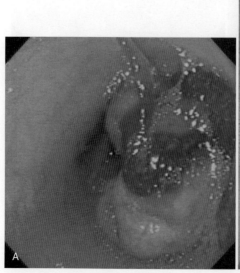
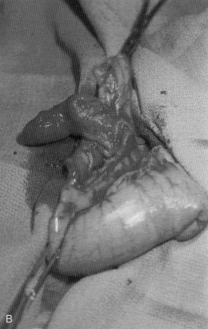

Figura 277.16 Inversão cecal (intussuscepção cecocólica) em cão jovem da raça Weimaraner. **A.** Visão endoscópica de um ceco ulcerado evertido no cólon proximal. **B.** Após a incisão no cólon proximal, o ceco evertido hemorrágico está exposto e pode ser removido por tiflectomia. (Cortesia de Alasdair Hotston-Moore.) (*Esta figura se encontra reproduzida em cores no Encarte.*)

são tratados com glicocorticoides. Isquemia localizada e aumento da pressão intraluminal de origem neurogênica parecem estar envolvidos, com os glicocorticoides reduzindo a produção de mucina e prejudicando a cura. A princípio, a ulceração do cólon causará hematoquezia, mas pode levar à perfuração e à peritonite séptica. O prognóstico é ruim.

DOENÇAS QUE CAUSAM OBSTRUÇÃO

Neoplasia no IG é a causa mais comum de obstrução do IG (ver anteriormente). Outros processos intramurais não neoplásicos, como intussuscepção, hematoma e estenose de fibrose podem causar obstrução. Granuloma PIF e ficomicose (ver anteriormente) devem ser incluídos na lista de diagnóstico diferencial. Corpos estranhos lineares e não lineares, além de compressão por uma próstata aumentada, também podem causar obstrução intraluminal e extraluminal, respectivamente.

Intussuscepção[165,168,258,538-558]

Uma intussuscepção é uma invaginação de um segmento do trato gastrintestinal (*intussusceptum*) no lúmen do segmento adjacente (*intussuscipiens*). A intussuscepção enterocólica representa a maioria dos casos relatados e pode ser dividida em três tipos: cecocólica (ou inversão cecal; ver acima), ileocólica e, mais raramente, ileocecal. Dessas três formas, a segunda é a mais encontrada na prática e aquela que mais causa obstrução. Fatores predisponentes incluem parasitismo intestinal, enterite viral, corpos estranhos e massas, podendo ser seguido por um episódio de diarreia aguda. No entanto, muitas intussuscepções ileocólicas são vistas em animais jovens e parecem idiopáticas, com a sugestão de que são subjacentes à uma incoordenação muscular intestinal, pois o sistema nervoso entérico não está totalmente desenvolvido. Intussuscepções em animais mais velhos quase sempre se desenvolvem em torno de uma lesão, como um tumor ou causas de peritonite focal (p. ex., perfuração ou deiscência de ferida).

Fisiopatologia

A invaginação seguida de intussuscepção do íleo para o cólon resulta em obstrução luminal e distensão do segmento intestinal proximal à intussuscepção. Uma vez que o mesentério e o suprimento de sangue estão incluídos no segmento invaginante, um comprometimento vascular pode ocorrer, o que inicialmente leva a edema, hemorragia intramural e, às vezes, isquemia e necrose do intestino.

Exame clínico

Os sinais clínicos de intussuscepção ileocólica são vômito intermitentes, perda progressiva de apetite, diarreia sanguinolenta mucoide e uma massa cilíndrica palpável no abdome cranial. Dor abdominal não é um achado consistente. A maioria dos casos é aguda, mas a intussuscepção crônica é possível, e os animais afetados podem eventualmente sucumbir aos efeitos da anorexia ou perda de sangue, em vez da desidratação (Figura 227.17 A e B).

Diagnóstico

Com algumas intussuscepções ileocólicas, o *intussusceptum* pode eventualmente se projetar pelo ânus e deve ser diferenciado de um prolapso retal. Uma sonda romba passada entre o segmento protuberante e o esfíncter anal é indicativa: se ela pode ser passada cranial ao púbis sem atingir o fórnice, o intestino protuberante é a ponta de uma intussuscepção. Achados radiográficos abdominais podem ser suspeitos de uma intussuscepção, mas a ultrassonografia abdominal é o método preferido de diagnóstico. O aparecimento de uma massa semelhante a um alvo consistindo em dois ou mais anéis concêntricos hiperecoicos e hipoecoicos em seção transversal, ou

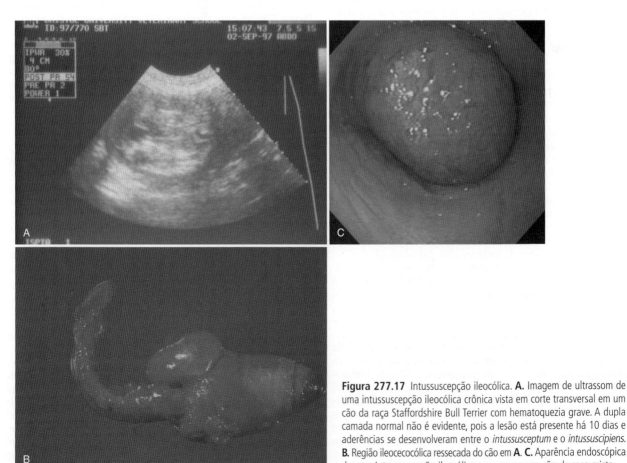

Figura 277.17 Intussuscepção ileocólica. **A.** Imagem de ultrassom de uma intussuscepção ileocólica crônica vista em corte transversal em um cão da raça Staffordshire Bull Terrier com hematoquezia grave. A dupla camada normal não é evidente, pois a lesão está presente há 10 dias e aderências se desenvolveram entre o *intussusceptum* e o *intussuscipiens*. **B.** Região ileocecocólica ressecada do cão em **A**. **C.** Aparência endoscópica de uma intussuscepção ileocólica precoce em um cão de raça mista.

múltiplas linhas paralelas hiperecoicas e hipoecoicas em seção longitudinal, é virtualmente patognomônico. A colonoscopia raramente é indicada, mas, se realizada, o *intussusceptum* pode ser visualizado (Figura 277.17 C).

Tratamento e prognóstico

O manejo cirúrgico da intussuscepção ileocólica envolve redução ou ressecção e anastomose. Se possível, a região ileocecocólica é preservada para reduzir o refluxo e a contaminação fecal do íleo. A síndrome do intestino curto ocorrerá se grandes extensões do ID tiverem de ser ressecadas (ver Capítulo 276). As complicações mais comuns após a cirurgia são recorrência, deiscência, peritonite, íleo paralítico e obstrução intestinal. A taxa de recorrência em cães é relatada como entre 11 e 20%, sendo mais provável se houver vazamento no local da anastomose que cause uma peritonite. Tentativas históricas de prevenir a recorrência pela administração de hioscina para induzir íleo paralítico podem apresentar um risco aumentado e um retorno precoce à nutrição enteral, e espera-se que a motilidade normal seja recomendada. Se houver recorrência, a enteroplicatura cirúrgica de alças intestinais pode ser realizada.

Estenose[176,472,477,559-562]

Uma estenose benigna do IG é rara em cães e gatos, e uma suspeita de neoplasia subjacente deve sempre ser considerada, a menos que haja uma história de cirurgia de IG anterior ou impactação de corpo estranho que poderia ter causado hematoma ou ulceração com subsequente fibrose. Estenoses inflamatórias foram relatadas em gatos. Lesões não acidentais também devem ser consideradas uma causa potencial. Uma constipação intestinal proximal à estenose ocorrerá, e o tratamento se dá por dilatação com balão ou implante de *stent* (ou estente).

Corpo estranho

Se um corpo estranho intestinal causar uma obstrução, é mais provável ocorrer no ID. Apenas ocasionalmente corpos estranhos obstruem o cólon, pois primeiro têm de passar pelo estreito ID e pelo esfíncter ileocólico.

SÍNDROME DO INTESTINO IRRITÁVEL[1,563-568]

Em humanos, a síndrome do intestino irritável (SII) é um distúrbio multifatorial funcional do trato GI caracterizado por aumento e diminuição da dor abdominal em associação com diarreia e/ou prisão de ventre. Problemas psicológicos subjacentes podem ser predisponentes, e os pacientes podem ter maior consciência da motilidade gastrintestinal, mas a SII também pode ocorrer após uma gastrenterite bacteriana aguda, quando o sistema nervoso entérico permanece interrompido por muitos meses. A condição pode ser gerenciada com analgésicos centrais, como antidepressivos tricíclicos ou inibidores seletivos da recaptação da serotonina, além de intervenções psicológicas.

Uma síndrome diarreica idiopática de IG foi caracterizada em cães e comparada com a SII humana. Porém, embora a diarreia mucoide e o tenesmo predominem sobre a constipação intestinal, pode ocorrer hematoquezia. No entanto, existem definições estritas (critérios de Roma III) para o diagnóstico de SII em humanos, e hematoquezia não deve estar presente. Assim, não está claro que os cães realmente sofram de SII. Ainda assim, todas as investigações em cães com essa síndrome são negativas para bactérias e outros patógenos, evidência histológica de colite e neoplasia do cólon, de modo que o termo "diarreia crônica idiopática do intestino grosso" tem sido usado, em vez de SII. Os cães afetados podem responder à alimentação com uma dieta altamente digestível, suplementada com fibra solúvel. Ansiolíticos, como Librax (clordiazepóxido com brometo de clidínio, um antimuscarínico), e antiespasmódicos, como hioscina, mebeverina, óleo de hortelã-pimenta, também

são relatados como tendo alguma eficácia, a despeito de haver uma suspeita de forte efeito placebo no tutor. Isso reduz o estresse no cão, que pode realmente ser a causa ou pelo menos exacerbar o problema.

CONSTIPAÇÃO INTESTINAL

A constipação intestinal e a obstipação são manifestações do mesmo problema, mas de gravidade diferente. A primeira é definida como evacuação infrequente ou difícil de fezes, mas não necessariamente implica uma perda permanente de função. Os pacientes podem sofrer de um ou dois episódios de constipação intestinal sem progressão posterior. Uma constipação intestinal intratável que se tornou refratária a cura ou controle é referida como obstipação e, portanto, implica uma perda permanente de função. Um paciente é presumido como obstipado somente após várias falhas de tratamentos consecutivos. O megacólon dilatado é o estágio final da disfunção do cólon, qualquer que seja a causa (ver Capítulo 42).

Animais constipados costumam apresentar disquezia – tentativas repetidas e malsucedidas de defecar ou dor ao defecar –, e às vezes o material fecal líquido pode vazar. Com obstipação e megacólon, o paciente pode desistir de tentar defecar, mas eventualmente fica indisposto com vômitos, anorexia e desidratação. O megacólon se desenvolve por meio dois mecanismos patológicos: dilatação e hipertrofia. O megacólon hipertrófico se desenvolve como consequência de lesões obstrutivas, como consolidação viciosa de fraturas pélvicas, tumores e corpos estranhos. Megacólon hipertrófico causado por constrição pélvica pode ser reversível com osteotomia pélvica precoce ou progredir para megacólon dilatado irreversível, se a terapia apropriada não for instituída. O megacólon dilatado pode ocorrer de modo secundário a anormalidades eletrolíticas, distúrbios neuromusculares, ou ser idiopático.

Vários fatores podem predispor à constipação intestinal (ver Figura 276.5 C; ver Capítulo 42), sendo os gatos hospitalizados particularmente de risco em razão da falta de atividade, da falta de vontade de defecar enquanto estão internados, da tendência a desenvolver desidratação, da hipopotassemia quando indispostos e da administração de opioides analgésicos. Causas específicas, como fratura pélvica e lesões neurológicas por tração da cauda equina, também são mais comuns em gatos. Prostatomegalia em cães machos intactos e hérnia perineal em cadelas são motivos mais comuns de constipação intestinal em cães, que também têm predisposição para comer ossos.

Uma revisão de casos publicados sugere que 96% dos casos de obstipação em gatos são contabilizados como megacólon idiopático (62%), estenose do canal pélvico (23%), lesão neural (6%) ou deformidade da medula espinal sacral em gatos da raça Manês (5%). Um menor número de casos foi relacionado com complicações da colopexia (1%) e neoplasia do cólon (1%). Hipoganglionose colônica ou aganglionose foi suspeitada, mas não comprovada, em outros 2% dos casos. Fatores endócrinos, como obesidade e hipotireoidismo, foram citados em vários casos, mas não necessariamente implicados como parte da patogênese do megacólon. Assim, a maioria dos casos é de origem idiopática, ortopédica ou neurológica.

Diagnóstico

A constipação intestinal e a obstipação costumam ser prontamente identificadas por palpação abdominal.

Um exame neurológico completo deve ser realizado com ênfase especial na função da medula espinal caudal, para identificar lesão da medula espinal, trauma do nervo pélvico e deformidade sacral da medula espinal em gatos da raça Manês (ver Capítulo 259). Gatos com prisão de ventre causada por disautonomia podem ter outros sinais de falha autonômica do sistema nervoso, como retenção urinária, regurgitação causada pelo megaesôfago, midríase, diminuição do lacrimejamento, prolapso da membrana nictitante e bradicardia.

O exame retal digital deve ser realizado com cuidado, sempre sob sedação ou anestesia em gatos. Uma má consolidação de fratura pélvica pode ser detectada ou identificar corpos, divertículos retais, estenoses, inflamação ou neoplasia.

Embora seja improvável que os pacientes apresentem alterações significativas em dados laboratoriais, um hemograma completo e um perfil de bioquímica sérica devem ser feitos em todos os pacientes com obstipação e megacólon em que uma causa física não possa ser encontrada. Causas da constipação intestinal metabólica, como desidratação, hipopotassemia e hipercalcemia, podem ser detectadas. A concentração basal de tiroxina sérica e outros testes de função da tireoide também devem ser considerados em animais com constipação intestinal recorrente e outros sinais consistentes com hipotireoidismo.

As radiografias devem ser feitas para caracterizar a gravidade da impactação do cólon e identificar fatores predisponentes, como material estranho radiopaco intraluminal – por exemplo, lascas de osso –, massas intraluminais ou extraluminais, fraturas pélvicas e anormalidades da coluna vertebral (Figura 277.18). Massas extraluminais podem ser avaliadas posteriormente por ultrassonografia e biopsia guiada, enquanto massas intraluminais são mais bem avaliadas por endoscopia após limpeza do material fecal (ver Capítulo 114).

Tratamento[45,171,175,569-577]

O plano terapêutico específico dependerá da gravidade da constipação intestinal e da causa subjacente. Os primeiros episódios de constipação intestinal costumam ser transitórios e se resolver sem terapia. Gatos hospitalizados devem ser mantidos hidratados e alimentados com dieta contendo fibras fermentáveis. Episódios leves a moderados ou recorrentes de constipação intestinal podem ser tratados, muitas vezes em regime ambulatorial, com modificação da dieta, enemas de água quente, orais ou supositórios laxantes, agentes procinéticos do cólon ou uma combinação dessas terapias (ver Capítulo 114). Casos graves geralmente requerem breves períodos de hospitalização para corrigir a desidratação e anormalidades metabólicas, bem como para evacuar fezes impactadas usando enemas de água, extração manual de fezes retidas, ou ambos. A terapia de acompanhamento nesses gatos é dirigida a corrigir fatores predisponentes e prevenir a recorrência. A colectomia subtotal se tornará necessária em gatos sofrendo de obstipação ou megacólon dilatado idiopáticos.

Remoção de fezes impactadas

Isso pode ser realizado por meio de supositórios, laxantes orais, enemas retais ou extração manual.

Supositórios retais

Os supositórios retais podem conter dioctil sulfossuccinato de sódio (DSS), um laxante emoliente também chamado de docusato de sódio; glicerol (sin. glicerina), um lubrificante laxante; ou bisacodil, um laxante estimulante. Seu uso requer um animal de estimação e tutor complacentes e podem ser usados isoladamente ou em conjunto com a terapia laxante oral como tratamento de primeira linha, ou como forma de prevenir a recorrência.

Laxantes

Os laxantes promovem a evacuação do intestino por estimulação do transporte de fluido e eletrólitos e/ou por motilidade propulsiva. Muitos produtos estão disponíveis, a maioria de laxantes formadores de massa contendo suplementos de fibra na dieta derivados de grãos de cereais, farelo de trigo ou Psyllium. Dietas suplementadas com fibra estão disponíveis comercialmente, ou o tutor do animal pode adicionar Psyllium, farelo de trigo ou abóbora aos alimentos enlatados.

Laxantes emolientes. Os laxantes emolientes são detergentes aniônicos que aumentam a solubilidade de água e lipídios na digesta, aumentando a absorção de lipídios e diminuindo a de água. O docusato de sódio está disponível em apresentação oral e em forma de enema. O docusato de cálcio ou sulfossuccinato de potássio é uma alternativa em alguns países.

Laxantes lubrificantes. Os laxantes lubrificantes incluem o óleo mineral ("parafina líquida") ou vaselina e uma combinação mais palatável de parafina branca e cera de abelha (Katalax). As propriedades lubrificantes desses agentes impedem a absorção de água do cólon e facilitam a passagem fecal. Esses efeitos são geralmente moderados, e, em geral, os lubrificantes são apenas benéficos na constipação intestinal leve. O uso de óleo mineral deve ser limitado à administração retal por causa do risco de pneumonia por aspiração lipoide com administração oral, sobretudo em gatos deprimidos ou debilitados, pois ele é insípido e pode ser inalado, em vez de engolido. Produtos de parafina branca são mais facilmente administrados por tutores de gatos, pois só precisam ser espalhados no animal em um local onde ele possa se lamber.

Laxantes hiperosmóticos. Os laxantes hiperosmóticos consistem em depolissacarídeos mal-absorvíveis (lactose, lactulose, lactitol), sais de magnésio (citrato, hidróxido, sulfato) e limpadores orais do cólon, como fosfato de sódio hipertônico e PEGs (ver preparação para colonoscopia). Lactulose e PEGs são os agentes mais eficazes nesse grupo. Os ácidos orgânicos produzidos da fermentação da lactulose estimulam a secreção de fluidos no cólon e a motilidade propulsora. Lactulose administrada em uma dosagem oral de 0,5 mℓ/kg a cada 8 a 12 horas deve produzir fezes moles em gatos. Muitos felinos com recorrência ou constipação intestinal crônica foram bem tratados assim, mas os casos leves podem ser gerenciados apenas com a adição de leite na dieta.

Laxantes estimulantes. Laxantes estimulantes como bisacodil, dantrona, fenolftaleína, óleo de rícino, cascara e sene são um grupo diversificado de agentes que estimulam a motilidade propulsora do cólon. O bisacodil, por exemplo, estimula a secreção de células epiteliais mediada por óxido nítrico e a despolarização neuronal mioentérica. A diarreia resulta do efeito combinado do aumento da secreção da mucosa e da propulsão colônica. O bisacodil, na dosagem de 5 mg por via oral, a cada 24 horas, é o laxante estimulante mais eficaz em gatos. A lubiprostana é um dos mais novos laxantes desenvolvidos para humanos, que aumenta a secreção do cólon, estimulando os canais de cloreto. Seu uso em animais não foi relatado.

Enemas

Os enemas podem ser necessários para episódios moderados ou graves de constipação intestinal. Água morna de torneira (5 a 10 mℓ/kg) ou soluções de enema incluindo solução salina isotônica quente (5 a 10 mℓ/kg), DSS (5 a 10 mℓ/gato), óleo mineral (5 a 10 mℓ/gato) ou lactulose (5 a 10 mℓ/gato) podem

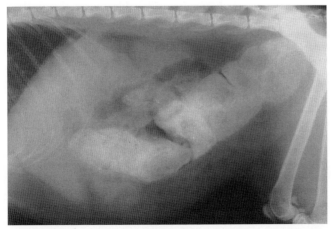

Figura 277.18 Radiografia abdominal lateral de gato com constipação intestinal grave causada por megacólon idiopático.

ser usadas. Todas elas devem ser administradas lentamente por meio de um cateter de borracha bem lubrificado ou uma sonda de alimentação de um balde de enema, ou usando uma bomba de Higginson, para que não seja aplicada pressão excessiva (ver Capítulo 114). Enemas contendo fosfato de sódio são contraindicados em gatos e cães pequenos por causa de sua propensão a induzir hipernatremia fatal, hiperfosfatemia e hipocalcemia.

Extração manual. A extração manual de fezes impactadas é necessária para casos que não respondem a laxantes ou enemas. Água morna ou solução salina é infundida no cólon, enquanto a massa é massageada suavemente por palpação abdominal. A extração digital das fezes do reto é, então, realizada. É frequentemente aconselhável evacuar toda a massa fecal durante um período de vários dias para reduzir os riscos de anestesia prolongada e de perfuração de uma parede colônica distendida e desvitalizada. Dispositivos do tipo "colher" para evacuar as fezes devem ser usados apenas com grande cautela.

Terapia preventiva[477,78]

Uma vez que as fezes impactadas tenham sido liberadas, é importante instituir medidas para prevenir a recorrência. Qualquer causa subjacente deve ser corrigida, se possível – por exemplo, osteotomia pélvica, dilatação de estenose ou colocação de stent (ver Capítulo 123) e castração para reduzir a prostatomegalia –, e quaisquer fatores predisponentes, como desidratação, falta de exercício, alimentação excessiva etc., devem ser evitados. Alimentação com uma dieta com adição de fibra e/ou leite é uma estratégia simples e muitas vezes eficaz, mas em alguns casos a intervenção farmacológica ainda é necessária.

Agentes procinéticos do cólon[71-73,567,579-595]

Estudos in vitro mostraram que a cisaprida estimula a contração da musculatura lisa do cólon felino. Embora isso ainda não tenha sido mostrado in vivo de modo conclusivo, um grande corpo de experiências observacionais sugere que a cisaprida seja eficaz na estimulação da motilidade propulsiva do cólon em constipação intestinal felina idiopática leve a moderada. Casos de obstipação e megacólon de longa data provavelmente não responderão. Porém, esse medicamento foi proibido em muitos países a partir do ano 2000, após relatos de efeitos colaterais cardíacos (QT prolongado) e morte súbita em humanos. A ranitidina e a nizatidina foram sugeridas como alternativas, uma vez que têm atividade pró-cinética, estimulando a atividade colinérgica in vitro, porém a experiência indica que não são muito eficazes in vivo.

O tegaserode, um potente agonista parcial dos receptores $5-HT_4$ e um agonista fraco dos receptores $5-HT_{1D}$, foi desenvolvido por ter efeitos procinéticos definidos no cólon canino, mas também foi retirado do mercado graças ao prolongamento do intervalo QT. A prucaloprida é ligada à cisaprida com uma atividade pró-cinética semelhante, contudo sem efeitos cardíacos, e está disponível na Europa. É um potente agonista do receptor $5-HT4$ que estimula as CMGs e a defecação em cães e gatos. A mosaprida, uma droga relacionada, não tem atividade no cólon e é tão ineficaz quanto a metoclopramida na estimulação da motilidade colônica.

A acotiamida facilita a atividade muscarínica da acetilcolina e foi demonstrado que estimula a atividade pós-prandial gastroduodenal e colônica em cães a uma dosagem de 30 mg/kg, tendo sido aprovada (Acofide) para uso em humanos na Ásia. Altas dosagens de mirtazapina também mostraram acelerar o esvaziamento gástrico e o trânsito no cólon, além dos efeitos estimulantes do apetite e antináusea mais conhecidos. Por fim, a instalação intracolônica de capsaicina, presente em grandes quantidades nas sementes e nos frutos carnosos das plantas do gênero Capsicum (pimentas), estimula a motilidade colônica e a defecação, mas, quando administrada oralmente, retarda o trânsito do ID.

Prognóstico

Muitos animais podem ter um ou dois episódios de constipação intestinal sem mais recorrência, enquanto outros podem progredir para insuficiência colônica completa. Gatos com constipação intestinal leve a moderada geralmente respondem a um tratamento conservador com modificação da dieta, laxantes emolientes ou hiperosmóticos e agentes procinéticos do cólon. O uso precoce de agentes procinético do cólon, além de um ou mais agentes laxantes, pode prevenir a progressão da constipação intestinal para obstipação e megacólon nesses animais, que de outra forma necessitariam de colectomia.

MEGACÓLON IDIOPÁTICO FELINO[143,596-602]

O megacólon idiopático é mais observado em gatos de meia idade (média: 5,8 anos), machos (70%), de pelo curto sem raça definida (46%), de pelo longo (15%) ou da raça Siamês (12%). Os afetados geralmente apresentam defecação reduzida, ausente ou dolorosa por um período variando de dias a semanas ou meses. Eles podem ser observados fazendo várias tentativas improdutivas de defecar na caixa de areia, ou apenas por sentar-se na caixa de areia por longo tempo. A impactação do cólon é um achado consistente no exame físico em gatos afetados. Outros sinais vão depender da gravidade e da cronicidade da obstipação e do megacólon, incluindo desidratação, perda de peso, debilitação, dor abdominal e linfadenopatia mesentérica leve a moderada.

A etiopatogenia do megacólon idiopático não está totalmente esclarecida, mas os gatos afetados têm perda permanente da estrutura e da função do cólon. A terapia (laxantes, procinéticos) pode ser eficaz no início, mas a maioria dos afetados requer colectomia. A patogênese do megacólon dilatado idiopático parece envolver distúrbios funcionais no músculo liso do cólon. A lesão pode começar no cólon descendente e progredir para envolver o cólon ascendente. Estudos in vitro mostram que o músculo liso do cólon obtido de gatos que sofrem de megacólon dilatado idiopático submetidos à colectomia desenvolvem menos estresse isométrico em resposta a neurotransmissores (acetilcolina, substância P, colecistocinina), despolarização da membrana (KCl) ou estimulação elétrica de campo, quando comparados com controles saudáveis.

A colectomia subtotal deve ser considerada em gatos refratários à terapia medicamentosa.[603-611] Eles quase sempre têm prognóstico favorável para recuperação após colectomia, em especial se a válvula ileocólica estiver preservada, embora diarreia leve a moderada possa persistir por semanas a meses no pós-operatório em alguns casos.

REFERÊNCIAS BIBLIOGRÁFICAS

As referências bibliográficas deste capítulo se encontram online no Ambiente de Aprendizagem.

CAPÍTULO 278

Doenças Anorretais

Stefan Unterer

A porção distal do trato digestivo, incluindo o canal anal e reto, é uma parte muito sensível do trato gastrintestinal (GI), e a irritação da mucosa retal e da área perianal frequentemente causam dor intensa, tenesmo e disquezia. Disfunções da região anorretal podem levar à incontinência fecal, que afeta as condições higiênicas e aspectos sociais da vida dos tutores dos animais de estimação e está associada à angústia clínica do paciente. O tratamento sintomático imediato e intenso, bem como uma investigação completa orientada para o problema, geralmente são indicados em pacientes com doença anorretal.

ANATOMIA

Estruturas anorretais incluem reto, canal anal, esfíncteres anais interno e externo, músculos do diafragma pélvico, bem como os sacos anais (*sparanal sinus*) e glândulas circum-anais (*glandulae circumanales*) (Figura 278.1). O reto começa na entrada pélvica. Antes de entrar no canal anal curto, torna-se dilatado para formar a ampola retal, que está ausente em gatos. O lúmen do canal anal está contraído na junção anorretal, onde dobras longitudinais da mucosa (mais proeminentes em cães do que em gatos) pressionam juntos para obstruir o orifício. A mucosa do canal anal é dividida em três zonas anulares consecutivas: colunares, intermediárias e cutâneas. Endoscopicamente visíveis, linfonodos pequenos e solitários (1 a 3 mm) são uma característica proeminente da mucosa retal. A continência fecal depende principalmente de dois esfíncteres: o anal interno (músculo liso circular espesso do intestino; contração máxima contínua sob controle involuntário) e o anal externo (músculo estriado; contração durante as fases de distensão retal sob controle voluntário).

Três áreas glandulares estão presentes nas regiões anorretal e perianal. As glândulas anais (*glandulae anales*) são glândulas tubuloalveolares que produzem uma secreção gordurosa e se abrem para o exterior nas zonas colunar e intermediária. As glândulas do seio paranal (*glandulae sinus paranalis*) situam-se na parede e se abrem para os seios paranais (sacos anais). Sua secreção fétida serosa a pastosa é importante para a marcação territorial. Os sacos anais estão localizados entre o músculo interior liso e o músculo estriado externo do ânus em cada lado do canal anal e aberto ventrolateral ao ânus através de uma abertura de 1 a 2 mm de largura. As aberturas são visíveis ou podem ser expostas puxando a pele de cada lado do ânus ventrolateralmente.

A parte retroperitoneal do reto e do trato anal é suportada por tecido conjuntivo e músculos do diafragma pélvico. O diafragma pélvico é composto de dois músculos esqueléticos (músculo elevador do ânus e coccígeo) e duas camadas de fáscia (fáscia externa e interna do diafragma pélvico). O par de músculos retococcígeos se separa da parte dorsolateral da camada longitudinal músculo liso retal e se estende até a quinta e sexta vértebras da cauda.[1] Os músculos coccígeos cruzam o

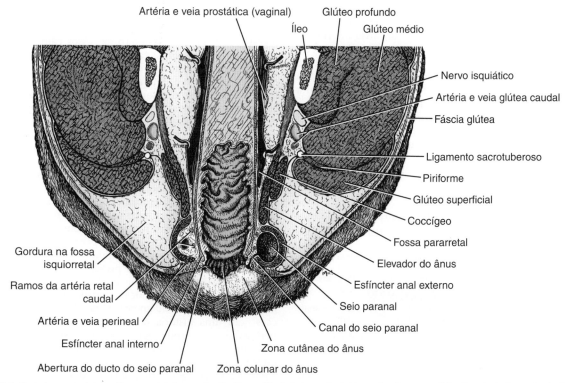

Figura 278.1 Corte transversal da região anorretal de um cão. (De Evans HE, de Lahunta A: *Guide to the dissection of the dog*, 8 ed., St. Louis, 2017, Saunders.)

reto lateralmente causando a sua compressão, enquanto o músculo retococcígeo ajuda a camada de músculo circular no movimento da coluna fecal para fora.[2] A drenagem linfática da pele anal ocorre através dos linfonodos inguinais superficiais, e os vasos linfáticos de tecidos mais profundos drenam para o grande linfonodo ilíaco medial.

O cólon descendente, o reto e o esfíncter de músculo liso do ânus são inervados por fibras simpáticas originadas dos segmentos da medula espinal L1-L4 ou L5 através dos nervos hipogástricos. A inervação simpática para o cólon descendente e reto é inibitória, ao passo que é facilitadora para o esfíncter anal interno. Fibras parassimpáticas originárias da medula espinal sacral inervam o cólon descendente e o reto através do nervo pélvico e estimulam a motilidade do cólon e do reto. Fibras somáticas da medula sacral inervam o bem definido músculo estriado do esfíncter anal externo através do nervo pudendo, levando a uma contração consciente do esfíncter. Fibras aferentes da parede retal, esfíncteres e períneo ascendem aos centros do tronco encefálico para a regulação do neurônio motor superior e ao córtex cerebral para a percepção consciente[3] (Figura 278.2).

Uma vez que a inervação do reto é semelhante à da bexiga urinária, disúria também pode estar associada a problemas neurológicos que causam doença anorretal.

FISIOLOGIA DA DEFECAÇÃO

A ingestão de alimentos pode estimular a defecação, induzindo a propagação de ondas de pressão, que movem o conteúdo intestinal para o reto (reflexo gastrocólico).[4] O aumento da pressão intrarretal causa o relaxamento reflexivo do esfíncter anal interno (inibição do reflexo retosfincteriano).[5,6] No entanto, as fibras aferentes da parede retal ascendem aos funículos dorsal e lateral até o centro do tronco encefálico para regulação do neurônio motor superior e ao córtex cerebral para percepção consciente. Antes da defecação, o reflexo de inibição retosfincteriana é suprimido, e a força do músculo estriado no esfíncter anal externo (mediado pela inervação somática da medula espinal sacral) é aumentada até que seja tomada a decisão consciente de iniciar a defecação.[7] Se a defecação for consciente, a pressão intrarretal suprimida diminui por meio do relaxamento do reto (i. e., acomodação retal). Isso permite que um volume maior de fezes seja mantido no reto em um nível inferior de pressão intraluminal (fase de armazenamento).[8] Volume fecal progressivamente crescente estimula impulsos progressivamente mais fortes para defecar. A defecação geralmente é precedida por contrações migratórias gigantes do cólon que produzem a maior força propulsora para evacuar material fecal do reto.[9,10] Idealmente, cães devem ser levados para uma caminhada de 20 a 30 min depois de se alimentar para ajudar a produzir movimento intestinal. O impulso para defecação origina-se no córtex cerebral e desce via trato motor através do tronco encefálico para os neurônios motores inferiores. A inervação parassimpática via nervo pélvico estimula a motilidade colônica e retal. A postura e o aumento da pressão intrapélvica pela contração dos músculos abdominais e diafragma facilitam a defecação. O relaxamento coordenado do esfíncter anal externo, mediado por fibras somáticas do plexo sacral e do ramo retal caudal do nervo pudendo, ocorrendo simultaneamente com o aumento da pressão intrarretal, causam a expulsão das fezes.

HISTÓRICO E EXAME FÍSICO EM PACIENTES COM SUSPEITA DE DOENÇA ANORRETAL

Pacientes com doença anorretal podem apresentar uma variedade de manifestações clínicas. Os sinais clínicos comuns incluem constipação intestinal, tenesmo, urgência para defecar, passagem de muco e hematoquezia/sangramento retal (ver Capítulo 42). Tenesmo anal (i. e., esforço para defecar) frequentemente é observado em casos obstrutivos e distúrbios inflamatórios da região anorretal. No entanto, o tenesmo também pode ser visto em pacientes com doenças urogenitais e frequentemente os tutores não conseguem diferenciar sinais GI de urogenitais. Perguntar sobre hábitos urinários, observando a postura do paciente durante o esforço e a palpação da uretra pélvica e próstata em cães machos, ajuda o veterinário a localizar o problema.

Um bom exame físico, incluindo exame completo de palpação abdominal e exame retal digital, é o primeiro passo na diferenciação entre obstrução do intestino grosso e inflamação, uma vez que o problema está localizado no trato GI inferior (ver Capítulo 2). Em distúrbios obstrutivos, o intestino normalmente está impactado fecalmente antes da estenose. A palpação abdominal frequentemente pode detectar um cólon impactado; no entanto, ocasionalmente radiografias abdominais são necessárias. Uma ampola retal fecalmente impactada pode ser identificada com o exame retal digital. Uma quantidade substancial de fezes no reto de um paciente com dificuldade de defecar é indicativo de constipação intestinal e, eventualmente, o exame retal pode identificar uma causa para a obstrução (p. ex., estenose retal ou massa, desvio do cólon devido a hérnia perineal, estenose de canal pélvico). Se nenhuma obstrução ou nenhum desvio da parede retal forem detectados, um distúrbio de motilidade ou ingestão de material estranho (p. ex., ossos, cama de gato) é uma causa frequente de impactação do cólon e da ampola retal.

A proctite – inflamação da mucosa colorretal – é a causa mais comum de tenesmo em cães e gatos. Deve ser suspeitada na presença de tenesmo, disquezia e/ou hematoquezia e na ausência de constipação intestinal. A presença simultânea de diarreia de intestino grosso sugere inflamação mais generalizada da mucosa do cólon. A duração dos sinais clínicos é importante, porque os sinais agudos frequentemente são autolimitados e não requerem uma avaliação aprofundada. Em doenças crônicas, os tutores devem ser questionados se um tratamento prévio já foi realizado e se uma melhora clínica foi observada com alterações na dieta e uso de antimicrobianos ou anti-inflamatórios/imunossupressores. Tenesmo crônico em um cão macho não castrado de meia-idade a idoso, juntamente com prisão de ventre e inchaço perianal, é típico de hérnia perineal. Diarreia paradoxal de intestino grosso causada por fluido e muco que contornam a massa fecal retida pode estar presente. Um exame retal digital com evaginação unilateral ou bilateral da parede retal sugere diagnóstico de hérnia perineal; cuidado deve ser tomado para não perfurar inadvertidamente a parede retal distendida. Em cães com uma história de tenesmo crônico devido a hérnia perineal e um episódio agudo de forte esforço ou dor na área retal, um encarceramento da bexiga urinária ou intestino pode estar presente. Deve-se suspeitar de bexiga urinária preenchida e retroflexionada se a hérnia não for redutível por pressão digital externa e uma estrutura firme e cheia de líquido for sentida.

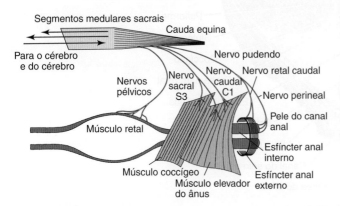

Figura 278.2 Controle neural da defecação. (De Strombeck DR, Guilford WG: Small animal gastroenterology, 2 ed., Davis, CA, 1990, Stonegate Publishing.)

A neoplasia retal pode causar tenesmo/disquezia devido à obstrução (tumores oclusivos ou fibroso) ou irritação da mucosa retal. Os tutores às vezes observam hematoquezia e sangue vermelho brilhante cobrindo a superfície das fezes formadas. Os tumores retais são muito fáceis de encontrar quando avançados; no entanto, nos estágios iniciais, um exame retal cuidadoso e metódico e às vezes a proctoscopia são necessários. Estenoses retais parciais podem facilmente não ser notadas em cães grandes; em raças gigantes, pode ser necessário inserir dois ou três dedos para ver se o ânus e reto podem expandir-se para seus diâmetros normais.

Distúrbios perianais podem causar tenesmo/disquezia devido a estenose anal (p. ex., neoplasia da glândula perianal, formação de estenose secundária à inflamação crônica ou fístula perianal), inflamação (p. ex., fístula perianal associada a colite, saculite da glândula anal) ou constipação intestinal em pacientes evitando defecação devido à dor. Lamber e esfregar a região perianal são sinais ainda mais específicos de irritação perianal. O diagnóstico geralmente é simples pelo exame da área perianal. Por causa da dor intensa, sedação ou anestesia geral às vezes são necessárias para avaliar completamente a gravidade da doença. Em cães da raça Pastor-Alemão que apresentam o diagnóstico de fístula perianal, este geralmente pode ser feito apenas por exame físico. Outros diagnósticos diferenciais para ulceração e fistulação perianal, como neoplasia e pitiose retal, devem ser considerados em qualquer raça (ver Capítulo 277). A saculite anal é uma doença relativamente comum, mas abscedação grave é infrequente. Palpação e compressão cuidadosa dos sacos anais enquanto um dedo é inserido no reto são importantes para distinguir um saco anal abscedado ou impactado de um tumor de saco anal.

Em animais com incontinência de reservatório (i. e., sensação retal alterada devido à inflamação), a defecação geralmente está associada a tenesmo e urgência. Em animais com incontinência de esfíncter (ausência de reconhecimento consciente da passagem de fezes) sem anormalidades aparentes do esfíncter anal, a disfunção da medula espinal sacrococcígea é muito provável. Uma avaliação neurológica, incluindo observação da marcha, avaliação do reflexo de retirada e do tônus muscular dos membros pélvicos, do reflexo perineal e tônus do esfíncter anal e avaliação da dor lombossacral, é indicada nesses casos.

Filhotes de cães e gatos com agenesia anorretal (ânus imperfurado) não podem defecar. Durante os primeiros dias pós-parto, o abdome distende-se progressivamente, e o animal torna-se inapetente e letárgico. Pacientes com estenose anal congênita e fístula retovaginal podem ser assintomáticos por várias semanas até que a constipação intestinal após o desmame da dieta líquida ocorra. Os animais afetados podem ficar inquietos, começar a apresentar esforço para defecação e mostrar um abdome aumentado e abaulamento do períneo.

DOENÇAS DO RETO

Proctite

A proctite – inflamação do ânus e reto – está mais comumente associada à colite (ver Capítulo 277) ou a distúrbios perianais inflamatórios, como fístulas perianais e saculite. A proctite localizada foi descrita em cães após irradiação pélvica.[11] Causas adicionais incluem lesão traumática (p. ex., corpo estranho) e reação da mucosa após prolapso retal. Os sinais clínicos da proctite geralmente incluem tenesmo, disquezia e hematoquezia. A urgência para defecar geralmente é um sinal proeminente; secreção de muco e, menos frequentemente, de pus pode ser observada. Um exame físico completo deve ser realizado. Um exame retal pode revelar evidências de infiltração neoplásica da parede retal ou do ânus, uma estenose retal e/ou uma hérnia perineal, e todas podem causar sinais clínicos semelhantes aos da proctite. O exame fecal (ver Capítulo 81) e a citologia retal

são úteis para detectar parasitas, e o aumento do número de leucócitos fecais sugere proctite infecciosa. A indicação para proctoscopia (ver Capítulo 113) e avaliação histológica da mucosa retal, que é necessária para um diagnóstico definitivo, depende da duração dos sinais clínicos e do sucesso do tratamento. A proctite aguda frequentemente é autolimitada ou responde a tratamento empírico com uma dieta de fácil digestão e medicamentos, como anti-helmínticos (p. ex., fembendazol; ver Capítulo 163), anti-inflamatórios focais de ação rápida (p. ex., espuma retal de budesonida) e analgésicos sistêmicos (p. ex., metamizol [dipirona], buprenorfina; ver Capítulos 126 e 166). Um aumento do número de leucócitos na avaliação citológica fecal/retal pode ser uma indicação para tratamento empírico com antibióticos (p. ex., amoxicilina + clavulanato, metronidazol; ver Capítulos 220 e 277); coprocultura de rotina raramente é útil.

Na proctite crônica que não responde à conduta citada, a proctoscopia e/ou colonoscopia, com avaliação histológica da mucosa colorretal, é indicada (ver Capítulo 113). A primeira biopsia, que deve ser feita com pinça estéril, deve ser submetida a cultura e teste de sensibilidade para E. coli, a fim de identificar um antibiótico apropriado em caso de colite/proctite granulomatosa causada por uma cepa aderente e invasiva de E. coli detectada histologicamente.[12] Colorações especiais (p. ex., metenamina de prata de Gomori, ácido periódico de Schiff) podem ser necessárias para detectar infecção fúngica invasiva.[13] Na proctite crônica idiopática, linfocítico-plasmocítica ou eosinofílica, drogas imunomoduladoras sistêmicas, como corticosteroides, aminossalicilatos (não em gatos) e/ou ciclosporina, podem ser utilizadas. Agentes tópicos administrados por via retal podem reduzir a dosagem necessária dos medicamentos sistêmicos. Medicamentos tópicos usados atualmente para proctite ulcerativa em humanos incluem espuma retal de budesonida ou hidrocortisona, bem como ácido 5-aminossalicílico e preparações retais de tacrolimo (ver Capítulo 277).[14]

Hérnia perineal

O diafragma pélvico dos cães está sujeito à herniação. Músculos fracos do diafragma pélvico (músculos coccígeos e levantadores do ânus) não fornecem um suporte forte para a parede retal. Os músculos tornam-se mais finos e alongados, resultando em distensão retal focal persistente e potencial impactação fecal. Edema perianal ou excessiva frouxidão ventrolateral no ânus podem estar presentes. Devido ao desvio retal, o material fecal frequentemente fica impactado no reto. A prevalência geral de hérnias perineais (HP) em cães é relativamente baixa (≈ 0,1 a 0,4%).[15] A HP canina ocorre predominantemente em cães machos não castrados de meia-idade a idosos e apenas ocasionalmente em cadelas.[16] HP em gatos é rara e geralmente secundária a problemas subjacentes, como uretrostomia perineal, megacólon, massas perineais ou trauma.[17,18] Predisposições de raça foram relatadas em Boston Terrier, Boxer, Corgi Irlandês, Pequinês, Collie, Poodle, Kelpie Australiano, Dachshund e Old English Sheepdog.[19,20]

Diagnóstico

A hérnia perineal geralmente pode ser diagnosticada através de histórico e exame clínicos. O exame retal vai revelar uma falta de suporte da parede retal com um desvio em direção ao lado da hérnia para cães com hérnia unilateral e uma dilatação de toda a ampola retal para cães com hérnia bilateral. A maioria dos cães com HP tem tenesmo crônico e edema perianal[21] (Figura 278.3) e normalmente são examinados por causa da constipação intestinal ou diarreia paradoxal do intestino grosso, conforme descrito anteriormente. O deslocamento caudal e a herniação da próstata, bexiga urinária e outros órgãos abdominais[21,22] podem levar a sinais clínicos dramáticos e ocorrem em 18 a 25% dos cães afetados.[20,21,23,24] Essas estruturas podem ficar estranguladas, levando a um abdome agudo (ver Capítulo 143).

Uma bexiga urinária retroflexionada e cheia deve ser suspeitada se a hérnia não for redutível por pressão digital externa e uma estrutura firme e cheia de líquido for sentida; a cistocentese através da parede perineal pode confirmar essa suspeita (ver a seguir). As radiografias abdominais podem revelar massas fecais, opacidade de tecidos moles devido a hérnia de bexiga ou próstata e alças cheias de ar do intestino delgado na área perineal (Figura 278.4).[17] Estudos de contraste positivos (p. ex., enema de bário) ou negativos (p. ex., insuflação de ar) do reto podem confirmar o diagnóstico e avaliar a gravidade e localização (uni versus bilateral) da HP. A ultrassonografia perianal pode avaliar o conteúdo da hérnia e identificar a retroflexão da bexiga urinária e herniação da próstata. Os estudos de imagem também são valiosos para identificar algumas doenças subjacentes, como obstrução colorretal (p. ex., massas intra e extraluminais) e prostática (p. ex., prostatite, cistos intra e paraprostáticos) e doenças do trato urinário inferior (p. ex., urolitíase e infiltração neoplásica).

O hemograma geralmente é normal, mas azotemia e hiperpotassemia são possíveis com obstrução pós-renal (p. ex., bexiga urinária retroflexionada); um leucograma inflamatório pode ser notado com necrose de órgãos encarcerados, prostatite ou bactérias translocadas através de uma parede retal danificada. Um banco de dados mínimo pode excluir distúrbios simultâneos antes de anestesia e cirurgia reparatória.

Patogênese

Em cães, diferenças anatômicas específicas de raça e sexo têm sido implicadas no desenvolvimento da HP.[25] A predisposição em cães braquicefálicos sugere uma fraqueza hereditária do

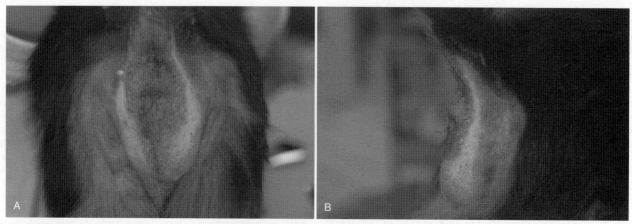

Figura 278.3 Hérnia perineal bilateral em cão (moderada à esquerda e grave à direita). (Cortesia do Dr. Pfeifer, Tierärztliche Klinik Nürnberg.)

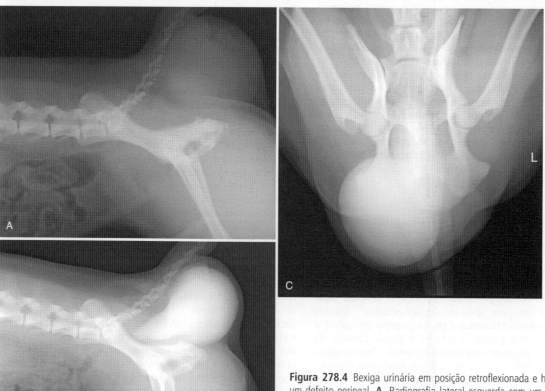

Figura 278.4 Bexiga urinária em posição retroflexionada e herniada devido a um defeito perineal. **A.** Radiografia lateral esquerda com um edema opaco de partes moles ventral às vértebras caudais. **B.** Visões lateral esquerda e (**C**) ventrodorsal de um cistograma de contraste positivo mostrando a bexiga urinária retroflexionada ventral às vértebras caudais. (Cortesia do Dr. Ohlerth, Vetsuisse Faculty, Universidade de Zurique, Suíça.)

diafragma pélvico nessas raças.[15] A descoberta de HP quase exclusivamente em cães machos intactos sugere uma base hormonal,[15] embora as concentrações séricas de testosterona e 17-beta estradiol não sejam diferentes em cães afetados e não afetados.[26] A maior incidência em cães machos em comparação com fêmeas tem sido associada a um músculo levantador do ânus mais fraco, e uma diminuição no número de receptores de andrógenos no músculos elevador do ânus e coccígeo foi proposta.[27] A relaxina afeta o metabolismo do colágeno, suavizando os componentes do tecido conjuntivo (p. ex., canal de parto).[28] A relaxina em machos é sintetizada principalmente na próstata e é secretada no plasma seminal.[29] Uma maior expressão de receptores de relaxina foi encontrada nos músculos do diafragma pélvico de cães com HP.[30,31] Fatores de crescimento (crescimento e diferenciação) do músculo esquelético também podem desempenhar um papel, porque o aumento da expressão do fator de crescimento epidérmico e caspase-3 ativa e a diminuição da expressão do fator de crescimento transformante alfa foram identificados no elevador do ânus de cães com HP.[32]

Tratamento

Pacientes com HP pequenas e sinais clínicos mínimos muitas vezes podem ser controlados com redutores da consistência fecal (p. ex., fibras dietéticas e lactulose), enemas periódicos (ver Capítulo 114) e remoção digital das fezes. Transtornos subjacentes que causam o aumento crônico da pressão intra-abdominal devem ser tratados e/ou descartados. Os proprietários devem ser avisados de que a progressão da doença é provável, o encarceramento de órgãos com hérnia é possível e os sinais podem ser agudos quando os órgãos encarcerados estão obstruídos ou isquêmicos, o que representa uma situação de emergência (ver Capítulo 150).

Depois de avaliar a condição física do paciente (sinais de doença sistêmica, bradicardia devido a hiperpotassemia) e situação metabólica e hematológica (azotemia, hiperpotassemia, hipoglicemia e anemia), a descompressão imediata da bexiga é indicada se o veterinário acredita que a bexiga está herniada. Uma cistocentese guiada por ultrassom da área perianal usando técnica asséptica é uma maneira útil de descomprimir a bexiga: é rápida e fácil de realizar, e a anestesia geralmente não é obrigatória. Concentrações maiores de potássio e creatinina no líquido aspirado em comparação com sangue também podem confirmar que o líquido aspirado é a urina. A bexiga urinária descomprimida frequentemente pode ser reposicionada por compressão digital externa, mas, se isso não for possível, o cateterismo pode manter a bexiga vazia até a correção cirúrgica da hérnia (ver Capítulos 105 e 106).

HP avançada (p. ex., HP recorrente, grande dilatação do saco herniário, doença prostática que requer omentalização prostática, e bexiga urinária retroflexionada) é uma indicação para cirurgia. Defeitos no diafragma pélvico podem ser fechados com sutura direta ou usando malha de tecidos autógenos ou sintéticos. As taxas de complicação pós-operatória relatadas de uma herniorrafia padrão variam de 28,6 a 61%, incluindo uma taxa de recorrência de 10 a 46%.[15] Atualmente, a transposição do músculo obturador interno é considerada a técnica mais confiável e tem taxas de sucesso a longo prazo > 90% em casos não complicados.[15,33] Uma abordagem cirúrgica de 2 etapas (pexia do cólon, bexiga urinária e ducto deferente; em seguida, retalho do músculo obturador interno) é recomendada para HP avançada/complicada e tem uma taxa de sucesso de 90%.[24,34] No entanto, um estudo retrospectivo recente relatou que a laparotomia não foi indicada em cães com HP e retroflexão da bexiga urinária porque o reposicionamento da bexiga pode ser realizado de forma confiável durante a cirurgia perineal. A retroflexão da bexiga urinária não aumentou significativamente a incidência de complicações pós-operatórias e não teve nenhum efeito no resultado a longo prazo.[21]

Material prostético, como tela de polipropileno,[35] submucosa de intestino delgado suína[36] e canina,[37] fáscia lata autóloga[38] e *tunica vaginalis*,[16] geralmente é necessário apenas para aqueles pacientes com HP recorrente com dimensões de hérnia que não permitem o fechamento por herniorrafia convencional. A *tunica vaginalis* autóloga pode ser colhida durante a castração.

A castração de rotina é recomendada como parte do tratamento da HP porque o risco de recorrência de HP para cães castrados é 2,7 vezes menor do que para cães não castrados.[19] A atrofia prostática torna a entrada pélvica mais larga (tornando a defecação mais fácil) e os níveis de relaxina são mais baixos.

O manejo clínico pré e pós-operatórios visa tratar e prevenir a infecção devido à translocação bacteriana através da parede retal danificada ou a infecção de ferida cirúrgica; manter as fezes amolecidas (p. ex., dieta enriquecida com psyllium, lactulose); prevenir tenesmo devido à dor; e tratar distúrbios (p. ex., colite crônica, prostatite, cistite) que predispõem à recorrência de HP (ver Capítulo 277).

Prognóstico

A elevada taxa de sucesso cirúrgica (> 90%) precisa ser considerada com cautela, já que recorrência de hérnia primária foi documentada até 4 anos após a cirurgia.[2] O prognóstico depende do tratamento bem-sucedido das causas subjacentes, da gravidade e da cronicidade da doença e da habilidade do cirurgião em realizar o reparo mais apropriado. Nos casos complicados com retroflexão da bexiga urinária, já foram relatadas taxas de mortalidade de até 30%.[20,25,39] As complicações pós-operatórias em 25 a 30% dos pacientes incluem lesão do nervo isquiático (ciático), incontinência fecal, infecção do local da cirurgia, prolapso retal com esforço excessivo, colocação incorreta de suturas no saco anal ou no lúmen retal, necrose da bexiga urinária e recorrência da hérnia primária.[15]

Neoplasia retal

A neoplasia retal é incomum em cães e gatos. Os sinais clínicos mais comuns incluem hematoquezia, tenesmo, disquezia e/ou fezes em formato de fita. Na maioria dos casos, uma massa pode ser palpada no toque retal.[40-42] Pólipos benignos, adenocarcinoma, leiomioma, leiomiossarcoma, linfoma, fibrossarcoma e tumores de células plasmáticas foram relatados.[40-43] Pólipos benignos podem se transformar em adenocarcinoma *in situ*.[44] O linfoma, o tumor mais comum em gatos, ocorre principalmente no intestino delgado ou na junção ileocólica, mas os gatos ocasionalmente desenvolvem adenocarcinoma intestinal.[45,46] A ocorrência é destacada em gatos da raça Siamês.[46,47] Cães das raças Collie e Pastor-Alemão podem ser predispostos a tumores intestinais, especialmente adenocarcinomas, carcinoma retal e pólipos,[48,49] enquanto a raça Dachshund Miniatura pode ser predisposta a doenças inflamatórias e pólipos retais.[50]

Diagnóstico

O diagnóstico requer citologia e/ou análise histopatológica de amostras obtidas endoscópica ou cirurgicamente (ver Capítulo 113). É fundamental obter tecido submucoso para distinguir lesões benignas de malignas. Isso pode ser feito endoscopicamente, com o devido treinamento, usando equipamento de biopsia rígida com pinça; alternativamente, biopsia de espessura total é necessária. Exames completos, incluindo ultrassonografia abdominal, radiografias torácicas, hemograma completo, perfil bioquímico sérico e urinálise, são recomendados antes da terapia. Isso se justifica porque a maioria dos cães afetados é de meia-idade a idosos e podem ter comorbidades. Além disso, o linfoma, por definição, é uma doença sistêmica, e metástase a partir de adenocarcinoma retal foi relatada.

Tratamento

A ressecção cirúrgica é o tratamento de escolha para massas retais localizadas, malignas ou benignas. Uma variedade de abordagens cirúrgicas foi descrita, incluindo *pull-through* retal, abordagem abdominal aberta ou transpélvica para massas benignas e malignas, e remoção endoscópica transretal de tumores benignos.[40,42,51-55]

Além da cirurgia, piroxicam, um medicamento anti-inflamatório não esteroide, pode ajudar a aliviar e reduzir os sinais clínicos associados a pólipos retais em alguns cães.[44]

Prognóstico

O tempo de sobrevivência varia amplamente, dependendo do tipo de tumor, estágio e técnica cirúrgica utilizada. Sobrevivência prolongada de muitos meses a anos após a remoção bem-sucedida de um tumor primário[40,52] e/ou quimioterapia de um linfoma retal[43] foi relatada.

Prolapso retal

Os prolapsos retais são classificados como: retal externo completo (prolapso retal de espessura total; parede retal externamente visível, forma mais comum); retal externo parcial (prolapso da mucosa; mucosa protuberante visível externamente, pode às vezes pode ser observada em pacientes durante episódios de tenesmo ou permanentemente em formas leves de prolapso retal) (Figura 278.5); ou intussuscepção retal interna (invaginação da parede retal; não visível externamente, ainda não descrito em pequenos animais).[56]

Diagnóstico

O prolapso retal pode ser detectado no exame físico; no entanto, para a seleção precisa do tratamento, a mucosa retal deve ser diferenciada de uma intussuscepção ileocólica que prolapsou pelo ânus.[57] A inserção cuidadosa de uma sonda romba e bem lubrificada entre a parede do reto e o tecido prolapsado será possível se houver uma intussuscepção, mas não em um prolapso retal.[58] A parede retal protuberante deve ser examinada em busca de infiltrados neoplásicos. Após o reposicionamento, ultrassonografia, radiografias com contraste negativo, ou endoscopia devem ser consideradas. Para a investigação de anormalidades congênitas complexas da parede do cólon (p. ex., duplicação do cólon), tomografia computadorizada com contraste negativo ou ressonância magnética podem ser úteis.[59] Técnicas de imagem da região abdominal, biopsias endoscópicas e urinálise podem identificar outras causas de esforço para defecação.

Patogênese

O prolapso retal geralmente é devido a um distúrbio urogenital ou gastrintestinal que produz esforço grave ou persistente. As causas mais comuns de prolapso retal são disquezia de colite grave ou proctite secundária devido a parasitas.[60] Outras causas incluem:

- Condições intestinais: neoplasia intestinal, corpo estranho, constipação intestinal e defeitos congênitos[40,61-64]

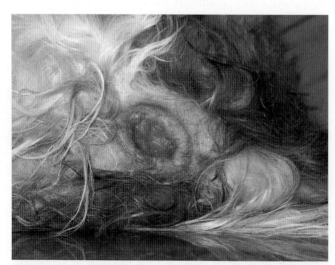

Figura 278.5 Prolapso retal da mucosa em um cão com colite/proctite. (Cortesia do Dr. Tomsa, Ennetseeklinik für Kleintiere, Suíça.) (*Esta figura se encontra reproduzida em cores no Encarte.*)

- Anormalidades anorretais: fístula perianal, saculite e correção cirúrgica de hérnia perineal sem colopexia[65]
- Incompetência do esfincter anal devido a problemas neurológicos ou disfunção muscular[66]
- Causas urogenitais: inflamação do trato urinário inferior, urolitíase, neoplasia cística ou uretral e distúrbios da próstata[62,67]
- Uma cistocele (protrusão da bexiga urinária para dentro da vagina) foi relatada[68]
- Anormalidades conformacionais (vulva recuada, estenose do vestíbulo vaginal) causando estrangúria.[69]

Tratamento

O tratamento deve ser imediato, para reduzir trauma adicional da mucosa e minimizar o desconforto. O manejo conservador inclui o tratamento das causas subjacentes do esforço crônico e tenesmo pós-cirúrgico. A cirurgia geralmente é indicada e três técnicas cirúrgicas incluem a sutura perianal em bolsa, colopexia e ressecção retal.[58,65] Para prolapso retal discreto com dano mínimo ao tecido, a mucosa deve ser limpa e reidratada com uma solução isotônica morna, lubrificada com um gel à base de água e reposicionada por manipulação digital suave. Uma sutura em bolsa de fumo é feita, deixando uma abertura grande o suficiente para permitir a passagem de fezes moles, mas sem mais prolapso; a colocação temporária de um tubo através do ânus durante essa sutura, e a remoção do tubo imediatamente após a ligadura estar completa, ajuda a prevenir o aperto excessivo.[58] A conduta terapêutica inclui a lactulose para manter as fezes amolecidas, corticosteroides tópicos (p. ex., espuma de hidrocortisona), corticosteroides sistêmicos (prednisolona 1 mg/kg PO a cada 24 horas), metronidazol e medicamentos/opioides analgésicos (p. ex., buprenorfina). A defecação deve ser adequada para evitar a constipação intestinal após a colocação da sutura.

A colopexia é útil quando o tecido estiver viável, se a redução manual do prolapso for difícil ou com prolapsos recorrentes.[34,70] Geralmente é realizada por celiotomia e pode ser combinada com outros procedimentos (p. ex., herniorrafia aposicional com hérnias perineais).[24,68,70,71] Uma laparoscopia minimamente invasiva é uma técnica alternativa.[72] A ressecção retal deve ser realizada apenas quando absolutamente necessária e com a compreensão total do tutor quanto aos riscos, pois pode resultar em complicações graves.[58] As indicações incluem mucosa necrótica e eliminação de tecido retal redundante. Uma técnica de implantação de uma tipoia de elastômero de silicone foi descrita para pacientes com anormalidades do esfíncter anal. O tecido fibroso resultante pode aumentar o tônus anal, evitando o prolapso retal durante a defecação.[66] O cuidado pós-operatório é semelhante ao prolapso retal, sendo também importante tratar as causas subjacentes.

Prognóstico

O prognóstico em formas brandas com uma causa subjacente tratável geralmente é bom. Em pacientes com recorrência e formas graves de prolapso retal que requerem procedimentos cirúrgicos complexos, o prognóstico é reservado. Complicações pós-operatórias incluem formação de estenose, incontinência e deiscência, o que pode ser fatal.

Estenose retal e anal

Estenoses retais e anais ocorrem quando o lúmen retal ou a abertura anal são comprimidos por tecido cicatricial de inflamação crônica, trauma ou câncer.[73-75] Uma estenose congênita também pode estreitar o canal anorretal.[76] Estenoses retais em cães são raras. As causas relatadas incluem: proctite/colite, estenose anastomótica pós-ressecção de massa neoplásica, inflamação perianal crônica, corpos estranhos, histoplasmose, malformação congênita[75] e uma complicação tardia da irradiação.[11] Estenoses retais e anais são incomuns em gatos.

Uma vez que as estenoses podem ser congênitas, inflamatórias ou neoplásicas, todas as idades podem ser afetadas. Cães da raça Pastor-Alemão são predispostos a fístulas perianais e doença intestinal inflamatória, que pode estar associada a estenoses anorretais.[77,78] Além desse caso, nenhuma predisposição por raça é relatada.[75] Estenoses podem ser assintomáticas até que o calibre luminal se torne pequeno o suficiente para causar obstrução. A maioria dos pacientes vai ao veterinário por causa do tenesmo decorrente de constipação intestinal.[75] Outros sinais clínicos podem incluir anorexia, dor abdominal e vômitos.[79] A diminuição da motilidade intestinal e a obstrução podem levar a supercrescimento secundário de bactérias intestinais e produção excessiva de gás manifestada como distensão abdominal, borborigmo e flatulência. Animais com obstrução parcial podem produzir fezes em fita. As queixas adicionais incluem hematoquezia, diarreia e sangramento retal.

Estenoses anorretais geralmente podem ser identificadas durante exame retal, que normalmente revela uma banda circunferencial fibrótica e firme, que não pode ser esticada.[75] Na estenose anorretal causada por doenças infiltrativas, a estenose do canal anorretal pode estar presente a uma distância maior (vários milímetros a centímetros), e às vezes uma massa assimétrica pode ser sentida. No entanto, alguns carcinomas colorretais formam estenoses que não podem ser distinguidos da estenose fibrosa benigna do intestino.[74] Às vezes, estenoses com um diâmetro luminal muito pequeno (p. ex., 1 a 2 mm) não podem passar por exame digital sem causar danos aos tecidos.

Diagnóstico

Embora as estenoses geralmente sejam detectadas por exame retal, diagnósticos adicionais caracterizam a lesão e identificam as causas subjacentes. Estudos radiográficos com contraste (ar e bário) avaliam a extensão e localização de estenoses retais.[73,75,76] O ultrassom pode detectar espessamento mural da parede retal, intumescimento de linfonodos abdominais e lesões metastáticas (a localização intrapélvica e gás colorretal podem limitar a visualização). Uma proctocolonoscopia (ver Capítulo 113) pode permitir a visualização da estenose, mas pode ser difícil de executar se ela estiver perto do ânus.[80] Quando uma estenose distal puder ser perpassada por um endoscópio de pequeno diâmetro, uma visão retroflexionada deve ser usada para avaliar a lesão (ver Capítulo 277). Biopsias diferenciam estenoses benignas de malignas.

Tratamento

O tratamento ideal depende da duração, tipo de tecido (fibrótico *vs.* muscular) e causa subjacente. A dilatação por balão repetida sob controle endoscópico ou fluoroscópico geralmente resolve anéis fibróticos benignos,[73,75] exercendo uma força radial no tecido e rompendo a estenose, rica em fibras de colágeno. Um a três procedimentos com 4 a 6 dias de intervalo aumentam gradualmente o diâmetro da estenose sem rompimentos excessivos, reduzindo, assim, a probabilidade de formação de estenose recorrente. O número de procedimentos depende do grau de contração recorrente do tecido e dos sinais clínicos. O tamanho do balão é baseado no diâmetro do orifício de estenose, grau de destruição do tecido e tamanho do paciente (p. ex., gatos e cães de raças pequenas: 10 a 18 mm; cães de raças de médio e grande portes: tamanho do balão em mm = peso em kg + 5). Injeções intralesionais concomitantes de triancinolona podem resultar em melhores taxas de sucesso porque os corticosteroides inibem a recuperação do tecido cicatricial.[73,81] *Bougienage* com um dilatador anal bem lubrificado pode ser mais fácil e mais barata em cães de raças de médio a grande portes e podem ser feitos em continuidade, diariamente, pelo tutor em casa para reduzir o risco de nova estenose. A colocação de *stent* metálico autoexpansível para alívio da obstrução do cólon é um tratamento paliativo não cirúrgico para pacientes com doença metastática ou sistêmica em que a ressecção cirúrgica não é possível nem garantida (ver Capítulo 123).[74,82] A correção cirúrgica é reservada para estenoses causadas por neoplasia anorretal, estenoses anorretais recorrentes após dilatação malsucedida e para grandes estenoses.[83,84] A amputação retal transanal *pull-through* (anastomose coloanal) para ressecção *em bloco* pode estar associada a uma alta incidência de complicações (p. ex., incontinência fecal, sangramento retal, deiscência e infecção).[55]

Os tratamentos adicionais incluem uma dieta de poucos resíduos, emolientes fecais por várias semanas e controle da dor durante a fase pós-operatória.

Prognóstico

Muitos pacientes com estenoses benignas podem ser tratados satisfatoriamente apenas pela dilatação.[75] Se a cirurgia for necessária, complicações pós-operatórias conferem um prognóstico reservado. Lesões malignas estão associadas a um prognóstico ruim, mas o tratamento paliativo pode melhorar a qualidade de vida.[74]

Malformações anorretais

A malformação anorretal mais frequentemente relatada em pequenos animais é a atresia do ânus, com uma prevalência

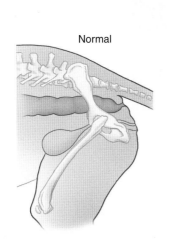
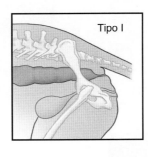
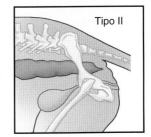
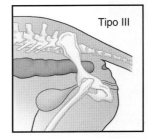
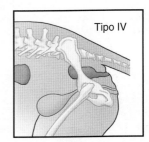

Figura 278.6 Tipos de atresia anal em cães: estenose anal congênita (Tipo I); ânus imperfurado isolado (Tipo II) ou combinado com a terminação mais cranial do reto como uma bolsa cega (Tipo III); e descontinuidade do reto proximal com desenvolvimento normal anal e retal terminal (Tipo IV). As áreas sombreadas em vermelho identificam o cólon e o reto. (Redesenhada de Vianna ML, Tobias KM: Atresia ani in the dog: a retrospective study. *J Am Anim Hosp Assoc* 41:317-322, 2005). (*Esta figura se encontra reproduzida em cores no Encarte.*)

relatada de ≈ 0,007% em cães. Como a correção cirúrgica é um desafio, e muitos cães e gatos afetados são eutanasiados no momento do diagnóstico, a verdadeira prevalência é difícil de determinar. Fêmeas e algumas raças caninas (Spitz Finlandês, Boston Terrier, Maltês, Chow Chow, Pointer Alemão de Pelo Curto, Poodle Miniatura, Poodle Toy e Schnauzer Miniatura) são predispostas.[85] Quatro tipos de atresia do ânus (Figura 278.6) incluem: Tipo I: estenose anal congênita (anel fibroso na abertura anal); Tipo II: ânus imperfurado isolado (apenas uma fina membrana sobre o ânus); Tipo III: ânus imperfurado combinado com terminação mais cranial do reto como uma bolsa cega (em cães ≥ 1 cm abaixo da extremidade terminal do reto e pele perineal); Tipo IV: descontinuidade do reto proximal com desenvolvimento retal terminal e anal normais. A cloaca embrionária representa uma comunicação entre os tratos gastrintestinal, urinário e reprodutivo, e anormalidades anorretais estão ocasionalmente associadas a malformações urogenitais; fístula retovaginal combinada com atresia do ânus tipo II é a mais comum de todas.[86-89] Malformações anorretais também podem estar associadas a outras anomalias congênitas (disgenesia sacrocaudal e hidrocefalia).[86]

Diagnóstico

O diagnóstico é baseado no histórico clínico e em sinais e achados do exame físico. Filhotes de cães e gatos com agenesia anorretal (ânus imperfurado) sem fístula não podem defecar. Mecônio e fezes se acumulam dentro do reto pós-parto, o abdome distende-se progressivamente e o filhote torna-se inapetente e letárgico. Pacientes com estenose anal congênita (atresia do ânus Tipo I) e fístulas retovaginais podem ser assintomáticos por várias semanas até que ocorra constipação intestinal após o desmame da dieta líquida.[90] Em cadelas ou gatas com passagem de fezes pelo trato urogenital, irritação vulvar e cistite vão se desenvolver.[89,91] Uma sonda com ponta de bola pode ser usada para explorar suavemente o ânus e determinar se o trato termina às cegas (*i. e.*, Tipo I e IV).[87] Anormalidades congênitas simultâneas podem incluir fenda palatina, fontanela aberta, hidrocefalia, deformação esquelética, onfalocele abdominal e defeitos cardíacos congênitos. As radiografias abdominais podem ajudar a determinar a extensão da atresia retal, o grau de dilatação do cólon e quaisquer deformidades sacrococcígeas; meio de contraste iodado infundido através da vagina ou fístula pode caracterizar o tipo de malformação anorretal. Urinálise com cultura de urina e teste de sensibilidade a antimicrobianos é indicada em todos os casos com uma comunicação entre o trato gastrintestinal e urinário.

Tratamento

A cirurgia é o tratamento de escolha para atresia anal, embora a estenose anal seja corrigida com *bougienage* e dilatação por balão[90] (Figura 278.7 e Capítulo 123). Todas as formas de ânus imperfurado (atresia do ânus tipos II-IV) exigem correção cirúrgica.[76,85,87] Uma técnica de retalho de fístula, descrita no tratamento da fístula retovaginal e atresia do ânus, reduz o risco de lesão iatrogênica do músculo esfíncter externo e sua inervação.[86] Recomenda-se analgesia pós-operatória e manutenção com dieta de poucos resíduos e emolientes fecais.

Prognóstico

O reparo cirúrgico e a dilatação por balão da atresia anal tipos I e II resultam em continência fecal na maioria dos casos.[85,87,90] O prognóstico para filhotes de cães e gatos com anomalias mais complexas (*i. e.*, atresia anal tipos II e IV, fístula retovaginal) é reservado. Deiscência da ferida pós-operatória, formação de estenose e incontinência são complicações comuns.[76]

Em contraste com gatos mais velhos com megacólon, que geralmente é irreversível, a função do cólon e do megacólon frequentemente melhora após a correção da atresia anal. Uma infecção do trato urinário ascendente que leve a dano renal crônico pode afetar o prognóstico geral.[86]

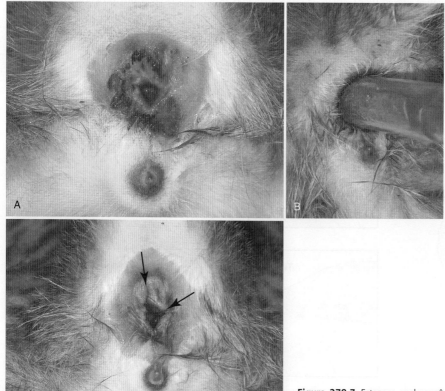

Figura 278.7 Estenose anal congênita em um filhote de gato de 8 semanas antes (**A**), durante (**B**) e após (**C**) dilatação do balão. Observe a ruptura do anel fibroso (*setas pretas*) depois do procedimento. (Cortesia do Dr. Tomsa, Ennetseeklinik für Kleintiere, Suíça, © GST | SVS.) (*Esta figura se encontra reproduzida em cores no Encarte.*)

Fístula perianal

A fístula perianal (FPA, furunculose anal) em cães é uma doença crônica inflamatória que causa ulceração e vias fistulosas nas áreas anal e perianal. Conforme a doença progride, a fistulização perianal pode se tornar extensa (Figura 278.8). Uma estenose anal pode se desenvolver. Suspeita-se de um mecanismo multifatorial imunomediado em hospedeiros geneticamente suscetíveis. A raça Pastor-Alemão é especialmente predisposta a FPA, representando > 80% dos casos.[92] Outras raças afetadas são Setter Irlandês, Labrador Retriever, Old English Sheepdog, Collie, Border Collie, Buldogue Inglês e Bouvier de Flandres.[92,93] Caudas de base ampla e caudas baixas são hipotetizadas como fatores que predispõem ao supercrescimento bacteriano e inflamação. A doença geralmente afeta cães de meia-idade, com idade média de 4 a 7 anos,[94] e não é relatada em gatos.

A apresentação da FPA varia consideravelmente. Os sinais clínicos iniciais podem incluir lambedura perineal persistente e, ao longo do tempo, disquezia, hematoquezia, tenesmo, secreção perianal purulenta, automutilação e incontinência fecal.[95,96] Os cães podem se apresentar com obstrução devido à cicatriz que causa estenose anal ou, inversamente, incontinência fecal devida aos músculos do esfíncter e nervos correspondentes danificados. Perda de peso e doença sistêmica podem ocorrer em pacientes gravemente afetados.[77,97-101] Sedação e analgesia muitas vezes são necessárias para um exame completo da área perianal para avaliar com precisão a gravidade (muitas vezes após tricotomia e limpeza) e realizar um exame retal digital com o mínimo de desconforto. O exame, incluindo avaliação dos sacos anais, visa detectar abscessos, determinar a extensão e interconexão de trechos fistulosos, avaliar qualquer envolvimento de estruturas adjacentes e registrar o número e o tamanho das aberturas da fístula. Tratos fistulosos devem ser lavados com solução salina estéril e sondados com um instrumento estéril não cortante. O esfíncter anal deve ser avaliado quanto ao espessamento e à evidência de estenose anorretal. Uma hérnia perineal associada confere um prognóstico pior.

Diagnóstico

O diagnóstico geralmente é baseado em sinais (principalmente associados a raça e idade), histórico e achados característicos do exame físico. Outras causas de fistulização (p. ex., abscedação crônica do saco anal, tumores perianais, trauma de mordidas ou corpos estranhos) devem ser descartadas. Colonoscopia e biopsias do cólon (ver Capítulo 113) podem ser indicadas, já que 50% dos cães com FPA têm colite concomitante.[96] A avaliação histopatológica do tecido pode descartar uma neoplasia. Fistulogramas podem ser úteis se a excisão cirúrgica dos tratos de drenagem for considerada; eles também podem documentar fistulas retocutâneas verdadeiras e raras. As radiografias abdominais são indicadas para procurar evidências de constipação intestinal, que pode ocorrer devido a estenose anorretal ou dor (ver Figura 278.8).

Patogênese

A doença de Crohn humana está associada a FPAs em 15 a 43% dos pacientes.[102] Por extrapolação, uma doença semelhante, multifatorial, imunomediada, com predisposição genética é suspeitada na FPA canina. A capacidade de resposta a terapia imunossupressora, as densas camadas histopatológicas de células plasmáticas e nódulos linfoides perivasculares, e uma expressão aumentada de citocinas mediadas por células Th1 (mRNA para IL-1-beta, IL-6, fator de necrose tumoral alfa, IL-8, IL-10 e fator de crescimento transformador beta) detectadas em biopsias dos tecidos da FPA dão suporte a essa hipótese.[103] A natureza ulcerativa da FPA canina pode ser devida a uma regulação positiva das enzimas metaloproteinases da matriz derivada de macrófagos (MPM), particularmente MPM-9 e MPM-13, que são endopeptidases dependentes de zinco capazes de degradar componentes da matriz extracelular.[104]

Acredita-se que a FPA canina tenha uma patogênese complexa envolvendo múltiplos fatores genéticos. Uma deficiência seletiva de imunoglobulina A (IgA) demonstrada em cães da raça Pastor-Alemão é um possível fator imunológico que leva à FPA.[105] Uma associação significativa de alelos do gene do complexo de histocompatibilidade canina de classe II (MHC) e FPAs foi descrita.[106] As moléculas de MHC de classe II são responsáveis pela apresentação de antígenos e subsequente ativação de células T.

Em humanos, polimorfismos de nucleotídio único (SNPs) no domínio de oligomerização de nucleotídio 2 (NOD2) desempenham um importante papel na etiologia da doença de Crohn.[107] Um estudo recente de análise mutacional identificou uma associação de 4 SNPs no exon 3 de NOD2 com a doença inflamatória intestinal em cães da raça Pastor-Alemão, mas em nenhuma outra raça canina (genótipos analisados em um modelo de sobredominância).[108] Finalmente, um estudo de associação de todo o genoma para identificar regiões nominalmente associadas ao FPA canino no Pastor-Alemão revelou que regiões dos genes ADAMTS16 e CTNND2 no cromossomo 34 eram mais significativamente associados à doença.[109] Pouco se sabe sobre a função de ADAMTS16, mas uma relação inversa entre a expressão de ADAMTS16 e MPM-13 foi encontrada em um estudo anterior.[110] MPM-13 é uma endopeptidase superexpressa na FPA canina. Ela apresenta um papel potencial na patogênese da doença de Crohn humana.[104,111] O gene CTNND2 codifica para a delta-catenina, possivelmente responsável pela desregulação da angiogênese.[109] Muitos outros fatores foram responsabilizados pela patogênese da PAF, incluindo reação alimentar adversa,[112] fatores anatômicos, como maior densidade de glândulas apócrinas na pele da região perianal,[113] fatores microambientais e higiênicos devido a caudas apertadas[95] e infecções bacterianas secundárias.[92,114]

Tratamento

Nem a terapia médica nem a cirúrgica geralmente são curativas. O objetivo principal da terapia é melhorar a qualidade de vida

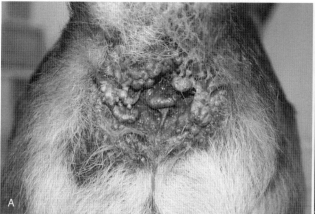
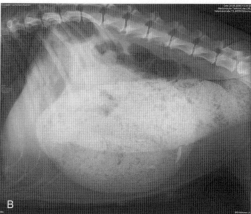

Figura 278.8 Fístula perianal grave em um cão Pastor-Alemão (**A**) associada à formação de estenose e constipação intestinal grave (**B**).

do paciente induzindo e mantendo a remissão. O manejo clínica é o tratamento atual de escolha. A cirurgia só é recomendada para fístulas incompletamente resolvidas após pelo menos 6 semanas de tratamento ou para tratamento de complicações. A terapia medicamentosa inclui imunossupressão, diminuição das populações bacterianas da área perianal, auxílio ao paciente para defecar, terapia dietética e manejo da dor.

Os pelos da área perianal devem ser removidos, devendo ser mantida seca e limpa diariamente com um antisséptico suave (p. ex., solução de clorexidina diluída, xampu antimicrobiano). Antibióticos eficazes contra bactérias anaeróbias (p. ex., metronidazol) devem ser administrados por várias semanas. Emolientes fecais (p. ex., psyllium, lactulose) ajudam a reduzir a dor durante a defecação e analgésicos que não afetam negativamente a motilidade GI (p. ex., dipirona, gabapentina) são indicados. Atenção à dieta é recomendada. O aumento da incidência de FPA em cães com reações alimentares adversas[112] e uma resposta benéfica a novas dietas de proteína em combinação com prednisolona têm sido relatados (ver Capítulo 178).[115] A ciclosporina (CsA), um inibidor da calcineurina, é o tratamento de escolha para FPA em cães da raça Pastor-Alemão.[116] Ela leva à inibição da proliferação e ativação de linfócitos T auxiliares e T citotóxicos.[117] A forma de microemulsão da CsA (Atopica, Elanco e Cyclavance® [no Brasil]), aprovada para dermatite atópica, é recomendada e oferece maior biodisponibilidade, além de menor variabilidade nas concentrações sanguíneas em comparação com outras formulações,[118] sendo administrada em dosagem de 4 a 8 mg/kg PO a cada 24 horas por 2 a 4 meses. Uma vez que os sinais clínicos melhorem substancialmente, a dosagem pode ser reduzida em aproximadamente 25% a cada 4 a 8 semanas com base na resposta clínica. A dosagem sérica de concentração da ciclosporina (ver Capítulo 165) é apenas recomendada com melhora clínica inadequada ou suspeita de toxicose (sinais gastrintestinais significativos, concentrações séricas de enzimas hepáticas > 3 vezes o normal, azotemia renal aguda). Uma forte correlação entre a concentração de ciclosporina no sangue e a eficácia clínica não foi caracterizada.[118] A coadministração de cetoconazol (5 a 10 mg/kg PO q 24 h) geralmente reduz pela metade a dose necessária de CsA via inibição competitiva das enzimas microssomais P450, que reduzem custos, uma vez que o cetoconazol é mais barato que a CsA. Essa terapia combinada produziu uma taxa de remissão de > 90% entre 9 e 16 semanas em diferentes estudos.[99-101] Uma dosagem anti-inflamatória de prednisolona (p. ex., 1 mg/kg PO a cada 24 horas, reduzida à mais baixa possível na melhora) pode ser um tratamento paliativo útil para aumentar o apetite e o bem-estar, e reduzir a inflamação. As dosagens imunossupressoras de prednisolona apenas melhoram cerca de um terço dos pacientes, e efeitos adversos indesejados são comuns.[115] A azatioprina tem sido usada como adjuvante dos glicocorticoides, mas os efeitos adversos podem incluir sinais gastrintestinais, supressão da medula óssea, hepatotoxicose e pancreatite.[119]

O tacrolimo, outro inibidor da calcineurina, é 10 a 100 vezes mais potente do que a CsA. Um estudo relatou resolução completa de lesões perianais em 5/10 cães, uma resposta parcial em 4/10 cães e nenhuma melhora em 1 cão.[98] Tacrolimo (0,1%) é aplicado na região perianal a cada 12 horas (usando luvas) na fase de indução, para reduzir a dosagem de medicamentos sistêmicos concomitantes. Após a resolução completa dos sinais clínicos, a aplicação pode ser reduzida para uma frequência mais baixa, que controle a inflamação.

Devido à alta taxa de complicações da cirurgia (i. e., até 70%)[120,121] e às altas taxas de sucesso com inibidores de calcineurina,[100,101] a cirurgia deve ser restrita à ressecção de vias de drenagem residuais e bolsas anais com abscesso, após várias semanas de tratamento médico intensivo.[97] A criocirurgia, excisão a laser e cauterização química foram relatadas, com taxas variáveis de sucesso.[122,123] Uma dilatação anal cautelosa pode ser necessária para o tratamento de estenose anal.

Prognóstico

Com tratamento médico intensivo, incluindo ciclosporina, metronidazol, limpeza local e tacrolimo tópico, muitos casos de doença leve a moderada atingem remissão completa. No entanto, terapia imunossupressora a longo prazo geralmente é necessária, mas restrições financeiras podem limitar o tratamento ideal. Casos graves podem exigir terapia cirúrgica, que pode resultar na resolução completa da FPA, porém com risco de complicações.

DOENÇAS DO SACO ANAL

Impactação, saculite e abscesso do saco anal

Desordens não neoplásicas do saco anal são relativamente comuns em cães, mas infrequentes em gatos. A impactação do saco anal foi o terceiro distúrbio de saúde mais prevalente registrado em cães que frequentaram clínicas veterinárias de cuidados primários na Inglaterra em um estudo.[124] A saculite anal e o abscesso do saco anal podem ser de difícil tratamento. A saculectomia é necessária em alguns casos com doença crônica e inflamação recorrente do saco anal. Estudos prévios relataram prurido perianal em > 95% dos cães com doença do saco anal,[125] enquanto outras causas incluem reações alimentares adversas e dermatite atópica canina.[126]

Em um estudo, cães das raças Chihuahua e Poodle Miniatura se mostraram mais predispostos a saculite anal, enquanto as raças Cavalier King Charles Spaniel e Labrador Retriever foram significativamente mais relatadas para doença do saco anal.[127]

Diagnóstico

O diagnóstico da doença do saco anal canino é baseado em sinais clínicos, exame físico e avaliação das secreções do saco anal. O conteúdo do saco anal varia em cor e consistência em cães normais, e não é uma base confiável para o diagnóstico de doença do saco anal.[126,128] A impactação do saco anal pode ser suspeitada se ele se mostrar dilatado e difícil de comprimir. Sacos anais inchados e doloridos sugerem saculite. O exame microscópico do conteúdo do saco anal é realizado com frequência. No entanto, um estudo prospectivo cego recente de avaliação citológica das secreções do saco anal não mostrou diferença significativa em relação a células inflamatórias e bactérias entre cães assintomáticos e cães com história típica de doença do saco anal.[125] O diagnóstico diferencial inclui neoplasia de saco anal ou perianal, infecção fúngica, fístula perianal e trauma.

Patogênese

A causa específica de impactação e saculite é desconhecida;[128] corpos estranhos são incomuns.[127] Substâncias com ação antimicrobiana, como lisozima, IgA, lactoferrina e o grupo de peptídios das betadefensinas são produtos das glândulas anais.[129] Alterações nesses produtos secretados podem reduzir a barreira de defesa microbiana, mudar a consistência do exsudado ou ambos. Fezes pastosas e/ou um pequeno ducto podem predispor à obstrução do saco anal e permitir a proliferação bacteriana. Escherichia coli, Enterococcus faecalis, Clostridium spp. e Proteus spp. são mais comumente encontrados na saculite.[130] A impactação, inflamação e abscedação do saco anal podem se desenvolver em associação a fístulas perianais.[77]

Tratamento

A impactação do saco anal é tratada pelo esvaziamento manual dos sacos anais e possivelmente lavagem com solução salina morna conforme necessário. Para a saculite sem abscedação, a instilação de um antibiótico tópico e pomada de corticosteroide após a lavagem podem ser suficientes. Tratamento antimicrobiano sistêmico por 2 a 3 semanas (p. ex., amoxicilina-clavulanato; cefalexina; ou sulfonamida-trimetoprima) em combinação com terapia local (p. ex., compressas frias, pomadas de corticosteroide) pode ser necessário em casos graves, resistentes ou recorrentes. Sacos anais abscedados (Figura 278.9) devem ser abertos cirurgicamente e lavados sob anestesia geral; compressas quentes aplicadas antes da cirurgia podem preparar o abscesso para ser aberto.

A remoção cirúrgica do saco anal deve ser considerada nos casos que não respondem satisfatoriamente ao tratamento. Técnicas fechadas são associadas a uma taxa de complicação menor em comparação com as técnicas abertas.[131] O manejo da dor e a prevenção das lambeduras da área perianal pelo cão são indicadas em todos os casos com inflamação substancial do saco anal.

Prognóstico

O prognóstico com impactação do saco anal e inflamação leve geralmente é bom. A maioria dos pacientes com inflamação substancial responde ao tratamento médico intensivo. A saculectomia anal tem uma taxa geral de complicação pós-operatória de 32%. Em um estudo, os cães com peso < 15 kg tiveram um risco aumentado de complicações pós-operatórias, incluindo prurido perineal, deiscência incisional, incontinência fecal temporária, constipação intestinal e diarreia. O risco de dano permanente do esfíncter anal parece ser muito baixo com técnica cirúrgica cuidadosa.[127]

Neoplasia perianal

Glândulas perianais, circum-anais ou hepatoides (assim chamadas porque, citológica e histologicamente, as células se assemelham aos hepatócitos) são consideradas glândulas sebáceas não secretoras, modificadas no cão.[132,133] Os gatos não têm um análogo às glândulas perianais caninas, e os adenomas e adenocarcinomas perianais são muito raros.

A maioria dos casos de adenoma perianal tem história de massa ou massas tumorais não dolorosas de crescimento lento. Os tumores podem ser únicos, múltiplos ou até difusos. Tipicamente são encontrados na área perianal sem pelos, mas podem se estender às regiões com pelos, ulcerar e infeccionar. Eles raramente aderem a estruturas mais profundas.[132] Os adenocarcinomas perianais normalmente crescem mais rapidamente, são maiores e mais firmes, tornam-se ulcerados e aderem aos tecidos subjacentes, em comparação com sua contrapartida benigna.[134] Doença maligna deve ser suspeitada em machos castrados com um diagnóstico de tumor perianal recorrente ou recém-diagnosticado, porque os adenocarcinomas não são dependentes de hormônio.

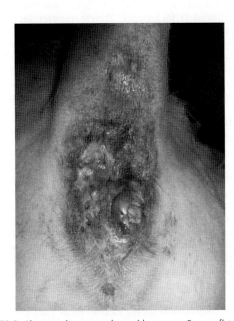

Figura 278.9 Abscesso do saco anal rompido em um cão com fístula perianal. (Cortesia do Dr. Schmitz, Universidade de Giessen, Alemanha.)

Diagnóstico

Uma avaliação geriátrica de rotina antes da anestesia, incluindo potencialmente radiografias torácicas e ultrassonografia abdominal, é desejável em um cão macho não castrado que apresente uma massa perianal altamente suspeita para adenoma perianal benigno. A aspiração por agulha fina para avaliação citológica pode não diferenciar tumores perianais benignos de malignos, mas pode descartar outras formas de câncer ou do desenvolvimento da massa. A avaliação histopatológica das amostras é recomendada. Metástase no adenocarcinoma perianal é relatada em 15% dos casos.[134]

Patogênese

Os adenomas perianais são as neoplasias perianais mais comuns (59 a 96% dos casos).[132,135] O desenvolvimento de tumor e a progressão são conduzidos por andrógenos e suprimidos por estrógenos. Cães machos não castrados mais velhos têm maior risco, com uma idade média de 10 anos.[136,137] Adenomas em cadelas são quase exclusivamente encontrados em fêmeas esterilizadas, em que o baixo nível de estrógeno não suprime a formação do tumor; relatos sugerem a secreção de testosterona das glândulas adrenais em casos raros de hiperadrenocorticismo.[138,139] Os adenocarcinomas da glândula perianal são menos comuns e representam 3 a 12% dos tumores perianais.[134]

Tratamento

Mais de 90% dos cães machos não castrados são curados com castração e remoção de massa tumoral, sendo este o tratamento de escolha para lesões benignas.[132,136] A cirurgia é recomendada em machos com tumores ulcerados ou recorrentes e em cadelas. Além de técnicas cirúrgicas padrão, criocirurgia e *laser* de dióxido de carbono para remoção da massa tumoral foram relatados.[140,141] No entanto, a avaliação da margem para invasividade, que é uma característica marcante dos adenocarcinomas perianais, não é possível com essas técnicas.[142] Para adenocarcinomas perianais, a remoção cirúrgica completa com margens adequadas é indicada.[136] Como a recorrência local é comum no adenocarcinoma, uma biópsia incisional para planejar a ressecção cirúrgica radical é encorajada quando esse diagnóstico é sugerido. A radioterapia pós-operatória pode melhorar o controle local, mas faltam dados sobre o assunto.

Prognóstico

Os adenomas perianais têm um bom prognóstico após cirurgia e castração, enquanto para adenocarcinomas o prognóstico é pior.[132,134,136] Em uma série de 41 cães, tumores < 5 cm de diâmetro (estágio T2) foram associados a uma taxa de controle de > 60% em 2 anos. A detecção de metástase no momento do diagnóstico foi negativamente relacionada à sobrevivência. Em um estudo, o tempo de sobrevivência mediana para cães com linfonodo ou metástase a distância foi de apenas 7 meses, mas o tratamento intensivo não foi tentado em 5/6 cães.[134]

Neoplasia do saco anal

Adenocarcinomas de glândulas apócrinas dos sacos anais são raros, representando aproximadamente 17% de todos os tumores na região perianal e 2% de todos os tumores de pele e subcutâneos.[133,142] Esse tumor é raro em gatos, embora possa ser mais comum em animais da raça Siamês.[143-148] A idade mediana relatada é de 11 anos em cães e 12 anos em gatos. Não há predisposição por gênero.[135,149-151] Para identificação e tratamento antecipados, um exame retal e perianal completo deve ser rotina para todo cão adulto atendido clinicamente.[152-154]

Os adenocarcinomas de glândula apócrina do saco anal (AGASACA) geralmente afetam um saco anal, mas os tumores bilaterais têm sido relatados.[152-155] Esses tumores podem ser muito agressivos, e elevadas taxas de metástase no momento do diagnóstico (média de 50%, variação 46 a 96%) foram relatadas. A metástase é encontrada mais comumente em nódulos linfáticos sublombares/pélvicos de modo precoce ou nos pulmões e ossos lombares/pélvicos mais tardiamente na doença.[135,149-151,153-156] Um estudo em cães da raça Cocker Spaniel Inglês, uma raça de alto risco, mostrou associação entre o desenvolvimento do tumor e um haplótipo do complexo histocompatibilidade principal (alelo DLA-DQB1), sugerindo um fator genético no desenvolvimento do tumor.[157]

Os sinais clínicos em cães com AGASACA podem ser devidos à presença física de massa tumoral primária, metástases para linfonodos regionais ou hipercalcemia paraneoplásica (ver Capítulo 352). Os animais podem apresentar evidências de dor ao defecar, hematoquezia e/ou secreção inflamada dos sacos anais. Em alguns casos, os problemas causados por linfonodos sublombares severamente dilatados, como fezes achatadas ou esforço para defecar, são dominantes. Poliúria e polidipsia, anorexia, letargia ou vômito podem ser causados por hipercalcemia paraneoplásica, que é mediada pela secreção tumoral de peptídio relacionado ao hormônio da paratireoide.[149,150] Aproximadamente 27% dos cães com AGASACA têm níveis elevados de cálcio sérico (ver Capítulo 69). Em até 39% dos cães, o tumor primário foi um achado incidental no exame físico.[150] Como cães, gatos afetados podem apresentar tenesmo, constipação intestinal, esfregar-se no chão, presença de uma massa ou secreção hemorrágica.[143,146,147] A hipercalcemia paraneoplásica não é comumente relatada em gatos.[143]

Diagnóstico

Uma massa firme e discreta na área do saco anal, linfadenomegalia sublombar, poliúria e polidipsia são altamente sugestivas. Tumores dos sacos anais podem tornar-se secundariamente inflamados e infectados. O diagnóstico definitivo é feito por citologia ou histopatologia. Uma vez que AGASACA tem uma taxa muito alta de metástase, o estadiamento deve incluir radiografias torácicas e ultrassonografia ou radiografia abdominal. A avaliação ultrassonográfica dos linfonodos é superior às radiografias simples e pode identificar outros locais potenciais de metástase abdominal.[158] Pacientes com claudicação ou dor óssea devem ser avaliados radiograficamente ou por cintilografia nuclear para evidência de metástase óssea. Um exame retal cuidadoso, hemograma completo, painel bioquímico sérico e urinálise são recomendados. O manejo clínico da hipercalcemia ou da função renal prejudicada pode ser necessário antes da cirurgia porque a hipercalcemia pode resultar em lesão renal (ver Capítulos 322 e 352). As mesmas diretrizes para o estadiamento de tumores de saco anal em cães se aplicam a pacientes felinos com suspeita de AGASACA.

Tratamento e prognóstico

A remoção cirúrgica abrangente do tumor primário e gânglios linfáticos sublombares metastáticos aumentados isoladamente ou em combinação com quimioterapia adjuvante e/ou radioterapia permite um tempo médio de sobrevivência de 16 a 18 meses.[150,151] Até cães com doença metastática podem ter uma boa qualidade de vida por meses. A ressecção cirúrgica agressiva de grandes tumores apresenta o risco potencial de causar incontinência fecal. Fatores prognósticos negativos incluem grande tamanho do tumor primário,[150,151] presença de metástases em linfonodos,[151] presença de metástases a distância,[150,151] estágio clínico avançado,[151] não procurar cirurgia ou quimioterapia isoladamente[150] e nenhuma terapia.[151] Existem resultados conflitantes sobre o significado prognóstico da hipercalcemia em AGASACA.[149-151,153,154]

A radioterapia pode ser paliativa ou definitiva para doença não ressecável ou tratamento de linfonodos metastáticos (ver Capítulo 340).[159] A radioterapia definitiva é utilizada para o tratamento de doença microscópica após a remoção cirúrgica do tumor primário, visando prevenir a recorrência local.[153] Os efeitos colaterais podem incluir irritação ou ruptura intestinal, diarreia e dor à defecação a curto prazo e possivelmente estenose retal a longo prazo.[159]

Os agentes quimioterápicos mais comumente usados são a cisplatina, carboplatina, actinomicina D ou mitoxantrona.[149,151,153]

O fosfato de toceranibe, um inibidor da tirosinoquinase, mostrou eficácia moderada, com uma duração média de resposta de 19 a 23 semanas em 33 cães refratários às terapias anteriores.[160] Uma relação significativa entre um sistema de estadiamento modificado e a sobrevivência foi encontrada em um estudo de cães tratados prospectivamente de acordo com um algoritmo de gerenciamento predefinido.[151] Em gatos, tempos de sobrevivência e prognóstico conflitantes para essa doença são relatados. Um estudo de 39 gatos demonstrou um tempo médio de sobrevivência de 3 meses (intervalo de 0 a 23 meses) com 85% dos gatos sucumbindo à doença local ou metastática.[143]

INCONTINÊNCIA FECAL

A incontinência fecal é a passagem involuntária de fezes através do ânus, em contraste com a descarga anal de pequenas quantidades de muco, pus ou sangue. A continência depende de esfíncteres anais funcionais internos e externos. Uma sensação normal de distensão retal e capacidade de reservatório adequada do reto são necessárias para prevenir a incontinência fecal (incontinência de reservatório). Alterações anatômicas e doenças neurológicas podem ser responsáveis pela incontinência fecal. Um histórico detalhado é essencial para diferenciar incontinência de reservatório da incontinência de esfíncter. Animais com incontinência esfincteriana não têm consciência da passagem das fezes e normalmente não ficam em postura adequada para defecar. Com a incontinência esfincteriana, o gotejamento anal inconsciente pode ser agravado pelo aumento da pressão intra-abdominal (p. ex., tosse, excitação). Ver também Capítulo 42.

Em animais com incontinência de reservatório, a defecação é geralmente associada a tenesmo e urgência. A sensação retal alterada devido à inflamação (p. ex., proctite) pode produzir incontinência. Esses animais normalmente têm diarreia, hematoquezia e muco fecal.

Uma vez que a incontinência esfincteriana neurogênica comumente é associada à disfunção da cauda equina,[161-163] evidências de disfunção sacrococcígea do neurônio motor inferior devem ser avaliadas (ver Capítulo 266). A marcha é avaliada para ataxia; os membros pélvicos para diminuição dos reflexos de retirada e diminuição do tônus muscular; e a cauda para baixo, tônus reduzido e perda de sensação (ver Capítulo 259).[164] O reflexo perineal e o tônus do esfíncter anal podem ser reduzidos devido à disfunção do nervo sacral. A perda do reflexo do músculo detrusor pode produzir gotejamento de urina devido a transbordamento de uma bexiga cheia, caso em que a urina pode ser eliminada facilmente. Podem ocorrer incontinências fecal e urinária na síndrome da cauda equina, e o sinal mais comum dessa síndrome é a dor induzida pela palpação da manipulação da área lombossacral ou da cauda (ver Capítulo 266). Lesões graves (p. ex., aquelas que causam paraplegia) craniais à medula espinal sacral (i. e., disfunção do neurônio motor superior) podem causar perda do controle sobre a defecação.

Diagnóstico

Um exame neurológico completo geralmente revelará deficiências que sugerem razões neurogênicas e anatômicas para a incontinência. O reto e a área perianal devem ser avaliados cuidadosamente para causas não neurogênicas de incontinência. Com doença localizada na medula espinal sacrococcígea, as radiografias frequentemente identificam discopondilite, fraturas ou neoplasia, embora a tomografia computadorizada e a ressonância magnética sejam mais sensíveis,[165,166] especialmente para lesões compressivas da medula espinal não detectadas pela mielografia. Doença inflamatória da medula espinal podem ser identificadas com exame do líquido cefalorraquidiano (ver Capítulo 115), e anormalidades mioneurais podem ser detectadas por eletrodiagnóstico (ver Capítulo 117). A abordagem diagnóstica para incontinência de reservatório inclui exame fecal para parasitas (ver Capítulo 81) e proctoscopia/biopsia para diagnóstico de proctite ou infiltração neoplásica (ver Capítulo 113).

Patogênese

A defecação envolve atividade coordenada dos sistemas nervoso autônomo (parassimpático e simpático) e somático. Uma disfunção nos componentes sacrais dessa inervação causa incontinência esfincteriana neurogênica. Em animais jovens, anormalidades congênitas anorretais podem ser associadas à insuficiência do esfíncter anal (p. ex., atresia do ânus tipo I, fístula retovaginal). Em cães e gatos adultos, inflamação grave (p. ex., fístula perianal), infiltração neoplásica, trauma e procedimentos cirúrgicos perianais podem danificar o esfíncter anal ou sua inervação.

Tratamento e prognóstico

A laminectomia descompressiva é eficaz para a estenose lombossacral degenerativa causando síndrome da cauda equina em cães, e a incontinência fecal pode melhorar no pós-operatório. Um estudo retrospectivo de 69 cães mostrou que a incontinência fecal estava presente antes da cirurgia em 6% dos casos. Em geral, cachorros com incontinência urinária ou fecal têm um prognóstico pior do que cães que estavam continentes antes da cirurgia.[167] Devido à doença compressiva do disco toracolombar, uma prevalência de 6,8% de incontinência fecal permanente foi relatada. Cães com paraplegia antes da cirurgia tiveram maior frequência de incontinência em comparação com cães que deambulavam.[168] Incontinência fecal causada por lesões anorretais pós-operatórias e/ou traumáticas pode melhorar com o tempo. A incontinência fecal foi a complicação mais comum (42 de 74 cães) após cirurgia *pull-through* em cães com massas retais, sendo transitória em 19 e permanente em 23 cães.[55] Complicações pós-operatórias da defecação ocorreram em 9/62 cães após saculectomia anal.[127] Incontinência fecal ocorreu em 2/51 cães após o tratamento cirúrgico da fístula perianal.[169]

Novas técnicas cirúrgicas e estudos experimentais para pacientes com perda de função do esfíncter anal foram descritos, incluindo uma técnica de diafragma espiral retal,[170] implantação de uma tipoia de silicone de elastômero,[66] transposição de um retalho do músculo semitendinoso[171] e reinervação do esfíncter anal com a transferência do nervo motor femoral para o nervo pudendo.[172] A doença colorretal inflamatória pode causar incontinência e deve ser tratada (ver anteriormente neste capítulo e Capítulo 277). Os tratamentos incluem anti-helmínticos, dietas hipoalergênicas, antibióticos (p. ex., tilosina) e/ou anti-inflamatórios (p. ex., corticosteroides, sulfassalazina). Alguns pacientes com doença inflamatória intestinal podem responder a uma dieta rica em fibras. Outros se beneficiam com dietas de alta digestibilidade e poucos resíduos, que reduzem o volume fecal e a frequência de defecação. Administração de enemas de pequeno volume (ver Capítulo 114) para estimular a defecação periodicamente pode manter o cólon e o reto vazios e melhorar a continência em alguns casos. Loperamida (0,1 a 0,2 mg/kg PO a cada 8 horas), um opioide que retarda o trânsito do cólon e aumenta o tônus do esfíncter anal interno, pode ajudar a controlar a incontinência fecal em pacientes diarreicos. A loperamida não deve ser usada em cães com defeito *MDR1* (mutação no gene de resistência múltipla a medicamentos).

A incontinência fecal pode ser difícil de controlar. Apesar de não representar um problema de limitação de vida, alguns pacientes serão eutanasiados por inconveniência e aspectos de higiene.

REFERÊNCIAS BIBLIOGRÁFICAS

As referências bibliográficas deste capítulo se encontram online no Ambiente de Aprendizagem.

CAPÍTULO 279

Peritonite

Thandeka Roseann Ngwenyama e Rance K. Sellon

ANATOMIA E FISIOLOGIA DO PERITÔNIO

A cavidade peritoneal se estende do diafragma à pelve e é limitada pelas vértebras lombares, pela musculatura sublombar e pelos músculos oblíquo, transverso e reto do abdome. O diafragma tem três aberturas naturais (esofágica, cava e hiatos aórticos), bem como aberturas em forma de fenda emparelhadas dorsalmente que podem permitir o movimento de fluido ou ar entre a cavidade peritoneal e a pleural.[1,2] O peritônio, uma membrana serosa de origem mesodérmica embrionária, é composto por uma única camada de células mesoteliais ancoradas em uma membrana basal com uma camada mais profunda de tecido conjuntivo de células adiposas, macrófagos, linfócitos, fibroblastos e fibras elásticas de colágeno.[1,3-6] O peritônio parietal reveste a cavidade abdominal e reflete no peritônio visceral para cobrir os órgãos abdominais; os reflexos peritoneais formam os mesentérios, os omentos e os ligamentos abdominais. A cavidade peritoneal é um espaço entre o peritônio parietal e visceral.[1,2] O peritônio é altamente permeável à água e solutos de baixo peso molecular, permitindo a troca bidirecional entre a cavidade peritoneal e o plasma; uma membrana basal fenestrada permite que algumas partículas passem facilmente para dentro de vasos linfáticos.[5,7] Animais sadios contêm fluido peritoneal que consiste em < 1 mℓ/kg de um dialisado de plasma claro e cor de palha caracterizado como um transudato, com < 3 mil células nucleadas (monócitos, linfócitos e células mesoteliais)/$\mu\ell$ e < 2,5 g/dℓ (< 25 g/ℓ) de proteína (albumina).[5,8] As células mesoteliais produzem pequenas quantidades de surfactante para lubrificar os órgãos e evitar o atrito.[6] O peritônio é capaz tanto de absorção quando de exsudação; em um paciente normal, há um equilíbrio entre eles.[7] Mudanças na pressão intra-abdominal durante a respiração promovem a circulação do líquido peritoneal cranialmente ao longo do abdome ventral, depois dorsalmente ao longo da superfície diafragmática do fígado.[9] O fluido peritoneal drena via linfáticos diafragmáticos e do ducto torácico para os linfonodos do esterno e mediastinais.[1] Assim, a linfadenopatia esternal identificada em radiografias torácicas, provavelmente, reflete doença intra-abdominal. As defesas peritoneais inatas consistem no sistema complemento, neutrófilos, basófilos, mastócitos, linfócitos, macrófagos, células *natural killer*, drenagem linfática, tecido linfoide associado ao peritônio, capacidade de absorção e localização, e o omento, que tem atividade imunogênica.[10] A compartimentalização peritoneal de doenças resulta em maiores concentrações de citocinas inflamatórias e biomarcadores no fluido peritoneal do que no sangue periférico; o peritônio pode atuar como uma barreira para diminuir a absorção de substratos e criar esse gradiente.[11]

DEFINIÇÕES, CLASSIFICAÇÃO E FISIOPATOLOGIA

A peritonite, inflamação do peritônio, pode ser causada por etiologia não infecciosa ou infecciosa (Tabela 279.1). A lesão peritoneal provoca uma intensa reação inflamatória, resultando no acúmulo de citocinas inflamatórias na cavidade peritoneal, ativação do complemento, produção de imunoglobulinas, liberação de substâncias vasoativas e um desequilíbrio de mediadores inflamatórios e anti-inflamatórios. A inflamação resulta em vasodilatação, aumento da permeabilidade vascular, oclusão de estômatos peritoneais por fibrina e formação de aderências. A peritonite pode levar à síndrome de resposta inflamatória sistêmica (SRIS) e características clínicas associadas (ver Capítulo 132).[1,3]

A peritonite pode ser classificada em função da etiologia (primária vs. secundária vs. terciária), distribuição (focal ou difusa) e duração (aguda ou crônica).[1] A peritonite primária é causada por uma fonte extra-abdominal, como disseminação hematogênica, e provavelmente apresenta algum componente de imunocomprometimento. Outras rotas propostas são por translocação do trato gastrintestinal (GI), através das aberturas naturais do diafragma para o espaço pleural e da bolsa ovárica.[5,12] O melhor exemplo de peritonite primária em medicina veterinária é a forma efusiva da peritonite infecciosa felina (PIF) causada por propagação hematogênica do coronavírus entérico felino mutado (ver Capítulo 224). Outras causas relatadas de peritonite primária em medicina veterinária incluem infecção por bactérias, fungos e parasitas (Tabela 279.1).[12,13]

A peritonite secundária é causada por doença intra-abdominal séptica ou asséptica, e é o tipo mais comum em cães e gatos (ver Capítulo 143). Peritonite séptica secundária de extravasamento gastrintestinal ou ruptura causada por ulceração (administração de inibidor seletivo da ciclo-oxigenase-2),[14,15] doença infiltrativa, corpo estranho, obstrução, vazamento em partes de tubos de alimentação, neoplasia, trauma por penetração, dano isquêmico, torção, vólvulo ou deiscência de uma incisão cirúrgica anterior são comuns.[16-29] A origem mais frequente do extravasamento gastrintestinal relatada em cães é a deiscência de ferida cirúrgica,[18,29] embora perfuração por corpo estranho intestinal também tenha sido relatada como a causa mais comum.[20,25] Em um estudo, o extravasamento gastrintestinal em gatos foi associado principalmente à neoplasia,[24] enquanto outro estudo identificou trauma como a causa predominante.[26] A peritonite séptica costuma ser polimicrobiana, mas o microrganismo isolado mais frequentemente, independentemente da causa basal, é E. coli.[20,21]

A peritonite biliar desenvolve-se como consequência de trauma do trato biliar, colecistite necrosante e complicações pós-operatórias de cirurgia do trato biliar (p. ex., deiscência de uma incisão de colecistotomia);[30-33] a bile de cães normais é estéril, e a peritonite biliar séptica está associada a uma elevada taxa de mortalidade. As fontes propostas de bactérias incluem feridas abertas ou penetrantes, ruptura de uma vesícula biliar infectada, ascensão do trato GI, translocação de bactérias entéricas, ou endotoxemia e bacteriemia sistêmica e portal.[31,33] Trauma abdominal contuso com subsequente ruptura da bexiga é a causa mais comum de uroperitônio em cães e gatos (ver Capítulo 143). Outras causas de uroperitônio incluem ruptura secundária à obstrução uretral, neoplasia e iatrogênica (cateterismo uretral, pressão manual da bexiga, cistocentese, penetração inadvertida durante a cirurgia abdominal).[34-37]

A peritonite terciária é uma infecção intra-abdominal recorrente após a terapia inicial cirúrgica e antimicrobiana de uma peritonite bacteriana secundária.[3] Essa categoria é predominantemente reconhecida na medicina humana.

Tabela 279.1 Etiologia da peritonite (primária[12,13] vs. secundária[14-37]).	
CAUSAS PRIMÁRIAS	**EXEMPLOS**
Viral	Peritonite infecciosa felina (PIF)
Bacteriana	E. coli*, Enterococcus spp.*, Clostridium spp.*, Salmonella Typhimurium, Chlamydia felis, Propionibacterium, Bacillus, Staphylococcus, Bacteroides, Fusobacterium, Actinomyces, Morganella morganii, Peptostreptococcus spp.
Parasitária	Mesocestódios, Sparganum proliferum
Fúngica	Blastomyces, Histoplasma e Candida spp.
CAUSAS SECUNDÁRIAS	**EXEMPLOS**
Química	Ácido gástrico, bile, enzimas pancreáticas, urina, bário
Mecânica, corpo estranho	Sutura, pelos, compressas cirúrgicas (gossipiboma) Algodão, seda, linho, espiguetas de gramíneas
Amido, granulomatosa	Pó de luvas cirúrgicas (talco, amido de milho)
Parasitárias	Cestódeos
Protozoários	Neospora, Toxoplasma
Causas sépticas	
Origem gastrintestinal	Vazamento/ruptura (secundária a ulceração, obstrução de corpo estranho, neoplasia, trauma, torção com dano isquêmico ou deiscência de uma incisão cirúrgica anterior)
Origem hepatobiliar	Abscesso hepático, torção/isquemia do lobo hepático com colonização bacteriana, rompimento do trato biliar (causado por colecistite séptica necrosante, iatrogênica ou trauma contuso), pancreatite séptica necrosante ou abscesso pancreático
Origem urogenital	Uroperitônio séptico, abscesso renal, piometra, ruptura uterina, torção/isquemia uterina com colonização bacteriana, reprodução traumática, abscesso prostático
Origem hemolinfática	Abscesso esplênico, torção/isquemia esplênica com colonização bacteriana, abscesso do linfonodo mesentérico
Feridas penetrantes	Feridas de mordida, feridas de arma de fogo, trauma veicular
Cirúrgica iatrogênica	Contaminação peritoneal cirúrgica
Diálise peritoneal ou drenagem abdominal (sucção fechada, abdome aberto)	Se ascendente, infecção bacteriana/fúngica

*Agentes mais comuns.

ACHADOS HISTÓRICOS, SINAIS CLÍNICOS E EXAME FÍSICO

Os sinais podem ajudar a priorizar as prováveis causas de peritonite. Animais jovens são mais propensos a ter obstrução por corpo estranho ou doenças infecciosas, enquanto as neoplasias são mais prováveis em pacientes geriátricos. Em pacientes sexualmente intactos, prostatite e piometra são diferenciais. Cães de raças grandes e gigantes são predispostos a vólvulo intestinal e gástrico. As informações históricas pertinentes a serem coletadas em todos os casos incluem: exposição a toxinas, alimentação inadequada, possível ingestão de corpo estranho, outros animais da casa afetados, condições médicas preexistentes (p. ex., tumor de mastócitos), medicamentos atuais (drogas anti-inflamatórias não esteroides [AINEs], glicocorticoides), história de trauma ou cirurgia gastrintestinal recente, exposição a outros animais, progressão e duração dos sinais clínicos (agudos *versus* crônicos) e revisão dos sistemas.

Os sinais clínicos podem ser variáveis e não específicos, dependendo da causa. Os sinais podem incluir anorexia, letargia, depressão, fraqueza, colapso, vômito, diarreia, poliúria/polidipsia, disúria, anúria, hematúria e secreção vulvar ou prepucial. Em um estudo recente, apenas 48% dos gatos com peritonite tinham histórico de vômito; depressão/letargia e anorexia foram os mais achados comuns.[26] Anormalidades no exame físico podem incluir evidências de derrame peritoneal (abdome distendido, onda de fluido no balotamento [ver Capítulo 17]); sinais compatíveis com a síndrome da resposta inflamatória sistêmica (SIRS), como taquicardia/bradicardia, taquipneia, pirexia/hipotermia e leucocitose/leucopenia; e sinais clínicos compatíveis com estados progressivos de choque. Outras descobertas podem incluir feridas, hérnias, icterícia e dor abdominal. Cães são mais propensos do que os gatos a apresentarem sinais de dor abdominal.[5] Em dois estudos recentes, apenas cerca de metade dos gatos com peritonite exibiu sinais de dor abdominal.[24,26]

DIAGNÓSTICO

A história e o exame físico costumam orientar o diagnóstico inicial, mas a análise do fluido peritoneal é provavelmente o teste de diagnóstico mais determinante. A abdominocentese pode ser feita às cegas, se grandes volumes de fluido estão presentes, ou com orientação de ultrassom para volumes menores. Orientação por ultrassom, amostragem de quatro quadrantes, ou da lavagem peritoneal diagnóstica (ver Capítulo 90) aumentam a taxa de sucesso e rendimento. A análise do fluido peritoneal inclui avaliação da aparência bruta (cor, caráter), concentração de proteína, gravidade específica e exame citológico (ver Capítulo 74). Análise bioquímica (glicose, bilirrubina, creatinina, potássio) da efusão pode ajudar a diferenciar as causas subjacentes em alguns pacientes.

Na maioria dos pacientes com peritonite, o fluido será um exsudato (proteína > 3,5 g/dℓ [> 35 g/ℓ]; contagem de células nucleadas > 5.000/μℓ). O fluido de um abdome séptico é um exsudato com predominância de neutrófilos degenerados e organismos infecciosos, como bactérias intracelulares. A precisão do exame citológico do fluido para o diagnóstico de peritonite séptica variou de 57 a 100%;[5,21,38,39] uma terapia antibiótica anterior ou localização da coleta da amostra podem resultar em falsos negativos. A contagem de células nucleadas no fluido peritoneal é considerada uma das mais confiáveis variáveis para o diagnóstico de derrame séptico em cães e gatos.[38] Em um estudo, uma contagem de células nucleadas do fluido peritoneal (predominantemente neutrófilos) > 13.000 células/μℓ foi 86% sensível e 100% específico em cães, e 100% sensível e 100% específica em gatos para o diagnóstico de derrame séptico.[38] Uma diferença de mais de 20 mg/dℓ (> 1,1 mmol/ℓ) na glicose de amostras pareadas de sangue e líquido peritoneal foi 100% sensível e 100% específica para o diagnóstico de peritonite séptica em cães, e 86% sensível e 100% específico em gatos. Uma diferença de lactato menor que 2 mmol/ℓ entre o sangue e o fluido peritoneal foi preditiva de peritonite séptica em cães (63% de sensibilidade, 100% de especificidade); essa mesma associação não foi demonstrada em gatos.[38] Levin *et al.* descobriram que todos os cães com efusões sépticas tinham um lactato do líquido peritoneal maior que 2,5 mmol/ℓ.[39] A diferença de glicose e lactato entre o sangue e fluido peritoneal pode não ser tão confiável para o diagnóstico de peritonite séptica no pós-operatório ao avaliar líquido abdominal coletado de drenos de sucção fechados.[40]

Cães com neoplasia tiveram concentrações significativamente mais baixas de glicose e níveis mais elevados de lactato em seu fluido abdominal do que cães sem neoplasia.[41] As concentrações

de proteína do líquido peritoneal não distinguem de forma confiável efusão séptica e não séptica em cães ou gatos. Cultura bacteriana de microrganismos aeróbios e anaeróbios e perfil de sensibilidade de cepas isoladas de derrame abdominal obtido no momento do diagnóstico preliminar e antes de o início da antibioticoterapia são recomendados em casos de suspeita de peritonite séptica. Uroperitônio é diagnosticado se a concentração de creatinina no fluido peritoneal exceder a concentração sérica em mais de 2 vezes, ou se a concentração de potássio no fluido peritoneal excede a concentração de potássio sérico por um fator de mais de 1,4 (cães) ou 1,9 (gatos).[34-37] A peritonite biliar é diagnosticada se a concentração de bilirrubina no líquido peritoneal exceder a concentração de bilirrubina sérica em mais que 2 vezes; o exame citológico pode revelar pigmento biliar ou cristais.[31]

Um hemograma completo, perfil bioquímico sérico, gasometria arterial (ver Capítulo 128) e painel de coagulação (ver Capítulo 196) são recomendados para orientar o tratamento. Esses testes contribuem com informações de prognóstico, mas os resultados podem ser inespecíficos e variar com a etiologia. Anormalidades no hemograma completo podem incluir neutrofilia marcada com desvio à esquerda, alterações tóxicas e anemia, especialmente em gatos. Em um estudo de gatos com peritonite séptica, neutrófilos imaturos foi identificada em 64%, leucócitos tóxicos em 36% e anemia em 35%.[24] Leucopenia e neutrofilia acentuadas foram associadas a aumento da mortalidade em gatos.[42] A gravidade de uma mudança degenerativa à esquerda é significativamente associada ao desfecho (risco de morte ou eutanásia) em cães e gatos com peritonite séptica.[43,44]

Anormalidades comuns em perfis de bioquímica sérica e gasometria incluem acidose metabólica com hiperlactatemia; hipocalcemia; hiperpotassemia (uroperitônio); hiperglicemia seguida de hipoglicemia (gatos > cães > humanos); hipoalbuminemia; atividades de enzimas hepáticas elevadas e hiperbilirrubinemia e azotemia de origem pré-renal, renal (lesão renal aguda) ou pósrenal (uroperitônio). Concentração elevada de lactato plasmático na admissão, depuração fraca de lactato e hiperlactatemia pós-operatória persistente estão associadas a aumento da mortalidade e morbidade em cães com peritonite séptica (ver Capítulo 70).[45] A hipocalcemia é comum em pacientes graves, incluindo aqueles com peritonite séptica, mas o mecanismo fisiopatológico ainda não foi claramente estabelecido. Hipocalcemia persistente durante a hospitalização pode ser um indicador de prognóstico negativo em cães e gatos com peritonite séptica.[46,47] Pacientes com uroperitônio desenvolvem hiperpotassemia porque a urina, que é rica em potássio, acumula-se na cavidade abdominal e o potássio é reabsorvido na circulação sistêmica pelo peritônio; podem ocorrer arritmias cardíacas com risco de vida (ver Capítulo 248).[35,37] Efusões peritoniais têm sido associadas a uma diminuição da razão sódio: potássio (Na: K).[48,49] Os mecanismos propostos incluem a diminuição do volume circulante efetivo devido à perda de fluido rico em sódio e subsequente ativação do sistema da renina-angiotensina-aldosterona (SRRA) e liberação de hormônio antidiurético (ADH). A diminuição da liberação de sódio para os túbulos renais distais e a diminuição da caliurese podem diminuir a razão Na: K.[50] Anormalidades na concentração de glicose no sangue podem ser uma característica da peritonite. Em um estudo de gatos com peritonite séptica, a hipoglicemia foi identificada em 10, e hiperglicemia em 6, de 46 pacientes.[24] A hipoalbuminemia é comum na peritonite séptica e não séptica e tem sido relatada como uma complicação de drenagem peritoneal aberta em cães e gatos.[24] O aumento das atividades de alanina aminotransferase (ALT) e gamaglutamil transferase (GGT) está associado ao aumento da mortalidade em cães com peritonite difusa tratada com drenagem peritoneal aberta.[20] Hiperbilirrubinemia pode ser observada em cães e gatos com várias causas de peritonite, especialmente peritonite biliar ou pancreatite.

Na presença de bacteriúria e piúria em uma amostra de urina, devem-se solicitar cultura e antibiograma de urina, uma vez que as bactérias na urina podem ser semelhantes às encontradas no fluido peritoneal se ele for séptico. Com sepse grave, pode haver prolongamento dos tempos de coagulação (TP e TTPa), trombocitopenia, diminuição do fibrinogênio, elevação em produtos de degradação de fibrina e D-Dímeros, e/ou diminuição dos níveis de antitrombina (AT), compatível com coagulação intravascular disseminada (ver Capítulo 197). Deficiências das proteínas C e AT e hipercoagulabilidade parecem ser características compatíveis com a sepse canina de ocorrência natural e poderiam ser indicadores prognósticos úteis na peritonite séptica canina.[51] Testes auxiliares, como imunoensaios de lipase específica do pâncreas (PLI), podem ser úteis na avaliação da pancreatite (ver Capítulos 289, 290 e 291) como uma possível causa de peritonite.

As imagens abdominais podem ajudar no diagnóstico da peritonite. As radiografias de investigação podem mostrar perda local ou generalizada de detalhes, evidência de vólvulo ou torção, um corpo estranho GI ou evidência de obstrução mecânica, efeito de massa, prostatomegalia, piometra ou pneumoperitônio. Ruptura GI secundária a dilatação volvulogástrica, neoplasia, AINEs ou glicocorticoides foram responsáveis pela maioria dos casos de pneumoperitônio espontâneo em um estudo.[52] A radiografia de feixe horizontal é mais sensível para detecção de pequenos volumes de gás e pode ajudar a diferenciar as bolhas de gás sobrepostas ao trato GI.[52] Pneumoperitônio idiopático é um diagnóstico de exclusão quando a doença intra-abdominal está ausente e é considerada um distúrbio não cirúrgico.[53-56] A ultrassonografia abdominal pode mostrar derrame peritoneal localizado, definir uma etiologia subjacente da peritonite e ajuda a orientar a amostragem de fluido abdominal (ver Capítulos 88 e 89). A radiografia de contraste pode avaliar o trato gastrintestinal superior e avaliar a integridade de tubos de gastrostomia ou jejunostomia; urografia excretora ou cistouretrografia podem confirmar uroperitônio. Tomografia computadorizada de múltiplos detectores e aprimorada com contraste (CE-MDCT), quando disponível, pode ser realizada com segurança e com sucesso em pacientes com condições abdominais agudas, acordados ou levemente sedados[57] e podem diferenciar com precisão condições abdominais agudas cirúrgicas de não cirúrgicas em cães (ver Capítulo 143).[58]

TRATAMENTO

Estabilização médica

Os objetivos do tratamento médico são restaurar um volume de circulação satisfatório, corrigir distúrbios acidobásicos, equilibrar o balanço eletrolítico e minimizar a contaminação em progresso. Os pacientes podem se apresentar em vários graus de choque hipovolêmico (ver Capítulo 127) e requerem fluidoterapia com cristaloides e/ou coloides (ver Capítulo 129) e hemoderivados (ver Capítulo 130). Os objetivos durante as primeiras 6 horas de reidratação usando a abordagem da fluidoterapia dirigida por objetivos iniciais são: pressão arterial média (PAM) ≥ 65 mmHg (ver Capítulo 99), pressão venosa central (PVC) 8 a 12 mmHg (ver Capítulo 76), débito urinário ≥ 0,5 mℓ/kg/h (ver Capítulo 106), saturação venosa central de oxigênio ≥ 70% (ver Capítulo 98) e lactato < 2 mmol/dℓ (ver Capítulo 70).[59-62] A fluidoterapia é iniciada com pequenos *bolus* (10 a 20 mℓ/kg durante 5 a 15 min) de cristaloides isotônicos, exceto em doença cardíaca primária clinicamente significativa. Da mesma forma, coloides sintéticos podem ser administrados em dosagens de 5 mℓ/kg ao longo de 5 a 10 min e/ou solução salina hipertônica (cloreto de sódio 7 a 7,5%) administrada em 4 a 6 mℓ/kg.[63,64] Vasoativos, como a norepinefrina, epinefrina, vasopressina e dopamina são recomendados para choque que não responde à fluidoterapia; norepinefrina é o vasoconstritor de primeira linha para choque séptico.[65] Eletrólitos (potássio, fosfato, magnésio) e glicose podem ser suplementados se indicado. A administração

de albumina pode ser necessária em pacientes hipoalbuminêmicos com diminuição da pressão coloidosmótica (ver Capítulo 130). A necessidade de administrar grandes volumes de plasma para aumentar as concentrações de albumina circulante torna as fontes de albumina concentradas preferidas, a menos que não estejam disponíveis. A albumina sérica humana (soluções a 5 e 25%) tem sido transfundida com segurança em pacientes gravemente enfermos, incluindo aqueles com peritonite, para aumentar as concentrações de albumina e pressão sanguínea sistêmica.[66,67] A albumina canina liofilizada (5%) tem sido administrada em cães hipoalbuminêmicos após tratamento cirúrgico para peritonite séptica.[68]

O monitoramento intensivo pode ser necessário para pacientes hemodinamicamente instáveis. Cateteres arteriais (ver Capítulo 75) permitem a avaliação da gasometria e o monitoramento contínuo da pressão sanguínea. Cateteres venosos centrais jugulares, ou cateteres centrais inseridos perifericamente (ver Capítulo 76), permitem a medição da pressão venosa central e auxiliam na avaliação se um paciente recebeu um volume adequado de fluido ou está sobrecarregado de fluido. A medição de pressão venosa central pode ajudar a determinar quando os vasoconstritores são necessários além da fluidoterapia. Cateteres urinários (ver Capítulo 106) permitem a avaliação da produção de urina e o monitoramento das necessidades de fluidos, e podem ser usados para separação de urina em pacientes com uroperitônio. A administração de sangue total fresco, concentração de hemácias e plasma pode ser indicada em pacientes com anemia ou coagulopatias (ver Capítulo 130).

Início precoce e seleção apropriada de terapia antimicrobiana de amplo espectro são importantes na peritonite séptica. Os antimicrobianos devem ser, provavelmente, eficazes contra as bactérias que causam choque séptico (predominantemente *E. coli*, *Clostridium* spp. e *Enterococcus* spp.[21]), ter boa penetração em tecidos presumivelmente infectados e ser administrados por via intravenosa na primeira hora após a sepse grave ou o choque séptico terem sido reconhecidos (ver Capítulo 161). O controle da fonte deve ser tentado em 6 horas.[65] Após o início da terapia com antibióticos de amplo espectro, o regime de antibióticos deve ser revisto com base na condição do paciente e nos resultados da cultura e antibiograma, para reduzir a terapia o menor número de drogas e menor dosagem necessária (escalonamento do antibiótico).[65] Para infecção adquirida na comunidade sem evidência de insuficiência renal, é recomendada a combinação de amicacina (15 mg/kg IV a cada 24 horas) e clindamicina (12 mg/kg IV a cada 12 horas). Se houver evidência de insuficiência renal, é recomendada uma cefalosporina de terceira geração, como cefotaxima (22 mg/kg IV a cada 8 horas), no lugar da amicacina. Se a suspeita for infecção por *Enterococcus*, é recomendada a inclusão de ampicilina (22 mg/kg IV a cada 8 horas) em qualquer um dos regimes anteriores.[69]

Tratamento: estabilização cirúrgica

A necessidade de tratamento cirúrgico depende da causa base da peritonite. A intervenção cirúrgica imediata pode não ser necessária para peritonite bacteriana primária, idiopática, pneumoperitônio e uroperitônio.[12,13,37,53-56] Metas cirúrgicas para peritonite séptica são exploração abdominal, eliminação da fonte de contaminação, desbridamento de material necrótico, reparo, lavagem e drenagem. A colocação de um tubo de alimentação deve ser considerada durante a exploração cirúrgica inicial (ver Capítulo 82). O omento deve ser preservado para suas funções benéficas, incluindo drenagem de fluidos, adesão, angiogênese e atividade imunológica.[1] Não há diferença relatada no resultado do gerenciamento da drenagem da peritonite séptica aberta, fechada ou de sucção fechada.[20-23,29,70,71] O fechamento primário sem drenagem é recomendado se a fonte de contaminação puder ser controlada com reparo, desbridamento e lavagem.[22] A drenagem de abdome aberto e drenos de sucção fechados são recomendados se o desbridamento e a lavagem não puderem remover o material infeccioso e estranho, ou se a fonte de contaminação não puder ser reparada. O fechamento de um abdome aberto normalmente pode ser realizado 3 a 5 dias após a cirurgia inicial. Desvantagens da drenagem peritoneal aberta são perda de grandes quantidades de líquido e proteínas plasmáticas da cavidade peritoneal, evisceração de órgãos abdominais, infecções nosocomiais, necessidade de cuidados intensivos de enfermagem, adesão de vísceras ao material de bandagem, persistência da peritonite e sepse.[20,23] O fechamento assistido a vácuo tem sido usado com sucesso na medicina veterinária para o tratamento da peritonite séptica (Vídeo 279.1).[70,71]

CUIDADOS PÓS-OPERATÓRIOS

O manejo pós-operatório abrangente e monitoramento intensivo em pacientes criticamente enfermos com peritonite podem ser necessários. A colocação de um cateter arterial, cateter venoso central e cateter urinário permitirá um monitoramento mais adequado. Um cateter urinário pode ser usado para medir a pressão intra-abdominal, usando a técnica intravesicular, para prevenir a síndrome do compartimento abdominal.[72] O monitoramento da telemetria cardíaca fornece informações sobre a frequência cardíaca e arritmias cardíacas que possam necessitar de tratamento (ver Capítulo 248). O manejo da drenagem abdominal consiste em manter locais de saída limpos, monitorando e registrando o volume e o aspecto da drenagem, e exames citológicos em série do fluido. O clínico deve monitorar o fluido que "entra" e o que "sai" perdido na urina, curativos e drenagem, e ajustar a fluidoterapia adequadamente. A analgesia é predominantemente fornecida por uma taxa de infusão constante de opioides, mas analgesia multimodal com cetamina, lidocaína, anestésicos locais, dexmedetomidina e infusão peridural contínua pode ser necessária para controlar a dor (ver Capítulo 126). Nutrição enteral precoce via nasoesofágica, tubos de alimentação nasogástrica, esofagostomia ou gastrostomia são indicados em pacientes criticamente enfermos (ver Capítulo 82). Possíveis complicações da alimentação enteral incluem vômitos/regurgitação, diarreia, distúrbios eletrolíticos/acidobásicos e mau funcionamento do tubo de alimentação (obstrução, deslocamento, infecção do local de saída). A nutrição parenteral (ver Capítulo 189) pode ser fornecida através de uma veia central (nutrição parenteral total) ou veia periférica (nutrição parenteral periférica ou parcial). A nutrição parenteral está associada a maiores complicações metabólicas, e cuidados intensivos de enfermagem são necessários para administração asséptica.[73] Um estudo em cães que sobreviveram à peritonite séptica demonstrou que a nutrição precoce (dentro de 24 h após a hospitalização para ambas as vias parenteral e enteral) foi associada a uma duração de hospitalização significativamente menor (em torno de 1,6 dia).[74] Outros cuidados pós-operatórios específicos podem ser direcionados para o tratamento de complicações secundárias, incluindo anemia (ver Capítulo 198), síndrome da resposta inflamatória sistêmica (ver Capítulo 132), coagulopatia intravascular disseminada (ver Capítulo 197), pneumonia por aspiração (ver Capítulo 242), pancreatite (ver Capítulos 290 e 291), vasculite e disfunção de múltiplos órgãos (lesão renal aguda, disfunção hepática e colestase, síndrome da angústia respiratória aguda).

PROGNÓSTICO

O prognóstico associado à peritonite varia de acordo com a etiologia, espécie, população de pacientes, comorbidades e manejo clínico ou cirúrgico de casos. As taxas de sobrevivência geral para animais com peritonite séptica são relatadas entre 47 e 85% em cães[12,16,18,20-23,25,29,68-70] e 44 e 71% em gatos.[12,13,16,21,23,24,28] Indicadores de mau prognóstico na peritonite séptica incluem altas atividades de enzimas hepáticas séricas (GGT, ALT),[20] hipotensão refratária, colapso cardiovascular, coagulopatia intravascular disseminada, disfunção pulmonar e disfunção de múltiplos órgãos.[15,75] A taxa de sobrevivência geral para cães com peritonite séptica biliar é 27 a 45% e 87 a 100% para peritonite biliar não séptica.[30,31] A taxa de sobrevivência relatada em um estudo de gatos com uroperitônio sem lesões traumáticas concomitantes foi de aproximadamente 62%; não há estudos correspondentes para cães.[34] Um resultado favorável para pacientes com peritonite depende do reconhecimento precoce, estabilização médica intensiva, controle da fonte usando gerenciamento cirúrgico quando necessário e cuidados pós-operatórios abrangentes.

REFERÊNCIAS BIBLIOGRÁFICAS

As referências bibliográficas deste capítulo se encontram online no Ambiente de Aprendizagem.

SEÇÃO 19
Doenças Hepatobiliares

CAPÍTULO 280

Avaliação Diagnóstica da Função Hepática

Sarah Cocker e Keith Richter

INTRODUÇÃO

O fígado possui função fundamental em diversos processos biológicos essenciais à vida. As principais funções do fígado são: imunorregulação; armazenamento de vitaminas, oligoelementos minerais, glicogênio, sangue e triglicerídeos; detoxificação e excreção de toxinas e outras substâncias; funções digestivas; e metabolismo de carboidratos, lipídios, proteínas, vitaminas e hormônios endócrinos.[1] O fígado possui uma capacidade de regeneração notável após perda funcional significativa. O fígado de ratos pode se regenerar ao seu tamanho original após remoção de até 70% do órgão, dentro de 5 a 7 dias.[2] Entretanto, hepatopatias associadas a fibrose, inflamação ou infecções virais prejudicam esse processo regenerativo e a função hepática é deteriorada.[2] Como o fígado possui tamanha capacidade de regeneração, sintomas mais específicos de hepatopatias, tais como icterícia, ascite, tendências hemorrágicas, hipoglicemia e encefalopatia hepática (EH), geralmente não ocorrem até os estágios finais de um processo mórbido. Os sinais clínicos iniciais de hepatopatia, como êmese, diarreia, letargia, poliúria (PU), polidipsia (PD) e inapetência, são extremamente inespecíficos. Dessa forma, o diagnóstico de doenças hepatobiliares primárias pode ser desafiador. Uma abordagem lógica, que compreenda a resenha do paciente, bem como o histórico clínico, os achados de exame físico, as anormalidades bioquímicas e hematológicas, os resultados de exames de imagem e de amostras obtidas por meio de biopsia hepática, deve ser utilizada para a obtenção do diagnóstico.

RESENHA E HISTÓRICO CLÍNICO (ANAMNESE)

Predisposição racial

Para algumas hepatopatias existem fortes predisposições raciais que podem ajudar a levantar a suspeita de doença hepatobiliar, mesmo na presença de sinais iniciais inespecíficos, assim como suspeita de hepatopatias específicas. Em outras situações, o histórico é geralmente muito sugestivo de uma hepatopatia específica. Por exemplo, gatos de meia-idade com sobrepeso e histórico recente de perda de peso e anorexia devem levantar a suspeita de lipidose hepática felina (LHF).[3] O acúmulo de cobre

nos hepatócitos pode ser secundário ao aumento da ingestão, a anormalidades primárias no metabolismo hepático de cobre ou à alteração na excreção biliar de cobre.[4] Achados histopatológicos em pacientes com distúrbios hereditários de armazenamento de cobre mostram acúmulo de cobre na região centrolobular, enquanto em pacientes com acúmulo de cobre secundário à colestase, o cobre é encontrado no parênquima periporta.[4,5] Ao mesmo tempo que existem diversas raças predispostas à doença por acúmulo de cobre, como cães Labrador Retriever, Doberman Pinscher, Dálmata, Skye Terrier e West Highland White Terrier, a mutação específica do gene (COMMD1) somente foi constatada em cães da raça Bedlington Terrier.[4] O acúmulo de cobre nos hepatócitos pode começar em pacientes com menos de 1 ano de idade, mas eles não apresentam sinais clínicos até que estejam com pelo menos alguns anos de vida.[4] Nas raças Doberman e Labrador parece que as fêmeas são mais predispostas.[4] A doença por acúmulo de cobre também já foi diagnosticada em gatos, com possível predisposição nas raças Siamês e Pelo Curto Europeu.[4] A hepatite idiopática crônica já foi descrita como relacionada às raças Labrador Retriever, Poodle Standard, Doberman Pinscher, Cocker Spaniel Americano e Inglês, e Springer Spaniel Inglês (no Reino Unido).[4,6,7] Com frequência, a hepatite crônica é observada simultaneamente ao acúmulo de cobre em cães das raças Labrador e Doberman Pinscher. A amiloidose hepática já foi documentada em gatos Abissínios, Orientais e Siameses, bem como em cães Shar-pei chineses.[8,9]

Desvios (*shunts*) portossistêmicos

Desvios portossistêmicos (DPS) podem ser congênitos ou adquiridos (ver Capítulo 284). Os DPS congênitos geralmente ocorrem em um único vaso intra ou extra-hepático. Cães com DPS extra-hepático congênito geralmente são de raças puras de tamanho pequeno e *toy*. As raças mais comumente afetadas são Yorkshire Terrier, Bichon Havanês, Maltês, Dandie Dimont Terrier, Pug e Schnauzer.[10] A maioria dos DPS intra-hepáticos é observada em raças de cães de porte maior, sendo mais prevalente em Lébrel Irlandês, Labrador e Golden Retriever, Boiadeiro Australiano e Pastor-Australiano.[10] Em gatos, os DPS tendem a ser extra-hepáticos, e as raças mais acometidas incluem Gato Doméstico de Pelo Curto, Persa, Siamês, Himalaio e Birmanês.[10] A maioria dos animais com DPS congênito, por ocasião da consulta, tem menos que 1 ou 2 anos de idade, mas podem não manifestar sinais clínicos até que sejam muito mais velhos. Foi relatado que a idade média de animais com DPS extra-hepático adquirido múltiplo foi de 3 anos no momento da consulta. Esses animais normalmente possuem baixa estatura, com histórico de apatia ou letargia em alguns momentos. Eles podem ter um histórico de intolerância a anestésicos, perda de peso, ataxia e comportamento bizarro (cegueira intermitente, pressão da cabeça contra obstáculo imóvel, progressão obstinada em paredes ou cantos, andar compulsivo, latidos aleatórios ou agressividade).[10] A associação entre a ingestão da refeição e o início dos sintomas foi relatada em 30 a 50% dos pacientes.[11] Histórico de sintomas gastrintestinais, PU/PD e sintomas relativos ao trato urinário inferior também é relativamente comum. Em gatos, a coloração da íris pelo cobre, inapropriada para a raça, foi documentada (Figura 280.1).[12]

Outras hepatopatias

Pacientes com hipoplasia de veia porta (HPV) congênita sem a constatação macroscópica de *shunt* (também conhecida como displasia microvascular ou DMV) apresentam sinais mais tardiamente, raramente desenvolvem sinais clínicos e possuem excelente prognóstico a longo prazo (ver Capítulo 284). Cães das raças Maltese, Cairn e Yorkshire Terrier são raças predispostas à DMV.[13-15] A idade média desses pacientes no momento da consulta é de 3,25 anos, mas pode variar até 10 anos de idade.[13] A hepatopatia vacuolar progressiva é reconhecida como uma doença relacionada à raça em cães Scottish Terrier.[15,16] Um estudo recente demonstrou que a hepatopatia vacuolar nessa raça pode estar relacionada à esteroidogênese adenal e predisposição a carcinoma hepatocelular.[16]

Obtenção de informações gerais

Informações pertinentes sobre o histórico clínico incluem medicamentos utilizados atualmente, assim como exposição a drogas, toxinas, nutracêuticos e suplementos que podem ser mantidos em casa; o ambiente do paciente, que inclui períodos de supervisão a passeios; exposição a toxinas ambientais e microrganismos infecciosos; histórico de viagens; e estado vacinal. No Boxe 280.1 há uma lista de hepatotoxinas comuns. No Boxe 280.2 há uma lista de microrganismos infecciosos comuns que acometem o fígado. Gatos de meia-idade com sobrepeso e histórico recente de perda de peso e anorexia devem levantar suspeita de lipidose hepática felina (LHF).[3]

Boxe 280.1 Hepatotoxinas comuns

Agentes ambientais
Cicadáceas
Cogumelos do gênero *Amanita*
Aflatoxina
Algas verde-azuladas

Aditivos alimentares
Xilitol

Produtos químicos
Metais pesados
Arsênico

Fármacos
Paracetamol
Amiodarona
Azatioprina
Carprofeno
Cetoconazol
Corticosteroides
Diazepam (oral; gatos)
Dietilcarbamazina – oxibendazol
Doxiciclina
Estanozolol (gatos)
Fenazopiridina
Fenobarbital
Griseofulvina (gatos)
Halotano
Lomustina
Mebendazol
Metimazol (gatos)
Metotrexato
Mitotano
Nitrofurantoína
Sulfonamidas
Tetraciclinas
Tiacetarsamida
Zonisamida

Boxe 280.2 Microrganismos infecciosos que comumente afetam o fígado

- Bactérias
  - *Leptospira*
  - *Mycobacterium tuberculosis*
  - *Escherichia coli*
  - *Clostridium perfringens*
- Vírus
  - Adenovírus canino 1
- Fungos
  - *Blastomyces dermatitidis*
  - *Cryptococcus neoformans*
  - *Histoplasma capsulatum*
  - *Coccidioides immitis*
- Parasitas
  - *Platynosomum fastosum*
  - Toxoplasma
  - Schistosoma
  - Larva migrans.

ACHADOS DE EXAME FÍSICO

Icterícia

Uma das manifestações mais comuns de doenças hepatobiliares é a icterícia. As membranas mucosas mais acessíveis à inspeção em busca de icterícia ao exame físico são esclera, terceira pálpebra, palato mole e sublingual (Figura 280.2). Geralmente, a icterícia não pode ser detectada até que a concentração sérica de bilirrubina seja superior a 3 mg/dℓ (frequentemente até 5 mg/dℓ). Entretanto, o plasma visivelmente ictérico (observado em tubo capilar de hematócrito), ou soro sanguíneo, pode ser observado quando a concentração de bilirrubina estiver acima de 0,5 a 1 mg/dℓ. Uma discussão sobre bilirrubina é encontrada posteriormente neste capítulo.

Sintomas dermatológicos

A síndrome hepatocutânea é uma forma de dermatite necrolítica superficial relatada em alguns cães e gatos com hepatopatia (ver Capítulo 285). Tipicamente se manifesta em cães na forma de hiperqueratose e subsequente formação de crostas e fissuras nos coxins plantares. Eritema, erosões ou ulcerações, secreção serosa a purulenta, crostas e placas hiperqueratóticas podem ser

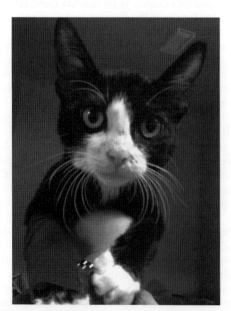

Figura 280.1 Gato com íris cuja cor se deve ao cobre, em caso de desvio portossistêmico congênito. (*Esta figura se encontra reproduzida em cores no Encarte.*)

observadas em outros locais, inclusive na pele perioral, perianal, perivulvar, prepucial e escrotal.[17] Em gatos, pode não surgir lesão nos coxins, como acontece em cães. Ulceração e formação de crostas em junções orais mucocutâneas e ulceração nas pinas, áreas perioculares, áreas interdigitais, parte ventral do abdome e região inguinal, com ou sem formação de crostas, são observadas em gatos.[17]

Ascite

Ascite é o acúmulo de líquido livre na cavidade abdominal (ver Capítulo 17). Cães e gatos com ascite grave podem apresentar distensão abdominal (Figura 280.3) e ter baloteamento positivo à palpação abdominal (ver Capítulo 17). Na hepatopatia, a ascite se deve tipicamente à hipertensão portal (HP), embora a diminuição da pressão oncótica vascular causada por hipoalbuminemia também possa participar de sua fisiopatogênese. A ascite também pode ser secundária à ruptura de vesícula biliar ou efusão oriunda de neoplasias hepáticas (inclusive hemoabdome). A ascite secundária unicamente à diminuição da pressão oncótica geralmente não ocorre até que a concentração sérica de albumina seja < 1,5 g/dℓ.[18] A hipertensão portal ocorre secundariamente ao aumento da resistência e/ou do fluxo sanguíneo na circulação porta.[19] As causas de HP são classificadas com base na localização anatômica como pré-hepáticas, intra-hepáticas ou pós-hepáticas.[19-24] As causas pré-hepáticas se devem ao aumento da resistência da veia porta extra-hepática e estão associadas à obstrução mural ou intraluminal (p. ex., atresia congênita ou fibrose, trombose, neoplasia) ou compressão extraluminal.[5,20,25-31] Fístulas arteriovenosas hepáticas também causam HP pré-hepática (ver Capítulo 284).[5,32-34] Pacientes com HP pré-hepática geralmente são jovens e apresentam ascite e sinais de encefalopatia hepática.[19] A HP intra-hepática ocorre em razão do aumento da resistência nos afluentes microscópicos da veia porta, sinusoides ou pequenas veias hepáticas.[19] A HP intra-hepática é ainda classificada em pré-sinusoidal, sinusoidal e pós-sinusoidal.[19] Hepatite crônica com fibrose ou cirrose é a causa mais comum de HP intra-hepática. A HP pós-hepática ocorre secundariamente à obstrução de veias hepáticas maiores, como a veia cava caudal pós-hepática ou do átrio direito.[19] Exemplos de HP pós-hepática incluem insuficiência cardíaca direita, doença pericárdica, hipertensão pulmonar e síndrome de Budd-Chiari.[35-38] O acúmulo de líquido ascítico secundário à HP pré-hepática e pré-sinusoidal, e possivelmente HP intra-hepática sinusoidal possui baixa concentração de proteína (< 2,5 g/dℓ), enquanto o acúmulo de fluido ascítico secundário à HP pós-hepática, pós-sinusoidal e sinusoidal intra-hepática tem alta concentração de proteína (> 2,5 g/dℓ).[19] A hipertensão portal também pode levar ao desenvolvimento de desvios (*shunts*) portossistêmicos adquiridos múltiplos (DPSAM) e encefalopatia hepática.[19]

Encefalopatia hepática

A encefalopatia hepática (EH) é uma disfunção cerebral secundária à disfunção hepática (ver Capítulos 281 e 284).[39] Esta síndrome ocorre menos comumente em gatos do que em cães.[18] A patogênese da EH é multifatorial e está associada a toxinas oriundas do trato gastrintestinal que desviam da metabolização hepática.[19] A amônia é uma das mais importantes dessas toxinas. Outros produtos tóxicos incriminados na patogênese da EH incluem aminoácidos aromáticos, ácidos biliares, benzodiazepínicos endógenos, ácido gama-aminobutírico, glutamina, fenol, ácidos graxos de cadeia curta, triptofano, diminuição do alfacetoglutarato e falsos neurotransmissores.[10] Existem duas formas de EH: aguda e crônica. A forma aguda é causada por insuficiência hepática fulminante. Os animais acometidos geralmente morrem em poucos dias e a encefalopatia é grave.[18] A forma crônica é muito mais comum do que a aguda e o prognóstico é melhor, contanto que a doença hepática primária seja reversível.[39,40] A forma crônica é secundária a uma lesão na circulação portossistêmica colateral (DPS múltiplo adquirido ou DPS congênito).[18] A EH crônica também pode ser observada em gatos com lipidose hepática, pois gatos não são capazes de sintetizar arginina no fígado e a sua depleção ocorre após jejum prolongado. A arginina é necessária para a conclusão do ciclo da ureia e sem ela a detoxificação da amônia é prejudicada.[18]

Causas raras de EH crônica são anormalidades metabólicas congênitas, nas quais uma das enzimas envolvidas na metabolização da amônia está anormal.[18] Os sinais clínicos iniciais da EH são sutis e incluem apatia, indiferença e diminuição do estado de alerta. Em casos de doença mais grave e avançada, os sinais incluem ataxia, andar em círculos, pressão da cabeça contra objeto imóvel, sialorreia, estupor e coma. Convulsões são incomuns, mas podem ser observadas simultaneamente a outros sintomas de EH.[18] O teste de intolerância à amônia pode ser utilizado como método auxiliar para confirmação do diagnóstico de EH, caso a concentração de amônia não seja conclusiva e ainda persista a suspeita de EH. A execução desse teste é discutida na seção sobre amônia neste capítulo. Esse teste não é útil em pacientes com altos valores basais de amônia, pois nesse caso já há comprovação de EH.[41]

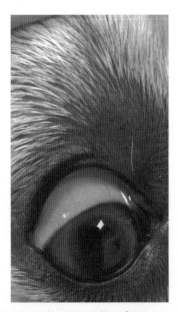

Figura 280.2 Cão com esclera ictérica. (*Esta figura se encontra reproduzida em cores no Encarte.*)

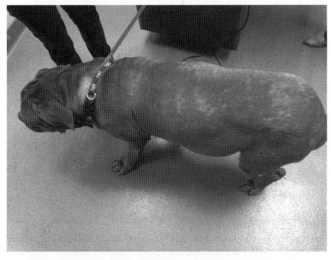

Figura 280.3 Cão com distensão abdominal causada por ascite.

AVALIAÇÃO LABORATORIAL DE DOENÇAS HEPATOBILIARES

Enzimas hepáticas (ver Capítulo 65)

Considerações gerais

A elevação da atividade sérica das enzimas hepáticas é frequentemente o primeiro achado que leva à suspeita da presença de doença hepatobiliar. As enzimas hepáticas avaliadas em perfis bioquímicos típicos incluem alanina aminotransferase (ALT), aspartato aminotransferase (AST), fosfatase alcalina (ALP) e gamaglutamil transpeptidase (ou transferase) (GGT). Essas enzimas refletem a integridade da membrana do hepatócito (ALT e AST), necrose do hepatócito ou do epitélio biliar (ALT e AST), colestase (ALP e GGT) ou mecanismo de indução (ALP e GGT).[42] O padrão de elevação de enzimas hepáticas pode ser útil para priorizar uma lista de diagnósticos diferenciais. As enzimas hepáticas são classificadas como enzimas de extravasamento hepatocelular (ALT, AST), o que indica lesão hepatocelular, e enzimas de indução (ALP, GGT), associadas ao aumento da síntese enzimática. A magnitude da elevação da enzima hepática é considerada discreta se for 5 vezes inferior ao maior valor de referência; moderada se o valor for 5 a 10 vezes superior ao maior valor da faixa de referência (ou de normalidade); e acentuadamente elevada se for mais que 10 vezes acima do maior valor da faixa de referência.[42] É importante lembrar que a atividade anormal de enzimas hepáticas é mais comum do que a presença de hepatopatias primárias, já que existem diversas outras condições clínicas que aumentam as atividades das enzimas hepáticas (Boxe 280.3). A elevação das atividades de enzimas hepáticas na ausência de lesão hepatobiliar pode ser consequência da administração exógena de corticosteroides ou de fenobarbital, aumento endógeno de corticosteroides, lesão em tecidos não hepáticos que também contêm essas enzimas (p. ex., isoenzima ALP óssea) e lesão secundária a dano em órgãos cuja drenagem sanguínea depende da veia porta, especialmente o trato gastrintestinal e o pâncreas. Este último processo é conhecido como hepatopatia reativa. Há também hepatopatias relevantes com atividades de enzimas hepáticas normais ou somente discretamente aumentadas. Estas incluem anormalidades vasculares (DPS e DMV), neoplasia hepática metastática (até metade desses casos podem ter atividades de enzimas hepáticas normais) e cirrose em estágio terminal (no qual há depleção enzimática).

Embora elevações nas atividades séricas de enzimas hepatobiliares sejam muito sensíveis na detecção de doenças hepatobiliares e a magnitude da elevação possa estar correlacionada ao grau de lesão, elas não são indicativas da capacidade funcional anabólica ou catabólica do fígado. Outros parâmetros bioquímicos e testes de função hepática precisam ser avaliados para determinar a capacidade funcional do fígado.

Boxe 280.3 Causas de elevação de enzimas hepáticas na ausência de doença hepatobiliar primária

Medicamento
Terapia glicocorticoide
Terapia com fenobarbital

Inflamação/Infecção
Pancreatite
Distúrbios gastrintestinais
Sepse
Infecções sistêmicas
Lesão muscular

Endocrinopatia
Hiperadrenocorticismo
Diabetes melito
Hipertireoidismo
Hipotireoidismo

Hipoxia
Insuficiência cardíaca congestiva
Status epilepticus
Hipotensão grave
Choque

Outras causas
Osteossarcoma ou outros tumores ósseos
Hemólise aguda grave
Síndrome pós-caval
Tumores mamários
Animal jovem em fase de crescimento
Erro laboratorial

Alanina aminotransferase e aspartato aminotransferase

Elevações nas atividades de ALT e AST ocorrem secundariamente ao extravasamento das enzimas a partir do hepatócito, após dano à sua membrana; assim, elas são denominadas enzimas de extravasamento hepatocelular. A meia-vida ($T_{1/2}$) da ALT é de 48 a 60 horas no cão e, presumivelmente, de cerca de 6 horas no gato.[43,44] A $T_{1/2}$ plasmática da AST é de aproximadamente 22 horas no cão e, de forma estimada, de 77 minutos no gato.[45,46] Normalmente, a atividade da ALT é mais elevada do que a atividade da AST, em parte devido a sua meia-vida mais longa. As enzimas de extravasamento hepatocelular estão presentes em altas concentrações no fígado, mas também em outros tecidos. A AST está presente em altas concentrações no fígado, no músculo e nas hemácias.[42] A ALT, entretanto, está presente essencialmente no fígado, em concentração muito maior do que no músculo.[42] Como a maior parte da ALT é encontrada no fígado, em comparação com outras enzimas hepatocelulares, é a mais específica das enzimas para lesão hepática. A avaliação da atividade sérica da creatinoquinase (CK) é geralmente útil para diferenciar elevações de ALT e AST devido à lesão muscular versus lesão hepática.[47] A atividade de CK aumenta rapidamente após lesão muscular, com valores máximos em aproximadamente 6 a 12 horas após a lesão, e decréscimo dentro de 24 a 48 horas, devido à sua curta meia-vida.[48] Elevações na atividade de AST são concomitantes às de ALT, mas em menor magnitude.[44] O aumento da atividade de AST acompanhado de ALT normal indica origem extra-hepática da enzima (músculo ou hemácia). Assim, se a atividade sérica de AST for maior do que a de ALT, a elevação da atividade sérica de CK corrobora a origem muscular de AST. Se a atividade sérica de CK for normal com um padrão de AST sérica maior do que de ALT sérica, a origem da AST de hemácias é outra possível explicação (como acontece em casos de hemólise in vitro ou in vivo).

A maior parte das enzimas ALT e AST está localizada na fração solúvel do citosol e cerca de 20% da AST é encontrada na mitocôndria.[42] A presença de uma fração de AST na mitocôndria é uma das razões pela qual sua atividade sérica é menos sensível do que a ALT na detecção de lesão hepática (além de sua meia-vida mais curta). Adicionalmente, como a AST é encontrada em alta concentração em outros órgãos, é menos específica do que a ALT no diagnóstico de lesões hepatocelulares. Os maiores incrementos de ALT ocorrem secundariamente à necrose hepatocelular e inflamação, enquanto elevações moderadas a graves podem ocorrer por conta de neoplasia hepática, doença do trato biliar (obstrutiva ou não obstrutiva) e cirrose.[42,49] Após lesão hepatocelular grave, a atividade de ALT geralmente aumenta de forma acentuada dentro de 24 a 48 horas, alcançando valores 10 a 100 vezes maiores do que o valor normal, com atividade máxima nos primeiros 5 dias após a lesão.[50-56] Na hepatopatia aguda, uma diminuição de 50% ou mais na atividade de ALT durante poucos dias (a meia-vida sérica da ALT) é considerada um bom sinal prognóstico.[42] É importante ressaltar, entretanto, que a diminuição das atividades de enzimas hepáticas pode representar uma diminuição na quantidade de hepatócitos viáveis durante hepatopatia crônica, intoxicação grave ou supressão de transaminase por toxinas (p. ex., microcistina, aflatoxina).[42] A hepatite crônica está associada a flutuações nas atividades de enzimas hepáticas. Conforme a lesão é sanada, a atividade sérica de ALT diminui, mas a de ALP pode aumentar devido ao processo proliferativo regenerativo.[42] Após necrose hepatocelular aguda grave, a atividade de AST aumenta sobremaneira nos primeiros 3 dias para valores 10 a 30 vezes acima da faixa de referência em cães, e até 50 vezes acima do valor de referência em gatos.[50,52,57] A administração de glicocorticoides a cães pode causar aumento discreto da atividade sérica de AST, que diminui várias semanas após a descontinuação da terapia glicocorticoide.[58]

Fosfatase alcalina

Ao contrário das enzimas hepáticas de extravasamento, a ALP está ligada a membranas celulares por ligações glicosil-fosfatidilinositol.[42] A liberação de ALP de sua ligação à membrana

CAPÍTULO 280 • Avaliação Diagnóstica da Função Hepática

celular é facilitada pela presença de ácidos biliares, que exercem um efeito semelhante a um detergente no local de ligação à membrana.[59,60] Incrementos na atividade sérica de ALT ocorrem secundariamente à nova síntese hepática ou eluição da enzima a partir da membrana celular. A elevação de ALP é a anormalidade mais comum no perfil bioquímico sérico de cães, e a das enzimas hepáticas é a que possui menor especificidade para doença hepatobiliar.[42] Em cães, a sensibilidade e a especificidade da elevação de ALP para doença hepatobiliar são de 80 e 51%, respectivamente.[44] Em cães, a fosfatase alcalina está presente em maior quantidade, em ordem decrescente, na mucosa intestinal, córtex renal, placenta, fígado e osso.[42] No gato é discutível quais tecidos contêm as maiores concentrações de ALP.[61-63] Existem três isoenzimas principais de ALP no soro sanguíneo de cães: de indução óssea (ALP-O), de indução hepática (ALP-H) e de indução por corticosteroides (ALP-C).[64-67] As isoenzimas intestinal, renal e placentária contribuem pouco, ou quase nada, para a elevação de FA no soro sanguíneo por apresentarem meias-vidas extremamente curtas.[42] Em cães adultos, a ALP-H e ALP-C são as principais responsáveis pela elevação da atividade sérica de ALP, enquanto em gatos adultos a isoenzima ALP-H é a principal.[42] A $T_{1/2}$ plasmática de ALP-H e ALP-C é de 70 horas no cão, enquanto a $T_{1/2}$ da isoenzima hepática é de somente 6 horas no gato.[61,68,69] Em cães, mas não em gatos, a atividade sérica total de ALP pode ser influenciada por esteroides exógenos ou endógenos e por alguns fármacos.[42] A mensuração da isoenzima específica ALP-C não é clinicamente útil para diferenciação entre doença hepatobiliar primária e efeitos de glicocorticoides endógenos ou exógenos, pois a atividade de ALP-C se eleva em várias hepatopatias primárias. Em gatos, a ALP é menos sensível (50%), porém mais específica (93%) para doenças hepatobiliares devido à sua curta meia-vida, pelo fato de que gatos não possuem ALP-C e porque os hepatócitos de felinos contêm menos ALP.[44] Elevações na atividade sérica de ALP-O se devem à sua liberação secundária ao crescimento e remodelamento ósseo em cães e gatos jovens, ou por condições patológicas, como osteomielite, osteossarcoma ou outros tumores ósseos, ou hiperparatireoidismo secundário renal.[42,61,64,69,70] A isoenzima ALP-O pode também contribuir significativamente para a elevação da atividade sérica de ALP notada em alguns gatos com hipertireoidismo.[63,70-72] Em cães, as maiores elevações da atividade sérica de ALP (até 100 vezes ou mais acima do normal) são observadas em distúrbios colestáticos, carcinoma hepatocelular grave, carcinoma de ductos biliares e após administração de glicocorticoides.[42]

Gamaglutamil transpeptidase (ou transferase)

Assim como a ALT, a GGT está ligada à membrana celular dos hepatócitos. A GGT em cães e gatos é encontrada em maiores concentrações nos rins e pâncreas, com menor quantidade no fígado, vesícula biliar, intestino, baço, coração, pulmões, músculo esquelético e eritrócitos.[73-75] A atividade sérica de GGT é majoritariamente oriunda do fígado, e o aumento de sua atividade sérica reflete o aumento da síntese hepática e eluição a partir da superfície da membrana celular.[42] Semelhante à sua influência na ALP, os glicocorticoides e outros indutores de enzimas microssomais podem estimular a produção de GGT em cães.[42] Em cães, a sensibilidade e especificidade da GGT para detecção de doenças hepatobiliares são de 50 e 87%, respectivamente.[44] Elevações concomitantes na atividade de ALP aumentam a especificidade para doença hepatobiliar a 94%.[44] Em gatos com doença hepática inflamatória, a GGT sérica é mais sensível (86%), porém menos específica do que a ALP.[44,76] Em gatos com lipidose hepática, em que a causa primária não está associada à doença hepatobiliar necrosante inflamatória, a magnitude do aumento da atividade sérica de ALP (em relação ao limite superior da faixa de valores normais) quase sempre é maior do que a magnitude do incremento da atividade sérica de GGT. Em contraste, gatos com doença hepatobiliar necrosante inflamatória, com ou sem lipidose hepática secundária, geralmente

a magnitude do aumento da atividade de GGT é maior do que a da elevação da atividade sérica de ALP.[42] Em cães neonatos a atividade de GGT pode se elevar após a ingestão de colostro; isso não ocorre em gatos.[77-79]

Parâmetros e testes de função hepática

Glicose

Hipoglicemia somente ocorre após perda aproximada de 75% da função hepática e é resultado da redução do estoque hepático de glicogênio, da gliconeogênese e da depuração da insulina (ver Capítulo 61).[44,47] A hipoglicemia também pode ser observada periodicamente em pacientes com desvio (*shunt*) portossistêmico (DPS). É importante lembrar que existem vários outros diagnósticos diferenciais para hipoglicemia que não seja insuficiência da síntese hepática, como hipoadrenocorticismo, sepse, menor captação em animais jovens em crescimento, toxinas (xilitol) com ou sem envolvimento hepático, insulinoma e outras neoplasias que causam síndrome paraneoplásica (ver Capítulo 352).

Nitrogênio ureico sanguíneo

No caso de diminuição significativa da função hepática ou de desvio (*shunt*) do sangue do fígado, a conversão de amônia em ureia diminui e pode-se constatar baixo teor de nitrogênio ureico sanguíneo (NUS)no perfil bioquímico.[44] Em pacientes com DPS o desvio anormal de sangue ao redor do fígado resulta em menor disponibilização de amônia ao fígado para entrada no ciclo da ureia, o que acarreta hiperamonemia e diminuição do teor de NUS.[47] Pacientes que recebem dieta com restrição proteica rigorosa e aqueles com anorexia podem também apresentar baixo conteúdo de NUS (ver Capítulo 62).

Proporção albumina/globulina

O fígado é responsável pela síntese de albumina. Na hepatopatia crônica pode ocorrer hipoalbuminemia após perda de aproximadamente 70% da função hepática.[44] Geralmente, quando a concentração sérica de albumina está baixa devido à hepatopatia avançada, a concentração sérica de globulinas permanece normal ou aumentada. Há raros relatos de hiperalbuminemia em pacientes com carcinoma hepatocelular.[80] O fígado é responsável pela síntese de alfaglobulina e betaglobulina, e estas podem estar diminuídas nas doenças hepatobiliares, mas a produção de gamaglobulina depende principalmente de linfócitos B e plasmócitos.[47] Hipoglobulinemia é observada principalmente quando ocorre perda gastrintestinal de proteínas, e não disfunção hepática. Hiperglobulinemia pode ser observada em pacientes com *shunt* (desvio) ou diminuição da massa tecidual hepática (menor quantidade de células de Kupffer) secundária à diminuição da filtração e depuração de toxinas e microrganismos oriundos da circulação porta (ver Capítulo 60).[47]

Colesterol

Na doença hepatobiliar a concentração sérica de colesterol pode ser variável (ver Capítulo 63). Doenças colestáticas estão tipicamente associadas à hipercolesterolemia, enquanto hipocolesterolemia pode ser constatada na hepatopatia em estágio terminal.[44]

Bilirrubina

A bilirrubina é o pigmento que dá à bile a cor amarelo-amaronzada.[18] A elevação da concentração de bilirrubina na circulação sanguínea sistêmica pode levar ao acúmulo do pigmento em tecidos e, em consequência, icterícia clínica (ver Figura 280.2). As causas de hiperbilirrubinemia são agrupadas em três principais categorias: aumento de produção (hemólise), também denominada como pré-hepática; presença de hepatopatia que causa conjugação e/ou excreção inadequada de bilirrubina; e causas pós-hepáticas (excreção biliar de bilirrubina anormal) (Figura 280.4).[18,44] A hiperbilirrubinemia também pode ser

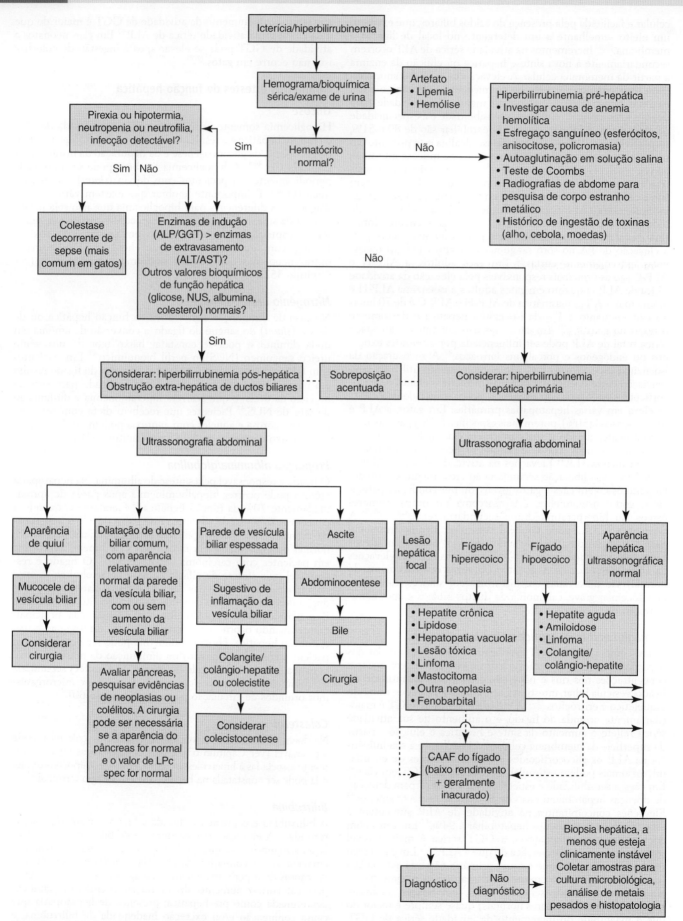

Figura 280.4 Algoritmo diagnóstico para hiperbilirrubinemia. *ALP*, fosfatase alcalina; *ALT*, alanina aminotransferase; *AST*, aspartato aminotransferase; *GGT*, gama-glutamil transferase; *LPc spec*, lipase pancreática canina específica; *NUS*, nitrogênio ureico sanguíneo.

causada por colestase relacionada à sepse, em que citocinas inibem a expressão de transportadores dos hepatócitos necessários para carrear bilirrubina, e pode ocorrer sem a presença de doença hepatobiliar.[44] A elevação discreta da concentração sérica de bilirrubina também pode ocorrer por artefatos de hemólise ou lipemia. A mensuração das concentrações séricas de bilirrubina direta (conjugada) ou indireta (não conjugada) não possui valor para diferenciação das causas de aumento da bilirrubina sérica. Os padrões de elevação de enzimas hepáticas também são de pouco valor para o clínico determinar se a elevação do teor de bilirrubina é secundária a causas hepáticas ou pós-hepáticas. Em vez disso, são necessários exames de imagem (mais comumente o exame ultrassonográfico) para a distinção entre causas hepáticas e pós-hepáticas de elevação da concentração sérica de bilirrubina.

Geralmente, as causas pré-hepáticas (hemólise) são detectadas quando há diminuição acentuada no volume globular (ou hematócrito) e/ou outras características marcantes de anemia hemolítica (como esferocitose e/ou teste de Coombs positivo). Aproximadamente 10% de todos os pacientes com hepatopatia apresentam icterícia clínica.[18] Em gatos com lipidose hepática, mais de 95% apresentam hiperbilirrubinemia.[3] Na obstrução extra-hepática de ductos biliares (OEHDB) total é possível notar fezes acólicas devido à ausência de estercobilina nas fezes.[18] Após a obstrução de ductos biliares, a bilirrubina conjugada no plasma se liga de forma covalente e irreversível à albumina (chamada de delta-bilirrubina), cuja meia-vida é de cerca de 2 semanas. Portanto, um paciente pode permanecer visivelmente ictérico durante várias semanas, apesar da resolução da obstrução do ducto biliar.[18] A concentração de bilirrubina não é influenciada por anormalidade na perfusão hepática; portanto, animais com DPS congênito não apresentam icterícia.[18]

Ácidos biliares

Os ácidos biliares são sintetizados pelo fígado exclusivamente a partir do colesterol, que é a principal via de excreção de colesterol.[18] Os ácidos biliares são então excretados para o trato biliar e armazenados na vesícula biliar. A colecistocinina é secretada pela mucosa duodenal em resposta à presença de gordura ou proteína na ingesta e atua como o principal estímulo para a contração da vesícula biliar.[81-84] A contração da vesícula biliar ocorre lentamente, ao longo de uma a duas horas.[18] Assim que a vesícula biliar contrai, os ácidos biliares são excretados no duodeno para ajudar a solubilizar os lipídios da dieta.[85] Em seguida, são reabsorvidos no íleo e transportados de volta para o fígado através da veia porta, onde > 95% dos ácidos biliares são removidos e o processo é novamente reiniciado.[85] Essa via é chamada de circulação êntero-hepática, e falhas nela devido à disfunção hepática ou shunt portossistêmico levam à elevação na concentração sérica de ácidos biliares. Incrementos na concentração sérica de ácidos biliares podem ser observados em casos de shunt portossistêmico, hepatopatia parenquimatosa e colestase.[86]

Uma estimativa da eficiência da circulação êntero-hepática pode ser obtida pela avaliação da concentração sérica de ácidos biliares. Geralmente obtém-se uma amostra de sangue após jejum de 12 horas (pré-prandial) e, em seguida, 2 horas após uma pequena refeição (pós-prandial).[44] Os valores limiares típicos para os teores de ácidos biliares pré e pós-prandiais são 15 mcmol/ℓ e 25 mcmol/ℓ, respectivamente. Foi relatado que elevações das concentrações de ácidos biliares pré e pós-prandiais são 99% sensíveis e 95 a 100% específicas para o diagnóstico de DPS em cães e gatos.[10,44] Um estudo que investigou a sensibilidade e a especificidade dos ácidos biliares em jejum para o diagnóstico de DPS constatou valores de 93 e 67% em cães, e 100 e 71% em gatos, respectivamente. Quando os valores limiares aumentaram para 58 mcmol/ℓ, em cães, e 34 mcmol/ℓ, em gatos, a sensibilidade não foi alterada em cães (91%) e foi menor em gatos (83%), mas a especificidade aumentou em ambas as espécies (84% em cães e 86% em gatos).[85]

Ao mesmo tempo que a mensuração de ácidos biliares é bastante útil no diagnóstico de DPS em cães e gatos, e cirrose em cães (sensibilidade de praticamente 100%), a sua utilidade é limitada para a triagem da maioria das doenças hepatobiliares (sensibilidade de 54 a 74%).[44] Valores pré-prandiais maiores que pós-prandiais podem ocorrer secundariamente à contração interdigestiva da vesícula biliar ou devido a anormalidades no esvaziamento gástrico, no trânsito intestinal ou na resposta à liberação de colecistocinina. Isso não tem relevância clínica, qualquer que seja o maior valor utilizado para interpretação. Valores pós-prandiais falsamente elevados podem ser decorrentes de lipemia. Valores pós-prandiais falsamente diminuídos podem ser resultado de falhas na liberação de colescistocinina, o que leva à inadequada contração da vesícula biliar, se a refeição contém teores inadequados de proteína ou de gordura.[44] Doenças de íleo graves ou sua ressecção prévia podem diminuir a reabsorção de ácidos biliares, diminuindo assim os valores pós-prandiais de ácidos biliares.[44] Quando utilizada como teste de função hepatobiliar, a magnitude da elevação da concentração sérica de ácidos biliares não possibilita diferenciar a categoria da doença, com exceção de que pacientes com hepatopatia vacuolar raramente apresentam elevação acentuada (superior a 75 a 100 mcmol/ℓ).

Amônia

A amônia é oriunda principalmente da ação de bactérias do cólon em subprodutos da proteína ingerida.[19] A amônia intestinal é absorvida e adentra a veia porta. Em estados saudáveis, a amônia é quase completamente removida da circulação porta durante uma passagem pelo fígado, por meio da conversão em ureia no ciclo da ureia.[18,85] O fígado possui uma capacidade enorme de reserva para detoxificação da amônia; portanto, geralmente ocorre encefalopatia hepática (EH) somente quando o sangue com alto teor de amônia desvia do fígado em razão da existência de desvio portossistêmico.[18] A hiperamonemia também pode ocorrer secundariamente a anormalidades do metabolismo no ciclo da ureia. Isso pode ser observado em gatos com anorexia e hepatopatia devido à carência de arginina, a qual é essencial como substrato para detoxificação da amônia no ciclo da ureia.[85] A insuficiência hepática deve causar uma redução de aproximadamente 70% na atividade do ciclo da ureia para que ocorra hiperamonemia.[12] A concentração plasmática de amônia normal em animais saudáveis é baixa (< 45 mcmol/ℓ).[18] É relatado que a sensibilidade e a especificidade da utilização de valor elevado da amônia em jejum, para o diagnóstico de DPS em cães, são de 98 e 89%, respectivamente.[87]

O manuseio da amostra é extremamente importante para a mensuração acurada da amônia. A concentração de amônia deve ser mensurada em um paciente em jejum, em amostra de sangue fresco sem hemólise coletado em tubos contendo heparina de lítio. As amostras devem ser centrifugadas, em centrífuga refrigerada, dentro de 30 minutos após a coleta e transferidas em gelo.[18,85] Se mantida em temperatura ambiente, a amônia é liberada espontaneamente a partir de fontes nitrogenadas.[18] A incerteza das mensurações de amônia por meio de métodos enzimáticos e a labilidade da amônia comprometem a utilização desse teste para o diagnóstico de EH.[3] Se há dúvida quanto aos valores de ácidos biliares e à concentração basal de amônia, pode-se realizar o teste de tolerância à amônia para melhor avaliar a presença de EH. Para a realização do teste de tolerância à amônia, administram-se 2 mℓ de solução de NH_4Cl 5%/kg, por via retal profunda (10 a 20 cm), por meio de um cateter flexível. Coletam-se uma amostra pré-administração da solução de NH_4Cl e amostras 20 e 40 minutos após a administração. Pacientes sem EH apresentam valores basais na faixa normal e incremento mínimo da concentração de amônia após o teste. Esse teste não é seguro em pacientes com valores basais de amônia > 150 mcmol/ℓ.[41]

Proteínas de coagulação

O fígado pode participar da hemostasia de várias maneiras. Primeiro, o fígado produz todos os fatores de coagulação, com exceção do subtipo de von Willebrand do fator VIII.[18,88] Segundo, a colestase pode prejudicar a absorção de vitaminas lipossolúveis, como a vitamina K.[47] Os fatores de coagulação dependentes da vitamina K são os fatores II, VII, IX, X, proteína C e proteína S.[89] A má absorção de vitamina K e a menor ativação dos fatores dependentes de vitamina K podem levar ao prolongamento do tempo de protrombina (TP), mas geralmente não causam coagulopatia clínica.[90,91] Essa é a anormalidade de coagulação mais comum em gatos com doença hepatobiliar.[92] Terceiro, várias proteínas inibidoras da coagulação, incluindo antitrombina III, proteína C e proteína S, são sintetizadas no fígado. Quarto, o represamento esplâncnico de sangue pode levar ao sequestro prolongado de plaquetas em seus locais de degradação no baço, o que pode induzir trombocitopenia. Isso é denominado de hiperesplenismo e ocorre secundariamente à hipertensão portal. O hiperesplenismo já foi documentado em seres humanos, mas até hoje não foi relatado em pacientes veterinários com hipertensão portal.[18,89] Quinto, alguns fatores de coagulação, como o fibrinogênio, atuam como reagentes de fase aguda e são produzidos em excesso por hepatócitos em casos de doença inflamatória ou neoplásica, o que leva ao maior consumo de fibrinogênio.[18] Isso geralmente ocorre em doenças hepáticas difusas associadas à necrose significativa de hepatócitos, como nas formas ativas de hepatite e linfoma hepático.[88] Por fim, algumas doenças hepatobiliares podem levar à coagulação intravascular disseminada (CID). Bioquimicamente isso consiste em baixa concentração de fibrinogênio, trombocitopenia, TP e TTPa (tempo de tromboplastina parcial ativada) prolongados e elevação das concentrações de produtos da degradação do fibrinogênio e de D-Dímero (ver Capítulo 197). Ao mesmo tempo que anormalidades nos testes de coagulação são comuns em cães e gatos com doença hepatobiliar, a ocorrência de hemorragias espontâneas é muito rara. Entretanto, a presença de anormalidades acentuadas de coagulação em pacientes com hepatopatia é um indicativo de prognóstico e parece ser reflexo da magnitude da insuficiência hepática funcional.[93]

A proteína C plasmática é uma glicoproteína ligada ao dissulfeto, com peso molecular semelhante ao da albumina. Como afirmado anteriormente, é sintetizada no fígado e circula como um zimogênio plasmático cuja $T_{1/2}$ é de aproximadamente 6 horas. Assim que ativada, a proteína C se liga à proteína S e, juntas, exercem seus efeitos anticoagulantes pela degradação dos fatores Va e VIIIa.[94] Em um estudo que avaliou a utilidade da proteína C plasmática na detecção de doença hepatobiliar e DPS em cães, foi observado que uma atividade de proteína C menor que 70% era comum em pacientes com DPS (88%), mas rara em pacientes com DMV (5%).[94]

Achados hematológicos

As alterações mais evidentes observadas no hemograma incluem microcitose (associada a distúrbios no transporte de ferro em pacientes com anormalidades vasculares), hemácias em alvo, poiquilocitose e corpúsculos de Heinz (gatos).[44] A anemia pode ser secundária à hemorragia causada por úlceras gastrintestinais observadas em hepatopatias avançadas, distúrbio hemorrágico ou anemia decorrente de doença crônica.[44] Alguns pacientes podem apresentar também discreta trombocitopenia.[44] Poiquilocitose é observada em 63% e anemia em 22% dos gatos atendidos com lipidose hepática.[3]

Exame de urina

Existem algumas poucas anormalidades que podem ser notadas no exame de urina, as quais podem ser compatíveis com a presença de hepatopatias (ver Capítulo 72). A maioria é inespecífica. O único achado específico de hepatopatias no exame de urina é a bilirrubinúria em gatos. A presença de bilirrubina na urina de gatos é sempre anormal e indica doença hepatobiliar ou hemolítica.[18] Em cães, entretanto, particularmente nos machos, o limiar para excreção de bilirrubina é baixo. Adicionalmente, seus rins possuem enzimas capazes de produzir bilirrubina a partir do radical heme e conjugá-la. Assim, a urina de cães saudáveis, especialmente machos, pode conter bilirrubina.[18] Gatos com lipidose hepática podem apresentar glóbulos de gordura refratários (lipidúria) no exame do sedimento urinário.[3] Cerca de metade dos cães com desvio portossistêmico apresenta cristais de biurato de amônia no exame do sedimento urinário.[18] Esses cristais também podem ser observados no sedimento urinário de gatos com desvio portossistêmico.[95] Isso ocorre em razão da menor conversão hepática do ácido úrico em alantoína e de amônia em ureia.[96] A amônia e o ácido úrico se agregam na urina ácida e formam cristais.[18] Estes são infrequentemente associados à insuficiência hepática devido a outras causas.[97] É importante lembrar, entretanto, que existem determinadas predisposições raciais para o desenvolvimento de cristais de biurato de amônia na ausência de doença hepatobiliar, como acontece em Dálmata, Buldogue Inglês e, possivelmente, gatos Siameses.[98-101] A densidade específica da urina em pacientes com doença hepatobiliar pode ser baixa. Isso supostamente se deve à perda da hipertonicidade medular renal (devido à baixa concentração de NUS), falhas na metabolização de hormônios (diminuição na metabolização do cortisol, o que ocasiona uma síndrome "semelhante à síndrome de Cushing"), além de polidipsia psicogênica, que também pode ter alguma participação.[102] Uma síndrome semelhante à de Fanconi (presença de glicosúria apesar de euglicemia, com ou sem proteinúria; ver Capítulo 326) recentemente foi reconhecida em alguns pacientes com hepatopatia por armazenamento de cobre secundário ao acúmulo de cobre nos túbulos renais.[103]

EXAMES DE IMAGEM DO FÍGADO

Radiografia

Em comparação com exames de imagem cintilográficos e ultrassonográficos, as radiografias abdominais laterais direitas demonstraram ter a maior correlação com o peso real do fígado em cães.[104,105] O tamanho do fígado pode ser determinado em radiografias por meio de mensuração do comprimento do órgão, com base na posição do eixo gástrico.[106-109] O eixo gástrico normal é descrito como perpendicular à coluna e paralelo à última costela.[110] Radiograficamente, a hepatomegalia se apresenta como margens hepáticas caudoventrais arredondadas ou rombas, extensão de margens hepáticas além do gradil costal e deslocamento do eixo gástrico.[106] Nas radiografias, a micro-hepatia é sugerida pelo deslocamento cranial do eixo gástrico e diminuição da distância entre o diafragma e o lúmen gástrico.[107] A posição do eixo gástrico pode ser afetada por outros fatores que não seja o tamanho do fígado; portanto, a aferição do comprimento hepático pode ser mais confiável na avaliação do tamanho do fígado.[108,109] Isso pode ser realizado pela mensuração do comprimento do órgão, em centímetros, com base no comprimento do eixo a partir da margem ventral e sua comparação com o comprimento de T11 (medido na altura do ponto médio, paralelo ao eixo longitudinal do corpo vertebral).[110] Relata-se que o comprimento normal do fígado é de 5,5 ± 0,8 vezes o comprimento de T11.[109] Estudo recente avaliou o comprimento hepático normal em cães Pequinês e constatou-se que o órgão é menor do que previamente afirmado em 4,64 vezes o comprimento de T11.[110] A perda de detalhe seroso é sugestiva de ascite.[19] Gás livre na região do fígado é compatível com ruptura de abscesso hepático ou colecistite enfisematosa (ver Capítulo 288).

Ultrassonografia

As características hepáticas típicas avaliadas durante o exame ultrassonográfico (ver Capítulo 88) do abdome incluem ecogenicidade e uniformidade do parênquima, estruturas vasculares, estruturas biliares e estimativa do tamanho do fígado.[111-115] Estas características são avaliadas para determinar: (1) presença de lesões focais; (2) arquitetura e estrutura hepática; (3) diâmetro do lúmen e espessura da parede dos ductos biliares extra e intra-hepáticos, e da vesícula biliar; (4) anormalidades vasculares, especialmente da veia porta, mas também a presença de fístula arteriovenosa; (5) presença de líquido livre no abdome; e (6) avaliação com ecodoppler da velocidade e direção do fluxo sanguíneo portal.[88] É importante lembrar que o fígado pode parecer inalterado no exame ultrassonográfico, mesmo na presença de doença grave.[116] Em um estudo que comparou os achados ultrassonográficos do fígado com o histopatológico do órgão, ao mesmo tempo que o exame ultrassonográfico sem indicação de alteração apresentou correlação estatisticamente significativa com a ausência de doença hepática, no exame histopatológico indicou que 63% desses pacientes tinham anormalidades no exame histopatológico.[117] Nesse estudo, a maioria dos cães com doença hepatobiliar e exame ultrassonográfico sem alteração foi diagnosticada com hepatopatia inflamatória ou lesões degenerativas. As alterações ultrassonográficas do fígado também não são preditivas da presença, ausência ou grau de fibrose hepática.[117] Pode-se observar parênquima hepático hiperecoico em casos de hepatite crônica, lipidose hepática, hepatopatia causada por esteroide, outras hepatopatias vacuolares, lesão tóxica, linfoma, mastocitoma, sarcoma histiocítico e tratamento com fenobarbital.[118] Para determinar se o fígado se apresenta hiperecoico, sua ecogenicidade deve ser comparada àquela da gordura falciforme ou baço, ambos devem normalmente ser mais hiperecoicos (mais brilhantes) do que o fígado. Parênquima hepático hipoecoico pode ser notado em casos de hepatite aguda, amiloidose, linfoma ou colangite/colângio-hepatite.[118]

O exame ultrassonográfico é bastante útil na avaliação de OEHDB (ver Capítulo 288). Neoplasias, pancreatite, colélitos, lama biliar, inflamação ou mucocele biliar podem causar OEHDB.[118] O ducto biliar comum pode medir até 3 mm de diâmetro em cães normais e até 4 mm de diâmetro em gatos normais.[119,120] O Doppler colorido pode ser utilizado para diferenciar estruturas biliares de vasculares. A vesícula biliar pode ter tamanho normal ou aumentado em casos de OEHDB. Portanto, a presença de vesícula biliar de tamanho normal não deve ser utilizada para descartar a possibilidade de OEHDB.[118] Em casos de colângio-hepatite as referências portais podem parecer proeminentes, as paredes da vesícula biliar e de ductos biliares podem parecer espessadas, e pode haver aumento da quantidade de lama na vesícula biliar.[118] A colecistite é indistinguível da colângio-hepatite ao exame ultrassonográfico.[118] Espessamento da parede da vesícula biliar também pode ser observado em casos de hepatite, líquido livre no peritônio e hipoproteinemia.[121] Em um estudo previamente mencionado, a identificação ultrassonográfica de espessamento da parede da vesícula biliar foi significativamente correlacionada à inflamação no exame histopatológico.[117] Colélitos são mais comuns em cães do que em gatos e surgem como estruturas hiperecoicas no interior da vesícula biliar ou de ductos biliares, os quais ocasionam sombreamento acústico.[118] A colecistite enfisematosa pode ser observada como presença de gás no trato biliar e pode ser devida à infecção pela bactéria *Escherichia coli* ou *Clostridium perfringens*, e também foi associada ao diabetes melito.[118]

As características ultrassonográficas de mucocele biliar incluem lama biliar imóvel que não se altera pela ação da gravidade e/ou bile ecogênica com padrão estrelado ou finamente estriado, também denominado padrão "semelhante a um quiuí" (ver Capítulo 288).[122] Não foi observada associação entre o padrão ultrassonográfico biliar e a probabilidade de ruptura colecística em um estudo com 14 cães com mucocele biliar.[123] Entretanto, outro estudo mostrou que um padrão estrelado incompleto foi estatisticamente mais comum em cães que apresentavam ruptura de vesícula biliar, embora isso não tenha sido patognomônico para ruptura da vesícula biliar nem ainda seja preditivo com base nos padrões ultrassonográficos biliares.[122]

Nesse estudo, a maioria dos cães não desenvolveu espessamento da parede da vesícula biliar, tampouco dilatação de ductos biliares extra-hepáticos. Quando ocorre ruptura da vesícula biliar, geralmente é diagnosticada diretamente pela observação da descontinuação da parede da vesícula biliar e indiretamente com base em evidências de alterações pericolecísticas, como gordura hiperecoica e acúmulo de líquido.[122] É relatado que a sensibilidade da ultrassonografia para o diagnóstico de ruptura de vesícula biliar seja de 85%.[124] É importante lembrar que a dilatação biliar nem sempre está associada à doença biliar ativa, pois o trato biliar de cães pode permanecer dilatado após a resolução da doença.[125]

A ultrassonografia pode ser útil no diagnóstico de DPS (ver Capítulo 284). A sensibilidade relatada para a identificação ultrassonográfica de DPSAM é de 67% comparada àquela do DPS congênito (90 a 100%),[126] embora a detecção de *shunt* seja muito dependente do operador e do equipamento. Em um estudo constatou-se fígado pequeno em 96% dos cães com doença vascular primária, e em 100% dos cães com DMV.[117] Relata-se que proporções veia porta:artéria aorta e veia porta:veia cava maiores ou iguais a 0,8 e 0,75, respectivamente, descartaram indubitavelmente a possibilidade de DPS extra-hepático.[126] Proporção veia porta:artéria aorta menor ou igual a 0,65 foi firmemente relatada em *shunts* (desvios) extra-hepáticos.[126] Urólitos e renomegalia são achados comuns em cães e gatos com DPS.[127-129] Em geral, desvios vasculares extra-hepáticos se originam da veia porta, esplênica, gástrica direita ou esquerda ou gastroepiploica.[126,130] Desvios portocavais desembocam na veia cava caudal e o local de entrada é caracterizado por fluxo turbulento no Doppler colorido e espectral.[118] Em casos de hipertensão portal e DPSAM, é possível notar ascite, mas é incomum em casos de DPSC.[30,131-133] Geralmente, DPSAM são visualizados na área perirrenal dorsal esquerda como um plexo de vasos esplênicos a renais pequenos e tortuosos.[5,126,134,135] Outros achados sugestivos de hipertensão portal incluem redução da velocidade do fluxo sanguíneo portal (< 10 cm/s), fluxo hepatofugal e dilatação da veia porta e da veia gonadal esquerda.[19] Fístulas arteriovenosas criam conexões entre a veia porta e as artérias hepáticas.[121]

A presença de uma massa hepática ao exame ultrassonográfico do abdome deve levar à suspeita de neoplasia (ver Capítulo 287). Um estudo conduzido por Murakami *et al.* relatou que cães com grandes massas hepáticas e efusão peritoneal tinham maior probabilidade de apresentar neoplasia hepática maligna.[136] Entretanto, o diagnóstico deve ser confirmado pelo exame histopatológico, já que existem diversas condições benignas que podem parecer semelhantes a massas ao exame ultrassonográfico, como degeneração, inflamação ou hiperplasia nodular.[117] Abscessos hepáticos podem ter uma aparência variável, semelhante a uma massa, ao exame ultrassonográfico e podem estar associados à presença de gás livre (artefatos de reverberação).[118] Lesões císticas surgem como estruturas cavitárias anecoicas que geralmente possuem margens claramente definidas; elas podem ter formato arredondado ou irregular e podem conter septos hiperecoicos.[118] Outras lesões hepáticas anecoicas incluem necrose e algumas neoplasias cavitárias. Granulomas podem ser secundários a uma ampla variedade de microrganismos infecciosos ou corpos estranhos e no exame ultrassonográfico se apresentam como lesões parenquimatosas hiperecoicas multifocais bem delimitadas.[118,121] A torção do lobo hepático é rara em cães. O lobo afetado se mostra hipoecoico e o Doppler colorido mostra redução ou ausência de fluxo sanguíneo no lobo.[118]

A ultrassonografia contrastada possibilita avaliar de maneira não invasiva os padrões de perfusão dos órgãos. É amplamente utilizada na tentativa de distinguir lesões malignas de benignas, sendo classificada como fase inicial e fase tardia. A fase inicial consiste em uma fase arterial (*wash-in*) e uma fase venosa portal (*wash-out*).[118] Durante as fases portal e tardia, todas as lesões benignas, com exceção de cistos e hemangiomas com trombose, exibem isoatenuação ou discreto ganho comparado ao tecido hepático circundante. Lesões hepáticas malignas mostram hipoatenuação ou não apresentam perfusão.[137] A sensibilidade e especificidade para diagnóstico e diferenciação de nódulos hepáticos benignos e malignos são de 100 e 94,1%, respectivamente.[118]

Outros exames de imagem

Tomografia computadorizada

A tomografia computadorizada (TC) pode ser útil para determinar o tamanho do fígado e diagnosticar lesões tumorais hepáticas e DPS. A exacerbação da massa tumoral pelo contraste pode ajudar na diferenciação entre lesões benignas e malignas.[118] A angiografia por TC possui sensibilidade de 96% e especificidade de 89% para o diagnóstico de DPS congênito em cães e tem probabilidade 5,5 vezes maior de determinar corretamente a presença ou ausência de DPS congênito do que a ultrassonografia abdominal.[138] A TC possui várias vantagens: não é um procedimento invasivo, é capaz de retratar de forma acurada a origem do vaso anômalo, possui o potencial para reconstruções tridimensionais e é menos dependente do operador do que a ultrassonografia.[118,139,140] As desvantagens incluem a necessidade de anestesia geral na maioria dos casos e a possibilidade de ocorrência de artefatos de movimentação, o que pode requerer a repetição da varredura ou do escaneamento.[118] A TC está se tornando rapidamente um dos métodos mais comumente utilizados de diagnóstico de DPS extra-hepático.

Ressonância magnética

Semelhante à TC, a ressonância magnética (RM) mostrou-se útil no diagnóstico de neoplasias hepáticas e DPS. Um estudo que investigou a utilidade da RM contrastada na distinção entre neoplasias benignas e malignas constatou que a RM foi acurada em 33 de 35 lesões, com sensibilidade e especificidade de 100 e 90%, respectivamente.[141] A sensibilidade e especificidade relatadas da angiografia por RM no diagnóstico de DPS congênito único foram de 79 e 100%, respectivamente.[142] A RM é raramente utilizada no diagnóstico de DPS, pois a angiografia por TC é capaz de fornecer detalhamento semelhante mais rapidamente e com um custo menor comparada à RM.[143]

Cintilografia portal utilizando tecnécio (^{99m}Tc)-enxofre coloidal

Tecnécio (^{99m}Tc)-enxofre coloidal são pequenas partículas coloidais que se localizam no sistema reticuloendotelial. Em cães normais, a maior parte do tecnécio (^{99m}Tc)-enxofre coloidal se localiza no fígado, enquanto em pacientes com DPS uma parte significativa se localiza no pulmão.[144] Esta técnica não é específica para DPS em cães, pois a captação nos pulmões ocorre por outras causas de insuficiência hepática; ademais, não pode ser utilizada em gatos para o diagnóstico de DPS porque em gatos normais ocorre captação pulmonar.[144,145]

Cintilografia portal por via retal

Esta técnica consiste na administração de um radionuclídeo (geralmente pertecnetato de sódio) no cólon. Em pacientes normais, o pertecnetato inicialmente é visualizado no fígado e então no coração. Em pacientes com DPS, o sangue portal que contém pertecnetato desvia do fígado, sendo visualizado inicialmente no coração.[146] Desvios de menor magnitude podem ter chegada simultânea do pertecnetato ao fígado e coração.[146] A análise quantitativa da cintilografia portal por via retal (CPPR) pode ser realizada em um computador que calcula a fração de desvio (FD), a qual é uma estimativa da porcentagem do sangue portal que desvia do fígado.[145,147] Cães normais devem ter uma FD < 5%. A maioria dos pacientes com DPS congênito apresenta FD > 60%, geralmente de 80 a 95%.[146] A principal desvantagem da CPPR é que mostra um mau detalhamento

anatômico, impossibilitando detectar o local exato e o tipo (congênito ou adquirido) do desvio, e os exames ocasionalmente podem não ser diagnósticos (geralmente devido à má absorção pelo cólon).[146] Em pacientes com DMV a CPPR é normal.[146]

Cintilografia portal transesplênica

A cintilografia portal transesplênica (CPTE) é realizada por ultrassom, com injeção de um radiofármaco (pertecnetato de sódio) na região central do parênquima esplênico.[146] As imagens resultantes são de melhor qualidade do que aquelas obtidas na CPPR.[148,149] Normalmente, o radiofármaco é rapidamente absorvido pelo baço em direção à veia esplênica, fluindo para a veia gástrica esquerda e então para a veia porta principal até chegar ao fígado. O radiofármaco passa pelos sinusoides hepáticos até a veia hepática, a veia cava caudal e, então, o coração.[146] A FD normal para cães é de aproximadamente 2,64%.[146] A visualização de vasos de desvio ocorre em 90% dos casos.[148,149] A cintilografia portal transesplênica pode distinguir entre desvios porto-ázigos e portocaval-espleno-caval e algumas vezes entre desvios congênitos e adquiridos.[146] Desvios portossistêmicos localizados caudais à entrada da veia esplênica na veia porta podem não ser observados por essa técnica.[146] À semelhança do que acontece na CPPR, os desvios de menor magnitude podem ter chegada simultânea do pertecnetato ao fígado e coração.[146] O tecnécio (^{99m}Tc)-mebrofenina pode ser utilizado como alternativa ao pertecnetato de sódio e facilitar a localização do desvio.[146] Assim como acontece com a CPPR, a CPTE não é útil no diagnóstico de DMV.[146]

COLETA DE AMOSTRAS DE FÍGADO

Aspiração com agulha fina

A aspiração com agulha fina (AAF) do fígado é muito menos invasiva, possui menos risco, apresenta resultados mais rápidos e é de menor custo do que a obtenção de amostras por meio de biopsia hepática (ver Capítulos 89 e 93). Esse procedimento geralmente pode ser realizado sem sedação, analgesia ou anestesia, a menos que o paciente seja agressivo ou relute à contenção. Anestésicos locais geralmente também não são utilizados. A aspiração do fígado com agulha fina é geralmente considerada segura, mas os tutores devem ser alertados quanto ao risco de hemorragia, embora raro. A aspiração do fígado com agulha fina deve ser guiada por ultrassom e com uma agulha calibre 22G a 25G. Frequentemente obtém-se menor contaminação com sangue pela rápida agitação da agulha sem a seringa ("técnica de máquina de costura") comparada à aspiração utilizando uma seringa. Em pacientes com doença difusa, devem ser coletados diversos aspirados de locais diferentes. A amostra coletada deve ser colocada em lâminas de vidro para confecção de esfregaços finos. Os autores recomendam corar uma a duas lâminas com coloração Diff-Quik no hospital e avaliar essas lâminas em microscopia óptica, a fim de pesquisar a presença de hepatócitos. Isso garante que uma amostra adequada tenha sido coletada antes do envio para exame citológico. Colorações específicas podem ser aplicadas às lâminas para pesquisar grânulos intra-hepáticos de cobre (corante rodanina ou ácido rubeânico), lipídios (corante Sudan) e glicogênio (coloração pelo ácido periódico de Schiff).[88]

As principais desvantagens do diagnóstico citológico em amostras obtidas por AAF do fígado são alta frequência de resultados não confiáveis devido à baixa celularidade e à presença de artefatos e ausência de arquitetura tecidual para avaliação das lesões.[150] A concordância geral entre o diagnóstico em exame citológico e exame histológico varia de 30 a 61%.[151,152] Estudo retrospectivo recente avaliou a acurácia do AAF guiado por ultrassom de lesões hepáticas focais e constatou maior sensibilidade para alterações vacuolares (57,9%), seguidas de

CAPÍTULO 280 • Avaliação Diagnóstica da Função Hepática

neoplasias (52%).[153] Esse estudo também mostrou que tumores de célula redonda (valor preditivo positivo [VPP] 75%) e carcinomas de origem não hepatocelular (VPP 85,7%) foram as neoplasias diagnosticadas mais prontamente no exame citológico. O VPP para o carcinoma hepatocelular foi de 100%. O estudo também verificou que apenas aproximadamente 50% dos pacientes com diagnóstico histopatológico de neoplasia tinham células neoplásicas detectadas no exame citológico. Esses achados sugerem que, ao mesmo tempo que o diagnóstico de neoplasias pela citologia seja muito provavelmente correto, o exame citológico, por si só, não pode ser utilizado para excluir o diagnóstico de neoplasias.

A citologia de amostras do fígado obtidas por AAF pode ser útil para confirmar o diagnóstico de lipidose hepática felina (ver Capítulo 284). A vacuolização hepatocelular difusa por triglicerídeos é característica dessa síndrome.[3] Entretanto, se a causa primária da lipidose hepática for uma hepatopatia primária, um diagnóstico definitivo pode não ser confirmado somente pela citologia, já que o diagnóstico citológico de doenças hepatobiliares pode ser notavelmente discordante de amostras obtidas por biopsia.[3]

Biopsia hepática

O diagnóstico da maioria das doenças hepatobiliares requer exame histopatológico do tecido hepático. Nas hepatopatias difusas, as amostras podem ser obtidas de diferentes locais, mas a lesão focal requer escolha mais seletiva do local de biopsia (ver Capítulos 89 e 95). Em casos de grandes lesões focais, as amostras devem ser coletadas na periferia da lesão, já que grandes massas teciduais podem apresentar um centro necrosado. Riscos da biopsia hepática incluem complicações anestésicas, especialmente em pacientes com hepatopatia avançada devido à incapacidade de metabolizar anestésicos, hemorragia, embolia gasosa (laparoscopia) e choque vagotônico.[3,88,154] O choque vagotônico está geralmente associado à biopsia com agulha e o risco é maior em pacientes que apresentam dilatação de ductos biliares e quando se utiliza agulha de biopsia automática de disparo rápido. Há pouca evidência objetiva de que a condição de coagulação avaliada por meio da mensuração de TP, TTPa, concentração de fibrinogênio, contagem plaquetária ou tempo de sangramento de mucosa oral (TSMO; ver Capítulo 80) está correlacionada com o risco de hemorragia após biopsia hepática.[155,156] A vitamina K1 e/ou plasma fresco congelado podem ser administrados antes da realização de biopsia hepática, caso o clínico esteja preocupado com o risco hemorrágico maior.

As três técnicas de biopsia hepática mais comumente utilizadas são biopsia com agulha, biopsia laparoscópica e biopsia cirúrgica. A anestesia geral é necessária para a cirurgia e laparoscopia, e pode ser necessária para alguns pacientes submetidos a biopsia com agulha. A biopsia com agulha possui limitações devido ao pequeno tamanho da amostra. Uma boa biopsia com agulha representa 1/50.000 de todo o fígado.[157] Recomenda-se agulha de calibre 14 G para cães de médio a grande porte, e 16 G para cães pequenos e gatos.[88] A biopsia com agulha pode ser realizada por via percutânea, guiada por ultrassom ou sob controle visual durante laparoscopia ou cirurgia. A técnica com agulha do tipo Tru-Cut é a mais amplamente utilizada e em geral pode ser realizada guiada por ultrassom.[88] Existem três tipos de agulhas do tipo Tru-Cut: manual, semiautomática e automática. Dispositivos manuais são de difícil manuseio e apenas recomendados em procedimentos com controle visual direto durante a cirurgia.[88,155] Os tipos semiautomático e automático são mais comumente utilizados. As principais desvantagens da biopsia hepática guiada por ultrassom incluem a necessidade de sedação ou anestesia de alguns pacientes, dificuldade de obtenção de imagens do fígado de pequeno tamanho, dificuldade de obtenção de tecido hepático em pacientes com fibrose e amostras cuja representatividade da doença hepática primária é questionável. Na maioria das vezes, essa acurácia

questionável se deve ao risco potencial de erro na obtenção das amostras. Esse método ainda resulta em um tamanho relativamente pequeno da amostra, bem como possível fragmentação de tecido fibroso, e pode não possibilitar a obtenção de amostras de anormalidades localizadas em outros lobos (em geral, o lobo medial ou lateral esquerdo são alvos de coleta devido à facilidade de obtenção de imagens). Em um estudo com 124 pacientes comparou-se a acurácia diagnóstica da biopsia com agulha Tru-Cut com a biopsia cirúrgica em cunha do fígado, considerada padrão-ouro.[158] A discordância geral entre os dois métodos foi de 53% em cães e 50% em gatos, com mais de 60% de discrepância em casos de hepatite crônica ou cirrose, colangite/colângio-hepatite, anomalias vasculares portossistêmicas, displasia microvascular, fibrose e anormalidades diversas. Essas anormalidades são mais comumente observadas em cães e gatos com doença hepatobiliar. A maior acurácia foi constatada em casos de neoplasia (80% de concordância). A utilização de agulha calibre 14 G em detrimento de agulha calibre 18 G pode reduzir essa discordância, já que aumenta o número de tríades portais coletadas. Um estudo recente que avaliou a biopsia hepática transjugular em cadáveres de cães relatou ser esta uma técnica viável. Entretanto, outros estudos são necessários antes que essa técnica possa ser recomendada na rotina clínica.[159]

A laparoscopia envolve a distensão da cavidade abdominal com gás, seguida de implantação de um telescópio rígido através de um portal (cânula) na parede do abdome, a fim de examinar os conteúdos da cavidade abdominal (ver Capítulo 91).[155] A pinça e outros instrumentos utilizados durante a biopsia são então introduzidos no abdome através de portais adjacentes, a fim de possibilitar uma inspeção mais minuciosa dos órgãos abdominais e a coleta de amostras por meio de biopsia.[88,155] Essa técnica permite a avaliação macroscópica de todo o fígado, sistema biliar extra-hepático e estruturas circundantes, ao mesmo tempo que obtém múltiplas grandes amostras do fígado (ver Capítulo 283). A capacidade de obtenção de diversas amostras reduz o risco de artefatos de coleta em casos de diversidade regional dentro do fígado. Adicionalmente, pela visualização direta do parênquima hepático, o clínico pode correlacionar os achados histopatológicos e os dados clínicos com a aparência macroscópica do fígado, possibilitando um diagnóstico mais confiável. Esse método também permite a visualização de tumores menores e irregularidades que podem não ser evidentes no exame ultrassonográfico. Há geralmente mínima hemorragia durante esse procedimento, mesmo em pacientes com coagulopatias in vitro. A utilização de uma pinça em "colher" ou oval geralmente resulta em diminuição marcante na quantidade de hemorragia quando comparada a biopsias com agulha. Qualquer hemorragia pode ser visualizada diretamente, até a formação de coágulo adequado. Se a hemorragia persistir, pode-se realizar pressão direta no local com uma pinça romba durante cinco minutos. Se o local continua a sangrar, pode-se aplicar eletrocautério no local da biopsia ou colocar um produto hemostático tópico (esponja hemostática) diretamente no local da biopsia, utilizando pinças laparoscópicas. As principais desvantagens da laparoscopia são a necessidade de anestesia geral, o maior custo e a necessidade de conhecimento técnico e equipamento apropriado. Em uma revisão não publicada, relata-se taxa de complicação decorrente de laparoscopia diagnóstica inferior a 2%.[88] A laparoscopia também pode ser utilizada para obter amostras por biopsia de outros órgãos além do fígado, como pâncreas, rim, baço, linfonodo e intestino, assim como para colecistocentese (aspiração da vesícula biliar).[88] As amostras de biopsia obtidas por laparoscopia são significativamente maiores (aproximadamente 5 × 10 mm) do que aquelas obtidas por biopsia com agulha, mas ainda assim são menores do que as amostras obtidas cirurgicamente (1 a 2 cm).[88]

Para a biopsia hepática, exclusivamente, raramente indica-se cirurgia, se há disponibilidade de laparoscopia. A laparotomia é indicada antes da laparoscopia quando há suspeita de obstrução de ductos biliares ou anomalia vascular, que podem necessitar de correção cirúrgica, além da obtenção de biopsia hepática, ou quando o paciente é submetido à cirurgia por uma questão não relacionada à sua doença hepatobiliar. A vantagem da cirurgia é a exposição de órgãos, a capacidade de manipular os tecidos, a possibilidade de obter uma amostra maior e a possibilidade de monitorar o local da biopsia em busca de possíveis hemorragias.[88] As principais desvantagens da cirurgia são maior estímulo à dor e tempo de recuperação pós-cirúrgico.

A World Small Animal Veterinary Association (WSAVA) definiu padrões para unificar os critérios diagnósticos e a nomenclatura das doenças hepáticas.[5] Durante a biopsia, os autores obtêm pelo menos quatro a cinco amostras de diferentes lobos hepáticos, para exame histopatológico, uma amostra para cultura microbiológica aeróbica e anaeróbica e uma para quantificação de cobre e outros metais pesados.[88] Pode ser necessária a obtenção de amostras adicionais para histopatologia ao utilizar técnica de biopsia com agulha, a fim de aumentar a probabilidade de obter um diagnóstico mais confiável.

REFERÊNCIAS BIBLIOGRÁFICAS

As referências bibliográficas deste capítulo se encontram online no Ambiente de Aprendizagem.

CAPÍTULO 281

Princípios Gerais do Tratamento de Hepatopatias

Jonathan Andrew Lidbury

Frequentemente é necessário que médicos-veterinários desenvolvam protocolos terapêuticos para cães e gatos com hepatopatias. Isso pode ser desafiador por uma série de razões. Primeiro, a eficácia de vários dos fármacos e nutracêuticos utilizados no tratamento de hepatopatias nessas espécies ainda não foi rigorosamente estabelecida.[1] Portanto, a decisão sobre a utilização desses produtos geralmente se baseia na existência de uma razão fisiopatológica justificável, em evidências inferidas a partir de estudos em humanos, na ausência de efeitos adversos perceptíveis, ou na combinação dessas razões. A ausência de evidências é preocupante; como profissionais, nós deveríamos aspirar à confirmação de eficácia e segurança dos fármacos que utilizamos pela realização de estudos clínicos aleatórios controlados com placebo. Adicionalmente, a etiologia primária de várias doenças hepáticas de cães e gatos ainda não foi bem estabelecida. Por exemplo, em vários casos, a causa primária da hepatite crônica canina não pode ser identificada.[2] Isso significa que estamos frequentemente limitados à provisão de terapia de suporte, em vez de tratamento definitivo. Por fim, em razão das limitações dos testes não invasivos atuais para doenças hepáticas, a avaliação da resposta do paciente à terapia pode ser desafiadora.

FÁRMACOS COMUMENTE UTILIZADOS NO TRATAMENTO DE HEPATOPATIAS

Fármacos citoprotetores (Tabela 281.1)

Em razão de sua localização funcional entre as circulações esplâncnica e sistêmica, de sua participação central na metabolização de fármacos e toxinas, assim como de sua grande população de macrófagos residentes (células de Kupffer), o fígado é suscetível a danos oxidativos.[3] A glutationa, um tripeptídio sintetizado a partir de L-glutamato, L-cisteína e glicina, é um antioxidante essencial armazenado principalmente nos hepatócitos.[4] Constatou-se baixa concentração hepática de glutationa em gatos com obstrução de ductos biliares extra-hepáticos, gatos com lipidose hepática e cães e gatos com hepatopatia necrosante inflamatória, o que sustenta a importância da lesão oxidativa em uma ampla variedade de doenças hepatobiliares de cães e gatos.[5]

S-adenosilmetionina

A S-adenosilmetionina (SAMe) possui participação fundamental na síntese da glutationa via transulfuração.[4] Portanto, a principal razão para o tratamento de cães e gatos com SAMe é que pode ajudar a prevenir o dano oxidativo por prevenir a depleção de glutationa hepática. Relata-se também que a SAMe possui propriedades anti-inflamatórias, modula a apoptose e é anticarcinogênica.[4] Em cães e gatos, na dose recomendada de 20 mg/kg/24 horas VO, com o estômago vazio, há raros relatos de efeitos colaterais após o uso de SAMe, exceto episódios ocasionais de êmese e diminuição do apetite.[6] Existem evidências limitadas sobre a eficácia de SAMe em cães e gatos. Primeiro, mostrou-se que a combinação de SAMe e silimarina inibe a produção de citocinas pró-inflamatórias e a ocorrência de estresse oxidativo em culturas celulares de hepatócitos de cães.[7] Segundo, a administração oral de SAMe melhorou a condição de oxirredução hepática e eritrocitária em gatos saudáveis.[8] Adicionalmente, um estudo com 12 cães saudáveis demonstrou que a administração de SAMe diminuiu o estresse oxidativo associado à administração de doses imunossupressoras de prednisona, embora tenha falhado em prevenir o desenvolvimento de alterações histológicas compatíveis com hepatopatia vacuolar.[9] Por fim, em um estudo com cães tratados com o quimioterápico lomustina, os animais suplementados com um produto contendo silimarina, SAMe e fosfatidilcolina (Denamarin®) apresentaram menor incremento das atividades séricas de alanina aminotransferase e fosfatase alcalina e da concentração sérica de bilirrubina do que aqueles que não foram suplementados, sugerindo um efeito hepatoprotetor.[10] Entretanto, são necessários testes clínicos adicionais para comprovar a eficácia de SAMe no tratamento de cães e gatos com hepatopatia. De uma perspectiva prática, em razão do importante papel da lesão oxidativa em modelos experimentais de hepatopatias e em pessoas com hepatopatias, o autor utiliza SAMe como tratamento adjuvante em uma ampla variedade de doenças hepáticas de cães e gatos. Estas incluem lesão hepática aguda causada por fármacos ou intoxicação em cães e gatos, hepatite crônica em cães, hepatite crônica associada ao cobre em cães e lipidose hepática felina.

Tabela 281.1 — Fármacos citoprotetores hepáticos.

FÁRMACO	CLASSE/MECANISMO DE AÇÃO	INDICAÇÕES SUGERIDAS	DOSE	EFEITOS COLATERAIS POSSÍVEIS	COMENTÁRIOS
S-adenosilmetionina	Antioxidante, anti-inflamatório, modulador da apoptose, anticarcinogênico	Lesão hepática aguda, hepatite crônica canina, lipidose hepática felina	20 mg/kg/24 h VO	Episódios ocasionais de êmese e diminuição do apetite	Forneça pelo menos 1 h antes da alimentação; utilize um produto de biodisponibilidade comprovada
N-acetilcisteína	Antioxidante	Lesão hepática aguda, lipidose hepática felina	140 mg/kg IV, inicialmente, seguida de 70 mg/kg a cada 8 a 12 h	Frequentemente provoca êmese, se administrada por via oral; bem tolerada quando administrada por via intravenosa	Utilize em substituição à S-adenosilmetionina em pacientes que não toleram medicamento VO; administre solução 10%, na diluição 1:2 ao longo de 20 min por meio de equipo com filtro não pirogênico de 0,25 mícron
Silimarina	Antioxidante, imunomodulador, antifibrótico, colerético	Lesão hepática aguda, hepatite crônica canina, lipidose hepática felina	5 a 10 mg/kg/24 h VO (combinada com fosfatidilcolina), em cães, e 10 mg/kg/24 h VO em gatos (combinada com fosfatidilcolina)	Geralmente bem tolerada	A fosfatidilcolina aumenta a absorção de silimarina; utilize um produto de biodisponibilidade comprovada
Vitamina E	Antioxidante	Lesão hepática aguda, hepatite crônica canina, lipidose hepática felina	10 a 15 UI de acetato de alfatocoferol/kg/24 h VO	Geralmente bem tolerada	O ideal é fornecer com alimento; a eficácia ainda não foi comprovada
Ácido ursodeoxicólico	Colerético, substitui ácidos biliares hidrofóbicos, antiapoptose	Colangite felina, hepatite crônica, mucocele biliar não cirúrgica	10 a 15 mg/kg/24 h VO	Diarreia ocasional	Não parece ter efeito importante no teste de ácidos biliares séricos

N-acetilcisteína

A N-acetilcisteína (NAC) é uma formulação de L-cisteína que ajuda a repor as concentrações intracelulares hepáticas de cisteína e glutationa, propiciando, assim, proteção contra lesão oxidativa.[3] A administração oral de NAC está frequentemente associada à êmese em cães e gatos.[6] Portanto, essa formulação é, em geral, administrada por via intravenosa, quando utilizada no tratamento de hepatopatias nessas espécies. Em um estudo com cães submetidos à ligadura de ductos biliares, a NAC melhorou os marcadores de circulação hepática e a condição de oxirredução.[11] Adicionalmente, um estudo recente demonstrou que a suplementação com NAC durante as primeiras 48 h de hospitalização estabilizou a concentração eritrocitária de glutationa em cães doentes.[12] Entretanto, os pesquisadores não conseguiram demonstrar um efeito benéfico da NAC em modelos experimentais de lesão hepática isquêmica e reperfusão, em cães.[13] A administração intravenosa de NAC demonstrou ser benéfica no tratamento de intoxicação por paracetamol em seres humanos e é um tratamento aceito, embora não criticamente avaliado para esse tipo de intoxicação em cães e gatos. A NAC é geralmente administrada como uma solução 10% diluída na proporção 1:2 em solução salina, na forma de *bolus*, por via intravenosa, ao longo de 20 minutos, por meio de um equipo com filtro não pirogênico de 0,25 mícron, na dose de 140 mg/kg, inicialmente, seguida de 70 mg/kg, a cada 8 a 12 horas.[6,14] Aventou-se a

possibilidade de que a administração durante um período prolongado poderia ocasionar prejuízo à metabolização da amônia no ciclo da ureia.[14] O autor considera a utilização desse fármaco como parte do tratamento inicial de cães e gatos com lesão hepática aguda causada por outros fármacos ou intoxicações e de gatos com lipidose hepática. Assim que esses pacientes consigam tolerar o uso de SAMe por via oral, a administração de NAC é descontinuada.

Silimarina

A silimarina é uma mistura de pelo menos 7 flavanolignanos e 1 flavonoide extraído da planta cardo-mariano.[15] A silibinina é o componente mais abundante e biologicamente ativo da silimarina.[16] Acredita-se que a silimarina tenha ação antioxidante por remover radicais livres e reduzir a lipoperoxidação.[17] Evidências experimentais e estudos em pacientes humanos sugerem vários outros potenciais benefícios. Primeiro, acredita-se que a silimarina apresente diversas ações anti-inflamatórias, incluindo supressão do fator de necrose tumoral alfa, interleucina 1 beta e fator nuclear kappa beta, e possa inibir o fibrosamento hepático por meio da redução da proliferação, migração e síntese do DNA de células estreladas hepáticas, além de redução da expressão do colágeno hepático.[18-20] Adicionalmente, foi demonstrado que a silimarina apresenta ação colerética em ratos.[21] Em doses comumente utilizadas, a silimarina não parece causar quaisquer efeitos colaterais.[18] Apesar da diminuição da atividade de enzimas do citocromo P-450, da enzima UDP-glicuronil-transferase e da redução do transporte da glicoproteína-P em seres humanos, a silimarina apresenta efeito limitado na farmacocinética de diversos fármacos *in vivo*. Entretanto, ainda se recomenda precaução ao administrar silimarina simultaneamente a medicamentos em pacientes humanos.[22] A biodisponibilidade da silimarina é maior quando combinada com a fosfatidilcolina, que atua como agente solubilizante.[23] Para essa forma do fármaco recomenda-se a dose de 5 a 10 mg/kg/24 horas via oral. Para as formas de menor biodisponibilidade de silimarina recomenda-se administrar a dose de 20 a 50 mg/kg/dia via oral, fracionada em intervalos de 6 a 8 h.[6] Entretanto, atualmente existem evidências limitadas que sustentam a eficácia desse nutracêutico na literatura veterinária. Foi demonstrado que uma combinação de SAMe e silimarina inibe a inflamação e o estresse oxidativo de hepatócitos de cães *in vitro*.[7] Em um estudo em que se administrou a toxina do cogumelo *Amanita phalloides* a cães da raça Beagle, todos os 11 cães tratados com silibinina por via intravenosa sobreviveram, enquanto 4 de 12 cães do grupo-controle morreram.[24] Portanto, é prudente administrar silimarina a cães e gatos intoxicados pela toxina de cogumelos do gênero *Amanita*. Outro estudo não constatou claras evidências de que a silimarina tenha efeito protetor após a ingestão de tetracloreto de carbono em cães.[25] Quando utilizada em combinação com SAMe e fosfatidilcolina, a silimarina mostrou ter ação hepatoprotetora quando foi administrado o quimioterápico lomustina.[10] Embora sejam necessários mais estudos clínicos para comprovar sua eficácia, o autor utiliza a silimarina em cães e gatos com lesão hepática aguda causada por fármacos/toxinas, em cães com hepatite crônica, em cães com hepatite crônica associada ao cobre e em gatos com lipidose hepática (ver Capítulos 282 a 286).

Vitamina E

A vitamina E é, na verdade, uma família de oito vitaminas lipossolúveis, sendo o alfatocoferol a biologicamente mais ativa.[1] A principal ação da vitamina E é antioxidante, que protege fosfolipídios de lesão oxidativa pela remoção de radicais livres.[26] Geralmente, a vitamina E é bem tolerada por cães e gatos e raramente notam-se efeitos colaterais.[6] O alfatocoferol é, em geral, administrado na dose de 10 a 15 UI/kg/24 horas via oral para cães e gatos. Alguns clínicos consideram a utilização desse suplemento como parte do protocolo terapêutico para cães e gatos com hepatopatias que podem causar danos oxidativos, como lesão hepática aguda causada por fármacos ou intoxicações, lipidose hepática felina, hepatite crônica e hepatite crônica causada pelo cobre.[6] Não existem atualmente evidências clínicas que comprovem a eficácia da vitamina E em cães ou gatos com hepatopatia. Entretanto, estudos recentes demonstraram efeito benéfico (melhora de sinais clínicos, marcadores de estresse oxidativo ou marcadores inflamatórios) em cães com dermatite atópica[27] ou doença articular degenerativa,[28] o que sugere que a vitamina E pode ser um antioxidante efetivo nessas espécies.

Ácido ursodeoxicólico

O ácido ursodeoxicólico (AUDC) é um ácido biliar hidrofílico que supostamente possui diversas propriedades benéficas: pode substituir ácidos biliares hidrofóbicos mais tóxicos no *pool* circulante,[29] possui ação colerética[30] que aumenta a excreção de toxinas endógenas na bile, tem efeito citoprotetor por inibir a apoptose de hepatócitos[31] e efeitos imunomoduladores, como supressão da expressão da interleucina 2.[32] É a única terapia aprovada pela Federal Drug Administration para tratamento da cirrose biliar em seres humanos.[33] Quando utilizada na dose de 10 a 15 mg/kg/24 horas via oral em cães e gatos, esse fármaco causa poucos efeitos colaterais, além de episódios ocasionais de diarreia.[6] Por conta de seu efeito colerético e da substituição de ácidos biliares hidrofóbicos mais tóxicos, existe uma razão por trás da utilização desse fármaco em cães e gatos com colestase intra e extra-hepática, como em casos de colangite em gatos. Em um estudo retrospectivo recente em gatos com colangite linfocítica, aqueles tratados com prednisolona sobreviveram por mais tempo do que aqueles tratados com AUDC.[34] Entretanto, esse estudo não provou que o AUDC não é efetivo no tratamento de colangite linfocítica felina, já que por motivos éticos o tratamento não foi comparado a um placebo. A utilização do AUDC em cães e gatos com obstrução total de ductos biliares é controversa, pois alguns clínicos se preocupam com a possibilidade de aumentar o risco de ruptura da vesícula biliar.[6] Outros clínicos se sentem seguros ao utilizar o AUDC nessa situação; estudos em ratos submetidos à ligadura de ductos biliares mostraram que, de fato, o AUDC tem efeito benéfico em marcadores de estresse oxidativo e apoptose.[35] Entretanto, é importante ressaltar que para a maioria dos cães e gatos com obstrução total de ductos biliares indica-se intervenção cirúrgica. Quando o paciente apresenta sinais clínicos discretos, ou ausentes, o AUDC algumas vezes é utilizado como parte do tratamento medicamentoso de mucocele biliar não obstrutiva em cães.[36] Ademais, devido aos seus supostos efeitos imunomoduladores e antiapoptose há uma razão teórica para a utilização do AUDC em cães com hepatite crônica, embora sua eficácia nessa condição ainda não tenha sido criticamente avaliada.

Fármacos anti-inflamatórios/imunossupressores

Corticosteroides

Os corticosteroides são utilizados no tratamento de doença hepática alcoólica[37] e hepatite autoimune,[38] mas em doses maiores podem aumentar a carga viral em pacientes humanos com infecção pelo vírus da hepatite C.[39] À medida que a prednisona inativa é transformada em prednisolona ativa pelo fígado, teoricamente faz mais sentido tratar cães com hepatopatia avançada com a última.[40] Entretanto, não é sabido se essa escolha faz qualquer diferença no resultado clínico. Gatos devem receber prednisolona em vez de prednisona. Embora o acúmulo de cobre no fígado seja uma importante causa de hepatite crônica, em grande número de cães com hepatite crônica não se detecta a causa primária.[2] Frequentemente, esses cães possuem inflamação hepática e necrose geralmente nas zonas periportais. Há uma associação entre hepatite crônica e alelos e haplótipos de antígeno leucocitário canino de classe II em cães das raças Doberman Pinscher[41] e English Springer Spaniel,[42] o que sustenta a participação de autoimunidade como causa de hepatite crônica nessas raças. Entretanto, são necessários estudos adicionais para determinar se a autoimunidade é uma causa de hepatite crônica nessas e em outras raças. Existem algumas evidências clínicas que sugerem que a prednisolona é um tratamento efetivo de hepatite crônica em cães. Um estudo retrospectivo com 151 cães com hepatite crônica de causas diversas constatou que os animais tratados com corticosteroides sobreviveram por mais tempo do que aqueles que não foram.[43] Entretanto, esses resultados devem ser interpretados com precaução, pois o planejamento retrospectivo desse estudo foi sujeito a tendências, pois os clínicos podiam ter decidido pelo uso de corticosteroides em cães que mais provavelmente teriam uma resposta favorável. Os resultados de um estudo retrospectivo não controlado mais recente em 36 cães com hepatite crônica idiopática indicaram que a inflamação hepática diminuiu e os parâmetros de coagulação retornaram ao normal após 6 semanas de tratamento com prednisolona, e em alguns cães o grau da fibrose hepática estabilizou ou melhorou. Entretanto, a maioria desses cães manifestou recidiva dos sinais clínicos ou doença residual no fim do tratamento.[44] Deve-se ressaltar também que os glicocorticoides frequentemente causam efeitos adversos, como poliúria/polidipsia, polifagia, respiração ofegante, alterações dermatológicas, e de maneira importante podem ter um efeito prejudicial no fígado, o que causa hepatopatia vacuolar e possivelmente estresse oxidativo.[8] São necessários estudos clínicos prospectivos controlados com placebo que avaliem a eficácia da prednisolona no tratamento de hepatite crônica idiopática canina antes de sua recomendação definitiva. O autor considera a realização de um teste terapêutico com prednisolona em cães com hepatite crônica que não tenham hepatite crônica associada ao cobre (com base na quantificação e coloração de cobre) e possuam cultura bacteriana hepática e/ou biliar negativa, especialmente se houver inflamação hepática moderada a grave no exame histológico de uma amostra obtida por biopsia hepática. Prednisolona/prednisona são em geral administradas na dose de 1 a 2 mg/kg/24 horas via oral, com descontinuação gradual do medicamento.[45] Já que a administração de glicocorticoides torna difícil a avaliação da resposta do paciente ao tratamento por meio de mensurações seriadas das atividades séricas de enzimas hepáticas, alguns clínicos recomendam repetição da biopsia hepática 6 semanas após o início do tratamento.[46] A prednisolona é frequentemente utilizada para tratar gatos com colangite linfocítica e colangite neutrofílica crônica, após cultura bacteriana biliar negativa e ausência de resposta ao teste terapêutico com antimicrobianos. Gatos com colangite linfocítica tratados com prednisolona sobreviveram por mais tempo do que aqueles tratados com AUDC.[34]

Azatioprina

A azatioprina é um análogo da purina ocasionalmente utilizada como imunossupressora em cães com hepatite crônica idiopática, em geral com o objetivo de possibilitar a utilização de doses menores de prednisolona/prednisona.[46] Para esse propósito recomenda-se a dose de 2 mg/kg/24 h VO durante 2 semanas e, em seguida, em intervalos de 48 h entre doses. Entretanto, a eficácia da azatioprina no tratamento de hepatite idiopática crônica canina ainda não foi avaliada; em estudo recente verificou-se que 5 de 34 cães (15%) tratados com esse fármaco supostamente desenvolveram hepatotoxicose.[47] A azatioprina não deve ser utilizada em gatos.

Ciclosporina

A ciclosporina é um inibidor de células T utilizada para induzir a remissão de hepatite autoimune em crianças.[48] Alguns poucos cães com hepatite idiopática crônica responderam bem ao tratamento com ciclosporina (5 mg/kg via oral, em intervalo de 12 a 24 horas), sem utilização concomitante de corticosteroides (comunicação não publicada, David Twedt e Allison Bradley). Entretanto, nessa situação, é necessária a avaliação crítica da eficácia e segurança do uso de ciclosporina antes que possa ser recomendada.

Medicamentos utilizados no tratamento de acúmulo de cobre no fígado

D-penicilamina

A D-penicilamina é um fármaco quelante que se liga ao cobre (e alguns outros metais pesados), possibilitando que seja metabolizado no fígado e excretado na urina. A penicilamina também pode ter ação antifibrótica, pois previne a formação de ligações cruzadas entre moléculas de colágeno;[49] ademais, pode ter propriedades imunomoduladoras.[50] Esse fármaco é indicado no tratamento de hepatite crônica associada ao cobre em cães.[51] A D-penicilamina é efetiva na redução da concentração hepática de cobre em cães da raça Bedlington Terrier, mas parece

necessário o tratamento por toda a vida, além de uma dieta com restrição de cobre.[52] O tratamento com D-penicilamina também mostrou-se efetivo na hepatite crônica associada ao cobre em cães das raças Labrador Retriever[53] e Doberman Pinscher.[54] Estudos farmacocinéticos desse fármaco, administrado na dose de 10 a 15 mg/kg/12 horas via oral, indicam que é mais bem absorvido quando fornecido com o estômago vazio.[55] Efeitos colaterais gastrintestinais são comuns em cães tratados com D-penicilamina. Quando ocorrem, pode ser necessária a redução da dose, administração com pequena quantidade de alimento ou descontinuação do medicamento.[51] A quelação prolongada pode causar deficiência de cobre, manifestada por anemia microcítica hipocrômica, anorexia, êmese e perda de peso.[52,56] Em seres humanos, a penicilamina foi associada a uma série de efeitos colaterais, como febre, erupções cutâneas, síndromes semelhantes ao lúpus, linfadenopatia, proteinúria, citopenias e teratogenicidade.[57] Em pessoas, a D-penicilamina também pode causar depleção de vitamina B6[58] e, embora isso nunca tenha sido relatado em cães, alguns clínicos suplementam essa vitamina durante o tratamento. Recentemente a quelação de cobre pela utilização de D-penicilamina foi relatada em 5 gatos presumivelmente com acúmulo de cobre hepático primário ou secundário. Notavelmente, um desses gatos desenvolveu anemia hemolítica, que foi resolvida após descontinuação da D-penicilamina.[59]

Trientina (2,2,2-Tetramina)

A trientina (2,2,2-tetramina) é outro agente quelante que pode ser utilizado em cães com hepatite crônica associada ao acúmulo de cobre. Esse fármaco quase sempre é uma segunda opção terapêutica em cães que não toleraram a D-penicilamina devido aos seus efeitos colaterais gastrintestinais. A trientina mostrou-se efetiva na elevação da taxa de excreção urinária de cobre em cães;[60] é utilizada em pacientes humanos com doença de Wilson.[61] A trientina pode remover mais cobre do *pool* circulante e menos do *pool* tecidual, comparada à D-penicilamina[61] e, portanto, pode ser uma boa escolha para cães com hemólise causada por alta concentração sérica de cobre. Esse fármaco é administrado na dose de 10 a 15 mg/kg/12 horas via oral e deve ser fornecido com o estômago vazio.[51] Supostamente, está associado a menos efeitos colaterais do que a D-penicilamina, embora ainda possam ocorrer êmese e anorexia; atualmente há poucos dados clínicos que justifiquem a sua utilização em cães.

Zinco

O zinco diminui a absorção gastrintestinal de cobre. Seu mecanismo de ação consiste na indução de aumento da síntese de metalotioneína pelos enterócitos. A metalotioneína se liga ao cobre com maior afinidade do que o zinco, impedindo assim que o cobre adentre a circulação. Quando as células intestinais morrem e sofrem descamação, o cobre dentro delas passa para as fezes.[61,62] Relata-se que a suplementação oral com acetato de zinco reduz a concentração hepática de cobre em cães com acúmulo de cobre hepático primário ao longo de vários anos, sem efeitos colaterais aparentes.[63] Em um estudo recente com cães da raça Labrador com hepatite crônica associada ao cobre, a terapia adjuvante com zinco não pareceu aumentar os efeitos da redução de cobre na dieta.[62] Assim que a terapia de quelação reduz a concentração hepática de cobre a um valor próximo ao normal, o zinco é comumente utilizado juntamente a dieta com restrição de cobre como tratamento de manutenção.[51] É interessante ressaltar que, por conta de sua eficácia e baixa taxa de efeitos adversos, o zinco tem sido recomendado como tratamento exclusivo às pessoas com doença de Wilson assintomática, em vez de agentes quelantes.[61] O zinco geralmente é administrado aos cães na dose de 5 a 10 mg de zinco elementar/kg/12 horas via oral, de preferência entre as refeições. Entretanto, algumas vezes é necessário fornecer ao animal uma pequena quantidade de alimento, já que o zinco pode causar êmese e náuseas.[51] O acetato de zinco é mais bem tolerado do que outras formas de zinco. Durante o tratamento deve-se monitorar a concentração plasmática de zinco. Em cães, a concentração plasmática normal de zinco varia de 70 a 200 mcg/dℓ. Concentrações ao redor de 200 mcg/dℓ parecem reduzir efetivamente a absorção de cobre;[63] concentrações que excedam 800 a 1.000 mcg/dℓ podem causar hemólise.[64] Rações comerciais formuladas para cães e gatos com hepatopatia geralmente são suplementadas com zinco.

RECOMENDAÇÕES TERAPÊUTICAS GERAIS

Lesão hepática aguda/Insuficiência hepática aguda

A lesão hepática aguda pode levar à insuficiência hepática aguda, a qual em humanos é caracterizada por aumento das concentrações séricas de bilirrubina, encefalopatia hepática e distúrbios de coagulação.[65] Ao tratar cães e gatos com lesão hepática aguda, é importante tratar a causa primária. Exemplos são a descontinuação de fármacos hepatotóxicos, indução de êmese em paciente que recentemente ingeriu uma substância hepatotóxica ou tratamento de leptospirose com doxiciclina. Entretanto, o tratamento específico da causa nem sempre é possível e, como o transplante hepático não é uma opção em cães e gatos, a terapia de suporte é crucial. Como a lesão oxidativa é geralmente um componente primário ou secundário da lesão hepática aguda, o tratamento com antioxidantes, inclusive SAMe, vitamina E e silimarina, é justificável.[6] Em pacientes que não toleram medicação oral, pode-se administrar NAC, por via intravenosa, em vez de SAMe. Como a síndrome de falência múltipla dos órgãos, a lesão renal aguda e a síndrome da angústia respiratória adquirida são complicações da insuficiência hepática aguda, portanto as funções de outros órgãos sistêmicos devem ser rigorosamente monitoradas. A fluidoterapia é frequentemente necessária; é preciso ter cautela ao tratar desidratação e anormalidades acido-básicas e eletrolíticas, já que estas podem precipitar a ocorrência de encefalopatia hepática (EH). Pacientes que apresentam êmese são beneficiados pelo tratamento com fármacos antieméticos, como a ondansetrona (0,2 mg/kg/8 a 12 horas por via intravenosa para cães e a cada 12 horas para gatos) e metoclopramida (1 a 2 mg/kg/dia por via intravenosa, como infusão contínua). O maropitant é metabolizado pelas enzimas hepáticas do citocromo P450, o que torna prudente diminuir a dose e/ou a frequência de administração ao utilizar esse fármaco em pacientes com insuficiência hepática. A ulceração gastroduodenal também é uma importante complicação da lesão hepática aguda e, em casos de suspeita desse quadro, recomenda-se o tratamento com omeprazol (0,5 a 1 mg/kg via oral, a cada 12 a 24 horas) ou pantoprazol (0,5 a 1 mg/kg, a cada 12 a 24 horas) e sucralfato (0,5 a 1 g/cão/8 h ou 0,5 g/gato/8 horas via oral). O edema cerebral é reconhecido como uma complicação da insuficiência hepática aguda em seres humanos,[65] e a EH também está associada a edema cerebral de baixo grau.[66] Se os sinais clínicos sugerem edema cerebral, como piora dos déficits neurológicos corticais, e aumento da pressão sanguínea sistêmica possivelmente devido à bradicardia, deve-se administrar manitol (0,5 a 1 g/kg via intravenosa).[67] A ligeira elevação da cabeça do paciente pode facilitar a drenagem venosa e ajudar a reduzir a pressão intracraniana. Pacientes humanos com insuficiência hepática aguda, por definição, apresentam coagulopatias, mas estas infrequentemente levam a hemorragias espontâneas. Portanto, em pacientes humanos recomenda-se que plasma e outros derivados do sangue devem ser reservados àquelas pessoas com hemorragia espontânea ou na preparação para procedimento invasivo.[65] Novas pesquisas são necessárias para determinar se essa recomendação é também apropriada para cães e gatos com insuficiência hepática aguda. Deve-se ter cuidado ao administrar concentrado de hemácias armazenadas a cães e gatos com lesão hepática aguda, já que pode ocorrer aumento substancial da concentração de amônia durante o armazenamento dessas hemácias.[68] Como os pacientes com lesão hepática aguda possuem algumas vezes deficiências de vitamina K devido à colestase, recomenda-se o tratamento com vitamina K (3 doses de 0,5 a 1,5 mg/kg SC, em intervalos de 12 horas). Sepse é uma complicação potencial em pacientes humanos com insuficiência hepática aguda.[69] A utilização profilática de antimicrobianos diminui a incidência de infecções, mas não demonstrou conferir maior tempo de sobrevida e pode propiciar o desenvolvimento de infecções resistentes a antimicrobianos.[70] Portanto, é recomendado que cães e gatos com insuficiência hepática aguda sejam ativamente avaliados em busca de sinais de infecção e antimicrobianos de amplo espectro somente sejam utilizados se houver suspeita de infecção bacteriana.

Hepatite crônica

A hepatite crônica é mais comum em cães do que em gatos, sendo estes mais acometidos por colangite. Embora os agentes hepatoprotetores descritos anteriormente sejam frequentemente utilizados e possam ser benéficos no tratamento de cães com hepatite crônica, eles não substituem o tratamento das causas primárias das hepatopatias. É necessária a biopsia hepática para diagnosticar hepatite crônica e tentar identificar a causa primária.[46]

O acúmulo de cobre é uma causa importante de hepatite crônica em cães, o que faz com que cortes histológicos do fígado devam rotineiramente ser corados para análise de cobre, e uma amostra de fígado obtida por biopsia, não fixada, deve ser enviada para análise quantitativa de cobre. Mesmo assim, a decisão sobre em quais casos deve-se iniciar a quelação de cobre nem sempre é simples (Figura 281.1). Para a maioria dos laboratórios, o valor de referência para a concentração hepática de cobre de cães saudáveis é < 400 μg/g de peso seco (ou matéria seca [MS]). Entretanto, 9 cães saudáveis de pesquisa alimentados com ração comercial padrão apresentaram concentração hepática de cobre de 199 a 997 mcg/g, enquanto cães errantes, que presumidamente se alimentavam com dieta à base de restos alimentares, tiveram concentração de 69 a 372 μg/g MS.[71] Isso pode ser explicado porque as rações comerciais de cães contêm mais cobre do que restos alimentares. Pode ocorrer acúmulo de cobre no fígado devido a defeitos hereditários na excreção de cobre ou secundariamente à colestase. Em cães com hepatopatia primária por acúmulo de cobre, esse mineral tende a se acumular na zona centrolobular do fígado em alta concentração, geralmente > 1.000 mcg/g MS. Quando o acúmulo de cobre ocorre secundariamente à colestase, ele tende a ocorrer nas zonas periportais do fígado, está associado a menor concentração de cobre, comumente < 750 μg/g MS, e em geral não requer quelação.[18,72] Com base em trabalhos que utilizaram cães da raça Bedlington Terrier, a maioria dos laboratórios relatou que a concentração > 1.500 μg/g MS é hepatotóxica.[73] Entretanto, esse valor pode representar um limiar muito alto para a iniciação da quelação em outras raças. Novas pesquisas são necessárias para definir exatamente quando é apropriado iniciar a terapia de quelação. A partir de uma perspectiva prática, mesmo se não há lesão primária, o acúmulo de cobre no fígado pode causar lesão oxidativa, com subsequentes necrose e inflamação. Portanto, o autor institui a terapia de quelação em cães com concentração hepática de cobre > 1.500 μg/g MS, independentemente da distribuição, e também quando essa concentração é > 750 μg/g MS, se há acúmulo de cobre centrolobular, especialmente em raças que sabidamente desenvolvem hepatopatia primária por acúmulo de

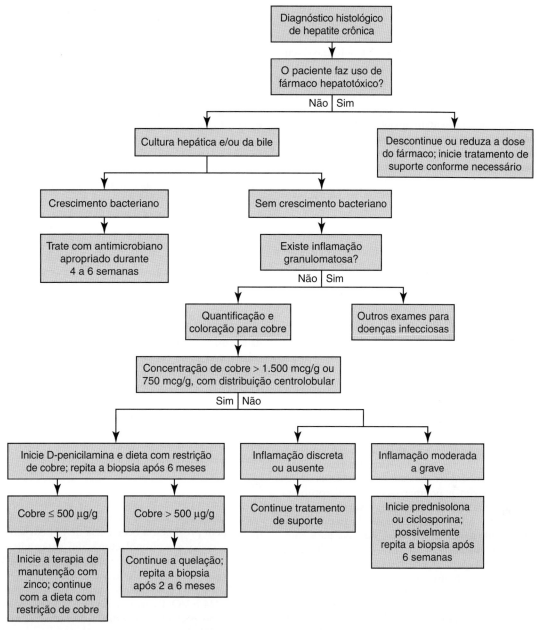

Figura 281.1 Tratamento de hepatite crônica canina. Esses pacientes também necessitam de terapia de suporte inespecífica que inclui agentes citoprotetores (ver Tabela 281.1) e, quando necessário, tratamento de complicações gastrintestinais causadas por hepatopatia, encefalopatia hepática ou ascite. Quando for diagnosticada hepatite granulomatosa, recomendam-se outros testes para doenças infecciosas, inclusive coloração histológica para bactérias e fungos, PCR para *Bartonella* spp., teste para esquistossomose canina, se geograficamente relevante, e possivelmente cultura para micobactéria.

cobre. Esses cães devem ser alimentados com dieta com restrição de cobre. Em estudo recente constatou-se que cães da raça Labrador Retriever com concentração hepática de cobre > 1.500 μg/g MS necessitaram de tratamento por pelo menos 10 meses para alcançar concentração hepática de cobre de 400 μg/g MS, e aqueles com concentração hepática de cobre inicial entre 1.000 μg/g MS e 1.500 μg/g MS necessitaram de tratamento por aproximadamente 6 meses.[53] A eficácia do tratamento é idealmente confirmada 6 meses após o início da quelação, por meio da mensuração da concentração de cobre em uma amostra de fígado obtida por biopsia. Para raças que não sejam Bedlington Terrier, é geralmente possível cessar a terapia de quelação e iniciar o tratamento de manutenção com zinco, ao mesmo tempo que se continua a dieta com restrição de cobre.

Infecções bacterianas aeróbicas e anaeróbicas devem sempre ser descartadas com base nos resultados da cultura microbiológica da bile e do tecido hepático. Quando é diagnosticada hepatite granulomatosa, recomendam-se outros testes para doenças infecciosas, inclusive coloração histológica para bactérias e fungos, reação em cadeia de polimerase (PCR) para *Bartonella* spp., teste para esquistossomose canina se geograficamente relevante e possivelmente cultura para micobactérias. Mesmo se esses microrganismos não forem identificados, pode ser prudente realizar testes terapêuticos com medicamentos efetivos contra eles, antes de iniciar a administração de fármacos imunossupressores. Se há suspeita de hepatite crônica causada por tratamento prolongado com um medicamento, como o fenobarbital, o fármaco é descontinuado, se possível. Se há um componente compatível com inflamação, especialmente de origem linfoplasmocítica, na ausência de uma causa primária tratável, deve-se realizar um teste terapêutico com prednisolona.[43] Assim que a prednisolona for iniciada, deve-se realizar avaliação seriada das atividades séricas das enzimas hepáticas, mas isso tem valor limitado no monitoramento da resposta à terapia. Portanto, recomenda-se a repetição da biopsia hepática 6 semanas após o início do tratamento para determinar se houve algum efeito benéfico.[44,46] Conforme discutido anteriormente, existe uma base fisiopatológica para o tratamento desses cães com SAMe, silimarina, AUDC e vitamina E.[6] A terapia de suporte geral é também importante para cães com hepatite crônica. Cães com hepatopatia, especialmente aqueles com hipertensão portal, apresentam maior risco de ulceração gastroduodenal.[74] Consequentemente, se confirmada a ulceração gastroduodenal ou há suspeita, deve-se iniciar o tratamento com omeprazol e sucralfato. Fármacos antieméticos também podem ser indicados. É importante o fornecimento de dieta adequada, de alta qualidade; cães com EH não necessitam ser alimentados com dieta com restrição de proteínas.[75]

Fibrose hepática

Não existem tratamentos comprovados para fibrose hepática em cães ou gatos, o que faz com que as recomendações seguintes sejam feitas com base em princípios fisiopatológicos e dados obtidos de outras espécies. A inflamação hepática crônica pode levar à ativação de miofibroblastos, inclusive células estreladas hepáticas e fibroblastos portais, que, por sua vez, podem causar fibrose hepática.[76] Quando possível, é fundamental o tratamento da causa primária da inflamação hepática. O tratamento com anti-inflamatórios/imunossupressores também é racional quando não é possível identificar/tratar com sucesso a causa primária da inflamação crônica. Em estudo previamente mencionado sobre cães com hepatite crônica idiopática constatou-se que, após o tratamento com prednisolona, a fibrose hepática foi resolvida em 14% dos animais e melhorou em outros 11%.[44] A lesão oxidativa também pode levar à ativação de células estreladas hepáticas,[77] o que faz com que antioxidantes, como SAMe e silimarina, possam também ser indicados. A colchicina se liga à tubulina, inibindo assim a polimerização de microtúbulos durante a mitose, o que impede, portanto, diversos processos celulares que incluem inflamação e fibrose. Entretanto, não existem evidências suficientes na literatura humana para comprovar a eficácia da colchicina no tratamento de fibrose hepática em pacientes com hepatopatia alcoólica e se sua utilização está associada à alta taxa de efeitos adversos.[78] Com exceção de alguns poucos relatos de caso,[79-81] a partir dos quais é difícil estabelecer um efeito positivo, a eficácia da colchicina ainda não foi avaliada em cães. Por conta disso e da alta incidência de efeitos colaterais gastrintestinais associados ao uso de colchicina, o autor não recomenda sua utilização. O uso terapêutico desse fármaco ainda não foi relatado em gatos, e esta espécie parece ser particularmente suscetível aos efeitos tóxicos da colchicina, que podem ser fatais.[82] Em ratos, o antagonista de receptores de angiotensina II, a losartana, demonstrou ter efeito antifibrótico no fígado. Entretanto, esses resultados ainda não foram positivamente reproduzidos em pacientes humanos,[83,84] e não existem estudos que avaliaram a eficácia desse medicamento no tratamento de fibrose hepática em cães ou gatos.

Encefalopatia hepática

É importante identificar e tratar os fatores que potencialmente precipitam a ocorrência de EH, como hemorragia gastrintestinal, infecção, desidratação, anormalidades eletrolíticas e alcalose, assim como administrar terapia de suporte.[85] Assim como em seres humanos,[86] a restrição rigorosa de proteínas não é mais recomendada para cães com EH, pois isso pode levar à desnutrição relacionada à hipoproteinemia.[75] Dietas à base de proteínas não oriundas da carne são geralmente recomendadas para cães com EH. Em um estudo em cães com desvio portossistêmico congênito alimentados com dois tipos de dieta com restrição de proteínas, uma com carne e outra com soja, verificou-se que ambas as dietas abrandaram a gravidade da EH. Entretanto, a melhora na concentração de amônia e nos parâmetros de coagulação foi significativamente maior em cães alimentados com dieta à base de soja.[87] Assim que os sintomas de EH são controlados com ração comercial de suporte hepático, recomenda-se a adição de proteína não oriunda da carne à dieta do paciente para ajudar a prevenir desnutrição relacionada à hipoproteinemia.[88] Gatos possuem maior necessidade de proteína na dieta do que os cães, pois não são capazes de regular o catabolismo proteico, mesmo quando a alimentação é suspensa.[89] Portanto, a restrição proteica grave é inapropriada para essa espécie. O laxante osmótico lactulose é comumente utilizado para tratar EH em cães e gatos. A lactulose pode ser administrada por via oral aos cães e gatos com EH crônica, na dose de 1 a 3 mℓ/10 kg de peso corporal, em intervalos de 6 a 8 horas. Em seguida, essa dose é ajustada até que o paciente defeque 3 ou 4 vezes/dia, com fezes amolecidas. Em pacientes com apoplexia ou coma, a lactulose pode ser administrada por via retal, após realização de enema com água morna.[67] A neomicina é um antibiótico aminoglicosídeo de baixa absorção que algumas vezes é utilizado no tratamento de cães e gatos com EH (20 mg/kg/8 horas via oral). A absorção gastrintestinal da neomicina é em geral muito baixa, mas a absorção sistêmica substancial pode causar ototoxicidade e nefrotoxicidade. Em seres humanos, a neomicina não é mais utilizada no tratamento de EH por essas razões.[90] O metronidazol é algumas vezes utilizado no tratamento de EH em cães e gatos (7,5 mg/kg VO, a cada 8 a 12 horas). O metronidazol é metabolizado no fígado e pode causar efeitos colaterais neurológicos que mimetizam aqueles da EH. Entretanto, estes são mais prováveis quando se utilizam doses maiores para esse propósito.

Ascite

O uso de furosemida pode causar desidratação/hipovolemia, hipopotassemia e alcalose metabólica hipoclorêmica, condições que podem precipitar a ocorrência de EH em seres humanos.[66] Por essa razão, a espironolactona, um antagonista do receptor de aldosterona, com dose inicial de 2 mg/kg/24 h VO, é preferida para o tratamento de ascite causada por hepatopatia em cães e gatos. Essa dose pode ser gradativamente aumentada para 4 mg/kg/24 h VO. Durante a diurese é prudente avaliar o peso corporal do paciente, a condição de hidratação/circulatória, o volume globular (ou hematócrito), a concentração sérica de creatinina e as concentrações séricas de eletrólitos. Se o tratamento com espironolactona não for efetivo, pode-se iniciar o uso de furosemida, em dose baixa (1 a 2 mg/kg/12 horas via oral).[91] Assim que a ascite é resolvida, é possível diminuir a dose do diurético. A restrição discreta de sódio na dieta também é aconselhável, e rações comerciais para cães e gatos com hepatopatia atendem a essa especificação. A abdominocentese terapêutica pode agravar a hipoalbuminemia e, portanto, deve ser reservada para animais refratários ao tratamento medicamentoso e/ou que apresentam comprometimento respiratório devido ao grande volume da ascite. Há relato de hipovolemia em seres humanos após a abdominocentese.[92] Portanto, em cães e gatos submetidos a esse procedimento, deve-se considerar a possibilidade de expansão simultânea da volemia com solução coloidal sintética ou plasma.[91]

REFERÊNCIAS BIBLIOGRÁFICAS

As referências bibliográficas deste capítulo se encontram online no Ambiente de Aprendizagem.

CAPÍTULO 282

Hepatopatias Inflamatórias/Infecciosas em Cães

Craig B. Webb

Hepatopatias em seres humanos são mais frequentemente causadas por infecção viral (hepatites A a E) ou alcoolismo.[1] O consumo crônico de álcool não é um problema em pacientes veterinários. Com o advento das vacinas contra adenovírus-2 canino (CAV-2), a hepatite infecciosa canina é agora uma causa rara de hepatopatia aguda em cães.[2] Duas doenças hepáticas menos comuns em seres humanos, a lipidose hepática não alcoólica e a hepatite autoimune, podem ser relevantes em animais em razão de potenciais semelhanças na fisiopatologia ou estratégias terapêuticas (ver Capítulo 280).[3] Mesmo na rotina de pacientes de pequeno porte, a localização primária de lesões hepáticas parece claramente distinta entre gatos e cães, sendo o sistema biliar predominantemente afetado em gatos, e o parênquima hepático é o alvo principal da doença em cães.

O grupo responsável pela padronização de doenças hepáticas da World Small Animal Veterinary Association padronizou a classificação e a nomenclatura das hepatopatias em cães e gatos.[4] A colangite (inflamação dos ductos biliares) é dividida em quatro grupos: colangite neutrofílica, colangite linfocítica, colangite destrutiva e colangite crônica associada à fasciolose hepática. As colangites neutrofílica e linfocítica são observadas quase exclusivamente em gatos, a fasciolose é diagnosticada predominantemente em gatos, enquanto a colangite destrutiva é uma rara condição em cães.[4] Inflamação portal, fibrose e proliferação de ductos biliares são achados histopatológicos frequentes em casos de colangite, mas a ultrassonografia do sistema biliar e avaliação citológica e cultura da bile são necessárias para o diagnóstico clínico mais confiável. As doenças hepáticas de gatos são abordadas no Capítulo 283.

A hepatite (inflamação do parênquima hepático), observada predominantemente em cães, é mais frequentemente classificada como aguda ou crônica.[5] A forma crônica é ainda caracterizada histopatologicamente de acordo com padrão, localização, tipo de infiltrado celular, gravidade e extensão da inflamação, bem como grau de apoptose e necrose de hepatócitos, fibrose, cirrose e perda de arquitetura.[6] Em cada uma dessas categorias incluem-se causas infecciosas de hepatopatias de cães, embora a hepatite infecciosa aguda possa incitar alterações progressivas que resultam em hepatite crônica após a morte do microrganismo infeccioso original. Hepatites granulomatosa, eosinofílica e lobular dissecante são três tipos histopatológicos adicionais, embora raros. A maioria dos casos de hepatite primária em cães, ao contrário da hepatite secundária ou reativa, é idiopática. Causas específicas de hepatite aguda em cães são listadas no Boxe 282.1. Com relação à hepatite crônica, a maioria dos casos também é idiopática, embora os diagnósticos diferenciais a serem considerados incluam infecções, toxinas, medicamentos, anormalidades metabólicas e doença imunomediada.[7]

HEPATITE AGUDA

À semelhança da pancreatite aguda, a hepatite aguda em cães pode ser rapidamente fatal, completamente reversível ou progredir para hepatite crônica com o passar do tempo. Nesses casos, o diagnóstico precoce e a intervenção intensiva, iniciando

---

Boxe 282.1 Causas de hepatite aguda em cães

Infecciosas
CAV-1 (adenovírus)
Leptospirose
Clostridium spp.
Erliquiose monocítica canina (*E. canis*)

Toxinas (ver Capítulo 152)
Micotoxinas, aflatoxinas
Cianobactérias – intoxicação por microcistina ("algas verde-azuladas" ou eflorescência de algas)
Cogumelos do gênero *Amanita*
Xilitol (substituto do açúcar)
Superdosagem de manganês (suplemento articular)
Ácido alfalipoico
Solventes orgânicos (CCl_4)

Fármacos
Carprofeno, paracetamol
Combinação sulfonamida-trimetoprima
Azatioprina
Amiodarona
Mitotano

Idiopática

---

com tratamento específico da causa incitante, se conhecida, são fundamentais para um resultado bem-sucedido. O início da manifestação clínica é súbito e pode incluir uma série de sintomas inespecíficos, como letargia, anorexia, êmese ou diarreia, febre, dor abdominal, poliúria e polidipsia e desidratação. Alguns cães podem apresentar icterícia; em poucos, se em algum, espera-se o desenvolvimento de ascite. Esses cães geralmente apresentam elevação acentuada da atividade sérica das enzimas hepáticas alanina aminotransferase (ALT) e fosfatase alcalina (ALP), com elevações variadas nas atividades séricas de gamaglutamil transferase (GGT) e aspartato aminotransferase (AST). Cães podem ou não apresentar hiperbilirrubinemia e diminuição da glicemia e das concentrações de colesterol ou nitrogênio ureico sanguíneo (NUS), dependendo, em parte, do momento e da gravidade da causa incitante. Em casos agudos raramente nota-se hipoalbuminemia; anormalidades de coagulação são improváveis, embora deva-se monitorar a hemostasia. O hemograma pode indicar estresse ou inflamação, enquanto o exame de urina pode indicar ausência de alteração. Um diagnóstico histopatológico é raramente sugerido em casos de hepatite aguda em que a causa incitante mais provável é esclarecida pelo histórico de exposição a fármacos e toxinas ou em diversos exames de sangue e sorológicos para pesquisa de microrganismos infecciosos.

Cães com hepatite infecciosa causada por CAV-1 apresentam sintomas agudos, como febre, letargia, anorexia, dor na porção cranial do abdome, melena, êmese, diarreia e anormalidades bioquímicas indicativas de envolvimento hepático e renal. Os cães podem desenvolver broncopneumonia, conjuntivite, fotofobia e opacidade de córnea ou "olho azul", resultado da uveíte anterior e edema de córnea (ver Capítulo 11). Com o advento de protocolos de vacinação efetiva que incluem o CAV-2 para induzir proteção cruzada sem patogenicidade, a prevalência dessa doença foi reduzida de forma significativa, embora não tenha sido eliminada.[2,8,9]

A leptospirose atualmente é a causa infecciosa mais comum de hepatite aguda em cães, embora historicamente a infecção tenha sido associada mais frequentemente à lesão renal aguda e menor envolvimento hepático (ver Capítulo 217).[10,11] A leptospirose canina, causada por sorovares de *Leptospira interrogans* ou *L. kirschneri*, também é uma importante zoonose e em casos suspeitos devem-se fazer isolamento apropriado e barreiras de proteção. Os sorovares mais prevalentes e os fatores de risco observados em cães afetados mudaram com o advento de diferentes protocolos vacinais e medicamentos, assim como a exposição e fatores ambientais.[12-15] Sinais clínicos comuns incluem êmese, letargia, icterícia, diarreia, poliúria/polidipsia e anorexia. Conjuntivite e uveíte podem ser observadas, assim como sintomas de pneumopatia e comprometimento respiratório, coagulopatia e vasculite. Cães geralmente apresentam febre, azotemia, elevação das atividades séricas de enzimas hepáticas, hiperbilirrubinemia, anormalidades eletrolíticas, leucocitose, trombocitopenia e possível prolongamento do tempo de coagulação. O exame de urina pode indicar hipostenúria, glicosúria e proteinúria, com presença de bilirrubina, hemácias e leucócitos.[16] A avaliação diagnóstica e recomendações terapêuticas[16] são apresentadas no Capítulo 217 e na Tabela 282.1.

Em um cão da raça Yorkshire Terrier levado à consulta por apresentar início agudo de êmese e diarreia, diagnosticou-se colângio-hepatite causada por *Clostridium* spp., por meio de colecistocentese guiada por ultrassom e cultura microbiológica da bile. As anormalidades bioquímicas eram compatíveis com colestase e no exame histopatológico constataram-se inflamação e necrose hepática. O cão foi tratado com sucesso com clindamicina, amoxicilina-clavulanato e ácido ursodeoxicólico.[17] *Clostridium piliforme* foi identificado em um filhote de cão que apresentava hepatite necrosante multifocal.[18] *Clostridium* spp. é um dos isolados mais comuns em culturas microbiológicas de bile em cães e gatos com doença hepatobiliar.[19]

Há um relato sobre um cão Pastor-Alemão adulto que apresentava sinais clínicos e anormalidades bioquímicas compatíveis com hepatite aguda, cujo diagnóstico foi de infecção por *Ehrlichia canis*; após a identificação de *E. canis* utilizando exames citológicos, imuno-histoquímicos e reação em cadeia de polimerase (PCR), o cão foi tratado com sucesso com terapia de suporte e doxiciclina.[20]

Hepatite aguda causada por aflatoxicose já foi diagnosticada em cães, após consumo de ração comercial contaminada. Os sinais clínicos eram compatíveis com doença hepática tóxica aguda; a constatação, no histórico clínico, da provável fonte de exposição deve levar a descontinuação e teste do produto. O tratamento é inespecífico e de suporte.[21,22]

A hepatite aguda causada por intoxicação pela microcistina de cianobactérias, após exposição à eflorescência de algas, em geral é fatal, mas vários cães já foram tratados com sucesso com uma combinação de NaCl 0,9%, KCl e dextrose, plasma fresco congelado e sangue total, S-adenosilmetionina (SAMe) e silibinina, vitaminas do complexo B, vitamina K, famotidina, penicilina G procaína e colestiramina oral, que sequestra ácidos biliares.[23-25]

A ingestão de cogumelos *Amanita* spp. causa inflamação, necrose e insuficiência hepática aguda em cães. O diagnóstico é frequentemente presuntivo baseado na exposição e nos sinais clínicos, embora a alfa-amanitina possa ser detectada em tecido hepático por meio de cromatografia líquida acoplada à espectrometria de massa.[26] Existem raros relatos de tratamento efetivo da intoxicação por cogumelo *Amanita*, mas na maioria das vezes a condição é fatal, mesmo com a administração de N-acetilcisteína e silibinina.[27]

Há relato de necrose hepatocelular após a administração de carprofeno em uma série de cães. Os sinais clínicos incluíam anorexia, êmese e icterícia. As anormalidades bioquímicas incluíam hiperbilirrubinemia e elevação da atividade de enzimas hepáticas. O exame de urina era compatível com doença tubular renal. A terapia de suporte resultou em resolução bem-sucedida em vários, mas não em todos os casos, e acredita-se que a intoxicação seja uma reação medicamentosa idiossincrática (ver Capítulo 169).[28,29]

Há relato de necrose hepática e insuficiência em quatro cães dentro de 1 mês após o início da administração da combinação sulfonamida-trimetoprima (STM). Todos esses pacientes morreram ou foram submetidos à eutanásia, apesar da terapia de suporte intensiva, e foi determinado que a hepatotoxicose causada pelo uso de STM mais provavelmente se trata de uma reação medicamentosa idiossincrática.[30]

Embora o acúmulo de cobre cause hepatite crônica, há um relato de insuficiência hepática aguda em um cão da raça Dálmata jovem causada pelo acúmulo excessivo de cobre no fígado.[31] Isso pode ser um indicativo de que a intoxicação por cobre envolve um componente genético nessa raça.

HEPATITE CRÔNICA

Em cães, a maioria dos casos de hepatite crônica é idiopática.[5,32] A etiologia mais comumente identificada como causa ou contribuinte à hepatite crônica é o acúmulo excessivo de cobre no fígado. Em pelo menos uma raça, o acúmulo de cobre é resultado direto de um defeito metabólico, enquanto em outras raças pode ser um epifenômeno, embora tratável. Pode haver progressão morfológica e clínica da hepatite aguda para hepatite crônica, mesmo com a eliminação da causa incitante original; nesse sentido, vários diagnósticos diferenciais para hepatite aguda (ver Boxe 282.1) podem ser incluídos como causas potenciais de hepatite crônica. Relata-se que algum mecanismo imunomediado também possa participar na etiologia da hepatite crônica em cães e, embora essa condição permaneça pouco definida, é frequentemente o alvo do tratamento da hepatite crônica.

Em cães, a manifestação clínica de hepatite crônica varia de aumento persistente das atividades de enzimas hepáticas até diminuição gradual na atividade, apetite e peso do animal, que podem ser atribuídos à "senilidade", até um início supostamente agudo de icterícia, anorexia, ascite e anormalidade do estado mental, indicativos de encefalopatia hepática. Anormalidades bioquímicas podem indicar redução significativa no metabolismo hepático, incluindo hipoglicemia, hipocolesterolemia, hipoalbuminemia, baixa concentração de NUS e hiperbilirrubinemia, juntamente com elevação das atividades de enzimas hepáticas. Por fim, as atividades de enzimas hepáticas podem ser normais, ou até mesmo abaixo dos valores de referência, em razão da perda grave de parênquima hepático (ver Boxe 280.3, no Capítulo 280). A diminuição dos fatores de coagulação normalmente produzidos pelo fígado pode ser clinicamente aparente, como hemorragia prolongada em um local de venopunção ou como prolongamento do tempo de coagulação (ver Capítulo 196). Em casos suspeitos de hepatite crônica, se não se constata aumento da concentração sérica de bilirrubina total, a avaliação das concentrações séricas de ácidos biliares pré e pós-prandial é uma excelente aferição da função hepática (ver Capítulo 280). Embora devam ser considerados diagnósticos diferenciais não hepáticos para a hiperbilirrubinemia, em cães o teste de ácidos biliares será anormal se a bilirrubina total estiver elevada de forma significativa em razão da hepatopatia, e os ácidos biliares são, portanto, um teste redundante nessa situação. Esses cães frequentemente apresentam poliúria, polidipsia e às vezes

CAPÍTULO 282 • Hepatopatias Inflamatórias/Infecciosas em Cães **1641**

Tabela 282.1 Considerações sobre o tratamento de hepatite aguda ou crônica em cães.

CONDIÇÃO/DOENÇA	TRATAMENTO	DOSE E CONSIDERAÇÕES*
Leptospirose	Doxiciclina	5 mg/kg/12 h VO ou IV durante 2 semanas
	Ampicilina	20 mg/kg/6 h IV no hospital
Enterobactérias: *E. coli*, *Enterococcus*, *Bacteroides*, *Streptococcus*, *Clostridium*	Ciprofloxacino Aminoglicosídeos Outros: enrofloxacino, clindamicina, cefalexina etc.	
Hepatite aguda	Plasmalyte®, Normosol®: cristaloide isotônico balanceado	Variável, baseada em diversos parâmetros
	Plasma fresco congelado: coloide, fatores de coagulação	Variável, baseada em diversos parâmetros
	Dextrose 2,5% + NaCl 0,45%: suplementação de líquido, hipoglicemia	Variável, baseada na glicemia
	Vitamina K1: fatores de coagulação dependentes de vitamina K	2,5 mg/kg/12 h SC, 1,6 mg/kg/24 h VO
	N-acetilcisteína: antioxidante, doador de metil, ↑ [Glu]	Dose única de 140 mg/kg IV; 70 mg/kg/6 h IV/VO
Encefalopatia hepática	Lactulose; ↓ pH do cólon, sequestra amônia, agente osmótico	Variável, baseada nos sintomas e na consistência das fezes, 5 a 30 mℓ VO ou enema
	Metronidazol: antibiótico, anaeróbicos	7,5 mg/kg/12 h VO
	Neomicina: antibiótico, baixa absorção	22 mg/kg/8 h VO
	S-adenosilmetionina: (SAMe) antioxidante, doador de metil, transulfuração	20 mg/kg/24 h VO
	Silimarina: intoxicação por cogumelo *Amanita*, antioxidante, anti-inflamatório, antifibrótico, hepatoprotetor	20 a 50 mg/kg/24 h VO
	Vitamina E: antioxidante na lipoperoxidação, antifibrótico	400 a 600 UI/24 h VO
	Vitaminas do complexo B	1 a 4 mℓ/cão/24 h SC IM IV
Cianotoxinas entéricas	Colestiramina: sequestra ácidos biliares	172 mg/kg/24 h VO
Hepatite crônica	Dieta: baixo conteúdo de Cu, adição de Zn e antioxidantes	Proteína: ↓ quantidade ↑ qualidade; ↑ CHO fermentáveis; ↓ Na
	Prednisolona: contraindicada na hepatite aguda	1 a 2 mg/kg/24 h VO; ajuste a dose de acordo com a resposta
	Azatioprina: imunossupressor antagonista da purina	2 mg/kg/24 VO, seguida de ajuste da dose
	Ciclosporina: imunossupressor celular	5 mg/kg/12 h VO
	Micofenolato de mofetila: inibição da síntese de purina	10 mg/kg/12 h VO
	Ácido ursodeoxicólico: ácido biliar hidrofílico, colerese, imunomodulação, ↑ produção de [Glu], citoprotetor	7,5 mg/kg/24 h VO ou 10 a 15 mg/kg/24 h VO
Acúmulo de cobre	D-penicilamina: quela Cu na circulação	5 a 15 mg/kg PO a cada 12 h, duas horas antes da alimentação, durante 6 meses, no mínimo
	Acetato de zinco: (35% de Zn elementar), impede a absorção de Cu	15 mg/kg/12 VO com alimento
	2,2,2-tetramina tetra-hidrocloreto (Trientina): quelante de Cu	5 a 15 mg/kg/12 h VO, 2 h antes da alimentação
	Tetratiomolibdato de amônio	20 mg/8 h VO
Fibrose	Colchicina	0,025 a 0,03 mg/kg/24 h VO
	Fosfatidilcolinas poli-insaturadas	50 a 100 mg/kg/24 h VO
Hipertensão portal	Espironolactona: diurético antagonista de aldosterona	1 a 2 mg/kg VO a cada 12 a 24 h
	Furosemida: diurético de alça	2 a 4 mg/kg VO ou IV a cada 8 a 12 h

*Aviso: Os clínicos devem sempre verificar as recomendações de doses com a informação mais atual disponível. *Glu*, glutationa; *IM*, intramuscular; *IV*, intravenosa; *SC*, subcutânea; *VO*, via oral.

hipostenúria. Outras anormalidades no exame de urina incluem hiperbilirrubinemia (0 a 1+, considerado normal em um cão) e cristalúria com cristais de biurato de amônio. O hemograma provavelmente indicaria leucograma de estresse ou inflamatório e poderia revelar anemia causada por doença crônica. De maneira alternativa, o hemograma poderia demonstrar anemia microcítica hipocrômica compatível com hemorragia gastrintestinal (GI) crônica secundária à hipertensão portal e edema intestinal. Os exames de imagem podem revelar fígado pequeno, brilhante e irregular com evidências de hipertensão portal ou desvios (shunts) adquiridos e ascite. O padrão-ouro para o diagnóstico e caracterização da hepatite crônica é a biopsia hepática. Infelizmente, esses cães frequentemente são atendidos quando a doença os torna maus candidatos à anestesia ou cirurgia. Mesmo a tentativa de biopsia hepática por via laparoscópica em cães com doença hepática crônica em estágio terminal poderia resultar em descompensação adicional da condição clínica. Entretanto, a biopsia hepática por laparoscopia (ver Capítulo 91) com exame histopatológico, análise de metais (cobre, ferro e zinco) e cultura microbiológica de tecido ou da bile é uma excelente oportunidade diagnóstica naqueles cães que estão relativamente estáveis, presumidamente em estágio mais precoce da doença, e possivelmente em condição clínica tratável ou pelo menos com um componente tratável, como o acúmulo de cobre. Em casos de hepatite crônica, a presença transitória de fibrose ou cirrose, que deformam o parênquima hepático, juntamente com necrose hepatocelular e inflamação mista, são ambas diagnósticas e, infelizmente, provavelmente prognósticas.

A hepatite aguda causada por toxinas (p. ex., aflatoxina) ou fármacos (p. ex., STM, anti-inflamatórios não esteroides) pode progredir para hepatite crônica com o passar do tempo, se o cão sobrevive ao dano inicial. Os fármacos que mais comumente causam hepatite crônica após administração por longo tempo são os anticonvulsivantes.[33,34] Embora a primidona seja raramente utilizada, há relatos de hepatotoxicose por fenitoína; o fenobarbital permanece a escolha comum para o tratamento de convulsões em cães.[35-37] Em cães, embora o fenobarbital supostamente induza produção da enzima hepática fosfatase alcalina (ALP), assim como os glicocorticoides, o exame histopatológico sugere que a elevação da atividade de ALT pela terapia com fenobarbital poderia ser decorrência do dano hepático.[38-40]

Assim como acontece com toxinas, as causas infecciosas de hepatite aguda podem ser a base para as alterações morfológicas que, por fim, progridem para hepatite crônica. Com o diagnóstico e tratamento precoces, vários cães com hepatite aguda causada por leptospirose se recuperam, ficam bem e, possivelmente, eliminam o microrganismo. Alguns desses cães podem desenvolver hepatite crônica muito mais tardiamente, com o passar do tempo, seja devido a uma infecção persistente de baixo grau, seja uma reação imunomediada contra a infecção original, seja uma continuação da resposta inflamatória. A identificação de causas infecciosas de hepatite crônica tem sido, de outra forma, desafiadora.[41,42] Em cães e gatos com inflamação hepática, os microrganismos mais comumente isolados da bile foram E. coli, Enterococcus spp., Bacteroides spp., Streptococcus spp. e Clostridium spp.[19] Helicobacter canis foi isolado do fígado de um cão com hepatite necrosante multifocal; todavia, Yersinia pseudotuberculosis, Salmonella spp., Clostridium piliforme, Campylobacter jejuni e riquétsias também são causas potenciais de hepatite infecciosa crônica.[43] A hepatite granulomatosa é uma forma de hepatite crônica na qual a etiologia frequentemente é infecciosa, incluindo micobactérias (ver Capítulo 212), fungos, larvas migrantes de nematódeos, Leishmania (ver Capítulo 221) e possivelmente Bartonella spp. (ver Capítulo 215).[44,45] A hepatite crônica com grande componente eosinofílico também pode ser causada por infecções parasitárias e larvas migrantes. O exame histopatológico e a cultura microbiana são componentes essenciais para o diagnóstico correto e um efetivo protocolo terapêutico. Fêmeas jovens da raça Springer Spaniel Inglês parecem predispostas a uma forma de hepatite crônica, na qual os achados histopatológicos são semelhantes àqueles da hepatite viral de seres humanos, mas até o momento nenhum vírus causal foi identificado.[46] Testes sorológicos, PCR e hibridização fluorescente in situ (HFIS) são tecnologias avançadas atualmente empregadas como ferramentas diagnósticas na busca por causas infecciosas da inflamação hepática. À medida que esta última tecnologia se torna mais prontamente disponível, é muito provável que esclareça a participação de bactérias na ocorrência de hepatite canina e, fazendo isso, ajuda a buscar antibioticoterapia específica naqueles casos em que é mais apropriada.

As terapias anti-inflamatória e imunossupressora geralmente são utilizadas no tratamento de hepatite crônica canina, frequentemente com bom efeito, de acordo com relatos informais. Isso sugere que em alguns desses casos há participação de algum componente imunomediado na etiologia ou progressão da doença. De forma ideal, um diagnóstico de uma condição imunomediada inclui a demonstração direta do componente do sistema imune responsável pela doença, mediada por anticorpos ou por células. Infelizmente, esse nível de especificidade raramente existe na medicina veterinária (p. ex., imuno-histoquímica e microscopia eletrônica, em caso de glomerulonefrite). Mais frequentemente, a evidência é circunstancial, como com a infiltração de linfócitos e plasmócitos em casos de doença intestinal inflamatória, a aglutinação de hemácias na anemia hemolítica imunomediada, ou a resposta acentuada a fármacos imunossupressores em casos de poliartrite imunomediada. Existem evidências circunstanciais também de um componente imunomediado na hepatite crônica canina, mas a resposta ao tratamento permanece o argumento clínico mais convincente para o uso contínuo de fármacos imunomoduladores em casos de hepatite crônica em cães.[47-51]

O acúmulo de cobre no fígado é o componente tratável mais comumente diagnosticado na hepatite crônica canina. O cobre (Cu) existe em uma série de formas, das quais o estado de oxidação cúprica (Cu^{2+}) provavelmente seja o responsável pela maior parte da hepatotoxicidade do cobre. O cobre é um componente fundamental no ciclo de redução e oxidação que gera radicais oxidativos que causam depleção das defesas antioxidantes hepáticas e causam danos a diversos componentes celulares.[52] Uma imensa quantidade de pesquisas em curso busca identificar o defeito ou marcador genético em uma série de raças, o defeito metabólico específico envolvido, o papel do cobre na dieta e o protocolo terapêutico mais efetivo para essa enfermidade.

A hepatopatia por acúmulo de cobre observada em cães da raça Bedlington Terrier é resultado de um defeito primário no metabolismo hepático de cobre, que ocasiona acúmulo excessivo de cobre nos lisossomos.[53,54] Pelo menos um defeito genético já foi identificado em animais Bedlington Terrier afetados por uma deleção no éxon 2 do gene COMMD 1 (gene MURR1 contendo o domínio do metabolismo do cobre); o padrão de herdabilidade parece ser autossômico recessivo.[55-58] A consequência metabólica dessa mutação é um defeito na capacidade de excretar cobre dos hepatócitos em direção aos canalículos biliares.[7,59,60] O papel do cobre na dieta e o dano oxidativo são discutidos com mais detalhes no Capítulo 285. O diagnóstico da intoxicação por cobre em cães da raça Bedlington é baseado em características histopatológicas e concentração e localização do cobre no fígado.[61,62] Nessa raça, o acúmulo de cobre hepático, os sinais clínicos, a diminuição da função hepática e os danos morfológicos são progressivos. A doença pode se manifestar como hepatopatia aguda ou, mais comumente, como doença hepática crônica, ambas clinicamente semelhantes a outras formas de hepatite aguda e crônica. Cães jovens da raça Bedlington Terrier podem apresentar um quadro pré-clínico assintomático, exceto com elevação das atividades de enzimas hepáticas. Raramente ocorre crise hemolítica aguda após intensa liberação de cobre do fígado para a circulação, o que pode ocorrer em qualquer cão com acúmulo excessivo de cobre hepático. O conteúdo normal de cobre hepático é < 400 ppm de matéria seca (MS), enquanto a concentração > 2.000 ppm resulta em doença funcional, morfológica e clínica. Cães da raça Bedlington Terrier apresentam acúmulo de cobre maior, até 50 vezes acima do normal, enquanto outras raças mais frequentemente apresentam valores 10 a 20 vezes acima do conteúdo normal. Em cães Bedlington Terrier homozigotos para o defeito genético, o acúmulo hepático de cobre pode começar com 8 a 12 semanas de idade, ou pode não ser evidente até 1 ano de idade e é progressivo. Em heterozigotos, pode haver um maior acúmulo ao redor dos 6 meses de idade, mas a concentração hepática de cobre é normal até os 15 meses de idade. Os clínicos não podem se basear na elevação das atividades séricas de enzimas hepáticas como marcador único da doença por acúmulo de cobre nessa raça, pois essas atividades podem ser normais em alguns casos. Esse padrão torna o teste genético uma importante ferramenta diagnóstica na tentativa de determinar quais indivíduos são afetados em uma idade jovem. O "teste de deleção TC" e "teste marcador TC" estão disponíveis no Veterinary Genetic Services e podem ajudar os criadores na tomada de decisões sobre acasalamentos.[63]

Até agora, Bedlington Terrier é a única raça na qual já foi identificada uma causa genética da hepatopatia por acúmulo de cobre. A possível herdabilidade da enfermidade em cães da raça Doberman Pinscher tem sido amplamente estudada, embora, assim como em várias raças, ainda não tenha sido estabelecido se o acúmulo de Cu é uma causa primária ou uma consequência secundária.[64-66] Em cães das raças West Highland White Terrier, Skye Terrier, Dálmata e Labrador Retriever pode ser uma condição familiar.[67-71] Um número crescente de outras raças apresenta acúmulo excessivo de cobre no fígado como causa ou consequência de sua condição. A prevalência crescente de intoxicação por cobre em cães de raças puras ou em mestiços destaca a provável importância de fatores ambientais, particularmente dietéticos, que contribuem de forma indubitável para esta condição.[72]

A distribuição do cobre hepático nos tecidos pode ajudar a diferenciar causas primárias de secundárias. Se o cobre é observado tanto em hepatócitos adjacentes ao tecido necrosado e inflamado quanto em hepatócitos distantes dessas lesões, sugere-se que o acúmulo de cobre é a causa primária da hepatopatia. Nesses casos, o acúmulo de cobre na zona 3 (centrolobular), assim como em nódulos regenerativos, e o grau de acúmulo em células de Kupffer e hepatócitos se correlacionam com a gravidade dos achados histopatológicos (ver Capítulo 285). Se o acúmulo de cobre é secundário a outra doença, em geral é encontrado na zona 1 (periporta), restrito àquelas áreas de tecido diretamente adjacentes à lesão celular, e não correlacionado com a gravidade da doença. Uma razão para a preferência pelo exame histopatológico de uma amostra de tecido em detrimento do exame citológico de aspirados hepáticos é a importância desses padrões zonais de distribuição. Mesmo os achados histopatológicos podem ser variáveis, desde a ausência de alterações celulares, com exceção do acúmulo de cobre na zona 3, até a presença de lipogranulomas e infiltrado inflamatório misto com cobre no citosol, ou fibrose, cirrose e perda da arquitetura hepática normal. O ácido rubeânico e a rodamina são corantes específicos de cobre, mas uma aferição quantitativa do cobre (espectroscopia de absorção atômica) é o ideal. Concentração de cobre > 400 ppm de MS é anormal, em vários casos de hepatite notam-se valores > 800 ppm, em casos graves > 1.500 ppm. O zinco e o ferro são os outros dois metais mais frequentemente quantificados em amostras obtidas por biopsia hepática. Ambos os metais possuem participações complexas nas doenças hepáticas, e ambos são potenciais alvos terapêuticos, com a suplementação com zinco e quelação do ferro, embora nenhum dos dois cause tanta preocupação como o acúmulo de cobre.[73]

TRATAMENTO

Até os dias atuais, existem, de forma surpreendente, poucas evidências sobre como basear as decisões terapêuticas em casos de inflamação hepática aguda ou crônica (ver Tabela 282.1). O primeiro alvo – tratamento da causa – é raramente uma opção, pois na maioria dos casos a causa incitante nunca é identificada e deve-se considerar como causa idiopática. Na ausência de um alvo específico, o foco da terapia se torna as anormalidades fisiopatológicas em curso e de suas consequências clínicas. Essas anormalidades incluem a extensão e a gravidade da inflamação e o tipo celular predominante envolvido; estase biliar; acúmulo de cobre; quantidade e extensão de fibrose, perda da arquitetura normal e progressão para cirrose e hipertensão portal; e a perda da função hepática.

Em casos de hepatite aguda secundária à ingestão de toxinas ou medicamentos, o agente incitante, se conhecido, é descontinuado imediatamente. Por conta do papel fundamental do fígado no metabolismo, a hepatotoxicose é um dos efeitos colaterais mais frequentemente listados para uma ampla variedade de medicamentos, bem como um alvo comum de toxinas e produtos metabólicos tóxicos. Deve-se obter uma anamnese cuidadosa e completa, incluindo todos os fármacos prescritos ou não, nutracêuticos, suplementos e petiscos, o que é parte fundamental da avaliação clínica. Também pode ocorrer intoxicação involuntária ou criminosa por meio da exposição a alimentos ou fatores ambientais, o que faz com que ambos devam ser questionados. A leptospirose é um diagnóstico diferencial particularmente importante em casos de hepatite aguda por conta do iminente risco zoonótico, do tempo e do esforço necessários para obter um diagnóstico definitivo e dos requerimentos terapêuticos mínimos e seguros (ver Capítulo 217). Mesmo em uma área de baixa prevalência e de exposição duvidosa, frequentemente são implementadas barreiras de proteção apropriadas e tratamento antimicrobiano assim que o paciente é hospitalizado, até o momento que a leptospirose possa ser excluída seguramente da lista de possíveis etiologias. Informações adicionais sobre manejo e tratamento de cães com leptospirose podem ser encontradas nas Declarações de Consenso de 2010 do ACVIM.[16]

A base do tratamento da inflamação hepática aguda é, de outro modo, a terapia de suporte, baseada em grande parte na condição clínica do paciente. A reposição de líquido é um componente fundamental para correção da desidratação (ver Capítulo 129), controle da condição acidobásica e do equilíbrio eletrolítico (ver Capítulo 128), manutenção da volemia, bem como da pressão sanguínea e da perfusão tecidual e dos órgãos (ver Capítulos 99 e 127) e suplementação de glicose. Em uma pesquisa sobre hepatite aguda idiopática constatou-se que antibióticos e ácido ursodeoxicólico foram as terapias mais frequentemente empregadas, enquanto prednisona, D-penicilamina e gliconato de zinco foram mais comumente administrados em casos de hepatite aguda causada pelo acúmulo de cobre.[5] A N-acetilcisteína atua como removedor de radicais livres e doador de radical metil; é utilizada em casos de hepatite aguda grave, a fim de aumentar a concentração hepática do antioxidante glutationa. Na hepatite aguda podem ser administrados diversos outros antioxidantes e precursores da glutationa, como SAMe, silimarina (silibinina) e vitamina E, embora a administração oral de medicamentos seja geralmente problemática na hepatite aguda.[74] O tratamento de suporte com coloides é controverso; contudo, o plasma ainda é utilizado em coagulopatias comprovadas. Nesses casos, antieméticos, redutores de acidez gástrica, protetores gástricos, estimulantes de apetite e analgésicos são possibilidades terapêuticas inespecíficas. Na maioria dos casos de hepatite aguda os glicocorticoides são contraindicados.

O tratamento de hepatite crônica também se baseia na condição clínica do paciente e, preferivelmente, nos achados histopatológicos padronizados pela WSAVA, na quantificação do cobre, nos resultados da cultura microbiológica e no monitoramento sequencial de parâmetros clínicos e bioquímicos. Se a causa for identificada, ela se torna o alvo específico, mas na maioria dos casos a doença é, novamente, idiopática.[75]

Pode ser necessária terapia antimicrobiana quando há suspeita de leptospirose; após resultado positivo de cultura bacteriana; em um cão febril com alterações hematológicas que incluem desvio à esquerda ou neutrófilos tóxicos; no caso de infiltrado hepático inflamatório supurativo; ou naqueles casos nos quais testes diagnósticos avançados, como HFIS, identificam um microrganismo-alvo em associação ao tecido inflamado. Nesses casos, a escolha do antibiótico costuma basear-se no desejo de cobrir um amplo espectro de possíveis microrganismos, ou é direcionada àqueles microrganismos frequentemente identificados em amostras de cultura positivas: *Escherichia coli*, *Enterococcus* spp., *Bacteroides* spp., *Streptococcus* spp. e *Clostridium* spp.[19] O conhecimento da sensibilidade a antibióticos (antibiograma) está se tornando componente fundamental para uma terapia efetiva em medicina veterinária. Relata-se que a maioria das enterobactérias isoladas de aspirados da vesícula biliar foi sensível a ciprofloxacino ou aos aminoglicosídeos; aminopenicilinas e cefalosporinas de primeira geração foram muito menos efetivas.[19] Doxiciclina, enrofloxacino, clindamicina, cefalexina, combinação amoxicilina-ácido clavulânico e marbofloxacino têm sido utilizados em casos de suspeita de hepatite bacteriana.

Antibióticos também são indicados em casos de encefalopatia hepática. Nesse caso, o objetivo é interferir no microbioma GI de tal forma que diminua a produção e, portanto, a absorção potencial de amônia. Assim, a escolha do antibiótico se baseia em sua atuação em componentes específicos do microbioma, como o metronidazol, ou com base no local predominante de ação, o trato GI, como a neomicina. A lactulose é outra terapia padrão para pacientes com sintomas de encefalopatia hepática, cujo objetivo é reduzir a absorção de amônia por meio da alteração do pH do conteúdo GI.[76,77]

O alvo da terapia do acúmulo de cobre no fígado é mais fortemente justificado em pacientes nos quais o conteúdo hepático real de cobre tenha sido quantificado em valores > 1.500 a 2.000 ppm. Com exceção de cães da raça Bedlington Terrier e talvez várias outras raças, o papel do acúmulo de cobre como anormalidade primária é menos claro e o uso indiscriminado de terapia quelante de cobre é mais problemático. Entretanto, em casos nos quais se constatou acúmulo hepático de cobre, estudos mostraram que a utilização a longo prazo da D-penicilamina é benéfica.[78,79] Uma dieta com baixo teor de cobre e suplementada com zinco também é comumente utilizada a fim de reduzir a exposição ao cobre, bem como remover esse mineral; é necessário tratamento durante meses e, de forma ideal, o acompanhamento inclui repetição da biopsia hepática e quantificação do cobre.[80-82] Se utilizada concomitantemente, a D-penicilamina pode quelar o zinco do sangue, reduzindo sua efetividade. A D-penicilamina pode causar efeitos colaterais GI substanciais. O cloridrato de trientina é uma alternativa como quelante de Cu, com evidências não publicadas de eficácia em uma série de cães, e o tetratiomolibdato de amônio, historicamente utilizado para intoxicação por cobre em ovelhas, está sendo pesquisado para uso em cães.[83,84]

A terapia que almeja a redução do dano oxidativo e a reposição da defesa antioxidante esgotada inclui, mais comumente, os nutracêuticos SAMe, silimarina (silibinina) e vitamina E. Embora a depleção das defesas antioxidantes tenha sido demonstrada em cães com doença hepática, estratégias efetivas de suplementação antioxidante são ainda baseadas predominantemente em considerações teóricas.[85]

O ursodiol (ácido ursodeoxicólico), um ácido biliar hidrofílico sintético, pode ter uma série de propriedades que seriam benéficas em casos de inflamação hepática. O ursodiol é um colerético utilizado frequentemente para combater a colestase e substituir ácidos biliares hidrofóbicos tóxicos, e pode ajudar a excluir o excesso de ferro ou cobre. O ursodiol pode ter propriedades imunomoduladoras e citoprotetoras, assim como capacidade de repor as defesas antioxidantes.[74]

Na inflamação hepática crônica na qual a fibrose progrediu para cirrose, é comum ocorrer hipertensão portal. A hipertensão portal, frequente em cães que também apresentam hipoalbuminemia, resulta em ascite, edema e ulceração do trato GI, e sintomas de encefalopatia hepática. O tratamento dos sintomas GI é inespecífico e de suporte, e inclui a utilização de sucralfato, bloqueadores H2 e inibidores da bomba de prótons. Plasma, coloides ou albumina humana podem ser utilizados para tentar manter a pressão oncótica vascular, mas essas terapias causam importantes efeitos colaterais. A espironolactona, em combinação com a furosemida, é uma abordagem medicamentosa para ascite, se o momento e os sinais clínicos permitirem; de outro modo, a abdominocentese terapêutica é utilizada em casos nos quais a ascite causa comprometimento cardiorrespiratório (ver Capítulo 90). Sintomas de encefalopatia hepática (EH) requerem intervenção dietética, com fornecimento de proteínas de alta qualidade, mas em menor quantidade, preferivelmente de origem vegetal, com fibras fermentáveis, e limitado conteúdo de gordura. A lactulose, administrada por via oral ou na forma de enema, é a terapia padrão para EH utilizada para acidificar o pH do cólon e reduzir a produção e absorção de amônia.

Inflamação ampla, sem evidência de infecção, infiltrado linfocítico-plasmocítico compatível com doença imunomediada, ou necessidade de tratar quadro importante de fibrose, são argumentos para utilização de corticosteroides em casos de hepatite crônica.[86] O tratamento contínuo com corticosteroides é contraindicado em casos de hepatite infecciosa, mas, por causa da incerteza diagnóstica, corticosteroides frequentemente são administrados simultaneamente com antibióticos no início do tratamento. Essa estratégia tem uma série de potenciais armadilhas e ressalta a importância de elaboração de um plano diagnóstico minucioso e de acompanhamento rigoroso para ajudar a direcionar o tratamento. A colchicina e o zinco também são utilizados na tentativa de retardar a progressão da fibrose; fármacos imunomoduladores adicionalmente utilizados, com certa frequência, incluem azatioprina, ciclosporina e micofenolato de mofetila.

RESUMO

Estão ocorrendo avanços importantes em nosso conhecimento sobre doenças hepáticas inflamatórias e infecciosas em cães. A padronização da interpretação histopatológica e da nomenclatura unificou o esquema de classificação das hepatopatias em cães. Avanços em curso nas técnicas moleculares e tecnologias diagnósticas, como PCR e HFIS, continuarão a ajudar a identificar e desvendar a etiologia primária de hepatopatias em cães. Por fim, novas fronteiras no tratamento, particularmente da hepatite crônica canina, incluem possibilidades excitantes, como transplante tecidual e terapia com células-tronco.[87,88]

REFERÊNCIAS BIBLIOGRÁFICAS

As referências bibliográficas deste capítulo se encontram online no Ambiente de Aprendizagem.

CAPÍTULO 283

Hepatopatias Inflamatórias/Infecciosas em Gatos

Marnin A. Forman

INTRODUÇÃO

Doenças hepatobiliares inflamatórias e infecciosas em gatos são causas comuns menos frequentes de morbidade e mortalidade.[1] Doença hepatobiliar inflamatória é uma das doenças hepáticas mais comuns em gatos nos EUA, no Reino Unido e na Europa.[2] Em um estudo, constatou-se que 45 de 175 biopsias hepáticas realizadas em gatos (26%) revelaram doença inflamatória.[3] Em gatos, duas hepatopatias inflamatórias comuns são colângio-hepatite (aguda [supurativa] e crônica [não supurativa ou mista]) e hepatite portal linfocítica.[3,4] Mais recentemente, o comitê de padronização da World Small Animal Veterinary Association (WSAVA) recomendou um sistema de classificação distinto para características histológicas de hepatite portal linfocítica e colangite linfocítica crônica[5] e um grupo internacionalmente aceito de terminologias diagnósticas para hepatopatias.[6] Esse esquema diferenciou inflamação de ductos biliares (colangite) em quatro categorias: colangite neutrofílica, colangite linfocítica, colangite destrutiva e colangite crônica associada à fasciolose.[6]

Doenças hepatobiliares infecciosas, diagnosticadas menos frequentemente, permanecem um importante diagnóstico diferencial ao formular protocolos terapêuticos. Há sobreposição na definição de doenças hepatobiliares infecciosas e inflamatórias, especialmente no caso de colangite neutrofílica. Já foram documentadas várias doenças hepáticas infecciosas primárias que resultam em inflamação secundária. Lipidose hepática felina, a doença hepática mais comum em gatos, é abordada no Capítulo 285. Doenças neoplásicas do fígado e hepatopatia causada por acúmulo de cobre no fígado são ocorrências possíveis e são brevemente discutidas (ver Capítulo 285). Os sinais clínicos apresentados, uma base de dados mínima e os exames de imagem podem ajudar a diferenciar doenças inflamatórias, infecciosas e neoplásicas, assim como lipidose hepática. Entretanto, o exame citológico ou histológico é essencial para obter o diagnóstico definitivo.

COLANGITE/COLÂNGIO-HEPATITE NEUTROFÍLICA

Definições

A colangite neutrofílica (CN) é mais comum em gatos do que em cães;[6] é subclassificada em colangite neutrofílica aguda (CNA) e colangite neutrofílica crônica (CNC).[1] A patogenia proposta consiste em infecção bacteriana intestinal ascendente.[1,7] Histologicamente, os neutrófilos são notados no lúmen do ducto biliar, intimamente associados ao ducto biliar, ou entre as células do epitélio biliar. Se a inflamação se estende além da placa limitante e em direção ao parênquima hepático, o diagnóstico é de colângio-hepatite (CH). A progressão da doença pode resultar em ruptura do ducto biliar e extravasamento de bile, necrose ou abscesso.[6]

Características clínicas e laboratoriais de rotina

Relatos iniciais sugeriam que gatos com doença neutrofílica aguda eram mais jovens e mais propensos a febre, perda de peso e neutrofilia com desvio à esquerda.[3,5,8] Mais recentemente, a sobreposição de achados clínicos e laboratoriais foi notada em gatos com doença aguda ou crônica.[1] Sinais clínicos comuns incluem letargia, êmese, perda de peso e diminuição do apetite. As anormalidades do exame físico não são comuns, mas consistem em febre (22%), icterícia (34%) e hepatomegalia (21%). Anormalidades no hemograma são detectadas em menos da metade dos gatos com CN e, quando presentes, incluem leucocitose (39%), neutrófilos bastonetes (33%) e anemia (34%). Gatos com colangite moderada à grave podem ter atividades séricas de enzimas hepáticas normais, mas incrementos na atividade da aspartato aminotransaminase (AST) foram notados em 98% dos gatos. Foram verificados aumentos variados nas atividades de alanina aminotransaminase (ALT) em 50 a 57%, fosfatase alcalina (ALP) em 14 a 48% e gamaglutamil transferase (GGT). Vários gatos com colangite possuem valores de enzimas hepáticas (ALT, ALP, GGT) dentro da faixa de referência, mas cerca de dois terços manifestam hiperbilirrubinemia.[3] Os parâmetros da função hepática foram infrequentemente anormais (hipoglicemia 7%, diminuição do nitrogênio ureico sanguíneo 0%, hipoalbuminemia 13% e hipercolesterolemia 6%).[1,3] A especificidade das concentrações séricas de ácidos biliares em jejum e pós-prandial, utilizando limites de 15 micromol/ℓ e 20 micromol/ℓ, respectivamente, foi maior do que a de teste enzimático e deve ser considerada quando há suspeita de hepatopatias em gatos com atividades enzimáticas e concentração de bilirrubina normais.[9] Com relação aos testes de coagulação, as anormalidades mais comuns citadas variaram e são mais provavelmente influenciadas pela população estudada e metodologia do teste.[10] Anormalidades incluíram prolongamento do tempo de protrombina (TP: 4 a 77% dos casos), prolongamento do tempo de tromboplastina parcial ativada (TTPa: 25 a 55%), redução das atividades dos fatores VII (68%) e XIII (31 a 78%, 75% em gatos com hepatopatia inflamatória) e aumento de PIVKA (75%), da concentração de D-Dímero (83%) e da atividade do inibidor alfa-2 da plasmina (67%) (ver Capítulo 196).[10-12]

Ultrassonografia e aspirado com agulha fina guiado por ultrassom

Anormalidades hepatobiliares são frequentemente detectadas durante o exame ultrassonográfico do abdome em gatos com CN, incluindo parênquima hiperecoico com ou sem hepatomegalia, distensão de ductos biliares ou da vesícula biliar e aumento de sedimento na vesícula biliar (ver Capítulo 88). Outras anormalidades comumente notadas em gatos com CN são aumento de volume do pâncreas, parênquima hipoecoico e parênquima peripancreático hiperecoico. Anormalidades do trato gastrintestinal (GI) incluem espessamento de parede e distensão por líquido.[1] Um estudo retrospectivo de diversas avaliações ultrassonográficas hepatobiliares (ecogenicidade e ecotextura do parênquima hepático, nitidez da veia porta, espessura da parede da vesícula biliar, diâmetro do ducto biliar e características do conteúdo da vesícula biliar) não conseguiu diferenciar gatos saudáveis daqueles com doença hepática infiltrativa difusa (inflamação, câncer ou lipidose).[13] Outro estudo não detectou qualquer característica para diferenciação das formas linfocítica e neutrofílica da colangite.[14] O diagnóstico de hepatopatia difusa baseado somente na ultrassonografia, com ou sem dados bioquímicos ou hematológicos de rotina, deve ser feito com cuidado, mesmo quando o exame é realizado por ultrassonografista habilidoso.[13]

O ultrassom não possibilita a coleta percutânea de amostras guiada, para exame citológico ou histológico (ver Capítulo 89). A avaliação citológica de amostra obtida por aspirado com agulha fina (AAF) possui vantagens distintas e limitações ao avaliar gatos com doenças hepáticas. Tem bom custo-benefício, é um procedimento prático, de realização relativamente fácil, fornece informação diagnóstica rápida quando comparado à histopatologia hepática, causa raras complicações, não necessita de muitos testes antes do procedimento (perfil de coagulação geralmente não é necessário) e pode ser em geral realizado sem anestesia ou sedação.[15] Quando guiado por ultrassom, o AAF pode ser útil do ponto de vista diagnóstico em gatos com doença difusa ou focal. A limitação importante da citologia hepática é o pequeno tamanho da amostra (células), que não reflete a morfologia da arquitetura do parênquima hepático e limita a capacidade de identificar corretamente a anormalidade hepática primária.[15] Em um estudo, verificou-se que somente 51% dos gatos apresentavam concordância de forma geral entre o diagnóstico citológico e o histopatológico. Doenças inflamatórias foram corretamente diagnosticadas em 27% dos casos.[16] Hepatopatias vacuolares tiveram a maior taxa de concordância, diagnosticadas corretamente em 83% dos casos.[16] Entretanto, 4 gatos com linfoma foram incorretamente diagnosticados como lipidose hepática na citologia de amostra obtida por AAF.[17] A questão levantada nesse relato foi a de que a citologia de amostra obtida por AAF pode não detectar lesões infiltrativas, particularmente se nodulares, multifocais ou periportais.[17] Embora o exame citológico de amostra obtida por AAF seja um procedimento diagnóstico útil, com vantagens, prefere-se uma abordagem diagnóstica lógica, por etapas, especialmente em gatos com doença não vacuolar, diagnóstico incerto ou diagnóstico citológico de lipidose hepática sem melhora da doença após o tratamento.[15,17]

Biopsia e cultura

Considerações gerais

Os resultados do exame histopatológico de gatos com doença hepática são classificados como focal, multifocal, zonal, localmente extenso ou panlobular difuso.[18] A colangite, inicialmente descrita como um processo difuso, é agora classificada como distribuição difusa ou limitada (focal, multifocal).[6,8,19] A gravidade da doença hepática indicada pela histopatologia varia entre os lobos hepáticos,[1] o que justifica a recomendação de obtenção de amostras por biopsia de diversos lobos hepáticos.[1]

Técnicas percutâneas guiadas por ultrassom e complicações

Agulhas de biopsia automática disparadas por mola são mais comumente utilizadas para obtenção de amostras por via percutânea, mas são utilizadas e recomendadas agulhas de biopsia manuais (ver Capítulo 89).[20] Biopsia realizada com agulha é um método rápido, de bom custo-benefício e minimamente invasivo para obter tecido hepático; entretanto, comparado a biopsias em cunha, essa técnica resulta em redução de um terço na área da superfície média da amostra da biopsia (Figura 283.1), o que pode resultar em erro de amostragem, perda de lesões patológicas e julgamento errôneo da gravidade da doença.[18] A fragmentação de amostras obtidas por biopsia com agulha, comum nesse tipo de procedimento, não causa interferência significativa na obtenção do diagnóstico.[18] Em gatos, embora a biopsia com agulha de calibre 18 G geralmente propicie obtenção de amostras muito pequenas, a agulha calibre 16 G possibilita a coleta de boas amostras.[15] A obtenção de amostras por biopsia com agulha supostamente está associada à baixa incidência de complicações.[18] Um relato mais recente mencionou complicações fatais que poderiam ter ocorrido devido à intensa vagotonia e choque ao utilizar instrumento de biopsia automático (Pro-Mag Ultra®). Essa complicação não foi observada com a utilização de um dispositivo semiautomático (agulha de biopsia VET-core®).[20] Hemorragia, a reação adversa mais comum, ocorre independentemente dos resultados de testes de coagulação prévios; a sua ocorrência é muito mais provável se o gato apresentar trombocitopenia ($\leq 80 \times 10^3$ plaquetas/$\mu\ell$) ou TTP ativada (TTPa) prolongada. Outras complicações menos frequentes consistem em coleta de tecidos não pretendidos (p. ex., grandes vasos sanguíneos, estruturas biliares, parede corporal, trato digestório, pâncreas, diafragma ou pulmão) e dor.[18,20-22] As principais complicações são em geral notadas dentro de 30 min a 1 h após a biopsia, mas podem ser detectadas até 10 h após o procedimento.[15,22]

Biopsia assistida por laparoscopia ou biopsia cirúrgica em cunha

A principal vantagem da biopsia assistida por laparoscopia ou da biopsia em cunha obtida por laparotomia é o maior tamanho da amostra, o que possibilita um diagnóstico mais acurado (ver Capítulo 91).[18] Pinças de biopsia laparoscópicas tipicamente propiciam amostras de cerca de 5 mm de diâmetro (45 mg de tecido hepático; Figura 283.2). Idealmente, as amostras obtidas cirurgicamente alcançam 2 cm de profundidade no tecido hepático.[15] As desvantagens da laparoscopia podem incluir o custo, as instalações necessárias, a necessidade de treinamento avançado

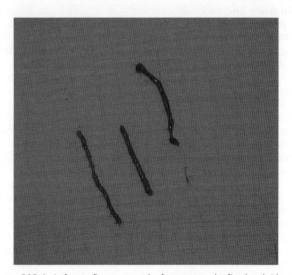

Figura 283.1 A fotografia mostra três fragmentos de fígado obtidos por biopsia hepática percutânea, guiada por ultrassom, utilizando-se dispositivo de biopsia com agulha calibre 16 G.

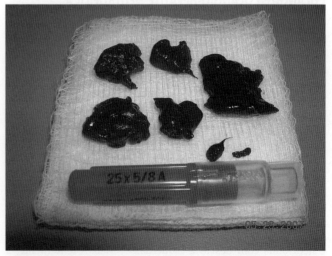

Figura 283.2 Fotografia com seis amostras de fígado obtidas por biopsia com pinça de biopsia em formato de copo por meio de laparoscopia.

do operador, tempo de procedimento mais longo (comparado ao da biopsia percutânea com agulha, mas geralmente é mais rápida do que a biopsia por laparotomia) e necessidade de anestesia geral. Em gatos as vantagens da biopsia por laparoscopia incluem a possibilidade de obtenção de amostra de maior tamanho, maior segurança em obter amostra do fígado, possibilidade de visualização de áreas anormais, alvos, no fígado para a amostragem, grau limitado de invasividade, oportunidade de obter amostras de biopsia não hepáticas (pâncreas, rins, baço, linfonodo e intestino) e possibilidade de aspiração da vesícula biliar (colecistocentese).[15] A visualização mais clara do órgão durante a laparoscopia permite a localização de pequenas lesões (< 0,5 cm) não facilmente observadas de outro modo.[15] Outras vantagens da biopsia por laparoscopia incluem rápida recuperação, menor tempo de internação, bem como baixas taxas de morbidade, infecção e dor pós-operatória (Figura 283.3).[15] Embora colecistectomia e colecistotomia assistida por laparoscopia tenham sido realizadas em gatos, elas não são procedimentos comuns.[23] A maioria das hepatopatias felinas (CN/CH) não requer cirurgia. A laparotomia cirúrgica convencional com realização de biopsia em cunha é indicada se o gato tiver uma anormalidade hepática primária ou for submetido à cirurgia abdominal concomitante, ou se a biopsia assistida por laparoscopia não for uma opção.

Cultura microbiológica

Culturas para bactérias aeróbicas e anaeróbicas podem ser bastante úteis na avaliação de gatos com doença hepatobiliar. Em um estudo constatou-se crescimento bacteriano em 36% das amostras de bile e 14% das amostras de tecido hepático, e 83% dos gatos tinham uma única espécie de bactéria.[24] Amostras de bile podem ser obtidas por meio de colecistocentese percutânea guiada por ultrassom, colecistocentese assistida por laparoscopia ou mediante cirurgia (ver Capítulos 88 e 89).[25] Complicações incomuns incluem ruptura de vesícula biliar e peritonite biliar.[5,25] Gatos com CN podem ter evidências de inflamação neutrofílica na bile. *E. coli*, sozinha ou em combinação com bactérias anaeróbicas facultativas ou obrigatórias, é o microrganismo mais comum em culturas de bile, mas também é possível encontrar outros microrganismos, inclusive da família Enterobacteriaceae (*Salmonella enterica, Klebsiella, Enterobacter*), bem como espécies de *Streptococcus, Enterococcus, Actinomyces, Acinetobacter, Pasteurella, Clostridium* e *Bacteroides*.[5] Em uma minoria de gatos com CN/CH foram isoladas bactérias em cultura aeróbica ou anaeróbica.[4] A utilização de testes mais modernos, como hibridização por fluorescência *in situ* (HFIS), pode ser mais sensível para detecção de infecções bacterianas.[7] Infecções ascendentes causadas por bactérias entéricas são a fonte mais provável dessas infecções; entretanto, é possível a disseminação hematógena.[5,7] A entrada dupla única do ducto biliar comum e do ducto pancreático na papila duodenal principal aumenta o risco de refluxo de conteúdo entérico e/ou pancreático.[5] A ocorrência de pancreatite e colangite pode estar associada a essa condição anatômica.[1]

Tratamento e prognóstico

Antibióticos

Antibióticos representam a terapia primária para CN/CH (Tabela 283.1).[26] De forma ideal, os antibióticos são escolhidos com base nos resultados de cultura bacteriana e antibiograma. Frequentemente, entretanto, inicia-se o tratamento com antibiótico empiricamente até que os resultados da cultura microbiológica estejam disponíveis. Os antibióticos devem ser efetivos contra bactérias entéricas aeróbicas e anaeróbicas, e excretados de forma ativa na bile. Antibióticos comumente utilizados incluem ampicilina, as combinações amoxicilina-clavulanato de potássio (Clavamox®), ampicilina-sulbactam (Unasyn®), ticarcilina dissódica-clavulanato de potássio (Timentin®) e metronidazol. Antibióticos menos frequentemente utilizados incluem cloranfenicol, tetraciclina e eritromicina. Sugere-se terapia durante 2 meses, mas a duração mais efetiva não é conhecida.[4]

Terapias inespecíficas

Alguns gatos com CN/CH estão em estado grave e necessitam de terapia para desidratação (ver Capítulo 129), anormalidades de eletrólitos séricos (ver Capítulos 67 a 69), coagulopatias (ver Capítulo 197), e/ou hipotensão (ver Capítulo 159). Outros gatos podem ser beneficiados com a utilização de estimulantes de apetite (mirtazapina, cipro-heptadina; ver Tabela 283.1) se apresentarem baixo grau de inapetência. A inapetência persistente pode ser tratada com a implantação de um tubo de alimentação enteral (tubo de esofagostomia ou tubo gástrico; ver Capítulo 82). A restrição proteica é somente necessária em gatos com encefalopatia hepática; de outra forma, uma dieta altamente digestível, com conteúdo moderado de gordura é frequentemente preferida (ver Capítulo 180).[27] A encefalopatia hepática é menos comum em gatos acometidos por hepatopatias adquiridas. Se presente, pode ser tratada com lactulose e/ou antibióticos (ver Capítulos 281 e 284). Outras terapias inespecíficas incluem controle da náuseas e/ou êmese, diminuição da produção de ácido gástrico e alívio da dor (mais comumente notada em casos de pancreatite). A cirurgia provavelmente é necessária para gatos com obstrução biliar total e para alguns gatos com coleólitos (Figura 283.4). Embora nas doenças obstrutivas tenha sido realizado desvio biliar-intestinal (*i. e.*, colecistoduodenostomia ou colecistojejunostomia), a taxa de morbidade pós-cirúrgica é alta.[28] Técnicas alternativas têm sido propostas e incluem colocação de *stent* no colédoco (ver Capítulos 120 e 123).[29] Aparentemente, entretanto, gatos apresentam maior morbidade após implante de *stent* no colédoco do que cães.[29] Portanto, o ácido ursodeoxicólico (Actigall®) frequentemente é administrado por suas propriedades anti-inflamatórias, imunomoduladoras e antifibróticas. O ácido ursodeoxicólico aumenta a natureza líquida das secreções biliares, mas os benefícios da sua utilização devem ser balanceados contra o risco de obstrução biliar ou de formação de coleólitos. Em gatos com colangite aguda o prognóstico é bom, com sobrevida superior a 1 ano.[3,5] Prognósticos ruins estão relacionados, mais provavelmente, a doenças concomitantes, como pancreatite, doença intestinal inflamatória e, em menor grau, nefrite.[3,30,31]

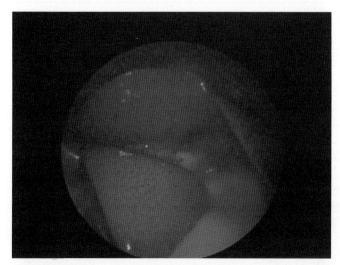

Figura 283.3 Imagem laparoscópica do mesmo gato da Figura 283.1 mostra uma aparência relativamente normal do fígado, exceto pelas margens hepáticas arredondadas. (*Esta figura se encontra reproduzida em cores no Encarte.*)

Tabela 283.1 Terapias medicamentosas para doenças hepáticas de gatos.

TRATAMENTO	DOSE
Fluidoterapia (ver Capítulo 129)	
Cristaloides isotônicos: ou seja, solução de NaCl 0,9%	Choque: 45 a 55 mℓ/kg/h IV; corrigir desidratação Manutenção: 40 a 45 mℓ/kg/dia IV
Coloides sintéticos: Hetastarch®, dextrana 70	Dose única de 2 a 5 mℓ/kg IV; se necessário, 10 mℓ/kg/dia IV TIC
Transfusão de plasma fresco congelado	10 a 40 mℓ/kg IV ao longo de 24 h
Fármacos anti-hipotensivos	
Cloridrato de dopamina	5 a 15 mcg/kg/min IV TIC
Cloridrato de dobutamina	0,2 a 2 mcg/kg/min IV TIC
Epinefrina	0,5 a 2 mcg/kg/min IV TIC
Norepinefrina	0,5 a 2 mcg/kg/min IV TIC
Vasopressina	0,01 a 0,04 UI/min IV (em pacientes em choque por vasodilatação que não respondem à reanimação hídrica e catecolaminas)
Antibióticos	
Ampicilina	20 a 40 mg/kg IV, a cada 6 a 8 h
Amoxicilina	10 a 20 mg/kg/12 h VO IV SC
Amoxicilina + ácido clavulânico (Clavamox®)	10 a 20 mg/kg/8 h VO
Ampicilina + sulbactam (Unasyn®)	20 a 40 mg/kg IV, a cada 8 a 12 h
Ticarcilina dissódica + clavulanato de potássio (Timentin®)	40 a 60 mg/kg IV, a cada 6 a 8 h
Metronidazol (Flagyl®)	15 mg/kg/12 h VO IV
Cloranfenicol	10 a 20 mg/kg/12 h VO IV IM SC
Tetraciclina	7 mg/kg/12 h IV, IM
Eritromicina	10 a 20 mg/kg/8 h VO IV
Estimulantes de apetite	
Mirtazapina (Remeron®)	3,75 mg (1/4 de comprimido de 15 mg) VO, a cada 24 a 72 h
Cipro-heptadina (Periactin®)	2 a 4 mg/gato VO, a cada 12 a 24 h
Diazepam (Valium®)	1 a 4 mg/gato VO, a cada 12 a 24 h
Terapia para náuseas/êmese	
Ranitidina	0,5 a 2 mg/kg/12 h VO IV
Famotidina	0,5 a 1 mg/kg VO IV SC, IM, a cada 12 a 24 h
Metoclopramida	0,2 a 0,4 mg/kg/8 h VO SC, IM* 1 a 2 mg/kg/dia IV TIC
Clorpromazina	0,5 mg/kg IV IM SC, a cada 6 a 8 h
Mesilatato de dolasetrona	0,6 a 1 mg/kg/12 h VO IV SC
Ondansetrona	0,1 a 1 mg/kg IV (lentamente) SC IM ou VO, a cada 6 a 12 h
Citrato de maropitant	1 mg/kg/24 h SC VO
Controle da dor	
Buprenorfina	0,005 a 0,01 mg/kg IV, IM, a cada 4 a 8 h
Butorfanol	0,2 a 0,4 mg/kg IM, cada 2 a 4 h
Medicamentos diversos	
Cobalamina (vitamina B_{12})	250 mcg/gato SC, semanalmente
Prednisolona	2,2 a 4,4 mg/kg/24 h VO 1 a 2 mg/kg/12 h VO
Ácido ursodeoxicólico (Actigall®)	10 a 15 mg/kg/24 h VO
Vitamina K_1	5 mg/gato IM, cada 24 a 48 h
Lactulose	0,5 a 1 mℓ/kg/8 h VO
Neomicina	20 mg/kg VO, a cada 8 a 12 h
Azatioprina	0,3 mg/kg VO, a cada 48 a 72 h
Metotrexato	0,4 mg/gato, dose total administrada em 1 dia, em 3 doses fracionadas Repita a cada 7 a 10 dias. Administre juntamente com ácido ursodeoxicólico (15 mg/kg/24 h VO) e folato (0,25 mg/kg/24 h VO)
Ciclosporina	3 a 4 mg/kg/12 h VO
Praziquantel	20 mg/kg/24 h SC ou IM, 3 a 5 dias consecutivos

*Considere terapia alternativa; menos efetiva em gatos. *IM*, intramuscular; *IV*, intravenosa; *SC*, subcutâneo; *TIC*, taxa de infusão contínua; *VO*, via oral.

COLANGITE LINFOCÍTICA

Considerações gerais
Os sinais clínicos e a avaliação diagnóstica de casos de colangite linfocítica (CL) são revisados na seção "Colangite neutrofílica/Colângio-hepatite", com algumas poucas exceções. Além de náuseas, êmese, letargia (apatia) e inapetência, os gatos com CL geralmente desenvolvem perda de peso gradual e icterícia (Figura 283.5).[32] Em contraste com a CN/CH, a anormalidade bioquímica mais consistente em gatos com CL é hipergamaglobulinemia; entretanto, incrementos nas atividades de enzimas hepáticas e da concentração de bilirrubina total são detectados em alguns gatos.[32]

Patogenia
A patogenia da CL supostamente era consequência da infecção bacteriana crônica em gatos com CN.[8] Estudos recentes utilizando HFIS constataram poucas evidências que sustentam a colonização bacteriana como um componente da etiopatogenia. Em vez disso, mecanismos imunomediados têm sido propostos.[7,33] Entretanto, um estudo provocativo em gatos, utilizando reação em cadeia de polimerase (PCR), detectou DNA de *Helicobacter* spp. em 26% dos gatos com CL (16% em animais do grupo-controle) e sugeriu a participação de *H. pylori* na etiologia de CL felina.[34] Em condição experimental, induziu-se CL mediante inoculação em gatos livres de patógenos específicos com sangue de gato infectado com *Bartonella Henselae* e/ou *Bartonella clarridgeiae*.[35]

Histologicamente, a CL é caracterizada por agregados densos de linfócitos ao redor dos ductos biliares, que não invadem o epitélio biliar. Os linfócitos podem ser detectados no lúmen biliar (ao contrário do que acontece na CN).[6] O principal diagnóstico diferencial é o linfoma hepático. Além das características histopatológicas, a imunofenotipagem (linfócito B e linfócito T) e o teste PCR para rearranjo do gene receptor de linfócito T (RCT) mostraram-se auxiliares para diferenciar CL de linfoma hepático. Predileção por ductos biliares, ductopenia, fibrose peribiliar, agregados portais de linfócitos B, lipogranulomas portais e RCT policlonais são características da CL.[6,33]

Tratamento e prognóstico
As terapias específicas e inespecíficas para CL e CN/CH são semelhantes (ver Tabela 283.1).[4] Vários gatos são tratados com antibióticos enquanto esperam os resultados histopatológicos e da cultura microbiológica. Quando causas infecciosas já foram excluídas e/ou os gatos não responderam ao tratamento com antibióticos, recomenda-se terapia imunossupressora, assumindo que a lesão hepática seja imunomediada.[4] A prednisolona, a primeira escolha como terapia imunossupressora, resulta em sobrevida mais longa comparativamente a de gatos submetidos ao tratamento com ácido ursodeoxicólico.[32] Além de suas propriedades imunossupressoras, a prednisolona pode limitar a lesão hepatocelular e aumentar o apetite. Com base na resposta terapêutica (resolução dos sinais clínicos) e em valores do perfil bioquímico sérico, a dose de prednisolona pode ser diminuída lentamente, mas muitos gatos necessitam de terapia a longo prazo.[4] A duração ótima do tratamento ainda não foi determinada. Aumentos persistentes ou progressivos das atividades de ALT e/ou ALP e da concentração sérica de bilirrubina total sugerem que o tratamento tem sido inadequado.[4] Em gatos que não respondem ao tratamento, é importante assegurar que não tenham linfoma subclínico. Em gatos com confirmação de CL/CH resistente a prednisona, as terapias alternativas incluem azatioprina, metotrexato e ciclosporina.[4] Em gatos com CL o prognóstico é bom e provavelmente melhor do que o de gatos com CN/CH. Em um estudo, notou-se sobrevida média de 795 dias, com taxas de sobrevida de 1, 2 e 3 anos de 74, 56 e 35%, respectivamente.[32] Gatos de raças puras com CL podem ser mais predispostos a sobrevida mais curta do que gatos da raça Doméstico de Pelo Curto.[32]

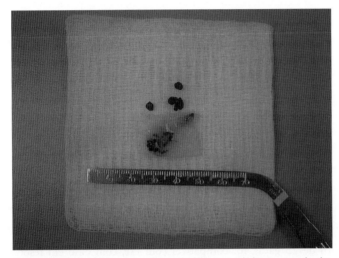

Figura 283.4 Fotografia mostra diversos colélitos no colédoco, causando obstrução parcial do ducto comum removido de um gato macho, castrado, com 14 anos de idade, da raça Doméstico de Pelo Curto, com grave colecistite linfocítica e neutrofílica.

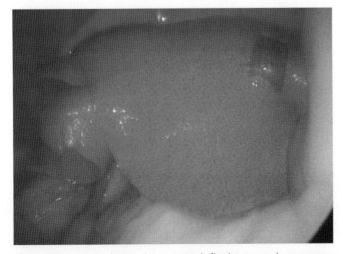

Figura 283.5 Imagem laparoscópica mostrando fígado aumentado e macroscopicamente amarelado, sugestivo de lipidose hepática; entretanto, a histopatologia revelou moderada colangite linfocítica e neutrofílica crônica e moderada lipidose hepática difusa. (*Esta figura se encontra reproduzida, em cores, no Encarte.*)

DOENÇAS HEPATOBILIARES INFECCIOSAS

Infecção bacteriana
Comparadas a doenças hepatobiliares inflamatórias, as doenças hepatobiliares infecciosas de gatos são relatadas menos frequentemente. Nota-se infecção em cerca de 15% dos gatos com doença hepatobiliar.[1,36] Infecções bacterianas são mais comuns em casos de CN/CH. Mesmo que os gatos sejam reservatórios naturais de *Bartonella henselae*, a peliose hepática causada por essa bactéria não é observada em gatos.[37] A patogenia proposta é de uma infecção secundária causada por bactéria intestinal ascendente. Tanto micro quanto macroabscessos hepáticos já foram relatados em gatos. Outros fatores envolvidos na patogenia incluem trauma, alteração do fluxo sanguíneo, torção de lobo hepático, infecção extra-hepática, sepse, condições de imunossupressão clínica e neoplasias.[38] A ultrassonografia possibilita a detecção e o diagnóstico de abscessos hepáticos, mediante exame citológico de amostra obtida por AAF e cultura microbiológica

(ver Capítulos 88 e 89). Resultados de culturas bacterianas aeróbicas e anaeróbicas em gatos com abscessos hepáticos são semelhantes àqueles de gatos com CN/CH, com isolados clinicamente raros de *Klebsiella, Listeria, Salmonella, Brucella, Yersinia pseudotuberculosis, Actinomyces, Nocardia* e *Pasteurella*.[38] O crescimento de diversas bactérias é detectado em mais de 50% dos gatos com abscessos solitários.[38,39] Devido à frequência de crescimento multibacteriano, a terapia antimicrobiana de amplo espectro deve ser direcionada a bactérias aeróbicas e anaeróbicas, independentemente dos resultados da cultura anaeróbica, sendo administrada por pelo menos 6 semanas.[38] Abscessos focais podem necessitar de drenagem cirúrgica ou hepatectomia parcial. A drenagem percutânea de abscessos hepáticos guiada por ultrassom tem sido relatada em cães[40] e utilizada com sucesso em gatos. Em um único estudo com 14 gatos que apresentavam abscessos hepáticos, a taxa de mortalidade geral foi de 79%. Os sobreviventes foram submetidos à hepatectomia parcial seguida de tratamento medicamentoso.[39] *Mycobacterium* spp. raramente causa infecção hepática em gatos (ver Capítulo 212). A histopatologia pode revelar doença granulomatosa extensa.[38]

Platinossomose

A colangite crônica tem sido associada à fasciolose hepática, a partir de infecção pelo grupo *Platynosomum* (*P. fastosum, P. concinnum* e *P. illiciens*; e podem ser sinônimos de *P. planicipitus, Dicrocelium concinnum, D. lanceolatum* var. *symmetricum* e *Concinnum*) e *Amphimerus pseudofelineus*.[41,42] O *Platynosomum fastosum*, prevalente em regiões tropicais e subtropicais das Américas do Norte, do Sul e Central, bem como do Caribe e de regiões da África e Ásia, é um pequeno trematódeo hepático detectado em ductos biliares e vesícula biliar de gatos.[42] Lagartos, caramujos terrestres e isópodos são implicados como hospedeiros intermediários/paratênicos.[42] Platinossomose ou "envenenamento por lagartos" é o nome dado a essa doença causada por essa infecção. Os gatos infectados provavelmente adquirem o parasita pela ingestão de lagartos infectados. Os sinais clínicos podem variar de ausentes a graves. Os sintomas são secundários à obstrução do trato biliar e insuficiência hepática.[42] Outros sinais clínicos e a avaliação diagnóstica de *P. fastosum* são revisados na seção "Colangite neutrofílica/Colângio-hepatite". O hemograma pode indicar eosinofilia em gatos com infestação maciça. Ovos embrionados (ovos marrom-dourados [sem corante], medindo 34 a 50 × 23 a 35 μ e com parede espessa) são excretados nas fezes de gatos infectados; exceções são os gatos com obstrução total de ductos biliares.[42] Infestações por parasitas adultos (lanceolado, coberto por uma fina cutícula, medindo 2,9 a 8 mm de comprimento × 0,9 a 2,5 mm de largura, ventosa oral subterminal e ventosa ventral) podem ser detectados na bile ou no fígado, na vesícula biliar e/ou nos ductos biliares. O tratamento mais efetivo consiste na administração de praziquantel.[42] Em gatos com obstrução de ductos biliares, recomenda-se terapia de suporte agressiva e desvio biliar-intestinal (*i. e.*, colecistoduodenostomia ou colecistojejunostomia) ou implantação de *stent* no colédoco (ver Capítulo 123).

Infecções virais

Vírus da leucemia felina

Gatos persistentemente infectados pelo vírus da leucemia felina (FeLV) frequentemente desenvolvem o complexo leucemia/linfoma ou fibrossarcoma. Eles também desenvolvem um amplo espectro de doenças não neoplásicas.[43] Em um estudo *post mortem*, constatou-se que 77% dos gatos positivos para FeLV apresentavam doenças não neoplásicas associadas ao FeLV e 23% desenvolveram câncer.[43] Nesse estudo, verificou-se que 25% dos gatos com icterícia eram positivos ao FeLV e 8% dos gatos infectados pelo vírus estavam ictéricos. A histopatologia de gatos infectados pelo FeLV revelou degeneração hepática descrita como dissociação celular, fígado gorduroso e necrose

focal. A doença hepática gordurosa e necrose hepática focal foram significativamente mais comuns nos gatos infectados por FeLV. A patogenia da lesão hepática associada à infecção por FeLV é desconhecida, mas pode ser, em parte, secundária à anemia.[43] Ver Capítulo 223.

Calicivírus felino

Mutações virulentas de calicivírus felino (CVF) raramente causam infecção hepática em gatos, com altas taxas de morbidade e mortalidade.[44] O CVF é altamente infeccioso e causa doença aguda do trato respiratório superior e da cavidade bucal; um vírus mutante foi identificado. Vários gatos infectados pelo CVF mutante morreram com sinais clínicos caracterizados por icterícia, edema, doença do trato respiratório superior, dermatite ulcerativa, febre, claudicação, afonia e inapetência.[44] A histopatologia hepática revelou necrose hepatocelular disseminada com discreta infiltração inflamatória em microscopia óptica. O antígeno do CVF nas células parenquimatosas e nas células de Kupffer pode ser detectado por exame imuno-histoquímico. No interior dos hepatócitos podem ser observadas partículas semelhantes ao calicivírus em microscopia eletrônica.[44] O tratamento envolve terapia de suporte agressiva e quarentena rigorosa para evitar a contaminação de gatos saudáveis, mesmo se vacinados.[44] Ver Capítulo 229.

Peritonite infecciosa felina

A peritonite infecciosa felina (PIF), uma infecção causada por coronavírus mutante, causa doença clínica com alta taxa de mortalidade assim que surgem os sinais clínicos. Raramente, gatos infectados sobrevivem semanas, meses ou anos.[45] A PIF é mais prevalente em gatos com menos de 3 anos de idade (especialmente aqueles com 4 a 16 meses de idade).[45] Hiperbilirrubinemia e hiperbilirrubinúria são comuns em gatos com PIF, devido à maior taxa de hemólise e destruição e reciclagem mais lenta de bilirrubina e biliverdina. Esses animais em geral não apresentam aumento das atividades de enzimas hepáticas. A PIF hepática primária não é comum.[45] A avaliação diagnóstica da PIF é revisada no Capítulo 224. O resultado de exame de amostras de fígado obtidas por biopsia percutânea guiada por ultrassom e da citologia de amostras hepáticas obtidas por AAF, em 16 de 25 gatos, foi compatível com PIF, com base em lesões piogranulomatosas intraparenquimatosas e/ou peri-hepatite fibrinosa. O antígeno do coronavírus felino foi detectado em 6 gatos. De 22 gatos, em 14 (64%) os achados citológicos foram compatíveis com PIF, com base na constatação de inflamação piogranulomatosa de alta celularidade. Seu fígado frequentemente tinha lesões histológicas compatíveis com PIF, mesmo na ausência de alterações macroscópicas.[46]

Vírus da imunodeficiência felina

O vírus da imunodeficiência felina (FIV), um lentivírus, foi isolado em gatos em todo o mundo (ver Capítulo 222). O FIV está associado a citopenias e câncer.[47,48] Na ausência de doenças concomitantes, o FIV raramente causa doença hepática. Em uma população experimental de 20 gatos livres de patógenos específicos infectados por FIV, somente um desenvolveu doença hepática primária.[48] Esse gato desenvolveu colangite, hiperplasia de ductos biliares, fibrose peribiliar e microabscessos. Um segundo gato desenvolveu linfoma hepático-renal. Também foi relatado que alguns gatos com FIV apresentavam degeneração hepática generalizada.[48] Gatos experimentalmente infectados por FIV e depois desafiados com *Toxoplasma gondii* desenvolveram toxoplasmose aguda generalizada, incluindo necrose hepática multifocal a coalescente.[48] Taquizoítos de *T. gondii* foram ocasionalmente detectados.[48] Em um estudo post mortem de gatos com toxoplasmose diagnosticada histologicamente, constatou-se que 70% de 90 amostras de fígado examinadas apresentavam *Toxoplasma gondii*.[49]

INFECÇÃO FÚNGICA

Os fungos *Histoplasma capsulatum* (ver Capítulo 233), *Coccidioides immitis* (ver Capítulo 232), *Blastomyces dermatitidis* (ver Capítulo 233), *Aspergillus* sp. (ver Capítulo 235), *Cryptococcus* sp. (ver Capítulo 231) e *Sporothrix schenckii* (ver Capítulo 236) podem, raramente, causar doença hepatobiliar infecciosa primária ou disseminada.[38] *Histoplasma capsulatum* é a segunda doença fúngica sistêmica mais comum em gatos e provavelmente a infecção fúngica hepática mais comum. Em gatos com doença disseminada ocorre envolvimento do fígado, juntamente com baço, trato gastrintestinal, ossos e medula óssea, tegumento e olhos.[50] O diagnóstico definitivo é obtido pela detecção de microrganismos no exame citopatológico ou em cultura microbiológica. O tratamento de escolha é o itraconazol, na dose de

5 a 10 mg/kg/12 horas via oral por um tempo mínimo de 4 a 6 meses.[50] Em algumas regiões, ocorrem infecções epidêmicas por *Sporothrix schenckii* em gatos, cães e seres humanos. Em um pequeno estudo, verificou-se que todos os gatos avaliados (n = 10) com esporotricose apresentavam *S. schenckii* detectado no exame histopatológico ou na cultura microbiológica do fígado. Todos esses gatos foram tratados com itraconazol; entretanto, em 60% a doença progrediu.[40]

REFERÊNCIAS BIBLIOGRÁFICAS

As referências bibliográficas deste capítulo se encontram online no Ambiente de Aprendizagem.

CAPÍTULO 284

Anomalias Vasculares Hepáticas

Chick Weisse e Allyson C. Berent

Desvios (*shunts*) portossistêmicos (DPSs) são anomalias vasculares que conectam a veia porta à circulação sistêmica, desviando dos sinusoides e do parênquima hepático.[1-6] Eles são considerados a anormalidade congênita hepatobiliar mais comum. Normalmente, a drenagem do sangue venoso oriundo do baço, do pâncreas, do estômago e do intestino adentra a veia porta, perfunde o fígado através da rede de sinusoides e drena através das veias hepáticas para a veia cava caudal (VCC).[3] O sangue do sistema porta carreia várias substâncias ao fígado, inclusive hormônios tróficos (intestinais e pancreáticos), nutrientes, produtos bacterianos e toxinas oriundas dos intestinos.[1,2,6] O fígado do feto possui função limitada para processar esses produtos, e um grande vaso de desvio, o ducto venoso, desvia a circulação hepática como um mecanismo protetor.[3,6] Esse vaso sanguíneo fetal, localizado no lado esquerdo do fígado, normalmente se fecha aos 3 a 10 dias de idade.[3,4,7] O fechamento é iniciado pelas alterações de pressão sanguínea após cessar o fluxo venoso umbilical; tromboxano ou diversos compostos adrenérgicos podem estimular a contração da musculatura do ducto venoso e auxiliar no fechamento do vaso.[3,5,6-8] Caso o ducto venoso permaneça patente (ou aberto), ou caso exista alguma outra comunicação congênita, tem-se um DPS. Quando o sangue desvia do fígado, fatores tróficos (particularmente insulina e glucagon) não estão disponíveis para estimular o crescimento do fígado, resultando em baixo desenvolvimento hepático, déficit na síntese de proteínas, disfunção reticuloendotelial, alteração nos metabolismos de gordura e proteínas, atrofia hepática e, eventualmente, insuficiência hepática.

Os sinais clínicos estão associados ao volume e à origem do sangue desviado do fígado, resultando em anormalidades da função hepática, encefalopatia hepática (EH), sintomas gastrintestinais (GI) crônicos, sintomas de trato urinário inferior, coagulopatias e retardo do crescimento.[2,3,5,6,9] Esses problemas se devem ao acúmulo de toxinas exógenas e endógenas no organismo, que, em geral, são metabolizadas ou excretadas pelo fígado, assim como insuficiência da função hepática normal (p. ex., gliconeogênese, ciclo da ureia, ciclo do ácido úrico, glicogenólise).[2,6,9-12]

EMBRIOLOGIA

As veias do abdome são embriologicamente oriundas das veias umbilical, vitelínica e cardinal caudal (Figura 284.1). As veias vitelínicas pareadas se originam do saco vitelínico e formam a veia hepática esquerda, os sinusoides hepáticos, a porção hepática da VCC, a veia porta pré-hepática e seus vasos afluentes.[7] Os sistemas vitelínico e umbilical se combinam para formar o ducto venoso e o ramo esquerdo da veia porta. As veias do abdome não portal, renal e gonadal são oriundas do sistema venoso cardinal. As veias cardinais caudais formam a VCC caudal ao fígado e a veia ázigos.[3,7] Em animais normais, os segmentos pré e intra-hepáticos da VCC se juntam na comunicação entre os sistemas cardinal e vitelínico. Há diversas comunicações portocavais e porto-ázigos não funcionais no feto, mas não são patentes em adultos, a menos que ocorra hipertensão portal, originando diversos desvios (*shunts*) extra-hepáticos adquiridos. Quando erros de desenvolvimento criam comunicações anormais entre esses dois sistemas, surgem desvios portossistêmicos extra-hepáticos (DPSEHs) congênitos.[7] A patência anormal do vaso, ou outro desenvolvimento anormal no sistema venoso vitelínico, resulta em DPS intra-hepático (DPSIH) congênito, cuja maioria não é necessariamente subsequente a um ducto venoso patente, sendo a causa dos outros DPSIHs ou DPSEHs divisionais esquerdos, direitos e centrais atualmente desconhecida.

ANATOMIA/CLASSIFICAÇÃO

A veia porta é formada pela confluência das veias mesentéricas cranial e caudal, fornecendo até 80% do sangue e 50% do conteúdo de oxigênio ao fígado, sendo o restante provido pelo sangue arterial hepático.[3,5,6,13] O sangue oriundo do trato GI, baço e pâncreas é drenado por suas respectivas veias, que se unem à veia porta. No cão, esta adentra o fígado e se ramifica em vasos esquerdo e direito, que irrigam os diversos lobos hepáticos. O ramo direito principal irriga o processo lateral direito e o processo caudado do lobo caudado, e o ramo principal esquerdo irriga todos os outros lobos, dando origem ao ramo

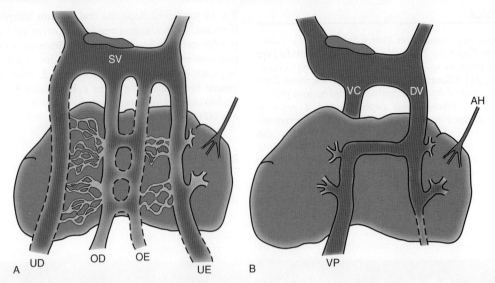

Figura 284.1 A. Anatomia vascular do fígado do feto. **B.** Alterações de desenvolvimento nos vasos sanguíneos do fígado do feto. As veias onfalomesentéricas (vitelínicas) originam a veia porta pré-hepática. Partes da veia umbilical esquerda e veias vitelínicas formam o ducto venoso (DV). *AH*, artéria hepática; *EU*, veia umbilical esquerda; *OD*, veia onfalomesentérica (vitelínica) direita; *OE*, veia onfalomesentérica (vitelínica) esquerda; *SV*, seio venoso; *UD*, veia umbilical direita; *VC*, veia cava; *VP*, veia porta. (Cortesia da Dra. Pamela Whiting.)

central, que supre o lobo medial direito.[3,13] No gato, a veia porta é dividida diretamente em ramos esquerdo, central e direito.[3,5,13] A veia porta se ramifica em vênulas menores onde o sangue adentra o parênquima através da tríade portal. Esse sangue segue através dos sinusoides hepáticos, é purificado no sistema reticuloendotelial e, então, é drenado em direção às veias centrais, que formam as vênulas hepáticas maiores e, finalmente, as veias hepáticas que desembocam na VCC. Quando o trajeto é interrompido por um vaso anômalo, o sangue é desviado do fígado e segue a via de menor resistência, alcançando a circulação sistêmica, sem ter passado pela circulação hepática.

A classificação mais recente das anomalias vasculares hepáticas sugere três categorias (Boxe 284.1): (1) DPSIHs e DPSEHs congênitos; (2) anormalidades associadas ao fluxo sanguíneo hepático anormal ou à hipertensão portal, atualmente denominadas *hipoplasia da veia porta* (HVP) *primária*; e (3) anormalidades do fluxo de saída. A segunda categoria, HVP, permanece controversa e inclui condições que poderiam ou não resultar em hipertensão portal. Estas são *HVP com hipertensão portal* (hipertensão portal não cirrótica [HPNC]/fibrose hepatoportal[14]/fibrose hepática idiopática[15]/doença veno-oclusiva[16]/hepatopatia crônica idiopática/hepatopatia não fibrosante[17]) e *HVP sem hipertensão portal* (anteriormente denominada *displasia microvascular* [DMV]).[18,19]

Boxe 284.1 Tipos de doença vascular hepática

Congênita (desvios portossistêmicos congênitos)
- Desvios vasculares portossistêmicos
  - Intra-hepáticos (DPSIHs)
  - Extra-hepáticos (DPSEHs)
- Hipoplasia da veia porta (HVP) primária
  - HVP com hipertensão portal (p. ex., hipertensão portal não cirrótica [HPNC])
  - HVP sem hipertensão portal (denominada anteriormente displasia microvascular [DMV])
- Distúrbios no fluxo de saída.

Adquirida (desvios portossistêmicos adquiridos)
- Desvios portossistêmicos múltiplos
  - Secundários à cirrose hepática (cirrose)
  - Secundários a malformações arteriovenosas hepáticas (MAVHs)

DPSs podem ser congênitos ou adquiridos. O desvio congênito é relatado em 0,18% dos cães e 0,05% de cães sem raça definida.[20] O DPS congênito mais comumente ocorre como um único vaso que origina comunicação vascular direta entre a irrigação venosa portal e a circulação venosa sistêmica (VCC ou veia ázigos), o que costuma ocorrer como uma comunicação intra ou extra-hepática única (80%). Em casos raros, alguns animais possuem duas ou mais comunicações congênitas.[21] Existem diversos tipos de DPS congênito tanto em cães quanto em gatos, incluindo desvios portocavais intra-hepáticos, desvios portocavais extra-hepáticos, desvios porto-ázigos extra-hepáticos, atresia de veia porta com anastomoses portocavais múltiplas resultantes, malformações arteriovenosas hepáticas (MAVHs), causando patência induzida por hipertensão portal nas anastomoses portossistêmicas, e DPS microintra-hepático (HVP sem hipertensão portal, denominada anteriormente DMV).[2,5,22-26] Aproximadamente 25 a 33% dos DPSs congênitos são intra-hepáticos tanto em cães como em gatos. DPSEHs únicos, sendo o desvio portocaval solitário principal o mais comum, representam 66 a 75% dos DPSs únicos congênitos em ambas as espécies.[1-4,26] A maioria dos DPSIHs ocorre em cães de raças de maior porte, ao passo que a maioria dos DPSEHs ocorre em raças de menor porte.[26] Alguns DPSEHs, como os desvios esplenocavais, podem estar associados a sinais clínicos menos graves, pois o sangue esplênico não tem origem GI e menor quantidade de sangue do sistema porta é desviada do fígado. Em geral, cães com DPSIHs possuem o maior volume de sangue portal desviado, manifestando sinais clínicos mais precoces, ou sintomas mais graves.[1,2,27,28]

Desvios adquiridos (20%) ocorrem com mais frequência secundários à hipertensão portal crônica, na qual o aumento da pressão portal leva à abertura dos vasos sanguíneos vestigiais fetais, o que é visto como anomalias congênitas, uma vez que esses vasos fornecem uma saída para a hipertensão portal. Em geral, os desvios adquiridos são múltiplos, tortuosos, extra-hepáticos e localizados próximo aos rins.[22-24] As causas mais comuns de desvios extra-hepáticos adquiridos são fibrose hepática (cirrose), HVP com hipertensão portal (HPNC)[23] ou MAVHs.[24]

A HVP com hipertensão portal, ou HPNC, foi descrita em várias raças de cães.[23,29] Essa condição é diagnosticada quando há hipertensão portal intra-abdominal, com uma veia portal patente e um fígado não cirrótico. A causa subjacente é desconhecida, com especulações de malformações vasculares intra-hepáticas difusas sérias, resultando em hipertensão portal e DPSEHs múltiplos.

A HVP sem hipertensão portal, anteriormente denominada DMV, é uma malformação microscópica da vasculatura hepática.[25,28] É caracterizada por pequenos vasos portais intra-hepáticos, hiperplasia do endotélio portal, dilatação da veia porta, vasos sanguíneos intralobulares juvenis aleatórios e hipertrofia venosa central e fibrose. Essas lesões podem possibilitar comunicações anormais entre as circulações porta e sistêmica, em nível microvascular. Isso pode ocorrer como doença isolada ou em combinação com DPS macroscópico. Cinquenta e oito por cento dos cães e oitenta e sete por cento dos gatos com HVP apresentam DPS congênito macroscópico concomitante.[18] Os sinais clínicos em cães com HVP podem ser semelhantes àqueles verificados em animais com DPS; entretanto, quando ocorre HVP sem desvio macroscópico, os sintomas costumam ser menos graves, ocorrem mais tardiamente e resultam em melhor prognóstico a longo prazo apenas com tratamento medicamentoso.

A MAVH é uma condição rara que envolve diversas comunicações arteriais de alta pressão e venosas de baixa pressão. Essa anormalidade, anteriormente denominada *fístula arteriovenosa hepática*, é mais apropriadamente nomeada como uma malformação, já que a maioria é composta por diversas comunicações (malformação) em vez de uma comunicação única (fístula). Em geral são congênitas e já foram descritas em cães e gatos.[24,30] Em geral, um ramo da artéria hepática se comunica diretamente com a veia porta por meio de múltiplos (dezenas a centenas de) vasos de desvio aberrantes. A alta pressão ocasiona fluxo sanguíneo hepatofugal e arterialização da veia porta; a hipertensão portal resultante, que origina diversos desvios extra-hepáticos para descomprimir o sistema, está associada, com frequência, à ascite. O prognóstico a longo prazo de MAVH é pior que o de DPS ou HVP, anormalidades mais comuns.[2,3,24]

ENCEFALOPATIA HEPÁTICA

A maioria dos sinais clínicos associados aos DPSs se deve à encefalopatia hepática, uma síndrome neuropsiquiátrica que envolve uma série de anormalidades neurológicas, a qual ocorre quando da perda de mais de 70% da função hepática.[10-12,31-37] A encefalopatia hepática é discutida com mais detalhes nos Capítulos 280 a 283 e 285.

AVALIAÇÃO DIAGNÓSTICA

Resenha

Os DPSEHs congênitos são observados mais comumente em cães de raças pequenas/toy: em um amplo estudo de casos, as raças Yorkshire Terrier, Bichon havanês, Maltês, Dandie Dinmont Terrier, Pug e Schnauzer Miniatura apresentaram razão de probabilidade de serem acometidas superior a 19.[5,20,26] Suspeita-se que o DPS seja hereditário em cães Yorkshire Terrier, que apresentam razão de probabilidade para DPS 35,9 vezes maior do que aquela verificada em todas as outras raças juntas.[20,38] No cão Maltês, suspeita-se de um modo recessivo de penetrância parcial de hereditariedade tanto para DPS macroscópico quanto para HVP.[39] Em gatos, os DPSEHs são mais comumente detectados,[3,38] embora os DPSIHs sejam relatados.[40-41] As raças Doméstico de Pelo Curto, Persa, Siamês, Himalaia e Birmanês são as mais representadas.[4,41-44] Desvios intra-hepáticos ocorrem mais em raças de cães de grande porte, incluindo Lébrel Irlandês, Retriever (Labrador, Golden), Boiadeiro Australiano e Pastor-Australiano.[3,4,45-47] Os DPSIHs divisionais esquerdos vêm sendo considerados hereditários no Lébrel Irlandês,[48,49] ao passo que os DPSIHs divisionais direitos acometem mais cães da raça Boiadeiro Australiano, machos, na Austrália.[47,50] Relata-se que cães da raça Cairn Terrier apresentam HVP hereditária, uma característica supostamente hereditária autossômica; em um relato, consta que cães da raça Yorkshire Terrier também foram bastante acometidos por DMV/HVP.[25,28] Em um recente relato[51] com cães com desvios portossistêmicos congênitos (DPSCs) ou adquiridos (DPSAs), os cães acometidos por DPSA eram mais idosos, mais pesados, com pior condição corporal e mais provavelmente tinham ascite, mas com menos probabilidade de manifestarem sintomas relativos ao sistema nervoso central (SNC) do que aqueles com DPSC.

Histórico clínico

A maioria dos cães e gatos com DPSs manifesta sintomas de doença crônica ou aguda antes de 1 ou 2 anos de idade, embora alguns tenham mais que 10 anos.[26,52] O DPS é muito mais comum em cães do que em gatos. Os DPSEHs adquiridos múltiplos em cães são diagnosticados em idade média de 3 anos (variação: 7 meses a 7 anos),[22] sendo a idade média de cães diagnosticados com HVP de 3,25 anos (variação: até os 10 anos de idade).[2,25] Em cães, não há clara predisposição por gênero, sendo os gatos machos mais propensos a essa condição.[1,26] O histórico tipicamente sugere que o animal "não se desenvolveu" desde o nascimento, possui baixa estatura (ou seja, o refugo da ninhada), apresenta perda de peso (11% dos casos) ou incapacidade em ganhá-lo, possui intolerância anestésica, apresenta períodos de apatia ou letargia, bem como "comportamento bizarro" (41 a 90% ficam alheios ao ambiente, pressionando a cabeça contra objetos imóveis, parados em frente a paredes ou cantos, com latidos aleatórios, cegueira intermitente, andar compulsivo ou agressividade).[1,2,5,26,53] Alguns animais apresentam histórico de disúria.[2,54] Poliúria e polidipsia (PU/PD) são comuns em cães, possivelmente devido ao baixo gradiente de concentração medular decorrente da baixa concentração de nitrogênio ureico sanguíneo (NUS), aumento do fluxo sanguíneo renal, elevação da secreção do hormônio adrenocorticotrófico (ACTH, *adrenocorticotropic hormone*) e hipercortisolismo associado e polidipsia psicogênica por encefalopatia hepática.[3,5,6,55] Nota-se ascite em 75% dos cães com MAVHs,[24] podendo ser observada em casos de DPS venoso-venoso se a hipoalbuminemia for grave. Essa complicação é observada em casos concomitantes de enteropatia com perda de proteína, quase sempre associada a ulceração/hemorragia GI ou doença intestinal inflamatória com ou sem linfangiectasia.

Sinais clínicos/exame físico

Os três sistemas corporais mais comumente afetados são SNC, GI e urinário.[2,3,5,26] Os sintomas de encefalopatia hepática podem ser óbvios ou bastante brandos, estando, em geral, associados a comportamento anômalo (ver também Capítulo 9). Os sintomas relativos ao de SNC mais evidentes incluem ataxia, obnubilação, andar compulsivo, andar em círculos, convulsões, latidos aleatórios e coma.[3,7,22,53] A manifestação de sintomas relacionados com a alimentação foi relatada em somente 30 a 50% dos animais de companhia.[5] Sintomas GI (êmese, diarreia, anorexia, pica e/ou hemorragia GI/melena/hematêmese) ocorrem em ≈ 30% dos cães, mas são menos frequentes em gatos.[5,22,26,41] Ptialismo, supostamente uma manifestação de encefalopatia hepática ou lesão GI, é muito comum em gatos (75%).[5,6,41,53,56] Hemorragia GI ocorre com mais frequência em cães de raças de grande porte com DPSIH, antes do reparo dessa lesão (≈ 30%), do que em cães com DPSEH.[57] Alguns animais (20 a 50%) apresentam sinais clínicos de doença do trato urinário inferior: hematúria, estrangúria, polaquiuria ou obstrução de uretra.[2] Devido à menor produção de ureia, à maior produção de amônia e à diminuição da metabolização do ácido úrico, é comum a formação de cálculos de urato de amônio (em 30 a 35,8% dos animais comprovadamente com DPSs, inclusive gatos[58]), podendo estar associada a infecções bacterianas do trato urinário.[26,54,58] Gatos com DPS e urolitíase pela formação de cristais de urato tendem a ser mais jovens (2 *versus* 7 anos) do que aqueles com urolitíase por cristais de urato sem DPS diagnosticado.[58]

A morfologia do desvio (*shunt*) pode estar associada aos sinais clínicos. Em uma série de casos, notaram-se sinais clínicos pré-operatórios em 88% dos cães com DPSC portocaval, comparados a 58% daqueles com DPSC porto-ázigos.[59] Sinais clínicos também foram mais comuns quando o desvio situava-se caudal ao fígado (91%), comparado aos animais que o apresentava entre o fígado e o diafragma (67%).[59] Os sintomas relativos ao SNC foram mais frequentes em casos de DPSCs, sendo os sintomas urinários mais comuns em casos de origem na veia gástrica direita, quando comparados a animais com origem do desvio na veia gastresplênica.[59] Em casos de DPSEH, os desvios espleno-frênicos e espleno-ázigos foram mais comumente observados em cães idosos do que desvios gastrocaval direito e espleno-caval.[60]

Defeitos congênitos concomitantes são comuns em animais com DPSs. Estes incluem criptorquidismo (30% dos gatos, machos, em um estudo[61] e 50% dos cães, machos, em outro[62]), sopros cardíacos que poderiam ser sopros inocentes em animais jovens ou indicar defeitos cardíacos congênitos,[3,5,53,61] e íris de cor de cobre, anormais para a raça, particularmente em gatos.[63]

Animais com HVP sem desvios macrovasculares manifestam sinais clínicos semelhantes àqueles descritos anteriormente. Em geral, esses cães e gatos são idosos, com sintomas muitas vezes discretos ou inexistentes.[5,25] A HVP com hipertensão portal é diagnosticada quando há hipertensão portal intra-abdominal, com veia porta patente, embora pequena, e fígado sem cirrose. Cães de raças puras são mais predispostos, particularmente Doberman pinscher (27% dos casos). A maioria dos cães apresenta menos de 4 anos de idade e pesa mais que 10 kg.[23] Os sinais clínicos são semelhantes aos de DPS ou cirrose hepática com hipertensão portal concomitante, resultando em ascite (60% dos casos), PU/PD, lesão GI, encefalopatia hepática e perda de peso, associados a DPSEHs múltiplos (Figura 284.2).

Os sinais clínicos associados a malformações arteriovenosas hepáticas (MAVHs) podem ser agudos ou crônicos. Na maioria dos animais, faz-se o diagnóstico no primeiro ano de vida, estando os sinais clínicos associados a DPSEHs múltiplos por hipertensão portal ou ascite. Cães de todos os portes e um pequeno número de gatos foram diagnosticados com a lesão.[5,24] Sintomas GI são comuns, e vários cães apresentam retardo do crescimento e letargia.[24] Ascite foi documentada em ≈ 75% dos cães, em menor escala do que se suspeitava, presumivelmente devido à descompressão do sistema porta pelos desvios (*shunts*) adquiridos nos outros 25% dos animais (Figura 284.3). Em um estudo, foram documentados sopros cardíacos em 20% dos cães com MAVHs.[24] Sinais de encefalopatia hepática costumam ser menos relatados em casos de MAVHs. Em alguns animais, o som de fluxo sanguíneo turbulento (sopro) pode ser auscultado na região hepática.

Achados clinicopatológicos

Alterações hematológicas quase sempre incluem anemia microcítica normocrômica arregenerativa discreta a moderada. Esferócitos, em cães, e poiquilócitos, em gatos, são comumente verificados na avaliação morfológica.[64] A causa da anemia microcítica não é completamente compreendida, embora estudos sugiram anormalidade no mecanismo de transporte de ferro, diminuição da concentração sérica de ferro, menor capacidade total de ligação ao ferro e aumento do armazenamento hepático de ferro nas células de Kupffer, o que poderia sugerir sequestro desse mineral.[65,66] A microcitose foi relatada, com ou sem anemia, em 60 a 72% dos cães, mas somente em ≈ 30% dos gatos.[3,65,66] Em geral, há melhora da microcitose depois de corrigido o desvio, o que não é observado de modo rotineiro em cães com HVP/DMV.[5,25] A leucocitose, devido à inadequada depuração de endotoxinas hepáticas e bactérias da circulação

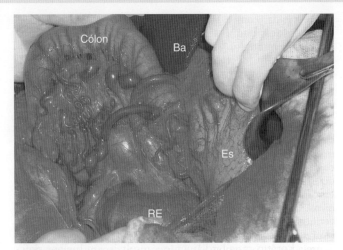

Figura 284.2 Cirurgia exploratória de um cão com hipertensão portal não cirrótica. Note os múltiplos desvios (*shunts*) portossistêmicos extra-hepáticos adquiridos na região do rim esquerdo e grandes veias dilatadas/tortuosas por todo o abdome, secundariamente à hipertensão portal. *Ba*, baço; *Es*, estômago; *RE*, rim esquerdo.

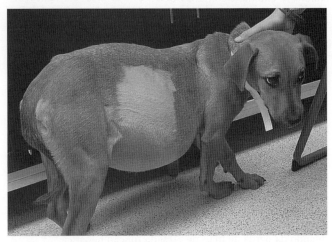

Figura 284.3 Cão jovem com ascite causada por malformação arteriovenosa hepática. Note a caquexia muscular dorsal associada à desnutrição.

portal, tem sido associada a mau prognóstico.[1,2,26,45,67] Monocitose e elevação da concentração de proteína-C reativa são mais comumente associadas à encefalopatia hepática.[36]

Anormalidades no perfil bioquímico sérico são extremamente comuns em animais com DPSs. A maioria delas se deve à menor síntese hepática: baixa concentração de albumina (50%), baixo teor de NUS (70%), hipocolesterolemia e hipoglicemia. Em gatos, a hipoalbuminemia é incomum, mas baixas concentrações de NUS e creatinina,[42,56] assim como atividades séricas de enzimas hepáticas, são comuns. Estas envolvem, em geral, incrementos discretos a moderados (duas a três vezes) de fosfatase alcalina e alanina aminotransferase.[64] Essas anormalidades são típicas de qualquer anomalia vascular hepática. A propósito, a concentração sérica de fosfatase alcalina é, em geral, maior do que a de alanina aminotransferase em cães com DPS, provavelmente em virtude da contribuição da isoenzima óssea em animais em fase de crescimento ou da lesão de organelas de hepatócitos e da maior liberação ou menor eliminação de fosfatase alcalina de canalículos.[5,64] Em um estudo, constatou-se que é mais provável que cães com DPSA tiveram menor valor de volume globular (ou hematócrito), maior valor de volume corpuscular médio e maior atividade de alanina aminotransferase do que cães com DPSC.[51] Em 81% dos cães com DPSC, o volume renal e a taxa de filtração glomerular estavam aumentados de maneira anormal antes da atenuação do desvio, com diminuição significativa após a ligação deste.[55] Isso poderia explicar, em parte, o motivo pelo qual são observadas baixas concentrações de NUS e creatinina no perfil bioquímico sérico.[55] A alta concentração de ácido hialurônico em cães com DPSC, supostamente causada pela menor taxa de depuração hepática, melhorou após a redução do desvio.[68] Isso sugere que a mensuração do teor de ácido hialurônico pode ser um bom teste de função hepática, inclusive para avaliação do sucesso da redução do desvio em cães com DPSC.

Em casos de DPSC, as anormalidades no exame de urina incluem baixa densidade urinária (> 50% apresentam hipostenúria ou isostenúria) e cristalúria com cristais de biurato de amônio.[3,5,8,53] A baixa densidade urinária provavelmente se deve à polidipsia, assim como à baixa concentração medular em razão da baixa concentração de NUS subsequente ao deficiente ciclo da ureia. Hiperamonúria, também resultante do deficiente ciclo da ureia hepático, combinada à hiperuricacidemia devido à deficiência na metabolização hepática de purina e pirimidina (ciclo do ácido úrico), resulta em excessiva excreção renal de amônia e urato. Esses compostos podem sofrer precipitação e originar cristais ou cálculos no rim ou na bexiga (cálculos foram observados em 30 a 36% dos casos).[8,12,26,54] A cristalúria por cristais de biurato de amônio é comum e pode ser observada em 26 a 57% dos cães e 16 a 42% dos gatos afetados.[54,58,62,69,70] Animais do sexo masculino, idosos, com histórico de tratamento medicamentoso antes da avaliação, mas sem morfologia de desvio portossistêmico, parecem ser condições associadas à urolitíase em cães com DPSEH congênito.[54] Proteinúria é comum em cães com DPS, supostamente secundária à glomerulopatia (p. ex., esclerose glomerular, fibrose glomerular, glomerulonefrite membranoproliferativa; ver Capítulo 325).[71] Aventa-se a possibilidade de que essa relação entre hepatopatia grave e glomerulonefrite, já observada em seres humanos, se deva ao acúmulo de antígenos nos rins, que, de outro modo, seriam depurados pelo fígado com circulação porta normal, resultando em glomerulonefrite imunomediada.[72]

Testes de função hepática

A mensuração da concentração sérica de ácidos biliares em jejum (12 horas) e 2 horas após a refeição é o exame preferido para avaliação da função hepática em animais com suspeita de DPS. Os ácidos biliares são sintetizados no fígado a partir do colesterol e, após conjugação, são secretados nos canalículos biliares e armazenados na vesícula biliar, até que sejam liberados no duodeno. Eles auxiliam na absorção de lipídios, por emulsificar a gordura intestinal e sua metabolização, são reabsorvidos a partir do íleo, transportados para o sistema biliar e captados pelos hepatócitos, para sua recirculação.[73-76] Ao mensurar a concentração sérica de ácidos biliares, faz-se a avaliação de todas as etapas – produção, excreção e recirculação êntero-hepática desses ácidos. Essas aferições podem ser influenciadas pelo momento de contração da vesícula biliar, pela taxa de transporte intestinal, pelo grau de desconjugação dos ácidos biliares no intestino delgado, pela taxa e eficiência da absorção de ácidos biliares no íleo, pelo fluxo sanguíneo portal e pela função de captação pelos hepatócitos e pelo transporte canalicular. Em alguns estudos, relata-se que a sensibilidade da elevação da concentração pós-prandial de ácidos biliares é de 100% para a detecção de DPS em cães e gatos.[73-76] Outros estudos sugerem que a sensibilidade de amostras pareadas é de 100%, mas não em amostras individuais. Um pequeno subgrupo de animais afetados apresenta concentração pós-prandial de ácidos biliares normal, com elevação em amostras obtidas em jejum, e um número ainda maior de pacientes apresenta concentração de ácidos biliares normal, em jejum, e elevada em amostra pós-prandial.[26,74] Cães da raça Maltês normais podem ter alta concentração de ácidos biliares, sem evidência de disfunção hepatocelular.[50] Outros resultados falso-positivos não relacionados com DPS se devem ao momento inapropriado da coleta da amostra, outras doenças hepatobiliares/colestase,

terapia glicocorticoide ou anticonvulsivante, colapso de traqueia, convulsões e doença GI.[6,64,75,77] Resultados falsamente baixos podem ocorrer por retardo na absorção intestinal devido ao prolongamento do tempo de transporte intestinal, ausência de contração da vesícula biliar, inadequada ingestão alimentar/ retardo no esvaziamento gástrico e má absorção ou má digestão. A contração da vesícula biliar pode ocorrer entre as refeições, resultando em maior concentração de ácidos biliares em amostra obtida no período pré-prandial do que no pós-prandial. A elevação persistente da concentração de ácidos biliares verificada em animais com DPS se deve ao desvio de ácidos biliares reabsorvidos para a circulação sistêmica.[6,64,75]

Quando há suspeita de resultado falso-negativo, pode-se realizar o teste de tolerância à amônia. Duas amostras são avaliadas: obtidas antes e 30 minutos após a administração de cloreto de amônio (100 mg/kg; dose máxima de 3 g), por meio de tubo nasogástrico, cápsula oral ou infusão por enema de cólon. Relata-se que, na insuficiência hepática, a sensibilidade desse teste é de 95 a 100%.[8,78,79] O teste deve ser realizado com cuidado, sendo contraindicado em animais com encefalopatia hepática.[79] A principal fonte de amônia no sangue se deve a sua absorção do trato GI: > 75% é gerada pelo metabolismo de bactérias do cólon.[6,12,53] O sangue portal fornece amônia aos hepatócitos, onde é convertida em ureia, no ciclo desta. Em animais com DPS ou outras deficiências hepáticas essa conversão não ocorre de maneira eficiente, resultando em aumento da concentração de amônia. A separação do plasma e a análise laboratorial precisam ser feitas dentro de 20 minutos após a coleta da amostra, o que torna esse teste problemático. Em gatos com hiperamonemia e encefalopatia hepática, relatou-se um erro inato na metabolização da amônia devido à deficiência enzimática (da enzima ornitina transcarbamilase) no ciclo da ureia.[80] Outras causas de hiperamonemia em animais jovens incluem acidemia metilmalônica, outras deficiências enzimáticas no ciclo da ureia e hiperamonemia induzida por obstrução de uretra.[5,80] Essas condições não estão associadas a DPS.

A concentração de amônia não é tão sensível (62 a 88% dos animais com DPS apresentam concentração anormal) quanto à mensuração de ácidos biliares, especialmente após jejum prolongado ou tratamento medicamentoso efetivo da encefalopatia hepática.[6,26,50,62] Foram documentados teores basais de amônia falso-positivos (em filhotes de cães Lébrel irlandês), bem como falso-negativos, tornando a elevação da concentração de amônia um indicativo, mas não diagnóstico de DPS.[26,79,81] A mensuração da concentração sanguínea de amônia 6 horas após a refeição aumentou a sensibilidade de detecção de 62 para 91%, em cães com DPS.[82] Elevações em quaisquer desses testes de função hepática são sugestivas de insuficiência hepática, mas não comprovam o diagnóstico de DPS.

Perfis de coagulação

A maioria dos cães com DPS apresenta tempo de coagulação prolongado (ver Capítulo 196), embora hemorragias espontâneas sejam raras e não costumem ocorrer até que uma intervenção cirúrgica seja realizada.[83,84] Em um estudo, constatou-se que a taxa de mortalidade pós-cirúrgica foi maior naqueles cães que tiveram agravamento importante de coagulopatia após a cirurgia.[85] Como as células parenquimatosas hepáticas sintetizam a maioria dos fatores de coagulação (I, II, V, IX, X, XI, XIII [e VIII pelo endotélio vascular hepático]), os animais com insuficiência hepática, como acontece em casos de DPS, teriam, em tese, algumas deficiências desses fatores, com coagulopatias resultantes. O prolongamento do tempo de protrombina (TP) e/ou do tempo de tromboplastina parcial ativada (TTPa) ocorrem após ≈ 65 a 80% de perda desses fatores.[6,12,83] O fígado também regula a coagulação pela depuração de fatores ativados, o que faz com que possa ocorrer a regeneração de fatores inativados e fibrinolíticos.[84,86,87] Animais com doenças hepáticas crônicas, assim como em casos de DPS, tipicamente apresentam somente prolongamento de TTPa, ao passo que aqueles com doença hepática aguda podem ter prolongamentos tanto do TP como do TTPa.[86] O TTPa prolongado em casos de DPS supostamente se deve a anormalidade na síntese hepática, anormalidades qualitativas e depuração de fatores de coagulação.[83-85] A propósito, a deficiência de fatores inclui aqueles envolvidos nas vias comum (II, V e X) e extrínseca (VII) da coagulação, levando à expectativa de prolongamento também do TP. Uma possível explicação é a deficiência do fator XII, que pode causar prolongamento do TTPa apenas sem hemorragias evidentes.

Cães com DPS apresentam contagem de plaquetas anormalmente baixa no período pré-cirúrgico, que piora no período pós-cirúrgico (média: 161.000/µℓ).[83] Nenhuma diminuição relatada na contagem de plaquetas foi baixa o suficiente para causar hemorragia clínica. Isso pode justificar a possibilidade de coagulopatia pós-cirúrgica por consumo excessivo. De forma geral, em um estudo, verificou-se que o perfil de coagulação (TP, TTPa e contagem de plaquetas) retornou ao normal em 6 semanas após a correção cirúrgica do DPS, mas não em animais que tinham desvios persistentes.[83]

Em alguns cães com DPSC, os parâmetros de coagulação e a tromboelastografia revelaram anormalidades hemostáticas consistentes com marcadores de coagulopatia e condição de hipercoagulação concomitante.[88] Nesse estudo, foi observado que uma condição de hipercoagulação seria 40 vezes mais provável quando associada à encefalopatia hepática clínica.[88]

Derrame abdominal

Ascite raramente é observada em cães com DPS congênito único, a menos que ocorra hipoproteinemia e hemorragia GI graves ou hipertensão portal associada a MAVH, HPNC ou DPSEHs múltiplos adquiridos (hepatopatia crônica/cirrose). Em geral, o derrame em qualquer uma dessas condições é um transudato puro, claro e relativamente acelular, com teor de proteína total < 2,5 g/dℓ, densidade < 1,017 e < 1.000 células nucleadas/µℓ.[64]

Histopatologia

A maioria dos cães com DPSC apresenta proliferação microscópica de ductos biliares, hipoplasia de veias afluentes portais intra-hepáticas, atrofia hepatocelular (lobular), proliferação ou duplicação arteriolar, lipidose e alterações vacuolares citoplasmáticas (lipogranulomas), hipertrofia de musculatura lisa, aumento de vasos linfáticos ao redor das veias centrais e hipertrofia de células de Ito e de células de Kupffer.[6,89-92]

Alguns animais possuem evidências de fibrose discreta ao redor das veias centrais e alguns poucos têm sinais de necrose ou inflamação.[6,89] Em uma avaliação de dados histopatológicos comparados ao prognóstico em cães com DPSC, não houve associação significativa em termos estatísticos entre características histológicas e tempos de sobrevida.[89] Sob o aspecto histórico, características histológicas associadas a um mau prognóstico incluíram fibrose, hiperplasia biliar e necrose.[5,6,90] Alguns cães com DPS possuem lesões focais, que consistem em pigmentos citoplasmáticos marrons em células de Kupffer e/ou macrófagos (ceroide e hemossiderina) e vacúolos lipídicos denominados *lipogranulomas*,[92] alterações essas que vêm sendo associadas de maneira inconsistente ao prognóstico.[89,92,93]

Outro estudo avaliou as lesões histopatológicas hepáticas relacionadas com os achados clínicos e a capacidade de reduzir o desvio (*shunt*) por completo em cães com DPSC.[94] A ausência de veias portais identificáveis (36% dos cães) foi associada ao aumento da proliferação arteriolar hepática e à diminuição da tolerância à redução cirúrgica completa e da opacificação dos vasos portais intra-hepáticos no exame de portovenografia. A redução cirúgica do DPSC resultou em significantes alterações clínicas, bioquímicas séricas e portovenográficas indicativas de melhora da função hepática, mas somente alterações sutis na reavaliação histológica hepática.[94]

Em um estudo com cães com DPSEH congênito, maiores volumes do fígado estavam associados a menos gotículas de lipídios por ponto de tecido à histopatologia.[93] O número de lipogranulomas estava associado de maneira positiva à idade, mas a existência de lipidose hepática e lipogranulomas não demonstrou efeito no desenvolvimento de desvios adquiridos ou na magnitude do aumento do volume hepático depois da atenuação do desvio.[93] Um estudo com 40 gatos com DPS, avaliados antes e depois da análise histopatológica de atenuação cirúrgica, demonstrou hipoplasia da veia porta e hiperplasia arteriolar em todas as amostras.[95] Em quantidades variáveis, foram observados inchaço do hepatócito, com alteração macro (30%) e microvesicular vacuolar (50%), fibrose (42,5%) e hiperplasia biliar (20%), e hemossiderina no interior das células de Kupffer (5%). Gatos com alterações macrovesiculares vacuolares eram, de maneira significativa, mais velhos (média de idade: 18,5 *versus* 8,5 meses). Nas amostras de biopsia de acompanhamento depois da atenuação parcial, não houve diferenças significativas nas características histopatológicas, embora a vasculatura intra-hepática tenha melhorado à portovenografia.[95]

Cães com HVP, sem (DMV) ou com (HPNC) hipertensão portal, compartilham alterações histopatológicas hepáticas observadas em cães com DPSC. Essas síndromes podem, portanto, ser confundidas histologicamente se não forem fornecidos o histórico e os sinais clínicos corretos.[23,25,29] Cães com HPNC costumam apresentar fibrose mais significativa, que se estende em direção ao parênquima, sobretudo ao longo dos tratos portais ou até mesmo em regiões de transição a outras áreas portais ou veias centrais.[23]

Os achados histopatológicos de cães com MAVH cujas biopsias foram coletadas dos lobos hepáticos não envolvidos na comunicação arteriovenosa são, em geral, semelhantes àqueles com desvio venoso-venoso. O tecido hepático em íntima proximidade com a malformação costuma possuir vênulas portais amplamente dilatadas, hiperplasia arteriolar acentuada, proliferação muscular e capilarização sinusoidal. Algumas veias portais possuem evidências de formação de trombos e recanalização.[5,24]

Cães com encefalopatia hepática podem ter alterações histopatológicas no SNC, que incluem polimicrocavitação do tronco encefálico, núcleos cerebelares ou córtex cerebral e hipertrofia e hiperplasia dos astrócitos protoplasmáticos corticais cerebrais.[3,8]

Diagnóstico por imagem

Diversas modalidades de imagem podem ser utilizadas para o diagnóstico de DPS. Radiografias abdominais simples costumam mostrar micro-hepatia (60 a 100% dos cães, 50% dos gatos) e renomegalia bilateral.[3,5] Em cães com HVP, o tamanho do fígado e dos rins pode ser normal à radiografia.[5,25] Cálculos radiopacos marginalmente podem ser observados na bexiga, na uretra, nos ureteres e/ou nos rins. Estes são, de modo geral, cálculos de biurato de amônio associados com cristais de sais de cálcio ou estruvita; esses cálculos também podem ser radiolucentes. Para diagnosticar de modo definitivo um desvio macroscópico utilizando-se modalidades de imagem contemporâneas, podem ser necessárias ultrassonografia abdominal, cintilografia, angiografia (portal ou arterial), angiografia por tomografia computadorizada (ATC) ou angiografia por ressonância magnética (ARM).

Ultrassonografia de abdome

A ultrassonografia é a ferramenta diagnóstica mais amplamente utilizada nos casos de DPS, vez que não é invasiva, não exige anestesia geral (embora a sedação torne os achados de DPSEH mais confiáveis em diversas circunstâncias) e não necessita de licença/manuseio especial (em comparação à cintilografia). Diminuição do número de veias hepáticas e portais, fígado subjetivamente pequeno e um vaso anômalo são verificados com mais frequência em casos de DPS congênito (Figura 284.4). Relata-se que DPSEHs são mais difíceis de diagnosticar na

CAPÍTULO 284 • Anomalias Vasculares Hepáticas

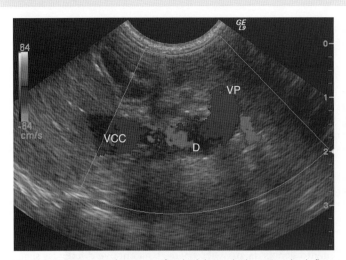

Figura 284.4 Imagem ultrassonográfica de abdome, obtida em Doppler de fluxo colorido, mostrando um desvio (*shunt*) portossistêmico extra-hepático. Note a comunicação anormal entre a veia porta (*VP*), o vaso do desvio (*D*) e a veia cava caudal (*VCC*). (*Esta figura se encontra reproduzida em cores no Encarte.*)

ultrassonografia em virtude do pequeno tamanho do paciente e dos vasos, da localização variável e da existência de gás nos intestinos e pulmões. DPSEHs múltiplos costumam ser mais difíceis de localizar, estando, em geral, próximos ao rim esquerdo. A sensibilidade para detecção de desvios (*shunts*) variou de 74 a 95%, e a especificidade, de 67 a 100%.[96-98] Em um estudo, a distinção correta entre DPSIH e DPSEH foi possível em 92% dos casos. A sensibilidade é maior em casos de DPSIH (95 a 100%) do que de DPSEH, devido à presença de parênquima hepático ao redor do vaso do desvio (*shunt*) e ao diâmetro tipicamente maior do vaso intra-hepático do desvio e da veia porta associada.[96] A qualidade dos resultados dependem do operador e de sua experiência. As imagens obtidas em Doppler de fluxo colorido e de onda pulsada são úteis para identificação de alterações na direção do fluxo, pois MAVHs classicamente possuem fluxo hepatofugal, e desvios venoso-venosos, fluxo hepatopetal através da veia porta (Figura 284.5). A velocidade do fluxo portal foi maior ou variável em 53% dos cães com DPSEH e em 92% daqueles com DPSIH.[5] Cães e gatos comprovadamente com DPSEH apresentam menor valor da razão do tamanho entre a veia porta e a artéria aorta. A ultrassonografia também é útil para detectar urólitos em cães e gatos com anomalias vasculares hepáticas, pois esses cálculos quase sempre são radiolucentes.[96,99,100]

A venografia com contraste por ultrassonografia envolve a administração percutânea de uma mistura de solução salina homogeneizada e 1 mℓ de sangue heparinizado autólogo em direção ao baço, guiada por ultrassom.[101] Ao visualizar a veia cava, a veia porta e o átrio direito de cães com DPSC, é possível diferenciar desvios intra de extra-hepáticos, dependendo do local de entrada das microbolhas em direção à VCC. Desvios porto-ázigos e portocaval também podem ser diferenciados dessa forma.[101]

Cintilografia

A cintilografia transcolônica pela utilização do radioisótopo tecnécio (^{99m}Tc) na forma de pertecnetato é um método útil e não invasivo de detecção de DPS.[100] Administra-se um *bolus* do radioisótopo no cólon, por via retal, e realiza-se a varredura do paciente com uma câmera gama. O isótopo normalmente é absorvido e drenado, nessa ordem, pelas veias do cólon e, então, pela veia mesentérica caudal, pela veia porta, pelo fígado e pelo coração. Havendo DPS, o isótopo alcança o coração, desviando-se do fígado, e então retorna a esse órgão pela circulação arterial (Figura 284.6).[100] Se houver desvio, uma fração dele pode ser calculada, obtendo-se uma estimativa da porcentagem de sangue portal que se desvia do fígado. Uma fração < 15% é considerada normal; a maioria dos cães com DPS apresenta fração > 60 a 80%. Alguns gatos (52% em um estudo) possuem fração inferior a dos cães.[102] Há variação considerável (absorção variável no cólon, variabilidade do operador, conteúdo de fezes no cólon), o que faz com que comparações em momentos diferentes sejam difíceis e não devam ser utilizadas para avalição do sucesso pós-cirúrgico.[103] Se o isótopo for administrado em uma parte "muito à frente" do reto pode ocorrer absorção diretamente na VCC, resultando em fração de desvio falsamente elevada. A meia-vida do tecnécio, na forma de pertecnetato, é de 6 horas, o que faz

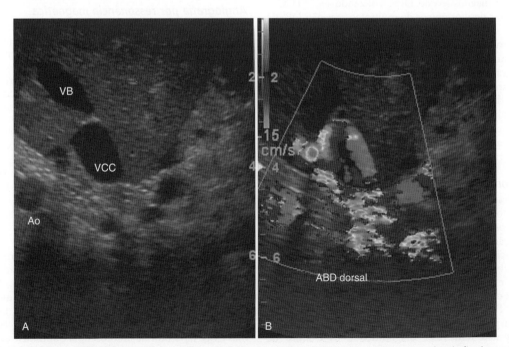

Figura 284.5 Ultrassonografia de abdome de um cão com malformação arteriovenosa hepática. **A.** Imagem ultrassonográfica do fígado mostrando vasculatura irregular entre a artéria aorta (*Ao*) e a veia cava caudal (*VCC*). **B.** Doppler colorido do fluxo sanguíneo turbulento na veia porta e desvios (*shunts*) adquiridos. *ABD*, abdome; *VB*, vesícula biliar. (*A figura B encontra-se reproduzida em cores no Encarte.*)

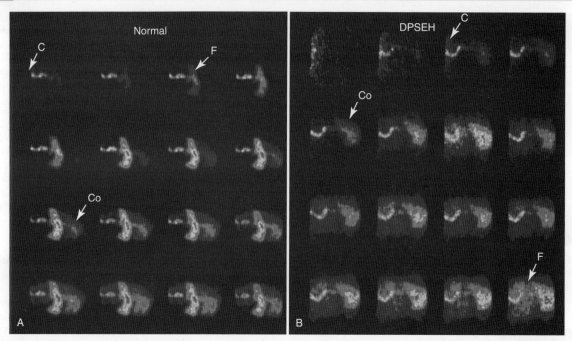

Figura 284.6 Cintilografia portal transcolônica utilizando tecnécio (^{99m}Tc) na forma de pertecnetato. **A.** Cintilografia de um cão normal. A série de imagens mostra (da esquerda para a direita) o fluxo do radionuclídeo desde o cólon (*C*), onde é, de maneira inicial, rapidamente absorvido, até a veia porta, perfundindo o fígado (*F*) e alcançando posteriormente o coração (*Co*). Compare com as imagens mostradas em **B**, de um cão com desvio portossistêmico extra-hepático (*DPSEH*); note o nucleotídio alcançando o coração (*Co*), antes do fígado (*F*), indicando desvio portossistêmico. (Cortesia da Dra. Lillian Aronson.) (*Esta figura se encontra reproduzida em cores no Encarte.*)

com que animais devam ser isolados por, pelo menos, 24 horas após o procedimento. A cintilografia não fornece informações morfológicas quanto ao tipo ou à localização do desvio, não distingue DPSIH de DPSEH e não pode diferencia desvios simples de múltiplos. A cintilografia pode ser normal ou anormal em cães com DMV/HVP. Frações de desvio podem ser inferiores em cães com DMV do que naqueles com DPS macroscópico. A estimativa da fração de desvio não é exata, sendo sujeita à variação inter e intraoperador. A utilização de cintilografia portal transesplênica no diagnóstico de DPS, utilizando-se ^{99m}TCO$_4^-$, ajudou a distinguir desvios únicos de múltiplos, mas não DPSIH de DPSEH, não sendo, portanto, utilizada de modo rotineiro.[104]

Um estudo recente correlacionou o volume do fígado, a anatomia do sistema vascular portal em ATC, a perfusão hepática e a cintilografia em cães com DPSC antes e após a redução com constritor ameroide.[105] Na cintilografia, notou-se correlação entre a redução da perfusão arterial hepática e a fração de desvio portal com o volume do fígado, e ambos foram indicadores de redução bem-sucedida do desvio. Adicionalmente, os cães cuja vasculatura portal não era visível na ATC no período pré-cirúrgico o foi no período pós-cirúrgico.[105]

Angiografia por tomografia computadorizada

A ATC é o padrão-ouro para avaliação do sistema venoso portal em seres humanos.[106] Não é invasiva, é um procedimento rápido e mostra todos os vasos afluentes e as ramificações portais após uma única injeção de contraste venoso periférico. Pode ser utilizada com acurácia em qualquer espécie, seja qual foro tamanho de animal, possibilitando a manipulação maior da imagem após a conclusão do exame. A ATC de dupla fase fornece uma avaliação completa da vasculatura portal e hepática, sendo considerada superior à TC de fase única.[107] Esse exame é mais útil em animais com suspeita de DPSIH e MAVH, ou para os quais a ultrassonografia não tem valor diagnóstico e os exames de imagem mais invasivos, como a portografia, não são recomendados (Figura 284.7). A ATC é útil para o planejamento pré-procedimento, tanto em abordagens cirúrgicas quanto radiológicas intervencionistas (RI), em casos de DPSIH ou MAVH, pela redução da dissecção ou manipulação hepática excessiva durante a cirurgia e minimização da dose de contraste durante o procedimento RI.

Um estudo recente em cães com DPSEH utilizando ATC constatou que a ela propiciou visão geral excelente da anatomia do desvio, além de informações sobre diversos vasos afluentes que poderiam passar despercebidos durante a exploração cirúrgica.[108]

Angiografia por ressonância magnética

A ARM também pode fornecer imagens tridimensionais pré-cirúrgicas do desvio (*shunt*), auxiliando no planejamento pré-procedimento (Figura 284.8). As imagens obtidas em ATC de dupla fase possibilitam interpretação relativamente fácil, fornecem detalhamento superior (particularmente em varredura por TC de múltiplos cortes [*multislice*] mais modernas) e custam menos do que a ARM. Em um estudo, constatou-se que as imagens obtidas em RM sem angiografia com uso do contraste gadolínio foram menos promissoras, com sensibilidade de 63 a 79%, embora tenha sido descrita especificidade de até 97%.[5] A ARM com contraste (ARM-C) pode detectar DPSEH e DPSIH[109] e teve valor diagnóstico em anomalias vasculares portais em 16 de 17 cães, incluindo DPSIH (n = 13), DPSEH (n = 2), MAVH (n = 1) e sem desvio (n = 1).[110]

Portovenografia

A portografia/portovenografia não é comumente realizada devido à disponibilidade de outras modalidades de imagem menos invasivas (ultrassonografia, cintilografia, ATC/ARM). A portografia mesentérica cirúrgica é o teste angiográfico mais comumente realizado para documentação de DPS em cães e gatos. Ela permite a visualização de um desvio (*shunt*) do vaso, mas exige laparotomia, fluoroscopia e administração intravenosa (IV) de contraste (Figura 284.9). A sensibilidade da portografia transcirúrgica é de 85 a 100% e depende do posicionamento do paciente e da subtração digital da imagem fluoroscópica.[3-5]

CAPÍTULO 284 • Anomalias Vasculares Hepáticas 1659

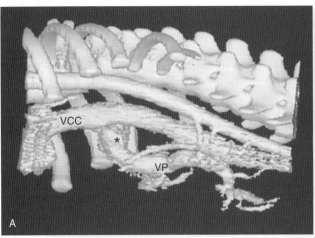
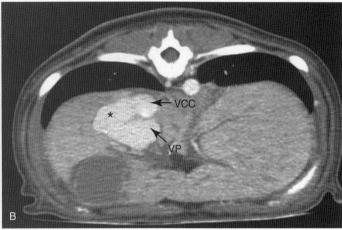

Figura 284.7 Angiografia por tomografia computadorizada (ATC) de um cão jovem com desvio (*shunt*) portossistêmico intra-hepático divisional direito. **A.** Reconstrução tridimensional do desvio (cranial à esquerda). A veia porta (*VP*) pode ser visualizada desembocando no desvio (*asterisco*), o qual adentra a veia cava caudal (*VCC*). **B.** Imagem angiográfica TC axial de fase dupla; na imagem, o lado direito do cão está à esquerda. Note o contraste evidenciando a comunicação entre a VP e a VCC através do desvio.

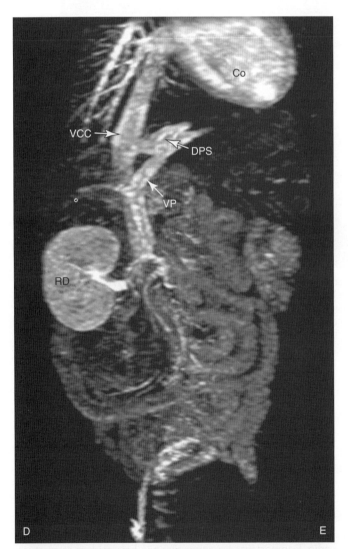

Figura 284.8 Angiograma por ressonância magnética em um cão jovem com desvio (*shunt*) portossistêmico intra-hepático divisional esquerdo. Note o realce do contraste na veia cava caudal (*VCC*), que se comunica com a veia porta (*VP*) através do vaso anormal do desvio portossistêmico (*DPS*). *Co*, coração; *RD*, rim direito.

Classicamente, a diferenciação entre DPSIH e DPSEH por meio de portografia baseia-se no local onde o *shunt* desvia da veia porta. Se esse local for cranial à 13ª vértebra torácica, o desvio é tipicamente intra-hepático; mas, caso seja caudal a ela, é, em geral, extra-hepático.

Uma alternativa à venografia portal cirúrgica é a venografia esplênica percutânea guiada por ultrassom. Sob o guia ultrassonográfico, injeta-se um *bolus* de ≈ 2 a 4 mℓ de ioexol (240 a 360 mg/mℓ)/kg na veia esplênica. Utiliza-se fluoroscopia ou radiografia para a obtenção de imagens da drenagem venosa esplênica através da veia porta, com a detecção do fluxo venoso hepático ou sistêmico (Figura 284.10). Entretanto, nessa técnica, o DPSEH localizado caudalmente pode passar despercebido, se o ramo portal se comunica com a VCC em uma posição mais caudal do que a veia esplênica.[111]

A injeção de contraste na artéria mesentérica, procedimento conhecido como *arteriograma mesentérico cranial* com via de acesso através da artéria femoral, não costuma ser utilizada devido a diversas alternativas menos invasivas.

DIAGNÓSTICOS DIFERENCIAIS

Em qualquer animal com suspeita de DPS congênito, devem-se excluir condições que causem sinais clínicos semelhantes (p. ex., parasitismo GI, hipoadrenocorticismo, enteropatia com perda de proteína, outras hepatopatias primárias, DMV/HVP, HPNC e MAVH). Se as concentrações de ácidos biliares forem sugestivas de DPS, é necessária a diferenciação entre DMV, HPNC, MAVH e DPS, notavelmente por modalidades de exames de imagens diagnósticas mencionadas anteriormente. Foi documentado que a concentração plasmática de proteína C ajuda a diferenciar a DMV de DPS (a concentração de proteína C foi > 70% em 80% dos cães com DMV e baixa em cães com DPS).[112] Se ainda assim houver forte suspeita de DPS macroscópico, mas este permanecer não identificado, deve-se então realizar biopsia hepática com ou sem mensuração da pressão no sistema porta para diagnosticar diversas formas de HVP. Se MAVH não for diagnosticada em um cão jovem com ascite e evidências clinicopatológicas de disfunção hepática, então é possível que haja HPNC, sendo necessário o exame histológico do tecido hepático para excluir a possibilidade de outras doenças hepáticas graves e direcionar o tratamento. Outras hepatopatias (hepatite crônica, cirrose ou leptospirose) podem causar sinais clínicos semelhantes, mas são mais comuns em cães idosos,

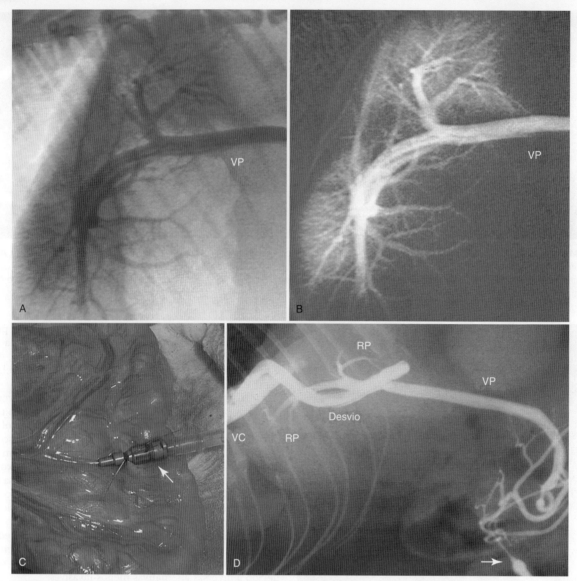

Figura 284.9 A. Portograma com contraste positivo em um cão com perfusão portal normal mostrando veia porta (*VP*) bem desenvolvida e ramificação portal. **B.** Subtração digital do portograma do mesmo cão mostrando melhor visualização da anatomia vascular. **C.** Jejuno com um cateter diâmetro 22-G fixado em uma veia jejunal para portografia e aferições da pressão portal. **D.** Portograma mesentérico realizado com cateter jejunal (*seta*) mostrando VP e ramos portais (*RP*) hipoplásicos, bem como desvio (*shunt*) portossistêmico (desvio) adentrando a veia cava (*VC*) caudal.

sendo, com frequência, acompanhadas de hiperbilirrubinemia. Se forem detectadas hiperamonemia e encefalopatia hepática em um animal sem evidência de DPS, deve-se realizar a avalição metabólica em amostra de urina à busca de evidência de deficiência de ornitina transcarbamilase ou de outras anormalidades metabólicas relacionadas com o ciclo da ureia.[80]

TRATAMENTO

Tratamento clínico

Deve-se tentar o tratamento clínico (Tabela 284.1) de animais com anomalias portovasculares antes da correção cirúrgica ou por radiologia intervencionista (RI) do DPS, em casos de DMV ou HPNC ou de desvios macrovasculares nos quais a cirurgia não é possível ou foi recusada. O tratamento clínico objetiva controlar os sinais clínicos associados ao desvio, mas não trata a diminuição da perfusão hepática subjacente. Quando um cão ou gato com sintomas de encefalopatia hepática é examinado, é necessária sua rápida estabilização clínica; devem ser implementados procedimentos intensivos para reduzir a concentração de amônia até um valor próximo ao normal. Nada deve ser administrado ao animal por via oral até que ele esteja alerta e consciente. Pode ser necessária fluidoterapia IV para repor e manter a hidratação, especialmente se o animal for incapaz de beber ou estiver desidratado. A solução de Ringer com lactato costuma ser evitada devido à necessidade de conversão hepática do lactato em bicarbonato. Em geral, a suplementação com potássio é necessária devido à depleção deste causada por diarreia crônica ou menor absorção desse eletrólito; ademais, a hipopotassemia pode contribuir para a encefalopatia hepática.[10,53]

A acidose metabólica (ver Capítulo 128) pode contribuir para a encefalopatia hepática e deve ser corrigida lentamente mediante fluidoterapia e, em casos raros, com bicarbonato de sódio. É importante assegurar que não haja acidose respiratória concomitante antes da terapia com bicarbonato de sódio. A glicose deve ser suplementada juntamente com solução de uso IV, particularmente em filhotes com DPS, nos quais a reserva de glicogênio e a neoglicogênese são mínimas. A terapia para encefalopatia hepática aguda grave consiste em restrição total de alimentação por via oral (VO), administração de enema com

CAPÍTULO 284 • Anomalias Vasculares Hepáticas 1661

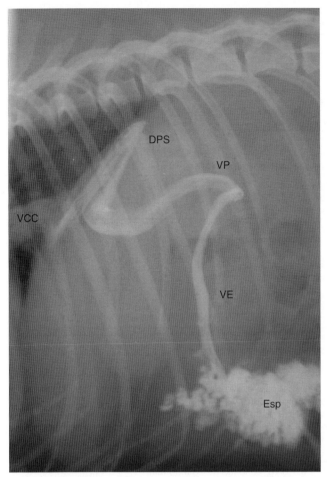

Figura 284.10 Portograma esplênico percutâneo guiado por ultrassom em um cão mostrando captação de contraste esplênico (*Esp*), veia esplênica (*VE*), veia porta (*VP*) e desvio (*shunt*) portossistêmico (*DPS*) adentrando a veia cava caudal (*VCC*). Note a óbvia ausência de perfusão hepática. (Cortesia do Dr. Skye Stanley.)

água aquecida e/ou lactulose (ver Capítulo 114), terapia oral com lactulose, tratamento antimicrobiano (metronidazol, ampicilina ou neomicina) e terapia anticonvulsivante, se necessário (ver Tabela 284.1). O ácido gama-aminobutírico (GABA) e seus receptores foram incriminados na patogênese da encefalopatia hepática.[10] A utilização de um antagonista de benzodiazepínicos, como o flumazenil (0,02 mg/kg IV, até obter o efeito desejado), mostrou ser benéfica em seres humanos em estado de coma causado por encefalopatia hepática. O manitol deve ser administrado aos animais com encefalopatia hepática grave ou após episódio convulsivo (ver Capítulo 148).[10] Em seres humanos, relata-se associação entre encefalopatia hepática e edema cerebral.[2,10]

Em geral, o controle de convulsões é iniciado com a administração de baixa dose de midazolam (um benzodiazepínico preferido ao diazepam devido à ausência do propilenoglicol, como veículo, o qual exige metabolização hepática). Assim que as convulsões forem controladas, pode-se administrar fenobarbital, brometo de potássio, brometo de sódio ou levetiracetam (ver Tabela 284.1 e Capítulos 35 e 260). Um estudo constatou que número significativamente menor (0/42) de cães tratados previamente com levetiracetam (20 mg/kg/8 h VO, por um período mínimo de 24 h, no período pré-cirúrgico) manifestou convulsão no período pós-cirúrgico, após redução do DPS, ao passo que 4/84 (5%) daqueles não tratados previamente com esse fármaco apresentaram convulsões.[113] Em três cães com estado de mal epiléptico (*status epilepticus*) após redução do DPS, verificou-se que um *bolus* de propofol em taxa de infusão contínua, combinado com fenobarbital, propiciou recuperação e alta hospitalar em todos os cães após 7 a 9 dias, sem sintomas recorrentes relativos ao SNC.[114]

A lactulose, um dissacarídeo metabolizado por bactérias do cólon em ácidos orgânicos, pode ser administrada por meio de enema ou por via oral. Ela promove a acidificação do conteúdo do cólon, retendo a amônia na forma de amônio, ao mesmo tempo em que diminui o número de bactérias e as elimina juntamente com o amônio nas fezes. O efeito osmótico resulta em catarse, reduzindo o tempo de trânsito fecal e a exposição das bactérias para proliferação e produção de amônia. Antibióticos, como metronidazol, neomicina ou ampicilina, diminuem o número de bactérias GI, permitindo uma redução ainda maior na produção de amônia. O metronidazol e a ampicilina também diminuem o risco de translocação bacteriana e infecções sistêmicas. Em animais com sinais de hemorragia ou anemia, a transfusão de concentrado de hemácias, sangue total ou plasma fresco congelado pode ser benéfica (ver Capítulo 130). Se houver evidências de encefalopatia hepática, dá-se preferência ao sangue total fresco, já que o sangue armazenado contém menor quantidade de fatores de coagulação e alta concentração de amônia, agravando potencialmente o quadro clínico da encefalopatia hepática.

O manejo nutricional é importante, sobretudo em animais jovens com má condição corporal. As dietas devem ser prontamente digestíveis, conter proteína de alto valor biológico (suficiente para atender às necessidades do animal, mas não para causar encefalopatia hepática), suprir, de modo suficiente, ácidos graxos essenciais, ter boa palatabilidade e atender às necessidades mínimas de vitaminas e minerais. Proteínas do leite e de vegetais possuem menor quantidade de aminoácidos aromáticos (tirosina e fenilalanina) e maior quantidade de aminoácidos de cadeias ramificadas, como valina, leucina e isoleucina. É menos provável que essas fontes causem encefalopatia hepática.[2,10] O conteúdo proteico de 18 a 22%, para cães, e 30 a 35%, para gatos (com base na matéria seca), deve ser o objetivo, com preferência por proteínas lácteas ou vegetais.

Sangramento gástrico/ulceração devem ser tratados com inibidor do receptor de histamina (famotidina), inibidor da bomba de próton (omeprazol) +/– com sucralfato. Animais com DPSIH têm predisposição a desenvolver úlceras GI (Figura 284.11).[57-115] Ácido gástrico vitalício e terapia supressora em cães com DPSIH diminuíram a morbidade associada ao sangramento GI. Os anti-inflamatórios não esteroidais (AINEs) devem ser evitados em qualquer cão com doença hepática, sobretudo naqueles com DPSIH, vez que esses fármacos podem perpetuar a ulceração GI.

Podem ocorrer ascite e fibrose em animais com MAVH e HPNC, mas raramente em casos de DPS, a menos que haja hipoalbuminemia grave. Se a ascite ocorrer devido à baixa pressão oncótica, deve-se recomendar terapia com coloide. Caso a ascite se deva à hipertensão portal, indica-se terapia diurética e dieta com baixo teor de sódio (ver Capítulo 183). Fontes adicionais de sódio (particularmente petiscos) podem exacerbar a ascite e, portanto, devem ser evitadas. A espironolactona é o diurético de escolha inicial devido a sua ação poupadora de potássio. A furosemida também pode ser necessária, mas deve ser utilizada com precaução, pois potencializa, ainda mais, a hipopotassemia. Em algumas situações, é necessária a abdominocentese terapêutica para deixar o animal mais confortável e facilitar a ventilação pulmonar (ver Capítulo 90). Sob o aspecto teórico, diversos fármacos podem reduzir a formação de tecido conjuntivo e a fibrose hepática: prednisona (1 mg/kg/24 h VO), D-penicilamina (10 a 15 mg/kg/12 h VO) e colchicina (0,03 mg/kg/24 h VO).

A terapia nutracêutica de suporte é recomendada para diversas doenças hepáticas, mas não é necessária em anomalias portovasculares que podem ser reparadas com cirurgia ou de forma intervencionista. Para aqueles animais que não possuem alternativa corretiva (DMV, HPNC, DPSEHs múltiplos) ou quando os

Tabela 284.1 Tratamento clínico recomendado para desvio (*shunt*) portossistêmico.

CONDIÇÃO	TRATAMENTO

Translocação bacteriana/diminuição da absorção de subprodutos bacterianos (amônia)	Enema de limpeza com água aquecida ou solução de lactulose a 30%, na dose de 5 a 10 mℓ/kg (ver Capítulo 114)
	Lactulose oral: 0,5 a 1 mℓ/kg VO, a cada 6 a 8 h, até induzir 2 a 3 defecações diárias com fezes amolecidas
	Antibióticos
	  Metronidazol: 7,5 mg/kg/12 h IV ou VO
	  Ampicilina: 22 mg/kg/6 h IV
	  Neomicina: 22 mg/kg/8 h VO (evite se houver qualquer evidência de hemorragia intestinal, ulcerações ou doença renal)

Coagulopatia (sintomática; pós-cirúrgica)	Plasma fresco congelado: 10 a 15 mℓ/kg ao longo de 2 a 3 h (ver Capítulo 130) Vitamina K$_1$: 3 doses de 1,5 a 2 mg/kg/12 h por via subcutânea (SC) ou intramuscular (IM), em e, então, a cada 24 h (ver Capítulo 197)

Úlcera gastrintestinal (muito comum em casos de DPSIH – inicie o tratamento antes da intervenção) (muito comum em casos de MAVH devido à hipertensão portal)	Supressores da acidez gástrica
	  Famotidina: 0,5 a 1 mg/kg/12 h IV ou VO
	  Omeprazol: 0,5 a 1 mg/kg VO, a cada 12 a 24 h
	  Esomeprazol: 0,5 mg/kg IV, a cada 12 a 24 h
	  Misoprostol: 2 a 3 mg/kg/12 h VO
	Protetor de mucosa
	  Sucralfato: 1 g/25 kg/8 h VO
	Tratar a coagulopatia

Controle de convulsões	Evite benzodiazepínicos*
	Fenobarbital (4 doses de 4 mg/kg IV, a cada 3 a 6 h)
	Brometo de potássio (KBr): deve ser evitado em gatos porque causa broncospasmo
	  Dose de ataque: 400 a 600 mg/kg/dia fracionada em 1 a 5 dias VO, com alimento; se necessário, pode ser administrada VR
	  Manutenção: 20 a 30 mg/kg/24 h VO
	  O KBr pode ser administrado por via IV, se necessário
	Propofol: 1 a 3,5 mg/kg, na forma de *bolus* IV, seguido de TIC de 0,01 a 0,25 mg/kg/min*
	Levetiracetam: 20 mg/kg/8 h (até 60 mg/kg/8 h) VO ou IV (*não há dados de literatura baseados em evidências que sustentem essa abordagem)

Redução de edema cerebral	Manitol: *bolus* de 0,5 a 1 g/kg, ao longo de 20 a 30 min
Suporte nutricional	Restrição proteica moderada de 18 a 22%, para cães, e 30 a 35%, para gatos (com base na matéria seca); proteínas lácteas ou vegetais são as preferidas Suplementação com vitaminas do complexo B (1 mℓ/ℓ de solução IV) Suplementação polivitamínica
Terapia hepatoprotetora (para doenças crônicas não relacionadas com DMV, HPNC, DPSEHs etc.)	S-adenosil-L-metionina: 17 a 22 mg/kg/dia VO Ácido ursodesoxicólico: 10 a 15 mg/kg/dia VO Vitamina E: 15 UI/kg/dia VO Cardo-mariano (silimarina): 8-20 mg/kg VO, fracionada a cada 8 h L-carnitina: 250 a 500 mg/dia VO (gatos)

*Há controvérsias. *DMV*, displasia microvascular; *DPSEHs*, desvios portossistêmicos extra-hepáticos múltiplos; *DPSIH*, desvio portossistêmico intra-hepático; *HPNC*, hipertensão portal não cirrótica; *MAVH*, malformação arteriovenosa hepática; *TIC*, taxa de infusão contínua.

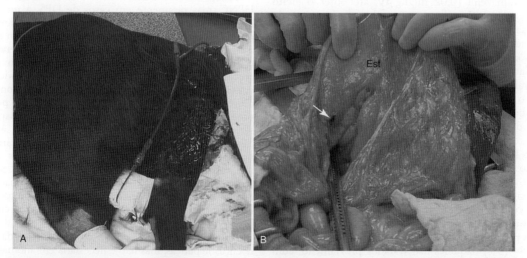

Figura 284.11 Cão da raça Labrador com desvio portossistêmico intra-hepático e úlcera gastrintestinal concomitante. **A.** Hematoquezia intensa e melena que necessitaram de transfusão de concentrado de hemácias. **B.** Laparotomia exploratória no mesmo cão mostrando úlcera perfurada (*seta*) no antro pilórico do estômago (*Est*). (*Esta figura se encontra reproduzida em cores no Encarte.*)

desvios permanecem patentes (p. ex., MAVHs, vários DPSIHs), alguns nutracêuticos podem ser úteis, incluindo S-adenosil-L-metionina (SAMe), ácido ursodesoxicólico, vitamina E e cardo-mariano/silimarina (ver Tabela 284.1). SAMe possui propriedades hepatoprotetoras, antioxidantes e anti-inflamatórias. É importante na estrutura, fluidez e função da membrana. Ela também auxilia na metabolização da glutationa (GSH), que participa em diversos processos metabólicos e possui um papel crítico nos mecanismos de detoxificação da célula. A depleção da GSH hepática pode causar efeitos tóxicos indiretos nessas células, pelo aumento do estresse oxidativo, sobretudo em gatos. A vitamina E é outro antioxidante que pode ser recomendado para prevenir e minimizar a lipoperoxidação nos hepatócitos. O ácido ursodesoxicólico é recomendado para a maioria das hepatopatias inflamatórias, oxidativas e colestáticas, quase sempre utilizado em casos de HPNC. Ele possui propriedades anti-inflamatórias, imunomoduladoras e antifibróticas, além de aumentar a fluidez das secreções biliares, promovendo colerese e diminuindo os efeitos tóxicos dos ácidos biliares hidrofóbicos nos hepatócitos. A silimarina é o extrato ativo do cardo-mariano. Há uma abundância de dados relativos a modelos experimentais *in vivo* e *in vitro* demonstrando as propriedades antioxidantes e removedoras de radicais livres da silimarina.[10] Especificamente, ela demonstrou inibir a peroxidação lipídica de hepatócitos e membranas microssomais e proteger contra danos de genes pela supressão do peróxido de hidrogênio, superóxido e lipo-oxigenase. A silimarina também aumenta o conteúdo hepático de GSH, parece retardar a formação hepática de colágeno e possui efeitos hepatoprotetores por meio da inibição da função das células de Kupffer. O cardo-mariano possui baixa toxicidade e poucos efeitos colaterais.

Resultados após tratamento clínico exclusivo

Em seres humanos com DPS congênito, o prognóstico a longo prazo sem a cirurgia é excelente, segundo relatos. Em medicina veterinária, um relato descreve 27 cães com DPSC avaliados após tratamento clínico exclusivo de longa duração; 14/27 (51,8%) animais foram submetidos à eutanásia, com um tempo de sobrevida médio (TSM) de 9,9 meses (idade média no momento da eutanásia: 20 meses); 4/27 (14,8%) não foram acompanhados; e 9/27 (33%) sobreviveram por longo tempo, com TSM de 56,9 meses (4,7 anos; com variação de 5 meses a > 7 anos) com vários destes ainda vivos no momento da avaliação.[45] Dos 27 cães, 9 apresentavam DPSEH, 17 tinham DPSIH e 1 era portador de um quadro complexo. Essa distribuição provavelmente ocorre devido ao fato de que mais veterinários estão indecisos em tratar cirurgicamente DPSIH do que DPSEH, devido às complicações relatadas e às dificuldades técnicas. Cães com DPSIH submetidos exclusivamente ao tratamento clínico manifestaram sintomas relativos ao SNC de mesma intensidade ou mais frequentemente, sinais clínicos GI menos frequentes e sintomas relativos ao trato urinário tão frequente quando antes do tratamento. Ao contrário, cães com DPSEH tiveram sinais clínicos de ocorrência semelhante ou em menor frequência quando medicados.[45] Cães submetidos a tratamento medicamentoso tiveram declínio significativo no teor de proteína total e nas atividades de fosfatase alcalina e alanina aminotransferase. A longo prazo, não foram constatadas alterações significativas nas concentrações de ácidos biliares, NUS e albumina nem no volume corpuscular médio (VCM). Onze de dezessete (64,7%) cães com DPSIH foram submetidos à eutanásia, em geral devido ao descontrole dos sintomas de encefalopatia hepática, assim como 3/9 (33%) daqueles com DPSEH.

Indicadores prognósticos do tratamento clínico de cães com DPSC incluem idade no início dos sinais clínicos (maior sobrevida em cães idosos) e concentração de NUS (valores maiores foram associados à sobrevida mais longa); não se constatou correlação entre as concentrações séricas de ácidos biliares, proteína total e albumina, bem como as atividades de fosfatase alcalina e alanina aminotransferase, o VCM e o tempo de sobrevida. De forma geral, poderia ser esperado que > 50% dos cães tratados clinicamente seriam submetidos à eutanásia dentro de 10 meses após o diagnóstico e ≈ 33% poderiam sobreviver a longo prazo somente com tratamento clínico, embora os sinais clínicos não cessem necessariamente. A eutanásia é mais frequente por conta dos sintomas persistentes de encefalopatia hepática e, em alguns casos, devido à fibrose hepática progressiva e à subsequente hipertensão portal.[63] Um segundo estudo de cães com DPSC observou que 24/27 cães (88%) tratados somente de forma medicamentosa morreram ou foram submetidos à eutanásia, comparados a 21/97 cães (21,6%) tratados com cirurgia.[116] Nesse estudo, a sobrevida não foi influenciada pela idade ou pela morfologia do desvio (*shunt*). Considerando essas estatísticas, a redução cirúrgica ou intervencionista, quando possível, é o tratamento de escolha para casos de DPS congênito.[116,117]

Tratamento cirúrgico

Tratamento pré-cirúrgico do paciente

Vários animais se apresentam debilitados, em má condição corporal e neurologicamente instáveis antes da anestesia e cirurgia. Na rotina, recomenda-se o tratamento clínico intensivo, conforme descrito anteriormente, mesmo em animais assintomáticos. Após o diagnóstico, o animal pode ser liberado e retornar para cirurgia semanas a meses depois. Nenhum momento para a realização da cirurgia foi definido como ideal, mas a maioria dos cirurgiões prefere realizar inicialmente tratamento medicamentoso, a fim de melhorar os sinais clínicos, controlar a encefalopatia e ganhar peso antes da intervenção. Além do risco potencialmente reduzido de convulsões no período pós-cirúrgico, os animais menores debilitados possuem risco de hipotermia, hipoglicemia e complicações associadas à hemorragia transcirúrgica, no período perioperatório. A utilização da terapia anticonvulsivante pré-cirúrgica permanece um procedimento controverso, quase sempre empregada em pacientes que apresentam encefalopatia hepática. Evidências preliminares mostram que o tratamento prévio com levetiracetam pode diminuir o risco de convulsões no período pós-cirúrgico e aumentar a sobrevida (ver anteriormente).[113,118] Ainda não está claro se os anticonvulsivantes devem ser empregados de modo rotineiro no período pré-cirúrgico, enquanto o paciente estiver recebendo terapia medicamentosa apropriada.

Há relatos de anestesia geral para animais com doença hepática.[119] Em resumo, deve-se evitar o uso de anestésicos que se ligam fortemente às proteínas plasmáticas ou que dependem de metabolização hepática. Além disso, o fornecimento de glicose costuma ser iniciado após a anestesia, pois esses animais quase sempre estão magros, debilitados e em jejum antes da cirurgia. Após a indução da anestesia (ver Capítulo 130), administra-se, de modo geral, uma solução coloide (particularmente em casos de DPSIH). Em pequenos animais, embora o plasma possa ser utilizado sem custo exagerado os autores preferem administrar coloides sintéticos (1 a 2 mℓ/kg/h IV), quando possível, a fim de reduzir o risco de reações induzidas por transfusão sanguínea e trombose perioperatória do DPS manipulado, que poderiam, em teoria, resultar de administração excessiva de plasma. Além disso, uma vez que esses pacientes não apresentam, de modo rotineiro, condição clínica que predisponha à hipocoagulação, e mais dados suportariam esse estado, a utilização do plasma como suporte coloidal não deveria ser recomendada de modo rotineiro. Recomenda-se o uso de antibióticos no período perioperatório a esses pacientes, que são jovens e imunologicamente incompetentes, assim como o fato de que está sendo utilizado um implante. Muitos já receberam antibióticos como parte do protocolo de tratamento clínico pré-cirúrgico. Avaliações do tipo sanguíneo e do perfil de coagulação são obtidas rotineiramente, sobretudo em casos de DPSIH, seja qual for o risco de hemorragia.

A tricotomia deve ser ampla e incluir o tórax (particularmente em casos de DPSIH tratado cirurgicamente ou quando a anatomia do desvio for ainda desconhecida no período pré-cirúrgico), a fim de preparar o animal para possível esternotomia caudal. A tricotomia da região ventral do pescoço pode ser útil quando se faz a cateterização da veia jugular, pois, no período transcirúrgico, ocasionalmente faz-se a mensuração da pressão venosa central. Deve-se prever a ocorrência de hipotermia; pode-se utilizar ar ou líquido aquecido ou cobertor, com ou sem garrafas de água aquecidas. As garrafas de água esfriam rápido, de forma que devem ser substituídas regularmente. Em casos de procedimentos intervencionais, deve-se realizar tricotomia tanto da região da veia jugular (DPSIH) quanto da artéria femoral (MAVH), para facilitar o acesso ao vaso sanguíneo.

Cirurgia

O objetivo da cirurgia em caso de DPS é recompor o vaso anormal, a fim de restabelecer o fluxo sanguíneo através do parênquima hepático. A redução total do desvio permanece o objetivo da cirurgia, pois a sua oclusão parcial tem um prognóstico pior.[91,120] Infelizmente, a maioria dos animais acometidos apresenta desenvolvimento do sistema porta insuficiente para possibilitar a ligadura completa do desvio (*shunt*) agudo à cirurgia, e ≈ 32 a 52% dos cães com DPSEH e < 15% daqueles com DPSIH toleram a recomposição completa do desvio (Figura 284.12).[91,120-122] Portanto, permanece um balanço delicado: redução do desvio para aumentar a pressão sanguínea portal o suficiente para estimular o desenvolvimento de perfusão portal, sem causar hipertensão portal excessiva. Caso ocorra hipertensão portal aguda, o paciente pode desenvolver ascite, congestão intestinal, diarreia, hipoxemia e, possivelmente, necrose intestinal. Caso ocorra hipertensão portal crônica, quando do não desenvolvimento da vasculatura portal, pode haver DPSs adquiridos múltiplos. A introdução de dispositivos de oclusão progressiva pode reduzir o risco de hipertensão portal aguda, mas ainda é incerto se eles reduzem o desenvolvimento de hipertensão portal crônica e subsequentes desvios adquiridos múltiplos. Supostamente, 40 a 50% dos cães desenvolveram novamente sinais clínicos após ligadura parcial de DPSEH meses a anos após a cirurgia (não incluindo dispositivos de oclusão gradativa).[26,120,123] Não está claro se esses cães tiveram um pior prognóstico por conta da oclusão parcial ou da redução do desenvolvimento vascular portal no momento da cirurgia, que impediram a redução aguda completa. Ademais, é incerto se esses cães apresentavam desvio persistente ou desenvolveram DPSs adquiridos.[91]

Após detecção e dissecção cuidadosa, o desvio (*shunt*) é isolado e aplica-se uma sutura circundante o mais próximo possível da circulação sistêmica (ao final do desvio).

A oclusão do desvio neste local garante que todos os vasos do sistema porta que se juntam ao desvio também são ocluídos. O posicionamento da oclusão no lado da veia porta do desvio (origem do desvio) pode permitir a continuação do desvio ao redor do fígado se quaisquer ramos vasculares auxiliares forem negligenciados. O procedimento cirúrgico foi descrito em detalhes em outras publicações.[123-131] É importante ressaltar que, após a oclusão temporária do desvio, uma pressão portal transcirúrgica > 9 a 10 cm de água acima da pressão em repouso (pré-ligadura) ou pressão absoluta > 17 a 24 cm de água foram associadas a maiores complicações pós-cirúrgicas.[91,132,133] Sinais clínicos também têm sido utilizados para determinar se a oclusão completa aguda do desvio pode ser tolerada. Em um estudo, constatou-se que 11 de 12 cães que não apresentavam encefalopatia com sinais clínicos atribuíveis somente à urolitíase por urólitos de biurato de amônio toleraram com segurança a oclusão completa.[134] Animais com aplasia portal aparentemente sobrevivem devido à perfusão arterial hepática, quase sempre detectadas em exame de amostra obtida por biopsia hepática que relata proliferação arteriolar hepática.[89,90] É mais provável que haja um amplo espectro de tamanhos do desvio e desenvolvimento vascular portal nesses animais, o que poderia explicar o motivo pelo qual parte dos pacientes com DPS manifesta sinais clínicos mínimos e pode viver por longo tempo com ou sem terapia medicamentosa.

Ao realizar cirurgia, recomenda-se exploração abdominal completa, pois animais com uma anormalidade congênita costumam possuir outras. A bexiga deve ser palpada com cuidado, a fim de detectar a cálculos que devem ser removidos. Recomenda-se castração, assim como biopsia hepática, embora um estudo tenha relatado que não é possível predizer o diagnóstico com base apenas nos resultados de biopsia, antes da ligadura.[89] Os autores não realizam biopsia hepática como rotina; entretanto, ela pode ser indicada quando um desvio macroscópico não puder ser identificado após a cirurgia ou a portografia.

Desvios portossistêmicos extra-hepáticos

Após a detecção de DPSEH, o cirurgião pode decidir se é possível realizar oclusão completa pela utilização de aferições da pressão portal, venografia porta e/ou inspeção visual. Se for

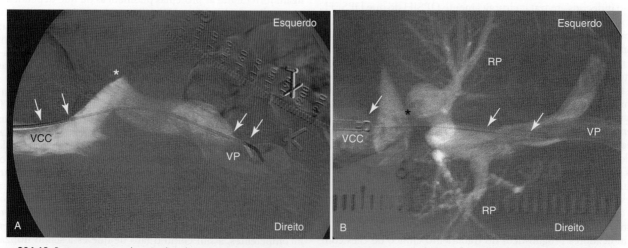

Figura 284.12 Portogramas por subtração digital transjugular percutâneos realizados em dois cães com desvios (*shunts*) portossistêmicos intra-hepáticos divisionais esquerdos mostrando alteração nos vasos sanguíneos do sistema porta (ambos os cães em posição ventrodorsal, com a cabeça voltada para a esquerda). **A.** Portograma com cateter (*setas*) através do desvio (*asterisco*) e na veia porta (*VP*) mostrando o desvio que adentra a veia cava caudal (*VCC*) e sem perfusão portal evidente. **B.** Portograma com cateter (*setas*) através do desvio (*asterisco*) e na VP mostrando boa perfusão portal via ramificações portais (*RP*) desenvolvidas em todo o fígado.

possível a oclusão completa aguda do desvio, é recomendada; entretanto, a oclusão completa pode aumentar o risco do procedimento.[91,120]

Dispositivos de oclusão gradual, como constritores ameroides (CAs) e faixas de celofane (FCs), alteram a forma de tratamento da maioria dos DPSEHs. Sob o aspecto histórico, acreditava-se que a caseína higroscópica em CAs absorvia aos poucos o líquido peritoneal, resultando em expansão concêntrica, e não excêntrica, devido ao anel de aço inoxidável circundante (Figura 284.13). Essa oclusão completa do desvio ocorreu em 6/12 cães após 1 mês e em outros 3/12 até os 7 meses de cirurgia.[128] Entretanto, diferentes resultados, inclusive oclusão parcial e trombose, foram notados em casos de implantação de CAs nas veias ilíacas dos cães.[135] Ademais, se a oclusão do desvio for muito rápida (ou se for afetada pela quantidade de dissecções necessárias para a implantação do CA, o peso dele na veia de paredes finas do DPS, a repetição de nova esterilização de um CA,[136] ou o tamanho ou a extensão da reação tecidual ao redor do CA[137]), pode ocorrer DPSs adquiridos múltiplos, conforme relatado em 17% dos cães após implantação do CA.[127,128] As taxas relatadas de complicações são de 7 a 20% e de mortalidade, de 0 a 17% após implantação do CA em casos de DPSEH, com resultados bons a excelentes em 94% dos cães e sobrevida média estimada de 152 meses.[26,127,128,138,139] Cães com oclusão incompleta do desvio podem ainda ter um bom prognóstico: o fluxo mantido com o desvio após implantação do CA foi detectado em 21% dos pacientes em um estudo com resultados bons a excelentes.[138] Em comparação à ligadura com fios, o uso de CA demonstrou reduzir o tempo cirúrgico, assim como a taxa de complicações transcirúrgicas.[138,140] Após implantação de CA em cães com DPSEH, a varredura por ATC e a perfusão mostram menor volume hepático pré-cirúrgico e maior incremento subsequente do volume; notou-se correlação entre a perfusão arterial hepática e a cintilografia portal com a oclusão bem-sucedida do desvio.[105]

As FCs têm sido avaliadas como um implante alternativo para oclusão gradual do DPSEH. Esse material de baixo custo é derivado de celulose de plantas e, em geral, obtido de pacotes de cigarros ou de presentes, além de ser inflamatório e causar fibrose progressiva ao redor dos vasos. O material é facilmente esterilizado e armazenado, leve (não torce o DPS) e requer menor dissecção ao redor do desvio. Evidências recentes sugerem que a maioria dos "materiais de celofane" disponíveis no mercado, na verdade, não são como celofane, vez que apresentam estriações visíveis (confirmadas em espectroscopia de infravermelho).[141] A oclusão mais progressiva obtida com FC em estudos experimentais[126] supostamente reduz a ocorrência de DPS adquirido.

Após dissecção e isolamento do desvio, uma peça de celofane dobrada em três camadas, com ≈ 3 a 4 mm de diâmetro, é posicionada ao redor do desvio e fixada com hemoclipes (Figura 284.14). A oclusão completa do desvio parece ser possível sem a oclusão inicial do desvio durante a implantação; na verdade, a oclusão parcial no momento da colocação da FC pode estar associada ao desenvolvimento de DPSA.[142]

Após a implantação de FC em casos de DPSEH, a taxa de complicação é ≈ 10 a 13% e a taxa de mortalidade, de 3 a 9%, com resultados bons a excelentes em ≈ 84% dos cães.[142,143] Entretanto, DPSAs múltiplos foram demonstrados em 3/16 cães (19%) com elevadas frações de desvio 6 semanas após a implantação de FC.[144] De forma geral, pela revisão da literatura, parece que vários cães com DPS podem manifestar resolução dos sinais clínicos mesmo com a persistência do desvio.[121,138,139,144]

Desvios portossistêmicos intra-hepáticos

Cães e gatos com DPSIH apresentam uma situação muito mais complexa. Em geral, esses desvios são muito maiores, localizados no parênquima hepático, e costumam não ser detectados de imediato. Locais de consistência macia podem ser sentidos, de modo ocasional, no lobo hepático acometido, onde o geralmente grande DPSIH está localizado, o que pode não ajudar a identificar a localização ideal de dissecção. Quando os desvios divisionais esquerdos são tratados mediante cirurgia, comumente utiliza-se abordagem pós-hepática (cranial ao fígado), pois, em geral, eles adentram a veia hepática esquerda, que, por sua vez, desemboca na VCC, na altura do diafragma. Em caso de desvios divisionais direito e central, que, em geral, desembocam na VCC, na região intra-hepática, quase sempre a abordagem cirúrgica é pré-hepática (caudal ao fígado), a fim de dissecar o ramo contribuinte da veia porta (que tipicamente é muito maior do que o ramo da veia porta esquerdo). Diversos procedimentos pré-cirúrgicos (ATC, ARM) e transcirúrgicos (portovenografia) podem ajudar a identificar a anatomia do desvio. Opções cirúrgicas incluem dissecção cirúrgica e oclusão do desvio por meio de sutura, CA, FC ou oclusor hidráulico (OH), oclusão completa do DPSIH com criação de um enxerto de veia jugular do DPSEH, oclusão temporária do influxo hepático por dissecção intravascular e embolização percutânea transvenosa com mola, através da veia jugular (descrita com detalhes no Capítulo 123).[2,57,132,143,145-151]

As taxas de complicações cirúrgicas são substancialmente maiores em casos de DPSIH (29 a 77%), quando comparadas às de DPSEH.[123,152] As taxas de mortalidade são de 6 a 23%, após ligadura, ou 0 a 9%, após implantação de CA, com resultados bons a excelentes em ≈ 75 a 100% dos cães, após ligadura, e ≈ 70 a 90%, após colocação de CA.[147,153,154] Resultados bons

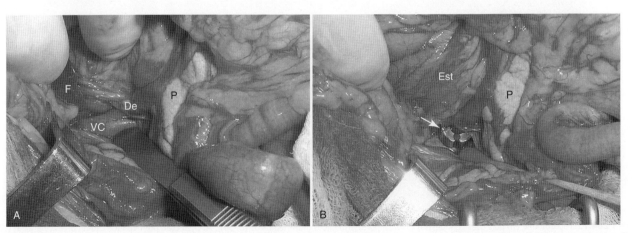

Figura 284.13 Laparotomia em um cão com desvio (shunt) portossistêmico extra-hepático (DPSEH). **A.** DPSEH esplenocaval (De) adentrando a veia cava (VC), visualizado no abdome dorsal direito entre o fígado (F) e o pâncreas (P). **B.** O mesmo cão após implantação de um constritor ameroide (seta) no término do desvio na VC. Est, estômago.

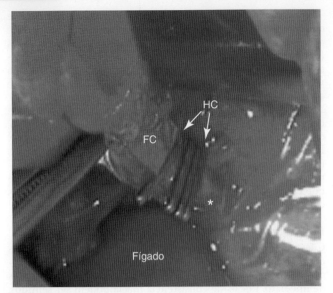

Figura 284.14 Laparotomia em um cão com desvio (*shunt*) portossistêmico extra-hepático após implantação de uma faixa de celofane (*FC*) ao redor do desvio (*asterisco*); a FC foi fixada no local por quatro hemoclipes (*HC*). (Cortesia do Dr. Eric Monnet.) (*Esta figura se encontra reproduzida em cores no Encarte.*)

a excelentes foram relatados em somente 50% dos cães tratados com FC, com taxa de complicação perioperatória de 55% e taxa de mortalidade perioperatória de 27%.[143]

A persistência do desvio e a insegurança do uso de dispositivos de oclusão progressiva levaram à pesquisa de OH, um manguito de silicone ajustável posicionado ao redor do DPSIH e conectado a um tubo, e uma via de acesso vascular posicionada SC no momento da cirurgia (Figura 284.15). Esse dispositivo pode ser inflado de modo manual com solução salina utilizando-se uma agulha de Huber introduzida por via transcutânea no local de acesso, com o cão acordado, semanas a meses depois da implantação, conforme necessário, para inflar devagar o manguito e ocluir o desvio de maneira progressiva.[155] A sobrevida imediata foi de 100% para 10 cães submetidos à oclusão de desvios intra-hepáticos por meio de OH, com taxa de complicação transcirúrgica de 20%; em 3 de 10 cães, foram necessárias revisões cirúrgicas antes da realização de modificações do dispositivo. Em 8 cães, foram documentadas resolução dos sinais clínicos e sobrevida por longo tempo,[155] mas houve suspeita de persistência do desvio, DPSA e/ou disfunção hepática com base na elevação persistente do teor de ácidos biliares (4/8) e em resultados positivos na cintilografia (5/8), 2 semanas após a oclusão completa por meio de OH.[21,147,155,156]

Complicações após oclusão do desvio postossistêmico

Complicações transcirúrgicas costumam estar associadas a complicações anestésicas ou hemorragia durante a dissecção do desvio. Complicações pós-cirúrgicas associadas ao DPS incluem, em geral, anormalidades neurológicas, hipertensão portal aguda e persistência do desvio (do desvio original ou pelo desenvolvimento de DPSA). Convulsões no período pós-cirúrgico não associadas a encefalopatia hepática ou hipoglicemia foram relatadas em até 12% dos cães.[118] Em um estudo, a administração de fenobarbital no período pré-cirúrgico parece ter reduzido a gravidade, mas não a ocorrência, de sequelas neurológicas após o tratamento cirúrgico do desvio.[118] Em outro, verificou-se que o uso de levetiracetam, na dose de 20 mg/kg/8 h VO, ao longo de ≥ 24 h, no período pré-cirúrgico, reduziu de forma significativa a ocorrência de convulsões no período pós-cirúrgico, em cães com DPSEH.[113] Em cães e gatos, ocorrem convulsões no período pós-cirúrgico, independem do tipo de oclusão realizada, podem ocorrer dias depois e não parecem ser causadas pela encefalopatia hepática original. Relatos sobre a possibilidade de animais idosos serem mais sujeitos a convulsões são conflitantes.[118,157,158] Explicações possíveis incluem a descontinuação abrupta de benzodiazepínicos endógenos ou alterações nas concentrações ou razões de aminoácidos cerebrais.[10,11,159] Todos os pacientes submetidos ao tratamento cirúrgico de DPS devem ser monitorados rigorosamente em busca de sequelas neurológicas. Não há consenso sobre um algoritmo para o tratamento desses sintomas; entretanto, o manejo intensivo deve ser instituído de imediato, com terapia anticonvulsivante e/ou *bolus* de propofol (1 a 3,5 mg/kg IV), seguido de taxa de infusão contínua (TIC) de propofol IV (0,1 a 0,2 mg/kg/min, ou mais).[160] Dá-se preferência à dose de ataque de fenobarbital porque os níveis plasmáticos terapêuticos podem ser alcançados de maneira rápida e podem ser monitorados sem demora. A preocupação sobre a utilização de um medicamento potencialmente hepatotóxico em um paciente com DPS é menos preocupante quando a expectativa é pelo uso a curto prazo. É difícil controlar animais em decúbito, sedados e possivelmente comatosos com brometo de potássio, sendo as concentrações de levetiracetam ainda não bem conhecidas ou mensuráveis em cães.

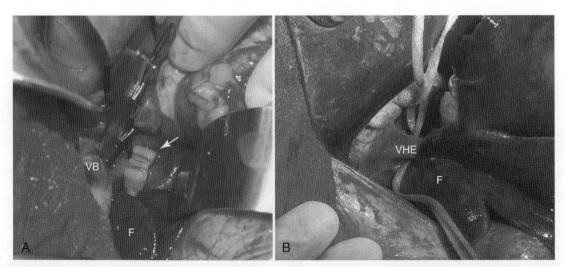

Figura 284.15 Laparotomia em dois cães com desvios (*shunts*) portossistêmicos intra-hepáticos (*DPSIH*). **A.** Dissecção pré-hepática caudal à vesícula biliar (*VB*) e ao fígado (*F*) de um DPSIH divisional direito após implantação de um oclusor hidráulico (*seta*) fixado no local com sutura com fio de polipropileno. **B.** Dissecção pós-hepática da veia hepática esquerda (*VHE*), entre o fígado e o diafragma, em um caso de DPSIH divisional esquerdo, antes da sutura. (**A.** Cortesia do Dr. Chris Adin.) (*Esta figura se encontra reproduzida em cores no Encarte.*)

Alguns animais podem necessitar de ventilação e outros podem demorar semanas, ou mais, para se recuperar. Foi relatado que a acepromazina ajuda a diminuir a atividade convulsiva em cães sem DPS, ao contrário do que se supunha sobre esse fármaco diminuir o limiar convulsivo.[161] Ela tem sido utilizada em baixa dose (0,005 a 0,01 mg/kg IV) para convulsões após procedimentos. De forma geral, o prognóstico é considerado ruim; entretanto, vários animais podem se recuperar com o passar do tempo e com tratamento de suporte agressivo. A recuperação pode não ser completa e alguns pacientes ainda podem manifestar algum grau de disfunção neurológica a longo prazo. Relatos descreveram 6 de 10 cães e 9/11 que se recuperaram por completo após disfunção neurológica pós-ligadura, embora em alguns a recuperação não tenha sido total.[118,143]

Algum grau de hipertensão portal pode ocorrer após oclusão parcial súbita ou completa do desvio, caracterizada por ascite discreta, com ou sem drenagem incisional. Entretanto, formas que representam ameaça à vida são relativamente incomuns, sobretudo pela introdução de dispositivos de oclusão progressiva. Sintomas pós-cirúrgicos preocupantes incluem êmese, distensão abdominal, ascite progressiva, dor abdominal e hipotensão. Estes podem ocasionar choque e coagulação intravascular disseminada. Nos cães e gatos que não respondem ao tratamento de suporte intensivo inicial, recomenda-se a remoção imediata do dispositivo de oclusão; entretanto, quando do surgimento dos sinais clínicos, a recuperação do paciente é muito incomum. A utilização de anticoagulantes e/ou trombolíticos no período pós-cirúrgico, a fim de prevenir ou tratar essas situações, não foi avaliada de maneira suficiente. Em geral, a hipertensão portal não tem sido um problema na técnica de embolização percutânea transvenosa com mola para casos de DPSIH.[21] Isso provavelmente se deve ao fato de que a oclusão do desvio ocorre na região pós-sinusoide, no orifício do desvio na VCC. Elevação na pressão gerada nessa localização parece ser aliviada pela presença de desvios venosos intra-hepáticos colaterais antes (em pressão inferior) que ocorra hipertensão portal pré-sinusoidal. Isso possui o efeito duplo de redução do risco de complicações secundárias à hipertensão portal, bem como da probabilidade de restabelecimento completo do fluxo portal hepático sem certo grau de desvio, o que pode ser uma compensação razoável entre risco e benefício, com provável ocorrência com qualquer tipo de oclusão de DPSIH realizada nesse local. É provável que esse fenômeno também explique a persistência de anormalidades nas avaliações clínicas, bioquímicas e cintilográficas verificadas em casos de oclusão completa do desvio no momento do procedimento, pelo emprego de técnicas de oclusão do desvio.[21]

Hipoglicemia (ver Capítulo 61) e hipotermia (ver Capítulo 49) pós-cirúrgica podem, em geral, ser prevenidas por meio de cuidado apropriado do paciente. Recentemente, relatou-se hipoglicemia em 44% dos cães submetidos ao tratamento cirúrgico de DPSEH e aproximadamente um terço não respondeu à suplementação com dextrose. Alguns desses animais podem responder à administração suprafisiológica de glicocorticoides (dose única de 0,1 a 0,2 mg de dexametasona/kg IV), assim como à aceleração da recuperação anestésica. Uma insuficiência glicocorticoide relativa (ver Capítulo 133) ainda não foi documentada nesses animais.[162]

A recidiva ou persistência dos sinais clínicos é a complicação mais comum a longo prazo observada após o tratamento de DPS. Vários relatos não mencionam acompanhamento a longo prazo suficiente para conhecer a real ocorrência desses problemas. A recidiva de sinais clínicos sugere que: o desvio original permanece patente; outro desvio estava presente originalmente; fez-se a oclusão de um vaso sanguíneo incorreto; vários desvios adquiridos se desenvolveram; há doença parenquimatosa hepática ou doença neurológica concomitante. Os testes bioquímicos séricos, inclusive os de função hepática, podem confirmar essa suspeita, mas são necessários exames de imagem adicionais para identificar a causa. Se os exames de imagem confirmarem a oclusão do desvio sem DPSA, um diagnóstico presuntivo de HVP/DMV pode ser feito.

Cães com DPSIH apresentam uma complicação potencial adicional distinta, porém importante: grave ulceração e hemorragia GI, a causa mais comum de morbidade e mortalidade a longo prazo verificada em uma série de casos.[21] Após a introdução da terapia de supressão vitalícia da acidez gástrica em cães com DPSIH, a taxa de mortalidade relativa à ulceração GI nos casos que atendemos diminuiu de 25 para 3,2%. Há diversas teorias para a ocorrência tão comum de ulceração GI em cães com DPSIH (p. ex., hipergastrinemia, anormalidade no fluxo sanguíneo GI, hipoprostaglandinemia, comprometimento da integridade da mucosa, produção anormal de muco, reposição anormal de células). Hipergastrinemia não parece ser a causa.

Tratamento cirúrgico de desvios portossistêmicos em gatos

O tratamento perioperatório de gatos é semelhante ao mencionado para cães; entretanto, uma maior frequência de sinais neurológicos, tanto no período pré-operatório quanto no pós-cirúrgico, apesar de terapia medicamentosa apropriada, resultou na utilização de terapia anticonvulsivante no período pré-cirúrgico, em gatos. Pode-se utilizar levetiracetam ou fenobarbital, devido a complicações respiratórias potenciais associadas ao uso de brometo de potássio. O tratamento cirúrgico de DPS em gatos é tecnicamente semelhante ao de cães, em termos de identificação do desvio e métodos de oclusão. Embora alguns cirurgiões utilizem ligadura por meio de sutura, a maioria usa CA ou FC em gatos, mesmo havendo algumas preocupações quanto à resposta inflamatória a tais dispositivos nessa espécie suficientes para resultar consistentemente em fibrose progressiva e oclusão do desvio.

Assim como acontece em cães, a taxa de mortalidade perioperatória em gatos com DPSEH é baixa.[56,163,164] Duas diferenças críticas entre o tratamento de DPS em gatos (comparado a cães) são: alta taxa de complicações perioperatórias e pior resultado a longo prazo, sobretudo devido às sequelas neurológicas. Após ligação por meio de sutura, relata-se taxa de complicações de aproximadamente 37 a 60% (sequelas neurológicas) e de 8 a 77% após a implantação de CA, bem como em um quinto e três nonos dos gatos após o uso de FC.[56,143,163-166] Os sinais neurológicos incluem convulsões em 8 a 33% dos gatos e cegueira central (geralmente transitória) em até 44% dos pacientes.[52,143,163-165] Recentemente demonstrou-se que escores menores (redução da perfusão portal) verificados na portografia intraoperatória mesentérica estão associados à maior incidência de complicações neurológicas após a oclusão do desvio.[166] Mais recentemente, foi descrita uma classificação diferente de desvios espleno-sistêmicos em gatos, predominantemente detectados em gatas castradas idosas quase sempre com doença hepática concomitante, que pode estar associada à hipertensão portal; essa é uma população de pacientes com DPS diferente e, portanto, os tratamentos variam de acordo com o quadro clínico.[167]

Os resultados de estudos devem ser interpretados com cautela devido a diferentes períodos de acompanhamento dos pacientes; entretanto, resultados razoáveis a excelentes foram relatados em 75% dos gatos após ligadura por meio de sutura, 25 a 75% após implantação de CA e 66 e 100% (5/5) após implantação de FC.[52,143,163-165] Vários gatos apresentam boa resposta clínica, embora persistam sinais bioquímicos de disfunção hepática: em cerca de 33 a 66% dos gatos, os testes de função hepática estavam anormais e, em 57%, havia persistência do desvio no período pós-cirúrgico.[143,163,164] O contrário também é verdadeiro, porque alguns gatos com disfunção persistente do

SNC apresentaram resultados normais nos testes de função hepática.[56] Nesse mesmo relato, aproximadamente um terço dos gatos foi submetido à eutanásia dentro de 1 ano devido à disfunção persistente do SNC após a implantação de CA, apesar de a maioria ter apresentado resultados normais em testes de função hepática.[56] DPSIHs são raros em gatos, fato que dificulta a previsão de recuperação. Neles, o DPSIH pode ser tratado de forma semelhante, com uso de sutura, CA, FC ou embolização transvenosa com mola.[56,143,145,163,164]

Tratamento cirúrgico e intervencionista de malformações arteriovenosas hepáticas

MAVHs são anomalias vasculares raras que envolvem múltiplas comunicações arteriais com a veia porta (Figura 284.16). Como elas costumam envolver diversas comunicações (e não apenas uma) com um nicho, ou "ninho", central, o termo *malformação* em vez de *fístula* é mais apropriado. Em geral, essas comunicações são oriundas da artéria hepática, mas também pode haver envolvimento da artéria gastroduodenal, da artéria gástrica esquerda e das artérias frênicas. Angiografia, ATC ou ARM ajudam a identificar a origem e o trajeto desses numerosos vasos (Figura 284.17). Devido ao desvio do sangue arterial de alta pressão para a veia porta, ocorre grave hipertensão portal crônica (geralmente com subsequente ascite importante), que resulta em múltiplos DPSAs na tentativa de aliviar a tensão na veia porta, conforme discutido em detalhes, anteriormente. DPSAs múltiplos foram observados em todos os cães com MAVH.

O tratamento de MAVH consiste em lobectomia hepática, ligadura da artéria nutriente ou embolização com cola das artérias anormais guiada por fluoroscopia.[24,168] A maioria das MAVHs está localizada nos lobos hepáticos direito ou central, e 25% delas envolveu dois lobos. A lobectomia pode ser desafiadora, por conta da vascularização e da proximidade à vesícula biliar e à VCC (Figura 284.18). Na lobectomia parcial, recomenda-se a oclusão temporária da veia porta e da artéria celíaca (e frequentemente da artéria mesentérica cranial), a fim de reduzir a hemorragia intraoperatória.[168] Além disso, a lobectomia pode ser contraindicada se a MAVH envolver a maior parte do parênquima hepático, pois a massa hepática remanescente após a ressecção da malformação arteriovenosa (MAV) pode não possibilitar função hepática suficiente. O procedimento de embolização da MAVH com cola, é descrito no Capítulo 123. Mais recentemente, os autores pesquisaram a oclusão venosa da MAVH, já que essas anomalias vasculares lembram as grandes MAVs pélvicas em seres humanos, que podem ser beneficiados com a embolização venosa (em vez de arterial). O conceito é de que uma única via proximal que drena a região imediatamente distal ao nicho da MAV propicia oclusão, a qual pode ser mais segura e efetiva do que a tentativa de embolização de inúmeras pequenas artérias que irrigam os ramos proximais ao nicho. Embora essa abordagem seja promissora, somente um único caso foi tratado dessa forma até o momento.[169]

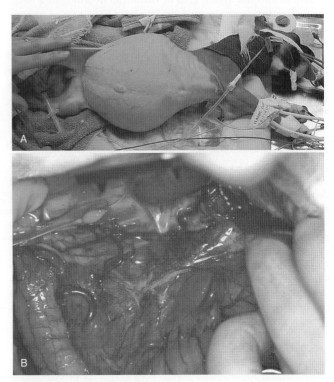

Figura 284.16 Filhote de cão da raça Boxer com malformação arteriovenosa hepática. **A.** Imagem pré-cirúrgica mostrando séria distensão abdominal devido à ascite e caquexia muscular acentuada. **B.** Imagem transcirúrgica após a remoção do líquido abdominal mostrando múltiplos desvios portossistêmicos extra-hepáticos adquiridos, resultantes da grave hipertensão portal. (*Esta figura se encontra reproduzida em cores no Encarte.*)

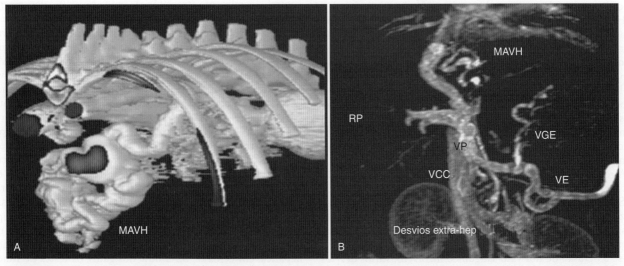

Figura 284.17 A. Angiograma por tomografia computadorizada reconstruído tridimensionalmente de um cão com malformação arteriovenosa hepática (*MAVH*). **B.** Angiograma por ressonância magnética de um outro cão com MAVH mostrando a veia gástrica esquerda (*VGE*), a veia esplênica (*VE*), a veia porta (*VP*), os ramos portais (*RP*), a veia cava caudal (*VCC*) e múltiplos desvios portossistêmicos extra-hepáticos (desvios extra-hepáticos) adquiridos.

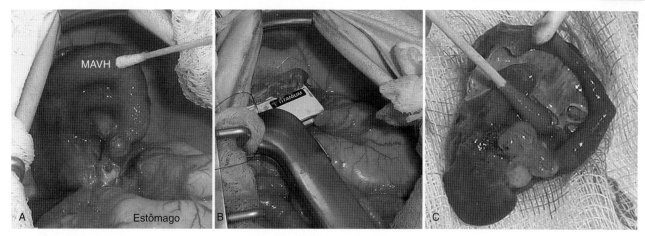

Figura 284.18 Laparotomia em um filhote de cão da raça Boxer com malformação arteriovenosa hepática (*MAVH*). **A.** Grande MAVH vascular, malformação da vesícula biliar e mínima porção normal de parênquima hepático. **B.** Grampeador toracoabdominal, sobre a base da MAVH, após grampeamento e excisão do lobo envolvido. **C.** MAVH seccionada após excisão, mostrando dilatações vasculares no parênquima. (*Esta figura se encontra reproduzida em cores no Encarte.*)

Complicações da cirurgia incluem hemorragia, hipertensão portal, hipotensão sistêmica, bradicardia e formação de trombos venosos portais ou mesentéricos.[24] A sobrevivência perioperatória foi de 100% em cães submetidos à embolização com cola, com ou sem hepatectomia parcial, e de 75 a 91% naqueles submetidos somente à cirurgia.[24] O resultado a longo prazo foi de razoável a bom em 38 a 57% dos cães tratados apenas com a cirurgia e de 100% para um pequeno número de cães submetidos à embolização com cola. De forma geral, 75% dos cães continuam a necessitar de controle dietético ou tratamento medicamentoso dos sinais clínicos devido à persistência do DPSEH adquirido.[24] Pode ocorrer a recidiva das comunicações arteriovenosas, bem como dos sinais clínicos, com a necessidade de procedimentos de embolização adicionais. A sobrevida a longo prazo é considerada razoável a boa com essa técnica intervencionista, mas muito poucos casos foram tratados dessa forma para se ter certeza.

Cuidados pós-cirúrgicos

Após tratamento cirúrgico ou intervencionista, os pacientes são mantidos em fluidoterapia IV até que estejam se alimentando ou ingerindo água. A dextrose é adicionada à solução de uso IV quando a glicemia estiver < 80 mg/dℓ. Os pacientes são monitorados por conta da hipoglicemia (ver Capítulo 61), da hipotermia (ver Capítulo 49), do retardo da recuperação anestésica, da hemorragia (ver Capítulo 135), das convulsões (ver Capítulo 35) e dos sintomas de hipertensão portal. Em geral, os animais necessitam de analgésicos opioides, como a buprenorfina, durante 1 a 3 dias após a cirurgia, embora nenhum analgésico tenha sido necessário após embolização com mola do DPS. Pode ser necessária a sedação com baixa dose (0,005 a 0,02 mg/kg IV) de acepromazina se os cães estiverem vocalizando ou comprimindo o abdome, já que essas atividades aumentam a pressão portal. A acepromazina não parece precipitar convulsões em cães com desvio (e pode até preveni-las); entretanto, não deve ser utilizada em animais com hipotensão.[161]

Após a cirurgia, institui-se dieta restrita a proteínas, uso de antibióticos e lactulose até que a função hepática melhore. Os protocolos de descontinuação dos medicamentos variam entre os cirurgiões, não sendo definido um que seja ideal. A descontinuação dos medicamentos pode ser ainda mais retardada quando se implantam dispositivos de oclusão gradativa, sobretudo após uso de FC, que ocasiona oclusão mais lenta. Perfis bioquímicos são avaliados 1 mês após a cirurgia. Se os parâmetros da função hepática estiverem normais, o tratamento medicamentoso é descontinuado ao longo de 2 a 4 semanas. Com 3 meses, os ácidos biliares são avaliados em cães e gatos com DPSEH. Essa abordagem não é utilizada de rotina em cães com DPSIH ou naqueles com MAVH, principalmente se o paciente estiver clinicamente bem e seja possível cessar o tratamento medicamentoso, pois é comum a persistência do desvio; em vez disso, nesses pacientes, são monitoradas as concentrações de proteína C, bem como os valores do hemograma e dos testes bioquímicos, antes e depois do procedimento.[112] Se as concentrações de ácidos biliares estiverem moderadamente aumentadas, os animais são reavaliados 5 a 7 meses após a cirurgia. Alguns clínicos recomendam suplementação com silimarina (cardomariano) ou S-adenosil-L-metionina, em razão de seus efeitos hepatoprotetores e antioxidantes (ver Tabela 284.1); são raros os testes clínicos de eficácia em animais com HVP ou DPS congênito.[171]

De modo geral, os pacientes são submetidos à descontinuação da terapia medicamentosa 1 mês após o tratamento radiológico intervencionista, processo esse que demora aproximadamente 1 a 2 meses, iniciando com o metronidazol e, então, a lactulose, seguida de transição para uma dieta de manutenção de adultos (ver Capítulo 180). Se isso tudo for bem tolerado, a concentração de proteína C e os valores do hemograma (volume corpuscular médio) e dos testes bioquímicos (albumina, NUS, colesterol, glicose) melhorarem e não ocorrer recidiva dos sinais clínicos, então a resposta é considerada boa, independente dos valores dos ácidos biliares. Já foi demonstrado várias vezes que o retorno da concentração de ácidos biliares ao valor normal após a oclusão do DPS não está necessariamente relacionado com a recuperação a longo prazo.[26,83,120,152]

PROGNÓSTICO

Os indicadores de prognóstico, resultados e sobrevida estão descritos na Tabela 284.2.[170]

Tabela 284.2 Prognóstico relatado para anomalias vasculares hepáticas.

ANOMALIA VASCULAR HEPÁTICA	PROGNÓSTICO
Tratamento clínico[45]	O **prognóstico** para o tratamento clínico exclusivo é **reservado a ruim** devido à progressão da atrofia hepática e dos sinais clínicos **Indicadores prognósticos** para animais submetidos apenas ao tratamento medicamentoso: idade no início dos sinais clínicos (idosos → sobrevida mais longa), NUS (maiores teores → sobrevida mais longa). Não há correlação entre o tempo de sobrevida e os teores séricos de ácidos biliares, proteína total, albumina, fosfatase alcalina, alanina aminotransferase ou VCM
DPSEH[26,52,67,83,121,125,138,142,143]	**Taxa de mortalidade:** 2 a 32% (ligadura), 7% (implantação de constritor ameroide), 6 a 9% (faixa de celofane) **Idade:** mostrou-se que *não* está associada à recuperação a longo prazo; cães idosos (> 4 anos) tiveram recuperação tão boa quanto cães mais jovens, no momento da cirurgia A **causa de morte** mais comum após oclusão do DPS é a persistência de sintomas neurológicos graves. Outras causas incluem hemorragia transcirúrgica, coagulopatia pós-cirúrgica, hipertensão portal e gastrenterite hemorrágica Em cães submetidos à **implantação de constritor ameroide**, a hipoalbuminemia pré-cirúrgica foi associada à persistência do desvio após a cirurgia **Outros fatores:** hipoalbuminemia ou leucocitose pré-cirúrgica, ocorrência de convulsões após a cirurgia e persistência do desvio 6 a 10 semanas após a cirurgia são relatados como indicadores de prognóstico ruim a longo prazo
DPSIH[21,46,67,120,123,132,133,143,152,153,172-174]	**Tempos de sobrevida média** relatados variam de 1 a 3 anos **Melhor recuperação a curto prazo e menor riscos de complicações** foram associados ao peso corporal (> 10 kg) e às concentrações séricas de proteína total (> 4 g/dℓ), albumina (> 2,6 g/dℓ) e NUS (> 7,4 g/dℓ) **Melhor sobrevida a longo prazo** foi associada a maiores valores de HCT e proteína total (> 4 g/dℓ) **Pior recuperação a longo prazo** foi associada a hipoalbuminemia ou leucocitose no período pré-cirúrgico, ocorrência de convulsões após a cirurgia e persistência do desvio 6 a 10 semanas após a cirurgia **Complicações pós-cirúrgicas** foram relatadas em até 77% dos casos cirúrgicos, com taxa de mortalidade a curto prazo de 11 a 28% **Taxa de mortalidade geral** varia de 23 a 63,6%. Em cães com DPSIH, o retorno da concentração sérica de ácidos biliares pós-cirúrgica ao normal **não** foi associado à sobrevida em curto ou longo prazo (permaneceu elevada em cães com melhora dos sinais clínicos, independentemente de a ligadura ser completa ou parcial) **A taxa de mortalidade perioperatória durante o procedimento de ETPM** diminuiu para < 5%, com taxa de mortalidade a longo prazo < 30% (< 15%, desde que se inicie terapia supressora de acidez gástrica vitalícia) **Ulceração e hemorragia gastrintestinal (GI)** são as causas mais comuns de morbidade e mortalidade a longo prazo nesses pacientes. Com a terapia de supressão de acidez gástrica vitalícia, a taxa de mortalidade por ulceração GI diminuiu de 25 para 3,2%
MAVH[24,169]	**Sobrevida:** cães com MAVH tiveram taxa de sobrevida no período periprocedimento de 100% após embolização com cola, com ou sem hepatectomia, e 75 a 91% quando tratados somente com cirurgia **Recuperação a longo prazo** é razoável a boa em 38 a 57% dos cães (cirurgia somente) e próximo a 70% (embolização com cola). Quando surgem vasos colaterais, pode ser necessária a embolização seriada. De forma geral, 75% dos cães continuam a necessitar de controle dietético ou tratamento clínico, independentemente da abordagem. É possível que esses pacientes sejam beneficiados pela implantação de faixa de celofane na veia cava, se o sistema porta estiver bem desenvolvido
DMV/HVP[25]	**Sobrevida:** 22/24 (92%) pacientes tiveram boa sobrevida a longo prazo ou morreram por motivos não relacionadas com a DMV
HPNC[23]	**Sobrevida:** 13/33 pacientes sobreviveram a longo prazo (40%), mas vários foram submetidos à eutanásia devido aos achados durante a cirurgia, sem tentativa de tratamento clínico. O prognóstico geral deve ser considerado favorável
DPS em gatos[5,41,42,56,145,163,164,175,176]	**Taxa de mortalidade perioperatória:** 0 a 23% após oclusão **Complicações pós-cirúrgicas** são relatadas em até 75% dos gatos. As mais comuns são disfunções neurológicas, que incluem convulsões generalizadas e cegueira central, as quais podem regredir alguns meses após a cirurgia **Recuperação.** Em gatos sobreviventes disponíveis para acompanhamento, verificou-se recuperação a longo prazo boa ou excelente em 66 a 80% dos animais submetidos a diversas técnicas de oclusão do desvio. Recuperação excelente foi relatada em 25% dos gatos com persistência do desvio; do contrário, anormalidades neurológicas contínuas ou recorrentes foram relatadas em 57% dos gatos, com cintilografia ou testes de função hepática normais. A persistência do desvio é comum em gatos após o procedimento, provavelmente devido ao desenvolvimento de DPSEHs múltiplos Apesar de maior taxa de complicações em gatos, a taxa de mortalidade é baixa, considerada favorável quando comparada à de cães

Continua

Tabela 284.2 Prognóstico relatado para anomalias vasculares hepáticas. (*Continuação*)	
ANOMALIA VASCULAR HEPÁTICA	PROGNÓSTICO
DPS adquirido[3,5,22,23,173]	**Ligadura de desvios individuais não** é considerada apropriada ou efetiva, já que tipicamente alivia a hipertensão portal Tentou-se **a utilização de bandagem na veia cava** (constrição cirúrgica da veia cava caudal, cranial ao DPSEH), para redirecionar o fluxo sanguíneo para a veia porta. Complicações que podem ocorrer incluem ascite, edema de membros pélvicos, desenvolvimento de outros desvios porto-ázigos e persistência de má perfusão portal. Nesses casos, a sobrevida foi semelhante aos animais submetidos ao tratamento medicamentoso **A ocorrência de DPSEHs múltiplos foi relatada após implantação de ameroide**, tanto em cães como em gatos, em quase 10 a 20% dos casos de DPSEH congênito único. O tratamento deve almejar o controle dos sinais clínicos de encefalopatia hepática e retardar a progressão da hepatopatia (tipicamente fibrose hepática)

DMV, displasia microvascular; *DPS*, desvio portossistêmico; *DPSEH*, desvio portossistêmico extra-hepático; *DPSIH*, desvio portossistêmico intra-hepático; *ETPM*, embolização transvenosa percutânea com mola; *HCT*, hematócrito; *HPNC*, hipertensão portal não cirrótica; *HVP*, hipoplasia venosa portal; *MAVH*, malformação arteriovenosa hepática; *NUS*, nitrogênio ureico sanguíneo; *VCM*, volume corpuscular médio.

REFERÊNCIAS BIBLIOGRÁFICAS

As referências bibliográficas deste capítulo se encontram online no Ambiente de Aprendizagem.

CAPÍTULO 285

Doenças Metabólicas Hepáticas

Penny J. Watson

INTRODUÇÃO

O fígado está centralmente envolvido em várias vias metabólicas de cães e gatos (ver Capítulos 280 e 281). Portanto, não é surpreendente que esse órgão seja afetado por diversas doenças metabólicas. Existem notáveis diferenças entre as espécies em várias das vias metabólicas hepáticas particularmente marcantes entre gatos e cães. Isso pode explicar, em parte, o motivo pelo qual doenças metabólicas observadas em cães e gatos costumam ser muito diferentes.

Hepatopatia metabólica pode ser definida como qualquer dano ao fígado devido ao acúmulo de produtos de vias metabólicas normais ou anormais. Isso compreende condições, ou causas, primárias e secundárias, com a existência de uma sobreposição entre essas duas. Por exemplo, um acúmulo secundário clinicamente insignificante de gordura (esteatose) devido à hiperlipidemia familiar primária em um cão pode estar associado ao desenvolvimento de mucocele biliar e estase biliar clinicamente relevante. O acúmulo de cobre também pode resultar em hepatopatia primária na verdadeira doença de armazenamento de cobre ou ser secundário à sobrecarga dietética e à estase biliar, mas, em ambos os casos, o acúmulo de cobre pode causar necrose de hepatócitos, principalmente se acompanhado de outra condição patológica, como intoxicação por fármacos anti-inflamatórios não esteroides.

HEPATOPATIAS VACUOLARES, ESTEATOSE, HIPERLIPIDEMIA E LIPIDOSE HEPÁTICA FELINA

Introdução

As hepatopatias metabólicas predominantemente secundárias mais comuns em pequenos animais são as vacuolares, nas quais ocorre acúmulo de gordura (esteatose), de glicogênio ou de água nos hepatócitos (edema hepatocelular, ou inchaço turvo).[1] Existem características histológicas que ajudam a diferenciar os tipos de vacuolização (Figura 285.1), o que pode ser desafiador, sendo necessárias colorações especiais para obter um diagnóstico

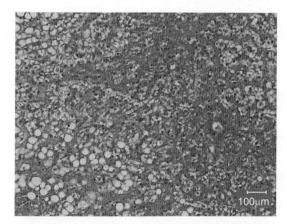

Figura 285.1 Corte histológico do fígado de um cão da raça Cavalier King Charles Spaniel de 9 nove anos de idade, com doença de valva mitral, mostrando vacuolização de hepatócitos, característica tanto de alteração hidrópica (vacúolos pequenos; lado direito da figura) quanto de esteatose (células com citoplasma claro; lado esquerdo da figura). São necessárias colorações especiais para a confirmação. O cão estava recebendo diversos medicamentos para cardiopatia e dieta com alto teor de gordura, mas a causa da vacuolização era incerta. Coloração com hematoxilina e eosina; ×100. (Cortesia do Departamento de Patologia; Departamento de Medicina Veterinária; Universidade de Cambridge, Reino Unido.) (*Esta figura se encontra reproduzida, em cores, no Encarte.*)

correto (ácido periódico de Schiff [PAS, *periodic acid-Schiff*] para glicogênio, e óleo vermelho O, para gordura). Em cães e gatos, várias doenças do armazenamento lisossomal também ocasionam vacuolização de hepatócitos. Ocorre inchaço turvo quando os hepatócitos são lesionados e menos capazes de manter a homeostase de líquidos. Se o edema do hepatócito for sério e crônico, pode causar morte do hepatócito, fibrose e até mesmo cirrose.

Várias anormalidades podem causar hepatopatia vacuolar, como a hipoxia hepática associada à insuficiência cardíaca congestiva direita ou à intoxicação (Boxe 285.1). A deficiência congênita grave de cobalamina também foi relatada como causa de vacuolização espumosa de hepatócitos, lipogranulomas, necrose celular individual e discreta fibrose em cães, possivelmente devido à hiper-homocisteinemia secundária.[2] Portanto, a "hepatopatia vacuolar" não é um diagnóstico e nem sempre ocorre devido ao excesso de glicocorticoides; em vez disso, esse achado histológico deve desencadear uma busca por intoxicação ou doença primária (ver Capítulo 286). O processo nem sempre é benigno e reversível; em cães, há relatos de progressão para disfunção hepática evidente e morte,[3] sendo possível a predisposição ao carcinoma hepatocelular em seres humanos[4] e em cães da raça Scottish Terrier.[5]

Hepatopatia esteroide

A hepatopatia distinta observada em cães que recebem glicocorticoides exógenos ou com hiperadrenocorticismo foi inicialmente relatada em 1977.[6] Em geral, os hepatócitos se tornam vacuolizados com incrementos marcantes do glicogênio citoplasmático, ou até mesmo nuclear.[1] A vacuolização se inicia na região centrolobular (zona 3) e se torna generalizada quando crônica.[7] O aumento marcante da atividade sérica de fosfatase alcalina é único em cães e pode ser resultado do retardo da depuração da isoenzima fosfatase alcalina intestinal, devido à hiperglicosilação hepática sob influência de glicocorticoides, embora seja desconhecido o motivo pelo qual isso ocorre em cães e em mais nenhuma outra espécie.[8]

Tradicionalmente, a hepatopatia esteroide tem sido considerada benigna em cães. Entretanto, a associação relatada entre hepatopatia semelhante àquela causada por glicogênio e remodelamento hepático e carcinoma em cães Scottish Terrier, e entre hiperadrenocorticismo e mucocele biliar, sugere que todas as hepatopatias vacuolares de cães devem ser levadas mais a sério, sobretudo quando crônicas e sérias.

O tratamento mais efetivo para hepatopatia esteroide é a remoção da fonte de glicocorticoides exógenos ou endógenos. Quando isso não for possível, recomendam-se antioxidantes (ver Capítulo 281). A administração de S-adenosilmetionina a

cães com hepatopatia induzida por esteroides aumentou a concentração de glutationa hepática total e causou efeito benéfico na proporção glutationa oxidada:glutationa total nos hepatócitos, mas não influenciou a aparência histológica dos vacúolos.[9]

Hepatopatia vacuolar semelhante àquela causada por glicogênio em cães Scottish Terrier

Uma forma particular de hepatopatia vacuolar idiopática em Scottish Terrier foi relatada nos EUA e na França. É caracterizada por um aumento marcante na atividade sérica de fosfatase alcalina e um risco aparentemente maior de carcinoma hepatocelular.[5,10,11] A síndrome é mais comum em cães de meia-idade (idade mediana, 8 anos [variação 1 a 14 anos]; idade média, 8,3 anos), embora cães com carcinoma hepatocelular sejam idosos. Não há predileção sexual. Há, em geral, uma elevação moderada a marcante da atividade sérica de fosfatase alcalina e aumento mais discreto de alanina aminotransferase; quase metade dos cães afetados manifesta sinais clínicos sugestivos de hiperadrenocorticismo (hepatomegalia; abdome abaulado; polidipsia e poliúria). Entretanto, os resultados dos testes de função adrenal são variáveis: há uma resposta inconsistente do cortisol no teste de estimulação por hormônio adrenocorticotrófico (ACTH, *adrenocorticotropic hormone*) e no teste de supressão com baixa dose de dexametasona, e em um estudo constatou-se que 5/7 cães apresentaram proporção cortisol:creatinina urinária normal(ver também Capítulo 306).[5] As anormalidades endócrinas mais consistentes em cães afetados consistem em aumento de progesterona e androstenediona após estimulação com ACTH. Em 26% dos casos, o exame ultrassonográfico mostra aumento das glândulas adrenais. Mucocele biliar foi relatada em 16% dos casos.[5] Na ultrassonografia, o fígado possui, com mais frequência, uma aparência mosqueada ou grosseira. O desenvolvimento de nódulos hipoecoicos parece retratar histologicamente a morte de hepatócitos e colapso.[5] Os cães acometidos parecem responder mal aos tratamentos tradicionais de hiperadrenocorticismo, verificando-se efeitos colaterais graves causados pelo uso de mitotano ou cetoconazol e ineficácia do trilostano. As recomendações terapêuticas atuais são, portanto, incertas, além do monitoramento ultrassonográfico regular em busca de desenvolvimento de massas hepatocelulares ou mucocele e cirurgia, conforme necessário. Faz sentido também fornecer aos cães acometidos suplementos antioxidantes, sobretudo S-adenosilmetionina, dada a redução na concentração da glutationa oxidada relatada após suplementação com essa substância em outras hepatopatias vacuolares em cães.[9,12]

Esteatose hepática

O acúmulo de gordura nos hepatócitos é denominado *esteatose* (ou lipidose ou degeneração gordurosa por patologistas veterinários). Esteatose é o termo preferido, já que é utilizada em livros-texto de toxicologia e medicina humana, além de evitar confusão com a síndrome clínica de lipidose hepática em gatos.[1] Nos cortes teciduais de rotina fixados em formalina, a gordura é visualizada como vacúolos claros no citoplasma, pois os lipídios são perdidos durante o processamento da amostra de tecido. A demonstração de gordura com o uso de corantes especiais exige cortes congelados. A esteatose microvesicular consiste em múltiplos vacúolos menores do que o núcleo celular; é típica no diabete melito em cães (ver Figura 285.1). A esteatose macrovesicular consiste em vacúolos maiores que costumam deslocar o núcleo para a periferia da célula. De modo geral, a lipidose hepática felina está associada a uma mistura de esteatose micro e macrovesicular[1] (Figura 285.2).

Em cães, a esteatose pode ser decorrência de lesão ao hepatócito (degeneração gordurosa), assim como de aflatoxicose.[13] Em gatos, a intoxicação crônica por vitamina A resulta em hipertrofia das células estreladas hepáticas, preenchidas por gordura, com ou sem esteatose hepatocelular e fibrose.[1,14] Esteatose também foi relatada em cães com desvio (*shunt*)

Boxe 285.1 Causas de hepatopatias vacuolares primárias e secundárias em cães e gatos

Hepatopatia esteroidal e anormalidade turva
- Hepatopatia esteroidal – secundária a altas concentrações de corticosteroides circulantes (exógenos ou endógenos)
- Hepatopatia vacuolar de cães Scottish Terrier (sobreposição com hepatopatia esteroidal?)
- Deficiência ou intoxicação, p. ex., grave deficiência de cobalamina em cães
- Secundária a dano hepático causado por outra enfermidade, p. ex., insuficiência cardíaca congestiva, neoplasia, outra doença hepatobiliar, doença gastrointestinal, doença renal, doença infecciosa.

Esteatose
- Lipidose hepática felina – primária ou secundária
- Intoxicação – p. ex., aflatoxina (cães); intoxicação por vitamina A (gatos)
- Secundária à hiperlipidemia familiar canina
- Secundária à endocrinopatia: hipotireoidismo e diabetes melito (cães); ocasionalmente hipertireoidismo (gatos).

CAPÍTULO 285 • Doenças Metabólicas Hepáticas

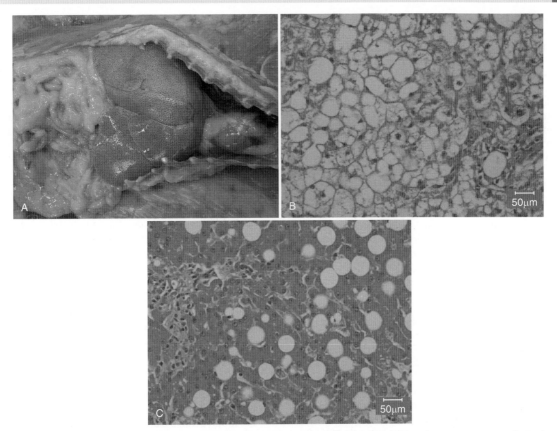

Figura 285.2 A. Aparência macroscópica do fígado pós-morte de um gato que morreu em decorrência de lipidose hepática. Note a aparência alaranjada pálida do fígado. **B.** Corte histológico do fígado do mesmo gato da figura A mostrando esteatose acentuada em hepatócitos. Coloração com hematoxilina e eosina; ×200. **C.** Corte histológico de outro gato mostrando células de Ito (estreladas) proeminentes. Note as células grandes com citoplasma pálido e núcleo posicionado na periferia. Os hepatócitos circundantes parecem normais. Essa é uma resposta comum a danos hepáticos ou a alto teor de vitamina A na dieta, não devendo ser confundida com lipidose hepática. (Cortesia de Fernando Constantino-Casas, Departamento de Patologia; Departamento de Medicina Veterinária; Universidade de Cambridge, Reino Unido.) (*Esta figura se encontra reproduzida, em cores, no encarte.*)

portossistêmico congênito, embora aparentemente não tenha significado prognóstico após a oclusão do desvio.[15,16] Em cães e gatos, a esteatose em hepatócitos também ocorre secundariamente a uma série de anormalidades primárias ou secundárias da metabolização de gordura (ver Capítulo 182). Em gatos com lipidose hepática, esse acúmulo de gordura é grave o suficiente para inibir a função dos hepatócitos e causar insuficiência hepática aguda reversível (ver Lipidose hepática felina, a seguir). Entretanto, em cães, embora a esteatose hepática possa se tornar muito grave em algumas doenças, como no diabetes melito, não se acredita que resulte em doença hepática inflamatória e insuficiência hepática. Isso difere do que ocorre em seres humanos, nos quais a doença hepática não alcoólica e a esteato-hepatite são causas cada vez mais importantes de hepatopatia progressiva, cirrose e insuficiência hepática. A metabolização de gordura é muito diferente entre cães e seres humanos (ver Capítulo 182) – notavelmente, os cães são muito resistentes à aterosclerose e não desenvolvem a tríade hiperlipidemia, hipertensão e diabetes tipo 2, conhecida em seres humanos como síndrome metabólica.[17] Isso pode explicar, em parte, o motivo pelo qual os cães são tão resistentes à insuficiência hepática progressiva causada por esteatose.

Lipidose hepática felina

Introdução

A lipidose hepática felina (LHF) foi inicialmente relatada em 1977 em dois gatos, nos EUA.[18] Vários relatos se seguiram nesse país, mas a ocorrência da doença permaneceu incomum na Europa. Entretanto, mais recentemente, o diagnóstico de LHF aumentou na Europa, onde a doença secundária parece ser mais comum do que a doença idiopática primária. As razões para essa mudança epidemiológica são incertas. LHF é definida como um "envolvimento difuso de > 50% de hepatócitos com vacúolos citoplasmáticos compatíveis com a aparência de lipídios".[19] Gatos são propensos a desenvolver esteatose hepática discreta a moderada quando apresentam anorexia por qualquer razão e, também, em resposta a danos hepáticos tóxicos. É importante diferenciar essa esteatose discreta da verdadeira lipidose hepática. É também importante diferenciar lipidose em hepatócitos da proliferação de células de Ito (ver Figura 285.2).

Fisiopatologia

Embora a fisiopatologia ainda não seja bem compreendida, obesidade, anorexia e estresse são considerados importantes fatores predisponentes. LHF é relatada em duas formas: idiopáticas primária e secundária. A forma primária é verificada em gatos com sobrepeso que permaneceram em jejum por longo período, mas não sem que haja detecção de doença primária. O tempo de jejum e o grau de obesidade necessários para causar a doença parecem ser variáveis. Em um estudo, gatos desenvolveram lipidose hepática após mais de 25% de perda de peso.[19] Em outro estudo, seis gatos de laboratório obesos desenvolveram LHF após 6 a 7 semanas de anorexia e perda de 30 a 40% do peso corporal.[20] LHF secundária está associada a outra doença, sobretudo colangite, pancreatite, doença intestinal inflamatória, neoplasia, diabetes melito ou hipertireoidismo.[19,21,22] Tanto na doença primária quanto na secundária, considera-se que a combinação de jejum e estresse aumenta a lipólise periférica e que há um efeito de gargalo no fígado, de tal forma que os lipídios mobilizados se tornam aprisionados, com saída reduzida. Gatos com LHF possuem elevados teores circulantes de triglicerídeos e ácidos graxos não esterificados, compatíveis com lipólise de gordura periférica e redução da função da lipase hormônio-sensível.[23] O conteúdo de triglicerídeos do fígado de um gato normal é de 1%; em um gato com LHF, aumenta para 43%[24] (ver Figura 285.2). Eles também possuem maior concentração sérica de beta-hidroxibutirato do que os gatos normais, indicando cetogênese hepática.[25] O gato ainda é capaz de mobilizar triglicerídeos de origem hepática, em certo grau, conforme demonstrado por estudos que constataram aumento significativo de lipoproteínas de densidade muito baixa no soro de gatos com LHF.[25] É proposto que eles não podem remover triglicerídeos de forma rápida o suficiente para compensar o aumento acentuado na mobilização. A razão para o desequilíbrio permanece incerta, assim como a razão pela qual alguns gatos parecem ser mais suscetíveis do que outros. Foi sugerido que a combinação de deficiência de proteínas e balanço negativo de nitrogênio, causada pelo jejum, reduz a capacidade de produção de apoproteínas, para a saída de gordura do fígado, e que as deficiências de taurina e carnitina contribuem na patogênese da doença, embora evidências experimentais para esses efeitos sejam limitadas.

A concentração circulante de insulina em gatos com LHF é normal ou reduzida, sugerindo que aqueles acometidos não são resistentes à insulina,[23,26] o que também contrasta com a doença do fígado gorduroso não alcoólico (DFGNA) verificada em seres humanos. Em gatos, quando a obesidade é induzida de modo experimental, eles desenvolvem resistência à insulina e apresentam alta concentração desse hormônio, durante a anorexia, e desenvolvimento de LHF, situação essa substituída por baixo teor de insulina. É também notável que são necessários vários meses para induzir obesidade em gatos por meio de manipulação dietética, mas somente algumas poucas semanas de jejum em um gato obeso para causar LHF.[27] Um estudo recente demonstrou que gatos afetados possuem altas concentrações de adiponectina e leptina,[26] o que também contrasta com o que acontece em seres humanos acometidos por DFGNA, na qual ocorre diminuição na concentração de adiponectina. Altas concentrações de leptina devem resultar em redução do conteúdo de lipídios em tecidos não adiposos, como o fígado, o que faz pensar que os gatos acometidos sejam resistentes à leptina.

A esteatose exagerada e marcante nos hepatócitos interfere na atividade metabólica das células e causa colestase secundária devido à compressão de pequenos canalículos biliares intrahepáticos. Dessa forma, a consequência é uma forma de insuficiência hepática aguda (potencialmente reversível), com sinais clínicos graves e efeitos na função hepática. Essa síndrome clínica aguda, associada à lipidose hepática em gatos, está em contraste acentuado com o observado em seres humanos e cães, nos quais ocorre esteatose hepática, sem resultar em insuficiência hepática. Os sinais clínicos em seres humanos somente ocorrem em um estágio tardio da enfermidade, quando ela se torna inflamatória (esteato-hepatite).

Resenha e achados clínicos
Estudos clínicos mencionam maior prevalência de LHF em gatas mais jovens ou de meia-idade. É relatado que a maioria dos gatos afetados, mas não todos, era obesa antes do início de um período de anorexia, seguido da doença. A forma da doença idiopática tende a ser mais frequente em animais jovens do que a doença secundária.[19,23] Os sinais clínicos são típicos de insuficiência hepática aguda, com êmese, anorexia, fraqueza e perda de peso. Há ocorrência de sialorreia e depressão, provavelmente como manifestações de encefalopatia hepática, ao passo que outras são incomuns. Ao exame físico, os gatos acometidos costumam apresentar hepatomegalia palpável e icterícia. Desidratação é comum e evidências de perda de peso recente costumam ser aparentes, com perda da massa corporal que recobre a coluna vertebral, mas com retenção de gordura nas regiões inguinal e abdominal, típica de perda de peso em gatos. De modo geral, o coxim de gordura falciforme é mantido e pode ser observado em radiografias do abdome.

Diagnóstico
Baseia-se em resultados de amostras obtidas por biopsia hepática, mas o histórico e os achados clinicopatológicos e os resultados de exames de imagem típicos aumentam o índice de suspeita de LHF. Os resultados do perfil bioquímico sérico tipicamente revelam elevações moderadas a acentuadas na concentração de bilirrubina e nas atividades de fosfatase alcalina e alanina aminotransferase; em casos de doença primária, a atividade de gamaglutamil transferase (GGT) costuma ser normal. A constatação de elevação marcante nas atividades de fosfatase alcalina, com atividade de GGT normal ou discretamente elevada em um gato, aumenta o índice de suspeita de LHF, em vez de doença do trato biliar.[19] Entretanto, um gato com LHF secundária grave também pode apresentar atividade de GGT bastante elevada, caso tenha doença concomitante acompanhada de estase biliar (p. ex., pancreatite, colangite). Hipopotassemia é um achado comum, devido à anorexia prolongada e à êmese, sendo relatada como um indicador de mau prognóstico.[19] Hiperglicemia é usual (40 a 50% dos gatos), mas, em geral, transitória.[19,23] Entretanto, já que o diabetes melito é relatado como um fator predisponente à LHF secundária, isso deve ser diferenciado de maneira cuidadosa, por meio da mensuração da concentração sérica de frutosamina e de mensurações seriadas da glicemia durante o tratamento. Ademais, se o gato apresentar cetose, é provável que ele tenha diabetes melito. Em cerca de metade dos gatos afetados, nota-se tempo de coagulação prolongado, mas os relatos de hemorragias clinicamente relevantes são raros.[19]

De modo geral, o exame ultrassonográfico do abdome mostra um fígado difusamente hiperecoico, mais hiperecoico do que gordura falciforme adjacente. A visualização de vasos sanguíneos hepáticos pode ser reduzida. A ultrassonografia também possibilita a avaliação de outros órgãos, em busca de doenças concomitantes, sobretudo o pâncreas. Em um estudo que avaliou a acurácia diagnóstica da ultrassonografia em doenças hepáticas de cães e gatos, a LHF teve a maior acurácia, com um diagnóstico correto em 50 a 71% dos casos, dependendo do ultrassonografista.[28] Gatos obesos sem lipidose podem apresentar fígado hiperecoico,[29] de tal forma que a aparência ultrassonográfica deve ser interpretada em conjunto com achados clínicos e clinicopatológicos.

O diagnóstico definitivo requer avaliação histológica de uma amostra obtida por biopsia tecidual. O ideal é realizar biopsia guiada por ultrassom (ver Capítulo 89) ou biopsia em cunha (ver Capítulo 91) para excluir a possibilidade de doenças primárias relevantes. A aspiração com agulha fina (AAF), com exame citológico de esfregaços, não foi fidedigna em alguns casos, podendo, inclusive, levar a um falso diagnóstico de LHF em um gato com linfoma hepático ou colangite.[30,31] Nesses casos, é provável que haja LHF, mas como uma alteração secundária à doença hepática primária grave. Entretanto, a realização da biopsia requer normalização do tempo de coagulação e de anestesia geral, o que representa um risco maior ao gato com doença aguda. Pode-se realizar, rapidamente e de forma segura, AAF do fígado guiada por ultrassom ou AAF cega guiada pelo dedo, se houver hepatomegalia palpável. A aspiração às cegas deve ser realizada no lado esquerdo, a fim de evitar a punção da vesícula biliar. Se as características citológicas dos esfregaços forem fortemente sugestivas de LHF, o gato pode ser tratado de maneira apropriada, inclusive com alimentação intensiva. Se o gato não responder ao tratamento conforme o esperado, então deve-se realizar biopsia hepática assim que ele estiver clinicamente estável. O clínico e o tutor devem estar cientes do maior risco de biopsia hepática em gatos com LHF: inicialmente, o tempo de coagulação deve ser normalizado e, se a biopsia for guiada por ultrassom deve-se evitar a utilização de dispositivos de biopsia semiautomáticos, pois já há relatos de mortes de gatos quando da utilização desses aparatos.[32] Laparoscopia ou laparotomia para obtenção de biopsia em cunha são as técnicas preferidas, sobretudo porque o fígado pode ser monitorado em busca de hemorragias e o pâncreas e outros órgãos podem também ser inspecionados em busca de anormalidades. Na lipidose hepática, o fígado é friável. Em um estudo com 195 cães e 51 gatos submetidos a diversas biopsias de órgãos abdominais em uma instituição, apenas 3 tiveram complicações importantes depois do procedimento: 2 eram gatos e ambos tinham LHF.[33]

Tratamento

O fator mais importante que influencia o prognóstico em gatos com LHF é o início precoce de alimentação intensiva, que, em geral, exige algum tipo de tubo de alimentação (ver Capítulo 82). Sem alimentação assistida, a taxa de mortalidade em gatos afetados chega a 90%, ao passo que, com a instituição de manejo dietético intensivo, ela diminui para 40% ou menos.[19] Por não serem efetivos o suficiente, orexígenos não são indicados aos gatos com LHF, uma vez estes não voltam a se alimentar por si mesmos de forma segura. Em um estudo, o uso imediato de tubo de alimentação resultou em sobrevivência de 6/7 gatos (86%).[20] Outro estudo constatou que a taxa de mortalidade foi discretamente maior em gatos com LHF secundária, comparada à LHF primária, que poderia refletir o retardo no uso de tubo de alimentação.[19] É igualmente importante iniciar quanto antes o manejo nutricional intensivo tanto em gatos com doença secundária quanto naqueles com doença primária. Entretanto, também é interessante identificar e tratar qualquer doença primária nesses gatos.

O uso de tubo de alimentação pode ser iniciado dentro de 12 horas, assim que os desequilíbrios hidreletrolíticos tenham sido corrigidos (ver Capítulos 82 e 180). O tubo nasoesofágico é útil a curto prazo, porque possui a vantagem de não necessitar de anestesia geral para sua colocação. Entretanto, há necessidade de um tubo mais permanente, como o de esofagostomia ou gastrostomia, assim que o gato estiver estabilizado, já que o retorno à ingestão voluntária de alimento demora, pelo menos, 12 a 16 dias ou mais.[20] A alimentação deve ser introduzida lentamente, utilizando-se uma dieta com o maior conteúdo possível de proteína. As dietas com alto teor proteico são as mais efetivas na redução da gordura hepática, na LHF induzida experimentalmente.[34] Em gatos, ocorre redução significativa do volume gástrico após jejum prolongado.[35]

Na fase aguda da doença os gatos quase sempre necessitam fluidoterapia intravenosa (ver Capítulo 129) para reverter a desidratação e corrigir as anormalidades eletrolíticas, particularmente a hipopotassemia (ver Capítulo 68). A adição de cloreto de potássio no tubo de alimentação também é uma escolha acertada, podendo ser necessária a inclusão de fosfato de potássio ou fosfato de sódio quando as concentrações séricas de eletrólitos diminuírem após o início da alimentação. A síndrome da realimentação foi relatada em um gato com LHF alimentado por meio de tubo, com redução súbita das concentrações séricas de potássio e fósforo, resultando em hemólise, de tal forma que esses parâmetros devem ser monitorados com cuidado em gatos afetados.[36] Alguns autores também recomendam a adição de outros nutrientes no tubo de alimentação, como vitaminas do complexo B, carnitina e taurina, mas não há evidência de que seja necessária a inclusão rotineira de nutrientes extras às dietas de gatos em cuidado crítico. Entretanto, é aconselhável mensurar a concentração sérica de cobalamina em gatos acometidos, uma vez que ela pode estar baixa, sobretudo em gatos com doença gastrintestinal concomitante. No caso de deficiência, recomenda-se a suplementação parenteral de cobalamina. Existem fortes evidências de que os gatos afetados apresentam lesões oxidativas sistêmicas e hepáticas; portanto, recomenda-se a suplementação com antioxidantes, como S-adenosilmetionina (20 mg/kg/24 h VO, com estômago vazio, ou 100 a 400 mg/gato/dia) e vitamina E (dose ideal incerta, mas 100 UI/dia VO é adequada).[12] Os gatos acometidos quase sempre apresentam tempo de coagulação prolongado, que se normaliza após o tratamento parenteral com vitamina K. Também pode ser necessário tratamento de suporte: antiemético, se o gato estiver vomitando, sendo o maropitant a escolha ideal porque

também possui ação antináusea. Podem ser necessários procinéticos se houver retardo do esvaziamento gástrico após alimentação por meio de tubo. A ranitidina é uma boa escolha inicial, por conta de sua ação procinética colinérgica e pela possibilidade de ser administrada por via intravenosa.

Um pequeno número de gatos pode desenvolver encefalopatia hepática clinicamente relevante, condição que requer tratamento. Esse aspecto do tratamento é discutido nos Capítulos 281, 283 e 284. A orientação atual para o tratamento de gatos com LHF e encefalopatia hepática é não alimentá-los com dieta restrita em proteína, mas sim reduzir a quantidade fornecida; alimente-os com refeições menores, mais frequentemente, e institua tratamento de qualquer doença inflamatória concomitante.

Hiperlipidemia canina

A hiperlipidemia é definida como aumento na concentração sérica, seja de triglicerídeos, seja de colesterol, ou de ambos.[37-55] Anormalidades de lipídios são discutidas no Capítulo 182.

Mucocele de vesícula biliar

Mucocele de vesícula biliar consiste em hiperplasia mucinosa cística da parede da vesícula biliar com acúmulo de muco espesso.[41,56-64] Inicialmente relatada em cães em 1995,[56] ela é incomum, mas parece ser cada vez mais frequente e está associada a hepatopatias vacuolares.[57] Essa anormalidade é abordada no Capítulo 288.

DERMATITE NECROLÍTICA SUPERFICIAL

Introdução e fisiopatologia

A dermatite necrolítica superficial (síndrome hepatocutânea, necrose epidérmica metabólica, eritema migratório necrolítico) é uma hepatopatia incomum, mas muito caraterística, supostamente secundária a uma anormalidade metabólica subjacente. As alterações hepáticas e cutâneas resultantes são características e muito mais graves e sérias do que aquelas associadas a hepatopatias vacuolares secundárias comuns, relatadas em várias endocrinopatias. Em seres humanos, a maioria das pessoas possui tumor secretor de glucagon e diabetes melito concomitante. Há relatos de alguns poucos cães com glucagonomas, geralmente metastáticos,[65-67] e um caso em um cão com insulinoma.[68] Entretanto, na maioria dos casos em cães não há tumor detectável, a concentração sérica de glucagon está normal e a causa não é identificada. Dermatite necrolítica superficial também foi relatada em 11 cães tratados com fenobarbital,[69] embora nesse estudo retrospectivo a contribuição do antiepiléptico na ocorrência da doença tenha sido incerta e a resposta à interrupção do tratamento, não conhecida.

As características marcantes são os achados histológicos típicos verificados em amostras obtidas por biopsia cutânea e pela aparência característica do fígado no exame ultrassonográfico. A patogênese subjacente das lesões cutâneas parece envolver deficiências de aminoácidos. Baixas concentrações séricas de aminoácidos foram observadas em todos os cães acometidos examinados.[66,67,70] Deficiências de zinco e ácidos graxos também são incriminadas e, em seres humanos, deficiências múltiplas foram identificadas, inclusive de vitaminas do complexo B. Sugere-se que as deficiências ocorram devido à atividade metabólica hepática exacerbada sob estímulo da maior atividade do glucagon ou a algum estímulo não identificado em cães com concentração normal desse hormônio.[71]

Manifestação clínica

A dermatite necrolítica superficial costuma acometer cães idosos de raças de pequeno porte, embora já tenha sido relatada em diversas raças, inclusive Golden Retriever e Border Collie. Em um estudo, constatou-se que 75% dos animais afetados eram machos, com ambas idades médias e medianas de 10 anos, e variação de 5 a 15 anos.[70] De modo geral, os cães afetados são levados à consulta em decorrência das lesões cutâneas: as típicas são hiperqueratóticas, eritematosas e crostosas, particularmente em extremidades (regiões de coxins, nariz, periorbital e perianal), ao redor da genitália, e, quase sempre, em áreas de pontos de pressão. Com frequência, as lesões desenvolvem fissuras, são infectadas secundariamente por bactérias dolorosas. Cães podem também apresentar sintomas de diabetes melito, que ocorre entre 25 e 40% dos casos, embora geralmente ocorra em um estágio posterior da doença. Em seres humanos, sugere-se que o diabetes melito se desenvolva devido à acentuada resistência à insulina causada pela alta concentração circulante de glucagon. Em cães com concentração normal de glucagon, a causa do diabetes melito é incerta. O atendimento clínico por conta de sintomas relacionados com a hepatopatia é incomum. Em casos acompanhados de glucagonoma, os cães podem também ser atendidos com sinais clínicos de neoplasia metastática.

Cães com dermatite necrolítica superficial, associada ao tratamento com fenobarbital, também são idosos, com idade mediana de 10 anos. Em um estudo, verificou-se que os cães vinham recebendo fenobarbital por um período médio de 6 anos antes do desenvolvimento das lesões.[69]

Diagnóstico

O diagnóstico é definido com base nos resultados de exames de amostras obtidas por biopsia cutânea, pela exclusão de outras causas e pela aparência típica do fígado em exames de imagem e na avaliação histológica. Amostras de biopsia cutânea indicam hiperqueratose paraqueratótica típica, com edema inter e intracelular, o que resulta em uma clássica aparência "vermelha, branca e azul" nos cortes de pele corados com hematoxilina e eosina. O único diagnóstico diferencial para essa enfermidade é a dermatose responsiva ao zinco, que pode ser excluída com base na raça e no histórico dietético (ver Capítulos 10 e 186).

No perfil bioquímico sérico, é comum notar elevações nas atividades de fosfatase alcalina e alanina aminotransferase, e cerca de metade dos casos relatados refere hipoalbuminemia, sugestiva de balanço negativo de nitrogênio. Hiperglicemia e glicosúria são constatadas naqueles casos acompanhados de diabetes melito.

A ultrassonografia hepática mostra uma aparência semelhante a queijo suíço, muito característica, com nódulos hipoecoicos de tamanhos variados circundados por bordas hiperecoicas,[72] o que, à histologia, corresponde a áreas nodulares de hepatócitos normais envolvidos por zonas de parênquima colapsado com hepatócitos vacuolizados. No caso de glucagonoma ou outro tumor pancreático, é possível visualizar a neoplasia primária e as metástases no exame ultrassonográfico, mas, para identificar o tipo de tumor, é necessário o exame histológico de amostras submetidas à coloração imuno-histoquímica.

Tratamento

Na maioria dos cães, o prognóstico de dermatite necrolítica superficial é ruim, com relatos frequentes de morte ou eutanásia dentro de 6 meses após o diagnóstico. A cura é muito incomum; há um relato de resolução das lesões cutâneas após remoção completa do tumor pancreático. Outro caso de glucagonoma metastático foi controlado por 6 semanas com injeções subcutâneas de octreotida, embora o cão tenha sido então submetido à eutanásia em razão dos sintomas relativos ao tumor.[65] Ainda não se sabe se a descontinuação da terapia com fenobarbital e a substituição por um anticonvulsivante alternativo resolveriam a dermatite necrolítica superficial naqueles casos associados ao uso de fenobarbital.

Na maioria dos casos nos quais não foi identificada a causa primária faz-se tratamento de suporte. O procedimento mais importante é o suprimento amplo de aminoácidos, pois a doença está associada à deficiência desses elementos. Dietas hepáticas exclusivas, portanto, não são indicadas, já que possuem teor restrito de proteínas. O ideal é fornecer uma dieta de alta qualidade, de alta digestibilidade e com alto teor de proteínas, como um alimento formulado para doença gastrintestinal ou para o período de convalescência. A suplementação extra com zinco e ácidos graxos essenciais também costuma ser recomendada. Alguns autores relatam administração parenteral semanal de aminoácidos, embora existam muito poucos casos tratados para fornecer evidências da eficácia dessa abordagem. O fornecimento de gemas de ovos demonstrou ser benéfico a seres humanos e em um cão alimentado com uma gema de ovo por dia juntamente com dieta de suporte hepático, ácidos graxos essenciais e colchicina. As lesões cutâneas cessaram e o cão estava bem 22 meses após o atendimento clínico.[73]

O tratamento de suporte das lesões cutâneas deve incluir antibióticos apropriados para as infecções secundárias, xampu e analgesia. Se possível, evite o uso de corticosteroides, em razão do risco de precipitação de diabetes melito.

Dermatite necrolítica superficial em gatos

A dermatite necrolítica superficial em gatos é muito menos comumente relatada em gatos do que em cães. Dos 5 casos relatados, 3 pacientes apresentavam tumores pancreáticos, sugerindo um mecanismo fisiopatológico semelhante àquele mencionado para seres humanos.[74,75] Os sinais clínicos e o diagnóstico são semelhantes aos verificados em cães.

HEPATOPATIAS CAUSADAS POR ARMAZENAMENTO ANORMAL OU NORMAL EXCESSIVO DE METAL OU METABÓLITO

Cobre e o fígado

O acúmulo excessivo de cobre no fígado é uma importante causa de hepatite crônica em cães[76-79] e, em menor grau, em gatos.[80,81] Essa anormalidade é descrita nos Capítulos 281 e 282.

Sobrecarga de ferro: hemocromatose

A sobrecarga de ferro no fígado, ou hemocromatose, também pode ser primária ou secundária. Como o ferro não é excretado na bile, caso haja aumento da absorção intestinal, excreção anormal ou aumento do armazenamento hepático desse mineral secundário à hemólise, haverá a ocorrência de doenças secundárias.

A hemocromatose primária é relativamente comum em seres humanos; é uma condição hereditária autossômica recessiva. Mais de 90% dos casos no norte da Europa se devem a uma mutação, a qual pode ser rastreada em ancestrais célticos. O ferro se acumula na região periporta, ocasionando fibrose e lesões hepáticas. Isso contrasta com relatos em cães e gatos, nos quais a sobrecarga de ferro é mais comumente relatada no fígado, mas é sempre secundária e não parece resultar em lesão, a menos que o aumento de ferro seja acentuado ou acompanhado de outros metais. Em um estudo, relata-se que o incremento de ferro no fígado de cães somente resultou em lesões quando combinado ao aumento no conteúdo de cobre.[78] É possível induzir, na prática, hemocromatose clinicamente relevante em cães, por meio de sobrecarga marcante de ferro na dieta;[82] lesões hepáticas também foram relatadas em cães com alta concentração hepática de ferro, associada à anemia hemolítica causada por deficiência da enzima piruvato quinase[83] e repetidas transfusões sanguíneas terapêuticas.[84] Em todos esses casos, as lesões hepáticas foram semelhantes àquelas observadas em seres humanos com hemocromatose, com sobrecarga de hemossiderina em macrófagos e células de Kupffer, degeneração hepatocelular e fibrose periporta, que progride para fibrose e cirrose. Portanto, não há dúvida de que o excesso de ferro é prejudicial ao fígado. Entretanto, isso é raro em cães e gatos. Relatos anedóticos de hemocromatose em ninhadas de cães da raça Yorkshire Terrier, no Reino Unido e nos EUA, não foram confirmados na forma de publicações.

DEFICIÊNCIA DE ALFA₁-ANTITRIPSINA

A deficiência de alfa$_1$-antitripsina foi sugerida como causa de doença hepática em cães na Suécia, particularmente naqueles da raça Cocker Spaniel, em 1994.[85] Entretanto, não há outros relatos na literatura veterinária desde 1982 e os estudos originais descreveram uma síndrome muito diferente daquela causada pela deficiência de alfa$_1$-antitripsina em seres humanos, o que faz com que a contribuição potencial da deficiência de alfa$_1$-antitripsina para a ocorrência de hepatopatias em cães permaneça sem comprovação.

A alfa$_1$-antitripsina é uma elastase neutrofílica sintetizada no fígado. A deficiência de alfa$_1$-antitripsina causa uma doença comum em seres humanos, resultando em hepatopatias em alguns pacientes acometidos, sendo o enfisema o sinal clínico predominante, como resultado da atividade descontrolada da elastase neutrofílica nas paredes alveolares; somente um pequeno número de indivíduos manifesta doença hepática. De modo geral, as pessoas acometidas apresentam sintomas durante a infância, de forma semelhante à doença de armazenamento lisossomal, com hepatite por células gigantes e grânulos resistentes à diástase PAS-positivos nos hepatócitos.

Em cães, foram identificadas três formas de alfa$_1$-antitripsina por meio de foco isoelétrico, denominadas rápida, intermediária e lenta.[85] A forma intermediária foi mais comum em cães da raça Cocker spaniel com hepatite crônica, embora, em outro estudo, não tenha sido identificada em todos com essa doneça.[85] Alguns cães também apresentavam inclusões globulares no retículo endoplasmático. Entretanto, na maioria dos cães a concentração sérica de alfa$_1$-antitripsina estava normal ou aumentada. Em cães, é possível mensurar as concentrações de alfa$_1$-antitripsina no soro e nas fezes,[86] mas a deficiência no soro é extremamente rara nessa espécie. O teste fecal é muito mais frequentemente utilizado como teste para enteropatia com perda de proteína.

A mensuração de alfa$_1$-antitripsina foi validada para gatos, e a alfa$_1$-antitripsina fecal parece estar aumentada em casos de enteropatia com perda de proteína nessa espécie.[87] Não há relato de deficiência de alfa$_1$-antitripsina no soro, tampouco de hepatopatia associada a essa deficiência, em gatos.

AMILOIDOSE

Amiloide é uma proteína complexa que pode existir em duas formas: a forma solúvel "normal" e a forma de fibrilas autoagregadas "anormal", com folhetos betapregueados. É o acúmulo da forma agregada que causa a doença. A amiloidose pode ser sistêmica ou local, bem como familiar ou adquirida (esporádica). Existem diversas proteínas amiloides associadas a diferentes doenças. Algumas são encontradas em órgãos únicos, como a forma relatada em ilhotas pancreáticas de humanos e felinos, enquanto outras são mais generalizadas. A forma generalizada mais comum relatada em pequenos animais é a amiloide A sérica (AAS), que em geral é secundária à doença inflamatória. A AAS é uma proteína de fase aguda sintetizada nos hepatócitos, sendo sua transcrição regulada por citocinas. Juntamente com a proteína C reativa, é a proteína de fase aguda produzida em maior quantidade em caso de inflamação. É necessário que ocorra aumento de AAS para o desenvolvimento de amiloidose; contudo, nem todos os indivíduos com aumento de AAS desenvolverão a doença: a razão pela qual alguns animais desenvolvem amiloidose e outros não é pouco compreendida, mas provavelmente envolve uma interação de predisposição genética e fatores ambientais desencadeantes.

A amiloidose causada pela amiloide AL, que é uma cadeia leve de imunoglobulina G monoclonal, é raramente relatada em pequenos animais, embora tenha sido descrita em associação à doença traqueal em cães e ao plasmocitoma extramedular, tanto em cães como em gatos. Nesse tipo de amiloidose, o envolvimento hepático parece não ser importante.

Amiloidose hepática felina

Introdução e resenha

O tropismo tecidual da AAS varia entre cães e gatos, assim como entre indivíduos e raças. A amiloidose hepática, na qual o fígado é o principal local de importância clínica, é descrita mais comumente em gatos. Nessa espécie, a amiloidose é mais comumente familiar e sistêmica (associada à AAS), embora possa ser esporádica. Em gatos Abissínios, essa anormalidade costuma se manifestar como doença renal crônica, com maior envolvimento da medula renal do que do glomérulo (ver Capítulo 324). Em gatos Abissínios, quase sempre há o envolvimento do fígado, o que não costuma ser a causa dos sinais clínicos ou da morte. Entretanto, gatos Siameses com amiloidose apresentam, com frequência, envolvimento hepático; na literatura veterinária, a maioria predominante refere-se a gatos dessa raça. A amiloidose hepática também foi relatada em gatos Domésticos de Pelo Curto (DPC), orientais de pelo curto e em um gato Devon Rex.[88-91] Em geral, os casos são observados em adultos jovens. Estudos da estrutura e dos genes que codificam a AAS de gatos mostraram que tanto os gatos Siameses quanto os Abissínios produzem uma variação muito limitada de tipos de AAS, quando comparados aos gatos DPC. Foram identificadas moléculas distintas de AAS em gatos Abissínios e Siameses, mas ainda não se sabe se essas diferenças são importantes para os diferentes tropismos teciduais nas diferentes raças.[90,92]

Manifestação clínica

Gatos com amiloidose hepática mais comumente são levados à consulta por conta de hemorragia intra-abdominal aguda por ruptura do fígado muito friável, o que causa anemia e hipotensão que podem ser fatais. Casos não fatais são submetidos à autotransfusão e se recuperam lentamente, mas podem apresentar recidivas.[91] Os gatos também podem apresentar icterícia e hepatomegalia como achados clínicos principais. Ao exame físico, é comum notar hepatomegalia, também devendo almejar a identificação de qualquer doença inflamatória concomitante, como gengivite crônica ou doença do trato respiratório superior, que podem predispor à produção de AAS.

Diagnóstico

O diagnóstico definitivo se baseia em achados histológicos em amostras obtidas por biopsia hepática, realizada somente após cuidadosa avaliação do tempo de coagulação. A amiloidose não é diagnosticada de forma confiável por AAF e citologia, embora esses procedimentos tenham sido relatados como diagnósticos em um caso da doença em cão.[93] Achados clinicopatológicos e ultrassonográficos propiciam informações auxiliares, mas não são diagnósticos. Gatos com amiloidose predominantemente hepática quase sempre apresentam elevação de atividades de enzimas hepáticas e da concentração de bilirrubina e anemia. Observam-se aumentos discretos a acentuados na atividade de alanina aminotransferase e de globulinas, mas as atividades de enzimas biliares raramente se elevam. Azotemia é observada em alguns, mas não em todos os gatos.[91] Os gatos podem ter doenças inflamatórias concomitantes, o que complica o cenário hematológico: relata-se que um gato com amiloidose hepática também apresentava peritonite infecciosa felina (PIF) como comorbidade.[91] À ultrassonografia, mostra-se hepatomegalia com trato biliar normal e aumento difuso da ecogenicidade hepática. PIF, linfoma e lipidose hepática são possibilidades que devem ser descartadas.

Tratamento

Até o momento não há tratamento efetivo para amiloidose hepática felina. A terapia de suporte e o controle da doença inflamatória sistêmica concomitante é o procedimento-padrão atual para os gatos acometidos. A colchicina é utilizada em cães da raça Shar-pei e em seres humanos com febre familiar do Mediterrâneo,

SEÇÃO 19 • Doenças Hepatobiliares

mas não há relato de seu uso em gatos; provavelmente a sua toxicidade é um fator limitante nessa espécie. Tratamentos que bloqueiam a interleucina beta-1 estão sendo testados em seres humanos, mas ainda não foram relatados em pequenos animais.

Amiloidose canina

Os cães, assim como os gatos, sofrem mais os efeitos renais da amiloide A sérica. Eles são mais comumente levados à consulta com nefropatia com perda de proteína, como resultado de doença predominantemente glomerular (ver Capítulo 325). Há dois principais grupos de amiloidose canina: a forma observada em diversas raças de cães, relativamente comum e que acomete, de modo predominante, animais idosos e raramente afeta outros órgãos além dos rins; e a doença multissistêmica diagnosticada em cães da raça Shar-pei chineses, que pode afetar o fígado.[94]

A doença em cães Shar-pei chineses causa episódios recorrentes de febre e edema articular, semelhante à febre do Mediterrâneo em seres humanos (ver Capítulo 203). O envolvimento hepático primário não é comum, mas foi relatado em quatro cães, nos quais era a causa predominante dos sinais clíncos:[93,95,96] três fêmeas e um macho, todos castrados. Eles foram levados à consulta por apresentarem anorexia e letargia, bem como anormalidades no perfil bioquímico sérico sugestivas de doença colestática. Um deles apresentou ruptura de fígado espontânea. Todos os casos foram diagnosticados por meio de biopsia hepática, embora o diagnóstico de amiloidose hepática por AAF e

citologia também tenha sido relatado em um cão Shar-pei.[93] Os cães acometidos por essa condição são tratados com colchicina (ver Capítulo 281).

DOENÇAS DO ARMAZENAMENTO LISOSSOMAL E O FÍGADO

Um grande número de doenças do armazenamento lisossomal relatadas em cães[1] (e em seres humanos) resulta em vacúolos nos hepatócitos e, às vezes, em hepatomegalia. Entretanto, os sinais clínicos predominantes em geral não são hepáticos, mas sim neurológicos e esqueléticos (ver Capítulo 260). A exceção é a doença do armazenamento de lipídios (doença do armazenamento de ésteres de colesterol), relatada em um pequeno grupo familiar de cães da raça Fox Terrier, na Alemanha, e na qual o sinal clínico predominante era hepatosplenomegalia devido ao acúmulo de lipídios e de cristais de colesterol no fígado e no baço.[97] O prognóstico em cães acometidos é incerto, mas foi considerada uma doença benigna em seres humanos.

REFERÊNCIAS BIBLIOGRÁFICAS

As referências bibliográficas deste capítulo se encontram online no Ambiente de Aprendizagem.

CAPÍTULO 286

Doenças Hepatotóxicas

Lauren A. Trepanier

INTRODUÇÃO

O fígado é um alvo comum de intoxicação por xenobióticos. É o local de biotransformação de primeira passagem de vários compostos absorvidos por via oral, alguns dos quais podem gerar metabólitos reativos. São reconhecidas duas principais categorias de hepatotoxicidade induzida por fármacos.

A primeira é citotóxica, devido à toxicose hepática do composto original ou de um metabólito gerado; em geral, esse mecanismo leva a um padrão hepatocelular de lesão hepática devido à necrose de hepatócitos. O segundo mecanismo é a colestase, que pode ocorrer quando compostos inibem ou diminuem a função de bombas transportadoras das membranas sinusoidais ou canaliculares, interferindo, assim, no efluxo de sais biliares e na função dos hepatócitos. Um padrão colestático pode também resultar de dano mitocondrial, levando à esteatose, como observado na doença hepática alcoólica em seres humanos.[1] Em seres humanos, esses padrões são definidos utilizando-se um valor "R" baseado nas atividades séricas de alanina aminotransferase (ALT) e fosfatase alcalina (ALP), em que R = (ALT/limite superior de normalidade)/(ALP/limite superior de normalidade). Valor de R > 5 indica lesão hepatocelular, R < 2, lesão colestática e R de 2 a 5 representa um padrão misto.[2]

A hepatotoxicidade também pode ser classificada como dose-dependente ou idiossincrática, embora possa haver sobreposição entre as duas. Na hepatotoxicidade dose-dependente, ou intrínseca, a toxicidade aumenta com a elevação da dose em uma ou mais espécies, com o acometimento de praticamente todos os membros de uma população ou espécie em caso de

dose suficientemente alta. A hepatotoxicidade dose-dependente pode ser causada pelo composto original ou por um metabólito gerado seguramente na espécie tratada (Figura 286.1). Essas reações são relativamente previsíveis e o monitoramento terapêutico do fármaco pode ser útil para prevenção. É preciso reduzir a dose, mas, em geral, não há necessidade de descontinuação permanente do fármaco (Boxe 286.1).

Boxe 286.1 Fármacos e compostos químicos comumente associados à hepatotoxicidade dose-dependente em cães (C) ou gatos (G)

Paracetamol (C, G)

Aflatoxina (C, G)

Cogumelos *Amanita* (C, G)

Amiodarona (C)

Azatioprina (C)

Antifúngicos azóis (C, G)

Lomustina (C)

Cicadáceas (sagu-de-jardim) (C)[92]

Glipizida (G)[93]

Fenazopiridina (predomínio de rabdomiólise)[94]

Fenobarbital (C)

Fenitoína (C)[95]

Primidona (C)[95]

Xilitol (C)

A hepatotoxicidade idiossincrática é mais difícil de prever, já que as reações ocorrem somente em pequena proporção dos pacientes expostos (Boxe 286.2). A intoxicação não se agrava com o aumento da dose na população geral (portanto, elas não são consideradas "dose-dependentes"), mas a toxicidade pode aumentar com a elevação da dose em indivíduos suscetíveis. A toxicidade idiossincrática é quase sempre causada por metabólitos reativos variavelmente gerados pelos indivíduos. Esses metabólitos reativos podem causar estresse oxidativo, dano mitocondrial ou formação de haptenos que desencadeiam uma resposta imunológica humoral ou mediada por linfócitos T (ou células T) (Figura 286.2). Embora as reações hepatotóxicas idiossincráticas sejam algumas vezes denominadas hipersensibilidades a fármacos, elas podem ou não envolver uma resposta imune adaptativa. A hepatotoxicidade idiossincrática costuma requerer a descontinuação do fármaco suspeito, e medicamentos relacionados estruturalmente podem causar reação semelhante. Ver também o Capítulo 169.

Boxe 286.2 Fármacos mais comumente associados à hepatotoxicidade idiossincrática em cães (C) ou gatos (G)

Carprofeno (C)
Diazepam (G)
Mitotano (C)[96]
Metimazol (G)
Sulfonamidas potencializadas (C)
Zonisamida (C)[97,98]

HEPATOTOXICIDADES INDUZIDAS POR FÁRMACOS DOSE-DEPENDENTES

Paracetamol

O paracetamol é uma clássica hepatotoxina dose-dependente em várias espécies. Em cães, este fármaco pode ser utilizado com segurança como antipirético e analgésico, na dose de 10 a 15 mg/kg/8 h VO, sem a toxicidade gastrintestinal dos fármacos anti-inflamatórios não esteroides (AINEs)-padrão. Entretanto, doses > 150 a 250 mg/kg causam necrose hepática centrolobular

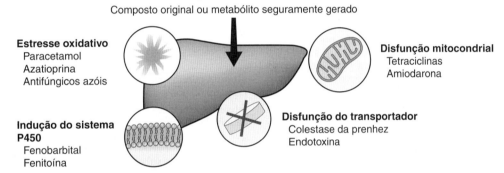

Figura 286.1 A hepatotoxicidade dose-dependente associada a fármacos costuma ser causada pelo medicamento original ou por um metabólito consistentemente gerado. Fármacos podem inibir ou reduzir a ação de bombas transportadoras e causar colestase funcional, como pode ocorrer com metabólitos de hormônios endógenos durante a prenhez. Vários fármacos levam à formação de metabólitos reativos causadores de estresse oxidativo; exemplos incluem paracetamol, azatioprina e antifúngicos azóis. Na intoxicação causada por esses compostos, a suplementação com antioxidante pode ser efetiva no tratamento ou na prevenção da hepatotoxicidade. Fármacos que interferem na função mitocondrial podem ocasionar esteatose pela inibição da betaoxidação de ácidos graxos ou levar a dano hepatocelular mais grave devido à anormalidade na respiração celular. Por fim, os fármacos que atuam como indutores do sistema P450, como o fenobarbital, podem atuar como mediadores da hepatotoxicidade por bioativação crônica de toxinas ambientais.

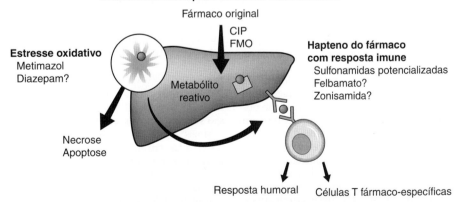

Figura 286.2 Embora a patogênese de diversas hepatotoxicidades idiossincráticas não esteja esclarecida, o mecanismo mais comumente demonstrado é a geração de metabólitos reativos, que leva ao estresse oxidativo e/ou à formação de haptenos. Os metabólitos reativos são tipicamente gerados localmente no fígado pelas vias citocromo P450 (CIP), flavina mono-oxigenase (FMO) ou outras. Esses metabólitos podem se ligar a importantes proteínas e causar anormalidades na função dos hepatócitos, ou gerar espécies reativas de oxigênio, que danificam a membrana dos hepatócitos. Produtos de adição de fármaco-proteína também podem ser processados e apresentados ao sistema imune em associação a moléculas do complexo principal de histocompatibilidade (MHC, *major histocompatibility complex*). Na presença de um sinal de "perigo", como o estresse oxidativo, a apresentação de peptídios ligados a fármacos pode levar à expansão clonal de células T fármaco-específicas e/ou à geração de anticorpos fármaco-específicos cujos alvos são proteínas dos hepatócitos.

aguda.[3] Em gatos, a toxicidade hematológica, caracterizada por metemoglobinemia e cianose, parece predominar sobre a toxicidade hepática direta.[4] Gatos são muito mais sensíveis à toxicidade por paracetamol devido à carência da expressão de UGT1A6, a enzima que propicia a glicuronidação do paracetamol,[5] e possivelmente também devido à menor expressão do transportador ABCG2, que atua na excreção do sulfato de paracetamol, em seres humanos.[6]

O paracetamol é bioativado em seu metabólito reativo, a NAPQI (N-acetil-p-benzoquinona imina), que é detoxificada pela conjugação com glutationa. Isso explica a razão do tratamento de dose excessiva ("superdosagem") com o protocolo terapêutico-padrão do precursor da glutationa, N-acetilcisteína (dose de ataque de 140 mg/kg IV, seguida de 7 doses de 70 mg/kg/6 h). Embora a N-acetilcisteína seja mais efetiva em seres humanos quando administrada dentro de 8 horas após a ingestão de paracetamol, esse antídoto ainda possui efeitos benéficos na sobrevida quando administrada muito mais tardiamente, no curso da intoxicação.[3]

A S-adenosil-L-metionina (SAMe) também pode ser utilizada na intoxicação de cães que podem tolerar o uso de medicamento oral; o protocolo utilizado bem-sucedido consiste na dose de ataque de 40 mg/kg VO, seguida de 20 mg/kg/24 h VO durante 7 dias.[7] A cimetidina é recomendada para inibir a oxidação do paracetamol em NAPQI; entretanto, esse fármaco não atua na geração de NAPQI *in vitro*,[8] e não é efetivo em seres humanos que receberam dose excessiva de paracetamol. Portanto, a cimetidina não é recomendada.[3] Para cães e gatos com metemoglobinemia concomitante à intoxicação por paracetamol, o ascorbato (vitamina C; 30 mg/kg SC ou IV, a cada 6 a 8 horas) pode ser efetivo para restabelecer a função da hemoglobina.[9] Entretanto, a eficácia do ascorbato em cães e gatos intoxicados por paracetamol jamais foi avaliada.

Fenobarbital

A hepatotoxicidade pelo fenobarbital parece depender de doses cumulativas, com possíveis fatores moduladores individuais. Os sintomas tipicamente surgem após 1 ano ou mais de tratamento com esse medicamento, estando a duração da administração associada ao grau de lesão histológica em cães epilépticos.[10] A manifestação clínica pode variar de elevação subclínica na concentração sérica de ácidos biliares até insuficiência hepática fulminante.[11] Os achados histológicos típicos em cães com sinais clínicos são fibrose portal em ponte, hiperplasia de ductos biliares e regeneração nodular. Não se constatou correlação entre doses maiores de fenobarbital ou concentração sérica do fármaco com anormalidade na concentração sérica de ácidos biliares em cães epilépticos; entretanto, o quadro clínico de alguns cães com hepatotoxicidade por fenobarbital pode melhorar após a redução da dose do fármaco.[11]

Um possível mecanismo da hepatotoxicidade por fenobarbital é a indução de enzimas do sistema citocromo P450, com bioativação secundária e hepatotoxicidade por outros fármacos, componentes da dieta ou toxinas ambientais.[10] Por exemplo, o fenobarbital aumenta a hepatotoxicidade do tetracloreto de carbono em cães,[12] do clorofórmio em ratos[13] e do paracetamol em hepatócitos de humanos.[14] Portanto, a hepatotoxicidade por fenobarbital pode ser modulada por exposições ambientais, em alguns cães. É interessante ressaltar que o fenobarbital não causa indução enzimática[15] ou hepatotoxicidade em gatos.

Na ocorrência de sintomas de hepatotoxicidade em cães durante o tratamento prolongado com fenobarbital, este deve ser descontinuado ou a dose diminuída, com adição de outro anticonvulsivante (ver Capítulos 35 e 260). Por exemplo, pode ser substituído pelo brometo de potássio (KBr), com dose de manutenção de 40 a 60 mg/kg/24 h via oral, e o fenobarbital pode ser então descontinuado em um período curto, de 1 a 3 semanas. Na maioria dos cães, é possível prever hepatotoxicidade clinicamente relevante por meio de mensurações seriadas da concentração sérica de ácidos biliares, da concentração de fenobarbital e do perfil da função hepática, idealmente a cada 6 meses. Deve-se evitar concentração sérica de fenobarbital > 40 mg/μℓ, já que isso pode ser um fator de risco para hepatotoxicidade.[11] Ademais, hiperbilirrubinemia, o surgimento de hipoalbuminemia ou a elevação da atividade sérica incompatível de ALT > ALP são clinicamente relevantes. Ademais, a constatação recente de sedação induzida por uma dose estável de fenobarbital pode indicar anormalidade na depuração hepática do fármaco, sendo uma indicação para a mensuração da concentração de ácidos biliares.

Antifúngicos azóis

Cetoconazol, itraconazol e fluconazol podem causar aumento da atividade sérica de ALT em cães, embora sinais clínicos, como icterícia, sejam incomuns.[16,17] Elevação discreta e clinicamente irrelevante na atividade de ALT também já foi relatada em gatos tratados com itraconazol e fluconazol.[18,19] Em cães com blastomicose, alta dose de itraconazol (10 mg/kg/dia VO) foi associada a maior risco de anormalidade na atividade de ALT do que a dose de 5 mg/kg/dia VO, sem diferença na eficácia terapêutica.[20] Ademais, relata-se correlação entre a elevação das atividades séricas de ALT e ALP e a concentração plasmática de itraconazol, o que sustenta a possibilidade de um mecanismo dose-dependente.

Em modelos experimentais com animais, a hepatotoxicidade do cetoconazol é atribuída a um metabólito oxidativo, o N-deacetil cetoconazol, que se liga de modo covalente a proteínas hepáticas e causa depleção de glutationa.[21,22] Em geral, o fluconazol parece ser menos hepatotóxico do que o cetoconazol ou o itraconazol, tanto em seres humanos como em modelos experimentais com animais.[23-25] Em cães com blastomicose, notamos elevação da atividade sérica de ALT em 26% dos animais tratados com itraconazol (aumento médio: 2,7 vezes) e em 17% daqueles com fluconazol (aumento médio: 1,5 vezes).[17] Embora não se tenha constatado diferença estatística, na rotina clínica temos observado aumento da atividade sérica de ALT durante o tratamento com itraconazol, que diminui após substituição pelo fluconazol, durante o tratamento de blastomicose em cães.

Hepatopatias subclínicas durante terapia com antifúngicos azóis são comuns o suficiente para justificar o monitoramento de rotina.[17,20] Se novos incrementos nas enzimas hepáticas forem notados (particularmente da ALT), indica-se uma redução da dose do antifúngico, precedida por um período de repouso, dependendo da gravidade. Quando a administração do fármaco é iniciada em dose baixa, deve-se repetir o monitoramento clínico e bioquímico sérico após 1 semana e fazer reavaliações subsequentes. Para cães que desenvolvem hepatotoxicidade pelo itraconazol, pode-se substitui-lo pelo fluconazol, com cuidadoso monitoramento de acompanhamento. Com base nos dados obtidos em modelos de hepatotoxicidade em roedores, também pode ser instituído tratamento concomitante com precursores da glutationa, como a SAMe, em cães que apresentam elevação das atividades de enzimas hepáticas causada por antifúngicos azóis.

Azatioprina

A azatioprina pode aumentar a atividade sérica de ALT e/ou ALP em cerca de 20% dos cães;[26] em geral, essas anormalidades são subclínicas, mas, em alguns cães, estão associadas a icterícia e sinais clínicos.[27] Anormalidades de enzimas hepáticas são observadas, em média, 14 dias (variação de 9 a 52 dias) após o início da administração de azatioprina, que é significativamente mais cedo do que a típica ocorrência de citopenias (em média, 53 dias).[26]

Em modelos animais, a lesão hepática causada pela azatioprina está relacionada com a geração de metabólitos oxidativos e a depleção de antioxidantes hepáticos,[28,29] e pode ser prevenida pelo tratamento experimental prévio com N-acetilcisteína.[30] Os metabólitos oxidativos da azatioprina são gerados pela xantina oxidase; de fato, tem-se utilizado o alopurinol, um inibidor da xantina oxidase, para prevenir a hepatotoxicidade induzida pela azatioprina em pacientes humanos.[28] Entretanto, esse procedimento requer monitoramento cuidadoso dos metabólitos da azatioprina, a fim de evitar a exacerbação da mielossupressão; ademais, não é recomendada aos cães.

Cães tratados com azatioprina devem ser monitorados de modo rotineiro em busca de aumento de atividades de enzimas hepáticas, especialmente nas primeiras 2 a 8 semanas de tratamento.[26] A administração concomitante de glicocorticoides pode dificultar a interpretação das atividades das enzimas hepáticas; entretanto, a elevação incompatível da atividade sérica de ALT em relação com a ALP ou até mesmo incrementos sutis na concentração sérica de bilirrubina são causas de preocupação. Em cães, os fatores de risco para hepatotoxicidade por azatioprina não são claros, mas parece que cães da raça Pastor-Alemão são mais sujeitos a essas enzimopatias.[26] Após a redução da dose de azatioprina, as atividades das enzimas hepáticas podem se estabilizar ou normalizar. Em cães, a suplementação com precursores da glutationa pode ser efetiva na prevenção ou reversão da hepatotoxicidade por azatioprina mas ainda precisa ser avaliada.

Amiodarona
A amiodarona causa hepatotoxicidade clinicamente relevante em aproximadamente 45% dos cães submetidos ao tratamento de fibrilação atrial refratária e arritmias ventriculares, depois de um período médio de 16 semanas após o início da terapia de manutenção.[31,32] Tipicamente, nota-se aumento predominante na atividade de ALT, com ou sem hiperbilirrubinemia. Em alguns cães, a hepatopatia pode ser acompanhada de neutropenia.[31] Essas anormalidades costumam regredir 1 a 3 meses após a descontinuação do fármaco.

Em modelos animais, a toxicidade foi atribuída a dois metabólitos oxidativos: a mono-N-desetilamiodarona (MDEA) e a di-N-desetilamiodarona (DDEA), os quais geram espécies reativas de oxigênio que desacoplam a fosforilação oxidativa e causam dano mitocondrial.[33] Em seres humanos, esses metabólitos são gerados pela enzima CYP3A4, podendo sua geração ser inibida in vitro pelo cetoconazol.[33]

Em razão da prevalência da hepatotoxicidade e da neutropenia, recomendam-se hemograma e perfil bioquímico sérico basais em todos os cães antes do início da terapia com amiodarona, com reavaliação das enzimas hepáticas após dose de ataque e mensalmente durante o tratamento.[32] A constatação de aumentos substanciais da atividade sérica de ALT é indica a necessidade de redução da dose ou descontinuação do fármaco.

Lomustina
A lomustina (CCNU) é um composto alquilante utilizado como agente quimioterápico único em cães com mastocitoma, linfoma, sarcoma histiocítico e outras neoplasias. Entretanto, a lomustina está associada a aumento importante na atividade sérica de ALT (> 5 vezes do valor basal) em aproximadamente 29% dos cães tratados.[34,35] A elevação da atividade enzimática pode ser súbita, sendo mais comum após 1 a 3 doses de lomustina, quando administrada em intervalos de 3 a 4 semanas. Cães também pode desenvolver hiperbilirrubinemia moderada. O risco de elevação de ALT é maior em cães da raça Boxer e naqueles mais jovens (≤ 5 anos de idade).[34]

Os sinais clínicos de hepatotoxicidade são constatados em uma população estimada em 6% dos cães tratados com lomustina; são mais comumente notados após, em média, 4 doses e estão associados a alta dose cumulativa (em média, 350 mg/m²).[36] A avaliação histopatológica do fígado mostra agregados portais de células de Kupffer preenchidas por hemossiderina, aumento dos núcleos de hepatócitos e vacuolização destes.[34,36]

O(s) mecanismo(s) envolvido(s) na hepatotoxicidade por lomustina não é(são) conhecido(s). Em pacientes humanos, a hepatotoxicidade não é um efeito colateral comum da lomustina; contudo, ratos tratados com lomustina manifestam sintomas de hepatotoxicidade; o padrão colestático e a ocorrência das lesões de canalículos biliares parecem ser diferentes daqueles observados em cães.[37]

A redução da dose ou descontinuação do fármaco (em caso de marcante elevação enzimática) ocasiona redução na atividade de ALT na maioria dos cães. Entretanto, a descontinuação da quimioterapia por lomustina não é aconselhável em cães que apresentam neoplasia. Alguns cães que, no início, apresentavam doença hepática avançada (ascite e desvios [shunts] adquiridos) foram submetidos à eutanásia; portanto, recomenda-se o monitoramento das enzimas hepáticas em todos os cães tratados com lomustina. Em um estudo aleatório controlado com placebo verificou-se que a combinação de SAMe e com silibina foi efetiva na redução da incidência e gravidade da hepatopatia causada por lomustina em cães com diversos tumores.[38] Portanto, esse suplemento deve ser utilizado como terapia adjuvante em todos os cães tratados com lomustina.

Tetraciclinas
Historicamente, a administração intravenosa de altas doses de tetraciclina é associada à esteatose microvesicular em pacientes humanos, sobretudo em mulheres grávidas.[39] O mecanismo parece envolver a inibição da betaoxidação de ácidos graxos nas mitocôndrias dos hepatócitos, assim como da secreção de lipoproteína hepática.[39,40] Embora a tetraciclina iniba a betaoxidação de ácidos graxos em hepatócitos de cães in vitro,[41] não existem evidências histológicas de esteatose após o uso de tetraciclina ou doxiciclina em cães.

Em um estudo retrospectivo com 386 cães tratados com doxiciclina (dose média de 16 mg/kg/dia), notou-se que 36 a 39% deles apresentaram aumento da atividade sérica de ALT ou de ALP para a faixa anormal durante o tratamento. As elevações nas atividades séricas foram de até 23 vezes para ALT e de até 16 vezes para ALP.[42] Entretanto, nenhum grupo-controle foi acompanhado, e as atividades das enzimas hepáticas foram mensuradas a critério do clínico, de tal forma que outras causas de aumento de enzimas não puderam ser descartadas. Em razão da utilização disseminada da doxiciclina e da ausência de relato de hepatopatia com sinais clínicos, esses achados são surpreendentes e necessitam de avaliação adicional.

HEPATOTOXICIDADES IDIOSSINCRÁTICAS INDUZIDAS POR FÁRMACOS

Sulfonamidas potencializadas
Sulfonamidas potencializadas são os antimicrobianos mais comumente associados à hepatotoxicidade idiossincrática em cães. Foram incriminadas as combinações trimetoprima-sulfadiazina, ormetoprima-sulfadimetoxina e sulfametoxazol-trimetoprima genérico. Em geral, os sinais clínicos são observados 5 a 30 dias após o início da administração de sulfonamidas, com período médio de 12 dias.[43] Em alguns cães, o padrão hepatocelular pode progredir ao longo de vários dias para um padrão colestático. Necrose hepática é a lesão histológica predominante. Os sintomas podem incluir, também, febre (55% dos casos), neutropenia transitória, trombocitopenia, anemia hemolítica, poliartropatia, proteinúria, ceratoconjuntivite seca, lesões cutâneas ou uveíte.[43] Cães da raça Doberman são predispostos à toxicidade idiossincrática por sulfonamidas, embora artropatia e glomerulonefropatia, e não hepatotoxicidade, sejam tipicamente relatadas nessa raça.[44,45]

Os antimicrobianos do grupo das sulfonamidas são oxidados e originam metabólitos nitrosos, que se ligam de forma covalente a proteínas e atuam como haptenos. Em seres humanos, a toxicidade idiossincrática por sulfonamidas é terminantemente imunomediada, com documentação de anticorpos antifármaco e células T específicas para o fármaco e seu metabólito. Se as sulfonamidas potencializadas precisarem ser prescritas, o cliente deve ser orientado a perceber qualquer sinal discreto de doença. A não descontinuação do uso de antimicrobianos do grupo das sulfonamidas no momento do desenvolvimento inicial de sintomas adversos pode levar à morte do paciente.

Embora antídotos específicos para a hipersensibilidade às sulfonamidas não tenham sido avaliados, este autor recomenda a suplementação com um precursor da glutationa (SAMe ou N-acetilcisteína, utilizando-se os mesmos protocolos empregados na intoxicação por paracetamol, descritos anteriormente) e ascorbato (30 mg/kg/8 h IV [dose empírica]), com base em nossos achados de que, tanto a glutationa quanto o ascorbato, podem reverter a formação de haptenos do metabólito nitroso para microssomos hepáticos de cães, in vitro (Lavergne & Trepanier, resultados não publicados). Glicocorticoides não são recomendados durante o estágio agudo da necrose hepática por conta do risco potencial de exacerbar a encefalopatia hepática ou a translocação de bactérias, mas, com base em nossa experiência, eles podem ser utilizados na condição subaguda, particularmente caso haja persistência de um padrão colestático após a descontinuação do fármaco e do tratamento de suporte.

Carprofeno

A potencial hepatotoxicidade do carprofeno é bem reconhecida entre os clínicos veterinários, com incidência estimada pelo fabricante de 1,4 casos para cada 10 mil cães tratados (0,05%). Os sinais clínicos de insuficiência hepática aguda são notados 5 a 30 dias após o início da administração; em média, 19 dias.[46,47] Os sinais clínicos foram até mesmo observados em um cão não tratado que ingeriu fezes de outro tratado com carprofeno, no ambiente doméstico.[48]

Em todos os cães relatados, verifica-se um padrão hepatocelular predominante ou um padrão misto.[46-48] É importante ressaltar que nenhum cão apresentava aumento da atividade de ALP na ausência de aumento concomitante clinicamente significativo de ALT. Necrose hepática em ponte é o achado histopatológico predominante. Embora, no relato inicial, houvesse maior número de cães da raça Labrador retriever predisposto,[46] é mais provável que esse predomínio se deva à maior preferência dessa raça pelos proprietários e seus riscos de osteoartrite, já que não foi possível reproduzir a síndrome em cães da raça Labrador sob condições controladas (Comunicação pessoal, Pfizer Animal Health).

Em razão da baixa incidência e do início súbito da hepatotoxicidade idiossincrática causada por carprofeno em cães, o monitoramento de rotina das enzimas hepáticas não é uma abordagem eficiente para prevenir a intoxicação clínica. É mais importante orientar os tutores no sentido de observar sinais sutis de doença durante a administração de AINEs, que incluem inapetência, êmese, diarreia, letargia ou urina de coloração escura. Ao notar os sinais clínicos, os cães devem ser prontamente avaliados. A constatação de atividade de ALT normal em face da doença clínica essencialmente descarta a possibilidade de hepatotoxicidade por carprofeno; se esta for diagnosticada, deve-se controlar a dor induzida pela inflamação com o uso de um AINE estruturalmente diferente, mas somente após recuperação total.

Metimazol

Cerca de 1 a 2% dos gatos com hipertireoidismo submetidos ao tratamento com metimazol, um medicamento antitireoidiano, manifestam evidências clínicas de hepatopatia com icterícia,[49] tipicamente no primeiro mês de tratamento. Essas alterações são distintas de incrementos "inocentes" das atividades séricas de ALT e ALP observadas em casos de hipertireoidismo não tratado. A hepatopatia pode ter um padrão predominantemente hepatocelular ou colestático, com ou sem hiperbilirrubinemia. Essas reações costumam ser reversíveis após descontinuação do fármaco, mas podem ser fatais se não detectadas de imediato.

Em modelos animais, a hepatotoxicidade por metimazol se manifesta como elevação da atividade sérica de ALT e necrose hepática centrolobular dose-dependente, na presença de depleção de glutationa.[50] A hepatotoxicidade é atribuída a um metabólito oxidativo, a N-metiltioureia, que é diretamente gerada pela flavina mono-oxigenase.[51] Essa via metabólica ainda precisa ser avaliada em gatos.

Gatos tratados com metimazol devem ser avaliados em busca de aumento das atividades séricas de ALT e ALP, caso os animais apresentem letargia ou anorexia. Caso os gatos desenvolvam sinais clínicos adversos, deve-se descartar a possibilidade de toxicidade idiossincrática (hepatopatia, discrasia sanguínea ou escoriação facial) por meio de exame físico, hemograma e perfil bioquímico sérico. Esses eventos adversos idiossincráticos requerem a descontinuação do metimazol, dado o risco de progressão para manifestações mais graves.[49] A administração transdérmica de metimazol não parece evitar a toxicidade idiossincrática, inclusive a hepatotoxicidade.[52] Dada a participação da depleção de glutationa na hepatotoxicidade causada por metimazol em modelos experimentais, a eficácia dos precursores da glutationa precisa ser avaliada no tratamento dessa reação adversa ao fármaco.

Diazepam

O diazepam representa uma clássica idiossincrasia em gatos, inicialmente reconhecida e relatada em meados dos anos 1990.[53-55] Relata-se que os gatos manifestaram sinais clínicos de anorexia e sedação evidente 5 ou mais dias após o início da administração, com progressão para icterícia e insuficiência hepática evidente. Os exames de sangue indicaram aumento marcante das atividades de ALT em todos os gatos. Em amostras obtidas por biopsia hepática, notou-se necrose hepática centrolobular evidente, com discreta a marcante hiperplasia de ductos biliares.[53] Hipoglicemia relativa foi um achado comum. Os gatos acometidos eram tipicamente saudáveis antes da administração oral de diazepam por conta de problemas comportamentais. A síndrome da hepatotoxicidade por diazepam em gatos foi relatada tanto após o uso do diazepam genérico quanto de marcas patenteadas,[53] mas não foi observada após administração parenteral de diazepam como medicação pré-anestésica.

Infelizmente, o mecanismo envolvido nessa reação adversa ao fármaco, potencialmente fatal, não foi pesquisado. Em ratos, doses diárias comparáveis de diazepam, por longo tempo, causaram alterações necróticas, mas sem a manifestação fulminante observada em gatos.[56] Síndrome clínica semelhante não foi relatada em seres humanos.

Desde então, em encontros veterinários on-line (Veterinary Information Network), surgiram relatos subsequentes de hepatotoxicidade por diazepam em gatos submetidos à administração oral desse fármaco para controle de convulsões ou espasmo uretral. Embora a toxicidade pareça ser relativamente rara, existem fármacos alternativos mais seguros para transtornos comportamentais, convulsões e espasmo uretral em gatos. Isso torna a administração oral de diazepam de longa duração uma primeira escolha inapropriada nessa espécie, particularmente sem uma discussão clara sobre os riscos e as alternativas com o tutor.

HEPATOTOXINAS PRESENTES NO DOMICÍLIO E NO AMBIENTE

Aflatoxinas

Aflatoxinas são produzidas por Aspergillus spp. e podem ser encontradas no milho, no amendoim ou na soja mofados; ração para animais de companhia contaminada; e sementes consumidas por pássaros selvagens.[57] Em vários mamíferos, inclusive cães e gatos, a aflatoxina B1 é uma hepatotoxina dose-dependente.[58] A aflatoxina B1 é bioativada por enzimas do citocromo P450 em metabólitos epóxidos eletrofílicos que levam à produção de adutores de proteínas e DNA e depleção de glutationa.[59] Recentemente foram relatados vários grandes surtos de hepatotoxicidade causados por aflatoxina presente em ração comercial para cães, com a morte de mais de uma centena deles.[57,60]

Os sinais clínicos da hepatotoxicidade causada por aflatoxina são típicos de insuficiência hepática aguda e pode ocorrer morte hiperaguda.[60,61] A sensibilidade da redução das concentrações séricas de proteína C, antitrombina e colesterol parece maior do que o aumento das atividades de enzimas hepáticas ou da concentração de bilirrubina no curso inicial da doença.[60] Como esperado, hiperbilirrubinemia, hipoalbuminemia e hipocolesterolemia são indicadores ruins de prognóstico. O achado histopatológico mais evidente é a vacuolização lipídica difusa em hepatócitos, em combinação com fibrose e hiperplasia de ductos biliares; em casos de exposição crônica, também pode ser observada cirrose.[60,62] É importante ressaltar que a necrose hepática maciça não é uma característica da aflatoxicose em cães.

Caso haja suspeita de hepatotoxicidade por aflatoxina em um paciente, deve-se obter um cuidadoso histórico sobre a dieta fornecida nas 8 semanas anteriores ao início dos sintomas, pois alguns cães manifestam sinais clínicos da doença somente após exposição subcrônica.[61] Os tutores podem relatar relutância do animal em consumir uma nova marca de ração para cães ou a ração de um novo pacote quando inicialmente introduzida.[63,64] Amostras de alimentos (diversas latas fechadas ou 1 kg de alimento seco) devem ser reservadas para análise de aflatoxina B1,[63] e amostras do conteúdo do vômito, de soro e de urina devem ser guardadas para análise do metabólito M1 da aflatoxina B1.[62] Além disso, a embalagem ou rótulo do produto e o número do lote devem ser documentados, e tanto o fabricante da ração quanto a Agência Nacional de Vigilância Sanitária (Anvisa) devem ser contatados. O prognóstico é reservado, e somente cerca de um terço dos cães acometidos sobrevive após tratamento intensivo da insuficiência hepática.[60,61]

Xilitol

O adoçante artificial xilitol é encontrado em gomas de mascar sem açúcar, rebuçados, guloseimas assadas, creme dental, *spray* nasal e até mesmo em suspensões de fármacos e fórmulas de nutrição parenteral total. Quando ingerido por cães em dose de 0,15 g/kg, ou mais, o xilitol causa intoxicação aguda, caracterizada por liberação de insulina e sinais clínicos de hipoglicemia dentro de 30 a 60 minutos (ver também Capítulo 152).[65] Em alguns cães, isso pode ser acompanhado de necrose hepática aguda 6 a 72 horas após a exposição, algumas vezes ocasionando coagulopatia de consumo e insuficiência hepática fulminante.[65,66] Entretanto, nem todos os cães que desenvolvem hepatopatia possuem evidências de hipoglicemia prévia. O mecanismo da hepatopatia causada por xilitol não é conhecido, mas pode ocorrer devido à interferência no metabolismo intermediário ou estresse oxidativo concomitante.[65] Em outras espécies, a ingestão de xilitol não causa hepatopatia, mas a administração intravenosa de altas doses leva à depleção hepática de adenosina trifosfato (ATP) em seres humanos;[67] ademais, foi associada à hiperbilirrubinemia (aparentemente sem aumento das atividades das transaminases), em pessoas.[68]

Em cães que sabidamente ingeriram xilitol deve ser induzida êmese (ver Capítulo 151), mas é contraindicada quando se constatam sinais de hipoglicemia. Carvão ativado não é contraindicado, mas pode não adsorver o xilitol de maneira efetiva.[69] Os cães devem ser monitorados ainda mais, em busca de sinais de dano hepatocelular por até 72 horas após a ingestão, com a provável indicação do tratamento precoce com um precursor da glutationa (SAMe ou N-acetilcisteína).[65,66]

Cogumelos *Amanita*

A cicuta-verde (*Amanita phalloides*) é encontrada em toda a América do Norte; nos EUA está concentrada nas florestas da costa oeste, de Los Angeles a Vancouver, e da costa leste, de Maryland ao Maine.[70] Esses fungos contêm amatoxinas, notavelmente alfa-amanitina, que são altamente tóxicas aos humanos e a outros mamíferos. As amatoxinas inibem a RNA-polimerase,[71,72] o que leva à diminuição da geração de RNA mensageiro (RNAm), interrupção da síntese proteica e necrose de células metabolicamente ativas, inclusive células das criptas intestinais, hepatócitos e células dos túbulos renais.[73,74]

Os cães podem ser expostos a *Amanita* spp. enquanto procuram alimentos em florestas. Os sinais clínicos de êmese, hematoquezia e dor abdominal ocorrem dentro de 6 a 24 horas após

a ingestão, acompanhados de séria hipoglicemia após 24 a 48 horas, causada pela liberação de insulina estimulada pela alfa-amantina.[75] Por fim, ocorre necrose hepática maciça e necrose tubular renal após 36 a 84 horas.[73] A ingestão de mais de um ou dois cogumelos pode ser fatal para um cão adulto.

A silibina, encontrada no cardo-mariano, inibe a captação de amatoxina pelos hepatócitos *in vitro*, mediada pelo transportador OATP1B3.[76,77] Notavelmente, relata-se que a silibina (50 mg/kg VO) evitou a morte de cães quando administrada 5 e 24 horas após a intoxicação experimental por *Amanita*.[78] Outros inibidores do OATP1B3 incluem, em ordem decrescente de potência, ciclosporina A, rifampicina, montelucaste, penicilina G e fosfato de prednisolona;[77] ademais, a penicilina G também protegeu contra toxicidade por alfa-amantina em modelos experimentais com roedores.[79]

O diagnóstico definitivo de aflatoxicose pode ser confirmado pela detecção de alfa-amantina na urina, no soro ou plasma e no rim ou fígado, embora fragmentos do cogumelo também possam ser encontrados no vômito ou no conteúdo gástrico.[73] Caso seja possível obter uma amostra do cogumelo suspeito, a página da web da North American Mycological Association pode fornecer os nomes de voluntários espalhados por todo o país que podem auxiliar na identificação do cogumelo. Qualquer quantidade de cogumelo selvagem ingerido por um cão deve ser considerada preocupante, e os clínicos devem fazer contato telefônico com órgão de controle de intoxicação animal de sua região em busca de orientações específicas.[80]

Algas verde-azuladas

Algas verde-azuladas, que, na verdade, não são algas verdadeiras, mas sim cianobactérias fotossintéticas, proliferam em águas mornas paradas e ricas em nutrientes. Os gêneros que produzem hepatotoxinas incluem *Microcystis aeruginosa* (encontradas em lagos de água doce, tanques e reservatórios) e *Nodularia spumigena* (encontrada em águas salobras e oceânicas). As cianotoxinas microcistina e nodularina inibem as enzimas serina/treonina fosfatases no fígado,[81] com subsequente hiperfosforilação e anormalidades de proteínas do citoesqueleto. Isso causa dissociação do hepatócito, necrose hepática e depleção da glutationa.[82,83]

Os cães podem ser expostos ao ingerir ou nadar em águas mornas paradas com "espuma" verde-azulada visível ou "eflorescência de alga", ou ao ingerir o "tapete" de espuma no solo.[84] Cães podem desenvolver sinais de doença aguda e insuficiência hepática dentro de horas após a ingestão. A exposição à nodularina também pode causar necrose tubular renal proximal e lesão renal anúrica,[85,86] cuja manifestação clínica pode se assemelhar à leptospirose aguda.

O diagnóstico pode ser confirmado por meio de exame citológico do conteúdo do vômito[84] e análise toxicológica da água, do vômito, das fezes ou das amostras do fígado, em busca de nodularina ou microcistina.[86-88] Embora a hepatotoxicidade possa ser rapidamente fatal, há relato de cães que sobreviveram após tratamento de suporte intensivo, incluindo precursores da glutationa (ver anteriormente).[89] Além disso, a colestiramina pode se ligar fortemente à cianotoxina no intestino, havendo um único relato de caso de resposta clínica e sobrevivência após medicação (170 mg de colestiramina/kg/24 h VO) de um cão com intoxicação comprovada por microcistina.[90]

Sagu-de-jardim

O sagu-de-jardim (ou palmeira-sagu; *Cycas revoluta, Cycas circinalis* e *Zamia floridana*) são plantas cicadófitas encontradas em regiões subtropicais. Nos EUA, as intoxicações são observadas predominantemente nos estados do sudeste, onde as sementes caem no solo no início da primavera.[91] As sementes são mais tóxicas, mas a ingestão de raízes e folhas também pode causar sinais clínicos.[92] O princípio tóxico, a cicasina, é bioativado em metilazoximetanol por bactérias intestinais; esse metabólito ocasiona toxicidade gastrintestinal e hepática.

Os sintomas gastrintestinais podem ser notados dentro de minutos a horas após a ingestão, enquanto os sinais bioquímicos de hiperbilirrubinemia e aumento das atividades de enzimas hepatocelulares e colestáticas podem não ocorrer antes de 24 a 48 horas.[92] Sintomas neurológicos, como ataxia, déficit proprioceptivo ou convulsões, são observados em 20 a 50% dos cães intoxicados por cicadófitas.[91,92] O exame histopatológico mostra lesões hepáticas que incluem hemorragia centrolobular e necrose, com colapso de estroma, em cães mais gravemente acometidos.[91]

As taxas de mortalidade podem chegar a 50%,[91,92] com a recomendação de monitoramento intensivo e de suporte. A administração de carvão ativado aumenta a sobrevida.[91]

REFERÊNCIAS BIBLIOGRÁFICAS

As referências bibliográficas deste capítulo se encontram online no Ambiente de Aprendizagem.

CAPÍTULO 287

Neoplasias Hepáticas

Nick Bexfield

INTRODUÇÃO

Prevalência

Tumores do fígado e da árvore biliar em cães e gatos podem ser primários ou metastáticos. Tumores primários são relativamente incomuns, representando 0,6 a 1,5% de todas as neoplasias em cães.[1-3] Tumores hepáticos primários representam cerca de 1 a 3% de todas as neoplasias em gatos, mas até cerca de 7% de todos os tumores não hematopoéticos.[4,5] Em cães, as neoplasias metastáticas são aproximadamente três vezes mais frequentes do que os tumores hepáticos primários e costumam ser oriundas mais comumente do baço, do trato gastrintestinal (GI) e do pâncreas.[3,6] Tumores primários são mais comuns em gatos, mas, em cães, geralmente são malignos.[1,3,5,7,8] Embora a incidência máxima de neoplasias hepatobiliares primárias ocorra aos 10 a 12 anos de idade em ambas as espécies, os gatos desenvolvem tumores hepáticos malignos em uma idade mais jovem do que tumores benignos.[3,6,8-11]

Tecidos de origem e morfologia tumorais primários

Existem quatro tipos teciduais gerais dos quais os tumores hepáticos primários são derivados: hepatocelular, ducto biliar, neuroendócrino e mesenquimal. Os tipos morfológicos de tumores hepáticos primários são maciços, nodulares e difusos.[1] Tumor "maciço" é definido como uma massa tecidual solitária grande confinada a um lobo hepático; tumores "nodulares" são multifocais e podem envolver múltiplos lobos; e tumor "difuso" consiste em nódulos multifocais ou coalescentes que afetam todos os lobos ou em substituição difusa do parênquima hepático.[4,12] O fígado também pode ser acometido por outras doenças neoplásicas, inclusive linfoma (ver Capítulo 344), mastocitose sistêmica (ver Capítulo 349) e histiocitose maligna (ver Capítulo 350).[5,12]

Cães

Os tumores hepáticos primários mais comuns em cães são adenoma e carcinoma hepatocelular. Adenoma de ductos biliares e carcinoma são observados com menos frequência.[1] Fibromas, fibrossarcomas, hemangiomas e hemangiossarcomas são neoplasias hepáticas primárias relativamente incomuns em cães. Em um estudo, faz-se a diferenciação de 106 neoplasias hepáticas primárias de cães, em grupos bem definidos, com base em colorações histopatológicas e imuno-histoquímicas, em busca de marcadores representativos de linhagens hepatocíticas e colangiocíticas (ducto biliar).[13] Os resultados mostraram que 77% eram tumores hepatocelulares, 9%, neoplasias de ductos biliares e 3%, tumores hepáticos neuroendócrinos.[13]

Gatos

Adenomas de ductos biliares são os tumores hepatobiliares primários mais comuns em gatos (> 50%).[8,10,14-16] Em um relato de 61 tumores hepáticos primários de gatos, classificados em grupos bem definidos, com base em avaliações histopatológicas e imuno-histoquímicas, constataram-se 41% de tumores de ductos biliares, 34% de neoplasias hepatocelulares e 13% de tumores hepáticos neuroendócrinos.[17] Nesse último estudo, todos os tumores de ductos biliares eram carcinomas, não sendo identificado nenhum adenoma de ductos biliares. Estudos adicionais que utilizem imuno-histoquímica podem propiciar melhor conhecimento dos tumores hepáticos primários de cães e gatos.

Hiperplasia nodular: um importante diagnóstico diferencial para qualquer tumor hepático

A hiperplasia hepática nodular é relativamente comum, sendo detectada em 15 a 60% dos cães idosos.[5] A hiperplasia nodular também ocorre em gatos idosos e pode resultar em nódulos únicos ou múltiplos; quase sempre é detectada como um achado acidental durante laparotomia ou no exame pós-morte.[17,18] Em geral, a hiperplasia nodular é difusa, com uma "aparência clássica" de neoplasia hepática. Assim, antes da condenação de um cão ou gato, deve-se realizar exame histológico.

PATOLOGIA

Tumores hepatocelulares

Carcinoma hepatocelular (CHC)

O CHC é o tumor hepático mais comum em cães, correspondendo a > 50% dos casos em alguns estudos. É o segundo tumor mais comum em gatos.[1,4,5,8,10,12-14] A idade média dos cães afetados é de 12 anos; > 80% dos cães possuem > 10 anos de idade.[1,2,19] Embora a maioria dos estudos não tenha conseguido identificar predisposição racial ou sexual, em um relato consta que 16% dos cães acometidos eram da raça Schnauzer Miniatura.[1,2,13,19] Morfologicamente, 53 a 83% dos CHCs são maciços, 16 a 25%, nodulares e até 19%, difusos.[1,12] Os lobos lateral e medial esquerdo e o lobo caudado estão envolvidos em até dois terços dos cães com CHC maciço.[1,2,19,20] Metástase é mais comum em cães com

CHC nodular ou difuso; locais comuns de metástase são os linfonodos regionais, o peritônio e os pulmões.[1,12,14] A taxa de metástases varia de 0 a 37%, em cães com CHC maciço e 93 a 100% em cães com CHC nodular ou difuso.[1,2,8,10,12,14,19,20]

Adenomas hepatocelulares (hepatomas)

Em cães, os hepatomas são, em geral, achados acidentais na necropsia e raramente causam sinais clínicos, a menos que rompam e causem hemorragia.[12] Em gatos, o adenoma hepatocelular ocorre com mais frequência do que o CHC.[14] Em cães e gatos, adenomas podem ser encontrados como massas abdominais claramente palpáveis, por vezes pedunculadas. Deve haver cuidado ao distinguir a doença benigna da doença metastática. Adenomas solitários podem se tornar bastante grandes e invadir outros órgãos. O hepatoblastoma é raro e somente relatado em um cão.[21]

Linhagens tumorais

Com base em colorações histopatológicas e imuno-histoquímicas em busca de marcadores representativos de linhagens hepatocíticas e colangiocíticas, os tumores hepatocelulares de cães podem ser classificados em três subgrupos, cada qual com características morfológicas e imuno-histoquímicas específicas.[13] De longe, o maior subgrupo foi composto por tumores hepatocelulares, com 0 a 5% de positividade para queratina 19 (K19), provavelmente oriunda de hepatócitos maduros, os quais foram bem diferenciados e não tinham evidência de metástase.[13] O segundo grupo consistia em tumores com > 5% de positividade para K19, os quais eram pouco diferenciados e havia metástases intra-hepáticas e/ou distantes. Estes apresentavam características de células progenitoras hepáticas (CPHs), sem diferenciação adicional de linhagens colangiocíticas ou hepatocelulares, e podem ser oriundos de CPHs ou da desdiferenciação de hepatócitos maduros. O terceiro grupo, pequeno, apresentou uma posição intermediária quanto à coloração para K19 e malignidade. Em estudo semelhante em gatos, o exame histopatológico e imuno-histoquímico classificou 21 de 61 tumores hepáticos primários como de origem hepatocelular, e estes foram subdivididos em adenomas (n = 18) e carcinomas (n = 3).[17] Todos os carcinomas hepatocelulares tiveram evidências de metástases intra-hepáticas e/ou distantes.[17]

Tumores de ductos biliares

Em cães e gatos, há dois tipos de tumores de ductos biliares: carcinoma e adenoma. Estudos prévios relataram que o carcinoma de ductos biliares, ou colangiocarcinoma, é o tumor hepático maligno não hematopoético mais comum em gatos e o segundo mais comum em cães (Figura 287.1).[1,8,10,12,14] Em estudo recente no qual tumores hepáticos primários de gatos foram classificados com base em colorações histopatológicas e imuno-histoquímicas em busca de marcadores representativos de linhagens hepatocíticas e colangiocíticas, os tumores de ductos biliares (100% dos quais eram malignos) foram os mais comuns.[17] Relatos prévios sugeriram que carcinomas de ductos biliares correspondem a 22 a 41% de todos os tumores hepáticos malignos, em cães.[1,6] Entretanto, em outro estudo constatou-se uma frequência relativamente baixa (9%) de tumores de ductos biliares em cães.[13] Nesse estudo, todos os carcinomas de ductos biliares testaram positivo para marcadores imuno-histoquímicos, sugerindo que eram oriundos de colangiócitos diferenciados produtores de mucina, normalmente presentes em ductos biliares maiores.[13]

Em cães, sugeriu-se predileção racial por Labrador Retriever[22] e predisposição sexual para fêmeas, para tumores de ductos biliares.[1,23,24] Não há predisposição racial ou sexual aparente para casos de carcinoma de ductos biliares em gatos, nos quais 37 a 46% são maciços, até 54%, nodulares e 17 a 54%, difusos.[1,12,22,24] Carcinomas de ductos biliares podem ser intra, extra-hepáticos ou localizados no interior da vesícula biliar. Localizações intra-hepáticas são mais comuns em cães, enquanto uma distribuição igual entre tumores intra e extra-hepáticos foi relatada em gatos.[1,14] Carcinoma de ductos biliares localizados na vesícula biliar é raro em cães e gatos; é um câncer agressivo, com taxa de metástases de até 88% em cães e 78% em gatos. A metástase se instala com mais frequência em linfonodos regionais e pulmões.[1,8,10,14,22,24] Em um estudo, constatou-se que todos os tumores de ductos biliares de gatos apresentavam crescimento infiltrativo ou invasão vascular, juntamente com metástases intra-hepáticas e/ou distantes. Três tumores foram associados à doença hepática cística congênita do tipo adulto.[17] Relatou-se que 67 a 80% dos gatos, apresentavam metástase intraperitoneal e carcinomatose.[8,10]

Os adenomas benignos dos ductos biliares, devido à sua aparência cística, também são denominados cistadenomas biliares ou hepatobiliares. Eles podem ser únicos ou múltiplos e, em geral, não causam sinais clínicos até que estejam grandes e comprimindo órgãos adjacentes.[15,16,25] Em gatos, eles corresponderam a mais de 50% de todos os tumores hepatobiliares primários.[5,8,10,14,15,25] Entretanto, em estudo recente utilizando colorações histopatológicas e imuno-histoquímicas em busca de marcadores representativos para linhagens hepatocíticas e colangiocíticas, verificou-se que nenhum dos 61 tumores hepáticos primários, em gatos, era adenoma.[17] Em outros relatos, gatos machos parecem ser predispostos, embora não tenha sido relatada nenhuma predisposição racial clara.[15,16] Em estudo semelhante utilizando histopatologia e imuno-histoquímica, nenhum adenoma biliar foi detectado em 106 cães com tumores hepáticos primários.[13]

Tumores neuroendócrinos

Tumores neuroendócrinos, também conhecidos como carcinoides hepáticos, surgem a partir de células neuroectodérmicas e são raramente relatados em cães e gatos.[1,10,12-14,26,27] Em um estudo, notou-se que a frequência de carcinomas neuroendócrinos em cães (3%) e gatos (13%) foi relativamente baixa.[13,17] Colorações imuno-histoquímicas utilizadas na identificação de tumores neuroendócrinos humanos são úteis para a determinação da origem celular.[13,17,26,27] Em geral, eles são intra-hepáticos, embora também tenham sido relatados tumores neuroendócrinos da vesícula biliar.[26,28-30] Eles tendem a ocorrer em uma idade mais jovem do que outros tumores hepatobiliares, em média, aos 7 anos de idade.[1,29] Tumores neuroendócrinos hepáticos primários são biologicamente agressivos e, em geral, não é possível sua ressecção cirúrgica devido à natureza difusa.[1,26,29] Locais frequentes de metástases incluem os linfonodos regionais, o peritônio e os pulmões; outros locais relatados são o coração, o baço, os rins, as glândulas adrenais e o pâncreas.[29]

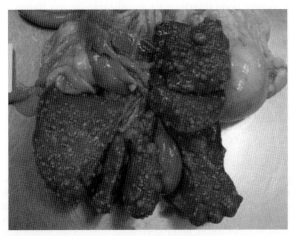

Figura 287.1 Aparência macroscópica de colangiocarcinoma hepático primário difuso em uma cadela da raça Cavalier King Charles Spaniel de 7 anos de idade. O animal foi atendido em estado de coma, com grave encefalopatia hepática. (*Esta figura se encontra reproduzida, em cores, no Encarte.*)

Tumores mesenquimais e outros

Em gatos e cães, os tumores primários de origem mesenquimal são raros.[1,8,10,12,14,31] Em dois estudos recentes de 106 tumores hepáticos primários em cães e 61 em gatos, não se detectou nenhum tumor mesenquimal,[13,17] com a identificação mais frequente de hemangiossarcoma, leiomiossarcoma e fibrossarcoma. Outros sarcomas relatados incluem rabdomiossarcoma, lipossarcoma, osteossarcoma, condrossarcoma e mesenquimoma maligno.[1,8,10,12,14,31-36] Hemangiossarcoma é o tumor mesenquimal hepático primário mais frequentemente relatado em gatos e o leiomiossarcoma o mais comum em cães. Os tipos morfológicos maciço e nodular foram relatados em 33 e 67% dos casos, respectivamente.[1,31] Machos parecem propensos a tumores mesenquimais, sem predisposição racial conhecida.[1] Tumores mesenquimais hepáticos são biologicamente agressivos, com metástases pulmonares e esplênicas relatadas em 86 a 100% dos cães.[1,31] Em geral, cães com sarcoma histiocítico disseminado possuem envolvimento hepático.[37-39] Mielolipoma é um tumor hepatobiliar benigno de gatos; pode ser único ou multifocal.[4,5,40,41] Histologicamente, esses tumores são compostos de tecido adiposo misturado a elementos hematopoéticos normais, quase sempre benignos.

SINAIS CLÍNICOS E ACHADOS DE EXAME FÍSICO

Os sinais clínicos de neoplasias hepáticas costumam ser vagos, inespecíficos e incluem letargia, inapetência, perda de peso, êmese, poliúria/polidipsia, pirexia e ascite.[5] De maneira incomum, sinais neurológicos podem ocorrer devido a hipoglicemia paraneoplásica, encefalopatia hepática ou metástase no sistema nervoso central,[1,26,27,42,43] sendo descrita, em um cão, fraqueza devido à *myasthenia gravis* associada ao CHC.[44] Icterícia é mais comum em cães com carcinoma de ductos biliares e tumor neuroendócrino difuso.[1,12,24] De maneira relativa, os sinais clínicos possuem pouco valor para diferenciação entre tumores hepáticos primários ou metastáticos e doenças hepáticas não neoplásicas. Aproximadamente 50% dos gatos e 25% dos cães com tumores hepatobiliares não manifestam sinais clínicos. Muitos são diagnosticados com tumor hepático somente quando da constatação da elevação nas atividades de enzimas hepáticas.[5] De modo geral, o exame físico não indica alteração, exceção feita à palpação de uma massa abdominal cranial ou hepatomegalia em até 75% dos cães e gatos com tumor hepático. A alopecia paraneoplásica foi relatada em um gato com CHC em estágio avançado.[45]

DIAGNÓSTICO

Patologia clínica

Hematologia e testes de coagulação

Os achados clinicopatológicos costumam ser inespecíficos. O exame hematológico pode indicar anemia não regenerativa discreta devido à doença crônica, sequestro ou hemólise, ou à carência de ferro.[5,46] Leucocitose com neutrofilia pode ser observada em casos de inflamação ou necrose associada a neoplasias.[1,2,19,20] Trombocitose é observada em aproximadamente 50% dos cães com CHC maciço.[20] Hemangiossarcomas hepáticos primários ou metastáticos podem resultar em anemia regenerativa e trombocitopenia.[5] Tempo de coagulação prolongado é uma consequência potencial de qualquer doença hepática, embora raramente tenha relevância clínica, a menos que a insuficiência hepática seja consequência de doença difusa. Cerca de 20% dos cães com CHC extenso ou avançado apresentam tempo de coagulação prolongado (ver Capítulos 196 e 197).[19,20] Animais com hemangiossarcoma hepático são sujeitos ao desenvolvimento de coagulação intravascular disseminada (CID).[47]

Bioquímica sérica

As atividades de enzimas hepáticas estão comumente aumentadas em cães e gatos com tumores hepatobiliares e indicam dano do epitélio hepatocelular ou biliar ou estase biliar.[5,48] Entretanto, o aumento da atividade de enzimas hepáticas não é específico de neoplasias hepáticas e não reflete o grau de envolvimento neoplásico do fígado. Comparados aos tumores hepáticos metastáticos, é mais provável que os tumores hepáticos primários resultem em hipoproteinemia, hipoglicemia e aumento das atividades séricas de fosfatase alcalina (ALP) e alanina aminotransferase (ALT), com menos probabilidade de causarem hiperbilirrubinemia.[3,48] Em cães, uma proporção aspartato aminotransferase:alanina aminotransferase (AST:ALT) inferior a 1 foi consistente com CHC ou carcinoma de ductos biliares, em um estudo, enquanto uma proporção maior esteja mais provavelmente associada a tumores neuroendócrinos ou mesenquimais.[1]

Testes de função hepática

Há relato de elevada concentração sérica de ácidos biliares, uma anormalidade inespecífica em 50 a 75% dos cães e 33% dos gatos com tumores hepáticos. Embora as neoplasias biliares sejam mais comuns em gatos, somente 33% deles apresentam icterícia. Outras alterações bioquímicas podem incluir hipercalcemia, hiperglobulinemia e hipoglicemia,[1] que pode ser observada como um efeito paraneoplásico em virtude do consumo de glicose pela grande massa tumoral ou como reflexo da produção de uma substância semelhante à insulina (ver Capítulo 352).[42,43] Hipoalbuminemia, mais comum em cães do que em gatos, pode refletir uma resposta de fase aguda negativa, catabolismo e baixo consumo nutricional, ou insuficiência hepática. O aumento da atividade sérica da lipase pancreática (LP) foi relatado em 6 cães com neoplasia pancreática ou hepática.[49] Há aumento da alfafetoproteína (AFP), uma glicoproteína produzida por hepatócitos fetais, neoplásicos ou em regeneração em cerca de 75% dos cães com CHC e em 55% com carcinoma de ductos biliares.[50,51] Em cães, a concentração sérica de AFP diminui após a remoção cirúrgica do CHC.[52] Entretanto, os cães possuem diversas fontes potenciais de AFP, tanto neoplásicas quanto não neoplásicas, limitando a sua utilidade como marcador diagnóstico ou terapêutico.[50,51] Nenhum estudo foi realizado para avaliar AFP em gatos com tumor hepático.

Exames de imagem

Radiologia

Os exames de imagem são valiosos para o diagnóstico, estadiamento e planejamento cirúrgico de animais com tumores hepatobiliares. Radiografias de abdome podem detectar um tumor abdominal cranial, com deslocamento caudal e lateral do estômago. Ascite pode interferir na visualização de um tumor.[5,19,23] Ocasionalmente, verifica-se mineralização distrófica de uma neoplasia ou da árvore biliar.[4] A importância da avaliação de radiografias de tórax é considerada crucial para excluir a possibilidade de doença metastática.

Ultrassonografia (US) abdominal

A US abdominal (ver Capítulo 88) tem diversas vantagens em relação às radiografias do abdome em animais com hepatopatia. Pode ser realizada para determinar a existência de uma neoplasia hepática e para identificá-la como tumor maciço, nodular ou difuso.[5,53-55] Na doença focal, a US pode ser utilizada para determinar o tamanho, a localização e a relação da neoplasia com as estruturas circundantes. Entretanto, para a detecção de lesões tumorais, a sensibilidade varia amplamente e depende da habilidade do operador, do equipamento e do tipo de tumor.[55,56] Tumores difusos costumam ser observados como nódulos ou massas parenquimatosas hipoecoicas, heterogêneas ou multifocais, sendo menos comum que as lesões tumorais apareçam difusamente hiperecoicas ou, às vezes, normais.[57] Um componente cístico pode ser observado em cistadenomas biliares ou hemangiossarcomas hepáticos. Entretanto, deve-se ter cuidado com massas hepáticas visualizada na US, já que estudo recente mostrou grande variação na aparência ultrassonográfica em todos os tipos de hepatopatias em cães. Não foi possível associar a aparência ultrassonográfica com o diagnóstico histológico.[57] As características ultrassonográficas mais prevalentes foram lesões hepáticas multifocais em 63% dos cães com hemangiossarcoma e em 43% com CHC. Lesões na forma de alvo, associadas à malignidade, foram identificadas em 67% dos casos.[57] A avaliação de lesões tumorais por Doppler (fluxo colorido) pode mostrar padrões de vascularização que ajudam a distinguir neoplasias de outras lesões benignas.[5,58] O índice de perfusão pelo Doppler pode ser útil na avaliação de linfonodos e do fígado em busca de metástases.[59] A US contrastada pode ajudar a diferenciar lesões benignas de malignas.[60-62]

Tomografia computadorizada (TC) ou ressonância magnética (RM)

Técnicas de obtenção de imagem avançadas podem ser úteis no diagnóstico e estadiamento de tumores hepáticos. Em cães, a RM de lesões focais hepáticas ou esplênicas teve alta sensibilidade (100%) e especificidade (90%) na diferenciação de neoplasias malignas de benignas. Os resultados da RM identificaram corretamente o CHC.[63] Em seres humanos, TC e RM são excelentes técnicas para detectar pequenas lesões hepáticas e determinar a relação entre os tumores hepáticos e as estruturas circundantes.[32] A RM fornece contraste superior de tecidos moles e provavelmente propicia melhor detecção, quantificação e localização da lesão, quando comparada à TC.

Aspiração com agulha fina (AAF) e biopsia

Resultados de exames de imagem e patologia clínica tipicamente não fornecem diagnóstico definitivo em pacientes com neoplasias hepáticas. A obtenção de amostras para citologia e/ou histologia pode ser vital para o fornecimento de informações adicionais e, em vários casos, do diagnóstico definitivo. As exceções podem ser os casos de tumores hepáticos solitários ou maciços, quando a ressecção cirúrgica é realizada sem o diagnóstico histológico pré-cirúrgico, pois a cirurgia pode, por si só, propiciar diagnóstico e tratamento. As amostras podem ser coletadas por meio de AAF ou biopsia com agulha guiada por US (ver Capítulo 89) ou por meio de laparoscopia (ver Capítulo 91) ou de laparotomia. Antes de qualquer biopsia, recomenda-se a obtenção do perfil de coagulação (ver Capítulo 196). Hemorragia discreta a moderada é uma complicação relativamente frequente (cerca de 5%).[53,55,56,64] O paciente deve ser submetido a anestesia geral ou sedação profunda para evitar que ele se movimente durante a biopsia com agulha.

A principal desvantagem do exame citológico de amostra obtida por AAF é sua limitada acurácia diagnóstica. Em um estudo, verificou-se que a concordância entre a citologia e a histopatologia foi de cerca de 30% em cães e de 50% em gatos.[65] No caso de lesões focais, a AAF pode ser útil e não necessitar biopsia. Em cães com lesões hepáticas focais, a sensibilidade do exame citológico em amostra obtida por AAF guiada por ultrassom, comparada ao exame histopatológico para a detecção de neoplasias, foi de 52%. A citologia teve o maior valor preditivo positivo quando a lesão era neoplásica (87%).[66] Em geral, a AAF para o diagnóstico de neoplasias hepáticas difusas é mais confiável.[67] Técnicas mais invasivas, como laparoscopia e laparotomia, também podem ser utilizadas para obtenção de amostra de tecido para o diagnóstico definitivo ou estadiamento. Além disso, deve-se realizar US de acompanhamento várias horas após a biopsia, a fim de verificar se há hemorragia no local em que ela foi realizada. É ideal que haja o monitoramento pós-cirúrgico cuidadoso por 24 horas.

TRATAMENTO

Carcinoma hepatocelular solitário

A ressecção cirúrgica, em geral, lobectomia, é recomendada para a maioria dos tumores hepáticos primários solitários que não ocasionaram metástase, especialmente em cães com CHC maciço.[20] Em casos raros, a cirurgia é uma opção para a maioria dos tumores hepatobiliares nodulares ou difusos, dada a impossibilidade da ressecção completa. Entretanto, às vezes, faz-se a ressecção local de nódulos primários ou metastáticos, quando se considera provável a melhora dos sinais clínicos, como a redução potencial de hemorragias com risco à vida do paciente. Deve-se realizar desvio da árvore biliar (anastomoses entericobiliares) no caso de lesões obstrutivas que envolvam as estruturas biliares extra-hepáticas, dada a possibilidade de resultados paliativos a longo prazo, vez que a oclusão da árvore biliar crônica resulta em cirrose. Exames de imagem avançados antes da ressecção cirúrgica dos tumores hepáticos podem avaliar com precisão a localização e extensão da neoplasia. A preparação pré-cirúrgica de pacientes para lobectomia hepática inclui a correção de hipovolemia, anormalidades eletrolíticas, anemia e déficit de fatores de coagulação. Em 42 cães com CHC maciço submetidos à lobectomia hepática, a taxa de mortalidade transcirúrgica foi de cerca de 5% e a taxa de complicações, de quase 30%.[20] As complicações após a ressecção cirúrgica incluem hemorragia, comprometimento vascular, redução da função hepática e hipoglicemia.[4,20,69]

Carcinoma hepatocelular nodular ou difuso

A radioterapia não tem destaque no o tratamento de tumores hepáticos, vez que, como o fígado é delicadamente sensível até mesmo quando se trata de baixa dose de radiação, há dificuldade para limitar a exposição tecidual.[5] Em pessoas, o CHC é considerado resistente à quimioterapia", com taxa de resposta < 20%.[32] De modo geral, a quimioterapia pós-cirúrgica adjuvante não propicia benefícios significativos em cães ou gatos com tumores hepáticos primários. Entretanto, a terapia exclusiva com gencitabina é utilizada em cães com CHC (4 maciços, 10 nodulares e 4 difusos). O tempo de sobrevida médio foi de 983 dias.[70] Em um estudo, notou-se que um quarto dos cães com CHC maciço tratados com mitoxantrona apresentaram resolução completa da lesão.[71] Nenhuma informação desse tipo está disponível sobre o uso de gencitabina ou mitoxantrona em gatos.

Embora o transplante hepático, a administração direcionada de quimioterápicos (quimioterapia intra-arterial), a quimioembolização transarterial e os protocolos imunoterapêuticos que utilizam antígenos específicos do tumor tenham sido utilizados em seres humanos com CHC, essas opções não foram exploradas de maneira ampla em animais.[72,73] A embolização às cegas e a quimioembolização foram consideradas de eficácia moderada no tratamento de um número limitado de cães com CHC não passível de ressecção (ver Capítulo 125).[74,75] A lobectomia hepática é recomendada aos gatos com adenoma único de ductos biliares ou lesões múltiplas confinadas a um ou dois lobos.[8,10,15,16,25] A lobectomia é também recomendada aos gatos e cães com carcinoma maciço de ductos biliares.

Carcinomas nodulares ou difusos de ductos biliares

Não há opção terapêutica efetiva conhecida para animais com essas neoplasias, vez que a ressecção cirúrgica não é possível e esses tumores não são sensíveis à radioterapia ou à quimioterapia.[5] Como a maioria dos tumores neuroendócrinos é nodular ou difusa, além de não possuir comportamento agressivo, em geral, eles não são amenizados com a ressecção cirúrgica, não havendo relatos sobre o uso de rádio ou quimioterapia para esse tipo de tumor em cães ou gatos.

Tumores mesenquimais maciços solitários e outros

Recomenda-se lobectomia em casos de tumores mesenquimais solitários e maciços, embora muitos já tenham ocasionado metástase no momento do diagnóstico.[1,31] A radioterapia costuma ter eficácia limitada em tumores mesenquimais hepáticos primários, existindo poucos relatos de uso de quimioterapia no tratamento dessas neoplasias hepáticas. Com base na resposta de tumores mesenquimais em outros locais à quimioterapia, é provável que tumores hepáticos mesenquimais primários respondam mal a esse procedimento. Entretanto, pode-se utilizar quimioterapia adjuvante em casos de hemangiossarcoma visceral.[76-78] Há poucos relatos sobre as opções terapêuticas para tumores hepáticos primários incomuns, embora a lobectomia hepática seja recomendada para gatos com mielolipoma hepático primário único.[5] Linfoma hepático (ver Capítulo 344), mastocitose sistêmica (ver Capítulo 349) e histiocitose maligna (ver Capítulo 350) podem ser tratados por quimioterapia sistêmica.[5]

PROGNÓSTICO

Cães

Fatores prognósticos para cães com CHC maciço incluem localização do tumor, atividades séricas de ALT e AST e proporções fosfatase alcalina (ALP):AST e ALT:AST.[20] O subtipo histopatológico do CHC e as características anaplásicas também podem influenciar na predição de metástases e no prognóstico. Não foi possível obter tempo de sobrevida médio de 42 cães com CHC maciço tratados por meio de lobectomia hepática, após mais de 1.460 dias de acompanhamento.[20] Em comparação, o tempo de sobrevida médio foi de somente 270 dias em cães tratados de forma conservadora, e estes tiveram probabilidade 15 vezes maior de morrer em decorrência de causas relacionadas com o tumor do que os cães tratados com cirurgia.[20] Embora a localização de um CHC maciço possa aumentar o risco cirúrgico, ela não interfere na recuperação de cães que sobrevivem à cirurgia. O prognóstico para cães com CHC maciço é bom, sendo relatada recidiva local do tumor em 0 a 13%, após lobectomia.[19,20] Entretanto, foi relatado que a doença metastática em outras regiões do fígado ou outros órgãos chegou a 37%.[19,20] Em contraste, já que a ressecção cirúrgica costuma não ser possível, o prognóstico para cães com CHC dos tipos nodular e difuso é ruim.

Gatos

Em gatos com adenoma de ductos biliares passível de ressecção cirúrgica, o prognóstico é excelente, sem relato de recidiva local ou progressão para malignidade.[8,15,25] Entretanto, a sobrevida de gatos e cães com carcinoma maciço de ductos biliares tratados por ressecção cirúrgica é curta: a maioria dos pacientes morre dentro de 6 meses em decorrência de recidiva local ou doença metastática.[5,8] O prognóstico para tumores neuroendócrinos hepáticos primários é ruim, já que são raramente passíveis de ressecção; ademais, no momento do diagnóstico geralmente já ocorreu metástase a linfonodos regionais, peritônio e pulmões.[1,29] Apesar de a ressecção cirúrgica ser uma opção para alguns tumores hepáticos mesenquimais primários, como no momento do diagnóstico já há metástase, o prognóstico, novamente, é ruim.[1,31] Entretanto, essa estratégica pode propiciar melhora nos efeitos de ocupação de espaço do tumor ou impedir que ocorra hemorragia com risco à vida do paciente. O prognóstico para gatos com mielolipoma hepático primário é excelente, com sobrevida longa e sem relato de recidiva local.[4,41]

REFERÊNCIAS BIBLIOGRÁFICAS

As referências bibliográficas deste capítulo se encontram online no Ambiente de Aprendizagem.

CAPÍTULO 288

Doenças da Vesícula Biliar e do Sistema Biliar Extra-hepático

Ale Aguirre

ANATOMIA E FISIOLOGIA

A vesícula biliar é um órgão em formato de lágrima situado na região cranioventral do abdome, entre os lobos hepáticos medial direito e quadrado. A vesícula biliar é um reservatório onde a bile é armazenada, modificada e, por fim, excretada. A bile é formada nos hepatócitos e ativamente secretada nos canalículos biliares. A partir deles, a bile flui para os ductos intralobulares e, por fim, aos ductos lobares, que originam os ductos hepáticos esquerdo e direito. O ducto cístico é um ramo do ducto hepático e segue em direção à vesícula biliar, sendo um importante ponto de referência para distinguir os ductos hepáticos contínuos do ducto biliar comum (Figura 288.1). Há uma variação substancial no número de ductos hepáticos e de suas anastomoses com os ductos hepáticos comum e cístico.[1-3] Em alguns gatos, constatou-se vesícula biliar bilobada dupla.[4]

A bile contém colesterol, lecitina, fosfolipídios e sais biliares, emulsifica a gordura e neutraliza o ácido presente no alimento parcialmente digerido. A contração da vesícula biliar libera a bile no ducto biliar comum, que adentra o duodeno através do esfíncter de Oddi. No cão, o ducto biliar comum se une ao ducto pancreático menor e ambos desembocam, separadamente, na

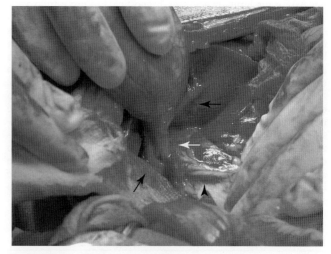

Figura 288.1 Fotografia da vesícula biliar e da árvore (ou trato) biliar. O ducto cístico (*seta branca*) é um importante ponto de referência porque une a vesícula biliar à árvore biliar e separa os ductos hepáticos mais proximais (*setas pretas*) do ducto biliar comum mais distal (*ponta de seta preta*).

papila duodenal principal.[5] No gato, o ducto biliar comum se funde com o ducto pancreático principal, antes de adentrar o duodeno.[1]

Veja o algoritmo para doenças da vesícula biliar e do sistema biliar extra-hepático (Figura 288.2).

COLELITÍASE E COLEDOCOLITÍASE

Etiologia

Colélitos, ou cálculos biliares, são uma das anormalidades mais comumente reconhecidas na vesícula biliar.[6,7] Cadelas idosas são predispostas a essa doença, sendo as raças de cães mais comumente acometidas Schnauzer e Poodle Miniaturas. No cão, foram relatados colélitos de colesterol, bilirrubina e mistos.[6] Cálculos com matriz de cálcio são raros devido à capacidade de a vesícula biliar de cães absorver cálcio livre na bile.[2,8] Em gatos, os colélitos contêm colesterol, derivados da bilirrubina e sais de cálcio.[9]

A origem dos colélitos é apenas parcialmente compreendida, sendo evidente a variação entre espécies. O colesterol é altamente hidrofóbico e necessita de transporte em micelas para permanecer suspenso na solução. Quando ocorre desequilíbrio entre sais biliares e colesterol, a bile se torna mais viscosa, levando à formação de cálculos biliares. Diversas anormalidades podem ocasionar colelitíase. Estas incluem discinesia da vesícula biliar, hipercolesterolemia, hipertrigliceridemia, hiperbilirrubinemia, doenças endócrinas e anormalidades de absorção e transporte de colesterol na vesícula biliar. Também há predisposição de raças e espécies.[10]

Os coledocólitos, cálculos no ducto biliar comum, podem ser primários ou secundários. Cálculos primários se formam diretamente no ducto biliar comum. Cálculos secundários são mais comuns e são formados na vesícula biliar, passando posteriormente para o ducto biliar comum.

Sinais clínicos

Em casos de colélitos, é possível uma série de sinais clínicos. Vários pequenos animais são assintomáticos. Em casos mais graves, pode ocorrer ruptura da vesícula biliar ou do ducto biliar, causando peritonite biliar.[11] Os sinais clínicos mais consistentes em que os animais são levados para atendimento são dor abdominal, êmese, anorexia e icterícia. Deve-se ter cuidado ao interpretar os sinais clínicos, já que diversas anormalidades abdominais, como pancreatite, gastrenterite, corpo estranho gastrintestinal e neoplasias, se manifestam de forma semelhante.[2,6,7]

Diagnóstico

Em casos de colelitíase, os achados laboratoriais variam amplamente, sendo o Leucograma de estresse o mais comum. Entretanto, leucocitose com neutrofilia e desvio à esquerda é típica em pacientes com ruptura biliar. Em pacientes com doença crônica, nota-se anemia não regenerativa discreta a moderada. Quase sempre constata-se aumento da concentração de bilirrubina total e das atividades de fosfatase alcalina (ALP) e gamaglutamil transferase (GGT). Bilirrubinúria costuma ser evidente e, com frequência, precede a icterícia clínica. Devido à curta meia-vida da ALP no gato (6 horas, comparada a 72 horas em cães), até mesmo incrementos discretos são significativos.[2,12] As elevações das atividades de alanina aminotransferase (ALT) e aspartato aminotransferase (AST), quando presentes, são menos marcantes do que as de ALP e GGT. Hipercolesterolemia discreta ocorre em casos de

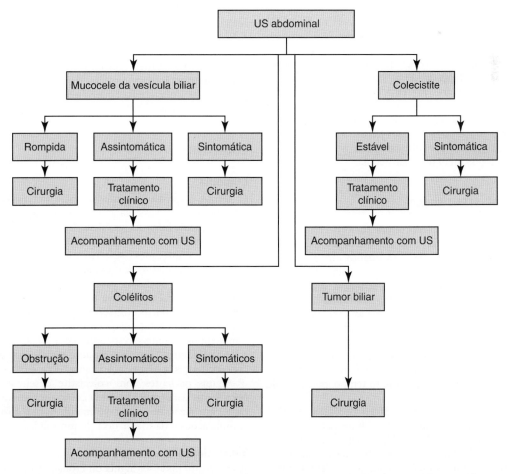

Figura 288.2 Algoritmo para doenças da vesícula biliar e do sistema biliar extra-hepático. *US*, ultrassonografia.

colestase e elevações intensas, observadas em casos de obstrução biliar. Em caso de sepse ou endotoxemia, pode ocorrer hipoalbuminemia e hipoglicemia.[2,6,7]

De modo geral, radiografias de abdome possuem limitado valor diagnóstico, já que a maioria dos cálculos contém teor de cálcio insuficiente para ser visualizada. Se o forem, eles são observados como estruturas radiopacas únicas ou múltiplas na região cranioventral do abdome, em projeções laterais, e na região cranial direita do abdome, em projeções ventrodorsais.[6]

A ultrassonografia é a modalidade diagnóstica de escolha. Um ultrassonografista experiente pode detectar cálculos biliares, espessamento da parede da vesícula biliar, dilatação da árvore biliar ou líquido pericolecístico.[6,13-15] A dilatação de ductos extra-hepáticos pode ser evidente dentro de 24 a 48 horas após obstrução total, enquanto a dilatação de ductos intra-hepáticos demora 5 a 7 dias para ocorrer.[13] Em gatos, um ducto biliar comum maior que 5 mm é indicativo de obstrução biliar extra-hepática.[14] Estudos ultrassonográficos para pesquisa de contração da vesícula biliar utilizando-se Lipofundin® e eritromicina vêm sendo realizados e podem auxiliar na detecção de obstrução biliar.[16-20]

Tratamento

A terapia de dissolução medicamentosa de colélitos que causam obstrução aguda raramente é efetiva. O tratamento consiste em cuidados de suporte até que o(s) cálculo(s) seja(m) excretado(s). A administração de soluções de uso intravenoso e de antibióticos e analgésicos é benéfica aos pacientes com obstrução biliar discreta a moderada. Em pacientes com doença obstrutiva grave, é fundamental o restabelecimento do fluxo no trato biliar, sendo obtido de forma mais efetiva por meio de cirurgia. Múltiplos procedimentos cirúrgicos já foram descritos. Em geral, colélitos alojados nos ductos biliares podem ser removidos após colecistectomia, mas, às vezes, faz-se necessária a coledocotomia. Colecistectomias e coledocotomias ocasionam menores taxas de morbidade e mortalidade e são, portanto, os tratamentos de escolha.[21] Em contraste, outros procedimentos podem ser necessários, dependendo de vários fatores, incluindo viabilidade dos ductos biliares, presença de constrições e localização da obstrução biliar, mas estes costumam causar maior taxa de mortalidade.[5,22,23] Há técnicas de desvio biliar minimamente invasivas, que incluem drenagem trans-hepática ou transabdominal percutânea guiada por ultrassom ou implantação de cateter percutâneo por meio de laparoscopia.[24,25]

IMPLANTAÇÃO DE STENT BILIAR

A implantação de stent no colédoco, por meio de cirurgia ou endoscopia, está revolucionando o tratamento de anormalidades biliares extra-hepáticas tanto em cães quanto em gatos (ver Capítulo 123).[26-29] Há dois tipos gerais de stent biliar. O stent de plástico (poliuretano) é utilizado para facilitar a drenagem e manter o fluxo na árvore biliar. Em geral, essa prótese plástica é expelida de maneira espontânea após semanas a meses ou pode ser removida por meio de endoscopia, caso queira (Vídeo 288.1). O stent metálico, capaz de se expandir, é considerado mais permanente e geralmente reservado para doença recorrente ou neoplasia do ducto biliar (Figura 288.3). Ambos os tipos de stent foram implantados com sucesso, por muito tempo, por meio de cirurgia aberta.[26,27,29]

A colangiopancreatografia retrógrada endoscópica (CPRE) consiste na combinação de endoscopia e fluoroscopia; é um procedimento de avaliação da árvore biliar menos invasivo (ver Capítulo 123). Novos relatos demonstraram sua utilidade em pacientes clínicos.[28-32] Um endoscópio com visão lateral é introduzido até o duodeno proximal, possibilitando a visualização direta da papila duodenal maior. Um cateter utilizado em esfincterotomia e um fio-guia são introduzidos através do endoscópio em direção à papila duodenal maior. O fluoroscópio é utilizado para monitorar o avanço do fio-guia. Assim que se obtém acesso ao ducto biliar comum, injeta-se o contraste e monitora-se, por meio de fluoroscópio, a fase CPRE do procedimento. Constrições (ou estenoses), cálculos e neoplasias malignas são visualizados com experiência. Realiza-se esfincterotomia para abrir o esfíncter de Oddi e facilitar o avanço de outros instrumentos. Cálculos ou sedimentos, se presentes, podem ser removidos pela limpeza do ducto biliar por meio de balão. Ademais, pode-se realizar a dilatação de constrições e tumores para restabelecer o fluxo de bile, a fim de manter a patência da árvore biliar, pode-se implantar um stent no ducto biliar comum por meio de endoscópio (ver Vídeo 288.1). Complicações são infrequentes, mas podem incluir pancreatite, perfuração de duodeno ou de ducto biliar, colangite/colângio-hepatite bacteriana e estenose causada pelo stent.[28,29,33]

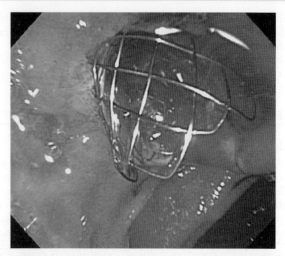

Figura 288.3 Fotografia obtida após implantação de stent biliar metálico por meio de endoscopia, em caso de obstrução recorrente do ducto biliar comum distal em um cão da raça Pastor-Alemão.

COLECISTITE

Etiologia

O termo colecistite é utilizado para definir tanto condições inflamatórias da vesícula biliar quanto sintomas relacionados com a vesícula biliar na ausência de cálculos biliares.[34] O termo compreende uma ampla variedade de doenças agudas e crônicas, com ou sem infecções bacterianas ou parasitárias. A origem da colecistite em animais de companhia não foi esclarecida. Fatores predisponentes incluem estase biliar, mucocele de vesícula biliar, doenças bacterianas ou parasitárias ascendentes e neoplasias biliares.[34] Infarto e disseminação hematógena de bactérias também podem estar envolvidos. Em gatos, as infecções bacterianas supostamente são secundárias à inflamação e não seriam o fator incitante.[35] Em alguns pacientes, são detectados colélitos concomitantes, mas a relação causal é desconhecida.[2,6,36]

Alguns pacientes com colecistite desenvolvem colecistite necrosante, geralmente referida como uma condição mórbida à parte, em razão de sua grave manifestação, do maior risco de complicações e da maior taxa de mortalidade.

Sinais clínicos

A colecistite pode ser aguda ou crônica. Com frequência, casos discretos são assintomáticos. Em casos de colecistite aguda moderada a grave, predominam anorexia, êmese, dor abdominal e febre. A presença de icterícia é variável. A colecistite crônica é muito mais difícil de diagnosticar. Sinais clínicos podem incluir anorexia intermitente, êmese e perda de peso progressiva. Pode ocorrer dor abdominal, porém de difícil detecção durante o exame físico. Em casos de colecistite, ocorre efusão abdominal devido à ruptura de vesícula biliar e peritonite biliar.

Diagnóstico

À semelhança do que acontece na colelitíase, os achados laboratoriais variam amplamente em casos de colecistite. A maioria das alterações clinicopatológicas é compatível com colestase ou doença biliar pós-hepática.[2,36] Em gatos com colecistite, as elevações das atividades de ALT, ALP e da concentração de bilirrubina total se correlacionam bem com alterações ultrassonográficas, com maior potencial de significado clínico.[37]

Aspirados de efusão tipicamente resultam em líquido amarelo-esverdeado sugestivo de bile.[38,39] A análise da efusão biliosa é caracterizada por inflamação supurativa, com ou sem pigmento biliar. Bactérias intra e extracelulares são comuns. A concentração de proteína total varia de 2,9 a 5,6 g/dℓ. Se o conteúdo de bilirrubina na efusão for maior do que o dobro daquele do sangue circulante, então há ruptura biliar.[38,39]

As características radiográficas variam e podem incluir diminuição do detalhamento da membrana serosa, compatível com efusão abdominal, colélitos ou enfisema da vesícula biliar.[39] Em animais de companhia, atualmente o diagnóstico ultrassonográfico é o procedimento padrão-ouro.[13] A ultrassonografia revela fielmente a presença de sedimento suspenso, colélitos, espessamento da parede da vesícula biliar, obstrução biliar extra-hepática e enfisema da vesícula biliar (Figura 288.4). Lama biliar hiperecoica na vesícula biliar ou na árvore biliar extra-hepática é particularmente preocupante em gatos; em geral, indica colecistite.[14,37,40] Diferentemente, em cães idosos a lama biliar é um achado comum, geralmente irrelevante.[41] Em gatos, espessura da parede da vesícula biliar maior que 1 mm indica com segurança a presença de doença da vesícula biliar.[42] Líquido pericolecístico e aderências de omento, se detectados, são sugestivos de perfuração.[15] As efusões abdominais são prontamente detectadas e podem conter materiais particulados.

Tratamento

Aos pacientes com colecistite, há disponibilidade tanto de tratamento clínico quanto o cirúrgico.[2,6,36,43] O tratamento clínico de rotina inclui antimicrobianos, soluções de uso intravenoso (IV) e analgésicos. A colecistocentese é útil tanto como procedimento diagnóstico quanto terapêutico.[44] Dá-se preferência à abordagem trans-hepática, já que o fígado propicia compressão interna no local da drenagem. O risco do procedimento é mínimo quando a vesícula biliar é drenada por completo, limitando a possibilidade de vazamento. A peritonite biliar e o colapso vasovagal são complicações relatadas. Culturas bacterianas positivas foram encontradas em 62% dos pacientes com colecistite. *Escherichia coli*, *Enterococcus* spp., *Bacteroides* spp., *Streptococcus* spp., *Clostridium* spp. e *Helicobacter* spp. foram os isolados mais comuns.[35,45] Os resultados do antibiograma revelaram que 80% dos microrganismos eram sensíveis a ciprofloxacino e aos aminoglicosídeos. A eficácia das penicilinas e cefalosporinas de primeira geração é menos confiável.[45] A escolha de antibióticos deve se basear em resultados de testes de sensibilidade antimicrobiana (antibiograma), quando possível, e o tratamento mantido por, no mínimo, 1 mês e, se necessário, por mais tempo, a fim de garantir a cura apropriada. Em casos graves de colecistite ou em pacientes com peritonite biliar, a colecistectomia é o tratamento preferido, já que remove imediatamente a principal fonte de infecção.[36,39] Os estudos ultrassonográficos de contração da vesícula biliar podem auxiliar na tomada de decisão sobre a escolha de tratamento medicamentoso ou cirúrgico.[16-20]

COLECISTITE ENFISEMATOSA

A colecistite enfisematosa é uma manifestação rara da colecistite aguda complicada por microrganismos produtores de gás,[11,46-50] que pode se acumular no lúmen, na parede ou nos tecidos pericolecísticos. É uma rara condição mórbida nos cães e extremamente rara em gatos. Há relato de associação com diabetes melito no cão.[48]

Os sinais clínicos e resultados de exames clinicopatológicos são semelhantes aos da colecistite. À radiografia, a doença é caracterizada por opacidade esférica a ovoide sobreposta sobre a silhueta hepática.[46-48] Na ultrassonografia, a interface do gás é visualizada na região da vesícula biliar, com variável sombreamento distal. A parede da vesícula biliar, o sedimento ecogênico e o líquido podem ser ocultos, dependendo do grau de reverberação.[46-48] Aderências, líquido pericolecístico localizado ou efusão ecogênica generalizada costumam estar relacionados à ruptura biliar.[15] A tomografia computadorizada (TC) é ideal para o diagnóstico, já que possibilita a visualização direta do gás no lúmen da vesícula biliar, da parede e nos ductos biliares.[34] A intervenção cirúrgica é mais apropriada devido ao alto risco de ruptura da vesícula biliar e peritonite séptica.[36,39,46-48] Microrganismos anaeróbicos são mais comumente isolados e incluem *E. coli* e *Clostridium perfringens*.[48] Em geral, fluoroquinolonas, metronidazol e cloranfenicol são utilizados, já que alcançam altas concentrações na bile e são altamente efetivos contra anaeróbicos. No exame histopatológico, notam-se, com frequência, colecistite necrosante e pequenos abscessos bacterianos na parede da vesícula biliar.[36,48] Caso o paciente sobreviva ao período perioperatório, há possibilidade de um prognóstico favorável. De modo geral, a morte dele deve-se à sepse, ao choque ou à peritonite.

NEOPLASIAS BILIARES

Em cães e gatos, os tumores primários da vesícula e da árvore biliares são extremamente raros, ainda que esteja havendo aumento do número de casos relatados.[2,51-57] Cistadenomas e adenocarcinomas biliares (colangiocarcinoma) são tumores da árvore biliar bem conhecidos.[58] Recentemente, o linfoma de

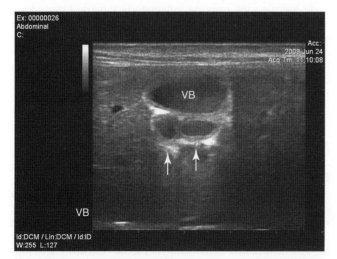

Figura 288.4 Imagem ultrassonográfica de um gato com colecistite. Há espessamento da parede da vesícula biliar (*VB*) e o lúmen está preenchido com material particulado hiperecoico. O ducto biliar comum está dilatado e tortuoso (*setas*).

grandes células em cães, assim como o linfoma de pequenas células e carcinomas neuroendócrinos em gatos, foi diagnosticado devido à melhora das capacidades diagnósticas.[54-57]

Cistadenoma biliar

Cistadenoma biliar ocorre com certa frequência em gatos idosos; é raro em cães. Mais comumente, é oriundo de ductos biliares intra-hepáticos e, com menos frequência, de ductos biliares extra-hepáticos.[53] Em gatos, ele responde por mais de 50% de todos os tumores hepatobiliares,[51] com uma predisposição por machos.[53] Ele pode ser único ou multifocal e envolver um ou mais lobos hepáticos. A transformação maligna foi observada em alguns gatos.[51]

Cistadenoma biliar é, em geral, um achado acidental em gato idoso,[51-53] com ausência de alterações hematológicas. Elevações discretas nas atividades das transaminases hepáticas em triagem de rotina podem ser a única alteração. Poucos sinais clínicos são notados e, se presentes, estão associados à ocupação de espaço pela neoplasia. Aspirados de cistadenomas guiados por ultrassom tipicamente revelam um líquido claro a amarelo, com celularidade variável. O diagnóstico definitivo é mais bem obtido em amostras coletadas por meio de biopsia tecidual com agulha, biopsia laparoscópica em cunha ou por cirurgia aberta.

Cistadenomas multifocais pequenos devem ser monitorados por ultrassonografia; a ressecção cirúrgica é raramente necessária. Grandes cistadenomas podem necessitar de cirurgia, sendo o prognóstico favorável, mesmo quando a ressecção é parcial.[51,53]

Carcinoma biliar (colangiocarcinoma)

O carcinoma biliar é o tumor hepatobiliar mais comum em gatos e o segundo em cães.[51] Provavelmente, o carcinoma biliar surge de ductos intra-hepáticos em cães; entretanto, gatos podem apresentar tumores intra e extra-hepático. Cães da raça Labrador Retriever e cadelas supostamente têm mais predisposição a ele.[51] Carcinoma biliar na vesícula biliar é extremamente raro em ambas as espécies.

A maioria dos carcinomas biliares é formada por neoplasias de crescimento lento, que, de início, são localmente agressivos. De modo geral, tumores estão em estágio avançado no momento do diagnóstico, já que os sinais clínicos raramente ocorrem antes do início da obstrução biliar. Pacientes com adenocarcinoma biliar em estágio avançado costumam manifestar letargia, êmese, perda de peso e icterícia.[59] Por ocasião do diagnóstico, é comum notar doença metastática. Em gatos, a colangite parasitária crônica pode levar a adenocarcinoma biliar.[60]

A ressecção cirúrgica é o tratamento de escolha para adenocarcinoma biliar, quando o tumor ou os tumores estiverem confinados a um único lobo e não houver evidências de doença metastática.[51,59] O prognóstico de adenocarcinoma biliar difuso é ruim. Técnicas de desvio biliar utilizando-se diversos *stents* foram pesquisadas em doenças não malignas, sendo atualmente avaliadas em tumores não passíveis de ressecção.[26,27] A embolização arterial percutânea e a quimioembolização de tumores hepáticos foram realizadas em um pequeno número de pacientes, sendo tais procedimentos cada vez mais utilizados.[61]

DOENÇAS PARASITÁRIAS DO SISTEMA BILIAR

Etiologia

Algumas espécies de parasitas infectam prontamente a árvore (ou trato) biliar e o fígado de gatos (*Platynosomum fastosum*, *Platynosomum concinnum* e *Amphimerus pseudofelineus*).[2,60,62-65] Os ovos dos parasitas são excretados nas fezes desses animais. Um caramujo, primeiro hospedeiro, ingere os ovos e, em seguida, um segundo hospedeiro, anfíbio ou réptil, como sapo, lagartixa

ou lagarto, ingere o caramujo. Os gatos ingerem o segundo hospedeiro intermediário para manter o ciclo. Aqueles que saem de casa para caçar são os mais predispostos, sobretudo se habitarem a região sudeste dos EUA, do Caribe ou do Havaí.[2] Não existe predileção racial ou sexual. Colangite bacteriana, colângio-hepatite, fibrose de ducto, obstrução biliar extra-hepática, insuficiência hepática e morte são sequelas conhecidas da colângite parasitária.[2,60,62,63,65] Pesquisa recente mostrou que o parasitismo biliar crônico pode ocasionar colangiocarcinoma.[60]

Sinais clínicos

Os sinais clínicos da doença biliar parasitária dependem do grau de lesão hepática e obstrução biliar. Vários gatos são portadores assintomáticos. Perda de peso, anorexia e êmese são as queixas mais comuns em gatos sintomáticos. Icterícia e distensão abdominal podem ser notadas durante o exame físico, em regiões endêmicas do país.[2,62,63]

Diagnóstico

Em geral, os resultados do hemograma são inespecíficos, mas podem indicar leucograma de estresse ou neutrofilia por neutrófilos segmentados. Eosinofilia, se presente, é sugestiva de infecção parasitária. Os resultados dos exames bioquímicos são variáveis, mas é possível notar elevação das atividades de enzimas hepáticas e da concentração de bilirrubina total, particularmente se o paciente estiver em estado crítico. O teste de sedimentação fecal (ver Capítulo 81) é o método mais confiável para confirmação do diagnóstico.[2] Em geral, radiografias de abdome não mostram alterações ou podem revelar hepatomegalia. A dilatação de ductos, cistos hepáticos e obstrução biliar são bem documentados e são prontamente observados na ultrassonografia abdominal. Aspiração e citologia da bile são úteis para identificar ovos do parasita se o exame coproparasitológico for negativo.[63,65] Amostras obtidas por biopsia hepática podem conter parasitas e/ou ovos.[62,63]

Tratamento

A administração de anti-helmínticos é o tratamento de escolha. O praziquantel, na dose única de 20 mg/kg ou 1 vez/dia, por 3 dias consecutivos, é efetivo na eliminação do parasita.[2] Podem ser necessárias doses de até 40 mg/kg, 1 vez/dia, durante 3 dias, particularmente em casos de infecção por *A. pseudofelineus*.[64] O ursodiol pode ser útil como agente colerético e como anti-inflamatório, mas não existem estudos controlados que demonstrem benefícios definitivos. A morte súbita de vários parasitas pode induzir uma resposta inflamatória intensa. Esteroides e anti-histamínicos, administrados antes do tratamento, podem ajudar a limitar a cascata inflamatória.[63] Pacientes atendidos com obstrução biliar quase sempre necessitam de cirurgia. Antibióticos são indicados aos pacientes com colangite neutrofílica detectada no exame histopatológico. O prognóstico em pacientes que necessitam de cirurgia e naqueles com extenso envolvimento hepático é reservado.[2,62,63]

MUCOCELE BILIAR

Etiologia

Mucocele biliar é definida como a presença de bile semissólida ou material mucoide inerte no interior da vesícula biliar.[66-70] A mucocele se tornou uma das doenças biliares mais preeminentes do cão. A expansão da mucocele no lúmen da vesícula biliar supostamente causa estiramento da parede vesicular e interrupção do fluxo sanguíneo, resultando em necrose por pressão na parede e subsequente peritonite biliar.[66,68,69] Fatores predisponentes incluem dislipidemias, distúrbios de motilidade da vesícula biliar, endocrinopatias e administração exógena de esteroides.[68] Predisposições raciais incluem cães das raças Shetland Sheepdog, Cocker Spaniel e Schnauzer Miniatura.[66,68,70] Mucocele ocorre mais comumente em cães idosos. A idade mediana é de 10 anos, com variação de 3 a 17 anos.[66,68-70] Complicações potenciais da mucocele incluem obstrução de ductos biliares extra-hepáticos, colecistite, colecistite necrosante, peritonite biliar e pancreatite.

Avanços recentes propõem etiologias da mucocele. O hiperadrenocorticismo sabidamente aumenta sobremaneira o risco de ocorrência de mucocele.[71] Pesquisas recentes constataram que altas doses de esteroides exógenos resultam em concentração significativamente maior de ácidos biliares não conjugados no trato biliar extra-hepático.[72] Ácidos biliares não conjugados são mais hidrofóbicos; quando em conteúdo excessivo, causam lesão do epitélio biliar. A secreção de mucina aumenta como resultado da lesão e, por fim, ocasiona hiperplasia mucinosa, uma das características histológicas que definem a mucocele.[73-75] Hipotireoidismo também foi sugerido como um mecanismo de formação de mucocele. Foi estabelecido que o fluxo da bile é reduzido em seres humanos com hipotireoidismo. Com baixa concentração de tiroxina, ocorre prejuízo ao relaxamento do esfíncter de Oddi, alteração da metabolização hepática de colesterol e diminuição na secreção biliar.[76,77] Supostamente a mucina se organiza e solidifica sob essas condições. É interessante observar que os xenobióticos foram recém-incriminados como causa de produção de mucocele. Verificou-se que cães Shetland Sheepdog tratados com produtos antipulgas à base de imidacloprida estavam mais predispostos à mucocele do que os membros da raça não tratados com o fármaco. Outras raças não mostraram a mesma sensibilidade aos achados específicos verificados na raça Shetland Sheepdog.[78]

O diagnóstico de mucocele biliar em gatos é crescente.[79-81] Supostamente, estase biliar é o mecanismo fisiopatológico predominante, já que as endocrinopatias são menos comuns. Estima-se que 12% dos gatos apresentam anormalidades biliares congênitas, o que pode sugerir uma questão estrutural ou de drenagem congênita que predisponha ao desenvolvimento de mucocele e outras doenças biliares nessa espécie.[82]

Sinais clínicos

Ao que tudo indica, a mucocele biliar se desenvolve devagar e, portanto, a manifestação clínica varia amplamente. O maior conhecimento sobre a doença facilitou a detecção de mucocele acidental na ultrassonografia abdominal. De maneira alternativa, pacientes podem ser atendidos com sinais de abdome agudo, associados a obstrução de ductos biliares extra-hepáticos, pancreatite ou peritonite biliar. Pacientes sintomáticos costumam ser levados à consulta por apresentarem êmese, anorexia, letargia e dor abdominal. A febre está comumente associada a colecistite bacteriana ou peritonite biliar. Nota-se icterícia em aproximadamente 40% dos pacientes.[66,69,70]

Diagnóstico

Anormalidades clinicopatológicas de rotina são, em geral, indistinguíveis de outras doenças hepatobiliares, com predomínio da elevação da atividade da enzima fosfatase alcalina (ALP).[66-70] Quase sempre, nota-se elevação das atividades de ALT e GGT e da concentração de bilirrubina total, particularmente em pacientes sintomáticos. Ocorre aumento marcante da concentração de colesterol em pacientes com obstrução de ductos biliares. Leucocitose com neutrofilia, com desvio à esquerda, é verificada mais comumente em caso de peritonite biliar, colecistite bacteriana ou colângio-hepatite bacteriana.

Radiografias de abdome são úteis para exclusão de outras doenças hepatobiliares, mas não para o diagnóstico definitivo de pacientes com mucocele. A ultrassonografia continua sendo o exame padrão-ouro para a detecção de mucocele de vesícula biliar.[66-70] Alterações ultrassonográficas são geralmente realçadas por camadas de contraste no interior da vesícula biliar (Figura 288.5 e Vídeo 288.2). Na mucocele imatura, a lama biliar hiperecoica pode estar suspensa ou dependente da gravidade. Há líquido anecoico, ou bile líquida, em quantidades variáveis. Uma borda anecoica ou hipoecoica (camada de mucina) separa a lama biliar da parede da vesícula biliar. Linhas de fratura costumam ser visíveis na camada de mucina e tipicamente formam uma aparência estrelada ou estriada,[66] que, em geral, é referida como um quiuí. Na mucocele biliar madura, uma borda anecoica ou hipoecoica é o achado predominante, estando a lama biliar, em geral, localizada na região central e inerte. Fragmentos de mucina e colélitos podem ser observados suspensos na vesícula biliar, alojados nos ductos biliares comuns ou císticos, e, em raros casos, livres na cavidade abdominal. A parede da vesícula biliar pode estar normal ou difusamente espessada. Líquido e gordura hiperecoica podem ser visualizados próximo à vesícula biliar, sugerindo sua ruptura ou peritonite localizada.[15] É importante ressaltar que a aparência da mucocele pode variar amplamente e o padrão ultrassonográfico nem sempre se correlaciona com a gravidade da doença.[82]

À histologia, a mucocele é caracterizada por hiperplasia mucinosa cística da mucosa da vesícula biliar, com mucina gelatinosa espessa aderida à superfície luminal.[66,68-70] Pode ocorrer colecistite linfoplasmocítica ou neutrofílica, ou uma combinação de ambas.

Tratamento

A correção cirúrgica é indicada a vários pacientes; é essencial quando há peritonite biliar.[66,68-70] A colecistectomia é o procedimento curativo mais comum. No caso de mucocele não complicada, pode ser realizada por meio de laparoscopia.[83] Culturas de microrganismos aeróbicos e anaeróbicos são essenciais no momento da cirurgia, já que 9 a 66% dos pacientes apresentam infecções bacterianas concomitantes.[66,70] Bactérias podem incluir *Enterococcus* spp., *Enterobacter* spp., *E. coli*, *Staphylococcus* spp. e *Streptococcus* spp.[66,68,69]

No caso de mucocele biliar, a terapia medicamentosa foi efetiva em alguns pacientes, sobretudo naqueles com hipotireoidismo.[66-68]

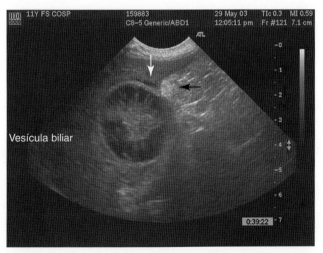

Figura 288.5 Imagem ultrassonográfica de mucocele biliar madura em um cão da raça Cocker Spaniel exibindo aparência estrelada. A camada de mucina é hipoecoica, ao passo que a bile ecogênica está situada na região central. Há um pequeno volume de efusão (*seta branca*) e a gordura adjacente é hiperecoica (*seta preta*). Ambas as características são sugestivas de ruptura de vesícula biliar. Note a semelhança com um quiuí cortado.

Uma terapia que combina fármaco colerético e antibiótico é mais frequentemente utilizada. Fármacos coleréticos, como ursodiol e S-adenosil-L-metionina (SAMe), alteram o microambiente da vesícula biliar e aumentam o fluxo de bile. O ursodiol é um ácido biliar hidrofílico que diminui a secreção de mucina do epitélio biliar e reduz a formação de cristais de colesterol.[84] Pacientes com obstrução biliar merecem cuidado especial, pois os medicamentos coleréticos podem causar ruptura da vesícula ou do trato biliar. O ideal é escolher o antibiótico com base nos resultados da cultura microbiológica da bile e do teste de sensibilidade antimicrobiana (antibiograma). Entretanto, a terapia empírica contra bactérias anaeróbicas é uma escolha lógica. O tratamento deve ser mantido durante, no mínimo, 4 a 8 semanas.[42-44] Ademais, dieta com baixo teor de gordura provavelmente é benéfica.[67,68]

O prognóstico a longo prazo para pacientes com mucocele biliar é muito variável. Pacientes com peritonite séptica e biliar apresentam a maior taxa de mortalidade. Pacientes estáveis, com mucocele não rompida, apresentam o prognóstico mais favorável. A taxa de mortalidade perioperatória varia de 22 a 40%.[66,70] O prognóstico é excelente para os pacientes que sobrevivem ao período perioperatório.[66,68-70] Recomenda-se sempre a avaliação e o tratamento de doenças endócrinas concomitantes.

REFERÊNCIAS BIBLIOGRÁFICAS

As referências bibliográficas deste capítulo se encontram online no Ambiente de Aprendizagem.

SEÇÃO 20
Doenças Pancreáticas

CAPÍTULO 289

Pancreatite: Etiologia e Fisiopatologia

Thomas Spillmann

A pancreatite aguda (PA) em cães e gatos é definida como uma inflamação pancreática completamente reversível, caracterizada pela presença de edema, infiltrado neutrofílico e necrose, no exame histológico. A doença pode ser local ou ocasionar síndrome da resposta inflamatória sistêmica (SRIS; ver Capítulo 132) e insuficiência múltipla de órgãos, possivelmente fatal.[1-6] A pancreatite crônica (PC) é caracterizada pela inflamação continuada (linfocítica/linfoplasmocítica), com alterações irreversíveis, como fibrose. A progressão clínica da PC pode ser subclínica ou recorrente, com episódios de doença mais ou menos graves, como acontece na agudização da pancreatite crônica. Em alguns casos, a perda de tecido pancreático reduz a função exócrina e/ou endócrina do pâncreas.[1-6] Em cães e gatos, a pancreatite se manifesta com uma ampla variedade de sinais clínicos que se sobrepõem não somente a doenças não pancreáticas, mas também à PA e à PC (ver Capítulos 290 e 291).[4,5] Ademais, os sinais clínicos e os resultados de testes laboratoriais e da ultrassonografia abdominal podem ser conflitantes.[3-8] A diferenciação morfológica da inflamação pancreática é, entretanto, raramente realizada, apesar da comprovada segurança e validade da aspiração com agulha fina guiada por ultrassom (ver Capítulo 89) e da biopsia pancreática cirúrgica ou laparoscópica (ver Capítulo 91).[9-14] O valor diagnóstico do procedimento é, todavia, influenciado por uma distribuição desigual da inflamação pancreática.[1,2]

A etiologia da pancreatite aguda e crônica permanece desconhecida, ou idiopática. Diversos fatores de risco foram propostos tanto para cães quanto para gatos, a maioria deles baseada em estudos experimentais, analogias com medicina humana e relatos de casos.

Predisposição racial foi documentada em estudos retrospectivos e de casos controlados. Cães da raça Schnauzer Miniatura, assim como Yorkshire e outras raças Terrier, parecem predispostos à PA.[15-19] A maioria dos gatos com pancreatite supurativa e necrótica aguda é da raça Doméstico de Pelo Curto.[20,21] A PC parece afetar mais comumente cães das raças Cavalier King Charles Spaniel, English Cocker Spaniel, Boxer e Collie.[22-24]

Associações genéticas com o gene tripsinogênio catiônico (PRSS1), o gene regulador da condutância transmembrana na fibrose cística (CFTR) e o gene inibidor da serina protease Kazal-tipo 1 (SPINK1) foram documentadas em seres humanos. Em cães, não foi observada associação entre a pancreatite e as mutações no gene PRSS1 ou gene CFTR. O papel das variantes do gene SPINK1 em cães Schnauzer Miniatura permanece controverso.[16,17,25,26] Até o momento não há tais estudos em gatos.

Associação ao gênero parece possível em cães com PA. Estudos retrospectivos parcialmente controlados propuseram que a castração (machos/fêmeas) ou o gênero masculino são fatores de risco.[18,19,27] Avaliações pós-morte em cães com PC revelaram que, em fêmeas, não se constatou maior risco relativo para a doença, apesar do acometimento de um número maior delas.[22]

Hipertrigliceridemia e obesidade foram consideradas importantes fatores de risco para pancreatite canina.[27] Estudos prospectivos de casos controlados em cães Schnauzer Miniatura revelaram que cães com histórico de pancreatite tinham cinco vezes mais chance de apresentar hipertrigliceridemia. Em cães com concentração sérica de triglicerídeos $\geq$ 862 mg/dℓ ($\geq$ 9,7 mmol/ℓ), verificou-se uma probabilidade 4,5 vezes maior de apresentar valor no teste de imunorreatividade da lipase pancreática (ILP) sérica compatível com pancreatite.[15,28] Um estudo prospectivo transversal em cães com sobrepeso e naqueles obesos mostrou associação entre hipertrigliceridemia com aumento acentuado da concentração sérica de ILP, mas sem desenvolvimento de pancreatite clínica.[29]

Imprudências dietéticas, incluindo acesso ao lixo e a sobras de refeições, foram consideradas fatores de risco para PA em cães, em um estudo retrospectivo controlado e em um relato de caso.[27,30] Embora dieta com alto teor de gordura tenha sido proposta como fator de risco para pancreatite, essa associação jamais foi documentada de forma confiável.

Infecções sabidamente estão associadas à PA em cães e gatos. Em cães com babesiose, a PA foi documentada em vários estudos retrospectivos e parece ser de valor prognóstico quanto à sobrevivência do paciente.[31-34] A erliquiose monocítica canina não causa PA em cães da raça Beagle infectados experimentalmente, mas os cães com doença de ocorrência natural podem apresentar aumento da concentração sérica de ILP, sem pancreatite clinicamente aparente.[35] A ocorrência de PA, juntamente com erliquiose granulocítica e leishmaniose, foi mencionada em dois relatos de caso, sugerindo uma complicação individual, em vez de sequela regular dessas infecções.[36,37] Pancreatite bacteriana ou séptica não foi relatada até hoje. Entretanto, a translocação de bactérias ao pâncreas foi induzida experimentalmente em cães e gatos.[38-40] Recentemente, a colonização bacteriana foi documentada no pâncreas de gatos com pancreatite de ocorrência natural, a hibridização in situ por fluorescência indicando colonização mais frequente em casos de pancreatite moderada a grave do que na pancreatite branda.[41,42] A obstrução de ductos biliares pode exacerbar a pancreatite e prejudicar a capacidade de excreção de bactérias em gatos com fibrose pancreática e anormalidades na papila principal devido à terminação conjunta do ducto biliar comum e do ducto pancreático nessa espécie.[6,42,43] Entretanto, resultados bem-sucedidos em cultura de bactérias (*Enterococcus hirae*) foram relatados somente em um gato com colangite ascendente e pancreatite.[44] A inflamação concomitante de pâncreas, fígado e intestino é considerada uma sequela frequente em gatos, mas a relação causa-efeito ainda não foi esclarecida.[42] Há relato de infecção por uma cepa de calicivírus felino altamente virulenta em casos graves de PA em duas séries de casos independentes.[45,46] A infecção do pâncreas e do fígado por trematódeos raramente foi envolvida na ocorrência de pancreatite felina, sendo documentada apenas em relatos ocasionais.[47-50] *Toxoplasma gondii* e *Bartonella* spp. não parecem causar pancreatite em gatos. Estudo recente não constatou associação significativa entre a concentração sérica de ILP em gatos e a presença de anticorpos contra os patógenos.[51]

Reações farmacológicas parecem ser idiossincráticas, em vez de verdadeiros fatores de risco, conforme proposto para as sulfonamidas potencializadas (ver Capítulo 286).[52,53] Fármacos amplamente mencionados em relatos ocasionais de casos de PA incluem azatioprina, L-asparaginase, antimoniato de meglumina, N-metil-glucamina e clomipramina.[54-62] Estudos prospectivos não revelaram evidências de pancreatite em cães que receberam L-asparaginase para tratamento de linfoma ou antimoniato de meglumina para tratamento de leishmaniose.[58,59] Em um estudo retrospectivo, verificou-se que o tratamento com fenobarbital/brometo de potássio supostamente causou pancreatite em até 10% dos cães tratados.[63] Isso foi sustentado pela constatação de elevação da concentração sérica de ILP e de hipertrigliceridemia em cães tratados com esses fármacos antiepilépticos.[64,65] Em gatos, a hipercalcemia experimental aguda induziu PA após infusão arterial, mas não após infusão venosa periférica de gluconato de cálcio.[66-68] Não existem relatos de hipercalcemia de ocorrência natural associada à PA em gatos. Injeções de colecistocinina-8 e ceruleína podem induzir PA em cães.[69-71]

Intoxicações parecem ser causas raras de PA; a intoxicação por zinco foi mencionada em diversos relatos de caso.[72-75] Acidentes ofídicos podem ter importância regional, conforme relatado em casos de envenenamento fatal por *Vipera xanthina palestinae*, acompanhado de pancreatite necrótica aguda (ver Capítulo 156).[76] A intoxicação por organofosforados foi pesquisada em estudos experimentais que demonstraram que o pâncreas de cães, mas não o de gatos, é sensível ao composto (ver Capítulo 152). Ao contrário de cães, parece que os gatos não possuem quantidade abundante de butirilcolinesterase fixada no tecido pancreático.[77,78] Em gatos, a intoxicação por lírio-da-páscoa é altamente nefrotóxica e o efeito pancreatotóxico se limita à degeneração de células acinares, sem inflamação (ver Capítulo 155).[79]

Doenças endócrinas associadas à PA em cães incluem hiperadrenocorticismo (ver Capítulo 306), hipotireoidismo (ver Capítulo 299) e diabetes melito (ver Capítulo 304), inclusive cetoacidose diabética.[19,80-82] Em cães e gatos, a PC é considerada uma causa, e não uma consequência, do diabetes melito.[4,83,84]

Traumas e intervenções cirúrgicas ou minimamente invasivas também são possíveis fatores de risco. A pancreatite traumática pode decorrer da síndrome da queda de grande altura, em gatos.[85] Cirurgias prévias, que não castrações, foram associadas ao aumento da razão de probabilidade (RP = 21,1) para pancreatite em gatos.[27] A colangiopancreatografia retrógrada endoscópica (CPRE) pode causar PA (ver Capítulo 123). Cães e gatos podem apresentar elevação transitória nas atividades e concentrações séricas de enzimas pancreáticas após CPRE, sem sinais clínicos de pancreatite,[46,86-90] o que pode ser causado por inflamação subclínica.[91]

A fisiopatologia da pancreatite aguda tem sido foco de revisões recentes, minuciosas e relevantes.[3,5,6,42,92-94] Modelos animais para experimentação são a principal base para o conhecimento atual sobre eventos subcelulares que ocasionam destruição de células acinares, assim como fatores que promovem respostas inflamatórias complexas locais e sistêmicas.[92-94] A PA e a necrose pancreática aguda são sugeridas como respostas ao mesmo estímulo, mas com diferente progressão clínica e consequências. Portanto, a PA discreta é uma condição localizada, com recuperação total sem complicação. Diferentemente, a PA grave, com necrose, pode ser localizada, mas também causar SRIS, resultando na síndrome da disfunção múltipla de órgãos (SDMO) e morte.[3,5,92-94]

O principal fator que inicia a inflamação pancreática parece ser a ativação da tripsina no interior das células acinares, causada por três situações básicas: (1) bloqueio do ápice da célula acinar no ducto pancreático, levando à colocalização e à fusão dos grânulos de zimogênio e lisossômicos; (2) estresse oxidativo; ou (3) hipotensão. O mecanismo de autodefesa contra a tripsina ativada consiste em sua neutralização por um inibidor pancreático da secreção de tripsina intracelular, o qual é saturado quando da ativação de mais de 10% da tripsina,[3,93] que, por sua vez, ativa outras proenzimas inativas normalmente armazenadas em grânulos de zimogênio. A liberação de enzimas digestivas ativadas no tecido pancreático causa, de início, inflamação local com migração de neutrófilos ao pâncreas. Isso é acompanhado de produção subsequente de espécies reativas de oxigênio e óxido nítrico, o que contribui para a inflamação.[3,93] O desvio de apoptose para necrose supostamente é causado por neutrófilos, juntamente com a endotelina-1 e a fosfolipase A3.[3,93] O comprometimento da microcirculação pancreática e o aumento da permeabilidade vascular contribuem para o edema e a necrose pancreática; a pancreatite necrosante resulta em uma redução progressiva de capilares não responsiva à reanimação volêmica.[93] A inflamação local adicional e a SRIS são causadas por uma combinação de diferentes vias inflamatórias, com o envolvimento de uma grande variedade de mediadores, como o fator de necrose tumoral-alfa, interleucina (IL)-1beta, IL-6, IL-10, fator de ativação plaquetária, molécula de adesão intercelular-1, CD40L, componente do complemento C5a, quimiocinas, substância P e sulfito de hidrogênio, assim como os sistemas cinina-calicreína e renina-angiotensina-aldosterona.[93,94] De possível valor clínico são as descobertas de que os receptores da substância P pancreática e neurocinina (NK)-1 são altamente suprarregulados em ratos com PA induzida, e que camundongos *knockout* (geneticamente manipulados) deficientes em receptores NK-1 são protegidos contra PA e lesão pulmonar associada.[95,96] Receptores NK-1 também parecem atuar como mediadores de dor pancreática em camundongos e seu bloqueio protege camundongos com sepse contra lesão pulmonar.[97,98] A utilidade dos antagonistas de receptores de NK-1 no tratamento de cães e gatos com PA ainda deve ser estudada.[93]

O desenvolvimento de complicações sistêmicas pode ser resumido como a seguinte cadeia de eventos: a PA causa SRIS, que resulta em SDMO. Características de SDMO que necessitam de atenção especial em seres humanos e são parcialmente documentadas em cães e gatos com PA incluem lesão pulmonar aguda (ver Capítulo 242), doença renal aguda e uremia (ver Capítulo 322), coagulação intravascular disseminada (ver Capítulo 197) e arritmias cardíacas (ver Capítulo 248).[93,98-101] Complicações locais após PA incluem acúmulo de líquido pancreático, pseudocistos e bolsões necróticos predispostos a infecções em seres humanos. Relatos de caso em cães e gatos, entretanto, descreveram somente complicações assépticas.[93,102-104]

Pancreatite crônica supostamente é uma complicação tardia da PA ou consequência de inflamação imunomediada crônica, conforme proposto para a PC destrutiva de ductos verificada em cães da raça English Cocker Spaniel.[4,5,24,93] Em gatos, a PC é considerada mais comum do que a PA.[6] Em cães e gatos, a PC é caracterizada por perda de tecido pancreático devido à fibrose, que pode, em seu estágio final, levar à insuficiência pancreática exócrina (IPE) e/ou ao diabetes melito.[4,5,6,23,42,105,106] Em cães, a IPE é, entretanto, mais frequentemente causada por atrofia acinar pancreática, que envolve outro mecanismo fisiopatológico (ver Capítulo 292).[107] A progressão clínica da PC varia de doença subclínica até episódios recorrentes de agudização de pancreatite crônica. O mecanismo fisiopatológico envolvido ainda precisa ser elucidado. Supostamente o aumento da pressão no ducto pancreático pode ser um fator contribuinte para a agudização da pancreatite crônica. As anormalidades do ducto pancreático são uma característica da PC em seres humanos também documentadas após colangiopancreatografia por ressonância magnética em gatos com PC induzida ou de ocorrência natural.[108-110]

REFERÊNCIAS BIBLIOGRÁFICAS

As referências bibliográficas deste capítulo se encontram online no Ambiente de Aprendizagem.

CAPÍTULO 290

Pancreatite em Cães: Diagnóstico e Tratamento

Jörg M. Steiner

INTRODUÇÃO

Em cães, atualmente a pancreatite é reconhecida como uma doença comum. Em um estudo com mais de 200 cães que morreram ou foram submetidos à eutanásia por uma ampla variedade de motivos, e que foram submetidos à avaliação necroscópica, verificou-se que mais de 8% apresentavam evidências macroscópicas de pancreatite.[1] Ademais, aproximadamente 50% deles tinham lesões microscópicas sugestivas de pancreatite crônica e aproximadamente 30%, de pancreatite aguda.[2] Esse estudo elevou a conscientização de clínicos para casos de pancreatite de forma dramática, mas muitos casos da doença, especialmente aqueles subclínicos, permanecem sem diagnóstico, sendo desconhecidas as consequências das falhas em diagnosticar pancreatite subclínica. Entretanto, as consequências conhecidas da pancreatite crônica discreta são exacerbação aguda da doença crônica, diabetes melito e insuficiência pancreática exócrina. Assim, o diagnóstico de pancreatite, mesmo em casos de doença crônica discreta, seria, dessa forma, benéfico ao clínico veterinário, ao animal e ao tutor.

DIAGNÓSTICO

Manifestação clínica

A manifestação clínica de cães com pancreatite pode variar bastante. Vários cães, sobretudo aqueles com doença crônica, são assintomáticos, ao passo que alguns apresentam sinais clínicos inespecíficos e outros manifestam, ainda, sinais clínicos de doença grave e complicações sistêmicas. Os sinais clínicos clássicos associados à pancreatite aguda grave em cães incluem êmese, dor abdominal, letargia e desidratação.[3] Alguns pacientes podem ter diarreia e outros, febre.[3] As complicações sistêmicas da pancreatite estão associadas a sinais clínicos de determinada complicação específica. Por exemplo, a lesão renal pode estar associada a oligúria, anúria ou até mesmo poliúria; a insuficiência pulmonar, ao aumento da frequência e do esforço respiratório; a encefalopatia pancreática, a sintomas neurológicos; e a coagulação intravascular disseminada, por sua vez, a diátese hemorrágica. Diferentemente, pacientes com doença crônica branda podem manifestar apenas sinais clínicos inespecíficos, como hiporexia ou anorexia, letargia ou alterações comportamentais.[4]

Diagnóstico por imagem

A pancreatite pode estar associada a alterações radiográficas, como diminuição do contraste no abdome cranial e deslocamento de órgãos abdominais.[3] Entretanto, essas alterações são subjetivas e a radiografia abdominal não é um exame sensível, tampouco específico, para o diagnóstico de pancreatite em cães. Entretanto, a radiografia de abdome é importante em cães com suspeita de pancreatite para descartar outros diagnósticos diferenciais, como corpo estranho gastrintestinal em paciente com episódios agudos de êmese e dor abdominal. A ultrassonografia abdominal pode ser muito útil no diagnóstico de pancreatite em cães, mas possui importantes limitações.

A sensibilidade da ultrassonografia abdominal depende de vários fatores, inclusive resolução do equipamento, habilidade do operador, nível de suspeita do ultrassonografista, mas, de forma mais importante, da gravidade da doença. Em cães com pancreatite aguda grave, a necrose pancreática é evidenciada por áreas hipoecoicas no pâncreas.[3] Outros achados ultrassonográficos em cães com pancreatite incluem aumento do pâncreas, efusão peritoneal, gordura peripancreática ou mesentérica hiperecoica, aumento da papila duodenal ou dilatação do ducto pancreático.[3] Alguns pacientes com pancreatite crônica podem apresentar pâncreas hiperecoico devido à fibrose pancreática.[5] A especificidade da ultrassonografia abdominal é limitada por outras lesões que ocasionam as mesmas alterações ultrassonográficas, ou semelhantes, como aquelas observadas em pacientes com pancreatite (Vídeos 290.1 e 290.2). Por exemplo, qualquer doença que leve à efusão abdominal tem o potencial de ser interpretada de maneira errônea como pancreatite.[5] O aumento do pâncreas também pode ser devido à hipertensão portal.[6] Por fim, a hiperplasia pancreática nodular, uma condição extremamente comum em cães idosos e supostamente não associada a casos atuais ou prévios de pancreatite, pode ocasionar alterações de ecogenicidade, que podem ser interpretadas de maneira errônea como pancreatite.[7] Assim, o sucesso do diagnóstico depende da utilização criteriosa dessa modalidade de exame por um ultrassonografista experiente.

Tomografia computadorizada e ressonância magnética do abdome são procedimentos de rotina em pessoas com suspeita de pancreatite, mas historicamente ambas foram consideradas carentes de sensibilidade no diagnóstico de pancreatite no cão.[8] Entretanto, estudos mais recentes sugeriram que a acurácia diagnóstica dessas modalidades diagnósticas pode ser melhorada.[9,10]

Patologia clínica geral

Uma ampla variedade de alterações hematológicas e bioquímicas séricas foi relatada em cães com pancreatite aguda grave.[3] Entretanto, essas alterações devem ser interpretadas como manifestações da condição sistêmica do paciente e como indicativo de potenciais complicações sistêmicas, e não como indicação direta de inflamação pancreática. Ademais, achados nos perfis hematológico e bioquímico sérico podem ajudar a direcionar o clínico a diagnósticos diferenciais alternativos e devem, dessa forma, ser considerados cruciais para a triagem de qualquer cão com suspeita de pancreatite.

Atividade sérica da amilase

Amilases são enzimas que catalisam a hidrólise de carboidratos complexos e são sintetizadas e secretadas por diferentes tipos celulares do organismo, inclusive células acinares pancreáticas. Enquanto alguns cães com pancreatite espontânea demonstram incrementos na atividade sérica de amilase, vários outros não o fazem. Ademais, como as amilases são sintetizadas e secretadas por outros tecidos, o aumento na atividade sérica de amilase também pode ser observado em diversas outras condições.[11] Assim, a mensuração da atividade sérica de amilase tem pouco valor no diagnóstico de pancreatite em cães.

Atividade sérica de lipase total

A lipase hidrolisa lipídios, como os triglicerídeos, que são lipídios apolares muito importantes para o armazenamento de energia corporal a longo prazo. Como resultado, os triglicerídeos precisam ser transferidos para dentro e para fora das células de modo rotineiro, e, como estes são completamente apolares, eles devem, a princípio, ser hidrolisados em produtos de lipólise mais polares, como glicerol, monoglicerídeos, diglicerídeos e ácidos graxos. Esse é o motivo pelo qual existem várias lipases diferentes no corpo, incluindo lipase gástrica, lipase pancreática, lipase hepática e lipase hormônio-sensível. O número exato de lipases no organismo é desconhecido, mas existem várias; enquanto algumas delas apresentam semelhanças estruturais, muitas somente compartilham funções (i. e., atividade lipolítica). A atividade sérica de lipase total pode ser mensurada por diversas diferentes metodologias, todas elas utilizando um substrato diferente. Vários testes utilizam o 1,2-diacilglicerol como substrato. Estes apresentam especificidade limitada (aproximadamente 50%) para o pâncreas exócrino e sensibilidade limitada (também de aproximadamente 50%) para pancreatite canina.[11] Nos últimos 20 anos, tem-se utilizado um substrato sintético, a resorufina (GPPR), como substrato alternativo tanto em medicina humana como em veterinária. Embora alguns estudos possam sugerir maior especificidade para o pâncreas exócrino do que os testes que utilizam 1,2-diacilglicerol, outros estudos não confirmaram esses achados.[12,13] Embora a utilidade clínica geral dos testes baseados no GPPR seja provavelmente melhor do que aquela baseada no 1,2-diacilglicerol, mais estudos são necessários para confirmar esses resultados, vez que esse substrato não é, de forma alguma, específico para o pâncreas exócrino em cães. Ademais, foi descrito um teste rápido que utiliza a trioleína como substrato.[14] Entretanto, até o momento o único estudo disponível mostra que esse teste se correlaciona com o teste da imunorreatividade da lipase pancreática sérica, quando mensurada exclusivamente em amostras de soro sanguíneo não lipêmicas, ictéricas ou hemolisadas, alterações bastante comuns em cães com pancreatite.[14] Além disso, esse teste não é específico para o pâncreas exócrino.

Imunorreatividade semelhante à tripsina

A imunorreatividade semelhante à tripsina (TLI) é específica para a função pancreática exócrina. Entretanto, a sensibilidade da TLI sérica para pancreatite em cães é muito menor do que aquela da imunorreatividade da lipase pancreática sérica de cães (PLIc) ou da ultrassonografia abdominal.[15] Isso ocorre provavelmente devido ao fato de que o tripsinogênio, que é a forma de tripsina presente em quantidade ínfima no soro sanguíneo sob condições fisiológicas, é uma molécula muito pequena, sendo assim rapidamente removida do espaço vascular por meio da excreção renal. Na pancreatite o tripsinogênio é ativado em tripsina de maneira prematura, mas esta é logo removida do soro por inibidores da proteinase. Entretanto, deve-se ressaltar que a TLIc continua sendo o teste de escolha para o diagnóstico de insuficiência pancreática exócrina (IPE; ver Capítulo 292).

Imunorreatividade da lipase pancreática

Há disponibilidade de um teste específico para a mensuração da imunorreatividade da lipase pancreática em cães (PLIc, agora mensurada por Spec LPc®, IDEXX Laboratories, Westbrook, Maine).[16] Esse teste baseia-se na detecção da lipase pancreática pela utilização de um anticorpo específico, sendo, dessa forma, o único a mensurar exclusivamente a lipase pancreática. Isso foi confirmado por meio de imunoistoquímica, a qual demonstrou que, de todos os tecidos avaliados, somente as células acinares pancreáticas foram coradas para lipase pancreática.[17] Ademais, a PLIc foi mensurada em um grupo de cães com IPE, mostrando concentrações séricas indetectáveis ou seriamente diminuídas de PLIc em todos os cães.[18] Em outro estudo, a PLIc sérica foi avaliada em cães saudáveis submetidos à eutanásia em um abrigo de animais, mostrando especificidade da concentração sérica de PLIc (mensurada pelo Spec LPc) de 97,5%.[19] Notou-se aumento significativo da concentração sérica de PLIc em cães com doença renal crônica experimentalmente induzida, mas a maioria dos cães apresentava concentração sérica de PLIc no intervalo de referência e nenhum dos cães tinha concentração séricas de PLIc acima do valor de corte recomendado para pancreatite.[20] Além disso, a administração oral de prednisona a longo prazo não influenciou a concentração sérica de PLIc.[21]

Diversos estudos clínicos avaliaram a sensibilidade da concentração sérica de PLIc no diagnóstico de pancreatite em cães. No geral, a sensibilidade depende da gravidade da doença, mas a maioria dos estudos relata sensibilidade superior a 80% em cães com pancreatite clínica aguda e sensibilidade acima de 60% em cães com pancreatite branda.[15,22-24] Estes dados mostram que atualmente a concentração sérica de PLIc é a informação diagnóstica mais sensível disponível para pancreatite canina, embora, assim como verificado na maioria dos testes diagnósticos em medicina veterinária ou humana, a sensibilidade seja inferior a 100%, sendo necessária a interpretação cuidadosa juntamente com as informações do histórico do paciente, de outros dados clínicos e da mensuração da concentração sérica de PLIc para obter o diagnóstico correto.

Ademais, há disponibilidade de um teste rápido para mensuração semiquantitativa da PLIc (SNAP LPc®, IDEXX Laboratories, Westbrook, Maine),[24] que é útil para excluir a possibilidade de pancreatite em cães com sinais clínicos sugestivos da doença, quando o teste é negativo.

Além disso, um teste com resultado positivo sugere pancreatite. Todavia, uma amostra de soro sanguíneo também deve ser enviada ao laboratório para mensuração de PLIc (pelo Spec LPc), a fim de confirmar o diagnóstico e obter um valor basal que possa ser então utilizado para monitorar a progressão da doença.

Deve ser feita menção especial a cães que não manifestaram sinais clínicos ou apresentaram apenas sintomas não comumente associados à pancreatite, mas com concentração sérica de PLIc indicativa de diagnóstico de pancreatite (Figura 290.1). A primeira questão requer uma discussão aprofundada com o tutor, de modo a garantir que não há nenhum sinal clínico sutil (p. ex., alteração de comportamento, apetite fastidioso ou outro). Na ausência de tais sinais, a PLIc dever ser reavaliada após 10 a 14 dias. Se, nesse período, o valor de PLIc tiver diminuído, não é necessário nenhum outro exame. Se, entretanto, o valor de PLIc permanecer alto, o paciente deve ser avaliado para

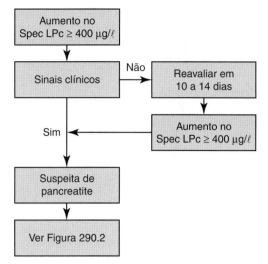

Figura 290.1 Algoritmo para cães com aumento do valor no Spec LPc.

quaisquer fatores de risco de pancreatite crônica, mediante a mensuração das concentrações séricas de triglicerídeos e cálcio e do esclarecimento sobre o histórico de fármacos administrados pelo tutor. Se for identificado um fator de risco, o paciente deve ser tratado de acordo. Entretanto, mesmo se nenhum desses fatores de risco puder ser identificado, exames e tratamento adicionais são justificáveis, a fim de prevenir complicações a longo prazo causadas pela pancreatite crônica branda.

Citologia e histopatologia

A avaliação citológica de uma amostra obtida por aspirado com agulha fina do pâncreas (ver Capítulo 89) é um ótimo procedimento para confirmar o diagnóstico de pancreatite. Diversos estudos demonstraram que há pouco risco na obtenção de aspirado com agulha fina do pâncreas.[25] A existência de células acinares pancreáticas confirma a aspiração bem-sucedida do pâncreas, ao passo que a de células inflamatórias no mesmo aspirado confirma inflamação pancreática.[26] Entretanto, em pacientes com necrose pancreática grave, podem ser aspirados apenas restos celulares e a avaliação citológica pode ser inconclusiva. Além disso, a ausência de células inflamatórias no infiltrado não descarta a possibilidade de pancreatite, pois as lesões inflamatórias podem ser muito localizadas.[1]

Tradicionalmente, a avaliação histopatológica de uma amostra obtida por biopsia pancreática é considerada o procedimento diagnóstico definitivo de pancreatite. A biopsia de pâncreas pode ser realizada durante laparotomia exploratória ou laparoscopia (ver Capítulo 91).[27,28] Pancreatite pode ser sugerida com facilidade pela aparência macroscópica do pâncreas, em alguns casos, e a avaliação histopatológica pode confirmar o diagnóstico em definitivo.[22,28] Entretanto, a ausência de pancreatite não pode ser comprovada pela histopatologia, mesmo quando se obtêm várias amostras. Em caso de pancreatite crônica branda, as lesões podem ser muito localizadas.[1] Também, deve-se ressaltar que, ao mesmo tempo em que uma biopsia pancreática, por si só, não esteja associada a muitas complicações, vários pacientes com pancreatite grave possuem alto risco anestésico e potencial de hipotensão; a anestesia é considerada um fator de risco para o agravamento de pancreatite.[28]

TRATAMENTO DE PANCREATITE AGUDA GRAVE

Por fim, as pancreatites aguda e crônica podem somente ser diferenciadas conclusivamente com base no exame histopatológico (i. e., a pancreatite crônica é caracterizada por alterações irreversíveis, como atrofia e fibrose pancreáticas). Todavia, é provável que muitos, se não a maioria, dos animais com pancreatite aguda branda não são levados para atendimento veterinário; ademais, a maioria dos casos de pancreatite crônica é discreta.

Tratamento etiológico

Sempre que possível, a causa da doença deve ser eliminada ou tratada. Entretanto, isso pode ser difícil, já que a maioria dos casos de pancreatite canina é considerada idiopática. Diversas causas e fatores de risco de pancreatite canina foram identificados, sendo a imprudência dietética um deles.[29] Além disso, a hipertrigliceridemia grave é considerada um fator de risco para a doença; em um estudo, constatou-se que concentração sérica de triglicerídeos acima de 850 mg/dℓ (aproximadamente 9,6 mmol/ℓ) foram associadas a aumento significativo do risco de pancreatite em cães da raça Schnauzer Miniatura.[30,31] A pancreatite é especialmente comum nessa raça e, recentemente, três mutações diferentes no gene *SPINK-1* foram identificadas em cães acometidos.[32] Embora mutações desse gene também sejam associadas à pancreatite hereditária em seres humanos, a mutação no gene *SPINK-1* não é causa comum de pancreatite hereditária em seres humanos. Traumas contundentes externos (p. ex., devido a acidentes automobilísticos) podem, também, causar pancreatite em cães. Trauma cirúrgico pode causar pancreatite, mas pacientes humanos submetidos à cirurgia de órgãos distantes do pâncreas também demonstraram maior risco dessa condição, sugerindo que a hipoperfusão do pâncreas durante a anestesia pode ser uma preocupação maior do que o próprio manuseio cirúrgico.[33] Em raras situações, relata-se suspeita de que microrganismos infecciosos, inclusive *Babesia canis* e *Leishmania infantis*, causem pancreatite.[34,35] Vários compostos farmacêuticos foram incriminados como causas de pancreatite em seres humanos, sendo a maioria deles a causa de pancreatite devido a uma reação idiossincrática não previsível ou dose-dependente.[36] Em cães, existem certas evidências de que brometo de potássio, fenobarbital, cálcio e L-asparaginase podem causar pancreatite, mas diversos fármacos podem ser responsáveis por casos isolados.[37-39] Um histórico minucioso é importante para identificar muitos dos fatores de risco mencionados, inclusive histórico de trauma ou imprudência dietética. Além disso, um histórico detalhado dos fármacos utilizados pode identificar algum que tenha sido descrito como potencial fator de risco para pancreatite. Se o paciente estiver sendo submetido a algum tratamento, deve ser avaliado com cuidado, para verificar se ele precisa dessa medicação específica ou se o fármaco pode ser descontinuado ou substituído por outro medicamento. O hemograma e o perfil bioquímico sérico, incluindo triglicerídeos e cálcio, podem fornecer informações sobre a possível etiologia.

Tratamento de suporte

A fluidoterapia agressiva é a base do tratamento de suporte para cães com a forma grave de pancreatite (ver Capítulo 129). Desequilíbrios hidreletrolíticos e ácido-base precisam ser avaliados e corrigidos o mais precocemente possível. Isso é muito importante, pois complicações sistêmicas estão associadas ao agravamento dessas condições e várias delas, assim que estabelecidas, são difíceis, ou até impossíveis, de tratar. Estudos recentes em seres humanos demonstraram que diferenças mínimas na concentração de nitrogênio ureico sanguíneo (NUS), no momento da admissão no hospital, bem como alterações mínimas no NUS durante as primeiras 24 a 48 horas após a internação, podem ter impacto dramático na recuperação de pacientes com pancreatite aguda.[40]

Tradicionalmente, a alimentação é retirada de cães com pancreatite, mas, nos últimos 10 anos, essa prática vem sendo questionada com base em experiências em seres humanos.[41] Há boas evidências em seres humanos com pancreatite grave de que a alimentação é crucial para equilibrar os efeitos catabólicos da doença.[42] Além disso, foi demonstrado em diversos estudos que a nutrição enteral é superior à nutrição parenteral.[43] Um estudo recente fez observações semelhantes em cães.[44] Embora não haja diferença nas taxas de mortalidade de cães alimentados por meio de tubo de esofagostomia ou com dieta parenteral total, os primeiros melhoraram significativamente mais rápido do que os cães alimentados por via parenteral.[44]

Ademais, estudos em seres humanos demonstraram que a alimentação que adentra o trato digestivo antes da papila duodenal não está associada a piores resultados, quando comparada a pacientes alimentados por meio de tubo de jejunostomia.[45] Assim, de forma geral, cães com pancreatite devem ser alimentados sempre que possível,[45] com a escolha de uma dieta com teor ultrabaixo de gordura. Se os pacientes não tiverem apetite, deve-se tentar alimentação por um tubo de gastrostomia, esofagostomia ou nasogástrico (ver Capítulo 82).[45] Se o paciente apresenta episódios graves de êmese (i. e., êmese consistente mesmo com terapia antiemética agressiva), deve-se implantar um tubo de jejunostomia ou alimentá-lo por meio de dieta parenteral parcial ou total.[45]

Analgesia

Dor abdominal é o principal sinal clínico em pacientes humanos com pancreatite aguda ou crônica; é descrita em mais de 90% dos pacientes humanos (ver Capítulo 143).[46] A dor abdominal nem sempre é notada em cães com pancreatite. Em um relato, somente 58% dos cães com pancreatite grave a tinham.[3]

Entretanto, pode parecer improvável que a dor abdominal ocorra com menos frequência em cães do que em seres humanos, e parece ser mais plausível que a dor permaneça sem ser detectada em vários pacientes caninos. Dessa forma, deve-se admitir dor abdominal, com a utilização de analgésicos em todos os cães com pancreatite (ver Capítulo 126). Meperidina, tartarato de butorfanol, buprenorfina, morfina, fentanila, metadona, ou combinações de diversos fármacos analgésicos, todos em doses-padrão, podem ser utilizados em pacientes hospitalizados.

Antieméticos

A terapia antiemética (ver Capítulo 39) é importante no tratamento de pacientes com pancreatite grave, não somente porque náuseas e êmese são incapacitantes, mas também porque esses sintomas podem impedir um suporte nutricional adequado. O maropitant, um antagonista de receptores neurocinina-1 (NK-1), é o fármaco de escolha como agente antiemético para cães com pancreatite grave.[47] Ele atua em nível central, inibindo a substância P no sistema nervoso central, e, assim, bloqueia os estímulos periféricos e centrais do vômito. O maropitant é administrado por via subcutânea, na dose de 1 mg/kg/24 h. Assim que o paciente não apresente mais episódios de êmese, o fármaco pode ser administrado por via oral, na dose de 2 mg/kg/24 h. Embora a êmese, em vários pacientes, possa ser tratada com sucesso somente com o maropitant, a adição de um antagonista do receptor 5-HT$_3$, como a ondansetrona, pode ter efeito sinérgico. De forma semelhante ao maropitant, os antagonistas de 5-HT$_3$ atuam em receptores periféricos e central, e também bloqueiam estímulos periféricos e centrais do vômito. A ondansetrona é utilizada na dose de 0,1 a 0,2 mg/kg, via IV lenta, a cada 6 a 12 horas. Cessado o vômito, o fármaco pode ser administrado por via oral. Outros antagonistas de 5-HT$_3$ também estão disponíveis. Metoclopramida não é um antiemético potente e, em geral, não é suficiente para cães com pancreatite grave.

Inibidores da proteinase

Com base no conhecimento da fisiopatologia da pancreatite aguda, os inibidores da proteinase têm sido, por longo tempo, o centro de novas estratégias terapêuticas para pancreatite. Infelizmente, nenhum estudo foi capaz de demonstrar evidências fortes de que os inibidores da proteinase sejam efetivos em cães com pancreatite de ocorrência natural, o que contrasta com a pancreatite experimental em cães, na qual o inibidor da proteinase Trasylol® demonstrou prevenir a morte, quando administrado ao mesmo tempo da indução da pancreatite.[48] É provável que isso ocorra pelo fato de que, enquanto a ativação prematura do tripsinogênio em tripsina possui um papel na patogênese inicial da pancreatite, não parece ser importante na progressão e no desenvolvimento das complicações sistêmicas.

Plasma fresco congelado

O plasma fresco congelado e o sangue total fresco contêm macroglobulinas alfa-$_2$, albumina e fatores anticoagulantes e coagulantes (ver Capítulo 130). Em estudos clínicos em paciente humanos com pancreatite aguda, não houve benefício da administração do plasma.[49] Estudo recente em cães sugeriu, inclusive, que a administração de plasma fresco congelado está associada ao agravamento do quadro clínico.[50] Entretanto, o estudo foi retrospectivo e é possível que os pacientes com doença mais grave e com mais complicações recebam plasma.[50] De forma anedótica, acredita-se que o plasma fresco congelado seja útil em cães com formas graves de pancreatite. Mais estudos são necessários para responder a essa questão em definitivo.

Antibióticos

Em contraste a seres humanos, cães com pancreatite raramente apresentam complicações por infecções bacterianas. Além disso, mesmo que elas ocorram com frequência em pacientes humanos com pancreatite e sejam estimadas como responsáveis por aproximadamente 25 a 50% de todas as mortes associadas à pancreatite aguda, até o momento não foi comprovada uma vantagem evidente do uso de antibióticos na rotina.[51,52] Portanto, a utilização de fármacos antibióticos deve ser limitada àqueles cães que manifestarem complicação por infecção bacteriana (p. ex., pneumonia por aspiração, necrose com infecção) ou quando houver forte suspeita de complicação de origem infecciosa.

Anti-inflamatórios

Glicocorticoides não mostraram ser benéficos em pacientes humanos com pancreatite grave sem pancreatite autoimune, devendo a utilização deles ser limitada a pacientes caninos com pancreatite e choque cardiovascular. Fármacos anti-inflamatórios não esteroides foram incriminados como causas potenciais de pancreatite; ademais, não propiciaram nenhum benefício em estudos humanos.

Outras estratégias terapêuticas

Várias outras estratégias terapêuticas foram avaliadas, seja em modelos experimentais de pancreatite, seja em testes clínicos. Entretanto, nenhum efeito benéfico consistente pôde ser demonstrado para qualquer uma delas. Muitos estudos avaliaram o benefício de diversos antioxidantes em pacientes com pancreatite aguda grave, mas nenhum dos estudos controlados foi capaz de demonstrar algum benefício.[53] Um estudo avaliou a utilização de um probiótico em pacientes com pancreatite aguda grave, mas o resultado foi pior em pacientes tratados do que naqueles não tratados com ele.[54] Além disso, fármacos antiácidos e antissecretórios (i. e., anticolinérgicos, calcitonina, glucagon, somatostatina) não demonstraram nenhum resultado promissor. De início, o tratamento com inibidores do fator de ativação plaquetária (IFAP) mostrou resultados promissores, mas um grande estudo multicêntrico internacional não constatou benefício algum.[55,56] A dopamina mostrou-se útil na prevenção da progressão da pancreatite em gatos com pancreatite induzida experimentalmente, quando administrada dentro de 12 horas após o início da doença.[57] Embora esse limite de tempo possa impedir que a dopamina seja efetiva na terapia de rotina da pancreatite, os pacientes submetidos à anestesia podem se beneficiar do tratamento com esse medicamento.

Intervenção cirúrgica

Na pancreatite humana, o tratamento de pacientes com pancreatite aguda grave se tornou cada vez mais conservador nos últimos

30 anos.[58] Embora, em termos históricos, a necrosectomia ou a lavagem abdominal tenham sido consideradas úteis, essas intervenções atualmente são consideradas prejudiciais ao paciente. As únicas situações nas quais a intervenção cirúrgica parece indicada em cães com pancreatite grave seriam aquelas acompanhadas de foco de necrose infeccionado ou outro tipo de acúmulo de líquido infectado (alguns dos quais foram previamente denominados como abscessos pancreáticos, mas esse termo não é mais utilizado na pancreatologia humana). A maioria dos pacientes com obstrução biliar secundária não apresenta obstrução total e a ruptura de ducto biliar é rara. Assim, a intervenção cirúrgica é raramente necessária e pode comprovadamente ser prejudicial a um paciente já debilitado.[59]

TRATAMENTO DA PANCREATITE CRÔNICA BRANDA

Vários cães com pancreatite manifestam a forma branda de pancreatite crônica (Figura 290.2).

TRATAMENTO DA CAUSA

Assim como nos casos de pancreatite aguda, o tratamento da causa da pancreatite crônica branda é também uma questão fundamental. Para esse propósito, diversos fatores de risco devem ser estimados, incluindo avaliação da hipertrigliceridemia e hipercalcemia do paciente e obtenção de um histórico detalhado sobre os fármacos administrados. Além disso, o paciente deve ser avaliado em busca de quaisquer possíveis doenças concomitantes que possam influenciar o tratamento, como doença intestinal inflamatória, hepatite crônica e diabetes melito. Embora o diagnóstico definitivo de tais enfermidades concomitantes possa ser desafiador, o clínico deve buscar evidências razoáveis para tais condições complicadoras, inclusive com mensuração da glicemia, das concentrações séricas cobalamina e folato e das atividades séricas de enzimas hepáticas. Outros exames podem ser necessários se quaisquer anormalidades forem identificadas e o tratamento geral do paciente precisar ser ajustado a elas. Ademais, o paciente deve ser minuciosamente avaliado para determinar se há necessidade de terapia antiemética e/ou analgésica. Se o paciente não apresentar nenhum sinal clínico, a analgesia pode não ser justificada. No entanto, apesar de não apresentar quaisquer sinais de desconforto abdominal, mas não estiver bem, podem ser administrados analgésicos leves, como butorfanol ou tramadol, por via oral (ver Capítulo 356). Desconforto abdominal evidente pode requerer o uso de adesivos de fentanila (ver Capítulo 126). Qualquer sinal de êmese ou náuseas (i. e., hiporexia, anorexia, sialorreia, engasgo) pode necessitar da utilização de um antiemético efetivo, como o maropitant e/ou um antagonista de 5-HT_3 (ver Capítulo 39). Doses-padrão são utilizadas por via oral durante cerca de 5 dias, o que, espera-se, seja um

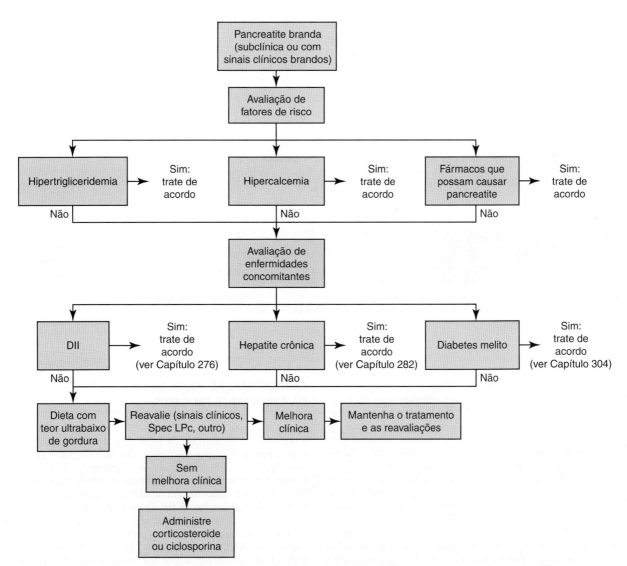

Figura 290.2 Algoritmo para tratamento de pancreatite branda. *DII*, doença intestinal inflamatória; *Spec LPc*, lipase pancreática canina.

tempo suficiente para que a pancreatite melhore e o sinais clínicos associados sejam amenizados. Cães com pancreatite crônica branda devem receber uma dieta com teor ultrabaixo de gordura, com menos de 20 g de gordura/1.000 kcal (ver Capítulo 179). Além disso, é crucial discutir com o tutor o conteúdo de gordura na dieta e lembrá-lo de que guloseimas também podem conter quantidade relevante de gordura. Dessa forma, é importante substituí-las por guloseimas com baixo teor de gordura, como vegetais e frutas, seguindo as mesmas recomendações mencionadas anteriormente, ou guloseimas preparadas na própria casa (p. ex., com base em dietas com teor ultrabaixo de gordura). Alguns pacientes podem ter enfermidades concomitantes que também podem necessitar de dieta especial, como hipersensibilidade alimentar (ver Capítulos 178 e 186) ou doença renal crônica (ver Capítulo 184). Na maioria desses pacientes, as necessidades dietéticas para pancreatite são mais importantes do que a condição concomitante, já que a pancreatite pode levar à exacerbação aguda mais rapidamente do que a anormalidade concomitante. Uma alternativa é consultar um nutrólogo veterinário para a formulação de uma dieta caseira que atenda às necessidades dietéticas tanto para a pancreatite como para a condição concomitante. Inicialmente, o paciente deve ser reavaliado a cada 2 ou 3 semanas, a fim de avaliar os sinais clínicos e mensurar a concentração sérica de lipase pancreática no Spec LPc. Assim que a condição clínica melhorar ou estabilizar, a frequência de reavaliações pode ser diminuída com base em cada paciente.

Nas últimas duas décadas, uma nova forma de pancreatite, a autoimune, foi descrita em seres humanos; é caracterizada por um infiltrado linfocítico-plasmocitário no pâncras.[60] Seres humanos com pancreatite autoimune respondem de maneira favorável à administração de corticosteroides. Recentemente, surgiram algumas publicações descrevendo pancreatite crônica em cães da raça English Cocker Spaniel com algumas das características da pancreatite autoimune humana.[61,62] Além disso, vários clínicos começaram a tratar com cautela cães com pancreatite crônica fazendo uso de corticosteroides quando estes não respondem a outros tratamentos, sendo observados benefícios com essa estratégia terapêutica em uma série de casos. O

autor utiliza um protocolo terapêutico que envolve a mensuração da concentração basal de lipase pancreática no Spec LPc e tratamento do paciente com 2 mg de prednisona/kg/12 h VO, durante 5 dias, seguido de 1 mg/kg/12 h VO, durante outros 5 a 7 dias, e, então, reavalia os sinais clínicos e, mais uma vez, mensura lipase pancreática no Spec LPc. Se houver melhora dos sinais clínicos ou se o valor obtido no Spec LPc estiver diminuído de maneira significativa, reduz-se gradativamente a dose de prednisona. Além disso, há relato de tratamento efetivo de um cão com pancreatite crônica com ciclosporina; está sendo realizado um teste clínico a respeito do procedimento.[63] O autor mensura a concentração sérica basal de lipase pancreática no Spec LPc e, então, utiliza dose de 5 mg de Atopica®/kg/24 h, VO, durante 3 semanas; depois disso, faz nova avaliação a fim de avaliar a condição clínica do paciente e mensurar, novamente, a lipase pancreática no Spec LPc. O tratamento é mantido a longo prazo, com base nos critérios mencionados anteriormente. Entretanto, outros estudos são necessários antes que essas estratégias terapêuticas possam ser recomendadas para uso mais rotineiro em cães.

Prognóstico

O prognóstico para cães com pancreatite está diretamente relacionado com a gravidade da doença, da extensão da necrose pancreática, da ocorrência de complicações sistêmicas e pancreáticas, da duração da doença e da existência de doença concomitante. Diversos sistemas prognósticos foram desenvolvidos para prever o resultado em pacientes humanos com pancreatite, logo após a admissão hospitalar.[64-66] Todos eles almejam identificar de antemão pacientes em alto risco e tratá-los de maneira intensiva. Vários desses sistemas de prognóstico foram adaptados e avaliados em cães.[67,68] Infelizmente, nenhum deles mostrou-se útil em condições clínicas de rotina.

REFERÊNCIAS BIBLIOGRÁFICAS

As referências bibliográficas deste capítulo se encontram online no Ambiente de Aprendizagem.

CAPÍTULO 291

Pancreatite em Gatos: Diagnóstico e Tratamento

Craig G. Ruaux

Em gatos, nossa compreensão e nosso reconhecimento de doenças inflamatórias do pâncreas sofreram uma alteração considerável em um período de tempo relativamente curto. Ainda no final dos anos 1990, a pancreatite em gatos era tida como uma doença relativamente incomum, tendo a pancreatite crônica suposta "importância clínica limitada".[1] Atualmente sabemos que a pancreatite é a doença mais comum do pâncreas exócrino em gatos,[2] sendo a pancreatite crônica comum como doença primária e comorbidade que acompanha várias outras doenças do gato.[3-5] Em grande parte, esse enorme conhecimento adquirido relativo à doença se deve à melhora marcante nas modalidades de diagnóstico por imagem, nos métodos de exames químicos minimamente invasivos e no simples reconhecimento de que as manifestações clínicas da doença pancreática no gato são bastante diferentes daquelas observadas no cão.

CARACTERIZAÇÃO HISTOLÓGICA DA PANCREATITE EM GATOS

Como a pancreatite é, por definição, uma doença inflamatória, a documentação objetiva da existência de inflamação no parênquima pancreático por meio de avaliação histopatológica é ainda considerada padrão-ouro para o diagnóstico dessa doença.[6-8] Foram descritos sistemas de pontuação histológicos para avaliação do tipo e grau de gravidade da pancreatite no gato.[6] A maioria dos autores faz distinção entre pancreatite aguda (caracterizada por edema intersticial, infiltração neutrofílica e possível necrose da gordura mesentérica) e pancreatite crônica (caracterizada por infiltração linfocítica, fibrose e degeneração acinar cística), ao descrever a doença inflamatória do pâncreas do gato.[1,6] Entretanto, é comum que cortes histológicos do pâncreas

CAPÍTULO 291 • Pancreatite em Gatos: Diagnóstico e Tratamento

mostrem um padrão misto de infiltração; ademais, a distribuição das lesões no pâncreas de gatos pode ser irregular, conforme descrito em cães.[9]

Alguns relatos sugerem que a inflamação pancreática crônica (particularmente infiltrado linfocítico e/ou fibrose) é bastante comum no gato doméstico. Em um estudo que avaliou 115 gatos submetidos à necropsia, independentemente da causa, foram observadas evidências de pancreatite em 67% dos gatos doentes e em 45% daqueles clinicamente normais (i. e., gatos sem histórico de doença, que morreram, em geral, por conta de trauma).[6] A pancreatite crônica foi o achado mais comum, sendo observada em 60% de todas as amostras; um pouco mais de 50% delas apresentavam somente pancreatite crônica. No mesmo grupo de gatos, constatou-se pancreatite aguda em 18 casos (15,7%): 7 demonstraram somente pancreatite aguda e 11, uma mistura de alterações agudas e crônicas. Em estudo recente que avaliou indicações e complicações da biopsia pancreática, detectou-se pancreatite crônica ou "crônica agudizada" em 10/19 gatos, enquanto em outros dois casos identificou-se "pancreatite" sem especificação entre aguda e crônica, perfazendo um total de 12/19 (63%) dos casos nos quais a inflamação pancreática foi identificada em gatos com suspeita clínica de doença pancreática.[10] É interessante ressaltar que, nesse estudo, a frequência com que os cães foram diagnosticados com lesões pancreáticas em comparação aos gatos foi menor.

SINAIS CLÍNICOS DE PANCREATITE EM GATOS

Um dos grandes desafios no tratamento de gatos com pancreatite é a natureza incerta dos sinais clínicos tipicamente manifestados neles. Com base na agregação dos dados de três estudos envolvendo uma variedade de diagnósticos histológicos de base e gravidade aparente da doença, os sinais clínicos mais comuns de pancreatite no gato são redução do apetite, letargia, desidratação e êmese (Tabela 291.1). Dor abdominal, um sinal clínico muito comum de pancreatite no cão, é muito menos frequentemente constatada no gato. A avaliação acurada de dor abdominal no gato (ver Capítulo 126) pode ser muito difícil, podendo, assim, a frequência verdadeira desse problema nesses animais com pancreatite ser subestimada;[11] entretanto, a importante observação de que a dor abdominal é raramente valorizada por clínicos que avaliam gatos com pancreatite é verdadeira. Dada a natureza inespecífica dos sinais clínicos de pancreatite no gato, essa doença deve ser considerada no diagnóstico diferencial de qualquer felino com êmese, anorexia/hiporexia ou letargia, nos quais outra causa mais provável não foi identificada. Em gatos, não é possível distinguir pancreatite aguda de pancreatite crônica com base na manifestação clínica, na duração

dos sinais clínicos ou na gravidade aparente da doença.[2,12,13] Em gatos, embora a doença pancreática crônica seja comumente considerada menos grave do que a pancreatite aguda,[13] ambas podem ocorrer com complicações ou comorbidades que causam riscos potenciais à vida do paciente, não sendo particularmente útil, do ponto de vista clínico, a tentativa de diferenciá-las.

ABORDAGEM DIAGNÓSTICA DE GATO COM SUSPEITA DE PANCREATITE

Exames bioquímicos e hemograma de rotina

Anormalidades bioquímicas e hematológicas são comuns em gatos com pancreatite, mas não existem anormalidades ou padrões individuais de achados que sejam específicos para pancreatite nessa espécie. As anormalidades que costumam ser observadas incluem leucocitose, neutrofilia com desvio à esquerda, elevação das atividades de alanina aminotransferase (ALT) e fosfatase alcalina (ALP) e da concentração de bilirrubina, azotemia, hipercolesterolemia, hipoalbuminemia, hipopotassemia, hipocalcemia e hiperglicemia.[11-14] Com frequência, a hipocalcemia está associada a doenças necrosantes mais graves e justifica terapia mais intensiva (ver a seguir).[11,14,15]

Em gatos, embora nenhum padrão específico de resultados no perfil bioquímico de rotina sugira pancreatite, os exames de patologia clínica de rotina continuam sendo parte importante do plano diagnóstico e do protocolo terapêutico. O reconhecimento de anormalidades bioquímicas séricas, particularmente elevação de atividades de enzimas hepáticas e da concentração de bilirrubina, bem como de anormalidades eletrolíticas, é parte importante do planejamento terapêutico e de suma importância no reconhecimento precoce de comorbidades comuns, como lipidose hepática (ver Capítulo 285) e diabetes melito (ver Capítulo 305), que necessitam de intervenções adicionais.

Testes diagnósticos específicos para o pâncreas

Em gatos com pancreatite, a combinação de ausência de achados bioquímicos específicos, natureza incerta dos sinais clínicos e presença variável de dor abdominal torna a busca por testes diagnósticos sensíveis, específicos e minimamente invasivos para pancreatite algo de grande interesse e importância. É ainda comum que vários laboratórios de referência e analisadores bioquímicos de uso domiciliar forneçam estimativas de atividades catalíticas séricas de amilase e lipase no perfil bioquímico de rotina tanto para cães quanto para gatos (ver Capítulo 64). Essas atividades enzimáticas são amplamente consideradas como de baixa ou nenhuma utilidade diagnóstica na avaliação da doença pancreática de gatos.[2,11-13,16,17] Além disso, foram relatados graus

Tabela 291.1 — Histórico e sinais clínicos comuns de pancreatite em gatos agregados com base em três estudos diferentes.[1,12,28]

SINAL CLÍNICO	ESTUDO				TOTAL	PREVALÊNCIA GERAL
	STOCKHAUS *ET AL.*[28]	FERRERI *ET AL.*[12] (PAN)	FERRERI *ET AL.*[12] (PC)	HILL & WINKLE[1]		
Número de gatos	33	30	33	40	136	
Inapetência	32 (97%)	19 (63%)	23 (70%)	39 (98%)	113	83%
Letargia	33 (100%)	15 (50%)	17 (52%)	40 (100%)	105	77%
Desidratação	24 (73%)	10 (33%)	17 (51%)	37 (93%)	88	65%
Êmese	18 (55%)	13 (43%)	13 (39%)	14 (35%)	58	43%
Icterícia	6 (18%)	5 (16%)	8 (24%)	21 (53%)	40	29%
Perda de peso	3 (9%)	12 (40%)	7 (21%)	NE	22	16%
Dor abdominal	17 (52%)	NE	NE	10 (25%)		

Gatos de um estudo (Ferreri *et al.*[12]) estão subdivididos em pancreatite aguda necrosante (*PAN*, n = 30) e pancreatite crônica não supurativa (*PC*, n = 33). A prevalência geral está arredondada para o valor percentual inteiro mais próximo. *NE*, não especificado.

muito altos de variabilidade interinstrumental e entre os instrumentos para esses (e muitos outros) analitos da patologia clínica de gatos;[18,19] assim, a mensuração das atividades tradicionais de amilase e lipase, seja qual for o laboratório, possui utilidade questionável na avaliação do paciente felino.

O pâncreas é uma fonte de diversas proteínas e peptídios unicamente sintetizados nesse órgão. Várias dessas proteínas (ver Capítulo 271) receberam pelo menos alguma atenção como testes diagnósticos para pancreatite em gatos, incluindo tripsinogênio felino (TLIf),[20] o peptídio de ativação da tripsina[21] e a lipase específica do pâncreas (PLIf e Spec LPf) (ver Capítulo 289).[22] O pressuposto de base desses testes é de que, em geral, há somente quantidades muito pequenas dessas proteínas na circulação (quase sempre em concentrações limítrofes ou abaixo do limite de detecção do teste), mas, havendo disfunção celular acinar, essas proteínas extravasam para o interstício e a circulação, onde podem ser detectadas. A detecção de concentrações aumentadas dessas proteínas é, dessa forma, considerada evidência de anormalidades celulares acinares e tida como compatível com diagnóstico de pancreatite.[8,13]

A sensibilidade e a utilidade clínica reais de TLIf e PLIf/Spec LPf foram avaliadas em diversos estudos. A utilização de uma concentração sérica de TLIf > 100 mg/ℓ como um valor limiar para o diagnóstico de pancreatite fez com que sensibilidades com variações de aproximadamente 28 a 64% tenham sido relatadas por vários autores para o diagnóstico de pancreatite aguda ou crônica em gatos.[20,21,23] Esses estudos são bastante variáveis em termos de número de pacientes, delineamento do estudo e métodos diagnósticos adicionais utilizados, tornando questionável, dessa forma, a comparação direta das sensibilidades relatadas. Independentemente, a maior sensibilidade relatada, de aproximadamente 64%, é subótima, na melhor das hipóteses, tendo em vista que foi obtida em um grupo relativamente pequeno (n = 10) de gatos com fortes evidências de doença pancreática relevante (seja por alterações ultrassonográficas características, seja por confirmação histológica em amostra obtida por biopsia pancreática). Uma concentração sérica normal de TLIf não descarta de modo confiável a doença pancreática em gatos.[24] A especificidade da elevação da concentração de TLIf também foi questionada por alguns autores que detectaram alta concentração de TLIf em gatos sem fortes evidências de doença pancreática, bem como na existência de outras doenças relevante, como doença intestinal inflamatória, linfoma gastrintestinal e azotemia.[23,25] Uma interpretação alternativa desses dados, apoiados pela observação de que a doença pancreática no gato costuma ser acompanhada de sinais clínicos vagos ou "silenciosos" e de que é uma comorbidade comum a várias doenças, seria a probabilidade de doença pancreática concomitante em muitos desses casos.

Relata-se a detecção de alta concentração sérica de lipase pancreática felina específica (PLIf ou Spec LPf) possui maior sensibilidade e especificidade do que a TLIf. Em um estudo, no qual a sensibilidade e a especificidade gerais obtidas foram de 28 e 82%, respectivamente, a sensibilidade e especificidade gerais da PLIf foi de 67 e 67%, respectivamente.[26] No mesmo estudo, a sensibilidade da PLIf para o diagnóstico de pancreatite "moderada a grave" foi de 100%. Um estudo maior (n = 182 gatos) com o teste Spec LPf relatou sensibilidade geral para esse teste de 79%, com especificidade de 82% para a detecção de pancreatite nesse grupo de animais.[27] De forma geral, atualmente o teste Spec LPf possui a maior sensibilidade e especificidade relatadas entre qualquer modalidade diagnóstica para detecção de pancreatite em gatos.[24] No momento, a mensuração de Spec LPf como marcador prognóstico e parâmetro de monitoramento para recuperação tem recebido atenção limitada.[28] A elevação no Spec LPf para valor > 20 mg/ℓ foi associada a um prognóstico pior em gatos hospitalizados com pancreatite. Nenhum dado na literatura indica que elevação maior no Spec LPf esteja associada a uma resposta pior à terapia de gatos com pancreatite crônica, desde que seja realizado tratamento apropriado das comorbidades.

A baixa sensibilidade e especificidade dos testes tradicionais que mensuram as atividades de amilase e lipase para o diagnóstico de pancreatite, em todas as espécies, pode ser parcialmente explicada pela baixa especificidade do substrato para a maioria dos testes catalíticos. Os substratos utilizados nesses testes variam em termos de seletividade para lipase pancreática, com alguns substratos demonstrando seletividade muito maior para a lipase de origem pancreática na circulação. O éster 1-2-o-dilauril-*rac*-glicero-3-ácido glutárico-(6'-metilresorufina) (DGGR) é um substrato da lipase com especificidade relativamente alta para lipase pancreática.[29] Esse teste foi avaliado e validado para gato doméstico.[30] A concordância geral entre os testes de lipase DGGR e Spec LPf foi alta, com coeficiente kappa de Cohen entre 0,60 (concordância moderada) e 0,75 (concordância substancial), em limiares variados aplicados para valores de DGGR-lipase e Spec LPf, para o diagnóstico de pancreatite.[30] Nesse mesmo estudo com 251 gatos com suspeita clínica de pancreatite, constatou-se que a atividade de DGGR-lipase > 26 U/ℓ tinha sensibilidade de 48% e especificidade de 63%, enquanto a Spec LPf > 5,3 mg/ℓ tinha sensibilidade de 57% e especificidade de 63%.[30] Esse estudo sugere que a atividade de DGGR-lipase pode ter alguma utilidade clínica na avaliação de gatos; entretanto, isso seria dependente da utilização do substrato específico em qualquer que seja o sistema analítico utilizado. Informações com relação aos substratos de fato utilizados por vários laboratórios de referência e sistemas bioquímicos de uso domiciliar comumente encontrados na prática veterinária não estão prontamente disponíveis neste momento.

Diagnóstico por imagem

Alterações em radiografias simples que acompanham a pancreatite aguda no gato são semelhantes àquelas descritas em cães, e incluem redução do contraste abdominal, dilatação de alças intestinais e efusão pleural. Esses sinais são sutis, inespecíficos e demonstram baixas sensibilidades (28 a 50% para redução do contraste abdominal, 24 a 42% para dilatação intestinal, 20 a 29% para efusão pleural).[1,12,20,31,32] Em gatos com pancreatite crônica, os achados em radiografias simples não são bem caracterizados.

A disponibilidade crescente de ultrassonografia abdominal de alta resolução em animais de companhia (ver Capítulo 88) melhorou de forma considerável a utilização do diagnóstico por imagem para caracterização da doença pancreática no gato. Nessa espécie, foram descritas a aparência ultrassonográfica do pâncreas normal e alterações compatíveis com doença pancreática (Figura 291.1).[12,32-34] Aumento do volume pancreático, gordura abdominal e mesentérica hiperecoica, alteração da ecogenicidade do parênquima (mais comumente hipoecoico ou com padrão misto), efusão abdominal, cistos ou pseudocistos pancreáticos, corrugação do duodeno e dilatação do ducto pancreático são considerados achados consistentes com pancreatite em gatos com sinais clínicos compatíveis.[12,23,32,35] Ao mesmo tempo em que esses achados são indicadores confiavelmente específicos de doença pancreática, sua sensibilidade para diagnóstico acurado da pancreatite confirmada à histologia é bastante variável, sendo relatada sensibilidade de ≈ 11 a 80%.[12,23,26] A sensibilidade da ultrassonografia abdominal para a detecção da doença pancreática de gatos parece depender bastante do operador.[32] Diversas publicações recentes mencionam pesquisas relativas ao grau de concordância entre os achados de ultrassonografia abdominal e os exames minimamente invasivos específicos do pâncreas (Spec LPf e atividade de DGGR-lipase).[35,36] Dada a variável e a quase sempre baixa sensibilidade da ultrassonografia abdominal para o diagnóstico de pancreatite em gatos, esse exame não pode ser utilizado de forma confiável como um teste de "exclusão" para essa doença. Entretanto, informações significativas adicionais úteis para o tratamento desses casos costumam ser obtidas, sobretudo na triagem de comorbidades, como colangite/colangio-hepatite, ou existência de doenças extrapancreáticas que poderiam explicar os sinais

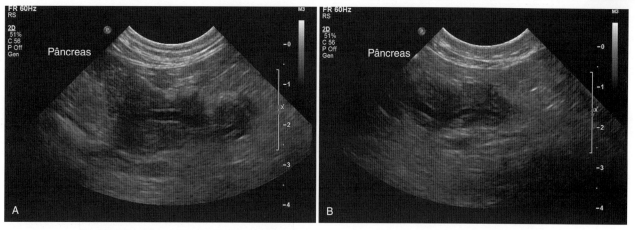

Figura 291.1 Imagens de ultrassonografia abdominal de rotina do pâncreas de um gato atendido com início agudo de letargia, inapetência e febre. O pâncreas está aumentado e hipo a heteroecoico e a gordura mesentérica circundante está hipoecoica. O ducto pancreático está proeminente e com diâmetro aumentado (aproximadamente 4 mm). Esses achados são compatíveis com pancreatite aguda.

clínicos. Dessa forma, a ultrassonografia abdominal, realizada por um operador bem treinado e experiente, é recomendada a todos os gatos nos quais há suspeita clínica de pancreatite.

Relato recente menciona a utilização de ultrassonografia endoscópica em gatos, incluindo grupos-controle saudáveis e gatos com diagnóstico de pancreatite.[37] Embora esse estudo tenha demonstrado que a técnica seja executável no gato, e a visualização de todo o pâncreas tenha parecido melhor pela técnica endoscópica, a ultrassonografia endoscópica não alterou o diagnóstico nessa espécie.

Modalidades de imagem de melhor definição, como a tomografia computadorizada, receberam alguma atenção em gatos com pancreatite.[20,36,38] Nesses estudos, ou a sensibilidade foi baixa, ou não foram apreciadas alterações na aparência pancreática entre os grupos normal e sintomático. A combinação do alto custo da tomografia computadorizada e da necessidade de sedação profunda ou anestesia para esse procedimento influencia sobremaneira a utilização da tomografia computadorizada na avaliação e no diagnóstico de pancreatite no gato.

Biopsia pancreática e histopatologia

Como mencionado anteriormente, a maioria das fontes considera a detecção histológica de inflamação pancreática como o teste diagnóstico padrão-ouro para pancreatite, seja qual for a espécie.[10,24] A biopsia pancreática no gato não é um procedimento comum na rotina clínica veterinária, provavelmente por ser uma abordagem invasiva por celiotomia/laparotomia, bem como pela preocupação contínua de que a manipulação cirúrgica do pâncreas possa resultar em pancreatite pós-cirúrgica.[7] Um estudo retrospectivo recente demonstrou que a biopsia pancreática propicia, em geral, informações úteis do ponto de vista diagnóstico, uma vez que biopsias de 14/19 gatos com suspeita clínica de pancreatite demonstraram, pelo menos, algum grau de anormalidade histológica.[10] Nesse estudo, a pancreatite crônica foi a anormalidade mais comumente detectada em gatos.

Técnicas laparoscópicas para visualização e biopsia de órgãos abdominais, incluindo o pâncreas, são menos invasivas do que a laparotomia exploratória, e demonstraram ser seguras em gatos clinicamente sadios (ver Capítulo 91).[39,40] Um estudo retrospectivo recente relatou que somente 9/13 gatos submetidos à laparoscopia para avaliação de sinais compatíveis com pancreatite foram, de fato, submetidos à biopsia pancreática, ainda que no mesmo relato não se tenham constatado complicações pós-cirúrgicas (n = 31 casos).[7] Em relato mais recente,[10] complicações pós-cirúrgicas foram observadas em 10/43 cães e gatos após biopsia cirúrgica do pâncreas; 5/10 casos demonstraram sinais de pancreatite pós-cirúrgica. Em gatos, 3/19 animais demonstraram alguma evidência de sinais pós-cirúrgicos que poderiam ser considerados sugestivos de pancreatite.

Ao mesmo tempo em que a biopsia cirúrgica de pâncreas de gatos é subutilizada e a taxa de complicações relatadas na literatura até o momento baixa sejam argumentos para o uso mais frequente dessa modalidade, alguns pontos fracos da biopsia pancreática precisam ser reconhecidos. No cão, lesões pancreáticas costumam apresentar distribuição irregular, sendo necessárias múltiplas amostras obtidas por biopsia para que essa técnica propicie resultado mais útil.[9] Embora estudos semelhantes não tenham sido publicados em gatos, é razoável assumir que a distribuição de lesões pancreáticas pode ser semelhantemente irregular nessa espécie, e a avaliação de uma única amostra obtida por biopsia (comum em caso de biopsia por laparoscopia) pode resultar em achados falso-negativos. Mesmo utilizando técnica laparoscópica, a biopsia cirúrgica do pâncreas é invasiva e cara, com a necessidade de equipamento especializado, além de habilidade. A biopsia cirúrgica requer anestesia, o que pode ser um alto risco em pacientes hemodinamicamente instáveis com quadro clínico mais grave; portanto, a maior utilização desse procedimento provavelmente seja em gatos com pancreatite crônica.[7,24,40]

ABORDAGEM TERAPÊUTICA EM GATO COM SUSPEITA DE PANCREATITE

Uma abordagem racional para avaliação inicial, planejamento terapêutico e manejo de um gato com suspeita de pancreatite é apresentada na Figura 291.2. Já que a pancreatite "aguda" necrosante e a pancreatite não necrosante "crônica" do gato não podem ser distinguidas com base em achados clínicos, exame de imagem abdominal, exames bioquímicos ou resultados de testes pancreáticos específicos, e a biopsia pancreática é ainda um procedimento relativamente incomum, a etapa inicial necessária ao diagnóstico desses casos é a avaliação do estado clínico geral do paciente e a gravidade aparente da doença. Gatos com suspeita de pancreatite atendidos com dor abdominal intensa, taquipneia, taquicardia, febre importante, colapso ou outra evidência de síndrome inflamatória sistêmica ou choque circulatório devem ser considerados portadores de doença grave necessitando, portanto, de cuidado hospitalar imediato e intensivo. A existência de diversas anormalidades nos exames bioquímicos de triagem, sobretudo hipoalbuminemia e hipocalcemia, é um forte indicativo de doença grave com risco à vida do paciente.[11] Gatos atendidos com perda de peso, hiporexia, êmese ocasional e letargia, mas sem evidências imediatas

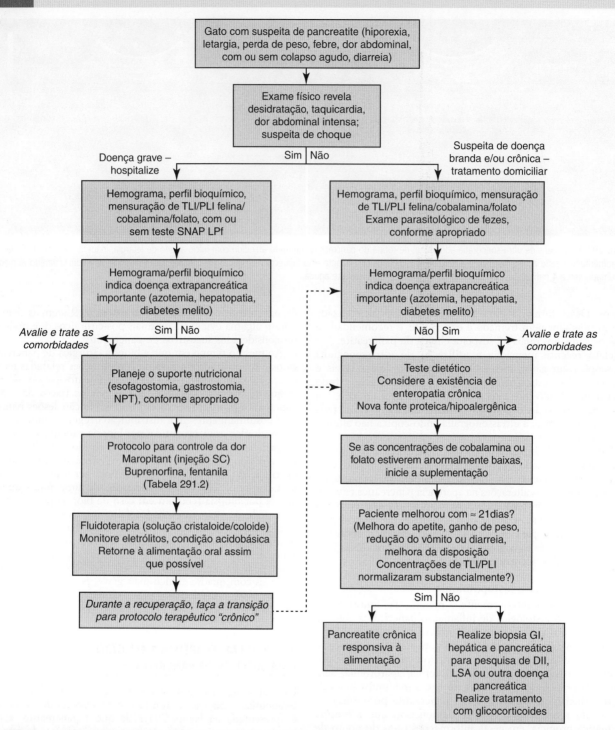

Figura 291.2 Protocolo terapêutico e manejo de gato com suspeita de pancreatite. *DII*, doença intestinal inflamatória; *GI*, gastrintestinal; *LSA*, linfoma; *NPT*, nutrição parenteral total; *PLI*, lipase pancreática específica; *SC*, subcutânea; *TLI*, imunorreatividade semelhante à tripsina.

de comprometimento hemodinâmico significativo, são considerados portadores de doença menos grave, provavelmente crônica, e são tratados no ambiente domiciliar.

Gatos com doença grave necessitam terapia intensiva, incluindo fluidoterapia (ver Capítulo 129), analgesia efetiva (ver Capítulo 126) e planejamento precoce de suporte nutricional (ver Capítulos 82 e 189), dado o risco de lipidose hepática acompanhada de comorbidade. Os objetivos do tratamento consistem em repor a volemia, restaurar e manter a perfusão em órgãos-alvo (particularmente o pâncreas, já que a isquemia pancreática é um tem um papel importante no desenvolvimento de pancreatite necrosante[13]) e restaurar e manter a pressão oncótica coloidal plasmática.

Em geral, soluções coloides, como amidos sintéticos à base de hidroxietil, são benéficas na reanimação inicial desses pacientes. Também pode ser utilizado plasma fresco congelado de gato, o que provavelmente propicia suporte oncótico ao mesmo tempo em que repõe proteínas que participam na cascata de coagulação (ver Capítulo 130); entretanto, existem poucas informações na literatura veterinária com relação à utilização do plasma em casos de pancreatite grave em gatos. Em nossa clínica, costumamos utilizar nesses gatos uma combinação de soluções coloides sintéticas e soluções cristaloides para reanimação inicial e manutenção da volemia. Nesses gatos, deve-se prever a ocorrência de anormalidades eletrolíticas relevantes, sobretudo hipopotassemia e hipocalcemia.[2,11] A suplementação

CAPÍTULO 291 • Pancreatite em Gatos: Diagnóstico e Tratamento

com potássio é administrada em combinação com soluções cristaloides, após diretrizes rotineiras para concentrações baseadas em determinações seriadas das concentrações séricas de potássio (ver Capítulos 68 e 129).

Analgesia efetiva e controle do vômito são importantes aspectos do tratamento da pancreatite grave em todas as espécies, inclusive em gatos. Uma seleção de medicamentos frequentemente úteis no tratamento de pancreatite em gatos está resumida na Tabela 291.2. Em geral, o controle da dor por narcóticos é indicado a gatos com pancreatite suficientemente grave que justifique hospitalização. Adesivo transdérmico de fentanila (25 µg/h) pode ser muito efetivo para analgesia mais prolongada (até 72 horas), sem necessidade de manuseio frequente e injeções nesses pacientes, mas é necessário tratamento inicial com um medicamento injetável ou de uso sublingual (comumente buprenorfina), já que pode demorar até 12 horas para que seja obtida concentração terapêutica de fentanila.[2] O maropitant, um antagonista do receptor neuroquinase-1, é um efetivo antiemético e

Tabela 291.2 — Medicamentos mais utilizados no tratamento de gatos com pancreatite.

CLASSE	FÁRMACO	MECANISMO	PRINCIPAL INDICAÇÃO	DOSE E VIA	NOTAS SOBRE ADMINISTRAÇÃO
Analgésico	Buprenorfina	Opioide	Aguda grave	0,01 a 0,02 mg/kg SC IM IV, TM	Agonista/antagonista misto
	Fentanila	Opioide	Aguda grave	Adesivo transdérmico: 25 µg/h 5 µg/kg *bolus* IV, TIC 2 a 4 µg/kg/h	Ajuste a dose até fazer efeito; inicie com doses baixas em pacientes críticos
	Butorfanol	Opioide	Aguda grave	0,1 a 0,5 mg/kg SC IM IV	
Antiemético Antináuseas	Maropitant	Antagonista de receptor neurocinina-1	Aguda grave Crônica	1 mg/kg/24 h SC 1 mg/kg/24 h VO	Também propicia alguma analgesia. Pode ser útil no tratamento domiciliar de doença crônica agudizada
	Dolasetrona, ondansetrona	Antagonista de receptor 5-HT$_3$	Aguda grave	0,8 a 1 mg/kg/24 h IV	Pode-se usar em combinação com maropitant, metoclopramida
	Metoclopramida	Antagonista de receptor dopaminérgico D$_2$	Aguda grave	0,2 a 0,5 mg/kg VO SC, IM, a cada 6 a 8 h 1 a 2 mg/kg/24 h TIC	Uso recomendado na forma de TIC, em pacientes críticos
Supressor de acidez gástrica	Omeprazol	Inibidor da bomba de prótons	Aguda grave	1 a 1,3 mg/kg/12 h VO	Em gatos, é necessária a administração a cada 12 h para controle efetivo do pH gástrico[48,49]
	Pantoprazol	Inibidor da bomba de prótons	Aguda grave	0,7 a 1 mg/kg/12 h IV	Útil em pacientes nos quais o vômito não está controlado
	Ranitidina	Antagonista de receptor histamínico H$_2$	Aguda grave	3,5 mg/kg/12 h VO	Utilizado principalmente por sua ação procinética, NÃO como supressor efetivo de ácido, em gatos
Anti-inflamatórios	Prednisolona, prednisona	Glicocorticoide	Crônica	2 a 4 mg/kg/dia VO, reduzindo a dose em 0,5 mg/kg a cada 14 dias	Ajuste a dose até obter a menor dose efetiva. A resistência insulínica pode limitar a utilidade em gatos diabéticos/pré-diabéticos. Vários gatos apresentam baixa resposta à prednisona (inefetiva)
	Ciclosporina A	Inibição da calcineurina	Crônica	5 mg/kg VO, a cada 12 a 24 h	Utilize em pacientes mal controlados ou naqueles com histórico de diabetes melito
	Clorambucila	Fármaco alquilante	Crônica	0,1 a 0,2 mg/kg/dia VO, ou 0,15 a 0,3 mg/kg/72 h VO	Utilize em pacientes mal controlados ou naqueles com histórico de diabetes melito. Monitore quanto à possibilidade de mielossupressão. Ajuste a dose até obter a mínima efetiva durante vários meses
Estimulantes do apetite	Mirtazapina	Antidepressivo tricíclico	Aguda grave Crônica	3,75 mg/gato/72 h VO	Dose representa um quarto de um comprimido de 15 mg
	Cipro-heptadina	Antagonista de receptor histamínico H$_1$ e 5 HT	Crônica	1 a 4 mg/gato/dia VO	Eficácia questionável

IM, via intramuscular; *IV*, via intravenosa; *SC*, via subcutânea; *TIC*, taxa de infusão IV constante; *TM*, transmucosa; *VO*, via oral.

SEÇÃO 20 • Doenças Pancreáticas

possui efeitos antinociceptivos nas vísceras.[41] A combinação de maropitant com um antagonista de receptor 5-HT$_3$, como a ondansetrona ou a dolasetrona (Tabela 291.2), propicia controle efetivo de êmese e náuseas nesses pacientes, com necessidade mínima de manuseios repetidos durante o dia.

As comorbidades extrapancreáticas, particularmente doenças hepáticas e diabetes melito devem ser pesquisadas e tratadas de maneira apropriada, inclusive com reintrodução precoce da alimentação, conforme apropriado. Embora existam dados limitados disponíveis com relação a gatos e nutrição enteral precoce em casos de pancreatite grave, nossa experiência clínica diz que ela costuma ser bem tolerada e benéfica. Tanto em seres humanos como em cães, existem cada vez mais evidências de que o retorno precoce à nutrição enteral está associado a melhor recuperação, menor tempo de hospitalização e baixa frequência de efeitos colaterais.[42-44]

Gatos com suspeita clínica de pancreatite crônica são tratados basicamente da mesma maneira que aqueles com enteropatia crônica ou doença intestinal inflamatória (ver Capítulo 276).

Não há como distinguir pancreatite crônica, como uma enfermidade solitária, de doença inflamatória multissistêmica (denominada doença inflamatória felina ou "triadite").[5,45] Inicialmente, recomenda-se a modificação dietética, com a utilização de uma nova fonte de proteína ou dieta hipoalergênica. Ao contrário de cães, nos quais a restrição de gordura é fundamental para o controle da maioria dos casos de pancreatite crônica, o mesmo não aplica aos gatos, devido às altas necessidades constitutivas para o ácido aracdônico.[46,47] Muitos respondem à modificação da dieta; para aqueles que não, é de bom senso usar tratamento anti-inflamatório ou imunomodulador, considerando que não há nenhuma outra comorbidade que contraindicaria a utilização desses medicamentos.

REFERÊNCIAS BIBLIOGRÁFICAS

As referências bibliográficas deste capítulo se encontram online no Ambiente de Aprendizagem.

CAPÍTULO 292

Insuficiência Pancreática Exócrina

Jörg M. Steiner

INTRODUÇÃO E DEFINIÇÃO

A insuficiência pancreática exócrina (IPE) consiste em uma síndrome caracterizada pela síntese e secreção insuficientes de enzimas digestivas pelo pâncreas exócrino. A causa mais comum de IPE é a ausência absoluta de células acinares pancreáticas devido à destruição de células acinares, na pancreatite crônica (tanto em cães quanto em gatos) ou à depleção de células acinares devido à atrofia acinar pancreática (cães). Em ambos os casos, há carência de todas as enzimas digestivas pancreáticas. Em raros casos, pode haver falta de uma única enzima, que, mesmo se total, costuma não causar sinais clínicos. Entretanto, a deficiência isolada de lipase pancreática foi relatada como causa de sinais clínicos de IPE em seres humanos e em um cão.[1,2] Outra causa infrequente de IPE é a obstrução do ducto pancreático, seja por um tumor, seja por lesão cirúrgica, condição que pode levar à ausência de enzimas digestivas no lúmen do intestino delgado, apesar da produção acinar normal. Hipoplasia ou aplasia pancreática também pode causar sinais clínicos de IPE. Pode haver tal suspeita quando o paciente é diagnostica com essa condição em uma idade muito jovem (Figuras 292.1 e 292.2), mas até o momento nenhum caso foi demonstrado de forma conclusiva em filhote de cão ou gato.

ETIOLOGIA

Em cães e gatos, a causa mais comum de IPE é pancreatite crônica, que supostamente é o motivo dessa insuficiência em quase 100% dos gatos e em aproximadamente 50% dos cães, nos quais os outros cerca de 50% de casos se devem à atrofia acinar pancreática (AAP), que costuma ser observada de maneira exclusiva em cães das raças Pastor-Alemão, Rough-Coated Collie e Eurasiana.[3,4] Diversos estudos sugerem que a AAP é uma anormalidade hereditária autossômica recessiva no cão Pastor-Alemão e, também, no cão Eurasiano.[5-7] Entretanto, a busca por um marcador genético para essa doença não foi bem-sucedida, embora o sequenciamento de todo o genoma canino com a utilização de um conjunto de marcadores microssatélites e variantes genéticas SNPs (*single nucleotide polimorphisms*), tenha revelado diversas regiões que parecem estar associadas a essa condição.[8] De forma interessante, um estudo de acasalamento de um macho Pastor-Alemão com uma fêmea igualmente acometidos resultou apenas em 2 filhotes acometidos de uma ninhada de 6 animais, sugerindo fortemente indício contra a herdabilidade como uma característica autossômica recessiva simples.[9] Assim, é provável que essa condição seja poligênica.[10]

PATOGÊNESE

Enzimas digestivas ou pré-formas inativas de enzimas digestivas (*i. e.*, zimogênios) que participam da digestão de todos os principais componentes alimentares são secretadas por células acinares pancreáticas. Na ausência dessas células, seja qual for a causa, ocorre má digestão. Entretanto, é importante ressaltar que o trato gastrintestinal (GI) é altamente redundante e que há, em geral, mais de uma enzima digestiva para a mesma função digestiva. Por exemplo, a lipase pancreática é fundamental para a digestão de gordura, mas o estômago também sintetiza e secreta lipase gástrica, que é responsável por uma fração significativa da digestão normal de gordura, no cão.[11] Além disso, em termos fisiológicos, o pâncreas exócrino possui uma grande capacidade de reserva, e estimou-se que os sinais clínicos de IPE somente surgem quando há perda de mais de 90% da função pancreática exócrina.

A má digestão leva à presença de componentes alimentares não digeridos no lúmen intestinal, o que pode causar diarreia, proliferação de microbiota do intestino delgado e perda de peso.

Entretanto, suspeita-se que os sinais clínicos não ocorram somente devido à má digestão, mas que a IPE também ocasione má absorção. Essa teoria surgiu devido à ausência de fatores tróficos normalmente secretados pelo pâncreas exócrino que ajudam a manter a normalidade da mucosa GI.

O pâncreas exócrino também é a principal fonte de fator intrínseco em cães e gatos.[3] Em acentuado contraste com seres humanos, nos quais o fator intrínseco é secretado, sobretudo, pela mucosa gástrica, em cães e gatos o fator intrínseco se origina, em especial, no pâncreas exócrino (ver Capítulo 271).[12] Em um estudo, verificou-se que 82% dos cães com IPE apresentavam diminuição da concentração sérica de cobalamina, 36% dos quais com hipocobalaminemia marcante.[13] Todos os gatos com IPE mencionados na literatura apresentavam hipocobalaminemia.[14-16]

MANIFESTAÇÃO CLÍNICA

A IPE pode ser subclínica; duas grandes séries de casos relativos a cães da raça Pastor-Alemão detectaram vários animais com diminuição marcante no valor da imunorreatividade semelhante à tripsina (TLI), no soro sanguíneo, sem quaisquer sinais clínicos.[7,17] Alguns dos cães foram submetidos à laparotomia exploratória e notou-se que a massa tecidual pancreática estava intensamente diminuída.[17] O sinal clínico mais comum relatado em cães e gatos com IPE é perda de peso (Figuras 292.3 e 292.4).[15,18] Fezes amolecidas também costumam ser observadas (Figura 292.5), mas diarreia líquida é bastante incomum.[15,18] Muitas vezes, os pacientes possuem pelame de má qualidade e relata-se que os cães com IPE apresentam borborigmos e maior flatulência.[18] Vários cães e gatos com IPE manifestam aumento do apetite; os cães podem até mesmo manifestar coprofagia ou pica.[18] Em gatos, pode-se notar sujidades oleosas no pelame da região perineal, o que não é um achado comum.[15]

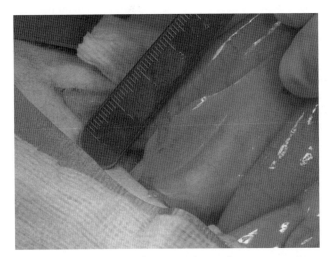

Figura 292.1 Suspeita de hipoplasia pancreática. A figura mostra o pâncreas de um gato diagnosticado com insuficiência pancreática exócrina em idade muito jovem (menos de 3 meses), durante castração de rotina. Note que o pâncreas parece extremamente pequeno, sugerindo atrofia ou hipoplasia pancreática.

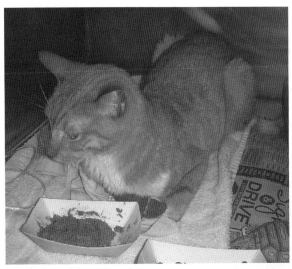

Figura 292.3 A fotografia mostra Theo, um gato castrado com 4 anos de idade, diagnosticado com insuficiência pancreática exócrina (IPE). Note a aparência magra dele. (Cortesia de Dr. Kenneth Jones, Jones Animal Hospital, Santa Mônica, Califórnia; Reimpressa de Steiner JM: Exocrine pancreatic insufficiency. In August JR, editor: *Consultations in feline internal medicine*, St. Louis, 2010, Saunders Elsevier, p. 225-231.)

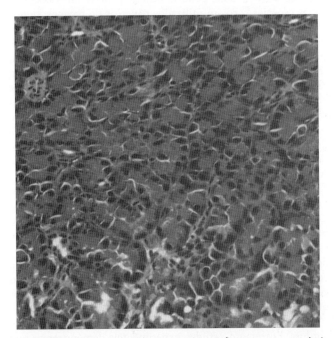

Figura 292.2 Suspeita de hipoplasia pancreática. A figura mostra a aparência histopatológica do pâncreas de um gato diagnosticado com insuficiência pancreática exócrina em idade muito jovem. Note que a estrutura acinar parece normal e não há evidência de inflamação ou de fibrose, sugerindo hipoplasia pancreática. (*Esta figura se encontra reproduzida em cores no Encarte.*)

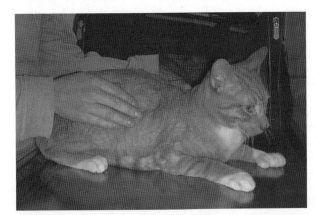

Figura 292.4 Gato com insuficiência pancreática exócrina tratado. Essa figura mostra Theo, o gato da Figura 292.3, 2 meses após o início da terapia de reposição enzimática. Durante esse período, Theo havia ganhado quase 1,3 kg e, segundo relatos, estava mais ativo. (Cortesia de Dr. Kenneth Jones, Jones Animal Hospital, Santa Mônica, Califórnia; Reimpressa de Steiner JM: Exocrine pancreatic insufficiency. In August JR, editor: *Consultations in feline internal medicine*, St. Louis, 2010, Saunders Elsevier, p. 225-231.)

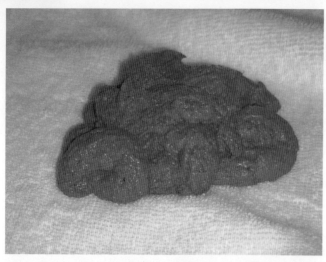

Figura 292.5 Grande amostra de fezes de gato com insuficiência pancreática exócrina (IPE) (paciente mostrado na Figura 292.3). Note a consistência amolecida e a coloração marrom-clara típicas. Além disso, a amostra de fezes parece conter partículas de alimento não digeridas. (Cortesia de Dr. Kenneth Jones, Jones Animal Hospital, Santa Mônica, Califórnia; Reimpressa de Steiner JM: Exocrine pancreatic insufficiency. In August JR, editor: *Consultations in feline internal medicine*, St. Louis, 2010, Saunders Elsevier, p. 225-231.) (*Esta figura se encontra reproduzida em cores no Encarte.*)

DIAGNÓSTICO

A mensuração de de TLI sérica é o teste diagnóstico de escolha para cães e gatos com suspeita de IPE. A concentração sérica é aferida por um teste espécie-específico para TLI, que mensura as concentrações de tripsinogênio catiônico, tripsina catiônica e algumas moléculas de tripsina catiônica ligadas a moléculas inibidoras de proteinases. Sob condições fisiológicas, somente uma pequena quantidade de tripsinogênio sintetizado pelas células acinares pancreáticas é liberada no compartimento vascular. Como tripsinogênio e tripsina são moléculas bastante pequenas, elas são rapidamente excretadas pelos rins. Portanto, somente se houver funcionamento normal do pâncreas é que uma pequena quantidade de tripsinogênio pode ser detectada no soro (Vídeo 292.1). Ao contrário, em pacientes com IPE, seja qual for a causa, a quantidade de tripsinogênio liberada na circulação sanguínea encontra-se acentuadamente diminuída (valores de corte atuais para o diagnóstico de IPE: 2,5 µg/ℓ, em cães, e 8 µg/ℓ, em gatos) ou indetectáveis (ver Vídeo 292.1). De forma geral, a TLI sérica é altamente sensível e específica para o diagnóstico de IPE em cães e gatos. Entretanto, há dois cenários especiais, em que a TLI sérica pode estar normal, mesmo no paciente com IPE. O primeiro cenário é a deficiência exclusiva de lipase pancreática, descrita em um cão.[2] A segunda situação em que a concentração de TLI sérica pode estar normal em um paciente com IPE é a obstrução de ducto pancreático. Tais casos ainda não foram descritos na literatura, com a identificação de um único cão com essa enfermidade (Hill S, comunicação pessoal, 2007).

Existem outros testes recomendados para a avaliação da função pancreática exócrina, incluindo o teste de turbidez plasmática, o teste do ácido para-amino benzoico e a atividade proteolítica fecal; entretanto, nenhum deles é considerado útil no diagnóstico de IPE em cães e gatos.[19,20] Além disso, há um exame de fezes para mensuração de elastase pancreática atualmente comercializado na Europa. Estudos iniciais mostraram sensibilidade e especificidade aceitáveis do teste, mas o valor preditivo positivo estimado foi menor que 60%.[21,22] Em outro, a concentração fecal de elastase mostrou estar associada a uma alta taxa de resultados falso-positivos (23%) no teste.[23] Assim, o diagnóstico de IPE com base na concentração fecal de elastase acentuadamente diminuída deve ser comprovado pela aferição da concentração sérica de TLI, a fim de evitar um diagnóstico errôneo de IPE.

TRATAMENTO

A reposição de enzimas pancreáticas é a base do tratamento de IPE.[24,25] A reposição de enzimas pancreáticas pode ser feita por meio de diversas opções.[26] O extrato pancreático desidratado obtido do pâncreas de suínos é, de longe, o meio mais comum e efetivo de reposição de enzimas pancreáticas. A terapia é iniciada com 1 colher de chá de extrato desidratado para cada 10 kg de peso corporal na refeição. Assim que o paciente tiver respondido por completo à terapia, a dose pode ser gradativamente diminuída, até obter a dose mínima efetiva. É importante ressaltar que a atividade enzimática do produto pode variar de lote para lote, com a variação discreta da dose mínima efetiva com o passar do tempo. Enzimas pancreáticas também estão disponíveis na forma de comprimidos e cápsulas, mas estudos em seres humanos e cães demonstraram que o pó é preferível a outras formulações.[25,27] Complicações da suplementação enzimática são raras, mas um estudo relatou que 3 de 25 cães tratados com suplementos de enzimas pancreáticas desenvolveram hemorragia oral.[28] Quando dessa ocorrência, deve-se avaliar o perfil de coagulação, a fim de excluir a possibilidade de coagulopatia responsiva à vitamina K, condição relatada em dois gatos com IPE.[29] No caso de perfil de coagulação normal, a dose de enzimas pancreáticas deve ser diminuída. Dois cães do estudo citado anteriormente continuaram bem após a diminuição da dose, mas em um deles ocorreu recidiva dos sinais clínicos.[28] Se o paciente se recusar a consumir o pó pancreático misturado à alimentação ou no raro caso de alergia alimentar ao pó pancreático de origem suína, pode-se utilizar pâncreas fresco cru de várias espécies.[25] Foram utilizados pâncreas de bovinos, suínos, ovinos e de animais de caça. Aproximadamente 30 a 90 gramas de pâncreas cru substituem 1 colher de chá de extrato pancreático desidratado. O pâncreas deve ser cortado em pedaços finos, fracionados em porções suficientes para uma refeição e imediatamente congelado. O tecido pancreático congelado permanece com sua atividade enzimática durante longo período. Questões foram levantadas sobre a potencial ameaça de contaminação do pâncreas cru congelado. Em teoria, o consumo de pâncreas cru de bovinos e ovinos implica o risco de transmissão de encefalopatia espongiforme bovina, ao passo que o pâncreas cru de suínos, o risco de transmissão de pseudorraiva (doença de Aujeszky). Entretanto, esse risco é mais ou menos acadêmico, já que o pó pancreático desidratado pode ter exatamente o mesmo perigo. O pâncreas de animais de caça e de ovinos pode estar infestado por *Echinococcus* spp., podendo esse parasita potencialmente causar doença relevante e até mesmo morte. Esse risco deve, dessa forma, ser discutido com o tutor antes do início da terapia com pâncreas cru dessas fontes. A pré-incubação do alimento com extrato pancreático não parece ser necessária para obter uma resposta terapêutica.

Alguns autores recomendam uma dieta com baixo teor de gordura. Entretanto, estudos experimentais demonstraram que a digestibilidade da gordura em cães tratados com suplementos pancreáticos não retorna ao normal, sugerindo que a restrição de gordura somente aumentaria o risco de deficiências de vitaminas lipossolúveis e ácidos graxos essenciais.[30] Um estudo não demonstrou nenhum benefício da alimentação com dietas com restrição de gordura em cães com IPE.[13] Além disso, dois outros não revelaram efeito significativo da dieta na eficácia terapêutica em cães com IPE.[31,32] Portanto, o autor acredita que uma dieta de manutenção de alta qualidade seria a melhor indicação. Entretanto, dietas com alto conteúdo de fibras devem ser evitadas, já que podem interferir na absorção de gordura.

Como mencionado anteriormente, vários pacientes com IPE possuem deficiência de cobalamina e, dessa forma, todo cão e gato com IPE deve ser avaliado em busca de possível deficiência de cobalamina. Embora a mensuração da concentração sérica de cobalamina não propicie uma estimativa do conteúdo de cobalamina em nível celular, a mensuração do ácido metilmalônico (AMM) no soro é mais cara e somente disponível em alguns locais; assim, a mensuração da concentração sérica de cobalamina é considerada o exame de rotina para avaliação da concentração de cobalamina em cães e gatos. Com base nas aferições de cobalamina e AMM em grande número de cães e gatos, atualmente recomenda-se suplementar qualquer paciente com IPE, caso apresente concentração sérica de cobalamina inferior a 400 ng/ℓ. Tradicionalmente, a cobalamina é suplementada por meio de injeções semanais de cianocobalamina (250 μg em gatos e 250 a 1.500 μg em cães, baseadas no peso corporal aproximado) por via subcutânea. Em casos raros, utiliza-se hidroxocobalamina. As doses são administradas semanalmente, durante 6 semanas, e então uma dose adicional após 1 mês, com reavaliação da concentração sérica de cobalamina depois de 1 mês. Existem alguns dados preliminares que podem sugerir que a suplementação oral diária é igualmente efetiva, o que precisa ser comprovado por estudo prospectivo antes de utilizar essa modalidade terapêutica de modo rotineiro.[33] Vários pacientes com IPE tratados de maneira apropriada apresentam concentração sérica de cobalamina normal ou até mesmo acima do normal no momento da reavaliação, com a descontinuação da suplementação com cobalamina, mas vários outros requerem suplementação por toda a vida. Demostrou-se diminuição das concentrações séricas da maioria das vitaminas lipossolúveis em cães com IPE, o que também pode ser considerado no caso dos gatos.[31] Entretanto, a suplementação sistemática com vitaminas lipossolúveis não foi pesquisada nesses pacientes, podendo a suplementação excessiva causar efeitos colaterais. Relatos anedóticos de suplementação com vitamina E (400 a 500 UI/24 h VO durante 1 mês) estão disponíveis, mas o efeito benéfico de tal terapia ainda não foi avaliado.

Vários pacientes com IPE respondem bem à terapia de reposição enzimática e suplementação com cobalamina, se indicada. Entretanto, alguns podem não responder de maneira adequada à terapia-padrão. Causas potenciais de falhas no tratamento devem ser avaliadas. O tipo, a formulação e a dose do suplemento enzimático devem ser revisados; se houver qualquer suspeita de que a reposição enzimática possa ser insuficiente, o protocolo deve ser ajustado de acordo. Além disso, pacientes devem ser avaliados em busca de doenças concomitantes, como doença intestinal inflamatória (ver Capítulo 276), diabetes melito (ver Capítulos 304 e 305) ou disbiose de intestino delgado (ver Capítulo 276). Se não houver evidências de nenhuma doença concomitante, pode-se tentar um teste terapêutico com um fármaco antimicrobiano. O tratamento de escolha envolve a administração de tilosina (Tylan® – pó, na dose de 25 mg/kg/12 h VO, durante 6 a 8 semanas), mas outros antibióticos, como metronidazol, também podem ser utilizados.

Caso os pacientes ainda não tenham respondido ao tratamento, pode-se tentar a terapia antiácida. Uma grande parte da lipase pancreática suplementada por via oral é irreversivelmente destruída pelo baixo pH gástrico.[34] O aumento do pH no estômago faz com que essa perda da enzima possa ser diminuída, obtendo-se melhor resposta terapêutica. Entretanto, deve-se ressaltar que, ao mesmo tempo em que o aumento do pH gástrico reduz a quantidade de lipase pancreática destruída durante a passagem pelo estômago, também aumenta a quantidade de lipase gástrica destruída e o resultado pode não levar a uma alteração significativa na digestibilidade de gordura. Entretanto, pode-se tentar um teste com omeprazol, na dose de 0,7 a 1 mg/kg/12 h, VO, que pode causar melhora significativa.

Se nenhuma dessas medidas levar ao controle dos sinais clínicos, a diminuição do conteúdo de gordura na dieta pode ser efetiva. Entretanto, como mencionado anteriormente, a alimentação com dieta com baixo teor de gordura pode estar associada a complicações, devendo ser utilizada somente como último recurso.

PROGNÓSTICO

Tradicionalmente, a IPE foi considerada uma condição vitalícia, já que se considera que as células acinares pancreáticas não se regeneram. Entretanto, existem dados experimentais que podem sugerir alguma capacidade regenerativa dessas células.[35] Além disso, há relatos anedóticos isolados de pacientes com IPE que melhoraram e não precisaram mais de suplementação enzimática. Um estudo avaliou fatores prognósticos para cães com IPE.[13] Nele, o único fator associado a prognóstico ruim foi a acentuada hipocobalaminemia, com sobrevida média de 1.346 dias, comparada a de 2.709 dias (p = 0,012) de cães sem hipocobalaminemia marcante.[13] De forma geral, a maioria dos cães e gatos com IPE pode ser tratada com sucesso, com qualidade e expectativa de vida normais.

REFERÊNCIAS BIBLIOGRÁFICAS

As referências bibliográficas deste capítulo se encontram online no Ambiente de Aprendizagem.

CAPÍTULO 293

Neoplasia do Pâncreas Exócrino

Peter Bennett

INCIDÊNCIA E ORIGEM

A ocorrência de tumores do pâncreas exócrino, em geral detectados em cães idosos, pode ser maior em cadelas da raça Airedale Terrier.[1-5] Em geral, a prevalência de carcinoma pancreático tem sido variavelmente descrita como incomum a rara.[1,3,6-10] Taxas estimadas de cerca de 18 e 12 por 100 mil pacientes em idade de risco foram relatadas em cães e gatos, respectivamente.[5] Hiperplasia benigna e adenomas são incomuns, de pouca relevância clínica e mais frequentemente descritos como um achado incidental em exames pós-morte, em gatos.[4,8,11-13]

O carcinoma pancreático é uma das causas mais comuns de morte relacionada com câncer em pessoas e mostrou pouca melhora nos resultados nos últimos 40 anos.[14] Tumores do pâncreas exócrino malignos se originam em ductos pancreáticos ou estruturas acinares. Em cães, os tumores do pâncreas exócrino malignos possuem, em geral, origem acinar, enquanto em homens (e possivelmente em gatos) eles são mais frequentemente oriundos dos ductos.[4,10,12,15,16] Alguns tumores possuem características teciduais acinares e ductais.[17] Estudos demonstraram que células de carcinomas pancreáticos exibem tamanha plasticidade que a origem não pode ser prontamente determinada por meio de exame histológico de rotina.[18,19] Células neoplásicas pancreáticas mistas, com características exócrinas e endócrinas, foram relatadas em cães e gatos.[20,21] Carcinossarcoma foi diagnosticado em um gato.[22]

ETIOLOGIA E FISIOPATOLOGIA

Em cães ou gatos, não se identificou uma causa etiológica para neoplasias pancreáticas, mas a injeção do carcinógeno metilnitronitrosoguanidina em ductos pancreáticos de cães normais levou ao desenvolvimento de carcinoma do pâncreas exócrino.[23] Em pessoas, relata-se associação entre a ocorrência dessa neoplasia com dieta com alto teor de gordura, tabagismo, alcoolismo, pancreatite crônica e exposição a carcinógenos industriais ou quimioterapia com fármacos alquilantes.[24,25] Casos da neoplasia com doenças neoplásicas e inflamatórias concomitantes são relatados.[25] Um gato jovem da raça Bengal com pseudocistos pancreáticos desenvolveu carcinoma do pâncreas exócrino dentro de 6 meses.[26] O início precoce de carcinoma do pâncreas exócrino foi relatado em dois cães da raça Collie Cinza com hematopoese cíclica, mas a relação entre as duas condições é desconhecida.[27] Mutações K-ras foram identificadas em pessoas e cães com câncer do pâncreas exócrino.[28-30]

Embora o comportamento biológico dos carcinomas pancreáticos possa ser variável, eles costumam ser agressivos, com invasão local e metástases detectadas no momento do diagnóstico.[1,2,10,12,31] Duodeno, linfonodos regionais, fígado e pulmões são os locais mais comuns de metástases.[8] A carcinomatose abdominal provavelmente surge da disseminação direta de células cancerígenas na cavidade peritoneal.[32] A maioria dos relatos de caso descreve progressão rápida desde o momento do diagnóstico, mas há exceções.[33] Uma série de cães com uma variante hialinizante do carcinoma pancreático teve melhores resultados do que os comumente relatados; um cão com doença metastática no momento do diagnóstico sobreviveu 15 meses sem tratamento.[34] A agressividade do carcinoma do pâncreas exócrino e a resistência dele à terapia parecem associadas, em parte, à rede vascular limitada, que contribui para hipoxia e escasso suprimento de nutrientes. Uma complexa reprogramação de vias metabólicas possibilita que a célula cancerígena sobreviva. A tentativa de almejar tais vias desreguladas pode propiciar um meio de melhorar a recuperação do paciente (ver Capítulo 338).[14]

SINAIS CLÍNICOS E EXAME FÍSICO

Pacientes com neoplasia do pâncreas exócrino manifestam uma ampla variedade de sintomas.[13,35] Sinais clínicos vagos e inespecíficos incluem redução do apetite, perda de peso, diarreia e desconforto abdominal. Alguns animais apresentam sintomas compatíveis com pancreatite aguda: náuseas, êmese, anorexia e dor abdominal (ver Capítulos 290 e 291).[9,12,36-40] Pode-se notar efusão abdominal.[40] Dor, comum em pessoas, não é um sinal proeminente em cães ou gatos.[16] A duração dos sintomas pode variar de dias a meses.[13,35]

Gatos podem apresentar alopecia extensa, mais evidente na parte ventral do abdome, mas, algumas vezes, pode envolver os membros e as patas; tal alopecia paraneoplásica foi observada em outras neoplasias internas (ver Capítulo 352).[41-45] Metástases ósseas são incomuns, mas, havendo, podem causar dor ou claudicação.[38] Esteatite necrosante multifocal foi relatada em alguns cães e em um gato, ocasionando múltiplas massas teciduais subcutâneas, febre e fístulas drenantes.[46,47] Há relatos de poliúria e polidipsia secundárias à hipercalcemia paraneoplásica; um cão desenvolveu lesão metastática na hipófise, levando a diabetes insípido central.[48,49] Dois cães, um com adenoma e o outro com carcinoma, tiveram uma combinação de paniculite, poliartrite e osteomielite.[50]

Em geral, animais com adenoma pancreático não manifestam sinais clínicos, a menos que o tumor cause ascite, se estiver ocasionando obstrução, ou, em gatos, que possa ser grande o suficiente para ser palpado.[51] Carcinomas pancreáticos também podem ser palpáveis.[52] A dor é variável e não observada com tanta frequência como em pessoas.[53] A palpação da massa tumoral pode induzir náuseas. A compressão do ducto biliar extra-hepático pode levar à icterícia (Figura 293.1). Cerca de 10% dos casos de obstrução biliar extra-hepática ocorrem devido a carcinomas de pâncreas exócrino.[54] Evidências de perda de peso são observadas em alguns pacientes. Em gatos com alopecia, a pele parece brilhante e delgada.

DIAGNÓSTICO

Resultados de exames hematológicos, perfil bioquímico sérico e exame de urina de rotina

Em geral, os resultados de exames hematológicos de rotina são inespecíficos.[8] Anemia não regenerativa discreta a moderada pode ser observada, como acontece em qualquer doença crônica. Os valores dos leucócitos podem estar normais ou, se houver significativa inflamação peritumoral, verifica-se neutrofilia com desvio à esquerda.[12,55] A menos que haja hemorragia significativa, a contagem de plaquetas geralmente é normal. Há relato de trombocitopenia em casos de metástase em medula óssea.[55]

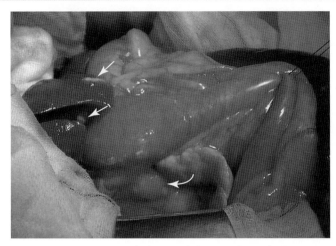

Figura 293.1 Essa imagem obtida no período transcirúrgico de cão com carcinoma pancreático mostra um pequeno (1 cm) tumor (*seta curva*) causador de obstrução do ducto biliar comum. A cirurgia de derivação propiciou 5 meses de boa qualidade de vida. Lesões metastáticas são vistas no fígado (*setas retas*).

Os resultados de exames bioquímicos séricos podem incluir valores de amilase e lipase aumentados. A concentração de lipase pode estar acentuadamente elevada.[2,50,56] Incrementos marcantes da lipase, juntamente com alteração mínima da concentração de amilase, devem levar à suspeita de neoplasia pancreática ou hepática.[56] A concentração de bilirrubina e as atividades de enzimas hepáticas podem estar aumentadas secundariamente à obstrução do ducto biliar comum ou a metástases hepáticas (ver Capítulos 53 e 65).[2] As alterações nos parâmetros de função hepática podem ser mais evidentes do que as de marcadores de doença pancreática.[1] Hipercalcemia foi relatada em alguns cães acometidos.[48] De modo geral, o exame de urina não indica alteração, a menos que haja glicosúria. Nem o diabetes melito nem a insuficiência pancreática exócrina estão associados a tumores pancreáticos em cães ou gatos.[1,8,57] Entretanto, essas condições podem ocorrer em simultâneo. Foram relatados casos de dois gatos com diabetes melito e carcinoma do pâncreas exócrino concomitantes, mas ambos apresentavam hiperadrenocorticismo.[58] Em recente revisão sobre carcinomas exócrinos em gatos, verificou-se que 5/34 tinham diabetes melito.[40]

Exames de imagem

As alterações verificadas em radiografias de abdome costumam ser mínimas, mas é possível visualizar o efeito de massa com deslocamento do duodeno e/ou perda do detalhamento seroso devido à ascite.[1,38,59] Um efeito de massa pode ser observado em gatos com hiperplasia nodular ou adenoma.[51] A doença pulmonar nodular pode ser observada em casos de metástases pulmonares. A ultrassonografia é útil para o diagnóstico de carcinoma pancreático, com sensibilidade maior do que a radiografia (ver Capítulo 88).[60] Mesmo na ultrassonografia, a diferenciação entre carcinoma inicial e pancreatite crônica ou hiperplasia nodular pode ser difícil.[61] O pâncreas, em geral, parece maior do que o usual e pode estar hipoecoico ou com uma aparência mista. Lesões císticas são incomuns em cães e gatos. A gordura circundante pode estar normal ou ter hiperecogenicidade típica de pancreatite. O aumento de linfonodos regionais é comum.[51] O fígado deve ser examinado com cuidado em busca de lesões nodulares, que podem ser hipoecoicas, hiperecoicas ou mistas, inclusive lesões em forma de alvo. Se a ascite for resultado de carcinomatose, as lesões peritoneais, de modo geral, não são visualizadas.[32] Lesões em massa, inclusive pseudocistos e abscessos, algumas vezes observadas após pancreatite aguda, podem estar grandes o suficiente para serem palpadas em cães e devem ser diferenciadas de lesões neoplásicas.[62,63] A utilização de agentes de contraste durante a ultrassonografia pode ajudar a diferenciar a pancreatite crônica do carcinoma pancreático. O contraste também pode facilitar a detecção de metástases hepáticas.[64] A ultrassonografia contrastada, em cães, pode facilitar na diferenciação de tumores do pâncreas exócrino daqueles do pâncreas endócrino.[65] Em pessoas, a ultrassonografia endoscópica melhora a visualização do pâncreas.[66] Não existem estudos comparativos das sensibilidades da tomografia computadorizada (TC) e da ultrassonografia em cães e gatos, mas a TC é considerada superior em pessoas.[25] A TC também é mais sensível para detecção de metástases. Não parece haver vantagem no uso de ressonância magnética (RM) para neoplasias pancreáticas, em seres humanos.[67]

Aspiração com agulha fina, citologia e biopsia

A citologia (ver Capítulo 93) propicia um valor preditivo positivo razoavelmente bom, mas um valor preditivo negativo moderado a ruim.[9,35,68,69] O risco de complicações após aspiração com agulha fina (AAF) em seres humanos é baixo.[68] Células atípicas podem ser detectadas em líquido ascítico.[2,35] Lesões císticas, que não costumam ser notadas em cães ou gatos, podem ser, de certa forma, comuns em seres humanos. O exame de líquido cístico obtido por AAF indicou menor taxa de resultados falso-negativos do que amostras obtidas durante cirurgia ou por biopsia.[70] A citologia pode ser útil para o diagnóstico de metástases oriundas de neoplasias distantes ao pâncreas, como o linfoma.[17]

Biopsia e histopatologia são padrão-ouro para o diagnóstico de neoplasia pancreática.[36] As amostras podem ser obtidas utilizando-se agulha de biopsia guiada por ultrassonografia ou durante exploração cirúrgica (ver Capítulos 89 e 91).[35] Assim como acontece no exame citológico, se as amostras de biopsia forem obtidas de locais de metástase, em geral não é possível identificar em definitivo o tecido de origem como sendo o pâncreas. Os resultados de biopsia podem ser descritos como consistentes em casos de carcinoma pancreático. A utilização de colorações imunoistoquímicas para amilase e carboxipeptidase pode ajudar a determinar se as lesões metastáticas são de origem pancreática.[71] Em gatos com alopecia, as lesões são caracterizadas pela presença de folículos no final da fase telógena, com moderada hiperplasia epidérmica, hiperqueratose e dermatite superficial e perivascular.[44] Essas lesões são semelhantes àquelas observadas em casos de hiperadrenocorticismo, mas a fragilidade cutânea não é uma característica.[44]

TRATAMENTO

Quando da possibilidade de ressecção, a cirurgia propicia melhor resultado a longo prazo, em pessoas acometidas. Os resultados podem ser semelhantes em cães e gatos, mas é provável que a cirurgia não seja curativa, dada a alta taxa de metástases antes do diagnóstico.[1,8,9] A cura é possível, mas requer uma lesão passível de extirpação total; em seres humanos, é mais provável se não houver acometimento dos linfonodos regionais.[72] Pancreatectomia total e subtotal foi descrita em cães normais com morbidade aceitável e tratamento a longo prazo com insulina e suplementação com enzimas pancreáticas (ver Capítulos 293, 304 e 305).[73] Existem poucos relatos de cirurgia pancreática em gatos.[74] Em vários animais, a cirurgia pode ser paliativa, pois alivia a obstrução.[36] Diversas técnicas estão sendo avaliadas em seres humanos devido aos maus resultados cirúrgicos, ainda persistentes.[66,75]

A implantação de *stent* no ducto biliar comum pode aliviar a obstrução (ver Capítulo 123), enquanto a obstrução duodenal pode ser aliviada pela técnica Billroth tipo II. Ambos os procedimentos são considerados paliativos, tendo sido utilizados em seres humanos em combinação com outros tratamentos.[66]

Relata-se baixa resposta do carcinoma pancreático à quimioterapia em seres humanos, assim como em cães e gatos. A gencitabina é o fármaco quimioterápico de escolha para as pessoas acometidas, tendo sido utilizada como terapia exclusiva ou em combinação com carboplatina, em gatos e cães com carcinoma do pâncreas exócrino.[40,76,77] Testes pré-clínicos com fármacos específicos, especialmente inibidores da tirosinoquinase, foram promissores, o que não foi traduzido em utilidade clínica. Pequenos avanços na sobrevida foram observados quando o inibidor da tirosinoquinase, o erlotinibe, que bloqueia o receptor do fator de crescimento epidérmico, foi administrado juntamente com o quimioterápico gencitabina.[76] Relata-se o uso de radioterapia, como parte da terapia transcirúrgica, em seres humanos. Cães normais tratados durante a cirurgia com a técnica de Billroth tiveram altas taxas de morbidade e de mortalidade.[78] A utilização de fármacos anti-inflamatórios não esteroides em pacientes com carcinoma do pâncreas exócrino pode ter valor limitado. Em um estudo que pesquisou a expressão de ciclo-oxigenase-2 em carcinomas de gatos, constatou-se coloração positiva somente em 25% dos casos.[79]

PROGNÓSTICO

De forma geral, o prognóstico para pacientes com carcinoma do pâncreas exócrino é muito ruim. Em gatos, a sobrevida média geral foi de 97 dias.[40] Notou-se aumento da sobrevida para uma mediana de 165 dias em gatos tratados com cirurgia ou quimioterapia, em comparação àqueles submetidos à terapia paliativa ou que tinham efusão abdominal. A sobrevida média foi de 26 e 30 dias, respectivamente.[40] Em 8 gatos relatados, a maioria morreu ou foi submetida à eutanásia dentro de 1 semana após o diagnóstico.[13]

REFERÊNCIAS BIBLIOGRÁFICAS

As referências bibliográficas deste capítulo se encontram online no Ambiente de Aprendizagem.

SEÇÃO 21
Doenças Endócrinas

CAPÍTULO 294

Anormalidades Relativas ao Hormônio de Crescimento em Gatos

Stijn J. M. Niessen

HIPOSSOMATOTROPISMO FELINO

Prevalência

O hormônio do crescimento (GH, *growth hormone*) é crucialmente importante em razão de suas ações anabólicas diretas e indiretas. A carência de GH durante o crescimento, a fase anabólica mais importante da vida de um animal, causa consequências patológicas dramáticas. O hipossomatotropismo felino congênito (HFC; "nanismo hipofisário") parece raro, já que há somente alguns poucos relatos de gatos acometidos.[1,2] O hipossomatotropismo felino adquirido (HFA) também é raramente documentado, com a exceção de decréscimos documentados, assintomáticos, verificados após hipofisectomia para remoção de tumor hipofisário.

Causas

O HFC é completamente descrito em cães, nos quais essa condição pode representar a falha primária na diferenciação completa da ectoderme craniofaríngea da bolsa de Rathke em uma hipófise anterior (adeno-hipófise) funcional saudável; foram incriminadas mutações no gene *LHX3*, que codifica fatores de transcrição essenciais ao desenvolvimento da hipófise (ver Capítulos 20 e 295).[3] A(s) causa(s) em gatos é(são) desconhecida(s), embora deficiências semelhantes possam ser relevantes. Há relato de associação com hidrocefalia congênita, em um gato.[2] O HFA pode ser consequência de uma condição que causa anormalidade na produção normal do lobo hipofisário anterior e na secreção do GH, inclusive doenças inflamatórias, infecciosas, imunomediadas, traumáticas (inclusive iatrogênica, após hipofisectomia) ou neoplásicas.[1]

Manifestação clínica

Hipossomatotropismo felino congênito

No caso de um filhote de gato com deficiência de GH, uma consulta com um médico-veterinário é agendada quando da observação de crescimento retardado do animal com 1 a 2 meses de vida. Isso se torna mais óbvio quando os irmãos da ninhada estão disponíveis para comparação (Figura 294.1). O período pós-natal inicial de 1 a 2 meses é determinado, em sua maior parte, geneticamente e, portanto, parece normal. Questões surgem quando a segunda fase de crescimento, influenciada pelo GH, não se concretiza.[1] Se houver deficiência exclusiva de GH (estando os outros hormônios hipofisários normais), a baixa estatura será proporcional (nanismo proporcional). Se um filhote de gato apresenta deficiência de outros hormônios da adeno-hipófise, especialmente do hormônio tireoestimulante, as proporções podem estar bem distorcidas. As características físicas do hipotireoidismo congênito em filhotes de gatos podem incluir contorno corpulento largo, como observado em casos de hipotireoidismo congênito exclusivo (ver Capítulos 299 e 300).[1] O HFC também pode causar retenção prolongada de dentes decíduos. O pelame dos gatos afetados é, com frequência, seco e opaco, com potencial para retenção de pelos secundários e ausência concomitante de pelos primários ou longos.[1,2] Há relato de edema bilateral da córnea devido à redução na densidade celular do endotélio corneal e de camadas de epitélio celular da córnea, em um gato

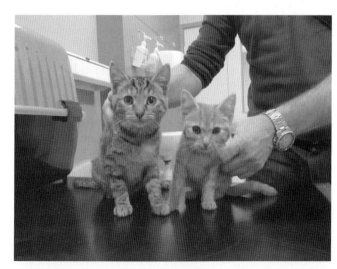

Figura 294.1 Dois filhotes de gatos Domésticos de Pelo Curto, irmãos, com 5 meses de vida; o gato à direita foi atendido por apresentar retardo do crescimento e baixa estatura proporcional e foi diagnosticado com hipossomatotropismo congênito, com base na constatação de concentração sérica indetectável de IGF-1 e exclusão de causas mais comuns de retardo do crescimento. (Cortesia da Dra. Ruth Gostelow, Royal Veterinary College.)

com suspeita de hipotireoidismo.[2] Outras manifestações incluem fraqueza generalizada e letargia. A hipoglicemia pode estar associada ao aumento da sensibilidade insulínica causado pela ausência dos efeitos anti-insulínicos do GH ou meramente relacionada com a natureza frágil de um pequeno filhote fraco com limitada capacidade gliconeogênica.

Hipossomatotropismo felino adquirido

Não há relato de HFA em gatos.[1] Após concluída a fase de crescimento, é provável que as consequências clínicas da deficiência de GH sejam sutis, possivelmente muito brandas para serem notadas por tutores ou veterinários. Seres humanos com deficiência de GH adquirida que apresentam os primeiros sintomas na vida adulta apresentam maiores taxas de morbidade e de mortalidade, em conjunto com a piora na qualidade de vida.[4-6] Com o aumento da experiência com hipofisectomia para tratamento de hipersomatotropismo felino e de outros tumores hipofisários, o HFA pode se tornar uma questão relevante. Entretanto, em nossa experiência com gatos que apresentavam concentração sérica subnormal de fator do crescimento semelhante à insulina-1 (IGF-1, *insulin-like growth fator-1*), não constatamos consequências clínicas claramente deletérias após hipofisectomia.

Diagnóstico

O diagnóstico de hipossomatotropismo felino congênito (HFC) deve se basear em um cenário clínico sugestivo e exclusão de causas mais comuns de nanismo proporcional, que incluem hepatopatia (particularmente desvio [*shunt*] portossistêmico), desnutrição, doença gastrintestinal, renal ou cardiovascular ou expectativa de crescimento inapropriada. O diagnóstico pode ser confirmado pela constatação de concentração sérica de GH abaixo do valor de referência, obtidos aleatoriamente. Entretanto, testes de GH felino confiáveis raramente estão disponíveis no mercado. Quando disponíveis, os resultados obtidos em gatos saudáveis e naqueles com HFC podem se sobrepor, em parte porque o GH, como todos os hormônios da adeno-hipófise, é secretado de forma pulsátil.[7] Testes de estimulação (provocativos), padrão-ouro para o diagnóstico de deficiência de GH em seres humanos e cães, ainda não foram validados para os gatos.

Uma alternativa ao teste baseado no GH é a obtenção de concentração sérica baixa ou indetectável de IGF-1. A síntese hepática de IGF-1 é induzida, sobretudo, pelo GH, sua secreção não é pulsátil e os resultados refletem as concentrações de GH nas 24 horas precedentes. Os clínicos devem ter em mente que determinadas doenças e fármacos podem influenciar os resultados de GH e IGF-1, ocasionando falsa impressão de deficiências. Por exemplo, o IGF-1, principalmente sintetizado no fígado, pode estar diminuído em casos de disfunção hepática. Diminuições moderadas, mas não graves, na concentração de IGF-1 foram relatadas em gatos com linfoma, diabetes melito recém-diagnosticado e doença renal.[7,8] As concentrações séricas de IGF-1 também estão relacionadas com o tamanho corporal, o que pode ser relevante em filhotes de baixa estatura. Relata-se que um filhote macho de 7 meses de vida com hipotireoidismo congênito e crescimento retardado desproporcional apresentava concentração sérica de IGF-1 moderadamente diminuída, que retornou à normalidade após 6 semanas de terapia de reposição com hormônio da tireoide.[9]

Tratamento e prognóstico

A terapia de reposição com GH ainda não foi descrita em gatos, embora provavelmente seja semelhante àquela utilizada em cães (ver Capítulo 295). Já que não há teste de GH felino disponível no mercado, há dúvida sobre a produção de anticorpos ao utilizar GH de outras espécies (suíno, humano). Deficiências concomitantes de hormônios hipofisários, se presentes, devem ser tratadas. Se a reposição de GH for muito dispendiosa ou indesejável (um efeito adverso importante é o desenvolvimento de diabetes melito), o tratamento das deficiências concomitantes

de hormônios pituitários (se presentes) pode ser a única estratégia de tratamento. Progestágenos vêm sendo empregados para induzir secreção de GH pela glândula mamária em cães (ver Capítulo 295), mas não aumentaram a concentração de GH ou IGF-1 em gatos, apesar de a expressão de genes de GH felino no tecido mamário ter sido submetida a alterações fibroadenomatosas induzidas por progestágenos.[10,11]

Dada a constatação de ausência de resposta clínica significativa, a terapia de reposição de GH para casos de HFA póshipofisectomia não tem sido realizada. Um ajuste na ingestão calórica diária parece apropriado em gatos com diminuição comprovada de IGF-1 ou GH, pois a deficiência de GH em seres humanos causa aumento da quantidade de tecido adiposo (especialmente na região abdominal).[4] Em nossa experiência, há risco de obesidade em gatos submetidos, com sucesso, à hipofisectomia.

Há poucos relatos de gatos com deficiência de GH submetidos ao tratamento. Isso impede a avaliação completa de alternativas terapêuticas ou de prognóstico de HFC felino. Se não tratada, essa anormalidade parece ter um prognóstico ruim, com expectativa de vida mais curta e desenvolvimento de doenças infecciosas, degenerativas ou neurológicas.[1,2]

HIPERSOMATOTROPISMO FELINO

Considerações gerais

Embora a deficiência de GH pareça ser um problema clínico somente em filhotes e gatos jovens com anormalidade de crescimento, a possibilidade de hipersomatotropismo felino (HSFe; acromegalia) deve ser considerada em qualquer gato de meiaidade a idoso com diabetes melito, cujo excesso causa resistência à insulina e subsequente diabetes melito pela redução de receptores de insulina, interferindo em uma gama de processos pósreceptor de insulina, e outros mecanismos.[12]

Prevalência

O HSFe é uma doença primária relativamente comum de diabetes melito felino. As taxas de prevalência variam de 18 a 32%, com potencial para variações geográficas e/ou diferenças nos métodos de recrutamento ou triagem.[12-15] No maior estudo de triagem realizado até o momento, com 1.221 gatos, no Reino Unido, o recrutamento foi iniciado pelo oferecimento de mensurações gratuitas de frutosamina em gatos com diabetes melito. A amostra de soro sanguíneo foi utilizada para mensurar a concentração de IGF-1 e, se extremamente elevada, foram oferecidos testes confirmatórios (inclusive tomografia computadorizada [TC] contrastada da hipófise). Com base nas 1.221 amostras testadas para IGF-1 (IGF-1 > 1.000 ng/mℓ foi o valor de corte arbitrário), verificou-se que 319 gatos (26%) foram considerados suspeitos e 95% deles foram confirmados como portadores de HSFe.[15] Com base nesses dados de prevalência e em testes de triagem precedentes para doenças menos comuns (p. ex., infecção do trato urinário no diabetes melito felino; prevalência estimada de 12%), recomenda-se que os gatos com a doença recentemente diagnosticada sejam avaliados quanto à possibilidade de HSFe (Figura 294.2).[16] A triagem de todos os animais recém-diagnosticados com diabetes é de bom senso, ao se considerar as graves implicações do HSFe concomitante, Alterando-se o tratamento, o potencial para remissão do diabetes e o prognóstico.

Causas

Considerações gerais

O HSFe é causado por uma transformação neoplásica de acidófilos (somatotrofos) na adeno-hipófise, levando ao aumento da frequência e amplitude dos padrões de secreção pulsátil de GH. Esses tumores, em sua maioria, são adenomas; todavia, há relatos

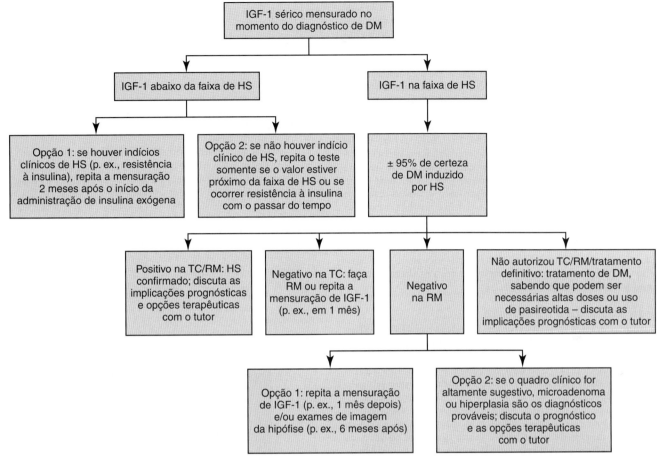

Figura 294.2 Possível abordagem para triagem de gatos recém-diagnosticados com diabetes para hipersomatotropismo (HS). *DM*, diabetes melito; *IGF-1*, fator de crescimento semelhante à insulina-1; *RM*, ressonância magnética; *TC*, tomografia computadorizada.

de um pequeno número de carcinomas hipofisários e algumas hiperplasias não neoplásicas.[12,17] A causa do desenvolvimento do tumor não é compreendida; foram propostos fatores ambientais e genéticos.

Causas ambientais

Contaminantes organo-halogenados foram incriminados como causas de doenças oncogênicas endócrinas em diversas espécies, inclusive seres humanos e gatos.[18-24] Eles são produtos químicos persistentes e bioacumulativos encontrados em pesticidas organoclorados, substâncias químicas industriais (como bifenilos policlorados [BPCs]) e retardantes de chama bromados (RCBs) adicionados a materiais que reduzem o risco de inflamação (como éteres difenil polibromados [EDPBs]). Gatos e seres humanos são continuamente expostos a tais agentes químicos, pelo menos em parte, via contaminação alimentar e domiciliar (poeira). Esta pode ser especialmente relevante em gatos, devido ao intenso comportamento de lambedura dos pelos (*grooming*). Em um relato, foram detectadas concentrações significativamente maiores de todos os contaminantes estudados, em gatos com HSFe, quando comparados às de gatos com diabetes melito primário e com as daqueles sem endocrinopatia.[18] Dados também sugeriram que o HSFe pode reduzir a capacidade de um gato metabolizar substâncias químicas persistentes, como BPCs. Contaminantes semelhantes foram incriminados na ocorrência de hipertireoidismo felino (ver Capítulo 301).[19-22]

Causas genéticas

Adenomas pituitários humanos foram considerados de origem monoclonal, sugerindo que se formam como consequência de uma mutação somática celular única adquirida.[25] Foi então demonstrado que um mecanismo adicional para o desenvolvimento de adenoma hipofisário secretor de GH envolveu mutações de linhagens germinativas que inativam genes supressores tumorais.[26-30] Mutações da proteína de interação com o receptor de aril-hidrocarboneto, uma proteína supressora tumoral, foram demonstradas em até 40% de pessoas com adenoma secretor de GH familiar ou espontâneo isolado. O aril-hidrocarboneto está envolvido em uma gama de ações, que incluem ativação de enzimas que metabolizam xenobióticos, tornando a ligação previamente discutida com a exposição e o acúmulo de contaminantes organo-halogenados ainda mais interessante.[27-30] Em um estudo com DNA genômico (sem grupo-controle), constatou-se que 2 de 10 gatos com HSFe apresentavam apenas um polimorfismo de nucleotídio único não conservador no éxon 1 do gene *AIP* (AIP:c.9 G > T), sugerindo que alguns gatos podem ser geneticamente predispostos ao desenvolvimento de HSFe.[31]

Manifestações clínicas

Sintomas iniciais de HSFe

Os sinais clínicos iniciais em gatos com HSFe são determinados, em parte, pelo momento da preocupação do tutor. A maioria dos gatos finalmente diagnosticados como HSFe é primeiro observada por um veterinário após o tutor se preocupar com poliúria e polidipsia (PU/PD) secundárias ao diabetes melito e os efeitos osmóticos da glicosúria. Em geral, inicia-se o tratamento com insulina, que pode amenizar efetivamente os sinais clínicos em alguns gatos (inclusive com remissão diabética temporária). Entretanto, na maioria dos pacientes é difícil obter controle glicêmico razoável. Somente alguns gatos com HSFe não apresentam diabetes melito concomitante. Esses gatos podem ter anormalidades de acromegalia fenotípicas, descritas nesta seção, e/ou polifagia extrema. Em um estudo com 319 gatos com suspeita de HSFe, verificou-se idade média de 11,3 anos (variação 4 a 19), sendo 70% machos castrados. Embora tenham sido incluídas diversas raças, 87% eram gatos Domésticos de Pelo Curto.[15] Essas observações são semelhantes àquelas verificadas em gatos com diabetes melito primário e não são úteis para aumentar o índice de suspeita de HSFe. O peso corporal e a concentração de frutosamina foram significativamente maiores em gatos com IGF-1 na faixa de hipersomatotropismo (comparados àqueles com IGF-1 < 1.000 ng/mℓ), apesar de doses diárias de insulina significativamente maiores (média de 15 UI/dia versus 6 UI/dia).[15] Entretanto, os gatos com HSFe apresentaram variações no peso corporal, pequenas a grandes, e na necessidade de insulina (moderada a alta). Dados sugerem que se deve suspeitar de HSFe ao se notar ganho de peso em um gato com controle diabético subótimo ou quando se constatar resistência à insulina inexplicável. Alterações fenotípicas características eventualmente ocorrem como consequência dos efeitos anabólicos de GH e IGF-1 e são somente óbvios quando o gato teve a doença por um período de vida mais longo. Somente 24% dos clínicos indicaram forte suspeita de HSFe antes que seus pacientes fossem diagnosticados como portadores dessa condição.[15]

Sinais associados a HSFe crônico

Quando a doença se torna crônica, os gatos com HSFe podem manifestar sinais clínicos "clássicos" (Boxe 294.1). A incidência relativamente alta (53%) de estridor no trato respiratório superior de gatos com HSFe se deve ao edema tecidual. Em geral, a nasofaringe mais estreita faz com que o tutor note que seu gato está "roncando."[17,32] O aumento da largura da cabeça e características faciais largas (Figura 294.3) podem ser as características mais óbvias ao exame físico. Entretanto, essas alterações podem ser sutis e difíceis de observar por conta dos pelos da face, da variação conformacional relacionada com a raça e da tendência de os tutores não notarem alterações que se desenvolvem de forma bastante gradual. Em resumo, a presença das chamadas alterações físicas típicas pode ajudar o clínico, embora a ausência delas não deva diminuir a suspeita de HSFe, especialmente em gatos com diabetes melito. Ademais, parece mais apropriado utilizar o termo "hipersomatotropismo", e não acromegalia, pois esse último implica incorretamente que os gatos acometidos devam ter alterações fenotípicas características.

Diagnóstico

Concentrações séricas ou plasmáticas de GH e IGF-1

Para a maioria dos veterinários, a mensuração da concentração sérica de IGF-1 total é o meio mais viável e acessível de triagem de HSFe.[17] Felizmente, foi demonstrado que o valor preditivo positivo de uma concentração de IGF-1 > 1.000 ng/mℓ foi o respeitável valor de 95% em radioimunoensaio.[15,17] Entretanto, recomenda-se aos leitores utilizar apenas faixas de valores de referência elaboradas por laboratórios independentes e específicos. Foi validado um teste ELISA (ensaio de imunoabsorção enzimática) para IGF-1.[33]

O problema de amostras de sangue obtidas aleatoriamente para mensuração da concentração de IGF-1 como teste de triagem para HSFe é que a síntese hepática de IGF-1 depende de concentração adequada de insulina na circulação porta. Tal insulina pode estar deficiente em gatos recém-diagnosticados com diabetes melito, resultando em resultado falso-negativo para IGF-1 em cerca de 9% dos gatos não tratados. Adicionalmente, relatou-se em gatos diabéticos sem HSFe aumento da concentração de IGF-1.[17] Além disso, existem diferenças nos testes para determinação de IGF-1.[34] Todos esses fatores devem ser considerados ao se fazer a triagem de HSFe em gatos com diabetes melito (Figura 294.2). Endocentrações séricas de IGF-1 são úteis como marcadores da eficácia terapêutica pós-hipofisectomia, mas não são adequadamente sensíveis para documentar diminuições menos marcantes de GH que podem

Boxe 294.1 Possíveis sinais clínicos observados em gatos com hipersomatotropismo

1. Sintomas associados a diabetes melito (poliúria, polidipsia, polifagia)
2. Ganho de peso, apesar de controle diabético subótimo (embora a perda de peso também seja possível)
3. Polifagia, independentemente do controle diabético (possivelmente extrema)
4. Estridor inspiratório (ronco)*
5. Características faciais largas* (Figura 294.3)
6. Prognatismo inferior (protrusão da mandíbula)* (Figura 294.3)
7. Patas "achatadas" (aumento distal dos membros/patas)*
8. Aumento abdominal com organomegalia*
9. Problemas de mobilidade devido à artropatia* e/ou à neuropatia diabética
10. Resistência à insulina (necessidade de dose de insulina exógena superior a 1,5 UI/kg)
11. Sopro cardíaco e insuficiência cardíaca congestiva*
12. Sintomas relativos ao sistema nervoso central (p. ex., andar em círculos, cegueira, convulsões, depressão)*

*Geralmente presente apenas na doença crônica; sinais clínicos não estão presentes de modo consistente.

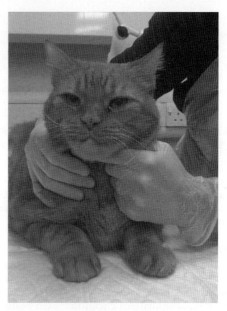

Figura 294.3 Gato Doméstico de Pelo Curto de 11 anos com diabetes melito causado por hipersomatotropismo. Podem-se notar características faciais largas, embora não tenham sido notadas pelo tutor. Essas alterações faciais tendem a estar presentes somente quando há hipersomatotropismo por um longo tempo.

ocorrer após radioterapia.[17] Os testes para mensurar GH disponíveis no mercado permanecem indefiníveis, apesar de todos os gatos testados para HSFe terem mostrado elevação acima do intervalo de referência.[7] No momento, os testes de supressão do GH (geralmente utilizando glicose, por via oral), considerados padrão-ouro para o diagnóstico de hipersomatotropismo humano, não foram considerados úteis aos gato.[7,17]

Exames de sangue alternativos

Já que o HSFe está associado ao crescimento tecidual, foi avaliado o pró-peptídio pró-colágeno sérico tipo III (PIIIP), um indicador periférico da substituição (turnover) do colágeno.[35] O PIIIP sérico mediano foi cinco vezes maior em gatos com diabetes melito induzido por HSFe, quando comparado ao de gatos com diabetes melito primário. A concentração sérica de grelina, um secretagogo de GH, foi menor em casos de HSFe quando comparada a de gatos saudáveis, mas os resultados foram semelhantes àqueles de gatos com diabetes melito primário.[36] O monitoramento da concentração sérica de grelina pode ser útil na avaliação do tratamento. Incrementos significativos foram documentados após radioterapia efetiva em casos de HSFe, enquanto as alterações no IGF-1 não foram significativas.[36]

Tomografia computadorizada (TC) e ressonância magnética (RM)

A confirmação de HSFe por meio de exames de imagem avançados é recomendada e geralmente útil, já que se nota aumento da hipófise com a utilização de RM ou TC com contraste (Figura 294.4). Entretanto, a ausência de massa tumoral ou tumefação não deve ser interpretada como exclusão da possibilidade de HSFe. Pode haver microadenoma e hiperplasia acidófila, podendo ser mais comuns do que atualmente diagnosticados. Já que os gatos são diagnosticados mais precocemente no curso da doença, espera-se encontrar menor prevalência de massas tumorais visualizadas em exames de imagem avançados. Em casos mais crônicos, a TC pode mostrar prognatismo inferior associado ao HSFe (cerca de 25% dos gatos acometidos), malformações da articulação temporomandibular e aumento da espessura da pele, de tecidos subcutâneos e do osso calvário.[32]

Tratamento e prognóstico

Hipofisectomia

Com a experiência contínua adquirida com a hipofisectomia em medicina veterinária, tal procedimento é reconhecido como tratamento "padrão-ouro" para HSFe, já que não há contraindicação.[37,38] As contraindicações, ainda em avaliação, incluem um tamanho particularmente grande do tumor, comorbidades significativas que impedem uma recuperação anestésica e pós-cirúrgica segura (particularmente em casos de doença renal ou cardiovascular significativa) ou a oposição do tutor à cirurgia. O comprometimento financeiro com a cirurgia pode ser um obstáculo; é importante que o tutor seja conscientizado sobre o custo da insulinoterapia ou radioterapia ineficiente.

Em nossa experiência, os tumores hipofisários são abordados pela base do crânio; o neurocirurgião faz a cirurgia através da boca e nasofaringe do gato (abordagem transfenoidal; faz-se a incisão no palato mole). Aproximadamente 85% dos gatos apresentam remissão do diabetes dentro de 2 meses após a cirurgia e o restante manifesta bom controle glicêmico com doses de insulina mais convencionais. Essas respostas mostram a enorme resiliência das células beta do pâncreas dos gatos, que parecem se recuperar após meses ou até mesmo anos de séria resistência à insulina. Em nossa experiência, a taxa de mortalidade peri e pós-cirúrgica é de cerca de 10%, o que é um risco aceitável para a maioria dos tutores de gatos, especialmente dada a escassez de alternativas terapêuticas efetivas. Após a cirurgia, os gatos são tratados com baixas doses de hidrocortisona e levotiroxina (ambas por toda a vida) e acetato de desmopressina (que pode ser descontinuado na maioria dos gatos). A terapia de reposição de GH não é considerada necessária (ver discussão prévia sobre HFA).

Tratamento clínico

Análogos da somatostatina (SST) e agonistas de dopamina não se mostraram efetivos.[17] Felizmente, a pasireotida, um novo análogo da SST que se liga a vários receptores, com alta afinidade pelos subtipos 1, 2, 3 e 5 do receptor de SST, recentemente demonstrou suprimir de forma efetiva a somatotropina em gatos com HSFe e diabetes melito concomitante.[39,40] Gatos tratados tiveram diminuição significativa no valor médio da glicemia durante 12 horas e nas concentrações séricas de IGF-1, de frutosamina e na necessidade de insulina. Foram testadas uma forma injetável de curta ação, a cada 12 horas, e uma forma injetável de longa ação de administração mensal. Aproximadamente 25% dos gatos tratados com a forma de administração mensal apresentaram remissão do diabetes. As desvantagens incluem efeitos colaterais gastrintestinais discretos (fezes amolecidas/diarreia) e o custo do tratamento.

Radioterapia

Embora a eficácia da radioterapia tenha sido inicialmente sugerida como ótima, mesmo o uso de tecnologia estereotáxica ou *gamma-knife* não obteve resultado semelhante à hipofisectomia.[17,41-45] O efeito da radioterapia mostrou-se particularmente imprevisível quanto à recuperação; quando deve-se esperar uma recuperação; em qual extensão a radioterapia altera a necessidade de insulina; e por quanto tempo persistirão os efeitos dela. A falta de resposta em termos de normalização da concentração de IGF-1 coloca ainda mais dúvidas sobre a real eficácia do procedimento, mesmo em gatos que necessitam menor dose de insulina.[36] Na verdade, as alterações relacionadas com o HSFe progrediram, mesmo quando se obtém melhora ou resolução do diabetes melito.[45] A radioterapia ainda pode servir como um procedimento útil para redução do tumor e ser utilizada em gatos com uma grande massa pituitária que implica maior risco cirúrgico, ou quando não se permite hipofisectomia nem tratamento com pasireotida.

Tratamento somente do diabetes melito

Se as opções terapêuticas definitivas forem recusadas pelos tutores, a única opção terapêutica que resta (com exceção da eutanásia) é o tratamento exclusivamente do diabetes melito secundário. O protocolo terapêutico é o mesmo recomendado para diabetes melito primário (ver Capítulo 305); todavia, frequentemente são necessárias altas doses de insulina para obter uma qualidade de vida aceitável. Alguns clínicos sugerem que as doses de insulina não devem exceder um determinado nível, mas nossa experiência indica que a utilização de doses extremamente altas é, algumas vezes, a única forma de obter uma qualidade de vida aceitável. A utilização da insulinoterapia em altas doses significa que os tutores precisam estar preparados para, e de fato precisam aceitar, a possibilidade de hipoglicemia iatrogênica; mas essa ocorrência parece rara. O tumor hipofisário mantém seu padrão secretório pulsátil de GH, o que explica os episódios de redução de GH e aumento da sensibilidade à insulina.

Doses apropriadas de insulina devem ser obtidas mediante aumento gradativo da dose, conforme necessário, geralmente aumentando até 1 UI/injeção/gato/semana. O ideal é obter curvas glicêmicas periódicas, juntamente com a avaliação

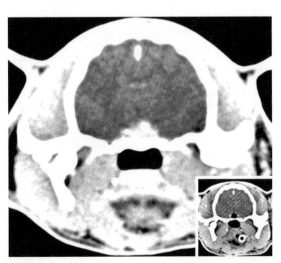

Figura 294.4 Imagem do cérebro de um gato diabético com hipersomatotropismo obtida em tomografia computadorizada (TC). A hipófise aumentada pode ser vista na base do crânio, estendendo-se além da borda dorsal da sela túrcica e mostrando captação heterogênea de contraste. *Detalhe:* imagem de TC do mesmo gato após hipofisectomia bem-sucedida. A pituitária é alcançada através da nasofaringe, após incisão do palato mole. O gato apresentou remissão do diabetes 2 semanas após o procedimento.

cuidadosa da condição clínica. Se a dose de insulina for aumentada de maneira muito rápida, há risco maior de ocorrência do efeito Somogyi. Sequelas negativas das alterações de acromegalia progressivas podem exigir atenção, inclusive o tratamento de artropatia (ver Capítulos 203 e 353), insuficiência cardíaca congestiva (ver Capítulo 247) ou doença renal crônica (ver Capítulo 324). Os sintomas relativos ao sistema nervoso central (p. ex., convulsões, cegueira, depressão) devido à expansão da massa tumoral hipofisária são raros, dada a natureza de crescimento lento. Entretanto, podem ocorrer sintomas que podem justificar o uso de protocolos terapêuticos paliativos adicionais (ver Capítulo 260). As avaliações regulares da qualidade de vida devem ser planejadas; se a resposta terapêutica se mostrar insatisfatória, recomenda-se eutanásia (ver Capítulo 7).[46] Isso é especialmente importante nos gatos cujo diabetes melito não pode ser controlado ou naqueles que manifestam polifagia extrema induzida por GH. A fluoxetina tem sido utilizada para diminuir esse sintoma, com eficácia variável.

REFERÊNCIAS BIBLIOGRÁFICAS

As referências bibliográficas deste capítulo se encontram online no Ambiente de Aprendizagem.

CAPÍTULO 295

Anormalidades Relativas ao Hormônio de Crescimento em Cães

Hans S. Kooistra

HORMÔNIO DO CRESCIMENTO

Fontes

O hormônio do crescimento (GH, do inglês *growth hormone*) é um polipeptídio de cadeia única, bastante grande, que contém 190 aminoácidos. A sequência de aminoácidos do GH varia consideravelmente entre as espécies, mas o GH em cães e suínos é idêntico.[1] Hormônios da adeno-hipófise (hipófise anterior ou lobo anterior da hipófise), inclusive GH, são secretados em pulsos rítmicos separados por períodos intermitentes de baixa produção. A secreção hipofisária de GH é regulada, principalmente, por ações opostas do peptídio hipotalâmico estimulador, o hormônio liberador de GH (GHRH, do inglês *growth hormone releasing hormone*), e do peptídio hipotalâmico inibidor, a somatostatina (Figura 295.1). Os pulsos de GH refletem, de maneira predominante, a liberação pulsátil de GHRH, enquanto as concentrações entre os pulsos são controladas, principalmente, pela somatostatina. A síntese e a secreção de GH também podem ser estimuladas por secretagogos que não o GHRH, que atuam em receptores que não de GHRH. O ligante endógeno para esses receptores é a grelina, sintetizada e secretada no estômago.[2] Em cães jovens, a grelina é mais potente do que o GHRH no estímulo da síntese e secreção de GH.[3] Além disso, ela estimula o consumo de alimentos, assim como o esvaziamento gástrico e intestinal. O jejum e a ingestão alimentar estão associados a maior e menor concentrações circulantes de grelina, respectivamente.[4]

Em cães, o GH é sintetizado em tecidos hipofisários e mamários. A administração de progestágenos pode aumentar a concentração plasmática de GH em cães, mas essa secreção não é pulsátil, sensível ao GHRH e inibida pela somatostatina. Ademais, a concentração plasmática de GH induzida por progestágenos não diminui após hipofisectomia, indicando que esse GH é oriundo de um local extra-hipofisário. Assim, ele é sintetizado em focos do epitélio de ducto mamário hiperplásico.[5] O GH mamário é bioquimicamente idêntico ao GH hipofisário, e o gene que codifica o GH mamário é idêntico àquele da hipófise.[6]

O padrão típico de secreção pulsátil do GH é alterado durante a fase lútea (diestro) de cadelas saudáveis, com maior concentração basal e menos pulsos. O GH mamário induzido pela progesterona pode suprimir parcialmente a secreção hipofisária de GH. Assim, a síntese de GH mamário é normal durante o diestro em cadelas saudáveis, provavelmente induzindo a proliferação do tecido mamário em preparação para a lactação, por meio de ações autócrina e parácrina locais.[7] Concentrações relevantes de GH foram detectadas na secreção de glândulas mamárias de cadelas, principalmente no colostro.[8] O GH do colostro pode promover o desenvolvimento gastrintestinal do neonato. A produção mamária de GH induzida por progestágenos pode também participar no desenvolvimento de tumores da glândula mamária ou na progressão do tumor.

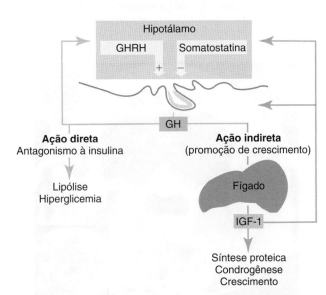

Figura 295.1 A secreção hipofisária do hormônio do crescimento (GH) está sob controle hipotalâmico, inibindo-a (somatostatina) ou estimulando-a (hormônio liberador de GH [GHRH]); também é modulada por meio de controle de retroalimentação (*feedback*) negativa do fator de crescimento semelhante à insulina-1 (IGF-1) e do próprio GH. As ações catabólicas (diabetogênicas) diretas do GH são mostradas no lado esquerdo da figura e as ações anabólicas indiretas, no lado direito. (Redesenhada de Rijnberk A, Kooistra HS, editors: *Clinical endocrinology of dogs and cats*, 2 ed., Hannover, Alemanha, 2010, Schlütersche.)

Ações fisiológicas

As ações do GH circulante podem ser divididas em duas principais categorias: ações catabólicas rápidas e ações anabólicas lentas (longa ação) (ver Figura 295.1). As ações rápidas se devem principalmente ao antagonismo à insulina, resultando em aumento da lipólise, gliconeogênese, restrição do transporte de glicose através de membranas celulares e hiperglicemia. As ações anabólicas lentas são mediadas por fatores de crescimento semelhantes à insulina (IGFs) produzidos em uma série de tecidos (sobretudo no fígado), os quais possuem sequência cerca de 50% semelhante à insulina. Esses IGFs atuam como promotores de crescimento parácrinos e autócrinos locais. Ao contrário da insulina, os IGFs se ligam a proteínas de ligação (IGFPLs), o que prolonga a meia-vida e é compatível com ações promotoras de crescimento a longo prazo. Os IGFs são importantes determinantes da regulação do tamanho corporal, pelo estímulo à síntese de proteínas, à condrogênese e ao crescimento.

A distinção das ações biológicas opostas do GH não é estrita ou absoluta. Existem evidências de que o GH exerça efeito promotor de crescimento não somente por meio de IGFs, mas também diretamente em células-alvo. O GH pode ser o principal determinante do tamanho corporal. Parece que cães jovens de raças de grande porte passam por períodos mais longos de alta liberação de GH (i. e., hipersomatotropismo juvenil) do que cães jovens de raças de pequeno porte.[9] Por outro lado, existe uma forte correlação linear entre a concentração plasmática de IGF-1 e o tamanho corporal. Ademais, há relato de um haplótipo de polimorfismo de nucleotídio único de IGF-1 como importante fator no tamanho definitivo do corpo de cães.[10] O IGF-1 tem efeito inibidor na liberação de GH, impedindo diretamente a secreção e indiretamente pelo estímulo à liberação de somatostatina. O GH também suprime a síntese e a secreção de GHRH no hipotálamo (ver Figura 295.1).

ACROMEGALIA

Patogênese

A acromegalia é uma síndrome de crescimento excessivo de ossos e tecidos moles e resistência à insulina, devido à secreção prolongada e excessiva de GH. Em cães de meia-idade e idosos, a progesterona endógena (fase lútea do ciclo estral) ou os progestágenos exógenos podem causar excesso de GH devido à secreção mamária de GH. A acromegalia também foi relatada em um cão com um tumor mamário produtor de GH.[11] Em cães, o hipotireoidismo está associado ao aumento das concentrações plasmáticas de GH e IGF-1.[12,13] Em cães, raramente um adenoma somatotrofo hipofisário pode causar acromegalia, ao contrário do que ocorre em gatos, que apresentam uma frequência muito maior dessa condição (ver Capítulo 296).[14]

Manifestações clínicas

Os sintomas de hipersecreção de GH tendem a surgir lentamente e, em geral, incluem edema de tecidos moles da cabeça, do pescoço e do abdome. Em alguns cães com acromegalia, a hipertrofia grave dos tecidos moles da boca e faringe pode causar roncos e até mesmo dispneia (Figura 295.2). Proliferação de cartilagem articular, reação periosteal periarticular e espondilose deformante podem resultar em rigidez de membros ao caminhar, dificuldade em se levantar e rigidez do pescoço. Quase sempre, os cães acometidos apresentam poliúria e, algumas vezes, polifagia. Em geral, a poliúria se dá sem glicosúria, mas pode ocorrer diabetes melito devido à resistência à insulina. O exame físico pode revelar pregas cutâneas espessas, especialmente no pescoço; prognatismo; e amplos espaços interdentais (ver Figura 295.2). O excesso de GH por longo tempo também pode ocasionar aumento generalizado do tamanho de órgãos e subsequente distensão abdominal. Os exames laboratoriais, de modo geral, indicam hiperglicemia. É possível que o aumento da atividade sérica da fosfatase alcalina decorra da atividade glicocorticoide intrínseca

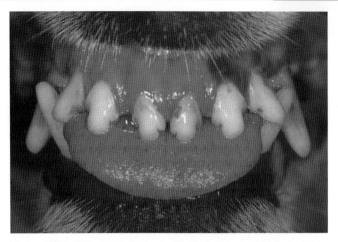

Figura 295.2 Boca de um cão da raça Beagle de 4 anos com excesso de hormônio do crescimento induzido por progestágenos. Note a hiperplasia da gengiva, o alargamento dos espaços interdentais e a língua relativamente grande.

dos progestágenos. Cães da raça Pastor-Alemão parecem predispostos à acromegalia.[15] A acromegalia secundária ao hipotireoidismo tende a ser muito mais branda do que outros tipos. Grandes adenomas de somatotrofos compressivos podem causar sintomas relativos ao sistema nervoso central.

Já que o IGF-1 plasmático se liga a proteínas plasmáticas, sua concentração não oscila de forma tão ampla como a do GH. Além disso, a sequência de aminoácidos do IGF-1 é menos espécie-específica e, assim, a sua concentração pode ser mensurada por testes heterólogos (humanos). Por conta da forte correlação linear entre a concentração plasmática de IGF-1 e o tamanho corporal, são necessários intervalos de referência específicos para as raças.[16] Se o excesso de GH for notado em um cão não submetido ao tratamento com progesterona ou progestágenos, ele deve ser testado para hipotireoidismo. Exames de imagem avançados da região hipofisária podem revelar a presença de adenoma de somatotrofos.

Diagnóstico

Em cães com acromegalia, quase sempre a concentração plasmática basal de GH excede os valores da faixa de referência, mas pode não ser anormal se a anormalidade for discreta ou se a doença estiver na fase inicial. O aumento da concentração de GH, por si só, pode ser decorrência de coleta da amostra logo após o pulso de secreção de GH de uma hipófise normal. O diagnóstico de acromegalia é indicado quando a administração de GHRH (1 μg/kg por via intravenosa [IV]) não estimular a secreção de GH ou se a aplicação de somatostatina (10 μg/kg IV) não suprimir o GH. Como a sequência de aminoácidos do GH varia entre as espécies, deve-se utilizar um teste homólogo espécie-específico para a mensuração do GH. Testes de GH não estão amplamente disponíveis no mercado.

Tratamento

Em cães, a acromegalia induzida pela progesterona pode ser tratada de maneira efetiva mediante ovariectomia. Se o excesso de GH não causar depleção total das células beta pancreáticas, a ovariectomia pode prevenir ou reverter o diabetes melito. Cães com excesso de GH induzido por progestágenos devem ter aqueles fármacos descontinuados. A administração de bloqueadores de receptores de progesterona, como o aglepristone, diminui de forma significativa as concentrações plasmáticas de GH e IGF-1 em cães com acromegalia induzida por progestágenos.[17] O tratamento de cães com hipotireoidismo primário com levotiroxina resulta em normalização das concentrações plasmáticas de GH e IGF-1.[12]

Em cães com acromegalia devido a adenoma de somatotrofo, o tratamento deve ser direcionado ao tumor hipofisário.

Opções terapêuticas incluem tratamento medicamentoso, radioterapia e hipofisectomia. O tratamento medicamentoso com análogos da somatostatina de longa ação (caros), como octreotida e lanreotida, abranda os sintomas, normaliza a concentração plasmática de IGF-1 e reduz o tamanho do tumor em cerca de 50% em pessoas com acromegalia. Os antagonistas de receptores de GH desenvolvidos para uso em seres humanos, como o pegvisomanto, também podem ser efetivos em cães. A radiação pode diminuir o tamanho do tumor hipofisário. As desvantagens da radioterapia incluem secreção excessiva persistente de GH, apesar da diminuição do tamanho, disponibilidade limitada, maior tempo de hospitalização, anestesias frequentes, custo e possibilidade de recidiva caso uma resposta inicial seja observada. A hipofisectomia transfenoidal foi realizada com sucesso em cães com hipercortisolismo devido a um adenoma corticotrofo e em gatos com acromegalia causada por adenoma de somatotrofo.[18] A experiência em cães com acromegalia é limitada.

NANISMO HIPOFISÁRIO

Patogênese
Qualquer defeito na organogênese da hipófise pode causar deficiências de hormônios hipofisários, isoladas ou combinadas.

A deficiência congênita de GH, ou nanismo hipofisário, é o exemplo mais evidente de deficiência de hormônio pituitária. A deficiência congênita de GH foi descrita em diversas raças de cães. A condição é observada mais frequentemente como uma anormalidade hereditária autossômica recessiva simples em cães da raça Pastor-Alemão. Pesquisas genealógicas indicam que a origem do gene recessivo é uma mutação ocorrida por volta de 1940, com a detecção de vários cães campeões carreadores.[19,20] Cães anões da raça Pastor-Alemão tipicamente apresentam deficiências combinadas de GH, hormônio tireoestimulante (TSH, do inglês *thyroid stimulating hormone*) e prolactina, anormalidade na liberação de gonadotropinas e secreção normal de hormônio adrenocorticotrófico (ACTH, do inglês *adrenocorticotropic hormone*) (Figura 295.3).[21] A deficiência congênita de GH supostamente resulta da atrofia por compressão da adeno-hipófise devido à formação de cisto na bolsa de Rathke. De fato, existem cistos hipofisários na maioria dos cães anões da raça Pastor-Alemão.[21] Entretanto, cães anões jovens da raça Pastor-Alemão podem não ter ou apresentar apenas um pequeno cisto e poucas evidências de atrofia por compressão da hipófise.[21] Ademais, a preservação da secreção de ACTH vai contra a formação de cistos na bolsa de Rathke como causa primária do nanismo hipofisário.

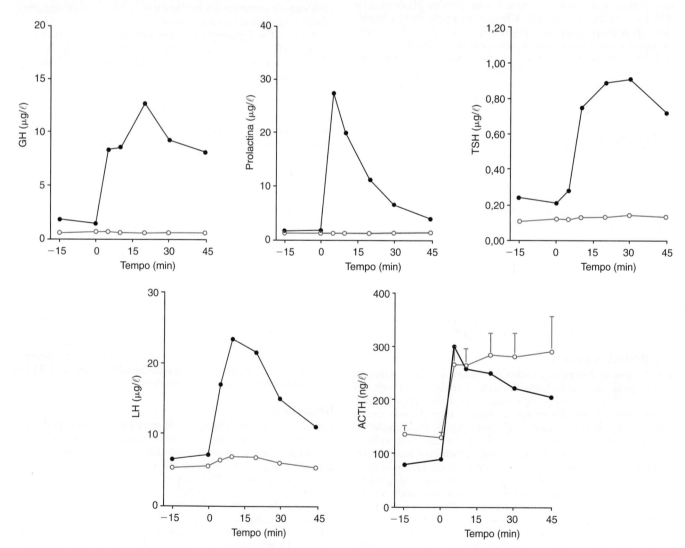

Figura 295.3 Resultados de uma combinação de testes da função da adeno-hipófise (média e DP) em 8 cães da raça Pastor-Alemão com nanismo (○) e em oito cães saudáveis da raça Beagle (●). *ACTH*, hormônio adrenocorticotrófico; *GH*, hormônio do crescimento; *LH*, hormônio luteinizante; *TSH*, hormônio tireoestimulante. (De Kooistra HS, Voorhout G, Mol JA, et al.: Combined pituitary hormone deficiency in German Shepherd Dogs with dwarfism. *Domest Anim Endocrinol* 19:177, 2000. Com gentil permissão de Domestic Animal Endocrinology.)

Estudos genéticos demonstraram que o nanismo hipofisário se deve a uma mutação no gene *LHX3*.[22] O LHX3 é um membro da família do homeodomínio da proteína LIM de fatores de transcrição que se ligam ao DNA. Em seres humanos e ratos, os defeitos moleculares no gene *LHX3* resultam em déficits de todos os hormônios da adeno-hipófise, com exceção do ACTH. Esses achados são idênticos ao fenótipo endócrino dos cães anões da raça Pastor-Alemão. A análise do íntron 5 do *LHX3* revelou que, nos anões, ocorre deleção de um das seis repetições do par de bases 7 (bp), reduzindo o tamanho do íntron a somente 68 bp, resultando em divisão defeituosa do *LHX3*.[22] Esse defeito genético também é a causa de nanismo hipofisário em cães das raças Saarloo Wolfdog e Czechoslovakian Wolfdog; ambas são raças híbridas de cães e lobos oriundos do Pastor-Alemão.[23] A triagem de alguns cães Saarloo Wolfdog e Czechoslovakian Wolfdog clinicamente saudáveis mostrou que 31 e 21%, respectivamente, são portadores do defeito genético. Esses resultados indicam que o nanismo hipofisário é uma anormalidade relevante e enfatiza a necessidade de realização de exames. O nanismo hipofisário e seus defeitos do DNA associados costumam ser incompatíveis com a vida, o que explica o motivo pelo qual a condição é incomum.

Manifestações clínicas

O nanismo hipofisário pode ocasionar uma ampla gama de manifestações clínicas.[24] Animais com nanismo hipofisário são levados à consulta veterinária aos 2 a 5 meses de vida, por conta do retardo de crescimento proporcional, retenção de pelos lanosos ou secundários e ausência de pelos primários ou longos (Figura 295.4). Os pelos lanosos se desprendem com facilidade e pode haver desenvolvimento gradativo de alopecia no tronco, com início em pontos de fricção, poupando a cabeça e as extremidades. A pele se torna progressivamente hiperpigmentada e escamosa. Infecções bacterianas secundárias são comuns. Os anões costumam ter um espelho nasal pontudo, semelhante ao de uma raposa. Devido à liberação prejudicada de gonadotrofina, quase sempre os anões machos apresentam criptorquidismo uni ou bilateral e as fêmeas comumente não ovulam devido à ausência do pico do hormônio luteinizante. A mutação em *LHX3* também está associada a malformações da articulação atlantoaxial, o que pode levar à instabilidade e à compressão dinâmica da medula espinal cervical.[25] Em geral, animais com nanismo hipofisário são ativos e alertas, mas a inapetência e a diminuição da atividade costumam ocorrer com cerca de 2 a 3 anos de idade devido ao hipotireoidismo secundário e à disfunção renal.

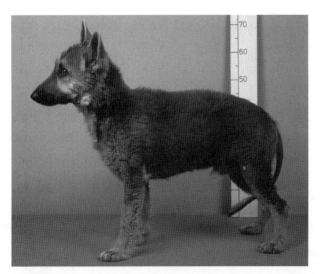

Figura 295.4 Cão da raça Pastor-Alemão de 6 meses de vida com retardo de crescimento, retenção de pelos secundários (pelame de filhote) e ausência de pelos primários, devido ao nanismo hipofisário.

Diagnóstico

Embora os sinais clínicos de nanismo hipofisário possam ser óbvios, outras causas endócrinas e não endócrinas de retardo do crescimento e/ou da alopecia devem ser excluídas. Nenhuma anormalidade, com exceção da elevação na concentração sérica de creatinina, é notada no exame laboratorial de rotina de cães com nanismo hipofisário de ocorrência natural.[21] A deficiência de GH (com ou sem deficiência de hormônio tireoideano) causa desenvolvimento glomerular anormal e disfunção renal. É comum notar baixa concentração plasmática de IGF-1 e TSH e baixa concentração sérica de T_4. Entretanto, baixa concentração de IGF-1 não propicia o diagnóstico definitivo de nanismo hipofisário.

Como os valores plasmáticos basais de GH podem também estar baixos em animais saudáveis, o diagnóstico definitivo da deficiência de GH deve se basear em resultados de testes de estimulação. Para esse propósito, pode ser utilizado GHRH (1 μg/kg) ou fármacos alfa-adrenérgicos, como a clonidina (10 μg/kg) ou xilazina (100 μg/kg). A concentração plasmática de GH deve ser mensurada imediatamente antes da administração por via intravenosa do estimulante e 20 a 30 min depois. Em cães saudáveis, a concentração plasmática de GH deve aumentar, pelo menos, duas a quatro vezes após a estimulação. Em cães com nanismo hipofisário não ocorre elevação significativa no conteúdo circulante de GH (ver Figura 295.3). A estimulação supra-hipofisária com hormônio liberador de corticotrofina (CRH, do inglês *corticotropina-releasing hormone*), hormônio liberador de tireotrofina (TRH, do inglês *thyrotropin-releasing hormone*) ou hormônio liberador de gonadotrofina (GnRH, do inglês *gonadotropina-releasing hormone*) pode revelar a existência de outras deficiências de hormônios hipofisários.[21] Concentração plasmática de GH superior a 5 μg/ℓ, 20 minutos após a administração por via intravenosa de 2 μg de grelina/kg, exclui a possibilidade de nanismo hipofisário.[26]

Exames de imagem da área hipofisária (tomografia computadorizada ou ressonância magnética) costumam revelar a existência de cistos hipofisários em cães com deficiência congênita de GH.[21] Apesar da presença de cistos, a maioria dos cães jovens com nanismo hipofisário tem a hipófise extremamente pequena, compatível com hipoplasia hipofisária (i. e., ausência de células endócrinas na adeno-hipófise). O tamanho do cisto aumenta gradativamente com o passar do tempo.[27] Quando os cistos são grandes, o tamanho da hipófise também pode aumentar. Como cães saudáveis podem ter cistos hipofisários, o diagnóstico definitivo do nanismo hipofisário não pode se basear somente na presença de cistos hipofisários.

Foi desenvolvido um teste de DNA para auxiliar na detecção da mutação *LHX3*.[22,23] A disponibilidade desse teste não somente possibilita um diagnóstico apropriado de cães com deficiência congênita de GH, mas também permite que os criadores impeçam o nascimento de anões, testando a condição de portador de potenciais animais reprodutores e planejando o correto programa de acasalamento.

Tratamento

Não há disponibilidade de GH canino. Tentativas foram feitas para tratar cães com deficiência congênita de GH utilizando GH heterólogo. A formação de anticorpos impede a utilização do GH recombinante humano.[28] A administração de GH suíno não resulta na formação de anticorpos, pois a sequência de aminoácidos do GH suíno é idêntica à do GH canino.[1] A dose subcutânea (SC) de GH suíno recomendada, de 0,1 a 0,3 UI 3 vezes/semana, pode resultar em excesso de GH e efeitos colaterais, como diabetes melito. Portanto, recomenda-se o monitoramento das concentrações plasmáticas de GH e de glicose 3 vezes/semana, durante o tratamento. O uso de doses a longo prazo deve ser determinado com base em mensurações da concentração plasmática de IGF-1. O crescimento linear causado pela administração de GH suíno depende da condição das placas de crescimento quando do início do tratamento. Em geral, nota-se resposta benéfica na pele e no crescimento de pelos lanosos dentro de 6 a 8 semanas após o início da terapia, mas o crescimento dos pelos longos é variável.

A demonstração da capacidade de os progestágenos induzirem expressão do gene GH na glândula mamária de cadelas, com subsequente secreção de GH na circulação sistêmica, levantou a possibilidade do tratamento da deficiência congênita de GH com progestágenos. O tratamento de cães jovens anões da raça Pastor-Alemão com injeções SC de 2,5 a 5 mg de acetato de medroxi-progesterona/kg, inicialmente em intervalos de 3 semanas e, em seguida, de 6 semanas, resultou em algum aumento do tamanho corporal e desenvolvimento de pelame de adulto. Em paralelo às melhoras físicas, constatou-se elevação brusca na concentração plasmática de IGF-1 simultânea ao aumento da concentração plasmáticas de GH, mas sem exceder o limite superior de normalidade da faixa de referência.[27] Relata-se que o tratamento de cães com nanismo hipofisário com proligestona resultou no desenvolvimento de pelame de adulto, aumentou o peso corporal e elevou a concentração plasmática de IGF-1.[29] Entretanto, a administração de progestágenos pode causar períodos recorrentes de piodermite pruriginosa, mau desenvolvimento esquelético, desenvolvimento de tumores mamários, acromegalia, diabetes melito e hiperplasia endometrial cística. Assim como acontece no tratamento utilizando GH suíno, é importante monitorar as concentrações plasmáticas de GH, IGF-1 e glicose. Cadelas devem ser submetidas à ovário-histerectomia antes do início do tratamento com progestágeno. O tratamento com levotiroxina deve ser iniciado assim que houver evidências de hipotireoidismo secundário.

Prognóstico

O prognóstico a longo prazo de cães anões da raça Pastor-Alemão não tratados quase sempre é reservado. Aos 3 a 5 anos, esses cães se tornam apáticos, magros e com áreas de alopecia. Essas alterações podem ocorrer devido à perda progressiva da função hipofisária, à expansão contínua dos cistos hipofisários e à insuficiência renal progressiva. Nesse estágio, os tutores costumam recorrer à eutanásia. Embora o prognóstico melhore consideravelmente quando os cães anões são tratados de maneira apropriada com levotiroxina e GH suíno ou progestágeno, seu prognóstico ainda permanece reservado.

Deficiência de hormônio do crescimento adquirida

Além de cães e gatos que desenvolvem deficiência de hormônio do crescimento adquirida após hipofisectomia eletiva a fim de remover um tumor e aqueles que a desenvolvem após lesão cerebral traumática, existem relatos de cães adultos que desenvolvem deficiência de GH de ocorrência natural.[30] Foi proposto que a deficiência de GH pode explicar algumas formas de alopecia em cães das raças Spitz alemão, Poodle Miniatura, Chow-chow, Keeshond e outros, descrita em cães de ambos os gêneros, castrados ou não, e de qualquer idade. Entretanto, a condição é mais comumente diagnosticada em cães com 1 a 3 anos. Nesses animais, a alopecia costuma envolver o tronco, a região posterior das coxas, o períneo e o pescoço; em geral, a pele se torna escura. A alopecia não parece ser atribuível a quaisquer doenças endócrinas que sabidamente resultem em atrofia cutânea e perda de pelos (i. e., hipotireoidismo, hipercortisolismo ou hiperestrogenismo devido a tumor testicular). Embora o tratamento com GH heterólogo[31] ou acetato de medroxiprogesterona[32] tenha mostrado resultado ruim a moderado, a condição foi denominada "deficiência de GH de início adulto" e "dermatose responsiva ao GH".

Incertezas sobre a participação do GH na ocorrência dessa condição são ainda mais exemplificadas por outros nomes, como "alopecia responsiva à castração", "alopecia responsiva à "biopsia" e "alopecia X".[31,32] A enfermidade ainda não está bem definida porque um terço dos cães apresenta resposta normal no teste de estimulação com GH. Ainda, em alguns animais com resposta normal à estimulação, o tratamento com GH foi efetivo. Em outros, medidas aparentemente não relacionadas, como castração ou administração de testosterona, foram acompanhadas de surgimento de um novo pelame.[33] Quando os testes de estimulação com GH foram realizados em cães da raça Spitz alemão com alopecia e em um grupo-controle, sem alopecia, verificou-se que a concentração circulante média de GH não aumentou de maneira significativa em ambos os grupos.[34] Assim, a associação entre algumas formas dessa alopecia de início na vida adulta e a menor secreção de GH não é bem aceita. Não é provável que haja verdadeira deficiência de GH, já que a concentração plasmática de IGF-1 situa-se invariavelmente na faixa de variação normal.[31]

REFERÊNCIAS BIBLIOGRÁFICAS

As referências bibliográficas deste capítulo se encontram online no Ambiente de Aprendizagem.

CAPÍTULO 296

Diabetes Insípido

Robert E. Shiel

FISIOLOGIA

Fonte e estrutura da vasopressina

A vasopressina arginina (AVP, do inglês *arginine vasopressina*), o principal hormônio responsável pela homeostase hídrica, é um pequeno peptídio derivado de um precursor maior dentro de neurônios magnocelulares dos núcleos paraventricular e supraóptico do hipotálamo.[1,2] A pré-pró-vasopressina é constituída de peptídio-sinal e de polipeptídios que posteriormente formam AVP, neurofisina-2 e a glicoproteína copeptina.

Após clivagem do peptídio-sinal, a pró-vasopressina é transportada para o retículo endoplasmático. A neurofisina-2 é necessária para o correto processamento, transporte, clivagem e pode proteger a AVP contra degradação enzimática. A função da copeptina é desconhecida. O pró-hormônio é armazenado em grânulos neurossecretores antes do transporte axonal através do trato hipotalâmico-neuro-hipofisário e conservado na neuro-hipófise (hipófise posterior ou lobo posterior da hipófise). A clivagem enzimática, até formação de moléculas constituintes, ocorre durante o transporte e armazenamento.

Estímulos para secreção

Em resposta a um estímulo para liberação de AVP, é gerado um potencial de ação no corpo celular hipotalâmico, que se propaga ao longo do axônio até a neuro-hipófise, resultando em exocitose do conteúdo do grânulo cálcio-dependente e liberação dos três produtos. Como a neuro-hipófise não possui barreira hematencefálica e contém vasos capilares fenestrados, a entrada na circulação sistêmica é rápida.[3] O principal estímulo para liberação de AVP é o aumento da osmolalidade (OSM) plasmática. Diversos órgãos circunventriculares, inclusive o órgão subfórnix e o órgão vascular da lâmina terminal, atuam como osmorreceptores capazes de alterar a secreção de AVP e a sede.[4] Além disso, neurônios magnocelulares podem ser diretamente estimulados por alteração na concentração plasmática de sódio (Na^+).[5] Um incremento de 1% na OSM plasmática é suficiente para estimular a liberação de AVP. Em cães, como a meia-vida da AVP é estimada como sendo menor que 6 minutos, uma diminuição na OSM plasmática é rapidamente seguida de redução na secreção de AVP.[6] A volemia é controlada, sobretudo, pelo sistema renina-angiotensina-aldosterona. Entretanto, barorreceptores arteriais de alta pressão presentes no seio carotídeo e no arco aórtico e receptores de volume de baixa pressão nos átrios e no sistema venoso pulmonar podem inibir a secreção de AVP pela ação dos nervos glossofaríngeo e vago.[2] Uma diminuição de 10 a 15% na volemia ou na pressão sanguínea pode reduzir esse estímulo inibidor, resultando em secreção de AVP. Outros fatores que influenciam a secreção de AVP incluem estresse, náuseas, dor, doença cerebral estrutural, terapia com determinados fármacos, hipoglicemia e atividade física. A ingestão hídrica, associada à diminuição na secreção de AVP antes da alteração da OSM plasmática, pode ser mediada por receptores de volume ou de osmolalidade faríngeos.[7,8]

Interação de mecanismos reguladores e diversos locais de ação da vasopressina arginina

Os mecanismos reguladores são altamente interativos. Por exemplo, o aumento da concentração de angiotensina II pode estimular a secreção de AVP e a sede pelo órgão subfórnix, enquanto barorreceptores podem estimular a liberação de renina e AVP.[4] De maneira semelhante, peptídios natriuréticos contribuem para a regulação do balanço de Na^+ e o equilíbrio hídrico. O peptídio natriurético cerebral (tipo B) tem ação inibitória na liberação de renina, aldosterona e AVP. AVP e angiotensina II possuem efeitos estimulatórios na liberação do peptídio natriurético atrial (PNA).[9,10]

As ações da AVP são mediadas por uma série de receptores associados à proteína-G. Na ausência de AVP, as superfícies celulares do lúmen dos ductos coletores renais principais possuem mínima permeabilidade à água. A ligação da AVP aos receptores basolaterais V2 aumenta a concentração de monofosfato cíclico de adenosina e ativa a proteinoquinase A, uma via de fosforilação que causa fusão da aquaporina-2, que contém vesículas intracitoplasmáticas (conhecidas como agregóforos), com as membranas celulares apicais. O aumento resultante da expressão de aquaporina-2 aumenta a permeabilidade e reabsorção hídrica mediante o movimento passivo de moléculas do lúmen tubular hipotônico até o córtex isotônico e/ou interstício medular hipertônico. Assim que o estímulo do receptor cessa, as aquaporinas são novamente internalizadas e armazenadas nos agregóforos por um mecanismo mediado pela clatrina. A estimulação de neurônios magnocelulares também aumenta a síntese de AVP; entretanto, há um retardo de várias horas antes que a AVP recém-formada esteja pronta para liberação. Por essa razão, quantidade relativamente grande de AVP é armazenada na neuro-hipófise. A liberação de AVP não é restrita às terminações nervosas e intumescências axonais contidas na neuro-hipófise; a liberação pode ocorrer de vários locais do neurônio, inclusive o corpo celular e dendritos e soma hipotalâmicos, e axônios não dilatados.

A ação da AVP vai além do controle do equilíbrio hídrico. A ligação a receptor V2 pode induzir à liberação do fator de von Willebrand, ativador do plasminogênio tecidual, e do peptídio natriurético atrial. A AVP também estimula a síntese de óxido nítrico e aumenta a concentração circulante do fator de coagulação VIII. A ativação de receptores V1a causa contração do músculo liso vascular, glicogenólise e ativação plaquetária. A ligação a receptores V1b, na adeno-hipófise (ou hipófise anterior), atua sinergicamente com o hormônio liberador de corticotrofina para estimular a liberação de ACTH. A estimulação de receptores V1b em outros tecidos endócrinos pode aumentar a secreção de catecolaminas e insulina. A AVP também foi identificada como um importante neurotransmissor e mediador químico no cérebro, com ações fundamentais em diversas áreas, incluindo recuperação da memória, aprendizado, manutenção do ciclo circadiano e comportamento social.

FISIOPATOLOGIA DO DIABETES INSÍPIDO

Considerações gerais

O diabetes insípido está associado à diminuição da produção ou ação da AVP. Embora raro em cães e gatos, a doença é bem descrita, sendo um importante diferencial para poliúria e polidipsia (PU/PD), particularmente quando grave.

Diabetes insípido central

O diabetes insípido central é caracterizado por deficiência total ou parcial de AVP. Em seres humanos, a transecção traumática do pedúnculo hipofisário ou a cirurgia da hipófise podem causar um padrão conhecido como diabetes insípido trifásico.[2,27,28] O primeiro estágio é o diabetes insípido agudo devido ao colapso do axônio e à incapacidade de liberar AVP. O segundo estágio, a fase antidiurética, se deve à liberação descontrolada de grandes reservas da neuro-hipófise. O terceiro estágio surge após a depleção das reservas de AVP e recidiva do diabetes insípido central. Essa terceira fase pode ser permanente, mas pode ocorrer recuperação parcial e deficiência subclínica devido à capacidade de liberação de AVP por componentes neuronais remanescentes.

O diabetes insípido central também pode ser causado por mutações no gene *AVP* de seres humanos, afetando, em geral, o peptídio-sinal ou a neurofisina.[2] É provável que precursores mutantes sejam retidos no retículo endoplasmático, o que explica a diminuição de AVP e a toxicidade celular observada em alguns casos. Tais causas genéticas não foram pesquisadas em cães ou gatos, mas diabetes insípido central congênito foi descrito em ninhadas de cães da raça Afghan Hound.[15] Há relatos de cães e gatos jovens com diabetes insípido central parcial ou total.[11,20,25]

Em cães e gatos, a ocorrência de diabetes insípido central deveu-se mais comumente a defeitos estruturais no hipotálamo e/ou na neuro-hipófise. A neoplasia de hipófise é mais frequentemente incriminada em cães e o trauma, em gatos; entretanto, diversas outras causas são descritas (Boxe 296.1).[11-26] O padrão trifásico descrito em algumas pessoas não foi observado em cães ou gatos, mas a hipofisectomia em cães com hiperadrenocorticismo hipófise-dependente ocasiona diabetes insípido central prolongado (mais de 2 semanas após a cirurgia) em 53% dos cães. Aproximadamente 42% deles necessitam tratamento permanente.[29] Alterações durante o período pós-cirúrgico inicial não são bem caracterizadas devido à suplementação frequente de cães com AVP sintético após a cirurgia, mas o diabetes insípido central foi mais provável em cães com aumento hipofisário e menos comum em gatos após hipofisectomia.[30] O diabetes insípido central idiopático foi relatado tanto em cães como em gatos. Exames de imagem avançados não foram realizados em muitos desses animais e a possibilidade de doença subjacente não foi excluída.

Boxe 296.1 Causas de diabetes insípido central e nefrogênico em cães e gatos

Idiopáticas
Trauma
Neoplasia
  Craniofaringioma
  Meningioma
  Adenoma ou carcinoma cromófobo
  Linfoma
  Neoplasia metastática
Cirurgia
Anormalidades congênitas
Infecção
Inflamação
Cistos

Diabetes insípido nefrogênico

O diabetes insípido nefrogênico é caracterizado pela diminuição da ação da AVP nos rins. Diabetes insípido nefrogênico secundário é uma característica de diversas anormalidades (ver Capítulo 45), inclusive hiperadrenocorticismo (ver Capítulo 306), piometra (ver Capítulo 316), hipercalcemia (ver Capítulos 69 e 297), hiponatremia (ver Capítulos 67 e 309), pielonefrite (ver Capítulo 327) e hepatopatia (ver Capítulo 284). diabetes insípido nefrogênico primário (familiar) é um raro distúrbio genético associado a alterações qualitativas ou quantitativas na expressão da aquaporina-2. Em seres humanos com diabetes insípido nefrogênico familiar, foram detectadas mutações específicas nos genes do receptor V2 e da aquaporina-2; mais de 90% dos pacientes apresentam mutação no cromossomo X (ligada ao sexo) do gene do receptor V2.[31] Cerca de 10% dessas pessoas supostamente desenvolvem mutações *de novo*. Mutações autossômicas da aquaporina-2 são menos comuns.

Suspeitou-se de diabetes insípido nefrogênico primário em uma ninhada de cães da raça Husky siberiano, nos quais 3 de 4 machos apresentavam quantidade normal de receptores V2 na medula interna, mas com capacidade de ligação à AVP dez vezes menor.[32] Como os sinais clínicos eram restritos aos machos, incriminou-se o envolvimento do gene do receptor V2, também localizado no cromossomo X de cães. Há relatos de casos isolados de diabetes insípido nefrogênico primário,[33-35] mas não em gatos.

CARACTERÍSTICAS CLÍNICAS

Resenha

O diabetes insípido pode ocorrer em qualquer idade e em qualquer raça. A resenha depende muito da causa primária. Neoplasias são mais prováveis em animais idosos e doença congênita em jovens. Os sinais clínicos podem ser agudos ou progredir gradativamente durante semanas a meses.

Sinais clínicos

Classicamente, o diabetes insípido está associado a poliúria e polidipsia (PU/PD) significativas e consumo de água comumente estimada pelos tutores como 5 a 20 vezes acima do normal. Animais podem apresentar sede contínua e preferir água a alimentos, o que pode ocasionar perda de peso. A ingestão de grande volume de água pode levar à êmese. Quase sempre a PU significativa causa noctúria e incontinência urinária por fluxo exagerado. Anormalidades neurológicas são comuns em cães com neoplasia de hipotálamo ou de hipófise (ver Capítulo 259). Em um estudo, constatou-se que 7 de 17 cães com diabetes insípido central desenvolveram sinais neurológicos 2 semanas a 12 meses após o diagnóstico inicial.[11] Os sintomas incluíam convulsões, obnubilação, alterações comportamentais e tremores. Anormalidades neurológicas também podem ocorrer caso não seja fornecida água ao animal ou caso ele não consiga beber. A desidratação hipertônica resultante pode levar à desidratação celular e à manifestação de anorexia, fraqueza, ataxia, convulsões e morte. A desidratação hipertônica também pode causar desmielinização osmótica. Da mesma forma, sinais neurológicos podem ocorrer em animais com livre acesso à água após período de restrição hídrica. Isso pode causar rápida diminuição da OSM plasmática e edema cerebral.

Sinais clínicos associados a anormalidades endócrinas podem também ser observados. Por exemplo, cães com tumor cromófobo hipofisário funcional e hipercortisolismo secundário podem apresentar apenas sintomas de hiperadrenocorticismo. Da mesma forma, defeitos estruturais hipotalâmicos e hipofisários ou hipofisectomia podem levar a sinais clínicos associados ao hipotireoidismo central ou, menos comumente, ao hipoadrenocorticismo secundário.[36] Podem ocorrer deficiência de hormônio do crescimento e de gonadotrofina, mas sem sinais clínicos. Deficiências endócrinas persistentes são comuns em seres humanos após traumatismo cranioencefálico.[37] Em cães e gatos, tais deficiências podem ser subclínicas e não diagnosticadas.[12,24,38]

Exames de rotina

Exames clinicopatológicos de rotina podem não revelar anormalidade em animais com diabetes insípido central, desde que não haja restrição de água e outros distúrbios. Pode ocorrer diminuição da concentração de ureia devido à diluição medular renal e à menor reabsorção dependente de AVP. Caso tenha havido restrição hídrica, é possível notar alterações indicativas de desidratação, incluindo elevação do valor do hematócrito e da concentração de proteína, Na^+ ou cloreto, assim como azotemia pré-renal. Em cães acometidos, a OSM sérica pode estar normal ou aumentada. Hipostenúria é o único achado clinicopatológico consistente em animais com diabetes insípido central total ou diabetes insípido nefrogênico. No diabetes insípido central parcial, pode-se observar isostenúria ou urina minimamente concentrada. Em um estudo, detectou-se cistite bacteriana em 4 de 17 cães.[11] Em todos os casos, deve-se realizar cultura bacteriana para excluir a possibilidade de pielonefrite como causa de diabetes insípido nefrogênico secundário.

EXAMES CONFIRMATÓRIOS

Diabetes insípido central e nefrogênico
versus polidipsia primária

Não há um único teste que apresente excelente sensibilidade e especificidade para o diagnóstico de diabetes insípido. Devido aos efeitos de diversas condições na liberação e ação de AVP, é essencial excluir outras causas de PU/PD antes de buscar o diagnóstico de diabetes insípido. Vários métodos estão disponíveis para distinguir diabetes insípido central, diabetes insípido nefrogênico primário e polidipsia primária. De modo geral, o diabetes insípido nefrogênico primário pode ser excluído com base nos sinais clínicos. Entretanto, a distinção entre diabetes insípido central e polidipsia primária pode ser desafiadora, sendo a interpretação do teste complicada pelo conhecimento incompleto dos mecanismos fisiopatológicos envolvidos nessas condições. Por exemplo, a secreção de AVP não é normal na maioria das pessoas com polidipsia primária, com taxas e momentos alterados para liberação de AVP.[39,40] É incerto se essas alterações representam um mecanismo de retroalimentação (*feedback*) negativa na liberação de AVP em resposta à hiper-hidratação crônica ou se há anormalidades primárias no controle de AVP, enquanto distúrbios de osmorreceptores podem afetar simultaneamente a regulação da sede e a secreção de AVP. De forma semelhante, a resposta de AVP e a capacidade de concentração da urina em cães com polidipsia primária foi caracterizada como exagerada, subnormal ou não linear.[41,42] Isso é ainda mais complicado pela natureza pulsátil e variável da secreção de AVP em cães e pelos efeitos potenciais da hiper ou hipo-hidratação crônica na secreção e ação da AVP.[43]

Teste de privação hídrica modificado

Indicações e fase 1

O teste de privação hídrica modificado é o teste auxiliar mais comumente recomendado para diferenciar diabetes insípido central, diabetes insípido nefrogênico e polidipsia primária (Figura 296.1). Ele é demorado e pode estar associado a risco, mesmo se realizado de forma apropriada. A fase 1 do teste envolve um período de 3 a 5 dias de restrição hídrica progressiva. Na teoria, isso possibilita o restabelecimento de certo gradiente de concentração medular renal, provavelmente diminuído em animais com PU/PD crônica. Devem ser fornecidos alimentos secos e o volume total de água estimado, fracionado e fornecido em várias pequenas porções, conforme for possível, a fim de evitar períodos prolongados de privação total de água. Embora geralmente realizado em casa, é possível que a desidratação hipertônica e sintomas associados ocorram durante essa fase de restrição hídrica. Portanto, os tutores devem ser orientados quanto aos potenciais efeitos adversos da restrição hídrica e monitorar o peso corporal e o comportamento do animal. A desidratação hipertônica é mais provável em animais com PU significativa. Portanto, pode ser prudente hospitalizar tais animais para observação.

Fase 2

A água é completamente retirada para iniciar a fase 2. O monitoramento adequado é essencial porque rapidamente pode ocorrer desidratação hipertônica com risco de morte. O teste é iniciado no início da manhã para possibilitar a observação próxima do paciente durante todo o dia. Uma balança confiável é essencial, já que o animal deve ser pesado, pelo menos, a cada 60 minutos, após o início da fase 2. Também, é essencial a habilidade em monitorar as concentrações séricas de eletrólitos, nitrogênio ureico sanguíneo, hematócrito e proteína total pelo menos a cada 60 minutos. O teste de privação hídrica modificado deve ser descontinuado se o animal manifestar apatia, letargia e azotemia ou se a concentração sérica de Na^+ aumentar de modo excessivo. A OSM e a densidade urinária, ao se esvaziar a bexiga a cada momento, devem ser monitoradas a cada 30 a 60 minutos. A privação hídrica é mantida até que ocorra perda de 3 a 5% do peso corporal ou até que a densidade urinária exceda 1,025. Na maioria dos animais com diabetes insípido central completo ou diabetes insípido nefrogênico primário, esse ponto final é alcançado dentro de 3 a 10 horas. Entretanto, em animais com diabetes insípido central parcial ou polidipsia primária pode demorar um tempo consideravelmente maior. Se a densidade urinária aumentar para um valor acima de 1,025, o diagnóstico de polidipsia primária pode ser confirmado e o teste, descontinuado.

Fase 3

Essa fase começa assim que o animal tiver perdido 3 a 5% do peso corporal e submetido à administração de desmopressina (1-desamino-8-D-arginina vasopressina [DDAVP]), um análogo sintético da AVP (2 a 10 μg por via intravenosa [IV]). Volumes hídricos de manutenção podem ser administrados por via IV durante esse estágio para diminuir a probabilidade de desidratação progressiva. A densidade urinária é monitorada a cada 30 minutos durante 2 horas e, então, a cada hora durante 8 horas, e, se necessário, após 12 e 24 horas. A concentração urinária

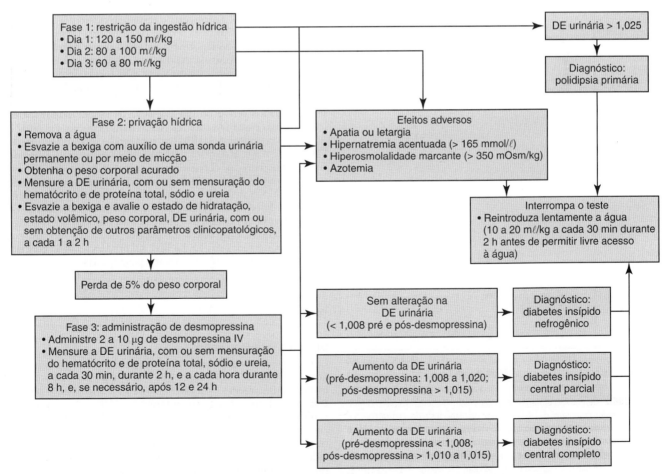

Figura 296.1 Algoritmo para realização do teste de privação hídrica modificado. *DE*, densidade específica.

máxima é tipicamente observada após 4 a 8 horas; entretanto, o teste pode ser descontinuado mais cedo se a densidade da urina aumentar para um valor acima de 1,015. Após a conclusão do teste, a água deve ser reintroduzida gradativamente, com cerca de 10 a 20 mℓ/kg a cada 30 minutos por, pelo menos, 2 horas, antes de permitir livre acesso à água. Se o animal começa a beber água compulsivamente, o livre acesso deve ser descontinuado de imediato para evitar êmese e risco de desidratação grave.

Interpretação do teste

A interpretação dos resultados do teste pode ser desafiadora. A polidipsia primária é caracterizada por aumento da densidade urinária em resposta apenas à restrição hídrica. Entretanto, a incapacidade em restabelecer o gradiente de concentração medular renal pode resultar em resposta incompleta. O aumento da densidade urinária após administração de DDAVP é compatível com diabetes insípido central, enquanto a ausência de resposta sugere diabetes insípido nefrogênico. diabetes insípido central parcial pode estar associado à concentração limitada em resposta à restrição hídrica e ao aumento adicional da densidade urinária após administração de DDAVP (Figura 296.2). Entretanto, em alguns casos de diabetes insípido central parcial, desidratação grave pode estimular a secreção máxima de AVP e incapacidade de responder à DDAVP.

Teste terapêutico com desmopressina (DDAVP)

Uma alternativa simples ao teste de privação hídrica modificado é o teste terapêutico com DDAVP. A ingestão hídrica diária média é determinada pelo tutor antes do início do teste. A desmopressina é administrada durante 5 a 7 dias e a resposta avaliada ao notar alterações na ingestão hídrica. Pode-se mensurar a densidade urinária para confirmar a opinião subjetiva do tutor. Em cães com diabetes insípido central, nota-se, tipicamente, diminuição marcante da ingestão hídrica e aumento da densidade urinária. Cães com diabetes insípido nefrogênico primário e aqueles com polidipsia primária não respondem ao teste. Antes da administração inicial de DDAVP, é fundamental a exclusão de outras causas de PU/PD. Respostas parciais podem ser observadas em animais com diabetes insípido nefrogênico secundário ou polidipsia primária. Entre as vantagens do teste terapêutico, incluem-se menor risco de desidratação grave com risco de morte, menor necessidade de monitoramento intensivo e possibilidade de realizar o teste sem hospitalização. Embora efeitos adversos associados ao uso de DDAVP sejam raros, a administração desse fármaco a um animal com aumento persistente da ingestão de água devido à polidipsia primária pode, em teoria, resultar em intoxicação hídrica e hiponatremia.

Outros testes

A mensuração de AVP tem pouco valor diagnóstico devido à natureza pulsátil e variável da secreção de AVP. As amostras requerem manuseio cuidadoso e os testes validados não estão amplamente disponíveis. O teste de infusão de solução salina hipertônica já foi considerado o método padrão-ouro para diferenciar diabetes insípido central, diabetes insípido nefrogênico e polidipsia primária. O teste baseia-se na resposta da AVP à infusão de solução de cloreto de sódio a 20%. A resposta diminuída da AVP é considerada compatível com diabetes insípido nefrogênico central. Uma resposta normal ou exagerada da AVP sem aumento correspondente da densidade urinária indica diabetes insípido nefrogênico, enquanto uma resposta normal da AVP com elevação apropriada da densidade urinária sugere polidipsia primária. Entretanto, o teste não diferencia, de forma confiável, diabetes insípido central de polidipsia primária.

A expressão da aquaporina-2 na urina mostrou refletir intimamente as alterações na exposição à AVP em cães saudáveis, mas não foi utilizada clinicamente. De forma semelhante, a concentração plasmática de copeptina, o c-terminal do precursor de AVP, mostrou estar correlacionada à secreção de AVP em seres humanos, sendo útil na avaliação de suspeita de diabetes insípido, mas esse marcador não foi avaliado em cães ou gatos.[44] Ressonância magnética (RM) e tomografia computadorizada (TC) podem ser úteis para detectar lesões estruturais hipofisárias e hipotalâmicas, como aquelas causadas por neoplasias ou traumatismos.[45,46] Em seres humanos, na RM, a constatação de sinais de hiperintensidade na sela túrcica supostamente representam fosfolipídios ou grânulos secretórios na neuro-hipófise e estão ausentes na maioria dos pacientes acometidos por diabetes insípido central. Em cães, a intensidade da neuro-hipófise em imagens ponderadas em T1, na RM, foi proporcional ao conteúdo de AVP. Entretanto, não foram pesquisadas alterações em situações clínicas.

TRATAMENTO

Diabetes insípido central

O tratamento do diabetes insípido central pode não ser necessário em todos os casos, desde que o acesso à água esteja disponível continuamente e a PU/PD não seja angustiante para o animal ou tutor. O análogo sintético da AVP, a desmopressina (DDAVP), pode ser utilizado em casos de diabetes insípido central completo ou parcial. Embora seja um potente agonista do receptor V2, não há relato de expansão excessiva da volemia e de hiponatremia com o uso de protocolos terapêuticos atualmente recomendados para cães com diabetes insípido central. A DDAVP tem mínimos efeitos nos receptores V1a e não há

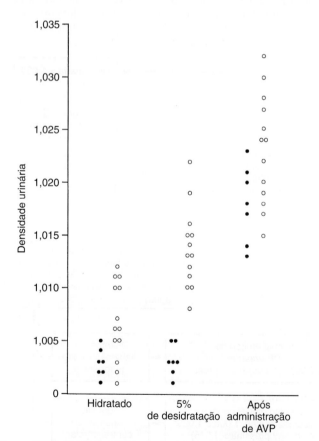

Figura 296.2 Densidade urinária de 7 cães com diabetes insípido central (círculo fechado) completo e 13 cães com diabetes insípido central parcial (círculo aberto) no início (hidratado), no fim da fase II (desidratação de 5%) e no final da fase III (após administração de arginina vasopressina [AVP]) do teste de privação hídrica modificado. Note a semelhança nas respostas da densidade urinária e da osmolalidade urinária. (De Feldman EC, Nelson RW, Reusch CE, et al.: Canine & feline endocrinology, 4 ed., St. Louis, 2015, Elsevier, Inc.)

relato de hipertensão como efeito adverso. A administração de DDAVP é efetiva no controle dos sinais clínicos, na maioria dos animais. A dose ótima e a frequência de administração se baseiam em informações anedóticas e os protocolos terapêuticos, na resposta individual apropriada. Em cães, a DDAVP, disponível como solução intranasal para seres humanos, é comumente administrada em doses empíricas. As doses variaram de 1 a 4 gotas (cerca de 1,5 a 5 µg/gota) instiladas no saco conjuntival ou no nariz, em intervalos de 8 a 24 h. Como alternativa, pode-se administrar preparação injetável, na dose de 2 a 5 µg, a cada 12 a 24 h. A forma de comprimido pode ser administrada na dose de 100 µg, em intervalos de 12 a 24 h. Embora estudos experimentais tenham demonstrado aumento da concentração plasmática de desmopressina dose-dependente, após administração oral do fármaco, a resposta terapêutica é variável. Em gatos, há relato de administração oral (25 a 50 µg, a cada 8 a 12 h) SC (4 µg/24 h) e conjuntival (1 gota/12 h). Tanto em cães como em gatos, a dose e o intervalo entre as doses devem ser ajustados de modo a obter o controle adequado, em cada indivíduo. A resposta ao tratamento é rápida; se o tratamento for descontinuado, nota-se rápido retorno da PU. Alguns tutores podem optar pelo tratamento apenas durante a noite, para diminuir a probabilidade de noctúria.

Diabetes insípido nefrogênico

O diabetes insípido nefrogênico primário é extremamente raro em cães e gatos. A maioria das recomendações terapêuticas foi extrapolada de seres humanos, cuja minoria sofre com efeitos antidiuréticos parciais relacionados com altas doses de DDAVP.

Diuréticos tiazídicos diminuem a absorção de Na^+ nos túbulos distais, resultando em diminuição da volemia e subsequente redução da taxa de filtração glomerular, com aumento na reabsorção de Na^+ e água nos túbulos proximais. Como resultado, diminui a disponibilidade de água no túbulo distal e, assim, a perda de água. Efeitos adicionais podem incluir redução da taxa de filtração glomerular mediada pela resposta de retroalimentação (*feedback*) tubuloglomerular e suprarregulação dos efeitos na expressão do transportador de Na^+ distal e da aquaporina-2.[47-49] Para diminuir ainda mais o conteúdo de solutos na urina, recomenda-se uma dieta com baixos teores de Na^+ e de proteína. Fármacos anti-inflamatórios não esteroides (AINEs) podem ter efeito sinérgico; entretanto, é comum a ocorrência de efeitos adversos.[50] Também podem ser utilizados diuréticos que poupam potássio, a fim de auxiliar na prevenção de hipopotassemia iatrogênica. Tem-se utilizada clorpropamida, embora em geral para o tratamento de diabetes insípido central parcial. Seu modo de ação não é conhecido, embora evidências sugiram que pode atuar estimulando receptores de AVP e liberando a sinalização de receptor constitutivo.[51] Diuréticos tiazídicos foram administrados a cães com diabetes insípido nefrogênico primário. O efeito foi variável, com redução do volume de urina em até 50% na minoria dos casos.[33-35] Em cães e gatos, a dose de hidroclorotiazida recomendada é de 2,5 a 5 mg/kg/12 h VO.

PROGNÓSTICO

O prognóstico para cães com diabetes insípido central é variável, dependendo da causa. Casos idiopáticos e traumáticos podem ser controlados com sucesso durante vários anos, enquanto aqueles que envolvem neoplasias hipotalâmicas ou hipofisárias possuem prognóstico pior. Em uma série de casos, verificou-se que 7 de 17 cães permaneciam vivos 18 a 72 meses após o diagnóstico.[11] Os 10 cães restantes morreram ou foram submetidos à eutanásia 1 semana a 2 anos após o diagnóstico, mais comumente por conta do desenvolvimento de sinais neurológicos.

REFERÊNCIAS BIBLIOGRÁFICAS

As referências bibliográficas deste capítulo se encontram online no Ambiente de Aprendizagem.

CAPÍTULO **297**

Hiperparatireoidismo Primário

Barbara J. Skelly

HOMEOSTASE DO CÁLCIO EM CÃES E GATOS

Função do cálcio

O cálcio (Ca), elemento mais abundante no corpo devido à sua presença nos ossos, é necessário para diversos processos fisiológicos, como a transmissão de vários sinais recebidos nas superfícies celulares para o compartimento intracelular, condução do estímulo nervoso, transmissão neuromuscular, contração muscular, coagulação sanguínea, secreção hormonal e metabolização do glicogênio hepático. Efeitos adversos nos sistemas orgânicos são notados quando ocorrem anormalidades na homeostase do Ca. O esqueleto atua como um reservatório de Ca para correção de diminuição na concentração sérica desse elemento. O Ca pode ser excretado ou absorvido nos rins e no intestino delgado. O receptor sensível ao cálcio (CaSR, do inglês *Ca sensing receptor*), responsável por garantir que a concentração circulante de Ca seja mantida dentro de uma faixa limitada, é uma proteína-G presente na glândula paratireoide, rins, cartilagens e ossos.[1] Interações entre o CaSR e o paratormônio (PTH, do inglês *parathyroid hormone*), sintetizado e secretado pela glândula paratireoide, podem interferir direta ou indiretamente nos ossos, no trato gastrintestinal (GI) e nos rins, de modo a manter a concentração circulante de Ca em uma estreita faixa de referência.[2]

Mensuração do cálcio e sua regulação no soro sanguíneo

O cálcio, em comum com outros eletrólitos importantes, é regulado intimamente para manter estreitos intervalos de referência. As concentrações séricas de cálcio total (tCa) são, em geral, de cerca de 2,3 a 2,8 mmol/ℓ (9,2 a 11,2 mg/dℓ), em cães, e 2,1 a 2,5 mmol/ℓ (8,4 a 10 mg/dℓ), em gatos. Os intervalos de referência variam entre os laboratórios. Sempre que houver problema com esse eletrólito, recomenda-se a mensuração tanto da concentração de tCa quanto de Ca ionizado (iCa), a forma biologicamente ativa do eletrólito. Cerca de 50% da concentração de tCa é representada por iCa, aproximadamente 40% ligados a proteínas (albumina e pequena taxa com globulina) e menos de 10% formam complexos com ânions, como bicarbonato ou citrato. Para a mensuração de tCa no soro sanguíneo ou no plasma heparinizado, utilizam-se métodos espectrofotométricos. Os anticoagulantes citrato, ácido etilenodiaminotetracético (EDTA) e oxalato não são recomendados porque eles causam quelação do cálcio. Hemólise e lipemia podem aumentar falsamente a concentração aferida de tCa. A hipoproteinemia diminui a concentração aferida de tCa, mas não interfere na concentração aferida de iCa. Clinicamente, a concentração sérica de Ca mais importante é a do iCa, obtida pelo método do eletrodo de íon-específico. Entretanto, a proporção de iCa em uma amostra pode ser alterada pelo manuseio da amostra. Quando as amostras são armazenadas, a metabolização das hemácias aumenta a concentração sanguínea de ácido láctico e, assim, o pH do soro diminui e a fração de iCa aumenta. Diferentemente, quando as amostras são expostas ao ar, ocorre perda de dióxido de carbono (CO_2) e, assim, o pH aumenta e a fração de iCa diminui.

Controle da concentração sérica de cálcio

Os principais fatores que controlam a concentração circulante de Ca são: hormônio da paratireoide (paratormônio [PTH, do inglês *parathyroid hormone*]), proteína relacionada com o paratormônio (PTHrP, do inglês *parathyroid hormone-related protein*), vitamina D (vitamina D_3, calcitriol, 1,25-$[OH]_2$-colecalciferol) e calcitonina. O CaSR regula as concentrações extracelulares de Ca. A hipercalcemia ativa o CaSR, reduzindo a síntese e secreção de PTH. A hipocalcemia inativa o CaSR, aumenta a secreção de PTH e da expressão do gene do *PTH* e estimula a proliferação celular das glândulas paratireoides. A homeostase do Ca sofre alteração quando a atividade do CaSR é anormal ou quando há interferência de alguma doença.

Paratormônio

Descrição e função

O paratormônio (PTH, do inglês *parathyroid hormone*) é um hormônio polipeptídico pequeno (contém 84 aminoácidos) sintetizado e secretado nas glândulas paratireoides. Cães e gatos possuem quatro glândulas paratireoides (dois pares). Um par está incrustado ou estreitamente associado a cada lobo da tireoide (Figura 297.1). Em geral, as glândulas craniais, "externas", estão situadas fora da cápsula da tireoide e as glândulas caudais, "internas", no tecido tireoidiano. As glândulas paratireoides consistem em cordões de aglomerados de células ao redor de capilares (Figura 297.2). As células principais da paratireoide sintetizam PTH, o que aumenta as concentrações séricas de Ca (tanto tCa quanto iCa) e diminui a concentração sérica de fósforo, seja direta, seja indiretamente, por meio de três principais órgãos-alvo: ossos, rins ou trato GI (Figura 297.3). O PTH é continuamente sintetizado por células principais e metabolizado com rapidez. Grânulos secretórios presentes no interior das células principais contêm hormônio ativo intacto, inclusive o aminoácido-34, N-terminal biologicamente ativo e as porções carboxiterminais necessárias para a atividade do PTH.[2-4] Quando a concentração sérica de Ca diminui, a taxa de degradação dos grânulos secretórios é reduzida. De forma contrária, quando a concentração sérica de Ca aumenta, a taxa de degradação se eleva. A vitamina D influencia a dinâmica da síntese e secreção de PTH: alta concentração de vitamina D retarda a transcrição do gene do *PTH* e reduz a taxa de síntese do hormônio. Alta concentração de fósforo reduz a avaria do PTH e aumenta a secreção do hormônio.

Testes para mensuração de paratormônio

O PTH e seus fragmentos clivados da molécula intacta são circulantes. Para avaliação confiável da função da paratireoide, deve-se mensurar o PTH intacto, que é biologicamente ativo (aminoácidos 1 a 84).[5,6] Os testes desenvolvidos para mensuração do PTH são sensíveis e específicos. Testes mais antigos utilizavam anticorpos direcionados ao C-terminal (aminoácidos 39 a 84) e ao N-terminal (aminoácidos 12 a 24, ou 26 a 32). Entretanto, os resultados desses testes incluíam concentrações

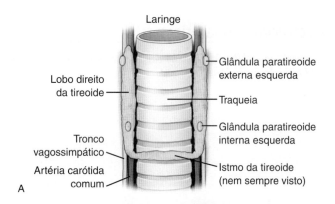

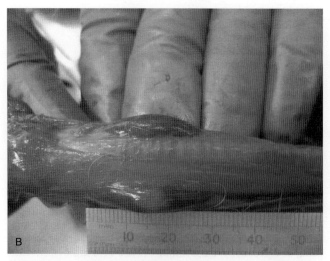

Figura 297.1 A. Representação esquemática da localização anatômica das glândulas paratireoides. **B.** Amostra patológica macroscópica mostrando a região cervical ventral de um gato, após dissecção, com aumento de glândula paratireoide. (Cortesia de Fernando Constantino-Casas.)

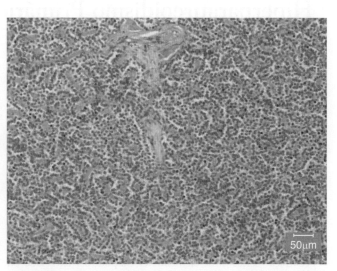

Figura 297.2 Aparência histológica da glândula paratireoide de um cão saudável mostrando cordões ou aglomerados de células ao redor dos capilares. Coloração com hematoxilina e eosina, barra = 50 micrômetros. (Cortesia de Fernando Constantino-Casas.) (*Esta figura se encontra reproduzida em cores no Encarte.*)

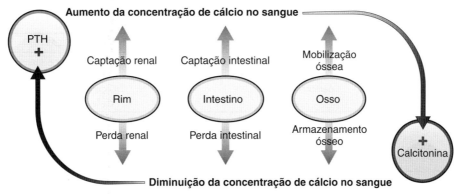

Figura 297.3 Homeostase do cálcio. A liberação de paratormônio (*PTH*) aumenta a captação de cálcio nos rins e no intestino, além de estimular sua mobilização dos ossos.

de certos fragmentos clivados entre os aminoácidos 1 e 12. Exames atuais (geralmente ELISA) utilizam combinações de anticorpos, que somente mensuram o hormônio intacto.[7] Há disponibilidade de um teste ELISA específico para cães, mas que também foi validado para gatos. Alguns laboratórios validaram testes de PTH específicos para humanos, para uso em cães e gatos.[8,9] Já que a disponibilidade do teste é variável, novos métodos devem ser validados para a espécie de interesse. Para a mensuração de PTH, prefere-se amostra de plasma coletado em EDTA. Considerando que o PTH é lábil, as amostras devem ser imediatamente centrifugadas e congeladas até que sejam analisadas. O laboratório deve fornecer informações sobre o manuseio da amostra; vários deles fornecem pacotes para o congelamento para envio da amostra. O intervalo de referência para o PTH é de aproximadamente 20 a 65 pg/mℓ, no cão, e < 25 pg/mℓ, no gato, mas podem diferir, dependendo do laboratório e do método de teste utilizado.

Proteína relacionada com o paratormônio

Descrição e função

A proteína relacionada com o paratormônio (PTHrP, do inglês *parathyroid hormone-related protein*) é fundamental para a homeostase do cálcio no feto. Após o nascimento, a PTHrP se torna praticamente indetectável em animais saudáveis. Comprovou-se que o aumento da concentração de PTHrP causa hipercalcemia humoral maligna (HHM).[10] A PTHrP possui os mesmos efeitos fisiológicos do PTH, aumentando as concentrações de tCa e iCa e diminuindo a concentração séricas de fósforo. A mensuração de PTHrP é um teste auxiliar de diagnóstico importante e útil para avaliação de cães e gatos com hipercalcemia, particularmente quando há suspeita de neoplasia. A constatação de concentração normal ou baixa de PTHrP não exclui em definitivo a possibilidade de doença neoplásica, enquanto concentração elevada está, em geral, associada a neoplasia maligna (ver Capítulo 352).

Mensuração da proteína relacionada com o paratormônio

A PTHrP pode ser mensurada de forma confiável utilizando-se testes imunorradiométricos (IRMA) ou radioimunoensaios de N-terminal (RIEs) em dois sítios. Várias formas circulantes de PTHrP, além do hormônio intacto PTHrP (aminoácido 1 a 141), possuem atividade biológica. Estas incluem um fragmento N-terminal de aminoácido 1 a 36 e um fragmento N-terminal e região média de aminoácido 1 a 86. A participação dessas diferentes formas não é completamente compreendida. Assim como o PTH, a PTHrP não é estável, é mensurada, de preferência, em amostra de plasma coletado em EDTA e as amostras devem ser manuseadas conforme descrito para o PTH. Em cães e gatos, o intervalo de referência para PTHrP geralmente é < 0,5 pmol/ℓ.

Vitamina D (vitamina D$_3$, calcitriol, 1,25-[OH]$_2$-colecalciferol)

A síntese do colecalciferol, hidroxilado no fígado para produzir 25-OH-colecalciferol (25-OH vitamina D, ou calcidiol) e não rigorosamente controlada, propicia uma reserva de vitamina D inativa pronta para ativação em 1,25-(OH)$_2$-vitamina D, ou calcitriol. Essa etapa é controlada, ocorre nos rins e sua síntese é estimulada pelo PTH via alfa-1-hidroxilase e suprimida por alta concentração de fósforo. O 25-OH-colecalciferol também pode ser catabolizado por meio de 24-hidroxilação e, então, excretado. A vitamina D (25 e 1,25-[OH]$_2$ D) pode ser mensurada em gatos e cães, por laboratórios veterinários especializados.

Calcitonina

A calcitonina, um peptídio sintetizado por células C da glândula tireoide, reduz a concentração sérica de Ca e possui funções que limitam a hipercalcemia pós-prandial. Embora a calcitonina possa contrabalancear os efeitos do PTH, sua função é relativamente menor. Após tireoidectomia e paratireoidectomia total, a consequência clínica é a hipocalcemia devido ao hipoparatireoidismo, e não a hipercalcemia devido à deficiência de calcitonina. De forma semelhante, quando há neoplasia de células C (carcinoma tireoidiano medular) e produção excessiva de calcitonina, a homeostase do cálcio não é prejudicada. Em seres humanos, é improvável que a liberação de calcitonina pela ação do CaSR estimulada pelo Ca contribua de forma substancial na homeostase do Ca. Em geral, a calcitonina não é mensurada em pacientes com anormalidades na concentração de Ca, e não havendo teste disponível no mercado.

Como esses hormônios atuam em conjunto para manter a homeostase do cálcio?

O PTH é o principal regulador da homeostase do cálcio. O PTH aumenta a concentração sérica de Ca pela elevação da reabsorção devido ao incremento do número de osteoclastos nas superfícies ósseas, pelo aumento da absorção tubular renal de Ca nos túbulos contorcidos distais e na alça ascendente de Henle e pelo aumento na hidroxilação da 25-OH vitamina D em 1,25-(OH)$_2$ vitamina D, que aumenta a absorção de Ca no intestino delgado.[2,3]

DIAGNÓSTICOS DIFERENCIAIS DE HIPERCALCEMIA EM CÃES

A hipercalcemia pode ser causada pelo acesso a agentes exógenos que alteram a concentração de Ca ou ser resultado de anormalidades em um dos mecanismos homeostáticos endógenos (Tabela 297.1; ver Capítulo 69). As abordagens utilizadas no plano diagnóstico sistemático de cães clinicamente estáveis ou naqueles com hipercalcemia são revisadas na Figura 297.4.

Tabela 297.1 Classificação, causa e características de diversas condições hipercalcêmicas.

CLASSIFICAÇÃO	CAUSA	CARACTERÍSTICAS
Paratireoide-dependente	Hiperparatireoidismo primário (hiperplasia, adenocarcinoma ou adenoma de paratireoide)	Valor de PTH no intervalo de referência ou aumentado tCa e iCa elevados PO_4 baixo ou no limite inferior de normalidade
	Doença renal crônica	PTH elevado tCa discretamente elevado iCa em geral normal PO_4 elevado
Paratireoide-independente	Câncer (linfoma, adenocarcinoma de saco anal, outros carcinomas, timoma, mieloma múltiplo, neoplasia óssea primária ou metastática)	PTH normal ou diminuído PTHrP pode estar elevado; nem todos os tumores associados à hipercalcemia produzem PTHrP Lesões osteolíticas
Vitamina D-dependente	Iatrogênica (suplementação com óleo de fígado de bacalhau etc.) Plantas (glicosídeos de calcitriol encontrados em frutos e vegetais de beladona, vegetais e flores de jasmim e outras plantas) Intoxicação por rodenticidas (colecalciferol) Creme antipsoríase (calcipotriol e calcipotrieno)	PTH suprimido tCa e iCa elevados PO_4 elevado Vitamina D pode estar elevada, dependendo da forma ingerida
Doença granulomatosa dependente da produção local de vitamina D	Paniculite Blastomicose Outras doenças granulomatosas	Pode ser difícil caracterizar devido à etiologia desconhecida da hipercalcemia. Algumas vezes, a vitamina D elevada é incriminada.[54–56] Também há relato de PTHrP elevado[57]
Mecanismo desconhecido	Hipoadrenocorticismo (doença de Addison) Hipercalcemia idiopática felina (HIF)	Associado à ausência de alterações mensuráveis nas moléculas-chave

iCa, cálcio ionizado; *PTH*, paratormônio; *PTHrP*, proteína relacionada com o paratormônio; *tCa*, cálcio total.

HIPERPARATIREOIDISMO PRIMÁRIO EM CÃES

Definição

O hiperparatireoidismo primário (HPTP), uma condição incomum em cães e rara em gatos, deve ser considerado entre as possíveis causas de hipercalcemia, sobretudo em cães idosos relativamente assintomáticos.[12-14] O HPTP é caracterizado por hipercalcemia e concentração inapropriadamente alta de PTH (seja dentro, seja acima do intervalo de referência), sem outra causa subjacente identificável (Figura 297.5).

Causa

HPTP ocorre após uma ou mais glândulas paratireoides começarem a funcionar de forma autônoma. O hiperparatireoidismo secundário ocorre após anormalidade não endócrina da homeostase do Ca, associada a doença renal crônica ou deficiência crônica de Ca na dieta. Em geral, o HPTP é causado por adenoma solitário, carcinoma ou hiperplasia adenomatosa em uma glândula paratireoide. Em < 10% dos cães com HPTP, nota-se mais de uma glândula envolvida. Em uma série de casos de cães submetidos à cirurgia, constatou-se que 87% tinham adenoma solitário, 8%, hiperplasia e 5%, carcinoma.[15] Tecido paratireoidiano metastático funcional foi relatado somente em 1 de centenas de cães com HPTP mencionados na literatura veterinária.[16]

Como consequência da alteração patológica em uma ou mais glândulas paratireoides, ocorre secreção excessiva persistente de PTH, seja qual for a concentração sérica de Ca. Quando o hiperparatireoidismo é primário, em geral uma glândula afetada é a fonte de secreção autônoma de PTH. O hiperparatireoidismo secundário, quase sempre se deve à hiperplasia de mais de uma glândula paratireoide em resposta a estímulos mais generalizados para produção de PTH. Na realidade, a diferenciação entre HPTP e secundário pode ser difícil. A avaliação histológica de

glândulas paratireoides extirpadas raramente revela evidências claras e definitivas de serem benignas ou malignas. A hiperplasia pode não afetar as glândulas de forma uniforme e, embora mais associada com frequência à doença secundária, foi descrita como causa de HPTP em gatos e cães.[14,17,18]

Comparações com hiperparatireoidismo primário humano

Em seres humanos, o HPTP pode ocorrer esporadicamente ou estar associado a uma síndrome que inclui outras doenças endócrinas ou neoplásicas. Foi observado que o HPTP esporádico é iniciado por mutações somáticas no gene *MEN1* (a mutação genética verificada em casos de neoplasias endócrinas múltiplas) em aproximadamente 35% dos casos. Outras mutações ocorrem em baixas frequências.[19,20] Formas não esporádicas da doença incluem hiperparatireoidismo familiar isolado, a única manifestação não sindrômica (HFI, OMIM[a]:145000), hipercalcemia familiar hipocalciúrica (HFH, OMIM:145980), neoplasias endócrinas múltiplas tipo 1 (NEM1, OMIM:131100) e tipo 2A (NEM2A, OMIM:171400) e síndrome do hiperparatireoidismo/tumor de mandíbula (HPT-TM, OMIM:145001). Genes distintos estão associados à HFH (receptor sensível ao cálcio [CaSR], proteína-2 adaptadora [AP2S1], subunidade-alfa 11 da proteína-G [GNA11]), NEM1 (*MEN1*, codificando um supressor tumoral), NEM2 *(RET)* e HPT-TM (*HRPT2*, codificação de parafibromina, outro supressor tumoral).[21-24] Mutações nesses genes não estão incriminadas em todos os casos clínicos, sugerindo que outros *locus* podem estar envolvidos. O HFI foi associado a mutações em três genes – *MEN1, CaSR* e *HRPT2*.[25,26]

---

[a]N.R.T.: *Online Mendelian Inheritance in Man*, base de dados que relaciona as doenças humanas e os respectivos genes.

O diagnóstico de HFI é confirmado se os critérios diagnósticos para qualquer um dos outros fenótipos não forem detectados em testes genéticos-padrão não moleculares. Em pacientes humanos com HFI, os genes *MEN1* e *CaSR* são avaliados de início, já que o *HRPT2* é uma causa menos comum da doença.[26,27] Keeshond é a única raça de cães na qual constatou-se predisposição familiar ao HPTP. Cães dessa raça foram submetidos a estudo com abordagem de um gene candidato.[28,29] Mutações nos genes *MEN1*, *CaSR* e *HRPT2* foram descartadas como causas de PHPT em cães da raça Keeshond. Apesar de utilizar uma análise de associação genômica ampla nessa raça, ainda não se definiu a mutação causadora.

Resenha

HPTP é uma doença de cães idosos (idade média de 11,2 anos; variação de 6 a 17 anos), sem aparente predisposição sexual.[15] Em uma revisão, verificou-se que cães da raça Keeshond tiveram maior razão de probabilidade associada à raça, de 50,7.[28,30,31]

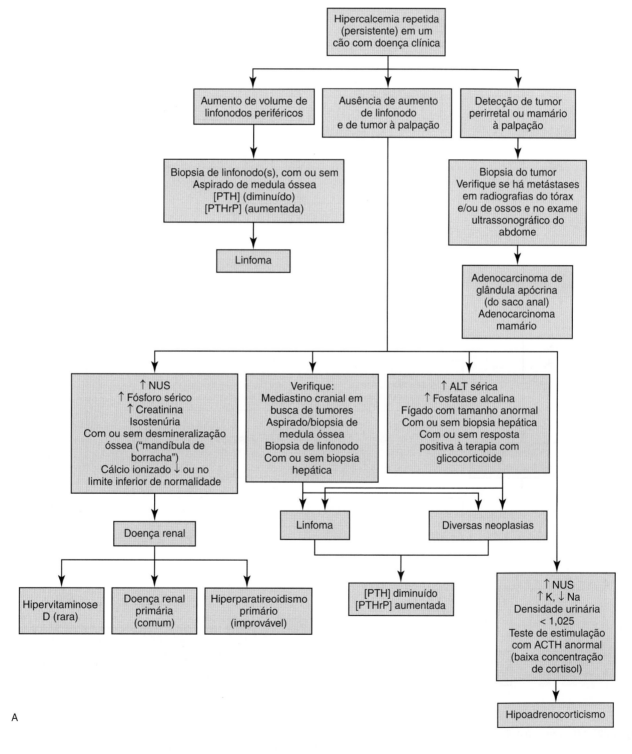

Figura 297.4 A. Algoritmo para avaliação de um cão hipercalcêmico doente.

Continua

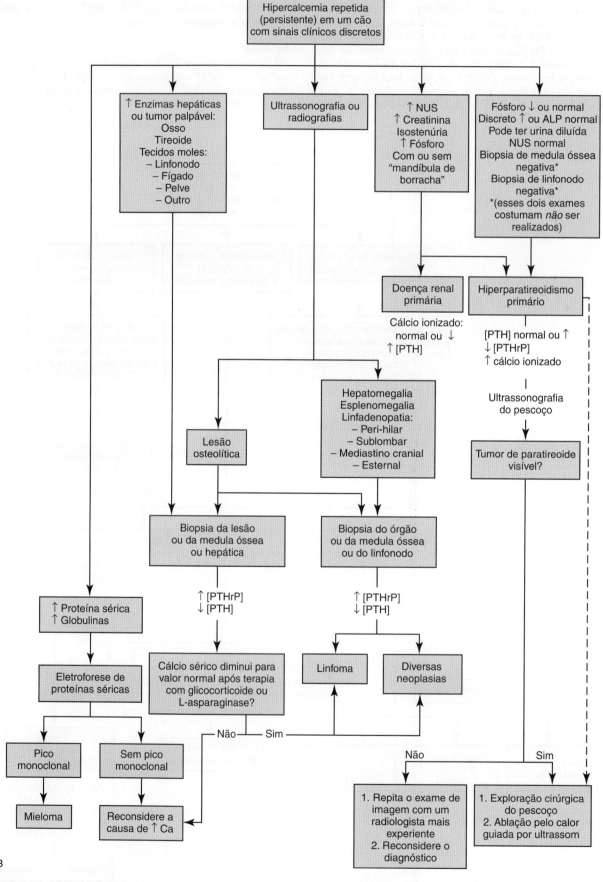

Figura 297.4 (Continuação) B. Algoritmo para avaliação de um cão com hipercalcemia, mas sem sinais clínicos graves ou preocupantes. *ACTH*, hormônio adrenocorticotrófico; *ALP*, fosfatase alcalina sérica; *ALT*, alanina aminotransferase; *NUS*, nitrogênio ureico sanguíneo; *PTH*, paratormônio; *PTHrP*, proteína relacionada com o paratormônio. (De Feldman EC, Nelson RW, Reusch CE, et al.: *Canine and feline endocrinology*, 4 ed., St. Louis, 2015, Elsevier.)

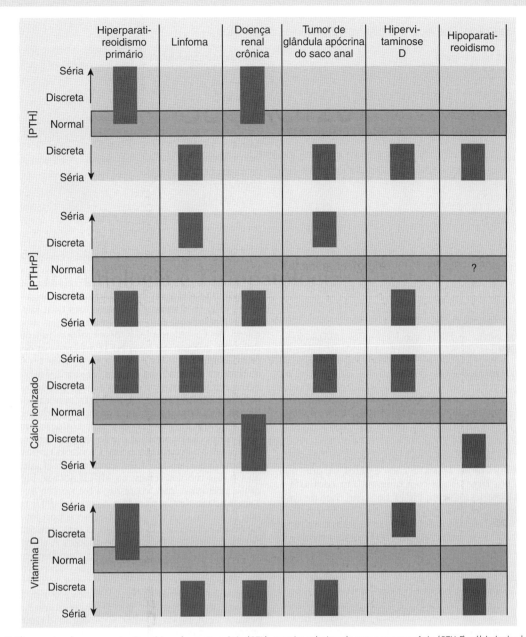

Figura 297.5 Gráfico mostrando as concentrações séricas de paratormônio (*PTH*), proteína relacionada com o paratormônio (*PTHrP*), cálcio ionizado e vitamina D nas causas mais comuns de hipercalcemia em cães. (De Feldman EC, Nelson RW, Reusch CE, et al.: *Canine and feline endocrinology*, 4 ed., St. Louis, 2015, Saunders.)

Gatos são acometidos com menos frequência, e não há informações sobre predisposição racial disponíveis. HPTP neonatal foi relatado em uma ninhada de filhotes da raça Pastor-Alemão, o que parece ter sido um evento isolado.[17]

Histórico e sinais clínicos

Considerações gerais

HPTP não é uma doença dramática; ao contrário, é lentamente progressiva, insidiosa e branda (Boxe 297.1). Já que os cães acometidos tendem a ser idosos, vários sinais clínicos são atribuídos simplesmente ao envelhecimento por tutores que podem não buscar aconselhamento veterinário até que seja tardio na evolução da doença. Em geral, a hipercalcemia é um achado fortuito quando as amostras de sangue são obtidas por outras razões. De 210 cães com HPTP, notou-se que 42% foram identificados como hipercalcêmicos quando atendidos por outras razões, como acompanhamento geriátrico de rotina, ou quando foram realizados exames de sangue pré-anestésicos para procedimentos, como tratamento dentário.[30] Pode haver uma associação entre tutores de cães preocupados com a possibilidade de dor mandibular ou dificuldade em mastigar alimentos duros e HPTP, sobretudo em cães da raça Keeshond. A razão mais comum para a busca por aconselhamento veterinário foi a ocorrência de sinais clínicos relacionados com a urolitíase (polaquiúria, estrangúria e hematúria) ou infecção do trato urinário (50% dos 210 casos).[30] A urolitíase pode causar obstrução aguda do fluxo urinário em cães com HPTP (ver Capítulos 107 e 331).

Poliúria, polidipsia e outros sintomas (ver Boxe 297.1)

Menos de 10% dos tutores de cães com HPTP notaram a ocorrência de poliúria e polidipsia (PU/PD); isso é um número surpreendentemente pequeno, dado que o Ca antagoniza os efeitos da vasopressina (hormônio antidiurético [ADH, *antidiuretic hormone*]) nos ductos coletores dos rins e a hipercalcemia inibe a captação tubular de sódio e cloreto, inibindo ainda mais os mecanismos de concentração urinária. Os cães acometidos apresentam PU, com PD compensatória secundária. Esse sinal clínico pode ser subestimado pelos tutores de cães, pois a progressão é gradativa e, talvez, a noctúria e a incontinência nesses

Boxe 297.1 Sinais clínicos de hipercalcemia/hiperparatireoidismo primário

Sintomas renais e do trato urinário
Poliúria
Polidipsia
Incontinência urinária
Estrangúria
Polaquiúria
Urolitíase

Sintomas gastrintestinais
Êmese*
Inapetência
Constipação intestinal

Sintomas neuromusculares
Depressão
Intolerância ao exercício
Tremores*
Contrações musculares*
Convulsões*

Outros
Dor de dente
Dificuldade em se alimentar
Marcha rígida*
Claudicação*

*Incomum a raro.

animais idosos seja simplesmente tolerada. Em geral, cães com HPTP possuem baixo nível de atividade, parecem indiferentes e podem parecer deprimidos. Novamente, esses sinais podem ser atribuídos ao envelhecimento e algumas vezes não mencionados até depois do tratamento efetivo, quando é descrito, com frequência, que os cães "rejuvenesceram".

Em pessoas, os sinais de HPTP são lembrados utilizando-se o mnemônico "cálculos, ossos, desconforto abdominal, constipação intestinal e queixas psiquiátricas".[b] (Algumas pessoas com HPTP apresentam depressão e/ou debilidade em decorrência de dor óssea. O termo *thrones* do mnemônico refere-se à constipação intestinal comumente notada em pessoas com HPTP. Entretanto, a literatura atual sugere que essa visão clássica está mudando, já que mais pacientes são diagnosticados apesar de poucos sintomas (ou nenhum), com a progressão da doença, em geral, de forma benigna, mesmo sem tratamento.[32,33] Ainda é incerto se isso também se aplica a cães e gatos, já que não existem estudos em larga escala com animais. Em contraste à experiência com cães, pessoas com HPTP possuem risco de crise hipercalcêmica incomum e com potencial risco de morte. Essa síndrome está associada à rápida deterioração funcional multiorgânica e a uma taxa de mortalidade de 100%, se não tratada.[34] Não existem relatos dessa síndrome em medicina veterinária, mas há um espectro de gravidade e progressão da doença nos cães diagnosticados com HPTP. Cada cão deve ser avaliado individualmente, analisando-se a necessidade de intervenção. Sintomas GI incluem inapetência, êmese e constipação intestinal. Esses sinais clínicos podem ser secundários a hipoexcitabilidade e dismotilidade do músculo liso intestinal induzidas pelo Ca.

Formação de cálculos nos rins e no trato urinário

Além de causar PU e PD compensatória, a hipercalcemia devido ao HPTP pode aumentar o risco de insuficiência renal, que acomete alguns cães com HPTP, mas outros, não. Em cães com HPTP, a concentração de fósforo deve estar no limite inferior de normalidade ou abaixo dos valores do intervalo de referência. Se esse não for o caso, a insuficiência renal pode estar em andamento, mesmo antes da detecção de azotemia evidente. Nesses casos, recomenda-se monitoramento mais frequente e o prognóstico é mais reservado. Foi sugerido que o cálculo do produto entre Ca × fósforo pode ajudar a predizer a probabilidade de insuficiência renal; cães portadores de HPTP com baixa concentração de fósforo e produto Ca × fósforo relativamente baixo supostamente possuem menor risco. Em um grande estudo de caso com 210 cães, constatou-se que o risco de insuficiência renal foi baixo, enquanto em uma série menor de casos (29 cães) aproximadamente 25 animais desenvolveram doença renal crônica. Nesse estudo, o produto Ca × fósforo foi um mau preditor de doença renal.[35] Uma população geneticamente homogênea de cães da raça Keeshond possibilita a investigação de doença renal crônica naqueles indivíduos portadores da mutação ligada ao HPTP. Se não tratados, alguns cães com HPTP continuam a ter função renal normal, mesmo com hipercalcemia prolongada e, em alguns casos, séria (> 4 mmol/ℓ). Outros cães com HPTP sucumbem à insuficiência renal com elevação muito mais modesta da concentração de Ca. Alguns cães desenvolvem nefrólitos e urolitíase. Relata-se que um cão com HPTP morreu em decorrência de um grande nefrólito e insuficiência renal após ter sido considerado efetivo o tratamento da doença (Figura 297.6). Assim, está claro que a predição da recuperação a longo prazo, com ou sem tratamento, é muito problemática. No tratamento de hipercalcemia, é preferível errar por excesso de cautela; ademais, deve-se evitar atraso no tratamento para proteger a função renal.

A formação de urólitos é comum em cães com HPTP devido ao aumento da concentração de Ca filtrado pelos rins e excretado na urina (ver Capítulo 331). Embora o PTH aumente a absorção de Ca dos túbulos renais, no HPTP nota-se hipercalciúria marcante, presumivelmente porque a reabsorção de Ca não se iguala à quantidade de Ca filtrado. Cães com HPTP também apresentam aumento da excreção de fósforo e, portanto, a urina deles é supersaturada com Ca e fósforo, o que aumenta a precipitação desses minerais e a formação de cálculos. A absorção intestinal de oxalato da dieta diminui quando há abundante quantidade de Ca intraluminal, pois o oxalato de Ca não é absorvível pelo intestino. Se a absorção intestinal de Ca aumentar, acontece o mesmo com a absorção de oxalato. Nessa situação, o rim filtra mais Ca e oxalato, novamente levando à supersaturação da urina. Em pessoas com hipercalcemia, a avaliação da quantidade de Ca excretado na urina é comumente feita pela aferição da proporção cálcio:creatinina na urina, estudos esses estudos não amplamente realizados em animais (ver Capítulo 73).

Exame físico

Achados relevantes no exame físico são poucos e inespecíficos (ver Boxe 297.1). Eles podem incluir rigidez e anormalidades da marcha, letargia, fraqueza e caquexia muscular. Poucas informações são obtidas pela palpação da área ventral do pescoço, já que os tumores de paratireoide costumam ser muito pequenos para tal.

Cálcio total, cálcio ionizado, fósforo, paratormônio, proteína relacionada com o paratormônio

tCa e iCa

Ao se detectar hipercalcemia, devem-se avaliar as concentrações de iCa, fósforo, PTH e PTHrP. A principal característica do HPTP é o aumento das concentrações de tCa e iCa, enquanto o teor de PTH situa-se dentro ou acima do intervalo de referência. Em um estudo com 210 cães com HPTP, notou-se que a concentração média de tCa era de 3,6 mmol/ℓ (14,5 mg/dℓ).[30] Houve variação na gravidade da hipercalcemia: aumento discreto em 52% dos cães (> 3 a ≤ 3,5 mmol/ℓ, > 12 a ≤ 14 mg/dℓ), aumento moderado em 30% (> 3,5 a < 4 mmol/ℓ, > 14 a < 16 mg/dℓ), aumento grave em 12% (> 4 a ≤ 4,5 mmol/ℓ, > 16 a

---

[b]N.R.T.: Na tradução para o português, perde-se a rima que facilita a memorização: "*stones, bones, abdominal groans, thrones and psychiatric moans.*"

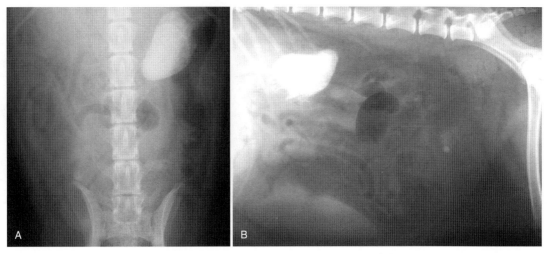

Figura 297.6 Radiografias de abdome nas projeções ventrodorsal (**A**) e lateral (**B**) mostrando um grande nefrólito no rim esquerdo e múltiplos urocistólitos menores.

< 18 mg/dℓ), e hipercalcemia grave (> 4,5 mmol/ℓ, > 18 mg/dℓ) em 6% dos animais. Nos 210 cães, as concentrações de iCa acompanharam as concentrações de tCa. A concentração plasmática média de iCa foi 1,71 mmol/ℓ (variação de 1,22 a 2,41 mmol/ℓ, intervalo de referência de 1,12 a 1,41 mmol/ℓ).

A gravidade da hipercalcemia provavelmente depende da duração da doença. Em geral, cães da raça Keeshond de famílias com HPTP começam a apresentar discreta hipercalcemia (até 3,5 mmol/ℓ, 14 mg/dℓ) aos 6 a 8 anos, condição que se agrava gradativamente ao longo dos anos seguintes. Alguns cães não tratados continuam a apresentar concentração elevada de Ca até que se instala hipercalcemia grave (> 4 a < 4,5 mmol/ℓ, > 16 a < 18,5 mg/dℓ). Após esse valor, ocorre certa estabilização e a concentração não continua a se elevar de modo marcante, à semelhança do que acontece em seres humanos. Cães da raça Keeshond com 13 a 15 anos, não tratados, mantiveram hipercalcemia grave até o momento da morte devido a outras doenças. Como a base genética para HPTP em outras raças não é conhecida, não está claro o quão reproduzível é esse padrão entre as raças, mas em todas elas a doença parece lenta e insidiosa. Cães acometidos não são considerados doentes pelos tutores.

Fósforo

HPTP, hipercalcemia e função renal normal causam hipofosfatemia, um achado incomum em cães (Boxe 297.2). O PTH inibe a reabsorção renal de fósforo e a concentração sérica desse eletrólito situa-se no limite inferior do intervalo de referência ou abaixo dele. No estudo com 210 cães com HPTP, constatou-se concentração sérica média de fósforo de 2,8 mg/dℓ (0,9 mmol/ℓ; com variação de 1,3 a 6,1 mg/dℓ, 0,4 a 1,9 mmol/ℓ; intervalo de referência de 3 a 6,2 mg/dℓ, 0,9 a 2 mmol/ℓ).

Paratormônio

Em cães com hipercalcemia comprovada, a concentração circulante de PTH deve ser avaliada após confirmação de elevação nas concentrações de tCa e iCa e a exclusão de causas mais óbvias (linfoma). Se um cão hipercalcêmico apresenta concentração de PTH com valor na metade superior n ou acima do intervalo de referência (i. e., na metade superior do intervalo de referência, > 35 pg/mℓ para cães, com intervalo de referência de 20 a 65 pg/mℓ), isso é anormal e compatível com HPTP. Na maioria dos casos de hipercalcemia não causada por HPTP, as concentrações de tCa e iCa estão aumentadas, estando a de PTH diminuída ou indetectável.

Proteína relacionada com o paratormônio

Em geral, a concentração de PTH é mensurada juntamente com a de PTHrP. Se o HPTP não for a causa da hipercalcemia, o valor de PTHrP pode ajudar na redução da lista de diagnósticos diferenciais, a fim de incluir neoplasias malignas que podem não ter sido identificadas. O intervalo de referência para PTHrP é, em geral, < 0,5 pmol/ℓ tanto em cães quanto em gatos.

Outros exames bioquímicos, hemograma, exame de urina

Exames bioquímicos séricos, que não sejam Ca e fósforo, estão, em geral, normais em cães com HPTP. Já que os cães hipercalcêmicos podem ter risco de lesões renais, devem-se mensurar as concentrações de nitrogênio ureico sanguíneo, creatinina e fósforo, que podem estar aumentadas devido à lesão renal pre-existente ou fatores pré-renais.

Isso pode complicar o diagnóstico, já que alterações associadas a HPTP e insuficiência renal secundária podem simular aquelas da doença renal primária, com elevação secundária de PTH e hipercalcemia (Tabela 297.2). Parâmetros hematológicos não indicam alterações consistentes, embora possa ser detectada anemia por doença crônica se a hipercalcemia o for. Como a hipercalcemia causa diabetes insípido nefrogênico secundário, espera-se densidade urinária < 1,020 e alguns pacientes apresentam hipostenúria. Hematúria, proteinúria, bacteriúria, piúria e cristalúria são achados comuns.

Boxe 297.2 Causas de hipofosfatemia

Diminuição da absorção intestinal de fósforo
Diminuição da ingestão dietética
Má absorção/esteatorreia
Êmese/diarreia
Antiácidos quelantes de fósforo
Deficiência da vitamina D

Aumento da excreção urinária de fósforo
Hiperparatireoidismo primário
Diabetes melito, com ou sem cetoacidose
Hiperadrenocorticismo (de ocorrência natural/iatrogênico)
Síndrome de Fanconi (anormalidades nos túbulos renais)
Administração de diuréticos ou bicarbonato
Recuperação de hipotermia
Hiperaldosteronismo
Administração intensiva de soluções parenterais
Hipercalcemia maligna (estágio inicial)

Desvios transcelulares de fósforo
Administração de insulina
Administração parenteral de glicose
Alimentação excessiva
Alcalose respiratória

Tabela 297.2 Comparação entre as características clinicopatológicas de hiperparatireoidismo primário (HPTP) e hiperparatireoidismo secundário renal.

	HIPERPARATIREOIDISMO PRIMÁRIO	HIPERPARATIREOIDISMO SECUNDÁRIO RENAL
Cálcio total	↑	↓ ou normal ou ↑
Cálcio ionizado	↑	↓ ou normal
Fósforo	↓	↑
PTH	↑ ou no limite superior	↑ ou no limite superior
PTHrP	Normal	Normal

PTH, paratormônio; PTHrP, proteína relacionada com o paratormônio.

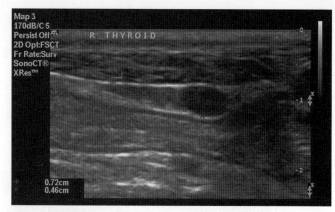

Figura 297.7 Ultrassonografia mostrando a aparência típica de adenoma de paratireoide.

Diagnóstico por imagem

A ultrassonografia da região ventral do pescoço é a modalidade de imagem mais útil na avaliação de um cão com suspeita de HPTP; em 90 a 95% deles, são detectados nódulos na paratireoide por radiologistas experientes.[30] Um transdutor de alta frequência, de 7,5 a 10 MHz, é necessário para uma resolução de imagem adequada. Em cães e gatos saudáveis, as glândulas paratireoides em geral possuem < 3 mm em seu maior diâmetro; elas são detectadas somente em centros de excelência e por profissionais experientes. Quando há hiperplasia ou aumento de volume e adenoma, ou carcinoma nas glândulas paratireoides, as imagens mostram nódulos hipoecoicos com diâmetro de 2 a 20 mm, redondos a ovais, dentro ou próximos do tecido tireoidiano (Figura 297.7).[36] Nódulos na tireoide foram detectados por acaso na ultrassonografia cervical em 14 de 91 (15%) cães avaliados por conta de hipercalcemia.[37] O achado de um nódulo tireoidiano pode complicar o diagnóstico, porque pode não representar a origem da hipercalcemia, mas indicar diversos problemas. Em cães, avaliou-se o uso de cintilografia, com a administração de tecnécio-sestamibi[99m], como um exame auxiliar para detecção da paratireoide; mas, ao contrário do que ocorre em seres humanos, constatou-se carência de sensibilidade e especificidade e, portanto, não é recomendada.[38] Recomendam-se radiografias simples ou ultrassonografia do abdome à busca de quaisquer anormalidades, inclusive cálculos renais ou vesicais que contenham cálcio. Raramente, nota-se extensa calcificação renal (ver Figura 297.6).

Testes genéticos para hiperparatireoidismo primário em cães da raça Keeshond

Há disponibilidade de um teste genético para HPTP familiar em cães da raça Keeshond, que almeja identificar cães dessa raça portadores do alelo que sofreu mutação, responsável pela doença autossômica dominante. O teste está disponível no Animal Health Diagnostic Center, na Cornell University, e os detalhes estão disponíveis em: https://ahdc.vet.cornell.edu/Sects/Molec/PHPTtesting.cfm. Já que a base molecular para esse teste ainda não foi revisada por pares, a sensibilidade e a especificidade não são conhecidas. É recomendado que criadores de cães da raça Keeshond estejam cientes do genótipo da linhagem de seus animais e que eles obtenham a progênie de cães não testados. Os cães em risco devem ser monitorados periodicamente quanto à ocorrência de hipercalcemia, em geral notada aos 6 a 8 anos. Entretanto, o HPTP pode ocorrer de maneira precoce ou tardia ou, então, jamais se manifestar durante toda a vida do cão.

CONTROLE PRÉ-TERAPÊUTICO DE HIPERCALCEMIA

Terapia hídrica

A terapia emergencial para hipercalcemia é raramente necessária em cães com HPTP, a menos que a concentração de Ca seja considerada "séria" a "grave". Alguns veterinários acreditam que praticamente nenhum cão com HPTP necessita algum tipo de terapia antes do tratamento específico de HPTP, seja qual for o grau de hipercalcemia. Outros sugerem que a hipercalcemia séria a grave seja tratada na tentativa de diminuir a concentração sérica de Ca enquanto aguardam os resultados dos exames. Como, em geral, os testes para PTH e PTHrP são realizados em laboratórios especializados, pode haver um atraso entre a obtenção de um diagnóstico presuntivo de HPTP e a confirmação desse diagnóstico. A lesão renal causada por hipercalcemia persistente devido ao HPTP é bastante incomum, mas impossível de prever (ver Capítulo 324). Todos os animais acometidos devem ser considerados em risco, se houver hipercalcemia significante.

O intuito da terapia hídrica (ver Capítulo 129) é exacerbar a excreção renal de Ca e minimizar sua reabsorção óssea. É o fator fundamental para o controle de hipercalcemia. A diurese induzida pela administração de solução de cloreto de sódio a 0,9%, na dose de 5 a 10 mℓ/kg/h, deve aumentar a excreção renal de Ca e diminuir sua concentração sérica. O objetivo da terapia hídrica é corrigir qualquer desidratação ou déficit volêmico e expandir o volume extracelular para aumentar a taxa de filtração glomerular. O cloreto de sódio é a solução preferida, pois o íon sódio compete com o íon Ca e reduz a reabsorção tubular. Quando um animal é considerado satisfatoriamente hidratado, a furosemida (2 mg/kg VO, a cada 8 a 12 horas) pode aumentar ainda mais a excreção renal de Ca. Ao utilizar alta dose de solução de cloreto de sódio, sobretudo em conjunto com a furosemida, deve-se evitar a indução de hipopotassemia. Se a terapia hídrica não reduzir a concentração sérica de Ca, podem-se administrar glicocorticoide, bifosfonato, calcitonina ou plicamicina.

Glicocorticoides

Os glicocorticoides não influenciam muito a concentração sérica de Ca de cães com HPTP e raramente reduzem o valor mensurado. A utilização de glicocorticoides (na dose de aproximadamente 1 mg de prednisolona/kg ou equivalente) com intuito de reduzir a concentração sérica de Ca deve ser restrita àqueles cães claramente diagnosticados, mas nos quais há atraso no tratamento; eles são mais efetivos quando administrados aos animais com hipercalcemia maligna. Os glicocorticoides causam rápida lise tumoral e reduzem a síntese e secreção de PTHrP. Eles exacerbam a excreção renal de Ca bem como diminuem a absorção intestinal e a reabsorção óssea de cálcio. Quando utilizados em pacientes sem comprovação do diagnóstico podem mascarar e dificultar o diagnóstico de neoplasias.

Bifosfonatos

Os bifosfonatos diminuem a reabsorção óssea por inibir a atividade osteoclástica e induzir apoptose de osteoclastos. Diversos bifosfonatos já foram empregados. Aqueles utilizados majoritariamente incluem fármacos de uso oral (clodronato, etidronato, alendronato) e injeção intravenosa (IV) de pamidronato. Embora o uso de medicamento oral seja prático para os tutores, essa via não é muito efetiva, pois < 1% da dose é absorvida.[39] A infusão IV de pamidronato é mais confiável (1,3 a 2 mg/kg, em 150 ml de solução salina a 0,9%, administrada ao longo de 2 horas). A ação do pamidronato, aproximadamente cem vezes mais potente do que o etidronato, pode durar até 3 semanas. A dose pode ser repetida conforme necessário. Esse fármaco é geralmente bem tolerado[40], mas pode causar efeitos colaterais GI e hipocalcemia, sobretudo se em dose excessiva. O pamidronato vem sendo utilizado com mais frequência para tratar pessoas com hipercalcemia maligna, mas um bifosfonato mais potente, o zoledronato, atualmente supera o pamidronato como fármaco de escolha. A ação do zoledronato é 100 a 850 vezes maior do que a do pamidronato, vez que pode ser infundida com mais rapidez, mas ainda não foi muito utilizado em cães.[41]

Calcitonina

A calcitonina de salmão está disponível no mercado e, assim como os bifosfonatos, inibe não só a atividade osteoclástica, mas também a reabsorção renal de Ca. É útil como tratamento emergencial para diminuir a concentração de Ca, mas possui a desvantagem de necessitar, após a infusão IV inicial (4 UI/kg), de terapia de manutenção diária (4 a 8 UI/kg por via subcutânea [SC], a cada 12 a 24 horas).[42] A calcitonina pode causar anorexia e êmese, é cara e raramente utilizada. Os animais podem se tornar resistentes à ação da calcitonina após alguns dias de tratamento.

Plicamicina (mitramicina)

Há poucos relatos de uso desse fármaco em cães. Sugeriu-se dose de 25 μg/kg IV, em solução de dextrose a 5%, ao longo de 2 a 4 horas, em intervalos de 2 a 4 semanas.[43]

Cinacalcete

Esse fármaco é um calcimimético; atua diretamente no receptor sensível ao Ca, podendo controlar as concentrações de Ca, fósforo e PTH em pacientes humanos submetidos à diálise. Foi sugerido que esse fármaco pode ser útil em cães e gatos com hipercalcemia, sobretudo em gatos com hipercalcemia idiopática, mas não existem dados que suportem sua utilização.

OPÇÕES TERAPÊUTICAS DEFINITIVAS

Paratireoidectomia cirúrgica

A cirurgia é o tratamento de escolha em várias instituições de referência, especialmente se o nódulo da paratireoide for grande (> 10 mm, em seu maior diâmetro).[44] A boa visualização de cada lobo da tireoide é essencial durante a exploração cirúrgica do pescoço, obtida com a utilização de uma abordagem pela linha média ventral. Adenoma de paratireoide, carcinoma ou glândulas hiperplásicas são facilmente diferenciados de glândulas paratireoides normais, em geral com aparência mais escura e de maior tamanho (Figura 297.8). Quando as glândulas paratireoides internas estão afetadas, elas podem ser detectadas por meio de palpação e ser vistas na parte ventral ou dorsal da glândula tireoide. A detecção de tecido de paratireoide anormal, isolado e com ação autônoma pode ser auxiliada amplamente se sua localização tiver sido previamente identificada na ultrassonografia.

Adenomas de paratireoide podem ser removidos por meio da dissecção da glândula aumentada, a partir do tecido tireoidiano adjacente, ou mediante tireoidectomia parcial, na qual o nódulo da paratireoide e parte da glândula tireoide são removidos em bloco. Em cães com HPTP, somente uma glândula costuma ser afetada. Se mais de uma estiver aumentada, então até três glândulas podem ser removidas de uma só vez. Pelo menos uma glândula paratireoide deve ser mantida *in situ*, de modo a manter a homeostase do Ca. Quando várias glândulas estão aumentadas, é mais provável que elas sejam hiperplásicas, e não adenomatosas, e, portanto, deve-se suspeitar de hiperparatireoidismo secundário, e não do tipo primário.

Foram descritas técnicas transcirúrgicas para determinar se a remoção do tecido paratireoidiano anormal funcional foi bem-sucedida.[45] Em um estudo, amostras foram obtidas antes, durante e após a cirurgia (20 minutos após a remoção do adenoma), a fim de avaliar a cinética das concentrações de PTH e confirmar a remoção do tecido funcional. Todos os cães desse estudo apresentaram diminuição significativa da concentração de PTH nas amostras obtidas antes e após a cirurgia e aumento da concentração de PTH em momentos em que houve manipulação da glândula paratireoide. Isso pode ajudar na identificação cirúrgica da paratireoide, mas somente de forma retrospectiva, já que a análise das amostras, na maioria dos centros veterinários, não é feita no local e, inevitavelmente, envolve um atraso de vários dias.

Ablação percutânea com etanol guiada por ultrassom

Para que os nódulos da paratireoide sejam tratados de maneira efetiva com o uso de injeção de etanol, eles devem ser identificados em exame ultrassonográfico e apresentarem > 3 mm no seu maior diâmetro, de forma que uma agulha calibre 27 G possa ser introduzida com segurança no nódulo. Os animais devem ser submetidos à anestesia geral. O etanol causa necrose de coagulação e trombose no nódulo da paratireoide.[46] O sucesso depende do profissional, já que a habilidade é necessária para a introdução correta da agulha e para a injeção, de forma que a artéria carótida e o tronco vagossimpático, intimamente associados, não sofram nenhum tipo de comprometimento. Ao se comparar três técnicas de tratamento de HPTP, constatou-se que a ablação por etanol foi a menos efetiva, obtendo-se resultado positivo em 13/18 procedimentos (72%), em comparação

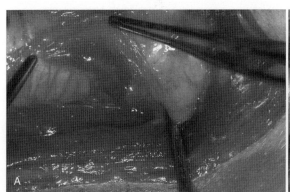 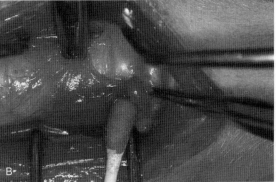

Figura 297.8 Fotografias transcirúrgicas obtidas durante a remoção de adenoma de paratireoide. **A.** A glândula tireoide está exposta. **B.** A extremidade do cotonete está em contato com a glândula paratireoide aumentada. (Cortesia de Ed Friend.)

a 45/48 (94%) no caso de cirurgia e 44/49 (90%) quando se realizou ablação pelo calor.[44] Entretanto, somente um pequeno número de casos foi tratado por ablação por etanol; em relato mais recente, menciona-se taxa de sucesso > 90% em 30 cães.[47]

Ablação pelo calor percutânea guiada por ultrassom

Essa técnica é a menos frequentemente utilizada das três, porque poucas instituições possuem os equipamentos necessários. A técnica envolve a introdução de uma agulha individual conectada a uma unidade de radiofrequência no nódulo da paratireoide, a qual é ligada e a voltagem ajustada para induzir necrose térmica visível na ponta da agulha.[48] O cão é anestesiado e posicionado em uma placa de aterramento do eletrocautério. Em seguida, introduz-se um cateter de demora calibre 20 G no nódulo da paratireoide. Em geral, no início aplica-se radiofrequência de 10 watts, que é aumentada gradativamente conforme necessário, até que toda a glândula se torne hiperecoica (Vídeo 297.1).

CONSIDERAÇÕES PRÉ-TRATAMENTO E PÓS-TRATAMENTO

Vitamina D

Quando o HPTP é tratado com sucesso, a concentração sérica de PTH e, portanto, de Ca deve diminuir rapidamente e, em alguns casos, pode ocorrer um episódio de hipocalcemia, o que costuma acontecer quando a concentração de Ca antes do tratamento estiver séria ou gravemente elevada por algum tempo antes do tratamento. Em cães, é difícil prever maior risco de ocorrência de episódio de hipocalcemia.[49-50] Em geral, a hipocalcemia é mais provavelmente observada se o valor do tCa antes do tratamento for > 3,5 mmol/ℓ (14 mg/dℓ) ou se o de iCa for > 1,80 mmol/ℓ, ao longo de alguns meses, embora isso seja variável. Também, a rapidez na qual a concentração de iCa diminui é fundamental para o surgimento de sinais clínicos. Ocasionalmente (raramente), podem ser observados sinais clínicos de hipocalcemia (fasciculações musculares, vocalização, respiração ofegante e tetania; ver Capítulo 298) em animais cuja concentração de Ca diminui de forma aguda, mas ainda com valor na faixa de normalidade ou abaixo do intervalo de referência.

A presença de adenoma de paratireoide com função autônoma faz com que glândulas paratireoides previamente normais se atrofiem, tornando-as incapazes de sustentar imediatamente a homeostase normal do Ca após a remoção do tecido anormal. Esse efeito pode ser mais pronunciado se mais de uma glândula paratireoide for removida. Tal episódio pode ser evitado pela administração oral de vitamina D, com ou sem Ca, no período pós-tratamento imediato, ou quando a concentração de Ca estiver moderada a seriamente elevada, pelo início da suplementação de cálcio e vitamina D, 12 a 24 horas antes do tratamento. A vitamina D está disponível em diversas preparações, sendo importante utilizar uma que tenha início relativamente rápido de ação ou o momento do início do tratamento terá de ser mais precoce. As duas preparações recomendadas com mais frequência são calcitriol e alfacalcidol. O calcitriol (1,25-di-hidroxicolecalciferol) é a vitamina D ativa e não requer metabolização para ser efetiva. Possui rápido início de ação (1 a 4 dias) e meia-vida curta. Espera-se que os efeitos tóxicos cessem em 2 a 7 dias. Esse fármaco está disponível na forma de cápsulas de 0,25 ou 0,5 µg. A dose utilizada é de 20 a 30 ng/kg/12 h VO.[51] O alfacalcidol é uma formulação também comumente utilizada. A 25-hidroxilação hepática, necessária antes que esse fármaco se torne ativo, ocorre de maneira rápida, de forma relativamente descontrolada. Não há diferença significativa no tempo necessário para obter o efeito máximo, quando comparado ao calcitriol. O fármaco está disponível como cápsulas de 0,25, 0,5 e 1 µg e na forma de suspensão (2 µg/mℓ), na dose de 0,01 a 0,03 µg/kg/24 h. Entretanto, essas *doses são variáveis e devem ser ajustadas*, para mais ou para menos, conforme necessário, para cada animal.

Cálcio

A vitamina D pode ser administrada com ou sem suplementação oral de Ca. Três opções de Ca são: gliconato de Ca, lactato de Ca e carbonato de Ca. As doses são calculadas com base no conteúdo de cálcio *elementar* de cada preparação (25 a 50 mg/kg/dia, fracionadas em intervalos de 8 ou 12 h), e *não* com base no conteúdo em miligramas do comprimido. Dessa forma, as doses são as mesmas, pois o conteúdo de Ca elementar foi levado em consideração (p. ex., 1 mg de Ca elementar = 11,2 mg de gliconato de Ca, 7,7 mg de lactato de Ca ou 2,5 mg de carbonato de Ca). Com frequência (sobretudo quando a hipocalcemia pós-cirúrgica for grave e sintomática), a suplementação com Ca é utilizada para estabilização a curto prazo do paciente. A longo prazo, é raramente necessário utilizar a suplementação de Ca porque a maioria das rações de animais contém quantidade mais que suficiente de Ca. A administração de vitamina D é muito importante, pois possibilita a absorção do Ca da dieta.

Tratamento emergencial em curto prazo da hipocalcemia

A suplementação IV de Ca pode ser necessária para cães que se tornam seriamente hipocalcêmicos após o tratamento, sintomáticos ou assintomáticos. Os sinais clínicos de hipocalcemia estão listados no Boxe 297.3 e são descritos no Capítulo 298. Cães hospitalizados e que não estejam realizando atividade física ou submetidos a estresse exagerado podem estar clinicamente estáveis, com concentração de Ca abaixo dos valores da faixa de normalidade, mas ficam melhor quando suplementados e monitorados com cuidado, na tentativa de evitar um episódio de hipocalcemia. Quando ocorre um episódio hipocalcêmico o tratamento preferido é a administração por via intravenosa de solução de gliconato de Ca a 10%. Cães sintomáticos (com tetania) podem ser tratados com 0,5 a 1,5 mℓ/kg IV lenta, ao longo de 20 a 30 minutos, até que os sinais clínicos tenham sido atenuados e o cão considerado clinicamente estável. Durante a infusão, o ideal é que se realize eletrocardiograma para monitorar a atividade cardíaca. Se necessário, pode-se aferir o pulso, como um monitoramento menos sensível. A infusão IV de Ca deve ser interrompida caso ocorra elevação do segmento ST, encurtamento de QT ou arritmias.

Depois disso, devem-se administrar 10 a 15 mg/kg/h (10 a 15 mℓ/kg, ao longo de 24 horas), em taxa de infusão constante (TIC), até que o tratamento oral possa ser seguramente iniciado. O Ca aplicado por via IV pode ser irritante vascular cáustico, que leva à tromboflebite se a concentração de Ca infundida for mantida em um nível alto por um período longo (mais de 1 a 2 dias). O cateter IV deve ser inspecionado de maneira contínua, verificando-se sua patência e eficácia, na tentativa de evitar extravasamento da solução de Ca para fora da veia. Isso também pode resultar em extenso dano tecidual (Figura 297.9).

Boxe 297.3 Sintomas de hipocalcemia

Sintomas associados à excitabilidade neuromuscular
Fasciculações ou tremores musculares
Rubor facial, mordedura de patas
Hipersensibilidade a estímulos externos
Marcha rígida
Convulsões tetânicas
Parada respiratória

Alterações de comportamento
Agitação
Ansiedade
Vocalização
Agressividade

Outros
Respiração ofegante
Hipertermia

Há opiniões variadas quanto à administração subcutânea (SC) de Ca. A formação de abscessos e úlceras cutâneas estéreis foi relatada em alguns cães após administração por via subcutânea de alguns sais de Ca.[13] Entretanto, alguns autores recomendam que o gliconato de Ca seja administrado por essa via porque é muito menos provável que cause algum problema. Embora seja verdade que o gliconato de Ca possa ser administrado por via SC, sem efeitos adversos, ele pode causar úlceras cutâneas importantes. Por essa razão, são recomendadas somente as vias de administração por via intravenosa e oral (Tabela 297.3). Quando a concentração de tCa antes do tratamento for > 3,5 mmol/ℓ (14 mg/dℓ) ou de iCa > 1,8 mmol/ℓ, sobretudo quando o aumento da concentração de tCa ou iCa for sério (> 4 mmol/ℓ, 16 mg/dℓ; > 2 mmol/ℓ), é aconselhável iniciar a suplementação com vitamina D, 24 a 36 horas antes do tratamento, para que retarde a diminuição da concentração de Ca após o tratamento e evite hipocalcemia grave. Esse tratamento é sempre um malabarismo, já que não é aconselhável exacerbar a hipercalcemia preexistente. Entretanto, dado o conhecido atraso no início da ação das preparações de vitamina D, o pré-tratamento por 1 dia não é considerado prejudicial.

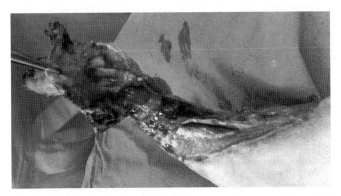

Figura 297.9 Fotografia do membro pélvico de um cão da raça Bichon Frisé que recebeu gliconato de cálcio pela veia safena durante vários dias e desenvolveu tromboflebite grave e desprendimento tecidual, como consequências dos efeitos irritantes do cálcio. (Cortesia de Christina Strand Thomsen e James Warland.)

PROGNÓSTICO

O prognóstico em curto e médio prazos (< 2 anos) para HPTP é excelente em todas as raças de cães. Em todas, com exceção da raça Keeshond, o prognóstico a longo prazo também parece bom. Em cães da raça Keeshond, como acontece em várias formas de HPTP em seres humanos, a recidiva é uma possibilidade eminente. Isso não é surpreendente em pessoas, dados os mecanismos de patogênese da doença e a participação de genes supressores tumorais no desenvolvimento de hiperparatireoidismo. Em seres humanos, quando se faz o tratamento cirúrgico de HPTP realiza-se paratireoidectomia subtotal, na qual somente uma pequena quantidade de tecido paratireoidiano permanece *in situ*, para manutenção da homeostase do cálcio. Cães da raça Keeshond possuem predisposição genética para o desenvolvimento de adenomas de paratireoide. Após a remoção de um deles, podem surgir outros se o cão viver por tempo suficiente. Cães dessa raça que tiveram HPTP devem ser monitorados por toda a vida, verificando possível recidiva da doença, sobretudo se a primeira cirurgia tiver sido realizada em idade relativamente jovem (< 9 anos). Uma abordagem alternativa para cães da raça Keeshond com HPTP hereditário é a remoção das glândulas paratireoides, deixando apenas uma, por ocasião da primeira cirurgia. Na experiência do autor, isso pode resultar em séria hipocalcemia pós-cirúrgica, o que, em alguns casos, exige terapia suplementar vitalícia, para seu controle. Relata-se que um cão Keeshond inicialmente tratado com sucesso aos 10 anos apresentou recidiva de hipercalcemia aos 11 anos e meio de idade e foi submetido a uma segunda cirurgia. Embora tenham permanecido duas glândulas paratireoides, esse cão nunca mais foi capaz de manter uma concentração sérica normal de cálcio e recebeu vitamina D até que morreu por outra causa, vários anos depois. Essa recuperação variável à cirurgia e a necessidade de cálcio suplementar torna o controle da doença efetivo no complexo período perioperatório em cães da raça Keeshond, especialmente por apresentarem muitas dificuldades a longo prazo.

HIPERPARATIREOIDISMO PRIMÁRIO EM GATOS

O HPTP foi relatado em poucos gatos de meia-idade a idosos. Os sinais clínicos relatados incluíam êmese, PU/PD, perda de

Tabela 297.3 Fármacos à base de cálcio e vitamina D disponíveis para o tratamento de hipocalcemia.

	FÁRMACO	DOSE	PRECAUÇÕES
Aguda	Gliconato de cálcio a 10%	0,5 a 1,5 mℓ/kg, ao longo de 20 a 30 min	Monitore a função cardíaca por meio de auscultação, palpação do pulso ou eletrocardiograma, em busca de bradicardia, intervalo QT mais curto e elevação do segmento ST
	Borogliconato de cálcio a 10%	0,5 a 1 mℓ/kg, ao longo de 20 a 30 min	
	Cloreto de cálcio a 10%	0,16 a 0,5 mℓ/kg, ao longo de 20 a 30 min	
Subaguda	Gliconato de cálcio a 10%	10 a 15 mℓ/kg, ao longo de 24 h, em solução de NaCl a 0,9%	Não administre SC
	Borogliconato de cálcio a 10%	6 a 9 mℓ/kg, ao longo de 24 h, em solução de NaCl a 0,9%	
	Cloreto de cálcio a 10%	3 a 5 mℓ/kg, ao longo de 24 h, em solução de NaCl a 0,9%	
Crônica	Carbonato de cálcio Gliconato de cálcio Lactato de cálcio	25 a 50 mg de cálcio *elementar**/kg	Pode ser interrompido assim que a dose de vitamina D adequada for obtida
	Calcitriol	20 a 30 ng/kg/dia VO, fracionada em 2 vezes/dia	Tempo para obter efeito máximo < 4 dias
	Alfacalcidol	0,01 a 0,03 µg/kg/dia	Tempo para obter efeito máximo < 4 dias
	Di-hidrotaquisterol	0,02 a 0,03 mg/kg/dia, reduzindo para 0,01 a 0,02 mg/kg a cada 24 a 48 h, conforme necessário	Tempo para obter efeito máximo < 7 dias

*1 mg cálcio = 11,2 mg de gliconato de cálcio = 7,7 mg de lactato de cálcio = 2,5 mg de carbonato de cálcio. *NaCl*, cloreto de sódio.

SEÇÃO 21 • Doenças Endócrinas

peso e tumor cervical palpável.[52] Embora a glândula paratireoide anormal possa não ser palpável, à semelhança do que ocorre em cães, a doença da paratireoide costuma estar associada a estruturas císticas que tornam a presença do tumor mais evidente. Como o hipertireoidismo é uma causa muito mais comum de neoplasia cervical palpável em gatos, inicialmente deve-se excluir tal possibilidade. PU/PD podem ser mais brandas em gatos e a densidade urinária pode não estar alterada de maneira significativa, a menos que o gato apresente insuficiência renal concomitante.[14] Os gatos, assim como os cães, podem também desenvolver urolitíase com cálcio.[53] Em gatos, o tratamento preferido para HPTP é a remoção do tecido paratireoidiano anormal.[12] Assim como mencionado para os cães, o sucesso terapêutico é muito maior quando se realiza ultrassonografia antes da cirurgia, para a detecção de tumor(es) de paratireoide. O prognóstico a longo prazo é bom, após a cirurgia. Outros protocolos terapêuticos não foram relatados em gatos. Em gatos, pode ser necessário o tratamento com Ca e análogos da vitamina D devido ao desenvolvimento de hipocalcemia após a remoção da glândula paratireoide. Há menos informações disponíveis em gatos sobre quando prescrever a administração de cálcio e vitamina D para evitar um episódio hipocalcêmico pós-cirúrgico, mas aplicam-se os mesmos princípios descritos para os cães. Novamente, é difícil prever quais pacientes necessitarão de suplementação e por quanto tempo.

REFERÊNCIAS BIBLIOGRÁFICAS

As referências bibliográficas deste capítulo se encontram online no Ambiente de Aprendizagem.

CAPÍTULO 298

Hipoparatireoidismo

Patty Lathan

CONTEXTO HISTÓRICO

As glândulas paratireoides foram inicialmente detectadas em rinocerontes indianos, por Richard Owen, em 1850. Ivar Sandstrom foi o primeiro a nomear e a descrevê-las, em 1880, enquanto Giuilo Vassale e Francesco Generali relataram, em 1900, que a paratireoidectomia completa resultara em tetania.[1] O hipoparatireoidismo de ocorrência natural foi inicialmente descrito em cães, em 1966, e em gatos, em 1990.[2,3] O hipoparatireoidismo primário idiopático permanece uma doença extremamente incomum tanto em cães como em gatos.

FISIOPATOLOGIA

A fisiologia normal da paratireoide é apresentada no Capítulo 297. A carência de paratormônio (PTH, *parathyroid hormone*) ou de sua ação resulta em hipocalcemia e hiperfosfatemia, por meio de uma combinação de mecanismos: diminuição da reabsorção óssea de cálcio (Ca; ver Capítulo 69), o que causa menor liberação de Ca e fósforo (PO_4) na circulação sanguínea, menor absorção de Ca e PO_4 no intestino delgado e menor reabsorção de Ca e menor excreção de PO_4 através dos túbulos renais. Os efeitos renais do PTH são os fatores que mais influenciam a concentração sérica de PO_4. A carência de PTH ocasiona elevação da concentração de PO_4. Em indivíduos sadios, o Ca estabiliza as membranas dos neurônios por limitar a permeabilidade ao sódio (Na) e despolarização da membrana. Entretanto, na hipocalcemia os neurônios, tanto do sistema nervoso central quanto do sistema nervoso periférico, se tornam hiperexcitáveis, ocasionando os sintomas comuns de convulsões, tremores/fasciculações musculares e marcha rígida (devido à dor e/ou à tetania muscular).

ETIOLOGIA

A hipocalcemia mais grave em cães e gatos sem histórico de trauma ou cirurgia cervical é classificada como hipoparatireoidismo primário idiopático. Entretanto, em alguns pacientes há suspeita de etiologia imunomediada, já que as glândulas paratireoides podem ser vistas como muito pequenas na necropsia; a histologia revela, com frequência, quantidade acentuadamente diminuída de células parenquimatosas, infiltração de linfócitos e, em menor grau, de plasmócitos e neutrófilos.[4-6] A resolução do hipoparatireoidismo, em um cão submetido à terapia imunossupressora, sustenta a possibilidade de um mecanismo imunomediado como causa da doença, em alguns pacientes.[7]

MANIFESTAÇÕES CLÍNICAS EM CÃES

Resenha

No momento do diagnóstico, a idade dos cães com hipoparatireoidismo primário varia de 6 semanas a 13 anos (média: cerca de 6 anos), sendo as fêmeas de cães das raças Schnauzer Miniatura, Poodle, Pastor-Alemão e Terrier predispostas.[4,5,8,9] Cães da raça São Bernardo são os mais acometidos na Austrália e na Nova Zelândia.[8,10]

Sinais clínicos

A maioria dos sinais clínicos associados ao hipoparatireoidismo está relacionada com "tetania" ou "hiperexcitabilidade" neuromuscular. Convulsões, tremores musculares, fasciculações musculares e marcha rígida são relatados na maioria dos cães, notando-se abertura e fechamento descontrolados da mandíbula em cerca de metade dos cães com fasciculações (Vídeo 298.1).[4,8] Respiração ofegante, esfregação da face, mordidas nas patas e alterações de comportamento (como inquietude, ansiedade e agressividade) são frequentemente identificadas ao questionar tutores atentos. Esses sintomas podem ser explicados pelas cãibras e dor musculares ou pela sensação de tremores musculares.[4,8] Nessa condição, nota-se ataxia ou andar em círculos. Sinais inespecíficos incluem inapetência, êmese, "fraqueza", letargia e diarreia. A duração dos sinais clínicos antes do diagnóstico varia de algumas poucas horas a 1 ano ou mais (mediana: cerca de 2 semanas).[4,8] Em geral, sintomas neuromusculares se tornam mais graves com o passar do tempo, são episódicos e exacerbados por atividade física ou excitação. Praticamente todos os sinais clínicos associados ao hipoparatireoidismo cessam após o tratamento.

Exame físico

Ao exame físico, nota-se que os cães com hipoparatireoidismo primário costumam apresentar hipertermia, tensão, ansiedade, irritabilidade, marcha rígida, podendo rosnar ou atacar após serem tocados ou palpados. Por exemplo, o animal pode apresentar abdome tenso devido à dor em músculos abdominais ou em outro local, ou o cão pode estar prevendo sensação de dor porque carícias podem lhe ter causado cãibras musculares e dor no passado. Cães podem, algumas vezes, se tornar agressivos ou não aceitar carícias, particularmente na cabeça. Em alguns cães, a auscultação torácica revela taquiarritmias. Na primeira consulta ou após o início do tratamento, é possível notar catarata lenticular que surge como pequeno ponto ou linha de opacidade nas regiões subcapsulares corticais anterior e posterior(ver Capítulo 11). O mecanismo da formação da catarata é incerto, mas não parece prejudicar a visão.[4,8,11]

MANIFESTAÇÕES CLÍNICAS EM GATOS

Diferentemente do que ocorre em cães, os gatos machos são sujeitos ao hipoparatireoidismo primário. Os sinais clínicos em gatos são semelhantes àqueles mencionados em cães, mas os felinos apresentam inapetência e letargia com maior frequência. A catarata lenticular e/ou o prolapso de terceira pálpebra são observados em alguns gatos.[3,11-13] Um gato com insuficiência miocárdica e achados ecocardiográficos compatíveis com cardiomiopatia dilatada apresentou resolução das alterações cardíacas após tratamento do hipoparatireoidismo.[14]

AVALIAÇÃO DIAGNÓSTICA EM CÃES E GATOS

Bioquímica sérica, hemograma, exame de urina, eletrocardiograma

No momento do diagnóstico (Figura 298.1), é observada hipocalcemia em todos os animais de companhia com hipoparatireoidismo e, em quase todos, hiperfosfatemia. Em animais de companhia com hipocalcemia grave, recomenda-se a repetição da mensuração da concentração de cálcio total (tCa), simplesmente porque a condição é incomum, sobretudo se os sinais clínicos não forem consistentes. A coleta de sangue em tubo com ácido etilenodiaminotetracético (EDTA) ("tampa roxa") ou até mesmo a contaminação da agulha com EDTA antes da transferência do sangue para outro tubo pode diminuir artificialmente o conteúdo de Ca devido sua ligação ao EDTA. Como o Ca ionizado (iCa) é a forma biologicamente ativa, sua mensuração pode fornecer uma representação mais acurada da gravidade da hipocalcemia. Em animais com hipoparatireoidismo, as diminuições em tCa e iCa tendem a ser semelhantes quanto à gravidade. Na ausência de hipoalbuminemia, se a aferição do iCa não for possível, a demonstração repetida de baixas concentrações de tCa em um paciente com sinais clínicos compatíveis é, em geral, adequada para confirmar a hipocalcemia. Os sinais clínicos de hipocalcemia não costumam ser observados até que a concentração de tCa seja < 7 mg/dℓ ou a c de iCa < 0,8 mmol/ℓ. Em caso de hipocalcemia aguda, podem ocorrer sintomas com valores maiores. Pacientes com hipoparatireoidismo podem ter diminuição marcante da concentração de tCa (tão baixas quanto

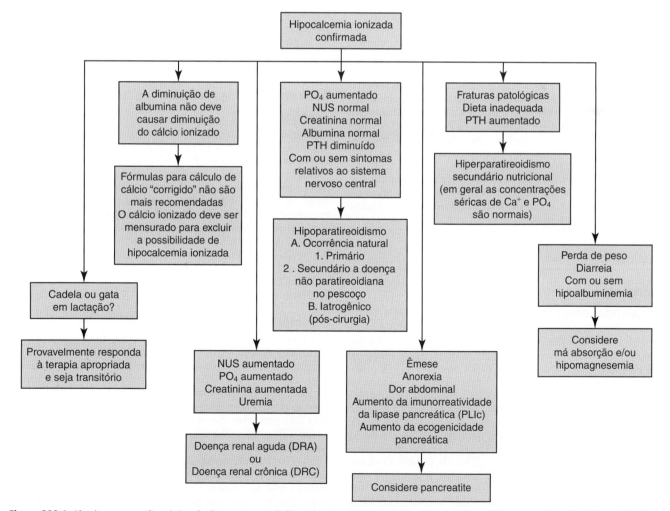

Figura 298.1 Algoritmo para o diagnóstico de diversas causas de hipocalcemia. *NUS*, nitrogênio ureico sanguíneo; *PTH*, paratormônio. (De Feldman EC, Nelson RW, Reusch CE, et al.: *Canine and feline endocrinology*, 4 ed., St. Louis, 2015, Saunders.)

2,7 mg/dℓ).[4,8] Já que cães e gatos não exibem sinais clínicos, considera-se que a doença progrediu tão cronicamente que houve certa adaptação fisiológica.[11]

Hipomagnesemia (Mg; ver Capítulo 68) foi documentada em cães da raça Yorkshire Terrier com hipocalcemia e enteropatia com perda de proteína concomitantes. Baixa concentração de magnésio pode contribuir para a diminuição da secreção de PTH.[15] Entretanto, a concentração de magnésio é normal na maioria dos cães com hipoparatireoidismo primário e somente discreta a moderadamente diminuída em alguns. Como esses cães se recuperam sem suplementação de magnésio, a relevância desse achado é desconhecida.[4,11] O conjunto de resultados de exames bioquímicos séricos, hemograma e exame de urina não indica alteração em animais com hipoparatireoidismo primário. O aumento da atividade da enzima creatinoquinase foi relatado em um gato e um cão, e seria esperado em qualquer animal com atividade muscular excessiva.[14,16] A hipocalcemia induz duração prolongada dos potenciais de ação cardíacos no eletrocardiograma, resultando em prolongamento do segmento ST e, subsequentemente, do intervalo Q-T (ver Capítulo 248).[8]

Paratormônio

O diagnóstico de hipoparatireoidismo primário requer a constatação de baixa concentração de Ca e concentração inapropriadamente baixa de PTH. Devido à rigorosa regulação do Ca, a concentração de PTH deveria estar aumentada, acima do valor de referência, em animais saudáveis com hipocalcemia. Assim, as concentrações séricas de PTH em cães e gatos com hipoparatireoidismo primário podem estar baixas ou no limite inferior da faixa de normalidade.

DIAGNÓSTICOS DIFERENCIAIS

O diagnóstico diferencial de hipocalcemia inclui algumas poucas condições comuns e uma série de causas incomuns. As enfermidades relacionadas com a glândula paratireoide incluem anormalidades primárias da glândula, como destruição imunomediada, destruição idiopática, remoção cirúrgica e raras condições em seres humanos ainda não relatadas em cães ou gatos (ver Capítulo 69). Condições incomumente associadas à hipocalcemia são hipomagnesemia, doença renal aguda (DRA), doença renal crônica (DRC), pancreatite, diabetes melito, eclâmpsia, síndrome de má absorção, obstrução do trato urinário e uso de enema que contenha fósforo. Hipoalbuminemia causa redução não relevante do tCa, mas não do iCa, por conta da ligação à albumina. Outras diversas causas foram observadas (ver Capítulo 69).

TRATAMENTO

Tratamento emergencial

Terapia intravenosa intensiva

Cães com hipocalcemia grave devem ser tratados inicialmente com gliconato de cálcio, na forma de *bolus* IV, e mantidos em taxa de infusão contínua (TIC) de gliconato de cálcio (em geral adicionado a soluções de uso IV) (ver Capítulo 146). A suplementação oral com Ca é também fornecida até que o calcitriol (1,25-di-hidrocolecalciferol; 1,25-di-hidrovitamina D_3; vitamina D_3 ativa) faça efeito, para o controle a longo prazo. De início, um cão ou gato com tetania deve ser submetido à infusão IV lenta de gliconato de cálcio a 10%, na dose de 0,5 a 1,5 mℓ/kg (5 a 15 mg/kg), ao longo de 10 a 15 min. Lembre-se de que o gliconato de cálcio a 10% contém 9,3 mg de Ca/mℓ. O eletrocardiograma deve ser monitorado durante a infusão e esta descontinuada caso se constatem bradicardia, contrações ventriculares prematuras ou encurtamento do intervalo QT. Assim que o eletrocardiograma se normalizar, a infusão pode ser reiniciada, mas à taxa mais lenta. O cloreto de cálcio não deve ser

utilizado em cães e gatos, pois é extremamente cáustico e pode causar úlcera tecidual, caso ocorra extravasamento vascular. Após a administração do *bolus* inicial de gliconato de cálcio, deve-se reavaliar a concentração sérica de tCa ou iCa. Na maioria dos animais, nota-se melhora significativa dos sinais clínicos, bem antes da normalização da concentração de Ca.

Após a estabilização clínica, deve-se adicionar o gliconato de cálcio a qualquer solução de uso IV de manutenção e administrá-lo na dose de 2,5 a 3,5 mg/kg/h (0,3 a 0,4 mℓ/kg/h), lembrando, novamente, que o gliconato de cálcio contém 9,3 mg de Ca/mℓ.[17] A repetição de *bolus* somente é recomendada quando há sintomas agudos de tetania. A concentração de Ca deve ser mensurada 1 ou 2 vezes/dia, nos primeiros dias, e a taxa de infusão ajustada de acordo com a necessidade. Após suplementação oral de Ca e vitamina D (calcitriol) e estabilização da concentração sérica de Ca, a suplementação de Ca pode ser diminuída.

Tratamento subcutâneo conservador

Tem-se utilizado tratamento subcutâneo (SC) com gliconato de cálcio como alternativa à taxa de infusão constante (TIC). Embora incomum, a administração por via subcutânea de Ca pode causar morbidades significativas por causar lesão tecidual (resultou na morte de um cão), não sendo mais recomendada. Se, por qualquer razão, não for possível o uso de TIC, os tutores devem ser orientados quanto às complicações potenciais da administração por via subcutânea de Ca. Calcinose cutânea foi relatada em dois cães e um gato, após administração por via subcutânea de gliconato de cálcio.[8,16,18] Um protocolo para tratamento SC consiste no fornecimento da mesma dose, via SC, inicialmente administrada na forma de *bolus* IV, diluindo-se uma parte de gliconato de cálcio para uma parte de solução cristaloide, em intervalos de 6 a 8 h. Reduz-se a dose e a frequência de administração à medida que o uso oral de Ca e calcitriol começa a fazer efeito.[17]

Tratamento de longa duração

Contexto geral

No hipoparatireoidismo primário, o Ca não pode ser obtido de ossos ou da dieta sem PTH ou vitamina D, tampouco é reabsorvido nos rins. Como o PTH não está disponível no mercado, análogos da vitamina D de uso oral são fundamentais no tratamento de longa duração do hipoparatireoidismo. A suplementação oral com Ca pode ser utilizada precocemente no tratamento e, de modo geral, descontinuada após algumas semanas se o cão ou gato estiver se alimentando bem, pois o Ca da dieta deve ser suficiente para suprir as necessidades diárias. As opções atualmente disponíveis para a suplementação da vitamina D incluem calcitriol e ergocalciferol (vitamina D_2). O di-hidrotaquisterol, um análogo sintético da vitamina D, não está mais disponível no mercado.

Calcitriol

É a forma ativa da vitamina D_3, com um tempo muito mais curto para induzir efeito máximo (1 a 4 dias) e menos tempo necessário para regressão de intoxicação (1 a 7 dias) do que o ergocalciferol (5 a 21 dias e 1 a 18 semanas, respectivamente). Dessa forma, prefere-se o calcitriol ao ergocalciferol, a menos que limitações financeiras impeçam sua utilização (ver Capítulo 297 para alternativas ao calcitriol).[11] A dose inicial de calcitriol (20 a 40 ng/kg/dia, 0,02 a 0,04 µg/kg/dia) é em geral fornecida durante 2 a 4 dias e, então, diminuída para 10 a 20 ng/kg/dia (0,01 a 0,02 µg/kg/dia). Quando se utilizam formulações disponíveis no mercado, a dosagem de calcitriol pode ser um desafio, pois as cápsulas em gel somente estão disponíveis em concentrações limitadas (0,25 µg e 0,5 µg), as quais não são práticas para o uso em cães e gatos. Com base em observações clínicas, as formulações obtidas em farmácias de manipulação não se mostraram compatíveis. Assim, para cada paciente, o produto deve ser obtido sempre da mesma farmácia de manipulação de referência e não utilizado após o prazo de validade.

Ergocalciferol

A dose inicial de ergocalciferol é de 4.000 a 6.000 UI/kg/dia. Assim que a concentração de Ca tiver se estabilizado em 8 a 9,5 mg/dℓ, a dose pode ser geralmente diminuída para dias alternados. A partir desse momento, deve-se determinar a frequência da dose, com base no monitoramento. A concentração de Ca deve, então, ser monitorada semanalmente e a dose ajustada conforme necessário.[11]

Administração oral de cálcio

A suplementação oral de Ca deve também ser fornecida inicialmente, mas pode, de modo geral, ser ajustada e descontinuada dentro de 1 semana após o início do calcitriol. A dose inicial, fracionada, em gatos é de 0,5 a 1 g/dia. Em cães, administra-se 1 a 4 g/dia, em doses fracionadas. Podem ser utilizados gliconato de cálcio e lactato de cálcio, mas o carbonato de cálcio é, com mais frequência, escolhido devido à disponibilidade. É importante estabelecer a dose com base no conteúdo de Ca elementar. Carbonato de cálcio, gliconato de cálcio e lactato de cálcio têm, respectivamente, 40, 9 e 13% de Ca elementar (1 g de carbonato de cálcio contém 400 mg de Ca elementar).[19]

Objetivo do tratamento

O objetivo é manter a concentração séricas de Ca um pouco abaixo do limite inferior do valor de referência (cerca de 8 a 9,5 mg/dℓ). Essa é uma concentração alta o suficiente para prevenir os sinais clínicos de hipocalcemia e diminuir o grau de calciurese devido à carência de PTH; ademais, é baixa o suficiente para evitar intoxicação por vitamina D: hipercalcemia, hiperfosfatemia e DRA. Assim que a concentração sérica de Ca aumenta para 7,5 a 8 mg/dℓ, após administração oral de vitamina D e Ca, e o paciente estiver se alimentando bem e ingerindo água, eles recebem alta hospitalar. A princípio, reavaliações devem ocorrer a cada 2 a 3 dias. Assim que a concentração sérica de Ca tiver se estabilizado, os intervalos de reavaliações podem ser progressivamente prolongados, até uma vez a cada 2 a 3 meses. Os tutores devem ser orientados a retornar se ocorrerem quaisquer sinais de hipocalcemia ou hipercalcemia. Esta deve ser tratada pela descontinuação da administração de vitamina D até que a concentração de Ca se normalize; terapia adicional, inclusive de soluções de uso IV e furosemida, é quase sempre desnecessária.

PROGNÓSTICO

O prognóstico de cães e gatos com hipoparatireoidismo, com tutores capazes e dedicados, é excelente. Os tutores devem ser lembrados de que essa doença requer tratamento de longa duração e frequente monitoramento, a fim de ajudar a prevenir hipocalcemia ou hipercalcemia. A maioria dos cães e gatos morre em decorrência de causas não relacionadas com o hipoparatireoidismo, quando se faz tratamento apropriado.[4,8,11]

REFERÊNCIAS BIBLIOGRÁFICAS

As referências bibliográficas deste capítulo se encontram online no Ambiente de Aprendizagem.

CAPÍTULO 299

Hipotireoidismo em Cães

Carmel T. Mooney

INTRODUÇÃO

Hipotireoidismo é a doença tireoidiana mais comum e uma das anormalidades endócrinas de maior prevalência em cães, estimada em 0,2 a 0,8%.[1-3] Uma pesquisa com cães segurados da Suécia, entretanto, sugeriu uma prevalência menor, de 0,07%.[4] Essa pode ser uma taxa mais acurada, já que não é influenciada por uma população que procura atendimento e inclui um grande número de animais de linhagem mais provavelmente acometidos por hipotireoidismo.[5]

FISIOLOGIA

A glândula tireoide dos cães consiste em dois lobos separados, um em cada lado da traqueia. Cada lobo é composto por folículos microscópicos delimitados por uma camada única de epitélio tireoidiano. O lúmen de cada folículo contém coloide, uma substância de armazenamento de tireoglobulina secretada pelas células foliculares. A tireoglobulina é uma grande glicoproteína que contém iodotirosinas, componentes de hormônios tireoidianos. A maior parte das etapas envolvidas na síntese de hormônios tireoidianos é catalisada pela enzima tireoide peroxidase (TPO).

A principal função da glândula tireoide é produzir hormônios tireoidianos ativos – 3,5,3',5'-L-tetraiodotironina (tiroxina, T_4) e 3,5,3'-L-triiodotironina (triiodotironina, T_3) (Figura 299.1). Quase todos esses hormônios estão ligados a proteínas na circulação sanguínea. Aproximadamente 60% do T_4 está ligado à globulina ligadora de tiroxina, 17% à transtirretina, 12% à albumina e 11% a diversas frações de lipoproteínas.[6] A ligação do T_3 é semelhante. As afinidades de ligação dos hormônios tireoidianos são menores em cães do que em seres humanos e, consequentemente, em cães as concentrações totais são menores, as frações livres maiores (estimadas em aproximadamente 0,1 a 0,3% para T_4 e 1% para T_3) e meias-vidas séricas mais curtas (10 a 16 horas para T_4 e 5 a 6 horas para T_3). Somente a fração livre é metabolicamente ativa, com a porção ligada à proteína servindo como um reservatório passivo para controlar o fornecimento de hormônio aos tecidos. O T_3 é aproximadamente três a cinco vezes mais potente do que o T_4. Até 60% do T_3 não é produzido pela glândula tireoide, mas sim pela monodesiodação periférica do anel externo do T_4, uma etapa que pode ser autorregulada. A desiodação do anel interno resulta na formação de T_3 reverso metabolicamente inativo (rT_3).

Os hormônios tireoidianos atuam na maioria dos tecidos do organismo, amplamente pela interação com receptores nucleares

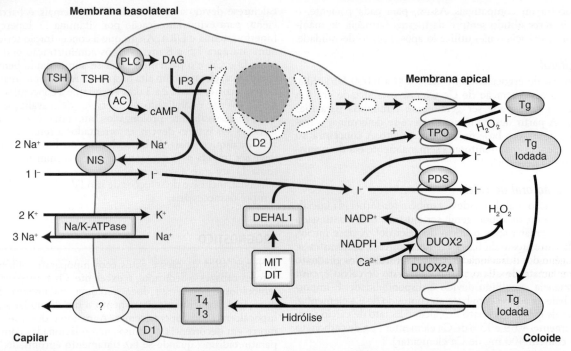

Figura 299.1 Síntese de hormônios tireoidianos. Ilustração esquemática de uma célula folicular da tireoidiana mostrando os principais mecanismos de transporte tireoidiano de iodeto e síntese do hormônio tireoidiano. *AC*, adenilciclase; *cAMP*, adenosina monofosfato cíclico; *ATPase*, adenosina trifosfatase; *D1*, deiodinase tireoidiana tipo 1; *D2*, deiodinase tireoidiana tipo 2; *DAG*, diacilglicerol; *DEHAL1*, iodotirosina desalogenase 1 (1YD); *DIT*, diiodotirosina; *DUOX*, oxidase dupla; *IP3*, inositol trifosfato; *MIT*, monoiodotirosina; *NADP*, forma oxidada da nicotinamida adenosina dinucleotídio fosfato; *NADPH*, forma reduzida da nicotinamida adenosina dinucleotídio fosfato; *NIS*, cotransportador de sódio-iodeto; *PDS*, pendrina (SLC26A4); *PLC*, fosfolipase C; T_3, triiodotironina; T_4, tiroxina; *Tg*, tireoglobulina; *TPO*, peroxidase tireoidiana; *TSHR*, receptor de tireotropina. (De Salvatore D, Davies TF, Schlumberger MJ et al.: Thyroid physiology and diagnostic evaluation of patients with thyroid disorders. In Melmed S, Polonsky KS, Larsen PR et al., editors: *Williams textbook of endocrinology*, 12 ed., Philadelphia, 2011, Elsevier, p. 327-361.)

específicos, para modificar a expressão de uma diversa gama de genes. Portanto, os hormônios tireoidianos influenciam múltiplos processos metabólicos, a partir da regulação da demanda mitocondrial de oxigênio para o controle da síntese proteica. Alguns efeitos podem ocorrer dentro de minutos a horas, mas outros podem demorar semanas a meses. A produção do hormônio tireoidiano é controlada, principalmente, por um mecanismo de retroalimentação (*feedback*) negativo (Figura 299.2). O hipotálamo secreta o hormônio liberador de tireotrofina (TRH, do inglês *thyrotropin-releasing hormone*), que estimula células específicas da adeno-hipófise (lobo anterior da hipófise) a induzir a síntese e a secreção de tireotrofina (hormônio tireoestimulante [TSH, do inglês *tyroid-stimulating hormone*]). O TSH promove o aprisionamento do iodeto na tireoide, bem como a síntese e a liberação de hormônios tireoidianos.

O excesso de T_4 livre (T_4L) e T_3 induz um mecanismo de *feedback* negativo no hipotálamo e na adeno-hipófise, diminuindo a síntese e a liberação de TRH e TSH e, subsequentemente, a produção de hormônio tireoidiano. Os hormônios tireoidianos possuem uma influência importante na taxa metabólica, no crescimento, no desenvolvimento do sistema nervoso central (SNC) e na renovação tecidual. Além disso, possuem efeitos inotrópico e cronotrópico positivos no coração, são necessários para a síntese e metabolização de colesterol e estimulam a eritropoese. Quando deficientes, o espectro de anormalidades possíveis é extenso.

PATOGÊNESE DO HIPOTIREOIDISMO

Considerações gerais

O hipotireoidismo resulta da diminuição da produção de T_4 e T_3. Pode surgir por conta de uma anormalidade em qualquer etapa do eixo hipotálamo-hipófise-tireoide. É denominado

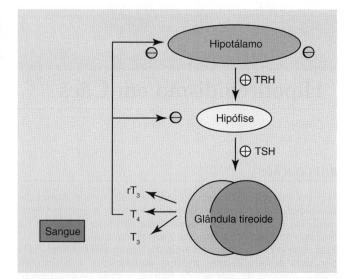

Figura 299.2 Regulação das concentrações de hormônios tireoidianos. As concentrações dos hormônios tireoidianos são controladas pelo eixo hipotálamo-hipófise-tireoide, que atua como um ramo do mecanismo de *feedback* negativo. A tireotrofina (TSH) estimula a síntese e a liberação de T_4 e menor quantidade de T_3 pela glândula tireoide. O T_3 intracelular, derivado da desiodação de T_4 na hipófise, reduz a síntese e a secreção de TSH, sendo o principal determinante da concentração de TSH. O hormônio liberador de tireotrofina (TRH), secretado pelo hipotálamo, modula a liberação de TSH pela hipófise. O aumento das concentrações dos hormônios tireoidianos também, supostamente, reduz a síntese e a secreção de TSH. Hormônios que inibem a secreção de TSH incluem dopamina, somatostatina, serotonina e glicocorticoides. TRH, prostaglandinas e agonistas alfa-adrenérgicos aumentam a secreção de TSH. (De Scott-Moncrieff CR: Hypothyroidism. In Ettinger SJ, Feldman EC, editors: *Textbook of veterinary internal medicine*, 7 ed., St. Louis, 2010, Elsevier, p. 1751-1761.)

primário ou central (incluindo secundário e terciário), dependendo de onde a lesão primária se situa: na glândula tireoide (primário), hipófise (secundário) ou hipotálamo (terciário). É também descrito como congênito ou adquirido, dependendo da idade na qual se desenvolve.

Hipotireoidismo congênito

O hipotireoidismo congênito é significativamente menos comum do que o adquirido. Ele resulta de hipoplasia ou aplasia da tireoide, disgenesia ou disormonogênese. O hipotireoidismo congênito pode ser mais prevalente do que atualmente se pensa, porque alguns indivíduos são subdiagnosticados e outros morrem ao nascimento ou logo depois dele. O hipotireoidismo central (resultante da deficiência de TSH ou TRH) foi relatado esporadicamente em uma família de cães da raça Schnauzer gigante.[7-11] A deficiência de TSH é comum em casos de nanismo hipofisário; há relatos de cães com disgenesia de tireoide.[12-14] Hipotireoidismo congênito acompanhado de bócio, como resultado de disormonogênese e deficiência de TPO, foi relatado esporadicamente como uma anomalia autossômica recessiva com penetrância completa em cães das raças Toy Fox e Rat Terrier, para os quais há disponibilidade de testes genéticos.[15-17] Diferentes mutações com fenótipo semelhante foram relatadas em cães das raças Tenterfield Terrier, Spanish Water Dog e Papillon.[18-20] O hipotireoidismo congênito pode ser constatado em filhotes de cadelas alimentadas com dieta deficiente em iodo ou submetidas à administração de diversos fármacos, ou em filhotes expostos à deficiência ou ao excesso de iodo quando jovens.[21-23]

Hipotireoidismo adquirido

Central

O hipotireoidismo central (deficiência de TRH ou TSH) é raro, sendo responsável por menos de 5% dos cães com hipotireoidismo. Neoplasias de hipófise e hipofisectomia cirúrgica responderam pela vasta maioria dos casos relatados, sendo as deficiências pós-traumáticas as causas menos comuns.[24-26] Há relato de um cão com hipotireoidismo terciário relacionado com a neoplasia, mas isso é tão incomum que as indicações clínicas para a diferenciação entre doença secundária e terciária parecem incomuns.[27] Hipotireoidismo secundário é uma doença potencial, incomum e reversível causada pelo excesso de glicocorticoides.[28,29] O hipotireoidismo central resulta em degeneração atrófica da tireoide, caracterizada por distensão de folículos por coloide e epitélio circundante achatado, alterações bastante diferentes daquelas associadas ao hipotireoidismo primário.[11]

Primário

Na enorme maioria de cães, a doença tireoidiana primária adquirida é a causa de hipotireoidismo. À histologia, a tireoidite linfocítica e a atrofia de tireoide são igualmente comuns. A tireoidite linfocítica é uma doença autoimune destrutiva caracterizada por infiltração multifocal ou difusa da glândula tireoide por linfócitos, macrófagos e plasmócitos, bem como pela substituição progressiva do tecido tireoidiano por tecido conjuntivo fibroso.[30,31] Está associada à inflamação sistêmica e a uma dominante resposta imune celular.[32] Diferentemente, a atrofia idiopática é descrita como um processo degenerativo com mínimas alterações inflamatórias e substituição gradativa do tecido tireoidiano por tecido adiposo e conjuntivo.[30] Alguns pesquisadores acreditam que a atrofia idiopática é o estágio final da tireoidite linfocítica e que está associada a semelhantes marcadores de inflamação.[32] Independentemente, a causa incitante dessas condições é incerta.

É necessária a biopsia da tireoide para o diagnóstico definitivo de tireoidite linfocítica, mas sua existência pode ser inferida pela demonstração de autoanticorpos circulantes contra antígenos tireoidianos, como tireoglobulina, T_4, T_3 e tireoide peroxidase. Autoanticorpos antitireoglobulina (TgAAs) são mais comuns,

enquanto os outros raramente ocorrem isoladamente.[33-35] Testes para TgAA, amplamente disponíveis, apresentam excelente sensibilidade e especificidade diagnóstica.[36-38] Aproximadamente 50% dos cães com hipotireoidismo possuem TgAAs circulantes, correspondendo à frequência da tireoidite linfocítica.[35,39-44] A tireoidite linfocítica é lentamente progressiva; causa sintomas de hipotireoidismo após destruição de aproximadamente 75% da glândula. A progressão dela pode ser dividida em quatro estágios (Tabela 299.1). Neles, a velocidade de progressão é variável, e nem todos os cães desenvolvem hipotireoidismo funcional. Aproximadamente 20% dos cães eutireóideos positivos para TgAA desenvolvem evidências hormonais de disfunção tireoidiana dentro de 1 ano após o teste, mas somente 5% desenvolvem sinais clínicos de hipotireoidismo.[45] A maioria dos cães permanece positiva para TgAA e assintomática; um pequeno número deles apresenta resultados negativos, posteriormente, sem evidência de disfunção tireoidiana. Alguns cães com hipotireoidismo e positivos para TgAA se tornam negativos, o que sustenta o conceito de que a atrofia da tireoide representa um estágio final da tireoidite linfocítica. Em teoria, a destruição total do tecido tireoidiano leva à redução da estimulação imune, à ausência de tireoidite histológica e à conversão para negatividade aos autoanticorpos. Há relato de progressão histopatológica de tireoidite linfocítica em atrofia folicular.[46] Ademais, cães eutireóideos e positivos para TgAA (tireoidite silenciosa/subclínica) são mais jovens do que os cães com hipotireoidismo e positivos para TgAA e do que aqueles com hipotireoidismo e negativos para TgAA.[42] A proporção de cães com hipotireoidismo e positivos ou negativos para TgAA varia dependendo da raça, com diferentes taxas de progressão da doença ou diferentes suscetibilidades.

As predisposições raciais relatadas, juntamente com a natureza familiar do hipotireoidismo em cães de raças puras, são compatíveis com um forte componente hereditário na ocorrência da doença.[47] Algumas raças apresentam alta prevalência de positividade para TgAA e aumento significativo do risco de desenvolvimento do hipotireoidismo. Essas raças incluem, mas não se limitam a, Setter inglês, Golden Retriever, Rhodesian Ridgeback, Cocker Spaniel e Boxer.[42] O hipotireoidismo familiar é também reconhecido em colônias de cães das raças Dogue Alemão, Beagle e Borzoi, e, na Suécia, em cães Hovawart e Schnauzer gigante.[40,46,48,49] Diversos fatores de risco, genéticos e ambientais, foram incriminados no desenvolvimento da doença

Tabela 299.1	Estágios progressivos da tireoidite linfocítica.			
	HISTOPATOLOGIA DO TECIDO TIREOIDIANO	**TESTE PARA TgAA**	**CONCENTRAÇÕES DE HORMÔNIOS TIREOIDIANOS**	
			TSH	**T_4/T_3**
Silencioso	Maior parte normal, infiltração discreta	Positivo	Normal	Normal
Subclínico	Infiltração mais evidente	Positivo	Aumentada	Normal
Clínico	> 75% substituído	Positivo	Aumentada	Diminuída
	Tecido tireoidiano mínimo, infiltração limitada	Negativo	Aumentada ou diminuída	Diminuída

T_3, triiodotironina; T_4, tiroxina; *TgAA*, autoanticorpos antitireoglobulina; *TSH*, hormônio tireoestimulante (tireotrofina). (De Mooney CT: Canine hypothyroidism. A review of the aetiology and diagnosis. *N Z Vet J* 59:105-114, 2011.)
Esse sistema de classificação é amplamente baseado em estudos que avaliam indiretamente a tireoidite linfocítica, por meio da mensuração da concentração de autoanticorpos antitireoglobulina circulantes.

tireoidiana autoimune em seres humanos, mas constatações semelhantes são menos claras em cães. Nestes, haplótipos e alelos específicos do antígeno leucocitário canino (DLA, do inglês *dog leukocyte antigen*), do complexo de histocompatibilidade principal (MHC, do inglês *major histocompatibility complex*), conferem maior suscetibilidade ao hipotireoidismo em diversas raças: Doberman pinscher, Rhodesian Ridgeback, Setter inglês e Schnauzer gigante.[50-53] Relatos pessoais sugerem a associação entre protocolos de vacinação intensivos e desenvolvimento de doença autoimune, de forma geral, e de tireoidite em particular, mas tal suposição não foi comprovada em pesquisas sobre tireoidite em cães da raça Beagle.[54] A estação do ano (verão *versus* inverno) e a região geográfica (diferentes estados dos EUA) podem influenciar a prevalência da doença, por mecanismos desconhecidos.[42]

MANIFESTAÇÕES CLÍNICAS

Resenha

Hipotireoidismo pode acometer cães de qualquer raça, mas, em geral, afeta os animais de raças puras listados. A idade média no momento do diagnóstico é de aproximadamente 7 anos e varia de 0,5 a 15 anos. É um diagnóstico incomum em cães com menos de 2 anos. Raças predispostas à tireoidite linfocítica tendem a desenvolver hipotireoidismo em uma idade mais precoce. Machos não castrados e fêmeas castradas podem ser mais sujeitos a hipotireoidismo.[1-3]

Sinais clínicos

Características gerais

O hipotireoidismo causa uma série de sinais clínicos (Tabela 299.2). O início do hipotireoidismo é insidioso, e, como não há características patognomônicas, ele é incluído como diagnóstico diferencial de doenças comuns e incomuns. Os sinais clínicos mais frequentes estão relacionados com anormalidades metabólicas e dermatológicas, que ocorrem concomitantemente em cerca de 70% dos cães acometidos. Quase sempre as características dermatológicas são mais evidentes e preocupantes para os tutores. Menos comumente, há relatos de sintomas cardiovasculares, neuromusculares, reprodutivos, oftalmológicos e/ou gastrintestinais.

Características metabólicas

Redução da taxa metabólica é uma ocorrência típica.[55] Sinais clínicos associados, notados em cerca de 80% dos cães, incluem

Tabela 299.2 Anormalidades clínicas associadas ao hipotireoidismo.

Sintomas metabólicos	Letargia
	Obesidade ou ganho de peso
	Intolerância ao exercício
	Intolerância ao frio
Sintomas dermatológicos	Alopecia
	Pelame seco/de baixa qualidade
	Hiperpigmentação cutânea
	Piodermite
	Seborreia
Outras anormalidades	Diversas neuropatias, doença vestibular central, coma mixedematoso, miopatia subclínica, distrofia corneal lipídica, bradicardia, nanismo desproporcional, diminuição da fertilidade, problemas relacionados com o parto, diminuição da produção de lágrimas

letargia, ganho de peso, intolerância ao exercício, retardo mental, intolerância ao frio, fraqueza generalizada e tremores.[1,2] Embora 40 a 50% dos cães acometidos estejam acima do peso ou obesos, o hipotireoidismo é a causa de obesidade em somente uma minoria deles.

Características dermatológicas

Hormônios tireoidianos têm importante participação na manutenção do crescimento dos pelos e em respostas imunes humorais e celulares. Anormalidades dermatológicas ocorrem em até 80% dos cães com hipotireoidismo e podem ser extensas.[1,2,56] Aa alterações incluem adelgaçamento dos pelos, pelame grosseiro e seco, alopecia com envolvimento frequente dos flancos e das coxas e falha no crescimento dos pelos após a tosa. O hipotireoidismo está classicamente associado a uma "alopecia endócrina" não pruriginosa, simétrica e bilateral, com tendência a poupar a cabeça e as extremidades. A alopecia costuma ser notada em áreas corporais de fricção. Estas incluem o pescoço, em cães que usam coleiras; as extremidades laterais, em cães de grande porte; e a cauda, resultando na denominada "cauda de rato" do cão com hipotireoidismo. Pode ocorrer alopecia focal, multifocal e assimétrica. Embora supostamente a alopecia que acomete o plano nasal esteja altamente associada ao hipotireoidismo, ela é um achado inespecífico. Em alguns poucos cães, ocorre retenção do pelame, que se torna opaco e geralmente mais claro por conta do descoramento ambiental. Outros sinais de hipotireoidismo incluem pele seca e com bastante descamação, seborreia, otite, hiperpigmentação e infecções bacterianas secundárias (embora a piodermite seja relatada em < 10% dos cães acometidos). Também há relato de infecção causada por *Malassezia*. Pode haver prurido caso ocorram infecções ou piodermite. Pode haver suspeita de hipotireoidismo, particularmente se o tratamento-padrão for ineficaz.

Em seres humanos, o hipotireoidismo está associado ao acúmulo de ácido hialurônico na derme (mixedema), resultando em aparência de pele inchada, sem sinal de Godet positivo, pálida e fria ao toque. O mixedema também ocorre em cães, sendo mais evidente na cabeça, e dá origem à "expressão facial trágica" em razão do espessamento dos lábios da pele sobre a fronte e da ptose palpebral. Raramente, pode ocorrer vesiculação mucinosa.[57] Alterações histológicas comuns associadas ao hipotireoidismo também são observadas em outras anormalidades endócrinas, incluindo predominância de pelos em fase telógena e folículos telógenos sem pelos (folículos querogênicos).[58,59] Embora também haja relato de hiperpigmentação e presença de folículos atróficos e distróficos, eles são menos comuns quando comparados a outras anormalidades endócrinas. Espessamento da derme e músculos eretores do pelo vacuolizados são considerados achados mais específicos de hipotireoidismo.[59] Dermatite com infecção secundária pode obscurecer esses achados.

Características cardiovasculares

Os hormônios tireoidianos apresentam efeito inotrópico positivo direto, o que estimula a função do miocárdio e aumenta a resposta ao estímulo adrenérgico. Em teoria, o hipotireoidismo pode causar problemas relevantes à função cardíaca, o que é raro acontecer. Em relatos com grande número de cães com hipotireoidismo, anormalidades cardíacas foram raramente relatadas, com exceção de cães (aproximadamente 15%) com bradicardia assintomática.[1,2] No eletrocardiograma, o hipotireoidismo está associado a onda R de baixa amplitude, onda T invertida, bradicardia sinusal e, ocasionalmente, bloqueio atrioventricular de primeiro grau ou, mais raramente, de segundo grau.[60,61] O hipotireoidismo é uma possível causa de bradiarritmia, particularmente quando há outros sinais clínicos compatíveis.

No ecocardiograma de um cão com hipotireoidismo, nota-se diminuição reversível da fração de encurtamento e discreto aumento do diâmetro sistólico final do ventrículo esquerdo, sugestivo de comprometimento da função miocárdica.

Existem alguns poucos relatos de insuficiência cardíaca congestiva e disfunção do miocárdio com fibrilação atrial, que respondem parcial ou completamente à terapia cardíaca apropriada e/ou à suplementação com hormônio tireoidiano.[62-64] Entretanto, é incerto se o hipotireoidismo foi a causa, um achado acidental ou se ele é capaz de exacerbar uma cardiomiopatia subclínica subjacente. Estudos maiores focaram em cardiomiopatias dilatadas específicas de algumas raças. A prevalência de hipotireoidismo não é maior em cães da raça Doberman com cardiomiopatia dilatada (com ou sem insuficiência cardíaca congestiva), comparada àquela de pacientes com doença não cardíaca.[65] Pode haver uma relação causal entre hipotireoidismo e cardiomiopatia dilatada, já que nem todos os cães do grupo não cardíaco foram submetidos ao ecocardiograma. Alguns poderiam ser portadores de doença subclínica. Outro estudo não conseguiu demonstrar uma associação entre hipotireoidismo e cardiomiopatia em cães Doberman, mas há maior risco de hipotireoidismo em cães dessa raça com cardiomiopatia dilatada.[66] Esses resultados podem refletir predisposições independentes para essas doenças ou ser uma via comum em suas patogêneses.

Em seres humanos, a aterosclerose é uma complicação conhecida da hipercolesterolemia e por anormalidades lipídicas induzidas pelo hipotireoidismo. A aterosclerose é rara em cães, presumivelmente por conta de diferenças em sua composição lipoproteica e no metabolismo (ver Capítulo 182). Entre o número limitado de casos relatados no exame pós-morte parece ser comum a ocorrência de hipotireoidismo, bem como de diabetes melito.[67,68] A concentração de colesterol é consistentemente maior em cães que desenvolvem aterosclerose, mas os padrões específicos de hiperlipidemia ainda não foram elucidados. As consequências clínicas da aterosclerose são incertas, mas sabe-se que pode acometer os sistemas cardiovascular e nervoso. Existem poucos relatos de tromboembolia aórtica e aterosclerose grave associadas ao hipotireoidismo.[62,69] Há relato de efusão pericárdica baseada em colesterol em um cão com hipotireoidismo.[70]

Características neuromusculares

Diversos distúrbios neurológicos foram associados ao hipotireoidismo, desde a disfunção de um ou vários nervos cranianos até neuropatias periféricas generalizadas e doença do SNC. Embora o hipotireoidismo possa interferir na função neurológica em razão do acúmulo de mucopolissacarídeos, do comprometimento do transporte axonal ou da aterosclerose, são evidências limitadas de um efeito causal direto. Relatos de síndrome de Horner, paralisia do nervo facial e paralisia de laringe causadas por hipotireoidismo não são confiáveis devido a questões relacionadas com o diagnóstico.[71-73] Paralisia do nervo facial, paralisia de laringe, megaesôfago, doença vestibular periférica e disfunção do neurônio motor inferior (fraqueza generalizada, déficit proprioceptivo, diminuição de reflexos segmentares com progressão potencial para paraparesia ou tetraparesia) foram descritos em cães com hipotireoidismo.[1,2,74,75] Há relato de acalasia cricofaríngea responsiva a hormônio tireoidiano.[76]

Embora a indução experimental de hipotireoidismo não reflita de forma acurada a progressão insidiosa da doença de ocorrência natural, a disfunção neurológica é rara após ablação da tireoide com iodo radioativo.[77] Em cães com hipotireoidismo, uma anormalidade concomitante pode ser responsável pelos sintomas neurológicos. Em outros, é difícil avaliar a resposta à suplementação com hormônio tireoidiano, porque outros tratamentos podem ter sido empregados ou porque pode ter ocorrido cura espontânea da condição neurológica. Embora seja esperada uma resposta razoável à suplementação com hormônio tireoidiano na disfunção neurológica induzida por hipotireoidismo, somente uma minoria dos cães com megaesôfago exibe resposta clínica ou radiográfica evidente.[74,78] De fato, o hipotireoidismo não é um fator de risco significativo para o desenvolvimento de megaesôfago.[79] De forma semelhante, a miastenia *gravis* tem sido associada ao hipotireoidismo, mas pode ser uma doença imunomediada concomitante.[2,80,81]

Relatos de doença do SNC no hipotireoidismo são menos comuns, mas talvez seja menos branda. A disfunção vestibular central é uma complicação rara, mas reversível, mesmo se não houver outros sintomas de hipotireoidismo.[82,83] Mecanismos potenciais envolvidos incluem doença vascular aterosclerótica causadora de infarto cerebral e/ou anormalidades metabólicas diretamente devido à deficiência de hormônios tireoidianos. Aterosclerose no SNC foi descrita em um cão e suspeita na raça Labrador Retriever com doença neurológica e séria hiperlipidemia.[84,85] O hipotireoidismo também foi associado ao coma mixedematoso, uma sequela com risco de morte caracterizada por obnubilação profunda, estupor, fraqueza, hipotermia (frequentemente sem tremor), hipoventilação, bradicardia e hipotensão.[86-88] Em vários pacientes há evidências de fatores precipitantes: cirurgia, insuficiência cardíaca, tratamentos farmacológicos ou sepse fulminante. Convulsões foram descritas em um cão portador de hipotireoidismo com aterosclerose, mas o hipotireoidismo somente foi diagnosticado em cerca de 3% dos cães com convulsões associadas a causas metabólicas ou tóxicas.[89,90]

Talvez a associação mais controversa entre hipotireoidismo e sistema nervoso esteja relacionada com o comportamento (ver Capítulo 9). Existem poucas evidências que sustentem a afirmação de que o hipotireoidismo é responsável por comportamento agressivo. Os poucos relatos de casos de agressividade relacionada à dominância e o medo em cães com hipotireoidismo foram, de modo geral, comportamentos de longa data que não cessaram por completo após suplementação com hormônio tireoidiano.[91-93] A prevalência de hipotireoidismo em cães com problemas de comportamento é baixa e não é maior do que a de cães sem tal problema.[94,95]

Pode ser difícil distinguir sinais clínicos causados por neuropatias (ver Capítulo 268) daqueles ocasionados por miopatias (ver Capítulo 354). Miopatias decorrentes de hipotireoidismo podem causar anormalidades da marcha, fraqueza e intolerância ao exercício (ver Capítulo 31). De maneira experimental, o hipotireoidismo pode causar hiperpotassemia induzida pelo exercício, que pode contribuir para o menor desempenho e menor resistência.[96] Em situações nas quais o hipotireoidismo experimental não causou neuropatia, não houve evidências bioquímicas, eletrofisiológicas e morfológicas de miopatia.[97] À histologia, as miopatias costumam ser caracterizadas por inclusões de bastões de nemalina, aumento de miofibras do tipo I, diminuição de fibras do tipo II, degeneração anormal de mitocôndrias e miofibras com depleção substancial de carnitina livre no músculo esquelético.[97] A miopatia por bastões de nemalina foi associada a sinais clínicos, inclusive com envolvimento cardíaco, em dois cães.[98,99]

Características oftalmológicas (ver Capítulo 11)

O hipotireoidismo, devido à hiperlipidemia, pode resultar em arco lipoide. Embora não seja comum, já foi bem descrito, particularmente em cães da raça Pastor-Alemão.[100] A associação entre ceratoconjuntivite seca e hipotireoidismo é especulativa. No hipotireoidismo experimental, o teste lacrimal de Schirmer, a pressão intraocular e o exame oftalmoscópico permaneceram inalterados por até 17 semanas. Nenhuma anormalidade histológica foi notada após a necropsia.[101] A redução da produção de lágrimas foi relatada em cães com hipotireoidismo, condição que pode exacerbar outras doenças oculares subjacentes.[102]

Características reprodutivas

Diversas anormalidades reprodutivas foram atribuídas ao hipotireoidismo. A indução experimental de hipotireoidismo em cadelas, a curto prazo (mediana de 19 semanas), resultou no prolongamento do parto e redução da sobrevida de filhotes, sem afetar o intervalo interestro, a fertilidade, o tamanho da ninhada ou a duração da gestação.[103] O hipotireoidismo mais crônico (pelo menos por 40 semanas) resultou em diminuição da fertilidade, aumento da mortalidade periparto e menor peso ao nascimento, sem interferir no intervalo interestro, na duração da gestação ou no comportamento reprodutivo.[104] O hipotireoidismo induzido experimentalmente não está associado a nenhum efeito nos índices reprodutivos de machos (contagem de espermatozoides, diâmetro escrotal, motilidade/morfologia dos espermatozoides, libido) durante um período de 2 anos.[105] Pesquisa com cinco raças de cães (Dogue Alemão, Dogue de Bordeaux, Mastiff Inglês, Leonberger e Golden Retriever) não constatou associação entre infertilidade e hipotireoidismo, mas a prevalência de hipotireoidismo foi muito baixa para se obter conclusões acuradas.[106] Há relato de um cão com hipotireoidismo, hiperprolactinemia e galactorreia.[107] Testes de função hipofisária em cães com hipotireoidismo indicaram que hiperprolactinemia é somente provável em cadelas não castradas.[108]

Outras características

Há relatos pessoais de constipação intestinal, êmese e diarreia associadas ao hipotireoidismo, mas carecem de evidências.[1,2] Pessoas com hipotireoidismo frequentemente apresentam constipação intestinal devido à diminuição da atividade peristáltica gastrintestinal (GI).[109] Sugere-se que a diarreia associada ao crescimento excessivo de bactérias no intestino delgado se deve, possivelmente, à redução da motilidade intestinal.[110] Uma associação entre mucocele biliar e hipotireoidismo foi proposta, mas não comprovada.[111,112] O hipotireoidismo não está associado à doença renal aguda ou crônica, tampouco à poliúria/polidipsia, exceto em casos raros de glomerulonefrite associada à tireoidite.[113] Em pacientes com hipotireoidismo, constatou-se diminuição na taxa de filtração glomerular, mas sua importância clínica não é conhecida.[114,115] Foi sugerido, mas não demonstrado, que cães com hipotireoidismo necessitam de menor dose de anestésico para um dado efeito e que o manejo deles durante a anestesia é mais difícil. Experimentalmente, verificou-se que os efeitos cardiovasculares e a concentração alveolar mínima de isoflurano não foram diferentes em cães com hipotireoidismo, quando comparados aos cães saudáveis.[116,117]

Hipotireoidismo congênito

Cães acometidos no início da vida podem desenvolver quaisquer sinais notados em adultos com hipotireoidismo. Entretanto, os cães com hipotireoidismo congênito apresentam nanismo desproporcional evidente. Filhotes acometidos parecem normais ao nascimento, mas os sintomas costumam se tornar evidentes ao redor de 8 semanas de idade. Os animais acometidos possuem crânio desproporcionalmente largo, macroglossia, retardo da erupção dentária, tronco quadrado e membros curtos.[20] Essas características ajudam a diferenciar essa doença do nanismo pituitário e suas características proporcionais. Pode-se notar constipação intestinal; em geral, o distúrbio mental é óbvio. Bócio pode ou não ser evidente, dependendo da causa primária. Quando presente, o bócio pode causar disfagia/dispneia, por ação mecânica. À radiografia, o retardo da maturação esquelética e a disgenesia epifisária são achados comuns e podem eventualmente causar doença articular degenerativa ou outras anormalidades ortopédicas.[13,118]

Síndromes de imunoendocrinopatias

A maioria das doenças endócrinas autoimunes em seres humanos ocorre isoladamente, mas existem situações em que duas ou mais doenças ocorrem simultaneamente ou em sequência. A síndrome poliendócrina autoimune do tipo 1 (SPA-1) é um raro distúrbio autossômico recessivo caracterizado pela tríade candidíase mucocutânea, doença tireoidiana autoimune e doença de Addison. Essas pessoas apresentam maior suscetibilidade a outras doenças autoimunes.[119] A doença poliendócrina autoimune do tipo 2 (SPA-2) é mais comum, menos bem definida e está associada à agregação e à suscetibilidade familiar determinada por diversos fatores genéticos.[119] Anteriormente conhecida como doença autoimune poliglandular ou síndrome de Schmidt, é geralmente definida pelo desenvolvimento de duas ou mais das seguintes anormalidades: doença de Addison, doença de Graves, tireoidite autoimune, diabetes melito tipo 1A, hipogonadismo primário, miastenia *gravis* e doença celíaca. A doença de Addison, simultânea ao diabetes melito tipo 1 (52% dos pacientes) ou ao hipotireoidismo (69% dos pacientes), é a ocorrência mais comum.[120,121]

Essas anormalidades são bem menos definidas em cães. Relatos de caso único e série de casos descreveram combinações que simulam a condição em humanos, inclusive hipotireoidismo e diabetes melito,[1-3,122-124] hipotireoidismo e hipoadrenocorticismo,[3,125-133] juntamente com adeno-hipofisite,[134] hipotireoidismo, hipoadrenocorticismo, diabetes melito e hipoparatireoidismo,[128] hipotireoidismo e miastenia *gravis*,[2,80,81] e, ocasionalmente, outras doenças autoimunes.[135] A prevalência de diabetes melito em cães com hipotireoidismo foi estimada em 1,2 a 10%, enquanto a prevalência de hipotireoidismo em cães diabéticos é estimada em 4%.[1,3,124] A prevalência de hipoadrenocorticismo em cães com hipotireoidismo varia de 1 a 3% enquanto a prevalência de hipotireoidismo em cães com hipoadrenocorticismo é de cerca de 4%.[2,3,128] Deve-se suspeitar de hipotireoidismo em cães com hipoadrenocorticismo, sobretudo quando houver baixa resposta à terapia mineralocorticoide, hiponatremia persistente ou bradicardia, hipercolesterolemia inapropriada ou outros sinais clínicos que sustentem a suspeita.[129] Em um estudo de 35 cães com duas ou mais anormalidades endócrinas concomitantes, a combinação de hipotireoidismo e diabetes melito (29%) foi mais comum do que a de hipotireoidismo e hipoadrenocorticismo (23%).[136]

Sem dúvida, existem dificuldades em confirmar com exatidão o hipotireoidismo em cães portadores de outras doenças. As combinações são todas potencialmente imunomediadas e podem estar relacionadas geneticamente; contudo, há outras explicações possíveis. Clinicamente, o hipotireoidismo foi reconhecido como causa incomum de resistência à insulina em cães diabéticos.[122] Sabe-se que ele induz resistência à insulina em modelos experimentais, em cães. A tolerância à glicose deles é mantida pelo aumento compensatório da secreção de insulina.[137,138] Embora a obesidade possa ter um papel parcial na resistência, outros fatores associados à deficiência de hormônios tireoidianos também podem ser importantes.[137] Os casos de hipotireoidismo de ocorrências natural e experimental foram associados ao excesso de hormônio do crescimento (ou IGF-1), talvez devido à transdiferenciação de células hipofisárias somatotróficas em tireosomatotropos.[108,137,139-141] O excesso de hormônio do crescimento é altamente diabetogênico.[142] Relata-se que um cão com hipotireoidismo, acromegalia e diabetes melito reverteu o quadro após suplementação com hormônio tireoidiano.[143] Estudos genéticos e clínicos adicionais são necessários para investigar completamente a existência de anormalidades poliendócrinas autoimunes em cães.

ROTINA CLINICOPATOLÓGICA

Considerações gerais

Diversas alterações hematológicas e bioquímicas são descritas como "comuns" em cães com hipotireoidiamo, mas nenhuma é específica. A presença delas propicia evidências que sustentam o diagnóstico de hipotireoidismo, mas, de forma mais importante, elas podem auxiliar na inclusão ou exclusão de doenças não tireoidianas; estas podem ser responsáveis pelos sinais clínicos do paciente ou interferir na interpretação dos testes de função tireoidiana. As anormalidades mais frequentes no hipotireoidismo incluem anemia, hipercolesterolemia, hipertrigliceridemia, aumento da atividade da creatinoquinase (CK) e diminuição da concentração de frutosamina.

Hemograma

No hipotireoidismo, a anemia é tipicamente normocítica normocrômica discreta. É notada em 32 a 44% dos casos.[1,2,144] É raro os valores do volume globular (hematócrito) estarem abaixo de 25%, o que indica uma anemia não frequentemente detectada ao exame físico. Denominada, em geral, anemia "fisiológica", é provável que seja o resultado da diminuição da produção de eritropoetina e ausência de efeito estimulatório de hormônios tireoidianos na medula óssea.[145] Cães com hipotireoidismo não anêmicos costumam apresentar contagem de hemácias no menor quartil do intervalo de referência. Aumento da contagem de leucócitos é extremamente incomum em cães com hipotireoidismo.

O hipotireoidismo foi associado ao aumento da contagem de plaquetas de pequeno tamanho, resultado de uma relação inversa entre trombopoese e eritropoese.[148] Há relatos pessoais de que o surgimento frequente de hematomas está associado a hipotireoidismo, talvez como resultado da diminuição da concentração plasmática do antígeno do fator de von Willebrand (vWf:Ag).[149] Entretanto, o hipotireoidismo não está associado ao prolongamento do tempo de sangramento da mucosa bucal ou a alteração significativa na concentração de vWf:Ag, as quais diminuem após suplementação com hormônio tireoidiano.[150,151] A associação entre hipotireoidismo e doença de von Willebrand provavelmente reflete predisposições raciais para ambas as condições. A suplementação de cães da raça Doberman eutireóideos com doença de von Willebrand com hormônios tireoidianos não influencia a concentração ou atividade do vWf:Ag no plasma.[152]

Perfil bioquímico sérico

Nota-se hipercolesterolemia em aproximadamente 75% dos cães com hipotireoidismo, quase sempre acompanhada de hipertrigliceridemia.[1,2,144] Quanto maior a concentração de colesterol, mais provável que o cão tenha hipotireoidismo. Os hormônios tireoidianos estimulam a síntese, mobilização e degradação de lipídios. A degradação é mais seriamente afetada no hipotireoidismo, resultando no acúmulo de lipídios. As mensurações de lipoproteínas plasmáticas de cães com hipotireoidismo mostram aumento das concentrações de lipoproteínas de baixa densidade, lipoproteínas de densidade muito baixa e lipoproteínas de alta densidade.[146] O aumento da atividade de CK é verificado em 18 a 35% dos cães com hipotireoidismo, mas não costuma exceder o dobro do limite superior do intervalo de referência.[1,2] Quase sempre considerada resultado da diminuição da metabolização ou excreção, a miopatia induzida por hipotireoidismo pode também ser responsável pelas alterações na atividade de CK.[97] Nota-se aumento da concentração de frutosamina em 36 a 82% dos casos, presumivelmente devido à redução da renovação de proteínas corporais, e não à significante hiperglicemia crônica.[1,147] Esse aumento pode interferir no monitoramento do tratamento de cães diabéticos portadores de hipotireoidismo. Incrementos discretos nas atividades das enzimas hepáticas, sobretudo fosfatase alcalina e gamaglutamil transferase, são constatados em até 30% dos cães com hipotireoidismo, talvez devido à discreta deposição de lipídios no fígado.[1,2] Se as atividades enzimáticas estiverem acentuadamente aumentadas, deve-se considerar outra anormalidade primária.

TESTES DA FUNÇÃO DA TIREOIDE

Considerações gerais

Embora amplamente melhorada nos últimos anos, a capacidade de diagnosticar com acurácia o hipotireoidismo pode ser um desafio. Diversos testes estão disponíveis e suas recomendações de uso e interpretações são variáveis. Exames comumente utilizados incluem T_4 total (T_4t), T_3 total (T_3t), T_4 livre (T_4L), TSH canino (TSHc) e presença de TgAA, T_4AA e T_3AA. Testes para T_3 livre e T_3 reverso (T_3r) estão disponíveis, mas não são utilizados no diagnóstico. Testes de função dinâmicos incluem testes de estimulação por TRH e TSH. A glândula tireoide pode ser avaliada por ultrassonografia, tomografia computadorizada (TC), ressonância magnética (RM) ou por cintilografia qualitativa e quantitativa da tireoide. Nem todos os testes avaliam diretamente

a função tireoidiana, mas podem fornecer evidências indiretas de anormalidades na tireoide. Dos testes disponíveis, nenhum deles apresenta sensibilidade diagnóstica de 100%. De maneira importante, há diversos fatores não tireoidianos que podem influenciar os resultados dos testes da função da tireoide, interferindo negativamente na especificidade diagnóstica.

Fatores não tireoidianos que influenciam as concentrações de hormônios tireoidianos

Raça, sexo, idade, estado reprodutivo, condição corporal e atividade física sabidamente afetam de forma significativa as concentrações de hormônios tireoidianos. De forma importante, doenças não tireoidianas e terapias farmacológicas prévias e atuais podem alterar os resultados dos exames. A metodologia do teste pode influenciar a acurácia e a confiabilidade dos resultados obtidos.

Metodologias dos testes

Testes para mensuração de hormônios tireoidianos totais

Os testes de hormônios tireoidianos totais mensuram as concentrações circulantes de hormônios livres e daqueles ligados a proteínas. Radioimunoensaio (RIE) ainda é a técnica de referência-padrão para mensuração de T_4t e T_3t. Foram desenvolvidos testes que incluem métodos não isotópicos e o mais utilizado em pesquisa: a combinação de cromatografia líquida e espectrometria de massa (HPLCMS). Os testes RIE são menos caros e utilizam menor volume de amostra, mas estão sujeitos a restrições devido à radiação e não podem ser completamente automatizados. Métodos não isotópicos podem ser completamente automatizados (preferidos por laboratórios comerciais) ou desenvolvidos para uso no próprio laboratório. Esses métodos utilizam enzimas, quimioluminescência ou fluorescência, em vez de radioisótopos, como emissores de sinais. Podem ser quantitativos (preferidos) ou semiquantitativos.

Há uma concordância razoável entre as diferentes metodologias de testes para T_4t, mesmo quando se utiliza RIE desenvolvido para humanos, se modificado de forma a possibilitar a mensuração de baixas concentrações observadas em cães.[153-155] Diferentes concentrações ocorrem com diferentes tipos de exames, enfatizando a necessidade de intervalos de referência específicos para o método e o laboratório. Relatos casuais indicam que valores errôneos são mais prováveis com métodos enzimáticos ou de fluorescência. Métodos enzimáticos são considerados menos acurados.[156] As concentrações de T3t são semelhantes em seres humanos e cães, de tal forma que testes desenvolvidos para humanos não necessitam de modificações.

Tanto os resultados de T_4t como de T_3t podem ser influenciados por autoanticorpos, os quais podem aumentar ou diminuir falsamente os resultados, dependendo do teste e do sistema de separação utilizados. Autoanticorpos aumentam os valores mensurados em sistemas que utilizam hormônio ligado ao anticorpo para estimar as concentrações hormonais, assim como a maioria dos sistemas de testes utilizados comumente para mensuração de T_4t. Quando há T_4AA, o valor mensurado pode estar dentro ou acima do intervalo de referência. Se a estimativa da concentração hormonal se basear na fração hormonal não ligada, os autoanticorpos falsamente diminuem os resultados. Alguns testes de T3t são, dessa forma, afetados, com concentrações que se tornam indetectáveis.

Existem alguns poucos estudos que avaliam de forma objetiva o efeito de autoanticorpos nos resultados dos testes. Uma pesquisa não constatou diferença entre as concentrações de T_4t mensuradas por quimioluminescência e por HPLC (teoricamente livre da interferência de autoanticorpos) em cães positivos para T_4AA, com concentrações de T_4t dentro do intervalo de referência.[157] Entretanto, somente duas das amostras foram avaliadas e a função da tireoide de cada paciente era incerta. Outros pesquisadores sugerem que a concentração de T_4t esteja abaixo, dentro ou acima do intervalo de referência em aproximadamente 54, 34 e 12% de cães com hipotireoidismo e positivos para T4AA, respectivamente (PA Graham, comunicação pessoal). Resultados dentro ou acima do intervalo de referência de T4t foram relatados em diversos animais com hipotireoidismo e sabidamente positivos para TgAA.[158]

Hormônio livre (não ligado)

Concentrações circulantes de T_4L são semelhantes em seres humanos e cães. Dessa forma, testes utilizados para seres humanos podem ser empregados em cães sem modificação. Os métodos baseados em diálise de equilíbrio e ultrafiltração são, em geral, considerados padrão-ouro para mensuração da concentração de T_4L. Tais métodos envolvem a separação da fração de T_4L, seguida de sua estimativa por meio de RIE altamente sensível. Esses testes, utilizados por grandes laboratórios comerciais, são laboriosos e caros. Entretanto, a mensuração acurada de T_4L por outros métodos é controversa. Os testes utilizados com mais frequência utilizam análogos de hormônios com estruturas moleculares semelhantes ao T_4, e considera-se que não reagem com proteínas de ligação, sendo, assim, capazes de competir com o T_4L presente na amostra. Em seres humanos, eles supostamente estimam meramente a concentração de T_4L, com pouca vantagem em relação ao teste de T_4t. A utilização desses testes é considerada mais problemática na mensuração mais acurada da concentração de T_4L em pacientes com distúrbios associados a proteínas de ligação aos hormônios tireoidianos anormais, doenças não tireoidianas, altas concentrações de ácidos graxos livres e autoanticorpos contra hormônios da tireoide.[159]

Em comparação às técnicas que utilizam diálise de equilíbrio, as concentrações de T_4L em cães são significativamente menores, quando se utilizam diferentes análogos diretos de T_4L no RIE, sobretudo em pacientes com doenças não tireoidianas.[160] A acurácia e a concordância entre quimioluminescência direta e diálise de equilíbrio como testes para T_4L foram relatadas como adequadas ou limitantes.[161,162] Entretanto, a mensuração combinada de T_4t e T_4L por métodos análogos adiciona pouca informação diagnóstica, quando comparada a testes individuais para cada um dos hormônios, sugerindo que os testes podem não mensurar a concentração de T_4L.[163] Esses ensaios, assim como o de T_4t, são influenciados pela presença de T_4AA.[158]

Testes para hormônio tireoestimulante

A avaliação do TSH requer um teste espécie-específico. Testes por quimioluminescência e imunorradiométricos para TSH específico de cães (TSHc) estão disponíveis e apresentam correlação razoável.[164] Esses testes falham em detectar baixa concentração, o que é menos importante em cães com hipotireoidismo primário, já que eles devem apresentar alta concentração de TSHc. Entretanto, essa limitação pode ter implicações no diagnóstico do hipotireoidismo central ou na avaliação de dose excessiva em cães tratados com hormônio tireoidiano.

Testes para autoanticorpo antitireoglobulina

Métodos de teste espécie-específicos para TgAA canino estão disponíveis no mercado. O teste foi modificado para minimizar a ligação não específica à IgG, reduzindo, assim, a taxa de resultados falso-positivos e equivocados, previamente relatados. A presença de T_3AAs e T_4AAs pode ser inferida se resultados discordantes do hormônio total forem detectados em cães positivos para TgAA. Eles também podem ser especificamente mensurados em alguns laboratórios especializados.

Armazenamento e interferências

A maioria dos hormônios tireoidianos e o TSHc são relativamente estáveis, em amostras armazenadas. Entretanto, há aumento significativo da concentração de T_4L se a amostra for mantida em temperatura ambiente por longo tempo. Recomenda-se centrifugação, transporte sob refrigeração e mensuração o mais breve possível das amostras. Em geral, hemólise, lipemia e hiperbilirrubinemia não interferem nos resultados do RIE, o que não pode ser garantido para métodos não isotópicos.[165] A lipemia intensa pode aumentar falsamente a concentração de T_4L, quando mensurada por diálise de equilíbrio.[166]

Fatores fisiológicos

Momento da coleta, idade e sexo. O momento da coleta não é importante, já que, em cães, não se constatou interferência do ritmo circadiano na secreção de hormônios tireoidianos. No entanto, ocorrem oscilações ocasionais que podem causar falso resultado subnormal.[167-169] A concentração de T_4t diminui com a idade e pode estar abaixo dos intervalos de referência em cães idosos.[170] Diferentemente, cães com menos de 3 meses de vida apresentam valores duas a cinco vezes maior do que adultos. De modo variável, sexo e fase do ciclo estral são relatados como fatores que afetam as concentrações de hormônios tireoidianos, mas sem relevância clínica.

Raça e atividade física. Pesquisas iniciais sugeriram que as concentrações de hormônios tireoidianos eram menores em cães de maior porte, mas essas observações eram provavelmente relacionadas com a raça, e não com o tamanho do animal.[171] Os cães lebreiros (Sighthound), por exemplo, sabidamente apresentam concentrações de hormônios tireoidianos circulantes relativamente baixas. A magnitude e os hormônios afetados variam entre as raças. Valores de T_4t abaixo dos intervalos-padrão de referência são notados em cerca de 90% dos cães Greyhound, 75% dos Basenji, 65% do Sloughi, 55% dos Saluki, 25% dos Whippet, e somente em 5% dos Scottish Deerhound.[172-177] Em vários animais, as concentrações são tão baixas (no limite ou abaixo da detecção do teste) que não é possível calcular o intervalo de referência específico para a raça. Baixos valores de T_3t são observados em cães Saluki e Irish Wolfhound, mas não em Greyhound.[172,175,178] A concentrações de T_4L pode ser baixa em Greyhound e Irish Wolfhound, mas não em cães Whippet.[172,175,176,178] A concentração de T_4t também é baixa em cães das raças Dogue de Bordeaux e Schnauzer gigante.[171,179] A concentração de TSH não parece ser tão influenciada pela raça. Treinamento e atividade física intensa estão associados à diminuição nas concentrações de hormônios tireoidianos, mas breve exercício pouco influencia.[176,180-183]

Doenças não tireoidianas. Doenças podem induzir profundas alterações nas concentrações de hormônios tireoidianos, em seres humanos (Tabela 299.3). Anteriormente denominada "síndrome do eutireóideo doente", síndrome de T_3 baixo" e "doença clínica com baixo valor de T_4", o termo "síndrome da doença não

---

Tabela 299.3 Efeito de doenças não tireoidianas nas concentrações séricas de hormônios tireoidianos e da tireotrofina.

	HORMÔNIO			
GRAVIDADE DA DOENÇA	**T$_3$T**	**T$_4$T**	**T$_4$L**	**TSH**
Discreta	↓	↔	↔	↔
Moderada	↓↓	↓	↔↓↑	↔↓
Grave	↓↓↓	↓↓	↔↓	↓↓
Recuperação	↓↔	↓↔	↔↓	↑↔

T_3, tri-iodotironina; T_4, tiroxina; TSH, hormônio tireoestimulante (tireotrofina); ↓, diminuição da concentração; ↔, a concentração permanece a mesma; ↑, aumento da concentração. (De Mooney CT: Canine hypothyroidism. A review of the aetiology and diagnosis. *N Z Vet J* 59:105-114, 2011.)

Esses efeitos são amplamente conhecidos para T_3 e T_4. No caso do TSH, os dados superam os de seres humanos. A maior parte das pesquisas relacionadas com cães não incriminou qualquer efeito da doença no valor de TSH, o que é complicado por conta da incapacidade de que o teste atualmente utilizado detecte concentração baixa e suprimida. O número de setas indica a gravidade crescente.

tireoidiana" é atualmente utilizado para descrever alterações nas concentrações de hormônios tireoidianos secundárias a doenças agudas ou crônicas. Existem numerosos mecanismos potenciais para essa condição, incluindo redução da conversão periférica de T_4 em T_3, redução da afinidade de ligação às proteínas de ligação ao hormônio tireoidiano, alteração na metabolização do hormônio tireoidiano, alterações na expressão ou função dos receptores do hormônio tireoidiano ou alteração das funções do hipotálamo/hipófise. A anormalidade mais comum associada à síndrome da doença não tireoidiana em seres humanos é a supressão da concentração circulante de T_3t, com valor de T_4t dentro do intervalo de referência.[184] Conforme a doença se agrava, ocorre supressão tanto de T_3 como de T_4 total, o que está associado a menor chance de recuperação. As concentrações de T_4L e TSH são menos afetadas, mas, em doenças graves, pode-se observar a supressão de ambos. Ocasionalmente, aumentos transitórios no T_4L são observados. A concentração de TSH circulante pode aumentar durante a fase de recuperação da doença.

Concentrações diminuídas de hormônios tireoidianos foram relatadas em uma ampla variedade de doenças que afetam diversos sistemas do organismo.[185-197] Os mecanismos envolvidos ainda não foram elucidados, mas um estudo preliminar constatou diminuição na concentração de transtirretina, embora, provavelmente, tenha importância mínima.[198] Infusões de interleucina-2 recombinante induziram alterações semelhantes àquelas ocorridas em doenças não tireoidianas, em modelos experimentais em cães.[199] Em um estudo abrangente de doenças não tireoideinas em cães, a redução simultânea em T_3t e T_4t a acompanhou somente em T_3t. A supressão isolada de T_4t foi incomum.[188] Diminuições maiores em T_4t e T_3t foram associadas a doenças mais graves e pior prognóstico.[186-188,200-202] Em geral, concentrações de T_4L (por diálise de equilíbrio) se mantêm nos intervalos de referência, em todas as doenças, com exceção das mais graves[187,188] e no hiperadrenocorticismo.[28,187,188] Ocasionalmente, nota-se aumento de T_4L, embora mal definido.[203,204] A compreensão da influência da doença na concentração de TSHc é dificultada pela baixa sensibilidade dos testes atuais, já que valores normais não podem ser distinguidos dos baixos. Incrementos sabidamente ocorrem na fase de recuperação de doenças.[203,204] Não se deve esperar alteração nas concentrações de hormônios tireoidianos em doenças menos graves e, se presente, deve-se pensar em outra explicação. Concentrações de hormônios tireoidianos não são afetadas por osteoartrite, alopecia sazonal de flanco recidivante, dermatite atópica ou piodermite.[205-208]

Tratamento farmacológico

Diversos fármacos sabidamente alteram as concentrações de hormônios tireoidianos, que variam somente de T_4t até uma condição que simula hipotireoidismo primário (Tabela 299.4). Os fármacos que causam tais alterações incluem, mas não se limitam a, glicocorticoides, fenobarbital, ácido acetilsalicílico, cetoprofeno, carprofeno, clomipramina e antimicrobianos à base de sulfonamidas.[209-213] Para muitos, a dose e a duração do tratamento ditam a magnitude do efeito. Sulfonamidas merecem menção especial, já que podem induzir hipotireoidismo e até mesmo coma mixedematoso por conta da capacidade de inibir, de modo reversível, a TPO.[214-218] Em cães doentes tratados com medicamentos supressores da tireoide, espera-se redução adicional de cerca de 15% na concentração de T_4t.[188] O efeito de diversos outros fármacos ainda não foi especificamente avaliado em cães, mas eles podem ser considerados fatores passíveis de afetar as concentrações hormonais, até que se prove o contrário. As concentrações de hormônios tireoidianos se normalizam assim que o tratamento é interrompido. Para vários fármacos, inclusive tiroxina, recomenda-se, pelo menos, um período de descontinuação de 6 semanas antes da realização de testes de função tireoidiana, talvez mais prolongado após tratamento com sulfonamidas.[209,218,219]

| Tabela 299.4 | Efeito do tratamento farmacológico nas concentrações séricas de hormônios tireoidianos e da tireotrofina. |

	HORMÔNIO		
FÁRMACO	**T_4T**	**T_4L**	**TSH**
Prednisona/prednisolona	↓↔	↓↔	↔↓
Fenobarbital	↓↔	↓↔	↔↑ (↓)*
Brometo de potássio	↔	↔	↔
Sulfonamidas	↓	↓	↑
Propranolol	↔	↔	↔
Clomipramina	↓	↓	↔
Ácido acetilsalicílico	↓	↓↔	↔
Cetoprofeno	↓	↔	↔
Carprofeno	↓↔	↓↔	↔↓
Deracoxibe	↔	↔	↔

*Fenobarbital foi associado com aumento significativo da concentração de TSH. Entretanto, os valores raramente excedem o limite superior do intervalo de referência. O aumento do TSH é inesperadamente baixo, comparado à diminuição das concentrações dos hormônios tireoidianos, o que pode indicar um efeito supressor desse fármaco no TSH. T_4, tiroxina; *TSH*, hormônio tireoestimulante (tireotrofina). (De Mooney CT: Canine hypothyroidism. A review of the aetiology and diagnosis. *N Z Vet J* 59:105-114, 2011. Dados compilados das referências 209 a 218.)

| Tabela 299.5 | Sensibilidade e especificidade das concentrações de hormônios tireoidianos, tireotrofina e autoanticorpos antitireoglobulina no diagnóstico de hipotireoidismo. |

	T_4T	**T_4L**	**TSH**	**TgAA**
Sensibilidade	89 a 100%	80 a 98%	58 a 87%	91 a 100%
Especificidade	73 a 82%	78 a 94%	82 a 100%	94 a 100%

T_4, tiroxina; *TgAA*, autoanticorpos antitireoglobulina; *TSH*, hormônio tireoestimulante (tireotrofina). (Dados compilados das referências 36 a 38, 189, 192, 194, 220, 221.)

Diagnóstico de hipotireoidismo: testes hormonais basais

Considerações gerais

Os diversos testes diagnósticos utilizados na investigação do hipotireoidismo estão resumidos na Tabela 299.5.[36-38,189,194,220,221]

Concentração de T_3t

A mensuração de T_3t tem valor limitado no diagnóstico de hipotireoidismo devido à sua baixa sensibilidade. Os valores de T_3t se mantêm acima ou no intervalo de referência em até 90% dos cães com hipotireoidismo.[192] Esses achados podem estar relacionados com maior secreção de T_3 pela glândula tireoide ou pela conversão periférica de T_4, à medida que diminui a função tireoidiana. Isso representa potencial benefício a curto prazo para o indivíduo, já que o T_3 é o mais potente dos hormônios tireoidianos ativos. Dependendo do sistema utilizado no exame, a presença de T_3AA pode também aumentar falsamente a concentração obtida. T_3AAs estão presentes em > 5% das amostras de cães com suspeita de hipotireoidismo.[34] Embora isso pareça pouco, há T_3AAs em > 40% dos cães com hipotireoidismo e positivos para TgAA.[42] A especificidade de T_3t no diagnóstico de hipotireoidismo também é baixa. Valores baixos são comuns em determinadas raças, em associação a doenças não tireoidianas, e após administração de diversos fármacos. O único valor da mensuração de T_3t refere-se a raças de cães que sabidamente apresentam T_4t baixo, mas que mantêm a concentração de T_3t nos intervalos de referência, como acontece em cães Greyhound.[172]

Concentração de T_4t

Na maioria dos cães com hipotireoidismo, nota-se diminuição da concentração de T_4t circulante. Sua sensibilidade diagnóstica é excelente, sendo frequentemente recomendada como teste de triagem. Valores situados no intervalo de referência costumam ser utilizados para excluir a possibilidade de hipotireoidismo, mas os T_4AAs podem causar falso aumento desse valor, estando presentes em < 2% das amostras de cães com suspeita de hipotireoidismo, mas o número de cães com T_4AAs aumenta para 14% naqueles com hipotireoidismo e positivos para TgAA.[34,42] Isso diminui a sensibilidade diagnóstica e significa que não se pode excluir a possibilidade de hipotireoidismo, seja por um valor situado no do intervalo de referência, seja aumentado de T_4t. Uma preocupação ainda maior quanto a confiar somente no T_4t é sua baixa especificidade, devido a diversos fatores não tireoidianos, que resultam em redução de sua concentração em animais eutireóideos. Esses fatores incluem raça, idade, doenças não tireoidianas e terapias farmacológicas. O T_4t jamais deve ser utilizado como único teste diagnóstico para hipotireoidismo em cães.[175]

Concentração de T_4L

Na maioria dos cães com hipotireoidismo, o valor de T_4L é inferior àquele do intervalo de referência. É incerto o motivo pelo qual um pequeno número de cães com hipotireoidismo apresenta valor no limite inferior da faixa de referência, mas isso diminui a sensibilidade diagnóstica. Entretanto, a concentração de T_4L (por diálise de equilíbrio) é menos afetada por fatores extratireoidianos do que a de T_4t. Assim, sua especificidade diagnóstica para hipotireoidismo é alta. A mensuração da concentração de T_4L é, portanto, considerada o teste individual mais acurado para o diagnóstico de hipotireoidismo.[220]

Concentração de TSHc

Espera-se aumento da concentração de TSHc em cães com hipotireoidismo primário devido à ausência de um mecanismo de *feedback* negativo para o hormônio tireoidiano. Entretanto, o teste de TSHc apresenta apenas sensibilidade moderada como teste diagnóstico porque os valores de um número significativo de cães com hipotireoidismo situam-se no intervalo de referência. Talvez uma parte dos cães com hipotireoidismo tenha doença central, em vez de mediada pela tireoide, o que é improvável, pois os valores estão quase sempre dentro dos intervalos de referência, em vez de diminuídos ou no limite de detecção do teste. Em cães com hipotireoidismo, ocorrem oscilações aleatórias na concentração de TSHc, dentro dos intervalos de referência, mas essa é uma explicação improvável para todos os casos dos baixos valores verificados.[222,223]

Em estudos experimentais, há evidências de que a secreção hipofisária de TSH diminui em casos de hipotireoidismo crônico, presumivelmente como resultado de dessensibilização do receptor de TRH. Isso poderia acontecer na doença de ocorrência natural.[108,139-141] Embora possa ser uma explicação plausível para valores de TSHc no intervalo de referência em alguns cães com hipotireoidismo, pode-se argumentar que poucos têm a doença por um período necessário para induzir tais alterações. É possível que valores altos de TSHc sejam suprimidos no hipotireoidismo por conta de doenças não tireoidianas concomitantes ou por tratamento farmacológico.[220] Sugeriu-se que os testes atuais não mensuram todos os possíveis isômeros do TSHc. Embora a sensibilidade diagnóstica desse teste seja baixa, a mensuração da concentração de TSHc tem especificidade diagnóstica relativamente boa. Valores altos são menos comumente observados em cães eutireóideos, já que o TSHc não é amplamente afetado por doenças não tireoidianas ou por fármacos, com exceção das sulfonamidas. Valores altos são, entretanto, uma característica do hipotireoidismo silencioso e subclínico.[42]

Autoanticorpos antitireoglobulina

Resultados positivos para TgAA estão associados à tireoidite linfocítica, mas podem estar presentes na circulação muito antes do surgimento dos sinais clínicos de hipotireoidismo, no cão.[42] Assim, os TgAAs não fornecem informações sobre a função da tireoide. A positividade para TgAA, incomum em cães com doença não tireoidiana, é sugestiva de doença subjacente.[38,43,224] Um teste positivo para TgAA sustenta, indiretamente, o diagnóstico de hipotireoidismo.

Testes hormonais basais no contexto de informação clínica

Como já discutido, a sensibilidade e a especificidade menores que o ideal dos testes disponíveis dificultam a confirmação confiável do diagnóstico de hipotireoidismo, e esse diagnóstico jamais deve se basear apenas nos resultados dos testes. Em vez disso, os exames devem ser realizados em cães que provavelmente tenham a doença: aqueles que possuam dados epidemiológicos apropriados com características clínicas e clinicopatológicas que sustentam o diagnóstico, após exclusão de doenças não tireoidianas relevantes e sem histórico recente de uso de medicamentos supressores da tireoide (Figura 299.3). Então, deve-se optar por uma combinação de testes com alta sensibilidade/baixa especificidade e alta especificidade/baixa sensibilidade, o que reduz as suas limitações. As mensurações simultâneas de T_4t e TSHc propiciam melhor custo-benefício e estão amplamente disponíveis. A mensuração de T_4L pode ser reservada aos cães cuja concentração de T_4t provavelmente esteja sendo influenciada por doenças concomitantes ou terapias farmacológicas. A mensuração de TgAA serve como teste de triagem para a potencial influência do T_4AA e fornece informações sobre a patogênese.

Diagnóstico de hipotireoidismo: utilização de testes de estimulação (provocativos)

Indicações

Anteriormente, os testes de estimulação com TSH e TRH eram recomendados de modo rotineiro como auxiliares na confirmação do diagnóstico de hipotireoidismo. Atualmente esses testes devem ser reservados aos cães cujo diagnóstico não pôde ser confirmado com base nos sinais clínicos e testes basais. Os testes de estimulação também podem ser utilizados para avaliar o desempenho do teste quando da necessidade de um método confiável e independente de diferenciação de hipotireoidismo e eutireoidismo.

Estimulação com hormônio tireoestimulante

O teste de estimulação com TSH foi considerado "padrão-ouro" no diagnóstico de hipotireoidismo em cães. Em estudos iniciais, utilizava-se TSH de bovinos, não mais disponível. Resultados semelhantes são obtidos com o uso de TSH recombinante humano (TSHrh).[225] As doses IV recomendadas são 50 a 75 µg/cão ou 100 µg para cães com mais de 20 kg, obtendo-se amostras antes e 6 horas após a administração.[226-228] Sugeriu-se uma dose de 150 µg/cão para distinguir, de forma mais acurada, hipotireoidismo de doença não tireoidiana.[229] Diferentemente do que ocorria com o TSH de bovinos, não foram relatadas reações adversas, mesmo após repetidas doses. O TSHrh reconstituído pode ser armazenado em temperatura de 4°C, durante 4 semanas, ou de −20°C, por até 12 semanas, sem perda do valor biológico, possibilitando o uso de múltiplas doses de um mesmo frasco, com redução dos gastos.[227,230] Os critérios de interpretação são variáveis.[231] Em geral, em cães eutireóideos a concentração de T_4t aumenta mais de 1,5 vezes a concentração basal, com valor absoluto > 30 nmol/ℓ. Em cães com hipotireoidismo, a estimulação é mínima, com valor de T_4t pós-TSH < 20 mmol/ℓ. Alguns cães apresentam valor que não se enquadra em nenhuma categoria, difícil de interpretar.

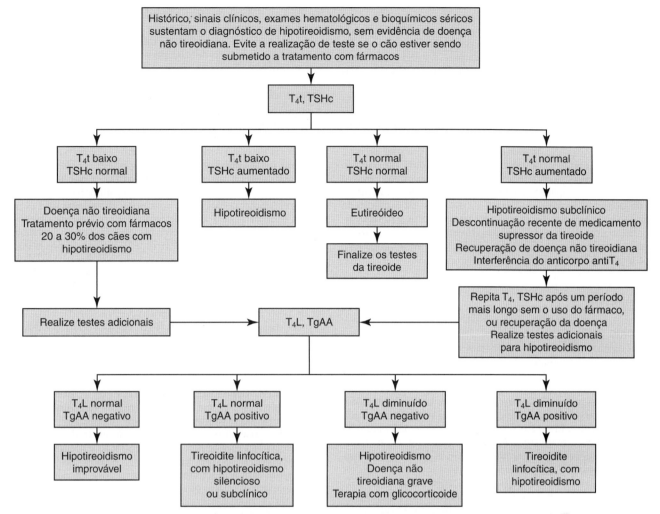

Figura 299.3 Algoritmo para o diagnóstico de hipotireoidismo em cães. T_4, tiroxina; *TgAA*, autoanticorpos antitireoglobulina; *TSHc*, hormônio tireoestimulante canino. (De Mooney CT: Canine hypothyroidism. A review of the aetiology and diagnosis. *N Z Vet J* 59:105-114, 2011.)

Estimulação com hormônio liberador de tireotrofina

O teste de resposta ao TRH, no qual a concentração de T_4t é mensurada antes e após a administração de TRH, foi outrora recomendado como alternativa útil ao teste de estimulação com TSH. Infelizmente, o teste de resposta ao TRH é considerado menos confiável do que a maioria dos outros testes basais atualmente disponíveis. Na melhor das hipóteses, uma boa resposta ao TRH pode excluir a possibilidade de hipotireoidismo de forma confiável. Entretanto, a ausência de resposta de T_4 ao TRH não confirma hipotireoidismo, sendo um achado comum em uma ampla variedade de doenças não tireoidianas em cães que receberam alguns medicamentos e naqueles saudáveis.[232]

Pode-se avaliar a resposta do TSHc ao TRH.[140] Baixa dose (10 μg/kg) de TRH induz pico de estimulação hipofisária cerca de 20 minutos após administração por via intravenosa, ao mesmo tempo em que os efeitos colaterais são minimizados. Seres humanos com hipotireoidismo primário apresentam resposta exagerada e prolongada do TSH ao TRH. No entanto, embora ocorra resposta limitada de TSH ao TRH em cães com hipotireoidismo, o teste acrescenta pouca informação àquela obtida pelos testes de hormônios tireoidianos basais.[233] A estimulação com TRH é amplamente limitada às pesquisas.

Diagnóstico por imagem

Considerações gerais

Os exames de imagem da tireoide estão bem definidos para o diagnóstico de gatos com hipertireoidismo e cães com neoplasia de tireoide.[234,235] Teoricamente menos influenciada por doenças não tireoidianas ou por fármacos, a interpretação de algumas técnicas de imagem é semelhante àquela do TgAA. Assim, os exames de imagem podem fornecer informações sobre a aparência macroscópica, e não da função da tireoide.

Ultrassonografia

Em geral, cada lobo da tireoide é descrito como fusiforme, em imagem longitudinal, e triangular, em imagem transversa, com cápsula lisa e ecogenicidade homogênea, sendo iso ou hiperecoico em comparação ao músculo esternotireóideo adjacente, em cães saudáveis e naqueles com doenças não tireoidianas. Os lobos da tireoide de cães com hipotireoidismo apresentam ecogenicidade significativamente menor, não são homogêneos, mas sim delimitados de forma irregular, pequenos e mais arredondados.[185,236,237] Qualquer uma dessas alterações pode estar presente em cães com hipotireoidismo, e a aparência dos lobos pode diferir. Entretanto, pode haver diferenças nas imagens obtidas na ultrassonografia da tireoide, dependendo da raça;[238] além disso, dependem da habilidade, da experiência e do parecer do operador.

Exames de imagem avançados

TC e RM dos lobos da tireoide de cães saudáveis foram descritas.[239,240] Comparações com cães portadores de hipotireoidismo ainda não foram publicadas. Dado o seu custo e a necessidade de anestesia, os exames de imagem avançados têm uso limitado.

Varredura com tecnécio-[99m]

O uso de tecnécio-[99m] (na forma de pertecnetato; $^{99m}TcO_4^-$) para o cálculo quantitativo da captação pela glândula tireoide foi sugerido como a técnica mais acurada para distinguir cães com hipotireoidismo primário daqueles com doenças não tireoidianas.[241] Os valores de captação em cães com hipotireoidismo variam de 0,03 a 0,26% e, em animais eutireoídeos com baixa concentração de T_4t, de 0,39 a 1,86%. Entretanto, essas diferenças marcantes não são uniformemente aceitas, já que os glicocorticoides, em particular, parecem diminuir a captação de tecnécio pela tireoide, ocasionando resultados questionáveis.[242] Em seres humanos, constatou-se alteração da captação do radioisótopo associada a diversas doenças não tireoidianas e medicamentos. A aparência cintilográfica da doença inflamatória da tireoide é variável. Entretanto, a avaliação da captação de tecnécio pela tireoide foi promissora para confirmação de eutireoidismo em cães Greyhound, para investigação de hipotireoidismo central e diferenciação entre disgenesia e disormonogênese, no hipotireoidismo congênito.[235,243]

TRATAMENTO

Contexto geral

Cães com hipotireoidismo necessitam de terapia de reposição de hormônio tireoidiano durante toda a vida. Extratos de tireoide "naturais" ou desidratados são rústicos e não confiáveis quando comparados aos produtos sintéticos, que são mais previsíveis e possuem maior prazo de validade. O T_4 sintético é o tratamento de escolha, já que é o principal produto secretado pela glândula tireoide e é o pró-hormônio fisiológico para o T_3 metabolicamente mais ativo. A administração de T_3 se desvia desse processo fisiológico normal, aumentando o risco de tireotoxicose. Como o T_3 possui meia-vida mais curta, ele deve ser administrado várias vezes ao dia e pode causar deficiência de T_4 no cérebro e na hipófise, embora as consequências sejam incertas. Produtos de uso humano com uma combinação de T_4 e T_3 não são recomendados para cães, já que a proporção é inapropriada, resultando em excesso de T_3. O T_4 está amplamente disponível como medicamentos originais e genéricos, na forma de comprimido ou líquido para administração oral.

Suplementação com T_4

Dose

A secreção diária total de T_4 em cães foi estimada em cerca de 2,5 µg/kg.[244] Entretanto, quando essa quantidade de T_4 é fornecida por via IV ou SC para cães submetidos à tireoidectomia e à paratireoidectomia, sua concentração circulante permanece extremamente baixa.[245] É necessária uma dose IV quatro vezes maior para normalizar a concentração de T_4, e doses orais ainda maiores. A necessidade oral pode ser explicada pelo fato de a absorção GI de T_4 ser estimada em somente 10 a 50% da quantidade administrada por via oral, sendo desconhecidas as razões para a necessidade de alta dose IV.[244] A má absorção GI está presumivelmente relacionada com o conteúdo intraluminal, os fatores dietéticos e as bactérias intestinais que se ligam ao T_4 e reduzem sua disponibilidade, quase sempre reduzida pela metade quando administrada com alimento.[246] Isso não implica que todos os cães devam estar em jejum antes da administração de T_4; em vez disso, a associação temporal entre alimentação e administração oral deve ser padronizada para cada animal, particularmente no dia do monitoramento. A variação de componentes da dieta pode influenciar a absorção de T_4. Portanto, recomenda-se o fornecimento de uma dieta compatível.[247] A biodisponibilidade também varia dependendo do fármaco à base de T_4 utilizado. Ocorre maior variação na biodisponibilidade com produtos genéricos, mas também com produtos patenteados (originais).[248] Em um estudo, notou-se que a biodisponibilidade de uma formulação líquida de uso oral foi aproximadamente o dobro daquela de um comprimido, mas, em outro, foi comparável ao utilizar diferentes fármacos, indicando que nem todos os produtos podem ser utilizados de forma intercambiável.[246,249]

Frequência

A farmacocinética do T_4 é semelhante em cães com hipotireoidismo e naqueles saudáveis.[250] Quando administrado por via oral (seja 1 ou 2 vezes/dia), o T_4 é rapidamente absorvido, com ocorrência de concentração máxima em cerca de 3 a 5 horas e, em geral, meia-vida sérica de 9 a 15 horas.[246,250,251] Doses maiores estão associadas a meias-vidas mais curtas, o que sugere uma cinética dose-dependente.[251] Em grande número de cães com hipotireoidismo, constatou-se concentração máxima de T_4 cerca de 4 a 6 horas após a administração.[248] Rapidamente obtém-se concentração plasmática estável, possibilitando avaliação precoce da eficácia (p. ex., dentro de 2 semanas) após o início do tratamento.[246]

A dose e a frequência de administração ótimas de T_4 para cães com hipotireoidismo permanece de certa forma controversa. Há recomendação de dose diária total de 0,02 a 0,04 mg/kg de peso corporal, com administração fracionada, uma, 2 ou 3 vezes/dia. A maioria dos estudos publicados avaliou a dose de 0,02 mg/kg, 1 vez/dia, com a premissa de que a meia-vida sérica de T_4 não necessariamente reflete seu efeito biológico.[55,252,253] Esse protocolo foi efetivo, embora tenha sido necessário aumento da dose em cerca de 35% dos cães.[253] Essa porcentagem pode ser diminuída dependendo da preparação de T_4 utilizada e da garantia de consistência com os períodos de alimentação.[252] Nesse protocolo, o número de cães que necessitam redução da dose é de cerca de 6 a 10%. A dose administrada 2 vezes/dia está associada a menor pico de concentração e menor oscilação na concentração de T_4t circulante.[248] A dose de 20 µg/kg, 2 vezes/dia, também foi efetiva, mas não pode exceder a 1 vez/dia. Não existem relatos que avaliem o número de cães nos quais os ajustes de dose são necessários pela utilização da dose de 2 vezes/dia. É importante ressaltar que o efeito de uma determinada dose de T_4 varia em cada indivíduo. Dessa forma, o monitoramento clínico, clinicopatológico e hormonal é de crucial importância na determinação da dose e da frequência de administração de T_4 a cada cão, o que pode necessitar vários ajustes. Uma vantagem prática da escolha da dose 1 vez/dia pode estar relacionada com o maior comprometimento do tutor, já que a terapia deve ser feita pelo resto da vida.

Resposta clínica

Cães com hipotireoidismo tratados de maneira adequada não devem manifestar sinais clínicos da doença, lembrando que a melhora pode levar semanas a meses até que se torne aparente. Em geral, alterações metabólicas, como obnubilação e letargia, são as primeiras a melhorar dentro de dias após o início da terapia, e espera-se uma perda de peso de 10% nos primeiros meses. Melhoras dermatológicas são esperadas dentro de 1 mês após o início do tratamento, mas podem demorar 2 a 3 meses até que haja normalização, quase sempre com uma fase de aumento da perda de peso, precedida do reinício do crescimento dos pelos. A melhora dos sintomas neurológicos pode demorar até 6 meses.[254]

Resposta clinicopatológica

A normalização das alterações clinicopatológicas associadas ao hipotireoidismo ocorrem, em geral, em paralelo à resposta clínica.[253] As concentrações séricas de colesterol e triglicerídeos costumam diminuir de maneira drástica, enquanto a contagem de hemácias aumenta de maneira progressiva durante os 3 primeiros meses de terapia de reposição com hormônio tireoidiano. A concentração de frutosamina diminui de maneira significativa, conforme aumenta a renovação (turnover) proteica.[147,253] A terapia de reposição com hormônio tireoidiano reverte com rapidez as alterações induzidas pelo hipotireoidismo na adiponectina, na leptina e na taxa de filtração glomerular.[115,255]

Monitoramento

O objetivo principal do monitoramento terapêutico é compreender a satisfação do tutor com a resposta ao tratamento, juntamente com a detecção do pico da concentração de T_4t circulante. A resposta efetiva em cães tratados 1 vez/dia está associada a um pico da concentração de T_4t mediano (6 horas após a administração) de aproximadamente 4 µg/dℓ (50 nmol/ℓ).[55,253] Valores inferiores a 2,7 µg/dℓ (35 nmol/ℓ) costumam estar associados a uma resposta clínica inadequada, indicando-se aumento da dose. Ocasionalmente ocorre pico da concentração de T_4t excessivamente elevado, acima de 7 µg/dℓ (> 90 nmol/ℓ). Embora cães costumem ser resistentes à tireotoxicose clínica grave, esse valor deve levar à pronta diminuição da dose. A administração dela 2 vezes/dia faz com que o valor de T_4t situe-se no limite superior de normalidade ou um pouco acima do intervalo de referência, 4 a 6 horas após a administração, e esteja no intervalo de referência antes da próxima dose. Em termos gerais, ao se dobrar a dose de T_4 administrada, aumenta-se o pico da concentração de T_4t circulante em cerca de 50 a 60%, por conta da biodisponibilidade e farmacocinética dose-dependentes.[248,251] Embora isso possa ser utilizado para definir a exata magnitude da alteração de dose, é mais em geral ditada pela concentração do hormônio no próximo comprimido disponível, quando se utiliza esse modo de administração. O ajuste da dose mais acurado pode ser possível utilizando-se a formulação líquida.

A mensuração de TSHc possibilita uma avaliação a longo prazo da adequação do tratamento, diferentemente da mensuração de T_4t, que somente fornece informações relacionadas com o tratamento naquele dia em especial.[253] A mensuração de TSHc ajuda a detectar o mau comprometimento de tutores nos casos em que existe um esforço particular para administrar a medicação nos dias correspondentes à visita de monitoramento. Infelizmente, em cães com hipotireoidismo que não apresentaram aumento na concentração de TSHc antes do tratamento, a mensuração durante a terapia de reposição com hormônio tireoidiano não possui valor algum. Além disso, a concentração de TSHc circulante pode ser altamente sensível aos efeitos da terapia de reposição com hormônio tireoidiano, de tal forma que pode ocorrer supressão de TSHc sem a obtenção de um controle clínico ideal. As limitações dos atuais testes de TSHc não possibilitam a detecção de suplementação hormonal excessiva.

Dose excessiva

Os cães parecem ser particularmente resistentes aos efeitos tireotóxicos da suplementação excessiva com T_4.[252,253] Alguns necessitam de até 20 vezes a dose-padrão de T_4 para manifestarem tireotoxicose clínica. Os sinais clínicos de tireotoxicose incluem polidipsia, poliúria, polifagia, respiração ofegante, perda de peso, hiperatividade, taquicardia e hipertermia. A maioria dos sintomas deve cessar dentro de alguns dias após a descontinuação da terapia. Em geral, a concentração correspondente de T_4t está acima de 7 µg/dℓ (> 90 nmol/ℓ). O desenvolvimento de tireotoxicose foi relatado em um cão por conta da ingestão de fezes de um animal contactante suplementado.[256]

Introdução gradual da suplementação com T_4

A introdução gradual da suplementação (25 a 50% da dose inicial) foi recomendada em cães com doenças concomitantes, como cardiopatias, hipoadrenocorticismo e diabetes melito. Entretanto, a administração da dose de 20 µg/kg, 1 vez/dia, não foi associada a efeitos adversos em cães com essas doenças, conferindo outra vantagem desse protocolo terapêutico.[253]

Falha na resposta terapêutica

Uma falha na resposta à terapia em geral se deve à incapacidade em obter concentração de hormônio tireoidiano circulante e, em geral, responde ao ajuste da dose. Entretanto, a utilização de T_3 pode ser necessária em cães com anormalidade na absorção de T_4 e doença GI concomitantes. A falha em obter a resposta clínica esperada quando as concentrações de hormônios tireoidianos estão adequadas deve levar à investigação imediata de outra doença subjacente. Doses anti-inflamatórias diárias de prednisolona, mas não em dias alternados, em cães com hipotireoidismo diminuem a concentração de T_4t; entretanto, ajustes da dose não são necessários, já que a concentração de T_4L permanece inalterada.[257]

Mixedema

O coma mixedematoso está associado a uma redução significativa da taxa metabólica e, potencialmente, hipovolemia/desidratação. Nem a via de administração oral tampouco a SC/IM é adequada, pelo menos de início. Nesses cães, deve-se administrar T_4 por via IV, na dose de 5 µg/kg/12 h. Ocorrida a estabilização, pode-se iniciar a administração oral. Resolução do estado mental anormal, deambulação e hipotensão sistólica devem ser esperadas dentro de 30 horas.[86,88]

Tratamentos anedóticos

O T_4, potencialmente, possui diversos efeitos farmacológicos não relacionados com os seus efeitos fisiológicos, quando suplementado em casos de insuficiência tireoidiana. Como consequência, existem relatos anedóticos, mas raramente comprovados, da utilização de T_4 em diversas situações clínicas, incluindo a utilização de T_4 para melhorar a qualidade do pelame.[58] A terapia de reposição com hormônio tireoidiano foi utilizada em cães com agressividade direcionada ao tutor e com concentração do hormônio tireoidiano no menor valor da faixa de normalidade, sem nenhum efeito significativo.[258] Em seres humanos, o tratamento de pacientes com síndrome da doença não tireoidiana com T_4 é controverso, com evidências persuasivas limitadas de que tal procedimento melhore a resposta terapêutica, exceto em pacientes com cardiopatia.[184] Em cães, a adição de T_4 à terapia-padrão para insuficiência cardíaca congestiva devido à insuficiência do miocárdio não melhora a sobrevida, em comparação ao uso de placebo (ver Capítulo 133).[259] Da mesma forma, a suplementação com T_4 não altera o desenvolvimento de complicações cardíacas decorrentes da terapia crônica com doxorrubicina, em cães.[260]

PROGNÓSTICO

De modo geral, o prognóstico para cães com hipotireoidismo é excelente.

REFERÊNCIAS BIBLIOGRÁFICAS

As referências bibliográficas deste capítulo se encontram online no Ambiente de Aprendizagem.

CAPÍTULO 300

Hipotireoidismo em Gatos

Sylvie Daminet

ETIOLOGIA

Considerações gerais

Em gatos, há relatos de hipotireoidismo iatrogênico, congênito e espontâneo, de ocorrência natural, com início na idade adulta. É mais provável que veterinários sejam confrontados com hipotireoidismo *iatrogênico*, cujo potencial impacto na função renal merece atenção particular. Embora tenham sido relatados alguns poucos casos bem documentados de hipotireoidismo felino *congênito*, o hipotireoidismo *espontâneo* na fase adulta foi diagnosticado apenas em casos raros.

Hipotireoidismo iatrogênico

O hipotireoidismo iatrogênico é uma consequência bem reconhecida secundária ao tratamento de gatos com hipertireoidismo (ver Capítulo 301). Pode resultar de dose excessiva de fármaco antitireoidiano, tireoidectomia bilateral ou terapia com iodo radioativo (^{131}I). A tireoidectomia unilateral pode resultar em hipotireoidismo transitório. A administração de medicamentos antitireoidianos comumente leva à concentração sérica de tiroxina total (T_4t) abaixo do intervalo de referência, quase sempre sem sinais clínicos, talvez porque a concentração de triiodotironina total (T_3t) (o hormônio ativo) esteja, de modo geral, normal.

O hipertireoidismo, causado, em geral, por tecido tireoidiano anormal com função autônoma, suprime cronicamente a liberação endógena do hormônio tireoestimulante (TSH, do inglês *thyroid stimulating hormone*) da hipófise e, por fim, ocasiona atrofia do tecido tireoidiano normal. Após tratamento do hipertireoidismo com ^{131}I (ver Capítulo 301), a combinação de destruição de células previamente hiperativas, em conjunto com a lenta recuperação, induz a produção hormonal pelo tecido tireoidiano atrofiado "normal" e pode levar a um período de hipotireoidismo transitório. Essa simples explicação para a patogênese do hipotireoidismo iatrogênico é semelhante à do hipotireoidismo transitório, que surge após cirurgia ou até mesmo o tratamento medicamentoso. Em gatos com hipertireoidismo, assim que a concentração de T_4t diminui, a concentração de TSH deve aumentar. O TSH, por sua vez, estimula as células da tireoide atrofiada a funcionar. Após o tratamento com ^{131}I ou após tireoidectomia, é comum um período transitório de hipotireoidismo iatrogênico.[2] Gatos com hipertireoidismo e com função renal normal e com hipotireoidismo transitório após tratamento em geral não manifestam sinais clínicos de hipotireoidismo, sem necessidade de suplementação hormonal. Na verdade, a administração de terapia tireoidiana retarda a recuperação das células atrofiadas. A incidência de hipotireoidismo após terapia com iodo radioativo provavelmente depende, pelo menos em parte, da dose de ^{131}I administrada, da duração do acompanhamento e dos critérios utilizados para definir a condição de baixa função tireoidiana. Dessa forma, a incidência relatada varia de incomum, com 5%, a comum, com 83%.[2,3] Gatos com captação cintilográfica por ambos os lobos da tireoide, em varredura com pertecnetato, parecem predispostos ao desenvolvimento de hipotireoidismo após tratamento com ^{131}I.[3]

Hipotireoidismo congênito

De forma geral, o hipotireoidismo primário congênito pode ser classificado em duas principais categorias: *disormonogênese tireoidiana* (um defeito na biossíntese de hormônios tireoidianos) e *dismorfogênese tireoidiana* (um defeito no desenvolvimento anatômico da tireoide, em geral descrito como hipoplasia ou aplasia). Ambas as formas em seres humanos ocorrem provavelmente devido a uma anomalia genética hereditária autossômica recessiva. A disormonogênese é uma condição na qual ocorre redução da síntese de hormônio tireoidiano, diminuição do *feedback* negativo para a hipófise (e hipotálamo), aumento da secreção de TSH, hiperplasia da glândula tireoide e aumento da tireoide (bócio). A disormonogênese, associada a anormalidades na ação da peroxidase tireoidiana e na organificação do iodo, foi descrita em gatos de uma família das raças Doméstico de Pelo Curto e Abissínio.[4,5] A dismorfogênese não causa aumento da tireoide, tendo sido documentada em gatos com parentesco, cuja condição é compatível com hereditariedade autossômica recessiva.[6] O hipotireoidismo secundário à resistência ao TSH foi sugerido em uma família de gatos Japoneses.[7] Em gatos, ainda não há relato de deficiência do hipotálamo ou da hipófise, com hipotireoidismo secundário congênito (hipotireoidismo central).

Hipotireoidismo em idade adulta

Somente alguns poucos gatos bem documentados com hipotireoidismo primário adquirido *espontâneo* (de ocorrência natural) foram descritos.[8-10] Características histopatológicas de suas glândulas tireoides foram diversas. Elas incluem infiltração linfocítica acentuada, atrofia idiopática e bócio hiperplásico difuso, com relato de hipotireoidismo secundário devido a trauma cefálico.[11]

MANIFESTAÇÕES CLÍNICAS

Considerações gerais

As manifestações clínicas mais comuns das formas iatrogênica, congênita e adquirida em idade adulta do hipotireoidismo em gatos são destacadas na Tabela 300.1 e ilustradas na Figura 300.1 e no Vídeo 300.1. Embora muitos sinais de hipotireoidismo em gatos sejam semelhantes àqueles considerados típicos em cães hipotireóideos (ver Capítulo 299), existem diferenças. Por exemplo, poucos gatos com hipotireoidismos, independentemente da etiologia, desenvolvem alopecia não pruriginosa bilateral simétrica grave. Inapetência e retardo mental marcante costumam ser observados. Filhotes com hipotireoidismo congênito podem desenvolver constipação intestinal grave.

Hipotireoidismo em idade adulta (iatrogênico e espontâneo)

Letargia, inapetência e alterações cutâneas são sinais clínicos comuns, que podem ser graves. Sintomas dermatológicos são caracterizados por pelame opaco, seco e desgrenhado (possivelmente com nós) e seborreia seca. Alopecia auricular pode ocorrer em alguns gatos. Os pelos se desprendem com facilidade, sendo possível que o crescimento de novos pelos após a tosa seja ruim. Hipotermia e bradicardia são ocasionalmente notadas ao exame físico. No hipotireoidismo em idade adulta de ocorrência natural, os sintomas são quase sempre marcantes, talvez como resultado do baixo índice de suspeita do profissional. Assim, a doença não é diagnosticada até que seja grave. Face inchada, presumivelmente devido ao mixedema, foi relatada em um gato.[8]

CAPÍTULO 300 • Hipotireoidismo em Gatos   1759

Tabela 300.1 Características clínicas mais importantes em casos de hipotireoidismo iatrogênico, congênito e de ocorrência natural em idade adulta, em gatos.

	HIPOTIREOIDISMO IATROGÊNICO	HIPOTIREOIDISMO CONGÊNITO	HIPOTIREOIDISMO DE OCORRÊNCIA NATURAL EM IDADE ADULTA
Letargia	+	+ (Pode incluir retardo mental)	+ (Pode incluir retardo mental)
Ganho de peso ou obesidade	+	+	+
Inapetência	+	+	+*
Constipação intestinal	+	+* (Pode incluir megacólon)	+
Bócio	− ou +	Possível	−
Nanismo desproporcional	−	+*	−
Fechamento retardado das placas de crescimento (à radiografia)	−	+*	−
Sintomas dermatológicos (especialmente seborreia e fácil desprendimento de pelos)	+	+	+*

*Indica que é uma característica importante. As características clínicas podem ser discretas ou graves. +, Em geral presente; −, ausente. (De Mooney CT, Peterson ME, editors: *Manual of canine and feline endocrinology*, 3 ed., Gloucestershire, England, 2011, British Small Animal Veterinary Association, p. 111-115.)

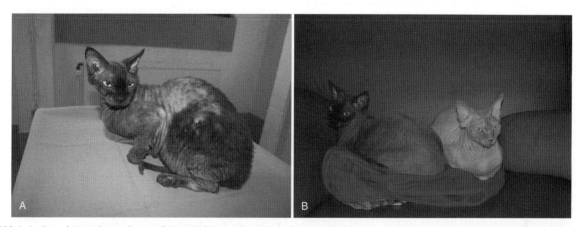

Figura 300.1 A. Gato da raça Devon Rex macho, castrado, com 5 anos, com histórico de letargia, retardo mental e inapetência. O gato também apresentava diabetes melito e baixa concentração sérica de T_4t, bem como aumento de hormônio tireoestimulante canino, o que confirmou o diagnóstico de hipotireoidismo primário. Esse gato também tinha pelame seborreico, cujos pelos se desprendiam com facilidade. Note a otite ceruminosa bilateral. **B.** Mesmo paciente de **A**, 1 ano antes do início dos sinais clínicos de hipotireoidismo. (Cortesia de E. Mercier e S. Daminet.)

Hipotireoidismo congênito

Muitos dos sintomas observados no hipotireoidismo de ocorrência em idade adulta também podem ser observados em filhotes acometidos. Já que o hormônio tireoidiano é essencial para o desenvolvimento pós-natal normal do esqueleto e do sistema nervoso, os filhotes com hipotireoidismo congênito apresentam nanismo desproporcional evidente e anormalidades neurológicas, parecendo, em geral, normais ao nascimento. O crescimento retardado, quando comparado ao de companheiros de ninhada, costuma se tornar evidente aos 2 meses de vida, com desenvolvimento de nanismo desproporcional nos meses seguintes. Os sintomas consistem em cabeça grande e larga, orelhas pequenas, corpo arredondado e pescoço e membros curtos. Os filhotes acometidos parecem letárgicos, podendo manifestar episódios recorrentes graves de constipação intestinal. Algumas vezes, a letargia e o retardo do crescimento podem não ser reconhecidos pelos tutores, que levam o gato para atendimento veterinário por conta da constipação intestinal recorrente. Convulsões foram relatadas como um problema importante em dois companheiros de ninhada com hipotireoidismo congênito.[6] Gatos acometidos possuem pelos que cobrem todo o corpo, cujo pelame é composto, sobretudo, por pelos secundários, com poucos deles longos. Os dentes são subdesenvolvidos e retardos na erupção dentária e na substituição dos dentes decíduos são comuns. Ao exame físico, podem ser detectados hipotermia, bradicardia e, algumas vezes, bócio palpável (com defeitos de organificação).

A sobrevida de filhotes acometidos não tratados depende amplamente da etiologia do hipotireoidismo congênito. É provável que vários filhotes acometidos morram sem diagnóstico, como portadores da "síndrome do definhamento do filhote". Filhotes acometidos podem morrer dentro de alguns meses, enquanto aqueles com anormalidades parciais na atividade da peroxidase podem viver até a fase adulta sem nunca manifestar sinais clínicos evidentes da doença.

DIAGNÓSTICO

Considerações gerais

Em gatos, o diagnóstico de hipotireoidismo pode ser desafiador, independentemente da causa primária. Assim como em cães, um diagnóstico presuntivo pode ser feito com base na combinação de características clínicas compatíveis e anormalidades notadas nos resultados de exames laboratoriais de rotina (anemia e hipercolesterolemia). A confirmação do diagnóstico de hipotireoidismo requer testes hormonais ou cintilografia da tireoide. Mesmo gatos com *hipotireoidismo iatrogênico* apresentam poucas "dicas" para o diagnóstico, apesar do histórico recente do tratamento de hipertireoidismo. Assim como acontece em indivíduos idosos, condições concomitantes são comuns (p. ex., doença renal crônica), potencialmente causando a chamada "síndrome do eutireóideo doente" (ver Capítulo 299). Da mesma forma, a redução da atividade e/ou do ganho de peso após o tratamento pode enganar o tutor ou o veterinário. Por um lado, essas alterações são esperadas com a resolução do hipertireoidismo; mas, por outro, elas podem indicar a existência de outras doenças ou de hipotireoidismo. Assim, de certa forma, os sinais clínicos de hipotireoidismo iatrogênico e aqueles esperados com o retorno ao estado eutireóideo podem se sobrepor.

Tratamento de hiperadrenocorticismo seguido de hipotireoidismo ou azotemia

Após terapia com ^{131}I, vários gatos desenvolvem diminuição acentuada, mas transitória, na concentração de T_4t, abaixo do normal, seguida de retorno ao eutireoidismo dentro de 3 a 6 meses. Na maioria dos gatos tratados para hipertireoidismo, com função renal normal, o hipotireoidismo transitório não é clinicamente relevante e não necessita ser tratado. É aconselhável esperar 3 a 6 meses após terapia com ^{131}I antes de confirmar o diagnóstico de hipotireoidismo iatrogênico *permanente*, especialmente se os sinais clínicos do hipotireoidismo não forem convincentes e o gato não manifestar azotemia.

Existe risco de sérios impactos negativos do hipotireoidismo na função renal (ver Capítulo 301), especialmente em gatos com doença renal preexistente.[1,12,13] Gatos com hipotireoidismo iatrogênico (após terapia com ^{131}I ou tireoidectomia) e azotemia devem ser imediatamente tratados com suplementação por levotiroxina, pois tal procedimento aumenta a taxa de filtração glomerular, melhora a função renal e reduz a gravidade da azotemia. Caso um gato com hipertireoidismo desenvolva azotemia enquanto recebe medicação antitireoidiana, a dose do medicamento deve ser ajustada ou descontinuada. Relata-se que o hipotireoidismo iatrogênico agrava a azotemia e reduz a expectativa de vida em gatos com doença renal crônica (DRC) preexistente.[1] Recomenda-se a administração de levotiroxina imediatamente após hospitalização para terapia com ^{131}I.[14] Resultados preliminares em gatos com hipertireoidismo e DRC em estágio 2 ou 3, definido pela International Renal Interest Society (IRIS), sugerem que o tratamento de hipotireoidismo iatrogênico é benéfico para evitar o agravamento da azotemia.[14] Ainda, um protocolo que utiliza doses ultrabaixas de ^{131}I (1 a 2 mCi) foi efetivo no restabelecimento da condição de eutireoidismo, sem induzir hipotireoidismo iatrogênico (3%) em gatos com hipertireoidismo brando, com pequenos nódulos na tireoide.[15]

Hipotireoidismo espontâneo (congênito e de ocorrência em idade adulta)

O *hipotireoidismo espontâneo (congênito e de ocorrência em idade adulta)* é provavelmente subdiagnosticado, mas permanece sendo raro. Filhotes costumam parecer normais ao nascimento e o início das características típicas, como nanismo desproporcional, ocorre, em geral, mais tardiamente. Alguns filhotes morrem precocemente ou podem ser diagnosticados de modo errôneo como portadores de megacólon idiopático ou de alguma outra anomalia congênita.

Características clinicopatológicas de rotina

A incidência de anemia normocítica normocrômica discreta e/ou hipercolesterolemia em gatos com hipotireoidismo não é conhecida, mas é observada com mais frequência em gatos com a doença iatrogênica. No hipotireoidismo congênito essas alterações são inconsistentes.[6]

Concentrações hormonais (Figura 300.2)

Tiroxina total (T_4t)

Baixas concentrações circulantes de T_4t são esperadas em qualquer gato com hipotireoidismo. A constatação de concentração de T_4t no intervalo de referência sustenta fortemente a condição de eutireoidismo e exclui seguramente a preocupação com hipotireoidismo. Entretanto, assim como acontece em cães, o T_4t pode estar suprimido por doenças não tireoidianas; quanto mais grave a doença, menor a concentração de T_4t. Portanto, a diminuição da concentração de T_4t é uma informação sensível, mas não específica, e não deve ser considerada como diagnóstica de hipotireoidismo. Além disso, uma série de fármacos demonstrou suprimir de forma significativa a concentração de T_4t em cães,[17] o que ainda não foi pesquisado em gatos. Como o diagnóstico de hipotireoidismo primário espontâneo não deve se basear somente na concentração basal de T_4t, recomenda-se mensuração da concentração sérica de TSH canino (TSHc), teste de resposta ao TSH recombinante humano (TSHrh) ou cintilografia da tireoide, para confirmar o diagnóstico da doença.

Tiroxina livre (T_4L)

Ao contrário do observado em cães, é incerto o benefício da mensuração da concentração de T_4L, comparado ao da mensuração de T_4t, como testes auxiliares de diagnóstico em gatos. Espera-se baixa concentração de T_4L (em diálise de equilíbrio) em gatos com hipotireoidismo, mas também na presença de doença não tireoidiana. Entretanto, relata-se aumento da concentração de T_4L em gatos eutireoideos com doenças não tireoidianas.[16,18]

Tireotrofina (TSH) endógena

Em cães com hipotireoidismo, o aumento da concentração sérica de TSH pode confirmar hipotireoidismo primário (de origem na glândula tireoide). Ainda não há disponibilidade de teste específico para mensuração de TSH em gatos. Entretanto, relata-se o uso do teste imunorradiométrico canino, em gatos.[19] Notou-se aumento da concentração de TSHc em dois gatos com hipotireoidismo primário de ocorrência em idade adulta.[9,10] Gatos com hipotireoidismo iatrogênico devem também apresentar aumento da concentração sérica de TSHc.[1,20,21] A utilização de TSHc (e espera-se, em breve, o uso de TSH felino) deve ser útil para diferenciar hipotireoidismo primário congênito do secundário (deficiência de TSH).

Testes de função tireoidiana dinâmicos

O teste de resposta ao TSHrh foi descrito em gatos para distinguir doença não tireoidiana do hipotireoidismo iatrogênico, após terapia com ^{131}I.[22] Embora avaliado em um número limitado de gatos, parece ser uma alternativa valiosa ao TSH bovino para o teste de estimulação. Em gatos, para realizar o teste de estimulação por TSHrh obtém-se uma amostra de sangue para mensuração da concentração basal de T_4t. Em seguida, administram-se 25 µg de TSHrh, por via IV, e, finalmente, uma segunda amostra de sangue é obtida 6 horas depois. O TSHrh está disponível no mercado como Thyrogen® (Genzyme Corporation, Países Baixos); o conteúdo do frasco pode ser fracionado e armazenado congelado, conforme previamente descrito, para viabilizar esse teste.[22,23]

Diagnóstico por imagem

Radiografia

Assim como mencionado para cães (ver Capítulo 299), a radiografia pode ser particularmente útil no diagnóstico de hipotireoidismo congênito. Várias das alterações observadas são praticamente patognomônicas. As radiografias mostram retardo do desenvolvimento esquelético, sobretudo disgenesia epifisária dos corpos vertebrais e ossos longos.

Cintilografia da tireoide

A captação de tecnécio, na forma de pertecnetato ($^{99m}TcO_4^-$), pelos lobos tireoidianos é um procedimento sensível e específico para o diagnóstico de hipotireoidismo em cães e gatos (ver Capítulo 301), sendo um exame promissor para se tornar uma importante ferramenta para o diagnóstico de hipotireoidismo

CAPÍTULO 300 • Hipotireoidismo em Gatos

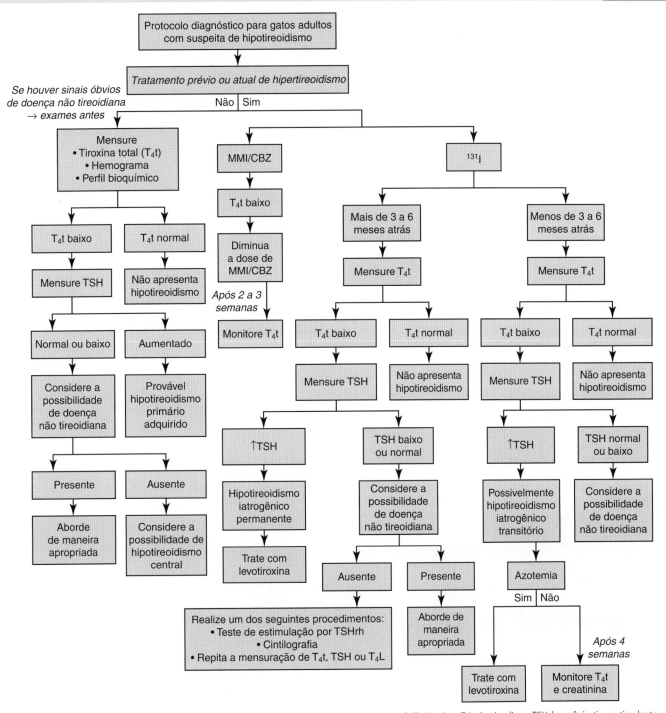

Figura 300.2 Diagnóstico de hipotireoidismo em gatos adultos. *CBZ*, carbimazol; *MMI*, metimazol; T_4, tiroxina; T_4L, tiroxina livre; *TSH*, hormônio tireoestimulante; *TSHrh*, hormônio tireoestimulante recombinante humano.

em gatos. Pode ser especialmente útil em gatos nos quais o diagnóstico é duvidoso, como naqueles com doença concomitante (síndrome do eutireóideo doente). O achado esperado no hipotireoidismo de ocorrência na idade adulta é redução ou ausência de captação de $^{99m}TcO_4^-$ pela glândula tireoide (Figura 300.3). A cintilografia da tireoide foi utilizada como técnica não invasiva para confirmar o diagnóstico de hipotireoidismo espontâneo em um gato.[9]

Ademais, a cintilografia com uso de ^{123}I pode ser um teste diagnóstico útil para esclarecer o mecanismo primário do hipotireoidismo congênito. Em caso de dismorfogênese, espera-se ausência de captação de ^{123}I., a qual pode estar normal em caso de deficiência de peroxidase tireoidiana. Entretanto, a organificação (incorporação do iodo) é deficiente, sendo observada a liberação anormal de ^{123}I após administração de perclorato (teste de excreção do perclorato).

Veterinários costumam utilizar o teste terapêutico com levotiroxina como ferramenta diagnóstica para hipotireoidismo. Infelizmente, a resposta positiva ao tratamento não significa que o gato tenha, na verdade, hipotireoidismo. A combinação das mensurações de T_4t e TSHc provavelmente é o método mais eficiente e econômico para o diagnóstico de hipotireoidismo primário. Quando há dúvida quanto os resultados, outros testes diagnósticos, como o de estimulação por TSHrh ou cintilografia, devem ser considerados antes de iniciar o teste terapêutico com levotiroxina.

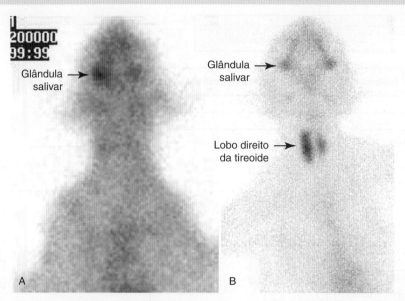

Figura 300.3 A. Imagem de projeção ventral de varredura cintilográfica da tireoide de um gato com hipotireoidismo primário em idade adulta. Note a captação de pertecnetato nas glândulas salivares (*seta*) e ausência de captação na região cervical (tireoide). **B.** Para propósitos de ilustração, essa figura mostra o aumento da captação de pertecnetato na glândula tireoide de um gato com hipertireoidismo. (Imagens de K. Peremans.)

TRATAMENTO

Embora dados farmacocinéticos estejam somente disponíveis em gatos saudáveis, a dose oral recomendada para suplementação de tiroxina varia de 100 μg/gato/24 h a 10 a 20 μg/kg/24 h. Dados preliminares recentes sugerem que o tratamento com intervalos entre doses de 12 horas (0,075 mg/12 h) com estômago vazio pode ser mais efetivo.[24] Assim como mencionado para cães, os gatos acometidos devem ser reavaliados após 4 a 8 semanas. Ajustes adicionais da dose devem se basear na resposta clínica e no monitoramento terapêutico da concentração de T_4t após a medicação. Com tratamento apropriado, o prognóstico de hipotireoidismo adquirido é excelente. No hipotireoidismo congênito o prognóstico é reservado e depende muito da causa primária do hipotireoidismo e da idade por ocasião do diagnóstico.

REFERÊNCIAS BIBLIOGRÁFICAS

As referências bibliográficas deste capítulo se encontram online no Ambiente de Aprendizagem.

CAPÍTULO 301

Hipertireoidismo Felino

Thomas K. Graves

Desde sua primeira descrição na literatura veterinária há apenas 35 anos, o hipertireoidismo se tornou a doença endócrina mais comum de gatos domésticos e uma das mais importantes na prática felina. Existem diversas estimativas de prevalência da doença na América do Norte e na Europa, o que indica que a incidência da condição parece ser crescente.[1-3] A prevalência geral do hipertireoidismo felino (HTF) é de 2 a 4% e, pelo menos, de 6% em gatos com mais de 9 anos. De acordo com algumas estimativas, quase 10% dos gatos geriátricos desenvolverão essa doença.

FISIOPATOLOGIA

Condições de hipertireoidismo humano (doença de Graves e bócio nodular tóxico)

Hormônios tireoidianos controlam a taxa metabólica do organismo (a fisiologia tireoidiana é revisada no Capítulo 299). O aumento das concentrações sistêmicas de hormônios tireoidianos leva a um estado hipermetabólico responsável pelas anormalidades observadas no hipertireoidismo. Em pessoas com doença de Graves – a forma mais comum de hipertireoidismo –, a condição é o resultado de autoanticorpos que ativam receptores de tirotrofina (TSH, do inglês *thyroid stimulating hormone*), que, por sua vez, levam à síntese e à secreção excessiva de hormônios tireoidianos. Ainda não foram identificadas evidências de uma causa imunomediada em gatos, cuja condição tireoidiana é quase sempre considerada análoga ao bócio nodular tóxico humano (doença de Plummer).[4,5] O bócio nodular tóxico e o HTF compartilham algumas características histopatológicas: ambos são causados pela hiperplasia adenomatosa do tecido tireoidiano, fazendo com que os nódulos secretem hormônios tireoidianos de modo autônomo, o que escapa do controle do hipotálamo e da hipófise. Esses nódulos raramente mostram características de malignidade e são considerados tumores endócrinos benignos. Embora exista certa controvérsia na literatura, a doença de Plummer é supostamente causada por mutações

CAPÍTULO 301 • Hipertireoidismo Felino

ativadas no receptor de TSH ou de suas moléculas de sinalização em cascata, levando à alta secreção constitutiva do hormônio tireoidiano.[6]

Hipertireoidismo felino

Existem resultados conflitantes na literatura, mas foram identificadas mutações do receptor de TSH em alguns gatos hipertireóideos, assim como na subunidade alfa da adenosina monofosfato cíclico (cAMP) de ativação da proteína G.[7,8] Também foram demonstradas diminuições na expressão da proteína G inibitória em casos de bócio felino, o que poderia diminuir a capacidade de inibir a produção de cAMP, resultando em secreção sustentada de hormônio tireoidiano em excesso.[9] Esse é provavelmente um dos vários fatores que podem contribuir para o desenvolvimento de HTF. Existem muitos estudos que implicam substâncias bociogênicas na alimentação, com a implicação de determinados tipos de alimentos enlatados felinos em alguns poucos estudos epidemiológicos de HTF, cuja associação continua a ser estudada.[10,11] Sugeriu-se que concentrações amplamente discrepantes de iodo em dietas comerciais felinas poderiam ser responsáveis pelos níveis de estimulação de TSH variados e pelo desenvolvimento de nódulos tireoidianos em gatos.[11]

A presença de éteres difenílicos polibromados (EDPBs) em alimentos enlatados e no ambiente doméstico do gato também foi sugerida como fator importante na etiopatogenia do HTF.[12,13] EDPBs são utilizados como retardantes de chama em grande número de produtos domésticos, podendo estar em altas concentrações na poeira doméstica ingerida pelos gatos durante a auto-higienização (*self-grooming*). Os distúrbios tireoidianos causados por EDPBs são postulados como causa de secreção crônica e excessiva de TSH, o que poderia levar a um efeito hipertrófico da glândula tireoide e, eventualmente, resultar em hiperplasia adenomatosa ou neoplasia. Uma associação entre EDPBs e HTF ainda não foi comprovada, em parte em razão da falta de um teste de TSH felino confiável e de dificuldades do estudo dos efeitos de desreguladores endócrinos sobre a expectativa de vida dos gatos.

Doença tireoidiana uni e bilateral e histologia

Em gatos, os nódulos tireoidianos hiperfuncionais afetam mais comumente ambos os lobos da glândula tireoide, sendo a doença unilateral observada em menos de um terço dos casos[14] e doença assimétrica bilateral, em mais de 50% dos gatos com HTF. A doença ectópica é relativamente incomum, ocorrendo em cerca de 4% dos gatos. Uma pequena porcentagem de gatos com HTF foi diagnosticada com adenocarcinoma tireoidiano funcional.[14-16] A incidência do carcinoma tireoidiano foi estimada em 1 a 2%, o que é questionável, pois a histologia costuma não estar disponível em gatos acometidos.

CARACTERÍSTICAS CLÍNICAS

Epidemiologia

Os maiores estudos dos achados clínicos em gatos com HTF foram publicados décadas atrás.[17-19] Os médicos-veterinários se tornaram cada vez mais conscientes e mais bem preparados para diagnosticar a doença. Assim, algumas descrições clínicas anteriormente publicadas costumam não ser mais encontradas.[17-19] O HTF é uma doença de gatos de meia-idade e idosos, sem predileção racial ou sexual clara. Em nossa revisão com 160 gatos com HTF observados na Universidade de Illinois, a idade média ao diagnóstico (12,5 anos) está de acordo com relatos iniciais, que sugerem 12 a 13 anos, com uma variação de 4 a 20 anos.[17-19]

Histórico (sinais clínicos)

Comuns

Os sinais clínicos de HTF são variáveis, o que reflete a natureza generalizada e multissistêmica da doença. Em decorrência de sua alta prevalência, é comum a triagem rotineira com exames de hormônios tireoidianos séricos basais em gatos de meia-idade ou idosos. Em geral, o diagnóstico de HTF é confirmado em gatos com sinais clínicos sutis (ou ausentes). Sinais clínicos comuns (Tabela 301.1) incluem perda de peso, polifagia, hiperatividade, êmese, diarreia, poliúria/polidipsia (PU/PD), interrupção do hábito de se lamber e alterações comportamentais, sendo comum qualquer combinação de sinais clínicos e graus variados de gravidade. A perda de peso é o sinal clínico mais comum de HTF. Com frequência, gatos acometidos possuem má condição corporal e aparência desgrenhada. Apesar da idade, os gatos com HTF podem parecer hiperativos, agressivos ou exibir sinais de ansiedade, sendo comuns distúrbios relacionados com o prejuízo à tolerância ao estresse e respiração ofegante.

Incomuns

Embora a hiperatividade e o aumento do apetite sejam comuns, uma pequena porcentagem de gatos com HTF é letárgica, alheia ao ambiente e hiporéxica. Essa condição incomum é referida como hipertireoidismo "apático". Em seres humanos, o hipertireoidismo apático – também denominado hipertireoidismo assintomático – ocorre, sobretudo, nos idosos, em associação a doenças concomitantes e/ou terapias que causem letargia e diminuição do apetite.[20,21] Entretanto, essa condição já foi descrita em pacientes mais jovens.[22] O mecanismo do HTF apático ainda não foi estabelecido. Uma associação entre estados mórbidos subjacentes e HTF apático ainda não foi publicada.

Palpação da tireoide

Um ou mais nódulos tireoidianos costumam ser palpáveis no HTF. Foram descritas técnicas diferentes para palpação da glândula tireoide felina. A técnica mais comum e eficaz é realizada com o o gato sentado, estendendo-se a cabeça para exposição do pescoço ventral (Figura 301.1, Vídeo 301.1). Enquanto se estendem a cabeça e o pescoço do gato com uma mão, desliza-se tanto o polegar quanto o dedo indicador da outra – com pressão moderada desde a laringe, na direção caudal, até a entrada torácica – diversas vezes em um movimento de inspeção lento. O aumento da glândula tireoide será sentido como um deslizar do tecido nodular sob a ponta do dedo. Nódulos podem ser sentidos em um ou ambos os lados da traqueia. Esse método de palpação é

Tabela 301.1	Porcentagem de cada achado clínico entre gatos hipertireóideos.		
ACHADOS DO HISTÓRICO (%)		**ACHADOS DO EXAME FÍSICO (%)**	
Perda de peso	88	Bócio	83
Polifagia	49	Magreza	65
Êmese	44	Sopro cardíaco	54
PU/PD	36	Taquicardia	42
Hiperatividade	31	Ritmo de galope	15
Diminuição do apetite	16	Agressividade	15
Diarreia	15	Pelame desgrenhado	9
Letargia	12	Onicogrifose	6
Fraqueza	12	Alopecia	3
Dispneia	10	ICC	2
Respiração ofegante	9	Ventroflexão do pescoço	1
Grande volume fecal	8		
Anorexia	7		

ICC, insuficiência cardíaca congestiva; *PU/PD*, poliúria/polidipsia. De Broussard JD, Peterson ME,.Fox PR: Changes in clinical and laboratory findings in cats with hyperthyroidism from 1983 to 1993. *J Am Vet Med Assoc* 206:302, 1995.

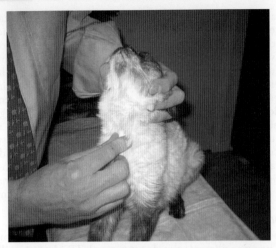

Figura 301.1 Técnica apropriada para palpação da glândula tireoide felina. Note que o polegar distal e o indicador devem ser estendidos para propiciar o maior contato possível com a superfície do pescoço ventral do gato.

bem tolerado pela maioria dos gatos. Nódulos cervicais ventrais também são palpáveis em vários gatos não hipertireoideos.[23,24] Em um estudo, havia nódulos cervicais ventrais palpáveis em quase 70% de gatos eutireóideos com suspeita de HTF.[25] O significado clínico – se houver – desses nódulos é desconhecido. Em alguns gatos, eles podem representar adenomas benignos não funcionais de origem tireoidiana ou paratireoidiana.[23] Tais nódulos podem ou não progredir para doença endócrina. Enquanto gatos com HTF tendem a ter bócio palpável maior do que aqueles sem a doença, ainda não foi estabelecida clara relação entre a palpação tireoidiana e a atividade funcional da glândula tireoide felina.

Exame geral

Muitos dos sinais descritos por tutores também são óbvios ao exame físico. Alguns gatos com HTF são periódica ou persistentemente resistentes à contenção, podendo a utilização de uma cesta aberta relaxar alguns deles e, assim, permitir o exame mais minucioso (ver Capítulo 2). Não é recomendada a contenção com força ou firme de qualquer gato, já que pode resultar em sinais graves em gatos com HTF. Perda de peso – o sinal clínico mais comum – pode estar associada à diminuição da elasticidade da pele. De modo geral, esses gatos não estão desidratados, mas podem facilmente sofrer sobrecarga volêmica se avaliados de maneira errônea como se precisassem de fluidoterapia.

Sistema cardiovascular

Coração

Sopro cardíaco sistólico, taquicardia e ritmo de galope são comuns em gatos com HTF, ocorrendo em 54, 42 e 15% deles, respectivamente. A insuficiência cardíaca congestiva evidente é diagnosticada em aproximadamente 2% dos gatos com HTF. O hormônio tireoidiano, principalmente a triiodotironina (T_3), possui uma ampla gama de efeitos cardíacos.[26] Ele possui efeito cronotrópico positivo, provoca um tempo de condução atrioventricular mais curto e aumenta a resposta dos receptores miocárdicos beta-adrenérgicos. Os efeitos inotrópicos positivos dos hormônios tireoidianos (tanto T_3 como tiroxina [T_4]) ocorrem em razão das alterações nas atividades dos canais iônicos e do aumento das atividades de isoenzimas cardíacas de miosina. A hipertrofia miocárdica é comum em gatos com HTF e resultado da maior expressão de proteínas miocárdicas e, talvez, da hipertrofia miocárdica hipertensiva concomitante.

Pressão sanguínea

A associação entre HTF e hipertensão é, de certa forma, delicada. O reconhecimento da hipertensão em gatos com HTF não é claro. A mensuração da pressão sanguínea é razoavelmente confiável em gatos saudáveis, pela utilização da oscilometria ou ultrassonografia por Doppler (ver Capítulo 99). Ambas se correlacionam bem com as aferições intra-arteriais.[27,28] O "efeito do jaleco branco" nem sempre é reconhecido em gatos, mas pode ser mais evidente naqueles com HTF intolerantes ao estresse. De início, supunha-se que a prevalência da hipertensão em gatos com HTF era alta. Uma publicação identificou prevalência de 87%, cuja definição de "hipertensão" pode ter sido irrealisticamente baixa.[29] Embora o estudo tenha sido bem controlado, com gatos hipertireóideos comparados aos normais e àqueles com doença renal crônica (DRC), relatos posteriores identificaram taxas de prevalência de 5 e 20%.[30,31] Mostrou-se "efeito do jaleco branco" significativo em gatos com HTF, sem diminuição na pressão sanguínea após tratamento.[30] Curiosamente, foi observado aumento da ocorrência da hipertensão em gatos após tratamento do HTF.[31]

A hipertensão raramente ocorre em seres humanos hipertireóideos, e, quando associada à tireotoxicose, ela é, em geral, apenas sistólica. Os hormônios tireoidianos causam diminuição acentuada na resistência vascular periférica. Os efeitos hemodinâmicos da tireotoxicose incluem aumento da frequência cardíaca e do volume sistólico. Foi proposto que o aumento da frequência cardíaca é o somatório da pressão nas artérias periféricas, resultando em hipertensão sistólica geral.[32] Ainda não se sabe se isso também ocorre ou não em gatos com HTF. Foi relatado que aqueles com HTF apresentam hipertensão diastólica, possivelmente relacionada com a DRC subjacente. Ademais, bloqueadores beta-adrenérgicos são efetivos no tratamento de seres humanos hipertireóideos com hipertensão sistólica, mas o efeito do atenolol sobre a hipertensão em gatos hipertireóideos é inconsistente.[33] É difícil saber se o hipertireoidismo felino causa hipertensão. Há uma associação entre as duas, mas causa e efeito ainda não foram estabelecidos, e a hipertensão pode não ser comum. Em um estudo, apenas 5 de 30 gatos com hipertensão tinham HTF.[34] Em um estudo de gatos com retinopatia hipertensiva, somente 5 de 69 gatos eram hipertireóideos.[35]

Sistema urinário

Poliúria e polidipsia (PU/PD) são observadas em mais de um terço dos gatos com HTF, e vários mecanismos podem explicar esse efeito. Seres humanos com hipertireoidismo apresentam resposta exagerada à sede quando da ocorrência de pequenas alterações na osmolalidade plasmática, em comparação a indivíduos eutireóideos. Isso levou os investigadores a propor a polidipsia primária como causa de poliúria no hipertireoidismo.[36] A menor ativação dos canais de aquaporinas nos túbulos renais, associada aos hormônios tireoidianos, e o aumento da excreção tubular de solutos também foram implicados como possíveis causas de poliúria primária no hipertireoidismo.[37] Nenhum dos mecanismos foi examinado em gatos com HTF, mas poderia haver atuação de ambos ou um deles.

Hormônios tireoidianos afetam uma ampla gama de processos fisiológicos que ocorrem nos rins.[38-40] Como afetam o débito cardíaco e o tônus vascular periférico, eles exercem impacto sobre o fluxo sanguíneo renal e a função glomerular. O conceito de aumento do fluxo sanguíneo renal no HTF é sustentado pela diminuição induzida por hormônios tireoidianos na resistência vascular sistêmica, que causa relaxamento da musculatura lisa dentro dos capilares. Além disso, o relaxamento da musculatura lisa se segue à ação de vasodilatadores locais, ao aumento da responsividade à acetilcolina e à diminuição da resposta à endotelina.

No córtex renal, o excesso de hormônios tireoidianos é acompanhado pelo aumento da atividade da óxido nítrico sintase (causando aumento da vasodilatação) e do número de receptores beta-adrenérgicos e pela diminuição da resistência vascular. Essas ações podem levar à ativação do sistema renina-angiotensina-aldosterona. A diminuição da resistência arteriolar aferente e o aumento da pressão hidrostática elevam a taxa de filtração glomerular (TFG). Existem também múltiplos efeitos do hormônio tireoidiano sobre a função tubular renal, incluindo aumento da ativação dos canais de cloreto e reabsorção do íon cloreto em túbulos proximais e na alça de Henle. Isso, por sua vez, diminui a carga de cloreto percebida na mácula densa do túbulo distal e aumenta tanto a retroalimentação tubuloglomerular quanto a filtração glomerular. O excesso de hormônios tireoidianos aumenta a atividade de sódio-potássio ATPase e a troca de sódio por hidrogênio, levando ao aumento da troca de Na^+/Ca^{++} e à reabsorção tubular do íon cálcio. A associação entre hipertireoidismo e discreta hipercalcemia, embora não documentada em gatos, foi reconhecida durante muitas décadas em pessoas com tireotoxicose. O oposto – a hipocalcemia – foi relatada em gatos com HTF.[41,42] O hormônio tireoidiano diminui as concentrações de creatinina sérica, pelo aumento de sua secreção tubular, elevando a TFG e diminuindo a massa de músculo esquelético. A creatinina sérica, derivada da quebra de creatinina e fosfocreatinina nos músculos, é inversamente proporcional à massa muscular. Apesar dos mecanismos que poderiam diminuir as concentrações séricas de creatinina em gatos com HTF, quase 25% estão azotêmicos no momento do diagnóstico. Embora o aumento do nitrogênio ureico sérico tenha sido observado em 26% dos gatos com HTF, e da creatinina em 23%, esses achados provavelmente refletem a realidade de ambas as condições serem comuns em gatos.[18]

Sistema gastrintestinal
Êmese e diarreia são comuns em gatos com HTF (ver Tabela 301.1). Em pessoas não gestantes com tireotoxicose, a êmese é incomum, supostamente causada pelo estímulo à zona deflagradora de quimiorreceptores ou relacionada com a estase gástrica causada pelo hormônio tireoideano.[43,44] O mecanismo da hiperêmese no HTF não está claro. A tireotoxicose altera as contrações musculares do intestino delgado, aumenta a motilidade intestinal e diminui de maneira acentuada o tempo de trânsito entre boca e ceco, contribuindo para a diarreia, comum no hipertireoidismo.[45,46]

AVALIAÇÃO DIAGNÓSTICA DE ROTINA

Urinálise
Não existem achados na urinálise específicos para HTF. Entretanto, gatos hipertireóideos quase sempre são isostenúricos, conforme discutido anteriormente. Como os gatos com HTF podem apresentar DRC, diabetes melito ou uma miríade de outras condições, a urinálise é essencial (ver Capítulo 72).

Hemograma
Eritrocitose discreta é notada em aproximadamente metade dos gatos com HTF. Como a "anemia da doença crônica" é esperada em gatos idosos doentes, um hematócrito no limite superior ou discretamente aumentado deve alertar o clínico sobre possível HTF, mesmo se as concentrações séricas de hormônios tireoidianos estiverem normais. O aumento da demanda celular por oxigênio é um mecanismo estabelecido da eritropoese induzida por eritropoetina e hormônios tireoidianos no hipertireoidismo.[47,48] O hormônio tireoidiano pode atuar diretamente sobre a medula óssea. Eosinopenia e linfopenia são anormalidades adicionais do hemograma em gatos com HTF, ocorrendo em 34 e 40% deles, respectivamente.[18]

Bioquímica sérica
O aumento da atividade de enzimas hepáticas é comum em gatos hipertireoideos.[17-19] Mais de 80% daqueles com HTF apresentam aumento da atividade de alanina aminotransferase e mais da metade, das atividades da fosfatase alcalina. As causas para essas alterações são multifatoriais e, provavelmente, relacionadas com estresse metabólico hepático, congestão passiva, toxicidade direta do hormônio tireoidiano e outros fatores. Cerca de um quarto dos gatos hipertireóideos são azotêmicos no momento do diagnóstico. Alguns deles podem ter azotemia pré-renal, sendo comum doença renal concomitante.

CONFIRMAÇÃO DO DIAGNÓSTICO

Testes de tiroxina total e livre, T_3 e hormônio tireoestimulante

Exames de sangue disponíveis e utilização do T_4T como teste de triagem
Ensaios de hormônios tireoidianos, incluindo testes para tiroxina total (T_4t), triiodotironina total (T_3t) e, em menor extensão, T_4 livre (T_4L), estão amplamente disponíveis (Figuras 301.2 e 301.3). A mensuração da tireotrofina sérica (hormônio tireoestimulante [TSH]) não é muito utilizada em gatos, mas pode ter valor diagnóstico, ao contrário da aferição das concentrações séricas basais de T_3t, em razão do alto grau de sobreposição entre gatos normais, os com HTF e aqueles com doença não tireoidiana.[49,50] O teste de triagem mais comumente utilizado é a aferição da concentração sérica de T_4t. O resultado acima dos intervalos de referência confirma o diagnóstico em mais de 91% dos gatos com HTF.[50]

Tiroxina total dentro dos limites de referência?
O achado de uma concentração sérica normal de T_4t não exclui o diagnóstico de HTF. Um número relativamente alto de gatos hipertireóideos apresenta resultados basais séricos de T_4t normais ou no limite superior, um fenômeno conhecido como "hipertireoidismo oculto", com diversas explicações possíveis. A princípio, os hormônios tireoidianos flutuam diariamente no HTF.[51] Até mesmo gatos com HTF grave apresentam concentrações de T_4t que ocasionalmente diminuem quanto aos valores de referência durante alguns dias, em algum momento (ver Figura 301.2). Portanto, a abordagem mais simples para um gato com forte suspeita de HTF, mas no qual a concentração de T_4t está normal, é simplesmente reavaliar o T_4t em outro dia. Outra explicação possível para o achado de concentração sérica normal de T_4t em um gato com HTF é a existência de doença não tireoidiana (Tabela 301.2). Quase todas as doenças concomitantes podem diminuir as concentrações séricas de T_4t, causando resultados falso-negativos em HTF.

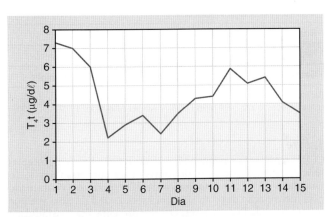

Figura 301.2 Flutuação diária das concentrações séricas de T_4t em um gato com hipertireoidismo durante um período de 15 dias. A flutuação dentro do intervalo normal (*área sombreada*) pode explicar o fenômeno de hipertireoidismo oculto em alguns gatos. (Dados de Peterson ME, Graves TK, Cavanagh I: Serum thyroid hormone concentrations fluctuate in cats with hyperthyroidism. *J Vet Intern Med* 1:142, 1987.)

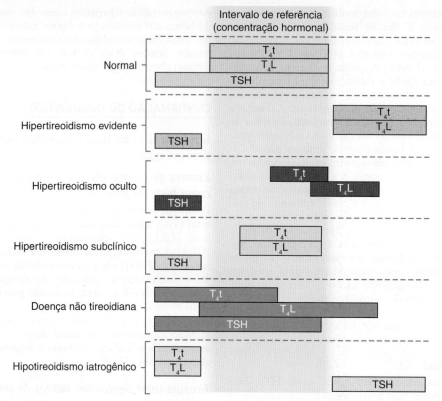

Figura 301.3 Distribuição provável das concentrações séricas de T₄t, T₄L e TSH em gatos normais e naqueles com hipertireoidismo evidente, hipertireoidismo oculto, hipertireoidismo subclínico, doença não tireoidiana e hipotireoidismo iatrogênico. Os intervalos normais de referência para todos os três hormônios estão representados pelas áreas sombreadas. (Baseada em dados publicados nas referências 3, 50, 51, 52, 53, 54, 55 e 57.)

Tabela 301.2 Concentrações séricas médias de tiroxina total (T₄t) em gatos normais e naqueles com diversas doenças não tireoidianas.

DOENÇA	MÉDIA DO T₄T
Diabetes melito	4 nmol/ℓ
Hepatopatia	8 nmol/ℓ
Doença renal crônica (DRC)	10 nmol/ℓ
Neoplasia sistêmica	12 nmol/ℓ
Insuficiência cardíaca congestiva	11 nmol/ℓ
Doença inflamatória intestinal	18 nmol/ℓ
Doença inflamatória das vias respiratórias	14 nmol/ℓ
Neoplasia focal	16 nmol/ℓ
Gatos normais	24 nmol/ℓ

De Peterson ME, Gamble DE: Effect of nonthyroidal illness on serum thyroxine concentrations in cats: 494 cases (1988). *J Am Vet Med Assoc* 197:1203, 1990.

T₄ livre

O T₄L representa a pequena fração de T₄t não ligada a proteínas séricas, estando, portanto, disponível para conversão em T₃ (o hormônio ativo). O diagnóstico de HTF pode ser confirmado pela mensuração das concentrações séricas de T₄L, uma vez que o teste é validado para gatos. O T₄L apresenta alta sensibilidade para HTF, sendo positivo em mais de 98% dos gatos com HTF.[50] É possível que o achado mais importante seja o aumento das concentrações séricas de T₄L em 95% dos gatos com hipertireoidismo oculto.[50] Mesmo que a sensibilidade do T₄L pareça ser maior do que a do T₄t, não é recomendado como teste de triagem diagnóstica de primeira linha para HTF, em razão da baixa especificidade e do valor preditivo positivo baixo. Até 12% dos gatos com doença não tireoidiana apresentam aumento das concentrações séricas de T₄L, indicando que determinada aferição de T₄L pode ser interpretada apenas no contexto dos sinais clínicos e resultados de urinálise, hemograma, perfil bioquímico sérico e T₄t.[49,52]

Além de sua menor especificidade, os testes de T₄L tendem a ser caros e as metodologias dos exames podem ser controversas. Existem muitos tipos de ensaios utilizados para T₄L, devendo-se utilizar métodos de exames corretos. Basicamente, existem dois tipos gerais de testes para T₄L. No ensaio de uma etapa, o T₄L é mensurado no plasma ou soro na presença de T₄ ligado à proteína. No ensaio de duas etapas, técnicas como as de diálise ou ultracentrifugação são utilizadas para separar o T₄L da amostra no primeiro passo, com a utilização, então, de um teste altamente sensível para T₄L. Ao mesmo tempo em que o método de diálise de equilíbrio para avaliação do T₄L é válido, são escassos os estudos publicados para embasar a recomendação de que somente esse tipo de ensaio deva ser utilizado.

Uso combinado de T₄ total e livre

Embora um estudo tenha indicado que a combinação de T₄t e T₄L séricos não melhorou a acurácia diagnóstica quando comparado a qualquer um dos testes utilizados isoladamente,[53] a combinação pode ainda ser útil em alguns indivíduos. Gatos com doença não tireoidiana e aumento do T₄L supostamente apresentarão baixa concentração sérica de T₄t, ao passo que aqueles com HTF oculto manifestarão, em teoria, aumento do T₄L e T₄t normal ou no limite superior. Entretanto, concentrações de T₄t abaixo do ponto médio dos valores de referência foram relatadas em gatos com HTF oculto.[51]

TSH sérico

Em uma série de gatos com HTF e DRC, as concentrações séricas de TSH estavam baixas em todos eles.[54] Os valores de

TSH são utilizados para descrever o "hipertireoidismo subclínico" em gatos também.[3,55] No HTF subclínico, as concentrações basais séricas de hormônios tireoidianos, incluindo T_4L, estão normais, enquanto o TSH sérico está baixo. Gatos com essa constelação de resultados hormonais possuem maior probabilidade de evidências histológicas de hiperplasia nodular e/ou adenoma da glândula tireoide.[55] É mais provável que esses gatos desenvolvam HTF dentro de um período mais curto do que aqueles com concentrações séricas normais de TSH.[3] Entretanto, não há ampla disponibilidade de ensaios confiáveis para mensuração de TSH felino. Utilizam-se ensaios para TSH canino, mas, ao se empregar TSH felino recombinante, o teste canino detecta $\leq 40\%$ do TSH felino, dificultando a interpretação de concentrações baixas.[56] O achado de resultados aumentados de TSH sérico pode ser mais útil, pois pode indicar hipotireoidismo iatrogênico após tratamento de hipertireoidismo.[57]

Teste de supressão por T_3

Indicações

Em gatos com sinais clínicos de HTF, mas com resultados equivocados de hormônios tireoidianos basais, pode-se utilizar o teste de supressão por T_3.[58,59] Gatos com HTF podem ter nódulos tireoidianos autonomamente funcionais que secretam hormônios tireoidianos, seja qual for o controle hipofisário. Dessa forma, espera-se que a secreção hipofisária de TSH seja cronicamente suprimida. Em gatos normais, a administração de T_3 exógeno suprime a secreção hipofisária de TSH e, em seguida, causa queda na concentração sérica de T_4t. Em gatos com HTF, entretanto, a administração de T_3 exógeno possui pouco ou nenhum efeito sobre as concentrações séricas de T_4t. O teste de supressão por T_3 diferencia de forma confiável gatos com hipertireoidismo oculto daqueles com função tireoidiana normal. O teste demora 2 dias para ficar pronto e exige duas visitas hospitalares para coleta de sangue, o que pode ser inconveniente.

Protocolo e interpretação

O sangue é coletado e o soro, separado e armazenado congelado ou refrigerado antes da administração de 7 doses de T_3 (liotironina sódica). No início do dia após coleta inicial de sangue, o T_3 é administrado (25 µg/gato/8 h por via oral (VO), durante 2 dias). Na manhã do dia 3, o gato é submetido à sétima dose de T_3 e, então, retorna à clínica para coleta de amostra de sangue pós-T_3. Tanto as amostras pré como pós-T_3 são avaliadas para T_4t e T_3t com os mesmos ensaios a fim de mitigar a variação intratestes. Se os tutores tiverem conseguido administrar o T_3, a concentração sérica de T_3t será maior na segunda amostra (a única razão para mensuração do T_3t). Em gatos saudáveis, as concentrações séricas de T_4t são suprimidas pelo T_3 exógeno, ao passo que em gatos com HTF decréscimos no T_4t sérico são discretos ou ausentes. Existe pouca ou nenhuma sobreposição entre as concentrações séricas de T_4t pós-T_3 ao se comparar gatos eutireóideos e hipertireóideos. O teste de supressão por T_3 pode ser valioso para o diagnóstico de HTF em gatos com resultados normais de testes de hormônios tireoidianos basais.

Teste de estimulação por hormônio liberador de tireotrofina

Quando administrado por via intravenosa (IV) a gatos saudáveis, o TRH causa aumentos consistentes nas concentrações séricas de T_4t, em geral de duas vezes. Em gatos com HTF, a elevação pós-TRH é discreta ou ausente, tornando o exame uma ferramenta potencialmente útil para o diagnóstico de HTF oculto.[60] Esse teste é realizado pela mensuração das concentrações séricas de T_4t antes e 4 h depois da administração por via intravenosa de TRH (0,1 mg/kg); gatos normais e aqueles com HTF apresentam elevação no $T_4t > 60\%$ e $< 50\%$, respectivamente.[60] Ao mesmo tempo que esse exame pode ser utilizado para o diagnóstico de HTF em gatos com concentrações séricas de T_4t

normais em repouso, ele possui desvantagens significativas. Embora disponível em alguns países, a comercialização do TRH foi banida do mercado norte-americano em 2002, não podendo o TRH utilizado em pesquisas laboratoriais ser recomendado para pacientes clínicos.[61] Um relato sugeriu acurácia diagnóstica limitada do teste de estimulação por TRH em gatos com doenças concomitantes, um grupo que pode incluir aqueles com a forma oculta de HTF.[62] A administração do TRH costuma ocasionar reações colinérgicas graves e mediadas pelo sistema nervoso central.[63-66] Dentro de segundos após a administração do TRH, em geral os gatos exibem sinais transitórios, porém graves, de salivação, taquipneia, micção, náuseas, êmese e diarreia.

Cintilografia tireoidiana

A captação pela glândula tireoide do pertecnetato ou iodo radioativo é extremamente sensível para o diagnóstico de HTF.[67] Tanto a captação tireoidiana de pertecnetato quanto a relação tireoide-glândula salivar podem ser calculadas. Ambas se correlacionam fortemente com a hipertiroxinemia. A utilização desses testes é limitada pela disponibilidade. Em estudo recente de larga escala dos resultados de cintilografia tireoidiana no HTF, quase 99% dos gatos apresentavam relação tireoide-glândula salivar $> 1,5$ quando comparados à relação daqueles saudáveis < 1 (Figura 301.4). A relação tireoide-plano de fundo é menos sensível do que a tireoide-glândula salivar. Como esses exames precisam de instalações sofisticadas, sedação e administração de um agente radioativo, a cintilografia tireoidiana não é comumente utilizada para confirmar o diagnóstico de HTF. Seu maior valor pode estar na avaliação pré-cirúrgica de gatos submetidos à tireoidectomia, pois pode ser utilizado para identificação de doença unil ou bilateral, doença ectópica, doença intratorácica, podendo levantar suspeitas de carcinoma tireoidiano.

TRATAMENTO

Contexto geral e prognóstico

Se não tratado, hipertireoidismo costuma progredir para comprometimento metabólico grave, cardiopatia e morte. Embora os tempos de sobrevida no HTF sem tratamento não tenham sido relatados, os tempos médios de sobrevida para gatos tratados com iodo radioativo variaram de 2 a mais de 5 anos (Tabela 301.3).[68-70] Embora gatas aparentemente sobrevivam por mais tempo do que machos após o tratamento para HTF, ambos podem viver por bastante tempo. O HTF pode ser tratado com fármacos antitireoidianos (tioureilenos), iodo radioativo, tireoidectomia cirúrgica ou com a eliminação de iodo da dieta (Tabela 301.4). Os efeitos colaterais estão associados a todos os tratamentos para HTF e incluem, após resolução deste, insuficiência renal e hipotireoidismo.

Tabela 301.3 Efeito da idade e do gênero no diagnóstico em taxas de sobrevida em 5 anos em gatos com hipertireoidismo.

IDADE AO DIAGNÓSTICO	GÊNERO	SOBREVIDA EM 5 ANOS (%)
10 anos	F	42
	M	28
13 anos	F	25
	M	13
16 anos	F	11
	M	4

Dados de Slater MR, Geller S, Rogers K: Long-term health and predictors of survival for hyperthyroid cats treated with iodine 131. *J Vet Intern Med* 15:47, 2001.

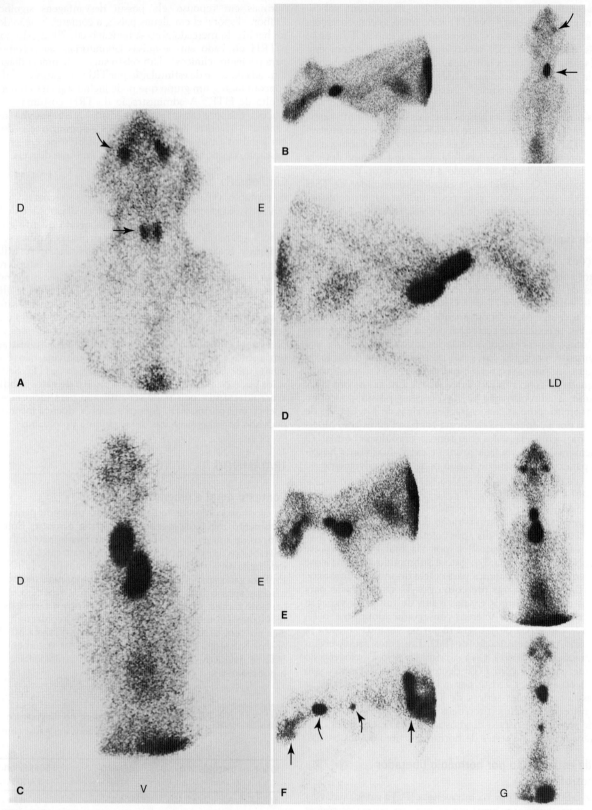

Figura 301.4 A. Varredura da tireoide (tecnécio-^{99m} [Tc^{99m}] radioativo) de um gato normal. Note o tamanho semelhante e a densidade dos lobos tireoidianos (*seta reta*) e das glândulas salivares (*seta curva*). **B.** Varredura da tireoide por Tc^{99m} de um gato com tireotoxicose e tumor tireoidiano unilateral. Note a densidade da tireoide (*seta reta*) comparada àquela das glândulas salivares (*seta curva*). **C e D.** Varredura da tireoide por Tc^{99m} de um gato com tireotoxicose e tireoides hiperfuncionais adenomatosas simétricas bilaterais. **E.** Varredura da tireoide por Tc^{99m} de um gato com tireotoxicose e tireoides hiperfuncionais adenomatosas assimétricas bilaterais. **F e G.** Projeções lateral e dorsoventral de uma varredura da tireoide por Tc^{99m} de um gato com tireotoxicose e tireoides hiperfuncionais adenomatosas assimétricas bilaterais. Note que essa varredura mostra a tireoide maior acima da menor, e não a massa maior mais comum descendendo ainda mais e em geral localizada abaixo da massa menor (C a E). **F e G.** Note a tireoide grande no pescoço (*seta curva da esquerda*); o pequeno tecido tireoidiano adenomatoso no mediastino anterior (*seta curva da direita*); as glândulas salivares e a saliva, que concentram pertecnetato (*seta reta da esquerda*); e a mucosa gástrica, que concentra pertecnetato (*seta reta da direita*). (De Feldman EC, Nelson RW, Reusch CE et al.: *Canine and feline endocrinology and reproduction*, 4 ed., St. Louis, 2015, Saunders.)

CAPÍTULO 301 • Hipertireoidismo Felino

Tabela 301.4 Comparação das considerações terapêuticas para hipertireoidismo felino.

	FÁRMACOS TIOUREILENOS	IODO RADIOATIVO	TIREOIDECTOMIA
Custo inicial	Baixo	Alto	Alto
Custo a longo prazo	Moderado	Baixo	Baixo
Anestesia	Jamais	Algumas vezes	Sempre
Facilidade de uso	Fácil	Moderada	Difícil
Recorrência	Comum	Rara	Moderada
Tempo para eutireoidismo	2 a 4 semanas	Imediato	2 a 4 semanas
Hospitalização	Nenhuma	3 a 10 dias	1 a 3 dias
Discrasias sanguíneas	Raras	Jamais	Jamais
Hipocalcemia	Jamais	Jamais	Comum
Reações adversas gastrintestinais	Comuns	Jamais	Jamais

Fármacos antitireoidianos tioureilenos

Ação

O metimazol é o fármaco mais comumente utilizado para o tratamento do HTF, estando disponível e aprovado para utilização em gatos nos EUA, ao passo que, tanto o metimazol como o carbimazol, um "profármaco" do metimazol, estão aprovados para uso na Europa. Um terceiro fármaco antitireoidiano, propiltiouracila, está disponível, mas raramente é utilizado em razão de relatos iniciais de anemia hemolítica e trombocitopenia.[71,72] Tioureilenos inibem as tireoperoxidases das células foliculares tireoidianas, dificultando a iodação de resíduos tirosil na tireoglobulina e o acoplamento dos resíduos tirosil em T_4 e T_3. Esses fármacos diminuem a produção do hormônio tireoidiano, acabam com os estoques celulares foliculares de hormônio préfabricado, diminuem as concentrações circulantes de hormônio tireoidiano e revertem a tireotoxicose.

Administração oral

Como o grau de tireotoxicose varia de paciente para paciente, fármacos antitireoidianos devem ser ajustados de acordo com as necessidades individuais.[73] A dose inicial recomendada de metimazol é de aproximadamente 2,5 mg/gato/12 h, VO. O carbimazol, disponível em formulação de liberação prolongada, é iniciado a 10 ou 15 mg VO, 1 vez/dia. Ajustes de dose devem se basear na resposta ao tratamento. Caso a dose do fármaco antitireoidiano tenha sido adequada, o eutireoidismo deve retornar dentro de 2 a 3 semanas. Confere-se à maioria dos gatos a dose de 2,5 mg/12 h, VO, de metimazol; doses eficazes relatadas variaram de 2,5 a 20 mg/dia para o metimazol e 10 a 20 mg/dia para o carbimazol de liberação prolongada. De forma geral, as doses devem ser ajustadas para alcançar uma concentração sérica basal de T_4t que esteja dentro ou abaixo do meio do intervalo de referência para T_4t. Não existe resolução consistente dos sinais clínicos em gatos tratados com metimazol com concentrações séricas de T_4 no limite superior.[74] Embora alguns pesquisadores tenham sugerido que doses maiores de metimazol, 1 vez/dia, possam ser substituídas pelo protocolo recomendado a cada 12 horas, o metimazol, quando administrado 1 vez/dia, não é tão efetivo.[75]

Transdérmico

Embora os fármacos antitireoidianos orais sejam, em geral, bem tolerados pelos gatos e pelos tutores que precisam administrar os comprimidos, alguns animais não podem ser tratados dessa forma,[76] uma vez que alguns gatos apresentam reações adversas gastrintestinais e alguns tutores são incapazes de administrar a medicação. Em tais casos, o metimazol transdérmico pode ser utilizado.[77,78] Formulações transdérmicas são tipicamente produzidas por farmácias de manipulação, devendo-se haver o cuidado

Tabela 301.5 Frequência de reações adversas suspeitas com risco de morte ao metimazol.

	METIMAZOL ORAL (%)	METIMAZOL TRANSDÉRMICO (%)
Hepatopatia	2,6	4
Diátese hemorrágica	2,5	Não relatada
Trombocitopenia	2,8	8
Agranulocitose	2,7	6,1

Outras reações adversas suspeitas relatadas incluem relatos de caso de miastenia *gravis* e anemia aplásica. (Adaptada de Daminet S, Kooistra HS, Fracassi F *et al.*: Best practice for the pharmacological management of hyperthyroid cats with antithyroid drugs. *J Small Anim Pract* 55:4, 2014.)

para garantir a qualidade e a consistência (ver Capítulo 168). Doses efetivas de metimazol transdérmico não diferem de maneira significativa das formulações orais, com a observação de algumas considerações. Antes de tudo, existem evidências que sugerem maior tempo para alcançar o eutireoidismo (4 semanas) com o metimazol transdérmico.[78] É razoável, portanto, iniciar o monitoramento de T_4t posteriormente. Ademais, tutores devem ser aconselhados a utilizar luvas ao administrar o metimazol transdérmico, a fim de evitar contato com a pele. O metimazol é muito mais potente em pessoas do que em gatos, já o metimazol transdérmico é altamente eficaz para o tratamento de pessoas com hipertireoide, o que faz com que mesmo quantidades pequenas possam ter alguma consequência sobre o tutor.[79] A resposta ao metimazol transdérmico é menos consistente do que com o fármaco oral para alcançar as concentrações séricas de T_4t dentro do intervalo de referência.[80]

Reações adversas graves

Reações adversas indesejadas são comuns ao tratar gatos com fármacos antitireoidianos. Como algumas delas podem causar risco de morte (Tabela 301.5), é importante, a princípio, monitorar os gatos de perto. Em geral, as reações adversas ocorrem dentro dos 3 primeiros meses após o início do tratamento, período esse recomendado para monitorar os gatos de perto.[74] Reações adversas com risco de morte incluem agranulocitose, trombocitopenia, hepatopatia grave e hemorragia não associada à trombocitopenia. Se ocorrer alguma dessas reações, o fármaco antitireoidiano utilizado deve ser interrompido imediatamente. A taxa de mortalidade por essas reações adversas ao fármaco é alta. Essas reações adversas graves observadas após terapia com metimazol não são relatadas com o carbimazol, mas elas ainda podem ocorrer. Faz pouco sentido que os perfis de reações adversas possam ser muito

SEÇÃO 21 • Doenças Endócrinas

diferentes entre os dois medicamentos, pois o carbimazol é metabolizado em metimazol a fim de exercer seu efeito terapêutico. É importante também notar que, ao mesmo tempo que as reações adversas gastrintestinais são menos comuns em gatos tratados pela via transdérmica, o risco de reações adversas com risco de morte certamente não é amenizado pela troca da terapia oral para transdérmica, o que pode até ser pior. Nenhum estudo coeso comparando as reações adversas dos fármacos antitireoidianos designados aleatoriamente para tratar HTF foi concluído, de forma que é difícil comparar esses fármacos.

Reações adversas comuns e discretas

As reações adversas mais comuns observadas com fármacos antitireoidianos não causam risco de morte, mas podem ser razões para a falha terapêutica (Tabela 301.6). Sinais gastrintestinais, incluindo náuseas, êmese, letargia e diarreia, são comuns. O carbimazol aparentemente apresenta maior risco de efeitos colaterais gastrintestinais.[73] Leucopenia, eosinofilia e linfocitose foram observadas. Essas alterações devem ser monitoradas, já que, em geral, cessam apesar da continuação do tratamento. A leucopenia discreta observada após o uso de tioureileno pode ser preocupante, pelo receio de agranulocitose, mas a interrupção do tratamento costuma não ser necessária. Escoriação em face, uma reação grave sem risco de morte, é observada em alguns gatos tratados com fármacos antitireoidianos. Considera-se que gatos provavelmente sofram de prurido facial como reação farmacológica, já que eles se arranham em excesso, provocando feridas passíveis de sangramento na face, na cabeça e no pescoço. Essa reação adversa ao fármaco exige a interrupção do tratamento com o medicamento antitireoidiano. Quando um fármaco antitireoidiano, que provoca reações adversas, mas não causa risco de morte, precisa ser interrompido, não há como se prever reações posteriores com o fármaco.

Comprometimento do tutor

Uma das principais desvantagens da utilização do metimazol ou do carbimazol para o manejo a longo prazo do HTF é a necessidade do comprometimento prolongado por parte do tutor. Como os fármacos antitireoidianos não "curam" a condição clínica, eles devem ser administrados durante toda a vida do gato, o que pode ser difícil para alguns tutores. Além disso, a doença tende a avançar apesar do tratamento com medicamentos antitireoidianos, o que, em geral, exige o aumento na dose do fármaco com o passar do tempo, a fim de manter o eutireoidismo. Embora as razões não sejam claras, um estudo indicou que gatos tratados somente com metimazol apresentaram menos da metade da sobrevida média quando comparados àqueles tratados com iodo radioativo ou aos tratados, a princípio, com metimazol e, eventualmente, com iodo radioativo.[69] Isso pode não ter nada a ver com o tratamento, mas sim com a condição dos gatos e os meios financeiros dos tutores ao selecionar o tratamento.

Iodo radioativo

Visão geral

A utilização do iodo radioativo (^{131}I) pode ser o tratamento de escolha para HTF.[70,81] Hormônios tireoidianos e tireoglobulina são as únicas moléculas orgânicas iodadas no corpo, de forma que qualquer iodo ingerido ou injetado é recolhido pelo simporte sódio-iodeto das células epiteliais foliculares tireoidianas. Assim, isótopos radioativos de iodo estão concentrados na glândula tireoide, onde suas partículas beta exercem lesão tecidual local significativa, destruindo o tecido tireoidiano hiperativo. O tecido normal adjacente pode certamente também ser afetado, mas o iodo radioativo é administrado em doses que têm por objetivo alcançar o eutireoidismo.

Dose, protocolo e reações adversas

Diversos métodos são utilizados para o cálculo da dose do iodo radioativo necessário para tratar o HTF. A utilização de estudos cinéticos sobre traços de iodo radioativo é o método mais complexo para determinação da dose. Alguns clínicos utilizam uma dose fixa de ^{131}I para todos os gatos, tipicamente de 4 a 5 mCi. Um terceiro método para determinação da dose de iodo radioativo utiliza uma rubrica de pontuação que emprega tamanho da glândula tireoide, sinais clínicos e T_4t sérico.[70] Nenhum método apresenta uma vantagem clara. Diferentes métodos para administração de iodo radioativo incluem as vias intravenosa, subcutânea e oral.[81] É comum que gatos com HTF sejam tratados com terapia farmacológica antitireoidiana antes da escolha da terapia por iodo radioativo. Os radioterapeutas frequentemente recomendam que a utilização do metimazol seja descontinuada por um período específico antes da administração do iodo radioativo, mas essa prática é questionável. Em um relato de preditivos de resposta para a terapia por iodo radioativo, não houve diferença nos resultados do tratamento ao comparar gatos cujo metimazol foi retirado 5 dias antes ou depois antes do tratamento.[82] Outras reações adversas à terapia por iodo radioativo, que não a insuficiência renal após o tratamento e, algumas vezes, o hipotireoidismo, são raras. Disfagia transitória, provavelmente decorrente da inflamação induzida pela radiação na glândula tireoide, raramente foi relatada.[70]

A escolha do paciente é importante ao considerar a terapia por iodo radioativo, cuja maioria dos gatos tolera sem problemas. Como esses animais ficarão alojados em ambiente isolado por motivos de segurança pela radiação, gatos com condições médicas concomitantes que necessitem de observação ou tratamentos frequentes são candidatos ruins, assim como aqueles que sofrem de ansiedade extrema decorrente da separação da família. O período de hospitalização para gatos submetidos à terapia por iodo radioativo costuma variar de 3 a 10 dias, dependendo das exigências individuais de licenciamento nas dependências de radiação da instituição.

Tireoidectomia cirúrgica

Quando realizada por um cirurgião hábil e experiente, os resultados da tireoidectomia cirúrgica costumam ser satisfatórios para a resolução permanente do HTF com poucas complicações (Figura 301.5).[16] As complicações cirúrgicas incluíram hipocalcemia transitória (em razão da remoção ou lesão das glândulas paratireoides ou de sua irrigação sanguínea) em 6% dos gatos e morte dentro de 3 dias após a cirurgia em 3%. O desenvolvimento de hipocalcemia é a razão mais importante para monitorar gatos durante 2 a 3 dias no período pós-cirúrgico no

---

Tabela 301.6 Frequência de reações adversas suspeitas sem risco de morte ao metimazol e ao carbimazol.

	METIMAZOL ORAL (%)	METIMAZOL TRANSDÉRMICO (%)	CARBIMAZOL ORAL (%)
Sinais gastrintestinais (êmese, anorexia)	22	3,7	33
Anomalidades hematológicas discretas (leucopenia, eosinofilia, linfocitose)	16,4	Não relatadas	34,9
Escoriações faciais	4	8	11,6

Adaptada de Daminet S, Kooistra HS, Fracassi F et al.: Best practice for the pharmacological management of hyperthyroid cats with antithyroid drugs. J Small Anim Pract 55:4, 2014.

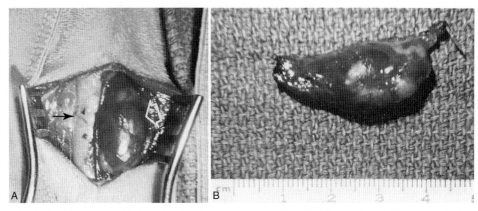

Figura 301.5 A. Fotografia da tireoide (*seta vazada*) durante a cirurgia em um gato com hipertireoidismo unilateral. Note a traqueia (*seta sólida*). **B.** O adenoma solitário após completa excisão. (De Feldman EC, Nelson RW: *Canine and feline endocrinology and reproduction*, 3 ed., St. Louis, 2004, Saunders.)

hospital. Se ocorrer hipocalcemia, ela é tratada com suplementação de cálcio e vitamina D (ver Capítulo 298), sendo quase sempre transitória. Um argumento contrário à tireoidectomia cirúrgica como tratamento do HTF é o risco anestésico. Portanto, quase sempre se recomenda que, antes da tireoidectomia cirúrgica, os gatos sejam tratados com fármacos antitireoidianos, a fim de alcançar o eutireoidismo. Ao mesmo tempo que é lógico, não existem relatos que suportem essa recomendação.

Manejo dietético

Contexto geral

Uma dieta restrita em iodo para o tratamento do HTF (ração úmida) está disponível no mercado. O iodo é necessário para a produção do hormônio tireoidiano. Espera-se que a restrição estrita do iodo da dieta reduza as concentrações do hormônio tireoidiano. Dados iniciais sobre a eficácia dessa dieta estiveram disponíveis apenas na forma de resumo, de autoria do fabricante, o que levantou questões quanto à efetividade dela para o controle da hipertiroxinemia e seus sinais clínicos. Houve questões também sobre as possíveis reações adversas da deficiência de iodo em gatos. Um estudo prospectivo não controlado, financiado pelo fabricante da dieta, fornece respostas a algumas dessas questões.[83]

Eficácia

Muitos gatos com HTF, alguns anteriormente tratados com uma modalidade diferente e alguns recém-diagnosticados, foram alimentados com uma dieta restrita em iodo durante 8 semanas em um estudo recente. Os sinais clínicos do HTF, conforme relatado por tutores ou clínicos de atendimento primário, melhoraram de maneira significativa na quarta semana de manejo dietético. Nenhum efeito adverso foi observado. Concentrações séricas de T$_4$t diminuíram para o intervalo de referência em 68% dos gatos na quarta semana e em 75% dos gatos na oitava semana. As concentrações séricas de T$_4$t, entretanto, permaneceram na faixa superior do intervalo de referência. Relações entre o limite superior da concentração normal do T$_4$t e valor mensurado foram de 0,91 e 0,69 na quarta e oitava semanas, respectivamente. Alguns poderiam considerar questionável que o hipertireoidismo clínico seria resolvido quando as concentrações de T$_4$t permanecessem no limite superior do intervalo de referência. Gatos apresentam reversão dos sinais de forma mais consistente, por exemplo, quando as concentrações séricas de T$_4$t pós-metimazol estiverem na metade inferior do intervalo normal.[74] Um resultado irrefutável, com base no estudo de van der Kooij *et al.*, é de que não houve diminuição das concentrações séricas de creatinina ou ureia nitrogenada nos gatos alimentados com a dieta restrita em iodo. Isso poderia ter implicações importantes para gatos que desenvolvem insuficiência renal após o tratamento do hipertireoidismo; de maneira controversa, ela poderia ser visualizada como evidência adicional de que a terapia dietética não foi efetiva.

Recomendação

Se uma dieta restrita em iodo for escolhida para tratar o HTF, os seguintes pontos devem ser levados em consideração. Primeiro, como pouco iodo é necessário para manter a função tireoidiana, pode-se oferecer apenas uma dieta restrita em iodo. Todos os outros alimentos, petiscos ou presas capturadas provavelmente teriam teor de iodo suficiente para contrabalançar os efeitos da dieta. Segundo, gatos com HTF em abrigos com vários animais devem ser alimentados à parte ou todos, sem exceção, com a dieta restrita em iodo. Em gatos normais ou hipertireóideos, não foram relatados possíveis efeitos deletérios da restrição de iodo a longo prazo.

Outras terapias

Diversas outras terapias foram descritas para hipertireoidismo felino. Estudou-se o tratamento não cirúrgico de nódulos tireoidianos pela utilização de ablação pelo calor por radiofrequência percutânea guiada pelo ultrassom ou injeção intratireoidiana de etanol.[84-86] Essas técnicas apresentam eficácia e segurança questionáveis, não sendo, portanto, recomendadas. O ácido iopanoico, um agente de contraste administrado por via oral utilizado na colecistografia, foi avaliado até certo grau para a utilização no tratamento do HTF. Ao mesmo tempo que pode diminuir as concentrações séricas do hormônio tireoidiano, a utilização a longo prazo não é recomendada em razão do efeito transitório do fármaco.[87]

INSUFICIÊNCIA RENAL PÓS-TRATAMENTO

Visão geral

A maioria dos gatos tratados para hipertireoidismo eventualmente desenvolve doença renal crônica (DRC; ver Capítulo 324) e morre de insuficiência renal.[68,69] Neles, o tratamento do HTF pode ter efeito deletério sobre a função renal, provavelmente porque o HTF pode mascarar a DRC subjacente preexistente.[88-93] O tratamento do HTF, seja qual for a modalidade, causa queda consistente, e algumas vezes desastrosa, da TFG e desenvolvimento de DRC evidente. Estimativas da prevalência de DRC após tratamento do HTF variam: em um estudo, foi de 15% durante um período de 8 meses e, em outro, de 60% durante um período de 6 meses.[93,94]

Previsão da insuficiência renal pós-tratamento

Os parâmetros clínicos pré-tratamento que poderiam ajudar a prever o desenvolvimento de insuficiência renal pós-tratamento no HTF não são convincentes.[93,95] Existe uma convicção comum de que gatos com urina bem concentrada (densidade específica > 1,035) possuem função renal adequada e menor risco de insuficiência renal pós-tratamento,[96,97] o que não é embasado por evidências. Em um relato, 20 gatos com HTF que desenvolveram insuficiência renal evidente dentro de 6 meses após o tratamento com iodo radioativo foram comparados a 19 gatos no período pós-tratamento, nos quais não ocorreu insuficiência renal evidente.[95] Dez dos vinte gatos que desenvolveram azotemia (50%) tinham mensurações de densidade específica urinária antes do tratamento maiores que 1,035. Três desses gatos tinham mensurações de densidade específica acima de 1,050. Portanto, a densidade específica urinária não deve ser utilizada como um preditivo do estado renal pós-tratamento em gatos hipertireóideos.

Pode ser imprudente tratar o hipertireoidismo em um gato com função renal questionável. Isso levou à recomendação de que gatos com problemas na função renal sejam, a princípio, tratados com metimazol, pois seus efeitos podem ser reversíveis. Um estudo mostrou diminuições consistentes na TFG após tratamento com metimazol para HTF. A reversão desse efeito foi notada quando a terapia com metimazol foi interrompida em um gato.[89] Ao mesmo tempo que parece lógico escolher um tratamento reversível para HTF e avaliar a resposta renal à terapia antes do tratamento com iodo radioativo ou cirurgia, não existem estudos que confirmem os benefícios dessa estratégia. Quando a insuficiência renal é diagnosticada em um gato previamente tratado para HTF, os clínicos devem tentar balancear os tratamentos para HTF e insuficiência renal.

Tratamento da insuficiência renal pós-tratamento

Clínicos que tratam gatos com insuficiência renal evidente após tratamento para HTF podem considerar a suplementação por hormônio tireoidiano como meio de restaurar o fluxo sanguíneo renal e aumentar a TFG. Existem evidências que sugerem que o hipotireoidismo iatrogênico contribui para o desenvolvimento de insuficiência renal após tratamento para HTF.[93] Naquele estudo, o desenvolvimento de azotemia não afetou os tempos de sobrevida de gatos eutireóideos após tratamento de HTF. Entretanto, gatos tanto hipotireóideos quanto azotêmicos após o tratamento do HTF sobreviveram por um período mais curto, sugerindo que o hipotireoidismo iatrogênico poderia contribuir para o desenvolvimento da azotemia em gatos tratados para HTF.

Como o hipotireoidismo iatrogênico foi associado à diminuição da sobrevida e da azotemia em gatos com HTF, foram estudados os efeitos renais da redução de doses de carbimazol ou metimazol para alcançar o eutireoidismo.[94] A restauração do eutireoidismo foi acompanhada por diminuição nas concentrações séricas e do peso corporal e incrementos de frequência cardíaca, hematócrito e atividades séricas de fosfatase alcalina. Assim, a diminuição na massa muscular pode ter contribuído para o declínio das concentrações séricas de creatinina. As outras alterações são compatíveis com HTF descontrolado. Em um estudo não publicado, acompanhamos gatos tratados com tiroxina após insuficiência renal pós-tratamento e observamos resultados desencorajadores. O tratamento com tiroxina resultou em aumento na concentração de T_4t no soro, conforme esperado, mas não houve diminuição significativa nos teores de nitrogênio ureico sanguíneo ou da creatinina. O peso e a condição corporal permaneceram inalterados em nosso pequeno grupo de gatos.

REFERÊNCIAS BIBLIOGRÁFICAS

As referências bibliográficas deste capítulo se encontram online no Ambiente de Aprendizagem.

CAPÍTULO 302

Hipertireoidismo Canino

Cynthia R. Ward

Diferentemente do observado em gatos, o hipertireoidismo é uma condição clínica incomum em cães, que quase sempre surge de um tumor tireoidiano funcional e maligno que secreta hormônio tireoidiano em excesso. Em geral, tumores tireoidianos são massas cervicais facilmente palpáveis. Não é comum que o fornecimento de dietas cruas que contenham tecido glandular tireoide cause hipertireoidismo clínico.

PATOGÊNESE

Câncer tireoidiano de ocorrência natural

O câncer tireoidiano apresenta prevalência de 1 a 4% de todas as neoplasias relatadas em cães e é o tumor neuroendócrino mais comum. Tumores tireoidianos caninos costumam ser malignos. Dez a trinta por cento dos tumores tireoidianos caninos são adenomas benignos.[1,2] Adenomas tipicamente pequenos e não funcionais, em geral, não são diagnosticados até que observados como um achado acidental de necropsia. Entretanto, com o aumento da utilização da ultrassonografia cervical, são notadas massas tireoidianas descobertas por acaso.[41] O tamanho não é um fator preditivo de malignidade.[1] Tumores tireoidianos de maior relevância clínica são carcinomas, sejam de origem de células foliculares, sejam de células medulares; estes também denominados carcinomas de *células parafoliculares* ou de *células-C*. Carcinomas de células foliculares – que compõem aproximadamente 70% dos tumores tireoidianos caninos – surgem de células foliculares da tireoide coradas para tireoglobulina na imunoistoquímica. Carcinomas tireoidianos medulares – que compõem aproximadamente 30% dos tumores – surgem de células parafoliculares produtoras de calcitonina e são coradas para anticorpos contra calcitonina na imunoistoquímica.[3-5]

Hipertireoidismo iatrogênico

Os sinais clínicos de hipertireoidismo podem ser observados em cães sem doença primária da glândula tireoide. O hipertireoidismo iatrogênico pode ocorrer quando um cão é suplementado em excesso com levotiroxina para tratamento do hipotireoidismo ou por ingestão acidental. De forma geral, cães parecem resistentes à manifestação de sinais de hipertireoidismo caso haja pouco excesso de hormônio tireoidiano exógeno. Relatos recentes implicaram fontes alimentares, incluindo alimentos crus ou dietas desidratadas não cozidas que contenham tecido tireoidiano, como causa de tireotoxicose em cães.[6,7] Os cães descritos nesses estudos apresentavam sinais clínicos de hipertireoidismo, que foram resolvidos quando da remoção do alimento suspeito.

Papel do hormônio tireoestimulante no desenvolvimento tumoral

A etiologia do carcinoma tireoidiano canino é desconhecida. Em seres humanos, os fatores de risco incluem exposição à radiação e ausência de ingestão dietética de iodo.[8] Indivíduos que sofrem com a falta de iodo na dieta ou que consomem alimentos que o bloqueiam apresentam diminuição do *feedback* negativo hipofisário e excesso de secreção de hormônio tireoestimulante (TSH, do inglês *thyroid stimulating hormone*) (ver Capítulo 299). O TSH estimula diretamente a mitogênese de células tireoidianas, síntese hormonal, e foi postulado como envolvido na transformação neoplásica tireoidiana (Figura 302.1). Outras evidências do excesso da atividade de TSH causadoras do desenvolvimento de neoplasias tireoidianas são as mutações no receptor de TSH, que mostraram causar bócio nodular tóxico benigno em seres humanos.[9] Ademais, o aumento das concentrações de TSH mostrou induzir angiogênese em linhagens de células neoplásicas tireoidianas, o que pode ser relevante para o desenvolvimento do tumor de tireoide em cães.[10] Aproximadamente 50% dos cães da raça Beagle com tireoidite linfocítica induzida e não tratada e aumento das concentrações de TSH desenvolveram tumores tireoidianos. Os carcinomas foram mais comuns que os adenomas.[11] Assim, a exposição crônica ao excesso de TSH pode causar desregulação do crescimento e função celulares em cães. Uma relação familiar no desenvolvimento do carcinoma tireoidiano também foi mostrada na colônia de cães Beagle pela análise de pares de irmãos.

Etiologia genética do desenvolvimento tumoral

Diversas anormalidades genéticas nas proteínas de transdução do sinal celular foram descritas como agentes causadores do carcinoma tireoidiano humano. Estas incluem mutações pontuais no gene *ras* e anormalidades na via PI3 K/Akt (ver Figura 302.1). Essas vias de transdução de sinal são acopladas aos receptores de superfície tirosinoquinase e receptores acoplados à proteína G, como o receptor de TSH. No carcinoma de células foliculares humano, anormalidades na via PI3 K/Akt foram implicadas.[12] Genes importantes nessa via são os fatores de crescimento endotelial vascular *VEGFR-1* e *VEGFR-2*. O fator de crescimento endotelial vascular (VEGF, do inglês *vascular endothelial growth fator*) é um alvo para ativação da angiogênese pelo TSH nas linhagens de células neoplásicas tireoidianas.[13] Em 74 cães com neoplasia tireoidiana, a coloração imunoistoquímica revelou VEGF em carcinomas de células foliculares e medulares, embasando o papel de fator angiogênico no desenvolvimento do carcinoma tireoidiano.[14] Uma vez que as células do carcinoma tireoidiano canino se ligam ao TSH de maneira normal, isso pode explicar o efeito da exposição crônica ao excesso de TSH, ao contribuir para a transformação neoplásica observada em cães de uma colônia de cães da raça Beagle.[11,15]

Estudos de anormalidades genéticas em moléculas de sinalização em células tumorais caninas são limitados. Foram observadas mutações pontuais de p53, um gene supressor tumoral, em apenas 1 de 23 cães com carcinoma tireoidiano.[13] Em 59 daqueles com essa condição, a expressão de mRNA de diversos genes na via PI3 K/Akt foi maior do que daqueles no tecido tireoidiano canino normal.[16] Ademais, foram documentadas mutações *missense* do K-RAS que causariam ativação desregulada. A análise de microarranjo, ao comparar expressão genética do tumor tireoidiano e tireoide normal em cães, identificou expressões diferenciais de osteopontina, uma proteína expressa em excesso em carcinomas de células foliculares em seres humanos e implicada na ativação da via PI3 K/Akt. Isso foi observado em todos os 5 cães com tumores tireoidianos, mas também em 4 eutireóideos.[17] Anormalidades moleculares nas vias mitogênicas são um componente provável da patogênese do carcinoma tireoidiano canino.

EPIDEMIOLOGIA

A idade média de cães com carcinoma tireoidiano varia de 9 a 11 anos.[3,18-22] Um estudo sugeriu que a idade mediana pode, de certa forma, ser maior: dos 10 aos 15 anos.[2] Não existe predileção sexual. Raças que podem ser predispostas ao carcinoma tireoidiano incluem cães Golden Retriever, Beagle, Boxer e Husky Siberiano.[2,3] Foram relatados carcinomas tireoidianos medulares em uma família de cães sem raça definida com influência do Malamute do Alasca na linhagem.[23]

HISTÓRICO CLÍNICO

A queixa principal inicial para a maioria dos cães com carcinoma tireoidiano é a descoberta de um tumor cervical pelo tutor. A maioria dos animais é diagnosticada dentro de 1 a 2 meses após a descoberta dele; entretanto, pode haver atrasos de 1 a 2 anos.[37] À palpação, tumores tireoidianos costumam ser firmes, indolores, móveis ou fixos. A "mobilidade" é um fator importante não só no estadiamento do tumor, mas também para a previsão do sucesso cirúrgico (Tabela 302.1). Tanto o lobo tireoidiano direito

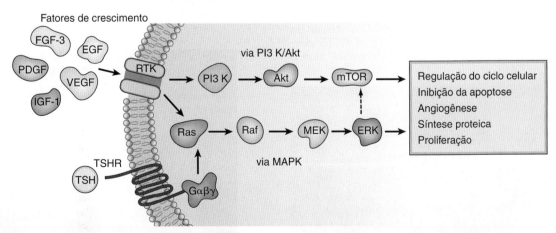

Figura 302.1 Visão geral simplificada da via de sinalização PI3 K/Akt/mTOR. Em geral, a suprarregulação dessa via é observada em células tumorais e, supostamente, tem papel na patogênese do carcinoma tireoidiano canino. *EGF*, fator de crescimento epidérmico; *ERK*, quinase regulada por sinal extracelular; *FGF-3*, fator de crescimento de fibroblastos-3; *IGF-1*, fator de crescimento semelhante à insulina-1; *MAPK*, proteinoquinase ativada por mitógeno; *MEK*, quinase MAPK/ERK; *mTOR*, alvo da rapamicina mecânico (ou mamífero); *PDGF*, fator de crescimento derivado de plaquetas; *PI3 K*, fosfoinositídeo quinase-3; *RTK*, receptor tirosinoquinase; *TSH*, hormônio tireoestimulante; *TSHR*, receptor de TSH; *VEGF*, fator de crescimento endotelial vascular. (Ilustração por Katie Yost, MS. ©2015 The University of Georgia Research Foundation, Inc.)

como o esquerdo podem estar envolvidos igualmente no desenvolvimento tumoral, podendo os tumores ser bilaterais.[19,21] A sedação pode ajudar na palpação completa da área, mas, em geral, não é necessária. Linfonodos periféricos regionais devem também ser palpados com cuidado em busca de aumento do tamanho ou dor. Pode haver suspeita de carcinomas tireoidianos ectópicos se visualizado um edema indolor em qualquer localização desde a língua até a entrada torácica.[39]

A maioria dos carcinomas tireoidianos não é funcional. Os sinais clínicos, portanto, estão em geral associados à ocupação do espaço pelo tumor. Estes incluem dificuldade de deglutição, disfonia, tosse, dispneia ou edema reconhecível de cabeça ou membro torácico.[3,18,24] A dispneia também pode ocorrer em razão da disseminação do tumor metastático para os pulmões. Foi relatado que carcinomas tireoidianos invadem os principais vasos sanguíneos, o que causa hemorragia local e torácica.[25] Carcinomas tireoidianos ectópicos foram relatados no mediastino, na base do coração e na região sublingual; portanto, os sinais clínicos podem estar relacionados com o tamanho tumoral nessas áreas ou a invasão desses tecidos.[26-33] Em cães, a condição do hormônio tireoidiano pode variar com carcinoma tireoidiano; aproximadamente 10% são hipertireóideos.[22,34-36] Cães hipertireóideos quase sempre mostram sinais clássicos de êmese, diarreia, perda de peso, hiperatividade, respiração ofegante, poliúria/polidipsia e hipertensão sistêmica (Figura 302.2; ver Capítulo 301).

DIAGNÓSTICO

Diagnósticos diferenciais

A maioria dos cães com carcinoma tireoidiano é levada ao médico-veterinário após o tutor notar a existência de um tumor cervical. Entretanto, sinais de hipertireoidismo podem ser a primeira alteração observada por alguns tutores. Nesses cães, em geral, massa é sentido um tumor cervical palpável ao exame físico. Diagnósticos diferenciais incluem aumento de linfonodos, glândula salivar, granuloma, abscesso ou corpo estranho. Assim, um plano diagnóstico completo deve ser delineado, com a tentativa da realização de uma avaliação mais profunda do tumor cervical.

Exames laboratoriais

Se houver um tumor tireoidiano, o exame de sangue pode revelar hipercalcemia paraneoplásica (ver Capítulo 352).[38] A densidade urinária quase sempre é < 1,020 se um cão for hipercalcêmico e/ou hipertireóideo. Para determinar a função tumoral, as concentrações de T_4 total sérico (T_4t), T_4 livre (T_4L) por diálise de equilíbrio e de TSH canino (TSHc) devem ser avaliadas, assim como os anticorpos antiT$_4$. Se houver um tumor tireoidiano, em geral haverá aumento tanto do T_4t como do T_4L. O TSHc deve estar diminuído em decorrência do *feedback* negativo causado pelo excesso de hormônio tireoidiano (ver Capítulo 299). Autoanticorpos antiT$_4$ que possam interferir em determinados procedimentos do teste não devem ser mensurados.

Diagnóstico por imagem

Em geral, radiografias simples confirmam a existência de um tumor de tecidos moles que desvia ou comprime a traqueia, a laringe e/ou o esôfago. A ultrassonografia, uma modalidade de triagem rápida, não invasiva e confiável para definição de tumores tireoidianos, pode fornecer detalhes adicionais sobre a vascularização e/ou invasão de outras estruturas (Figura 302.3).[40] Contudo, os clínicos devem interpretar os achados ultrassonográficos com cautela, já que podem ser identificados tumores tireoidianos sem significado clínico. Em 14 de 91 cães hipercalcêmicos (15%) sem tumor cervical palpável, identificou-se um total de 15 massas tireoidianas ao exame ultrassonográfico: 2 eram carcinomas de tireoide e 13 provavelmente eram cistos sem significado clínico ou nódulos benignos.[41] A tomografia computadorizada (TC) pode fornecer informações adicionais com relação à natureza das massas tireoidianas, especialmente invasão dos tecidos adjacentes (Figura 302.4).[39,42] Em um estudo com 23 cães com suspeita de carcinoma tireoidiano, a TC teve a maior especificidade (100%) e a ressonância magnética (RM), a maior sensibilidade (93%) para o diagnóstico dessa neoplasia.[40] A TC também permite a avaliação dos pulmões em busca de possíveis metástases. Recomenda-se que a TC ou a RM seja realizada para estadiamento tumoral e antes da possível cirurgia.

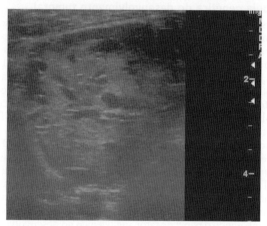

Figura 302.3 Ultrassonografia de carcinoma tireoidiano canino. Projeção transversa da área cervical direita mostrando uma massa tireoidiana diagnosticada como um carcinoma. (Cortesia do Dr. Scott Secrest.)

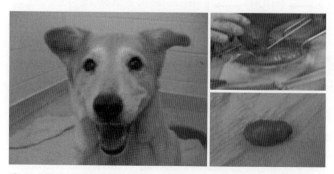

Figura 302.2 Cadela de 10 anos castrada, sem raça definida, foi diagnosticada com carcinoma tireoidiano funcional. Os sinais clínicos dela incluíam perda de peso, poliúria, polidipsia, respiração ofegante e hiperatividade, com elevação do T_4 sérico. Um carcinoma tireoidiano bem encapsulado foi removido, com a resolução da tireotoxicose após a cirurgia.

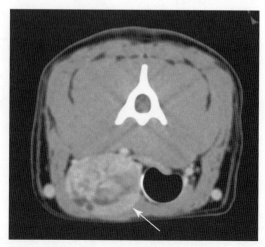

Figura 302.4 Imagem por tomografia computadorizada de carcinoma tireoidiano do lado direito (*seta*). (Cortesia do Dr. Scott Secrest.)

A cintilografia é uma modalidade de imagem efetiva que auxilia no diagnóstico e no estadiamento do carcinoma tireoidiano. O ^{99m}Tc-pertecnetato (^{99m}TcO$_4$) utiliza o transportador sódio-iodeto relativamente específico presente na tireoide e nas glândulas salivares. Já que a proteína transportadora está suprarregulada, à medida que a atividade da glândula tireoide aumenta, os níveis de captação do radionuclídeo podem estar correlacionados com a função tireoidiana. Portanto, a cintilografia é sensível para identificação de alguns carcinomas tireoidianos e, potencialmente, de tecido ectópico e/ou metastático (Figuras 302.5 e 302.6).[32] O padrão de captação do radionuclídeo não pode ser correlacionado com a histologia do tumor, mas predizer o grau de distúrbios capsulares e invasão tecidual local.[19,43] Essa informação pode ser útil ao prever a possibilidade de ressecção cirúrgica e prognóstico a longo prazo, já que carcinomas tireoidianos invasivos apresentam um pior prognóstico.[44] A cintilografia não é sensível para identificação de metástases pulmonares, sendo inferior às radiografias torácicas simples e à TC para estadiamento.[3,19,43] O ^{123}I pode ser superior ao ^{99m}TcO$_4$ para a cintilografia, já que a relação entre o tecido-alvo e o plano de fundo favorece a captação específica pelo tecido tireoidiano. Entretanto, a menor radioatividade do composto requer tempos mais longos de aquisição da imagem, o que pode não ser prático.[43]

Histologia

O diagnóstico definitivo do carcinoma tireoidiano exige a identificação de células malignas em um exame citológico ou, de preferência, histológico. A citologia por aspiração com agulha fina (AAF) costuma ser utilizada para o diagnóstico definitivo do carcinoma tireoidiano em seres humanos,[8] sendo menos confiável para o carcinoma tireoidiano canino (ver Capítulo 93). Como os carcinomas tireoidianos são bastante vascularizados, amostras obtidas por AAF geralmente contêm poucas células, mas grande quantidade de sangue.[22] Entretanto, dependendo do tutor ou das restrições do paciente, a citologia por AAF pode fornecer um método diagnóstico barato e não invasivo.[45] A orientação por ultrassonografia é recomendada em casos de AAF, para evitar áreas bastante vascularizadas.

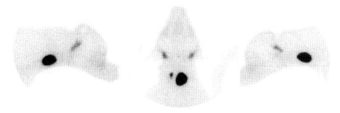

Figura 302.5 Imagens cintilográficas de cão com carcinoma tireoidiano funcional. Note o aumento da captação no lobo esquerdo da glândula tireoide, com captação mínima do lado direito. Isso indica diminuição da atividade da tireoide direita, em resposta à supressão do hormônio tireoestimulante causada pela secreção excessiva desregulada do tumor. (Cortesia do Dr. Gregory Daniel.)

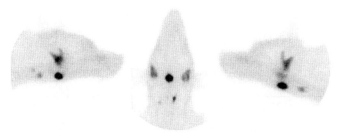

Figura 302.6 Imagens cintilográficas de cão com carcinoma tireoidiano ectópico sublingual. Note o aumento da captação na área sublingual, com captação mínima nas glândulas tireoides. (Cortesia do Dr. Gregory Daniel.)

A histologia é o padrão-ouro pelo qual carcinomas tireoidianos são diagnosticados. Para tumores pequenos e não invasivos, a biopsia excisional pode ser diagnóstica e ser terapêutica. De modo geral, tumores tireoidianos caninos são bem ou moderadamente diferenciados.[1,3,20] A malignidade é definida pela existência de invasão capsular ou vascular. Ao contrário dos seres humanos, o subtipo histológico não parece carrear significado prognóstico em cães com tumores tireoidianos bem diferenciados.[3,20,22] Portanto, é crucial determinar as qualidades invasivas do tumor para o prognóstico. Já que os tumores tireoidianos são bastante vascularizados, a hipótese de que a identificação de microvasos é prognóstica tem sido proposta. Entretanto, a densidade de microvasos não mostrou auxiliar na predição de metástases ou sobrevida.[21] A imunoistoquímica é essencial para determinação da origem de carcinoma tireoidianos.

ESTADIAMENTO

Tumores tireoidianos caninos são estadiados com base no tamanho do tumor primário e na identificação de disseminação aos linfonodos regionais ou metástases a distância (ver Tabela 302.1). Recomenda-se o estadiamento completo de cães com carcinoma tireoidiano, de forma que opções terapêuticas e prognóstico possam ser apresentados aos tutores.

TRATAMENTO

Cirurgia

Para carcinomas de tireoide solitários, bem encapsulados e móveis, recomenda-se a excisão cirúrgica (ver Figura 302.2).[20,24] A remoção do tumor reduz não apenas a carga tumoral, como também pode aliviar a compressão dos tecidos adjacentes. Tumores invasivos são menos passíveis de excisão cirúrgica. Estruturas adjacentes invadidas por tumores tireoidianos incluem nervo laríngeo recorrente, artéria carótida, veia jugular, laringe, traqueia ou esôfago. Essas estruturas podem ser ainda mais lesadas caso haja a tentativa de excisão cirúrgica. Além disso, como os carcinomas tireoidianos são bastante vascularizados, a hemorragia extensa pode resultar de uma cirurgia mal planejada ou por distúrbios hemorrágicos coexistentes,[22] devendo-se empregar exames de imagem avançados antes da cirurgia para determinar a extensão da invasão. Outras complicações potenciais da cirurgia incluem hipocalcemia, pela

Tabela 302.1 Estadiamento clínico de tumores tireoidianos caninos.

ESTÁGIO	DIÂMETRO DO TUMOR PRIMÁRIO	ENVOLVIMENTO DE LINFONODOS REGIONAIS	METÁSTASE A DISTÂNCIA
I	< 2 cm; a ou b	Não	Não
II	Sem evidências de tumor (doença microscópica)	Ipsilateral	Não
	< 2 cm; a ou b	Ipsilateral	Não
	2 a 5 cm; a ou b	Nenhum ou ipsilateral; a	Não
III	> 5 cm	Nenhum	Não
	Qualquer tamanho	Ipsilateral ou bilateral; b	Não
IV	Qualquer tamanho	Nenhum	Sim

Subestágio a = tumor ou linfonodos móveis; subestágio b = tumor ou linfonodos fixos a estruturas adjacentes. (Adaptada de Owen LN, editor: *TNM classification of tumours in domestic animals*, Geneva, IL, 1980, World Health Organization, p. 51-52.)

remoção das glândulas paratireoides, ou distúrbios do seu suprimento sanguíneo, o que seria bastante raro caso fosse realizada tireoidectomia unilateral. Pode-se tentar a tireoidectomia bilateral naqueles casos incomuns nos quais há carcinomas discretos e móveis em ambas as tireoides. Nesses casos, as glândulas paratireoides devem ser preservadas pelo cirurgião ou o tecido paratireoidiano removido, triturado e reimplantado em uma localização que não o pescoço.[46,47] A maioria dos cães submetidos à tireoidectomia bilateral necessita de reposição do hormônio tireoidiano por toda a vida, a fim de tratar o hipotireoidismo iatrogênico (Tabela 302.2). Se nenhum tecido paratireoidiano for preservado, os cães podem ser tratados com sucesso com terapia com calcitriol a longo prazo, a fim de corrigir o hipoparatireoidismo (ver Tabela 302.2; ver também Capítulos 297 e 298). Entretanto, como o tratamento a longo prazo do hipoparatireoidismo é difícil, deve, se possível, ser evitado. O tempo de sobrevida médio para cães após tireoidectomia unilateral é de aproximadamente 3 anos, sendo semelhante para tireoidectomia bilateral: de 30 a 39 meses.[46,47] Se possível, recomenda-se também a remoção de carcinoma tireoidiano ectópico. Descreveu-se uma técnica cirúrgica que envolveu a ressecção parcial do aparelho hioide durante excisão cirúrgica de carcinomas tireoidianos cervicais ectópicos em 5 cães, 4 dos quais sobreviveram pelo menos 20 meses após a cirurgia.[33]

Radiação com feixe externo

Em cães com tumor tireoidiano aderido e fixo em razão da extensa invasão local, a cirurgia não costuma ser uma opção razoável. A radioterapia deve ser considerada como terapia principal para o controle local ou como meio de reduzir o tamanho tumoral, de forma que a cirurgia possa ser uma opção futura. A radiação por feixe externo é mais comumente utilizada em cães com carcinoma tireoidiano.[21,48,49] Em 25 cães com carcinomas tireoidianos sem possibilidade de ressecção e sem metástases visíveis, o intervalo livre de progressão médio foi de 45 meses após radioterapia.[21] As taxas de sobrevida livres de progressão em 1 e 3 anos foram de 80 e 72%, respectivamente. O tempo para a redução máxima do tumor foi bastante variável: de 8 a 22 meses. Em um estudo com 8 cães, o tempo de sobrevida médio foi de 24,5 meses após radioterapia; nenhum animal apresentou novo crescimento do tumor primário, mas 4 morreram por doença metastática.[48] Efeitos colaterais agudos da radioterapia incluem inflamação do esôfago, traqueia ou laringe, resultando em disfagia; tosse ou rouquidão; e alopecia e eritema no local da radiação, os quais ocorreram em aproximadamente metade dos cães tratados, mas cessaram na maioria deles em 2 a 3 semanas. Podem ocorrer reações adversas tardias, como alopecia permanente, tosse seca crônica e fibrose cutânea.[21]

Em cães com doença metastática, a radioterapia por feixe externo pode ocasionar diminuição do tumor primário. Ela se beneficia da natureza de crescimento geralmente lento de carcinomas tireoidianos, de forma que qualquer procedimento para redução da carga tumoral é benéfico. Em 13 cães com doença metastática que receberam radiação fracionada semanalmente, o crescimento tumoral foi interrompido em todos eles, com a diminuição de 10 tumores em pelo menos 50%.[49] O tempo de sobrevida médio foi de aproximadamente 8 meses, incluindo os cães com metástases pulmonares previamente identificadas.

Terapia por radionuclídeo

A terapia por iodo radioativo (^{131}I) é comumente utilizada no período pós-cirúrgico em seres humanos com carcinomas tireoidianos.[8] Ela é eficaz no fornecimento de doses altas de radioatividade de partículas beta à glândula tireoide, sendo utilizada para destruir carcinomas microscópicos em qualquer lugar do

Tabela 302.2	Medicamentos utilizados para tratamento de suporte do hipertireoidismo canino.			
FÁRMACO	**CLASSE**	**INDICAÇÃO**	**DOSE**	**MONITORAMENTO**
Metimazol	Antitireoidiano	Tireotoxicose	2,5 a 5 mg/12 a 24 h VO Ajuste a dose de acordo com as concentrações séricas de T_4	T_4 sérico 1 a 2 semanas após o início da medicação
Atenolol	Bloqueador beta-adrenérgico	Prevenção da crise tireotóxica	0,25 a 1 mg/kg/12 h VO	Pressão sanguínea
Propranolol	Bloqueador beta-adrenérgico	Prevenção da crise tireotóxica	0,1 a 0,2 mg/kg/8 h VO	Pressão sanguínea
Enalapril ou benazepril	Inibidores da enzima conversora de angiotensina (ECA)	Hipertensão tireotóxica	0,25 a 0,5 mg/kg/12 a 24 h VO	Pressão sanguínea
Anlodipino	Bloqueador dos canais de cálcio	Hipertensão tireotóxica	0,1 a 0,5 mg/kg/24 h VO	Pressão sanguínea
Pamidronato	Bifosfonato	Hipercalcemia paraneoplásica	1 a 2 mg/kg IV diluído em 250 mℓ de solução de NaCl a 0,9% e administrado durante 2 horas, a cada 3 a 4 semanas	Parâmetros de função renal e cálcio sérico
Alendronato	Bifosfonato	Hipercalcemia paraneoplásica	0,5 a 1 mg/kg/24 h VO	Erosões esofágicas e cálcio sérico
Calcitriol	Análogo da vitamina D	Hipocalcemia pós-cirúrgica	0,03 a 0,06 µg/kg/dia	Efeito máximo em 2 a 4 dias. Monitore o cálcio sérico
Levotiroxina	Suplementação tireoidiana	Hipotireoidismo pós-cirúrgico	0,022 mg/kg/12 a 24 h	Monitore o T_4 sérico

IV, via intravenosa; *NaCl*, cloreto de sódio; *VO*, via oral.

corpo. Há aumento da captação de ^{131}I pelo tratamento com TSH, que, em geral, é administrado imediatamente antes do ^{131}I, o qual mostrou ser captado pelas células do carcinoma de tireoide, embora em níveis menores do que as células tireoidianas normais.[50] O ^{131}I tem sido efetivo no tratamento de cães com carcinoma de tireoide em estágios II a IV.[44,51,52] A comparação direta dos estudos é difícil, em razão dos diferentes protocolos de dosagem do ^{131}I, da ausência ou existência de tratamento concomitante com TSH, das muitas terapias adjuntas e de diferentes avaliações hormonais antes do tratamento. Entretanto, em 100 cães, os tempos de sobrevida médio variaram de 12 a 34 meses e foram mais longos naqueles submetidos ao ^{131}I como adjuvante à cirurgia.[44,52] A efetividade do tratamento por [131]I não foi correlacionada à condição tireoidiana nesses estudos. Um efeito colateral grave da terapia por ^{131}I inclui a supressão irreversível da medula óssea, observada em cães submetidos a doses ≥ 0,2 GBq/kg ou 5,5 mCi/kg.[51,52]

Embora o ^{131}I se mostre promissor no tratamento de carcinomas tireoidianos, especialmente como adjuvante à cirurgia, o manuseio de grandes quantidades de radioatividade e o fornecimento de áreas de isolamento apropriadas para abrigar cães radioativos permanecem problemáticos. Em seres humanos, o TSH é administrado de rotina com o ^{131}I, a fim de diminuir a dose do iodo. A utilização de TSH recombinante humano sobre a captação do iodo radioativo em 9 cães com tumores tireoidianos foi relatada utilizando-se o isótopo ^{123}I, com uma meia-vida mais curta do que a do [131]I. A administração do TSH não teve efeito sobre a captação do ^{123}I nas glândulas tireoides desses 9 cães.[53]

Quimioterapia

Existem poucos estudos que examinam o papel dos agentes quimioterápicos no tratamento do carcinoma tireoidiano canino, provavelmente porque os resultados iniciais foram decepcionantes. Doxorrubicina, cisplatina e mitoxantrona foram utilizadas em um número pequeno de cães com neoplasias de tireoide.[54-57] Destas, a cisplatina mostrou ter o melhor efeito, com sobrevida média de 11 meses. O melhor efeito desses fármacos provavelmente ocorra contra doença metastática microscópica, sendo necessários novos estudos para mostrar a possível efetividade como terapia adjuvante.

Terapia médica de suporte

Aproximadamente 10% dos carcinomas tireoidianos caninos são funcionais e secretam, de maneira sistemática, excesso de hormônio tireoidiano.[22,34-36] Cães acometidos podem apresentar sinais clássicos de hipertireoidismo, incluindo poliúria, polidipsia, hiperatividade, perda de peso, hipertensão, polifagia e taquicardia. A tireotoxicose deve ser tratada antes que o cão seja submetido à anestesia para técnicas avançadas de imagem ou para cirurgia. Ademais, o hipertireoidismo em cães com tumores tireoidianos funcionais que não podem sofrer ressecção deve ser tratado para aumentar a longevidade e a qualidade de vida. O hipertireoidismo pode ser tratado com metimazol, à semelhança do que ocorre com os gatos (dose = 2,5 a 5 mg/cão VO, a cada 12 ou 24 horas). Os teores séricos de T_4 devem ser monitorados 1 a 2 semanas após o início da terapia, com o início de ajustes adequados. O tratamento é eficaz em controlar os sinais clínicos com efeitos colaterais insignificantes. Em cães hipertireóideos submetidos à anestesia ou à cirurgia, um bloqueador beta-adrenérgico, como o atenolol, deve ser considerado uma noite antes e no dia do procedimento, a fim de evitar taquicardias relacionadas com potencial crise tireotóxica (ver Tabela 302.2 e Capítulo 301).[58]

Cães hipertireóideos também podem apresentar hipertensão sistêmica significativa (ver Capítulo 99).[36] Embora a remoção do tumor tireoidiano funcional possa normalizar a pressão sanguínea, a hipertensão sistêmica deve ser tratada em cães com tumores sem possibilidade de ressecção ou naqueles com carcinoma tireoidiano metastático funcional (ver Capítulo 158). Anti-hipertensivos, como inibidores da ECA e/ou anlodipino, podem ser utilizados para tais pacientes. A hipercalcemia paraneoplásica pode também ocorrer em casos raros de carcinoma tireoidiano (ver Capítulo 352).[38] Fármacos que diminuem os teores de cálcio, como o pamidronato ou o alendronato, podem ser utilizados para tratar tais casos, caso a carga tumoral não possa ser diminuída (ver Tabela 302.2 e Capítulos 297 e 298).

REFERÊNCIAS BIBLIOGRÁFICAS

As referências bibliográficas deste capítulo se encontram online no Ambiente de Aprendizagem.

CAPÍTULO 303

Tumores Secretores de Insulina

Johan P. Schoeman

Insulinoma é um tumor secretor de insulina de células beta pancreáticas. A secreção excessiva desse hormônio causa sinais clínicos de hipoglicemia, uma condição incomum em cães e rara em gatos. O foco deste capítulo será no insulinoma canino, descrito pela primeira vez em um cão, em 1935.[1]

PATOLOGIA

Células beta pancreáticas secretoras de insulina compreendem aproximadamente 70% das células das ilhotas de Langerhans. Em consequência, tumores de células beta são as neoplasias mais comuns de células de ilhotas caninas. A maioria dos insulinomas caninos é maligna; em um relato que utilizou imunoistoquímica,

17 de 18 eram carcinomas e 1, adenoma.[2] Aproximadamente 80% dos insulinomas são solitários, localizados em um ramo pancreático, e não no corpo do pâncreas (Figura 303.1).[3-5] Ocasionalmente, nenhum nódulo discreto é observado durante a avaliação macroscópica pancreática, havendo a necessidade de histologia para identificação do tumor.

A taxa de lesões metastáticas detectadas em 179 cães de diferentes estudos variou de 45 a 64%. Ela é maior em estudos que se baseiam na necropsia, em comparação àqueles que utilizam amostras obtidas cirurgicamente.[3,6,7] De acordo com a Organização Mundial da Saúde (OMS), o estadiamento clínico de tumores pancreáticos define o estágio I como $T_1N_0M_0$ (existência de um tumor primário e ausência de metástases em linfonodos regionais ou distantes), estágio II como $T_1N_1M_0$ e

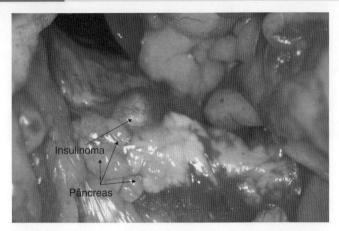

Figura 303.1 Insulinoma solitário circundado por tecido pancreático. (Cortesia da Dra. Lillian Aronson.) (*Esta figura se encontra reproduzida em cores no Encarte.*)

estágio III como $T_1N_1M_1$ ou $T_1N_0M_1$. A maioria dos cães com insulinoma apresenta a doença em estágio II ou III, sendo os locais mais comuns de metástases os linfonodos regionais e o fígado. A doença metastática possui distribuição ilimitada.[8] Embora a etiologia do insulinoma não seja conhecida, a produção local do hormônio de crescimento (GH, *growth hormone*), não associada ao aumento das concentrações plasmáticas de GH, foi documentada no insulinoma canino primário e metastático, possivelmente promovendo proliferação de células da ilhota por mecanismos parácrinos e autócrinos.[9]

FISIOPATOLOGIA

A proliferação neoplásica de células beta pancreáticas causa secreção autônoma excessiva da insulina e resulta em hipoglicemia. Os mecanismos compensatórios mais importantes para hipoglicemia são a inibição da secreção de insulina e a estimulação de secreção de hormônios contrarregulatórios. A glicose, o regulador principal da secreção de insulina, entra nas células beta pancreáticas e é metabolizada em ATP, fechando os canais de K^+ sensíveis a ele. O fechamento resulta em diminuição do efluxo de K^+, despolarização de células beta, abertura dos canais de Ca^{2+} voltagem-dependentes e exocitose da insulina. Em animais saudáveis, a secreção de insulina é completamente inibida quando a glicemia é menor que 80 mg/dℓ. Entretanto, a secreção de insulina por células beta pancreáticas, independentemente da glicemia, persiste apesar da hipoglicemia e representa uma das principais características bioquímicas do insulinoma: concentrações sanguíneas de insulina altas ou normais, apesar da hipoglicemia. Os quatro hormônios contrarregulatórios secretados em resposta à hipoglicemia são glucagon, catecolaminas, GH e glicocorticoides. Destes, o glucagon e as catecolaminas são os mais importantes nas respostas a curto prazo à hipoglicemia.

CARACTERÍSTICAS CLÍNICAS

Epidemiologia
A idade média de cães com insulinoma é de 9 anos, com variação de 3 a 15. Embora qualquer raça de cão possa desenvolver insulinoma, ele foi relatado com maior frequência em cães de raças de portes médio e grande. Estudos controlados do risco racial para insulinoma ainda não foram publicados, não existindo predileção sexual aparente para a doença.

Sinais clínicos
Os sinais clínicos ocorrem em razão do efeito da hipoglicemia sobre o sistema nervoso central (neuroglicopenia) ou da liberação de catecolaminas induzida pela hipoglicemia. A glicose é a fonte única mais importante de energia para o cérebro. Como tanto o armazenamento de carboidratos como a capacidade cerebral de utilizar outros combustíveis são limitados, a função depende de um suprimento contínuo de glicose. Os sinais clínicos atribuíveis à neuroglicopenia incluem convulsões, colapso, fraqueza, ataxia, desorientação, retardo mental e distúrbios visuais. Sinais clínicos relacionados com a liberação excessiva de catecolaminas e estimulação do sistema nervoso simpático incluem tremores, fome e agressividade.

A gravidade dos sinais clínicos está parcialmente correlacionada ao nadir da glicemia. A hipoglicemia grave pode, finalmente, resultar em coma e morte. Entretanto, sinais clínicos também podem estar relacionados com a duração e a velocidade com a qual a hipoglicemia ocorre, pois diminuições graduais na glicemia têm menor probabilidade de estimular a secreção de catecolaminas. Ocasionalmente, os sinais clínicos são episódicos, pois a secreção de hormônios contrarregulatórios aumenta a glicemia, resolvendo de forma transitória os sinais neuroglicopênicos. A alimentação pode aliviar os sinais clínicos caso restaure a glicemia a níveis normais. Entretanto, ela pode exacerbar, de forma rebote, os sinais clínicos, pelo maior estímulo de secreção insulínica. Ademais, jejum, exercício ou excitação podem piorar os sinais clínicos, pela diminuição da glicemia ou pelo aumento da estimulação simpática. Os sinais clínicos relatados em 198 cães, com base em diversos estudos, estão listados na Tabela 303.1. Embora a maioria deles apresente mais de um desses sinais clínicos, alguns cães não têm nenhum. A duração relatada dos sinais clínicos antes do diagnóstico varia de 1 dia a 3 anos.

EXAME FÍSICO

O exame físico não apresenta alterações na maioria dos cães com insulinoma.[4,6,10] Os cães podem estar acima do peso em razão dos efeitos anabólicos da insulina. Alterações pós-ictais podem ser aparentes se a convulsão tiver ocorrido recentemente. Polineuropatia periférica, caracterizada por paresia posterior ou tetraparesia e diminuição ou ausência de reflexos apendiculares, foi descrita em 13 cães com insulinoma.[8,11,12] A etiologia dessa neuropatia periférica, associada ao insulinoma, não é conhecida, mas pode ocorrer com distúrbio imunomediado paraneoplásico não relacionado com as alterações metabólicas do insulinoma.[12]

DIAGNÓSTICOS DIFERENCIAIS

Os diagnósticos diferenciais para hipoglicemia podem ser separados naqueles associados à secreção excessiva de insulina ou fatores semelhantes à insulina, naqueles causados pela diminuição da produção de glicose, em outros causados em razão do consumo excessivo de glicose, situação ocasional associada a um fármaco ou hipotéticos. Distúrbios nos quais o mecanismo mais importante para hipoglicemia é a secreção em excesso da insulina ou fatores semelhantes à insulina incluem insulinoma, tumor extrapancreático (*i. e.*, tumores hepáticos) ou hiperplasia de células beta. Condições associadas à diminuição da produção de glicose incluem hipoadrenocorticismo (ver Capítulo 309), hipopituitarismo (ver Capítulo 295), deficiência de GH (ver Capítulo 295), insuficiência hepática (ver Capítulos 280 e 285) e doenças de armazenamento de glicogênio (ver Capítulo 260). Neonatos e raças toy podem apresentar distúrbios na produção de glicose. Jejum, desnutrição ou prenhez também podem resultar em hipoglicemia. O excesso de consumo de glicose pode ocorrer na sepse ou no exercício extremo (especialmente em cães de caça). Alguns dos muitos fármacos relatados, passíveis de induzir hipoglicemia em seres humanos, incluem insulina, hipoglicemiantes orais (p. ex., sulfonilureia), salicilatos (p. ex.,

CAPÍTULO 303 • Tumores Secretores de Insulina

Tabela 303.1 Sinais clínicos decorrentes de insulinomas relatados em 198 cães com base em diversos estudos.[3-5,7,8,10]

SINAL CLÍNICO	NÚMERO (%) DE 198 CÃES
Convulsão	95 (48)
Colapso	79 (40)
Fraqueza generalizada	74 (37)
Tremores/contração muscular	40 (20)
Ataxia	48 (20)
Intolerância ao exercício	30 (15)
Fraqueza de membros pélvicos	28 (14)
Desorientação/comportamento bizarro/histeria	19 (10)
Polifagia	16 (8)
Poliúria e polidipsia	16 (8)
Estupor/letargia	12 (6)
Convulsões focais faciais	6 (3)
Obesidade ou ganho de peso	6 (3)
Cegueira	5 (2,5)
Anorexia	5 (2,5)
Diarreia	4 (2)
Inclinação de cabeça	2 (1)
Agressividade	2 (1)

ácido acetilsalicílico), paracetamol, betabloqueadores (p. ex., propranolol), agonistas beta-2, etanol, inibidores da monoamina oxidase, antidepressivos tricíclicos (p. ex., amitriptilina), inibidores da enzima conversora de angiotensina (p. ex., captopril), antibióticos (p. ex., tetraciclina), sobredose de lidocaína e lítio. A hipoglicemia fictícia pode ocorrer quando as hemácias não são imediatamente separadas do soro ou em animais com policitemia grave ou leucocitose.

AVALIAÇÃO DIAGNÓSTICA

Concentrações séricas de glicose e insulina

Uma abordagem algorítmica para a hipoglicemia é mostrada na Figura 303.2. A suspeita clínica de insulinoma começa com a documentação dos sinais clínicos apropriados, hipoglicemia (glicemia menor que 60 mg/dℓ), e hiperinsulinemia concomitante (concentrações séricas de insulina dentro ou acima do intervalo de referência).[13] A identificação de um tumor pancreático, com estudos de imagem, pode fortalecer essa suspeita. O diagnóstico de insulinoma é confirmado pelo exame histológico e pela coloração imunoistoquímica da massa pancreática.

Além da hipoglicemia descoberta quase sempre ao acaso, o hemograma, o perfil bioquímico e a urinálise costumam estar normais.[4,7] Embora a hipoglicemia seja observada em amostras obtidas aleatoriamente de cães com insulinoma, especialmente se a coleta for repetida, é importante notar que alguns animais são euglicêmicos.[7,14] Hipopotassemia discreta e aumento das atividades da fosfatase alcalina e/ou da alanina aminotransferase foram documentados.[5,7] Quando há suspeita de insulinoma em um cão euglicêmico, ele deve ser monitorado de perto, em busca de hipoglicemia, quando em jejum. A glicemia deve ser mensurada a cada 30 a 60 minutos. Na maioria dos cães com insulinoma, a hipoglicemia (glicemia < 60 mg/dℓ) ocorre dentro de 12 horas após a refeição anterior.

O soro para mensuração da concentração de insulina deve ser submetido na mesma amostra na qual a hipoglicemia foi documentada. Um número extremamente limitado de cães com insulinoma não apresenta hipoglicemia, mesmo após mensurações repetidas ou jejum prolongado de 48 a 72 horas.[7] A frutosamina baixa é utilizada para fortalecer a suspeita clínica de insulinoma em diversos cães com euglicemia.[14] A concentração de hemoglobina A1 c glicada é baixa em alguns animais, mas não em todos os cães com insulinoma.[15] A repetição das mensurações séricas de insulina também pode auxiliar no diagnóstico. Um estudo do insulinoma canino identificou que 76% dos cães apresentaram aumento da concentração sérica de insulina, quando aferida uma vez, e 91%, quando aferida duas vezes.[7]

Razões e outros testes

Outros testes foram descritos para o diagnóstico de insulinoma em cães euglicêmicos com concentrações séricas normais de insulina. As razões entre insulina e glicose e glicose e insulina não são recomendadas em razão da baixa sensibilidade, já a relação corrigida entre insulina e glicose não o é em razão da baixa especificidade. Foram descritos testes adicionais de tolerância e estimulação, mas não são aconselhados em decorrência da utilidade questionável e/ou dos efeitos adversos potencialmente fatais da hipoglicemia.

Diagnóstico por imagem

Radiografias e ultrassonografia

A maioria dos cães com insulinoma não apresenta alterações nas radiografias torácicas e abdominais.[4,6,8,16] Ao combinar resultados de estudos nos quais a ultrassonografia abdominal foi realizada, houve a identificação de um tumor pancreático em 49 de 87 (56%) cães. Metástases abdominais foram notadas em 17 (19%).[3,5,8,16] Embora a ultrassonografia abdominal possa ser útil para dar suporte à suspeita clínica de tumor pancreático e metástases, foram descritos resultados falso-positivos e falso-negativos (Figura 303.3). Recentemente, o emprego da ultrassonografia foi bem-sucedido em discriminar insulinomas de carcinomas pancreáticos.[17,18]

Exames de imagem avançados

Uma técnica de imagem ótima para identificação do insulinoma em seres humanos ainda precisa ser identificada.[19] Entretanto, a TC de multidetecção por secção fina, fase dupla e de alta qualidade do pâncreas é efetiva para identificação de tumor pancreático na maioria dos casos.[19] Em seres humanos, a ultrassonografia intraductal e transcirúrgica (não amplamente disponível) é mais sensível do que a TC para a detecção de pequenos insulinomas (diâmetro de 1 a 3 mm).[19] A utilização da TC foi relatada em um pequeno número de cães com insulinoma, mas sua sensibilidade ainda precisa ser determinada.[20-22] Em um estudo, 14 insulinomas foram visualizados por ultrassonografia, TC e TC por emissão de fóton único. As imagens por TC identificaram corretamente o maior número de tumores (10/14, 71%).[22]

Em outro estudo, foi detectado, em um de cada três cães com insulinoma, um tumor pela TC por angiografia (TCA) em fase dupla, e, em dois, não foi constatado um tumor pancreático pela ultrassonografia.[20] Em dois desses cães, houve forte realce do insulinoma, notado apenas durante a fase arterial do estudo, destacando o valor da fase dupla (Figuras 303.4 a 303.6).[20] A administração intravenosa (IV) de somatostatina sintética marcada radioativamente, seguida da cintilografia do corpo inteiro, possui valor limitado para visualização de insulinomas em pessoas, provavelmente em razão do baixo número de receptores de somatostatina expressos em insulinomas humanos.[19] A cintilografia com receptores de somatostatina foi relatada em um pequeno número de cães com insulinoma.[23,24] Focos anormais de atividade foram observados 1 a 24 horas após administração do radioligante, mas a localização precisa do tumor foi obtida apenas em 1 de 5 cães.[24]

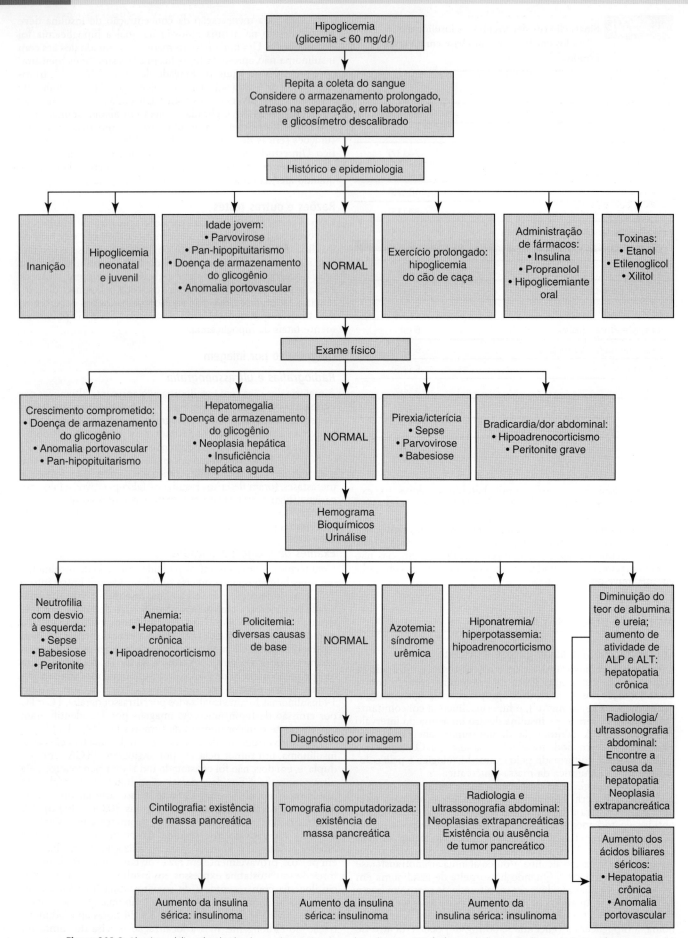

Figura 303.2 Algoritmo delineador da abordagem diagnóstica para a hipoglicemia. *ALP*, fosfatase alcalina; *ALT*, alanina aminotransferase.

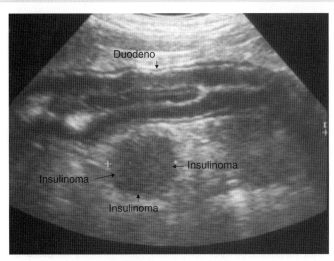

Figura 303.3 Ultrassonografia abdominal de insulinoma hipoecoico redondo, circunscrito por tecido pancreático. O duodeno é visualizado acima do pâncreas. (Cortesia do Dr. Wilfried Mai.)

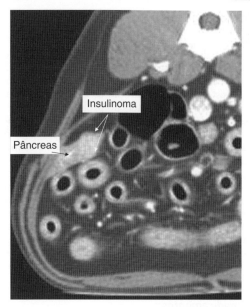

Figura 303.5 Angiografia por tomografia computadorizada (TC) em fase dupla durante a fase venosa do estudo. Há um ligeiro realce do insulinoma. (Cortesia do Dr. Wilfried Mai.)

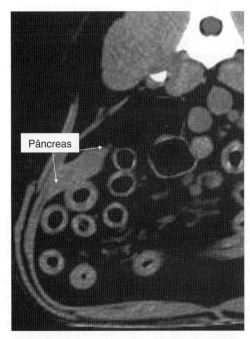

Figura 303.4 Angiografia por tomografia computadorizada (TC) antes da administração do contraste. Um insulinoma ainda não é visível dentro do pâncreas. (Cortesia do Dr. Wilfried Mai.)

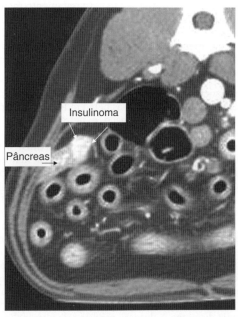

Figura 303.6 Angiografia por tomografia computadorizada (TC) em fase dupla durante a fase arterial do estudo. Há um forte realce do insulinoma. (Cortesia do Dr. Wilfried Mai.)

TRATAMENTO

Hipoglicemia aguda

Durante uma crise hipoglicêmica aguda, deve-se administrar dextrose a 50% como *bolus* lento (0,5 g/kg, IV, diluído em uma relação de 1:3 em solução de NaCl a 0,9%). O *bolus* deve ser seguido de taxa de infusão contínua (TIC) IV de solução de dextrose a 2,5 a 5%. Deve-se administrar a menor quantidade de glicose necessária com cautela, pois ela estimula a secreção de insulina. Isso pode causar hipoglicemia rebote e um círculo vicioso difícil de quebrar. A administração de dextrose deve ser interrompida quando da cessação dos sinais clínicos, mesmo se houver persistência de hipoglicemia discreta. Na maioria dos cães, a neuroglicopenia cessará após administração da dextrose. Entretanto, se o animal não responder somente à administração de dextrose, dexametasona (0,1 mg/kg/12 h IV) e/ou análogos da somatostatina (10 a 50 µg/8 a 12 h SC) podem ser administrados.

Em casos graves, o animal pode ser beneficiado pela sedação com diazepam ou pentobarbital durante várias horas, para resolver a atividade convulsiva. A hipoxia cerebral pode levar a edema cerebral e, havendo suspeita, pode ser tratado com manitol (1 g/kg IV administrado como uma solução a 20%, na taxa de 2 mℓ/kg/h) e furosemida (1 a 2 mg/kg/4 h IV) (ver Capítulo 148).[25]

Uma TIC IV de glucagon (5 a 13 ng/kg/min, com ou sem dextrose a 10% concomitante) foi relatada em um cão com hipoglicemia associada ao insulinoma. Os sinais clínicos atribuídos à hipoglicemia cessaram dentro de 20 minutos, com a resolução da hipoglicemia dentro de 1 hora. O glucagon aumenta a glicemia, pela promoção da glicogenólise e gliconeogênese, bem como a secreção de insulina, e os animais assim tratados também necessitam de monitoramento constante em busca de piora ou de hipoglicemia rebote.[26]

Cuidado em longo prazo

Cirurgia

O tratamento de eleição a longo prazo para o insulinoma é a ressecção cirúrgica do tumor e de metástases óbvias.[5] Dois cães foram submetidos à ressecção bem-sucedida de trombos tumorais que se estenderam em direção às veias pancreaticoduodenais.[27] Um cão apresentou intervalo prolongado livre da doença após ressecção do tumor primário, apesar das lesões metastáticas.[28] A exploração cirúrgica e a biopsia de um tumor pancreático podem confirmar o diagnóstico e auxiliar na estimativa do tempo de sobrevida.[10] Quando ocorre hiperglicemia pós-cirúrgica, ela costuma ser transitória e cessar assim que as células β normais, suprimidas pela secreção autônoma de insulina de células neoplásicas, recobrarem a função. Aproximadamente 10% dos cães com insulinoma desenvolvem diabetes melito após remoção do tumor e necessitam de insulina exógena por um período completamente imprevisível (1 a 37 meses).[6,7,10] Outras complicações pós-cirúrgicas incluem pancreatite, cetoacidose diabética, retardo na cicatrização de feridas, arritmias ou parada cardíaca, hemorragia, sepse e leucopenia.[3,5,7]

Terapia medicamentosa

Conceito geral. Essa revisão sobre a terapia medicamentosa é limitada a agentes cuja utilização tenha sido relatada em cães com insulinoma de ocorrência natural. O uso de medicamentos adicionais é discutido em outras seções.[25] O tratamento medicamentoso pode ser indicado antes da cirurgia, no período pós-cirúrgico, caso necessário, e em cães nos quais a cirurgia não é realizada. A terapia medicamentosa pode ser dividida em terapia citotóxica direcionada à destruição das células beta secretoras de insulina e em tratamento que vise ao alívio da hipoglicemia.

Estreptozocina. A estreptozocina, um antibiótico nitrosureia, destrói seletivamente células beta em localizações pancreáticas ou metastáticas. O fármaco é nefrotóxico em cães. A diurese com salina diminui o tempo de contato do fármaco com as células epiteliais tubulares renais e pode reduzir o risco de nefrotoxicose. Em um estudo com 17 cães, a maioria deles submetida à ressecção incompleta de lesões macroscópicas, foi realizado tratamento com NaCl a 0,9% (18 mℓ/kg/h IV) durante 3 horas antes, 2 horas durante e 2 horas depois da infusão de estreptozocina (500 mg/m^2), administrada a cada 3 semanas durante 5 ciclos. Butorfanol (0,4 mg/kg, por via intramuscular [IM]) foi administrado imediatamente após o tratamento com estreptozocina como um antiemético, mas êmese ainda foi observada em aproximadamente um terço dos tratamentos. Outros efeitos colaterais incluíram diabetes melito; hipoglicemia transitória e convulsões; hiperglicemia transitória; aumento transitório na atividade de ALT; azotemia; trombocitopenia ou neutropenia discretas. A duração mediana da normoglicemia em cães tratados com estreptozocina foi de 163 dias, o que não foi diferente, em termos estatísticos, do que aquela observada em cães tratados com cirurgia ou medicamento.[8] Em um estudo com 19 cães, utilizou-se a mesma dose e protocolo com a salina, mas em um intervalo intensificado de 2 semanas. Infelizmente, 8/19 desenvolveram diabetes melito e 2/19 apresentaram nefrotoxicidade, com intervalo de progressão livre mediano semelhante (196 dias).[29] Outros estudos são necessários antes da recomendação da terapia com estreptozocina.

Terapias comuns. As principais formas para aliviar a hipoglicemia incluem modificação dietética e tratamento com prednisona, diazóxido ou somatostatina sintética. Recomendam-se pequenas refeições, porém frequentes (a cada 4 a 6 horas), ricas em proteínas, gorduras e carboidratos complexos (ver Capítulo 181). Açúcares simples (presentes em alimentos úmidos de cães e soluções IV) devem ser evitados. A prednisona, o fármaco menos caro e mais comumente utilizado, aumenta a glicemia, pelo aumento da gliconeogênese e da atividade da glicose 6-fosfatase, ao mesmo tempo que diminui a captação da glicose sanguínea

pelos tecidos e estimula a secreção de glucagon. Glicocorticoides podem ser administrados por via intravenosa durante uma crise hipoglicêmica aguda, como a dexametasona. Em geral, a prednisona é utilizada quando um cão está estável, administrada em dose oral inicial de aproximadamente 0,5 mg/kg/dia. As doses podem ser aumentadas de maneira gradativa, conforme necessário, até que o fármaco não seja mais percebido como redutor de episódios convulsivos ou que ocorram sinais intoleráveis de hiperadrenocorticismo iatrogênico (poliúria/polidipsia).[10,25]

Diazóxido. O diazóxido é um derivado benzotiadiazínico cuja principal ação é inibir o fechamento dos canais de K$^+$ dependentes de ATP das células beta pancreáticas, evitando a despolarização e inibindo a abertura de canais de Ca^{2+} voltagem-dependentes. A diminuição do influxo de Ca^{2+} resulta em diminuição da exocitose de vesículas secretórias que contêm insulina. O diazóxido também aumenta a glicemia, pelo estímulo à glicogenólise e à gliconeogênese e pela inibição da captação tecidual de glicose.[30] Aproximadamente 70% dos cães apresentam uma resposta às doses de diazóxido de 10 a 40 mg/kg/dia VO, divididas a cada 8 a 12 h. Mais uma vez, é importante iniciar com a menor dose, aumentando-a gradativamente, conforme necessário.[7] Em cães, efeitos colaterais não são comuns. Eles incluem ptialismo, êmese e anorexia. Limitações adicionais da terapia com diazóxido incluem disponibilidade limitada e custo considerável.

Octreotida. A octreotida é um análogo sintético de longa ação da somatostatina, cujo modo primário de ação é a inibição da secreção de insulina por meio da sua afinidade de ligação a qualquer um dos cinco subtipos de receptores de somatostatina presentes em tumores secretores de insulina. Cães mostram resposta variável à octreotida, provavelmente em razão da inibição variável da secreção de glucagon e GH pela octreotida.[31] Se a supressão da secreção de glucagon e GH for de maior magnitude e duração, quando comparada à da secreção de insulina, a octreotida pode, de fato, piorar a hipoglicemia. Ao mesmo tempo que alguns insulinomas caninos podem não ter receptores de somatostatina, 12 cães com insulinoma tratados com dose única de octreotida de 50 µg/cão por via subcutânea (SC) (peso mediano de 23 kg) apresentaram diminuição na concentração plasmática de insulina, sem alteração das concentrações de glucagon, hormônio do crescimento e hormônio adrenocorticotrófico.[32] Esses achados justificam os estudos que utilizam a octreotida de longa ação em cães com insulinoma. Nenhum efeito colateral adverso foi relatado. Em pessoas, eles incluem dor discreta no local da injeção (amenizada se a solução for aquecida antes da administração), náuseas, êmese, dor abdominal, constipação intestinal ou esteatorreia.

PROGNÓSTICO

O tempo de sobrevida mediano de 142 cães submetidos à pancreatectomia parcial, relatado em diferentes estudos, foi de 12 a 14 meses, com variação de 0 dias a 5 anos.[3-5,7,10] Cães com doença clínica em estágio I têm intervalo livre de doença significativamente mais longo; em aproximadamente 50%, a normoglicemia deve voltar 14 meses após o período pós-cirúrgico, quando comparados a apenas 20% de cães em estágio clínico II ou III.[6] Além disso, cães jovens e aqueles com hipoglicemia pós-cirúrgica persistente apresentam pior prognóstico.[6] Em contrapartida, cães com hiperglicemia pós-cirúrgica ou normoglicemia apresentam prognóstico significativamente melhor.[3] Um estudo relatou tempo de sobrevida mediano de 785 dias em 19 cães com insulinoma submetidos à pancreatectomia parcial, que melhoraram para 1.316 dias no subgrupo de cães que também receberam prednisona.[33] É mais provável que esses tempos de sobrevida sejam atribuíveis à detecção precoce, aos protocolos de ressecção tumoral mais radicais e à terapia medicamentosa mantida após recidiva. Mostrou-se também que o tamanho tumoral e a taxa mitótica, conforme demonstrado pelo índice Ki67 (um marcador de proliferação), atuam como marcadores prognósticos significativos no insulinoma canino,[34] o que foi acompanhado por um estudo de imunoistoquímica por microarranjo tecidual, que corroborou os achados anteriores em 32 amostras de insulinoma. A análise multivariável mostrou que o tamanho tumoral e o índice Ki67 mantiveram o poder preditivo para o tempo de sobrevida, assim como o tamanho tumoral para o intervalo livre da doença.[35] Em contrapartida, idade, sexo, peso corporal, sinais clínicos e sua duração, detecção ultrassonográfica da massa pancreática, localização do tumor, presença macroscópica de doença metastática e concentração de glicose ou insulina no sangue não foram significativamente associados ao prognóstico.

NEOPLASIA DE CÉLULAS DA ILHOTA SECRETORAS DE INSULINA NO GATO

O insulinoma felino é raro, tendo sido relatado em 7 gatos, com variação de idade entre 12 e 17 anos. Três deles eram Siameses e cinco, machos castrados.[25,36-38] O histórico e os sinais clínicos são semelhantes àqueles relatados em cães com insulinoma. O diagnóstico baseia-se na identificação do aumento da concentração sérica de insulina no momento da hipoglicemia e é auxiliado por ultrassonografia abdominal e histologia.[38] A imunoistoquímica do insulinoma felino revelou expressão de insulina, cromogranina A e somatostatina, sem expressão de glucagon ou polipeptídio pancreático.[39] Deve haver cautela ao utilizar um ensaio para insulina validado para gatos. A terapia consiste em ressecção cirúrgica do tumor pancreático e das metástases, seguida do tratamento com prednisona e refeições frequentes, porém pequenas. A utilização do diazóxido ou da octreotida não foi relatada em gatos.

REFERÊNCIAS BIBLIOGRÁFICAS

As referências bibliográficas deste capítulo se encontram online no Ambiente de Aprendizagem.

CAPÍTULO 304

Diabetes Melito Canino

Federico Fracassi

INTRODUÇÃO

O diabetes melito (DM) é um distúrbio endócrino comum, caracterizado por hiperglicemia crônica resultante de deficiência na produção, ação, ou ambas, de insulina. Em cães, a prevalência do DM foi estimada em aproximadamente 1% de cães em instituições especializadas e de aproximadamente 0,3% em clínicos gerais.[1-4] A incidência relatada do DM em uma população de 182.087 cães atendidos na Suécia foi de aproximadamente 13 casos por 10 mil (0,13%) cães em idade de risco.[5]

CLASSIFICAÇÃO E ETIOLOGIA

Tipos de diabetes melito

Existem duas formas predominantes de DM em pessoas, outrora referidas como DM de "início juvenil" e "início adulto". Esses termos foram atualizados para "insulinodependente" (DMID) e "não insulinodependente" (DMNID). Atualmente, são empregados os termos DM tipos 1 e 2: o tipo 1 explica a condição para cerca de 10% dos seres humanos diabéticos e o tipo 2, quase idêntico ao "DMNID" prévio, é utilizado para definir a condição em cerca de 90% das pessoas com DM no mundo todo.[6] A forma mais comum de DM em cães lembra a condição humana do tipo 1, caracterizada por hipoinsulinemia permanente, sem aumento das concentrações de insulina sérica endógena ou peptídio-C após administração de um secretagogo da insulina (p. ex., glicose, glucagon, aminoácidos) e a necessidade absoluta de insulina exógena para controlar a glicemia, evitar cetoacidose e sobreviver.[7] Com raras exceções, todos os cães diabéticos necessitam de terapia insulínica exógena para tratar a hiperglicemia.[8]

Histologia e possíveis causas primárias

Observações histológicas comuns no tecido pancreático de cães com DM incluem redução do número e tamanho das ilhotas pancreáticas, diminuição do número de células beta dentro das ilhotas e vacuolização, aumento e degeneração de células beta.[9,10] A causa de base da disfunção/destruição da célula beta pancreática em cães não foi estabelecida. Em seres humanos e cães, o DM é, sem dúvida, uma doença multifatorial que envolve fatores genéticos e ambientais (Boxe 304.1).[8,11-15]

O conceito de predisposição genética baseou-se em associações familiares, análises de pedigree de cães da raça Keeshond e diversas outras raças e estudos genômicos para identificar a suscetibilidade e haplótipos de complexos de histocompatibilidade principais protetores.[1,5,16] Uma série de genes ligados à suscetibilidade ao DM em pessoas também está associada ao aumento do risco em cães.[17] O DM canino tem sido associado aos genes de classe II (antígeno leucocitário canino [DLA, do inglês *dog leukocyte antigen*]) do complexo de histocompatibilidade principal (MHC, do inglês *major histocompatibility complex*). Haplótipos e genótipos semelhantes foram identificados nas raças mais suscetíveis. Uma região com um número variável de repetição em tandem (VNTR, do inglês *variable number of tandem repeats*), assim como diversos polimorfismos, foi identificada no gene da insulina canino, com alguns alelos associados à suscetibilidade ou à resistência ao DM de uma maneira raça-específica.[17]

A Associação Americana de Diabetes recomendou a subcategorização do DM tipo 1 humano (DMT1) em tipos 1A (imunomediado) e 1B (deficiência insulínica idiopática grave).[18] O DM tipo 1A é caracterizado por infiltrado linfocítico das ilhotas, conhecido como insulinite, e pela presença de autoanticorpos séricos a componentes pancreáticos (insulina, descarboxilase 65 do ácido glutâmico [GAD65] intracelular ou antígeno-2 do insulinoma [IA-2]) antes do desenvolvimento da hiperglicemia (Figura 304.1).[19] Um componente imunomediado foi implicado no desenvolvimento do DM canino. Infiltrado linfocítico de ilhotas pancreáticas foi relatado, com a identificação de anticorpos direcionados contra células das ilhotas, insulina, proinsulina, GAD65 e IA-2 em cães com DM.[20-24] Apesar desses estudos, o papel da autoimunidade na

Boxe 304.1 Fatores potenciais envolvidos na etiopatogenia do diabetes melito canino

Deficiência insulínica

Em cães, a deficiência insulínica é caracterizada pela perda de células beta. A etiologia da deficiência/destruição das células beta em cães diabéticos é atualmente desconhecida, mas uma série de processos mórbidos supostamente está envolvida:
- Hipoplasia/abiotrofia congênita de células beta
- Destruição imunomediada de células beta
- Perda de células beta associadas à pancreatite
- Exaustão/toxicidade pela glicose de células beta como consequência de resistência insulínica prolongada.

Resistência insulínica

Em geral, a resistência insulínica resulta de antagonismo da função insulínica por outros hormônios, e pode ser exacerbada pela presença de infecções ou inflamação:
- Diestro/prenhez
- Doença hormonal concomitante
  - Síndrome de Cushing
  - Hipotireoidismo
  - Acromegalia
- Iatrogênica
  - Glicocorticoides
  - Progestágenos
- Intolerância ao carboidrato associada à obesidade
- Infecção
- Doença concomitante
- Insuficiência renal
- Cardiopatia
- Hiperlipidemia
- Déficits de receptores de insulina, como aqueles observados em seres humanos, poderiam existir em pacientes diabéticos caninos, embora ainda não tenham sido relatados.

Adaptada de Davison LJ: Canine diabetes mellitus. In Mooney CT, Peterson ME: *BSAVA manual of canine and feline endocrinology*, 4 ed., Gloucester, England, 2012, British Small Animal Veterinary Association, p. 117.

patogênese do DM canino permanece incerto. Um estudo recente não observou evidências de etiologia autoimune das ilhotas.[9] Ao contrário do DMT1 humano, que ocorre principalmente na adolescência e no início da vida adulta, cães costumam ser diagnosticados na meia-idade ou na velhice.[25] Foi proposto que o DM canino se assemelha mais intimamente a pessoas com "diabetes autoimune latente dos adultos" (DALA).[11,26]

Causas secundárias

O DM pode ocorrer secundariamente a distúrbios do pâncreas exócrino ou qualquer processo que lesione o pâncreas de maneira difusa, mais notavelmente a pancreatite.[27] A incidência de pancreatite identificável à histologia, quase sempre grave, em cães diabéticos varia de 30 a 40% e supostamente contribui para o desenvolvimento de DM e cetoacidose diabética.[28-30] A perda da função de células beta é irreversível em cães com DM, sendo necessário terapia insulínica por toda a vida para sobrevivência. O DM transitório ou reversível é extremamente incomum em cães, quase sempre reconhecido em diabéticos subclínicos com condição antagonista à insulina concomitante (i. e., diestro, prenhez) ou que foram submetidos a um fármaco antagonista da insulina (i. e., glicocorticoides). Após o estro, todas as cadelas normais (gestantes ou não) entram na fase luteal, dominada pela progesterona (diestro), do ciclo ovariano. O diestro dura 60 a 90 dias, e ocorre a cada 6 a 12 meses. A progesterona (Pg) estimula a secreção do hormônio de crescimento (GH, do inglês *growth hormone*) pelo tecido mamário. Tanto a Pg como o GH antagonizam os efeitos da insulina.[31] Fêmeas idosas são frequentemente diagnosticadas com DM enquanto em diestro (gestantes ou não), quando as concentrações séricas de Pg e GH estão aumentadas.[32-34] O tratamento com ovário-histerectomia remove a fonte de Pg e, por sua vez, o estímulo para secreção de GH. Se uma população adequada de células beta funcionais ainda estiver presente no pâncreas, a hiperglicemia pode ser resolvida sem insulinoterapia. A incapacidade de corrigir rapidamente a resistência insulínica resulta quase sempre em perda progressiva de células beta e maior probabilidade de dependência permanente de insulina.[33]

"Período de lua de mel"

Um "período de lua de mel" ocorre em alguns cães com DM recém-diagnosticado, caracterizado por controle glicêmico excelente em resposta a pequenas doses de insulina (< 0,2 UI/kg/

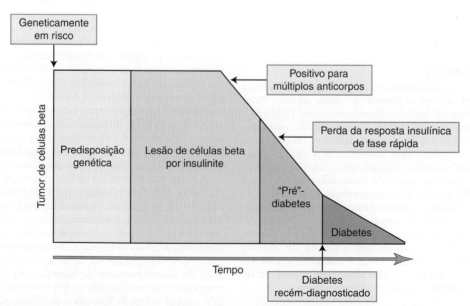

Figura 304.1 Estágios hipotéticos no desenvolvimento de diabetes tipo 1 em seres humanos, começando com a suscetibilidade genética e terminando com a disfunção completa de células beta. (De Eisenbarth GS et al.: Type 1 diabetes mellitus. In: Kronenberg HM, Melmed S, Polonsky KS et al., editors: *Williams textbook of endocrinology*, 11 ed., Philadelphia, 2008, Saunders Elsevier, p. 1398.)

injeção), presumivelmente em razão da função residual de células beta. Tipicamente, o controle glicêmico nesses cães se torna mais difícil, sendo necessário aumentar as doses de insulina meses após o início do tratamento, à medida que aquelas células beta funcionais residuais morrem e não são substituídas. A secreção endógena de insulina diminui.[35] O DMNID ou tipo 2 é raro em cães, estando quase sempre associado à condição ou ao tratamento concomitante de antagonismo à insulina. A resistência insulínica induzida pela obesidade foi documentada em cães, embora a progressão para o DM tipo 2 ainda não tenha sido mostrada.[36]

FISIOPATOLOGIA

O diabetes melito é resultado da deficiência relativa ou absoluta da secreção de insulina pelas células beta pancreáticas. A deficiência insulínica, por sua vez, causa diminuição da utilização tecidual de glicose, aminoácidos e ácidos graxos, glicogenólise e gliconeogênese hepáticas aceleradas e acúmulo de glicose na circulação, o que causa hiperglicemia.[37] Nem a absorção intestinal de glicose nem a entrada de glicose nos eritrócitos, nos rins ou no cérebro não são afetadas. A glicosúria ocorre à medida que a capacidade tubular renal para reabsorção de glicose é excedida, em geral quando a glicemia é > 180 a 220 mg/dℓ. A diurese osmótica induzida pela glicose resultante causa poliúria (PU), perda de água e ativação do mecanismo de sede (polidipsia; PD). O balanço calórico negativo resultante da incapacidade de utilizar glicose, certa perda de calorias pela glicosúria e catabolismo tecidual levam à polifagia.

A fisiologia das consequências do DM é praticamente idêntica àquela da inanição. O metabolismo proteico é desviado para diminuição na síntese e no incremento na proteólise. Esses aminoácidos disponíveis aumentam a gliconeogênese hepática – uma boa resposta à inanição –, mas, no DM, contribui ainda mais para a hiperglicemia ao custo de balanço negativo do nitrogênio, perda de massa muscular e possível caquexia.[38] A falta contínua de insulina e glicose intracelular acelera então o catabolismo lipídico, com mobilização de triglicerídeos, o que leva ao aumento dos teores de ácidos graxos livres (AGLs) plasmáticos. Os AGLs são transportados ao fígado, onde são submetidos à betaoxidação em acetil CoA, cuja quantidade pode exceder a necessidade da produção de ATP pela oxidação no ciclo de Krebs. A acetil CoA é, portanto, metabolizada em seus produtos alternativos: os corpos cetônicos. Novamente, em resposta à inanição, as cetonas são uma fonte aceitável a curto prazo para obtenção de energia. Em casos de inanição prolongada ou no DM, a produção de corpos cetônicos em excesso pode levar à cetose e, em diabéticos, à cetoacidose. O aumento da concentração hepática de ácidos graxos aumenta a síntese hepática de triglicerídeos e lipoproteínas de muito baixa densidade (VLDL, do inglês *very low density lipoproteins*), o que causa hiperlipidemia e lipidose hepática (ver Capítulo 285).

EPIDEMIOLOGIA

O DM é mais comumente diagnosticado em cães de meia-idade e idosos, com 5 a 12 anos.[1,3,5] Raramente, o DM foi relatado em cães jovens.[3,39] O pico de prevalência vai de 7 a 10 anos, e a maioria dos estudos, mas não todos, sugere maior risco em fêmeas.[1,3-5,40] Diferenças regionais na popularidade de raças ou na variação racial em campanhas de castração podem influenciar a predisposição sexual dentro de uma população, embora também haja variação das associações identificadas entre castração e diagnóstico de DM. Sugeriu-se predisposição genética a favor ou contra o desenvolvimento de DM em cães (Tabela 304.1) Por exemplo, cães Boxer raramente são relatados em estudos epidemiológicos sobre DM, visto que podem ter uma das menores incidências da doença. Diferenças genéticas dentro da mesma

Tabela 304.1 Riscos de desenvolvimento de diabetes melito de acordo com a raça.

RAÇAS EM ALTO RISCO	RAZÃO DE PROBABILIDADE	RAÇAS EM BAIXO RISCO	RAZÃO DE PROBABILIDADE
Terrier Australiano	9,39	Pastor-Alemão	0,18
Schnauzer	5,85	Collie	0,21
Schnauzer Miniatura	5,10	Pastor de Shetland	0,21
Bichon Frisé	3,03	Golden Retriever	0,28
Spitz	2,90	Cocker Spaniel	0,35
Fox Terrier	2,68	Pastor-Australiano	0,44
Poodle Miniatura	2,49	Labrador Retriever	0,45
Samoieda	2,42	Doberman Pinscher	0,49
Cairn Terrier	2,26	Boston Terrier	0,51
Keeshond	2,23	Rottweiler	0,51
Maltês	1,79	Basset Hound	0,56
Poodle Toy	1,76	Setter Inglês	0,60
Lhasa Apso	1,54	Beagle	0,64
Yorkshire Terrier	1,44	Setter Irlandês	0,67

Derivada da análise do Veterinary Medical Database (VMDB) de 1970 a 1993. O VMDB compreende registros médicos de 24 escolas de medicina veterinária nos EUA e no Canadá. Os registros de caso do VMDB analisados incluíram aqueles das primeiras visitas hospitalares de 6.078 cães com diagnóstico de diabetes melito e 5.922 cães randomicamente selecionados com atendimentos hospitalares de qualquer diagnóstico que não fosse diabetes melito, atendidos nas mesmas escolas veterinárias, no mesmo ano. Somente raças com mais de 25 casos de diabetes melito foram incluídas. (De Guptill L *et al.*: Is canine diabetes on the increase? In *Recent advances in clinical management of diabetes* mellitus, Dayton, Ohio, 1999, Iams Company, p. 24.)

raça em decorrência de diferentes linhagens sanguíneas também impactam as predisposições. Por exemplo, o Elkhound sueco e norueguês, o Terrier australiano e o Samoieda apresentam maior incidência de DM na Suécia, ao passo que cães das raças Setter irlandês e inglês são os principais representantes na Itália.[2,5]

ANAMNESE

O histórico típico de um cão com DM inclui os sinais clínicos clássicos de poliúria/polidipsia/polifagia (PU/PD/PF) e perda de peso. PU/PD são constantes em cães diabéticos. A PF pode ser diminuída por uma condição concomitante que diminua o apetite (p. ex., pancreatite, cetose, cetoacidose diabética). A perda de peso pode não ser notada em cães recém-diabéticos. As razões mais comuns para cães com DM não diagnosticado serem levados ao veterinário são a necessidade de urinar durante a noite ou dentro de casa. Caso o cão possua livre acesso a ambientes externos para urinar, o tutor pode consultar o veterinário quanto a questões relacionadas com perda de peso, aumento acentuado do apetite, cegueira súbita causada por formação de catarata (Figura 304.2) ou sinais associados à cetoacidose diabética (p. ex., letargia, anorexia, êmese, fraqueza). O tempo do início dos sinais clínicos até o desenvolvimento de cetoacidose diabética é imprevisível, variando de dias a meses, e pode depender do tipo e da gravidade de distúrbios concomitantes, o que causa resistência insulínica e/ou estimulação à produção de cetonas.

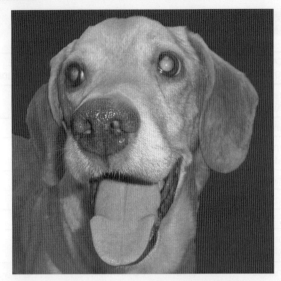

Figura 304.2 Catarata completa bilateral secundária ao diabetes melito causando cegueira em um cão. (*Esta figura se encontra reproduzida em cores no Encarte.*)

EXAME FÍSICO

Em cães com DM recém-diagnosticado, anormalidades detectadas ao exame físico dependem da duração da doença, da existência de distúrbios concomitantes e se houve estabelecimento da cetoacidose diabética. Um exame físico minucioso é de crucial importância, sobretudo para detectar questões decorrentes de uma doença concomitante. Cães com DM descomplicado costumam estar em boa condição, podendo não haver alterações ao exame físico. Cães diabéticos estar acima (obesos) ou abaixo do peso ou dentro da faixa de normalidade. A letargia pode ser evidente. O pelame de cães com DM recém-diagnosticado ou mal controlado pode ser opaco. Hepatomegalia em razão da lipidose hepática induzida pelo diabetes é comumente palpável. Catarata também é comum. Pode haver uveíte anterior e ceratoconjuntivite seca. Os sinais neurológicos comumente observados em gatos diabéticos (p. ex., fraqueza em membros pélvicos, ataxia, posição plantígrada) não são comuns em cães.

DIAGNÓSTICO

O diagnóstico do diabetes melito é confirmado com base nos sinais clínicos apropriados, na hiperglicemia em jejum persistente (> 200 mg/dℓ) e na glicosúria concomitante. Tanto a hiperglicemia persistente quanto a glicosúria são de importância fundamental para o diagnóstico do DM. A hiperglicemia distingue o DM da glicosúria renal primária, e a glicosúria separa o DM de outras causas de hiperglicemia (Boxe 304.2). Hiperglicemia discreta, com concentrações abaixo do limiar renal (> 100 e < 180 mg/dℓ), é assintomática e quase sempre observada como um achado acidental. O DM é bastante improvável se um cão tiver hiperglicemia discreta sem glicosúria. A hiperglicemia induzida pelo estresse é comum em gatos, mas rara em cães. Indica-se avaliação diagnóstica para distúrbios que causem resistência insulínica se a hiperglicemia discreta persistir em um cão em jejum, sem estresse, sem a indicação de insulinoterapia, uma vez que não há DM clínico. Evidências concomitantes de cetonúria estabelecem o diagnóstico de cetose diabética, ao passo que cetonúria e acidose metabólica, com aumento do ânion *gap*, um diagnóstico de cetoacidose diabética. Concentrações de cetona no sangue podem ser avaliadas com uma gota de sangue, utilizando-se um sensor eletroquímico portátil para 3-beta-hidroxibutirato (3-HB). Concentrações sanguíneas baixas a moderadas de 3-BH costumam indicar cetose diabética, ao passo que valores maiores (> 3,8 mmol/ℓ) sugerem cetoacidose diabética (ver Capítulo 142).[41]

Boxe 304.2 Causas de hiperglicemia e glicosúria em cães

Causas de hiperglicemia
Diabetes melito
Estresse, agressividade, excitação, nervosismo, medo (bastante incomum)
Pancreatite
Pós-prandial (dietas que contenham monossacarídeos, dissacarídeos e propilenoglicol)
Antagonismo hormonal:
- Síndrome de Cushing
- Diestro
- Feocromocitoma
- Acromegalia.

Iatrogênico:
- Glicocorticoides
- Progestágenos
- Diuréticos tiazídicos
- Sedativos alfa-2 agonistas
- Fluidos que contenham dextrose
- Solução de nutrição parenteral.

Trauma encefálico

Causas de glicosúria
Diabetes melito
Disfunção tubular renal:
- Síndrome de Fanconi
- Glicosúria renal primária
- Lesão renal aguda (p. ex., leptospirose)
- Nefrotoxinas.

Iatrogênico:
- Fluidos que contenham dextrose

Causas de glicosúria falso-positivas:
- Glicose no frasco de coleta do tutor para urina (p. ex., pote de geleia)
- Vitamina C ou pigmento na urina pode afetar os resultados da fita reagente para análise urinária.

Assim que o DM for diagnosticado, é de extrema importância avaliar minuciosamente a saúde geral de um cão. O clínico deve identificar qualquer pista para uma condição que possa ter contribuído para o desenvolvimento da doença (p. ex., síndrome de Cushing [ver Capítulo 306], hipotireoidismo [ver Capítulo 299], pancreatite [ver Capítulo 290]) ou que possa representar uma consequência do DM (p. ex., perda de peso, fraqueza, infecção de trato urinário). A avaliação laboratorial mínima em um cão recém-diagnosticado com DM deve incluir hemograma, perfil bioquímico sérico, com inclusão de concentração de frutosamina, e urinálise com urocultura. Concentrações séricas de Pg devem ser avaliadas em qualquer fêmea diabética inteira. A ultrassonografia abdominal (ver Capítulo 88) é indicada para avaliação de pacientes em busca de evidências de pancreatite, aumento adrenal, tumores, piometra, cistos ovarianos e outras questões. Em decorrência da prevalência relativamente alta da pancreatite, deve-se considerar a imunorreatividade da lipase pancreática (PLIc), especialmente se a ultrassonografia não estiver disponível. Outros exames, incluindo radiografias torácicas, podem ser indicados (Boxe 304.3).

QUESTÕES TERAPÊUTICAS

Planos e objetivos terapêuticos

Em cães, o tratamento bem-sucedido de DM requer comprometimento do tutor e excelente interação entre este e a equipe veterinária. O "tutor" pode ser uma ou várias pessoas, enquanto a equipe veterinária envolvida no cuidado a longo prazo desses cães deve incluir médicos-veterinários, técnicos e equipe não técnica. O tutor deve ser educado com cuidado no que se refere ao DM, sobre como essa doença é tratada de maneira diferente

Boxe 304.3 Anormalidades clinicopatológicas comumente observadas em cães com diabetes melito descomplicado

Hemograma
1. Quase sempre normal
2. Leucocitose neutrofílica ou neutrófilos tóxicos podem ser observados se houver pancreatite ou infecção

Painel bioquímico
1. Hiperglicemia
2. Hipercolesterolemia
3. Hipertrigliceridemia (lipemia)
4. Aumento da atividade da alanina aminotransferase (em geral, < 500 UI/ℓ)
5. Aumento da atividade da fosfatase alcalina (em geral, < 500 UI/ℓ)

Urinálise
1. Densidade urinária > 1,025
2. Glicosúria
3. Cetonúria variável
4. Proteinúria
5. Bacteriúria

Testes auxiliares
1. Hiperlipasemia, se houver pancreatite
2. Imunorreatividade tripsina-*like* sérica em geral normal
   a. Baixa em casos de insuficiência pancreática exócrina
3. Imunorreatividade de lipase pancreática em geral normal
   a. Alta em casos de pancreatite aguda
   b. Normal a alta em casos de pancreatite crônica
4. Concentração de insulina basal sérica variável
   a. Diabetes melito insulinodependente: baixa, normal
   b. Induzido por resistência insulínica: baixa, normal, aumentada

em cães quando comparada a pessoas e os objetivos da terapia. O estabelecimento e a concordância sobre a definição de "sucesso terapêutico" são extremamente importantes. Para a maioria dos veterinários, o objetivo primário no manejo a longo prazo do DM deve ser a satisfação do tutor com o estado do cão, o que quase sempre é alcançado caso a PU possa ser eliminada ou reduzida de maneira significativa, o peso corporal esteja estável e aceitável, a PF seja tolerável e o cão interaja normalmente com outros na casa. Tutores informados e envolvidos no tratamento dos cães parecem ter maior sucesso e satisfação ao providenciar cuidados. É fundamental que m tutor bastante motivado trabalhe com o veterinário. Cães com DM tipicamente necessitam de duas injeções diárias de insulina e uma rotina relativamente fixa. Os tutores devem estar dispostos não só quanto à administração, mas também ter reservas suficientes para insulina, insumos, testes necessários para o manejo do DM com o passar do tempo, assim como para possíveis períodos intermitentes de hospitalização.[42] É importante fornecer informações detalhadas aos tutores sobre todos os aspectos técnicos do DM e viabilizar o pronto acesso ao tratamento, se necessário. Ademais, o tratamento deve seguir um protocolo preciso e compreensível (Boxe 304.4).

Iniciação da insulinoterapia

Assim que diagnosticado, deve-se começar o tratamento do DM. Cães em boa condição e com apetite excelente podem ser tratados como "diabéticos descomplicados", mesmo na presença de cetonúria. Os objetivos da terapia são reduzir ou resolver os sinais clínicos, evitar as complicações a curto prazo (p. ex., hipoglicemia, cetoacidose diabética), atingir as áreas previamente discutidas de melhora clínica e ter uma boa qualidade de vida. Em cães com DM, isso pode ser alcançado com insulinoterapia exógena, dieta apropriada, exercício, prevenção ou controle de distúrbios concomitantes inflamatórios, infecciosos, neoplásicos

ou hormonais e prevenção de fármacos antagonistas da insulina (ver Capítulo 358). Não é recomendado esperar por glicemias normais ou próximas do normal, dado o risco de hipoglicemia, uma complicação comum, séria e com potencial risco de morte, quase sempre o resultado de insulinoterapia em excesso. A maioria dos cães diabéticos é descrita como em bom estado se as glicemias forem mantidas entre 90 mg/dℓ e 250 mg/dℓ.

Educação do tutor

É de fundamental importância educar os tutores quanto ao tratamento bem-sucedido de um cão com DM (ver Capítulo 79). Estes devem estar familiarizados com os sinais clínicos do DM e conscientes sobre as alterações na ingestão hídrica, no débito urinário, no apetite e no peso corporal. Inapetência, êmese, diarreia ou letargia incomum são sempre preocupantes e merecem uma consulta veterinária. A princípio, a insulina deve ser administrada após a refeição, para evitar o dilema de tê-la administrado a um cão que se recusa a comer. Deve-se enfatizar que a consistência no tempo das injeções, das refeições, do tipo e da quantidade de comida e do exercício facilitarão o controle do DM. Os tutores devem conhecer os sinais de hipoglicemia e cetoacidose diabética. Infelizmente, vários cães com DM se tornam cegos pela formação de catarata (ver Figura 304.2), o que pode ocorrer, apesar dos melhores esforços do tutor para um controle excelente.

Ao mesmo tempo que os tutores são fundamentais para o bom controle do DM, as decisões com relação à insulina, à dose e à frequência de administração devem sempre ser feitas pelo tutor/equipe veterinária. A insulina deve ser armazenada em um refrigerador, com o frasco em pé, e homogeneizada de maneira correta.

Vetsulin®/Caninsulin® devem ser agitadas, algumas insulinas não necessitam de homogeneização e outras devem ser gentilmente roladas entre as mãos. Os tutores devem utilizar seringas apropriadas (40 UI/mℓ para insulinas veterinárias e 100 UI/mℓ para insulinas humanas), aprender a eliminar bolhas de ar e administrar a insulina por via subcutânea, sob a parede lateral do tórax. Deve-se evitar a utilização de seringas não equiparadas com base nas tabelas de conversão para insulinas 40 UI e 100 UI/mℓ ou o cálculo próprio do tutor, para não haver confusão. Em geral, seringas de insulina de 40 UI possuem escalas em mililitros e unidades; o tutor deve ser instruído a utilizar as escalas de unidades. A técnica de administração deve ser demonstrada até que o tutor se sinta confortável (a prática em casa com uma banana madura pode ser benéfica). Se uma caneta de administração de insulina for utilizada, os tutores devem ser especificamente treinados com essa ferramenta. Instruções escritas são úteis. Tutores de cães diabéticos devem ser encorajados a manter registros detalhados de glicemia, glicosúria, cetonas da urina e quaisquer alterações em outros parâmetros dos cães.

Recomendações dietéticas (ver Capítulo 181)

O alimento fornecido a cães com DM deve ser palatável, para garantir consumo regular. Dietas devem ser completas em termos nutricionais, devendo-se ter consistência diária com relação à composição, aos ingredientes e às calorias. Esses fatores aumentam a chance de necessidades consistentes tanto da insulina quanto da resposta. É ideal que a condição corporal próxima do ideal seja atingida e mantida. Um cão com DM pode estar em sobrepeso ou abaixo do peso. Em ambas as condições, o peso próximo do ideal é um objetivo razoável. Por ser um hormônio anabólico, diabéticos tratados com insulina ganham peso com facilidade. Já que é anabólica, fazer com que um cão obeso com DM perca peso é muito mais difícil. Entretanto, a resistência insulínica induzida pela obesidade foi documentada em cães, havendo melhora da tolerância à glicose com a perda de peso.[43] As dietas para perda de peso devem ser consideradas para cães diabéticos obesos, já que costumam ser ricas em fibras insolúveis, com baixos níveis de gordura e densidade calórica diminuída. Tais dietas não devem ser

SEÇÃO 21 • Doenças Endócrinas

Boxe 304.4 Protocolo para o manejo de cães diabéticos

- Diagnóstico do diabetes melito (histórico, exame físico, hiperglicemia, glicosúria, frutosamina aumentada)
- Avaliação laboratorial de rotina (hemograma, bioquímica sérica, urinálise, urocultura)
- Ultrassonografia abdominal, imunorreatividade da lipase pancreática canina, se indicado
- Interrupção de fármacos diabetogênicos
- Administração de insulinas de ação intermediária/longa (Caninsulin®/Vetsulin®, NPH, Lantus): 0,25 UI/kg/12 h SC
- Instituição do tratamento para problemas concomitantes (p. ex., infecção do trato urinário)
- Prescreva uma dieta "diabética" comercial. Alimente o cão com 2 refeições de mesma proporção, logo antes de cada injeção de insulina. Se em sobrepeso, a meta é de 1 a 2% de perda de peso por semana. Dietas com alto teor de fibras e de baixa caloria não devem ser fornecidas para cães diabéticos magros ou emaciados, até que o controle glicêmico esteja estabelecido e um peso corporal normal seja obtido utilizando-se dieta com alto nível calórico e com baixo teor de fibras, desenvolvida para manutenção. Recomendações dietéticas para distúrbios concomitantes (p. ex., doença renal crônica, alergia alimentar, pancreatite) possuem prioridade sobre uma dieta diabética específica
- Instruções ao tutor (requer pelo menos 1 h)
  - Em casos de fêmeas inteiras, marque a castração. Esse procedimento deve ser feito o mais rápido possível
  - Forneça instruções por escrito.

Reavaliação 1 semana após o diagnóstico
- Histórico, exame físico, peso corporal
  - Administração de alimento e insulina na clínica. Para cães que se recusam a comer no local, a comida e a insulina devem ser administradas em casa e a curva glicêmica iniciada logo após a chegada à clínica (o mais cedo possível)
- Aferição da glicose a cada 1 a 2 h pelo restante do dia
- Frutosamina
- Ajuste da dose de insulina, se necessário: 10 a 25%.

Reavaliação 2 a 3 semanas após o diagnóstico
- Repita todos os passos realizados na primeira reavaliação (histórico, exame físico, peso corporal, curva glicêmica, frutosamina, ajuste da dose)
- Introdução ao monitoramento doméstico e instrução quanto a todos os aspectos técnicos relevantes (requer pelo menos meia hora)
- O tutor deve aferir a glicemia em jejum 2 vezes/semana e realizar curva glicêmica duas vezes ao mês.

Reavaliação 6 a 8 semanas após o diagnóstico
- Repita todos os procedimentos realizados na primeira reavaliação (histórico, exame físico, peso corporal, curva glicêmica, frutosamina, ajuste da dose). A curva glicêmica pode não ser necessária se o cão parecer clinicamente bem, se a glicemia mensurada próximo ao momento da administração da insulina for de 180 a 250 mg/dℓ e a frutosamina estiver entre 350 μmol/ℓ e 450 μmol/ℓ
- A técnica de administração do tutor deve ser avaliada para aqueles que fazem monitoramento doméstico.

Reavaliação 10 a 12 semanas após o diagnóstico
- Repita todos os procedimentos realizados 6 a 8 semanas após o diagnóstico.

Outras reavaliações a cada 4 meses
- Repita todos os procedimentos realizados 6 a 8 semanas após o diagnóstico.

Objetivos da terapia
- Sinais clínicos: resolução da poliúria/polidipsia e polifagia, peso corporal normal
- Glicemia: é ideal que esteja entre 250 mg/dℓ (antes da administração de insulina) e 90 mg/dℓ (nadir)
- Concentração de frutosamina: é ideal que esteja entre 350 μmol/ℓ e 450 μmol/ℓ. (atenção: a concentração de frutosamina é a variável menos importante para avaliação do controle metabólico).

---

fornecidas a cães diabéticos abaixo do peso. Assim que o controle glicêmico for estabelecido e um peso corporal próximo ao normal alcançado, deve-se considerar o fornecimento de uma dieta consistente densa em calorias e com baixos teores de fibras desenvolvida para manutenção.[37]

Diversas dietas de prescrição comerciais estão disponíveis para cães diabéticos. Para minimizar a hiperglicemia pós-prandial, nenhuma deve conter quantidades significativas de açúcares simples. As calorias devem consistir, principalmente, em carboidratos complexos e proteínas. A quantidade de gordura na dieta deve ser minimizada, a fim de evitar o aumento de colesterol, triglicerídeos, glicerol livre e ácidos graxos livres circulantes.[44] A gordura da dieta pode contribuir diretamente para a resistência insulínica, promover produção de glicose hepática e, em cães saudáveis, suprimir a função das células beta.[45,46] A gordura da dieta deve ser particularmente restrita a qualquer cão com histórico de pancreatite ou hiperlipidemia persistente.

Diversos estudos, mas não todos, que avaliam o papel de dietas ricas em fibras no manejo de cães com DM demonstraram que maiores teores de fibras na dieta melhoram o controle glicêmico.[47-49] Um estudo não conseguiu mostrar benefícios do fornecimento de uma dieta rica em fibras para cães diabéticos com peso normal.[44] A maioria das dietas para DM contém uma combinação de fibras solúveis e insolúveis. Complicações comuns do fornecimento de dietas ricas em fibras incluem aumento da frequência de defecações (fibras insolúveis); constipação intestinal e obstipação (fibras insolúveis); fezes moles a aquosas (fibras solúveis); e flatulência excessiva (fibras solúveis).[37] Problemas com a palatabilidade, que, em geral, resultam

da troca de dietas de maneira muito rápida, podem ser evitados em muitos pacientes pela transição gradativa de uma dieta para outra. Com o passar do tempo, cães podem se tornar menos interessados em dietas ricas em fibras e a palatabilidade pode ser maior pela adição de carne cozida moída. A dieta também deve levar em consideração condições concomitantes (i. e., doença inflamatória intestinal, doença renal crônica, alergia/intolerância alimentar), que podem ter prioridade sobre uma dieta específica para DM.

Para simplificar o tratamento, a maioria dos cães com DM deve ser alimentada diariamente com duas refeições de mesma proporção, a cada 12 horas aproximadamente, antes da administração da insulina, evitando-se, dessa forma, que o animal se recuse a comer depois do recebimento do medicamento. Em cães com apetite inalterado, o alimento pode ser oferecido imediatamente após a administração da insulina, o que ajuda o animal a associar a injeção desagradável com a refeição mais agradável. A alimentação à vontade pode ser benéfica para alguns gatos diabéticos, mas não é recomendada para cães. Cães enjoados devem ser alimentados no momento da administração da insulina, disponibilizando-se as sombras de comida durante todo o dia.

Exercícios

Por facilitar o manejo do DM canino, exercícios consistentes devem ser encorajados (ver Capítulos 355 e 359). A atividade física diminui a glicemia, pelo aumento da absorção de insulina do local de injeção, do fluxo sanguíneo e da distribuição de insulina aos músculos exercitados, pelo estímulo à translocação (i. e., suprarregulação) dos transportadores de glicose (principalmente

GLUT-4) em células musculares e pelo aumento da eliminação de glicose das concentrações basais de insulina.[50,51] O período e a quantidade de exercício diário devem ser compatíveis com o momento das refeições e da insulina. Por exemplo, não é apropriado para um cão diabético se exercitar pouco ou simplesmente não se exercitar ou durante a semana e, então, fazê-lo em excesso durante os fins de semana. Como o exercício extenuante e esporádico pode induzir hipoglicemia, ele deve ser evitado. No dia em que um cão com DM estiver envolvido em exercício intenso ou incomum (*i. e.*, caça), é importante reduzir a dose matutina da insulina. A redução percentual necessária para prevenir a hipoglicemia não é previsível; dessa forma, uma redução inicial de 50% é razoável. Ajustes adicionais devem se basear na experiência com questões como hipoglicemia sintomática ou PU durante ou depois do exercício. Os tutores de cães com DM devem sempre ter uma fonte de glicose prontamente disponível, caso sinais de hipoglicemia sejam observados ao realizar uma atividade física.

INSULINA

Visão geral

Vários tipos de insulina são utilizados para tratamento a longo prazo do DM. Com base na duração de ação e potência, eles incluem insulinas de ação intermediária (lenta, protamina neutra de Hagedorn [NPH]) e longa (insulina protamina zíncica [PZI], insulina glargina, insulina detemir) (Tabela 304.2). A insulina lenta (Vetsulin®, Caninsulin®) é uma insulina zíncica de origem suína de 40 UI/ml, com 30% de insulina amorfa de ação curta e 70% de insulina microcristalina de longa ação. A NPH (100 UI/ml; Humulin N®, Novolin N®) é uma insulina humana recombinante, em geral administrada a cada 12 h. A hiperglicemia pós-prandial pode ocorrer em cães bem regulados.[58] Uma insulina PZI de longa ação de 40 UI/ml, produzida com insulina humana recombinante, é aprovada para utilização em gatos (ProZinc®). Essa insulina pode ser útil para alguns cães nos quais a duração das insulinas de ação intermediária seja muito curta.[54] As insulinas glargina e detemir são análogos de insulina sintéticos de longa ação, desenvolvidos para manter concentrações basais de insulina em pessoas diabéticas, com a crescente utilização em cães.

Análogos da insulina

Análogos da insulina são modificados a partir de peptídios de insulina humana, possuem efeitos fisiológicos semelhantes e são comumente utilizados no tratamento de gatos e cães diabéticos.[59]

O aminoácido asparagina na insulina humana é substituído pela glicina na posição A21, com a adição de duas moléculas de arginina com cargas positivas ao terminal-C da cadeia B para criar a insulina glargina (Lantus®).[60] Essa estrutura resulta em baixa solubilidade aquosa em pH neutro, mas solubilidade completa em pH 4. A solução ácida da glargina injetada no meio com pH neutro do tecido SC forma microprecipitados de análogos da insulina que retardam a absorção e atrasam o início da ação. O resultado é um suprimento basal relativamente constante e sem pico de insulina.[60] Em razão da importância do pH, a glargina jamais deve ser diluída ou misturada com qualquer solução que possa alterar o pH. Em cães, a insulina glargina se mostrou segura e eficaz no controle glicêmico bom a moderado.[55,56]

O aminoácido treonina, na posição 30 da cadeia B, foi removido e um ácido graxo com 14 carbonos (ácido mirístico) foi ligado ao aminoácido lisina na posição 29 da cadeia B para criar a insulina detemir (Levemir®). Essas modificações permitem que a insulina se ligue de forma reversível à albumina, retardando a absorção e prolongando seu efeito metabólico consistente por até 24 horas em pessoas.[61] Em cães, a insulina detemir é aproximadamente quatro vezes mais potente quando comparada a outras preparações de insulina. A insulina detemir, administrada por via SC, a cada 12 h, é um tratamento potencial para cães com DM. Em razão da maior potência dessa insulina em cães, doses menores são necessárias para controlar a glicemia. Recomenda-se uma dose inicial de 0,1 UI/kg, a cada 12 h. A insulina detemir deve ser utilizada com cautela, especialmente em pequenos animais.[57] A utilização de diluentes especificamente desenvolvidos para essa insulina permite o fornecimento seguro de doses pequenas.

Armazenamento, homogeneização e diluição da insulina

O congelamento ou o aquecimento inativam a insulina. Embora o armazenamento da insulina em temperatura ambiente seja aceitável, os tutores devem ser instruídos a acondicioná-la na porta da geladeira, para manter um ambiente estável e consistente, de frasco para frasco, bem como de paciente para paciente. Alguns veterinários recomendam substituir a insulina a cada mês, a fim de evitar a inativação ou contaminação. Entretanto, o "tempo de prateleira" da insulina produzida comercialmente, armazenada e manuseada de maneira correta, é muito mais longo do que as recomendações do fabricante. Problemas com a perda da potência ou esterilidade da insulina são extremamente raros. A substituição mensal rotineira não é recomendada. Embora tenha sido afirmado que agitar em vez de homogeneizar gentilmente inativaria a insulina, estudos recentes mostram mais uma

Tabela 304.2	Preparações de insulina comumente utilizadas para o tratamento do diabetes melito descomplicado em cães.						
INSULINA	PRODUTO	ORIGEM	CONCENTRAÇÃO (UI/ml)	DURAÇÃO DO EFEITO (horas)	FREQUÊNCIA DE ADMINISTRAÇÃO	DOSE INICIAL (UI/kg/injeção)	DOSE (UI/KG) DE INSULINA MEDIANA (VARIAÇÃO) POR INJEÇÃO POR KG DE PESO CORPORAL PARA OBTENÇÃO DO CONTROLE GLICÊMICO (UI/kg/injeção)
Lenta	Vetsulin®/ Caninsulin®	Porcina	40	8 a 14	A cada 12 h	0,25	0,8 (0,3 a 1,4)[52]
NPH	Humulin N®/ Novolin N®	Recombinante humana	100	4 a 10	A cada 12 h	0,25	0,8 (0,4 a 1,9)*[53] 0,4 (0,3 a 0,8)†[53]
PZI	ProZinc®	Recombinante humana	40	10 a 16	A cada 12 h	0,25 a 0,5	0,9 (0,4 a 1,5)[54]
Glargina	Lantus®	Recombinante humana	100	8 a 16	A cada 12 h (a cada 24 h)	0,3	0,6 (0,1 a 1,1)[55] 0,5 (0,32 a 0,67)[56]
Detemir	Levemir®	Recombinante humana	100	8 a 16	A cada 12 h (a cada 24 h)	0,1	0,12 (0,05 a 0,34)[57]

*Cães com < 15 kg. †Cães com > 15 kg. *NPH*, protamina neutra de Hagedorn; *PZI*, insulina protamina zíncica.

vez que ela é resistente à destruição dessa forma. Para consistência, entretanto, é sugerido rolar gentilmente a maioria dos produtos veterinários entre as mãos. Tanto a Vetsulin® quanto a Caninsulin® devem ser "vigorosamente agitadas", até que seja observada uma suspensão homogênea, uniformemente leitosa. A diluição da insulina pode ser bastante útil em cães pequenos, sobretudo ao utilizar a detemir, que é quatro vezes mais potente que as outras insulinas. Apenas soluções diluentes fornecidas pelo fabricante devem ser utilizadas. É importante enfatizar que a insulina glargina é pH-dependente e não deve ser diluída.

Canetas de aplicação de insulina

Canetas aplicadoras, desenvolvidas para uso em pessoas diabéticas, devem facilitar a mensuração e a administração da insulina, tornando-as menos dolorosas e mais precisas. As canetas de aplicação de insulina mostraram diminuir a ansiedade, o desconforto e o constrangimento social associados à administração de insulina.[62] Informações limitadas estão disponíveis sobre a utilização desses dispositivos em cães. A insulina porcina lenta é o único produto veterinário de insulina comercializado com uma caneta. Elas estão disponíveis em dois tamanhos: uma dose máxima de 8 UI, VetPen® (0,5 a 8 UI), com incrementos de dose de 0,5 UI; e uma dose máxima de 16 UI, VetPen® (1 a 16 UI), com incrementos de 1 UI. Os tutores que optarem pela utilização desse aparato devem ser treinados quanto à montagem (Vídeo 304.1) e à utilização (Vídeo 304.2).

Recomendações iniciais da insulina

O tratamento do DM canino exige insulina exógena para manter o controle glicêmico. Em cães com DM recém-diagnosticada, as primeiras insulinas em geral recomendadas são aquelas do grupo de ação intermediário, como a lenta (Vetsulin®/Caninsulin®) ou NPH recombinante humana. Em ambas as situações, o clínico deve iniciar com uma dose de aproximadamente 0,25 UI/kg/12 h SC. Essa abordagem conservadora deve ser suficiente para evitar a hipoglicemia sintomática ou o efeito Somogyi (hiperglicemia de rebote). Cães podem ser hospitalizados durante 1 a 2 dias para completar a avaliação diagnóstica e iniciar a terapia. A glicemia deve ser verificada 2 a 3 vezes/dia para identificar hipoglicemia, se presente. Se a glicemia diminuir < 80 mg/dℓ, a dose da insulina deve ser reduzida. Entretanto, não é recomendado aumentar a dose se a glicemia permanecer alta, pois a ação da insulina pode melhorar após alguns poucos dias (o chamado equilíbrio).[38] A insulinoterapia pode ser iniciada no ambulatório, que é menos dispendiosa e considerada mais eficaz por alguns.

FÊMEAS EM DIESTRO

Cadelas inteiras diagnosticadas com DM devem ser submetidas à ovário-histerectomia o mais cedo possível; o ideal é que seja 1 a 3 dias após o início da insulina.[38] A ovário-histerectomia é mais importante se a cadela estiver em diestro e sob a influência de Pg, pois a cirurgia reduzirá a resistência insulínica pela eliminação da Pg e, em alguns poucos cães, a remissão do DM pode ocorrer após alguns dias ou semanas.[63] Todas as cadelas inteiras com DM devem ser castradas, mesmo se não houver relação óbvia estabelecida entre o diestro e o início do DM. Após a castração, o controle glicêmico deve ser monitorado de perto, com ajustes apropriados na dose de insulina. Embora a castração não leve à remissão do DM na maioria dos cães, ela impede a secreção de GH derivado da glândula mamária induzida pela Pg em ciclos subsequentes, a resistência insulínica e a descompensação preocupante. Se a castração não for possível, a administração do antagonista do receptor de Pg – aglepristone – pode reduzir a resistência insulínica.[64]

CONDIÇÕES CONCOMITANTES

Condições inflamatórias, infecciosas, neoplásicas e metabólicas concomitantes são comuns em cães recém-diagnosticados com DM, podem interferir na responsividade tecidual à insulina e causar um impacto negativo sobre o manejo do DM. De forma semelhante, glicocorticoides e Pgs reduzem a sensibilidade à insulina (Capítulo 358). Distúrbios concomitantes e fármacos diabetogênicos podem causar resistência à insulina pela alteração do metabolismo de insulina (questões pré-receptores), diminuição da concentração ou afinidade de ligação aos receptores de insulina na membrana celular (questões receptores), interferência na cascata de sinalização de receptores de insulina (questões pós-receptores) ou qualquer uma dessas combinações.[37] A resistência insulínica pode ser discreta (p. ex., obesidade) a grave (p. ex., síndrome de Cushing) ou variar (p. ex., pancreatite crônica) (Tabela 304.3).

A avaliação minuciosa (histórico, exame físico e exames hospitalares) de cães recém-diagnosticados com DM é extremamente importante. A identificação e o tratamento de doenças concomitantes são parte fundamental para o manejo bem-sucedido do DM. Algumas condições (p. ex., pancreatite crônica) não são, assim como o DM, resolvidas em definitivo e exigem manejo a longo prazo. Os tutores devem ser informados que o tratamento do DM, por si só, pode ser desafiador. Condições concomitantes podem dificultar ainda mais o sucesso terapêutico. Monitoramento frequente e ajustes da dose são quase sempre necessários. A administração de glicocorticoides ou Pgs deve ser interrompida e, se possível, medicamentos alternativos devem ser utilizados (ver Capítulo 358). Se os glicocorticoides forem absolutamente necessários, a dose e a frequência devem ser mantidas o mais baixo possível. A consistência na dose e na frequência facilitará a obtenção do controle.

Tabela 304.3	Causas reconhecidas de ineficácia aparente da insulina ou resistência insulínica em cães diabéticos.	
CAUDADAS PELA INSULINOTERAPIA	**DISTÚRBIOS TIPICAMENTE CAUSADORES DE RESISTÊNCIA INSULÍNICA GRAVE**	**DISTÚRBIOS TIPICAMENTE CAUSADORES DE RESISTÊNCIA INSULÍNICA DISCRETA OU FLUTUANTE**
Insulina inativa	Síndrome de Cushing	Obesidade
Insulina diluída	Diestro em fêmeas inteiras	Infecções
Técnica de administração imprópria	Tumor adrenocortical secretor de progesterona	Hipotireoidismo
Dose inadequada	Fármacos diabetogênicos	Inflamações crônicas
Efeito de Somogyi	Glicocorticoides	Pancreatite crônica
Frequência inadequada de administração de insulina	Progestágenos	Doença inflamatória intestinal
Distúrbios na absorção de insulina		Doença da cavidade oral
Anticorpos anti-insulina		Doença renal crônica
		Doença hepatobiliar
		Cardiopatia
		Hipertireoidismo
		Insuficiência pancreática exócrina
		Hiperlipidemia
		Neoplasia
		Glucagonoma
		Feocromocitoma

De Feldman EC, Nelson RW, Reusch C: *Canine and feline endocrinology*, 4 ed., St. Louis, 2015, Saunders.

MONITORAMENTO DO DIABETES MELITO

Visão geral
O cuidado a longo prazo de diabéticos e os ajustes nas medicações devem se basear, principalmente, nas observações do tutor suplementadas por exames hospitalares periódicos. As avaliações hospitalares devem incluir peso corporal, exame físico e concentrações de glicose e frutosamina séricas. A princípio, os teores de glicose e curvas glicêmicas devem ser realizados na clínica. Em seguida, se treinados de maneira adequada, os tutores, em sua maioria, estarão aptos a realizar o monitoramento doméstico, pela aferição da glicose capilar com um glicosímetro portátil.

Frequência de avaliações hospitalares (ver Boxe 304.4)
Membros da equipe veterinária e tutores devem ter ciência de que costuma ser necessário 1 a 3 meses antes que o controle glicêmico razoável e estável seja alcançado. Em alguns, o processo é direto e leva pouco tempo, ao passo que, em outros, ajustes na insulina e outros fatores nunca cessam. O monitoramento periódico é utilizado para ajudar a garantir o tratamento seguro e eficaz. Inicialmente, reavaliações são recomendadas com 1, 2 a 3, 6 a 8 e 10 a 12 semanas após o diagnóstico. Cães costumam, então, ser examinados aproximadamente a cada 4 meses, ou conforme necessário.

Histórico clínico e exame físico
Os parâmetros mais relevantes para avaliação do controle glicêmico são o parecer do tutor com relação ao animal, especificamente sobre o estado da PU/PD/PF, do peso corporal e da saúde geral. O peso corporal é enfatizado, já que os diabéticos, por conta das doses altas de insulina, tendem a ganhar peso. Diabéticos bem controlados possuem peso corporal estável, próximo ao ideal. Achados objetivos ao exame físico são utilizados em conjunto com o parecer do tutor. Caso ele esteja satisfeito com o peso corporal estável e o exame físico compatível com bom controle glicêmico do animal, são recomendados apenas outros exames para evitar sobredoses. Os tutores devem relatar especificamente qualquer possível episódio hipoglicêmico (p. ex., fraqueza, ataxia, "parecer intoxicado"). A persistência ou recidiva dos sinais clínicos ou a alteração indesejada no peso são sugestivas de mau controle glicêmico ou presença de doença concomitante. A concentração sérica de frutosamina e as curvas glicêmicas podem ajudar a caracterizar a questão, direcionar as alterações no tratamento e indicar a necessidade de exames adicionais.

Frutosamina sérica
As frutosaminas são proteínas glicadas produzidas por reações não enzimáticas irreversíveis entre a glicose e as proteínas plasmáticas presentes na circulação.[65] Estima-se que as concentrações de frutosamina em cães sejam determinadas pela glicemia média durante as 2 a 3 semanas prévias. A frutosamina sérica não é afetada por alterações agudas na glicemia. Níveis médios maiores de glicose resultam em quantidades mais altas de frutosaminas no sangue. O excelente controle glicêmico, definido como glicemia próxima do normal na maior parte do tempo, resulta em concentrações de frutosamina dentro ou somente discretamente acima dos valores de referência. Níveis menores de frutosamina, independentemente da glicemia, foram observados em casos de hipoproteinemia, azotemia, hipoalbuminemia, hiperlipidemia e hemólise.[66,67] O aumento das concentrações séricas de frutosaminas foi observado em casos de hipotireoidismo e em 2 cães com hiperglobulinemia causada por mieloma múltiplo.[68,69] Cada laboratório deve gerar um intervalo de referência, mas a maior parte varia de aproximadamente 200 a 360 μmol/ℓ.

Na maioria dos cães diabéticos recém-diagnosticados, os níveis de frutosamina são > 400 μmol/ℓ, com alguns podendo chegar a 1.500 μmol/ℓ. É importante lembrar que nem a normoglicemia nem as concentrações normais de frutosamina devem ser o alvo terapêutico ao tratar cães com DM. A glicemia, em cães diabéticos bem controlados, flutua entre o normal e discretamente acima do limiar renal. Em geral, cães bem controlados apresentam certa glicosúria e são moderadamente hiperglicêmicos durante o dia. Assim, as frutosaminas séricas dentro dos intervalos de referência (especialmente na metade inferior) são mais sugestivas de episódios prolongados de hipoglicemia decorrente da sobredose de insulina. Concentrações séricas de frutosamina de 360 a 450 μmol/ℓ sugerem bom controle glicêmico, 450 a 550 μmol/ℓ, controle moderado e > 550 μmol/ℓ, mau controle do DM.

O aumento das concentrações de frutosamina, mesmo se acima de 550 μmol/ℓ, não ajuda a identificar uma causa para o mau controle glicêmico. Todas as possíveis causas devem ser consideradas. Estas incluem subdose da insulina, curta duração do efeito da insulina, erros na preparação ou administração da insulina, dieta imprópria, qualquer doença que sabidamente cause resistência insulínica e efeito Somogyi (ver Tabela 304.3). A concentração sérica de frutosamina jamais deve ser utilizada como indicador único do controle glicêmico, mas, sim, interpretada em conjunto com o parecer do tutor, os sinais clínicos, o peso corporal e a glicemia. A discrepância entre a concentração de frutosamina e a situação clínica/perfil glicêmico é observada algumas vezes. Por exemplo, uma concentração alta de frutosamina sugere controle ineficaz. Mas, se o cão estiver clinicamente bem, com a glicemia dentro da faixa desejada, o clínico deve manter a terapia atual e fazer uma nova avaliação. A discrepância entre as concentrações de frutosamina e a situação clínica pode permanecer ambígua, havendo diferenças individuais com relação à glicação da proteína.[70] Em alguns, a frutosamina não é útil.

Monitoramento da glicosúria
O monitoramento diário pelo tutor da urina em busca de açúcar e cetonas pode ser útil. A maioria dos diabéticos possui quantidades variadas de glicose em praticamente todas as amostras de urina, com um ocasional negativo. A ausência persistente do açúcar pode ser um indicativo de sobredose de insulina ou controle excelente. A cetonúria sugere controle inadequado e descompensação. Ao visualizar cetonas na urina de um animal que raramente as tem, o tutor deve contactar o veterinário. Em geral, as decisões baseiam-se na condição do cão. Os tutores não devem ajustar a dose da insulina com base na glicosúria da manhã, o que costuma levar à sobredose e aumentar a probabilidade de hipoglicemia induzida pela insulina, seguida de hiperglicemia (efeito Somogyi). O excesso de glicose na urina pode ser causado por diversas questões.

Glicemia única
Uma única aferição da glicemia raramente é útil para o monitoramento do DM, com exceção do achado de um resultado baixo, sempre indicativo de sobredose. Aferições glicêmicas únicas podem ser suficientes quando o tutor acredita que o cão está praticamente assintomático, o exame físico não apresenta alterações e os teores séricos de frutosamina estão entre 360 e 450 μmol/ℓ. Em tais casos, glicemia entre 180 mg/dℓ e 250 mg/dℓ, próxima ao horário da administração da insulina, é compatível com bom controle glicêmico, não sendo necessárias, de modo geral, mensurações adicionais.

Glicosímetros portáteis
Durante a fase inicial de ajuste e nas subsequentes de manejo a longo prazo da terapia, se os sinais de DM persistirem, recidivarem ou os teores de frutosamina estiverem altos, mensurações glicêmicas únicas devem ser evitadas e uma curva glicêmica, obtida. Curvas glicêmicas seriadas podem fornecer diretrizes para realizar ajustes racionais da insulinoterapia. Em geral, a glicemia é medida com o uso de um glicosímetro portátil. Para evitar múltiplas venopunções, o clínico deve coletar sangue da

orelha (Vídeos 304.3 e 304.4; ver Capítulo 79).[71] Diversos glicosímetros portáteis estão disponíveis, cuja acurácia varia de maneira considerável quando utilizados em cães, já que foram desenvolvidos para seres humanos,[71-75] mas alguns deles são suficientemente acurados e precisos para monitorar a glicemia canina. Entretanto, a maioria fornece resultados inferiores, quando comparados aos métodos de referência dos laboratórios. Esse viés pode resultar em diagnóstico incorreto da hipoglicemia ou no conceito equivocado de que o controle glicêmico do animal está melhor do que o de fato. O glicosímetro AlphaTRAK® (Abbott Animal Health) foi especialmente desenvolvido para utilização em cães e gatos, sendo mais acurado e preciso do que os glicosímetros portáteis desenvolvidos para seres humanos.[73] As vantagens adicionais do AlphaTRAK® são o pequeno volume de sangue necessário (0,3 µℓ) e a amplitude dos valores aferidos (20 a 750 mg/dℓ). Em contrapartida, o AlphaTRAK® tende a superestimar os valores da glicemia, potencialmente omitindo a hipoglicemia. O glicosímetro é menos acurado em cães com hematócrito abaixo de 30%.[76] Se houver qualquer dúvida com relação à acurácia, as mensurações podem ser comparadas com os resultados laboratoriais.

Curvas glicêmicas e ajustes da dose de insulina

Ao coletar uma curva glicêmica, o cão deve ser observado no início da manhã e as glicemias coletadas a cada 1 a 2 horas durante todo o dia. O clínico deve iniciar logo antes da primeira administração de insulina e continuar até que a próxima dose seja aplicada. Um estudo recente não conseguiu identificar diferenças relevantes na glicemia durante o dia em comparação à noite, já que a maioria dos cães responde bem à mesma dose de insulina nos dois períodos.[77] Se houver suspeita de diferentes glicemias durante o dia *versus* a noite (p. ex., glicemias boas e controle dos sinais clínicos durante o dia, mas PU/PD durante a noite), deve-se considerar uma curva glicêmica de 24 horas ou a utilização de um dispositivo de monitoramento contínuo da glicemia.[37]

Ao realizar uma curva glicêmica, devem-se manter os horários da insulina e da alimentação estipulados pelo tutor. O apetite ruim pode afetar sobremaneira os resultados da curva glicêmica. O alimento e a insulina podem ser administrados na clínica após a mensuração da primeira glicemia. Se um cão se recusar a se alimentar no local, deve-se suspender a curva glicêmica. Em seguida, o tutor deve alimentar o cão em casa, administrar a insulina e, então, levá-lo para a clínica o mais rápido possível, a fim de iniciar a avaliação da curva glicêmica, que permitirá que o clínico determine se a insulina administrada é efetiva e identifique o nadir da glicose, o momento do pico de efeito da insulina, a duração do efeito dela e o grau de flutuação das glicemias. Se o DM estiver bem controlado, as glicemias devem estar entre 90 mg/dℓ e 250 a 300 mg/dℓ (Figura 304.3). A eficácia da insulina é avaliada, em parte, pela determinação da diferença entre a maior e a menor glicemia. Uma pequena diferença (p. ex., 50 mg/dℓ) é aceitável se a maior glicemia registrada for < 220 mg/dℓ, mas não é aceitável se for > 300 mg/dℓ.[38] Os parâmetros mais importantes são o nadir da glicose e a duração do efeito da insulina.

É ideal que o nadir da glicose esteja entre 90 mg/dℓ e 150 mg/dℓ, vez que um menor pode ser causado por sobredose de insulina, sobreposição excessiva da ação da insulina (comum se forem utilizados análogos da insulina de longa ação), período prolongados sem alimentação (o cão se recusa a comer no hospital) ou exercício extenuante. Um nadir da glicose < 160 mg/dℓ pode ser causado por dose insuficiente de insulina, resistência insulínica, fase contrarregulatória do efeito Somogyi, estresse e problemas técnicos atribuídos aos tutores. Em um cão já tratado com altas doses (p. ex., > 1,5 UI/kg por injeção), erros do tutor, resistência insulínica e efeito Somogyi são os principais diagnósticos diferenciais.

A duração da ação da insulina pode ser determinada se o nadir da glicose se enquadrar na variação desejada. A duração é definida como o tempo desde a administração, passando pelo nadir de glicose, até chegar ao ponto em que a glicemia excede 250 mg/dℓ. Quando a duração for muito breve (p. ex., < 8 horas), os sinais de DM costumam se manifestar. Quando a duração for muito longa (p. ex., > 14 horas), o risco de hipoglicemia ou efeito Somogyi é maior. A duração da ação pode ser alterada com mudanças na dieta. O clínico pode alterar para um produto de insulina com perfil de ação diferente. A realização da curva glicêmica em dias consecutivos não é recomendada, porque promove hiperglicemia induzida pelo estresse.

Jamais se deve admitir que as curvas glicêmicas sejam reprodutíveis. As variações diárias e a condição diabética, por si só, raramente são estáticas. As variações incluem as quantidades tanto de insulina recolhida na seringa a cada aplicação quanto de insulina absorvida a cada administração, bem como as interações entre insulina, dieta, exercício, estresse, excitação, presença de distúrbios concomitantes e secreção de hormônios

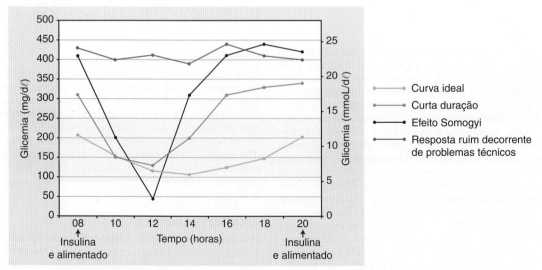

Figura 304.3 Curvas glicêmicas representativas em cães tratados com insulina de ação intermediária, a cada 12 h. A área azul é a faixa preferida da glicemia em cães diabéticos tratados (90 a 250 mg/dℓ). Linha verde: curva ideal. Linha laranja: duração curta da insulina. Linha azul: efeito Somogyi, com contrarregulação após diminuição rápida da glicemia. Linha vermelha: resposta ruim em razão de problemas técnicos, fase contrarregulatória do efeito Somogyi, resistência insulínica, má absorção de insulina ou anticorpos contra ela. (Adaptada de Reusch CE, Robben JH, Kooistra HS: Endocrine pancreas. In Rijnberk A, Kooistra HS, editors: *Clinical endocrinology of dogs and cats*, 2 ed., Hannover, Germany, 2010, Schlütersche, p. 165.) (*Esta figura se encontra reproduzida em cores no Encarte.*)

contrarregulatórios (p. ex., glucagon, epinefrina, cortisol, hormônio do crescimento). Todos esses fatores mudam com o tempo e alteram as chances de curvas glicêmicas reproduzíveis. A falta de consistência nos resultados da curva glicêmica pode criar frustrações, a menos que esperadas, é comum e reflete qualquer variável que poderia alterar a glicemia. Quando a alteração da dose parecer apropriada, ela não deve exceder 10 a 25%. Entretanto, na hipoglicemia documentada ou suspeita, a dose deve ser diminuída em, pelo menos, 50%. As doses de insulina não devem ser modificadas com frequência maior do que a cada 5 a 7 dias, exceto em casos de hipoglicemia.

Monitoramento doméstico

Os tutores devem ser encorajados a avaliar o DM do cão diariamente (ver seção anterior). Inicialmente, o peso corporal deve ser aferido e registrado a cada semana. É recomendável que a mensuração da glicose com glicosímetros portáteis, utilizando-se sangue capilar, seja feita em casa. O sangue capilar pode ser obtido com o uso de lancetas em vários locais: o aspecto interno da pina é um bom local para amostras capilares (ver Vídeo 304.4; ver também Capítulo 79); boas alternativas são a mucosa oral (Vídeo 304.5) ou o coxim da pata (Vídeo 304.6).[78] Os tutores devem estar intimamente familiarizados com os glicosímetros portáteis, mas o acesso ao suporte veterinário deve estar disponível. Um bom momento para a introdução do conceito de monitoramento doméstico é após 3 a 4 semanas de tratamento. Nesse momento, o cliente estará, de certa forma, familiarizado com o DM e compreenderá o tempo necessário para o cuidado da doença. Assim que estiver familiarizado com o procedimento, o tutor poderá realizar a curva glicêmica, pela mensuração da glicemia pela manhã, antes de fornecer tanto a insulina com o alimento, e, então, a cada 2 horas, até que a próxima injeção seja aplicada. Em casa, a interpretação da curva glicêmica deve ser a mesma daquela realizada no hospital. Um problema que pode ser previsto diz respeito àqueles tutores muito zelosos, que, ao monitorar a glicemia com muita frequência, começam a interpretar os resultados e ajustar a dose da insulina sem consultar o veterinário, uma prática que quase sempre leva a confusão, pior controle do DM e aumento do risco de sobredose.

Monitoramento glicêmico contínuo

Os sistemas de monitoramento contínuo da glicemia (SMCGs), utilizados de modo rotineiro para pessoas com DM, estão começando a ser usados em cães.[79] Esses sistemas permitem que a glicemia seja monitorada sem a necessidade de coletas repetidas de sangue. O SMCG mensura a glicose intersticial em vez da glicemia. O fluido intersticial é facilmente acessível e os resultados são praticamente os mesmos da glicemia.[79-81] O SMCG utilizado com mais frequência (Guardian REAL-time®) afere a glicose intersticial com um pequeno sensor flexível inserido na pele, no espaço SC, e fixado a ela com fita. O sensor, conectado a um transmissor e também fixado com fita, envia dados por rede sem fio a uma distância máxima de até 3 metros para um monitor do tamanho de um pager. Os dados são coletados a cada 10 segundos e o valor médio da glicose computado a cada 5 minutos. Os dados podem ser baixados para um computador, para análise.

Dispositivos de SMCG possuem algumas limitações. Eles precisam ser calibrados 2 a 3 vezes/dia, o que exige amostras de sangue. Os sensores são bastante caros e podem ser utilizados somente por alguns dias. O monitor demonstra as concentrações de glicose de 40 a 400 mg/dℓ; concentrações fora dessa variação são registradas de maneira correta, mas precisam ser baixadas para que sejam visualizadas. Um novo SMCG (FreeStyleLibre®, da Abbott) produzido para seres humanos possui sensores extremamente pequenos, não precisa de calibração, é barato e o sensor pode ser utilizado por até 14 dias (Figura 304.4). Um estudo recente mostrou que esse SMCG é acurado em casos de hiperglicemia e euglicemia, mas menos preciso se a glicemia estiver < 100 mg/dℓ.[81a] O SMCG pode fornecer uma percepção sobre os teores de glicose durante todo o dia e ajudar a identificar flutuações, episódios de hipoglicemia e tendências que podem, de outra forma, passar despercebidas.[70]

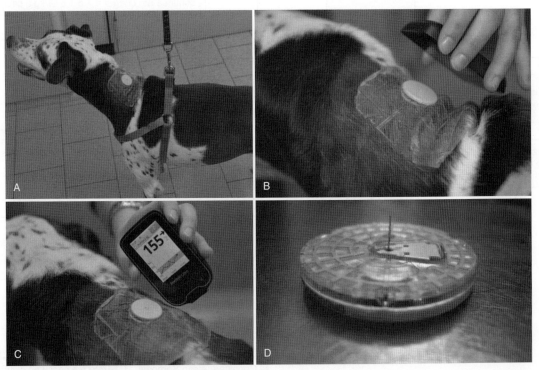

Figura 304.4 Uso de sistema de monitoramento contínuo de glicose (SMCG), FreeStyle Libre®, em um cão. **A.** O sensor subcutâneo é implantado na área cervical dorsal e fixado com uma fita adesiva. Nessa foto, ele está implantado por 12 dias (a repilação do pelo abaixo do adesivo é evidente). **B.** O adesivo do sensor deve ser "escaneado" com o leitor para obtenção dos valores da glicose em tempo real. Isso pode ser feito segurando-se o leitor a 4 cm do sensor. O adesivo do sensor armazena até 8 horas de dados de glicose naquele momento (valores são obtidos a cada minuto). **C.** Teores de glicose são mostrados em tempo real. Aqui a glicose é de 155 mg/dℓ. **D.** Sensor removido 14 dias após a implantação.

CONDIÇÕES CAUSADORAS DE PERSISTÊNCIA OU RECIDIVA DOS SINAIS CLÍNICOS

Visão geral

A persistência ou recidiva dos sinais clínicos é um problema frequente em qualquer cão com DM. A recidiva dos sinais pode ser observada a qualquer momento. Causas comuns incluem questões técnicas na administração da insulina, utilização do tipo incorreto (para esse paciente) e dose ou frequência de administração menor que a ideal. Outros problemas comuns são a responsividade da insulina causada por distúrbios concomitantes inflamatórios, infecciosos, neoplásicos ou hormonais (Figura 304.5).

Questões técnicas

Razões comuns para o controle glicêmico ruim são erros no manuseio ou na administração da insulina. Especificamente,

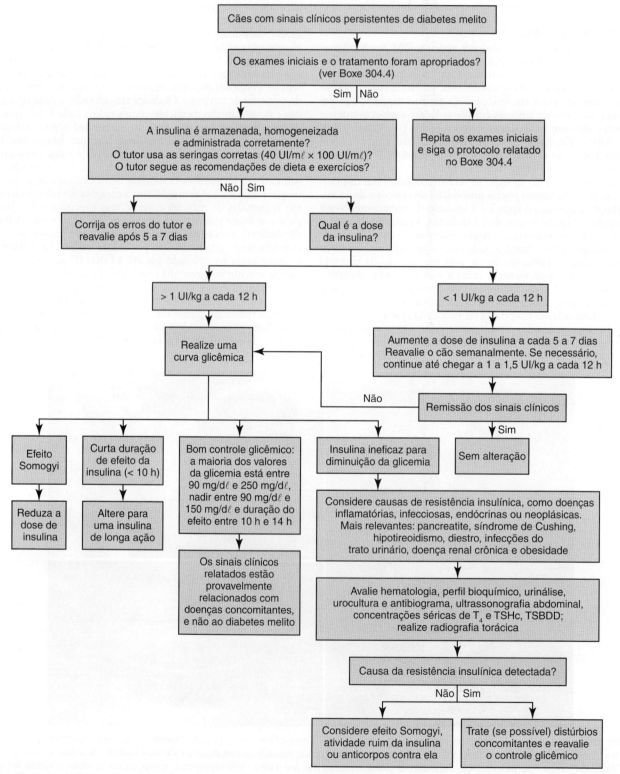

Figura 304.5 Algoritmo para abordagem de cão com sinais clínicos persistentes de diabetes melito. T_4, tiroxina; *TSBDD*, teste de supressão por baixa dose de dexametasona; *TSHc*, hormônio tireoestimulante canino.

incapacidade de homogeneizar a preparação de maneira correta; utilização de diluente impróprio; emprego de insulina congelada, aquecida ou fora do prazo de validade; técnica de injeção incorreta, utilizando-se uma seringa ou caneta de aplicação de insulina; ou dose inapropriada de insulina ou tamanho da seringa (40 UI/mℓ *versus* 100 UI/mℓ é um erro frequente). Esses problemas podem ser identificados pela avaliação cuidadosa do histórico e das solicitações ao tutor para que leve a insulina e a caneta de aplicação ou seringa para as consultas. Caso surjam essas questões, o veterinário ou técnico pode observar todo o procedimento, fornecendo assistência até que o tutor domine a técnica.

Subdose de insulina

A maioria dos cães é bem controlada com doses de insulina ≤ 1 UI/kg por administração por via subcutânea, a cada 12 horas. Se a dose de insulina for consideravelmente menor do que 1 UI/kg por administração e o cão estiver recebendo insulina a cada 12 h, a subdose pode explicar o mau controle glicêmico. Nessa situação, a dose deve ser gradativamente aumentada em 10 a 25% por semana.

Sobredose de insulina e contrarregulação da glicose (efeito Somogyi)

O efeito Somogyi é definido como hiperglicemia de rebote, causado pela resposta fisiológica à hipoglicemia, que induz secreção de hormônios contrarregulatórios. Na resposta aguda, o glucagon e a epinefrina são secretados. Eles, por sua vez, estimulam a resposta de ação mais prolongada pela secreção de cortisol e GH. Essa "contrarregulação" ocorre quando a glicemia está < 65 mg/dℓ, embora também possa acontecer quando de sua queda rápida (em 2 a 3 horas), independentemente do nadir.[82] Os sinais clínicos decorrentes da hipoglicemia não são observados em todos os casos, ao passo que os sinais de resposta hiperglicêmica (PU/PD) são óbvios. Assim, um histórico cíclico de dias de bom controle, seguido de vários dias de controle ruim, deve levantar a suspeita de efeito Somogyi.

O diagnóstico exige evidências de hipoglicemia ou queda rápida de glicose, seguidas, dentro de horas, de hiperglicemia (> 300 mg/dℓ). Concentrações séricas de frutosamina são imprevisíveis, mas costumam estar aumentadas (> 500 μmol/ℓ). A hiperglicemia de rebote e a resistência insulínica podem persistir por 24 a 72 horas. O diagnóstico pode ser difícil e exigir várias curvas glicêmicas, mais bem conduzidas em casa utilizando-se um glicosímetro portátil ou SMCG. Algumas vezes não é fácil diferenciar efeito Somogyi da duração curta de efeito da insulina. Se o Somogyi tiver sido documentado ou supostamente ocorrido, a dose de insulina deverá ser arbitrariamente reduzida aos poucos (1 a 5 UI, dependendo do tamanho do cão e da dose da insulina), devendo o tutor monitorar os sinais clínicos do cão durante os próximos 2 a 5 dias. Se não for observada nenhuma alteração, devem-se tentar reduções de dose adicionais. Se os sinais clínicos piorarem, deve-se considerar uma causa diferente para a inefetividade (*i. e.*, curta duração do efeito de insulina; ver Tabela 304.3).

Curta duração de ação da insulina

Em alguns cães diabéticos, o efeito das insulinas NPH e lenta pode durar menos do que 8 horas (ver Figura 304.3). Como resultado, a hiperglicemia significativa (acima do limiar renal de aproximadamente 200 mg/dℓ) pode permanecer por horas a cada dia. Os tutores de cães cuja insulina não dura o suficiente costumam relatar PU/PD. A questão pode ser mostrada em uma curva glicêmica. O tratamento envolve a troca por uma insulina de longa ação, a cada 12 h (*i. e.*, PZI, glargina ou detemir; ver Tabela 304.2).

Duração prolongada do efeito da insulina

Podem ocorrer problemas com duração prolongada de ação caso a insulina dure mais do que 12 horas; nesses casos, insulinas administradas a cada 12 horas se sobrepõem e aumentam o risco

de hipoglicemia, que, por sua vez, poderia levar ao efeito Somogyi e a sinais clínicos causados por hipoglicemia, hiperglicemia ou ambas. A duração prolongada da ação da insulina costuma ser observada quando o nadir da glicose ocorre 10 ou mais horas após a administração. As opções terapêuticas incluem diminuição da frequência de administração, de a cada 12 horas para a cada 24 horas, ao se utilizar as insulinas detemir ou glargina. O clínico também pode considerar a alteração da insulina para uma de duração de ação mais curta.

Anticorpos anti-insulina

As insulinas canina, porcina e humana são semelhantes. O desenvolvimento de anticorpos anti-insulina significativos não é comum em cães com DM tratados com insulina porcina ou recombinante humana.[22] Insulinas canina e bovina, entretanto, diferem de maneira significativa. Anticorpos contra a insulina foram identificados em 40 a 65% dos cães tratados com insulina bovina/porcina ou 100% daqueles tratados com insulina de fonte bovina.[83,84] A existência de anticorpos anti-insulina pode alterar a farmacocinética e/ou farmacodinâmica da insulina exógena. O resultado costuma ser resposta errática à insulina, mau controle da glicemia, incapacidade de controlar o DM por longos períodos, necessidade de ajustes frequentes da dose da insulina e, ocasionalmente, desenvolvimento de resistência à insulina.[37] A insulina bovina, amplamente utilizada no passado para tratar o DM canino, não é mais utilizada, diminuindo a incidência de anticorpos anti-insulina. Embora incomuns, anticorpos contra insulina podem se desenvolver em cães tratados com insulina recombinante humana, devendo ser considerados como causa possível de mau controle glicêmico se não for identificada nenhuma outra explicação.[37] A documentação de anticorpos anti-insulina séricos deve utilizar ensaios validados para cães. A troca por uma insulina de fonte 100% porcina deve ser considerada se anticorpos anti-insulina forem identificados em um cão diabético mal controlado.

Distúrbios concomitantes causadores de resistência à insulina

Na maioria dos cães com DM, as doses de insulina podem ser reguladas ≤ 1 UI/kg, a cada 12 h. Em cães com demandas maiores de insulina, deve-se suspeitar de distúrbios concomitantes após o descarte de "problemas técnicos", efeito Somogyi ou curta duração de ação da insulina. Nenhuma dose de insulina define claramente resistência insulínica. Propôs-se que a resistência insulínica deve ser sugerida quando o controle glicêmico for ruim, apesar de doses de insulina > 1,5 UI/kg, a cada 12 h, quando altas doses (> 1,5 UI/kg) forem necessárias para manter a glicemia < 300 mg/dℓ ou quando o controle glicêmico for errático, com o ajuste contínuo da dose da insulina.[37] Qualquer distúrbio inflamatório, infeccioso, neoplásico ou endócrino pode causar resistência insulínica, assim como a obesidade e vários medicamentos, especialmente glicocorticoides e progestágenos.

A resistência insulínica é mais comumente causada pela administração de glicocorticoides, diestro, hipotireoidismo, pancreatite crônica, doença renal crônica, infecções, neoplasia, hiperlipidemia, obesidade grave e síndrome de Cushing. Os locais mais comuns de infecção são na região oral (dental) e no trato urinário. Outras causas menos comuns de resistência insulínica são insuficiência pancreática exócrina, cardiopatia, insuficiência hepática, glucagonoma e feocromocitoma (ver Tabela 304.3).

Anamnese e exame físico são os primeiros "testes" mais importantes na tentativa de identificar distúrbios concomitantes. Na maioria das situações, um plano diagnóstico completo, incluindo hemograma, perfil bioquímico sérico, urinálise com cultura bacteriana, ultrassonografia abdominal e radiografias torácicas, deve ser considerado como "triagens" iniciais para doenças concomitantes. Quando indicado, o clínico pode considerar um teste de supressão por dose baixa de dexametasona, concentração sérica de progesterona (em fêmeas inteiras), teste de função tireoidiana, imunorreatividade sérica da lipase pancreática (PLIc), imunorreatividade sérica tripsina-*like* (TLI) e tomografia computadorizada ou ressonância magnética (tumor hipofisário).

COMPLICAÇÕES EM LONGO PRAZO DO DIABETES MELITO

Hipoglicemia

A hipoglicemia é uma complicação extremamente comum da insulinoterapia, sendo raramente fatal.[85] A hipoglicemia pode ocorrer em decorrência de grandes incrementos na dose da insulina, aumento súbito na sensibilidade à insulina em razão do tratamento ou da melhora de distúrbios concomitantes (p. ex., tratamento do hipotireoidismo), sobredose de insulina inadvertida, controle glicêmico excessivamente rigoroso, sobre-posição excessiva da ação da insulina em cães que recebem insulina a cada 12 h, exercício em excesso e inapetência resultante de sobredose relativa de insulina. Sinais de hipoglicemia incluem letargia, fraqueza, ataxia e aumento do apetite. A maioria dos tutores descreve a hipoglicemia como se o cão parecesse intoxicado. Caso ele não seja alimentado, com a consequente progressão da hipoglicemia, podem ocorrer convulsões, coma e morte.

A hipoglicemia sintomática deve ser tratada com glicose administrada como alimento rico em açúcar. Se o cão não puder se alimentar, a glicose pode ser aplicada nas membranas mucosas orais, na forma de gel ou solução de glicose (xarope Karo®), onde pode ser diretamente absorvido. Assim que recuperado, o cão deve ser alimentado.[42] Cães em colapso devem ser submetidos à administração por via intravenosa de dextrose imediatamente, na forma de *bolus* inicial IV de 1 mℓ/kg de dextrose a 33%, seguida de infusão de dextrose a 5%. As taxas podem ser alteradas, se necessário. Após a hipoglicemia sintomática, os tutores devem ser instruídos a interromper a insulina até que a glicosúria ocorra novamente e, então, administrar 25 a 50% menos dela. Em seguida, a dose de insulina deve ser ajustada, conforme necessário, para melhorar a resposta clínica e as mensurações da glicemia.[37] O tratamento da hipoglicemia assintomática também exige a redução da dose de insulina de cerca de 10 a 20% ou a substituição por uma que possua um efeito de duração mais curta.

Complicações oculares

A formação de catarata é a complicação a longo prazo mais comum em cães diabéticos (ver Figura 304.2). Um estudo de coorte retrospectivo com 132 cães diabéticos atendidos em um hospital universitário especializado observou a formação de catarata em 14% daqueles com DM no momento do diagnóstico. Nesse estudo, o intervalo de tempo para que 25, 50, 75 e 80 da população do estudo desenvolvesse catarata foi de apenas 60, 170, 370 e 470 dias, respectivamente.[86] A catarata supostamente ocorre como resultado da alteração da relação osmótica na lente induzida pelo acúmulo intracelular de sorbitol e galactitol, ocasionado após o metabolismo de glicose e galactose por enzimas dentro da lente. O acúmulo de sorbitol e galactitol nas células da lente aumenta a osmolaridade intracelular, causa influxo de líquido com edema subsequente e ruptura das fibras da lente, o que leva ao desenvolvimento da catarata.[87] Uma vez iniciada a formação da catarata, ela é irreversível e pode evoluir bastante rápido. A cegueira pode ser evitada pela remoção da lente anormal. A visão é restaurada em 80 a 90% dos cães com DM submetidos à remoção da catarata.[88,89] Outras complicações oculares do diabetes podem incluir uveíte, ceratoconjuntivite seca, conjuntivite bacteriana e retinopatia diabética.

Neuropatia diabética

Embora descrita em cães, sua prevalência é desconhecida.[90-93] A neuropatia subclínica parece ser mais comum. Sinais clínicos de neuropatia diabética (fraqueza, atrofia muscular, hiporreflexia, hipotonia) são os mais comumente reconhecidos em cães diabéticos durante 5 anos ou mais.[37,93] A neuropatia diabética em cães é, sobretudo, uma polineuropatia distal, caracterizada por desmielinização segmentar e degeneração axonal.

Nefropatia diabética

Há relatos ocasionais de nefropatia diabética em cães diabéticos, mas sua relevância clínica permanece desconhecida. Alterações microscópicas podem incluir glomerulonefropatias membranosas com fusão dos processos podais, espessamento da membrana basal glomerular e tubular, aumento no material de matriz mesangial, presença de depósitos subendoteliais, fibrose glomerular e glomerulosclerose.[94,95] A microalbuminúria é utilizada como um marcador precoce para o desenvolvimento da nefropatia diabética em seres humanos. Em um estudo, o aumento da albumina da urina foi observado em 11 (55%) de 20 cães com DM, com mais da metade apresentando aumentos concomitantes na relação proteína-creatinina urinária.[96] Resultados semelhantes foram observados em um estudo no qual a proteinúria, a pressão sanguínea e a retinopatia diabética foram monitoradas durante um período de acompanhamento de 2 anos. Nenhum efeito significativo do tempo desde o diagnóstico ou controle glicêmico foi detectado para qualquer uma das medidas examinadas.[97] O valor preditivo e a relevância clínica da microalbuminúria em cães diabéticos ainda precisam ser esclarecidos. Na maioria dos cães com DM, a doença renal crônica supostamente ocorre como uma condição independente.[37]

PROGNÓSTICO

O prognóstico para cães diagnosticados com DM depende, em parte, do comprometimento do tutor para com o tratamento da doença, da facilidade de regulação da glicemia, da presença e reversibilidade de distúrbios concomitantes e da prevenção de complicações crônicas associadas ao estado diabético. Em um grande estudo envolvendo cães segurados na Suécia, 347 sobreviveram pelo menos 30 dias após a primeira queixa do DM. A proporção daqueles que sobreviveram 1, 2 e 3 anos foi de 40, 36 e 33%, respectivamente,[5] existindo uma taxa de mortalidade relativamente alta durante os 6 primeiros meses de tratamento em razão das doenças concomitantes, como cetoacidose, pancreatite ou infecções. O consenso é de que cães diabéticos bem controlados, que sobrevivem aos primeiros 6 meses de tratamento, possuem expectativa de vida semelhante àqueles não diabéticos de mesma idade, sexo e raça.

REFERÊNCIAS BIBLIOGRÁFICAS

As referências bibliográficas deste capítulo se encontram online no Ambiente de Aprendizagem.

CAPÍTULO 305

Diabetes Melito Felino

Jacquie Rand e Susan A. Gottlieb

PATOGÊNESE

Tipos de diabetes melito

O diabetes melito (DM) é caracterizado por hiperglicemia persistente causada por secreção insuficiente de insulina pelas células beta pancreáticas. Os mecanismos envolvidos na incapacidade das células beta pancreáticas formam a base para classificação dos tipos de DM. As classificações atuais utilizadas no DM humano, quase sempre aceitas na medicina veterinária, envolvem quatro tipos: 1, 2, gestacional e outros específicos.[1] O DM tipo 1 em pessoas segue a destruição imunomediada de células beta com predisposições genéticas e gatilhos ambientais, levando a uma deficiência absoluta de insulina.[1] O DM tipo 1 é raro em gatos, com base nos estudos histológicos e na ausência de autoanticorpos circulantes anticélulas beta.[2,3] Entretanto, os sinais clínicos, os achados histológicos e os anticorpos nas células das ilhotas compatíveis com o DM tipo 1 foram relatados em um filhote de gato com 5 meses de vida.[4] O DM tipo 2 é caracterizado por resistência insulínica com falha concomitante das células beta em montar uma resposta compensatória adequada, a fim de manter a euglicemia.[1] O tipo 2 é a forma mais comum de DM em gatos, com base nos fatores de risco (idade avançada e obesidade), características clínicas e endócrinas (resistência insulínica, secreção insulínica variável e remissão) e histologia das ilhotas (vacuolização das ilhotas e depósito amiloide).[5-7] O DM tipo 2 parece corresponder a cerca de 80 a 90% dos gatos examinados em serviços veterinários de cuidado primário em países ocidentais, com base nas taxas de remissão e outras características clínicas e fenotípicas.[8,9] O DM gestacional é inicialmente diagnosticado durante a gestação, mas não foi relatado em gatos, embora o tenha sido em cães.[1,10,11]

Outros tipos específicos de DM em gatos incluem a perda de ilhotas pancreáticas em razão de pancreatite ou neoplasia. Em gatos, a resistência insulínica e o DM podem ocorrer secundariamente ao hipersomatotropismo (acromegalia; ver Capítulo 294) ou ao hiperadrenocorticismo (HAC) (síndrome de Cushing; ver Capítulo 307).[2,12-15] Esses "outros" tipos de DM felino provavelmente representam menos de 20% dos casos observados nos locais de atendimento primário, mas podem ser mais representados em instituições especializadas. Em geral, a acromegalia começa clinicamente como um DM mal controlado, apesar do uso de doses de insulina consideradas adequadas.[15,16] O adenocarcinoma pancreático é relatado em 8 a 19% dos felinos diabéticos submetidos à eutanásia em instituições de atendimento terciário.[2,12] A pancreatite (ver Capítulo 291) se apresenta no momento do diagnóstico do DM em até 60% dos gatos, com base em achados bioquímicos e de exames de imagem, embora os sinais clínicos não sejam frequentes.[17-19] À histologia, a maioria das lesões é compatível com pancreatite crônica, enquanto a pancreatite aguda ou subaguda necrosante é a causa de mortalidade.[2,20] Na maioria dos gatos, a pancreatite não parece ser suficientemente grave para causar DM, mas pode contribuir com a perda de células beta e reduzir a probabilidade de remissão do DM.[19,20]

Prevalência e fatores de risco

Estimativas com relação à prevalência do DM felino variam em aproximadamente 0,25 a 1%.[21-25] Diversos estudos da Austrália e do Reino Unido atribuem uma prevalência de cerca de 1 para 200 gatos (0,5%).[23,24,26] Nos EUA, a prevalência relatada em hospitais-escola veterinários aumentou de 1 em 1.250 (0,08%), em 1970, para 1 em 81 (1,2%), em 1999.[25] Não se sabe se esse aumento aparente da prevalência ocorreu em razão de fatores como a obesidade.[25] Raças com maior suscetibilidade ao DM incluem o Birmanês, na Austrália, na Nova Zelândia e no Reino Unido; e o Maine Coon, o Azul russo e o Siamês, nos EUA.[23,24,27-29] O Birmanês possui frequência de DM cerca de 4 vezes maior do que outros gatos; cerca de 10% dos gatos com 8 anos ou mais têm DM. O(s) gene(s) envolvido(s) nesse processo parece(m) autossômico(s), e não ligado(s) ao sexo, com poucos sinais de ação gênica dominante com penetração completa.[22-24,27,30]

Diabetes tipo 2

Seres humanos versus *gatos*

O DM humano tipo 2 apresenta etiologia complexa, é causado por fatores genéticos e interações ambientais e o risco aumenta com o passar dos anos.[1] De forma semelhante, os fatores de risco para o DM felino incluem idade, gênero masculino (a relação macho:fêmea é de 1,5:1), obesidade, falta de atividade física, confinamento doméstico, raça e administração de esteroides ou acetato de megestrol repetida ou de longa ação.[21,24,25,31] A maioria desses fatores diminui a sensibilidade à insulina e aumenta a demanda sobre as células beta para produzir insulina.[32-34] Em seres humanos, o DM tipo 2 é uma doença poligênica com hereditariedade complexa, embora variantes genéticas correspondam a < 10% do risco geral, destacando a importância dos fatores ambientais.[35] Cerca de 60 *locus* gênicos estão associados ao DM tipo 2, a maioria envolvida com a biologia da célula beta, refletindo o significado da falha da célula beta na patogênese.[36,37] Em gatos domésticos, o polimorfismo no gene receptor de melanocortina 4 *(Mc4R)* está associado ao DM em animais com sobrepeso, de forma semelhante ao observado em seres humanos.[38] Em pessoas, a mutação desse gene aumenta o apetite e a obesidade, já, em gatos, parece estar associada à progressão para o DM,[38] sendo esse polimorfismo 3,7 vezes mais provável naqueles animais com sobrepeso com DM em comparação àqueles com sobrepeso não diabéticos, mas não foi observada diferença entre obesos e gatos magros não diabéticos.

Em seres humanos, alguns *locus* genéticos, associados ao maior risco para síndrome metabólica, estão localizados dentro de genes sabidamente associados ao metabolismo lipídico.[39] Gatos Birmaneses parecem ser propensos à desregulação do metabolismo lipídico; gatos Birmaneses magros mostram padrões de expressão genética semelhantes a gatos domésticos obesos.[40] Em gatos, as características clínicas do DM são semelhantes a DM atípico observado em afro-americanos e asiáticos: sinais clássicos de poliúria, polidipsia (PU/PD) e perda de peso, com concentrações glicêmicas relativamente altas. Eles são suscetíveis à cetose, mas podem sofrer remissão dentro de algumas semanas após o início da insulinoterapia. Pacientes possuem o fenótipo tipo 2 e histórico familiar de DM.[41,42,42a] O DM atípico está associado a uma série de *locus* genéticos.[43-45]

Resistência insulínica

O DM tipo 2 é uma doença multifacetada, caracterizada por insuficiência de células beta e resistência insulínica.[35] A sensibilidade insulínica, definida como a capacidade de uma dada concentração de insulina diminuir a glicemia, é determinada geneticamente em pessoas. A sensibilidade insulínica diminui com a obesidade, a falta de atividade física e é um efeito colateral da administração de glicocorticoides e progestágenos.[32,46-50] A redução da sensibilidade insulínica (resistência) é a característica principal do DM tipo 2. Gatos com DM são cerca de seis vezes menos sensíveis à insulina do que o normal, causando aumento da produção da glicose hepática e redução da utilização de glicose em tecidos periféricos.[7,51] Em gatos, cada quilo de aumento no peso corporal acima do ideal causa cerca de 30% de diminuição da sensibilidade insulínica e um ganho de 44% reduz a sensibilidade insulínica e a efetividade da glicose (capacidade de a glicose aumentar sua própria captação celular e suprimir a produção endógena) em 50%.[32,47,52] Embora não se saiba se a sensibilidade insulínica é determinada geneticamente, gatos magros com baixa sensibilidade à insulina subjacente apresentam maior risco de desenvolvimento de intolerância à glicose por obesidade.[32]

Secreção de insulina reduzida

A redução da secreção de insulina secundária à falha de células beta é a segunda característica importante do DM tipo 2. Em indivíduos saudáveis, células beta respondem à troca de requerimentos e sofrem hipertrofia e hiperplasia para atender às maiores demandas, como em casos de obesidade.[53] Entretanto, em uma minoria de pacientes obesos, ocorre falha das células beta. Processos associados à obesidade (distúrbios do metabolismo de glicose, ácidos graxos e aminoácidos) danificam as células beta, o que reduz sua capacidade secretória.[35] A obesidade e o DM tipo 2 estão associados à inflamação crônica, que aumenta as citocinas e a infiltração de células imunes em tecidos envolvidos na homeostase energética (gordura, fígado, músculo, ilhotas pancreáticas).[35] Tais infiltrados foram relatados em gatos com DM e obesos.[19,54-57] A citocina inflamatória interleucina-1 beta, bem como sua expressão, estava aumentada em modelos de gatos hiperglicêmicos/obesos.[58] A falha das células beta não é completamente compreendida, especialmente em estágios iniciais. Diversos mecanismos afetam de maneira adversa as células beta e prejudicam a secreção de insulina, por diminuição da expressão do gene dela e redução da capacidade de as células beta proliferarem em resposta à maior demanda. Esses fatores contribuem para a morte das células beta.[35,59] A toxicidade das fibrilas intracelulares alteradas e polimerizadas (oligômeros) do polipeptídio amiloide das ilhotas (IAPP, do inglês *islet amyloid polypeptide*) e a glicolipotoxicidade estão envolvidas no desencadeamento de alguns desses mecanismos. Há evidências de que tanto a deposição amiloide de ilhotas de oligômeros alterados de IAPP (Figuras 305.1 e 305.2) e a glicotoxicidade diminuem não só os números de células beta, como a função delas em gatos.[6,60-63] Embora não seja uma causa inicial de falha de células beta, a hiperglicemia crônica possui um papel central na disfunção de células beta e na incapacidade progressiva de secretar insulina.[62-64] Em gatos, a toxicidade por glicose é dose-dependente. Em concentrações persistentes de glicose de 540 mg/dℓ (30 mmol/ℓ), as concentrações de insulina são reduzidas a valores basais dentro de 3 a 7 dias, com ocorrência de cetonemia dentro de 10 a 30 dias após deficiência acentuada de insulina.[62,63] O aumento de ácidos graxos livres também reduz a função de células beta, predominantemente observado na presença de alta glicose (glicolipotoxicidade).[62,64]

Amilina e polipeptídio amiloide da ilhota

A deposição de amilina ou IAPP alteradas é típica de DM tipo 2 em seres humanos e gatos.[6,58,60,61,65] A amilina ou IAPP é um hormônio que modula a ação da insulina, é cossecretado com a ela e quantidades maiores são secretadas por indivíduos com resistência insulínica.[61] Em seres humanos e gatos, a amilina pode ser dobrada em folhetos com pregas beta e formar oligômeros de amilina polimerizados e dobrados de maneira errônea, que atuam como agregados intracelulares tóxicos e fibrilas. Eles contribuem para a inflamação da ilhota e morte das células beta.[60,61,65] O depósito amiloide da ilhota é maior em modelos felinos de hiperinsulinemia devido à resistência insulínica e está associado ao DM evidente.[66] O depósito amiloide da ilhota e os oligômeros ou fibrilas de IAPP intracelulares tóxicos, como contribuintes da insuficiência de células beta, podem explicar o motivo pelo qual seres humanos e gatos são singularmente suscetíveis ao DM tipo 2, enquanto cães obesos e outras espécies não o desenvolvem.

Dano oxidativo

O estresse oxidativo e as modificações provavelmente possuem um papel central na disfunção das células beta, que possuem capacidade antioxidante limitada e são suscetíveis ao estresse oxidativo.[67] A glico e a lipotoxicidade estão associadas a modificações oxidativas para células beta, por produção excessiva de espécies reativas de oxigênio secundária ao aumento da respiração celular.[68,69] A princípio, a indução da proteína-2 desacoplada

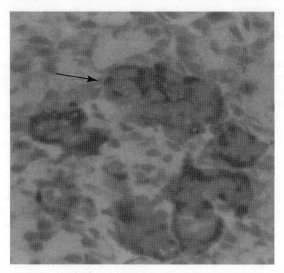

Figura 305.1 A *seta* indica uma ilhota pancreática normal com tecido exócrino circundante. As células beta estão coradas na ilhota para mostrar o hormônio amilina (polipeptídio amiloide da ilhota [IAPP]). (Cortesia de T. Lutz, Dr. Med. Vet., PhD, University of Zurich, Switzerland. In Rand JS, Martin GJ: Management of feline diabetes mellitus. *Vet Clin North Am Small Anim Pract* 31[5]:881-913, 2001.) (*Esta figura se encontra reproduzida em cores no Encarte.*)

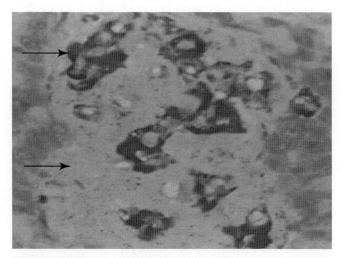

Figura 305.2 Ilhota pancreática de um gato diabético mostrando extenso depósito amiloide (*seta inferior*) substituindo células beta (*seta superior*). (Cortesia de T. Lutz, Dr. Med. Vet., PhD, University of Zurich, Switzerland. In Rand JS, Martin GJ: Management of feline diabetes mellitus. *Vet Clin North Am Small Anim Pract.* 31[5]:881-913, 2001.) (*Esta figura se encontra reproduzida em cores no Encarte.*)

(UCP-2, do inglês *uncoupling protein-2*) é utilizada pelas células beta como mecanismo protetor contra respiração mitocondrial excessiva. Entretanto, a ativação da UCP-2 causa aumento da geração de radicais livres de oxigênio e estresse oxidativo,[70] que diminui a produção de insulina e amilina ao mesmo tempo que aumenta as vias pró-inflamatórias ou apoptóticas, como fator nuclear kappa B (NF-κB) e c-JUN N-terminal quinase (JNK).[67,71,72]

DIAGNÓSTICO

Glicemia, tolerância à glicose e diagnóstico do diabetes melito evidente

A glicosúria ocorre assim que a glicemia excede a capacidade tubular proximal para reabsorção do filtrado glomerular (aproximadamente 250 a 290 mg/dℓ ou 14 a 16 mmol/ℓ).[73,74] A perda de glicose na urina contribui para a redução de peso e o estímulo do apetite, mas não a ponto de ser tão significativa como a incapacidade de acesso celular à glicose para função normal. As perdas hídricas causadas pela diurese osmótica da glicose estimulam a polidipsia, a fim de manter o balanço hídrico. Assim, os sinais clínicos clássicos de DM resultam de poliúria, polidipsia, polifagia e perda de peso. Em gatos, o limite superior para a glicemia é de aproximadamente 113 a 117 mg/dℓ (6,3 a 6,5 mmol/ℓ) após utilização do glicosímetro portátil e hospitalização por uma noite e jejum de 18 a 24 horas.[75,76] Concentrações persistentemente acima dessa faixa devem ser consideradas pré-DM, a menos que o DM evidente seja confirmado. Valores ≥ 180 a 288 mg/dℓ (≥ 10 a 16 mmol/ℓ) foram relatados como diagnósticos para DM evidente.[77,78]

O valor da glicose estabelecido estatisticamente em gatos idosos (≥ 8 anos) é < 176 mg/dℓ (< 9,8 mmol/ℓ), 2 horas após a administração de 0,5 g/kg de glicose, ou < 117 mg/dℓ (< 6,5 mmol/ℓ), 3 horas após administração de 1 g/kg de glicose, mensurado em um teste de tolerância à glicose simplificado.[75,76] Ao utilizar esses critérios, 20% dos gatos obesos ≥ 8 anos são intolerantes à glicose.[75] É recomendado que a glicemia aferida a cada 2 horas seja ajustada para baixo em 1,8 mg/dℓ (0,1 mmol/ℓ) para cada unidade de escore de condição corporal acima de 5 de 9, para explicar a sobredose relativa de glicose em gatos obesos.[79] A tolerância anormal à glicose é mais bem confirmada por um teste repetido.

Tolerância prejudicada à glicose e pré-diabetes melito

Seres humanos com concentrações glicêmicas acima do normal, mas abaixo do DM em jejum ou depois de 2 horas do teste de tolerância à glicose (TTG), são classificados como portadores de distúrbios da glicose em jejum ou tolerância prejudicada à glicose, respectivamente.[1,80] Eles são considerados pré-diabéticos e com maior risco de desenvolvimento de DM tipo 2 (5 a 10% progridem para DM evidente/ano).[1,80-83] Mais de 50% das pessoas com DM não são diagnosticadas e 3 a 4 vezes mais possuem pré-DM não diagnosticado.[1,80,84] O número de gatos não diagnosticados com DM pode ser grande. Se identificadas antes da progressão para o DM evidente, as pessoas costumam ter o controle glicêmico razoável, com perda de peso, manejo dietético e exercício.[80] Doze a vinte e seis por cento das pessoas nos EUA, na Europa e na Austrália possuem alteração da glicose em jejum, um percentual que aumenta para 39% com 65 anos de idade.

Alterações da glicose em jejum raramente são diagnosticadas em gatos. A hiperglicemia discreta quase sempre é atribuída ao estresse causado pelo trajeto à clínica, o "efeito do jaleco branco", à contenção ou à doença.[81,84-86] Assim como em pessoas, a identificação e o tratamento do pré-DM ou do DM subclínico em gatos podem atrasar ou impedir a progressão para o DM evidente. A maioria dos gatos em remissão do DM continua a ter distúrbios do metabolismo de glicose compatíveis com pré-DM e alto risco de recidiva.[76] Gatos em remissão do DM, com

concentrações normais da glicose em jejum e tolerância normal à glicose, não desenvolvem DM dentro de 12 meses. Entretanto, houve recidiva do DM 9 meses após o teste em 67% dos gatos com tolerância à glicose moderadamente alterada (> 252 mg/dℓ; > 14 mmol/ℓ após 3 h durante um TTG com administração de 1 g/kg por via intravenosa [IV]) e em 100% daqueles com alteração moderada da glicose em jejum (≥ 135 a 162 mg/dℓ; ≥ 7,5 a 9 mmol/ℓ).[76] É improvável que a glicemia abaixo do limiar renal (250 a 290 mg/dℓ; 14-16 mmol/ℓ), mas acima do ponto para DM (180 mg/dℓ; 10 mmol/ℓ), cause sinais clínicos e seja classificada como DM subclínico.[73] Gatos assintomáticos, com concentrações glicêmicas persistentemente acima de 117 mg/dℓ (6,5 mmol/ℓ), podem evitar o DM evidente ou provavelmente se beneficiariam de uma dieta com baixos níveis de carboidratos, perda de peso e, talvez, com sensibilizantes insulínicos, como o darglitazone.[87]

Resultados de triagem da glicemia (ver Capítulo 61)

Quando o sangue é obtido logo após a chegada à clínica, uma glicemia normal de triagem deve ser < 166 mg/dℓ (9,2 mmol/ℓ). Esse valor acima do normal ocorre em razão do efeito confundidor do estresse sobre a glicemia em gatos, capaz de aumentar de maneira acentuada a glicemia minutos depois do evento estressante.[88] Em alguns gatos, o pico das concentrações de glicose ocorre 10 minutos após o estresse agudo e não retorna aos teores basais durante > 3 horas.[85] Em alguns gatos, o estresse, por si só, aumenta a concentração de glicose em uma média de 74 mg/dℓ (4,1 mmol/ℓ) e até 195 mg/dℓ (10,8 mmol/ℓ) em 10 minutos. Esse aumento ocorre em paralelo ao das concentrações de lactato e norepinefrina.[85] Em razão dos efeitos do estresse, a glicemia de triagem pode não ser um preditivo útil da recidiva do DM em gatos em remissão, por conta dos efeitos confundidores provocados pelo estresse da viagem e pelo manuseio e, em outros, pelos efeitos ocasionados pela alimentação (Figura 305.3).[76] Gatos idosos com glicemia > 117 mg/dℓ (> 6,5 mmol/ℓ) devem ser internados, testados novamente 4 e 24 horas depois e tratados de maneira apropriada com base nos resultados dos exames (Figura 305.4).

Cetose diabética e cetoacidose diabética (ver Capítulo 142)

No momento do diagnóstico do DM, 12 a 37% dos gatos possuem cetoacidose diabético (CAD) e alguns estão em cetose, mas não em acidose (CD).[2,77] A CAD pode ser desencadeada por doenças concomitantes (especialmente infecções), cujos sinais incluem depressão, êmese e anorexia.[89] A cetose pode ocorrer durante um período de 10 a 30 dias, assim que o gato se tornar acentuadamente insulinopênico, sem necessariamente necessitar de uma doença concomitante.[63] Assim que em cetose e sem insulinoterapia, a CAD progride de maneira rápida. Pequenas doses de insulina podem prevenir a acidose, mesmo que haja persistência da hiperglicemia.[63] Dezesseis dias após indução experimental de hiperglicemia em gatos saudáveis (540 mg/dℓ; 30 mmol/ℓ), a cetonemia por beta-hidroxibutirato (> 0,5 mmol/ℓ) foi evidente. A cetonemia não ocorreu com glicemias de 306 mg/dℓ (17 mmol/ℓ), o que reflete o efeito protetor da insulina.[63] A cetonúria por beta-hidroxibutirato ocorreu após hiperglicemia acentuada persistente por uma média de 23 dias, embora tempos individuais tenham variado amplamente, assim como o limiar renal (19,6 mg/dℓ, variação de 3,1 a 40,6 mg/dℓ; 1,88 mmol/ℓ, variação de 0,3 a 3,9 mmol/ℓ). A cetonúria foi detectada após 5 dias com tiras para urinálise, que aferiram acetoacetato e acetona. No dia 27, a maioria dos gatos apresentava hálito cetônico e lipemia evidente. Com base nesse estudo, quando as glicemias estiverem < 360 mg/dℓ (< 20 mmol/ℓ), é improvável que o beta-hidroxibutirato esteja aumentado (> 10 mg/dℓ; > 1 mmol/ℓ), não devendo, portanto, ser utilizado como base para diferenciar a hiperglicemia por estresse do diabetes.

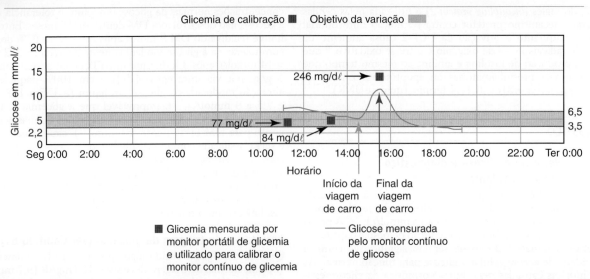

Figura 305.3 Monitoramento intermitente portátil da glicemia (Abbott AlphaTRAK®) e monitoramento contínuo da glicemia (Medronics iPro®) em um gato clinicamente saudável durante um trajeto de carro de 60 minutos entre a clínica e a casa. As glicemias aumentaram de forma constante de 84 mg/dℓ (4,7 mmol/ℓ) para 245 mg/dℓ (13,6 mmol/ℓ) e diminuíram até o normal durante um período semelhante.

Frutosamina

A frutosamina é produzida por uma reação não enzimática entre a glicose e os grupos amina de proteínas plasmáticas, sendo uma medida útil no controle glicêmico para gatos nos quais não há possibilidade de monitoramento doméstico ou hospitalar, podendo também auxiliar no diagnóstico do DM.[90] Quando a hiperglicemia (306 ou 540 mg/dℓ; 17 ou 30 mmol/ℓ) foi induzida experimentalmente em gatos, as concentrações de frutosamina aumentaram acima do valor de referência (331 µmol/ℓ) dentro de 3 a 5 dias. Entretanto, o nível médio de frutosamina não aumentou acima de 350 µmol/ℓ quando a glicemia foi mantida em 306 mg/dℓ (17 mmol/ℓ) durante 6 semanas.[91] Em gatos, a concentração de frutosamina provavelmente reflete a concentração glicêmica média da semana anterior. Apenas alterações > 33 µmol/ℓ em um indivíduo provavelmente terão significado.[91] A frutosamina não deve ser utilizada para diferenciar a hiperglicemia por estresse do DM quando a glicemia for ≤ 360 mg/dℓ (20 mmol/ℓ). A diferenciação deve se basear em concentrações seriadas da glicemia e, se presentes, glicosúria e sinais clínicos. Para uma dada glicemia, as frutosaminas plasmáticas variam amplamente entre indivíduos felinos. Há ocorrência de resultados falso-positivos (gatos normais com teores altos de frutosamina) e resultados falso-negativos (gatos com DM com teores normais de frutosamina), inclusive em gatos diabéticos com hipertireoidismo.[90,92,92a]

OBJETIVOS DA TERAPIA E REMISSÃO DO DIABETES

Diabetes recém-diagnosticado

Controle glicêmico estrito

No DM recém-diagnosticado, o objetivo da terapia é manter tanto a glicemia dentro ou próximo do normal (72 a < 180 mg/dℓ; 4 a < 10 mmol/ℓ) quanto evitar a hipoglicemia clínica. O controle glicêmico excelente para resolução da glicotoxicidade, alcançado precocemente em gatos com DM recém-diagnosticado, aumenta a probabilidade de "remissão" do DM, definida como euglicemia persistente por, pelo menos, 2 a 4 semanas, sem necessidade de insulinoterapia exógena ou hipoglicemiantes orais.[8,76,93] Por exemplo, 84% dos gatos com DM recém-diagnosticado, submetidos a um protocolo com controle glicêmico rigoroso, alcançaram remissão dentro de 6 meses, quando comparados a apenas 35% (p < 0,001) que não foram submetidos a controle glicêmico estrito instituído por, pelo menos, 6 meses.[94]

Remissão

Fatores relacionados associados à remissão do DM incluem dieta com baixos níveis de carboidratos (12% versus 26% de energia), insulina de longa ação (glargina versus PZI ou lenta), maior idade, menor dose máxima de insulina (dose máxima média de glargina de 0,4 UI/kg versus 0,7 UI/kg ou < 3 UI/gato versus > 3 UI/gato), instituição precoce do controle glicêmico estrito (< 6 meses versus ≥ 6 meses), administração recente de corticosteroides, ausência de neuropatia, menores glicemias médias após tratamento com insulina e menores concentrações de colesterol.[8,93-96] Gatos idosos que desenvolvem DM possuem maiores taxas de remissão, possivelmente sugerindo uma progressão mais lenta da doença.[93] Glicemia média < 288 mg/dℓ (< 16 mmol/ℓ), após 17 dias de tratamento com glargina, foi associada, de maneira significativa, à remissão.[8]

Embora a remissão seja relatada com uma variedade de fármacos hipoglicemiantes orais, terapias com insulina, protocolos de insulinoterapia e dietas, as maiores taxas de remissão (> 80%) o são em gatos diabéticos recém-diagnosticados tratados com protocolo cujo objetivo era alcançar glicemias normais ou próximas disso, ao utilizar insulina de longa ação (glargina ou detemir), dieta com baixos níveis de carboidrato (≤ 6% de energia oriunda de carboidratos), monitoramento frequente hospitalar ou doméstico da glicemia e ajustes de dose apropriados da insulina, fazendo uso de um protocolo de dose que almeje o controle glicêmico estrito.[8,94,97] Entretanto, não são conhecidas contribuições de pequenos números de casos, ausência de estudos duplo-cego ou confiança na interpretação dos tutores.[98]

Administração de corticosteroides

A administração de corticosteroides 6 meses antes do diagnóstico de DM está associada a maiores taxas de remissão.[94] Em seres humanos, o DM induzido por fármacos é considerado um "outro tipo específico", distinto do tipo 2. Pode ser mais fácil reverter esse processo fisiopatológico subjacente ou a administração de esteroides pode desmascarar os defeitos de células beta associados a outra doença, como DM tipo 2 ou pancreatite, resultando na busca do tratamento imediato pelo tutor (ver Capítulo 358).[1]

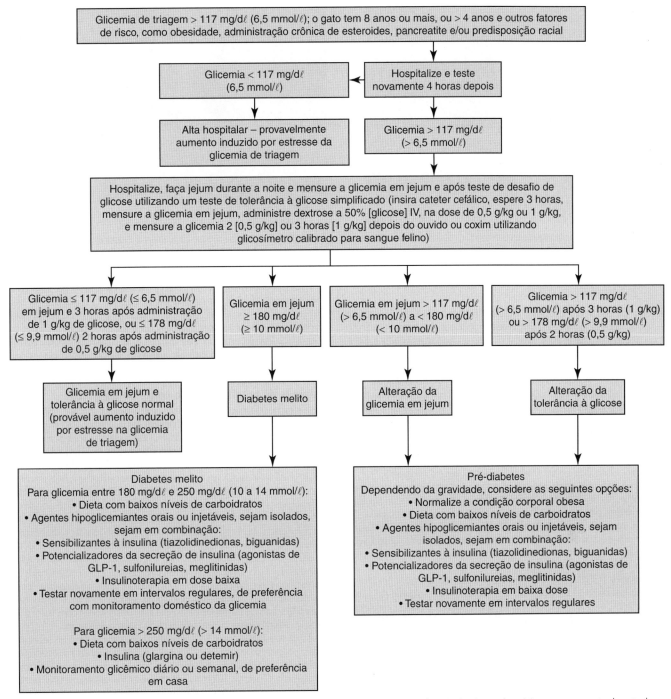

Figura 305.4 Algoritmo para processo diagnóstico e tratamento de gatos com 8 anos ou mais com glicemia de triagem (sem jejum e no momento de entrada na clínica) > 117 mg/dℓ (6,5 mmol/ℓ). *GLP-1*, peptídio semelhante ao glucagon-1.

Neuropatia periférica (NP)

No momento do diagnóstico do DM, a neuropatia periférica (NP) está associada à menor probabilidade de remissão (Figura 305.5 e Vídeos 12.2, 305.1 e 305.2), estando presente em 79% dos gatos que não atingiram remissão apesar da implementação de um protocolo que almejasse o controle glicêmico intensivo.[94] Como a neuropatia surge tardiamente na evolução da doença, é provável que esses gatos tivessem DM crônico, com maior dano às células beta.[94]

Diabetes melito em longo prazo sem remissão

Gatos tratados por mais de 6 meses sem alcançar a remissão do DM possuem objetivos terapêuticos discretamente diferentes: controlar os sinais clínicos e evitar, ao mesmo tempo, a hipoglicemia clínica. A remissão pode ser notada em um pequeno número de gatos, mesmo após 2 anos ou mais de insulinoterapia, caso tenha sido implementado um controle glicêmico rigoroso.

Recidiva

A maioria dos gatos em remissão do DM não possui função normal das células beta ou insulina suficiente para manter a tolerância normal quando desafiados com glicose, devendo, portanto, continuar a serem considerados pré-diabéticos. Aproximadamente 76% apresentam distúrbio evidente da tolerância à glicose após o teste de desafio e 19%, alteração das glicemias em jejum (discreta hiperglicemia persistente > 117 mg/dℓ a < 180 mg/dℓ; > 6,5 a < 10 mmol).[76] Um número reduzido de células das ilhotas pancreáticas é histologicamente evidente,

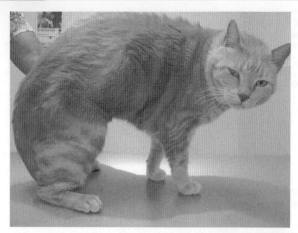

Figura 305.5 Posição plantígrada e/ou fraqueza muscular observadas em uma proporção significativa de gatos diabéticos recém-diagnosticados, estando associadas de maneira negativa à probabilidade de remissão diabética. (Fotografia com permissão de R. Marshall.)

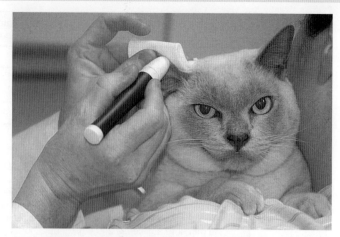

Figura 305.6 Coleta de sangue da orelha para monitoramento doméstico da glicemia. (Fotografia de Mia Reeve-Johnson.)

apesar da remissão do DM, incluindo diminuição da densidade de células beta, quando comparada à de gatos do grupo-controle (1,4% em comparação a 2,6%).[96] Aproximadamente 25 a 30% dos gatos em remissão do DM recidivam, necessitando novamente da insulina exógena, e < 25% atingem uma segunda remissão.[76,93,94] O monitoramento doméstico da glicemia e o teste de tolerância à glicose podem ser utilizados para identificar gatos em risco de recidiva. Glicemia em jejum de ≥ 135 mg/dℓ (≥ 7,5 mmol/ℓ) e moderada alteração da tolerância à glicose com ≥ 5 horas de retorno à glicemia ≤ 117 mg/dℓ (≤ 6,5 mmol/ℓ) ou glicemia > 252 mg/dℓ (> 14 mmol/ℓ) após 3 horas durante um teste de tolerância à glicose (1 g/kg dextrose IV) foram associadas à recidiva dentro de 9 meses após atingir a remissão.[76]

A remissão foi mais longa em gatos com maior peso corporal no momento do diagnóstico, possivelmente indicando que aqueles com menor peso corporal tinham duração mais prolongada do DM e menor quantidade de células beta funcionais.[93] Assim como em pessoas pré-diabéticas, fármacos que melhoram a sensibilidade à insulina (tiazolidinedionas, biguanidas) também o fazem com a secreção dela (agonistas do peptídio semelhante ao glucagon-1 [GLP-1], sulfonilureias, meglitinidas), ou a insulinoterapia em baixa dose pode ter um papel no tratamento de gatos com alteração da tolerância à glicose ou aumento da glicemia em jejum, a fim de reduzir a probabilidade de recidiva do DM.[80]

MONITORAMENTO DA RESPOSTA AO TRATAMENTO

Glicemia, frutosamina

O objetivo da terapia é atingir glicemias consistentemente normais ou próximas do normal (3 a 10 mmol/ℓ), a fim de maximizar as chances de remissão, minimizar os sinais clínicos da hiperglicemia e evitar hipoglicemia. O monitoramento dos sinais clínicos (ingestão hídrica, peso corporal, apetite) é útil, mas um indicador relativamente insensível do controle glicêmico, sobretudo quando as glicemias estão abaixo do limiar renal (252 a 288 mg/dℓ; 14-16 mmol/ℓ). A frutosamina é um indicador útil do controle glicêmico durante a semana anterior, mas há variações em diferentes testes com relação à metodologia e aos intervalos de referência (321 a 400 μmol/ℓ), o que faz com que as comparações seriadas do gato sejam mais úteis.[76,91,99,100] A mensuração do consumo hídrico doméstico está mais intimamente correlacionada à glicemia média em um período de 24 horas do que a concentração de frutosamina.[101]

Para maximizar a probabilidade de remissão do DM, a glicemia é a variável mais útil para ajuste da dose de insulina, especialmente quando próxima do normal. A glicemia é mais bem mensurada com um glicosímetro portátil calibrado para gatos e com sangue colhido da orelha ou do coxim (Figura 305.6; ver Capítulo 79). Como a hiperglicemia por estresse pode ser imprevisível e levar à confusão, recomenda-se o monitoramento doméstico da glicemia, o que é mais apropriado antes da administração da insulina, a fim de impedir a sobredose quando a glicemia estiver próxima do intervalo normal.

Sistemas de monitoramento contínuo da glicose

Os sistemas de monitoramento contínuo da glicose (SMCGs) facilitam a identificação de hiperglicemia e hipoglicemia e são utilizados principalmente para monitoramento da glicemia em gatos hospitalizados. Com a crescente disponibilidade de unidades mais compactas, as quais fornecem 6 a 7 dias de dados, elas serão cada vez mais utilizadas para o monitoramento doméstico.[102-104] Os SMCGs reduzem o número de amostras de sangue necessárias durante o monitoramento intensivo, direcionam a dose de insulina para regulação mais estrita, são úteis para flutuações entre hiperglicemia e hipoglicemia de gatos diabéticos difíceis de estabilizar e auxiliam na identificação da ação de insulina de curta duração e hiperglicemia de rebote (efeito Somogyi).[102] As unidades fornecem dados em tempo real ou retrospectivos. As unidades compactas são adequadas para monitoramento doméstico, sendo as unidades em tempo real mais utilizadas no ambiente hospitalar, onde fornecem informações imediatas para o ajuste de cada dose de insulina.

As desvantagens dos SMCGs atuais são consideráveis: eles são caros, requerem calibração 2 a três 3 por dia, com mensurações glicêmicas obtidas por outros métodos, a variação da glicemia mensurada é menor do que da maioria dos glicosímetros portáteis, a faixa de transmissão das unidades sem fio é restrita e a vida útil do sensor é finita (necessitando de reposição em 3 a 7 dias). Os sensores podem ser implantados no flanco, no tórax lateral, no espaço interescapular, na prega lateral do cotovelo ou no pescoço dorsal. O posicionamento no pescoço fornece a melhor leitura de dados contínuos (Figura 305.7, Vídeo 305.3).[102,104,105] Dependendo da atividade esperada do gato, pode ser necessário fixar o monitor no local com cola tecidual, fita ou bandagem.[102]

INSULINOTERAPIA

A insulina exógena é o tratamento mais efetivo e confiável para obtenção de excelente controle glicêmico.[8,106] Existem vários tipos disponíveis de insulina para o tratamento.

Insulina lenta (Caninsulin/Vetsulin®, Merck Animal Health)

A insulina lenta (Vetsulin Caninsulin®) é uma insulina de ação intermediária, derivada de suínos, de 40 UI/mℓ, que consiste em

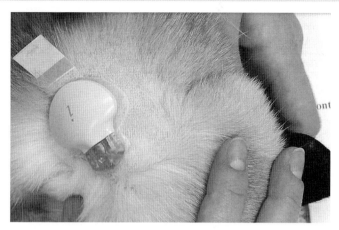

Figura 305.7 Monitor contínuo de glicemia (Medronics iPro®) após implantação e antes da fixação no local.

30% de semilenta amorfa (curta ação) e 70% de ultralenta cristalina (longa ação).[107] A concentração de 40 UI/ml difere das insulinas de 100 UI/ml registradas para utilização em seres humanos e algumas registradas para uso veterinário. Para evitar erros na dose, é importante que as seringas apropriadas de 40 UI/ml não sejam trocadas de forma inadvertida por seringas de 100 UI/ml. Doses iniciais para insulina lenta são de 0,25 a 0,5 UI/kg de peso corporal por via subcutânea (SC), a cada 12 horas, e não devem exceder 3 UI/gato.[108] Em um estudo de 12 meses com 25 gatos (15 recém-diagnosticados), considerou-se que 84% apresentavam resposta boa ou excelente ao tratamento, com base na satisfação do tutor e na resolução dos sinais clínicos, e 28% alcançaram a remissão do DM dentro de 16 semanas após o início do tratamento.[109] A dose inicial mediana foi de 0,5 UI/kg SC, a cada 12 h, e não mudou de maneira significativa durante a evolução do estudo. Em um outro com 46 gatos diabéticos (39 recém-diagnosticados), controle bom a excelente foi alcançado em 72%, com base na resolução dos sinais clínicos, e 15% obtiveram remissão dentro de 20 semanas.[110] Os sinais clínicos de hipoglicemia foram evidentes em 20% dos gatos, e a maioria ocorreu em doses maiores do que 0,5 UI/kg ou 3 UI/gato.[110]

Depois de administrada insulina lenta a gatos diabéticos, o nadir da glicemia costuma ocorrer em cerca de 3 a 6 horas (média de 4 horas), com o retorno da glicemia aos valores pré-administração entre 8 e 10 horas (chamado de retorno aos níveis basais ou duração de ação).[110,111] Em razão dessa duração de ação relativamente curta, mesmo com a administração a cada 12 horas, a hiperglicemia ocorre, de modo geral, durante várias horas, 2 vezes/dia (antes de cada injeção).[111,112] Como resultado, mesmo que nadires apropriados sejam alcançados, a glicemia quase sempre é alta ($\geq$ 360 mg/dl; $\geq$ 20 mmol/l) antes de cada aplicação de insulina, tornando essa a quarta escolha de insulina em gatos. A hiperglicemia acentuada 2 vezes/dia provavelmente contribui para as menores taxas de remissão em gatos tratados com insulina lenta, quando comparados aos tratados com insulina de longa ação. A dose de insulina deve ser ajustada com base no nadir das glicemias, para atingir concentrações dentro do intervalo normal. Não se deve basear a dose na glicemia no momento da aplicação de insulina, a menos que a concentração seja < 360 mg/dl (< 20 mmol/l), o que indica que a ação da insulina é mais longa do que 12 h ou, mais frequentemente, o retorno da secreção endógena de insulina e remissão iminente.[113]

Insulina protamina zíncica

A insulina protamina zíncica (PZI) possui a adição de protamina e zinco para prolongar sua duração de ação.[114] Ao mesmo tempo que não está disponível para uso em seres humanos desde os anos 1990, ela ainda é utilizada em gatos nos EUA e no Reino Unido. De origem animal, é agora uma PZI recombinante humana (ProZinc®, Boehringer Ingelheim).[115,116] A ProZinc® apresenta concentração de 40 UI/ml, devendo, portanto, o uso de seringas apropriadas de insulina ser discutido com o tutor para evitar o uso inadvertido de seringas de 100 UI/ml e doses incorretas. Algumas farmácias de manipulação nos EUA fornecem PZI de origem bovina para uso veterinário, mas, em um estudo, somente 1 de 12 farmácias fabricou de maneira consistente a PZI capaz de atender às especificações necessárias da farmacopeia dos EUA.[117] A dose inicial recomendada é de 1 a 3 UI/gato ou 0,25 a 0,5 unidades/kg de peso corporal ideal, com a dose verdadeira escolhida com base na gravidade dos sinais clínicos e na hiperglicemia (Tabela 305.1).[8,118]

De 133 gatos diabéticos tratados com PZI (120 recém-diagnosticados e 13 previamente tratados com outra insulina), 85% obtiveram bom controle dentro de 45 dias, com base na melhora dos sinais clínicos, na estabilização do peso corporal e na redução da glicemia média 9 horas após administração de PZI e/ou redução da concentração sérica de frutosamina.[116] A hipoglicemia bioquímica foi identificada em 64% dos gatos, embora apenas 2 tivessem sinais clínicos. Em um estudo de gatos diabéticos recém-diagnosticados, três oitavos alcançaram a remissão em 112 dias, o que não foi significativamente diferente da taxa de remissão de dois oitavos obtida em gatos tratados com insulina lenta.[8] Em gatos saudáveis, a PZI resulta em uma curva glicêmica bifásica. O primeiro nadir ocorre em cerca de 4 horas (variação de 1,5 a 8 horas) e um segundo, em 14 horas (variação de 6 a 24 horas). A duração média de ação é de 21 horas (variação de 9 a > 24 horas).[119] Em gatos diabéticos, o primeiro nadir da glicemia ocorreu em 5 a 7 horas.[116] Essa é nossa terceira escolha para DM em gatos.

Glargina (Lantus®, Sanofi-Aventis, proteção da patente vencida em fevereiro de 2015)

A glargina (100 UI/ml) é um análogo de insulina humana de longa ação. A asparagina, na posição A21, é substituída por glicina, e duas argininas são adicionadas à cadeia B nas posições 31 e 32, daí o seu nome.[120] Essas alterações resultam em uma insulina solúvel em soluções ácidas, mas que forma microprecipitados no pH neutro de tecidos SC, prolongando sua liberação.[120,121] Em seres humanos, a glargina fornece concentrações basais de insulina durante 24 horas, sendo utilizada, em geral, em conjunto com insulina de curta ação administrada no momento da alimentação, para simular os padrões normais de secreção endócrina de insulina.[120] Ao utilizar o método de grampo euglicêmico em gatos saudáveis, a glargina teve duração de ação de 10 horas (6,6 a 13 horas).[122] Entretanto, ao utilizar o teste de resposta à insulina em gatos saudáveis, o nadir da glicose foi alcançado 14 horas (10 a 24 horas) após administração de glargina, e a duração de ação foi de 22 horas (12 a > 24 horas).[119] Em gatos saudáveis, a duração de ação é significativamente mais longa do que a insulina lenta (10 horas, variação de 5 a 24+), embora semelhante à PZI (21 horas, variação de 9 a 24+).[119] Em gatos saudáveis, não se observou nenhuma diferença significativa na duração de ação ao comparar doses de 0,5 UI/kg SC, a cada 24 h e 0,25 UI/kg SC, a cada 12 h.[123]

Recomenda-se que a glargina (a cada 12 h) seja utilizada como insulina única para gatos com DM, em conjunto com uma dieta com baixos níveis de carboidrato, a fim de minimizar incrementos pós-prandiais da glicemia.[119] A aplicação a cada 12 horas facilita a sobreposição da ação da insulina de uma injeção para a próxima, resultando em efeitos compatíveis de diminuição da glicose durante 24 horas, o que aumenta as chances de remissão do DM.[119,122,123] É importante ressaltar que o controle glicêmico não foi significativamente diferente entre a glargina administrada 1 vez/dia e a lenta, administrada 2 vezes/dia.[124] As doses iniciais recomendadas são de 0,25 UI/kg de peso corporal ideal SC, se a glicemia for < 360 mg/dl (< 20 mmol/l), ou 0,5 UI/kg (máximo de 3 UI/gato) SC, se a glicemia for maior (Tabelas 305.1 e 305.2).[8,94,118] Caso não se pretenda realizar o monitoramento da glicemia na primeira semana de terapia,

SEÇÃO 21 • Doenças Endócrinas

Tabela 305.1	Protocolo de dose de glargina, detemir ou insulina protamina zíncica, monitoramento de glicose a cada 1 a 2 semanas utilizando-se um glicosímetro calibrado para gatos (p. ex., AlphaTRAK®, da Abbott Animal Health).
PARÂMETRO UTILIZADO PARA AJUSTE DA DOSE	**ALTERAÇÃO NA DOSE**
Inicie com 0,5 UI/kg, SC, a cada 12 h se a glicemia for > 360 mg/dℓ (> 20 mmol/ℓ) ou 0,25 UI/kg, SC, a cada 12 h de peso corporal ideal se a glicemia for menor Não aumente na primeira semana, a menos que ocorra resposta mínima à insulina, mas diminua, se necessário. Monitore a resposta à terapia durante os 3 primeiros dias Se não houver monitoramento na primeira semana, inicie com 1 UI/gato, SC, a cada 12 h	
Se a glicemia pré-insulina for > 216 mg/dℓ (> 12 mmol/ℓ), desde que o nadir não esteja na faixa hipoglicêmica OU Se o nadir da glicemia for > 180 mg/dℓ (> 10 mmol/ℓ)	Aumente em 0,25 a 1 UI, dependendo da dose total de insulina (maior ou menor que 3 UI/gato) e do grau de hiperglicemia (o quão próximo de 180 mg/dℓ estiver a glicemia [10 mmol/ℓ])
Se a glicemia pré-insulina for ≥ 180 a ≤ 216 mg/dℓ (≥ 10 a ≤ 12 mmol/ℓ) OU Se o nadir da glicemia for de 90 a 160 mg/dℓ (5 a 9 mmol/ℓ)	Mesma dose
Se o nadir da glicemia for de 63 a < 72 mg/dℓ (3,5 a < 5 mmol/ℓ)	Utilize o nadir da glicose, a água ingerida, a glicose na urina e a próxima glicemia pré-insulina para determinar se a dose de insulina deve ser diminuída ou mantida
Se a glicemia pré-insulina for < 180 mg/dℓ (< 10 mmol/ℓ) OU Se o nadir da glicemia for < 63 mg/dℓ (< 3,5 mmol/ℓ)	Reduza em 0,25 a 1 UI, dependendo da dose total de insulina (maior ou menor que 3 UI/gato) e do grau de hiperglicemia (o quão próximo de 180 mg/dℓ estiver a glicemia [10 mmol/ℓ]) Se a dose total for de 0,5 a 1 UI, a cada 12 h, mude para a cada 24 h Se a dose total for de 0,5 a 1 UI, a cada 24 h, interrompa a insulina e verifique a possibilidade de remissão diabética
Se forem observados sinais clínicos da hipoglicemia	Reduza em 50%

Ao utilizar um glicosímetro calibrado para sangue humano equivalente a plasma, diminua a concentração-alvo de glicemia em 9 mg/dℓ; 0,5 mmol/ℓ.[8,94,97]

recomenda-se uma dose inicial de 1 UI/gato, embora essa abordagem possa retardar a resolução dos sinais clínicos. Ao realizar a transição de outra insulina para a glargina, se a dose for < 3 UI, o clínico deve utilizar a mesma dose. Para doses ≥ 3 UI, recomenda-se a dose conservadora: por exemplo, começar com 50 a 66% da dose, mas aumentar dentro de 48 a 72 horas se o controle não for adequado.[125]

Glicemias médias significativamente menores no décimo sétimo dia e taxas de remissão significativamente maiores foram alcançadas em 16 semanas de tratamento com glargina (8/8 gatos), em comparação à insulina lenta (2/8) e à PZI (3/8) no DM recém-diagnosticado, alimentados com uma dieta com baixos teores de carboidrato (6% de energia de carboidratos) e administração de insulina a cada 12 horas.[8] Oitenta e quatro por cento de 55 gatos diabéticos alcançaram remissão dentro de 6 meses do diagnóstico após terem sido tratados com glargina e com a utilização de um protocolo que visou atingir a euglicemia.[94]

Em seres humanos com DM tipos 1 e 2, são relatados menos episódios hipoglicêmicos com a glargina, quando comparados a insulinas de ação mais curta.[126,127] Ao mesmo tempo que a hipoglicemia bioquímica (< 54 mg/dℓ ou < 3 mmol/ℓ) ocorre em gatos diabéticos recém-diagnosticados tratados com glargina, nenhum dos 8 gatos desenvolveu sinais clínicos, comparados a 2 tratados com insulina lenta e 1 com PZI.[8] Em um estudo maior com 55 gatos tratados com glargina e um protocolo que visou à euglicemia, a hipoglicemia bioquímica (< 50 mg/dℓ ou < 2,8 mmol/ℓ) foi frequente quando mensurada com um glicosímetro calibrado para sangue total em seres humanos, embora um gato tenha desenvolvido sinais discretos de hipoglicemia clínica (inquietude).[94] Glargina é nossa primeira escolha em gatos e também pode ser utilizada para o tratamento de cetoacidose diabética (ver Capítulo 142).[128]

Detemir (Levemir®, NovoNordisk)

Detemir (ver Capítulo 304) é um análogo da insulina humana de longa ação (100 UI/mℓ). O aminoácido treonina em B30 é removido e um ácido graxo miristoil, com 14 carbonos, é ligado de forma covalente à lisina na posição B29.[121] A ação prolongada da detemir é resultado da absorção lenta para o sangue, uma vez que, após administração, ela se autoassocia em hexâmeros e di-hexâmeros, que também se ligam de forma reversível à albumina, prolongando o tempo de permanência no local da injeção. Ocorre alguma retenção adicional na circulação, associada à ligação à albumina.[121,129,130] No DM humano tipo 2, detemir e glargina são semelhantes em ação, mas a detemir apresenta efeito menos variável.[130] Ao mesmo tempo que a dose a cada 24 horas é adequada em seres humanos para fornecer concentrações basais de insulina, a duração de ação em gatos saudáveis, utilizando-se método do grampo euglicêmico, é mais curta, com recomendação da aplicação a cada 12 horas.[122] A detemir apresenta início de ação discretamente posterior comparado à glargina (1,8 h, variação de 1,1 a 2,5 versus 1,3 h, variação 0,9 a 1,6) em gatos saudáveis utilizando o método do grampo euglicêmico. A duração de ação (11,7 h, variação de 9,1 a 14 comparada a 10 h, variação de 6,6 a 13) e o final de ação (13,5 h, variação de 11 a 16 comparada a 11,3 h, variação de 8 a 14,5) não foram significativamente diferentes da glargina, mas houve menor variabilidade entre gatos do que com a glargina.[122]

As doses iniciais e os protocolos para aumento de dose são os mesmos da glargina (ver Tabelas 305.1 e 305.2).[97,118] A princípio, a maioria dos gatos requer cerca de 25 a 30% menos detemir do que glargina (1,75 UI comparado a 2,5 UI), embora doses finais possam ser semelhantes.[94,97] Gatos podem apresentar sensibilidade inicial à detemir, que é transitória e costuma durar por 24 a 48 horas. Portanto, caso se opte pela alteração da glargina ou de outra insulina, inicie com cerca de metade da atual dose de insulina e aumente dentro de 48 horas, se ocorrer diminuição insuficiente da glicose. Aumente a dose a cada 3 a 7 dias, até que a glicemia esteja controlada. De forma semelhante aos achados nos gatos tratados com glargina, a remissão ocorreu em 81% daqueles tratados com detemir dentro de 6 meses do diagnóstico e um protocolo que visou à euglicemia,

CAPÍTULO 305 • Diabetes Melito Felino

Tabela 305.2 Protocolo de dose da glargina ou detemir e monitoramento intensivo doméstico da glicemia (mínimo de 3 mensurações ao dia com média de 5) durante período de estabilização (6 a 12 semanas), utilizando-se um glicosímetro calibrado equivalente ao plasma para gatos (p. ex., AlphaTRAK®, da Abbott Animal Health).[94]

PARÂMETRO UTILIZADO PARA AJUSTE DA DOSE	ALTERAÇÃO NA DOSE
Fase 1: dose inicial e primeiros 3 dias de glargina	
Inicie com 0,25 UI/kg de peso corporal ideal SC, a cada 12 h, OU Se o gato tiver recebido outra insulina anteriormente, aumente ou reduza a dose inicial, levando essa informação em consideração. A glargina possui potência menor do que a insulina lenta ou PZI na maioria dos gatos	
Gatos com histórico de desenvolvimento de cetonas e glicemia > 300 mg/dℓ (> 17 mmol/ℓ) após 24 a 48 h do início da insulina	Aumente em 0,5 UI
Se o nadir da glicemia for < 72 mg/dℓ (< 4 mmol/ℓ) e não houver sinais clínicos de hipoglicemia	Reduza a dose em 0,25 a 0,5 UI, dependendo se o gato estiver em doses baixas ou altas de insulina (maior ou menor do que 3 UI/gato) e da gravidade da hipoglicemia
Fase 2: aumento da dose	
Se o nadir da glicemia for > 300 mg/dℓ (> 16,6 mmol/ℓ)	Aumente a cada 3 dias, em 0,5 UI
Se o nadir da glicemia for de 200 a 300 mg/dℓ (11,1 a 16,6 mmol/ℓ)	Aumente a cada 3 dias, em 0,25 a 0,5 UI, dependendo se o gato estiver em doses baixas ou altas de insulina e da gravidade da hiperglicemia
Se o nadir da glicemia for de 117 a < 200 mg/dℓ (6,5 a < 11 mmol/ℓ) e o pico for > 200 mg/dℓ (> 11 mmol/ℓ)	Aumente a cada 5 a 7 dias, em 0,25 a 0,5 UI, dependendo se o gato estiver em doses baixas ou altas de insulina e da gravidade da hiperglicemia
Se o nadir da glicemia for < 63 ou < 72 mg/dℓ (< 3,5 ou < 4 mmol/ℓ)	Concentração verdadeira utilizada para diminuir a dose depende da frequência de monitoramento e resposta prévia a alterações da dose de insulina, quando a glicemia estiver ao redor do limite inferior da faixa normal. Reduza a dose em 0,25 a 0,5 UI, dependendo se o gato estiver em doses baixas ou altas de insulina. Se ocorrerem sinais clínicos de hipoglicemia, reduza a dose em 0,5 a > 1 UI, dependendo da gravidade
Se a glicemia, no momento da próxima aplicação de insulina, for de 72 a 117 mg/dℓ (4 a 6,5 mmol/ℓ)	Inicialmente, teste qual dos métodos alternativos é mais compatível àquele gato: a. Alimente o gato e reduza a dose em 0,25 a 0,5 UI, dependendo se o gato estiver em doses baixas ou altas de insulina b. Alimente o gato, espere 1 a 2 h e, quando a glicemia aumentar para > 117 mg/dℓ (> 6,5 mmol/ℓ), forneça a dose normal. Se a glicemia não aumentar dentro de 1 a 2 h, reduza a dose em 0,25 UI ou 0,5 UI (como descrito anteriormente) c. Divida a dose: alimente o gato e forneça a maior parte da dose imediatamente. Então, administre o restante da dose 1 a 2 h depois, quando a glicemia tiver aumentado para > 117 mg/dℓ (> 6,5 mmol/ℓ) Se todos esses métodos levarem ao aumento da glicemia, forneça a dose completa se a glicemia pré-insulina for de 72 a 117 mg/dℓ (4 a 6,5 mmol/ℓ) e observe com atenção os sinais de hipoglicemia. De forma geral, para a maioria dos gatos os melhores resultados na fase 2 ocorrem quando a insulina é quantificada da forma mais consistente possível, fornecendo-se a dose completa normal no momento regular da administração
Fase 3: manutenção da dose. Almeje manter a glicemia dentro da faixa de 72 a 200 mg/dℓ (4 a 11 mmol/ℓ) durante todo o dia	
Se o nadir da glicemia for < 63 ou 70 mg/dℓ (< 3,5 ou 4 mmol/ℓ)	Reduza a dose em 0,25 a 0,5 UI, dependendo se o gato estiver em doses baixas ou altas de insulina
Se o nadir ou pico da glicemia for > 200 mg/dℓ (> 11 mmol/ℓ)	Aumente a dose em 0,25 a 0,5 UI, dependendo se o gato estiver em doses baixas ou altas de insulina e do grau de hiperglicemia
Fase 4: redução da dose. Diminua a dose de insulina lentamente em 0,25 a 0,5 UI, dependendo da dose	
Quando a menor glicemia do gato for, de maneira regular (todo dia, por pelo menos 1 semana), entre 63 mg/dℓ e 117 mg/dℓ (4 a 6,5 mmol/ℓ) e, de modo geral, abaixo de 117 mg/dℓ (6,5 mmol/ℓ)	Reduza a dose em 0,25 a 0,5 UI, dependendo se o gato estiver em doses baixas ou altas de insulina
Se o nadir da glicemia for de 55 a < 63 mg/dℓ (3 e < 4 mmol/ℓ), pelo menos em três momentos em dias separados	Reduza a dose em 0,25 a 0,5 UI, dependendo se o gato estiver em doses baixas ou altas de insulina
Se o nadir for < 55 mg/dℓ (< 3 mmol/ℓ) uma vez	Reduza a dose imediatamente em 0,25 a 0,5 UI, dependendo se o gato estiver em doses baixas ou altas de insulina
Se o pico da glicemia for > 200 mg/dℓ (> 11 mmol/ℓ)	Aumente imediatamente a dose de insulina para a última dose efetiva
Fase 5: remissão. Euglicemia durante o mínimo de 14 dias sem insulina. Monitore a glicemia, pelo menos duas a três vezes ao dia durante 14 dias, para garantir que permaneça ≤ 117 mg/dℓ (≤ 6,5 mmol/ℓ); então, 1 a 2 vezes/semana depois. Se a glicemia aumentar para 117 a < 180 mg/dℓ (6,5 a < 10 mmol/ℓ), institua outra terapia, como sensibilizantes insulínicos ou agonistas de GLP-1, para manter a glicemia ≤ 117 mg/dℓ (≤ 6,5 mmol/ℓ); se ≥ 180 mg/dℓ (≥ 10 mmol/ℓ), reinstitua a insulina 1 a 2 vezes/dia, dependendo da gravidade da hiperglicemia	

SEÇÃO 21 • Doenças Endócrinas

enquanto esse dado foi de somente 42% caso o controle glicêmico tenha sido retardado por 6 meses ou mais.[97] A detemir é nossa segunda opção de insulina em razão da menor experiência, mas gatos tratados com glargina, com controle ruim, especialmente de curta duração de ação, devem ser testados com a detemir enquanto se buscam por doenças concomitantes.

Armazenamento da insulina

O tempo de prateleira recomendado pelo fabricante em temperatura ambiente, após abertura, é de 28 dias para glargina e de 6 semanas para detemir. Entretanto, elas são relativamente estáveis em solução, e vários tutores de gatos com DM utilizam-nas efetivamente refrigeradas durante 6 meses ou mais. Os períodos de validade curtos em frascos de medicação injetável de uso múltiplo, mesmo se houver conservantes, decorre da avaliação da *Food and Drug Admnistration* (FDA) sobre o risco de contaminação bacteriana, que é extremamente baixo. As preparações de glargina e detemir contêm o preservativo antimicrobiano metacresol, que é bacteriostático e mais efetivo em temperatura ambiente. Os tutores devem ser instruídos a descartar imediatamente a insulina com aparência turva ou mudança de coloração.

Administração de doses pequenas de glargina e detemir

A administração de doses pequenas utilizando-se insulinas de 100 UI/mℓ (detemir ou glargina) pode ser problemática e limitar sua utilização quando forem necessárias doses menores que 1 UI. Canetas de aplicação são recomendadas para doses menores do que 2 UI, pois fornecem maior acurácia, estabilidade e minimizam o risco de contaminação bacteriana, quando comparadas à insulina diluída.[131-133] Canetas de aplicação de insulina, como a HumaPen Luxura HD® (Eli Lilly) e a NovoPen Junior® (EUA)/Demi® (outros países) (NovoNordisk), fornecem doses de insulina acuradas e precisas em incrementos de 0,5 UI (ver Capítulo 304). Entretanto, em alguns gatos, particularmente naqueles entrando em remissão e recuperando alguma função das células beta, os ajustes de dose podem ser necessários em incrementos menores do que 0,5 UI.

A detemir pode ser diluída utilizando-se um meio especial para tal, disponibilizada pela NovoNordisk, mas, em alguns países, o fabricante não o fornecerá a veterinários. A detemir também pode ser diluída em água ou salina estéril, o que também dilui o aditivo antimicrobiano (metacresol).[134] Minimize o risco de contaminação bacteriana com a diluição imediata antes de cada administração. Se diluída em um frasco e mantida refrigerada, descarte a insulina após 30 dias. A potência pode ser afetada de maneira adversa com a utilização desse método. Nem a diluição nem a homogeneização com outras insulinas são recomendadas para a glargina. Entretanto, em seres humanos com DM a mistura da glargina com outras insulinas tem sido bem-sucedida, apesar da formação de um precipitado turvo na seringa.[135] A diluição tanto da detemir (1:10) como da glargina (1:100) com salina é relatada para o tratamento de DM neonatal humana transitória, para facilitar a administração de doses muito pequenas, embora o efeito da diluição sobre a eficácia ou a estabilidade ainda não tenha sido relatado em seres humanos ou gatos.[134]

Escolha da insulina

Antes da disponibilidade da insulina de longa ação, os objetivos do tratamento de gatos com DM eram resolver os sinais clínicos e melhorar a qualidade e a duração de vida. Dadas as altas taxas de remissão do DM ao utilizar insulinas de longa ação, dietas com baixos níveis de carboidrato e protocolos que visavam a glicemias normais ou próximas ao normal, a insulina deve ser escolhida a fim de maximizar essa oportunidade. A remissão do DM possui vantagens de bem-estar, custo para os tutores e qualidade de vida para ambos. A glargina e a detemir estão associadas a maiores taxas de remissão em gatos com DM recém-diagnosticado. Estas devem ser as insulinas de primeira escolha para um gato com DM recém-diagnosticado. Entretanto, nem a glargina nem a detemir

estão registradas para uso em gatos. Em alguns países, as leis exigem o uso de produtos aprovados inicialmente para medicina veterinária e só depois permitem o uso diferente do indicado na bula da glargina ou da detemir caso haja falha no tratamento. Caso o uso de insulinas veterinárias registradas seja obrigatório legalmente, a PZI é recomendada, mas está disponível somente em um número limitado de países.

DIETA

Contexto geral

O papel da dieta no tratamento e na prevenção do DM é inquestionável (ver Capítulo 181). Dietas comerciais felinas com alimento seco derivam até 60% de energia dos carboidratos (média de 41%).[25,136,137] Gatos são carnívoros natos; com base na metanálise de dados de 27 estudos de presas naturais de gatos ferais, a ingestão de energia média diária é de cerca de 2% de carboidratos (extrato livre de nitrogênio), 52% de proteína bruta e 46% de gordura bruta.[138] Gatos são relativamente intolerantes à glicose quando comparados a cães e seres humanos.[1,139-141] Existem evidências de que gatos limitam a ingestão quando os níveis de carboidratos são > 40% de energia metabolizável (EM).[139,142-145]

Papel da dieta na prevenção do diabetes

Gatos com sobrepeso apresentam risco 4,6 vezes maior de DM do que aqueles com condição corporal ideal, sendo a obesidade o fator de risco adquirido mais importante (ver Capítulo 176).[24,77] Aproximadamente 25 a 63% dos gatos estão acima do peso ou obesos e 20% daqueles obesos com mais de 8 anos são pré-diabéticos, com alteração da tolerância à glicose ou da glicose em jejum.[75,146-150] Em gatos, seres humanos e cães, o carboidrato é o principal macronutriente a determinar a magnitude do aumento pós-prandial da glicose e da insulina plasmáticas.[151-153] Tanto em gatos magros alimentados com refeições ou à vontade, o carboidrato resulta em glicemias pós-prandiais significativamente maiores do que as quantidades equivalentes (% EM) de proteína ou gordura. O pico da glicemia foi de 151 mg/dℓ (8 mmol/ℓ) ou 31% maior para uma dieta rica em carboidratos (47% de carboidratos da EM, 12,9 g/100 kcal) do que para uma rica em proteínas (46% de proteínas de EM, 37% de carboidratos de EM, 7,1 g/100 kcal), com um pico de 115 mg/dℓ (6 mmol/ℓ) (p < 0,001). As concentrações pós-prandiais de insulina apresentaram tendência semelhante.[153] Existe também uma tendência consistente de que as concentrações de glicose e insulina sejam menores para a dieta rica em proteína quando comparada àquela rica em gordura (ambas com 27% de carboidratos da EM).

É importante ressaltar que a magnitude e a duração da hiperglicemia pós-prandial são exacerbadas pelo ganho de peso.[32,154] Em gatos com sobrepeso alimentados com uma dieta disponível no mercado, rica em carboidratos (51% da EM; 14,5 g/100 g/kcal), as concentrações pós-prandiais médias de glicose durante 24 horas foram de 119 ± desvio padrão de 18 mg/dℓ (6,6 ± 1 mmol/ℓ) e os picos de glicemia chegaram a 241 mg/dℓ (13,4 mmol/ℓ) e na faixa do DM para gatos.[77,154] O fornecimento de dietas ricas em gordura que excedem as necessidades de energia de manutenção está associado à obesidade e, portanto, aumenta o risco de DM.[150,155,156] Um estudo comparou alimentos úmidos e secos e observou que gatos alimentados somente com dietas úmidas (com maiores níveis de gordura e menores de carboidratos) tiveram risco três vezes maior de DM, enquanto o fornecimento somente de dietas secas (maiores níveis de carboidratos, menores níveis de gordura) foi associado ao risco duas vezes maior, sugerindo que o efeito adverso da obesidade oriundo de uma dieta com maiores níveis de gordura seja um risco maior para o DM, embora a ingestão maior de carboidratos também o aumente, presumivelmente pela elevação da glicemia pós-prandial.[24] Ao mesmo tempo que dietas ricas em carboidrato (≥ 50% da EM) possam conter proteína insuficiente para gatos, é improvável que dietas com níveis moderados de carboidratos (20 a 30% da EM) sejam prejudiciais para adultos jovens e magros com função normal das células beta. Entretanto, dietas com ≤ 12% de energia oriunda de carboidratos são indicadas para gatos com risco maior de DM. A partir do momento que a idade é um fator de risco para DM, gatos idosos com outros fatores de risco (raça, uso de corticosteroides, obesidade) poderiam se beneficiar de uma dieta com baixos níveis de carboidratos, para minimizar a secreção de insulina necessária para manter a euglicemia.[157]

Papel da dieta no tratamento do diabetes (ver Capítulo 181)

O objetivo principal do tratamento do DM felino é alcançar a remissão. A minimização de carboidratos (CHO) da dieta reduz a demanda sobre as células beta pancreáticas para produzir insulina. Dados oriundos de uma série de estudos em gatos com DM indicam que dietas com baixos níveis de carboidratos (≤ 13% da EM; < 4 g/100 kcal da EM) podem melhorar o controle glicêmico, reduzir a concentração da frutosamina e aumentar a probabilidade de remissão do diabetes.[8,94,95,97,158,159] Quando 63 gatos diabéticos foram alimentados durante 16 semanas (11 recém-diagnosticados e 52 previamente diagnosticados), uma dieta com baixos níveis de carboidratos e fibras (12% da EM; 3,5 g de CHO/100 kcal) resultou em taxas de remissão significativamente maiores (68% *versus* 41%) e melhor controle glicêmico, com base na resolução dos sinais clínicos e das concentrações séricas de frutosamina < 400 µmol/ℓ (81% *versus* 56%), quando comparada a uma dieta com níveis moderados de carboidrato e altos de fibras (7,6 g de CHO/100 kcal, 26% da EM).[95] Não existem estudos relatados que comparem dietas de ≤ 6% da EM com 12% da EM.[98] Entretanto, as maiores taxas de remissão relatadas (> 80%) estão associadas à utilização de uma dieta restrita em carboidratos (< 6% da EM), combinada a protocolos de insulina que almejam atingir glicemias normais ou próximas disso.[8,94,97] Em gatos diabéticos obesos a longo prazo que não perderam peso ou atingiram remissão com manejo apropriado, a remissão do DM é improvável. A prioridade deve então ser atingir uma condição corporal ideal, a fim de reduzir o risco de outras comorbidades associadas à obesidade em gatos.

A normalização da condição corporal e da massa muscular são objetivos dietéticos, sendo importante a perda de peso controlada pela restrição energética.[157] Embora a remissão possa ocorrer antes de perda de peso significativa, a obtenção de condição corporal ideal é provavelmente importante para manutenção da remissão e melhoria da sensibilidade insulínica.[47,93,94] Uma dieta compatível para perda de peso para um gato com DM possui gordura < 4 g/100 kcal, carboidratos < 3 g/100 kcal e proteína > 10 g/kcal; entretanto, a ingestão de energia deve também ser controlada.[157] Alimentos enlatados ajudam a diminuir a ingestão de energia e peso corporal, pois a umidade aumenta o volume e a hidratação do alimento.[160]

A doença renal crônica (DRC) é relatada em 26 a 62% de gatos com DM (ver Capítulo 324).[94,97] Quantidades controladas de proteína e restrição do fósforo melhoram o tempo de sobrevida em gatos com DRC e, portanto, dietas diabéticas com teores altos de proteína e baixos de carboidratos provavelmente são contraindicadas, especialmente em gatos no estágio 2 ou 3 da DRC, pela Sociedade Internacional de Interesse Renal (IRIS) (ver Capítulo 184).[161] Se um gato tiver bom apetite, a administração de acarbose, com dieta renal de prescrição de níveis moderados de carboidratos, pode auxiliar na redução da glicemia pós-prandial.[162] Dietas com níveis ultrabaixos de carboidratos à base de produtos hortifrutigranjeiros (≤ 2% da EM), sobretudo peixe ou carne, costumam possuir níveis consideravelmente mais altos de fósforo do que as dietas de prescrição veterinárias disponíveis desenvolvidas para DM felino, devendo, portanto, ser evitadas na DRC.

HIPOGLICEMIANTES ORAIS

Conceito geral

Medicamentos hipoglicemiantes orais podem ser utilizados como terapia exclusiva em diabéticos com insulina endógena suficiente para manter a euglicemia ou combinados à insulinoterapia. Os fármacos orais atuam pela estimulação da secreção de insulina pelas células beta pancreáticas, aumentando a sensibilidade insulínica nos tecidos ou retardando a absorção intestinal de glicose.[163] De forma geral, a menos que o cliente opte pela eutanásia, os medicamentos hipoglicemiantes orais não são recomendados como agentes exclusivos em gatos com DM recém-diagnosticado com sinais evidentes, pois o controle glicêmico deles é muito melhor com a insulina.[8,106,173] Entretanto, hipoglicemiantes orais podem ser efetivos no tratamento do DM subclínico ou pré-diabetes em gatos, bem como em alguns deles, quando combinados à insulinoterapia.

Sulfonilureias

As sulfonilureias estimulam a secreção de insulina pelas células beta pancreáticas, pela ligação a ATPases, que, sequencialmente, fecham os canais de potássio (K) e abrem os canais de cálcio (Ca) nas membranas celulares. O influxo resultante aumenta as concentrações de cálcio intracelulares, desencadeando a liberação da insulina armazenada.[164,165] A glipizida é a sulfonilureia utilizada com maior frequência em gatos. Ela melhorou os sinais em 30% daqueles com DM, e 15% apresentaram controle bom a excelente com base em glicemias próximas do normal, resolução dos sinais clínicos e ausência de glicosúria.[106,166] Entretanto, 56% apresentaram piora da glicemia e necessitaram de insulina.[106] A remissão do DM foi relatada em apenas 12% dos gatos recém-diagnosticados tratados com glipizida.[106] Os gatos mais propensos a responder não são cetônicos, apresentam sinais discretos de DM, condição corporal aceitável e boa saúde.[167] A dose inicial recomendada é de 2,5 mg por via oral (VO), a cada 12 horas, com alimento, que pode ser aumentada para 5 mg VO, a cada 12 horas, caso não seja observada melhora no controle glicêmico.[166,167] Em 5 a 10% dos gatos, o controle glicêmico se torna inadequado dentro de semanas a anos, necessitando de insulinoterapia.[166,168]

Meglitinidas

Esses fármacos também estimulam a secreção de insulina pela ligação a ATPases nas células beta pancreáticas em locais diferentes do que as sulfonilureias e desencadeiam a mesma cascata de reações, ocorrendo efeitos sinérgicos quando da combinação dos dois.[164,169] O efeito da meglitinida nateglinida sobre a glicemia e a secreção insulínica foi comparado ao da sulfonilureia glimepirida em gatos saudáveis após utilização de teste de tolerância à glicose de 0,5 g/kg IV. A nateglinida teve início de ação mais rápido (20 minutos *versus* 60 minutos), mas duração de ação mais curta (60 minutos *versus* 180 minutos).[170]

Biguanidas

As biguanidas apresentam efeito sensibilizante à insulina que necessita de células beta funcionais, já que aumentam a resposta hepática e de tecidos periféricos à insulina, diminuindo, assim, a produção de glicose e aumentando a captação dela.[169-171] Embora o mecanismo de ação exato seja desconhecido, elas interrompem os processos oxidativos mitocondriais no fígado e corrigem desequilíbrios no metabolismo intracelular do cálcio nos tecidos periféricos.[172] A metformina, a única biguanida disponível no mercado, foi administrada a 5 gatos com DM recém-diagnosticado (glicemias médias de 487 mg/dℓ ou 27 mmol/ℓ); 1 de 5 apresentava concentrações séricas de insulina mensuráveis antes do tratamento, sendo esse o único gato que alcançou bom controle glicêmico (glicemia média de 167 mg/dℓ ou 9,3 mmol/ℓ). Esse gato necessitou de uma dose de 50 mg VO, a cada 12 horas, durante > 8 semanas.[173]

Tiazolidinediona

Tiazolidinedionas (TZDs) se ligam ao receptor gama ativado pelo proliferador do peroxissoma no núcleo e alteram a expressão gênica, levando a maior sensibilidade insulínica no tecido adiposo, no músculo e no fígado,[174,175] o que diminui a gliconeogênese hepática e aumenta o metabolismo da glicose no músculo, resultando em diminuição das glicemias em jejum.[174] O darglitazone aumentou as concentrações de insulina em gatos obesos durante um teste de tolerância à glicose IV, mas não normalizou seu padrão de secreção da insulina.[87]

Inibidores da alfaglicosidase

Fármacos como a acarbose reduzem a glicemia pós-prandial pela inibição da ação das dissacaridases da borda em escova ligadas à membrana (glicoamilase, sucrase, isomaltase, maltase) no intestino delgado. Ao retardar a quebra de carboidratos complexos, eles tornam a absorção intestinal de glicose mais lenta e reduzem o pico da glicemia pós-prandial.[166,169] Em gatos saudáveis, a acarbose, administrada na dose de 25 mg/gato VO, a cada 24 h, com refeição com altos níveis de carboidrato (50% de energia oriunda de carboidratos), reduziu de forma significativa as glicemias médias nas primeiras 12 horas, em comparação a gatos alimentados somente com a refeição (91 mg/dℓ ou 5,1 mmol/ℓ versus 106 mg/dℓ ou 5,9 mmol.[162] Entretanto, as glicemias não foram significativamente menores (93 mg/dℓ ou 5,2 mmol/ℓ) do que em gatos com refeições com baixos níveis de carboidrato (6% de energia oriunda de carboidratos) e não houve diferença nas glicemias médias quando foi fornecida uma dieta com baixos níveis de carboidratos, com ou sem acarbose.[162] O efeito de diminuição da glicose foi evidente apenas nas primeiras 12 horas após administração de acarbose e foi minimamente efetivo em gatos que fazem múltiplas refeições pequenas. Em gatos com DRC, nos quais uma dieta pobre em proteínas e com níveis moderados de carboidratos é indicada, a acarbose pode ser utilizada para diminuir a absorção de glicose do trato gastrintestinal. Entretanto, como a acarbose é mais efetiva quando os gatos se alimentam dentro de um curto período de tempo após a administração, é provável que seja minimamente efetiva naqueles no estágio 3 ou 4 da DRC pela IRIS, que possuem pouco apetite e consomem pequenas quantidades de alimento várias vezes ao dia. A acarbose, administrada na dose de 12,5 mg/gato VO, a cada 12 h, com uma dieta com baixos níveis de carboidrato, não foi associada a maiores reduções nos requerimentos medianos de insulina ou controle glicêmico do que gatos alimentados somente com dieta pobre em carboidratos (redução da dose de 5 UI/gato SC, a cada 12 horas para 1 UI/gato SC, a cada 12 h).[159]

Oligoelementos

Cromo, vanádio e tungstênio podem melhorar a sensibilidade insulínica. O cromo é um cofator para a função da insulina, que aumenta o transporte de glicose ao fígado, ao tecido adiposo e ao músculo.[169] A suplementação oral, em doses maiores que 300 ppb, resultou em melhora da tolerância à glicose, com doses de 600 ppb levando à diminuição significativa da glicemia (139 mg/dℓ ou 7,7 mmol/ℓ, em comparação a 150 mg/dℓ ou 8,3 mmol/ℓ) em gatos saudáveis com peso normal.[176] Doses menores que 100 μg em gatos obesos não tiveram efeito sobre a tolerância à glicose.[177] O vanádio, na dose de 0,2 mg/kg/dia, reduziu a glicemia e a concentração sérica de frutosamina e melhorou os sinais clínicos (poliúria e polidipsia) em gatos com DM na fase inicial.[178] Em gatos diabéticos tratados com PZI, a suplementação com vanádio, na dose de 45 mg/gato/dia, melhorou o controle glicêmico, com um requerimento médio de insulina de 3 UI em gatos suplementados com vanádio comparados a 5 UI naqueles tratados somente com PZI.[179]

TERAPIAS NOVAS E EMERGENTES

Terapias baseadas em incretinas

Incretinas são hormônios gastrintestinais (ver Capítulo 310) rapidamente liberados em resposta à ingestão alimentar, que estimulam a síntese e a liberação de insulina, ao mesmo tempo que suprimem a secreção de glucagon.[180] Elas incluem o peptídio semelhante ao glucagon-1 (GLP-1), secretado pelas células L na porção distal do trato intestinal, que se liga aos receptores acoplados à proteína G nas células alfa e beta pancreáticas.[180-182] O GLP-1 também aumenta a sobrevida da célula beta, retarda o esvaziamento gástrico e suprime o apetite.[181,182] O GLP-1 possui meia-vida curta e é degradado pela dipeptidilpeptidase-4 (DPP-4), encontrada em vários tecidos e no plasma. Dentro do intestino, ela degrada o GLP-1 pela clivagem da molécula e diminuição da afinidade pelo receptor.[181,183] As concentrações de GLP-1 estão reduzidas em gatos obesos e seres humanos após desafio à glicose. O efeito insulinotrópico do GLP-1 está reduzido em casos de DM humano tipo 2.[184-187]

Fármacos adicionais incluem agonistas de GLP-1 resistentes à degradação pela DPP-4 e inibidores da DDP-4.[185,188] Como as ações do GLP-1 dependem da glicose, a hipoglicemia é rara.[186] A exenatida (duas vezes/dia) e a exenatida de liberação prolongada (1 vez/semana) são preparações injetáveis de agonistas de GLP-1 utilizadas como terapia adjuvante ou exclusiva no DM humano tipo 2.[186] Em gatos saudáveis, a exenatida (1 μg/kg) aumentou a insulina em 2,4 vezes dentro de 15 minutos durante um grampo hiperglicêmico isoglicêmico.[189] Durante um teste de resposta à refeição em gatos saudáveis, doses de 2 μg/kg (exenatida) e 200 μg/kg (liberação prolongada) foram as melhores doses, aumentando as concentrações de insulina em 330 e 178%, respectivamente.[190] Em gatos saudáveis, a resposta da insulina após uma refeição foi semelhante em comparação à exenatida, à exenatida de liberação prolongada e ao inibidor de DPP-4 sitagliptina.[191] Efeitos gastrintestinais discretos transitórios (êmese e diarreia) foram observados com os três fármacos. Em gatos com DM recém-diagnosticado tratados com glargina e dieta pobre em carboidratos, os também tratados com exenatida de liberação prolongada apresentaram melhor controle glicêmico, menores doses de insulina e maiores taxas de remissão (44% versus 25%), comparados àqueles tratados com placebo.[192] Efeitos adversos discretos e transitórios incluíram redução do apetite, náuseas e êmese.

Amilina

A amilina, cossecretada com a insulina pelas células beta pancreáticas, suprime a secreção de glucagon, retarda o esvaziamento gástrico e promove saciedade.[193,194] No DM, diminuições da produção de amilina estão associadas à disfunção e à perda de células beta pancreáticas.[193,195] Em pacientes humanos com DM tipos 1 e 2 fazendo uso de insulina, o análogo sintético da amilina, a pramlintida, injetada na hora da refeição, diminuiu a glicemia pós-prandial, a dose da insulina e a ingestão de energia, aumentou a saciedade pós-prandial e induziu perda de peso.[194,196,197] Em gatos saudáveis, a amilina, administrada 5 minutos antes do início de um teste de estimulação por arginina IV (0,2 g/kg), de um teste de tolerância à glicose IV (0,5 g/kg) ou de um teste de resposta à refeição, causou diminuição nas concentrações plasmáticas de glucagon e insulina nos testes de tolerância à arginina e à glicose IV.[198]

Insulina inteligente

Um produto sintético da insulina desenvolvido para ser de longa ação e responsivo a concentrações de glicose mostrou atividades semelhantes àquelas do pâncreas saudável de ratos. A adição de um domínio alifático à insulina facilita as interações hidrofóbicas e fornece tempo de permanência mais longo no sangue. Uma molécula de ácido fenilborônico (AFB) se liga reversivelmente à glicose, resultando em ativação da insulina apenas quando a glicemia estiver alta.[199] Testes clínicos estão inacabados.

GATOS DIABÉTICOS MAL CONTROLADOS

Diagnósticos diferenciais

Ao mesmo tempo que o bom controle glicêmico ou a remissão são atingidos na maioria dos gatos diabéticos assim que a insulinoterapia apropriada e o monitoramento são instituídos, alguns gatos são difíceis de controlar, quase sempre necessitando de doses altas de insulina. A incapacidade em obter controle clínico e glicêmico do DM pode ocorrer em razão do mau comprometimento do tutor ou da técnica de administração, da insulina ou da dose inapropriadas (dose e/ou frequência) ou das doenças subjacentes que contribuem para a resistência insulínica.

Armazenamento, homogeneização, seringas

O armazenamento inapropriado da insulina, levando a perda de potência, administração incorreta (p. ex., técnica ruim de injeção, com algumas bolhas de ar na seringa) ou dose irregular, pode contribuir para o mau controle glicêmico.[74] A homogeneização inadequada da suspensão da insulina lenta pode resultar em dose errática, porque as concentrações de insulina variam em cada dose, o que deve ser descartado pela conversa com clientes antes de investigações adicionais. Esses fatores podem ser facilmente retificados com instruções apropriadas. Erros na dose de insulina podem ocorrer quando um tipo de seringa é alterado por outro e o tutor continua a dosar a insulina com base nas graduações do corpo da seringa. Por exemplo, se um gato que recebe insulina lenta porcina (40 UI/ml, Vetsulin/Caninsulin®, Intervet), normalmente aplicada com seringas de 40 UI/ml (1 graduação = 0,025 ml), tiver o tipo de seringa alterada de forma inadvertida para seringas de 0,3 ml, 100 UI/ml (1 graduação = 0,01 ml), resultará em administração somente de 40% da dose. Erros semelhantes ocorrem quando seringas de 0,3 ml são acidentalmente entregues a um cliente que utiliza seringas de insulina de 1 ml (1 graduação = 0,02 ml). Entretanto, se a substituição for ao contrário, pode parecer que há aumento da sensibilidade à insulina, levando à hipoglicemia.

Duração curta de ação da insulina

Em gatos tratados com insulinas de ação intermediária, como a lenta, a duração de ação pode ser muito curta para manter diminuições prolongadas na glicemia, mesmo quando administradas a cada 12 horas.[111,119] O nadir da glicemia é alcançado 3 a 5 horas após administração da insulina lenta porcina em gatos com DM, com o retorno das glicemias aos níveis basais dentro de 9 a 10 horas.[110,111] Portanto, na maioria dos gatos tratados a cada 12 horas com insulina lenta porcina não há efeito de diminuição da glicose pela insulina exógena durante 2 a 3 horas antes da aplicação da insulina. A presença contínua das concentrações basais de insulina é importante para supressão da gliconeogênese hepática.[200] A duração curta de ação provavelmente explica a hiperglicemia acentuada (≥ 360 mg/dl; 20 mmol/l) antes de cada administração de insulina em vários gatos tratados com a insulina lenta, mesmo quando há boa diminuição da glicose após administração da insulina, com a obtenção de concentrações apropriadas de nadir. As mensurações seriadas da glicemia, especialmente se aferidas em casa, podem ajudar a identificar esse problema. Nesses gatos, a alteração para insulina de ação mais longa, como a glargina ou a detemir, costuma resolver o controle ruim.

Doença subjacente

Contexto geral

Doenças subjacentes podem contribuir para resistência insulínica e mau controle, apesar do bom comprometimento do

cliente e da seleção e da dose apropriadas da insulina. Testes adicionais devem ser oferecidos se as doses de insulina excederem 1 a 1,5 UI/kg, a cada 12 h, e o controle glicêmico permanecer ruim (glicemia média > 270 mg/dl ou > 15 mmol/l).

Acromegalia

A acromegalia, ou hipersomatotropismo, resulta do aumento da produção do hormônio do crescimento (GH, *growth hormone*), tipicamente devido a um adenoma hipofisário (ver Capítulo 294). O aumento do GH causa defeitos pós-receptores na ação da insulina em tecidos-alvo. Essa resistência insulínica pode ser extrema.[14] Apesar de hiperplasia substancial de células beta, a resistência insulínica pode exceder a capacidade secretória da insulina para manter a euglicemia, o que resulta em DM concomitante.[14] A secreção do fator de crescimento semelhante à insulina-1 (IGF-1, do inglês *insulina-like growth factor 1*) também aumenta, o que medeia as alterações anabólicas associadas.[201] Em gatos, sinais clínicos comuns de acromegalia incluem poliúria e polidipsia, polifagia e ganho de peso. Aumento dos órgãos abdominais, sopro cardíaco sistólico, alargamento das características faciais, prognatismo inferior, patas grandes e estridor respiratório também podem ocorrer conforme a doença progride. A princípio, vários gatos com acromegalia parecem normais.[16] A acromegalia, com seus efeitos anabólicos, deve ser considerada como diagnóstico diferencial de qualquer gato com controle ruim do DM, com peso corporal estável ou crescente.[14,202] A acromegalia é a doença subjacente mais comum em gatos com controle ruim do DM, correspondendo talvez a 25 a 30%.[15,201,203] Uma pequena minoria de gatos diabéticos acromegálicos responde, a princípio, à insulina e, ocasionalmente, chega a atingir a remissão. Entretanto, gatos acromegálicos, de modo geral, necessitam mais do dobro da insulina do que aqueles diabéticos sem acromegalia, com doses medianas de 7 UI, a cada 12 horas (variação 1 a 35 UI), e algumas doses são tão altas (20 a > 70 UI) que induziriam hipoglicemia fatal na maioria dos gatos com DM.[16,201]

O exame de IGF-1 é o teste diagnóstico mais comumente utilizado para acromegalia, com concentrações tipicamente acima de > 1.000 mg/ml em gatos acometidos.[201] Uma vez que a produção de IGF-1 depende da estimulação de receptores hepáticos de GH pela insulina, a insulinopenia presente no momento do diagnóstico do DM pode diminuir os resultados de maneira falsa. Recomenda-se que o exame de IGF-1 seja adiado até 6 a 8 semanas após o início da insulinoterapia.[16] Em termos práticos, é raro identificar resistência insulínica antes de 6 semanas após o início da terapia, pois a dose de insulina é aumentada lentamente, sendo algumas semanas necessárias antes que a resistência possa ser reconhecida. Exames de imagem intracranianos por ressonância magnética ou tomografia computadorizada também são úteis para a confirmação do diagnóstico, sobretudo se for considerado o tratamento terapêutico. As opções terapêuticas incluem terapia paliativa com insulina, cirurgia, radioterapia e tratamento medicamentoso. A hipofisectomia cirúrgica possui altas taxas de sucesso, e a maioria dos gatos alcança a remissão diabética.[204,205] A radioterapia pode reduzir o tamanho tumoral e a secreção hormonal, mas não normaliza as concentrações de GH e IGF-1.[16,202,206] Tanto o tratamento cirúrgico como a radioterapia são limitados por sua disponibilidade geográfica. Embora as opções medicamentosas não tenham tido sucesso previamente, em um relato recente um novo análogo da somatostatina (Pasireotide, Novartis) reduziu as necessidades de insulina em gatos acromegálicos, mas é excessivamente caro.[16] A terapia paliativa com altas doses de insulina é uma abordagem conservadora e provavelmente o método mais comum utilizado. Em alguns gatos, pode ter moderado sucesso no controle dos sinais clínicos de DM por um período. Recomenda-se o monitoramento doméstico da glicemia caso doses de insulina cada vez maiores estejam sendo utilizadas para controlar a glicemia, em razão da flutuação na secreção de GH e, portanto, da glicemia.

Hiperadrenocorticismo, glucagonoma

O HAC é caracterizado pelo excesso de glicocorticoides endógenos causado pela secreção crescente do hormônio adrenocorticotrófico (ACTH, do inglês *adrenocorticotropic hormone*) por um tumor hipofisário funcional e, subsequentemente, do cortisol pelas adrenais, ou por um tumor funcional do córtex adrenal que aumenta a secreção de glicocorticoides (ver Capítulo 307).[16] Os glicocorticoides induzem o DM pelos distúrbios à sensibilidade insulínica, pela diminuição da captação de glicose pelos tecidos periféricos e pelo aumento da gliconeogênese hepática, e podem inibir a secreção de insulina pelas células beta pancreáticas.[16] O excesso de concentrações de cortisol costuma levar ao acúmulo de gordura abdominal, que também é um fator predisponente para resistência insulínica e DM.[207-209] Cerca de 80% dos gatos com HAC possuem DM no momento do diagnóstico.[202] O HAC é uma causa menos comum de resistência insulínica do que a acromegalia, e raramente resulta em doses de insulina tão altas.[16] Existe uma preocupação de que o DM mal controlado possa aumentar a atividade do eixo hipotálamo-hipófise-adrenal dos gatos, o que poderia ocasionar resultados de testes anormais. Entretanto, um teste de supressão por baixa dose de dexametasona, realizado em 22 gatos diabéticos 6 semanas após o início da insulinoterapia, mostrou supressão completa em 4 e 8 horas em 20 gatos, independentemente do controle glicêmico, concluindo que esse é um teste viável para gatos diabéticos. Os dois gatos restantes tinham HAC.[210]

O glucagon é um antagonista da insulina. Seria esperado que tumores que produzem glucagon induzam ou piorem o DM.

Pancreatite

A pancreatite pode destruir as células beta pancreáticas, causar perda de função e diminuir a sensibilidade tecidual à insulina (ver Capítulos 289 e 291).[18,202] Ela pode piorar o controle glicêmico, diminuir a probabilidade de remissão do DM ou estar associada à recidiva da doença.[19,76] A pancreatite pode ser difícil de diagnosticar, devendo-se basear na interpretação dos sinais clínicos, ultrassonográficos e resultados do teste de imunorreatividade sérica da lipase pancreática felina (PLIf). Embora poucos gatos com DM tenham sinais clínicos de pancreatite, cerca de 60% apresentam achados bioquímicos e de exames de imagem compatíveis no momento do diagnóstico.[2,19] Entretanto, evidências histológicas de pancreatite também são comuns em gatos não diabéticos (14 a 67%). O número de neutrófilos, macrófagos, linfócitos T e B e índices de pancreatite não foram diferentes em gatos diabéticos e não diabéticos, tornando a relevância clínica dos achados motivo de debate.[17,19,55,211]

A pancreatite foi diagnosticada apenas em 14% dos gatos diabéticos investigados por mau controle glicêmico.[2] Gatos diabéticos, com evidências histológicas pós-morte de pancreatite crônica, apresentaram concentrações glicêmicas médias maiores do que aqueles sem lesões histológicas, o que não foi significativo nem havia diferença entre o tempo de sobrevida médio entre os dois grupos.[2] A porcentagem de gatos com DM (83%), com aumento do PLIf acima de 11 mmol/ℓ, foi maior do que para gatos não diabéticos (66%), mas não houve associação significativa entre as concentrações de PLIf em gatos diabéticos e o controle glicêmico deles.[212] Em 17% dos gatos diabéticos, o PLIf estava acentuadamente aumentado (> 50 μg/ℓ), enquanto havia apenas incrementos moderados (20 a 50 μg/ℓ) ou discretos (12 a 20 μg/ℓ) em gatos não diabéticos.[212] Gatos diabéticos com pancreatite crônica podem se beneficiar da budesonida, da ciclosporina (5 mg/kg VO, a cada 12 a 24 h) ou do clorambucila (2 mg/gato VO, a cada 48 a 72 h) se a pancreatite recidivar frequentemente e estiver associada a controle glicêmico ruim e resistência insulínica.[18,213] Gatos diagnosticados com pancreatite aguda próximo ao momento do início do DM podem alcançar remissão e alguns podem retornar à tolerância normal à glicose com resolução da doença.[18,76] Entretanto, a pancreatite necrosante aguda pode ser a causa de mortalidade em gatos diabéticos.[2]

Hipertireoidismo, infecções do trato urinário, outras condições

A alteração da tolerância à glicose foi relatada em gatos hipertireóideos, mas nos diabéticos a resistência insulínica não costuma ser apreciada clinicamente (ver Capítulo 301).[214] Infecções do trato urinário (ITU), cavidade oral, pele ou outros órgãos podem contribuir para resistência insulínica.[202] Diminuição da tolerância à glicose, resistência insulínica e hiperinsulinemia ocorrem como efeitos colaterais de infecções bacterianas em seres humanos.[215,216] Cerca de 12 a 13% dos gatos diabéticos têm ITU (mais frequentemente por *E. coli*), talvez em razão da diminuição da concentração urinária e da glicosúria (ver Capítulo 330).[217,218] Pessoas com DM possuem maior risco de ITU fúngica (*Candida albicans* ou *C. glabrata*), o que foi relatado em gatos.[219,220]

Doença renal crônica

A nefropatia diabética, caracterizada principalmente por doença glomerular, é diagnosticada em 20 a 40% das pessoas diabéticas.[196] A hiperglicemia altera a anatomia microvascular e causa lesão glomerular por alteração do fluxo sanguíneo, permeabilidade vascular, perda celular e diminuição da produção de fatores tróficos.[221] Embora a DRC seja comum em gatos idosos, a nefropatia diabética é um achado histológico incomum (ver Capítulo 324). Entretanto, 50% dos gatos diabéticos apresentavam alterações glomerulares compatíveis com aquelas observadas em pessoas diabéticas e 33%, alterações tubulointersticiais.[222] Em gatos não diabéticos com DRC, lesões glomerulares foram identificadas em 15% e doença tubulointersticial, em 70%.[223] Em seres humanos, a nefropatia diabética começa com microalbuminemia e progride para proteinúria evidente.[196] A microalbuminemia e a relação proteína/creatinina urinária foram significativamente maiores em gatos com DM (70 e 70%, respectivamente), comparados àqueles saudáveis do grupo-controle (18 e 9%, respectivamente).[224,225] São necessárias pesquisas para estudar a importância da proteinúria em gatos com DM. Ureia e glicose eram significativamente maiores em gatos com remissão do DM quando comparados àqueles do grupo-controle, mesmo após exclusão de gatos com DRC em estágio ≥ 2 pela IRIS. Pode ocorrer aumento na ureia, pois é um subproduto do ciclo da glicose-alanina. O piruvato no músculo é convertido em alanina e transportado até o fígado, onde é convertido em piruvato, liberando ureia. O piruvato é um substrato para gliconeogênese, que provavelmente contribui para a discreta hiperglicemia nesses gatos.[226]

HIPOGLICEMIA

Diagnóstico e tratamento

Fisiologia e sinais

A hipoglicemia é uma potencial complicação da insulinoterapia em qualquer diabético (ver Capítulos 61 e 303). Em gatos, a glicose baixa pode ser uma questão principalmente bioquímica, assintomática ou sintomática. Sinais de hipoglicemia variavelmente surgem em glicemias < 60 mg/dℓ (< 3,5 mmol/ℓ), e a hipoglicemia grave (≤ 18 mg/dℓ ou 1 mmol/ℓ) causa risco de morte.[227,228] O cérebro é incapaz de sintetizar ou armazenar glicose. Ele necessita de um suprimento contínuo de sangue, e as células não requerem insulina para sua utilização.[227-230] Em gatos, os sinais clínicos de hipoglicemia incluem letargia, tremores, depressão, ataxia ou, em casos graves, convulsões e coma. Em pessoas, episódios repetidos de hipoglicemia podem alterar as respostas compensatórias e resultar em inconsciência hipoglicêmica. Há ausência dos sinais clínicos iniciais preocupantes, como tremores, normalmente desencadeados em resposta à liberação de epinefrina. Nesses indivíduos, o início súbito de convulsões ou coma está associado à glicopenia neuronal.[231]

Uma condição semelhante relatada em cães pode ocorrer em gatos.[89,232] Em seres humanos, os valores limítrofes para hipoglicemia bioquímica foram determinados com base nos limiares para ativação do glucagon e epinefrina (< 70 mg/dℓ ou < 3,9 mmol/ℓ).[231] Em gatos, as glicemias < 50 ou 54 mg/dℓ (< 2,8 ou 3 mmol/ℓ) são utilizadas como indicadores de hipoglicemia bioquímica quando mensuradas com glicosímetro calibrado para sangue total humano.[8,94] Quando mensurada com um glicosímetro calibrado para sangue felino, o limite inferior foi de 50 mg/dℓ (2,8 mmol/ℓ) em gatos em jejum e hospitalizados por uma noite.[76]

No DM, a hipoglicemia iatrogênica ocorre em razão da sobredose de insulina, sobretudo em gatos que estão recuperando a capacidade de sintetizar e secretar a insulina endógena, isto é, em remissão iminente.[8] Nesse cenário, há o risco de se administrar muita insulina quando as glicemias não estiverem mais altas. Outras causas comuns de sobredose que levam à hipoglicemia incluem erros na extração da insulina para a seringa ou quando da utilização incorreta de uma seringa incorreta. Tais erros podem causar riscos de morte e não ser detectados até que ocorra hipoglicemia grave. O hipotálamo contém neurônios sensíveis à glicose que detectam e respondem à hipo ou à hiperglicemia.[227] A compensação rápida para a hipoglicemia ocorre pela inibição da produção de insulina, ao mesmo tempo que são estimulados o glucagon pancreático e a epinefrina adrenal.[228] A diminuição da insulina pancreática não pode ocorrer no DM, já que foi administrada de forma exógena.[231] O glucagon aumenta a glicólise hepática e a gliconeogênese. A epinefrina atua no fígado e nos rins para aumentar a produção de glicose.[200,228] Entretanto, a produção de glucagon pelas células alfa pancreáticas, em resposta à hipoglicemia, pode estar ausente ou diminuída no DM, secundariamente à ausência de sinalização das células beta pancreáticas.[229]

Tratamento

Se possível, gatos hipoglicêmicos devem ser alimentados com uma refeição rica em carboidratos (> 35% de energia oriunda de carboidratos) e a insulinoterapia descontinuada até que a hiperglicemia recidive (recomendações variam de > 117 a > 216 mg/dℓ; > 6,5 mmol/ℓ a > 12 mmol/ℓ). Doses subsequentes de insulina devem ser reduzidas em 25 a 50%.[89,233] Se ocorrerem sinais mais graves – como ataxia –, um xarope à base de glicose, desenvolvido para pacientes diabéticos humanos ou veterinários, pode ser administrado por via oral ou misturado ao alimento (forneça 0,5 a 1 g e repita 15 a 20 min depois, se necessário). Mel ou xarope de bordo podem ser utilizados em emergências domésticas, mas dá-se preferência ao xarope Karo® (xarope de milho com glicose a 15 a 20%). Em uma emergência, antes ou durante o transporte ao hospital, uma pessoa pode esfregar soluções que contenham glicose nas gengivas ou administrá-las como enema.[227,234] Em geral, o tratamento hospitalar consiste em um *bolus* inicial IV de dextrose (0,5 g/kg), seguido de infusão contínua (IC) de dextrose a 2,5%, até que a glicemia normal ou aumentada seja mantida.[227,234]

Em pessoas com DM e hipoglicemia grave, a injeção de glucagon pode ser utilizada para estimular a gliconeogênese hepática e a glicólise.[228] O glucagon vem sendo utilizado com sucesso em cães com hipoglicemia refratária ou convulsões associadas a sobredose de insulina, insulinoma e hipoglicemia paraneoplásica (ver Capítulo 303).[235,236] Em um gato, o glucagon melhorou de forma acentuada os sinais neurológicos que haviam persistido após euglicemia restaurada por infusão de dextrose.[235] Não foi observado nenhum efeito adverso da infusão. O glucagon para injeção (frasco de 1 mg) está disponível prontamente,

é reconstituído com o diluente do fabricante e suas instruções para uso devem ser seguidas. Ele pode ser adicionado a 1.000 mℓ de NaCl a 0,9% (e não a qualquer infusão de dextrose), administrado por via intravenosa como um *bolus* inicial de 50 mg/kg e, então, como IC, na taxa de 10 a 15 ng/kg/min. A dose pode necessitar de ajustes de até 40 ng/kg/min.[235]

Efeito Somogyi (hipoglicemia induzida pela insulina com hiperglicemia de rebote)

A hipoglicemia decorrente da sobredose de insulina pode desencadear uma resposta contrarregulatória que leva a uma hiperglicemia rebote, conhecida como o efeito Somogyi.[89,237] Um estudo recente de 10.767 curvas glicêmicas de 55 gatos tratados com protocolo intensivo de insulina glargina observou que, ao mesmo tempo que a hipoglicemia bioquímica ocorreu com frequência (93%), somente 0,42% das curvas glicêmicas foram compatíveis com hiperglicemia de rebote (< 50 mg/dℓ ou < 2,8 mmol/ℓ, seguidas de > 300 mg/dℓ ou > 16,7 mmol/ℓ dentro de 4 a 10 h).[238] Diversos estudos em pessoas com DM concluíram que a hiperglicemia de rebote é rara e não está associada a maios níveis de GH, cortisol ou glucagon, mas está inversamente correlacionada com as concentrações de insulina.[239-243] Portanto, a maioria dos casos de hiperglicemia de rebote aparente resulta da deficiência relativa de insulina, e não da resposta a hormônios antagonistas.

Embora a dose de qualquer insulina deva ser reduzida se um gato desenvolver hipoglicemia assintomática, ela não deve ser reduzida na suposição de um efeito Somogyi, quando as glicemias estiverem altas e pouco responsivas à insulina. Nas semanas iniciais da insulinoterapia, é comum haver flutuação das glicemias, o que costuma ser resolvido com o tempo e doses consistentes, mas pode ser atribuído de maneira errônea à hiperglicemia de rebote.

RESUMO

Em resumo, na prática veterinária geral, o DM afeta aproximadamente 1 em 200 gatos, a maioria dos quais possui o DM tipo 2. Há a ocorrência de outros tipos de DM, e a acromegalia parece comum em gatos mal controlados. Os objetivos da terapia envolvem a implementação precoce de controle glicêmico rigoroso para maximizar a probabilidade de remissão, ao mesmo tempo que a hipoglicemia clínica é evitada. As maiores taxas de remissão relatadas envolvem o uso de insulina de longa ação (glargina ou detemir), uma dieta com baixos níveis de carboidrato (≤ 6% de energia oriunda de carboidratos), o monitoramento frequente da glicemia, de preferência em casa, e o ajuste apropriado da dose da insulina visando a glicemias normais ou próximas disso. A maioria dos gatos em remissão do DM apresenta homeostase anormal da glicose e devem ser considerados pré-DM. A recidiva diabética ocorre em 25 a 30% dos gatos dentro de 1 a 2 anos, sendo mais provável naqueles com glicemias moderadamente alteradas (≥ 135 a 162 mg/dℓ; 7,5 a 9 mmol/ℓ). O monitoramento doméstico contínuo da glicemia é recomendado para gatos em remissão, para detectar a deterioração precoce na homeostase da glicemia e facilitar a implementação precoce da terapia apropriada.

REFERÊNCIAS BIBLIOGRÁFICAS

As referências bibliográficas deste capítulo se encontram online no Ambiente de Aprendizagem.

CAPÍTULO 306

Hiperadrenocorticismo Canino

Dolores Pérez-Alenza e Carlos Melián

Em 1932, o dr. Harvey Cushing descreveu sinais clínicos em pessoas com adenomas basofílicos hipofisários. Os tumores provavelmente produziam hormônio adrenocorticotrófico em excesso (corticotrofina [ACTH, do inglês *adrenocorticotropic hormone*]), causando estimulação excessiva do córtex adrenal, hiperplasia adrenocortical bilateral secundária e excesso crônico na concentração sérica de cortisol, uma "característica fundamental" do hiperadrenocorticismo (HAC, do inglês *hyperadrenocorticism*). A causa mais comum do HAC canino de ocorrência natural é o hiperadrenocorticismo hipófise-dependente (HHD), no qual um adenoma hipofisário funcional (raramente, um carcinoma) secreta ACTH autônoma e excessivamente e ocasiona as mesmas alterações já descritas. Um distúrbio hipotalâmico que causa hiperplasia hipofisária ainda não foi documentado em cães. A produção ectópica (não hipofisária) do ACTH em excesso foi descrita em cães, mas é extremamente rara. A segunda causa mais comum do HAC canino é um tumor adrenocortical funcional (TAF; adenoma ou carcinoma), que produz, de maneira autônoma, cortisol em excesso. Os leitores devem se lembrar de que, em cães, a causa mais comum de "síndrome de Cushing" é iatrogênica, já que a utilização de glicocorticoides é comum no tratamento de uma série de condições neoplásicas, inflamatórias ou imunomediadas (ver Capítulos 164 e 165).

FISIOLOGIA DO EIXO HIPOTÁLAMO-HIPÓFISE-ADRENAL

Hipotálamo

O hipotálamo possui o controle primário da função hipofisária. A hipófise regula a função adrenocortical e a secreção de cortisol. O hormônio liberador de corticotrofina (CRH, do inglês *corticotropina-releasing hormone*), um polipeptídio com 41 aminoácidos, apresenta meia-vida plasmática de aproximadamente 1 hora. O sistema porta hipotálamo-hipofisário libera CRH para a hipófise anterior, onde estimula os corticotrofos a secretar ACTH. A estimulação da secreção hipotalâmica de CRH é mediada por citocinas (interleucinas-1 e 6 e fator de necrose tumoral-alfa), leptina, dopamina, arginina-vasopressina (AVP) e angiotensina II. A inibição do CRH é mediada por glicocorticoides e somatostatina. Os glicocorticoides são os reguladores dominantes do *feedback* negativo do CRH. O ACTH (peso molecular: 4.500 dáltons), um hormônio peptídio com uma cadeia única de 39 aminoácidos, é clivado a partir da molécula precursora, a pró-opiomelanocortina (POMC). O ACTH canino e o humano diferem pelo aminoácido residual na posição 37. Os aminoácidos 1 a 18 da região terminal da molécula de ACTH são responsáveis por sua atividade biológica. Outros fragmentos do POMC são biologicamente ativos; betalipoproteína (beta-LPH), betaendorfina, hormônio estimulante de melanócitos (MSH, do inglês *melanocyte-stimulating hormone*) alfa e gama, unindo o peptídio (peptídio J), e fragmento N-terminal.[2,3]

Hipófise

Existem três unidades funcionais na hipófise canina: a hipófise anterior (formada por *pars infundibularis* e *pars distalis*); o lobo intermediário (*pars intermedia*); e a hipófise posterior (neuro-hipófise). Um produto da *pars distalis*, o ACTH (de forma menos importante, beta-LPH), é estimulado principalmente pelo CRH e suprimido, sobretudo, por glicocorticoides (cortisol). A *pars intermedia* contém células "A", que produzem MSH-alfa e peptídio do lobo intermediário semelhante à corticotrofina (CLIP, do inglês *corticotropin-like intermediate lobe peptide*), e células "B", que sintetizam POMC clivado em ACTH e beta-LPH. As células "B" são reguladas, em parte, pela inibição dopaminérgica tônica.[4-6] A secreção do beta-LPH e da betaendorfina é semelhante àquela do ACTH; estresse e hipoglicemia aumentam sua secreção, enquanto glicocorticoides suprimem-na. As betaendorfinas podem atuar como "opiáceos endógenos", sugerindo um papel no alívio da dor; a fisiologia do beta-LPH é desconhecida. O MSH está envolvido na secreção de melanina (melanogênese) por melanócitos na pele e nos pelos. A hipoglicemia aumenta os teores plasmáticos de fragmentos N-terminais, mas seu papel é desconhecido. Em seres humanos, tanto o CRH como o ACTH são secretados de forma pulsátil com ritmo diurno que resulta em um pico antes de acordar pela manhã. Em cães, o ACTH também é secretado de forma pulsátil, com 6 a 12 picos diários. Um ritmo diurno ainda não foi identificado. A secreção de ACTH é regulada por CRH, resposta ao estresse, inibição do *feedback* pelo cortisol e fatores imunológicos. Estressantes físicos, emocionais e químicos, como dor, trauma, hipoxemia, hipoglicemia aguda, exposição ao frio, cirurgias e pirógenos, estimulam a secreção de ACTH e cortisol.

Córtex adrenal

O córtex adrenal possui três camadas (zonas) distintas: a zona glomerular externa, a zona fasciculada média e a zona reticular interna. A síntese da maioria dos esteroides adrenais é mediada por enzimas do sistema citocromo P450 oxigenase. Em razão de diferenças nessas enzimas, o córtex adrenal funciona como unidades diferentes. A zona glomerular externa, a única fonte de mineralocorticoides (principalmente aldosterona), é deficiente em atividade de 17-alfa-hidroxilase e incapaz de sintetizar cortisol ou andrógenos. A síntese de aldosterona é regulada principalmente pelo sistema renina-angiotensina e concentrações séricas de potássio. O ACTH possui um papel diminuto.

As zonas fasciculada e reticular do córtex funcionam de forma semelhante com relação à produção de cortisol e andrógenos. Somente células nessas zonas possuem atividade de 17-alfa-hidroxilase e podem sintetizar 17-alfa-hidroxipregnenolona e 17-alfa-hidroxiprogesterona, precursores do cortisol e dos andrógenos adrenais. Essas duas zonas são reguladas principalmente pelo ACTH, que estimula a síntese rápida e secreção de cortisol (e andrógenos). A estimulação crônica pelo ACTH leva à hiperplasia adrenocortical. A deficiência crônica de ACTH resulta em diminuição da esteroidogênese e atrofia adrenocortical (ver Capítulo 309).

PATOGÊNESE

Hiperadrenocorticismo hipófise-dependente

Cerca de 80 a 85% dos cães com HAC de ocorrência natural possuem HHD: a secreção excessiva de ACTH hipofisário (> 90% possuem um tumor hipofisário detectável), hiperplasia adrenocortical bilateral e secreção excessiva crônica de glicocorticoides (Figura 306.1).[7] Tumores hipofisários podem surgir da

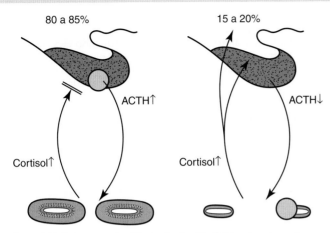

Figura 306.1 Esquema simplificado do eixo hipofisário-adrenal em cães com hiperadrenocorticismo hipófise-dependente (*esquerda*) e com tumor adrenal funcional (*direita*). ACTH, hormônio adrenocorticotrófico.

pars distalis (cerca de 70%) ou da *pars intermedia* (aproximadamente 30%).[7] Enquanto a secreção de ACTH na *pars intermedia* relativamente avascular é regulada, em parte, pelo CRH, a atividade da *pars intermedia* é controlada principalmente por fibras dopaminérgicas e serotoninérgicas dos centros superiores. As células predominantes da *pars intermedia* (células A) são imunocoradas intensivamente para alfa-MSH e fracamente para ACTH, enquanto as células B da *pars intermedia* coram fortemente para ACTH e fracamente para alfa-MSH. A intensa coloração por ACTH das células B da *pars intermedia* é semelhante às características de coloração das células da *pars distalis* produtoras de ACTH.[7,8]

Tumores hipofisários costumam ser classificados, à histologia, como adenomas (bem delimitados do parênquima adjacente), adenomas invasivos (apresentando invasão local do parênquima cerebral ou estruturas adjacentes) ou carcinoma (com metástases a distância intra ou extracranianas).[9] Vinte de trinta e três cães com tumores hipofisários apresentavam um adenoma em um estudo e 80%, HAC; 11/33 apresentavam um carcinoma invasivo e 45%, HAC; e 2/33 apresentavam HAC e um carcinoma.[9] Já que tumores hipofisários grandes tendem a ser resistentes ao *feedback* negativo pela dexametasona, o tamanho do tumor hipofisário pode estar relacionado com o grau de insensibilidade do *feedback* a glicocorticoides do tumor. Tumores que se originam na *pars intermedia* podem crescer mais do que aqueles na *pars distalis*, mas tumores hipofisários nem sempre mantêm suas características de origem. Tumores de cães com HHD não podem ser facilmente distinguidos como se originários da *pars distalis* ou da *pars intermedia*, mesmo com níveis plasmáticos de alfa-MSH ou resistência à dexametasona.[10-12] A hiperplasia hipofisária também é mencionada como causa de HHD em cães; entretanto, ainda não existe prova de tal condição.

Os dois mecanismos propostos com relação à patogênese dos tumores hipofisários incluem (1) uma teoria hipotalâmica e (2) uma teoria monoclonal.[13] A teoria hipotalâmica, que não é aceita amplamente, afirma que a estimulação crônica dos corticotrofos hipofisários pelo CRH hipotalâmico e pela vasopressina, em conjunto com defeitos adquiridos de receptores de glicocorticoides, leva à ação inibitória inferior do cortisol. Ademais, a neurodegeneração dopaminérgica em animais idosos ou a menor expressão de receptores de dopamina contribuem para a diminuição de ações de *feedback* do cortisol. Essa inibição reduzida poderia levar a secreção excessiva de ACTH, hiperplasia hipofisária e, eventualmente, transformação neoplásica de alguns corticotrofos, em razão de uma mutação somática.

A teoria hipofisária sugere que o tumor é a causa principal de HAC e se desenvolveu após mutação somática de um corticotrofo, criando um clone tumoral.[13] Essa teoria é amplamente aceita e apoiada, em parte, pelas baixas concentrações de CRH relatadas em cães com HHD, em conjunto com estudos que mostram que quase todos os adenomas corticotrofos são monoclonais.[14,15] A ocorrência de HHD em uma família de 7 cães da raça Dandie Dinmont Terrier também reforça essa teoria.[16] Adenomas corticotrofos caninos provavelmente contêm células-tronco que impulsionam o crescimento tumoral e são resultado de um processo com vários estágios de gênese tumoral, sendo o primeiro a mutação somática que precede a expansão clonal do tumor.[17]

Tumores adrenocorticais funcionais

Cerca de 15 a 20% dos cães com HAC de ocorrência natural possuem tumor adrenocortical que secreta, de maneira autônoma, quantidades excessivas de cortisol. As concentrações plasmáticas circulantes de CRH hipotalâmico e ACTH são suprimidas pelo cortisol do tumor, causando atrofia da adrenal oposta não envolvida e das células não neoplásicas na adrenal que contém o tumor. Nenhuma característica clínica ou bioquímica permite que cães com TAF decorrente de adenoma sejam discriminados daqueles com carcinoma.[18] É mais provável que os tumores adrenais > 2 cm de diâmetro e aqueles que invadem a vasculatura regional sejam carcinomas. A malignidade é confirmada se metástases a distância parecem semelhantes à histologia. A citologia não é confiável em discriminar tumores benignos de malignos, e mesmo a diferenciação histológica pode ser difícil. A malignidade é mais provável em tumores que romperam a cápsula ou invadiram a vasculatura.[19] Em geral, TAFs são unilaterais, sem tendência óbvia com relação ao lado. Tumores adrenocorticais bilaterais já foram descritos. Alguns poucos cães tiveram um tumor adrenal secretor de cortisol em uma glândula e um feocromocitoma (ver Capítulo 311) na outra.

A secreção de cortisol por TAFs é episódica, aleatória, independe do controle do ACTH e suprime a síntese e secreção de ACTH. O papel dos receptores de ACTH (ACTHR) na secreção do cortisol pelo TAF pode ser limitado. Alguns cães com um TAF não apresentam resposta do cortisol ao ACTH administrado de forma exógena, outras apresentam resposta normal e há ainda aqueles que possuem respostas exageradas. A suprarregulação das enzimas esteroidogênicas não parece estar envolvida na patogênese do TAF, mas a infrarregulação dos ACTHRs pode estar relacionada com a malignidade.[20] A expressão ectópica de proteínas receptoras de polipeptídio inibitório gástrico (GIP, do inglês *gastric inhibitory polypeptide*) e vasopressina 2 (V2), observadas na zona fasciculada de TAFs, pode ter papel na patogênese tumoral.[21] O fator esteroidogênico 1 (SF1, do inglês *steroidogenic fator 1*), associado à patogênese de tumores adrenais em seres humanos, é expresso em TAFs caninos e pode ser usado como marcador prognóstico ou alvo terapêutico.[22]

Hiperadrenocorticismo hipófise-dependente e tumor adrenocortical funcional concomitantes, hiperplasia nodular, secreção ectópica de hormônio adrenocorticotrófico

A coexistência de tumores hipofisários e adrenais foi descrita em 17 cães cada qual com um tumor adrenocortical e hiperplasia adrenal contralateral; 10 cães tinham um adenoma adrenocortical; 4, adenomas corticais adrenais bilaterais e 3, um carcinoma adrenal.[23] Lesões hipofisárias incluíram um microadenoma cromofóbico em 12, macroadenoma hipofisário em 4 e um carcinoma hipofisário em 1 cão. É possível que tais tumores adrenais tenham sofrido transformação de hiperplasia inicial. Cães com HHD costumam desenvolver hiperplasia adrenocortical bilateral simétrica. Entretanto, alguns podem desenvolver hiperplasia *nodular* adrenocortical, na qual uma ou ambas as glândulas podem ter um ou vários nódulos de tamanhos variados. Com o passar do tempo, pode ser difícil de distinguir tais nódulos de tumores adrenocorticais.

A *secreção ectópica de ACTH*, derivada de qualquer um de uma série de tipos tumorais, é responsável por aproximadamente 15% de pessoas com HAC.[24] A condição ectópica de

HAC pode ser mais grave clinicamente do que HHD. Carcinomas de células pulmonares pequenos são a causa mais comum de secreção ectópica de ACTH em seres humanos, mas foram associados a tumores carcinoides (*i. e.*, do pulmão, dos brônquios, do intestino, do fígado, do pâncreas e do ovário), timoma, tumores de células de ilhotas pancreáticas, neuroblastoma olfatório, carcinoma medular da tireoide e feocromocitoma.

A síndrome do ACTH ectópico é uma causa extremamente rara de HAC em cães. Um cão Pastor-Alemão de 8 anos com secreção ectópica de ACTH, que supostamente, a princípio, tinha HHD, foi tratado com hipofisectomia transesfenoidal, mas teve recidiva dos sinais clínicos, concentrações plasmáticas de ACTH e relações anormais de corticoide:creatinina urinária, com a detecção de um tumor pancreático com envolvimento hepático. A avaliação histológica revelou um tumor neuroendócrino, considerado fonte de secreção ectópica de ACTH. O cão foi tratado e respondeu bem ao trilostano.[25]

EPIDEMIOLOGIA

O hiperadrenocorticismo é relativamente comum em cães idosos. Em um estudo durante um período de 15 anos em um hospital-escola veterinário, o HAC foi diagnosticado em mais de 1 a cada 100 cães, excedendo as estimativas prévias de 1 a 2/1.000.[26,27] Esse aparente crescimento da prevalência da doença pode ter ocorrido devido ao aumento na expectativa de vida dos cães e do conhecimento sobre a doença e à realidade de que o estudo foi concluído em um centro de atendimento especializado.

SINAIS CLÍNICOS

O HAC de ocorrência natural é mais comumente diagnosticado em cães de meia-idade a idosos. No momento do diagnóstico, a idade varia de 6 meses a 20 anos, com idade média de 11 anos. Nessa ocasião, quase todos os cães com HAC têm mais do que 6 anos[28,29] e mais de 75% dos com HHD e 90% daqueles com TAF têm mais de 9 anos. O HAC é um distúrbio sem predisposição racial significativa.[27] O HHD tende a ocorrer em cães menores: Poodle, Teckel, raças Terrier. Aproximadamente 75% dos cães com HHD pesam menos que 20 kg, ao passo que quase 50% daqueles com TAF, mais de 20 kg. A predileção sexual em cães com HAC é possível, sendo 60 a 65% fêmeas.[29]

MANIFESTAÇÕES CLÍNICAS

Contexto geral

A maioria das anormalidades clínicas e laboratoriais em cães com HAC é causada por excesso crônico de cortisol. Em alguns poucos cães, os sinais podem ser causados por crescimento tumoral hipofisário ou adrenal e/ou invasão, metástases, diabetes melito (DM), hipertensão sistêmica ou tromboembolia. Os sinais clínicos são consequência da combinação dos efeitos gliconeogênico, imunossupressor, anti-inflamatório, catabólico proteico e lipolítico dos glicocorticoides. O HHD não pode ser distinguido do TAF com base nos sinais clínicos nem na duração.[30] Os sinais variam de sutis a bastante graves. Alguns cães possuem HAC confirmado após acompanhamento do progresso com o passar do tempo. Por conta do maior conhecimento do HAC pelos médicos-veterinários, os cães estão sendo avaliados em fases mais precoces da doença, quando as manifestações clínicas podem ser discretas.[30]

Histórico clínico

Duração

Em geral, o HAC é uma doença crônica e progressiva. Os sinais clínicos podem estar presentes há meses, já que esses cães

costumam estar em boa condição e com um excelente apetite. Os tutores podem atribuir os sinais iniciais ao envelhecimento normal e buscar ajuda veterinária apenas quando eles se tornarem intoleráveis: poliúria (urinar pela casa) ou polifagia (roubar comida, comer lixo, chamar a atenção de forma contínua e, ocasionalmente, atacar ou proteger a comida de forma agressiva).

Questões a considerar

O primeiro passo para suspeitar que um cão possa ter HAC é sempre baseado no histórico. Os sinais clínicos notados pelo tutor devem ser obtidos com cuidado. O clínico deve evitar "conduzir o tutor". Em vez de perguntar se o animal está bebendo água ou urinando em excesso, é preferível questionar vagamente sobre a ingestão hídrica e o débito urinário. Também, é importante conhecer os sinais não compatíveis com HAC (p. ex., êmese, diarreia, anorexia ou dor) para evitar realizar testes para HAC em cães com doenças não adrenais.[30] O histórico de medicamentos pode ser extremamente importante, incluindo fármacos tópicos, já que os sinais clínicos da síndrome de Cushing iatrogênica e de ocorrência natural são idênticos. Diversos medicamentos (p. ex., anticonvulsivantes, diuréticos etc.) apresentam efeitos colaterais que simulam HAC. Algumas das questões mais importantes quando há a suspeita de HAC incluem: (1) Seu cão foi submetido a algum tratamento recente ou está sendo atualmente?; (2) Como é a ingestão hídrica, a produção de urina e o apetite do seu cão agora, em comparação há 12 meses?; (3) Seu cão pode pular dos móveis ou para fora do carro; se "sim", ele pode pular para dentro do carro ou em cima dos móveis? Se "não", há quanto tempo?; (4) Como é a respiração do seu cão (ofegante em repouso)?; e (5) O seu cão está dormindo mais? Cães com HAC podem ter um ou vários sinais clínicos, cada um dos quais variando em intensidade. Tanto a polidipsia/poliúria (PU/PD; o sinal clínico mais comum) ou a alopecia, sugestivas de uma endocrinopatia, podem ser os únicos sinais clínicos em alguns cães com HAC.

Sinais comuns

As observações clássicas do tutor incluem PU/PD, polifagia (PF), ganho de peso aparente (abdome abaulado), fraqueza muscular, respiração ofegante e perda de peso (Tabela 306.1). PU/PD é observado em cerca de 90% dos cães com HAC. A PU provavelmente se deve ao aumento das taxas de filtração glomerular e à inibição da ação do hormônio antidiurético (ADH, do inglês *antidiuretic hormone*), em nível tubular renal, levando à diminuição na reabsorção hídrica tubular renal. O ADH exógeno causa redução dramática na PU/PD, sugerindo que a interferência do cortisol, com a liberação de ADH, é responsável por essas manifestações.[29] Infecções do trato urinário (ITUs) são comuns em cães com HAC e provavelmente ocorrem por efeitos imunossupressores do

Tabela 306.1	Manifestações clínicas do hiperadrenocorticismo canino no momento do atendimento inicial.	
COMUNS	**MENOS COMUNS**	**INCOMUNS**
Polidipsia	Letargia	Tromboembolia
Poliúria	Hiperpigmentação	Ruptura ligamentar
Polifagia	Comedões	Paralisia de nervo
Respiração ofegante	Pele delgada	facial
Distensão abdominal	Crescimento ruim do	Pseudomiotonia
Alopecia endócrina	pelo	Diabetes melito
Hepatomegalia	Extravasamento	resistente à
Fraqueza muscular	urinário	insulina
Hipertensão sistêmica	Atrofia testicular	
	Anestro persistente	

Adaptada de Behrend EN, Kooistra HS, Nelson R *et al.*: Diagnosis of spontaneous canine hyperadrenocorticism: 2012 ACVIM consensus statement (small animal). *J Vet Intern Med* 27:1292, 2013.

excesso de cortisol, diminuição das propriedades bactericidas da urina diluída e retenção urinária, sobretudo em cães que vivem em ambientes internos. Vários cães com PU desenvolvem um grau de diminuição do tônus vesical, o que pode levar à incontinência por fluxo excessivo. Entretanto, sinais de polaquiuria, hematúria e estrangúria não são comuns, talvez em razão das ações anti-inflamatórias do cortisol.

Apetite, aparência, força muscular, respiração

A maioria dos cães com HAC tem excelente apetite ou PF, uma resposta direta e única dos cães aos glicocorticoides. Mesmo que alguns com HAC apresentem ganho de peso, a maioria tem uma aparência de abdome abaulado (Figura 306.2), que simula o ganho de peso. Cinco a dez por cento dos cães com HAC desenvolvem diabetes melito (DM, ver neste capítulo "Perfil bioquímico sérico: glicemia" e no Capítulo 304) e podem apresentar perda de peso (Figura 306.3). O abdome pendular é secundário à fraqueza da musculatura abdominal, associado ao aumento do peso do conteúdo abdominal em razão da hepatomegalia, uma bexiga excessivamente distendida, e da redistribuição da gordura periférica para o mesentério. As concentrações de leptina são significativamente maiores em cães obesos com HAC do que nos obesos saudáveis, o que pode ser um fator para

tal.[31] A fraqueza muscular é bastante comum, resultando da degeneração muscular secundária aos efeitos catabólicos dos glicocorticoides. Não é frequente que a fraqueza muscular seja tão profunda a ponto de os cães não poderem se levantar e ter dificuldade em se manter em pé. A respiração ofegante excessiva é comum e atribuída à diminuição da complacência pulmonar, à fraqueza dos músculos respiratórios, à hipertensão pulmonar ou aos efeitos diretos do cortisol sobre o centro respiratório. Os sinais podem ser exacerbados por excitação ou exercício. A doença tromboembólica pulmonar, uma complicação rara do HAC, também pode causar dificuldade respiratória moderada a grave (ver Capítulo 243). Evidências radiográficas de mineralização pulmonar são comuns em cães com HAC e podem contribuir para a hipoxemia em alguns casos.[32]

Sistema nervoso central

Sinais do sistema nervoso central (SNC) ocorrem em 10 a 25% dos cães com HHD em razão da "síndrome do macrotumor hipofisário", um tumor que invade e comprime tecidos dorsais à sela túrcica. Letargia moderada a grave é o distúrbio mais comum, mas outros sinais incluem inapetência ou até mesmo anorexia, estupor, andar em círculos, andar a esmo (Vídeo 306.1), ataxia, alterações comportamentais e convulsões.

Sinais incomuns/miotonia

Sinais clínicos menos comuns em cães com HAC são frouxidão ligamentar, que pode levar à ruptura e à claudicação (Figura 306.4), paralisia uni ou bilateral de nervo facial, anestro, atrofia testicular ou tromboembolia decorrente da hipercoagulabilidade.[30] Tumores adrenais podem invadir a veia frênico-abdominal, a veia cava caudal, ou ambas, causando a formação de trombos. É muito incomum que tumores causem hemorragia abdominal ou retroperitoneal ou edema de membros pélvicos. Em casos raros, cães com HAC desenvolvem miopatia, caracterizada por contração muscular persistente e ativa após interrupção de esforço voluntário, conhecido como pseudomiotonia de Cushing. Ela costuma afetar os membros pélvicos, causando marcha rígida (Vídeo 306.2) ou, em casos mais avançados, incapacidade de andar (Figura 306.5). O diagnóstico pode ser confirmado por eletromiografia (ver Capítulo 117), na qual são notadas descargas miotônicas bizarras e de alta frequência. A histologia muscular revela miopatia degenerativa não inflamatória.

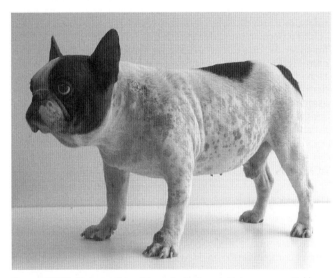

Figura 306.2 Abdome distendido e sinais dermatológicos em um Buldogue Francês com hiperadrenocorticismo hipofisário.

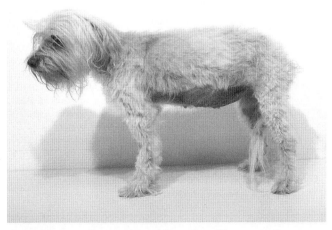

Figura 306.3 Atrofia muscular e abdome distendido em um cão sem raça definida com hiperadrenocorticismo e diabetes melito.

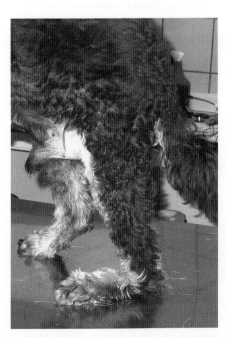

Figura 306.4 Posição plantígrada decorrente da frouxidão ligamentar grave em um cão sem raça definida com hiperadrenocorticismo hipofisário.

EXAME FÍSICO

Características comuns
Distensão abdominal é a característica mais comum no exame físico de cães com HAC. A alopecia endócrina bilateral simétrica de tronco é comum. A princípio, o pelame se torna opaco e seco, mas, com o passar do tempo, a pele se torna hipotônica, podendo ocorrer sinais, como a incapacidade de o pelo crescer após a tosa, comedões, suscetibilidade aumentada a hematomas, hiperpigmentação e alterações seborreicas. Alguns cães têm alopecia grave, que poupa apenas a cabeça e as extremidades distais. A pele delgada e o sistema imune suprimido predispõem os cães com HAC à piodermite, presente em cerca de 50% dos animais com HAC.

Calcinose cutânea
Essa é uma condição dermatológica incomum, mas característica em cães com síndrome de Cushing de ocorrência natural ou iatrogênica (ver Capítulo 10 e Figura 306.6). É caracterizada por placas irregulares sobre ou sob a pele, causadas por depósito distrófico de cálcio (Ca) e localizadas nas áreas temporais da cabeça, da linha média dorsal, do pescoço, do abdome ventral ou das áreas inguinais. As atividades gliconeogênicas e catabólicas proteicas do cortisol estão envolvidas na patogênese da calcinose cutânea, na qual o rearranjo de estruturas moleculares de proteínas leva à formação de uma matriz orgânica que atrai e se liga ao cálcio, formando cristais de apatita.[33]

Cães não castrados
Atrofia testicular e anestro em fêmeas são sequelas menos comuns do HAC. O *feedback* negativo do cortisol sobre a hipófise diminui a síntese e a secreção de FSH e LH. Machos costumam possuir testículos pequenos, de consistência macia, e esponjosos bilateralmente, enquanto fêmeas estão em anestro, cuja duração pode ser indicativa da duração do HAC.

Doença aguda
Ocasionalmente, cães com HAC podem desenvolver sinais agudos de letargia grave, fraqueza, palidez nas membranas mucosas e dor. Embora rara, essa complicação pode ocorrer como consequência da ruptura de um tumor adrenal em razão da hemorragia intra-abdominal ou retroperitoneal aguda, sendo um dos poucos cenários (em conjunto com a tromboembolia pulmonar, que também é rara) no qual um cão com HAC pode apresentar uma condição aguda, com risco de morte.[34]

Síndrome da degeneração retiniana adquirida súbita
Uma associação entre síndrome da degeneração retiniana adquirida súbita, um distúrbio retiniano idiopático que causa cegueira súbita e permanente em cães adultos (ver Capítulo 11), e HAC foi sugerida, mas faltam evidências.[35] A perda de visão em cães com HHD, ao mesmo tempo que é bastante incomum, é relacionada com o aumento de concentrações séricas de triglicerídeos ou alterações no fluxo vascular retiniano.[36] A cegueira, associada ao aumento da interleucina-6 e à diminuição das concentrações de óxido nítrico, afetam de maneira adversa o fluxo sanguíneo e aumentam o risco de perda de visão.[37]

ACHADOS CLINICOPATOLÓGICOS (TABELA 306.2)

Contexto geral
Deve-se suspeitar do diagnóstico de HAC inicialmente pelas observações do tutor, com ou sem alterações físicas. Testes endócrinos devem ser realizados apenas quando os sinais clínicos forem compatíveis com HAC.[30] Com uma suspeita clínica de

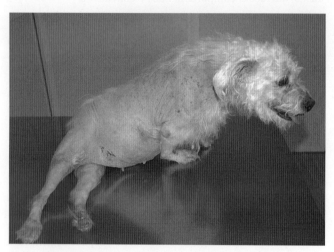

Figura 306.5 Cão sem raça definida com hiperadrenocorticismo causando sinais clínicos avançados, inclusive pseudomiotonia.

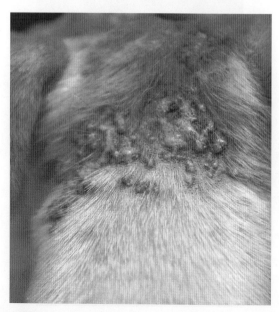

Figura 306.6 Calcinose cutânea grave em um cão sem raça definida com hiperadrenocorticismo. (*Esta figura se encontra reproduzida em cores no Encarte.*)

| Tabela 306.2 | Anormalidades laboratoriais comuns em cães com hiperadrenocorticismo. |

HEMOGRAMA	PAINEL BIOQUÍMICO SÉRICO	URINÁLISE
Leucocitose neutrofílica	Aumento da fosfatase alcalina	Densidade específica ≤ 1,018 a 1,020
Linfopenia	Aumento da alanina aminotransferase	Proteinúria
Eosinopenia	Hipercolesterolemia	Infecções do trato urinário (quase sempre sem evidências de inflamação)
Trombocitose	Hipertrigliceridemia	
Eritrocitose discreta	Hiperglicemia (discreta e não associada a diabetes melito)	

Adaptada de Behrend EN, Kooistra HS, Nelson R et al.: Diagnosis of spontaneous canine hyperadrenocorticism: 2012 ACVIM consensus statement (*small animal*). *J Vet Intern Med* 27:1292, 2013.

HAC, os resultados de hemograma, perfil bioquímico sérico, urinálise com cultura e ultrassonografia abdominal devem ser revisados antes de considerar os exames hormonais. Diversas alterações são comuns, mas nenhuma é patognomônica para HAC. A ausência de anormalidades não descarta o HAC.

Hemograma
Linfopenia decorrente de linfocitólise esteroide, eosinopenia causada pelo sequestro na medula óssea, neutrofilia e monocitose, em razão da maior demarginação capilar esteroide, são comuns em cães com HAC. Juntas, essas alterações de leucócitos são chamadas de "leucograma de estresse", mas não são específicas. Outras alterações do hemograma associadas ao HAC incluem aumento das contagens plaquetárias e eritrocitose discreta (estimulação direta da medula óssea ou questões ventilatórias).

Perfil bioquímico sérico

Fosfatase alcalina sérica, alanina aminotransferase, colesterol, triglicerídeos
Incrementos na atividade de fosfatase alcalina (ALP) são a anormalidade laboratorial mais consistente, observada em 85 a 95% dos cães com HAC. Em muitos, os aumentos são acentuados (> 10 vezes acima do intervalo de referência), mas os resultados não são específicos (observados em inúmeras condições). A ALP jamais deve ser considerada um exame de triagem para o HAC, uma vez que não existe correlação entre atividade da ALP e gravidade do HAC, resposta à terapia ou prognóstico.[38] Quase toda a ALP em cães com HAC é uma isoenzima hepática induzida por esteroides (FAS), uma resposta única da isoenzima em cães. A FAS normal pode ajudar a descartar HAC.[39,40] As atividades da alanina aminotransferase (ALT) costumam estar discreta a moderadamente aumentadas em cães com HAC. Esses aumentos podem ocorrer em razão do dano causado por hepatócitos edemaciados, acúmulo de glicogênio, interferência no fluxo sanguíneo hepático ou necrose hepatocelular. Aumentos discretos a moderados nas concentrações de colesterol e triglicerídeos são observados em > 50% dos cães com HAC.

Glicemia
A discreta hiperglicemia em jejum (abaixo do limiar necessário para que a glicose apareça na urina) é comum em cães com HAC. O DM evidente (glicose > 250 mg/dℓ e glicosúria) não é comum, ocorrendo em cerca de 5% dos cães com HAC. Os glicocorticoides aumentam a gliconeogênese hepática e diminuem a utilização periférica de glicose, pela interferência na ação da insulina em nível celular (defeitos do receptor e do pós-receptor). A expressão gênica das moléculas de sinalização da insulina (pós-receptor) é suprimida em cães com HAC.[41] A hiperinsulinemia induzida pelo hipercortisolismo, para manter a tolerância aos carboidratos, quase sempre não é adequada para normalizar completamente a glicemia em todos os cães.[42] A hiperinsulinemia e a resistência insulínica estão provavelmente relacionadas com gordura abdominal e adipocinas, já que cães obesos com HAC apresentam concentrações maiores de leptina e insulina quando comparados aos saudáveis obesos. Concentrações de leptina e insulina diminuem com o tratamento com trilostano.[31] Outras adipocinas e fatores relacionados (adiponectina, tumor de necrose tumoralalfa, interleucina-6) não são diferentes.[31] Cães com HAC e DM costumam ser resistentes à insulina. O teste adrenocortical pode ser considerado em cães com DM e resposta persistentemente insatisfatória a doses altas de insulina. Entretanto, o leitor é encorajado a apreciar as numerosas explicações potenciais para um cão diabético parecer resistente à insulina (ver Capítulo 304). Nesse contexto, o HAC é uma explicação incomum.[30]

Nitrogênio ureico sanguíneo, fosfato (PO$_4$), cálcio, ácidos biliares, pâncreas
Aproximadamente 30 a 50% dos cães com HAC possuem nitrogênio ureico sanguíneo (NUS) abaixo dos intervalos de referência,

em razão da diurese. A azotemia é incomum em cães com HAC e, se presente, é uma indicação para não tratar o HAC, segundo alguns autores. A hipofosfatemia pode ocorrer em cães com HAC, devido ao aumento da excreção urinária. Também há aumento do Ca urinário, o que pode resultar em hiperparatireoidismo secundário e hiperfosfatemia em > 40%.[38,43,44] Os resultados dos testes dos ácidos biliares podem estar discretamente aumentados em até 30% dos cães com HAC.[45] Cães com HAC, sem pancreatite clínica, possuem níveis maiores de imunorreatividade lipase pancreática canina (PLIc) do que aqueles saudáveis, mas a especificidade é baixa (45 a 65%, dependendo da técnica). O aumento da PLIc em cães com HAC deve ser interpretado com cautela (ver Capítulo 290).[46]

Parâmetros de coagulação
A tromboembolia pulmonar (ver Capítulo 243) é uma complicação reconhecida em cães com HAC, talvez em razão de um estado de hipercoagulabilidade subjacente (ver Capítulo 196). Ao mesmo tempo que não é completamente compreendida, o aumento dos fatores pró-coagulantes (II, V, VII, IX, X, XII e fibrinogênio) e a diminuição da antitrombina foram descritos em um estudo. Em outro, porém, não foi identificada nenhuma diferença nos parâmetros de coagulação após a utilização de testes viscoelásticos com sangue total.[47,48] A diminuição dos níveis de antitrombina e o aumento da agregação plaquetária foram observados em cães tratados com prednisona.[49] Ademais, observou-se uma tendência de hipercoagulabilidade, definida como o achado de, pelo menos, uma anormalidade em um painel de coagulação utilizando tromboelastografia e perfis de coagulação, em > 80% dos cães com HAC.[50,51] As anormalidades mais comuns incluem tempos de protrombina (TP) mais curtos, maiores concentrações de fibrinogênio e aumento dos complexos trombina-antitrombina. Entre os parâmetros tromboelastográficos, foram documentados maior ângulo (MA) máximo da trombina, aumento dos ângulos alfa e valores menores de k.[50-52] A maioria dessas anormalidades persiste apesar do tratamento com trilostano.[52] Comorbidades (hipertensão, hipercolesterolemia, DM) poderiam estar associadas à hipercoagulabilidade. A correlação entre pressão sanguínea e concentração de colesterol ou de triglicerídeos não foi observada em nenhum resultado de teste de coagulação.[50]

Urinálise (ver Capítulo 72)
A maioria dos cães com HAC apresenta PU e densidade específica urinária < 1,020 (em geral, < 1,012), mas sem observância de glicose. A proteinúria é comum, com relações proteína:creatinina urinárias (UP:C) em geral não maiores do que 1 para 6. A UP:C foi < 1 em cerca de 45% e > 0,5 em cerca de 70% dos cães com HAC não tratado,[53-56] com persistência da proteinúria em cerca de 20 a 40% daqueles com HAC.[53-55] As taxas de filtração glomerular antes do tratamento estão aumentadas em cerca de 60% dos cães com HAC, as quais diminuem com a terapia.[55] Assim, a UP:C deve ser inicialmente mensurada em cães com HAC e monitorada durante o tratamento em cães proteinúricos. Cães com HAC são predispostos à ITU em razão da imunossupressão e da retenção urinária. Aproximadamente 40 a 50% dos cães com síndrome de Cushing apresentam ITU no momento da avaliação inicial.[57] Entretanto, em razão dos efeitos anti-inflamatórios do hipercortisolismo crônico, muitos desses cães não apresentam sinais clínicos ou alterações na urinálise sugestivas de ITU e, portanto, a urocultura é recomendada com uma amostra obtida por cistocentese.

Testes de função tireoidiana
Cães com HAC e aqueles com hipotireoidismo podem ter certa sobreposição em resultados clínicos e laboratoriais, incluindo alopecia, ganho de peso, letargia e hipercolesterolemia. Cães com HAC apresentam polifagia, enquanto os hipotireóideos, diminuição do apetite. As concentrações séricas de tiroxina total

SEÇÃO 21 • Doenças Endócrinas

(T_4t) e livre (T_4L) costumam estar diminuídas em cães com HAC,[58-60] com o aumento das concentrações de T_4L em alguns animais.[58-60] Alterações na ligação do hormônio tireoidiano sérico ou no metabolismo hormonal periférico podem contribuir para tal. Cães com HAC com concentrações diminuídas dos hormônios tireoidianos tendem a apresentar concentrações normais ou diminuídas do hormônio tireoestimulante circulante (TSHc), enquanto cães hipotireóideos possuem resultados normais a aumentados. O eixo hipotálamo-hipófise-tireoide está suprimido pelo excesso de cortisol, havendo o aumento das concentrações de TSHc após tratamento bem-sucedido.[59]

DIAGNÓSTICO POR IMAGEM

Radiografias torácicas

Cães com suspeita ou confirmação de HAC devem ser avaliados com radiografias torácicas em busca de lesões metastáticas e para avaliar o paciente por qualquer questão que não seja suspeita. Achados comuns inespecíficos em cães com HAC incluem padrão pulmonar intersticial em muitos e brônquios ou anéis traqueais mineralizados em um menor número.[20]

Cães com HAC e tromboembolia pulmonar (TEP), o que é raro, apesar do "estado de hipercoagulabilidade" desses animais, podem apresentar campos pulmonares hipovascularizados (áreas de aumento da radiolucência decorrente da diminuição da perfusão distal a um trombo) ou infiltrados pulmonares alveolares, que correspondem a áreas de atelectasia, hemorragia ou infarto. Aumento da artéria pulmonar principal, cardiomegalia do coração direito e efusão pleural foram relatados em cães com TEP.

Radiografias abdominais

Distensão abdominal, contraste radiográfico excelente em razão da deposição de gordura abdominal, hepatomegalia e distensão vesical são comumente observadas em cães com HAC. Urólitos com cálcio são ocasionalmente identificados.[61] Cerca de metade dos adenomas adrenais e carcinomas sofre calcificação, permitindo sua visualização, mas não indicando seu potencial maligno.[62] Relatou-se calcificação distrófica na pele, na pelve renal, no fígado, na mucosa gástrica ou em ramos da aorta abdominal em cães com HAC. A osteopenia é discreta e sem importância clínica. A avaliação radiográfica da densidade óssea não é sensível.[63]

Ultrassonografia

Hiperadrenocorticismo hipófise-dependente

A ultrassonografia abdominal completa, inclusive com a visualização de ambas as glândulas adrenais, é um auxílio diagnóstico valioso para a avaliação de cães com suspeita de HAC (ver Capítulo 88). A ultrassonografia pode ser útil para diferenciação do HHD do TAF. Se um tumor adrenal for visualizado, a ultrassonografia deve ser utilizada para avaliar o tamanho, a natureza invasiva e possíveis metástases. Ela também pode ajudar a avaliar sequelas do HAC (cálculos urinários, mucocele de vesícula biliar etc.) e para descartar condições não relacionadas com a adrenal (Vídeo 306.3). As glândulas adrenais são normalmente órgãos bilobados, hipoecoicos, achatados, localizados craniomedialmente aos rins. A espessura da glândula adrenal é considerada o indicador mais confiável do aumento; um limite de 7,4 mm – independentemente do tamanho ou da raça do cão – foi utilizado como limite superior de normalidade.[64,65] Entretanto, estudos recentes mostraram que o limiar do intervalo de referência varia de acordo com a raça e o tamanho corporal. O limite superior da altura do polo adrenal caudal, em um plano longitudinal, é de 5,4 mm (esquerda) e 6,7 mm (direita) em cães das raças Yorkshire Terrier e 7,9 mm (esquerda) e 9,5 mm (direita) para Labrador Retriever.[66] As glândulas adrenais de cães idosos tendem a ser maiores do que aquelas de cães

mais jovens.[67] A maioria de cães com HHD possui adrenomegalia bilateralmente simétrica, embora pelo menos 25% tenham glândulas de tamanho normal.[68] Em alguns cães com HHD, o aumento adrenal pode ser assimétrico devido à hiperplasia nodular, sendo mais difícil de interpretar (Vídeo 306.4). O tamanho da glândula adrenal não deve ser utilizado para o diagnóstico de HAC, em razão da sobreposição entre cães normais, cães doentes e aqueles com HAC.[64,65]

Tumor adrenocortical funcional

A ultrassonografia pode ser útil na visualização de um TAF e invasão vascular ou tecidual local. Deve-se suspeitar de tumor adrenal caso a glândula esteja aumentada, irregular (com perda de seu formato normal de amendoim) ou invadindo ou comprimindo estruturas adjacentes. A ecogenicidade de um TAF varia de aparência sólida a cística mista. O achado de assimetria moderada, atrofia adrenocortical contralateral (espessura da adrenal < 4 a 5 mm), destruição da arquitetura tecidual normal ou alguma combinação dessas é compatível com um TAF. A ultrassonografia possui limitações: é difícil diferenciar hiperplasia nodular bilateral de tumores adrenais bilaterais, tumores benignos não podem ser distinguidos de malignos e um TAF não pode ser distinguido de um feocromocitoma, um aldosteronoma, um tumor metastático ou um tumor adrenal não funcional.

Ultrassonografia contrastada

A ultrassonografia contrastada é um método não invasivo para quantificação de padrões vasculares da glândula adrenal em cães.[69,70] Em cães com HHD, há aumento d fluxo sanguíneo adrenal e do volume, não havendo semelhanças dos padrões de perfusão com aqueles de cães do grupo-controle, sendo necessários, portanto, mais estudos a respeito.

Tomografia computadorizada, ressonância magnética e "síndrome do macrotumor"

Tumores hipofisários > 1 cm de diâmetro (macroadenomas ou macroadenocarcinomas) são relativamente fáceis de visualizar, seja pela tomografia computadorizada (TC), seja pela ressonância magnética (RM). Tumores menores, que chegam a 1 cm em seu diâmetro maior, podem ser identificadas por imagem de TC, mas a RM é mais sensível para visualização de microadenomas hipofisários. Cinquenta e seis por cento dos cães com HHD possuem hipófise de aparência normal à TC.[71] A TC ou a RM deve ser realizada em cães com HHD e sinais de SNC. Os sinais associados a um grande tumor hipofisário podem ser vagos ou graves. Sinais sutis vagos incluem letargia, inapetência e retardo mental. Entre os vários sinais mais preocupantes, estão obnubilação grave, olhar perdido (ver Vídeo 306.1), anorexia completa, andar em círculos e alterações no comportamento. Sessenta e seis por cento dos cães com HHD com sinais neurológicos apresentavam tumor hipofisário detectável. Entretanto, > 70% daqueles com anormalidades neurológicas apresentavam tumor hipofisário detectável e 20%, macrotumor (i. e., um tumor ≥ 10 mm de comprimento).[72]

Varredura abdominal por tomografia computadorizada ou ressonância magnética e tumor adrenal identificado ao acaso

A TC e a RM são consideradas modalidades acuradas e confiáveis para visualização de glândulas adrenais. Com a TC ou a RM, podem-se identificar a localização do tumor adrenal, a existência de invasão vascular ou tecidual e metástases a distância. A TC pode ajudar a diferenciar HHD de TAF.[71] Um tumor adrenal visualizado ao acaso (incidentaloma adrenal, ver Capítulo 308) é detectado em uma pequena porcentagem de pessoas ou cães submetidos a exames de imagem abdominais,[73-75] sendo a maioria deles benigna e não funcional.

TESTES ENDÓCRINOS

Contexto geral dos testes de triagem e discriminação

Os testes endócrinos são essenciais para o diagnóstico de HAC, mas os resultados deles devem ser utilizados apenas para confirmar uma forte suspeita clínica. Indicações para a busca pelo diagnóstico de HAC incluem histórico sugestivo de HAC, visualização de macrotumor hipofisário ou tumor adrenal, cão diabético com resistência insulínica não atribuída a outra causa ou hipertensão persistente.[30] Muitas doenças afetam os resultados dos exames para HAC. Dessa forma, os testes devem ser evitados em cães com doença não adrenal moderada a grave. Ademais, é extremamente raro recomendar a terapia para HAC em qualquer cão doente por uma condição que não seja o HAC. Assim que ele for confirmado, os clínicos podem então tentar discriminar o HHD do TAF.

Os testes de triagem mais comumente utilizados para distinguir cães com e sem HAC incluem a relação corticoide:creatinina urinária (RC:CU), o teste de estimulação por ACTH (TEACTH) e o teste de supressão com baixa dose de dexametasona (TSBDD). Nenhum deles possui 100% de acurácia, e cada um apresenta vantagens e desvantagens. Como esses testes foram introduzidos na medicina veterinária anos atrás, os intervalos de referência e os valores limiares devem ser periodicamente reestabelecidos por laboratório.[30] Testes utilizados para discriminar o HHD do TAF incluem o TSBDD, o teste de supressão com alta dose de dexametasona (TSADD), o TSBDD utilizando a RC:CU, a mensuração das concentrações de ACTH e os exames de imagem por ultrassonografia, tomografia computadorizada e RM das adrenais.

Distinção de cães com e sem hiperadrenocorticismo (testes de triagem)

Relação corticoide:creatinina urinária

A excreção urinária de corticoides, determinada em uma amostra matinal, é o reflexo da secreção glicocorticoide adrenal durante um período de várias horas, anulando as questões relacionadas com as flutuações de concentrações sanguíneas. Diversos estudos mostraram que a RC:CU é um teste de triagem sensível (quase 100%), mas com baixa especificidade (20-77%).[76-79] Em razão da sua sensibilidade, a RC:CU é um bom teste para descartar o HAC, já que um resultado normal torna o diagnóstico extremamente improvável. Já que a RC:CU não é específica e sofre aumento em cães com muitas condições, outros testes são necessários se ela estiver aumentada em um cão com suspeita de HAC. De preferência, a urina é obtida em casa, pelo menos 2 dias depois da visita ao veterinário, para evitar o efeito do estresse.[80] Cães com HHD tendem a apresentar valores maiores de RC:CU do que aqueles com TAF; se > 100 (intervalo de referência, < 10), a probabilidade de HHD é de 90%.[81] A RC:CU requer pouco tempo e não é invasiva. A determinação da RC:CU basal pode ser realizada em conjunto com um TSADD, permitindo a avaliação da produção de cortisol e a sensibilidade da glândula adrenal à administração exógena de glicocorticoides.[30]

Cortisol do pelo

Foi relatado que as concentrações de cortisol do pelo são maiores em cães com HAC, comparadas a de cães sadios do grupo-controle.[82,83] Essa técnica não invasiva poderia ser considerada um teste de triagem para o HAC em cães, mas outros estudos são necessários.

Teste de estimulação por ACTH

O TEACTH avalia a resposta adrenocortical à estimulação máxima por ACTH, é um teste da reserva da glândula adrenal e o exame de escolha para identificação de HAC iatrogênico (Figura 306.7). Cães com HAC de ocorrência natural podem

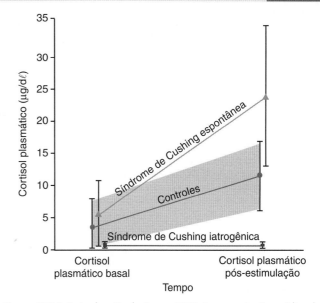

Figura 306.7 Teste de estimulação por ACTH. As concentrações médias do cortisol plasmático pelo radioimunoensaio (± 2 desvios padrões), determinadas antes e 1 hora após a administração de hormônio adrenocorticotrófico sintético em cães do grupo-controle, nos com hiperadrenocorticismo espontâneo e naqueles com hiperadrenocorticismo iatrogênico.

apresentar resposta normal ou exagerada ao ACTH exógeno e aqueles com síndrome de Cushing iatrogênica, resposta subnormal. A sensibilidade do teste de estimulação por ACTH é de 85% para o diagnóstico de HHD e 60% para o de TAF, sendo a especificidade de 85 a 90%.[84]

Diversos protocolos do teste foram descritos utilizando-se um peptídio sintético com os primeiros 24 aminoácidos do ACTH (Cortrosyn®, Synacthen®, Nuvacthen®) ou gel aquoso de ACTH porcino (Acthar Gel®, Questcor Pharmaceuticals, Inc., Union City, CA, EUA; indisponível em alguns países). A maioria recomenda a obtenção do sangue antes e 1 hora após administração de 250 μg/cão ou 5 μg/kg do ACTH por via intramuscular (IM) ou intravenosa (IV).[85,86] O ACTH reconstituído pode ser armazenado em seringas plásticas a −20°C durante 6 meses.[87] Em cães saudáveis, tetracosactida de depósito (250 μg/kg IM) e cosintropina (5 μg/kg IV) produziram respostas semelhantes após 60 minutos.[88] Ao utilizar o gel de ACTH, são obtidas amostras do plasma ou soro para o cortisol antes e 1 a 2 horas após a injeção IM de 2,2 UI/kg. A sensibilidade relativamente baixa dos resultados do TEACTH, em conjunto com a disponibilidade limitada e o custo crescente do ACTH sintético, reduziram sua utilização. Os resultados do TEACTH não podem diferenciar o HHD do TAF. Apesar de sua sensibilidade relativamente baixa, ele é menos afetado por doenças não adrenais, não consome muito tempo e é o único teste capaz de diferenciar HAC iatrogênico de HAC de ocorrência natural.

HAC "atípico" e TEACTH

Outro uso potencial do TEACTH é para cães com suspeita de HAC "atípico". O HAC "atípico" ou "oculto" refere-se a um cão com sinais clínicos, exame físico e achados clinicopatológicos compatíveis com HAC, mas com resultados de TSBDD, RC:CU e TEACTH dentro dos intervalos de referência. Foi sugerido que esses cães possuem um desarranjo da via de síntese de esteroides, que leva a concentrações anormalmente altas do precursor, mas com concentrações normais de cortisol. A mensuração da 17-hidroxiprogesterona (17-OH-P), um precursor do cortisol, antes e após o TEACTH pode ajudar a diagnosticar essa forma rara de HAC pela documentação de uma resposta exagerada da 17-OH-P ao ACTH.[89,90] Entretanto, os resultados do TEACTH devem ser interpretados com cuidado, uma vez que resultados

SEÇÃO 21 • Doenças Endócrinas

falso-positivos foram documentados em cães com doença não adrenal e sem evidências de HAC.[91] O diagnóstico de HAC "atípico" tem sido questionado. Cães com HAC discreto ou precoce com exames "normais", utilizando valores atuais limítrofes, podem ser diagnosticados pela utilização de valores de referência revisados. Ademais, como pode existir sensibilidade variável ao cortisol, alguns cães com alta sensibilidade podem mostrar sinais clínicos de HAC em concentrações menores de cortisol do que outros.[30,92]

Teste de supressão com baixa dose de dexametasona

O TSBDD é considerado o "teste de escolha" para confirmação de um diagnóstico de HAC de ocorrência natural em cães.[30,93] A resposta normal do eixo hipofisário-adrenocortical ao *feedback* negativo, associado à dexametasona exógena (um glicocorticoide), é a supressão do ACTH, que causa diminuição da secreção do cortisol. Cães com HAC são anormalmente resistentes à supressão por dexametasona. A sensibilidade do TSBDD é excelente. Os resultados são compatíveis com HAC em cerca de 90 a 95% de cães com HHD e em praticamente 100% daqueles com TAF. Ao mesmo tempo que a sensibilidade do TSBDD é excelente, a especificidade pode ser de 40 a 50%, especialmente quando da avaliação em uma população de cães com doença não adrenal.[79] Assim, o diagnóstico de HAC jamais deve se basear unicamente nos resultados do TSBDD, com o adiamento do exame em qualquer cão doente. O teste não é útil na detecção de HAC iatrogênico, é afetado por mais variáveis do que o TEACTH, requer 8 horas (ou 3 dias, caso seja utilizado o protocolo de RC:CU; veja a seguir) e não fornece informações úteis sobre o monitoramento do tratamento.

Amostras séricas ou plasmáticas são coletadas para aferição do cortisol antes, 4 e 8 horas após administração de dexametasona. Pode-se administrar dexametasona em polietilenoglicol (0,015 mg/kg, IV ou IM) ou fosfato sódico de dexametasona (0,01 mg/kg, IV) com resultados equivalentes (Figura 306.8).[29] Resultados confiáveis podem não ser obtidos em cães sob estresse ou tratados com fenobarbital. Em um cão com sinais clínicos de HAC, a ausência de supressão adequada do cortisol é compatível com o diagnóstico. Os resultados de cortisol basal e 8 horas após dexametasona são utilizados como porção de "triagem" da interpretação. Os resultados da amostra obtida após 4 horas podem ser úteis para discriminação do HHD e do TAF. Aproximadamente 30% dos cães com HHD exibem supressão sérica de cortisol com 4 horas ($< 1,4$ μg/dℓ ou < 40 nmol/ℓ), com concentração maior de cortisol com 8 horas. Esse padrão de escape ou em "V" é compatível com HHD, não sendo necessários outros testes discriminatórios.[84] Também é mais provável que cães com concentração sérica de cortisol com 4 ou 8 horas, que tenha diminuído para menos que 50% da concentração sérica basal de cortisol (pré-dexametasona), apresentem HHD. Aproximadamente 65% dos cães com HHD mostram supressão com a utilização de um desses três critérios.[93] A incapacidade em suprimir (cortisol em 4 e 8 h $> 1,4$ μg/dℓ e > 50% da concentração basal de cortisol) é compatível com diagnóstico de HAC, mas não é útil para discriminar HHD e TAF. A interpretação do TSBDD deve se basear em valores de referência atualizados e valores limítrofes estabelecidos por laboratório.

RC:CU/TSBDD combinados

O TSBDD pode ser realizado pela obtenção de urina para RC:CU, e não pela utilização do cortisol sérico ou plasmático.[94] Com esse protocolo, o tutor coleta amostras de urina em duas manhãs consecutivas, por volta das 8 horas, para RCCUs basais. Após coleta da segunda amostra, o tutor administra 0,01 mg/kg de dexametasona VO. A bexiga do cão deve ser esvaziada voluntariamente ou por cateterismo às 14 horas. Uma terceira e última amostra de urina é coletada às 16 horas, 8 horas após a administração da dexametasona. Os resultados sugerem que a supressão > 50% na RC:CU média e a diminuição na relação a < 10 seriam esperadas em cães saudáveis.[94] Em teoria, cães com HAC não apresentariam supressão.

Testes de discriminação em cães com hiperadrenocorticismo (hiperadrenocorticismo hipófise-dependente *versus* tumor adrenocortical funcional)

Teste de supressão com baixa dose de dexametasona

O TSBDD pode auxiliar na discriminação entre HHD e TAF. Os resultados são compatíveis com HHD se um dos três critérios for atingido: (1) concentração de cortisol com 4 h $< 1,4$ μg/dℓ; (2) concentração de cortisol com 4 h < 50% da concentração basal; (3) concentração de cortisol com 8 horas < 50% da concentração basal, mas ≥ 1 μg/dℓ. Aproximadamente 65% dos cães com HHD de ocorrência natural atendem a, pelo menos, um desses critérios.[93] Entretanto, valores limítrofes atualizados também são necessários. A resistência à dexametasona, na qual nenhum desses critérios é alcançado, é observada em 35% dos cães com HHD e em praticamente todos os pacientes com TAF. Nesses cães, outro teste de discriminação é indicado.

Teste de supressão por alta dose de dexametasona

A maioria dos cães com HHD apresenta certa resistência à supressão durante o TSBDD, mas doses maiores de dexametasona podem superar essa resistência. Do contrário, em razão da supressão crônica do ACTH hipofisário em cães com TAF secretor de cortisol, a administração da dexametasona, independentemente da dose, deixa de suprimir as concentrações de cortisol.[93] O protocolo recomendado para TSADD envolve a coleta do sangue antes e 4 ou 8 horas após administração de 0,1 a 1 mg/kg de dexametasona (IV ou IM). A dexametasona em polietilenoglicol ou o fosfato sódico de dexametasona podem ser utilizados com resultados equivalentes.

Em geral, a demonstração de diminuição na concentração de cortisol para teores $< 1,4$ μg/dℓ (40 nmol/ℓ) é considerada diagnóstica de HHD e exclui a possibilidade de TAF. A interpretação dos resultados também deve se basear nos valores de referência do laboratório para ambas as doses e a dexametasona utilizada. A ausência de supressão não é diagnóstica para um TAF, já que aproximadamente 35% dos cães com HHD não mostram supressão do cortisol. Evidências sugerem que é menos provável que cães com grandes tumores hipofisários mostrem resposta, independentemente da dose.[95] Em cães com HAC confirmado que não apresentam supressão pelo TSADD, ainda existe risco maior de HHD do que TAF.

A maioria dos cães com HHD que mostram supressão do cortisol no TSADD também o mostram no TSBDD. Os resultados do TSADD forneceram informações adicionais em apenas cerca de 10% que não suprimiram no TSBDD.[93] Portanto, é útil realizar um TSBDD de rotina em cães com suspeita de HAC. Entretanto, quando a resistência à dexametasona é mostrada no TSBDD, seria mais eficiente realizar outro teste para diferenciação, como exames de imagem da adrenal ou mensuração do ACTH endógeno.

RC:CU/TSADD combinados

Essa combinação pode ser utilizada como o teste endócrino inicial na avaliação de um cão com HAC. Uma amostra de urina é coletada em três manhãs consecutivas, em casa, para RC:CU. Após a coleta da segunda amostra, o tutor administra 0,1 mg/kg de dexametasona VO, ao cão, 3 vezes, em intervalos de 8 horas. A RC:CU basal média é calculada com base nos dois primeiros resultados. Se houver aumento da RC:CU basal, compatível com HAC, há probabilidade de HHD, caso o terceiro resultado da UC:CR seja < 50% do nível basal.[81]

ACTH endógeno (ACTHe)

A mensuração da concentração basal de ACTHe possui pouco valor como teste de triagem para HAC, mas pode ser útil para discriminar o HHD do TAF, após confirmação do HAC. Existe pouca sobreposição nas concentrações de ACTHe em resultados de cães com HHD quando comparados àqueles com TAF.[96]

CAPÍTULO 306 • Hiperadrenocorticismo Canino

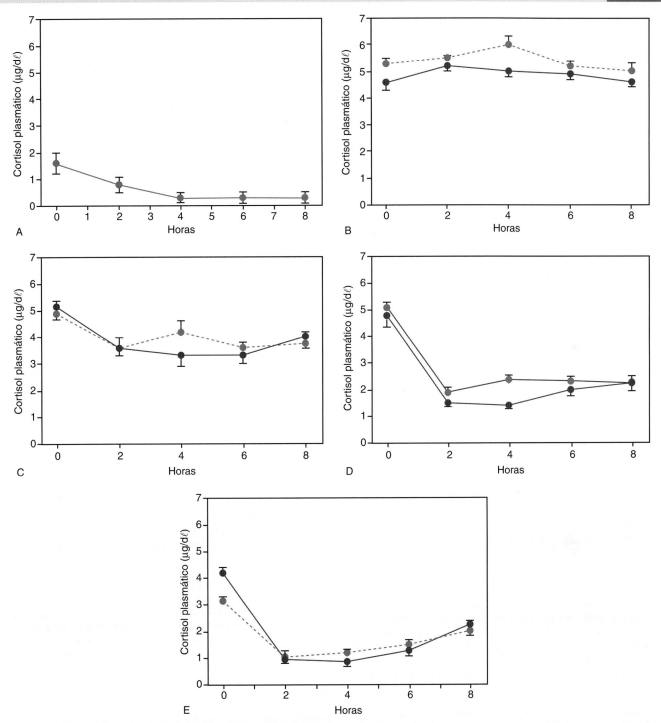

Figura 306.8 A. Concentrações plasmáticas médias do cortisol antes e após administração de uma baixa dose de dexametasona em 27 cães normais. **B.** Quarenta e oito cães com tumores adrenocorticais. **C.** Cento e trinta com hiperadrenocorticismo hipófise-dependente (HHD). **D.** Aqueles entre os 178 com síndrome de Cushing, que apresentavam, pelo menos, concentração plasmática de cortisol menor que 1,4 µg/dℓ após administração de dexametasona (total, 54; todos tinham HHD). **E.** Aqueles entre os 178 com síndrome de Cushing, que, após administração de dexametasona, apresentaram, pelo menos, diminuição da concentração plasmática de cortisol para menos que 50% da concentração basal (total, 95; todos tinham HHD). Note as duas curvas dos gráficos B, C, D e E. Elas representam a utilização de fosfato sódico de dexametasona (*linha tracejada*) e dexametasona em polietilenoglicol (*linha sólida*). Não é observada nenhuma diferença significativa nos resultados com esses produtos de dexametasona. (De Feldman EC, Nelson RW: *Canine and feline endocrinology and reproduction*, 2 ed., Philadelphia, 1996, Saunders, p. 227.)

As concentrações de ACTHe estão normais ou aumentadas em cães com HHD (p. ex., > 40 pg/mℓ ou > 8,8 pmol/ℓ) e quase sempre baixas ou indetectáveis (p. ex., < 20 pg/mℓ ou < 4,4 pmol/ℓ) naqueles com TAF ou HAC iatrogênico. Aproximadamente 20% dos cães com HAC possuem resultados de ACTHe obtidos de forma aleatória em uma faixa não diagnóstica (20 a 40 pg/mℓ). Neles, o teste pode ser repetido ou um exame de imagem indicado.

A coleta, o manuseio e a realização do exame com as amostras para resultados confiáveis do ACTHe podem ser difíceis e caros. As amostras devem ser coletadas em tubos de heparina ou ácido etilenodiaminotetracético (EDTA) e centrifugadas de imediato. O plasma é então colocado em tubos de plástico ou polipropileno (o ACTH se aderirá ao vidro) e imediatamente congelado até que o exame seja realizado. As amostras de plasma devem ser enviadas em gelo seco por serviço de entrega noturno. Se tais condições não forem viáveis, a aprotinina, um inibidor de protease, pode ser adicionada ao tubo de EDTA como preservativo para ACTH; em tais casos, a amostra pode ser enviada refrigerada em bolsas térmicas, não sendo necessário o congelamento.[97]

Avaliação ultrassonográfica do abdome e das glândulas adrenais

Espera-se um aumento simétrico bilateral em cães com HHD e, naqueles com TAF, um tumor adrenal solitário e atrofia da glândula contralateral. Entretanto, alguns cães com HHD possuem glândulas adrenais de aparência normal, enquanto outros apresentam hiperplasia nodular assimétrica, que pode ser confundida com um tumor adrenal. Alguns cães com tumores adrenais possuem glândula contralateral de aparência normal. A espessura máxima da glândula menor é útil para diferenciar tumores adrenais (< 5 mm) de hiperplasia assimétrica (> 5 mm).

Tomografia computadorizada e ressonância magnética

De modo geral, a ultrassonografia é aceitável para avaliação das adrenais em busca de um tumor, enquanto a TC e a RM são as únicas modalidades disponíveis para visualização de um tumor hipofisário. Os resultados de TC e RM não podem ser utilizados para substituir os testes de função endócrina. Cerca de 50% dos tumores hipofisários não são visíveis em ambas as modalidades e nenhuma pode determinar a função.[45] Adenomas invasivos, observados pela TC ou RM, possuem altura média (1,8 ± 0,7 cm) significativamente maior do que os não invasivos.[9] Em cães, os tumores hipofisários costumam se expandir dorsalmente, em razão da resistência mínima encontrada na sela diafragmática incompleta. O crescimento pode resultar em invaginação em direção ao terceiro ventrículo e comprimir e/ou invadir o hipotálamo. O quiasma óptico, rostral à hipófise, raramente é impactado por um tumor hipofisário em expansão, poupando a visão.

O tamanho da hipófise depende da raça e da variação individual. Em cães saudáveis, as mensurações tomográficas da hipófise revelaram tamanhos de 3,2 a 5,1 mm (altura), 4,2 a 6,9 mm (largura) e 3,6 a 7,2 mm (comprimento).[98] O primeiro sinal de alargamento da hipófise é um aumento na altura (extensão dorsal em direção à região suprasselar), que é provável quando o contorno dorsal da glândula sofre protrusão acima da extensão suprasselar das cisternas intercrurais, reconhecido com facilidade em exames de TC.[95] De forma alternativa, a relação entre a altura hipofisária e a área cerebral, mensurada em uma imagem através do centro da hipófise (relação H:C), pode ser utilizada para discriminar um tamanho hipofisário aumentado (relação H:C > 0,31) ou normal (H:C ≤ 0,31).[98]

Tumores grandes costumam ser detectados com facilidade em imagens tomográficas contrastadas, por conta do tamanho e formato alterado. Em 50 a 60% dos cães com HHD, pode-se detectar um tumor hipofisário à TC. Quarenta a cinquenta por cento dos cães com HHD possuem um tumor menor (< 3 a 4 mm), não visível, apesar do ganho com contraste. Modalidades tomográficas que utilizam uma série de varreduras transversas no centro da hipófise durante e após rápida injeção IV do meio de contraste (TC "dinâmica") podem, quase sempre, ajudar a distinguir a hipófise posterior da anterior, em razão de diferenças na vascularização. Em cães normais, observa-se não só um ganho precoce e intenso da hipófise posterior central ("*flush* hipofisário"), assim como um mais fraco e discretamente retardado da glândula anterior periférica. O deslocamento ou a distorção do *flush* hipofisário pode revelar a existência de pequenos tumores.[99]

Embora a TC e a RM sejam efetivas na identificação de grandes tumores hipofisários, a RM é superior no que diz respeito à definição da completa extensão tumoral e seus efeitos sobre as estruturas circundantes, parecendo mais acurada na identificação de pequenos tumores. O tamanho, o sinal e o ganho de contraste, característicos da RM da hipófise canina

normal, já foram descritos. Um estudo observou que cerca de 50% dos cães com HHD sem sinais neurológicos apresentam um tumor hipofisário que pode ser visualizado em exames de RM, variando de 4 a 12 mm de tamanho.[100,101]

TRATAMENTO

Considerações terapêuticas

A escolha do tratamento para um cão com HAC depende de diversos fatores: HHD *versus* TAF, gravidade da condição, existência de complicações do HAC ou doenças concomitantes, tratamentos disponíveis, eficácia da terapia, efeitos adversos e preferências do médico-veterinário e do tutor. O custo e a necessidade de acompanhamentos frequentes podem ser considerações essenciais. É importante lembrar, entretanto, que nem todos os cães com HAC, especialmente aqueles com HHD, precisam de tratamento imediato. Já que nenhum dos exames de triagem ou diferenciação para HAC é perfeito, não se deve tratar um cão sem sinais ou com apenas sinais clínicos mínimos, apesar de testes bioquímicos e/ou endócrinos anormais compatíveis com HAC.[30] Como o tratamento do HAC jamais é benigno, ele não deve ser iniciado, a menos que o cão mostre sinais clínicos inequívocos da condição. Esses fatores são ainda mais enfatizados com os objetivos da terapia sendo, principalmente, a melhora clínica percebida pelo tutor.

Contexto geral do tratamento do hiperadrenocorticismo hipófise-dependente

O HHD pode ser tratado de forma medicamentosa ou cirúrgica. A hipofisectomia é o tratamento de escolha em seres humanos com HHD e bem descrita em cães. A hipofisectomia não é amplamente utilizada, em razão do número limitado de cirurgiões com experiência, seus efeitos colaterais relacionados e o sucesso obtido com as terapias medicamentosas. A maioria dos cães com HHD é tratada com fármacos que inibem a síntese de hormônios adrenocorticais (*i. e.*, trilostano ou cetoconazol) ou que causem necrose parcial ou completa do córtex adrenal (*i. e.*, mitotano). Um medicamento que supostamente diminui a secreção de ACTH (selegilina) não é eficaz.

Ao mesmo tempo que o trilostano se tornou o tratamento de escolha para cães com HAC, o uso do mitotano também tem sido bem-sucedido na resolução das anormalidades clínicas e bioquímicas do HAC. Tanto o trilostano como o mitotano já causaram efeitos colaterais adversos sérios. Ambos os medicamentos diminuem o cortisol plasmático e aumentam a secreção do ACTH, o que pode aumentar o crescimento tumoral hipofisário.[102-104] Cães com macroadenomas hipofisários podem se beneficiar da radioterapia, que pode diminuir o tamanho tumoral e reduzir os sinais neurológicos. Por um lado, o tratamento do HHD envolve altos custos e requer monitoramento periódico; por outro, a maioria dos cães possui resposta boa ou excelente ao tratamento.

Terapia com trilostano

Histórico clínico e farmacologia

O uso do trilostano para o tratamento do HHD canino foi relatado pela primeira vez em 1998, e diversos estudos confirmaram sua eficácia clínica para o tratamento de cães com HAC.[102,103,105-117] O trilostano é um análogo esteroide sintético que atua como inibidor competitivo da enzima 3-beta-hidroxiesteroide desidrogenase (3-beta-HSD), que catalisa a conversão adrenocortical de pregnenolona em progesterona. A inibição da ação dessa enzima bloqueia a síntese de cortisol e, em menor extensão, da aldosterona (Figura 306.9).[106] O trilostano alcança picos de concentrações < 2 horas após a administração e é completamente metabolizado em 10 a 18 horas A inibição pelo trilostano da 3-beta-HSD é confirmada por diminuição nas

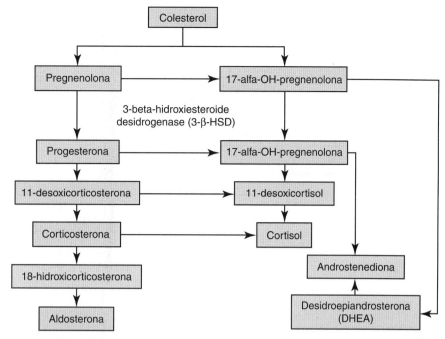

Figura 306.9 Vias biossintéticas de mineralocorticoides, glicocorticoides e andrógenos no córtex adrenal. A *3-beta-hidroxiesteroide desidrogenase*, que converte pregnenolona em progesterona e desidroepiandrosterona em androstenediona, é bloqueada pelo trilostano.

concentrações plasmáticas de cortisol, com aumentos concomitantes na 17-alfa-OH-pregnenolona. As concentrações de 17-alfa-OH-progesterona não mudam, sugerindo que o trilostano também pode inibir a 11-beta-hidroxilase, influenciando a interconversão do cortisol ativo em cortisona inativa pela 11-beta-hidroxiesteroide desidrogenase (11-beta-HSD).[102] O mRNA da glândula adrenal e a expressão proteica de 11-beta-HSD tipo 1 estão aumentados, enquanto o mRNA e a expressão proteica de 11-beta-HSD tipo 2, diminuídos.[118]

Dose inicial e frequência de administração

Dose, frequência de administração e protocolos de monitoramento para o trilostano continuam a ser avaliados. Doses utilizadas em estudos iniciais (de até 50 mg/kg/dia) eram maiores do que as recomendações atuais. As doses iniciais recomendadas pelo fabricante variam de 3 a 6,7 mg/kg, VO, a cada 24 h, dependendo do peso corporal. Entretanto, diversos estudos mostraram que doses de 0,2 a 1 mg/kg, VO, a cada 12 h, são efetivas e podem causar menos efeitos colaterais adversos.[113,114,116,117] Conforme o peso corporal aumenta, as doses necessárias de trilostano diminuem.[113,114] A dose inicial de trilostano deve se basear no peso corporal e na frequência planejada de administração. Em cães com HAC, há variação da duração da supressão do cortisol causada pelo trilostano. Na maioria, as concentrações de cortisol foram suprimidas por < 12 horas, o que explica o porquê de os protocolos a cada 24 horas não serem efetivos em todos os cães.[105,108] A proporção de cães que mostram bom controle do HAC melhora com a administração a cada 12 horas.[108,109,113,115-117] Também, com os protocolos a cada 12 horas, a dose diária total necessária para bom controle é, em geral, inferior.[108,109,113-117] Um estudo que avaliou o tempo de sobrevida de cães com HHD tratados com trilostano a cada 12 horas observou maiores tempos de sobrevida médios (900 dias) do que os relatados em um estudo que avaliou cães tratados a cada 24 horas (662 dias).[110,111] Mesmo que a maioria dos cães com HAC esteja bem controlada com a administração a cada 12 ou 24 horas, alguns respondem bem ao trilostano administrado a cada 8 horas.[108,113]

Recomenda-se uma dose inicial de 0,5 a 1 mg/kg VO, 2 vezes/dia. Protocolos com uma administração diária (1 a 2 mg/kg) devem ser reservados para tutores que recusam a alternativa a cada 12 horas. Embora doses iniciais baixas possam prolongar o tempo necessário para controlar os sinais clínicos, elas são cada vez mais adequadas, ao mesmo tempo que reduzem o risco de sobredose.[108] Alguns cães não apresentam boa resposta clínica ao tratamento a cada 24 horas, apesar de os resultados dos exames indicarem supressão adequada do cortisol no pico do efeito do trilostano. Neles, deve-se considerar a administração a cada 12 horas (ver a utilização da densidade urinária). Independentemente da dose inicial selecionada e da frequência de administração, o tratamento deve ser individualizado às necessidades do paciente e do tutor.

Avaliação da resposta ao trilostano e ajustes de dose

Espera-se que cães tratados com trilostano necessitem de ajustes de dose, com base na resposta clínica e/ou nos resultados de exames. Dentro de 7 a 10 dias após o início do trilostano, os tutores devem notar aumento da atividade e diminuição de PU/PD/PF. Dos três parâmetros, a PF pode diminuir mais lentamente, após várias semanas. Problemas dermatológicos podem levar meses para cessar por completo. A princípio, o pelame de alguns cães parece piorar, conforme o pelo e a pele seca mortos vão caindo, criando uma piora da alopecia e descamação grave.

Os ajustes terapêuticos devem se basear em sinais clínicos (PU), hemograma, perfil bioquímico sérico e resultados do TEACTH (Figura 306.10). Os resultados do TEACTH refletem a reserva adrenocortical, sendo o teste mais objetivo, específico e sensível para a avaliação da resposta terapêutica.[102,119-121] É extremamente importante relacionar os TEACTHs ao tempo de administração do trilostano. Recomendações incluem iniciar o teste para coincidir com o pico (2 a 3 horas após a administração) ou a baixa (logo antes de administrar a próxima dose) da ação do trilostano. Em um estudo que comparou os resultados do TEACTH realizado 2 ou 4 horas após a administração do trilostano, o efeito máximo na maioria dos cães (menor concentração de cortisol) foi detectado ao iniciar o teste 2 horas após a administração.[121] Os resultados desse estudo também ressaltam a importância da consistência do momento do TEACTH, que pode ser iniciado 8 a 12 horas após a administração em cães tratados a cada 12 horas, a fim de avaliar os efeitos da baixa e da duração da ação.[108,109] O início do TEACTH 24 horas após a administração pode documentar, de forma semelhante, a duração de ação do trilostano, se este for administrado 1 vez/dia.

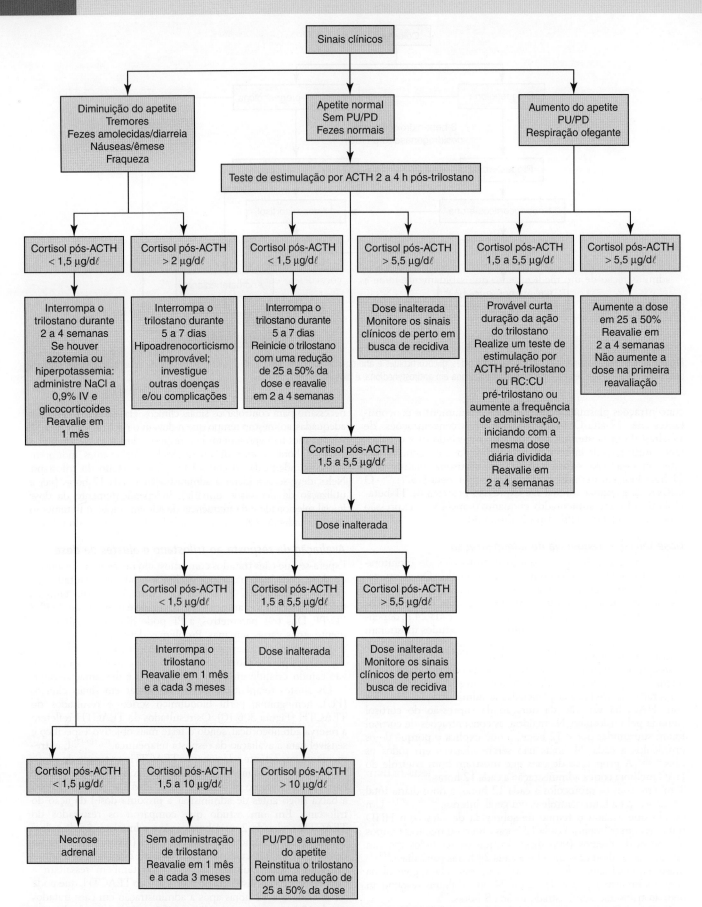

Figura 306.10 Algoritmo para monitoramento de cães com hiperadrenocorticismo tratados com trilostano. Se o teste de estimulação por ACTH for realizado 8 a 12 h após a administração, a interpretação do resultado será diferente, com uma faixa ideal de cortisol pós-ACTH entre 2 μg/dℓ e 10 μg/dℓ. Os cães devem ser reavaliados 2 a 4 semanas após qualquer ajuste de dose. Assim que for obtido um bom controle da doença, o paciente deve ser avaliado a cada 3 meses. *ACTH*, hormônio adrenocorticotrófico; *PU/PD*, poliúria/polidipsia; *RC:CU*, relação cortisol:creatinina urinária.

Reações adversas ao trilostano

O trilostano é bem tolerado pela maioria dos cães. Os efeitos adversos, se presentes, costumam ser discretos e causados pelas baixas concentrações de cortisol e/ou aldosterona. Alguns cães podem desenvolver letargia e diminuição do apetite dentro de poucos dias após o início da terapia. Os efeitos adversos graves incluem depressão, anorexia, êmese, diarreia, tremores, perda de peso, obnubilação e morte. Se um cão tratado com trilostano apresentar sinais preocupantes, o fármaco deve ser descontinuado de imediato, com a avaliação dos eletrólitos séricos, dos parâmetros renais, da glicemia e da pressão sanguínea.[107,109,110] Um TEACTH pode ser realizado, embora os resultados possam não ser úteis para o manejo de doença aguda grave ou crise.

Necrose adrenocortical induzida pelo trilostano

Assim que ocorrer sobredose pelo trilostano, pode haver supressão da função adrenal de cães durante dias, meses ou por mais tempo.[109] Hipoadrenocorticismo prolongado não é esperado após a administração de um medicamento que sabidamente inibe as enzimas adrenocorticais por menos que 12 horas, mas foram documentados graus variados de necrose adrenocortical e hemorragia causados pelo trilostano, especialmente dentro da zona fasciculada.[122] O hipocortisolismo prolongado pode ocorrer com ou sem deficiência de mineralocorticoides. Efeitos adversos preocupantes foram documentados com início em dias, meses ou anos após o início do tratamento em até 25% dos cães tratados com trilostano.[109,123] Um estudo com ratos submetidos a doses crescentes de trilostano mostrou que concentrações de ACTHe com aumento secundário podem ser responsáveis pela necrose adrenal.[124] Portanto, ao se evitar o hipocortisolismo, podem-se prevenir sinais e diminuir os riscos de necrose adrenal. A consideração dessas complicações potencialmente graves é extremamente importante para monitorar com cuidados cães que recebem trilostano, bem como realizar as avaliações recomendadas, mesmo que um cão esteja respondendo bem clinicamente.

Dose do trilostano em longo prazo e ajustes da frequência

Cães submetidos ao trilostano devem ser avaliados após 10 a 15 dias de tratamento e novamente após 1 mês, 3 meses e a cada 3 a 6 meses depois. Em cada reavaliação, devem-se obter histórico completo e exame físico. Hemograma e painel bioquímico sérico com eletrólitos podem ser indicados. Além disso, o clínico deve realizar um TEACTH a cada visita. O teste deve ser iniciado 2 a 4 horas após administração do trilostano, com a manutenção desse intervalo em todas as reavaliações subsequentes. Os ajustes de dose devem se basear na resposta clínica e nos resultados dos testes de rotina e endócrinos (ver Figura 306.10). Uma concentração de cortisol pós-ACTH de 1,5 a 5,5 mg/dℓ (41 a 152 nmol/ℓ) é considerada adequada quando o TEACTH for realizado com 2 a 4 horas após a administração.[125,126] O objetivo principal da primeira reavaliação é evitar a sobredose. A dose do trilostano não deve ser aumentada na primeira avaliação, mesmo que os sinais clínicos não tenham melhorado e a concentração pós-ACTH esteja acima de 5,5 µg/dℓ. Após a primeira reavaliação, se os sinais clínicos de HAC persistirem e o cortisol pós-TEACTH estiver > 5,5 µg/dℓ, a dose do trilostano deve ser aumentada. Se um cão submetido à administração de trilostano a cada 12 ou 24 horas estiver indo bem clinicamente, mas a concentração de cortisol pós-TEACTH estiver < 1,5 µg/dℓ, o trilostano deve ser interrompido durante 5 a 7 dias e, então, reiniciado com uma dose 25 a 50% inferior. Se, após outras 2 a 4 semanas, os valores de cortisol sérico permanecerem baixos, o trilostano deve ser descontinuado por tempo indeterminado e o TEACTH reagendado periodicamente a cada alguns meses ou sempre que o proprietário observar recidiva dos sinais. O trilostano deve ser reiniciado apenas se os sinais clínicos de HAC recidivarem e os teores de cortisol pós-TEACTH estiverem novamente aumentados.

Dose do trilostano em longo prazo e ajustes da dose utilizando a urina

O médico-veterinário pode utilizar a urina obtida antes da administração do trilostano para auxiliar nos ajustes a longo prazo. Nesse cenário, os resultados do TEACTH são utilizados para determinar a *dose* do trilostano e a densidade urinária utilizada para determinar a *frequência*. Por exemplo, se um cão continuar a apresentar PU/PD, densidade urinária antes da administração < 1,020 (sem glicosúria) e concentração sérica de cortisol pós-TEACTH > 1,5 e < 5,5 µg/dℓ, deve-se aumentar a frequência de administração.[104,108,113]

Hipocortisolismo

Se forem observados sinais clínicos compatíveis com hipocortisolismo, o trilostano deve ser interrompido enquanto da realização e avaliação do TEACTH e do perfil bioquímico sérico. Se o hipocortisolismo for confirmado, mas os eletrólitos séricos estiverem normais, o clínico deve interromper o trilostano, administrar glicocorticoides, conforme necessário, e repetir o TEACTH 2 a 4 semanas depois. Com base nesses resultados, pode ser necessário reinstituir o trilostano se o cão começar a mostrar sinais clínicos de HAC e a concentração de cortisol pós-TEACTH for > 10 µg/dℓ. Se o hipoadrenocorticismo persistir, a necrose adrenal é provável. Se o hipoadrenocorticismo for confirmado em conjunto com a hiperpotassemia e/ou a hiponatremia, o clínico deve interromper o trilostano por, pelo menos, 1 mês e tratar como uma crise adissoniana (ver Capítulo 309). Os TEACTHs devem ser repetidos após 1 mês e, então, a cada 3 a 6 meses para determinar quando o tratamento para a doença de Addison pode ser interrompido e se a terapia com trilostano deve ser reiniciada.

Uso dos teores de cortisol em baixa e/ou ultrassonografia

A avaliação do cortisol basal no pico de ação do trilostano (em geral, de 2 a 4 horas após a administração) tem sido estudada como uma ferramenta de monitoramento em cães com HAC e para detectar o hipocortisolismo (cortisol < 1,5 µg/dℓ). Uma concentração de cortisol basal 2 a 4 horas após a administração de 1,5 a 4,4 µg/dℓ de trilostano é considerada indicativa de controle adequado. Essa abordagem não é amplamente aceita, em parte por conta da considerável sobreposição entre controle excessivo, adequado e inadequado. Os TEACTHs são considerados muito mais informativos do que a avaliação do cortisol basal.[119,120]

Há alteração da aparência ultrassonográfica das glândulas adrenais com o tratamento com trilostano, quase sempre em razão dos incrementos na secreção de ACTH secundários à redução do *feedback* negativo ao cortisol.[118,127,128] Um aumento acentuado na ecogenicidade da zona externa também foi descrito. O córtex adrenal pequeno e heteroecoico pode ser indicativo de necrose.[123]

Terapias alternativas

Uma vacina com ACTH recombinante resultou na produção de anticorpos contra o ACTH em cães saudáveis; entretanto, o efeito sobre o eixo hipofisário-adrenal é sutil e transitório.[145] O receptor do fator de crescimento epidérmico (EGFR, do inglês *epidermal growth fator receptor*) é proposto como alvo terapêutico para tumores secretores de ACTH em cães.[146]

Tratamento cirúrgico do hiperadrenocorticismo hipófise-dependente (hipofisectomia)

A remoção cirúrgica transesfenoidal do tumor hipofisário que causa o HHD é o tratamento de escolha para seres humanos, enquanto é utilizada a hipofisectomia cirúrgica completa em cães.[7,147,148] Após hipofisectomia em cães com HHD, a fração livre de recidiva estimada em 1 ano foi de 90%. As taxas de sobrevida estimadas em 1, 2, 3 e 4 anos (86, 83, 80, 79%, respectivamente) são comparadas, de modo favorável, aos resultados observados em cães tratados com mitotano ou trilostano.[148]

Complicações associadas à hipofisectomia incluem diabetes insípido permanente ou prolongado, hipotireoidismo secundário, redução transitória ou interrupção da produção lacrimal, hipernatremia pós-cirúrgica discreta transitória e recidiva do HHD meses depois. As falhas terapêuticas incluíram mortalidade relacionada com o procedimento e hipofisectomias incompletas. O diabetes insípido central ocorreu com mais frequência em cães com aumento da hipófise, em comparação àqueles sem. Fatores relacionados com o aumento do risco de morte são idade avançada, grande tumor hipofisário e aumento das concentrações plasmáticas de ACTHe. Fatores associados à recidiva da doença foram grande tumor hipofisário, osso esfenoide espesso, alta relação cortisol:creatinina urinária e aumento das concentrações plasmáticas de alfa-MSH antes da cirurgia.[148] Uma modificação da abordagem transesfenoidal, utilizando-se a localização tomográfica da sela túrcica com um sistema de telescopia por vídeo de alta definição, vem sendo utilizada em cães com HAC. A taxa relatada de sobrevida em 1 ano foi > 80%.[149]

Radioterapia para hiperadrenocorticismo hipófise-dependente

Redução do tamanho do tumor

A radioterapia por cobalto-60 tem o potencial de reduzir de modo considerável o tamanho de um tumor hipofisário visível em cães com HHD sem sinais neurológicos.[150] Em um estudo, 6 cães receberam doses de radiação de 44 Gy divididas em 11 frações iguais utilizando-se uma unidade de telecobalto-60. As concentrações plasmáticas de ACTHe diminuíram momentaneamente em todos os cães; entretanto, os sinais clínicos de HAC foram resolvidos em somente 3/6 cães e recidivaram em 2 daqueles 3. Um ano após a radioterapia, nenhum tumor foi visualizado em 4 cães, com a diminuição de 25% em 2. Nenhum cão desenvolveu anormalidades neurológicas. Para cães com grandes tumores hipofisários, a experiência com a radioterapia é variável.[45,151,152] Em 24 cães com macrotumores hipofisários e sinais neurológicos tratados com radiação por megavoltagem (48 Gy durante 4 semanas em uma programação em dias alternados de 4 Gy/fração), foi observada uma correlação significativa entre tamanho relativo do tumor (i. e., tamanho do tumor com relação ao tamanho do calvário), gravidade dos sinais neurológicos e remissão desses sinais após radioterapia.[151] Com o aumento da gravidade dos sinais neurológicos, o prognóstico piorou. Esse foi o fator prognóstico mais confiável. Como a radioterapia é mais efetiva em cães com tumores relativamente pequenos, o tratamento precoce deve melhorar o prognóstico e a longevidade. Recomendou-se que cães com tumores hipofisários iguais ou maiores que 8 mm, na sua maior altura vertical, sejam submetidos à radioterapia como forma de terapia inicial.[45] Como ela encolhe os tumores de maneira efetiva, mas é muito menos bem-sucedida em resolver a HAC clínica, o uso do tratamento medicamentoso deve ser antecipado. Existem poucas complicações. As desvantagens da radioterapia incluem o custo e a disponibilidade.

Resposta clínica

Tumores hipofisários são relativamente sensíveis à radioterapia. Pode-se observar a melhora considerável e relativamente rápida em alguns cães, apesar dos sinais neurológicos iniciais graves. Em geral, o prognóstico e a gravidade dos sinais clínicos estão inversamente relacionados: cães com sinais neurológicos graves e um tumor > 20 mm em seu maior diâmetro apresentam prognóstico muito pior do que aqueles com sinais mais discretos e um tumor < 20 mm.

Ao mesmo tempo que alguns cães melhoraram durante a radioterapia, outros precisaram de semanas ou meses para tal. Portanto, os tutores devem ser encorajados a permitir que os cães levem muitos meses para responder ao tratamento.

Resposta endócrina

Na maioria dos cães com HHD, a radioterapia exerce pouco ou nenhum efeito ou somente uma influência transitória sobre a natureza secretora do tumor. Portanto, o tratamento medicamentoso costuma ser necessário para o controle do HAC, apesar do encolhimento do tumor. A recidiva dos sinais neurológicos semanas a anos depois é possível, mas rara. Em tais cães, a deterioração pode ser rápida. A TC ou a RM poderiam ser recomendadas para cada cão diagnosticado como HHD, mas especialmente para aqueles que apresentam resistência à dexametasona no TSBDD ou no TSADD. A radioterapia é aconselhável para cães com tumores > 7 mm, independentemente da presença ou da ausência de sinais neurológicos.[150]

Radiocirurgia estereotática (RCE)

A RCE fornece uma grande dose de radiação a um alvo bem definido e vem sendo utilizada em cães com tumores hipofisários.[153] O tratamento por RCE requer apenas um único procedimento anestésico, possui menos reações adversas agudas e os tempos de sobrevida em estudos iniciais parecem comparáveis à radioterapia convencional.

Tratamento: tumores adrenocorticais funcionais

Contexto geral

O tratamento ideal para cães com TAF causador de HAC é a remoção cirúrgica do tumor. A cirurgia pode ser terapêutica, permanente e requerer terapia a longo prazo. Entretanto, alguns cães com TAF são tratados com medicamentos. As razões para a terapia medicamentosa incluem: melhorar a condição clínica do paciente antes da cirurgia, um tumor inoperável, metástases no momento do diagnóstico, ser um mau candidato à cirurgia ou decisão do tutor. O fármaco adrenocorticolítico mitotano (o,p'-DDD) pode ser utilizado na tentativa de destruir o tumor, o que é raramente é alcançado.[154] O trilostano é eficaz para o controle dos sinais de HAC, melhorando a qualidade de vida, e os tempos de sobrevida são semelhantes àqueles obtidos com a cirurgia ou o emprego de mitotano.[155,156] Em cães diagnosticados com TAF, o trilostano pré-cirúrgico (0,2 a 1 mg/kg VO, a cada 12 h) é recomendado para a resolução dos sinais clínicos e anormalidades laboratoriais (que poderiam demorar 1 a 2 meses). A cirurgia é então realizada em um indivíduo mais sadio.

Adrenalectomia

A adrenalectomia cirúrgica é considerada o tratamento de escolha para tumores adrenais. A adrenalectomia, por celiotomia ou laparoscopia, é tecnicamente desafiadora, devendo ser realizada por um cirurgião experiente. Complicações pós-cirúrgicas, incluindo pancreatite, pneumonia, tromboembolia pulmonar, lesão renal aguda/oligúria/anúria, sepse, coagulação intravascular disseminada e hipoadrenocorticismo, são preocupantes, mas menos comuns após pré-tratamento apropriado.[45] Complicações trans e pós-cirúrgicas foram relatadas em uma porcentagem bastante variável de cães com TAF.[157-162] À medida que a habilidade cirúrgica e o manejo do paciente melhoram, as taxas de morbidade e mortalidade diminuem. A mortalidade perioperatória (13,5 a 30%) está diminuindo; espera-se que o uso de tecnologia minimamente invasiva (laparoscopia) diminua ainda mais a mortalidade e a morbidade.[157-162]

Fatores prognósticos

Em uma revisão de cães com TAF tratados com adrenalectomia, tamanho do tumor (≥ 5 cm), metástases a distância e trombose venosa (veia cava) foram associados a um prognóstico pior.[161] Em um outro, a invasão da veia cava caudal foi associada a uma maior taxa de mortalidade cirúrgica, mas não afetou o prognóstico a longo prazo.[162] O tempo de sobrevida mediano de cães com TAF submetidos à adrenalectomia é de cerca de 2 a 4 anos.[160-162] É importante lembrar que a idade média ao diagnóstico é de cerca de 11 anos.

Pré-cirúrgico

Antes da adrenalectomia, o HAC deve ser tratado e controlado com trilostano. Imediatamente antes da cirurgia, os resultados do hemograma, do perfil bioquímico sérico e das radiografias torácicas devem ser avaliados. A repetição da ultrassonografia é útil não apenas para a visualização do tumor, mas também para a pesquisa de evidências de metástases ou trombose venosa tumoral (Vídeo 306.5). A ultrassonografia possui sensibilidade relatada de 100% e especificidade de 96% na identificação correta de metástases abdominais.[163] A secreção autônoma de cortisol pelo tumor resulta em atrofia da glândula contralateral, sendo assim necessária a suplementação com glicocorticoide nos períodos trans e pós-cirúrgico. Fluidos IV devem ser administrados em uma taxa de manutenção no início da anestesia, durante a cirurgia e no período pós-cirúrgico (ver Capítulo 129). Assim que o cirurgião reconhecer o tumor adrenal, a dexametasona deve ser colocada em um frasco de infusão IV, na dose de 0,05 a 0,1 mg/kg, e administrada durante um período de 6 horas. Ela deve ser administrada 2 a 3 vezes/dia, até que a medicação oral possa ser tolerada.[29] A hidrocortisona, com atividade glicocorticoide e mineralocorticoide, pode substituir a dexametasona. Durante a cirurgia, a hidrocortisona pode ser administrada por via intravenosa (4 a 5 mg/kg) e, depois, 1 mg/kg IV, a cada 6 horas, até que a medicação oral seja tolerada. Um TEACTH, concluído na manhã após a cirurgia e cerca de 8 horas após a última dose de dexametasona, ajuda a determinar se o tumor foi completamente excisado (concentrações séricas baixas de cortisol antes e após ACTH) e a necessidade de manutenção da suplementação com glicocorticoide.

Pós-cirúrgico

O monitoramento intensivo pós-cirúrgico é essencial para prevenção ou resposta a complicações. A hiperpotassemia e/ou a hiponatremia devem ser tratadas com mineralocorticoides (ver Capítulo 309): fludrocortisona oral (0,01 a 0,02 mg/kg, a cada 12 h) ou pivalato de desoxicorticosterona IM (2,2 mg/kg por via subcutânea [SC], a cada 21 a 25 dias). Anormalidades eletrolíticas podem refletir as deficiências mineralocorticoides e, de modo geral, são, mas não sempre, transitórias, com duração de apenas alguns poucos dias. Antibióticos, analgesia e heparina (75 UI/kg, SC, a cada 8 h) são recomendados.[162] O tratamento pré-cirúrgico com trilostano, durante 1 ou 2 meses, pode suspender a necessidade de heparina. A prednisona oral deve ser considerada para todos os cães cujos resultados pós-cirúrgicos do TEACTH estavam abaixo do normal. Uma dose inicial de 0,5 mg/kg, VO, a cada 12 h, durante 3 dias, e então ajustada para 0,2 mg/kg/dia, durante 2 a 4 semanas. Resultados de um TEACTH realizado nesse momento, e meses depois, devem ser utilizados para determinar a necessidade de manutenção da suplementação com glicocorticoide.

Tratamento medicamentoso de tumores adrenocorticais: mitotano

Quando o paciente não é um bom candidato à cirurgia adrenal, o mitotano é uma opção alternativa para tentar a destruição completa ou parcial do tumor adrenal. Cães com TAF podem ser tratados com o protocolo padrão do mitotano previamente descrito para cães com HHD (ver tratamento com mitotano para HHD), mas em uma dose diária de 50 a 75 mg/kg VO. Um teste de estimulação por ACTH é realizado a cada 10 a 14 dias para avaliar a reserva adrenal. Administra-se um glicocorticoide oral (p. ex., prednisona ou prednisolona, 0,2 mg/kg/dia) durante todo o período de administração do mitotano, a fim de tentar evitar sinais clínicos de hipoadrenocorticismo. A administração diária do mitotano (dose de ataque) é mantida nessa dose ou aumentada até que os teores de cortisol desejados sejam alcançados ou ocorra intolerância ao fármaco. Em cães com TAF, esse período de ataque costuma ser mais longo, em comparação àqueles com HHD, com dose de indução de mitotano cumulativa até 10 vezes

maior do que em cães com HHD. Assim que as concentrações adequadas de cortisol pós-ACTH forem alcançadas, a dose de manutenção do mitotano é iniciada em 75 a 100 mg/kg, VO, semanalmente, em doses divididas, em conjunto com a suplementação diária de glicocorticoide. Em cães com tumores adrenais, uma dose de manutenção de mitotano também costuma ser maior do que 100 mg/kg, sendo comuns recidivas durante o tratamento (mais de 60% dos cães).[164] O trilostano é preferido ao mitotano, pois é mais eficaz no controle dos sinais clínicos. Os efeitos adversos relacionados com o mitotano, observados em até 60% dos cães tratados, incluem anorexia, fraqueza, êmese, diarreia e letargia, os quais podem ocorrer em razão do desenvolvimento de hipoadrenocorticismo; mas, em aproximadamente 50% deles, ocorrem em razão da toxicidade direta do fármaco.[164] Se ocorrerem reações adversas, o fármaco deve ser interrompido e o cão avaliado o mais rápido possível, já que pode ocorrer deficiência completa de glicocorticoides e mineralocorticoides (doença de Addison). Se houver suspeita de intoxicação, o mitotano deve ser descontinuado e reiniciado 5 a 7 dias depois, com uma dose 25 a 50% menor. Pode-se tentar a reinstituição da dose de manutenção maior posteriormente, o que costuma resultar em recidiva das reações adversas. Nessa situação, um tratamento diferente (trilostano) pode ser escolhido.

Tratamento medicamentoso do TAF: trilostano

Demonstrou-se eficácia do trilostano no controle dos sinais clínicos de hipercortisolismo em cães com TAF.[155,156,165,166] Ademais, o tempo de sobrevida de cães com TAF tratados com trilostano (mediana 11,5 a 14 meses) é semelhante àquele observado naqueles tratados com mitotano (mediana 3 a 15,6 meses).[155,156] Assim, o trilostano é o melhor tratamento medicamentoso para cães com TAF.

COMPLICAÇÕES E CONDIÇÕES CONCOMITANTES ASSOCIADAS AO HIPERADRENOCORTICISMO

Tumores hipofisários grandes

Definições

Aproximadamente 50% dos cães com HHD apresentam tumor visível nos exames de TC ou RM no momento do diagnóstico. Sinais neurológicos causados pela expansão de um tumor hipofisário são observados em aproximadamente 15 a 20% dos cães com HHD, incluindo um pequeno número dos quais com sinais, quando inicialmente diagnosticados com HAC. A maioria o é algum tempo após o início do tratamento.[100] A melhora do tratamento medicamentoso a longo prazo de cães com HHD pode simplesmente fornecer tempo suficiente para que tumores menores, que representam a maioria dos casos no momento do diagnóstico de HHD, se expandam a ponto de causar sinais clínicos. A maioria dos cães com HHD, com sinais causados por um grande tumor, foi tratada de forma medicamentosa por mais de 6 meses, e alguns por mais do que vários anos. Tumores hipofisários costumam ser categorizados de acordo com o tamanho: macrotumores ($\geq$ 10 mm no seu maior diâmetro) ou microtumores (< 10 mm). Essas designações arbitrárias, entretanto, possuem pouca utilidade clínica.[72] Manifestações clínicas de um tumor hipofisário em crescimento não correspondem somente ao tamanho, mas podem estar relacionadas com a velocidade de crescimento, o tamanho da cavidade craniana ou a existência de inflamação peritumoral, edema ou hemorragia. Parece mais apropriado utilizar o termo "macrotumor" para descrever tumores visíveis por meios de TC ou RM e "microtumor" para aqueles visualizados apenas por microscopia.[45]

Sinais, diagnóstico, tratamento

O início dos sinais neurológicos pode preceder, coincidir ou seguir (mais comumente) o diagnóstico e o tratamento medicamentoso a longo prazo do HAC. Em geral, os sinais clínicos iniciais associados a um tumor hipofisário em expansão são diminuições sutis no apetite e alterações no comportamento notadas apenas por alguém extremamente familiarizado com o cão. Outros sinais de início lento e progressivo são apatia, indiferença ao ambiente, inquietude, perda de interesse em atividades normais, episódios de desorientação aparente e perda grave do apetite e de peso. Posteriormente no curso da doença, os sinais podem incluir ataxia, andar compulsivo, andar em círculos, estupor e convulsões. A confirmação antes da morte de um tumor hipofisário requer exames de imagem avançados, como TC ou RM. A radioterapia ou a hipofisectomia são opções terapêuticas disponíveis, discutidas anteriormente (ver Tratamento cirúrgico do hiperadrenocorticismo hipófise-dependente).

Hipertensão

Há hipertensão sistêmica, definida como pressão sanguínea sistólica maior que 160 mmHg (ver Capítulo 99), em 38 a 86% dos cães com HAC não tratado (ver Capítulo 157).[55,167] A hipertensão sistêmica pode levar à proteinúria, quase sempre observada em cães com HAC (44 a 68%). Ambas podem melhorar ou cessar após o tratamento, mas nenhuma das condições é resolvida em todos os cães tratados.[55] As taxas de filtração glomerular estão aumentadas antes do tratamento e diminuem com a terapia para HHD. A persistência de proteinúria ou hipertensão após o tratamento bem-sucedido do HAC deve justificar a atenção.[55] As concentrações plasmáticas de aldosterona podem contribuir para hipertensão em cães com HAC não tratado. Entretanto, diversos estudos observaram que teores de aldosterona costumam estar abaixo do normal em cães com

HHD, porém altos naqueles com TAF.[167,168] Mais estudos são necessários para elucidar o mecanismo da hipertensão em cães com HAC. A proteinúria e a hipertensão sistêmica (presentes em até 80% dos cães com HAC não tratado) são fatores importantes no desenvolvimento e na progressão da doença renal crônica, devendo ser monitoradas em cães com HAC com hipertensão persistente, apesar do bom controle dessa condição.

Diabetes melito (ver Capítulo 304)

O diagnóstico de HAC em cães já diagnosticados com diabetes melito (DM) não deve ser complicado, assumindo que os sinais clássicos de HAC sejam observados. Por exemplo, PU (com densidade urinária < 1,008), alopecia bilateral simétrica, abdome abaulado, pele delgada, respiração ofegante, calcinose cutânea e NUS baixo são típicos de HAC, mas não de DM. Já que os sinais mais comuns de DM são os mesmos que aqueles do HAC (PU/PD/PF), o diagnóstico em diabéticos mal controlados com apenas esses sinais deve ser questionado. O uso apropriado de testes de triagem aumenta sua sensibilidade e especificidade, mas eles nunca devem ser utilizados como o único indicador de HAC. O diagnóstico ultrassonográfico de adrenomegalia é inespecífico. Nenhum auxílio diagnóstico é tão sensível e específico como o histórico e o exame físico.

REFERÊNCIAS BIBLIOGRÁFICAS

As referências bibliográficas deste capítulo se encontram online no Ambiente de Aprendizagem.

CAPÍTULO 307

Hiperadrenocorticismo Felino

Ian K. Ramsey e Michael E. Herrtage

INTRODUÇÃO

O hiperadrenocorticismo (HAC; síndrome de Cushing) felino é menos comum, porém mais grave e desafiador em diagnosticar ou tratar do que o HAC canino. O HAC felino possui um prognóstico pior do que a condição em cães. Ao contrário do que acontece com os cães, o HAC felino está fortemente associado a diabetes melito (DM) e/ou síndrome da hiperfragilidade cutânea, podendo ambas as condições complicar o tratamento. A fisiopatologia básica e outros aspectos do HAC felino são semelhantes ao canino (ver Capítulo 306). O foco deste capítulo está na condição clínica resultante da produção crônica excessiva de cortisol ou outros hormônios com ação semelhante a ele. Gatos com tumores adrenocorticais secretores de progesterona podem apresentar sinais clínicos compatíveis com HAC felino (ver Capítulo 308).[1,2] Alguns tumores adrenocorticais podem causar hiperaldosteronismo primário (ver Capítulo 308).

FISIOPATOLOGIA

O HAC felino é um distúrbio multissistêmico resultante da produção excessiva de cortisol pelo córtex adrenal. Existem relatos de caso únicos que descrevem gatos com HAC e muitas

séries de casos que, em conjunto, totalizam mais de 100.[3-24] Tanto o HAC hipófise-dependente (HHD) – causado pela secreção excessiva pela hipófise do hormônio adrenocorticotrófico (ACTH, do inglês *adrenocorticotropic hormone*) – como o HAC adrenal-dependente (HAD) – causado por um tumor adrenocortical funcional – foram relatados em gatos.[4] Aproximadamente 85% dos gatos com HAC de ocorrência natural possuem HHD e os 15% restantes HAD. HAD pode ser causado por um tumor adrenocortical benigno ou maligno. Relatou-se um pequeno número de gatos com tumores hipofisários multi-hormonais, incluindo tumores secretores de ACTH causadores de HHD.[18,25-28] O HAC iatrogênico foi descrito em gatos, associado à administração de glicocorticoides ou progestágenos.[29-31] O progestágeno acetato de megestrol, um esteroide particularmente potente em gatos, pode causar supressão adrenocortical prolongada após descontinuação.[32]

SINAIS CLÍNICOS

Contexto geral

Muitos dos gatos inicialmente diagnosticados com HAC apresentaram sinais clínicos consideráveis e óbvios, presentes durante vários meses antes do diagnóstico. Atualmente, o HAC felino está se tornando mais bem reconhecido, com variações na apresentação clínica e distúrbios bioquímicos associado mais bem apreciados.[6] O diagnóstico mais precoce pode evitar sinais clínicos graves, sobretudo na população felina diabética (Tabela 307.1 e Figura 307.1).

Idade, raça e sexo

O HAC felino é mais comum em gatos de meia-idade a idosos (a idade mediana em diversos estudos foi de 9,5 a 13 anos; variação de 3 a 15 anos). Parece não haver predileção sexual ou racial.

Alterações cutâneas

Manifestações cutâneas do HAC felino incluem alopecia de tronco e abdome, mas com muito menos frequência do que em cães. Um pelame desgrenhado e seborreico é comum. A pele delgada é predisposta a úlceras induzidas por trauma, hematomas e infecções secundárias bacterianas ou fúngicas (Figuras 307.2 e 307.3). A pele hiperfrágil costuma causar aflição em tutores e clínicos desavisados. Gatos com HAC devem sempre ser tratados com cautela (Figuras 307.4 e 307.5). A calcinose cutânea ainda não foi relatada no HAC de ocorrência natural ou iatrogênica.

Tabela 307.1 Frequência aproximada de achados clínicos no hiperadrenocorticismo felino.

ACHADOS	FREQUÊNCIA (%)
Diabetes melito concomitante	79
Poliúria/polidipsia	79
Polifagia	60
Distensão abdominal	54
Alopecia/falha no crescimento do pelo	43
Hiperfragilidade cutânea/úlceras espontâneas	40
Perda de peso/atrofia muscular	31
Fraqueza/letargia	29
Ganho de peso/obesidade	23
Pelame ruim (seco, seborreico etc.)	15

Com base nos dados fornecidos em sete séries de casos publicadas com um total combinado de 77 casos.[3-6,8-10] Note que três dessas séries (um total de 30 casos) foram selecionadas por modalidade terapêutica; entretanto, não houve diferença aparente nos sinais apresentados.

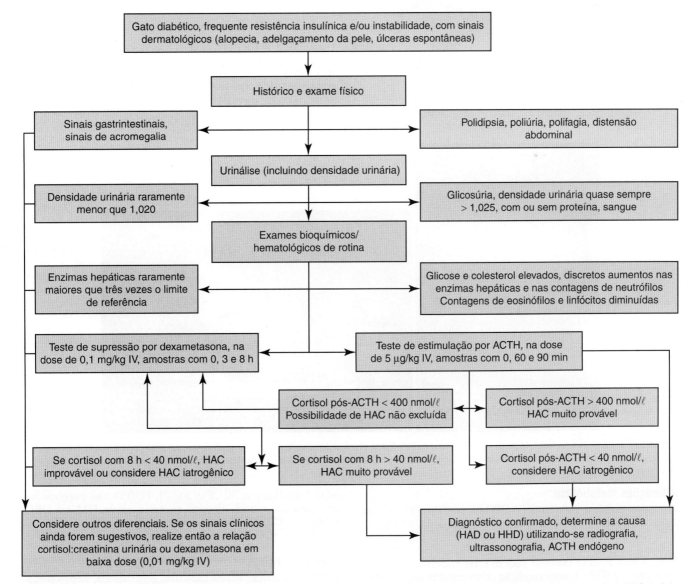

Figura 307.1 Abordagem diagnóstica a um gato com suspeita de hiperadrenocorticismo. Note que 400 nmol/ℓ = 14,5 µg/dℓ e 40 nmol/ℓ = 1,4 µg/dℓ. ACTH, hormônio adrenocorticotrófico; HAC, hiperadrenocorticismo; HAD, hiperadrenocorticismo adrenal-dependente; HHD, hiperadrenocorticismo hipófise-dependente.

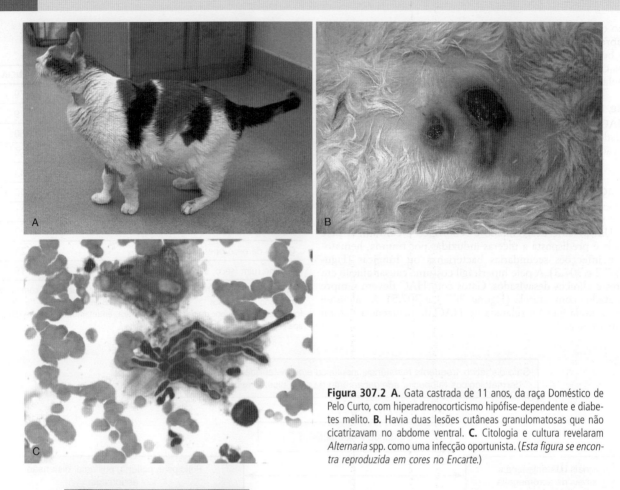

Figura 307.2 A. Gata castrada de 11 anos, da raça Doméstico de Pelo Curto, com hiperadrenocorticismo hipófise-dependente e diabetes melito. **B.** Havia duas lesões cutâneas granulomatosas que não cicatrizavam no abdome ventral. **C.** Citologia e cultura revelaram *Alternaria* spp. como uma infecção oportunista. (*Esta figura se encontra reproduzida em cores no Encarte.*)

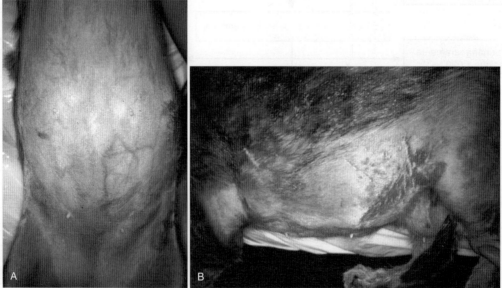

Figura 307.3 Gata castrada com 5 anos, da raça Doméstico de Pelo Curto, com hiperadrenocorticismo hipófise-dependente. Existe extensa alopecia ventral (**A**) e fragilidade cutânea evidenciada por cicatrizes oriundas de reparos cirúrgicos de úlceras cutâneas (**B**). (*Esta figura se encontra reproduzida em cores no Encarte.*)

Alterações metabólicas

Em gatos, poliúria, polidipsia (PU/PD) e polifagia (PF) são os sinais metabólicos mais comumente relatados de HAC. PU/PD e PF costumam estar associadas ao DM induzido por glicocorticoides, com consequente glicosúria e diurese osmótica. No HAC felino, PU/PD também podem estar associadas à doença renal crônica (DRC), uma condição concomitante rara em cães com HAC. A perda de peso pode ser observada no HAC felino, mas alguns gatos apresentam ganho de peso, apesar do DM mal controlado (Figuras 307.6 e 307.7). PU/PD não parecem ser uma característica da doença na ausência de DM ou DRC. Assim, PU/PD não podem ser utilizadas para reconhecer os estágios iniciais da doença.

Alterações físicas

Abdome pendular, atrofia muscular generalizada, hepatomegalia e ganho de peso são comuns. Uma minoria de gatos acometidos perde peso e alguns possuem a língua menos áspera.

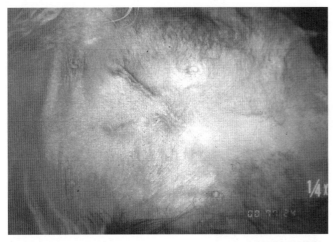

Figura 307.4 Gato Doméstico de Pelo Longo, de 10 anos, pele delgada frágil e alopecia ventral abdominal. (*Esta figura se encontra reproduzida em cores no Encarte.*)

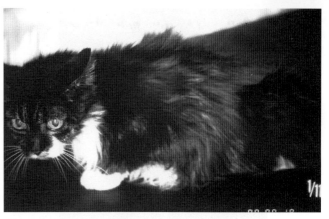

Figura 307.6 Gato Doméstico de Pelo Longo, de 10 anos, com hiperadrenocorticismo, diabetes e perda de peso significativa. O pelame está em más condições.

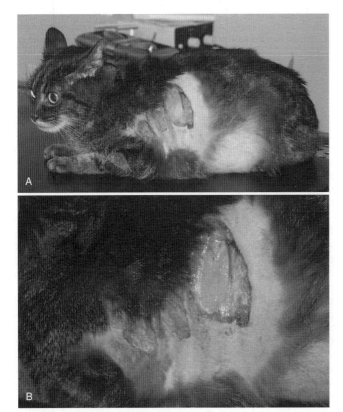

Figura 307.5 Gata castrada de 9 anos, da raça Doméstico de Pelo Curto, com hiperadrenocorticismo hipófise-dependente. **A.** Úlceras cutâneas espontâneas. **B.** Imagem aproximada. (*Esta figura se encontra reproduzida em cores no Encarte.*)

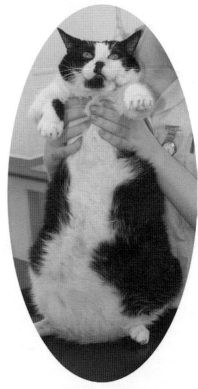

Figura 307.7 Gata castrada de 9 anos, da raça Doméstico de Pelo Curto, com hiperadrenocorticismo hipófise-dependente. Ela está obesa, com abdome pendular (peso corporal de 10 kg), apesar de cetoacidose diabética e pancreatite.

Ocasionalmente, são observadas úlceras ao longo da periferia da língua (Figura 307.8), embora não tenham sido relatadas em nenhuma série de casos.

DOENÇAS CONCOMITANTES

A maioria dos gatos diagnosticados com HAC também apresenta DM; em uma série de casos, 27 de 30.[10] Diversas outras séricas indicaram que uma maioria, mas não todos os gatos com HAC, possui DM concomitante.[6,9]

Gatos com DM e HAC concomitantes costumam ser resistentes à insulina, necessitando de grandes doses diárias de insulina ($\approx$ 2 unidades/kg) para controlar a hiperglicemia e a glicosúria.[3,6]

Vários gatos com HAC desenvolvem infecções, algumas vezes incomuns, mas quase sempre difíceis de resolver.[3,8,10,16] Essa aparente predisposição a infecções sugere que gatos com HAC sejam mais imunossuprimidos do que cães com essa condição ou que, por conta tanto da pele frágil quanto do DM e de outras condições concomitantes, haja aumento da gravidade de infecções.

Gatos com HAC podem ter DRC concomitante (ver Capítulo 324). Não existem evidências de correlação direta entre as duas condições nem que a presença de uma dificulta o tratamento da outra.[10] A incidência de gatos com ambas as condições é muito maior do que de cães com HAC. A maioria dos gatos com HAC, com densidade urinária < 1,020. também apresentava DRC. Gatos com HAC também podem desenvolver pancreatite (ver Capítulo 291), mas o efeito do aumento das concentrações de cortisol sobre a imunorreatividade da lipase pancreática felina (PLIf) ainda não foi investigado. Diferentemente do que se

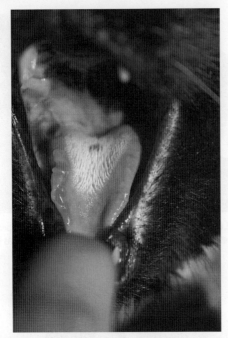

Figura 307.8 Úlcera na língua de um gato com hiperadrenocorticismo. As papilas (cerdas) na língua eram mais macias do que o normal.

Tabela 307.2 Frequência aproximada de achados clinicopatológicos no hiperadrenocorticismo felino.

ACHADOS	FREQUÊNCIA
Bioquímicos	
Hiperglicemia	> 43 de 47 (> 91%)
Hipercolesterolemia	> 16 de 31 (> 51%)
Aumento da alanina aminotransferase	16 de 45 (35%)
Aumento da fosfatase alcalina	11 de 46 (24%)
Urinálise	
Glicosúria	> 41 de 47 (> 87%)
Densidade urinária < 1,030	10 de 28 (36%)
Proteinúria	23 de 29 (79%)
Hematológicos	
Anemia	16 de 44 (36%)
Neutrofilia	21 de 39 (54%)
Linfopenia	26 de 45 (58%)
Eosinófilos indetectáveis	7 de 11 (63%)

Oriundos de dados fornecidos em quatro séries publicadas de casos não selecionados, com um total combinado de 47 casos.[3,4,6,10]

presume acontecer com os cães, a PLIf pode não ser um indicador confiável de pancreatite em gatos com HAC,[10,33] sendo 20% deles hipertensos (ver Capítulo 99), menos comum do que no HAC canino.[10,34] A cegueira aguda decorrente do deslocamento bilateral de retina foi relatada em um gato hipertenso com HAC (ver Capítulo 157).[22]

EXAMES LABORATORIAIS GERAIS E DE IMAGEM

Bioquímica sérica, hemograma, urinálise

Hiperglicemia, observada em aproximadamente 80% dos gatos com HAC, é a anormalidade laboratorial mais comum. A maior parte desses gatos também tem DM evidente, mas costuma haver hiperglicemia mesmo naqueles que não o apresentam (Tabela 307.2). A hipercolesterolemia foi relatada em cerca de 50% dos gatos com HAC, provavelmente relacionada com DM mal controlado e aumento da lipólise. Em uma revisão, > 50% dos gatos com HAC também apresentavam aumentos do nitrogênio ureico sanguíneo (NUS) e > 25% nas concentrações de NUS e creatinina.[35] Ao contrário de cães, gatos não apresentam a isoenzima induzida por esteroides da fosfatase alcalina (ALP), cuja meia-vida felina é mais curta. Há aumentos discretos na atividade de ALP em cerca de 30% dos gatos com HAC. Incrementos na ALP e na enzima hepatocelular alanina aminotransferase (ALT) estão provavelmente relacionadas com o DM. A distribuição dos leucócitos esperada na hipercortisolemia, na linfopenia, na eosinopenia e na neutrofilia ocorre de forma incompatível em gatos com HAC. Apesar de uma diurese induzida pela glicose em casos de HAC e DM, gatos não diabéticos com HAC parecem capazes de manter as densidades urinárias > 1,020. Em comparação a cães com HAC, gatos tendem a ter alterações físicas mais consideráveis e clinicopatológicas menos acentuadas.

Exames diagnósticos de imagem

Visão geral

Avanços no diagnóstico por imagem melhoraram a capacidade dos médicos-veterinários em identificar um tumor hipofisário ou aumento adrenal bilateral em gatos com HHD e tumores adrenais em gatos com HAD, assim como invasão de vasos ou órgãos, quase sempre por um tumor adrenal maligno. Essa informação pode ser utilizada para delinear o tratamento para cada indivíduo. Entretanto, a identificação de um tumor hipofisário ou adrenal não necessariamente indica a função. Portanto, o diagnóstico por imagem deve sempre ser interpretado dentro do contexto dos sinais clínicos e resultados de testes endócrinos.

Radiografia

A avaliação radiográfica do tórax e do abdome é aconselhável a todos os gatos com suspeita ou comprovação de HAC. Embora a informação "diagnóstica" seja obtida apenas no pequeno número de gatos nos quais o aumento adrenal pode ser detectado (Figura 307.9), radiografias simples torácicas e abdominais podem permitir a identificação de anormalidades concomitantes, que podem alterar o plano terapêutico e/ou prognóstico. Costuma haver realce do contraste abdominal pelo aumento acentuado da gordura intra-abdominal. Nem a osteopenia induzida por esteroides nem os urólitos com cálcio foram relatados em gatos com HAC. Em gatos com HAC, a atividade do hormônio paratireoidiano não foi relatada.[36] Em cães, a mineralização adrenal está quase sempre associada a neoplasias adrenais benignas ou malignas. Entretanto, a calcificação adrenal pode ser um achado benigno e acidental em gatos idosos (Figura 307.10).

Ultrassonografia abdominal

A utilização de equipamentos de ultrassonografia de alta resolução e um ultrassonografista experiente costumam identificar ambas as adrenais na maioria dos gatos saudáveis (ver Capítulo 88). As melhores imagens de adrenal são obtidas pela varredura, com o emprego de abordagens lateral intercostal direita e esquerda e abdominal. A glândula adrenal direita é mais difícil de identificar em razão da localização cranial mais profunda sob as costelas. Glândulas adrenais felinas normais são ovais a bilobadas e hipoecoicas, quando comparadas aos tecidos adjacentes. A medula adrenal saudável pode ser discretamente hiperecoica, quando comparada ao córtex, mas nem sempre é claramente visível. Glândulas adrenais felinas saudáveis possuem aproximadamente 4,5 a 13,7 mm de comprimento e 2,9 a 5,3 mm de espessura.[37]

CAPÍTULO 307 • Hiperadrenocorticismo Felino 1833

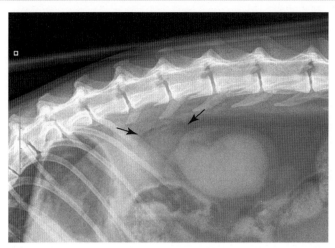

Figura 307.9 Radiografia abdominal lateral direita de Gato Doméstico de Pelo Curto, de 12 anos, castrado, com hiperadrenocorticismo decorrente de um tumor adrenal (*setas*).

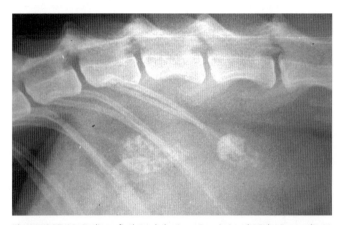

Figura 307.10 Radiografia lateral de Gato Doméstico de Pelo Curto, de 10 anos, com glândulas adrenais calcificadas. Isso pode ser um achado acidental em gatos idosos, não necessariamente associado à função adrenal anormal.

O desafio para o ultrassonografista é distinguir glândulas normais daquelas hiperplásicas ou neoplásicas. Embora as glândulas adrenais de gatos com HHD tenham sido caracterizadas como simetricamente aumentadas e de conformação normal, o diagnóstico de hiperplasia adrenal pode ser subjetivo. Adrenais hiperplásicas tendem a ser maiores e mais fáceis de identificar do que glândulas saudáveis, mas ainda devem ter um padrão hipoecoico homogêneo (Figura 307.11). A ultrassonografia pode aumentar a suspeita da existência de um tumor adrenal (Figura 307.12). Apesar de terem sido relatados tumores adrenais bilaterais, eles são raros.[2,3] Tumores adrenais malignos possuem propensão a invadir vasos sanguíneos próximos e tecidos circundantes. Assim, deve-se realizar a avaliação ultrassonográfica minuciosa dos vasos adjacentes e tecidos. Se um tumor adrenal for identificado, o fígado, o baço e os rins também devem ser examinados com cuidado em busca de evidências de metástases.

Tomografia computadorizada e ressonância magnética

Imagens por tomografia computadorizada (TC) e ressonância magnética (RM) provaram ser úteis no diagnóstico de tumores e hiperplasia adrenais e tumores hipofisários. A TC abdominal contrastada também pode ajudar a identificar a invasão tumoral da veia cava caudal ou de outros vasos sanguíneos ou aderências na área do tumor. Essas considerações compreendem algumas das necessárias para o planejamento cirúrgico de gatos para os quais a adrenalectomia é uma opção.

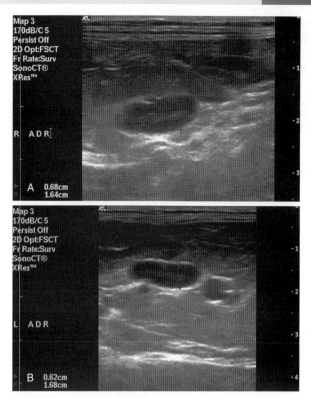

Figura 307.11 Ultrassonografias da glândula adrenal direita (**A**) e esquerda (**B**) de uma gata de 10 anos, da raça Doméstico de Pelo Curto, com hiperadrenocorticismo e diabetes melito. As glândulas adrenais estão aumentadas, com espessura maior que 0,53 cm (> 5,3 mm), e apresentam formato normal e tamanho semelhante, indicando que a causa é hipófise-dependente.

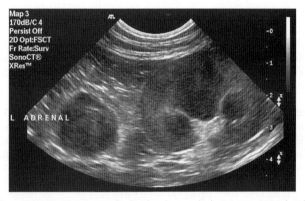

Figura 307.12 Ultrassonografia da adrenal esquerda de Gato Doméstico de Pelo Curto, castrado, de 12 anos, com hiperadrenocorticismo, mostrando uma lesão compatível com tumor adrenal, cuja causa é adrenal-dependente.

Não é clara a correlação entre tamanho do tumor hipofisário e presença ou desenvolvimento de sinais neurológicos. Naqueles gatos com sinais neurológicos, a avaliação por RM ou TC do cérebro é essencial, caso a cirurgia hipofisária ou a radioterapia for considerada.

TESTES ENDÓCRINOS

Visão geral (ver Figura 307.1)

O "melhor teste" para confirmação do diagnóstico do HAC felino ainda não foi estabelecido. Concentrações basais de cortisol têm pouca utilidade na avaliação da função adrenal em gatos, sendo, portanto, essencial o exame dinâmico (Tabela 307.3). A mensuração do cortisol no plasma felino ainda não foi sujeita

SEÇÃO 21 • Doenças Endócrinas

Tabela 307.3 Frequência aproximada de achados endócrinos no hiperadrenocorticismo felino.

TESTE	CRITÉRIOS PARA DIAGNÓSTICO DE HIPERADRENOCORTICISMO	FREQUÊNCIA
Teste de estimulação por ACTH	Cortisol 60 ou 90 min pós-ACTH maior que 400 nmol/ℓ (14,5 μg/dℓ)	28 de 39 (71%)
Teste de triagem de supressão por baixa dose (0,01 mg/kg/IV) de dexametasona positivo (maior que 27 nmol/ℓ [1 μg/dℓ])	8 h pós-dexametasona maior que 27 nmol/ℓ (1 μg/dℓ)	25 de 26 (96%)
Teste de supressão por dexametasona (0,1 mg/kg/IV)	8 h pós-dexametasona maior que 27 nmol/ℓ (1 μg/dℓ)	38 de 45 (84%)
ACTH endógeno	Maior que 20 pg/mℓ (= 4,4 pmol/ℓ) para diagnosticar HHD	14 de 19 (73%)
Ultrassonografia abdominal	Adrenomegalia bilateral ou adrenais simétricas (HHD) Tumor adrenal (HAD)	49 de 53 (92%)

Oriundos de dados fornecidos em oito séries de casos publicadas, com um combinado total de 84 casos.[3-10] Note que quatro dessas séries (total de 37 casos) foram selecionadas pela modalidade terapêutica.

a tantas análises quanto a concentração em cães. Mesmo adotando metodologias semelhantes, valores de referência gerados em laboratórios diferentes, utilizando máquinas diferentes, não podem ser utilizados de forma intercambiável.[38,39] Os clínicos devem, sempre que possível, utilizar valores de referência específicos do laboratório e consultar o pessoal antes de utilizar valores de outros laboratórios ou literatura para interpretação do teste.

Teste de estimulação por hormônio adrenocorticotrófico

O teste de estimulação por hormônio adrenocorticotrófico (TEACTH) pode ser útil para o diagnóstico de HAC felino. Entretanto, o pico da resposta é variável em gatos, tanto no que diz respeito ao momento quanto à magnitude. Devem-se obter amostras em 60 e 90 minutos após administração de tetracosactrina, na dose de 5 μg/kg ou 0,125 mg/gato IV.[40,41] A sensibilidade relatada do teste varia de 56 a 80%.[3,6,8,10] Gatos normais e aqueles com doenças crônicas raramente apresentam cortisol pós-ACTH > 400 nmol/ℓ (> 14,5 μg/dℓ).[42] Entretanto, algumas condições (p. ex., hipertireoidismo) podem resultar em concentrações pós-ACTH de cortisol de até 600 nmol/ℓ (21,7 μg/dℓ). Assim como no cão, os valores de cortisol > 600 nmol/ℓ (> 21,7 μg/dℓ) são bastante sugestivos, e valores entre 400 nmol/ℓ e 600 nmol/ℓ (14,5 e 21,7 μg/dℓ) dão suporte ao diagnóstico de HAC, no contexto dos sinais clínicos apropriados. Entretanto, gatos com HAC tendem a apresentar concentrações de cortisol menores do que cães com essa condição e raramente possuem concentrações de cortisol pós-ACTH > 800 nmol/ℓ (> 29 μg/dℓ). Um resultado do TEACTH dentro do intervalo de referência do laboratório não descarta o diagnóstico de HAC felino.

Testes de supressão por dexametasona

Tanto o grau quanto a duração da supressão adrenocortical causada pela dexametasona variam entre gatos saudáveis. Em geral, o teste de supressão por dexametasona (TSD) em "baixa dose" utiliza uma dose maior (0,1 mg/kg IV) em gatos do que

em cães. Em gatos saudáveis, as concentrações séricas de cortisol são suprimidas de forma confiável com essa dose e o exame é excelente se utilizado como um teste de triagem para distinguir gatos com HAC daqueles que não apresentam a condição. Entretanto, o teste também é utilizado para ajudar a discriminar o HAD do HHD sem evidências de que esse é um uso apropriado.[3,5,42] É importante salientar que as concentrações de cortisol após administração de 0,1 mg/kg de dexametasona são suprimidas em gatos com DM, mas não naqueles com HAC e DM, independentemente do controle glicêmico.[43] O TSD com 0,1 mg/kg apresenta boa especificidade. Entretanto, embora o cortisol não seja suprimido em 3 a 4 horas e 8 horas em gatos com HAD, há a supressão em alguns com HHD com 8 horas, reduzindo a sensibilidade. Recomenda-se que o TSD com baixa dose, utilizando-se a "dose canina" padrão (0,01 mg/kg IV; com amostras de sangue obtidas antes e 8 horas após a administração), seja utilizado para "triar" gatos para HAC.[3] Entretanto, 20% dos gatos saudáveis não suprimem após administração de 0,01 mg/kg.[44] Assim, o aumento da sensibilidade é compensado pela falta de especificidade. Esse "TSD em baixa dose" pode ser útil em determinadas circunstâncias, já que a "supressão normal" tornaria o diagnóstico de HAC bastante improvável. Da mesma forma, se um gato estiver apresentando sinais clínicos de HAC e uma "resposta normal" no TSD com dose de 0,1 mg/kg, então o teste com 0,01 mg/kg pode ser indicado. Em um estudo, quatro gatos realizaram ambos os testes de dexametasona, cujos resultados não alteraram o diagnóstico em nenhum dos animais.[10]

Relação corticoide:creatinina urinária

A urina deve ser sempre coletada em casa (e não no ambiente hospitalar), já que qualquer situação estressante pode aumentar a relação. Quase todos os gatos com HAC testarão positivo (boa sensibilidade), com a observação de resultados de testes falso-positivos naqueles com doença não adrenal (baixa especificidade).[45] É importante ressaltar que gatos hipertireóideos costumam apresentar aumento nos resultados na relação corticoide:creatinina urinária (RC:CU).[42,46] Assim, a RC:CU deve ser considerada como de baixa especificidade em um grupo de gatos com suspeita de HAC. Sabe-se que existem diferenças consideráveis entre testes para corticoides urinários no cão. Uma vez que isso também pode ser verdadeiro com relação à validade do teste para gatos, os resultados podem variar de acordo com o ensaio; assim, deve-se gerar uma referência individual para um teste específico, em vez de utilizar valores de referência publicados.[47,48]

Outros exames

Um protocolo combinado de TSD/TEACTH foi sugerido para gatos; entretanto, ele não foi suficientemente validado para que fosse recomendado. As concentrações de hormônios tireoidianos costumam estar normais em gatos com HAC, o que é importante, já que o hipertireoidismo pode ser considerado em qualquer animal com PU/PD e perda de peso. Em um estudo, 4 de 25 gatos com HAC apresentavam baixos teores de tiroxina.[10] Foi sugerido que os precursores de ACTH endógeno (pró-opiomelanocortina [POMC] e pró-ACTH) podem ser úteis na identificação de gatos com HHD.[49] Entretanto, tais testes ainda não estão amplamente disponíveis.

Testes para distinguir hiperadrenocorticismo hipófise-dependente de hiperadrenocorticismo adrenal-dependente

A confiabilidade de qualquer teste para distinguir gatos com HHD daqueles com HAD ainda não foi avaliada. As concentrações plasmáticas de ACTH endógeno devem estar normais ou aumentadas em gatos com HHD e baixas ou indetectáveis naqueles com um tumor adrenal. Esse teste parecer ser útil para distinguir o HHD do HAD, desde que o diagnóstico do HAC felino já tenha sido confirmado. Entretanto, é essencial que

CAPÍTULO 307 • Hiperadrenocorticismo Felino

qualquer exame seja validado para gatos.[9,10] Radiografia, ultrassonografia, TC e RM podem ser extremamente úteis para distinguir HHD do HAD.[3,6,7,49]

TRATAMENTO

Sempre que possível, gatos com HAC devem ser tratados. Haverá provável melhora do controle diabético caso o tratamento seja bem-sucedido, com a redução do risco de consequências adversas graves do HAC crônico (p. ex., hiperfragilidade cutânea e infecções incomuns ou difíceis de tratar).

Cirurgia

Hiperadrenocorticismo adrenal-dependente

Sempre que possível, tumores adrenais devem ser removidos cirurgicamente. Exames de imagem acurados por ultrassonografia abdominal ou TC contrastada devem ser empregados, se disponíveis, para avaliar invasões de vasos importantes ou rins. O hipoadrenocorticismo pós-cirúrgico é comum e requer tratamento com fludrocortisona ou pivalato de desoxicorticosterona (embora não tenha sido relatado). Prednisolona, necessária inicialmente, costuma ser ajustada com o passar do tempo. Gatos diabéticos podem sofrer remissão nos meses após a cirurgia. Aqueles que permanecerem diabéticos costumam necessitar de doses de insulina muito menores.[5] Relatou-se adrenalectomia por laparoscopia bem-sucedida, que deve ser considerada para o tratamento de neoplasia adrenal funcional unilateral em gatos quando os exames de imagem descartarem invasão intravascular e doença metastática.[50]

Hiperadrenocorticismo hipófise-dependente

Opções cirúrgicas para o HHD incluem hipofisectomia transesfenoidal e adrenalectomia bilateral.[5,7] Gatos cujo tratamento foi bem-sucedido para ambas as modalidades necessitam de terapia medicamentosa posteriormente. A hipofisectomia transesfenoidal é o único tratamento definitivo para HHD. O primeiro relato de 7 gatos com HHD submetidos à hipofisectomia transesfenoidal incluiu 2 que morreram dentro de semanas. Entretanto, o tratamento foi eficaz nos 5 sobreviventes. Com maior experiência no tratamento de doenças concomitantes e no fechamento cuidadoso do palato mole, haverá melhora nas taxas de sucesso.[7,51] É necessário tratamento pós-cirúrgico para o diabetes melito central (ver Capítulo 296). A reposição mineralocorticoide e glicocorticoide é em geral necessária durante várias semanas. Apesar das altas taxas de remissão iniciais em cães com HHD após hipofisectomia, a recidiva em aproximadamente 25% é preocupante.[52] Taxas semelhantes de recidiva podem ser observadas em gatos, embora não existam estudos publicados. A morbidade e a mortalidade parecem menores para gatos submetidos à adrenalectomia bilateral do que para cães; entretanto, complicações são frequentes.[5,6] A resolução ou a melhora do estado diabético pode ser observada nos meses após a cirurgia, mas prednisolona e fludrocortisona a longo prazo são necessárias. Dessa forma, a cirurgia não é uma opção razoável para gatos difíceis de medicar por via oral. Deve-se notar que as feridas cutâneas causadas por ulceração espontânea devem ser fechadas. Um dos autores observou que a cola tecidual é efetiva, evitando, assim, a necessidade de anestesia e risco maior de ulceração. A sutura também é possível.

Tratamento medicamentoso

Trilostano

O uso do trilostano, um inibidor competitivo da 3-beta-hidroxiesteroide desidrogenase, tem sido eficaz no tratamento de gatos com HAC.[8,9] Dos 20 gatos em duas séries, 17 sobreviveram por mais de 3 meses e vários por mais de 1 ano. Isso é muito melhor do que com qualquer outro tratamento medicamentoso.

Não existem estudos farmacocinéticos do trilostano ou de seus metabólitos em gatos; entretanto, com base em um caso no qual o cortisol foi mensurado sequencialmente, parece que o efeito sobre a produção desse hormônio é rápido, com duração de ação < 12 horas.[8] Fabricantes não recomendam que o trilostano seja utilizado se houver hepatopatia ou nefropatia concomitantes.

O trilostano deve ser administrado em uma dose inicial de 1 a 2 mg/kg, VO, a cada 24 horas. Entretanto, pareceria lógico administrá-lo na mesma frequência que a insulina. Se a insulina e o trilostano estiverem sendo utilizados 2 vezes/dia, a dose do trilostano também deve ser dividida, administrando-o em uma dose de 0,5 a 1 mg/kg, VO, a cada 12 horas. A reformulação costuma ser necessária. O trilostano parece ser bem tolerado e a melhora geralmente é observada em semanas.[9] Em uma série de 9 gatos com HAC e DM tratados com trilostano, os requerimentos de dose de insulina diminuíram, em média, em 36% em 6 gatos. Em um, houve aumento do requerimento da dose de insulina, sem ocorrência da remissão do DM.[9] Complicações importantes que podem ocorrer com o uso do trilostano incluem anorexia, letargia, hiponatremia e/ou hiperpotassemia.

Não existem critérios publicados que avaliem de forma crítica qualquer método para monitorar a resposta terapêutica. Embora o TEACTH seja utilizado com frequência, as concentrações desejadas de cortisol e o momento do teste foram estimados de cães. Entretanto, o tratamento de gatos com o trilostano tem sido bem-sucedido com a utilização desses valores.[8,9] De forma geral, o objetivo é uma concentração de cortisol pós-TEACTH, 4 h após a administração de trilostano, maior que 40 nmol/ℓ (> 1,4 µg/dℓ) e abaixo de aproximadamente 140 nmol/ℓ (5 µg/dℓ). Entretanto, atualmente os resultados do TEACTH mostraram ser preditivos não confiáveis do estado clínico de cães com HAC tratados com trilostano. Portanto, recomenda-se monitorar de perto o histórico e o exame físico como parâmetros críticos durante o tratamento.

Outras opções medicamentosas

O mitotano parece ser bem tolerado por gatos, apesar da sensibilidade aos hidrocarbonetos clorados.[11] Entretanto, o mitotano é frequentemente ineficaz no controle dos sinais clínicos do HAC felino.[3] Um caso relatado no qual foi administrada uma dose de 50 mg/kg/dia, VO, durante 1 semana e, então, 50 mg/kg/semana VO, foi bem controlado durante 40 semanas antes do desenvolvimento de sinais compatíveis com hipoadrenocorticismo.[12]

Se o trilostano e o mitotano estiverem indisponíveis ou forem ineficazes, outros inibidores da síntese esteroide podem ser utilizados. Metirapona, um inibidor da enzima 11-beta-hidroxilase que converte 11-desoxicortisol em cortisol, provou ser efetiva, pelo menos momentaneamente, no controle dos sinais clínicos e na supressão da produção de cortisol em um gato (65 mg/kg, VO, a cada 12 horas).[14] Ainda não foi determinado se a terapia a longo prazo com metirapona pode controlar o HAC felino ou se as concentrações crescentes de ACTH eventualmente quebram o bloqueio. Parece, entretanto, potencialmente útil para a estabilização pré-cirúrgica.[13]

O cetoconazol, um antifúngico imidazólico, é um inibidor da esteroidogênese em seres humanos e cães, mas ineficaz em gatos. Sua segurança tem sido questionada por conta dos relatos comuns de anorexia, perda de peso, êmese e diarreia. Hepatotoxicidade e trombocitopenia também foram notadas.[53,54] O cetoconazol não está mais disponível em algumas partes do mundo, tendo sido substituído pelo itraconazol. Não existem relatos do uso deste para o HAC felino.

Radioterapia hipofisária

Para gatos com sinais neurológicos associados a um grande tumor hipofisário, a radioterapia hipofisária pode se mostrar benéfica. Em um relato, houve melhora dos sinais neurológicos e endócrinos após radioterapia em sete gatos com HAC ou acromegalia causados por grandes tumores hipofisários.[55] A sobrevida mediana

SEÇÃO 21 • Doenças Endócrinas

foi de 17,4 meses, sem relatos da avaliação detalhada de alterações no estado endócrino. A radioterapia hipofisária tem sido associada à melhora do controle diabético em gatos com acromegalia, mas não foi relatado progresso semelhante no controle diabético naqueles com HAC.[56]

PROGNÓSTICO

O HAC felino não tratado ou não responsivo é um distúrbio progressivo com prognóstico reservado. Em geral, esses gatos morrem de infecções graves, DM descontrolado ou são submetidos à eutanásia. Com a terapia apropriada, gatos com adenomas adrenais ou HHD parecem ter prognóstico bom a excelente. Muitos dos gatos diabéticos com HAC felino precisam de menos insulina para tratar o diabetes. A remissão completa do DM pode ocorrer naqueles gatos submetidos ao tratamento definitivo eficaz para HAC.

REFERÊNCIAS BIBLIOGRÁFICAS

As referências bibliográficas deste capítulo se encontram online no Ambiente de Aprendizagem.

CAPÍTULO 308

Tumores Adrenocorticais Não Secretores de Cortisol e Incidentalomas

Ellen N. Behrend

INTRODUÇÃO

Em razão do uso comum de ultrassonografia abdominal, está havendo o reconhecimento mais frequente de tumores adrenais não secretores de cortisol e. Um tumor adrenal não é necessariamente um tumor adrenal (TA) primário, e nem todos os TAs são secretores de cortisol. Possibilidades não tumorais incluem hiperplasia nodular, cisto, abscesso, hematoma e granuloma. Em um estudo, 27% dos TAs caninos e 60% dos felinos eram lesões metastáticas.[1] Carcinomas pulmonares, mamários, prostáticos, gástricos, pancreáticos e melanomas apresentaram as maiores taxas de metástases em glândulas adrenais em cães. Um TA primário pode ser benigno ou maligno e pode ou não ser funcional (*i. e.*, secretar hormônio); mielolipomas ou lipomas podem ocorrer no córtex adrenal. Tumores funcionais secretam esteroides do córtex ou hormônios adrenérgicos da medula, isto é, um feocromocitoma (ver Capítulo 311). Dos TAs primários, aproximadamente 75% são adrenocorticais e 25% possuem origem neuroendócrina.[2]

INCIDENTALOMA

Apresentação clínica

A ultrassonografia é empregada de rotina para a avaliação de estruturas de tecidos moles abdominais (ver Capítulo 88). Em certas circunstâncias, observa-se um tumor adrenal aparentemente acidental, isto é, um "incidentaloma", definido como um "aumento focal da glândula adrenal em pacientes sem evidências prévias de doença adrenal". Deve-se suspeitar de TA quando houver perda do formato típico de uma glândula adrenal, independentemente do tamanho, assimetria no formato e no tamanho entre as glândulas adrenais ou o tumor parecer infiltrado na veia frênico-abdominal, na veia cava ou nos tecidos moles adjacentes (ver Figuras 306.9, no Capítulo 306, e 307.9 a 307.12, no Capítulo 307). A incidência de tumores adrenais acidentais é estimada em 4% em cães em geral, mas, em um estudo, aqueles com tumor adrenal acidental eram significativamente idosos e mais pesados do que os animais do grupo-controle.[3] Apenas 17% dos cães com tumor adrenal acidental

tinham menos que 9 anos e peso mediano de 21 kg, comparado aos 14 kg do grupo-controle. Em gatos, a incidência de incidentalomas adrenais é desconhecida. Como primeiro passo, a ultrassonografia abdominal deve ser repetida para garantir que tumor seja observado de maneira consistente (Figura 308.1). Assim que o tumor adrenal acidental for confirmado, uma série de diferenciais, conforme discutido, precisa ser considerada. Muitos fatores influenciam a agressividade da abordagem diagnóstica e terapêutica, que são gravidade de problemas concomitantes, razão original para realização de ultrassonografia abdominal, idade, probabilidade de a massa secretar hormônios de forma ativa e/ou maligna, tamanho e invasividade do tumor e desejos do cliente.

Abordagem diagnóstica

Base de dados iniciais

Resultados do histórico, do exame físico e dos exames de sangue e urina de rotina devem ser avaliados em busca de evidências de hipercortisolismo (ver Capítulos 306 e 307), hiperaldosteronismo, feocromocitoma (ver Capítulo 311) ou excesso de hormônios sexuais. Os testes apropriados devem ser realizados conforme indicado. Os tumores secretores de aldosterona e de hormônios sexuais são discutidos neste capítulo.

Avaliação da neoplasia pela ultrassonografia

Embora 14 a 30% dos tumores adrenais acidentais sejam malignos, é difícil determinar se um, em particular, é neoplásico e/ou maligno.[3] Esses diagnósticos requerem avaliação histológica. Embora a citologia tenha 90 a 100% de acurácia para diferenciação da origem cortical ou medular, não é um meio confiável para distinguir lesões benignas de malignas.[4] Os exames de imagem podem ser úteis, mas devem ser interpretados com cuidado. Características que não ajudam a diferenciar adenomas e carcinomas adrenais são a mineralização ou ecogenicidade à ultrassonografia. Tanto adenomas como carcinomas podem conter densidades minerais ou surgir como um tumor cranial ao rim (ver Figuras 307.9 e 307.10, no Capítulo 307). Ao mesmo tempo que mineralizações difusas e mal definidas costumam estar associadas a neoplasias adrenais, as mineralizações discretas

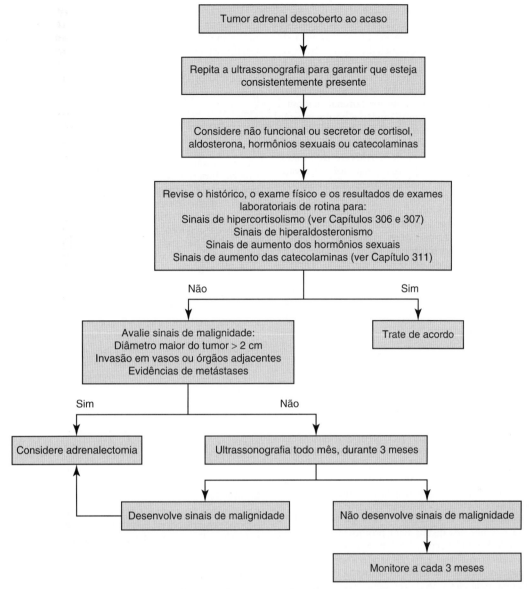

Figura 308.1 Abordagem diagnóstica e terapêutica para um incidentaloma.

e bem delimitadas ocorrem em animais clinicamente normais e podem ser uma alteração distrófica.[5] Na ultrassonografia, tanto TAs benignos como malignos podem ser hipo, iso ou hiperecoicos, comparados ao córtex renal, ou possuir ecogenicidade mista.

Radiografias torácicas e coleta guiada por ultrassonografia

Evidências de metástases podem ser identificadas em radiografias torácicas. Suspeitas de metástases para órgãos abdominais, especialmente o fígado, podem ser visualizadas e confirmadas por biopsia guiada por ultrassonografia (ver Capítulo 89). Se o maior diâmetro do TA for > 2 cm, os riscos de malignidade e crescimento são maiores.[3,6] Evidências de invasão em tecidos adjacentes e/ou veia cava são sugestivas de carcinoma. A natureza invasiva de tumores, entretanto, pode não ser observado.[7] Em 34 de 36 cães com TAs, a ultrassonografia foi 100% sensível e 96% específica para identificação de um trombo tumoral dentro da veia cava caudal. Entretanto, quando todas as formas de invasão vascular foram avaliadas, incluindo a invasão da parede vascular sem um trombo concomitante, a sensibilidade e a especificidade foram de 76 e 96%, respectivamente.[8] A existência de vasos tortuosos e heterogeneidade de ganho de contraste, pela avaliação ultrassonográfica contrastada, pode também ser marcador de malignidade.[9]

Tomografia computadorizada

Na tomografia computadorizada (TC) abdominal, má demarcação glandular, ganho irregular de contraste e textura não homogênea são evidências de malignidade.[10] A invasão vascular pode ser detectada pela utilização de TC com alta acurácia, embora não perfeita.[11-13] Em um estudo, a invasão vascular foi identificada de maneira correta utilizando-se a TC contrastada em 11 de 12 cães. A sensibilidade e a especificidade da TC contrastada para invasão vascular, comparadas à cirurgia ou à necropsia, foram de 92 e 100%, respectivamente. Em um cão, a invasão da veia frênico-abdominal não foi identificada pela TC.[11] Em contrapartida, glândulas adrenais aumentadas podem se aderir ou comprimir a veia cava, sugerindo invasão, quando esta não ocorre.[10]

Considere adrenalectomia a qualquer momento em que ocorrerem sinais de malignidade

Tratamento e acompanhamento

Se houver suspeita de tumor adrenal acidental maligno, a adrenalectomia é recomendada. Se os sinais clínicos, o exame físico ou os resultados dos exames de sangue e urina de rotina não forem compatíveis com um TA funcional, não existirem evidências de invasão tecidual ou vascular ou de malignidade e o tumor for < 2 cm no seu maior diâmetro, sugere-se uma abordagem conservadora não cirúrgica. A princípio, recomenda-se o monitoramento mensal ultrassonográfico para determinar se o tumor está crescendo ou alterando de aparência. O crescimento de tumores adrenais acidentais é imprevisível. Em um estudo de 7 cães com tumor adrenal acidental, 3 dos tumores suspeitos não foram identificados com mais de 4 meses depois da repetição da ultrassonografia e nenhum crescimento foi detectado após mais de 6 meses em 2 cães. Em 1 cão, o tumor adrenal acidental cresceu de 1,6 a 2,5 cm em seu maior diâmetro e houve invasão da veia cava em 10 meses. Em 1 cão, o tumor adrenal acidental cresceu de 2,5 a 3,1 cm em seu maior diâmetro, dentro de 8 meses.[3] Em 9 cães com TA secretor de hormônios que não o cortisol, acompanhados durante 12 meses, não foi observada nenhuma alteração em 7 animais. Os dois tumores que cresceram medeiam, originalmente, 2 e 2,5 cm de comprimento.[6]

Se um tumor adrenal acidental não aumentar de tamanho após 3 meses, o intervalo entre as avaliações ultrassonográficas pode ser maior. Entretanto, se ele estiver crescendo, alterando de aparência, comprimindo ou infiltrando vasos sanguíneos circundantes ou tecidos moles, ou se ocorrerem sinais clínicos associados à secreção excessiva de hormônios, a adrenalectomia pode ser justificada. Para TAs não secretores de cortisol, a sobrevida mediana sem cirurgia em 14 cães foi de 29,8 ± 8,9 meses (variação de 1 a 96 meses). Tamanhos tumorais maiores foram associados à sobrevida mais curta.[6]

TUMORES ADRENAIS SECRETORES DE ALDOSTERONA

A aldosterona é o principal mineralocorticoide sintetizado e secretado pela zona glomerular, a zona mais externa do córtex adrenal. Suas funções primárias são a regulação das concentrações séricas de sódio (Na) e potássio (K), além da homeostase do fluido intravascular. Aumentos no K sérico estimulam diretamente a secreção de aldosterona. Diminuições na pressão sanguínea, identificadas principalmente dentro dos rins, estimulam a síntese e a liberação de renina, que, por meio da angiotensina II, estimulam a secreção de aldosterona, isto é, do sistema renina-angiotensina-aldosterona (SRAA; ver Capítulo 246). A aldosterona atua nos néfrons distais para promover reabsorção de Na e excreção de K e hidrogênio. Ao conservar o Na, a aldosterona conserva indiretamente a água, elevando a volemia e, por sua vez, a pressão sanguínea; ela também aumenta diretamente a pressão sanguínea, pela elevação da resistência periférica total (ver Capítulo 157) A aldosterona também é sintetizada no coração, no cérebro e nos tecidos vasculares, onde pode ter ações parácrinas ou autócrinas.[14]

O hiperaldosteronismo pode ser primário ou secundário. O hiperaldosteronismo primário (HAP) é definido como uma secreção autônoma de aldosterona por células adrenocorticais. É caracterizado por excesso de aldosterona circulante e, através do *feedback* negativo, supressão da renina. O hiperaldosteronismo secundário é o resultado de uma condição, por exemplo, insuficiência cardíaca ou doença renal crônica (DRC), que estimula o SRAA. Assim, está associado ao aumento das concentrações de renina.

TUMORES SECRETORES DE ALDOSTERONA EM FELINOS

Definições de hiperaldosteronismo primário relacionado e não relacionado com um tumor

O HAP felino foi relatado pela primeira vez em 1983,[15] e tem sido cada vez mais diagnosticado nos últimos 20 anos. Gatos com um TA causador de HAP, isto é, um aldosteronoma, costumam possuir um adenoma ou carcinoma cortical unilateral, com relatos de adenomas adrenais bilaterais.[16] A incidência de tumores malignos excede a de benignos.[17] O HAP não relacionado com tumores (ver Capítulo 324) já foi descrito.[18-20]

Gatos acometidos possuem hiperplasia adrenocortical bilateral e a maioria apresenta evidências de DRC. Alguns gatos apresentam hiperplasia nodular da zona glomerular, esclerose arteriolar renal, esclerose glomerular, atrofia tubular e fibrose intersticial.

Epidemiologia e histórico de hiperaldosteronismo primário relacionado com tumores

Não existe predisposição racial aparente para o aldosteronoma felino. A idade mediana ao diagnóstico é de aproximadamente 13 anos, tendo a maioria > 10. Ambos os sexos são representados, e a maioria dos gatos acometidos é castrado.[21] Os sinais clínicos estão relacionados, principalmente, com hipopotassemia ou hipertensão sistêmica, sendo os mais comuns fraqueza persistente e progressiva, isto é, "polimiopatia "hipopotassêmica",[17] quase sempre observada quando a concentração sérica de K está < 3 mmol/ℓ. Ventroflexão cervical, fraqueza de membros pélvicos (algumas vezes com posição plantígrada), dificuldade em pular, apatia e ataxia são queixas comuns dos tutores. Alguns poucos gatos apresentaram rigidez de membros, disfagia ou colapso, com relatos de sinais episódicos e de início agudo.[18] A insuficiência respiratória secundária à fraqueza de músculos respiratórios é rara.[22,23] Tutores podem notar cegueira aguda e/ou alteração súbita na coloração do olho, decorrente, em geral, de hemorragia intraocular ou descolamento de retina (ver Capítulo 11) secundária à hipertensão (ver Capítulo 157). Na ocasião, a hipertensão pode causar convulsões, ataxia ou alterações comportamentais como resultado de edema do sistema nervoso central, hemorragia ou isquemia.[21] Poliúria e polidipsia (PU/PD) ocorrem em < 20% dos gatos com HAP.[21] Alguns deles apresentaram excesso de progestágenos concomitante, o que pode causar PU/PD.[24,25] A hipopotassemia pode causar diabetes insípido nefrogênico reversível e PU/PD. O apetite é variável, podendo estar aumentado, normal ou diminuído. A polifagia pode ser um sinal de excesso concomitante de outro hormônio, por exemplo, a progesterona.

Exame físico

Os achados do exame físico costumam estar relacionados com hipopotassemia (ver Capítulo 68) ou hipertensão (ver Capítulo 157). Em geral, a fraqueza é aparente. Evidências de hipertensão incluem vasos retinianos tortuosos e descolamento de retina, hemorragia e/ou edema (ver Capítulo 11). Sinais clínicos compatíveis com excesso de glicocorticoides ou progestágenos incluem fragilidade cutânea, alopecia e abdome pendular (ver Capítulo 307). Sopros cardíacos, ritmos de galope ou arritmias podem ser auscultados secundariamente à hipertrofia ventricular esquerda, uma sequela da hipertensão (ver Capítulo 55).

Diagnóstico

Exames laboratoriais de rotina

A única anormalidade típica dos exames laboratoriais de rotina é a hipopotassemia (ver Capítulo 68). A maioria dos gatos com aldosteronoma apresentou hipopotassemia moderada a grave, possivelmente porque o HAP não é considerado até que seja documentada hipopotassemia persistente, especialmente apesar da suplementação por K.[17] Um aumento da excreção fracionada urinária de K pode confirmar a etiologia renal da hipopotassemia (ver Capítulo 73). Em decorrência de um fenômeno de "escape da aldosterona", a hipernatremia é incomum no HAP. A hipertensão e a expansão volêmica podem sobrepor os efeitos poupadores de sódio da aldosterona e causar natriurese (ver Capítulo 73). Em geral, há aumento da atividade de creatinoquinase (CK; ver Capítulo 66) em razão da miopatia hipopotassêmica, mas sua gravidade é variável. A alcalose metabólica é comum, provavelmente em razão da excreção do íon hidrogênio mediada por aldosterona,[17] que deve ser considerada em qualquer gato com hipertensão não explicada, especialmente se refratária ao tratamento. Cerca de 85% dos gatos afetados são persistentemente hipertensos.[14]

Exames de imagem

A radiologia costuma não ser útil, mas um grande tumor pode ser visível em exames abdominais (ver Figura 307.9, no Capítulo 307). Há calcificação adrenal em aproximadamente 33% dos gatos idosos e saudáveis, o que não deve ser superestimado (ver Figura 307.10, no Capítulo 307). Metástases pulmonares são incomuns. Do contrário, a ultrassonografia é bastante útil. Todos os gatos relatados com aldosteronoma apresentaram um TA detectado à ultrassonografia (ver Figuras 307.11 e 307.12, no Capítulo 307) e alguns poucos TA bilateral, com a visualização de somente um dos dois tumores.[16,26] A glândula adrenal contralateral deve ser avaliada, já que uma diminuição no tamanho sugere que o TA é funcional e secretor de glicocorticoides ou progestágenos.[25] Apesar de incomuns, há ocorrência de tumores bilaterais,[16] devendo-se buscar evidências de malignidade. A ausência de invasão aparente em tecidos circundantes ou vasculatura deve ser vista com cuidado, já que a ultrassonografia não foi capaz de identificar invasões vasculares existentes em alguns gatos com aldosteronoma.[26,27] A TC e a ressonância magnética (RM) abdominais podem ser utilizadas, mas os relatos são limitados.[16,27] A citologia do tumor adrenal pode ser útil na determinação da origem, mas não da função ou da natureza maligna *versus* benigna.[28]

Aldosterona sérica

Ao mesmo tempo que a existência de um TA em um gato com hipopotassemia persistente e/ou hipertensão é altamente indicativa de aldosteronoma, a confirmação se baseia na demonstração do aumento das concentrações basais de aldosterona. Em geral, os testes estão disponíveis, não sendo necessário nenhum manuseio especial da amostra. Até hoje, as concentrações de aldosterona estavam aumentadas em todos os gatos relatados com aldosteronoma. As maiores concentrações de aldosterona ocorrem em casos de TA. Entretanto, as concentrações de aldosterona relatadas para casos de hiperaldosteronismo primário e secundário se sobrepõem. Concentrações > 1.000 pmol/ℓ foram relatadas em casos de HAP secundário, sobretudo em gatos com DRC. Além disso, como as suspeitas de HAP estão se tornando mais comuns, é provável que o teste ocorra em fases mais precoces da evolução da doença. No início da doença, espera-se que, em alguns gatos com HAP, as concentrações de aldosterona estejam dentro do limite superior dos valores de referência.

Atividade plasmática da renina

Já que o aumento das concentrações de aldosterona não é 100% específico para o diagnóstico de aldosteronoma, devem-se descartar doenças que causem hiperaldosteronismo secundário. Gatos hipertensos podem apresentar concentrações elevadas de aldosterona.[29] É difícil distinguir HAP de DRC, já que elas costumam coexistir. A DRC pode causar hiperaldosteronismo e vice-versa. É ideal que a atividade plasmática da renina (APR) e a concentrações de aldosterona sejam avaliadas em uma amostra. Em gatos com HAP, a APR está abaixo ou dentro dos valores de referência, pois o hiperaldosteronismo e a hipertensão exercem *feedback* negativo que diminui a APR. No hiperaldosteronismo secundário, como em casos de DRC, a APR está aumentada. Infelizmente, um teste felino para APR não está atualmente disponível no mercado nos EUA; ademais, eles necessitam de um grande volume de plasma, devendo essa substância separada ser congelada de imediato.

Outros testes endócrinos

Outros testes passíveis de confirmar HAD, além da APR, estão sob investigação. Em teoria, a mensuração da relação entre aldosterona e creatinina urinária (RA:CU) fornece um reflexo das concentrações de aldosterona com o passar do tempo, enquanto o sangue, a concentração em um único momento. Entretanto, em 9 gatos com HAP, apenas 3 apresentaram aumento da RA:CU.[19] Um teste que necessita da administração de fludrocortisona, um corticosteroide sintético com atividade mineralocorticoide, também está sob investigação, já que a

administração oral de mineralocorticoides (0,05 mg/kg, VO, a cada 12 h × 96 h) suprime de forma significativa a secreção de aldosterona (a mediana foi de 78% com base no nível basal) em gatos saudáveis.[19,30] Um gato com aldosteronoma metastático confirmado apresentou aumento da RA:CU após a administração da fludrocortisona.[30] Em gatos hipertensos, o diagnóstico de HAP, com ou sem hipopotassemia, pode ser excluído se a RA:CU no dia 4 suprimir > 50% do nível basal.[19]

Assim, a supressão por fludrocortisona possui méritos como um teste diagnóstico para HAP felino. Entretanto, a urina não é a via de excreção dos principais metabólitos da aldosterona em gatos, e a concentração urinária da aldosterona pode não refletir de forma acurada as concentrações sanguíneas.[31] De fato, em um estudo, as concentrações plasmáticas basais de aldosterona separaram de maneira mais clara gatos com e sem HAP do que a RA:CU.[19] Além disso, a coleta de urina de gatos em uma situação hospitalar costuma exigir cistocentese, o que pode ser difícil quando se trata de tamanho vesical insuficiente ou um gato não colaborativo. A coleta de urina em casa pode ser incômoda ou impossível, e a administração por via oral de fludrocortisona, 2 vezes/dia, durante 4 dias, desafiadora. Ademais, a fludrocortisona pode suprimir as concentrações séricas de K abaixo dos valores de referência e causar fraqueza muscular.[19] Em gatos saudáveis, a administração de apenas 3 doses de fludrocortisona (0,05 mg/kg, VO, a cada 12 h) suprimiu de forma significativa a concentração sérica de aldosterona, mas são necessários outros estudos em gatos com HAP para determinar a utilidade do teste.[32] Em razão da atividade glicocorticoide da fludrocortisona, 3 doses já são suficientes para suprimir de forma significativa as concentrações de cortisol; assim, poderiam ocorrer sinais de deficiência de glicocorticoide após conclusão do teste de supressão.[32]

Em conclusão, a suspeita de aldosteronoma surge pela identificação de hipopotassemia e hipertensão (Figura 308.2). A elevação da concentração plasmática de aldosterona e a identificação de um tumor discreto dentro da adrenal são necessárias para o diagnóstico. Confirmação histopatológica da origem do tumor, resolução dos sinais clínicos e normalização das concentrações de aldosterona no período pós-cirúrgico servem para confirmar ainda mais o diagnóstico.

Tratamento e prognóstico

A adrenalectomia por celiotomia ou laparoscopia é o tratamento de escolha para o aldosteronoma felino.[27,33] A adrenalectomia unilateral é potencialmente terapêutica; entretanto, por ser um procedimento desafiador de alto risco, deve ser realizado somente por cirurgiões experientes, em um hospital com uma unidade de cuidados intensivos (UCI) bem equipada, além de observação e cuidados durante 24 horas. No período pré-cirúrgico, a hipopotassemia deve ser corrigida pela administração oral e/ou parenteral de potássio. A avaliação de trombos e metástases tumorais é imperativa. A existência de trombos tumorais pode aumentar a possibilidade de complicações. Metástases podem diminuir as chances de sobrevida, e a cirurgia não será terapêutica. Além disso, a possibilidade de o tumor secretar um hormônio que não a aldosterona deve ser considerada e testada, conforme indicado. Se um glicocorticoide ou progestágeno for secretado, a adrenalectomia pode causar deficiência transitória de cortisol (ver Capítulo 307).

Na teoria, a secreção autônoma de aldosterona por um TA deveria suprimir as células normais da zona glomerular dentro da glândula adrenal contralateral, com a possível ocorrência de hipoaldosteronismo no período pós-cirúrgico. As concentrações séricas de eletrólitos devem ser monitoradas com frequência e a fluidoterapia IV ajustada de acordo, a fim de manter as concentrações séricas de K e Na dentro ou próximas dos intervalos de referência. Costuma não ser necessária a administração de um mineralocorticoide sintético no período pós-cirúrgico para tratar o hipoaldosteronismo.

Em relatos anteriores, as complicações perioperatórias ocorreram em 8 de 17 casos, incluindo letargia, anorexia, êmese, disfagia, hipertermia, infecções do trato respiratório superior, hemorragias

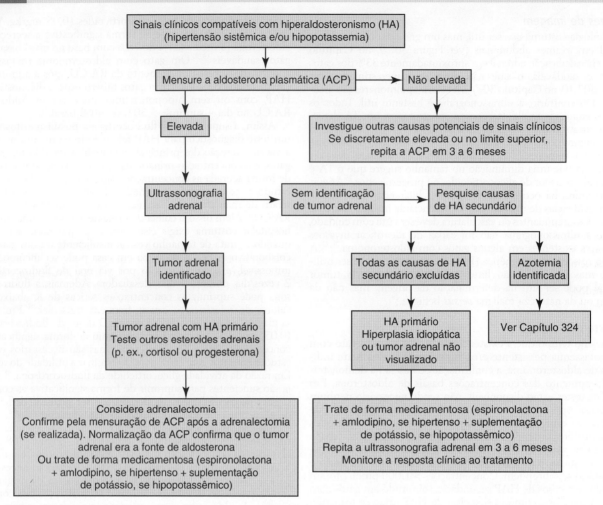

Figura 308.2 Abordagem diagnóstica para hiperaldosteronismo em gatos quando da indisponibilidade de um teste para atividade plasmática da renina (APR). (Adaptada, com autorização, de Refsal KR, Harvey AM: Primary hyperaldosteronism. In August JR, editor: *Consultations in feline internal medicine*, vol. 6, St. Louis, 2010, Saunders, Figura 24.9 B, p. 262.)

intra-abdominais trans ou pós-cirúrgicas, lesão renal aguda, sepse e suspeita de tromboembolia. Em 6 desses 8 gatos, o resultado foi fatal.[14,27] Em um relato mais recente, apenas 2 de 10 gatos com aldosteronoma tiveram um resultado fatal.[27] A média de dias de hospitalização perioperatória para todos os gatos foi de 5 dias. Dois foram submetidos à eutanásia 2 e 10 dias após a cirurgia, em razão de complicações cirúrgicas (um também possuía uma massa pancreática). A hemorragia não foi prevista por tipo tumoral, localização, tamanho ou invasão vascular. Dos 8 gatos que receberam alta do hospital, houve normalização da pressão sanguínea e das concentrações séricas de K, sem a necessidade de terapia a longo prazo. O tempo de anestesia longo foi associado de forma significativa à diminuição da sobrevida. A sobrevida mediana foi de 1.297 dias (variação de 2 a 1.582 dias). Não houve diferença significativa na duração da sobrevida em comparação a animais com adenoma (mediana, 1.329 dias) e aqueles com adenocarcinoma (248 dias; p = 0,2), mas o número de gatos foi pequeno. A cegueira decorrente do descolamento de retina pode ser resolvida com o passar do tempo (ver Capítulo 11). Não foram identificadas mortes após a alta hospitalar em razão do TA. Entretanto, 2 gatos foram submetidos à eutanásia devido à DRC, o que pode ter sido exacerbado pelo HAP.[27]

Gatos não submetidos à cirurgia podem ser tratados de forma medicamentosa para controlar a hipopotassemia e/ou a hipertensão sistêmica. A suplementação com potássio (2 a 6 mEq VO, a cada 12 h) tem sido efetiva. O besilato de amlodipino (0,625 a 1,25 mg/gato VO, a cada 24 h) é o tratamento de eleição para diminuir a pressão sanguínea (ver Capítulo 158). Podem-se utilizar até 2,5 mg se a pressão sanguínea não for controlada;

entretanto, a hipertensão pode se tornar refratária à medicação. A espironolactona, um antagonista competitivo do receptor de aldosterona, pode ser utilizado (2 a 4 mg/kg VO, a cada 24 horas) para diminuir tanto a pressão sanguínea como para aumentar o teor de K. Doses acima de 4 mg/kg podem causar anorexia, êmese e diarreia. O tratamento clínico resultou em tempos de sobrevida de 7 meses a 984 dias em 4 gatos, mas outro sobreviveu apenas por 50 dias em razão da falta de comprometimento do tutor.[17]

TUMORES SECRETORES DE ALDOSTERONA EM CÃES

Contexto geral e sinais clínicos

Em cães, o HAP é, de modo geral, causado por adenoma ou carcinoma solitário unilateral, sendo raro o diagnóstico de a hiperplasia adrenocortical idiopática bilateral.[34-37] O hiperaldosteronismo primário é uma doença de cães de meia-idade a idosos, e as queixas comuns dos tutores incluem letargia, anorexia, fraqueza e PU/PD. Ademais, assim como gatos com aldosteronoma, é incomum a ocorrência de tumores que secretam tanto mineralocorticoides como glicocorticoides,[35-37] o que faz com que possam ocorrer sinais clínicos e alterações laboratoriais compatíveis com excesso de glicocorticoides.

Diagnóstico

A existência de hipopotassemia e uma concentração sérica de Na no limite superior ou discretamente acima do intervalo de referência, em conjunto com o achado de um TA à ultrassonografia, deve aumentar suspeita de HAP. Alguns tumores secretores de aldosterona são bastante pequenos e não observados à ultrassonografia. De forma alternativa, pode ocorrer hiperplasia adrenocortical idiopática. Outros achados compatíveis com o diagnóstico de HAP incluem hipertensão sistêmica e alcalose metabólica. A confirmação de um aldosteronoma requer a documentação de aumento da concentração basal plasmática de aldosterona e APR suprimida, em conjunto com a exclusão de outras causas de hipopotassemia. Em cães com aldosteronoma, as concentrações de aldosterona são > 3.000 pmol/ℓ. Infelizmente, um teste para APR canino não está disponível atualmente. Os exames de urina, como a RA:CU, podem ter valor diagnóstico limitado ou ausente em cães. As principais formas de aldosterona presentes na urina humana são aldosterona livre, aldosterona-18-glicuronídeo e tetra-hidroaldosterona.[38] *Kits* disponíveis para mensuração de aldosterona detectam aldosterona livre e aldosterona-18-glicuronídeo (após hidrólise ácida do glicuronídeo). A urina canina contém menos aldosterona-18-glicuronídeo do que a humana e, ao contrário de gatos e seres humanos, não contém aldosterona livre detectável.[31]

Tratamento

A adrenalectomia unilateral é o tratamento de escolha para um tumor adrenal solitário, especialmente se não houver evidência de metástase a distância, invasão vascular ou infiltração nos rins ou na parede abdominal. Potássio oral, bloqueadores de receptores de mineralocorticoides (espironolactona) e fármacos anti-hipertensivos (amlodipino) devem ser administrados até que a cirurgia possa ser realizada. A terapia medicamentosa é indicada para o manejo a longo prazo do HAP, quando a adrenalectomia não for realizada, e para cães com suspeita de hiperplasia adrenocortical idiopática.

As concentrações séricas de eletrólitos devem ser monitoradas com frequência no período pós-cirúrgico e a fluidoterapia IV ajustada para manter as concentrações séricas de K e Na dentro ou próximas dos intervalos de referência. Se a hipopotassemia persistir, a suplementação oral de K pode ser iniciada. As concentrações séricas de magnésio ionizado devem ser monitoradas e a hipomagnesemia tratada, especialmente se a hipopotassemia for refratária à fluidoterapia IV (ver Capítulo 68). Mineralocorticoides (acetato de fludrocortisona oral ou pivalato de desoxicorticosterona injetável) devem ser administrados se a hiperpotassemia e a hiponatremia persistirem por mais de 72 horas, o que é raramente necessário. Apenas uma aplicação de pivalato de desoxicorticosterona costuma ser necessária; se a administração diária de acetato de fludrocortisona for empregada, ela pode ser normalmente ajustada e descontinuada dentro de 1 semana. Em geral, a hipertensão sistêmica melhora ou é resolvida dentro de 48 a 72 horas da adrenalectomia. A medicação anti-hipertensiva deve ser iniciada se a hipertensão persistir. Tentativas de suspender as medicações anti-hipertensivas devem ser iniciadas durante o mês seguinte. A terapia de reposição por glicocorticoides costuma não ser indicada no período pós-cirúrgico, a menos que o tumor esteja secretando um glicocorticoide. Um teste de estimulação por ACTH pode ser realizado 6 a 8 horas após a adrenalectomia, a fim de avaliar a função da glândula adrenal remanescente (ver Capítulo 306).

Prognóstico

A remoção cirúrgica de um adenoma apresenta prognóstico excelente, que é reservado a cães com carcinoma. Se existirem locais de metástases, costuma haver a persistência ou a recidiva de hiperaldosteronismo, hipopotassemia e sinais clínicos associados. Entretanto, esses tumores podem ter crescimento lento e a recidiva pode não ocorrer por mais de 1 ano. O manejo da recidiva com metastasectomia pode ser eficaz.[37] O prognóstico para hiperplasia adrenocortical idiopática é desconhecido e depende da efetividade da terapia medicamentosa. Em teoria, a adrenalectomia bilateral pode oferecer a cura, mas glicocorticoides e mineralocorticoides seriam necessários durante toda a vida.

TUMORES SECRETORES DE MINERALOCORTICOIDES QUE NÃO A ALDOSTERONA

Tumores que secretam mineralocorticoides que não a aldosterona, por exemplo, desoxicorticosterona, são raros.[39-41] Achados clínicos são os mesmos do HAP, mas as concentrações de aldosterona estão baixas. Como não existe nenhum teste disponível no mercado para mensuração de desoxicorticosterona, o diagnóstico seria presuntivo com base na constelação de resultados de exames diagnósticos.

TUMORES ADRENAIS SECRETORES DE HORMÔNIOS SEXUAIS

Contexto geral

Tumores adrenocorticais possuem o potencial de sintetizar e secretar uma série de esteroides que não o cortisol e a aldosterona. A secreção em excesso de hormônios sexuais por tumores pode estar associada a vias biossintéticas aberrantes e/ou deficiências enzimáticas. Progestágenos podem se ligar a receptores glicocorticoides ou deslocar o cortisol de sua proteína de ligação, aumentando as concentrações séricas de cortisol livre.[42,43] Em cães, os progestágenos suprimem a secreção endógena de ACTH e causam atrofia adrenal, ações essas compatíveis com a atividade glicocorticoide.[44]

Tumores adrenocorticais secretores de hormônios sexuais em felinos

Informações clínicas

Foi descrito um pequeno número de gatos com TA secretor de hormônios sexuais.[24,25,45-48] Houve variação de idade em 6 gatos: de 7 a 15 anos; 2 fêmeas e 4 machos, ambos castrados. As raças incluíram Doméstico de Pelo Longo e Curto, além do Himalaio. Relatou-se uma fêmea castrada de 14 anos, da raça Doméstico de Pelo Curto, com aumento adrenal bilateral e produção excessiva de estradiol e testosterona.[49] A produção em excesso de um progestágeno (p. ex., progesterona ou 17-hidroxiprogesterona) pode causar sinais de excesso de cortisol, como pelame de má qualidade, atrofia dérmica e fragilidade cutânea. Três dos quatro gatos com tumor secretor de progesterona apresentavam diabetes melito, sendo mal regulado em dois.[24,25,45,46] A produção excessiva de andrógenos pode causar alteração no odor da urina, no comportamento de micção em jato, na agressividade e no desenvolvimento de espículas penianas.[47,49] A hiperestrogenemia pode causar comportamento estral cíclico e aumento vulvar.[48,49] O tipo tumoral foi conhecido em 5 gatos: 1 adenoma e 4 carcinomas.[24,25,45-48]

Diagnóstico

A suspeita de um tumor secretor de hormônios sexuais começa com os sinais clínicos. Nenhum resultado de exames de rotina, por exemplo, hemograma ou perfil bioquímico sérico, auxiliará no diagnóstico. O achado de um TA na ultrassonografia deve aumentar a suspeita. Assim como em casos de aldosteronomas, tumores secretores de hormônios sexuais costumam ser observados à ultrassonografia. Em um gato, entretanto, o tumor havia substituído o tecido normal, observando-se apenas aumento discreto e formato arredondado à ultrassonografia.[48] Devem-se buscar por sinais de malignidade, como a obtenção de radiografias.

O diagnóstico definitivo da funcionalidade do tumor e do tipo do hormônio secretado é feito, na maioria das vezes, com a utilização do teste de estimulação por ACTH (125 µg cosintropina IV por gato), com sangue coletado antes e 1 hora após a aplicação.[24,25,45-48] Cortisol e hormônios sexuais são mensurados pré e pós-ACTH. Se um progestágeno for secretado, as concentrações de cortisol estarão no limite inferior ou abaixo do intervalo de referência. Assim, se um gato com aparente

SEÇÃO 21 • Doenças Endócrinas

hipercortisolismo não apresentar anormalidades esperadas nos testes para hiperadrenocorticismo, é razoável a consideração de um distúrbio que envolva hormônios sexuais. O estradiol não aumenta após administração de ACTH. Em um gato com tumor secretor de estrógenos, a concentração basal de estradiol estava aumentada, mas o valor pós-ACTH, não.[48]

Tratamento e prognóstico

A remoção cirúrgica ou laparoscópica de um TA é o tratamento de escolha. O prognóstico pode depender da existência de metástases, remoção bem-sucedida do tumor e estabilidade do paciente no período pré-cirúrgico. Se a secreção de cortisol estiver sendo suprimida pelo tumor, a reposição por glicocorticoides deve ser realizada no período pós-cirúrgico. O hiperprogesteronismo pode causar alterações, como pele delgada, tornando o gato um mau candidato à cirurgia.[46] Quatro gatos com TA secretor de hormônios sexuais foram submetidos à adrenalectomia. Um gato morreu em razão de causas desconhecidas 3 dias após a cirurgia.[24] Um gato foi submetido à eutanásia 10 meses após a cirurgia com DRC e 2 não foram acompanhados com 8 semanas e 12 meses após a cirurgia.[45,47,48] A aminoglutetimida foi o único tratamento medicamentoso testado para o controle da secreção de hormônios sexuais por um TA, cuja resposta foi transitória.[46] O trilostano foi utilizado para controlar a secreção de hormônios sexuais em um gato com hiperplasia adrenal bilateral. Após aproximadamente 6 meses, houve retorno dos sinais clínicos, sem a busca de nenhuma avaliação adicional ou tratamento.[49]

Tumores adrenocorticais secretores de hormônios sexuais em cães

Informações clínicas

Relatou-se um pequeno número de cães com TAs secretores de hormônios sexuais, mas nenhum com sinais clínicos de hiperestrogenemia ou hiperandrogenemia.[50-53] Dois cães com TA, uma Labradora de 11 anos e um Poodle Miniatura de 9, ambos castrados, apresentaram sinais clínicos de hiperadrenocorticismo, apesar de concentrações séricas de cortisol acentuadamente suprimidas após aplicação de ACTH.[52] Assim, os sinais clínicos ocorreram provavelmente em razão da hiperprogesteronemia. Ambos os cães possuíam PU/PD e polifagia. Um também apresentou alterações na coloração do pelame, ganho de peso, aumento da respiração ofegante e da região abdominal. Em outros cães com tumores secretores de hormônios sexuais, os sinais clínicos não foram delineados, mas as queixas presentes eram compatíveis com hipercortisolismo.[50,51,53]

Diagnóstico

A suspeita de um TA secretor de hormônios sexuais surgirá com os sinais clínicos. A indicação primária para mensuração dos hormônios sexuais é o achado de concentrações de cortisol abaixo dos intervalos de referência em um cão testado para hiperadrenocorticismo pelo teste de estimulação por ACTH ou teste de supressão por baixa dose de dexametasona (ver Capítulo 306).[52,53] Se glicocorticoides exógenos, em qualquer forma, ou medicação que altere a síntese de cortisol (p. ex., cetoconazol) forem descartados, pode haver um TA secretor de hormônios sexuais. O achado ultrassonográfico de um TA dá ainda mais suporte ao diagnóstico, mas a ausência de um tumor adrenal detectado não descarta o diagnóstico.

Para documentar elevações de hormônios sexuais, um teste de estimulação por ACTH deve ser realizado (ver Capítulo 306). Hormônios sexuais são mensurados em amostras coletadas antes e 1 hora após a administração de ACTH. Entretanto, as concentrações de hormônios sexuais devem ser interpretadas com cautela. Para o estradiol, existe uma ampla variabilidade no mesmo indivíduo e entre cães; concentrações basais randômicas de estradiol em determinados cães costumam exceder os valores de referência.[54] Vários cães sem hiperadrenocorticismo podem apresentar concentrações de hormônios sexuais de até 40 a 50% acima dos intervalos de referência.[55-57] Em 6 cães com feocromocitoma ou TA não funcional, as concentrações de androstenediona, progesterona, 17-hidroxiprogesterona, testosterona e/ou estradiol estavam aumentadas.[58]

Tratamento e prognóstico

A adrenalectomia, em teoria, é o tratamento de eleição. Entretanto, informações detalhadas estão disponíveis apenas para dois cães com TA secretor de hormônios sexuais. Um cão foi submetido à adrenalectomia e ficou bem por, pelo menos, 13 meses após a cirurgia. Um segundo foi tratado de forma medicamentosa com mitotano por aproximadamente 20 dias, em uma dose diária de 47 mg/kg, sem resposta, e os tutores não quiseram outras terapias. Dada a resistência do TA em geral ao mitotano, a falta de resposta não é surpreendente, dadas a dose e a curta duração do tratamento.

REFERÊNCIAS BIBLIOGRÁFICAS

As referências bibliográficas deste capítulo se encontram online no Ambiente de Aprendizagem.

CAPÍTULO 309

Hipoadrenocorticismo

Rebecka S. Hess

INTRODUÇÃO

Em 1855, o dr. Thomas Addison relatou pela primeira vez uma doença da "cápsula suprarrenal" (córtex adrenal) em uma série de casos, descrevendo 11 pessoas com o que é agora conhecido como hipoadrenocorticismo (HA) ou doença de Addison.[1] O córtex adrenal é dividido em três camadas: a zona glomerular, mais externa; a zona fasciculada, média e mais ampla; e a zona reticular, mais interna. O córtex adrenal secreta glicocorticoides e mineralocorticoides, essenciais para a sobrevivência. Portanto, a hipofunção ou a disfunção do córtex adrenal, como aquela observada no HA, pode causar risco de morte. Os glicocorticoides são secretados pelas três camadas corticais, enquanto a aldosterona, o mineralocorticoide mais importante, o é pela zona glomerular, a única zona que contém aldosterona sintase. A fisiologia adrenal básica é discutida no Capítulo 306.

O hipoadrenocorticismo é comum em cães e raro em gatos. Portanto, a discussão adiante aborda cães, sendo seguida de uma discussão breve de HA em gatos.

FISIOPATOLOGIA

Em seres humanos, o HA é um distúrbio autoimune raro. A maioria dos pacientes possui anticorpos contra a enzima esteroidogênica 21-hidroxilase, presente nas três camadas corticais adrenais.[2] Esses anticorpos supostamente levam à destruição do córtex adrenal.[3] A presença de anticorpos contra a 21-hidroxilase ou outros autoanticorpos adrenais em cães com HA de ocorrência natural ainda não foi documentada em número suficiente para dar suporte à teoria de que os anticorpos sejam a causa.[4] Entretanto, a adrenalite linfoplasmocítica e a atrofia adrenocortical foram documentadas em alguns cães com HA, o que sugere que a doença seja imunomediada.[5] Cães que desenvolvem tanto HA quanto hipotireoidismo sustentam o conceito de um processo imunomediado sistêmico.[6] A inflamação adrenal linfocítica e a formação de autoanticorpos precedem a atrofia de outras glândulas endócrinas (como a glândula tireoide). Por fim, algumas das características genéticas da doença envolvem a função imune.

O conceito de um componente genético envolvido na etiologia do HA canino é suportado pelo fato de que determinadas raças sabidamente apresentam um maior risco. O HA familiar foi relatado em algumas raças (Leonberger e Spitz alemão), tendo o Dogue Alemão maior risco quando comparado a outros cães.[7-9] Um estudo sobre hereditariedade da doença em cães da raça Bearded Collie revelou que o modo não foi autossômico dominante e que mais de um gene principal estava envolvido na fisiopatologia da doença.[10] Entretanto, em cães Poodle standard e Cão-d'Água Português, a hereditariedade parece ser influenciada por um único *locus* com efeito principal, sendo o modo autossômico recessivo.[11-13] No Cão-d'Água Português e no Springer Spaniel, dois genes com função imune – o complexo de histocompatibilidade principal para antígenos leucocitários caninos e a proteína 4 associada ao linfócito T citotóxico – são relatados como associados ao HA.[10,14] Um terceiro gene de função imune, *PTPN22*, é expresso de modo excessivo em cães da raça Cocker Spaniel com HA.[15]

Relatou-se que o complexo de histocompatibilidade principal possui um papel na etiologia do HA nos cães Nova Scotia Duck Tolling Retriever, Cocker Spaniel, Labrador Retriever, West Highland White Terrier, Bearded Collie e Poodle Standard.[14,16,17] Entretanto, as metodologias empregadas em alguns desses estudos foram questionadas, havendo a necessidade de mais estudos.[18] É possível que a etiologia genética da doença seja diferente entre as raças. É importante ressaltar que ainda não está claro se qualquer uma dessas diferenças genéticas é responsável pela formação de autoanticorpos antiadrenais e atrofia dos córtex adrenais.

CLASSIFICAÇÃO

Hipoadrenocorticismo primário

O HA primário é a forma mais comum da doença. Ela envolve a incapacidade direta do córtex adrenal e o HA clássico, a diminuição na secreção de glicocorticoides e mineralocorticoides pelas glândulas adrenais. O *HA primário atípico* é um termo utilizado para descrever a incapacidade direta do córtex adrenal, na qual a secreção do cortisol está ausente, mas as concentrações de sódio (Na) e potássio (K) ainda estão normais.[19] Alguns cães são inicialmente diagnosticados apenas com deficiência glicocorticoide, com base nas concentrações normais de Na e K, mas desenvolvem hiponatremia e hiperpotassemia com o passar do tempo.[7,19,20] Nesses cães, o HA "atípico" é transitório. Entretanto, outros cães diagnosticados como portadores de HA atípico mantêm concentrações normais de Na e K durante anos.[19,20] É interessante notar que alguns cães com HA documentado, com concentrações normais de Na e K, apresentam concentrações baixas de aldosterona, sugerindo que, nesses cães, a manutenção da concentração de eletrólitos não depende completamente da aldosterona.[20] Se, em cães, o HA for, de fato, uma condição imunomediada decorrente de anticorpos anti-21-hidroxilase, é possível que a destruição da zona glomerular – a zona produtora de aldosterona – seja retardada quando comparada à destruição das outras duas zonas, pois suas concentrações de 21-hidroxilase são as menores das três.

O HA primário, seja típico, seja atípico, ocorre como resultado de atrofia do córtex adrenal (Figura 309.1). Raramente, o HA ocorre secundariamente a um processo infiltrativo que destrói o córtex adrenal. A neoplasia é a causa mais comum dessa condição rara, embora tuberculose, doença fúngica, outras doenças granulomatosas ou infecciosas e infartos sejam possíveis.[21-23] Foi relatado um caso raro de HA, no qual a depleção de aldosterona precedeu a de glicocorticoide.[24] O HA primário iatrogênico transitório ou permanente pode ser causado por fármacos utilizados para tratar o hiperadrenocorticismo (Lysodren® ou trilostano; ver Capítulo 306). O hipoaldosteronismo isolado (sem deficiência glicocorticoide) foi relatado, mas é extremamente raro.

Hipoadrenocorticismo secundário

O HA secundário é raro. Ocorre em razão da falha dentro do hipotálamo ou da hipófise, em decorrência de neoplasias, inflamações, infecções, infartos ou traumas, causando distúrbios na secreção do hormônio adrenocorticotrófico (ACTH, do inglês *adrenocorticotropic hormone*) pela hipófise ou diminuição da secreção do hormônio liberador de corticotrofina (CRH, do inglês *corticotropina-releasing hormone*) pelo hipotálamo.[25-28] Assim como a maioria das doenças de sistema nervoso central (SNC), sinais neurológicos e outros déficits hormonais seriam esperados, mas o HA secundário idiopático enigmático foi relatado em cães sem sinais neurológicos e sobrevida a longo prazo apenas com a terapia glicocorticoide. Como a secreção de aldosterona é regulada majoritariamente pelo sistema renina-angiotensina-aldosterona (SRAA), e não pelo ACTH ou pelo CRH, essa condição envolve somente a deficiência glicocorticoide, com concentrações normais de Na e K. Ao contrário do HA primário atípico, no qual Na e K também estão normais, no HA secundário as concentrações de ACTH estão baixas (ver Figura 309.1). O HA secundário iatrogênico pode ocorrer após hipofisectomia ou administração de esteroides a longo prazo (ver Figura 309.1).[29] Esteroides exógenos suprimem a secreção de ACTH, havendo necessidade de tempo para que aquelas células recuperem a função após interrupção da administração de esteroides. Essa é a razão pela qual a administração de glicocorticoides deve ser sempre diminuída gradativamente, permitindo que as células secretoras de ACTH, e então as células adrenocorticais, retornem à função normal.

IDENTIFICAÇÃO, HISTÓRICO, SINAIS, EXAME FÍSICO

Idade

O HA é uma doença de cães jovens a de meia-idade, com idade mediana aproximada ao diagnóstico de 3 a 4 anos. Entretanto, a variação da idade ao diagnóstico é ampla: 2 meses a 12 anos (Tabela 309.1). Fêmeas podem ter maior risco para a doença.[7,30] O hipoadrenocorticismo pode ocorrer em qualquer raça, mas foi discutida a predisposição genética específica em algumas. Golden Retriever, Yorkshire Terrier, Pit Bull, Chihuahua e Lhasa Apso apresentam risco menor.[31]

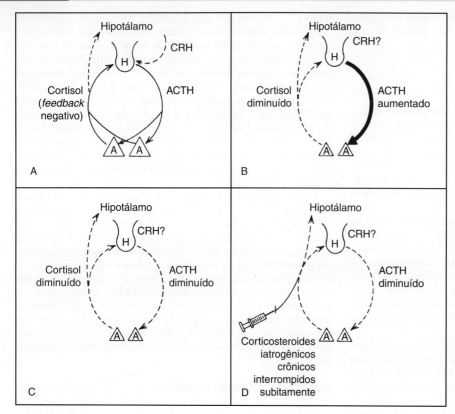

Figura 309.1 O eixo hipófise-adrenal em cães normais (**A**); nos com perda de função adrenocortical e excesso de secreção de hormônio adrenocorticotrófico (ACTH), em razão da ausência de *feedback* negativo (a forma mais comum de hipoadrenocorticismo) (**B**); naqueles com incapacidade de secretar ACTH e atrofia secundária do córtex adrenal, especificamente a zona fasciculada e a zona reticular (**C**); e naqueles tratados de maneira crônica com glicocorticoides exógenos em excesso, causando insuficiência na secreção hipofisária de ACTH e atrofia secundária do córtex adrenal (**D**). *A*, adrenal; *CRH*, fator (hormônio) liberador de corticotrofina; *H*, hipófise. (De Feldman EC, Nelson RW, Reusch CE, Scott-Moncrieff JCR: *Canine and feline endocrinology and reproduction*, 4 ed., St. Louis, 2015, Saunders.)

Histórico e sinais clínicos

Histórico em geral

Cães com HA podem apresentar um ou mais dos seguintes sinais clínicos, com diversos graus de gravidade: anorexia, perda de peso, êmese, diarreia, letargia, fraqueza, poliúria (PU), polidipsia (PD), tremores e, em casos extremos, colapso (ver Tabela 309.1). A maioria dos sinais clínicos é atribuída à falta de cortisol, podendo ser discretos, vagos e melhorar e piorar durante um período, até que um tutor astuto busque por cuidados veterinários ou o cão sofra rápida deterioração que necessite de intervenção emergencial. Algumas vezes circunstâncias estressantes, como uma cirurgia ou a estadia em um canil, podem levar um cão com "HA oculto" compensado no limite, com pouca reserva adrenocortical e capacidade limitada, a recair em uma crise.

Papel dos glicocorticoides e mineralocorticoides

Glicocorticoides são importantes na manutenção da barreira mucosa gástrica, que protege a mucosa gastrintestinal (GI) do conteúdo ácido. Os glicocorticoides também ajudam a manter a pressão sanguínea, a temperatura corporal e as concentrações de glicose.[32] Se a barreira mucosa GI for ineficaz em razão do HA, é comum a ocorrência de anorexia, êmese, diarreia e perda de peso subsequente, mas hematêmese e hematoquezia, não (ver Tabela 309.1). Em um estudo de cães admitidos para cuidado intensivo com necessidade de reanimação volêmica IV, hematêmese, melena e hematoquezia foram significativamente menos comuns naqueles com HA, quando comparados aos sem HA. Nesse mesmo estudo, fraqueza e letargia foram significativamente mais comuns em cães com HA.[30] Letargia, fraqueza, tremores e colapso podem ocorrer em decorrência da hipoglicemia, caso a glicose seja sintetizada de forma inadequada em razão da falta de glicocorticoides, que mediam o catabolismo de glicogênio e a síntese de glicose pela gliconeogênese em condições estressantes ou de jejum. A PU é atribuída à falta de mineralocorticoides. A deficiência de aldosterona causa perda de Na pela urina, que atua como um agente osmótico, levando à diurese osmótica. A PD é compensatória para a PU em uma tentativa de manter a hidratação.

Exame físico

As anormalidades do exame físico variam de discretas a graves e podem incluir: pulso fraco, desidratação, hipotensão, bradicardia, fraqueza muscular, condição corporal magra, dor abdominal e, em casos extremos, choque hipovolêmico ou hipotensivo ou convulsões (ver Capítulo 2). Em cães com HA, a desidratação ocorre em razão das perdas urinárias de Na, da diurese osmótica consequente e, então, da doença, que interfere na ingestão hídrica. Entre os cães que necessitaram de reanimação volêmica IV, os com HA possuem menor pressão sanguínea sistólica, quando comparados nos àqueles nos quais o diagnóstico de HA foi excluído. A pressão sanguínea sistólica média (ver Capítulo 99) em 53 cães com HA foi de 90 mmHg (variação de 40 a 150 mmHg; ver Tabela 309.1). A hipotensão é atribuída à ausência de glicocorticoides e seu papel importante na manutenção da pressão sanguínea normal (ver Capítulo 159).[33] A bradicardia é atribuída à hiperpotassemia. Quando a concentração de K no fluido extracelular cardíaco está anormalmente alta, o gradiente de concentração entre os compartimentos intra e extracelular diminui e o K é retido nas células. A corrente de K para fora, necessária para a fase 3 de repolarização rápida final do potencial de ação cardíaco, diminui, levando à bradicardia (ver Capítulo 248). A dor abdominal supostamente ocorre em razão da ausência de efeitos gastroprotetores dos glicocorticoides.

DIAGNÓSTICO

Contexto geral

A suspeita de HA começa com o histórico, os sinais clínicos e os achados de exame físico. A interpretação cuidadosa do hemograma e do perfil bioquímico deve ser útil para decidir quando buscar por um exame que avalie o eixo da adrenal. O diagnóstico de HA pode ser confirmado com resultados de um teste de estimulação por ACTH (TEACTH). A avaliação do eixo adrenal fica pronta em apenas 1 a 2 horas. Urinálise e urocultura devem ser consideradas ao avaliar qualquer cão com PU/PD. Análise fecal para detecção de parasitas, cultura bacteriana fecal para

Tabela 309.1 Comparação das características clínicas e dos achados do hemograma em cães doentes com e sem hipoadrenocorticismo.

VARIÁVEL	53 CÃES COM HIPOADRENOCORTICISMO	110 CÃES NOS QUAIS HOUVE SUSPEITA DE HIPOADRENOCORTICISMO E EXCLUSÃO	P
Idade (anos)	4,8 (0,6 a 11,8)	6,8 (0,4 a 16)	0,07
Êmese, com ou sem diarreia	43 (81%)	88 (80%)	0,87
Hematêmese ou melena, com ou sem hematoquezia	6 (11%)	28 (26%)	0,04
Depressão, fraqueza ou letargia	51 (96%)	85 (77%)	0,002
Dor abdominal	14 (26%)	45 (41%)	0,07
Pressão sanguínea sistólica (mmHg)	90 (40 a 150)	140 (50 a 210)	< 0,001
Duração da hospitalização (horas)	49 (16 a 240)	66 (3 a 312)	0,02
Sobreviveu à alta hospitalar	52 (98%)	100 (91%)	0,11
Hematócrito (VR: 40,3 a 60,3%)	46,1 (20,1 a 68,8)	42,2 (14,1 a 61,5)	0,006
Leucócitos (VR: 5,3 a 19,8 células × $10^3/\mu\ell$)	11,7 (5,6 a 31,2)	12,6 (0,9 a 64,2)	0,87
Neutrófilos (VR: 3,1 a 14,6 células × $10^3/\mu\ell$)	7,75 (2,77 a 25,90)	9,87 (0,68 a 53,93)	0,007
Linfócitos (VR: 0,9 a 5,5 células × $10^3/\mu\ell$)	2,38 (0,80 a 8,20)	1,07 (0 a 6)	< 0,001
Eosinófilos (VR: 0 a 1,6 células × $10^3/\mu\ell$)	0,57 (0 a 4)	0,12 (0 a 7)	< 0,001
Relação neutrófilos:linfócitos	3 (0,76 a 14,59)	9,51 (1,23 a 95,15)	< 0,001

Dados são expressos como mediana (variação) ou número (frequência). O hipoadrenocorticismo seria diagnosticado caso a concentração sérica de cortisol fosse ≤ 1 µg/dℓ 1 h após administração de hormônio adrenocorticotrófico (ACTH). O diagnóstico de hipoadrenocorticismo seria excluído caso a concentração sérica basal de cortisol fosse > 2 µg/dℓ ou se a concentração sérica de cortisol após administração exógena de ACTH fosse > 5 µg/dℓ.[30]

Salmonella e *Campylobacter* e radiografias abdominais podem ser justificadas para avaliação da anorexia, êmese ou diarreia. Se houver suspeita de pancreatite aguda, a ultrassonografia abdominal e a mensuração da concentração de lipase pancreática podem ser necessárias. Quando forem notadas arritmias, eletrocardiograma e radiografias torácicas podem ser valiosos.

Hemograma

Um estudo com 53 cães com HA, comparados a 110 doentes do grupo-controle, destacou algumas diferenças úteis entre achados do hemograma em cães com e sem HA.[30] Enquanto o leucograma de cães com HA estava dentro dos limites de referência, aqueles com HA apresentaram menor contagem de neutrófilos e maior de linfócitos e eosinófilos do que os doentes sem HA (ver Tabela 309.1). Uma contagem absoluta de linfócitos > 2.000 células/mcℓ foi aproximadamente 58% sensível e 85% específica como ferramenta de triagem para HA.[30]

Perfil bioquímico sérico de rotina

Contexto geral

O perfil bioquímico pode não revelar anormalidades ou apresentar diversas discretas ou graves. A maioria das observadas nos testes laboratoriais iniciais em cães com HA se resolve dentro de horas a dias após o início do tratamento. Anormalidades bioquímicas graves raramente são irreversíveis. Isso é importante ao discutir os possíveis resultados com um tutor antes do estabelecimento do cuidado intensivo ou diagnóstico definitivo. Ao contrário de outras doenças, azotemia grave, aumento das atividades de enzimas hepáticas e outros parâmetros alterados são quase sempre completamente reversíveis com o tratamento.

Valores de eletrólitos, renais e ácido-base

Muitas anormalidades eletrolíticas, inclusive hiponatremia, hiperpotassemia, hipocloremia, hipercalcemia (hiperCa) e acidose discreta, são comuns em cães com HA. A hiponatremia e a hiperpotassemia foram documentadas em > 80% dos cães com HA em razão da deficiência de aldosterona.[7,31] A utilização da relação Na:K permite que o clínico use ambas as mensurações ao decidir sobre a realização do teste para HA. Quando limiares

> 27 ou 28 são utilizados como valores de referência para Na:K, aproximadamente 95% dos cães são identificados de maneira correta como portadores ou não de HA.[7] Quando a relação Na:K for < 24, é bastante provável que o resultado do TEACTH confirme o HA.[7] A utilização da contagem linfocitária e da relação Na:K como ferramentas de triagem maximiza a probabilidade de tomar a decisão correta com relação à realização de um TEACTH. As contagens linfocitárias são afetadas por glicocorticoides e a relação Na:K é influenciada pelos mineralocorticoides.

A azotemia pré-renal é comum em cães com HA secundário à hipovolemia e à desidratação. A desidratação grave pode levar à lesão renal aguda, mas, na maioria dos cães com HA, os parâmetros renais retornam rápida e completamente aos valores de referência com a terapia. Não existem evidências que sugiram que qualquer lesão renal permanente acompanhe uma crise hipovolêmica com risco de morte como resultado de HA. Como a aldosterona facilita a excreção urinária do íon hidrogênio, a deficiência mineralocorticoide leva à acidemia em cerca de 60% dos cães com HA.[7,34] Há hipocloremia em 40 a 60% dos cães com HA, provavelmente porque o Na e o cloreto (Cl) são cotransportados do sangue para a urina.[7,31,35] A hipercalcemia foi relatada como um aumento no Ca total (tCa) e, menos comumente, como um aumento no Ca ionizado (iCa). A fisiopatologia da hipercalcemia em cães com HA não é completamente compreendida, mas não parece relacionada com a alteração das concentrações do hormônio paratireoidiano, a proteína relacionada com o hormônio paratireoidiano ou a 1,25-di-hidroxivitamina D sérica.[36,37] Os glicocorticoides facilitam a calciurese, cuja deficiência pode levar à retenção de Ca e à hipercalcemia. Também é possível que a acidemia contribua para o aumento na concentração de iCa, já que um excesso de íons hidrogênio carregados positivamente compete pela ligação com albumina e desloca os íons Ca carregados positivamente.

Glicose, colesterol, albumina, enzimas hepáticas e urinálise

A hipoglicemia ocorre em < 20% dos cães com HA e tende a ser discreta quando presente. Bastante incomum, a hipoglicemia pode causar risco de morte e convulsões,[38] sendo provavelmente o resultado da deficiência de cortisol, o que diminui a quebra do glicogênio e da gliconeogênese. O aumento da secreção de insulina não parece ser a causa de hipoglicemia.[39] O extravasamento de enzimas citosólicas é atribuído à baixa perfusão e à lesão isquêmica aos hepatócitos. A hipoalbuminemia e a hipocolesterolemia não são comuns, mas provavelmente ocorrem em razão da isquemia aguda do trato GI, e não pela disfunção hepática.[7,31] A urinálise costuma revelar isostenúria em razão da perda de Na e PU resultante.

Outros exames

A extensão e o foco de outros testes dependem dos sinais clínicos do indivíduo. Cães com letargia discreta com curso crescente e decrescente, inapetência e perda de peso serão avaliados de modo diferente daqueles criticamente doentes, com êmese aguda grave e desidratação. Testes adicionais são realizados para identificar uma série de possíveis condições em ambos os cenários. Em cães com HA, urocultura, exame coproparasitológico e culturas fecais costumam estar negativos. Em geral, as Radiografias abdominais são normais, embora alguns cães com HA tenham sido descritos como portadores de micro-hepatia. Em cães com bradicardia, um eletrocardiograma pode revelar ausência completa de ondas P, intervalos QRS largos e ondas T altas e, possivelmente, certo grau de bloqueio cardíaco, compatível com hiperpotassemia (Figura 309.2). Radiografias torácicas podem revelar microcardia decorrente da hipovolemia grave (Figura 309.3). Megaesôfago, relatado de forma anedótica em seres humanos com HA, ainda não foi estabelecido como secundário ao HA em cães. Se houver suspeita de pancreatite aguda, a ultrassonografia abdominal e a quantificação de lipase pancreática podem ser necessárias. A ultrassonografia não deve ser utilizada para avaliar a função adrenal, mas a espessura das glândulas adrenais em cães com HA costuma ser < 3 mm.[40]

Testes do eixo adrenal

Teste de estimulação por ACTH (TEACTH)

A confirmação do diagnóstico de HA requer testes de função da glândula adrenal. As funções glicocorticoides e mineralocorticoides são investigadas de maneira independente, e o TEACTH é o teste de escolha para o diagnóstico de HA, que pode ser realizado pela mensuração das concentrações séricas de cortisol antes e 1 hora após a administração de 5 µg/kg de ACTH sintético IV.[41] Como o volume de ACTH é pequeno, é necessário ter cautela para garantir a administração por via intravenosa. Se administrado acidentalmente por via SC, o ACTH não estimulará as glândulas adrenais e poderá levar a resultados errôneos do teste. Como o ACTH sintético é caro, alguns clínicos guardam o excesso para reduzir o custo ao cliente. Após reconstituição com salina a 0,9%, o ACTH pode ser refrigerado ou congelado. A refrigeração (4 a 8°C) por até 60 dias foi relatada para uso em seres humanos. Nossa experiência sugere utilizar o ACTH sintético refrigerado dentro de 14 dias ou o ACTH previamente congelado (a –20°C em seringas plásticas) dentro de 6 meses.[42,43]

Em um cão com função adrenal normal, a injeção de ACTH deve resultar em pico de secreção de cortisol pelas glândulas adrenais. Portanto, espera-se que a concentração sérica de cortisol antes da administração de ACTH esteja entre 0,5 µg/dℓ e 6 µg/dℓ e, após o TEACTH, > 2 µg/dℓ. Em um cão com HA, as adrenais foram destruídas e são incapazes de obter uma resposta apropriada ao ACTH. Na maioria dos cães com HA, as concentrações séricas de cortisol antes e após o TEACTH são < 1 µg/dℓ (indetectáveis; Figura 309.4). Um pequeno número de cães com HA pode apresentar concentrações séricas de cortisol entre 1 µg/dℓ e 2 µg/dℓ após o TEACTH; entretanto, o diagnóstico de HA com concentração sérica de cortisol > 1 µg/dℓ pós-ACTH deve ser feito com cautela e somente quando todos os outros diagnósticos diferenciais tiverem sido excluídos.

Relação cortisol:ACTH endógeno (C:ACTHe)

O custo do ACTH sintético e a falta de disponibilidade em alguns países levou a estudos que investigassem outras opções para o diagnóstico de HA. Ao mesmo tempo que a maioria dos cães com HA possui concentrações séricas de cortisol em repouso (basais) < 1 µg/dℓ, isso também pode ocorrer em alguns poucos cães sem HA. Assim, o cortisol em repouso, por si só, não pode ser utilizado para diagnosticar HA.[44,45] O C:ACTHe é promissor como auxílio diagnóstico para o diagnóstico de HA, com a necessidade de apenas uma amostra sanguínea, além de ter se mostrado significativamente inferior em cães com HA, quando comparados aos saudáveis, sem sobreposição com os resultados da relação.[46] Em um estudo de C:ACTHe em 15 cães com HA comparados a 5 com doença não adrenal, nos quais houve suspeita de HA e exclusão, não houve novamente sobreposição entre os resultados da relação dos dois grupos.[47] Em 5 dos 15 cães com HA, entretanto, houve mensuramento do ACTHe após a administração do ACTH exógeno.[47] Um número maior de cães deve ser estudado antes que esse teste possa ser recomendado para o diagnóstico definitivo de HA.

Avaliação mineralocorticoide

A avaliação das concentrações séricas de Na e K é um reflexo indireto, mas bom, da função da aldosterona. A relação entre a concentração plasmática de aldosterona e a atividade plasmática da renina em cães com HA foi investigada e mostrou ser significativamente inferior à de cães saudáveis, sem sobreposição.[46] Entretanto, a sobreposição foi observada entre concentrações plasmáticas individuais de aldosterona e atividades plasmáticas de renina, indicando que os resultados de testes individuais são menos específicos do que sua relação.[46] Ainda deve ser elucidado se a relação pode ser utilizada para confirmar o diagnóstico de HA.

Concentrações basais de cortisol

Ao mesmo tempo que não são úteis para o diagnóstico de HA, as concentrações basais de cortisol o são como um teste simples de triagem para excluir o HA de qualquer lista de diagnósticos diferenciais. É provável que cães com concentrações basais de cortisol > 2 µg/dℓ não tenham HA.[44] Esse teste é particularmente útil em cães com relações Na:K normais, com suspeita apenas de deficiência glicocorticoide.

HIPOADRENOCORTICISMO SECUNDÁRIO E HIPOALDOSTERONISMO ISOLADO

Raramente, cães apresentam HA "secundário" causado por deficiência de ACTH hipofisário. As concentrações de ACTHe desses cães estão baixas, enquanto as concentrações séricas de Na e K devem estar dentro dos intervalos de referência. A regulação de Na e K é controlada, principalmente, pela renina e pela angiotensina, e não pela hipófise ou pelo hipotálamo. Na instância singular de hipoaldosteronismo isolado, as concentrações de cortisol antes e após o TEACTH estão normais. Esses cães podem ser identificados pela combinação de hiperpotassemia, hiponatremia, baixa atividade plasmática de renina e baixas concentrações de aldosterona antes e após TEACTH.[48]

DOENÇA CRÍTICA

Uma revisão da resposta do eixo hipotálamo-hipófise-adrenal à doença crítica e o efeito da condição sobre o teste estão no Capítulo 133.

DIAGNÓSTICOS DIFERENCIAIS

O termo *"doença de pseudoAddison"* é utilizado para descrever condições que se assemelham à doença de Addison em seus resultados

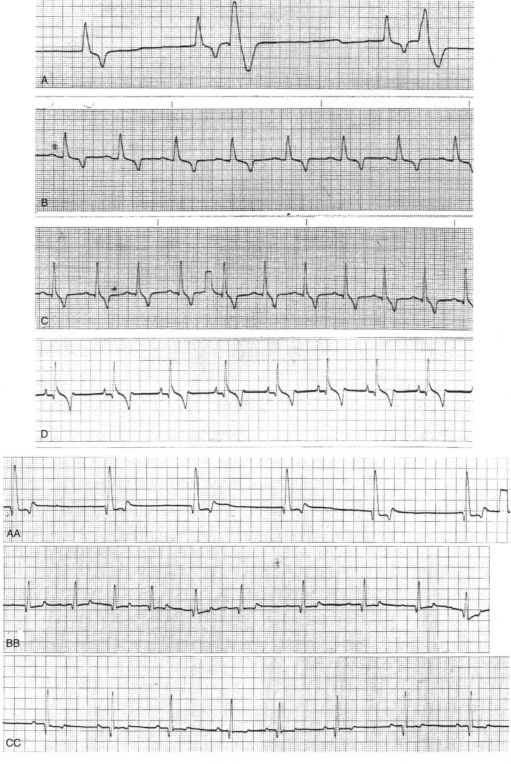

Figura 309.2 Segmentos seriados do eletrocardiograma (ECG) obtidos de dois cães com hipoadrenocorticismo e hiperpotassemia. **A** e **AA** ilustram o efeito de hiperpotassemia grave, com o cão em **A** com concentrações séricas de potássio de 8,6 mEq/ℓ e o em **AA** com mensuração de 9,4 mEq/ℓ. Note a falta de ondas P visíveis, os complexos QRS baixos e largos e as ondas T, as quais não possuem amplitude excessiva. O ECG em **A** também revela duas instâncias de um complexo QRS de aparência bizarra após um complexo QRS de aparência mais normal em um intervalo R-R mais curto (i. e., dois batimentos prematuros de aparência mais bizarra). Esses representam complexos ventriculares prematuros que poderiam ser resultado de acidemia, hipoxia miocárdica ou outros desequilíbrios metabólicos. **B** e **BB** são ECGs dos mesmos cães, como em **A** e **AA**, respectivamente. Eles foram obtidos aproximadamente 1 h após instituição da salina normal intravenosa como único tratamento. As concentrações séricas de potássio tinham diminuído para 7,6 mEq/ℓ e 7,9 mEq/ℓ, respectivamente. Dois fatores importantes a serem notados: (1) a melhora é observada em cada caso, com o retorno das ondas P, uma frequência cardíaca mais rápida e o desaparecimento de batimentos de escape ventricular; e (2) anormalidades ainda estão presentes, mais obviamente os intervalos P-R prolongados (bloqueio cardíaco de primeiro grau), que, por si só, sugerem hiperpotassemia, sobretudo quando associados a um complexo QRS alargado e intervalo Q-T curto. Existem diversas outras causas de prolongamento de intervalo P-R. Em **C** e **CC**, as concentrações séricas de potássio são consideravelmente inferiores, 6,2 mEq/ℓ e 5,9 mEq/ℓ, respectivamente. O intervalo P-R e as ondas P, QRS e T possuem duração mais curta, e as ondas R são mais altas. **D**. ECG do cão em **A**; a concentração sérica de potássio é de 5,6 mEq/ℓ, com a observação de uma onda T mais espiculada. (De Feldman EC, Nelson RW, Reusch CE et al.: *Canine and feline endocrinology and reproduction*, 4 ed., St. Louis, 2015, Saunders.)

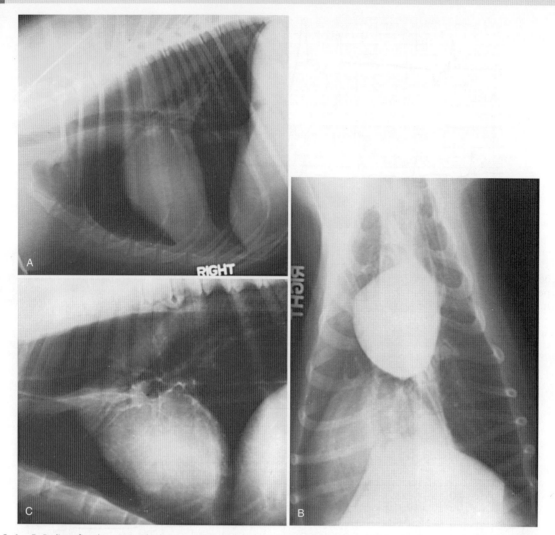

Figura 309.3 A e B. Radiografias de um cão Rhodesian Ridgeback de 3 anos levado ao hospital em estado semelhante ao de choque, secundário ao hipoadrenocorticismo. Note o coração pequeno em ambas as projeções e a pequena vasculatura pulmonar decorrente do baixo débito cardíaco. **C.** Projeção torácica lateral da radiografia de um cão de 5 anos com hipoadrenocorticismo e microcardia, veia cava caudal achatada e esôfago dilatado preenchido por ar. A dilatação esofágica, que pode estar associada ao hipoadrenocorticismo, foi resolvida com terapia hormonal apropriada para a doença primária. (De Feldman EC, Nelson RW, Reusch CE et al.: *Canine and feline endocrinology and reproduction*, 4 ed., St. Louis, 2015, Saunders.)

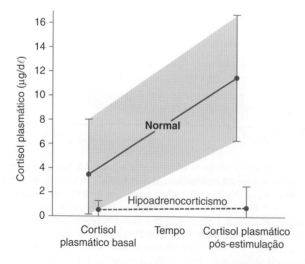

Figura 309.4 Concentrações plasmáticas de cortisol por radioimunoensaio antes e após estimulação por ACTH exógeno em cães normais e naqueles com hipoadrenocorticismo. Os intervalos são médias ± 2 desvios padrões. (De Feldman EC, Nelson RW: *Canine and feline endocrinology and reproduction*, 3 ed., St. Louis, 2004, Saunders.)

clínicos e/ou clinicopatológicos, o que é especialmente verdadeiro em casos de hiperpotassemia e hiponatremia concomitantes. Algumas doenças GI graves (especialmente tricuríase e salmonelose), doenças periparturientes e quilotórax estão entre as condições que podem simular o HA.[49-52] Os resultados do TEACTH devem discriminar o HA de outras condições. Os diagnósticos diferenciais para PU/PD (ver Capítulo 45), azotemia (ver Capítulo 62), isostenúria (ver Capítulo 72), eosinofilia (ver Capítulo 58), hiperpotassemia (ver Capítulo 68), hiponatremia (ver Capítulo 67), hipercalcemia (ver Capítulo 69), hipoglicemia (ver Capítulo 61), aumento das enzimas hepáticas (ver Capítulo 65), hipocolesterolemia (ver Capítulo 63), hipoalbuminemia (ver Capítulo 60) e acidemia (ver Capítulo 128) são abordados em seus respectivos capítulos.

TRATAMENTO

Crise aguda de hipoadrenocorticismo

Contexto geral e fluidoterapia
A fluidoterapia é o único componente mais importante e vital da terapia (ver Capítulo 129). Embora nenhum estudo tenha direcionado ainda as escolhas específicas de fluido, recomenda-se a solução de NaCl a 0,9% (salina), pois contém mais Na e Cl

CAPÍTULO 309 • Hipoadrenocorticismo

e menos K do que outros fluidos cristaloides. Questões podem ser levantadas com relação ao pH relativamente baixo da salina, mas o significado clínico da hiponatremia e da hiperpotassemia sem dúvida compensa o risco de acidose iatrogênica. Qualquer acidose associada ao HA costuma ser discreta e corrigida dentro de 12 a 24 horas da administração por via intravenosa da salina, em geral com o emprego de glicose e insulina. A dexametasona raramente é administrada nos estágios hiperagudos da terapia, a fim de iniciar e concluir o TEACTH. O tratamento com bicarbonato não é indicado.

Sódio (Na) e potássio (K)

A hiponatremia aguda e profunda pode causar edema cerebral. A correção rápida da hiponatremia também pode resultar em desvios osmóticos potencialmente fatais. Recomenda-se que os indivíduos hiponatrêmicos tenham a concentração sérica de Na aumentada em cerca de 1 a 2 mEq/ℓ nas primeiras 2 a 3 horas de tratamento e em cerca de 8 a 12 mEq/ℓ durante as primeiras 24 horas.[53] Durante as primeiras poucas horas de tratamento, as concentrações de Na e K devem ser mensuradas a cada 2 a 6 horas, dependendo da gravidade das anormalidades eletrolíticas e do estado clínico dos cães. Em geral, a hiperpotassemia aumenta de maneira considerável e, algumas vezes, é resolvida somente com solução salina IV intensiva.

Glicose, insulina, pivalato de desoxicorticosterona, bicarbonato

Se a hiperpotassemia grave persistir após 6 a 8 horas de fluidoterapia ou se a bradicardia for profunda, pode-se administrar dextrose IV. A glicose estimula a secreção de insulina, que move o K do fluido extracelular para as células, diminuindo de imediato as concentrações circulantes de K. Se a administração de dextrose, por si só, não conseguir diminuir o K, a insulina IV pode ser administrada com segurança se a glicemia estiver acima de 200 mg/dℓ. Quando a insulina for administrada, a glicose deve ser monitorada de perto para garantir que a hipoglicemia possa ser rapidamente identificada e tratada, se necessário. A hipoglicemia grave (glicemia < 60 mg/dℓ) no atendimento ou após a administração de insulina deve ser abordada com glicose adequada, adicionada à salina IV para criar uma solução de dextrose a 5%. De modo alternativo, pode-se administrar um *bolus* de dextrose (0,25 a 0,5 g/kg, diluído 1:3) IV. É importante lembrar que a administração de glicose pode causar hiperglicemia transitória. A hiperglicemia, por sua vez, faz com que as concentrações séricas de Na estejam baixas, pois a concentração crescente de glicose resulta em desvio de fluido para o espaço extracelular, diluindo o Na. Em seres humanos, sugeriu-se diminuição de cerca de 1 mEq/ℓ na concentração sérica mensurada de sódio para cada aumento de 62 mg/dℓ na glicemia acima do normal. Por fim, assim que o cão for reidratado, se a hiperpotassemia e a hiponatremia persistirem, o TEACTH for concluído e outros diagnósticos diferenciais importantes excluídos, os cães devem ser tratados com pivalato de desoxicorticosterona por via intramuscular (IM) ou subcutânea (SC) (2,2 mg/kg) para prover reposição mineralocorticoide efetiva a longo prazo. No evento muito improvável de acidose grave (pH < 7,1) não corrigida pela fluidoterapia, o bicarbonato pode ser administrado em incrementos de um quarto (0,3 × déficit de base × peso corporal em kg), a cada 20 minutos, enquanto o pH venoso é monitorado.

Terapia glicocorticoide

Em geral, não é necessário administrar glicocorticoides no estágio agudo do tratamento, sendo possível esperar, pelo menos, pela 1 hora necessária para completar o TEACTH. Como os resultados do TEACTH podem ditar o tratamento por toda a vida, é melhor evitar questões do tratamento glicocorticoide iniciado antes desse teste ou durante ele. Assim que o tratamento glicocorticoide for iniciado, ele deve ser gradativamente retirado. Cães não devem receber prednisona oral por, pelo menos, 48 horas antes de um TEACTH. Caso os glicocorticoides

sejam considerados vitais antes da realização do TEACTH, a dá-se preferência à dexametasona IV, que possui início de ação rápido e não interfere nos testes de cortisol se o TEACTH for realizado subsequentemente. Ao mesmo tempo que a dexametasona não possui reação cruzada com os testes de cortisol, ela suprime a secreção hipofisária de ACTH e CRH do hipotálamo, o que pode causar impacto nos resultados do TEACTH.

Terapia em longo prazo

Contexto geral

O tratamento a longo prazo começa após a hidratação de um cão com HA, a descontinuação da fluidoterapia, a normalização das concentrações séricas de eletrólitos e a interrupção do quadro de êmese, diarreia ou anorexia. Esse estágio de tratamento começa, em geral, 24 a 48 horas após admissão em consequência de uma crise, ou em um paciente tratado no ambiente domiciliar, se o diagnóstico for estabelecido. O tratamento a longo prazo consiste em suplementação mineralocorticoide e glicocorticoide. Em cães com concentrações séricas normais de Na e K, apenas glicocorticoides são necessários.

Glicocorticoides

Glicocorticoides podem ser suplementados com prednisona, o glicocorticoide mais comumente utilizado, ou acetato de fludrocortisona. Imediatamente após uma crise aguda, a prednisona pode ser administrada em uma dose relativamente alta de 0,5 mg/kg VO, a cada 12 h, durante 2 a 3 dias. Após esses primeiros dias, a dose da prednisona pode ser rapidamente diminuída para as necessidades fisiológicas (0,1 a 0,2 mg/kg VO, a cada 12 a 24 h). Muitos cães necessitam de doses muito menores para se manterem bem. Baixas doses devem evitar polifagia, ganho de peso, PU/PD e outros efeitos colaterais adversos tipicamente causados por glicocorticoides em cães. A identificação da "melhor" dose é um procedimento que se baseia em tentativa e erro. Se houver recidiva de letargia, anorexia, êmese e diarreia, a dose de prednisona pode ser aumentada. Os tutores devem ter prednisona extra disponível para uma crise ou como forma de se precaver de situações estressantes (viagem, canil, convidados em casa). Nessas situações, os tutores são instruídos a fornecer doses maiores de prednisona (0,5 mg/kg). O acetato de fludrocortisona contém tanto glicocorticoides como mineralocorticoides. Entretanto, é difícil suplementar ambos os hormônios de maneira apropriada com esse fármaco. Alguns cães desenvolvem efeitos colaterais induzidos por glicocorticoides típicos quando submetidos à fludrocortisona suficiente para corrigir as anormalidades eletrolíticas. Outros necessitam de prednisona, além de fludrocortisona, para impedir sinais clínicos GI compatíveis com HA.

Mineralocorticoides

Mineralocorticoides podem ser suplementados com pivalato de desoxicorticosterona ou acetato de fludrocortisona. O pivalato de desoxicorticosterona é administrado por via subcutânea aproximadamente a cada 25 dias.[a] A dose recomendada é de 2,2 mg/kg, a cada 25 dias, mas a experiência clínica e os relatos sugerem que o pivalato de desoxicorticosterona pode ser eficaz em manter as concentrações séricas normais de Na e K em doses menores e/ou quando administrado com menos frequência.[54] O clínico deve começar o tratamento na dose constante da bula, de 2,2 mg/kg SC, mensurando o Na e o K séricos 14 e 25 dias depois. Se a relação Na:K estiver acima de 32 no dia 14, a próxima dose de pivalato

---

[a]Nota do editor.: Recentemente, o pivalato de desoxicorticosterona comercialmente disponível na Europa (e talvez em outros locais) parece ser bem mais potente e de duração mais longa do que qualquer relato prévio indicaria. Médicos-veterinários são encorajados a consultar especialistas na área para compreender se houve mudança na dose e/ou na frequência de administração do pivalato de desoxicorticosterona desde a publicação deste livro-texto.

de desoxicorticosterona pode ser diminuída em cerca de 10% (2 mg/kg). Se a relação Na:K estiver acima de 32 no dia 25, a injeção de pivalato de desoxicorticosterona pode ser adiada por, pelo menos, 5 dias, momento no qual o processo é repetido. Assim que a concentração sérica de Na começar a diminuir ou a concentração de K aumentar, o pivalato de desoxicorticosterona deve ser administrado. O novo intervalo entre as injeções pode ser mantido. Se o intervalo entre as injeções for aumentado, a relação Na:K deve ser mensurada no meio e no fim desse novo intervalo, com um objetivo de 29 a 32. A dose é aumentada ou o intervalo diminuído se < 28 e o oposto > 32. Esse processo deve ser repetido várias vezes durante os primeiros meses (Figura 309.5).

A fludrocortisona é administrada por via oral, na forma de comprimido, 2 vezes/dia (0,01 mg/kg VO, a cada 12 h).[55] A dose deve ser ajustada pela avaliação da concentração sérica de Na e K a cada 5 dias e aumentada até que a relação Na:K esteja acima de 28. O tratamento de cães com pivalato de desoxicorticosterona e prednisona permite a suplementação eficaz de glicocorticoides e mineralocorticoides, separadamente. Um estudo recente também relatou que o pivalato de desoxicorticosterona foi mais efetivo do que a fludrocortisona na diminuição da atividade plasmática da renina, aumentando o Na e diminuindo o K em cães com HA.[56]

Monitoramento

O protocolo terapêutico recomendado para monitoramento e ajuste da dose de pivalato de desoxicorticosterona requer idas frequentes ao médico-veterinário. Embora haja gastos, os custos do tratamento de uma segunda crise por HA ou dos fármacos utilizados também são significativos. Por fim, é menos caro determinar as doses necessárias. Se o clínico puder fornecer uma dose menor, menos frequentemente, será melhor para o cão e menos caro para o tutor. Os tutores devem manter em mente que uma "dose perfeita" pode mudar por muitas razões. A reavaliação das concentrações de Na e K é necessária a cada alguns meses, mesmo em cães bem regulados.

As doses de glicocorticoides devem ser ajustadas, conforme necessário, para que o cão pareça estável e saudável. O clínico quer evitar sinais e alterações bioquímicas de hipo ou hiperadrenocorticismo. O monitoramento do tratamento mineralocorticoide é realizado pela mensuração da relação Na:K, conforme descrito. A atividade plasmática da renina também pode ser utilizada para monitorar o tratamento mineralocorticoide; entretanto, o exame não está amplamente disponível.[56] Os tutores devem monitorar os cães com cuidado e relatar qualquer sinal clínico preocupante, especialmente aqueles

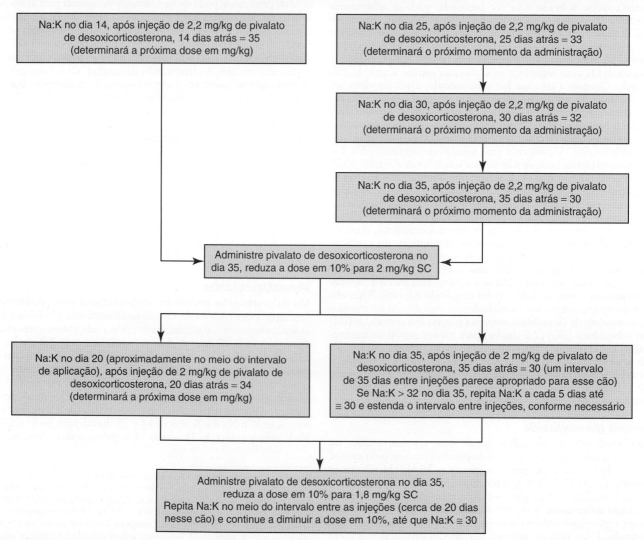

Figura 309.5 Algoritmo descrevendo o uso e os ajustes necessários do pivalato de desoxicorticosterona para o tratamento de cães com hipoadrenocorticismo.

sugestivos de excesso ou falta de glicocorticoides. PU/PD podem ocorrer em cães tratados para HA por diversas razões, e a identificação da causa específica pode ser desafiadora. O pivalato de desoxicorticosterona pode causar PU/PD sem ocasionar qualquer aumento no Na sérico. Glicocorticoides específicos ou fludrocortisona podem causar PU/PD. Assim, PU/PD são sinais de HA e de hiperadrenocorticismo. Ademais, qualquer cão pode desenvolver outra das várias condições que causam PU/PD. Portanto, essa questão relativamente comum deve ser avaliada com cautela.

É importante lembrar que cães diagnosticados com HA atípico podem progredir bem para um estado no qual haja deficiência de mineralocorticoides. Portanto, a avaliação periódica das concentrações de Na e K deve ser considerada de suma importância.

Prognóstico

O prognóstico para HA é excelente, desde que a crise aguda seja tratada de maneira eficaz e o diagnóstico estabelecido. A maioria dos cães com HA que necessita de fluidoterapia IV recebe alta hospitalar cerca de 48 horas após a admissão (ver Tabela 309.1).

HIPOADRENOCORTICISMO FELINO

O hipoadrenocorticismo é extremamente raro em gatos, mas, pelos poucos casos publicados, esses animais parecem ter sinais clínicos, achados de exame físico e anormalidades clinicopatológicas semelhantes aos observados em cães com HA.[57] HA típico espontâneo e atípico, HA iatrogênico associado à suspensão de esteroides e invasão neoplásica das adrenais foram relatados.[57-60] Documentou-se também pseudo-hipoadrenocorticismo com hiponatremia e hiperpotassemia em 4 gatos com efusão peritoneal.[61] Deve-se suspeitar de HA felino após a exclusão dos distúrbios mais comuns, com suporte diagnóstico dos achados clinicopatológicos. Em gatos, o protocolo para o TEACHT é diferente do que aquele em cães (ver Capítulo 306). O tratamento baseia-se na suplementação glicocorticoide e mineralocorticoide após tratamento da crise aguda. Para gatos com HA, o prognóstico não parece ser tão bom quanto para cães.[57]

REFERÊNCIAS BIBLIOGRÁFICAS

As referências bibliográficas deste capítulo se encontram online no Ambiente de Aprendizagem.

CAPÍTULO 310

Endocrinologia Gastrintestinal

Thomas Schermerhorn

INTRODUÇÃO

Segundo algumas estimativas, o trato gastrintestinal (GI) é o maior órgão endócrino do organismo. As funções endócrinas do pâncreas e do trato GI são diversas e envolvem mais de 30 hormônios responsáveis pela integração e coordenação de processos fisiológicos que regulam o apetite, a digestão e o metabolismo energético.[1] Esses são hormônios verdadeiros, que entram na circulação sanguínea para atuar em órgãos-alvo distantes do seu local de origem. Alguns produtos possuem funções parácrinas ou atuam como neurotransmissores. Alguns hormônios apresentam múltiplas isoformas e outros causam ações diferentes, dependendo do tecido-alvo. A diversidade bioquímica dos hormônios produzidos pelo trato GI e pâncreas é tão ampla como as funções que eles regulam, resultando em uma endocrinologia clínica complexa. Dentro de algumas famílias de hormônios – como gastrina e glucagon –, a maior diversidade é decorrente da produção de mRNA com *splicing* alternativo e produção de pré-pró-hormônios por genes específicos, que então sofrem várias modificações pós-translacionais para produzir uma série de produtos proteicos relacionados estruturalmente, mas distintos em termos funcionais. A exploração minuciosa dos mecanismos genéticos, bioquímicos e fisiológicos que regulam esses hormônios complexos está além do escopo deste capítulo, mas uma breve revisão permite a discussão de síndromes clínicas associadas a anormalidades da produção de hormônios intestinais. Vários hormônios GI e pancreáticos compartilham semelhanças bioquímicas e estruturais que permitem a classificação em muitas famílias de hormônios (Tabela 310.1). A partir de uma perspectiva clínica, as famílias da secretina, insulina e gastrina estão entre as mais relevantes. Outros hormônios que causam síndromes definidas em seres humanos, como a serotonina,

possuem papéis menos definidos em animais. Alguns, como a grelina e o peptídio semelhante ao glucagon-1 (GLP-1), podem atuar como emergentes no tratamento de distúrbios endócrinos (ver Capítulos 304 e 305).

HORMÔNIOS PANCREÁTICOS E INTESTINAIS

Essa família de hormônios inclui diversos produtos de origem GI ou das ilhotas pancreáticas. Membros clinicamente importantes da família da secretina incluem secretina, glucagon, peptídio semelhante ao glucagon (GLP) e peptídio inibitório gástrico (GIP). Outros hormônios importantes nesse grupo incluem gastrina, colecistocinina (CCK), somatostatina, motilina, grelina e serotonina.

Secretina

A secretina, um hormônio peptídico produzido pelas células S localizadas principalmente no duodeno, é liberada em resposta aos íons hidrogênio (H^+) contidos nas secreções gástricas.[2] Assim como outros hormônios intestinais (p. ex., CCK), a secretina circula em uma das várias formas moleculares dimensionadas (com a descrição de polipeptídios com 27, 28, 30 e 71 aminoácidos). Cada polipeptídio pode servir para uma função discretamente diferente. As principais ações endócrinas da secretina são a estimulação de líquido com bicarbonato e bile, respectivamente, pelas células ductais pancreáticas e pelo epitélio biliar. Outros efeitos incluem inibição da secreção de gastrina, produção de ácido gástrico e motilidade GI. A expressão de secretina ou de seu receptor foi relatada em neurônios do sistema nervoso central (SNC), coração e pulmões, mas mais estudos são necessários para definir o papel nesses locais não entéricos.

Tabela 310.1 | Visão geral dos hormônios gastrintestinais importantes.

SUBSTÂNCIA	ESTÍMULO FISIOLÓGICO	TECIDO-ALVO	EFEITOS FISIOLÓGICOS
Gastrina	Distensão gástrica Peptídios intraluminais	Células parietais e principais gástricas Células acinares pancreáticas Tecido gástrico, intestinal, pancreático	Secreção ácida e de pepsinogênio Secreção de enzimas pancreáticas Efeito trófico: crescimento
Colecistocinina	Nutrientes no duodeno (ácidos graxos, aminoácidos) Íon hidrogênio (H^+)	Vesícula biliar Esfíncter de Oddi Células acinares pancreáticas Estômago	Contração Relaxamento Secreção enzimática Efeito trófico: crescimento pancreático Inibe o esvaziamento gástrico
Secretina	Ácidos graxos intraduodenais Íon hidrogênio (H^+)	Células ductais (pâncreas) Árvore biliar Duodeno	Estimula a secreção de bicarbonato e água
Peptídio semelhante ao glucagon-1 (GLP-1)	Ácidos graxos intraluminais (duodeno e íleo)	Ilhotas pancreáticas de Langerhans (células beta) Estômago	Efeito da incretina: estimula a secreção de insulina na presença de glicose Inibe o esvaziamento gástrico
Peptídio inibitório gástrico (GIP)	Nutrientes no duodeno (ácidos graxos, glicose, aminoácidos)	Trato gastrintestinal (estômago, duodeno, jejuno, íleo)	
Somatostatina	Nutrientes (lipídios e proteínas) Bile	Estômago Vesícula biliar Pâncreas Intestino	Inibe a secreção ácida e de pepsinogênio Inibição da contração da vesícula biliar Inibição da secreção de insulina e exócrina Inibição da motilidade intestinal; diminuição da absorção de nutrientes
Motilina	Nutrientes (lipídios) Íon hidrogênio (H^+)	Intestino	Coordena o complexo migratório de motilidade (CMM) Coordena as secreções gástrica, pancreática e biliar
Grelina	Nutrientes (proteína)	Hipófise	Modula o hormônio do crescimento

Glucagon, peptídio semelhante ao glucagon e peptídio inibitório gástrico

O glucagon das células alfa das ilhotas pancreáticas e enteroglucagons das células GI L são produtos do mesmo gene. A diversidade dentro dessa família de peptídios surge do processamento específico tecidual de transcrições de genes primários. Nas células alfa das ilhotas, os RNAms primários codificam glucagon, enquanto nas células L aqueles derivados do mesmo gene, GLP, GIP, enteroglucagon e glicentina.[3] Glucagon, um hormônio vital na homeostase energética e no metabolismo de nutrientes, possui ações que geralmente balanceiam as ações anabólicas da insulina. O glucagon é o principal estímulo hormonal para a glicogenólise hepática e a gliconeogênese, ações opostas àquelas da insulina. GLP (GLP-1 e GLP-2) e GIP são enteroglucagons conhecidos como incretinas, porque suas ações incrementam a secreção de insulina induzida por nutrientes. Das incretinas, a GLP-1 é o secretagogo mais potente da insulina, tendo sido estudada extensivamente como adjuvante terapêutico potencial para o diabetes melito (DM). GLP-1 e GLP-2 são liberados pelas células L em resposta aos nutrientes intraluminais, e eles também modulam a absorção intestinal de glicose pela inibição da motilidade gástrica e pela suprarregulação mediada pela GLP-2 dos transportadores de glicose.[4,5]

Gastrina

A gastrina, sintetizada e secretada por células G neuroendócrinas localizadas no antro gástrico e no duodeno, é estimulada pela proteína ingerida e distensão gástrica e inibida por pH intraluminal baixo (< 3). A gastrina circula em diversas formas moleculares diferentes, que variam em peso molecular (p. ex., gastrina-34, 17 e 14), que se ligam a superfícies de tecidos-alvo.[6] A gastrina-34 é a principal gastrina circulante, mas a 17, menos abundante, possui efeitos biológicos mais potentes sobre a secreção ácida gástrica, a ação biológica primária desse hormônio. A gastrina atua em conjunto com a acetilcolina das terminações nervosas parassimpáticas autonômicas e histamina para regular a secreção de H^+ pelas células parietais gástricas. A gastrina possui efeitos tróficos sobre o epitélio gástrico e estimula o fluxo sanguíneo da mucosa, a liberação de pepsinogênio e a motilidade antral, além de influenciar a produção enzimática pancreática e possuir efeitos tróficos sobre o tecido pancreático e duodenal.

Colecistocinina

A colecistocinina (CCK), sintetizada pelas células I localizadas no duodeno e no jejuno, é liberada em resposta a uma série de substâncias que entram no duodeno, especialmente H^+, ácidos graxos e aminoácidos.[7] Durante a síntese, a transcrição de CCK é submetida a um processamento, que resulta em uma série de isoformas circulantes. Das sete isoformas identificadas de CCK, CCK-33, CCK-39 e CCK-58 são responsáveis pelos principais efeitos GI. CCK-8, expressa em neurônios, serve como um neurotransmissor peptídico no sistema nervoso entérico. Outras isoformas, como CCK-5, CCK-12 e CCK-63, possuem funções de menor importância GI. As principais ações da CCK incluem estimulação da contração da vesícula biliar e secreção enzimática pancreática, ambas mediadas por neurônios colinérgicos pré-sinápticos. A CCK também atua para coordenar a função digestória geral, incluindo a estimulação da secreção de fluido pancreático (na presença de níveis estimulatórios de secretina), a inibição do esvaziamento gástrico, o relaxamento do esfíncter de Oddi e a estimulação do crescimento pancreático.

Somatostatina

O peptídio somatostatina é sintetizado no hipotálamo, nas células delta das ilhotas pancreáticas, nas células D GI e nos subgrupos de neurônios no SNC e no sistema nervoso entérico. Células D intestinais liberam somatostatina em resposta aos nutrientes (gorduras e proteínas) e bile no lúmen intestinal. Os efeitos endócrinos, parácrinos e neurotransmissores da somatostatina inibem: ácidos gástricos, pepsinogênio, contração da vesícula biliar, secreção de insulina, função exócrina pancreática, motilidade GI e absorção de nutrientes (aminoácidos e glicose).[8]

Motilina

A motilina, um hormônio peptídico sintetizado nas células GI, está estruturalmente relacionada com a grelina. A secreção é cíclica, a depender se em jejum ou alimentado, mas suas principais ações endócrinas ocorrem durante o jejum. Entre as refeições, a motilina inicia e coordena os complexos migratórios de motilidade (CMMs), que servem para limpar os intestinos em estados interdigestivos. Depois de comer, a motilina é liberada em resposta ao ácido gástrico (H^+) ou aos lipídios que entram no intestino delgado. No estado alimentado, a motilina serve para coordenar as secreções gástrica, pancreática e biliar.[9]

Grelina

O hormônio grelina, estruturalmente relacionado com a motilina, foi recentemente identificado como um mediador importante do apetite e do metabolismo energético.[10] A grelina, sintetizada e secretada no estômago, estimula o apetite, o crescimento de adipócitos, além de síntese e secreção hipofisária de hormônio do crescimento (GH, *growth hormone*). A grelina fornece uma ligação entre nutrientes dietéticos, energia calórica e o eixo hipofisário-GH, vital para a regulação do crescimento.

Serotonina

Serotonina (5-hidroxitriptamina [5-HT]) é um neuropeptídio e hormônio localizado dentro dos neurônios entéricos e das células enterocromafins distribuídas por todo o trato GI. A 5-HT de origem enterocromafim atua como um agente endócrino e parácrino para estimular a contração da musculatura lisa GI e a secreção intestinal.[11]

INSULINOMA

Tumores neuroendócrinos, raramente diagnosticados em cães e gatos, costumam estar localizados no pâncreas, onde eles surgem das células das ilhotas (tumores de células das ilhotas; ver Capítulo 303). Lesões metastáticas são comuns no mesentério, no intestino e no fígado. O insulinoma não é comum, mas é o tumor neuroendócrino mais relatado em cães e raro em gatos (ver Capítulo 303).[12-15] O pâncreas é a localização mais frequente para a formação de insulinomas, mas esses tumores também podem ser encontrados em localizações mesentéricas, esplênicas e hepáticas. Não está claro se insulinomas não pancreáticos representam tumores primários ou metastáticos. Insulinomas causam aumentos flutuantes nas concentrações circulantes de insulina que não estão sob controle fisiológico. Como resultado, animais com insulinoma apresentam hipoglicemia episódica. O foco deste capítulo está no gastrinoma, no glucagonoma e em outras condições menos comuns.

GASTRINOMA

Contexto geral

Gastrinoma é um tumor não comum em cães e gatos,[16-20] não tendo sido publicado nenhum estudo em larga escala do gastrinoma canino ou felino. A produção excessiva de gastrina por gastrinomas pode levar à síndrome de Zollinger-Ellison, clinicamente associada à hipertrofia antral gástrica, à hiperacidez e à ulceração.[21] O tratamento envolve a remoção cirúrgica. A terapia de suporte é direcionada à supressão da produção de ácidos gástricos.

Epidemiologia e sinais clínicos

A literatura veterinária cita menos de 50 casos de gastrinoma em cães e gatos, sendo a maioria em cães. Em cães, a idade média ao diagnóstico é de cerca de 8 anos e, em gatos, quando um pouco mais velhos. Observações frequentes dos tutores incluem êmese, diarreia e perda de peso. Questões menos frequentes incluem dor abdominal aparente, hemorragia GI, polidipsia e constipação intestinal. A hiperacidez induzida pela gastrina pode levar a esofagite por refluxo, com regurgitação resultante, e cólica esofágica (ver Capítulo 273). Gastropatia, caracterizada por hipertrofia mucosa, ulceração mucosa e, em casos graves, obstrução da via de saída, leva à êmese e à perda de peso. A diarreia pode ocorrer em razão dos efeitos inibitórios da gastrina sobre a absorção hídrica intestinal. Gastrinomas, quase sempre bastante pequenos, não são costumam ser detectados durante a palpação abdominal. Os achados de exame físico dependem do estágio da doença. Sinais, se presentes, não são específicos. No início da doença, o exame físico, em geral, é perfeito. Animais com esofagite, ulceração ou perfuração gástrica apresentam dor à palpação esofágica ou abdominal, evidências de desidratação, febre e sinais de choque.

Achados laboratoriais

O gastrinoma não está associado a alterações específicas no hemograma ou nos painéis bioquímicos séricos. Achados não específicos de leucocitose, neutrofilia com desvio à esquerda, anemia e pan-hipoproteinemia causada pela inflamação e pela perda de sangue podem ser secundários a ulcerações gástricas. Outras anormalidades bioquímicas relatadas incluem hipoalbuminúria, hipopotassemia, hipocloremia, hiponatremia, alcalose metabólica, hiperbilirrubinemia e aumento das atividades de enzimas hepáticas. Alterações bioquímicas podem não ser causadas pelo gastrinoma, por si só, mas podem ocorrer secundariamente a consequências da hipergastrinemia, como êmese crônica, diarreia ou metástase hepática. Alguns cães com gastrinoma apresentavam distúrbios concomitantes (mielofibrose, obstrução de ductos biliares) que contribuíram para as alterações clinicopatológicas. Alguns gastrinomas podem produzir e secretar hormônios além da gastrina; relatou-se secreção concomitante de insulina e hormônio adrenocorticotrófico (ACTH, do inglês *adrenocorticotropic hormone*).

Exames diagnósticos de imagem de rotina

A ultrassonografia (ver Capítulo 88) é geralmente mais útil do que a radiografia na avaliação diagnóstica para o gastrinoma. A ultrassonografia abdominal, mais eficiente para detecção de um tumor pancreático do que as radiografias, pode revelar alterações gástricas compatíveis com ulceração, hipertrofia de pregas e mucosa e espessamento das paredes gástricas. A ultrassonografia pode também permitir a detecção de metástases para locais extrapancreáticos, como fígado ou linfonodos. Em geral, a radiografia simples não é útil ou revela apenas alterações inespecíficas. A utilização de radiografa contrastada, descrita em diversos relatos de caso, identificou hipertrofia de pregas gástricas, estreitamento do antro em razão da hipertrofia e defeitos da mucosa causados pela ulceração. A endoscopia – de valor limitado para obtenção do diagnóstico definitivo – pode fornecer informações úteis com relação a inflamação e ulceração esofágica, pregas gástricas proeminentes, hipertrofia antral, ulceração gástrica e duodenal e hipersecreção de fluido gástrico (ver Capítulo 113). A biopsia endoscópica pode permitir a caracterização histológica de alterações GI, mas provavelmente não fornecerá o diagnóstico definitivo de gastrinoma.

Diagnóstico

Contexto geral

Uma gama de opções de testes está disponível, incluindo mensuração das concentrações séricas de gastrina, produção ácida basal, estimulação da secreção de gastrina por secretina e cálcio e exames de imagem do tumor utilizando-se somatostatina marcada para localização cintilográfica. Esses estudos não são comuns em cães e gatos.

Mensurações basais: concentrações séricas de gastrina e pH gástrico

As concentrações séricas de gastrina costumam estar aumentadas em pessoas e cães com gastrinoma. Em seres humanos, os teores séricos de gastrina > 1.000 ng/ℓ, em conjunto com pH gástrico < 2,5, são considerados diagnósticos para gastrinoma. Esse pareamento das mensurações de gastrina e ácidos gástricos não tem sido utilizado extensivamente na medicina veterinária. As concentrações séricas de gastrina em cães com gastrinomas confirmados histologicamente variaram diversas vezes acima do limite superior de referência, mas nenhum limiar específico foi estabelecido. Em cães e gatos, as concentrações sanguíneas de gastrina podem estar aumentadas na doença renal, nas gastropatias, nas hepatopatias e com a utilização de fármacos que inibem a produção de ácidos gástricos. Mensurações de pH e/ou secreção de ácidos gástricos, relatados em alguns poucos cães com gastrinoma, apontaram pH gástrico baixo. A mensuração da concentração sérica de gastrina não pode ser utilizada como um teste único para confirmação do gastrinoma, mesmo se alta. Tais resultados são mais úteis quando a suspeita clínica para gastrinoma é alta e outros distúrbios que poderiam causar hipergastrinemia já foram descartados.

Testes provocativos

Testes provocativos medem a liberação de gastrina em resposta à secretina ou ao cálcio (Ca). Nem a injeção de secretina nem a de Ca levam ao aumento da concentração de gastrina em indivíduos normais, mas ambos causam liberação de gastrina por gastrinomas. O teste de estimulação por secretina é o teste provocativo mais frequentemente empregado em pessoas, mas a experiência com esse teste em animais é bastante limitada. O princípio do teste se baseia na responsividade aumentada do tecido do gastrinoma à secretina. Um protocolo utilizado em cães envolveu a obtenção de amostras séricas antes e 2, 5, 10 e 20 minutos após a injeção IV de secretina (2 a 4 UI/kg).[22] Um protocolo alternativo envolve a obtenção de amostras antes e 2, 5, 10, 30 e 60 minutos após a injeção IV de 2 UI/kg de secretina.[23] Amostras dos períodos de 2 e 5 minutos são mais úteis para o diagnóstico de gastrinoma, já que a resposta do tumor à secretina injetada é, em geral, rápida e de meia-vida curta. Seres humanos com gastrinoma apresentam aumento de cerca de duas vezes na gastrina após injeção de secretina. Embora relatos de testes de estimulação por secretina em cães sejam escassos, os resultados foram semelhantes àqueles relatados em seres humanos. Entretanto, nem todos os cães com gastrinoma mostraram aumento da gastrina maior que duas vezes acima do nível basal.[22]

Pode-se dar preferência ao teste de estimulação por Ca, uma alternativa para a estimulação à secretina, pois, além de não ser cara, está amplamente disponível. Efeitos cardíacos adversos durante a infusão são uma desvantagem importante, necessitando de precauções apropriadas (ver Capítulo 298). O protocolo descrito inclui amostras séricas coletadas antes e 15, 30, 60 e 90 minutos após infusão IV de Ca (2 mg/kg IV, administrado durante 1 minuto).[24] A secreção máxima de gastrina foi detectada com 60 minutos. Em geral, seres humanos com gastrinoma apresentam aumento de duas vezes das concentrações séricas de gastrina após estimulação, assim como os poucos cães com gastrinoma confirmado.

Patologia

De modo geral, gastrinomas são nódulos neoplásicos solitários localizados no pâncreas, havendo o relato de diversos tumores. No cão, o tumor está mais frequentemente localizado no ramo direito ou no corpo do pâncreas, sendo comuns metástases no momento do diagnóstico. Lesões metastáticas podem ser identificadas em locais não pancreáticos (linfonodos, mesentério, superfícies peritoneais, baço e fígado) em até 85% dos casos. Microscopicamente, gastrinomas são carcinomas com origem em células endócrinas que coram pela imunoistoquímica. Em estudos ultraestruturais, a identificação de grânulos intracelulares específicos pode permitir o diagnóstico definitivo de gastrinoma. Embora raramente realizadas, as mensurações de hormônios em extratos de tecido tumoral também podem ser utilizadas para confirmar a produção de gastrina. É comum a ulceração GI secundária à hipergastrinemia, podendo afetar o esôfago, o estômago e o intestino e resultar em perfuração e peritonite. A hipertrofia da parede gástrica foi relatada. Distúrbios endócrinos adicionais observados em alguns cães incluem carcinoma tireoidiano e hiperplasia adrenal.

GLUCAGONOMA

Contexto geral

O glucagonoma é um tumor endócrino raro relatado em vários cães[25-27] e em um único gato.[28] Ele surge de células alfa neuroendócrinas nas ilhotas pancreáticas. As concentrações circulantes de glucagon em excesso ocorrem em razão da secreção autônoma que induz a gliconeogênese hepática e glicogenólise, que, por sua vez, causam resistência insulínica, intolerância à glicose e, em alguns casos, DM evidente. O tratamento definitivo é alcançado pela remoção cirúrgica do glucagonoma. O eritema migratório necrolítico (EMN), uma condição dermatológica caracterizada por crostas e erupções cutâneas, é considerado patognomônico para o glucagonoma em pessoas.[29] Em cães, essa condição tem sido observada em casos de glucagonoma, mas está mais comumente associada à hepatopatia (ver Capítulos 10 e 285).[30]

Identificação e sinais clínicos

No momento do diagnóstico, os poucos cães descritos como portadores de glucagonoma eram de meia-idade ou idosos, e o gato tinha 6 anos. Em conjunto com sinais inespecíficos, como letargia e hiporexia, alguns poucos tutores dos cães se queixaram das erosões cutâneas que não cicatrizavam e das úlceras. A distribuição das lesões e o envolvimento de locais mucocutâneos são também compatíveis com dermatopatias autoimunes. Lesões relatadas envolvem lábios, nariz, orelhas, espelho nasal, coxins, ventre, região inguinal e extremidades (Figura 310.1). Cães com DM descompensado no momento do diagnóstico apresentaram polidipsia, poliúria e perda de peso. A insulinoterapia pode ser relativamente ineficaz para o controle da hiperglicemia, necessitando de doses altas.

Achados laboratoriais

Muitas anormalidades laboratoriais inespecíficas foram relatadas em cães com glucagonoma, mas nenhuma específica. O aumento das atividades séricas de alanina aminotransferase (ALT) e fosfatase alcalina (ALF), em conjunto com diminuições do teor de albumina, nitrogênio ureico sanguíneo (NUS) e colesterol, foi identificado em alguns cães com EMN e glucagonoma. Ao considerar um diagnóstico de glucagonoma, é válido lembrar que parâmetros hepáticos anormais em cães com glucagonoma simulam hepatopatias primárias, uma causa mais comum de EMN em cães. Testes de função hepática, como teores de ácidos biliares e amônia sanguínea, estão normais em cães com glucagonoma, mas podem ser importantes ao investigar a possibilidade de hepatopatia.

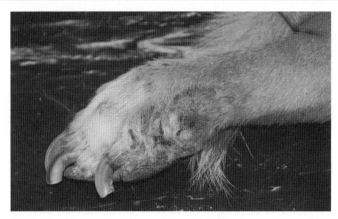

Figura 310.1 Lesões por eritema migratório necrolítico na pata e nos coxins de um cão com glucagonoma. (*Esta figura se encontra reproduzida em cores no Encarte.*)

Diagnóstico por imagem

A ultrassonografia abdominal (ver Capítulo 88) é mais sensível do que a radiografia para detecção da massa pancreática, não havendo a detecção de tumores na maioria dos cães com relatos de glucagonoma. A avaliação por tomografia computadorizada (TC) identificou um tumor pancreático em um cão. Anormalidades na aparência ultrassonográfica do fígado eram frequentemente observadas em cães com glucagonoma, mas não foi observado nenhum padrão compatível. Em cães com EMN, é importante lembrar que hepatopatias são causas mais comuns do que o glucagonoma. À ultrassonografia, anormalidades hepáticas devem ser avaliadas no contexto de um animal ter ou não hepatopatia primária ou glucagonoma.

Diagnóstico

O diagnóstico definitivo do glucagonoma se baseia na identificação de hiperglucagonemia, notada na maioria dos cães com glucagonoma previamente relatado. A hiperglucagonemia em cães acometidos mostrou variabilidade, com variação de elevações de aproximadamente 1,5 a 15 vezes acima do limite superior do valor de referência. Nenhuma concentração sérica é diagnóstica de glucagonoma, mas concentrações séricas > 1.000 ng/ℓ são o são em seres humanos. Como o glucagon sérico pode aumentar em distúrbios que não o glucagonoma, o diagnóstico é confirmado de maneira apropriada apenas quando a hiperglucagonemia ocorre em associação aos sinais clínicos relacionados com o excesso do hormônio. Os esforços diagnósticos podem ser complicados pela ausência de testes séricos disponíveis no mercado para o glucagon canino e felino. A mensuração dos aminoácidos plasmáticos pode fornecer suporte ao diagnóstico de glucagonoma. A hiperglucagonemia estimula a gliconeogênese hepática, acelera a quebra de aminoácidos e diminui as concentrações plasmáticas destes. Concentrações de arginina, histidina e lisina estavam reduzidas em todos os cães com glucagonoma nos quais as mensurações foram realizadas.

Patologia

Em geral, o glucagonoma pancreático é uma neoplasia solitária que pode surgir de qualquer região do pâncreas (ramos, corpo); relatos sugerem que a metástase é comum em cães. O fígado foi o local primário de metástase na maioria, embora a metástase linfática tenha sido observada. Nódulos metastáticos podem ser funcionais (metástase hepática foi o único local onde a produção de glucagon foi documentada em um cão com glucagonoma), sugerindo que a remoção cirúrgica incompleta das metástases poderia resultar em sinais persistentes. Por convenção, esses tumores são corados para glucagon, quando examinados pela imunoistoquímica. Pode-se detectar a expressão de outros hormônios das ilhotas e marcadores neuroendócrinos.

A maioria dos cães com glucagonoma exibiu coloração celular positiva para diversos hormônios, embora não esteja claro se esses tumores secretam hormônios que não o glucagon.

OUTROS TUMORES NEUROENDÓCRINOS

Carcinoides

Tumores neuroendócrinos que secretam substâncias vasoativas, como a 5-HT (também conhecida como serotonina) ou cininas, são conhecidos como tumores carcinoides. Esses tumores podem surgir de células neuroendócrinas localizadas no epitélio da árvore bronquial, pulmão, sistema biliar, trato GI e outros locais. Em pessoas, a "síndrome carcinoide" é caracterizada por diarreia aquosa, desconforto abdominal, cãibras abdominais, broncoconstrição e hiperemia de bochechas e testa ("rubor facial"). Tumores carcinoides são raros em cães e gatos. A maior parte das informações sobre esses tumores vem de descrições de casos isolados.[31] Em cães, carcinoides foram encontrados no estômago, no duodeno, no jejuno, na região ileocólica, no cólon e no reto.[32-36] Com base em alguns poucos relatos em gatos, localizações incluíram fígado, pâncreas e trato GI.[37,38] Metástases em linfonodos e outros locais, incluindo pulmões, foram comuns. A maioria dos carcinoides relatados em cães e gatos causam sinais relacionados com a presença física do tumor e não parecem ser funcionais. A síndrome carcinoide não foi relatada em gatos e o único cão relatado não apresentou concentrações elevadas de substâncias vasoativas, como 5-HT ou cininas.[39] O diagnóstico de carcinoide costuma ser confirmado pós-morte, mas, quando identificado antes da morte, a remoção cirúrgica é recomendada. A remoção do tumor pode melhorar os sinais que resultam de sua presença física (p. ex., obstrução intestinal), embora a alta frequência de metástases torne improvável a remoção completa do tumor. No único relato de caso de síndrome carcinoide suspeita em um cão, a remoção do tumor resultou em melhora ou resolução dos sinais clínicos.[39] As concentrações séricas de 5-HT e outras substâncias vasoativas podem ser mensuradas para confirmar a suspeita de carcinoide em pessoas, mas esses exames não foram realizados em animais. A avaliação histológica do tecido tumoral é necessária para confirmação do diagnóstico.

Polipeptidoma pancreático

O polipeptidoma pancreático é um tumor neuroendócrino mal compreendido que se dá como parte da síndrome da neoplasia endócrina múltipla (NEM) em pessoas, mas também com ocorrência esporádica em seres humanos e com relatos em cães.[24] Muitos tumores neuroendócrinos funcionais originários das ilhotas pancreáticas coram para diversos hormônios peptídicos, incluindo o polipeptídio pancreático (PP). Quando o principal hormônio proteico expresso é o PP, o tumor é designado como polipeptidoma pancreático. Os sinais clínicos associados ao excesso de secreção de PP são mínimos, e a maioria dos polipeptidomas pancreáticos são considerados não funcionais.[40] Houve suspeita de que uma minoria de polipeptidomas pancreáticos humanos produzia sinais clínicos relacionados com a liberação tumoral de PP. Sinais relatados com excesso de PP incluem dor abdominal e diarreia. Alguns haviam sofrido de pancreatite. Em um cão, o aumento das concentrações plasmáticas de PP estava associado a êmese crônica, úlceras duodenais e evidência de gastrite hipertrófica, o qual também apresentou um adenocarcinoma pancreático, que corou para PP e insulina, mas não para outros peptídios tipicamente produzidos por tumores neuroendócrinos pancreáticos caninos (gastrina, glucagon ou somatostatina).[24]

REFERÊNCIAS BIBLIOGRÁFICAS

As referências bibliográficas deste capítulo se encontram online no Ambiente de Aprendizagem.

CAPÍTULO 311

Feocromocitoma

Sara Galac

CONTEXTO GERAL E DEFINIÇÃO

O feocromocitoma é um tumor neuroendócrino produtor de catecolaminas que surge das células cromafins da medula adrenal,[1] considerado maligno. As manifestações são diversas e podem simular aquelas de várias condições que quase sempre resultam em erros e atrasos do diagnóstico. Não é surpreendente que o feocromocitoma tenha ganhado, dessa forma, o título de "grande imitador". A percepção do clínico quanto ao feocromocitoma representa um passo inicial crucial ao realizar o diagnóstico, mas evidências bioquímicas de produção excessiva de catecolaminas e exames de imagem são necessários para confirmação.[2,3] A maioria dos feocromocitomas é unilateral, mas ocasionalmente ambas as adrenais são acometidas. O feocromocitoma pode coexistir com outras neoplasias endócrinas, como tumor adrenocortical secretor de cortisol, tumor hipofisário secretor de hormônio adrenocorticotrófico (ACTH, *adrenocorticotropic hormone*), tumor tireoidiano, insulinoma ou tumor ou hiperplasia paratireoidiana.[4-8] Em cães, a etiologia do feocromocitoma é amplamente desconhecida. Recentemente, a análise de mutações demonstrou uma mutação *missense* da subunidade D succinato desidrogenase (*SDHD, succinate dehydrogenase subunit D*).[9] Em seres humanos, a mutação da linhagem germinativa da *SDHD* costuma se apresentar nas formas familiares do feocromocitoma, além de mutações em *SDHD, NF1, RET1* e *VHL*.[10,11] Há uma grande homologia de sequência entre *SDHD* canina e humana, e, em teoria, essa mutação poderia ser responsável pelo desenvolvimento de feocromocitoma em cães.[9]

FISIOLOGIA

A medula adrenal é originada do sistema nervoso simpático, mas sem os axônios e dendritos dos neurônios. As células medulares, chamadas de feocromócitos ou células cromafins, liberam epinefrina e norepinefrina na corrente sanguínea. A medula é altamente vascularizada e diretamente conectada ao sistema aórtico abdominal. Existe íntima relação vascular entre a medula e o córtex. O sangue que flui da zona reticular deixa a glândula pelos vasos na medula. A inervação e a vascularização singulares da medula adrenal são a base da resposta de "luta ou fuga".[12]

Catecolaminas (epinefrina e norepinefrina) são sintetizadas a partir do aminoácido tirosina por uma série de modificações (Figura 311.1). Quando a tirosina entra nas células cromafins, é convertida em L-di-hidroxifenilalanina pela enzima tirosina hidroxilase. Esse primeiro passo na via é o sinal comprometido com o limitante da velocidade e inibido pelo *feedback* pela norepinefrina. A depleção intracelular de catecolaminas aumenta rapidamente a atividade da enzima, enquanto o aumento dos teores de catecolaminas leva à diminuição da sua regulação.[13] Na maioria dos neurônios pós-ganglionares simpáticos, a norepinefrina é o produto final. Entretanto, a medula adrenal expressa uma enzima adicional não presente nos neurônios adrenérgicos: a feniletanolamina-N-metiltransferase (PNMT).[12] Como apenas a medula adrenal é exposta a altos teores de cortisol (em razão do fluxo sanguíneo centrípeto oriundo do córtex), a indução da expressão do gene *PNMT* é permitida. Esse mecanismo fisiológico precisa ser levado em consideração nos procedimentos diagnósticos para feocromocitoma.[14] Dentro da medula adrenal, a norepinefrina é liberada pelas vesículas cromafins para o citoplasma e convertida em epinefrina. A quantidade de epinefrina e norepinefrina armazenada varia de espécie para espécie. Em cães, as catecolaminas costumam incluir mais epinefrina (70%) e menos norepinefrina (30%). As porcentagens são de 60 e 40%, em gatos, e 80 e 20% em seres humanos.[15]

Catecolaminas são liberadas por exocitose após estimulação das células cromafins pela acetilcolina, oriunda do sistema nervoso simpático. O sinal de liberação é desencadeado por fatores estressantes, como ansiedade, medo, dor, trauma, hemorragia ou outras perdas de fluido, alterações no pH sanguíneo, hipoglicemia ou exposição ao calor ou ao frio excessivo. A meia-vida plasmática

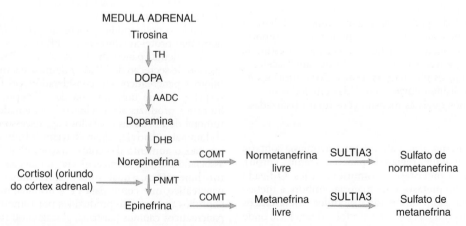

Figura 311.1 Representação esquemática da síntese de catecolaminas e do metabolismo na glândula adrenal. A tirosina é convertida em L-di-hidroxifenilalanina (*DOPA*) pela enzima tirosina hidroxilase (*TH*), e o metabolismo subsequente para dopamina é orquestrado pela enzima aromática L-aminoácido descarboxilase (*AADC*). Dopamina é convertida pela enzima dopamina beta-hidroxilase (*DHB*) em norepinefrina, que é finalmente convertida em epinefrina pela enzima PNMT, estimulada pelo cortisol oriundo do córtex adrenal. As catecolaminas são metabolizadas pela enzima catecol-O-metiltransferase (*COMT*) e podem ser mensuradas como normetanefrina livre e normetanefrinas no plasma. A conjugação da normetanefrina e metanefrina pela enzima sulfotransferase (*SULTIA3*) ocorre no trato gastrintestinal, nos rins e no fígado, e as metanefrinas conjugadas com sulfato podem ser mensuradas na urina.

das catecolaminas circulantes é curta, e sua inativação começa dentro de alguns minutos.[16,17] Elas são metabolizadas no fígado e nos rins, mas também podem ser inativadas por desconjugação no trato gastrintestinal (GI). Além desse metabolismo extra-adrenal das catecolaminas circulantes, existe um metabolismo contínuo da norepinefrina e epinefrina dentro da medula adrenal em razão do extravasamento de norepinefrina e epinefrina de seus grânulos de armazenamento, o que leva à produção substancial intracelular de metabólitos O-metilados, metanefrina (MN) e normetanefrina (NMN) (ver Figura 311.1). Esses processos metabólicos dentro da medula independem de liberação exocitótica das catecolaminas e representam a fonte primária de MN e NMN circulantes. Em seres humanos, aproximadamente 93% do MN e 25 a 40% do NMN circulantes são derivados do metabolismo das catecolaminas dentro das células cromafins adrenais. Existe uma concepção errônea de que os estoques vesiculares de catecolaminas existem em um estado estático até que um estímulo evoque a liberação para o espaço extracelular.[13] Em vez disso, os estoques vesiculares estão em um equilíbrio altamente dinâmico com as catecolaminas no citoplasma circundante. O transporte ativo rápido do citoplasma para as vesículas contrabalanceia o extravasamento externo passivo das vesículas. Embora apenas uma pequena fração das catecolaminas no citoplasma escape do sequestro vesicular, ela permanece como uma fonte importante de metabólitos de catecolaminas.[18] As catecolaminas ativam os receptores adrenérgicos acoplados à proteína-G, que são divididos em tipos alfa e beta e seus subtipos. Há ima visão geral da localização dos receptores e sua relevância fisiológica na Tabela 311.1.

MANIFESTAÇÕES CLÍNICAS

Epidemiologia

O feocromocitoma é diagnosticado mais frequentemente em cães idosos (média: 11 anos).[5,7,19] Não existe predileção sexual

Tabela 311.1 Tipos e subtipos de catecolaminas, localização tecidual e efeitos.

ÓRGÃO/TECIDO	TIPO DE RECEPTOR	EFEITO
Sistema cardiovascular	Beta-1	Aumento da frequência cardíaca e contratilidade
	Alfa-2	Vasoconstrição
	Beta-2	Vasodilatação das arteríolas do músculo esquelético, artérias coronarianas e todas as veias
Músculos bronquiais	Beta-2	Relaxamento
Trato gastrintestinal	Beta-2	Diminuição da motilidade
Ilhotas pancreáticas	Alfa-2	Diminuição na secreção de insulina e glucagon
	Beta-2	Aumento na secreção de insulina e glucagon
Fígado	Beta-2	Aumento na glicogenólise e gliconeogênese
Tecido adiposo	Beta-2	Aumento na lipólise
Bexiga urinária	Alfa-2	Aumento do tônus do esfíncter
	Beta-2	Relaxamento do músculo detrusor
Olho	Alfa-1	Midríase

Adaptada de Galac S, Reusch C, Kooistra H et al.: Adrenals. In Rijnberk A, Kooistra HS, editors: Clinical endocrinology of dogs and cats, 2 ed., Hannover, 2010, Schlütersche, p. 140.

ou racial aparente. A descrição frequente de feocromocitoma em algumas raças (Rhodesian Ridgeback, Labrador Retriever, Boxer, Golden Retriever, raças Terrier) reflete sua popularidade mais do que seu risco relativo à doença.[15,20] Em gatos, o feocromocitoma é considerado extremamente raro; somente três casos foram relatados na literatura veterinária.[21-23]

Sinais clínicos

Sinais clínicos associados ao feocromocitoma estão relacionados com as ações diretas das catecolaminas secretadas e/ou da ocupação de espaço ou natureza invasiva do tumor adrenal. A secreção hormonal pelo tumor é esporádica e imprevisível. Manifestações clínicas decorrentes do excesso de catecolaminas circulantes variam de maneira considerável. Cães com feocromocitoma mais frequentemente apresentam episódios intermitentes de colapso, fraqueza e/ou respiração ofegante.[5,7,19] Os episódios são paroxísticos e podem ocorrer diversas vezes/dia ou por semana ou apenas em intervalos de semanas a meses. Eles podem ser discretos ou causar risco de morte, bem como progredir com o passar do tempo. Manifestações clínicas relacionadas com o excesso de catecolaminas podem ser categorizadas como segue[15]:

- Sistema cardiorrespiratório e/ou hipertensão sistêmica: taquipneia, respiração ofegante, taquicardia, arritmias, colapso, palidez de mucosas, hemorragia nasal, gengival ou ocular, cegueira aguda
- Sistema neuromuscular: fraqueza, ansiedade, andar compulsivo, tremores musculares, convulsões
- Inespecíficos: anorexia, perda de peso, letargia
- Diversos: poliúria/polidipsia, êmese, diarreia, dor abdominal.

Grandes feocromocitomas podem se tornar invasivos, já que a estrutura heterogênea os torna predispostos a episódios de hemorragias e necrose. As manifestações clínicas de um feocromocitoma adrenal que ocupa espaço podem estar relacionadas com:

- Invasão da veia cava pelo tumor: ascite, edema de membro pélvico, distensão das veias epigástricas caudais
- Invasão da aorta pelo tumor (tromboembolia aórtica) membros pélvicos doloridos e fracos, paraparesia, ausência de pulso femoral, extremidades distais frias[5,24]
- Ruptura espontânea do tumor: hemorragia retroperitoneal (letargia, taquipneia, taquicardia, fraqueza, mucosas pálidas, dor abdominal).[25]

Em cães, feocromocitomas podem metastatizar para o fígado, os rins, o baço, os linfonodos regionais, os pulmões, o coração, os ossos e o sistema nervoso central. A doença metastática pode causar sinais clínicos específicos dos órgãos. Em cães, foram relatados diversas vezes paresia decorrente de metástases dentro do canal vertebral e claudicação, edema e dor em razão de metástases ósseas.[26-28]

O exame físico costuma estar normal. Quando da existência de sinais, respiração ofegante e taquipneia são mais comuns, seguidos de fraqueza, taquicardia e arritmias cardíacas.[7,29,30] Entretanto, os achados do exame físico dependem amplamente da existência ou não da atividade secretora pelo tumor. Esse caleidoscópio de manifestações clínicas e o diagnóstico infrequente do feocromocitoma exigem um alto nível de percepção clínica para o diagnóstico; de outra forma, essa condição pode ser facilmente negligenciada.

AVALIAÇÃO DIAGNÓSTICA

Contexto geral

Feocromocitoma é um desafio diagnóstico (Figura 311.2). A suspeita inicial poderia seguir o achado fortuito de um tumor adrenal durante os exames de imagem, comumente mencionada como "incidentaloma" (ver Capítulo 308). A confirmação desse diagnóstico, entretanto, requer evidências bioquímicas da produção

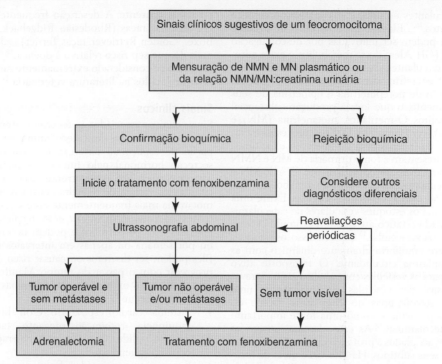

Figura 311.2 Algoritmo de uma abordagem diagnóstica para o feocromocitoma.

excessiva de catecolaminas.[31] Houve melhora considerável do diagnóstico veterinário de feocromocitoma com a introdução de testes para metabólitos plasmáticos e urinários das catecolaminas, NMN e MN.[15] Não existem, pelo menos ainda, diretrizes geralmente aceitas para um "teste de escolha" ou para algoritmos utilizados para confirmação, localização ou exclusão do diagnóstico de feocromocitoma.

Patologia clínica

Nenhuma anormalidade específica no hemograma, no painel bioquímico sérico ou na urinálise levantaria a suspeita de feocromocitoma.[15] Muitas anormalidades identificadas nos resultados de exames de sangue e de urina de rotina são causadas por distúrbios concomitantes comumente presentes em cães com feocromocitoma. Elevações nas atividades séricas de enzimas hepáticas foram relatadas em 10 a 25% dos cães com feocromocitoma,[7] mas valores anormais podem ser secundários a hipertensão sistêmica e alterações na perfusão hepática ou ser causados por uma série de doenças concomitantes potenciais. O hemograma costuma estar normal. Hiperglicemia foi relatada em aproximadamente 20% dos cães com feocromocitoma. Proteinúria, resultado da glomerulopatia hipertensiva ou doença concomitante, também é observada em aproximadamente 20%.[5,7] Hipostenúria/isostenúria podem ocorrer em razão do efeito inibitório das catecolaminas circulantes, especialmente da norepinefrina, sobre a secreção e atividade do hormônio antidiurético (ADH, *antidiuretic hormone*).[15]

Pressão sanguínea sistêmica

Embora a hipertensão arterial seja uma das principais características da doença, é detectada apenas em aproximadamente 50% dos cães com feocromocitoma no momento da avaliação.[15] Diversos padrões de hipertensão foram descritos em seres humanos com feocromocitoma.[2,16] Eles podem apresentar hipertensão persistente e estável ou hipertensão/normotensão com picos paroxísticos de hipertensão extrema; cerca de 10% são normotensos. Sugeriu-se que tais padrões variáveis de pressão sanguínea também existem em cães, o que precisa de confirmação em muitos pacientes.[32] Mensuração, preferivelmente repetida, da pressão sanguínea arterial sistêmica (ver Capítulo 99) é indicada a qualquer cão com suspeita de feocromocitoma, pois a hipertensão requer tratamento imediato (ver Capítulo 158). Em contrapartida, a falha em documentar a hipertensão sistêmica não descarta o feocromocitoma.

Diagnóstico por imagem

Contexto geral

Os exames de imagem fornecem informações importantes sobre tamanho e estrutura adrenais, envolvimento uni ou bilateral e contato com órgãos vizinhos e vasos sanguíneos ou invasão deles.[1,30] Com base nos critérios seletivos, os exames de imagem podem fornecer uma estimativa de malignidade potencial e ser extremamente úteis na seleção da melhor abordagem terapêutica, mas não podem prever o tipo histológico do tumor adrenal.

Radiologia

Radiografias abdominais possuem pouco valor para visualização do feocromocitoma, pois, ao contrário de tumores corticais, eles não costumam ser mineralizados.[30] Radiografias torácicas foram recomendadas antes da adrenalectomia para avaliar metástases, mas têm sido amplamente substituídas pela tomografia computadorizada (TC).[30,33,34] Anormalidades em radiografias torácicas podem incluir cardiomegalia generalizada, sobrecarga ventricular direita ou esquerda, congestão e edema pulmonares, presumivelmente resultantes da hipertensão sistêmica.

Ultrassonografia abdominal

Feocromocitomas podem ser visualizados como nódulos de poucos milímetros de diâmetro ou como tumores heterogêneos com diâmetro > 10 cm. A ecogenicidade deles pode ser hipoecoica ou heterogênea, e grandes tumores podem ter arquitetura multilobular e/ou multicística, com focos anecoicos de necrose e hemorragia. Não existe observação ultrassonográfica considerada patognomônica para feocromocitoma.[30,35] A maioria dos feocromocitomas é composta por tumores adrenais unilaterais e aumentados, com adrenal contralateral com tamanho e formato normais. Entretanto, como há ocorrência de feocromocitomas bilaterais, é desafiador diferenciá-los de hiperplasia adrenocortical. Foi feita uma tentativa de diferenciar tipos tumorais adrenais com a utilização de ultrassonografia contrastada.[36] Em feocromocitomas, não há ganho de contraste em áreas necróticas ou hemorrágicas ou cistos, mas o mesmo ocorre em carcinomas adrenocorticais. O diagnóstico diferencial mais importante está entre neoplasia cortical e medular, as quais não podem ser discriminadas por ultrassonografia. Relata-se que feocromocitomas invadem estruturas adjacentes e vasos sanguíneos mais frequentemente do que outros tipos de tumor adrenal. A invasão da veia cava ocorre em 15 a 55% dos feocromocitomas, com a probabilidade de os tumores da adrenal direita invadirem a veia cava caudal.[29,37,38] O comportamento invasivo não necessariamente indica malignidade; em vez disso, pode representar expansão do tumor em direção a áreas de menor resistência.[2]

Tomografia computadorizada e ressonância magnética

Os exames de imagem por TC são considerados mais acurados do que a ultrassonografia abdominal para a detecção de invasão luminal vascular por tumores adrenais.[30,33,39] A presença e a extensão da invasão vascular influenciam a escolha da terapia, sendo, portanto, importantes. Feocromocitomas possuem aparência variável nas imagens tomográficas, com focos múltiplos de baixa atenuação interpostos com áreas hiperatenuantes altamente vascularizadas, especialmente em grandes tumores.[30,39] Essas características, típicas de hemorragia e necrose, não são específicas para feocromocitoma e são mais prováveis quando tumores adrenais alcançam determinado tamanho. Um benefício adicional do exame por TC é que a imagem abdominal pode ser combinada com a pesquisa torácica por metástases. A utilização de um meio de contraste IV é controversa em pacientes com suspeita de feocromocitoma. Em pessoas, um meio de contraste iônico pode estimular a liberação de catecolaminas e induzir uma crise hipertensiva.[40,41] Embora tais complicações com meio de contraste iônico não tenham sido relatadas em cães com feocromocitoma, dá-se preferência aos meios de contraste não iônicos, pois não exercem tal efeito sobre as catecolaminas. De forma alternativa, o exame por RM pode ser realizado sem qualquer agente de contraste IV. A sensibilidade e a especificidade da TC e da RM em feocromocitomas são comparáveis em seres humanos,[42] mas ainda não existem até hoje relatos de varredura por RM de feocromocitomas em cães.

Exames de imagem nuclear

Em pessoas, a indicação primária para exames de imagem nuclear é para detectar qualquer extensão do feocromocitoma não identificada pelos exames de imagem anatômicos (TC ou RM), como tumores bilaterais ou múltiplos ou metástases.[31] O procedimento de escolha é a cintilografia utilizando ^{123}I-MIBG (metaiodobenzilguanidina), um radiofármaco que compete com a norepinefrina pela captação e pelo armazenamento em grânulos neurossecretórios das células catecolaminas, revelando, assim, o tecido medular funcional, com relatos de sua utilização em cães.[43] A tomografia por emissão de pósitrons (PET, do inglês *pósitron emission tomography*) com ^{18}F-MIBG (fluorobenzilguanidina) é reservada para tumores de crescimento rápido sem diferenciação, nos quais a captação de ^{123}I-MIBG é negativa. Existe pouca experiência com imagens funcionais de feocromocitoma em cães.[44]

Biopsia por aspiração percutânea com agulha fina

A utilização da citologia é direta na discriminação entre tumores adrenais corticais primários e aqueles de origem medular.[45] Ao mesmo tempo que grandes estudos de caso seriam necessários para confirmar a confiabilidade dessa abordagem, a questão permanece sobre se os benefícios desse procedimento superam os seus riscos. A biopsia adrenal pode, potencialmente, ter complicações fatais associadas à liberação de catecolaminas; dessa forma, a biopsia por aspiração com agulha fina é sugerida em pessoas somente após descartar a possibilidade de feocromocitoma.[46,47] Embora relatos publicados na literatura veterinária

não tenham descrito complicações, eles ainda são poucos. Questões sobre os riscos associados a esse procedimento permanecem. Dado que os achados citológicos não costumam alterar as estratégias de manejo e não podem discriminar tumores adrenais primários benignos de malignos, essa abordagem permanece controversa.

Tumor adrenal descoberto ao acaso

A prevalência do feocromocitoma em cães com massa adrenal identificada fortuitamente em um estudo de imagem é desconhecida (ver Capítulos 306, 308 e 310). Já que cães com feocromocitoma podem ter uma pletora de sinais clínicos e passar facilmente despercebidos, a avaliação de feocromocitomas é recomendada para um cão com um tumor adrenal descoberto ao acaso. Isso é enfatizado quando há suspeita do fenótipo de heterogeneidade, calcificação, margens irregulares, invasão local e/ou áreas de necrose no exame de imagem. Se o diagnóstico do feocromocitoma não puder ser confirmado, mas existir forte suspeita de malignidade no exame de imagem, o teste endócrino para excesso de cortisol e aldosterona deve ser realizado antes da adrenalectomia. Aqui, o propósito do teste é antecipar a suplementação hormonal pós-cirúrgica apropriada. A confirmação de malignidade é difícil, mesmo à histopatologia. Portanto, o exame de imagem pode fornecer apenas uma suspeita. Em situações clínicas, quando há ausência de alterações estruturais no tumor adrenal, recomenda-se o monitoramento do tamanho dele, com intervalos de 3 a 6 meses. Embora nenhum tamanho tenha sido identificado como limiar para confirmar ou excluir a malignidade, um aumento no tamanho de massas adrenais – se corroborado por outras características de imagem e/ou clínicas – é uma indicação para adrenalectomia.

Testes bioquímicos

Contexto geral

A demonstração bioquímica da produção excessiva de catecolaminas é essencial para o diagnóstico do feocromocitoma.[31,48] Em geral, as avaliações bioquímicas incluem mensuração das catecolaminas plasmáticas e urinárias e de seus metabólitos, MN e NMN, as chamadas metanefrinas.[3] O princípio da mensuração de metanefrinas baseia-se no metabolismo intramedular de catecolaminas. A produção de metanefrinas em células tumorais é autônoma e contínua. As concentrações de metanefrinas refletem de forma mais acurada o tumor do que as concentrações de catecolaminas, as quais são secretadas de maneira episódica.[13] Em seres humanos, a mensuração de metanefrinas fracionadas na urina ou metanefrinas livres no plasma fornece melhor sensibilidade diagnóstica do que mensurações urinárias ou plasmáticas das catecolaminas (epinefrina e norepinefrina) e outros metabólitos das catecolaminas.[3,48]

Catecolaminas urinárias

Em cães, a mensuração de catecolaminas urinárias deve ser realizada em uma amostra de uma única micção, com concentrações expressas como relação à concentração de creatinina na mesma amostra.[32,49] A relação NMN:creatinina urinária possui maior sensibilidade do que as relações entre MN, epinefrina ou norepinefrina com a creatinina.[49] Enquanto as relações urinárias entre epinefrina/norepinefrina e creatinina tenham sido sobrepostas em certo grau entre cães saudáveis e aqueles com feocromocitoma, a NMN urinária foi consistentemente maior naqueles pacientes com feocromocitoma. Isso poderia indicar que a maioria dos feocromocitomas produz norepinefrina, que é metabolizada em NMN e liberada continuamente na circulação, enquanto a norepinefrina é secretada somente de forma paroxística.[31,50] Com relação às mensurações urinárias de NMN, a mensuração da NMN livre plasmática foi superior à mensuração da MN livre no diagnóstico do feocromocitoma.[51,52] Não existe consenso sobre a avaliação do plasma *versus* urina; entretanto, de acordo com os últimos estudos, a relação urinária entre

NMN e creatinina é mais confiável.[52] Além da acessibilidade ao exame e experiência pessoal, a disponibilidade de valores de referência pode influenciar se o clínico deve utilizar plasma ou urina para esses exames. Por exemplo, NMN e MN livres plasmáticas são muito maiores em cães saudáveis do que em seres humanos, não se devendo subestimar a importância de valores de referência espécie-específicos.

Fármacos e condições passíveis de interferência

Um aspecto importante do diagnóstico bioquímico do feocromocitoma é a interferência de certos fármacos com as mensurações de catecolaminas e seus metabólitos.[17] As fenoxibenzaminas aumentam as concentrações de norepinefrina e NMN em pessoas. Em cães com suspeita de feocromocitoma, o exame deve ser concluído antes de qualquer tratamento. Glicocorticoides endógenos e exógenos possuem interações fisiológicas com catecolaminas e aumentam sua produção.[13] Além disso, existem semelhanças nas características clínicas do feocromocitoma e do hiperadrenocorticismo, tornando sua diferenciação ainda mais desafiadora. A discriminação entre os dois grupos foi novamente superior para a NMN, mas houve certa sobreposição dos valores de NMN no plasma e na urina entre os grupos. Em pessoas, recomenda-se um valor limiar quatro vezes acima do limite superior normal para distinguir resultados positivos verdadeiros de falso-positivos em pacientes com hipercortisolismo, com a proposta de uma regra semelhante para cães.[49] São necessários mais estudos para confirmar essa informação.

Inibina sérica

A mensuração das concentrações séricas de inibina pode ser útil. A inibina deve ser indetectável em cães com feocromocitoma, mas não naqueles com hiperadrenocorticismo.[53] Esse exame não é aplicável a cães sexualmente inteiros, pois não se pode distinguir a inibina sérica gonadal da adrenocortical.

TRATAMENTO

Contexto geral

A adrenalectomia é o melhor tratamento para um cão com feocromocitoma.[15,54] A remoção do tumor adrenal reverterá os sinais clínicos e sintomas associados à liberação de catecolaminas e evitará as complicações do crescimento descontrolado do tumor. Complicações que ocorrem durante e após a cirurgia são efeitos induzidos pelas catecolaminas, que são graves e causam risco de morte potencial. Os pré-requisitos para o sucesso são tratamento clínico pré-cirúrgico, anestesista experiente e cuidado pós-cirúrgico intensivo.[1] Se o tumor for inoperável ou a cirurgia não puder ser realizada por distúrbios concomitantes ou por outras razões, o tratamento clínico é indicado para bloquear a resposta alfa-adrenérgica às catecolaminas circulantes.[29] O tratamento medicamentoso não parece alterar a secreção ou o crescimento dos feocromocitomas.

Manejo pré-cirúrgico

O objetivo do tratamento clínico é prevenir as complicações induzidas pelas catecolaminas: crise hipertensiva, arritmias cardíacas, edema pulmonar e isquemia cardíaca. A fenoxibenzamina é um antagonista de receptores alfa-adrenérgicos que se liga de forma irreversível aos receptores adrenérgicos alfa-$_1$ e alfa-$_2$ e bloqueia a resposta alfa-adrenérgica à epinefrina e à norepinefrina circulantes.[55] Como a fenoxibenzamina possui uma longa duração de ação, picos de catecolaminas circulantes não podem superar a inibição. Em cães pré-tratados com fenoxibenzamina, a taxa de mortalidade após a adrenalectomia foi significativamente menor do que em cães não tratados.[29] A recomendação atual é iniciar com uma dose de 0,25 mg/kg VO, a cada 12 horas, e aumentá-la gradativamente a cada alguns dias, até que a dose final de 1 mg/kg seja alcançada. Durante esse período, o cão deve ser monitorado em busca de sinais clínicos de hipotensão (letargia, fraqueza ou síncope) ou outros efeitos adversos (êmese, taquicardia) e a dose ajustada, se necessário.[15] O pré-tratamento com fenoxibenzamina deve ser iniciado pelo menos 2 semanas antes da adrenalectomia. Entretanto, a dose e a duração ótimas do tratamento ainda não foram estabelecidas. Em pacientes com taquiarritmia, o bloqueio de receptores beta-adrenérgicos deve ser adicionado ao bloqueio de receptores alfa (p. ex., atenolol, 0,2 a 1 mg/kg, VO, a cada 12 a 24 horas). Essa adição, entretanto, jamais deve ser iniciada antes do bloqueio dos receptores alfa-adrenérgicos, já que a perda da vasodilatação mediada por receptores beta-adrenérgicos deixa a estimulação por receptores alfa-adrenérgicos sem oposição, o que poderia resultar em crises hipertensivas.

Cirurgia

A adrenalectomia deve ser realizada somente por um cirurgião experiente e em instalações adequadas. É essencial a comunicação estreita entre o cirurgião e o anestesista, pois a manipulação do tumor pode causar um pico de liberação de catecolaminas, levando a hipertensão, taquicardia e arritmias. O anestesista deve ser capaz de antecipar esses estágios críticos pelo aprofundamento da anestesia em curso. Se isso não for suficiente, um antagonista alfa-adrenérgico de curta duração pode ser administrado para combater a hipertensão. Um antagonista beta-1 de ação ultracurta pode ser adicionado se a taquicardia persistir.[15] A adrenalectomia laparoscópica tem ganhado popularidade. Estudos observacionais mostraram recuperação mais rápida, tempos de hospitalização mais curtos, menores complicações da cicatrização e tempos cirúrgicos mais curtos comparados à laparotomia.[56,57] O tamanho do tumor adrenal e a extensão da invasão vascular são os critérios mais importantes ao se decidir entre laparoscopia ou laparotomia aberta. Tumores de até 5 cm de diâmetro e sem invasão da veia cava caudal são passíveis de laparoscopia, enquanto a adrenalectomia aberta é indicada se houver invasão da veia cava. A remoção do trombo tumoral e a trombectomia são possíveis e não associadas a maior morbidade e mortalidade com uma abordagem apropriada da equipe.[34,58-60] Entretanto, um trombo tumoral extenso está associado a maior mortalidade pós-cirúrgica.[29]

No período pós-cirúrgico, os pacientes devem ser mantidos sob vigilância contínua por, pelo menos, 48 horas. As complicações incluem arritmias cardíacas (ver Capítulos 141 e 248), dificuldade respiratória (ver Capítulo 139), hemorragia (ver Capítulos 135 e 197) e hipertensão (ver Capítulos 157 e 158). Hipotensão (ver Capítulo 159) também é possível em razão da queda abrupta nas catecolaminas circulantes após remoção do tumor, na presença contínua do bloqueio do receptor alfa-adrenérgico (pela fenoxibenzamina).

Terapia medicamentosa

Em cães com feocromocitoma sem possibilidade de ressecção, metástases, doenças concomitantes graves e/ou restrições dos tutores, o tratamento medicamentoso com fenoxibenzamina é utilizado.[15] O protocolo de manejo pré-cirúrgico é aplicado e, se houver taquiarritmias, um antagonista seletivo beta-1 pode ser adicionado após administração de um bloqueador alfa-adrenérgico por, pelo menos, alguns dias. Ainda existem dados insuficientes para apreciação da sobrevida de cães que recebem apenas o tratamento medicamentoso.

HISTOPATOLOGIA

O diagnóstico definitivo do feocromocitoma baseia-se no exame histológico. Feocromocitomas consistem em células neoplásicas arranjadas em lóbulos apoiados por fino estroma fibrovascular. As células neoplásicas são redondas a poliédricas, com citoplasma eosinofílico a basofílico e núcleos hipercromáticos com atividade mitótica variável.[7,30] Pode haver compressão da arquitetura da zona cortical adrenal, assim como necrose e hemorragia, especialmente em casos de tumores grandes. A diferenciação entre tumor adrenal cortical e medular é feita pela imunoistoquímica. Marcadores neuroendócrinos são corados, sendo a cromogranina A a mais comumente utilizada.[61] Ela costuma estar presente em grânulos de cromatina nas células da medula, mas não em células corticais adrenais, o que a torna um marcador ideal. A diferenciação entre feocromocitoma benigno e maligno com base na histopatologia não é confiável. A presença de metástases é o único indicador confiável de malignidade,[62] enquanto o significado de invasão capsular e vascular por trombos tumorais permanece controverso.[62,63]

PROGNÓSTICO

Tamanho do tumor, sua atividade endócrina, invasão vascular e presença de metástases podem afetar o prognóstico. Com relação à remoção cirúrgica, há influência tanto do pré-tratamento com o bloqueador alfa-2-adrenérgico fenoxibenzamina como da extensão da invasão vascular. Fatores prognósticos adicionais envolvem idade, bem-estar geral e doenças concomitantes.

REFERÊNCIAS BIBLIOGRÁFICAS

As referências bibliográficas deste capítulo se encontram online no Ambiente de Aprendizagem.

SEÇÃO 22
Doenças Reprodutivas

CAPÍTULO 312

Endocrinologia Reprodutiva e Manejo Reprodutivo da Cadela

Stefano Romagnoli e Cheryl Lopate

CICLO REPRODUTIVO

O ciclo reprodutivo canino foi dividido historicamente em quatro estágios: proestro (atraente para o macho, mas relutante em aceitar a monta), estro (receptiva à cobertura), diestro (fase luteal/progestacional seguinte à reprodução) e anestro (quiescência reprodutiva). Essa classificação, proposta em 1900 por Heape, baseia-se no comportamento reprodutivo e está relacionada com as alterações clínicas da genitália externa de cadelas, sem levar em conta a boa interação dos hormônios reprodutivos.[1] Apesar da abundância de ferramentas de diagnóstico disponíveis atualmente, a classificação de Heape permanece válida e continua a ser usada tanto em ambientes científicos quanto em clínicos. O termo *estro* pode ser compreendido por alguns, mas criadores e proprietários de cães costumam empregar o termo *cio* em referência a toda a fase folicular (proestro + estro). O termo *cio permanente* é usado para denotar o período de reprodução (estro). O termo *diestro* não abrange por completo a fase luteal canina, que começa no início do estro devido à luteinização pré-ovulatória. No entanto, o diestro é considerado um termo apropriado para indicar o período durante o qual os corpos lúteos (CLs) caninos secretam ativamente a progesterona (P4) e a cadela não está mais disposta a procriar. Em animais de produção, o termo *metaestro* refere-se a todo o tempo em que uma fêmea está sob a influência de CLs e inclui o período de desenvolvimento inicial de CLs (mas imaturos), com pouca ou nenhuma produção sérica de P4.

Sazonalidade dos ciclos estrais e intervalos interestrais

Em geral, a cadela é considerada uma espécie monoéstrica (apenas um estro é concluído durante cada ciclo reprodutivo) e não sazonal (a ocorrência de estro não é influenciada pela estação do ano). Animais domésticos alojados dentro de casa tendem a ciclar em qualquer mês do ano,[2] embora a atividade cíclica baseada em estimativas em dados de registro de ninhada do *American Kennel Club* mostre picos no final do inverno e na primavera.[3] Tais picos de atividade cíclica durante a primavera têm sido observados em cadelas Beagle alojadas ao ar livre no norte da Europa e curiosamente relatados em outras de climas temperados. A sazonalidade da reprodução canina tem sido objeto de debate com base na sazonalidade (um ciclo anual) de lobos, dingos e Basenjis.[4,5] Embora a maioria das raças de cães domésticos pareça ter perdido sua fotorresponsividade, a influência do fotoperíodo na função hipotalâmica-hipofisária da cadela é mostrada por um ritmo anual de secreção de prolactina (PRL) em cães mestiços, alojados constantemente ao ar livre.[6] A seleção genética para desempenho e aparência externa pode ter diluído o efeito da estação, que pode permanecer em algumas cadelas e em algumas linhagens específicas dentro das raças. Do ponto de vista prático, a primavera deve ser sempre considerada como a época do ano em que a probabilidade de a cadela iniciar a atividade reprodutiva é maior.

O intervalo entre o início de ciclos estrais caninos consecutivos (intervalo interestral) varia muito entre as raças e dentro delas. A grande maioria de cães puros e mestiços cicla a cada 5 ½ a 6 ½ meses, com algumas exceções notáveis: Basenji e Mastiff tibetano ciclam uma vez ao ano e algumas cadelas Collie têm ciclos a cada 9 a 11 meses. Algumas linhagens de Pastor-Alemão, Doberman, Rottweiler, Labrador Retriever, Basset Hound e Cocker Spaniel ciclam três vezes ao ano.[7-14] Variações nos intervalos interestrais são, provavelmente, decorrentes de diferenças genéticas na duração do anestro.[7] Em geral, parece haver correlação negativa entre o tamanho do corpo e a frequência do ciclo. Cadelas de porte grande têm menos ciclos estrais no ano quando comparadas às raças menores. Cães > 6 anos de idade tendem a ter a duração de intervalo progressivamente mais longo. Ainda é discutível se a gestação, seguida de parto e lactação, aumenta a duração do interestro, sendo imprevisível o início do proestro em indivíduos.[2,9-11]

Proestro

Definição, mudanças e sinais induzidos por estrógeno (Tabela 312.1)

O termo *proestro* descreve a fase de transição entre a quiescência reprodutiva e o início do comportamento da reprodução. O início do proestro geralmente é sinalizado pelo aparecimento de corrimento vaginal com sangue, com duração média de 9 dias, mas que pode variar de alguns dias a quase 4 semanas.[11,12] O proestro se inicia com o desenvolvimento de folículos ovarianos e a secreção de seu principal produto: 17-betaestradiol (E2), que aumenta progressivamente ao longo do proestro, com pico

SEÇÃO 22 • Doenças Reprodutivas

| Tabela 312.1 | Relação entre citologia (1° dia do diestro citológico), comportamento (fim da aceitação do macho) e parâmetros endócrinos *versus* surgimento do pico do hormônio luteinizante (LH), ovulação, fechamento da cérvice e início do diestro na cadela. |

	1° DIA DO DIESTRO CITOLÓGICO (DIAS)	FIM DA ACEITAÇÃO DO MACHO (DIAS)	CONCENTRAÇÃO SÉRICA DE PROGESTERONA (ng/mℓ)
Pico de LH	−7 a −10	+6 a +19	2
Ovulação	−5 a −8	+3 a +10	4 a 10
Fechamento da cérvice	−2 a 0	−1 a +3	≈ 25 ou mais
1° dia do diestro citológico		−2 a +2	≥ 19 a 25

A progesterona sérica (P4) é a forma mais confiável para classificar a fase do ciclo, mas as informações de uma única amostra podem não permitir um estadiamento preciso em casos específicos, a menos que a citologia vaginal e/ou o comportamento sejam avaliados em conjunto. A citologia vaginal, isoladamente, é mais confiável do que o comportamento por si só, mas a avaliação do comportamento pode se tornar importante ao avaliar os dados de P4 sérica, se o esfregaço vaginal não puder ser coletado.

de concentrações de 50 a 120 pg/mℓ.[13,14] O aumento das concentrações séricas de E2 aumenta o fluxo sanguíneo para o sistema reprodutivo, afetando o endométrio (causando o crescimento e a ramificação das glândulas endometriais, com consequente aumento da espessura de todo o endométrio), a cérvice (causando relaxamento cervical e secreção de muco), a vagina (causando o crescimento das dobras da mucosa, aumento da elasticidade e secreção de muco) e a vulva (causando aumento da espessura da mucosa, edema e turgidez), mas não parece envolver o tecido mamário.[14,15] O *status* hormonal e as mudanças na perfusão vascular durante o proestro fazem com que a secreção vaginal e as glândulas adanais liberem feromônios potentes para atrais machos.[16,17] A reprodução não é aceita pela cadela em proestro. Se ela estiver no início ou no meio do proestro, ela pode participar normalmente de atividades que precedem a cobertura, mas, muitas vezes, recusa veementemente qualquer aproximação maior, ao desviar de cães machos ou rosnar para eles. No final do proestro, a cadela pode rejeitar a reprodução simplesmente sentando ou deitando.

Endoscopia e corrimento vaginal

O corrimento vaginal sanguinolento observado no proestro resulta, principalmente, de hemácias, mas também da diapedese de leucócitos através de capilares endometriais intactos no lúmen uterino, fluindo então através da cérvice em razão das contrações miometriais e, por fim, misturando-se com fluidos cervicovaginais. A pulsatilidade da secreção de E2 canina torna os testes séricos menos úteis do que a citologia vaginal, que é um excelente indicativo da secreção de E2 em 24 horas por folículos em maturação (ver Capítulos 44 e 119). Esfregaços vaginais de cadelas no início do proestro contêm predominantemente hemácias, alguns leucócitos e, sobretudo, células epiteliais não queratinizadas (parabasais, intermediárias pequenas e grandes). Na maioria das cadelas, o número de hemácias diminui durante a progressão do proestro para o estro (tornando a aparência da secreção vulvar progressivamente menos sangrenta), enquanto a proporção entre células queratinizadas e não queratinizadas aumenta de maneira progressiva, atingindo valores de 30 a 50% ao final do proestro. O E2 faz com que a mucosa vaginal se torne edemaciada e rosada e apareça na vaginoscopia – durante o proestro e início do estro – com pregas vaginais arredondadas e edemaciadas, com algum fluido tingido de sangue (ver Capítulo 119).[18] A cérvice canina também está edemaciada e palpável, por via abdominal, do final do proestro em diante. Como a cérvice normalmente não é palpável durante o anestro, a examinação dela pode ser um sinal indireto de que a cadela está no cio. Além disso, o útero fica dilatado e mais facilmente identificável à palpação abdominal.

Perfil hormonal (ver Tabela 312.1)

Após o aumento inicial de estrógeno, responsável pelos sinais clínicos do proestro, as concentrações séricas de E2 continuam a aumentar, com pico ao final do proestro. Esse pico e a sua redução subsequente marcam o final do proestro e, provavelmente, contribuem para estimular a onda de LH, o início do estro e a ovulação. Embora o hormônio mais importante no proestro canino seja o E2, com efeitos clínicos relevantes no comportamento e no sistema reprodutivo, as concentrações crescentes de outros hormônios reprodutivos também desempenham um papel. Durante as 24 a 48 h finais do proestro, a progesterona sérica (P4) aumenta de > 0,5 ng/mℓ para cerca de 1 ng/m, o que indica o início do desenvolvimento do tecido luteal dentro da parede dos folículos caninos em maturação. Esse aumento inicial da P4 sérica, denominada *luteinização pré-ovulatória*, é uma peculiaridade dos caninos e é também valioso no estadiamento da ovulação.[19,20]

No final do anestro, as concentrações séricas do hormônio luteinizante (LH, *luteinizing hormone*) sérico e do hormônio foliculoestimulante (FSH, *follicle stimulating hormone*) aumentam acima dos níveis basais para valores aproximados de 1 a 6 e 150.300 ng/mℓ, respectivamente (Figuras 312.1 e 312.2). A produção de E2 pelos folículos terciários codominantes em crescimento estimula a hipófise, sem promover liberação suficiente de LH-FSH para causar luteinização pré-ovulatória. Os valores de LH e FSH diminuem conforme o proestro progride, em razão do *feedback* negativo de E2 e inibina, e permanecem baixos até o final do proestro. Apesar do decréscimo nos valores de LH-FSH no início do proestro, o crescimento folicular contínuo provavelmente indica que o desenvolvimento folicular em cães é autônomo.[21] As concentrações de andrógenos (testosterona e androstenediona) aumentam no final do proestro, alcançando níveis comparáveis ao pico de LH (10 a 25 ng/mℓ) de machos adultos inteiros.[22] Apesar da observação ocasional de comportamento masculino ou de monta em algumas cadelas, não foi feita nenhuma correlação entre tais valores de andrógenos (que podem refletir as etapas intermediárias de conversão entre progesterona e estrógeno) e a expressão do comportamento estral na cadela.

Estro

Definição e sinais

Estro é a fase em que ocorrem tanto a reprodução quanto a ovulação (Figura 312.3). Os sinais clínicos do proestro permanecem evidentes durante o estro, embora apresentem ligeira tendência de mudança: a vulva ainda é maior do que o normal, mas torna-se mais macia enquanto a secreção vulvar torna-se progressivamente menos sanguinolenta e mais pálida. Tanto a cérvice quanto o útero são palpáveis por via abdominal. Os sinais comportamentais de receptividade aumentam de intensidade durante o estro, assim como as cadelas no estro aceitam os machos interessados, são receptivas a brincadeiras e a serem cobertas. Os sinais mais claros e consistentes da fase folicular (proestro + estro) são "exposição do

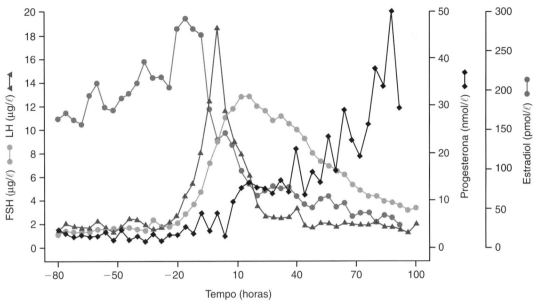

Figura 312.1 Diagrama do perfil hormonal típico de um cão que progride do final do proestro para o estro. *FSH*, hormônio foliculoestimulante; *LH*, hormônio luteinizante. (Adaptada de Schaefers-Okkens AC: The ovaries. In Rijnberk A, editor: *Clinical endocrinology of dogs and cats*, Dordrecht, Holanda, 1996, Kluwer Academic.) (*Esta figura se encontra reproduzida em cores no Encarte.*)

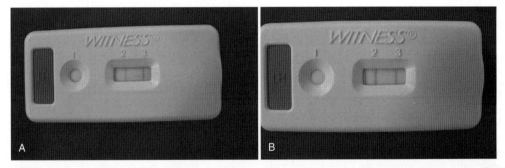

Figura 312.2 A. Teste negativo do hormônio luteinizante (LH). Linha de controle à direita, linha da amostra à esquerda. **B.** Teste positivo de LH. Linha de controle à direita, linha da amostra à esquerda.

clítoris" (inclinação da vulva para cima, quando o aspecto dorsal da pele vulvar é tocado), enrijecimento dos membros pélvicos (quando a pele em qualquer lado da vulva é tocada) e "sinalização da cauda" (desvio vertical ou contralateral da cauda, quando a pele vulvar é tocada em ambos os lados). Esses sinais são exibidos quase sempre totalmente durante o estro e podem ser observados perto do final do proestro em algumas fêmeas. O início da "sinalização" indica o início de estro, a vontade em reproduzir, e coincide com o pico de LH no primeiro dia do estro. Ocasionalmente, as cadelas podem permanecer não receptivas à cobertura durante todo o estro, apesar de nenhum outro achado anormal. Em cadelas Beagle, o fechamento da cérvice ocorreu 5 +/− 1 dias após a ovulação ou tão cedo quanto 1 dia antes do final do estro, com concentrações séricas de P4 em média 25 +/− 4 ng/mℓ.[23]

A duração média (9 dias) e o intervalo (4 a 24 dias) do estro canino baseiam-se no número de dias que as cadelas estão dispostas a reproduzir por ciclo.[9,24] Há uma notável variação em padrões de comportamento reprodutivo em cães. Embora raro, uma cadela em estro pode recusar-se a ser coberta por um macho específico, porque ela é dominante, ou em razão de uma aparente antipatia, o que pode levar o tutor a pensar que a cadela ainda não está no estro ou já saiu dele. Assim, a duração do estro, avaliada por observação clínica, pode não estar totalmente correta e pode explicar discrepâncias entre a citologia vaginal e o comportamento. Algumas cadelas podem começar a reproduzir 2 a 3 dias antes até 4 a 5 dias após atingir > 50% de queratinização em seu esfregaço vaginal.[25,26]

Endoscopia e citologia vaginal (ver Tabela 312.1)

O padrão de queratinização de > 50% células epiteliais vaginais (células superficiais nucleadas e anucleadas) reflete o início da receptividade sexual na maioria das cadelas. Essa porcentagem de células superficiais presentes na citologia vaginal não é sensível nem específica, pois pode aparecer pela primeira vez tão cedo quanto 6 dias antes ou tão tarde quanto 4 dias após a cadela estar disposta a reproduzir.[27] O "estro completo" é diagnosticado quando > 70% das células epiteliais vaginais aparecem queratinizadas (ver Capítulos 44 e 119).[28] O efeito da diminuição das concentrações de E2 pode ser observado na rápida reabsorção do edema da mucosa vaginal. Na endoscopia, dobras da mucosa vaginal parecem secas, brancas e enrugadas. Esse padrão é descrito como "crenulação" e uma prova indireta da diminuição de E2.[18]

Perfil hormonal (ver Tabela 312.1)

Os três principais padrões hormonais do estro são o pico de LH, a redução nas concentrações de E2 (a partir do pico alcançado ao final do proestro) e as concentrações crescentes de P4. Coincidindo com ou poucas horas após o pico das concentrações de E2 no proestro, há aumento rápido da secreção pituitária de LH a partir de concentrações basais para valores de 10 a 22 ng/mℓ, mantido naquela concentração sérica por aproximadamente 24 h. A duração da onda de LH pode ser tão breve quanto 18 a 96 h.[20,26,29-32] A ovulação ocorre cerca de 2 dias após o início da onda de LH e continua dentro de um desvio padrão estreito a partir dessa data.[12] O saldo final e o sinergismo de E2, P4 e LH

SEÇÃO 22 • Doenças Reprodutivas

desempenham papéis fundamentais no comportamento reprodutivo. O E2 secretado durante o proestro "prepara o sistema" e a P4 secretada na ovulação "ativa o sistema." A receptividade total parece ser desencadeada pela diminuição coincidente de E2 e aumento de P4.[33,34] A diminuição de E2 provavelmente desempenha o papel principal, já que é isso que realmente causa o pico de LH, enquanto o aumento da P4 parece realçar e sincronizar o comportamento estral da cadela.[35]

As concentrações séricas de P4 aumentam de valores < 1 ng/ml no final do proestro para cerca de 2 ng/ml no dia do pico de LH, atingindo valores de 4 a 10 ng/ml 2 dias depois, quando a ovulação está ocorrendo e os oócitos primários estão sendo liberado nos ovidutos, onde passam por sua fase final de maturação. O aumento inicial de P4 sérica > 2 ng/ml costuma coincidir com o pico de LH, embora em algumas cadelas possa ocorrer até 20 h depois.[32] Durante o processo ovulatório, as concentrações séricas de P4 se elevam rapidamente, com aumentos diários de 3 a 10 ng/ml ou mais. A magnitude desse aumento deve-se ao número de folículos ovulados, ao tamanho folicular, à quantidade de tecido luteal em desenvolvimento e a quanto de P4 é produzida por CL. Aumentos < 3 ng/ml/dia devem ser motivo de preocupação, pois podem sugerir falha na ovulação, com a obtenção de amostras adicionais nos próximos 1 a 2 dias.

Após o término do processo ovulatório e a maturação final do CL, as concentrações séricas de P4 continuam a aumentar durante as 2 primeiras semanas após o estro para valores na faixa de 15 a 60 ou mais ng/ml.

Uso dos resultados do ensaio de P4 no soro para o momento da ovulação (Tabela 312.2; ver Figura 312.3)

Os resultados do ensaio de P4 no soro podem ajudar a distinguir cadelas no início do estro (que podem não atingir a melhor taxa de concepção ou até não conceber se cobertas por um macho de baixa fertilidade) daquelas que estão ovulando e são mais férteis. Os resultados do ensaio podem confirmar a ovulação e o estágio do ciclo estral de forma confiável de 2 dias antes até 2 dias após a ovulação, um momento em que as concentrações de P4 aumentam de 1 a 2 ng/ml para > 10 a 12 ng/ml. No entanto, a análise de uma única amostra de P4 sérica coletada no pico ou após o início do pico de LH é menos informativa sobre o número de dias decorridos desde o início da ovulação em razão de variações individuais, de raça ou de idade. Os resultados de P4 no soro são comparáveis, independentemente do radioimunoensaio (RIA), do imunoensaio quimioluminescente (CLIA) ou do ensaio imunofluorescente ligado à enzima (ELFA).[26,36,37] Se for usado um ensaio humano, deve-se tomar cuidado e calibrá-lo para soro canino. Diferenças espécie-específicas no grau de ligação hormonal a proteínas transportadoras no soro podem alterar os resultados em até 20%. Os ensaios devem ser validados em uma base semestral/anual ou a cada mil a três mil amostras executadas por laboratórios veterinários comerciais que utilizam *kits* hormonais comercializados para uso humano. Em geral, é necessário um fator de conversão ao usar um sistema ELFA humano.[37]

Tabela 312.2	Concentrações de progesterona e eventos foliculares associados.

ATIVIDADE FOLICULAR/ ENDÓCRINA	CONCENTRAÇÃO DE PROGESTERONA (ALCANCE ng/ml)
Linha de base	< 0,5
Desenvolvimento folicular inicial	0,5 a 1,3
Pico de LH	1,3 a 1,9
Início da ovulação	4 a 8 média (alcance 4 a 10)
Pós-ovulação	> 10 ng/ml

Combinação entre observação de comportamento, citologia vaginal e análise de hormônios séricos

A análise de E2 sérico não é usada em razão da sua pulsatilidade. No entanto, a citologia vaginal permanece um excelente teste biológico para E2. Dados da citologia vaginal, combinados às concentrações séricas de P4 e à avaliação comportamental, são fundamentais para o estadiamento do ciclo estral e a identificação da ovulação. No entanto, cada uma dessas ferramentas, isoladamente, não é muito confiável. Comportamento estral, citologia vaginal e amostras séricas de P4 permanecem como os três pilares fundamentais para o manejo reprodutivo, bem como para determinar a duração do estro e excluir as condições ovarianas (cistos ovarianos/neoplasia). Testes de diagnóstico adicionais (como ensaio de LH, ultrassonografia ovariana, vaginoscopia) podem ser úteis em melhorar a precisão do estro e do estágio da ovulação, se forem usados de forma consistente, desenvolvendo perícia. Impedometria e arborização do muco cervical não são precisas no momento da ovulação (ver Tabela 312.1).

Diestro

Definição e sinais

O diestro, definido como a fase luteal ou progestacional do ciclo, costuma suceder a ovulação e durar precisamente 8 semanas em gestantes e 6 a 10 semanas nas não gestantes. A vulva, que se torna menos edemaciada e inchada durante os últimos dias de estro, continua a diminuir durante a primeira semana ou mais de diestro. Há pouca ou nenhuma secreção vulvar com sangue e cães machos não são atraídos. A mucosa vaginal parece plana, fina, seca e de coloração rosa a vermelha, com capilares facilmente visíveis na vaginoscopia (ver Capítulo 119). A cérvice é palpável nos primeiros dias de diestro, enquanto o útero permanece nessa condição e pode aumentar de tamanho sob a influência de P4.

Citologia vaginal, comportamento

Clinicamente, o primeiro dia de diestro (D1) é definido como o primeiro dia em que uma cadela se recusa a reproduzir ou como o dia em que é verificada uma mudança repentina na citologia vaginal: células vaginais epiteliais queratinizadas diminuem de 70 a 100% para < 30% na citologia, substituídas por células epiteliais intermediárias pequenas e grandes e células parabasais. Leucócitos, ausentes nos esfregaços de citologia após os primeiros dias do proestro e durante o estro, reaparecem (ver Capítulo 119). Essas mudanças costumam ocorrer dentro de 24 h após o início do diestro, embora qualquer uma delas possa ser observada pela primeira vez dentro de um intervalo de 4 dias; a vontade de reproduzir pode cessar 1 a 2 dias antes ou persistir 1 a 2 após o início do "diestro citológico". Mudanças na citologia vaginal podem ocorrer 5 a 8 dias após a ovulação e 7 a 10 após o pico de LH (ver Tabela 312.1).

A observação de D1 em um esfregaço vaginal indica que o estro já terminou e que provavelmente é tarde demais para atingir taxas ideais de concepção (tamanho normal da ninhada) usando-se a monta natural.

No entanto, taxas de fertilidade de 5 a 40% foram relatadas em cães Beagle, quando a monta natural ocorreu entre D1 e D3. Embora o tamanho da ninhada seja provavelmente menor com a reprodução natural no início do diestro, o tamanho normal da ninhada ainda pode ser alcançado usando-se a deposição de sêmen intrauterino durante esse mesmo período.[23] Clinicamente, D1 pode ser considerado o final da primeira semana de gestação: portanto, em cadelas gestantes o intervalo entre D1 e o parto é de aproximadamente 57 + 2 dias.[38]

O comportamento reprodutivo não é tão confiável quanto a citologia vaginal na determinação de D1. A concentração de P4 não deve ser útil, pois ela aumenta progressivamente durante o estro, com tendência a continuar durante as primeiras semanas de diestro. Mesmo assim, a avaliação comportamental jamais

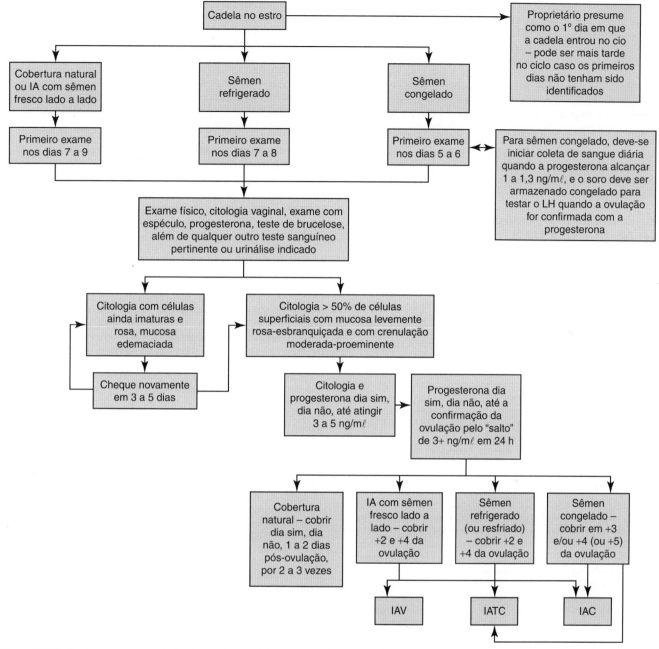

Figura 312.3 Algoritmo com recomendações do manejo reprodutivo para taxas de gestação ideias em cadelas saudáveis. *IA*, inseminação artificial; *IAC*, inseminação artificial cirúrgica; *IATC*, inseminação artificial transcervical; *IAV*, inseminação artificial vaginal.

deve ser desconsiderada, especialmente quando se discute a progressão do estro para diestro. Os criadores devem sempre ser encorajados a identificar o primeiro dia em que uma cadela se recusa a procriar (ou reproduzir), pois essa informação é usada na determinação da duração do estro e pode ajudar na indicação do tempo de ovulação. No entanto, é aconselhável perguntar se a recusa em reproduzir foi observada ou presumida com base em outros critérios. Os criadores devem ser instruídos e encorajados a estabelecer datas de início e término da aceitação do macho, observando o comportamento das cadelas, quando trazidas a um macho inteiro em uma observação diária.

Perfil hormonal

As concentrações séricas de P4 continuam a aumentar, alcançando valores de pico de 15 a 90 ng/mℓ, aproximadamente 2 a 4 semanas durante a fase luteal. Posteriormente, inicia-se um declínio gradual na P4 sérica em cadelas gestantes e não gestantes. Em geral, a diminuição da P4 não chega a < 5 ng/mℓ até a última semana em cadelas gestantes e jamais diminui abaixo de 2 ng/mℓ até 24 a 36 h pré-parto.

O suporte luteotrófico para os CLs caninos parece originar-se na hipófise, sendo a PRL considerada o fator mais importante para a produção de P4 ovariana canina. O LH tem um papel estimulatório, e não permissivo.[39-41] A PRL começa a ser secretada durante a 4ª semana da fase luteal, assim que a concentração sérica de P4 começa a diminuir.[42] As ações da PRL canina incluem suporte à síntese de P4 ovariana e desenvolvimento do tecido mamário, independentemente de gestação, mas de maior magnitude em cadelas gestantes. As concentrações séricas de PRL são significativamente maiores em cadelas gestantes quando comparadas às não gestantes após aproximadamente 35 dias pós-pico de LH. A administração de PRL para cadelas durante a fase lútea causa aumento na secreção de P4.[43-45] Os CLs de cadelas gestantes produzem mais P4 do que as das não gestantes.

Uma vez que o metabolismo de P4 é maior em cadelas gestantes, as diferenças entre as gestantes e as não gestantes nem sempre são óbvias.[14,20,29,46] O aumento na produção de P4 ovariana observada em cadelas gestantes após a implantação pode ser mediado por uma relaxina específica da gestação secretada pelos ovários durante o diestro. Durante a gestação, os sinciciotrofoblastos placentários caninos contribuem para o início da secreção de PRL.[47,48] A relaxina atua inibindo a contratilidade miometrial e promovendo a modificação da cérvice no final da gestação, em preparação para o parto.[49] Os papéis do estradiol, da testosterona e da androstenediona produzidos durante a fase lútea pelos CLs[22,50-52] não são claros. Provavelmente a concentração desses hormônios é o resultado de etapas intermediárias na síntese de P4, sendo, atualmente, a medição deles considerada de pouco ou nenhum uso clínico.

Monitoramento da progesterona e da gestação (ver Tabelas 312.1 e 312.2)

A magnitude da concentração de P4 alcançada durante as primeiras 3 semanas após D1 pode depender da raça, da idade, da saúde, do grau de estresse ambiental e social e, talvez, do nível de endogamia. Não há dados homogêneos sobre a concentração de P4 no soro canino nas diferentes raças e categorias de idade durante a gestação, evitando o fornecimento de diretrizes confiáveis sobre os valores "normais" de P4 sérica durante a fase luteal canina ou "limiares mínimos" de P4 sérica abaixo das concentrações nas quais a intervenção pode ser justificada (p. ex., manutenção da gestação com P4 exógeno). Curiosamente, a concentração mínima de P4 para manter a gestação durante as semanas 3 a 7 é provavelmente > 15 ng/mℓ. Em uma gestação de alto risco ou em uma cadela com histórico recorrente de perdas de gestação, concentrações de P4 < 15 ng/mℓ podem indicar a necessidade de P4 exógeno.[53]

No final da fase lútea, o fim da produção de P4 ovariana ocorre de maneira abrupta (dentro de 24 a 36 h) em gestantes e gradualmente (ao longo de 1 a 2 semanas) em cadelas não gestantes.[11,39,42]

O efeito luteolítico da prostaglandina F2-alfa endógena (PGF2-alfa) desempenha papel primordial no encerramento da atividade lútea em cadelas gestantes. Como não há aumento na secreção de PGF2-alfa em cadelas não gestantes, os CLs funcionam por mais tempo e são lisados por um processo imunomediado conduzido por citocinas derivadas de leucócitos (interleucinas [IL]-8, IL-10, IL-12, fator de necrose tumoral alfa e fator de crescimento transformante beta-1), que estão cada vez mais presentes dentro do tecido luteal canino ao longo do diestro.[50,54] Em cadelas gestantes, a queda abrupta na P4 sérica ao final da fase luteal desencadeia uma diminuição na temperatura corporal e um aumento de PRL sérica. Uma diminuição de cerca de 1 a 2°C na temperatura retal, após o declínio no P4 sérica, costuma ser observada em cadelas que estão dando à luz ou após o tratamento com uma PGF2-alfa ou aglepristone, embora o fim da fase luteal não seja relatado em cadelas não gestantes, em razão da diminuição gradual da P4 sérica.[55]

Prolactina, progesterona e parto

O aumento na concentração sérica de PRL é imediato e vigoroso antes do parto, como consequência da luteólise pré-parto súbita, enquanto o aumento é mais sutil em fêmeas não gestantes, novamente em razão do desaparecimento mais lento do CL.[56] Independentemente de gestação, a secreção de PRL no final da fase lútea tem pouco efeito sobre os CLs, mas estimula o início da lactação e o comportamento materno. Em cães, a estrita interdependência entre P4 e PRL tem várias implicações práticas: o uso de fármacos inibidores da prolactina (agonistas da dopamina ou antagonistas da serotonina) a qualquer momento a partir do meio da gestação (quando as concentrações de P4 ainda são altas) causará luteólise e aborto,[57] enquanto na queda de P4 a qualquer momento (i. e., seguindo-se a um tratamento luteolítico ou com o bloqueador do receptor de progesterona,

ovariectomia em diestro, interrupção de um tratamento à base de progesterona etc.) haverá aumento na PRL sérica, seguida de secreção de leite e exibição de comportamento materno. O monitoramento das concentrações séricas de PRL não é usado comumente, apesar da aplicação clínica potencial no monitoramento da gestação ou pseudogestação. No entanto, o monitoramento das concentrações séricas de P4 é uma ferramenta fundamental na reprodução canina para detectar a ovulação e para o tratamento de cadelas com insuficiência luteal, gestação prolongada, distocia ou cesariana eletiva.

Efeitos da progesterona e do hormônio do crescimento

Outra implicação clinicamente relevante da produção de P4 ovariana durante o diestro é a secreção de GH pela glândula mamária,[58] um processo fisiológico normal. Sob a influência de P4, as células epiteliais do ducto mamário secretam GH, aumentando os teores séricos basais de GH, e, em seguida, fazem retroalimentação negativa para suprimir secreção hipofisária de GH normal e pulsátil.[59] O GH mamário promove a proliferação normal das glândulas mamárias, por meio de efeitos autócrinos/parácrinos locais, prepara o endométrio para implantação, promovendo (com a P4 ovariana) hiperplasia do epitélio uterino, e causa resistência à insulina. Esse último efeito pode ter evoluído para evitar a hipoglicemia durante a gestação, uma vez que os predadores costumavam prolongar os intervalos entre as refeições. Claramente, esses efeitos do GH na cadela carreiam um risco potencial de causar ou agravar condições clínicas, como doenças mamárias e uterinas, bem como diabetes. Portanto, conforme o caso, algumas cadelas podem se beneficiar de monitoramento cuidadoso clínico, hormonal, ultrassonográfico uterino e, particularmente, bioquímico sérico durante o diestro, no caso de suspeita de diabetes melito.[60,61] Há evidências também de que o GH mamário se concentra no colostro, estimulando, assim, o desenvolvimento gástrico e intestinal de recém-nascidos lactentes.[62]

Pseudogestação

O efeito mais comum das ações combinadas de P4 e GH é o desenvolvimento mamário durante a segunda metade da fase luteal, seguido do início da lactação (assim que a P4 cai e a PRL atinge o pico), que ocorre tanto em cadelas gestantes quanto não gestantes, embora com muito menos intensidade no último grupo. Em cadelas não gestantes, a ocorrência de desenvolvimento mamário, lactação e exibição de comportamento materno é referida como pseudogestação ou pseudociese, uma condição parafisiológica. Em lobos, a pseudogestação é benéfica, pois, caso uma fêmea morra ou esteja impossibilitada de amamentar a ninhada após o parto, permite que outro membro da matilha assuma esse papel. Uma vez que a secreção de PRL ocorre normalmente em cadelas gestantes e não gestantes, a pseudogestação é considerada um fenômeno normal. Essa condição sofre remissão espontânea, mas torna-se evidente quando a secreção hormonal é alta, causando lactação persistente e forte comportamento materno, duas condições que levam a cadela a ficar nervosa, adotar objetos inanimados e se tornar anoréxica. Quando necessário, essa condição pode ser tratada com drogas inibidoras de prolactina, como cabergolina (5 µg/kg VO, a cada 24 h), metergolina (0,5 mg/kg VO, a cada 12 h) ou bromocriptina (20 a 50 µg/kg VO, a cada 12 h).

Anestro

Definição e sinais

Em cadelas, não há diferenças comportamentais no diestro e no anestro, com exceção dos primeiros dias de diestro citológico, durante os quais algumas cadelas ainda podem atrair machos e ocasionalmente reproduzir. Nesses últimos dias, a transição clínica, metabólica e comportamental do diestro para o anestro é suave e desprovida de quaisquer sinais clínicos relevantes. Assim como no diestro, a vulva é pequena, não há nenhuma secreção vulvar e cães machos não são atraídos.

Na vaginoscopia, a mucosa vaginal é seca e fina, plana e de coloração rosa-avermelhada a vermelho-escura, com capilares prontamente visíveis. Como consequência, o anestro não pode ser diferenciado do diestro tendo-se como base o comportamento reprodutivo. O anestro varia de tão curto quanto 2 até > 9 meses, o que explica a diferença nos intervalos interestro entre indivíduos. Embora a P4 do diestro seja uma fonte potencial de problemas clínicos em cadelas com risco de piometra, neoplasia mamária ou diabetes, o anestro não é caracterizado por tais problemas, uma vez que os ovários não secretam quantidades significativas de E2 ou P4. É importante instruir os proprietários quanto essas diferenças, uma vez que eles devem estar cientes das doenças associadas ao diestro.

Perfil hormonal

O anestro é definido como o período com o início de concentrações séricas de P4 < 1 ng/mℓ. Uma concentração sérica de P4 exata, definida como basal, ainda é uma questão a ser estudada. O tecido luteal em funcionamento é considerado ausente quando P4 é < 1 ng/mℓ. Cadelas em anestro apresentam concentrações de P4 sérica < 0,7 ng/mℓ, geralmente < 0,3 a 0,5 ng/mℓ. Concentrações < 0,3 ng/mℓ podem ser um requisito para estimular o início do proestro.[11] Essa baixa (e talvez progressiva diminuição) na concentração sérica de P4 persiste por 1 a 6 meses na maioria das cadelas saudáveis, aumentando apenas após a luteinização pré-ovulatória, que ocorre no final do proestro do ciclo seguinte. Durante o início ao meio do anestro, as concentrações de E2 também são baixas: 5 a 10 ng/mℓ.[30] Em razão desse padrão de baixa secreção ovariana de esteroides, os primeiros 1 a 2 meses após o final do diestro podem ser referenciados como anestro inicial ou "profundo", em razão da baixa sensibilidade dos ovários caninos ao hormônio liberador de gonadotrofina (GnRH, do inglês *gonadotropina-releasing hormone*).

À medida que o anestro progride, há aumento no número e na amplitude dos pulsos de GnRH hipotalâmicos, paralelamente ao aumento da responsividade à hipófise e ao aumento na sensibilidade ovariana às gonadotrofinas, com o desenvolvimento de receptores de FSH e LH,[63] o que é seguido de episódios de secreção de E2, que aumentam os receptores hipotalâmicos de estrógeno e estabelecem um ciclo de *feedback* positivo.[64,65] Essa interação de eventos do eixo hipotálamo-hipófise-ovário no final do anestro confirma as observações anteriores de elevações ocasionais dos teores de E2-25-50 ng/mℓ durante os 2 meses anteriores ao início da proestro.[25,30,66] No final do anestro, o aumento nas concentrações de E2 está associado a uma ligeira queratinização vaginal, sem edema vulvar ou secreção vulvar serossanguinolenta.[30] A secreção de GnRH, seguida de maiores concentrações séricas de FSH e LH, são dois fatores-chave no início do proestro, conforme comprovado pela administração de GnRH em pulsos ou por implante subcutâneo (SC) ou de produtos baseados em LH ou FSH que possam induzir o proestro.[67]

Dopamina e indução do estro

Estudos do papel das vias dopaminérgicas na retomada da ciclicidade na cadela envolveram três circuitos cerebrais principais: as vias mesolímbica, mesocortical e nigroestriatal, que inervam o sistema límbico (memória, comportamento), o córtex frontal (controle cognitivo, resposta emocional) e o núcleo estriado (controle motor), respectivamente. Uma quarta via dopaminérgica é a tuberoinfundibular, que conecta o hipotálamo à hipófise, onde influencia a secreção de hormônios, como a PRL. As observações de que os agonistas da dopamina reduzem as concentrações de PRL sérica e encurtam o anestro levaram à conclusão de que os dois eventos estavam relacionados: essa redução da PRL era importante para indução do estro na cadela.[68] Entretanto, fármacos agonistas não dopaminérgicos redutores de PRL não encurtam o anestro quando usados em doses farmacológicas, o qual pode ser alcançado com o uso de agonistas da dopamina em doses muito baixas para suprimir as concentrações de PRL.[69,70] Na cadela, a ativação da via tuberoinfundibular neural,

ao se administrar um agonista da dopamina, é seguida da retomada das concentrações séricas basais de FSH e LH, que simulam o ambiente fisiológico do anestro tardio, seguido do início do proestro. Agonistas da dopamina, como bromocriptina (20 µg/kg VO, a cada 12 h) e cabergolina (5 µg/kg/dia VO, ou tão baixo quanto 0,6 µg/kg/dia), encurtam a duração do anestro (induzindo, assim, o estro) na cadela, com o aumento da eficácia conforme ela avança mais para o meio ou o final do anestro.[70-72]

Útero em anestro

A involução uterina requer a descamação do revestimento endometrial, seguida de sua regeneração completa, prerrequisito fundamental para maximizar as chances de fertilização no ciclo seguinte. Quando o parto e o descolamento da membrana fetal ocorrem normalmente após parto, o reparo endometrial tem início imediato; mas, para que seja concluído, requer aproximadamente 143 a 155 dias após o início do estro. Em cadelas nulíparas, esse processo se completa aproximadamente 2 semanas antes.[73]

PADRÕES IRREGULARES DA CICLICIDADE OVARIANA

Importância do histórico completo

As cadelas podem apresentar padrões irregulares em qualquer estágio do ciclo. Algumas preocupações de proprietários podem ser decorrentes da falta de compreensão do que é considerado "normal". Portanto, os clínicos sempre devem rever cuidadosamente o máximo possível de dados do histórico com o tutor. Deve-se verificar a(s) data(s) de início do proestro e aceite/recusa do macho, bem como o tempo e o padrão da secreção vulvar. Qualquer perfil sérico de P4 anterior pode ser bastante valioso. A ocorrência de sinais comportamentais ou mamários de pseudociese (indicando que a ovulação ocorreu 1 a 2 meses antes) deve ser observada.

Proestro ou estro prolongado

Falha ovulatória

Há grande variação na duração da fase folicular canina. Tanto o proestro quanto o estro podem duram poucos dias até 24.[9,11,12,24] Raramente foram relatadas fases foliculares com duração de até 40 dias, devendo-se tomar cuidado para diferenciar ciclos normais, porém incomuns, de anormalidades verdadeiras, como *split heat* (cio cortado) ou aumento lento da P4. A ovulação normal é resultado de um processo complexo que requer estrógeno folicular suficiente para estimular a liberação de GnRH hipotalâmico, que faz com que a hipófise libere LH suficiente para causar a luteinização normal dos folículos pré-ovulatórios. A interrupção em qualquer etapa decorrente de estresse ambiental, manejo, social ou de saúde pode prejudicar a ovulação. O diagnóstico anovulatório baseia-se nas concentrações séricas de LH e P4 que não excedem 2 e 10 ng/mℓ, respectivamente, usando-se um ensaio quantitativo (CLIA, RIA ou ELFA) de amostras de soro coletadas diariamente ou, menos indicado, em dias alternados durante o proestro e o estro. Os ensaios quantitativos de LH não são amplamente acessíveis. O uso de testes qualitativos é menos indicado, uma vez que o pico de LH pode ter < 24 h de duração, e até mesmo os testes diários podem não ser frequentes o suficiente. Uma vez que as concentrações séricas de LH em cadelas anovulatórias jamais foram relatadas, a extensão e a quantidade de secreção de LH nelas são desconhecidas. Portanto, o valor do ensaio quantitativo de LH para diagnosticar a falha ovulatória é questionável, embora o LH sérico possa não alcançar a concentração ovulatória típica de 4 a 10 ng/mℓ. Dessa forma, a falha ovulatória normalmente é documentada quando a progesterona jamais excede 10 ng/mℓ.

As cadelas que experimentam um ciclo anovulatório costumam apresentar padrões normais de queratinização vaginal, atraem machos e quase sempre aceitam a monta. No entanto, a P4 sérica não aumenta > 10 ng/mℓ.[74,75] A falha ovulatória é rara;

estima-se que ocorra em aproximadamente 1% das cadelas acompanhadas no manejo reprodutivo.[74] Curiosamente, os autores observaram falha ovulatória mais frequentemente em cadelas de médio a grande porte (p. ex., Pastor-Alemão, Boiadeiro de Bernese, Labrador Retriever, Bullmastiff). Em teoria, a anovulação poderia ser tratada com GnRH, gonadotrofina coriônica humana (hCG, do inglês *human chorionic gonadotropina*) ou deslorelina, mas faltam estudos científicos que usam esses fármacos para esse fim. O potencial em interromper a função ovariana normal não deve ser subestimado. Em razão da incidência rara, a anovulação pode ser considerada uma perturbação fisiológica. Uma vez que os estressores potenciais são identificados e removidos, seria provavelmente mais sensato esperar (ou talvez induzir) o próximo cio, em vez de tratar uma cadela anovulatória com hormônios.

Aumento lento de P4

A luteinização pré-ovulatória de folículos ovarianos maduros causa aumento nas concentrações séricas de P4 marginais (1 a 2 ng/mℓ) antes e durante o pico de LH. O pico de LH, então, causa progressão constante da luteinização da parede folicular após a ovulação, com concentrações séricas de P4 atingindo 4 a 10 ng/mℓ em 48 h. O não aumento nas concentrações, com a permanência dos teores séricos de P4 em valores compatíveis com o estágio de pico de LH, indica anormalidade no processo ovulatório, definida como aumento lento de P4.[75] Quando a P4 sérica sobe lentamente, a concentração permanecerá nos valores correspondentes ao pico de LH (2 ng/mℓ) de alguns dias a 7, mas eventualmente esse patamar é seguido de aumento dos valores compatíveis com ovulação.

Existem poucas informações na incidência e na etiologia dessa doença. As causas para o aumento lento de P4 incluem muito pouco estrógeno para estimular a liberação de GnRH hipotalâmico, muito pouco LH hipofisário ou atraso na resposta folicular ao LH ou simplesmente maior pré-luteinização de folículos pré-ovulatórios antes do pico de LH. Em cadelas normais, a duração do pico de LH pode ser de até 96 h.[20,26,29-32] Portanto, é possível que cadelas com um período de platô de 3 a 4 dias na P4 sérica possam ter apresentado aumento longo e lento no LH, com ocorrência do pico de P4 em uma concentração de aproximadamente 3 a 4 ng/mℓ, em vez dos habituais 1,3 a 2 ng/mℓ. Foi mostrado que o primeiro dia da ovulação começa logo após o LH ser > 1 ng/mℓ. Retrospectivamente, contando-se para trás desde o parto, o dia estimado do pico de LH pode ser encontrado no início ou no final do platô de P4.[75]

Embora cadelas com aumento lento de P4 acabem ovulando e, portanto, possam reproduzir, o manejo reprodutivo desses animais é mais complicado, pois pode exigir o monitoramento repetido das concentrações séricas de P4 e, possivelmente, LH também. Portanto, quando há suspeita ou confirmação de aumento lento da P4, deve-se evitar o uso de sêmen resfriado ou congelado ou viagens de longas distâncias para encontrar um reprodutor, devendo a cadela ser coberta com um macho local. Ademais, pode ser difícil estabelecer a data de cobertura com base nas concentrações séricas de P4, devendo esta ser confirmada com ultrassonografia entre 25 e 35 dias a partir da primeira cobertura.[76]

Split heat

Split heat é definido como uma fase folicular curta, frequentemente com sinais típicos de proestro ou até mesmo com aceitação do macho por período curto, mas sem aumento das concentrações séricas de P4 acima de valores basais. Esses ciclos anovulatórios curtos são seguidos de um ciclo ovulatório em cerca de 50% das cadelas, em até 3 meses. Nas outras, podem ocorrer ciclos normais após um intervalo interestro normal (para essa raça).[74] O *split heat* pode recidivar, conforme observado em cadelas com histórico de intervalos interestrais curtos (< 3 meses).

Embora os intervalos interestrais curtos possam ser ocasionados por uma fase luteal insuficiente, sempre que uma cadela apresentar histórico de intervalo interestro curto o manejo reprodutivo deve ser cuidadosamente revisado, levando-se em consideração a possibilidade de *split heat*, cujas causas são consideradas as mesmas da falha ovulatória e do aumento lento de P4: baixa secreção de estrógeno, baixa liberação de GnRH hipotalâmico, baixa liberação de LH hipofisário e falha dos folículos na resposta ao LH. Deve-se considerar com cuidado a decisão de tratar ou não uma cadela com *split heat* com um indutor de ovulação, pois não há informações sobre a eficácia de quaisquer tratamentos sugeridos. Em cadelas com histórico de intervalos interestrais curtos que apresentam *split heat*, o uso de mibolerona na dose sugerida para supressão do estro é recomendado para prolongar o intervalo interestro a 6 meses.[75,77] Nessas cadelas, a gestação pode ser alcançada se o perfil de progesterona pós-mibolerona for normal.[75]

Hipoluteoidismo

Também chamada de insuficiência luteal, luteólise prematura ou fase luteal insuficiente, o *hipoluteoidismo* é definido como uma falha da P4 luteal em se manter nas concentrações necessárias por um período apropriado, normalmente 63 dias a partir da ovulação, para manutenção da gestação. As concentrações séricas de P4 podem diminuir para < 2 ng/mℓ logo após a ovulação (no final do estro) ou a qualquer momento durante o diestro. Embora rara, a insuficiência lútea foi relatada em cadelas gestantes, mas não em não gestantes.[78-82] Causas da insuficiência lútea canina não foram relatadas. Em mulheres no primeiro trimestre, a insuficiência lútea pode ser decorrente da doença ovariana policística. Distúrbios relacionados com a tireoide e a prolactina foram mostrados, possivelmente decorrentes do uso de análogos de GnRH na reprodução assistida. A luteólise prematura foi relatada em cadelas tratadas com deslorelina para induzir o estro, porém faltam informações sobre outras causas dessa condição, potencialmente endócrinas ou relacionadas com o estresse.[83-85]

Em cadelas cobertas, o diagnóstico de insuficiência luteal requer diagnóstico elaborado para descartar outras causas potenciais de baixa concentração de P4: por exemplo, sofrimento ou morte fetais podem resultar na diminuição da concentração de P4 como uma resposta fisiológica normal; portanto, devem-se descartar a viabilidade fetal e as condições bacterianas ou virais que afetam a saúde fetal ou materna.[86] Em cadelas cobertas nas quais o hipoluteoidismo é uma preocupação, a P4 sérica sempre deve ser testada após a confirmação da gestação pela ultrassonografia de rotina. A análise das concentrações séricas de P4, ao se descobrir na ultrassonografia de rotina que a cadela não está gestante, ajuda a descartar a insuficiência lútea.

O nascimento de ninhadas saudáveis em cadelas gestantes com insuficiência luteal usando-se progesterona parenteral oleosa (2 mg/kg por via intramuscular [IM], a cada 3 dias [intervalo 2 a 4]),[75,78] acetato de megestrol oral (2,2 mg/kg, a cada 48 h, do dia 25 em diante),[80] alitrembolona (0,088 mg/kg VO, diariamente)[82] e acetato de medroxiprogesterona (0,1 mg/kg VO, diariamente) se deu de forma bem-sucedida.[53,81] Os autores têm utilizado com sucesso cápsulas orais de progesterona micronizada (Prometrium Merck; 100 mg/cão ou 5 mg/kg, a cada 12 h). No decorrer do tratamento, as concentrações séricas de P4 devem ser avaliadas a cada 2 a 3 dias. Estima-se que seja necessário medicação adicional se as concentrações séricas de P4 caírem < 15 ng/mℓ durante as 3 a 7 semanas de gestação ou < 5 ng/mℓ nas semanas 8 e 9. Ao suplementar com uma progesterona que possa ser monitorada por meio de testes sanguíneos, o ideal é tentar manter um perfil normal de progesterona durante a segunda metade da gestação, com valores máximos de 15 a 20 ng/mℓ por volta do meio da gravidez, seguido de um declínio lento a 5 ng/mℓ durante a última semana de gestação. Toda suplementação deve ser interrompida 2 a 3 dias antes da data de parto normal prevista para a cadela. Durante o primeiro mês de gestação, prefere-se o uso de compostos naturais de progesterona, por reduzir o risco de malformações fetais congênitas. O uso de compostos sintéticos é considerado seguro na segunda metade da gestação,[87] tendo a vantagem de a concentração da P4 sérica do paciente refletir a produção endógena.

Estro persistente

Manifestações de comportamento estral persistentes podem ser iatrogênicas (*i. e.*, decorrentes do tratamento com agonistas de GnRH ou estrógenos) ou ocorrer naturalmente durante o estro.[88,89] Esse último geralmente é decorrente de anormalidades na função ovariana, caracterizada por comportamento estral, esfregaço vaginal totalmente queratinizado e baixas concentrações séricas de P4 (pré-ovulatórias) que persistem por > 21 dias. As causas de estro persistente podem ser falha ovulatória, síndrome do "aumento lento de P4" ou condições como cisto folicular ovariano ou tumores de células da granulosa. O diagnóstico do estro persistente pode ser um desafio quando, em razão da anovulação ou do aumento lento de P4, é necessária uma avaliação criteriosa do histórico, pois essas condições podem não ser percebidas antes da apresentação, enquanto as anormalidades ovarianas (cistos foliculares ou neoplasia ovariana) são facilmente diagnosticadas por ultrassonografia.

Além da sugestão de que o estro persistente pode se resolver de maneira natural, o tratamento não foi descrito. Preparações hormonais que estimulem o crescimento folicular (p. ex., gonadotrofina coriônica equina) não devem ser utilizadas, pois podem aumentar a secreção de estradiol, aumentando o risco de aplasia medular e/ou piometra. O uso de hCG (22 UI/kg, IM, 1 vez/dia, por 3 dias) foi relatado como eficaz em finalizar o estro por desencadear o início do diestro ou anestro.[90] Usamos uma combinação de hCG (500 a 1.000 UI, IM, 2 doses, 48 h de intervalo) e GnRH (1,5 µg/kg, IM, a cada 24 h × 4 dias; ou colocação de um implante de deslorelina de 2,1 mg até que a luteinização fosse detectada: progesterona > 5 ng/mℓ). Raramente ocorreu ovulação. Mais comumente, a luteinização de folículos ou de cistos foliculares permite à cadela sair do estro. A ovulação fértil é improvável, pois os oócitos estão degenerados no momento em que o diagnóstico é feito e a terapia iniciada. A inseminação ou a reprodução não devem ser realizadas.

O prognóstico da fertilidade após o estro persistente é relatado como desfavorável. Se precedido por um intervalo interestral normal, pode ainda valer a pena tentar cobertura natural no estro seguinte. Foi relatada piometra em uma cadela com estro persistente após tratamento bem-sucedido com hCG. A ovariohisterectomia é sempre considerada uma opção de sucesso para a resolução.

Intervalos interestrais curtos

Os intervalos interestrais variam entre raças e dentro delas. Intervalos de 4 meses entre cios consecutivos são considerados normais em algumas linhagens de Pastor-Alemão, Rottweiler, Akita, Labrador Retriever, Cocker Spaniel e Basset Hound, apesar dos intervalos interestrais mais comuns serem de aproximadamente 6 meses. Intervalos interestrais curtos nessas e em outras cadelas individuais são descritos ocasionalmente.[53,91] Cadelas com intervalos interestrais curtos apresentam uma tendência a funções luteais curtas.[91] A incidência dessa condição é desconhecida, mas pode ocorrer em até 5 a 10% das cadelas saudáveis. As causas de intervalos interestrais curtos são desconhecidas, porém o papel da produção ovariana de progesterona parece ser relevante. Foi sugerido que é necessário "um aumento suficiente de progesterona em amplitude e duração para o reconhecimento de um ciclo pelo hipotálamo e o estabelecimento de um anestro de duração adequada (> 3 meses) para um intervalo interestral normal".[75] Um estudo subsequente concluiu que cadelas com intervalos interestrais curtos apresentam tendência à função lútea deficiente.[91] Portanto, é provável que haja relação direta entre a duração do diestro e a do anestro.

O anestro desempenha papel importante na involução uterina e na retomada da ciclicidade. Em cadelas não paridas, o reparo endometrial é concluído cerca de 135 dias após o início do estro. A amplitude e o número dos pulsos hipotalâmicos de GnRH e a responsividade ovariana e pituitária aumentam conforme o anestro progride.[32,73] Um anestro curto encurtará a duração do intervalo interestral, afetando de maneira negativa a fertilidade do ciclo subsequente, por impedir a conclusão do reparo normal do endométrio e/ou uma resposta normal do eixo hipotálamo-hipófise-ovário. A fertilidade após um intervalo interestral curto pode ser menor. Em termos diagnósticos, o cariótipo deve ser considerado anormalidade cromossômica, já que pode causar intervalos interestrais curtos e infertilidade.[92,93] Foi descrito o tratamento bem-sucedido com a administração diária de mibolerona por, pelo menos, 30 dias antes do próximo ciclo previsto, conforme necessário.

MANEJO REPRODUTIVO

Pré-cobertura

Idade à primeira cobertura

A idade recomendada para a primeira cobertura depende da raça, do uso, da saúde e das preferências do proprietário.

Recomenda-se que raças pequenas e miniaturas tenham > 18 meses de idade e as médias e gigantes, > 24 meses. Essas recomendações devem permitir a maturidade e o crescimento da cadela antes de emprenhar. Embora, na maioria das raças, a puberdade possa ocorrer muito antes dessas idades, o desenvolvimento físico e psicológico não está completo e os efeitos negativos da gestação são permanentes.

Testes genéticos

Os testes necessários variam com a raça e podem incluir varredura radiográfica (p. ex., OFA e PennHIP), avaliação especializada (p. ex., cardiologia, oftalmologia) e triagem genética de esfregaços de sangue, cabelo ou bochecha (p. ex., OptiGen, PennGen, VetGen) (ver Capítulos 3 e 4).[94] Se o resultado dos testes genéticos gerar preocupações, o criador deve considerá-las. Como não existe cão perfeito, há momentos em que a reprodução de um animal com um distúrbio genético pode ser aceitável, a fim de introduzir características específicas desejáveis na linhagem sanguínea ou da raça. Uma avaliação criteriosa de acasalamento para esses indivíduos pode reduzir o risco de transmissão do distúrbio para a prole (*i. e.*, cruzar um animal acometido com um sem doenças).

Saúde geral e teste de Brucella

Recomendam-se hemograma e análises bioquímicas séricas e urinálise, sobretudo em cadelas reprodutoras > 4 anos de idade. Especificamente, as cadelas devem ser rastreadas para doença renal, uma vez que as artérias renais e ovarianas surgem dos mesmos vasos e a gestação pode desviar o sangue dos rins em favor do útero gravídico. Urinálise, microalbuminúria e/ou razão proteína:creatinina são recomendadas em cadelas idosas. Outros testes específicos podem depender do local onde a cadela reside (*i. e.*, titulação de carrapatos, teste de dirofilariose). Em geral, o teste da tireoide não é necessário, a menos que haja sinais clínicos, uma vez que foi documentado que o hipotireoidismo tem pouco impacto na fertilidade (os estágios 2 e 3 podem afetar a duração do parto).[95-103] Uma vez que a tireoidite autoimune pode ter uma origem de base genética, cadelas com doença da tireoide devem ser avaliadas. Aquelas com hipotireoidismo clínico decorrente da atrofia idiopática da tireoide podem ser submetidas à reprodução após o tratamento com a reposição do hormônio da tireoide e a confirmação de uma resposta aceitável, com o controle mensal das concentrações da tireoide durante a gestação, uma vez que ela afeta o metabolismo e pode aumentar a demanda por suplementação da tireoide. Tanto a cadela quanto o macho devem ser testados para brucelose dentro de 8 semanas da reprodução (ver Capítulo 213).[104-106] A brucelose pode ser disseminada por contato de aerossol ou reprodução. Os testes de triagem incluem o teste rápido de aglutinação em lâmina (RSAT, do inglês *rapid slide agglutination test*), o ensaio imunoenzimático (ELISA, do inglês *enzyme-linked immunosorbent assay*) e o teste de aglutinação em tubo (TAT, do inglês *tube agglutination test*). Se positivo, podem-se fazer teste confirmatório (teste de imunodifusão em gel de ágar [IDGA], hemoculturas e reação em cadeia da polimerase [PCR, do inglês *polymerase chain reaction*]).

Exame físico

Antes da reprodução, deve-se realizar um exame físico completo da cadela e do cão, para garantir que ambos estejam saudáveis e que a cadela seja capaz de levar a gestação a termo (ver Capítulo 2). Deve-se dar atenção especial à condição corporal. Cadelas obesas apresentam redução das taxas de ovulação, diminuição da resistência e maior dificuldade em respirar no final da gestação, quando o útero gestante comprime o diafragma. Cadelas com sobrepeso (ver Capítulo 176) têm maior incidência de inércia uterina e distocias obstrutivas em razão do aumento da gordura pélvica. Machos obesos podem não ter resistência ou capacidade para realizar monta natural. A insulação escrotal pela gordura pode afetar a qualidade do sêmen. As glândulas mamárias devem ser palpadas em busca de tumores ou outras anormalidades, com a realização de um exame digital vaginal para descartar estenoses vestíbulo-vaginais, septos, hímen remanescente, estenoses vulvares, tumores vaginais ou cistos ou outros impedimentos à cobertura ou ao parto.

Momento da ovulação e manejo do sêmen

O momento da ovulação é recomendado para todos os cruzamentos, a fim de minimizar as coberturas necessárias, preservar os espermatozoides, maximizar o uso de machos, reduzir o número de espermatozoides inseminados em cadelas predispostas à endometrite induzida por cobertura, melhorar as taxas de concepção, maximizar o tamanho da ninhada e permitir a determinação de uma janela de data de parto (ver Tabelas 312.1 e 312.2; ver também Figuras 312.1 a 312.3). É importante saber a data do parto para cesarianas de emergência ou eletivas, para a gestão da gestação de alto risco e para a prestação de cuidados durante o parto pela equipe veterinária e pelos cuidadores. Para coberturas com sêmen fresco, o momento da ovulação não precisa ser monitorado tão de perto quanto para o sêmen resfriado ou congelado, pois o espermatozoide sobrevive por longos períodos no sêmen fresco, ao contrário do sêmen resfriado ou congelado. Ainda, o acesso ilimitado ao macho deve maximizar as taxas de concepção. Em situações nas quais o macho está sendo utilizado com várias fêmeas ao mesmo tempo, é indicado o monitoramento mais estrito para maximizar a quantidade de espermatozoides para cada cobertura. As coberturas com sêmen congelado exigem maior precisão quanto ao momento da ovulação, porque o espermatozoide sobrevive por pouco tempo, geralmente apenas 8 a 12 h, tornando imperativo que todos os oócitos tenham sido ovulados e estejam maduros o suficiente para serem fertilizados próximo à ovulação.

Comportamentos e mudanças físicas

As melhores taxas de concepção são alcançadas combinando-se avaliação do comportamento com as alterações físicas, anatomia perineal, citologia vaginal, espéculo vaginal, concentrações de P4 e dosagem de LH (ver Capítulo 119). Essas técnicas complementares oferecem maior chance de determinar com precisão o período fértil pelo tempo do início da ovulação. Embora haja um padrão típico na maioria das cadelas, há exceções quanto às normais saudáveis. No início do proestro (e às vezes por até 1 mês antes), os machos são atraídos para a área perineal e para locais onde ela urina. Os comportamentos de marcação de urina aumentam conforme a cadela se aproxima e entra no proestro. Os lábios vulvares começarão a inchar, com início da secreção vulvar, que, a princípio, é acompanhada de sangue vermelho/marrom-escuro. A fonte dessa secreção é o útero, devido ao aumento da fragilidade capilar, como resultado do aumento das concentrações de estrógeno. Conforme a cadela progride do proestro para o estro, o sangramento diminui e a secreção torna-se mais pálida. Algumas cadelas param de sangrar durante o período fértil, enquanto outras sangrarão durante todo o período até o diestro.

Conforme a cadela se aproxima do período fértil, o edema vulvar diminui, resultando em amolecimento dos lábios vulvares e permitindo a introdução. As cadelas com uma vulva infantil ou encapuzada podem melhorar a conformação durante o estro ou a abertura vulvar pode continuar a dificultar a reprodução natural.

O comportamento reprodutivo da cadela e o maior interesse do macho coincidem com as mudanças na proporção de estrógeno (E2):progesterona (P4). As concentrações de E2 começam a diminuir antes do rápido aumento de P4, tornando a cadela receptiva. Aquelas com ciclos atípicos (estro ou proestro curto ou longo) podem não correlacionar de maneira apropriada o comportamento receptivo com o período fértil, o que pode ser confundido por criadores que acreditam que o macho pode determinar a ovulação da cadela. No entanto, em razão da sobrevivência do espermatozoide no trato reprodutivo da cadela por até 11 dias, a cobertura até 7 a 10 dias antes da ovulação ainda pode resultar em gestação.[107-109] Caso o criador acredite que a cadela tenha sido coberta no momento da ovulação, quando, no entanto, ela o foi muito antes, a data calculada para o parto (baseada nas datas de cobertura) será significativamente mais cedo. Por essas razões, os veterinários devem ter muita cautela ao determinar as datas previstas de parto a partir das datas de cobertura. Como regra geral, a data adequada pode ser entre 54 e 72 ± 2 dias a partir de uma data qualquer de cobertura.

Uso da citologia vaginal

As lâminas de citologia vaginal (ver Capítulo 119) devem ser empregadas a partir de 5 a 8 dias após o início de secreção sanguinolenta na cadela ou antes naquelas com histórico de ovulação precoce. Algumas cadelas podem não sangrar muito e, em outras, pode haver acúmulo de sangue na vagina cranial. Outras podem, ainda, lamber meticulosamente a região perineal e permanecer livres de sangue, podendo, às vezes, os primeiros dias do ciclo passar despercebidos por proprietários desatentos ou inexperientes. Se houver edema e interesse do macho por vários dias, a realização de citologia precoce (e exame de espéculo) garantirá que os estágios iniciais do ciclo não passem despercebidos. A citologia deverá ser feita a cada 2 a 4 dias, até que haja pelo menos 50% das células superficiais, momento em que deve ser adicionado o teste da P4. O uso de citologia vaginal deve ser continuado pelo menos a cada 2 a 4 dias, para garantir que o ciclo esteja progredindo normalmente. Anormalidades do ciclo serão observadas, sobretudo, na citologia, muito antes de os resultados endócrinos indicarem qualquer preocupação (p. ex., *split heat* ou ciclos anovulatórios). A citologia vaginal também poderá ser utilizada para documentar o dia 1 do diestro, o qual é tão útil quanto a progesterona na determinação de uma data de parto da cadela, especialmente se o dia da ovulação passar.

Uso do exame de espéculo vaginal

O exame do espéculo pode ser realizado simplesmente usando-se um otoscópio e um cone de otoscópio limpo, devendo ser realizado toda vez que uma citologia for obtida (ver Capítulos 44 e 119). A progressão de uma mucosa rosa edemaciada no início do proestro para uma branca e proeminentemente crenulada é outro indicador de progressão normal do ciclo. A taxa em que as mudanças ocorrem é um indicador de desenvolvimento e maturação dos folículos do ciclo. Essas mudanças, combinadas com a citologia, a concentração de P4 e as alterações comportamentais, ajudam o profissional a determinar quando a cadela deverá ser examinada quanto ao momento da ovulação. Assim que confirmada, a continuação na feitura de exames de espéculo e citologia poderá ajudar a determinar o primeiro dia de diestro, conforme a mucosa começa a achatar e se tornar rosada nesse dia de transição.

Monitoramento da progesterona (P4)

No início do proestro, as concentrações de P4 são basais; normalmente < 1 ng/mℓ (quando relatado em nmol/ℓ, dividir por 3,14). À medida que os folículos se tornam maduros, pequenos pulsos de LH começam a causar a pré-luteinização da parede folicular, resultando em aumento lento, mas gradual, da P4. Uma vez que os folículos estejam maduros, a onda de LH pré-ovulatória é estimulada. Em geral, o pico de LH é provável quando a P4 é o dobro da basal (ver Tabelas 312.1 e 312.2). Uma vez ocorrida a ovulação, há rápido aumento das concentrações de P4 por 2 a 3 semanas. O aumento de P4 entre o pico de LH e a ovulação é mais gradual do que o após a ovulação. Algumas cadelas apresentam platô de P4 entre 2 ng/mℓ e 8 ng/mℓ por um ou mais dias, tornando crítico o monitoramento da P4 até a ovulação ser confirmada por um aumento de 3 ng/mℓ ou mais em um período de 24 h. É importante lembrar que a ovulação não ocorre em nenhum valor específico de P4, mas, sim, é confirmada por um aumento rápido e progressivo, normalmente de 3 ng/mℓ ou mais, em um período de 24 h, uma vez que alcança aproximadamente 4 a 10 ng/mℓ.

Depois do aumento inicial pós-ovulação, as mudanças diárias podem ser mais rápidas ou mais lentas. Ocasionalmente, a P4 pode aumentar apenas 2 a 2,5 ng/mℓ no(s) dia(s) pós-ovulação, podendo ser útil a inclusão de teste de LH para essas cadelas. O teste P4 pode ser feito com menor frequência no início/meio do proestro (a cada 3 a 5 dias). Quando a citologia indicar que a maioria das células é superficial, o teste de P4 deve ser feito com maior frequência. Uma vez que a progesterona atingir o intervalo de ovulação (3 a 5 ng/mℓ), recomenda-se o teste dia sim, dia não.

Monitoramento do hormônio luteinizante

O hormônio luteinizante (LH, do inglês *luteinizing hormone*) é liberado, a princípio, em pequenos pulsos durante o meio do proestro, seguido de um grande aumento pré-ovulatório no final do proestro e início do estro, com duração de 12 a 96 h. O pico de LH normalmente é alcançado 2 dias após a ovulação. Em razão da variabilidade na duração da onda de LH, são necessárias coletas diárias de sangue para a detecção, sendo seu início considerado o evento motivador da ovulação. Então, mesmo que o pico tenha duração de 2 a 3 dias, é correto usar o primeiro dia como "dia 0" no momento da ovulação. Normalmente, o teste de LH é realizado usando-se um ensaio de fluxo de membrana (Witness® LH, Zoetis Corp; ver Figura 312.2). O *kit* de teste interno é útil pois permite a interpretação da intensidade de mudança de cor em relação ao controle, além de reduzir o tempo de resposta, o que pode ser bastante limitante. Em algumas, o pico de LH deve ser identificado levando-se em consideração os dados de P4. Lembre-se de que um pico de LH não garante a ovulação. Então, é fundamental confirmá-la avaliando-se sempre as concentrações de P4. Ao se esperar até que a ovulação seja confirmada, reduz-se o número de testes de LH a serem executados.

Inseminação artificial
Ver Capítulo 118.

Frequência de inseminação
Deve-se realizar a monta natural ou o usar sêmen fresco ou fresco resfriado uma ou duas vezes, começando 2 dias após a ovulação (4 dias pós-LH) e novamente 2 dias depois. Inseminações simples planejadas (incluindo inseminação cirúrgica) costumam ser realizadas do meio para o final do período fértil. As coberturas com sêmen congelado devem ser realizadas somente após a maturação completa de todos os oócitos; dia 3 ou 4 pós-ovulação (dias 5 ou 6 pós-pico de LH).

Estratégias para cobertura indesejada (Figuras 312.4 e 312.5)

Confirmação da gestação
Se ocorrer um acasalamento acidental, o ideal é examinar a cadela o mais rápido possível pela citologia vaginal e concentração sérica de P4, o que permite o preparo do ciclo e ajuda a determinar a possibilidade de estabelecimento da gestação. Se a cadela tiver sido coberta recentemente, os espermatozoides

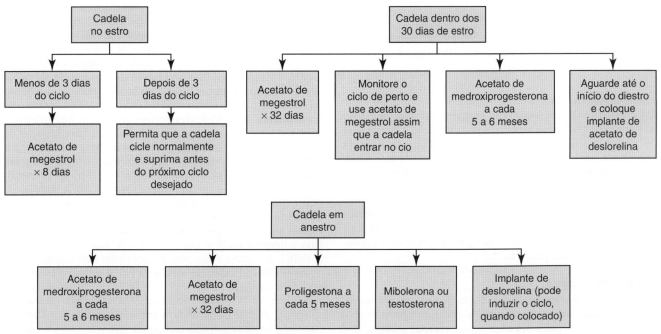

Figura 312.4 Algoritmo com alternativa para a supressão do estro.

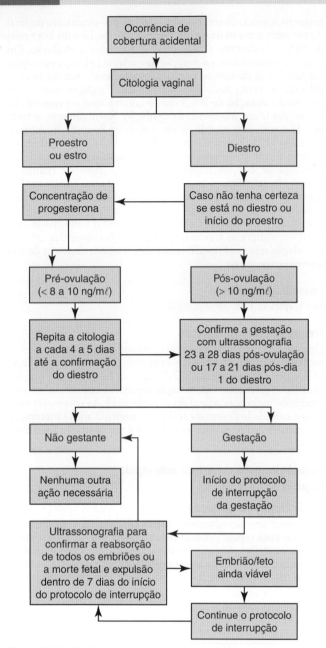

Figura 312.5 Algoritmo com recomendações para interrupção da gestação em cadelas após cobertura indesejada.

costumam ser vistos na citologia vaginal. Se ela estiver no início do proestro ou diestro, a gestação é improvável; mas, se estiver no estro e tiver sido realmente coberta, a gestação é bem provável. Antes de iniciar a interrupção da gestação, esta deve ser confirmada (ver Capítulo 315). Apenas cerca de 60% das cadelas atendidas para a interrupção da gravidez estão prenhes após uma cobertura indesejada, provavelmente por suspeita não confirmada de acasalamento. A palpação, mesmo feita por clínicos experientes, não é perfeita. Assim, a gestação deve ser confirmada por ultrassonografia (assim que completar 19 dias pós-LH), teste de relaxina (100% de acurácia > 30 dias de gestação) ou radiografias (após o dia 43 pós-LH).[110-115]

Tratamento cirúrgico

As cadelas não destinadas à reprodução devem ser submetidas à ovário-histerectomia (esterilizadas) a qualquer momento após cobertura acidental, independentemente de ela estar gestante.[110-118] O risco cirúrgico é baixo e a ovariectomia pode ser considerada para cadelas muito jovens em estro ou diestro inicial, mas qualquer uma com uma possível doença uterina ou que tenha tido um ciclo estral deve ser submetida à ovário-histerectomia, já que a permanência do útero pode resultar em granuloma de coto ou piometra. Cadelas castradas no meio ou final do diestro podem desenvolver pseudociese devido ao declínio abrupto de P4. Se a lactação for excessiva, o uso de agentes antiprolactina pode ser considerado.

Razões para a interrupção da gestação, histórico

Os proprietários podem desejar interromper a gestação do animal por inúmeras razões: doença na cadela que ameace sua vida se a gestação continuar; cobertura acidental indesejada; ou cobertura não intencional de animais jovens ou consanguíneos. Com a maioria dos protocolos de interrupção da gestação, o intervalo interestral pode ser encurtado, já que o diestro o foi efetivamente. Foram recomendados inúmeros protocolos para a interrupção da gestação, dependendo do estágio da gestação.[110-117,119-134] A P4, sintetizada e secretada pelos CLs, é necessária para a manutenção da gestação na cadela.[135-137] Os CLs são sustentados pelo LH e pela PRL.[41,118] A maioria dos protocolos envolve a supressão da produção de um ou de ambos ou o impedimento de que a P4 se ligue aos receptores uterinos. Nos últimos 10 dias de gestação, as cadelas abortarão fetos vivos, exigindo monitoramento do veterinário ou do dono, suporte ou eutanásia humanitária de fetos prematuros. Se o estágio da gestação for desconhecido, recomenda-se a feitura de exames ultrassonográficos seriados em intervalos semanais, começando 3 semanas após a cobertura da cadela, até que a gestação possa ser confirmada ou refutada com segurança. O número de exames dependerá da experiência do operador, das instalações, do tamanho do paciente e da preparação (tricotomia, gel lubrificante, posicionamento, frequência respiratória).

Prostaglandinas (PGF2-alfa)

Esses compostos podem ser usados individualmente ou em combinação para interrupção da gestação sem que afete a fertilidade futura.[110-118] A PGF2-alfa inicia a luteólise e promove a limpeza uterina,[110-118,138-148] podendo ser usada logo nos dias 8 a 10 do diestro, porém a gestação ainda não pode ser confirmada. A gestação pode ser considerada "bem provável" caso tenha sido observada cobertura e a citologia vaginal for compatível com o estro.[142,147] A PGF2-alfa pode ser administrada a cada 12 ou 48 h, dependendo do protocolo e do uso natural ou sintético do produto (Tabela 312.3). Mostrou-se que baixas doses são tão eficazes quanto as usadas anteriormente, mas causam muito menos efeitos colaterais.[147-149] Quando iniciada no começo do diestro, a terapia com PGF2-alfa deve ser continuada até que a luteólise seja completa, enquanto, no final da gestação, o término do tratamento é o esvaziamento total do útero. CLs caninos são notadamente resilientes; eles podem retomar a função após a aparente luteólise completa.[110-118,149] Assim, a concentração de P4 deve ser < 1,5 ng/mℓ na conclusão da terapia e 48 a 72 h depois, para garantir que a gestação não seja mantida. Em geral, a luteólise requer pelo menos 7 dias durante os primeiros 30 dias de gestação e apenas 4 dias após o dia 30. A inclusão de PGE1 (misoprostol) diariamente na cérvice, começando no momento da PGF2-alfa e continuando até que o corrimento vaginal seja notado, pode reduzir o número de dias necessários para a limpeza uterina, por facilitar o relaxamento da cérvice. A PGE1, no entanto, não tem propriedades luteolíticas.[150]

As reações adversas causadas pela PGF2-alfa são variadas e a gravidade depende da dose.[110-115,118,139-141,143,151] Cadelas tornam-se tolerantes à PGF2-alfa quando ela é administrada de maneira contínua. A PGF2-alfa afeta a musculatura lisa e os efeitos colaterais comuns incluem taquipneia, broncoconstrição, hipersalivação, náuseas, êmese, defecação e bradicardia. Altas doses

CAPÍTULO 312 • Endocrinologia Reprodutiva e Manejo Reprodutivo da Cadela

Tabela 312.3 Protocolos de fármacos para interrupção da gestação.

FÁRMACO 1	DOSE	DURAÇÃO	FÁRMACO 2	DOSE	DURAÇÃO
PGF2-alfa natural	10 a 50 µg/kg SC, a cada 8 a 12 h	4 a 7+ dias			
PGF2-alfa natural	10 a 50 µg/kg SC, a cada 12 h	4 a 7+ dias	Cabergolina	5 µg/kg VO, a cada 24 h	7 a 10 dias
PGF2-alfa natural	10 a 50 µg/kg SC, a cada 12 h	4 a 7+ dias	Bromocriptina	10 a 20 µg/kg VO, a cada 12 h	10 dias
PGF2-alfa natural	10 a 50 µg/kg SC, a cada 12 h	4 a 7+ dias	Aglepristone	10 mg/kg SC: 2 doses em um intervalo de 24 h	Se a gestação ainda for viável em 7 a 10 dias, repetir a 3ª dose
Cloprostenol	1 µg/kg SC, a cada 48 h	3 a 4 doses (6 a 8 dias)			
Cloprostenol	1 µg/kg SC, a cada 48 h	1 a 3 doses	Cabergolina	5 µg/kg VO, a cada 24 h	7 a 10 dias
Cloprostenol	1 µg/kg SC, a cada 48 h	2 a 3 doses	Bromocriptina	10 a 20 µg/kg VO, a cada 12 h	10 dias
Cloprostenol	1 µg/kg SC, a cada 48 h	2 a 3 doses	Aglepristone	10 mg/kg SC: 2 doses em um intervalo de 24 h	Se a gestação ainda for viável em 7 a 10 dias, repetir a 3ª dose
Aglepristone	10 mg/kg SC: 2 doses em um intervalo de 24 h	Se a gestação ainda for viável em 7 a 10 dias, repetir a 3ª dose			
Dexametasona	200 µg/kg VO, a cada 12 h	10 a 12 dias: continuar até que o abortamento esteja completo			

podem causar incoordenação motora leve e depressão do sistema nervoso central. Os efeitos dos análogos da PGF2-alfa, que têm maior afinidade para se ligar aos receptores PGF2-alfa, são mais pronunciados do que os da PGF2-alfa natural; assim, a frequência da dose é menor.[110,114,144,145,148] Em cães braquicefálicos, deve-se ter cuidado extremo, já que a broncoconstrição e a taquipneia podem ser fatais. A administração de atropina, brometo de prifínio ou metopimazina 15 min antes da injeção de PGF2-alfa minimiza tanto os efeitos na musculatura lisa quanto os colaterais negativos em mais de 50% dos cães.[151]

Agonistas do receptor de dopamina

A bromocriptina e a cabergolina, derivados alcaloides com atividade agonista do receptor de dopamina, inibem a síntese de PRL luteotrófica.[68,110-118,152-155] A secreção de PRL começa no meio da gestação. Assim, os agonistas do receptor de dopamina são úteis após 30 a 35 dias de gestação. Qualquer uma das medicações pode causar a interrupção da gestação, mas a duração do tratamento é muito menor com PGF2-alfa simultânea (ver Tabela 312.3). O benefício da terapia adicional de agonistas do receptor de dopamina é que o desenvolvimento da glândula mamária também é suprimido. A lactação é improvável se a gestação for interrompida com a combinação de PGF2-alfa e agonistas do receptor de dopamina.[153,154] A bromocriptina causa mais êmese e anorexia. Esse tratamento não afeta a fertilidade nos ciclos subsequentes.

Dexametasona

A dexametasona (independentemente da via de administração) induz o aborto quando administrada por 10 dias ou mais em cadelas gestantes (ver Tabela 312.3).[156-158] A morte fetal começa 5 a 9 dias após o início da terapia, porém alguns fetos podem permanecer viáveis por até 12 dias. Esse medicamento não deve ser utilizado no final da gestação, porque pode induzir o parto de fetos vivos. Se o tratamento for iniciado antes do dia 40, ocorre reabsorção fetal, enquanto, após o dia 40, aborto. É fundamental que a terapia seja continuada até a confirmação da morte de todos os fetos; caso contrário, a gestação pode continuar a termo e os fetos podem desenvolver palatosquise ou queilosquise (fenda palatina ou lábio leporino). Os efeitos colaterais incluem polidipsia, poliúria e anorexia, que duram por todo o tratamento. A fertilidade nos ciclos subsequentes, curiosamente, não é afetada por essas medicações.

Antagonistas do receptor de progesterona

O uso da mifepristona (RU486) e do aglepristone (RU534) foi bem-sucedido na interrupção da gestação (ver Tabela 312.3). Esses fármacos têm três vezes mais afinidade aos receptores uterinos em comparação à P4,[159-162] uma leve atividade antiglicocorticoide e não reduzem as concentrações séricas de P4. O aglepristone está disponível no mercado para administração por via subcutânea (< 5 mℓ/injeção) na Europa, na América do Sul, no Canadá, na Austrália e na Ásia, mas não nos EUA, sem autorização especial. Uma vez que o fármaco tem uma base oleosa, os locais de injeção devem ser massageados para facilitar a absorção e reduzir a irritação local. Esses medicamentos podem ser administrados do dia 1 do diestro até o dia 45 da gestação. Se administrado após o dia 45, podem nascer fetos vivos e prematuros. No início da gestação, antes do dia 30, geralmente os fetos são reabsorvidos. Entre os dias 30 e 45, pode ser observada secreção vaginal sanguinolenta ou expulsão de fetos mortos. Esses medicamentos não devem ser usados em pacientes com hipoadrenocorticismo, diabetes melito, doença pulmonar obstrutiva crônica, endocardite ou doença hepática. Os efeitos colaterais podem incluir irritação local nos locais de injeção, anorexia, êmese, diarreia, excitação ou depressão. Após a interrupção da gestação, pode ocorrer pseudociese.

Acetato de megestrol

Cadelas cobertas nos primeiros 2 a 3 dias do estro podem ter a supressão do ciclo por meio da administração de 2,2 mg/kg de acetato de megestrol por 8 dias.[114] Há algum risco de piometra ou endometrite quando cadelas adultas ou mais velhas são tratadas com essa medicação, e é improvável que cadelas adultas jovens saudáveis desenvolvam qualquer condição uterina (ver Capítulos 315 e 316). É importante confirmar a interrupção do ciclo (sem ocorrência da ovulação), pois, se ele progredir, a cadela pode ficar gestante e o cliente pode não reconhecer isso até o final da gestação, quando os protocolos de interrupção podem não ser mais possíveis ou resultar no parto de fetos vivos.

Estrógenos

Os estrógenos têm sido usados historicamente para interrupção da gestação.[163-169] Atualmente, o uso deles é contraindicado, pois existem outras opções eficazes com efeitos colaterais menos significativos e graves. Os estrógenos, quando administrados no início da gestação, podem afetar o movimento do oócito ou do embrião pelo oviduto e dentro do útero, alterar o ambiente do oviduto, causando a degeneração do oócito, ser diretamente embriotóxicos ou interferirem na implantação do embrião. Os estrógenos aumentam a contratilidade uterina e relaxam a cérvice. Os efeitos colaterais incluem aplasia da medula óssea, hiperplasia endometrial cística, piometra e supressão da fertilidade futura por meio dos efeitos a longo prazo sobre a secreção de gonadotrofina. Os estrógenos não são mais considerados seguros para interrupção da gestação.

Citrato de tamoxifeno

Provavelmente interrompe a gestação por meio de sua atividade estrogênica, ao alterar o tempo de trânsito do embrião pelos ovidutos ou interferir na implantação.[170] Essa medicação pode ser efetiva quando administrada durante o proestro até o dia 15 do diestro, mas não depois. Os efeitos colaterais negativos incluem cistos ovarianos, endometrite ou piometra.

MANIPULAÇÃO DO CICLO REPRODUTIVO CANINO

Supressão do estro

A manipulação do ciclo reprodutivo inclui a realização da supressão do estro, definida como a interrupção ou redução da atividade em progresso. Assim, a *supressão do estro* é usada para tratar cadelas no proestro/estro (para interromper o cio). Os termos *prevenção ou adiamento do estro* para cadelas em anestro envolvem o evitamento do proestro/estro por completo. As indicações para essas duas condições distinguem as preocupações dos proprietários dos fármacos necessários. A supressão do estro costuma ser solicitada de maneira súbita em cadelas de exposição, corrida ou caça, uma preocupação quase emergencial. Assim sendo, uma vez terminado o evento esportivo ou a exposição durante o qual o proestro ocorra, a cadela pode voltar a ciclar novamente, o que torna a supressão um tratamento a curto prazo. Portanto, os progestágenos de curta ação são preferidos.

Atualmente, o único progestágeno disponível de curta ação no mercado veterinário é o acetato de megestrol, vendido como um fármaco oral na maioria dos países europeus, na Austrália, na América do Sul e em outros lugares. O acetato de megestrol tem meia-vida de algumas horas e afinidade por receptores de P4 15 a 25 vezes maior do que a atividade endógena da P4, mas também notável afinidade por receptores andrógenos (75%) e glicocorticoides (37%), respectivamente.[171,172] O acetato de megestrol provavelmente atua nos ovários e no eixo hipotalâmico-hipofisário. Ele suprime não só a função hipofisária, como também a atividade ovariana, fazendo com que a atividade do ciclo cesse. Quando administrado por 8 dias consecutivos (2,2 mg/kg/dia) no início (nos 3 primeiros dias) do proestro, o acetato de megestrol é eficaz na supressão do cio de 92 a 97% das cadelas tratadas em 3 a 8 dias.[173-175] A eficácia pode não ser tão boa em cadelas com períodos de proestro muito curtos ou longos.[173-175] O intervalo do tratamento ao retorno do estro dura, em média, 4 a 6 (variação 1 a 9) meses e, em geral, a fertilidade pós-tratamento é normal.[174,175] Deve-se evitar o tratamento de cadelas por três ou mais ciclos consecutivos ou no estro de fêmeas púberes. A proligestona, uma progestina de longa ação, é comercializada para a supressão do estro em uma única administração de 10 a 33 mg/kg SC (a dose varia inversamente com o peso corporal).[176] Enquanto a proligestona é eficaz no adiamento do estro, há pouca informação sobre seu uso para a supressão do estro na cadela.

Em cadelas jovens e saudáveis, o uso de acetato de megestrol na dose anteriormente mencionada pode estimular o apetite e diminuir a atividade (causando, assim, ganho de peso). Alguns cães apresentam aumento mamário e endometrial leves, o que não é preocupante.[175,177] A evidência de piometra foi relatada em 0,8% das 389 cadelas tratadas com acetato de megestrol, não havendo aumento da incidência de neoplasia mamária em um levantamento com 700 animais.[173,175] O acetato de megestrol é diabetogênico e pode causar supressão adrenocortical, mas apenas se forem usadas doses maiores que 2,2 mg/kg/dia VO, e/ou a duração do tratamento for superior a 8 dias.[178-180] Quando usado em doses baixas (ver seção posterior), o acetato de megestrol pode ser administrado diariamente por até 1 ano sem efeitos adversos.[172] Em razão das ações endócrinas, o acetato de megestrol é contraindicado a cadelas diabéticas ou àquelas com histórico de doença mamária, uterina ou hepática.

Adiamento do estro com acetato de megestrol

Visão geral

O adiamento do estro é usado, em geral, por um período de 6 a 18 meses, quando se tenta evitar que uma cadela entre em proestro/estro ou se torne gestante. A administração de progestina faz com que a cadela entre em fase luteal artificial, que bloqueia a ciclicidade, via *feedback* negativo, por meio da supressão da liberação de LH e FSH. A administração de progestina reduz receptores de estrogênio do tecido-alvo, promove o crescimento e a secreção endometrial, causa fechamento cervical, altera o transporte de gametas, diminui a motilidade dentro do trato reprodutivo e suprime a ovulação.[21] O efeito antiovulatório das progestinas na onda de LH depende do momento da administração: se administrado no pico de E2 ou logo após, a ovulação pode ser estimulada, enquanto o mesmo tratamento vários dias ou muito antes do pico de E2 o suprime.[176] O acetato de medroxiprogesterona altera a secreção de inibina e ativina e o E2 ovariano canino, inibindo o pico pré-ovulatório de FSH-LH hipofisário.[181,182] À medida que o anestro avança, o adiamento induzido por progestinas é menos efetivo. Portanto, o tratamento com progestina no início/meio do anestro é mais eficaz e causa retorno posterior à atividade cíclica, quando comparado ao no anestro tardio, quase sempre caracterizado por um efeito mais curto.

Protocolos

O acetato de megestrol (0,55 mg/kg/dia VO, por 32 dias) suprimiu de maneira efetiva o estro em 199 cadelas em anestro tardio; 98% não mostraram atividade cíclica ao longo do tratamento.[173] Essa dose de supressão de estro tornou-se bastante popular. Entretanto, doses diárias bem mais baixas (0,01 a 0,05 mg/kg VO, por 32 dias) são efetivas na prevenção da atividade cíclica por até 1 ano.[172] O efeito do início do acetato de megestrol em diferentes momentos dentro do anestro não ficou claro.[172] O retorno ao cio após a administração de acetato de megestrol em 5 cadelas foi de 218 dias (intervalo de 116 a 311) com a dose de 0,05 mg/kg/dia, por 94 dias em 5 cadelas (intervalo de 22 a 243) com a dose de 0,01 mg/kg/dia e de 120 a 180 dias em 199 cadelas (intervalo de 30 a 210) com o protocolo de 0,55 mg/kg/dia durante 32 dias[172,173].

Reações adversas

As reações adversas associadas ao adiamento do estro com acetato de megestrol são semelhantes às relatadas para supressão do estro, embora a dose de acetato de megestrol para o adiamento do estro seja muito mais baixa, com menor risco de efeitos colaterais. No estudo de dose baixa, não foi fornecida nenhuma informação a respeito dos efeitos colaterais do tratamento com acetato de megestrol.[172] Em gatos tratados com doses baixas de acetato de megestrol (2,5 mg/semana VO, por 30 semanas), os efeitos colaterais mais comuns foram aumento do apetite e do peso corporal, mudança de temperamento e aumento mamário.[183] A curto prazo, o uso de doses intermediárias (2,5 mg/dia, por algumas semanas) pode provocar supressão da adrenocortical e/ou diabetes melito, possivelmente reversíveis, enquanto, a longo prazo, doses altas (2,5 mg/dia, por meses, ou 2,5 mg/semana, por anos) podem ocasionar alterações potencialmente não reversíveis endócrinas, uterinas e das glândulas mamárias.[183] Embora os relatos de reações adversas em cães induzidas pelo acetato de megestrol não gerem grandes preocupações, há indícios de que alguns casos se desenvolvam de maneira preocupante.

Adiamento do estro com acetato de medroxiprogesterona

Protocolos

O acetato de medroxiprogesterona tem sido usado em cães por muitos anos, com grande quantidade de informações científicas disponíveis sobre sua eficácia e reações adversas. A afinidade do receptor de acetato de medroxiprogesterona é menor que a do acetato de megestrol: é apenas 5 vezes mais potente que a P4 e sua afinidade por receptores andrógenos e glicocorticoides é 100 e 1.000 vezes menor do que o de acetato de megestrol. No entanto, o acetato de medroxiprogesterona tem meia-vida mais longa: 12 a 17 h após a administração oral ou 40 a 50 dias quando administrado por via parenteral. Uma vez que as injeções são necessárias apenas duas vezes ao ano para cadelas em anestro, acetato de medroxiprogesterona tem sido usado para adiamento prolongado em doses de 2 mg/kg/3 meses, 3 mg/kg/4 meses ou 2,5 mg/kg/5 meses SC.[176,177,184] No entanto, doses mais baixas provavelmente são eficazes. Administração de acetato de medroxiprogesterona (1,5 mg/kg) a cada 13 semanas inibiu a ovulação em cadelas Beagle.[185] Além disso, 5 cadelas Beagle adultas tratadas diariamente com acetato de medroxiprogesterona oral (0,05 mg/kg) não apresentaram estro durante todo o período de 365 dias de tratamento.[172]

Reações adversas

A relação entre a dose de acetato de medroxiprogesterona e as reações adversas é provável em cães, com doses mais baixas apenas controlando ciclicidade e comportamento e as mais altas podendo causar efeitos uterinos, mamários e endócrinos de longa duração. Estudos epidemiológicos mostraram maior risco de tumores mamários malignos em cadelas tratadas por períodos longos com acetato de medroxiprogesterona.[186] Infelizmente, os relatos sobre as reações adversas causadas pelo acetato de medroxiprogesterona foram vagos e independentes da dose ou duração do tratamento. Resultados de estudos de toxicidade crônica do acetato de medroxiprogesterona em cães podem superestimar alguns efeitos colaterais.[177,185,187-189] O acetato de medroxiprogesterona atua no mesmo tecido-alvo que o acetato de megestrol, ou seja, útero, glândula mamária, sistema endócrino, metabolismo basal e apetite. O tratamento parenteral com doses < 2 mg/kg, a cada 5 a 6 meses, pode provavelmente ser utilizado com segurança em cadelas jovens e adultas saudáveis por mais de 1 ano (i. e., até 3 administrações consecutivas). Recomendam-se períodos de tratamento mais curtos para cadelas de meia-idade ou mais velhas com alterações no útero e nas glândulas mamárias relacionadas com a idade. Doses mais baixas podem estar associadas ao retorno precoce ao estro; no entanto, isso seria compensado por um menor risco de saúde para cadelas tratadas. Doses > 2,5 mg/kg ou aquelas administradas em frequência maior do que a cada 5 meses são muito altas e não devem ser usadas, já que aumentam o risco de nódulos mamários (benignos e/ou malignos), hiperplasia endometrial cística, resistência à insulina e secreção mamária de GH levando à acromegalia.[182,190,191]

Adiamento do estro com proligestona

Visão geral

Proligestona é um progestágeno injetável comercializado para uso em pequenos animais na Europa, com indicação para adiamento do estro, devendo ser administrada na dose de 10 (para cadelas de grande porte) a 33 (para cadelas de pequeno porte) mg/kg aos 0, 3 e 7 meses e depois a cada 5 meses. A eficácia desse protocolo é relatada como > 95%.[177,192] Durante a administração crônica, podem ocorrer cios repentinos, embora pouco seja conhecido sobre a sua incidência. Embora, a princípio, se tenha pensado se tratar de uma ação progestacional e do eixo hipotálamo-hipofisário-gonadal mais leve em comparação ao acetato de megestrol e ao acetato de medroxiprogesterona, estudos posteriores demonstraram que os mesmos efeitos colaterais dessas duas substâncias podem ser observados com o uso da proligestona.[177] Durante a administração crônica de proligestona em cães, foram relatadas a estimulação do endométrio, levando à hiperplasia endometrial cística e à piometra, e a hipertrofia mamária acompanhada de secreção de GH, levando à acromegalia, embora notoriamente em uma dose superior à normal, 5 a 10 mg/kg SC, a cada 3 semanas.

A incidência de piometra e/ou tumores mamários ao usar protocolo normal é relatada como baixa ou irrelevante.[193] O intervalo do tratamento à atividade do ciclo após o tratamento com proligestona pode ser de 3 a 9 meses.[177]

Adiamento do estro com andrógenos

A testosterona e seus derivados estão amplamente disponíveis. Estanozolol e medicamentos à base de decanoato de nandrolona estão disponíveis para uso veterinário na Europa, na América do Norte e em outros lugares. As indicações não reprodutivas foram descritas, mas a ação no ciclo reprodutivo canino não foi investigada com precisão. Concentrações prolongadas e elevadas de andrógenos administradas a homens causam *feedback* negativo para o eixo hipotálamo-hipofisário, reduzindo a secreção hipofisária de LH e FSH e também se ligando a receptores andrógenos.

Podem ocorrer ações semelhantes em cadelas que receberam andrógenos, com supressão hipofisária e consequentes diminuições em resposta a E2, uma vez que também se ligam a receptores andrógenos nos tecidos-alvo E2.[176] Formulações parenterais de propionato de testosterona (100 mg/cão/semana) ou ésteres de testosterona mistos (25 mg/kg, a cada 4 a 6 semanas) ou formulações orais de metiltestosterona (0,25 a 0,5 mg/kg/dia ou 25 mg/cão/semana) são comumente usados para adiar o estro em galgos de corrida. Uma formulação de depósito de cipionato de testosterona (2 mg/kg, IM) tem sido eficaz no adiamento do estro por 239 dias em 4/5 cadelas tratadas.[194] Para aumentar a eficácia, o tratamento deve ser iniciado pelo menos 1 mês antes do início do proestro.[195] O retorno ao estro, após a retirada do tratamento, pode variar de 1 mês a anos.

Mibolerona, um andrógeno sintético comercializado na América do Norte, é uma formulação oral, de uso diário, para adiar a atividade cíclica em cadelas por até 3 anos. No entanto, o tratamento por mais de 2 anos não é recomendado. A dose depende da raça e do peso corporal. Cães Pastores-Alemães e mestiços de Pastor-Alemão devem receber a dose máxima (180 μg/dia), enquanto os da raça Bedlington Terrier não devem ser tratados em razão da história de disfunção hepática. Outras raças de cães podem ser tratadas com base no peso corporal; as cadelas de < 12, 12 a 23, 23 a 45 e com mais de 45 kg devem receber 30, 60, 120 e 180 μg/dia, respectivamente. O intervalo do tratamento ao estro seguinte é de aproximadamente 2 meses (7 a 200 dias).

Qualquer andrógeno pode causar aumento da massa muscular, hipertrofia clitoriana (potencialmente irreversível após terapia prolongada), latido grave, mudança de temperamento (agressividade) e comportamento de monta. O anestro deve ser sempre confirmado e a gestação descartada (para evitar o risco de potencial masculinização de fetos femininos) antes de administrar um andrógeno.[196]

INDUÇÃO DO ESTRO

Visão geral

A indução do estro pode ser solicitada ao tentar encurtar um intervalo interestro normal ou mais longo do que o normal, podendo ser alcançada com gonadotrofinas, agonistas da dopamina ou agonistas de GnRH. Enquanto a supressão ou o adiamento do estro é relativamente fácil, a indução do estro é um desafio, em razão da inconsistência na resposta aos diferentes tratamentos. Em cadelas, tentaram-se muitos tratamentos com resultados variáveis e, muitas vezes, insatisfatórios (ao considerar a taxa de gestação e o tamanho da ninhada), incluindo LH e FSH isoladamente ou combinados, gonadotrofina coriônica equina, assim como estrógenos e naloxona.[67] O uso de fármacos antiprolactínicos, agonistas de GnRH e agonistas da dopamina, é caracterizado por resultados satisfatórios, com preferência na clínica prática.

Agonistas dopaminérgicos

Quando administrados diariamente em sua dose antigalactogênica normal, iniciando no anestro, os agonistas da dopamina, como a cabergolina (5 μg/kg VO, a cada 24 h) e a bromocriptina (20 a 50 μg/kg VO, a cada 12 h), podem encurtar a duração do anestro, antecipando, assim, o início do proestro.[71,197,198]

Doses baixas de cabergolina (0,6 μg/kg) têm sido usadas com sucesso,[70] assim como os antagonistas da serotonina para induzir o cio, mas apenas em doses mais altas do que o normal (metergolina, 0,56 a 1,2 mg/kg, IM, a cada 72 h até o proestro); uma dose alta de metergolina exercerá efeitos agonistas da dopamina em oposição à dose antigalactogênica normal de 0,5 mg/kg, que não pode encurtar o anestro.[69,199,200] A duração do tratamento com agonistas da dopamina por 2 a 4 semanas normalmente é suficiente para induzir o início do proestro, embora ocasionalmente algumas cadelas possam não responder até os 35 ou 40+ dias de terapia. Não há dados suficientes sobre a porcentagem de cadelas responsivas e qual a duração máxima da administração durante a qual o tratamento deve ser interrompido. Foram relatadas taxas de sucesso de 50 a 80% e possíveis diferenças raciais na eficácia dos agonistas da dopamina para o término do anestro. O tratamento deve ser continuado até o meio do proestro. A fertilidade de um ciclo induzido com um agonista da dopamina é considerada normal. Uma vez que o estro se torne evidente, o uso de hCG não parece ajudar de maneira significativa.[70]

Agonistas de hormônio liberador de gonadotrofina

Quando usados em cadelas em anestro, os agonistas de GnRH, como a deslorelina (na dose de 1,05 mg, 2,1 mg ou 4,7 mg) induzem a retomada da ciclicidade dentro de 2 a 9 dias.[83,85,201,202] O intervalo entre o início do proestro e a ovulação pode ser mais curto em cadelas induzidas com deslorelina do que naquelas com ciclos espontâneos; no entanto, todos os outros parâmetros de fertilidade parecem estar normais.[83,85,202] Em razão do conhecido efeito supressor do implante de deslorelina na secreção de progesterona por volta do meio da gestação,[83-85,201] o implante administrado para induzir o estro deve ser removido entre o início do proestro e a ovulação, a fim de evitar a perda da gestação pela luteólise prematura.[83,85,203] A colocação de um implante em um local de fácil acesso, como a área periumbilical, a mucosa vestibular ou o lado medial do membro, ajuda a localizá-lo e removê-lo rapidamente na hora apropriada. A deslorelina tende a ser mais eficaz quando administrada tardiamente, em comparação ao anestro precoce, e, em geral, é considerada um fármaco muito seguro e eficaz para induzir o estro fértil na cadela. Cadelas tratadas no final do anestro mostram cio dentro de 4,2 +/- 1,4 dias em 97% dos casos, a ovulação ocorre em 83% dos casos e, de forma bastante constante, 12 +/- 3 dias após o tratamento e a taxa de gestação é de aproximadamente 70%.[85] No entanto, a necessidade de agir de forma invasiva para alcançar a remoção precoce, a fim de evitar a falha luteal prematura, permanece duvidosa. Além disso, há relatos de cios prolongados e ciclos anovulatórios.[84,85,201,204,205] Para evitar a estimulação ovariana desnecessária, os implantes devem ser removidos no mais tardar 15 dias após o tratamento, ainda que a cadela não tenha ovulado.[85]

REFERÊNCIAS BIBLIOGRÁFICAS

As referências bibliográficas deste capítulo se encontram online no Ambiente de Aprendizagem.

CAPÍTULO 313

Efeito a Longo Prazo da Esterilização e da Castração na Saúde de Cães e Gatos

Hilde de Rooster e Nathalie Porters

HISTÓRICO

Gonadectomia cirúrgica (*i. e.*, a remoção de ovários em fêmeas ou testículos em machos) continua sendo o método de esterilização mais eficiente, além de ser o único permanente e de fácil aplicação no controle da reprodução de animais de companhia.[1] A castração é o procedimento cirúrgico mais comum na prática clínica em pequenos animais.[2] A castração eletiva, no entanto, ainda é proibida em alguns países, mas na maioria é muito bem-aceita e geralmente vista como segura e benéfica para a saúde animal.

Veterinários têm o papel importante de informar o proprietário dos animais sobre os benefícios e riscos da gonadectomia, apesar de a idade ótima para a realização da gonadectomia não ser conhecida. Nesse debate, uma distinção deve ser feita entre animais abandonados (população) e aqueles de proprietários (indivíduos). Tradicionalmente, a gonadectomia eletiva em cães e gatos é realizada entre 6 e 9 meses de idade apesar da falta de evidências sobre essa recomendação.[3,4] Uma vez que muitos gatos entram na puberdade antes dos 6 meses de idade, fêmeas podem ficar gestantes antes da castração. Em cães, o momento do seu primeiro cio depende do tamanho e da raça. O primeiro cio parece ser o melhor ponto para dirigir a decisão do que a idade. Gonadectomia pré-puberdade (GPP), definida como gonadectomia realizada antes dos 4 meses de idade ou da maturidade sexual, tem sido realizada para animais de abrigo, primeiro nos EUA, depois no Reino Unido e mais recentemente em outros países.[5-16] A literatura apresenta poucos estudos que avaliam os efeitos em curto e longo prazo da castração em várias idades. As informações em geral comparam o *status* de esterilização ao momento da doença, em vez de comparar gonadectomia pediátrica *versus* em idade tradicional. Em estudos em que a idade no momento da cirurgia foi avaliada, a interpretação dos dados é complicada pela variação nas definições usadas por grupos de cães como tendo sido castrados "cedo" ou "tarde" na vida. Uma comparação entre castração pré e pós-puberdade revelaria dados mais relevantes sobre riscos e benefícios.

ANESTESIA E CIRURGIA

A gonadectomia eletiva deveria ser realizada apenas em animais que podem passar pelo procedimento com segurança, reduzindo riscos ou complicações.[7,17,18] Particularmente em animais de abrigo, doenças infecciosas são as principais causas de problemas de saúde e mortalidade pouco após GPP.[4,19] Filhotes de gatos e cães são mais vulneráveis a doenças infecciosas que adultos imunizados, e suas respostas a vacinação são normalmente desconhecidas devido à presença de anticorpos maternais (ver Capítulo 208).[20] Sugere-se que a gonadectomia seja adiada até que animais de proprietários sejam completamente vacinados.[15,18,21]

Diferentes protocolos anestésicos foram provados seguros e efetivos para a gonadectomia de filhotes de gatos e cães.[9,15,17,22-26]

Comparados a adultos, filhotes de cães e gatos têm sistemas e órgãos imaturos, colocando-os em alto risco de hipoglicemia, hipotermia, bradicardia, hipotensão e hipoxia.[12,17,27-29]

Essas diferenças fisiológicas são importantes no planejamento anestésico e cirúrgico. Enquanto protocolos para gonadectomia em animais pediátricos são similares aos usados em adultos, seus tecidos imaturos são mais frágeis e até mesmo uma perda sanguínea mínima pode rapidamente se tornar preocupante.[4,9,15,17]

SAÚDE A LONGO PRAZO

Apesar da alta prevalência de gonadectomia (em animais jovens) na prática veterinária, existem poucos estudos de qualidade e peso adequados que avaliam o efeito da gonadectomia, assim como a idade e o momento de realização da gonadectomia, sobre a saúde e doença em cães e gatos. Evidências sobre riscos de várias doenças seguidas da castração são geralmente pobres, dadas as dificuldades práticas de controlar variáveis confundidoras. A maioria dos dados é obtida através da pesquisa de dados e assim relatam a diferença em contas simples. O *status* de castração de animais doentes não é adequadamente comparado ao *status* da população hospitalar geral. Além disso, variáveis confundidoras não são levadas em consideração. Proprietários de animais castrados podem levar seus animais com maior frequência ao veterinário, aumentando a probabilidade de diagnóstico da doença. Similarmente, animais castrados têm vida mais longa e mais tempo para desenvolver condições relacionadas à idade. É aceitável que a gonadectomia (em animais jovens) não apenas influencia o trato genital, mas também outros sistemas orgânicos. A maioria das vantagens na saúde de animais castrados supera as desvantagens em potencial (ver Capítulo 319).

BENEFÍCIOS

Social

Um benefício social da gonadectomia eletiva é a contribuição no controle populacional e bem-estar animal.[3] Filhotes indesejados contribuem para o aumento do número de animais entrando em abrigos de animais, juntando-se a populações selvagens, ou sendo mortos.[30-32] Animais castrados têm menor risco de ser abandonados em abrigos.[32-35]

Saúde

A gonadectomia em cães e gatos é acompanhada por uma gama de benefícios de saúde, primeiro por reduzir o risco de muitas doenças no trato genital que aparecem mais tarde na vida. A remoção de ambas as gônadas elimina completamente doenças relacionadas à gestação e ao parto assim como de doenças ovarianas (cistos, neoplasias) em fêmeas de cães e gatos. Similarmente, doenças testiculares são eliminadas em machos castrados. A ovário-histerectomia eletiva (esterilização) elimina qualquer possibilidade de hiperplasia endometrial cística, piometra ou neoplasia uterina. A castração eletiva também diminui a incidência de vaginite, prolapso vaginal, pseudociese e hipertrofia mamária felina. Machos castrados reduzem a possibilidade de desenvolver hiperplasia prostática benigna e prostatites. O momento da retirada dos ovários também é associado a menor risco de câncer mamário.[3,36] Risco de desenvolver carcinoma mamário felino é drasticamente reduzido em gatos castrados antes de 1 ano de vida.[37] Estudos iniciais com tumores de glândulas mamárias em caninos relataram risco significativamente menor de transformação maligna por GPP, mas uma revisão sistemática recente encontrou poucas evidências que sugerem tal efeito protetivo.[38,39] Outros estudos em cães com câncer em glândula mamária demonstraram um efeito positivo na sobrevida quando a castração é realizada no momento da mastectomia.[40] Outras vantagens substanciais da gonadectomia na saúde incluem incidência reduzida de doenças associadas às andanças e um risco diminuído de transmissão de doenças infecciosas por causa da redução da cópula e brigas entre machos.[41] Qualquer vantagem associada à castração deve ser mais estudada em relação a efeitos posteriores adicionais à gonadectomia pré *versus* pós-puberdade.

DETRIMENTOS EM POTENCIAL

Desordens urogenitais não neoplásicas

Genitália externa

Hormônios gonadais são responsáveis pelo desenvolvimento normal da genitália externa em cães e gatos.[42-44] Gatas castradas com 7 semanas ou 7 meses apresentam vulva menor comparadas a de gatas sexualmente intactas aos 12 meses de idade.[43] Observações similares têm sido feitas para cadelas.[44] Exposição peniana completa foi impossível em gatos machos GPP e possível em apenas 60% dos gatos gonadectomizados aos 7 meses.[42] Assim como em cães machos, castração precoce resultou em prepúcios menores.[44] Não há evidência de significância clínica dessas diferenças anatômicas.

Diâmetro uretral

É uma preocupação que a gonadectomia (pré-púbere) possa resultar em uretras de menores diâmetros em cães e gatos machos, aumentando o risco de obstrução uretral (ver Capítulo 335).[44,45] Estudos têm falhado em demonstrar redução uretral em gatos machos não castrados *versus* castrados em idades diferentes.[42,46] Em estudos de grupos a longo prazo, nenhuma correlação foi encontrada entre idade da gonadectomia e incidência de doença do trato reprodutivo baixo em felinos (FLUTD) em ambos os sexos.[11,19,47] Mesmo assim, gonadectomia em qualquer idade em gatos tem sido descrita repetidamente como um dos fatores de risco potenciais para FLUTD.[48-51] Não foi relatada sequela clínica da castração em uretra de cães machos enquanto dados conflitantes foram relatados sobre o risco de cistite em cadelas. Mais cadelas gonadectomizadas do que não castradas mostraram cistite persistente em um estudo.[52] Muitos estudos demonstraram que cálculos vesicais foram mais frequentemente observados em cães castrados *versus* não castrados (ver Capítulo 331).[53] Dois estudos mostraram conclusões diferentes sobre GPP influenciando a probabilidade do desenvolvimento de cistite tardia na vida quando comparado à idade tradicional dos cães gonadectomizados.[47,54]

Incontinência

Menos de 1% das cadelas inteiras desenvolvem incontinência urinária adquirida (IUA) em algum momento da vida (ver Capítulo 335).[55,56] No entanto, IUA em cadelas castradas varia de 2 a 20%.[57] Quando cadelas castradas entre 12 semanas e 6 meses de idade foram comparadas a cadelas castradas pós-púberes, raça e tamanho em vez de idade à castração no momento da gonadectomia, houve associação a taxas observadas de incontinência.[58] Em um estudo de caso-controle, cadelas castradas pré-púberes foram menos propensas ao desenvolvimento de incontinência urinária do que cadelas castradas mais tarde na vida.[59] A baixa incidência foi também observada por outros, embora sinais clínicos mais distintos de incontinência urinária foram observados em cadelas afetadas castradas pré-puberdade.[60]

Crescimento esquelético

Existem evidências amplas de que as fises fecham após a puberdade.[44,61,62] A falta dos hormônios gonadotróficos afeta negativamente o fechamento de fises específicas.[43,44,63-67] Alguns têm concluído que esse atraso, especialmente observado após GPP, pode resultar em ossos mais longos.[65,66] Em paralelo, sugeriu-se que as placas de crescimento afetadas podem ser mais suscetíveis a lesões e fraturas.[43,44,66,68] A relevância clínica do fechamento tardio das fises após GPP comparado com a idade tradicional de realização da gonadectomia é largamente questionada.[11,19,47] A maioria dos gatos com fratura de fise capital femoral era de machos obesos.[66,69] Uma vez que a gonadectomia aumenta a incidência da obesidade, a gonadectomia deve ser um fator de risco independente.

Em cães, displasia de quadril (DQ) e doença do ligamento crucial cranial (DLCC) têm sido associadas à castração (ver Capítulo 353).[70-72] Supõe-se que o fechamento assimétrico de placas de crescimento pode causar deformidade e relaxamento das articulações do quadril e do joelho.[44,73] Cães machos castrados são considerados mais suscetíveis a ter DQ e cães castrados cedo são vistos como de alto risco.[47,70,74] Tanto machos quanto fêmeas castrados têm maior probabilidade de desenvolver DLCC.[70,74] Assim, não parece haver evidências da diferença de um risco de desenvolver DLCC entre cães pré e pós-púberes castrados.[47,54] Ambas condições ortopédicas, no entanto, têm desenvolvimento multifatorial. Bagagem genética, predisposição racial e obesidade estão entre os fatores que podem influenciar o risco de desenvolvimento dessas desordens ortopédicas.[75]

Sobrepeso e obesidade

É normal encontrar animais de companhia acima do peso. Gonadectomia é um dos maiores fatores de risco para o desenvolvimento de sobrepeso (ver Capítulo 176).[76-84] Algumas raças de cães parecem mais predispostas ao ganho de peso após a castração.[85] O risco de desenvolver sobrepeso não foi diferente com relação à idade da gonadectomia.[86] Surpreendentemente, alguns sugerem que cães castrados pré-púberes são menos suscetíveis ao ganho de peso excessivo que cães castrados em idade mais tardia.[47] Novas percepções mais objetivas em gatos desafiam as sugestões prévias.[87] Dada a contribuição potencial de obesidade para muitas outras condições, o papel dos veterinários de instruir com muito cuidado os proprietários para evitar o ganho de peso excessivo após a gonadectomia (em jovens) pela restrição energética quando atingem a maturidade é crucial.[77,86,88,89]

Neoplasias (ver Capítulos 344 a 351)

Em cães, o aumento na prevalência de uma variedade de doenças neoplásicas atribuídas à gonadectomia implica que os hormônios gonadais podem ter qualidades protetivas contra a proliferação neoplásica em determinados tecidos.[90-92] O papel da retirada dos hormônios reprodutivos sobre a fisiopatologia de determinada doença neoplásica ainda permanece amplamente desconhecida. O fato de que algumas raças de cães individualmente possam ter predisposição variável a complicações dificulta ainda mais a interpretação de resultados. Para gatos, somente dados equivalentes e isolados de análises de riscos para condições neoplásicas foram obtidos. Carcinoma de próstata é relativamente incomum em cães castrados e inteiros (ver Capítulo 337). No entanto, uma incidência significantemente maior de câncer de próstata é descrita em cães castrados.[92-94] Em contraste, foi relatado que a castração pré-púbere em cães machos reduz o risco de doença neoplásica na próstata.[95] Um aumento na prevalência de câncer de bexiga em cães tem sido notado em cães machos e fêmeas castrados.[93] Nenhum dos estudos separou cães pelo momento da realização da gonadectomia antes ou depois da puberdade.

Supõe-se que o desenvolvimento do linfoma canino é suprimido pelos hormônios gonadais endógenos em cadelas inteiras. Machos inteiros e especialmente os castrados de ambos os gêneros apresentam risco alto.[91] Em cães da raça Golden Retriever, um estudo focado nas implicações de saúde relacionadas à castração demonstrou que machos castrados antes de 1 ano de idade são aproximadamente 3 vezes mais suscetíveis a desenvolver linfoma quando comparados a machos inteiros (ver Capítulo 344). Nenhum cão castrado quando mais velho desenvolveu linfoma.[74] Gatos castrados apresentam risco aumentado de linfoma intestinal, mas isso pode ser um reflexo direto da idade em vez do *status* de neutralização.[96]

Constatou-se que a gonadectomia em cães de ambos os gêneros está correlacionada com um aumento em 2 vezes no risco de desenvolvimento de osteossarcoma (ver Capítulo 348).[97] Um estudo de grupos de Rottweilers, uma raça predisposta, indicou que a gonadectomia realizada antes de 1 ano de idade resultou em aumento do risco.[90] Embora isso possa sugerir um efeito protetivo dos hormônios gonadais, nada se sabe sobre um possível mecanismo.

Comparadas com fêmeas caninas inteiras, cadelas gonadectomizadas apresentaram aumento significativo do risco de ter hemangiossarcoma esplênico e/ou cardíaco (ver Capítulo 347), mas diferenças equivalentes foram menos óbvias em machos.[98,99] Em Golden Retrievers, nenhuma diferença na taxa de doenças foi aparente entre fêmeas inteiras e castradas cedo, mas cadelas castradas acima de 1 ano de idade apresentaram aumento significativo do risco.[74] Em estudos sobre mastocitoma cutâneo canino (ver Capítulo 349), a castração foi identificada como um fator de risco em fêmeas.[74,100]

Outras doenças (endócrinas, reprodutivas, imunomediadas)

Reação à vacina, asma e pele

Em estudos em cães e gatos, reações de hipersensibilidade após a vacinação foram mais comuns em cães castrados.[101,102] Levantou-se a hipótese de que a falta de retroalimentação negativa pelos hormônios gonadais aumentam a secreção de hormônios pituitários, influenciando a resposta imune à vacinação. Sugere-se que a castração antes de 5,5 meses esteja associada à redução na incidência de asma e gengivite em felinos comparada a gatos submetidos à castração entre 5,5 e 12 meses de idade.[47] Outro estudo de grupos, no entanto, não observou um aumento significativo na incidência de desordens no sistema tegumentar (incluindo pequenas alergias de pele) entre animais castrados antes e depois de 24 semanas de vida.[11] Com base em achados recentes, também é improvável que a idade à gonadectomia esteja associada a problemas de hipersensibilidade de pele em felinos.[19]

Diabetes melito

A castração é associada a risco aumentado de diabetes em cães e gatos de ambos os gêneros; no entanto, o peso não foi considerado (ver Capítulos 304 e 305). A castração de cadelas previne o diabetes melito induzida pela progesterona (muito rara), mas aumenta o risco de diabetes melito por consequência da obesidade.[103,104] Em gatos castrados, o risco maior de diabetes pode ser reflexo do risco aumentado pela obesidade em vez da castração.[105] Obesidade e castração são associadas à redução da sensibilidade à insulina.[106]

Outras condições

Dados conflitantes sobre a incidência e prevalência de muitas outras condições patológicas e longevidade após a castração tem sido relatados. Cães castrados podem apresentar maior risco de hipotireoidismo.[107,108] Similarmente, pancreatite aguda foi diagnosticada mais frequentemente em animais castrados que em inteiros.[109,110] Embora longevidade excepcional tenha sido citada em cadelas inteiras da raça Rottweiler, a maioria dos estudos sugere que animais castrados vivem mais.[111-114] Um ponto metodológico importante sobre os efeitos potenciais do *status* de castração sobre a vida útil é que os animais são grosseiramente categorizados como castrados e inteiros com base na presença da gônada no momento da morte, sem indicação quanto ao momento em que a castração ocorreu.[115]

SUMÁRIO

As decisões sobre a gonadectomia eletiva (pré-púbere) em um animal individual dependem de vários fatores. Em gatos, sob uma perspectiva de controle populacional, é vital que a castração seja realizada antes que eles possam se reproduzir. Isso implica que filhotes e gatos em abrigos sejam castrados antes da adoção. Gatos de proprietários, sem intenção de uso para reprodução, devem ser castrados por volta de 4 meses de idade, desde que estejam adequadamente vacinados. Consequências danosas relacionadas à castração em gatos são extremamente raras.

A decisão para cães é muito menos clara. Para um cão com proprietário, inúmeros fatores interagem com as variáveis e são avaliados ao determinar o melhor momento para realizar a castração. Cadelas inteiras apresentam risco comum e sério de desenvolvimento de doenças (tumores de glândulas mamárias, piometra) que podem ser reduzidas ou prevenidas com sucesso pela castração eletiva. É ideal que elas sejam castradas antes ou logo depois do primeiro cio. Em cães machos, os benefícios na saúde pela castração eletiva são muito menos óbvios e podem pesar menos que os prejuízos potenciais. Vulnerabilidades específicas de algumas raças devem ser cuidadosamente consideradas na decisão sobre a castração.

Deveria ser fácil para veterinários promover a educação dos clientes sobre sua responsabilidade social, como pela população de cães e gatos, pelos cuidados com o animal individualmente, assim como pela alteração na incidência de doenças; entretanto, tudo isso é muito complexo. Mais pesquisas prospectivas são necessárias, não apenas para quantificar incidências de doenças relevantes clinicamente, mas também para identificar variáveis que trazem confusão e podem influenciar nos riscos observados.

REFERÊNCIAS BIBLIOGRÁFICAS

As referências bibliográficas deste capítulo se encontram online no Ambiente de Aprendizagem.

CAPÍTULO 314

Reprodução Felina Clínica

Eva Agneta Axnér

SAZONALIDADE

O gato doméstico apresenta atividade reprodutiva sazonal de dia longo porque o aumento das horas de luz no dia estimula a ciclicidade.[1,2] A duração da estação reprodutiva se diferencia de acordo com o local geográfico, sem sazonalidade próxima a linha do equador.[1] Gatos individualmente mantidos sob fotoperíodos idênticos, no entanto, mostram grande variação no período de estação reprodutiva e número de ciclos estrais.[3] Também existem diferenças entre raças com uma tendência para reprodução sazonal. Por exemplo, gatos Persas têm uma sazonalidade mais pronunciada que os gatos Birmaneses. Condições de manejo podem afetar também os ciclos, uma vez que a luz artificial pode interferir na sazonalidade. Para estimular o estro, as gatas podem ser mantidas em um ambiente de luz controlada com pelo menos 12 a 14 meses de luz cada dia.[2] Atividade estral será finalizada quando a luz diária cair para abaixo de 8 horas.[2] O efeito da estação ou da duração do dia na reprodução do macho é menos pronunciada, mas há flutuações sazonais na atividade testicular e qualidade espermática. Machos em geral procriam ao longo de todo o ano, embora a qualidade do esperma possa ser inferior na estação não reprodutiva.[4,5]

PUBERDADE

O primeiro estro em geral ocorre entre 4 e 21 meses de idade nas fêmeas felinas. A gestação, no entanto, tem sido observada, ocasionalmente em fêmeas jovens de 4 meses de idade.[6-8] Como os ciclos são sazonais, a idade à puberdade é afetada pelo mês do nascimento. As fêmeas podem entrar no primeiro cio na primeira estação de monta após terem nascido ou no segundo ano.[3] A puberdade é menos óbvia em machos. Os testículos já sofreram descida para a bolsa escrotal ao nascimento ou com poucos dias.[9] A espermatogênese é em geral estabelecida aos 6 a 8 meses e a puberdade é associada a um aumento no peso testicular e na concentração da testosterona sérica.[10,11] A idade da primeira monta, porém, pode ser afetada por vários fatores.[12] Características dependentes secundárias a andrógenos se desenvolvem em machos em associação com a produção crescente de androgênios. Machos maduros apresentam espículas penianas bem desenvolvidas (Figura 314.1). Essas espículas regridem após a castração quando a testosterona cai a níveis basais. Em filhotes, o prepúcio é um pouco aderido ao pênis e se solta parcialmente ao redor dos 5 meses de idade. O pênis e o prepúcio são separados sob a influência de andrógenos.[12] Se o macho é castrado antes da puberdade, a aderência pode então ser mantida (ver Capítulo 313).[13] Outras características físicas de machos não castrados maduros incluem pele grossa, bochechas bem desenvolvidas e marcação territorial com urina. A urina de machos inteiros tem um odor forte dependente de andrógeno. A tendência e a idade de marcação territorial com urina variam. Durante a puberdade, o comportamento territorialista e a tendência de brigar com outros machos intactos também aumentam.[14]

CICLO ESTRAL

Gatas são poliéstricas sazonais. Embora gatas sejam consideradas ovuladoras induzidas, a ovulação espontânea pode ocorrer ocasionalmente. O ciclo pode ser dividido de acordo com a atividade ovariana.

Fase folicular (proestro e estro)

A fase folicular é caracterizada pelo estágio do ciclo estral em que existem folículos ativos nos ovários e aumento das concentrações de estradiol séricas (Figuras 314.2 e 314.3). O estabelecimento da fase folicular é abrupto e pode ser subdividido em proestro e estro. O proestro é em geral menor que 1 dia de duração, não é mais longo que 2 dias e pode não ser observado. O proestro inicia com o desenvolvimento de folículos ovarianos e a gata apresenta comportamento de estro, mas não aceita a

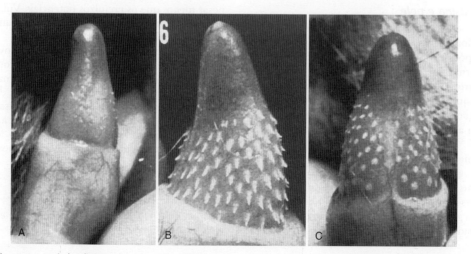

Figura 314.1 Pênis felino mostra espículas distintas do macho inteiro (**B**) que estão ausentes no macho castrado (**A**). Espículas começam a atrofiar dentro de semanas da castração (**C**). (De Aronson LR, Cooper ML: Penile spines of the domestic cat: their endocrine behavior relations. *Anat Rec* 157:71-78, 1967; usada com permissão.)

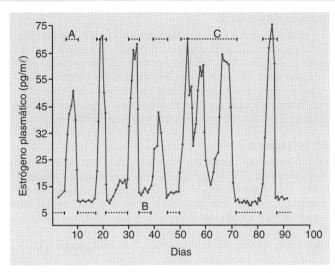

Figura 314.2 Concentrações de estrógeno plasmático ao longo de vários ciclos estrais na gata. Estrógeno plasmático alto (**A**) está presente durante o comportamento de estro e baixo (**B**) durante o intervalo interestro. Estrógeno plasmático pode não retornar a níveis basais entre ciclos e pode causar um aparente prolongamento do comportamento de estro (**C**). (De Feldman EC, Nelson RW: *Canine and feline endocrinology and reproduction*, 3 ed., St. Louis, 2004, Elsevier; usada com permissão.)

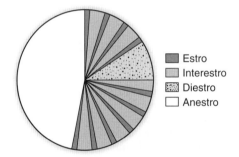

Figura 314.3 O padrão reprodutivo na gata doméstica não gestante durante 12 meses. Em média, na gata, a estação reprodutiva acontece durante o fotoperíodo de dias longos. Na ausência de ovulação, ocorre a atresia folicular e não há aumento da progesterona sérica. Após a ovulação espontânea ou uma cobertura estéril, a progesterona sérica é aumentada e a gata entra em diestro. Um período de diestro geralmente prolonga o ciclo. A variabilidade individual é, no entanto, muito ampla em algumas gatas cíclicas mais ou menos durante o ano, enquanto outras gatas podem somente entrar em estro 1 ou 2 vezes ao ano.

monta. Concentrações aumentadas de estradiol sérico induzem comportamento estral, definido como o período em que a fêmea permite o acasalamento. Folículos ovarianos em geral atingem o tamanho de 2 a 3 mm de diâmetro ao início do estro.[15] O comportamento de estro típico inclui vocalização, lordose com abaixamento do tórax, elevação da pelve, deflexão da cauda para o lado, fricção e rolamentos. Quando a fêmea demonstra lordose, ela frequentemente faz movimentos de pedalar com as patas traseiras. Uma quantidade escassa de descarga vaginal clara pode ser observada. O dia específico de comportamento estral em relação à maturação folicular varia.[16] A duração do estro é em geral de 5 a 8 dias, mas pode ser mais curto, como 2 dias, e mais longo, até 19 dias.[16,17]

A citologia vaginal pode ser usada para diagnosticar a fase folicular (Vídeo 314.1). A concentração elevada do estradiol sérico causa espessamento e queratinização do epitélio vaginal. A fim de fazer um esfregaço vaginal, a gata é contida firmemente pela nuca, e um *swab* de algodão umidificado com solução fisiológica é inserido pela abertura vulvar, avançado pelo vestíbulo da vagina, rotacionado e retirado. Um esfregaço com > 80% de células cornificadas indica que o estradiol sérico está acima de concentrações basais (Figura 314.4). O aumento inicial do estradiol sérico frequentemente precede o comportamento do estro e a queratinização vaginal dia a dia.[16]

Interestro

O interestro é definido como um período inativo entre dois períodos de estros durante a estação ativa. Se a gata não ovula, os folículos ovarianos regridem e o estradiol sérico retorna às concentrações basais. O comportamento de estro finaliza e os ovários ficam em um estágio de inatividade. A duração do interestro pode ser curta, de 2 dias, mas varia ao redor de 1 a 2 semanas (ver Figuras 314.2 e 314.3).

Diestro sem gestação (pseudogestação)

O diestro, a fase lútea, é o estágio no qual os corpos lúteos ativos nos ovários sintetizam e secretam progesterona. Essa fase pode ocorrer após uma cobertura estéril ou uma ovulação espontânea. A progesterona sérica aumenta acima das concentrações basais (> 3 nmol/ℓ). A duração da fase lútea não gestante (pseudogestação) varia de 4 a 8 semanas, com uma média de 38 dias (ver Figura 314.3).[18]

Anestro

O anestro é um período mais longo sem atividade cíclica. Os ovários estão inativos e as concentrações de progesterona e estradiol séricas estão basais (ver Figura 314.3). Não há definição que caracterize a diferença de tamanho entre as fases de interestro e anestro. O anestro geralmente inicia quando a duração das horas

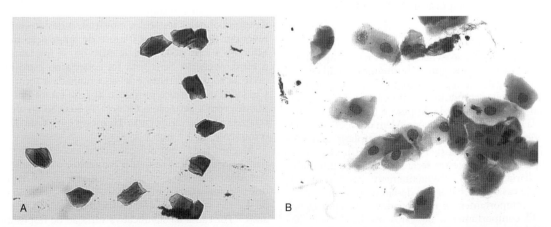

Figura 314.4 Citologia vaginal. Hemacolor. **A.** Aumento de 20×. Células queratinizadas de gata em estro. **B.** Aumento de 40×. Células intermediárias de uma gata que não está em estro. Note o núcleo granulado com células queratinizadas em **A**.

de luz diária diminui, mas existem variações individuais significantes na duração e momento do anestro. Muitas gatas permanecem em anestro em verões mornos a quentes.

Duração do ciclo estral

A duração do ciclo estral completo (*i. e.*, do dia 1 do estro até o dia 1 do próximo estro) varia em cada indivíduo. Em parte, a variação depende se as gatas ovularam ou não. Normalmente, a gata entra em estro toda segunda ou terceira semana durante a estação reprodutiva (ver Figuras 314.2 e 314.3). O intervalo interestro pode, no entanto, ser curto, apenas 2 dias, em uma gata normal. Se a gata ovula, o ciclo em geral tem de 6 a 10 semanas de duração por causa da pseudogestação e do efeito supressivo da progesterona sobre a atividade folicular.[18] Um período de anestro prolonga o tempo entre os períodos de estro. Algumas gatas têm ciclos mais ou menos ao longo do ano, enquanto outras gatas têm ciclos apenas 1 ou 2 vezes ao ano.

COBERTURA E OVULAÇÃO

Considerando que gatos são territorialistas, é aconselhável que a cobertura ocorra no "território" do macho.[19] No entanto, algumas vezes a chance de sucesso é melhor se o macho é movido para o território da fêmea, especialmente se a fêmea parece amedrontada. O macho inicia a cobertura agarrando a gata pela nuca, frequentemente induzindo uma lordose ainda mais pronunciada. A introdução é rápida e finaliza quando a gata emite uma vocalização característica. A não ser que o macho rapidamente se retire, a fêmea pode atacá-lo. Ela então inicia a reação pós-coito típica: rolamento intenso no chão e lambedura da área genital. A cobertura será repetida quando a gata permitir. A cobertura em geral estimula a liberação do hormônio liberador de gonadotrofinas (GnRH) pelo hipotálamo que, em retorno, induz a liberação do hormônio pituitário, o hormônio luteinizante (LH). Muitas coberturas podem ser requeridas para alcançar o limiar de LH necessário para induzir a ovulação.[20] Folículos não estão sempre maduros nos primeiros dias de comportamento de estro. Assim, é aconselhável não separar os gatos antes de 3 a 4 dias de estro para garantir que a ovulação ocorra. Uma vez que o limiar de LH secretado foi alcançado, todos os folículos maduros vão ovular. A ovulação é completada 25 a 32 horas após a cobertura.[21] Os oócitos podem ser fertilizados até 49 horas após a indução da ovulação.[22]

GESTAÇÃO E PARTO (VER CAPÍTULO 315)

Controle permanente e temporário de reprodução

Castração

Os gatos em que não há interesse na reprodução devem ser castrados ou esterilizados. Isso evita ninhadas não planejadas e comportamentos relacionados com os hormônios gonadais (ver Capítulo 313). Em gatis de reprodução, também há a necessidade de um controle reprodutivo temporário. Ciclos estrais frequentes são associados à perda de peso e isso torna difícil a manutenção da gata em boas condições. Além disso, ciclos repetidos predispõem o aumento do risco de hiperplasia endometrial cística (HEC) e piometra (ver Capítulo 316). O método mais natural para suprimir o estro seria a redução de disponibilidade de luz diária, mas isso é frequentemente complicado em um ambiente de casa. Pode haver um desejo de reduzir temporariamente os comportamentos relacionados com andrógenos em machos. O comportamento de gatos machos, particularmente esguichar a urina, frequentemente torna difícil manter um gato inteiro livre dentro de casa como um pet.

Indução da ovulação

A ovulação aumenta o intervalo interestro (ver Figuras 314.2 e 314.3) e pode ser induzida pela estimulação vaginal com um *swab* de algodão. Algumas gatas podem ter sua ovulação induzida enquanto são acariciadas. Alguns machos castrados continuam a cobrir e alguns criadores os mantêm com fêmeas em estro para prolongar o intervalo interestro. O risco de piometra deve ser considerado quando uma fase lútea é induzida.

Progestágenos

Os progestágenos usados em gatos incluem o acetato de medroxiprogesterona (MPA), proligestona e o acetato de megestrol (MA). Sua disponibilidade para uso veterinário varia. Outros progestágenos sem indicação para gatos têm sido usados, mas faltam estudos detalhados sobre seus efeitos e efeitos colaterais. Dependendo da atividade do ingrediente e da dose, o risco de efeitos e os efeitos colaterais variam.[23] A proligestona está disponível apenas para aplicação IM, enquanto MAP e MA estão disponíveis para uso oral em tabletes e em formulação de depósito para administração por via intramuscular.[23] Para fêmeas em reprodução, os tabletes de ação curta são preferíveis, uma vez que a duração do efeito do tratamento é fácil de ser controlado. Progestágenos têm sido usados também para suprimir o comportamento de machos pelas suas ações antiandrogênicas. Embora a qualidade espermática reduza como um resultado do tratamento com progestágenos, machos podem, em geral, produzir novas ninhadas.

Efeitos colaterais potenciais incluem o desenvolvimento de HEC, piometra, hipertrofia mamária, acromegalia, diabetes melito e tumores mamários. Alterações de pele nos locais de injeção, incluindo descoloração, alopecia, atrofia de pele e calcinose circunscrita, têm sido reportadas.[23-27] Recomenda-se que a administração de progestágenos inicie durante o interestro ou nas fases de anestro em doses suficientemente altas para suprimir completamente o estro, mas baixas o suficiente para evitar os efeitos colaterais. Também é melhor evitar o tratamento por longos períodos, uma vez que efeitos colaterais sejam provavelmente dependentes de doses totais. A gestação deve ser descartada antes de iniciar o tratamento porque progestágenos podem masculinizar fetos e inibir o parto. Embora a administração de progestágenos possa induzir efeitos colaterais indesejáveis, a atividade estral frequente e regular pode não ser a melhor alternativa.

Agonistas GnRH

Embora não licenciados para gatos, implantes de liberação lenta de GnRH têm sido estudados e comumente usados como uma supressão reversível da fertilidade em gatos.[27] Após a estimulação inicial, o implante promove supressão da secreção de FSH e LH, o que, em contrapartida, suprime testosterona e produção de estradiol pelos testículos e ovários. A deslorrelina está disponível em implantes de 4,7 mg e de longa ação de 9,4 mg. O estímulo inicial pode induzir estro ou, se implantados durante o estro, ovulação. Se a gata foi coberta no estro induzido, ela pode se tornar gestante e levar a ninhada a termo ou abortar. Cuidados maternais e produção de leite estarão ausentes se elas mantiverem a gestação a termo.[27] A duração do efeito tem sido relatada e pode variar entre 16 meses e mais de 37 meses com o implante de 4,7 mg.

Machos, após a estimulação inicial, exibem supressão da espermatogênese, volume testicular reduzido e concentrações basais de testosterona sérica. Espículas penianas regridem e machos tratados se comportam como gatos castrados. A duração do implante de 4,7 mg varia entre 430 e 705 dias, mas pode ser acima de 3 anos.[27] Por causa da significativa variação de resposta e reversibilidade da infertilidade, os proprietários devem ser informados que as gestações podem ocorrer apesar do tratamento. De modo a serem capazes de reduzir a duração do efeito do tratamento, os implantes em geral são colocados SC na área umbilical para facilitar a remoção.

Melatonina

Embora não licenciado para uso em gatos, um implante de 18 mg licenciado para ovelhas (Melovine, CEVA Sante Animal, Libourne, França) tem sido usado para curtos períodos (2 a 4 meses) de reversibilidade da supressão do estro em gatas. A duração do efeito é maior quando o implante é colocado durante o interestro.[28] Nenhum efeito colateral foi relatado.[28,29]

INTERRUPÇÃO DA GESTAÇÃO

A interrupção médica da gestação deve sempre ser seguida pela ultrassonografia 7 a 10 dias após o tratamento para confirmar o efeito do tratamento.

Ovário-histerectomia (castração)

O método mais comum de interrupção da gestação em gatos é a castração, preferencialmente o mais cedo possível durante a gestação.

Aborto medicamentoso

Bloqueio de receptores de progesterona

Gatas que se pretende manter na reprodução podem ter o aborto induzido medicamentosamente. Não há, no entanto, nenhuma droga licenciada para esse propósito em gatos. Aglepristona (Alizine, Virbac S.A., França) está licenciada em muitos países para a indução do aborto em cadelas e é efetivo em gatas pelo bloqueio dos receptores de progesterona. Duas injeções de 10 a 15 mg/kg SC, são dadas em um intervalo de 24 horas.[30,31] A eficácia é de 100% em gestação recente, mas é menor ($\approx$ 88%) em gestações no meio do seu desenvolvimento.[30,31] Efeitos colaterais são mais comuns e mais pronunciados em gestações terço médias ou finais comparados ao tratamento de gestações iniciais e podem incluir anorexia, aborto parcial, nenhum efeito, retenção de fetos mortos, retenção de membranas placentárias, descarga vaginal, infecção uterina e edema no local de aplicação de injeções. O tratamento pode ser iniciado no dia da cobertura e deve ser feito o mais cedo possível, preferivelmente antes da implantação. O tratamento iniciado no dia 45 da gestação induziu o aborto em 4/6 gatas (67%), mas o tratamento não é indicado após o dia 45.[32] O tratamento tardio na gata reduz a eficácia e aumenta o risco de liberação de filhotes prematuros vivos.

Cabergolina

Cabergolina, um agonista dopaminérgico, pode ser usado para bloquear a prolactina. É licenciada em alguns países para bloquear a produção de leite em cadelas e gatas e para tratar cadelas com pseudogestação. A prolactina é um luteotrófico necessário para a segunda metade da gestação na gata, e a administração de um agonista dopaminérgico após esse período causa uma queda na concentração de progesterona sérica e subsequente interrupção da gestação. O tratamento pode ser iniciado após o dia 30 da gestação. A combinação da cabergolina com o cloprostenol é mais eficiente que a cabergolina sozinha. O tratamento diário pode ser iniciado no dia 25 (5 mcg/kg de cabergolina VO a cada 24 h) por 7 a 10 dias até a interrupção da gestação, combinada com cloprostenol 2,5 mcg/kg, SC, nos dias 1, 3 e 5. Iniciar o tratamento após o dia 48 não é recomendado, uma vez que isso pode resultar no nascimento de filhotes vivos prematuros que vão ficar famintos porque a lactação foi suprimida.[33] Outros agonistas dopaminérgicos são associados a mais efeitos colaterais que a cabergolina.

Prostaglandinas

A PGF2-alfa, usada para interromper a gestação em gatas, é um luteolítico e induz a contração uterina. Seu fraco efeito luteolítico, não efetivo em gatos como em muitas outras espécies, explica por que as doses relativamente altas são requeridas para a interrupção da gestação. A dose de PGF2-alfa natural (2 mg/gata IM a cada 24 h por 5 dias) iniciada aproximadamente no dia 33 após a cobertura induziu o aborto em 4/4 gatas.[34] Efeitos colaterais incluem náuseas, vômito e diarreia. Por causa desses efeitos colaterais, combinar o tratamento com a cabergolina, conforme descrito, é recomendado para permitir o uso de doses baixas com poucos efeitos colaterais.

Estrógenos e glicocorticoides

Nem estrógenos nem glicocorticoides são recomendados para a interrupção da gestação por causa da escassez de documentação, risco potencial de efeitos colaterais e a disponibilidade de alternativas melhores.

ANORMALIDADES DO CICLO ESTRAL

Estro prolongado

Comportamento de estro de duração de 16 a 19 dias é provavelmente indicativo de anormalidades ovarianas. No entanto, algumas vezes, as gatas demonstram comportamento semelhante ao estro na ausência do aumento das concentrações séricas de estradiol.[16] A citologia vaginal pode ser usada para distinguir um estro verdadeiro de um comportamento semelhante ao estro na ausência do estradiol elevado. A secreção prolongada do estradiol causada por desordens ovarianas deve ser diferenciada de um ciclo normal com um intervalo interestro curto antes de iniciar o tratamento. Cistos foliculares ou tumores ovarianos funcionais podem ser secretores de estrógeno e causar aumentos crônicos (ver Capítulo 351).

O ultrassom (US) não pode ser usado para diagnosticar cistos produtores de hormônios, uma vez que podem existir outros tipos de cistos dentro ou próximo do ovário e sem significância clínica (p. ex., cistos de *rete ovarii* e ducto mesonéfrico remanescentes). A produção de hormônios pode ser confirmada com citologia vaginal (ver Figura 314.4). A ovário-histerectomia é o tratamento de escolha para cistos ovarianos. No entanto, tratamento médico pode ser realizado em gatas com valor para reprodução. A indução da ovulação com gonadotrofina coriônica humana (hCG; 250 UI, IM a cada 24 h por 2 dias) pode causar luteinização cística.[35] Tratamentos com progestágenos de curta duração (acetato de medroxiprogesterona) é uma alternativa que em geral causa atrofia cística. No entanto, o risco de induzir doença uterina deve ser considerado antes de o tratamento médico ser iniciado. Remoção cirúrgica dos cistos pode ser uma alternativa para uma avaliação da gata em reprodução.[36]

Anestro primário

A puberdade pode ocorrer mais tarde, aos 21 meses de idade. Se a gata não exibe estro antes dos 2 anos de idade, o anestro primário é suspeitado. Alterações de desenvolvimento são incomuns em gatas, mas podem causar o anestro primário. Hermafroditismo, monossomia do cromossomo X, pseudo-hermafroditismo e defeito de receptores de andrógeno têm sido relatados. Cariotipagem e laparotomia para avaliar os órgãos reprodutivos internos e histologia de gônadas podem ser requeridas para o diagnóstico definitivo. Algumas vezes, genitália externa ambígua pode levantar a suspeita de uma desordem de desenvolvimento.[37]

Anestro secundário

Algumas gatas sadias apresentam um ou dois ciclos estrais por ano. A razão mais comum para o anestro prolongado é a quantidade de luz insuficiente. Desordens endócrinas como uma causa de anestro prolongado não tem sido descrita. Anestro iatrogênico pode ser causado pela administração ou exposição de progesterona ou agonistas-GnRH de ação longa.

Ovariectomia prévia

Se o histórico da gata for desconhecido, o *status* reprodutivo pode ser observado pela avaliação do estradiol após o estímulo com buserelina, medição de concentrações séricas de LH, ou avaliação do hormônio antimülleriano (HAM).[38-40] A medida do LH é facilmente realizada em laboratórios, apresenta alta sensibilidade e especificidade, mas não é tão confiável quanto os outros dois testes. Fêmeas inteiras apresentam baixas concentrações de LH sérico, enquanto fêmeas castradas apresentam concentrações aumentadas, devido à ausência de retroalimentação negativa. Medições de LH são mais bem realizadas com a citologia vaginal para excluir estro, que pode causar aumento das concentrações de LH em fêmeas inteiras. Ambos os falsos negativos e falsos positivos podem ocorrer. Estradiol sérico basal não é útil, uma vez que as concentrações séricas em fêmeas não castradas e castradas são semelhantes. No entanto, 120 minutos após a injeção de 0,4 mcg/kg IM de buserelina, fêmeas inteiras apresentam aumento das concentrações do estradiol sérico não observada em fêmeas castradas.[38] Em fêmeas, o hormônio antimülleriano é unicamente produzido pelas células da granulosa e é basal em fêmeas castradas e acima do basal em fêmeas inteiras.[40] A avaliação do HAM é, portanto, um teste confiável para determinar a presença dos ovários.

Indução do estro

O melhor e mais natural método de induzir o estro é aumentar a quantidade de luz diária em um ambiente de luz controlado. Isso pode ser feito cobrindo as janelas durante o período escuro do fotoperíodo, ou então o estímulo das mudanças na luz externa pode ser mais forte que a luz artificial interna. O contato com fêmeas cíclicas ou o odor de machos também podem ter um efeito estimulante. A indução farmacológica pode ser realizada pela aplicação de eCG (100 a 150 UI IM). Altas doses podem causar hiperestimulação ovariana.[41] Injeções repetidas com FSH também induzem o estro, mas podem ser menos práticas que o eCG. A indução farmacológica do estro não pode ser alcançada em gatas pré-púberes. O diestro deve ser descartado antes do tratamento pela confirmação das concentrações basais de progesterona séricas.

Estro silencioso

O comportamento de estro é em geral muito óbvio, mas algumas vezes pode ser vago ou ausente, mesmo em fêmeas com ondas foliculares normais (ver Figura 314.2).[16] O estro silencioso pode ser diagnosticado com amostras repetidas de citologia vaginal. No entanto, para isso, pode ser necessário coletar amostras frequentes, de 2 a 3 vezes na semana, para que seja possível detectar o estro.

DISTÚRBIOS UTERINOS E TUMORES VAGINAIS

Ver Capítulos 316 e 351.

PROBLEMAS RELACIONADOS ÀS GLÂNDULAS MAMÁRIAS

Tumores de glândulas mamárias
Ver Capítulo 351.

Mastite
Ver Capítulo 315.

Hiperplasia mamária

Um aumento mamário anormal, conhecido como hipertrofia mamária felina, hiperplasia mamária ou hiperplasia fibroadenomatosa mamária, é uma condição não neoplásica. Ela é progesterona-dependente, sendo as mais afetadas as fêmeas não castradas jovens que tenham ovulado ou gatas que tenham sido tratadas com progestágenos.[42] Poucos foram os relatos de gatas que não tinham tido exposição prévia a progesterona ou progestágenos exógenos.[43,44] Embora a condição seja em geral benigna, isso pode se tornar fatal devido a necrose e infecção generalizada. Enquanto a remissão espontânea é possível, o tratamento pode ser necessário. A ovário-histerectomia em fêmeas intactas que ovularam remove a fonte de progesterona e resulta em regressão do tecido mamário. Isso pode, no entanto, levar um longo período, como 5 a 6 meses, até a condição de completa regressão. A remoção da glândula mamária afetada tem sido recomendada, mas a cirurgia pode ser difícil em casos avançados. Embora não licenciado para gatas, o tratamento com o bloqueador de progesterona aglepristone (Alizina, Virbac S.A., França; 10 a 20 mg/kg SC, 1 vez/semana) causa remissão.[44] Uma resposta marcante pode ser esperada em 1 a 2 semanas com remissão completa após 4 semanas.[44] É importante lembrar que o tratamento com aglepristone interrompe qualquer gestação.

PROBLEMAS NA COBERTURA

A maioria dos problemas no momento da cobertura está relacionada ao manejo e ao temperamento, e não a condições patológicas. Preferências por parceiros, insegurança e fêmea em proestro ou na fase de interestro em vez do estro são causas potenciais de falhas na cobertura. Se mais de um macho é mantido na mesma área, o macho dominante pode suprimir a cobertura dos machos subordinados.[19] Um frênulo persistente pode tornar impossível para o macho cobrir e é facilmente corrigido. Não se sabe se a condição é hereditária.[45] Anéis de pelos penianos podem causar problemas na cobertura em machos de pelo longo e são facilmente removidos, uma vez identificados. Gatos com problemas de cobertura por causa de baixa libido devem ser removidos da reprodução para evitar o mesmo problema em gerações futuras.

FALHAS DE CONCEPÇÃO COM ESTRO E COBERTURA APARENTEMENTE NORMAL

Anovulação

Se a gata retornar ao estro 2 a 3 semanas após a cobertura, é mais provável que a ovulação tenha falhado. A cobertura muito cedo no estro ou poucas coberturas podem resultar em anovulação. Não é sempre óbvio se a gata realmente cruza. Falha de cobertura é aparentemente a causa mais comum de anovulação. Falha de ovulação pode ser confirmada com uma amostra de progesterona 1 a 3 semanas após a cobertura (Figura 314.5).

Anormalidades de desenvolvimento

O desenvolvimento anormal do ducto mülleriano pode causar aplasia da vagina cranial e ausência de cérvice, resultando em falha no transporte espermático.[46,47]

Nutrição

Dietas insuficientes em taurina, araquidonato ou cobre são associadas à baixa taxa de concepção.[48-50] Com o aumento do uso de dietas feitas em casa, incluindo dietas com alimentos crus, existe um risco de desequilíbrios nutricionais, assim como a ingestão de patógenos transmitidos pelo alimento (ver Capítulo 192).

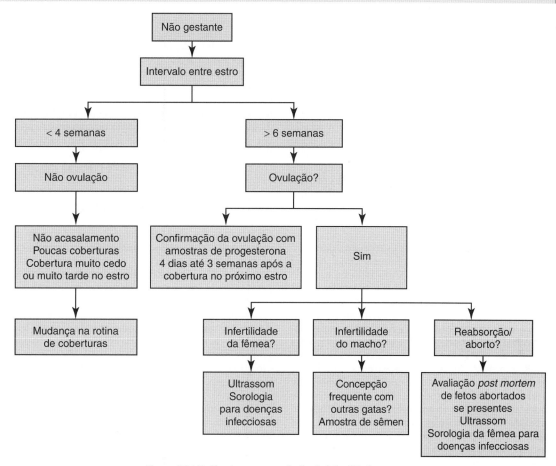

Figura 314.5 Algoritmo para avaliação da infertilidade em gatos.

Aberrações cromossômicas
Aberrações cromossômicas têm sido identificadas como uma causa de falha gestacional, mas são extremamente difíceis de ser diagnosticas sob condições clínicas.[51]

Estresse
O estresse pode aumentar a síntese e a secreção de hormônios de estresse, incluindo catecolaminas, glicocorticoides e progesterona. Embora o estresse não seja uma causa comprovada de problemas de fertilidade em gatos, perfis hormonais anormais associados ao estresse são conhecidos por interferir na gestação inicial em outras espécies.

Causas infecciosas de infertilidade e subfertilidade
Ver Capítulo 317.

INFERTILIDADE NO GATO MACHO

Qualidade seminal pobre
Qualidade seminal pobre pode ser devida a condições congênitas em machos com hipoplasia testicular ou adquirida em machos com degeneração testicular. No macho com qualidade seminal pobre causada por degeneração testicular, a condição pode aumentar enquanto o prognóstico para a hipoplasia testicular é pobre.[4,45] As duas condições não podem ser distinguidas sempre clinicamente ou até mesmo histologicamente. Um macho que previamente tenha produzido filhos, no entanto, provavelmente apresenta um prognóstico melhor do que um macho sem fertilidade prévia comprovada. Testículos pequenos e azoospermia completa são sinais desfavoráveis. Desordens cromossômicas em gatos machos têm sido mais descritas em machos escama de tartaruga. Tanto os com pelos vermelhos quanto os com pelos não vermelhos estão ligados ao cromossomo X extra necessário para o padrão de pelagem de escama de tartaruga. Embora esse padrão de pelagem seja de desordem cromossômica, o cromossomo X extra ocorre também em machos com outras cores de pelagem.[45]

Desordens de pênis
A hipospadia é uma condição congênita rara com localização anormal da abertura da uretra e já foi descrita em gatos.[52] Priapismo e ereção dolorosa persistente são pouco comuns e normalmente requerem amputação peniana devido às lesões isquêmicas.[53]

Criptorquidismo
O criptorquidismo é o resultado da falha de um ou ambos os testículos de descer para o escroto. Embora os testículos normalmente desçam ao nascimento em gatos, eles podem mover-se livremente para cima e para baixo do canal inguinal antes da puberdade. O diagnóstico definitivo não deve ser feito antes de um gato atingir pelo menos 6 meses de vida. Foi relatado que a incidência é de 1,3 a 1,9% em todos os gatos machos, com uma apresentação maior em Persas.[54-56] O criptorquidismo unilateral é mais comum (83 a 90% dos casos) do que bilateral e a localização inguinal é a mais comum.[54,55] A castração bilateral é recomendada uma vez que esses machos devem ser removidos dos programas de reprodução e para evitar comportamentos de macho. Não é sabido se o criptorquidismo aumenta o risco de neoplasia testicular em gatos, uma vez que existem poucos casos de neoplasia testicular descritos. A ultrassonografia pode ser usada para localizar testículos retidos.[57] Quando a história do gato é desconhecida, a inspeção do pênis para a presença de espículas penianas ou avaliação do HAM sérico distingue criptorquidismo bilateral de machos previamente castrados.[40] Poliorquidismo (testículo extra) e monorquidismo (ausência do testículo) são extremamente raros.[55,58]

SEÇÃO 22 • Doenças Reprodutivas

COLETA DE SÊMEN

A maioria, mas não todos os gatos machos reprodutores em uma colônia de gato, pode ser treinada para a coleta de sêmen. O sêmen é coletado com uma vagina artificial personalizada e permite-se que o macho monte uma fêmea em estro.[22] Em uma situação clínica, é improvável que a coleta de sêmen com uma vagina artificial tenha sucesso. A eletroejaculação sob anestesia ou cateterização uretral sob sedação profunda com um alfa-2-agonista são alternativas que não requerem treinamento prévio nem a necessidade de manter o macho em seu próprio território.[59,60] Para o método de cateterização uretral, um cateter urinário de ponta aberta é inserido aproximadamente 9 cm para dentro da uretra em um macho que está sedado profundamente com um alfa-2-agonista, e então o cateter é retirado. O fluido seminal se acumula no cateter e pode ser levado para dentro de um pequeno tubo de teste.[59]

O volume de sêmen e o número de espermatozoides são baixos quando comparados a cães. O volume seminal normal em geral varia de 10 a 200 mcℓ e é afetado pelo método de coleta. Volumes maiores são coletados com eletroejaculação em comparação com outros métodos. O número de espermatozoides varia de 3 milhões a 150 milhões, com maiores valores quando coletados com vagina artificial. A morfologia espermática é muito variável entre machos individualmente, com uma grande quantidade de machos que produz alta proporção de espermatozoides anormais. Morfologia espermática pode ser variável entre ejaculados de um mesmo indivíduo. Parece que machos reprodutores podem produzir altas proporções de espermatozoides anormais sem serem inférteis, dependendo do tipo de anormalidades espermáticas. No entanto, machos com fertilidade ruim frequentemente apresentam alto número de anormalidades espermáticas originadas dos testículos ou podem ser completamente azoospérmicos.[4]

INSEMINAÇÃO ARTIFICIAL

A inseminação artificial não é um procedimento rotineiro no gato. No entanto, a demanda pelos proprietários de gatos tem crescido, e métodos de preservação de sêmen e inseminação intrauterina têm avançado. Na ausência de estímulo de cobertura, a ovulação pode ser induzida com hCG (75 a 100 UI, IM). A determinação do momento ideal para a indução da ovulação é complicada devido às variações individuais entre gatas saudáveis, mas a maioria das gatas responde no dia 3 ou 4 do estro. O ultrassom pode ser usado para acompanhar a maturação oocitária para um momento mais exato, com a indução da ovulação quando pelo menos um folículo ovariano tenha alcançado 3 mm de diâmetro.[15] O sêmen fresco pode ser depositado na região cranial da vagina usando um cateter "tom cat" fino com extremidades abertas. O sêmen congelado deve ser depositado dentro do útero para melhores resultados.[61] A inseminação vaginal pode ser realizada sem sedação ou anestesia, dependendo do temperamento da gata, enquanto a inseminação intrauterina requer anestesia. A deposição intrauterina cirúrgica pode ser usada, mas os métodos de deposição transcervical têm sido desenvolvidos e devem ser considerados como alternativa de primeira escolha.[61]

AVALIAÇÃO ANTES DA REPRODUÇÃO

Os registros dos gatos frequentemente requerem que gatos em reprodução tenham documentos demonstrando que não apresentam hérnia umbilical e os machos apresentam testículos desenvolvidos e normais. Esses critérios devem ser aplicados para animais em reprodução, sendo ou não requisitos para o registro. Também existem recomendações específicas para cada raça sobre testes de doenças hereditárias.[62] Gatos reprodutores devem ser testados rotineiramente para vírus da leucemia felina (FeLV) e da imunodeficiência felina e somente gatos negativos podem contatar outros gatos no gatil. Vacinas contra FeLV não são 100% efetivas e não previnem a infecção (ver Capítulo 223). Sendo assim, é preferível fazer testagens rotineiras em vez da vacinação.[63] Testes rotineiros para outras doenças infecciosas também podem ser garantidos em algumas circunstâncias, mas a estratégia de manejo de um teste positivo para agentes difundidos na população deve ser considerada antes. Para algumas raças, como Rex, Pelo Curto Inglês e Sagrado da Birmânia, testes de sangue em grupo antes da estação reprodutiva são recomendados para evitar a isoeritrólise felina fetal.

Aumentar o número de vacinas essenciais traz benefícios para gatis de reprodução antes de cada cobertura para aumentar o número de anticorpos que serão transferidos para os filhotes pelo colostro e proteger os fetos de infecções (ver Capítulo 208). A vacinação durante a gestação, no entanto, não é recomendada.

REFERÊNCIAS BIBLIOGRÁFICAS

As referências bibliográficas deste capítulo se encontram online no Ambiente de Aprendizagem.

CAPÍTULO 315

Problemas na Gestação, no Parto e no Periparto em Cães e Gatos

Autumn P. Davidson

O período do periparto se inicia aproximadamente 9 semanas antes do parto (pré-parto) e continua por cerca de 30 a 45 dias pós-parto até o desmame. O diagnóstico de problemas nas periparturientes primeiro requer a diferenciação de eventos normais. O tratamento eficiente depende, então, tanto do diagnóstico temporal quanto da intervenção terapêutica. O período do periparto pode ser associado à alta morbidade e até mesmo à mortalidade para a parturiente e os neonatos.

PERITONITE PELO SÊMEN

Um diagnóstico diferencial comum para uma cadela sexualmente intacta com sinais agudos de dor abdominal deve incluir piometra, ruptura uterina e torção uterina. Peritonite aguda secundária à deposição de sêmen dentro da cavidade abdominal, uma condição extremamente rara, deve ser considerada entre as condições que possivelmente podem causar esses sinais em cadelas no estro. Normalmente essas cadelas têm histórico recente de exposição a machos intactos ou inseminação artificial. O sêmen é forçado para dentro do útero durante o bloqueio copulatório devido ao grande volume de fluido prostático na fração final do ejaculado canino. Normalmente, o sêmen não entra na cavidade peritoneal de cadelas após a cobertura. No entanto, se a cobertura for com um cão muito maior ou se a cadela apresentar um útero doente, o sêmen poderá ser forçado para dentro da cavidade peritoneal por meio de trauma ou pelas tubas uterinas. A deposição intraperitoneal do sêmen pode causar uma peritonite supurativa e uma resposta inflamatória sistêmica porque o fluido prostático contém grande quantidade de antígenos não próprios. A estabilização seguida pela exploração por laparotomia e lavagem do abdome são indicadas. A inspeção da vagina e do útero à procura de perfuração deve ser cuidadosamente realizada. Essa síndrome apresenta alta morbidade e mortalidade.

HIPEREMESE *GRAVIDARUM*

Cadelas podem apresentar uma perda de apetite transitória e, algumas vezes, vômito durante as segunda e terceira semanas de gestação. Enquanto isso se resolve, em geral, espontaneamente, anorexia persistente pode impedir uma nutrição adequada durante a gestação. Metoclopramida (0,1 a 0,2 mg/kg VO ou SC a cada 12 horas) pode ajudar. Antieméticos alternativos podem ser seguros ou recomendados em cadelas gestantes. Clínicos devem avaliar riscos e benefícios. Em casos incomuns, alimentação forçada deve ser empregada.

VASCULITE: TROMBOSE NA GESTAÇÃO

A gestação resulta em um estado de hipercoagulação, o qual se torna problemático em pessoas com pró-trombose genética. Hipercoagulabilidade já foi documentada em cadelas gestantes. Cadelas afetadas estão em risco tanto para trombose arterial quanto para venosa, conforme evidenciado pelos níveis elevados de D-Dímero (ver Capítulo 196). O ultrassom (US) pode ser usado para documentar trombose, mais comumente envolvendo a veia cava caudal e causando congestão venosa de membros pélvicos (Vídeo 315.1).

A terapia antitrombótica com heparina de baixo peso molecular é utilizada em mulheres, mas não tem sido avaliada em cadelas gestantes. O aborto devido à hemorragia placentária ou fetal é um risco. A varfarina é contraindicada em gestantes, uma vez que atravessa a placenta. O ácido acetilsalicílico causa defeitos congênitos (fenda palatina). Acredita-se que a condição seja hereditária em mulheres; cadelas afetadas devem ser removidas da reprodução.

EDEMA GESTACIONAL

Edema acentuado na região distal dos membros pélvicos, nas glândulas mamárias caudais e no períneo é, ocasionalmente, observado em cadelas de raças de grande porte com grandes ninhadas e concentrações de albumina séricas normais. A trombose venal deve ser excluída com o US Doppler. A hiperplasia vaginal pode ocorrer a termo e ser confundida com o edema gestacional (ver Capítulo 146). O estradiol normal médio aumenta próximo ao termo da gestação, pode induzir a formação de hiperplasia vaginal (mais comumente vista durante o estro) e comprometer o canal do parto, o que é uma indicação para a cesariana eletiva. Hiperplasia vaginal pode ser confirmada pelo exame digital da vagina e achado de uma massa originada na região cranial à papila uretral. Se o edema gestacional for confirmado, exercícios leves (caminhada ou natação) podem ajudar. O uso de diuréticos não é aconselhado porque complicações têm sido observadas (poliúria fetal, desidratação) e há suspeita de teratogenia. Edema grave do períneo pode ser causa de distocia.

PERDA GESTACIONAL

Visão geral

O aborto de todos ou alguns filhotes de uma ninhada pode resultar de trauma, infecção, condições metabólicas ou degenerativas. Perda embrionária precoce não é em geral reconhecida porque a reabsorção ocorre. Perda fetal no meio da gestação, de 21 a 30 dias de gestação, pode ser reconhecida com US (Figura 315.1). Perda gestacional tardia (> 40 dias) em geral causa aborto reconhecível. Causas infecciosas de reabsorção na cadela incluem *Brucella canis*, *Toxoplasma gondii*, *Neospora caninum*, herpes-vírus-1 canino, vírus minuto canino, também conhecido como parvovirus canino tipo 1, *Cryptosporidium canis* ou qualquer bactéria oportunista ascendente.[1,2] Causas infecciosas de reabsorção/aborto na gata são em geral virais: vírus da leucemia, vírus panleucopenia, herpes-vírus e vírus da imunodeficiência. Reabsorção/aborto pode também ser devido ao protozoário *Toxoplasma gondii* ou a várias bactérias: *Streptococcus* spp., *Escherichia coli*, *Campylobacter* spp. e *Salmonella* spp.[2,3]

Brucelose

É incomum a brucelose canina (ver Capítulo 213) causar aborto/reabsorção, o que pode acontecer cedo (antes de 20 dias) na gestação resultando em reabsorção fetal ou mais comumente (75%) na gestação tardia (geralmente 45 a 59 dias) resultando em aborto. Qualquer cadela com perda gestacional não explicada deve ser examinada para *Brucella*. Técnicas de sorologia, cultura de tecidos ou sangue, histologia e reação da cadeia de polimerase (PCR) são apropriadas para o diagnóstico. Uma avaliação sorológica positiva é detectável em muitos cães infectados com 8 a 12 semanas. Uma vez que a incubação varia de 2 a 12 semanas, há uma janela de tempo na qual um indivíduo infectado pode iludir diagnósticos sorológicos. A interpretação correta de um resultado sorológico é crítica para realizar um diagnóstico acurado. A triagem sorológica é sensível, mas não é específica: alta taxa de falsos positivos ocorre porque a superfície de antígenos de *B. canis* faz forte reação cruzada com anticorpos de várias espécies de bactérias não patogênicas. Pode haver 50 a 60% de falsos positivos por causa de reação cruzada com anticorpos de *Bordetella* spp., *Pseudomonas* spp., *Moraxella* spp. e *B. ovis*. Falsos negativos são raros, a não ser que o teste seja realizado muito cedo na infecção. Teste confirmatório é necessário por causa da alta incidência de falsos positivos. Por essa

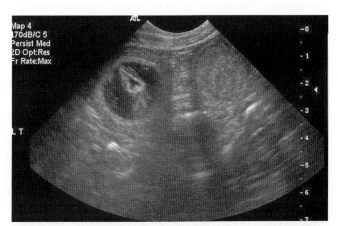

Figura 315.1 Imagem ultrassonográfica de um feto canino normal no meio da gestação (*esquerda*) e reabsorção fetal (*direita*). A reabsorção não tem estruturas ou membranas fetais reconhecíveis e não tem fluido alantoide.

razão, a testagem é recomendada pelo menos 1 mês antes da data prevista para início da estação reprodutiva. Um falso-negativo pode ocorrer se um cão ou uma cadela infectados recentemente estão há menos de 8 semanas pós-exposição à infecção e o título não se tornou positivo ainda. Entretanto, um teste negativo é em geral indicativo de um cão verdadeiramente negativo. Cães e cadelas infectados devem ser removidos de programas de reprodução e colocados em quarentena.

A erradicação de situações de doenças em canis não têm sucesso sem a remoção (abate) de todos os cães infectados (corrente ou historicamente).

Herpes-vírus canino

Os sinais clínicos da infecção por herpes-vírus canino 1 (ver Capítulo 228) em cães adultos são leves, as suspeitas de uma infecção no canil frequentemente se inicia com mortes neonatais e/ou doenças em filhotes. Quando a infecção ocorre, os problemas dependem do estágio da gestação. Infecção em estágios iniciais causa morte fetal e mumificação; no meio da gestação, pode resultar em aborto; em estágios mais tardios, nascimento prematuro. Em doenças de ocorrência natural, filhotes em geral nascem aparentemente saudáveis, mas ficam doentes e morrem durante as primeiras semanas pós-parto. Normalmente, a imunidade na cadela é desenvolvida e até aquelas que perderam as ninhadas por causa da infecção por herpes-vírus podem, mais tarde, dar à luz ninhadas normais.[4,5] Até recentemente, o tratamento da infecção por herpes-vírus canino em neonatos tem sido ingrata, e a recuperação pode ser associada a danos cardíacos e neurológicos. O tratamento com soro imune vindo de parturientes afetadas é ineficiente em filhotes infectados. O aciclovir é um agente antiviral com atividade contra a variedade de vírus que incluem o herpes simples. Seu uso em medicina veterinária não é bem estabelecida e deve ser usado somente em situações de indicação e com cautela. A segurança e eficiência em humanos com menos de 2 semanas de idade não são estabelecidas. A dosagem (20 mg/kg VO a cada 6 horas, por 7 dias) é extrapolada da dose humana. A vacinação canina para herpes-vírus pode estar disponível, mas a indicação e a eficácia permanecem não fundamentadas.

Infecções em gatos

A triagem viral apropriada em gatis deve reduzir a incidência da associação do vírus à perda gestacional. O aborto na infecção viral em gatas está relacionado à doença sistêmica e não ao impacto direto no trato reprodutivo. A infecção pela panleucopenia felina durante o início da gestação causa subfertilidade e reabsorção; infecção na gestação média é geralmente associada ao aborto ou mumificação fetal. A clássica panleucopenia fetal associada à hipoplasia cerebelar neonatal (ver Capítulo 225) manifesta-se clinicamente como tremores e incoordenação em neonatos e é associada à infecção em gestação tardia. A leucemia felina e/ou gatas infectadas com imunodeficiência viral exibem subfertilidade, interrupção do desenvolvimento fetal, absorção, natimortos e/ou filhotes de gatos com baixo peso ao nascimento. Gatas com infecção por *Toxoplasma gondii*, especialmente se imunocomprometidas, podem produzir natimortos ou filhotes de gatos com baixo peso ao nascimento.

Perda gestacional tardia

A perda gestacional tardia pode ocorrer como resultado de um parto pré-termo ou prematuro. Tanto o hipoluteísmo quanto a atividade uterina inapropriada acompanhados pelas mudanças na cérvice têm sido implicados na fisiopatologia do nascimento pré-termo em cães e gatos. O parto prematuro é definido como mudanças na atividade uterina e cervical que levam à perda da gestação via reabsorção ou aborto antes do termo, para o qual causas metabólicas, infecciosas, congênitas, traumáticas ou tóxicas foram identificadas. O parto prematuro está associado a níveis de progesterona < 2 ng/mℓ e o diagnóstico

retrospectivo é frequente após a avaliação da parturiente e dos fetos ter sido realizada por causa das perdas gestacionais. Essa avaliação deve incluir avaliação metabólica da parturiente para doenças sistêmicas e infecciosas. Histopatologia e cultura dos fetos expelidos e placenta devem ser realizadas. A nutrição do canil/gatil, medicações e fatores ambientais devem ser avaliados. A parturiente que experiencia atividade miometrial prematura em uma gestação pode ou não ter o mesmo problema em gestações subsequentes.

Parto prematuro

Visão geral da experiência humana

Em mulheres, partos prematuros ocorrem em 10 a 12% das gestações humanas, mas isso representa 80% de morbidade e mortalidade fetais. O diagnóstico de partos prematuros requer avaliação da contratilidade uterina pela tocodinamometria, fibronectina fetal e medição transvaginal do comprimento da cérvice com US. Juntos, esses parâmetros têm valores preditivos altos. Mulheres que tiveram partos prematuros são consideradas de risco para o mesmo problema em gestações subsequentes. Antibióticos, hidratação e repouso não trazem benefícios. Se a intervenção é indicada, agentes tocolíticos são defendidos. Contraindicações aos tocolíticos incluem pré-eclâmpsia grave, descolamento de placenta, infecção intrauterina, anormalidades cromossômicas ou congênitas, dilatação cervical avançada e evidência de comprometimento fetal ou insuficiência placentária. Agentes tocolíticos inibem contração miometrial e incluem betamiméticos (terbutalina, ritodrina), sulfato de magnésio, bloqueadores de canais de cálcio e inibidores da síntese de prostaglandina (indometacina, cetorolaco, sulindaco).

Testes clínicos em pessoas que receberam compostos progestágenos profiláticos não ajudaram suficientemente. Com base na metanálise, a prevenção do parto pré-termo ou a prevenção do abortamento recorrente parecem ser feitas com o uso do metabólito natural de progesterona, caproato 17 alfa-hidroxiprogesterona (17 P). A manutenção da gestante canina ou felina requer níveis de progesterona > 1 a 2 ng/mℓ e durante a gestação normal são de 15 a 90 ng/mℓ, declinando gradualmente durante a segunda metade da gestação até o decréscimo abrupto para concentrações basais a termo (em geral o dia antes ou o dia após o parto). A progesterona promove o desenvolvimento do tecido endometrial glandular, a inibição da contratilidade miometrial (causa relaxamento da musculatura lisa miometrial), bloqueia a ação da ocitocina, inibe a formação de junções *gap* e inibe a função dos leucócitos no útero. Em muitas espécies, mudanças na progesterona ou na relação progesterona: estrógeno na placenta, decídua ou membranas fetais são importantes para iniciar o parto. Antagonistas da progesterona administrados a termo podem resultar em uma taxa aumentada do aborto espontâneo.

Hipoluteísmo em cães e gatos

Na cadela, os corpos lúteos ovarianos são a única fonte de progesterona. Em gatas, a produção placentária de progesterona ocorre na segunda metade da gestação. A função luteal canina é autônoma no início da gestação, mas suportada por hormônios luteotróficos (LH e prolactina) depois da segunda semana de gestação. Hipoluteísmo, falha primária luteal que ocorre antes do termo da gestação, não é uma causa documentada de abortos, mas a indução do aborto requer redução dos níveis de progesterona plasmática < 2 ng/mℓ. O diagnóstico da perda gestacional causada pela luteólise prematura é difícil, requer documentação de níveis inadequados de progesterona plasmática antes do aborto para o qual nenhuma outra causa foi encontrada. Para medição dos níveis precisos de progesterona, especialmente no alcance crítico 1 a 3 ng/mℓ, o uso de *kits* de teste rápido de ELISA não é acurado. Para baixas concentrações, laboratórios comerciais são mais eficazes. Alguns laboratórios oferecem resposta rápida (< 8 horas), facilitando o diagnóstico.

CAPÍTULO 315 • Problemas na Gestação, no Parto e no Periparto em Cães e Gatos

Os níveis de progesterona diminuem em resposta à morte fetal; assim, a documentação de níveis baixos de progesterona após um aborto não estabelece um diagnóstico de hipoluteísmo. Progesterona dada para a manutenção da gestação a parturientes com anormalidades fetais primárias, placentite ou infecção intrauterina pode causar crescimento fetal continuado com a possibilidade de distocia e sepse. A administração de muita progesterona para manter a gestação em uma parturiente necessitando da terapia pode atrasar o parto, impactar na lactação, colocar em perigo a vida de cadelas e fetos, e pode masculinizar fetos femininos. Parturientes com níveis de progesterona baixa e histórico de perdas de gestação a termo sem patologia aparente também podem ser avaliadas para atividade miometrial prematura no meio da gestação, usando tocodinamometria. A síntese de prostaglandinas do endométrio e da placenta em associação à atividade miometrial prematura pode resultar secundariamente em luteólise.

A atividade uterina prematura que coloca em perigo a sobrevivência fetal foi identificada antes da luteólise completa ocorrer, e a intervenção é indicada se a gestação é normal de outra forma.[6] Agentes tocolíticos, sozinhos ou em combinação com a progesterona, reduzem a atividade miometrial. Terbutalina (Brethine, Ciba Geigy; 0,03 mg/kg VO a cada 8 h) é usada para suprimir a contratilidade uterina em cadelas e gatas com histórico de perdas prematuras de outras gestações normais. Idealmente, a dose é titulada para efeito usando tocodinamometria e é descontinuada 24 horas antes do termo. A suplementação da progesterona somente é aconselhada em gestação tardia se a progesterona estiver < 2 a 3 ng/mℓ para evitar consequências teratogênicas. A progesterona sérica pode ser monitorada apenas quando suplementada com a produção natural (progesterona oleosa, 2 ng/kg IM a cada 72 h). O altrenogeste (Regumate, Merck Animal Health), um progestágeno sintético usado em éguas, é administrado por via oral na dose de 0,09 mg/kg a cada 24 h. Ambas as formas de suplementação devem ser descontinuadas de modo oportuno para prevenir interferência com o parto normal. Em geral, produtos sintéticos orais são interrompidos dentro de 24 horas da data prevista para o parto e o formulário de deposição injetável 72 horas antes. Esse protocolo requer acurácia na determinação prévia da ovulação (esperado que o parto ocorra 64 a 66 dias do pico do LH ou aumento inicial na progesterona, ou 56 a 58 dias do primeiro dia do diestro citológico). A identificação menos acurada da duração gestacional pode ser tentada com datas da cobertura (58 a 72 dias da primeira cobertura), radiografia ou US. Cadelas e gatas manejadas com sucesso para irritabilidade uterina ou parto prematuro frequentemente têm inércia uterina e requerem cesariana.

CONDIÇÕES METABÓLICAS

Observações gerais

O volume sanguíneo aumenta em 40% durante a gestação, fornecendo adequada reserva para repor sangue e fluidos perdidos no parto. O aumento no volume plasmático causa hemodiluição e o hematócrito esperado é em geral de 30 a 35% ao termo. Débito cardíaco aumentado é causado pela frequência cardíaca aumentada e pelo volume ejetado. A capacidade funcional residual do pulmão é diminuída pelo deslocamento cranial do diafragma pelo útero gravídico. O consumo de oxigênio durante a gestação aumenta em 20%. Cadelas gestantes podem ter esvaziamento gástrico atrasado, deslocamento do estômago e risco aumentado de refluxo gastresofágico. Sinais de acromegalia podem ocorrer na cadela secundários ao excesso de progesterona induzindo a secreção de hormônio de crescimento (GH).[7] Diabetes melito gestacional é raro na cadela e na gata e, quando presente, é atribuído aos efeitos anti-insulina da progesterona (mediados pelo nível elevado de hormônio de crescimento, ver

Capítulos 304 e 305). Grandes fetos que predispõem à distocia podem ser resultado de sua insulina aumentada em resposta à hiperglicemia maternal. No entanto, não é comum cadelas diabéticas levarem uma ninhada a termo.

Toxemia da gestação

A toxemia da gestação na cadela ocorre como resultado do metabolismo de carboidratos alterado na gestação tardia resultando em cetonúria sem glicosúria ou hiperglicemia. É mais comum devido à nutrição fraca (falta de nutrição ou apetite reduzido devido a outro fator) durante a última metade da gestação. Lipidose hepática pode ocorrer (ver Capítulo 285). A melhora no plano nutricional pode resolver a condição, mas o término da gestação pode ser indicado em muitos casos.

Eclâmpsia e hipocalcemia

Definição

Tetania puerperal ou eclâmpsia, uma hipocalcemia limitante à vida (ver Capítulo 146), ocorre mais comumente em cadelas durante as primeiras 4 semanas pós-parto, mas pode ocorrer nas últimas semanas de gestação e também em gatas. A condição é causada pela depleção do cálcio ionizado (iCa) no compartimento extracelular devido a nutrição perinatal imprópria, suplementação inapropriada de Ca, ou sérias perdas no leite.[8,9] Parturientes pequenas com ninhadas grandes apresentam maior risco. Suplementação excessiva de Ca pré-natal aumenta o risco de eclâmpsia pela supressão da liberação de paratormônio, interferindo no mecanismo normal do metabolismo do Ca e utiliza o Ca dietético.

Profilaxia

Uma dieta comercial balanceada de crescimento (filhotes) sem suplementação adicional de vitaminas ou minerais pode ser dada durante a segunda metade da gestação e durante a lactação. Queijo *cottage* e produtos similares devem ser evitados. Eles interrompem o balanço normal do fósforo-magnésio dietéticos. Condições metabólicas que favorecem a ligação da proteína do Ca sérico e promovem ou exacerbam a hipocalcemia incluem alcalose da hiperpneia durante o parto. Hipoglicemia e hipertermia também podem ocorrer.

Sinais e tratamento

Os sinais que precedem o desenvolvimento de contrações musculares tônico-clônicas (não são convulsões) incluem mudanças comportamentais, salivação, prurido facial e distal, marcha rígida, dor no membro, ataxia, hipertermia e taquicardia. A intervenção terapêutica, iniciada imediatamente após o reconhecimento dos sinais de tetania sem esperar pela confirmação bioquímica, inclui imediata infusão IV lenta de gliconato de Ca 10% (1 a 20 mℓ [0,5 mℓ/kg]) até o resultado (ver Capítulo 298). Monitoramento cardíaco para detecção de bradicardia ou arritmia deve acompanhar a administração e, se detectadas, é indicado interromper temporariamente o tratamento e uma redução subsequente da taxa de infusão. O manitol pode ser indicado para inflamação e edema. Corticosteroides não são indicados porque eles promovem calciúria, reduzem absorção de Ca pelo intestino e prejudicam a mobilização óssea. A hipoglicemia deve ser corrigida se presente. A resolução da hipocalcemia em geral também resolve a hipertermia. Uma vez que os sinais neurológicos são controlados, o volume de gliconato de Ca dado IV deve ser dado SC diluído em 50% com solução fisiológica. Isso pode ser repetido a cada 6 a 8 h até que a parturiente esteja estável e capaz de receber a suplementação oral. Esforços para diminuir as perdas pela lactação pela parturiente e a melhora no seu plano de nutrição são indicados. Se a resposta à terapia for eficaz, a amamentação poderá ser gradualmente reinstituída até que os neonatos possam ser amamentados com segurança, em geral bem cedo (3 semanas). Suplementação

SEÇÃO 22 • Doenças Reprodutivas

concorrente com leite para reposição para cadela/gata é encorajada. A administração de Ca durante a lactação, mas não na gestação, pode ser realizada em parturientes com histórico de eclâmpsia recorrente (carbonato de Ca 500 a 4.000 mg/parturiente/dia VO, divididos).

DISTOCIA

Objetivo do diagnóstico e manejo

O envolvimento veterinário na obstetrícia de cães e gatos tem vários objetivos: aumentar neonatos vivos (minimizando natimortos resultantes das dificuldades no processo de parto), minimizar morbidade e mortalidade na parturiente e promover sobrevivência aumentada de neonatos durante a primeira semana de vida. A sobrevivência de neonatos está diretamente relacionada à qualidade do parto. Distocia (ver Capítulo 146) é definida como a dificuldade na liberação normal do neonato do útero pela vagina e vários critérios são aplicados para identificar essa condição (Boxe 315.1 e Figura 315.2). A distocia deve ser diagnosticada em momento oportuno para intervenção médica ou cirúrgica a fim de melhorar o prognóstico. A causa de distocia deve ser identificada para guiar as decisões terapêuticas.

Parto normal

Gestação

Clínicos são comumente questionados se cadelas ou gatas na gestação estão a termo e se elas estão prontas para parir uma ninhada, e então intervir se o parto não foi iniciado. A determinação acurada da duração da gestação é difícil se inúmeras cópulas ocorreram e o momento da ovulação não foi determinado. A gestação prolongada é uma forma de distocia. O cálculo da gestação na cadela é mais difícil que na gata, porque cadelas apresentam ovulação espontânea. A gestação normal na cadela é de 56 a 58 dias desde o primeiro dia do diestro (detectado pela citologia vaginal seriada, definida como o primeiro dia que a citologia retorna a ≤ 50% de células cornificadas/superficiais; ver Capítulo 119), 64 a 66 dias do aumento inicial da progesterona

acima da linha base (geralmente > 2 ng/mℓ), ou 58 a 72 dias a partir da primeira cobertura. Predizer a duração da gestação sem a detecção prévia da ovulação é difícil por causa da potencial disparidade entre comportamento de estro e o momento atual da concepção em cadelas e da duração do sêmen viável no trato reprodutivo da fêmea (> 7 dias).

As datas de cobertura não estão intimamente correlacionadas com as datas de parto. Adicionalmente, sinais clínicos da finalização da gestação não são específicos: a aparência radiográfica da mineralização do esqueleto fetal varia ao termo, o tamanho do feto varia com a raça e o tamanho da ninhada, e a queda característica na temperatura corporal (tipicamente < 99°F [< 37,2°C]) varia e pode não ser detectada em todas as cadelas. Raça, paridade e tamanho da ninhada podem também influenciar a duração da gestação.[10] Uma vez que a gata apresenta ovulação induzida (a ovulação ocorre 24 a 36 horas após o coito), a duração da gestação pode ser prevista com maior acurácia a partir da data de cobertura, assumindo que as coberturas ocorrem em um número de dias limitado. A duração da gestação em gatas varia entre 52 e 74 dias (média de 65 a 66 dias), medida do primeiro ao último dia de cobertura. Por causa do prognóstico ruim de filhotes prematuros, é melhor que a intervenção seja adiada até que o estágio I do parto seja iniciado, ou que a gestação prolongada esteja confirmada (ver Figura 315.2).

Parto

Geralmente as cadelas entram no estágio I do parto dentro de 24 h do declínio da progesterona sérica < 2 a 5 ng/mℓ devido à liberação da prostaglandina e é comumente associado a uma queda transitória na temperatura corporal (< 99°F; < 37,2°C). As gatas, em geral, entram no estágio I do parto 24 horas após os níveis da progesterona sérica caírem para < 2 ng/mℓ. O monitoramento seriado dos níveis de progesterona sérica para impedir o parto é problemático porque *kits* internos para resultados rápidos são inerentemente menos acurados entre 2 e 5 ng/mℓ e porque um declínio rápido nos níveis de progesterona pode ocorrer ao longo de um período de algumas horas. Laboratórios comerciais que oferecem progesterona quantitativa por quimiluminescência geralmente têm um tempo de resposta de 12 a 14 horas, não sendo suficientemente rápido para permitir a decisão sobre a necessidade imediata de uma intervenção obstétrica.

O estágio I do parto na cadela normalmente dura de 12 a 14 horas. Durante esse tempo o útero tem contrações miometriais de frequência e força crescentes, causando a dilatação cervical. Esforços abdominais (contrações externas visíveis) não são em geral evidentes durante o estágio I do parto, mas cadelas podem exibir mudanças na disposição e no comportamento, tornam-se reclusas, não descansam, formam ninho de maneira intermitente, frequentemente se negam a comer e algumas vezes vomitam. Podem ficar ofegantes e tremendo. A secreção vaginal deve ser clara e aquosa. O estágio II normal na cadela inicia quando o esforço abdominal externo pode ser visualizado. Contrações miometriais culminam na liberação do neonato. A apresentação do feto na cérvice desencadeia o reflexo de Ferguson, promovendo a liberação de ocitocina endógena a partir do hipotálamo. Normalmente, o parto não dura mais que 1 a 2 horas entre filhotes, embora grandes variações existam. A expulsão pode levar de 1 a > 24 h, mas em geral menos. A secreção vaginal pode ser clara, serosa ou hemorrágica, ou verde (uteroverdina). Cadelas geralmente continuam a fazer ninho entre expulsões e podem amamentar e cuidar de neonatos intermitentemente. Ter anorexia, estar ofegante e tremer é comum. O estágio III do parto é definido como a expulsão da placenta. Cadelas frequentemente alteram entre os estágios II e III do parto até que todos os filhotes tenham sido expulsos. Os estágios do parto na gata são similarmente definidos. É relatado que o estágio I do parto na gata dura pelo menos de 4 a 24 horas, e os estágios II e III de 2 a 72 horas, embora a completa expulsão dos neonatos dentro de 24 horas seja esperada com gatas normais.

Boxe 315.1 Pistas para reconhecer a distocia

Falha em iniciar estágio do parto I a termo (gestação prolongada):
- > 72 dias a partir da primeira cobertura
- > 64 a 66 dias a partir da data do pico de LH ou do aumento inicial de progesterona (1,5 a 2,5 ng/mℓ)
- > 56 a 58 dias a partir do dia 1 do diestro (a citologia vaginal do primeiro dia tem < 50% de células superficiais; a cadela geralmente não é receptiva ao macho nessa data).

Falha ao entrar no estágio I > 24 h após a queda de temperatura < 99°F (< 37,2°C) ou quando a progesterona < 2,0 ng/mℓ

Falha em prosseguir para o estágio II após 24 h no estágio I

Falha ao parir todos em tempo hábil (6 a 8 h); fortes contrações abdominais por > 1 h sem parto (não é possível avaliar as contrações uterinas sem tocodinamometria); contrações abdominais fracas > 4 a 6 h

Sofrimento fetal ou materno (natimortos, dificuldade de ressuscitar os neonatos, cadela exausta/fraca, dolorida ou em choque)

Hemorragia vaginal abundante

Uteroverdina sem expulsão imediata, indicando descolamento de placenta

Histórico de distocia irreversível (raças condrodistróficas, anormalidades pélvicas, estenoses vaginais, massas ou hiperplasia)

Anormalidades radiográficas: obstrução, mau posicionamento, gás intrauterino/fetal sugerindo morte fetal, feto(s) superdimensionado(s)

Bradicardia fetal persistente (FC < 170 a 200 bpm)

De Feldman EC, Nelson RW: *Canine and feline endocrinology and reproduction*, 3 ed., St. Louis, 2003, Saunders.

CAPÍTULO 315 • Problemas na Gestação, no Parto e no Periparto em Cães e Gatos

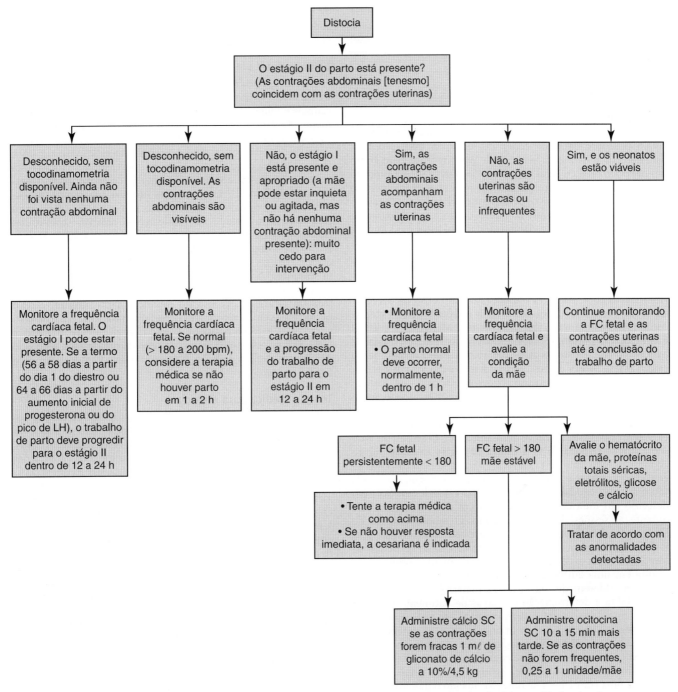

Figura 315.2 Algoritmo para diagnóstico e manejo da distocia. *FC*, frequência cardíaca; *LH*, hormônio luteinizante; *SC*, via subcutânea.

Causas de distocia

Fatores maternos

A inércia uterina é a causa mais comum de distocia. A inércia uterina primária resulta em falha na expulsão de qualquer neonato a termo e suas causas são multifatoriais, incluindo componentes genéticos e defeitos metabólicos ao nível celular.[11] Ocorre uma falha intrínseca para estabelecer contratilidade miometrial funcional de nível progressivo. A inércia uterina secundária é a finalização do parto após um ou mais neonatos terem sido expulsos, mas não a ninhada inteira. Isso pode resultar de causas metabólicas, anatômicas (obstrutivas) ou genéticas. Anormalidades no canal de parto, como restrições vaginais, estenose de trauma pélvico prévio, estenose em determinadas raças e massas intravaginal ou intrauterina, podem causar distocia obstrutiva. Na maioria dos casos, anormalidades no canal podem ser detectadas no exame pré-cobertura e resolvidas ou evitadas pela cesariana eletiva (C). As causas do comprometimento que tornam a parturiente incapaz de completar a expulsão incluem hipocalcemia (ver Capítulo 69), hipoglicemia (ver Capítulo 61), reação inflamatória sistêmica (ver Capítulo 132), sepse (ver Capítulo 132) e hipotensão (devido a hemorragia e choque; ver Capítulo 159).

Fatores fetais

Fatores fetais que contribuem para a distocia mais comumente envolvem incompatibilidade do tamanho fetal e materno, anormalidades fetais e mau posicionamento e/ou má postura fetais. A gestação prolongada com ninhadas de pequenos tamanhos pode causar distocia devido a feto(s) de tamanho muito grande. Anormalidades fetais devido a hidrocefalia e anasarca similarmente também podem ser causas de distocias. A má posição (o ventre do feto proximal ao dorso da parturiente) e má postura fetal (flexão de pescoço e junções escapuloumerais mais comumente) promovem distocia, uma vez que o feto não pode ficar transverso no canal de parto mole.

Diagnóstico (ver Figura 315.2 e Boxe 315.1)

Visão geral

O clínico deve obter rapidamente um histórico cuidadoso e detalhado sobre datas de cobertura, qualquer avaliação feita para detectar a ovulação, histórico de parto recente, bem como um histórico médico geral. O exame físico deve ser endereçado ao *status* geral da paciente, assim como inclui um exame pélvico digital e/ou vaginoscópico para permeabilidade do canal do parto, avaliação do tamanho da ninhada e do feto (radiografia é mais usada), avaliação da viabilidade fetal (o ideal é o Doppler ou ultrassom em tempo real) e atividade uterina (tocodinamometria é mais útil).

Monitoramento fetal e uterino

Abordagens correntes para o monitoramento obstétrico veterinário envolvem o uso de dispositivos de monitoramento externo, como tocodinamometria (Healthdyne Inc., Marietta, GA, EUA) e um Doppler portátil (Sonicaid, Oxford Instruments, England) para detectar e registrar a atividade uterina e taxa de batimento cardíaco fetal. Esses dispositivos podem ser usados em casa ou na clínica veterinária. Seu uso requer que o pelo seja cortado da região caudal da caixa torácica e sobre a região do útero gravídico do flanco lateral para permitir o contato próprio do sensor uterino e Doppler fetal. O sensor uterino detecta mudanças nas pressões intrauterina e intra-amniótica. O sensor, passado sobre a área raspada da gata/cadela na região caudolateral do abdome usando uma cinta elástica, é em geral bem tolerado. O gravador do sensor é usado em uma pequena mochila colocada sobre a região caudal do ombro. Cadelas/gatas devem ficar em descanso em uma cama de parto ou em um caixote ou baia durante as sessões de monitoramento. O monitoramento de Doppler fetal é realizado bilateralmente com uma unidade portátil com cadelas/gatas em decúbito lateral, usando gel de ultrassom. Direcionar o Doppler perpendicularmente sobre o feto resulta em uma amplificação característica dos sons cardíacos fetais, que diferem de sons arteriais maternais ou cardíacos, a qual habilita a determinação das taxas de batimento cardíaco fetal. A interpretação do padrão contrátil em tiras produzidas pelo monitor uterino requer treinamento e experiência. Os dados são transferidos por modem para a equipe obstétrica treinada que posteriormente se comunicará com o clínico veterinário responsável e o cliente. As imagens são feitas 2 vezes/dia, cada uma com 1 hora de duração, quando o monitoramento residencial é realizado, de forma intermitente em cadelas ou gatas em casa conforme indicado durante o trabalho de parto ativo; ou na clínica veterinária por períodos mais curtos de tempo (mínimo de 20 minutos) quando os pacientes estão sendo avaliados por suspeita de distocia.

O útero canino e o felino têm cada um seu padrão de contratilidade, variando em frequência e força antes e durante os estágios diferentes do parto. Tarde na gestação, o útero pode contrair uma ou duas horas antes de o estágio I do parto ser iniciado. Assim, sessões normais podem se mostrar sem atividade. Durante os estágios I e II do parto, as contrações uterinas variam em frequência de 0 a 12 por hora e em força de 15 a 40 mmHg, com picos acima de 60 mmHg. As contrações durante a atividade do parto podem variar de 2 a 5 min de duração. Padrões reconhecíveis existem durante o pré-parto e parto ativo (estágios I-III). Aberrações na contratilidade uterina podem ser detectadas durante o monitoramento. A inércia uterina pode ser determinada até quando fatores externos e abdominais são vistos. Padrões

de partos anormais e disfuncionais podem ser fracos ou prolongados, e frequentemente são associados ao estresse fetal. A conclusão do parto pode ser avaliada via tocodinamometria.

Estresse fetal via monitoramento

A presença de estresse fetal é detectada pela desaceleração da frequência cardíaca. A frequência cardíaca normal de fetos caninos e felinos ao termo é de 170 a 230 bpm (bpm) ou pelo menos $4\times$ a frequência cardíaca materna. No período periparturiente, o débito cardíaco fetal é principalmente dependente da taxa quando o ventrículo direito está relativamente duro (baixa complacência) e o sistema nervoso autônomo está imaturo (resposta inotrópica mínima às catecolaminas). Desacelerações associadas às contrações uterinas sugerem incompatibilidade no tamanho entre o feto e a parturiente ou mau posicionamento fetal. As acelerações normais transitórias ocorrem com o movimento fetal. A frequência cardíaca de fetos ≤ 150 a 160 bpm indica estresse, taxas ≤ 130 bpm estão associadas à baixa sobrevivência se não expulsos dentro de 30 a 60 minutos. A frequência cardíaca fetal ≤ 100 bpm indica a necessidade de expulsão imediata dos neonatos (medicamentosa ou cirúrgica). O uso do monitoramento uterino e fetal permite ao clínico veterinário detectar e monitorar o parto, bem como manejar medicamentosa ou cirurgicamente o parto à vista. Em um estabelecimento de reprodução de cães, a taxa de natimortos declina de 9,2 a 2,5% com o uso do monitoramento fetal e uterino.

Terapia médica para distocia

A terapia medicamentosa para distocia, administração de gliconato de Ca e ocitocina, pode ser direcionada e sob medida com base nos resultados do monitoramento (ver Capítulo 146). Geralmente, a aplicação de Ca aumenta a força das contrações miometriais, enquanto a ocitocina aumenta sua frequência. O Ca é dado antes da ocitocina na maioria dos casos, a fim de melhorar a força de contração antes de aumentar a frequência. O gliconato de Ca (solução 10% com 0,465 mEq Ca/mℓ; 1 mℓ/5,5 kg SC [Fujisawa Inc., EUA]) é dado como indicativo, notando a força de contração uterina, em geral a cada 4 a 6 horas. A ocitocina (10 USP unidades/mℓ; American Pharmaceutical Partners Inc., Los Angeles, California, EUA) é efetiva, iniciando-se com 0,25 unidades SC ou IM no máximo de 2 unidades por cadela ou gata. Altas doses de ocitocina, ou *bolus* IV, podem causar tetania, contrações uterinas ineficientes, que podem comprometer a suplementação fetal de oxigênio pela compressão da placenta. A frequência da administração de ocitocina é ditada pelo padrão de parto e é geralmente dada, aproximadamente, a cada 30 a 60 minutos. Adicionalmente, a ação da ocitocina parece ser melhorada quando dada 15 minutos após o Ca. A maioria das cadelas/gatas está eucalcêmica, sugerindo que o benefício do Ca está ao nível celular ou subcelular.

Terapia cirúrgica (cesariana)

Indicações

A cirurgia é indicada se uma cadela ou gata falha em responder ao manejo médico ou se um estresse fetal é evidenciado apesar do aumento da contratilidade uterina (sugerindo incompatibilidade do canal do parto materno ao tamanho do feto, mau posicionamento fetal ou má postura incompatíveis com a expulsão vaginal), ou se padrões contráteis aberrantes são notados pelo monitoramento vaginal. A cesariana bem orquestrada é resultado do estabelecimento e da coordenação de protocolos anestésicos e de reanimação neonatal com uma ótima avaliação pré-operatória da parturiente. Sempre deve ser lembrado que a parturiente pode estar debilitada e requerer manejo anestésico cuidadoso, pode ter pouco tempo para a preparação pré-anestésica rotineira, e ela pode ter sido alimentada recentemente. Pelo menos,

CAPÍTULO 315 • Problemas na Gestação, no Parto e no Periparto em Cães e Gatos

hematócrito, sólidos totais, Ca sérico e níveis de glicose devem ser avaliados no pré-operatório. O suporte de fluidoterapia IV é indicado (5 a 10 mℓ/kg/h; ver Capítulo 129).

Agentes anestésicos e pré-anestésicos

Protocolos de bloqueios espinais são descritos no Capítulo 146. A atropina não é aconselhada como pré-medicação porque atravessa a placenta, bloqueia a resposta fetal bradicárdica adaptativa para hipoxemia e relaxa o esfíncter esofágico inferior, tornando a aspiração maternal mais provável. No entanto, o uso de um anticolinérgico é indicado para a parturiente por causa da estimulação vagal antecipada durante a manipulação uterina. O glicopirrolato (0,01 a 0,02 mg/kg SC) não atravessa a placenta e é preferido. A maioria das parturientes não precisa de tranquilização pré-anestesia, o que tem um efeito depressor do útero. Os tranquilizantes fenotiazínicos são transportados rapidamente através da placenta. Agonistas alfa 2-adrenorreceptores (dexmedetomidina, xilazina) e opioides são contraindicados por causa do grave efeito depressor cardiorrespiratório. Se a tranquilização é necessária em uma parturiente intratável, sedativos narcóticos são preferíveis, uma vez que seus efeitos podem ser revertidos (naloxano 1 a 10 mcg/kg IV ou IM) durante a reanimação neonatal (ver Vídeo 146.1). Metoclopramida (0,1 a 0,2 mg/kg) pode ser administrada por via subcutânea ou IM antes da indução da anestesia, reduzindo o risco de vômito. A pré-oxigenação por máscara (5 a 10 minutos) é sempre indicada (ver Capítulo 131). A preparação inicial do abdome pode ser iniciada durante esse momento. Para a indução da anestesia, agentes dissociativos, como quetamina e barbitúricos, são evitados porque podem ser profundamente depressores de fetos. O propofol (6 mg/kg IV para efeito) parece ser mais útil; sua rápida redistribuição limita os fatores fetais depois da expulsão. A alfaxalona (Alfaxan, Jurox) a 1,5 a 4,5 mg/kg IV (canino) e 2,2 a 9,7 mg/kg IV (felino) é usada como agente indutor para a cesariana, mas a depressão fetal e neonatal ocorre, e estudos em gestantes e em lactantes são necessários. A indução por máscara causa mais hipoxemia fetal e maternal que o propofol.

Para a manutenção da anestesia, agentes voláteis são preferíveis, especialmente aqueles com baixos coeficientes de partição (isoflurano e sevoflurano). Esses agentes mostram captura e eliminação rápidas, e podem ter melhores margens cardiovasculares de segurança que outros agentes solúveis (halotano). O óxido nítrico pode ser usado para reduzir a dose de outros agentes anestésicos, que é transferida rapidamente através da placenta e, embora apresente efeitos mínimos sobre o feto no útero, pode resultar em significante hipoxia por difusão após a expulsão. O uso de um anestésico local (bupivacaína 2 mg/kg) por bloqueio em linha na pele e tecido SC antes da incisão permite uma entrada mais rápida para o abdome, enquanto é feita a transição da parturiente da indução com propofol para a manutenção inalatória e ajuda a diminuir o desconforto pós-operatório.

Cirurgia/ovário-histerectomia

A ovário-histerectomia (OH) no momento da cesariana é uma opção para o cirurgião e o proprietário, mas resulta em tempo anestésico ampliado, amamentação neonatal atrasada e aumenta a chance de perda sanguínea materna. A OH deve ser adiada se possível. Acredita-se que a ação do estrógeno em um modelo permissivo para receptores de prolactina nas glândulas mamárias faz com que a remoção dos ovários seja indesejável. Se a viabilidade uterina é questionável, a OH deve ser realizada. Em uma parturiente normal, o útero vai começar a involuir rapidamente após a remoção dos fetos, mas, se não for o caso, a ocitocina pode ser administrada (0,25 a 1 unidade por parturiente) para facilitar a involução, ajudando a reduzir qualquer sangramento e promovendo a descida do leite. A cesariana eletiva é comum em pessoas (> 50% de partos nos EUA). Os criadores

podem requerer a cesariana eletiva quando apreensivos sobre o processo de parto. Existem prós e contras para considerar quando aconselhar clientes sobre a cesariana eletiva. Indicações para a cesariana eletiva incluem filhote único, fetos muito grandes, raças braquicefálicas ou hidrocefálicas, ou inabilidade histórica para o parto vaginal. Sessenta por cento das cadelas submetidas a cesariana podem parir pela via vaginal em gestações subsequentes.

Pós-cirúrgico

O desconforto deve ser previsto na parturiente; uma vez que os fetos foram removidos, analgesia narcótica deve ser administrada a ela. No período pós-operatório, não é aconselhável o uso de anti-inflamatórios não esteroides em razão de seu metabolismo incerto para o aleitamento dos neonatos com metabolismos renal e hepático imaturos. Analgesia narcótica é preferível. Narcóticos orais, como o tramadol, 10 mg/kg/dia VO em doses fragmentadas, oferecem analgesia excelente para cadelas em amamentação com a mínima sedação do neonato. Em todos os casos, os clientes devem ser advertidos a monitorar de perto a cadela no pós-parto até o comportamento materno normal se estabelecer. Pós-cesariana, as cadelas podem ficar desajeitadas, desatentas e até agressivas com os filhotes. O mecanismo normal da ligação materna tem sido superado pela cirurgia, e o cuidado neonatal normalmente fica normal com o tempo.

Período pós-parto imediato

Normalmente, parturientes se mantêm próximo aos seus filhotes durante as primeiras 2 semanas pós-parto, saindo por curtos períodos da caixa de parto; se sair, apenas para comer ou defecar/urinar. Elas devem estar alerta e felizes de ficar com seus filhotes. Algumas parturientes protetoras podem se mostrar agressivas com outros animais da casa ou pessoas, no início. Tal comportamento tende a sumir após 1 a 2 semanas de lactação. A lactação é, provavelmente, a maior demanda nutricional e calórica da fêmea ao longo da vida. Perda de peso e desidratação têm que ser evitadas porque é perigoso para a cadela e têm um impacto negativo na lactação. Comida e água devem ficar à vontade. Algumas vezes, tanto a água quanto a comida devem ser colocadas dentro da caixa da cadela nervosa. Anorexia parcial pode ser exibida durante as últimas semanas de gestação e no período pós-parto imediato, mas o apetite deve retornar e aumentar com a progressão da lactação. Inapetência durante as últimas semanas de lactação pode ser devida a deslocamento ou compressão de órgãos (estômago) pelo útero gravídico. Anorexia parcial no pós-parto recente é notada após o consumo da placenta, causando lesões digestivas. Diarreia pode ser secundária na cadela que recebeu mais alimento ou alimento mais rico que o de costume. Também pode ocorrer supercrescimento bacteriano secundário à má assimilação de carboidratos. Eflúvio acentuado no pós-parto é normal em cadelas, geralmente ocorre em 4 a 6 semanas após o parto e poupa apenas a cabeça. É mais frequente que aqueles que ocorrem em conjunto com o ciclo estral típico. Os proprietários devem ser informados de que esse não é um problema, desde que seja notado junto à perda de peso tipicamente associada à lactação.

A temperatura corporal da parturiente pode estar levemente aumentada (< 103°F [< 39,4°C]) no período pós-parto imediato, refletindo a inflamação normal associada ao parto. Ela deve voltar ao normal dentro de 24 a 48 horas. Se uma cesariana foi realizada, fica difícil diferenciar a febre causada por um processo inflamatório pós-cirúrgico de outra provocada por alguma doença. Exame físico e contagem sanguínea completa podem ajudar. O corrimento normal do pós-parto é de cor vermelho-tijolo, sem odor, e diminui ao longo de vários dias a semanas (involução uterina e processo de reparação que ocorre em até 16 semanas na cadela). As glândulas mamárias não devem estar doloridas, quentes, eritematosas ou duras. Elas devem ser simétricas e moderadamente firmes. O leite normal tem cor cinza a branca e consistência aquosa.

Comportamento maternal inapropriado

O comportamento materno apropriado é crítico para a sobrevivência neonatal e inclui atenção, proteção, facilitação da amamentação, juntar os neonatos e higiene. Embora o comportamento materno seja instintivo, pode ser negativamente influenciado pelas drogas anestésicas, dor, estresse e interferência humana. A ligação maternal é mediada por feromônios, iniciada no parto. O parto deve ocorrer em lugar quieto, com sons familiares, com a mínima interferência humana, porém com adequada supervisão. Parturientes com bom instinto materno exibem cuidado quando entram ou se movem dentro da caixa de parto para não pisar ou deitar e traumatizar os neonatos. Um guarda-corpo dentro da caixa de parto ajuda a evitar o sufocamento dos filhotes.

O reflexo neuroendócrino que regula a contração de células mioepiteliais das glândulas mamárias e subsequente ejeção do leite é mediado pela ocitocina e ativado pela sucção neonatal. Durante o estresse, a epinefrina induz vasoconstrição, bloqueando a entrada da ocitocina na glândula mamária e prevenindo a queda no leite. Uma cadela nervosa e agitada tem pouco leite disponível. Tranquilizantes antagonistas da dopamina, com mínima interferência na prolactina (acepromazina 0,01 a 0,02 mg/kg VO a cada 6 a 24 horas), podem ser dados na dose efetiva mais baixa para minimizar a sedação neonatal. Isso pode melhorar o comportamento materno e a disponibilidade de leite em cadelas nervosas. O empilhamento dos neonatos próximo do corpo da parturiente facilita a manutenção da temperatura corporal apropriada (neonatos não termorregulam/tremem até 4 semanas de idade) e torna a amamentação imediatamente disponível. O comportamento materno normal inclui a delicada recuperação do neonato que se tornar disperso e isolado na caixa. A limpeza dos neonatos imediatamente seguida do parto estimula suas funções cardiovasculares e pulmonares e remove líquidos amnióticos. Parturientes que demonstram pouco interesse na reanimação de neonatos podem ter comportamento maternal fraco ao longo do período pós-parto. A limpeza maternal também estimula o reflexo neonatal para urinar e defecar, além de manter o pelo do neonato limpo e seco. Ocasionalmente, o comportamento protetor excessivo ou agressão maternal induzida pelo medo pode acontecer. A tranquilização leve da parturiente pode ajudar, mas a transmissão de drogas pelo leite para o neonato pode ser problemática. Benzodiazepínicos, agonistas do GABA, são melhores que fenotiazínicos para agressão induzida por medo (diazepam 0,55 a 2,2 mg/kg VO a cada 8 a 12 horas).

DOENÇAS UTERINAS

Ruptura e prolapso uterino

O prolapso completo ou parcial do útero é incomum em cadelas e raro em gatas (Figura 315.3). O diagnóstico é baseado na palpação de uma massa tubular firme saliente pela vulva no pós-parto e uma inabilidade de identificar o útero com o US abdominal. A hiperplasia vaginal e o prolapso devem ser excluídos pelo exame físico, vaginoscopia, ou radiografia com contraste (ver Capítulo 146). Tecidos prolapsados podem estar macerados e/ou infeccionados por exposição e contaminação. O tamanho da maioria das cadelas e gatas impede o reposicionamento manual; laparotomia e OH são em geral indicadas.

A ruptura do útero ocorre mais comumente em cadelas com ninhadas bem grandes que pode causar estiramento e afinamento da parede uterina, especialmente em cadelas multíparas com distocia. A ruptura pode ocorrer também com o uso inapropriado de agentes ecbólicos (Figura 315.4). A laparotomia imediata é indicada para recuperar fetos, reparar ou

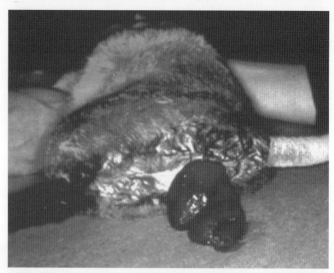

Figura 315.3 Prolapso uterino felino associado à distocia. (*Esta figura se encontra reproduzida em cores no Encarte.*)

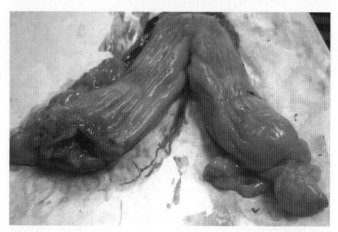

Figura 315.4 Ruptura do corno esquerdo cranial secundária ao uso de ocitocina em uma distocia obstrutiva.

remover o útero e a cultura/lavagem da cavidade abdominal. O útero deve ser cuidadosamente examinado em qualquer cesariana para detectar ruptura e áreas de fragilidade. A peritonite (ver Capítulo 279) pode resultar de um pequeno rasgo uterino. A histerectomia unilateral pode ser considerada se a área lesionada for limitada e a matriz for valiosa para um programa de reprodução.

Subinvolução de sítios da placenta

Uma secreção vaginal persistente serossanguinolenta a hemorrágica além de 16 semanas pós-parto pode indicar subinvolução de sítios da placenta (SIPS), uma condição na qual células trofoblásticas fetais persistem no miométrio (elas devem degenerar), falha na trombose de vasos endometriais, prevenção de involução uterina normal e existência de regiões interplacentárias normais. Massas eosinofílicas de colágeno e glândulas endometriais dilatadas sobressaem dentro do lúmen uterino e vaza sangue. A causa não é conhecida, a perda de sangue é em geral mínima, a infecção intrauterina em geral não está presente e a fertilidade não é afetada. O tratamento geralmente não é necessário, uma vez que a recuperação é espontânea e os sintomas são leves.

Se o sangramento vaginal pela SIPS é copioso e causa anemia, as desordens hemorrágicas (prováveis defeitos na via intrínseca ou trombocitopenia/trombocitopatias), trauma, neoplasia do trato geniturinário, metrite e proestro, devem ser descartadas.

CAPÍTULO 315 • Problemas na Gestação, no Parto e no Periparto em Cães e Gatos

Citologia vaginal, vaginoscopia, testes de coagulação e US abdominal devem ser considerados. O benefício de prostaglandinas, ocitocina ou outros ecbólicos é questionável e não provado. O valor preventivo de minidoses de ocitocina dadas no período pós-parto imediato também não é provado, mas pode ser prejudicial. A laparotomia e a OH são curativas se a perda de sangue é significante ou problemática para o proprietário. O exame histológico do útero é indicado para confirmar o diagnóstico.

Metrite

Metrite, uma infecção aguda séria do endométrio no pós-parto, deve ser suspeitada se a cadela apresentar letargia, anorexia, queda na lactação, febre, secreção vaginal fétida e/ou cuidado materno ruim. A metrite pode ser precedida por distocia, manipulação obstétrica contaminada, fetos retidos e/ou retenção de placenta. Mudanças hematológicas e bioquímicas frequentemente sugerem septicemia, inflamação sistêmica e endotoxemia. Citologia vaginal mostra uma secreção séptica hemorrágica à purulenta. O US abdominal é excelente para a avaliação da parede uterina e os conteúdos intrauterinos para o material fetal e placentário. A metrite é caracterizada por um endométrio ecogênico plissado com fluido no lúmen. Uma cultura da vagina cranial é mais representativa da flora intrauterina e deve ser submetida tanto à cultura/sensibilidade aeróbica quanto anaeróbica, permitindo avaliação retrospectiva da terapia com antibiótico empiricamente selecionada. A ascensão bacteriana do trato geniturinário baixo é mais comum que a disseminação hematógena. *Escherichia coli* é a causa mais comum em cadelas e gatas.

A terapia consiste em fluido IV e suporte eletrolítico, antibióticos apropriados e evacuação uterina usando prostaglandina F_{2alpha} (0,1 a 0,2 mg/kg SC a cada 12 a 24 h) ou cloprostenol (1 a 3 mcg/kg SC a cada 12 a 24 h) por 3 a 5 dias ou até a evacuação do útero ser completa e a cadela ou gata ficar estável. A cefalexina (10 a 20 mg/kg VO a cada 8 a 12 h) ou amoxicilina com clavulanato (14 mg/kg VO a cada 12 h) são seguras para neonatos e usadas quando cultura e sensibilidade estão pendentes. Muitas parturientes afetadas podem ser manejadas sob uma base ambulatória, permitindo que a amamentação neonatal continue em casa. A OH pode ser indicada se ocorrer peritonite e a resposta aos medicamentos for ruim. É pouco provável que a ocitocina promova uma evacuação uterina efetiva quando administrada > 24 a 48 horas pós-parto. Os filhotes devem ser cuidados se a parturiente estiver seriamente doente. A metrite pode se tornar crônica e causar infertilidade. A retenção de placenta, normalmente, não é um problema, se 1 a 2 dias depois do parto sem complicações.

DOENÇAS MAMÁRIAS: AGALAXIA, GALACTOSTASIA, MASTITE

Agalaxia

A agalaxia é definida como falha na oferta de leite para os neonatos. Agalaxia primária, falha no desenvolvimento mamário durante a gestação, resultando em falha na produção de leite, é incomum, e um defeito no eixo pituitária-ovário-glândula mamária é suspeitada. O uso de componentes de progesterona na gestação tardia pode interferir na lactação. Agalaxia secundária, uma falha na disponibilidade de leite devido à falha na ejeção ou descida, é mais comum. O desenvolvimento mamário é acentuado, mas o leite não pode ser imediatamente expelido através dos esfíncteres das tetas. A produção de colostro no período pós-parto imediato não deve ser confundida com agalaxia. A agalaxia pode ocorrer secundária a parto prematuro, estresse, má nutrição, debilidade, dor, metrite ou mastite. O tratamento inclui suplementação de leite para os neonatos, encorajamento da sucção neonatal, oferecimento de ótima nutrição e água para a parturiente, e resolução de qualquer doença que esteja presente. Se detectada cedo, a descida do leite pode frequentemente ser induzida farmacologicamente com minidose de ocitocina (0,25 a 1 unidade SC a cada 2 h). Neonatos são removidos por 10 a 30 minutos antes da injeção, então são encorajados a sugar. O proprietário pode delicadamente "apertar" a glândula. Metoclopramida (0,1 a 0,2 mg/kg SC a cada 12 h) pode promover liberação de prolactina. A descida do leite é notada em geral dentro de 24 horas.

Galactostasia

A galactostasia resulta no ingurgitamento e edema da glândula mamária com desconforto, que interfere na amamentação e pode ser autoperpetuante. Pode ocorrer secundária a tetas invertidas ou imperfuradas, falha na rotação de amamentação, perda da ninhada, uma ninhada pequena não usual, ou raramente uma pseudociese. O encorajamento da sucção ou delicadamente fazer uma evacuação manual das glândulas afetadas é indicado. Se a galactostasia ocorrer durante o desmame, o uso de cabergolina 2,5 a 5 mcg/kg/dia VO por 4 a 6 dias poder ser útil.

Mastite

A mastite é uma inflamação séptica de uma ou de múltiplas glândulas mamárias. Pode ser aguda e grave ou crônica de baixo grau. Coliformes, *Staphylococcus* e *Streptococcus* são muito comumente isolados de cadelas e gatas. A origem da bactéria é cutânea, exógena ou hematógena. A mastite pode ser associada à metrite. Desconforto mamário leve e calor, galactostasia, inflamação cutânea e massa intramamária palpável são os primeiros sinais. O leite pode ser vermelho ou marrom devido às células sanguíneas vermelhas e células sanguíneas brancas. Algumas cadelas exibem dor, relutância a amamentar ou deitar, anorexia e letargia. Febre pode ser recorrente e preceder outros sinais clínicos. Casos avançados podem progredir para choque séptico com abscesso ou necrose em glândulas. O diagnóstico é baseado no exame físico. A contagem de células de leite em cadelas não é preditivo de mastite. A cultura e sensibilidade do leite coletado assepticamente de glândulas afetadas permitem avaliação retrospectiva de seleção de antibióticos.

A terapia deve incluir antibióticos e fisioterapia leve. Analgésicos podem ser indicados; neonatos toleram analgesia por opioides na parturiente. Cefalexina (10 a 20 mg/kg VO a cada 8 a 12 h) e amoxicilina com clavulanato (14 mg/kg VO a cada 12 h) são aconselhadas e seguras para os neonatos. A antiobioticoterapia pode ser garantida até o desmame e pode impedir amamentação posterior se a condição forçar o uso da droga potencialmente tóxica aos neonatos. Compressas mornas ou terapia de hidromassagem da glândula afetada com ordenha suave do leite pode ajudar a evitar a formação de abscesso e/ou ruptura. Necrose grave garante mastectomia quando a parturiente é estabilizada, com manejo agressivo de feridas. O ultrassom pode guiar o manejo do abscesso em desenvolvimento. A terapia antiprolactina (cabergolina 1,5 a 5 mcg/kg/dia VO dividida a cada 12 h) pode ser indicada se grave e reduzir a lactação se o desmame for oportuno. O desmame inicial não é indicado uma vez que este promove galactostasia. Não há evidências de que a amamentação em glândulas afetadas seja problemática para os neonatos, mas eles tendem a evitar as glândulas se o leite não for produzido de imediato. A glândula afetada deve ser protegida de traumas nas bordas da caixa ou de traumas causados pelas unhas dos neonatos. A mastite pode reaparecer em lactações subsequentes independentemente das medidas preventivas tomadas; antibióticos profiláticos não são recomendados; entretanto, é indicada uma boa higiene e evitar a galactostasia.

REFERÊNCIAS BIBLIOGRÁFICAS

As referências bibliográficas deste capítulo se encontram online no Ambiente de Aprendizagem.

CAPÍTULO 316

Piometra e Hiperplasia Endometrial Cística

Annika Bergström

DEFINIÇÃO

A hiperplasia endometrial cística (HEC) e a piometra são os distúrbios uterinos mais frequentes em cadelas de meia-idade e inteiras mais velhas. A HEC inclui o desenvolvimento de cistos patológicos e o espessamento do endométrio, o que é uma resposta anormal do útero canino e do felino a longos períodos repetidos de altas concentrações de progesterona sérica durante as fases luteais do ciclo estral, embora cadelas em anestro possam ser diagnosticadas com piometra,[1] uma doença caracterizada por material purulento dentro do útero. Cadelas ovariectomizadas bilateralmente não desenvolvem piometra, uma vez que são necessários esteroides ovarianos. A piometra pode ser fatal, especialmente nos casos em que a cérvice está fechada.

EPIDEMIOLOGIA

A HEC e a piometra são comuns em cadelas inteiras, em razão de longos períodos de alta concentração de progesterona sérica. As gatas também são acometidas, mas não tão frequentemente quanto as cadelas. A piometra costuma ser diagnosticada em certas raças, como Rough Collie, Rottweiler, Cavalier King Charles Spaniel, Golden Retriever, Bernese Mountain Dog[2,3] e em aproximadamente 15% de todas as cadelas Beagle.[4] Em algumas raças, a incidência de piometra aos 10 anos de idade chega a 50%. Em média, aproximadamente 25% de todas as cadelas inteiras a desenvolvem nessa idade.[2] A incidência de HEC é maior em gatas de rua que vivem em colônia do que nas de rua que vivem sozinhas. As gatas de rua têm maior número de células intersticiais ovarianas de significado desconhecido. Em gatas > 5 anos de idade, a frequência de HEC foi de aproximadamente 90%; nas de 2 a 4 anos, cerca de 30% apresentaram evidência histológica desse distúrbio.[5] A piometra é mais comum em gatas > 7 anos de idade. Nas atendidas por planos veterinários, a taxa de risco de incidência foi de 17/10 mil gatas sob risco por ano, com as da raça Sphinx correndo maior risco (433/10 mil gatas sob risco por ano). Nesse estudo, a mortalidade foi de aproximadamente 6%.[6]

FISIOPATOLOGIA

Hormônios associados à hiperplasia endometrial cística e à piometra

Durante o ciclo estral canino, o útero está sob a influência do estrógeno, por um período relativamente curto, e da progesterona, por 9 a 12 semanas após a ovulação, independentemente da gestação, o que resulta em aumento do crescimento endometrial, secreções glandulares e inibição da drenagem pelo estímulo do fechamento da cérvice (ver Capítulo 312). A progesterona também diminui as contrações miometriais e inibe a atividade leucocitária no endométrio, aumentando o risco de crescimento bacteriano.[7] O período de diestro cria um ambiente uterino excelente para o desenvolvimento das bactérias.[8] A HEC, na qual o endométrio torna-se espesso em razão de um maior número de glândulas císticas, desenvolve-se após repetidas fases luteais e devido ao aumento da idade em todas as cadelas.[1] Não há diferenças significativas nas concentrações séricas hormonais em cadelas que desenvolvem piometra em comparação às saudáveis (ver Capítulo 312). Portanto, foi sugerido que os receptores uterinos hormonais podem desempenhar um papel na patogênese da piometra.[9-11] Em cadelas com HEC, estudos de receptores uterinos de estrógeno e progesterona não forneceram resultados consistentes.[12-14]

Classicamente, a HEC é considerada precursora da piometra. Uma hipótese alternativa é que uma infecção bacteriana de baixo grau dentro do útero cause a proliferação endometrial e a HEC. Nem todas as cadelas com HEC desenvolvem piometra, mas há aquelas que podem desenvolvê-la sem que seja precedida pela HEC.[15] Cadelas clinicamente saudáveis podem apresentar alterações uterinas, por exemplo, aquelas com HEC podem acumular muco estéril, líquido seroso ou hemorrágico sem sinais de doença.[16] Em geral, a piometra se desenvolve durante o diestro, quando há aumento da concentração sérica de progesterona e os ovários costumam apresentar corpos lúteos (Figura 316.1). Embora menos comum, a piometra em gatas também se desenvolve secundariamente à sensibilização uterina pela progesterona, não sendo, de modo geral, diagnosticadas com HEC. Com base na histopatologia e na análise hormonal, 40 a 57% das gatas com piometra ou endometrite estavam na fase luteal e 43% daquelas com piometra se encontravam na fase folicular.[17]

Menos comumente, foi descrita hiperplasia endometrial pseudoplacentacional (deciduoma), uma forma de HEC,[18,19] a qual representa a placentação da fase luteal, semelhante à histologia normal do endométrio nos locais de placentação na gestação normal.[19]

Bactérias associadas à piometra

Durante o estro, as bactérias da flora vaginal normal podem ascender ao útero através da cérvice aberta, incluindo *Escherichia coli* (a mais comum), *Streptococcus* spp., *Enterobacter* spp., *Proteus* spp., *Klebsiella* spp. e *Pseudomonas* spp. A *E. coli* pode

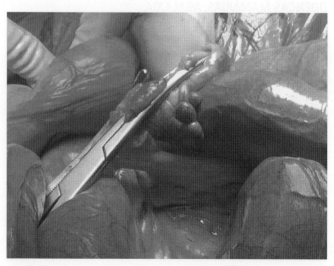

Figura 316.1 Corpos lúteos visíveis nessa cadela com piometra submetida a ovário-histerectomia.

se aderir a receptores específicos no endométrio e no miométrio.[8] As endotoxinas bacterianas podem causar lesões a vários órgãos, o que é especialmente verdadeiro para a endotoxina do lipopolissacarídeo de *E. coli*. A polidipsia observada em cadelas com piometra é um mecanismo compensatório para repor a água perdida pelos rins (ver Capítulo 45). As endotoxinas bacterianas prejudicam a capacidade da alça de Henle de reabsorver sódio e cloreto. As endotoxinas da *E. coli* têm também a capacidade de causar insensibilidade ao hormônio antidiurético (ADH, do inglês *antidiuretic hormone*), o que causa perda adicional da capacidade de concentração urinária (ver Capítulo 296).[8]

Hiperplasia endometrial cística

A infertilidade é o único sinal clínico associado à HEC. Se ela progredir para um útero repleto de líquido, o principal sinal pode ser semelhante ao de uma cadela ou gata com piometra: secreção vaginal. Podem ser observadas poliúria, polidipsia e diminuição da higidez. Não foi reconhecido nenhum tratamento médico para a HEC.

Piometra

Em cadelas e gatas, os fatores de risco para o desenvolvimento de piometra incluem o uso de progestágenos para a supressão do estro ou estrógeno para a indução do estro ou a interrupção da gestação.[3,9,14,20] O estrógeno regula de maneira positiva os receptores endometriais de progesterona e estrógeno.

SINAIS CLÍNICOS E DIAGNÓSTICO

Tempo e sinais

A piometra em cadelas costuma se desenvolver de 4 semanas a 4 meses após o estro, durante o diestro, quando a dominância da progesterona é necessária para a manutenção da gestação.[21] Em geral, as cadelas são de meia-idade ou mais velhas, mas essa condição é diagnosticada em qualquer idade. Em um estudo com gatas, a idade média para o desenvolvimento de piometra foi de 32 meses e em 8 semanas após o estro.[22] Como a piometra é comum, ela deve ser sempre incluída como um possível diagnóstico se uma cadela ou gata inteira estiver doente. O útero pode estar ligeiramente aumentado de tamanho ou bastante dilatado (Figura 316.2). Os diagnósticos diferenciais com aparência similar no exame ultrassonográfico são hidrometra, mucometra e hemometra não letais[16].

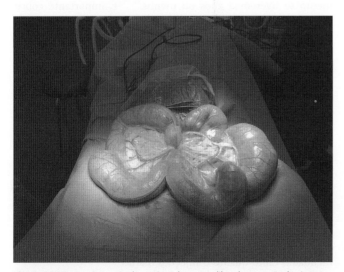

Figura 316.2 Exteriorização de um útero bastante dilatado em razão de piometra, antes da remoção cirúrgica. O risco de ruptura e peritonite séptica é iminente.

Em geral, a piometra resulta em secreção vaginal se a cérvice estiver aberta, permitindo a drenagem de fluido uterino hemorrágico, serossanguinolento ou mucopurulento. Se a ela permanecer fechada, não há secreção vaginal e o conteúdo uterino pode aumentar de volume, resultando em risco de ruptura uterina e peritonite se não reconhecida e tratada em tempo hábil. Cadelas e gatas com piometra cervical fechada costumam apresentar inapetência, obnubilação, letargia, poliúria, polidipsia e distensão abdominal,[21] podendo haver febre. Podem ocorrer septicemia, toxemia, síndrome da resposta inflamatória sistêmica, CID, choque e morte (ver Capítulos 132, 146, 207 e 279). Os sinais clínicos potenciais incluem taquicardia, tempo de preenchimento capilar prolongado e pulsos femorais fracos.[16] A taxa de resposta inflamatória sistêmica correlaciona-se positivamente com a duração do período de sinais clínicos, indicando que um atraso no tratamento leva à rápida progressão da doença clínica.[23]

Alguns animais de estimação podem desenvolver resposta inflamatória sistêmica secundária a uveíte (ver Capítulo 11), dores articulares (ver Capítulo 203) e edemaciamento das articulações. A palpação abdominal pode revelar um útero dilatado de difícil exploração. É extremamente recomendada a palpação cuidadosa para prevenir a ruptura uterina. Em razão da gravidade da inflamação e da endotoxemia, algumas cadelas estão muito doentes, apesar de terem o útero relativamente pequeno ou ligeiramente distendido. Nas cadelas, recomenda-se exame vaginal para excluir doença vaginal, por exemplo, neoplasia, como a causa da secreção vaginal. Em gatas, os sinais clínicos mais comuns são secreção vaginal, anorexia e letargia.[24]

Recomendações de exames laboratoriais e de imagem

Hemograma

Dependendo da gravidade da doença, algumas cadelas podem apresentar parâmetros sanguíneos normais. A maioria daquelas com piometra apresenta alterações acentuadas no hemograma que se correlacionam com infecção grave e/ou inflamação crônica. Observou-se anemia normocítica normocrômica em aproximadamente 70% das cadelas com piometra, provavelmente causada por diminuição da eritropoese.[25] A diminuição das concentrações de ferro secundárias à inflamação crônica pode diminuir a eritropoese. Efeitos tóxicos na medula óssea decorrentes da sepse podem suprimi-la ainda mais. É comum um aumento acentuado na contagem total de leucócitos na piometra, mas significativamente menor em cadelas com HEC.[26,27] Leucocitose com neutrofilia grave, desvio à esquerda e monocitose são vistos com frequência. Cadelas com piometra cervical fechada apresentam maior número de leucócitos.[8] Em doença grave, a endotoxemia pode progredir de modo a suprimir a medula óssea e levar à neutropenia, especialmente porque os neutrófilos continuam a inundar o útero. Leucopenia, febre e hipotermia são fatores preditores de peritonite em cadelas com piometra. Naquelas com leucopenia, o risco de peritonite é 18 vezes maior e o tempo de internação, 3,5.[31]

Biomarcadores e bioquímica sérica

Em geral, a atividade da fosfatase alcalina (ALP) sérica, a globulina e a proteína total aumentam em cadelas com piometra. A proteína C reativa e o amiloide A sérico podem ser marcadores que ajudam a distinguir a piometra da HEC.[26] Em razão da colestase intra-hepática, podem ocorrer aumentos na ALP, na bilirrubina e no colesterol.[28] A azotemia pré-renal ocorre secundariamente à desidratação e a azotemia renal pode ser resultado da lesão tubular reversível. As concentrações séricas do fator do crescimento semelhante à insulina-1 (IGF-1, *insulin-like growth fator-1*) e de ferro são mais baixas em cadelas com piometra, secundariamente à resposta inflamatória. A proteína C reativa e o amiloide A sérico são mais altos em cadelas com piometra e o amiloide A sérico provavelmente o é em gatas essa

SEÇÃO 22 • Doenças Reprodutivas

afecção. Esses biomarcadores podem ser usados para identificar sepse em cadelas com piometra, já que são significativamente mais baixos nas saudáveis e com HEC.[26,29,30]

A proteína C reativa também pode ser um marcador útil para a avaliação de complicaçõespós-operatórias.[29,32,33] A concentração de lactato sérico pré-operatório não foi relacionada com a síndrome da resposta inflamatória sistêmica nem com a hospitalização prolongada.[34] A mensuração repetida do lactato sérico pode ser recomendada a cadelas gravemente enfermas com piometra, para garantir que o consumo de energia celular seja recuperado (ver Capítulo 70). A PGF2-alfa plasmática está aumentada tanto em cadelas como em gatas com piometra, em comparação aos animais saudáveis.[35,36] O aumento das prostaglandinas plasmáticas provavelmente se origina da síntese endometrial decorrente da estimulação de endotoxinas bacterianas.

Exames de imagem

As modalidades mais comumente usadas para confirmar o diagnóstico de piometra são a ultrassonografia abdominal (ver Capítulo 88) ou a radiografia. A ultrassonografia é o teste mais sensível e específico que pode também ajudar a diferenciar piometra de mucometra. Na piometra, a parede uterina é espessa e o lúmen distendido com fluido heterogêneo seroso a viscoso. Na mucometra, o líquido uterino é mais uniformemente hipoecoico. Outras modalidades de diagnóstico podem ser usadas, como a tomografia computadorizada e a ressonância magnética, mas geralmente não são necessárias.

Cultura bacteriana

As amostras bacterianas mais comuns no útero de cadelas e gatas com piometra são *Escherichia coli*. A sensibilidade bacteriana aos antimicrobianos geralmente é alta, com base em um estudo no qual apenas 10% das amostras de *E. coli* provenientes de piometra uterina eram resistentes à amoxicilina.[37] Amostras obtidas com um *swab* estéril da vagina cranial podem ser úteis para piometras de cérvice aberta tratadas clinicamente, porém as bactérias vaginais podem ser diferentes daquelas do útero. A importância clínica de amostras bacterianas obtidas da bursa ovariana não está clara. Essas amostras podem ser positivas em cadelas saudáveis e naquelas com mucometra. Ainda, apenas cerca de metade das amostras bacterianas da bursa ovariana de cadelas com piometra foi a mesma daquela recuperada do útero infeccionado.[38]

Urinálise

Pode ocorrer infecção do trato urinário (ITU) simultaneamente à piometra, com isolados bacterianos idênticos (ver Capítulo 330).[39,40] Após o tratamento cirúrgico da piometra, a ITU costuma se resolver de maneira espontânea. A cistocentese não é recomendada a cadelas com piometra em razão do risco de perfuração do útero purulento, mas pode ser realizada no intraoperatório de maneira controlada. Proteinúria pode ser vista em algumas cadelas em razão da deposição de imunocomplexos nos glomérulos, mas, em geral, se resolve com a resolução da condição.[8] A densidade urinária pode estar normal, diminuída ou aumentada, dependendo da endotoxemia, do estado de hidratação, dos efeitos da interferência de *E. coli* com ação do ADH em nível tubular renal e da presença de ITU.

TRATAMENTO

Estabilização inicial

A cadela ou gata com piometra pode necessitar de tratamento emergencial antes ou durante o manejo cirúrgico, incluindo terapia com fluidos (ver Capítulo 129) e tratamento da acidose (ver Capítulo 128), distúrbios eletrolíticos (ver Capítulos 67 a 69) e hipoglicemia (ver Capítulo 62). A endotoxemia é abordada com fluidoterapia agressiva (ver Capítulo 146). A terapia

antimicrobiana deve ser direcionada contra a *E. coli*, sendo a amoxicilina eficaz em 90% dos casos (ver Capítulo 161).[37] Se for observada resistência à amoxicilina no teste de sensibilidade, deve-se escolher um antibiótico apropriado diferente. Os antimicrobianos não são recomendados para cadelas e gatas estáveis, desde que a origem da infecção seja removida cirurgicamente (ovário-histerectomia). Uma vez que 15% das cadelas com piometra apresentaram hemocultura positiva, todas aquelas com sinais clínicos de septicemia e febre devem ser tratadas com antimicrobianos no perioperatório.[41] Em casos de peritonite séptica decorrente do vazamento de pus para o abdome (ver Capítulo 279), deve-se continuar com os antimicrobianos por 10 dias. Nos outros casos, eles não são administrados ou, então, interrompidos após a cirurgia.

A gravidade da doença correlaciona-se com o nível de toxinas bacterianas que causam sinais clínicos, sendo a fluidoterapia adequada um componente essencial do tratamento. Se as cadelas apresentarem taquiarritmia ventricular concomitante, a incitação de anormalidades deve ser manejada e o tratamento antiarrítmico considerado (ver Capítulo 248). Em cadelas tratadas clinicamente, os antimicrobianos são administrados até que o útero pareça normal à ultrassonografia, geralmente após cerca de 3 semanas. A terapia antimicrobiana pode agravar a endotoxemia, já que os lipopolissacarídeos são liberados quando da morte das bactérias,[42] daí a importância do monitoramento constante e da fluidoterapia adequada.

Tratamento clínico

Histórico e seleção de caso

A cirurgia é o tratamento de eleição para a piometra. O tratamento clínico para piometra é recomendado apenas a cadelas reprodutoras estáveis sem sinais de sepse, endotoxemia, hipotermia ou febre (Figura 316.3). Além disso, apenas aquelas sem disfunção hepática ou renal devem ser tratadas clinicamente. É extremamente importante monitorar de perto esses animais durante o tratamento, já que eles podem desenvolver peritonite ou endotoxemia. Cadelas com a cérvice fechada devem ser tratadas cirurgicamente, apesar de algumas recomendações contrárias.[43,44] Antes de recomendar o tratamento clínico, deve-se considerar o risco elevado de piometra na prole da cadela sob tratamento. Provavelmente existem fatores genéticos para o desenvolvimento dessa doença, já que algumas raças são conhecidas por serem mais predispostas a ela (ver anteriormente).

O prognóstico após o tratamento clínico depende da existência e da gravidade da metrite, se a cérvice estava fechada ou aberta e da ocorrência de cistos cervicais ou endometriais. As cadelas têm maior probabilidade de emprenhar após o tratamento se tiverem 5 anos ou menos.[44,45] É importante cobrir essas cadelas no primeiro ou segundo estro após o término do tratamento clínico. A terapia antimicrobiana é administrada simultaneamente e deve se basear na cultura vaginal obtida com um *swab* estéril. A ultrassonografia é usada para avaliar os efeitos do tratamento clínico semanalmente (Tabela 316.1).

Prostaglandinas

As prostaglandinas estimulam a dilatação cervical e aumentam a atividade miometrial, o que leva à expulsão de conteúdo uterino. Depois da administração de prostaglandinas várias vezes, dá-se a lise dos corpos lúteos, que são a única fonte de progesterona e, à medida que ocorre a lise, as concentrações de progesterona declinam a níveis basais (anestro) (ver Capítulo 312). As prostaglandinas sintéticas causam menos reações adversas, mas podem ser menos eficazes do que as prostaglandinas naturais.[44] Para diminuir os efeitos adversos destas, podem-se usar doses mais baixas, com o aumento gradual delas (ver Tabela 316.1).[46] Dependendo do protocolo, podem ser recomendadas tanto quanto 5 injeções diárias.[1]

Os efeitos colaterais das prostaglandinas podem ser moderados a graves e incluem respiração ofegante, náuseas, êmese,

CAPÍTULO 316 • Piometra e Hiperplasia Endometrial Cística

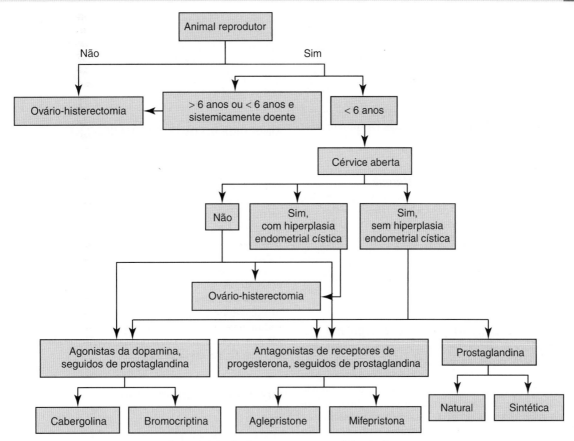

Figura 316.3 Algoritmo para tratamento clínico da piometra.

Tabela 316.1 Protocolos de tratamento clínico em cadelas e gatas diagnosticadas com piometra.

TRATAMENTO CLÍNICO	DOSE (INJEÇÕES SC)	EFEITO	REFERÊNCIA
PGF2-alfa natural (dinoprostona)	Dia 1: 0,1 mg/kg a cada 24 h Dia 2: 0,2 mg/kg a cada 24 h Dias 3 a 7: 0,25 mg/kg a cada 24 h Gata: Dias 1 a 3 (5): 0,1 ou 0,25 mg/kg a cada 12 ou 24 h	64 a 100% de sucesso, dependendo da duração do tratamento Gata: 95% de sucesso	8, 22
PGF2-alfa sintética (cloprostenol)	Dias 1 a 7: 1 a 2,5 µg/kg × 1 Gata: Dias 1 a 3: 5 µg/kg a cada 24 h	75 a 90% de sucesso, dependendo da duração do tratamento 5/5 gatas saudáveis	63, 64
Bloqueador de receptores de progesterona (aglepristone)	Dias 1, 2 e 7/8: 10 mg/kg a cada 24 h Dias 1 e 2, 7 e 8: 10 mg/kg a cada 24 h Gata: Dias 1, 2, 7, 14: 10 mg/kg a cada 24 h	93% de sucesso 10% de reincidência 75% de sucesso 48% de reincidência 9/10 gatas saudáveis	49 a 51
Combinação: aglepristone (A) e cloprostenol (C)	A: Dias 1, 2 e 8: 10 mg/kg a cada 24 h C: Dias 3 a 7: 1 µg/kg a cada 24 h C: Dias 3, 5, 8, 10, 12: 1 µg/kg a cada 24 h Piometra com cérvice aberta e fechada	85% de sucesso 13 a 20% de reincidência em 1 ano	43, 52

Todas as injeções são administradas por via subcutânea (SC).

diarreia e salivação. Para reduzir o risco de anorexia e náuseas, as prostaglandinas devem ser administradas antes da alimentação. Sempre há risco de ruptura uterina, especialmente em uma piometra de cérvice fechada. A cadela ou gata medicada deve ser mantida na clínica pelo menos 4 horas após o tratamento, mas pode ficar em casa durante a noite entre as injeções.[8] A recidiva após o tratamento é comum; em um estudo, 4 de 10 cadelas tratadas desenvolveram piometra após o estro subsequente.[47] Em gatas, as prostaglandinas têm sido usadas com sucesso no tratamento da piometra e são consideradas uma alternativa à cirurgia. Oitenta e um por cento daquelas tratadas gestaram uma ninhada após um tratamento bem-sucedido.[22] Curiosamente, a prostaglandina E (misoprostol), administrada por via intravaginal, tem sido utilizada no tratamento da piometra em cadelas, já que induz o relaxamento da cérvice.[48]

Bloqueador de receptores de progesterona (aglepristone)

Uma vez que o aglepristone pode abrir a cérvice fechada, ele é usado para o tratamento de gestação indesejada em cadelas e gatas, assim como para a piometra nesses animais.[49-51]

Esse produto não está disponível comercialmente nos EUA ou no Canadá, mas é usado na Europa. Os efeitos adversos são menos graves do que os com prostaglandinas e incluem inquietação, perda de apetite, diarreia e cólicas abdominais. A taxa de sucesso em cadelas é de aproximadamente 75% para recuperação tanto a longo prazo quanto da fertilidade; também foi relatado sucesso quando empregado em gatas.[43,49,51] O risco de recidiva de piometra é maior em cadelas com cistos ovarianos e/ou cistos endometriais.[50] As cadelas e gatas costumam ficar em casa entre as injeções.

Combinação de prostaglandinas e bloqueadores de receptores de progesterona

A combinação desses fármacos diminui os efeitos adversos e melhora os resultados, com 84% das cadelas clinicamente saudáveis após o tratamento fazendo uso de um protocolo que incluiu ambos os agentes.[52] A prostaglandina é um agente uterotônico mais eficaz, resultando em diminuição mais rápida do diâmetro luminal e da progesterona em comparação ao uso isolado do aglepristone. Quando o cloprostenol é administrado em conjunto com o aglepristone, uma dose baixa é usada com pouco ou nenhum efeito colateral (1 µg/kg).[44]

Agonistas da dopamina (prostaglandina, cabergolina)

Esses agentes reduzem rapidamente a concentração plasmática de progesterona em razão da luteólise rápida[53,54] provocada clinicamente, que pode ser usada para induzir o parto e para tratar a piometra. O efeito é esperado em 48 horas após o início tratamento, que inclui prostaglandinas, prostaglandinas e bloqueadores de receptores de progesterona ou prostaglandinas e agonistas da dopamina. Se o efeito do tratamento clínico for malsucedido, deve-se recomendar a ovário-histerectomia.

Drenagem transcervical

A drenagem do útero doente foi realizada com cateteres colocados no lúmen uterino através da cérvice até a vagina.[55] O uso de cateterismo endoscópico transcervical para diagnóstico, inseminação artificial ou drenagem uterina tem sido sugerido para cadelas e gatas, mas na piometra é incomum.[56-58]

Tratamento cirúrgico: ovário-histerectomia

Visão geral

A ovário-histerectomia é o tratamento recomendado para a piometra. Após a estabilização pré-operatória, a cirurgia é realizada assim que o animal estiver estável. Em casos de septicemia decorrente da infecção uterina, a cirurgia deve ser realizada rapidamente e, portanto, a fluidoterapia agressiva é necessária (ver Capítulos 129 e 146). Se o útero estiver rompido, o abdome é lavado com 200 a 300 mℓ/kg de fluido, com a recomendação de drenagem fechada por sucção (ver Capítulo 279). Em cadelas e gatas, a sobrevivência após lavagem peritoneal aberta e drenagem fechada por sucção é de 70% na peritonite séptica.[59,60] A drenagem fechada por sucção é fácil de usar e não requer anestesia repetida, como no caso da lavagem peritoneal aberta.

Complicações cirúrgicas/anestésicas

As complicações pós-operatórias incluem hemorragia, peritonite, infecções de feridas, fístulas no trato e questões relacionadas com a anestesia. Em cadelas com síndrome da resposta inflamatória sistêmica e sepse, como pode haver o desenvolvimento de arritmias ventriculares, o eletrocardiograma deve ser monitorado de perto no período pós-operatório. Pode ocorrer sepse pós-operatória, e tanto a proteína C reativa quanto o IGF-1 podem ser marcadores úteis para avaliação no período pós-operatório.[29,32]

SÍNDROME DO OVÁRIO REMANESCENTE

A síndrome do ovário remanescente pode ocorrer após a ovário-histerectomia e é resultado da remoção cirúrgica malsucedida de todo o tecido ovariano (ver Capítulo 319). Se, apesar da ovário-histerectomia, o animal começar a mostrar comportamento de estro, deve-se realizar ultrassonografia abdominal em busca de tecido ovariano. Também são recomendados ensaios hormonais para estradiol, progesterona e hormônio luteinizante, em conjunto com esfregaços vaginais para verificar a existência de células cornificadas e, assim, confirmar tecido ovariano remanescente. A síndrome do ovário remanescente pode ser mais comum em cadelas, já que o tecido ovariano está localizado mais profundamente e é mais difícil de ser alcançado durante o procedimento cirúrgico em comparação às gatas. Em cadelas e gatas, o tecido ovariano remanescente pode ser tratado por cirurgia aberta ou laparoscopia.[61]

PIOMETRA DE COTO UTERINO

Em cadelas e gatas, a piometra de coto uterino tem apresentação clínica semelhante à piometra, com exceção da ovário-histerectomia, realizada anteriormente. O tecido ovariano remanescente é comumente visto no abdome após cirurgia em casos de piometra de coto. A ultrassonografia pode ser utilizada para diagnóstico e revelará áreas de preenchimento de fluido na região cervical. O procedimento é cirúrgico e inclui o tratamento do abscesso cervical, bem como a remoção de quaisquer restos de tecido ovariano.[62]

PROGNÓSTICO

Cadelas e gatas com HEC ou piometra de baixo grau sem síndrome da resposta inflamatória sistêmica ou sepse apresentam bom prognóstico após a ovário-histerectomia. O diagnóstico é reservado a animais gravemente doentes, mas a maioria deles sobrevive com fluidoterapia agressiva pré-operatória e intervenção cirúrgica rápida. Após tratamento clínico em animais estáveis sem sinais de sepse, endotoxemia, hipotermia ou febre, o prognóstico é bom e as chances de recuperação da fertilidade são consideradas boas, especialmente em animais mais jovens.[1] No entanto, o risco de recidiva é alto após o tratamento clínico.

REFERÊNCIAS BIBLIOGRÁFICAS

As referências bibliográficas deste capítulo se encontram online no Ambiente de Aprendizagem.

CAPÍTULO 317

Outras Causas Infecciosas de Infertilidade e Subfertilidade em Cães e Gatos

Sophie Alexandra Grundy

INTRODUÇÃO

Geralmente, as doenças infecciosas podem ser identificadas por meio de cultura, reação em cadeia da polimerase (PCR) ou histologia (ver Capítulo 207). Os obstáculos para a obtenção de um diagnóstico definitivo de doenças infecciosas dos órgãos reprodutivos na prática clínica incluem a falta de amostra, o custo e as interpretações desafiadoras. Portanto, é difícil de estabelecer o verdadeiro impacto das doenças infecciosas no desempenho reprodutivo canino e felino. As técnicas de PCR aumentam a disponibilidade de triagem diagnóstica de multi-patógenos com custo reduzido, mas a coleta de amostras, a seleção do local da amostra e o controle de qualidade do laboratório têm potencial para impactar os valores preditivos positivos e negativos. Os resultados podem ser confusos, pois os patógenos reprodutivos também podem ser considerados "microbiota normal" em animais de estimação saudáveis. Painéis de diagnóstico que combinam cultura, PCR e histopatologia fornecem uma oportunidade para entender a verdadeira relação entre doenças infecciosas e desempenho reprodutivo em cães e gatos. A educação do cliente sobre as opções de teste disponíveis e os requisitos da amostra são componentes essenciais do processo de diagnóstico, pois normalmente são os clientes que têm maior acesso aos tipos de tecido, como a placenta ou um feto abortado.

COLETA, TIPO E LOCAL DE AMOSTRA

Existem 4 principais categorias de patógenos reprodutivos infecciosos: bacterianos, virais, protozoários e fúngicos. Qualquer um desses pode causar "tempestades" semelhantes de falha reprodutiva em uma população reprodutiva. Todos os casos de perda reprodutiva beneficiam-se da coleta adequada de amostras para cultura, histologia e PCR.[1] O PCR, de grande valor diagnóstico para identificação de doenças infecciosas, permite a identificação rápida de patógenos e é altamente sensível. Como resultado, é importante considerar os protocolos de coleta de amostra. Muitos patógenos reprodutivos são onipresentes ambientalmente e encontrados normalmente nas microbiotas oral, genital, urinária ou gastrintestinal. A interpretação deve ser feita de acordo com o contexto do ambiente, o tipo de amostra, a localização e o método de coleta. Todas as amostras para PCR e cultura devem ser coletadas da maneira mais estéril possível para evitar contaminação. Aplicadores com ponta de algodão com haste de plástico, luvas, instrumentos estéreis e uma superfície limpa são recomendados ao coletar as amostras. As amostras devem ser refrigeradas até o envio.[2]

O tecido placentário pode ser extremamente útil para compreender as questões reprodutivas em cadelas e gatas gestantes. A placenta pode ser considerada o guardião da imunidade do feto em desenvolvimento. Ao coletar a amostra da placenta, deve ser feita uma preparação de lâmina para o rastreamento imediato de *Brucella canis* e *Campylobacter jejuni*. Devem ser coletadas duas amostras do tecido: uma para fixação em formalina e outra para PCR. Se disponíveis, as amostras de rim, fígado, baço e pulmão fetais também devem ser coletadas em duplicata: uma para fixação de formalina e outra para PCR. Uma amostra do fígado fetal ou um esfregaço do abdome são ideais para cultura bacteriana. Devem ser coletados da mãe sangue total com EDTA e soro, além de um esfregaço vaginal para PCR. As amostras de PCR devem ser mantidas refrigeradas.

Ao pesquisar infecções reprodutivas por patógenos em machos, devem-se realizar a cultura do sêmen e, preferencialmente, a contagem de colônias comparada à cultura uretral (ver Capítulo 318). Amostras do ejaculado também podem ser enviadas para triagem de doenças infecciosas por PCR. Várias combinações de cultura, PCR e histologia estão disponíveis em laboratórios particulares e universitários. Esses painéis ou pacotes de testes combinados oferecem uma opção econômica para a triagem de vários patógenos.

CULTURA VAGINAL PRÉ-COBERTURA

Microbiota normal

É comum ser solicitada a realização de uma cultura bacteriana da abóbada vaginal como uma triagem pré-cobertura. Há uma tendência incorreta de presumir que uma cultura vaginal positiva é anormal e indicativa de um útero infectado e anormal.[3-11] Alguns criadores acreditam incorretamente que o canal vaginal normal é estéril e exigem uma cultura pré-cobertura negativa antes de permitir a cobertura natural. No entanto, o canal vaginal normal tem populações de bactérias aeróbias e anaeróbias, e 60 a 100% das cadelas saudáveis têm culturas vaginais positivas.[3-10] Considerando a exposição anatômica a bactérias orais e gastrintestinais, os isolados vaginais comuns de cadelas incluem *Enterococcus faecalis*, *Escherichia coli*, *Klebsiella pneumoniae*, *Proteus mirabilis*, *Pasteurella multocida* e bactérias associadas à pele (*Streptococcus* spp. e *Staphylococci* spp.) (Tabela 317.1).[3-10]

Embora as culturas bacterianas sejam normalmente limitadas a aeróbios, os anaeróbios também estão incluídos entre a flora vaginal normal (*Bacteroides* spp., *Peptostreptococcus* spp., *Clostridium* spp.).[9] Embora existam frequências relativas ligeiramente diferentes para cada isolado, os "organismos normais" são consistentes através dos estudos.[3-10] Os tipos de bactérias isoladas por cadela saudável são relativamente estáveis durante o ciclo reprodutivo, mas a contagem e o número de isolados tendem a aumentar durante o proestro e o estro.[4,5] Durante o proestro e o estro, foi demonstrado que a população bacteriana uterina reflete a população bacteriana vaginal, provavelmente devido ao relaxamento da cérvice e às alterações hormonais que diminuem as respostas imunes uterinas.[4] Durante o diestro e o anestro, as populações bacterianas uterinas geralmente desaparecem, tornando-se raro isolar bactérias durante esse período.[4,8]

SEÇÃO 22 • Doenças Reprodutivas

Tabela 317.1 Frequência de isolados bacterianos vaginais em cadelas saudáveis em estudos selecionados, 1978-2012.

ORGANISMO BACTERIANO	PORCENTAGEM POSITIVA DE ISOLADOS BACTERIANOS (CADELAS SAUDÁVEIS) POR ESTUDO						
	Ling, 1978[10]	Odsbaldiston, 1972[11]	Hirsch, 1977[3]	Olson, 1978[6]	Baba, 1983[9]	Bjurstrom, 1992[8]	Gropetti, 2012[5]
Arcanobacterium pyogenes							2,9
Bacillus spp.				3,7			
Bacteroidaceae spp.		10			55		
Corynebacterium spp.	35		6	2,5		40,7	
Enterococci		10				44,1	
Enterococcus faecalis			4				23,5
Escherichia coli	25	50	22	18,5	23	84,7	2,9
Haemophilus		10					
Klebsiella pneumoniae							2,9
Moraxella spp.	10						
Mycoplasma spp.	30				43	59,3	
Pasteurella spp. *Pasteurella multocida*	5			9,9	34	67,8 98,3	8,8
Peptococcaceae (*Clostridium* spp.)					27		
Proteus spp.	5*		6*	4,9	9	25,4*	2,9*
Pseudomonas aeruginosa	5	10	2				
Staphylococci spp. coagulase-positiva	70	10	13	6,2	20		2,9
Staphylococci spp. coagulase-negativa	5		6	6,2	4	22,0	
Streptococcus spp.		10			52		2,9
Beta-hemolítico	35		9	14,8	89,8		20,6
Streptococci "viridans"	20		14	13,6		55,9	26,4

*Proteus mirabilis. As bactérias em linhas sombreadas indicam que são isoladas com maior frequência em todos os estudos.

Cultura vaginal durante proestro e estro

Frequentemente são levantadas preocupações específicas com relação a culturas positivas de *E. coli* ou *Streptococcus* spp., pois estão comumente associadas a piometra, mastite e septicemia neonatal. No entanto, a grande maioria das culturas vaginais de cadelas saudáveis é positiva para *E. coli*.[4,6,8,12] Um estudo associou cultura vaginal positiva para *Streptococcus* spp. no proestro à *diminuição do risco* de infecção uterina durante o diestro.[5]

Com anos de suporte da literatura, não há evidências que sustentem a cultura de rotina ou o tratamento com antibióticos de uma cadela assintomática com uma cultura vaginal positiva pré-cobertura. Estudos futuros quantificando os níveis microbianos da microbiota vaginal normal podem ser usados para definir as populações bacterianas vaginais patogênicas. Uma vez que a citologia vaginal é frequentemente avaliada durante o proestro de cadelas (ver Capítulos 119 e 312) e normalmente revela um grande número de bactérias ou bactérias fagocitadas, os tutores podem solicitar tratamento para essas bactérias. No entanto, não há correlação entre bactérias vaginais (fagocitadas ou não), neutrófilos vaginais e fertilidade em cadelas assintomáticas.[5] As bactérias no canal vaginal são normais e as bactérias observadas citologicamente não são razões válidas para o tratamento antimicrobiano durante o proestro. Os tutores devem ser informados de que a maioria das cadelas submetidas a culturas vaginais pré-cobertura está em proestro ou estro, momento em que se *espera* que os resultados sejam positivos. Embora possa

haver pressão dos proprietários da cadela ou do cão reprodutor para tratar uma cadela com cultura vaginal positiva com antibióticos antes da cobertura, deve-se também observar a crescente evidência de que o uso indiscriminado de antimicrobianos em cadelas reprodutoras está correlacionado à indução de bactérias resistentes que podem alterar a microbiota vaginal e promover o crescimento de populações de bactérias patogênicas. Isso coloca canis e neonatos em maior risco e não melhora o desempenho reprodutivo.[13-15] Quando uma cadela com cultura positiva pré-cobertura deve ser tratada? Como regra geral, o tratamento durante o proestro deve ser considerado para uma cadela que exibe uma secreção vaginal claramente anormal e com crescimento significativo de uma única espécie bacteriana normal pura ou isolado bacteriano atípico.

CULTURA E SECREÇÃO VAGINAL

As culturas bacterianas da secreção vaginal geralmente diferem da microbiota normal apenas no que diz respeito ao número de bactérias isoladas.[3] Em cadelas ou gatas sintomáticas, o tratamento é recomendado para uma única bactéria isolada presente em números elevados, normalmente de 3+ a 4+ em uma escala de 4 pontos.[3,16] A escolha do antimicrobiano deve ser feita levando-se em consideração a sensibilidade e a concentração inibitória mínima (CIM).

MYCOPLASMA E UREAPLASMA

Culturas vaginais positivas para *Mycoplasma* são comuns em cadelas e não têm importância clínica no que diz respeito à fertilidade. Em cães reprodutores, entretanto, a cultura positiva de *Mycoplasma pode* estar associada à infertilidade se a contagem de cultura quantificada do sêmen for 2 log$_{10}$[a] vezes maior do que a da uretra.[22] Muitos estudos que avaliaram culturas vaginais caninas não comentam sobre *Mycoplasma*. *Mycoplasma* spp. não crescem facilmente em condições de cultura aeróbia padrão.[4-6,17] Quando avaliadas especificamente, as taxas de cultura vaginal de *Mycoplasma* e *Ureaplasma* positivas em cadelas saudáveis são altas, como 88 e 50%, respectivamente; quando presente, o *Ureaplasma* está geralmente associado ao *Mycoplasma*.[18-20] Em um estudo, as taxas de cultura vaginal positiva para *Ureaplasma* foram maiores em cadelas com secreção vaginal (75%), mas não houve relação significativa entre *Mycoplasma*, *Ureaplasma* e fertilidade.[19] Setenta e dois por cento a 84% das amostras de sêmen de cães reprodutores saudáveis foram positivas na cultura para *Mycoplasma*.[19] Embora presente em alguns casos de orquite canina, o *Mycoplasma* não é isolado com maior frequência em cães inférteis.[17,19,21] Geralmente, *Ureaplasma* não está presente no prepúcio ou sêmen de machos férteis, mas é encontrado em cerca de 70% dos machos inférteis, comumente isolado em associação com *Mycoplasma*.[19] Tanto para a cadela quanto para o cão, *Mycoplasma canis* é o isolado mais frequente. Nos machos, o *Mycoplasma cynos* também é observado.[19] As fêmeas geralmente têm várias espécies identificadas.[18-20] A avaliação de sêmen simultânea é recomendada.

CAMPYLOBACTER JEJUNI

Campylobacter jejuni foi relatado em associação ao aborto na cadela.[23-25] Em todos os casos, a característica clássica é o aborto tardio ou a morte fetal intrauterina cerca de 1 semana antes da data prevista para o parto. As cadelas também podem apresentar secreção vaginal hemorrágica.[23-25] Ninhadas inteiras podem ser abortadas, mas o parto parcial de ninhadas vivas também é relatado. Como os fetos ainda não estão a termo, eles podem nascer vivos, mas não são viáveis com menos de 61 (fêmeas) ou 62 (machos) dias de gestação com o dia 0 definido pelo pico de hormônio luteinizante.[26] Um diferencial importante para essa apresentação clínica é *Brucella canis* (ver Capítulo 213), a principal causa de aborto bacteriano em cães. Deve-se usar equipamento de proteção individual na avaliação desses casos, devido ao potencial zoonótico de ambos os organismos. O diagnóstico é baseado na cultura bacteriana positiva ou no PCR positivo, da placenta *e* fígado fetal, ou pulmão.[23-25] O tratamento bem-sucedido é raro.

LEPTOSPIROSE

Organismos da leptospira induzem inflamação uterina acentuada e o aborto é o sinal reprodutivo mais comum de infecção por leptospira na cadela.[27,28] Há retorno à fertilidade após o tratamento bem-sucedido. Em cães reprodutores, a vasculite induzida por leptospirose pode causar ruptura da barreira hematotesticular e qualquer cão reprodutor diagnosticado com leptospirose deve ter o sêmen avaliado inicialmente 65 dias após a recuperação para avaliar o potencial reprodutivo (ver Capítulo 217).

OUTRAS BACTÉRIAS

Tanto a *Salmonella* quanto a *Listeria* são relatadas como causa de doenças do trato reprodutivo na cadela e na gata. A *Salmonella* é causa incomum de perda reprodutiva e está mais frequentemente associada a doenças sistêmicas.[29] A *Listeria* foi relatada, na literatura, como causa de aborto, mas é considerada um patógeno incomum.[30] *Bartonella* spp. têm sido associadas a perdas reprodutivas em condições experimentais, mas isso é difícil de provar em casos clínicos devido às dificuldades para isolar o organismo (ver Capítulos 215 e 216).[31]

PATÓGENOS VIRAIS

Os patógenos virais são uma consideração importante ao avaliar as perdas reprodutivas na cadela e na gata, pois podem atravessar a placenta, infectar o embrião ou o feto, além de debilitar a mãe.[32] Muitas infecções virais podem ser confirmadas por PCR em amostras de tecido em combinação com histologia. Para uma discussão aprofundada dos principais patógenos virais, o leitor deve consultar as discussões individuais na seção de doenças infecciosas (ver Capítulos 222 a 225 e 229).

Embora o herpes-vírus (ver Capítulos 227 e 228) esteja sendo revisto, vale destacar que o impacto reprodutivo do herpes-vírus canino (HVC) é extremamente difícil de definir como resultado de sua latência, baixa imunogenicidade, produção de anticorpos de curta duração e transitória excreção viral.[33] As flutuações dos hormônios reprodutivos parecem alterar a reativação viral, mas não está claro como isso afeta o curso da doença clínica.[33,34] De fato, dado que não há diferença na titulação de anticorpos entre cadelas saudáveis e aquelas com anormalidades reprodutivas, além de taxas de recuperação zero de PCR vaginal em canis com doença endêmica, a perda reprodutiva devido ao HVC é extremamente difícil de documentar, a menos que esteja associada à perda neonatal.[33-35] Quando disponível, a vacinação é recomendada 10 dias após a cobertura e novamente 6 semanas depois, pois acredita-se que títulos mais elevados de anticorpos no diestro podem proteger contra a falha reprodutiva.[33,36] Foi descrito um tratamento médico bem-sucedido de HVC neonatal usando aciclovir (ver Capítulo 162).[37]

PATÓGENOS PROTOZOÁRIOS

O *Toxoplasma* pode estar associado à perda reprodutiva na gata principalmente devido aos efeitos sistêmicos da doença na mãe.[12] Sabe-se que a transmissão transplacentária de *Neospora* ocorre na cadela, mas o impacto desse organismo no desempenho reprodutivo não é claro.[12] Foi relatado um único caso de aborto associado a *Leishmania* na literatura.[38] O leitor é encaminhado para o Capítulo 221 para uma discussão aprofundada da doença protozoária.

REFERÊNCIAS BIBLIOGRÁFICAS

As referências bibliográficas deste capítulo se encontram online no Ambiente de Aprendizagem.

---

[a]2 log$_{10}$ refere-se a uma diferença de 100 vezes entre a contagem microbiana quantificada ou uma diferença de 99% na população bacteriana.

CAPÍTULO 318

Exame de Saúde Reprodutiva e Distúrbios de Reprodução em Cães Machos

Gary C.W. England e Lúcia Daniel Machado da Silva

EXAME DA SAÚDE REPRODUTIVA

Visão geral

O exame de saúde reprodutiva (ESR) é comumente realizado para acessar a fertilidade em cães jovens antes do acasalamento, monitorar a fertilidade durante a vida reprodutiva, garantir fertilidade em animais com idade avançada, investigar possíveis infertilidades, monitorar a recuperação depois da doença reprodutiva, e como parte da preservação do sêmen e programa de inseminação artificial. Realizar o ESR também pode ser importante antes da compra.

Comportamento e saúde

Veterinários comumente focam no trato reprodutivo quando estão realizando o ESR. Outros acessos de saúde geral e temperamento devem ser incluídos também. Alguns podem recomendar testes genéticos ou outros. Isso requer conhecimento de muitos problemas comportamentais relevantes e condições que podem ser reavaliadas em outras seções deste livro ou *sites* úteis, como o Centro de Informações de Saúde Canina (*www.caninehealthinfo.org*), uma base de dados centralizada em saúde canina patrocinada pela Fundação Ortopédica para Animais.

Exame da genitália externa e interna

O pênis

O pênis e o prepúcio devem ser examinados para garantir a escolha por animais que possam reproduzir normalmente e com ausência de doenças. O exame é mais bem realizado antes da introdução da cadela para rufiação. Baixo volume de descarga prepucial mucopurulenta é comum e normal. O prepúcio deve cobrir o comprimento do pênis, e o pênis deve ser relativamente fácil de ser exposto pelo prepúcio; em cães experientes isso pode iniciar a ejaculação que deve ser antecipada para que o sêmen possa ser coletado se isso ocorrer. A pele do pênis deve ser macia, sem lesões vesiculares e papulares. No entanto, nódulos linfoides que aparecem na base do pênis são comuns e normais, especialmente quando há descarga prepucial. O pênis pode ser palpado através do prepúcio e a palpação deve ser suave e não dolorosa. A uretra pode ser palpada caudalmente ao longo do períneo até o ânus.

O escroto e os testículos

A pele do escroto não deve ter lesões. O espessamento de pele ou a evidência de que o animal está com coceira podem indicar lesão escrotal (testicular) prévia. O pescoço do escroto deve ser palpado para permitir a identificação do canal deferente e confirmar a ausência de hérnia inguinal. Os testículos são posicionados quase horizontalmente, e um pode estar posicionado levemente cranial. Eles devem ser móveis dentro do escroto, de tamanho similar e firmes, mas não duros. O tamanho dos testículos está relacionado com a massa corporal; por exemplo, cada testículo em um cão de 15 kg saudável é aproximadamente 3 × 2 × 1,5 cm. O corpo do epidídimo corre ao longo da superfície dorsal dos testículos, e a cauda do epidídimo está no polo caudal.

A próstata

A próstata é a glândula acessória única. Se normal, ela pode ser facilmente palpada pelo reto como uma estrutura dividida em dois lobos simétricos (cada um de 2 cm de diâmetro aproximadamente) por um sulco longitudinal central. A próstata deve ter uma textura firme, não dolorosa e móvel dentro da pelve.

Avaliação da libido

O comportamento do macho quando introduzido à fêmea no estro e a cobertura são frequentemente avaliados no ESR. Isso pode oferecer informações úteis quanto à "infertilidade" causada por problemas comportamentais, experiências negativas prévias, ou dor ao coito. Cães machos e fêmeas sadios brincam quando são apresentados pela primeira vez, ocasionalmente incluindo a monta da fêmea. Nesse momento o cão pode ejacular um pequeno volume de líquido transparente. Essa é a primeira fração do ejaculado e não contém espermatozoides. O cão vai continuar a montar, fazer movimentos de propulsão e desmontar até que sua posição permita que o pênis penetre a vagina. Após a penetração, o cão atinge a ereção completa, continua os movimentos de propulsão e a segunda fração do ejaculado (rica em espermatozoides) é ejetada. Uma vez que os movimentos de propulsão tenham diminuído, o cão faz um giro de 180° e desmonta enquanto o pênis não muda de posição, mantendo-se dentro da vagina. O cão e a cadela agora ficam em pé rabo a rabo (isso é chamado de laço copulatório) enquanto a terceira fração (prostática) é ejaculada. O laço dura em média 20 minutos, mas varia consideravelmente entre cães e podem ser curtos, cerca de 5 minutos, ou mais longos, mais de 60 minutos.

Coleta de sêmen e avaliação

Coleta do ejaculado

A coleta de sêmen é simples, amostras podem ser coletadas por estimulação manual do pênis com ou sem uma cadela no cio para rufiar (Vídeo 318.1). O cão primeiro atinge uma ereção parcial e então mostra os movimentos de propulsão durante os quais a primeira e a segunda frações do ejaculado são ejetadas. Quando os movimentos de propulsão finalizam a segunda fração (fração rica) do ejaculado, ela continua sendo ejetada por pouco tempo. A partir de então os cães levantam uma de suas patas traseiras (como no laço copulatório) e é necessário virar o pênis para que gire em uma direção caudal entre os membros posteriores enquanto a terceira fração (prostática) é ejetada. As três frações podem ser coletadas separadamente usando um funil de plástico acoplado diretamente a um tubo. Uma vez que muitos materiais são tóxicos para o espermatozoide canino, todos os tubos, seringas e pipetas devem ser cuidadosamente testados antes do seu uso na rotina. Os equipamentos de coleta devem ser limpos e secos. Após a coleta do sêmen, amostras devem ser mantidas aquecidas, uma vez que a refrigeração pode reduzir a motilidade e dar a falsa impressão de baixa qualidade espermática. Existem inúmeros aspectos da avaliação do sêmen, conforme detalhado a seguir.

Volume, cor, concentração e contagem total de espermatozoides no ejaculado

O volume é medido com o uso de um tubo graduado ou uma pipeta. É importante fazer uma medida acurada do volume da segunda fração para permitir o cálculo da contagem total de espermatozoides. Em um cão de porte médio, os volumes aproximados por fração são cerca de 0,5 a 2 mℓ (primeira fração; normalmente clara e transparente), 0,5 a 1,5 mℓ (segunda fração; normalmente branca ou com uma cor cremosa) e 15 a 20 mℓ (terceira fração; normalmente clara e transparente), embora comumente a terceira fração não seja coletada inteira (Figura 318.1). Exames citológicos do centrifugado e esfregaços corados podem ajudar a estabilizar a natureza de qualquer contaminação.

É comum medir a concentração do sêmen por meio do hemocitômetro. Um pequeno volume da segunda fração é diluída em uma taxa padrão para permitir a contagem espermática. Água destilada com detergente é comumente utilizada como um diluente para matar espermatozoides e prevenir aglomerados. O sêmen diluído é colocado dentro da câmara e o número de espermatozoides é contado; o fator de diluição é então usado para calcular a concentração inicial de espermatozoides. No entanto, o número total de espermatozoides é uma medida mais útil que a concentração. A contagem total de espermatozoides (CTE) é o número total de espermatozoides dentro do ejaculado e é calculado pela multiplicação do volume da segunda fração pela concentração espermática. CTE é mais significativa que a concentração e o volume. Cães normais produzem 300 a 1.000 $\times 10^6$ espermatozoides em cada ejaculado. Uma vez que há um *pool* de espermatozoides armazenado dentro do epidídimo, alguns dos quais são removidos a cada ejaculação, o número de espermatozoides no ejaculado é determinado pelo número de espermatozoides armazenados e a frequência de ejaculados (ejaculações frequentes vão esvaziar o reservatório epididimal). Se coletado diariamente por 4 a 5 dias, o número de espermatozoides presentes no ejaculado é indicado pela produção diária de espermatozoides. Em cães normais, existe uma boa correlação entre produção espermática diária e os volumes dos testículos e a largura do escroto.

Motilidade espermática

A motilidade espermática é comumente avaliada subjetivamente, embora em centros de referência haja um aumento no uso das análises computadorizadas. Para uma avaliação subjetiva, uma gota de sêmen é colocada em uma lâmina de microscopia aquecida, coberta com uma lamínula e mantida a 30 a 35°C. A avaliação em baixas temperaturas pode gerar resultados errôneos.

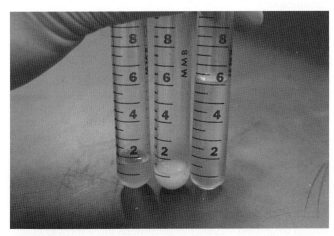

Figura 318.1 Frações do ejaculado canino. A primeira (*esquerda*), originária da glândula prostática, não contém espermatozoides; a segunda (*no meio*) é rica em espermatozoides; e a terceira (*direita*) é novamente originária da próstata e não contém espermatozoides.

A motilidade decresce ao longo do tempo quando a lâmina é deixada na mesa do microscópio (provavelmente devido ao efeito da luz e à queda de temperatura). Amostras devem então ser avaliadas rapidamente. Subjetivamente, a porcentagem de espermatozoides dentro de cada uma das cinco categorias são:
- Categoria 0: não há espermatozoides móveis
- Categoria I: espermatozoides móveis, mas não estão com movimentos progressivos
- Categoria II: espermatozoides móveis, mas com movimentos progressivos fracos
- Categoria III: espermatozoides móveis, com movimentos progressivos moderados
- Categoria IV: espermatozoides móveis, com movimentos progressivos rápidos.

O uso desse critério mostra que cães normais apresentam mais de 70% de espermatozoides na categoria IV e 90% de motilidade total (soma das categorias I-IV).

Morfologia espermática

Um método simples para avaliar a morfologia espermática e a integridade da membrana é o uso da combinação de eosina e nigrosina. O sêmen é diluído 1:5 em um volume base de coloração de nigrosina/eosina e então uma gota é transferida para uma lâmina, um esfregaço é feito seco. Os espermatozoides ficam com silhueta nigrosina azul-roxa; espermatozoides brancos são classificados como vivos (estes espermatozoides têm membranas intactas, o que previne a entrada da eosina para dentro da célula espermática) e espermatozoides rosa são classificados como mortos. Os esfregaços devem ser examinados em um aumento de 100x com óleo de imersão e pelo menos 100 espermatozoides classificados conforme as características de coloração e morfologia. A maioria dos cães férteis tem mais de 60% de espermatozoides vivos e com morfologia normal.

Os espermatozoides normais têm uma aparência típica (Figura 318.2), e uma variedade de métodos é usada para classificar o espermatozoide anormal. É comum a classificação de acordo com as anormalidades ocorridas durante (a) espermatogênese (anormalidades primárias), (b) fase de desenvolvimento epididimal (anormalidades secundárias), ou (c) coleta e processamento (anormalidades terciárias). No entanto, um sistema proposto recentemente descreve as anormalidades dos espermatozoides como sendo compensáveis (anormalidades que impedem que o espermatozoide chegue ao oócito) ou não compensáveis. O termo compensável indica que a anormalidade não impede espermatozoides normais de fertilizarem o oócito; basta ter espermatozoides normais suficientes para que os espermatozoides anormais sejam compensados. Anormalidades compensáveis incluem cabeça disforme, defeitos de cauda, espermatozoides imóveis e imaturos. Outras anormalidades espermáticas são descritas como não compensáveis, uma vez que esses espermatozoides podem alcançar o oócito e desencadear a despolarização oocitária, mas após isso ocorre falha na fertilização ou falha posterior no desenvolvimento embrionário. Dessa maneira, esses espermatozoides efetivamente bloqueiam outros espermatozoides normais de realizarem uma fertilização normal. Grande número de espermatozoides normais não consegue compensar as anormalidades espermáticas presentes. Espermatozoides com cabeça sutilmente disforme ou vacúolos nucleares são típicos de anormalidades não compensáveis. Outros sistemas de classificação usam terminologias que descrevem as mudanças gerais na qualidade do sêmen; por exemplo, oligozoospermia é o termo usado para descrever um ejaculado que contém baixo número de espermatozoides morfologicamente normais. Esse tipo de sistema pode então ser subdividido conforme a descrição de anormalidades predominantes (como de acrossoma, pescoço, peça intermediária, cauda) e a consideração dessas significâncias. Esse método pode não ser aplicável quando existem formas anormais múltiplas em vez de um ou dois tipos predominantes.

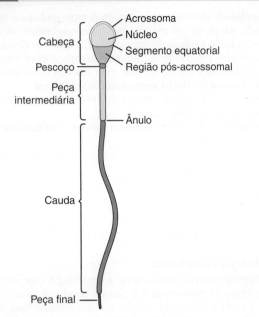

Figura 318.2 Representação esquemática da morfologia do espermatozoide normal.

Outros tipos de células no ejaculado

Os ejaculados deveriam ser avaliados para a identificação da presença de células não espermáticas. Os esfregaços hematológicos comuns podem ser usados em preparações secas ou amostras concentradas pela centrifugação, para ajudar na detecção de condições prostáticas. Isso também pode auxiliar a confirmar azoospermia quando células espermatogênicas podem ser encontradas. O número médio de neutrófilos é comum, em geral originados do prepúcio (Figura 318.3).

Teste úmido hiposmótico

O teste úmido hiposmótico é considerado um teste de integridade da membrana de espermatozoides funcionais. Espermatozoides normais, expostos a um meio hiposmótico, absorvem a água e desenvolvem caudas enroladas/dobradas. Dessa maneira, simplesmente contar a porcentagem de espermatozoides com caudas dobradas quando expostos a um meio hiposmótico pode ser considerado um marco de função de membrana. A maioria das amostras normais apresenta mais de 70% de espermatozoides com caudas dobradas usando esse método.

Ligação espermatozoide-oócito ou ensaio de penetração

Esses testes avaliam a ligação ou penetração do oócito pelo espermatozoide. Um número predeterminado de espermatozoides é incubado com oócitos homólogos ou oócitos de *hamsters* (que permitem a penetração da maioria dos espermatozoides), e o número de oócitos ligados ou penetrados é contado após um tempo específico. Isso permite a avaliação da habilidade de os espermatozoides terem a reação acrossomal, mudarem suas características de motilidade (tornam-se hiper-reativos) e se ligarem para penetrar os oócitos.

Amostras arquivadas

Após as amostras serem avaliadas, é prudente arquivar uma porção para comparação com avaliações futuras. Amostras podem ser preservadas na diluição 1:1 com solução salina tamponada seguida do armazenamento em frasco selado. Isso permite que amostras sejam armazenadas a temperatura ambiente por muitos anos sem mudanças substanciais na morfologia espermática ou nas características de coloração.

Predição da fertilidade

Visão geral

É difícil predizer a fertilidade com precisão por causa da ampla variedade de características seminais vistas em animais férteis. Amplas faixas de normalidade foram descritas (Tabela 318.1) e sêmens dentro desses limites são considerados provavelmente férteis, desde que a libido e a habilidade copulatória estejam normais. Em muitos cães, uma ou mais avaliações podem estar no limite. Se um cão pouco à vontade ejacula uma amostra pobre, é indicado repetir o exame, uma vez que a ejaculação pode ter sido incompleta. Se a amostra está um pouco fora da variação normal, o cão ainda deve ser considerado de fertilidade normal se o regime de cobrição é ajustado (*i. e.*: aumentar a frequência de coberturas em uma janela curta após a ovulação). Quando uma amostra não contém espermatozoides (é azoospérmica), uma segunda amostra deve ser coletada ou uma tentativa feita para estabelecer se a ejaculação de fato ocorreu pela medição da concentração da fosfatase alcalina.

Concentração da fosfatase alcalina seminal

Grandes quantidades de fosfatase alcalina (FA), produzidas pelo epidídimo, estão presentes em ejaculados normais (> 5.000 IU/ℓ). Amostras azoospérmicas com aumento de concentração da FA (5.000 a 20.000 IU/ℓ) são verdadeiramente azoospérmicas, enquanto aquelas com baixas concentrações de FA (< 5.000 IU/ℓ) representam ejaculação incompleta, ejaculação retrógrada ou obstrução de epidídimo ou do canal deferente. Se espermatozoides não são encontrados em coletas repetidas, a urina deve ser avaliada para pesquisa da presença de espermatozoides e, se positiva, o diagnóstico de ejaculação retrógrada deve ser considerado.

Exame ultrassonográfico do trato reprodutivo

Visão geral

O exame ultrassonográfico (US) do trato reprodutivo deve ser um componente de rotina do ESR. O uso do US Doppler colorido e pulsátil pode ser considerado para avaliação da perfusão vascular testicular e prostática. Um pequeno número de estudos descreveu o uso do US com contraste para detecção de desordens reprodutivas.

Ultrassonografia escrotal

O exame do escroto pode ser realizado com o uso de transdutores lineares ou setoriais de alta frequência após aplicação de grande quantidade de gel de US. É prudente não cortar o pelo do escroto, uma vez que isso frequentemente resulta em irritação e autotrauma secundário seguido por lambeduras incessantes. O exame do pescoço do escroto pode ser realizado para eliminar hérnia escrotal. Os testículos e epidídimos são em geral examinados nos planos sagital, transverso e frontal (dorsal). Os epidídimos são mais facilmente identificados usando o plano longitudinal com o

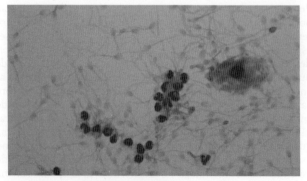

Figura 318.3 Contaminantes no sêmen podem ser identificados em muitos casos usando colorações hematológicas. Aqui aglomerados de neutrófilos do prepúcio são identificados entre grande número de espermatozoides (o espermatozoide não cora bem quando colorações hematológicas são usadas). (*Esta figura se encontra reproduzida em cores no Encarte.*)

CAPÍTULO 318 • Exame de Saúde Reprodutiva e Distúrbios de Reprodução em Cães Machos

Tabela 318.1 Características seminais de cães férteis.

	PROGRESSIVA, CATEGORIA IV, MOTILIDADE (%)	VOLUME DA SEGUNDA FRAÇÃO RICA EM ESPERMATOZOIDES (mℓ)	CONCENTRAÇÃO DE ESPERMATOZOIDES DA SEGUNDA FRAÇÃO ($\times 10^6$/mℓ)	ESPERMATOZOIDES TOTAIS NO EJACULADO ($\times 10^6$)	ESPERMATOZOIDES NORMAIS VIVOS (%)
Média	82	1,2	330	410	74
Variação	40 a 95	0,3 a 3,3	50 a 820	36 a 1.980	50 a 92

transdutor posicionado na superfície ventral dos testículos; dessa maneira, a seção longitudinal tubular do corpo do epidídimo e a aparência triangular da cauda do epidídimo podem ser facilmente identificadas na superfície dorsal dos testículos.

O parênquima testicular normal é relativamente hipoecoico com pontos ecogênicos difusos e regulares, os quais representam uma extensão do mediastino fibroso responsável por suportar o parênquima. O mediastino aparece como uma imagem ecogênica linear que se estende do polo cranial ao caudal quando a imagem é feita no plano longitudinal e como um círculo ecogênico de aproximadamente 2 mm quando a imagem é formada no plano transversal. Sombras acústicas são comuns na região distal do mediastino testicular. Os testículos são limitados pelas túnicas testicular e vaginal, o que parece uma linha única ecogênica, a não ser que haja hidrocele e líquido, o que cria uma linha dupla. Os epidídimos são hipoecoicos e pontilhados quando comparados com o parênquima testicular. Testículos que parecem mais heterogêneos são frequentemente associados à qualidade de sêmen inferior, assim como aqueles que têm uma aparência geral mais hipoecoica ou hiperecoica. O US pode ser usado como uma medida acurada do tamanho testicular e para calcular o volume testicular. Normalmente há boa relação entre volume testicular e tamanho corporal e relação geral entre tamanho testicular e qualidade seminal. O US Doppler pulsátil é utilizado para medir perfusão sanguínea da artéria testicular. Diferenças foram identificadas na comparação entre cães em idade pré-púbere e púbere, assim como cães férteis e inférteis. O Doppler colorido também pode auxiliar na identificação de aumento da perfusão associado a condições patológicas. De maneira similar, US com contraste (técnica em que microbolhas são injetadas dentro das veias) pode ser utilizado para documentar com acurácia a perfusão vascular e destacar as lesões.

PRÓSTATA (VER CAPÍTULO 337)

Avaliação endócrina

A avaliação dos hormônios reprodutivos circulantes é de valor limitado. A administração de hormônio liberador de gonadotrofina exógeno estimula o aumento do hormônio luteinizante (LH) dentro de 30 minutos e aumenta a testosterona em 60 minutos. A administração da gonadotrofina coriônica humana (hCG; atividade semelhante à do LH) resulta no aumento da testosterona. Esses testes são aplicados para detectar a presença de tecido testicular e não são usados para mudanças súbitas na pituitária ou na função testicular. A concentração basal dos hormônios em cães varia consideravelmente ao longo do dia. As concentrações plasmáticas de testosterona em cães saudáveis inteiros são em geral > 4ng/mℓ (14 nmol/ℓ) e cães castrados apresentam concentrações de testosterona < 2 ng/mℓ (7 nmol/ℓ). Cães com espermatogênese prejudicada em geral apresentam resultados normais, assim como cães com criptorquidismo bilateral também. As concentrações do LH e do hormônio folículo estimulante (FSH) variam acentuadamente ao longo do dia e há limitadas informações sobre os valores normais e como eles mudam em várias condições. As concentrações de LH e FSH podem estar aumentadas em cães com problemas na espermatogênese, mas os resultados flutuam.

Pesquisas de infecção bacteriana

Proprietários e criadores podem ter dúvidas sobre pesquisas de rotina de pais e mães sobre patógenos bacterianos venéreos. Em países onde *Brucella canis* é endêmica, a pesquisa por este organismo é crucial antes de ser iniciada a reprodução (ver Capítulo 213). É particularmente importante que as fêmeas sejam avaliadas, uma vez que elas podem ser portadoras assintomáticas. A história pode revelar infecção aguda prévia que originou orquite ou epididimite, as quais, por sua vez, causam sinais sistêmicos de doença, dor, descarga e perda de libido. Infecção crônica pode levar à degeneração testicular, embora em alguns cães a fertilidade seja recuperada após a fase aguda de infecção. Anormalidades espermáticas múltiplas e aglutinação de espermatozoides podem ser detectadas. A *Brucella canis* pode ser isolada do sêmen de cães infectados.

Além da *Brucella canis*, não há evidência de que outra bactéria seja um patógeno venéreo em cães. Todos os cães têm uma microbiota comensal residente e essas bactérias podem mudar. Bactérias comumente isoladas incluem *Streptococcus* hemolítica, outros *Streptococcus*, *Staphylococcus*, *Escherichia coli* e outras. Muitos cães apresentam uma microbiota mista com 2 a 5 diferentes espécies presentes. Pesquisas de rotina são desnecessárias e o uso de antibióticos para bactérias comensais não seguem os guias de melhores práticas.

Pesquisa de vírus

Cães reprodutores podem se infectar com herpes-vírus canino e, com reativação, podem ser notadas no pênis e na superfície do prepúcio lesões vermelhas pequenas e aumentadas, algumas vezes ulceradas. Os vírus podem ser detectados por PCR oferecido por muitos laboratórios comerciais. Vacina contra herpesvírus canino não parece proteger cães da infecção nem a reduzir a recrudescência viral (ver Capítulo 228).

Cariótipo

Anormalidades grosseiras de mau desenvolvimento da genitália podem ser um indicativo de problemas genéticos que podem ser identificados com estudos de cromossomos por sangue EDTA, que pode ser cultivado e examinado. Cães normais possuem 78 cromossomos: 38 pares de autossomos acrocêntricos e 2 cromossomos sexuais metacêntricos.

Aspiração testicular por agulha fina e biopsia

A aspiração por agulha fina (AAF) testicular pode ser útil se houver anormalidades grosseiras testiculares ou se uma lesão focal puder ser vista por US (ver Capítulos 87 e 93). Aspiração guiada por US é particularmente útil para uma coleta precisa de amostra. O cão deve ser sedado antes da colocação da agulha de 20 G ligada a uma seringa para dentro da região de interesse. A biopsia permite a avaliação da espermatogênese e detecção de células neoplásicas e inflamatórias. No entanto, a biopsia é invasiva e pode causar alterações testiculares graves; portanto, não é recomendada.

Avaliação prostática adicional

Métodos adicionais para exame da próstata incluem citologia de líquidos prostáticos, AAF e biopsia (ver Capítulo 111). A primeira e a terceira frações do ejaculado canino são primariamente prostáticas e podem ser coletadas por estimulação manual. Cada fase do ejaculado pode ser coletado separadamente, levado à cultura e avaliado citologicamente. Se um ejaculado não pode ser obtido, o líquido prostático pode ser obtido pela massagem da próstata pela via transretal, enquanto lavados são realizados simultaneamente na uretra prostática com 5 a 10 ml de solução salina. Um cateter uretral pode ser colocado de maneira simples até o nível da glândula prostática e por onde é realizada a sucção para a recuperação de células para o exame citológico. A AAF da próstata pode ser feita pela via transabdominal, especialmente se a glândula for grande. Se a próstata permanece dentro do canal pélvico, a via perineal é requerida (ver Capítulo 337). Ambas as técnicas podem ser acompanhadas do uso do US como guia. A esterase prostática específica canina (EPEC) é uma protease serina encontrada nas células epiteliais prostáticas normais, no líquido prostático e no soro ou plasma. As concentrações da EPEC são altas em cães idosos e podem ser marcadores de hiperplasia prostática benigna (HPB). A HPB é uma mudança normal em decorrência da idade nos cães e frequentemente não apresenta sinais clínicos.

PUBERDADE, FERTILIDADE E DESORDENS CLÍNICAS

Visão geral

As concentrações da testosterona plasmática alcançam níveis normais para adultos com a maturação das células de Leydig após aproximadamente 5 meses de idade. Raças grandes tipicamente demonstram características sexuais secundárias mais tardiamente que raças pequenas. Machos de tamanho médio alcançam a puberdade ao redor de 10 a 12 meses e podem ejacular espermatozoides normais. O número total de espermatozoides no ejaculado aumenta e atinge um platô por volta dos 2 anos de idade. Aproximadamente 80 a 90% das coberturas entre machos e fêmeas férteis normais resultam em gestação. A opinião veterinária pode ser buscada para machos que apresentam falha em gerar ninhadas com duas ou mais cadelas sadias. Se o cão não é usado frequentemente, o reconhecimento de possíveis problemas pode ser atrasado. É interessante considerar a ESR como rotina a cada 12 meses.

Baixa libido, falha em atingir ereção ou introdução

Baixa libido é uma causa incomum de infertilidade em cães mais comumente observada em machos idosos ou naqueles com hipogonadismo. A baixa libido não está associada à baixa testosterona na ausência de doença testicular óbvia. A suplementação de testosterona exógena não é recomendada para aumentar a libido em cães, uma vez que pode suprimir a função pituitária e reduzir a qualidade do sêmen. Causas comuns de baixa libido aparente incluem a inexperiência do macho, manejo reprodutivo fraco, ou a fêmea ser trazida ao macho em momento inapropriado. Alguns cães podem ter sido previamente reprimidos quando mostraram interesse nas cadelas e isso pode ter resultado em um bloqueio fisiológico para a expressão normal do comportamento sexual de machos. Alguns cães são beneficiados se colocados para cobrir uma cadela experiente e quieta.

Raramente cães falham em ter uma ereção por baixa libido ou desinteresse em fêmeas e são relutantes a cobrir. Nesses cães até mesmo o estímulo manual do pênis falha na estimulação da ereção. Trauma prévio (fratura de osso peniano) pode causar falha do corpo cavernoso no preenchimento com sangue, resultando em falha erétil completa ou parcial. Anormalidades podem ser detectadas pela observação do pênis durante a tentativa de coleta de sêmen. Tratamentos extrabula com sildenafila não são úteis. Algumas vezes é melhor coletar o sêmen para inseminação artificial da cadela. Falha para alcançar a introdução normal pode ser o resultado de anormalidades do pênis ou prepúcio, de doença que causa dor e impede a introdução, ou de anormalidades do trato reprodutivo feminino caudal que impedem a introdução.

Pênis, prepúcio e anormalidades relacionadas

Frênulo persistente do pênis

Falha na ruptura do frênulo peniano na puberdade pode resultar em um desvio ventral do pênis durante a ereção e falha na cópula. Em alguns cães, a tração do frênulo causa dor ou leva ao sangramento da pele do pênis. O frênulo (que é normalmente avascular) pode ser incisionado para permitir uma cura efetiva. Uma vez que essa pode ser uma característica herdada, deve ser considerada antes da introdução dos machos na reprodução.

Fratura de pênis

Fratura traumática do osso peniano em geral causa edema agudo, hemorragia uretral e disúria. Após a cicatrização pode haver dor residual, desvio do pênis, ou anormalidades de ereção. Isso pode resultar na inabilidade para atingir uma introdução normal. Alguns desses machos nunca mais alcançarão um coito normal, e a reprodução deve ser assistida pelo uso da coleta de sêmen e inseminação artificial.

Hiperplasia linfoide

Pequenos nódulos linfoides de 1 a 2 mm de diâmetro são comumente presentes nas glândulas caudais na região do reflexo prepucial na base do pênis e são especialmente comuns em cães com descarga prepucial mucopurulenta. Essa descarga é em geral normal e associada a crescimento bacteriano comensal dentro do prepúcio. Ocasionalmente esses nódulos linfoides podem ser numerosos ou particularmente protuberantes e traumatizados quando o prepúcio é retraído no momento da cobertura ou coleta de sêmen. Hiperplasia linfoide extensiva pode causar dor e sangramento durante o coito, mas em geral eles não previnem a cobertura.

Neoplasia peniana

Os tumores de pênis são raros. Carcinomas de células escamosas são mais comuns; eles se espalham localmente e metastatizam para os linfonodos inguinais. Hemorragia de neoplasias ulceradas pode ser o primeiro sinal clínico, embora em geral ocorra lambedura frequente do pênis. Quando as lesões são grandes, podem impedir a introdução. Cirurgias radicais de ressecção são indicadas na ausência de metástase. Tumor venéreo transmissível (TVT; ver Capítulo 351) é uma possibilidade, mas uma massa não é sempre presente. O diagnóstico de TVT é importante, uma vez que a transmissão de células de indivíduos infectados semeia a mucosa genital do recipiente. Animais não devem ser usados para a reprodução se qualquer tecido tumoral ativo estiver presente. Espalhar para a cavidade oral e nasal é comum por causa da lambedura. A maioria dos cães é curada com quimioterapia.

Fimose

Um orifício prepucial anormal pequeno pode ocorrer tanto por consequência de alterações congênitas como por resultado de trauma ou inflamação. Isso pode acarretar uma estreita passagem de urina durante a micção, e o gotejamento de urina dentro do prepúcio pode resultar e causar balanopostite. Cães afetados não são capazes de copular e mostram sinais de dor durante a ereção e introdução. Alargamento cirúrgico do orifício é em geral curativo.

Dor musculoesquelética que impede a introdução

Alguns cães podem ser incapazes de copular em razão da dor musculoesquelética causada por problemas de coluna ou ortopédicos (ver Capítulo 353). Em doenças não hereditárias, alguns

CAPÍTULO 318 • Exame de Saúde Reprodutiva e Distúrbios de Reprodução em Cães Machos

machos podem acasalar após a aplicação de agentes anti-inflamatórios, mas outros podem requer coleta de sêmen e inseminação artificial.

Causas femininas de falha na introdução

Várias anormalidades no trato reprodutivo caudal das cadelas podem impedir a introdução. Um exame cuidadoso da cadela para a presença de hipoplasia vulvar, restrições vaginais ou hiperplasia vaginal deve ser rotineiramente realizado antes da cobertura. A detecção desses problemas é importante, uma vez que a tentativa da cobertura pode causar sofrimento e dor tanto ao cão como à cadela, e isso pode resultar em problemas fisiológicos que inibem futuras coberturas.

Falha na emissão do ejaculado

Ejaculação retrógrada

A ejaculação retrógrada, rara em cães, é em geral uma condição neurológica que causa deposição do sêmen dentro da bexiga em vez da emissão do sêmen. Em cães mais aflitos, nenhum ejaculado é visto embora alguns eliminem pequeno volume da segunda fração do ejaculado. Lavagem da bexiga com solução fisiológica após a cobertura pode ser diagnóstica. Alguns cães com ejaculação retrógrada podem ser manejados pela prevenção da micção previamente à cobertura ou a coleta de sêmen, e outros respondem a agentes simpatominérgicos (fenilpropanolamina). Em cães não responsivos, a bexiga pode ser esvaziada de urina, parcialmente preenchida com solução fisiológica antes de ser estimulados, e a lavagem da bexiga é feita depois. A coleta de sêmen realizada dessa maneira pode ser usada para inseminação artificial.

Obstrução tubular

A obstrução do trato genital tubular pode ser resultado da ausência do sêmen no ejaculado, embora na maioria dos casos a condição seja unilateral e resulte em baixo número de espermatozoides no ejaculado em vez da ausência completa. Se bilateral, há uma óbvia lesão do escroto, testículos ou epidídimos, e é raro que um cão apresente apenas azoospermia obstrutiva. Causas potenciais incluem inflamação aguda, granuloma espermático, neoplasia, vasectomia prévia e aplasia segmentar. Com lesões bilaterais, ejaculados são azoospérmicos, não há presença de espermatozoides na urina, e a concentração de fosfatase alcalina é baixa.

Falha na ejaculação

Falha na ejaculação pode ser o resultado de problemas fisiológicos similares aos relatados em baixa libido e mais comumente em cães jovens, inexperientes, ou que experienciaram dor durante a introdução. Eles exibem falha na excitação e podem falhar no desenvolvimento completo da ereção (o laço copulatório está em geral ausente). Paciência e uso de uma cadela experiente podem sobrepor esses problemas. A rufiação do cão por um tempo antes da cobertura pode aumentar a excitação e ajudar a superar o problema.

Qualidade de sêmen ruim

Visão geral

Um dos aspectos mais importantes da investigação de infertilidade é a performance de uma avaliação de sêmen detalhada, uma vez que certas características da qualidade do sêmen predizem capacidade fertilizante. Conforme discutido, é possível classificar as anormalidades seminais de acordo com a origem, independentemente de serem compensáveis ou não, ou usando a terminologia que descreve as mudanças gerais na qualidade do sêmen.

Hemospermia

Ejaculados sanguinolentos ou vermelhos são relativamente comuns em cães. Em geral, sangue é notado na fração prostática (primeira ou terceira) do ejaculado. Ocasionalmente, eritrócitos são identificadas microscopicamente quando não vistos grosseiramente. Uma vez que a próstata é a única glândula acessória do cão macho, o sangramento ou a descoloração é claramente sempre associada a uma doença prostática, comumente HPB. Presença de sangue exige melhor avaliação da próstata (ver Capítulo 337). Se a contaminação da segunda fração é significante e o sêmen será utilizado para inseminação artificial, este deve passar por centrifugação, remoção do líquido que contém eritrócitos e ressuspensão dos espermatozoides em meio diluente.

Urospermia

A primeira fração do ejaculado lava a uretra de resquícios de urina, *debris* celulares, e é eliminada antes da introdução. Assim, é comum encontrar urina na primeira fração e, se ocorrer a mistura com a segunda fração, pode levar a um efeito tóxico. A contaminação da segunda fração com a primeira deve ser evitada e, se ocorrer, o sêmen deve ser diluído em meio centrifugado, o sobrenadante deve ser removido e os espermatozoides ressuspensos em um novo meio.

Azoospermia

Visão geral

Aparentemente, ejaculados normais que não contenham espermatozoides representam sinais de azoospermia. Existem várias explicações. Diagnósticos frequentemente requerem exames bioquímicos e citológicos do ejaculado, exame de US e aspiração por agulha fina do testículo (Figura 318.4). Causas comuns incluem disfunções gonadais adquiridas, ejaculação incompleta, falha de emissão (ver anteriormente) e disfunções gonadais congênitas.

Disfunção gonadal adquirida

A disfunção gonadal adquirida representa > 55% dos machos "inférteis". A condição deve ser chamada de perda espermatogênica ou degeneração testicular. Muitos desses cães foram previamente férteis, mas desenvolveram redução da fertilidade (ambos por redução do número de cadelas prenhas e pelo decréscimo do tamanho das ninhadas) antes de desenvolver azoospermia. Em algumas raças (Labrador Retriever, Welch Springer Spaniel), o problema ocorre dentro de algumas linhagens específicas e pode ter uma etiologia imunomediada. No Beagle, uma relação entre orquite degenerativa focal e tireoide foi estabelecida. Em muitos, a exposição não reconhecida a toxinas ou o uso de drogas que causam azoospermia levam à degeneração testicular. A maioria dos cães azoospérmicos apresenta ejaculados com concentrações de fosfatase alcalina normais, confirmando a ejaculação sem a presença de espermatozoides. Normalmente há mudanças no tamanho do testículo, calcificação e fibrose são notadas pelo US do parênquima testicular. A AAF e a citologia podem ser úteis. Na maioria o prognóstico de fertilidade não traz esperanças. No entanto, azoospermia é reversível com descanso sexual na maioria dos cães. A etiologia não é entendida, embora esses cães não tenham testículos pequenos ou evidências US de doenças. É plausível que uma ejaculação incompleta tenha ocorrido. Esses cães devem ser reexaminados após um período de descanso sexual antes do diagnóstico irreversível de azoospermia.

Ejaculação incompleta

Machos nervosos inexperientes comumente têm uma ejaculação incompleta ou falha na ejaculação. O diagnóstico depende da idade, história de cobertura, observação da cobertura, coleta de amostras de sêmen e detecção de baixas concentrações da fosfatase alcalina. O exame de urina após centrifugação pode ser útil para distinguir essas duas condições, uma vez que cães sem obstrução podem ter espermatozoides presentes dentro da bexiga, mas não a condição patológica de ejaculação retrógrada.

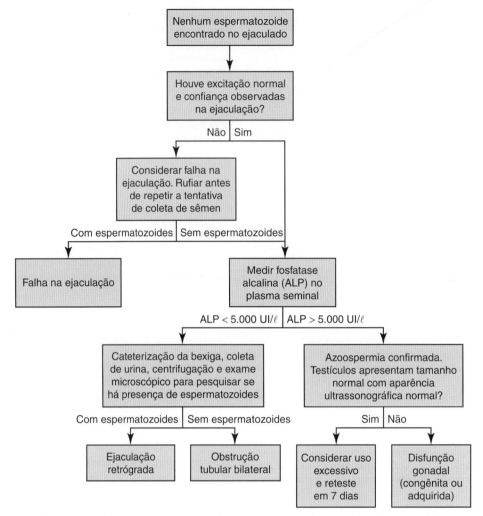

Figura 318.4 Algoritmo para investigação de cães com ausência de espermatozoides no ejaculado.

Essa é uma observação comum em cães normais. Ejaculação incompleta pode ser tratada por meio de mudanças nas práticas de cobertura para melhorar a experiência dos cães e pela rufiação do cão por um tempo mais longo antes da cobertura. Permitir que o cão possa cobrir uma cadela experiente pode aumentar sua performance.

Disfunção gonadal congênita

Disfunção gonadal congênita é em geral vista em cães que são fenotipicamente machos, mas com anormalidades cromossômicas (síndromes XXY ou XX-machos). Esses cães em geral têm ausência de espermatogênese, assim são relativamente fáceis de serem diagnosticados uma vez que é comum haver hipoplasia testicular no exame. Os testículos são palpáveis, porém menores e flácidos. Eles são em geral hiperecoicos no US.

Falha na emissão

A ejaculação retrógrada e a obstrução tubular (se bilateral) podem resultar em azoospermia conforme discutido anteriormente.

Oligozoospermia

Definição

Oligozoospermia é o termo usado para descrever ejaculados que contêm baixo número de espermatozoides morfologicamente normais. É incomum em cães e pode ocorrer como resultado de ejaculação incompleta, uso excessivo, ou ejaculação retrógrada.

Ejaculação incompleta

Ejaculação incompleta causada por inexperiência ou uma cobertura dolorosa prévia é provavelmente a causa mais comum de oligozoospermia. Nesses casos devem ter um baixo número de espermatozoides normais dentro do ejaculado. A condição pode ser diagnosticada e manejada conforme descrito anteriormente.

Uso excessivo

Frequentemente, cães idosos podem ter oligozoospermia se forem usados frequentemente na reprodução. É provável que a produção diária de espermatozoides e ejaculações frequentes esgotem as reservas espermáticas extragonadais. O descanso sexual pode permitir um aumento na reserva para alcançar números apropriados. A qualidade do sêmen de cães começa a declinar aproximadamente a partir dos 7 anos de idade. O manejo cuidadoso do tempo de cobertura é requerido em cães idosos para garantir que números apropriados de espermatozoides estejam disponíveis para fertilização.

Ejaculação retrógrada

Na ejaculação retrógrada, um volume pequeno da segunda fração do ejaculado pode ser coletado e que contém baixo número de espermatozoides normais. É incomum e na maioria dos casos há uma ausência completa de espermatozoides. Essa condição pode ser diagnosticada e tratada conforme discutido previamente.

Teratozoospermia

Teratozoospermia é a presença de espermatozoides com morfologia anormal. Em muitos casos, tais anormalidades morfológicas resultam em motilidade prejudicada de tal forma que teratozoospermia e astenozoospermia ocorrem simultaneamente. Existe pouca informação sobre anormalidades espermáticas específicas e fertilidade em cães.

Grande número de espermatozoides com anormalidade de peças intermediárias, anormalidades de base da cabeça/peça intermediária e edema de peça intermediária foi relatado em cães inférteis. Espermatozoides com defeitos de peça intermediária e deformidade de acrossoma também são associados à infecção experimental de *Brucella canis*. Não há ligação direta que explique por que essas anormalidades de espermatozoides causam infertilidade. Em cães, isso não é especialmente importante enquanto as anormalidades associadas à infertilidade são reconhecidas. Em alguns cães, várias anormalidades podem ser vistas. Em geral, quando > 40% dos espermatozoides são morfologicamente anormais, existe um declínio na fertilidade. As causas de teratozoospermia não são frequentemente determinadas. Muitos cães estão em estágios recentes de degeneração testicular após um dano e mais tarde se tornam azoospérmicos. A avaliação repetida do sêmen após aproximadamente 2 meses deve permitir avaliar a progressão do processo da doença a ser estabelecida. Em alguns casos, teratozoospermia é vista em cães mais velhos como resultado de mudanças degenerativas nos testículos em decorrência da senilidade.

Astenozoospermia

A astenozoospermia se refere à morfologia normal do espermatozoide, mas motilidade reduzida. Conforme previamente descrito, o monitoramento cuidadoso da motilidade é necessário para garantir a detecção. Amostras de sêmen refrigerado frequentemente apresentam espermatozoides com motilidade reduzida. Outras causas incluem doença imunomediada e contaminação do ejaculado. A última não é uma condição de infertilidade.

Aglutinação espermática

Anticorpos antiespermatozoides podem causar aglutinação e motilidade baixa. Embora a causa de tal produção de anticorpos seja em geral desconhecida, demonstrou-se em infecções experimentais com *Brucella canis*. Na maioria dos cães, o prognóstico de infertilidade é reservado.

Contaminação do ejaculado

A contaminação do ejaculado com componentes tóxicos (água, urina, certos plásticos, alguns lubrificantes, resíduos de agentes esterilizantes e forro de látex da vagina artificial) pode reduzir a motilidade ou produzir imobilidade espermática sem mudanças morfológicas óbvias. Avaliação cuidadosa dos métodos de coleta de sêmen e da manipulação deve ser empreendida.

Normospermia

Existem muitos cães que parecem inférteis apesar de terem qualidade espermática normal. Em muitos, existem problemas anatômicos, físicos ou fisiológicos que previnem o cortejo normal, introdução e ejaculação. Alguns sugerem que uma cultura seminal positiva e/ou mudanças em pH, bioquímica ou celularidade do líquido prostático ou plasma seminal podem influenciar a fertilidade. Em geral, no entanto, quando existem tais mudanças no ejaculado, também existem mudanças secundárias na morfologia espermática que influenciam na fertilidade.

CAPÍTULO 319

Distúrbios Reprodutivos em Cães ou Cadelas Castrados

Autumn P. Davidson

INTRODUÇÃO

Os distúrbios médicos do trato reprodutivo não se limitam a cães machos e fêmeas não castrados. Os distúrbios geniturinários ocorrem em cães castrados de ambos os sexos e diversas condições médicas podem ser atribuídas à presença de gônadas remanescentes após um procedimento de castração incompleta. Os benefícios da castração em cães de estimação são bem documentados. A identificação e o manejo adequado dos distúrbios relacionados à castração são importantes na medicina veterinária.

INCONTINÊNCIA URINÁRIA NA CADELA OVARIECTOMIZADA

A incontinência urinária é uma complicação comum e previsível da ovariectomia na cadela (ver Capítulo 333). Em cães castrados mais velhos, a incontinência urinária é menos comum e geralmente relacionada à mielopatia, em vez do hipogonadismo.

A incompetência do esfíncter uretral que resulta na incontinência urinária ocorre mais comumente em cadelas ovariectomizadas maiores (> 20 kg) com mais de 8 anos de idade; o momento da ovariectomia não interfere, a menos que o cão tenha < 12 semanas.[1] O diagnóstico diferencial inclui a incontinência por transbordamento devido à isostenúria ou hipostenúria (ver Capítulo 45), a infecção do trato urinário (ver Capítulo 330), a ectopia não diagnosticada, a micção comportamental ou submissa e os distúrbios inflamatórios ou neoplásicos do trato geniturinário (ver Capítulo 351).

O perfil quantitativo da pressão uretral é "padrão-ouro" para o diagnóstico de distúrbios uretrais, mas normalmente não está disponível (ver Capítulo 335). A incontinência urinária é problemática para cães domésticos e aumenta a incidência de infecção do trato urinário (ITU) causada por bactérias ascendentes.

Uma vez diagnosticada, geralmente por um processo eliminatório, a terapia para a incontinência urinária associada à incompetência do esfíncter uretral envolve a reposição de estrógeno (os estrógenos sensibilizam os receptores adrenérgicos alfa-1 do esfíncter uretral para norepinefrina), fenilpropanolamina (um simpaticomimético que melhora o tônus uretral por meio dos receptores adrenérgicos alfa-1), ou a combinação dos dois, uma vez que seus efeitos são sinérgicos (ver Capítulo 333).[1] Para cães com tratamento médico ineficiente, a implantação de colágeno periuretral por endoscopia pode melhorar a condição por semanas a meses, mas a disponibilidade é limitada. As opções cirúrgicas incluem a colpossuspensão, o dobramento uretral, o *sling* transobturatório vaginal e a colocação de oclusor hidráulico uretral (ver Capítulo 124); todos mostraram benefícios em um pequeno número de casos (ver Capítulo 335).

VESTIBULOVAGINITE CRÔNICA

Histórico
Cadelas com vestibulovaginite crônica podem ter um quadro de secreção vulvar purulenta ou mucosa a hemorrágica (ver Capítulo 44) e, geralmente, sinais de desconforto (lambedura, fuga e polaciúria). A dermatite vulvar e perivulvar está frequentemente presente e pode ser grave. A condição é observada em cadelas ovariectomizadas de qualquer idade, meses a anos após a esterilização. Geralmente, o histórico inclui várias tentativas terapêuticas sem resolução, embora possam ocorrer melhorias transitórias. Normalmente, a duração é de semanas a meses, mas às vezes perdura por anos.

Etiologia
A etiologia da vestibulovaginite crônica é multifatorial. A causa primária pode ser mascarada e/ou exacerbada por terapias comuns: o uso de antimicrobianos por tempo prolongado, automutilação e duchas. A biopsia da mucosa vaginal com frequência mostra inflamação linfoplasmocitária inespecífica, porém, às vezes, a inflamação é supurativa (neutrofílica) ou eosinofílica. Culturas vaginais podem mostrar crescimento excessivo de espécies bacterianas atípicas, muitas vezes resistentes (culturas gram-negativas puras, *Pseudomonas* spp.), especialmente se foram usados antibióticos extensivamente. Ocasionalmente, um supercrescimento de levedura é identificado. A vestibulovaginite bacteriana primária é rara. Estenoses vaginais são comumente identificadas, mas raramente contribuem e geralmente representam má interpretação do estreitamento normal na junção vestibulovaginal em uma cadela virgem. As verdadeiras estenoses vaginais circunferenciais são craniais à papila uretral e, portanto, não contribuem para o acúmulo de urina. As anomalias vaginais dorsoventrais septadas também são geralmente posicionadas craniais à papila uretral. Ambas podem interferir na cobertura ou no parto, mas é improvável que contribuam para a vestibulovaginite na cadela ovariectomizada. A vaginite juvenil ("filhote") e a ovariectomia previamente ao primeiro ciclo estral não predispõem à vestibulovaginite crônica no adulto.[2] Muitas são classificadas como idiopáticas.

Avaliação clínica

Exame físico, testes laboratoriais, imagem
O exame físico (EF) da área vulvovaginal sem sedação/analgesia deve ser evitado devido à dor ou ao medo. Recomenda-se uma base de dados mínima, incluindo hemograma completo, análises químicas do soro, urinálise (UA, de preferência obtida por cistocentese) e cultura de urina. A radiografia (vaginograma/uretrograma/cistograma/PIV) e/ou a ultrassonografia (US) de todo o trato geniturinário podem ser úteis na identificação de anormalidades e no diagnóstico diferencial (ver Capítulo 88). O exame de preferência é a US, pois não requer anestesia e pode ser realizada a avaliação de todo o abdome, com foco particular no trato geniturinário, incluindo os antigos sítios ovarianos e o coto uterino (Figura 319.1).[3]

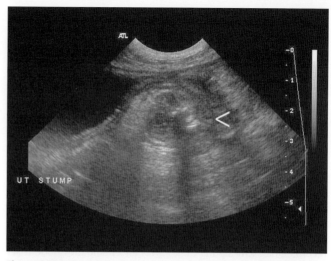

Figura 319.1 Imagem de ultrassom transversal de um coto ovariano anormal; a seta indica um corpo estranho ecogênico (aresta de planta).

Exame endoscópico
Quando não são identificadas anormalidades na US (i. e., granuloma de coto uterino, cistite crônica, urolitíase, lesões trigonais), deve-se considerar um exame vaginal completo sob sedação adequada (pesada) ou anestesia (ver Capítulos 44 e 119). Deve-se usar um equipamento endoscópico que permita a avaliação de toda a abóbada vaginal. Um cistouretroscópio rígido com infusão de solução salina é o ideal. Otoscópios e espéculos vaginais não permitem adequada avaliação de toda a abóbada vaginal. Os proctoscópios pediátricos carecem da sensibilidade ótica dos cistouretroscópios. A avaliação vaginoscópica deve incluir a visualização da vulva externa, da fossa clitoriana, do vestíbulo, da papila uretral ± uretra/bexiga urinária, junção vestibulovaginal, vagina e região caudal da cérvice (ver Capítulos 108 e 119).[4] A aparência e a saúde da mucosa em todo o trato, a presença de massas, de corpos estranhos e a fonte de qualquer secreção devem ser determinadas. Se for identificado um estreitamento vaginal ou um acentuado estreitamento da junção vestibulovaginal, é importante observar se a inflamação vaginal secundária à retenção de secreções está presente cranial à restrição. Se a vagina cranial é normal, a estenose ou o estreitamento provavelmente não contribuem para a vaginite vestibular (Figuras 319.2 a 319.4).

Citologia, biopsia e cultura
A citologia da secreção vulvar, a citologia da mucosa vaginal, culturas vaginais aeróbicas e a biopsia da mucosa vaginal afetada podem ajudar na melhor compreensão dessa condição (ver Capítulo 119). A interpretação das culturas vaginais deve levar em consideração as terapias antimicrobianas anteriores que podem afetar a microbiota vaginal normal (bactérias gram-negativas e positivas, incluindo *Mycoplasma* spp.). A identificação de qualquer anormalidade anatômica que possa contribuir é importante (estenoses significativas, lesões de massa, dobras vulvares dorsais ou laterais redundantes, anomalia anatômica ureteral). É útil examinar a cadela em posição normal de pé, para avaliar a anatomia externa com precisão (dobras vulvares?), após urinar, e novamente após decúbito (urina acumulada e quente?). Muitas vezes, esse exame completo só ocorre após a cadela ser sedada ou anestesiada (Figuras 319.5 e 319.6). A presença de acúmulo de urina na abóbada vaginal pode ser mal interpretada. A presença de dobras vulvares redundantes pode ser de difícil visualização se a cadela estiver posicionada esternal ou dorsalmente.

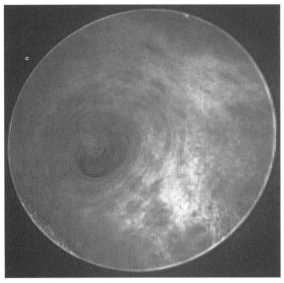

Figura 319.2 Imagem vaginoscópica de vaginite idiopática crônica; a mucosa vaginal é friável e eritêmica. (*Esta figura se encontra reproduzida em cores no Encarte.*)

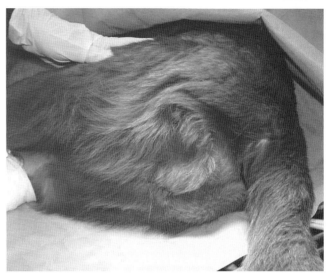

Figura 319.5 Dobras vulvares laterais e dorsais redundantes em uma cadela com vaginite crônica.

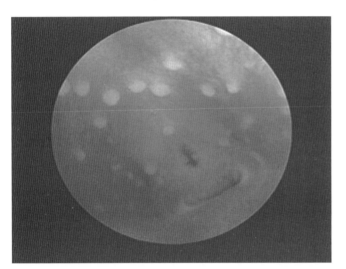

Figura 319.3 Imagem vaginoscópica de folículos linfoides na mucosa vaginal. (*Esta figura se encontra reproduzida em cores no Encarte.*)

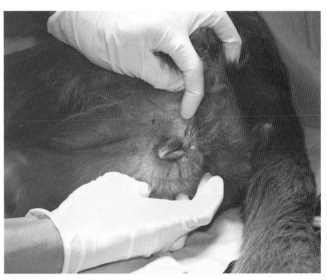

Figura 319.6 Acentuada dermatite perivulvar visível pela retração das dobras redundantes na mesma cadela vista na Figura 319.5.

Tratamento

Diretrizes gerais

O manejo da maioria das cadelas é feito com a interrupção de qualquer irrigação/ducha tópica, a prevenção da automutilação com colar elisabetano e o início de terapia antimicrobiana apenas quando indicada pela interpretação adequada da cultura e dos testes de sensibilidade. A terapia antimicrobiana deve ser limitada a cadelas com patógenos que têm a flora normal deslocada (p. ex., *Pseudomonas* spp.). A analgesia e a terapia anti-inflamatória são indicadas na maioria dos casos. Os AINEs são superiores aos corticosteroides porque estes aumentam o risco de ITU. Os narcóticos, como o tramadol (2 a 5 mg/kg VO a cada 8 h) e a gabapentina (10 a 60 mg/kg dividido VO a cada 8 a 12 h), podem ser benéficos para uma analgesia adequada.

Condições específicas

Se for identificada uma causa específica de vaginite crônica, a resolução pode ser direta. A identificação e remoção de corpos estranhos devem ser curativas (Figura 319.7). Se as anormalidades anatômicas (dobras vulvares laterais ou dorsais redundantes,

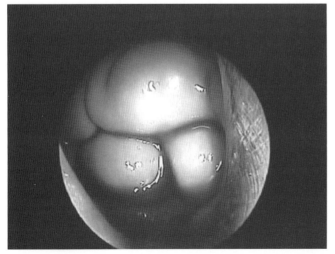

Figura 319.4 Imagem vaginoscópica de hemorragia proveniente do coto uterino via cérvice. (*Esta figura se encontra reproduzida em cores no Encarte.*)

estenose vaginal significativa, coto uterino granulomatoso) contribuíram ou causaram a condição, indica-se a correção cirúrgica e um cuidadoso pós-operatório (Figura 319.8).[5-7] O manejo adequado da infecção crônica do trato urinário, se identificada, deve resolver a vaginite associada. A cirurgia e/ou a quimioterapia podem ser indicadas para massas urogenitais ou neoplasias (Figura 319.9).

Idiopática

A condição é idiopática se a causa não puder ser diferenciada de anatômica, corpo estranho, infecciosa, granulomatosa ou neoplásica. A terapia com reposição de estrógeno oral frequentemente é útil ao estabelecer a integridade normal da mucosa e eventual normalização da abóbada vaginal. A vaginite idiopática em cadelas ovariectomizadas é semelhante à vaginite por depleção de estrógeno pós-menopausa em mulheres. As mulheres melhoram com a aplicação intravaginal de estrógeno, o que é difícil na cadela.[8] O estrógeno oral (Estriol, Incurin, Merck ou dietilestilbestrol combinado, DES) é recomendado; a dose é empírica e geralmente a mesma usada para incontinência urinária devido à incompetência do esfíncter uretral (Estriol 0,5 a 2 mg/cadela VO a cada 24 a 48+ h; DES 0,20 a 1 mg/cadela VO a cada 48 a 72 h). São necessárias várias semanas de terapia antes que a melhora seja observada. Os efeitos colaterais são incomuns: a superdosagem resulta em sinais de proestro/estro (atraindo cães machos, edema vulvar); se for seguida a dosagem recomendada, a mielossupressão é altamente improvável. Os analgésicos e anti-inflamatórios devem ser continuados até que seja estabelecido um efeito do estrógeno com alívio. A citologia vaginal ou a vaginoscopia (ver Capítulo 119) podem confirmar o efeito do estrógeno (Figura 319.10 e Vídeo 319.1).

TOXICOSE DE ESTRÓGENO NA CADELA OVARIECTOMIZADA

Sinais e fontes de estrógeno

O hiperestrogenismo causa sinais comportamentais e/ou físicos de estro em uma cadela. As fontes de estrógeno em uma cadela castrada são limitadas. As fontes endógenas de estrógeno incluem tecido ovariano residual (síndrome do ovário remanescente [SOR]) ou doença da glândula adrenal. O estrógeno exógeno normalmente resulta do consumo de produtos transdérmicos de reposição hormonal humana, mas também pode ocorrer pela superdosagem de estrógeno prescrito pelo veterinário para a incontinência urinária. O excesso de estrógeno em uma cadela castrada causa atração de cães machos, edema da vulva, secreção vulvar mucoide a sanguinolenta, interação passiva com cães machos, sinalização e, às vezes, cobertura. A secreção sanguinolenta associada ao estrógeno é de origem uterina, indicando a presença do útero ou de um coto uterino. O excesso de estrógeno crônico pode causar alopecia simétrica, ginecomastia e/ou lactação.

Síndrome do ovário remanescente

Etiologia

A SOR é relatada como responsável por cerca de 17% das complicações pós-ovariectomia/ovário-histerectomia porque

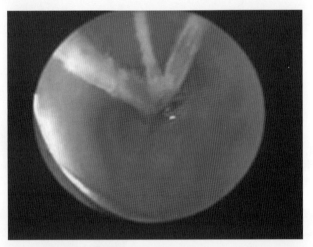

Figura 319.7 Imagem vaginoscópica de uma aresta de planta embutida no orifício cervical caudal. (*Esta figura se encontra reproduzida em cores no Encarte.*)

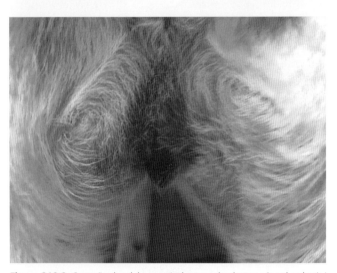

Figura 319.8 Correção das dobras perivulvares redundantes pós-vulvoplastia/episioplastia.

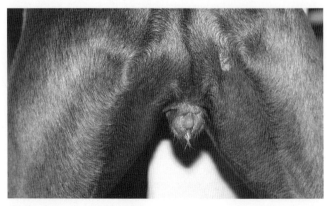

Figura 319.9 Hiperplasia clitoriana que contribui para vulvite/vaginite crônica. (*Esta figura se encontra reproduzida em cores no Encarte.*)

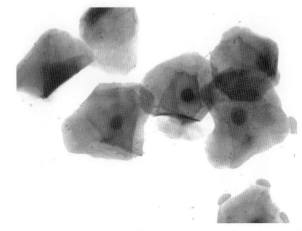

Figura 319.10 Citologia vaginal demonstra a influência do estrógeno: células da mucosa vaginal superficial.

um ou ambos os ovários não foram completamente removidos. Não há nenhuma correlação com a idade na cirurgia, dificuldade na cirurgia, obesidade da cadela, ou experiência do cirurgião. A presença de tecido ovariano anatomicamente anormal (fragmentação no ligamento largo) é possível, mas bastante incomum. Um "ovário supranumerário" é extremamente raro. Experimentalmente, a funcionalidade pode retornar ao tecido ovariano removido de seu suprimento vascular e recolocado para dentro ou sobre a parede abdominal lateral. Não foi relatada nenhuma predisposição racial ou distribuição geográfica para essa condição.

Sinais

Os sinais de um ciclo estral geralmente ocorrem meses a anos após a ovariectomia/ovário-histerectomia, mas podem começar dentro de dias. Os sinais de proestro duram em média 9 dias. Os sinais de estro duram em média 9 dias; se a ovulação ocorrer, segue-se o diestro (influência da progesterona) com duração de 45 a 60 dias. O intervalo médio entre os sinais dos ciclos estrais é de 7 meses (ver Capítulo 312). Destaca-se que, se houver um ovário remanescente funcional, os sinais normalmente são cíclicos ou periódicos (a cada 5 a 8 meses) em vez de constantes. Quando uma cadela está sob influência da progesterona, pode-se desenvolver a piometra de coto causando uma secreção vulvar purulenta (ver Capítulos 142 e 316). Sinais constantes do efeito de estrógeno sugerem uma fonte exógena, geralmente um produto hormonal transdérmico de uso humano. Outras possibilidades são a doença no ovário remanescente (cisto folicular, neoplasia funcional) ou, raramente, doença da glândula da adrenal.[10] O clínico deve considerar múltiplas variáveis.

Teste e diagnóstico (Figura 319.11)

Deve ser realizado um banco de dados mínimo que inclua hemograma completo, perfil bioquímico e urinálise com cultura, mas geralmente não são dignos de nota. É incomum, mas pode ser observada anemia crônica por perda de sangue se a hemorragia for profunda. Foi observada a perda crônica de sangue em cães com neoplasia ovariana, cistos foliculares, distúrbio de sangramento ou outra doença sistêmica. É possível que ocorra a pancitopenia devido à intoxicação por estrógeno (ver Capítulos 52 e 54). A citologia vaginal identificará o efeito do estrógeno: a cornificação da mucosa vaginal é um bioensaio para as concentrações plasmáticas elevadas de estradiol (ver Figura 319.10 e Capítulo 119). Uma concentração de progesterona sérica > 2 ng/mℓ (mensurada 1 a 3 semanas após o comportamento de estro) é compatível com o tecido luteal funcional e com a SOR. Para fins de diagnóstico, podem ser usados GnRH (50 mcg IM), hCG (400 UI IV) ou hCG (1.000 UI: 1/2 IV, 1/2 IM) para induzir a ovulação ou a luteinização, mas, em razão da natureza refratária do ovário remanescente, isso é raramente informativo. O teste com qualquer uma das drogas envolve a avaliação da concentração sérica de progesterona 2 a 3 semanas após a administração. Um resultado positivo do hormônio antimülleriano (HAM), agora disponível comercialmente (MOFA), em uma cadela > 6 meses de idade (pós-púbere) indica a presença de tecido ovariano.[11] É o teste de escolha para a triagem. A exposição ao estrógeno exógeno não afeta os resultados do HAM, permitindo a diferenciação do ovário remanescente da toxicidade estrogênica exógena. Em cadelas ovariectomizadas, os resultados dos ensaios do hormônio luteinizante (Witness LH, Zoetis) estão aumentados (> 1 ng/mℓ) devido à ausência de *feedback* negativo. No entanto, quando um resultado positivo é obtido, aconselha-se repetir o teste em 24 horas para descartar a detecção do pico de LH de 12 a 24 horas em uma cadela inteira no estro (ela deveria ter uma citologia vaginal representativa; ver Capítulos 119 e 312). Se os resultados são positivos com vários dias de intervalo, indica-se a gonadectomia completa ou total. Um teste negativo (< 1 ng/ℓ) é encontrado em cadelas inteiras, a menos que seja realizado no momento do pico de LH durante o proestro.[12] A exposição ao estrógeno exógeno em uma cadela gonadectomizada pode fazer com que o LH se torne falso negativo.

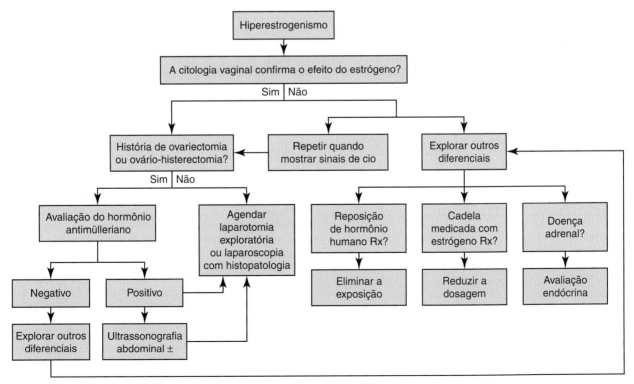

Figura 319.11 Algoritmo para diagnosticar a causa do hiperestrogenismo.

A US pode ser usada como suporte ao diagnóstico da SOR inicialmente suspeitada pelo histórico, sinais clínicos, citologia vaginal e um HAM positivo (ver Capítulo 88). A imagem deve começar em um plano sagital ligeiramente caudolateral aos rins (onde é esperado o tecido ovariano remanescente).

O tecido ovariano remanescente pode ser visível apenas durante na fase folicular (estruturas císticas, anecoicas) ou na fase luteal (estruturas císticas hipoecoicas ou isoecoicas) (Figura 319.12, Vídeos 319.2 e 319.3). O tecido ovariano ectópico pode ser difícil de ser localizado e a visualização da imagem com US requer experiência. Quando positivo, pode-se ter mais confiança ao propor a laparotomia. As glândulas adrenais devem ser avaliadas ao mesmo tempo quanto ao tamanho e à forma (ver Capítulo 308).[3]

Tratamento cirúrgico

A laparotomia exploratória, com o objetivo de remover o tecido ovariano residual, confirma e resolve o problema. A identificação de tecido ovariano residual é facilitada pela presença de folículos ativos ou corpos lúteos resultantes; o clínico deve agendar o procedimento cirúrgico quando os sinais clínicos estiverem presentes. Como houve a remoção parcial ou total do útero, as preocupações usuais sobre a realização de cirurgia em uma cadela com estro são atenuadas. Todo o tecido ovariano visível deve ser removido e avaliado histologicamente. Se não for identificado nenhum tecido ovariano visível, todo o tecido residual nos pedículos ovarianos deve ser ressecado e submetido à histologia. Se houver transformação neoplásica, a histopatologia é importante. Um granuloma de coto ou uma piometra devem ser removidos. A remoção do tecido luteal funcional pode induzir sinais transitórios de pseudogestação em cadelas no pós-operatório devido ao aumento resultante na prolactina (ver Capítulo 315). Se for intenso, pode-se administrar terapia antiprolactina (cabergolina; Galastop 2,5 mcg/kg VO a cada 24 h por 4 a 6 dias). A remoção bem-sucedida do tecido ovariano remanescente deve resultar na cessação dos sinais clínicos de estro, mesmo se houver doença ovariana.

Tratamento médico

A terapia médica é frequentemente solicitada por clientes que não desejam realizar um segundo procedimento cirúrgico. Os compostos progestacionais ou androgênicos usados para suprimir a atividade ovariana folicular não são recomendados em razão dos efeitos colaterais indesejáveis (neoplasia mamária, diabetes melito, comportamento indesejável). Quando aperfeiçoada e comercialmente disponível nos EUA, a imunocontracepção ou a administração de agonistas de GnRH oferece uma alternativa viável à laparotomia. Em cadelas que receberam ou consumiram estrógeno, evitar a exposição ao estrógeno deve levar à resolução dos sinais clínicos em 2 a 4 semanas (Figura 319.13).[13] Geralmente, os proprietários desconhecem que a medicação com produtos transdérmicos fica ativa após o consumo por animais de estimação.

ADENOCARCINOMA PROSTÁTICO

Visão geral

O adenocarcinoma prostático é uma doença de cães machos geralmente castrados e com mais de 10 anos de idade (ver Capítulos 337 e 351). Ele apresenta um prognóstico desfavorável. O adenocarcinoma prostático origina-se da porção glandular da próstata; outros tipos de tumor prostático incluem fibrossarcoma, leiomiossarcoma, carcinoma de células transicionais (CCT) e carcinoma de células escamosas. O CCT e o adenocarcinoma prostático (ACA) são as doenças malignas primárias mais comuns da próstata. O CCT origina-se do epitélio de transição que se estende desde a bexiga até a próstata ou do uroepitélio da uretra prostática. A maioria dos adenocarcinomas

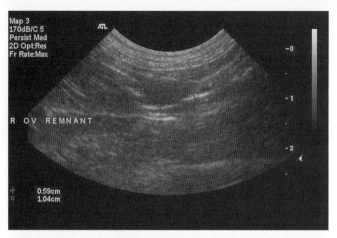

Figura 319.12 Imagem ultrassonográfica sagital de um ovário remanescente que mostra uma estrutura folicular hipoecoica discreta (cursores).

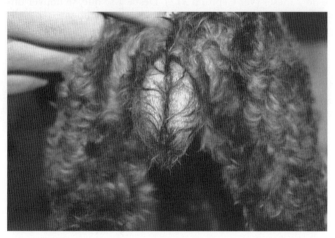

Figura 319.13 Aumento vulvar em uma filhote ovariectomizada sem raça definida de 12 semanas de idade, resultante de exposição à terapia de reposição hormonal transdérmica pelo proprietário.

prostáticos não expressa receptores de andrógeno e não parece ser influenciada por andrógenos. Em contraste, a castração (especialmente < 1 ano de idade) parece ser um fator de risco para o seu desenvolvimento. A hiperplasia benigna prostática anterior não é um fator de risco para a neoplasia de próstata.[14,15]

Achados clínicos e testagem

Estrangúria, disúria, tenesmo, fezes pequenas, dor lombar e anormalidades na marcha são sinais clínicos comuns. Os tumores são frequentemente detectados após a disseminação metastática, pois os sinais clínicos ocorrem tardiamente e a triagem precoce não está disponível. No exame retal, uma próstata grande (especialmente se o cão é castrado), assimétrica, irregular e dolorosa pode ser identificada. Comumente, os cães afetados têm dor abdominal, dor lombossacral e/ou linfadenopatia sublombar. A anorexia e a perda de peso associada reduzem a condição corporal. O hemograma completo e os achados do perfil químico refletem a doença crônica e a inflamação. Se a massa for obstrutiva, poderá ocorrer azotemia pós-renal causando hidroureter e hidronefrose. Ocorre elevação da fosfatase alcalina em ≈ 50% dos cães, talvez associada a metástases ósseas axiais. Na urinálise, podem ser notadas hematúria, piúria, bacteriúria e células de transição atípicas (ver Capítulo 72). A ITU é uma comorbidade comum (ver Capítulo 330). As células de transição malignas aparecem semelhantes às células de transição reativas, tornando a biopsia importante. As radiografias torácicas são indicadas para triagem da metástase pulmonar.

As radiografias da coluna lombar podem mostrar metástase nas vértebras. A mineralização da próstata aumentada e/ou linfadenomegalia sublombar é sugestiva de malignidade da doença.

A US abdominal é uma ferramenta diagnóstica valiosa, que permite a avaliação de parênquima prostático, linfáticos regionais, extensão da bexiga urinária, obstrução uretral ou trigonal e presença de hidroureter e hidronefrose. São comuns o parênquima prostático hiperecoico focal ou multifocal com assimetria, contorno irregular da cápsula e mineralização. Devido à necrose e hemorragia, podem estar presentes regiões cavitárias e uma acentuada linfadenomegalia sublombar (Figura 319.14).[16] A US e a biopsia ou aspiração por agulha fina (AAF) guiada por US (ver Capítulos 89 e 93) são úteis, mas o risco de disseminação do tumor torna preferível a biopsia aberta. A histopatologia (em vez da citologia) geralmente é necessária para diferenciar o tipo de tumor.

Tratamento (ver Capítulos 337 e 351)

A terapia com AINEs, muitas vezes em combinação com analgésicos orais, pode prolongar a vida. A quimioterapia (carboplatina, cisplatina, doxorrubicina, gencitabina) pode melhorar os sinais, mas a cura é improvável. A prostatectomia pode prolongar a vida se o câncer estiver confinado à cápsula prostática, mas há uma alta taxa de complicações (incontinência, estenose uretral). A radiação paliativa e/ou *stent* uretral oferecem alívio a curto prazo. Para tenesmos, são indicados laxantes. Bisfosfonatos IV, como pamidronato (0,65 a 2 mg/kg IV, infusão lenta com NaCl a 0,9% por mais de 2 h), podem ajudar no alívio da dor de metástases esqueléticas.

METAPLASIA ESCAMOSA PROSTÁTICA

A metaplasia escamosa da próstata ocorre como consequência do hiperestrogenismo, seja de origem endógena (tumor de células de Sertoli funcional, disfunção da glândula adrenal) ou exógena (terapia para hiperplasia benigna da próstata, consumo inadvertido de medicação com hormônio transdérmico pelo proprietário). A metaplasia escamosa epitelial prostática é acompanhada por estase secretora e potencial para cistos intraprostáticos. A glândula prostática geralmente é grande para um cão castrado e firme à palpação. A compressão da uretra e do cólon pode causar disúria e tenesmo. Outros achados físicos típicos de hiperestrogenismo podem estar presentes: atratividade para machos, ginecomastia, alopecia simétrica, hiperpigmentação e prepúcio pendular. A presença de um testículo abdominal (criptorquidia) deve ser descartada por meio de US se ambos os testículos não forem palpáveis. A intoxicação da medula óssea por estrógeno pode causar palidez das membranas mucosas (anemia; ver Capítulo 52), petéquias ou hemorragia (trombocitopenia; ver Capítulo 54) e febre (secundária à neutropenia). Deve ser feito um histórico criterioso com relação à possível exposição a medicamentos de hormônio transdérmico humano ou terapia anterior proposital com estrógeno para prostatomegalia.

Para a mielotoxicose e a saúde geral, devem-se avaliar hemograma completo, perfil químico sérico e urinálise/cultura. As alterações são variáveis, dependendo da duração da exposição, dose e do tempo entre a causa e o teste. Nas primeiras 2 a 3 semanas, tanto a trombocitopenia quanto a trombocitose podem ser observadas com anemia progressiva e leucocitose (a contagem de leucócitos pode exceder 100.000/mcℓ). Após 3 semanas, podem ser observadas a pancitopenia e a anemia aplásica. A hematúria pode ocorrer devido à trombocitopenia ou ao sangramento prostático. Sob influência do estrógeno, as células epiteliais escamosas podem ser vistas na urina ou reconhecidas em amostras da mucosa prepucial.

Em um cão castrado sem testículos escrotais, deve-se realizar US abdominal para a pesquisa de um testículo criptorquídeo transformado em maligno ou uma próstata incomum, aumentada, cavitária e hiperecogênica. Concentrações séricas baixas do hormônio luteinizante (LH, Zoetis) podem indicar a presença de tecido testicular. Se com a US for descoberto um testículo abdominal com uma massa parenquimatosa ou uma próstata aumentada, as amostras de AAF ou biopsia podem fornecer evidências citológicas de neoplasia testicular funcional ou metaplasia escamosa epitelial prostática (ver Capítulos 89 e 93). A terapia é direcionada pelos achados clínicos, mas é importante interromper a exposição ou a terapia de estrógeno exógeno. Se for um criptorquídeo, a castração deve ser recomendada. A infecção prostática concomitante ou abscesso podem estar presentes e devem ser tratados apropriadamente (ver Capítulo 337).

PRIAPISMO

Definição e etiologia

O priapismo é uma ereção peniana persistente sem estimulação sexual e categorizada como não isquêmica (arterial, fluxo alto) ou isquêmica (veno-oclusivo, baixo fluxo), que ocorre mais comumente em cães castrados (Figura 319.15). O priapismo isquêmico é bem doloroso e considerado uma emergência, já que pode resultar rapidamente em necrose. Qualquer forma pode resultar em trauma significativo para o tecido peniano (ver Capítulo 146).[17] A castração de um cão com priapismo não é útil, já que a condição não é mediada pela testosterona. O priapismo deve ser diferenciado da parafimose, que ocorre mais comumente em cães machos inteiros após a coleta de sêmen ou masturbação e resulta da constrição do pênis ereto pela abertura prepucial (Figura 319.16). O priapismo também deve ser diferenciado de outras causas de edema peniano, como hematoma, trauma ou lesões de massa (Figuras 319.17 e 319.18). Os hematomas penianos geralmente se formam como resultado de um trauma ou distúrbios hemorrágicos. A inspeção visual simples e a palpação do pênis geralmente são suficientes para diferenciar essas condições, mas os exames US e/ou Doppler colorido podem ajudar ainda mais a diferenciar esses distúrbios do priapismo (Figura 319.19). A US do períneo e do corpo inteiro do pênis pode ajudar na identificação de neoplasia, fratura do osso peniano, hematoma ou tromboembolia (Vídeos 319.4 e 319.5).

A ereção canina é mediada pelo nervo pélvico, que surge principalmente do primeiro e segundo nervos sacrais (S1-S2) e é composta por fibras nervosas parassimpáticas. O estímulo do nervo pélvico causa ereção pelo aumento da pressão arterial do pênis, inibindo parcialmente a drenagem venosa e dilatando as artérias penianas. O nervo pudendo, que surge dos nervos sacrais S1-S3, também está envolvido, estimulando a contração dos

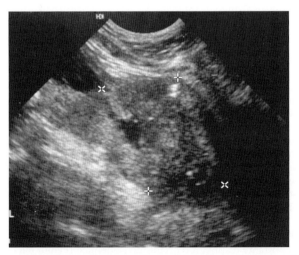

Figura 319.14 Imagem ultrassonográfica sagital de adenocarcinoma prostático (*cursores*); a mineralização é evidente.

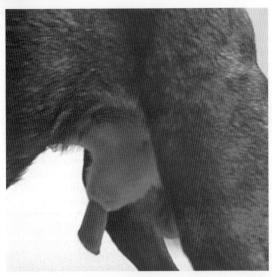

Figura 319.15 Priapismo em um Boston Terrier castrado; observe que o bulbo da glande está dentro do prepúcio.

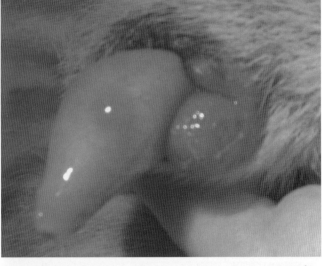

Figura 319.18 Linfoma que envolve a mucosa peniana canina e causa efeito de massa.

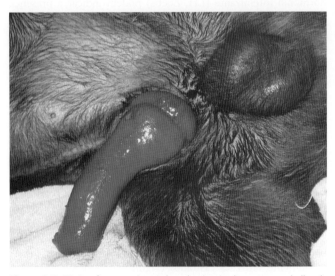

Figura 319.16 Parafimose após a coleta de sêmen; observe que o bulbo da glande está fora do prepúcio.

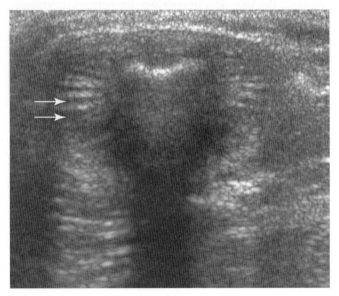

Figura 319.19 Priapismo; imagem ultrassonográfica transversal do pênis canino nos níveis do bulbo da glande (as *setas* indicam acúmulo de sangue).

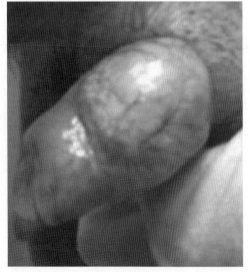

Figura 319.17 Ruptura da túnica albugínea que causa efeito de massa no pênis canino.

músculos extrínsecos do pênis. O nervo hipogástrico, um nervo simpático originado dos segmentos da medula espinal lombar L1-L4, também pode ter um papel regulador. O nervo hipogástrico é responsável pela secreção de fluido prostático e ejaculação. A estimulação das fibras da cadeia simpática aumenta a resistência arterial, diminui a pressão do corpo cavernoso, diminui a resistência venosa e inibe as ereções. A inibição simpática do processo erétil é mediada pelo sistema alfa-1 adrenérgico.[18] O priapismo verdadeiro (qualquer uma das formas) pode estar associado a distúrbios vasculares (eferentes ou aferentes), neuropatia, ou mielopatia (lombossacral). Uma hipótese sobre a fisiopatologia do priapismo sugere a neuroestimulação dissinérgica do fluxo de entrada e saída dos vasos sanguíneos penianos causando vasospasmos ou espasmos da musculatura lisa. Essa desregulação pode ocorrer no nível do pênis, do SNC (medula espinal), ou do sistema nervoso periférico.

Diagnóstico e tratamento

É importante distinguir o priapismo isquêmico (evolui para gangrena) do não isquêmico, assim como identificar e tratar a causa subjacente. Se confirmado como isquêmico, deve-se realizar, sob sedação ou anestesia, a imediata aspiração dos corpos cavernosos com ou sem irrigação (ver Capítulo 146). As injeções intracavernosas de fenilefrina podem ser consideradas, mas apresentam alguns riscos, pois não foram determinadas as dosagens adequadas para cães e gatos. Portanto, é importante começar com baixas doses (1 a 3 mcg/kg) e monitorar o cardiovascular. É importante fornecer lubrificação para limitar danos teciduais secundários à exposição e escoriação. É indicado o uso de colar elizabetano. Se a drenagem intracavernosa e as injeções não forem bem-sucedidas ou se houver lesão tecidual significativa, a amputação peniana e a uretrostomia perineal podem ser necessárias.

O priapismo não isquêmico pode se resolver espontaneamente, mas pode levar horas a dias. Portanto, recomendam-se a terapia conservativa com analgésicos, proteção da integridade peniana por meio de lubrificação e o uso de um colar elizabetano. A sedação com uma droga fenotiazínica pode ser útil.

Diversos medicamentos sistêmicos têm benefício potencial, embora existam poucos dados controlados em relação à eficácia. A gabapentina (10 a 60 mg/kg VO diariamente, divididos a cada 8 a 12 h), a terbutalina (1,25 a 5 mg/cão VO a cada 8 a 12 h) ou a efedrina (1 a 2,5 mg/kg VO a cada 12 h) podem ser tentadas. Recomenda-se aumentar a dosagem incrementalmente. Se a detumescência não for alcançada com um desses medicamentos após alguns dias de tratamento, a solução pode ser trocá-lo por outro.

REFERÊNCIAS BIBLIOGRÁFICAS

As referências bibliográficas deste capítulo se encontram online no Ambiente de Aprendizagem.

CAPÍTULO 320

Cuidados dos Neonatos durante o Período Pós-Parto

Margret L. Casal

DEFINIÇÕES

Nas mulheres, o "período pós-parto" é definido como as 6 a 8 primeiras semanas seguintes ao parto. Durante esse período, o útero retorna ao seu tamanho normal de não gestante. Esse é também o período de tempo durante o qual ocorre a maioria das mortes neonatais.[1,2] Na medicina veterinária, o período pósparto é descrito como o período de cerca de 2 (secreção dos lóquios) a 8 semanas (o tempo que o útero leva para retornar ao seu tamanho normal macroscopicamente).[3-6] O foco deste capítulo é o período de tempo mais crítico para os neonatos: as primeiras 2 a 3 semanas de vida.

PRÉ-PARTO

A criação de neonatos saudáveis começa antes de eles nascerem. O exame físico da mãe e do pai deve ser realizado e é uma oportunidade para identificar possíveis problemas infecciosos ou genéticos (ver Capítulo 2). Em raças puras, pode-se considerar a triagem genética (ver Capítulos 3 e 4). A cadela e o reprodutor devem ser rastreados para *Brucella* (ver Capítulo 213), e a gata e o gato para os vírus da leucemia felina (ver Capítulo 223) e imunodeficiência felina (ver Capítulo 222). Devem ser realizados exames de fezes (ver Capítulo 81) e tanto o pai quanto a mãe devem estar em dia com o controle parasitário (ver Capítulo 163) e vacinal (ver Capítulo 208). A dieta da mãe deve ser ajustada para atender às demandas da gestação e o seu peso corporal monitorado, uma vez que as taxas de mortalidade são mais altas em ninhadas de gatas e cadelas abaixo ou acima do peso (Capítulo 315). Os alimentos crus não são recomendados durante a gestação devido à possível exposição a bactérias (p. ex., *Salmonella* spp.) ou parasitas (p. ex., *Toxoplasma gondii*) (ver Capítulo 192).[7,8] A maioria das dietas comerciais é adequada e pode ser complementada com comida para filhote de cão ou gato durante o último trimestre. A adição de vitaminas ou outros suplementos é desnecessária e pode ser prejudicial. O excesso de vitamina A, por exemplo, pode causar defeitos na linha média de fetos. A administração de vacinas vivas modificadas durante a gestação também pode causar defeitos fetais ou doença ativa. O fembendazol é seguro para a vermifugação de cadelas durante a gestação para reduzir a transmissão transplacentária de *Toxocara canis* e o pamoato de pirantel em gatas para diminuir a liberação de *Toxascaris leonina*.

PERÍODO PÓS-PARTO IMEDIATO

O estresse deve ser minimizado com o fornecimento de local para parto/amamentação com uma caixa limpa e seca e pela redução do tráfego de humanos e animais para evitar a introdução de doenças infecciosas. A caixa de parto ou de amamentação deve ser feita de um material que possa ser facilmente higienizado, como aço inoxidável ou plástico. A roupa de cama deve ser lavável (cobertores, toalhas) ou descartável (jornais, fraldas). Outros materiais que podem ser necessários incluem um substituto do leite apropriado para a espécie, tubos de alimentação, balança de precisão, termômetros digitais que possam medir temperaturas baixas, como 32°C (89,5°F), garrafas/luvas de água quente ou mantas térmicas, estetoscópio, bolsas de líquido (Ringer ou NaCl a 0,9%), equipo, agulhas, seringas, propés e desinfetante para as mãos (ver Capítulo 171). Os aparelhos para aquecimento devem ser usados com cautela, pois os neonatos podem não ser capazes de escapar se a temperatura estiver muito alta. Os propés e os desinfetantes para as mãos são usados para minimizar a chance de transmissão de doenças nos canis ou gatis.

A temperatura ambiente para os neonatos deve ser relativamente alta (29,5 a 32,2°C; 85 a 90°F), pois os neonatos não conseguem regular sua temperatura corporal. Durante a primeira semana de vida, a temperatura deve ser ajustada para 24 a 26,7°C (75 a 80°F) para raças de cães e gatos com pelo. Raças sem pelo (p. ex., cão Pelado Mexicano, gatos Sphinx) podem exigir um ambiente com temperaturas ligeiramente mais elevadas. A baixa temperatura corporal interfere na função imune celular. A manutenção da temperatura ambiente adequada diminui a morbidade. Para evitar o ressecamento da pele, os níveis de umidade devem ser mantidos em cerca de 55 a 65%; a umidade mais alta é propícia a doenças infecciosas. A equipe do gatil e do canil deve cuidar primeiro dos animais mais jovens para diminuir a transmissão de doenças infecciosas a essa subpopulação mais vulnerável.

AVALIAÇÃO E CUIDADO COM OS NEONATOS

Visão geral

Depois que toda a ninhada tiver nascido, deve-se examinar cada neonato, incluindo teste de reflexos básicos (endireitamento, procura, sucção, reflexo lombar), verificação de fenda palatina, hérnia umbilical, fontanela aberta, atresia anal, simetria, tônus muscular e quaisquer outros defeitos congênitos graves. Os neonatos devem ser identificados individualmente, e todos os achados registrados em seus respectivos prontuários. Durante as três primeiras semanas de vida os pesos corporais devem ser registrados diariamente, já que a redução do ganho de peso, a falta de ganho de peso ou a perda de peso podem ser os primeiros sinais de doença. A observação diária e os exames físicos rápidos são importantes para reconhecer o surgimento de sinais de doenças, como sepse, infecção por trás das pálpebras fechadas, diarreia, mudança na atividade mental, desidratação e hipotermia. Geralmente, é difícil determinar a causa de doenças em neonatos que não sejam lesão resultante de um trauma. A maioria apresenta perda de peso, hipotermia, hipoglicemia e/ou desidratação. As lesões podem resultar de um esmagamento acidental pela mãe, de cuidados excessivos da mãe ou do homem, ou mordida pela mãe ou por outro animal. As feridas são tratadas adequadamente e são administrados antibióticos (penicilinas, cefalosporinas) seguros para a faixa etária.[9]

Hidratação

Os neonatos possuem maior conteúdo de água corporal ($\approx$ 80%) e são incapazes de concentrar a urina. A desidratação é sempre uma preocupação a ser evitada. A autorregulação do fluxo sanguíneo renal, ainda não desenvolvido, resulta em diminuição da taxa de filtração glomerular. Os mecanismos compensatórios, como o aumento da frequência cardíaca e a contratilidade cardíaca em resposta à desidratação, são limitados em neonatos. As suas altas taxas metabólicas e perdas insensíveis (evaporação e respiração) contribuem para a necessidade de fluidos, e a desidratação pode se desenvolver rapidamente. Mesmo uma desidratação leve pode comprometer a saúde e precisa ser tratada imediatamente. A verificação da umidade das membranas mucosas orais permite melhor avaliação da hidratação do que o turgor da pele, a qual ocorre mais tarde em neonatos do que em adultos. Os sinais clínicos incluem membranas mucosas pegajosas a secas (desidratação 5 a 7%), membranas mucosas muito secas somadas a uma perceptível diminuição na elasticidade da pele (10% desidratação) e colapso circulatório (mais de 12% de desidratação). As causas mais comuns de desidratação são diarreia, vômito, inapetência, fome e negligência.

Em casos leves, os líquidos podem ser administrados por via subcutânea, em que a absorção é lenta e a probabilidade de sobrecarregar o sistema é menor. O ideal é que os líquidos sejam administrados por via intravenosa através da veia jugular ou cefálica (ver Capítulo 129). Na ausência de acesso IV, podem ser colocados cateteres intraósseos (IO) no fêmur ou no úmero, usando uma agulha 18 a 22 G ou uma agulha espinal 20 G × 3,75 cm (ver Capítulo 77).

No local do acesso, injeta-se uma pequena quantidade de lidocaína (menos de 0,5 mℓ) infiltrando os tecidos cutâneo, subcutâneo e periósteo. A área deve ser preparada assepticamente. O acesso ao canal medular é obtido através da fossa trocantérica para o fêmur ou através do tubérculo maior no úmero. As necessidades da fluidoterapia de manutenção são altas 80 a 100 mℓ/kg/dia (3 a 4 mℓ/kg/h), mas os volumes totais administrados são pequenos e a sobrecarga de volume ocorre rapidamente devido à incapacidade do neonato para processar rapidamente os fluidos.

Em desidratação moderada a grave ou choque, podem ser administrados 30 a 40 mℓ/kg de cristaloides isotônicos em *bolus* durante 5 a 10 minutos. Antes da administração, os líquidos devem ser aquecidos, mas não superior a 1°C (2,2°F) acima da temperatura corporal. Os equipos podem passar por um banho de água morna ou sob uma manta de aquecimento para evitar o resfriamento. Uma vez estabilizados, os neonatos podem ser mantidos a 6 mℓ/kg/h com 50% do déficit adicionado acima de 6 horas (déficit = BW × % de desidratação) para reidratação. Os pulmões devem ser auscultados com frequência para garantir que não haja sobrecarga de volume.

Hipotermia

Os neonatos são incapazes de regular a temperatura corporal. A hipotermia pode ser grave e causada por negligência materna ou diminuição do metabolismo por diversos motivos.[10] Seja qual for a causa, ela deve ser tratada imediatamente após a obtenção de amostras para o diagnóstico. A hipotermia resulta em diminuição da motilidade intestinal, o que pode levar ao íleo. A alimentação por sonda ou a alimentação forçada em neonatos podem causar aspiração seguida por pneumonia ou edema, resultando no aumento da pressão intratorácica e em dificuldade respiratória. Neonatos com dor ou dificuldade respiratória muitas vezes engolem ar e pioram o edema. Esse círculo vicioso pode resultar em distúrbio circulatório e morte. Além disso, a hipotermia inibe a função imune celular, aumentando a suscetibilidade à infecção.

A hipotermia em um cão ou gato neonato é definida como a temperatura corporal abaixo de 34,4°C (94°F) no nascimento, abaixo de 35,6°C (96°F) com 1 a 3 dias de idade, ou abaixo de 37,2°C (99°F) com 1 semana de idade. Neonatos hipotérmicos com temperatura corporal acima de 31,1°C (88°F) podem apresentar inquietação, choro contínuo, membranas mucosas vermelhas e pele fria ao toque. O tônus muscular pode ser aceitável, mas a frequência respiratória deve estar acima de 40/minuto e a frequência cardíaca acima de 200/minuto. Em temperaturas corporais na faixa de 29,4°C (85°F), os neonatos parecem letárgicos e incoordenados, mas respondem aos estímulos. Notam-se umidade e pequenas bolhas de saliva nas comissuras labiais. A frequência cardíaca cai para menos de 50/minuto e a frequência respiratória fica entre 20 e 25/minuto. Os sons abdominais estão ausentes e o metabolismo é bastante reduzido, resultando em hipoglicemia. Os neonatos com temperatura corporal abaixo de 21°C (70°F) podem estar em coma, mas deve-se tentar o tratamento se responderem aos métodos extremos de excitação.

Conforme descrito, os neonatos afetados devem ser mantidos secos, hidratados e lentamente aquecidos, não aumentando a temperatura a mais de 1°C (2,2°F) por hora. Se o neonato for prematuro (e/ou de baixo peso ao nascer), a umidade e a temperatura podem ser brevemente aumentadas para 85 a 90% e 29,5 a 32,2°C (85 a 90°F), respectivamente. A temperatura e a umidade mais altas ajudam a manter a temperatura corporal central do neonato, a hidratação e o metabolismo. O superaquecimento deve ser evitado e a posição corporal do neonato deve ser alterada com frequência para reduzir o vômito e, portanto, a aspiração. Incubadoras de oxigênio e incubadoras neonatais humanas fornecem oxigênio e ar quente para reaquecer os neonatos com segurança e rapidez.

CAPÍTULO 320 • Cuidados dos Neonatos durante o Período Pós-Parto

Em hipotermia grave, podem ser administrados líquidos quentes por via intravenosa ou por cateter intraósseo. Se aquecidos muito rapidamente, os neonatos podem sofrer prostração pelo calor. Os sinais clínicos incluem aumento do esforço e da frequência respiratória, cianose, diarreia e, por fim, convulsões. Frequentemente, ocorrem condições de risco de vida se a temperatura corporal for elevada a mais de 2°C (4,5°F) por hora. O superaquecimento pode ser corrigido com banhos de ar frio e água morna. No entanto, falência de órgãos retardada e morte ainda podem ocorrer, apesar da resposta positiva inicial. Podem ocorrer queimaduras na pele se os neonatos não conseguirem escapar de uma fonte de calor. O tratamento consiste na aplicação local de vaselina para prevenir desidratação, cristaloides IV e antibióticos sistêmicos ou orais. As queimaduras requerem uma grande quantidade de energia para a cicatrização e, portanto, deve ser fornecida suplementação calórica 2 a 4 vezes para manutenção.

Hipoglicemia

A hipoglicemia, definida como glicose sérica < 30 mg/dℓ (alguns sugerem < 75 mg/dℓ), é a causa mais comum de convulsões neonatais. Outros sinais clínicos incluem tremores, choro, irritabilidade, entorpecimento, letargia, coma e estupor. São causas comuns de hipoglicemia em neonatos fome, negligência e erros inatos do metabolismo, como a doença de armazenamento de glicogênio, desvios portossistêmicos e hipopituitarismo. A terapia consiste na administração de dextrose IV a 0,5 a 1 g/kg como solução de dextrose 2,5 a 5% em Ringer com lactato ou solução salina normal. A osmolalidade de soluções com alta dextrose (> 5%) pode ser cáustica e causar flebite. Se necessário, a dextrose pode ser aplicada diretamente nas membranas mucosas orais. Os mecanismos reguladores não estão totalmente desenvolvidos em neonatos; portanto, os níveis de glicose sanguínea, durante a terapia, devem ser monitorados de perto para evitar hipo ou hiperglicemia. No entanto, não se deve remover mais do que 5% do volume de sangue semanalmente, ou seja, não mais do que 0,5 mℓ de sangue/100 g de peso corporal. O sangue colhido deve ser cuidadosamente limitado.

Alimentação

Se um neonato não estiver ganhando ou mantendo o peso corporal, a suplementação pode ser necessária (ver Capítulo 171).[10] Os neonatos caninos e felinos devem ser capazes de ingerir as necessidades diárias de calorias e líquidos em quatro a cinco mamadas. Espera-se que os filhotes ganhem aproximadamente 2,2 gramas por quilograma do peso adulto previsto por semana. Os filhotes felinos geralmente nascem com 80 a 120 g e devem ganhar 70 a 100 g por semana. No entanto, é comum que os neonatos percam ou mantenham peso durante o primeiro ou segundo dia de vida. Contanto que estejam vigorosos e mamando, nenhum tratamento é necessário. Devem ser usados somente os substitutos de leite apropriados para a espécie. Os problemas mais comuns com a suplementação são a alimentação excessiva ou insuficiente. A superalimentação de substitutos do leite quase sempre resulta em diarreia, e a subalimentação pode resultar em desidratação e ganho de peso insuficiente. As fórmulas caseiras e muitos substitutos comerciais do leite que contêm leite de vaca podem ser deficientes em fatores de crescimento, aminoácidos e outros nutrientes essenciais. A densidade calórica da fórmula costuma ser alta, mas o conteúdo de líquidos é baixo. Portanto, as necessidades de líquido podem não ser atendidas, apesar de os requisitos de energia serem atendidos. Se forem possíveis várias mamadas ao longo do dia, a diluição da fórmula para atender às necessidades calóricas e de líquidos pode resolver o problema. Se necessário, o leite pode ser de alta densidade calórica e podem ser administrados líquidos

SC. Os neonatos devem ser estimulados a urinar e a defecar após cada alimentação, pela massagem da área anogenital com uma bola de algodão úmida. Nesse momento, a falta de permeabilidade anal ou diarreia pode ser observada. Urina altamente concentrada pode ser indicativa de desidratação. A constipação intestinal também pode ser observada, sugerindo o preparo inadequado do substituto do leite ou o hipotireoidismo em filhotes felinos.

Para garantir o ganho de peso, os neonatos devem ser pesados diariamente durante as três primeiras semanas de vida. Os neonatos nunca devem receber suplementos se a temperatura corporal estiver abaixo de 35,6°C (96°F), pois o trato intestinal fica lento e pode ocorrer aspiração. A alimentação pode ser iniciada se ruídos intestinais estiverem presentes. A alimentação suplementar pode ser fornecida por meio de sonda ou da colocação de um neonato com uma mãe substituta. Neste último caso, pode ser necessário esfregar o neonato junto aos outros filhotes da ninhada (ou mesmo em suas fezes) para induzir a ama de leite a adotar e a cuidar do órfão.

Alguns neonatos podem ser alimentados com mamadeira para atender às suas necessidades (ver Capítulo 171). Para isso, o neonato é mantido na vertical, permitindo a colocação das patas dianteiras na mamadeira ou na mão da pessoa. Deve-se conceder tempo suficiente ao neonato para engolir e respirar entre os goles; caso contrário, eles tendem a engolir ar ou aspirar. A alimentação por sonda é uma maneira conveniente de suplementar o recém-nascido com necessidades nutricionais, especialmente se houver malformações ou se o neonato estiver fraco.[10] Quantidades exatas de alimento podem ser oferecidas e isso pode tomar menos tempo se múltiplos neonatos precisarem ser suplementados. Dependendo do tamanho do neonato, pode ser utilizado um tubo de alimentação de plástico de 5 ou 8 F para alimentação por tubo. Para determinar o comprimento necessário do tubo e para que a ponta do tubo repouse logo após o esfíncter esofágico inferior, o tubo de alimentação é colocado ao longo do lado do neonato desde a ponta do nariz até a última costela. É feita uma marca em três quartos do comprimento mensurado da ponta do tubo de alimentação e isso indicará a parte do tubo de alimentação a ser colocada. A correta colocação da sonda é indicada pela pressão negativa ao puxar o êmbolo da seringa, pela vocalização do neonato e pelo fato de o neonato ter engolido a sonda.

A alimentação deve ocorrer na dosagem e taxa indicadas na embalagem do sucedâneo do leite. Às vezes, pode ser necessário diluir. O conteúdo calórico e fluido do leite canino, felino, bovino e caprino são indicados na Tabela 320.1.

Tabela 320.1	Teor de nutrientes do leite de diferentes espécies.			
	LEITE DE CADELA	LEITE DE GATA	LEITE DE VACA	LEITE DE CABRA
Conteúdo líquido (%)	77,3	79	87,7	87
Gordura (%)	9,5	8,5	3,6	4,1
Proteína (%)	7,5	7,5	3,3	3,6
Lactose (%)	3,3	4	4,7	4
ME kcal/100 mℓ leite	146	121	64	69

Adaptada de Casal ML: Management of orphan puppies and kittens. In Lopate C, editor: *Management of pregnant and neonatal dogs, cats, and exotic pets*, Ames, IA, 2012, Wiley Blackwell, p. 207-216.
Observe as diferenças na energia metabolizável (EM) entre as diferentes espécies. Ao misturar leite de vaca ou de cabra como substituto do leite para os neonatos, é importante estar ciente de que, a fim de cobrir as necessidades de energia, as concentrações de lactose serão muito altas e causarão diarreia. Os substitutos do leite comerciais são a melhor escolha.

SÍNDROME DO DEFINHAMENTO NEONATAL

A síndrome do definhamento neonatal não é um diagnóstico, mas sim uma condição clínica caracterizada por anorexia, letargia, emagrecimento, defeitos do nascimento e morte.[11] Os neonatos podem ser muito fracos ao nascimento para mamar, o que resulta em desidratação, hipotermia, hipoglicemia e morte dentro de horas a dias.[12] O diagnóstico da causa subjacente começa com histórico completo (ver Capítulo 1), incluindo informações sobre a gata ou a cadela, o ambiente, a ingestão de colostro, os substitutos do leite e quaisquer medicamentos administrados.[13] Após um minucioso exame físico (ver Capítulo 2), podem ser tomadas decisões a respeito da necessidade de exames de sangue e urina. Pode ser necessário estabilizar o paciente antes de completar o exame físico e buscar o diagnóstico. Se possível, os resultados dos exames de sangue, urinálise e/ou radiografias devem ser comparados aos controles normais de mesma idade. Nos neonatos com suspeita de doença congênita ou genética, uma cuidadosa revisão do *pedigree* e um histórico detalhado das ninhadas anteriores podem ser úteis.[14] Se forem afetados vários neonatos em uma ninhada, pode ser necessário realizar a eutanásia do neonato mais doente da ninhada e submetê-lo à necropsia para melhor entender a causa da doença.[15]

REFERÊNCIAS BIBLIOGRÁFICAS

As referências bibliográficas deste capítulo se encontram online no Ambiente de aprendizagem.

SEÇÃO 23
Doenças Renais

CAPÍTULO 321

Abordagem Clínica e Avaliação Laboratorial da Doença Renal

Harriet M. Syme e Rosanne Jepson

INTRODUÇÃO

A função dos rins é regular o volume e a composição do fluido extracelular pela formação da urina, o que é alcançado pela formação de um ultrafiltrado plasmático pela passagem de solutos, pequenas proteínas e outros constituintes não celulares do sangue através da barreira de filtração glomerular. O volume do ultrafiltrado formado é determinado, principalmente, pelo número de néfrons funcionais, mas também é afetado pela pressão hidrostática dentro do tufo capilar glomerular. Após a filtração, a composição desse fluido é alterada de acordo com as necessidades fisiológicas do animal, pela secreção e reabsorção de solutos e água, conforme passa ao longo do néfron. Em um animal saudável, sob condições fisiológicas normais, menos de 1% do fluido filtrado pelo glomérulo eventualmente será excretado como urina.

A doença renal pode influenciar esses processos em uma série de formas diferentes, a qual é mais frequentemente diagnosticada quando da diminuição da taxa de filtração glomerular (TFG) (reconhecida, em geral, como azotemia), em um paciente com doença renal crônica (DRC) ou lesão renal aguda. Essas síndromes são discutidas em detalhes nos Capítulos 322 e 324, respectivamente. A doença renal também pode ser reconhecida quando um paciente desenvolve proteinúria em razão da lesão à barreira de filtração glomerular (ver Capítulo 325). Os defeitos tubulares renais podem resultar em alteração da composição da urina (e, como consequência, do plasma) (ver Capítulo 326) ou urolitíase (ver Capítulos 331 e 332). Ademais, o rim possui uma série de funções endócrinas e é fundamental para a manutenção da pressão sanguínea (ver Capítulo 157).

ABORDAGEM CLÍNICA

A investigação de um paciente para doença renal pode ser iniciada pelos problemas clínicos existentes (poliúria/polidipsia, sinais relacionados com uremia, palpação renal anormal, edema ou ascite) ou após realização de exames de sangue de rotina e urinálise em um paciente com sinais inespecíficos (p. ex., depressão e anorexia) ou no qual foram realizados testes de triagem para "bem-estar".

Histórico clínico

Tutores de pacientes com DRC em geral relatarão que o animal está ingerindo água e/ou urinando mais do que o normal. A polidipsia foi definida como ingestão > 100 mℓ/kg/dia em cães (e talvez metade dessa quantidade em gatos), mas, mesmo que esse limiar não seja excedido, um aumento relatado na sede pode ainda ser significativo. O volume de urina produzido raramente é quantificado, mas os tutores podem notar aumento ou que a urina está mais diluída do que o normal. É importante diferenciar poliúria de polaquiuria (com pequeno volume), disúria e incontinência urinária, que costumam ser atribuíveis a problemas do trato urinário inferior, e não dos rins. Entretanto, é bastante comum que a doença coexista nos tratos urinários inferior e superior (p. ex., a poliúria exacerbará a incontinência urinária, a pielonefrite geralmente resultará de infecções ascendentes do trato urinário e as lesões obstrutivas, de azotemia pós-renal), o que faz com que esses problemas possam ter relevância. Existem muitas causas potenciais de poliúria e polidipsia (ver Capítulo 45), das quais a doença renal é apenas uma, e um histórico médico completo deve ser obtido para tentar excluir ao máximo alguns desses diagnósticos diferenciais e confirmar a existência da doença renal. A redução do apetite ou a perda de peso pode ser relatada em pacientes com doença renal, mas que também ocorre em muitas outras doenças. Sinais atribuídos à hipertensão sistêmica (hifema, midríase, cegueira) podem ser relatados pelos tutores de gatos com DRC, mas muito menos comuns em cães.[1-3]

O histórico em pacientes com insuficiência renal aguda (IRA) pode ser muito inespecífico (letargia, inapetência), mas tipicamente possui curta duração. Em algumas situações, os pacientes terão longo histórico relacionado com a condição clínica que os predispôs ao desenvolvimento de IRA, e essa cronicidade pode causar confusão na diferenciação entre doença aguda e crônica. Ocasionalmente, pacientes com IRA terão histórico de ingestão conhecida de toxinas ou de medicamentos prescritos potencialmente nefrotóxicos.

Exame físico

Um exame físico completo deve ser realizado em todos os pacientes com doença renal (ver Capítulo 2). Os rins devem ser avaliados quanto ao tamanho e aos contornos e se a palpação leva a sinais de desconforto. Os rins de gatos são facilmente palpados, mas costumam ser de difícil identificação conclusiva em cães. O tamanho da bexiga pode ser importante: se estiver grande em um paciente que tenha acabado de urinar, sugere poliúria; se túrgida, pode indicar obstrução; e, se estiver vazia em um paciente que tenha acabado de urinar, pode indicar oligúria.

O estado de hidratação pode ser anormal em pacientes com doença renal com desidratação e/ou hipovolemia, algumas vezes como consequência da poliúria ou contribuindo para o desenvolvimento da IRA. Edema e/ou ascite são características de síndrome nefrótica, mas também podem ocorrer como consequência de hiper-hidratação em pacientes que estejam oligúricos ou anúricos. Gatos são particularmente vulneráveis ao desenvolvimento de efusão pleural por hiper-hidratação e podem ser tornar dispneicos.

Pacientes com doença crônica podem estar em condição corporal ruim. Quando a DRC ocorre em animais jovens e em fase de crescimento, pode haver deformidades da maxila e mandíbula ("mandíbula de borracha" decorrente da osteodistrofia fibrosa), embora essa apresentação seja incomum. Animais idosos ocasionalmente sofrem fraturas patológicas em razão de distúrbios minerais e ósseos relacionados com a DRC. As membranas mucosas podem estar pálidas em pacientes com DRC, como resultado de anemia. Pode haver ulceração urêmica da mucosa oral (Figura 321.1) e necrose de ponta de língua se a azotemia for grave, mas não diferem entre doença renal aguda e crônica.

A pressão sanguínea deve ser aferida em todos os pacientes com nefropatia (ver Capítulo 99). É ideal que o exame de fundo de olho seja realizado em todos os pacientes, sobretudo em qualquer cão ou gato com pressão sistólica maior que 160 mmHg (ver Capítulo 11).

Diferenciação entre doença aguda e crônica

A doença renal crônica (DRC) costuma ser definida como um problema presente por um período de tempo definido (em geral, 2 a 3 meses ou mais); entretanto, conceitualmente, pode ser mais útil considerar a DRC como uma condição caracterizada por perda permanente de néfrons funcionais. A condição é irreversível, sem qualquer possibilidade de recuperação verdadeira, embora os néfrons remanescentes possam hipertrofiar e hiperfiltrar. Portanto, é vital diferenciar pacientes com DRC daqueles com IRA, nos quais a recuperação é possível (ver Capítulo 322), já que o tratamento desses dois grupos de pacientes é muito diferente.

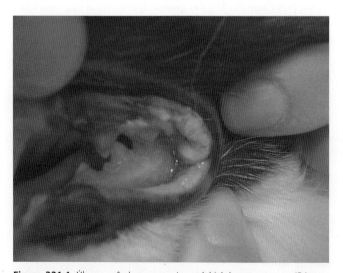

Figura 321.1 Úlceras urêmicas na comissura labial de um gato com IRA, que cicatrizaram quando da melhora da azotemia, ocorrida como resultado de ingestão de lírio (Cortesia de Helen Wilson). (*Esta figura se encontra reproduzida em cores no Encarte.*)

Em geral, a diferenciação de doença aguda de crônica é feita facilmente com base no histórico e nos achados de exame físico do paciente. Um histórico a longo prazo de poliúria e polidipsia costuma estar presente em cães e gatos com DRC, embora ocasionalmente os tutores não reconheçam isso. A perda de peso decorrente da hiporexia pode ser uma característica do histórico do paciente ou da má condição corporal ou do pelame evidentes ao exame físico, caso a doença seja crônica. Entretanto, essas características não estão invariavelmente presentes e podem, algumas vezes, ter causas alternativas, caso o paciente tenha mais de uma doença.

O tamanho e o formato renal podem fornecer pistas valiosas para diferenciar a azotemia aguda (tamanho normal ou aumentado, formato normal, ocasionalmente sensação de turgidez anormal) da crônica (pequeno e/ou de formato irregular). A palpação renal costuma ser mais informativa em gatos do que em cães. O diagnóstico por imagem pode ser utilizado para fornecer informações adicionais, o que permite uma avaliação mais objetiva do tamanho e do contorno renal, em conjunto com a avaliação em busca de mineralização e perda de arquitetura interna, alterações compatíveis com cronicidade.

Pode haver anemia não regenerativa em pacientes com DRC (ver Capítulo 199). As causas são multifatoriais, mas a deficiência relativa de eritropoetina supostamente é a mais importante. A anemia também pode ocorrer em pacientes com IRA por uma série de razões: por exemplo, pacientes em hiper-hidratação, com leptospirose ou hipoadrenocorticismo podem estar anêmicos. Além disso, hemorragia ou hemólise resultando em hipoxia/hipotensão podem servir como causa incitante de IRA. A identificação da anemia não deve, portanto, ser considerada indicativa de que, invariavelmente, sua natureza é crônica. Principalmente se a anemia for regenerativa (ver Capítulo 198), devem-se sugerir causas alternativas para ela e possível IRA.

A hiperpotassemia está mais frequentemente associada à IRA, sobretudo a causas pós-renais de azotemia. Ela pode, entretanto, ocorrer ocasionalmente em cães com DRC que estão sendo alimentados com dietas renais, especialmente se forem tratados concomitantemente com inibidores da enzima conversora de angiotensina (ECA) ou bloqueadores dos receptores de angiotensina.[4] A urinálise completa, além de mandatória na investigação da azotemia, pode fornecer pistas valiosas para a causa de base (ver Capítulo 72); por exemplo, piúria, bacteriúria e cilindros leucocitários seriam compatíveis com pielonefrite, cristais de monoidrato de oxalato de cálcio sugerem intoxicação por etilenoglicol e glicosúria indica disfunção tubular proximal. Entretanto, a pielonefrite e a disfunção tubular proximal podem ser de natureza aguda ou crônica. Grandes números de cilindros granulares e cilindros de células tubulares epiteliais renais são indicativos de necrose tubular aguda.

Em uma pequena proporção de casos com azotemia recém-diagnosticada, após revisão cuidadosa do histórico e do exame físico, avaliação ultrassonográfica dos rins e exames rotineiros hematológicos, bioquímicos e urinálise, a natureza aguda ou crônica do problema permanece incerta. Esse cenário pode ocorrer quando um paciente não mostra evidências de doença crônica, mas sua azotemia não melhora de maneira substancial após manejo apropriado de suporte para IRA presumida. Nesses casos em especial, testes adicionais úteis para diferenciação de doença aguda de crônica incluem radiografia da mandíbula/maxila, para pesquisar a perda da lâmina dura ao redor dos dentes;[5,6] exame ultrassonográfico das glândulas paratireoides, para detectar hipertrofia compatível com estimulação crônica;[7] e, pelo menos em teoria, mensuração da hemoglobina carbamilada (que reflete a concentração predominante de ureia), embora testes para tal finalidade não estejam atualmente disponíveis no mercado.[8,9] A biopsia renal (discutida adiante) também é ocasionalmente utilizada para diferenciar a doença aguda da crônica.

Diferenciação entre azotemias pré-renal, renal e pós-renal

A distinção entre causas pré-renais e renais de azotemia é mais frequentemente feita com base na mensuração da densidade urinária, que, caso seja maior do que 1,030 em um cão ou 1,035 em um gato, então a azotemia é considerada de origem pré-renal. Entretanto, há diversas ressalvas para essas regras. Gatos com doença renal crônica (DRC) algumas vezes manterão a capacidade significativa de concentração da urina (> 1,035 ou até mesmo 1,040), mesmo que azotêmicos. A urina concentrada foi documentada em gatos após nefrectomias parciais (7/8).[10] Cães e gatos com doença glomerular primária também mantêm, algumas vezes, a capacidade de concentração urinária, mesmo que tenham desenvolvido azotemia. Ao contrário, é importante considerar que o paciente somente será capaz de concentrar a urina em face da azotemia pré-renal se os mecanismos para tal dos ductos tubulares/coletores estiverem intactos. Se houver falta de hipertonicidade medular (p. ex., em paciente com hipoadrenocorticismo ou que esteja sendo alimentado com dieta muita restrita em proteínas) ou interferência na função tubular (pacientes submetidos a diuréticos) ou de ductos coletores (pacientes com causas primárias ou secundárias de diabetes insípido), a formação de urina concentrada não será possível, mesmo que a azotemia seja pré-renal. Nesses pacientes, a natureza pré-renal da azotemia é confirmada pela administração de fluidos intravenosos (ou redução da dose de diuréticos) e documentação da resolução.

Em geral, há suspeita de azotemia pós-renal com base no histórico e exame físico do paciente, com sinais atribuídos à obstrução ou à ruptura do trato urinário inferior (ver Capítulos 150 e 335). Os exames de imagem também podem ser informativos, particularmente em pacientes com obstrução parcial ou ureteral unilateral, nos quais os sinais clínicos são menos obviamente indicativos do problema. Se houver líquido livre retroperitoneal ou na cavidade peritoneal, então uma amostra deve ser coletada para análise; a concentração de creatinina no líquido maior que o dobro do sangue é compatível com ruptura do trato urinário. Por ser um irritante químico, a urina faz com que as inflamações assépticas neutrofílicas sejam comuns, mas a quantidade de hemorragia e inflamação associada é variável.[11]

Avaliação da gravidade da doença

A International Renal Interest Society (IRIS) desenvolveu um esquema de estadiamento para a DRC, subsequentemente endossado pela Society for Nephrology and Urology, em 2006, o qual é amplamente utilizado nos dias de hoje (ver Capítulo 324). Mais recentemente foi desenvolvido um sistema de graduação para IRA (ver Tabela 322.1, no Capítulo 322).

DIAGNÓSTICO LABORATORIAL

Avaliação da função renal

Taxa de filtração glomerular

A avaliação direta da taxa de filtração glomerular (TFG) é o padrão-ouro para avaliação da função de filtração e excreção do rim.[12-14]

A avaliação da TFG pode ser benéfica em uma série de situações importantes, que incluem a avaliação da função renal em pacientes com suspeita de doenças renais não azotêmicas (p. ex., paciente não azotêmico apresentando poliúria e polidipsia ou densidade urinária persistentemente baixa), nos quais o clínico deseja excluir a doença renal como causa de base para os sinais apresentados. A TFG pode ser útil como ferramenta de triagem para pacientes nos quais a doença renal incipiente é esperada (p. ex., raças com nefropatias conhecidas de início juvenil ou adulto) ou naqueles submetidos à administração de medicamentos potencialmente nefrotóxicos, nos quais a detecção da redução da função renal poderia levar à alteração da abordagem

terapêutica. A mensuração da TFG também pode ser útil a pacientes com doença renal nos quais a estimativa da redução da função renal seja necessária, a fim de ajustar a dose de medicações sujeitas à excreção renal. Atualmente, não existem evidências que apoiem o uso rotineiro da avaliação de TFG em pacientes com DRC azotêmica, nos quais a creatinina é um marcador substituto apropriado da função renal.

Diversas metodologias têm sido avaliadas e validadas tanto em cães como em gatos para avaliação direta da TFG, incluindo avaliação da depuração urinária e plasmática. Marcadores da TFG devem ter uma série de características importantes: eles devem ser livremente filtrados no glomérulo, não circular ligados às proteínas plasmáticas, não sofrer reabsorção ou secreção pelos túbulos e não alterar, por si sós, a TFG ou serem tóxicos aos rins.

As mensurações da TFG, seja qual for a metodologia, exigem padronização antes da interpretação, considerando, principalmente, os efeitos potenciais do peso corporal, da raça, do sexo e da idade. A mais comumente utilizada é de que a TFG seja expressa em termos de peso corporal, embora, com isso, se assuma a linearidade da relação entre peso corporal e TFG. Embora valores exatos variem dependendo da metodologia utilizada, e comparações diretas devam ser realizadas apenas entre métodos idênticos, a TFG tipicamente é de 3,5 a 4,5 mℓ/min/kg para cães e 2,5 a 3,5 mℓ/min/kg para gatos. Entretanto, em razão da escala metabólica, o peso corporal pode não ser um padrão apropriado, sobretudo em cães com < 10 kg ou > 50 kg. Embora parâmetros alternativos para padronização, como área de superfície corporal (ASC) e volume de fluido extracelular (VFEC),[15,16] possam parecer atraentes, a melhor fórmula para o cálculo da área de superfície corporal ainda tem de ser determinada.[17] Estudos com cães sugerem que a padronização para ASC pode ser preferível em detrimento do peso corporal.[18-23] A TFG, conforme avaliada pela depuração da creatinina endógena, foi previamente documentada como maior em filhotes de cães e gatos.[24-26] Em cães machos, a creatinina é ativamente secretada em pequenas quantidades pelo túbulo renal, potencialmente superestimando a TFG quando avaliada pela depuração da creatinina.[27]

Depuração renal ou urinária

A depuração renal ou urinária está relacionada com a taxa na qual uma substância filtrada é removida de certo volume de plasma pelos rins na urina, fornecendo informações acerca da quantidade do marcador que aparece na urina por unidade de tempo. A análise da depuração urinária requer a avaliação de uma quantidade da substância – seja exógena, seja endógena – tanto no plasma como na urina (ver Capítulo 73) durante um determinado período. A depuração urinária é calculada utilizando-se a seguinte fórmula: $D = (Uv \times Uc)/Pc$, em que D = depuração (mℓ/minuto), Uv é a taxa de fluxo urinário (mℓ/minuto), Uc é a concentração do soluto na urina e Pc é a concentração do soluto no plasma. A depuração urinária requer a implantação de uma sonda urinária (ver Capítulo 105) e esvaziamento vesical repetido e completo durante um período de coleta de urina de 12 a 24 horas, embora tenham sido descritos protocolos de amostragem/coleta mais curtos.[28-30] Toda urina deve ser coletada durante todo o período do estudo, já que, se isso não for feito, haverá subestimação da TFG. A depuração urinária da inulina tem sido considerada o método padrão-ouro para estimativa da TFG, mas a disponibilidade limitada dessa substância e dos laboratórios que a quantificam e a dificuldade relativa de realização da coleta completa da urina fazem com que seja rara a utilização desse método clinicamente.[28,30-37] Metodologias alternativas utilizam depuração renal de creatinina ou ioexol endógenos ou exógenos.[29,38]

Depuração plasmática

É uma metodologia mais frequentemente utilizada na prática clínica, já que evita a necessidade de coleta da urina. Devem-se obter amostras em determinados momentos com acurácia, a fim de evitar erros no cálculo da ASC. Marcadores de depuração plasmática utilizados incluem inulina, creatinina exógena, ioexol e radiomarcadores, como o iodo-hipurato de sódio [^{125}I], o [51]Cr-ácido etilenodiaminotetracético (EDTA) e o [99m]Tc-ácido dietilenotriaminopentacético (DTPA). Embora a depuração urinária da inulina seja considerada padrão-ouro, ela não é recomendada, já que até 40% dela é excretada por vias não renais no cão,[32] ainda não tendo sido estudada a depuração extrarrenal da inulina no gato.

A TFG determinada pela depuração plasmática é calculada utilizando-se a equação $Dep_{plasmática} = D/ASC$, em que D = dose da substância administrada e ASC, a área sob a curva da concentração plasmática *versus* tempo (ver Capítulo 160). A ASC é determinada pela obtenção da concentração plasmática da substância em intervalos determinados múltiplos durante um período predeterminado de tempo. Uma série de modelos farmacocinéticos diferentes pode ser utilizada para determinar a ASC, dependendo do analito e da frequência de amostragem. Modelos farmacocinéticos de um, dois ou diversos compartimentos, bem como aqueles sem compartimento, foram previamente utilizados para estimativa da ASC em estudos veterinários sobre TFG. O número de compartimentos ou modelo utilizado tem impacto sobre o cálculo da ASC e, portanto, da TFG calculada resultante.[45] Protocolos múltiplos de amostragem podem ser menos que o ideal, sobretudo em pacientes pequenos ou anêmicos. Portanto, muitos estudos focaram recentemente na validação de protocolos de amostragem limitada ou de amostra única, que fornecem uma abordagem mais simples de avaliação da TFG pela depuração plasmática na clínica.

Métodos de uma única amostra para estimativa da TFG também foram avaliados em cães[22,23,74] e gatos[22,23,72] utilizando-se abordagens de regressão linear ou não linear para determinar o melhor momento para uma única amostra, com base em métodos com múltiplas amostras.[79] A avaliação verdadeira da TFG utilizando-se um método de amostra única exige que o volume de distribuição seja conhecido e que a amostra seja coletada no momento que houver mistura completa do marcador com o volume de distribuição.[79-82] Recentemente avaliada no gato, tal abordagem sugere que o melhor momento para obtenção da amostra seja 180 minutos após a administração do marcador ioexol.[83] Embora isso seja aplicável para a maioria dos gatos nos quais a mensuração da TFG seja clinicamente necessária (*i. e.*, gatos com TFG próxima do normal), o momento da amostragem precisaria ser adiado para qualquer gato que sabidamente tenha baixa TFG.[83]

Metodologias alternativas para a avaliação da taxa de filtração glomerular

- **Marcadores radioisótopos:** uma das principais vantagens da avaliação de um radiomarcador é o potencial de realizar a cintilografia renal utilizando-se uma câmera gama, o que permite a avaliação da TFG global e renal individual pela mensuração da porcentagem captada da dose do marcador por rim separadamente. Entretanto, dificuldades associadas à cintilografia renal incluem experiência da equipe em definir a área de interesse, necessidade de sedação/anestesia geral, ajuste para profundidade renal, disponibilidade de instalações apropriadas para cintilografia e hospitalização após o procedimento. Diversos estudos avaliaram a determinação cintilográfica nuclear da TFG em cães e gatos utilizando-se ^{51}Cr-EDTA e ^{99m}Tc-DTPA[31,35,75]
- **Tomografia computadorizada:** tem sido utilizada em conjunto com a administração de ioexol para fornecer uma estimativa da captação renal global e individual de maneira semelhante à cintilografia.[84-91] Em razão da facilidade de realização desses exames e da disponibilidade relativamente ampla da tomografia computadorizada, são necessários outros estudos que avaliem essa abordagem
- **Marcadores fluorescentes:** sinistrina é um polifrutano avaliado como um marcador potencial para depuração

plasmática.[92] Um estudo preliminar avaliou a sinistrina marcada por fluorescência como um marcador transcutâneo da TFG promissor para o futuro como metodologia não invasiva.[93] Outro estudo avaliou a fluorescência radiométrica por fibra ótica como método para TFG[94]

- **TFG estimada:** na medicina humana, a TFG é estimada de rotina com base na concentração plasmática de creatinina ou cistatina C (TFG estimada; TFGe) utilizando-se equações que levam em consideração outros fatores, como idade, sexo, raça e mensurações do peso corporal, que refletem a massa muscular.[95-97] Tais equações parecem oferecer vantagens em termos de avaliação da função renal quando comparadas apenas às concentrações plasmáticas de creatinina ou cistatina C. Até hoje, somente um estudo tentou formular tal equação para gatos, mas a TFGe não ofereceu benefícios substanciais sobre a utilização da creatinina plasmática como estimativa da TFG.[98]

Marcadores plasmáticos/séricos substitutos da taxa de filtração glomerular

Para a maioria dos pacientes, a avaliação inicial da função renal será realizada pela utilização de um marcador substituto da TFG, mais comumente a quantificação da ureia e da creatinina.

Ureia. A ureia é produzida a partir da amônia derivada dos aminoácidos, como parte do ciclo da ornitina dentro do fígado. Aminoácidos utilizados na produção da ureia podem ser originados de fontes proteicas endógenas ou exógenas. A ureia é filtrada no glomérulo, mas sofre reabsorção passiva dentro dos túbulos. O grau de reabsorção aumenta com taxas mais lentas de fluxo tubular, tipicamente identificadas em pacientes hipovolêmicos ou desidratados. A concentração plasmática/sérica de ureia é comumente relatada como nitrogênio ureico sanguíneo (NUS) nos EUA e como ureia em quaisquer outros lugares no mundo, o que potencialmente causa grande confusão, já que são necessárias duas etapas de conversão: primeiro de NUS em ureia e, então, das tradicionais unidades (mg/dℓ) para SI (mmol/ℓ).

Uma das principais limitações da ureia como marcador da função renal é que a produção e a excreção não são constantes e podem ser influenciadas por muitos fatores. É amplamente recomendado que tanto cães como gatos estejam em jejum de, no mínimo, 8 a 12 horas antes da avaliação das concentrações de ureia, para evitar os efeitos da ingestão proteica dietética sobre as concentrações de ureia. Condições associadas ao aumento do catabolismo proteico (p. ex., febre, queimaduras, infecções, inanição, hipertireoidismo) aumentam o teor de ureia.[99] Em particular, a hemorragia gastrintestinal superior é uma importante causa de elevação das concentrações de ureia e da relação ureia:creatinina em cães e gatos.[100] Em contrapartida, redução da função hepática, desvio portossistêmico e dietas pobres em proteína podem contribuir para a redução das concentrações de ureia. Fitas de testes reagentes estão disponíveis para avaliação rápida e barata da ureia, mostrando boa sensibilidade e especificidade em cães e gatos.[101]

Creatinina. A creatinina é o marcador substituto mais amplamente utilizado da TFG na prática clínica,[102] produzida a partir da desidratação da creatina e defosforilação da fosfocreatina no músculo. Contanto que a massa muscular permaneça estável, a creatinina é produzida em uma taxa diária constante. Entretanto, as concentrações de creatinina são afetadas pela massa corporal magra e, como tal, animais jovens e aqueles com massa muscular pobre terão concentrações proporcionalmente inferiores de creatinina plasmática/sérica do que indivíduos maduros ou bem musculosos.[103] Estudos sugerem que as concentrações plasmáticas de creatinina aumentam gradativamente durante o primeiro ano de vida em cães e, então, permanecem estáveis ou aumentam moderadamente até 8 a 10 anos,[102] enquanto em filhotes de gatos as concentrações de creatinina são relativamente altas ao nascimento, mas semelhantes ou inferiores ao valores em adultos até as 8 semanas de vida.[104] Foi documentado que Galgos possuem maiores concentrações de creatinina do que outras raças, provavelmente como consequência da musculatura.[105] Em gatos, foram relatadas diferenças relacionadas com raças, principalmente a de que Birmaneses possuem maiores concentrações plasmáticas de creatinina.[106-108] Não existe efeito aparente do sexo sobre a creatinina plasmática no gato ou cão. A creatinina é livremente filtrada no glomérulo e muito fracamente secretada nos túbulos renais em cães, sobretudo em machos, mas essa informação é de significado clínico insignificante, mesmo em um paciente com função renal reduzida.[32,41,46,109]

Relata-se que as concentrações séricas de creatinina estejam entre 5 $\mu mol/\ell$ e 10 $\mu mol/\ell$ (0,05 a 0,1 mg/dℓ) maiores do que no plasma. A creatinina é menos influenciada por ingestão recente de proteínas do que a ureia. Entretanto, estudos que avaliam o efeito da alimentação sobre as concentrações de creatinina têm sido variáveis, vez que uns relatam que a administração de carne crua ou cozida leva a incrementos por até 12 horas no período pós-prandial, enquanto outros indicam diminuição ou ausência de alterações após alimentação com dietas comerciais.[110-112] Todavia, é preferível avaliar o teor de creatinina em um paciente em jejum por 8 a 12 horas.

No laboratório, as concentrações de creatinina costumam ser mensuradas pelo método inespecífico de Jaffe (com base na formação de um cromógeno amarelo-alaranjado quando a creatinina é misturada ao íon picrato em condições alcalinas) ou por técnicas enzimáticas específicas. Cromógenos que não a creatinina podem interferir na mensuração da creatinina ao utilizar a reação de Jaffe.[113,114] Entretanto, o grau relativo de interferência diminui em pacientes com doença renal, já que há aumento da concentração verdadeira de creatinina. Métodos enzimáticos não são afetados por cromógenos que não a creatinina, mas podem ser influenciados por hiperbilirrubinemia.[113] Os intervalos de referência relatados do laboratório podem variar amplamente, sendo sempre importante, portanto, comparar os resultados com o intervalo de referência relevante; o ideal é que as amostras comparativas do mesmo paciente sejam analisadas no mesmo laboratório ou com a utilização do mesmo analisador.[115]

A creatinina possui uma relação exponencial com a TFG (Figura 321.2),[116] o que significa que, em pacientes com uma TFG próxima do normal, ela é um marcador insensível da função renal, já que alterações na TFG resultam apenas em um incremento relativamente pequeno na concentração plasmática de creatinina. A relação entre creatinina e TFG é válida somente em pacientes nos quais a função renal esteja estável. A magnitude da alteração nas concentrações de creatinina e ureia não pode ser utilizada para determinar se a azotemia possui origem pré-renal, renal ou pós-renal ou, ainda, o potencial para reversibilidade da azotemia.

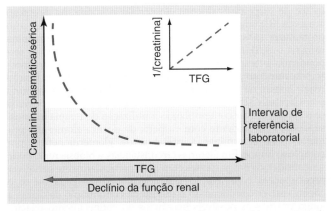

Figura 321.2 A creatinina mostra uma relação exponencial com a taxa de filtração glomerular (TFG) (*linha tracejada*) quando plotada diretamente, enquanto a relação entre a recíproca da creatinina plotada contra a TFG se aproxima de uma linha reta (*detalhe*).

Dimetilarginina simétrica. A dimetilarginina simétrica (SDMA, do inglês *symmetric dimethylarginine*) é um derivado dimetilado da arginina produzido a partir da metilação intranuclear de resíduos L-arginina pela metiltransferase da proteína arginina, em conjunto com seu estereoisômero dimetilarginina assimétrica (ADMA, do inglês *asymmetric dimethylarginine*). A SDMA é excretada principalmente por filtração renal, indicando que possui características necessárias para um marcador endógeno da função renal.[117] A SDMA plasmática mostrou ter boa correlação com a concentração plasmática de creatinina.[118,119] Em gatos azotêmicos e não azotêmicos, mostrou-se uma relação linear entre o recíproco da SDMA (1/SDMA) e a TFG, avaliada pela depuração plasmática do ioexol de forma semelhante ao recíproco da creatinina (1/creatinina).[120] Estudos sugerem que as concentrações de SDMA são menos influenciadas pela massa muscular corporal do que a creatinina plasmática.[103,119,121] Estudos preliminares sugerem que a SDMA pode ser um marcador mais sensível do declínio precoce da função renal em gatos.[122] A avaliação da SDMA não parece ser afetada pelo fornecimento de uma dieta renal suplementada com óleo de peixe ou L-carnitina no cão.[121] Entretanto, outros estudos ainda são necessários para determinar o efeito da doença concomitante sobre esse novo marcador. Historicamente, a avaliação da SDMA tem sido limitada pela necessidade de quantificação por cromatografia líquida acoplada à espectrometria de massa. Entretanto, o desenvolvimento recente de um imunoensaio disponível comercialmente tem tornado esse marcador amplamente disponível como teste diagnóstico clínico (ver Capítulo 324).[123]

Cistatina C. É uma proteína de baixo peso molecular (13 quilodáltons [kDa]) que atua como inibidor de proteinase e é produzida em uma taxa constante, pois é codificada por um gene de manutenção intracelular.[124,125] A cistatina C não está ligada às proteínas plasmáticas e é livremente filtrada no glomérulo.[126] Entretanto, ao contrário de outros marcadores, ela é reabsorvida por endocitose mediada por megalina dentro dos túbulos proximais e catabolizada.[126-128] Não ocorre secreção tubular de cistatina C, que, na medicina humana, foi proposta como um marcador mais sensível da TFG do que a concentração plasmática de creatinina.[129] Ademais, como a cistatina C urinária é tipicamente muito baixa, uma concentração aumentada dela pode indicar disfunção tubular.[130] Diversos estudos avaliaram o uso potencial de cistatina C em cães e gatos. Entretanto, até hoje esses estudos não mostraram superioridade consistente sobre a creatinina e fatores confundidores podem limitar a utilidade desse marcador na prática.[124] De fato, dois estudos recentes indicam que a cistatina C sérica não é um marcador útil para identificação da redução da função renal no gato.[124a,b]

Avaliação da proteinúria

Proteinúria é o termo utilizado para descrever quantidades aumentadas de proteína na urina. Contanto que causas de proteinúria pré-renais (p. ex., proteínas de Bence Jones) e pós-renais (inflamação do trato urinário inferior) possam ser excluídas, a proteinúria pode ser considerada de origem renal. A barreira de filtração glomerular, composta por endotélio capilar glomerular, membrana basal e podócitos epiteliais, limita a passagem de proteínas de peso molecular médio e alto do sangue para o filtrado glomerular, com típica retenção da albumina (69 kDa) e de proteínas maiores. Proteínas que sofrem filtração em pacientes saudáveis são efetivamente reabsorvidas por endocitose mediada por megalina e cubulina dentro das células tubulares proximais, de tal forma que a magnitude da proteinúria é tipicamente baixa, a qual pode ser originada da alteração na estrutura ou função da barreira de filtração glomerular, proteinúria glomerular ou ocorrer em razão da redução da capacidade de as células tubulares proximais reabsorverem proteínas – proteinúria tubular. A proteinúria deve ser avaliada em todos os pacientes com DRC como parte do esquema de estadiamento da IRIS (ver Capítulo 324). Em outros pacientes, a proteinúria pode ser investigada quando um resultado positivo for obtido em uma fita reagente de urina ou a nefropatia perdedora de proteínas for um diferencial clínico em um paciente com efusão cavitária ou edemas periféricos sugestivos de síndrome nefrótica ou hipoalbuminemia, especialmente quando a concentração de globulina for normal. Diversas metodologias estão disponíveis para a avaliação da proteinúria.

Fita reagente de urina bioquímica colorimétrica

Fitas reagentes de urina são as mais frequentemente utilizadas como teste de triagem para detecção de proteinúria. Elas tipicamente possuem maior sensibilidade para albuminúria do que outras proteínas urinárias com limite inferior de detecção de 30 mg/dℓ. De forma geral, essas fitas apresentam sensibilidade razoável (> 80%), mas especificidade muito baixa, sobretudo em gatos.[149,150] Resultados falso-negativos podem ocorrer em casos de proteinúria de Bence Jones ou em urinas diluídas ou ácidas. Resultados falso-positivos são relatados mais comumente em gatos e podem ser consequência de urina alcalina ou altamente concentrada, piúria/hematúria ou a realização da leitura em um intervalo de tempo incorreto.[149,151,152] Dadas as limitações desse teste, em qualquer paciente para o qual haja questões relacionadas com a presença de proteinúria, a avaliação adicional da relação proteína:creatinina urinária é necessária.

Teste do ácido sulfossalicílico

É realizado em alguns laboratórios diagnósticos como um teste confirmatório, com limite relatado de detecção de 5 mg/dℓ.[151,153] Ao contrário das fitas reagentes de urina, o teste do ácido sulfossalicílico pode detectar globulinas e proteínas de Bence Jones na urina.

Microalbuminúria

É definida como uma concentração de albumina > 1 mg/dℓ, mas abaixo daquela tipicamente detectável nas fitas reagentes de urina, < 30 mg/dℓ.[151] A microalbuminúria pode ser mensurada por testes semiquantitativos rápidos espécie-específicos ou por técnicas de ELISA espécie-específicas. Semelhantemente às concentrações de proteína da urina, a albumina da urina, quando quantificada, deve ser padronizada com relação à concentração urinária de creatinina, para fornecer uma relação de albumina à creatinina na urina, ou à densidade urinária de 1,010. A pesquisa de microalbuminúria pode ser considerada em pacientes nos quais há preocupações com relação a um resultado falso-negativo em um exame de rotina por fita reagente de urina, quando a proteinúria em baixo nível pode ser preditiva do início de doença glomerular hereditária, em pacientes geriátricos, nos quais há o desejo de um teste de triagem mais sensível, ou para o monitoramento de microalbuminúria já conhecida. A interpretação de microalbuminúria é importante, já que a presença dela pode ser afetada por causas pós-renais. Entretanto, o efeito da hematúria e piúria sobre a microalbuminúria é variável. Estudos sugerem que é improvável que as concentrações de microalbuminúria excedam 1 mg/dℓ até que a urina esteja macroscopicamente hematúrica (> 250 hemácias/campo) e que, em um grupo de 70 amostras de urina com piúria (> 5 leucócitos/campo), 67% apresentavam concentrações insignificantes de albumina urinária.[154] Qualquer resultado positivo deve ser repetido após 7 a 14 dias, para garantir que esse seja um achado verdadeiro e persistente. Resultados discordantes sugerem que o primeiro provavelmente tenha sido um fenômeno transitório, mas, se ambos forem positivos, isso então dá suporte à necessidade de monitoramento ou avaliação contínua da relação proteína:creatinina urinária.

Relação proteína:creatinina urinária

As relações proteína:creatinina urinária são o método mais comumente utilizado para quantificação da proteinúria. Uma relação proteína:creatinina urinária > 0,4 no gato e > 0,5 no cão corresponde a concentrações urinárias de albumina > 30 mg/dℓ,

considerada anormal se for um achado persistente ($\geq$ 3 ocasiões com $\geq$ 2 semanas de intervalo).[155] A relação proteína:creatinina urinária > 2 é fortemente sugestiva de doença glomerular de base, embora outras etiologias não possam ser excluídas sem a biópsia renal.[155-157] Estudos mostraram que relações proteína:creatinina urinária pontuais se correlacionam bem com a quantificação de proteína urinária em 24 horas, invalidando a necessidade de coleta de urina durante 24 horas em pacientes clínicos.[158-160] A relação proteína:creatinina urinária $\geq$ 0,2 tanto no cão quanto no gato apresenta um bom nível de especificidade para detecção de microalbuminúria (> 1 mg/dℓ) de 98,6 e 90,8%, respectivamente. Entretanto, a sensibilidade da relação proteína:creatinina urinária para detectar um baixo nível de microalbuminúria não é tão boa: de 47,9% no cão e 32,7% no gato.[149] Entretanto, um outro estudo em felinos sugeriu que a relação proteína:creatinina urinária teve bons resultados, com sensibilidade de 84,6% e especificidade de 81,8% quando comparada a um resultado positivo em uma fita semiquantitativa para determinação de microalbuminúria.[150]

Estudos recentes mostram que existem poucas diferenças no resultado da relação proteína:creatinina urinária obtida de uma amostra do jato médio de urina coletada por micção espontânea quando comparada à cistocentese.[161,162] Entretanto, um estudo mostrou que, em cães, os valores de relação proteína:creatinina urinária obtidos em um ambiente hospitalar podem ser maiores do que em casa.[163] Estudos sugerem que é improvável que a relação proteína:creatinina urinária seja influenciada pela hematúria, a menos que evidente (> 250 hemácias/campo), e que o efeito da piúria provavelmente seja mínimo na maioria dos pacientes.[154] Parece haver pouca variabilidade interlaboratorial ao avaliar a relação proteína:creatinina urinária com três metodologias e reagentes diferentes.[164] Entretanto, um estudo que avaliou cães com nefropatia hereditária ligada ao cromossomo X relatou variabilidade individual diária considerável. Esse estudo apoiou o fato de que a relação proteína:creatinina urinária deve mudar em 35% para pacientes com relação proteína:creatinina urinária $\approx$ 12 e em 80% para aqueles com relação proteína:creatinina urinária $\approx$ 0,5 para que reflita uma alteração verdadeira na relação proteína:creatinina urinária, e não pela variabilidade diária.[165] Ademais, enquanto uma amostra pode ser suficiente para avaliação da relação proteína:creatinina urinária < 4 em cães, devem-se avaliar não só > de 2 amostras de pacientes com a proteinúria mais acentuada (relação proteína:creatinina urinária > 4), como também realizar uma média, a fim de fornecer uma representação verdadeira da magnitude da proteinúria.[165] O armazenamento de um volume equivalente a três amostras de urina é um modo semelhante e com maior custo-benefício para avaliar a proteinúria em pacientes apresentando relação proteína:creatinina urinária > 4.[166]

Biopsia renal

A biopsia renal costuma ser realizada em pacientes com alto índice de suspeita de doença glomerular primária. As diretrizes atuais da IRIS sugerem que ela seja considerada em pacientes com proteinúria substancial persistente (relação proteína:creatinina urinária > 3,5), naqueles nos quais a proteinúria não esteja respondendo à terapia antiproteinúria ou, então, se ele estiver mostrando aumento progressivo da proteinúria ou declínio da função renal, apesar da instituição da terapia-padrão para proteinúria (ver Capítulo 325). A biopsia renal também pode ser considerada se o clínico estiver contemplando a utilização de terapia imunossupressora em paciente com suspeita de doença glomerular primária, para determinar a presença de glomerulonefrite por complexo imune. Em algumas circunstâncias, a biopsia renal pode ser considerada em pacientes com IRA, particularmente se houver preocupações com relação a glomerulonefrite aguda ou se o cliente estiver considerando o mérito da continuação da diálise a longo prazo e os possíveis benefícios do conhecimento relacionado com evidências de uma resposta regenerativa dentro do parênquima renal remanescente. Entretanto, na maioria das situações, a biopsia renal não levaria a uma identificação definitiva da etiologia da IRA.

Uma investigação diagnóstica minuciosa deve ser sempre realizada antes da realização da biopsia renal, a fim de avaliar a possibilidade de qualquer processo mórbido como causa de base que contribua para a proteinúria do paciente (p. ex., doença neoplásica ou infecciosa como etiologia), para documentar que a proteinúria seja um achado persistente, e para garantir que não possa ser atribuída a origens pré ou pós-renais (ver Capítulo 325).[157] Considerações importantes para pacientes submetidos à biopsia renal devem incluir o controle da hipertensão sistêmica, quando presente (ver Capítulos 99 e 157), interrupção de terapia antitrombótica por um período mínimo de 72 horas antes do procedimento e avaliação da hemostasia (contagem plaquetária, tempo de tromboplastina parcial ativada, tempo de protrombina, tromboelastografia, tempo de sangramento de mucosa oral [ver Capítulo 80], tipagem sanguínea). Contraindicações para a biopsia renal incluem DRC em estágio renal IV pela IRIS, quando é improvável que o grau de gravidade da doença renal de base seja reversível, independentemente dos achados da biopsia renal, pacientes com doença tubulointersticial primária nos quais não exista índice de suspeita para doença glomerular responsiva à terapia imunossupressora, evidências de hidronefrose, pielonefrite, distúrbios hemostáticos e abscessos renais.

Também não há sentido em realizar uma biopsia renal em pacientes com alto índice de suspeita para amiloidose ou nefropatia hereditária, dado que, até hoje, não existem evidências de que eles responderão aos agentes imunossupressores.

Muitos métodos estão disponíveis para biopsia renal, incluindo Tru-Cut® guiada pelo ultrassom (ver Capítulo 89), biopsia laparoscópica (ver Capítulo 91), cirurgia por laparoscopia e laparotomia exploratória completa com Tru-Cut® ou biopsia por cunha cirúrgica.[167-169] Independentemente da técnica utilizada, é importante garantir que a biopsia seja obtida somente do tecido cortical (Figura 321.3), o que garante que não apenas a área de interesse esteja disponível para avaliação (i. e., glomérulos localizados dentro do córtex), como também haja redução do risco de hemorragia substancial, que pode ocorrer se a junção corticomedular for atravessada em razão da localização das artérias arqueadas dentro dessa região. Para garantir que o dispositivo permaneça dentro do tecido cortical, deve-se, particularmente, ter precaução ao utilizar um dispositivo de biopsia Tru-Cut® associado a uma abordagem por laparoscopia ou laparotomia exploratória completa. Foi documentado que o número de glomérulos obtidos foi significativamente maior quando da utilização de um dispositivo de biopsia Tru-Cut® de calibre 14 G, em comparação a um de 18 G – seja por laparoscopia, seja guiada por ultrassom –, com aumento evidente dos artefatos nas amostras de biopsia com calibre 18 G.[170] Entretanto, na maioria dos pacientes, um dispositivo de biopsia Tru-Cut® calibre 18 G obterá uma amostra satisfatória, embora nos grandes possa-se preferir a utilização de um de 16 G,[168] com a obtenção de, no mínimo, duas peças de 10 mm de comprimento de tecido cortical. Em situações nas quais a peça de tecido cortical seja menor que 10 mm ou que haja preocupação com a presença substancial de artefatos, então uma terceira amostra deve ser obtida.[168] Independentemente da metodologia, contanto que o operador seja experiente, biopsias renais satisfatórias podem ser obtidas tanto em gatos (86,2%) como em cães (87,6%).[171] É mais provável que as amostras tenham qualidade satisfatória quando coletadas sob anestesia geral, que permite, principalmente, o controle da respiração de pacientes submetidos à biopsia renal guiada por ultrassom com Tru-Cut®, embora também seja relatado que esse procedimento é realizado com sucesso sob sedação profunda.[168]

Após o procedimento, a amostra de biopsia renal deve ser manuseada com cuidado para evitar artefatos por esmagamento ou manuseio; o ideal é que seja mantida em solução salina. A confirmação de glomérulos nas amostras pode ser constatada pela avaliação sob aumento 10× a 40×.[168] Elas devem ser cuidadosamente divididas para avaliação por microscopia óptica (fixado em formol), microscopia por transmissão eletrônica (MTE, glutaraldeído) e imunofluorescência (meio de Michel).[168]

Em razão da natureza especializada da interpretação da biopsia renal, quando possível, as amostras devem ser revisadas por um nefropatologista veterinário especialista (Boxe 321.1). A microscopia óptica não deve ser restrita à hematoxilina e à eosina, mas também incorporar a avaliação com tricrômico de Masson para identificar colágeno e tecido conjuntivo. A hematoxilina por ácido periódico de Schiff destaca a junção entre os compartimentos teciduais (p. ex., tubular, cápsula de Bowman e membrana basal capilar); a prata metenamina de Jones cora as estruturas finas da membrana basal glomerular, o que é útil para a identificação de depósitos de complexos imunes; e o vermelho Congo identifica substância amiloide.[172,173] Um estudo recente indicou que em aproximadamente 27,4% dos casos, a MTE foi necessária para confirmar ou realizar o diagnóstico de glomerulonefrite mediada por imunocomplexos, o que seria outrora classificado inapropriadamente com base somente na microscopia óptica.[156] Quando são identificados depósitos de imunocomplexos, a imunofluorescência pode ser utilizada subsequentemente para determinar sua origem com anticorpos direcionados contra IgG, IgA, IgM, C1q, C3 e cadeias leves lambda e kappa.[168,172,173]

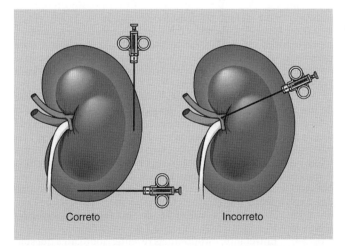

Figura 321.3 Demonstração da técnica de biopsia renal mostrando a colocação correta e incorreta do instrumento de biopsia no rim. (Cortesia da Dra. Shelly Vaden, North Carolina University, Raleigh, N.C.)

Boxe 321.1 Prestadores de serviço de biopsia renal pela Associação Mundial de Médicos-Veterinários de Pequenos Animais (WSAVA)

International Veterinary Renal Pathology Services
Dra. Rachel Cianciolo (telefone: 614-292-9717, e-mail: rachel.cianciolo@cvm.osu.edu)
The Ohio State University
301 Goss Laboratory
1925 Coffey Road
Columbus, Ohio 43210
Obs.: Substituiu o serviço previamente prestado em Texas A & M pelo Dr. George Lees

Dr. Luca Aresu (e-mail: luca.aresu@unipd.it)
European Veterinary Renal Pathology Service
Department of Comparative Biomedicine and Food Science
University of Padova
Viale dell'Università 16
Legnaro (Pádua)
35020, Itália
Obs.: Substituiu o serviço previamente prestado em Utrecht

Estudos que avaliam o efeito da repetição da biopsia renal sobre a função renal de cães e gatos saudáveis não documentaram impacto significativo sobre a TFG.[174,175] Entretanto, foram relatadas complicações em 13,4% dos cães e 18,9% dos gatos.[171] Fatores associados ao aumento do risco no momento da biopsia renal incluem pacientes de pequeno porte (< 5 kg), azotemia grave (creatinina sérica > 5 mg/dℓ) e evidências de distúrbios hemostáticos.[171] Hemorragia é relatada em 9,9% dos cães e 16,9% dos gatos, devendo ser tratada de maneira agressiva quando identificada. Outras complicações relatadas incluem hematúria evidente (4,2% dos cães e 3,1% dos gatos), embora hematúria microscópica possa ser mais comum, hidronefrose (0,4% dos cães e 3,1% dos gatos) e morte (2,5% dos cães e 3,1% dos gatos).[171,176] Infartos lineares são comumente observados após biopsia renal em cães e gatos.[171]

Aspirados renais com agulha fina raramente são esclarecedores em pacientes nos quais existe alto índice de suspeita de glomerulopatia primária. Entretanto, para doenças de base inflamatória, neoplásica primária ou metastática (p. ex., linfoma), essa pode ser uma alternativa de baixo risco, quando comparada à biopsia renal, já que fornece diagnóstico citológico em 78% dos casos de linfoma renal canino.[177]

Avaliação da hipercoagulabilidade na doença glomerular

A *hipoalbuminemia* pode ser identificada em pacientes com proteinúria moderada a marcante, sendo um componente da síndrome nefrótica em conjunto com hipercolesterolemia, proteinúria e efusão cavitária ou edema periférico (ver Capítulo 60). Tradicionalmente, o desenvolvimento de um estado de hipercoagulabilidade em pacientes com glomerulopatia é atribuído à perda de *antitrombina*, que possui peso molecular comparável à albumina e pode, portanto, ser excretada pela urina. Entretanto, a associação entre a proteinúria e as concentrações de antitrombina é fraca. A *tromboelastografia* (TEG) fornece uma avaliação total do estado de coagulação. Diversos artigos de revisão cobrem os princípios desse teste diagnóstico.[178-180] Cães com doença glomerular, incluindo aqueles com síndrome nefrótica, foram identificados com estado de hipercoagulabilidade com base na tromboelastografia.[181,182] Um estudo inicial sugeriu que cães com doença glomerular e nefropatia perdedora de proteínas apresentaram antitrombina significativamente inferior e proteína C significativamente superior a de cães com outras doenças sistêmicas.[181] Entretanto, um estudo mais recente avaliando 28 cães com nefropatia perdedora de proteínas (relação proteína:creatinina urinária > 2) mostrou que, embora esses animais estivessem em hipercoagulabilidade de acordo com os parâmetros da TEG, não houve associação entre ela, a relação proteína:creatinina urinária, a antitrombina ou as concentrações séricas de albumina.[182] Esse estudo indica que nem a magnitude da hipoalbuminemia nem as concentrações de antitrombina ou a magnitude da proteinúria podem ser utilizadas como preditivos do risco de complicações trombóticas em cães com doença glomerular ou para direcionar a terapia antitrombótica. Em tais pacientes, pode ser necessária uma avaliação minuciosa do sistema de coagulação.[182] Para informações sobre o tratamento da hipercoagulabilidade na doença glomerular, ver os Capítulos 196, 197 e 325.[183]

Testes genéticos na doença renal

Uma série de raças de cães e gatos sabidamente possui mutações genéticas causadoras de doença renal subjacente (ver Capítulo 328). Para algumas dessas condições, estão disponíveis testes genéticos em laboratórios comerciais. Como até hoje não foi identificada nenhuma condição glomerular hereditária que se beneficie da terapia imunossupressora, a realização de um teste genético apropriado relacionado com a raça poderia ajudar na prevenção da necessidade da biopsia renal. Uma origem genética para distúrbios tubulares diversos (p. ex., cistinúria, hiperoxalúria, hiperuricosúria) foi identificada e pode agora ser testada.[184-187] À medida que o campo da genética canina e felina se expande e novas tecnologias se tornam cada vez mais disponíveis, nossa compreensão sobre as mutações genéticas de base como causa de condições renais em cães e gatos provavelmente se tornará mais ampla.[188]

Urinálise

A urinálise (ver Capítulo 72) é um componente importante da avaliação da função renal, particularmente em termos de capacidade de concentração urinária, função glomerular e tubular, e da existência de infecções do trato urinário, as quais, em determinadas situações, podem ascender até afetar o parênquima renal e resultar em pielonefrite. A avaliação bioquímica da função renal deve ser sempre realizada concomitantemente à urinálise.

Capacidade de concentração urinária

A capacidade de concentração urinária é, em determinadas situações, espécie-específica, podendo o gato, por exemplo, atingir maior concentração urinária do que o cão. A maior parte da água é reabsorvida dentro dos túbulos proximais, da alça de Henle e no início do túbulo contorcido distal ($\approx$ 85%). O restante é reabsorvido no final do túbulo distal e pelos ductos coletores, sob o controle do hormônio antidiurético (ADH, do inglês *antidiuretic hormone*), outrora denominado arginina vasopressina (AVP), o que facilita a inserção dos canais hídricos de aquaporinas 2. A liberação de ADH é controlada pela osmolaridade plasmática e também pela volemia, capacitando a concentração e a diluição da urina de forma ativa. A reabsorção hídrica ocasionada pelo ADH depende do gradiente de concentração medular mantido pelo sistema multiplicador contracorrente.

A urina normal contém predominantemente moléculas de baixo peso molecular (p. ex., eletrólitos e ureia). A **osmolalidade urinária** é a concentração de moléculas osmoticamente ativas dissolvidas na urina, dependentes somente do número de moléculas e não relacionadas com o seu tamanho ou peso molecular, sendo relatada como osmoles por quilograma (Osm/kg) (ver Capítulo 73). A osmolalidade urinária (U_{Osm}) é mensurada em laboratórios, utilizando-se osmômetros de ponto de depressão de congelamento com base no princípio de que cada mol de soluto dissolvido diminuirá o congelamento em 1,86°C. A relação entre osmolalidade e densidade específica é considerada linear,[189] sendo, portanto, a densidade urinária mensurada por refratômetro manual mais frequentemente utilizada como uma aproximação da osmolalidade urinária na prática clínica. O termo *isostenúria* é utilizado para definir a densidade urinária entre 1.,008 e 1,015 (osmolalidade urinária de 300 mOsm/kg) e indica que a urina possui a mesma concentração de solutos que o filtrado glomerular e o plasma. O termo **hipostenúria** é utilizado para definir a densidade urinária < 1,008 (U_{Osm} < 300 mOsm/kg), indicando diluição tubular ativa, enquanto a **hiperstenúria**, um termo raramente utilizado, implicaria uma densidade urinária > 1,015 (U_{Osm} > 300 mOsm/kg). As fitas reagentes de urina não são uma metodologia confiável para avaliação da densidade urinária.[190]

A **densidade urinária** é avaliada tipicamente pela utilização de um refratômetro manual e definida como a relação entre o peso do volume de líquido e o peso de um volume igual de água destilada, a depender do número, do tamanho e do peso das partículas na urina.[191] Estudos iniciais sugerem que a urina felina possui um índice refratário superior à humana ou a canina e que a utilização de refratômetros desenvolvidos para uso humano levaria a resultados falsamente altos,[191] o que levou ao desenvolvimento de refratômetros específicos para felinos ou, de modo alternativo, à utilização de um **fator de conversão felino** (0,846 × densidade específica no refratômetro médico) + 0,154.[191] Entretanto, estudos mais recentes abordam a questão dessa diferença entre as espécies.[192-194] Aqueles que avaliam refratômetros digitais e ópticos análogos sugerem que os resultados provavelmente são comparáveis em cães e gatos.[194,195]

CAPÍTULO 321 • Abordagem Clínica e Avaliação Laboratorial da Doença Renal

Outros fatores endógenos que podem influenciar a densidade urinária incluem proteinúria ou glicosúria graves, que resultarão em superestimativa discreta da densidade urinária. Cada grama de proteína e de glicose por decilitro aumenta a densidade urinária em 0,003 a 0,005 e em 0,004 a 0,005, respectivamente.[196] Substâncias administradas exogenamente que aumentam as mensurações da densidade urinária incluem coloides, manitol e ioexol.[197]

Em pacientes com função renal normal, a concentração de urina é muito variável. Um paciente com função renal normal que esteja desidratado ou apresente azotemia pré-renal prevista apresentará concentração urinária máxima a fim de preservar a volemia, com densidade urinária > 1,030 no cão e > 1,035 no gato.

O **teste de privação hídrica (TPH)** é utilizado como um exame de resposta tubular à AVP em pacientes com poliúria e polidipsia, quando todos os diferenciais tiverem sido excluídos, com exceção de diabetes insípido nefrogênico ou central e polidipsia psicogênica (ver Capítulo 296).[203] O TPH de qualquer paciente que esteja azotêmico ou tenha desenvolvido azotemia pré-renal em face da urina diluída de maneira inapropriada (densidade urinária < 1,030) deve, na realidade, ser descartado e o animal submetido a restrição hídrica.

Marcadores de disfunção/dano tubular

Uma série de marcadores pode fornecer informações sobre a alteração ou perda aparente da função tubular e ser importante na avaliação de determinadas doenças renais agudas e crônicas.

Glicosúria

A glicose filtrada é quase completamente reabsorvida dentro das células tubulares proximais pelos transportadores SGLT2 (e, em menor extensão, SGLT1), não devendo ser identificada na urina de cães ou gatos saudáveis. A glicosúria é identificada se o limiar máximo tubular renal para absorção de glicose (180 mg/dℓ; 10 mmol/ℓ no cão e 300 mg/dℓ; 16,6 mmol/ℓ no gato) for excedido. A glicosúria é mais comumente identificada em pacientes que apresentam hiperglicemia concomitante (ver Capítulo 61); entretanto, a glicosúria primária renal em face da euglicemia indica alteração na função tubular renal. A glicosúria renal foi identificada como um distúrbio tubular renal único ou complexo. No último, pode haver aumento da excreção de outras moléculas (p. ex., aminoácidos, fosfato, bicarbonato e eletrólitos), podendo ser hereditária (p. ex., síndrome de Fanconi [ver Capítulo 328]) ou adquirida (ver Capítulos 322 e 326). A glicosúria pode ser identificada utilizando-se uma tira de teste colorimétrica, com base na reação enzimática de oxidase da glicose. Determinados antibióticos, como a ciprofloxacina,[204,205] ao utilizar a reação de oxidase da glicose, e penicilinas e cefalosporinas,[205,206] ao fazer uso de reagentes à base de sulfato de cobre, podem fornecer resultados falso-positivos em uma fita reagente de urina na avaliação da glicose, devido a propriedades de redução do açúcar.

Fração de excreção (FE) de eletrólitos é a fração da quantidade de um eletrólito mensurado filtrada e excretada pela urina (ver Capítulo 73). A determinação da FE costuma exigir a coleta de urina durante um período prolongado (≈ 24 horas); o ideal é que o paciente esteja posicionado em uma gaiola metabólica ou sondado, para garantir a coleta completa da urina. Entretanto, como é amplamente impraticável no contexto clínico, a avaliação pontual da FE de eletrólitos é, portanto, mais comumente utilizada. A avaliação pontual da FE pode ser calculada utilizando-se a seguinte fórmula:

$$\% \text{ FE} = [(\text{Concentração urinária de E}) \times (\text{Concentração plasmática de creatinina})/(\text{Concentração urinária de creatinina}) \times (\text{Concentração plasmática de E})] \times 100$$

Eletrólitos não ligados a proteínas são livremente filtrados no glomérulo e, então, reabsorvidos dentro dos túbulos. A reabsorção de solutos conservados (p. ex., aminoácidos e glicose) dentro do túbulo proximal é praticamente completa (> 99%), de tal forma que a fração de excreção em animais saudáveis é < 1%. Entretanto, para solutos como o sódio e o potássio, ocorre aproximadamente dois terços da reabsorção, independentemente das necessidades corporais (túbulos proximal e distal e alça de Henle), sendo o restante excretado ou reabsorvido, dependendo da regulação hormonal homeostática (p. ex., aldosterona). De forma semelhante, a reabsorção de cálcio (túbulos proximal e distal) é rigorosamente regulada pelo paratormônio, e a reabsorção de fósforo (túbulos proximal e distal) é controlada pela combinação do paratormônio e do complexo fator de crescimento de fibroblastos 23/alfa-Klotho.[207]

Diversos fatores exógenos e endógenos influenciam a FE de eletrólitos, como idade, raça, ingestão alimentar, composição dietética, exercícios, taxa de ultrafiltração, *status* de solutos e volemia do indivíduo, função renal e administração de fármacos.[12,208] O cálculo da FE de eletrólitos a partir de uma amostra pontual é, na melhor das hipóteses, uma avaliação superficial da excreção urinária em 24 h dos eletrólitos de cães e gatos, como consequência de imprecisões ao utilizar a creatinina como um marcador da TFG, flutuações nas concentrações urinárias de eletrólitos devido à alteração dietética e ritmos circadianos.[208-211] Não existem intervalos de referência claramente definidos para FE de eletrólitos, embora sejam relatados valores considerados normais.[208] A FE de eletrólitos é raramente utilizada clinicamente na medicina veterinária, em razão da variabilidade marcante inter e intrapacientes (ver Capítulo 73).

Para pacientes nos quais a quantificação da FE de eletrólitos estiver sendo considerada, sugere-se uma dieta padronizada por um período mínimo de 1 semana, a fim de prevenir o efeito de flutuações dietéticas e que o paciente tenha sido normalmente hidratado durante vários dias.[12] A FE da maioria dos eletrólitos aumenta à medida que a TFG diminui, o que limita o valor desse teste em pacientes clínicos com disfunção renal.[12,208] Isso pode ser consequência da resposta compensatória e hipertrofia dos néfrons remanescentes, o que permite o aumento da reabsorção, apesar de redução substancial do tumor renal funcional. Recentemente, entretanto, a avaliação seriada da FE do sódio tem sido relatada como um indicador potencialmente prognóstico do resultado da IRA.[212]

Aminoacidúria ocorre quando aminoácidos, que normalmente são efetiva e completamente reabsorvidos pelas células dos túbulos proximais (> 99%), são identificados na urina. Isso pode ocorrer em razão do excesso de concentrações circulantes de um dado aminoácido, o que leva às concentrações do filtrado a exceder a reabsorção tubular máxima por meio de um defeito intrínseco no mecanismo de reabsorção tubular, ou da incapacidade de processamento intracelular ou mecanismos de transporte na superfície basolateral da célula tubular proximal. A aminoacidúria pode ser um achado isolado em razão de um defeito em uma proteína de transporte individual, por exemplo, cistinúria, embora outros aminoácidos possam estar envolvidos (lisina, glicina, ornitina e arginina), e hiperuricosúria, ou ser parte de um distúrbio tubular renal complexo, como a síndrome de Fanconi, que pode ser hereditária (p. ex., Basenji) ou adquirida (p. ex., IRA) (ver Capítulo 326). O perfil de aminoácidos da urina, o qual pode indicar um distúrbio tubular renal primário ou secundário, está atualmente disponível na Universidade da Pensilvânia (PennGen).

Avaliação acidobásica e do pH urinário

O rim está intrinsecamente envolvido na homeostase ácido-base, sendo o túbulo proximal responsável pela absorção de íons hidrogênio e bicarbonato, mas o túbulo distal está estrategicamente localizado para a regulação homeostática da secreção do íon hidrogênio e o ajuste do pH urinário.[207] A avaliação do *status* ácido-base pela hemogasometria (ver Capítulo 128) pode ser importante no manejo de pacientes com DRC (ver Capítulo 324) e IRA (ver Capítulo 322), nos quais a acidose metabólica pode ser identificada. Ademais, a acidose tubular renal é um grupo raro de distúrbios que levam à acidose metabólica, quando a avaliação do *status* ácido-base e do pH urinário são fundamentais para alcançar o diagnóstico (ver Capítulo 326).

Em cães e gatos, o pH urinário é variável e pode ser influenciado por uma série de fatores externos e internos, incluindo dieta, medicações ou distúrbios ácido-base subjacentes. O pH urinário pode ser avaliado por testes de fitas reagentes bioquímicas ou pela utilização de um medidor de pH manual calibrado. Fitas reagentes bioquímicas são utilizadas de rotina para a avaliação do pH urinário na prática clínica, embora estudos tenham mostrado que elas são acuradas apenas dentro de variação ± 0,5 do pH e, portanto, quando a avaliação acurada dele for necessária, devem-se usar medidores calibrados de pH.[213-215]

Marcadores de lesão tubular

Nos últimos anos, tem havido interesse considerável no desenvolvimento de biomarcadores modernos de lesão tubular que poderiam ser utilizados para a detecção precoce da IRA e/ou DRC antes do início da azotemia evidente. Tais biomarcadores ofereceriam a oportunidade de interferir clinicamente em um ponto mais precoce e também apresentar potencial prognóstico. Até hoje, a maioria desses marcadores é utilizada em situações experimentais ou de pesquisa, não estando amplamente disponíveis no mercado. Estudos iniciais que avaliam nefrotoxinas (p. ex., gentamicina) tiveram como foco o papel das **enzimas urinárias** (p. ex., N-acetil-betad-glicosaminidase, gamaglutamil transferase, lactato desidrogenase, fosfatase alcalina, alanina aminopeptidase e a enzima específica felina, cauxina), que, quando liberadas na urina a partir de sua localização na borda em escova, indicam dano tubular regional. Mais recentemente, estudos exploraram o uso de **proteínas de baixo peso molecular** (BPM < 35 kDa; por exemplo, proteína de ligação ao retinol, beta$_2$-microglobulina, alfa$_1$-microglobulina), que são livremente filtradas no glomérulo e reabsorvidas por endocitose mediada por megalina e cubulina. O dano tubular reduz a capacidade para essa reabsorção e, dessa forma, concentrações aumentadas de proteínas de BPM são esperadas na urina de animais com doença tubular primária. Marcadores alternativos incluem **proteínas tubulares** (p. ex., lipocalina associada à gelatinase neutrofílica [NGAL, do inglês *neutrophil gelatinase-associated lipocalin*], lesão renal 1 [KIM1, do inglês *kidney injury 1*] e clusterina) ou **marcadores inflamatórios** (IL-8), os quais novamente informam a ocorrência de dano tubular direto ou processos inflamatórios durante a lesão renal.[216,217] Destes, a NGAL tem recebido maior atenção como marcador potencial de IRA (ver Capítulo 322). Estudos mais recentes que avaliam a DRC em gatos começaram a explorar a excreção urinária de **marcadores pró-fibróticos**, como o fator transformador de crescimento-beta,[218] e potenciais **marcadores de hipoxia** (p. ex., fator de crescimento endotelial vascular). Para todos os marcadores urinários, é importante que as concentrações mensuradas ou atividades enzimáticas sejam relatadas em associação às concentrações de creatinina urinária ou à densidade urinária padronizada para corresponder ao volume urinário.

Indicadores de doença renal na urinálise

A urinálise de rotina consiste na avaliação da densidade urinária a fim de que se faça uma avaliação da capacidade de concentração (ver anteriormente), avaliação da fita reagente bioquímica (ver anteriormente para discussão com relação à avaliação do pH, da glicosúria e da proteína), avaliação microscópica do sedimento e urocultura. A coleta da urina para análise é abordada no Capítulo 105. Em relação especificamente à doença renal, a urinálise é benéfica para detecção da redução da capacidade de concentração urinária (ver densidade urinária anteriormente), infecções do trato urinário e pielonefrite secundária (ver Capítulo 327), identificação de hematúria, que pode ter origem renal, indicadores de IRA (p. ex., formação de cilindros ou cristais de monoidrato de oxalato de cálcio em pacientes intoxicados por etilenoglicol) e pode fornecer uma indicação com relação à disfunção tubular, seja por alteração no pH, seja por presença de glicosúria e proteinúria ou de determinados tipos de cristais na avaliação do sedimento (p. ex., cistinúria). O ideal é que a urinálise seja sempre realizada com uma amostra fresca avaliada em temperatura ambiente. A metodologia utilizada para coleta da urina deve ser considerada ao interpretar os achados laboratoriais. A urina deve inicialmente ser avaliada em termos de aparência visual (ver Capítulo 77), incluindo coloração, odor e turbidez. Os leitores são direcionados para diversas revisões abrangentes sobre a realização da urinálise completa e fatores pré e pós-analíticos que podem influenciar os resultados.[249-251]

Hematúria

O número excessivo de hemácias na urina é conhecido como hematúria, que pode ser microscópica (detectável somente pela fita reagente ou avaliação microscópica) ou macroscópica (grosseiramente visível). Existem muitas causas potenciais para hematúria de origem renal, embora causas relacionadas com o trato urinário inferior (p. ex., infecção do trato urinário) e sistêmicas (p. ex., coagulopatia) sejam mais comumente identificadas, devendo ser diferenciadas da hematúria como consequência de doença com origem no trato genital (ver Capítulo 47). Baixos níveis de hemácias podem ser identificados na urina normal do cão e gato, com valores tipicamente < 5 hemácias/campo na amostra coletada por micção espontânea. Entretanto, números maiores podem ser identificados em pacientes nos quais a urina é coletada por cateterização ou cistocentese (< 20 hemácias/campo). Ocasionalmente, cilindros eritrocitários podem ser formados e, se identificados na urina, implicam origem renal da hemorragia (p. ex., hematúria renal idiopática).

Piúria

Envolve o aumento de leucócitos na urina (Figura 321.4) e é mais provavelmente identificada em pacientes com inflamação e infecção do trato urinário (ver Capítulo 350) ou infecção bacteriana ascendente aos rins, resultando em pielonefrite (ver Capítulo 327).

Entretanto, a presença de piúria, por si só, não pode ser utilizada para diferenciar se a infecção está localizada no trato urinário inferior ou no superior, a menos que os cilindros celulares identificados sejam leucocitários (Figura 321.5), indicando envolvimento renal, ou que a amostra tenha sido obtida diretamente da pelve renal pela realização de pielocentese.

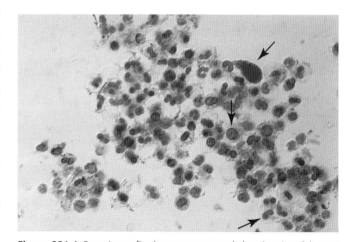

Figura 321.4 Fotomicrografia de amostra anormal de urina. Leucócitos na urina estão sujeitos a alterações degenerativas que podem dificultar a identificação. Eles podem encolher na urina concentrada ou edemaciar na urina diluída. Agregados de leucócitos estão frequentemente associados a infecções. Há células epiteliais de transição ocasionais nesse campo (*duas setas no topo*), com a observação de um neutrófilo com núcleo polimorfonuclear e citoplasma edemaciado (*seta no campo inferior*). (*Esta figura se encontra reproduzida em cores no Encarte.*)

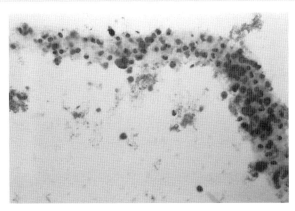

Figura 321.5 Fotomicrografia de um cilindro leucocitário na urina. Neutrófilos podem ser observados dentro desse cilindro, sugerindo pielonefrite. (*Esta figura se encontra reproduzida em cores no Encarte.*)

achados concomitantes da urinálise (p. ex., presença de sedimento ativo), resultados quantitativos da cultura (expressos em unidades formadoras de colônia/mℓ de urina), assim como os sinais clínicos do paciente antes do diagnóstico da infecção do trato urinário e a administração de antibioticoterapia.[255] Mais informações com relação ao diagnóstico e ao tratamento de infecções do trato urinário inferior e pielonefrite são fornecidas nos Capítulos 327 e 330, respectivamente.[263-268]

Cristalúria

No contexto da doença renal, a cristalúria pode fornecer informações sobre alterações na função tubular. A presença de cristalúria na urina de cães e gatos depende do pH urinário, da

Células epiteliais

Tanto células epiteliais escamosas como de transição podem ser identificadas no sedimento urinário, sendo o baixo número delas considerado normal. Células epiteliais escamosas (Figura 321.6) podem ser observadas em maior número em amostras coletadas por micção espontânea e cateterismo, com significado clínico limitado com relação à doença renal, já que provavelmente refletem contaminação oriunda da uretra ou vagina. Células epiteliais de transição são derivadas do urotélio e podem ser originadas da pelve renal até a uretra e, portanto, poderiam refletir lesão renal (Figura 321.7). Elas são células de tamanho variável, mas tipicamente menores com terminações cônicas (células caudadas) quando originadas da pelve renal (Figura 321.8). Entretanto, uma origem renal definitiva pode ser determinada apenas se as células epiteliais formarem cilindros celulares epiteliais (Figura 321.9), confirmando a origem tubular.

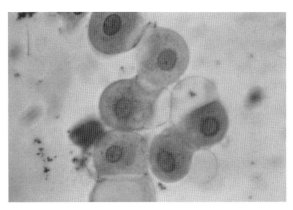

Figura 321.7 Fotomicrografia de um feixe de células epiteliais de transição na urina. (*Esta figura se encontra reproduzida em cores no Encarte.*)

Bacteriúria

Tradicionalmente, foi considerado que a urina dentro da bexiga está em um ambiente estéril, enquanto a uretra distal e o trato genital podem alojar bactérias. Entretanto, como esse não é necessariamente o caso, pode ocorrer bacteriúria subclínica, que se refere à identificação de bactérias na urina por uroculturas positivas de uma amostra coletada por cistocentese na ausência de evidências clínicas de infecção do trato urinário.[254,255] Em cães e gatos, a prevalência da bacteriúria subclínica é baixa em indivíduos saudáveis (2 a 9%),[256-259] mas pode ser maior (até 30%) em pacientes com doença concomitante (p. ex., hipertireoidismo, diabetes melito e doença renal crônica).[260-262] Os clínicos devem, portanto, considerar com cuidado o método escolhido para coleta da amostra (i. e., cistocentese, cateterismo, micção espontânea),

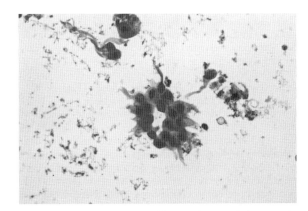

Figura 321.8 Fotomicrografia de células epiteliais caudadas na urina. As caudas, nessas células epiteliais pequenas, sugerem que elas se originaram na pelve renal. (*Esta figura se encontra reproduzida em cores no Encarte.*)

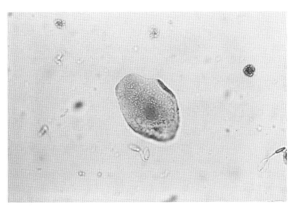

Figura 321.6 Fotomicrografia de uma célula epitelial escamosa na urina. Observe o núcleo pequeno, o formato celular irregular e a dobra da margem citoplasmática em algumas áreas. (*Esta figura se encontra reproduzida em cores no Encarte.*)

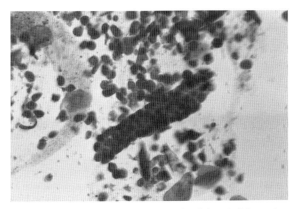

Figura 321.9 Fotomicrografia de um cilindro de célula epitelial na urina, com a identificação de pequenas células epiteliais renais nele. (*Esta figura se encontra reproduzida em cores no Encarte.*)

temperatura e do período de tempo entre a coleta e avaliação e a concentração de solutos que podem formar cristais. A cristalúria pode ser identificada na ausência de urolitíase, podendo determinados tipos (estruvita, fosfato amorfo, oxalato de cálcio) ser um fenômeno normal em cães e gatos. A formação *in vitro* da cristalúria mostrou ocorrer em 30% das amostras, com ocorrência mais provável em casos de armazenamento prolongado (24 h > 6 h); a refrigeração aumenta tanto o número quanto o tamanho dos cristais identificados.[269] Igualmente, a urolitíase pode ser detectada sem qualquer evidência de cristalúria (ver Capítulos 331, 332 e 334).[250]

Cilindrúria (formação de cilindros)

Os cilindros podem ser identificados nas avaliações do sedimento urinário como estruturas cilíndricas alongadas, cuja presença implica, de imediato, uma origem renal do dano, já que eles são tipicamente formados dentro do ramo ascendente da alça de Henle e do ducto coletor, onde as taxas de fluxo tubular são mais lentas. A presença de cilindros dentro da urina é denominada cilindrúria. Raros cilindros hialinos ou granulosos podem estar normais em cães e gatos, mas a presença de grandes números ou de cilindros celulares é sempre anormal e implica dano renal tubular. Os cilindros podem ser classificados como hialinos, granulosos, céreos, gordurosos, celulares (epiteliais, leucocitários, hemáticos), podem conter cristais e/ou microrganismos ou ter origem mista.

Cilindros hialinos são compostos inteiramente por material proteináceo (mucoproteína, proteína de Tamm-Horsfall/uromodulina, albumina) e possuem aparência cilíndrica descolorida (Figura 321.10). Pequenos números podem ser identificados em indivíduos após exercício extremo ou febre, mas, mais comumente, na urina de pacientes com proteinúria acentuada.

Entretanto, eles podem passar despercebidos se houver atraso na avaliação do sedimento ou em urinas alcalinas ou diluídas devido à dissolução. Se células epiteliais forem aprisionadas dentro da mucoproteína, são então denominados **cilindros epiteliais** (ver Figura 321.9), nos quais as células são claramente visíveis e implicam a presença de dano celular tubular direto (p. ex., por intoxicação por gentamicina). **Cilindros granulosos** (Figuras 321.11 e 321.12) são identificados quando há degradação parcial dos componentes celulares de um cilindro, tipicamente indicativos de lesão tubular renal isquêmica ou nefrotóxica. **Cilindros céreos** (Figura 321.13) ocorrem em situações nas quais houve degradação celular completa, deixando um cilindro que possui uma textura lisa, cérea. Cilindros céreos são formados durante períodos prolongados de estase tubular, são relativamente estáveis e descritos quase sempre como contorcidos, com terminações rombas. **Cilindros gordurosos** são raramente identificados, mas, quando presentes, podem implicar um distúrbio no metabolismo lipídico (p. ex., diabetes melito ou síndrome nefrótica). **Cilindros eritrocitários** indicam hemorragia renal acentuada (p. ex., após biopsia renal ou em casos de hematúria renal idiopática), enquanto

cilindros leucocitários (ver Figura 321.5) podem ser identificados em casos de inflamação renal acentuada (p. ex., pielonefrite) ou de necrose tubular aguda.

Bilirrubinúria
Ver Capítulo 53.

Cetonúria
Ver Capítulo 142.

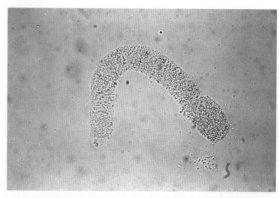

Figura 321.11 Fotomicrografia de um cilindro finamente granuloso na urina.

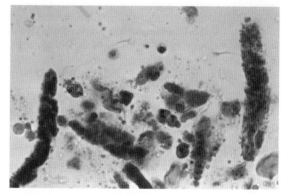

Figura 321.12 Fotomicrografia de cilindros grosseiramente granulosos na urina, vários dos quais observados nesse campo; o cilindro à direita contém grânulos grosseiros, enquanto o da extrema esquerda é um cilindro celular em degeneração. (*Esta figura se encontra reproduzida em cores no Encarte.*)

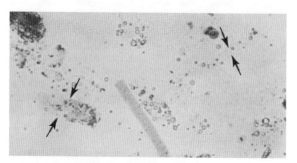

Figura 321.10 Fotomicrografia de cilindros hialinos na urina. Observe a natureza transparente desses cilindros (*entre setas*), não visualizados com facilidade por conta da densidade óptica muito baixa, o que traz a necessidade de baixa iluminação para visualização. O cilindro mais escuro no centro do campo é um cilindro céreo, havendo várias gotículas de lipídios no fundo.

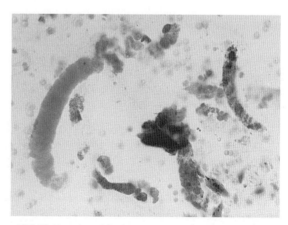

Figura 321.13 Fotomicrografia de uma amostra de urina com cilindros céreos e granulosos. O cilindro à esquerda é céreo, enquanto os outros são granulosos. Note que o cilindro céreo é translúcido, enquanto os cilindros hialinos são transparentes. Cilindros céreos são quebradiços e quase sempre possuem rachaduras ou terminações rompidas.

Parasitas

Raramente ovos de parasitas de *Stephanurus dentatus*, *Capillaria plica* (Figura 321.14), *Capillaria felis* e *Dioctophyma renale* podem ser identificados na urina, assim como microfilárias de *Dirofilaria immitis* no sedimento urinário canino.[250]

DIAGNÓSTICO POR IMAGEM

Em geral, o diagnóstico por imagem constitui uma parte integral do plano diagnóstico do cão ou gato com doença renal. Diversas modalidades de imagem estão disponíveis, cada qual com vantagens e limitações inerentes, que devem ser consideradas quando do alinhamento de um plano diagnóstico para um determinado paciente. Detalhes da técnica e os achados de imagem normais não são descritos com profundidade; para mais informações, os leitores são encaminhados para textos de diagnóstico por imagem e revisões apropriadas.[270-275]

Radiologia e tomografia computadorizada

Radiografias simples podem ser utilizadas para fornecer informações sobre o tamanho dos rins. Para descrever a variação de acordo com o peso corporal, o comprimento desse órgão costuma ser avaliado como uma relação ao comprimento da segunda vértebra lombar em uma projeção ventrodorsal; os valores de referência para a relação mais frequentemente citados são de 2,5 a 3,5 para o cão[276] e 2,4 a 3 para o gato,[277] embora diversos estudos tenham observado que o tamanho renal em animais normais possa se estender além desses limites, o que faz com que essas mensurações devam ser interpretadas com cautela.[278,279] O volume renal pode ser estimado de forma acurada com base em imagens de tomografia computadoriza (TC), utilizando-se o método de contagem de voxel.[280]

Radiografias também fornecem certas informações sobre o contorno renal. Entretanto, a ultrassonografia e as técnicas avançadas de imagem são, de modo geral, atualmente utilizadas em detrimento à radiografia para essa avaliação, em razão das informações adicionais fornecidas com relação à arquitetura renal interna. Cálculos renais e uretéricos são quase sempre radiopacos e, consequentemente, visíveis em radiografias abdominais. Entretanto, mesmo urólitos de composição mineral tipicamente radiopacos (oxalato de cálcio, estruvita e fosfato de cálcio) podem não ser visíveis se os cálculos forem muito pequenos, um problema particular em cálculos ureterais felinos (ver Capítulo 329). Algumas vezes, a mineralização distrófica e a nefrocalcinose são visíveis à radiografia, se as alterações forem extensas, mas são mais frequentemente detectadas à ultrassonografia.

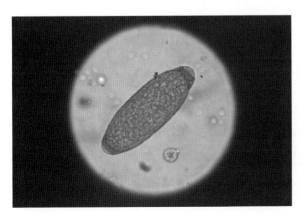

Figura 321.14 Ovo de *Capillaria plica* identificado na urina de um cão com sinais clínicos de polaquiúria. (Reproduzida, com autorização gentil de Alice Hughes.)

Urografia excretora (urografia intravenosa) pode ser realizada a fim de fornecer informações adicionais sobre o sistema coletor renal (pelve renal, ureteres, junção ureterovesical), como nos exames de um paciente com suspeita de obstrução do trato urinário, ruptura ou incontinência urinária (ver Capítulo 329). Embora também possa fornecer informações com relação ao número renal, ao tamanho, ao contorno e à arquitetura interna, a urografia excretora tem sido amplamente substituída pela ultrassonografia e outras modalidades de imagem, sendo raramente utilizada para esse propósito principal.

A imagem por TC dos rins pode ser selecionada em detrimento de outras modalidades de imagem, quando o foco de interesse for a pelve renal e o ureter (em geral por questões de obstrução ou ectopia ureteral)[281,282] ou houver um tumor dentro do rim ou próximo a ele.[283-287] Foram descritos padrões trifásicos da captação de contraste e excreção em cães submetidos a exames de TC,[288] assim como técnicas para angiografia tomográfica para a caracterização da anatomia vascular antes da doação dos rins para transplante.[289,290]

Ultrassonografia

É uma modalidade de imagem diagnóstica útil na investigação da doença renal, já que pode fornecer informações anatômicas importantes com relação ao tamanho, ao formato e à arquitetura interna renal. Deve-se reconhecer também, entretanto, que a aparência dos rins pode estar completamente normal, mesmo quando houver doença renal significativa.

No cão, as dimensões renais estão correlacionadas com o peso corporal, embora o volume renal esteja, de fato, relacionado de forma linear com o peso corporal, e a relação com o comprimento renal (o qual é determinado com mais frequência clinicamente) se afaste da linearidade em pacientes com menos de 10 kg.[291] Métodos para indexação do comprimento renal, com relação ao diâmetro aórtico[292] ou ao comprimento do corpo de L5,[293] têm sido propostos como métodos alternativos para avaliação do tamanho renal, mas não apresentam utilização disseminada. A avaliação subjetiva do tamanho renal é comum, mas, uma vez que a variabilidade geral do tamanho renal seja enorme, a validade dessa abordagem parece duvidosa. Em geral, o tamanho renal normal em gatos é considerado entre 3 e 4,5 cm,[294] embora possa ser maior nos machos inteiros,[295] e estudos recentes sugerem que comprimentos renais de até 5 cm sejam comuns, mesmo em animais castrados.[296-298] Pode ocorrer aumento renal difuso, com arquitetura renal interna relativamente normal, em razão de hipertrofia compensatória, IRA por diversas causas, amiloidose, linfoma, desvios portossistêmicos e acromegalia.[271,299-302] Rins pequenos são observados em casos de hipoplasia ou displasia renal, doença renal crônica em estágio terminal de diversas etiologias e como sequela de obstrução ureteral crônica.[271,303-307]

Os rins costumam ser menos ecogênicos que o fígado e o baço, o que pode variar com a frequência do transdutor utilizada.[308] Ademais, vacúolos de gordura no epitélio tubular renal supostamente afetam a ecogenicidade dos rins felinos, resultando em iso ou hiperecogenicidade do tecido cortical renal em gatos saudáveis com relação ao parênquima hepático adjacente.[309] O aumento difuso na ecogenicidade cortical é um indicador muito inespecífico de doença renal, que foi relatado em associação a glomerulonefrite, pielonefrite, leptospirose, necrose tubular aguda, doença renal em estágio final, peritonite infecciosa felina, nefrocalcinose, linfoma renal e outros tumores e intoxicação por etilenoglicol.[300,303,310-316] Na intoxicação por etilenoglicol, o aumento na ecogenicidade é quase sempre dramático e pode sugerir o diagnóstico, mas, para os outros distúrbios, o incremento na ecogenicidade é em geral não discriminatório.[275] Observou-se que alterações na ecogenicidade estão correlacionadas somente de forma fraca com os achados histológicos.[317] Aumento da ecogenicidade renal costuma ser observado em associação à ausência de definição corticomedular, que é outro achado muito inespecífico comumente associado à DRC, seja qual for a etiologia subjacente. Em um estudo de cães jovens com displasia renal, a perda de definição corticomedular e o aumento da ecogenicidade refletiram a gravidade das alterações histopatológicas renais, mesmo na ausência de azotemia.[318]

Lesões focais são mais fáceis de identificar pela ultrassonografia renal; as císticas possuem contorno arredondado a oval, conteúdos livres de ecogenicidade, paredes delgadas e mostram forte ganho acústico distal. Em geral, cistos únicos e simples são achados acidentais. Lesões pequenas múltiplas semelhantes a cistos podem ser observadas em casos de doença renal em estágio terminal; se ocorrerem em razão de lesões glomérulocísticas, podem estar confinadas ao córtex renal.[319] Determinadas doenças familiares podem resultar em lesões císticas na junção corticomedular especificamente,[320,321] podendo haver outros cistos no córtex e na medula. A doença renal policística (DRP) autossômica dominante é comumente observada em gatos da raça Persa e outras relacionadas[322-324] e ocasionalmente em cães,[325-327] resultando em múltiplos cistos de tamanho variado disseminados por todo o córtex e a medula (ver Capítulo 328). Se as lesões císticas possuírem paredes espessas ou irregulares, septações internas ou se o conteúdo não for completamente anecoico, então outros distúrbios, como hematomas, abscessos e tumores, devem ser considerados diagnósticos diferenciais.[271,275,286,328-331]

Tumores sólidos renais são comumente neoplásicos e podem ser hipo, iso ou hiperecoicos com relação ao parênquima renal circundante ou ter padrão misto.[273,274,300,330,332] A aparência dessas lesões não é característica do tipo tumoral; dessa forma, aspirado ou biopsia são necessários para diferenciação. Granulomas, hematomas calcificados ou abscessos são diagnósticos diferenciais potenciais para esse tipo de lesão, mas muito menos comuns do que tumores. A princípio, um infarto renal agudo pode parecer iso ou hipoecoico e, assim, ser confundido com um tumor, que costuma ser diagnosticado em estágio crônico, resultando em lesões hiperecoicas em formato de cunha, que são mais extensas em direção à superfície externa do rim.[273-275]

O fluido ao redor do rim pode ser subcapsular ou perirrenal, o que pode ser de difícil diferenciação. Pequenos volumes de fluido podem ser acúmulos de urina, sangue, transudato ou exsudato, observados em casos de extravasamento de urina, IRA, obstrução ureteral, abscessos renais, hemorragia ou neoplasia.[274,275,313,333,334] Um grande volume de fluido anecoico provavelmente representa um pseudocisto perinéfrico, o que é mais comum em gatos do que em cães, quase sempre observado em associação à DRC, podendo ser uni ou bilateral.[335,336] O espessamento subcapsular hipoecoico simulando acúmulo de fluido é uma aparência relativamente comum de linfoma renal em gatos.[337] A demonstração do fluxo sanguíneo dentro da região subcapsular utilizando-se o Doppler mostra que se trata de acúmulo celular, e não fluido.

Algumas vezes, há uma linha hiperecoica distinta paralela à junção corticomedular: o chamado sinal do aro medular, considerado uma variante normal em gatos.[309] Embora, quando inicialmente relatado, esse achado estivesse associado à doença renal em cães,[338-340] ele também é considerado por muitos como uma variante normal, sobretudo quando observado na ausência de outros sinais da doença.[341] Mais recentemente, foi sugerido que a medula externa pode estar relativamente hiperecoica em cães, sobretudo naqueles de raças de pequeno porte, o que pode ser confundido com o verdadeiro sinal do aro medular (não localizado diretamente adjacente ao córtex renal, mas discretamente distanciado dele, dentro da medula).[342] Ademais, relatou-se uma banda difusa de tecido hiperecoico dentro da medula interna de alguns cães com leptospirose aguda[313] (Figura 321.15).

Em cães e gatos normais, a urina não pode ser visualizada dentro da pelve renal; entretanto, equipamentos ultrassonográficos atuais

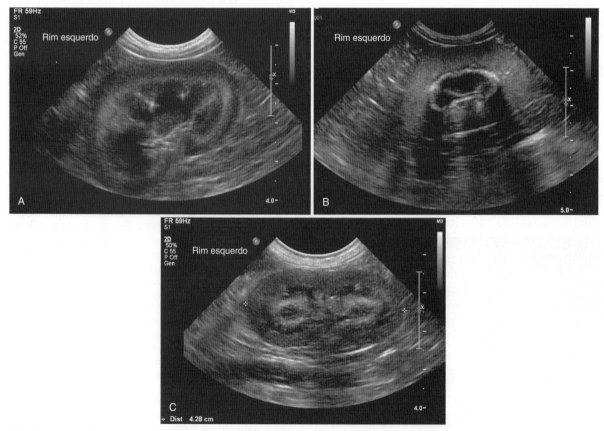

Figura 321.15 Imagens ultrassonográficas em eixo longo dos rins de três cães diferentes: **A.** Medula externa hiperecoica de um Cocker Spaniel não azotêmico. **B.** Sinal de aro medular em um cão com intoxicação por etilenoglicol. **C.** Sinal de banda medular na medula interna de um cão com IRA decorrente de leptospirose. (De Hart DV, Winter MD, Conway J et al.: Ultrasound appearance of the outer medulla in dogs without renal dysfunction. *Vet Radiol Ultrasound* 54:652-658, 2013.)

de alta resolução permitem a detecção de pielectasia discreta durante a diurese, que[343,344] pode ser assimétrica. O diagnóstico diferencial para dilatação pélvica renal, portanto, inclui todas as doenças renais poliúricas, assim como lesões obstrutivas e pielonefrite.[312,344,345] Nem sempre há alterações ultrassonográficas em pacientes com pielonefrite, entretanto as relatadas, além da pielectasia, incluem aumento da ecogenicidade da medula e/ou córtex renal e hiperecogenicidade do revestimento mucoso da pelve renal.[271,275,312] Quando a razão para a dilatação pélvica for incerta,

a pielografia renal anterógrada percutânea guiada por ultrassom pode ser utilizada para identificar e caracterizar em definitivo a obstrução ureteral (ver Capítulo 329).[346,347]

REFERÊNCIAS BIBLIOGRÁFICAS

As referências bibliográficas deste capítulo se encontram online no Ambiente de Aprendizagem.

CAPÍTULO 322

Lesão Renal Aguda

Cathy E. Langston

INTRODUÇÃO

Os rins têm alto risco de insulto isquêmico e nefrotóxico em razão de uma série de fatores, incluindo a alta proporção de débito cardíaco do rim (20%) em comparação com o peso corporal total (0,5%), alta demanda metabólica, e potencial concentração de nefrotoxinas nas células epiteliais tubulares.[1,2] A lesão renal aguda (LRA) corresponde de 1 a 4% das admissões hospitalares, complica uma porcentagem estimada de 7 a 36% dos episódios de internação em pessoas, e complica os quadros de sepse em uma taxa ainda maior (47%).[3-9] A incidência de LRA naturalmente adquirida em animais é desconhecida, mas seus efeitos podem ser devastadores. A LRA ocorreu em 15 a 22% dos cães e gatos hospitalizados, especificamente em 12% dos cães com sepse abdominal em um estudo, e até mesmo a lesão renal menor aumenta a mortalidade em pessoas e animais.[10-14] Em diversos estudos de doenças não renais, o aumento das concentrações de ureia nitrogenada sanguínea (UNS) ou creatinina séricas foram associadas de forma inconsistente com a mortalidade.[15-20]

DEFINIÇÃO E ESTADIAMENTO DA LESÃO RENAL AGUDA

Clássica *versus* mais branda

A LRA tem sido definida como um aumento na creatinina sérica acima do limite superior do valor de referência, na ausência de cronicidade.[21-23] Essa definição é sensível, mas não específica. A LRA não é somente um declínio rápido na função renal; está frequentemente associada à retenção de catabólitos urêmicos, desarranjo do estado volêmico, desequilíbrios eletrolíticos e distúrbios ácido-básicos. Um aumento de > 0,3 mg/dℓ ou > 25% de incremento da creatinina basal são duas das várias definições da LRA utilizadas em pessoas para detectar lesão renal sutil.[24,25] Como a creatinina é mal correlacionada com a taxa de filtração glomerular (TFG) em baixos níveis de disfunção, tais alterações na creatinina podem representar uma dramática diminuição na função renal, mas ainda permanecer dentro do intervalo de referência (ver Capítulo 62). Esses incrementos podem não se encaixar na definição clássica, mas eles representam LRA, no fato de que mesmo alterações discretas possuem implicações prognósticas.[13]

Estadiamento da lesão renal aguda

Diversos esquemas de estadiamento têm sido aplicados para a LRA em pessoas e animais. Em um estudo retrospectivo de cães em cuidado intensivo, o desenvolvimento de até mesmo um baixo nível de LRA (aumento da creatinina de ≥ 0,3 mg/dℓ ou 1,5 a 2 vezes o valor basal da creatinina) foi associado à maior mortalidade do que quadros sem LRA (58 *vs.* 16%).[10] Em outro estudo de cães e gatos hospitalizados e tratados em casa, cães, mas não gatos, que permaneceram não azotêmicos com um aumento na creatinina de ≥ 0,3 mg/dℓ tiveram mortalidade em 90 dias 3 vezes maior quando comparados àqueles nos quais a creatinina não sofreu alteração.[11] Tanto em cães quanto em gatos que desenvolveram LRA, a mortalidade foi três vezes maior com 30 e 90 dias, comparados a quadros sem LRA.[11] Por conta das inconsistências na definição de IRA, um esquema de estadiamento foi adotado pela International Renal Interest Society (IRIS), no qual critérios separados são baseados em alterações na creatinina, doença renal preexistente e débito urinário (Tabela 322.1).[26]

ETIOLOGIA

Categorias

As causas de LRA foram, classicamente, divididas em: causas hemodinâmicas (pré-renal), renais intrínsecas e pós-renais (Figura 322.1). Conceitualmente, cada categoria é distinta, mas podem se sobrepor em um indivíduo, o que complica a distinção do papel de cada uma. Danos renais extrínsecos persistentes podem levar a um dano renal intrínseco, pois são pontos diferentes em continuidade. O termo *uremia aguda* compreende as alterações bioquímicas induzidas por todas as categorias. Em pessoas, é estimado que 20 a 80% das uremias agudas tenham causas hemodinâmicas, 5 a 15% apresentem causas pós-renais e 10 a 45% sejam resultado de insuficiência renal intrínseca. As causas intrínsecas mais comuns são isquêmicas e por nefrotoxinas, com incidências menores de doenças de grandes vasos, microvasculatura, glomerular ou túbulo-intersticial aguda.[27-29] Em pessoas, a uremia aguda no momento da admissão hospitalar ocorre graças a causas hemodinâmicas em 70% dos casos, é resultado de uma única condição sem envolvimento de outros órgãos e costuma ter prognóstico bom. A uremia aguda que ocorre no hospital costuma ser causada por múltiplos insultos, tem envolvimento sistêmico de múltiplos órgãos, está associado a causas hemodinâmicas em 40% dos casos e, geralmente, apresenta prognóstico pior.[6,30,31]

Tabela 322.1	Esquema de classificação da lesão renal aguda pela IRIS.[200]	
ESTADIAMENTO DA LRA	**CREATININA SANGUÍNEA (mg/dℓ)**	**DESCRIÇÃO CLÍNICA**
Grau I	< 1,6	IRA não azotêmica: a. IRA documentada: (evidências históricas, clínicas, laboratoriais ou de exames de imagem de IRA, oligúria/anúria clínica, responsividade volêmica*) e/ou b. Aumento progressivo não azotêmico na creatinina sanguínea; ≥ 0,3 mg/dℓ (≥ 26,4 mcmol/ℓ) dentro de 48 h c. Oligúria mensurada (< 1 mℓ/kg/h) ou anúria durante 6 h
Grau II	1,7 a 2,5	IRA discreta: a. IRA documentada e azotemia estática ou progressiva b. Aumento azotêmico progressivo na creatinina sanguínea; ≥ 0,3 mg/dℓ (≥ 26,4 mcmol/ℓ) dentro de 48 h, ou responsividade volêmica* c. Oligúria mensurada (< 1 mℓ/kg/h) ou anúria durante 6 h
Grau III Grau IV Grau V	2,6 a 5,0 5,1 a 10,0 > 10,0	IRA moderada a grave: a. IRA documentada e aumento das gravidades de azotemia e insuficiência renal funcional

*Volume responsivo é um aumento na produção de urina a > 1 mℓ/kg/h durante 6 horas e/ou diminuição da creatinina sérica até os níveis basais em 48 horas. IRIS, International Renal Interest Society; LRA, lesão renal aguda.

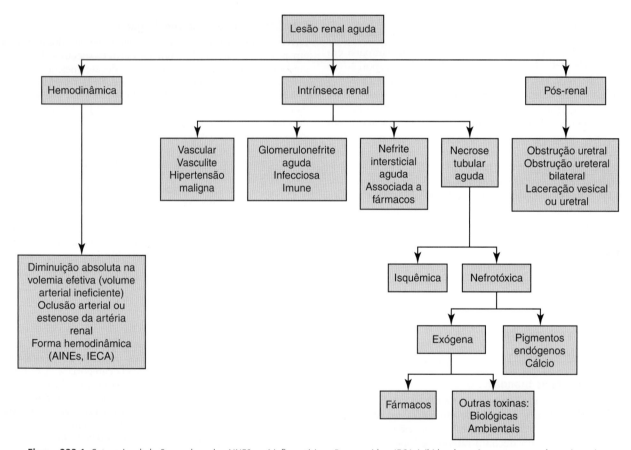

Figura 322.1 Categorias de lesão renal aguda. *AINES,* anti-inflamatórios não esteroides; *IECA,* inibidor da enzima conversora de angiotensina.

Azotemia responsiva ao volume (azotemia hemodinâmica)

Fornecimento insuficiente de sangue aos rins funcionais pode causar distúrbios da depuração de solutos e toxinas urêmicas. Enquanto essa condição costuma ser denominada de azotemia pré-renal, diferentes terminologias têm sido sugeridas para ajudar a esclarecer a causa desse fenômeno, incluindo azotemia hemodinâmica, azotemia transitória e azotemia responsiva ao volume.[32-36] Qualquer processo que diminua o fluxo sanguíneo renal, incluindo desidratação, hipovolemia, hipotensão, diminuição do volume circulante efetivo (i. e., insuficiência cardíaca, cirrose hepática, síndrome nefrótica), anestesia, hipoadrenocorticismo, trauma, cirurgia, choque (hipovolêmico, hemorrágico, hipotensivo, séptico), intermação, hipoalbuminemia ou hipoperfusão renal (i. e., secundário a fármacos anti-inflamatórios não esteroidais, inibidores da enzima conversora de angiotensina [ECA]), pode contribuir para esse distúrbio funcional.

A azotemia hemodinâmica é caracterizada por aumento dos níveis de UNS e creatinina em conjunto com uma densidade urinária específica concentrada. A fração de excreção do sódio (Na) na urina quase sempre é baixa, com exceção dos estados ávidos por Na, como a insuficiência cardíaca congestiva, insuficiência hepática e síndrome nefrótica (ver Capítulo 73).[37] A azotemia hemodinâmica é caracterizada por rápida reversão quando a condição de base é corrigida (*i. e.*, repondo os déficits hídricos e mantendo a pressão sanguínea arterial média acima de 80 mmHg).[36,38,39] Se esses fatores hemodinâmicos não forem abordados rapidamente, o paciente pode progredir para um estado não responsivo a volume. Em um estudo em pessoas, a azotemia transitória resolvida em 1 dia dobrou as probabilidades de mortalidade comparada a quadros sem azotemia. A azotemia hemodinâmica pode ser renomeada como LRA transitória.[33-35] Ao mesmo tempo que vários animais com má perfusão renal (p. ex., desidratação, hipotensão) respondem a fluidos IV, alguns não o fazem (p. ex., insuficiência cardíaca congestiva, sepse).[36] Embora a redução do fluxo sanguíneo renal e isquemia venham sendo considerados contribuintes importantes para a patogenia da LRA, a hipoperfusão renal por si só (80% de redução do fluxo sanguíneo renal durante 2 horas) não induziu LRA sustentada.[40] Respostas inflamatórias locais e sistêmicas, alterações na distribuição do fluxo sanguíneo intrarrenal, disfunção microcirculatória e hemodinâmica glomerular contribuem para a disfunção renal.[41] Esses fatores não são corrigidos pela fluidoterapia.

Insuficiência renal intrínseca

Contribuintes

A insuficiência renal intrínseca pode acompanhar o dano a qualquer setor do rim: glomérulos, túbulos, interstício ou vasos. Mais comumente, a insuficiência renal intrínseca acompanha o dano isquêmico ou tóxico tubular (Tabela 322.2). A isquemia, em geral oriunda de hipoperfusão, é a causa mais comum de insuficiência renal intrínseca em pessoas.[30,42] Em conjunto, as causas hemodinâmicas e intrínsecas renais correspondem por 70 a 75% dos casos de LRA.[6,43] A obstrução prolongada (> 1 semana) pode também levar à insuficiência renal intrínseca.[39] Múltiplos fatores podem estar presentes e pode ser difícil determinar a contribuição relativa de cada um. Contribuintes específicos para a insuficiência renal intrínseca por isquemia incluem progressão da azotemia hemodinâmica, hipotensão, hipovolemia, colapso circulatório, vasoconstrição renal excessiva, ou doença vascular renal (trombose, coagulação intravascular disseminada, ou estenose), queimaduras cutâneas extensas e reações transfusionais. Uma variedade de doenças infecciosas pode levar à LRA. A pielonefrite bacteriana costuma ser causada por infecção ascendente oriunda do trato urinário inferior, mas a infecção pode ter origem hematógena (ver Capítulo 327). A maioria das infecções do trato urinário (ITUs; 74%) é causada por organismos gram-negativos.[44,45] *Escherichia coli* é o mais comum e corresponde a 37 a 45% de ITUs, enquanto organismos gram-positivos correspondendo a 25 a 30%.[44,45] Condições predisponentes para o desenvolvimento de pielonefrite incluem endocardite bacteriana, discoespondilite e piometra.[44]

Leptospirose

A leptospirose (ver Capítulo 217) é causada por diversos sorovares de *Leptospira interrogans* ou por *Leptospira kirschneri* sorovar grippotyphosa. É uma bactéria filamentosa e móvel. Cada sorovar é mantido por um ou mais hospedeiros naturais. Sorovares clinicamente importantes e seus hospedeiros naturais na América do Norte incluem canicola (cão), icterohaemorrhagiae (rato), grippotyphosa (roedores, guaxinim, gambás), hardjo (vaca), e bratislava (rato, suíno, equino potencialmente). Espécies adaptadas ao hospedeiro quase sempre não desenvolvem a doença a partir do sorovar que carreiam, mas a infecção em um hospedeiro incidental pode causar a doença na forma grave. O método primário de transmissão é pela água contaminada com urina, embora solo, pastos e alimentos contaminados com urina também sejam vias de exposição. Organismos podem penetrar as membranas mucosas, pele úmida ou macerada, ou pele intacta. A exposição à urina, sangue ou saliva também pode transmitir a doença. O organismo prefere um ambiente quente, úmido e alcalino, e mais provavelmente estará presente em água estagnada ou de curso lento. Um aumento na incidência é comum após períodos de alagamento. O pico de incidência em cães ocorre de julho a novembro.[46-50] Cães machos adultos de raças de grande porte com acesso à rua mais provavelmente contrairão leptospirose, embora um estudo recente tenha observado que cães menores (< 7 kg) tiveram a maior prevalência, talvez porque esse grupo foi menos frequentemente vacinado.[46-48,51-53] A intussuscepção do intestino delgado foi notada em cães filhotes e adultos com IRA induzida por leptospirose.[54] Embora fosse sugerido que gatos tradicionalmente eram resistentes à leptospirose, gatos com doença renal mais provavelmente eram soropositivos do que gatos sem doença renal.[55] Uma IRA rapidamente progressiva com síndrome nefrótica tem sido reconhecida m cães com sorologia positiva para *Borrelia burgdorferi*. Apesar da terapia agressiva, vários pacientes não respondem.

Nefrotoxinas

Existe uma ampla gama de causas nefrotóxicas de IRA (Tabela 322.3; ver Capítulos 152 a 156). As causas mais comuns de nefrotoxicidade em cães são o etilenoglicol, fármacos anti-inflamatórios não esteroidais (AINEs), colecalciferol e aminoglicosídeos.[56] As causas mais comuns em gatos são etilenoglicol, colecalciferol e lírio.[56] O aumento da utilização de AINEs para o manejo perioperatório da dor pode aumentar a

---

Tabela 322.2	Causas de insuficiência renal aguda intrínseca.

EVENTOS ISQUÊMICOS	DOENÇAS RENAIS PRIMÁRIAS	DOENÇAS SECUNDÁRIAS COM MANIFESTAÇÃO RENAL	NEFROTOXINAS
Choque (hipovolêmico, hemorrágico, hipotensivo, séptico)	Infecciosa (pielonefrite, leptospirose, borreliose)	Infecciosa (peritonite infecciosa felina, babesiose, leishmaniose, endocardite bacteriana)	Toxinas exógenas Fármacos Toxinas endógenas
Diminuição do débito cardíaco (insuficiência cardíaca congestiva, arritmias, parada cardíaca, tamponamento cardíaco)	Imunomediada (glomerulonefrite aguda, LES, rejeição de transplante renal, vasculite)	Síndrome da resposta inflamatória sistêmica, sepse, falência múltipla de órgãos, coagulopatia intravascular disseminada	
Anestesia profunda/cirurgia extensa	Neoplasia (linfoma)	Pancreatite	
Trauma		Síndrome hepatorrenal	
Hipertermia/hipotermia		Hipertensão maligna	
Queimaduras cutâneas extensas			
Reação transfusional			
Trombose vascular renal/CID			
Hiperviscosidade/policitemia			
AINEs			

AINEs, anti-inflamatórios não esteroidais; *CID*, coagulação intravascular disseminada; *LES*, lúpus eritematoso sistêmico.

Tabela 322.3 Nefrotoxinas.[56,201]

CLASSE DO AGENTE	EXEMPLOS
Antibacterianos	Aminoglicosídeos, cefalosporinas (cefaloridina, cefazolina, cefalotina), penicilinas, sulfonamidas, fluoroquinolonas, tetraciclinas, vancomicina, carbapenemas, aztreonam, rifampicina, nafcilina, polimixina
Antiprotozoários	Sulfametoxazol-trimetoprima, sulfadiazina, tiacetarsamida, pentamidina, dapsona
Antifúngicos	Anfotericina B
Antivirais	Aciclovir, foscarnet
Quimioterápicos	Cis ou carboplatina, doxorrubicina, azatioprina, metotrexato
Imunossupressores	Ciclosporina, interleucina-2
Anti-inflamatórios não esteroidais	Todos
Inibidores da enzima conversora de angiotensina	Todos
Diuréticos	Todos
Agentes de contraste	
Terapêuticos diversos	Alopurinol, cimetidina, apomorfina, Dextrana 40, penicilamina, EDTA, estreptoquinase, metoxifluorano, antidepressivos tricíclicos, agentes que diminuem os lipídios, antagonistas do cálcio, análogos da vitamina D3 (medicações para psoríase), lítio, acidificantes urinários que contêm fósforo
Metais pesados	Mercúrio, urânio, chumbo, sais de bismuto, crômio, arsênio, ouro, cádmio, tálio, cobre, prata, níquel, antimônio
Compostos orgânicos	Etilenoglicol, clorofórmio, pesticidas, herbicidas, solventes, tetracloreto de carbono e outros hidrocarbonetos clorados
Toxinas diversas	Nitrato de gálio, bisfosfonatos, cogumelos, uvas, passas, veneno de serpente, veneno de abelha, lírios, rodenticidas que contêm vitamina D3, fluoreto de sódio, fertilizante à base de superfosfato
Toxinas endógenas	Hemoglobina, mioglobina

incidência de IRA. Doenças renais agudas primárias incluem condições imunes, neoplásicas ou degenerativas. Doenças sistêmicas podem causar IRA por afetar a hemodinâmica renal ou criar uma resposta inflamatória sistêmica. Doenças sistêmicas associadas à IRA incluem peritonite infecciosa felina, pancreatite, sepse, síndrome da resposta inflamatória sistêmica, falência múltipla de órgãos, coagulação intravascular disseminada, anemia hemolítica, hipertermia, insuficiência cardíaca e hiperviscosidade.

Lesão renal aguda pós-renal

A azotemia pós-renal é causada por extravasamento de urina dentro do tecido ou por obstrução uretral. Obstruções podem ocorrer na uretra, em ambos os ureteres, ou em um ureter com um rim funcional solitário (ver Capítulos 329 a 332 e 335). A obstrução urinária diminui a depuração renal por uma combinação de eventos neuro-humorais e aumento da pressão retrógrada no rim. Um aumento na pressão no sistema coletor após obstrução altera o equilíbrio das pressões hidrostática e oncótica, e diminui a TFG. A azotemia é rapidamente revertida pelo alívio da obstrução, embora a obstrução a longo prazo possa levar à insuficiência renal intrínseca.

A ureterolitíase em gatos é cada vez mais frequente, comumente observada como uma uremia grave aguda em um gato que estava aparentemente sadio.[57] A azotemia secundária ao extravasamento é rapidamente revertida fornecendo drenagem da urina do corpo, seja por cateter peritoneal em casos de uroabdome ou desvio urinário (i. e., sonda uretral ou *stent* que se estende acima e abaixo do local de ruptura). A urina é cáustica e inflamatória. Pode levar à peritonite estéril (ver Capítulo 143). O extravasamento de urina no abdome em um animal com uma ITU pode levar a uma peritonite séptica, uma emergência cirúrgica (ver Capítulo 279).

AS QUATRO FASES DA LESÃO RENAL AGUDA

A IRA começa sem sinais clínicos como um insulto isquêmico ou nefrotóxico, e continua até que uma alteração definível na função renal (aumento na UNS ou creatinina; diminuição do débito urinário). A duração de tempo necessária para observar alterações é variável, dependendo da natureza e gravidade do insulto.[58] Durante esse estágio, a intervenção precoce pode impedir a progressão. O segundo estágio é uma extensão do primeiro, com manutenção da hipoxia e respostas inflamatórias que propagam o dano renal.[59] Estruturas corticais (túbulo proximal e alça de Henle) são predispostas a danos tóxicos e isquêmicos porque recebem 90% do fluxo sanguíneo renal e são altamente metabólicas. A hipoxia leva a uma diminuição no ATP que, por sua vez, prejudica a bomba Na^+-K^+ com subsequente edema celular e morte.[60] Após a lesão celular tubular, há perda das superfícies celulares apical e basal da borda em escova, provavelmente causada por aumento no cálcio citosólico (Ca).[61] A lesão subletal pode progredir para morte celular. A intervenção pode não obter sucesso nessa fase.

A fase 3 é a fase de manutenção, que em geral dura de 1 a 3 semanas.[58] O débito urinário pode estar aumentado ou diminuído e a urina se assemelha ao ultrafiltrado, com poucas modificações pelos processos tubulares. Nesse estágio, uma quantidade crítica de dano irreversível já ocorreu. A quarta fase, de recuperação, é anunciada por um aumento no débito urinário que pode ou não estar acompanhado por uma diminuição do Na urinário porque os túbulos proximais e ramos ascendentes das alças de Henle têm reduções no número de transportadores de Na e proteínas aquaporinas-2.[58,62] Durante esse período, perdas extremas de Na levam à depleção volêmica que podem retardar ou interromper a recuperação renal. A regeneração e reparo do tecido renal podem levar semanas a meses.

DIAGNÓSTICO

Apresentação clínica
Animais com IRA costumam apresentar < 1 semana de anorexia, letargia, náuseas ou êmese, diarreia, oligúria/polidipsia (PU/PD) ou oligúria/anúria, e fraqueza. Animais com exposição a uma nefrotoxina podem não ter outros achados de histórico significativos. A ingestão de lírios por gatos pode estar associada a episódios de êmese de folhas ou outras partes da planta. Os sinais agudos de sistema nervoso central (SNC) podem estar presentes no início da evolução da intoxicação por etilenoglicol (ver Capítulo 152) em cães e gatos. O exame físico pode revelar graus variados de hidratação, quase sempre boa condição corporal, halitose urêmica ou ulceração oral com uremia grave, dor renal (dor abdominal específica ou inespecífica), aumento renal, taquicardia ou bradicardia.

Avaliação laboratorial
A avaliação clínica laboratorial costuma incluir hematologia (hemograma), urinálise e bioquímicos séricos. Anormalidades podem incluir azotemia (elevação de UNS, creatinina), aumento do fosfato, acidose metabólica, hipocalcemia e/ou hipo- ou hiperpotassemia. A anemia pode acompanhar a perda sanguínea, se ocorrer sangramento gastrintestinal (GI). A urinálise pode revelar isostenúria ou uma densidade urinária específica minimamente concentrada (< 1,035), proteinúria e glicosúria. Cilindros no sedimento urinário (ver Capítulo 72) indicam dano renal em andamento, mas são frágeis e podem sofrer desintegração se a avaliação for retardada (assim como durante o envio de amostras a um laboratório). Hemácias, leucócitos ou bactérias podem estar presentes. Cristais de oxalato cálcio podem indicar podem indicar intoxicação por etilenoglicol (ver Capítulo 152). A urocultura pode revelar uma pielonefrite bacteriana (raramente fúngica) como causa da LRA.

Diagnóstico por imagem
Radiografias podem demonstrar rins normais ou aumentados e/ou nefrólitos/ureterólitos. A ultrassonografia abdominal pode revelar rins normais ou aumentados (ver Capítulo 88). Em casos de intoxicação por etilenoglicol, os rins podem parecer hiperecoicos. O acúmulo perirrenal de fluido pode ser observado em casos de leptospirose em cães, linfoma em gatos e outras condições. A hidronefrose pode indicar obstrução ou pielonefrite. A dilatação pélvica renal discreta pode ocorrer após fluidoterapia agressiva. A dilatação ureteral discreta que se estende minimamente após a pelve renal suporta a inflamação associada à pielonefrite. Um ureter dilatado pode ser atribuído a uma obstrução por cálculo (frequentemente difícil de visualizar). Pielografia ou tomografia computadorizada (TC) intravenosa (IV) ou anterógrada podem demarcar melhor a obstrução ureteral (Figura 322.2).

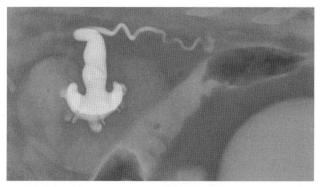

Figura 322.2 Pielografia anterógrada demonstra dilatação da pelve renal e ureter proximal. O contraste pode ser observado no ureter por vários centímetros, mas o ureter não pode ser visualizado até a bexiga. A bexiga contém contraste oriundo do rim contralateral.

Aspirado por agulha fina renal e biopsia
Aspirado por agulha fina
A aspirado por agulha fina (AAF) renal (ver Capítulos 89 e 93) pode ser útil para o estabelecimento do diagnóstico de linfoma renal. A AAF, utilizando uma agulha de diâmetro 22 ou 25, guiado ou não por ultrassonografia, pode ser realizada com sedação pesada. O risco de hemorragia é baixo. O linfoma renal pode ser confirmado pela citologia, mas a incapacidade em confirmar ainda o deixa como possibilidade. A citologia por AAF não pode diagnosticar definitivamente a maioria das outras condições.

Biopsia
A biopsia percutânea guiada pelo ultrassom pode ser realizada após administração de um anestésico de rápida ação ao animal (ver Capítulo 89). A agulha de biopsia é direcionada pela curvatura maior do rim em direção ao córtex, ou pelo córtex e pela medula em direção ao polo renal. A pelve renal e vasos maiores devem ser evitados. As vantagens desse procedimento incluem evitar a formação de ferida cirúrgica e realização de anestesia geral, mas as desvantagens incluem o pequeno tamanho da amostra e a incapacidade de controlar o sangramento. A biopsia por agulha laparoscópica (ver Capítulo 91) ou biopsia cirúrgica em cunha por meio de uma incisão laparoscópica no flanco quase sempre fornece amostra suficiente para o diagnóstico acurado. A biopsia renal pode identificar um diagnóstico específico (i. e., intoxicação por etilenoglicol, linfoma renal, leptospirose), ou pode revelar necrose tubular aguda – um achado patológico específico, mas que é causado por várias condições. O risco de hemorragia quando a uremia é grave é alto por conta da trombocitopatias (ver Capítulo 197).

Testes específicos da função renal
Creatinina sérica e taxa de filtração glomerular
A creatinina sérica é provavelmente uma das mensurações mais comumente utilizadas de função renal na medicina clínica, mas é um marcador insensível para a disfunção renal discreta (ver Capítulos 62, 321 e 324). Somente pequenas alterações na creatinina sérica ocorrem apesar de grandes diminuições na TFG quando a função renal estiver próxima do normal, enquanto pequenas alterações na TFG levam a grandes alterações na creatinina sérica quando a função estiver severamente comprometida (Figura 322.3). Em pessoas, equações de fatoração em diferentes variáveis (i. e., idade, gênero, etnia) foram desenvolvidas para estimar a TFG a partir da creatinina sérica, para evitar o ônus da mensuração da TFG, mas equações semelhantes não foram consideradas úteis na medicina veterinária. Valores normais para TFG em cães variam pelo tamanho e raça.[63,64] Existem métodos úteis para mensuração da TFG, incluindo depuração plasmática (iohexol, creatinina exógena), depuração urinária (creatinina endógena ou exógena) ou cintilografia renal.

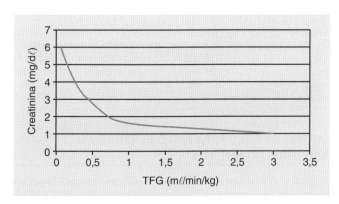

Figura 322.3 Taxa de filtração glomerular (*TFG*) e concentração de creatinina sérica.

Excreção fracionada de sódio

A excreção fracionada de sódio (EF_{Na}) (ver Capítulo 73) pode ser utilizada para ajudar a diferenciar azotemia hemodinâmica da azotemia renal intrínseca e é calculada a partir da equação:

$$EF_{Na} = [(Na\ urina \times creatinina\ plasma)]/$$
$$(Na\ plasma \times creatinina\ urina)/\times 100$$

Em casos de azotemia hemodinâmica e depleção volêmica, os rins conservam Na efetivamente, resultando em uma excreção fracionada < 1%. Em casos de dano renal intrínseco, a EF_{Na} será maior. Os resultados são difíceis de avaliar com doenças concorrentes que podem prejudicar a capacidade de concentração da urina, ou pelo uso de diuréticos. A reabsorção fracionada da ureia tem sido avaliada para ajudar a distinguir a azotemia renal hemodinâmica da intrínseca, mas não possui especificidade.[65,66]

Biomarcadores

Biomarcadores de função renal mais sensíveis do que a creatinina estão sendo buscados.[67] De modo ideal, um painel de biomarcadores seria capaz de detectar a disfunção renal muito mais precocemente (quando intervenções mais provavelmente são efetivas), distinguir doença aguda da crônica, fornecer alguma indicação da duração e gravidade, e ser prognóstico. A cistatina C se correlaciona com a TFG melhor do que a creatinina sérica em cães, e provavelmente estará elevada antes da creatinina no início da doença renal.[68] Entretanto, a cistatina C ainda não foi avaliada em cães com LRA. A gamaglutamil transpeptidase (GGT) e N-acetil-beta-D-glicosaminidase (NAG) são biomarcadores urinários de dano tubular (ou intersticial) e estão elevados na doença renal inicial (ver Capítulo 321).[69] A lipocalina associada à gelatinase neutrofílica aumenta antes da creatinina na IRA e parece útil para diferenciação entre doença renal aguda e crônica (DRC).[70-73] O fator de crescimento de fibroblastos-23 e dimetilarginina simétrica (SDMA) estão também sendo avaliadas como marcadores precoces de doença renal (ver Capítulo 324).

Testes para doenças específicas

Testes diagnósticos específicos estão disponíveis para determinadas causas de IRA. O teste rápido para etilenoglicol pode ser realizado com um *kit* de teste comercialmente disponível (ver Capítulo 152). Resultados falso-positivos são possíveis se fármacos contendo propilenoglicol (p. ex., etomidato, diazepam, carvão ativado) forem administrados. Resultados falso-negativos são possíveis em gatos por conta do limite inferior de detecção do kit (50 mg/dℓ). A determinação de concentrações sanguíneas de determinados fármacos está disponível para determinar se há concentração tóxica e para monitorar a resposta à terapia. A leptospirose (ver Capítulo 217), doença de Lyme (ver Capítulo 211), febre maculosa (infecção por *Rickettsia rickettsii*; ver Capítulo 218) podem causar insuficiência renal oligúrica. Sinais de vasculite, poliartrite, meningite e trombocitopenia discreta são prováveis em casos de LRA. *Ehrlichia canis* pode causar um espectro semelhante de sinais clínicos, embora lesões renais sejam mais prováveis decorrentes de dano glomerular com proteinúria do que por LRA.

FATORES DE RISCO PARA LESÃO RENAL AGUDA ADQUIRIDA NO HOSPITAL

A LRA que se desenvolve antes da avaliação veterinária consequente de uma causa única (*i. e.*, ingestão de nefrotoxina por um animal previamente sadio). Diversos fatores de risco aumentam o risco de LRA. Em animais com fatores de risco preexistentes,

é prudente a atenção cuidadosa para evitar ou minimizar outros riscos (Boxe 322.1). Em um estudo retrospectivo de 29 cães com LRA adquirida no hospital, 72% foram expostos a uma nefrotoxina, 69% tinham > 7 anos, 41% tinham doença cardíaca crônica (ver Capítulo 357), 35% tinham doença renal preexistente, 31% tinham neoplasia, 28% tinham febre e 14% tinham sido submetidos à anestesia.[22] O estudo não incluiu dados sobre o estado de hidratação, o que faz com que a contribuição dos efeitos hemodinâmicos não possa ser determinada. A depleção volêmica é um fator predisponente significativo para o desenvolvimento de LRA adquirida no hospital.[1,37] A depleção volêmica exacerba a hipoperfusão renal e aumenta o risco de LRA pós-cirúrgica.[74] Como os três principais determinantes fisiológicos do fluxo sanguíneo renal são débito cardíaco, volume intravascular e pressão de perfusão renal, a atenção a todos é necessária, embora a LRA possa ocorrer mesmo se todos estes parâmetros estiverem normais.[75,76] Se houver hipotensão e o animal estiver euvolêmico, agentes vasopressores podem ser necessários, mas há risco de causar vasoconstrição intrarrenal.[1,77]

Sepse (ver Capítulo 132)

Em pessoas com sepse, a norepinefrina demonstrou ser mais eficaz para melhorar a pressão sanguínea, causar diurese e diminuir a mortalidade quando comparada à dopamina em doses altas.[77,78] A vasopressina arginina, um potente agente vasopressor,

---

> **Boxe 322.1** Fatores de risco para a lesão renal aguda adquirida no hospital[1,22,60,199]
>
> **Condições clínicas**
> Hipoperfusão
>   Depleção volêmica
>   Hipoalbuminemia ou diminuição da POC
>   Diminuição do débito cardíaco
>   Hipotensão sistêmica
>   Aumento da viscosidade sanguínea
> Anormalidades eletrolíticas
> Acidose
> Hipertensão sistêmica
> Febre
> Sepse
> Anestesia
> Cirurgia
> Choque
> Falência múltipla dos órgãos
> Torção gástrica
> Fármacos nefrotóxicos, especialmente:
>   Meio de contraste (potencializado por hiponatremia)
>   AINEs (potencializado por anestesia, depleção de sódio ou volêmica, sepse, ICC, síndrome nefrótica, hepatopatia)
>   Combinações de fármacos nefrotóxicos (aminoglicosídeos + furosemida, IECA + diurético)
>
> **Doenças preexistentes**
> Insuficiência renal
> Pancreatite
> Insuficiência hepática
> Diabetes melito
> Doença cardiovascular
> Mieloma múltiplo
> Trauma
> Queimaduras extensas
> Idade avançada
> Vasculite
> Febre
> Neoplasia

AINEs, fármacos anti-inflamatórios não esteroidais; *ICC*, insuficiência cardíaca congestiva; *IECA*, inibidor da enzima conversora de angiotensina; *POC*, pressão osmótica coloidal.

é recomendada para pacientes que estão hipotensos apesar da norepinefrina.[77] A vasopressina causa mais constrição arteriolar eferente enquanto a norepinefrina possui maior efeito sobre a arteríola aferente. A vasopressina foi mais efetiva para redução da progressão da LRA quando comparada à norepinefrina em pacientes com choque séptico.[79] A manutenção do débito cardíaco adequado e prevenção de vasoconstrição periférica demonstrou diminuir o risco de LRA.[80] Em pacientes de alto risco, evite o uso de qualquer fármaco potencialmente nefrotóxico. Protocolos anestésicos devem focar em evitar a hipotensão e manter a volemia normal e pressão. Distúrbios eletrolíticos demonstraram aumentar o risco de LRA. O baixo Na potencializa a LRA induzida por meio de contraste. Hipopotassemia, acidose metabólica, hipocalcemia e hipomagnesemia aumentam a nefrotoxicidade por gentamicina.[1] O controle estrito da hiperglicemia pela insulinoterapia diminui a LRA em pessoas não diabéticas em estado crítico de doenças.[75,81]

Aminoglicosídeos

Aminoglicosídeos são comumente associados à nefrotoxicidade em cães e gatos porque eles não são metabolizados, possuem baixo peso molecular e são hidrossolúveis (ver Capítulo 161). Estes fatores levam à quase completa excreção exclusiva na urina.[82] Eles são facilmente ionizados em complexos catiônicos que se ligam a locais aniônicos nas células epiteliais do túbulo proximal, são então internalizados por pinocitose, o que leva a concentrações corticais renais 10 vezes daquela do plasma e pode causar dano tubular renal.[82] Fatores que aumentam o risco de intoxicação incluem uso prolongado (> 5 dias), elevação os níveis mínimos (> 2 μg/mℓ para gentamicina e tobramicina, > 5 μg/mℓ para amicacina), doença renal preexistente, desidratação, hipopotassemia, hipocalcemia, hipomagnesemia, acidose metabólica, idade, administração concorrente de fármacos nefrotóxicos, administração de diuréticos e terapia antiprostaglandina.[1,83]

A intoxicação por aminoglicosídeos pode ser reduzida pela posologia menos frequente.[1] A eficácia de aminoglicosídeos é determinada pelo pico da concentração (6 a 10 μg/mℓ para gentamicina, 25 a 30 μg/mℓ para amicacina), mas a intoxicação está intimamente correlacionada às concentrações mínimas.[83] A frequência de administração 1 vez/dia em vez de três vezes diárias pode atingir níveis sanguíneos terapêuticos, resulta em níveis mínimos inferiores, mas ainda efetivos, e diminui a incidência de IRA de 24 a 5%.[74,83-85] O monitoramento diário de sedimentos da urina fresca em busca de proteínas ou cilindros pode dar um indicativo de dano renal antes do início da azotemia (ver Capítulo 72). Se um animal estiver azotêmico antes da terapia, um regime terapêutico alternativo deve ser escolhido ou o intervalo de doses prolongado por um fator relacionado à creatinina sérica (i. e., se a creatinina sérica for de 4 mg/dℓ, aumente o intervalo de 8 horas × 4 para 32 horas), se o fármaco dever ser utilizado.[82]

Outros antibióticos

A administração de tetraciclinas vencidas pode causar uma síndrome semelhante a de Fanconi (glicosúria, aminoacidúria, hiperfosfatemia) por causa do acúmulo de metabólitos na mitocôndria que interferem com enzimas oxidativas tubulares proximais.[2] Penicilinas não são diretamente nefrotóxicas, mas elas podem induzir uma reação de hipersensibilidade porque os derivados das penicilinas podem atuar como um hapteno.[83] As sulfonamidas atuam causando cristais intratubulares, exacerbadas por dano renal, débito urinário menor e maior acidez urinária.[83]

Fármacos anti-inflamatórios não esteroidais

Os AINEs inibem a enzima ciclo-oxigenase (COX), que atua sobre o ácido araquidônico para formar prostaglandinas (ver Capítulo 164). AINEs possuem um baixo potencial de nefrotoxicidade em pacientes saudáveis pós-cirúrgicos.[84,86] A função renal é mais dependente da síntese de prostaglandinas em situações nas quais o fluxo sanguíneo pode estar diminuído, como durante anestesias, cirurgias, depleção de Na ou volêmica, hipotensão, sepse, insuficiência cardíaca congestiva, síndrome nefrótica, hepatopatia, doença renal preexistente, idade avançada ou terapia concomitante com fármacos (especialmente outros AINEs). Isso ocorre porque a prostaglandina predominante nos rins causa dilatação arteriolar aferente, que mantém o fluxo sanguíneo renal e contrabalanceia os efeitos da vasoconstrição sistêmica.[87] Pelo bloqueio da produção de prostaglandinas, os AINEs carreiam maior risco de intoxicação nessas situações.[1,87]

As duas isoformas de ciclo-oxigenase são a COX-1 e COX-2. As isoformas da COX-1 são constitutivamente expressas em todo o corpo e são responsáveis pela geração de prostaglandinas envolvidas nas funções fisiológicas rotineiras. As enzimas COX-2 são rapidamente induzidas nos locais da inflamação. Inibidores seletivos da COX-2 deveriam ter bom efeito clínico com menores efeitos adversos GI do que inibidores não seletivos da COX. Entretanto, a COX-2 pode ser constitutivamente expresso nos rins, e a expressão pode ser maior por uma série de situações que levam à diminuição do volume circulante verdadeiro ou efetivo.[88] AINEs seletivos da COX-2 parecem não ser mais seguros para os rins do que os AINEs não seletivos.[86,88] A utilização de AINEs no período perioperatório em gatos tem sido associada à IRA mesmo quando doses estavam dentro da faixa recomendada.[89] O prognóstico para intoxicação por AINEs é favorável se reconhecida precocemente.[56,87]

Substâncias nefrotóxica devem ser evitadas se possível em pacientes com fatores de risco para LRA.[80] Diuréticos devem ser evitados se houver azotemia hemodinâmica.[80] Fármacos menos nefrotóxicos devem ser utilizados preferencialmente, como anfotericina B lipídica emulsificada ou lipossomal em vez da anfotericina B regular, ou carboplatina em vez da cisplatina.[84,90-96] Se o fármaco nefrotóxico deve ser administrado, expansão volêmica modesta pode diminuir a nefrotoxicidade em casos selecionados, incluindo a utilização de agentes de contraste, anfotericina, cisplatina e fármacos que induzem cristalúria.[84,97-99] A expansão volêmica e natriurese ajudam a prevenir a IRA em alguns casos.[1]

MONITORAMENTO

Visão geral e hidratação

Qualquer animal em estado crítico possui risco de desenvolver LRA e parâmetros apropriados devem ser monitorados. Aqueles com fatores de risco específicos adicionais podem necessitar de monitoramento específico. O monitoramento pode permitir a otimização de parâmetros hemodinâmicos, supervisão das complicações urêmicas comuns e avaliação da resposta à terapia.[100] A frequência de monitoramento depende da gravidade da doença.

O monitoramento do estado de hidratação é um processo contínuo primordial para planos apropriados de fluidoterapia (ver Capítulo 129). Ferramentas acuradas prontamente disponíveis para avaliar a volemia ainda não são viáveis na prática veterinária, mas a volemia pode ser mensurada utilizando técnicas de diluição do indicador, marcadores radioativos, espectroscopia por bioimpedância ou outros métodos. Apesar da falta de dados objetivos precisos, existem várias formas para estimar a hidratação. A diminuição do turgor cutâneo pode indicar desidratação (5% de peso corporal ou mais), recente perda de peso ou perda da elasticidade por conta do envelhecimento. Membranas mucosas secas ou enoftalmia também sugerem desidratação, embora animais urêmicos possam ter xerostomia. A hiperidratação pode causar umedecimento de membranas mucosas, aumento da elasticidade cutânea (pesada ou gelatinosa), tremores, náuseas, êmese, inquietude, secreção nasal serosa, quemose, taquipneia, tosse, dispneia, crepitação pulmonar e edema, efusão pleural, ascite, diarreia ou edema subcutâneo (SC) (especialmente do espaço intermandibular e calcâneo).[39,101] Entretanto, animais com baixa pressão osmótica coloidal (*i. e.*, hipoalbuminemia) ou alterações na permeabilidade vascular podem parecer hiperidratados com base na avaliação do turgor cutâneo, ainda possuem depleção volêmica intravascular. O peso corporal deve ser mensurado 3 a 4 vezes/dia com base na mesma escala para monitorar o balanço hídrico. Alterações no peso corporal durante a hospitalização refletem primariamente alterações no conteúdo hídrico corporal. Um animal doente pode perder até 0,5 a 1% de peso corporal por dia por conta de anorexia; alterações em excesso dessa quantidade são causadas por alterações no estado volêmico.[102]

Pressão sanguínea, hematócrito, sólidos totais, pressão venosa central

Como a hipertensão ou hipotensão podem ser prejudiciais à função renal, o monitoramento da pressão sanguínea pode ser crítico (ver Capítulos 157 a 159). Métodos oscilométricos ou a tecnologia por Doppler são mensurações indiretas comumente utilizadas (ver Capítulo 99). A mensuração direta é mais acurada para avaliação da pressão sanguínea, mas não é frequentemente utilizada porque envolve a cateterização arterial. A pressão sanguínea < 80 mmHg é insuficiente para manter a perfusão renal adequada e deve ser imediatamente abordada para evitar danos renais maiores.[39] Um aumento na pressão sanguínea pode indicar um ganho de fluido; ao contrário, uma diminuição na pressão sanguínea pode indicar uma perda hídrica líquida. Por conta da alta porcentagem de pacientes com hipertensão (80% de cães com LRA grave, 20 a 30% dos cães e gatos com DRC), tendências das pressões em vez dos valores absolutos são de maior utilidade para avaliação de alterações no estado de hidratação.[39,103-105] De forma semelhante, tendências no hematócrito e sólidos totais pode refletir alterações na volemia na ausência de hemorragias ou transfusões sanguíneas. Como cada parâmetro é impactado por aspectos além do estado de hidratação, estes fatores devem ser visualizados agregados. Tem sido sugerido que a mensuração da pressão venosa central por um cateter IV central (ver Capítulo 76) ajuda a determinar o estado volêmico, mas não prevê a responsividade ao volume já que existe uma série de fatores que o impactam.[106,107]

Monitoramento cardíaco, acidobásico, débito urinário

O monitoramento do débito cardíaco necessita de um cateter na artéria pulmonar, equipamento especial e é raramente utilizado.[108] O eletrocardiograma (ECG) é a única ferramenta que permite o reconhecimento de arritmias que podem causar risco de morte devido à diminuição do débito cardíaco (ver Capítulo 103). O ECG pode ser utilizado para auxiliar no reconhecimento de distúrbios de condução causados por hiperpotassemia (ver Capítulo 248). O ecocardiograma pode ser utilizado para avaliar a performance miocárdica e pode fornecer informações sobre o estado volêmico pela avaliação do volume da câmara (ver Capítulo 104). A análise da hemogasometria venosa é útil para determinação do estado acidobásico (ver Capítulos 75 e 128). Anormalidades eletrolíticas são um fator de risco e um efeito da IRA. Portanto, o monitoramento regular eletrolítico é aconselhado. Concentrações de UNS e creatinina são facilmente mensuradas, mas são marcadores insensíveis da disfunção renal precoce, pois a TFG deve ser menor do que 75% do normal para que estes valores estejam elevados.

A importância do monitoramento do débito urinário e composição não pode ser subestimada. A produção de urina em um animal saudável é de cerca de 1 a 2 mℓ/kg/h e uma diminuição pode ser uma resposta renal apropriada à hipovolemia ou uma alteração patológica na função renal. A IRA pode também causar poliúria (> 2 mℓ/kg/h). Métodos para determinação do volume urinário incluem a implantação de um cateter urinário permanente com sistema de coleta fechado, coleta de urina por micção natural, gaiola metabólica ou pesar a cama ou caixa de areia da gaiola (1 mℓ de urina = 1 g; ver Capítulos 105 e 106). Uma sonda permanente é mais precisa, embora questões

técnicas, como o extravasamento de urina ao redor da sonda ou desconexão inadvertida, possam causar mensurações incorretas. O risco de uma ITU iatrogênica pode ser menor se for dada atenção cuidadosa à higiene da sonda, incluindo a limpeza das porções externas da sonda com antisséptico múltiplas vezes/dia e troca diária da bolsa de coleta e equipo.[109] A coleta completa da urina por micção natural é difícil por conta da falta de cooperação do animal ou incontinência. Uma escala acurada é necessária para mensurar pequenos volumes de urina em gatos e cães pequenos, mas o ato de pesar a cama ou caixa de areia da gaiola antes e após a utilização pode fornecer uma avaliação adequada. Perdas de fluido por êmese e diarreia costumam ser estimadas. Outras perdas (drenagem de ascite ou efusão pleural) ou sucção da sonda nasogástrica devem ser mensuradas. Quando ocorreu o dano renal, os cilindros urinários podem surgir antes do aumento dos níveis de ureia e creatinina. Portanto, o sedimento urinário deve ser avaliado diariamente em animais que recebem aminoglicosídeos ou outros potenciais medicamentos nefrotóxicos (ver Capítulo 72).

PREVENÇÃO

A prevenção da LRA envolve evitar ou minorar os fatores de risco ao utilizar fármacos renoprotetores. Agentes de contraste causam vasoconstrição da circulação renal.[80] A incidência de nefrotoxicidade induzida por contraste é difícil de estimar, mas pode chegar a até 30% em pessoas com fatores de risco preexistentes, mas em menos do que 10% das pessoas sem fatores de risco.[110,111] Relatos de LRA induzida por meio de contraste em cães são raros.[112] Estudos que avaliam a incidência de efeitos adversos dos agentes de contraste radiográficos iodados em cães e gatos não observaram insuficiência renal pós-contraste, mas o pequeno número de animais avaliados e o atraso entre a administração do contraste e avaliação pós-contraste da UNS e creatinina (média de 38 a 60 dias para cães, 3 a 105 dias para gatos) prejudicam a avaliação acurada.[113,114] Dos três gatos avaliados dentro de 3 dias após receber um agente de contraste iodado (não iônico), dois tiveram incrementos na UNS e creatinina pós-contraste, mas ambos estavam sendo avaliados por conta da obstrução ureteral e estavam azotêmicos antes da administração do contraste.[114]

A diurese salina antes da administração diminui a toxicidade.[80] Recomendações para a prevenção da IRA induzida por agente de contraste em pacientes críticos agudamente incluem expansão volêmica rápida e agressiva antes da realização do estudo radiográfico, evitar o manitol e a furosemida, utilizar uma baixa dose de contraste ou um agente não iônico.[74,84] Embora a utilização da acetilcisteína não tenha provado ser efetiva, por conta de seu baixo custo e poucos efeitos colaterais, sua utilização poderia ser considerada.[74,115]

Não existem evidências de que o tratamento profilático com furosemida protege contra a LRA adquirida no hospital.[116] Estudos demonstraram efeitos deletérios da administração profilática de diuréticos de alça em pacientes predispostos à LRA, apesar de razões teóricas para utilização da furosemida para prevenir a LRA.[77,117] Bloqueadores dos canais de cálcio têm sido utilizados para prevenir a LRA em pessoas que recebem transplantes, mas não previnem a LRA em situações sem transplante.[116,118] O fenoldopam, um agonista seletivo de receptor dopaminérgico-1 (DA-1), pode dilatar artérias renais, inibir a atividade da Na$^+$/K$^+$-ATPase, inibir a angiotensina II e inibir o hormônio antidiurético.[119] Ele não possui atividade em receptores DA-2, alfa- ou beta-adrenérgicos, de forma que não causa vasoconstrição, taquicardia ou arritmias algumas vezes observadas pelo uso da dopamina.[58,116] O fenoldopam manteve o fluxo sanguíneo renal em um modelo experimental de hipovolemia em cães, sugerindo que pode ter um efeito renoprotetor na lesão isquêmica aguda.[120,121] Em um estudo de gatos saudáveis, o efeito diurético e o aumento transitório da TFG foram notados 4 a

CAPÍTULO 322 • Lesão Renal Aguda **1947**

6 horas após uma infusão de 2 horas de fenoldopam. Um dos seis gatos teve uma diminuição na TFG 2 horas após a infusão.[119] Vários outros agentes terapêuticos têm sido investigados para utilização potencial para casos de LRA, incluindo peptídio natriurético atrial, teofilina, fatores de crescimento semelhantes à insulina, anticorpos contra moléculas de adesão, removedores de radicais livres de oxigênio, infusão de aminoácidos e prostaglandinas. Nenhum destes provou ser seguro ou efetivo para pessoas.[43] Em um modelo experimental da LRA isquêmica em ratos, uma única dose de eritropoetina ou darbopoietina administrada 6 horas após o insulto isquêmico inibiu de forma significativa a morte celular apoptótica subsequente, aumentou a regeneração epitelial tubular, minimizou a gravidade da disfunção renal e promoveu recuperação funcional renal mais rápida, mas os resultados dos testes clínicos não estão disponíveis.[122]

TRATAMENTO

Objetivos

Os objetivos terapêuticos para o paciente com LRA almejam limitar danos renais maiores e aumentar a recuperação celular. Estratégias para melhorar o fornecimento de oxigênio renal, reduzir a demanda metabólica e manter o débito urinário utilizadas para prevenir a LRA são igualmente importantes no tratamento. A limitação de respostas citotóxicas e inflamatórias, e promoção da regeneração das células tubulares é desejável.[116] O tratamento obtém maior sucesso durante as fases de indução e extensão, e o sucesso diminui assim que as fases de manutenção e posteriores foram alcançadas. Portanto, o reconhecimento imediato do processo mórbido e instituição de terapia específica são importantes.

Estratégias terapêuticas de fluido

Fontes de perdas

A terapia mais efetiva da LRA é o manejo cuidadoso do balanço hídrico, que envolve avaliação minuciosa da hidratação, um plano terapêutico personalizado com relação à fluidoterapia para o paciente específico, e reavaliação repetida e frequente do equilíbrio hidreletrolítico, com alterações apropriadas no plano terapêutico em resposta a alterações no estado do paciente (ver Capítulo 129). Perdas hídricas normais consistem em perdas insensíveis e sensíveis. Perdas insensíveis não são conscientemente percebidas, como a água perdida pela respiração, fezes ou sudorese. A sudorese é negligível em cães e gatos. Existe variação na perda hídrica respiratória em cães (normal: ≈ 22 mℓ/kg/dia) já que eles podem perder quantidades consideráveis pela ofegância. A principal fonte de perda hídrica sensível é a urina; outros incluem êmese, diarreia, drenagem de cavidades corporais, queimaduras etc. Em animais saudáveis, perdas são repostas pelo consumo de água e alimento, mas o animal doente não consome quantidades adequadas tipicamente. Em casos de doença renal, o volume urinário está frequentemente alto, baixo ou inapropriado.

Fluidoterapia tradicional

Em geral, o clínico administra fluidos IV para corrigir a desidratação e então utiliza taxas agressivas de administração de fluido para forçar a diurese. Se a azotemia não for resolvida, o clínico então aumenta a taxa de fluido. Entretanto, evidências agora implicam que essa abordagem pode de fato piorar a função renal e prejudicar a capacidade de recuperação. Em um estudo de cães submetidos à anestesia e cirurgia em casos de reparo do ligamento cruzado cranial com administração de solução de lactato de Ringer (SRL) na taxa de 10 mℓ/kg/h, a TFG e débito urinário não aumentaram, mas o peso corporal aumentou a partir de uma média de 32,6 kg para uma média de 33,7 kg. Estes cães estavam sistemicamente normais e embora alguns tenham recebido carprofeno, ele não teve efeito sobre os parâmetros renais e hídricos.[123] Após administração de fluidos cristaloides, 80% se movem em direção ao interstício, causando edema intersticial, que leva à piora da difusão de oxigênio e metabólitos, e pode piorar o resultado renal e geral.[124,125] Os rins são fisiologicamente adaptados para conservar Na e fluido, e não excretar excessos.[125] Em pacientes saudáveis, pode levar dias para aquele fluido ser excretado.[124,126]

Abordagem revisada da fluidoterapia

A fluidoterapia pode ser melhor considerada como um processo de três passos: (1) reanimação aguda para restaurar volume intravascular efetivo, perfusão de órgãos e oxigenação tecidual, causando um equilíbrio hídrico positivo; (2) manutenção da homeostase do volume intravascular sem acúmulo de fluido; e (3) remoção de fluido durante a convalescência para remover volume hemodinamicamente desnecessário.[127]

Choque hipovolêmico

Alguns animais com IRA são atendidos em choque hipovolêmico (ver Capítulo 127), com sinais de letargia, hipotensão (pressão sanguínea sistólica < 80 mmHg; ver Capítulos 99 e 159), má perfusão (extremidades frias, mucosas pálidas/acinzentadas com tempo de preenchimento capilar lento), hipotermia, ou taquicardia.[128] A terapia imediata é necessária para prevenir danos maiores aos órgãos com cristaloides administrados na taxa de 60 a 90 mℓ/kg para cães e 45 a 60 mℓ/kg para gatos (ver Capítulo 129). Cerca de 25% daquele volume são administrados durante 5 a 15 minutos.[129] Se os parâmetros hemodinâmicos não melhorarem suficientemente com essa primeira dose, uma segunda dose igual deve ser administrada. Esforços agressivos de fluidos são mantidos até que o paciente esteja hemodinamicamente são e tenha perfusão tecidual adequada. Em cães em choque ressuscitados a desfechos tradicionais (frequência cardíaca, pressão arterial média, débito urinário), 38% tiveram diminuição persistente da saturação venosa central de oxigênio, sugerindo que eles tiveram choque oculto, apesar de parâmetros de perfusão aparentemente normais.[130]

A reanimação adequada avaliada pelo cumprimento de objetivos identificáveis diminui a morbidade renal quando comparada à utilização de doses padrões de reanimação em pessoas.[100] É almejado atingir a correção dos parâmetros de perfusão dentro de 6 horas após a terapia direcionada ao objetivo. Após terapia precoce e agressiva para desfechos fisiológicos mensuráveis, o volume de fluido administrado durante essa fase de reanimação pode ser alto, mas menos é fornecido subsequentemente, de tal forma que o volume total administrado durante a hospitalização é o mesmo após terapia direcionada ao objetivo quando comparada à terapia convencional, mas a mortalidade e incidência de IRA são menores após terapia direcionada ao objetivo.[131]

Reidratação

O volume de fluidos que precisam ser administrados para corrigir a desidratação é calculado a partir de uma fórmula: peso corporal (em kg) × % estimada de desidratação* = déficit de fluido em L. Como a desidratação < 5% não pode ser detectada clinicamente, os animais que parecem hidratados (mas não hiperidratados) devem receber cerca de 5% do seu peso corporal em fluidos durante 2 a 4 horas para reverter rapidamente qualquer dano renal mantido pela má perfusão e para avaliar rapidamente o débito urinário. Fluidos podem ser administrados durante um período mais longo se o comprometimento cardiovascular impedir a administração rápida de fluidos. Se um *bolus* de fluido foi utilizado para reanimação inicial, aquele volume é subtraído do déficit de desidratação. A manutenção de perfusão renal adequada, pela correção da desidratação/depleção volêmica e restauração da pressão sanguínea e débito cardíaco, é essencial.

---

*Como decimal (p. ex., para 7%, use 0,07).

SEÇÃO 23 • Doenças Renais

Fluidoterapia de "manutenção"

Visão geral

Em geral estimada em cerca de 66 mℓ/kg/dia, a dose de fluido de "manutenção" presume débito urinário "normal" sem perdas excessivas (i. e., êmese, diarreia). O débito urinário em um animal com LRA pode ou não ser "normal". Mesmo que o débito urinário seja normal (0,5 a 2 mℓ/kg/h), rins lesados podem não ser capazes de alterar o volume para excretar uma carga de fluido. Estes pacientes possuem oligúria relativa. O fornecimento de fluidos IV acima das necessidades de "manutenção" por muito tempo tem sido advogada como um método de diurese forçada, para promover remoção de toxinas e lavar cilindros tubulares. Enquanto valorosa em determinadas situações (p. ex., nefropatia por agentes de contraste), essa abordagem é agora considerada como subótima.[125] Não somente a fluidoterapia agressiva não é útil, como a sobrecarga volêmica repetidamente demonstrou piorar os resultados porque não aumentam o fornecimento de oxigênio renal apesar de melhorar o débito cardíaco e fluxo sanguíneo renal.[41,132,133] A manutenção da hidratação ótima ao mesmo tempo que se evita assiduamente a hiper- ou sub-hidratação é um dos desafios mais importantes e difíceis no tratamento da LRA.

Balanço hídrico

O método de "balanço hídrico" de administração de fluido ajuda a manter um balanço hídrico apropriado por equiparar o volume administrado ao volume excretado. É útil para todas as situações de LRA, incluindo LRA com anúria/oligúria, oligúria relativa e PU. Esse método de determinação de taxa de fluido não leva em conta a desidratação e deve somente ser utilizado após concluir a reidratação. Os três componentes de cálculo de volume são perdas insensíveis (perda de fluido pela respiração e fezes normais; 22 mℓ/kg/dia), perdas urinárias (calculadas pela mensuração verdadeira), e perdas contínuas (i. e., estimadas pela êmese, diarreia, drenagem de cavidades corporais). Se uma bomba de infusão não estiver disponível, a dose de fluido pode ser determinada pelo cálculo de necessidades insensíveis diárias de fluido e divisão pelo intervalo de administração (i. e., se ajustar a taxa de fluido para 4 vezes/dia, dividindo a necessidade diária de fluido por 4); para esse volume, a quantidade de urina produzida nas 6 horas prévias (ou intervalo apropriado) e um volume estimado de outras perdas devem ser adicionados. Se uma bomba de infusão estiver disponível, as necessidades insensíveis diárias de fluido podem ser calculadas e divididas por 24 para calcular uma taxa por hora. Para isso, o volume do débito urinário em cada hora durante o intervalo de monitoramento prévio deve ser adicionado, mais uma estimativa das perdas contínuas (Boxe 322.2). Outros fluidos administrados que devem ser incluídos no cálculo incluem medicamentos, transfusões e nutrição. Pacientes em anúria devem receber fluidos para repor somente as perdas insensíveis. Se o paciente estiver hiperidratado, a perda insensível deve ser descartada. A hiperidratação em um paciente anúrico ou incapacidade de induzir diurese em um paciente oligúrico ou anúrico é uma indicação para diálise, que é a única outra opção terapêutica efetiva (ver adiante e no Capítulo 110).

Quando o paciente for estabilizado e estiver adentrando a fase de recuperação, qualquer fluido acumulado deve gradativamente ser removido pela diminuição do volume administrado para um volume menor do que o excretado. Se houve acúmulo excessivo de fluido, diuréticos podem acelerar a remoção de fluido. Diuréticos são inefetivos para prevenir ou tratar a IRA, e embora um estudo tenha observado menor mortalidade em pacientes com IRA que receberam maiores doses de furosemida, esse efeito não foi significativo ao controlar o balanço hídrico.[116,117,134-137] Em outras palavras, o benefício da furosemida foi controlar a sobrecarga de fluido associada com piores resultados.[137] Em alguns animais, a PU profunda ocorre durante a recuperação, o que pode levar à desidratação e pior da perfusão renal se o volume de fluidos administrado for inadequado. Naquelas situações, a fluidoterapia IV é mantida até que o paciente possa manter a hidratação adequada com fluidos enterais (por ingestão voluntária ou sonda de alimentação; ver Capítulo 82) e SC. Pode levar semanas para obter novamente a capacidade suficiente de concentração urinária para diminuir gradativamente os fluidos IV em casos mais extremos.

Tipo de fluido

Escolhas Dos vários tipos de fluido disponíveis, uma solução poliônica balanceada (i. e., SRL, Plasmalyte®) é apropriada na maioria das situações (ver Capítulo 129). Fluidos com concentrações de cloreto próximas das do plasma (i. e., SRL, Plasmalyte®, com 98 a 111 mEq/ℓ) estão associados a menor incidência de IRA quando comparados a fluidos com maiores concentrações de cloreto (i. e., salina 0,9%, 150 mEq/ℓ), embora não tenha sido observado efeito sobre a mortalidade.[138-140] Conforme uma maior concentração de cloreto é apresentada ao túbulo distal, a mácula densa induzirá vasoconstrição arteriolar aferente renal.[141] A salina fisiológica (NaCl 0,9%) é indicada em casos de hiponatremia, mas fluidos com menor concentração de Na são mais apropriados em casos de maiores concentrações de Na (i. e., NaCl 0,45% com dextrose 2,5%, SRL com meia força com dextrose 2,5%). A dextrose 5% em água (D5W) é raramente apropriada como escolha de fluido único, mas pode ser combinado à SRL ou salina 0,9% para fazer soluções de ½- ou ¾ de força de Na (25 mℓ de SRL + 25 mℓ D5W = 50 mℓ de SRL ½-força + 2,5% dextrose).

Soluções coloidais (i. e., amido de hidroxietila) têm sido recomendadas em casos de hipotensão persistente ou se houver hipoalbuminemia (p. ex., nefropatia com perda de proteína, doenças associadas à vasculite, ou graves perdas GI ou hemorragia), em uma dose de 20 mℓ/kg/dia. Apesar de relatos iniciais de que coloides poderiam expandir o volume vascular com menores dores do que os cristaloides, relatos recentes refutam esse achado. Em um grande estudo em situações de cuidado intensivo humano, o grupo do hetastarch recebeu menos fluido do que o grupo da salina, e teve um menor balanço hídrico positivo (921 ± 1069 mℓ vs. 982 ± 1161 mℓ, p = 0,03), mas o efeito poupador de fluido foi menor do que o previsto.[142,143] Coloides rapidamente escapam do compartimento vascular, assim como cristaloides.[132,144] O hetastarsch está associado a um risco maior de LRA e mortalidade em pacientes doentes em estado crítico; o licenciamento foi restrito na Europa e a US Food and Drug Administration (FDA) aprovou um alerta sobre a utilização em pacientes sépticos.[145-149] Uma alternativa aos coloides sintéticos é a albumina humana, mas esse produto causa o risco de anafilaxia (ver Capítulo 130).[150,151]

Oligúria e anúria

Definições

Uma diminuição da produção de urina pode ocorrer por causas hemodinâmicas, intrínsecas renais ou pós-renais. Uma resposta

---

> **Boxe 322.2** Exemplos de cálculos para fluidoterapia in-and-out
>
> **Exemplos de cálculos sem bomba de infusão**
> 4,5 kg gato × 22 mℓ/kg/dia = 100 mℓ/dia
>   100 mℓ/dia ÷ 4 = 25 mℓ por 6 h
>   30 mℓ de débito urinário durante 6 h prévias
>   Episódios de êmese cerca de 3 vezes/dia (≈ 8 mℓ em cada vez) = 6 mℓ durante 6 h
> 25 + 30 + 6 mℓ = 61 mℓ para administrar durante as próximas 6 h
>
> **Exemplos de cálculos com bomba de infusão**
> 4,5 kg × 22 mℓ/kg/dia = 100 mℓ/dia
>   100 mℓ/dia ÷ 24 = 4 mℓ/h
>   30 mℓ de débito urinário durante 6 h prévias ÷ 6 = 5 mℓ/h
>   Episódios de êmese cerca de 3 vezes/dia (≈ 8 mℓ cada vez) = 1 mℓ/h
> 4 + 5 + 1 = 10 mℓ/h

renal apropriada contra a perfusão renal inadequada por hipovolemia ou hipotensão inclui retenção hídrica com diminuição concomitante do volume urinário. A perfusão renal deve ser otimizada antes de determinar se a oligúria é patológica ou fisiológica. Um volume de fluido igual a 3 a 5% do peso corporal deve ser administrado a pacientes que parecem normalmente hidratados porque menos que 5% de desidratação não pode ser detectada clinicamente. Em animais que estão claramente em hipervolemia, essa administração de fluido não é necessária. Rins saudáveis podem autorregular o fluxo sanguíneo renal em pressões de perfusão entre 80 e 180 mmHg, mas a perfusão pode ser mais linear em rins lesados.[38,102] A pressão arterial média deve ser mantida acima de 60 a 80 mmHg, ou a pressão sistólica acima de 80 a 100 mmHg quando mensurada pela tecnologia Doppler (ver Capítulo 99). A anúria aparente pode ser causada pela obstrução do trato urinário ou extravasamento de urina para os tecidos peritoneais, retroperitoneais ou SC, e devem ser excluídos antes de determinar que a ausência de urina é resultado de um dano renal intrínseco. A anúria é definida essencialmente como a ausência de produção de urina.[39] Vários valores têm sido utilizados para definir a oligúria, incluindo < 0,25 mℓ/kg/h, < 0,5 mℓ/kg/h, e < 1 a 2 mℓ/kg/h.[39] Em um animal hidratado e bem perfundido, < 1,0 mℓ/kg/h pode ser considerada oligúria absoluta e volumes de urina de 1 a 2 mℓ/kg/h em um animal em fluidoterapia agressiva é considerado oligúria relativa.[39,102] O volume de urina acima de 2 mℓ/kg/h é considerado PU.

Avaliação da ação diurética

Não existem evidências de que os diuréticos melhoram o resultado da IRA. A capacidade de responder aos diuréticos pode ser um marcador de lesão renal menos grave e melhor prognóstico. Em pessoas, o aumento do débito urinário pela utilização de diuréticos retarda o encaminhamento para diálise, talvez inapropriadamente.[135] Entretanto, na medicina veterinária, onde a diálise não está disponível tão prontamente para controlar o estado hídrico, um aumento no débito urinário pela utilização de diuréticos pode permitir o aumento no volume de outras medicações ou nutrição, e pode ser justificada mesmo sem melhora na função renal. A sobrecarga volêmica tem sido associada a um resultado pior.[152-157]

Manitol/glicose

O manitol é um diurético osmótico que causa expansão do volume extracelular e inibe a reabsorção renal de Na pela inibição da renina. O manitol também aumenta o fluxo tubular, o que pode aliviar as obstruções intratubulares por cilindros e debris. O manitol diminui a resistência vascular e edema celular; aumenta o fluxo sanguíneo renal, TFG e excreção de solutos; protege da congestão vascular e agregação de hemácias; remove radicais livres; induz a produção de prostaglandina intrarrenal e vasodilatação; e induz a liberação de peptídio natriurético atrial.[39,58,102,158] Manitol pode atenuar o influxo de Ca para a mitocôndria de células renais lesadas de modo subletal, diminuindo assim o risco de progressão da lesão para dano letal. Apesar de vantagens teóricas, nenhum estudo randomizado demonstrou uma resposta clínica melhor pela utilização do manitol e expansão volêmica do que somente por expansão volêmica em pessoas ou gatos saudáveis.[58,159] O manitol deve ser administrado como um *bolus* lento IV de 0,25 a 1 g/kg. Se a produção de urina aumentar, pode ser administrado em uma taxa de infusão contínua (CRI) de 1 a 2 mg/kg/min IV ou 0,25 a 0,5 g/kg a cada 4 a 6 h (ver Capítulo 78).[39] Doses em excesso de 2 a 4 g/kg/dia podem causar LRA. O manitol não deve ser administrado a pacientes que estejam desidratados, porque exacerbará ainda mais a desidratação intracelular. Por outro lado, também é contraindicado se houver hiperidratação, e pode piorar quadros de edema pulmonar. A dextrose hipertônica pode ser utilizada como um diurético osmótico, se o manitol não estiver disponível. A dose total diária de 22 a 66 mℓ/kg de solução de dextrose a 20% deve causar hiperglicemia e glicosúria.[160]

Diuréticos de alça

Diuréticos de alça (furosemida) podem aumentar o fluxo urinário sem incrementar a TFG.[58,77,84,159,161] Apesar do aumento no débito urinário, diuréticos de alça não melhoram o resultado, sugerindo que aqueles que respondem possuem insuficiência renal menos grave, resultando em melhor resultado para recuperação independentemente da terapia farmacológica.[58,77,84,161,162] Por exemplo, pessoas que poderiam ter convertido insuficiência renal oligúrica em não oligúria tiveram melhores escores APACHE e maior depuração da creatinina antes do tratamento, sugerindo que eles tiveram lesão renal menos grave.[162] Por conta da percepção de que existe uma baixa taxa de complicação associada aos diuréticos de alça, eles frequentemente são utilizados apesar da ausência de benefícios comprovados. Diuréticos de alça inibem a bomba Na^+-$2Cl^-$-K^+ na membrana celular luminal da alça de Henle, diminuindo o transporte transcelular de Na. A atividade basal da Na^+/K^+-ATPase se torna desnecessária e o consumo medular de oxigênio diminui, o que pode proteger o rim de lesões maiores.[162,163] A quantidade de dano estrutural ao ramo ascendente espesso da alça de Henle diminui após a administração de furosemida quando avaliada em rins perfundidos isolados.[163] Diuréticos de alça também possuem efeitos vasodilatadores renais.[116]

Apesar dessas razões teóricas para utilizar diuréticos de alça, um estudo retrospectivo em pessoas demonstrou um risco maior de morte ou incapacidade de recuperação renal em um grupo de tratamento com furosemida. Potenciais explicações incluíram os efeitos prejudiciais do fármaco, atraso no reconhecimento da gravidade de insuficiência renal com subsequente atraso no início da diálise, ou utilização preferencial de diuréticos de alça em pacientes com uma evolução mais grave da doença.[77,135] Diuréticos de alça podem tornar o manejo hídrico mais fácil em pessoas, sem alterar o resultado.[162] Indicações estabelecidas para a utilização de furosemida na medicina veterinária incluem tratamento da hiperidratação ou hiperpotassemia.[39] A furosemida não deve ser administrada a pacientes com LRA induzida por aminoglicosídeos.[102]

Um aumento no débito urinário deve ser aparente 20 a 60 minutos após uma dose IV de furosemida de 2 a 6 mg/kg. Ototoxicidade foi relatada em altas doses em pessoas, e doses de 10 a 50 mg/kg podem causar efeitos adversos em animais (apatia e anorexia em gatos; hipotensão, apatia, ataxia em cães).[102] Se não houver resposta a altas doses, a terapia deve ser descontinuada. Se uma resposta ocorre, essa dose pode ser administrada a cada 6 a 8 horas ou até que a sobrecarga de volume tenha sido corrigida. A CRI fornece diurese mais sustentada com doses cumulativas menores de furosemida quando comparada a infusões repetidas em *bolus*.[77] Em pessoas, o tempo até o efeito máximo com uma dose de ataque e CRI é de 1 hora, e sem a dose de ataque é de 3 horas. A dose em pessoas é de cerca de 0,01 a 0,15 mg/kg/h, sendo que alguns relatos utilizam doses que chegam a até 0,75 mg/kg/h.[164] Em cães normais, 0,66 mg/kg/h resultou em diurese, e doses de 0,25 a 1 mg/kg/h têm sido utilizadas em cães e gatos com insuficiência renal de ocorrência natural.[39,165,166] Como desequilíbrios hidreletrolíticos podem ocorrer rapidamente se ocorrer diurese, o monitoramento frequente é necessário.

Dopamina/fenoldopam

Foi demonstrado que a dopamina tornou alguns pacientes humanos oligúricos em não oligúricos, mas não aumenta a TFG ou melhora o resultado.[58,84,167,168] Por conta da falta de eficácia e efeitos colaterais associados à dopamina, ela não é mais recomendada para o tratamento da insuficiência renal oligúrica, exceto para o controle pressor.[39,169] O fenoldopam, um agonista seletivo de receptor DA-1, aumenta o débito urinário.[58,116] Seus efeitos sobre a TFG e resultado renal não são conhecidos.

Antagonistas de canais de cálcio

Antagonistas dos canais de cálcio presumivelmente revertem a vasoconstrição renal por causar vasodilatação predominantemente pré-glomerular, inibir a vasoconstrição induzida por mecanismos de retroalimentação túbulo-glomerular, causar natriurese independente da TG e diminuir o dano renal após o transplante.[170] Embora os resultados de um estudo que utilizou o diltiazem em adição à terapia-padrão em cães com LRA por leptospirose não tenham sido significativos, existiu uma tendência para o aumento do débito urinário e resolução mais completa da azotemia.[170]

Terapia de reposição renal

Indicações

A terapia de reposição renal é utilizada para pacientes que não respondem ao tratamento medicamentoso (Figura 322.4; ver Capítulo 110). O momento apropriado para instituir a terapia dialítica não está claramente estabelecido, embora a hiperpotassemia intratável, sobrecarga volêmica com risco de morte ou sinais urêmicos persistentes não sejam controversos (Boxes 322.3 e 322.4). A instituição precoce da diálise em pessoas pode melhorar o resultado comparada ao início tardio na evolução da doença. O início da diálise em um nível inferior de hiperidratação melhora o resultado em pacientes pediátricos.[103] O transplante renal não é um procedimento emergencial (ver Capítulo 323). Se um gato com IRA for estabilizado, mas não recuperar a função renal, o transplante pode ser considerado.

Diálise peritoneal

A diálise peritoneal é raramente utilizada para a LRA em pessoas doentes em estado crítico, mas é mais prontamente disponível para animais do que a hemodiálise ou hemofiltração.[171] A diálise peritoneal remove toxinas urêmicas por difusão a partir da membrana peritoneal para o dialisato infundido no abdome, e então é drenado. Os materiais necessários são prontamente disponíveis, mas o procedimento é demorado (ver Capítulo 109). Complicações comuns incluem oclusão do cateter e peritonite. Resultados semelhantes à hemodiálise foram documentados em gatos tratados com diálise peritoneal, sendo que 10 de 22 gatos sobreviveram até a alta hospitalar, mas os resultados históricos pela diálise peritoneal em cães são menos favoráveis (26% de sobrevida).[172-174]

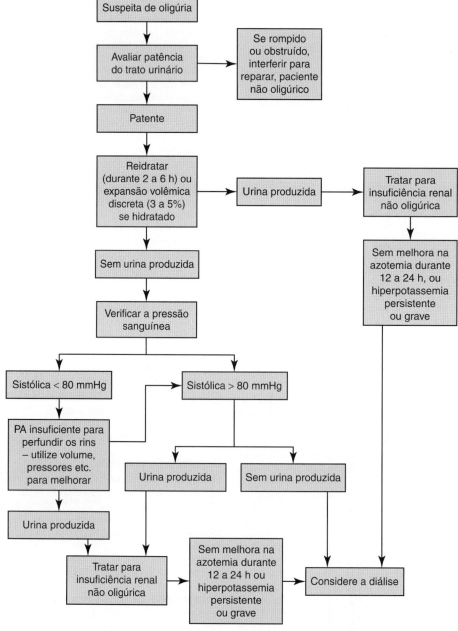

Figura 322.4 Algoritmo para o tratamento da IRA. *PA*, pressão arterial.

Boxe 322.3 Indicações para terapia de reposição renal

Produção urinária inadequada
Edema pulmonar com risco de morte ou sobrecarga hídrica
Hiperpotassemia ou outro distúrbio hidreletrolítico ou ácido-básico com risco de morte
Azotemia progressiva/sem remissão
Insuficiência cardíaca congestiva resistente a diuréticos ou hiperidratação grave na ausência de doença renal
Intoxicação aguda/superdosagem de medicamentos com substância que deve ser removida por diálise

Boxe 322.4 Características do paciente para terapia de reposição renal

≥ 2,5 kg
Pressão sanguínea sistólica ≥ 80 mmHg
Tratável

Terapia de reposição renal extracorpórea

A terapia de reposição renal extracorpórea (TRRE) (ver Capítulo 110; Vídeo 322.1) inclui a hemodiálise intermitente (HDI) e terapia de reposição renal contínua (TRRC). A TRRE remove toxinas urêmicas a partir da circulação sanguínea por difusão e/ou convecção. Durante o tratamento, o sangue do paciente é continuamente carreado até o dialisador pelo equipo de descarte (circuito extracorpóreo) e então retorna. O dialisador, ou rim artificial, contém uma membrana porosa cujo tamanho e carga determinam quais partículas são filtradas. Moléculas de tamanho pequeno a médio em alta concentração, como ureia e creatinina, são difundidas pelos poros para uma solução de dialisato no lado oposto da membrana. Grandes moléculas, como a albumina e células, são muito grandes para passar pelos poros. Eletrólitos, como o Na, podem passar facilmente pela membrana. Assim, soluções de dialisato possuem concentrações eletrolíticas fisiológicas para impedir perda significativa. A ultrafiltração remove fluido do paciente pela criação de um gradiente de pressão hidrostática entre o compartimento sanguíneo e o compartimento do dialisato. Solutos dissolvidos no fluido são então removidos por depuração convectiva. Se um grande volume de fluido for removido para atingir a depuração adequada do soluto por convecção, o fluido e infundido para o circuito extracorpóreo para evitar desidratação. Existem diversos modelos e fabricantes de máquinas de diálise, mas cada um deve ser capaz de circular o sangue no circuito extracorpóreo, circular o dialisato ou fluido de reposição e controlar precisamente a ultrafiltração.

A HDI envolve o rápido fluxo sanguíneo e rápido fluxo de dialisato para remoção eficiente de toxinas urêmicas e fluido, permitindo que os tratamentos ocorrem em determinados intervalos. Um regime poderia incluir várias horas por tratamento, 3 a 4 vezes/semana. Máquinas desenvolvidas para HDI são capazes de suprir o grande volume de dialisato necessário para misturar água purificada com soluções eletrolíticas concentradas. Concentrações de Na e bicarbonato podem ser independentemente ajustadas e adaptadas às necessidades do paciente. Por conta da complexidade do equipamento e da possibilidade de alterações agudas no estado do paciente durante o tratamento, a HDI quase sempre é realizada por equipe de diálise especialmente treinada. A TRRC pode ser realizada até que a recuperação renal ocorra ou até que o animal esteja estável e possa sofrer a transição para HDI. O dialisato estéril pré-embalado é utilizado com estas máquinas, e soluções com várias concentrações de solutos (i. e., Na, K, bicarbonato) estão disponíveis. As taxas de fluxo de dialisato são muito mais lentas em TRRC (até 8 ℓ/h) comparadas à HDI (20 a 50 ℓ/h), mas a duração do tratamento é mais longa. A escolha da modalidade, seja HDI ou TRRC, não demonstrou afetar o resultado.[84,171] Tanto a HDI como a TRRC necessitam de acesso vascular. Para o tratamento a curto prazo, cateteres de lúmen duplo, posicionados de forma percutânea com um fio-guia (técnica de Seldinger; ver Capítulo 76) ou por mínima exposição cirúrgica do vaso, são utilizados. Estes cateteres podem ser implantados com um anestésico local e sedação discreta.

Anticoagulantes

Certa forma de anticoagulação é necessária durante a diálise para prevenir a trombose no circuito extracorpóreo. A heparina não fracionada é comumente utilizada e é monitorada pelo tempo de coagulação ativado. Com anticoagulação regional por citrato, este é administrado como uma CRI no circuito extracorpóreo e se liga ao Ca para prevenir a coagulação no circuito. Como a anticoagulação ocorre fora do paciente, as complicações hemorrágicas associadas à anticoagulação são mínimas. O cloreto de cálcio é administrado por um cateter central IV, ou peplo circuito extracorpóreo bem no local onde o sangue está reentrando no corpo, para impedir a hipocalcemia no paciente.

Complicações

Complicações encontradas durante o manejo dialítico podem ser resultado do procedimento de diálise ou da insuficiência renal subjacente. A síndrome do desequilíbrio da diálise é uma condição caracterizada por um rápido declínio na osmolalidade sanguínea causada pela rápida remoção dos osmoles (especialmente ureia) pela diálise, o que leva a sinais de SNC (p. ex., convulsões, alterações comportamentais). Em pequenos animais, a remoção do volume de sangue necessário para preencher o circuito de diálise pode resultar em hipotensão. A hemorragia relacionada à anticoagulação por heparina mais provavelmente ocorrerá durante os primeiros tratamentos por diálise, enquanto a resposta individual à heparina está sendo determinada, e em sessões prolongadas (> 6 horas). A trombose na ponta do cateter de diálise no átrio direito é comum em cateteres implantados durante 3 semanas, o que prejudica o fluxo sanguíneo adequado.

TRATAMENTO DA OBSTRUÇÃO URETERAL

A obstrução ureteral é uma causa relativamente frequente de LRA em gatos (ver Capítulo 329). Alguns cálculos ureterais passam para a bexiga dentro de horas a dias, mas se não, o alívio da obstrução é necessário para recobrar a função renal. É esperado que obstruções que persistem por 7 dias reduzam permanentemente a função renal em um terço e, após 40 dias, nenhum retorno da função é esperado. O alívio pode ser fornecido por ureterotomia cirúrgica, colocação de um *stent* ureteral, ou implantação de um dispositivo de desvio ureteral, que envolve a conexão de uma sonda de nefrostomia no rim com uma sonda de cistostomia posicionada na bexiga (ver Capítulo 124). Gatos muito doentes para anestesia podem ser beneficiados pela diálise (peritoneal ou extracorpórea). Uma alternativa à diálise é a implantação de uma sonda percutânea de nefropielostomia, que deve resolver a azotemia dentro de alguns dias se for pós-renal, mas um procedimento definitivo para remoção ou desvio da obstrução será eventualmente necessário.[175,176]

TRATAMENTO DE DOENÇAS ESPECÍFICAS

Antimicrobianos

Derivados da penicilina e doxiciclina são uma escolha inicial excelente para cães com leptospirose (ver Capítulo 217), embora penicilinas não eliminem o estado portador. A doxiciclina e eritromicina são efetivas conta o estado portador. O tratamento deve ser mantido por pelo menos 4 semanas. *Borrelia burgdorferi* pode

SEÇÃO 23 • Doenças Renais

ser tratada com doxiciclina (ver Capítulo 211). A pielonefrite costuma ser causada por bactérias gram-negativas, contra as quais as fluorquinolonas possuem bom espectro e boa penetração em tecido renal. A ampicilina, amoxicilina, amoxicilina-ácido clavulânico ou cefalosporinas podem ser efetivas. Fármacos do grupo da sulfa-trimetoprima são efetivos contra *E. coli* e bactérias gram-positivas. Sulfonamidas não atingem concentrações intrarrenais efetivas; somente o componente trimetoprima é efetivo. Aminoglicosídeos devem ser evitados graças a uma potencial nefrotoxicidade. O tratamento da pielonefrite deve ser mantido por pelo menos 4 a 6 semanas. A urina deve ser cultivada 3 a 7 dias após a conclusão da antibioticoterapia e repetida em 1 mês, se negativa. Se a cultura for positiva, o tratamento é indicado por mais 4 semanas com antibiótico apropriado.

Outros medicamentos

A utilização do fomepizol ou etanol para intoxicação por etilenoglicol deve ser iniciada dentro de 8 h após a ingestão (ver Capítulo 152). Além de melhorar a perfusão renal com a fluidoterapia, a intoxicação por AINEs pode ser tratada com misoprostol, um análogo da prostaglandina E (1 a 3 µg/kg PO a cada 6 a 8 horas). Ao tratar a intoxicação por aminoglicosídeos, a ticarcilina e carbenicilina formarão complexos com os aminoglicosídeos, prevenindo assim a captação renal, e pode ser um tratamento inicial após doses excessivas.[83] A alcalinização urinária é recomendada para intoxicação por sulfonamidas e nefropatia por pigmentos.[80,83] A manutenção de altas taxas de fluxo urinário com manitol e fluidoterapia em altos volumes podem também ser benéfica.

TRATAMENTO DAS COMPLICAÇÕES URÊMICAS

Hiperpotassemia

Terapias agudas

A excreção renal é o principal mecanismo para remoção de K do corpo (ver Capítulo 68). A hiperpotassemia crônica é improvável quando a função renal estiver normal. A hiperpotassemia, possivelmente com risco de morte, é mais provável em casos de LRA oligúrica ou anúrica quando comparada à PU.[102] O aumento do K extracelular altera o potencial elétrico das células excitáveis. Alterações ECG típicas incluem bradicardia, ondas T altas e espiculadas, intervalo QT curto, complexo QRS largo e uma onda P pequena, ampla ou ausente. A hiperpotassemia grave pode levar ao ritmo sinoventricular, fibrilação ventricular ou parada atrial. A fraqueza muscular pode estar presente em casos de concentração sérica de K > 8 mEq/ℓ.[177] Um animal com alterações ECG suspeitas pode necessitar de terapia emergencial antes que os resultados do K sérico estejam disponíveis. O gliconato de Ca 10% (0,5 a 1 mℓ/kg IV até fazer efeito, administrado lentamente) pode ser utilizado em situações críticas para restaurar a excitabilidade da membrana cardíaca, mas não diminui as concentrações de K. Durante a infusão, o ECG deve ser monitorado e a taxa diminuída ou interrompida se as arritmias piorarem. Os efeitos cardíacos devem ser aparentes dentro de minutos, mas a duração do efeito é menor do que 1 hora.[178] O fornecimento de Ca aumenta o risco de mineralização de tecidos moles se a hiperfosfatemia ocorrer.

Insulina, glicose, bicarbonato

Diversos métodos podem ser utilizados para movimentar o K a partir do espaço extracelular para intracelular. A insulina regular (0,5 unidade/kg IV) causa um efeito dentro de 20 a 30 minutos. A dextrose (1 a 2 g por unidade de insulina administrada como *bolus* IV, depois 1 a 2 g por unidade de insulina em fluidos IV administrados durante 4 a 6 horas) é necessária para impedir a hipoglicemia quando a insulina for utilizada. A dextrose induz

a liberação de insulina endógena em pacientes não diabéticos e pode ser utilizada sem administração concorrente de insulina para controlar hiperpotassemia discreta à moderada, em uma dose de 0,25 a 0,5 g/kg IV.

A acidose metabólica por ácidos minerais (p. ex., NH_4Cl, HCl), mas não por ácidos orgânicos (p. ex., ácido láctico, cetoácidos) faz com que o K seja direcionado das células para o espaço extracelular e circulação conforme os íons hidrogênio adentram as células. A correção da acidose mineral metabólica com bicarbonato faz cm que o K retorne às células conforme o H^+ é combinado com o HCO_3^- e removido. A dose de bicarbonato de Na utilizado para tratar a hiperpotassemia é baseada no cálculo do déficit de base (de forma ideal), ou uma dose fixa de 1 a 2 mEq/kg IV durante 10 a 20 minutos. O bicarbonato de Na é contraindicado se a pressão parcial de dióxido de carbono (P_{CO_2}) estiver aumentada ou se houver alcalose metabólica, já que pode causar hipernatremia ou acidose paradoxal de SNC. Se a concentração de Ca ionizado estiver baixa, a dextrose é preferida em detrimento do bicarbonato porque a alcalemia exacerba a hipocalcemia (ver Capítulo 69).[102]

Albuterol, resinas de trocas e fármacos para evitar

O beta-agonista albuterol tem sido utilizado para tratar a hiperpotassemia em pessoas porque direciona o K para as células.[102] A resina de troca de cátions, poliestireno-sulfonato de sódio, pode ser administrada por via oral ou por enema (dose: 2 g/kg a cada 6 a 8 horas como uma suspensão em sorbitol 20%).[39] Essa se liga ao K no trato GI, libera Na, demora várias vezes para atuar e inclui efeitos colaterais como hipernatremia e constipação intestinal. Os efeitos de diminuição do K destes fármacos, com exceção do poliestireno-sulfonato, são temporários. As concentrações séricas de K sobem gradativamente dentro de várias horas de administração, a menos que a produção de urina seja induzida. Assim que a produção de urina é retomada, mesmo que mínima, as concentrações séricas de K quase sempre diminuem. A diálise peritoneal ou hemodiálise podem ser necessárias para controlar finalmente o K se persistirem a oligúria ou anúria. Fármacos que contribuem para a hiperpotassemia devem ser evitados, incluindo betabloqueadores inespecíficos, digoxina, inibidores da ECA, antagonistas de receptores de angiotensina, fármacos anti-inflamatórios não esteroidais, diuréticos poupadores de potássio (espironolactona, amilorida, trianetereno), altas doses de trimetoprima, ciclosporina e nutrição parenteral total (NPT).[69]

Hipopotassemia

O K baixo pode ocorrer em casos de LRA por conta das excessivas perdas urinárias devido à PU, utilização de diuréticos ou perdas devido êmese ou diarreia. A quantidade de cloreto de K adicionada aos fluidos IV deve ser baseada na concentração sérica (ver Capítulo 68). A suplementação oral com K (1 a 3 mEq/kg/dia) pode ser utilizada para animais que estejam se alimentando ou que possuem sonda de nutrição. A concentração sérica de K deve ser monitorada frequentemente para evitar hiperpotassemia ou hipopotassemia.

Sódio (Na)

As concentrações séricas de Na podem estar normais, aumentadas ou diminuídas na IRA (ver Capítulo 67). A hipernatremia antes da fluidoterapia indica excessiva perda de água livre. A administração de bicarbonato de Na ou salina hipertônica pode causar hipernatremia. A hiponatremia pode indicar perdas devido à excessiva excreção urinária, êmese, diarreia ou hiponatremia dilucional transitória após administração de manitol, dextrose hipertônica ou soluções coloidais. Soluções com baixas concentrações de Na (dextrose 5%, NPT, formulações enterais) podem causar hiponatremia. Em várias situações, a desidratação inicial segue as perdas hídricas isonatrêmicas e uma concentração normal de Na.[39,102] Os sinais clínicos são improváveis, a

Acidose metabólica

A acidose metabólica é comum na LRA. A carga diária de H^+ é excretada com NH_3 como NH_4^+ ou com fosfato como $H_2PO_4^-$ (ver Capítulo 128). Os rins falhando são incapazes de excretar H^+ ou reabsorver HCO_3^-. A acidose pode ser piorada pela acidose láctica pela desidratação e má perfusão. A terapia intravenosa com bicarbonato de Na pode ser considerada se a acidose persistir após correção da desidratação e, em geral, é revertida para animais com um pH menor que 7,2 ou $HCO_3 < 12$ mEq/ℓ. O tratamento com bicarbonato de Na é voltado para causar a combinação do ácido (H^+) com (HCO_3^-) para formar H_2CO_3, que é dissociado em H_2O e CO_2. Se os pulmões forem incapazes de eliminar o CO_2, a reação não ocorre. A administração de bicarbonato, entretanto, pode aumentar a P_{CO_2} e levar à acidose paradoxal de SNC. Como o CO_2 é altamente difusível, a rápida movimentação a partir da circulação para o SNC faz com que haja a conversão em ácido (H^+) naquele ambiente. O tratamento com bicarbonato de Na também é contraindicado em casos de hipernatremia. As doses de bicarbonato são calculadas a partir da fórmula: $0,3 \times$ peso corporal (kg) $\times$ déficit de base, na qual o déficit de base $= 24 - HCO_3$ do paciente. Forneça ¼ a ½ diretamente IV, e uma dose adicional de ¼ a ½ nos fluidos IV durante as próximas 2 a 6 horas. Ajuste quaisquer doses subsequentes com base na avaliação seriada das determinações hemogasométricas. Os agentes alcalinizantes orais podem ser utilizados assim que a ingestão oral seja possível. O citrato de K (40 a 75 mg/kg PO a cada 12 horas) almeja a acidose metabólica e hipopotassemia. O bicarbonato de Na oral (8 a 12 mg/kg PO a cada 12 horas) é mais palatável na forma de comprimido comparado ao pós. As doses devem ser ajustadas com base na necessidade.

Cálcio (Ca) e magnésio (Mg)

Hipocalcemia

Uma das várias causas de distúrbios do Ca em animais com IRA inclui uma diminuição aguda na filtração glomerular, o que leva ao aumento abrupto do fósforo, que por sua vez causa hipocalcemia aguda devido à lei de ação de massas (ver Capítulo 69). Diminuições do Ca estimulam a síntese e secreção do hormônio paratireoideano, que aumenta os níveis de Ca de volta aos níveis normais. A acidose metabólica aumenta a fração de Ca ionizado (iCa). A hipocalcemia sintomática (tetania) ocorre infrequentemente em casos de IRA. A hipocalcemia pode ser mais grave em casos de LRA induzida por anticongelantes (ver Capítulo 152), pois anticongelantes com fosfato podem causar hiperfosfatemia grave aguda enquanto o etilenoglicol é convertido em oxalato, o qual forma complexos com o Ca. O tratamento com Ca aumenta o risco de mineralização de tecidos moles em animais hiperfosfatêmicos. A dose mínima de gliconato de Ca que controla os sinais clínicos deve ser utilizada quando necessária. O gliconato de Ca 10% pode ser utilizado (dose: 0,5 a 1,5 mℓ/kg IV durante 20 a 30 minutos). Assim como ao tratar a hiperpotassemia, é importante monitorar o ECG durante a infusão.

Hipercalcemia

A hipercalcemia, com base nas concentrações séricas de Ca total, costuma ser discreta e associada à iCa normal sem necessidade de tratamento. Se o iCa estiver aumentado, isso pode ser resolvido pela fluidoterapia. Fluidos que contêm Ca (como o SRL) devem ser evitados. A salina (NaCl 0,9%) é um fluido ideal porque o conteúdo de Na aumenta a calciurese. A furosemida também promove excreção urinária de Ca. A terapia com bicarbonato de Na diminui o iCa conforme mais Ca se liga às proteínas séricas. A hipercalcemia por insuficiência renal não é responsiva a glicocorticoides.[180] A calcitonina ou bifosfonatos poderiam ser considerados se a hipercalcemia for grave, embora bifosfonatos possam induzir insuficiência renal.[180]

Magnésio (Mg)

Como os rins são a via primária de excreção, as concentrações de Mg podem estar aumentadas na IRA, mas a terapia específica, em geral, não é necessária (ver Capítulo 68). O Mg, tal qual observado em alguns quelantes de fosfato, deve ser evitado. A hipomagnesemia pode ocorrer em casos de PU e insuficiência renal. A hipopotassemia pode ser refratária à terapia se houver hipomagnesemia concorrente. O sulfato de Mg ou cloreto de Mg podem ser administrados por via intravenosa. Diversas formas estão disponíveis para suplementação oral.[181]

Fósforo (PO₄)

O PO_4 da dieta é prontamente absorvido no trato GI e excretado pelos rins (ver Capítulo 69). A diminuição da excreção comumente leva à hiperfosfatemia, tanto na LRA como na DRC. A fluidoterapia intravenosa pode controlar parcialmente as concentrações de PO_4 por abordar o componente hemodinâmico e melhorar o fluxo sanguíneo renal. Não existem tratamentos específicos para diminuir o PO_4 sérico na IRA, exceto pela terapia de reposição renal. Os quelantes de PO_4 impedem a absorção a partir dos alimentos. Os quelantes orais de PO_4 podem ser adicionados quando a nutrição enteral for iniciada. O hidróxido de alumínio ou carbonato de alumínio é administrado em doses de 30 a 90 mg/kg/dia, divididas com as refeições. O acetato de Ca (60 a 90 mg/kg/dia) e carbonato de Ca podem causar hipercalcemia e devem ser evitados em casos de hipercalcemia. O carbonato de Ca combinado com quitosana é um produto veterinário para quelar o PO_4.

Hipertensão

A hipertensão é uma complicação comum da LRA, afetando 37% dos cães no momento da admissão e chegando até 80% durante a hospitalização (ver Capítulos 157 e 158).[105] A carga progressiva de volume como resultado da fluidoterapia IV pode contribuir para a incidência e gravidade da hipertensão. A hipertensão aguda pode causar danos oculares (descolamento de retina, hifema, edema retinal; ver Capítulo 11). Os sinais de SNC ocorrem pela hemorragia (ver Capítulo 260), anormalidades cardíacas (ver Capítulo 253), ou progressão do dano renal. O tratamento é indicado se a pressão sanguínea sistólica for > 180 mmHg. Animais com LRA e hipervolemia podem também ter hipertensão que responde à diminuição da sobrecarga volêmica. Se medicamentos anti-hipertensivos forem necessários, o objetivo é diminuir a pressão sistólica para < 180 mmHg, mas evitando diminuições acentuadas. O amlodipino (0,18 a 0,3 mg/kg PO a cada 24 horas para gatos, 0,2 a 0,4 mg/kg PO a cada 24 horas para cães) pode ocasionar uma resposta dentro de 24 a 48 horas. Se a pressão sanguínea não melhorar dentro de algumas horas, doses adicionais podem ser administradas em cães, até uma dose máxima de 1 mg/kg/dia.[105] Inibidores da ECA costumam ser evitados em casos de IRA porque podem diminuir a perfusão renal por causar constrição arteriolar aferente. Se o controle imediato da hipertensão for necessário, o início da ação da hidralazina (2,5 mg/gato PO ou SC em uma administração, 0,5 a 3 mg/kg PO a cada 12 horas para cães) é de 15 minutos (SC) a 1 hora (PO). A pressão sanguínea deve ser monitorada intimamente após a administração (ver Capítulo 99).

Distúrbios hematológicos

A anemia pode ocorrer em casos de IRA por conta da hemorragia GI, repetidas coletas de sangue, ou diluição associada à sobrecarga volêmica. Se os sinais clínicos de anemia estiverem presentes (*i. e.*, taquicardia, sopro cardíaco, fraqueza, letargia, anorexia), a transfusão sanguínea é indicada (ver Capítulo 130). A transfusão com papa de hemácias é preferida em detrimento do sangue total se o animal estiver em hipervolemia e/ou oligúrico. Não existe grau absoluto de anemia que dite a transfusão. Critérios mais liberais quase sempre são usados se a anemia ocorrer de forma aguda. Os produtos recombinantes da eritropoetina podem aumentar a produção de hemácias durante 1 semana. Eles têm sido utilizados quando a anemia for antecipada, para diminuir eventuais requerimentos transfusionais, embora existam riscos de reações imunológicas. A uremia induz defeitos de função plaquetária. O tempo de sangramento de mucosa oral (ver Capítulo 80) estará prolongado apesar de um perfil de coagulação normal. A desmopressina (1-desamino-8-arginina vasopressina [DDAVP]; ver Capítulos 201 e 296) é utilizada em pessoas urêmicas com hemorragia ativa, mas esse tratamento ainda não foi avaliado em animais. A duração da atividade em pessoas é curta (menor que 24 horas) e seria considerada imediatamente antes de procedimentos invasivos.[182]

Distúrbios gastrintestinais e pancreatite

Complicações gastrintestinais (GI) (anorexia, náuseas, êmese, íleo paralítico) ocorrem comumente em casos de LRA, com hemorragia em 10 a 30% das pessoas afetadas.[80] Os bloqueadores da histamina ou antagonistas da bomba de prótons são comumente utilizados na IRA para inibir a secreção ácida gástrica. Como alguns desses fármacos são excretados pelos rins, a dose e frequência devem ser ajustados. Antieméticos são frequentemente necessários (ver Capítulo 39). Modificadores da motilidade são indicados se houver íleo paralítico. Se houver evidências de ulceração GI (p. ex., hematêmese, melena, relação UNS:creatinina aumentada, pan-hipoproteinemia com anemia aguda), um protetor gástrico (sucralfato) deve ser administrado (Tabela 322.4). A pancreatite é comum em casos de IRA (ver Capítulos 290 e 291). Antieméticos, analgésicos e suporte nutricional precoce (parenteral [ver Capítulo 189] se a êmese não estiver controlada, por sonda enteral [ver Capítulo 82] se o paciente estiver em anorexia, mas sem êmese) são recomendados.

Suporte nutricional

A IRA é uma condição altamente catabólica. Embora difícil de identificar claramente a contribuição do manejo nutricional para o resultado, o estado nutricional ruim é um importante fator para o aumento da morbidade e mortalidade.[183] A alimentação enteral precoce pode ajudar a preservar a integridade da mucosa GI.[184] Embora dietas renais (redução do PO_4 e proteína de alta

---

Tabela 322.4 Fármacos comuns utilizados para tratar sinais gastrintestinais na uremia.*

FÁRMACO	INDICAÇÃO	DOSE-CÃES	DOSE-GATOS	AJUSTE PARA INSUFICIÊNCIA RENAL E COMENTÁRIOS
Famotidina	Diminuir a acidez	0,5 a 1 mg/kg PO IM IV a cada 12 a 24 h	0,25 a 0,5 mg/kg PO SC a cada 24 h	Prolongar o intervalo ou diminuir a dose
Ranitidina	Diminuir a acidez, modificador da motilidade	0,5 a 2 mg/kg PO IV a cada 8 a 12 h	0,5 a 2,5 mg/kg PO SC IM IV a cada 12 h	Prolongar o intervalo ou diminuir a dose
Cimetidina	Diminuir a acidez	5 a 10 mg/kg PO IM IV a cada 4 a 6 h	5 a 10 mg/kg PO IM IV (lento) a cada 6 a 8 h	Prolongar o intervalo ou diminuir a dose
Omeprazol	Diminuir a acidez	0,5 a 1 mg/kg PO a cada 24 h	0,7 mg/kg PO a cada 24 h	Não abrir as cápsulas
Pantoprazol	Diminuir a acidez	0,5 a 1 mg/kg IV (durante 15 min) a cada 24 h	0,5 a 1 mg/kg IV (durante 15 min) a cada 24 h	
Metoclopramida	Antiemético, modificador da motilidade	0,1 a 0,5 mg/kg PO SC IM a cada 6 a 8 h, 0,01 a 0,02 mg/kg/h CRI	0,2 a 0,4 mg/kg SC a cada 6 a 8 h ou 0,01 a 0,02 mg/kg/h CRI	Diminuir a dose
Ondansetrona	Antiemético	0,1 mg/kg PO a cada 12 a 24 h	0,1 mg/kg PO a cada 6 a 8 h, 0,1 a 0,3 g/kg IV a cada 6 a 8 h	
Dolasetrona	Antiemético	0,5 mg/kg PO SC IV a cada 24 h	0,5 mg/kg PO SC IV a cada 24 h	
Maropitant	Antiemético	2 mg/kg PO a cada 24 h ou 1 mg/kg SC a cada 24 h durante 5 dias	1 mg/kg PO SC diariamente durante 5 dias	
Mirtazapina	Antiemético, estimulante de apetite	1,1 a 1,3 mg/kg PO a cada 24 h	1,88 mg por gato PO a cada 48 h	
Clorpromazina	Antiemético	0,2 a 0,5 mg/kg IM SC a cada 6 a 8 h	0,2 a 0,5 mg/kg IM SC a cada 8 h	
Proclorperazina	Antiemético	0,1 a 0,5 mg/kg IM SC a cada 8 a 12 h		
Sucralfato	Protetor gástrico	0,5 a 1 g PO a cada 6 a 8 h	0,25 g/gato PO a cada 8 h	
Misoprostol	Análogo citoprotetor da PGE	1 a 3 mcg/kg PO a cada 6 a 12 h		
Cisaprida	Modificador da motilidade	0,1 a 0,5 mg/kg PO a cada 8 a 12 h	2,5 a 5 mg/gato PO a cada 8 a 12 h	

*A maioria desses fármacos não foi ainda aprovada para utilização no cão ou gato. *CRI*, taxa de infusão contínua; *PGE*, prostaglandina E.

qualidade) sejam indicadas para o tratamento da DRC, a dieta ideal para IRA não é conhecida (ver Capítulo 184).[185,186] Na ausência de informações, dietas enterais para animais ou pessoas doentes em estado crítico têm sido utilizadas.[102] A anorexia é comum no paciente hospitalizado com insuficiência renal (ver Capítulo 23). Se o apetite não retornar dentro de poucos dias de terapia, a colocação de uma sonda de alimentação (ver Capítulo 82) pode permitir a administração de uma quantidade apropriada da dieta desejada, fácil administração de medicações orais, e é fortemente recomendada em animais que não consomem voluntariamente as calorias adequadas. Se o vômito impedir a alimentação enteral, a nutrição parenteral parcial ou NPT podem ser utilizadas (ver Capítulo 189).

Na suplementação enteral ou parenteral, o volume que pode ser administrado possivelmente será limitado em pacientes anúricos ou oligúricos. A maioria das dietas líquidas compatíveis para utilização por sonda nasoesofágica ou nasogástrica tem densidade calórica ao redor de 1 kcal/mℓ.[187] A provisão de 100% dos requerimentos basais de energia geralmente exigirá um volume de cerca do dobro dos requerimentos hídricos insensíveis. Fórmulas comuns para cálculo da nutrição parenteral total também utilizam o dobro dos requerimentos hídricos insensíveis.[188] A necessidade para suporte nutricional é uma indicação para remoção do fluido por diálise no paciente oligúrico. A suplementação com glutamina pode melhorar a sobrevida em pacientes humanos em LRA, mas mais pesquisas são necessárias.[189]

Infecções

Infecções ocorrem em 30 a 70% das pessoas com LRA por conta das defesas prejudicadas secundariamente à uremia, combinada à utilização de antibioticoterapia.[80] Os locais primários de infecção incluem o trato urinário, locais onde defeitos ocorrem nas barreiras normais (p. ex., cateteres IV), e trato respiratório.[80] A taxa de infecção em pacientes veterinários com LRA é desconhecida, mas a taxa de infecções em cães e gatos submetidos à hemodiálise (predominantemente para LRA) é de pelo menos 25%.

PROGNÓSTICO

A mortalidade da LRA é alta tanto em casos adquiridos no hospital como na comunidade. Em cães com discreto aumento na creatinina (< 50% aumento a partir dos níveis basais ou aumento ≥ 0,3 mg/dℓ, mas não azotêmicos), a mortalidade foi de 55 a 58%. Em cães e gatos que desenvolveram LRA mais grave no hospital, a mortalidade foi de 44 a 61% em cães e 58 a 73% em gatos.[10,11,22] A taxa de mortalidade em cães com LRA adquirida na comunidade foi de 56%.[21] As taxas de mortalidade em gatos com LRA adquirida na comunidade foram de 47 a 64%.[23,190] A taxa de mortalidade em pessoas é de cerca de 50%.[191] A diminuição da produção de urina é um fator prognóstico ruim em cães e gatos com LRA.[22,23] A gravidade da azotemia não foi preditiva do resultado na maioria dos estudos de gatos ou cães com LRA, enquanto um aumento inicial grave da creatinina sérica foi associado à incapacidade de recuperação em casos de LRA em um estudo com cães.[21-23,192,193] Em uma série de casos de gatos com LRA, para o incremento de cada

| Tabela 322.5 | Taxas de sobrevida para diversas etiologias da IRA.[2,23,52,202] | |

CATEGORIA	MANEJO SEM DIÁLISE	HEMODIÁLISE
Obstrutiva (gatos)	91%	70 a 75%
Infecciosa	82%	58 a 86%
Metabólica/hemodinâmica	66%	56 a 72%
Outra	50%	29 a 56%
Tóxica	43 a 69%	18 a 35%

unidade do potássio sérico, em mEq/ℓ, houve uma diminuição de 57% na chance de sobrevida.[23] Em outro estudo, menores temperaturas corporais, albumina sérica e lactato desidrogenase foram preditivos de mortalidade.[190] Dos gatos que sobrevivem ao episódio de LRA, cerca de metade recebeu alta com uma concentração sérica normal de creatinina. A outra metade dos sobreviventes tiveram azotemia persistente.[23] Em cães com LRA, 24 de 99 desenvolveram DRC (24 de 43 sobreviventes).[21] A etiologia da doença é um fator prognóstico em casos de LRA (Tabela 322.5). Em um estudo, 50% dos gatos com uma causa nefrotóxica ou outra qualquer sobreviveram, enquanto 75% daqueles com isquemia sobreviveram.[23] Em cães com LRA adquirida no hospital, 43% com exposição a substâncias nefrotóxicas sobreviveram, embora não tenha sido observada associação entre o tipo de insulto renal e o resultado nesse estudo.[22]

De forma geral, 40 a 60% dos pacientes com IRS tratados com hemodiálise sobrevivem, uma conquista notável, tendo em vista que a população de pacientes compreende animais que não respondem à terapia medicamentosa convencional.[194,195] A taxa de sobrevida para casos de LRA por causas infecciosas foi de cerca de 58 a 100%.[192,193,196,197] Causas hemodinâmicas e metabólicas tiveram taxa de sobrevida de 40 a 72%.[193,198] Somente 20 a 40% dos pacientes com LRA por causas tóxicas sobrevivem.[192,193] Dos pacientes que recebem hemodiálise e não sobrevivem, cerca de metade desses morrem ou são eutanasiados por conta de condições extrarrenais (p. ex., pancreatite, complicações respiratórias). Cerca de um terço dos pacientes que não sobrevivem são eutanasiados por conta de incapacidade de recuperação da função renal. Sinais urêmicos persistentes, complicações da diálise e causas desconhecidas correspondem pelas mortes restantes de pacientes. Assim como pacientes tratados de forma medicamentosa, aproximadamente metade tem o retorno da função renal (definido pela concentração sérica normal de creatinina) e metade possuem DRC persistente.

REFERÊNCIAS BIBLIOGRÁFICAS

As referências bibliográficas deste capítulo se encontram online no Ambiente de Aprendizagem.

CAPÍTULO 323

Transplante Renal

Chad W. Schmiedt

TRANSPLANTE RENAL EM GATOS

Seleção do candidato

O receptor ideal do aloenxerto renal são gatos com doença renal crônica (DRC) significativa e compensada que, de outra forma, são saudáveis. O melhor momento para o transplante com relação ao estágio da doença renal é desconhecido, mas o adiamento até que o animal esteja no estágio terminal da uremia não é desejável, pois o grau de azotemia é um fator de risco conhecido para resultados ruins.[1,2] Por outro lado, o transplante renal em felinos com DRC assintomático em estágio inicial também não é o ideal, em razão do longo tempo de sobrevida em casos de manejo medicamentoso e do risco perioperatório. Diversos centros utilizam um nível mínimo de creatinina sérica de 4,0 mg/dℓ como limiar para maximizar as oportunidades benéficas do tratamento medicamentoso e mitigar o risco perioperatório em gatos minimamente afetados.

Tem sido observado que gatos idosos têm menor sobrevida após o transplante quando comparados com os mais jovens.[1,2] Entretanto, felinos velhos sem outras comorbidades significativas podem passar por melhora substancial da qualidade de vida após o transplante. Portanto, esses animais podem estar aptos para o transplante e devem ser considerados sob a luz de sua completa situação clínica.

Antes do transplante, uma avaliação sistêmica minuciosa é realizada para aumentar a chance de sucesso e garantir que o rim do doador não seja desperdiçado. Os critérios variam um pouco entre os centros de transplante e devem ser confirmados em cada local, mas, em geral, os testes necessários estão listados no Boxe 323.1. Condições que descartam um gato para o transplante incluem infecções pelo vírus da imunodeficiência felina (FIV) ou da leucemia felina (FeLV), cardiopatia moderada à grave, neoplasia, pielonefrite, outras comorbidades significativas ou a incapacidade dos tutores para medicar ou obter cuidado veterinário. Problemas que inviabilizam o transplante até serem solucionados incluem hipertensão sistêmica, hipertireoidismo, infecções ativas e doença periodontal.

Gatos nos quais os veterinários suspeitam de infecção latente podem ser submetidos a testes com ciclosporina durante 1 a 3 meses antes do transplante. O objetivo de um exame com ciclosporina é atingir concentrações sanguíneas terapêuticas da substância (300 a 500 ng/mℓ) e monitorar infecções antes do procedimento definitivo. Animais com DRC secundária ou concomitante à urolitíase por oxalato podem ainda ser submetidos ao transplante renal com bons resultados, embora a nefrolitíase por oxalato de cálcio no aloenxerto seja possível.[3]

Seleção do doador

Doadores de rins devem ser gatos jovens ($\approx$ 1 a 2 anos) sem doenças. Programas de transplante exigem que os tutores do receptor adotem gatos doadores. A fonte dos doadores pode ser o gatil do receptor, um abrigo ou sociedade humanitária, uma colônia intramural no centro de transplante ou vendedores classe A licenciados pela USDA – o último é mais comum, já que gatos para criação minimizam os riscos potenciais da transmissão da doença. Candidatos a doador devem ser minuciosamente avaliados em busca de doenças. A transmissão da doença

---

> **Boxe 323.1** Testes gerais necessários antes do transplante renal
>
> - Hemograma e perfil bioquímico sérico
> - Urinálise e cultura
> - Relação proteína:creatinina urinária
> - Mensuração da pressão sanguínea
> - Concentração sérica de hormônio tireoideano (T$_4$)
> - Testes de doenças infecciosas
>   - Imunodeficiência viral felina
>   - Leucemia viral felina
>   - IgG e IgM para *Toxoplasma*
>   - Títulos ± para coronavírus
>   - Títulos ± para *Mycoplasma*
>   - *Western blot* ± para *Bartonella*
> - Ecocardiograma
> - Radiografias abdominais e torácicas
> - Ultrassom abdominal
> - Tipo sanguíneo
> - Avaliação odontológica

---

pelo rim doado é possível.[4,5] Para otimizar o planejamento cirúrgico, imagens transversas podem ser utilizadas para investigar a vasculatura renal do dador antes da cirurgia.[6]

Em especial na Europa, há questões éticas sobre o transplante renal felino, particularmente sobre o uso de gatos saudáveis como doadores.[7] Critérios rigorosos para os receptores, impactando positivamente a qualidade de vida dos receptores, e a realocação de felinos de abrigos ou de gatis criadores com tutores devotos podem mitigar questões relacionadas com a remoção do rim de um gato doador. Um estudo que acompanhou 16 doadores renais, 2 a 5 anos após a nefrectomia unilateral, observou a preservação da função renal e eritropoética em 14 deles, enquanto dois desenvolveram urina diluída e proteinúria.[8]

Cirurgia

Detalhes da técnica cirúrgica variam entre cirurgiões, porém os resultados a longo prazo têm sido relativamente consistentes, sugerindo que as consequências são mínimas.[1,2] A menos que haja indicação, os dois rins nativos não são removidos. Aloenxertos são implantados em uma localização heterotrópica caudal aos rins nativos. A artéria renal é anastomosada de forma término-lateral com a aorta, e a veia renal é anastomosada de forma término-lateral com a veia cava caudal.

Existem duas estratégias para o momento anestésico e cirúrgico ideal ao doador e receptor renal. Com a técnica simultânea de transplante, doador e receptor são anestesiados ao mesmo tempo.[9] Duas equipes cirúrgicas trabalham lado a lado e coordenam a retirada do doador e o implante no receptor. Nela, o tempo de isquemia geral é reduzido, assim como o estresse cirúrgico suportado por um único cirurgião, que realiza tanto a retirada quanto o implante. Por outro lado, no transplante sequencial, o rim é retirado do doador, lavado e armazenado em uma solução fria de sacarose-fosfato, sendo implantado no doador, em geral, poucas horas após a retirada.[2] O tempo mais prolongado de armazenamento isquêmico frio em gatos utilizando sacarose-fosfato é de 7 horas.[10]

As vantagens da estratégia sequencial incluem a exigência de apenas uma equipe anestésica, cirúrgica, e efeitos protetores da isquemia pelo frio para a redução da lesão celular.[11] Apesar do tempo isquêmico mais prolongado, o resfriamento do aloenxerto reduz o dano celular associado ao período isquêmico lesivo pelo calor. A solução de sacarose-fosfato reduz significativamente a lesão isquêmica pelo frio, em comparação com a lavagem com solução salina.[12] A despeito da estratégia de transplante, o objetivo é limiar o tempo de isquemia pelo calor – isto é, o tempo de anastomose vascular – para 60 minutos ou menos. Na técnica simultânea, o tempo de isquemia pelo calor começa no momento da retira do órgão; na técnica sequencial, quando o aloenxerto é removido da solução de armazenamento do órgão. A isquemia pelo calor termina quando o fluxo sanguíneo é restaurado para o aloenxerto.

Após a liberação das pinças vasculares e a restauração do fluxo sanguíneo para o aloenxerto, o ureter é implantado na bexiga do hospedeiro. Há duas técnicas principais empregadas para a neoureterocistostomia. Na de aposição mucosa, o ureter sofre transecção próximo à junção ureterovesical do doador durante o procedimento de remoção do órgão. O ureter é encurtado, e a porção distal que sofreu transecção é espatulada. A mucosa ureteral é suturada na mucosa vesical do receptor por técnicas intra ou extravesicais.[13] A segunda técnica é a da papila ureteral, na qual a do doador é removida com o ureter e suturada em uma localização extravesical à bexiga e serosa do receptor.[14]

Imunossupressão

Após transplante renal, a ciclosporina microemulsificada e a prednisolona são mais usadas para imunossupressão (ver Capítulo 165). Em gatos, a dose recomendada iniciada de ciclosporina é de 4 mg/kg PO a cada 12 horas, sendo ajustada com base nos níveis sanguíneos totais. A concentração-alvo no sangue nos 3 a 6 meses pós-transplante é $\approx$ 500 ng/mℓ, sendo reduzida para $\approx$ 300 ng/mℓ com o passar do tempo. De forma importante, a ciclosporina microemulsificada ou modificada deve ser prescrita, pois apresenta maior biodisponibilidade e eficácia quando comparada com a ciclosporina não emulsificada.[15] O cetoconazol tem sido usado para a inibição do metabolismo da ciclosporina e a permissão de uma única dose diária, o que pode ser importante para alguns tutores (ver Capítulo 165).[16] A absorção gastrintestinal de ciclosporina varia de forma significativa entre gatos; portanto, a dose deve ser baseada na concentração sanguínea do indivíduo, a qual é monitorada com frequência (semanalmente) logo após o transplante, até que a dose oral apropriada seja identificada. A periodicidade do monitoramento é estendida com o passar do tempo, com um intervalo máximo de 3 meses. Em felinos com má absorção da ciclosporina microemulsificada, o tratamento com a vitamina B pode aumentar a absorção.[17]

A prednisolona em baixa dose (0,25 a 0,5 mg/kg PO a cada 12 horas) também é usada frequentemente e pode ser mantida por um longo tempo se bem tolerada e necessária, ou reduzida e descontinuada se ocorrerem complicações. Outros regimes imunossupressores têm sido descritos de modo experimental em gatos após o transplante renal[18] ou sugeridos como opções com base em experimentos *in vitro*.[19]

Complicações

Diversas complicações agudas são previsíveis, dadas as manipulações cirúrgicas necessárias, e incluem hemorragia, tromboembolismo e uroabdome. Estudos ultrassonográficos por Doppler ou ultrassonografia contrastada são realizados rotineiramente no período pós-cirúrgico, a fim de avaliar o fluxo sanguíneo dentro do aloenxerto (Vídeo 323.1). No período perioperatório, gatos receptores podem se tornar hipotensos, se hipovolêmicos secundariamente à hemorragia da anastomose. Transfusões sanguíneas perioperatórias devem ser administradas se o animal apresentar anemia moderada à grave e/ou sintomática (ver Capítulo 130). O retorno ao normal da concentração de eritropoetina e a resolução concomitante da anemia são extremamente variáveis.[20]

A maioria dos gatos retornará a um hematócrito acima de 28% em torno de 1 mês após o transplante.[20] Na ausência de hemorragia pós-cirúrgica ativa, a heparina em baixa dose (125 UI/kg SC a cada 8 horas) é utilizada por mais ou menos 5 dias após o transplante, de modo a minimizar o risco de tromboembolismo.

Hipertensão sistêmica grave tem sido relatada de forma aguda depois de transplante renal e está associada a sinais clínicos neurológicos (ver Capítulo 157).[21] Em um estudo, 21/34 gatos se tornaram severamente hipertensos (pressão sanguínea sistólica $\geq$ 170 mmHg), tendo o tratamento com hidralazina reduzido as complicações neurológicas, em comparação com uma coorte histórica (ver Capítulo 158).[21,22] Nos receptores felinos de transplantes renais, a dose inicial típica de hidralazina para o tratamento de hipertensão grave é de 1 mg/gato SC. A pressão sanguínea do doador, então, é monitorada por 15 a 20 minutos para observar a redução (ver Capítulo 99). Se não houver melhora, incrementos adicionais de 1 a 2,5 mg são administrados a cada 15 minutos, até uma dose total máxima de 5 mg.

Função retardada do enxerto é um termo utilizado para descrever a ausência de função em um aloenxerto com fluxo sanguíneo normal e sem evidências de obstrução urinária pós-renal. Tem sido definida na literatura veterinária como uma concentração sérica de creatinina $\geq$ 3 mg/dℓ, 3 dias após o transplante, e foi relatada em 5 de 60 gatos submetidos ao transplante renal.[2] A função retardada do enxerto é uma consequência de lesão ao enxerto pré, peri ou transcirúrgico. Por exemplo, em humanos, aloenxertos coletados de doadores idosos, diabéticos ou hipertensos, cadáveres sem atividade cardíaca, cirurgias de transplante com tempos isquêmicos prolongados ou aloenxertos com obstrução ureteral pós-cirúrgica têm maior risco de função retardada do enxerto.[23] Aloenxertos com função retardada muitas vezes desenvolverão função normal, mas têm risco maior de perda precoce e tardia do aloenxerto.[23] Questões sobre a qualidade marginal dos rins do doador não são importantes em transplantes veterinários por conta de nossa capacidade em selecionar doadores saudáveis. Assim, fatores de risco relevantes no transplante veterinário para o retardo da função do enxerto se relacionam com lesão isquêmica transcirúrgica ou complicações pós-cirúrgicas, como constrição ureteral, trombose etc.

Uma reação aguda de rejeição é caracterizada por aumento palpável do aloenxerto, hipertermia ou hipotermia, apatia, anorexia, perda de peso e de função do aloenxerto. Gatos afetados podem ser assintomáticos.[24] Se eles forem submetidos ao transplante renal e não receberem tratamento imunossupressor, o tempo de sobrevida médio é de 23 dias.[24] Em um exame ultrassonográfico, um aloenxerto que sofre rejeição aguda apresenta uma área transversa aumentada e perda da definição da junção corticomedular, por conta do aumento da ecogenicidade da medula (Figura 323.1).[25] Pode também haver fluido perirrenal ou peritoneal. O índice resistivo costuma ser mensurado em aloenxertos renais, mas não demonstrou ser um indicador sensível de rejeição do aloenxerto.[25,26] Alterações na mensuração ultrassonográfica do tamanho do aloenxerto renal (comprimento, largura, área transversa) têm sido associadas à disfunção do aloenxerto.[26] Uma biopsia do aloenxerto raramente é necessária, e um atraso no tratamento até confirmação da biopsia pode ser desastroso. Baixa concentração sanguínea de ciclosporina, azotemia, leucocitose, alterações ultrassonográficas características, ausência de infecção ativa e paciente em estado geral ruim suportam a pesquisa do diagnóstico de rejeição do aloenxerto.

Em geral, uma reação de rejeição aguda pode ser controlada e revertida pela administração intravenosa de doses imunossupressoras de corticosteroides, ciclosporina e fluidoterapia. A terapia deve ser mantida até que a concentração sérica de creatinina estabilize, o que costuma levar vários dias. O aloenxerto pode recuperar a função basal, dependendo de quão rapidamente a reação de rejeição é diagnosticada e tratada de modo eficaz. Muitas vezes, mesmo após tratamento com sucesso, há certa perda de função, aumento da antigenicidade do enxerto e maior risco de futuras reações de rejeição.[27]

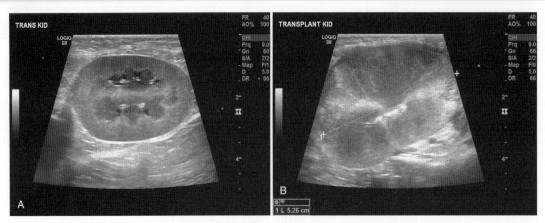

Figura 323.1 A. Imagem ultrassonográfica sagital normal de um aloenxerto renal 1 dia após transplante renal em gato. **B.** O mesmo rim de **A** sofrendo uma reação aguda de rejeição. O aloenxerto é maior e tem ecotextura heterogênea com perda de definição da junção corticomedular.

Complicações crônicas são comuns após transplante renal, o que exige manejo pós-cirúrgico dedicado. Uma reação de rejeição aguda retardada pode ocorrer em qualquer momento depois da cirurgia se o regime imunossupressor for descontinuado, a medicação for administrada incorretamente ou houver alteração da absorção do fármaco secundariamente à doença gastrintestinal ou alteração da dieta. A avaliação frequente das concentrações sanguíneas de ciclosporina é indicada para minimizar o risco de rejeição aguda retardada do aloenxerto.

A perda crônica e gradativa da função do aloenxerto é um problema importante no transplante renal, sobretudo em humanos. Historicamente, essa condição foi chamada de *rejeição crônica*. No entanto, de um tempo para cá, vem-se usando *nefropatia crônica do aloenxerto*, *disfunção crônica do aloenxerto* e, mais recentemente, *fibrose intersticial* e *atrofia tubular* para descrever a condição ligada às lesões histopatológicas principais.[27] Alterações características da nefropatia crônica do aloenxerto humano têm sido descritas conforme relacionadas com os aloenxertos renais felinos.[28] Cerca de 70% dos aloenxertos felinos avaliados tiveram evidências histológicas de nefropatia crônica do aloenxerto.[28]

Por conta da necessidade de imunossupressão crônica, os receptores do transplante têm maior risco de infecções, que podem ser recidivantes, uma recrudescência de uma infecção latente ou transmitidas ao receptor pelo aloenxerto. Infecções depois de transplante renal foram relatadas em 25 a 36% dos pacientes.[2,29] A maioria é bacteriana, mas virais, fúngicas, protozoáricas e micobacterianas também foram relatadas.[2,29] Uroabdome e diabetes melito foram identificadas como fatores de risco para infecções pós-transplante em gatos.[2,29] A transmissão de toxoplasmose por aloenxerto e recrudescência da toxoplasmose em receptores de transplante felinos foi relatada. O tratamento da toxoplasmose ativa em gatos imunossuprimidos, em geral, não obtém sucesso, sendo importante uma avaliação minuciosa para essa doença antes da cirurgia.[4,5]

Após o transplante renal, gatos têm risco mais ou menos 6 vezes maior de desenvolver câncer, quando comparados com aqueles da mesma idade saudáveis.[30-33] Esse problema é bem reconhecido em pessoas após transplante de órgãos sólidos e está relacionado com a estimulação antigênica crônica do aloenxerto e a influência imunossupressora e oncogênica de vários regimes imunossupressores.[34,35] A ciclosporina pode promover oncogênese por diversos mecanismos, incluindo promoção da angiogênese tumoral, inibição do reparo do DNA, inibição da apoptose e síntese do fator transformados de crescimento-beta (TGF-beta).[36,37] Em gatos, assim como em humanos, o linfoma é a neoplasia maligna mais comum após transplante renal e é comumente um linfoma de células B, difuso, de médio a alto grau (ver Capítulo 344).[30,32,33] A sobrevida depois do diagnóstico muitas vezes é baixa, com tempos de sobrevida médios relatados entre 2 e 15 dias.[30-32]

A fibrose peritoneal tem sido relatada em gatos após o transplante renal.[38,39] A fibrose retroperitoneal foi relatada em 21% dos felinos transplantados,[38] mas não é relatada com frequência em outras séries de casos.[1,2] Clinicamente, a condição é caracterizada por sinais inespecíficos, como letargia, anorexia e azotemia. O aloenxerto e o ureter associado se tornam enclausurados em uma cápsula fibrótica, que resulta em obstrução ureteral, azotemia pós-renal, hidroureter e hidronefrose.[39] A condição ocorre em uma média de 62 dias após o transplante, e os fatores de risco são desconhecidos.[39] O tratamento é o desbridamento cirúrgico do tecido cicatricial e ureterólise, ou liberação cirúrgica do ureter pela cicatriz retroperitoneal. A recorrência ocorreu em 6 de 25 gatos submetidos à cirurgia e tratados por nova ureterólise.[39] O tratamento profilático transcirúrgico com carboximetilcelulose tem sido sugerido como forma de minimizar a formação de aderências.[39]

Após o transplante renal, a nutrição deve ser ajustada de acordo com as necessidades de cada paciente. Se cálculos urinários estiverem presentes antes do transplante, uma dieta apropriada deve ser selecionada para preveni-los no aloenxerto (ver Capítulo 324). A manutenção de gatos em uma dieta renal pós-transplante poderia aumentar a probabilidade de obesidade, em razão do maior conteúdo de carboidratos. A seleção de uma dieta com menores níveis de carboidratos, como uma sênior, e o frequente monitoramento do peso podem ajudar a minimizar o ganho de peso. O diabetes melito é comum em receptores de transplante felinos, e a obesidade predisporá os pacientes ao seu desenvolvimento. Os receptores de transplante têm probabilidade 5,4 vezes maior de se tornar diabéticos, quando comparados com gatos controle com DRC, e a ocorrência de diabetes resulta em um aumento de 2,4 vezes na mortalidade.[40] Fatores de risco para o desenvolvimento de diabetes na população felina transplantada são desconhecidos.

Resultados

Após o transplante, a sobrevida em 6 meses é de aproximadamente 60 a 65%, e, em 3 anos, de cerca de 40%.[1,2] Quando essas estatísticas são consideradas para gatos liberados do hospital, a sobrevida em 6 meses aumenta substancialmente para 84%, e, em 3 anos, para 45%.[2]

Embora pareça óbvio, gatos mais velhos têm sido associados a menores tempos de sobrevida.[1,2] Outros fatores supostamente associados à sobrevida geral incluem azotemia pré-cirúrgica, peso corporal, concentração pós-cirúrgica de creatinina, percentual de declínio da creatinina com base nos níveis pré-cirúrgicos, pressão sanguínea arterial derivada do Doppler e doença infecciosa pré-cirúrgica.[2] Mais trabalhos são necessários para validar esses fatores de risco em outras populações de pacientes.

REFERÊNCIAS BIBLIOGRÁFICAS

As referências bibliográficas deste capítulo se encontram online no Ambiente de Aprendizagem.

CAPÍTULO 324

Doença Renal Crônica

David James Polzin

VISÃO GERAL DA DOENÇA RENAL CRÔNICA

Definições

A doença renal crônica (DRC) é a forma mais comumente reconhecida de doença renal em cães e gatos. É definida como anormalidades estruturais e/ou funcionais de um ou ambos os rins que estiveram continuamente presentes por 3 meses ou mais. As descrições arcaicas *insuficiência renal* e *falência renal* não foram uniformemente e adequadamente definidas; portanto, elas foram substituídas por um sistema de estadiamento de DRC desenvolvido pela International Renal Interest Society (IRIS; *www.iris-kidney.com*). O sistema de estadiamento da DRC pela IRIS fornece especificidade com relação à extensão da disfunção renal e reconhecimento da amplitude completa da DRC estrutural e funcional. Os rins de cães e gatos com DRC possuem reduções permanentes no seu número de néfrons funcionais. Embora a estrutura e função renal não sejam consistentemente paralelas, doenças renais primárias em geral demonstram evidências de desarranjos estruturas e funcionais.

A apresentação clínica de pacientes com DRC tipicamente reflete a extensão da redução da função renal, e não o impacto das lesões estruturais.

Na maioria das situações, a DRC é irreversível e progressiva, mesmo após tratamento. Entretanto, é comum que a azotemia pré-renal ou pós-renal, ou doenças renais ativas (chamadas de doenças renais crônicas agudizadas) coexistam com a DRC. Ao contrário da DRC, estas complicações podem ser reversíveis (p. ex., pielonefrite, obstrução ureteral, desidratação etc.). Após correção de doenças primárias reversíveis e/ou condições pré-renais ou pós-renais, não deve ser esperada melhora adicional da função renal, pois mecanismos compensatórios e adaptativos desenvolvidos para manter a função renal já ocorreram amplamente, alterações que promovem perda progressiva de néfrons remanescentes e da função renal. Esta característica da DRC (denominada "progressão espontânea da DRC") foi explicada pela "hipótese perde e ganha", que afirma que a consequência da maximização da função renal residual pelos processos adaptativos renais a fim de manter a homeostase resulta em um perde-e-ganha do dano permanente aos néfrons remanescentes. Assim, não é necessário para o processo inicial da doença persistir para que o declínio progressivo da função renal continue.

A DRC costuma causar um declínio lento, mas inexoravelmente progressivo da função. Em alguns pacientes, este padrão segue um declínio quase linear, enquanto em outros o padrão é caracterizado por períodos de relativa estabilidade seguidos por episódios de declínio abrupto da função renal. Alguns pacientes podem ter períodos múltiplos de função renal estável e uma série de declínios abruptos antes de sucumbir para a DRC. Entretanto, exceções para este padrão progressivo são reconhecidas, particularmente entre um conjunto substancial de gatos que possuem função renal estável durante anos. Em um estudo recente, somente 101 de 213 (47%) gatos com DRC demonstraram evidências de aumento progressivo nos valores séricos de creatinina.[1] Este padrão de estabilidade também pode ser observado em alguns cães jovens com displasia renal. A menos que ocorra maiores lesões renais ou que a DRC esteja em estágio avançado, a rápida deterioração da função renal remanescente é atípica. Em vez disso, a função renal frequentemente permanece

estável ou sofre declínio em meses a anos.[2,3] Assim, independente da causa incitante, a DRC é uma doença irreversível e lentamente progressiva. Ao mesmo tempo que nenhum tratamento pode corrigir as lesões renais irreversíveis existentes da DRC, as consequências clínicas e bioquímicas da redução da função renal podem frequentemente ser amenizadas pela terapia de suporte, e a evolução progressiva natural da DRC pode ser retardada por intervenção terapêutica.

Prevalência e populações afetadas

Prevalência geral

A prevalência da doença renal tem sido estimada variando entre 0,5 e 7% em cães e entre 1,6 e 20% em gatos.[4] Entretanto, tem sido sugerido que uma estimativa razoável da prevalência geral da DRC na prática geral em pequenos animais nos EUA seria de 1 a 3% de gatos e 0,5 a 1,5% de cães.[5] Um estudo estimou a prevalência da DRC em cães do Reino Unido em 0,02 a 1,44%.[6] Dos cães estudados nesse relato, 95/136 (63,6%) eram dos estágios III ou IV de DRC da IRIS, enquanto 37/136 (26,6%) tinham concentrações de ureia nitrogenada sanguínea (BUN) de 112,0 mg/dℓ ou acima.

Gatos

Embora frequentemente considerada uma doença de animais idosos, a DRC ocorre com frequência variada em cães e gatos de todas as idades. Em um estudo retrospectivo de gatos com DRC, 53% dos gatos afetados tinham acima de 7 anos, mas a variação de idade foi de 9 meses a 22 anos.[7] Em um estudo sobre a distribuição etária da doença renal em gatos a partir de dados submetidos ao *Veterinary Medical Data Base* na Purdue University entre 1980 e 1990, 37% dos gatos com diagnóstico de "insuficiência renal" tinham menos de 10 anos, 31% dos gatos tinham entre 10 e 15 anos, e 32% dos gatos eram mais velhos que 15 anos.[8] De forma semelhante, em um estudo de gatos com DRC relatado em 1988, a idade média deles era de 12,6 anos com uma variação de 1 a 26 anos.[3,9] A idade média entre 45 gatos do grupo-controle nesse estudo foi de 10 anos. Durante os anos 1990, a prevalência da doença renal entre gatos de todas as idades foi de 16 casos para cada mil gatos examinados, e entre gatos com mais de 15 anos, 153 por mil.[7] Em um estudo de gatos com mais de 9 anos, 30,5% dos gatos desenvolveram azotemia dentro de 12 meses.[10] Gatos da raça Maine Coon, Abissínio, Siamês, Azul Russo e Birmanês foram relatados de forma desproporcional como afetados.

Cães

Cães do Reino Unido com 12 anos ou mais tiveram 5,5 vezes chances maiores, e cães entre quatro e 7 anos tiveram 0,22 vezes a probabilidade de desenvolver DRC quando comparados a cães entre 7 e 12 anos.[6] No mesmo estudo, cães das raças Cocker Spaniel e Cavalier King Charles Spaniel tiveram maiores probabilidades de DRC comparados a cães sem raça definida. Entretanto, cães de raças puras não demonstraram aumento da probabilidade da DRC, seja de forma geral ou para aqueles com menos de 5 anos. Uma associação entre DRC e menor peso corporal foi previamente relatada em cães, mas tal associação não foi observada no estudo do Reino Unido.[6,11] Embora a DRC aparentemente ocorra menos comumente em cães do que em gatos, a incidência aumenta com o avanço da idade em ambos. Com base em dados submetidos de 1983 a 1992 ao *Veterinary Medical Data Base* na Purdue University, 18% dos cães com diagnóstico de "insuficiência renal" tinham menos de 4 anos, 17% tinham entre 4 e 7 anos, 20% tinham entre sete e 19 anos, e 45% tinham mais de 10 anos. A prevalência de um diagnóstico de "insuficiência renal" entre cães de todas as idades foi de nove casos para cada mil cães examinados. A prevalência de "insuficiência renal" entre cães entre sete e 10 anos foi de 12,5 por mil cães examinados, para cães entre 10 e 15 anos foi de 24 por mil, e entre cães com mais de 15 anos foi de 57 por mil. Mais recentemente, a prevalência da DRC em cães observada na prática geral foi estimada em até 1,5%.[5] A observação de maiores probabilidades de DRC com o avanço da idade é consistente com a teoria da progressão da DRC desde o dano renal inicial subclínico até a doença clínica.

Causas de doença renal crônica

Suspeita inicial

A maioria dos cães e gatos é inicialmente suspeita de ser paciente com DRC após notar aumento da concentração sérica de creatinina. Os valores séricos de creatinina acima dos valores de referência implicam que a taxa de filtração glomerular (TFG) diminuiu em 75% ou mais e que pelo menos 75% dos néfrons em ambos os rins foram lesados ou perdidos. Assim, o diagnóstico de DR em cães e gatos é reconhecido relativamente tardiamente na evolução da doença. Tipicamente, os rins são pequenos porque néfrons perdidos são substituídos por tecido cicatricial e inflamação crônica, fato que não fornece muitas diretrizes sobre a origem etiológica da lesão (Figura 324.1). Além disso, os néfrons remanescentes refletem modificações adaptativas e compensatórias que podem interferir no estabelecimento da origem etiológica da DRC. Assim, a base etiológica da doença renal não é em geral determinada. Talvez a detecção mais precoce da DRC (p. ex., da DRC em estágio I da IRIS) poderia fornecer uma oportunidade de estabelecimento da(s) doença(s) incitantes responsáveis pela DRC.

Cães

A DRC pode iniciar com uma variedade de diferentes condições familiares, congênitas ou adquiridas. Os achados da biopsia em 37 cães com azotemia renal primária revelou que 58% tinham nefrite tubulointersticial crônica, 28% tinham uma glomerulonefropatias, e foi observada amiloidose em 6%, embora estimativas anteriores sugeriram que a doença glomerular pode corresponder a mais de 50% da DRC em cães.[12,13] Durante a última década, a ocorrência da doença glomerular parece ter aumentado substancialmente em áreas geográficas selecionadas em razão do aumento da proeminência de determinadas doenças infecciosas, como a borreliose nos EUA (ver Capítulo 211) e leishmaniose na Europa (ver Capítulo 221).[14] Muitos desses cães possuem ou desenvolvem DRC; entretanto, uma mensuração acurada da prevalência da doença glomerular em cães ainda não foi estabelecida. A proporção de DRCs devido à doença glomerular é confundida por cães afetados com diversas síndromes renais concorrentes, incluindo DRC, lesão renal aguda (IRA), síndrome nefrótica ou proteinúria isolada (inicialmente em estágio I de DRC pela IRIS).

Gatos

Em gatos com DRC, 70% tinham nefrite tubulointersticial, glomerulonefropatias foi observada em 15%, linfoma em 11% e amiloidose em 2%. Assim como em cães, a(s) causa(s) incitante(s) da DRC frequentemente não podem ser determinadas. A base etiológica das doenças no túbulo-interstício tem sido especialmente elusiva. Glomerulonefropatias têm sido ligadas a uma série de processos inflamatórios neoplásicos, metabólicos, e infecciosos e não infecciosos.[15] Diversos agentes infecciosos são propostos como possíveis fatores promotores de prevalência severamente alta da DRC felina. O vírus da imunodeficiência felina (FIV) tem sido ligado à doença renal em gatos, embora poucos com DRC sejam positivos para FIV.[16,17] Um morbilivírus felino tem sido associado com lesões tubulointersticiais em gatos.[18] As vacinas do herpes-vírus felino tipo 1, calicivírus e o vírus da panleucopenia cultivadas em cultura de tecido felino e administradas por via subcutânea em filhotes de gatos induzem anticorpos antitecido-renal-felino no soro, levantando questões de que as vacinações podem ter um papel no desenvolvimento da DRC.[19-21] Ao mesmo tempo que essas causas têm sido propostas como possíveis causas de DRC felina, elas permanecem amplamente infundadas.

Surgiu a hipótese de que pelo menos em alguns gatos, a doença renal pode ser um mecanismo adaptativo associado ao envelhecimento normal.[22] O início precoce das alterações tubulointersticiais renais ocorre em gatos adultos mais jovens, e isso tem sido proposto como uma adaptação defensiva. Além disso, ao mesmo tempo que gatos idosos sucumbiram à doença renal evidente com maior frequência, gatos com alterações tubulointersticiais renais possuíram durações de vida mais prolongadas independentemente da causa da morte. Maior encurtamento de telômeros foi notado em gatos com DRC em suas células epiteliais tubulares proximais e distais do que em gatos saudáveis jovens ou geriátricos.[23] O encurtamento de telômeros não foi detectado em amostras de pele ou fígado de nenhum dos gatos, sugerindo que é específico dos rins. Foi concluído que a DRC felina está associada a telômeros encurtados e aumento da senescência celular em rins afetados, o que pode apresentar futuros alvos para terapia intervencionista.

Terapias específicas

Apesar da irreversibilidade das lesões renais generalizadas associadas à DRC, é importante formular planos diagnósticos a fim de tentar identificar a causa de base e determinar se ainda está ativa. Embora terapias específicas direcionadas a eliminar ou controlar a causa primária em geral não alterem substancialmente as lesões renais existentes, é importante no contexto de minimizar danos adicionais aos néfrons. Doenças renais potencialmente amenizáveis à terapia específica incluem pielonefrite bacteriana, uropatia obstrutiva, nefrolitíase, linfoma renal (particularmente em gatos), nefropatia hipercalcêmica, pseudocistos perinéfricos e algumas glomerulopatias.

Prognóstico da doença renal crônica

Fatores que influenciam

Vários fatores influenciam o prognóstico da DRC, tanto favoravelmente como desfavoravelmente, incluindo a qualidade do

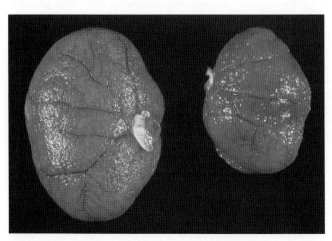

Figura 324.1 Rins pequenos, irregulares e com perfurações finas de um gato com doença renal crônica. A assimetria do tamanho entre esses rins pode refletir diferenças na gravidade da doença e efeitos da hipertrofia compensatória.

cuidado médico fornecido e o nível de comprometimento do tutor. O prognóstico frequentemente influencia uma questão de tratamento do tutor e comprometimento nas recomendações seguintes. Portanto, é importante fornecer o prognóstico mais acurado possível, melhor estabelecido após revisão dos resultados de uma avaliação minuciosa. Fatores a serem considerados ao estabelecer um prognóstico para animais com DRC incluem: (1) a natureza da doença renal primária, (2) gravidade e duração dos sinais clínicos e complicações da uremia, (3) probabilidade de melhora da função renal (reversibilidade, primariamente de condições renais primárias pré-renais, renais, pós-renais e recém-adquiridas), (4) gravidade do distúrbio funcional renal intrínseco, (5) taxa de progressão da disfunção renal com ou sem terapia, e (6) idade do paciente. Ao mesmo tempo que os sinais urêmicos podem ser um preditor razoável do prognóstico a curto prazo em alguns indivíduos, complicações pré-renais, pós-renais e renais ativas podem ser instigadores dos sinais e podem ser reversíveis. A fim de estabelecer de forma mais acurada o prognóstico relacionado à DRC subjacente, complicações pré-renais, pós-renais e ativas (p. ex., pielonefrite) devem ser inicialmente tratadas. O sistema de estadiamento da DRC pela IRIS é um guia útil para fornecer um prognóstico preliminar. Gatos com DRC sobrevivem mais tempo do que cães.

Prognóstico de gatos com doença renal crônica
Em um estudo retrospectivo, o tempo e sobrevida mediano para 211 gatos com DRC e concentrações séricas de creatinina entre 2,3 e 3,8 mg/dℓ foi de 771 dias.[24] Entretanto, a sobrevida variou de forma significativa de acordo com o estágio da DRC pela IRIS. Gatos com DRC em estágio II pela IRIS tiveram um tempo de sobrevida mediano de 1.151 dias com intervalo de confiança (IC) 95% de 1.014 a 1.565 dias. Como estes dados somente incluem um subgrupo de gatos em estágio II de DRC pela IRIS, as durações da sobrevida poderiam ter sido mais prolongadas se todos os gatos em estágio II tivessem sido incluídos (1,6 a 2,3 mg/dℓ). A expectativa de vida mediana para gatos com DRC em estágio III pela IRIS foi de 679 dias (IC 95%: 445 a 910 dias) e foi de 35 dias para gatos em estágio IV de DRC pela IRIS (IC 95%: 21 a 99 dias). Nesse estudo, o fosfato (PO_4) sérico e os estágios da IRIS foram os únicos parâmetros basais que afetam de forma significativa o tempo de sobrevida. Entretanto, a gravidade da proteinúria também influencia a sobrevida.[25-27] A hipertensão não parece ser um determinante primário da sobrevida em gatos com DRC, mas afeta a gravidade da proteinúria. Ambas as questões podem ser mascaradas pelo efeito da terapia anti-hipertensiva.[25,26]

Ao contrário de pessoas e cães, a terapia com amlodipino da hipertensão em gatos está associada a uma redução da proteinúria, o que influencia a sobrevida estratificada pelo estadiamento da IRIS.[27] A anemia demonstrou ser um indicador prognóstico em alguns, mas não em todos os estudos. A desidratação e terapia podem confundir o uso do hematócrito como um indicador prognóstico. Em um estudo, a perda de peso foi o indicador mais confiável de deterioração clínica em gatos com DRC, e a nefrolitíase foi identificada como um fator de comorbidade comum em gatos com DRC.[1] Em um estudo de casos controlados de 14 gatos com DRC em estágios II e III, a nefrolitíase não associada à obstrução urinária não foi associada ao aumento das taxas de mortalidade ou na taxa de progressão da doença.[29]

Prognóstico de cães com doença renal crônica
Em 228 cães diagnosticados como portadores de DRC por clínicas de atendimento geral, seu tempo de sobrevida mediano desde o diagnóstico foi de 226 dias (IC 95%: 112 a 326 dias).[6] Durante o estudo, 118/228 (52%) cães morreram, 99/118 foram eutanasiados. O estágio de DRC pela IRIS e a concentração de BUN influenciaram de forma significativa sua sobrevida. Comparados aos estágios I e II da DRC pela IRIS, cães com DRC em estágio III pela IRIS tiveram 2,6 vezes e em estágio IV tiveram 4,7 vezes a mortalidade. Cães com concentrações de BUN $\geq$ 112 mg/dℓ no momento do diagnóstico inicial tiveram 7,8 (IC 95%: 2,6 a 22,7) vezes a taxa de mortalidade devido à DRC do que cães com valores de BUN < 44,8 mg/dℓ.

O tratamento da DRC em cães parece afetar o prognóstico. Em um estudo clínico de 38 cães com DRC espontânea, a concentração sérica de creatinina média não pareceu influenciar a sobrevida quando cães foram alimentados com uma dieta renal e a sobrevida mediana para 21 cães com uma concentração média de creatinina sérica de 3,3 mg/dℓ foi de 615 dias. A sobrevida mediana para os cães nesse grupo com valores séricos de creatinina entre 2,0 e 3,1 mg/dℓ foi também de 615 dias.[2] Entretanto, em 17 cães que tiveram uma concentração sérica de creatinina de 3,7 mg/dℓ e foram alimentados com uma dieta de manutenção, a sobrevida mediana foi de 252 dias, e naqueles com valores séricos de creatinina entre 2,0 e 3,1 mg/dℓ, foi de 461 dias. Menos informações têm sido relatadas sobre o prognóstico e fatores de risco para cães *versus* gatos com DRC. A proteinúria foi identificada como um fator de risco para o desenvolvimento de sinais clínicos de uremia e para morte em cães com DRC.[30] Em um estudo, a proteinúria teve um efeito progressivamente adverso sobre o resultado: o risco de morte devido à DRC aumentou em 60% para cada unidade da relação proteína:creatinina urinária (RUPC) acima de 1.

A hipertensão arterial (ver Capítulo 157) foi identificada como um fator de risco para mortalidade em cães com DRC, mas assim como em gatos, efeitos adversos da hipertensão em cães podem ser mediados, pelo menos em parte, pela proteinúria.[31] Cães com DRC e as maiores pressões sanguíneas sistólicas basais possuem um maior declínio da função renal com o passar do tempo, possuem maior risco de crises urêmicas e morte. Ao mesmo tempo que isso não prova uma relação de causa e efeito entre hipertensão e doença renal progressiva, sugere que os valores iniciais de pressão sanguínea devem ser considerados ao formular um prognóstico para cães com DRC. Maiores escores de condição corporal (ver Capítulo 170) estão associados a um melhor prognóstico (maior tempo de sobrevida) em cães com DRC.[32] De forma semelhante, a obesidade está associada à maior sobrevida em seres humanos com DRC, consistente com um papel significativo da inanição sobre o resultado (ver Capítulos 176 e 177).

Doenças congênitas/familiares
Comparada à velocidade de progressão da DRC em cães de meia-idade a idosos com doença renal adquirida, a DRC pode progredir mais lentamente em vários cães com nefropatias congênitas ou familiares não caracterizadas por proteinúria (displasia renal; ver Capítulo 328). Uma velocidade de progressão comparavelmente mais lenta também foi observada em cães jovens com DRC adquirida (p. ex., após exposição a nefrotoxinas). Vários desses cães parecem resistentes notavelmente ao desenvolvimento de sinais clínicos de uremia apesar de elevações substanciais nas concentrações séricas de creatinina e ureia nitrogenada.

CONSEQUÊNCIAS CLÍNICAS DA DOENÇA RENAL CRÔNICA

Uremia

Definição
A uremia é a síndrome clínica que resulta da perda das funções renais. Distúrbios das funções glomerulares, tubulares e endócrinas renais levam à retenção de metabólitos tóxicos, alterações no volume e composição de fluidos corporais, e excessos ou deficiências de alguns hormônios. Os sinais clínicos de uremia refletem o efeito líquido desses desarranjos por todo organismo. Uma definição alternativa de uremia é "os efeitos mórbidos da insuficiência renal que ainda não podemos explicar."[33,34] A patogênese de algumas anormalidades previamente relacionadas como parte da síndrome urêmica é agora compreendida (p. ex., hipertensão devido à sobrecarga volêmica, anemia devido à

deficiência de eritropoetina [EPO]), de forma que não seriam mais consideradas como parte da síndrome urêmica pela utilização dessa definição mais moderna e restritiva.

Sinais clínicos

Os sinais clínicos mais provavelmente levam à consulta veterinária são poliúria e polidipsia (PU/PD). Os sinais clínicos mais proeminentes de uremia estão relacionados ao trato gastrintestinal (GI): anorexia, náuseas, êmese, ulcerações orais, estomatite, necrose das margens da língua, halitose (hálito urêmico), diarreia, melena e hematoquesia. Outros achados clínicos em cães e gatos com DRC podem incluir: perda de peso, caquexia muscular, hipotermia, letargia, fraqueza, tremores musculares, pericardite urêmica e pneumonite, hipertensão, alteração do comportamento (encefalopatia urêmica ou hipertensiva), osteodistrofia renal e diáteses hemorrágicas. Em um estudo, os sinais mais comuns de DRC foram êmese (50%), PU/PD (44%), alteração do apetite (40%), diarreia/melena (37%), perda de peso/caquexia (29%), letargia/depressão (22%), incontinência urinária (20%), halitose (12%) e anemia (4%).[6]

Patogênese

A patogênese dos sinais específicos da uremia é variavelmente compreendida. De forma geral, três mecanismos principais estão envolvidos: (1) excreção alterada de eletrólitos e água, (2) excreção reduzida de solutos orgânicos (*i. e.*, toxinas urêmicas), e (3) alteração da síntese de hormônios renais. Estas alterações afetam virtualmente todo sistema orgânico, produzindo dessa forma a síndrome urêmica. Mais de 70 sinais clínicos foram identificados em pessoas urêmicas.

Excreção alterada de eletrólitos e água

Uma função primária dos rins é manter o balanço hídrico e eletrolítico. A excreção de água e eletrólitos deve acomodar alterações na ingestão. Conforma a taxa de filtração glomerular (TFG) declina com a evolução da doença renal, a necessidade de excreção de água e eletrólitos permanece a mesma, a menos que a ingestão seja modificada. Conforme a TFG declina, a carga excretora de eletrólitos e água por néfron remanescente aumenta substancialmente, mas a excreção de várias substâncias pode ser mantida por meio de reduções concomitantes no grau de reabsorção tubular. Se a TFG diminui em três quartos, os néfrons remanescentes devem excretar cada um quatro vezes mais sódio (Na). Assim, a manutenção do balanço hídrico e eletrolítico requer que mais água e eletrólitos sejam excretados por néfron remanescente. Para o Na, potássio (K) e água, um estado estável pode ser mantido mesmo que a TFG possa ser reduzida em mais de 80%.[35] Embora os rins possuam capacidade marcante de manter o balanço hídrico e eletrolítico bem mesmo em estágios avançados da doença, mecanismos compensatórios são limitados e finalmente falham na doença em estágio terminal. Os mecanismos compensatórios para alguns eletrólitos são mais efetivos para manutenção do equilíbrio. Por exemplo, a excreção adaptativa de PO_4 é menos efetiva do que a excreção adaptada de Na. Se a ingestão de PO_4 permanecer inalterada e a TFG declinar, a necessidade para excreção de PO_4 pode exceder as taxas diárias máximas adaptativas de excreção de PO_4, e o PO_4 começa a acumular, levando à hiperfosfatemia progressiva (hiperPO_4). Manifestações clínicas de distúrbios da excreção de água e eletrólitos podem incluir edema, hipertensão, hipoNa, hiperK, acidose metabólica e hiperPO_4.

Excreção reduzida de solutos orgânicos

Embora a ureia e a creatinina sejam mais conhecidos, os rins excretam uma ampla variedade de solutos orgânicos (ver Capítulo 62). Vários desses solutos são manuseados primariamente pela filtração glomerular, mas a secreção tubular renal e reabsorção podem afetar a excreção renal final. Uma importante diferença entre manuseio renal de solutos orgânicos e manuseio

renal de eletrólitos e água é que a excreção de solutos orgânicos não é geralmente ativamente regulada e as concentrações sanguíneas começam a subir após o declínio inicial da TFG, e continuam a aumentar progressivamente conforme a função renal continua a declinar.[33,34] Quando a TFG declina a níveis próximos de 10% do normal, os sinais clínicos podem começar a surgir, em geral atribuídos às concentrações aumentadas de solutos orgânicos. Entretanto, a presença de uma maior concentração de uma substância não comprova que seja uma toxina urêmica. Entretanto, a possibilidade de que solutos urêmicos possam de fato ser contribuintes para a síndrome urêmico é suportada pela observação de que algumas anormalidades urêmicas são transferíveis em casos de soro ou plasma urêmico. Anormalidades que têm sido dessa forma demonstradas incluem: inibição da Na-K adenosina trifosfatase (ATPase), inibição da função plaquetária, disfunção leucocitária, perda de assimetria lipídica da membrana do eritrócito, e resistência insulínica.

Mais de 100 potenciais solutos urêmicos foram listados pelo grupo European Uremic Toxin Work (EUTox).[33,34] Entretanto, tem sido difícil confirmar as substâncias como toxinas urêmicas verdadeiras. Foi sugerido que a maioria dos solutos urêmicos retidos seja provavelmente atóxica, e aqueles que são tóxicos podem somente exercer seus efeitos quando presentes em combinação com outros solutos urêmicos. A ureia e creatinina, por si só, não são toxinas urêmicas. Entretanto, a concentração plasmática de ureia supostamente é um bom reflexo das concentrações sistêmicas de vários solutos urêmicos. Assim, a demonstração de que o tratamento diminui as concentrações de ureia por si só não é evidência conclusiva de redução da toxicidade urêmica (ver Capítulo 62).

Além dos distúrbios de excreção, várias moléculas de tamanho médio e diversas citocinas e fatores de crescimento se acumulam na DRC porque a capacidade do rim para catabolizar várias substâncias também está prejudicada. Além disso, os níveis plasmáticos de vários hormônios polipeptídicos, incluindo o paratormônio (PTH), insulina, glucagon, hormônio luteinizante e prolactina, aumentam em pacientes com DRC por conta do distúrbio do catabolismo renal, assim como pelo aumento da secreção glandular.

Alteração da síntese de hormônios renais

Os rins normalmente produzem uma série de hormônios essenciais, incluindo calcitriol (vitamina D; 1,25-di-hidroxicolecalciferol), EPO, prostaglandinas, quininas e renina. Em particular, o calcitriol e EPO possuem papéis bem estabelecidos na patogênese de consequências clinicamente importantes da DRC grave. O calcitriol, a forma mais metabolicamente ativa da vitamina D, é essencial para o metabolismo de Ca e esquelético. Deficiências de vitamina D podem resultar em hiperparatireoidismo secundário renal e osteodistrofia renal. O PTH tem sido identificados como uma toxina urêmica, embora as consequências do hiperparatireoidismo além do seu papel na osteodistrofia renal na DRC sejam mal estabelecidas. Ademais, a maioria das células possui receptores para calcitriol e a ativação inadequada desses receptores pode contribuir para os sinais clínicos da uremia. Aparentemente a restauração de níveis adequados de calcitriol em cães e seres humanos com DRC pode retardar a progressão da doença renal e prolongar a sobrevida.[36] A deficiência de EPO está associada à anemia arregenerativa que pode promover fraqueza, letargia e hiporexia.

Consequências gastrintestinais

Anorexia, êmese

Complicações GI são os sinais clínicos mais comuns e óbvios de uremia. Os sinais clínicos podem incluir náuseas, êmese (ver Capítulo 39), redução do apetite (ver Capítulo 23), estomatite, ulceração GI, diarreia e colite (ver Capítulo 40). A diminuição do apetite e perda de peso são achados inespecíficos que podem preceder outros sinais de uremia em cães e gatos. O apetite pode ser seletivo para determinados alimentos e pode ter momentos de melhora e piora. Os fatores que promovem perda de peso e desnutrição incluem anorexia, náuseas, êmese e a subsequente redução na ingestão de nutrientes, desarranjos hormonais e metabólicos, e fatores catabólicos relacionados à uremia, particularmente acidose. A anorexia parece ser de origem multifatorial. Estudos que utilizaram modelos roedores sugerem que uma molécula média, o "fator anoréxico", talvez um peptídio, no plasma pode suprimir o apetite.[37] A elevação das concentrações séricas de leptina também tem sido implicada como um fator que contribui para a anorexia.[38] Os episódios de êmese são frequentes, mas inconsistentes na uremia e podem resultar dos efeitos de toxinas urêmicas não identificadas sobre a zona de gatilho quimiorreceptor emética medular e da gastrenterite urêmica. A gravidade do vômito está correlacionada variavelmente com a magnitude da azotemia. Como a gastrite urêmica pode ser ulcerativa, pode ocorrer hematêmese. Embora a êmese supostamente seja mais frequente em cães urêmicos, ela ocorre em cerca de 25 a 33% dos gatos urêmicos.[3] A êmese pode prejudicar a PD compensatória, aumentando o risco de desidratação e exacerbando a azotemia pré-renal e os sinais clínicos da uremia.

Gastropatia urêmica

Definição. A gastropatia urêmica e seus sinais clínicos associados parecem ser mais comuns em cães do que em gatos.[39] Em cães é caracterizada microscopicamente pela mineralização dos vasos sanguíneos mucosos e submucosos, edema e atrofia glandular.[39] A mineralização parece estar relacionada ao produto $Ca \times PO_4$. O aumento dos níveis de gastrina devido à redução da depuração renal pode ter um papel no desenvolvimento da gastropatia urêmica.[40] Gatos com DRC também possuem níveis elevados de gastrina que pioram com a gravidade da DRC.[40] A gastrina induz a secreção de ácido gástrico diretamente pelo estímulo de receptores localizados nas células parietais gástricas, assim como pelo aumento da liberação de histamina por mastócitos na mucosa gástrica. O aumento da liberação de histamina também pode promover ulceração GI e necrose isquêmica da mucosa por meio de um mecanismo vascular caracterizado por pequena dilatação de vênulas e capilares, aumento da permeabilidade endotelial e trombose intravascular.[41] Entretanto, a hiperacidez gástrica não foi documentada em cães ou gatos urêmicos, e a necrose da mucosa e ulceração parecem achados incomuns na gastropatia urêmica em cães.[39]

Em um estudo recente de 37 gatos com DRC, a ulceração gástrica, edema, mineralização vascular e hemorragia não foram observadas; entretanto, 16/37 (43%) dos gatos tinham fibrose gástrica de gravidade variável e 14/37 (38%) dos gatos tinham paredes gástricas mineralizadas.[42] A mineralização gástrica foi restrita a gatos nos estágios III e IV da DRC pela IRIS. O aumento dos produtos $Ca-PO_4$ esteve correlacionado com a gravidade da doença. Os níveis séricos de gastrina foram significativamente maiores em gatos com DRC quando comparados a gatos não azotêmicos, mas o aumento das concentrações de gastrina não foi associado à ulceração gástrica. Ao mesmo tempo que a inapetência ocorreu em 84% (26/31) e a êmese ocorreu em 45% (14/31) dos gatos com DRC, uma relação significativa não foi aparente entre estes sinais clínicos e lesões gástricas, e não houve relação significativa entre sinais clínicos e concentrações de gastrina. Gatos com mineralização gástrica tinham apetites ruins, sugerindo que os sinais clínicos de náuseas e êmese em gatos com DRC mais provavelmente ocorrem graças aos efeitos das toxinas urêmicas sobre a zona de gatilho quimiorreceptora do que por lesões patológicas da parede gástrica.

Disfagia. Em um estudo de 80 gatos com DRC espontânea, a disfagia e desconforto oral ocorrem em cerca de 8% dos gatos urêmicos e 38% dos gatos em estágio final da DRC.[3] A doença periodontal foi observada em 31% dos gatos urêmicos e 35% em estágio final da DRC. A halitose foi relatada em cerca de 8%

dos gatos em ambos os grupos. DRC moderada à grave pode resultar em estomatite urêmica caracterizada por membranas mucosas secas (xerostomia), ulcerações orais (particularmente localizadas na mucosa oral e língua), descoloração amarronzada da superfície dorsal da língua, necrose e maceração da porção anterior da língua (associada à necrose fibrinoide e arterite), e hálito de odor urêmico. A degradação da ureia em amônia por urease bacteriana pode contribuir para estes sinais. A higiene oral ruim e doença dentária podem exacerbar o início e gravidade da estomatite urêmica.

Enterocolite urêmica. A enterocolite causa diarreia e ocorre em cães e gatos com uremia grave. É tipicamente menos dramática e menos comum do que a gastrite urêmica. Em um estudo, a diarreia não foi relatada por tutores de 80 gatos com DRC espontânea.[3] Quando presente, a enterocolite urêmica é frequentemente hemorrágica, embora esta hemorragia GI possa inicialmente passar desapercebida. Ela também pode ser complicada pela intussuscepção. A enterocolite urêmica pode, pelo menos em parte, resultar do efeito irritante do aumento da produção de amônio no cólon associado a altas concentrações de ureia. Ao contrário da diarreia, a constipação intestinal é relativamente comum em gatos com DRC. Entretanto, ela parece ser primariamente uma manifestação de desidratação, e não de disfunção GI. Ela também pode ocorrer como uma complicação de agentes quelantes intestinais de PO_4.

Alteração da capacidade de concentração urinária, poliúria, polidipsia e noctúria

Entre as manifestações clínicas mais precoces e comuns da DRC estão a PU/PD, noctúria e incontinência urinária devido à redução da capacidade de concentração urinária (ver Capítulos 45 e 46). A PD foi o sinal clínico mais comum relatado em um estudo de 80 gatos com DRC. Os tutores de gatos reconheceram a PD mais frequentemente do que a PU. Embora os valores de densidade urinária específica de gatos em estágios II a IV de DRC estejam em geral abaixo de 1,035, alguns gatos parecem reter a capacidade adequada de concentração urinária (i. e., densidade específica > 1,035), especialmente no início da evolução da DRC. A diminuição da capacidade de concentração urinária resulta de diversos fatores, incluindo: aumento da carga de solutos por néfrons remanescentes (diurese por solutos), alteração da gênese do gradiente hipertônico da medula renal em razão dos distúrbios da arquitetura medular renal e do sistema multiplicador contracorrente pela doença, e alteração da responsividade renal ao hormônio antidiurético (ADH). A alteração da responsividade ao ADH pode resultar, pelo menos em parte, do aumento da taxa de fluxo tubular renal distal, que limita o equilíbrio entre o fluido tubular e o interstício medular hipertônico. Adicionalmente, a atividade da adenilciclase estimulada pelo ADH e permeabilidade hídrica no néfron distal pode ser alterada na uremia.[43] Conforme a capacidade de concentração urinária é perdida, o volume urinário é determinado pela carga diária de solutos da urina. A carga de solutos é predominantemente composta por sal e ureia, ambos os quais podem ser modificados pela alteração do conteúdo dietético de sal e proteína, respectivamente. Outros fatores importantes que podem influenciar o volume urinário são a sede (consumo hídrico) e administração terapêutica de fluidos. A PD é uma resposta compensatória à PU. Se a ingestão hídrica não consegue acompanhar as perdas hídricas urinárias, a desidratação ocorrerá por conta da incapacidade em conservar água pela concentração urinária. A desidratação subsequente à ingestão inadequada de fluidos é um problema comum em gatos com DRC. Alguns cães e gatos com DRC avançada possuem capacidade limitada de excretar a água ingerida, o que causa discreta hiponatremia.

Hipertensão arterial e consequências cardiovasculares

Os principais mecanismos que supostamente contribuem para a hipertensão na DRC incluem a retenção de fluidos, ativação do sistema renina-angiotensina-aldosterona (SRAA) e aumento da atividade do sistema nervoso simpático (ver Capítulo 157).[35,44] A hipertensão em seres humanos com DRC é predominantemente atribuída à expansão volêmica. A remoção de fluidos por diuréticos ou diálise elimina a hipertensão ou a torna mais responsiva a medicações.[35] De forma semelhante, a hemodiálise que inclui a remoção de fluidos em excesso (ultrafiltração) frequentemente tem reduzido ou normalizado a pressão sanguínea em cães e gatos que estavam hipertensos antes do tratamento. Nos casos que a expansão volêmica não é a causa para hipertensão em seres humanos com DRC, o aumento da atividade do SRAA parece ser um importante determinante da hipertensão. O aumento da liberação de renina é presumidamente secundário à doença vascular ou áreas focais de isquemia dentro dos rins doentes. Entretanto, um estudo em gatos relatou que gatos hipertensos frequentemente possuem aumento significativo das concentrações plasmáticas de aldosterona com diminuição das atividades plasmáticas de renina, e que a atividade plasmática de renina diminui com a terapia anti-hipertensiva, sugerindo que a retenção de sal e água pode ser uma importante causa para hipertensão. Isso pode também explicar, pelo menos em parte, o motivo pelo qual inibidores da enzima conversora de angiotensina (ECA) podem ser ineficazes como fármacos anti-hipertensivos em gatos com DRC.

A hipertensão pode ser primária (idiopática) ou secundária a doenças, como DRC. Em cães e gatos, a DRC é a causa mais comum para hipertensão secundária, enquanto a hipertensão primária parece ser incomum (ver Capítulo 157). É possível a hipertensão afetar de forma adversa o prognóstico a longo prazo em cães e gatos com DRC, pelo menos em parte por promover proteinúria.[31] A hipertensão arterial presumidamente está entre as complicações mais comuns a DRC; entretanto, a prevalência verdadeira da hipertensão arterial entre cães e gatos com DRC não é conhecida. Alguns estudos sugeriram que a hipertensão pode ser incomum em cães com DRC, enquanto outros estudos relataram que até 66% dos gatos e 50 a 93% dos cães com DRC possuem hipertensão.[6,31,46,47] Entretanto, outros estudos em cães sugerem que uma prevalência de 20 a 30% pode ser mais acurada.[25,48] Cães com doenças glomerulares podem ter maior risco de apresentarem pressões sanguíneas elevadas.[49] Um estudo estimou a prevalência de hipertensão sistólica em gatos com DRC em aproximadamente 13 a 28%.[46] A prevalência verdadeira e o impacto clínico da hipertensão permanece ainda a ser mais claramente estabelecida em cães e gatos, mas parece haver um consenso entre nefrologistas veterinários de que pressões sanguíneas elevadas podem levar à lesão de órgãos-alvo em cães e gatos com DRC e, portanto, justifica a detecção e tratamento.[50] Os sistemas mais comumente afetados pela elevação da pressão sanguínea incluem os olhos, rins, sistema nervoso e sistema cardiovascular.

A hipertensão está presente quando há elevação persistente da pressão sanguínea sistólica e/ou diastólica, ou quando um paciente previamente diagnosticado como hipertenso está recebendo medicação anti-hipertensiva (independentemente do nível atual da pressão sanguínea). É geralmente aceito que as mensurações da pressão sanguínea sistólica em gatos e cães acordados e não ansiosos não devem exceder cerca de 160 a 170 mmHg, e estes valores provavelmente representam uma estimativa razoável do limiar do tratamento. A fim de tornar a terminologia da pressão sanguínea mais familiar aos veterinários e tutores, a IRIS mudou sua terminologia para que seja semelhante àquela utilizada pela American Heart Association (Boxe 324.1).[b] Categorias desde "normotensos" até "hipertensão "grave" implicam sequencialmente lesão de risco mínimo, baixo, moderado ou alto ao órgão associada à hipertensão.[50]

---

[a]N.R.T.: Esta informação foi atualizada em 2019 (*http://www.iris-kidney.com/education/staging_system.html*).

Boxe 324.1 Estadiamento da doença renal crônica (DRC) pela International Renal Interest Society (IRIS) em cães e gatos

A. Estágio da DRC pela IRIS

ESTÁGIO	VALORES SÉRICOS DE CREATININA (mg/dℓ/mcmol/ℓ)	
	CÃES	GATOS
Estágio I	< 1,4/< 125	< 1,6/< 140
Estágio II	1,4 a 2,0/125 a 179	1,6 a 2,8/140 a 249
Estágio III	2,1 a 5,0/180 a 439	2,9 a 5,0/250 a 439
Estágio IV	> 5,0/> 440	> 5,0/> 440

B. Subclassificação de DRC pela IRIS por proteinúria (relação proteína:creatinina urinária)

CLASSIFICAÇÃO	RELAÇÃO PROTEÍNA:CREATININA URINÁRIA	
	CÃES	GATOS
Proteinúrico (P)	> 0,5	> 0,4
Proteinúrico limítrofe (PL)	0,2 a 0,5	0,2 a 0,4
Não proteinúrico (NP)	< 0,2	< 0,2

C. Subclassificação de DRC pela IRIS por estágios de pressão sanguínea para cães e gatos

CATEGORIA	PRESSÃO SANGUÍNEA	
	PRESSÃO SANGUÍNEA SISTÓLICA (mmHg)	PRESSÃO SANGUÍNEA DIASTÓLICA (mmHg)
Normotensão (N)	< 150	< 95
Hipertensão limítrofe (HL)	150 a 159	95 a 99
Hipertensão (H)	160 a 179	100 a 119
Hipertensão grave	≥ 180	≥ 120

Dados de http://iris-kidney.com/pdf/staging-of-ckd.pdf. © Copyright 2016 International Renal Interest Society.

Anemia

A anemia é comum em cães e gatos com DRC, embora sua magnitude seja geralmente discreta até os estágios avançados da DRC. Em seres humanos, o hematócrito começa a cair quando a TFG foi reduzida em cerca de 40% do normal, e dessa forma a gravidade da anemia é tipicamente proporcional à perda da função renal.[35] A anemia da DRC tipicamente é caracterizada como normocrômica, normocítica e arregenerativa (ver Capítulos 50 e 199). A biopsia de medula óssea (ver Capítulo 92) é tipicamente caracterizada por hipoplasia de precursores eritroides com pouca ou nenhuma interferência com a leucopoese normal e megacariocitopoese. Em esfregaços sanguíneos, hemácias espiculadas e deformadas (equinócitos) podem ser notadas. Os sinais clínicos de anemia incluem palidez das membranas mucosas, fadiga, indiferença ao ambiente, letargia, fraqueza e anorexia.

A causa primária para a anemia da DRC é a inadequada secreção de EPO pelos rins. A EPO é um hormônio glicoproteico produzido nos rins em resposta à diminuição do fornecimento de oxigênio. A EPO se liga a um receptor em progenitores eritroides, fazendo com que essas células se diferenciem em normoblastos e então em eritrócitos maduros. A produção inadequada de EPO resulta do declínio da massa funcional renal. Enquanto a localização precisa intrarrenal da produção de EPO tem sido elusiva, células endoteliais capilares peritubulares podem ser a localização mais provável.[35] O sensor renal de oxigênio é provavelmente uma proteína heme que sofre uma alteração conformacional em resposta à diminuição do fornecimento de oxigênio, o que aumenta o mRNA da EPO.[35] Fatores induzíveis pela hipoxia (FIH), e em particular o FIH-2, emergiram como o fator de transcrição que regula a síntese de EPO no rim e possui um papel crítico na regulação da captação intestinal do ferro.[51]

Pacientes anêmicos com DRC possuem uma deficiência de EPO relativa, e não absoluta, de forma que os níveis plasmáticos tipicamente excedem o faixa normal, mas estão baixos com relação à gravidade da anemia.[52] Gatos anêmicos com DRC possuem concentrações plasmáticas de EPO semelhantes a gatos normais.[53] Assim, as causas primárias para anemia da DRC são a produção renal insuficiente de EPO, duração de vida mais curta das hemácias, anormalidades nutricionais (notadamente deficiências de ferro, vitamina B12 e folato), fatores inibidores de EPO no plasma urêmico, perda de sangue e mielofibrose.

Hiperparatireoidismo secundário renal
Prevalência e fisiopatologia
Múltiplos fatores promovem o desenvolvimento do hiperparatireoidismo secundário renal (HPSR; ver Capítulos 69 e 297). A retenção de PO_4, uma consequência da diminuição da TFG, mesmo na insuficiência renal inicial está intimamente relacionada ao desenvolvimento de HPSR.[58,59] Incrementos no fator de crescimento de fibroblastos-23 (FGF-23), em resposta ao HPSR, também ocorrem precocemente na DRC. Como um hormônio fosfatúrico, a ação do FGF-23 é mitigar a retenção de PO_4 no início da evolução da DRC, mas também inibir a atividade da alfa-hidroxilase-1 renal, levando assim à diminuição dos níveis de calcitriol.[59] O declínio dos níveis de calcitriol está entre as alterações mais precoces que promove o desenvolvimento de HPSR. O HPSR está presente em um número estimado de 47% dos gatos assintomáticos somente com evidências bioquímicas de DRC. Ele ocorre antes da azotemia em alguns gatos, mesmo quando as concentrações séricas de PO_4 e Ca estão dentro dos valores de referência.[54-56] A prevalência geral do HPSR em gatos com DRC foi de cerca de 84% em um estudo e todos os pacientes com DRC em "estágio terminal" têm HPSR. De forma geral, os níveis plasmáticos de PTH aumentam conforme a concentração sérica de creatinina aumenta.[57]

Uma deficiência relativa de calcitriol foi descrita em cães com DRC, embora as concentrações absolutas estejam dentro dos valores de referência.[60] Surgiu uma hipótese de que a deficiência relativa ou absoluta de calcitriol possui um papel fundamental no desenvolvimento do HPSR.[61] O PTF promove a atividade da alfa-hidroxilase-1 renal e formação do calcitriol. Por sua vez, o calcitriol limita a síntese de PTH pela inibição por retroalimentação. A ausência dessa inibição normal por retroalimentação aumenta os níveis de PTH. Inicialmente, o HPSR aumenta a atividade da alfa-hidroxilase-1 apesar da manutenção da retenção de PO_4, restaurando dessa forma a produção de calcitriol ao normal. Entretanto, a normalização da produção de calcitriol ocorre às custas da persistência do aumento da atividade plasmática do PTH: um exemplo clássico da "hipótese perde-e-ganha". Conforme a DRC continua a progredir, a perda de células tubulares renais viáveis finalmente limita a síntese renal de calcitriol e as concentrações permanecem baixas. A deficiência de calcitriol leva à resistência esquelética contra a ação do PTH e eleva o limiar para supressão induzida pelo Ca da secreção do PTH. A resistência esquelética ao PTH limita a liberação esquelética de Ca, ao mesmo tempo que eleva o limiar para a secreção de PTH, o que permite que o HPSR persista mesmo quando as concentrações plasmáticas de Ca ionizado estejam normais ou elevadas.[57,61]

A retenção de PO_4 provavelmente promove o HPSR diretamente. A restrição de PO_4 em cães e pessoas com DRC demonstrou diminuir a secreção de PTH sem influenciar os níveis de calcitriol.[62-64] Em pessoas não tratadas com DRC discreta à moderada (concentração sérica de creatinina ≤ 3,0 mg/dℓ), as concentrações séricas de PO_4 estiveram diretamente correlacionadas ao PTH, independente das concentrações séricas de Ca ou calcitriol.[65] Esta correlação esteve presente apesar da maioria dos pacientes ter concentrações séricas de PO_4 dentro dos valores de referência. De forma importante a hiperfosfatemia evidente pode não ser um pré-requisito para que o fósforo tenha um efeito sobre a secreção de PTH. A redução dos níveis de calcitriol pode ter um efeito permissivo e/ou efeito direto adicional sobre a secreção de PTH nessa situação.[65]

Na DRC mais avançada, a presença de toxinas urêmicas parece impedir a inibição da proliferação de células paratireoideanas induzidas pelo calcitriol.[66] Nesse ponto, somente a concentração sérica de Ca se correlaciona com a atividade sérica de PTH.[65] A absorção GI alterada de Ca graças aos baixos níveis séricos de calcitriol provavelmente tenha um importante papel no HPSR. As concentrações sanguíneas de Ca ionizado (iCa) estão frequentemente reduzidas em gatos com DRC. Ao mesmo tempo que as concentrações de iCa foram relatadas como baixas a altas em cães com DRC em um estudo, > 50% dos gatos com DRC avançada em estágio final estavam hipocalcêmicos.[54,67]

Consequências clínicas
Embora o HPSR e a osteodistrofia renal sejam sequelas bem documentadas da DRC, a osteodistrofia renal é incomum em cães e gatos. Em cães, ela mais frequentemente ocorre nos animais imaturos, presumidamente porque o osso em crescimento metabolicamente ativo é mais suscetível aos efeitos adversos do HPSR. Por motivos inexplicados, os ossos do crânio e da mandíbula são em geral os mais severamente afetados e podem se tornar tão desmineralizados que os dentes se tornam móveis e alterações fibrosas se tornam óbvias, particularmente na maxila (Figura 324.2). A proliferação marcante do tecido

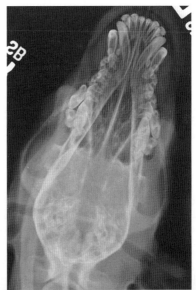
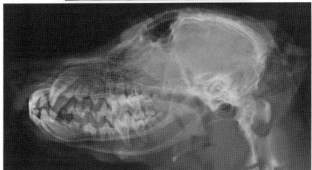

Figura 324.2 Radiografias de um cão jovem com DRC em estágio III, hiperparatireoidismo secundário renal e osteodistrofia renal. O cão foi trazido para atendimento com dor grave que estava localizada no crânio e particularmente na maxila e mandíbula. A avaliação patológica da estrutura óssea revelou osteodistrofia fibrosa-cística.

SEÇÃO 23 • Doenças Renais

conjuntivo associada à maxila pode causar distorção da face. Fraturas mandibulares são incomuns. Outras manifestações clínicas possíveis, embora incomuns, da osteodistrofia renal grave incluem lesões ósseas císticas, dor óssea e retardo do crescimento. Potenciais consequências não esqueléticas do HPSR incluem retardo mental e letargia, fraqueza, anorexia e aumento da incidência de infecções devido à imunodeficiência.[57] Os níveis excessivos de PTH podem também promover nefrocalcinose e consequente perda progressiva da função renal.

O HPSR pode estar associado ao aumento substancial das glândulas paratireoides (ver Capítulo 298). Isso possui importância cínica em gatos porque o hipertireoidismo é também comum e a palpação de uma massa cervical logicamente pode levantar a suspeita de doença tireoideana, e não da paratireoideana. Entretanto, em um relato, as glândulas paratireoides hiperplásicas eram palpáveis como massas paratraqueais em 11 de 80 gatos com DRC.[3] Deve haver cuidado para confirmar cada condição antes do início do tratamento.

Achados laboratoriais

Acidose metabólica

A acidose metabólica é relativamente comum na DRC, mas a acidose grave é primariamente notada naqueles com DRC avançada (ver Capítulo 128).[28,68] Um estudo sobre 59 gatos com DRC revelou que o pH sanguíneo < 7,27 foi observado em 10 de 19 gatos com azotemia grave, três de 20 gatos com azotemia moderada e nenhum de 20 gatos com azotemia discreta. A acidose metabólica não foi observada como um fator prognóstico em gatos ou cães com DRC.[24,26] Entretanto, a acidose metabólica é agora reconhecida como promotora da progressão da DRC em seres humanos, embora isso não tenha sido confirmado em cães ou gatos.[68-70]

Uma combinação de reabsorção tubular do bicarbonato filtrado e excreção de íons hidrogênio com amônia e tampões urinários, principalmente o PO_4, mantém o equilíbrio ácido-básico normal. Conforme a função renal declina, a excreção do íon hidrogênio é mantida amplamente pelo aumento da quantidade de amônio excretada pelos néfrons remanescentes. Conforme a quantidade de amônio excretada aumenta por néfron remanescente, a excreção total renal de amônio tipicamente não aumenta acima do normal. Em algum nível da DRC, a capacidade de aumentar a produção renal de amônia é perdida e ocorre a acidose metabólica. A diminuição da reciclagem medular de amônia por causa do dano renal estrutural pode também contribuir para a alteração da excreção de amônio.[28] A diminuição da filtração de ácidos tituláveis, como o PO_4 e compostos do sulfato, associada a distúrbios da secreção tubular renal de prótons também podem contribuir.[71]

Distúrbios na reabsorção tubular renal do bicarbonato filtrado não são típicos de cães e gatos com DRC, mas podem ocorrer em distúrbios tubulares selecionados, como a síndrome de Fanconi (ver Capítulo 326). A retenção de PO_4 e ácidos orgânicos (ácido úrico, ácido hipúrico, ácido láctico etc.) na DRC promove um aumento do ânion gap. Entretanto, a acidose hiperclorêmica (ânion gap normal), ânion gap alto ou acidoses mistas hiperclorêmicas com ânion gap alto podem ocorrer na DRC. A acidose hiperclorêmica é mais provável em pacientes menos severamente azotêmicos.

A acidose metabólica crônica pode causar anorexia, náuseas, êmese, letargia, fraqueza, perda de massa muscular, perda de peso e desnutrição. A acidificação da dieta de cães e gatos pode causar balanço negativo de Ca, desmineralização óssea ou balanço negativo do potássio, o que por sua vez por promover hipopotassemia, disfunção renal e depleção da taurina.[72] A acidose crônica pode promover desnutrição proteica apesar de adequada ingestão dietética.[68] O catabolismo proteico aumenta em pacientes com acidose, fornecendo uma fonte de nitrogênio para a síntese hepática de glutamina, o substrato para síntese renal de amônia.[73] Os efeitos combinados da redução da síntese proteica devido à uremia e proteólise acelerada devido à acidose

promove elevações na BUN, aumento da excreção do nitrogênio e balanço negativo do nitrogênio típicos de acidose urêmica. A terapia de alcalinização efetivamente reverte a quebra de proteínas associada à acidose e reverte vários sinais.

As necessidades de proteínas na dieta parecem ser semelhantes para pacientes normais e aqueles com DRC, a menos que a acidose urêmica esteja presente (ver Capítulo 184). Quando o status ácido-básico está normal, reduções adaptativas na degradação proteica do músculo esquelético protege aqueles que consomem dietas com baixos níveis de proteína contra perdas na massa corporal magra. A acidose metabólica bloqueia as respostas metabólicas contra a restrição proteica da dieta de duas formas: (1) ela estimula a degradação irreversível dos aminoácidos essenciais de cadeia ramificada, e (2) estimula a degradação da proteína no músculo.[73] Assim, a acidose pode limitar a capacidade dos pacientes em se adaptar à restrição proteica da dieta. A acidose metabólica também suprime a síntese de albumina em seres humanos e é capaz de reduzir a concentração da albumina sérica.

Azotemia, ureia nitrogenada sanguínea, creatinina

A azotemia é definida como o excesso de ureia ou outros compostos nitrogenados não proteicos no sangue (ver Capítulo 62). A perda da função renal leva ao acúmulo de uma ampla variedade de compostos não proteicos que contêm nitrogênio, incluindo ureia e creatinina. Vários produtos de degradação do catabolismo proteico são excretados por filtração glomerular. Assim, aqueles com DRC primária possuem distúrbios da capacidade de excretar catabólitos proteináceos amplamente por conta da redução marcante da TFG. Como esses compostos são derivados quase que completamente da degradação proteica, sua produção aumenta quando o conteúdo proteico da dieta aumenta. A ureia é sintetizada utilizando o nitrogênio derivado do catabolismo de aminoácidos e pode ser excretada pelos rins, retida na água do organismo ou metabolizada em amônia e aminoácidos mais dióxido de carbono por bactérias no trato GI. Independentemente da toxicidade *per se* da ureia, as concentrações de BUN estão tipicamente relacionadas ao conteúdo dietético proteico. Além disso, as concentrações de BUN tendem a estar correlacionadas razoavelmente bem com os sinais clínicos de uremia. Por propósitos práticos, a BUN pode assim ser vista como um marcador substituto das "toxinas urêmicas" retidas.

Além do aumento da ingestão proteica e declínio da função renal, as concentrações de BUN podem também estar aumentadas por hemorragia GI, aumento do catabolismo proteico, diminuição dos volumes urinários (graças a fatores pré-renais, como desidratação) e determinados fármacos (p. ex., glicocorticoides). As concentrações de BUN podem cair em casos de desvios portossistêmicos, insuficiência hepática, dietas com baixos níveis de proteína e inanição. Em algumas situações, uma BUN reduzida pode indicar desnutrição calórica proteica devido à ingestão inadequada como consequências de dietas formuladas inapropriadamente ou inapetência. Como muitos fatores extrarrenais influenciam a BUN, a creatinina é uma medida mais confiável da TFG na DRC. As concentrações de BUN e creatinina sérica devem ser utilizadas em conjunto na avaliação dos pacientes, particularmente naqueles que consomem dietas com restrição proteica. A relação entre a BUN e concentração sérica de creatinina deve diminuir quando a ingestão dietética proteica for reduzida. Em pacientes que consomem dietas com redução de proteínas, um aumento na relação entre BUN e concentrações séricas de creatinina pode sugerir baixa adequação à dieta, aumento do catabolismo proteico, hemorragia GI, desidratação, anorexia ou declínio da massa muscular.

Hiperfosfatemia

Os rins são responsáveis pela excreção de PO_4, sendo que a quantidade na urina representa aquela no filtrado glomerular menos a absorvida pelos túbulos (ver Capítulo 73). Se a ingestão dietética de PO_4 permanecer constante, um declínio na TFG leva à retenção e finalmente hiperfosfatemia. Entretanto, durante os estágios iniciais da DRC, o PO_4 sérico tipicamente permanece dentro dos limites de referência por conta dos decréscimos compensatórios na reabsorção pelos néfrons remanescentes. Essa adaptação tubular renal é uma consequência dos efeitos fosfatúricos do FGF-23 e PTH. Quando a TFG declina abaixo de cerca de 20% do normal, este efeito adaptativo alcança seu limite e ocorre hiperfosfatemia.

A consequência primária da retenção de PO_4 e hiperfosfatemia é a progressão da DRC. As concentrações séricas de PO_4 demonstraram estar diretamente ligadas à mortalidade em seres humanos, gatos e cães com DRC.[24,26,74,75] Um estudo recente em pessoas com DRC notou que cada incremento de 1 mg/dℓ no PO_4 sérico foi associado independentemente ao aumento do risco de insuficiência renal e mortalidade.[76] Concentrações plasmáticas mais altas de PO_4 demonstraram predizer a progressão em gatos com DRC em estágio III pela IRIS.[1] O produto Ca × PO_4 também possui uma tendência sobre o risco de mortalidade. Produtos > 72 possuem maior mortalidade relativa.[74] O risco de mortalidade associado à hiperfosfatemia pareceu ser independente dos níveis elevados de PTH, o que por si só pareceu ter somente uma fraca associação com a mortalidade. A análise do Ca não revelou correlação com o risco relativo de morte.

Hipercalcemia, hipocalcemia e hipermagnesemia
Concentrações de Ca total, ionizado e complexo ligado a proteínas variam amplamente em pacientes com DRC (ver Capítulos 67 a 69).[67] Incrementos no iCa foram detectados em 6% e diminuições em 26% de 80 gatos com DRC.[67] A concentração sanguínea média de iCa foi significativamente inferior em gatos com DRC do que em controles saudáveis; > 50% dos gatos com DRC avançada (estágio IV) estavam hipocalcêmicos. Entretanto, quando esses mesmos 80 gatos foram avaliadas as concentrações séricas de cálcio total (tCa), a hipercalcemia foi observada em 21% e hipocalcemia em 8%. Claramente, as concentrações séricas de tCa não refletem fielmente as concentrações de iCa em gatos com DRC. Discrepâncias semelhantes foram observadas em cães.[67,77] A acidose metabólica em casos de DRC não parece explicar as discrepâncias entre as concentrações de iCa e tCa em cães.[78] O mecanismo relacionado ao aumento do tCa sérico apesar de concentrações normais a reduzidas de iCa é provavelmente explicado pelo aumento das concentrações de cálcio em complexo com ânions orgânicos e inorgânicos retidos, como o citrato, PO_4 ou sulfato.[67] Por conta desse efeito, fórmulas desenvolvidas para "corrigir" as variações da albumina sérica não são úteis em cães e gatos com DRC.

A hipermagnesemia é comum na DRC porque os rins são os principais responsáveis pela excreção do magnésio (Mg).[54] Tipicamente na DRC, a ligação do Mg a proteínas é normal, a quantidade de Mg formando complexos está aumentada, e o Mg ionizado (iMg) pode estar aumentada, normal ou diminuída. Embora os mecanismos homeostáticos envolvidos no controle do Mg não sejam bem documentados, eles parecem se basear nos ossos, intestino e rins, como observado no controle do Ca e PO_4.

Hipopotassemia e doença renal crônica primária
Uma associação entre DRC e hipopotassemia foi descrita em gatos, mas é incomum em cães.[78,79] A restrição dietética de Na em gatos com DRC pode estar associada à inapropriada excreção de potássio pela urina que pode promover hipopotassemia.[48] A caliurese pode resultar da ativação do SRAA pela restrição dietética de Na. Outros fatores que podem promover hipopotassemia são a redução da ingestão alimentar e persistente desidratação em baixo grau, ambas as quais são comuns em gatos com DRC (ver Capítulo 68).

Enquanto a hipopotassemia continua a ser detectada em vários gatos com DRC, a fraqueza muscular é incomum. Provavelmente esta melhora é o resultado do aumento do conteúdo de K de dietas terapêuticas. Embora a fraqueza muscular generalizada tenha sido descrita como um sinal cardeal da hipopotassemia, a diminuição da função renal e anorexia são provavelmente explicações mais prováveis. Em vários gatos com DRC e hipopotassemia, a função renal melhora com a suplementação por K e restauração das concentrações normais de K, sugerindo que a hipopotassemia pode induzir um declínio reversível e funcional da TFG. De forma interessante, a função renal demonstrou estar afetada de forma adversa em gatos normais quando uma dieta acidificante com restrição de K foi fornecida, as duas condições possivelmente como aditivas.[82] Com base nesses resultados, surgiu a hipótese de que gatos com DRC possuem um ciclo autoperpetuante de perda urinária excessiva de K e depleção de K de todo organismo, provavelmente para diminuir ainda mais a função renal.

Hipopotassemia como causa de doença renal crônica
Existem evidências limitadas de que além de ser uma consequência da DRC, a hipopotassemia pode ser uma causa ou promotora de DRC progressiva em gatos. Em um estudo não controlado dos efeitos a longo prazo da alimentação de uma dieta restrita em K e acidificante, evidências de disfunção renal ocorreram em três de nove gatos, enquanto nefrite intersticial linfoplasmocítica e fibrose intersticial foram observadas em cinco de nove.[79] Entretanto, ainda não está claro se a depleção de K ou hipopotassemia precede o início da DRC. Em outro estudo, quatro de sete gatos com DRC induzida alimentados com uma dieta contendo 0,3% de K desenvolveram hipopotassemia, enquanto quatro gatos com função renal normal alimentados com a mesma dieta não.[80] De forma interessante, o conteúdo muscular de K em gatos normocalêmicos com DRC espontânea diminuiu, sugerindo que os déficits totais de K no organismo podem ocorrer bem antes do início da hipopotassemia.[81]

Hiperaldosteronismo primário em gatos como causa de doença renal crônica
O hiperaldosteronismo primário (HAP) foi descrito em alguns gatos idosos.[100,101] Esses gatos foram descritos como hipopotassêmicos graves frequentemente e associados à polimiopatia hipopotassêmica, e hipertensão que pode ser marcante, refratária e comumente associada a lesões retinais e cegueira (ver Capítulo 308). Ademais, gatos com HAP frequentemente parecem ter evidências concorrentes de doença renal. Como gatos com DRC podem também ter hipopotassemia concorrente e hipertensão, a discriminação de gatos com HAP e gato com DRC é importante.

Foi recomendado que o diagnóstico de HAP em gatos seja baseado nas concentrações plasmáticas de aldosterona (CPA), atividade plasmática de renina (APR) e o cálculo da relação entre aldosterona e renina (RAR).[101] É sugerido que a APR baixa e aumentos na CPA e na relação CPA:APR sejam considerados consistentes com o diagnóstico de HAP.[100,101] Entretanto, um estudo recente de 196 gatos com mais de 9 anos e sem diagnóstico de HAP relatou que a CPA está aumentada significativamente em gatos hipertensos azotêmicos comparados a gatos normotensos equiparados pela função renal.[45] Ademais, a APR estava significativamente inferior em gatos hipertensos comparados a gatos sem hipertensão e não azotêmicos, e a RAR estava significativamente maior em gatos azotêmicos e hipertensos. Esses dados sugerem que vários gatos com DRC e hipertensão possuem baixos valores de renina e alta APR. Os autores desse relato sugeriram que a partir do momento que o aumento da CPA não foi ocasionado pela APR, o aumento da CPA poderia ser dependente de tumor adrenal primário. Em outro estudo, a hiperplasia adrenocortical bilateral pode ser um achado "quase "onipresente" em gatos com mais de 9 anos (97%), e o estadiamento histopatológico da gravidade da lesão adrenal falhou em discriminar gatos normotensos e hipertensos.[102] Estes achados falham em confirmar que um distúrbio adrenal está levando à elevação da CPA em gatos hipertensos.

SEÇÃO 23 • Doenças Renais

Como os testes de CPA, APR e RAR possuem tendências semelhantes em gatos com DRC e gatos com HAP, a confirmação do diagnóstico de HAP deve ser abordada cuidadosamente. De forma geral, gatos com HAP provavelmente terão níveis maiores de CPA e RAR comparados àqueles observados em gatos com DRC, mas valores de corte claros ainda não foram validados. Como adenomas e carcinomas adrenais são responsáveis pela maioria dos casos relatados de HAP felino, exames de imagem das adrenais devem ser incluídos no plano diagnóstico.[100] Achados ultrassonográficos relatados em gatos com HAP incluem massas adrenais, e calcificação adrenal ou alterações na ecogenicidade adrenal. A tomografia computadorizada (TC) e ressonância magnética (RM) também podem ser utilizadas para visualizar as adrenais. Entretanto, a presença de lesões nas adrenais não comprova o HAP porque massas adrenais em gatos são frequentemente achados incidentais (ver Capítulo 308). A remoção cirúrgica da massa adrenal, quando possível, pode ser curativa.[100]

AVALIAÇÃO DIAGNÓSTICA

Visão geral
Testes diagnósticos apropriados facilitam o melhor tratamento e a acurácia do prognóstico. A avaliação possui seis objetivos: (1) confirmar a presença de doença renal, (2) diferenciar doença aguda de crônica, (3) estadiar a DRC, (4) identificar todas as complicações bioquímicas e hematológicas, (5) determinar o tipo e/ou causa de doença renal se possível, e (6) identificar a presença de quaisquer comorbidades (Tabela 324.1; ver Capítulos 62, 321 e 357).

Confirmação do diagnóstico de doença renal crônica

Definição
A doença renal é definida como uma anormalidade funcional ou estrutural em um ou ambos os rins. Doenças renais funcionais são mais comumente reconhecidas por azotemia ou outras anormalidades em exames, enquanto a doença renal estrutural pode ser palpada ou observada em estudos de imagem ou biopsia renal. Anormalidades são consideradas "marcadores" de doença renal e devem levar à investigação adicional imediata para determinar se são resultado de doença renal (Boxe 324.2).

Concentração sérica de creatinina
A concentração sérica de creatinina, um indicador da TFG, é o teste laboratorial primário utilizado para identificar alterações da função renal. Entretanto, é relativamente insensível para estimar a TFG até que uma redução substancial na função renal tenha ocorrido. Uma redução de 75% da TFG é necessária antes que os valores séricos de creatinina excedam consistentemente os intervalos de referência. A insensibilidade dos resultados da creatinina sérica resulta de pelo menos dois importantes fatores:

a relação inata entre TFG e creatinina sérica, e a compreensão de que condições que não a doença renal intrínseca podem causar aumento da concentração sérica de creatinina.

A relação entre creatinina sérica e TFG é tanta que cada vez que a TFG diminui pela metade, a concentração sérica de creatinina dobra. Por exemplo, se um cão possui creatinina basal de 0,5 mg/dℓ e sua TFG diminui em 50%, a creatinina sérica somente aumenta para 1,0 mg/dℓ, ainda bem dentro dos intervalos de referência. Se uma redução adicional de 50% na TFG (para 25% da TFG original), a creatinina subirá para cerca de 2,0 mg/dℓ, discretamente anormal e frequentemente reconhecida. Um declínio adicional de 50% na TFG (para 12,5% do normal) é refletido em uma creatinina sérica de cerca de 4,0 mg/dℓ. Assim, a inclinação da elevação da concentração sérica de creatinina se torna muito mais íngreme após ocorrência de uma perda substancial da TFG, mas é achatada durante grande parte da variação da TFG. Ocorre que quanto mais ampla a variação normal para a concentração sérica de creatinina menos sensível ela é para detecção de doença renal intrínseca. Entretanto, se a variação se torna muito estreita, a creatinina sérica perderá especificidade porque outros fatores podem influenciar o valor: massa muscular corporal, raça etc. Este dilema é intrínseco da natureza da creatinina sérica e limita sua utilizada para do diagnóstico de DRC precoce.

Concentração de ureia nitrogenada sanguínea
Embora a BUN tenha sido tradicionalmente tida como um indicador adicional para estimativa de alterações na TFG, ela é influenciada por vários fatores importantes que não estão

---

Tabela 324.1	Complicações e comorbidades na doença renal crônica (DRC).

COMPLICAÇÕES DA DRC	COMORBIDADES
Anemia	Cardiopatia
Hipertensão arterial	Doença articular degenerativa
Desidratação	Doenças dentárias e orais
Hiperparatireoidismo	Hipertireoidismo (gatos)
Hiperfosfatemia	Nefrólitos e ureterólitos
Hipocalcemia e hipercalcemia	Infecções do trato urinário
Hipopotassemia	
Desnutrição	
Acidose metabólica	
Sinais urêmicos	

Boxe 324.2 Marcadores de lesão renal

Marcadores sanguíneos*
Azotemia
Hiperfosfatemia
Hipoalbuminemia
Hiperpotassemia
Hipopotassemia
Acidose metabólica
Hipocalcemia
Hipercalcemia
Anemia hipoproliferativa
Hipoalbuminemia
Dimetilarginina simétrica (SDMA)

Marcadores urinários
Concentração urinária prejudicada
Diluição urinária prejudicada
Proteinúria
Cilindrúria
Hematúria
Piúria
pH urinário inapropriado
Glicose urinária inapropriada
Cistinúria
Bacteriúria

Marcadores em exames de imagem – Anormalidades no rim
Aumento ou diminuição do tamanho renal
Mineralização renal, nefrólitos ou ureterólitos
Formato renal anormal
Ausência de um rim
Ecotextura renal anormal pela ultrassonografia

Hipertensão arterial
Pressão sanguínea mensurada
Lesões retinais consistentes com hipertensão

*Deve haver a confirmação da origem renal dos marcadores para serem evidências de dano renal. SDMA, dimetilarginina simétrica.

relacionados à TFG, incluindo perfusão renal, ingestão proteica, hemorragia GI superior, intervalo de tempo entre a ingestão alimentar e coleta da amostra de sangue, fármacos (p. ex., corticosteroides), taxa de fluxo urinário e função hepática. Além disso, a excreção de ureia é o efeito líquido da filtração glomerular e reabsorção tubular renal. Assim, os valores de BUN podem divergir substancialmente daqueles das concentrações de creatinina sérica graças a fatores não relacionados à TFG.

A BUN pode ser melhor do que a creatinina como uma mensuração das toxinas urêmicas e assim tende a se correlacionar melhor do que a concentração sérica de creatinina com os sinais clínicos e prognóstico.[6] Entretanto, a interpretação dos valores de BUN pode ser complexa e mesmo enganosa. Um objetivo da restrição dietética proteica é diminuir os níveis de toxinas urêmicas e tal dieta tipicamente diminui a BUN, aparentemente uma alteração favorável. Entretanto, níveis inferiores de BUN podem ser observados quando pouco ou nenhum alimento é ingrido. A BUN baixa nessa situação pode ser mal interpretada como uma resposta favorável à terapia quando de fato é resultado de inanição. A mensuração simultânea da creatinina sérica e BUN demonstrou ter benefícios limitados comparada à mensuração somente da creatinina sérica.[83]

Azotemia versus uremia

Os termos *azotemia* e *uremia* não são intercambiáveis. A azotemia é definida como concentrações anormais de ureia, creatinina e outras substâncias não proteicas nitrogenadas no sangue, plasma ou soro. É um achado laboratorial que pode ter diversas causas fundamentalmente diferentes. Ela não implica a presença ou ausência de sinais clínicos. Como a azotemia pode ser causada por fatores que não estão diretamente relacionados ao sistema urinário e por anormalidades do trato urinário inferior não diretamente relacionadas aos rins, a *azotemia* não deve ser utilizada como sinônimo para doença renal ou uremia. A azotemia pode resultar de causas pré-renais, renais ou pós-renais. Como os compostos nitrogenados não proteicos (incluindo ureia e creatinina) são substâncias endógenas, incrementos anormais no soro podem ser causados por uma maior taxa de produção (pelo fígado para ureia; pelos músculos para a creatinina), ou por uma diminuição da taxa de perda (primariamente pelos rins). A azotemia pré-renal pode resultar de distúrbios da perfusão renal (p. ex., desidratação, insuficiência cardíaca, choque etc.) ou aumento da produção de compostos nitrogenados não proteicos. A azotemia pré-renal não é evidência de doença renal e pode ser corrigida pela eliminação da causa do distúrbio da perfusão renal ou do aumento da produção de compostos nitrogenados não proteicos.

A uremia é definida como a síndrome clínica polissistêmica que resulta da perda extensiva de funções renais. A doença renal pode estar presente se azotemia ou uremia. A azotemia pode ocorrer sem uremia ou doença renal (p. ex., azotemia pré-renal). A uremia não ocorre sem azotemia, mas a uremia pode ocorrer sem a doença renal (p. ex., extravasamento de urina dos ureteres ou bexiga em tecidos, que pode levar à azotemia e sinais urêmicos).

A azotemia renal confirma o diagnóstico de doença renal e é o resultado de diminuição da TFG consequente à doença ou lesão renal primária. Pode ou não ser reversível com o passar do tempo, mas não é resolvida em resposta à fluidoterapia. A capacidade de concentração da urina está prejudicada em cães e gatos com azotemia renal. Valores de densidade urinária específica menores que 1,030 em cães e menores que 1,035 em gatos são considerados como evidências de "concentração urinária inadequada" em pacientes azotêmicos ou desidratados. O achado de azotemia concorrente a valores de densidade urinária específica menores que 1,030 em cães e menores que 1,035 em gatos é altamente sugestivo de azotemia renal. Note que cães e gatos não azotêmicos com perfusão renal adequada (hidratação e fluxo sanguíneo renal normais) podem normalmente ter valores de densidade urinária abaixo de 1,030 ou 1,035, respectivamente. A azotemia renal e pré-renal podem ocorrer em

conjunto. Essa combinação deve ser considerada quando animais possuem azotemia e capacidade inadequada de concentração urinária (azotemia renal), mesmo que a fluidoterapia reduza parcialmente a magnitude da azotemia (o componente pré-renal da azotemia geral).

A azotemia pós-renal é resultado do fluxo urinário obstruído ou extravasamento de urina para uma cavidade corporal ou tecidos (p. ex., ruptura da bexiga). A densidade urinária específica não é útil para identificação de azotemia pós-renal. A distensão do sistema coletor urinário (ureter(es) e/ou bexiga) é sugestiva de azotemia pós-renal, assim como a urina na cavidade peritoneal ou tecidos ao redor do sistema urinário. Estudos de imagem contrastados do sistema coletor urinário podem ser utilizados para confirmar a obstrução ou extravasamento urinário. A correção da obstrução ou defeito urinário em geral resolve a azotemia. Entretanto, a obstrução urinária prolongada (principalmente por obstrução parcial) pode levar à lesão renal e azotemia renal. A azotemia pós-renal pode ocorrer concorrentemente à azotemia primária e/ou azotemia pré-renal.

Densidade urinária específica

A obtenção da densidade urinária específica (DUE) no mesmo momento que a concentração sérica de creatinina é fundamental para interpretação correta (ver Capítulos 62, 72 e 321). Como afirmado, a DUE é essencial para diferenciação imediata entre azotemia pré-renal e renal primária. Amostras de urina obtidas após administração de fluidos ou determinados medicamentos provavelmente estarão alteradas, eliminando assim o valor da DUE. De forma geral, a concentração sérica de creatinina é interpretada como consistente com azotemia primária quando a DUE for < 1,030 em cães e < 1,035 em gatos. Na maioria dos cães e vários gatos com DRC, os valores de DUE ficam entre 1,006 e 1,020 e, quando em estágios avançados de DRC, isostenúria (DUE = 1,008 a 1,012) é comum. O achado de isostenúria indica que os rins não estão modificando a concentração da urina a partir da concentração do plasma. Uma DUE < 1,006 não é consistente com azotemia renal porque concentrações abaixo de isostenúria necessitam de função renal adequada. Alguns gatos com DRC podem manter a capacidade substancial de concentração urinária (*i. e.*, 1,020 a 1,035, e ocasionalmente > 1,035). Uma maneira alternativa para diferenciação entre azotemia primária e pré-renal é repetir a concentração sérica de creatinina após um desafio apropriado de fluidoterapia IV que elimine a condição pré-renal. Se a azotemia for resolvida 24 a 48 horas após a administração de fluidos, o animal é considerado "responsivo a fluidos" e, portanto, a azotemia ocorreu por causas pré-renais.

Dimetilarginina simétrica na doença renal crônica

O processo de degradação proteica inclui a metilação da arginina e formação de numerosas moléculas, incluindo a dimetilarginina assimétrica (ADMA) e dimetilarginina simétrica (SDMA).[84] A ADMA é um inibidor endógeno de óxido nítrico sintase e está associada à disfunção endotelial, vasoconstrição e incrementos da pressão sanguínea. É depurada pelo fígado e rins. Ao contrário, o SDMA possui pouca ação fisiológica e ≥ 90% é eliminada pelos rins. A depuração renal ocorre por meio de filtração, sem reabsorção tubular.[85] As concentrações séricas de SDMA se correlacionam bem com a TFG em gatos e cães. Em cães com nefropatia hereditária ligada ao cromossomo X, o SDMA sérica esteve correlacionado tanto à creatinina como à TFG estimada pelo iohexol.[86] Em um modelo canino de DRC, o SDMA esteve melhor correlacionado à TFG do que à creatinina.[87] Em 69 gatos de tutores com DRC, as concentrações de SDMA estavam aumentadas e correlacionadas com a creatinina; SDMA também esteve bem correlacionado com uma faixa de TFGs em gatos idosos.[88,89]

O SDMA demonstrou ser um marcador para doença renal precoce em cães, gatos e seres humanos.[86,90,91] Cães com nefropatia hereditária ligada ao cromossomo X rapidamente progridem de normais ao nascimento para doença renal em estágio final. Em um grupo de cães com nefropatia hereditária ligada ao cromossomo X, as mensurações do SDMA sérico, creatinina e TFG estimada pela depuração do ioxehol foram acompanhadas durante a evolução da doença. O SDMA aumentou mais precocemente do que a creatinina. O valor de SDMA aumentou após declínios de 30% na TFG, enquanto a creatinina sérica não aumentou até perda de 50 a 50% da função renal. A creatinina foi avaliada tanto como um valor sérico único de corte como uma tendência com o passar do tempo, e em ambas as situações o SDMA provou ser um indicador mais precoce de perda da função renal.[86] O acompanhamento seriado da creatinina sérica aumenta sua sensibilidade para detecção da redução da função renal e é melhor do que uma mensuração única. Entretanto, o SDMA superou o acompanhamento seriado da creatinina e provou ser um melhor indicador da doença renal precoce. Estudos longitudinais retrospectivos em cães e gatos que desenvolveram DRC forneceram evidências maiores de que o SDMA sérico aumenta mais precocemente do que a creatinina. Dois estudos retrospectivos em cães e gatos conduzidos durante vários anos conforme eles desenvolveram DRC de ocorrência natural revelaram o aumento do SDMA antes da creatinina por uma média de 17 meses em gatos (variação de 1,5 a 48 meses) e 10,2 meses em cães (variação de 0,5 a 32 meses). O SDMA aumentou após um decréscimo de cerca de 40% na TFG (25% em um caso).[92]

O SDMA é útil para identificação e monitoramento da doença renal em pacientes sarcopênicos (ver Capítulo 177). Uma questão principal com a creatinina envolve sua relação com a massa muscular. O aumento da massa muscular promove a observação de maiores valores de creatinina enquanto a redução da massa muscular está associada a valores inferiores. Por exemplo, gatos idosos com DRC frequentemente desenvolvem grave sarcopenia. Por conta da perda de massa muscular, as concentrações séricas de creatinina estão baixas com relação à TFG e subestimam a gravidade da disfunção renal. Ao contrário, o SDMA é minimamente impactado pela massa muscular em cães e gatos.[86,91-95] Em um estudo em cães que comparou a massa corporal magra, idade, creatinina sérica e SDMA demonstrou que a massa magra e idade foram variáveis significativas para a creatinina, mas não para as concentrações de SDMA.[96] O SDMA é mais bem utilizado para complementar os exames renais existentes. As concentrações séricas de SDMA > 14 mcg/dℓ são anormais em cães e gatos. Incrementos nas concentrações séricas de SDMA e creatinina com concorrente urina inapropriadamente concentrada são consistentes com doença renal. O aumento do SDMA e uma concentração sérica de creatinina dentro dos limites de referência sugere doença renal inicial. Entretanto, aumentos persistentes no SDMA durante meses é uma evidência mais forte de doença renal. Aumentos persistentes do SDMA por mais de 3 meses em cães com creatinina sérica < 1,4 mg/dℓ ou gatos com creatinina sérica < 1,6 mg/dℓ são consistentes com diagnóstico de DRC em estágio I pela IRIS. Ao contrário da creatinina, o SDMA não é influenciado pela massa corporal magra e, portanto, será um melhor marcador de doença renal em animais com baixos escores de condição corporal. O painel da IRIS fornece diretrizes para utilização do SDMA para ajustar as recomendações terapêuticas em pacientes com baixos escores de condição corporal (ver sistema de estadiamento da DRC).

Doença renal aguda *versus* crônica

O diagnóstico de DRC requer a confirmação de doença renal e evidência de cronicidade. Na DRC, *crônico* significa uma perda irreversível e em geral progressiva da função renal e/ou estrutura. Nessa situação, a capacidade para compensação renal chegou ao máximo, que tipicamente reflete a duração de aproximadamente 3 meses ou mais. Ao contrário, a IRA (ver Capítulo 322) é potencialmente reversível, seja pela resolução de pelo menos parte da lesão renal, desenvolvimento de melhora compensatórias adaptativas na função renal, ou ambos. Assim, as consequências a curto e longo prazo da IRA e DRC são potencialmente bastante diferentes.

A *cronicidade* da DRC pode ser estimada a partir do histórico médico, achados de exame físico, alterações históricas nos achados laboratoriais ou alterações estruturais renais observadas por exames de imagem ou patologia renal. Perda de peso, PU, PD, hiporexia e outros sinais por cerca de 3 meses ou mais fornecem evidências substanciais de cronicidade. Da mesma forma, o *status* nutricional e qualidade do pelame em declínio são mais típicos de DRC do que de IRA. Aumentos documentados típicos na creatinina sérica durante um período ≥ 3 meses adiciona, suporte conclusivo para o diagnóstico de DRC. O critério de pelo menos 3 meses de redução da função renal é baseado na observação de que a hipertrofia compensatória renal pode continuar por um período após a IRA. A proteinúria persistente por 3 meses ou mais também suporta o diagnóstico de DRC. Ao mesmo tempo que as anemias arregenerativas (ver Capítulo 199) são típicas, elas não são diagnósticas porque condições não relacionadas podem causar anemia. Rins pequenos palpáveis ou de pequeno tamanho notado em exames de imagem fortemente suportam o diagnóstico de DRC; a perda de néfrons está em geral associada à fibrose. Em algumas situações, especialmente em gatos, um rim pode se tornar aumentado em associação a alterações compensatórias após encolhimento do rim devido à fibrose (ver Figura 324.1). Ao mesmo tempo que são incomuns, as alterações esqueléticas consistentes com osteodistrofia renal (ver Figura 324.2) podem confirmar a presença de DRC por conta do tempo necessário para seu desenvolvimento.

ESTADIAMENTO DA DOENÇA RENAL CRÔNICA

Visão geral

A International Renal Interest Society (IRIS) propôs um sistema com quatro estágios para estadiamento da DRC em cães e gatos baseado na função renal, proteinúria e pressão sanguínea (ver Boxe 324.1). Tal estadiamento facilita a aplicação de diretrizes apropriadas para o diagnóstico, prognóstico e tratamento. Embora os valores específicos utilizados para categorizar pacientes com DRC nesses estágios sejam baseados amplamente em dados observacionais, o estadiamento é, todavia, útil para o estabelecimento do prognóstico e tratamento de pacientes com DRC.[6,24]

Alinhamento do estágio de DRC pela IRIS e seu tratamento

O estadiamento da DRC é baseado na concentração sérica de creatinina do paciente. Como descrito, a creatinina sérica permanece a estimativa mais comumente utilizada da TFG em cães, gatos e seres humanos. Entretanto, sua especificidade e sensibilidade limitadas podem levar à classificação errônea. O estadiamento, portanto, deve ser baseado em um mínimo de dois valores de creatinina sérica obtidos quando o paciente estiver em jejum, bem hidratado e determinado durante um período de várias semanas. Se estável, é característico de DRC. O estado clínico geral deve ser considerado ao interpretar as concentrações séricas de creatinina e outros exames laboratoriais, e ao planejar o tratamento do paciente.

Variações entre laboratórios, características específicas do paciente (p. ex., raça, idade, gênero, condição corporal e massa corporal magra), e eventos transitórios pré-renais e pós-renais podem influenciar os valores séricos de creatinina. A redução da massa muscular é uma manifestação comum da DRC avançada e pode resultar em uma redução substancial da concentração sérica de creatinina relativa à verdadeira TFG, particularmente em gatos. A IRIS sugere que os valores de SDMA podem ser utilizados para modificar o estadiamento da DRC pela IRIS em cães e gatos nos quais a massa muscular corporal está acentuadamente reduzida (ver www.iris-kidney.com). Em animais em estágio II da DRC pela IRIS com baixos escores de condição corporal e uma concentração de SDMA ≥ 25 mcg/dℓ,[c] a extensão da disfunção renal provavelmente é subestimada e as recomendações terapêuticas listadas sob o estágio III de DRC pela IRIS devem ser consideradas. Em animais em estágio III da DRC pela IRIS com baixos escores de condição corporal e uma concentração de SDMA ≥ 45 mcg/dℓ,[d] a extensão da disfunção renal é provavelmente subestimada e as recomendações terapêuticas listadas sob o estágio IV da DRC pela IRIS devem ser consideradas.

O diagnóstico de DRC deve ser baseado na variação da creatinina sérica estabelecida para seu laboratório, e não no valor de corte da DRC em estágio II pela IRIS. Como valores de referência publicados para creatinina sérica são frequentemente amplos, entretanto, alguns animais classificados como portadores de azotemia renal discreta (estágio II) podem ter valores de creatinina sérica dentro dos valores de referência publicados. Para evitar o diagnóstico errôneo, é importante que evidências de DRC além do valor de creatinina sérica sejam buscados. Além disso, o maior tamanho corporal pode estar associado a um maior limite superior da creatinina sérica em cães. Estudos preliminares sugerem que essas limitações da concentração sérica de creatinina podem ser esclarecidas pela mensuração concorrente da concentração sérica de SDMA.

Descrições clínicas da doença renal crônica pela International Renal Interest Society

Estágios

O estágio I inclui cães e gatos não azotêmicos com DRC. O estágio II da DRC inclui cães e gatos que estão discretamente azotêmicos. A não ser pela PU/PD, animais em um desses estágios em geral não têm sinais clínicos de disfunção renal. Ocasionalmente, gatos e cães em estágio II possuem perda de peso ou inapetência. Entretanto, vários animais possuem sinais clínicos resultantes de suas lesões renais (p. ex., pielonefrite aguda, nefrolitíase). Aqueles com proteinúria marcante ou hipertensão sistêmica devido à DRC podem ter sinais clínicos relacionados a essas questões. A função renal está frequentemente estável ou lentamente progressiva por um período extensivo em cães e gatos não proteinúricos e não hipertensos com DRC em estágios I e II. Entretanto, quando ocorre a progressão, é importante determinar se o processo etiopatológico primário de base da DRC pode estar contribuindo para a progressão.[4] Pacientes com DRC em estágios I e II devem ser avaliados com o objetivo de identificar e fornecer tratamento específico para sua doença renal primária quando possível. Além disso, a função renal deve ser monitorada para possível progressão de sua DRC.

Animais com azotemia moderada são classificados como portadores de DRC em estágio III e eles podem ter sinais clínicos imputáveis à perda da função renal; entretanto, com terapia apropriada, eles tipicamente não possuem sinais clínicos de uremia evidente. Como a DRC em estágio III é tipicamente progressiva, além de identificar e tratar a DRC primária, a terapia alinhada para modificar fatores que promovem a progressão da DRC pode ser benéfica. A DRC em estágio IV inclui cães e gatos com azotemia grave (valores séricos de creatinina > 5,0 mg/dℓ) e, em geral, sinais clínicos de uremia. Iniciativas diagnósticas e terapêuticas nesse estágio incluem aquelas apropriadas para pacientes em estágio III, assim como a terapia desenvolvida para prevenir ou amenizar os sinais de uremia.

[b]N.R.T.: 35 pelas novas diretrizes (*http://www.iris-kidney.com/pdf/IRIS_Staging_of_CKD_modified_2019.pdf*).

[c]N.R.T.: 54 pelas novas diretrizes (*http://www.iris-kidney.com/pdf/IRIS_Staging_of_CKD_modified_2019.pdf*).

Subestadiamento dos estágios de doença renal crônica pela International Renal Interest Society

Como pode ser útil do ponto de vista terapêutico e prognóstico, o sistema de estadiamento da IRIS subclassifica ainda mais animais de acordo com a magnitude de sua proteinúria e/ou pressão sanguínea arterial. Antes de realizar uma RUPC, a urinálise e urocultura devem ser realizadas para descartar infecções, hemorragia ou inflamação como causa do aumento da RUPC. O sedimento urinário deve ser determinado como inativo antes de realizar a RUPC. A menos que acentuadamente elevada ou < 0,2, é recomendado que a RUPC seja reavaliada duas a três vezes durante pelo menos 2 semanas. A média dessas determinações deve ser utilizada para classificar o paciente como não proteinúrico, proteinúrico limítrofe ou proteinúrico (ver Boxe 324.1). A urina coletada em cada possui valores menores de RUPC do que amostras coletadas no hospital.[97] Animais com proteinúria limítrofe devem ser reavaliados após 2 meses. Em alguns animais, a classificação da proteinúria pode mudar devido à evolução da doença ou em resposta à terapia.

A pressão arterial sistêmica também deve ser determinada várias vezes durante diversas semanas (ver Boxe 324.1). A mensuração da pressão sanguínea deve ser realizada antes do exame físico ou coleta de sangue ou urina. Isso auxilia a minimizar a hipertensão do "jaleco branco". Idealmente, o animal é levado para uma sala de exame calma logo após chegar à clínica. O tutor e o animal não devem ser incomodados por cerca de 5 a 10 minutos para minimizar a ansiedade. Então um técnico veterinário treinado para realizar mensurações de pressão sanguínea deve calmamente adentrar a sala e obter 5 a 10 mensurações com a mínima contenção possível do animal. Os valores devem ser documentados em conjunto com a frequência cardíaca e comentários sobre o nível de ansiedade percebido do paciente.

Identificação de complicações clínicas, bioquímicas ou hematológicas da doença renal crônica

Histórico clínico e exame físico

Ao obter o histórico (ver Capítulo 1), o clínico deve buscar sinais clínicos que possam datar o início da doença renal (p. ex., PU, PD, perda de peso, hiporexia), informações sobre possíveis doenças congênitas ou hereditárias, evidências de infecções atuais ou prévias, neoplasias, doenças metabólicas, sinais ou distúrbios de trato urinário inferior, histórico de medicamentos (atuais e prévios), exposições a toxinas, dieta, apetite, e evidências de distúrbios renais prévios. O exame físico (ver Capítulo 2) deve enfatizar as condições dentárias e orais, exame retinal em busca de lesões hipertensivas, hidratação, edema, escore de condição corporal, avaliação da massa corporal magra, peso corporal acurado, qualidade do pelame, frequência e qualidade do pulso, palpação do trato urinário, dor óssea, temperatura corporal (uremia pode estar associada à baixa temperatura corporal) e exame retal. Em gatos, a área cervical deve ser cuidadosamente avaliada em busca de evidências de aumento tireoideano.

Testes recomendados

Uma vez que a maioria dos sistemas do organismo é afetada pela DRC e uremia, a base de dados diagnóstica inicial recomendada é ampla. O mínimo deve incluir o histórico médico, exame físico, pressão sanguínea arterial (ver Capítulo 99), hemograma, um painel bioquímico sérico completo com inclusão de eletrólitos séricos, status ácido-básico (concentração sérica de bicarbonato ou CO_2 total, ou hemogasometria), urinálise completa (ver Capítulo 72), urocultura, RUPC e radiografias abdominais simples e/ou ultrassonografia abdominal (de forma ideal, ambos). Em gatos, o exame de T4 deve ser descartado para descartar hipertireoidismo concorrente (ver Capítulo 301).

Biopsia renal

A biopsia e avaliação histológica do tecido obtido podem ser úteis para identificação da causa de doença renal (ver Capítulo 89). Entretanto, cães e gatos com DRC em estágios III e

IV da IRIS tipicamente possuem rins pequenos e fibrosados. Ademais, independentemente do estágio da DRC, a hipertensão e rins pequenos são contraindicações relativas à biopsia por conta dos riscos de hemorragia e perda de massa renal. Relatos recentes sobre os achados histopatológicos em gatos com DRC descreveram lesões renais e ligaram algumas dessas às características clinicopatológicas; entretanto, esses estudos não revelaram as origens etiopatológicas da DRC.[98,99] A indicação primária para biopsia é a proteinúria (ver Capítulo 325), nos quais os achados de biopsia podem influenciar o tratamento.

TRATAMENTO DA DOENÇA RENAL CRÔNICA

Visão geral e objetivos

O tratamento medicamentoso conservativo é padrão e a única opção realista para a maioria dos cães e gatos com DRC. Ele consiste em terapia de suporte e sintomática desenvolvida para amenizar os sinais clínicos, corrigir déficits ou excessos de fluido, assim como do balanço eletrolítico, acidobásico, endócrino e nutricional. A terapia deve minimizar as consequências clínicas e fisiológicas da redução da função renal e deve ser desenvolvida para retardar a perda progressiva da função renal. A terapia específica para a doença renal ativa e tratamento de comorbidades também pode ser indicada. A fim de melhor atingir esses objetivos, as recomendações terapêuticas devem ser individualizadas e baseadas em seu estado clínico e laboratorial individual. Como a DRC é progressiva e dinâmica, a avaliação seriada clínica e laboratorial do animal, e a modificação da terapia em resposta às alterações, é fundamental para o tratamento medicamentoso conservativo. O plano terapêutico deve levar em consideração o estágio de DRC pela IRIS de cada animal, sinais clínicos, fatores de risco para progressão, complicações existentes e comorbidades. A terapia administrada para doença renal ativa deve ser identificada. Apesar da irreversibilidade das lesões renais da DRC, a progressão pode ser retardada ou cessada com a terapia desenvolvida para eliminar doenças renais ativas. Assim, uma avaliação diagnóstica minuciosa deve incluir uma pesquisa para doença ativa que possa estar complicando a DRC.

O tratamento de pacientes com DRC requer comprometimento contínuo com o tutor. Assim, o manejo da DRC com sucesso é otimizado pelo desenvolvimento de um plano a longo prazo que inclui: (1) educação introdutória do tutor com relação à doença do animal e o tratamento, (2) um plano específico para monitoramento do progresso e resposta ao tratamento, e (3) facilitação contínua do comprometimento do tutor no plano terapêutico.[103] A incapacidade de incluir tutores na equipe que toma decisões frequentemente resulta em uma resposta terapêutica imperfeita. Um plano inicial bem desenvolvido para facilitar o sucesso inicial da implementação do plano terapêutico possui o potencial de melhorar amplamente o resultado clínico a longo prazo através da melhora do comprometimento (Boxe 324.3).

Fatores que provavelmente influenciam o sucesso de um plano terapêutico incluem: (1) atitude do tutor e aceitação do plano terapêutico, (2) paciência e algumas vezes criatividade para promover a aceitação do tutor e do animal dos tratamentos recomendados, e (3) manutenção do comprometimento contínuo do tutor ao plano terapêutico e conexão com a equipe veterinária para a duração da vida do animal. O primeiro passo para o desenvolvimento de um plano terapêutico a longo prazo para cães e gatos com DRC é desenvolver um plano terapêutico que funcione para o tutor assim como para o animal. Se um plano terapêutico for muito presente, consumir muito tempo, for caro ou se for percebido como um distúrbio na ligação entre humano e animal, provavelmente não terá sucesso.

O ponto final para a otimização do resultado a longo prazo de animais com DRC é um plano para acompanhamento ativo

---

> **Boxe 324.3** *Checklist* para o tratamento da doença renal crônica
>
> 1. Confirme que o paciente tenha doença renal
>   a. Testes de função renal (creatinina sérica, BUN, SDMA)
>   b. Urinálise, relação proteína:creatinina urinária, e/ou urocultura
>   c. Exames de imagem
> 2. Confirme que a doença renal é crônica
>   a. Histórico médico
>   b. Exame físico
>   c. Exames de imagem renal
> 3. Estabeleça o estágio da DRC pela IRIS do paciente (ver Boxe 324.1)
>   a. Dois valores de creatinina sérica em jejum em um paciente bem hidratado
>   b. Relação proteína:creatinina urinária (2 a 3 valores)
>   c. Pressão sanguínea arterial (2 a 3 valores)
> 4. Desenvolva um plano terapêutico para a DRC do paciente
>   a. Determine as opções terapêuticas apropriadas para o paciente
>   b. Priorize e selecione quais opções terapêuticas recomendar com base na prioridade médica e preferências do tutor (que podem incluir custos, demandas para o tutor e preferências dele)
> 5. Revise o plano terapêutico com o tutor e confirme a vontade de comprometimento com os tratamentos selecionados
> 6. Agende consulta(s) de acompanhamento para avaliar a resposta do paciente à terapia
> 7. Organize atualizações telefônicas regulares para avaliar a resposta à terapia e confirme a adequação e o comprometimento do tutor com o plano terapêutico
>   a. Avalie a compreensão do tutor sobre o plano terapêutico
>   b. Determine se o tutor está com problemas de adequação
>   c. Avalie a resposta do paciente à terapia e determine se o paciente precisa ser observado antes da próxima consulta agendada
>   i. Atividade
>   ii. Comportamento
>   iii. Apetite e quantificação da ingestão alimentar (e peso corporal, se disponível)
>   iv. Consumo hídrico
>   v. Percepção do tutor sobre o bem-estar do animal

---

iniciado pelo veterinário. Além do agendamento de visitas clínicas rotineiras, é altamente útil para um técnico veterinário familiarizado com o animal, tutor e plano terapêutico que mantenha contato com os cuidadores pelo menos semanalmente até que o tutor esteja confortável que o plano terapêutico está indo bem e todas as questões tenham sido satisfatoriamente respondidas. Razões para a manutenção da comunicação são encorajar e ensinar o cuidado com relação ao plano terapêutico, para avaliar a resposta à terapia, determinar se existem problemas com relação à adequação, e para decidir se quaisquer sinais alarmantes ocorreram indicando a necessidade de reavaliar o exame ou discussão por telefone com o veterinário.

Terapia dietética (ver Capítulo 184)

Visão geral

De todas as terapias utilizadas para tratar cães e gatos com DRC, as dietas renais possuem o maior benefício e a maioria das evidências que suporta sua efetividade.[103] Embora comumente chamadas de dietas "pobres em proteína", as dietas renais não deveriam ter baixos níveis de proteína de fato. As dietas renais deveriam ter outras modificações, incluindo redução de PO_4 e Na, vitaminas B adicionadas, aumento da densidade calórica, adição de fibras solúveis, um efeito neutro sobre o equilíbrio ácido-básico, e suplementação de ácidos graxos poli-insaturados ômega-3 e antioxidantes. Além disso, dietas renais felinas tipicamente contêm suplementação de K.

Fósforo dietético

A maioria das dietas de manutenção contém quantidades substanciais de PO_4. A hiperfosfatemia e hiperparatireoidismo ocorrem quando as dietas de manutenção são consumidas por cães e gatos com DRC. A proteína tipicamente contribui com uma quantidade substancial de PO_4 nos alimentos de animais, mas elas não são a única fonte. Estudos em cães e gatos com DRC ligaram a hiperfosfatemia à diminuição da sobrevida e lesões renais.[24,26,58,75] A limitação do PO_4 da dieta é indicada para cães e gatos em estágios II a IV da DRC pela IRIS.[104] Os benefícios da redução da ingestão de PO_4 incluem redução da retenção, menores níveis séricos de PO_4, diminuição do HPSR, retardo da progressão da DRC e redução da mortalidade.[58]

Ácidos graxos poli-insaturados ômega-3 e antioxidantes

O estresse oxidativo parece ter consequências adversas na doença renal crônica.[105] A suplementação dietética com ácidos graxos poli-insaturados (PUFAs) ômega-3 demonstrou ser benéfica em cães com DRC induzida.[106] Comparados a cães alimentados com dietas com altos níveis de gorduras saturadas ou PUFAs ômega-3, cães com DRC submetidos à administração de PUFAs ômega-3 tiveram menor mortalidade, melhor função renal, menores lesões renais, menor proteinúria e níveis de colesterol inferiores.[106] Estes benefícios podem ser o resultado de efeitos favoráveis sobre o metabolismo lipídico e hemodinâmica renal, supressão da inflamação e coagulação, redução da pressão sanguínea e ações antioxidantes.[107] Um estudo avaliou os efeitos da administração de PUFAs ômega-3 (relação entre ômega-6 e ômega-3 de 5:1) e antioxidantes dietéticos (vitamina E, carotenoides, luteína) sobre o declínio progressivo da TFG em cães com DRC induzida. Os resultados indicaram que tanto a suplementação por PUFA ômega-3 como antioxidantes foram benéficas.[108] Entretanto, a combinação dos dois pode ter tido benefícios sinérgicos. Assim, a suplementação dietética com PUFAs ômega-3 e antioxidantes é recomendada para cães e gatos com DRC. As quantidades e relação ômega-3:ômega-6 ótimas ainda não foram estabelecidas. Embora a terapia com PUFA ômega-3 e antioxidantes em gatos com DRC esteja indisponível, a suplementação com vitaminas E e C e betacarotenos reduz o estresse oxidativo em gatos.[109]

Proteína

Os produtos de degradação do catabolismo proteico supostamente contribuem para os sinais clínicos da uremia. Ao mesmo tempo que a quantidade de proteína fornecida a cães e gatos com DRC ainda não foi estabelecida, o consenso geral é que a limitação da ingestão proteica da dieta amenize os sinais clínicos da uremia na DRC e seja, portanto, indicada parta os estágios III e IV da DRC. Ao mesmo tempo que não é tida como uma toxina urêmica importante, a BUN é um marcador substituto para produtos de degradação nitrogenados não proteicos retidos e tipicamente se correlaciona melhor com os sinais clínicos do que a concentração sérica de creatinina. Entretanto, a redução da ingestão proteica da dieta em animais com DRC que não possuem sinais clínicos de uremia tem sido questionada. A limitação de sua ingestão proteica tem sido justificada por seu potencial em retardar a progressão da DRC.[110] Entretanto, alguns autores têm argumentado que a alta ingestão proteica na dieta não demonstrou de forma clara promover a progressão da DRC e pode ser necessária para manter a nutrição adequada. Entretanto, quando o consumo da dieta renal é adequado e a restrição proteica não é excessiva, dietas renais não causam desnutrição. Um argumento razoável adicional para recomendação de dietas renais no estágio II e início do estágio III da DRC pela IRIS é que pode ser mais fácil iniciar a conversão para dietas renais bem antes do início dos sinais clínicos de uremia.[104]

Terapia dietética – evidências de estudos clínicos

Cães. A efetividade da terapia dietética em minimizar episódios urêmicos e reduzir a mortalidade em cães e gatos com DRC de ocorrência natural foi estabelecida.[2,111,113] Estudos compararam uma dieta renal com PUFAs ômega-3 com uma dieta de manutenção prototípica. Dietas renais tinham proteína, PO_4 e Na limitados quando comparados a uma dieta de manutenção para adultos. Em cães, o risco de desenvolvimento de uma crise urêmica foi reduzido em cerca de 75% quando alimentados com uma dieta renal.[2] O intervalo mediano livre de sintomas em cães alimentados com uma dieta renal foi de 615 dias comparado a 252 dias em cães alimentados com uma dieta de manutenção para adultos. O risco de morte, independentemente da causa, foi reduzido em 66% e o risco de morte por causas renais foi reduzido em 69% para cães que consumiam uma dieta renal. O tempo de sobrevida mediano para cães que consumiam uma dieta renal foi de 594 dias comparado a 188 dias para cães que consumiam uma dieta de manutenção. Além disso, tutores que forneciam uma dieta renal relataram escores de qualidade de vida significativamente maiores para seus cães do que tutores que forneciam uma dieta de manutenção.

Gatos. Quarenta e cinco gatos com valores de creatinina sérica de 2,0 mg/dℓ a 4,5 mg/dℓ (estágios II e III de DRC pela IRIS) foram separados em dois grupos: 22 foram alimentados com uma dieta comercial renal e 23 foram alimentados com uma dieta de manutenção.[113] Os riscos de crises urêmicas e mortes por distúrbios renais foram reduzidos quando uma dieta renal foi fornecida. Entre os 22 gatos alimentados com uma dieta renal, não houve crises urêmicas ou mortes por distúrbios renais, e três mortes ocorreram por causas não renais durante 2 anos. Dos 23 gatos que consumiram uma dieta de manutenção, seis desenvolveram crises urêmicas e cinco morreram de causas renais. Dois estudos adicionais, um teste não randomizado e um estudo retrospectivo, suportam a efetividade de dietas renais em gatos com DRC.[9,112] O estudo clínico não randomizado comparou uma dieta renal manufaturada a uma situação sem alteração da dieta.[10] Ao mesmo tempo que não era randomizado ou cego, os resultados forneceram fortes evidências que suportam a eficácia de dietas renais felinas. Gatos alimentados com uma dieta renal (sobrevida média de 633 dias) viveram substancialmente por mais tempo do que gatos que consumiam suas dietas regulares (sobrevida média de 264 dias). Além disso, gatos alimentados com uma dieta renal tinham menores concentrações de BUN, PO_4 sérico e PTH. Um estudo realizado em 31 clínicas veterinárias nos Países Baixos comparou tempos de sobrevida para gatos alimentados com uma de sete dietas renais felinas comerciais a gatos alimentados com uma dieta de manutenção.[113] O tempo de sobrevida mediano para os gatos alimentados com uma dieta renal foi de 16 meses comparado a sete para gatos alimentados com suas dietas usuais. Ademais, o fornecimento de dietas renais diminui os níveis plasmáticos de PO_4 e FGF-23 comparado a gatos com DRC que consomem suas dietas usuais.[113] Incrementos nas concentrações de PO_4 e FGF-23 foram implicados como promotores da progressão de DRC.

Resumo. Os estudos clínicos descritos aqui claramente suportam a utilização de dietas renais para cães em estágios III e IV de DRC, e gatos com DRC em estágios II a IV. O valor das dietas renais em cães com DRC em estágio II ainda não foi criticamente avaliado, mas são benéficas para redução da magnitude da proteinúria.[114] Assim, dietas renais são recomendadas para todos os cães com doença renal proteinúrica.[115,116] Esses estudos não determinaram seletivamente os benefícios da modificação de componentes dietéticos individuais, mas relatam, em vez disso, os resultados de um "efeito da dieta".

Retenção de fósforo, hiperfosfatemia e hiperparatireoidismo secundário renal (HPSR)

Visão geral. Como a capacidade de excretar PO_4 diminui conforme a DRC progride, a ingestão deve ser reduzida em paralelo ao declínio da função renal (ver Capítulos 69 e 321). Se não, a retenção de PO_4, hiperfosfatemia e HPSR ocorrerão, aumentando o declínio progressivo na função renal e mortalidade.[35,58,117] A minimização da retenção e hiperfosfatemia é um importante objetivo terapêutico em cães e gatos com DRC porque parece retardar a progressão da DRC e prolongar a sobrevida.[58,75,118] Como a perfusão renal alterada aumenta as concentrações séricas de PO_4, o primeiro passo para correção da hiperfosfatemia é garantir que o animal esteja bem hidratado. Então, a minimização da retenção de PO_4 e hiperfosfatemia é promovida pela limitação do conteúdo dietético e/ou utilização de agentes orais que quelam PO_4 dentro dos intestinos.[119] A abordagem usual é iniciar com a terapia dietética renal. Agentes quelantes são utilizados quando uma dieta renal, por si só, não consegue normalizar a concentração sérica de PO_4 (Boxe 324.4). Dietas renais, por si só, em geral normalizam as concentrações séricas de PO_4 na maioria dos animais em estágio II da DRC e em vários animais em estágio III da DRC. Animais em estágio III avançado de DRC pela IRIS e estágio IV da DRC pela IRIS tipicamente são beneficiados pela administração de um quelante intestinal de PO_4 para atingir os objetivos.[57,118] Evidências atuais sugerem que o alvo principal é o PO_4 sérico, e não o PTH.

Restrição dietética de PO_4. Os objetivos do tratamento estão ligados ao estadiamento da DRC pela IRIS (ver Boxe 324.4). Valores de referência ou "normais" para a concentração sérica de PO_4 *não são o objetivo terapêutico* em animais com DRC. Quando a concentração sérica de PO_4 for maior do que o objetivo, ela deve ser considerada aumentada e a redução da sua concentração é em geral indicada para cães e gatos com estágios II a IV de DRC. A concentração sérica de PO_4 deve sempre ser avaliada após um jejum de 12 horas para evitar efeitos pós-prandiais e tais dietas requerem várias semanas para obtenção de resultados. Em gatos com DRC, o efeito dietético completo foi aparente após 28 a 49 dias.[118] As concentrações séricas de PO_4 devem ser reavaliadas 4 a 6 semanas após o início da dieta renal. Se dentro dos valores de referência, a dieta deve ser mantida e o PO_4 sérico reavaliado a cada 3 a 4 meses (a cada 4 a 6 meses pode ser adequado para cães e gatos em estágio II de DRC pela IRIS se dois resultados sequenciais estiverem dentro da faixa desejada). Se uma dieta renal por si só não faz com que o paciente atinja o valor almejado do PO_4 sérico após 4 a 6 semanas, a adição de um quelante intestinal é razoável.

Quelantes intestinais. Medicações que aprisionam o PO_4 no intestino impedem sua absorção. O quelante de PO_4 deve estar presente no intestino no mesmo momento que o alimento com seu PO_4. Os quelantes são mais efetivos quando administrados em conjunto com dietas restritas em PO_4 porque uma menor quantidade precisa ser quelada. O alto conteúdo dietético de PO_4 pode limitar amplamente a efetividade dos agentes quelantes ou substancialmente aumentar a dose necessária para atingir o efeito terapêutico desejado. A administração de 1.500 a 2.500 mg de carbonato de alumínio para cães com DRC moderada não conseguiu corrigir de forma consistente a hiperfosfatemia quando cães foram alimentados com dietas contendo

mais que 1% de PO_4 com base na matéria seca.[119] Como muitas dietas de manutenção para cães e gatos contêm altos níveis de PO_4, é improvável que os objetivos terapêuticos possam ser atingidos somente pela adição de agentes quelantes. A minimização da quantidade de PO_4 que precisa ser quelada é importante porque a administração de uma quantidade excessiva pode diminuir o apetite ou causar náuseas, êmese, diarreia e constipação intestinal.[120]

Agentes quelantes intestinais contendo alumínio na forma de sais de hidróxido, óxido ou carbonato têm sido a primeira escolha em cães e gatos porque são efetivos e baratos (Tabela 324.2).[121] Embora agentes quelantes à base de alumínio sejam em geral bem tolerados e seguros em cães e gatos, a intoxicação por alumínio foi relatada em cães com DRC avançada tratados com altas doses.[122] A intoxicação foi notada na forma de neuropatias cranianas, periféricas e juncionais. Os sinais clínicos incluíram fraqueza, ataxia, ausência de reflexos patelares, diminuição da propriocepção do membro pélvico, diminuição do reflexo de ameaça, obnubilação, tetraparesia e decúbito lateral. A microcitose foi também notada e pode ser útil na detecção precoce de intoxicação por alumínio. A terapia de quelação foi necessária para corrigir a intoxicação. Quelantes de PO_4 à base de alumínio podem diminuir a palatabilidade e causar constipação intestinal.

Agentes quelantes de PO_4 à base de cálcio são efetivos, mas podem causar hipercalcemia, especialmente quando o calcitriol for administrado também. Essa combinação deve ser evitada. Pessoas que são submetidas ao tratamento com quelantes de PO_4 sem Ca tiveram redução da mortalidade por todas as causas quando comparadas a pessoas submetidas a quelantes à base de Ca.[123] As concentrações de iCa devem ser monitoradas quando quelantes à base de Ca forem utilizados. O carbonato de lantânio e outros sais de lantânio parecem ser bastante efetivos em quelar o PO_4. Estes possuem menos efeitos colaterais porque o lantânio não é absorbido, reduzindo o risco de intoxicação quando comparado aos sais de alumínio. O lantânio é bem aceito e tolerado por gatos e o carbonato de lantânio demonstrou inibir a absorção intestinal de oxalato, impedindo a nefrocalcinose em um modelo murino.[124,125] O sevelamer, uma resina de troca de ânions, não é comumente utilizada em cães e gatos. Ao contrário da maioria dos quelantes de PO_4, o sevelamer não libera um cátion, mas pode causar acidose metabólica e hipercalcemia. Os sais de lantânio e cloridrato de sevelamer são geralmente muito mais caros do que os sais de Ca ou alumínio.

Tabela 324.2	**Agentes quelantes intestinais de fosfato.**
QUELANTE INTESTINAL DE FOSFATO	**DOSES RECOMENDADAS**
Hidróxido de alumínio (600 mg/5 mℓ)*	30 a 90 mg/kg/dia[†] PO
Carbonato de lantânio (500 mg/ comprimido palatável)	12,5 a 25 mg/kg/dia[†] PO
Carbonato de lantânio octaidratado (200 mg/mℓ)	2 mℓ PO no alimento 1 a 2 vezes/dia[†]
Carbonato de cálcio (500 mg/ comprimido)	30 mg/kg[†] PO
Quitosana e carbonato de cálcio (pó)	4,4 g/10 kg[†] PO
Cloridrato de sevelamer (400 mg/ comprimido)	33 a 54 mg/kg[†] PO

*O hidróxido de alumínio USP também está disponível como pó. [†]Dose diária deve ser dividida entre as refeições diárias (em geral 2 a 3 refeições/dia). O produto deve ser misturado no alimento ou administrado imediatamente antes ou após cada refeição.

Boxe 324.4 Objetivos terapêuticos recomendados para as concentrações séricas de fósforo		
ESTÁGIO DA IRIS	**CONCENTRAÇÃO-ALVO DO FÓSFORO SÉRICO**	
ESTÁGIO	**(mg/dℓ)**	**(mmol/dℓ)**
I	2,5 a 4,5	0,81 a 1,45
II	2,5 a 4,5	0,81 a 1,45
III	2,5 a 5,0	0,81 a 1,61
IV	2,5 a 6,0	0,81 a 1,94

Quando administrar agentes quelantes.
Agentes quelantes de PO_4 devem ser administrados no momento da refeição ou próximos a esse horário com o objetivo de quelar o PO_4 da dieta. A administração de quelantes não associada a refeições reduz acentuadamente sua efetividade. Agentes quelantes à base de Ca que são administrados entre as refeições atuam como um suplemento de Ca em vez de um quelante de PO_4. Os agentes devem ser administrados "até ter efeito", o que significa que as doses devem ser ajustadas desde a dose inicial para atingir a concentração sérica de PO_4 almejada sem doses excessivas. A terapia é em geral iniciada utilizando a menor dose recomendada e aumentada conforme necessário a cada 2 a 4 semanas. Se a dose excede substancialmente aquela recomendada, é melhor adicionar um agente quelante diferente em vez de arriscar uma superdosagem. Diferentes agentes quelantes podem ser combinados para minimizar o risco de superdosagem de um fármaco.

Desidratação e fluidoterapia

Visão geral
A prevenção e correção da desidratação é extremamente benéfica para cães e gatos com DRC (ver Capítulo 129). O balanço hídrico em animais com PU deve ser mantido pela PD compensatória e a desidratação ocorre se quantidades adequadas não são consumidas. Gatos com DRC parecem ser particularmente suscetíveis à desidratação crônica, talvez porque sua PD compensatória é inadequada. A falta de acesso à água de boa qualidade, algumas condições ambientais e doenças concorrentes que limitam a ingestão hídrica ou causam perdas de fluidos (p. ex., pirexia, êmese ou diarreia) podem levar à desidratação. Membranas orais secas e diminuição do turgor cutâneo são comuns na desidratação, mas esses achados podem confundir. A xerostomia (membranas orais secas) pode resultar da uremia. A perda de elasticidade cutânea é comum em cães e gatos que perderam peso, são idosos ou estão em mau estado nutricional. A desidratação crônica pode diminuir o apetite e/ou causar letargia, fraqueza, constipação intestinal, azotemia pré-renal e predisposição à IRA. A IRA em animais com DRC preexistente é uma causa comum de progressão da doença (ver também Capítulo 322). Os tutores de animais com DRC devem ser educados com relação a perdas episódicas de fluidos devido à êmese e diarreia que poderiam não causar problemas quando o animal estava saudável, mas podem causar deterioração sérica da função renal ou precipitar crises urêmicas quando o animal é afligido pela DRC.

Indicações
O clínico deve considerar administrar fluidos subcutâneos (SC) aos animais com DRC com sinais de desidratação crônica ou recorrente. Os benefícios da fluidoterapia SC incluem melhora do apetite, aumento da atividade e menos constipação intestinal. As recomendações com relação aos fluidos SC devem ser feitas caso a caso. Nem todo animal com DRC requer ou se beneficiará de tal terapia. Ao mesmo tempo que vários gatos com DRC parecem ser beneficiados pela fluidoterapia SC, menos cães necessitam dela. Ademais, a administração doméstica de fluidos SC não é apropriada para todos os tutores. Ao mesmo tempo que não é um procedimento caro, a administração por via subcutânea de fluido requer tempo e pode ser estressante para a relação entre tutor e animal. Ela também tem o potencial de promover hipernatremia, hipopotassemia, hipertensão e sobrecarga volêmica.

Escolha do fluido, volume, frequência
Em geral, uma solução eletrolítica balanceada (p. ex., solução de Ringer com lactato) é administrada por via subcutânea a cada 1 a 3 dias, conforme necessário. O volume administrado depende do peso do animal. A maioria dos gatos recebe cerca de 75 a 125 mℓ por dose. Se a resposta clínica não for excelente, a dose pode ser cuidadosamente aumentada, mas a sobrecarga volêmica deve ser evitada. Além disso, fluidos que contêm Na administrados por via SC não fornecem a água livre de eletrólitos que indivíduos saudáveis consomem. Portanto, é fisiologicamente mais apropriado fornecer água por uma sonda de alimentação, o que pode ser mais fácil do que SC para alguns clientes (ver Capítulo 82). Como o excesso de ingestão de Na pode prejudicar os rins, as recomendações para administração a longo prazo de Na em qualquer forma devem ser cuidadosamente consideradas.[126]

A resposta à fluidoterapia SC a longo prazo deve ser avaliada pela verificação frequente do estado de hidratação, sinais clínicos, pressão sanguínea, função renal e, possivelmente, valores de eletrólitos. Se uma melhora detectável nos sinais clínicos e/ou função renal não acompanhar a fluidoterapia, a necessidade para terapia a longo prazo deve ser reavaliada.

Manejo de sinais gastrintestinais da uremia

Terapia antiemética
Apetite seletivo, náuseas e êmese estão entre os sinais mais comuns de DRC e uremia. Com o passar do tempo, a complicação mais importante de DRC é a ingestão alimentar inadequada, o que torna a inanição o fator mais comum que leva à morte em cães e gatos com DRC. Complicações gástricas de uremia diferem em cães e gatos. Enquanto a gastrite urêmica com ulceração pode ocorrer em cães, gatos mais provavelmente terão fibrose gástrica e mineralização.[42] As lesões em cães supostamente são resultado de aumentos nas concentrações séricas de gastrina, o que estimula a hiperacidez gástrica. A utilização de bloqueadores H2 (p. ex., famotidina, ranitidina), inibidores da bomba de prótons (omeprazol, pantoprazol, esomeprazol) e sucralfato é recomendada para cães com inapetência, náuseas e êmese. Essas terapias aparentemente seriam inapropriadas em gatos com DRC. A utilização de inibidores da bomba de prótons foi ligada à IRA em pessoas idosas.[127]

Em cães e gatos, a ativação da zona de gatilho quimiorreceptor por toxinas urêmicas promove anorexia, náuseas e êmese. A uremia provavelmente possui efeitos diretos GI. A terapia antiemética é útil para o manejo de náuseas e êmese urêmica. A utilização de fármacos antieméticos não melhora diretamente o apetite, mas eles podem minimizar a perda de alimentos e fluidos pela êmese. O maropitant e a ondansetrona atuam sobre a zona de gatilho quimiorreceptor, assim como no intestino. O maropitant oral (4 mg/gato/dia durante 2 semanas) tem sido um antiemético efetivo para gatos em estágios II e III de DRC pela IRIS.[128] O maropitant pode ser utilizado em cães e gatos com DRC em uma dose de 1 a 2 mg/kg/dia PO ou 1 mg/kg/dia SC ou IV. O maropitant não é limitado a períodos de 5 dias de tratamento. Enquanto a ondansetrona demonstrou ser efetiva em seres humanos urêmicos, estudos farmacocinéticos indicaram má disponibilidade quando administrada por via oral com uma curta meia-vida em gatos e cães.[129] A ondansetrona (0,1 a 1 mg/kg SC) possui melhor disponibilidade e meia-vida mais prolongada em gatos.

Terapia orexígena
A mirtazapina (1,87 mg/gato PO a cada 48 h; 3,75 a 30 mg/cão PO a cada 24 horas) aumentou o apetite, atividade e peso corporal de forma significativa em gatos com DRC, ao mesmo tempo que diminuiu os episódios de êmese.[130] A superdosagem pode causar hiperexcitabilidade, tremores e vocalização. A Cipro-heptadina não pode ser utilizada concorrentemente com a mirtazapina. Um estudo em seis Beagles indicou que cães podem ter um diferente perfil farmacocinético comparado a gatos e seres humanos.[131]

Alimentação por esofagostomia (ver Capítulo 82)
A incapacidade em estabilizar um animal em um escore de condição corporal aceitável provavelmente afetará adversamente o resultado a longo prazo. A alimentação por sonda de

esofagostomia pode ser bastante benéfica para cães e gatos com declínio progressivo do peso corporal, apesar de todos os esforços para atingir a nutrição adequada. Sondas de esofagostomia são indolores, efetivas e convenientes para o fornecimento de alimentos, água e medicações para cães e gatos com DRC. É uma forma útil de estabilizar ou melhorar a nutrição, sinais clínicos, longevidade e satisfação do tutor. De forma geral, a colocação da sonda menos provavelmente será efetiva quando a decisão de proceder for adiada até que tenham ocorrido uremia e desnutrição avançadas.

Acidose metabólica

Diagnóstico

A acidose da DRC pode causar desnutrição, sinais clínicos de uremia e osteodistrofia renal (ver Capítulo 128).[75] Estudos em seres humanos e roedores sugerem que a acidose metabólica pode também causar progressão da DRC; entretanto, é incerto se isso está ligado aos baixos níveis séricos de bicarbonato, alta carga de ácidos na dieta ou ambos.[132,133] Enquanto dados não estão disponíveis para cães, a acidose metabólica afetou cerca de 15% dos gatos em estágio III de DRC pela IRIS e cerca de 53% em estágio IV de DRC pela IRIS.[28] Essas observações sugerem que somente uma minoria dos gatos com DRC em estágios II e III pela IRIS clinicamente estáveis provavelmente serão beneficiados pela terapia rotineira de alcalinização. Assim, a decisão de intervir com a terapia de alcalinização deve ser baseada em uma avaliação laboratorial do estado ácido-básico. Baixos valores séricos ou plasmáticos de CO_2 total obtidos por técnicas de análise automatizadas devem ser confirmados pela hemogasometria (ver Capítulo 128).[134] Ao considerar a terapia para acidose da DRC, o estado ácido-básico deve ser avaliado pela hemogasometria quando o animal estiver bem hidratado. A terapia oral para acidose deve ser considerada quando a hemogasometria confirmar que os valores plasmáticos de bicarbonato permanecem abaixo de 15 mmol/ℓ. Entretanto, a intervenção parenteral deve ser considerada para gatos com acidose metabólica e um pH sanguíneo < 7,10, a fim de aumentar o valor para níveis acima de 7,20.[135]

Tratamento

Opções terapêuticas para terapia de alcalinização incluem dietas renais, citrato de K e bicarbonato de Na. A maioria das dietas renais é neutra a discretamente alcalinizante. Se a terapia dietética por si só não conseguir amenizar a acidose metabólica, a terapia de alcalinização deve ser considerada. A solução de citrato de K fornece K e alcalinização, e em geral é mais palatável do que o bicarbonato de Na. A dose é feita até "fazer efeito", com doses iniciais de 40 a 60 mg/kg a cada 8 a 12 horas e um objetivo de manter as concentrações sanguíneas de bicarbonato dentro dos valores de referência. O bicarbonato de Na (dose inicial: 8 a 12 mg/kg a cada 8 a 12 horas) é geralmente não palatável, exceto quando administrado na forma de comprimidos. Estas medicações devem ser administradas em pequenas doses frequentemente para minimizar flutuações do pH sanguíneo. A resposta à terapia deve ser avaliada após 10 a 14 dias, antes da administração da droga, e a dose ajustada de acordo.

Distúrbios do potássio (hipopotassemia e hiperpotassemia)

Hipopotassemia (ver Capítulos 68 e 321)

A depleção de potássio (K) e hipopotassemia (hipoK) são relativamente comuns em gatos com DRC em estágios II e III, com ocorrências estimadas em 20 a 30%. É menos comum em gatos em estágio IV.[3,7,8] Gatos hipertensos possuem concentrações plasmáticas de potássio diminuídas de forma significativa.[46] A depleção total do K corporal é provavelmente mais comum do que a hipoK.[81] Ao contrário, a hipoK é incomum em cães com

DRC. Os mecanismos que são a base para o desenvolvimento da hipoK em gatos com DRC permanecem incertos, mas a ingestão inadequada, aumento da perda urinária e aumento da ativação do SRAA devido à desidratação crônica e/ou restrição dietética de sal podem desempenhar papeis.[48] Enquanto o aumento do conteúdo de K das dietas renais reduziu a incidência e gravidade de sinais clínicos evidentes de hipoK, ainda permanece como um achado laboratorial comum em gatos com DRC. É importante salientar que o agente anti-hipertensivo amlodipino pode promover hipoK em gatos com DRC.[136]

A hipoK e depleção de K podem afetar de forma adversa os rins e músculos de gatos com DRC. Dietas com baixos índices de K e altos níveis de ácidos foram implicadas como prejudiciais à função renal e promotoras do desenvolvimento de lesões tubulointersticiais linfoplasmocítica em gatos.[82-85] A depleção de K pode levar à redução do fluxo sanguíneo renal e TFG como consequência da vasoconstrição renal mediada pela angiotensina II e tromboxano. Ademais, a hipoK pode causar PU pela alteração da responsividade renal ao ADH (ver Capítulos 45 e 296) e por estimular os centros da sede cerebrais pela angiotensina II. A polimiopatia hipopotassêmica, caracterizada por fraqueza muscular generalizada e ventroflexão cervical, é uma complicação bem reconhecida da DRC em gatos, embora menos comumente observada atualmente devido talvez à suplementação de K de dietas renais.

Enquanto existe um consenso de que gatos com hipoK devem receber suplementação para corrigir ou prevenir consequências renais ou musculares da depleção de K e hipoK, o valor da suplementação "profilática" para gatos normocalêmicos ainda não foi estabelecido. A reposição oral é a via mais segura e preferida. A terapia parenteral é geralmente reservada para gatos que necessitam de reversão emergencial da hipoK ou para gatos que não podem ou não irão tolerar a terapia oral. Até 30 mEq/ℓ de cloreto de K pode ser adicionado aos fluidos com pretensão de administração por via subcutânea. A suplementação oral de K pode ser feita como sais de gliconato ou citrato; o cloreto de K não é recomendado porque não é palatável e é acidificante. A forma de gliconato (2 a 6 mEq/gato/dia) está disponível como comprimidos, gel flavorizado ou pó palatável. A acidose é um fator de risco importante para o desenvolvimento de hipoK e, portanto, também deve ser tratada. A solução de citrato (40 a 60 mg/kg/dia a cada 6 a 8 horas) é uma excelente alternativa com a vantagem de fornecer terapia alcalinizante simultânea. A fraqueza muscular em geral é resolvida dentro de 1 a 5 dias após o início da suplementação de K. A dose, a seguir, é ajustada com base na resposta clínica e concentrações séricas de K, que devem inicialmente ser monitoradas a cada 7 a 14 dias. Em gatos com polimiopatia hipopotassêmica, pode ser necessário monitorar as concentrações séricas a cada 24 a 48 horas inicialmente. É incerto se todos os gatos necessitam de suplementação a longo prazo de K.

A fluidoterapia intensa durante crises urêmicas, particularmente com fluidos deficientes em K, pode causar hipoK em gatos ou cães que não estavam hipopotassêmicos. Portanto, as concentrações séricas de K devem ser monitoradas durante a fluidoterapia e fluidos de manutenção devem ser suplementados com cloreto de K para prevenir hipopotassemia iatrogênica (concentrações de 13 a 20 mEq/ℓ são apropriadas para fluidos de manutenção). O K por via IV não deve ser administrado em taxas que excedam 0,5 mEq/kg/h.

Hiperpotassemia

A hiperpotassemia (hiperK) é incomum na DRC; entretanto, pode ocorrer em casos de DRC em estágio IV pela IRIS avançados (ver Capítulos 68 e 321). Ela tende a ocorrer quando o consumo alimentar atinge a ingestão calórica adequada, mais comumente por sonda de alimentação, e/ou pela utilização de inibidores da ECA ou bloqueadores de receptores de angiotensina (BRAs). A hiperK pode ser tratada pela redução do K da dieta ou pela prevenção da captação intestinal.[137] Resinas poliméricas

(p. ex., sulfato de poliestireno sódico) foram tidas como inadequadas. Em seres humanos com DRC, o ciclossilicato de zircônio sódico, um trocador catiônico altamente seletivo que se liga ao K dentro do intestino, demonstrou ser eficaz para amenizar a hiperK.[138]

Hipertensão arterial

Razões para a terapia

A DRC é a causa mais comumente reconhecida para hipertensão em cães e gatos. Ela foi ligada a complicações renais, oculares, neurológicas e cardíacas (ver Capítulo 157). A retinopatia ocorre em cerca de 60% dos gatos hipertensos e é a manifestação clínica mais comum deles.[139] Os sinais clínicos observados em gatos hipertensos incluem letargia, cegueira, hemorragia retinal, descolamento de retina, hemorragia cerebral, convulsões, estupor e hipertrofia ventricular.[140-142] Em um estudo, a retinopatia e encefalopatia hipertensiva foram relatadas em três de 14 cães com valores de pressão sanguínea acima de 180 mmHg.[46] A DRC preexistente aumenta supostamente a vulnerabilidade dos rins à lesão hipertensiva.[143] A hipertensão pode ser um fator de risco independente para a progressão da DRC em cães, embora a proteinúria não tenha sido incluída em um modelo estatístico utilizado para confirmar essa associação.[31] Entretanto, em gatos com DRC, a hipertensão está associada ao aumento da proteinúria em cães e gatos, e, como a proteinúria parece promover lesão renal em ambas as espécies, a diminuição da pressão sanguínea a fim de limitar a proteinúria é um objetivo apropriado.[35,144] Evidências clínicas de humanos, cães e gatos indicam que a redução farmacológica da pressão arterial (PA) provavelmente reduz o risco de lesão hipertensiva em órgãos. A hidralazina SC reduz a prevalência de convulsões que ocorrem como consequência da hipertensão após transplante renal (ver Capítulo 323).[141] Ademais, em um modelo induzido de doença renal hipertensiva, somente dois de 10 gatos que receberam a amlodipino desenvolveram evidências de lesões retinais comparados a sete de 10 gato que receberam placebo.[140]

Indicações para o tratamento

A indicação para terapia anti-hipertensiva é tratar e/ou prevenir o desenvolvimento de lesões em órgãos-alvo, incluindo os rins, olhos, cérebro e coração (ver Capítulo 158). Entretanto, é desconhecido o nível da PA no qual a lesão renal progressiva pode ser induzida. As recomendações da IRIS para o tratamento da hipertensão são baseados em estimativas de risco de desenvolvimento de lesão em órgão-alvo que ocorre em faixas específicas de PA em cães ou gatos com DRC. Cães e gatos com hipertensão discreta (pressões sistólicas entre 160 mmHg a 179 mmHg) devem ter a hipertensão confirmada com pelo menos três determinações em um período de 1 a 2 meses. O tratamento deve ser suspenso até que as mensurações estabeleçam que a hipertensão seja persistente. Em cães e gatos com hipertensão mais grave (pressões sistólicas acima de 180 mmHg), o período de espera deve ser reduzido e as duas reavaliações concluídas em 1 a 2 semanas. Entretanto, quando houver evidências de lesão em órgãos relacionada à hipertensão, ou se a pressão sanguínea sistólica estiver em níveis emergenciais (> 200 mmHg), a terapia anti-hipertensiva deve ser iniciada imediatamente. Esforços razoáveis devem ser feitos para minimizar o risco de que as elevações mensuradas na pressão sanguínea representem um efeito transitório do "jaleco branco", em vez de uma elevação sustentada.[145] Parece improvável que pressões sistólicas acima de 200 mmHg reflitam qualquer resposta de ansiedade. Note que algumas raças de cães, notadamente os galgos, podem ter intervalos de PA até 40 mmHg maiores do que aqueles fornecidos nas diretrizes, e as decisões sobre o diagnóstico e tratamento devem ser ajustadas de acordo. Evidências sugerem que cães e gatos com DRC podem ter maior risco de lesão renal adicional ou desenvolvimento de complicações associadas à PA elevada.[31,51,140-142] Animais nos estágios I até IV da DRC pela IRIS e hipertensão confirmada ou grave devem ser tratados.

Objetivos e diretrizes para o tratamento da hipertensão na doença renal crônica

O melhor desfecho para a terapia anti-hipertensiva ainda não foi estabelecido para cães e gatos com DRC (ver Capítulo 158). Na ausência de tal informação, o tratamento da hipertensão arterial deve ser iniciado com cautela com o objetivo de reduzir a PA para um nível *pelo menos* < 160/100 mmHg. Com exceção em animais com lesões neurológicas oculares ou neurológicas agudas e graves, a redução rápida na PA não é indicada. Cães com hipertensão podem necessitar de diversos ajustes de doses e fármacos, o que leva semanas a meses para atingir o controle satisfatório. Ao contrário, os gatos frequentemente respondem muito mais rápido. A redução da PA é um processo a longo prazo no qual a redução gradativa e sustentada deve ser o objetivo. Reduções súbitas ou graves na PA nunca são indicadas, pois é importante evitar hipotensão clínica. O tratamento deve ser feito passo a passo e ajustes realizados até que o desfecho terapêutico seja atingido (i. e., pressão sistólica < 160 mmHg). Ao mesmo tempo que ainda é incerto se a restrição do Na é efetiva em diminuir a PA em cães ou gatos com hipertensão, uma alteração gradativa para uma dieta com menores níveis de Na é recomendada no momento do início da intervenção farmacológica. Geralmente, evite iniciar a terapia anti-hipertensiva até que a hidratação esteja cuidadosamente restaurada a fim de evitar diminuições abruptas da PA e/ou perfusão renal. Inibidores da ECA, como o enalapril e benazepril, e o amlodipino, um bloqueador dos canais de Ca, são os pilares da terapia anti-hipertensiva em cães e gatos. Estes fármacos podem ter benefícios renoprotetores únicos e são, portanto, opções iniciais apropriadas para o tratamento da hipertensão na DRC.

Fármacos, doses e combinações

O tratamento deve iniciar com um inibidor da ECA fornecido em uma dose-padrão (Tabela 324.3). A dose pode necessitar ser progressivamente aumentada, com recomendação do dobro da dose máxima. Se o objetivo não for atingido apesar dos ajustes da dose, um bloqueador dos canais de Ca (amlodipino) deve ser implementado. Novamente, a dose pode ser aumentada até o dobro da dose máxima, conforme necessário. O BRA e/ou hidralazina podem ser adicionados se os outros fármacos não conseguiram atingir o objetivo. Pessoas tratadas para proteinúria com inibidores da ECA e um BRA, e não apenas com um deles, pode ter risco de desenvolvimento de hiperpotassemia, hipotensão e/ou insuficiência renal.[146] O clínico deve considerar a interrupção do inibidor da ECA antes da adição de um BRA, ou deve monitorar a possibilidade de hiperpotassemia, hipotensão e/ou azotemia progressiva. O tratamento deve começar com o bloqueador dos canais de Ca, o amlodipino. Se a dose inicial não conseguir normalizar a PA, poderá ser gradativamente aumentada para uma dose máxima de 1,25 mg/kg/dia PO. Se o fármaco anti-hipertensivo adicional for necessário, o clínico deve considerar a adição de um inibidor da ECA ao bloqueador dos canais de Ca. O tratamento da hipertensão arterial em geral deve ser feito por toda a vida. Assim que o tratamento conseguir atingir a PA almejada, o monitoramento é essencial para a manutenção do controle. Cães e gatos em terapia anti-hipertensiva devem ser monitorados com uma frequência de pelo menos 3 meses (ver Capítulo 158). A avaliação de lesões retinais secundárias à hipertensão (ver Capítulos 11 e 157) deve ser realizada no momento do monitoramento da PS (ver Capítulo 99). Ao utilizar o esquema médico passo-a-passo descrito, os ajustes da dose são realizados conforme necessidade para manter as PAs < 160/100 mmHg.

Incrementos na concentração sérica de creatinina, PA baixa e sinais clínicos de hipotensão devem motivar a reavaliação dos fármacos anti-hipertensivos e doses. Pequenos aumentos na creatinina sérica que não sejam progressivos podem ocorrer de forma segura com a terapia anti-hipertensiva. Entretanto, aumentos grandes ou progressivos da concentração de creatinina

Tabela 324.3	Fármacos utilizados para tratar a proteinúria e hipertensão em cães e gatos.	
FÁRMACO (MECANISMO)	DOSE INICIAL	ESQUEMA DE ESCALONAMENTO DA DOSE
Benazepril (inibidor da ECA)	0,5 mg/kg PO a cada 24 h	Aumente em 0,5 mg/kg/dia até o máximo de 2 mg/kg/dia
Enalapril (inibidor da ECA)	0,5 mg/kg PO a cada 24 h	Aumente em 0,5 mg/kg/dia até o máximo de 2 mg/kg/dia
Telmisartana (BRA)	1 mg/kg PO a cada 24 h	Aumente em 0,5 mg/kg/dia até o máximo de 2 mg/kg/dia
Losartana (BRA)	0,125 mg/kg/dia PO	0,25 mg/kg/dia em cães azotêmicos 0,5 a 1,0 mg/kg/dia PO em cães não azotêmicos
Amlodipino (BCC) Gatos	< 5 kg: 0,625 mg PO a cada 24 h/gatos ≥ 5 kg: dose inicial de 1,25 mg PO	Dobre a dose se a pressão sanguínea permanecer elevada (dose por gato)
Amlodipino (BCC) Cães	0,1 a 0,3 mg/kg PO a cada 24 h	Pode aumentar a dose até 0,75 mg/kg PO a cada 24 h até que a pressão sanguínea seja reduzida para a pressão almejada (PS sistólica < 160 mmHg)

BCC, bloqueador dos canais de cálcio; BRA, bloqueador do receptor de angiotensina; ECA, enzima conversora de angiotensina.

podem refletir problemas com o fármaco ou dose. Se a PA sistólica declinar persistentemente abaixo de 120 mmHg ou ocorrerem sinais de hipotensão, como fraqueza ou taquicardia, fármacos anti-hipertensivos e doses devem ser ajustados para aumentar a PA e amenizar os sinais clínicos.

Tratamento da anemia da doença renal crônica

Causas

A anemia da DRC pode ter um profundo efeito sobre a qualidade de vida. Até 65% dos gatos desenvolvem anemia conforme a DRC progride.[147] A anemia em animais com DRC frequentemente possui origem multifatorial. A causa primária para anemia é a produção inadequada de EPO. A perda sanguínea iatrogênica e espontânea, malnutrição (incluindo proteína, ferro, folato e talvez outros), inflamação/infecção crônica e redução da duração de vida das hemácias podem complicar e contribuir para a anemia. Coletas excessivas de sangue são preocupantes e devem ser evitadas. A incapacidade em identificar e corrigir estas complicações podem prejudicar os efeitos da reposição hormonal.

A perda sanguínea GI crônica de baixo grau pode causar anemia moderada à grave em animais com DRC que teriam, de outro modo, produção endógena suficiente de EPO para manter suas contagens eritrocitárias e hematócritos (HTs) na faixa subclínica. Esses animais podem ou não ter sinais GI evidentes ou melena. A deficiência de ferro e relações entre BUN e creatinina acima do esperado no contexto da dieta podem fornecer evidências indiretas de perda sanguínea oculta GI. A trombocitose e hemácias hipocrômicas são consistentes com deficiência de ferro e hemorragia GI. Por conta da dificuldade para confirmação da hemorragia GI, uma tentativa terapêutica com antagonistas de receptores H2 histamínicos ou bloqueadores H2 e sucralfato deve ser considerada. Melhoras do hematócrito e/ou apetite suportam o papel da hemorragia GI na origem da anemia. Ao mesmo tempo que as ulcerações gástricas são comuns em cães com DRC, elas não são comuns em gatos, nos quais a gastropatia urêmica parece ser diferente.[42]

Agentes estimulantes de eritrócitos

As formas mais efetivas para correção da anemia da DRC é a utilização de agentes estimulantes de eritrócitos (AEEs) para corrigir a deficiência de EPO na DRC. Excluindo os fatores que prejudicam sua efetividade, a administração de AEEs induz um aumento dose-dependente do HT. Em cães e gatos, o aumento do HT para o nível do limite inferior da faixa normal leva cerca de 2 a 8 semanas, dependendo do HT inicial e dose administrada. Conforme a anemia é corrigida, a maioria dos animais demonstra aumento do apetite, peso corporal, nível de energia e sociabilidade.[148] Os AEEs atualmente disponíveis incluem alfaepoietina, betaepoietina, alfadarbepoietina e ativadores

contínuos de receptores de EPO.[147] As principais diferenças entre esses produtos envolvem o grau de glicosilação. Isso afeta sua depuração renal e, portanto, influencia a duração de ação. A eficácia clínica entre esses produtos é relatada como semelhante em seres humanos. Os AEEs disponíveis são baseados na EPO humana. EPOs caninas e felinas compartilham 81,3 e 83,3% de homologia, respectivamente, com a EPO humana.[147] Esses níveis de homologia permitem que esses fármacos sejam efetivos em estimular substanciais incrementos do HT, tanto em cães como em gatos. Entretanto, durante a evolução da terapia, há risco de desenvolvimento de anticorpos anti-EPO, reconhecidos em cães e gatos, principalmente com a alfaepoietina.

Anticorpos induzidos por agentes estimulantes de eritrócitos

Aproximadamente 25 a 30% dos gatos e até 50% dos cães que recebem epoietina desenvolvem anticorpos anti-EPO neutralizantes; entretanto, nem todos os casos com anticorpos anti-EPO desenvolvem anemia.[148] Esses anticorpos reagem de forma cruzada com todos os AEEs, incluindo a EPO endógena do animal. O desenvolvimento de anticorpos anti-EPO pode suprimir de forma acentuada a eritropoese e resultar em aplasia pura de hemácias (APHs; ver Capítulo 199). Vários animais com APH se tornam dependentes de transfusão, embora se viverem por tempo suficiente, podem retornar a resposta à EPO endógena ao normal. Embora estudos controlados sobre o desenvolvimento de anticorpos direcionados ao AEE darbepoietina não estejam disponíveis, parece que esse produto é muito menos imunogênico quando comparado à R-HuEPO®.[149,150] É sugerido que a meia-vida mais longa da darbepoietina pode reduzir a carga de antígenos administrada comparada à R-HuEPO®, reduzindo assim o risco de formação de anticorpos.[147]

Outros efeitos adversos relacionados à eritropoetina

Ao mesmo tempo que o desenvolvimento de anticorpos anti-EPO é a reação adversa mais importante ligada aos AEEs, outros efeitos relatados em cães e gatos incluem hipertensão sistêmica, convulsões, reações nos locais de administração, êmese e febre.[148,149] A hipertensão pode ocorrer ou piorar por causa do aumento da resistência vascular periférica secundário ao aumento do fornecimento de oxigênio e reversão da vasodilatação induzida pela hipoxia crônica.

O aumento da viscosidade sanguínea graças ao aumento do HT supostamente é discreto. Convulsões, relatadas em cães e gatos tratados com rHuEPO, não são diretamente causadas por AEEs, mas estão sim relacionadas a adaptações compensatórias a aumentos na massa de hemácias.[148] Reações alérgicas incluindo reações cutâneas ou mucocutâneas, ou celulite, algumas fezes com febre e artralgia ocasionalmente ocorrem em cães e gatos no início da terapia com EPO.[148] Lesões geralmente são resolvidas dentro de alguns dias e a maioria não recidiva quando a terapia é reiniciada.

rHuEPO® versus darbepoietina

AEEs são indicados em cães e gatos com: (1) DRC avançada (estágios III e IV de DRC pela IRIS), (2) valores de HT abaixo de 22%, e (3) aqueles com sinais clínicos atribuídos à anemia: taquipneia, taquicardia, fraqueza e anorexia. Ao mesmo tempo que tanto o rHuEPO® como darbepoietina estão disponíveis, a darbepoietina é preferida para cães e gatos. As vantagens da darbepoietina sobre a epoietina incluem riscos aparentemente inferiores de formação de anticorpos anti-EPO e administração semanal. Um estudo relatou 56% (14/25) de gatos submetidos ao tratamento com darbepoietina que atingiram o HT almejado (25%). Os gatos que atingiram esse nível almejado sobreviveram por um tempo significativamente maior do que gatos que não responderam (média de 238 dias para os que responderam; 83 dias para os não sobreviventes).[149] Em outro estudo, sete de sete gatos com DRC atingiram o HT almejado (30%), e nenhum teve evidências de formação de anticorpos anti-EPO.[150]

Protocolo da darbepoietina

A darbepoietina é inicialmente administrada por via subcutânea (1 mcg/kg, semanalmente) e mantida até que o HT do animal atinja o limite inferior do valor de referência (gatos: 25 a 35%; cães: 37 a 42%). Assim que atingido, a dose de darbepoietina é reduzida em 20 a 25% ou a frequência da administração é diminuída para cada 2 semanas. A dose de manutenção pode então ser ajustada mensalmente, conforme necessário, para manter o HT dentro da faixa almejada. Como doses excessivas de AEE foram ligadas a resultados adversos em seres humanos, é recomendado que HTs anormalmente altos sejam evitados.[151] Inicialmente, as avaliações de exame físico e PA (ver Capítulo 99) devem ser realizadas semanalmente até que o HT almejado seja atingido e então mantidas mensalmente. Em geral, o HT aumenta cerca de 1 a 3% semanalmente; taxas mais rápidas de aumento devem ser evitadas por conta de uma associação com a hipertensão. Assim que estável, reavaliações devem ser conduzidas a cada 1 a 3 meses. É essencial que avaliações regulares de acompanhamento sejam mantidas enquanto continuar a terapia com darbepoietina.

Deficiência de ferro

Vários cães e gatos com DRC avançada possuem deficiência de ferro (Fe). O aumento do número de hemácias requer ferro, que deve ser administrado no início da terapia com AEE. Ao mesmo tempo que o Fe pode ser suplementado VO, é difícil fornecer quantidades adequadas sem causar complicações GI. Portanto, o Fe dextrana (50 mg/gato; 50 a 300 mg/cão) deve ser fornecido por injeções. Embora rato, o Fe dextrana pode causar uma reação anafilática, de forma que é prudente informar os tutores sobre essa possibilidade e observar o animal por um período de tempo após a administração. Se necessário, a dose de Fe pode ser repetida mensalmente.

Diversas causas de respostas discretas ou incapacidade de resolver a anemia com a terapia por AEE foram identificadas: deficiência de Fe, perdas contínuas GI, hemólise, doença inflamatória ou maligna concorrente, e sobrecarga de alumínio. Erros de tutores relacionados ao armazenamento do fármaco, manuseio ou administração podem causar respostas inadequadas. Se a anemia for corrigida com terapia por AEE, mas os valores de HT declinarem novamente, o desenvolvimento de anticorpos anti-EPO deve ser também considerado. A abordagem diagnóstica para a falha do tratamento com AEE deve considerar o histórico de administração de fármacos, exame físico, hemograma, perfil bioquímico sérico, cobalamina sérica e painel do Fe (Fe sérico, ferritina e saturação da transferrina), biopsia de medula óssea e exames de imagem (evidências de doenças infecciosas ou neoplásicas). Quando esses testes não conseguem identificar uma causa para a falha do tratamento em cães e gatos que inicialmente responderam à terapia com AEE, deve haver a suspeita de formação de anticorpos anti-EPO e a terapia com AEE deve ser interrompida.[104] Com exceção de um teste de anticorpos anti-EPO, as relações entre linhagens mieloide e eritroide da medula óssea podem fornecer o melhor método para determinar se a resistência ocorreu devido à formação de anticorpos. Quando a EPO é interrompida precocemente, os títulos de anticorpos podem declinar e a eritropoese suprimida pode ser revertida.

Terapia com calcitriol

Razão

O calcitriol (1,25-di-hidroxivitamina D), o metabólito mais ativo da vitamina D, resulta da hidroxilação renal da 25-hidroxivitamina D. Ele aumenta a captação GI de Ca e PO_4, inibe a síntese e secreção de PTH, suprime o crescimento da glândula paratireoide e ativa receptores celulares. Causas possíveis de redução dos níveis de calcitriol na DRC incluem retenção de PO_4, aumento dos níveis de FGF-23 e redução da massa renal. A retenção de PO_4 e hiperfosfatemia reduzem a produção de calcitriol pela inibição da atividade da alfa-1-hidroxilase renal, que converte o 25-hidroxicolecalciferol em calcitriol.[59] Conforme a DRC progride, a redução da massa renal limita ainda mais o número de células disponíveis para realizar a hidroxilação da 25-hidroxivitamina D. A terapia com calcitriol demonstrou reduzir os níveis de PTH em cães e gatos com DRC.[57,36] Embora o PTH tenha sido considerado como uma toxina urêmica responsável por vários sinais constitucionais ou uremia, os benefícios clínicos da redução de PTH não foram ainda conclusivamente documentados.[52,152] Os resultados de um estudo clínico indicaram que o calcitriol reduziu a mortalidade em cães com DRC nos estágios III e IV pelo retardo da progressão da DRC.[36] Pessoas com DRC tiveram benefícios semelhantes relacionados à sobrevida após serem tratados com calcitriol.[153] Entretanto, um estudo clínico semelhante em gatos revelou benefícios ambíguos para o calcitriol em relação à alteração da evolução da DRC. Nenhum estudo pode confirmar ou refutar a melhora relacionada ao fármaco proposta pelos sinais clínicos.

Diretrizes do tratamento

A terapia com calcitriol (2 a 3 ng/kg PO a cada 24 h) é indicada para cães com DRC nos estágios III e IV, e possivelmente naqueles em estágio II da DRC para retardar a deterioração progressiva da função renal, mas sua utilização em gatos permanece especulativa. Antes de administrar o calcitriol, nem o PO_4 sérico ou o iCa devem estar aumentados, já que o calcitriol aumenta a absorção GI de ambos. Ambos devem ser monitorados durante a terapia a fim de evitar a hiperfosfatemia e hipercalcemia ionizada. É incerto se cálculos renais que contenham Ca constituam uma contraindicação relativa à terapia com calcitriol. O tratamento por toda a vida é necessário para atingir o efeito desejado de redução da mortalidade renal. Como ele aumenta a absorção GI de Ca e PO_4, o calcitriol não deve ser administrado com refeições. O fornecimento do calcitriol durante a noite com estômago vazio reduz o risco de indução de hipercalcemia. Uma farmácia de manipulação é necessária para preparar formulações que podem ser utilizadas em cães e gatos, tendo em vista que a formulação humana é muito forte.

Superdosagem

A dose excessiva de calcitriol é perigosa e deve ser evitada devido à indução de hipercalcemia com possível lesão renal (nefropatia hipercalcêmica). A detecção precoce da hipercalcemia, se ocorrer, é indicada para limitar a extensão da lesão renal. Entretanto, a hipercalcemia após administração de vitamina D é imprevisível (i. e., pode ocorrer após dias a meses de tratamento). Portanto, o monitoramento contínuo das concentrações séricas de Ca, PO_4 e creatinina após 2, 5 e 8 semanas é necessário para detectar hiperCa, hiperPO$_4$, ou deterioração da função renal antes da ocorrência de dano renal irreversível. A hipercalcemia mais provavelmente ocorrerá quando a terapia com calcitriol for combinada com agentes quelantes de PO_4 que contenham Ca, particularmente o carbonato de Ca. Se as concentrações de PO_4 e iCa permanecerem bem controladas após 8 semanas de terapia com calcitriol, o monitoramento deve continuar a cada 1 a 2 meses. O produto das concentrações séricas de tCa × PO_4 não deve exceder 60; o objetivo é manter valores entre 42 e 52.[69]

O início de ação rápido do calcitriol (cerca de um dia) e curta duração de ação (meia-vida menor que um dia) permite o rápido controle da hipercalcemia indesejada pela sua interrupção completa. A terapia pode ser reinstituída com uma dose ou frequência de administração menores após as concentrações séricas de Ca e PO_4 voltarem aos níveis almejados. Quando a terapia com calcitriol for associada à hipercalcemia, a dose diária pode ser dobrada e administrada em dias alternados. Essa abordagem pode ser mais segura porque o efeito do calcitriol sobre o trato GI está relacionado à duração da exposição celular ao calcitriol. Quando a concentração plasmática de PTH estiver acentuadamente elevada ou quando a terapia padronizada com calcitriol não conseguir normalizar os níveis plasmáticos de PTH, a terapia em pulso com calcitriol é recomendada.[52] Nessa abordagem, os animais recebem 20 ng/kg de calcitriol PO 2 vezes/semana durante a noite com estômago vazio. A terapia em pulso é em geral utilizada por até 1 a 2 meses para suprimir a resistência do HPSR. Se obtiver sucesso, o calcitriol é então administrado em uma dose diária padronizada. Enquanto o calcitriol é efetivo em diminuir o PTH, a importância da mensuração das concentrações de PTH durante a terapia com calcitriol é incerta e os benefícios clínicos da supressão do HPSR permanecem sem comprovação. No estudo canino que confirmou os benefícios de sobrevida após a terapia com calcitriol, as doses foram aumentadas em até 5 ng/kg/dia (média: 1,9 ng/kg/dia) para diminuir os valores de PTH até a faixa normal, a menos que a hipercalcemia tenha ocorrido. Se ocorreu hipercalcemia, a dose de calcitriol foi reduzida.

Como minimizar a progressão da doença renal crônica

Todos os animais com DRC possuem risco de progressão da doença como consequência da doença renal primária, em associação a uma série de fatores secundários que podem promover doença renal progressiva, ou ambos. Um importante objetivo terapêutico para o tratamento de pacientes com DRC é minimizar ou prevenir a perda progressiva da função renal. O tratamento desenvolvido para limitar a progressão da doença renal pode envolver uma série de intervenções que incluem terapia dietética, minimização da proteinúria, controle da hipertensão e terapia com calcitriol. Uma hipótese recente propõe que a pressão sanguínea, proteinúria e fosfato podem de fato estar ligados aos seus efeitos sobre a progressão da DRC através, em parte, do sistema FGF-23/klotho e deficiência de calcitriol.[154] A efetividade da terapia dietética em prolongar a sobrevida de cães e gatos com DRC foi descrita. As dietas renais são claramente indicadas para cães com DRC em estágios III e IV, e em gatos com DRC em estágios II a IV. A proteinúria e hipertensão são fatores de risco bem estabelecidos para progressão da doença renal em seres humanos.[55,156] Estudos clínicos confirmaram que a proteinúria é um fator de risco para o aumento da mortalidade em cães e gatos.[25,31] Em cães, foi observado que o risco de um evento adverso (crise urêmica ou morte) aumenta em 1,5 vezes para cada 1 unidade de incremento da RUPC acima de 1,0.[31] A PA elevada foi relatada como um fator de risco para o aumento da mortalidade em cães, mas não em gatos.[31,144]

Tratamentos desenvolvidos para limitar a proteinúria e hipertensão demonstraram serem importantes para retardo da progressão da DRC em seres humanos. A evidência em cães e gatos é semelhante, embora de certa forma menos convincente. Em cães

com glomerulopatia, o tratamento com o inibidor da ECA enalapril reduziu de forma significativa a proteinúria, mas a duração do estudo foi muito breve para avaliar de forma adequada o valor renoprotetor da terapia.[157] Entretanto, em um estudo que examinou os efeitos do enalapril em cães Samoieda com nefrite hereditária, os cães tratados sobreviveram 1,36 vezes mais que cães não tratados. Em gatos com valores de RUPC maiores que 1,0, o tratamento com benazepril parecer estar associado a maiores tempos de sobrevida, embora o efeito não tenha atingido significância estatística. Em gatos com valores de RUPC menores que 1,0, os dados foram controversos.[26] Esse último achado é consistente com observações em seres humanos que sugerem que a magnitude dos benefícios obtidos pelos inibidores da ECA é proporcional à magnitude da redução na proteinúria.

O grupo de consenso sobre proteinúria da ACVIM sugeriu iniciar esforços com relação à redução da proteinúria glomerular em cães e gatos com estágios I a IV de DRC.[50] A intervenção terapêutica é indicada quando a RUPC for maior que 2,0 em cães e gatos com DRC em estágio I, e quando exceder 0,5 em cães e 0,4 em gatos com DRC em estágios II a IV. Agora é bem estabelecido em pessoas que a redução terapêutica da proteinúria pela supressão do SRAA ameniza os efeitos adversos da proteinúria sobre os rins. Evidências experimentais e clínicas confirmaram os efeitos benéficos do controle da PS em retardar a progressão de nefropatias diabéticas e não diabéticas em seres humanos.[155,158] Em um grande estudo clínico, o efeito renoprotetor da terapia anti-hipertensiva foi aumentado ainda mais pela manutenção da PA abaixo do valor almejado usual.[159] Como consequência, a PA "ideal" a ser obtida utilizando terapia anti-hipertensiva em pessoas com DRC depende das características clínicas do paciente. Fatores, como a presença ou ausência de proteinúria podem influenciar os objetivos da terapia. A terapia anti-hipertensiva foi mais efetiva em limitar a progressão da doença renal em pacientes com proteinúria. A maior redução da PA parece ser necessária para renoproteção equivalente com maiores níveis e proteinúria.[155,159] Estudos realizados em cães com DRC induzida indicam que a administração do inibidor da ECA enalapril limitou a hipertensão glomerular e sistêmica, proteinúria e lesões glomerulares e tubulointersticiais.[160] De forma interessante, o enalapril foi renoprotetor nesse estudo apesar do fato de que cães tinham somente hipertensão discreta e proteinúria relativamente modesta.

Os efeitos renoprotetores de inibidores da ECA não podem ser explicados inteiramente pelos seus efeitos somente sobre a pressão sanguínea. É provável que a renoproteção resulte em parte da supressão dos níveis renais de angiotensina II. Por conta do papel da angiotensina II na progressão da DRC, os bloqueadores de receptores de angiotensina também têm sido considerados para humanos com DRC.[161] Os bloqueadores de receptores de angiotensina e inibidores da ECA diferem no mecanismo pelo qual eles inibem a angiotensina II. Os inibidores da ECA bloqueiam a conversão de angiotensina I em angiotensina II. Entretanto, a formação de angiotensina II não é completamente inibida porque também ela pode ser gerada por uma via não dependente da ECA, como pela enzima quimase. Além disso, como a bradicinina é normalmente degradada pela ECA, a terapia com inibidores da ECA está associada a níveis elevados de bradicinina. A bradicinina é um vasodilatador que pode ter efeitos renoprotetores pela estimulação da produção de óxido nítrico. Os antagonistas de receptores de angiotensina bloqueiam o receptor tipo 1, mas deixam os efeitos sobre os receptores tipo 2 sem oposição, o que parece ser importante na vasodilatação. Em ratos com nefropatia, foi relatado que o antagonismo à angiotensina II normaliza a proteinúria, elimina a infiltração de células inflamatórias e ameniza as alterações estruturais glomerulares e tubulares.[162] Uma combinação de um antagonista de receptores de angiotensina e um inibidor da ECA foi sugerida como uma forma de maximizar o bloqueio do sistema renina-angiotensina por afetar tanto a biodisponibilidade da angiotensina II e por afetar sua atividade a nível do receptor.[163]

Cada tipo de fármaco demonstrou ser efetivo em reduzir a proteinúria e retardar a progressão da doença renal. Entretanto, em modelos experimentais e clínicos em seres humanos, a terapia de combinação demonstrou ser mais efetiva do que qualquer medicamento único.[161] Em seres humanos, não parece haver aumento em eventos de intoxicações ou adversos em casos de terapia de combinação.[158] Ainda precisa ser determinado para cães e gatos com DRC se a terapia de combinação é segura, efetiva e se fornece uma vantagem terapêutica. Entretanto, o bloqueador do receptor II de angiotensina losartana pode não atingir níveis sanguíneos efetivos, possivelmente devido à conversão inadequada para o metabólito ativo.[164] Não é sabido se o mesmo é verdadeiro para o irbesartana, mas doses recomendadas de irbesartana são muito maiores do que as recomendadas para seres humanos, sugerindo um problema potencial com relação à conversão desse fármaco também. O bloqueio do sistema renina-angiotensina limita tanto a angiotensina II como a aldosterona enquanto retarda a progressão da doença renal. Estudos recentes implicaram a aldosterona como um importante fator patogênico nesse processo.[165,166] O bloqueio seletivo da aldosterona, independente do bloqueio da renina-angiotensina, reduz a proteinúria e lesões glomerulares em gatos com doença renal experimental. Quando o bloqueio da SRAA ameniza a proteinúria e lesão glomerular, a reinfusão seletiva da aldosterona restaura a proteinúria e lesões glomerulares apesar do bloqueio mantido. Essa observação sugere um papel patogênico independente para a aldosterona como um mediador de doença renal progressiva. A aldosterona parece promover lesão renal progressiva por meio de efeitos hemodinâmicos e ações celulares diretas.[165] Parece possuir propriedades fibrogênicas nos rins, talvez em parte por promover a produção da citocina pró-fibrótica fator transformador de crescimento-beta (TGF-beta).[166] Estudos experimentais demonstraram que a eplerenona, um antagonista de receptores de aldosterona, pode atenuar a proteinúria e dano renal, independentemente de seu efeito sobre a pressão sanguínea. Ao mesmo tempo que inibidores da ECA inicialmente causam uma redução aguda na concentração de aldosterona, esse efeito não é sustentado. Foi proposto que a utilização de antagonistas de receptores de aldosterona em adição a inibidores de ECA terá benefícios adicionais ao proteger os rins.[165] Entretanto, o papel dessa forma de terapia ainda tem de ser estabelecido em cães e gatos. Conforme descrito acima, o calcitriol parece ter efeitos

renoprotetores em cães. Também foi relatado como renoprotetor em humanos com DRC. Os mecanismos de renoproteção ainda não foram completamente elucidados, mas podem incluir a ativação de receptores de vitamina D em diversos tecidos no organismo, melhora na viabilidade de podócitos, supressão do HPSR e supressão do SRAA.[117,153,167,168]

MONITORAMENTO DO PACIENTE

A resposta ao tratamento deve ser monitorada em intervalos apropriados de forma que o tratamento possa ser individualizado para necessidades específicas, e frequentemente variáveis do paciente. A base de dados obtida antes do início da terapia ou após correção de uma crise urêmica evidente deve ser utilizada como base para comparação do progresso do paciente. Essa avaliação deve ser repetida em intervalos apropriados. De forma geral, as avaliações a cada 2 a 4 semanas são sugeridas até que a resposta inicial à terapia possa ser estabelecida. Entretanto, a frequência de avaliação pode variar dependendo da gravidade da disfunção renal, complicações presentes no paciente, tratamentos aplicados e resposta ao tratamento. Pacientes que recebem terapia com EPO ou calcitriol necessitam de monitoramento frequente durante toda a vida. Após a resposta inicial à terapia, se houver, ter sido estabelecida, cães e gatos com DRC em estágio I podem necessitar de avaliação infrequentemente, a cada 6 a 12 meses, dependendo da natureza da doença. Por exemplo, cães em estágio I com proteinúria substancial podem necessitar de monitoramento muito mais frequente dependendo da evolução da doença. Gatos com DRC em estágio II tipicamente devem ser monitorados a cada 3 a 6 meses. Cães com DRC em estágio II, e cães e gatos com DRC em estágio III devem ser reavaliados a cada 2 a 4 meses, dependendo da estabilidade da função renal. Recomendações específicas para o monitoramento são descritas nas diversas seções sobre tratamento.

REFERÊNCIAS BIBLIOGRÁFICAS

As referências bibliográficas deste capítulo se encontram online no Ambiente de aprendizagem.

CAPÍTULO 325

Glomerulopatias

Shelly L. Vaden

Glomerulopatias são uma causa importante de doença renal em cães.[1] Em cães randomicamente selecionados, a prevalência de lesões glomerulares vai de 43 a 90%,[2] e a prevalência parece aumentar com a idade.[3] Glomerulopatias também ocorrem em gatos, embora sejam menos comuns. A glomerulonefrite por imunocomplexos (GNIC), amiloidose e glomeruloesclerose são consideradas como as doenças glomerulares mais comuns de cães, correspondendo a cerca de 84% das lesões descritas em um relato recente de 501 cães com doença glomerular (Boxe 325.1).[4] Foi feito progresso na tentativa de desenvolver uma compreensão mais profunda das diferentes apresentações clínicas das várias doenças glomerulares que ocorrem em cães; poucos estudos foram realizados em gatos.

As recomendações do consenso foram publicadas com relação à abordagem ao diagnóstico, terapia-padrão e tratamento imunossupressores para cães com suspeita de glomerulopatia.[5-9]

ESTRUTURA E FUNÇÃO GLOMERULAR NORMAL

O glomérulo é um leito capilar modificado que funciona como um filtro, através do qual um ultrafiltrado do plasma é formado.[10,11] A barreira de filtração é composta por três camadas: o endotélio fenestrado, membrana basal glomerular (MBG) e células epiteliais viscerais, ou podócitos (Figura 325.1). Diafragmas em fendas são junções celulares especializadas presentes

Boxe 325.1 Doenças glomerulares descritas em cães e gatos

Glomerulonefrite por imunocomplexos (GNIC)
  Membranosa*
  Membranoproliferativa
  Nefrite por lúpus
  Proliferativa (rara)
  Tipo crescente (rara)
  Nefropatia por IgA (rara)
Glomeruloesclerose
  Glomeruloesclerose segmentar focal
  Glomeruloesclerose global
Amiloidose
Nefrite hereditária
Glomerulopatia por alteração mínima (rara)

*Glomerulopatia membranosa é a doença glomerular mais comum em gatos; outras glomerulopatias parecem incomuns.

entre os podócitos que conectam as fendas de filtração. O filtrado passa através das fenestrações endoteliais, permeia a MBG e então passa através das fendas de filtração das células epiteliais e para o espaço urinário.[12] Essa estrutura complexa é livremente permeável à água e pequenos solutos dissolvidos, mas retém células e a maioria das macromoléculas, como proteínas. O principal determinante de passagem para o filtrado é o tamanho molecular; a carga iônica pode ter menor importância. As fendas epiteliais provavelmente fornecem resistência ao fluxo do líquido, enquanto a MBG é provavelmente o determinante primário da barreira seletiva ao tamanho por atuar como um gel modificado através do qual macromoléculas passam.[13] Pequenas moléculas, como a inulina (5.000 Daltons), passam livremente através do filtro. Substâncias são retidas com maior eficiência conforme possuem maior tamanho até aproximadamente 60 mil a 70 mil Daltons; somente pequenas quantidades de substâncias maiores do que isso são filtradas. A albumina, uma proteína carregada negativamente, com um peso molecular de 69 mil Daltons, é normalmente amplamente excluída do filtrado. No final, a albumina é impedida de passar para o filtrado. Por muito tempo se acreditou que a carga iônica também influencia a filtração, e que proteínas carregadas negativamente são retidas em maior extensão do que seria previsto somente pelo tamanho.[14] Os processos podais dos podócitos e os diafragmas em fenda entre eles, assim como a membrana basal e o endotélio, são ricos em glicoproteínas carregadas negativamente,

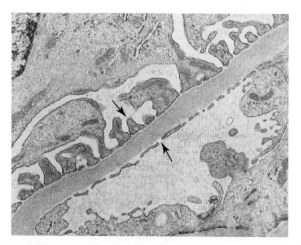

Figura 325.1 Micrografia eletrônica de uma parede capilar glomerular demonstrando a barreira de filtração composta por endotélio fenestrado, a membrana basal glomerular e a célula epitelial visceral (podócito). (Cortesia de J.C. Jennette, School of Medicine, University of North Carolina, Chapel Hill, NC.)

criando essa barreira de cargas. Esses poliânions supostamente possuem um importante papel na manutenção da permeabilidade glomerular normal e formato das células epiteliais viscerais. Apesar desse sistema de filtração complexo, pequenas quantidades de albumina e outras proteínas são normalmente observadas no filtrado. A degradação substancial dessas proteínas ocorre, resultando em excreção somente de fragmentos peptídios, que não são detectados por testes de proteína total rotineiros. Proteínas e fragmentos de peptídios podem também sofrer reabsorção no néfron distal até o glomérulo.[14]

ACHADOS CLÍNICOS

Epidemiologia

As glomerulopatias podem ocorrer em qualquer idade, mas parecem ser mais comuns em cães de meia-idade a idosos. A prevalência da microalbuminúria, um marcador de aumento da permeabilidade glomerular, aumenta conforme o cão envelhece, com aumentos mais acentuados observados além dos 6 anos.[15] A idade média de 375 cães com uma série de glomerulopatias relatadas em cinco estudos foi de 8,3 anos.[1,16-19] Cães com síndrome nefrótica (SN) podem ser acometidos com uma idade mais jovem (média de 6,2 anos).[20] Cães machos e fêmeas foram igualmente representados. Entretanto, a idade média e a predileção sexual observada em casos de glomerulopatias específicas variam de certa forma das medidas gerais. As doenças glomerulares frequentemente ocorrem secundariamente a outro processo mórbido. Doenças inflamatórias infecciosas e não infecciosas podem mais provavelmente acometer animais jovens e de meia-idade, enquanto neoplasias são mais comuns conforme os cães se tornam idosos. Doenças glomerulares familiares geralmente são manifestadas em uma idade mais jovem. Diversas raças de cães sabidamente possuem doenças glomerulares familiares (Tabela 325.1); várias dessas podem ter uma maior incidência de doenças glomerulares; entretanto, a possibilidade que essa maior representação reflita a popularidade dessas raças requer maior avaliação.[16,21]

Histórico clínico

Os sinais clínicos associados a glomerulopatias variam consideravelmente, dependendo da gravidade da proteinúria e da presença ou ausência de azotemia renal.[16,17,22] Vários animais com glomerulopatias são assintomáticos, e a proteinúria é detectada durante os exames de rotina. De forma alternativa, os animais podem manifestar sinais específicos relacionados à condição inflamatória, infecciosa ou neoplásica de base. Sinais de glomerulopatias podem ser inespecíficos (p. ex., perda de peso, letargia) ou consistentes com doença renal crônica ou uremia (poliúria, polidipsia, anorexia, êmese e halitose). A lesão renal aguda não é uma apresentação comum em animais com doença glomerular, mas ocorre em algumas ocasiões. Quando as perdas urinárias de proteína são graves, sinais de retenção de fluido (p. ex., aumento abdominal consistente com ascite, edema periférico) ou tromboembolismo (p. ex., dispneia, perda de função do membro) podem estar presentes. O dano hipertensivo ao sistema nervoso central (ver Capítulo 260), olhos (ver Capítulo 11), ou coração pode induzir uma série de sinais clínicos (ver Capítulo 157).

Achados de exame físico

O exame físico (ver Capítulo 2) é geralmente irretocável em cães com doença glomerular.[16,17,22] Evidências inespecíficas de doença sistêmica podem estar presentes (p. ex., má condição corporal ou pelame de má qualidade). Cães com doença renal avançada podem ter ulcerações orais, membranas mucosas pálidas ou desidratação. O edema subcutâneo ou ascite, ou ambos, são algumas vezes notados (ver capítulo18). Ocasionalmente, cães possuem evidências físicas de doença tromboembólica, como dispneia ou

Tabela 325.1	Lista de raças de cães e gatos com glomerulopatias familiares.
RAÇA	**GLOMERULOPATIA**
Gato Abissínio	Glomerulopatia proliferativa focal
Beagle	Amiloidose
Bernese Montanhês	Glomerulonefrite mesângio-capilar
Bullmastiff	Glomerulopatia
Bull Terrier	Nefrite hereditária
Cocker Spaniel (especialmente Inglês)	Nefrite hereditária
Dálmata	Nefrite hereditária
Doberman Pinscher	Glomeruloesclerose, atrofia glomerular cística
Foxhound Inglês	Amiloidose
Dogue de Bordeaux	Glomerulopatia juvenil progressiva
Greyhound	Vasculopatia glomerular e necrose
Terranova	Glomeruloesclerose
Welsh Corgi	Glomeruloesclerose, atrofia glomerular cística
Rottweiler	Glomerulopatia atrófica
Samoieda (raro)	Nefrite hereditária
Sharpei	Amiloidose
Soft Coaten Wheaten Terrier	Podocitopatia

diminuição do pulso periférico (ver Capítulo 256). Evidências de um processo predisponente inflamatório, infeccioso ou neoplásico podem ser detectadas durante o exame físico. Os rins dos animais afetados possuem tamanho variável. Animais com doença renal crônica geralmente têm rins pequenos, firmes e de formato irregular (ver Capítulo 324), enquanto aqueles com doenças de duração mais curta frequentemente possuem rins de tamanho normais ou ocasionalmente aumentados (ver Capítulo 322).

Achados clinicopatológicos e de imagem

A proteinúria é a principal característica da doença glomerular e é discutida no Capítulo 72. A avaliação minuciosa da proteinúria inclui a localização da fonte e avaliação da persistência e magnitude.[5] Uma relação proteína:creatinina urinária (RUPC) maior que 0,5 ou 0,4 em um cão ou gato, respectivamente, é anormal em uma amostra de urina livre de inflamação ou descoloração por hematúria (ou > 150 hemácias/ campo). Não existe um número mágico ou intervalo de números para a RUPC que seja diagnóstica para qualquer doença renal; a sobreposição nos intervalos esperados é muito ampla para ser clinicamente confiável.[23] Entretanto, quanto maior a magnitude da proteinúria, conforme avaliada pela RUPC, maior a probabilidade do animal ter doença glomerular. Em três estudos de albumina urinária em modelos caninos de doença glomerular, a microalbuminúria foi detectada antes de aumentos na RUPC, e a magnitude da microalbuminúria aumentou com o passar do tempo em cães que eventualmente desenvolveram RUPC aumentada.[24-26] Um cão com microalbuminúria persistente de magnitude crescente deve ser avaliado como um portador de um processo lesivo à barreira de

filtração glomerular e pode eventualmente desenvolver proteinúria evidente. Lesões glomerulares também foram identificadas em cães sem proteinúria.[27-29]

Isostenúria é um achado variável em cães e gatos com glomerulopatia. A presença de azotemia renal e uma capacidade de concentração intacta é indicativa de doença glomerular. Em um estudo, 37% dos cães com glomerulonefrite (GN) tinham densidades urinárias específicas acima de 1,035, e a isostenúria foi detectada somente em 29%.[17] Entretanto, em cães com amiloidose, a urina diluída (i. e. uma densidade urinária específica menor que 1,016) foi mais comum, ocorrendo em 63% comparados a somente 5,1% que demonstraram evidências de capacidade de concentração acima de 1,035.[22] A cilindrúria é comum em cães com glomerulopatia; cilindros são mais frequentemente hialinos, mas podem ser granulosos, céreos ou gordurosos (ver Capítulo 72). A proteinúria promove a precipitação da mucoproteína de Tamm-Horsfall, que por sua vez envelopa a proteína no lúmen tubular em um cilindro hialino, protegendo assim o epitélio tubular renal dos efeitos danosos das proteínas. Os cilindros granulares e céreos formam em casos de degeneração progressiva dos cilindros celulares, que são o resultado de células epiteliais tubulares danificadas. A hematúria renal ocorre por lesão glomerular em seres humanos e é mais comum em doenças específicas (p. ex., nefropatia por IgA, glomerulonefrite proliferativa mesangial), mas parece ser menos comum em cães com glomerulopatias.[11] Eritrócitos que passaram através do leito capilar glomerular anormal são frequentemente disformes; a morfologia de eritrócitos da urina pode ser utilizada para diferenciar a hematúria de origem glomerular daquela resultante de outras causas.

A hipoproteinemia causada por hipoalbuminemia ocorre em vários cães e gatos com glomerulopatia e é mais provável acometer animais com proteinúria grave. A hipoalbuminemia ocorreu em 60 e 70% dos cães com GN ou amiloidose, respectivamente.[17,22] Azotemia, hiperfosfatemia e acidose metabólica, consistentes com insuficiência renal, podem estar presentes em cães com doença grave. Dos cães com GN ou amiloidose, 53 e 26%, respectivamente, não estavam azotêmicos no momento do diagnóstico.[17,22] Anemia arregenerativa que ocorre secundariamente à doença renal crônica ou doença sistêmica é observada em vários animais afetados. Outras anormalidades hematológicas também podem refletir doenças sistêmicas concorrentes e possivelmente subjacentes. A trombocitose e hiperfibrinogenemia são achados comuns em cães com doença glomerular.

A síndrome nefrótica (SN) de hipoalbuminemia, proteinúria, hipercolesterolemia e edema, embora patognomônica de glomerulopatia, estava presente em somente 15% dos cães com GN em um estudo.[17] A SN incompleta (i. e., sem edema ou ascite) foi mais comum, ocorrendo em 49% dos cães.[17] É esperado que a SN ocorra mais comumente em doenças de cães associadas à proteinúria marcante, mas não foi associada a qualquer diagnóstico histológico em um estudo.[20]

A **síndrome nefrítica** é um termo que tem sido primariamente utilizado para descrever um conjunto de sinais que ocorrem secundariamente à inflamação renal, geralmente aguda, que se estende ao glomérulo. Em pessoas, essa síndrome é caracterizada por hematúria e cilindros hemáticos com um ou mais dos sinais seguintes: proteinúria subnefrótica, edema, hipertensão, azotemia e oligúria. Embora a síndrome nefrítica ainda não tenha sido completamente descrita em cães, talvez por conta da provável baixa prevalência de glomerulonefrites agudas em cães, é possível que cães com nefrite aguda por doença de Lyme possam ter uma síndrome "nefrítica-like" (ver Capítulo 211).

Em radiografias, os rins podem parecer normais ou pequenos e irregulares; alguns animais podem ter rins aumentados. Alterações semelhantes no formato e tamanho podem ser observadas com exames ultrassonográficos; o aumento da ecogenicidade do córtex e a perda da distinção corticomedular podem também ser notadas. A pelve renal pode estar discretamente dilatada se houver poliúria ou se estiverem sendo administrados fluidos.

As recomendações do consenso afirmam que a avaliação diagnóstica deve ser mais extensa para um cão com RUPC acima de 3,5 e/ou mais anormalidades clínicas como resultado de lesão glomerular para um cão com somente proteinúria discreta.[5] Uma avaliação extensa incluiria exames que facilitariam a detecção de doenças infecciosas, inflamatórias ou neoplasias subjacentes. Uma avaliação física minuciosa deve ser realizada; doenças da cavidade oral ou pele não devem ser subestimadas como potenciais distúrbios subjacentes (ver Capítulos 10 e 272). A citologia aspirativa deve ser realizada em todas as massas cutâneas e subcutâneas (ver Capítulo 86). Os exames sorológicos para doenças infecciosas regionais devem ser realizados. A avaliação poderia incluir exames para autoanticorpos (p. ex., anticorpo antinuclear, ANA) em animais com anormalidades extrarrenais (p. ex., trombocitopenia, poliartrite; ver Capítulo 205). Durante a avaliação radiográfica ou ultrassonográficas do abdome, deve ser dada atenção para outros órgãos a fim de detectar processos mórbidos extrarrenais (ver Capítulo 88). Radiografias torácicas, particularmente em cães de meia-idade a idosos, devem ser avaliados em busca de qualquer evidência de doenças neoplásicas.

Biopsia renal e diagnósticos histológicos

A biopsia renal fornece um diagnóstico definitivo de doença glomerular, mas pode não ser necessária se o tratamento de uma doença potencial subjacente leva à resolução da proteinúria e uma doença renal em estágio terminal já ocorre. Quando avaliada apropriadamente, os espécimes de biopsia renal podem fornecer informações clínicas importantes sobre o tipo e gravidade de lesões em cães e gatos com doença glomerular. De fato, a obtenção de um diagnóstico histológico acurado pode ser um dos fatores mais importantes para a obtenção de um tratamento exitoso do cão ou gato com glomerulopatia. Decisões clínicas relacionadas ao diagnóstico, tratamento e prognóstico podem ser feitas a partir das informações obtidas pela biopsia renal.

Obtenção e processamento do espécime de biopsia renal

O procedimento utilizado para obter um espécime de biopsia renal é discutido nos Capítulos 89 e 321. O procedimento de biopsia renal requer conhecimento e deve ser realizado somente por uma equipe experiente.[30] A hipertensão (ver Capítulo 157) e distúrbios de coagulação (ver Capítulo 196) devem ser controlados antes da biopsia. Quando um espécime for utilizado para avaliação da doença glomerular, somente o tecido cortical deve ser obtido; a biopsia da medula não é necessária e está associada a um risco maior de hemorragia, infarto e fibrose. A utilização de anestesia geral está associada à capacidade de obter espécimes de melhor qualidade. Uma amostra adequada de córtex possui um mínimo de cinco glomérulos quando examinada pela microscopia óptica, embora um glomérulo pode ser o necessário para realizar um diagnóstico definitivo em animais nos quais a doença é difusa (i. e., uma em que a maioria dos glomérulos está envolvida) e facilmente reconhecível (i. e., amiloidose).

Se um método percutâneo for utilizado para obtenção de um espécime de biopsia renal de um paciente com glomerulopatia, pelo menos duas amostras de qualidade do córtex renal (i. e., cada uma com mais de 10 mm de comprimento) devem ser obtidas, utilizando uma agulha de diâmetro 16 ou 18. Um microscópio de dissecção pode ser utilizado para verificar que amostras adequadas de biopsia foram obtidas. Uma amostra deve ser colocada em formalina, e a outra deve ser dividida em dois pedaços menores contendo glomérulos. Uma peça é colocada em uma solução fixadora compatível para microscopia eletrônica por transmissão (MET) (p. ex., formalina 4% mais glutaraldeído 1% em tampão fosfato sódico), e a outra peça é congelada para microscopia imunofluorescente (MIF). Ima alternativa à congelação é imergir o tecido em amônio sulfato-N-etil-maleimida (i. e., solução de Michel), que preserva as imunoglobulinas fixadas em tecidos. Biopsias em cunha devem ser divididas em uma forma semelhante; tecidos para MET devem ser triturados apropriadamente. O tecido para MET deve ser colocado em um fixador dentro de cinco minutos após a biopsia.

Cortes finos (2 a 4 mm) de tecidos integrados em parafina devem ser utilizados para microscopia óptica porque os cortes padronizados de 5 a 6 mm são muito espessos para avaliação adequada da celularidade glomerular e espessura da alça capilar.[10,23] A coloração por hematoxilina e eosina pode ser utilizada para avaliação inicial; entretanto, o ácido periódico de Schiff (PAS), que cora glicoproteínas, é a coloração preferida de vários nefropatologistas e é particularmente útil para demonstração de cicatrização intersticial e glomerular, e avaliação da MBG. A metenamina de prata cora especificamente a membrana basal dos túbulos, glomérulos e cápsula de Bowman. O tricrômio é útil para avaliação do mesângio e é a melhor coloração para microscopia óptica para visualização das imunoglobulinas. O Vermelho Congo pode ser utilizado para demonstrar a presença de amiloide. A MIF ou imuno-histoquímica devem incluir pelo menos colorações para imunoglobulina M (IgM), IgG, IgA e C3.

Avaliação do espécime de biopsia renal

Somente patologistas que possuam experiência na patologia renal devem avaliar espécimes de biopsia renal. A inclusão de MET e MIF não são somente viáveis, mas necessárias para determinação da presença ou ausência de imunocomplexos e realização de um diagnóstico morfológico acurado e clinicamente útil.[23] A limitação pela avaliação somente da microscopia óptica frequentemente permite apenas uma interpretação subjetiva da lesão glomerular. Um sistema de classificação padronizado para a caracterização das lesões glomerulares em cães foi proposto.[23]

O glomérulo norma contém quatro a oito lóbulos, cada um composto por capilares suportados por um núcleo centrolobular de matriz mesangial (Figura 325.2).[10,11] A MBG é delgada, delicada, positiva para PAS e argirofílica. O lúmen capilar glomerular é normalmente amplamente patente e delimitado por citoplasma de células endoteliais eosinofílicas (Figura 325.3). Deve haver somente um ou dois núcleos por região de célula mesangial. Células epiteliais parietais, células epiteliais viscerais, células endoteliais e células mesangiais compõem o glomérulo normal e podem facilmente ser identificadas por MET (ver Figura 325.1). As células epiteliais parietais achatadas delimitam a superfície interna da cápsula de Bowman. As células epiteliais viscerais (podócitos) delimitam a superfície externa das alças capilares e jazem sobre a MBG. Os podócitos, que são caracterizados por seus processos podais, formam a camada mais externa da parede capilar. As células endoteliais delimitam a superfície interna das alças capilares, com os núcleos dispostos na região centrolobular em direção ao mesângio. As fenestrações

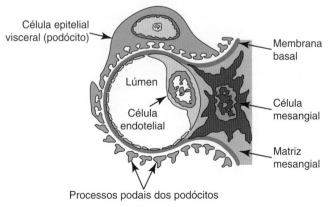

Figura 325.2 Diagrama esquemático demonstrando a composição de cada lóbulo em um capilar normal. (Cortesia de J.C. Jennette, School of Medicine, University of North Carolina, Chapel Hill, NC.)

do citoplasma da célula endotelial podem as visualizadas facilmente. A MBG normal deve ser aproximadamente da mesma espessura da base de um processo podal virado em 90°.

DOENÇAS GLOMERULARES

Várias doenças glomerulares afetam cães; um menor número parece afetar gatos (ver Boxe 325.1). A abordagem histórica de aglomerar essas sob o guarda-chuva de "GN" limitou os avanços da nossa compreensão e tratamento desses distúrbios. Uma abordagem mais adequada é tratar esses distúrbios como separados para o melhor da nossa capacidade. Essa seção destaca o que é conhecido sobre as doenças individuais em cães e gatos, com informações adicionais agrupadas a partir da riqueza de conhecimento sobre essas doenças em seres humanos. A lesão glomerular adquirida é resultado do dano contínuo após formação de imunocomplexos ou depósito (p. ex., nefropatia membranosa, NM; glomerulonefrite membranoproliferativa, GNMP) ou dano causado por fatores sistêmicos que afetam o glomérulo (p. ex., amiloidose). Em um grande estudo de 501 cães, 48,1% tinham GNIC.[4] Imunocomplexos que são depositados no glomérulo ou que são formados *in situ* iniciam o dano glomerular.[31] Mecanismos imunomediados celulares também são importantes na patogênese da inflamação glomerular. Assim que o dano glomerular foi iniciado, outros processos contribuem para a lesão glomerular, incluindo ativação do complemento e da cascata de coagulação, além de células residentes; o influxo de neutrófilos, monócitos e plaquetas; liberação de enzimas proteolíticas; síntese de citocinas ou outros fatores de crescimento; geração de mediadores lipídicos pró-inflamatórios; e alteração de fatores hemodinâmicos. Os mecanismos que determinam se o dano renal será progressivo ou o processo será resolvido são incertos.

Glomerulonefrite membranoproliferativa

A GNMP é uma das doenças glomerulares mais comuns em cães. Embora relatada em até 60% dos cães em diversos estudos, em um relato recente no qual as biópsias renais foram submetidas à extensa avaliação patológica, a GNMP foi identificada em 26% das 89 biópsias.[1,23,32] As lesões glomerulares mais provavelmente serão chamadas de GNMP quando a avaliação não incluir a utilização de MIF e ME; a incidência de GNMP é mais seguramente superestimada em estudos prévios.

Características clínicas

A idade média de cães com GNMP em um estudo foi de 10,5 anos.[19] Machos e fêmeas parecem ser igualmente afetados. Mesmo que a doença seja comum, nenhum estudo minucioso sobre GNMP como uma doença glomerular distinta foi realizado em cães. Em seres humanos, a doença é caracterizada por uma evolução lentamente progressiva, e cerca e 50% daqueles afetados desenvolvem SN. Em um estudo sobre SN em cães, 36% dos cães com GNMP tinham SN.[20] Em um estudo de cães, a GNMP foi associada à constelação mais grave de anormalidades clínicas; o grupo de cães com GNMP tinha a maior mediana de relação RUPC, a maior mediana de concentrações séricas de creatinina, as menores concentrações séricas de albumina e a maior frequência de hipertensão do que qualquer outro grupo.[23]

A GNMP foi identificada como uma doença familiar em cães da raça Bernese montanhês. Uma forma singular, rapidamente progressiva de GNMP que é acompanhada por necrose tubular e inflamação intersticial, e é uniformemente fatal foi relatada em associação à infecção por *Borrelia burgdorferi* em cães.[21] A idade média dos cães afetados foi de somente 5,6 anos. Labrador Retrievers e Golden Retrievers foram predispostos de forma significativa para o desenvolvimento dessa lesão.

Patogênese

A forma de GNMP identificada em cães se alinha mais intimamente à GNMP tipo I em pessoas, que também é chamada de *glomerulonefrite mesângio-capilar*, é geralmente induzida por doenças infecciosas e é caracterizada por acúmulo de imunocomplexos no lado subendotelial da MBG.[10,11] A GNMP foi associada a uma série de doenças infecciosas em cães. O acúmulo de imunocomplexos leva à ativação do complemento mediado por citocinas, expansão do mesângio e influxo de leucócitos.

Em seres humanos com GNMP, a diminuição do complemento é tão comum que essa doença é algumas vezes denominada como *glomerulonefrite hipocomplementêmica*. A hipocomplementemia parece ocorrer seja por aumento do consumo secundário à ativação de imunocomplexos da via clássica ou pela presença de autoanticorpos anticomplemento conhecidos como fatores nefríticos. De forma interessante, a GNMP tipo I também ocorrem em Spaniel Bretões e seres humanos com deficiência congênita de C3.[27] O papel patogênico da hipocomplementemia não é compreendido.

Caracterização histopatológica

A GNMP é diagnosticada quando tanto as alças capilares espessadas como a hipercelularidade mesangial (mais de três núcleos por região mesangial) estão presentes (Figura 325.4).[10,11,19,23] O glomérulo pode tomar uma aparência aumentada e segmentada ou lobulada. O mesângio ativado expande as paredes capilares

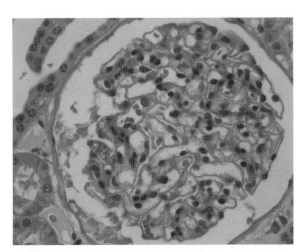

Figura 325.3 Glomérulo normal de um cão. Note que os lumens dos capilares estão amplamente patentes e as alças capilares são delgadas, frequentemente parecendo descontínuas. Não existe hipercelularidade. (*Esta figura se encontra reproduzida em cores no Encarte.*)

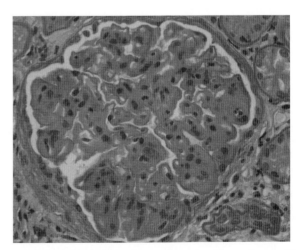

Figura 325.4 Glomérulo de um cão com glomerulonefrite membranoproliferativa (mesângio-capilar). Note as alças capilares espessadas e a hipercelularidade mesangial, que resultam na aparência segmentada e lobulada. (*Esta figura se encontra reproduzida em cores no Encarte.*)

e em direção ao espaço subendotelial, causando o contorno duplo, ou "trilho de trem", aparência da MBG que pode ser observada pela microscopia óptica. Pelo MIF, a deposição de imunocomplexos pode ser identificada em casos de GNMP conforme os depósitos granulares de C3 em combinação com IgG, IgM ou IgA, ou combinações dessas, na MBG ou mesângio, ou ambos. A MET também pode ser utilizada para identificar os depósitos imunes na GNMP.

Tratamento específico

O tratamento efetivo da doença subjacente infecciosa, inflamatória ou neoplásica é o pilar do tratamento de pacientes com GNMP (ver adiante). A terapia imunossupressora deve ser considerada em cães que possuem doença grave, persistente ou progressiva. Como a ativação de plaquetas parece estar envolvida na patogênese dessa doença, fármacos antiagregação plaquetária também devem ser fornecidos.[11]

Prognóstico

Dados específicos com relação ao prognóstico da GNMP em cães são escassos. Em pessoas, a azotemia, proteinúria grave, hipertensão sistêmica e lesões tubulointersticiais acentuadas no momento do atendimento são os preditores mais significativos de um resultado desfavorável.[11]

Nefropatia membranosa

A NM é outra doença glomerular comum em cães. Ao mesmo tempo que foi relatada em até 45% dos cães em diversos estudos, foi identificada em 26% das biopsias minuciosamente avaliadas em um estudo recente.[2,19,23,33-35] É a doença glomerular mais comum em gatos, nos quais outras formas de doença glomerular são incomuns.[36,37] A doença é algumas vezes denominada como *glomerulopatia* ou *nefropatia*, e não como GN, porque raramente existem evidências de uma resposta inflamatória no glomérulo ou interstício.

Características clínicas

A NM parece ser mais comuns em cães e gatos machos (relações aproximadas entre machos e fêmeas, 1,75:1 em cães e 6:1 em gatos). A idade média dos cães afetados a partir de quatro estudos foi de 8 anos, mas houve variação considerável (1 a 14 anos). A doença é mais comum em gatos mais jovens, com uma idade média aproximada de somente 3,6 anos (variação, 1 a 7 anos).[36] Não parece haver predileção racial, embora uma preponderância de Doberman Pinschers tenha sido observada em um relato. De forma interessante, quatro de cinco desses cães Dobermans tinham 3 anos ou menos, o que pode sugerir um padrão familiar.[34]

A proteinúria em animais com NM pode ser massiva.[29] Em um estudo de SN em cães, 38% dos cães com NM tinham SN.[20] A micro-hematúria é relatada em 30 a 40% dos humanos com NM, mas ainda não foi sistematicamente estudada em cães e gatos.[11] Gatos e cães com NM podem apresentar sinais de doença renal avançada. Vários gatos possuem rins normais a aumentados no momento do atendimento.

A NM possui quatro estágios ultraestruturais que estão correlacionados à evolução temporal da doença e apresentação clínica em cães, gatos e seres humanos.[10,11,34,36] Embora não sejam universalmente aceitas, existem algumas sugestões de que esses estágios estão relacionados aos resultados terapêuticos em seres humanos com NM, no fato de que pessoas podem ter maior probabilidade de responder ao tratamento apropriado se eles estiverem em um dos dois primeiros estágios. Estágios mais avançados em gatos e cães demonstraram estar correlacionados à azotemia mais grave, enquanto animais com doenças mais discretas mais provavelmente terão SN.[34,36] Em alguns casos, estágios diferentes foram observados dentro do mesmo espécime de biopsia.

Patogênese

Em seres humanos, a NM é considerada como primária (i. e., idiopática) ou secundária à outra doença; a doença primária é mais comum.[11] O achado de anticorpos no lado subepitelial é singular à NM e sugere que a ligação ocorre no lado urinário da MBG. A ativação subsequente do complemento e respostas de citocinas podem ser reduzidas, porque o local da reação é distante da circulação, o que contribui para a ausência de inflamação associada à NM.

Embora a patogênese exata desse distúrbio seja desconhecida, a NM primária é considerada como uma GNIC. Em humanos com NM primária, as evidências suportam que os imunocomplexos se formam *in situ*, quando anticorpos não ligados reagem com antígenos fixos do podócitos. Com relação a isso, a doença primária pode ser um distúrbio autoimune verdadeiro.

Imunocomplexos circulantes mais provavelmente possuem um papel maior em pacientes com doença secundária. A proteinúria provavelmente ocorre por meio de um mecanismo dependente do complemento, independente de células inflamatórias. O complexo complemento terminal (complexo de ataque à membrana C5b-9) tem sido implicado na patogênese dessa doença. O aumento das concentrações urinárias do complexo de ataque à membrana tem sido demonstrado em alguns, embora não em todos, os indivíduos com NM. A demonstração desse complexo pode ser mais provável no início do processo mórbido, quando a formação ativa de depósitos imunes ocorre. A miríade de irregularidades do sistema imune foi relatada em associação à NM em humanos (p. ex., alteração da relação entre CD4[+] e CD8[+], disfunção do receptor Fc e supressão da função celular), o que suporta um papel patogênico para um defeito imunológico subjacente. Essas irregularidades são talvez baseadas em uma suscetibilidade genética, uma teoria suportada por agrupamento familiar de NM em humanos.[10,11]

Caracterização histopatológica

A MBG normalmente de aparência rendilhada se torna uniformemente espessada e mais rígida como resultado da deposição de imunocomplexos nos espaços subepiteliais na NM (Figura 325.5).[10,19,23] Novo material na membrana basal se acumula ao redor dos depósitos imunes. Como os depósitos não são impregnados por prata, "pontas" podem ser identificadas do lado de fora da MBG quando uma coloração apropriada de prata é utilizada. Casos avançados podem demonstrar espessamento irregular e distorção das paredes capilares com alargamento ocasional do mesângio. MIF é útil para determinar o local de deposição de imunocomplexos. A coloração de imunocomplexos causa uma aparência de colar de pérolas por toda MBG e pode ser tão escura que pode ser difícil diferenciar de um padrão linear. Em casos secundários, os espaços mesangiais também são corados.

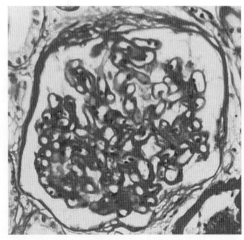

Figura 325.5 Glomérulo de um cão com nefropatia membranosa. Note as alças capilares espessadas, de aparência rígida, e a ausência de hipercelularidade. (Cortesia de J.L. Robertson, Virginia Maryland Regional College of Veterinary Medicine, Blacksburg, VA.) (*Esta figura se encontra reproduzida em cores no Encarte.*)

A MET deve ser utilizada para confirmar a localização dos depósitos imunes e caracterizar o estágio de progressão da doença (Figura 325.6).[11,23,34,36] A deposição de imunocomplexos, engolfamento progressivo dos complexos pela MBG circundante, e resolução eventual dos depósitos caracterizam os estágios. O estágio I possui depósitos imunes densos subepiteliais sem projeções adjacentes de material da membrana basal e somente espessamento mínimo da MBG. Projeções do material adjacente da MBG, ou pontas, são identificadas no estágio II. Essas projeções eventualmente circundam os depósitos imunes (estágio III). No estágio IV, a MBG está acentuadamente espessada, e as zonas elétron-lucentes já substituíram alguns ou todos os depósitos elétron-lucentes. Na doença em estágio IV avançado, algumas vezes denominada como estágio V, existe espessamento variável da MBG e resolução aparente dos depósitos elétron-densos. Algumas vezes o estadiamento é difícil porque vários estágios da doença podem estar presentes simultaneamente.

Tratamento específico

Além da identificação de processo mórbidos potencialmente incitantes e tratamento inespecífico da proteinúria, a terapia imunossupressora pode ser justificada em cães ou gatos com doença grave, persistente ou progressiva. Humanos afetados com situações clínicas semelhantes podem responder à terapia imunossupressora.[11] Mesmo quando o tratamento for efetivo, recidivas podem ocorrer. A utilização de terapia imunossupressora em cães e gatos com NM precisa ser estudada.

Prognóstico

Ainda que a NM pareça ser progressiva em alguns cães e gatos, a progressão pode ser lenta o suficiente que vários animais podem ter vidas relativamente normais. Em um estudo de 24 gatos com NM, 4 (17%) sobreviveram 4 a 10 meses, e 8 (33%) tiveram sobrevida a longo prazo de 2,5 a 6 anos; a remissão clínica ocorreu em 7 (29%) dos gatos. Corticosteroides foram administrados a três dos oito sobreviventes a longo prazo. Entretanto, 11 gatos (46%) morreram ou foram eutanasiados por conta de SN ou doença renal avançada logo após o diagnóstico.[37] Sobreviventes a longo prazo tinham somente deposição de IgG, deposição de C3 ou ambos; gatos que também tinham deposição de IgM ou IgA tiveram um período de sobrevida mais curto. Os estágios III e IV de NM, definidos pela presença de depósitos intramembranosos, foram associados a um prognóstico mais reservado.[37]

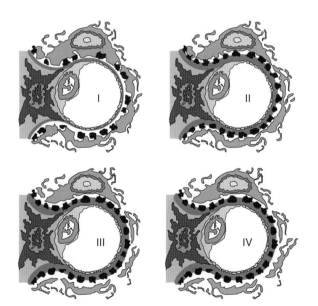

Figura 325.6 Estágios ultraestruturais na progressão da nefropatia membranosa. (Cortesia de J.C. Jennette, School of Medicine, University of North Carolina, Chapel Hill, NC.)

Os dados de sobrevida para cães parecem ser semelhantes ao que foi relatado em gatos, com sobrevidas relatadas variando de 4 dias a mais de 3 anos.[34] As remissões espontâneas foram relatadas. A remissão espontânea ocorre em 20 a 30% dos humanos com NM, enquanto 20 a 40% dos casos progridem para doença renal crônica.[11] O risco de progressão em humanos parece estar correlacionado com a magnitude da proteinúria e alteração da função renal; pacientes com o maior grau de proteinúria e azotemia mais provavelmente terão progressão mais rápida comparados a outros pacientes.

Glomerulonefrite proliferativa

A GN proliferativa, causada por proliferação endocapilar ou mesangial, correspondera a 2 a 16% das lesões glomerulares em cães em dois estudos, mas nenhum foi identificado em um estudo patológico recente, mais provavelmente porque diagnósticos incomuns foram excluídos.[19,23,32] Em humanos um diagnóstico patológico requer tanto uma descrição morfológica (p. ex., GN proliferativa mesangial) e uma designação específica da doença (p. ex., nefropatia por IgA, GN por lúpus).[10,11] Com a exceção da nefropatia por IgA, a GN proliferativa em cães não incluiu a designação específica da doença.[38,39]

Características clínicas

Cães com GN proliferativa relatados em dois estudos tinham em média entre 7 e 9 anos.[18,19] A proteinúria e azotemia renal foram os sinais mais comuns apresentados. A azotemia pode ser discreta ou moderada e aguda ou crônica. Embora a hematúria esteja associada a esse distúrbio em pessoas, sua presença em cães é desconhecida.[11]

Patogênese

A GN proliferativa é uma GNIC. A doença anti-MBG causa GN proliferativa em humanos, mas ainda não foi descrita no cão ou gato. A GN pós-infecciosa de humanos é uma forma de GN proliferativa que mais comumente ocorre após resolução de uma infecção estreptocócica. Infecções persistentes são causas mais prováveis de GNMP ou NM.[10]

Caracterização histopatológica

A GN proliferativa mesangial é caracterizada por hiperplasia de células mesangiais (mais que 4 células por área mesangial) que é frequentemente acompanhada por aumento da matriz mesangial (Figura 325.7).[10,19] A GN proliferativa endocapilar possui proliferação de células endoteliais com ou sem aumento da celularidade mesangial que ocorre parcialmente graças ao influxo de células mononucleares. A avaliação pela MIF revela depósitos granulares finos de IgG ou IgM, ou ambos, na MBG e mesângio. A MET localiza melhor os imunocomplexos. Como a GN proliferativa frequentemente ocorre secundariamente a doenças sistêmicas, os imunocomplexos são frequentemente identificados no mesângio, embora alguns complexos possam ser encontrados nas paredes capilares.

Tratamento específico

A origem potencial de imunocomplexos deve ser removida, e o tratamento inespecífico de doenças glomerulares deve ser seguido. A terapia imunossupressora pode ser justificada em animais com doença grave, persistente ou progressiva.

Prognóstico

Enquanto o prognóstico ainda não tenha sido completamente avaliado em cães a presença de azotemia avançada ou formação de crescentes estão provavelmente associados a um prognóstico pior.

Nefropatia por imunoglobulina A

Em diversos estudos de doença glomerular canina, a MIF demonstrou discreta à moderada frequência de positividade para IgA, sugestiva de nefropatia por IgA.[38,39] A IgA é

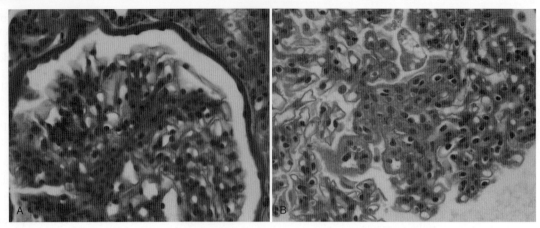

Figura 325.7 Glomérulo de cães com glomerulonefrite proliferativa. **A.** Glomerulonefrite proliferativa mesangial focal. **B.** Glomerulonefrite proliferativa endocapilar. (*Esta figura se encontra reproduzida em cores no Encarte.*)

predominantemente polimérica em cães e pode ser inespecificamente aprisionada no mesângio, mais do que a IgA monomérica, a forma predominante em humanos. O diagnóstico de nefropatia por IgA requer uma predominância de positividade para IgA na avaliação por MIF; depósitos concomitantes de IgG, IgM ou C3 podem estar presentes, mas devem ser menos intensos do que IgA. A GN proliferativa mesangial é a lesão microscópica esperada; alguns humanos não possuem quaisquer lesões glomerulares aparentes. Em um estudo de cães clinicamente normais com lesões glomerulares, 85% tinham depósitos de IgA.[28] Em outro estudo de 100 cães com e sem doença renal, 47 tinham deposição de IgA; em seis cães, a IgA foi a única imunoglobulina detectada.[39] O aumento da deposição de IgA foi associado à maior proliferação celular. Cães com doenças entéricas ou hepáticas tiveram a maior prevalência de deposição por IgA. A formação excessiva de imunocomplexos por IgA causada por doença entérica ou diminuição da depuração de complexos IgA em associação à hepatopatia foi proposta na patogênese da nefropatia por IgA secundária em humanos.[11]

A nefropatia por IgA foi descrita em três cães machos jovens à meia-idade (4 a 7 anos), com dados demográficos consistentes com aqueles de pessoas afetadas.[11,38] Os cães tinham proteinúria, graus variados de azotemia e episódios de hematúria. Cães foram domiciliados juntos, mas fatores ambientais predisponentes não foram identificados. O cão mais severamente afetado tinha hipertensão descontrolada e depósitos concomitantes de IgG ou IgM, ambos os quais são indicadores prognósticos negativos em humanos.

O tratamento de pacientes com nefropatia por IgA secundária deve ser direcionado ao tratamento da doença sistêmica associada e controle da hipertensão. O óleo de peixe rico em ácidos graxos ômega-3 administrado a humanos afetados resultou e, progressão retardada da doença renal, mas não levou à redução da proteinúria.[11]

Amiloidose

A amiloidose corresponde a aproximadamente 15% das lesões glomerulares em cães.[4] O termo amiloidose refere-se a um grupo diverso de doenças que possuem em comum a deposição extracelular de fibrilas formadas pela polimerização de proteínas com uma conformação de folheto pregueado.[40] A amiloidose reativa é a forma mais comum de amiloidose em cães e gatos, sendo que o cão é o animal doméstico mais comumente afetado por amiloidose. Com exceção do Sharpei Chinês, o amiloide é depositado primariamente nos glomérulos de cães afetados.[22,41] A amiloidose é relativamente incomum no gato, com exceção de gatos das raças Abissínio e Siamês (especialmente a variante colorida de pelo curto oriental).[42] Nos Abissínios, o amiloide é depositado primariamente na medula renal, embora o envolvimento glomerular tenha sido descrito.

Características clínicas

A amiloidose renal é mais comum em cães idosos. A idade média de cães afetados foi de 9,2 anos em um estudo, no qual 85% dos cães afetados tinham 7 anos ou mais.[22] Fêmeas parecem ser mais afetadas do que machos (a relação entre machos e fêmeas é de 1:1,7). Collies e Treeing Walker Coonhounds podem ter maior risco de ocorrência de amiloidose; o distúrbio é familiar em Sharpei Chineses e pode ser familiar em Beagles e Foxhounds Ingleses.[22,43]

Como a proteinúria associada à amiloidose pode ser massiva, vários animais trazidos ao veterinário estão em SN. Em um estudo da SN em cães, 56% dos cães com amiloidose tinham SN.[20] Entretanto, ao contrário da crença popular, cães com amiloidose não tinham RPCU ou concentrações séricas de creatinina maiores ou concentrações séricas inferiores de albumina do que cães em outros grupos de doenças.[23] Em outro estudo, seis de sete cães com amiloidose tinham proteinúria não seletiva, sugerindo uma perda acentuada das propriedades seletivas do tamanho da parede capilar glomerular.[29] Embora o amiloide possa ser depositado em outros sistemas de órgãos (fígado [ver Capítulo 285], baço, adrenais, trato gastrintestinal), sinais clínicos associados à deposição nestes órgãos são raros em cães. Doenças inflamatórias crônicas infecciosas ou não e neoplasias foram associadas à amiloidose reativa em 32 a 53% dos cães afetados; entretanto, vários cães e gatos com amiloidose reativa não tiveram processo inflamatório identificável no momento do atendimento.[16,22]

A amiloidose renal no Sharpei ocorre em uma idade mais precoce (idade média de 4,1 anos) do que em outros cães com amiloidose, mas assim como em outros cães, a doença é mais comum em fêmeas (relação entre machos e fêmeas de 1:2,5).[41] Em Sharpeis, o amiloide é mais comumente depositado na medula renal; somente 64% dos Sharpeis tinham envolvimento glomerular.[41] Como resultado, de 25 a 43% dos Sharpeis afetados tinham proteinúria. Cães afetados podem ter sinais de envolvimento de outros órgãos, particularmente o fígado (ver Capítulo 285). Vários Sharpeis possuem histórico de febre recorrente e edema das articulações tibiotársicas (comumente chamado de *febre do Sharpei* ou *síndrome do joelho inchado do Sharpei*; ver Capítulo 203) antes do desenvolvimento de amiloidose renal, sugerindo que esse pode ser um modelo animal de febre familiar do Mediterrâneo.

Patogênese

A proteína primária envolvida na formação de depósitos amiloides em cães e gatos é a proteína amiloide A (AA), que é formada pela polimerização da porção aminoterminal da proteína sérica amiloide A (SAA), um reagente de fase aguda.[40] A SAA é sintetizada e liberada por hepatócitos após estimulação deles por citocinas derivadas de macrófagos (p. ex., interleucina-1 [IL-1], IL-6, fator de necrose tumoral). Por conta dessa associação do amiloide A e doenças inflamatórias, essa forma de amiloidose tem sido denominada como amiloidose *reativa*, ou *secundária*.

Concentrações de SAA aumentam de cem a mil vezes após lesão tecidual. Embora as concentrações diminuam até níveis basais em 36 a 48 horas após a remoção do estímulo inflamatório, elas permanecem aumentadas se a inflamação persistir.[40] A inflamação crônica e incrementos persistentes ou prolongados nas concentrações de SAA são necessárias para o desenvolvimento de amiloidose reativa. Humanos com febre familiar do Mediterrâneo, uma doença semelhante àquela relatada em Sharpeis, possuem formação defeituosa de pirina, uma proteína envolvida na regulação de mediadores da inflamação.[44] Como somente uma pequena porcentagem de animais com inflamação crônica desenvolvem amiloidose, outros fatores devem estar envolvidos na patogênese.[40] Existem diversos polimorfos de SAA, e determinados polimorfos talvez sejam mais amiloidogênicos. Pode haver variações hereditárias ou adquiridas na capacidade de degradas SAA, um processo de dois passos que envolve proteases associadas à superfície celular contidas em monócitos. Um defeito no segundo passo desse processo pode predispor alguns indivíduos ao desenvolvimento de amiloidose. Foi demonstrado que a propriedade de degradação e AA do soro normal está diminuída em humanos com amiloidose reativa. Essa atividade esteve correlacionada às concentrações séricas de albumina; a hipoalbuminemia associada a processos inflamatórios ou amiloidose pode contribuir para a diminuição da atividade de degradação de AA. O aumento das concentrações de outras reagentes de fase aguda que são inibidores de proteases (p. ex., antitripsina e antiquimotripsina) também podem contribuir para a patogênese da amiloidose.

As concentrações de SAA estão aumentadas durante a fase pré-deposição, antes do surgimento dos depósitos teciduais de amiloide, mas podem persistir durante a fase de deposição. Abissínios com amiloidose renal possuem concentrações aumentadas de SAA.[40] Sharpeis Chineses com amiloidose renal possuem concentrações séricas aumentadas de IL-6, uma citocina que estimula a síntese e liberação de SAA.[45] A fase de deposição, durante a qual os depósitos amiloides surgem no tecido, é subdividida em duas fases. A fase rápida é caracterizada por rápidos aumentos na quantidade de amiloide, enquanto a fase platô e um momento quando pouca alteração líquida ocorre na deposição tecidual.

Caracterização histopatológica

A conformação preguada é responsável pelas propriedades características de coloração dos depósitos amiloides.[10] Quando o rim é avaliado por microscopia óptica convencional, os depósitos amiloides nos glomérulos parecem como material acelular que se expande em direção ao mesângio e MBGs, e com coloração eosinofílica homogeneamente com hematoxilina-eosina (Figura 325.8). Os depósitos glomerulares são mais frequentemente difusos e globais, mas às vezes são focais e segmentares. Os depósitos algumas vezes podem ser observados nas paredes de pequenos vasos sanguíneos, membranas basais tubulares e tecidos intersticiais. Quando corados com vermelho Congo e avaliados por microscopia óptica convencional, os depósitos amiloides tomam várias formas de vermelho, dependendo da quantidade de amiloide e da espessura do corte. Depósitos corados com vermelho Congo e avaliados por microscopia de polarização são birrefringentes e possuem uma coloração verde-maçã (Figura 325.9). A amiloidose reativa pode ser confirmada por descoloração dos depósitos amiloides corados por vermelho Congo por oxidação por permanganato de potássio. A MET não é necessária para confirmação do diagnóstico de amiloidose.

Tratamento específico

A configuração de folheto preguada das fibrilas amiloides leva à sua insolubilidade e resistência à proteólise, tornando o tratamento específico relativamente inefetivo. Em humanos com febre

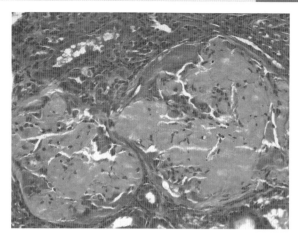

Figura 325.8 Amiloidose glomerular em um corte de biopsia renal canina corada com hematoxilina e eosina. (Cortesia de S.P. DiBartola, College of Veterinary Medicine, The Ohio State University, Columbus, OH.) (*Esta figura se encontra reproduzida em cores no Encarte.*)

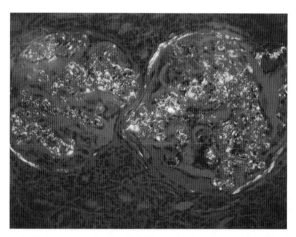

Figura 325.9 Corte corado com vermelho congo, demonstrando birrefringência típica de depósitos amiloides glomerulares. (Cortesia de S.P. DiBartola, College of Veterinary Medicine, The Ohio State University, Columbus, OH.) (*Esta figura se encontra reproduzida em cores no Encarte.*)

familiar do Mediterrâneo, a colchicina impediu o desenvolvimento de amiloidose renal mesmo em pacientes que continuaram a ter episódios febris recorrentes.[44,46] Isso levou à recomendação de que a colchicina seja utilizada no tratamento de Sharpeis com amiloidose renal. Idealmente, esse fármaco é administrado durante a fase de predeposição, na qual em Sharpeis é presumivelmente caracterizada por episódios recorrentes de febre e joelhos edemaciados. Entretanto, a administração de colchicina pode levar à remissão da proteinúria mesmo após o surgimento de depósitos amiloides. Nenhuma evidência suporta a efetividade da colchicina já que a amiloidose resultou em azotemia persistente ou hipoalbuminemia. Embora os efeitos do fármaco no tratamento da amiloidose não sejam completamente conhecidos, a colchicina prejudica a liberação de SAA dos hepatócitos se ligando aos microtúbulos e impedindo a secreção. Além disso, a colchicina pode impedir a produção de fator liberador de amiloide. A dose de colchicina utilizada é de 0,01 a 0,03 mg/kg administrada por via oral a cada 24 horas. Distúrbios gastrintestinais são o efeito colateral primário. A utilização de colchicina tem sido recomendada ocasionalmente para pessoas com amiloidose renal por causas que não a febre familiar do Mediterrâneo e justifica maiores avaliações em cães.

O dimetilsulfóxido (DMSO) demonstrou ser benéfico em um número limitado de cães com amiloidose renal, embora o benefício exato permaneça controverso.[46] Se administrado durante a fase de deposição rápida, o DMSO leva a uma diminuição nas concentrações de SAA e resolução dos depósitos teciduais. Entretanto, a quantidade de amiloide depositado nos rins de humanos se manteve inalterada após administração de DMSO, o que suporta a crença atual de que o DMSO não solubiliza fibrilas amiloides. Os efeitos anti-inflamatórios do DMSO podem causar alguns efeitos benéficos. A redução da fibrose intersticial e inflamação pode levar à melhora da função renal e redução da proteinúria. O DMSO possui um odor desagradável que pode causar baixo comprometimento do tutor. Ademais, esse fármaco pode contribuir para os sinais de náuseas e anorexia observados em alguns cães. A dose recomendada é de 90 mg/kg administrada por via oral ou subcutânea 3 vezes/semana. O DMSO deve ser diluído em água estéril na proporção de 1: 4 antes da administração para limitar a dor associada à injeção.

Prognóstico
O prognóstico para cães e gatos com amiloidose renal é geralmente reservado. Em um estudo de cães com amiloidose, 58% morreram ou foram eutanasiados no momento do diagnóstico. Nos cães remanescentes, a sobrevida variou de 2 a 20 meses; a sobrevida de 1 ano ou mais foi relatada em somente 8,5%.[40] A maior sobrevida foi observada em um cão tratado com DMSO.

Nefrite hereditária
O termo *nefrite hereditária* (NH) refere-se a um grupo diverso de doenças glomerulares hereditárias que são resultado de um defeito no colágeno da membrana basal (tipo IV).[47] Essas doenças são discutidas no Capítulo 328. Uma breve discussão sobre nefrite hereditária está incluída nesse capítulo porque deve ser considerada como um diagnóstico diferencial para qualquer cão com doença renal proteinúrica, particularmente se o cão for jovem.

Características clínicas
A nefrite hereditária foi relatada em diversas raças de cães. Uma forma recessiva autonômica da doença ocorre em Cocker Spaniels Ingleses e Springer Spaniels Ingleses, enquanto Bull Terriers e Dálmatas desenvolvem uma forma autossômica dominante.[47-51] Uma forma dominante ligada ao cromossomo X de NH foi escrita em Samoiedas e cães sem raça definida; fêmeas portadoras podem ter a doença na forma leve.[48] O relato em Samoiedas é de uma única ninhada; a doença não é considerada como comum nessa raça. A NH é caracterizada por proteinúria, hematúria renal e doença glomerular progressiva. Anormalidades de audição e oculares concorrentes, como descritas em humanos com NH, parecem ser incomuns em cães afetados, com a exceção do lenticone anterior, que ocorre em alguns Bull Terriers.[49]

Patogênese
A NH é resultado de uma mutação genética ou deleção no colágeno tipo IV, a proteína primária constituinte da MBG.[52,53] A presença de colágeno defeituoso leva à deterioração prematura da MBG e doença glomerular progressiva.

Caracterização histopatológica
Antes dos estudos com microscopia eletrônica em Cocker Spaniels Ingleses, as lesões renais eram descritas como hipoplasia cortical renal ou GN membranoproliferativa ou GN esclerosante. A MET é necessária para confirmar o diagnóstico de NH. A divisão multilaminar e fragmentação da MBG são observadas, frequentemente com depósitos intramembranosos elétron-densos.

Tratamento específico
Nenhum tratamento específico está disponível para cães afetados. A utilização de uma dieta formulada para as doenças renais e administração de inibidores da enzima conversora de angiotensina (ECA) provaram ser benéficas em cães afetados. A detecção precoce de NH através da triagem de cães de raças relevantes para microalbuminúria permite a intervenção terapêutica precoce, o que pode retardar a progressão da doença.[24]

Prognóstico
A velocidade de progressão é previsível em Samoiedas e Cocker Spaniel Ingleses, com doença renal terminal geralmente ocorrendo antes dos 2 anos.[47] Entretanto, a progressão da doença é mais variável em Bull Terriers e Dálmatas, sendo que alguns cães sobrevivem por até 10 anos.[49,50]

Doença por lesão mínima
Embora incomumente descrita em cães e gatos, a doença por lesão mínima (DLM) é uma causa comum de SN em humanos, especialmente em crianças.[11,54] Como a MET é necessária para o diagnóstico, a doença mais provavelmente é subdiagnosticada em cães e talvez em gatos. Em humanos, essa doença é algumas vezes denominada como doença nil, nefrose lipoide ou SN idiopática. Existem relatos isolados de cães que parecem ter DLM. Entretanto, existe somente um relato de caso bem descrito de DLM em um cão com SN.[54]

Características clínicas
A proteinúria é provavelmente de magnitude grave nessa doença, e a SN é comum.

Patogênese
Em humanos, a DLM é em geral idiopática, embora a doença secundária também ocorra. O aumento da produção de linfocinas por células T disfuncionais supostamente é responsável pelo aumento da permeabilidade da MBG.[11] A alteração primária é a perda da carga aniônica na parede capilar glomerular, levando ao colapso dos processos podais dos podócitos. Essa perda de seletividade de cargas é o evento crucial que leva à proteinúria. A proteinúria resultante é altamente seletiva; a albumina é a proteína primária perdida.

Caracterização histopatológica
Existe uma ausência de lesões microscópicas no glomérulo; por isso, o nome de DLM.[10] Ocasionalmente, a hipercelularidade discreta está presente. Algumas gotículas lipídicas podem estar presentes nos túbulos renais, mas não deve haver evidências de atrofia tubular ou fibrose intersticial. A deposição de imunoglobulinas é ausente quando avaliada por MIF; entretanto, pode haver aumento da coloração por vimentina, um marcador para células epiteliais glomerulares viscerais. O diagnóstico é confirmado por MET pela identificação de ocultação acentuada de processos podais (Figura 325.10). Em um estudo de lesões glomerulares em cães, 28 de 115 cães entraram na classificação da OMS de anormalidades glomerulares menores, mas somente um desses cães tinha DLM.[19] Portanto, a identificação de somente anormalidades glomerulares menores em um cão ou gato com proteinúria não confirma o diagnóstico de DLM.

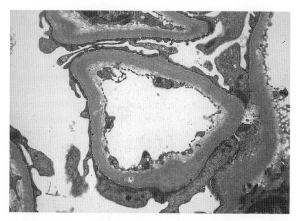

Figura 325.10 Micrografia eletrônica de uma alça capilar glomerular em um cão com doença por lesão mínima presumida. Ocorreu ocultação dos processos podais.

Tratamento específico
Uma importante razão para incluir a DLM na lista de diagnósticos diferenciais para cães com SN é a resposta aparentemente diferenciada da doença aos corticosteroides; a taxa esperada de resposta em humanos com DLM é de 80 a 90%.[11]

Prognóstico
O prognóstico para DLM em cães é desconhecido. Uma ou mais recidivas são observadas em 75 a 85% dos humanos afetados.[11]

Glomeruloesclerose
A glomeruloesclerose correspondeu a aproximadamente 20% das lesões glomerulares de cães em um grande estudo.[4] Enquanto a glomeruloesclerose frequentemente ocorre como uma lesão de estágio terminal em resposta à lesão glomerular, a glomeruloesclerose segmentar focal (GESF) é uma doença glomerular primária.[10] A prevalência de glomeruloesclerose aumenta com a idade, embora a porcentagem esperada de glomérulos esclerosados em cães de grupos de faixas etárias avançadas ainda não tenha sido completamente caracterizada. A glomeruloesclerose é um achado comum na nefropatia diabética de humanos. Embora a glomeruloesclerose e proteinúria possam ocorrer em cães com diabetes melito, a relevância clínica disso é desconhecida. A glomeruloesclerose pode ocorrer também após dano renal hipertensivo.

A GESF foi identificada em 29% das biopsias minuciosamente avaliadas em um estudo recente, tornando-a uma das doenças glomerulares mais comuns (Figura 325.11).[10,19,23] A GESF é diagnosticada no paciente proteinúrico que tem glomeruloesclerose segmentar em um glomérulo que é de outra forma normal, sem outras lesões glomerulares presentes que expliquem a esclerose. A avaliação por MIF deve ser negativa em pacientes afetados; entretanto, o aprisionamento inespecífico de imunoglobulinas e C3 pode ocorrer em áreas escleróticas.

Lesões tubulointersticiais associadas à doença glomerular
Proteinúria induz dano tubular, levando à perda progressiva de néfrons.[55] A proteinúria crônica pode levar à fibrose intersticial, degeneração tubular e atrofia e rarefação capilar peritubular. A proteinúria grave está associada a um resultado negativo do paciente em humanos com diversas doenças glomerulares; a urina de humanos proteinúricos demonstra mediadores de inflamação e fibrose renal, alguns dos quais são produzidos por túbulos renais expostos a várias proteínas.[55] Entretanto, a albumina provavelmente não é a culpada porque ratos e humanos com proteinúria altamente seletiva parecem ter menor risco de eventual dano tubulointersticial.

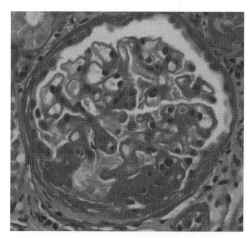

Figura 325.11 Glomérulo de um cão com uma lesão que lembra a glomeruloesclerose segmentar focal. Note a aparência relativamente normal dos cortes glomerulares que não estão esclerosados. (*Esta figura se encontra reproduzida em cores no Encarte.*)

A proteína nos túbulos é reabsorvida pelos túbulos proximais; as proteínas reabsorvidas são citotóxicas para as células epiteliais tubulares.[56,57] Nem somente as proteínas são citotóxicas, mas elas aumentam a sobrecarga das células epiteliais tubulares. Inicialmente, isso leva à hipertrofia compensatória das células epiteliais tubulares, mas eventualmente a célula não consegue lidar com o aumento da sobrecarga e morrerá. Certo dano também ocorre secundariamente à obstrução dos túbulos por cilindros de proteínas.[58] A lesão glomerular também resulta em diminuição da perfusão do interstício tubular e lesão adicional. Uma ligação direta ainda não foi estabelecida entre proteinúria e dano renal progressivo em cães, mas certamente existe em determinada extensão. Como a proteinúria pode ser um fator importante responsável pela doença renal progressiva em pacientes com doença glomerular, o tratamento agressivo da proteinúria deve ser considerado como um pilar do tratamento de cães e gatos cm doença glomerular.

TERAPIA-PADRÃO DA DOENÇA GLOMERULAR
Além do tratamento específico que poderia ser implementado em diversas doenças glomerulares, algumas intervenções terapêuticas são consideradas padrão para todos os cães com doença glomerular.[6] Essa terapia pode ser dividida em três categorias principais: (1) tratamento de potenciais processos mórbidos subjacentes, (2) redução da proteinúria, e (3) tratamento da uremia e outras complicações da doença renal generalizada (ver Capítulo 324).

A GNIC ou amiloidose ocorrem após uma reação imune ou inflamatória forte, potencialmente desorganizada, respectivamente, que ocorreu em resposta a um estímulo – frequentemente infeccioso, inflamatório ou neoplásico. De acordo, uma doença subjacente poderia ter iniciado a doença glomerular em até 63% dos cães afetados; uma avaliação minuciosa para doenças subjacentes é justificada. Algumas vezes, o agente incitante não é óbvio no primeiro atendimento porque a doença lesiva não está mais presente ou está oculta. A observação persistente e análise são necessárias, pois o processo mórbido causador pode se tornar óbvio nos meses seguintes após o atendimento. O passo inicial no tratamento de um cão ou gato proteinúrico é tratar e eliminar, se possível, qualquer doença predisponente potencial. Animais que são soropositivos para doenças infecciosas devem ser submetidos ao tratamento específico contra a infecção imediatamente, mesmo quando não houver evidências diretas de que a infecção está causando a proteinúria, e deve ser dada consideração para o tratamento imunossupressor utilizando as mesmas diretrizes apresentadas na discussão seguinte.[9] O cão deve ser subsequentemente avaliado para resolução da proteinúria, que pode ocorrer lentamente dentro de um período de meses. Se a proteinúria não cessar ou piorar, uma biopsia renal para determinar o diagnóstico histológico pode ser necessária.

Agentes antiproteinúricos devem ser considerados quando a RPCU estiver persistentemente acima de 0,5 em um cão; inibidores da ECA (p. ex., enalapril, benazepril) são os fármacos de escolha para a maioria dos cães afetados. O enalapril diminuiu de forma significativa a proteinúria e retardou o início ou a progressão da azotemia em cães com GN.[59] O tratamento de cães com doenças glomerulares com inibidores da ECA é agora considerado o tratamento de escolha.[59] Inibidores da ECA podem reduzir a proteinúria e preservar a função renal por diversos possíveis mecanismos. A diminuição da resistência arteriolar glomerular eferente causada pelos inibidores da ECA leva à diminuição da pressão hidrostática transcapilar glomerular e diminuição da proteinúria. Outros mecanismos propostos incluem redução da perda glomerular de heparan sulfato, diminuição do tamanho dos poros endoteliais dos capilares glomerulares, melhora do metabolismo de lipoproteínas, retardo do crescimento e proliferação mesangial glomerular, e inibição da degradação da bradicinina.[59] Tipicamente o enalapril ou benazepril (0,5 mg/kg administrados por via oral) é administrado 1 vez/dia, embora aproximadamente metade dos cães possam eventualmente precisar da administração 2 vezes/dia. A dose inicial pode ser gradativamente aumentada até atingir o alvo terapêutico de RPCU menor que 0,5 (objetivo ideal) ou uma redução maior que 50% do nível basal (objetivo alternativo). A concentração sérica de creatinina deve ser monitorada; é incomum que os cães tenham piora dose-limitante da azotemia (*i. e.*, aumento maior que 30% da creatinina sérica ou progressão da DRC em estágio IV pela IRIS) por conta da administração somente do inibidor da ECA. A hiperpotassemia é um efeito colateral comum em cães com doença glomerular que são ratados com um inibidor da ECA e pode ser controlada pela alimentação de uma dieta caseira com níveis reduzidos de potássio que tenha sido formulada por um nutrólogo veterinário.[60] Se ocorrer hiperpotassemia grave ou a proteinúria não for adequadamente controlada com um inibidor da ECA, um bloqueador do receptor de angiotensina (BRA; telmisartana, losartana) pode ser substituído ou adicionado. A terapia de combinação com um inibidor da ECA e um BRA pode levar à maior redução na proteinúria do que a monoterapia, seja com um inibidor da ECA ou com um BRA, mas deve ser utilizada com cautela e monitoramento cuidadoso do paciente até que os resultados de estudos controlados estejam disponíveis.[61]

O controle adequado da pressão arterial de cães hipertensos (ver Capítulo 158) pode também levar à redução da proteinúria e retardo da progressão da doença (ver Capítulo 157). Como os inibidores da ECA são agentes anti-hipertensivos relativamente fracos, agentes anti-hipertensivos adicionais (p. ex., amlodipino) podem ser necessários se a hipertensão (*i. e.*, pressão sanguínea sistólica maior que 160 mmHg) persistir após o início da terapia com inibidor da ECA.

Plaquetas e tromboxano podem ter um importante papel na patogênese da GN e inibidores da tromboxano-sintetase demonstraram diminuir a proteinúria em cães com GN experimentalmente induzida.[62] O ácido acetilsalicílico é um inibidor inespecífico da ciclo-oxigenase que pode ser utilizado para reduzir a inflamação glomerular e inibir a agregação plaquetária, o que pode ser um benefício adicionado de prevenir o tromboembolismo. Em teoria, baixas doses de ácido acetilsalicílico (1 a 5 mg/kg PO diariamente) podem ser utilizadas, mas o melhor protocolo com ácido acetilsalicílico para inibição plaquetária em cães é desconhecido. O clopidogrel (1,1 mg/kg PO a cada 24 h) também pode reduzir de forma efetiva a atividade plaquetária em cães, embora não existam evidências de que seja superior ao ácido acetilsalicílico.[63]

A recomendação do consenso da IRIS é fornecer dietas com níveis modificados de proteína para cães com glomerulopatia (ver Capítulo 184). A redução da proteína da dieta reduz a proteinúria e retarda a progressão da DRC.[64,65] Dietas não devem ser suplementadas com proteína, pois isso pode agravar as perdas proteicas urinárias. A melhor relação entre ácidos graxos poli-insaturados ômega-3 e 6 e restrição no sal e fósforo encontrados em dietas renais caninas também podem ser benéficas para cães com glomerulopatias. A suplementação com ácidos graxos ômega-3 demonstrou ser renoprotetora em cães com doença renal e amenizar a hipertensão, além de reduzir as concentrações séricas de triglicerídeos e colesterol em seres humanos com SN.[66] Esses efeitos positivos são em parte mediados através da geração de prostaglandinas de três séries. A restrição do sódio é benéfica no controle da hipertensão e retenção de fluidos.

TRATAMENTO IMUNOSSUPRESSOR DE CÃES COM GLOMERULOPATIA

A utilização de fármacos imunossupressores (ver Capítulo 165) no tratamento de cães com glomerulopatia ainda não foi completamente estudada e deve ainda ser considerada experimental.

Entretanto, as recomendações do consenso são de tratar cães que possuam glomerulopatia grave, persistente ou progressiva com evidências de patogênese imune ativa com base nos achados da biopsia.[7] O achado de depósitos elétron-densos em localizações subendoteliais, subepiteliais, intramembranosas ou mesangiais do glomérulo por ME ou demonstração de coloração imunofluorescente positiva e inequívoca para imunoglobulinas e/ou complemento em um imunocomplexos e padrão de membrana basal antiglomerular de deposição nas alças capilares periféricas, ou compartimento mesangial pela MIF fornece evidências convincentes para iniciar um teste da terapia imunossupressora.[7] Evidências prováveis de uma patogênese imune podem ser documentadas por LM com um dos seguintes achados: coloração granular vermelha das paredes capilares com Tricrômio de Masson, pontas ao longo da MBG ou orifícios dentro da MBG pela coloração metenamina prata de Jones. Esses achados seriam esperados em até 50% dos cães com doenças glomerulares.[23] Quando os resultados da biopsia renal não estão disponíveis, se torna mais difícil tomar uma decisão sobre a utilização de terapia imunossupressora porque aproximadamente 50% dos cães com doença glomerular **não** teriam patogênese relacionada ao sistema imune da doença. As recomendações do consenso são de considerar os fármacos imunossupressores no tratamento de cães com glomerulopatia quando a fonte de proteinúria for claramente de origem glomerular, ou os fármacos não forem de outro modo contraindicados, a raça do cão e idade de início da doença não forem sugestivas de nefropatia familiar, a amiloidose parecer improvável e a creatinina sérica for maior que > 3,0 mg/dℓ ou aumentar progressivamente, ou a albumina sérica for menor que 2,0 g/dℓ.[8]

Cães com doença mais grave ou taxas de progressão devem ser tratados mais agressivamente do que aqueles com doença mais estável. De acordo com a afirmação do consenso da IRIS,[7] a terapia com um único agente ou terapia de combinação para o rápido início da imunossupressão deve ser considerada em cães com alta magnitude de proteinúria com hipoalbuminemia, SN, ou azotemia rapidamente progressiva. O micofenolato, ou ciclofosfamida, com ou sem administração a curto prazo de glicocorticoides, foi sugerido como a primeira escolha. Os glicocorticoides devem ser imitados à terapia a curto prazo porque a proteinúria foi demonstrada em cães com excesso de corticosteroides e podem induzir lesões glomerulares, e a administração de prednisolona demonstrou aumentar de forma reversível a proteinúria em cães com nefrite hereditária.[17,67,68] Cães com doença estável ou mais lentamente progressiva que apresentam resposta somente parcial ou ausente à terapia-padrão podem ser submetidos ao tratamento com fármacos que possuem início de ação rápido ou mais retardado, como o micofenolato, clorambucila ou ciclofosfamida. A ciclosporina foi também sugerida como uma primeira escolha para cães estáveis ou lentamente progressivos; entretanto, esse é o único fármaco que tem sido estudo prospectivamente em cães com doença glomerular, e foi observado que não causava benefícios, embora tenha havido falhas nesse estudo.[69] Todos os cães tratados com terapia imunossupressora para a doença glomerular devem ser monitorados intimamente. O tratamento deve ser descontinuado ou ajustado se efeitos adversos aos fármacos ocorrerem. Na ausência de efeitos adversos, 8 a 12 semanas de terapia devem ser fornecidas antes de alterar o curso do tratamento. Se a resposta terapêutica não for excelente ao final de 8 a 12 semanas, um protocolo alternativo terapêutico deve ser considerado. Entretanto, se após 3 a 4 meses uma resposta terapêutica não for obtida, deve haver consideração sobre a descontinuação da administração de fármacos imunossupressores. Se após esse tempo uma resposta for notada, a dose do fármaco ou posologia deve ser ajustada para uma que mantenha a resposta sem piorar os sinais de proteinúria, azotemia ou sinais clínicos.[7]

Monitoramento do paciente

Cães com doença glomerular estável e DRC em estágio 1 ou 2 pela IRIS devem ser avaliados 3 a 14 dias após alterações na terapia, enquanto aqueles com doença instável ou DRC em estágio 3 ou 4 pela IRIS devem ser avaliados 3 a 5 dias após qualquer alteração na terapia. Se alterações terapêuticas não estão sendo feitas e os cães estão aparentemente estáveis, reavaliações padronizadas devem ser feitas a cada 3 meses. A RPCU, urinálise, peso corporal, escore de condição corporal, pressão sanguínea arterial sistêmica e concentrações séricas de albumina, creatinina e potássio devem ser incluídas nessas avaliações. Como as lesões histológicas não necessariamente são resolvidas mesmo que a função renal possa melhorar, a repetição de biopsias geralmente não é necessária.

A resposta à terapia historicamente tem sido focada em uma redução da proteinúria. Entretanto, é lógico também avaliar alterações nas concentrações séricas de creatinina e albumina. Uma resposta completa à terapia é definida como uma redução na RPCU para níveis menores que 0,5, uma redução na creatinina sérica para níveis menores que 1,4 mg/dℓ, ou um aumento sustentado na albumina sérica para níveis acima de 2,5 g/dℓ; enquanto uma resposta parcial é definida como uma redução maior que 50% na RPCU, uma redução sustentada maior que 25% na creatinina sérica ou redução sustentada maior que 50% na albumina sérica quando comparados aos níveis basais, ou aumento na albumina sérica para níveis acima de 2,0 a 2,5 g/dℓ.[7] Variações diárias na RPCU ocorrem na maioria dos cães com proteinúria glomerular, sendo que a variação maior ocorre em cães com RPCU acima de 4.[70] A alteração da proteinúria é mais acuradamente mensurada pela avaliação de tendências na RPCU com o passar do tempo Como existe maior variação em cães com RPCU acima de 4, devem ser consideradas duas a três RPCU seriadas ou mensuração da RPCU na urina que foi agrupada a partir de duas ou três coletas.

COMPLICAÇÕES DA DOENÇA GLOMERULAR

Complicações da proteinúria grave incluem formação de edema, hipertensão sistêmica, hipercoagulabilidade e tromboembolismo, hiperlipidemia, aumento do risco de infecções, alteração da farmacocinética (ver Capítulo 160), desnutrição, caquexia muscular (ver Capítulo 177), e anormalidades endócrinas.[58] A formação de edema, hipertensão sistêmica e hipercoagulabilidade são as complicações mais frequentemente reconhecidas em cães, e menos comumente em gatos com doença glomerular.

Formação de edema

Diversos fatores contribuem para a formação do edema em pacientes com SN (ver Capítulo 18).[58] Em formas graves de SN, diminuições da pressão oncótica plasmática permitem a transudação de fluido em direção aos espaços intersticiais. A diminuição resultante no volume plasmático efetivo leva ao aumento da atividade do sistema renina-angiotensina-aldosterona e retenção de água e sódio, e piora do edema. Entretanto, a maioria dos humanos com SN não apresenta hipovolemias ou aumento das atividades plasmáticas de renina ou aldosterona. Assim, a retenção primária de sódio deve também estar envolvida na patogênese do edema nesses pacientes. Mecanismos propostos na retenção de sódio primária renal incluem uma redução da taxa de filtração glomerular individual de néfrons com aumento da reabsorção tubular proximal e modificação induzida por citocinas da reabsorção distal, levando à resistência a fatores natriuréticos, incluindo o peptídeo natriurético atrial. Em humanos, acredita-se que os mecanismos de retenção primária renal de sódio são os determinantes mais importantes da formação de edema até que a concentração sérica de albumina diminua para níveis abaixo de 2 g/dℓ. Abaixo dessa concentração, a pressão plasmática oncótica está suficientemente reduzida para permitir a transudação do fluido a partir do compartimento vascular em direção ao espaço intersticial.[58] Cães podem ser mais resistentes à formação de edema, que geralmente não ocorre até que a concentração sérica de albumina esteja abaixo de 1,5 g/dℓ. O volume plasmático pode estar reduzido até esse nível, tornando a utilização de diuréticos no tratamento do edema relativamente ineficaz e também perigosa por conta do maior risco de lesão renal aguda e tromboembolismo.[58] Cães com glomerulopatia

devem ter avaliação cuidadosa do estado de hidratação e volume vascular antes e durante a fluidoterapia. Essa avaliação deve ser baseada em mensurações seriadas do peso corporal, turgor cutâneo, coloração e umidade de membranas mucosas, tempo de preenchimento capilar, temperatura de extremidades, frequência cardíaca, qualidade do pulso e pressão sanguínea sistólica. A utilização de diuréticos deve ser limitada a situações nas quais a ascite ou efusão pleural estejam prejudicando de forma crítica a função dos órgãos.[6] Quando indicada, a furosemida pode ser o fármaco de escolha para cães com edema pulmonar ou hiperpotassemia e a espironolactona para cães com efusão pleural ou abdominal.[6] A provisão de exercícios adequados também podem ajudar a reduzir a formação de edema ou ascite.

Hipertensão

A hipertensão sistêmica foi relatada em até 80% dos cães com glomerulopatia (ver Capítulo 157). A frequência da hipertensão em cada forma de glomerulopatia não foi ainda estabelecida completamente em cães, mas varia em humanos. Achados preliminares sugerem que uma maior frequência de hipertensão poderia ser observada em cães com GNMP.[23] O mecanismo primário de hipertensão em associação à SN supostamente envolve a expansão do volume plasmático em associação à retenção renal primária de sódio. Entretanto, a geração de diversos fatores vasoativos (p. ex., renina, angiotensina II, endotelina) está aumentada em pacientes humanos com SN e pode contribuir para a hipertensão. A deficiência de óxido nítrico pode também ter um papel importante no desenvolvimento da hipertensão.[58] A pressão sanguínea deve ser mensurada em todos os cães e gatos com glomerulopatia, pois a hipertensão descontrolada é um fator de risco para a lesão renal progressiva (ver Capítulo 157 para discussão completa sobre hipertensão).

Tromboembolismo

O tromboembolismo (ver Capítulo 256), talvez a complicação mais séria da glomerulopatia, foi relatada em 5% dos cães com GN, 14% dos cães com amiloidose, e 13% dos cães com todas as formas de doença glomerular.[16,17,22] Como os êmbolos podem ser difíceis de detectar, a prevalência de tromboembolismo em cães com glomerulopatia pode ser maior do que a indicada por esses estudos. O risco de tromboembolismo é maior em cães com proteinúria na faixa nefrótica e hipoalbuminemia. O tromboembolismo pulmonar é o mais comum, mas os êmbolos podem se alojar em outras artérias (p. ex., mesentérica, renal, ilíaca, braquial, coronária) ou veia portal (ver Capítulo 243 para discussão completa sobre tromboembolismo pulmonar).

Embora a perda urinária de antitrombina (AT) tenha ganhado a maior atenção na medicina veterinária, a patogênese do estado de hipercoagulabilidade é multifatorial.[58] A AT é um inibidor da serino protease que modula a geração de fibrina; a heparina catalisa essas reações. A AT (65 mil Daltons) é semelhante em carga e tamanho à albumina (69 mil Daltons); a atividade sérica da AT está intimamente correlacionada à concentração sérica de albumina. Estudos prévios sugeriram que essa correlação íntima pode ser utilizada para prever o tromboembolismo quando a concentração sérica de albumina for menor que 2 g/dℓ, quando seria esperado que a atividade sérica de AT III estivesse menor que 75% do normal.[16] Um estudo recente de tromboelastografia em cães com glomerulopatia não conseguiu suportar essa conclusão, demonstrando que a hipercoagulabilidade pode ocorrer antes que ocorram alterações na albumina sérica ou atividade de AT.[71] Isso ocorre porque a patogênese da hipercoagulabilidade é complexa; outros fatores estão envolvidos. A albumina se liga ao ácido araquidônico, que, se livre, estimularia a agregação plaquetária através da geração de prostaglandinas (i. e., tromboxano B2); a hipoalbuminemia está associada ao aumento da agregação plaquetária.[58] A hipercolesterolemia contribui para a hipersensibilidade plaquetária pela influência sobre a atividade da enzima associada à membrana e receptor através da alteração da composição da membrana. O papel da hipersensibilidade plaquetária no desenvolvimento de hipercoagulabilidade pode ser aumentado pela trombocitose, que ocorre em vários animais com doença glomerular. O aumento das concentrações de fibrinogênio (*i. e.*, acima de 300 mg/dℓ), que está frequentemente presente em pacientes com SN, leva ao aumento da formação de complexo de fibrina e hiperagregação plaquetária. O risco de tromboembolismo pode ser ainda maior pelo aumento das concentrações de alfa-2 macroglobulina; alfa-2 antiplasmina; citocinas pró-coagulantes; fatores de coagulação V, VII, VIII e X; aumento da viscosidade plasmática e pressão intersticial; diminuição das concentrações plasmáticas de plasminogênio; diminuição do volume plasmático e fluxo sanguíneo; lesão endotelial e infecções.[58]

Varfarina, ácido acetilsalicílico e clopidogrel têm sido utilizados na prevenção do tromboembolismo em cães com maior risco. A varfarina é altamente ligada a proteínas. É muito difícil ajustar a dose adequadamente para prolongar o tempo de protrombina apropriadamente (*i. e.*, 150% dos níveis basais) em cães com hipoalbuminemia, e sua utilização não é recomendada. De forma alternativa, o ácido acetilsalicílico em baixa dose é barata, fácil de administrar e possui o benefício extra de reduzir potencialmente a proteinúria. Tanto o ácido acetilsalicílico como o clopidogrel inibem a função plaquetária e não existe um benefício terapêutico claro de um agente sobre o outro. Em teoria, a heparina seria ineficaz em cães com redução da atividade de AT.

Hiperlipidemia

A hipercolesterolemia foi relatada em 79% dos cães com GN e 86% dos cães com amiloidose (ver Capítulo 182).[17,22] As concentrações de colesterol de até 749 mg/dℓ foram relatadas, embora a concentração média tenha sido de 325 mg/dℓ em 69 cães com GN e 350 mg/dℓ em 23 cães com amiloidose.[16,17]

Aumentos do colesterol plasmático total, lipoproteína de muito baixa densidade (VLDL) e lipoproteína de baixa densidade ocorrem.[72] A hiperlipidemia é variavelmente observada em humanos com SN e ainda não foi completamente estudada em cães A patogênese da hiperlipidemia em associação à SN é complexa.[72] A hipoalbuminemia estimula a síntese proteica hepática, incluindo a síntese de lipoproteínas, levando à hipercolesterolemia.[58] A concentração sérica de albumina e pressão plasmática oncótica estão inversamente correlacionadas à magnitude da hipercolesterolemia. Ainda é incerto se a hipoalbuminemia ou diminuição da pressão oncótica plasmática, ou ambos, induzem o aumento da síntese. Alterações no catabolismo lipídico também contribuem para o desenvolvimento de hiperlipidemia. O orosomucoide, também conhecida do glicoproteína ácida alfa-1, que tem um importante papel na manutenção da permeabilidade seletiva glomerular, é perdido na urina de pacientes com doença glomerular. Perdas urinárias de orosomucoide exacerbam a proteinúria, mas também contribuem para

a hiperlipidemia por causar indiretamente a diminuição da produção hepática de heparan sulfato, um cofator necessário para a função normal da lipoproteína-lipase.[72]

Algumas evidências suportam a teoria de que a hiperlipidemia descontrolada contribui para a lesão glomerular e tubulointersticial. A LDL e LDL oxidada podem alterar a função celular mesangial e aumentar a síntese de matriz mesangial, acelerando assim a formação de glomeruloesclerose.[58] A deposição de lipoproteínas glomerular e tubulointersticial e citotoxicidade induzida por lipoproteínas também contribuem para a lesão renal. De forma interessante, lesões glomerulares foram identificadas em gatos com deficiência da lipoproteína-lipase e Schnauzers Miniatura com hiperlipidemia.[7]

PROGNÓSTICO

O prognóstico para cães e gatos com doença glomerular é variável e mais provavelmente baseado em uma combinação de fatores, que incluem o diagnóstico histológico. Embora seja esperado que a doença progressiva ocorra em uma grande porcentagem de animais com doença glomerular, a remissão espontânea e resposta à terapia específica também podem ser esperadas. Ademais, a progressão da doença pode ser lenta o suficiente para que os animais levem vidas relativamente normais, especialmente quando o diagnóstico for estabelecido precocemente no processo da doença. Em humanos, a azotemia, proteinúria grave, hipertensão sistêmica e lesões tubulointersticiais acentuadas no momento do atendimento são os preditores mais significativos de um resultado desfavorável na maioria das formas de doenças glomerulares. Impressões clínicas sugerem que essas mesmas variáveis afetam o prognóstico em cães e gatos.

A sobrevida mediana de 53 cães com GN e amiloidose que não morreram ou foram eutanasiados logo após o atendimento foi de somente 28 dias, embora alguns cães sobreviveram por mais de 3 anos.[16] Cães com doença glomerular e SN tinham uma sobrevida mediana mais curta do que aqueles sem SN (12,5 *vs.* 104,5 dias, respectivamente).[20] A sobrevida de cães não azotêmicos (creatinina sérica < 1,5 mg/dℓ) com ou sem SN (51 *vs.* 605 dias, respectivamente) foi maior.[20] Mais estudos são necessários para caracterizar o histórico natural e prognóstico das várias doenças glomerulares em cães e gatos.

REFERÊNCIAS BIBLIOGRÁFICAS

As referências bibliográficas deste capítulo se encontram online no Ambiente de aprendizagem.

CAPÍTULO 326

Doenças Tubulares Renais

Marie E. Kerl

Túbulos renais controlam o equilíbrio hídrico corporal, excreção de fármacos, balanço ácido-básico e regulação de eletrólitos. Enquanto a taxa de filtração glomerular (TFG) é o principal determinante da função renal, os túbulos determinam a composição final da urina. O ultrafiltrado glomerular contém todos os solutos plasmáticos que são menores que 69 mil Daltons; portanto, toda glicose, aminoácidos e

eletrólitos filtrados são fornecidos aos túbulos pelo ultrafiltrado. A maior parte das substâncias filtradas é reabsorvida. Defeitos tubulares que causam falta de função são incomuns a raros. Eles podem ocorrer regionalmente ou globalmente nos túbulos e são congênitos ou adquiridos. Indicadores de perfis bioquímicos, hemogasometria e urinálise podem ser monitorados para avaliar a função tubular.

Os túbulos renais são descritos de acordo com a função e localização anatômica. O túbulo proximal recebe ultrafiltrado do espaço de Bowman e reabsorve 60 a 65% do ultrafiltrado, uma proporção que é mantida por meio de uma ampla variação de TFG. Essa propriedade é responsável pelo impedimento de que os segmentos mais distais dos néfrons sejam sobrecarregados por fornecimento excessivo de solutos. A absorção tubular é realizada por transporte ativo de sódio (Na^+), que por sua vez promove reabsorção passiva de outros solutos. O túbulo proximal também secreta ativamente alguns solutos (p. ex., ânions orgânicos, cátions e íons hidrogênio [H^+]).[1] Solutos não são reabsorvidos uniformemente; virtualmente toda glicose e aminoácidos filtrados são reabsorvidos, enquanto quantidades menores de bicarbonato (HCO_3^-), Na^+ e cloreto são reabsorvidos. A principal função da alça de Henle é reabsorver aproximadamente 30% do cloreto de sódio ($NaCl$) filtrado contra um gradiente de concentração para gerar um interstício medular concentrado e criar um ultrafiltrado que é hiposmolar em relação ao plasma.[2] O túbulo distal e os túbulos e ducto coletores são responsáveis pelo controle fino de eletrólitos, incluindo Na^+, potássio e cálcio; a regulação final do equilíbrio ácido-básico; e reabsorção hídrica para produzir uma urina concentrada.[3] Manifestações clínicas de distúrbios tubulares renais incluem formação de cálculos urinários, acidose metabólica, glicosúria, aminoacidúria, distúrbios eletrolíticos e incapacidade de concentração urinária.

CISTINÚRIA

A cistinúria é causada por defeitos tubulares proximais hereditários nos quais a reabsorção de determinados aminoácidos não essenciais falha. Desses aminoácidos, a cistina é relativamente insolúvel na urina, resultando na formação de cálculos vesicais na urina ácida.[4-6] Várias raças de cães foram relatadas com cistinúria, e raros relatos foram feitos para gatos.[7,8] As raças de cães relatadas com maior risco de formação de urólitos de cistina variam de certa forma com a localização geográfica, e incluem o Buldogue Inglês, Staffordshire Bull Terrier, Chihuahua, Terranova, Teckel, Welsh Corgi, Rottweiler, Pinscher Miniatura e Jack Russell Terrier.[9-11] Em um relato, o diagnóstico de cálculo de cistina em cães Terranova diminuiu para 38%, comparado a 71% identificados 10 anos antes.[11] A identificação de cálculos de cistina é rara em gatos.[12]

Padrões de hereditariedade para cistinúria variam em pessoas, e são classificados como tipo 1 e não tipo 1. A cistinúria do tipo 1 é caracterizada por um padrão hereditário autossômico recessivo, no qual portadores possuem concentrações normais de aminoácidos na urina. O não tipo 1 é caracterizado por um padrão hereditário autossômico dominante com penetrância incompleta. No não tipo 1, a incidência da formação de cálculos é limitada em indivíduos portadores com cistinúria. Defeitos nos genes *Slc3a1* e *Slc7a9* correspondem pela maioria dos defeitos genéticos associados à cistinúria em pessoas.[4,13] Semelhante a pessoas, cães com cistinúria possuem diferentes modos de hereditariedade. Cães Terranova e Labrador Retriever foram identificados com uma forma grave de cistinúria tipo 1 causada por uma mutação missense que foi identificada no éxon 2 do gene *Slc3a1*.[4,13,14] Mais recentemente, cães Pastores-Australianos foram identificados com uma forma autossômica dominante de cistinúria causada por uma deleção do par de bases 6 que remove duas moléculas de treonina no gene *Slc3a1*, e em Pinschers Miniatura causada por uma mutação missense em *Slc7a9*.[15] Testes genéticos estão disponíveis para a mutação em cães Terranova por diversos anos, talvez causando a diminuição da identificação de cálculos de cistina nessa raça.[11,14] O teste genético também está disponível para outras raças afetadas.[15]

A idade média de formação de cálculos é de 4,9 anos de forma geral para cálculos de cistina; entretanto, cães Terranova e Labrador Retriever são tipicamente afetados com até 4 a

6 meses.[4,11] O grau de cistinúria pode variar dentre os indivíduos, e pode diminuir com a idade.[5] Machos são mais representados em casos de cálculos de cistina com apresentação clínica, mas a cistinúria sem formação de cálculos foi relatada em fêmeas. Os sinais clínicos associados à formação de cálculos de cistina incluem estrangúria, polaquiuria e hematúria (ver Capítulo 331). Cães machos podem desenvolver obstrução uretral secundária. A avaliação do sedimento urinário revela cristalúria por cistina em alguns cães afetados, mas um hemograma e análise bioquímica sérica não auxiliam o diagnóstico. Exames de imagem podem identificar cálculos, mas o tamanho, formato e densidade radiográfica dos cálculos variam. A opacidade radiográfica dos cálculos de cistina é semelhante àquela dos cálculos de estruvita e sílica; portanto, cálculos maiores de cistina podem frequentemente serem visualizados em radiografias simples A ultrassonografia e uretrocistografia contrastada podem ser diagnósticos se radiografias simples não obtiverem resultados positivos.[16]

O tratamento envolve a remoção mecânica ou dissolução médica dos cálculos e tratamento clínico a longo prazo para prevenir a recidiva (ver Capítulos 107 e 331). O tratamento cirúrgico é indicado em animais com obstrução uretral. A análise quantitativa dos cálculos fornece um diagnóstico definitivo. Infecções bacterianas do trato urinário devem ser resolvidas com antibioticoterapia apropriada (ver Capítulo 330). As estratégias de dissolução e prevenção incluem fornecimento exclusivo de dietas com restrição proteica. A cistina é duas vezes mais solúvel em um pH de 7,8 do que 6,5; portanto a alcalinização urinária é desejada.[17] Algumas dietas restritas em proteína (p. ex., Prescription Diet Canine u/d®, Hill's Pet Nutrition, Topeka, KS) resultam na formação de urina alcalina, mas se a terapia dietética não mantiver o pH urinário em um nível desejado, o citrato de potássio oral é recomendado.[16] A indução de diurese (p. ex., pelo fornecimento de alimentos enlatados de baixa proteína ou pela adição de água ao alimento seco) provavelmente é benéfica.[5,16]

Terapias farmacológicas para reduzir a formação de cálculos de cistina incluem fármacos tióis como a D-penicilamina e 2-mercapto-propionilglicina (2-MPG) (tiopronina). A cistina é formada por uma ligação dissulfeto entre duas moléculas de cisteína. Fármacos tióis formam uma ligação dissulfeto com a cisteína para criar um complexo mais solúvel entre cistina e fármaco tiol. Embora ambos os fármacos sejam efetivos, a quelação de metais e efeitos colaterais gastrintestinais da D-penicilamina a tornam uma escolha menos desejável.[6] O 2-MPG (15 a 20 mg/kg PO a cada 12 horas) é o tratamento de escolha, em combinação com modificações dietéticas para dissolução e prevenção de cálculos de cistina.[5,6,18]

CARNITINÚRIA

A carnitina é um aminoácido não essencial que contém enxofre que funciona como um cofator enzimático necessário para transportar ácidos graxos geradores de energia a partir do citoplasma para a matriz mitocondrial. A deficiência persistente, que foi relatada em cães com cardiomiopatia dilatada (ver Capítulo 252), pode resultar da biossíntese defeituosa, captação ou retenção tecidual defeituosa ou excessiva excreção renal.[19,20] A carnitinúria foi relatada em cães com cistinúria.[19] Embora dietas com altos níveis de gordura e baixos níveis de proteína sejam recomendadas para o tratamento de cistinúria, dietas ricas em gordura aumentam a excreção renal de carnitina em humanos. Cães saudáveis que consomem dietas com baixos e altos níveis de gordura excretam quantidades semelhantes de carnitina; entretanto, cães cistinúricos com alterada reabsorção de aminoácidos poderiam excretar uma quantidade excessiva de carnitina se consumirem uma dieta rica em gordura.[19] A excreção crônica e excessiva de carnitina eventualmente resulta em deficiência de carnitina, levando à cardiomiopatia.

HIPERURICOSÚRIA

A hiperuricosúria é definida como uma quantidade excessiva de ácido úrico, um produto intermediário do metabolismo proteico, na urina. As porções de purina de ácidos nucleicos sofrem metabolismo para formar hipoxantina e xantina, que são oxidadas em ácido úrico pela xantina oxidase (XO). Na maioria dos mamíferos, o ácido úrico é metabolizado ainda em alantoína (um produto mais solúvel) pela uricase hepática (ver Capítulo 332). Em cães saudáveis, a alantoína é o produto metabólito primário que é excretado pelos rins, enquanto humanos e primatas excretam principalmente ácido úrico.[21] Determinadas doenças de ocorrência natural, como o hiperadrenocorticismo, câncer e doença renal crônica, podem alterar os padrões de excreção para esses metabólitos, resultando em maior excreção de xantina ou ácido úrico comparada à alantoína.[22] O metabolismo ou excreção anormal da purina corresponde pela hiperuricosúria em cães de determinadas raças com uma predisposição genética para formação de cálculos de urato, ou naqueles com hepatopatia subjacente. A raça canina que é mais comumente afetada pela hiperuricosúria é o Dálmata; entretanto, Buldogues Ingleses e Terrier Preto da Rússia também foram identificados.[9,11] Dálmatas são intermediários entre cães de outras raças e humanos com relação ao metabolismo das purinas, excretando aproximadamente metade a dois terços da alantoína comparada ao urato.[4] Em humanos, o ácido úrico na circulação pode precipitar nas articulações e causar a síndrome clínica de gota; entretanto, cães Dálmata possuem níveis séricos de ácido úrico mais semelhantes aos cães de outras raças do que pessoas e não desenvolvem gota.[23] Diferenças existem entre Dálmatas e cães de outras raças com relação ao manejo hepático e renal do ácido úrico. A enzima uricase, que converte ácido úrico em alantoína, é armazenada nos peroxissomos hepáticos. O ácido úrico deve ser transportado para os hepatócitos antes que possa ocorrer a conversão em alantoína. Dálmatas possuem quantidades normais de uricase comparadas a cães de outras raças, mas Dálmatas possuem anormalidades do transporte do ácido úrico através da membrana hepática, o que limita o metabolismo do ácido úrico.[24] O ácido úrico é secretado por filtração glomerular e reabsorvido no túbulo proximal; entretanto, Dálmatas parecem ter menor reabsorção tubular proximal do que cães de outras raças. Além disso, Dálmatas possuem secreção tubular distal ativa de uratos como resultado de um defeito de transporte da membrana.[4,25] O defeito, uma mutação de sentido errado (missense) no gene *Slc2a9* que codifica um transportador do ácido úrico, é hereditária como um traço autossômico recessivo para todos os portadores Dálmatas.[26] Manifestações clínicas ocorrem em 25% dos Dálmatas machos. Esse gene também foi identificado como anormal em Buldogues Ingleses e Terrier Pretos da Rússia afetados por hiperuricosúria.[27]

Cães com hepatopatia primária têm redução da conversão de ácido úrico em alantoína e de amônia em ureia. Esses defeitos metabólicos causam hiperuricúria e hiperamonemia.[28] Anomalias vasculares portais e displasia microvascular hepática foram mais comumente associadas à formação de cálculos de urato, embora qualquer disfunção hepática grave possa predispor à formação de cálculos (ver Capítulo 284).[29] Gatos foram relatados com urolitíase por urato. Ao mesmo tempo que alguns gatos com cálculos de urato foram diagnosticados com desvios portossistêmicos, a causa não é aparente em outros gatos.[30,31]

Sinais clínicos de urolitíase por urato são consistentes com doença do trato urinário inferior (ver Capítulo 331). Cães machos podem desenvolver obstrução uretral (ver Capítulo 107). Cães jovens ou de meia-idade são mais comumente afetados do que cães idosos.[9,11] Para Dálmatas, machos são mais frequentemente diagnosticados com cálculos urinários do que fêmeas.[11] Cães com hepatopatia primária não possuem predisposição sexual para formação de cálculos; entretanto, cães machos idosos são mais clinicamente afetados.[29] Gatos que desenvolvem cálculos urinários de urato e são diagnosticados com uma anomalia vascular hepática são geralmente mais jovens (menos que 2 anos) comparados àqueles não diagnosticados com anomalia vascular hepática (4 a 7 anos), e são castrados.[30,31] O diagnóstico definitivo dos cálculos vesicais depende da remoção dos cálculos e análise quantitativa. Os cálculos de urato são radiopacos em radiografias simples, mas podem ser visualizados por ultrassonografia abdominal ou cistografia por duplo contraste. Estudos de função hepática (p. ex., ácidos biliares séricos pré e pós-prandiais, avaliação da amônia sanguínea) são apropriados para cães que não sejam da raça Dálmata e para gatos. Cálculos de urato tipicamente são pequenos e lisos, e variam de coloração, de amarelo a verde a preto.[32]

O tratamento consiste na remoção dos cálculos ou dissolução, seguida pelo manejo clínico a longo prazo para impedir a recidiva. A terapia de dissolução inclui uma dieta calculolítica, medicação com inibidores da XO, alcalinização da urina, eliminação de infecções secundárias e indução de isostenúria.[32] Uma dieta com restrição de purina que tenha níveis baixos de minerais calculogênicos (p. ex., Prescription Diet Canine u/d®; Hill's Pet Nutrition, Topeka, KS) é recomendada.[25,33,34] O alopurinol, um inibidor sintético da XO, é utilizado para o tratamento e prevenção de urolitíase de urato em Dálmatas porque pode reduzir as concentrações séricas e urinárias de ácido úrico pelo bloqueio do metabolismo de hipoxantina e xantina em ácido úrico. O alopurinol deve ser administrado somente a cães que consomem uma dieta restrita em purinas, para evitar a formação de cálculos de hipoxantina e xantina, e a dose deve ser ajustada com base na redução da concentração de ácido úrico na urina.[32,34,35]

A alcalinização da urina reduz a produção tubular renal de amônia, diminuindo assim a produção de íons de amônio na urina, que formam complexos com o urato para formar cálculos. Agentes alcalinizantes (p. ex., bicarbonato de sódio oral [$NaHCO_3$] ou citrato de potássio) devem ser administrados em uma dose que mantenha o pH da urina próximo de 7,0 a 7,5.[32,34,35] A produção de urina diluída é atingida pelo fornecimento de dietas com restrição proteica que reduzam a capacidade de concentração medular renal.

A remoção mecânica dos cálculos deve ser considerada em animais com obstrução uretral ou aqueles que não respondem à terapia de dissolução. O tempo médio para dissolução dos cálculos de urato é de aproximadamente 3,5 meses (variação, 1 a 18 meses).[34] A dissolução algumas vezes ocorre após reparo definitivo de uma anomalia portovascular, mas os cálculos não desaparecem sem resolução dos defeitos hepáticos subjacentes.[35] Como as causas dos cálculos de urato diferem, a terapia com alopurinol não é recomendada para cães com defeitos hepáticos, e não deve ser utilizada em gatos.[35]

O prognóstico é moderado a reservado para recidiva dos cálculos em Dálmatas e o sucesso a longo prazo depende do comprometimento do tutor com relação ao manejo por toda a vida. Em cães com hepatopatia subjacente, o prognóstico é bom se a terapia definitiva para a hepatopatia existir, mas reservado a ruim em cães com hepatopatia irreparável.

HIPERXANTINÚRIA

Cálculos de xantina são raros. A xantina é derivada de purinas da dieta e é metabolizada em ácido úrico pela atividade da XO (ver Capítulo 332). A redução da conversão enzimática aumenta a excreção urinária de xantina, que possui solubilidade semelhante àquela do ácido úrico na urina. A maioria dos cães que formam cálculos com xantina está recebendo alopurinol, um inibidor da XO, para o tratamento de cálculos de urato; entretanto, os cálculos idiopáticos de xantina já foram relatados.[11,36] Urólitos de xantina são raros em gatos, e foram relatados em gatos que não estavam recebendo alopurinol.[36-38] A xantinúria congênita foi relatada em Cavalier King Charles Spaniels, e em um Teckel de pelo duro.[39-41] A prevenção consiste em monitorar a cristalúria por xantina em cães que recebem alopurinol para prevenir cálculos de urato, e ajustar a dose do alopurinol ao paciente.

GLICOSÚRIA RENAL

Sob condições normais, a glicose é livremente filtrada no glomérulo e reabsorvida nos túbulos proximais por difusão facilitada em um mecanismo de cotransporte com o Na^+. O mecanismo de transporte possui uma capacidade máxima que é excedida com concentrações de glicemia de 180 a 220 mg/dℓ (10 a 12,2 mmol/ℓ) em cães e 260 310 mg/dℓ (14,4 a 17,2 mmol/ℓ) em gatos.[42] Quando a glicemia excede o máximo do transporte renal (p. ex., hiperglicemia por estresse ou diabetes melito), ocorre glicosúria. Essa é a explicação mais comum para glicosúria. Raramente, os defeitos tubulares proximais causados por lesão tubular ou distúrbios hereditários podem causar glicosúria na ausência de hiperglicemia.[42-45]

A glicosúria renal primária é rara, mas foi relatada em Scottish Terriers, Basenjis, Elkhounds Noruegueses e cães sem raça definida.[42,46,47] A glicosúria persistente tipicamente ocasiona poliúria e polidipsia por diurese osmótica, embora alguns cães sejam assintomáticos. A avaliação seriada de glicemias ou da concentração de frutosamina devem ser considerados para diagnosticas definitivamente a glicosúria renal por descartar a hiperglicemia como causa de glicosúria.[48] Não existe cura para a glicosúria renal primária, mas o prognóstico a longo prazo é bom com ingestão apropriada de fluidos e controle de infecções renais concorrentes. Em alguns cães, a glicosúria renal é o sinal inicial da síndrome de Fanconi.

SÍNDROME DE FANCONI

Em humanos, a síndrome de Fanconi é um defeito hereditário tubular proximal que resulta em glicosúria, aminoacidúria, proteinúria, fosfatúria e hipofosfatemia. A síndrome de Fanconi também foi relatada em cães, e Basenjis são mais afetados.[44,45,49,50] A síndrome de Fanconi é hereditária em 10 a 30% de todos os Basenjis. Testes genéticos para essa síndrome se tornaram disponíveis em 2011.[51] A síndrome de Fanconi idiopática e hereditária foi relatada raramente em outras raças.

A síndrome de Fanconi adquirida foi relatada em associação a uma série de diferentes causas, incluindo administração de gentamicina, diversas intoxicações que causa necrose tubular aguda, e hipoparatireoidismo primário.[43,52-54] Recentemente, uma série de casos de síndrome de Fanconi adquirida em cães que consumiram petiscos desidratados à base de frango (*chicken jerky*) fabricados na China foram identificados.[55-59] A primeira documentação de síndrome de Fanconi adquirida em gatos foi relatada. Quatro gatos sendo tratados para linfoma alimentar ou doença inflamatória intestinal estavam recebendo tratamento com clorambucila. Ensaios metabólicos da urina confirmaram aminoacidúria e glicosúria, e glicosúria foi interrompida em três dos quatro gatos quando o clorambucila foi descontinuado.[60]

A síndrome de Fanconi causa excreção fracional anormal de vários solutos.[45] A absorção anormal de glicose, resultando em glicosúria e diurese osmótica, é o achado mais óbvio. Anormalidades de reabsorção de aminoácidos variam entre diferentes indivíduos, mas geralmente incluem absorção anormal de cistina. A absorção anormal de bicarbonato, sódio, potássio e urato também ocorrem. A isostenúria algumas vezes ocorre antes da glicosúria e diurese osmótica como resultado do diabetes insípido nefrogênico.[61]

O início dos sinais clínicos em Basenjis afetados tipicamente ocorre entre os 4 e 8 anos, e não existe predileção sexual.[45] Os sinais clínicos tipicamente incluem poliúria, polidipsia, perda de peso, pelame de má qualidade, fraqueza e desidratação. O diagnóstico antes do início dos sinais clínicos é possível se raças predispostas forem regularmente avaliadas para glicosuria.[45] Testes diagnósticos tipicamente revelam glicosúria, euglicemia e isostenúria. Conforme a doença progride, a acidose metabólica hiperclorêmica e insuficiência renal ocorrem. A hipopotassemia significativa clinicamente pode contribuir para a fraqueza muscular.

A progressão é variável; algumas raças afetadas desenvolvem insuficiência renal dentro de alguns meses do início dos sinais clínicos, enquanto outros permanecem estáveis durante anos.[45]

O tratamento é de suporte, pois não existe cura para os defeitos tubulares. O monitoramento para acidose metabólica, infecções do trato urinário e azotemia deve ser realizado regularmente. Os veterinários frequentemente são chamados a participar do protocolo de tratamento da síndrome de Fanconi desenvolvido por entusiastas da raça Basenji, conhecido como protocolo Gonto.[45] Esse protocolo envolve o monitoramento intensivo e tratamento de anormalidades eletrolíticas secundárias e acidose metabólica. Com esse protocolo, a perda crônica de bicarbonato no túbulo proximal que resulta em acidose metabólica é tratada pela administração de bicarbonato de sódio oral, 8 a 12 mg/kg PO a cada 12 horas. Esse método de alcalinização aumentará a carga de sódio e resulta em bicarbonatúria; entretanto, não existe informação na literatura revisada por pares dos efeitos a longo prazo da administração de bicarbonato em cães ou gatos com doença de ocorrência natural.

De forma alternativa, o tratamento da acidose metabólica crônica por doença tubular renal pode ser atingido pela administração de citrato de potássio na dose de 40 a 75 mg/kg PO a cada 12 horas. Os objetivos da alcalinização devem ser manter a [HCO_3^-] sérica em uma faixa normal ($\approx$ 18 a 24 mEq/ℓ), e a [K^+] sérica entre 4 e 6 mEq/ℓ. A insuficiência renal deve ser tratada com restrição proteica na dieta, fluidoterapia, antagonistas de receptores de histamina-2 e tratamento da hipertensão (ver Capítulo 324). O tratamento para a síndrome de Fanconi adquirida deve ser direcionado à resolução da causa de base do distúrbio e fornecimento de terapia de suporte. Em uma pesquisa concluída com tutores e veterinários de cães afetados pela síndrome de Fanconi para identificar alterações clínicas e bioquímicas, e o resultado do paciente a longo prazo, o tempo de sobrevida mediano após o diagnóstico foi de 5,25 anos (variação, 7 dias a 9,8 anos).[45] Além disso, 86% dos tutores relatou qualidade de vida como "excelente" a "boa" durante o tratamento a longo prazo.[45] De 29 cães, 17 morreram ou foram eutanasiados por motivos não relacionados à síndrome de Fanconi.[45]

ACIDOSE TUBULAR RENAL

Os túbulos renais regulam a homeostase acidobásica por meio de dois processos: (1) reabsorção de 80 a 90% do HCO_3^- filtrado no túbulo renal proximal, e (2) excreção de ácidos por métodos de titulação de tampões urinários e excreção do amônio no túbulo renal distal.[62] O termo acidose tubular renal (ATR) descreve raros distúrbios tubulares que levam à acidose metabólica hiperclorêmica. Diversos tipos de ATR foram descritos com base na área dos túbulos renais afetados. A ATR proximal (tipo II) ocorre como resultado da incapacidade dos túbulos proximais em impedir a perda de HCO_3^-, e a ATR distal (clássica, ou tipo I) ocorre como resultado da incapacidade do túbulo distal em excretar H^+. A ATR do tipo IV envolve a ATR distal e hiperpotassemia secundária ao hipoaldosteronismo ou deficiência de aldosterona. Os critérios diagnósticos únicos existem para cada tipo de ATR (Tabela 326.1).[63]

Um defeito no cotransportador $Na^+ - HCO_3^-$ da membrana basolateral, com extravasamento de HCO_3^- em direção ao lúmen tubular, resulta em ATR proximal.[64] Esse distúrbio pode ocorrer isolado ou como parte de outro defeito tubular (p. ex., síndrome de Fanconi).[63] Perdas contínuas causam redução da concentração plasmática de bicarbonato, mas a acidose metabólica associada é autolimitante, por conta de a capacidade do túbulo distal excretar ácido. Se o bicarbonato de sódio ($NaHCO_3$) oral for prescrito para normalizar a concentração plasmática de bicarbonato, a quantidade de HCO_3^- apresentada ao túbulo distal aumenta e sobrecarrega o sistema de tamponamento distal, resultando em bicarbonatúria acentuada.[63]

Tabela 326.1	Características clínicas de acidose tubular renal (ATR) proximal e distal.[63]	
CARACTERÍSTICA	ATR PROXIMAL	ATR DISTAL
Hipercalciúria	Sim	Sim
Hiperfosfatúria	Sim	Sim
Citrato urinário	Normal	Diminuído
Doença óssea	Menos grave	Mais grave
Nefrocalcinose	Não	Possível
Nefrolitíase	Não em geral	Sim
Hipopotassemia	Discreta	Discreta a grave
Perda de potássio	Pior pela terapia alcalinizante	Melhor pela terapia alcalinizante
Alcalinizantes necessários para o tratamento	> 11 mEq/kg/dia	< 4 mEq/kg/dia
Outros defeitos da função tubular proximal*	Sim	Não
Reduções do bicarbonato (HCO_3^-) plasmático	Moderadas	Variáveis
Excreção fracional de bicarbonato com concentração sérica normal	> 15%	< 15%
pH urinário durante acidemia	< 6,0	> 6,0
pH urinário após administração de cloreto de amônio	< 6,0	> 6,0

*Reabsorção diminuída de sódio, potássio, fosfato, ácido úrico, glicose e aminoácidos.

O diagnóstico de ATR proximal é baseado em um pH urinário ácido e acidose metabólica hiperclorêmica, com uma TFG normal mas com aumento do pH urinário e da excreção fracional de HCO_3^- (> 15%) após normalização da concentração plasmática de HCO_3^- com administração de alcalinizantes. A identificação de defeitos tubulares proximais concorrentes (p. ex., glicosuria euglicêmica, aminoacidúria) também ajuda a localizar a ATR proximal.[63] A perda de bicarbonato torna a acidose metabólica pela ATR proximal difícil de ser corrigida, e a terapia alcalinizante exacerba a perda de potássio. O citrato de potássio é melhor para a utilização crônica do que o bicarbonato de sódio.[63] Um comprimido de 540 mg de citrato de potássio fornece 5 mEq de potássio e 1,7 mEq de citrato, e seu metabolismo tende 5 mEq de HCO_3^-.[17]

A ATR distal causa distúrbios da acidificação urinária como resultado da secreção prejudicada de H^+ no túbulo distal.[62,63] Consequentemente, os rins são incapazes de acidificar maximamente a urina em resposta à acidose metabólica sistêmica. Sob condições normais, o túbulo distal é capaz de excretar íons H^+ contra um gradiente de concentração acentuado por conta da bomba íon hidrogênio – adenosina trifosfatase (H^+-ATPase). Esses segmentos tubulares possuem junções estreitas que resistem à volta do ácido, e eles são capazes de gerar amônia para capturar íons H^+ pela formação de íons amônio, que são subsequentemente excretados.[64]

A ATR distal tipo IV está associada ao hipoaldosteronismo ou antagonismo da aldosterona. A acidose mais provavelmente resulta da perda da estimulação pela aldosterona da H^+-ATPase e diminuição da absorção distal de Na^+. Essa síndrome não foi ainda caracterizada na medicina veterinária, mas deve ser considerada em animais com acidose metabólica hiperclorêmica e hipopotassemia.[62,63]

Características úteis para o diagnóstico de ATR distal incluem acidose metabólica hiperclorêmica com aumento do pH urinário (> 6,0). Ao contrário da ATR proximal, com sua acidose metabólica sistêmica relativamente discreta, a ATR distal pode ter uma acidose metabólica mais grave porque o túbulo distal não fornece capacidade de tamponamento. Características clínicas observadas em humanos com ATR distal incluem nefrolitíase, nefrocalcinose, desmineralização óssea, retardo do crescimento e hipopotassemia.[62,64] A ATR distal foi relatada em gatos com pielonefrite e em um gato com lipidose hepática, assim como em três cães com anemia hemolítica imunomediada, e em um cão com leptospirose e que estava recebendo terapia com zonisamida.[65-67] Um gato com ATR distal idiopática foi relatado.[68] O diagnóstico pode ser confirmado pela incapacidade em acidificar a urina com o teste do desafio com cloreto de amônio. Esse teste é realizado pela mensuração do pH urinário antes e em intervalos de uma hora durante seis horas após administração oral de 110 mg/kg de cloreto de amônio. Cães normais devem acidificar a urina para um pH de 5,0, e gatos para um pH de 5,5.

O tratamento para a ATR distal consiste na administração de uma fonte alcalinizante. Uma combinação de citrato de potássio e sódio, em uma dose que varia de 1 a 5 mEq/kg/dia, por via oral, dividida em duas doses, pode ser preferida em detrimento do HCO_3^- como fonte alcalinizante.

DIABETES INSÍPIDO NEFROGÊNICO

O termo diabetes insípido nefrogênico (DIN) descreve qualquer distúrbio no qual o mecanismo de concentração urinário é incapaz de responder ao hormônio antidiurético (ADH) para produzir urina concentrada. O ADH é produzido no hipotálamo, armazenado na neuro-hipófise e liberado na circulação em resposta à hiperosmolaridade ou hipovolemia.[69] Após a liberação, o ADH se liga aos receptores na membrana basolateral dos túbulos coletores renais e ductos coletores, tornando a superfície luminal tubular permeável à água livre, o que promove formação de uma urina que é mais concentrada do que o plasma. A DIN adquirida é uma causa comum de poliúria, porque pode resultar da interferência com o receptor causada por toxinas (p. ex., endotoxinas de *Escherichia coli*), fármacos (p. ex., glicocorticoides, quimioterápicos), condições metabólicas (p. ex., hipopotassemia, hipercalcemia), injúria ou perda tubular (p. ex., doença cística renal, pielonefrite bacteriana), ou alterações no gradiente de concentração medular (p. ex., diminuição da osmolaridade medular).[70] A DIN adquirida também foi identificada como a queixa inicial do atendimento que ocorreu 11 dias antes do desenvolvimento de insuficiência renal aguda por leptospirose.[71]

A DIN congênita é uma doença rara causada por uma deficiência de receptores de ADH. Os sinais clínicos, aparentes logo após o nascimento, incluem polidipsia e poliúria graves, e urina hipostenúrica (densidade específica de 1,001 a 1,005; osmolaridade < 200 mOsm/kg). O diagnóstico é baseado na incapacidade de concentrar a urina após teste de privação hídrica modificado, incapacidade de responder ao ADH exógeno, e exclusão de causas mais comuns de DIN.[69,72]

Tratamento da DIN adquirida deve ser direcionado em resolver a causa subjacente. A terapia da DIN congênita consiste em consumo hídrico livre, restrição dietética de sódio e proteínas, e/ou diuréticos tiazídicos (clorotiazida, 20 a 40 mg/kg PO a cada 12 horas; ou hidroclorotiazida, 2 mg/kg PO a cada 12 horas). A restrição dietética de sódio e proteínas reduz a quantidade de soluto presentes nos rins que deve ser excretada na urina a cada dia, reduzindo mais a perda hídrica obrigatória (ver Capítulo 184).[72] A adição de terapia diurética às restrições dietéticas resulta em desidratação discreta, aumento da captação de fluido e sódio no túbulo proximal, e redução de 20 a 50% do débito urinário.[72] Se o tratamento clínico não for uma opção para o cliente e a poliúria possa ser tolerada, o animal pode ser mantido somente em consumo hídrico livre. O diabetes insípido é discutido com mais detalhes no Capítulo 296.

Tabela 326.2 Biomarcadores urinários atualmente submetidos a estudo para determinar disfunções renais em cães.[75,76]

BIOMARCADOR	SEGMENTO DO NÉFRON	MECANISMO	COMENTÁRIOS
Proteínas de peso molecular intermediário/alto			
Albumina	G, TP	Extravasamento glomerular, diminuição da reabsorção	Amplamente disponível Inespecífica para localização da lesão (glomerular *vs.* tubular proximal)
Imunoglobulina A/G	G	Extravasamento glomerular	Sem vantagem diagnóstica sobre o monitoramento da relação proteína:creatinina urinária
Proteínas de baixo peso molecular			
Proteína de ligação ao retinol	TP	Diminuição da reabsorção	Estável na urina ácida e quando congelada Aumentos progressivos em casos de doença renal crônica Variação intraindividual ampla
Microglobulina alfa-1	TP	Diminuição da reabsorção	Estável em urina ácida Diminuída por hepatopatia
Microglobulina beta-2	TP	Diminuição da reabsorção	Bom preditor da TFG em cães Instável em urina ácida Insensível para monitorar progressão
Enzimas tubulares			
N-acetil-B-D-glicosaminidase (NAG)	TP, TD	Aumento da liberação	Pode ser mensurada em amostras de urina pontuais Afetada por outras doenças (p. ex., hipertireoidismo, diabetes melito), piúria e armazenamento a longo prazo
Gamaglutamil transferase (GGT)	TP	Aumento da liberação	Pode ser mensurada em amostras de urina pontuais Instável na urina ácida Hematúria e piúria podem causar interferência com no exame
Fosfatase alcalina (fração intestinal)	TP, TD	Aumento da liberação	
Lactato desidrogenase	TP	Aumento da liberação	
Lipocalina associada à gelatinase-neutrofílica	TP	Aumento da liberação	Estável em ciclos de congelamento e aquecimento Hematúria e piúria podem causar interferência com no exame Neoplasias, inflamações e infecções podem diminuir a especificidade

G, glomérulo; *TD*, túbulo distal; *TFG*, taxa de filtração glomerular; *TP*, túbulo proximal.

EVIDÊNCIAS DE LESÃO TUBULAR AGUDA UTILIZANDO BIOMARCADORES URINÁRIOS

A lesão tubular aguda (LTA) representa a fase inicial do desenvolvimento de dano renal estrutural e funcional, e precede o desenvolvimento de insuficiência renal aguda clinicamente aparente desde que os biomarcadores renais séricos não estejam tipicamente acima dos limites de referência (ver Capítulo 322). A iniciação da LTA ocorre por doenças de ocorrência natural (p. ex., insulto tóxico, isquemia renal, doença infecciosa), mas também pode ocorrer secundariamente a outras doenças críticas, secundariamente à resposta inflamatória sistêmica, ou por intervenção terapêutica com agentes nefrotóxicos.[73,74] A identificação precoce da LTA permitiria ao veterinário alterar a terapia para deter a lesão renal contínua, ou ser útil como indicador prognóstico ao lidar com os clientes. Os achados bioquímicos séricos, urinálise e avaliações de sedimento demonstraram ser indicadores relativamente insensíveis da necrose tubular aguda. O conceito de biomarcadores urinários refere-se à presença de substâncias bioquímicas na urina que forneceriam uma indicação de disfunção de células tubulares e morte.[75,76]

Exemplos de biomarcadores urinários comuns que estão atualmente em uso incluem a glicose e albumina urinárias. Biomarcadores novos atualmente submetidos à investigação estão em três categorias: biomarcadores de proteínas de alto peso molecular na circulação sistêmica, biomarcadores de proteínas de baixo peso molecular na circulação sistêmica ou aqueles constitutivamente expressos em diversas células renais, e biomarcadores enzimáticos (ver Capítulo 321).[75,76] Biomarcadores enzimáticos de maior interesse em pesquisas são grandes (> 80 kD) e são, portanto, somente expressos na urina a partir do extravasamento de células tubulares danificadas. Esses biomarcadores podem provar ter utilidade clínica maior porque as enzimas se tornam elevadas na urina antes do início da disfunção evidente, a análise é frequentemente mais simples do que de proteínas, e a quantidade ou relação com a creatinina de determinadas enzimas pode ser capaz de predizer o grau e severidade da injúria.[77-81] No futuro, painéis de biomarcadores poderiam ser úteis para localizar o sítio de lesão renal, determinar a gravidade e monitorar a progressão; entretanto, biomarcadores urinários requerem mais estudos para determinar a sensibilidade e especificidade para doenças particulares, e padronização de ensaios, antes de se tornarem disponíveis para uso clínico para veterinários atuantes. A Tabela 326.2 fornece um resumo de biomarcadores urinários estudados para LTA em cães.

REFERÊNCIAS BIBLIOGRÁFICAS

As referências bibliográficas deste capítulo se encontram online no Ambiente de aprendizagem.

CAPÍTULO 327

Pielonefrite

Astrid M. van Dongen

INTRODUÇÃO

A pielonefrite é uma inflamação que envolve a pelve renal, mas também o parênquima renal. Em animais de companhia, é em geral observada no contexto de uma infecção complicada do trato urinário graças a bactérias que ascenderam do trato urinário inferior (ver Capítulo 330).[1] Entretanto, diferentes vias de infecção (p. ex., hematógena) podem ocorrer, e outros agentes infecciosos, como fungos[2-4] e até mesmo infestações renais por nematódeos foram descritas.[5]

Essa doença é uma sequela comum em animais de companhia com condições predisponentes que comprometem a imunidade sistêmica, alteram significativamente a composição urinária ou prejudicam os mecanismos de defesa do hospedeiro do trato urinário (variando de anormalidades na micção, a anormalidades teciduais preexistentes no trato urinário superior). Se não tratada, a pielonefrite bacteriana dará origem a danos permanentes e progressivos do rim envolvido, pode causar um abscesso retroperitoneal[24] ou levar à septicemia.

O reconhecimento oportuno de pacientes afetados pode ser desafiador porque os sinais clínicos e achados diagnósticos algumas vezes são enganosamente discretos, especialmente se a pielonefrite for somente unilateral. Ademais, os sinais associados são inespecíficos e podem facilmente ser ocultados por aqueles que surgem de outras comorbidades. Da mesma forma, o tratamento desses pacientes é exigente, em geral necessitando de avaliações repetidas conforme complicações e/ou recidivas não são incomuns.

FISIOPATOLOGIA

Infecções ascendentes da uretra, através da bexiga e ureter até a pelve renal e tecido renal, são consideradas uma via muito mais provável em animais de companhia, em vez da via hematógena ou pelo sistema linfático (p. ex., no contexto de endocardite bacteriana ou discoespondilite). A colonização subsequente da pelve renal e estabelecimento do foco bacteriano na área medular do rim não é facilmente obtido e em geral requer morbidades adicionais (Boxe 327.1).

Fatores predisponentes (ver Boxe 327.1)

A pielonefrite bacteriana é citada como uma complicação em pacientes com uma doença sistêmica que prejudica o sistema imune, como o hiperadrenocorticismo em cães[6] ou gatos com infecção pelo vírus da imunodeficiência felina.[11] Glicosúria, seja de origem renal[12] ou por conta do diabetes melito[7,13] também está associada a infecções complicadas do trato urinário. Alterações estruturais dos rins,[10] acúmulo de material (p. ex., um coágulo ou nefrólito)[8] na pelve renal, e pielectasia devido à obstrução uretral, tornarão mais fácil a colonização por uropatógenos do trato urinário superior. De forma semelhante, distúrbios anatômicos como ureteres ectópicos[9] ou anormalidades funcionais, como ocorre no refluxo vesicoureteral (RVU)[14] podem facilitar a ascensão adicional de infecções do trato urinário. Para uma discussão mais detalhada dessas

---

Boxe 327.1 Comorbidades associadas à pielonefrite bacteriana

Imunocompetência sistêmica comprometedora
- Endócrinas
  - Hiperadrenocorticismo (espontâneo ou iatrogênico)
  - Diabetes melito
- Infecciosas
  - Vírus da imunodeficiência felina

Mecanismos locais de defesa prejudicados
- Rins
  - Cicatrização renal
  - Glicosúria renal
  - Pielectesia (devido à obstrução ureteral, nefrólitos, coágulos etc.)
- Ureter
  - Obstrução ureteral (urólito, constrição, pressão circunjacente etc.)
  - Ureter(es) ectópico(s)
- Bexiga
  - Refluxo vesicoureteral
  - Cistite bacteriana preexistente (bacteriúria oculta?)

Propriedades bacterianas de virulência
- Sobrevivência na urina
- Aderência ao uroepitélio
- Capacidade de residir no meio intracelular
- Formação de biofilme
- Desenvolvimento de resistência antimicrobiana

---

comorbidades, o leitor é encaminhado para capítulos relacionados ao hiperadrenocorticismo (ver Capítulos 306 e 307), diabetes melito (ver Capítulos 304 e 305), doença renal crônica (ver Capítulo 324), urolitíase (ver Capítulos 331 e 332), infecções do trato urinário inferior (ver Capítulo 330), e distúrbios de micção (ver Capítulo 333).

Além desses fatores relacionados ao hospedeiro, características bacterianas relacionadas à sua capacidade de persistir na urina, aderir ao uroepitélio, se relocar no meio intracelular, formar um biofilme, e desenvolver resistência antimicrobiana[19] também impactarão sua virulência.

Sequelas

A doença renal crônica preexistente estando ou não presente, lesão renal adicional provavelmente ocorrerá como consequência de pielonefrite. Dependendo da magnitude, essa lesão pode resultar em sinais clínicos adicionais (p. ex., poliúria/polidipsia) e alterações metabólicas que são mais graves.

No diagnóstico inicial, pode ser desafiador ou impossível determinar a proporção de azotemia causada por lesão renal aguda e não por doença renal crônica preexistente (comumente denominada como doença renal crônica agudizada). Contudo, durante o tratamento do paciente, é importante considerar e almejar tanto a doença renal crônica como a lesão renal aguda, se existirem, pois a melhora acentuada clínica e bioquímica pode ainda ocorrer em 1 a 3 meses após o tratamento exitoso de um processo agudo como pielonefrite.

DIAGNÓSTICO (BOXE 327.2)

Fatores ambientais devem ser considerados, já que esses podem ocasionar exposição a patógenos. Diferenças geográficas existem com relação à ocorrência de infecções fúngicas ou nematódeas, mas também podem ser aplicadas em um nível mais local, como exposição a uropatógenos (possivelmente multirresistentes) em uma situação hospitalar.[29]

Epidemiologia

Diferenças entre espécies podem ser consideradas porque infecções do trato urinário são relatadas mais comumente em cães do que em gatos. Entretanto, em casos de pielonefrite, haverá um maior impacto por predisposições sexual, etária e racial para as diversas comorbidades, como discutido na seção de fisiopatologia, anteriormente.

Histórico e queixa principal

O histórico médico com relação ao paciente com possível pielonefrite deve incluir questões para avaliar fatores de risco por meio de viagens, dieta, doenças prévias, medicações e históricos familiares sugestivos.

Sinais observados pelo tutor associados à pielonefrite podem variar desde postura corporal anormal sugestiva de dor abdominal, e diversas alterações na micção que incluem disúria, poliúria/polidipsia, e/ou urina macroscopicamente anormal. Esses são mais sugestivos de pielonefrite se coincidirem com sinais generalizados de apatia, êmese e/ou episódios febris recorrentes. Entretanto, nenhum desses é específico da pielonefrite, os quais podem permanecer até mesmo subclínicos.

Achados físicos

Pelas razões descritas anteriormente, o foco do exame físico precisa incluir sistemas e anormalidades possíveis associadas a

---

Boxe 327.2 Lista para pacientes com suspeita de pielonefrite

Diferenças geográficas/prevalências regionais
Dados de resenha (espécie, raça, sexo, predisposições associadas à idade para comorbidades)
Histórico
- Fatores de risco (viagens, dieta, históricos de casos e familiares, medicações)
- Sinais clínicos que envolvem o sistema urinário (disúria, poliúria, polidipsia, urina anormal)
- Sinais clínicos de doença sistêmica (febre, êmese)
Exame físico
- Dependendo de comorbidades
- Palpação abdominal (especialmente rins e áreas adjacentes)
Urinálise
- Densidade específica
- Fita (glicose, cetonas)
- Avaliação microscópica do sedimento
  - Cristais, cilindros, células (epiteliais, eritrócitos, leucócitos)
  - Agentes infecciosos (bactérias, leveduras, fungos, ovos)
- Avaliação microbiológica (cultura e antibiograma)
Hemograma (hematócrito, contagem e diferencial de leucócitos)
Perfil bioquímico sérico (azotemia, eletrólitos, outros baseados em comorbidades)
Diagnóstico por imagem
- Ultrassom abdominal
  - Rins, ureteres, bexiga
  - Pielocentese
- Radiografia contrastada (menos comumente realizada quando ultrassonografia de alta resolução com ultrassonografista experiente está disponível)
Outros baseados em comorbidades

---

comorbidades suspeitas (ver Boxe 327.1). Em todos os casos, a palpação abdominal minuciosa e cuidadosa é indicada. Em gatos, os rins são somente frouxamente ligados à parede abdominal dorsal, permitindo a avaliação adequada mesmo se o gato estiver tenso. A palpação de ambos os rins em cães frequentemente é difícil, mas uma avaliação ainda pode ser feita pelo julgamento da resposta à palpação nas regiões renais e perirrenais. A evidência repetida de desconforto poderia ser indicativa de dor renal e aumenta a justificativa para o diagnóstico por imagem.

Exames laboratoriais

A urinálise (ver Capítulo 72) não somente é essencial para o diagnóstico de pielonefrite, mas também fornecerá informações valiosas sobre possíveis comorbidades. Por sua vez, isso determina a necessidade de testes diagnósticos adicionais e é um elemento importante para direcionar o plano terapêutico. O método de coleta, volume da amostra e avaliação macroscópica devem ser notados, e ajudarão a interpretar o resultado final. Um exame de urina de rotina[15] geralmente inclui a determinação por refratômetro da densidade específica e análise pela fita em busca da presença pelo menos da glicose (combinada a cetonas) em vista dos fatores predisponentes.

A avaliação microscópica ajudará a distinguir hematúria de hemo-(mio-)globinúria e poderia dar pistas para auxiliar com a localização (cilindros, células epiteliais diferentes) e doenças subjacentes (p. ex., cristais, infecções). A avaliação do sedimento seco e corado[16] pode permitir a identificação de leucócitos e potenciais agentes causais (variando de bactérias, leveduras e fungos, a ovos de parasitas). A magnitude da proteinúria renal presumida, que é mensurada pela relação proteína:creatinina urinária, é melhor avaliada após tratamento da inflamação do trato urinário.[17]

Quando os dados epidemiológicos e do histórico poderiam ser indicativos de hiperadrenocorticismo, uma amostra de urina coletada em casa para avaliação da relação urinária entre cortisol e creatinina pode ser valiosa (ver Capítulo 306).[18]

Embora um diagnóstico definitivo de pielonefrite bacteriana possa somente ser estabelecido se de fato a cultura positiva de uma amostra coletada por pielocentese for observada, uma amostra de urina por cistocentese no contexto de histórico, exame físico e/ou alterações de imagem sugestivos é aceita. Preferivelmente, uma cultura bacteriana anaeróbica quantitativa e antibiograma é realizada, mas opções com melhor custo-benefício, como sistemas de fita de urina podem ser considerados.[20]

Hemograma

A avaliação do hematócrito não possui valor diagnóstico para a pielonefrite por si só, mas pode ter um impacto sobre o tratamento do paciente em vista da suspeita de comorbidades ou quando os achados durante o exame físico forem sugestivos de anemia ou eritrocitose.[22] De forma semelhante, pacientes com pielonefrite podem demonstrar contagens leucocitárias anormais que variam desde leucopenia à leucocitose (predominantemente neutrofílica). Se caracterizada por um desvio à esquerda, a leucocitose também pode ser indicativa de bacteriemia secundária.

Perfil bioquímico sérico

Seja causa, seja consequência, a função renal anormal é uma característica comum da pielonefrite refletida não somente em anormalidades urinárias, mas também por distúrbios eletrolíticos séricos e possivelmente pelo desenvolvimento de azotemia se ambos os rins estiverem envolvidos. Para aqueles pacientes que demonstram outras comorbidades, uma gama muito mais ampla de parâmetros pode ser interessante; por exemplo, em casos com glicosúria, os níveis glicêmicos também serão interessantes.

Diagnóstico por imagem

A ultrassonografia abdominal oferece um modo conveniente de avaliar a morfologia renal, incluindo a distinção corticomedular e diâmetro pélvico renal (Figura 327.1).[23] Também pode

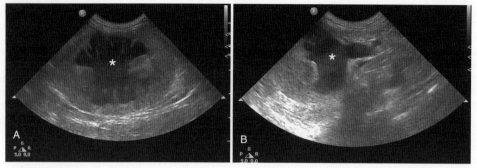

Figura 327.1 Imagens ultrassonográficas sagital (**A**) e transversal (**B**) de um rim com pielonefrite. A pelve renal está acentuadamente dilatada com fluido anecoico (*asteriscos*), e a estrutura do parênquima renal circundante está distorcida.

fornecer guia para a pielocentese percutânea e, dependendo do diâmetro uretral, experiência do operador e cooperação do paciente, até mesmo permitir a visualização do efluxo do ureter, identificação de uma obstrução, e/ou avaliação da localização de sua entrada na bexiga.

Radiografias simples fornecem informações limitadas, mas podem indicar a localização dos rins, a localização de estruturas adjacentes, e a presença de material com radiopacidade anormal (p. ex., calcificações) na região renal e/ou porções inferiores do trato urinário.

Com o auxílio do meio de contraste (administrado por via anterógrada ou retrógrada), a imagem radiográfica do sistema urinário pode ser amplamente melhorada para identificar distúrbios anatômicos (ureteres ectópicos) e funcionais, como refluxo vesicoureteral.

Tomografia computadorizada e ressonância magnética podem melhorar características específicas do trato urinário, fornecendo assim valor adicional nos casos em que permanecem dúvidas sobre a natureza ou grau de extensão do processo mórbido, mas tais modalidades geralmente não são necessárias para obtenção do diagnóstico de pielonefrite.

Embora as biopsias teciduais renais possam facilitar o diagnóstico de doença renal difusa, é muito menos provável que possam identificar adequadamente infiltrados muito localizados que predominantemente estão presentes na medula. Essa limitação, adicionada aos maiores riscos envolvidos na biopsia de tecido contaminado, significa que não é recomendado obter uma amostra de biopsia renal por método incisional ou em cunha em casos de qualquer infecção do trato urinário, incluindo pielonefrite bacteriana ativa.

TRATAMENTO DO PACIENTE

O plano terapêutico (Boxe 327.3) deve ser customizado de acordo com os achados do paciente porque raramente a pielonefrite é uma entidade isolada e o tratamento inacurado ou incompleto pode dar origem a complicações sérias ou até mesmo com risco de morte (por comorbidades maltratadas, pielonefrite descontrolada, ou ambos).

A maior prioridade deve ser dada para a estabilização respiratória e hemodinâmica se os achados forem indicativos de doença sistêmica grave. Isso em geral necessitará de hospitalização, e a combinação de fluidos IV e suporte eletrolítico com antibióticos parenterais. Em pacientes com pielonefrite em estado crítico, a seleção de antibióticos inicialmente é empírica (p. ex., ampicilina 20 mg/kg IV a cada 8 horas), e é baseada em padrões de suscetibilidade aplicáveis localmente[28] e regulações (p. ex., banindo o uso de antibióticos de último recurso, como fluorquinolonas e cefalosporinas de terceira geração se não fundamentado por resultados de cultura e antibiograma).

Boxe 327.3 Tratamento de pacientes com pielonefrite bacteriana

Estabilize se necessário (suporte hidreletrolítico, antibióticos IV)
Elimine ou reduza fatores/comorbidades predisponentes
Inicie antibioticoterapia, preferivelmente baseada em cultura e antibiograma (duração do tratamento: 3 a 4 semanas ou mais)
Acompanhamento
- Verifique a melhora clínica (primeira semana)?
- Verifique a urinálise antes do final do tratamento
- Reavalie a urinálise em busca da recidiva da infecção
  - 1 a 2 semanas após interrupção dos antibióticos
  - Quando os sinais clínicos surgirem
Avalie e monitore a função renal (e outras comorbidades)

Até onde for possível, medidas para tentar erradicar ou pelo menos reduzir os fatores predisponentes tratáveis devem ser tomadas (p. ex., início de tratamento do diabetes melito, ou início de medidas para normalizar a micção [ver Capítulo 333]).

Em pacientes que estão mais estáveis é apropriado considerar esperar os resultados do antibiograma *in vitro* antes de determinar qual antibiótico será utilizado, ou pelo menos reavaliar as escolhas terapêuticas prévias e seus resultados. Essa abordagem pode melhorar o resultado comparado a antibióticos empiricamente escolhidos, e (de forma ideal) também contribuem para deter o aumento na resistência antibiótica.[21] Além da sensibilidade *in vitro*, é válido também considerar a capacidade do antibiótico em penetrar no tecido renal. Custos e efeitos colaterais potenciais também devem ser levados em conta, assim como a duração prolongada do tratamento de pelo menos 3 a 4 semanas ou até por mais tempo, rotineiramente são apropriados em animais com infecções complicadas do trato urinário. Entretanto, as evidências que fundamentam esses esquemas prolongados de tempo são muito limitadas e atualmente sob análise em vista do aumento dos padrões e ocorrência de resistência antibiótica.[25]

Uma opção terapêutica alternativa relatada é a drenagem percutânea guiada por ultrassom com lavagem,[26] nos casos em que o tratamento localizado repetitivo com solução antisséptica eliminou com sucesso a infecção na pelve renal. A nefrectomia unilateral[27] como tratamento para pielonefrite deve ser vista como um último recurso quando, apesar de antibioticoterapia apropriada, recidivas ocorrem e um nicho bacteriano (p. ex., nefrólito) no rim é provável. É vital tentar garantir previamente que o rim remanescente terá função adequada. A azotemia persistente, portanto, poderia ser vista como uma contraindicação porque implica que ambos os rins estão debilitados. Em animais não azotêmicos, outros achados (p. ex., urinálise, achados ultrassonográficos renais) podem ser úteis, mas idealmente a cintilografia renal deve ser considerada para separar a função do rim esquerdo e do direito antes de considerar a nefrectomia.

Medidas adicionais para abordar a doença renal crônica devem ser priorizadas nesse estágio (ver Capítulo 324); mesmo quando

CAPÍTULO 328 • Doenças Renais Familiares e Congênitas de Gatos e Cães

é assumido que o paciente esteja clinicamente estável, ele/ela deve ser monitorado intimamente para garantir que a ingestão adequada de fluido e alimento. Se houver dúvidas, é melhor adiar qualquer alteração dietética que poderia influenciar adversamente, até que o apetite tenha melhorado satisfatoriamente.

Planos terapêuticos estabelecidos para pacientes com pielonefrite que já tinham doenças renais crônicas preexistentes poderiam necessitar de diversos ajustes (temporários) até que a estabilização e estágio sejam reconfirmados no acompanhamento, pois o controle ou eliminação da pielonefrite pode ter um papel discreto a importante na progressão da doença dependendo da gravidade da condição e resposta ao tratamento.

ACOMPANHAMENTO

Além de quaisquer doenças subjacentes, pacientes com pielonefrite devem ser considerados crônicos a menos que sejam comprovadamente de outro modo, significando que eles devem ter pelo menos um, e preferencialmente dois, atendimentos de acompanhamento.

O acompanhamento rotineiro por telefone é uma forma fácil para garantir melhora clínica, a qual deve ser notável ao tutor dentro de 1 semana se o tratamento for efetivo. Esse contato também pode render maior substanciação para uma visita de acompanhamento de fato ou pelo menos a submissão de amostra de urina para reavaliação. A urinálise para excluir infecções persistentes do trato urinário é realizada preferencialmente antes do final do tratamento, e poderia ser a melhor forma para garantir que a duração do tratamento seja de fato aceitável para determinado caso. Idealmente, a urinálise é também repetida após 1 a 2 semanas sem antibióticos e em qualquer momento depois que surgirem os sinais clínicos.

A avaliação microbiológica da urina permitirá a diferenciação entre recidiva (mesmo microrganismo está presente) ou reinfecção (diferente organismo está presente). Uma recidiva é mais indicativa de um nicho em algum outro lugar no trato urogenital que permite que o organismo persista e ressurja mesmo após um antibiótico apropriado, e essa informação possui importância clínica em termos de eliminar a causa incitante. A reinfecção em geral ocorre em animais imunocomprometidos (sistêmico ou localmente no trato urinário), e dessa forma, essa informação pode focar o plano diagnóstico e terapêutico mais especificamente.

Especialmente para aqueles pacientes que estavam azotêmicos no momento ou antes do diagnóstico, é válido reavaliar o paciente mais completamente pelo exame físico (incluindo mensuração da pressão sanguínea), urinálise (preferencialmente incluindo relação proteína:creatinina urinária), um perfil bioquímico sérico completo e hemograma.

Uma melhora na função renal frequentemente ocorre após o tratamento de uma lesão renal aguda como a pielonefrite. A realização de reavaliações em dois momentos após o tratamento exitoso da pielonefrite permite que o clínico identifique a presença e magnitude de tal melhora, e também determina o grau de perda de função residual (*i. e.*, estadiamento da doença renal crônica assim que a infecção for controlada).

Frequência e extensão do monitoramento adicional são altamente dependentes da situação clínica, e devem ser executadas mais prontamente em casos demonstrando uma exacerbação aguda, mas pode facilmente passar a períodos de 1 a 3 meses em animais estáveis.[30] Como a doença renal crônica é considerada como a origem e sequela de vários casos de pielonefrite, é recomendada a expansão da urinálise rotineira e cultura com a relação proteína:creatinina urinária, assim como o monitoramento da pressão sanguínea, hemograma e perfis bioquímicos séricos conforme clinicamente indicado.[30]

PROGNÓSTICO

O prognóstico é altamente dependente da eficácia do tratamento, de questões remanescentes que poderiam levar à recidiva/reinfecção, e a quantidade do dano que foi provocado sobre o tecido renal. A doença renal crônica é considerada como origem e sequela da pielonefrite, mas não necessariamente carreia um prognóstico pior, já que a morbidade é bastante variável e ligada ao estágio da doença. Pacientes com o estágio mais inicial que respondem bem ao tratamento antibacteriano podem permanecer estáveis durante períodos estendidos de tempo com uma excelente qualidade de vida.

REFERÊNCIAS BIBLIOGRÁFICAS

As referências bibliográficas deste capítulo se encontram online no Ambiente de aprendizagem.

CAPÍTULO 328

Doenças Renais Familiares e Congênitas de Gatos e Cães

Gilad Segev

INTRODUÇÃO

Doenças congênitas podem resultar de um distúrbio genético ou desenvolvimento anormal de órgãos durante a gestação; nomeadamente, distúrbios congênitos não são necessariamente hereditários. Doenças familiares estão presentes em uma prevalência relativamente alta em raças específicas, costumam desenvolver os sinais no início da vida e assumidamente têm uma base hereditária; entretanto, a última afirmação ainda tem de ser comprovada. Tanto em doenças congênitas como familiares, os sinais clínicos podem estar presentes ao nascimento ou se tornarem aparentes durante diversos estágios na vida (*i. e.*, um início tardio). Graças ao seu início tardio potencial, doenças congênitas e familiares devem ser suspeitas em animais que possuam sinais de doença renal crônica (DRC) em uma idade relativamente jovem (p. ex., < 5 anos). Doenças congênitas e familiares são mais prevalentes em cães quando comparados aos gatos e podem afetar diferentes localizações dentro do néfron (*i. e.*, glomérulo, túbulos, interstício). Essas doenças, muitas vezes, têm natureza progressiva e se tornam fatais, porém a taxa de progressão é bastante variável.

DOENÇAS DE DESENVOLVIMENTO

Definições

Agenesia renal, rins hipoplásicos

A agenesia renal é uma ausência completa de um ou ambos os rins. A agenesia bilateral foi já relatada, mas resulta em morte. A agenesia renal está frequentemente associada a outras anormalidades urogenitais congênitas, como a agenesia ureteral. A etiologia é desconhecida, mas a predisposição familiar foi sugerida em poucas raças, incluindo Beagles, Doberman Pinchers e Shetland Sheepdogs.[1-3] A agenesia renal unilateral é uma condição clinicamente silenciosa, dado que a função do rim contralateral esteja normal. Rins hipoplásicos são pequenos, e possuem um número reduzido de néfrons funcionais. A condição é frequentemente congênita e deve ser diferenciada da atrofia renal, que poderia ser secundária a outros distúrbios congênitos.[4] Os sinais clínicos e prognóstico dependem do grau de hipoplasia e da função renal geral.

Displasia renal

A displasia renal representa um grupo de anomalias de desenvolvimento, e é definida como uma diferenciação anormal do parênquima renal.[5] Macroscopicamente, os rins são indistinguíveis daqueles com DRC adquirida avançada. O achado mais consistente é a diferenciação inapropriada (comparada ao desenvolvimento do hospedeiro) de vários componentes do néfron. Por exemplo, podem ser observados néfrons imaturos (fetais) ao lado de néfrons normais. Os néfrons funcionais sofrem hipertrofia compensatória. Os glomérulos e túbulos fetais estão geralmente presentes em segmentos radiais, se estendendo desde a superfície do rim até a junção corticomedular. Achados histológicos adicionais incluem mesênquima imaturo persistente, ductos metanéfricos persistentes, proliferação epitelial tubular atípica e metaplasia disontogênica. Alterações secundárias podem também estar presentes e incluem nefrite intersticial, fibrose, mineralização, atrofia glomerular cística, cistos corticais e medulares e lipidose glomerular. A avaliação adequada é frequentemente dificultada pelas alterações secundárias mais dominantes. A displasia renal tem sido suspeita em várias raças. Em algumas raças, a doença tem sido muito caracterizada, mas em outras raças pode estar limitada a um único relato de caso ou série de casos (Tabela 328.1).[5-13] Relatos de nefropatia congênita em diversas raças (p. ex., Dogue Alemão, Yorkshire Terrier, Keeshond) provavelmente representaram a displasia renal.

Avaliação clínica

Achados clínicos e clinicopatológicos em cães com displasia renal são consistentes com DRC adquirida. Entretanto, alguns cães com displasia renal possuem poliúria e polidipsia (PU/PD) abundantes, talvez devido à diabetes insípido nefrogênica concorrente (ver Capítulos 45 e 296).[9] Alterações ultrassonográficas (US) são altamente variáveis, dependem da gravidade da doença, e não são necessariamente assimétricas. Essas incluem a diminuição da definição corticomedular e presença de manchas hiperecoicas multifocais dentro da medula renal, em conjunto com hiperecogenicidade medular generalizada.[14] O diagnóstico final é estabelecido pela avaliação de um grande número de glomérulos, muitas vezes necessitando de uma biopsia cirúrgica em cunha.[15]

Diretrizes para o estadiamento e tratamento

Diretrizes de estadiamento e tratamento para cães e gatos com doenças renais de desenvolvimento são semelhantes àquelas recomendadas para casos de DRC adquirida (ver Capítulo 324) com poucas modificações. A proteína da dieta deve ser intimamente avaliada em animais em crescimento. Animais com DRC congênita são frequentemente resilientes à azotemia e podem apresentar alguns poucos sinais clínicos mesmo em casos de doença avançada. Entretanto, o estadiamento completo e tratamento apropriado não devem ser retardados, já que um dos principais objetivos terapêuticos é retardar a velocidade de progressão da doença.

DOENÇAS GLOMERULARES

Visão geral

Diversas doenças glomerulares familiares e congênitas foram documentadas em algumas raças (Tabela 328.1). As mais comuns são nefrite hereditária e amiloidose. Os sinais clínicos dos animais afetados podem estar relacionados à nefropatia com perda de proteína (NPP) *per se*, ou à azotemia (ver Capítulos 62, 72, 324 e 325). A síndrome nefrótica (*i. e.*, proteinúria, hipoalbuminemia, hipercolesterolemia e edema/ascite) foi documentada em um grupo de cães. A hipertensão sistêmica (ver Capítulo 157) e tromboembolismo (ver Capítulos 243 e 256) também são complicações potenciais. A principal característica da doença glomerular é proteinúria; portanto, a detecção precoce requer urinálise (ver Capítulo 72), na ausência de testes genéticos (ver Capítulos 3 e 4).

Amiloidose

Definições

A amiloidose é um grupo heterogêneo de doenças caracterizado por deposição extracelular de proteínas insolúveis e fibrilares com uma conformação específica de folhetos pregueados.[16] A amiloidose hereditária é causada por genes mutantes que codificam proteínas variantes cuja estrutura as torna amiloidogênicas.[17] Proteínas amiloides podem se originar de múltiplos precursores e sua formação pode ser primária ou secundária (reativa). A amiloidose secundária é a forma mais comum em cães e gatos.[18] Apesar de suas origens diversas, todas proteínas amiloides possuem propriedades estruturais, físicas e químicas semelhantes, incluindo a formação de padrões de difração em raios X característica de agregados em folhetos, morfologia uniforme das fibrilas e padrões de formação fibrilar, e coloração específica com vermelho Congo e tioflavina T.[19] Em cães e gatos, as fibrilas de amiloidose renal são compostas por um fragmento N-terminal da proteína de fase aguda, a amiloide A sérica (ver Capítulo 325).

Amiloidose familiar

A amiloidose foi descrita em Sharpeis Chineses (SPCs), Beagles, Foxhounds Ingleses e gatos Abissínios.[20-22] A amiloidose é em sua maior parte reativa, e relativamente bem caracterizada em SPCs.[23] A febre familiar do Sharpei, caracterizada por episódios recorrentes de febre e concorrente edema de joelhos (ver Capítulo 203), provavelmente predispõe à amiloidose reativa sistêmica, semelhante à Febre Familiar do Mediterrâneo humana.[24,25] Depósitos são compostos pela proteína de fase aguda aminoterminal, amiloide A, produzida durante a inflamação como parte da resposta de fase aguda. O rim é o mais frequente e frequentemente o único local de deposição de amiloide. Existem diferenças notáveis entre amiloidose em SPCs e outras raças de cães. Primeiro, em SPCs (assim como em gatos Abissínios), as lesões medulares renais predominam, embora quando avançada, a deposição amiloide renal envolve todas as partes do néfron.[26,27] Em SPCs, a deposição amiloide é comumente notada em órgãos extrarrenais: baço, fígado, adrenais, pâncreas, submucosa gástrica e intestinal, miocárdio, tireoide, próstata e linfonodos.[16,27,28]

A doença tem um início clínico tardio. A maioria dos cães e gatos é levada para atendimento quando na meia-idade; entretanto, o diagnóstico é confirmado em uma faixa muito ampla de idades.[28] A maioria dos SPCs possui azotemia grave e não são trazidos para atendimento veterinário graças aos sinais

CAPÍTULO 328 • Doenças Renais Familiares e Congênitas de Gatos e Cães

Tabela 328.1 Doenças renais congênitas e familiares de cães e gatos.

DISTÚRBIO	RAÇAS AFETADAS	COMENTÁRIOS
Displasia renal	Lhasa Apso, Shih Tzu, WTPM, CKCS, Buldogue, Poodle Standard, Bull Mastiff, Cairn Terrier, Malamute do Alasca, Golden Retriever, Chow Chow, Cocker Spaniel, Kooikerhodje, Boxer, Sabujo Finlandês, Elkhound Norueguês, Schnauzer Miniatura	Em algumas raças (p. ex., Lhasa Apso, Shih Tzu) a doença é bem caracterizada e os critérios são completamente atingidos, enquanto em outras a doença é mal caracterizada, baseada em um único relato/série de casos. Outras raças são provavelmente afetadas
Glomerulopatias		
Amiloidose	Cães: Sharpei Chinês, Foxhound Inglês, Beagle Gatos: Abissínios	Possível autossômico recessivo em Sharpei Chinês[23]
Nefrite hereditária	Cocker Spaniel Inglês, Samoieda, Dálmata, Bull Terrier	
Podocitopatia	WTPM, Airedale Terriers	
GNMP	Cão Bernese Montanhês[59]	Deposição de imunocomplexos, hereditariedade autossômica recessiva sugerida
	Spaniel Bretão[60,61]	Deficiência congênita do terceiro componente do complemento (C3)
Glomerulopatia atrófica	Rottweiler[62]	Glomerulopatia membranosa atrófica difusa global com alterações degenerativas secundárias. Ambos os sexos são afetados e azotemia ocorre no primeiro ano de vida
Outras glomerulopatias	Welsh Corgi Pembroke,[63] Doberman Pinscher,[64] Wheaten Terrier de Pelo Macio, Bullmastiff,[65] Terranova[66]	
Doença renal policística	Cães: Bull Terrier, Cairn Terrier, WHWT Gatos: Persa, Himalaio, Azul Britânico	Pode estar presente em qualquer gato que tenha cruzamento com gatos Persas
Defeitos tubulares		
Glicosúria primária	Elkhound Norueguês[67]	
Cistinúria	Descrita em diversas raças de cães[68,69] e em gatos.[70] Raças comuns de cães incluem Buldogue Inglês, Terranova,[71,72] Teckel, Basset Hound, Rottweiler[73]	Defeito tubular proximal hereditário. Classificado como tipo 1 (autossômico recessivo) e não tipo 1 (autossômico dominante com penetrância incompleta). Predispõe a urólitos de cistina (ver Capítulo 331)
Hiperuricosúria	Dálmata,[68] Buldogue Inglês, Terrier Preto da Rússia	Defeito de transporte de membrana (autossômico recessivo). Cães Dálmatas também apresentam diminuição da reabsorção tubular proximal e secreção tubular distal ativa de uratos
Hiperxantinúria	Distúrbio congênito relatado no Cavalier King Charles Spaniel[74] e no Teckel de Pelo Longo[75]	
Síndrome de Fanconi	Basenjis[55-57]	
DIN congênita	Várias raças[76]	Deficiência do receptor do hormônio antidiurético no néfron distal e ductos coletores. Animais afetados apresentam profunda poliúria e polidipsia
Diversos		
Telangiectasia	Welsh Corgi Pembroke[77]	Hematúria evidente periódica tipicamente entre dois e 8 anos de idade
Nefropatia por refluxo com hipoplasia segmentar	Boxer[78,79]	Pielonefrite atrófica, não obstrutiva, graças ao refluxo vesicoureteral, causando hipoplasia renal
Cistoadenocarcinoma	Cães Pastores-Alemães[80]	Um traço autossômico dominante. Uma mutação no gene BHD foi suspeita.[81] A doença possui início tardio. Pode estar associada à dermatofibrose nodular concorrente e leiomiomas uterinos

CKCS, Cavalier King Charles Spaniel; GNMP, glomerulonefrite membranoproliferativa; WHWT, West Highland White Terrier; WTPM, Wheaten Terrier de Pelo Macio.

clínicos associados à NPP. A síndrome nefrótica é incomum é SPCs porque a deposição amiloide é predominantemente medular, o que causa dano intersticial antes do glomerular.[28] Consequentemente, comparada a outras raças, o grau de proteinúria em SPCs é inferior e o grau de azotemia é maior. A histologia é necessária para confirmar o diagnóstico. O prognóstico é pobre, entretanto os tempos de sobrevida variam substancialmente, dependendo do estágio da doença e do grau de azotemia.[28] Isso enfatiza a necessidade do diagnóstico precoce.

Nefrite hereditária

Definições

A nefrite hereditária, uma das doenças renais congênitas mais minuciosamente caracterizadas, é originada a partir de uma mutação genética que causa formação anormal de colágeno tipo IV. Normalmente, as membranas basais capilares glomerulares são compostas por uma rede de heterômeros de colágeno que contém cadeias alfa3-alfa4-alfa5. Uma mutação em um dos genes codificadores (COL4A3, COL4A4, COL4A5) resulta em cadeias formadas inapropriadamente incapazes de interagir com outras cadeiras para formar heterômeros alfa3-alfa4-alfa5.

Mutações demonstradas

Várias mutações e modos de hereditariedade foram descritos, incluindo ligado ao cromossomo X, autossômico recessivo e autossômico dominante. A nefrite hereditária ligada ao cromossomo X foi inicialmente relatada no Samoieda, com uma única substituição do nucleotídio no gene COL4A5 como a origem da mutação, causando cadeias alfa-5 anormais e montagem anormal do colágeno tipo IV. Isso resulta em divisão da membrana basal, que pode ser detectada por microscopia eletrônica no início da vida. A proteinúria é o primeiro indicador diagnóstico da doença e, em cães machos, pode ser detectada em até 3 meses de vida. A azotemia em machos ocorre e progride durante alguns meses até a morte com aproximadamente 1 ano de idade.[29] Fêmeas portadoras desenvolvem expressão em mosaico das cadeias alfa3-alfa4-alfa5. Assim como em machos, a proteinúria pode ser detectada no início da vida; entretanto, a azotemia progride em uma velocidade muito mais lenta e é aparente somente após alguns anos de idade.[30]

Em Cocker Spaniels Ingleses, a doença é autossômica recessiva e é originada de uma substituição de um único nucleotídio no gene COL4A4. Graças a esse modo de hereditariedade, machos e fêmeas são igualmente afetados. A proteinúria é detectada com poucos meses de vida, e a azotemia progride durante o primeiro e segundo anos de vida.[31,32] Uma mutação autossômica dominante foi descrita em cães Bull Terrier e Dálmatas, em sua maioria da Austrália.[33-35] A mutação genética subjacente ainda não foi caracterizada, mas todos os cães afetados possuem proteinúria. A apresentação clínica é altamente variável e a azotemia ocorre durante uma ampla gama de períodos de tempo, até se tornar aparente em vários meses ou com 7 a 8 anos de vida.[34,36] Consequentemente, cães com doença subclínica podem ser acasalados e a doença é difícil de erradicar.

Diagnóstico

O diagnóstico da nefrite hereditária é baseado na biopsia renal. Na nefrite hereditária ligada ao cromossomo X, a microscopia óptica revela características morfológicas da glomerulonefropatias membranoproliferativa. Nos distúrbios ligados ao cromossomo X e autossômicos recessivos, a imunocoloração da membrana basal glomerular demonstra o padrão anormal do colágeno tipo IV, mas nos Bull Terriers e Dálmatas, a imunocoloração demonstra um padrão normal do colágeno tipo IV, e o diagnóstico pode somente ser confirmado com base na avaliação microscópica eletrônica. Para alguns dos tipos de doença da nefrite hereditária, o teste genético está disponível.[37]

Podocitopatia e glomeruloesclerose

A nefropatia com perda de proteínas é diagnosticada em 10 a 15% dos Wheaten Terriers de Pelo Macio, com um modo complexo de hereditariedade.[38,39] A histologia das biopsias renais revela glomerulonefrite, glomeruloesclerose e evidências de degeneração e perda de podócitos. A doença possui um início tardio, com uma idade média de 6 anos.[39] Portanto, cães afetados são frequentemente acasalados antes de identificados como afetados. Os sinais clínicos em geral envolvem o trato intestinal assim como a NPP. Não existe marcador biológico disponível para identificação precoce; entretanto, o sequenciamento de genes candidatos em dois Airedale Terriers revelou alterações de um único nucleotídio nos genes intimamente ligados NPHS1 e KIRREL2, que codificam as proteínas da fenda diafragmática nefrina e Neph3/filtrina, respectivamente.[39,40]

DOENÇA RENAL POLICÍSTICA

Definições e raças afetadas

Caninos

A doença renal policística (DRP) foi relatada em cães e gatos. Raças caninas afetadas incluem o Bull Terrier, Cairn Terrier e West Highland White Terrier (WHWT). Uma mutação genética no gene policistina-1 (PKD1)[41,42] com um modo autossômico dominante de hereditariedade foi sugerida no Bull Terrier.[43] Um modo de herança autossômico recessivo foi sugerido no Cairn Terrier e no WHWT.[44,45] Cães Bull Terrier tiveram diminuída a função renal nos primeiros anos de vida, com cistos limitados aos rins. Cães das raças Cairn Terriers e WHWT desenvolvem sinais clínicos nos primeiros meses de vida, com múltiplos cistos em ambos os rins e fígado.

Felinos

A DRP é a doença felina genética mais comum que afeta gatos Persas e raças mistas, e é caracterizada por cistos renais, hepáticos e pancreáticos ocasionais. A prevalência relatada em gatos Persas é de aproximadamente 40% em todo o mundo.[46,47] O modo de hereditariedade é um defeito autossômico dominante que é originado a partir de uma mutação de um único nucleotídio (transversão C para A) no éxon 29 do gene PKD1, resultando em um códon de para prematuro.[48,49] Não foram identificados gatos homozigotos, o que suporta a sugestão de que a mutação é embrionária letal.[49] A DRP também foi descrita em gatos com ausência da mutação PKD1 e, portanto, outras mutações podem desencadear a DRP em gatos.[50] Cistos renais crescem lentamente, resultando em uma diminuição gradativa na quantidade do parênquima renal normal.

Sinais e diagnóstico

Os sinais clínicos são consistentes com DRC (ver Capítulo 324). Os rins estão em geral aumentados e irregulares ao exame físico. A detecção precoce pode ser feita pela utilização de ferramentas de testes genéticos (em gatos)[51,52] e ultrassonografia,[53] que demonstra diversos cistos corticais e medulares arredondados ou ovais, hipoecoicos a anecoicos, com até 7 semanas de vida.[54] Tanto em cães quanto em gatos, sua ausência aos 6 meses de vida está correlacionada à ausência de DRP.[48]

DISTÚRBIOS TUBULARES

Prevalência, definições

Defeitos tubulares são incomuns em cães e gatos. Distúrbios tubulares foram relatados como uma condição isolada ou podem acompanhar outros distúrbios renais hereditários ou familiares (ver Tabela 328.1). Distúrbios tubulares incluem glicosúria primária, aminoacidúria (p. ex., cistinúria), distúrbios eletrolíticos, distúrbios ácido-básicos (*i. e.*, acidose tubular renal proximal e distal), e distúrbios do metabolismo hídrico (*i. e.*, diabetes insípido nefrogênico).

Síndrome de Fanconi

A síndrome de Fanconi é um distúrbio familiar complexo em cães Basenji, com uma prevalência de pelo menos 10% e um modo de hereditariedade incerto (ver Capítulo 326).[55-57] O manuseio tubular renal da glicose, fosfato, sódio, potássio, ácido úrico, aminoácidos e bicarbonato pode ser prejudicado. Na urinálise, a glicosúria, proteinúria (em geral discreta) e baixa densidade urinária específica estão geralmente presentes. Em cães com doença avançada, azotemia, hipopotassemia e graus variados de acidose metabólica hiperclorêmica estão frequentemente presentes. Os sinais clínicos incluem poliúria e polidipsia, perda de peso e fraqueza. A maioria dos cães afetados é diagnosticada entre 4 e 8 anos de idade. A velocidade de progressão da doença é altamente variável, sendo que alguns cães têm duração de vida normal.[58]

CONDIÇÕES DIVERSAS

Existem diversos outros distúrbios renais que supostamente possuem base genética. Alguns desses estão limitados a um número muito pequeno de animais, são mal caracterizados, e a causa genética subjacente ainda não está determinada (ver Tabela 328.1).

REFERÊNCIAS BIBLIOGRÁFICAS

As referências bibliográficas deste capítulo se encontram online no Ambiente de aprendizagem.

SEÇÃO 24
Doenças do Trato Urinário Inferior

CAPÍTULO 329

Doenças de Ureter

Larry G. Adams

ANATOMIA E FISIOLOGIA DOS URETERES

Os ureteres são tubos fibromusculares que carreiam urina da pelve renal até a bexiga em um trajeto retroperitoneal. A parede do ureter é composta por camada adventícia externa, camadas muscular, submucosa e mucosa de epitélio de transição. A parede muscular do ureter consiste em camadas muscular longitudinal externa, circular média e longitudinal interna, com exceção da junção ureterovesicular (JUV), onde há apenas fibras longitudinais. Em cães, normalmente o diâmetro máximo do lúmen do ureter é menor que 2,7 mm, mesmo quando o animal é submetido à diurese hídrica.[1,2] Em gatos, o diâmetro normal do lúmen do ureter é de apenas 0,3 a 0,4 mm; portanto, mesmo pequenos ureterólitos ou restos celulares podem ocluir o ureter de gatos. Os ureteres adentram a bexiga na superfície serosa e formam um túnel através da parede vesical obliquamente até a superfície mucosa. O trajeto oblíquo do ureter intramural resulta em um efeito semelhante a uma válvula, conhecida como válvula vesicoureteral. A válvula vesicoureteral, juntamente com o peristaltismo do ureter e a complacência da bexiga, promove o fluxo unidirecional da urina, de modo a auxiliar na prevenção de infecções ascendentes ou de refluxo de urina aos rins (refluxo vesicoureteral). O ureter intramural possui uma conformação de gancho em J com a porção terminal virada de uma direção caudal para cranial antes de adentrar o trígono da bexiga. O grau de curvatura do ureter distal no trígono depende do grau de distensão da bexiga; maior distensão da bexiga resulta em maior grau de curvatura do ureter distal. O reconhecimento dessa curvatura é importante para a interpretação dos resultados de urografia excretora e para o acesso retrógrado aos ureteres durante a cistoscopia (ver Capítulo 108). Quando a bexiga está distendida excessivamente, as tentativas para colocação de guia urológico e cateter ureteral retrógrado até o ureter, por cistoscopia, são prejudicadas.

A inervação do ureter consiste em nervos simpáticos e parassimpáticos; entretanto, a inervação simpática parece ser mais importante para a contração ureteral mediada por mecanismo neurogênico.[3,4] Estudos mostraram a presença de receptores adrenérgicos alfa-1, alfa-2 e beta, bem como de receptores colinérgicos muscarínicos nos ureteres de cães.[4,5] Estudos semelhantes são escassos em gatos. Em cães, a densidade de locais de ligação aos receptores alfa-1 é significativamente maior do que a dos locais para outros tipos de receptor. Contudo, a inervação do ureter não é responsável pelo peristaltismo ureteral normal, que tem origem miogênica. O peristaltismo ureteral ocorre quando a urina entra no ureter, iniciando impulsos elétricos que precisam ser conduzidos entre as células de músculo liso. A atividade peristáltica normalmente é iniciada na pelve renal, e a urina é propelida em direção à bexiga. Como o peristaltismo do ureter normal tem origem miogênica, o peristaltismo ureteral persiste após o transplante. Durante a obstrução do ureter, ocorrem contrações espasmódicas mediadas por estímulo simpático, e a atividade peristáltica normal é inibida. A estimulação do ureter com agonistas alfa-adrenérgicos ocasiona contração do ureter; a estimulação com agonistas beta-adrenérgicos causa relaxamento do ureter.[3-5] Ademais, antagonistas alfa-1 adrenérgicos inibem o tônus basal do ureter, a frequência peristáltica e as contrações ureterais.[6] O entendimento da inervação do ureter pode contribuir para a escolha de medicamentos para o tratamento de doenças dos ureteres. Por exemplo, o tratamento farmacológico para facilitar o relaxamento do ureter para expulsão de ureterólitos pode incluir antagonistas alfa-adrenérgicos ou agonistas beta-2/beta-3 seletivos para relaxar os ureteres e reduzir o espasmo do ureter.[4,7,8]

ABORDAGEM DIAGNÓSTICA PARA DOENÇAS DE URETERES

Recomenda-se ao leitor consultar o Capítulo 321, no qual constam considerações gerais sobre o diagnóstico de doenças renais. Para cães e gatos com suspeita de doença de ureter, a avaliação diagnóstica deve incluir histórico clínico, exame físico, hemograma, perfil bioquímico sérico, exame de urina, urocultura e radiografias de abdome. As radiografias abdominais devem incluir todo o trato urinário, desde o diafragma até a porção mais caudal da uretra. A avaliação do trato urogenital por meio de ultrassonografia de abdome é um complemento útil às radiografias abdominais, quando disponível ao veterinário.

A avaliação do trato urogenital mediante ultrassonografia de abdome (juntamente com radiografias abdominais e uretrocistoscopia) tem substituído amplamente a urografia excretora no exame dos ureteres. A tomografia computadorizada (TC) com contraste também é útil para avaliação de anormalidades de ureter, como o delineamento da extensão e a localização de constrições ureterais, presença de ureterólitos, neoplasias de ureter ou lesões compressivas extramurais que causam obstrução do ureter. Se houver forte suspeita de obstrução de ureter com base em radiografias e ultrassonografia de abdome, pode-se

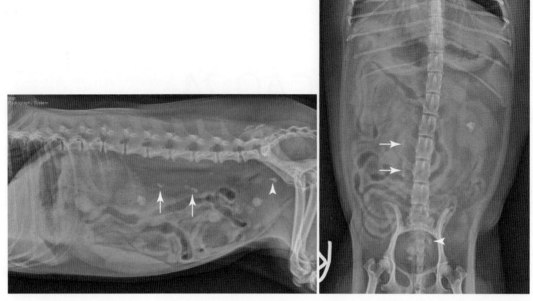

Figura 329.1 Radiografias lateral e ventrodorsal do abdome de cão mostram ureterólitos radiopacos no ureter direito (*setas*) e no ureter esquerdo distal (*ponta de seta*). Também há um nefrólito no lado esquerdo, e as margens do rim esquerdo estão irregulares. A ultrassonografia revelou dilatação moderadamente grave do ureter direito e da pelve renal proximal aos ureterólitos. Os ureterólitos distais do lado esquerdo passaram para a bexiga dentro de 24 horas após terapia hídrica IV.

realizar pielografia anterógrada durante procedimentos intervencionistas, como a implantação de endopróteses expansivas (*stent*) de ureter ou desvio subcutâneo do ureter (ver Capítulo 124), geralmente eliminando a necessidade de obtenção de imagens por TC ou outros exames contrastados, como a urografia excretora.[9]

URETERÓLITOS

Diagnóstico de ureterólitos

Ureterólitos resultam da migração de nefrólitos ou de fragmentos de nefrólitos para o ureter. À semelhança de urólitos em outras partes do trato urinário, os ureterólitos são diagnosticados com base em resultados de radiografias ou ultrassonografia. Ureterólitos radiopacos geralmente são visualizados na região retroperitoneal em radiografias do abdome (Figura 329.1), mas devem ser confirmados por outras modalidades de imagem antes de realizar qualquer tipo de intervenção. Alguns ureterólitos são radiolucentes e alguns ureterólitos radiopacos são muito pequenos para serem detectados em radiografias de abdome. A ultrassonografia geralmente é útil para detecção de ureterólitos ou de dilatação da pelve renal ou ureteral proximal aos ureterólitos que ocasionam obstrução (Figura 329.2).[10,11] A visualização direta dos ureterólitos frequentemente é possível em ultrassonografia (Figura 329.2); entretanto, em um estudo, a confirmação ultrassonográfica de ureterólitos não foi possível em 23% dos gatos examinados.[11] Embora informações semelhantes sobre cães com ureterólitos não tenham sido publicadas, os resultados são, provavelmente, semelhantes aos mencionados para gatos. A nefropielocentese guiada por ultrassom para pielografia anterógrada, mediante a administração de contraste na pelve renal, é uma opção minimamente invasiva para o diagnóstico de obstrução de ureter; no entanto, a técnica requer que a pelve renal esteja suficientemente dilatada para possibilitar a punção acurada da pelve com agulha.[12] Durante a nefropielocentese, a urina é aspirada da pelve renal, e então o contraste iodado é injetado na pelve em um volume aproximadamente igual à metade do volume aspirado. Radiografias seriadas ou fluoroscopia são utilizadas para monitorar a passagem do contraste, a fim de documentar a gravidade e o local da obstrução do ureter. A tomografia computadorizada (TC) obtida antes e depois da administração intravenosa do contraste pode ser utilizada para confirmar o número e a localização dos ureterólitos. A TC contrastada é preferida, em detrimento da nefropielocentese, principalmente quando não há dilatação suficiente da pelve renal. Imagens avançadas, como TC, frequentemente não são necessárias antes dos procedimentos intervencionistas porque a pielografia anterógrada é realizada como etapa inicial dos procedimentos intervencionistas, a fim de documentar e tratar a obstrução do ureter (ver Capítulo 124).[9]

Tratamento de ureterólitos

A remoção de ureterólitos é mais difícil do que a remoção de urólitos do trato urinário inferior. A dissolução medicamentosa

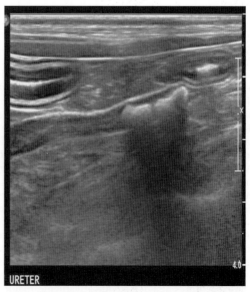

Figura 329.2 Imagem ultrassonográfica de dois ureterólitos obstrutivos, com distensão discreta do ureter proximal ao ureterólito. Note a sombra acústica criada pelos ureterólitos.

dos ureterólitos não é uma opção, sem a implantação de endoprótese expansiva (*stent*) de ureter, pois os ureterólitos não são continuamente banhados pela urina. Em ambos, cães e gatos, a composição mais comum dos ureterólitos envolve oxalato de cálcio; portanto, a maioria dos ureterólitos não é passível de dissolução. Recomenda-se o tratamento clínico conservador mediante monitoramento seriado dos ureterólitos, juntamente com administração intravenosa de fluidos e diuréticos (p. ex., manitol), pois há mínimo comprometimento da função renal e ausência de infecção, cólica renal ou dilatação de ureter progressiva.[13-15] Geralmente, cães e gatos com evidências de obstrução total por ureterólitos, com agravamento da azotemia ou evidência de pielonefrite, devem ser submetidos a tratamento minimamente invasivo, intervenção cirúrgica aberta ou litotripsia por onda de choque (LOC; apenas em cães).[9,13,16-20] Por conta de diversos fatores (tamanho do ureter, suscetibilidade à fragmentação por LOC, diferenças nas composições dos urólitos), a abordagem terapêutica para cães e gatos com ureterólitos é diferente para cada espécie.

Excreção espontânea de ureterólitos

O tamanho e a localização dos ureterólitos podem ajudar a determinar se há necessidade de intervenção. Em humanos, 68% dos ureterólitos com menos que 5 mm de diâmetro e 47% dos ureterólitos entre 5 e 10 mm são excretados espontaneamente.[21] A maioria dos ureterólitos excretados espontaneamente o faz dentro de 4 a 6 semanas. Em pessoas, a maioria dos ureterólitos com mais de 10 mm requer intervenção com LOC ou litotripsia a *laser* ureteroscópica para a remoção.[21] É difícil aplicar esses critérios específicos a cães e gatos por causa da ampla variação do peso corporal e do diâmetro do ureter, mas a taxa de excreção espontânea de ureterólitos parece ser muito menor em cães e gatos do que em humanos. Em um estudo experimental sobre ureterólitos artificiais em cães de caça, constatou-se que esferas sólidas com 2,8 mm de diâmetro ou mais fixaram-se firmemente no ureter; entretanto, esferas de 2,3 mm de diâmetro passaram para a bexiga dentro de 1 a 24 horas.[22] No entanto, esse estudo pode não ser aplicado a cães de menor porte com ureterólitos de excreção espontânea em razão de seu diâmetro ureteral menor. Da mesma forma, o diâmetro do lúmen do ureter normal do gato, de apenas 0,3 a 0,4 mm, resulta na incapacidade de excreção até mesmo de ureterólitos com menos de 1 a 2 milímetros na maioria dos gatos. Em um estudo de gatos com ureterólitos, o tratamento medicamentoso de gatos com ureterólitos obstrutivos foi relatado como efetivo em apenas 8 a 13% dos casos.[13] Ademais, dados recentes indicam que mais de 20% dos ureterólitos em gatos estão associados a constrições ureterais concomitantes; portanto, o sucesso do tratamento medicamentoso pode ser limitado por essas constrições.[17]

Tratamento medicamentoso expulsivo

O tratamento medicamentoso expulsivo (TME) pode ser importante no tratamento de ureterólitos obstrutivos. Os TME sugeridos consistem na administração por via intravenosa de fluidos, juntamente com diuréticos (p. ex., manitol), antagonistas alfa-adrenérgicos, agentes bloqueadores dos canais de cálcio (nifedipino), amitriptilina e glucagon. Em humanos, os critérios para utilização de TME *versus* procedimentos intervencionistas incluem o adequado controle da dor durante o TME, sem evidência de sepse, e adequada reserva renal.[21] Em cães e gatos, o TME mais aceito é a administração por via intravenosa de fluidos com diuréticos, a fim de aumentar o fluxo urinário e facilitar a excreção de ureterólitos, com monitoramento seriado de sua localização por meio de radiografias e ultrassonografia, juntamente com a administração do antagonista alfa-adrenérgico prazosina.[23,24]

Em pessoas, se um ureterólito permanece no mesmo local durante 2 semanas e se há aumento progressivo do ureter ou da pelve renal, se não é possível o alívio efetivo da dor, ou se a

função renal foi comprometida pela obstrução, recomendam-se técnicas intervencionistas em detrimento do TME,[21] e essa informação também pode ser aplicada a cães e gatos com ureterólitos. Se o animal for monitorado durante 2 semanas e o ureterólito não estiver deslocado distalmente, apesar do TME, algum tipo de intervenção pode também causar o deslocamento espontâneo em direção retrógrada, de volta para a pelve renal, e não em direção distal, para a bexiga.[25]

Em humanos, a metanálise de diversos estudos clínicos confirmou que antagonistas alfa-adrenérgicos facilitam a excreção de cálculos ureterais mais efetivamente do que outros medicamentos. O uso do antagonista alfa-adrenérgico tansulosina aumentou a taxa de excreção efetiva de ureterólitos em 29%, comparativamente aos pacientes do grupo-controle.[21] Em cães e gatos, a utilização do antagonista alfa-adrenérgico prazosina foi sugerida para TME como alternativa à tansulosina, mas estudos clínicos sobre a eficácia do TME são escassos nessas espécies.[24] Em gatos, a eficácia geral no TME é baixa e quase sempre há constrições ureterais concomitantes; portanto, o TME deve ser realizado por um período limitado (em geral 24 a 48 horas) e somente em gatos sem evidência de oligúria, azotemia grave, hidronefrose grave, sepse, hiperidratação ou hiperpotassemia. Em cães e gatos, os ureterólitos não obstrutivos (pelve renal < 4 a 5 mm) que não estão associados a infecções ou azotemia podem ser tratados de forma conservadora, com a utilização de TME durante 1 a 2 semanas, desde que a função renal esteja estável. Contudo, é necessário o monitoramento frequente em busca de complicações, como aumento progressivo do ureter ou da pelve renal, azotemia progressiva, oligúria e evidências de infecções do trato urinário (ITU) ou sepse, para prevenir a ocorrência de perda permanente da função renal do rim acometido.

Embora haja relatos clínicos empíricos de que o glucagon facilita a excreção de cálculos ureterais em gatos, o único estudo clínico sobre a administração de glucagon em gatos não mostrou qualquer benefício desse procedimento no tratamento de ureterólitos obstrutivos; ademais, notou-se incidência inaceitavelmente alta de efeitos colaterais.[26] Em razão da documentação de incidência inaceitável de efeitos colaterais e da ineficácia do glucagon, não se recomenda a administração desse medicamento a cães e gatos com ureterólitos.

Em um relato, menciona-se que a amitriptilina facilitou a excreção de tampão uretral em gatos machos com obstrução uretral.[27] Embora o título do artigo envolva cálculos uretrais, todos os gatos examinados pareciam apresentar *tampões* uretrais e, na verdade, não *urólitos*. Não há relato clínico que sustente a administração de amitriptilina como terapia expulsiva de ureterólitos em qualquer espécie; portanto, o seu uso para tal finalidade é desencorajado.

Tratamento de ureterólitos de estruvita em cães

Embora a vasta maioria dos urólitos em gatos seja de oxalato de cálcio, os nefrólitos e os ureterólitos de estruvita causados por infecções são o segundo tipo mais comum de urólitos no trato urinário superior de cães. Os achados clínicos que sustentam nefroureterólitos de estruvita incluem ITU causada por microrganismos produtores de urease (*Staphylococcus, Proteus, Klebsiella, Corynebacterium* e *Mycoplasma*), pH urinário alcalino, urólitos moderadamente radiopacos na pelve renal ou no ureter e cristalúria de estruvita. Em cães, embora os urólitos de estruvita no rim e na bexiga possam ser dissolvidos por meio de tratamento clínico, a obstrução do ureter por ureterólitos impede a dissolução medicamentosa efetiva e causa pionefrose obstrutiva, que frequentemente progride para urosepse.[28] Em cães com ureterólitos de estruvita obstrutivos, a obstrução deve ser corrigida antes de tentativas de dissolução medicamentosa.[28] Em humanos, o tratamento recomendado para pionefrose consiste na drenagem emergencial da urina infectada, juntamente com a implantação de endoprótese expansiva de ureter.[21] Em um relato recente em cães, menciona-se que a pionefrose obstrutiva foi tratada com

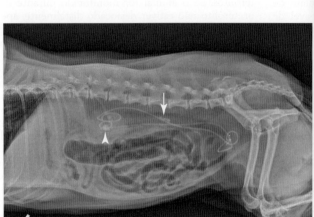 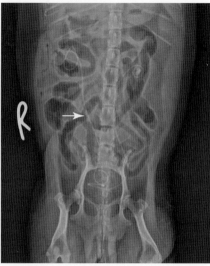

Figura 329.3 Radiografias de abdome mostram endopróteses expansivas (*stents*) de ureteres bilaterais após implantação por meio de cistoscopia retrógrada. Esse é o mesmo cão mostrado na Figura 329.1. Note os ureterólitos do lado direito ao longo da parte externa da endoprótese expansiva de ureter direita (*seta*) e o nefrólito do lado esquerdo (*ponta de seta*). O cão foi subsequentemente submetido a litotripsia por onda de choque para fragmentar o nefrólito e os ureterólitos; em seguida, as endopróteses expansivas e os fragmentos de urólitos foram removidos mediante cistoscopia.

sucesso por uma abordagem minimamente invasiva que consistia em lavagem retrógrada da pelve renal utilizando um cateter ureteral de extremidade aberta, combinada com implantação de endoprótese expansiva (*stent*) de ureter, guiada por cistoscopia.[28] Tanto a fluoroscopia quanto a cistoscopia são necessárias para essa abordagem (ver Capítulo 124). Assim que a crise inicial de pionefrose for efetivamente tratada mediante drenagem, implantação de endoprótese expansiva (*stent*) de ureter e terapia antimicrobiana IV, é possível a dissolução medicamentosa do ureterólito com a utilização de uma combinação de terapia antimicrobiana para ITU (com base nos resultados da urocultura) e ração para dissolução de estruvita, como Royal Canin Urinary SO®, Hill's Prescription diet s/d® ou c/d Multicare®, ou Purina Veterinary diet UR Urinary Ox/St Canine diet® (ver Capítulos 331 e 332). A dissolução medicamentosa de ureterólitos de estruvita não deve ser tentada sem a implantação concomitante de endoprótese expansiva de ureter, em razão do risco de obstrução, falha terapêutica e sepse. A dieta e o antibiótico devem ser mantidos até que as radiografias e a ultrassonografia documentem dissolução total dos urólitos. A preferência do autor é remover a endoprótese expansiva de ureter mediante cistoscopia ou realizar a substituição da endoprótese expansiva de ureter antes de descontinuar o uso de antibióticos.

Intervenções em casos de ureterólitos

Se cães e gatos com ureterólitos obstrutivos necessitam de intervenção, as opções incluem implantação de endoprótese expansiva (*stent*) de ureter, litotripsia por onda de choque (LOC), ureterotomia para remoção de ureterólitos, transecção do ureter e reimplantação de sua extremidade proximal à bexiga (ureteroneocistostomia), e implantação de derivação ureteral subcutânea (DUS). As taxas relativas de sucesso, indicações e complicações dessas técnicas variam de acordo com as espécies (ver Capítulo 124).

Endopróteses expansivas (stents) de ureter

A resolução da obstrução de ureter por ureterólitos é possível pela implantação de endopróteses expansivas (*stents*) de ureter por meio de cirurgia ou cistoscopia, para desviar a urina através dessa endoprótese, ao redor da obstrução do ureter. Em cães, os extensores ureterais podem ser colocados de forma retrógrada, até o ureter, em um guia metálico urológico, por meio de cistoscopia (Figura 329.3).[9,24,28] Em gatos, a implantação de endopróteses expansivas (*stent*) de ureter em geral requer cirurgia para sua implantação anterógrada mediante nefropielocentese; a implantação de endoprótese expansiva (*stent*) é muito mais difícil do que em cães.[17] As endopróteses expansivas (*stents*) podem ser utilizadas temporariamente ou mantidas por longo tempo. Em cadelas e gatas, se a endoprótese expansiva (*stent*) não é mais necessária para desviar a obstrução ureteral, ela pode ser facilmente removida por cistoscopia, pinçando a parte distal da endoprótese expansiva (*stent*) do ureter e tracionando-a cuidadosamente para removê-la através do ureter e da uretra. Em gatos, as endopróteses expansivas (*stents*) de ureter são em geral mantidas no ureter por longo tempo, embora em aproximadamente 20 a 25% dos gatos possa ser necessária sua substituição periódica.[17] Nas endopróteses expansivas internas, pode ocorrer agregação de minerais em sua parte externa e no seu interior, resultando em oclusão do ureter; isso requer a remoção da endoprótese expansiva ou a troca por uma nova (Figura 329.4).[16]

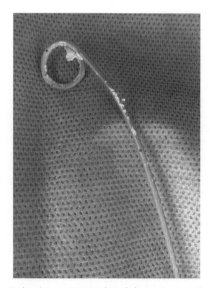

Figura 329.4 Endoprótese expansiva (*stent*) de ureter removida de um cão por causa da incrustação de depósitos de oxalato de cálcio, vistos na parte externa da endoprótese expansiva. Depósitos de minerais no interior da endoprótese expansiva resultaram em obstrução parcial do *stent*, por isso necessitam de troca.

Dispositivos de derivação (bypass) ureteral subcutânea

A implantação cirúrgica de um dispositivo de derivação ureteral subcutânea (DUS) para propiciar uma via para desviar a urina do ureter obstruído é um procedimento relativamente recente. Essa técnica rapidamente se tornou uma das opções preferidas para o tratamento de ureterólitos e constrições ureterais em gatos.[9] Comparada à cirurgia ureteral tradicional, a taxa de mortalidade perioperatória relativa à implantação de DUS é muito menor; relata-se que, após a implantação de DUS, 94% dos gatos sobreviveram por ocasião da alta hospitalar.[9] O prognóstico a longo prazo de gatos que receberam endoprótese expansiva de ureter e DUS está relacionado ao estágio da doença renal crônica (DRC) residual, após resolução da obstrução ureteral; gatos com DRC em estágios 1 a 2 sobrevivem significativamente por mais tempo do que gatos com DRC nos estágios 3 a 4.[20] Ver Capítulo 124 e referências para detalhes sobre procedimentos intervencionistas urológicos, como a implantação de endoprótese expansiva (*stent*) de ureter e DUS.[9,17,19,24]

Cirurgia de ureter

A ureterotomia cirúrgica aberta é uma opção para o tratamento de ureterólitos em cães e gatos.[13,29] Na opinião do autor, a ureterotomia ou ureteroneocistostomia são apropriadas apenas a cães e gatos com um único ureterólito, sem nefrólito concomitante ou constrição de ureter (em decorrência de ureterotomia). A cirurgia de ureter pode resultar em obstrução temporária do lúmen ureteral no período pós-cirúrgico por conta do edema de mucosa no local da ureterotomia; portanto, pode-se realizar desvio da urina por meio da implantação de endoprótese expansiva (*stent*) de ureter (ver texto anterior), a fim de auxiliar no tratamento de obstrução de ureter.[13,17,29] Como a ureterotomia e ureteroneocistostomia apresentam maiores taxas de mortalidade e de complicações cirúrgicas do que LOC e implantação de endoprótese expansiva de ureter ou DUS, o autor prefere esses procedimentos minimamente invasivos alternativos à ureterotomia ou ureteroneocistostomia.[9,13,17,19,20,29]

Litotripsia por ondas de choque em casos de ureterólitos

A litotripsia por ondas de choque é uma opção minimamente invasiva para fragmentação e remoção de nefrólitos e ureterólitos em cães, mas não em gatos.[16,30-32] Na LOC, os urólitos são fragmentados por ondas de choque geradas fora do corpo, que têm como alvos os urólitos, com a utilização de ultrassonografia ou fluoroscopia integrada (ver Capítulo 124). Em cães, aproximadamente 80% dos ureterólitos podem ser resolvidos por meio de LOC, embora cerca de 50% dos cães necessitem de duas ou mais sessões de LOC, que é uma taxa maior de necessidade de novo tratamento do que em cães com nefrólitos.[16,32] Esses dados são semelhantes às observações em humanos e aos modelos experimentais que confirmam que os ureterólitos compactados são mais difíceis de fragmentar comparativamente aos nefrólitos.[33,34] Essa dificuldade em fragmentar os ureterólitos em comparação com os nefrólitos parece ser devida a incapacidade de formação de bolhas de cavitação e colapso na superfície dos ureterólitos, se estiverem circundados pela parede do ureter e não por urina.[35,36] As vantagens da LOC consistem em ser um procedimento não invasivo e ter taxa de complicações em cães menor que 10%; a obstrução de ureter transitória causada por fragmentos de urólitos é a complicação mais comum.[16,32]

A implantação de endoprótese expansiva de ureter não é essencial para o tratamento de ureterólitos por meio de LOC, mas há vantagens que beneficiam a eficiência da LOC e o tratamento do paciente. A endoprótese expansiva de ureter possibilita o desvio imediato da urina da obstrução ureteral no local de instalação do ureterólito e impede dano renal adicional causado por uropatia obstrutiva (ver Figura 329.3). Como as endopróteses expansivas (*stents*) de ureter são radiopacas, elas facilitam o direcionamento dos ureterólitos durante a LOC.

Essas endopróteses de ureter também induzem dilatação passiva do ureter e, assim, aumentam o diâmetro do lúmen do ureter em aproximadamente 3 vezes.[37] Embora isso tenha a vantagem teórica de aumentar a eficiência da fragmentação do urólito, a implantação de endoprótese expansiva de ureter não é recomendada no tratamento por LOC de ureterólitos em humanos.[30] Todavia, endopróteses expansivas de ureter podem ser mais benéficas na LOC em cães, comparativamente aos humanos, por causa do menor diâmetro do ureter. A dilatação passiva do ureter também facilita a excreção dos fragmentos de nefrólitos e ureterólitos, após a remoção da endoprótese expansiva de ureter. A implantação dessa endoprótese de ureter pode também ser realizada para impedir a obstrução do ureter por fragmentos de ureterólitos, após LOC de nefrólitos ou ureterólitos maiores em cães (ver Figura 329.3).[16]

Diferentemente de cães, a LOC *não* é efetiva para fragmentação e remoção de ureterólitos em gatos.[16,32] Em razão do pequeno diâmetro do ureter de gatos, até mesmo fragmentos com menos de 1 mm não atravessam o ureter desses animais; em outras espécies, a LOC geralmente resulta em fragmentos de urólitos de 1 a 2 mm, ou mais. Além do menor diâmetro do ureter, os urólitos de oxalato de cálcio de gatos são mais resistentes à fragmentação, em comparação com urólitos de oxalato de cálcio de cães.[38] Em gatos clinicamente normais utilizados em pesquisa, o dano renal e a redução da função renal foram rotineiramente observados após aplicação de menos de 50% da "dose" de ondas de choque terapêutica normal utilizada em cães submetidos à LOC.[32] Em combinação, todos esses fatores resultam na recomendação de que a LOC *não* deve ser utilizada para tratamento de nefrólitos ou ureterólitos em gatos.

OBSTRUÇÃO DO URETER

Os sinais clínicos de obstrução do ureter podem não ser aparentes, a menos que ocorra obstrução bilateral ou obstrução unilateral simultânea à redução da função do rim contralateral. Os sinais clínicos de obstrução de ureter consistem em dor abdominal, também descrita como cólica ureteral (menos consistentemente observada do que em pessoas com obstrução de ureter), disúria (principalmente na obstrução da parte distal do ureter em gatos) e sintomas de anormalidades da função renal, como anorexia, êmese e oligúria. Pacientes com obstrução bilateral total do ureter manifestam sintomas de insuficiência renal oligúrica grave. A obstrução bilateral total do ureter pode levar à morte dentro de 48 a 72 horas. Várias obstruções de ureter são parciais, principalmente as associadas a ureterólitos.

A obstrução de ureter pode ser decorrência de causas intraluminais, intramurais ou extramurais. A obstrução intraluminal pode ocorrer como resultado de ureterólitos, coágulos ou outros restos teciduais intraluminais. Causas intramurais incluem constrição do ureter, estenose de ureter, edema de mucosa e neoplasia. A compressão extramural pode ser decorrência de ureteres circuncavais, tumores retroperitoneais, fibrose retroperitoneal, neoplasia de bexiga ou ligadura cirúrgica acidental do ureter durante ovário-histerectomia. O ureter circuncaval (ou ureter retrocaval) é uma anomalia congênita caracterizada por deslocamento ventral (ou duplicação) da veia cava caudal, que passa sobre o ureter, resultando em potencial compressão do ureter proximal, pois ele passa por trás da veia cava. O ureter direito é mais frequentemente acometido do que o ureter esquerdo. Em um estudo recente, constatou-se a presença de ureteres circuncavais em aproximadamente 1/3 dos gatos submetidos à necropsia e não estavam associados à obstrução óbvia dos ureteres.[39] Entretanto, em relatos clínicos de gatos com obstruções ureterais, os ureteres circuncavais pareceram estar associados à presença de constrições ureterais proximais ao local em que a veia cava passa sobre o ureter.[40,41] A diferença nesses dois relatos pode ter sido o fato de que a presença de ureteres circuncavais combinada até mesmo com pequenos ureterólitos pode resultar em constrições de ureteres. Os sinais clínicos e a recuperação de gatos com obstrução associada a ureteres circuncavais são semelhantes a outras causas de obstrução de ureter.[40] Constrições ureterais associadas a ureteres circuncavais podem ser mais efetivamente tratadas por meio de implantação de DUS, comparativamente à cirurgia ou implantação de endoprótese expansiva de ureter.[17,40] Em humanos, a estenose de ureter na junção ureteropélvica (JUP) é uma anormalidade comumente diagnosticada. A estenose do ureter na JUP foi recentemente relatada em um cão.[42] O cão foi tratado com sucesso por implantação de endoprótese expansiva de ureter mediante cistoscopia retrógrada. A estenose da JUP também foi relatada em um gato adulto, resultando em insuficiência renal grave por hidronefrose em estágio terminal.[43] A fibrose retroperitoneal como causa de obstrução de ureter extramural foi relatada em 29 de 138 (21%) gatos submetidos a transplante renal.[44] Todos os 29 gatos apresentavam azotemia causada por uropatia obstrutiva secundária à fibrose retroperitoneal. Realizou-se cirurgia para aliviar a obstrução do ureter em 25 dos 29 gatos; ocorreu recidiva da obstrução ureteral em seis gatos (22%).[44]

A neoplasia mais comum que resulta em obstrução de ureter em cães é o carcinoma de célula de transição que se desenvolve no trígono da bexiga (ver Capítulo 351). Neoplasia metastática pode também resultar em obstrução ureteral. Obstruções de ureter malignas podem ser desviadas mediante a implantação paliativa de endoprótese expansiva de ureter.[45] Como é difícil visualizar o orifício do ureter durante cistoscopia em cães com neoplasia extensa do trígono, nesses pacientes a endoprótese expansiva de ureter deve ser posicionada por via percutânea, mediante nefropielocentese anterógrada ou por meio de cirurgia aberta (ver Capítulo 124).[45]

Neoplasia primária do ureter é rara em cães e gatos. As neoplasias primárias do ureter são carcinoma de célula de transição, leiomioma, leiomiossarcoma, sarcoma, mastocitoma, papiloma benigno e pólipo fibroepitelial.[46-52] Pólipo fibroepitelial é o tipo mais comum de neoplasia primária de ureter em cães.[47,48] A ureteronefrectomia é o tratamento mais comumente relatado para neoplasia de ureter unilateral, mas a DUS ou a implantação de endoprótese expansiva de ureter podem ser alternativas possíveis em alguns casos.[47,48]

TRAUMATISMO DO URETER

Há raros relatos de traumatismo de ureteres em cães e gatos.[53,54] A lesão ureteral pode resultar de traumatismo abdominal obtuso, ferimentos penetrantes ou lesão iatrogênica durante cirurgia, como ligadura involuntária ou transecção do ureter durante ovário-histerectomia. Em um relato, constatou-se que a lesão de ureter resultante de traumatismo obtuso representou apenas 0,01% das admissões hospitalares de cães.[53]

A ruptura do ureter resulta no acúmulo de urina no espaço retroperitoneal, azotemia pós-renal, hiperpotassemia e acidose metabólica. Se o rim e o ureter contralaterais estiverem funcionando normalmente, o diagnóstico de ruptura de ureter pode ser retardado por vários dias. Se o ureter se romper próximo à junção ureterovesical ou se o retroperitônio for comprometido pelo traumatismo, pode ocorrer uroabdome. Também pode ocorrer ruptura de ureter como uma complicação incomum de ureterólitos.

A extensão e a localização da lesão de ureter e a função do rim contralateral determinam o tratamento da lesão ureteral. A ureteronefrectomia foi relatada como o tratamento mais comum para ruptura unilateral de ureter, desde que o rim e o ureter contralaterais apresentem funções normais.[53] Em cães com traumatismo na parte distal do ureter, a implantação da parte saudável do ureter acima do local lesionado (ureteroneocistostomia) é uma alternativa à ureteronefrectomia.[54] Para lacerações incompletas do ureter (< 50% da circunferência), o tratamento conservador por meio de desvio da urina frequentemente possibilita a cicatrização da lesão ureteral. A implantação de endoprótese expansiva de ureter por meio de cistoscopia ou cirurgia é uma opção minimamente invasiva para desvio da urina a fim de permitir a cicatrização de lacerações parciais de ureter (ver Capítulo 124).

Uma consequência incomum do traumatismo de ureter é a formação de um pseudocisto paraureteral, ou urinoma, que se desenvolve quando a urina que extravasou do ureter para o retroperitônio é encapsulada por uma espessa parede fibrosa.[55-57] A transecção involuntária do ureter durante ovário-histerectomia foi a causa de urinoma em um cão.[58] Pode ser necessária uma ureteronefrectomia para o tratamento de urinoma, desde que a função do rim contralateral seja normal.

ANORMALIDADES ANATÔMICAS

Anormalidades de ureter congênitas

Anormalidades de ureter congênitas incluem ureter ectópico, ureterocele, estenose da junção ureterovesicular (JUV), agenesia ureteral e duplicação do ureter.

A agenesia ureteral e a duplicação ureteral são raras em cães e gatos.[59-61] A agenesia ureteral resulta da falha no desenvolvimento do broto ureteral e pode ser completa ou segmentar. A agenesia de ureter está comumente associada à agenesia renal contralateral, pois o broto ureteral induz a proliferação e diferenciação do rim metanéfrico embrionário.[60] A duplicação de ureter ocorre quando mais de um broto ureteral se desenvolve a partir do mesmo ducto mesonéfrico ou quando ocorre divisão do broto ureteral.[59] A duplicação de ureter pode estar associada a rim duplo e ectopia ureteral.[59,61] A estenose congênita da JUV foi relatada em 10 cães; em 7 deles a estenose da JUV estava associada à abertura de ureter ectópico.[62] A estenose da JUV causa obstrução parcial da parte distal do ureter (Figura 329.5 C). A estenose de JUV foi corrigida com sucesso por meio de ablação por *laser* guiada por cistoscopia em todos os 10 cães.[62]

Ureteres ectópicos

Ureteres ectópicos são definidos como aberturas ureterais localizadas em qualquer local distal à localização normal do trígono (ver Capítulo 336).[63] Ureteres ectópicos podem ser unilaterais ou bilaterais e extramurais ou intramurais. Os ureteres ectópicos extramurais se desviam inteiramente da bexiga e são inseridos em uma localização distal. Ureteres ectópicos intramurais adentram a superfície serosa da bexiga em uma localização dorsolateral normal; porém, em vez da abertura no trígono, o ureter forma um túnel através da submucosa da bexiga e da uretra e desemboca no colo vesical distal à localização normal do trígono, uretra ou vestíbulo vaginal. Variações da configuração dos ureteres ectópicos intramurais incluem aberturas ureterais duplas, múltiplas aberturas fenestradas, duas aberturas ureterais intramurais em um único orifício e canais ureterais (Figura 329.5). Ureteres ectópicos comumente estão associados a outras anormalidades do trato urogenital, inclusive agenesia renal, hipoplasia renal, formato irregular dos rins, hidroureter, ureterocele, estenose de JUV, remanescências do úraco, bexiga pélvica, anormalidades da uretra e remanescências do septo paramesonéfrico.[62-68] As raças de maior risco de ocorrência de ureteres ectópicos são Husky Siberiano, Labrador Retriever, Golden Retriever, Terranova, Buldogue Inglês, West Highland White Terrier, Fox Terrier, Skye Terrier, Border Terrier, Griffon, Entlebucher Mountai e Poodle Miniatura e Toy.[68-70] As cadelas são muito mais comumente acometidas por ureteres ectópicos do que os cães machos. Ureteres ectópicos são menos comuns em gatos, comparativamente aos cães. Durante a cistoscopia ou urografia excretora, as aberturas dos ureteres em gatos normais parecem estar localizadas na uretra proximal; essa localização anormal não deve ser confundida com ureteres ectópicos.

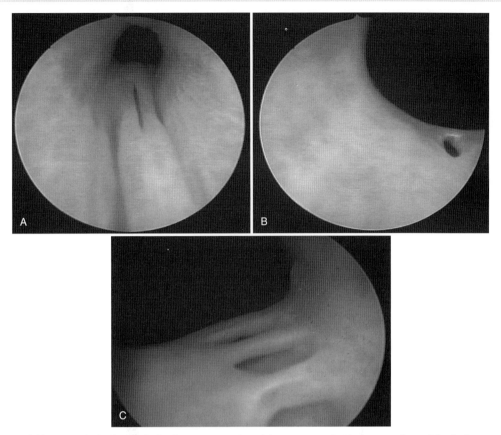

Figura 329.5 Imagens obtidas por meio de cistoscopia de aberturas ureterais ectópicas na uretra. **A.** Abertura semelhante à fenda do ureter ectópico direito na membrana uretral dorsal de um cão com ureteres ectópicos bilaterais. **B.** Abertura estenosada do ureter ectópico esquerdo na uretra proximal, distal à junção da bexiga e uretra (mesmo cão da Figura 329.5 A). **C.** Aberturas múltiplas de um ureter ectópico na uretra proximal de outro cão.

Embora historicamente o diagnóstico de ureteres ectópicos era confirmado por meio de urografia excretora, quando disponível, a cistoscopia se tornou o método preferido de diagnóstico (ver Figura 329.5). A ultrassonografia também tem sido sugerida como uma opção diagnóstica para detecção de ureteres ectópicos; entretanto, a ultrassonografia não detecta de forma acurada todos os ureteres ectópicos.[71] Estudos compararam a acurácia diagnóstica de urografia excretora, TC contrastada e cistoscopia para detecção de ureteres ectópicos.[63,72] As imagens obtidas em TC contrastada e cistoscopia foram as informações diagnósticas mais acuradas para detecção de ureteres ectópicos.[63,72] A cistoscopia tem a vantagem adicional de que ureteres ectópicos intramurais podem ser diagnosticados e corrigidos por meio de ablação por *laser* guiada por cistoscopia durante o mesmo procedimento anestésico.[73-75]

A ablação por *laser* da parede entre o lúmen da uretra e o lúmen do ureter intramural efetivamente desloca a abertura do ureter até o lúmen da bexiga, sem necessidade de cirurgia aberta (ver Capítulos 108 e 124). A ablação por *laser* guiada por cistoscopia dos ureteres ectópicos intramurais pode ser realizada utilizando *laser* hólmio: YAG ou diodo.[73-75] Os resultados parecem semelhantes aos obtidos na cirurgia para correção de ureteres ectópicos, embora não haja estudos publicados que comparem diretamente os resultados da correção cirúrgica e a ablação por *laser*. Cães com boa função uretral apresentam continência urinária após a correção por *laser* dos ureteres ectópicos, enquanto cães com incompetência uretral concomitante continuam a apresentar incontinência urinária, a menos que o tratamento da incompetência uretral concomitante seja efetivo.[73-75] Ureteres ectópicos extramurais não podem ser corrigidos por ablação por *laser* e necessitam de transecção cirúrgica e reimplantação na bexiga.

Ureterocele

Ureterocele é uma dilatação cística da parte terminal do ureter, que frequentemente apresenta protrusão em direção ao lúmen da bexiga (ver Capítulo 336).[76-80] Ureteroceles são classificadas em ortotópica (também denominada intravesical) se a abertura do ureter estiver em uma localização normal do trígono, ou ectópica se a abertura do ureter estiver distal à localização normal do trígono. A ureterocele pode causar uma série de sinais clínicos, conforme o tamanho e se o ureter é ectópico ou não. A incontinência urinária é o sintoma mais comum de ureterocele.[76,77] A ureterocele pode pressionar a bexiga e a uretra proximal, resultando em retenção urinária funcional, ou pode causar disúria, estrangúria e polaquiúria. Cães com ureterocele também podem apresentar ITU recidivante. Embora a ureterocele seja uma anormalidade congênita, alguns cães com ureterocele não manifestam sinais clínicos até tardiamente na vida.[76] A ureterocele pode estar associada a anormalidades de desenvolvimento ou adquiridas do trato urinário superior ou inferior, inclusive hidroureter e hidronefrose moderadas a graves, ureteres ectópicos e anomalias uretrais. Ureterocele é diagnosticada por meio de urografia excretora, cistoscopia ou ultrassonografia.

O tratamento de ureterocele depende do tipo e da extensão das anomalias concomitantes e se a abertura do ureter é ectópica ou não. A excisão cirúrgica da ureterocele com reimplantação do ureter tem sido recomendada em caso de ureterocele ectópica ou associada à obstrução do ureter.[76,80] O autor tratou com sucesso ureteroceles ectópicas intramurais mediante ablação por *laser* guiada por cistoscopia, em quatro cadelas, evitando assim a necessidade de cirurgia aberta. Também se pode fazer a incisão da ureterocele ortotópica por meio de cistoscopia, utilizando *laser* ou realizando cistotomia; entretanto, isso geralmente resulta em refluxo vesicoureteral, que pode contribuir para a ocorrência de pielonefrite, caso haja ITU também. Portanto, recomenda-se o tratamento efetivo da ITU antes da correção da ureterocele.

Fístula uretrorretal ou ureterovaginal

Fístulas entre a uretra e o reto ou entre o ureter e a vagina são condições incomuns em cães; podem ser congênitas ou adquiridas (ver Capítulo 336).[81-86] Fístulas ureterovaginais em geral se originam como resultado de ovário-histerectomia quando o ureter é acidentalmente incluído na sutura ao redor do coto vaginal. Fístulas uretrorretais podem ser congênitas ou podem ser adquiridas após traumatismo pélvico. Cães da raça Buldogue Inglês são os mais comumente acometidos por fístulas uretrorretais congênitas.[85,86] Sinais clínicos de fístulas uretrorretais

incluem eliminação de urina pelo ânus durante a micção e, mais comumente, ITU recidivante.[85,86] Incontinência urinária é o sinal clínico mais comum de fístula ureterovaginal em cadelas.[81,82] Recomenda-se a correção cirúrgica das fístulas uretrorretais ou ureterovaginais; porém, a correção cirúrgica de fístulas uretrorretais pode ser difícil por causa da localização intrapélvica e da ITU concomitante. Após a correção cirúrgica de fístula uretrorretal, é essencial a resolução da ITU secundária, que pode necessitar de terapia antimicrobiana por longo tempo.

REFERÊNCIAS BIBLIOGRÁFICAS

As referências bibliográficas deste capítulo se encontram online no Ambiente de Aprendizagem.

CAPÍTULO 330

Infecções do Trato Urinário Inferior

Michael W. Wood

INTRODUÇÃO

A causa de infecções do trato urinário (ITU) é multifatorial, depende da interface entre a virulência de um microrganismo e as alterações nas competências anatômicas, ambientais e imunológicas do hospedeiro. Mais comumente, os microrganismos envolvidos são bactérias uropatogênicas oriundas da flora intestinal que ascendem pelo trato urogenital distal em direção à uretra proximal e bexiga.[1-3] Em vários cães com defesas urinárias normais, as bactérias invasoras são eliminadas em 3 dias, sem necessidade de tratamento com antibiótico.[4] São os indivíduos com defesas comprometidas que apresentam maior risco de colonização e bacteriúria persistente (Boxe 330.1).

Outros microrganismos, como fungos, causam ITU em cerca de 1% de cães e gatos, mas não são discutidos neste capítulo. Por favor, consulte a 7ª edição desse livro-texto, Capítulo 313, de autoria de Barrak Pressler, para uma revisão sobre ITU não bacteriana.

CARACTERÍSTICAS DA INFECÇÃO

Bacteriúria assintomática

Definições tradicionais de ITU implicam aderência, multiplicação e persistência de microrganismos invasores no lúmen do trato urinário.[5,6] Com base em observações recentes em medicina humana e veterinária, a documentação microbiológica de bacteriúria não é equivalente ao diagnóstico de ITU. Nem toda bacteriúria está associada a sinais clínicos de infecção do trato urinário inferior (ITUI), como dor abdominal caudal, polaciúria, estrangúria, hematúria e disúria. Na medicina humana, indivíduos com bacteriúria persistente, mas sem sinais clínicos de ITUI, são denominados portadores de bacteriúria assintomática (BAS).[7] Em cães e gatos, o reconhecimento de sinais discretos de ITU é desafiador, e o termo bacteriúria subclínica (BSC) pode ser mais apropriado.[8]

Em pessoas, o tratamento de BAS não é recomendado em várias circunstâncias porque a erradicação da BAS não impede a recolonização futura da bexiga[9] e existe a hipótese de que a presença de cepas causadoras de BAS propicia certo grau de

---

Boxe 330.1 Defesas naturais e adquiridas do trato urinário inferior do hospedeiro

Micção normal
- Volume de urina adequado
- Micção frequente
- Micção completa
- Continência urinária

Estruturas anatômicas
- Zonas uretrais de alta pressão
- Características da superfície do urotélio
- Peristalse uretral
- Secreções prostáticas (fração antibacteriana e imunoglobulinas)
- Comprimento da uretra
- Valvas do flape ureterovesical
- Peristalse ureteral

Barreiras de defesa da mucosa
- Produção de anticorpos
- Camada superficial de glicosaminoglicanos
- Propriedades antimicrobianas intrínsecas da mucosa
- Esfoliação de células uroteliais
- Interferência bacteriana por microrganismos comensais do trato urogenital distal
- Imunidade inata da mucosa: receptores *toll-like* etc.

Propriedades antimicrobianas da urina
- pH urinário extremamente alto ou baixo
- Hiperosmolalidade
- Alta concentração de ureia
- Ácidos orgânicos
- Carboidratos de baixo peso molecular
- Mucoproteínas de Tamm-Horsfall
- Peptídios de defesa do hospedeiro (p. ex., defensinas)

Imunocompetência sistêmica
- Imunidade mediada por células
- Imunidade humoral

Adaptado de Osborne CA, Lees GE: Bacterial infections of the canine and feline urinary tract. In Osborne CA, Finco DR, editors: *Canine and feline nephrology and urology*, Baltimore, 1995, Williams & Wilkins, p. 759-797.

proteção contra a colonização do trato urinário por bactérias mais patogênicas.[10] Evidências que demonstram o benefício da BAS em medicina veterinária são escassas; entretanto, em pesquisas veterinárias limitadas, relata-se a prevalência de BAS de 2,1 a 8,9%, em cães,[11,12] e 10 a 28,8%, em gatos,[13,14] sendo *E. coli* e *Enterococcus faecalis* as bactérias mais comumente detectadas.[11-13]

Importância dos fatores de virulência e de *fitness* na infecção

A possibilidade de ocorrência de doença clínica pela colonização da bexiga depende, fundamentalmente, da expressão gênica da bactéria. As bactérias contêm ilhas genômicas que codificam fatores *fitness* (*i. e.*, capacidade de o microrganismo sobreviver e transmitir seu genótipo a seus descendentes, quando comparados com microrganismos competidores) que promovem comensalismo e/ou fatores de virulência e ditam a gravidade da ITU. A quantidade de material genético contido em uma bactéria é limitada; portanto, geralmente as bactérias evoluem por meio do aumento do fator de virulência ou *fitness*.[15] Consequentemente, bactérias com alto *fitness*, como genes de resistência a múltiplos antibióticos, são comumente encontradas em infecções crônicas que também possuem menor potencial de virulência.[16]

Genes de *fitness* e virulência possuem uma enorme plasticidade, e as bactérias constantemente se adaptam a alterações que ocorrem em seu microambiente.[17] Bactérias respondem a alterações na disponibilidade de nutrientes, osmolaridade e defesas do hospedeiro pela obtenção de material genético por transferência gênica horizontal, genes existentes mutantes e alteração da expressão de genes de virulência e antivirulência.[18] Várias cepas causadoras de BAS contêm genes de virulência não expressos; portanto, o fenótipo bacteriano atual não é necessariamente preditivo de patogenicidade futura, particularmente se o ambiente da bexiga está em fluxo.[15,19] Alguns genes são preditivos de virulência mais importantes do que outros, inclusive genes que codificam a produção de toxinas, como a hemolisina, ou a expressão de fímbrias de aderência uroepitelial.[20]

Moléculas de aderência bacteriana possuem diferentes afinidades por áreas do trato urinário. No caso de *E. coli* uropatogênica (ECUP), as fímbrias tipo 1, codificadas por genes *fim*, ligam-se ao alvo manose no urotélio[21] e são expressas por quase todas as bactérias que causam pielonefrite e cistite e por 77% das cepas causadoras de BAS.[22] Clinicamente, a presença de fímbrias tipo 1 quase sempre está associada à maior gravidade da infecção,[23] e elas são comumente observadas na superfície da ECUP durante a colonização inicial da bexiga.[24] Diferentemente, as fímbrias P, codificadas por genes *pap*, ligam-se aos receptores alfa-D-galactopiranosil-(1 a 4)-beta-D-galactopiranosida situados no trato urinário superior.[25] Essas moléculas de aderência são constatadas em 78% das cepas causadoras de pielonefrite, 22% das cepas que causam cistite e em apenas 15% das cepas assintomáticas.[22] Entre outros uropatógenos, as bactérias gram-negativas são, de longe, as que mais expressam moléculas de aderência semelhantes, com alta afinidade por tecido renal,[26] e, assim, microrganismos como *Streptococcus* spp. e *Enterococcus* spp. frequentemente não estão associados à ocorrência de pielonefrite.[27]

DIAGNÓSTICO DE INFECÇÃO DO TRATO URINÁRIO

Detecção de bacteriúria

A cultura microbiológica aeróbica ainda é o padrão-ouro para detecção de bacteriúria. A cultura quantitativa da urina identifica o microrganismo infectante específico e possibilita a contagem de colônias, ambos importantes, considerando a relevância clínica da bacteriúria. A urocultura também fornece informações para identificação de infecções persistentes e reinfecções, e pode fornecer algumas informações, como os medicamentos

que podem ser efetivos com base no microrganismo isolado. A urocultura não possibilita a distinção entre BAS e ITU; entretanto, o exame do sedimento urinário pode fornecer evidências de inflamação, tornando útil sua realização juntamente com esses dois testes diagnósticos (ver Capítulo 72).

Ao interpretar os resultados da urocultura e do exame do sedimento urinário, devem-se considerar os métodos de coleta e armazenamento da amostra. Ambos os testes diagnósticos são influenciados pelo tempo decorrido até o processamento, pela temperatura e pelo meio de armazenamento. Hemácias e leucócitos, assim como cilindros, podem ser destruídos na urina hipotônica ou alcalina deixada à temperatura ambiente durante apenas poucas horas. As bactérias podem iniciar a proliferação ou morrer caso a amostra de urina seja mantida sem refrigeração, ocorrendo resultado falso positivo ou falso negativo.[28] O exame do sedimento urinário e a urocultura devem ser realizados dentro de 30 minutos após a coleta, a fim de reduzir essas variáveis que confundem a interpretação. Se os exames precisam ser postergados, as amostras devem ser refrigeradas à temperatura de 4°C, e os testes realizados dentro de 24 horas.[28] Como alternativa, se o envio da amostra para urocultura depende de exames pendentes, o armazenamento da urina em um frasco com meio de conservação ou redutor, como o Port-a-cul® (BD Biosciences), ou meio de transporte Amies, pode prolongar o tempo de viabilidade da bactéria por até 72 horas, sem que haja proliferação bacteriana.[29,30]

Em algumas situações, o exame do sedimento urinário pode detectar bacteriúria. Bactérias com formato de bastonetes são prontamente detectadas quando a contagem de colônias excede 10 mil unidades formadoras de colônias (UFC)/mℓ, enquanto cocos são praticamente indetectáveis até que a contagem de UFC/mℓ alcance 100 mil colônias.[31] De modo geral, a sensibilidade e especificidade da detecção de bacteriúria no sedimento urinário não corado são de 75,9 e 56,7%, respectivamente.[32] A detecção de bacteriúria pode ser facilitada pela coloração do sedimento com novo azul de metileno, coloração de gram ou coloração de Wright modificada, aumentando a sensibilidade da detecção de bacteriúria para ≥ 83% e a especificidade para ≥ 98%.[32-35] Um teste de urina rápido com base na catalase, como o Accutest Uriscreen® (Jant Pharmaceuticals Co) também pode melhorar a sensibilidade da detecção de bacteriúria para 89%; no entanto, a reação cruzada entre bactérias e células somáticas, como leucócitos e células epiteliais, diminui a especificidade do exame para 71%.[36] Também pode ser difícil detectar bactérias catalase-negativas, como *Enterococcus* spp. e *Streptococcus* spp. Veja o Capítulo 72 para mais informações.

Epidemiologia da bacteriúria

O crescimento da maioria dos uropatógenos no meio de cultura fica aparente dentro de 18 a 24 horas após a incubação; contudo, alguns microrganismos, como *Corynebacterium* spp. e *Mycoplasma* spp., podem demorar 4 a 7 dias, respectivamente. Bactérias gram-negativas são mais comumente isoladas em cães, representando mais de 60% das culturas positivas. De modo geral, *E. coli* é isolada em 45 a 55% dos cães com bacteriúria, enquanto outros microrganismos gram-negativos, inclusive *Proteus* spp., *Pseudomonas aeruginosa* e *Klebsiella* spp., e as bactérias gram-positivas *Staphylococcus* spp., *Streptococcus* spp. e *Enterococcus* spp., são isolados em 2 a 14% das vezes.[37,38]

Em gatos, *E. coli* também é a causa mais comum da bacteriúria (37,3%), mas praticamente na metade das vezes ocorrem infecções gram-negativas e gram-positivas, e a bactéria gram-positiva *Enterococcus faecalis* está presente em 27% das amostras com urocultura positiva.[39] De modo geral, a incidência da bacteriúria é muito menor em gatos do que em cães, mas em ambas as espécies as fêmeas e os animais idosos são mais comumente acometidos.[32,37,39]

Bacteriúria relevante

Após a detecção de bacteriúria por meio de urocultura ou exame do sedimento urinário, o veterinário deve fazer a diferenciação entre contaminação e colonização da urina. Em cadelas, a flora vaginal normal pode conter várias cepas de bactérias uropatogênicas. Há predomínio de microrganismos gram-positivos, como *Enterococcus* spp., *Staphylococcus* spp. e *Streptococcus* spp., mas *E. coli*, *Proteus* spp. e *Pasteurella* spp. também são comuns, o que torna fundamental a escolha do método de coleta de urina e a contagem de colônias antes do diagnóstico de bacteriúria clinicamente relevante.[40-42]

Quando se detecta bacteriúria relevante, a constatação de piúria concomitante (> 3 a 5 leucócitos/campo de alta potência [hpf]) na urina de gatos ou cães é sugestivo de infecção, mesmo na ausência de sinais clínicos.[31] Isso não ocorre em pessoas, nas quais a BAS pode estar associada à piúria.[7] Dada a dificuldade para detecção de sinais clínicos discretos em cães e gatos, a definição veterinária para ITU peca pelo diagnóstico excessivo, de modo que infecções patogênicas discretas não sejam omitidas. Ocasionalmente, assim como em indivíduos com imunossupressão, um patógeno virulento pode colonizar o trato urinário sem causar sinais clínicos ou resposta inflamatória evidente (ver Capítulo 306).[43] Nessas situações, o clínico deve confiar em seu conhecimento sobre o microrganismo presente para decidir se há necessidade de intervenção.

TRATAMENTO DE INFECÇÃO DO TRATO URINÁRIO

Após o diagnóstico de ITU verdadeira, o tratamento com antimicrobianos ainda é a terapia padrão. Os protocolos terapêuticos variam dependendo do histórico prévio de ITU, doenças concomitantes, condição reprodutiva e espécie. Entretanto, em termos gerais, as estratégias terapêuticas para ITU envolvem duas grandes categorias: o tratamento de ITU não complicada e o tratamento de ITU complicada.

Infecção do trato urinário não complicada

Uma ITU não complicada, também conhecida como ITU simples, é definida como uma infecção de bexiga que ocorre em intervalo de não mais que um semestre em um cão saudável, com anatomia e função normais do trato urinário. Gatos e cães machos não castrados são exceções. Nesses pacientes, a ITU deve ser considerada complicada, já que cães não castrados podem apresentar prostatite simultaneamente e em gatos a ITU está comumente associada a uma doença sistêmica concomitante.[44-46]

Infecções não complicadas frequentemente estão associadas a sintomas graves relativos ao trato urinário inferior, de disúria, polaciúria e estrangúria, e necessitam de tratamento enquanto aguardam os resultados da urocultura. Ao escolher um antibiótico para uma infecção cuja sensibilidade da bactéria é desconhecida, devem-se considerar os padrões de resistência da população local, a concentração do antibiótico obtida na urina, o risco de eventos adversos e o custo do medicamento. Veterinários são encorajados a monitorar os padrões de resistência antimicrobiana em sua clínica, de modo a escolher um antibiótico com espectro e eficácia contra o agente etiológico suspeito. O antibiótico de primeira linha deve ter uma taxa de resistência local inferior a 10% para ITU não complicada (nem todas) diagnosticada na clínica. Os antibióticos de primeira linha sugeridos incluem amoxicilina, cefalexina ou a combinação sulfonamida-trimetoprima.[8]

Se os resultados do teste de sensibilidade antimicrobiana (antibiograma) do paciente revelam que a bactéria em questão é resistente ao antibiótico escolhido, mas o paciente apresentou melhora do quadro clínico, deve-se completar o tratamento com esse antibiótico, com monitoramento dos resultados do exame de urina e de cultura microbiológica realizados 3 a 5 dias após finalizar o tratamento, a fim de assegurar que a infecção foi erradicada. Alternativamente, se a bactéria que causa ITU é resistente ao antibiótico escolhido e não se constata melhora do quadro clínico, o antibiótico inicialmente escolhido deve ser descontinuado e o tratamento com um antibiótico apropriado deve ser iniciado.

Em medicina veterinária, a duração do tratamento recomendada para ITU não complicada é de 7 a 14 dias.[47,48] Entretanto, a terapia antimicrobiana de curta duração (menos de 3 dias) pode ser igualmente efetiva. As vantagens da terapia de curta duração incluem redução dos efeitos colaterais, maior comprometimento do tutor, redução dos custos e menor risco de desenvolvimento de resistência ao antibiótico, ao mesmo tempo que se mantém a eficácia clínica. Estudos recentes em cães indicaram que o tratamento de ITU não complicada com sulfametoxazol-trimetoprima ou altas doses de enrofloxacino, durante 3 dias, propiciou taxas de cura semelhantes àquelas do tratamento de 10 dias com cefalexina ou de 14 dias com amoxicilina-clavulanato.[49,50] Os protocolos terapêuticos de curta duração também reduzem o risco de reações de hipersensibilidade às sulfonamidas e de indução de cepas de bactérias mutantes resistentes às fluoroquinolonas quando se utilizam altas doses de enrofloxacino.[49,51] Apesar desses resultados, não se recomenda o uso de antibióticos de segunda linha, como amoxicilina-clavulanato, fluoroquinolonas e cefovecina no tratamento de ITU não complicada quando há a opção de tratamento com antibióticos de primeira linha.

Finalizado o tratamento de ITU não complicada, geralmente não há necessidade de testes diagnósticos ou monitoramento adicional. Também não há necessidade de terapia adjuvante e tratamento preventivo (ver a seguir).

Infecção do trato urinário complicada

ITU complicada implica que há anormalidades anatômicas, funcionais ou metabólicas subjacentes ou, ainda, comorbidades, seja impedindo a eliminação de uma infecção (persistente e recidiva), seja permitindo a reinfecção. O reconhecimento da causa primária e do local da colonização bacteriana é importante para evitar falha terapêutica ou recidiva da ITU.

Infecções persistentes

Infecções persistentes (refratárias) ocorrem quando a terapia antimicrobiana apropriada não consegue esterilizar a urina. Considerando que o antibiótico prescrito tenha sido administrado na dose e no período apropriados, as infecções persistentes indicam que a bactéria infectante desenvolveu resistência, o sistema imune do paciente está comprometido, ou a concentração urinária média (CUM) do antibiótico não foi capaz de atingir um valor pelo menos 4 vezes maior que a concentração inibitória mínima (CIM), capaz de impedir o crescimento bacteriano.[47,52]

Como a mensuração da concentração do medicamento na urina não é amplamente disponível, é necessário saber qual é o momento em que a excreção urinária do fármaco pode ser alterada, a fim de prevenir a ocorrência de infecções persistentes. Pode-se constatar baixa CUM de um antibiótico quando há diminuição da absorção intestinal de medicamentos administrados por via oral, comprometimento da perfusão sanguínea no tecido infectado, alteração na metabolização do medicamento, ou redução na capacidade de concentração da urina. Em resumo, nas infecções persistentes, é preciso avaliar a possibilidade de haver doença sistêmica, incluindo a avaliação funcional dos sistemas imune, gastrintestinal, hepático e renal. Se a anormalidade que resulta em infecção persistente não pode ser sanada, então é preciso ajustar a dose do antibiótico de modo a maximizar a CUM ou deve-se substituir o antibiótico.

Nas últimas décadas, com o aumento de ocorrência de ITU multirresistente, há uma população crescente de pacientes com infecções que não respondem ao tratamento com antibióticos de primeira ou de segunda linha. Têm-se proposto tratamentos alternativos, amplamente baseados em relatos de casos individuais e evidências pragmáticas. A administração de alta dose de amoxicilina/ácido clavulânico é um procedimento que utiliza a capacidade de concentração da urina para tratar infecções multirresistentes que, de outro modo, se mostram resistentes no teste de sensibilidade antimicrobiana (antibiograma).[53] Outra abordagem desvia das etapas de absorção, metabolização e excreção do antibiótico realizando a administração de antibióticos aminoglicosídeos diretamente na bexiga.[54-56]

Ocasionalmente, podem ser indicados procedimentos terapêuticos mais invasivos no tratamento de infecções persistentes, como a cistite crostosa. Associada primariamente à ITU causada por *Corynebacterium urealyticum*, a cistite crostosa se instala quando bactérias urease-positivas formam placas mineralizadas na mucosa ulcerada e inflamada do trato urinário.[57,58,58a] Deve-se suspeitar de cistite crostosa quando há infecção urease-positiva persistente em combinação com urina alcalina que contém cristais de estruvita. O diagnóstico pode ser auxiliado por ultrassonografia e cistoscopia, e quase sempre o tratamento requer terapia antimicrobiana apropriada, juntamente com acidificação da urina e desbridamento cirúrgico.[58]

Recidiva

A recidiva de ITU difere de uma infecção persistente pelo fato de que na recidiva a urina pode ser livre da infecção, mas há fontes de bactérias que continuam possibilitando a recolonização da urina pelo mesmo microrganismo dentro de alguns dias a semanas. Locais que podem albergar colônias de bactérias são rins, próstata, urólitos, vagina e, possivelmente, o urotélio.

O objetivo do tratamento de infecções recidivantes é identificar o local da infecção, de modo a assegurar a erradicação das bactérias na fonte de infecção. Em casos suspeitos de infecções teciduais, deve-se determinar a sensibilidade bacteriana com base na concentração plasmática atingível e na penetração do antibiótico no tecido, e não com base na CUM. Tradicionalmente, o período de tratamento é longo, com recomendação geral de 4 a 6 semanas. Entretanto, a melhor duração do tratamento para eliminar essas infecções é amplamente desconhecida. É possível que em determinadas circunstâncias a duração do tratamento possa ser seguramente reduzida (ver Capítulos 327, 331, 332 e 337).

A recidiva devido à formação de populações de bactérias intracelulares é um exemplo particular de ITU complicada, cuja relevância clínica é desconhecida em cães e gatos. Experimentalmente, as bactérias que possuem fímbrias do tipo 1, como *E. coli* e *Klebsiella pneumoniae*, passaram mais rapidamente para o meio intracelular durante a infecção.[59-61] Pequenos grupos de bactérias intracelulares podem atuar como fontes de bactérias intracelulares quiescentes (FBIQ) que colonizam novamente a bexiga semanas a meses depois, quando ocorre esfoliação de células uroteliais.[62-64] O tratamento com antibiótico, mesmo de longa duração, não é capaz de eliminar as FBIQ;[65] no entanto, relata-se que a administração intravesicular e intraperitoneal da forscolina, produzida pela planta *Coleus forskohlii*, reduziu a população de bactérias no urotélio, em um modelo de infecção intraurotelial em murinos.[66] A eficácia clínica do tratamento com forscolina não foi comprovada, sendo necessárias mais evidências antes de recomendar essa terapia para recidiva de ITU.

Reinfecção

A reinfecção ocorre quando há comprometimento dos mecanismos de defesa do hospedeiro que possibilita que novas cepas bacterianas colonizem a bexiga semanas a meses após uma ITU prévia (ver Boxe 330.1). Tanto na reinfecção quanto na recidiva, há um período em que a urina do paciente é estéril, tornando um desafio a diferenciação entre as duas quando espécies bacterianas semelhantes são isoladas em infecções subsequentes. A comparação dos padrões de sensibilidade antimicrobiana de infecções prévias e atuais frequentemente é utilizada como uma forma de diferenciar reinfecção de recidiva, mas diferentes cepas bacterianas podem ter perfis de sensibilidade semelhantes e o mesmo microrganismo infectante pode alterar a sua sensibilidade aos antibióticos, tornando esse procedimento não confiável.[67,68] A genotipagem utilizando eletroforese em gel de campo pulsado fornece evidências definitivas de reinfecção/recidiva.[68] A correta categorização da infecção como reinfecção ou recidiva é importante, já que a fisiopatologia e o tratamento necessário para reinfecção são diferentes daqueles da recidiva.

Se há suspeita de reinfecção, deve-se realizar uma avaliação sistêmica minuciosa do paciente. Quando possível, é feita avaliação da conformação da genitália externa, inclusive com exame digital, e da micção. A retenção de urina deve ser avaliada pela mensuração do volume residual na bexiga após a micção por meio de cateterismo ou estimativa ultrassonográfica.[69-71] O volume residual deve ser baixo, com valores comuns estimados em 0,1 a 0,4 mℓ/kg (Vídeo 330.1).[72,73] Exames avançados, que incluem exames radiográficos/contrastados, ultrassonografia, cistoscopia e perfil da pressão uretral, podem auxiliar na detecção de comprometimento dos mecanismos de defesa do hospedeiro, inclusive alterações anatômicas e mecânicas no trato urinário inferior.

O tratamento de reinfecções requer urocultura e antibiograma para nortear o tratamento. Tanto em cães quanto em gatos, a administração prévia de antibióticos é o principal fator de risco para o desenvolvimento de infecções multirresistentes;[74,75] portanto, pacientes com histórico de reinfecção apresentam maior risco de falha terapêutica quando se utiliza antibiótico escolhido empiricamente. Se no momento do diagnóstico da ITU os sinais clínicos são discretos, é prudente esperar os resultados do teste de sensibilidade antimicrobiana (antibiograma) antes do início do tratamento. Em situações nas quais o tratamento deve ser instituído imediatamente, deve-se optar por um antibiótico de primeira linha, conforme descrito anteriormente para ITU não complicada. Como cada reinfecção é causada pela recolonização por diferente cepa bacteriana, a duração dos tratamentos é semelhante em um paciente que apresenta repetidas infecções isoladas, sendo geralmente desnecessário um tratamento antimicrobiano de longa duração.

Tratamentos preventivos

Em mais de 25% dos cães não é possível detectar ou corrigir a anormalidade que possibilita a recolonização.[76] Nesses pacientes, o tratamento da reinfecção com antibióticos propicia apenas esterilização transitória da urina.[76,77] Um plano terapêutico efetivo, destinado à prevenção de ITU causada por microrganismo patogênico, seria a melhor opção terapêutica. Infelizmente, há poucas evidências clínicas de eficácia a longo prazo de quase todos os tratamentos preventivos. A maioria dos tratamentos mencionados a seguir é baseada em teorias, estudos *in vitro*, pequenas séries de casos ou relatos pragmáticos. A International Society for Companion Animal Infectious Diseases não recomenda qualquer das seguintes terapias nas diretrizes sobre tratamento de infecções do trato urinário publicadas em 2011.[8]

Em todos os planos terapêuticos preventivos a primeira etapa é a detecção de uma verdadeira ITU e então, se apropriada, a erradicação da infecção atual. Após esterilização da urina, os protocolos preventivos podem ser classificados em terapias que possibilitam que as bactérias permaneçam viáveis e em terapias que matam os microrganismos invasores. O tratamento efetivo com terapias que não utilizam antimicrobianos é mais atrativo porque não aplica pressões seletivas bactericidas, não induz resistência bacteriana e mantém viável a flora normal do paciente. As categorias de profilaxia sem o uso de antimicrobiano incluem inibição da aderência e interferência bacteriana, enquanto a profilaxia antimicrobiana frequentemente consiste na administração de antimicrobianos a longo prazo com doses modificadas.

Antiaderência

A base da terapêutica antiaderência é a inibição da capacidade de a bactéria se aderir ao urotélio, possibilitando que durante a micção ocorra excreção dos microrganismos invasores do trato urinário. Uma das terapias preventivas mais amplamente aceitas é o consumo de oxicocos e extrato de oxicocos. Proantocianidinas (PAC) com ligações tipo A isoladas de oxicocos possuem propriedades antibiofilme e podem impedir que ECUP com fímbrias, que causam pielonefrite, liguem-se às células uroepiteliais.[78-82] Em pacientes veterinários, são escassas as evidências *in vivo* de eficácia clínica de PAC, embora relata-se que a urina produzida por cães que consomem PAC reduz a aderência de *E. coli in vitro*.[83] Portanto, a utilização de PAC poderia ser efetiva na limitação da colonização do trato urinário por algumas cepas de bactérias que possuem fímbrias P.

A administração oral de D-manose é uma segunda opção de terapia antiaderência. A D-manose prejudica a aderência de bactérias no urotélio por inibir a interação entre as lectinas das extremidades das fímbrias tipo 1 com moléculas de carboidrato contidas nas células uroteliais.[84,85] Diversos estudos em roedores demonstraram diminuição da colonização por ECUP após incubação da bactéria juntamente com D-manose.[86-88] Embora permaneçam dúvidas sobre se a D-manose administrada por via oral é capaz de se concentrar na urina,[89] um estudo clínico recente em mulheres sugeriu que o consumo oral regular de D-manose pode reduzir a recidiva de ITU.[90] Evidências clínicas da eficácia desse procedimento em cães e gatos são escassas.

Uma terceira opção de terapia antiaderência envolve a utilização de glicosaminoglicanos (GAGs). Durante a ITU causada por *E. coli*, fatores de virulência produzidos por bactérias podem danificar a barreira protetora de GAG sobrejacente ao urotélio.[91,92] O intuito da terapia com GAG é que ocorra aderência de GAGs exógenos ao urotélio ou sua ligação a bactérias invasoras, impedindo a lesão induzida por esses microrganismos. Em pessoas, diversos estudos independentes demonstraram que a administração do GAG ácido hialurônico diretamente na bexiga reduz significativamente a taxa de recidiva de ITU;[93-95] contudo, em medicina veterinária, a eficácia da administração vesical de GAG para prevenir ITU ainda não foi comprovada.

Interferência bacteriana

A utilização de bactérias para prevenir ITU é baseada na suposição de que colônias de microrganismos não patogênicos estabelecidas no trato urinário alteram o microambiente, interrompendo a proliferação de bactérias colonizadoras patogênicas. Uma forma de interferência bacteriana envolve a administração de *E. coli* não patogênica na bexiga. Essa terapia almeja colonizar a bexiga com microrganismos que utilizam nutrientes locais, reduzindo a capacidade de colonização de uropatógenos.[96] Em pessoas com distúrbios de retenção urinária que causam reinfecções, a administração de *E. coli* 83972 na bexiga, a fim de induzir BAS, reduziu a ocorrência de reinfecções em até 50%.[97,98] Dois estudos que tentaram inocular *E. coli* 83972 na bexiga de cães saudáveis não foram capazes de estabelecer consistentemente a persistência de colônias;[99,100] entretanto, para o sucesso da colonização, pode ser necessária uma anormalidade, como a retenção urinária.

Um segundo método para alterar o microambiente urinário é a utilização de probióticos. *Lactobacillus* e outras bactérias produtoras de ácido láctico, teoricamente, diminuem o pH vaginal, inibindo, assim, a colonização de bactérias uropatogênicas.[101] Frequentemente, bactérias uropatogênicas colonizam a mucosa vaginal de mulheres com ITU recorrente.[101,102] A administração oral e vaginal de *Lactobacillus* aumentou a população de bactérias produtoras de ácido láctico na vagina, reduziu a quantidade de bactérias uropatogênicas isoladas e reduziu a taxa de recidiva de ITU.[103-105] Em cadelas, a importância de *Lactobacillus* como colonizador vaginal não é conhecida, já que esse microrganismo esporadicamente coloniza a cripta vaginal de cadelas castradas, normais e aquelas com ITU recidivante.[41] Cadelas suplementadas com bactérias produtoras de ácido láctico, por via oral, também não modificaram a população de bactérias vaginal, sugerindo que o suplemento oral de bactérias produtoras de ácido láctico possui utilidade limitada na prevenção de reinfecções em cães.[106]

Miscelânea de tratamentos preventivos sem uso de antimicrobianos

A administração de estrógenos ajuda a prevenir reinfecções em mulheres, alterando o microambiente urinário por induzir a multiplicação de *Lactobacillus* na vagina, diminuir o pH vaginal e restaurar a mucosa da uretra atrofiada.[107] Suplementos de estrógeno administrados por via oral e topicamente na vagina reduzem a taxa de ITU recorrente em mulheres após a menopausa.[108] Ainda não se sabe como esse tratamento é transferido a cães e gatos, mas pacientes com incompetência do mecanismo do esfíncter uretral subclínica podem ser beneficiados com a terapia com estrógenos (ver Capítulo 335).

Sais de metenamina são antissépticos urinários que originam formaldeído a partir da hexamina na urina ácida. Como é necessário pH urinário de 5,5 para a conversão de metenamina em concentração bacteriostática de formaldeído,[109,110] faz-se a administração concomitante de vitamina C e outros acidificantes urinários para obter esse pH baixo. Contraindicações ao uso da metenamina incluem ITU causada por bactérias urease-positivas e condições associadas à acidose metabólica, como doença renal crônica/uremia.[111] Uma revisão de Cochrane sugeriu que o hipurato de metenamina pode beneficiar as pessoas sem anormalidades apreciáveis do trato urinário, quando utilizado por 1 semana ou menos. A metenamina não parece efetiva em pacientes com bexiga neuropática e não há conhecimento de informações definitivas sobre sua efetividade a longo prazo.[112] O seu uso não é recomendado em medicina veterinária.

Terapias adicionais que parecem promissoras para o futuro incluem o desenvolvimento de anticorpos antibacterianos utilizando estratégias vacinais diversas[113,114] e a introdução de bacteriófagos capazes de danificar ECUP.[115] Algumas terapias vacinais atingiram eficácia modesta em testes clínicos realizados em pessoas e podem ser opções de tratamento profilático adicionais para prevenção da aderência e colonização de bactérias no urotélio.

Tratamento preventivo com antimicrobianos

Tanto em pacientes humanos quanto em veterinários, a utilização de profilaxia antibiótica a longo prazo, com dose modificada, é controversa.[8,116] Em estudos humanos, verificou-se que a profilaxia ativa reduziu a recorrência de infecções e esse procedimento pode ser útil em alguns animais que manifestam sinais clínicos graves.[111] Esse tratamento não previne infecções depois que ocorre descontinuação do antibiótico; ademais, pressões seletivas aplicadas a bactérias por tratamentos repetidos com antibióticos podem levar ao desenvolvimento de cepas de bactérias uropatogênicas multirresistentes e a falhas terapêuticas.[74,75,117]

A base da terapia profilática com antibióticos consiste na administração de 1/3 a 1/2 da dose total diária do antibiótico, geralmente à noite, após a última micção do dia. Durante a noite os antibióticos se concentram na urina, impedindo a colonização na urina. Os tratamentos diários são mantidos durante 6 meses, monitorados com cultura microbiológica mensal, a fim de assegurar que não ocorreu nova infecção. Após 6 meses, se a urina permanece estéril, os antibióticos podem ser descontinuados, e o tratamento repetido quando necessário.

REFERÊNCIAS BIBLIOGRÁFICAS

As referências bibliográficas deste capítulo se encontram online no Ambiente de Aprendizagem.

CAPÍTULO 331

Urolitíase no Trato Urinário Inferior de Cães

Jody P. Lulich e Carl A. Osborne

Urolitíase é um termo geral que se refere a causas e efeitos de cálculos em qualquer local do trato urinário. A urolitíase não deve ser vista conceitualmente como uma doença única, com uma única causa, mas sim como uma sequela de diversas anormalidades interativas. Assim, a síndrome da urolitíase pode ser definida como a ocorrência de fatores fisiopatológicos familiares, congênitos ou adquiridos, que em combinação aumentam progressivamente o risco de precipitação de metabólitos excretados na urina e formação de cálculos (i. e., urólitos; Figura 331.1).

DIAGNÓSTICO

Sintomas relativos ao trato urinário inferior (ver Capítulo 46) são indicações comuns na avaliação da presença de urólitos em cães. Exames de imagem são os exames mais utilizados para a confirmação do diagnóstico.[1] Ao realizar a radiografia de abdome, é importante obter imagem de todo o trato urinário, de modo a evitar que passe despercebida a possibilidade da presença de urólitos também em qualquer local do lúmen da uretra. Como pequenos urólitos, com menos de 2 mm de diâmetro, e alguns tipos de cálculos possuem baixa opacidade radiográfica (p. ex., urato, cistina), devem-se realizar ultrassonografia (US) de abdome, uretrocistografia contrastada ou outras técnicas mais sensíveis antes que se exclua completamente a possibilidade de urólitos serem a causa dos sinais clínicos. Essas modalidades de imagem também têm sido úteis para diferenciação de neoplasias uroteliais mineralizadas e corpos estranhos císticos formados a partir de urólitos. Embora a palpação do trato urinário inferior seja um método que carece de sensibilidade diagnóstica, esse procedimento diagnóstico simples não deve ser menosprezado. Em algumas situações, a palpação retal da uretra pélvica detectou urólitos que estavam ocultos pelos ossos pélvicos quando visualizados em radiografias ou eram inacessíveis à US de rotina.

O diagnóstico de urolitíase sem avaliar a composição do urólito não é suficiente para escolher um tratamento efetivo. Por exemplo, um cão com nefrólitos e cistólitos de estruvita induzidos por infecção não pode ser adequadamente tratado apenas por cistotomia. De forma semelhante, caso não se faça urocultura para bactérias aeróbicas antes da terapia, o tratamento com dieta terapêutica não será tão efetivo no controle da infecção subjacente. Em todos os casos de urólitos é fundamental que se façam a revisão de imagens apropriadas e o exame de urina de parte da amostra reservada para cultura bacteriana. Ademais, muitos pacientes necessitam de avaliação do perfil bioquímico sérico, especialmente aqueles com doença hepática ou obstrução de uretra.

ESTIMATIVA DA COMPOSIÇÃO MINERAL

Considerações gerais

A estimativa acurada da composição mineral de urólitos, antes de sua remoção, possibilita a elaboração de um protocolo terapêutico seguro e efetivo. Por exemplo, evitar o uso de medicamentos analgésicos não esteroides e de anestésicos metabolizados primariamente no fígado melhora a recuperação de cães com suspeita de urólitos de urato decorrentes de anomalias portovasculares hepáticas (ver Capítulo 284). Da mesma forma, alguns cães com suspeita de urólitos de cistina podem ser beneficiados pela castração no momento da remoção do urólito, a fim de minimizar a ocorrência de recidiva.[2] A constatação de cristalúria, o principal método de estimativa da composição do urólito, não é sensível, tampouco confiável.[3] Assim que os cálculos são formados, os cristais associados a eles quase sempre diminuem ou desaparecem da urina. Para estimar a composição do urólito de forma mais acurada, primeiramente devem ser obtidas radiografias simples, juntamente com informações quanto à prevalência do cálculo, à raça e ao sexo (Tabela 331.1). Essas informações, a identificação dos cristais e o pH da urina quase sempre são suficientes para estimar de forma confiável o principal componente da maioria dos urólitos.

Prevalência de urólito

O conhecimento da frequência na qual urólitos de diferentes tipos de minerais é diagnosticada é útil para estimar a composição do urólito. Em quase 70 mil urólitos de cães examinados, verificou-se que cálculos de oxalato de cálcio e estruvita representaram cerca de 80% dos urólitos. Notou-se predomínio de cálculo de oxalato de cálcio na América do Norte, Ásia e Europa, enquanto o cálculo de estruvita foi o mais comum na África, Austrália (mas não na Nova Zelândia) e América do Sul.[4] Nessa pesquisa, constatou-se que a maioria dos cães que tinham urólito de oxalato de cálcio era formada por machos (78%), e a maioria dos cães que apresentavam urólito de estruvita era formada por fêmeas (82%).

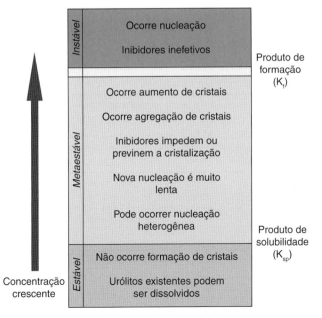

Figura 331.1 Estados de saturação relacionados à formação de cristais na urina.

Tabela 331.1 Estimativa da composição mineral dos urólitos de cães.

TIPO DE URÓLITO	PREVALÊNCIA (%)	APARÊNCIA RADIOGRÁFICA	RAÇAS COMUNS	SEXO % (NC/C)	CRISTALÚRIA	PH URINÁRIO
Oxalato de cálcio monoidratado	37,5	Radiopacidade moderada a marcante. Redondo, com superfície granular a irregular	Mestiços, Schnauzer Míni, Shih Tzu, Yorkshire Terrier, Chihuahua, Bichon (59,2%)	F-22 (3,2/18,8) M-76,8 (15,4/61,4)	Cristais em forma de halteres, estacas	< 6,5
Oxalato de cálcio di-hidratado	5,3	Radiopacidade moderada a marcante. Espiculado e rosetas com formato de estrela	Shih Tzu, Yorkshire Terrier, Schnauzer Míni, Bichon, Chihuahua	F-17,1 (2,3/14,8) M-81,4 (26,1/55,3)	Forma de envelope com cruz	< 6,5
Estruvita	36,8	Radiopacidade moderada a marcante. Redondo a facetado	Shih Tzu, Schnauzer Míni, Teckel, Pug, Bichon	F-82,2 (15,2/67) M-14,4 (7,2/7,2)	Em forma de prisma	> 7
Sais de urato	4,0	Radiolucente a marginalmente radiopaco. Redondo liso a aspecto de amora	Dálmata, mestiço, Yorkshire Terrier, Buldogue Inglês, Shih Tzu, Schnauzer Míni	F-19,2 (4,8/14,4) M-79,1 (25,1/54)	Amorfo, forma de glóbulos especulares com e sem espículas	≤ 6,5
Cistina	2,1	Radiolucente a marginalmente radiopaco. Redondo liso a aspecto de amora	Buldogue Inglês, mestiço, Chihuahua, Teckel, Buldogue Francês, Pitbull	F-0,9 (0,4/0,5) M-97,2 (76,8/20,4)	Em forma de hexágono	≤ 6,5
Sílica	0,4	Radiopacidade moderada a marcante. Formato de estrela com radiações geométricas com picos baixos a altos	Mestiço, Labrador Retriever, Shih Tzu, Pastor-Alemão, Chihuahua, Golden Retriever	F-6,7 (2,1/4,6) M-91,5 (37,3/54,2)		
Carbonato de fosfato de cálcio	0,5	Radiopacidade moderada a marcante. Redondo liso a facetado	Mestiço, Shih Tzu, Bichon, Pug, Schnauzer Míni, Chihuahua (57,2%)	F-77,8 (11,9/55,9) M-31,3 (13,8/17,5)	Amorfo	≥ 7,5
Brushita (fosfato de cálcio)	0,3	Radiopacidade baixa/moderada a marcante. Redondo liso	Shih Tzu, mestiço, Bichon, Yorkshire Terrier, Papillon, Maltês (71,3%)	F-32 (4,6/27,4) M-66,8 (31,4/35,4)	Amorfo	> 6,5
Apatita de CaP	0,1	Radiopacidade baixa/moderada a marcante. Redondo liso	Mestiço, Shih Tzu, Pug, Labrador Retriever, Teckel, Papillon (60,5%)	F-34,8 (4,6/30,2) M-62,8 (22,1/40,7)	Amorfo	> 6,5
Xantina	0,1	Radiolucente redondo a irregular	Mestiço, Dálmata, Labrador, não relatado, Cavalier KCS, Rottweiler (66,14%)	F-16,9 (7/16,9) M-81,7 (33,8/47,9)	Globular	
Composto	9,9	Cálculos maiores com camadas internas e externas de diferentes radiopacidades	Mestiço, Shih Tzu, Schnauzer Míni, Yorkshire Terrier, Bichon, Teckel (61,1%)	F-69,9 (13,8/56,1) M-28,7 (9,4/19,3)	Formas variáveis	
Misto	3,2	Variável	Mestiço, Shih Tzu, Schnauzer Míni, Bichon, Yorkshire Terrier, Pug (61,7%)	F-77,3 (14,3/63) M-21 (8,6/12,4)	Formas variáveis	

Míni, miniatura; *NC/C*, não castrado/castrado.

Aparência radiográfica dos urólitos

A aparência radiográfica dos urólitos (radiopacidade, uniformidade da radiopacidade, tamanho, formato e contorno) está altamente relacionada à sua composição; é um dos procedimentos mais confiáveis para estimar o tipo de urólito, antes da análise de sua composição (Figura 331.2).[5] Urólitos compostos de oxalato de cálcio, fosfato de cálcio e sílica são radiopacos. O cálculo de estruvita é moderadamente radiopaco, e os cálculos de cistina, urato e xantina comumente são radiolucentes. Urólitos radiopacos com menos de 2 mm podem ser difíceis de se visualizar em radiografias simples, necessitando de US ou uso de contraste para serem visualizados. Urólitos radiolucentes com mais de 5 mm podem ser vistos em radiografias simples. Um urólito cuja área central possua radiopacidade diferente daquela da camada externa é compatível com urólito composto. As mesmas generalidades radiográficas de urólitos não compostos se aplicam às camadas de urólitos compostos. O exame de urina geralmente é mais consistente na avaliação da composição da camada externa do cálculo.

Raça

Predisposição racial e anomalias genéticas hereditárias no processamento de precursores calculogênicos sustentam a importância da obtenção de informações epidemiológicas do paciente para auxiliar na estimativa da composição do urólito.[2,6,7] Embora tenham se detectado urólitos de oxalato de cálcio em mais de cem raças, 50% deles foram verificados em seis raças: Schnauzer Miniatura, Shih Tzu, Yorkshire Terrier, Chihuahua, Bichon Frisé e Maltês. Nessas raças de cães de pequeno porte e raças relacionadas, a prevalência de outros tipos de cálculos também é alta (ver Tabela 331.1). A ocorrência de urólitos de urato e cistina é maior em cães Buldogue Inglês.[8] A raça seria um fator preditivo mais confiável do tipo de urólito se houvesse uma relação tão consiste entre cães Dálmata e prevalência de cálculos de urato: 96% dos cães Dálmata que apresentam urólitos possuem cálculos de sais de urato.[9]

Exame de urina

O conhecimento do tipo de cristais na urina e do pH urinário pode ser útil no tratamento de cães com urolitíase, mas tais informações não são tão sensíveis ou específicas na predição da composição do urólito.[3] Assim que os cálculos são formados, é termodinamicamente mais favorável a deposição de minerais na superfície de um cálculo pré-formado do que a formação de novos cristais. Como resultado, os cristais são geralmente ausentes na urina de um animal com cálculo vesical. Quando presentes, os cristais podem não representar a composição do urólito, mas sim a influência do pH ou de fatores não relacionados ao urólito. Isso pode explicar por que são observados cristais de estruvita em cães com urólitos de oxalato de cálcio, na medida em que a urina é alcalinizada pela ação de medicamentos.

Remoção do urólito

A estimativa acurada da composição mineral de alguns urólitos pode ser difícil, especialmente daqueles cálculos mistos (i. e., não compostos por um mineral principal), compostos ou incomuns. Se o tamanho do urólito for menor que 3 mm, ele pode ser coletado durante a micção ou por remoção com sonda (Vídeo 331.1).[10] Durante a micção, os tutores podem posicionar um coador ou uma peneira de cozinha ou uma rede de pesca, de malha fina, no fluxo do jato de urina. Se tal procedimento não for bem-sucedido após várias tentativas, os urólitos podem ser extraídos com uma sonda de grande diâmetro, introduzida no cão em decúbito lateral esquerdo ou direito. Aplica-se anestésico local lubrificante na uretra; todavia, em alguns cães ansiosos, pode-se utilizar sedativo. Empregando-se uma técnica estéril, a extremidade da sonda urinária é introduzida na uretra distal e avançada até o trígono vesical. O local preciso pode ser determinado pela mensuração da distância por meio de radiografia. Conecta-se uma seringa à sonda e aplica-se suave pressão

negativa intermitente, à medida que a extremidade da sonda é removida da bexiga. Quando a extremidade da sonda urinária sai da bexiga e alcança a uretra, o fluxo de urina cessa. Então, avance a sonda em direção à bexiga e o fluxo de urina retorna quando a ponta da sonda adentra o trígono vesical. A extremidade da sonda também pode ser posicionada por meio de fluoroscopia ou guiada por US. Ao mesmo tempo que movimenta a bexiga, remova a urina remanescente e inspecione o conteúdo da seringa em busca de pequenos cálculos. Se não há cálculo, repita o procedimento administrando 5 mℓ de solução isotônica estéril/kg de peso corporal (até 50 mℓ quando se utiliza uma seringa de 60 mℓ) através da sonda e agite a bexiga durante o seu esvaziamento (Vídeos 331.2 e 331.3). O procedimento pode ser repetido até que os cálculos sejam extraídos. Envie os urólitos recuperados para análise quantitativa de minerais.

REMOÇÃO DE URÓLITO

Considerações gerais

A remoção de urólito tem sido classicamente uma atividade do cirurgião. Foram desenvolvidos procedimentos menos invasivos, e alguns podem ser realizados por qualquer veterinário (p. ex., dissolução medicamentosa e uro-hidropropulsão). Outros podem necessitar de treinamento avançado e material especial (p. ex., remoção com aparato na forma de cesta, litotripsia a *laser* [Figura 331.3], cistolitotomia percutânea; ver Capítulo 124).

Objetivos

Ao escolher um procedimento para remoção de urólitos, considere os seguintes objetivos focados no paciente:

1. Remover todos os cálculos e fragmentos. O risco de futura obstrução uretral pode ser devido à falha na remoção de todos os cálculos. A impossibilidade de remoção de todos os cálculos pode ocasionar sintomas contínuos de hematúria, estrangúria e disúria; a infecção do trato urinário também persiste. Assim, há necessidade de procedimentos adicionais para a extração do urólito.[11,12] Relata-se que cirurgia não remove consistentemente todos os cálculos. Em 128 cães submetidos à cirurgia para remoção de cálculos vesicais, apenas 19 (15%) apresentaram exames de imagem pós-cirúrgicos apropriados; detectou-se remoção incompleta de urólitos em 8 dos 19 cães (42%).[13] A eficácia da litotripsia a *laser* foi avaliada prospectivamente em 100 cães com urólitos de ocorrência natural, e a remoção incompleta foi detectada em 18 deles (9 com urólitos ≥ 3 mm, 7 com urólitos de 1 a 3 mm, e 3 com urólitos < 1 mm).[14]

2. Minimizar a lesão aos tecidos saudáveis. A vantagem de procedimentos não invasivos e minimamente invasivos é sua capacidade de preservar a anatomia normal. O fato de evitar a cirurgia ou mínimos transtornos aos tecidos provavelmente está associado a redução da taxa de infecções, redução da dor, menor tempo de hospitalização, retorno mais rápido à função, menor risco de complicações e menor extensão da cicatrização.[15]

3. Escolher procedimentos que provavelmente contribuam menos para a recidiva do urólito. A recidiva de urólitos após a remoção é comumente atribuída à falha do tratamento medicamentoso. Entretanto, quando foram analisados urólitos recorrentes em 1.733 cães, 163 (9,4%) foram atribuídos a um nicho no local de sutura.[16] Esses achados ressaltam o fato de que procedimentos cirúrgicos contribuem para a doença recorrente, que poderia ser evitada pelo emprego de técnicas minimamente invasivas.

Métodos de remoção de urólitos em animais assintomáticos

A remoção medicamentosa de urólitos assintomáticos compostos de estruvita consiste na acidificação da urina e no uso de antibióticos.[17,18] Cálculos de cistina são frequentemente tratados

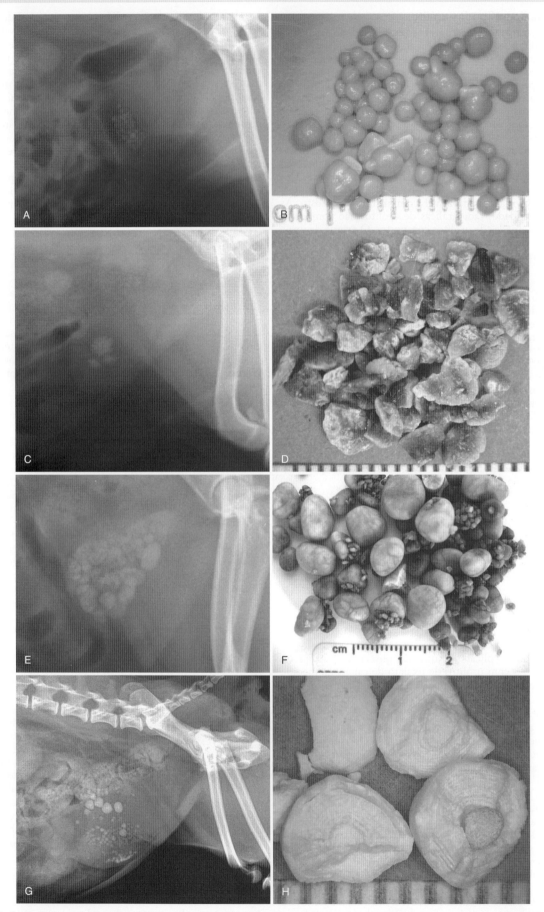

Figura 331.2 A e **B.** Urólitos de oxalato de cálcio monoidratado, antes e depois de uro-hidropropulsão. **C** e **D.** Urólitos de oxalato de cálcio di-hidratado, antes e depois de litotripsia. **E** e **F.** Urólitos de estruvita causados por infecção, antes e depois de cistotomia. **G** e **H.** Cálculos compostos com um centro de oxalato de cálcio e uma camada externa de estruvita, antes e depois de litotripsia a *laser*.

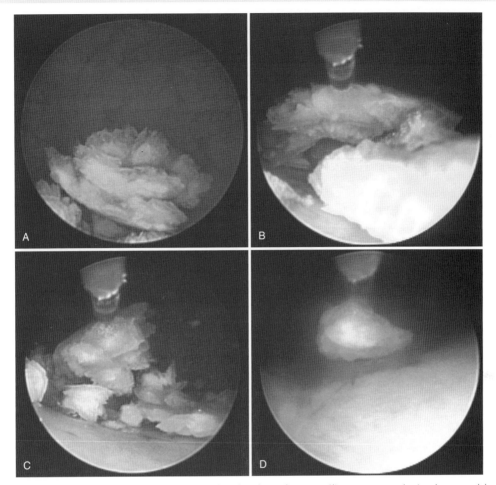

Figura 331.3 Visualizações cistoscópicas de um grande urólito de oxalato de cálcio e diversos urólitos menores na bexiga de uma cadela, antes (**A**) e durante (**B** a **D**) litotripsia a *laser*. **B.** Fibra de *laser* com ponteira de quartzo flexível com 550 μ de diâmetro posicionada próximo à superfície do urólito, que foi quebrado em dois fragmentos maiores. Note o feixe vermelho visível na superfície do urólito. **C.** Fragmentos do urólito de oxalato de cálcio após litotripsia a *laser* adicional. **D.** Note um pequeno fragmento adjacente à mucosa e que a energia do *laser* fragmenta o urólito sem dano à mucosa adjacente. Ocorre mínimo traumatismo na mucosa por conta das projeções pontiagudas do fragmento do urólito. (Reimpressa com permissão de Adams LG, Berent AC, Moore GE, Bagley DH: Use of *laser* lithotripsy for fragmentation of uroliths in dogs: 73 cases [2005-2006]. *J Am Vet Med Assoc* 232:1680-1687, 2008.) (*Esta figura se encontra reproduzida em cores no Encarte.*)

com prescrição de ração (Hill's u/d®).[19,20] Cálculos de urato são tratados com alopurinol e prescrição de ração (Hill's u/d®).[21] A ocorrência de cálculos de xantina causados por alopurinol requer a descontinuação desse medicamento. Deve-se tentar dissolver esses cálculos com o uso de medicamentos, a menos que tentativas prévias tenham sido ineficazes ou mal toleradas. Os urólitos podem ser monitorados e removidos assim que ocorrerem sintomas (Tabela 331.2). Urólitos assintomáticos pequenos o suficiente para passar através da uretra devem ser removidos por meio de uro-hidropropulsão (ver Vídeo 331.2) ou de remoção com um aparato semelhante a uma cesta (Vídeo 331.4).[14,22,23] Urólitos maiores devem ser deixados até que o paciente se torne sintomático. Os tutores devem ser orientados quanto aos sinais clínicos e planos de acompanhamento em caso de obstrução da uretra. Em animais cujo monitoramento do tutor não é confiável, pode ser melhor optar pela remoção do urólito antes do início da manifestação clínica da doença.

Métodos de remoção de urólitos em animais sintomáticos

Quando os urólitos causam sinais clínicos, quase sempre eles são muito grandes para ser removidos do trato urinário por meio de uro-hidropropulsão. Para aqueles cálculos passíveis de dissolução, inicialmente deve-se tentar a dissolução com medicamento. Se há obstrução da uretra, devem-se remover os cálculos para impedir nova obstrução. Tente remover todos os urólitos pela combinação de remoção com cesta (ver Vídeo 331.4), litotripsia a *laser* (Vídeos 331.5 e 331.6) e cistolitotomia percutânea (ver Capítulo 124).[14,24-29] Se esses procedimentos não estiverem disponíveis, os urólitos podem ser removidos por cistotomia depois que todos os uretrólitos tenham sido empurrados de volta à bexiga antes da cirurgia. Em razão da alta frequência de efeitos adversos associados à cirurgia da uretra (p. ex., constrição, infecções recorrentes do trato urinário etc.), não se recomenda uretrotomia ou uretrostomia, com exceção de condições especiais (p. ex., impossibilidade de o cliente arcar com gastos adicionais em caso de obstrução recorrente).[30]

PREVENÇÃO DE FORMAÇÃO DE URÓLITO (TABELA 331.3)

Oxalato de cálcio (CaC$_2$O$_4$)

A urolitíase causada por CaC$_2$O$_4$ é uma doença crônica, com alta taxa de recidiva (cerca de 50% em 2 anos).[30] Hipercalciúria parece ser o fator primário para a formação do cálculo; contudo, a escolha do tratamento efetivo pode ser um desafio porque (1) as verdadeiras causas são mal compreendidas; (2) não se sabe quais são os fatores de risco que mais contribuem para a ocorrência da doença; (3) os parâmetros da eficácia terapêutica, como a supersaturação relativa, são modelos matemáticos que

Tabela 331.2 — Métodos minimamente invasivos para remoção de cálculos.

MÉTODO	CANDIDATOS APROPRIADOS	CONTRAINDICAÇÃO RELATIVA	ABORDAGEM	CONCEPÇÕES ERRÔNEAS COMUNS
Micção espontânea	Pequenos urólitos (p. ex., < 2 a 3 mm) que podem passar facilmente pela uretra	Cães sintomáticos com urólitos cujo tamanho pode obstruir a uretra	Uma pequena peneira de cozinha ou rede de pesca posicionada sob o jato da urina do cão possibilita a coleta de cálculos excretados para análise	
Dissolução medicamentosa	Altamente efetiva para urólitos de estruvita, de xantina induzida por alopurinol e de cistina. Menos efetiva para cálculos de urato	Obstrução de uretra. Um único grande cálculo que ocupa quase toda a bexiga	No caso de urólito de estruvita causado por infecção, administre antibióticos durante todo o período de dissolução	Cães possuem maior risco de obstrução da uretra
Uro-hidropropulsão	Cálculos que provavelmente passam através da uretra; geralmente cálculos lisos com < 4 mm ou urólitos irregulares < 3 mm, mas isso é influenciado pelo tamanho do cão e de sua uretra. Cães com peso compatível para serem erguidos	Obstrução da uretra. Cistotomia recente. Constrição uretral	Evite o uso de anestésico que aumenta o tônus uretral (p. ex., dexmedetomidina). Utilize anestesia epidural caudal (lidocaína) para assegurar o relaxamento da uretra. Para relaxar ainda mais a uretra em cães anestesiados, administre 1 mg de propofol/kg IV imediatamente antes da massagem da bexiga. No caso de muitos cálculos irregulares, faça a remoção com um aparato semelhante a uma cesta, antes da uro-hidropropulsão	Um plano anestésico superficial é suficiente para relaxar a uretra. Um cálculo que se aloja na uretra é difícil de ser empurrado de volta à bexiga
Remoção do cálculo com um aparato semelhante a uma cesta	Cálculos ou fragmentos de cálculos que provavelmente passam através da uretra; geralmente urólitos lisos < 4 mm, mas isso é influenciado principalmente pelo tamanho do cão e de sua uretra		Posicione os cálculos de modo a passarem longitudinalmente através da uretra, com suas margens pontiagudas voltadas para o lado oposto à direção de retração. Utilize um tipo de cesta que permita o deslocamento dos urólitos, caso estejam presos no lúmen da uretra e precisem de reorientação ou reposicionamento	
Litotripsia intracorpórea a *laser*	Em machos com ≥ 6 kg e não mais que três cálculos que necessitam de litotripsia (i. e., entre 4 e 7 mm de diâmetro). Em fêmeas, sem restrição ao tamanho do cálculo, mas cálculos de estruvita devem ser dissolvidos com medicamentos. Todos os urólitos na uretra	Hematúria intensa reduz sobremaneira a visibilidade. Presença de um grande cálculo, a menos que sejam previstas mais de uma sessão de litotripsia para a remoção completa. Gatos machos e cães machos pequenos, nos quais não é possível passar a câmera através do lúmen uretral	Para melhorar a visibilidade no início e periodicamente, utilize uma sonda 8Fr para esvaziar a bexiga; em seguida, lave repetidas vezes com solução isotônica estéril. Evite o uso de anestésico que aumenta o tônus uretral (p. ex., dexmedetomidina). Aplique anestesia epidural caudal (lidocaína) para assegurar o relaxamento da uretra	Fragmentos do urólito são excretados durante a micção espontânea e não precisam ser removidos
Cistolitotomia percutânea	Machos com mais de três cálculos grandes (> 7 mm); contudo, pode ser realizada para todos os tipos se não há disponibilidade de litotripsia. Em fêmeas, a maioria dos cálculos pode ser removida por meio de litotripsia		Posicione um cateter Foley na uretra de tal forma que o balão inflado oclua a uretra proximal, a fim de minimizar a migração distal de cálculos	

Tabela 331.3 — Medicamentos comumente utilizados no tratamento de urolitíase em cães.

NOME	DOSE	MECANISMO DE AÇÃO	COMPLICAÇÕES ADVERSAS	INFORMAÇÕES ADICIONAIS
Alopurinol	Dissolução: 15 mg/kg/12 h Prevenção: 5 a 7 mg/kg a cada 12 a 24 h	Alopurinol e seu metabólito ativo oxipurinol inibem a xantina oxidase, impedindo a conversão de hipoxantina e xantina em ácido úrico	Urólitos de xantina Hipersensibilidade Nefropatia	Os inibidores mais recentes da xantina oxidase (Febuxostate®) não são análogos da purina e não necessitam de metabolização hepática para prolongar a sua ação
Citrato de potássio	75 mg/kg a cada 12 a 24 h, ajustada até obter pH urinário de 7 a 8	Aumenta a excreção renal de citrato que se liga ao cálcio e reduz a formação de oxalato de cálcio e sua aderência ao urotélio	Diminuição do apetite Hiperpotassemia	Forneça com alimento A maioria das formulações contém teor inapropriado de oxicoco, que pode aumentar o conteúdo de oxalato na urina. A maioria delas é formulada com dióxido de sílica, que pode contribuir para a recidiva de cálculos de sílica
dℓ-metionina	100 mg/kg/12 h	Acidificante urinário utilizado para aumentar a dissolução de estruvita em cães não tratados com rações terapêuticas	Diminuição do apetite Acidemia	Forneça com alimento
Vitamina B_6	2 a 4 mg/kg, a cada 24 a 48 h	Favorece a conversão de precursores de oxalato em glicina, minimizando a produção de oxalato		Recomendada apenas para cães que consomem alimentos deficientes em vitamina B_6
Hidroclorotiazida	2 mg/kg/12 h	Reduz a excreção urinária de cálcio por aumentar a reabsorção tubular renal desse mineral	Hipercalcemia Discreta desidratação	
Tiopronina (Thiola®)	Dissolução: 15 a 20 mg/kg/12 h Prevenção: 5 a 15 mg/kg/12 h	Liga-se à cisteína para formar um complexo mais solúvel do que o dímero da cisteína (i. e., cistina)	Proteinúria Trombocitopenia Anemia Pústulas	É difícil obter – consulte uma farmácia de manipulação

podem não apresentar boa correlação com a formação de urólito, especialmente quando avaliados em cães clinicamente saudáveis e sem urólitos.[32-34] Portanto, urólitos de CaC_2O_4 tendem a apresentar recidiva, apesar de nossos melhores esforços. Estratégias terapêuticas atuais para reduzir a quantidade de Ca na urina disponível para se ligar ao oxalato incluem apenas o fornecimento de alimentos com alta umidade (p. ex., enlatados, massas, caldos de carne), suficiente para propiciar densidade urinária < 1,020, bem como evitar o fornecimento de alimentos que causam acidificação da urina (< pH de 6,6 a 7). Dietas que induzem a produção de urina ácida em cães (pH < 6,6) foram associadas ao aumento da excreção de Ca e de urólitos de CaC_2O_4.[35,36] O veterinário pode administrar citrato de potássio ou outros sais de citrato para cães com urina consistentemente ácida. Adicione diurético, como hidroclorotiazida (2 mg/kg/12 h VO), ao protocolo terapêutico de cães com cristalúria persistente causada por CaC_2O_4x ou no caso de doença com alta taxa de recidiva.[37]

Foram desenvolvidas rações comerciais destinadas à prevenção de recidiva de cristalúria por CaC_2O_4, mas elas podem não ser ideais para todos os animais. Relata-se que a ração Hill's Prescription diet u/d® diminuiu a excreção de cálcio e de oxalato, bem como a taxa de recidiva de urolitíase por CaC_2O_4, em cães.[37] Essa ração possui baixos teores de sódio e proteína, propiciando a produção de urina com pH neutro a alcalino. Embora tenha passado pelos testes nutricionais da AAFCO, alguns nutricionistas consideram o conteúdo de proteína muito baixo. Se esse for o caso, forneça metade de Hill's Prescription diet u/d® e metade de um alimento sênior enlatado com conteúdo moderado de proteína, que não cause acidificação da urina (p. ex., Hill's Prescription diet g/d® ou Hill's Prescription diet c/d multicare®). Como a Hill's Prescription diet u/d® contém alto teor de gordura, os cães com hiperlipidemia hereditária (p. ex., alguns cães Schnauzer Miniatura) podem ser beneficiados com essa mistura. A Hill's Prescription diet w/d® é recomendada aos cães com urolitíase causada por CaC_2O_4 e que apresentam intolerância à gordura/lipídios ou anormalidades responsivas à gordura/lipídios (p. ex., histórico de pancreatite). Como essa dieta induz a produção de urina ácida, administre citrato de potássio para propiciar um pH urinário mais favorável (> 6,5). Relata-se que a ração Royal Canin SO® reduziu a supersaturação relativa de CaC_2O_4 em cães com urólitos compostos desse composto químico.[34] Como essa ração induz a acidificação da urina, é necessária a administração concomitante de citrato de potássio para obter um pH urinário mais favorável (> 6,5).

Estruvita

A maioria dos urólitos de estruvita é formada como consequência de infecções do trato urinário (ITU) causadas por bactérias que produzem urease. A urease é responsável pela conversão da ureia em amônia, que alcaliniza a urina e favorece a precipitação de estruvita. Portanto, o procedimento mais efetivo para minimizar as recidivas do urólito é prevenir futuras infecções do trato urinário (ver Capítulo 330; Figura 331.4). Diferentemente, quando não há infecção, previne-se efetivamente a formação de urólitos de estruvita mediante o fornecimento de rações terapêuticas (Hill's Prescription diet c/d multicare®, Royal Canin SO®, outras).

Cálculos de urato

Em cães, duas doenças distintas estão associadas à urolitíase por cálculo de urato: uma anormalidade hereditária do transportador de urato codificado pelo gene *SLC2A9* (Figura 331.5) e anomalia portovascular hepática (ver Capítulo 284).[7,38] Comum a ambas é o transporte ineficiente de ácido úrico para os hepatócitos, onde normalmente sofre oxidação enzimática, originando um produto final altamente hidrossolúvel, a alantoína. Em vez disso, são excretadas altas concentrações de ácido úrico na urina. A redução da taxa de recidiva da urolitíase é obtida pela diminuição da hiperuricosúria (p. ex., reduzir a ingestão dietética de purina e impedir a metabolização de precursores de urato) e pelo aumento da solubilidade do urato (*i. e.*, aumentar o pH urinário para 7 a 7,5). Foram formuladas diversas rações terapêuticas destinadas a reduzir a ingestão de purina (Purina HA®, Royal Canin UC® e Hill's Prescription diet u/d®).

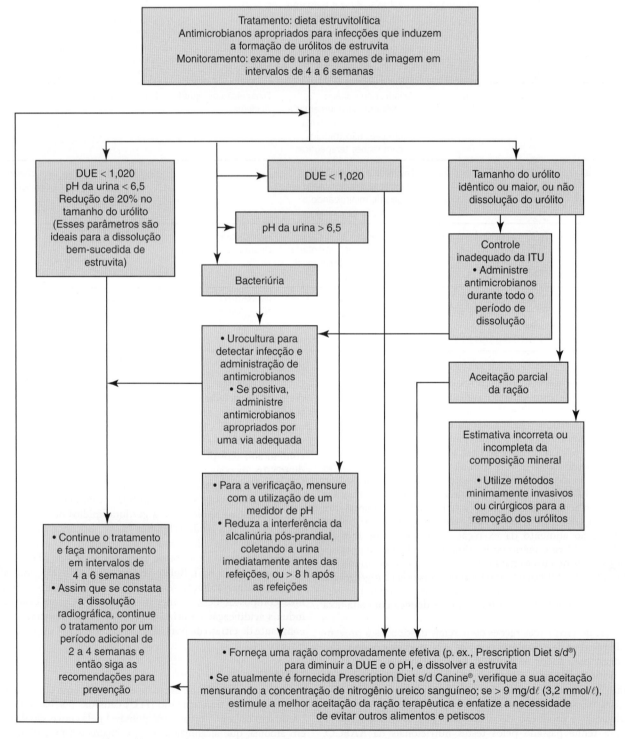

Figura 331.4 Dissolução de estruvita. *DUE*, densidade urinária específica; *ITU*, infecção do trato urinário.

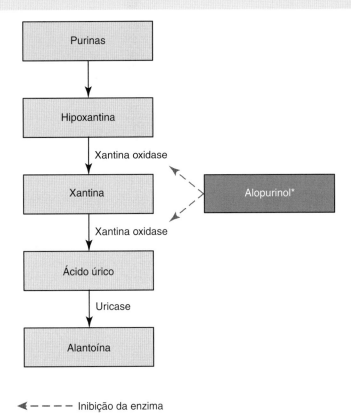

Figura 331.5 Via metabólica da degradação da purina em alantoína, mostrando o local de ação do alopurinol. *O principal metabólito do alopurinol, o oxipurinol, também inibe a xantina oxidase.

Forneça alimentos com alta umidade ou adicione água ao alimento, a fim de obter densidade urinária consistentemente baixa (< 1,020). Se o pH da urina estiver < 7, forneça citrato de potássio.

A prevenção de urólitos em cães com anomalias portovasculares é complicada. Comumente são administradas baixas doses de alopurinol (inibidor da xantina oxidase) aos cães que não apresentam doença hepática (p. ex., Dálmata, Buldogue etc.), a fim de reduzir a conversão de purinas em ácido úrico. Entretanto, é necessária função hepática suficiente para converter o alopurinol em seu análogo mais efetivo e de ação mais prolongada, o oxipurinol. Alimentos com baixo teor de purina/proteína e de proteínas vegetais de baixo valor biológico podem não ser ideais para os cães com hepatopatia. Por fim, geralmente a correção cirúrgica da anomalia vascular não é suficiente para prevenir a recidiva da urolitíase. Portanto, é importante fornecer quantidade suficiente de água e induzir a alcalinização da urina.

Cistina

Cistinúria é uma rara condição hereditária caracterizada por falha na reabsorção tubular renal de cistina (um aminoácido pouco solúvel; ver Capítulo 328). Os animais acometidos apresentam formação de urólitos de cistina recidivante. Para minimizar a recorrência do urólito, a melhor abordagem é aumentar o consumo de líquido, limitar a ingestão de proteína de origem animal, limitar a ingestão de sódio e alcalinizar a urina. A recidiva tem sido controlada apenas com a terapia farmacológica (Thiola®) e apenas com a terapia nutricional (Hill's Prescription diet u/d®).[19,21] Em algumas formas de cistinúria, a castração tem sido associada à redução da concentração urinária de cistina e prevenção de recidiva. Para identificar quais cães podem ser efetivamente tratados pela castração, mensure a concentração de cistina na urina antes e após a castração. Nesse grupo de cães, não se sabe se a castração, por si só, causa a dissolução do urólito.

Urólitos compostos

O urólito composto mais comum é formado por uma camada interna de CaC_2O_4 e uma camada externa de estruvita. Para prevenir recidiva, escolha a terapia nutricional para controlar o CaC_2O_4 e o tratamento antimicrobiano para controlar a estruvita. O segundo cálculo composto mais comum é formado por uma camada interna de estruvita e uma camada externa de carbonato/fosfato de cálcio. O controle da infecção do trato urinário previne a formação de ambos os minerais.

Urólitos de xantina

A xantinúria de ocorrência natural resulta de defeitos genéticos nas enzimas ou em cofatores que catalisam as etapas finais da degradação da purina. Para minimizar a recidiva do urólito, aumente o fornecimento de líquido, limite a ingestão de purina/proteína de origem animal e alcalinize a urina. Urólitos de xantina induzidos pelo alopurinol podem ser controlados pela descontinuação ou redução da dose de alopurinol, ao mesmo tempo que se reduz o consumo de purinas/proteínas.

Fosfato de cálcio

Urólitos de hidroxiapatita, fosfato de cálcio di-hidratado (brushita), ortofosfato tricálcico (whitlockite) e fosfato octacálcico são raros. As abordagens para prevenir a formação desses cálculos são as mesmas empregadas para urólitos de CaC_2O_4, a menos que estejam associados a anormalidades hipercalcêmicas, as quais, quando corrigidas, devem prevenir recidiva (ver Capítulos 69 e 297). Diferentemente, a prevenção de urólitos de carbonato/fosfato de cálcio depende de diagnóstico precoce e erradicação de infecções do trato urinário, ao mesmo tempo que se evitam protocolos nutricionais que estimulam a excreção de cálcio (p. ex., acidificação da urina).

Sílica

A causa de formação de urólitos de sílica é desconhecida, mas parece estar associada a três fontes: dióxido de silício encontrado como ingrediente inerte de vários comprimidos; consumo de grãos integrais, particularmente arroz, polpa de beterraba e soja; e utilização de água e alimentos de origem vegetal oriundos de locais geotérmicos ativos (vulcões, fontes termais, gêiseres). A substituição dessas fontes por outras com menor quantidade ou ausência de sílica e a recomendação de ingestão de alta quantidade de líquido devem reduzir a ocorrência de recidiva.

REFERÊNCIAS BIBLIOGRÁFICAS

As referências bibliográficas deste capítulo se encontram online no Ambiente de Aprendizagem.

CAPÍTULO 332

Urolitíase no Trato Urinário Inferior de Gatos

Mary Anna Labato

INTRODUÇÃO

Urolitíase é definida como a formação de urólitos (cálculos ou pedras) no lúmen do trato urinário. Urólitos podem variar em sua composição mineral.[1] Estudos recentes relataram que 7 a 28% dos gatos atendidos com sintomas relativos ao trato urinário inferior foram diagnosticados com urolitíase.[2-4] Em gatos, os tipos de urólitos mais comuns são os de estruvita (fosfato de amônio magnesiano) e de oxalato de cálcio (CaC_2O_4) (cada um respondendo por mais de 40% dos urólitos).[2-8] Urólitos de purina representam cerca de 5% dos casos; cerca de 7% dos urólitos são compostos por outras substâncias, como matriz, fosfato de cálcio, cálculos de sangue, cálculos compostos e aqueles induzidos por medicamentos[7,9] (Figura 332.1).

Sinais clínicos

Gatos com urólitos na bexiga, por ocasião da consulta, podem manifestar uma série de sintomas relativos ao trato urinário inferior. Estes incluem polaciúria, estrangúria, hematúria, periúria ou uma combinação desses sintomas. Quando um urólito se aloja na uretra, os sinais clínicos são relacionados à obstrução uretral (ver Capítulos 334 e 335). Esses sintomas não são específicos de urólitos; na lista de diagnósticos diferenciais, incluem-se infecções do trato urinário, cistite idiopática felina e neoplasias. Quase sempre os urólitos de bexiga não resultam em quaisquer sinais clínicos e são achados acidentais durante palpação abdominal, radiografias simples ou ultrassonografia do abdome.

Exames clínicos

Aos gatos atendidos com sinais clínicos sugestivos de urolitíase, um plano de diagnóstico básico mínimo consiste em hemograma e perfil bioquímico sérico. Na maioria das situações, os resultados desses exames situam-se na faixa de normalidade, mas podem revelar doenças subjacentes que podem predispor à formação de urólitos, como diabetes melito, doença renal crônica; ademais, os testes de função hepática podem sugerir uma anormalidade preexistente, como desvio portossistêmico. Em gatos geriátricos também devem ser mensuradas as concentrações de hormônios tireoidianos.

O exame de urina é essencial (ver Capítulo 72), embora possa haver urólitos sem cristalúria; além disso, esse exame não prediz de forma acurada o tipo de urólito. Cristalúria não é um achado consistente no exame de urina de gatos com urólitos. É importante determinar a densidade urinária, especialmente em gatos com histórico prévio de formação de urólitos. Nesses casos, é importante a produção de urina diluída, de forma que o conteúdo de minerais na urina não alcance o ponto de saturação para ocasionar a agregação de cristais e, por fim, a formação de cálculo. O pH da urina também influencia a formação de cristais. Estruvita, carbonato de cálcio e fosfato de cálcio (apatita) são menos solúveis em urina alcalina. Urato de amônio, sílica e cisteína são menos solúveis em urina ácida. As amostras de urina devem ser examinadas dentro de uma hora após a coleta, a fim de minimizar a cristalização *in vitro* dependente da temperatura e do tempo.[10] Caso haja sedimento ativo ou se a densidade urinária estiver baixa e a infecção for uma suspeita importante na lista de diagnósticos diferenciais, deve-se enviar a amostra para cultura microbiológica.

Deve-se realizar exame de imagem para confirmar a presença de urólitos. A projeção das radiografias simples deve incluir todo o sistema urinário. Os cálculos mineralizados que podem ser visualizados nas radiografias incluem os de CaC_2O_4, estruvita, apatita e sílica (Figura 332.2). A maioria dos urólitos de urato de amônio e cisteína não é mineralizada; assim, não visíveis em radiografias, a menos que sejam mistos com algum tipo de cálculo mineralizado. É necessária a cistouretrografia contrastada para visualizar esses urólitos.

A ultrassonografia de abdome é útil para detectar urólitos, tanto mineralizados quanto não mineralizados. Como uma modalidade diagnóstica, é capaz de detectar grandes cálculos não mineralizados, assim como os urólitos bem pequenos que podem frequentemente ser excretados com sucesso pelos pacientes (especialmente gatas) durante a micção (Figuras 332.3 e 332.4; Vídeo 332.1).

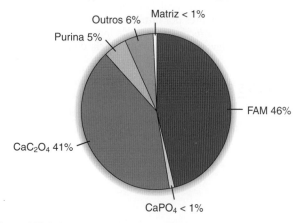

Figura 332.1 Composição mineral de urólitos de gatos – dados de 2013. CaC_2O_4, oxalato de cálcio; $CaPO_4$, fosfato de cálcio; *FAM*, fosfato de amônio magnesiano (estruvita). (De Minnesota Urolith Center.)

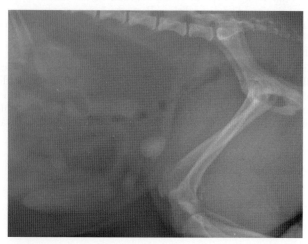

Figura 332.2 Radiografia simples de um urólito denso de mineral.

Princípios da análise da composição do cálculo

Há uma variedade de métodos disponíveis para analisar cálculos, disponibilizados por diversos laboratórios de diagnóstico (Boxe 332.1). Se o cálculo estiver disponível para análise, este deve ser enviado para exame. Os resultados auxiliam na tomada de decisões terapêuticas. A única situação em que não há necessidade de análise é quando os urólitos minerais densos respondem a dietas de dissolução, o que confirmaria o diagnóstico de urolitíase causada por cálculo de estruvita.

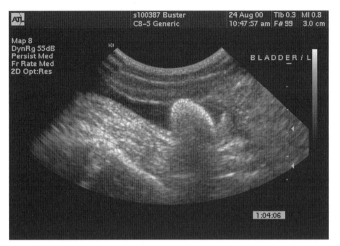

Figura 332.3 Imagem de cálculo de bexiga obtida em ultrassonografia de abdome.

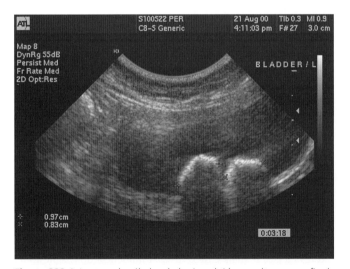

Figura 332.4 Imagem de cálculos de bexiga obtida em ultrassonografia de abdome.

Boxe 332.1 Laboratórios veterinários que realizam análise de cálculos urinários

Minnesota Urolith Center, University of Minnesota, http://www.cvm.umn.edu/depts/minnesotaurolithcenter/home.html

G.V. Ling Urinary Stone Analysis Laboratory, University of California, Davis, http://www.vetmed.ucdavis.edu/usal/index.cfm

Urolithiasis Laboratory, Houston, TX, http://urolithiasis-lab.com

Canadian Veterinary Urolith Centre, Guelph, Ontario, http://www.guelphlabservices.com

---

Lista não abrangente – verifique em seu laboratório outros locais que analisam urólitos.

Tratamento de urolitíase

A maioria dos urólitos de bexiga é removida cirurgicamente por meio de cistostomia de rotina (também comumente denominada cistotomia); entretanto, há uma série de métodos alternativos que podem ser empregados dependendo do número e tamanho dos urólitos. Uma abordagem cirúrgica menos invasiva envolve a realização de cistostomia guiada por laparoscopia, mas na maioria dos gatos é muito mais fácil realizar apenas cistotomia de rotina. Em gatas, se houver pequenos urólitos, de 1 a 3 mm, um método não invasivo indicado é a uro-hidropropulsão. Isso requer anestesia geral e o paciente deve ser submetido a um plano de inconsciência profundo. Introduz-se, assepticamente, uma sonda permanente (3 ou 5 Fr). Distende-se a bexiga com solução salina estéril até que esteja repleta, porém não tensa. O gato é então mantido em posição vertical, possibilitando que os urólitos sejam direcionados ao trígono e à uretra proximal. A sonda é removida e a bexiga massageada, ao mesmo tempo que a urina é coletada em um recipiente com um filtro ("filtro de cálculo") para reter os urólitos. Isso não deve ser tentado em gatos machos, a menos que tenham sido submetidos à uretrostomia perineal. As complicações causadas por esse procedimento incluem hematúria mínima e, como complicação relevante, ruptura de bexiga.[10]

UROLITÍASE CAUSADA POR CÁCULO DE PURINAS (URATO E XANTINA)

A prevalência de urólitos à base de purina tem sido relativamente estável ao longo dos anos, com relatos que variam de 3 a 10%.[11-13] Urólito de urato é o terceiro mais frequentemente relatado em gatos. O ácido úrico é um dos vários produtos de biodegradação oriundos da metabolização do nucleotídio purina. Em gatos, o urato de amônio é a forma mais comum de urólito de purina de ocorrência natural. Há poucas informações disponíveis sobre urólitos de urato nessa espécie animal. A forma do urólito de urato mais comumente identificada foi a de urato de amônio e hidrogênio[12] (Figura 332.5).

No estudo relatado por Appel *et al.* foram examinados urólitos de 10.083 gatos.[11] Constataram-se 398 animais com cálculos de urato (3,9%), dos quais a maioria era urato de amônio (385) e urólitos de ácido úrico (13). Os cálculos foram detectados em 58% dos machos e 41% das fêmeas. Nesse estudo em particular, a prevalência da urolitíase causada por cálculo de urato foi maior em gatos da raça Mau Egípcio (82%), à semelhança de outros relatos; ademais, a prevalência foi significativamente maior nas raças Birmanês (27%) e Siamês (13%) em comparação com outras raças.[11]

Há também uma relação entre a urolitíase causada por urato e a idade. A idade média de ocorrência de urolitíase por urato é menor do que a daqueles animais que apresentam cálculos que não sejam de urato. A ocorrência de urolitíase em gatos da raça Mau Egípcio parece ser significativamente maior em jovens, se comparada a todas as outras raças que desenvolvem cálculos.

A condições predisponentes à urolitíase causada por cálculo de urato incluem anomalias portovasculares (ver Capítulo 284), displasia microvascular (ver Capítulo 284) e qualquer forma de disfunção hepática grave (ver Capítulo 280). Além disso, pode ocorrer um defeito metabólico genético subjacente em algumas raças de gatos. Em gatos, a constatação de urolitíase causada por urato deve levar à imediata avaliação completa da função hepática e de anormalidades vasculares hepáticas.

Tratamento da urolitíase causada por cálculo de urato

A remoção cirúrgica de urólitos de urato ainda é o tratamento de escolha, até que sejam realizados outros estudos que confirmem a segurança e eficácia da dissolução medicamentosa desses urólitos em gatos. Para a prevenção de recidiva, recomenda-se uma dieta alcalinizante com restrição proteica. O alimento enlatado é

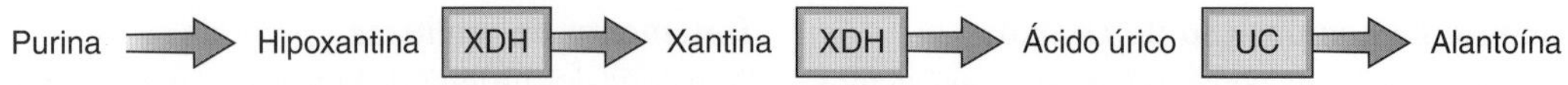

Purina ⟹ Hipoxantina | XDH | ⟹ Xantina | XDH | ⟹ Ácido úrico | UC | ⟹ Alantoína

Figura 332.5 Via metabólica da purina. *UC*, uricase; *XDH*, xantina desidrogenase.

preferível porque estimula o consumo de água. Recomenda-se ultrassonografia periódica do abdome para avaliar a possibilidade de recidiva, sendo preferida à cistografia de duplo contraste porque, geralmente, não requer sedação ou anestesia geral.

UROLITÍASE CAUSADA POR CÁLCULO DE XANTINA

A urolitíase causada por cálculo de xantina é incomum em gatos e está em geral associada à administração de alopurinol.[14,15] Há poucos relatos de casos de urólitos de xantina de ocorrência natural em gatos.[14,16,17] A urolitíase causada por xantina é um distúrbio raramente diagnosticado caracterizado pela deficiência da atividade da enzima xantina desidrogenase (XDH), observado em humanos e outros mamíferos. A deficiência de XDH induz a excreção urinária excessiva de xantina e hipoxantina. A hipoxantina é muito solúvel, mas a xantina é extremamente insolúvel na urina em qualquer pH.

Tratamento de urolitíase causada por cálculo de xantina

Não há protocolo medicamentoso para a dissolução de urólitos de xantina para os gatos. O tratamento de escolha é a remoção cirúrgica A prevenção envolve o fornecimento de uma dieta alcalinizante com restrição proteica e produção de urina diluída que garanta maior ingestão de água.

UROLITÍASE CAUSADA POR CÁLCULO DE CISTINA

A cistinúria felina foi primeiramente documentada em 1991.[18] Urólitos de cistina são raros e representam somente 0,1% de todos os urólitos detectados em gatos nos EUA e no Canadá.[6,13,18] A cistinúria é uma anormalidade hereditária do transporte renal de cistina e dos aminoácidos dibásicos ornitina, lisina e arginina (COLA). Esse erro inato do metabolismo leva à formação de cristais de cistina e, por fim, de urólitos. Recentemente, identificou-se cistinúria felina causada por uma mutação missense no gene *SLC3A1* em um Gato Doméstico de Pelo Curto macho que apresentava cálculos de cistina.[1] Existe um alto grau de heterogeneidade genética da cistinúria em cães e humanos; mais comumente, notam-se mutações no gene *SLC3A1*, que codifica uma proteína globular, com uma única extremidade transmembrana (rBAT).[19-21] O gene *SLC7A9* codifica uma proteína transportadora intramembranosa denominada proteína AT b[o,+]. O transportador de aminoácidos COLA é um heterotetrâmero formado a partir de 2 heterodímeros de AT b[o,+] e rBAT.[22] Na verdade, em gatos pode haver outras mutações responsáveis pela cistinúria que ainda não foram identificadas. A triagem de 5 outros gatos com cistinúria não detectou essa mutação.[19]

Urólitos de cistina foram diagnosticados em gatos com 4 meses a 12 anos de idade, com idade média de 3,6 anos. Parece não haver predisposição sexual ou racial. Embora a maioria dos gatos seja de raça Doméstico de Pelo Curto, os animais da raça Siamês parecem ser discretamente mais acometidos.[23] Embora nefrólitos de cistina tenham sido detectados em humanos e cães, até o momento todos os urólitos de cistina observados em gatos situavam-se no trato urinário inferior.

Além dos sintomas relativos ao trato urinário inferior, relata-se que os gatos com cistinúria apresentam salivação excessiva, letargia e convulsões. Esses sinais clínicos foram atribuídos à hiperamonemia secundária à absorção intestinal prejudicada e à excessiva excreção renal de COLA. Em gatos, a deficiência de arginina pode causar hiperamonemia. Gatos com cistinúria com distúrbios na absorção intestinal e reabsorção renal de arginina desenvolvem deficiência de arginina.

Tratamento de urólitos de cistina

Foram descritas opções terapêuticas medicamentosas, dietéticas e cirúrgicas para o tratamento de urólitos de cistina em pessoas e cães, mas ainda não foram descritas para gatos. A solubilidade da cistina aumenta o pH acima de 7,5; assim, é importante a alcalinização da urina com citrato de potássio (75 mg/kg/12 h VO), juntamente à ingestão adequada de água, para prevenir a formação de urólitos de cistina. A D-penicilamina e a 2-mercaptoproprionilglicina (2-MPG) são quelantes da cistina utilizados em cães e pessoas, mas não em gatos. A 2-MPG tem sido utilizada com segurança em gatos.[23] Também deve-se fornecer um alimento enlatado não acidificante, talvez suplementado com arginina.

Em cães com cistinúria tipo III (uma forma andrógeno-dependente), a castração de machos adultos parece ser curativa. Não é sabido se essa forma ocorre em gatos, mas a castração parece ser uma consideração lógica.

URÓLITOS DE SÍLICA E COMPOSTOS MISTOS

Em um laboratório de análise de urólitos, verificou-se que os cálculos contendo sílica corresponderam a aproximadamente 0,3% dos casos de gatos atendidos. Não pareceu haver predisposição racial ou sexual. Não há disponibilidade de ração para dissolução desses cálculos. Recomendações para prevenção desse tipo de urólito não estão bem estabelecidas. Em cães, recomenda-se uma dieta com baixo conteúdo de vegetais e maior teor de proteína animal e umidade. Em gatos, uma estratégia semelhante parece fazer sentido.

O Minnesota Urolith Center relatou a incidência de 6% de cálculos compostos mistos. Caso se tente inicialmente uma dieta de dissolução, como mencionado para cálculo de estruvita, e tal procedimento não pareça efetivo, é possível que haja outro tipo mineral no núcleo do urólito.

URÓLITOS DE ESTRUVITA

Em gatos, os urólitos de estruvita geralmente são formados em urina estéril. Isso é improvável em cães e humanos, nos quais os urólitos de estruvita são mais frequentemente associados a infecções por bactérias produtoras de urease. A fisiopatologia da formação de urólitos de estruvita não está completamente compreendida, mas provavelmente resulta da combinação de fatores raciais, sexuais e dietéticos. A influência do magnésio na formação de estruvita depende do pH urinário e da influência de íons, minerais e outros componentes da urina. Alcalúria está associada ao maior risco de formação de estruvita. A estruvita é mais solúvel na urina ácida (pH < 6,8). Fatores que podem estar associados à formação de urina alcalina, como dieta com baixo teor de proteína animal, acidose tubular renal distal ou histórico familiar de urólitos de estruvita, devem ser considerados em gatos com urolitíase causada por cálculo de estruvita.[23] O aumento das concentrações iônicas de minerais na urina é o fator estimulante para a formação de cristais. A urina persistentemente alcalina e a subsequente cristalúria por estruvita podem requerer a realização de cultura microbiológica da urina em busca de micróbios produtores de urease, inclusive *Staphylococcus* sp., *Proteus* sp. e *Ureaplasma* sp., mesmo que a urina da maioria dos gatos seja estéril.[24] Urólitos de estruvita estéreis são formados geralmente em gatos com 1 a 10 anos de idade. O Minnesota Urolith Center relatou que urólitos de estruvita representaram 46% de suas admissões.

Tratamento de urólitos de estruvita

A escolha do método terapêutico para urólito depende da experiência do veterinário, de fatores relacionados ao paciente e da preferência do proprietário. Diversas rações terapêuticas para dissolução de cálculos de estruvita são comercializadas; são formuladas para evitar excesso de magnésio e fósforo e manter o pH ácido da urina (isso aumenta a solubilidade da estruvita)[24] (Boxes 332.2 e 332.3). Rações de dissolução não foram associadas à obstrução da uretra, à medida que ocorre diminuição do tamanho dos urólitos. Ao fornecer uma ração formulada para dissolução, devem ser reavaliadas as radiografias de abdome 2 a 4 semanas após o início do fornecimento da ração. Nesse momento, os urólitos devem estar 33 a 100% menores. Em caso de alteração mínima no tamanho, a composição mineral do urólito pouco provavelmente é de estruvita ou as recomendações nutricionais não estão sendo seguidas pelos tutores. Após a constatação radiográfica da dissolução dos urólitos, a ração de dissolução deve ser mantida por um período adicional de 2 a 4 semanas. Na rara ocorrência de infecção concomitante do trato urinário, deve-se administrar um antibiótico apropriado durante todo o período de dissolução dos urólitos.

Em gatas e gatos submetidos a uretrostomia perineal, quando a quantidade de urólitos é baixa e o seu tamanho é menor que 4 mm, pode-se realizar uro-hidropropulsão, outro procedimento minimamente invasivo (ver Tratamento de urolitíase, mencionado anteriormente). Essa técnica propicia urólitos para análise e cultura microbiológica, bem como meio para remoção do urólito, especialmente se o gato manifesta sinais clínicos marcantes ou se os tutores optam por não utilizar uma ração de dissolução. A opção final de tratamento é a intervenção cirúrgica por meio de cistostomia ou cistostomia guiada por laparoscopia.

Prevenção de urólitos de estruvita

Estratégias de prevenção de urólitos de estruvita incluem procedimentos para diluição da urina, estimulando o gato a beber água ou aumentando o conteúdo hídrico da dieta. Isso induz micções frequentes e, assim, possibilita a excreção de cristais de estruvita ou de urólitos pequenos. Há disponibilidade de rações comerciais formuladas não somente para a dissolução do urólito, mas também para prevenção de sua recidiva (ver Boxe 322.3). Há várias vantagens quanto ao fornecimento de rações multipropósitos, incluindo a capacidade de fornecê-las a longo prazo como ração de manutenção, assim como o fato de que podem ser fornecidas a todos os outros gatos saudáveis do domicílio e, assim, aumentar o comprometimento do tutor. Geralmente, elas

---

> ### Boxe 332.2 Rações comercializadas apenas para dissolução e prevenção de cálculo de estruvita
>
> Hill's Prescription Diet s/d® enlatada e seca – apenas dissolução
> Iams Urinary-S Plus® enlatada e seca – apenas prevenção
>
> O Boxe não inclui todas as possibilidades dietéticas.

> ### Boxe 332.3 Rações comercializadas para dissolução e prevenção de cálculo de estruvita e prevenção de cálculo de oxalato de cálcio
>
> Hill's Prescription Diet c/d Multicare® enlatada e seca
> Hill's Prescription Diet Metabolic + Urinary® enlatada e seca
> Hill's Prescription Diet c/d Multicare Stress® enlatada e seca
> Royal Canin Veterinary Diets Urinary SO® enlatada e seca
> Royal Canin Veterinary Diets Moderate Calorie® enlatada e seca
> Royal Canin Veterinary Diets Olfactory Attraction® seca
> Purina Veterinary Diet UR St/Ox Urinary Formula® enlatada e seca
>
> O Boxe não inclui todas as possibilidades dietéticas.

---

são relativamente palatáveis e não há necessidade de um período de transição para os gatos aceitarem a mudança da dieta para uma ração formulada para prevenir a formação de urólitos.

URÓLITOS DE OXALATO DE CÁLCIO

Epidemiologia

Geralmente os gatos que apresentam urolitíase causada por oxalato de cálcio (CaC_2O_4) são de meia-idade a idosos, machos e castrados A raças de maior risco são Persa e Himalaio.

Sinais clínicos

Os sinais clínicos foram discutidos anteriormente neste capítulo. Incluem polaciúria, estrangúria, hematúria, periúria ou uma combinação deles. Gatos machos também podem apresentar obstrução da uretra secundária ao alojamento do urólito na uretra distal estreita. Nenhum desses sintomas é específico para urólitos, outros diagnósticos a serem descartados incluem cistite idiopática (ver Capítulo 334), infecções do trato urinário (ver Capítulo 330) e neoplasias (ver Capítulo 351). Ademais, os urólitos de bexiga podem ser achados incidentais sem que o gato manifeste qualquer sinal clínico.

Fisiopatologia

Os fatores químicos e físicos que influenciam a formação de cristais na urina são complexos, e muitas variáveis devem ser consideradas. Os dois principais fatores que interferem nesse processo são supersaturação da urina com materiais calculogênicos (cálcio e oxalato) e equilíbrio entre substâncias que estimulam e as que inibem a formação de CaC_2O_4. Quando a urina está supersaturada com cálcio e oxalato, a formação de cristais é mais provável; uma mensuração que reflete essa condição é a supersaturação relativa da urina (SRU). Essa mensuração é utilizada amplamente para avaliar o risco de formação de CaC_2O_4 em pessoas e está sendo utilizada também na medicina veterinária.[8,25]

Para avaliar a supersaturação de materiais calculogênicos na urina, analisou-se a importância relativa do conteúdo hídrico urinário, da concentração de cálcio e da concentração de oxalato. O conteúdo hídrico talvez seja a variável única mais importante que interfere na formação de CaC_2O_4. O aumento de água dilui a urina e aumenta o volume urinário, reduzindo, assim, a SRU de CaC_2O_4. A hiperoxalúria também é importante. A excreção urinária de oxalato depende da ingestão dietética, absorção intestinal, secreção tubular renal e taxa de síntese endógena. A absorção intestinal é influenciada por fatores que determinam a quantidade de oxalato livre no lúmen intestinal. O cálcio e o magnésio podem se ligar ao oxalato, originando complexos que são excretados, em vez de absorvidos A flora intestinal, como *Oxalobacter formigenes* e bactérias que produzem ácido láctico, pode degradar o oxalato e influenciar a fisiopatologia da doença. Relata-se que a hiperoxalúria decorrente da produção endógena excessiva é uma condição genética primária em pessoas, causada por anormalidades metabólitas; existe em duas formas (tipo I e tipo II). Alguns poucos casos de hiperoxalúria primária também foram relatados em gatos e parecem ser mais semelhantes à variante tipo II, observada em pessoas.[8,25,26]

Assim como a excreção de oxalato, a excreção urinária de cálcio depende da ingestão dietética, absorção intestinal e excreção tubular renal. A absorção intestinal de cálcio é semelhante à do oxalato pelo fato de que o cálcio é mal absorvido quando na forma de um complexo, mas é absorvido mais prontamente quando não está ligado a outra substância. Assim, o teor apropriado de ingestão de cálcio para minimizar a SRU de CaC_2O_4 na urina está relacionado à quantidade de oxalato presente, assim como a de outras substâncias com as quais pode formar complexos (p. ex., fosfato). A hipercalciúria também pode ser decorrência de hipercalcemia e anormalidades na reabsorção tubular de cálcio.

SEÇÃO 24 • Doenças do Trato Urinário Inferior

Diversas substâncias foram identificadas como indutoras ou inibidoras da formação de CaC_2O_4 na urina. As inibidoras incluem magnésio, citrato e pirofosfato, que formam complexos solúveis com o cálcio na urina e impedem a formação de cristais de oxalato. O citrato também pode diminuir o risco de formação de CaC_2O_4 pela alcalinização da urina. Proteínas, como a nefrocalcina e glicoproteína de Tamm-Horsfall, interferem na formação de cristais de CaC_2O_4 e podem ter uma participação adicional.

Há controvérsia quanto à importância do pH urinário na formação de CaC_2O_4. A solubilidade absoluta do CaC_2O_4 na urina é pouco influenciada em uma ampla faixa de pH, mas há várias razões para um baixo pH induzir a formação de CaC_2O_4: acidúria persistente está associada à acidose metabólica de baixo grau, que induz reabsorção de cálcio do osso e pode aumentar a excreção urinária de cálcio; a urina ácida pode diminuir a capacidade de o citrato e o pirofosfato atuarem como inibidores do CaC_2O_4; quando a urina é alcalina, ocorre maior reabsorção de cálcio no túbulo renal distal. Ademais, relata-se que o fornecimento de ração acidificante é um fator de risco para formação de CaC_2O_4 em gatos. Nessa espécie animal, o risco foi 3 vezes maior em indivíduos que receberam a ração, que induziu pH urinário de 5,99 a 6,15 em comparação com aqueles que receberam ração que induziu pH urinário de 6,5 a 6,9.[27] Estudos também avaliaram especificamente o efeito do pH sobre a SRU de CaC_2O_4, mas os resultados, até o momento, são conflitantes.

Diagnóstico

A avaliação clínica inicial de um gato com urolitíase causada por CaC_2O_4 deve incluir um exame minucioso em busca de qualquer causa primária. Hemograma, perfil bioquímico sérico, exame de urina e urocultura são considerados a base de dados mínima. O ideal é que o exame de urina seja realizado dentro de 60 minutos após a coleta, a fim de minimizar os efeitos do tempo e da temperatura na formação de cristais *in vitro*.[8] Deve-se mensurar a densidade urinária, e objetivos razoáveis para diminuir esse valor podem ser estabelecidos após a identificação do urólito. O pH urinário em gatos com cristais de CaC_2O_4 é variável, nem sempre são detectados cristais de CaC_2O_4 em gatos com urólitos que contêm CaC_2O_4.[8] Se a concentração de cálcio total está elevada, o teor de cálcio ionizado deve ser mensurado; havendo hipercalcemia, recomenda-se a mensuração do paratormônio (PTH), da proteína relacionada ao PTH e, possivelmente, da concentração sérica de vitamina D (ver Capítulo 297). Exames de imagem devem incluir tanto a radiografia quanto a ultrassonografia do abdome, pois em alguns casos os cálculos podem não ser vistos quando se utiliza apenas uma dessas modalidades. Como os cálculos de CaC_2O_4 possuem uma opacidade mineral, normalmente eles são facilmente observados em radiografias simples. Entretanto, a detecção de urólitos muito pequenos pode necessitar de ultrassonografia. Além disso, na ultrassonografia é difícil detectar urólitos alojados na uretra; dessa forma, exames de imagem do abdome caudal, incluindo a pelve, requerem a realização de radiografia.

Tratamento

Tratamentos cirúrgico e intervencionista

Até o momento não se conhece um protocolo terapêutico que dissolva urólitos de CaC_2O_4, e em vários casos o único tratamento efetivo é a remoção. A remoção do urólito pode ser feita por meio de cirurgia; métodos menos invasivos estão se tornando cada vez mais disponíveis, como a cistostomia percutânea guiada por laparoscopia, cistoscopia (em fêmeas com urólitos com menos de 3 mm de tamanho) e uro-hidropropulsão (em fêmeas e machos submetidos à uretrostomia perineal que apresentam urólitos com menos de 3 mm de tamanho). Se há informação de ocorrência prévia de urólitos, devem ser realizadas radiografias e ultrassonografia de abdome em intervalos de 2 a 3 meses.

Manejo dietético

Urólitos de CaC_2O_4 ocorrem em duas formas comuns, como CaC_2O_4 monoidratado (*whewellite*) e CaC_2O_4 di-hidratado (*weddellite*). As abordagens terapêuticas para essas duas formas são as mesmas.

É possível que a modificação dietética mais importante seja o aumento da ingestão hídrica e do volume urinário, ao mesmo tempo que diminui a densidade urinária. Estudos retrospectivos de gatos com urolitíase causada por CaC_2O_4 constataram risco significativamente menor de formação de CaC_2O_4 quanto maior era o teor de umidade na dieta.[27] O fornecimento de ração enlatada é a melhor forma de aumentar o conteúdo hídrico, mas alguns gatos não aceitam ração enlatada. Nesses casos, pode-se adicionar água ou caldos como suprimento de água. Bebedouros de água também podem ser úteis para aumentar a ingestão hídrica em gatos. Valores apropriados para densidade urinária de gatos são inferiores a 1,025; a obtenção de urina diluída em gatos pode ser muito difícil.

Há disponibilidade de diversas rações terapêuticas desenvolvidas para interferir na SRU do CaC_2O_4 e, pelo decréscimo da SRU, diminuir a probabilidade de recidiva do urólito. Essas rações geralmente possuem concentração discretamente maior de cloreto de sódio e discreta restrição proteica (ver Boxes 332.3 e 332.4). A suplementação de cloreto de sódio foi avaliada como um meio de aumentar o consumo hídrico, mas os resultados são controversos. O aumento do consumo de sódio aumenta a excreção urinária de cálcio e pode elevar o risco de urolitíase causada por CaC_2O_4. Entretanto, estudos prospectivos demonstraram que o aumento do conteúdo de sódio na dieta reduziu significativamente a SRU de CaC_2O_4 em gatos saudáveis e naqueles predispostos à formação de cálculos de CaC_2O_4.[28] Nesses estudos constatou-se que a excreção urinária diária *total* de cálcio aumentou, e aparentemente o efeito na SRU do CaC_2O_4 é compensado pelo aumento da ingestão hídrica e do volume de urina. Esses achados sugerem um benefício da suplementação de NaCl, mas são necessários estudos a longo prazo. A suplementação de sódio pode ser considerada quando se nota resposta inadequada à terapia dietética e urina não diluída, mas a escolha de pacientes para tal procedimento deve ser cuidadosa. Estudos a curto prazo em gatos não demonstraram efeitos adversos na função renal ou na pressão sanguínea, mas é preciso cuidado ao adicionar sal à dieta de gatos com doença renal ou hipertensão, até que estudos a longo prazo sejam realizados. Adicionalmente, dietas com alto teor de sódio são contraindicadas para animais cardiopatas.[25]

Historicamente, alto teor proteico na dieta tem sido associado a maior risco de formação de CaC_2O_4 porque pode induzir acidose e hipercalciúria. Entretanto, estudos retrospectivos em gatos constataram menor risco de formação de CaC_2O_4 com alto teor proteico na dieta.[25,29] De forma geral, a quantidade exata e o tipo de proteína ideais ainda precisam ser determinados, mas a maioria das rações formuladas para reduzir a ocorrência de urolitíase causada por CaC_2O_4 apresenta baixo conteúdo de proteína.

Outros nutrientes a serem considerados no manejo dietético de pacientes com urólitos de CaC_2O_4 são magnésio, citrato e fósforo. Supostamente, magnésio e fosfato (e citrato) presentes na urina atuam como inibidores da formação de urólito de CaC_2O_4 e não deve haver restrição na dieta. Ademais, não deve haver restrição de fósforo na dieta porque a concentração sérica

---

Boxe 332.4 Rações formuladas apenas para a prevenção de oxalato de cálcio

Iams Urinary-O Plus® enlatada e seca – apenas prevenção

O Boxe não inclui todas as possibilidades dietéticas.

de fósforo pode ativar a glândula paratireoide, resultando em aumento da concentração de vitamina D3 e aumento da absorção intestinal de cálcio.

Dietas acidificantes foram associadas a maior risco de formação de CaC_2O_4 em gatos, mas outros estudos mencionaram resultados conflitantes quanto à importância do pH urinário diário na prevenção de formação de CaC_2O_4. De forma geral, pode-se afirmar que o pH geralmente parece ser menos importante no controle da formação de cálculos de CaC_2O_4 do que no controle da formação de outros cálculos, como o de estruvita. Com base nas informações disponíveis, parece prudente evitar a acidificação significativa da urina. O valor-alvo inicial apropriado de pH urinário é, aproximadamente, 7; no entanto, com isso em mente, os valores-alvo de pH urinário obtidos com o fornecimento de quase todas as rações listadas nos Boxes 332.3 e 332.4 são ácidos. Isso ocorre porque o objetivo das rações Royal Canin Urinary SO® e Hill's Prescription Diet C/D Multicare® é prevenir urólitos tanto de CaC_2O_4 *quanto* de estruvita. Como no tratamento de cálculos de estruvita o controle do pH urinário é mais importante para a dissolução e prevenção do urólito do que no tratamento de cálculos de CaC_2O_4, o objetivo dessas rações é propiciar um pH inferior como parte da estratégia de prevenção de cálculo de estruvita. Apesar de ocasionarem urina discretamente ácida, todas as rações listadas são efetivas na formação de urina com baixa SRU de CaC_2O_4. Esse paradoxo aparente exemplifica a natureza complexa da urolitíase causada por CaC_2O_4, e vários fatores devem ser considerados ao formular uma ração apropriada. Com certeza, se os urólitos de CaC_2O_4 continuarem a ser um problema, apesar do fornecimento de uma ração apropriada, pode-se induzir a alcalinização da urina (ver a seguir), a fim de melhorar potencialmente o controle da formação de cálculos.[25]

Medicamentos

Fármacos podem ser adicionados ao protocolo terapêutico para urolitíase causada por CaC_2O_4 quando a terapia dietética, por si só, não é efetiva na prevenção do crescimento ou de recidiva de urólitos. O citrato de potássio tem sido utilizado efetivamente em pessoas como um agente alcalinizante urinário e também pode aumentar a ação inibidora do citrato na formação de CaC_2O_4. Contudo, até o momento, nenhum estudo demonstrou benefícios claros para o uso de citrato em gatos. Ademais, não há evidência de que a hipocitratúria seja um fator de risco para a formação de CaC_2O_4 em gatos. A dose de citrato de potássio recomendada é 75 mg/kg/12 h VO. Caso se faça o uso clínico de citrato de potássio como alcalinizante da urina, pode-se utilizar a dose inicial mencionada anteriormente, aumentando-a até obter pH próximo de 7. Quando esse fármaco é utilizado, deve-se monitorar a concentração sérica de potássio para evitar o desenvolvimento de hiperpotassemia. Outros estudos são necessários em gatos.

Os diuréticos tiazidas representam outra opção medicamentosa para reduzir a saturação de CaC_2O_4. Esses fármacos inibem o cotransportador de sódio-cloreto no túbulo renal distal e, assim, estimulam a reabsorção de cálcio e diminuem a excreção urinária de cálcio. Em um estudo com gatos saudáveis tratados com 1 mg de hidroclorotiazida/kg/12 h VO, verificou-se diminuição significativa da SRU urinária de CaOx.[30] Estudos sobre segurança e eficácia da administração a longo prazo são escassos.[25]

Monitoramento

A probabilidade de recidiva de urólitos de CaC_2O_4 varia entre estudos e, conforme foi relatada, pode ser de até aproximadamente 7% (esse percentual pode ser maior pelo fato de que a recidiva de urólitos nem sempre leva a uma análise repetida imediata). Dois estudos em gatos constataram diferentes resultados: registrou-se o reenvio de urólitos a partir de 7,1% de mais de 2 mil gatos acometidos no período de 5 anos (tempo médio de envio: 25 meses), enquanto 40% de um grupo de gatos com ureterólitos manifestou recidiva dentro de cerca de 1 ano.[25,31,32] Nenhum grupo do estudo reflete a população em risco. Se novos urólitos forem detectados antes que se tornem grandes, é possível utilizar tratamento menos invasivo, como uro-hidropropulsão. O tamanho do cálculo que pode ser expelido varia de acordo com a raça e o tamanho do animal, mas de forma geral os cálculos de bexiga menores que 5 mm em gatas e 1 mm em gatos são passíveis de retirada por meio de uro-hidropropulsão. A remoção de urólitos maiores requer um procedimento mais invasivo. Quatro semanas após o procedimento inicial, e então após 3 e 6 meses, seguidos de intervalos de 6 meses, recomenda-se a realização de radiografia ou ultrassonografia imediatamente após um procedimento de remoção, a fim de constatar a ausência de urólitos.

REFERÊNCIAS BIBLIOGRÁFICAS

As referências bibliográficas deste capítulo se encontram online no Ambiente de Aprendizagem.

CAPÍTULO 333

Doenças Relacionadas com a Micção Anormal

Julie K. Byron

INTRODUÇÃO

Fisiologia da micção

A principal finalidade do trato urinário inferior é armazenar urina e facilitar sua excreção no momento apropriado. Em 99% do tempo a bexiga armazena urina, enquanto a fase de esvaziamento representa apenas 1% do tempo. A coordenação de armazenamento e esvaziamento requer uma interação complexa entre os sistemas nervosos somático e autônomo, assim como a função normal dos órgãos e tecidos envolvidos.

Todos os três componentes do sistema nervoso periférico estão envolvidos no ciclo de micção (Tabela 333.1). Ademais, a micção consciente envolve a medula espinal lombar e sacral, assim como o tronco encefálico e o córtex cerebral.

Durante o preenchimento e armazenamento, a ativação de receptores de estiramento da parede vesical estimula um arco reflexo que aumenta o tônus da uretra e relaxa o músculo detrusor por meio de inervação simpática (Figura 333.1). No início da micção, os receptores de estiramento enviam sinais aferentes por meio de fibras mielinizadas do nervo pélvico até

| Tabela 333.1 | Componentes do sistema nervoso periférico envolvidos na micção. |

TIPO	LOCALIZAÇÃO	NERVO	FUNÇÃO QUANDO ESTIMULADO	FUNÇÃO QUANDO INIBIDO	FUNÇÃO QUANDO INAPROPRIADAMENTE ESTIMULADO	FUNÇÃO QUANDO INAPROPRIADAMENTE INIBIDO
Parassimpático (muscarínico M3)	Corpo vesical (detrusor)	Nervo pélvico (S1-S3)	Contração e esvaziamento da bexiga	Relaxamento do detrusor e preenchimento vesical	Bexiga hiperativa	Atonia vesical, retenção de urina
Simpático (adrenérgico beta-3)	Corpo vesical (detrusor)	Nervo hipogástrico (L1-L4)	Relaxamento do detrusor e preenchimento	Relaxamento do detrusor e micção	Retenção de urina	Diminuição da complacência vesical e aumento da pressão de preenchimento
Simpático (adrenérgico alfa-1)	Colo vesical/ uretra	Nervo hipogástrico (L1-L4)	Contração e continência	Micção	Retenção de urina	Uretra aberta, incontinência
Somático (nicotínico)	Uretra distal/ assoalho pélvico	Nervo pudendo (S1-S2)	Contração consciente/ reflexa e continência	Micção	Retenção de urina	Uretra aberta, incontinência

a medula espinal lombar cranial, ao centro pontino da micção, no cérebro. Se a condição for apropriada para micção, as vias parassimpáticas serão ativadas para estimular a contração do músculo liso da bexiga e os sinais parassimpáticos serão inibidos para propiciar o relaxamento da uretra (Figura 333.2).

Há também um arco reflexo uretral local que causa contração do músculo estriado ao redor da uretra mediada pelo sistema nervoso somático, em resposta ao aumento súbito da pressão abdominal e transferência da urina para a uretra, como acontece durante a tosse ou o espirro.

Além dos mecanismos neurológicos normais, diversos outros fatores são importantes para a função normal do ciclo de micção em cães e gatos. A integridade da musculatura lisa da uretra, da mucosa uretral, dos vasos sanguíneos associados e do suporte de tecidos conjuntivos também é importante.[1,2] Em fêmeas, o estrógeno parece ter uma influência significativa nesses tecidos.[3,4] Sua diminuição após a castração parece estar envolvida na incompetência do mecanismo do esfíncter uretral.[5,6] Em cães não castrados a hiperplasia de próstata pode ocasionar obstrução funcional da uretra e retenção urinária.

ANORMALIDADES DE ARMAZENAMENTO

Anormalidades de armazenamento se devem principalmente à incapacidade para manter o tônus uretral adequado em condição de pressão vesical normal. Isso pode ser decorrência de anormalidade anatômica ou de desenvolvimento, ou disfunção adquirida de medula espinal, bexiga ou uretra e tecidos circundantes. Anormalidades congênitas (ver Capítulo 336), como ureteres ectópicos ou malformação do seio urogenital, podem resultar em incontinência urinária inconsciente em jovens, enquanto a incontinência urinária adquirida, que inclui incompetência do mecanismo do esfíncter uretral (IMEU), do neurônio motor inferior da bexiga (NMIB) ou bexiga hiperativa (BHA) pode ocorrer tardiamente durante a vida (ver Capítulo 46).

Incompetência do mecanismo do esfíncter uretral

A incompetência do mecanismo do esfíncter uretral é a anormalidade de armazenamento da urina mais comum em cães.[7] O mecanismo do esfíncter uretral envolve a musculatura lisa da uretra, assim como os tecidos de sustentação circundantes, vasos

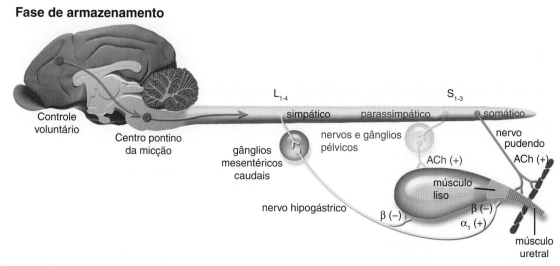

Figura 333.1 Inervação e vias de sinalização durante a fase de armazenamento de urina do ciclo da micção. *ACh*, receptores mediados por acetilcolina; *alfa*, receptores alfa-adrenérgicos; *beta*, receptores beta-adrenérgicos; L_{1-4}, segmentos 1 a 4 da medula espinal lombar; S_{1-3}, segmentos 1 a 3 da medula espinal sacral; *(+)*, estímulo da contração muscular; *(−)*, inibição da contração muscular. (De Tim Vojt. Reproduzida, com autorização, de The Ohio State University.)

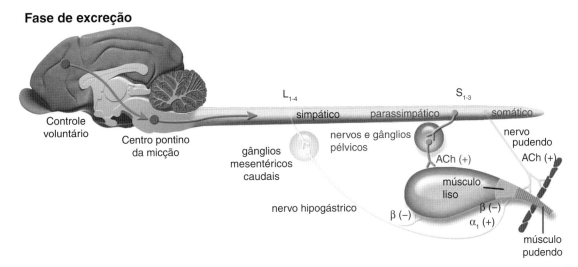

Figura 333.2 Inervação e vias de sinalização durante a fase de excreção de urina do ciclo de micção. *ACh*, receptores mediados por acetilcolina; *alfa*, receptores alfa-adrenérgicos; *beta*, receptores beta-adrenérgicos; L_{1-4}, segmentos 1 a 4 da medula espinal lombar; S_{1-3}, segmentos 1 a 3 da medula espinal sacral; *(+)*, estímulo da contração muscular; *(−)*, inibição da contração muscular. (De Tim Vojt. Reproduzida, com autorização, de The Ohio State University.)

sanguíneos da submucosa e urotélio. Supostamente, a IMEU resulta de falha nesse complexo por redução na responsividade e no tônus muscular, bem como alterações nos tecidos periuretrais. Em cadelas, essas alterações parecem estar associadas à redução no teor de estrógeno e ao aumento nas concentrações de hormônio foliculoestimulante e hormônio luteinizante após a castração – daí o termo "incontinência responsiva a hormônio".[8,9] A fisiopatologia de sua ocorrência em cães machos castrados é pouco compreendida; entretanto, há relato de aumento nos teores de hormônio foliculoestimulante e hormônio luteinizante em resposta à diminuição do teor de testosterona.[10,11]

A incompetência do mecanismo do esfíncter uretral é mais comum em cadelas castradas. É menos comum em machos castrados e rara em cães e gatos machos não castrados.[11] Parece acometer até 20% das fêmeas castradas e até 30% dos cães de raças de grande porte. Várias raças possuem maior risco, incluindo Dobermann Pinscher, Schnauzer Gigante, Old English Sheepdog, Rottweiler, Weimaraner e Boxer, mas qualquer raça pode ser afetada.[12] A literatura recente demonstrou maior risco de ocorrência de IMEU em cães castrados antes dos 3 meses de idade.[13,14] Outros estudos não constataram relação com a idade de castração,[15] e o melhor momento para castração, a fim de prevenir IMEU, permanece controverso (ver Capítulo 313). É possível que isso esteja relacionado ao desenvolvimento e à sensibilidade dos tecidos do esfíncter ao estrógeno e outros hormônios; no entanto, o mecanismo não é totalmente compreendido.

Fatores predisponentes, como bexiga pélvica, uretra curta e vulva retraída, também podem estar associados ao maior risco de ocorrência de IMEU; contudo, a presença de qualquer um desses fatores não necessariamente ocasiona incontinência. Uma redução na transmissão de pressão do abdome para a uretra proximal pode causar incontinência urinária em animais com uretra curta ou bexiga pélvica, por induzir um gradiente de pressão negativo da bexiga até a uretra. O extravasamento de urina observado em casos de vulva retraída ou "juvenil" pode estar relacionado ao represamento de urina no vestíbulo vulvar durante a micção, a qual extravasa em um momento posterior.

Manifestação clínica e diagnóstico de IMEU

A incontinência causada por IMEU frequentemente ocorre poucos anos após a castração, mas a idade de início é muito variável. Cães com IMEU em geral apresentam capacidade vesical normal e são capazes de urinar normalmente, com completo esvaziamento da bexiga. Embora a maioria desses cães seja saudável, os sinais clínicos podem se agravar sobremaneira quando há comorbidade, especialmente aquelas que causam poliúria. Em pacientes com poliúria, o aumento do volume de urina na bexiga pode levar ao aumento da pressão no já fragilizado mecanismo do esfíncter uretral e causar extravasamento de urina. A infecção do trato urinário inferior também pode agravar os sinais clínicos (ver Capítulo 330). Suspeita-se que IMEU e incontinência urinária de qualquer etiologia estão associadas a maior risco de infecção do trato urinário, mas não foram realizados estudos para avaliar completamente esse fato.

Tutores frequentemente buscam cuidados veterinários quando a frequência da incontinência se torna incômoda, embora na experiência do autor a incontinência possa estar presente há meses ou anos. É essencial estabelecer se o animal está urinando de modo inconsciente. Vários tutores se queixam de "incontinência" quando o animal apresenta micção submissa ou está urinando conscientemente em locais inapropriados (ver Capítulo 9). Cães com IMEU podem apresentar extravasamento de urina quando em decúbito, dormindo ou após esforço físico. Apesar de a excreção de urina ser involuntária, pode-se notar que os cães lambem mais constantemente a região perivulvar ou prepucial. A IMEU é uma condição adquirida, o que torna importante o questionamento do tutor quanto ao início dos sinais clínicos. Animais que manifestam incontinência urinária desde o nascimento ou antes da castração devem ser avaliados em busca de malformações congênitas, como ureteres ectópicos, antes de confirmar o diagnóstico de IMEU (ver Capítulo 336).

O exame físico desses animais é frequentemente normal, com exceção da mancha provocada pela urina na região perivulvar ou prepucial. Devem-se avaliar a conformação da vulva e a condição da pele perivulvar. A presença de dermatite perivulvar pode aumentar o risco de infecção do trato urinário. Em geral, a palpação retal e o exame da uretra são normais. Nota-se que a micção é normal e completa, com pouco ou nenhum volume de urina residual. A avaliação da presença de urina residual é essencial em cães machos com incontinência urinária, a fim de diferenciar IMEU de dissinergia uretral do detrusor, uma condição que causa esvaziamento incompleto da bexiga (ver adiante).

A constatação de incontinência urinária em uma cadela castrada e outrora saudável, sem incontinência, é frequentemente apropriada para o diagnóstico presuntivo de IMEU e teste terapêutico empírico. Devido à sua menor prevalência fora da população de cadelas castradas, as cadelas não castradas, os cães castrados ou não castrados e os gatos com históricos e sinais clínicos semelhantes devem ser submetidos à avaliação adicional antes da confirmação do diagnóstico de IMEU.

Devem ser realizados exame de urina e urocultura (ver Capítulo 72). A presença de isostenúria ou hipostenúria pode contribuir para a gravidade da incontinência e requer avaliação adicional em busca da causa primária. Conforme mencionado anteriormente, o risco de infecção do trato urinário em animais com IMEU ainda não foi avaliado, mas sua presença pode agravar os sintomas. Hemograma e perfil bioquímico sérico não são essenciais para o diagnóstico de IMEU, embora possam ser úteis na tomada de decisão terapêutica e são importantes na avaliação de animais com poliúria.

Se houver suspeita de anormalidades anatômicas, recomendam-se exames de imagem, como radiografia contrastada, ultrassonografia de abdome ou tomografia computadorizada contrastada. O exame cistoscópico do trato urinário inferior pode também ser necessário para avaliar a anatomia do trato urinário inferior e da vagina (ver Capítulo 108). Exames de diagnóstico avançados, como estudo urodinâmico, foram desenvolvidos para quantificar a pressão produzida ao longo da uretra, bem como a complacência e função do músculo detrusor da bexiga. Esses exames estão disponíveis em algumas instituições de referência e podem ser indicados a pacientes com sinais suspeitos e má resposta à terapia.

Tratamento medicamentoso da IMEU

A terapia medicamentosa da IMEU geralmente é considerada a primeira linha de tratamento; somente após falha ou intolerância à terapia medicamentosa é que se consideram as opções cirúrgicas. O tratamento clínico da IMEU em cadela castrada consiste em aumentar o número e a sensibilidade dos receptores alfa do esfíncter uretral ao estrógeno, ou no estímulo desses receptores com um alfa-agonista (Tabela 333.2).

Os estrógenos mais comumente utilizados são o dietilestilbestrol (DES) e o estriol (Incurin®, Merck Animal Health, Madison, NJ). Não há disponibilidade de DES no mercado, de forma que deve ser manipulado. O estriol parece ter uma taxa de resposta maior em cadelas do que o DES (89 e 65%, respectivamente).[16,17] Efeitos adversos associados ao uso do estrógeno estão relacionados à dose e incluem desenvolvimento da glândula mamária, edema vulvar e atratividade a machos.[16] Esses efeitos em geral diminuem após a redução da dose. Um evento adverso mais grave associado ao uso do estrógeno é a supressão irreversível da medula óssea (ver Capítulo 199).[18]

O monitoramento do hemograma em animais tratados com estrógeno é considerado imprescindível; entretanto, as doses que causam supressão da medula óssea são muito maiores do que as recomendadas para o tratamento de IMEU. O autor recomenda a realização do hemograma antes do início do tratamento com estrógeno, seguida de reavaliação 1 mês depois.

A fenilpropanolamina (PPA®, Proin, PRN Pharmacal, Pensacola, FL) é o alfa-agonista mais amplamente utilizado no tratamento da IMEU. A dose e a frequência necessárias para cada animal são muito variáveis e pode ser preciso o aumento da dose com o passar do tempo, a fim de manter a continência. Efeitos adversos associados à PPA incluem inquietude, agressividade, alterações nos padrões de sono e sintomas gastrintestinais. Esses efeitos são também em geral amenizados após a redução ou frequência da dose.[19,20] A resposta clínica à administração de PPA varia de 75 a 90%.[20,21] Frequentemente, tanto o estrógeno quanto a PPA são utilizados no mesmo paciente para tratamento de incontinência urinária grave ou refratária. Há relatos pragmáticos de maior eficácia quando utilizados simultaneamente, mas há poucas evidências publicadas que comprovam uma ação sinérgica.[22]

A fenilpropanolamina também quase sempre é utilizada em cães e gatos machos com IMEU. Além disso, cães machos castrados podem ser tratados com injeções mensais de cipionato de testosterona; porém, sua eficácia ainda não foi bem documentada. Embora cães machos com IMEU respondam melhor à PPA, a taxa de resposta é de apenas 43%, muito inferior à verificada em fêmeas.[11] Compostos à base de estrógeno não devem ser utilizados em machos devido ao risco de metaplasia prostática. Eles são raramente utilizados em gatos; ademais, em gatos tratados com estrógenos devem-se monitorar cuidadosamente as glândulas mamárias em busca de neoplasias.

Tratamento cirúrgico da IMEU

Em pacientes que não respondem à terapia medicamentosa, pode ser necessária intervenção cirúrgica. Tal procedimento deve ser recomendado quando o animal não responde ou não tolera o tratamento medicamentoso. Diversos procedimentos cirúrgicos têm sido utilizados para tratar IMEU, vários com o intuito de aumentar a transmissão de pressão abdominal à uretra proximal. Eles incluem colpossuspensão, fita vaginal transobturadora e uretropexia. Os resultados são variáveis e considerados de baixa eficácia a longo prazo, particularmente em animais cuja bexiga encontra-se em posição normal.[23] O procedimento cirúrgico mais promissor e comumente realizado para IMEU é a

---

Tabela 333.2 Fármacos frequentemente utilizados no tratamento de incompetência do mecanismo do esfíncter uretral.[38]

FÁRMACO	CLASSE	DOSE	EFEITOS COLATERAIS	PRECAUÇÃO
Fenilpropanolamina	Alfa-agonista	1 a 1,5 mg/kg/8 a 12 h VO	Hipertensão, agressividade, inquietude, transtornos gastrintestinais, ansiedade	Hipertensão, hiperadrenocorticismo, nefropatia
Dietilestilbestrol (DES)	Estrógeno	0,1 a 1 mg/cão/24 h VO, durante 5 a 7 dias, seguida de dose semanal ou conforme necessário	Mielossupressão (rara nessa dose), atratividade a machos, edema mamário/vulvar, alterações comportamentais	Machos (podem desenvolver metaplasia prostática)
Estrógeno conjugado	Estrógeno	0,02 mg/kg/24 h VO, durante 5 a 7 dias e, então, a intervalos de 2 a 4 dias, conforme necessário	Semelhantes aos mencionados para DES	Semelhantes às mencionadas para DES
Estriol	Estrógeno	2 mg/cão/24 h VO, durante 14 dias; em seguida, reduzir para 1 mg/24 h	Semelhantes aos mencionados para DES	Semelhantes às mencionadas para DES
Cipionato de testosterona	Andrógeno	2,2 mg/kg IM, a cada 4 a 8 semanas	Alteração comportamental, agressividade, adenoma perianal, hiperplasia de próstata	Cardiopatia, nefropatia, hepatopatia, prostatopatia

implantação de um esfíncter uretral artificial, que pode ser ajustado por meio de acesso subcutâneo (ver Capítulo 124). Estudos recentes demonstraram aumento significativo na continência em cães, machos e fêmeas, que não responderam à terapia medicamentosa para IMEU.[24-26]

Historicamente, têm-se utilizado compostos injetáveis para o preenchimento da uretra, principalmente colágeno bovino, a fim de aumentar a pressão uretral em repouso em cães com IMEU. Em 2009 os fabricantes do produto mais comumente utilizado o retiraram do mercado; dessa forma, no momento da elaboração deste capítulo, não havia disponibilidade de composto de preenchimento injetável para o tratamento de IMEU, com exceção de algum uso em pesquisa.

Anormalidade no neurônio motor inferior da bexiga

A incontinência urinária, como uma anormalidade de armazenamento de urina, também pode ocorrer secundariamente à lesão ou doença da medula espinal. Lesões da coluna vertebral, na região S1-S2, enfraquecem o músculo estriado do esfíncter. O comprometimento do arco reflexo local nesses segmentos torna fácil a compressão manual da bexiga, que pode se esvaziar com o aumento discreto da compressão abdominal. A identificação desses animais baseia-se na constatação de diminuição do tônus anal e de reflexo perineal fraco, bem como a bexiga facilmente manipulável (ver Capítulo 259). A maioria desses animais é incapaz de urinar voluntariamente e necessitam do uso intermitente de sonda ou cateter (ver Capítulo 105) ou da compressão manual da bexiga pelo tutor. A correção da lesão primária pode propiciar retorno parcial à função normal. Por causa da tendência de ocorrer esvaziamento incompleto da bexiga após sua compressão manual, esses animais apresentam maior risco de desenvolver infecção do trato urinário e devem ser cuidadosamente monitorados (ver Capítulo 330). Nesses pacientes tem sido utilizado betanecol, um agonista muscarínico, com o intuito de aumentar a contração do músculo detrusor; entretanto, a eficácia desse medicamento permanece controversa.[27,28]

Hiper-reflexia do músculo detrusor/bexiga hiperativa

A hiper-reflexia do músculo detrusor/bexiga hiperativa (BHA) é a forma mais comum de incontinência urinária em pessoas, mas tem sido mal caracterizada em animais de companhia. A real prevalência e importância da BHA como causa de incontinência urinária em cães e gatos é desconhecida. Em pessoas, a BHA é caracterizada por urgência súbita para urinar e perda involuntária da urina causada por episódios de contrações do músculo detrusor na presença de volume de urina na bexiga muito abaixo da capacidade vesical. Em cães, pode ser manifestada como perda da complacência e capacidade da bexiga e, em consequência, a necessidade de urinar mais frequentemente, sem poliúria ou inflamação do trato urinário inferior. A BHA pode ser uma causa da falha do tratamento em alguns cães tratados para suposta IMEU e, nesses animais, deve-se considerar a possibilidade de BHA. O diagnóstico de BHA em animais pode ser desafiador e só é definitivamente confirmado com a utilização de estudos urodinâmicos, como a cistometrografia. A resposta à terapia com fármacos antimuscarínicos quase sempre é utilizada para o diagnóstico presuntivo de BHA em animais. Os medicamentos mais comumente utilizados são oxibutinina e imipramina, esta última também possui ação alfa-agonista, aumentando potencialmente o tônus do esfíncter uretral. Efeitos adversos dessas medicações incluem anormalidades gastrintestinais, como diarreia e constipação intestinal, e sintomas parassimpatolíticos, como taquicardia e hipossialia.

ANORMALIDADES DE ESVAZIAMENTO

A incapacidade para esvaziar completamente a bexiga durante uma micção normal pode ser decorrência de obstrução funcional ou mecânica do fluxo urinário e da uretra, ou anormalidade do músculo detrusor que pode prejudicar a contração da bexiga. A incontinência por fluxo excessivo pode resultar da ausência de esvaziamento completo, geralmente quando o animal está em repouso. Um tutor pode não ser capaz de diferenciar tal condição daquela de um animal com anormalidade de armazenamento (p. ex., IMEU); cabe ao clínico determinar a doença primária de modo a instituir um protocolo terapêutico apropriado. A incapacidade de esvaziar completamente a bexiga é um fator de risco para ITU, e esses animais devem ser monitorados quanto à presença de infecção urinária.

Atonia do músculo detrusor

O esvaziamento completo da bexiga depende da contração normal do músculo detrusor. No animal normal, a bexiga relaxa durante o seu enchimento, com apenas discretos aumentos da pressão intravesical. À medida que ocorre o enchimento da bexiga, essa pressão aumenta até certo limiar, a partir do qual desencadeia a contração do músculo detrusor e o esvaziamento vesical. A perda da capacidade de contração adequada do detrusor pode resultar de anormalidades neurogênicas ou não neurogênicas. A lesão da medula espinal sacral (S1-S3) ou de nervos pélvicos pode ocasionar atonia vesical e quase sempre causa enfraquecimento do tônus uretral. Os animais acometidos geralmente apresentam diminuição do reflexo perineal e bexiga facilmente comprimida (NMIB). O tratamento da lesão primária, se possível, pode melhorar a atividade de micção. Entretanto, até que a função normal retorne, deve-se monitorar cuidadosamente a micção. Em cães machos faz-se o esvaziamento da bexiga por meio de compressão manual da bexiga ou com o uso de sonda ou cateter asséptico 2 a 4 vezes/dia no hospital ou no domicílio (ver Capítulo 105); em gatos e cadelas geralmente faz-se o esvaziamento mediante compressão manual da bexiga.

O dano direto ao músculo detrusor pode ser causado por distensão excessiva devido à obstrução mecânica ou funcional, aguda ou crônica, do fluxo de urina. As fibras musculares do detrusor transmitem potenciais de ação, os quais iniciam as contrações via junções íntimas. Após a distensão excessiva, essas junções são comprometidas, levando à ausência ou ineficácia da contração. A distensão excessiva pode ser aguda, como em casos de cistite felina obstrutiva idiopática em gato macho, ou crônica, como acontece em cão com obstrução funcional da uretra. A liberação da obstrução e a manutenção de um pequeno volume de urina na bexiga por até 2 semanas pode permitir que as junções se restabeleçam, retornando a função coordenada do músculo detrusor. Em geral, isso é controlado por meio do uso de cateter de demora ou cateterização estéril frequente da bexiga. O betanecol pode ser utilizado nesses pacientes para aumentar o estímulo à contração do detrusor, desde que o nervo pélvico esteja intacto. Outras medicações que demonstraram melhorar a função do detrusor são cisaprida e metoclopramida; contudo, a resposta entre os indivíduos é muito variável.[29,30] É essencial que a liberação de qualquer obstrução uretral, funcional ou mecânica, seja feita antes do início da terapia medicamentosa para melhorar a contração do detrusor.

Dissinergia detrusor-uretral

A obstrução funcional da uretra, ou dissinergia detrusor-uretral (DDU), é causada por anormalidade no arco reflexo que normalmente possibilita o relaxamento do esfíncter uretral no início da micção. A lesão supostamente ocorre no trato reticuloespinal, núcleo de Onuf ou gânglio mesentérico caudal e, provavelmente, implica a perda de sinais inibidores aos nervos pudendo e hipogástrico.[31] Não foi esclarecido se também há envolvimento de lesões aos nervos periféricos, às junções neuromusculares ou aos esfíncteres de músculo liso ou estriado.[32] Diferentemente do que acontece na anormalidade do "neurônio motor superior da bexiga", observada em animais com doença

SEÇÃO 24 • Doenças do Trato Urinário Inferior

de disco intervertebral toracolombar e outras lesões de medula espinal, o exame neurológico desses animais é tipicamente normal (ver Capítulo 259).

A DDU acomete principalmente cães machos de meia-idade de raças de grande porte ou gigante, embora cadelas e gatos possam ser afetados. Uma série de caso de 22 cães constatou idade média de 4,9 anos.[33] Os sinais clínicos são semelhantes àqueles verificados na obstrução mecânica da uretra. O animal frequentemente apresenta postura de micção e é capaz de produzir um jato de urina que rapidamente se torna atenuado ou cessa completamente. O animal pode continuar a manter a postura ou fazer várias tentativas de micção, mas sem esvaziar completamente a bexiga (Vídeo 333.1). A retenção de grande volume de urina residual geralmente ocasiona incontinência urinária por fluxo abundante e pode ser confundida com IMEU. Esse extravasamento pode ocorrer porque a hipertonicidade do esfíncter envolvido é frequentemente dinâmica e desencadeada pela ação de urinar. Em casos crônicos, pode ocorrer distensão excessiva da bexiga e subsequente atonia. Diferentemente do que acontece em animais com obstrução mecânica, em geral a cateterização desses cães é fácil (ver Capítulo 105); ademais a uretrografia contrastada pode ser normal ou revelar áreas de estreitamento da uretra (uretroespasmo).

O diagnóstico presuntivo de DDU é frequentemente obtido pela observação do ato de urinar de um cão com padrão de micção interrompida típico, constatação de grande volume de urina residual, fácil introdução de sonda urinária e exclusão da presença de obstrução mecânica. Em um estudo com 48 cães relatou-se volume de urina residual normal de 0,1 a 3,4 ml/kg de peso corporal, com média de 0,2 ml/kg (ver Capítulo 330 e Vídeo 330.1).[34] O autor utiliza como valor de referência < 0,5 ml/kg. Recomenda-se ultrassonografia para avaliar os ureteres e a pelve renal em busca de dilatações secundárias a obstrução crônica e refluxo ureterorrenal da urina.

O tratamento de esfíncter uretral hipertônico geralmente consiste em bloqueio alfa-adrenérgico com prazosina, um antagonista alfa-1 específico que atua nos esfíncteres uretrais interno e externo.[35] A tansulosina, que é específica para o subtipo alfa-1 presente no esfíncter uretral interno, também

tem sido efetiva nesses cães. Alguns cães requerem terapia adicional, caso o músculo estriado apresente comprometimento mais significante. Benzodiazepínicos, como o diazepam, ou outros relaxantes de músculo esquelético, inclusive acepromazina e metocarbamol, podem ser mais efetivos quando há envolvimento do esfíncter uretral externo. Comumente, administra-se diazepam 30 minutos antes da micção, a fim de reduzir a pressão no esfíncter uretral externo. O dantroleno e o baclofeno foram utilizados no passado como relaxantes de músculo esquelético; no entanto, o potencial para efeitos adversos diminuiu sua utilização em pacientes veterinários.[35,36] Em casos graves e refratários, pode ser necessária a cateterização estéril intermitente pelo tutor no domicílio (ver Capítulo 105). A terapia medicamentosa da atonia vesical associada deve ser iniciada após a liberação efetiva da obstrução funcional da uretra (Tabela 333.3). É necessário rigoroso monitoramento desses pacientes quanto ao volume de urina residual e à ocorrência de ITU, a fim de avaliar a eficácia do tratamento e prevenir complicações (ver Capítulo 330).

O prognóstico quanto à recuperação da micção normal é bom, mas a maioria dos cães necessita de tratamento para DDU por toda a vida. As tentativas de ajuste das medicações até obter a menor dose efetiva podem ser prejudicadas pela recidiva dos sinais clínicos após meses de micção normal.[33] O prognóstico parece ser pior em pacientes com atonia da bexiga ou ITU secundária à retenção de urina. Há relato empírico de que a extensão da uretra pode aliviar os sinais clínicos (ver Capítulo 124); entretanto, isso é considerado um procedimento de salvamento, com diversas complicações potenciais, sendo indicado apenas nos casos mais refratários.

Anormalidade no neurônio motor superior da bexiga

Lesões da medula espinal cranial até o segmento sacral geralmente causam obstrução funcional neurogênica da uretra. Isso ocasiona perda de sinais inibidores aos nervos hipogástrico e pudendo, condição que impede o relaxamento do esfíncter, necessário para a micção. Essa é a clássica "bexiga do neurônio motor superior", na qual o paciente é incapaz de urinar normalmente e é difícil a compressão manual da bexiga. Os pacientes

Tabela 333.3	Fármacos frequentemente utilizados para tratar anormalidades no esvaziamento da bexiga.[38]		
FÁRMACO	**CLASSE**	**DOSE**	**EFEITOS COLATERAIS/PRECAUÇÃO**
Prazosina	Antagonista-alfa$_1$, relaxante de músculo liso	1 mg/animal < 15 kg; 2 mg/animal > 15 kg; a cada 8 a 12 h VO	Hipotensão, fraqueza, síncope, transtornos gastrintestinais (GI)/ nefropatia, cardiopatia
Tansulosina*	Antagonista-alfa-1, relaxante de músculo liso	0,01 a 0,2 mg/kg/24 h VO	Hipotensão
Fenoxibenzamina	Antagonista alfa inespecífico, relaxante de músculo liso	Cão: 0,25 mg/kg/8 a 12 h Gato: 1,25 a 7,5 mg/gato/8 a 12 h VO	Hipotensão, taquicardia, miose/ hipotensão na primeira dose
Acepromazina	Antagonista alfa inespecífico, relaxante de músculo liso, ansiolítico	0,5 a 2,2 mg/kg/6 a 8 h VO	Sedação, hipotensão
Diazepam	Relaxante de músculo esquelético, ansiolítico	Cão: 0,5 a 2 mg/kg/8 h VO ou 30 min antes da micção	Sedação, ataxia/disfunção hepática, não utilizar em gatos
Metocarbamol	Relaxante de músculo esquelético	22 a 44 mg/kg/8 h VO	Sedação, fraqueza, hipersalivação
Baclofeno*	Relaxante de músculo esquelético	Cão: 1 a 2 mg/kg/8 h VO	Fraqueza, transtornos GI, não utilizar em gatos
Dantroleno	Relaxante de músculo esquelético	Cão: 1 a 5 mg/kg/8 h VO Gato:1 a 2 mg/kg/8 h VO	Fraqueza/hepatopatia
Betanecol	Parassimpatomimético	Cão: 2,5 a 15 mg/cão/8 h VO Gato: 1,25 a 5 mg/gato/8 h VO	Diarreia/obstrução GI ou uretral
Cisaprida	Procinético	Cão: 0,1 a 0,5 mg/kg/8 a 12 h VO Gato: 2,5 a 5 mg/gato/8 a 12 h VO	Ataxia, transtornos GI/obstrução GI

*De Lane IF, Westropp JL: Urinary incontinence and micturition disorders: pharmacologic management. *Kirk's current veterinary therapy*, 14 ed., St. Louis, 2009, Elsevier, p. 955-959.

mais comumente acometidos são aqueles com doença de disco intervertebral e paresia associada (ver Capítulo 266). Esses animais geralmente apresentam déficits neurológicos adicionais que incluem paresia e perda nociceptiva (ver Capítulo 259). O tratamento da lesão primária em geral leva ao retorno parcial ou completo da função normal de micção após dias a semanas. Até que a micção normal retorne, os pacientes são tratados da mesma forma que os casos de DDU, mediante bloqueio alfa-adrenérgico e compressão manual ou cateterização da bexiga. O monitoramento desses pacientes é crítico, pois há possibilidade de distensão excessiva da bexiga e ITU; também é importante o cuidado ambulatorial, particularmente pelo fato de que a incontinência urinária por fluxo excessivo que pode acompanhar esse procedimento pode causar lesões cutâneas nesses animais em decúbito.

Disautonomia

Disautonomia é uma condição rara que envolve a degeneração de neurônios dos gânglios nervosos autônomos, ocasionando disfunção simpática e parassimpática. Foi mais comumente relatada em cães e gatos no Reino Unido e na Escandinávia, mas poucos casos foram observados nos EUA em ambas as espécies.[37] A causa primária é desconhecida, mas a exposição a neurotoxinas é uma forte suspeita. Além dos achados clássicos de midríase irresponsiva e prolapso da glândula nictitante, as anormalidades observadas em casos de disautonomia podem variar desde íleo adinâmico e constipação intestinal até diminuição da função sistólica cardíaca. Esses cães e gatos frequentemente apresentam importante disfunção de micção e retenção urinária devido à atonia da bexiga e incontinência por fluxo excessivo secundária à incompetência do esfíncter uretral. Não há tratamento específico para disautonomia; a remissão espontânea é incomum. O prognóstico depende da gravidade dos sinais clínicos e do comprometimento das funções de órgãos específicos.

REFERÊNCIAS BIBLIOGRÁFICAS

As referências bibliográficas deste capítulo se encontram online no Ambiente de Aprendizagem.

CAPÍTULO 334

Cistite Idiopática Felina

C. A. Tony Buffington

INTRODUÇÃO

A cistite idiopática (intersticial) felina (CIF) é a causa mais comum de sintomas de trato urinário inferior (STUI) crônicos em gatos.[1] Nós estabelecemos o termo cistite intersticial felina[1] por causa das semelhanças entre a CIF e a cistite intersticial (CI) em humanos,[2] que quase sempre necessitavam de exame cistoscópico da bexiga para confirmar o diagnóstico. Neste capítulo, utilizamos o termo CIF para denominar a cistite idiopática, já que a cistoscopia não é mais necessária para confirmar o diagnóstico em humanos[3] e raramente está disponível (ou indicada) para gatos.

Além das etiologias "clássicas" dos STUI crônicos, recentemente propus uma causa relacionada ao sistema nervoso central para CIF em alguns gatos, a qual denominei síndrome de Pandora;[4] outros pesquisadores sugeriram uma etiologia semelhante em humanos.[5-7] Ademais, a periúria pode representar um comportamento de demarcação de terreno ou estar "relacionada a fatores ambientais ou sociais primários".[8] Os clínicos também devem considerar se estão diante de um episódio inicial ou de recidiva de uma doença crônica.[9,10]

EPIDEMIOLOGIA RECENTE

Em 2014, o Banfield State of Pet Health[11] relatou que a "cistite" (STUI) representou aproximadamente 5% dos diagnósticos em gatos com mais de 1 ano de idade levados para atendimento por apresentarem problema de saúde, e o Veterinary Pet Insurance relatou que "problemas de bexiga/trato urinário" foram as queixas mais comuns dos segurados, para gatos, em 2013.[12] A prevalência de doenças em gatos atendidos para avaliação de STUI parece ser da ordem de (% de casos): CIF, 55 a 73%; urolitíase, 10 a 20%; infecção microbiana, 1 a 25%[13-18] (não está clara, se houver, a participação de vírus na FIC[19]); e outras causas, 5 a 20%.

Um estudo retrospectivo controlado de casos de 2011[20] relatou que gatos com CIF apresentavam peso corporal e escore da condição corporal significativamente maiores; mais provavelmente eram mantidos em domicílios com vários gatos, mais nervosos e medrosos, mais predispostos a se esconder de visitantes desconhecidos, mais provavelmente utilizavam a caixa de excretas; segundo o tutor, consumiam menos água e tinham menor nível de atividade, menor comportamento de caça e menor acesso ao ambiente externo do que os gatos do grupo-controle. Das situações estressantes questionadas, somente a mudança de domicílio ocorreu com maior frequência em gatos com CIF. A ocorrência de piúria, hematúria e o aumento da proporção proteína: creatinina na urina foram significativamente maiores em machos com obstrução, comparados a machos sem obstrução, e a obstrução foi significativamente mais provável na presença de cristalúria por estruvita do que na ausência dessa condição. Ao mesmo tempo que esse achado sugeriu uma associação entre cristalúria por estruvita e obstrução em gatos machos com CIF, ele não pode esclarecer se a formação de cristais ocorreu antes, durante ou após o evento obstrutivo.

Na Noruega, em 2011 também foram relatados resultados de um estudo prospectivo relativo ao período de 2003 a 2007, sobre causas de STUI em 119 gatos enviados para atendimento primário (34 apresentavam obstrução).[21] Menciona-se que 65 gatos (55%) foram diagnosticados com CIF, 25 (21%) possuíam tampão uretral e 14 (12%) apresentavam infecção do trato urinário (ITU) bacteriana ou urolitíase. Em 63 gatos (62%) era o primeiro episódio de STUI, enquanto em 44 (38%) a doença era recorrente.

Um estudo de 2014[22] relatou que 302 gatos foram levados para atendimento na Clinic of Small Animal Medicine, Ludwig Maximilian University Munich, com sintomas de trato urinário inferior (STUI), entre 2000 e 2007. Os diagnósticos mais comuns foram de CIF (55%), ITU (18,9%), tampão uretral (10,3%), urolitíase (7%) e neoplasia (3,6%). Seis gatos (2%)

apresentavam cristalúria por estruvita grave, sem obstrução da uretra, e 9 gatos foram identificados com distúrbios neurogênicos (3%). Tampões uretrais foram significativamente mais frequentes em gatos com CIF do que naqueles com ITU; gatos com CIF e tampão uretral tinham pesos corporais significativamente maiores e eram significativamente mais jovens (< 10 anos de idade) do que os gatos com ITU ou neoplasia. Os machos eram mais predispostos do que as fêmeas ao desenvolvimento de CIF ou de tampão de uretra do que de ITU ou neoplasia. Não foram identificadas diferenças entre gatos afetados e não afetados quanto à distribuição racial, condições de vida, dieta, acesso ao ambiente externo, número de gatos no domicílio ou variações sazonais.

Os resultados de estudos epidemiológicos devem ser interpretados cuidadosamente. Tendências de seleção significantes (não intencionais), além da capacidade de identificar associações, mas não as causas, frequentemente ocorrem em animais levados para atendimento de um sinal clínico e com base nesse sintoma coleta-se a maioria das amostras. A determinação de prevalência e a distribuição das causas de STUI em nível populacional necessitam de um estudo com base na população, como foi realizado em humanos com CI e anormalidades relacionadas.[23] Outra abordagem potencialmente informativa seria um estudo longitudinal prospectivo, como o atualmente mencionado no Bristol Cats Study.[24]

FISIOPATOLOGIA

Como a queixa principal da maioria dos tutores de gatos com CIF são os STUI, por vários anos a maioria das pesquisas focou na detecção de anormalidades intraluminais ou intrínsecas da bexiga.[25-35] Conforme mencionado, a constatação de hemorragias petequiais na submucosa (glomerulações) por meio de cistoscopia é necessária para o diagnóstico de CI em humanos, mas essas lesões não são indicadores sensíveis ou específicos de IC[36] e já não fazem parte dos protocolos de diagnóstico.[37] Entretanto, a cistoscopia ainda pode ser utilizada para descartar a presença de doenças que podem "confundir" o diagnóstico em casos complicados.[3,38] Uma série de outros achados anormais na bexiga também foram relatados,[32,33,35,39-42] mas sua participação na etiopatogenia da CIF é desconhecida.

Gatos com CIF manifestam alterações da função nervosa sensorial.[4,43] Constatou-se aumento modesto na imunorreatividade da substância P (SP) em neurônios sensoriais[44] e hiperatividade do receptor de neurocinina-1 para SP[35] na bexiga de gatos com CIF e em pessoas com CI.[45,46] Contudo, os resultados de estudos clínicos com antagonistas da SP foram decepcionantes;[47] evidências recentes[48,49] sugerem que a SP pode abrandar a gravidade das reações inflamatórias, levando a pensar na possibilidade de que alterações observadas em pacientes poderiam refletir uma resposta protetora. Também foram detectadas anormalidades em corpos celulares ganglionares da raiz dorsal em toda a medula espinal lombossacra (L4-S3) de gatos com CIF.[50,51]

Até o momento, foram avaliados tratamentos que atuam nos neurônios sensoriais da bexiga sem sucesso. Estudos controlados com capsaicina e resiniferatoxina em pessoas com CI não constataram benefícios significativos comparativamente aos pacientes que receberam placebo.[52] Em 2006, um especialista concluiu: "A terapia por instilação intravesical basicamente não foi alterada nos últimos anos, mesmo com alguns estudos que não comprovaram a eficácia de alguns protocolos terapêuticos".[53] Isso continua a ocorrer;[54] em 2014[55] a eficácia do polissulfato de pentosana (Elmiron®, Janssen Scientific, Titusville, NJ) foi considerada equivalente à do placebo em pacientes humanos com CI, um achado relatado em gatos em 2009.[56]

Anormalidades do sistema de resposta ao estresse (SRS) central também foram detectadas.[4] A busca por alguns resultados anômalos em pesquisas com antagonista do fator liberador

de corticotropina[57] fez com que identificássemos zonas fasciculada e reticular significativamente menores nas glândulas adrenais de gatos com CIF comparativamente aos gatos saudáveis.[58] Até o momento, a explicação mais parcimoniosa para esses achados é a ocorrência de um evento estressante no início da vida, que permitiu que os glicocorticoides maternos cruzassem a placenta e inibissem a liberação fetal de ACTH.[59,60]

A ativação suficientemente intensa do SRS materno também pode causar outras alterações em sua ninhada.[61,62] Pesquisas recentes mostraram como processos de desenvolvimento evolutivos podem interagir com características ambientais, frequentemente transmitidos pela mãe através da placenta, na tentativa de equilibrar a fisiologia do organismo em desenvolvimento ao seu ambiente pós-natal. Um mecanismo notável que é a base desses efeitos é a modulação epigenética da expressão gênica.[63,64] Assim que o SRS se torna sensibilizado, ativações repetidas por eventos ambientais podem influenciar negativamente uma série de órgãos com base na suscetibilidade familiar (genética, epigenética). Além das anormalidades do TUI, gatos com CIF frequentemente apresentam uma série de outros problemas de saúde.[65-67] Embora esses problemas de saúde possam resultar de uma síndrome de dor vesical intensa crônica, eles frequentemente *precedem* o diagnóstico de CIF, tornando essa explicação improvável. Um padrão semelhante foi identificado em seres humanos.[68-70]

É importante ressaltar que o SRS pode ser ativado tanto perifericamente por fatores locais, como infecção ou inflamação ("ascendente"),[71] quanto centralmente pela percepção de uma ameaça ambiental externa ("descendente").[72,73] Ameaças ambientais externas podem ser físicas, psicológicas ou sociais e podem ser agudas ou crônicas. O aumento da atividade do SRS é comum em gatos confinados em ambientes não enriquecidos,[74] o que pode dificultar a interpretação clínica dos procedimentos diagnósticos devido à influência na temperatura corporal, nas frequências cardíaca e respiratória e na pressão sanguínea do gato;[75,76] ademais, pode influenciar a predisposição, precipitação ou perpetuação de uma série de problemas de saúde crônicos em gatos.[77] Adicionalmente, o aumento da sensibilidade da resposta à ameaça acústica, um reflexo do tronco encefálico que responde a estímulos altos inesperados,[78] foi detectado em gatos com CIF[79,80] e em pessoas com CI,[81] e é responsivo ao enriquecimento ambiental (EA) em gatos com CIF.[80]

A ativação do SRS pode aumentar o estímulo autônomo, principalmente o simpático, que, por sua vez, pode causar aumento agudo da permeabilidade epitelial e resultar em dano epitelial no caso de estímulo crônico.[82] Em gatos com CIF, relata-se que a exposição a fatores estressantes externos aumenta a concentração sanguínea de catecolaminas,[83,84] que aumenta ainda mais à medida que se mantém a exposição aos fatores estressantes,[84] possivelmente devido à dessensibilização de receptores alfa-2-adrenérgicos.[85,86] Diferentemente, a concentração plasmática de catecolaminas diminuiu em gatos saudáveis à medida que se acostumam aos fatores estressantes.[84]

Sabe-se muito bem que o estresse psicossocial crônico também estimula a inflamação sistêmica de baixo grau,[87-89] que pode resultar na expressão de comportamentos de doença.[90] Comportamentos de doença referem-se a combinações variáveis de êmese, diarreia, periúria, inapetência, febre, letargia, sonolência e exacerbação de comportamento semelhantes à dor, bem como diminuição da atividade geral, atividades relacionadas aos cuidados corporais (*grooming*) e interações sociais. Em gatos, os comportamentos de doença podem ser decorrências da ativação imune periférica *ou* central.[74,84,91] Em gatos, os fatores estressantes externos foram associados à exacerbação significativa dos comportamentos de doença, mais comumente manifestados como diminuição da ingestão de alimentos e da defecação, e aumento de defecações fora da caixa de excretas.[67] Assim, algumas das anormalidades mais comumente observadas em gatos de tutores, como apetite "caprichoso" e problemas com o uso da caixa de excretas, ocorrem após exposição a ameaças

CAPÍTULO 334 • Cistite Idiopática Felina 2043

externas em gatos com CIF e saudáveis, sugerindo que os clínicos deveriam incluir a participação de ameaças ambientais nos diagnósticos diferenciais de gatos levados à consulta por causa desses sintomas. É importante ressaltar que nós também observamos a resolução desses comportamentos em estudos laboratoriais[67] e clínicos[66] de gatos com CIF, em resposta à modificação ambiental multimodal (MAMO).

Resumo

A compreensão atual sobre a etiopatogenia da CIF se expandiu além da bexiga, para incluir as participações de influências do desenvolvimento, provavelmente mediadas por modulação epigenética da expressão gênica, e interações complexas entre indivíduos e seus ambientes. Ainda é preciso determinar como esses sistemas se comunicam e se manifestam como CIF em alguns gatos, mas não em outros. Fatores estressantes ambientais e comportamentais também estão associados a exacerbações dos sintomas de CIF e podem resultar em comportamentos de doença em gatos saudáveis e naqueles acometidos. O número e a variabilidade de anormalidades fisiológicas e comportamentais detectadas em gatos com CIF podem representar diferentes entidades mórbidas e/ou diferentes manifestações de um problema primário comum por causa da variação natural na ativação relativa às respostas neurais, endócrinas e imunes pelo SRS. Ao mesmo tempo que ainda muito tem de ser aprendido sobre CIF, essa perspectiva levou diretamente a aperfeiçoamentos no diagnóstico e nos princípios de tratamento que resultaram em melhores resultados clínicos.

DIAGNÓSTICO (VER CAPÍTULO 46)

Gatos de qualquer idade, raça ou sexo podem desenvolver CIF, embora seja diagnosticada mais comumente em gatos jovens e de meia-idade. A maioria dos gatos com STUI crônicos tem CIF, e a maioria dos gatos com CIF manifestou melhora dos sinais clínicos após alguns dias, mesmo sem tratamento,[10,20,67,92,93] de forma que o diagnóstico pode não ser necessário (mas pode sempre ser informado ao tutor) para gatos atendidos por apresentarem um primeiro episódio de STUI. Aos gatos com sintomas recorrentes recomenda-se avaliação adicional.

Uma radiografia de abdome que inclua todo o trato urinário pode detectar cálculos urinários radiopacos, e a realização de cistografia e uretrografia contrastadas pode detectar cálculos radiolucentes, lesões tumorais, coágulos sanguíneos ou constrições. Os resultados de exames contrastados da bexiga e da uretra geralmente são normais, embora em cerca de 15% dos casos ocorra espessamento difuso ou assimétrico da parede da bexiga.[34,94] Exames contrastados ou avaliação ultrassonográfica são indicados em gatos com mais de 10 anos de idade, quando a ocorrência de CIF é menos provável (ver Capítulo 332).

A ultrassonografia de abdome (ver Capítulo 88) possibilita a visualização de coágulos sanguíneos, pólipos, neoplasias e cálculos de cistina ou de urato de amônio, que são radiolucentes; contudo, não é ideal para o exame da uretra (p. ex., não é possível avaliar a maior parte da uretra de gatos machos); sempre se deve realizar radiografia, com ou sem contraste, para detectar cálculos ou tampões uretrais, se presentes.

Embora a maioria dos gatos com CIF não apresente ITU, em gatos com STUI crônicos deve-se realizar exame de urina completo (ver Capítulo 72) pelo menos uma vez (ver Capítulo 330); conforme mencionado anteriormente, a cistoscopia pode ser útil para excluir diagnósticos alternativos, mesmo que não seja útil para o diagnóstico de CIF (ver Capítulo 108).

TRATAMENTO

Recentes avanços terapêuticos para CIF refletem a perspectiva de que a CIF quase sempre representa um problema que afeta a bexiga mais do que um problema vesical. Se esses gatos apresentam SRS sensibilizado, as abordagens que almejem reduzir a ativação do SRS provavelmente são mais efetivas do que aquelas que não o fazem. Como as condições ambientais sabidamente afetam o comportamento e a saúde dos animais,[95] principalmente animais criados em cativeiro,[96] nós focamos os efeitos do enriquecimento ambiental (EA) na ocorrência de CIF por meio de adaptações de abordagens utilizadas em zoológicos e instalações de pesquisa.[97] Por essa perspectiva, o EA consiste em criar condições que permitam que o animal se sinta seguro, o que significa sustentar uma percepção do controle que excede sua percepção de ameaça. Essas condições incluem acesso a inovações apropriadas para a espécie, bem como atividades e interações com outros animais (inclusive pessoas). Nós definimos esses conceitos como modificação ambiental multimodal (MAMO),[98,99] os quais recentemente foram incluídos em diretrizes de EA profissionais.[100] O prognóstico da CIF depende do gato, da condição do domicílio e da capacidade e do comprometimento do tutor em implementar a MAMO. Em minha experiência com gatos portadores de CIF grave,[66,67,84] a implementação de EA efetivo leva à recuperação sem necessidade de tratamento farmacológico ou qualquer dieta especial em quase todos os pacientes.

O tratamento de CIF consiste em abordagens agudas e crônicas ao gato, tutor e ambiente. Conforme mencionado, na maioria dos gatos os sinais clínicos de STUI comumente cessam dentro de alguns dias. A menos que seja diagnosticada ITU concomitante, não se justifica o uso de antibiótico. Terapia analgésica pode ser apropriada para o controle de CIF aguda (descrita anteriormente). Os tutores de gatos outrora saudáveis, com menos de 10 anos de idade, podem ser orientados de que a causa mais comum dos sintomas de seus gatos seja CIF, sugerindo avaliações diagnósticas para excluir a possibilidade de outras enfermidades, se eles optarem por isso, e implementação de MAMO, a fim de facilitar a recuperação. O enriquecimento do ambiente da gaiola é útil para gatos hospitalizados, e recentes diretrizes[101] e recomendações[102] estão disponíveis.

A comunicação efetiva determina o resultado do tratamento por meio de MAMO.[98,103] Quando tutores compreendem que a implementação efetiva da MAMO pode diminuir a gravidade e a frequência de STUI e de sintomas de anormalidades concomitantes em seus gatos, o prognóstico é excelente.[66,67,84] MAMO consiste em educar o tutor acerca de seu gato, de forma geral; de CIF; do manejo efetivo dos recursos (alimento, água, áreas de repouso, caixa de excretas etc.); e das modificações no ambiente para reduzir a percepção de ameaças e de conflitos entre gatos em um domicílio onde há vários gatos. Diversos materiais informativos que podem ser recomendados aos tutores são fornecidos, na forma de folheto, ao tutor.

Há uma relação quadrática entre o ambiente e a saúde, sendo que os problemas ocorrem em condições inóspitas e caóticas;[77] assim, devem ser disponibilizados formulários que facilitem a avaliação do gato e de seus contactantes.[104,105] Além disso, sempre que possível prefiro utilizar uma abordagem de "tutor" (adesão) e não de "especialista" (complacência), a fim de auxiliar o tutor a alterar o trabalho de EA porque os tutores percebem que isso é de seu interesse.[106,107] Técnicos treinados também podem fazer esse trabalho efetiva e empaticamente.

Quando são sugeridas alterações, são oferecidas escolhas de recursos aos gatos para determinar suas preferências por alimentos e manejo de alimentação; água e bebedouro; caixa de excretas e substrato;[8] espaço; e maneiras de interação com pessoas e outros animais. A MAMO também fornece oportunidades para brincar e interações que são apropriadas para a espécie felina. Em domicílio com mais de um gato, devem-se aumentar o número e os locais dos recursos, a fim de criar um "ambiente de abundância", de modo a diminuir a competição por recursos que poderiam contribuir para a recidiva dos sintomas de CIF relacionados aos conflitos entre os gatos.

Alguns gatos são especialmente sensíveis a alterações nos horários de alimentação, horários de trabalho do tutor, adição ou saída de pessoas ou animais da casa e emoções do tutor, de forma que os transtornos em seus ambientes devem ser mínimos, realizados gradativamente e de acordo com as necessidades e limitações do gato. Embora o tema esteja além do escopo deste capítulo, as diretrizes detalhadas para a avaliação ambiental e implementação da MAMO estão disponíveis, de forma que possam ser utilizadas para informar as recomendações necessárias.[98-100]

Uma série de aspectos relativos à nutrição foi considerada para a inclusão em protocolos terapêuticos para gatos com STUI (ver Capítulo 185); poucos mostraram-se efetivos em gatos com CIF.[108] Por exemplo, foi proposto que a diluição da urina reduz o risco de recidiva dos sintomas em gatos com CIF,[109] mas estudos clínicos sobre CIF não constataram efeitos do teor de umidade da dieta;[10] ademais, tanto estudos laboratoriais quanto clínicos da MAMO, nos casos de CIF, relataram redução relevante na ocorrência de recidiva dos sintomas, sem diluição da urina,[66,67] de forma que qualquer efeito benéfico deve ser modesto.

Algumas rações de uso veterinário são comercializadas para animais com CIF. Os atributos desses alimentos incluem combinações variáveis de aumentos no conteúdo hídrico, a fim de reduzir a densidade urinária, e alterações nos conteúdos de minerais, cloreto de sódio, ácidos graxos ômega-3, antioxidantes, triptofano e alfacasozepina. Infelizmente, na literatura científica revisada por pares, não estão disponíveis resultados de estudos clínicos controlados de qualquer das rações atualmente comercializadas para gatos com CIF. Em um resumo de estudo de 2013 patrocinado por um fabricante de rações,[110] menciona-se que a taxa de recidiva em gatos alimentados com uma ração veterinária foi comparável àquela constatada em outros estudos,[10,56,66,67,93] enquanto a taxa de recidiva em gatos alimentados com uma ração comercial foi maior. Recomendações para EA foram fornecidas a todos os tutores, mas nenhum grupo tratado apenas com EA foi descrito, bem como um grupo de animais submetidos a "cuidados usuais". Lamentavelmente, a composição da ração veterinária atualmente disponível no mercado é diferente daquela da ração testada, de forma que os resultados não são clinicamente relevantes mesmo que sejam eventualmente publicados.

O triptofano, um aminoácido essencial, foi adicionado a algumas dietas com base no fato de que aumentaria a concentração de serotonina no sistema nervoso central, o que poderia, então, induzir um efeito ansiolítico. A maioria das pesquisas relativas aos efeitos do triptofano no humor consiste em estudos de seu fornecimento a curto prazo, embora com muito poucas, se quaisquer, evidências de efeitos benéficos a longo prazo.[111] Ademais, em gatos o triptofano fornecido na dieta pode não atuar na serotonina[112] e, mesmo se atuasse, alguém teria de demonstrar que isso levou a um resultado clínico desejado na população almejada, já que outros componentes da dieta podem influenciar a disponibilidade do triptofano. As rações também têm sido suplementadas com alfacasozepina, mas, pelo meu conhecimento, na literatura científica revisada por pares, não há informação sobre os efeitos desses alimentos em gatos com CIF.

A recomendação de alteração da dieta parece mais razoável quando o tutor ou o gato não aceita a dieta atualmente fornecida. Alguns tutores e gatos preferem alimentos secos e podem se opor à transição forçada para alimentos enlatados, principalmente quando a dieta tem pouco valor terapêutico comprovado. Não se recomendam as tentativas de alterar a composição da urina para minimizar a ocorrência de cristalúria em gatos com CIF não obstrutiva. Desconheço qualquer evidência publicada que sustente a ideia de que tipos comuns de cristais na urina do gato lesionam o urotélio ou agravam os STUI em gatos com CIF. Se uma alteração da dieta parece aconselhável, recomendo o fornecimento do novo alimento no momento da refeição, ao lado do alimento usual, em um recipiente diferente, para que o gato possa manifestar a sua preferência. Se o gato optar pelo novo alimento, o antigo pode ser descontinuado.

O manejo alimentar é outro aspecto do cuidado nutricional a ser considerado, desde que possa propiciar EA. O comportamento alimentar natural dos gatos inclui atividades predatórias, como perseguir e atacar. Esse comportamento pode ser estimulado escondendo pequenas quantidades de alimento ao redor da casa ou colocando o alimento em um comedouro a partir do qual o gato tenha que retirar pedaços individuais ou movimentar o comedouro para liberar a ração (se tal atividade for atrativa para o gato). Oportunidades para expressar comportamentos predatórios típicos da espécie são comumente disponibilizadas em felinos mantidos em cativeiro, a fim enriquecimento o ambiente[113-115] e, embora ainda não tenha sido estudado cuidadosamente em gatos domésticos, o ato de propiciar um "quebra-cabeça" com alimentos poderia beneficiar alguns gatos com CIF. A maioria dos gatos também parece preferir refeição individual em um local calmo, onde não são perturbados por outros animais, por movimentos súbitos ou pela atividade de um ducto de ar ou um eletrodoméstico que possa funcionar de modo inesperado.

Uma combinação de ferormônio facial felino sintético e valeriano (Feliway®; Ceva Sante Animale, Libourne, France) é comercializada como calmante para gatos, embora uma recente revisão sistemática tenha questionado sua eficácia.[116] O produto parece ser benéfico a alguns gatos, então recomendo um teste na forma de difusor domiciliar elétrico aos clientes. Um ou mais difusores podem ser posicionados onde o gato possa manifestar maior sinal de estresse: janelas, portas, móveis sujos ou caixas de excretas. O produto pode ser utilizado durante ou após a implementação de MAMO se o EA, por si só, não tiver possibilitado o controle suficiente dos sintomas.

Não se conhece a terapia analgésica mais efetiva para dor visceral crônica em gatos. Atualmente tratamos surtos ou episódios agudos com buprenorfina transmucosa oral, na dose de 10 a 20 µg/kg, 2 a 4 vezes/dia, por até 7 dias, frequentemente combinada com acepromazina (0,25 mg IM ou 2,5 mg [formulação injetável administrada por via oral] a cada 8 h), por até 4 dias. Há disponibilidade de preparações de buprenorfina de liberação prolongada, que podem propiciar níveis terapêuticos do fármaco por até 72 horas, para alívio da dor, após uma única injeção, mas desconheço qualquer relato de sua utilização em animais com CIF. Nossa abordagem ainda não foi testada em estudos controlados; o alívio aos gatos acometidos é apenas nossa impressão clínica. Administramos terapia analgésica por até 5 dias e recomendamos avaliações diagnósticas adicionais se os sinais clínicos não melhorarem significativamente. Analgésicos também podem ser utilizados quando ocorre recidiva dos sintomas antes do contato com o veterinário.

Também tem sido utilizado butorfanol, mas sua ação não é tão duradoura ou potente quanto a da buprenorfina;[117] adesivos de fentanila também têm sido utilizados em casos raros, nos quais a dor vesical foi considerada intensa. Relatos empíricos de uso de fármacos anti-inflamatórios não esteroides (AINEs), especialmente meloxicam e cetoprofeno, são abundantes, mas até o momento desconheço qualquer estudo publicado sobre segurança ou eficácia desses fármacos para casos de CIF. AINEs são aprovados para uso em gatos no controle preventivo da dor, em geral como dose única, antes de anestesia e cirurgia; o uso por longo tempo pode causar insuficiência renal intrínseca aguda, especialmente se o gato estiver desidratado por ocasião do uso desses medicamentos. A FDA recentemente solicitou a inclusão da seguinte informação na bula do meloxicam para gatos: "O uso repetido do meloxicam em gatos tem sido associado à insuficiência renal aguda e morte. Não administre dose injetável ou oral adicional de meloxicam aos gatos. Veja Contraindicações, Avisos e Precauções, para informações detalhadas". Robenacoxibe, um AINE de longa ação, recentemente se tornou disponível para uso em gatos; ainda não conheço relato de sua eficácia para gatos com CIF. Ademais, os AINEs não parecem propiciar alívio às pessoas com CI.[118]

Tentou-se uma série de outras abordagens farmacológicas para o tratamento de CIF, inclusive fármacos que alteram a contratilidade vesical/uretral, a fim de modificar o revestimento vesical e de alterar os perfis de neurotransmissores centrais.[109] Assim como mencionado para analgésicos, a eficácia da maioria desses fármacos ainda não foi avaliada em estudos clínicos controlados. Ademais, tem-se dado pouca importância aos potenciais efeitos negativos da administração crônica forçada de comprimidos aos gatos e, conforme mencionado, a resolução dos sinais clínicos tem sido repetidamente demonstrada, sem necessidade de tratamento farmacológico.[10,66,67,110,119]

Apesar de relatos empíricos ocasionais, não tenho conhecimento de publicação de estudo clínico com fármacos que alteram a contratilidade da bexiga ou da uretra em gatos com CIF; ademais, essa classe de fármacos não é efetiva em pessoas com CI. Até o momento, as pesquisas também não demonstraram benefício algum da suplementação oral de glucosamina[93] ou de polissulfato de pentosano por via oral[56] ou subcutânea[120] comparativamente ao uso de placebo para os pacientes com CIF (ou CI[55]). Dois antidepressivos tricíclicos, amitriptilina e clomipramina, têm sido utilizados para tratar gatos com CIF grave, embora nenhum deles seja especificamente indicado para esse propósito e devem ser utilizados com cautela.[10,17,109,121]

RESUMO

A causa mais comum de STUI em gatos é a CIF, que infelizmente continua sendo um diagnóstico de exclusão. Evidências convergentes obtidas em uma série de estudos sugere que a maioria dos casos de CIF é, mais provavelmente, um distúrbio que afeta a bexiga e não um anormalidade primária da bexiga, o que levou à hipótese da "síndrome de Pandora".[4] Como a CIF pode ser uma doença frustrante crônica, a orientação apropriada do proprietário, juntamente com a utilização de MAMO, analgésicos e possivelmente outros medicamentos podem, quase sempre, propiciar EA suficiente para possibilitar a recuperação clínica de casos agudos e crônicos da enfermidade.

Entretanto, além do tratamento, nós, veterinários, fizemos o juramento de utilizar nosso conhecimento científico e habilidades para proteger a saúde e o bem-estar animal, bem como prevenir e aliviar o sofrimento do animal. Em razão da comprovação dos efeitos do confinamento em gatos,[67,102,122,123] aconselho a implementação efetiva de EA, como cuidado de saúde preventivo, para todos os gatos, conforme necessário para sua saúde e seu bem-estar, assim como o fornecimento de dieta satisfatória, vacinação apropriada e controle de parasitas.

REFERÊNCIAS BIBLIOGRÁFICAS

As referências bibliográficas deste capítulo se encontram online no Ambiente de Aprendizagem.

CAPÍTULO 335

Doenças da Uretra

Joseph W. Bartges

As doenças da uretra são comuns em cães e gatos, quase sempre associadas a doenças da bexiga. Os sinais clínicos de doenças da uretra incluem polaciúria, estrangúria, periúria, hematúria (ver Capítulo 47), obstrução do fluxo urinário ou incontinência urinária (ver Capítulo 46). O exame físico deve incluir palpação da região perineal, exame retal (a uretra pélvica é palpável através da parede retal que segue dorsal aos ossos pélvicos) e exame da genitália externa. O exame de urina (ver Capítulo 72) é importante, já que pode indicar evidências de infecções ou neoplasias. Exames de imagem, como radiografia do abdome, uretrocistografia contrastada (ver Capítulo 124) e cistoscopia (ver Capítulo 108), podem ser necessários para o diagnóstico. O exame ultrassonográfico (US) da uretra é limitado pela pelve (ver Capítulo 88).

INCOMPETÊNCIA DO MECANISMO DO ESFÍNCTER DA URETRA

A incompetência do mecanismo do esfíncter da uretra (IMEU) degenerativa é a causa mais comum de incontinência urinária em cães; ocorre principalmente em fêmeas castradas vários anos após a ovário-histerectomia (ver Capítulo 333).[1,2] Os sinais clínicos incluem micção inconsciente, notando-se a presença de urina no local onde o cão deita; porém, enquanto acordado, a micção é normal e não ocorre incontinência. Em casos de incontinência urinária, é comum a ocorrência de infecção do trato urinário (ITU) causada por bactéria e frequentemente não está associada à presença de sedimento urinário ativo. A ITU agrava a incontinência urinária. Os tratamentos normalmente empregados consistem em medicamentos estrogênicos ou alfa-agonistas, sozinhos ou em combinação. Cães que não respondem a esses medicamentos podem ser submetidos à aplicação cirúrgica de agentes de preenchimento uretral ou implantação de um oclusor de uretra hidráulico.[1,3-5]

DOENÇA ANATÔMICA CONGÊNITA DA URETRA

Ureter ectópico

Definição

Ureter ectópico é incluído neste capítulo porque a incontinência urinária é decorrência da abertura anormal da uretra ou da vagina (ver Capítulo 336). Normalmente, os ureteres adentram a superfície caudal dorsolateral da bexiga e desembocam no trígono vesical após um curto trajeto intramural. O ureter ectópico consiste na terminação de um ou ambos os ureteres em um local que não é o normal e provavelmente se deve a uma anormalidade embriológica do broto ureteral a partir do ducto mesonéfrico. O grau de desvio do broto ureteral de sua posição normal determina o local da abertura ectópica. O ureter ectópico pode ser unilateral ou bilateral, intramural ou extramural.

A inserção do ureter ectópico extramural ocorre no trígono, distalmente a uretra, vagina ou vestíbulo em fêmeas, ou ao ducto deferente em machos. O ureter ectópico intramural se insere no trígono, mas adentra a parede da uretra até desembocar distalmente. Variações do ureter ectópico intramural incluem depressão ureteral, aberturas ureterais duplas, aberturas fenestradas múltiplas e dois ureteres intramurais que desembocam em um único orifício.[6] O ureter ectópico pode estar associado a outras anomalias congênitas do trato urogenital, inclusive agenesia, hipoplasia ou displasia renal; hidroureter; ureterocele; remanescências do úraco, bexiga pélvica; constrições vulvovaginais; e persistência de hímen.[7,8]

Resenha

Ureteres ectópicos (mais frequentemente bilaterais e intramurais) são mais comumente diagnosticados em cadelas jovens (idade mediana de 10 meses).[8,9] Machos com ureter ectópico quase sempre são um pouco mais velhos (cerca de 24 meses) quando diagnosticados. Presume-se que vários machos nunca são diagnosticados porque mantêm a continência urinária em razão do comprimento de sua uretra e do seu esfíncter uretral externo.[9] As raças que supostamente são mais predispostas à ocorrência de ureter ectópico são Husky Siberiano, Labrador Retriever, Golden Retriever, Terranova, Buldogue Inglês, West Highland White Terrier, Fox Terrier, Skye Terrier, Poodle Miniatura e Poodle Toy.[8] Na maioria dos casos, pode haver uma base genética, mas não está comprovada. Gatos são raramente diagnosticados com ureter ectópico.

Sinais clínicos e exame físico

Incontinência urinária intermitente ou contínua desde o nascimento ou desmame é o sinal clínico mais frequentemente relatado em cães com ureter ectópico. A maioria, entretanto, também parece urinar normalmente. Os achados no exame físico geralmente são pouco notáveis, com exceção da presença de pelos úmidos ou manchados por urina na região perivulvar ou prepucial. A assadura por urina pode causar dermatite secundária, e os tutores podem relatar lambedura frequente da região vulvar ou prepucial. Algumas cadelas desenvolvem vulvovaginite, constrição vulvovaginal ou persistência de hímen, condições que podem ser detectadas por meio de palpação digital ou vaginoscopia. Cerca de dois terços desses animais têm histórico de ITU.[6]

Diagnóstico

Deve-se realizar radiografia simples para avaliar o tamanho, o formato e a localização dos rins e da bexiga. Podem-se utilizar urografia excretora combinada com pneumocistografia, US de abdome, uretrocistografia contrastada com refluxo vesicoureteral, fluoroscopia ou tomografia computadorizada (TC) contrastada para o diagnóstico de ureter ectópico (Figura 335.1).[8,10] A uretrocistoscopia (ver Capítulo 108) é excelente, especialmente quando combinada com outros exames de imagem.[8] A dilatação do ureter ectópico é frequente, mas nem sempre presente.

Tratamento – cirurgia

Alguns cães podem responder parcial ou completamente aos fármacos utilizados para IMEU. Embora o tratamento medicamentoso possa ajudar no controle da incontinência urinária, prefere-se a correção cirúrgica ou ablação por *laser*. Um ureter ectópico extramural pode ser ligado em sua terminação distal e reimplantado na bexiga entre o ápice e o trígono vesical (neoureterocistostomia). No momento da cirurgia, deve-se obter amostra da parede da bexiga ou de urina da pelve renal para cultura microbiológica por causa da frequência de ITU bacteriana. Tradicionalmente, os ureteres ectópicos intramurais são tratados mediante a ligadura do segmento ureteral submucoso distal e criação de uma nova abertura ureteral no trígono da

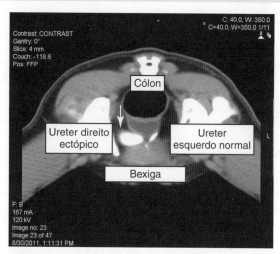

Figura 335.1 Imagem obtida em tomografia computadorizada (TC) excretora contrastada de uma cadela Poodle Standard, castrada, de 12 meses de idade, mostra ureter esquerdo normal, com fluxo de contraste em direção à bexiga, na altura do trígono vesical, e ureter direito dilatado que adentra a bexiga no trígono, mas forma um "túnel" na parte distal.

bexiga (neoureterostomia e reconstrução uretra-trígono); no entanto, em vários pacientes (44 a 67%), a incontinência urinária persiste porque o segmento intramural do ureter compromete a anatomia funcional do mecanismo do esfíncter uretral interno.[8,11,12]

Tratamento – laser

Pode-se utilizar ablação por *laser* transuretral para a correção de ureteres ectópicos intramurais (ver Capítulo 124). Um endoscópio rígido (em fêmeas) ou flexível (em machos) é introduzido de forma retrógrada na uretra; realiza-se uretrocistoscopia diagnóstica. Um cateter é introduzido no lúmen do ureter ectópico a fim de proteger a parede da uretra. Uma fibra a *laser*, diodo ou de preferência Hólmio:YAG, é introduzida através do canal de trabalho do cistoscópio e utilizada para a transecção da parede livre do ureter ectópico até que a abertura esteja o mais próximo possível da localização anatômica normal do trígono vesical.[13-16] Em casos de ureteres ectópicos intramurais, a incontinência urinária pode persistir porque pode haver comprometimento dos mecanismos do esfíncter uretral interno e da uretra proximal.[17] Após o procedimento a *laser*, parece que os cães são mais propensos à continência urinária do que após a cirurgia. Em cães com um rim que não pode ser recuperado por causa da hidronefrose ou pielonefrite, pode-se realizar nefroureterectomia.

Aplasia e hipoplasia da uretra

A aplasia uretral é uma anomalia congênita rara, caracterizada pela ausência total de uretra patente. A incontinência urinária está associada à ectopia dos ureteres.[18,19] Em gatas jovens, há relato de hipoplasia uretral, juntamente com incontinência urinária de início juvenil.[20-22] O diagnóstico é baseado nos sinais clínicos e exames de imagem. As características radiográficas consistem em encurtamento da uretra e aplasia vaginal. A hipoplasia uretral pode ser concomitante a outras anomalias congênitas e ITU bacteriana. Alguns cães respondem à terapia simpatomimética. A reconstrução cirúrgica do colo da bexiga pode melhorar ou resolver os sinais clínicos.[21,22]

Epispadia e hipospadia

Definições

Epispadia é um defeito congênito na face dorsal da uretra distal. A hipospadia é uma malposição ventral anômala do meato uretral.[23] Epispadia foi associada à extrofia da bexiga em uma cadela da raça Buldogue Inglês de 8 meses de idade.[24] Hipospadia é mais comumente observada em machos. Cães das raças Boston Terrier e Dálmata foram considerados os mais acometidos.[23,25] Também foi descrita em um gato Himalaio.[26] Ademais, foi relatada em um cão de trenó na Groenlândia, após potencial exposição intrauterina a 320 μg de organoclorado/dia (128 pg TEQ/kg/dia), valor 32 a 128 vezes acima das recomendações da Organização Mundial da Saúde (OMS) e do limiar para efeitos teratogênicos e reprodutivos.[27] A anomalia é rara e sua etiologia é incerta. Ela é classificada em glandular, peniana, escrotal, perineal ou anal, de acordo com a localização da abertura uretral, e pode ser considerada discreta, moderada ou grave. Na forma grave pode ocorrer subdesenvolvimento ou ausência do pênis, incapacidade de fusão do escroto e incapacidade de fechamento da uretra na região perineal. Outras anormalidades associadas à hipospadia são retenção de testículos, agenesia renal, defeitos ósseos ou anorretais, hérnia umbilical, hidrocefalia, incontinência urinária e ITU ascendente.[23,28] Pode-se realizar exame cromossômico para diferenciar hipospadia de hermafroditismo verdadeiro.[25]

Histórico, exame físico, diagnóstico e tratamento

Os cães acometidos são diagnosticados em várias idades; alguns não manifestam sinais clínicos, enquanto outros apresentam incontinência urinária, dermatite periuretral ou ITU bacteriana.[28,30] O diagnóstico frequentemente é baseado no exame físico. Cães machos afetados possuem um meato uretral ventral anormal que pode estar localizado em qualquer lugar ao longo da haste peniana, do escroto ou períneo, em geral associado à malformação do prepúcio e/ou pênis.[28,29] Em cadelas há relato de hipospadia juntamente com intersexo genético. Embriologicamente, a hipospadia resulta da fusão incompleta da prega urogenital. A presença de *osso peniano* em cães na maioria dos casos impede a reconstrução cirúrgica. A uretrostomia escrotal ou perineal combinada com a castração e remoção de vestígios prepuciais e tecidos penianos podem ter importância estética. Foram descritos encurtamento do pênis, amputação e reconstrução da uretra.[31-34] Uma técnica descreveu reconstrução significante, uretrostomia e amputação parcial do pênis. Essa técnica pode ser realizada na hipospadia glandular ou peniana, ou após ressecção da parte ventral do prepúcio distal, quando há tecido inadequado para sutura/fechamento simples em duas camadas.[35]

Malformações uretrogenitais

As malformações uretrogenitais são observadas em casos de intersexo; quase sempre o pseudo-hermafroditismo está associado à incontinência urinária.[36] Pseudo-hermafroditas possuem gônadas de um gênero e genitália externa de outro.[37] Ocorre em ambos os sexos, como resultado do desenvolvimento simultâneo de estruturas derivadas do ducto mülleriano (oviduto, útero e partes da vagina) e masculinização do seio urogenital. O fenótipo (aparência) depende do grau de masculinização do seio urogenital. A incontinência urinária provavelmente resulta da retenção de urina nas comunicações anômalas entre uretra e trato genital, que então extravasa passivamente.[38] A anomalia se manifesta no início da vida e pode ser acompanhada de ITU.[38] O diagnóstico é baseado nos sinais clínicos e exames de imagem. A incontinência urinária pode ser resolvida com correção cirúrgica.[36]

Foram descritos divertículos uretrais prostáticos em cães machos, juntamente com uretra intrapélvica anormalmente curta e ampla, colo vesical alargado e anomalias de ureteres.[39] Isso parece semelhante a uma condição descrita em um recém-nascido com membrana uretral posterior obstrutiva congênita, no qual uma membrana se estendeu em sentido proximal a partir do colículo seminal em direção ao colo da bexiga. Ao mesmo tempo que isso frequentemente resulta em doença renal crônica, um grau discreto de obstrução e de mecanismos protetores contra pressão foi relatado, que resulta em dilatação do utrículo prostático.[40]

Duplicação da uretra

A duplicação da uretra é uma anomalia congênita incomum descrita somente em cães jovens.[41-45] Por causa da íntima associação entre o desenvolvimento embrionário dos sistemas urogenital e gastrintestinal, a duplicação da uretra é quase sempre acompanhada de outras anomalias de duplicação. As anomalias resultam de divisão anormal da linha média sagital e subsequente desenvolvimento paralelo do intestino grosso, cloaca, reto ou seio urogenital.[46] Anomalias associadas dependem do estágio no qual ocorre a dismorfogênese. O exame físico pode revelar anormalidades anatômicas, incontinência urinária ou sinais clínicos associados à ITU bacteriana secundária. O diagnóstico é baseado nos achados de exame físico, exames de imagem e cirurgia exploratória. Em alguns casos, a duplicação da uretra pode ser passível de extirpação cirúrgica da estrutura duplicada; entretanto, em casos de duplicação extensa raramente se tenta a reconstrução cirúrgica.

Uretra ectópica

A uretra ectópica é caracterizada por posicionamento anormal do orifício uretral externo. Embriologicamente, a ectopia da uretra resulta da morfogênese anômala do seio urogenital, dos ductos paramesonéfricos (ductos müllerianos) ou mesonéfricos.[47] Os sinais clínicos dependem do local da terminação da uretra e de outras anomalias urogenitais concomitantes. Em uma fêmea da raça Buldogue Inglês de 21 meses de idade e com ectopia de ureter unilateral e uretra ectópica desembocando na parte distal da vagina, a incontinência urinária por toda a vida foi a característica clínica predominante.[48] Diferentemente, uma gata de 2 meses de idade da raça Doméstico de Pelo Curto, com uretra ectópica desembocando na parte ventral do reto, não apresentava incontinência urinária, mas o fluxo de urina saía pelo ânus.[49]

Fístulas uretrorretais, uretrovaginais e uretroperineais e divertículo uretral

Fístulas que conectam o lúmen uretral ao intestino grosso, vagina e região perineal foram descritas em cães e gatos.[44,50-57] Fístulas uretrorretais congênitas ocorrem por causa da falha na separação da cloaca fetal em segmento uretrovesical anterior e segmento posterior retal, pelo septo urorretal, resultando em comunicação permanente entre a uretra e o reto. Micropênis e fístula da linha média vestíbulo-perineal foram descritos em dois cães com incontinência urinária e considerados intersexos (cariótipo 78XX).[58] Também foi descrita como uma doença adquirida causada pela formação de abscessos prostáticos em um cão; todavia, pode ocorrer em decorrência de lesões traumáticas e doenças inflamatórias ou neoplásicas.[53,59] Machos parecem ser mais frequentemente afetados, e os cães da raça Buldogue Inglês parecem mais predispostos à fístula uretrorretal.[59] Os sinais clínicos se devem à passagem anormal de urina a partir da fístula durante a micção. Outros sintomas podem incluir diarreia, dermatite perineal e sinais clínicos associados à ITU bacteriana secundária. Fístulas foram associadas à urolitíase causada por estruvita induzida por infecção.[51,53,55] O diagnóstico é baseado em sinais clínicos e exames de imagem (Figura 335.2). O tratamento consiste em correção cirúrgica ou desvio da urina. A terapia conservadora (cateter urinário de demora, dieta com baixo teor de resíduos e antibióticos) foi efetiva em um cão com fístula uretrorretal secundária a um abscesso de próstata.[53]

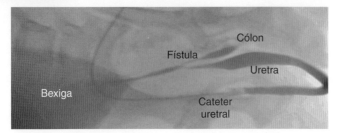

Figura 335.2 Uretrograma contrastado com a utilização de fluoroscópio mostra uma fístula uretrocolônica em um cão Buldogue Inglês, macho, não castrado, com 1 ano de idade.

Prolapso da uretra

Ocorre prolapso uretral quando a uretra distal sofre protrusão através do orifício uretral do pênis. O prolapso se apresenta como uma massa avermelhada ou roxa na extremidade do pênis em cães com menos de 5 anos de idade (Figura 335.3);[60] as raças Buldogue Inglês e Boston Terrier parecem predispostas.[61-63] O prolapso da uretra pode não estar associado a sinais clínicos ou o tutor pode notar apenas uma "massa" avermelhada a roxa na extremidade do pênis durante a micção; entretanto, o prolapso pode estar associado ao gotejamento de sangue, lambedura do prepúcio ou do pênis, ou sinais de doença do trato urinário inferior (ver Capítulos 44, 45 e 46). O diagnóstico é baseado no exame físico; o prolapso deve ser diferenciado de neoplasia. Se o prolapso da uretra estiver associado a sinais clínicos discretos, ou ausentes, pode não ser necessário tratamento.[64] O tratamento de prolapso da uretra consiste na tentativa de reduzir manualmente o tecido prolapsado; a lavagem com solução salina hipertônica pode facilitar a tentativa. Em seguida, faz-se a sutura em bolsa de tabaco frouxa; contudo, é comum a ocorrência de recidiva. A redução cirúrgica ou uretropexia é o tratamento preferido.[63]

Constrição e hipoplasia da uretra

Hipoplasia e constrições uretrais congênitas foram descritas em cães e gatos jovens.[21,65] Os sinais clínicos se devem à obstrução parcial ou total da uretra, no caso de constrição, ou incontinência urinária, no caso de hipoplasia (ver Capítulos 44 a 46). Sintomas sistêmicos, distensão ou ruptura da bexiga, incontinência por fluxo excessivo de urina, ITU bacteriana secundária ou hidronefrose podem acompanhar a obstrução do fluxo ou incontinência urinária em casos de hipoplasia da uretra. Há relato de incontinência urinária, hidroureter bilateral e hidronefrose em um cão Pastor-Alemão, macho, de 8 meses de idade, com constrição na parte média da uretra congênita.[65] O tratamento consiste em cirurgia. Se ocorrer constrição na uretra extrapélvica, pode-se realizar uretrostomia; se ocorrer na uretra intrapélvica ou intra-abdominal, então podem-se indicar ressecção da uretra e anastomose ou uretrostomia pré-púbica.[66,67] A dilatação da constrição da uretra também pode ser tentada com balão ou cateter introdutor Bougie. A incontinência urinária secundária à hipoplasia da uretra pode ser tratada por meio de cirurgia ou uso de um oclusor hidráulico uretral, com sucesso variável.[21]

Incontinência urinária congênita

Várias anomalias congênitas estão associadas à incontinência urinária. Além daquelas descritas em seções anteriores, o disrafismo espinal (malformações semelhantes a fendas na coluna e medula espinal resultantes de fechamento incompleto do tubo neural) causa incontinência urinária e fecal. IMEU congênita foi descrita em cães e gatos com hipoplasia uretral[21] ou em pseudo-hermafroditas com anormalidades neurogênicas;[38] no entanto, o ureter ectópico está mais comumente associado à incontinência urinária juvenil.[8,14,68]

DOENÇA URETRAL METABÓLICA – URETROLITÍASE E TAMPÕES URETRAIS DE MATRIZ CRISTALINA E OBSTRUÇÃO DA URETRA EM GATOS

Definições

A uropatia obstrutiva refere-se a anormalidades na estrutura e função do trato urinário causadas por comprometimentos do fluxo normal da urina e efeitos resultantes locais e sistêmicos desses comprometimentos.[69,70] A anormalidade do fluxo através da uretra, seja por obstrução física (Figura 335.4), seja por disfunção do músculo detrusor ou da uretra, é a causa dos sinais clínicos. Embora haja várias causas de obstrução uretral, a urolitíase é a mais comum em cães (ver Capítulo 331), sendo os tampões uretrais de matriz cristalina e os urólitos as causas mais comuns em gatos (ver Capítulo 332). Cerca de 10 a 20% dos gatos com sintomas relativos ao trato urinário inferior apresentam urolitíase ou tampões uretrais. Os urólitos de estruvita e oxalato de cálcio são os mais comumente relatados.[71] A maioria dos tampões uretrais contém grande quantidade de matriz (mucoproteína, contendo muco e restos de produtos inflamatórios), com quantidades variáveis de minerais. Os cristais são aprisionados na matriz. Supostamente, o muco é secretado pela bexiga e por células da mucosa uretral em resposta a um estímulo irritante ou inflamatório. A matriz

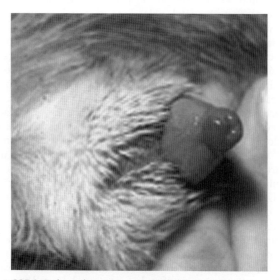

Figura 335.3 Prolapso da uretra em um cão Buldogue Inglês não castrado de 2 anos de idade.

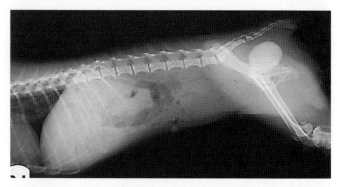

Figura 335.4 Imagem lateral do abdome, obtida em radiografia simples, de uma cadela da raça Yorkshire Terrier castrada, de 3 anos de idade, com obstrução da uretra causada por urólito de estruvita formado em razão da infecção e uroabdome ocasionado por ruptura da bexiga.

também contém tecido necrosado ou sangue, com ou sem células inflamatórias. Quase sempre os tampões uretrais de matriz cristalina se alojam na extremidade do pênis, onde há estreitamento da uretra, mas podem se alojar em qualquer local da uretra.

Consequências clínicas

As consequências clínicas da obstrução da uretra são, geralmente, mas nem sempre, associadas a sintomas de uremia. A obstrução parcial ou inicial do fluxo de urina pode não prejudicar a função renal o suficiente para causar uremia; entretanto, os sinais clínicos de uremia em geral surgem dentro de 24 h após a obstrução total da uretra. À medida que a massa renal funcional diminui ou que aumentam as pressões intravesical, ureteral e renal, ocorrem perda da capacidade de concentração da urina, aumento do volume de urina tubular renal e da pressão tubular, o que ocasiona azotemia e uremia. A detecção e remoção precoce da obstrução podem propiciar resolução imediata dos sintomas urêmicos, embora as anormalidades renais possam persistir por algum tempo. Ademais, a obstrução da uretra pode causar atonia do detrusor, lesão uretral, dano à mucosa da uretra e da bexiga, ITU ou ruptura de uretra ou bexiga.

Sinais clínicos, exame físico, resultados de exames laboratoriais

Os sintomas de uropatia obstrutiva variam dependendo de vários fatores: grau de comprometimento do fluxo urinário, duração da doença e presença de ITU bacteriana. Pacientes com obstrução da uretra podem ter ou não sinais clínicos prévios de doença do trato urinário inferior. Eles podem manifestar apenas sinais clínicos relativos ao trato urinário inferior, como disúria, hematúria, polaciúria, incapacidade de eliminar urina, ou dor (ver Capítulos 44, 45 e 46). Eles podem, porém, apresentar sintomas polissistêmicos de uremia: êmese, anorexia e obnubilação. Os tutores podem confundir animais com obstrução com aqueles com constipação intestinal, ou com dor abdominal ou nas costas.

O exame físico pode indicar um cão saudável ou um gravemente enfermo. É possível palpar uma bexiga grande e dolorosa. Bradicardia, hipotermia, palidez de membranas mucosas, tempo de preenchimento capilar prolongado, hiperpneia e halitose podem estar presentes. A extremidade do pênis pode estar roxoescura e edemaciada, e um ou mais urólitos podem ser palpados na uretra. Sempre que possível, deve-se realizar exame retal, a fim de excluir a possibilidade de um urólito na uretra pélvica ou obstrução da uretra por neoplasia ou doença de próstata. Devem ser coletadas amostras para a realização de hemograma, perfil bioquímico sérico, exame de urina e urocultura. Pode-se realizar cistocentese, com sucesso, mesmo em casos de obstrução uretral, desde que se tenha cuidado ao introduzir a agulha, direcionando sua extremidade no sentido do trígono, ao mesmo tempo que se mantém a bexiga estabilizada (ver Capítulo 105). Assim que ocorre a estabilização do animal, deve-se realizar radiografia simples do abdome. Podem ser realizados outros exames de imagem, como ultrassonografia (ver Capítulo 88), uretrocistografia contrastada ou uretrocistoscopia (ver Capítulo 108).

Tratamento – estabilização emergencial

As prioridades no tratamento de um paciente com obstrução da uretra dependem do grau de obstrução e da condição clínica geral do paciente. Se o animal estiver extremamente deprimido, deve-se fornecer oxigênio (ver Capítulo 131), introduzir um cateter IV (ver Capítulo 75) e obter amostras de sangue e de urina. Nos Capítulos 127, 129, 150 e 322 há uma revisão completa sobre o tratamento de tais emergências, inclusive fluidoterapia e correção de anormalidades eletrolíticas. Assim que estabilizado, o animal pode ser submetido à sedação ou anestesia, a fim de liberar a obstrução da uretra. Se o animal apresenta depressão intensa ou inconsciência, a liberação da obstrução da

uretra pode ser possível sem sedação ou anestesia. Em alguns cães machos, pode-se introduzir um cateter/sonda urinária, enquanto o cão estiver acordado, e os uretrólitos empurrados por meio de hidropropulsão em direção à bexiga sem sedação ou anestesia.

Vários protocolos estão disponíveis para facilitar a liberação da obstrução da uretra, inclusive: morfina (0,1 a 0,3 mg/kg IM), butorfanol (0,2 a 0,4 mg/kg IV ou IM), propofol (2 a 4 mg/kg IV), barbitúricos de curta ação (5 mg/kg IV), anestesia inalatória com isoflurano e cetamina (2,5 a 5 mg/kg IV), juntamente com diazepam (0,125 a 0,25 mg/kg IV) ou midazolam (0,125 a 0,25 mg/kg IV ou IM) ou acepromazina (0,05 a 0,1 mg/kg IV). A cistocentese, se necessária, deve ser realizada com a utilização de uma agulha de diâmetro 22 e comprimento de 1½ polegada, ou de um cateter de diâmetro 22 conectado a um equipo de extensão IV e torneira de 3 vias, a fim de descomprimir a bexiga e coletar as amostras necessárias. É importante estabilizar a agulha ou o cateter, a fim de evitar maiores danos à bexiga, ruptura vesical e uroabdome. A desobstrução da uretra deve ser realizada o mais rápido possível. Em gatos, um tampão uretral de matriz cristalina pode ser deslocado mediante massagem da parte distal do pênis, segurando-o entre o polegar e dedo indicador, e aplicando ligeira pressão na bexiga. Se a obstrução não for liberada, deve-se realizar hidropropulsão retrógrada.

Liberação de tampões uretrais de matriz cristalina em gatos (ver Capítulo 107)

Assim que estabilizado, o gato é posicionado em decúbito lateral ou dorsal e o pênis é exteriorizado da bainha prepucial puxando-a em direção caudodorsal e tornando a uretra reta. A extremidade do pênis e os tecidos periuretrais são cuidadosamente limpos e introduz-se com cuidado a ponta de um cateter de polipropileno TomCat® com abertura na extremidade, de calibre 3,5 French (Fr), lubrificado no orifício uretral externo, e o lúmen da uretra peniana é lavado com 12 mℓ de solução estéril (Vídeo 335.1). Esse procedimento geralmente é bem-sucedido ao lavar o material que causava obstrução de volta para a bexiga. Não lave a uretra com lidocaína, pois ela pode ser absorvida e se tornar tóxica. A massagem da uretra pélvica VR pode ajudar a deslocar o tampão.

Liberação de urólitos (ver Capítulo 107)

Retropulsão de urólitos em cães machos com obstrução

Os urólitos que causam obstrução da uretra devem ser submetidos à retropulsão em direção à bexiga, com a utilização de uma solução lubrificante estéril, composta de uma parte de lubrificante estéril e uma parte de água estéril.[75] O clínico pode colocar 15 mℓ de solução lubrificante estéril em uma seringa de 35 mℓ e 15 a 20 mℓ de solução estéril em outra seringa de 35 mℓ. Conecte as seringas a uma torneira de 3 vias, adicione a solução estéril à solução lubrificante e então passe a mistura para a frente e para trás, de uma seringa a outra, várias vezes. Como alternativa, adicione a solução estéril à solução lubrificante estéril em uma seringa e deixe em repouso durante 5 a 10 min. Submeta o cão ou o gato à anestesia ou sedação. Introduza um cateter de borracha (5 a 8 Fr), em cães, ou um cateter de polipropileno (3,5-Fr), em gatos, até o local da obstrução. Faça a infusão da mistura da solução lubrificante e com a solução estéril para lubrificar a uretra. Às vezes, isso é suficiente para empurrar os uretrólitos em direção à bexiga.

Se necessário, conecte uma seringa com fluido estéril à sonda uretral. Em seguida, oclua a porção proximal da uretra por meio de palpação retal, aplicando pressão digital para aprisionar a uretra contra o assoalho pélvico. Ao mesmo tempo, oclua a uretra peniana distal e infunda a solução estéril sob pressão. Quando a uretra estiver distendida, libere a oclusão da uretra pélvica. Frequentemente, à medida que os urólitos são empurrados em direção à bexiga, percebe-se uma sensação de "estalo" e a pessoa que realiza a palpação retal geralmente pode sentir a movimentação dos urólitos na direção cranial. Urólitos passíveis a esse procedimento incluem urato e cistina, por causa de sua textura lisa, a maioria dos cálculos de estruvita e alguns de oxalato de cálcio, pela textura da superfície. Esse procedimento não é efetivo se os urólitos estiverem incrustados na mucosa da uretra ou se houver uma constrição uretral proximal ao urólito. Um tratamento alternativo para uretrólitos é a litotripsia (ver Capítulo 124).[76-79]

Cadelas e gatos, machos ou fêmeas

Ocasionalmente, cadelas e gatos apresentam obstrução da uretra causada por urolitíase. Uretrólitos geralmente são palpáveis ao exame retal e podem ser empurrados para a bexiga utilizando uma combinação de cateterização da uretra e lavagem e movimentação digital do urólito VR.

Cateteres urinários de demora (ver Capítulo 106)

A decisão sobre a colocação de um cateter urinário de demora com sistema fechado depende da dificuldade de liberar a obstrução da uretra, do fluxo de urina obtido, da quantidade de cristais e/ou resíduos gelatinosos na urina após lavagem copiosa da bexiga, do grau de distensão excessiva da bexiga, da probabilidade de atonia do músculo detrusor, da gravidade da doença sistêmica e da causa da obstrução uretral. A administração de um antagonista de receptores alfa-2 (prazosina ou fenoxibenzamina) ajuda a diminuir o espasmo da uretra causado pela cateterização.[80,81] Dependendo da causa da obstrução uretral, deve-se realizar tratamento definitivo e adotar medidas preventivas apropriadas.[82] Durante o tempo de permanência do cateter urinário de demora, não se devem administrar antibióticos. Embora os antibióticos reduzam a ocorrência de ITU bacteriana, quando ocorrem infecções, elas exibem um maior grau de resistência antimicrobiana.[83] Em um estudo sobre cistite estéril induzida em gatos com cateter urinário permanente, constatou-se que alguns gatos tratados com amoxicilina desenvolveram cistite bacteriana, e as culturas bacterianas de amostras de rim obtidas durante a necropsia foram positivas.[84]

Complicações

Infecção bacteriana

A infecção bacteriana pode estar presente antes da obstrução da uretra ou ser introduzida durante os procedimentos utilizados para liberar a obstrução (ver Capítulo 330). A urina alcalina associada a infecções por microrganismos produtores de urease pode predispor à cristalúria por estruvita e urolitíase ou formação de tampões uretrais de matriz de estruvita. A erradicação da infecção é difícil enquanto persistir a estase urinária. Os sinais de infecção do trato urinário podem persistir após a liberação da obstrução da uretra. A obstrução do fluxo de urina predispõe o trato urinário superior a infecções bacterianas ascendentes por causa do refluxo vesicoureteral.

Anormalidade da micção

Após um período prolongado de retenção urinária, os animais podem ter dificuldade para esvaziar completamente a bexiga (ver Capítulo 333). Isso pode ocorrer em razão da diminuição da elasticidade vesical, lesão aos nervos, dano aos elementos contráteis, ou edema/inflamação uretral, resultando em espasmo uretral.[85] Atonia do detrusor, edema ou espasmo uretral podem persistir durante períodos imprevisíveis, dependendo da doença primária e do grau de dano irreversível causado pela obstrução da uretra, e isso pode influenciar a sobrevida.

Diurese pós-obstrução

A liberação da obstrução da uretra é acompanhada de alteração na capacidade de modular o equilíbrio hídrico e de sódio. Essa diurese pós-obstrução pode ser intensa e comprometer o estado de hidratação e o equilíbrio eletrolítico, além de necessitar de administração de solução de uso IV ou SC durante dias, a fim de evitar desidratação (ver Capítulo 322). A mensuração do débito urinário e do peso corporal após a liberação da obstrução da uretra ajuda a determinar o volume de líquido necessário para manter a hidratação.

Insuficiência renal intrínseca

Em casos de obstrução da uretra, embora a azotemia pós-renal ocorra mais comumente do que a azotemia renal, pode haver insuficiência renal primária (ver Capítulo 322). Fatores que podem contribuir para a ocorrência de insuficiência renal incluem perda do parênquima renal por causa da manutenção de pressão intrarrenal aumentada, produção de citocinas por leucócitos infiltrados no parênquima renal, desequilíbrios eletrolíticos, fibrose do parênquima renal lesionado e isquemia em razão da desidratação associada à obstrução uretral e diurese pós-obstrução.[86]

Morte

A uropatia obstrutiva que persiste por mais de 24 h quase sempre resulta em uremia pós-renal. A pressão retrógrada induzida pela obstrução prejudica a filtração glomerular, o fluxo sanguíneo renal e a função tubular.[87] Após a obstrução da uretra de gatos normais, constatou-se morte dos animais depois de 3 a 6 dias como consequência da insuficiência cardiopulmonar associada a desequilíbrios hidreletrolíticos ou insuficiência renal aguda oligúrica/anúrica.[73] O dano à superfície mucosa da bexiga e a presença de ITU bacteriana abrevia a sobrevida.

Prognóstico

O prognóstico para animais com obstrução da uretra depende da causa, da facilidade da desobstrução e do sucesso da terapia preventiva. Em um estudo com 45 gatos, machos, com obstrução da uretra, constatou-se recidiva da obstrução devido a urólitos ou tampões de matriz cristalina em cerca de um terço dos animais, recidiva dos sinais clínicos em cerca de metade e necessidade de eutanásia em 20%.[88] O principal componente mineral dos tampões uretrais de matriz cristalina em gatos é a estruvita; portanto, medidas preventivas devem incluir a modificação da dieta, a fim de prevenir a nova formação de cristais nesses gatos.

Caso não seja possível a liberação da obstrução (i. e., a desobstrução), se a obstrução for recorrente apesar do tratamento apropriado, ou se ocorrer trauma peniano durante a tentativa de desobstrução da uretra, deve-se realizar desvio cirúrgico do fluxo urinário (uretrostomia escrotal ou uretrostomia perineal).[89,90] As complicações da uretrostomia escrotal em cães consistem em hemorragia durante a cirurgia ou constrição no local após o procedimento. A uretrostomia perineal em gatos pode estar associada à formação de constrições, extravasamento de urina ou ITU bacteriana recorrente.[89,91-93] Na obstrução da uretra causada por neoplasia, podem ser utilizados extensores uretrais ou sonda/cateter de cistostomia (ver Capítulo 124).[94]

DOENÇA URETRAL NEOPLÁSICA

Neoplasia primária da uretra é incomum em cães e gatos. A extensão de neoplasias à uretra acontece em alguns casos de carcinoma de célula de transição da bexiga e de carcinoma de célula escamosa da próstata; contudo, há relatos de outras neoplasias.[95-104] O diagnóstico é obtido por meio de palpação da uretra VR, uretrografia contrastada, ou cistoscopia (Figuras 335.5 e 335.6). O tratamento consiste na remoção cirúrgica ou ablação a laser e/ou quimioterapia (ver Capítulo 351); também pode ser realizada a introdução de um extensor uretral para liberar a obstrução (Figura 335.7; ver Capítulo 124).[105-107]

CAPÍTULO 335 • Doenças da Uretra

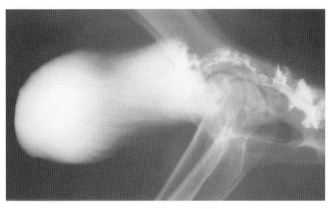

Figura 335.5 Uretrografia contrastada em uma cadela mestiça Chow-Chow, castrada, de 10 anos de idade, com carcinoma de célula de transição da uretra.

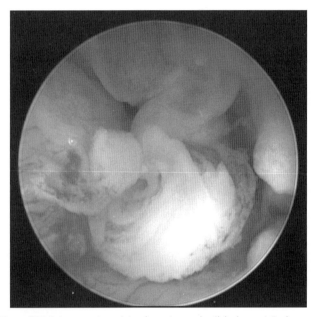

Figura 335.6 Imagem cistoscópica de carcinoma de célula de transição da uretra de uma cadela mestiça Staffordshire Terrier, castrada, com 10 anos de idade.

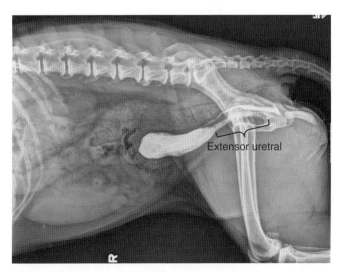

Figura 355.7 Vaginouretrocistografia contrastada lateral de uma cadela mestiça Staffordshire Terrier, castrada, de 10 anos de idade, com carcinoma de célula de transição da uretra (ver Figura 335.6), após introdução de extensor uretral metálico, capaz de se autoexpandir.

DOENÇA URETRAL IDIOPÁTICA – DISSINERGIA REFLEXA

Definições

Durante a micção normal, ocorrem contração do músculo detrusor e relaxamento da uretra. Isso resulta na excreção da urina. A dissinergia reflexa, também denominada *obstrução funcional da uretra* ou *dissinergia uretral do detrusor*, acontece quando não há coordenação entre a contração do detrusor e o relaxamento da uretra durante a micção; a uretra não relaxa ou se contrai antes do esvaziamento da bexiga (ver Capítulo 333). Clinicamente, os animais tentam urinar sem sucesso ou o início da micção resulta em um fluxo normal de urina, que é interrompido mesmo que o animal tente continuar a micção. Algumas vezes o jato normal cessa completamente ou diminui, ocasionando micção em jatos ou gotas de urina. Em mais de 50% dos cães não é possível identificar a causa da dissinergia reflexa. Essa anormalidade pode estar associada a lesões medulares craniais ao segundo segmento medular lombar. Hipoteticamente, as lesões que poderiam causar dissinergia reflexa incluem aquelas do trato reticuloespinal, do núcleo de Oluf ou do gânglio mesentérico caudal, bem como a perda de sinais inibidores aos nervos pudendo e hipogástrico.[108]

Resenha, sinais clínicos e diagnóstico

A dissinergia reflexa acomete principalmente cães machos de meia-idade, de raças de grande porte e gigantes, embora cadelas e gatos possam ser afetados.[109-113] Conforme mencionado, o animal assume postura de micção e frequentemente apresenta um bom fluxo de urina inicial que, subitamente, é interrompido ou se transforma em jatos ou gotas de urina, apesar de mantidas as tentativas de urinar. O volume de urina residual na bexiga é grande por causa da obstrução funcional uretral. Após a micção, considera-se que os cães devam ter volume de urina residual inferior a 0,5 mℓ de urina/kg de peso corporal.[114] Após a interrupção das tentativas de urinar, pode ocorrer extravasamento de urina, condição que mimetiza a incontinência urinária por fluxo excessivo. Isso ocorre porque a hipertonicidade do esfíncter uretral interno supostamente é desencadeada pela micção. Em casos crônicos, a distensão excessiva da bexiga pode ocasionar certo grau de atonia do músculo detrusor, resultando em grande volume de urina residual. O diagnóstico baseia-se em informações obtidas no histórico clínico e na observação da micção do animal. Exames de imagem podem revelar grande volume da bexiga após a micção, e a uretrografia contrastada pode mostrar incapacidade de dilatação adequada da uretra proximal ou espasmo uretral. É importante realizar um exame neurológico minucioso (ver Capítulo 259), embora a maioria dos pacientes não apresente déficits neurológicos. O único sinal clínico pode ser dor, por exemplo, dor cervical durante a manipulação.

Tratamento

O tratamento consiste em induzir relaxamento da uretra e, ocasionalmente, estimulação da contração da bexiga. Alfabloqueadores, como prazosina, tansulosina e fenoxibenzamina, reduzem o tônus do músculo liso do esfíncter uretral interno. O relaxamento do músculo esquelético do esfíncter uretral externo pelo uso de benzodiazepínicos ou outros relaxantes (acepromazina, metocarbamol, dantroleno) pode ser útil.[114-118] Pode ser necessária a cateterização urinária intermitente asséptica pelos tutores no domicílio (ver Capítulos 105 e 106). Pode-se utilizar um cateter de cistostomia para prevenir a distensão excessiva da bexiga e, em casos refratários, pode-se introduzir um extensor uretral na parte da uretra que apresenta constrição ou espasmo, com base na uretrografia contrastada (ver Capítulo 124).[109] O prognóstico quase sempre é moderado a bom; entretanto, geralmente os pacientes necessitam de tratamento por toda a vida, pois ocorrem recidivas. O prognóstico é pior quando há atonia do músculo detrusor e ITU recorrente.

DOENÇA URETRAL INFLAMATÓRIA/INFECCIOSA

Uretrite refere-se à inflamação da uretra. A inflamação pode ser primária ou secundária a outras anormalidades, inclusive traumatismo, urolitíase ou neoplasia.[96,119] A uretrite frequentemente ocorre em casos de cistite bacteriana em cães, ou cistite idiopática em gatos. A inflamação se deve ao comprometimento do revestimento urotelial e pode resultar em ulceração e erosão tecidual. A uretrite proliferativa pode ser secundária à infecção bacteriana crônica ou à doença imunomediada. A uretrite granulomatosa ou linfoplasmocítica causa hiperplasia epitelial, infiltração de linfócitos e plasmócitos e infecções bacterianas crônicas.[120]

Os sinais clínicos são compatíveis com doenças do trato urinário inferior (ver Capítulos 44 a 47). O diagnóstico é confirmado mediante palpação da uretra VR, uretrografia contrastada ou cistoscopia (ver Capítulo 108). A biopsia da uretra confirma a inflamação. O tratamento consiste em terapia antimicrobiana e, possivelmente, anti-inflamatórios se houver uretrite granulomatosa. Pode-se tentar terapia anti-inflamatória com prednisona (1 mg/kg/24 h VO), ciclofosfamida (2,2 mg/kg/24 h VO 4 dias por semana), ou piroxicam (0,3 mg/kg/24 h VO). Em casos de uretrite proliferativa, recomenda-se terapia anti-inflamatória, conforme descrita, ou terapia imunossupressora (2 mg de azatioprina/kg VO, a cada 24 a 48 h, ou 2 mg de prednisona/kg/24 h VO), combinada com terapia antimicrobiana. Havendo obstrução da uretra, pode ser necessário o uso de um cateter de cistostomia até que ocorra regressão da infiltração inflamatória e da obstrução da uretra.[94]

DOENÇA URETRAL TRAUMÁTICA

O trauma uretral pode ser causado por lesões por contusão ou penetrantes, especialmente durante cateterização urinária traumática (Figura 335.8).[121-124] O traumatismo causado por acidente automobilístico sem lesões perfurantes pode ocasionar lesão da uretra em razão de fraturas púbicas ou do osso peniano. Pode ocorrer traumatismo de uretra iatrogênico durante a cateterização urinária, especialmente quando se utiliza cateter de polipropileno rígido (ver Capítulos 105 e 106). Os sinais clínicos estão relacionados ao trato urinário inferior. A urina pode se acumular no tecido subcutâneo ou no abdome. Hematúria pode ser o único sintoma. O diagnóstico é confirmado pela uretrografia contrastada ou cistoscopia. O tratamento consiste na introdução de um cateter urinário de demora e correção cirúrgica ou desvio do fluxo de urina.[121,122,125,126] Se não for possível a restauração da uretra, pode ser necessária a uretrostomia.

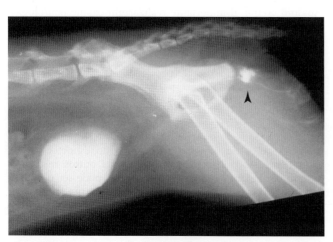

Figura 335.8 Perfuração da uretra (*ponta de seta preta*) causada por cateterização urinária forçada durante o procedimento para liberação de obstrução da uretra em um gato.

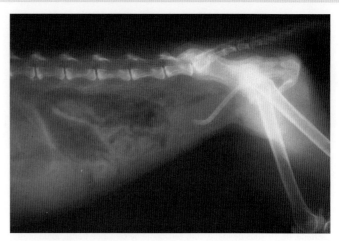

Figura 335.9 Incrustação mineralizada de um fragmento de cateter uretral retido em um gato castrado de 8 anos de idade.

CONSTRIÇÃO (ESTENOSE) DA URETRA

A constrição, ou estenose, uretral quase sempre é secundária a traumatismo uretral, especialmente durante a cateterização da uretra em gatos,[89,125] ou à cirurgia.[127,128] Clinicamente, cães e gatos com constrições uretrais apresentam esforço ao urinar, hematúria ou não conseguem urinar (ver Capítulos 44 a 47). Geralmente há histórico de evento traumático ou cirúrgico, embora a constrição da uretra possa ser decorrência de lesão neoplásica, como carcinoma de célula de transição. Se a constrição ocorre no local de um procedimento prévio de uretrostomia, o diagnóstico é confirmado por sua visualização na uretrografia contrastada, ou cistoscopia (ver Capítulo 108). O tratamento consiste em correção cirúrgica, dilatação do local da constrição ou introdução de um extensor uretral (ver Capítulo 124).[89,90,106,127,129,130]

CORPO ESTRANHO NA URETRA

Ocasionalmente, cães ou gatos com sinais clínicos de doença do trato urinário inferior e/ou obstrução uretral têm um corpo estranho na uretra. Entre os corpos estranhos relatados, incluem-se aparas de gramínea, bolinhas de chumbo, fragmento de palito de picolé migrante, que resultam na formação de urólitos de estruvita e urólitos de estruvita associado à agulha de costura.[131-134] Cateter uretral de demora pode atuar como corpo estranho, ocasionando sinais clínicos ou obstrução, caso o cão ou o gato mastigue a porção distal do cateter, o que resulta em retenção da porção proximal no lúmen do sistema urinário. Ele pode servir como um nicho de infecção ou incrustação (Figura 335.9). A remoção do corpo estranho resulta na resolução dos sinais clínicos, desde que não tenha ocorrido constrição uretral ou atonia do músculo detrusor. A prevenção do corpo estranho oriundo de fragmento de cateter retido consiste em assegurar que todo o cateter esteja presente quando removido pelo paciente ou pela equipe médica.

REFERÊNCIAS BIBLIOGRÁFICAS

As referências bibliográficas deste capítulo se encontram online no Ambiente de Aprendizagem.

CAPÍTULO 336

Doenças Congênitas do Trato Urinário Inferior

John M. Kruger, Joseph W. Bartges e Elizabeth A. Ballegeer

As anomalias congênitas do trato urinário de cães e gatos jovens podem ser decorrências de anormalidades hereditárias (genéticas) ou adquiridas que interferem na diferenciação e no crescimento do trato urinário em desenvolvimento ou de condições semelhantes que eventualmente interferem na estrutura ou função do sistema urinário já desenvolvido. A formação do sistema urinário depende de seu desenvolvimento sequencial e coordenado bem como da interação de tecidos embrionários múltiplos que envolvem a expressão de mais de 400 genes reguladores.[1-6] Apesar da extraordinária complexidade da organogênese do sistema urinário, anomalias congênitas da bexiga e da uretra são causas relativamente raras de doenças do trato urinário inferior.

ANOMALIAS DA JUNÇÃO URETEROVESICAL

Ureteres ectópicos (ectasia ureteral)

Ureteres ectópicos (UE) congênitos são caracterizados pela desembocadura de um ou de ambos os ureteres em um local diferente da parte craniolateral do trígono vesical.[7] A disembriogênese do broto ureteral e a falha da apoptose do ducto excretor comum durante a transposição do ureter resultam em aberturas ectópicas localizadas ao longo do trajeto de migração ureteral (condição denominada via ectópica).[8-11]

UE são classificados de acordo com o local da abertura anômala em relação ao colo vesical e o trajeto anatômico do ureter anômalo até a sua terminação. UE *intravesiculares* desembocam em locais caudais e mediais à sua posição normal na face craniolateral do trígono vesical, porém craniais ao colo da bexiga. UE *extravesiculares* desembocam em locais caudais ao ápice distal do trígono no colo vesical, uretra, útero ou vagina.[8,9,12-14] UE *intramurais* contactam a parede vesical normalmente, mas percorrem distalmente a submucosa através do trígono, antes de desembocarem na uretra ou na vagina (Figura 336.1).[7] UE intramurais também podem formar depressões ureterais, apresentar múltiplas aberturas ureterais ou não originar um orifício distal.[15] UE *extramurais* desviam totalmente da bexiga antes de desembocar na uretra, na vagina ou no útero (Figura 336.2). Cadelas parecem ser mais acometidas do que machos; entretanto, a prevalência de UE em machos pode estar subestimada.[8,14,16-18] A maioria dos UE verificada em cães, machos e fêmeas, é intramural e bilateral.[8,9,14,19-21] UE são considerados muito raros em gatos. Foram relatados apenas 31 casos de UE em gatos, dos quais 57% eram machos e 43% eram fêmeas.[20,22-40] Em gatos, a ampla maioria de UE é extramural, com prevalências semelhantes de malformações unilaterais (55%) e bilateral (45%). A uretra é o local mais comum de terminação de EU em cadelas e gatos. Em cães machos, a maioria dos UE desemboca no colo da bexiga ou na uretra pré-prostática.[8] Por causa da íntima relação entre o sistema de ductos metanéfricos e o desenvolvimento de órgãos urogenitais, os UE podem estar associados a outras anomalias congênitas concomitantes, como ectopia renal, aplasia/hipoplasia renal, ureterocele, remanescências de úraco, agenesia/hipoplasia de bexiga, agenesia ou ectopia uretral, incompetência do mecanismo do esfíncter uretral (ver Capítulo 333), malformações vestibulovaginais, fimose e criptorquidismo.[41,42]

Ureteres duplicados (duplos) associados à ectopia ureteral, hidroureter, hidronefrose e infecções do trato urinário também foram relatados em cães, machos e fêmeas, e em um gato.[28,43,44]

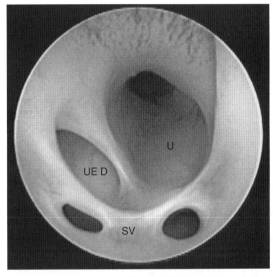

Figura 336.1 Imagem cistoscópica da uretra distal, vagina e vestíbulo em uma cadela da raça Husky Siberiano, castrada, de 2,5 anos de idade, com ureteres ectópicos intramurais bilaterais. Note a abertura do ureter ectópico intramural direito (*UE D*) na uretra distal (*U*) e um septo vaginal persistente (*SV*).

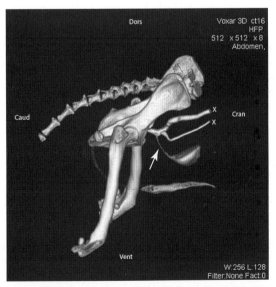

Figura 336.2 Imagem tridimensional reconstruída após urografia excretora por TC com contraste positivo obtida de um cão da raça Husky Siberiano, castrado, de 10 anos de idade, com histórico de 2 anos de incontinência urinária e ureteres ectópicos extramurais bilaterais. Note a dilatação dos ureteres ectópicos extramurais direito e esquerdo (*marcados por um X*), que adentram a uretra pré-prostática dorsal aproximadamente 1 cm caudal à junção vesicouretral. A *seta branca* mostra o contraste na uretra proximal com trajeto a partir da bexiga parcialmente distendida.

Estudos epidemiológicos na América do Norte e Europa detectaram maior prevalência de UE em cães das raças Border Terrier, Briard, Buldogue Inglês, Entlebucher Mountain Dog, Fox Terrier, Golden Retriever, Griffon, Labrador Retriever, Poodle Miniatura, Poodle Toy, Terranova, Husky Siberiano, Skye Terrier e West Highland White Terrier.[8,12,45-48] A alta predisposição dessas raças, a constatação de UE em cães com estreito parentesco e os resultados de análises de *pedigree* sugerem fortemente uma causa hereditária de UE.[12,14,45,49] Recentes estudos de genética de população confirmaram uma base hereditária para UE em Entlebucher Mountain Dog.[45] Entretanto, o modo específico de hereditariedade e a(s) mutação(ões) genética(s) envolvida(s) na ocorrência de UE nesta e em outras raças de cães ainda não foram relatados. Predisposições familiares ou raciais não foram identificadas em gatos com UE.[33]

Os sinais clínicos variam, dependendo do(s) local(is) da terminação do UE e da presença de outras anormalidades urogenitais concomitantes. Incontinência urinária é o sinal clínico predominante em cães e gatos afetados (ver Capítulo 46). Na maioria dos cães, a incontinência urinária quase sempre é detectada logo após o desmame, e sua gravidade pode variar desde gotejamento involuntário contínuo até incontinência intermitente durante períodos de repouso, excitação ou alterações na posição corporal. Entretanto, o início da incontinência urinária pode ser retardado em alguns cães, especialmente em machos.[8,12,14,17,18,50] Além disso, alguns cães, machos e fêmeas, e gatos afetados podem permanecer sem incontinência urinária.[8,12,14,40] Outros sinais clínicos podem incluir distensão abdominal, mancha nos pelos periuretrais, dermatite perivulvar e outros sintomas relativos ao trato urinário inferior (p. ex., polaciúria e disúria). A ectopia ureteral é frequentemente agravada por infecções do trato urinário concomitantes (ver Capítulo 330); essas infecções parecem menos comuns em gatos afetados.[15,30]

Embora a incontinência urinária em animais jovens seja altamente sugestiva de UE, outras causas congênitas e adquiridas de incontinência devem ser consideradas (ver Capítulo 333).[3] Radiografias simples e ultrassonografia do abdome possibilitam avaliar o tamanho, o formato e a localização dos rins, dos ureteres e da bexiga. A administração de diurético (1 mg de furosemida/kg IV) durante a ultrassonografia com Doppler colorido pode melhorar a sensibilidade dessa técnica e permitir a fenotipagem de cães como normais, com ectopia intravesicular ou com ectopia extravesicular (Vídeo 336.1).[45,51-53] Entretanto, o diagnóstico definitivo requer métodos diagnósticos adicionais, ou a combinação de métodos, incluindo urografia excretora (com ou sem pneumocistografia), vaginografia retrógrada, uretrografia, tomografia computadorizada (TC) com contraste, ou uretrocistoscopia (ver Capítulo 108).[8,9,12,42,53] A TC com contraste e a uretrocistoscopia parecem ser métodos mais confiáveis para a definição do diagnóstico, caracterizando a morfologia da abertura do ureter, e a identificação de outras anomalias urogenitais concomitantes (ver Figuras 336.1 e 336.2). A TC com contraste pode ter vantagens diagnósticas em cães machos, enquanto a uretrocistoscopia é considerada padrão-ouro em cadelas.[8,9,12,53]

O tratamento de incontinência urinária associada a UE requer a correção da(s) abertura(s) ureteral(is) anômala(s) e o tratamento de qualquer comorbidade que possa contribuir, como a incompetência do mecanismo do esfíncter uretral. Estratégias cirúrgicas empregadas para correção de UE incluem transecção e reimplantação do ureter (neoureterocistotomia), criação de um neostoma (neoureterostomia *in situ*), ou remoção completa do rim e de seu ureter (nefroureterectomia).[14,20,42,54] Na última década, a ablação a *laser* guiada por cistoscopia transuretral de UE intramural surgiu como uma alternativa minimamente invasiva à correção cirúrgica em cães (ver Capítulo 124).[18,19,21,55,56]

Nessa técnica, utiliza-se *laser* de hólmio:YAG ou de diodo para a transecção da parede livre do UE que está adjacente ao lúmen uretral, transpondo efetivamente a abertura ureteral para a bexiga (Vídeo 336.2). Independentemente da abordagem, é comum ocorrer incontinência urinária residual pós-procedimento, especialmente em cadelas, com taxa de incontinência residual de 30 a 75%.[14,21] O interessante é que em cães machos a correção cirúrgica ou a *laser* do UE pode estar associada a resultados mais favoráveis.[8,14,18] Cães com incontinência urinária pós-cirúrgica persistente podem apresentar simultaneamente incompetência do mecanismo do esfíncter urinário e podem se beneficiar do tratamento farmacológico com agonistas alfa-adrenérgicos, aplicações de agentes de preenchimento transuretral, ou implantação de um oclusor hidráulico uretral artificial (ver Capítulo 124).[57-64]

Ureterocele

Ureterocele é uma dilatação cística congênita do segmento submucoso terminal do ureter distal. *Ureterocele ortóptica (simples)* localiza-se no trígono da bexiga, com o orifício ureteral na posição normal. A ureterocele que acompanha ureter ectópico é classificada como *ureterocele ectópica*. As ureteroceles podem ser unilaterais ou bilaterais e quase sempre ectópicas.[8,14,65-67] A ureterocele tem sido mais comumente relatada em cadelas, mas também foi diagnosticada em cães machos e em um gato.[14,20,47,65-72] Pacientes com ureterocele ortóptica podem ser assintomáticos ou desenvolver sintomas relativos ao trato urinário inferior (i. e., disúria, estrangúria, polaciúria e hematúria).[67,72-76] Pacientes com ureterocele ectópica desenvolvem incontinência urinária. Além disso, tanto ureterocele ortóptica quanto ectópica estão frequentemente associadas a infecção concomitante do trato urinário e hidroureter ipsilateral, hidronefrose e disfunção renal.[65-78] O diagnóstico de ureterocele é baseado nos resultados de urografia excretora, TC com contraste, ultrassonografia, uretrocistoscopia ou celiotomia exploratória e cistotomia.[42,53] O tratamento de ureterocele consiste em aliviar os sinais clínicos mediante ablação transuretral a *laser* da ureterocele, ureterocelectomia, neoureterocistotomia ou ureteronefrectomia.[42,77]

ANOMALIAS DA BEXIGA

Agenesia e hipoplasia da bexiga

A agenesia ou hipoplasia da bexiga resulta em menor capacidade de armazenamento de urina e se manifesta como incontinência urinária.[17,30,79-81] A agenesia completa da bexiga é rara, mas foi relatada em uma cadela mestiça de 4 meses de idade que apresentava incontinência urinária.[79,80] Hipoplasia é mais comum em cães e gatos, e pode resultar do desenvolvimento embrionário anormal da bexiga ou de condições que limitam o enchimento vesical adequado durante o desenvolvimento fetal.[82] A ectopia ureteral está frequentemente associada à hipoplasia da bexiga, que pode contribuir para a incontinência urinária após a correção cirúrgica.[17,30,81] A capacidade de armazenamento da bexiga pode aumentar substancialmente vários meses após a correção do UE.[81,83]

Bexiga pélvica

A bexiga pélvica refere-se à bexiga que apresenta um trígono de formato obtuso, situado na região intrapélvica e associado a uma uretra curta.[84] Embora alguns cães afetados apresentem continência urinária, outros cães com bexiga pélvica manifestam incontinência refratária sem qualquer outra causa identificável.[84-87] A bexiga pélvica também tem sido associada a outras anomalidades do trato urinário inferior concomitantes.[84]

CAPÍTULO 336 • Doenças Congênitas do Trato Urinário Inferior

O diagnóstico de bexiga pélvica é definido por meio de radiografia com contraste. Como o grau de distensão vesical interfere diretamente na posição do trígono em relação ao arco pélvico, é necessária uma distensão adequada durante a uretrocistografia com contraste para avaliar a posição da bexiga. Se a bexiga pélvica estiver associada à incontinência urinária, pode-se tentar o tratamento farmacológico com agonistas alfa-adrenérgicos (ver Capítulo 333).[64] Se a incontinência urinária for refratária à terapia medicamentosa, podem-se realizar intervenção cirúrgica, aplicações de agentes de preenchimento uretral, ou implantação de um esfíncter uretral artificial (ver Capítulo 124).[59-63]

Extrofia

A extrofia refere-se à eversão da bexiga e, frequentemente, dos intestinos e da genitália externa através de defeitos da linha média na parede abdominal ventral.[88] Essa anormalidade rara foi relatada em uma cadela da raça Buldogue Inglês de 8 meses de idade que apresentava incontinência urinária e pielonefrite, bem como em um gato.[89,90] O tratamento consiste em cirurgia reconstrutiva.

Duplicação de bexiga

A duplicação total e parcial da bexiga, com e sem duplicação da uretra, foi relatada em cães e gatos jovens.[91-93] Os sinais clínicos podem incluir disúria, estrangúria, incontinência urinária e distensão abdominal. O diagnóstico é obtido por meio de exame físico e exames de imagem. O tratamento consiste em correção cirúrgica; entretanto, o sucesso depende do grau da malformação e a presença de outras anomalias congênitas.

Anomalias de úraco

As anomalias de úraco são ocorrências comuns em cães e gatos. O úraco é uma conexão fetal que possibilita a passagem de urina entre a bexiga em desenvolvimento e a placenta. Após o nascimento ele se atrofia completamente. No entanto, pode ocorrer persistência de remanescências macroscópicas ou microscópicas do úraco, como úraco patente ou como cistos ou divertículos uracais.[94,95]

Nota-se úraco patente quando o canal uracal permanece funcionalmente patente, resultando em perda inapropriada de urina através do umbigo.[69,96-99] O úraco patente quase sempre é acompanhado de onfalite, dermatite ventral e infecção do trato urinário. Raramente, pode-se notar uroabdome quando o úraco patente termina na cavidade abdominal.[100] Pode-se verificar cisto uracal quando o epitélio do úraco, em um segmento isolado do úraco patente, continua a secretar líquido.[95]

Nota-se divertículo vesicouracal quando uma parte do úraco localizada no vértice da bexiga não se fecha. As remanescências uracais são lúmens microscópicos delimitados por epitélio de transição presente no vértice vesical.[95] Em um estudo, constatou-se que aproximadamente 40% das bexigas de 80 gatos apresentavam divertículos microscópicos.[101] Divertículos microscópicos congênitos quase sempre são assintomáticos; entretanto, divertículos macroscópicos podem ser detectados em gatos e cães com remanescências uracais microscópicas após o início de doenças concomitantes adquiridas, mas não relacionadas, do trato urinário inferior (p. ex., infecção do trato urinário, urolitíase ou cistite idiopática).[102-105] Em gatos, vários divertículos macroscópicos desaparecem dentro de 2 a 3 semanas após o tratamento da doença adquirida e a resolução dos sinais clínicos.[103,104] Divertículos vesicouracais macroscópicos congênitos supostamente são causados por obstrução do fluxo de urina e surgem antes ou logo depois do nascimento. Em um estudo necroscópico de 50 cães sem sinais de doença do trato urinário, constatou-se que 30% dos cães apresentavam divertículos vesicouracais macroscópicos.[102] Divertículos macroscópicos persistentes aumentam o risco de infecção bacteriana do trato urinário e sinais clínicos associados de doença do trato urinário inferior.[106]

Divertículos vesicouracais são mais bem visualizados por meio de uretrocistografia com contraste positivo, ultrassonografia (ver Capítulo 88), ou cistoscopia (ver Capítulo 108). O tratamento dos divertículos vesicouracais depende do tamanho, do comportamento biológico e da associação com doença clínica. Vários divertículos macroscópicos associados à doença ativa do trato urinário inferior regridem com o tratamento bem-sucedido da doença adquirida.[103,104] Se os divertículos persistirem após terapia apropriada e estiverem associados à doença recorrente do trato urinário inferior, então justifica-se a realização de diverticulectomia.[105]

Divertículo do trígono vesical (parauretérico)

Os divertículos vesicais congênitos também podem surgir na região do trígono, presumivelmente como resultado de fraqueza inerente à musculatura vesical e subsequente herniação da mucosa da bexiga.[107] Supostos divertículos congênitos do trígono da bexiga foram detectados em dois cães da raça Pastor-Alemão levados à consulta por apresentarem hematúria, disúria, estrangúria e infecção do trato urinário.[108,109] O diagnóstico de divertículos do trígono é obtido por meio de cistografia com contraste positivo, ultrassonografia (ver Capítulo 88), cistoscopia (ver Capítulo 108) ou laparotomia exploratória. A diverticulectomia é indicada para resolver a estase urinária e reduzir o risco de infecção, urolitíase, obstrução e progressão para lesão maligna.

Fístula colovesical e comunicação uterovesical

Raramente, pode haver comunicação da bexiga com o cólon ou com o corno uterino.[32,33,110,111] As manifestações clínicas consistem em padrão anormal de micção (excreção simultânea de urina do prepúcio ou da vulva e do ânus), incontinência urinária, sintomas relativos ao trato urinário inferior e infecção do trato urinário. O tratamento se limita à correção cirúrgica.

Neoplasia vesical primária

Neoplasias de bexiga são raras em cães e gatos jovens.[112] Relata-se rabdomiossarcoma botrioide em cães de raças grandes com menos de 18 meses de idade, mas pode ocorrer em outros cães.[113-122] Rabdomiossarcomas botrioides são tumores mesenquimais embrionários que surgem a partir de células-tronco pluripotentes que se originam de remanescências da crista urogenital primitiva. São tumores infiltrativos que se projetam a partir do trígono em direção ao lúmen vesical como massas botrioides (que se assemelham a cachos de uva).[115] Os tumores podem estar associados a sintomas relativos ao trato urinário inferior, uropatia obstrutiva e osteoartropatia hipertrófica.[114,115] O tratamento consiste em cirurgia, com ou sem quimioterapia adicional.[123,124] Há relatos de metástases desse tumor aos tecidos locais (linfonodos, mesentério, omento, próstata) e a órgãos distantes (pulmão, fígado, rim, baço).[113,120,122]

ANOMALIAS DA URETRA

Aplasia e hipoplasia da uretra

A aplasia uretral é uma anomalia congênita rara caracterizada por ausência total de uretra patente. A incontinência está associada à ectopia do ureter.[69,125] A hipoplasia uretral foi descrita em gatas jovens e está associada à incontinência urinária de início em idade juvenil.[30,126,127] O diagnóstico é baseado nos sinais clínicos e em exames de imagem. As características radiográficas consistem em uretra curta e ausência de vagina. A hipoplasia uretral pode estar associada a outras anomalias congênitas e à infecção do trato urinário. Os animais acometidos podem responder à terapia alfa-adrenérgica; porém, em alguns casos, pode ser necessária a reconstrução cirúrgica do colo vesical para melhorar ou resolver os sinais clínicos.[126,127]

Epispadia e hipospadia

Epispadia é uma anomalia congênita na parte dorsal da uretra distal, e hipospadia refere-se à posição anormal ventral anômala do meato uretral.[128] Em uma cadela da raça Buldogue Inglês de 8 meses de idade, a epispadia estava associada à extrofia da bexiga.[89] A ocorrência de hipospadia é mais comum em cães, quase sempre em machos; as raças Boston Terrier e Dálmata são mais predispostas.[128-130] Há relato de hipospadia em um gato Himalaio.[131] Em cães machos acometidos, o meato uretral ventral anormal pode estar localizado em qualquer outro local ao longo da haste peniana, escroto ou períneo. Está em geral associado à malformação de prepúcio e pênis.[132,133] Hipospadia foi descrita em cadelas que apresentavam, simultaneamente, intersexualidade. Cães portadores da anomalia são atendidos com várias idades; podem ser assintomáticos ou apresentar sinais clínicos de incontinência urinária, dermatite periuretral ou infecção do trato urinário.[132,133] O diagnóstico é quase sempre baseado no exame físico. Em cães, na maioria dos casos, a presença de osso peniano impede a reconstrução cirúrgica. A uretrostomia escrotal ou perineal combinada à castração e remoção de tecidos prepuciais e penianos remanescentes pode ter importância estética. Também foram descritos encurtamento do pênis, amputação e reconstrução da uretra.[134-138]

Duplicação da uretra

A duplicação da uretra é uma anomalia congênita incomum diagnosticada em cães jovens, machos e fêmeas.[139-144] Por causa da estreita associação entre o desenvolvimento embrionário dos sistemas urogenital e gastrintestinal, a duplicação da uretra é frequentemente acompanhada de outras anomalias de duplicação que envolvem cólon descendente, reto, bexiga, vagina, vulva ou pênis. O exame de animais acometidos pode revelar anormalidades anatômicas, incontinência urinária ou sinais clínicos associados à infecção secundária do trato urinário.

O diagnóstico é baseado no exame físico, exames de imagem e cirurgia exploratória. Em alguns casos a duplicação da uretra pode ser passível de extirpação cirúrgica ou embolização da estrutura duplicada com cola de cianoacrilato.[139,144]

Uretra ectópica

A uretra ectópica é caracterizada pela posição anormal do orifício uretral externo. Os sinais clínicos dependem do local da terminação (desembocadura) da uretra anormal e de outras anomalias urogenitais concomitantes. A incontinência urinária por toda a vida foi a característica clínica predominante em uma cadela da raça Buldogue Inglês de 21 meses de idade com ectopia ureteral unilateral e uretra ectópica com terminação na parte distal da vagina.[145] Diferentemente, uma gata da raça Doméstico de Pelo Curto de 2 meses de idade com uretra ectópica terminando na parte ventral do reto não apresentava incontinência urinária, mas urinava através do ânus.[33]

Fístula uretrorretal, uretrovaginal e uretroperineal

Em cães e gatos há relatos de fístulas congênitas que conectavam o lúmen da uretra ao intestino grosso, vagina e períneo.[79,142,146-152] Cães machos parecem mais predispostos e naqueles da raça Buldogue Inglês parece ser mais comum a ocorrência de fístula uretrorretal.[153] O sinais clínicos se devem à passagem anormal de urina através da fístula durante a micção e podem incluir diarreia, dermatite perineal e sintomas associados à infecção secundária do trato urinário. Simultaneamente, têm-se detectado fístulas e urolitíase causada por cálculo de estruvita induzida por infecção.[79,149,151] O diagnóstico é baseado nos sinais clínicos e exames de imagem. O tratamento consiste em fistulectomia, desvio cirúrgico da urina e erradicação de infecção secundária do trato urinário (ver Capítulo 330).

Constrição uretral

Em cães e gatos jovens foram descritas supostas constrições (estenoses) congênitas da uretra.[127,154,155] Os sinais clínicos estão relacionados à obstrução parcial ou total da uretra e podem incluir estrangúria, polaciúria, micção demorada, distensão da bexiga, incontinência por fluxo urinário excessivo, hidroureter e hidronefrose. Em um cão Pastor-Alemão, macho, de 8 meses de idade, com constrição congênita na porção média da uretra, foram observadas incontinência urinária, hidroureter e hidronefrose bilaterais.[154] As constrições de uretra extrapélvicas podem ser tratadas por meio de uretrostomia, enquanto as constrições de uretra intrapélvicas ou intra-abdominais podem necessitar de ressecção da uretra e anastomose ou uretrostomia pré-púbica.[156,157] Como alternativa, as constrições uretrais podem ser tratadas mediante dilatação por cateter com balão guiada por cistoscopia ou fluoroscopia.[158-160]

Incompetência congênita do esfíncter uretral

A incompetência congênita do mecanismo do esfíncter uretral foi descrita em cães e gatos, e está frequentemente associada a outras malformações urogenitais (ureter ectópico, hipoplasia ou aplasia uretral, dilatação da uretra e divertículos na uretra prostática).[30,42,60,127,161] Contudo, em alguns pacientes jovens não castrados, pode haver incompetência congênita do mecanismo do esfíncter uretral na ausência de outras anomalias urogenitais congênitas. Embora a incontinência urinária possa diminuir ou ser resolvida com tratamento farmacológico, vários pacientes necessitam de intervenção cirúrgica adicional, aplicações de agentes de preenchimento uretral ou implantação de esfíncter uretral artificial (ver Capítulo 124).[57-64]

Malformações uretrogenitais

Malformações uretrogenitais associadas à intersexualidade, especialmente pseudo-hermafroditismo, estão frequentemente associadas à incontinência urinária.[162-164] Pseudo-hermafroditas possuem gônadas de um sexo e genitália externa que se assemelha àquela do sexo oposto.[165] Isso se deve ao desenvolvimento simultâneo de estruturas derivadas do ducto mülleriano (oviduto, útero e partes da vagina) e masculinização do seio urogenital. A aparência da genitália depende do grau de masculinização desse seio. A incontinência urinária é observada precocemente e pode ser acompanhada de infecção do trato urinário e outros sintomas relativos ao trato urinário inferior. Provavelmente, a incontinência urinária se deve à retenção de urina em comunicações anômalas entre a uretra e o trato genital, e subsequente extravasamento passivo de urina.[166] O diagnóstico é baseado nos sinais clínicos e exames de imagem. A incontinência urinária pode ser resolvida mediante correção cirúrgica.[162]

REFERÊNCIAS BIBLIOGRÁFICAS

As referências bibliográficas deste capítulo se encontram online no Ambiente de Aprendizagem.

CAPÍTULO 337

Doenças da Próstata

Michelle Anne Kutzler

Em cães, as principais doenças da próstata são hiperplasia prostática benigna (HPB), prostatite bacteriana aguda ou crônica, abscesso prostático, cistos paraprostáticos e neoplasia de próstata. Entre os estudos, as prevalências relatadas para doenças da próstata são muito variáveis, dependendo da idade e do estado reprodutivo da população. Provavelmente, os relatos são tendenciosos para HPB e prostatite, em países onde os cães raramente são castrados, e para neoplasias, em países onde a castração é um procedimento mais frequente. Em cães, estudos de manifestações clínicas de doença da próstata certamente não são representativos de sua real prevalência, dada a comum ocorrência de doença da próstata subclínica nessa espécie. Um estudo de cães que morreram devido a doenças não relacionadas à próstata indicou uma prevalência de 76% de doenças de próstata subclínica.[1] Em cães não castrados, manifestações sistêmicas graves sugestivas de sepse ou inflamação devem sempre levantar a suspeita de prostatite bacteriana aguda. A possibilidade de doença de próstata em cães castrados não deve ser descartada, já que a castração aumenta o risco de neoplasia de próstata, quando comparado a cães não castrados.[2]

Em gatos, a anatomia e localização da próstata difere de cães pelo fato de que esse órgão repousa sobre o arco cranial da pelve, no meio do trajeto entre a raiz do pênis e o colo da bexiga. A próstata consiste em dois lobos e recobre a uretra apenas dorsal e lateralmente.[3] Com base nessa localização, parece razoável esperar que, além dos sintomas relativos ao trato urinário inferior, podem ocorrer constipação intestinal e disquesia como consequências da obstrução parcial do intestino grosso pela próstata aumentada.[4]

Doenças da próstata são extremamente raras em gatos e incluem prostatite bacteriana crônica, abscesso prostático, metaplasia escamosa induzida por estrógeno, cistos paraprostáticos e neoplasia.[3,5-11] Apesar da raridade dessas doenças, ao se detectar aumento da próstata, devem ser realizados exames diagnósticos (p. ex., cistocentese, para coleta de amostra de urina para exame do sedimento urinário e para cultura microbiológica, e teste de sensibilidade antimicrobiana [antibiograma] [ver Capítulo 72]; e aspirado com agulha fina ou biopsia da próstata guiada por ultrassom, quando indicado [ver Capítulos 88, 89 e 111]). Em gatos, a doença de próstata deve ser incluída na lista de diagnósticos diferenciais para disquesia ou constipação intestinal, mesmo em animais castrados.

HIPERPLASIA PROSTÁTICA BENIGNA

Embora o crescimento normal da próstata seja alcançado em cerca de 2 anos de idade, as células da próstata sofrem hipertrofia e hiperplasia constantes sob a influência de andrógenos. O volume da próstata tende a aumentar com a idade e isso deve ser considerado normal em cães não castrados. Essa hiperplasia benigna espontânea é observada tanto em cães quanto em homens. Foi relatado que a HPB ocorre em 80% dos cães não castrados com mais de 5 anos de idade e 95% dos cães com mais de 9 anos de idade.[4,12] Entretanto, evidências histológicas de HPB podem ser constatadas em animais com até 2 anos de idade, com prevalência relatada de 16% nessa idade.[13] Além disso, a HPB parece acometer mais severamente os cães da raça Scottish Terrier do que de outras raças.[4]

Patogenia

O crescimento de células prostáticas é influenciado pela di-hidrotestosterona (DHT) (e em uma extensão muito menor pela testosterona), pelo beta-17-estradiol e por vários outros fatores de crescimento locais. Alterações na proporção andrógeno: estrógeno relacionadas à idade parecem importantes para o desenvolvimento de HPB. A DHT é o principal mediador da HPB, que promove crescimento de elementos estromais e glandulares.[12,14-17] A HPB pode progredir para HPB cística, bem como predispor os cães à prostatite bacteriana crônica, que pode progredir para cistite, epididimite e orquite. O estradiol pode induzir metaplasia de células epiteliais da próstata com obstrução glandular, retenção de líquido prostático e sangue, bem como formação de cistos parenquimatosos de tamanhos variados que podem ou não se comunicar com a uretra.[18] A estase progressiva da secreção e subsequente oclusão do ducto resulta na formação de múltiplas áreas cavitárias na próstata. Cistos parenquimatosos (intraprostáticos) geralmente se comunicam com a uretra, ao contrário de cistos paraprostáticos (ver adiante).[15,19]

Diagnóstico

Cães com HPB possuem uma próstata simetricamente aumentada, moderadamente firme e não dolorosa à palpação retal. A maioria dos cães acometidos não manifesta sinais clínicos evidentes.[15,20] A assimetria prostática pode ser detectada mediante palpação em cães com cistos prostáticos proeminentes, que frequentemente ocorrem na HPB cística. Os sinais clínicos surgem na maioria das vezes em estágios avançados da doença, quando a próstata aumentada comprime o cólon dorsalmente, e os cães apresentam dificuldade para defecar. Outros sintomas incluem secreção sanguinolenta na extremidade do pênis não relacionada à micção, hematúria, disúria, hematospermia e infertilidade. Como os cães com HPB são mais predispostos à prostatite bacteriana crônica, os sinais clínicos relacionados à dor abdominal caudal, marcha rígida, relutância em se movimentar e manifestações sistêmicas graves compatíveis com sepse podem dominar o cenário clínico. O diagnóstico definitivo de HPB requer biopsia da próstata, embora um diagnóstico presuntivo possa ser baseado na epidemiologia, no histórico clínico, no exame físico, na palpação retal e no exame do líquido prostático (ver Capítulo 111).[15] O líquido seminal de cães afetados contém sangue, com ou sem inflamação mononuclear mínima.[21] A cultura bacteriana quantitativa deve indicar menos de 100 bactérias/mℓ.[22] A ultrassonografia de abdome (ver Capítulo 88) confirma os achados do exame retal e mostra hipo ou hiperecogenicidade difusa discreta (Figura 337.1).[23,24] Os linfonodos sublombares não devem estar aumentados na HPB não complicada. O exame citológico (ver Capítulo 93) do aspirado obtido com agulha fina (ver Capítulo 89) pode mostrar características típicas de hipertrofia de células prostáticas, condição que aumenta ainda mais a suspeita de HPB.[25] A suspeita de HPB pode ser confirmada por teste terapêutico, utilizando supressão por andrógenos. As opções incluem acetato de osaterona (Ypozane®; disponível nos EUA), na dose de 0,25 a 0,5 mg/kg/24 h VO, durante 7 dias; relata-se que tal procedimento reduz o volume da próstata em ≈ 27% após 1 semana e em 40% após 2 semanas;[26] ou acetato de medroxiprogesterona (disponível nos EUA, em dose única de 3 a 4 mg/kg SC, que eliminou os sinais clínicos em 84% dos cães em 4 a

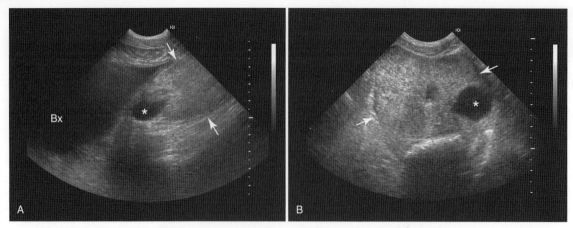

Figura 337.1 Imagens sagital (**A**) e transversa (**B**) da próstata (*entre setas*) com hiperplasia prostática benigna obtidas em ultrassonografia. Note o aumento de tamanho, a hipo e hiperecogenicidade discreta difusa, e um cisto intraprostático anecoico (*asterisco*). A bexiga (*Bx*) está à esquerda na imagem sagital.

6 semanas, sendo que 68% permaneceram livres dos sintomas por pelo menos 10 meses;[27] ou deslorelina (Suprelorin®; não disponível nos EUA), na forma de implante subcutâneo de 4,7 mg/cão, que reduziu o tamanho da próstata após 22 dias do início do tratamento, com resolução da HPB após 52 dias.[28] É difícil justificar um procedimento mais invasivo, como aspirado ou biopsia da próstata, quando métodos menos invasivos (ultrassonografia e teste terapêutico) sustentam fortemente o diagnóstico de HPB.[15] É importante compreender que a HPB é um achado incidental comum em cães de meia-idade a idosos, e esse diagnóstico deve ser interpretado com cautela em cães com sinais clínicos moderados a graves.

Tratamento

O objetivo do tratamento de cães com HPB é reduzir o tamanho da próstata, a fim de aliviar os sinais clínicos e diminuir o risco de complicações, como prostatite bacteriana crônica ou abscesso prostático. A *castração* é o tratamento de primeira escolha para a maioria dos cães. Ela causa rápida redução do volume prostático em 50% em 3 semanas e em 75% em 3 meses. Aproximadamente 3 semanas após a castração, a involução da próstata deve ser avaliada mediante palpação retal ou ultrassonografia, a fim de descartar a possibilidade de neoplasia ou abscesso concomitante anteriormente não detectados. Em cães reprodutores ou idosos, com maior risco anestésico, deve-se utilizar terapia de supressão reversível com andrógenos. Essas modalidades terapêuticas são seguras e práticas, mesmo para tratamento em médio e longo prazos.

A finasterida (Proscar®, Merck, na dose de 5 mg/cão/24 h VO [independentemente do peso corporal]) é um inibidor da alfa-5-redutase que bloqueia a conversão de testosterona em seu metabólito bioativo, a DHT. Esse tratamento resulta na diminuição do volume prostático em 50 a 70% em 2 a 4 semanas por meio de apoptose.[29,30] O volume do sêmen diminui, sem comprometer a qualidade do sêmen.[31] Embora ocorra diminuição da concentração de DHT, a concentração sérica de testosterona permanece inalterada. Portanto, os cães mantêm a libido e a fertilidade, e podem ser reprodutores efetivos.[32] Os sinais clínicos associados à HPB começam a melhorar após 1 semana de tratamento, e a maioria dos cães apresenta resolução total dos sintomas dentro de 4 semanas.[31] A próstata volta a ter aumento de tamanho, como havia na HPB, dentro de 8 semanas após a descontinuação do tratamento. Portanto, os protocolos terapêuticos devem ser mantidos por toda a vida reprodutiva do cão ou deve-se utilizar um esquema de 6 semanas de tratamento entremeado por um período de 6 semanas sem tratamento, por ser mais prático aos tutores. Nesses cães recomendam-se exames físicos regulares, inclusive palpação retal.

PROSTATITE BACTERIANA AGUDA

A prostatite aguda em geral é uma doença de cães adultos, não castrados ou recentemente castrados. Quase sempre é consequência de uma infecção ascendente em uma próstata hiperplásica, causada por bactérias aeróbicas que normalmente habitam a uretra,[3] embora possa ocorrer infecção hematógena.[33] A bactéria mais comumente identificada em cães é *Escherichia coli* (70%), seguida de *Staphylococcus* spp., *Klebsiella* spp., *Proteus mirabilis*, *Mycoplasma canis*, *Pseudomonas aeruginosa*, *Enterobacter* spp., *Streptococcus* spp., *Pasteurella* spp. e *Haemophilus* spp.[12] Há raros relatos de infecções causadas por bactérias anaeróbicas ou fungos, incluindo um cão com pitiose prostática.[33,34]

Diagnóstico

Cães com prostatite bacteriana aguda em geral manifestam sintomas de doença sistêmica, como depressão, anorexia, êmese e febre, bem como sinais clínicos mais específicos do órgão, como estrangúria ou tenesmo, dor abdominal caudal, secreção uretral/prepucial e marcha rígida ou hipermétrica. No exame retal, a próstata pode ter tamanho e formato normal à palpação, ou pode ser assimétrica, com superfície irregular. A próstata quase sempre é dolorosa à palpação.[23] Os cães acometidos geralmente apresentam quadro clínico grave. Os exames de sangue indicam inflamação sistêmica, inclusive neutrofilia com desvio à esquerda e neutrófilos com alterações tóxicas. O exame de urina (ver Capítulo 72) pode estar normal ou indicar hematúria, piúria e bacteriúria. A amostra de urina coletada por meio de cistocentese deve ser submetida à cultura microbiológica, já que ocorre fluxo retrógrado da secreção prostática à bexiga, de forma que há alta correlação entre os resultados das culturas de urina e do líquido prostático.[35] Nos exames de imagem (radiografia ou ultrassonografia [ver Capítulo 88]) para o diagnóstico de prostatite bacteriana aguda, nota-se prostatomegalia, que pode não ter sido palpável durante o exame retal. O aspirado com agulha fina guiado por ultrassom pode propiciar amostra de líquido prostático ou de parênquima para o exame citológico, e para cultura bacteriana e antibiograma; porém, por causa do risco de inoculação de bactérias ao longo do trajeto da agulha, o lavado prostático e a obtenção de amostra por meio de escova são alternativas mais seguras para a obtenção dessas amostras (ver Capítulo 111).[15]

Tratamento

A base do tratamento de prostatite bacteriana aguda é a terapia antimicrobiana apropriada, baseada nos resultados da cultura microbiológica e no antibiograma da urina e/ou do líquido prostático ou do parênquima. Como na prostatite bacteriana aguda a barreira hematoprostática está comprometida, ela não deve ser uma preocupação importante ao escolher um antibiótico. Entretanto, recomenda-se, quando possível, o início do tratamento diretamente com um antibiótico que tenha boa penetração no parênquima prostático, de forma que, assim que a barreira esteja restabelecida (após a fase aguda da infecção), não haja necessidade de alterar o antibiótico utilizado.[23] A barreira hematoprostática impede a difusão de fármacos ionizados e daqueles com baixa lipossolubilidade ou alta afinidade por proteínas.[16,36] Antibióticos básicos com pKa > 7 (p. ex., a combinação sulfametoxazol + trimetoprima e cloranfenicol) se difundem facilmente do sangue para o parênquima prostático. Como o pH do líquido prostático de cães normais é tipicamente ácido, o gradiente de pH entre o sangue e a próstata favorece o aprisionamento adicional de fármacos fracamente básicos que são ionizados no líquido prostático ácido.[12,37] As fluoroquinolonas são capazes de penetrar bem o parênquima prostático, independentemente do pH, e são, portanto, uma boa escolha para a terapia antimicrobiana empírica inicial, enquanto se aguardam os resultados da cultura microbiológica e do antibiograma.[38] Na dose de 5 mg/kg/12 h VO, a enrofloxacino atinge concentrações no líquido prostático e no parênquima que excedem a concentração inibitória mínima para a maioria dos patógenos.[38] A terapia antimicrobiana deve ser mantida por longo tempo (i. e., 4 a 6 semanas), de modo a reduzir o risco de formação de abscesso prostático. Amostras de urina e/ou líquido prostático devem ser novamente coletadas 2 a 3 semanas após o início do tratamento, enquanto o paciente ainda estiver sob tratamento, para confirmar a eficácia terapêutica (cultura negativa). A cultura também deve ser repetida 1 a 3 semanas após a descontinuação do uso de antibiótico.

O impacto potencial da prostatite bacteriana aguda não deve ser clinicamente subestimado, já que essa infecção pode progredir para sepse, inflamação sistêmica e comprometimento de vários órgãos (ver Capítulo 132). Os cães acometidos devem ser monitorados e tratados, se necessário, com solução de uso intravenoso (IV) (ver Capítulo 129), analgésicos (ver Capítulos 126 e 166) e cuidados de suporte. Após a fase aguda da infecção, pode-se realizar a castração como uma terapia adjuvante, a fim de reduzir o tamanho da próstata (e do volume de tecido infectado).[23] A castração não é recomendada durante a fase aguda da infecção, já que podem ser formados cordões espermáticos bastante fibrosados por causa da infecção bacteriana ascendente.[29] Inicialmente, deve-se utilizar terapia de supressão reversível com andrógenos, finasterida, até que a infecção esteja controlada e seja possível uma castração cirúrgica segura, ou a longo prazo (conforme descrito anteriormente) em casos de machos reprodutores nos quais a castração não é desejada.[12]

ABSCESSO PROSTÁTICO

A formação de abscesso prostático pode ser secundária à prostatite bacteriana aguda ou após metaplasia escamosa prostática induzida por estrógeno a partir de um cisto infeccionado.[35,40,41]

Diagnóstico

Os sinais clínicos de abscesso prostático são semelhantes àqueles da prostatite bacteriana aguda, incluindo sintomas de doença sistêmica, letargia, febre, dor à micção e defecação, e dor na região caudal do abdome.[15] Além do leucograma inflamatório, cães acometidos podem apresentar hipoglicemia induzida por sepse. O abscesso pode ser encapsulado e não ter contato direto com o sistema de ductos prostáticos. Portanto, a cultura bacteriana do líquido prostático pode fornecer resultado falso negativo.[42] A ultrassonografia (ver Capítulo 88) é importante para o diagnóstico e mostra uma ou mais lesões cavitárias hipoecoicas ou anecoicas no parênquima de uma próstata aumentada, com limites irregulares e formato assimétrico. O ultrassonografista experiente pode diferenciar abscesso de cisto não infeccionado, neoplasia cavitária ou hematoma.[43]

Podem ser observadas áreas hiperecoicas focais sugestivas de restos teciduais necrosados no interior do abscesso. Mesmo que clinicamente o abscesso prostático possa ser semelhante à pancreatite aguda, é importante obter o diagnóstico correto, já que o protocolo terapêutico é diferente.

Tratamento

O tratamento de abscesso prostático requer uma combinação de drenagem (ver adiante) e terapia antimicrobiana apropriada, já que apenas antibióticos não eliminam efetivamente a infecção. A isquemia local tende a impedir a penetração de antibióticos no abscesso e, diferentemente do que acontece na prostatite bacteriana aguda, a barreira hematoprostática comumente encontra-se íntegra.[39] Antibióticos que cruzam prontamente a barreira hematoprostática íntegra (p. ex., enrofloxacino, sulfonamida + trimetoprima, cloranfenicol) devem ser escolhidos e administrados durante 6 semanas após a drenagem. A próstata deve ser reavaliada por meio de ultrassonografia para assegurar que a cavidade do abscesso não esteja sendo novamente preenchida. À semelhança do tratamento mencionado da prostatite bacteriana aguda, o líquido prostático deve ser submetido à cultura microbiológica tanto durante o tratamento quanto 2 a 4 semanas após a descontinuação da terapia antimicrobiana. A castração e/ou terapia de supressão reversível com andrógenos devem ser realizadas para propiciar uma resolução mais rápida da infecção bacteriana.[44]

O abscesso deve ser drenado cirurgicamente ou por meio de aspiração percutânea guiada por ultrassom.[40,45] A drenagem percutânea guiada por ultrassom pode ser uma alternativa útil ao tratamento cirúrgico quando as lesões cavitárias são bem circunscritas e não há suspeita de neoplasia de próstata ou doença sistêmica concomitante. Durante a aspiração percutânea há um risco potencial de causar peritonite iatrogênica.[39] Além disso, mais de 50% dos cães submetidos à aspiração de abscesso prostático apresentaram recidiva do abscesso.[45] A instilação de solução de etanol 95% na cavidade do abscesso drenado foi utilizada com sucesso em um cão com doença recidivante.[40] A drenagem cirúrgica de um abscesso prostático deve incluir a técnica de omentalização ou marsupialização, com colocação de um dreno de Penrose. Em um estudo com 92 cães submetidos à última técnica, constatou-se que 22 cães morreram ou foram submetidos à eutanásia no período perioperatório imediato e apenas em 33 cães foram obtidos resultados bons a excelentes.[46] A técnica da omentalização resulta em menores taxas de recidiva, de mortalidade e de incontinência urinária, no período pós-operatório, comparativamente à técnica de marsupialização, motivo pelo qual a omentalização é preferida pelos cirurgiões.[39,47]

PROSTATITE BACTERIANA CRÔNICA

As infecções bacterianas crônicas da próstata são mais comuns do que infecções bacterianas agudas. Ambas acometem, principalmente, cães adultos não castrados ou infectados imediatamente antes da castração.[48] É difícil estimar a prevalência de prostatite bacteriana crônica porque até 35% dos cães não exibem sinais clínicos, tampouco apresentam leucograma inflamatório. Um estudo relatou prevalência de 24% de prostatite crônica subclínica em cães que morreram em razão de doenças não relacionadas à próstata.[1]

Diagnóstico

A queixa mais comum no atendimento de animais com prostatite bacteriana crônica é uma infecção recorrente do trato urinário, com persistência do mesmo patógeno, em um cão saudável não castrado ou recentemente castrado. A infecção persiste na próstata durante o tratamento antimicrobiano a curto prazo e isso ocasiona reinfecção do trato urinário após a descontinuação da terapia antimicrobiana.[23,49] Outros possíveis sinais clínicos incluem secreção uretral sanguinolenta independente da micção, assim como hematúria, anormalidade dos membros pélvicos durante a marcha ou desconforto ao se levantar.[50] Observações menos comuns mencionadas pelos tutores são sinais de dor testicular causados por epididimite ascendente ou infertilidade. Na palpação retal da próstata, os achados variam de normais para um cão adulto não castrado até, menos comumente, uma estrutura assimétrica, firme e irregular. A próstata em geral não é dolorida à palpação e isso pode levar à falsa impressão de que se pode excluir a presença de doença prostática.[23] O exame do líquido prostático (ver Capítulo 111) indica evidências de inflamação supurativa. Em mais de 70% dos cães com prostatite bacteriana crônica, a cultura microbiológica do líquido prostático detecta o crescimento de um único microrganismo.[16,51] O aspirado com agulha fina e/ou biopsia da próstata pode resultar em peritonite séptica (ver Capítulo 279) secundária à disseminação do microrganismo no trajeto da agulha, como foi relatada em casos de prostatite bacteriana aguda. No exame radiográfico, a próstata geralmente se apresenta normal. É possível verificar mineralização; porém, além de ser um achado inespecífico, é indistinguível de neoplasia.[23] Achados ultrassonográficos consistem em um padrão heterogêneo de ecogenicidade juntamente com um aumento focal ou difuso da ecogenicidade do parênquima e cavidades parenquimatosas hipoecoicas ou anecoicas (Figura 337.2).[52,53] Em casos de calcificação, fibrose ou presença de ar, pode-se observar sombreamento ultrassonográfico.[23]

Tratamento

O tratamento de prostatite bacteriana crônica é semelhante ao de infecções bacterianas agudas. Portanto, boas escolhas de antibióticos para casos de prostatite bacteriana crônica incluem a combinação sulfonamida + trimetoprima para a maioria das infecções causadas por bactérias aeróbicas, fluoroquinolonas para infecção por *Mycoplasma* spp. e cloranfenicol para infecção causada por bactérias anaeróbicas (ver seção sobre Prostatite bacteriana aguda, para explicação mais detalhada).[4,23,38] Assim como na prostatite bacteriana aguda, o tratamento antimicrobiano deve ser baseado nos resultados da cultura microbiológica e do antibiograma, e deve durar, no mínimo, 4 a 6 semanas, independentemente da resolução precoce dos sinais clínicos.[36] A castração propicia uma resolução significativamente mais rápida da infecção, comparativamente aos cães não castrados do grupo-controle.[44,54] Deve-se iniciar o tratamento com antibiótico 5 a 7 dias antes da castração, a fim de reduzir o risco de formação de cordões fibrosados.[15]

CISTOS PARAPROSTÁTICOS

Cistos paraprostáticos são remanescências do útero masculino preenchidas com líquido, que, quando presentes, situam-se fora do parênquima prostático.[55]

Diagnóstico

Os sinais clínicos estão relacionados ao tamanho do cisto e podem incluir disquesia e disúria por compressão extraluminal do cólon e uretra, respectivamente. Há relato de incontinência urinária em cães nos quais o cisto causava obstrução parcial da uretra com subsequente distensão excessiva da bexiga.[43] Dependendo do tamanho, é possível suspeitar de cistos paraprostáticos pela palpação do abdome; na palpação durante o exame retal, é possível perceber uma massa no canal pélvico.[55] Nas radiografias, quase sempre situam-se em posição craniolateral à próstata e tendem a deslocar a bexiga em direção cranioventral ou dorsal, e o cólon e o reto em direção dorsal (Figura 337.3). Características histopatológicas comuns incluem parede de tecido conjuntivo ou fibroso, com ou sem revestimento epitelial, e metaplasia óssea. Evidências radiográficas de mineralização de cistos são achados frequentes; um estudo relata a ocorrência em 50% dos

cães.[55] Cistos paraprostáticos mineralizados foram considerados como possível fator contribuinte ao desenvolvimento de hérnia perineal em cães.[56] No exame ultrassonográfico, geralmente os cistos paraprostáticos possuem halos hiperecoicos e conteúdo hipoanecoico ou anecoicos, às vezes com septações.

Tratamento

Embora a maioria dos cistos paraprostáticos não necessite de qualquer tratamento porque são achados incidentais, o tratamento de cistos causa sinais clínicos que consistem em desbridamento cirúrgico, omentalização, marsupialização e, se necessário, colocação de drenos cirúrgicos.[39] Em um estudo constatou-se que uma alternativa ao tratamento cirúrgico é a drenagem percutânea guiada por ultrassom, que está associada à menor taxa de morbidade, menor custo e melhor resultado, quando comparada à cirurgia.[45]

NEOPLASIA DE PRÓSTATA

Com exceção dos seres humanos, o cão é a única espécie que sabidamente apresenta incidência clinicamente relevante de câncer de próstata. Ambas as espécies compartilham várias semelhanças, e o cão serve como modelo experimental para a doença humana.[57,58] O adenocarcinoma é a neoplasia de próstata mais frequente em cães, porém mais da metade exibe heterogeneidade intratumoral.[58] O tumor pode surgir a partir de células do epitélio glandular ou de ductos da próstata, ou a partir do urotélio da uretra prostática, mas na maioria dos casos a origem celular exata ainda é desconhecida.[59] Outra neoplasia de próstata comum em cães é o carcinoma de célula de transição, oriundo da uretra prostática. Há raros relatos de outros tumores, como carcinoma sarcomatoide, hemangiossarcoma primário e metastático, e linfoma[60-63] (ver Capítulo 351).

Diagnóstico

Em cães, o diagnóstico específico de neoplasias de próstata pode ser desafiador, já que vários adenocarcinomas primários nessa espécie apresentam características morfológicas e microscópicas semelhantes àquelas de carcinoma de célula de transição.[59] De forma geral, em cães, as neoplasias de próstata são tumores epiteliais malignos que frequentemente apresentam estruturas semelhantes a glândulas ou ácinos e são, portanto, em geral classificados como adenocarcinomas.[64] Em cães, a maioria das neoplasias de próstata não expressa receptores androgênicos e não dependem de hormônio; portanto, não respondem à privação de andrógenos.[12,64] É importante ressaltar que, em cães, a castração aumenta significativamente o risco de desenvolvimento de neoplasias de próstata. Em um amplo estudo retrospectivo realizado em vários centros de referência, o risco de desenvolvimento de tumor de célula de transição na próstata de cães castrados foi 8 vezes maior do que em cães não castrados, e foi 2,1 vezes maior para o desenvolvimento de adenocarcinoma prostático.[65] Em termos de histologia, constatou-se que a castração aumenta a ocorrência de padrões de crescimento menos diferenciados no câncer de próstata em cães.[57] A castração não parece iniciar o surgimento do tumor, mas favorece sua progressão. Isso pode ser resultado da concentração suprafisiológica do hormônio luteinizante (LH), que persiste durante a vida do cão após a castração, como resultado da perda do mecanismo de retroalimentação negativo testicular. Os receptores de LH estão presentes no epitélio prostático humano,[66] mas ainda não foram pesquisados no tecido prostático normal ou neoplásico de cães. As predisposições raciais para neoplasias de próstata incluem cães mestiços e das raças Shetland Sheepdog, Scottish Terrier, Airedale Terrier e Dobermann Pinscher.[65]

Achados clínicos comuns em cães com neoplasias de próstata incluem disúria, hematúria macroscópica, disquesia, dor em membros pélvicos e ataxia.[64] Em estágios mais avançados,

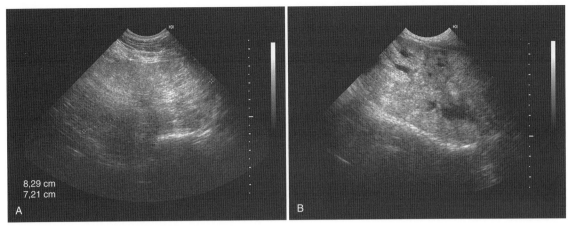

Figura 337.2 Imagens ultrassonográficas sagital (**A**) e transversa (**B**) da próstata de um cão com prostatite bacteriana crônica. Note o padrão heterogêneo de ecogenicidade mista, com aumento difuso da ecogenicidade do parênquima e cavidades parenquimatosas hipoecoicas a anecoicas (cistos intraprostáticos).

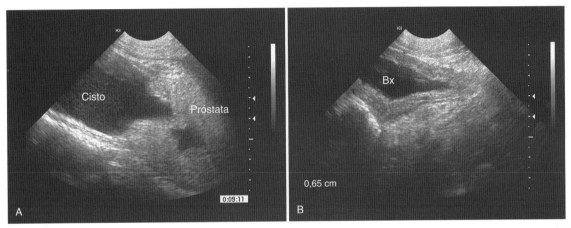

Figura 337.3 Imagens ultrassonográficas transversas da próstata com cisto paraprostático que se estende à superfície cranioventral da próstata (**A**) e a bexiga (*Bx*) quase vazia (espessura da parede de 0,65 cm, no limite normal de uma bexiga vazia) na superfície caudoventral da próstata (**B**).

notam-se sinais clínicos de síndromes paraneoplásicas, como letargia, anorexia, perda de peso e baixo escore da condição corporal. A disúria pode ser decorrência de prostatite concomitante ou de invasão local na uretra prostática, que resulta, ocasionalmente, em obstrução da uretra. Piúria e hematúria foram observadas em 62 e 66%, respectivamente, de 24 cães com câncer de próstata.[67] Por causa da natureza agressiva das neoplasias prostáticas em cães, a maioria dos animais, quando diagnosticados, apresenta doença em estágio avançado. Frequentemente, ocorre invasão local extensa e metástases viscerais disseminadas, com prevalência de até 80% no momento do diagnóstico.[67] Os locais mais comuns de metástases são os linfonodos sublombares e ilíacos, pulmões e ossos (principalmente as vértebras lombares e a pelve). Há relato de envolvimento do fígado, rins, baço e cérebro. A presença de tecido neoplásico na bexiga é uma manifestação comum de invasão local por células neoplásicas, o que também pode ser observado nos vasos linfáticos da próstata, no espaço perineural e na musculatura pélvica. Em cães, todas as neoplasias de próstata são consideradas altamente agressivas, com tendência a metástases disseminadas.

O diagnóstico de neoplasias de próstata em cães em geral é baseado no histórico, nos sinais clínicos, nos exames de imagem da próstata (ver Capítulo 88), no exame do líquido prostático (ver Capítulo 111), na citologia (ver Capítulo 93) e/ou na histopatologia. Alterações radiográficas podem incluir prostatomegalia, mineralização da próstata, evidências de linfadenomegalia regional e, possivelmente, evidências de metástases aos pulmões e ossos, especialmente vértebras lombares e pelve. Os achados ultrassonográficos podem incluir áreas hiperecoicas focais a difusas, mineralização e perda do contorno normal da próstata (Figura 337.4).[15] O aspirado com agulha fina percutâneo guiado por ultrassom é uma ferramenta diagnóstica viável para o diagnóstico citológico de neoplasias de próstata.[68] Entretanto, há um risco potencial de disseminação no trajeto da agulha na parede abdominal.[69] Essa complicação parece ser rara, mas a possibilidade não deve ser negligenciada, e o trajeto da agulha deve ser submetido à ressecção cirúrgica, se possível. O lavado prostático é uma alternativa valiosa ao aspirado com agulha (ver Capítulo 111).

Tratamento

De forma geral, a sobrevida da maioria dos cães com neoplasia de próstata clínica é curta, frequentemente varia de semanas a meses.[58] Em cães, como a maioria das neoplasias de próstata é agressiva e altamente metastática, o ideal é realizar terapias local e sistêmica. Contudo, no momento não há um protocolo terapêutico amplamente aceito; ademais, as opções terapêuticas são limitadas e muito pouco eficazes.[64] O piroxicam, um anti-inflamatório não esteroide, pode ser administrado na dose de 0,3 mg/kg/24 h VO; relata-se que reduziu com sucesso o tamanho de diversos carcinomas em cães.[70] Uma combinação de piroxicam com cisplatina (60 mg/m² IV, a cada 21 dias) resultou em remissão total ou parcial da neoplasia de bexiga em 71% dos cães, comparada à nenhuma remissão tumoral com o tratamento exclusivo com cisplatina (ver Capítulo 351).[71] A radioterapia não aumentou de forma significativa a sobrevida, e sua importância no tratamento de neoplasia da próstata em cães é incerta.

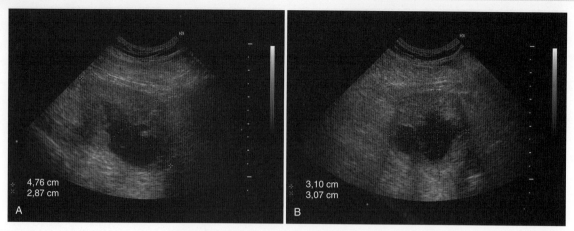

Figura 337.4 Imagens ultrassonográficas sagital (**A**) e transversa (**B**) de próstata com adenocarcinoma. Note o tamanho aumentado da próstata de um cão castrado, o aumento da ecogenicidade e a presença de cistos grandes e coalescentes com conteúdo luminal hipoecoico. A aparência ultrassonográfica do abscesso prostático pode ser semelhante àquela do adenocarcinoma de próstata. O diagnóstico deve ser confirmado por exame de uma amostra de líquido prostático e/ou biopsia prostática.

Outras opções terapêuticas incluem prostatectomia cirúrgica paliativa, parcial ou total.[72] Entretanto, tais abordagens estão associadas a sérios riscos de complicações e não necessariamente prolongam a sobrevida.[64] Outras opções terapêuticas paliativas podem ser benéficas e incluem o uso de bifosfonatos, para inibir os osteoclastos e auxiliar no controle de metástases ósseas (ver Capítulo 352).[73] A inibição da reabsorção óssea alivia a dor, reduz o risco de fratura e controla a hipercalcemia paraneoplásica.[64] Apesar de numerosas tentativas para melhorar o tratamento de neoplasias de próstata em cães, no momento o prognóstico é ruim.

REFERÊNCIAS BIBLIOGRÁFICAS

As referências bibliográficas deste capítulo se encontram online no Ambiente de Aprendizagem.

SEÇÃO 25
Câncer

CAPÍTULO 338

Características/Origem do Câncer

Chand Khanna e Amanda Foskett

Recentemente, tem aumentado muito nosso conhecimento sobre a biologia do câncer, junto com oportunidades para melhorar o diagnóstico e o tratamento da doença. Assim, é necessário que os clínicos tenham um sólido conhecimento da biologia básica do câncer e de como implementar melhores opções terapêuticas recentes e convencionais. É também importante integrar essa compreensão para utilizar apropriadamente os testes moleculares desenvolvidos recentemente para o diagnóstico e progressão do câncer.

Em 2000, Hanahan e Weinberg, laureados com o Prêmio Nobel, propuseram um modelo para compreender a complexidade do câncer, denominado como "Características do câncer".[1]

Um componente atrativo desse modelo proposto era sua estrutura coesa, que possibilitava considerar a complexidade e o número crescente de alterações moleculares identificadas em células cancerosas, bem como estabelecer como esses eventos contribuem, individualmente e coletivamente, para a origem do câncer. Em resumo, esse modelo sugeriu que apesar do grande número de alterações moleculares associadas ao câncer, todas elas poderiam ser compreendidas por sua contribuição a seis características fundamentais para o desenvolvimento de câncer. Essas características críticas foram denominadas como "características do câncer". Uma alteração molecular específica poderia contribuir para o surgimento de câncer, fornecendo a uma célula ou mais essas características; entretanto, é a aquisição de todas essas características que ocasiona o fenótipo completo do câncer. As peculiaridades ("características") que os autores priorizaram no modelo estão resumidas na Figura 338.1.

Uma consequência clínica importante desse modelo é que o tratamento efetivo do câncer deve priorizar alvos do câncer que são mais necessários para fornecer uma característica a uma célula. Em resumo, esse modelo possibilita a simplificação de milhares de genes ligados ao fenótipo do câncer em um conjunto simples de seis "características principais" que devem ser adquiridas, a fim de originar câncer a partir de uma célula normal. Ademais, esse modelo possibilita um foco nas características fundamentais do câncer, mais do que nas funções específicas de diversas alterações moleculares.

Dez anos após a publicação original desse modelo, propôs-se uma revisão que refinou as "características principais" mediante o esclarecimento de algumas características de progressão e metástase do câncer, e inclusão de "características de ativação" do câncer.[2]

O uso desse modelo permite que o clínico que foque nas características clínicas do fenótipo do câncer e não em uma longa lista de alterações genéticas moleculares. Ademais, ele fornece um esquema simples para caracterizar as contribuições advindas de diversas alterações moleculares.

CÂNCER, UMA DOENÇA GENÉTICA

Está claro, sob todos os pontos de vista, que o câncer é uma doença genética.[3,4] De fato, em relação à discussão anterior sobre as principais características do câncer, cada uma das seis características necessárias para o surgimento de câncer pode ser causada por alterações em genes. Dizer que o câncer é uma doença genética não significa que o câncer é uma doença hereditária, embora existam riscos familiares e, portanto, hereditários, associados à ocorrência de câncer.[5]

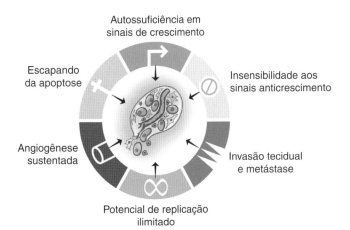

Figura 338.1 Seis características originais do câncer, conforme inicialmente elaboradas por Hanahan e Weinberg, em 2000. (De Hanahan D, Weinberg RA: The hallmarks of cancer. *Cell* 100[1]:57-70, 2000.)

A associação clássica entre câncer e genética envolve uma discussão sobre os genes promotores de tumores que se tornam hiperativos, denominados oncogenes, ou a perda de genes que normalmente limitam uma ou mais características do câncer, conhecidos como genes supressores de tumores. A ativação dos oncogenes ocorre por uma série de razões. Frequentemente, isso envolve uma mutação ou outra alteração estrutural que ativa um gene normal (um proto-oncogene) para se tornar uma oncogene associado ao câncer. O ganho de função observado em um oncogene é um evento dominante e, portanto, requer a alteração de somente um dos alelos do gene.[6,7] Por outro lado, a perda de um gene supressor de tumor é um evento recessivo e, portanto, requer a perda de ambos os alelos para que ocorra perda de função do gene supressor de tumor. Fato interessante é a perda de um gene supressor de tumor, o *P53*, que supostamente é a alteração genética mais comum observada em casos de câncer humano. De forma não surpreendente, a perda do *P53* também foi descrita em uma série de casos de câncer em medicina veterinária.[8-12] *P53* é um membro da família de genes descritos como genes de controle (gene *checkpoint*). *P53* e outros genes de controle atuam na "inspeção" do cenário genético de uma célula, de modo a determinar se há dano suficiente do DNA para impedir a divisão da célula, e seu progresso no ciclo celular (que se refere a uma série de etapas que possibilita a célula sofra mitose). O impedimento da divisão da célula permite que mecanismos de reparo do DNA reparem esse dano ao DNA identificado na célula. Se o dano do DNA for mais significativo, genes como *P53* não somente impedem a mitose, como também desviam a célula para uma via de morte celular programada (apoptose). Isso possibilita a eliminação dessa célula geneticamente alterada, impedindo-a, portanto, de contribuir potencialmente para uma característica do câncer. Portanto, a perda do *P53* e sua função de controle comprometem a capacidade das células adentrarem essa "via suicida/mortal" e, assim, aumenta o número de células geneticamente alteradas. A perda de dois alelos em um gene de supressão tumoral que, como mencionado, contribui para uma característica do câncer, frequentemente ocorre como resultado de um evento hereditário esporádico ("segundo golpe").

Nesse cenário, a primeira perda de um gene supressor tumoral é um risco familiar e a segunda perda é esporádica. A perda resultante desses dois alelos, frequentemente descrita como "golpe duplo", explica por que existem famílias com maior risco de tipos específicos de câncer. Isso foi inicialmente descrito por Knudson, na forma familiar e esporádica de retinoblastoma em humanos, que resulta da perda por golpe duplo do gene supressor tumoral do retinoblastoma (Rb).[13]

Historicamente, acreditava-se que a alteração genética que resultava na desregulação de um gene específico ocorria como uma alteração nos ácidos nucleicos que constituem aquele gene. É agora cada vez mais compreendido que essas alterações na função gênica podem ocorrer além de uma alteração específica no próprio gene. Esse conhecimento é incluído em um amplo campo da biologia do câncer denominado epigenética. Brevemente, a epigenética amplamente se refere a alterações nos elementos reguladores de um gene (denominados promotor ou intensificador do gene). De fato, alterações epigenéticas na função gênica podem ser um mecanismo mais comum da desregulação gênica associada ao câncer do que as alterações estruturais em um gene (*i. e.*, mutação). Fato interessante é que essas alterações epigenéticas na função gênica foram estreitamente relacionadas a diversos fatores de risco ambientais para ocorrência de câncer, além de outros fatores adquiridos.[14,15]

Telomerase e aquisição de potencial de replicação ilimitado

A aquisição de potencial de replicação ilimitado é uma característica do câncer; ela tem sido intimamente associada ao telômero e à telomerase. Telômeros são complexos proteicos do DNA especializados que recobrem as terminações dos cromossomos e mantêm a estabilidade genômica, impedindo a recombinação ou fusão com outros cromossomos. Cada telômero consiste em repetições seriadas de TTAGGG e várias proteínas relacionadas ao telômero. Em células normais, os telômeros se encurtam após cada divisão celular, condição conhecida como desgaste telomérico. A telomerase é uma transcriptase reversa capaz de realizar as repetições teloméricas terminais, estendendo assim o telômero e compensando o desgaste que ocorre durante a divisão celular.[16] Um conteúdo muito baixo é detectado em tecidos somáticos normais; entretanto, há alta concentração de telomerase em células germinativas e naquelas cancerosas, dando a elas potencial de proliferação a longo prazo. Algumas células cancerosas são capazes de manter o comprimento do telômero e sobreviver sem a telomerase.[17] Nessas situações, entram em ação mecanismos alternativos denominados coletivamente de alongamento alternativo de telômeros (AAT).[18,19] Esses mecanismos não são de todo compreendidos, mas são novos alvos terapêuticos ainda não descobertos (*i. e.*, ataxia telangiectasia e quinase relacionada à Rad3 [ATR]), que estão sendo alvos de novos fármacos anticâncer em cães.[20]

PROGRESSÃO TUMORAL E METÁSTASE

Para que as células cancerosas se disseminem a partir do tumor primário para locais secundários distantes, células individuais e grupos de células devem passar por uma série de mecanismos discretos associados à cascata metastática. Um estudo detalhado sobre a cascata metastática definiu recentemente as etapas críticas, que parecem ser as mais difíceis para a passagem bemsucedida das células cancerosas. Essas etapas representam *períodos singulares de vulnerabilidade* durante os quais os fatores estressantes celulares resultam na morte da maioria das células cancerosas e, especialmente, de células não metastáticas. Esses fatores estresses parecem ser maiores à medida que as células metastáticas interagem com o microambiente nos locais secundários de metástases. Apenas uma minoria das células cancerosas pode adaptar-se e sobreviver a essas condições vulneráveis durante a cascata metastática. De fato, o fenótipo metastático pode agora ser definido pela capacidade das células se adaptarem aos fatores estresses pelos quais passam durante esses períodos vulneráveis.[21-23] O conhecimento desses fatores estressantes e dos mecanismos pelos quais as células os vencem fornece uma oportunidade para a descoberta e desenvolvimento de terapias específicas para as metástases.

A metástase é um processo de várias etapas que resulta na disseminação de células tumorais, a partir de um local primário, até órgãos secundários distantes, e a eventual progressão da doença nesses locais secundários. Células cancerosas metastáticas são unicamente programadas para suportar e passar por fatores estresses celulares associados a cada etapa desse processo.

Com base em estudos sobre o fenótipo metastático das células do sarcoma em cães, roedores e humanos, acreditamos que um determinante comum de células cancerosas metastáticas é sua capacidade de resistir a esses fatores estresses.[24] Iniciando com nosso estudo sobre a ezrina, uma proteína associada a metástases, nós tomamos essa abordagem comparativa cruzada entre as espécies (murina, canina, humana) para o estudo das metástases como forma de desenvolver uma compreensão da metástase, que pode ser traduzida rapidamente ao clínico na forma de novos tratamentos.[24]

Dados recentes preliminares agora sugerem a distinção do retículo endoplasmático (RE) de células altamente metastáticas daquele de células com baixo poder de metástase. De fato, a resposta do RE em células altamente metastáticas parece levar a um efeito protetor que não é observado em células com baixo poder de metástase.[25] Esses dados sugerem que o RE e as suas respostas em células altamente metastáticas podem servir como alvos potenciais para novas terapias antimetastáticas. Estão sendo realizados estudos para a triagem e identificação de fármacos que almejam as vias de adaptação ao estresse do RE e que, dessa forma, podem ser úteis na prevenção da progressão metastática.

Angiogênese e o microambiente tumoral

A vasculatura tumoral e angiogênese têm sido estudadas extensivamente, especialmente como um alvo para o tratamento de câncer. A angiogênese tumoral refere-se à formação de vasos sanguíneos no microambiente tumoral mediante a germinação ou intussuscepção de vasos sanguíneos preexistentes. Isso é diferente da vasculogênese, ou formação de novos vasos sanguíneos, que ocorre durante a embriogênese. Os vasos sanguíneos no interior e ao redor de um tumor é de importância crítica, já que supre os nutrientes, fatores de crescimento, metabólitos, mediadores inflamatórios e oxigênio para a proliferação primária do tumor.[26] Os vasos sanguíneos tumorais também representam um meio para que as células tumorais adentrem os vasos sanguíneos e se disseminem para outras partes do corpo; ademais, possuem um papel vital na cascata metastática.

Em todos os tecidos ocorre angiogênese normal, sendo de particular importância na embriogênese e cicatrização de feridas. A hipoxia é o principal estimulante fisiológico para o desenvolvimento de vasos sanguíneos. Mecanismos sensores de hipoxia em tecidos com baixa perfusão sanguínea induzem a formação de novos vasos para suprir as necessidades metabólicas de células em um ambiente de hipoxia. As células respondem secretando fatores de crescimento pró-angiogênico, inclusive fator de crescimento do endotélio vascular (VEGF), fator de crescimento derivado de plaquetas (PDGF) e fator de crescimento de fibroblastos básico (bFGF), entre outros. Brevemente, esses fatores induzem a migração de células endoteliais presentes ao redor dos vasos sanguíneos em direção ao estímulo angiogênico e a formação de novos vasos. A geração de um novo suprimento sanguíneo a esses tecidos elimina o estímulo hipóxico e diminui a produção de VEGF.[27]

O microambiente tumoral muitas vezes não "obedece" a regras fisiológicas normais. Várias células cancerosas são capazes de induzir angiogênese na ausência de hipoxia. Diversos mecanismos foram incriminados como responsáveis por essa condição, inclusive a produção excessiva de VEGF e a regulação de outras citocinas estimulantes vasculares. Esse fenótipo foi associado à ativação de oncogenes, à perda de função de uma série de genes supressores tumorais e à regulação dos mecanismos de inibição da angiogênese. O microambiente tumoral também não possui as barreiras normais presentes em tecidos não cancerosos. Por exemplo, em tecidos cancerosos quase sempre há comprometimento da membrana basal e do tecido conjuntivo, criando uma interface alterada entre o tumor e os vasos sanguíneos, que pode influenciar o potencial metastático e o acesso aos nutrientes e a outros mediadores.[28]

Em medicina humana, foi desenvolvida uma infinidade de agentes terapêuticos com intuito de almejar várias etapas da via angiogênica.[29,30] Em medicina veterinária, também começaram a surgir no mercado medicamentos cujos alvos são pequenas moléculas. Especificamente, o Palladia® (toceranib) é um inibidor do receptor de tirosinoquinase (RTK) desenvolvido para atuar no gene *c-kit*, em mastocitomas. Esse fármaco também inibe as RTK do VEGF e de outras proteínas envolvidas na angiogênese. O toceranib é sabidamente efetivo contra uma série de tipos de câncer independentes do gene *c-kit*.[31] De fato, vários tipos tumorais expressam excessivamente VEGF ou PDGF, ou possuem sinalização aberrante ao VEGF, nos quais esse fármaco pode ter uma ação razoável.[32]

HIPÓTESE DA CÉLULA-TRONCO CANCEROSA

Sabe-se que no tecido canceroso há uma variedade de subpopulações de células, inclusive aquelas responsáveis pela rápida recidiva de um câncer após resposta inicial efetiva à terapia. A hipótese da célula-tronco cancerosa propõe que uma pequena, porém definida, população de células presentes no tumor é capaz de se autorrenovar e origem a células tumorais, tanto no local primário da neoplasia quanto em locais de metástases. Nesse ambiente heterogêneo, há um pequeno número de células de lenta divisão que diferem do resto da população celular do câncer, as quais são resistentes ao tratamento convencional. Aventa-se a possibilidade de que essa população de células seja a causa de recidiva da doença, apesar da resposta inicial efetiva ao tratamento (p. ex., quimioterapia, radiação ou cirurgia), ou de metástases distantes para outros locais do corpo, posteriormente, durante a progressão da doença.[33]

As células-tronco cancerosas (CTC) se tornaram uma área proeminente de interesse e pesquisa como um alvo potencial do tratamento contra o câncer. CTC foram inicialmente identificadas na leucemia mieloide aguda (LMA). Essas células foram caracterizadas por sua capacidade de autorrenovação e repopulação da medula óssea de camundongos com imunodeficiência combinada grave (IDCS), após transplante de células humanas de LMA e estimulação de citocinas *in vivo*.[34] Pesquisas posteriores identificaram uma hierarquia entre essas populações e descobriram marcadores celulares específicos, presentes somente nessa pequena população de CTC, que eram capazes de se diferenciar em células leucêmicas blásticas.[35] Diversos marcadores de CTC são agora identificados em uma série de tumores sólidos, inclusive câncer de mama,[36] colorretal,[37-39] pancreático,[40] hepatocelular,[41] ovariano[42] e de próstata,[43] entre vários outros, inclusive melanoma.[44] Marcadores específicos identificados nesses tipos tumorais foram relacionados ao prognóstico, à taxa metastática e à resposta ao tratamento, em pacientes oncológicos humanos, indicando que essas CTC podem ser um alvo útil para novos tratamento contra o câncer. Terapias variadas com atuação em vias celulares alteradas na população de células-tronco mostraram ser promissoras *in vitro* e em alguns testes clínicos.[45,46] A imunoterapia também tem sido utilizada para atuar em marcadores de superfície celular próprios das CTC, com eficácia variável, em estudos *in vitro* e *in vivo*[47] (ver Capítulo 341).

Embora novas terapias contra CTC ainda não sejam procedimentos de rotina comum na prática clínica, em medicina veterinária, esse procedimento apresenta uma nova e excitante abordagem que, provavelmente, beneficiará o paciente veterinário, no futuro.

REFERÊNCIAS BIBLIOGRÁFICAS

As referências bibliográficas deste capítulo se encontram online no Ambiente de Aprendizagem.

CAPÍTULO 339

Princípios e Práticas da Quimioterapia

Angela E. Frimberger e Antony S. Moore

A quimioterapia é a principal modalidade utilizada para tratar neoplasias sistêmicas, como neoplasias hematológicas e tumores sólidos metastáticos.

BIOLOGIA TUMORAL NA QUIMIOTERAPIA

Para o planejamento da quimioterapia é necessária uma boa compreensão sobre a biologia do tumor, discutida com detalhes no Capítulo 338.

A quimioterapia é mais efetiva em massa tumoral pequena. À medida que o tumor cresce, a taxa de crescimento diminui, ao passo que o tempo do ciclo celular aumenta, a heterogeneidade celular cresce (levando a um maior nível de resistência espontânea) e áreas de baixa perfusão sanguínea se maximizam. Assim, pode não ser possível a liberação de fármacos quimioterápicos nas células cancerosas em teores citotóxicos. Além disso, como a resistência à quimioterapia pode ocorrer por meio de mutações espontâneas que acontecem em cada ciclo de divisão celular em uma taxa intrínseca a cada neoplasia, a probabilidade de ocorrência de mutações que resultam em resistência ao fármaco está relacionada ao número de divisões celulares que ocorreram. Por fim, a citotoxicidade quimioterápica segue a cinética da morte fracionada. Por exemplo, se determinada dose do fármaco mata 4 log de células, então reduzirá um tumor de 10^{12} células para 10^8 células e um tumor de 10^{10} células para 10^6 células – ambas situações parecem propiciar resposta clínica total, pois geralmente 10^9 células é o limite de detecção clínica; entretanto, o último cenário é obviamente o preferível. Portanto, é mais vantajoso começar o tratamento de uma neoplasia com menor massa tumoral, e de forma geral, a quimioterapia será mais efetiva após a detecção precoce ou após um procedimento de citorredução ("remoção da maior parte possível do tumor"), por meio de cirurgia ou radioterapia.

ESTRATÉGIAS PARA QUIMIOTERAPIA

Ao realizar tratamento com quimioterápico é fundamental a comunicação entre o veterinário e o tutor. Essas comunicações devem ser francas e solidárias. Todas as opções devem ser apresentadas aos tutores, sem interferência das preferências dos tutores.

O diagnóstico definitivo do tipo de neoplasia, o estágio clínico da doença e a condição geral de saúde do paciente são importantes tanto no estabelecimento do prognóstico quanto na elaboração de um plano terapêutico. A triagem da condição geral de saúde é necessária para detectar outras enfermidades que possam influenciar a expectativa de vida (*i. e.*, outra doença sistêmica), condições que precisem ser resolvidas antes do início da quimioterapia (p. ex., infecção do trato urinário subclínica), ou condições que precisam ser consideradas ao planejar a quimioterapia (p. ex., doença cardíaca ou renal subclínica).

Estadiamento e avaliação geral da saúde

Todo paciente possui características individuais próprias, inclusive a metabolização e excreção dos fármacos; de modo semelhante, cada tipo de câncer apresenta características individuais. Os propósitos do estadiamento consistem em avaliar a extensão da doença e a saúde geral do animal – isso é importante para avaliar se a condição de saúde é apropriada para a terapia e para a triagem de condições não relacionadas ou secundárias que possam necessitar tratamento antes do início da terapia contra câncer ou que possam, separadamente, influenciar o prognóstico geral do animal. O estadiamento quase sempre tem significado prognóstico, que pode ajudar o veterinário e o tutor a tomar decisões apropriadas e racionais sobre o protocolo terapêutico. A maioria dos sistemas de estadiamento é baseada na avaliação de três importantes componentes da neoplasia maligna: o tamanho do tumor primário (T), a ocorrência de metástases aos linfonodos (N) e de metástases em locais distantes (M).

Objetivo do tratamento

Inicialmente, é importante estabelecer o objetivo do tratamento porque tal procedimento quase sempre define o curso da terapia. O objetivo da quimioterapia na oncologia humana é em geral curar o paciente; entretanto, em medicina veterinária, às vezes o tratamento paliativo pode ser o objetivo mais apropriado. Um diálogo contínuo e aberto permite que o tutor tome uma decisão apropriada e, por fim, propicia uma abordagem "em equipe" para o tratamento do câncer do animal.

Tratamento paliativo

O tratamento paliativo é definido como um procedimento que melhora da qualidade de vida e, possivelmente, a sobrevida, mas sem expectativa de cura do câncer. O tratamento paliativo é frequentemente apropriado quando o prognóstico é ruim e a toxicidade significativa da quimioterapia não é justificável, quando se espera apenas uma sobrevida breve. Para vários animais idosos, o diagnóstico de câncer é feito em um momento quando outras doenças podem limitar a sobrevida, mais do que o próprio câncer. Para esses animais, o cuidado paliativo pode ser mais apropriado, e deve-se considerar se o benefício da quimioterapia é maior do que o risco de intoxicação. É raramente efetivo o procedimento de iniciar o tratamento paliativo e depois alterar para uma abordagem mais agressiva. Entretanto, é comum iniciar o tratamento com intuito curativo e depois alterar para um tratamento paliativo.

Tratamento com intuito curativo

Cura é definida como a erradicação de todas as células tumorais, resultando em um estado permanente livre da doença; é o resultado ideal, embora nem sempre realista. A restrição das doses da quimioterapia para manter os efeitos colaterais dentro de uma condição clínica aceitável significa que quase sempre a cura é possível apenas em pequeno número de pacientes veterinários – por exemplo, 15% dos cães com linfoma e 20% dos cães com osteossarcoma, dada a terapia padrão de cuidados. Em cães e gatos que apresentam boa saúde e sem doença concomitante, e quando a quimioterapia mantém a possibilidade de controle prolongado do câncer com pouco risco de toxicidade, pode-se realizar quimioterapia com intenção curativa.

Quimioterapia combinada com outras modalidades terapêuticas

Na oncologia veterinária, a quimioterapia primária (quimioterapia como o tratamento único ou principal) é, em geral, reservada para neoplasias hematopoéticas (linfoma, leucemia, mieloma múltiplo). Para cães com tumores sólidos metastáticos (carcinoma e sarcoma), o uso exclusivo de quimioterapia raramente é curativo; é melhor considerada como tratamento paliativo.

A quimioterapia adjuvante é utilizada após a ressecção ou radiação de um tumor primário, a fim de retardar o progresso da doença metastática ou, possivelmente, propiciar a cura. Utiliza-se tal procedimento quando o animal apresenta risco significativo de recidiva ou metástase, mas antes que a progressão da doença seja clinicamente detectável – por exemplo, após amputação em cães com osteossarcoma. A quimioterapia adjuvante é efetiva porque é utilizada nos estágios iniciais do crescimento tumoral. Quando se faz a ressecção de uma neoplasia primária, os focos de micrometástases de células tumorais apresentam alta fração de crescimento e um pequeno número de células resistentes. A desvantagem da quimioterapia adjuvante é que os pacientes curados pela cirurgia são tratados desnecessariamente. Para tumores como osteossarcoma e hemangiossarcoma, em cães, e tumores mamários, em gatas, a porcentagem de cura cirúrgica é pequena, mas para animais com outros tumores, a decisão sobre os benefícios da quimioterapia pode ser mais difícil.

A *quimioterapia neoadjuvante* é utilizada antes das modalidades terapêuticas locais, como cirurgia ou radioterapia, com o objetivo de reduzir o tamanho do tumor primário e diminuir a extensão e os efeitos colaterais de outros tratamentos definitivos.

A *quimiorradioterapia* refere-se ao uso de fármacos quimioterápicos primariamente como sensibilizadores da radiação, e não por ter uma ação antineoplásica direta.

Classes de medicamentos e combinação de quimioterápicos

Vários padrões de protocolos de cuidados terapêuticos utilizam combinações de fármacos quimioterápicos. A compreensão dessa combinação de quimioterápicos requer o conhecimento das classes comuns de medicamentos em uso na oncologia veterinária.

Fármacos alquilantes (Tabela 339.1) criam ligações cruzadas no DNA, induzindo anormalidade na fita desse DNA. Uma característica interessante dessa classe de fármacos é a aparente ausência de resistência cruzada entre diferentes agentes alquilantes ou com outras classes de fármacos.

Antibióticos antineoplásicos (antraciclinas) (Tabela 339.2) atuam por meio da intercalação do DNA, interferindo com as topoisomerases e com outros mecanismos. Esses fármacos quase sempre apresentam resistência cruzada com outros medicamentos de sua classe e com fármacos de algumas outras classes, principalmente os inibidores da mitose, e são substratos para o surgimento de resistência a multifármacos (RMF).

Os inibidores da mitose (Tabela 339.3) atuam inibindo a montagem (alcaloides da vinca) ou desmontagem (paclitaxel) do fuso mitótico.

Compostos de platina (Tabela 339.4) criam ligações cruzadas no DNA. O mecanismo de ação é semelhante àquele dos agentes alquilantes, e não é observada nenhuma reação cruzada com outras classes de fármacos quimioterápicos.

Tabela 339.1 Agentes alquilantes comumente utilizados.

MEDICAMENTO (FÁRMACO)	APRESENTAÇÃO	EFEITOS COLATERAIS POTENCIAIS	DOSE/PROTOCOLO
Ciclofosfamida (Cytoxan®)	Comprimidos de 25 e 50 mg; frasco com 500 mg	Mielossupressão Cistite hemorrágica	250 mg/m² VO a cada 3 semanas 200 mg/m² IV a cada 3 semanas 50 mg/m²/VO a cada 48 h
Clorambucila (Leukeran®)	Comprimido de 2 mg (manter refrigerado)	Mielossupressão discreta, porém cumulativa	6 a 8 mg/m²/VO a cada 48 h 15 mg/m²/dia VO durante 4 dias, a cada 3 semanas
Melfalana (Alkeran®)	Comprimido de 2 mg (manter refrigerado)	Mielossupressão	1,5 mg/m²/dia VO durante 10 dias, seguido de "descanso" de 10 dias
Lomustina (CCNU®; Gleostine®)	Cápsulas de 5, 10, 40 e 100 mg	Mielossupressão, neutropenia e trombocitopenia retardada em cães; neutropenia retardada em gatos Toxicidade renal e hepática irreversível (incomum)	50 a 90 mg/m² VO a cada 4 a 6 semanas (cães) 50 mg/m² VO a cada 6 semanas (gatos)
Mecloretamina (Mustargen®)	Frasco com 10 mg	Mielossupressão Reação de extravasamento	No protocolo MOPP: 3 mg/m² IV (semanalmente)
Procarbazina (Matulane®)	Cápsula de 50 mg	Náuseas, anorexia, diarreia Mielossupressão	50 mg/m²/dia VO durante 14 dias (cães); 10 mg/gato/dia VO durante 14 dias
Dacarbazina (DTIC®)	Frasco com 200 mg	Mielossupressão Anorexia, êmese e diarreia	800 mg/m² em infusão IV lenta ao longo de 5 a 8 h, a cada 3 a 4 semanas (administra-se dolasetrona antes do tratamento)
Ifosfamida (Ifex®)	1 g, combinada com Mesna Frasco com 1 g	Mielossupressão Cistite hemorrágica (deve ser administrada com Mesna e protocolo de diurese) Toxicidade renal em gatos	375 mg/m² IV (cães) 900 mg/m² IV (gatos) Administrar a cada 3 semanas, em solução de NaCl 0,9%, com Mesna

Tabela 339.2 — Antibióticos antineoplásicos comumente utilizados.

MEDICAMENTO (FÁRMACO)	APRESENTAÇÃO	EFEITOS COLATERAIS POTENCIAIS	DOSE/PROTOCOLO
Doxorrubicina (Adriamycin®)	2 mg/mℓ Frascos com 10, 20, 50 e 200 mg	Mielossupressão Cardiotoxicidade cumulativa Anorexia, êmese, diarreia Reação alérgica Reação de extravasamento Toxicidade renal em gatos	30 mg/m² IV (cães grandes) 25 mg/m² ou 1 mg/kg IV (gatos e cães pequenos) Administrada a cada 2 a 3 semanas (a taxa de infusão IV não deve exceder a 2 mg/min)
Mitoxantrona (Novantrone®)	Frascos com 10 e 20 mg	Mielossupressão Efeitos gastrintestinais [GI] (incomuns)	5,5 a 6 mg/m² IV (cães) 6,5 mg/m² IV (gatos) Administrada a cada 3 semanas
Dactinomicina (actinomicina D, Cosmegen®)	Frasco com 0,5 mg	Mielossupressão Reação de extravasamento Diarreia, êmese	0,5 a 1 mg/m² IV Requer taxa de infusão lenta (até o momento não há relato de uso em gatos)
Bleomicina (Blenoxane®)	Frasco com 15 U (15 mg) NOTA: 1 U (Unidade USP) corresponde a 1.000 UI (Unidade Internacional), que corresponde à potência de 1 mg. Lembre que a potência de 1 mg é definida por bioensaio e não é idêntica ao peso seco de 1 mg (1 mg de peso seco de acordo com a unidade USP corresponde à potência de 1,5 a 2 mg)	Em humanos: reação alérgica, fibrose pulmonar	0,3 a 0,5 U/kg IV ou SC, semanalmente

Tabela 339.3 — Inibidores de mitose comumente utilizados.

MEDICAMENTO (FÁRMACO)	APRESENTAÇÃO	EFEITOS COLATERAIS POTENCIAIS	DOSE/PROTOCOLO
Vincristina (Oncovin®)	1 mg/mℓ	Mielossupressão discreta (relacionada à dose) Anorexia em gatos, raramente em cães (relacionada à dose) Neuropatia periférica (rara) Reação de extravasamento	0,5 a 0,75 mg/m² IV, semanalmente
Vimblastina (Velban®)	Frasco com 10 mg	Mielossupressão Neuropatia periférica (muito rara) Reação de extravasamento	3 mg/m² IV a cada 2 semanas (cães) 1,5 a 2 mg/m² IV a cada 2 semanas (gatos)
Vinorelbina (Navelbine®)	Frasco com 10 mg	Mielossupressão Neuropatia periférica (muito rara) Possível toxicidade renal em gatos Reação de extravasamento	15 a 18 mg/m² IV a cada 2 semanas (cães) 11,5 mg/m² IV, semanalmente (gatos)

Tabela 339.4 — Platinas utilizadas como agentes quimioterápicos.

MEDICAMENTO (FÁRMACO)	APRESENTAÇÃO	EFEITOS COLATERAIS POTENCIAIS	DOSE/PROTOCOLO
Cisplatina (Platinol®)	Frasco com 50 mg	Toxicidade renal Êmese e (menos comumente) diarreia Discretamente mielossupressora Edema pulmonar fatal em gatos	50 a 70 mg/m² IV, com diurese com salina 0,9% a cada 3 a 4 semanas NÃO UTILIZE EM GATOS
Carboplatina (Paraplatin®)	Frascos com 50, 150, 450 e 600 mg	Mielossupressão	250 a 300 mg/m² IV a cada 3 a 4 semanas (cães) 210 a 240 mg/m² IV a cada 4 semanas (gatos)

Antimetabólitos são análogos de metabólitos normais que são incorporados ao DNA, onde interferem na atividade enzimática, transcrição ou translação. Em doses para espécies veterinárias esses fármacos quase sempre causam toxicidade significativa e baixa eficácia e não são frequentemente utilizados em oncologia veterinária. A gencitabina é a mais utilizada em medicina veterinária; para esse fármaco, a taxa e o tempo de infusão são determinantes extremamente importantes da eficácia e efeitos colaterais, e a melhor dose e esquema de infusão ainda não foram determinados.

Uma importante classe de quimioterápicos recentes consiste em inibidores da tirosinoquinase (TKI). O uso desses quimioterápicos está em rápida expansão em oncologia humana; ademais essa classe contempla os primeiros quimioterápicos desenvolvidos especificamente para cães. Os dois fármacos dessa classe de uso veterinário são toceranibe (Palladia®) e masitinibe (Masivet®). Atualmente, a dose de toceranibe recomendada na bula (3,25 mg/kg/48 h VO) é considerada maior do que a clinicamente apropriada (2,5 a 2,75 mg/kg/48 h ou 3 vezes/ semana). Embora esses sejam novos fármacos empolgantes, e administrados por via oral, o risco de efeitos adversos dessa classe de fármacos é tão real quanto a de outros quimioterápicos. Monitoramento programado, ajustes de dose e cuidado de suporte são igualmente importantes.

Resistência tumoral a alguns fármacos quimioterápicos é comum, mesmo antes do início do tratamento. Ademais, as células tumorais adquirem resistência rapidamente após exposição a fármacos devido sua alta taxa de mutação. A combinação de quimioterápicos pode superar alguns problemas de resistência que interfere em diferentes vias metabólicas, em células resistentes a algum fármaco componente da combinação. Embora a combinação de quimioterápicos possa ser potencialmente mais tóxica às células normais, os padrões de toxicidade variam entre os fármacos (Tabela 339.5). A implantação de um protocolo criterioso de medicamentos quimioterápicos de forma que suas toxicidades não se sobreponham pode aumentar a morte de células tumorais sem a sobreposição de toxicidade combinada.

O protocolo quimioterápico desenvolvido é complexo e requer conhecimento detalhado dos medicamentos e de seus efeitos. Cada fármaco incluído deve ser pelo menos parcialmente efetivo contra o tumor-alvo, quando utilizado sozinho. Quando se administra uma combinação de fármacos no mesmo dia pode ser necessária a redução da dose de cada medicamento, de modo a obter maior intensidade da dose total (ver a seguir); entretanto, é preciso cuidado para não reduzir a dose de um medicamento altamente efetivo para possibilitar a administração de um segundo fármaco menos efetivo. Os medicamentos são então combinados levando em consideração tanto o mecanismo de ação quanto o perfil de toxicidade de cada um, para expor o tumor à maior concentração possível dos medicamentos e maximizar a intensidade da dose, enquanto se minimizam as toxicidades. Os protocolos mais seguros e efetivos são desenvolvidos por oncologistas veterinários.

Para reduzir o desenvolvimento de resistência aos fármacos, é importante não administrar medicamentos em doses subterapêuticas; deve-se fornecer a maior intensidade de dose possível. É também importante não modificar as doses ou o protocolo terapêutico planejados em antecipação à toxicidade que não ocorreu. Por exemplo, um cão que se tornou neutropênico após receber doxorrubicina não apresenta maior risco de mielossupressão induzida por outros quimioterápicos, como ciclofosfamida, de forma que as doses dos outros fármacos somente devem ser reduzidas se eles causarem toxicidade. Os cuidados de suporte, como o uso preventivo de antieméticos, também diminuem a necessidade de reduções de doses dos quimioterápicos. Por outro lado, se ocorre crescimento tumoral, não é um bom procedimento a continuação do mesmo protocolo terapêutico, nas mesmas doses. Em vez disso, deve-se administrar um protocolo alternativo, porém efetivo, utilizando medicamentos que não apresentam resistência cruzada.

Escolha dos medicamentos quimioterápicos

Dados publicados sobre a sensibilidade tumoral à quimioterapia estão mudando rapidamente. Embora haja disponibilidade de boas informações publicadas sobre cães com doenças mais comuns, informações sobre outras neoplasias frequentemente estão indisponíveis ou são baseadas em pequenas séries de casos. Ao contrário, para tumores raros que raramente causam metástases é difícil demonstrar eficácia adjuvante para qualquer tratamento quimioterápico. Mesmo quando há estudos concluídos, a publicação dos dados obtidos pode demorar; e os melhores recursos para os clínicos veterinários são informações de oncologistas veterinários, do Veterinary Cancer Society (*www.vetcancersociety.org*) e de bases de dados de literatura da internet, como Medline ou PubMed.

Além da eficácia, e possivelmente mais importante, a escolha definitiva de um medicamento (ou protocolo terapêutico) depende da toxicidade, da tolerância do tutor aos efeitos colaterais, dos objetivos do tratamento, do custo e do grau de conforto do veterinário em administrar a quimioterapia e propiciar cuidados de suporte.

Algumas considerações sobre a quimioterapia

Embora seja tentador pensar em protocolos quimioterápicos como uma "receita" para o tratamento de câncer, na verdade eles devem ser considerados como um guia. Os protocolos quimioterápicos veterinários são quase sempre simples, consistindo em um ou dois medicamentos quimioterápicos fornecidos em um intervalo que minimiza o risco de toxicidade, porém que mantém a maior intensidade de dose possível. Entretanto os protocolos para linfoma geralmente são complexos, com a combinação de diversos medicamentos (ver Capítulo 344).

Dose da quimioterapia

Como a citotoxicidade é o efeito desejado para a quimioterapia, vários medicamentos quimioterápicos possuem estreitas margens terapêuticas; ou seja, a dose tóxica é próxima da dose efetiva. Portanto, é importante que o cálculo das doses seja o mais acurado possível. Para alguns fármacos, a dose é baseada no "tamanho corporal metabólico" (área de superfície corporal [ASC, m^2]), e não no peso. Embora imperfeito, tal procedimento é baseado na generalização de que animais menores apresentam maior taxa metabólica e, portanto, devem receber uma dose maior, com base no peso corporal. Para alguns medicamentos (p. ex., doxorrubicina), a dose baseada na ASC não é apropriada, e cães e gatos pequenos devem receber dose menor do que a de cães maiores. Até que novas diretrizes estejam disponíveis, os veterinários devem se basear na dose indicada para os fármacos a ser utilizados e na tabela de conversão da ASC quando forem indicadas doses metabólicas.

Na oncologia humana, a dose pode ser adaptada a um indivíduo seja pelo monitoramento da concentração do fármaco,

Tabela 339.5	Potencial mielossupressor de alguns medicamentos quimioterápicos comumente utilizados.

ALTAMENTE MIELOSSUPRESSOR	MODERADAMENTE MIELOSSUPRESSOR	DISCRETAMENTE MIELOSSUPRESSOR
Doxorrubicina	Vincristina (0,75 mg/m²)*	Corticosteroides
Lomustina (CCNU)	Clorambucila	L-asparaginase*
Ciclofosfamida	Melfalana	Vincristina (0,5 mg/m²)*
Carboplatina	Metotrexato	Bleomicina
Vimblastina	Cisplatina	Estreptozotocina
Mitoxantrona	Hidroxiureia	
Vinorelbina	5-Fluoruracila	

*A combinação de vincristina e L-asparaginase pode ser altamente mielossupressora.

seja pelas características do paciente. Por exemplo, a dose apropriada de carboplatina pode ser calculada a partir de uma fórmula baseada na taxa de filtração glomerular (TFG) do paciente e na área sob a curva (AUC) desejadas. Esse tipo de cálculo não é em geral utilizado em oncologia veterinária; entretanto, são conhecidos princípios semelhantes: em pacientes com baixa TFG (aumento da concentração sérica de creatinina) deve-se reduzir a dose de carboplatina.

Evidências em oncologia humana e veterinária sugerem que a maior intensidade de dose propicia melhor resultado aos pacientes submetidos à quimioterapia. A intensidade da dose é expressa em mg do fármaco/m^2 por semana de terapia e pode ser modificada pelo ajuste da dose e/ou intervalo entre as doses ou sessões de quimioterapia.

Vias de administração

Os medicamentos quimioterápicos, em sua maioria, são administrados por via intravenosa (IV) ou por via oral (VO). Menos comumente, eles são administrados por via subcutânea (SC) ou intramuscular (IM). Às vezes, utilizam-se outras vias de administração. Para a maioria dos tratamentos quimioterápicos, a injeção por meio de um cateter que recobre a agulha (cateter *over-the-needle*), em um vaso sanguíneo periférico, é mais segura, reduzindo o risco de extravasamento do medicamento, mesmo quando é preciso injetar um pequeno volume do fármaco. Para infusões mais demoradas (mais de 30 minutos), provavelmente o risco de deslocamento de um cateter interno a uma agulha (cateter *through-the-needle*) é menor.

Quando são necessárias infusões por longo tempo, seja para o uso programado de medicamentos (como a gencitabina), seja para a administração de solução salina para diurese concomitante ao tratamento com fármacos nefrotóxicos (como a cisplatina ou a estreptozocina), recomenda-se o uso de uma bomba de infusão para assegurar diurese continuada e/ou até mesmo o fornecimento da dose do fármaco. Alterações em um desses fatores pode influenciar a eficácia da terapia e o risco de toxicidade.

O acesso vascular pode ser um problema em gatos e cães pequenos submetidos à quimioterapia. Como o risco de extravasamento é maior nesses animais, um acesso vascular implantável subcutâneo pode facilitar a aplicação do medicamento em horários programados e reduzir o estresse durante a administração do quimioterápico. Tal acesso pode ser mantido durante a terapia e, então, removido. O acesso vascular implantável deve ser colocado cirurgicamente, de forma semelhante a um cateter tunelizado, introduzindo-se uma bolsa subcutânea para a colocação do acesso venoso. Acessos venosos para uso veterinário estão disponíveis em Norfolk Vet Products®, Skokie, Illinois (*www.norfolkvetproducts.com*).

A maioria dos medicamentos de uso oral é administrada na forma de comprimidos ou cápsulas. Os comprimidos não devem ser fracionados por questão de segurança pessoal, e porque a distribuição do medicamento no comprimido pode não ser uniforme, ou o comprimido pode ser revestido (p. ex., clorambucila). Para pequenos animais, é possível a manipulação de fármacos de uso oral em cápsulas de tamanhos menores por uma farmácia de manipulação confiável, especialmente equipada para manuseio de produtos citotóxicos.

Cisplatina e carboplatina podem ser administradas aos cães na forma de infusão intracavitária, na cavidade pleural, pericárdica ou peritoneal; para tumores de bexiga pode elas podem ser administradas por via intravesical (ou seja, diretamente na bexiga).

A quimioterapia intralesional em geral envolve a suspensão de um medicamento quimioterápico em um veículo. Há relato de uso de cisplatina, bleomicina ou 5-fluoruracila em óleo de sésamo estéril ou em matriz de colágeno de bovinos. A mistura é injetada no tumor, propiciando uma alta exposição das células tumorais ao fármaco. Isso cânvolve concentrações sistêmicas mínimas de medicamentos, evitando o risco de toxicidade sistêmica. A quimioterapia intralesional é utilizada para tratar apenas tumores pequenos e facilmente acessíveis. Nesse procedimento,

deve-se ter muito cuidado para evitar a exposição da equipe médica, pois não raramente ocorre derramamento do fármaco; ademais pode ocorrer extravasamento do medicamento nos locais de aplicação.

Quimioterápicos de uso (5-fluoruracila – apenas para cães) estão disponíveis, mas raramente são utilizados por conta da toxicidade do fármaco e do risco de exposição às pessoas que aplicam o medicamento ou interagem com o cão. Alguns fármacos também podem ser administrados por via intra-arterial ou intratecal, em protocolos terapêuticos específicos; entretanto, isso é raramente utilizado em medicina veterinária.

A encapsulação do medicamento em lipossomos pode reduzir ou alterar a toxicidade de alguns fármacos quimioterápicos. A conjugação do lipossomo com polietilenoglicol reduz a depuração pelo sistema reticuloendotelial, originando lipossomos "ocultos" que permanecem mais tempo na circulação sanguínea. Há relato de que uma formulação de doxorrubicina encapsulada em lipossomos foi menos cardiotóxica em cães e gatos, mas resultou em uma nova toxicidade cutânea.

Quimioterapia metronômica

A quimioterapia metronômica utiliza pequenas doses de quimioterapia frequentes (em geral diárias ou em dias alternados), diferentemente da quimioterapia convencional que utiliza doses máximas toleradas em intervalos de semanas. Esse esquema de administração parece resultar em alteração no mecanismo de ação dos fármacos, de citotóxico para antiangiogênico (principalmente pela atuação em células endoteliais das neoplasias) e imunomodulador (principalmente pela inibição de células T reguladoras [Treg]). Os fármacos quimioterápicos escolhidos para uso metronômico quase sempre são administrados por via oral, como ciclofosfamida, clorambucila e lomustina (também denominada CCNU). Mais frequentemente, os inibidores da ciclo-oxigenase também são incluídos em combinações, a fim de exacerbar os efeitos antiangiogênico e imunomodulador. A quimioterapia metronômica tem se tornado popular em medicina veterinária porque quase sempre é bem tolerada, mas sua eficácia ainda não foi bem documentada na maioria das situações. Embora o tratamento seja geralmente menos dispendioso a curto prazo, comparado à quimioterapia convencional, vários animais necessitam formulações de fármacos disponíveis no mercado remanipulados para uso metronômico e isso pode ter um alto custo. Ademais, a quimioterapia metronômica quase sempre é mantida por um tempo muito longo (até anos), de forma que pode haver custos totais acumulados com o passar do tempo.

Apesar de sua popularidade, a maioria da literatura publicada sobre quimioterapia metronômica consiste em estudos retrospectivos relativamente pequenos, frequentemente em grupos de cães com tipos mistos de neoplasias. Assim, os dados são difíceis de interpretar e os resultados promissores preliminares ainda tem de ser acompanhados de evidências mais conclusivas da eficácia, na maioria das situações. Ocasionalmente, são constatadas boas respostas tumorais, mas a maioria da eficácia antitumoral relatada consiste em estabilidade da doença (entretanto, é razoável ressaltar que em oncologia veterinária há várias situações em que a estabilização da doença a longo prazo é de fato um benefício clínico significante).

Embora a quimioterapia metronômica seja geralmente considerada menos tóxica do que a quimioterapia convencional, ainda há risco de toxicidade, sendo importante um monitoramento cuidadoso. A quimioterapia metronômica com ciclofosfamida envolve um risco real de toxicidade urotelial, como acontece com a quimioterapia convencional com esse medicamento; os autores observaram que a administração de furosemida concomitante a cada dose de ciclofosfamida reduz sobremaneira esse risco, embora ainda o constatamos ocasionalmente e monitoramos cuidadosamente a ocorrência de hematúria microscópica. A quimioterapia metronômica com lomustina resultou em taxa de 30% de descontinuação da terapia por conta de sua toxicidade; portanto, essa abordagem terapêutica deve ser utilizada com cuidado. Obviamente, a adição de um medicamento anti-inflamatório não esteroide (AINE) em vários protocolos de quimioterapia metronômica também pode estar associado à toxicidade, como acontece com o uso de qualquer AINE (ver Capítulo 164). A quimioterapia metronômica com ciclofosfamida também parece ser moderadamente segura na maioria dos gatos, embora as evidências publicadas ainda contemplem um grupo pequeno e misto de gatos submetidos a acompanhamento clínico por um período relativamente curto.

Na opinião do autor, a quimioterapia metronômica com ciclofosfamida a longo prazo é provavelmente a melhor opção quimioterápica para sarcoma de tecidos moles que foram submetidos à ressecção incompleta, nos quais não é possível a extirpação completa e/ou uso de radiação. A quimioterapia metronômica pode também ser utilizada em outras situações nas quais os tutores do animal não aceitam a quimioterapia convencional, cirurgia e/ou radioterapia, quando já se tentou terapia convencional sem sucesso, ou como procedimento de "manutenção" após quimioterapia convencional adjuvante para tumores de risco particularmente alto. Entretanto, até que novas evidências estejam disponíveis, os autores sugerem que a quimioterapia metronômica seja considerada investigacional e não como terapia de primeira linha, na maioria das situações. Por fim, a segurança do tutor deve ser cuidadosamente considerada ao levar em conta o uso prolongado de medicamentos alquilantes no próprio domicílio; os tutores devem ser lembrados regularmente disso para não se tornarem displicentes com os procedimentos de segurança.

Quimioproteção

A administração de um segundo fármaco especificamente para minimizar a toxicidade de um quimioterápico aos órgãos do hospedeiro é denominada de *quimioproteção*.

Os quimioprotetores utilizados em oncologia humana e veterinária são a mesna e o dexrazoxano. A mesna reduz o risco de cistite associado à ifosfamida e a ciclofosfamida minimiza esse risco por se ligar a metabólitos tóxicos na urina. O dexrazoxano protege contra a cardiotoxicidade crônica associada à doxorrubicina e reduz a gravidade de lesão por extravasamento causada pela doxorrubicina, quando utilizada logo após o extravasamento.

CUIDADOS DE SUPORTE EM ANIMAIS SUBMETIDOS A QUIMIOTERAPIA

Os efeitos adversos da quimioterapia são discutidos com detalhes no Capítulo 343. Antes da administração da quimioterapia, as doses dos fármacos e suas toxicidades, assim como o protocolo de administração, devem ser revisados juntamente com o tutor. Após o tratamento, o animal deve ser monitorado no próprio domicílio, em busca de sinais de toxicidade. Na Figura 339.1 há um algoritmo para interpretação das contagens de neutrófilos após a quimioterapia.

A fim de que os animais mantenham a melhor qualidade de vida, e que as doses de quimioterápicos sejam mantidas em sua maior concentração, o veterinário deve, sempre que possível, utilizar cuidados de suporte proativos para prevenir ou tratar as toxicidades comuns. Avanços na prevenção e tratamento de dor e náuseas, assim como toxicidades órgão-específicas, como ocorrência de cistite, melhoram a capacidade do veterinário em fornecer doses apropriadas de quimioterápicos e alta qualidade de vida para os animais com câncer.

AVALIAÇÃO DA RESPOSTA TERAPÊUTICA

Para determinar se um dado tratamento é efetivo, é necessário avaliar a resposta terapêutica regularmente. Isso é importante

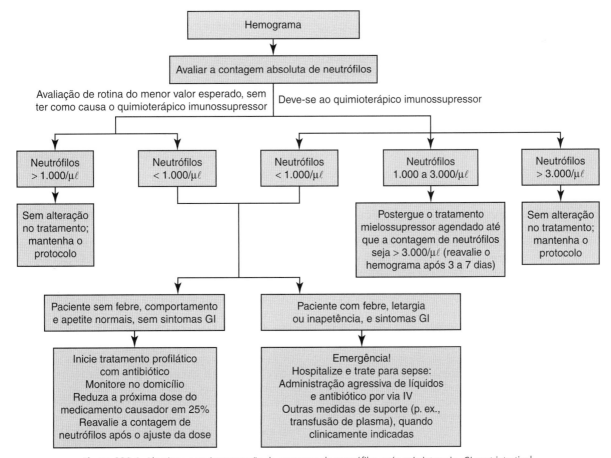

Figura 339.1 Algoritmo para interpretação da contagem de neutrófilos após quimioterapia. *GI*, gastrintestinal.

para evitar gastos desnecessários, toxicidade e progressão tumoral resultantes da continuidade da administração de um medicamento ineficaz. Os clínicos podem consultar os critérios do Veterinary Cooperative Oncology Group, para mensuração de tumores sólidos e linfonodos. A resposta ao tratamento pode então ser categorizada como remissão clínica/resposta completa (RC), resposta parcial (RP), doença estável (DE) ou doença progressiva (DP). Na literatura, a *taxa de resposta geral (TRR)* refere-se à combinação de RC e RP (outro termo utilizado na literatura mais recente, benefício clínico, refere-se à combinação de RC, RP e DE; embora haja várias situações clínicas nas quais a DE certamente é benéfica, é preciso cuidado ao ler relatos de testes terapêuticos que não comparam a TRR e o benefício clínico, já que não são equivalentes).

Resistência aos fármacos quimioterápicos

A resistência aos quimioterápicos pode ser intrínseca ou adquirida. Os fármacos podem ser fisicamente incapazes de atingir os tumores situados em locais de difícil acesso, como o sistema nervoso central, ou que apresentam baixa perfusão sanguínea. As células tumorais podem intrinsecamente conter poucos receptores para o medicamento ou, de alguma maneira, não serem suscetíveis ao seu mecanismo de ação (p. ex., células que possuem asparaginase sintetase são resistentes à L-asparaginase). Células neoplásicas podem desenvolver resistência espontânea aos fármacos por meio de mutações. Em cada divisão celular há risco de mutação para resistência; portanto, quanto maior o tumor (*i. e.*, quanto mais divisões celulares ele sofreu), maior a probabilidade de ocorrência de resistência. As células tumorais também podem desenvolver resistência a fármacos especificamente. A exposição a concentrações subletais do medicamento pode resultar em amplificação de gene responsável pela detoxificação de proteínas.

Embora a combinação de quimioterápicos possa minimizar a ocorrência de resistência a fármacos individuais, ela não evita a resistência cruzada entre diversos medicamentos quimioterápicos não relacionados. A proteína da bomba transmembrana (glicoproteína-P) está presente em alta quantidade em algumas células tumorais, e tanto sua prevalência quanto o seu conteúdo aumentam com a exposição ao quimioterápico. Esse fenômeno de resistência a múltiplos fármacos (RMF) envolve antraciclinas, inibidores da mitose e outros medicamentos. Agentes alquilantes, porém, não são substratos para a glicoproteína-P e representam a base do tratamento de pacientes com esse tipo de resistência a fármacos.

MANUSEIO SEGURO DO MEDICAMENTO QUIMIOTERÁPICO

A maioria dos medicamentos quimioterápicos é tóxica e mutagênica. Como a maioria deles é efetiva nas fases ativas do ciclo celular, a toxicidade relativa aos quimioterápicos é mais comum nos tecidos em renovação e quase sempre está relacionada à dose do medicamento. Isso tem implicações para o paciente (toxicidade e eficácia), assim como para a segurança do tutor do animal e da equipe veterinária ao manusear os medicamentos durante a administração e para os cuidados do paciente. Precauções devem ser tomadas ao manusear os fármacos quimioterápicos durante qualquer etapa, de preparação, administração e descarte de fármacos ou dejetos. Medicamentos alquilantes têm sido mais incriminados como os de maior risco às pessoas que os manuseiam. Dano aos órgãos e maior risco de perda fetal foram relatados em pessoas que manuseiam e administram quimioterápicos com cuidados inapropriados à segurança pessoal.

A administração apropriada de quimioterápicos foi abordada detalhadamente por vários autores. Brevemente, as regulações mantidas pela U.S. Occupational Safety and Health Administration (OSHA) devem ser seguidas, e os tutores, assim como toda a equipe que tem contato com os fármacos quimioterápicos, devem ser protegidos ao máximo. Atualmente, alguns países e estados possuem legislação específica para o uso de quimioterápicos na prática veterinária. É aconselhável entrar em contato com a autoridade responsável antes de elaborar o protocolo terapêutico. Deve-se manter um livro de registro do procedimento quimioterápico, que inclui a identificação de animais tratados e a equipe envolvida nos tratamentos, para monitorar as exposições. Os dados contidos na Ficha de Informação de Segurança de Produtos Químicos (FISPQ) para cada fármaco alertam para os perigos específicos à saúde, inclusive carcinogenicidade, principais meios de exposição, equipamentos de proteção, tratamento da equipe exposta de forma aguda, ativadores químicos, solubilidade, estabilidade, volatilidade e procedimentos específicos a serem tomados em caso de derramamento. A FISPQ deve ser requisitada, com envio inicial de qualquer medicamento quimioterápico; deve ser mantida arquivada em um local de fácil acesso. Deve-se manter um kit próprio para o caso de derramamento (disponível no mercado).

O ideal é utilizar uma capela de fluxo laminar vertical para preparar todos os fármacos quimioterápicos. Atualmente há dispositivos com sistema fechado de administração de fármacos, como Equashield® e PhaSeal® (Vídeo 339.1), em pequenas quantidades, compatíveis com a prática veterinária, e devem ser rotineiramente utilizados no manuseio de fármacos citotóxicos. Todos esses itens geralmente estão disponíveis em distribuidores de medicamentos quimioterápicos. Durante a administração parenteral, o uso de seringa com rosca diminui o risco de extravasamento ou derramamento do fármaco. Os medicamentos quimioterápicos devem ser armazenados em embalagem com fecho, e as seringas que contém o quimioterápico forem transportadas pelo hospital devem ser levadas nessas embalagens.

Riscos aos tutores de animais

Deve-se fornecer aos tutores uma ficha com informações sobre a segurança relativa à quimioterapia. Se os tutores estiverem administrando fármacos por via oral no domicílio, devem ser fornecidas luvas e embalagens com fecho para depositar os dejetos. Entretanto, a principal preocupação envolve pessoas que manuseiam os medicamentos (misturando e administrando), com menor risco àqueles que manuseiam fezes e urina no hospital e no domicílio.

Normas de segurança claras para tutores de animais que manuseiam líquidos corporais de pacientes submetidos à quimioterapia ainda não são totalmente explícitas e tendem a pecar por excesso de zelo. Portanto, supõe-se que o melhor é um período de 24 a 72 horas, por estar além do tempo de excreção dos principais metabólitos, após uma injeção na forma de *bolus*. A excreção de fármacos quimioterápicos e de seus metabólitos em líquidos corporais deve ser tratada com cuidado, mas não com pânico. A maioria dos tutores evita contato com urina e fezes do animal tratado, descuidando dos procedimentos higiênicos de rotina; entretanto, o contato acidental por uma única vez não é causa para alarme, quando seguido de lavagem normal. No caso de fármacos excretados na urina, o animal deve ser encorajado a urinar em um local onde a urina será rapidamente drenada, e qualquer urina em outras áreas deve ser manuseada e descartada como se faz com a urina de um paciente submetido à quimioterapia. Donos de animais grávidas devem consultar seus médicos antes de decidir pelo contato com seu animal tratado com quimioterápicos, e não devem manusear quaisquer medicamentos quimioterápicos.

CAPÍTULO 340

Princípios e Práticas de Radiologia Oncológica

Jessica Lawrence

INTRODUÇÃO

Considerações gerais

O câncer é a principal causa de morte natural em gatos e cães, e relata-se que sua prevalência pode estar aumentando.[1-3] *Câncer* é um termo abrangente que compreende várias doenças com diversos comportamentos biológicos, padrões de cuidados e prognósticos. Os veterinários são encorajados a obter conhecimentos a respeito do câncer, de modo a representar fontes de conhecimento para tutores e seus animais. A radioterapia começou no século 19, após a descrição de Roentgen sobre os raios X, em 1895, e a descoberta do elemento químico rádio por Marie e Pierre Curie, em 1898.[4-6] A *radiação oncológica* refere-se ao uso médico de radiação ionizante como parte do tratamento de câncer, matando ou controlando as células neoplásicas malignas. A radioterapia está disponível em várias instituições, tanto públicas quanto privadas.[7-9]

O propósito primário da radioterapia é propiciar controle de tumor local e/ou local-regional, embora às vezes seja recomendada radiação de metade do corpo ou de corpo inteiro. Dependendo da condição clínica, o intuito primário da radioterapia pode ser paliativo ou definitivo (potencialmente curativo), sendo comumente utilizada concomitante à cirurgia e/ou terapia sistêmica. Um dos principais desafios da radioterapia é atingir o tecido neoplásico com doses tumoricidas, ao mesmo tempo que o tecido normal é poupado. A maioria dos avanços na radiação oncológica, incluindo radioterapia de intensidade modulada (RTIM), radioterapia estereotáxica (RTE), radiocirurgia estereotáxica (RCE), e radioterapia guiada por imagem (RTGI), foca na melhora da capacidade em localizar o tumor almejado, administrar precisamente feixes de radiação alinhados e poupar estruturas normais para melhorar a tolerância geral e o resultado (Boxe 340.1). Os dois principais tipos da radioterapia são: radioterapia com intenção definitiva (intenção "curativa") e radioterapia com intenção paliativa. O objetivo da radioterapia com intenção definitiva é o controle a longo prazo (às vezes cura) de um tumor. O objetivo da radioterapia com intenção paliativa é amenizar os sintomas específicos causados por uma neoplasia (como hemorragia ou dor) (Boxe 340.2).

Considerações gerais sobre a seleção de pacientes veterinários para radioterapia

Candidatos

Cães e gatos (e, às vezes, outras espécies) devem ser avaliados cuidadosamente para assegurar que sejam bons candidatos para radioterapia. Assim que o tipo de tumor, o seu comportamento biológico e s extensão da doença sejam conhecidos, pode-se determinar a importância da radioterapia. A radioterapia exclusiva ou em combinação com a cirurgia pode ser apropriada para o tratamento de pacientes com doenças locais ou locais-regionais. A quimioterapia adjuvante pode ser administrada concomitante à radioterapia, dependendo do tipo de tumor. O planejamento prospectivo é melhor abordado ao envolver uma equipe que inclua clínico geral, cirurgião, oncologista clínico, radioterapeuta e o tutor. Essas pessoas são aquelas que tomam decisões sobre a melhor abordagem para o tratamento de uma neoplasia. Um protocolo terapêutico viável para um paciente pode não ser compatível para outro, mesmo quando o tumor é semelhante.

Estadiamento

Ao optar por radioterapia com intenção definitiva é importante o estadiamento do tumor mediante a determinação da extensão da lesão neoplásica, para saber se há doença localizada. Os testes diagnósticos tipicamente estão relacionados ao tipo do tumor primário e podem incluir hemograma, perfil bioquímico sérico, exame de urina, exame citológico de aspirado de linfonodos regionais, exames de imagem do tórax e/ou abdome e exames

---

Boxe 340.1 Terminologia radiológica comum

A terminologia relativa à radiação pode causar confusão e alguns termos podem ser utilizados como sinônimos, de forma imprecisa. A terminologia comum e as abreviações são fornecidas adiante, visando à melhor compreensão do leitor quanto aos termos comumente utilizados

- **Dose** – quantidade de radiação absorvida pelo paciente (Gray = Gy = 1 Joule/kg; o termo mais antigo "rad" não é utilizado)
- **Fração** – administração individual de radiação
- **Fracionamento** – a dose de radiação é dividida em frações ao longo de vários dias a semanas, dependendo da intenção do tratamento
- **Prescrição da radiação** – dose particular e número de frações prescritas para um tumor para determinado paciente
- **Radiação por feixe externo** – radiação liberada de fora do corpo por uma máquina que emite fótons de alta energia em um tumor
- **Radioterapia Conformacional 3D (RTC-3D)** – é o tipo de radioterapia conformacional baseada em imagens que melhora a distribuição da dose de radiação por toda a massa tumoral, o que pode limitar o dano ao tecido normal adjacente
- **Radioterapia de intensidade modulada (RTIM)** – melhor planejamento e liberação da radiação na qual a intensidade dos feixes de radiação

direcionados à massa tumoral alvo varia durante o tratamento, a fim de aumentar a semelhança de distribuição da dose de radiação no tumor, com uma rápida redução da dose de radiação às estruturas normais adjacentes

- **Radioterapia guiada por imagem (RTGI)** – imagem obtida imediatamente antes ou durante o tratamento, a fim de detectar erros no posicionamento do paciente e do tumor. A RTGI propicia garantia de nível de qualidade, pois os feixes de radiação são precisamente direcionados à massa tumoral
- **Radiocirurgia estereotáxica (RCE)** – consiste em um único tratamento que envolve uma grande fração (15 a 20 Gy), em geral utilizado para tratar tumores bem delimitados
- **Radioterapia estereotáxica (RTE)** – consiste em pequeno número de sessões (3 a 8) que envolve uma grande fração (10 a 20 Gy), utilizada para tratar pequenas lesões bem delimitadas
- **Plesioterapia** – radiação de "superfície" com penetração limitada (2 a 3 mm), em geral liberada por uma sonda de estrôncio-90 (^{90}Sr)
- **Braquiterapia** – radiação a curta distância (comumente radiação interna) em geral liberada de cápsulas radioativas.

Boxe 340.2 Resumo do protocolo de radioterapia (RT)

Protocolos de RT com intenção definitiva
- Geralmente, utiliza-se um grande número de frações/doses
- Baixa dose/fração
- Esperam-se efeitos colaterais agudos
- Geralmente é mais cara
- A intenção é obter controle a longo prazo ("curativa"), ao mesmo tempo que se limita a toxicidade tardia
- Baixo risco de toxicidade tardia clinicamente relevante

Protocolos de RT com intenção paliativa
- Menor número de frações/doses
- Alta dose/fração
- Poucos efeitos colaterais agudos
- Geralmente com custo moderado ao tutor
- A intenção é melhorar a qualidade de vida (melhora a função do órgão acometido, diminuindo a dor ou a hemorragia)
- Maior risco de toxicidade tardia clinicamente relevante

Protocolos de RT estereotáxica
- Menor número de frações/doses
- Alta dose/fração e dose total tumoricida
- Reduz a toxicidade aguda devido à presença de mínima quantidade de tecido normal na região submetida à alta dose
- Depende da verificação do posicionamento guiada por imagem
- Alto custo
- A intenção pode ser paliativa ou o controle a longo prazo, ao mesmo tempo que se limita a toxicidade ao tecido normal
- Aguardam-se resultados clínicos, em cães e gatos.

de imagem avançados. A tomografia computadorizada (TC) é um dos procedimentos mais úteis na avaliação da imagem de tumores, sendo fundamental para o planejamento da radioterapia auxiliada por computador. A ressonância magnética (RM) pode ser utilizada para o planejamento, em algumas situações. Os exames de imagem avançados podem possibilitar avaliações subjetivas iniciais quanto à extensão da doença, à localização de tecidos críticos próximos ou em um campo de tratamento potencial, e às possíveis opções terapêuticas razoáveis e aplicáveis. TC e/ou RM podem não ser indicadas antes da radioterapia, se os resultados não alterariam a terapia.

Orientação do tutor

Os tutores incluídos na equipe de tomadores de decisão devem compreender os custos, a frequência e a duração previstos com os tratamentos. Eles também devem ter conhecimento do risco de eventos adversos e dos resultados esperados. Os oncologistas radioterapeutas são capazes de estabelecer diversos aspectos da radioterapia, ou seja: (1) indicação de radioterapia com base em informações publicadas na literatura veterinária existente, (2) objetivo da radioterapia, (3) alvo da radioterapia (em geral, uma doença localizada pré-cirurgia ou pós-cirurgia), (4) tipo ou técnica de radioterapia, (5) dose planejada e protocolo de radioterapia, e (6) eventos adversos agudos e tardios esperados.

RADIOTERAPIA CLÍNICA

Aspectos práticos da radioterapia veterinária

Quando um paciente veterinário é submetido à radioterapia, é importante que o planejamento prospectivo propicie a melhor terapia e determine um método de posicionamento do paciente reprodutível e comprovado. Dessa forma, a radioterapia pode ser aplicada à massa tumoral almejado. O planejamento e a administração de tratamento avançado, como RTGI e RTE, dependem do posicionamento apropriado do paciente durante a liberação de cada fração, ou dose, de radiação. A diminuição das margens do volume-alvo planejado (PTV, do inglês *planning target volume*) é bem-sucedida quando se confirma o posicionamento apropriado antes de cada dose.

Ao contrário do que acontece na radioterapia oncológica em pessoas, os animais são anestesiados para realizar o planejamento terapêutico, bem como para a radioterapia, a fim de assegurar um posicionamento reprodutível e prolongado, para o tratamento. A maioria dos protocolos anestésicos consiste em anestésicos de rápida ação, que possibilitam rápida recuperação. Os pacientes submetidos à radioterapia típica são mantidos anestesiados por 60 a 90 minutos, para a primeira sessão, mas apenas 10 a 15 minutos para as sessões de radioterapia subsequentes. Os dispositivos de posicionamento, como colchões de imobilização, máscaras faciais, mordedores e cunhas de espuma, são frequentemente utilizados para obter uma posição de ajuste específica para o paciente e que possa ser repetida em cada sessão (Figura 340.1). Nem todos os tumores necessitam de amplo planejamento, mas geralmente quando há estruturas normais muito próximas ao alvo, o planejamento terapêutico 3D (em geral acompanhado de TC para obter informação sobre a densidade tecidual) auxilia na redução da toxicidade aos tecidos normais. As neoplasias de extremidades localizadas distantes de tecidos críticos raramente necessitam planejamento 3D, a menos que seja realizada radioterapia pré-cirúrgica ou haja preocupação quanto à extensão tumoral após a cirurgia.

Toxicidades teciduais

Terapia fracionada

Frequentemente, há preocupação quanto à toxicidade induzida por radiação na massa tecidual tratada. Antes do início da radioterapia é importante que se discuta minuciosamente as ocorrências próprias desse procedimento, com todos os envolvidos. A toxicidade terapêutica depende do esquema de fracionamento da radiação, do período de duração da radiação, e do tipo e volume de tecidos normais situados no campo de radiação. Como a radiação não discrimina os tipos de células, tanto em tecidos tumorais quanto naqueles normais, eles reagem de forma semelhante. Entretanto, a radiação terapêutica, o fracionamento

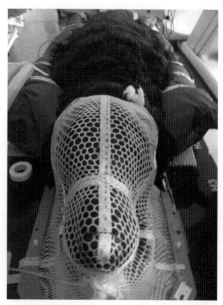

Figura 340.1 Paciente posicionado para tomografia computadorizada (TC), durante planejamento para radioterapia. A cabeça e o pescoço são posicionados sobre uma placa de plástico encaixada em um suporte de fibra de carbono posicionado na cabeça, fixado à mesa, enquanto o corpo é imobilizado em um colchão a vácuo. Utiliza-se uma máscara facial de acrílico para acomodar e fixar a cabeça ao encosto de cabeça e chassi. Utiliza-se alinhamento a *laser* para auxiliar no posicionamento em comum para TC e radioterapia.

e a técnica de liberação de radiação empregados tentam, em parte, explorar a diferença nas capacidades de reparo de tecidos normais e tumorais. Em geral, as células tumorais têm mecanismos de reparo danificados e maior número de células do ciclo celular devido sua maior taxa de proliferação. O tecido normal presente no campo de radiação é "dose-limitante" quanto à dose máxima que pode ser seguramente administrada. A dose fracionada, o esquema de tratamento e a dose total influenciam a tolerância tecidual normal.

A estrutura tecidual é importante porque o fracionamento da radiação reduz a toxicidade aos tecidos normais e pode melhorar a resposta geral de um tumor, comparativamente à administração de pequeno número de fracos, porém com alta dose por fração. A radiação administrada 1 ou 2 vezes/dia possibilita o reparo das células normais, mas não propicia tempo suficiente para o reparo de células tumorais. Isso permite que ocorra dano cumulativo no tumor exposto a repetidas frações.[4] Sempre, deve-se avaliar o benefício da probabilidade de controle da neoplasia frente à probabilidade de complicações. Em doses de radiação menores, a probabilidade de complicações é baixa e propicia uma chance moderada de controle do tumor, enquanto o aumento da dose propicia maior chance de controle do tumor, porém com maior risco de complicações no tecido normal (Figura 340.2).

Toxicidade aguda da radiação

Em geral, a toxicidade aguda da radiação é reversível, autolimitante, ocorre durante ou logo após a terapia, e os efeitos se limitam à área irradiada. Tecidos de rápida proliferação, como o epitelial, de membranas mucosas e tumorais são mais sujeitos à toxicidade aguda. Os tecidos que sofrem toxicidade aguda tendem a cicatrizar dentro de 2 a 4 semanas (Figura 340.3). O desconforto é esperado a curto prazo e a toxicidade aguda frequentemente não é prazerosa ao tutor, tampouco ao animal. As toxicidades agudas dependem da dose total de radiação administrada (quanto maior a dose, maior a toxicidade), mas também da duração e frequência do tratamento (em geral, tratamento mais curto aumenta a toxicidade) e da fração de dose (quanto maior a fração, maior a toxicidade). O tratamento quimioterápico concomitante à radiação pode aumentar a toxicidade aguda à radiação. Na oncologia veterinária não há disponibilidade de diretrizes sobre os fármacos envolvidos.[41] Os efeitos agudos são autolimitantes e na maioria dos casos as lesões cicatrizam sem intervenção médica, embora seja importante o uso de analgésico em pacientes submetidos à radioterapia.

No caso de toxicidade aguda grave inesperada, pode-se utilizar o tratamento cirúrgico padrão da lesão, de modo a assegurar que o local permaneça limpo e protegido. Poucos dados foram publicados quanto aos melhores métodos para tratar pacientes submetidos à radioterapia; ademais, não há diretrizes de consenso baseadas em evidências para a radiação oncológica.[42] Em uma pesquisa realizada em instituições veterinárias norte-americanas que lidam com radiação constatou-se que cerca de 75% delas utilizavam analgésicos e antibióticos por via oral, para tratar a dermatite causada pela radiação. Mas, há várias opiniões quanto às estratégias terapêuticas.[42] A equipe deve empregar métodos que evitam o agravamento maior das lesões, por lambedura, prurido ou fricção no local da radiação. No caso de lesões bucais, utilizam-se alimentos pastosos, enxaguantes bucais e, ocasionalmente, antibióticos (por via oral). Dada nossa consciência crescente sobre resistência antimicrobiana, em parte graças ao amplo uso indiscriminado de antibióticos de amplo espectro, por via oral, devem ser feitos esforços para determinar se métodos alternativos seriam úteis no tratamento da toxicidade por radiação.[43-45]

Efeitos adversos tardios

Efeitos adversos da radiação "tardios" surgem ≥ 6 meses após o término da radioterapia. Esses efeitos são determinados pelas estruturas presentes no campo irradiado. Efeitos adversos da radiação tardios tipicamente ocorrem em tecidos de proliferação lenta ou que não são renovados, como o coração, pulmões, rins, nervos, ossos e músculo. Também são verificados efeitos tardios diretamente relacionados aos efeitos colaterais agudos graves inesperados, que não se recuperam adequadamente. Esses tecidos que não se renovam são dose-limitantes. Assim, a dose prescrita para o tratamento da neoplasia deve manter uma taxa de efeitos tardios clinicamente relevantes menor que 5%. Na maioria dos casos o dano tecidual tardio é progressivo e irreversível e se deve ao dano vascular, inflamação crônica, fibrose, necrose e perda de células-tronco do tecido normal. Os efeitos tardios mais comuns são anormalidades estéticas, mas podem ocorrer toxicidade clinicamente relevante, como osteorradionecrose ou formação tumoral secundária, em caso de sobrevida longa (> 3 a 5 anos) após a radioterapia (Figura 340.4).[11] A probabilidade de ocorrência de efeitos da radiação tardios depende da quantidade da fração de radiação (quanto maior a fração, maior o risco de toxicidade tardia). A dose geral prescrita é também importante. Como os efeitos da radiação tardios quase sempre são irreversíveis, devem ser feitos esforços para evitar que ocorram (Tabela 340.1).

Protocolos terapêuticos paliativos *versus* definitivos (ver Boxe 340.2)

Os fatores que ditam a probabilidade de ocorrência de toxicidade tardia ajudam a escolher entre protocolos de radioterapia definitivos ou paliativos. É comum a recomendação de protocolos de radiação com intenção definitiva aos animais com bom prognóstico e maior probabilidade de sobrevida acima de 6 meses. Nesses tipos de protocolos a dose diária administrada é menor, de modo a "proteger" o tecido normal do desenvolvimento de toxicidades tardias relevantes, que poderiam influenciar negativamente a qualidade de vida. Protocolos paliativos são tipicamente reservados aos animais com prognóstico ruim. Os objetivos da terapia paliativa consistem em aliviar a dor associada à neoplasia, diminuir o tamanho de qualquer massa tumoral que ocasione obstrução (neoplasia de laringe ou que comprima o linfonodo ilíaco medial), e aliviar os sintomas debilitantes do câncer (hemorragia causada por uma grande massa tumoral ulcerada, na boca).

A radioterapia paliativa não visa prolongar a sobrevida, embora possa fazê-la indiretamente. Ela é prescrita para melhorar a qualidade de vida. Há diversos protocolos de radioterapia paliativa. Eles frequentemente envolvem radiação administrada 1 ou 2 vezes/semana, no total de três ou quatro doses, ou 4 ou 5 doses por dia. Como a dose de radiação aumenta em cada sessão, se os animais responderem bem ao tratamento e sobreviverem mais que 6 a 12 meses após o tratamento, há uma

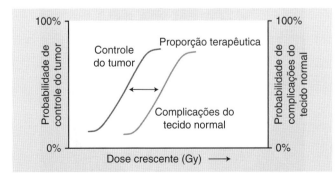

Figura 340.2 Proporção terapêutica descrita para radioterapia, na qual se considera o benefício da probabilidade de controle do tumor diante da probabilidade de complicações do tecido normal. Em doses de radiação menores a probabilidade de complicações é baixa, mas com probabilidade moderada de controle do tumor. O aumento da dose pode possibilitar maior chance de controle do tumor, mas com maior risco de complicações no tecido normal.

2076 SEÇÃO 25 • Câncer

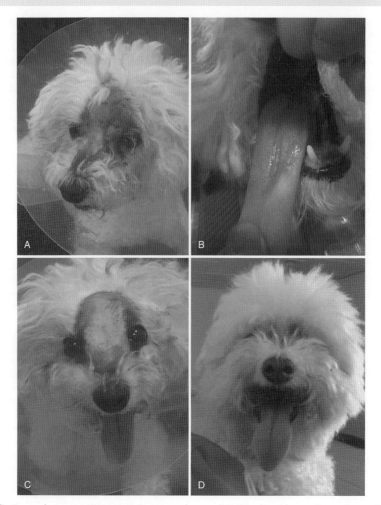

Figura 340.3 Toxicidade por radiação aguda em um cão com carcinoma nasal em estágio IV submetido a radioterapia com intenção definitiva. **A.** Descamação exsudativa aguda no campo irradiado, no final do tratamento. **B.** Inflamação aguda da mucosa da língua, que estava no campo irradiado. **C.** Cicatrização da descamação 2 semanas após a radioterapia. **D.** Efeitos adversos da radiação agudos completamente cicatrizados 16 meses após a radioterapia.

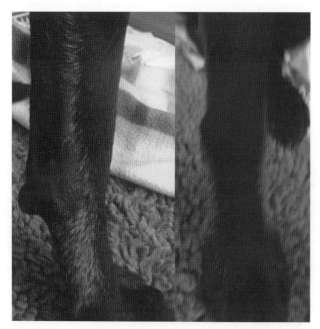

Figura 340.4 Toxicidade tardia por radiação após radioterapia com intenção definitiva de um sarcoma de tecido mole submetido a extirpação parcial. O campo de radiação é delimitado ao longo das faces lateral e caudal do membro, por alopecia e leucotriquia; a face dorsal do membro distal foi poupada para permitir a drenagem linfática.

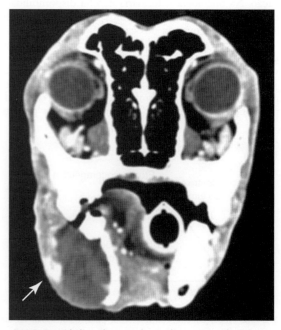

Figura 340.5 Toxicidade tardia por radiação clinicamente relevante em um cão submetido a radioterapia paliativa para linfoma gengival mandibular epiteliotrópico solitário. Surgiu osteossarcoma (*seta*) no campo de radiação 4 anos após o tratamento do linfoma; depois da realização de mandibulectomia, não se constatou evidência do linfoma em cortes histológicos.

Tabela 340.1 Possíveis toxicidades causadas pela radiação em cães e gatos.

PELE	TOXICIDADE AGUDA POR RADIAÇÃO	TOXICIDADE TARDIA POR RADIAÇÃO
Pele e tecido subcutâneo	Descamação exsudativa Alopecia	Fibrose e retração tecidual Úlcera que não cicatriza Leucotriquia Alopecia Tumor secundário (sarcoma)
Membros distais	Desprendimento de unha ou de coxim plantar	Neuropatia Fibrose e retração muscular
Medula espinal	Mielopatia transitória "aguda" retardada (rara)	Mielopatia Infarto Radiculopatia (síndrome do neurônio motor inferior)
Região cervical	Faringite Esofagite Traqueíte	Hipotireoidismo Constrição esofágica
Cavidade bucal	Mucosite	Doença periodontal Xerostomia (boca seca)
Cavidade nasal	Rinite Secreção nasal	Rinite crônica (secreção nasal)
Trato gastrintestinal (GI)	Gastrite, enterite ou gastrenterite Colite/proctite	Constrição
Olhos	Blefarite/blefarospasmo Conjuntivite Úlcera de córnea Ceratite Uveíte	Catarata Ceratoconjuntivite seca (CCS) Anormalidades na retina Cegueira
Cérebro	Encefalopatia (rara) Edema (raro) Efeitos sistêmicos: letargia, náuseas, êmese (rara)	Encefalopatia Infarto/hemorragia
Ossos		Osteorradionecrose Formação de tumor secundário (sarcoma)
Rins	Nefropatia aguda	Fibrose que progride para nefropatia

probabilidade maior de ocorrência de toxicidade tardia clinicamente relevante (Figura 340.5). RCE e RTE utilizam hipofracionamentos modestos, mas essas técnicas envolvem a administração precisa de radiação altamente conformacional em um pequeno alvo, minimizando a quantidade de tecido normal na região submetida à alta dose de radiação prescrita.[5] Dados clínicos em cães e gatos são limitados. Esse tipo de radiação tem sido utilizada para tumores sólidos: cerebrais, osteossarcoma canino, sarcomas vacinais em gatos e tumores nasais em cães.[46-52]

Radioterapia adjuvante

Considerações gerais

Como a morte celular segue cinéticas exponenciais, os tumores maiores necessitam de doses maiores de radiação para induzir uma resposta completa. De fato, diversos estudos demonstraram uma relação inversa entre a probabilidade de controle tumoral após radioterapia e o tamanho do tumor, em casos de mastocitomas, sarcomas de tecidos moles, neoplasias de hipófise e tumores bucais, em cães, e de carcinomas de célula escamosa de plano nasal e carcinomas de célula escamosa bucais, em gatos.[53-59] A radiação tende a ser mais efetiva na doença microscópica devido à natureza de crescimento dos tumores sólidos (crescimento Gompertziano) e a quebras na dupla fita de DNA de células tumorais, como alvos da terapia. Há exceções, na maioria dos tumores em animais a radioterapia é considerada mais efetiva no período pós-cirúrgico, quando as margens cirúrgicas não são extirpadas totalmente ou são estreitas, com risco de recidiva da neoplasia (Figura 340.6).

Na maioria dos casos, a radioterapia começa 10 a 20 dias após a cirurgia, possibilitando tempo para a cicatrização tecidual. O campo de radiação, então, inclui todas as áreas potencialmente contaminadas pela abordagem cirúrgica e áreas que provavelmente contenham doença microscópica. As vantagens da radioterapia pós-cirúrgica incluem: o estadiamento cirúrgico possibilita o ajuste de doses e volumes alvos de radiação; a radiação é mais efetiva na obtenção de controle a longo prazo ao atuar na doença microscópica; não prejudica a cicatrização pós-cirúrgica da ferida (embora isso seja raro em animais de companhia); e não há retardo na cirurgia, o que pode ter um benefício psicológico para pessoas com câncer (e potencialmente para os tutores).

Vantagens e desvantagens da realização de cirurgia antes da radioterapia

O estadiamento cirúrgico geralmente é considerado um dos melhores procedimentos para determinação da real extensão da neoplasia, pois as amostras são enviadas para exame histológico após a remoção da lesão. O cirurgião, portanto, possui um papel crítico quando se planeja radioterapia pós-cirúrgica. Antes da ressecção cirúrgica, é recomendável definir se a implantação de grampos ou marcadores radiopacos é útil para identificar as margens da excisão cirúrgica. A utilização de marcadores pode auxiliar no delineamento pós-cirúrgico do volume tumoral (VG e VTC) pretendido. Isso melhora a capacidade de exclusão do tecido normal.[60] Potenciais desvantagens da radioterapia pós-cirúrgica incluem: maior volume de tecido normal irradiado após a cirurgia, especialmente quando a cicatriz cirúrgica não

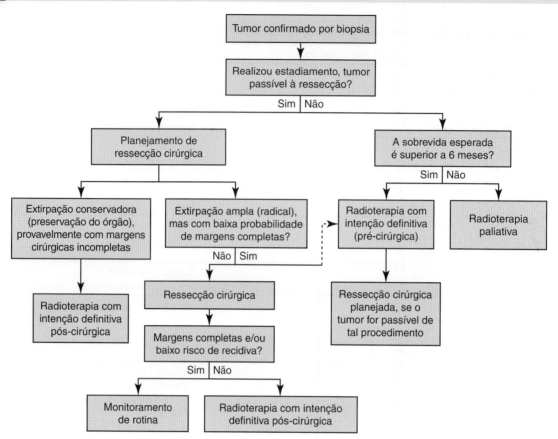

Figura 340.6 Algoritmo para a importância da radioterapia no tratamento oncológico de pacientes veterinários. A histologia, as características clínicas e o estadiamento do tumor, além de outros fatores, influenciam a tomada de decisão quanto à radioterapia definitiva. A radiação paliativa geralmente é realizada em pacientes com câncer em estágio avançado.

estiver bem alinhada ao leito tumoral; pode haver maior risco de disseminação de células tumorais durante a cirurgia; pode ocorrer alteração no suprimento sanguíneo às células tumorais residuais, criando um ambiente resistente à radiação e mais hipóxico, necessitando, assim, de dose total maior; se houver complicações cirúrgicas relacionadas à cicatrização da ferida, o tempo para o início da radioterapia pode ser retardado.

Radioterapia pré-cirúrgica

A radioterapia pré-cirúrgica é frequentemente recomendada para grandes tumores, quando não é sabido se o tumor pode ser seguramente e completamente extirpado, isto é, tumores de tireoide em cães ou sarcomas vacinais em gatos.[23-25,51,61-63] A radioterapia é geralmente prescrita em um protocolo de 3 a 4 semanas, seguido de um período de 2 a 4 semanas no qual qualquer lesão decorrente de toxicidade aguda deve cicatrizar, antes da cirurgia. Possíveis vantagens da realização de radioterapia pré-cirúrgica incluem: uso de menos radiação, talvez porque não houve alteração na vasculatura por manipulação cirúrgica; o campo de radiação é menor já que o volume tumoral e os alvos podem ser melhor definidos; não há retardo no início da radiação; e a extensão da cirurgia pode ser discretamente menor, dependendo da resposta ao tratamento.

Potenciais desvantagens da radioterapia pré-cirúrgica incluem: carência de estadiamento cirúrgico inicial, que pode prejudicar o planejamento da radioterapia; efeito deletério potencial na cicatrização pós-cirúrgica da lesão (embora isso não seja bem reconhecido em medicina veterinária, mesmo em casos nos quais a cirurgia é realizada meses após a radioterapia); e regiões hipóxicas em tumores volumosos mensuráveis podem inibir boas respostas celulares à radiação. Gatos com sarcoma vacinal quase sempre apresentam lesão extensa e altamente infiltrativa, por ocasião da consulta, tornando importante a realização de radioterapia pré-cirúrgica na diminuição dos potenciais efeitos da radiação tardios por possibilitar prescrição de menor dose total para o tratamento de uma lesão de volume menor. No caso de tumores não passíveis de ressecção, a radioterapia pré-cirúrgica pode originar um tumor menor (diminuir o grau de estadiamento), mais suscetível à extirpação. A decisão de realizar radioterapia pré-cirúrgica *versus* pós-cirúrgica deve ser tomada pela equipe.

Quimioterapia e radioterapia

A quimioterapia pode ser administrada simultaneamente à radiação graças ao comportamento biológico de alguns tumores, suas histologias tumorais subjacentes, ou como um sensibilizador à radiação. O grau de sinergismo entre os fármacos quimioterápicos e a radiação é extremamente variável. Em pessoas, alguns medicamentos interagem fortemente (doxorrubicina) e outros não demonstram sinergismo evidente (citosina-arabinosídeo). Até o momento, os esforços para avaliar os fármacos quimioterápicos, como a carboplatina e gencitabina, como sensibilizadores à radiação, em cães e gatos, foram desanimadores.[64,65] Embora muitos animais toleram quimioterapia e radioterapia concomitantes ou a combinação de inibidores da tirosinoquinase e radioterapia, é importante monitorar eventos adversos hematológicos, gastrintestinais ou da radiação inesperados.[41,64,66,67]

Tipos comuns de tumores tratados com radioterapia em oncologia veterinária

Vários tumores são responsivos à radiação; entretanto, a resposta final tende a ser variável e dependente de epidemiologia, histologia da neoplasia, localização, grau e/ou estágio da doença. É sempre importante lembrar que estruturas críticas normais adjacentes ao campo de radiação limitam a quantidade de radiação que pode ser administrada; ocasionalmente, as doses devem ser ajustadas para evitar dano relevante. Dependendo da condição clínica, a radioterapia também pode ser utilizada em outros tipos de tumores, como plasmocitoma solitário, linfoma solitário, tumor de glândula salivar, tumor do trato urinário distal, timoma e sarcoma histiocítico. A radioterapia paliativa pode ser empregada para a maioria dos tumores, assim como na tentativa de melhorar a disfunção ou aliviar a dor. No caso de neoplasias que respondem bem à radioterapia, uma nova sessão pode ser uma opção viável, mas depende do protocolo de radiação inicial, da dose total e do esquema de fracionamento, além da presença de tecidos normais muito próximos ao tumor recidivante ou progressivo. Dado os avanços tecnológicos relativos à radioterapia, é provável que a sua importância no tratamento de pacientes veterinários com câncer se tornará cada vez maior e integrado em abordagens multimodalidades.

REFERÊNCIAS BIBLIOGRÁFICAS

As referências bibliográficas deste capítulo se encontram online no Ambiente de Aprendizagem.

CAPÍTULO 341

Imunoterapia no Tratamento de Câncer

Barbara J. Biller

INTRODUÇÃO

Dentre as modalidades terapêuticas disponíveis para o tratamento de câncer, a imunoterapia possui o maior potencial para combater especificamente os tumores e poupar tecidos normais. É também única em sua capacidade de induzir uma resposta de memória a longo prazo, que pode prevenir a recidiva do tumor. Muitas pesquisas sobre câncer tradicionalmente visam o conhecimento de características da própria célula tumoral, como sinalização celular aberrante, persistência e ativação da invasão, e metástase. Mais recentemente, nota-se uma consciência crescente sobre a importância do hospedeiro e do microambiente tumoral na progressão do câncer (ver Capítulo 338); dentre os mais críticos desses fatores, inclui-se o sistema imune e sua resposta ao câncer.

A ideia de que o sistema imune possa controlar o câncer não é novidade. Em 1909, Ehrlich sugeriu que o câncer poderia ocorrer em uma "frequência esmagadora", em tese, pela função do sistema imune do paciente.[1] Na década de 1960, Burnet propôs que os linfócitos atuavam como vigilantes constantes de tecidos normais, eliminando células anormais por meio de um mecanismo que ele denominou *vigilância imune*.[1,2] A teoria de Burnet não foi amplamente aceita até a década de 1990, quando foram identificados antígenos associados à neoplasia e linfócitos específicos de tumores em pacientes humanos com câncer. Atualmente, sabe-se que quase todos os mecanismos imunes inatos e adaptativos conhecidos participam, em parte, do reconhecimento e do controle de tumores, ou, de modo inverso, auxiliam os tumores a evitar sua detecção.

CONSIDERAÇÕES GERAIS SOBRE IMUNOLOGIA TUMORAL

A dupla participação do sistema imune – em proteger contra o desenvolvimento tumoral e promover o seu crescimento – é ilustrada pelo mecanismo de *imunoedição*. Durante esse processo, o fenótipo das células neoplásicas evolui para escapar da detecção pelo sistema imune do hospedeiro. A imunoedição pode ser caracterizada por três etapas ou fases distintas. Na etapa inicial de vigilância imunológica (também conhecida como etapa de eliminação), as células alteradas são reconhecidas e eliminadas por meio da combinação de respostas imunes inatas e adaptativas (revisadas no Boxe 341.1). As poucas células que conseguem sobreviver entram em fase de equilíbrio, na qual há um balanço dinâmico entre eliminação e sobrevivência de células tumorais. Entretanto, na fase de escape final, a pressão imune constante e a instabilidade genética do tumor propiciam a expansão de uma população de células neoplásicas de baixa imunogenicidade, altamente imunossupressoras, que são bem preparadas para escapar de detecção adicional.[3]

O escape imune consiste em múltiplos mecanismos complexos, que podem ser classificados em duas amplas categorias. A primeira envolve a seleção de células tumorais de baixo grau de reconhecimento (como ausência de potentes antígenos tumorais ou perda de moléculas do complexo de histocompatibilidade principal) e alta capacidade de sobrevivência. A segunda envolve o desenvolvimento de um microambiente tumoral imunossupressor dominado pela produção de citocinas inibidoras (fator de transformação do crescimento beta [TGF-β] e interleucina [IL]-10) e o recrutamento de células imunes imunorreguladoras (como as células T reguladoras [Treg] e as células supressoras derivadas da linhagem mieloide [MDSC]). Em conjunto, essas alterações criam um microambiente tumoral que facilita a progressão do tumor, em vez de sua detecção.

O reconhecimento do impacto da imunoedição no câncer está melhorando a eficácia de terapias baseadas no sistema imune, muitas das quais provavelmente estarão mais amplamente disponíveis ao clínico veterinário nos próximos anos. Este capítulo destaca algumas das terapias mais promissoras sob avaliação em testes clínicos veterinários ou já utilizadas na prática. O capítulo revisa as imunoterapias que estimulam a imunidade de forma geral (imunoterapia tumoral inespecífica), assim como algumas abordagens específicas para tumores, como vacinas tumorais e anticorpos monoclonais (Figura 341.1).

IMUNOTERAPIA TUMORAL INESPECÍFICA

O objetivo da imunoterapia inespecífica é utilizar as armas inatas e adaptativas da resposta imune no reconhecimento e eliminação de células neoplásicas. De forma geral, a melhor estimulação da imunidade inata (mediada principalmente por células dendríticas e macrófagos) resulta em respostas imunes adaptativas mediadas por células (linfócitos) T e B mais efetivas.

> **Boxe 341.1** Principais células imunes envolvidas na estimulação e/ou inibição de respostas imunes antitumorais
>
> **Tipo de resposta**
> *Inata*
> Célula dendrítica (CD)
> - Inicia as respostas imunes adaptativas por meio da apresentação de antígenos e ativação de células-T; alguns subgrupos são imunossupressores no microambiente tumoral
>
> Neutrófilo associado ao tumor (TAN)
> - Pode recrutar Treg e sustentar a angiogênese tumoral
>
> Macrófagos
> - Fagócitos muito eficientes
>
> M1
> - Auxiliam na ativação de respostas antitumorais mediadas por células-T
>
> M2
> - Produzem citocinas imunossupressoras e facilitam a evasão tumoral
>
> Células supressoras derivadas de linhagem mieloide (MDSC)
> - Inibição direta e indireta de respostas imunes de células-T; recrutam Treg
>
> Célula *natural killer* (NK)
> - Dependente de perforina; morte direta de células tumorais reconhecidas como "estranhas"
>
> *Adaptativa: celular*
> Linfócito T citotóxico (LTC, CD8+ efetor)
> - Morte direta por meio de ativação e reconhecimento de antígenos tumorais
>
> CD8+ de memória
> - Novamente recrutados para proteger contra doenças recidivantes ou metastáticas
>
> Linfócito T Helper (Th)
> - Auxiliam (Th1) ou inibem (Th2, Th17) a função do LTC, dependendo do microambiente tumoral
>
> Th CD4+ (Th1, Th2, Th17)
>
> Linfócitos T reguladores (Treg)
> - Efeitos indiretos e diretos; recrutados para inibir outros efetores imunes, como LTC e CD
>
> *Adaptativa: humoral*
> Mediada por anticorpos (direta)
> - Reconhece células tumorais e induz apoptose
>
> Dependente do complemento (indireta)
> - Forma complexa de ataque à membrana que causa toxicidade à célula tumoral

Bacilo de Calmette e Guérin

Uma das formas de terapia inespecífica mais bem estudada é o modificador da resposta biológica (MRB), conhecido como bacilo de Calmette e Guérin (BCG). Trata-se de uma cepa modificada de *Mycobacterium bovis* inicialmente desenvolvida como vacina contra tuberculose no início do século 20. O contato direto do BCG com células malignas estimula a produção de diversas citocinas inflamatórias, incluindo interferona (IFN)-γ, IFN-α, IL-2, IL-6, IL-12 e fator de necrose tumoral (TNF)-α.[4] Essa resposta pró-inflamatória atrai e ativa neutrófilos, macrófagos e linfócitos T-citotóxicos, desencadeando a destruição de células tumorais e indução de linfócitos T de memória longa.[5]

A infusão de BCG na bexiga é uma das formas mais efetivas de tratamento de carcinoma urogenital de célula de transição em pessoas.[5] Embora o BCG tenha sido instilado na bexiga de cães e seja bem tolerado em baixa dose, constatou-se que não é efetivo no tratamento de carcinoma de célula de transição (CCT) canino, que tipicamente se manifesta como uma doença muito mais invasiva em cães quando comparada às pessoas.[6,7] O BCG também tem sido combinado à gonadotropina coriônica humana e administrado por via subcutânea para tratar mastocitoma em cães; verificou-se que foi tão efetivo quanto a quimioterapia exclusiva com vincristina, com menor ocorrência de efeitos colaterais, em um estudo clínico randomizado.[8] Outros estudos que avaliaram a administração de BCG em cães, isolada ou em combinação com outras terapias para carcinoma mamário, osteossarcoma e linfoma, não demonstraram benefícios terapêuticos.[9-11]

Tripeptídio muramil encapsulado em lipossomo

O dipeptídio muramil (MDP) é um componente imunoestimulador da parede celular do BCG modificado pela adição de um peptídio e por sua inclusão em membranas lipossômicas para resultar em tripeptídio muramil encapsulado em lipossomo (L-MTP-PE), um produto farmacêutico eficientemente carreado por monócitos e macrófagos que estimula uma cascata de respostas imunes antitumorais inatas e adaptativas no hospedeiro.[12] Com base em resultados de estudos clínicos em cães com osteossarcoma, hemangiossarcoma, melanoma e adenocarcinoma mamário, o L-MTP-PE foi utilizado em testes clínicos em humanos (majoritariamente crianças) com osteossarcoma.[13-15] Um estudo prospectivo aleatório de fase III demonstrou redução significativa no risco de morte por osteossarcoma quando o L-MTP-PE foi adicionado à quimioterapia sistêmica para o tratamento de doença local.[15] Pacientes com doença metastática ou recidivante também tiveram menor risco de

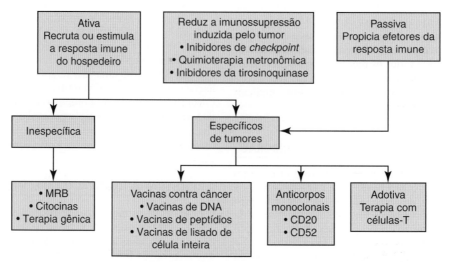

Figura 341.1 Imunoterapia para pacientes veterinários com câncer. Estão listadas as categorias e os mecanismos gerais de ação dos imunoterapêuticos mais utilizados em oncologia veterinária. Cada um é agrupado de acordo com o objetivo geral da terapia. *MRB*, modificadores da resposta biológica.

recidiva e morte quando o L-MTP-PE foi incluído no protocolo terapêutico. Igualmente conhecido como mifamurtida, o L-MTP-PE foi aprovado pela European Medical Association em 2009, como adjuvante à quimioterapia em crianças com osteossarcoma localizado. Nos EUA, o mifamurtida é considerado um medicamento órfão, mas atualmente não está disponível para uso veterinário. Se essa situação mudar, é provável que o fármaco terá de início um custo proibitivo, mas pode ser valioso na imunoterapia inespecífica de cães com osteossarcoma e outras neoplasias.

Terapia gênica e citocinas

Citocinas com propriedades imunoestimulantes, incluindo IL-2, IL-12, IL-15, IFN-gama e TNF-alfa, também são de interesse como imunoterápicos tumorais inespecíficos. Embora todas tenham sido avaliadas em pacientes veterinários, ao menos preliminarmente, a IL-12 parece mais promissora, porque pode almejar de forma efetiva os tecidos tumorais e, assim, evitar a toxicidade associada à administração sistêmica de citocinas. Em uma pesquisa clínica de cães com melanoma maligno, a IL-12, administrada por via subcutânea, se ligou a um anticorpo que visa áreas tumorais necrosadas. Essa estratégia resultou em mínimos efeitos tóxicos relevantes, bem como estimulou as atividades imunológicas e clínicas (taxa de resposta geral: cerca de 50%).[16]

Outra maneira de administrar citocinas consiste em terapia gênica, na qual as células do hospedeiro são submetidas à transfecção ou à transdução para expressar as proteínas recombinantes específicas de interesse. Por exemplo, o gene da IL-12 pode ser especificamente direcionado às células tumorais, desencadeando um ambiente local imunoestimulante. Essa abordagem pode ser particularmente útil no controle de grandes tumores, incluindo fibrossarcoma, carcinoma de célula escamosa e melanoma maligno, como evidenciado em vários estudos recentes que pesquisam a eficácia em gatos, cães e cavalos, respectivamente.[17-20]

IMUNOTERAPIA TUMORAL ESPECÍFICA

Mediante uma variedade de abordagens, o objetivo da imunoterapia tumoral específica é estimular uma resposta imune antitumoral que resulte na regressão clínica da neoplasia ou de suas metástases. Diferentemente da quimioterapia citotóxica, que induz rápida morte da célula tumoral, as respostas clínicas dependem do desenvolvimento de respostas imunes adaptativas que podem demorar vários meses ou mais para surgirem. Ademais, está cada vez mais evidente que uma resposta imune antitumoral, humoral ou celular não necessariamente está correlacionada à regressão do tumor. A constatação de "respostas mistas" é outro problema frequente na avaliação do resultado; esse fenômeno é caracterizado por diferentes respostas das metástases em diferentes tecidos do mesmo paciente. Fatores como esses representam desafios significantes ao delineamento de estudos clínicos que avaliam a imunoterapia tumoral específica, especialmente em termos de determinação da eficácia e de comparações entre os estudos. Para abordar alguns desses obstáculos, atualmente estão sendo avaliados os critérios da resposta específica relacionada ao sistema imune, juntamente aos métodos RECIST (do inglês, *response evaluation criteria in solid tumors*) mais tradicionais, a fim de obter uma série de padrões de resposta clínica mais abrangente e padronizar a avaliação de diversas respostas imunológicas.[21,22] Feito essas ressalvas, o restante desse capítulo se direciona a vacinas contra câncer e anticorpos monoclonais, duas formas de imunoterapia tumoral específica, com relevância particular à oncologia veterinária.

Vacinas contra câncer

Conforme descrito na Figura 341.1, há vários métodos de produção de vacinas contra câncer, inclusive aqueles que liberam antígenos tumorais específicos contra um alvo definido (vacinas de DNA e de peptídios) e aqueles que propiciam a exposição a uma gama de potenciais antígenos associados aos tumores que geralmente não são conhecidos (vacinas de lisados de células tumorais inteiras). Embora todas as abordagens apresentam prós e contras, em termos de preparação da vacina e a qualidade da resposta imune induzida, as vacinas contra câncer são versáteis e podem ser manuseadas para exacerbar fatores importantes da resposta imune ou para almejar tipos de tumores específicos ou até mesmo antígenos comuns a um espectro de neoplasias.

A única vacina contra câncer atualmente disponível no mercado para pacientes veterinários é a Oncept® (Merial Ltd, Duluth, MN), uma vacina xenogênica composta por ácidos nucleicos que contêm uma sequência de DNA que codifica a tirosinase humana. A tirosinase é uma glicoproteína intracelular essencial para a síntese de melanina, expressa em excesso na maioria dos tumores melanocíticos caninos.[23,24] Trabalhos anteriores mostraram evidências de atividades imunológicas e clínicas em cães com melanoma maligno na cavidade bucal e no dígito, levando à aprovação da vacina em 2010 para tratamento de melanoma maligno de cavidade bucal em estágios II e III.[25-28] Entretanto, mais recentemente, estudos relataram resultados conflitantes: alguns demonstraram melhores resultados em cães vacinados com Oncept®, enquanto outros não.[29-31] Embora para o melhor conhecimento da eficácia da Oncept® sejam necessárias pesquisas com estudos clínicos aleatórios mais abrangentes, a introdução de uma vacina contra câncer especificamente para cães foi um passo estimulante em direção à maior disponibilidade de imunoterapia para pacientes veterinários com câncer.

Em oncologia veterinária, há uma série de outras estratégias vacinais contra tumores sob investigação clínica. Uma das pesquisas mais intrigantes é o uso de *Listeria monocytogenes* atenuada, geneticamente modificada para expressar antígenos tumorais específicos. Quando o protótipo da vacina é administrado por via sistêmica, a bactéria *Listeria* infecta as células mieloides do paciente, que então induzem a expressão do antígeno desejado por células neoplásicas. Essa abordagem relata resultados promissores em modelos tumorais murinos e atualmente está sendo explorada utilizando o antígeno tumoral HER2/*neu* como alvo no osteossarcoma canino.[32-34]

Anticorpos monoclonais

Alguns dos avanços mais relevantes no tratamento de neoplasias em humanos tiveram como base o uso de anticorpos monoclonais (AcM) que almejam seletivamente as células malignas. Há um número crescente de AcM utilizados no tratamento de pacientes humanos com linfoma não Hodgkin e carcinoma de mama, próstata e cólon.[35] Vários AcM terapêuticos não são conjugados e atuam por meio de ligação a alvos específicos na superfície de células malignas, de modo a induzir apoptose. A apoptose ocorre através de efeitos diretos e indiretos, sendo estes tipicamente mediados pela ativação dos mecanismos efetores imunes secundários, como a citotoxicidade celular dependente de anticorpos (CCDA) ou a cascata do complemento. Os AcM também podem se ligar a toxinas, radioisótopos ou medicamentos quimioterápicos para causar a morte de células tumorais ou utilizados para inibir a imunossupressão induzida por tumores (p. ex., pela inibição de CTLA-4 ou PD-1, que limita as respostas imunes antitumorais mediadas por células-T).

Embora os AcM ainda não estejam disponíveis no mercado para uso em pacientes veterinários, vários deles estão sendo submetidos a estudos clínicos. Dados preliminares demonstraram que a adição de um AcM anti-CD20 (Aratana Therapeutics) ao protocolo COP ou à doxorrubicina prolongou a sobrevida, comparativamente a cães tratados apenas com quimioterapia.[36,37] Outro AcM, cujo alvo é o antígeno CD52 da célula T (Aratana Therapeutics), foi avaliado em cães com linfoma de células-T, mas a eficácia ainda não foi relatada. NV-01® (NexVet), um AcM que bloqueia a sinalização do fator de crescimento nervoso, recentemente foi testado em estudos clínicos em cães com osteoartrite. Além de sua eficácia como analgésico, constatou-se que o NV-01® reduziu a dor óssea em cães com osteossarcoma.[38] O NV-01® parece promissor para o controle de dor óssea e articular crônica de várias etiologias, tanto como terapia isolada quanto combinada a outros medicamentos. Prevê-se que esses e outros AcM estarão amplamente disponíveis nos próximos anos.

DESAFIOS PARA O FUTURO

Este capítulo fornece uma breve visão geral sobre a imunoterapia do câncer, focando nas estratégias mais frequentemente utilizadas em pacientes veterinários. Há outros procedimentos não abordados aqui, como a terapia adotiva de células-T ou administração de vírus oncolíticos, que também são promissores e estão sendo ativamente pesquisados. Independente da abordagem empregada, o sucesso da imunoterapia do câncer depende do desenvolvimento contínuo de terapias direcionadas à imunossupressão induzida pelo tumor. A aprovação recente pela U.S. Food and Drug Administration dos inibidores do *checkpoint* imune ipilimumabe e nivolumabe, que são AcM cujos alvos são CTLA-4 e PD-1 respectivamente, ilustra a consciência crescente dessa necessidade.

Pesquisas sobre as propriedades imunomoduladoras dos inibidores da tirosinoquinase (p. ex., fosfato de toceranib) e da quimioterapia metronômica são outros exemplos de esforços destinados a reduzir a imunossupressão. Em cães com uma série de tumores, constatou-se que a administração de toceranib ou de baixas doses diárias de ciclofosfamida reduziu a quantidade de Treg circulante.[39,40] De modo semelhante, as preparações lipossômicas do quimioterápico clodronato podem ser úteis na redução de MDSC em cães, devido aos efeitos do fármaco em macrófagos associados aos tumores.[41]

Apesar dos próximos desafios, o potencial para melhorar a recuperação clínica de pessoas e animais com câncer submetidos a imunoterapias modernas é significativo. Veterinários estão em posição única e criticamente importante para contribuir com esse esforço, por meio do seu trabalho com animais de companhia, tanto portadores de câncer quanto os de modelos de translação. À medida que aumenta rapidamente o nosso conhecimento sobre o microambiente tumoral e a nossa capacidade de direcioná-la, o uso clínico de imunoterapia anticâncer provavelmente se tornará uma rotina, como aconteceu com a radioterapia e a quimioterapia.

REFERÊNCIAS BIBLIOGRÁFICAS

As referências bibliográficas deste capítulo se encontram online no Ambiente de Aprendizagem.

CAPÍTULO 342

Terapia Molecular Dirigida

Cheryl London

INTRODUÇÃO

Avanços na biologia molecular, no sequenciamento do DNA e na bioinformática resultaram em uma caracterização muito mais detalhada da forma como os principais mecanismos-chave celulares são desregulados nas células neoplásicas. Em particular, o conhecimento da contribuição de proteínas que normalmente possuem importância fundamental na regulação da sobrevida celular, do crescimento, da diferenciação e da migração na biologia do tumor ajudou a estabelecer um quadro para o desenvolvimento de novos tratamentos que prejudicam o crescimento tumoral. Alvos relevantes para intervenção terapêutica incluem quinases, fatores de transcrição, proteínas que inibem a apoptose, proteínas de choque térmico e reguladores da exportação nuclear, entre outros. As duas abordagens mais comuns para atingir como alvo as proteínas celulares aberrantes são anticorpos monoclonais e inibidores de pequenas moléculas. Enquanto os anticorpos são direcionados principalmente às proteínas da superfície celular, os inibidores de pequenas moléculas podem interferir em proteínas da superfície celular, do citoplasma e do núcleo. Diversos inibidores de pequenas moléculas foram aprovados para o tratamento de neoplasias humanas e muitos outros estão sendo submetidos a testes clínicos. Em medicina veterinária, o uso de inibidores de pequenas moléculas é mais recente, com apenas dois inibidores, o toceranib e o masitinib, aprovados ou condicionalmente aprovados pela U.S. Food and Drug Administration (FDA) para uso em cães.[1,2] Esse capítulo discute o status atual dos inibidores de pequenos moléculas em oncologia clínica veterinária.

TOCERANIB

O fosfato de toceranib é um inibidor de pequenas moléculas biodisponível para uso oral, que inibe uma série de receptores de tirosinoquinases (RTK) da superfície celular, atuando como inibidor competitivo reversível da ligação com a adenosina trifosfato (ATP), impedindo a fosforilação e subsequente sinalização da cascata. O perfil inibitório do toceranib inclui RTK VEGFR2, PDGFR-beta e KIT.[2-5] Há estreita relação entre toceranib e sunitinib, que inibe a atividade de VEGFR2/3, PDGFR-alfa/beta, KIT, CSF1R, FLT-3 e RET.[6] Embora inicialmente tenha sido desenvolvido como um agente antiangiogênico, o amplo perfil de alvos do toceranib resulta também em atividade antitumoral direta. Ademais, está claro que o toceranib possui propriedades imunomoduladoras em cães com câncer, por meio da modulação por células-T reguladoras (Treg), contribuindo ainda mais para seus efeitos contra diversos tipos de neoplasias caninas.

Estudo clínico de fase 1

Inicialmente, o toceranib foi submetido a estudo clínico de fase 1 em 57 cães com uma série de neoplasias.[3] Respostas objetivas foram notadas em 16 cães (6 respostas completas [RC] e

10 respostas parciais [RP]), com doença estável (DE) em outros 15 cães, para uma atividade biológica geral de 54%. Com base no conhecimento do envolvimento da desregulação do KIT em mastocitomas caninos, a maior taxa de resposta foi observada nesta doença, sendo que 10 dos 11 cães com mutações do gene KIT exibiram benefícios clínicos. A dose máxima tolerada (DMT) foi estabelecida em 3,25 mg/kg a cada 48 horas por via oral (VO), e o perfil de eventos adversos observado foi principalmente relacionado ao trato gastrintestinal (GI), incluindo perda de apetite, diarreia e, menos comumente, vômito.

Estudo de campo central
Subsequentemente ao estudo clínico de fase 1, realizou-se um estudo clínico de campo aleatório controlado do toceranib com placebo em cães com mastocitomas de graus 2 e 3, sem possibilidade de ressecção.[2] Nesse estudo, a taxa de resposta para todos os 145 cães que receberam toceranib foi de 42,8% (21 RC, 41 RP), com outros 16 cães apresentando DE e atividade biológica geral de 60%. Os cães cujos mastocitomas apresentavam mutações do gene KIT tinham probabilidade duas vezes maior de responder ao tratamento com toceranib do que aqueles sem mutações, e cães sem metástases em linfonodos tiveram maior taxa de resposta do que aqueles com envolvimento de linfonodos. Esses dados foram a base para a aprovação subsequente do toceranib pela FDA, em 2009, para o tratamento de cães com mastocitoma.

Uso off-label (uso diferente do aprovado em bula)
Após sua aprovação, o toceranib foi utilizado off-label para tratar uma série de neoplasias em cães. Uma análise retrospectiva avaliou esse uso e constatou benefício clínico (RC, RP ou DE) em 63 de 85 (74%) cães com tumores sólidos, incluindo adenocarcinoma de saco anal (28/32; 8 RP, 20 DE), osteossarcoma metastático (11/23; 1 RP, 10 DE), carcinoma de tireoide (12/15; 4 RP, 8 DE), carcinoma de cabeça e pescoço (7/8; 1 RC, 5 RP, 1 DE) e carcinoma nasal (5/7; 1 RC, 4 DE).[7] A dose mediana de toceranib utilizada foi de 2,8 mg/kg, VO; 58,7% dos cães foram tratados com o medicamento 3 vezes/semana (segunda/quarta/sexta [S/Q/S]), e 74,6% receberam o tratamento durante 4 meses ou mais.

A sua ação também foi relatada em casos de linfangiossarcoma[8] e leucemia monocítica crônica,[9] além de vários outros relatos anedóticos de tipos de tumores individuais ainda não publicados. Isso indica que o toceranib pode ter uma ampla atividade antitumoral em cães.

Terapias combinadas
Piroxicam, um anti-inflamatório não esteroide misto, inibidor da ciclo-oxigenase (COX)-1/COX-2, mostrou-se efetivo no tratamento de carcinomas e frequentemente é incluído nos protocolos quimioterápicos metronômicos. Foi realizado um estudo de fase 1 em cães com câncer, a fim de estabelecer a segurança da administração concomitante da combinação toceranib/piroxicam[10] e foram observadas diversas respostas antitumorais. Constatou-se que a combinação das doses padronizadas para uso oral de ambos os fármacos (3,25 mg de toceranib/kg, a cada 48 horas VO, 0,3 mg de piroxicam/kg, a cada 24 horas VO) geralmente foi segura. Entretanto, os cães não foram monitorados para avaliar a ocorrência de efeitos colaterais GI após a administração por longo tempo. Portanto, o piroxicam é frequentemente administrado em intervalos de 48 h, alternando com o toceranib, para ajudar a reduzir o risco de toxicidade GI.

Para avaliar se a vimblastina e o toceranib poderiam ser combinados efetivamente, realizou-se um estudo clínico de fase 1 em cães com mastocitoma.[11] A toxicidade dose-limitante da combinação toceranib/vimblastina causou neutropenia, e a DMT da vimblastina foi de 1,6 mg/m^2, em semanas intercaladas, quando administrada juntamente com 3,25 mg de toceranib/kg, a cada 48 horas VO. Apesar da redução da vimblastina a taxa de resposta objetiva foi de 71%, sugerindo que há uma ação aditiva ou sinérgica quando os fármacos são administrados em combinação.

Para determinar se a combinação de radioterapia e uso de toceranib seria benéfica para mastocitoma canino, os cães com tumor sem possibilidade de ressecção foram tratados com prednisona, omeprazol, difenidramina e toceranib na dose de 2,75 mg/kg, S/Q/S, durante 1 semana antes de serem submetidos à radioterapia fracionada comum.[12] A taxa de resposta objetiva foi de 76,4% (58,8% RC, 17,6% RP) e o tempo de sobrevida médio não foi obtido, mesmo após um período de acompanhamento médio de 374 dias, sem relato de aumento da toxicidade pela radiação. Esses dados indicam que a combinação de radioterapia e toceranib propicia benefícios clínicos significativos em cães com mastocitoma sem possibilidade de ressecção. A combinação também parece ser benéfica para carcinoma nasal canino. Cães submetidos a 10 sessões de radiação (dose total de 42 Gy; ver Capítulo 340) e tratamento com toceranib tiveram um tempo de sobrevida médio de 615 dias, comparado a 371 dias de um controle histórico de tratamento semelhante, porém sem o uso de toceranib.[13]

Propriedades imunomoduladoras
A ciclofosfamida, em baixa dose, frequentemente é utilizada em protocolos quimioterápicos metronômicos, a fim de alterar o microambiente local por meio da modulação da angiogênese e da redução da quantidade de Treg imunossupressora. Para avaliar a ação do toceranib na função imune, cães com câncer receberam o fármaco em intervalos de 48 h, durante 2 semanas, período em que a baixa dose de ciclofosfamida foi adicionada ao protocolo terapêutico.[14] O toceranib reduziu de forma significativa a quantidade e o porcentagem de Treg no sangue periférico de cães tratados, com aumento concomitante da concentração sérica de interferona (IFN)-gama. Esses dados indicam que o toceranib pode ser efetivo em protocolos quimioterápicos metronômicos.

Toceranib na doença metastática microscópica
A eficácia do toceranib foi avaliada na doença metastática microscópica. Em um estudo, cães com osteossarcoma apendicular foram submetidos à amputação, seguida de quimioterapia com carboplatina, e então receberam, aleatoriamente, a combinação toceranib/piroxicam/ciclofosfamida ou piroxicam/ciclofosfamida (controle).[15] Não se constatou diferença na sobrevida livre de progressão da doença ou sobrevida geral, e esses resultados não diferiram de forma significativa dos dados históricos de cães submetidos à amputação e tratados somente com carboplatina. Em um segundo estudo, cães com hemangiossarcoma esplênico em estágio 1 ou 2 foram submetidos à esplenectomia e tratados com doxorrubicina.[16] Quando considerados livres da doença, após quimioterapia, receberam então toceranib. Quando comparados a um grupo-controle histórico tratado apenas com doxorrubicina, não se constatou melhora quanto à sobrevida livre de progressão da doença ou à sobrevida geral. Esses dados indicam que o toceranib provavelmente não propicia benefícios na doença metastática microscópica, na ausência de um indutor tumoral conhecido (i. e., mutação no gene KIT no mastocitoma).

Recomendações de dose atuais
Atualmente há evidências de que uma boa atividade biológica é obtida quando o tratamento é iniciado com dose inferior a 3,25 mg/kg de DMT e que cronogramas alternativos de dose são efetivos. Em um estudo de cães com tumores sólidos, constatou-se que doses de toceranib de 2,4 a 2,9 mg/kg a cada 48 horas VO, foram associadas a tempo de exposição ao medicamento considerado suficiente para a inibição do tumor, resultando em modulação de um marcador farmacodinâmico essencial, compatível com a inibição da sinalização de VEGFR.[17] É importante ressaltar que as doses menores foram associadas a um perfil de eventos adversos substancialmente menor, à dose de 3,25 mg/kg. Foram documentadas tanto RP quanto RC, e 35 de 40 cães continuaram o tratamento com toceranib durante 4 meses, em média.[17] Dados gerados a partir da análise retrospectiva do uso do toceranib em tumores sólidos indicaram que a administração do medicamento 3 vezes/semana pode ser

MASITINIB E IMATINIB

O mesilato de masitinib, condicionalmente aprovado em 2010, inibe a atividade de KIT, PDGFR e da quinase citoplasmática Lyn. Um amplo estudo clínico controlado com placebo foi realizado em mais de 200 cães com mastocitoma, nos quais o masitinib aumentou de forma significativa o tempo de progressão da neoplasia, comparativamente aos animais que receberam placebo, e o resultado foi melhor em cães com mastocitoma que apresentavam mutações no gene KIT.[1] O acompanhamento subsequente dos pacientes tratados com masitinib durante 2 anos identificou um maior número de pacientes com controle da doença a longo prazo, comparado àqueles tratados com placebo (40% *versus* 15% vivos após 2 anos).[18] Uma análise retrospectiva de cães com mastocitoma tratados com masitinib indicou taxa de resposta de aproximadamente 50%.[19] Embora o número de cães avaliados tenha sido pequeno, com manifestações variáveis da doença, esse estudo sugere que a atividade biológica do masitinib provavelmente é maior na doença primária do que na doença recidivante. O masitinib também foi efetivo no tratamento de linfoma de células-T em cães, embora nenhum estudo clínico tenha sido realizado em tal condição.

Ainda não há estudos específicos sobre o uso de mesilato de imatinibe (Gleevec®) em medicina veterinária, embora alguns poucos relatos tenham sido publicados com relação à sua utilização em cães e gatos. Nesses animais, o imatinibe foi bem tolerado, e foram observadas respostas antitumorais objetivas em cães com mastocitoma que carreavam os genes KIT mutante e do tipo selvagem.[20-22] Respostas também foram observadas em gatos com mastocitoma que apresentavam mutações no gene KIT.[23,24]

CONTROLE DE EVENTOS ADVERSOS CAUSADOS POR TOCERANIB E MASITINIB

Quase todos os inibidores de pequenas moléculas causam efeitos adversos; como as comorbidades subjacentes podem contribuir para a ocorrência desses efeitos, esforços devem ser feitos para melhorar a condição de saúde dos cães antes do uso desses medicamentos. Tanto para o toceranib quanto para o masitinib, os efeitos colaterais mais comuns estão relacionados ao trato GI, incluindo perda de apetite, diarreia e ocasionalmente vômito (ver Capítulo 343).[1-3,17,19] A administração de um supressor de ácido gástrico, principalmente o omeprazol, pode ser benéfica em mitigar o risco de úlcera GI, especialmente nos casos de mastocitoma. A inapetência é um efeito colateral relativamente comum e em geral responde aos medicamentos antináusea usuais (metoclopramida, ondansetrona, maropitant; ver Capítulo 39) ou à baixa dose de prednisona. Quanto ao controle de diarreia, a administração de metronidazol e/ou loperamida, juntamente a probióticos, quase sempre é benéfica. Tanto a nefropatia com perda de proteína (NPP; ver Capítulo 325) quanto a hipertensão sistêmica (ver Capítulo 157) têm sido associadas à administração de toceranib. A NPP geralmente é discreta à moderada e efetivamente tratada com enalapril, benazepril e/ou redução da dose do antineoplásico. De forma semelhante, a hipertensão pode ser tipicamente tratada com anlodipino. Relata-se que o masitinib causa NPP, embora raramente ocorra uma condição muito mais grave, às vezes fatal, de perda de proteína.[19,25] Foram constatados outros sinais de toxicidade, inclusive hepatotoxicidade, neutropenia e anemia, embora de rara ocorrência. A descontinuação do antineoplásico, redução da dose e modificação da posologia são procedimentos extremamente úteis para o controle dessas toxicidades.

OUTROS ALVOS MOLECULARES

Embora as quinases sejam o alvo mais comum da intervenção terapêutica, diversas outras proteínas são fundamentais para o crescimento e sobrevivência da célula tumoral. A proteína de choque térmico HSP90 é responsável pela maturação de diversas proteínas clientes, várias das quais são oncogenes (KIT, MET, BRAF, AKT). Inibidores da HSP90 impedem a maturação da proteína, resultando em sua degradação e na morte da célula tumoral. Em um estudo de fase 1, o inibidor de HSP90, STA-1474, mostrou boa atividade em cães portadores de uma série de tumores sólidos, principalmente mastocitoma.[26] Um estudo subsequente, que pesquisou o protocolo terapêutico em cães com mastocitoma, mostrou que a administração em 2 dias consecutivos foi mais efetiva para indução, respostas objetivas e infrarregulação sustentada do KIT (London *et al.*, não publicado). A exportina 1 (XPO1)[27] é o único exportador nuclear de vários supressores tumorais importantes e de proteínas reguladoras do crescimento.[28,29] Em neoplasias hematológicas e tumores sólidos, ocorre suprarregulação desse inibidor, frequentemente relacionada a prognóstico ruim. Em estudos clínicos nas fases 1 e 2, o KPT-335 (Verdinexor®), um inibidor de pequena molécula XPO1 biodisponível por via oral, foi efetivo em cães com linfoma de células T e B.[30] Há pesquisas clínicas em desenvolvimento para o uso de Verdinexor® no tratamento de linfoma canino.

A enzima histona desacetilase (HDAC) remove grupos acetil de proteínas histonas e regulam a transcrição gênica.[31] Inibidores de HDAC (HDACi) podem alterar a expressão de genes epigeneticamente silenciosos e, dessa forma, inibir a progressão tumoral.[32,33] O medicamento antiepiléptico ácido valproico é um HDACi efetivo em diversos modelos experimentais de tumores.[34-36] Em um estudo de fase 1, o ácido valproico foi administrado antes da doxorrubicina em cães com câncer.[37] Foram constatadas respostas objetivas, e algumas poucas ocorreram em tumores tradicionalmente resistentes à antraciclina; é importante ressaltar que a combinação foi segura e bem tolerada. Por fim, o RV1001 é um novo inibidor da pequena molécula fosfatidilinositol-3-quinase delta (PI3 K-delta) biodisponível por via oral, uma proteína de sinalização celular que sabidamente contribui para o crescimento tumoral. O RV1001 é efetivo contra PI3 K-delta em concentrações nanomolares baixas, com efeitos nas isoformas beta e gama, em baixas concentrações micromolares. Um estudo clínico de fase 1 com RV1001 em cães com linfoma de células T ou B inicial ou recidivante mostrou eficácia excelente, com taxa de resposta objetiva de 62% (3 RC, 10 RP).[38] A inibição de AKT foi demonstrada em amostras de tumores, dentro de duas horas após a administração de RV1001, mostrando rápida modulação do alvo. O RV1001 está sendo pesquisado para o tratamento do linfoma canino.

RESUMO

O desenvolvimento de inibidores de pequenas moléculas, cujos alvos são proteínas importantes para o crescimento e manutenção de neoplasias, transformou a terapia oncológica em humanos. Esses inibidores estão apenas começando a impactar a oncologia veterinária, com a disponibilidade de toceranib e masitinib, embora provavelmente outros medicamentos estarão disponíveis em breve. No futuro, a combinação de inibidores de pequenas moléculas com quimioterapia padrão e radioterapia provavelmente melhorará sobremaneira os resultados terapêuticos em pacientes veterinários com câncer.

REFERÊNCIAS BIBLIOGRÁFICAS

As referências bibliográficas deste capítulo se encontram online no Ambiente de Aprendizagem.

CAPÍTULO 343

Complicações da Terapia Antineoplásica

Louis-Philippe de Lorimier e Craig A. Clifford

INTRODUÇÃO

Tradicionalmente, por conta do mero objetivo de eliminar a maior quantidade possível de células cancerosas em cada dose administrada, a dose de medicamentos citotóxicos convencionais foi baseada no conceito de dose máxima tolerada (DMT), e não no modelo padrão de farmacocinética/farmacodinâmica (FC/FD) (ver Capítulo 160).[1] Com base nesse conceito, alguns efeitos colaterais são esperados e aceitos ("tolerados" pelo paciente) ao administrar uma dose inferior à DMT, e o que se considera "tolerado" é determinado com base na gravidade (estadiamento) dos efeitos colaterais observados.[2] Ao utilizar a terapia antineoplásica, sempre os potenciais benefícios devem superar os riscos, mas, mesmo com um conhecimento minucioso dos efeitos colaterais comuns, raramente é possível predizer de forma acurada como um indivíduo reagirá a um fármaco específico, até que tenha sido administrado (i. e., a própria DMT do paciente é desconhecida). A maioria dos medicamentos antineoplásicos possui faixas de doses que variam dependendo da doença tratada, da presença de comorbidades, da idade do paciente, dos resultados de exames de sangue anteriores ao tratamento (função dos órgãos), da espécie a ser tratada, da raça do paciente e da experiência do clínico.

A dose da maioria dos fármacos citotóxicos é expressa em mg/m^2, sendo o cálculo baseado na área de superfície corporal (ASC), presumivelmente um preditor mais apropriado da farmacocinética do medicamento. Entretanto, foram demonstradas limitações dessa abordagem, e o cálculo da dose baseado na ASC pode resultar em superdosagem em pacientes menores (menos de 10 a 15 kg) e possivelmente subdose em cães muito grandes.[3,4] Por esta razão, em pacientes menores, o cálculo da dose de alguns fármacos quimioterápicos pode ser mais confiável quando baseada no peso do animal, expressa em mg/kg, como comumente utilizado para carboplatina e doxorrubicina.

Corticosteroides são provavelmente a classe de fármacos antineoplásicos com o perfil de efeitos colaterais mais consistente, sendo a ocorrência de poliúria/polidipsia o efeito mais notável que influencia negativamente a qualidade de vida dos pacientes e dos tutores.

Novas classes terapêuticas de fármacos antineoplásicos estão surgindo (p. ex., inibidores da tirosinoquinase, vacinas terapêuticas, anticorpos monoclonais), e o conceito de DMT pode não ser o melhor para estabelecer as doses apropriadas para os novos tratamentos oncológicos. Para alguns desses fármacos mais recentes, pode-se avaliar a "inibição do alvo" in vivo para ajudar a definir a melhor dose que, em alguns casos, pode ser bem menor do que a DMT.[5] Geralmente, as complicações e os efeitos colaterais comuns da terapia antineoplásica são classificados por sistema; foi estabelecido um critério comum de terminologias e sistema de estadiamento.[2] Uma expressão utilizada por muito tempo para descrever as complicações mais comuns foi "BAG de efeitos colaterais", que significa efeitos colaterais na medula óssea (supressão [*bone marrow*, em inglês]), **a**lopecia e efeitos **g**astrintestinais. É óbvio que outros sistemas podem ser afetados.

MIELOSSUPRESSÃO

Os medicamentos quimioterápicos citotóxicos tradicionais são mielossupressores por natureza, já que rapidamente atuam em células em divisão. Dentre os agentes antineoplásicos, a enzima L-asparaginase é uma exceção, pelo fato de que, por si só, geralmente não causa mielossupressão. Tipicamente, os fármacos quimioterápicos convencionais podem causar vários graus de neutropenia e/ou trombocitopenia, já que neutrófilos e plaquetas possuem tempo de trânsito na medula óssea e meia-vida circulante curtos. No entanto, embora as hemácias apresentem tempo de trânsito na medula óssea e meia-vida circulante mais longos, pode ocorrer anemia resultante da quimioterapia em alguns indivíduos, especialmente naqueles submetidos a protocolos terapêuticos mais longos, com múltiplos medicamentos. A gravidade das citopenias é graduada de 1 a 4.[2]

Nos linfomas, algumas citopenias podem ser detectadas no momento do diagnóstico, antes do início de qualquer terapia, especialmente anemia (quase sempre não regenerativa causada por doença crônica) e trombocitopenia (frequentemente com um componente imunomediado ou resultante de infiltração na medula óssea). Anemia e trombocitopenia são também comuns no momento do diagnóstico de hemangiossarcoma visceral; a anemia regenerativa, causada por hemorragia interna e microangiopatia, e a trombocitopenia, resultante do consumo e destruição de plaquetas, geralmente se resolvem após a cirurgia (i. e., esplenectomia) e antes do início da quimioterapia.

Em linfomas de alto grau e leucemias agudas, pode ocorrer mieloftise e haver citopenias mais marcantes no momento do diagnóstico ou após a quimioterapia. Essa é uma situação na qual a L-asparaginase e os corticosteroides podem ser mais úteis no início do tratamento, devido à ausência de efeitos mielossupressores.

O nadir, ou a menor contagem celular após o tratamento, varia em função dos fármacos quimioterápicos utilizados. Mais frequentemente, é verificado por volta de 6 a 8 dias após a administração de fármacos citotóxicos comumente utilizados, inclusive alcaloides da vinca (vincristina, vimblastina, vinorelbina), doxorrubicina, mitoxantrona e alquilantes (ciclofosfamida, lomustina em cães), em altas doses pulsadas. Com o uso de carboplatina, o nadir é verificado por volta de 14 dias após o tratamento em cães, e 14 ou até mais de 25 dias, em gatos.[6,7] O nadir também é imprevisível quando se utiliza lomustina em gatos, ocorrendo entre 7 e 28 dias após sua administração, dependendo do indivíduo e da dose utilizada.[8]

Mesmo que todos os medicamentos citotóxicos possam resultar em neutropenia, dependendo da dose utilizada, os fármacos mais comumente associados a neutropenia clinicamente relevante em cães e gatos são carboplatina, doxorrubicina, lomustina, mitoxantrona, vimblastina e vinorelbina. Vincristina e ciclofosfamida geralmente são consideradas menos mielossupressoras; entretanto, ambas podem resultar em neutropenia grave (grau 4) quando utilizadas na maior dose da faixa de variação recomendada ou em indivíduos que são intrinsicamente mais sensíveis.[9] Pode-se notar neutropenia mais marcante quando a vincristina é administrada simultaneamente à

L-asparaginase. É importante ressaltar que os cães com mutação no gene ABCB1-1 delta (MDR-1) sabidamente apresentam maior risco de efeitos colaterais causados por vários fármacos e agentes quimioterápicos, incluindo alcaloides da vinca (vincristina, vimblastina, vinorelbina), doxorrubicina, mitoxantrona, taxanos e dactinomicina.[10,11] As raças que mais comumente apresentam a mutação são Collie (de pelos crespos ou lisos), Pastor-Australiano (miniatura ou padrão), McNab, Silken Windhound, Whippet de Pelo Longo, Shetland Sheepdog e Pastor-Alemão, para nomear alguns.[12] Para consultar listas completas e atualizadas sobre raças em risco e fármacos que causam problema, ou para informações sobre testes genéticos, visite o site do Washington State University Veterinary Clinical Pharmacology Laboratory (*http://vcpl.vetmed.wsu.edu/*). Cães das raças previamente mencionadas devem ser testados para determinar seu status de mutação; em indivíduos portadores da mutação, é necessária a redução da dose dos fármacos quimioterápicos que causam problema. É importante ressaltar que recentemente foram descritas mutações em ABCB1-1 delta em gatos e que podem influenciar a sensibilidade à quimioterapia e a outros fármacos nos gatos afetados.[13]

Deve-se realizar hemograma completo antes da administração de uma dose pulsada de um agente citotóxico em qualquer paciente. Em geral, um fármaco potencialmente mielossupressor não deve ser administrado quando a contagem de neutrófilos for inferior a 2.000/μl ou se a contagem de plaquetas for menor que 75.000/μl. Quando ocorre citopenia que impede a administração segura da quimioterapia, o tratamento deve ser postergado por 2 a 7 dias, e deve-se repetir o hemograma. Quando há necessidade de adiamento, a contagem de dias deve ser baseada na linhagem celular em questão (p. ex., menor tempo em casos de neutropenia, já que o tempo de trânsito na medula óssea é mais curto).

Por conta das razões discutidas anteriormente, sempre deve-se repetir o hemograma a cada 7 dias e, ocasionalmente, 14 dias após a terapia, a fim de monitorar e documentar o momento da menor contagem celular. Há maior risco de infecção sistêmica (sepse neutropênica) quando a contagem de neutrófilos é inferior a 1.000/μl. Geralmente recomenda-se terapia antibacteriana profilática por via oral (VO), aos pacientes com neutropenia que não manifestam sinais clínicos de doença (*i. e.*, febre, letargia); as escolhas comuns são sulfametoxazol/trimetoprima (15 a 30 mg/kg VO, a cada 12 h), amoxicilina/ácido clavulânico (13 a 15 mg/kg VO, a cada 12 h) e cefalexina (22 a 25 mg/kg VO, 12 h). Os tutores devem ser orientados a monitorar o seu animal em casa (comportamento geral, apetite, temperatura corporal). Em uma ampla maioria dos casos, a neutropenia em cães se resolve dentro de 2 a 5 dias, e geralmente nota-se leucocitose neutrofílica de rebote após a recuperação da medula. Em gatos, a recuperação de episódios de neutropenia pode demorar mais tempo (7 a 14 dias ou mais), principalmente após terapia com lomustina e carboplatina. Após um episódio de neutropenia grave (inferior a 1.000 neutrófilos/μl), a dose do medicamento que o causou deve ser reduzida em 10 a 20% em tratamentos subsequentes, a fim de diminuir o risco de complicações graves. É importante saber que a neutropenia, sendo um indicador da DMT, alcançada ou almejada, pode estar associada a um melhor prognóstico (duração da remissão e sobrevida) em cães e em pessoas com linfoma.[14] Por fim, a tentativa de evitar a todo custo um episódio neutropênico pode ser prejudicial ao paciente e favorecer a resistência e recidiva precoces.

Fármacos citotóxicos que afetam o trato gastrintestinal (GI) e a medula óssea apresentam maior risco de causar episódios sépticos neutropênicos, provavelmente por conta do maior risco de translocação de bactérias oriundas do trato GI. Dois estudos demonstraram que os fatores câncer risco para o desenvolvimento de sepse em cães, após quimioterapia, incluem menor peso corporal, diagnóstico de linfoma e administração de doxorrubicina ou vincristina.[15,16]

Episódios neutropênicos graves que resultam em sinais clínicos de doença, em geral incluindo febre, letargia e anorexia, devem ser tratados agressivamente, com hospitalização do paciente e monitoramento mais intensivo, a fim de prevenir sepse. Isso inclui um amplo monitoramento da glicemia e das concentrações de lactato e eletrólitos, bem como o estreito monitoramento dos parâmetros clínicos do paciente, como pressão sanguínea (ver Capítulo 99), temperatura corporal etc. No caso de sepse, deve-se realizar tratamento de suporte (ver Capítulo 132). Quando presentes, os sintomas digestivos devem ser tratados (ver adiante), bem como outros achados no perfil bioquímico sérico (p. ex., desequilíbrios eletrolíticos) ou em exames complementares. É óbvio que seria excelente realizar hemocultura, mas raramente é necessária ou compensadora, já que a maioria dos episódios sépticos neutropênicos responde rápida e efetivamente à terapia empírica agressiva, sendo a recuperação da medula o fator mais crucial.

O uso de fatores estimulantes de colônia (p. ex., rhG-CSF) é controverso, e seu benefício é questionável na maioria dos pacientes, uma vez que provavelmente há alta concentração endógena de G-CSF canino durante o episódio neutropênico. Ademais, um estudo recente demonstrou que os cães com episódio séptico neutropênico que receberam rhG-CSF apresentaram maior risco de tempo de hospitalização mais longo e de morte no hospital.[16] Na maioria dos pacientes com episódios de sepse neutropênica não complicados, a febre diminui rapidamente, dentro de horas, após o início do tratamento de suporte, e o paciente recebe alta hospitalar, evitando o risco de infecção nosocomial. Um estudo de 70 casos de cães com episódios sépticos neutropênicos causados por quimioterapia constatou uma taxa de mortalidade de 8,5%.[16]

Os gatos parecem desenvolver sepse neutropênica verdadeira muito menos comumente do que os cães, mesmo que nessa espécie a menor contagem celular frequentemente persista por mais tempo.

Quase sempre ocorre trombocitopenia transitória após a administração de quimioterápicos citotóxicos. Isso é mais comum com o uso de carboplatina, lomustina, dacarbazina, melfalana, dactinomicina, citosina-arabinosídeo e doxorrubicina. Raramente notam-se sinais clínicos quando a contagem de plaquetas é superior a 25.000/μl, mas os pacientes com trombocitopenia grave devem ser monitorados por conta da ocorrência de equimoses, petéquias e hemorragias (GI, gengival, epistaxe) e para evitar traumatismo. Alguns quimioterápicos alquilantes, inclusive lomustina, melfalana e clorambucila, podem causar trombocitopenia cumulativa, às vezes não totalmente reversível, após tratamento prolongado.[17] Devem ser realizados hemogramas regulares, e o fármaco deve ser descontinuado se há tendência de diminuição da contagem de plaquetas ou se essa contagem for inferior a 100.000 a 125.000 plaquetas/μl. O uso de medicamentos trombopoéticos é controverso e mal documentado até o momento.

Foram desenvolvidas e comercializadas duas tirosinoquinases de administração oral, fosfato de toceranib (Palladia®) e mesilato de masitinib (Kinavet-CA1®, Masivet®) para o tratamento de mastocitoma em cães. Mesmo não sendo consideradas verdadeiramente mielossupressoras como os agentes citotóxicos tradicionais, é possível notar citopenias com o uso de ambos os inibidores da tirosinoquinase aprovados para uso veterinário, secundárias à inibição da sinalização de crescimento celular, inclusive neutropenia, trombocitopenia e anemia.[18-21] Mais frequentemente, essas citopenias são discretas e reversíveis, mas às vezes podem ser graves o suficiente para justificar o adiamento do tratamento ("feriado do fármaco"), até que as contagens celulares retornem ao normal.

COMPLICAÇÕES DERMATOLÓGICAS

Alopecia, alterações na pigmentação

A alopecia causada por quimioterapia é uma complicação comum em pessoas e, embora seja um efeito colateral estético, traz um importante impacto psicológico negativo para vários pacientes. A perda de peso após a quimioterapia é um problema pequeno na oncologia veterinária, mas em algumas raças de cães que apresentam crescimento contínuo de pelos pode ocorrer perda de pelos maior que o usual ou manifestarem alopecia real, parcial ou total. As raças mais comumente afetadas são Maltês, Bichon Frisé, Poodle, alguns tipos de Terrier, Shih-tzu e Old English Sheepdog. Esse efeito colateral não impacta negativamente a qualidade de vida e é reversível assim que o tratamento for descontinuado (Figura 343.1). Às vezes, os gatos podem perder as vibrissas ou pelos faciais (mais tipicamente) quando submetidos à quimioterapia.

Alterações de pigmentação transitórias, mais frequentemente despigmentação, foram relatadas em cães tratados com fosfato de toceranib (Palladia®), sobretudo no nariz, coxins plantares, lábios e, menos comumente, todo o pelame.[19] Essa complicação, à semelhança da alopecia, parece ser puramente estética e não tem impactos negativos na qualidade de vida. Pode ser decorrência da inibição da proteína KIT, interferindo negativamente nos melanócitos cutâneos, e regride após a descontinuação do medicamento.

Extravasamento do medicamento

Alguns fármacos quimioterápicos causam irritação local quando administrados no espaço perivascular e incluem platinas (carboplatina e cisplatina), dacarbazina, mitoxantrona e taxanos. A reação local causada pelo extravasamento desses medicamentos é discreta à moderada e causa certo grau de desconforto, eritema, formação de crostas e edema. Os medicamentos verdadeiramente vesicantes são os alcaloides da vinca (vincristina, vimblastina, vinorelbina), antraciclinas (doxorrubicina, epirrubicina), dactinomicina e mecloretamina e causam lesão tecidual mais grave, quando há extravasamento perivascular.

É melhor prevenir a ocorrência de lesões por extravasamento do que tratá-las. A punção de uma veia que ainda não tenha sido utilizada por mais de 48 horas e a introdução asséptica de um cateter longo (ver Capítulo 75) logo antes da administração do quimioterápico reduzem o risco de extravasamento. Deve-se evitar o uso de bomba de infusão, preferindo a simples ação da gravidade ou seringa manual. Durante a administração do quimioterápico, recomenda-se o uso mínimo de bandagens, de modo a possibilitar a máxima visualização possível do cateter e do local de seu acesso cutâneo. Se ou quando se constata extravasamento do quimioterápico, a sua administração deve ser imediatamente descontinuada, e aplica-se pressão negativa ao cateter, à medida que ele é cuidadosamente extraído, para remover o máximo possível de medicamento que extravasou no espaço perivascular. Deve-se evitar bandagem oclusiva.

No caso de extravasamento de alcaloides da vinca (vincristina, vimblastina e vinorelbina), recomenda-se a aplicação de compressas quentes durante 15 a 20 min, 4 vezes/dia, por 2 a 3 dias. Alguns profissionais recomendam a instilação de solução salina estéril (5 a 10 mℓ) ao redor do local do extravasamento, com intuito de diluir o medicamento vesicante presente nos tecidos locais. Outros sugerem a administração tópica de dimetil sulfóxido (DMSO), às vezes misturado a um corticosteroide, após a aplicação de calor, mas a eficácia dessas abordagens é questionável. A infiltração local de hialuronidase foi descrita e pode ajudar a reduzir a gravidade da lesão tecidual local causada pelos alcaloides da vinca, mas a distribuição errática do fármaco dificulta seu uso consistente.[22] Em geral, o extravasamento de alcaloides da vinca resulta em dano tecidual discreto a moderado, menos comumente grave, e cicatriza por completo após 2 a 3 semanas, sem sequelas permanentes (Figura 343.2).

O extravasamento de doxorrubicina, epirrubicina ou dactinomicina é uma condição mais séria, que pode resultar em lesão tecidual local muito grave, às vezes progredindo para necrose dissecante nos tecidos profundos e, eventualmente, necessitando desbridamento cirúrgico ou, quando a lesão parece irreversível, amputação do membro (Figura 343.3). Diferentemente do recomendado para o extravasamento de alcaloides da vinca, no caso de extravasamento desses quimioterápicos indica-se a aplicação de compressas frias no local da lesão, durante 15 a 20 minutos, 4 vezes/dia, por 2 a 3 dias. Mais uma vez, o benefício da aplicação tópica de DMSO é questionável, mas a administração intravenosa oportuna de dexrazoxano, um quelante de ferro, pode ajudar a reduzir de forma marcante – e às vezes prevenir completamente – a extensão da lesão tecidual local.[23,24] O dexrazoxano é utilizado em dose 10 vezes maior do que a dose de doxorrubicina (p. ex., 300 mg/m^2, se o cão recebeu 30 mg de doxorrubicina/m^2), administrada por via intravenosa o mais precocemente possível após ocorrência do extravasamento, sendo o ideal repetir a dose após 24 e 48 horas. Em estudos com ratos, constatou-se benefício quando utilizado até seis horas após o extravasamento.

Extravasamentos de mecloretamina podem ser tratados com solução de tiossulfato de sódio 2,5%, um doador de enxofre, injetada diretamente nos tecidos onde ocorreu extravasamento (aplica-se o mesmo volume daquele da mecloretamina administrada).

Em todos os casos de extravasamento, deve-se fornecer analgesia apropriada mediante o uso de anti-inflamatórios não esteroides ou corticosteroides (ver Capítulo 164) e analgésicos adjuvantes (ver Capítulos 126 e 166). Às vezes, o uso de antibióticos pode ser benéfico quando há suspeita ou confirmação de infecção bacteriana secundária. Vale ressaltar a importância da prevenção de autotraumatismo sempre (p. ex., uso de colar elizabetano).

Eritrodisestesia palmoplantar

Também conhecida como "síndrome mão-pé" em pessoas, a eritrodisestesia palmoplantar (EPP) é frequentemente causada por toxicidade dermatológica associada à administração intravenosa de doxorrubicina lipossômica em cães e gatos.[25-29] Pode se manifestar como desconforto, eritema, alopecia e ulceração na axila, na região inguinal e na pele ao redor dos coxins plantares, em cães, e como alopecia focal no queixo e membros, em gatos.[25-29] Embora a EPP seja autolimitante, o desconforto pode ser intenso o suficiente para justificar o adiamento ou a descontinuação do tratamento. A administração oral simultânea de piridoxina (vitamina B6; 50 mg, VO, a cada 8 h) reduz sobremaneira a gravidade das lesões em cães com EPP.[26]

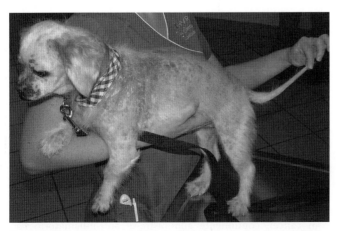

Figura 343.1 Alopecia causada por quimioterapia em cão da raça Shih-tzu submetido ao tratamento para linfoma.

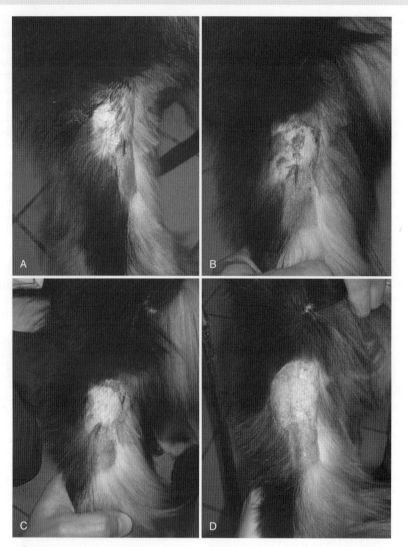

Figura 343.2 Lesão discreta causada por extravasamento de vincristina em um cão da raça Bernese Mountain, submetido ao tratamento de linfoma, mostrando a progressão da lesão nos dias 5 (**A**) e 10 (**B**), e então melhora nos dias 13 (**C**) e 17 (**D**).

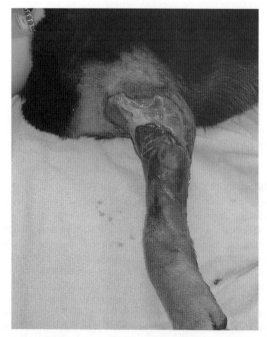

Figura 343.3 Lesão grave causada por extravasamento em cão da raça Rottweiler com osteossarcoma, tratado com doxorrubicina 12 dias antes.

COMPLICAÇÕES GASTRINTESTINAIS

Efeitos colaterais GI causados por terapia antineoplásica são frequentemente os mais temidos por pacientes oncológicos humanos e pelos tutores de animais com câncer, e por boas razões, já que eles sempre impactam negativamente a qualidade de vida. A toxicidade pode ser em decorrência do dano direto às células das criptas intestinais em fase de rápida divisão ou pela estimulação da zona de gatilho quimiorreceptora (ZGQ) no bulbo, através de neurotransmissores como a serotonina e a substância P, que se ligam aos receptores $5\text{-}HT_3$ e NK_1, respectivamente. A êmese pela estimulação da ZGQ é um sintoma agudo, que geralmente ocorre dentro de 24 horas após a administração de fármacos, e os quimioterápicos mais comumente incriminados são cisplatina (de longe o mais emetogênico), dacarbazina, estreptozotocina, doxorrubicina e mecloretamina. Anorexia, náuseas, êmese e diarreia causadas por toxicidade aos enterócitos imaturos geralmente ocorrem 1 a 5 dias após a administração do medicamento, e os fármacos mais incriminados como causas dos sinais clínicos são doxorrubicina, epirrubicina, dactinomicina, mitoxantrona, dacarbazina, alcaloides da vinca e taxanos. Os inibidores da tirosinoquinase, toceranib e masitinib podem causar irritação GI direta, resultando em anorexia, náuseas, êmese, diarreia ou hematoquesia. Em animais com câncer, comumente administra-se anti-inflamatório não esteroide (AINE) como analgésico e por seus conhecidos efeitos antineoplásicos. O potencial para irritação GI existe, e pode ser exacerbado quando o medicamento não seletivo piroxicam é combinado com alguns quimioterápicos citotóxicos.[30,31] A gravidade dos efeitos colaterais GI é graduada de 1 a 4.

A vincristina, em razão de seu efeito neurotóxico na função motora entérica, pode causar paralisia temporária do íleo (cães e gatos) e, ocasionalmente, constipação intestinal (gatos), nos dias seguintes à administração. Como resultado, pode ocorrer desconforto abdominal, anorexia, náuseas ou êmese, e os pacientes podem ser beneficiados com o tratamento com o fármaco procinético metoclopramida (0,3 a 0,5 mg/kg VO ou SC, a cada 8 horas). Em animais com câncer que não toleram a vincristina por conta de seus efeitos na motilidade intestinal, a substituição pela vimblastina pode ser uma opção.[31]

A anorexia induzida pela quimioterapia pode ser controlada com o fornecimento de alimentos mais palatáveis e, quando necessário, também pode ser utilizado estímulo farmacológico do apetite (ver Capítulo 23). Fármacos comumente utilizados incluem cipro-heptadina (cães: 0,2 mg/kg VO, cada 12 a 24 h; gatos: 2 a 4 mg VO, cada 12 a 24 h) e mirtazapina (cães: 0,5 mg/kg VO, a cada 24 h; gatos: 0,5 mg/kg VO, a cada 24 a 72 h).[33] Corticosteroides geralmente não são considerados boas escolhas como estimulantes do apetite, em razão de seus efeitos catabólicos, mas podem ser utilizados em baixa dose (p. ex., 0,5 mg de prednisona/kg VO, a cada 24 h; 0,05 mg de dexametasona/kg VO, a cada 24 h), a curto prazo, se não contraindicados. Oxazepam e acetato de megestrol têm sido utilizados ocasionalmente como estimulante do apetite em animais; é uma escolha comum em pessoas com caquexia secundária ao câncer, mas atualmente é raro recomendar esses medicamentos para tal finalidade. A administração intravenosa de baixas doses de propofol aumentou de forma significativa o consumo de alimentos em cães saudáveis, sem causar sedação excessiva, mas o efeito desejado não durou por tempo suficiente (15 minutos) para torná-lo clinicamente útil.[34] Um novo orexígeno aprovado para uso veterinário, a capromorelina, logo se tornará disponível como uma opção para animais com anorexia. Náuseas é uma causa subjacente comum da anorexia e pode ocasionar êmese quando suficientemente intensa. A orientação dos tutores sobre como reconhecer a ocorrência de náuseas em seu animal é crucial. Os sinais podem incluir perda de apetite, salivação excessiva, lambedura dos lábios, virar a cabeça quando se oferece o alimento e êmese. O fornecimento de alimentos mais palatáveis a um animal com náuseas pode agravar a sensação, o que não é recomendado. O tratamento das náuseas verdadeira ou suspeita é crucial, mesmo quando não for relatada êmese, e pode ajudar a melhorar o apetite. Os fármacos recomendados para o tratamento são praticamente os mesmos utilizados para êmese (ver adiante e Capítulo 39).

A êmese discreta (menos de 3 episódios em 24 horas) pode ser controlada mediante restrição alimentar durante 12 a 24 horas, seguida de introdução gradativa de refeições pequenas e frequentes de uma dieta leve. Se ocorrer êmese com o estômago vazio (p. ex., pela manhã), o uso de fármacos supressores de ácidos gástricos pode ser benéfico, incluindo famotidina (0,5 a 1 mg/kg, intravenoso [IV] ou VO, a cada 12 h) e omeprazol (0,5 a 1 mg/kg VO, a cada 24 h). Em casos de êmese moderada, justifica-se o uso de antieméticos; nos casos mais graves, recomenda-se terapia de suporte com soluções cristaloides de uso parenteral. O antiemético de ação central maropitant, um inibidor do receptor de neurocinina 1 (NK$_1$), foi aprovado para uso em cães para prevenir a êmese associada à cisplatina; ademais, mostrou-se efetivo na redução de êmese após administração de doxorrubicina.[35-37] Maropitant pode ser utilizado tanto em cães (1 mg/kg, IV ou SC, a cada 24 h; 2 mg/kg VO, a cada 24 h) quanto em gatos (1 mg/kg IV SC VO, a cada 24 h).[35-38] Outros antieméticos incluem metoclopramida; os antagonistas do receptor 5-HT$_3$, ondansetrona (0,5 a 1 mg/kg IV ou VO, a cada 12 a 24 h) e dolasetrona (0,5 a 1 mg/kg SC ou IV, a cada 12 a 24 h), e proclorperazina (0,1 a 0,5 mg/kg IV IM SC, a cada 8 h; 0,5 a 1 mg/kg VO, a cada 8 a 12 h). Embora

os antiácidos não tenham ação antiemética direta, o seu uso pode ser benéfico em pacientes com náuseas graves e êmese. Quadros graves de êmese necessitam terapia hídrica de suporte e monitoramento do perfil bioquímico sérico, que incluem avaliação do equilíbrio eletrolítico e ácido-base. Em casos mais graves, também pode ser necessária nutrição parenteral. Para administração subsequente de fármacos antineoplásicos que resultam em quadros moderados a graves de êmese, deve-se reduzir a dose (em 10 a 20%) e implementar uma abordagem preventiva. Em casos mais graves, pode ser necessária a alteração do protocolo terapêutico.

Ao tratar mastocitomas macroscópicos, alguns dos sinais clínicos GI podem ser decorrentes da elevada histaminemia, da acidez excessiva após degranulação espontânea ou da terapia citotóxica.[39,40] O alto teor de histamina, em razão da ligação aos receptores H2 nas células parietais, resulta em secreção excessiva de ácido clorídrico, diminuição do pH estomacal e irritação gástrica.

Os casos de diarreia discreta ou fezes amolecidas podem ser controlados pelo fornecimento de dieta leve altamente digestível. Em casos de diarreia mais intensa causada por quimioterapia em cães sem mutação de MDR-1, pode-se administrar loperamida (0,1 mg/kg VO, a cada 8 a 12 h).[41,42] Os antibióticos metronidazol (15 mg/kg VO, a cada 12 h) e tilosina (10 a 20 mg/kg VO, a cada 12 h) também são escolhas comuns. A utilização de argila natural para tratar diarreia induzida por quimioterapia mostrou-se benéfica.[43] Atualmente, os probióticos são utilizados na rotina clínica para tratar diarreia aguda ou crônica e podem ser combinados com outras terapias antidiarreicas (ver Capítulos 40, 167 e 178). Um estudo que avaliou o efeito do maropitant na prevenção de êmese induzida por doxorrubicina fortuitamente observou que também reduziu de forma significativa a frequência e gravidade da diarreia em cães tratados, comparativamente àqueles que receberam placebo.[37] Outro estudo controlado com placebo avaliou o uso profilático de sulfadiazina-trimetoprima (STM) em cães com osteossarcoma e linfoma tratados com doxorrubicina.[44] Os cães tratados (grupo STM) tiveram uma taxa de hospitalização significativamente menor e menor frequência e gravidade da toxicidade GI, quando comparados ao grupo placebo.[44]

Discretas toxicidades GI não necessitam modificação da dose. Toxicidades moderadas a graves podem necessitar hospitalização para terapia de suporte e sintomática, e as doses subsequentes devem ser reduzidas em 10 a 25% ou o protocolo terapêutico alterado, além de terapia profilática mais agressiva (antieméticos, antidiarreicos).

LETARGIA

Talvez um dos efeitos colaterais mais comuns e sub-relatados da terapia antineoplásica em animais, a letargia discreta, seja geralmente autolimitante. Fármacos mais comumente associados a algum grau de fadiga nos dias seguintes ao tratamento também quase sempre são mielossupressores e incluem doxorrubicina, carboplatina e lomustina, para nomear somente os mais comuns.

É importante distinguir entre a fadiga como efeito colateral temporário e reversível causada pela terapia e a letargia secundária a náuseas, anemia, dor ou progressão do tumor, já que essas causas subjacentes devem ser especificamente abordadas; todavia, em geral a letargia causada por quimioterapia, por si só, não requer intervenção. Após a primeira dose de vincristina administrada a um paciente submetido pela primeira vez à quimioterapia para linfoma, não é raro observar letargia discreta autolimitante de curta duração (geralmente 2 a 3 dias), enquanto bilhões de células do linfoma estão morrendo rapidamente, resultando em consumo de energia significativo pela grande quantidade de macrófagos ativados. Poucas semanas depois, o mesmo paciente com linfoma agora em regressão parcial (volume tumoral muito menor), recebendo uma segunda dose de vincristina idêntica à primeira, pode não manifestar fadiga alguma.

Quando a letargia é moderada à grave, devem ser realizados testes diagnósticos adicionais para excluir a possibilidade de citopenias, progressão da doença ou anormalidades concomitantes. A letargia extrema observada 24 a 48 horas após quimioterapia agressiva administrada pela primeira vez em um paciente com linfoma ou leucemia linfoblástica, com extensa morte tumoral, pode ser secundária à incomum síndrome da lise tumoral aguda (SLTA; ver Capítulo 344).

CARDIOTOXICIDADE

A cardiotoxicidade causada por quimioterapia é incomum, mas bem descrita em animais e principalmente associada ao uso de doxorrubicina. Outros medicamentos (p. ex., mitoxantrona e epirrubicina) foram desenvolvidos com a esperança de apresentar um perfil de eficácia semelhante, porém com menor risco de cardiotoxicidade. Ademais, foi demonstrado, em cães, que a forma lipossômica da doxorrubicina resulta em risco muito menor de cardiotoxicidade cumulativa.[45]

Há dois tipos de cardiotoxicidade induzida pela doxorrubicina: aguda ou cumulativa. A toxicidade aguda se manifesta como arritmias ventriculares transitórias que ocorrem durante a infusão intravenosa, secundária à liberação espontânea de histamina e catecolaminas, e geralmente não tem relevância clínica. A cardiotoxicidade cumulativa, mais grave, é resultado do dano permanente aos cardiomiócitos, especificamente da lesão oxidativa ao retículo sarcoplasmático, ocasionando redução da contratilidade, com ou sem arritmia, e insuficiência cardíaca congestiva irreversível (ver Capítulos 247 e 252).

Em cães sem doença miocárdica subjacente, o risco de cardiotoxicidade permanente é maior em casos de doses cumulativas superiores a 180 a 240 mg/m^2. A relação custo-benefício deve ser levada em consideração ao tratar cães com miocardiopatia subjacente ou com doses cumulativas que excedam 240 mg/m^2. Assim, as opções consistem no uso de um quimioterápico de menor cardiotoxicidade ou na administração intravenosa concomitante de dexrazoxano (na dose 10 vezes maior que a dose da doxorrubicina), um quelante de ferro que sabidamente reduz o risco de cardiotoxicidade causada pela doxorrubicina em cães e pessoas.[46,47]

HEPATOTOXICIDADE

A lomustina (CCNU) é conhecida por ser hepatotóxica aos cães; nota-se aumento da atividade sérica de alanina aminotransferase (ALT), um indicador de lesão hepatocelular, em até 86% dos cães tratados.[48-54] Essa hepatotoxicidade é cumulativa e em geral irreversível. Ademais, raramente pode ocorrer insuficiência hepática aguda após uma única sessão de quimioterapia. Além do hemograma pré-tratamento, deve-se monitorar a ALT antes de cada dose de lomustina; a elevação de ALT mais de três vezes acima do limite superior de normalidade deve bastar para postergar ou descontinuar o tratamento, a menos que os benefícios da terapia continuada claramente se sobreponham aos riscos. Um estudo clínico prospectivo aleatório avaliou a administração concomitante de hepatoprotetores, combinando S-adenosilmetionina e silibina com lomustina, em cães com câncer.[54] Constatou-se redução da taxa e gravidade das elevações de enzimas hepáticas em cães que receberam hepatoprotetores, comparativamente aos cães tratados somente com lomustina.[54] Em outro estudo, cães tratados com lomustina receberam o nutracêutico ácido alfalipoico como hepatoprotetor, mas não foi possível tirar conclusões quanto à eficácia desse procedimento devido à falta de um grupo controle.[55] Como regra geral, recomenda-se o uso concomitante de hepatoprotetores em cães tratados com lomustina. A hepatotoxicidade em gatos que recebem lomustina parece ser muito menos comum.[56] A gravidade das elevações das atividades das enzimas hepáticas e da concentração de bilirrubina é graduada de 1 a 4.

Elevações na atividade sérica de ALT são também relatadas após a administração de estreptozotocina em cães com insulinoma.[57]

A vincristina não é hepatotóxica, mas, assim como outros quimioterápicos, é excretada principalmente por via biliar. Em pacientes com colestase acentuada, como às vezes pode acontecer na infiltração hepática por linfoma, a vincristina deve ser temporariamente evitada ou utilizada em doses menores, em razão do aumento do risco de toxicidade devido sua longa meia-vida circulante.

Mesmo que não possam ser consideradas hepatotoxicidades verdadeiras, a elevação da atividade de fosfatase alcalina induzida por corticosteroides e a hepatopatia vacuolar são comumente associadas ao uso de corticosteroides em cães portadores ou não de câncer (ver Capítulo 285). Elevações discretas a moderadas reversíveis das atividades de enzimas hepáticas são relatadas com relativa frequência após o uso dos inibidores da tirosinoquinase aprovados para uso veterinário, toceranib e masitinib; em caso de tratamento prolongado, recomenda-se o monitoramento dessas atividades enzimáticas.[19,58]

NEUROTOXICIDADE

Comparativamente aos pacientes humanos, a neurotoxicidade é incomum em pacientes veterinários oncológicos. A vincristina sabidamente causa sintomas GI em animais (íleo adinâmico e constipação intestinal, em gatos) devido a seus efeitos neurotóxicos na função motora entérica, porém muito raramente causa neuropatia periférica semelhante à toxicidade dose-limitante observada em pessoas.[59] O risco de neurotoxicidade central pela vincristina, em geral extremamente baixo, pode ser maior em cães homozigotos para a mutação ABCB1-1 delta.[60]

Quando utilizado na dose padrão (150 mg/m^2 IV), o antimetabólito 5-fluoruracila (5-FU) raramente causa sintomas de neurotoxicidade com relevância clínica em cães.[61] Ele é, entretanto, extremamente neurotóxico aos cães após exposições acidentais a doses maiores; ademais, o 5-FU é absolutamente contraindicado aos gatos por ocasionar neurotoxicidade fatal.[62,63]

É raro o quimioterápico alquilante clorambucila, especialmente quando fornecido em protocolo terapêutico com altas doses administradas na forma pulsada, causar mioclonia reversível e convulsões em gatos e cães.[64,65] Sabidamente, o clorambucila também causa efeitos neurotóxicos na forma de alterações de humor e convulsões, em pessoas.[66,67] Em pessoas, a mecloretamina raramente causa diminuição reversível da capacidade auditiva ou perda da audição; entretanto, há relatos anedóticos de surdez parcialmente reversível em gatos.[68]

TOXICIDADE AO TRATO URINÁRIO

Nefrotoxicidade

Alguns fármacos quimioterápicos sabidamente são nefrotóxicos e requerem diurese salina intensa para reduzir o risco de nefropatia, em animais. Esses medicamentos incluem cisplatina (apenas aos cães), ifosfamida (cães e gatos) e estreptozocina (cães).[57,69-71] Animais com câncer e com confirmação ou suspeita de nefropatia não devem ser tratados com esses fármacos, devido à alta relação custo-benefício. Recomenda-se o estreito monitoramento dos parâmetros da função renal; a sua administração deve ser descontinuada caso seja constatada elevação da concentração de creatinina. A gravidade das elevações das concentrações de nitrogênio ureico sanguíneo (NUS) e de creatinina é graduada de 1 a 4.

Relata-se que a doxorrubicina apresenta potencial nefrotóxico em gatos, especialmente quando administrada na dose comum a cães.[72] Constatou-se que esse medicamento pode ser seguramente administrado na dose de 22 a 25 mg/m^2, e relata-se que a dose muito baixa (1 mg/kg) recomendada após o estudo inicial da toxicidade pode representar uma redução muito exagerada.[73] Em gatos tratados com doxorrubicina, deve-se monitorar os indicadores de função renal; ademais, recomenda-se prudência. Além da hepatotoxicidade previamente mencionada, a lomustina (CCNU) pode também ser nefrotóxica aos cães, seja administrada em alta dose pulsada, seja em protocolo metronômico de baixa dose.[53,74]

Os anti-inflamatórios não esteroides (AINE), inclusive o piroxicam e vários medicamentos aprovados para uso veterinário, são conhecidos por seu potencial nefrotóxico, independentemente de sua seletividade pela ciclo-oxigenase (COX)-2. Eles são comumente administrados em animais com câncer, tanto por suas propriedades analgésicas quanto por seus potenciais antineoplásicos. O seu uso deve ser criterioso e com monitoramento regular, sobretudo ao combiná-lo com outros medicamentos potencialmente nefrotóxicos, quando o seu uso é prolongado ou quando o paciente apresenta função renal questionável ou diminuída. A combinação de AINE com cisplatina é muito tóxica e deve ser desencorajada.[75-77]

Os bifosfonatos consistem em uma classe de fármacos utilizados em pacientes oncológicos devido a sua ação inibidora de osteoclastos, o que é benéfico no tratamento de dor óssea osteolítica e hipercalcemia. Eles geralmente são muito bem tolerados, mas tanto o pamidronato quanto o zoledronato, dois aminobifosfonatos potentes de uso intravenoso e clinicamente úteis, demonstraram potencial para nefrotoxicidade em estudos toxicológicos pré-clínicos. Estudos clínicos em cães com câncer demonstraram que os bifosfonatos podem ser seguramente administrados tanto em cães quanto em gatos, isolados ou combinados com outros medicamentos antineoplásicos.[78-85] A duração da infusão parece influenciar sua nefrotoxicidade, e o pamidronato (cães: 1 a 2 mg/kg, IV; gatos: 1 a 1,5 mg/kg, IV) deve ser administrado ao longo de duas horas, enquanto o zoledronato (cães: 0,15 a 0,25 mg/kg; gatos: 0,15 a 0,2 mg/kg) requer infusão mais curta de 15 minutos; ambos devem ser administrados em solução salina 0,9%.[78-85]

Relata-se que o mesilato de masitinib, um inibidor da tirosinoquinase, causa nefropatia com perda de proteína (NPP) em até 10% dos animais tratados e, em alguns casos, resulta em proteinúria severa.[20,21,86] Parâmetros de função renal, concentração sérica de albumina, exame de urina e relação proteína:creatinina na urina devem ser monitorados, e a administração do medicamento deve ser descontinuada em caso de proteinúria progressiva. A NPP induzida pelo fármaco parece ser reversível na maioria dos casos, se diagnosticada precocemente e com a remoção do agente causador.[20,21,86]

A carboplatina, diferentemente da cisplatina, não é nefrotóxica em doses clinicamente úteis. Estudos em gatos confirmaram que o ideal seria a administração de dose individualizada, baseada na taxa de filtração glomerular e na área sob a curva farmacocinética.[87-89]

Toxicidade urotelial

A cistite hemorrágica estéril (CHE) é uma complicação bem reconhecida, causada pela administração de ciclofosfamida e ifosfamida, sendo que a irritação direta do urotélio é principalmente causada pela acroleína, um metabólito inativo. Em cães, o risco de CHE pode variar de acordo com o protocolo de administração da ciclofosfamida e de doses cumulativas, e a administração simultânea de furosemida ou do composto que contém o grupo tiol, a mesna, reduz significativamente esse risco.[90-94] Gatos podem ser predispostos à CHE, mas é preciso cautela quando há fatores predisponentes presentes, inclusive cistite idiopática felina.

Em cães, se não for possível o uso de mesna juntamente a doses padrões de ciclofosfamida, recomenda-se o uso concomitante de ifosfamida ou de altas doses (mieloablativas) de ciclofosfamida, pois ambas resultam em alta taxa de CHE grave.[70,71,95-97] Ifosfamida, como previamente mencionado, também requer diurese salina, a fim de reduzir o risco de nefrotoxicidade.

Há relatos anedóticos de diversas estratégias terapêuticas para CHE. É imperativo, primeira e primordialmente, descontinuar a administração do medicamento causador por tempo indefinido, bem como confirmar CHE e excluir outros diagnósticos diferenciais (infecção do trato urinário, cristalúria, tumor de bexiga etc.).

Os sintomas de CHE geralmente tendem a melhorar assim que a causa é removida, mas em casos graves a recuperação clínica pode demorar semanas ou meses. O diagnóstico precoce, quando se confirma hematúria microscópica sem sinais clínicos detectáveis, seguida da descontinuação do medicamento, pode aumentar as chances de resolução rápida de CHE.

Tipicamente, em casos de CHE, utiliza-se com mais frequência a terapia sintomática que, quase sempre, consiste na administração de AINE, para amenizar o desconforto e a inflamação, e de oxibutinina (cães: 0,2 a 0,3 mg/kg VO, a cada 8 a 12 h) para abrandar a intensidade dos espasmos musculares. Alguns profissionais recomendam o uso de glicosaminoglicano polissulfatado (Adequan®) ou polissulfato de pentosana (Cartrophen Vet®), para auxiliar no restabelecimento da camada protetora da camada mucosa da bexiga. Em casos mais graves, pode ser necessário o uso de analgésicos adjuvantes; há relatos anedóticos de que os fármacos utilizados para tratar cistite idiopática (ver Capítulo 334) podem ser úteis, inclusive amitriptilina (1 a 2 mg/kg, VO, a cada 12 a 24 h) e gabapentina (8 a 15 mg/kg, VO, a cada 8 a 12 h). Em casos raros, mais extremos e refratários, pode ser necessária cirurgia mediante desbridamento ou cistectomia parcial. Há relato de tratamento medicamentoso para esses casos graves, que consiste na instilação de formalina diluída na bexiga, um procedimento que resultou na melhora dos sinais clínicos nos poucos casos relatados.[98,99]

REAÇÕES DE HIPERSENSIBILIDADE

Reações de hipersensibilidade (ver Capítulo 137) não são comuns, mas sua ocorrência é bem conhecida após administração de uma série de medicamentos quimioterápicos. Pode ocorrer uma verdadeira reação anafilática tipo I, mediada por IgE, após administração de L-asparaginase, sendo o risco maior quando utilizadas doses crescentes. A recomendação é que nunca se deve administrar L-asparaginase por via intravenosa, dando preferência às vias intramuscular e subcutâneas em cães e gatos, respectivamente, e tratamento prévio com difenidramina (1 a 2 mg/kg, IM ou SC), 15 minutos antes da administração do quimioterápico.

A doxorrubicina pode causar reação anafilactoide, acompanhada de hipotensão e taquicardia, ocasionada pela liberação espontânea de histamina por mastócitos por meio de um mecanismo não mediado por IgE.[100] Essa liberação de histamina, que também causa arritmia cardíaca, pode ser mais intensa em casos de administração mais rápida do antineoplásico; então, a recomendação geral é administrá-la na forma de infusão de curta duração (15 a 30 minutos). Ao seguir essa recomendação, o pré-tratamento com difenidramina ou dexametasona pode nem sempre ser necessário.

Por fim, alguns medicamentos quimioterápicos podem causar reações de hipersensibilidade cutânea relativamente graves mediadas por seus veículos inertes, em animais. As reações consistem em prurido, rubor, urticária e edema facial.[101-103] Elas foram relatadas após o uso de paclitaxel (gatos e cães) e etoposido (cães) devido aos seus veículos, Cremophor EL® e polissorbato-80, respectivamente, e relata-se a ocorrência de tais reações apesar de pré-medicação agressiva.[100-103] Métodos de administração ou formulações mais recentes podem ajudar a minimizar o risco de tais reações, inclusive a forma micelar de paclitaxel ou a administração por via subcutânea.[104-106]

TOXICIDADES ESPECÍFICAS E INCOMUNS

Em gatos, a administração intravenosa de cisplatina causa edema pulmonar grave fatal e, portanto, é absolutamente contraindicada, diferentemente do uso intralesional ocasional em baixa dose.

A fibrose pulmonar pode ser uma complicação causada por altas doses cumulativas de bleomicina em cães, mas é um problema clínico incomum na rotina.[107] Em gatos, altas doses cumulativas de lomustina podem resultar em hipertensão e fibrose pulmonarde.[108] A fibrose pulmonar pode também ser uma complicação incomum em cães tratados com o recente quimioterápico rabacfosadina (VDC-1101), sob avaliação pela FDA para aprovação para o tratamento de linfoma canino.[109]

A estreptozocina é um quimioterápico especialmente tóxico às células beta do pâncreas, sendo utilizada somente para tratar insulinoma em pessoas e cães. Uma complicação potencial esperada é a diabetes melito, em razão da ablação total das células beta; em um estudo prospectivo recente, foi constatada em 42% dos cães tratados.[57]

Há relato de pancreatite em baixa porcentagem de cães tratados com fosfato de toceranib.[19] A relação causa-efeito e o mecanismo de ocorrência primário ainda não foram estabelecidos. Recomendam-se testes diagnósticos apropriados quando um cão tratado com fosfato de toceranib apresentar sinais clínicos compatíveis com possível pancreatite.

A claudicação, mais provavelmente causada por cãibras musculares, foi associada ao uso do fosfato de toceranib em cães.[19] Tipicamente, a claudicação é discreta, com desvio do peso corporal de um membro para o outro e se resolve com uma breve descontinuação do fármaco (1 a 2 doses) e uma terapia analgésica apropriada. É importante ressaltar que raramente ocorre recidiva da claudicação após o reinício do tratamento com toceranib.

REFERÊNCIAS BIBLIOGRÁFICAS

As referências bibliográficas deste capítulo se encontram online no Ambiente de Aprendizagem.

CAPÍTULO 344

Tumores Hematopoéticos

David M. Vail

LINFOMA

O linfoma é o tumor hematopoético mais comum em cães e gatos; é definido como uma proliferação de células linfoides malignas principalmente nos linfonodos e órgãos viscerais sólidos, como fígado e baço. O linfoma é uma categorização indefinida de um grupo amplo e variado de diversos subtipos de câncer oriundos de células linfoides. A subcategorização de vários tipos de linfoma em cães e gatos está se tornando mais disponível, e finalmente é possível indicar um prognóstico mais acurado e um tratamento mais individualizado.

Etiologia

A etiologia do linfoma em animais de companhia é mal compreendida. Diversos fatores etiológicos foram pesquisados, inclusive genéticos e moleculares,[1-31] infecciosos,[32-42] ambientais[43-54] e imunológicos.[55-61] Embora diversas aberrações genéticas e moleculares tenham sido documentadas em cães e gatos, a relevância clínica e terapêutica desses fatores estão atualmente sob investigação e, portanto, ficam além do escopo deste capítulo; recomenda-se ao leitor interessado consultar os artigos originais listados nas referências bibliográficas.

Embora algumas variedades incomuns de linfoma em gatos tenham sido associadas, direta e indiretamente, ao vírus da leucemia felina (FeLV) e ao vírus da imunodeficiência felina (FIV), respectivamente, não há evidências fortes de uma etiologia por retrovírus em cães. Em cães e gatos foram incriminados como causas de linfoma distúrbios da função imune, inclusive terapia imunossupressora (p. ex., terapia de transplante renal) e doença inflamatória crônica, como dermatite atópica e linfoma cutâneo. Ademais, em um estudo, sugere-se a associação entre infecção gástrica por *Helicobacter* e linfoma de tecido linfoide associado à mucosa gástrica (TLAM) em gatos[62] e, talvez, em cães;[34] como essa síndrome é reconhecida em pessoas, justificam-se pesquisas adicionais.

Classificação

Foram avaliados diversos esquemas de classificação de linfoma, inclusive aqueles baseados na localização anatômica, no estadiamento clínico recomendado pela Organização Mundial da Saúde (OMS) (Tabela 344.1), no fenótipo histológico/citológico/imune e no genótipo.

Tabela 344.1 Estadiamento clínico do linfoma de animais domésticos, segundo a Organização Mundial da Saúde (OMS).

ESTÁGIO	CRITÉRIOS
I	Um único linfonodo
II	Vários linfonodos regionais
III	Linfadenopatia generalizada
IV	Envolvimento hepático e/ou esplênico (com ou sem estágio III)
V	Envolvimento da medula óssea ou sangue e/ou qualquer órgão não linfoide (com ou sem estágios I a IV)
Subestágio a	Sem sinais clínicos da doença
Subestágio b	Com sinais clínicos da doença

Adaptada de World Health Organization: *TNM classification of tumors in domestic animals*, Geneva, 1980, World Health Organization.

Classificação em cães

Nos cães, 80 a 85% dos casos são do tipo anatômico multicêntrico, em linfonodos periféricos, em estágio III ou IV da OMS. Menos frequentemente, são observadas localizações externas aos linfonodos, dos tipos alimentar (≈ 7%), cutâneo (≈ 6%), mediastinal (≈ 3%) e miscelânea de locais extranodais (no sistema nervoso central [SNC], ossos, coração, cavidade nasal e ocular primário). Conforme mencionado, "linfoma" é realmente um termo generalista que consiste em um grupo variado de diversos subtipos de câncer que surgem a partir de células linfoides. Atualmente, avanços nas classificações por meio de citometria de fluxo e exames histopatológico, imunofenotípico e genotípico estão fornecendo dados que podem permitir a subclassificação dessa doença em grupos importantes do ponto de vista prognóstico, o que pode finalmente resultar em recomendações terapêuticas mais personalizadas. O esquema de classificação histológico mais comumente aplicado é o da OMS, baseado em imunofenótipo e fenótipo histológico.[63] A maioria dos casos (≈ 80%) assemelha-se ao linfoma não Hodgkin (LNH) intermediário ou de alto grau em humanos. A maioria dos casos de linfoma canino consiste no imunofenótipo de células B, sendo que aproximadamente 25 a 30% são oriundos de células T. Aplicando a classificação da OMS, Valli et al. relataram que os cinco subtipos de linfoma mais comuns em cães (representando aproximadamente 80% dos casos), em ordem decrescente de frequência, são linfoma difuso de células B grandes (LDCBG), linfoma periférico de células T ainda não especificado, linfoma de zona T nodal, linfoma linfoblástico T e linfoma de zona marginal.[64] O LDCBG pode ser ainda classificado em subtipos diferentes do ponto de vista prognóstico, como centro germinativo e centro pós-germinativo, de acordo com o perfil da expressão gênica.[23] O diagnóstico/classificação de amostras clínicas por meio de citometria de fluxo e métodos histopatológicos, para fins de prognóstico e tratamento, são discutidos subsequentemente. Também há formas indolentes de linfoma (p. ex., de zona T e de zona marginal).[63-69]

Classificação em gatos

Atualmente, a maioria dos linfomas de gatos é classificada com base em sua localização anatômica, representada por formas indolentes de células pequenas/baixo grau ou fenótipos de células grandes/grau intermediário. Nessa espécie, a prevalência geral de linfoma parece estar aumentando, e a maior prevalência se deve ao aumento no número e na frequência relativa do tipo anatômico alimentar (e, em particular, o intestinal) do linfoma.[70-78] A epidemiologia típica para gatos com linfoma não pode ser afirmada uniformemente, já que varia amplamente com base na localização anatômica e na condição de positividade ao FeLV; portanto, será discutida individualmente em textos específicos sobre localização e na Tabela 344.2.[35,79-86] Em geral, a raça Siamês parece mais predisposta, principalmente para um tipo de linfoma mediastinal não associado ao FeLV em uma população mais jovem (mediana de 3 anos).[87] Duas formas distintas de linfoma merecem atenção especial. O linfoma linfocítico granular grande, um tumor de células redondas granulares, em geral envolve o trato intestinal e vísceras abdominais; como regra, há envolvimento sistêmico.[88-91] Os gatos afetados em geral são negativos para FeLV/FIV, e uma predominância do imunofenótipo de células T CD3+/CD8+ ou célula NK sugere sua origem no epitélio do intestino delgado. Também foi caracterizado um segundo tipo distinto, que se assemelha ao linfoma de Hodgkin em humanos.[92-94] Essa forma tipicamente envolve linfonodos solitários ou regionais da cabeça e pescoço, e, com base em suas características imunofenotípicas, os tumores são classificados como linfomas de células B, com abundância de células T. Histologicamente, os linfonodos podem ser ofuscados por linfócitos pequenos a blásticos nodulares ou difusos, com células bizarras ou multinucleadas características (células semelhantes a células de Reed-Sternberg). Não foi comprovada a sua relação com FeLV ou FIV.

Manifestação e sinais clínicos

Linfoma multicêntrico canino

O linfoma acomete principalmente cães de meia-idade a idosos. Não há predileção sexual, e há várias diferenças raciais. A prevalência de alguns imunofenótipos de linfoma varia com a raça.[16] A maioria dos casos ocorre em cães relativamente saudáveis (subestágio a), com linfadenopatia generalizada incidental (Figura 344.1). Em cães com a doença em subestágio b, os sinais clínicos são inespecíficos e podem incluir inapetência, perda de peso e letargia. A hipercalcemia paraneoplásica (ver Capítulo 352) pode resultar em sintomas de poliúria e polidipsia (ver Capítulo 45). Na doença em estágio V, se o envolvimento da medula óssea for marcante, citopenias periféricas podem resultar em manifestações que refletem sepse neutropênica, hemorragia trombocitopênica ou anemia.

Tabela 344.2 Características gerais das formas anatômicas de linfoma mais comumente encontradas em gatos.*

FORMA ANATÔMICA[†]	FREQUÊNCIA RELATIVA[‡]	IDADE MÉDIA (ANOS)	ANTÍGENO DO FELV	CÉLULAS B	CÉLULAS T	PROGNÓSTICO GERAL
Alimentar/gastrintestinal[§]						
Células pequenas/baixo grau	Comum	13	Raro	Rara	Comum	Bom
Intermediário/células grandes	Moderada	10	Raro	Comum	Rara	Ruim
Nasal	Incomum	9,5	Raro	Comum	Incomum	Bom
Mediastinal	Incomum	2 a 4	Comum	Incomum	Comum	Moderado-ruim
Linfonodos periféricos	Incomum	7	Incomum	Moderada	Moderada	Moderado-ruim
Laríngeo/traqueal	Incomum	9	Raro	DI	DI	Bom-moderado
Renal	Rara	9	Raro	Comum	Incomum	Moderado-ruim
SNC	Rara	4 a 10	Raro	DI	DI	Ruim
Cutâneo	Rara	10 a 13	Raro	Rara	Comum	Moderado
Hepático (puro)	Rara	12	Raro	Incomum	Comum	Ruim

*Dados podem incluir sobreposição ou mistura de localizações e representar a "era pós-FeLV". [†]Como o local primário de manifestação, e não disseminação ou progressão. [‡]Comum: mais de 50% das manifestações clínicas; moderado: 20 a 50% das manifestações clínicas; incomum: 5 a 20% das manifestações clínicas; raro: menos de 5% das manifestações clínicas. [§]Inclui aqueles relatados como "intra-abdominais", nos quais o intestino é um componente documentado. *DI*, dados insuficientes; *FeLV*, vírus da leucemia felina; *SNC*, sistema nervoso central.

Linfoma canino em outras localizações

A manifestação e sinais clínicos associados de linfoma refletem a forma anatômica presente em cada caso. Podem ocorrer *formas alimentares* com sintomas específicos do trato gastrintestinal (p. ex., êmese [ver Capítulo 39], diarreia [ver Capítulo 40], perda de peso [ver Capítulo 19], inapetência [ver Capítulo 23]). Podem ocorrer formas mediastinais com sintomas respiratórios (dispneia [ver Capítulo 28], abafamento de bulhas cardíacas) ou com síndrome pré-cava caracterizada por edema, com sinal de Godet (ver Capítulo 18) na cabeça, pescoço e membros torácicos, devido à compressão da veia cava cranial pelo tumor (Figura 344.2). Quase metade dos casos de linfoma mediastinal estão associados à hipercalcemia paraneoplásica,[95] resultando em polidipsia e poliúria como queixas do proprietário durante o atendimento.

O *linfoma cutâneo* tem sido denominado "grande imitador", devido a sua propensão em ocorrer em diversas formas. Lesões cutâneas únicas ou múltiplas são possíveis e conseguem surgir como placas eczematosas discretas ou tumores nodulares mais marcantes (Figura 344.3). As lesões podem ou não ser pruriginosas e se localizar em qualquer parte da pele e na cavidade bucal.

As localizações diversas do linfoma resultam em sintomas atribuíveis à sua localização (claudicação no caso de lesões ósseas e comprometimento neurológico em caso de linfoma no SNC).

Linfoma felino

Não foram detectadas consistentemente predileção sexual; entretanto, a prevalência pode ser maior na raça Siamês.[87] Em geral, é mais provável que os gatos manifestem doença clínica do que os cães; 75% ou mais dos animais apresentam sintomas do subestágio b, refletindo, em parte, a alta frequência de envolvimento gastrintestinal. Gatos com linfoma alimentar ou linfoma linfocítico granular grande apresentam graus variáveis de perda de peso (ver Capítulo 19), pelos emaranhados, inapetência (ver Capítulo 23), diarreia crônica (ver Capítulo 40) e êmese (ver Capítulo 39). Gatos com doença mediastinal quase sempre apresentam angústia respiratória grave (ver Capítulo 139), secundária à massa tumoral intratorácica ou à presença de efusão pleural significativa (ver Capítulo 244). Gatos com linfoma renal podem apresentar poliúria/polidipsia secundárias à insuficiência renal. No caso de linfoma nasal, espirros (ver Capítulo 27), secreção nasal serossanguinolenta crônica, exoftalmia e deformidade facial são sintomas comuns. Gatos com linfoma no SNC podem apresentar sinais clínicos constitucionais (anorexia e letargia) e sintomas relacionados a lesões intracranianas e/ou lesões medulares. Gatos com linfoma associado ao FeLV mais provavelmente apresentam anemia. Gatos com linfoma de Hodgkin com frequência apresentam aumento de um único linfonodo mandibular ou cervical; fora isso, se mostram clinicamente sadios (subestágio a).

Diagnóstico

Em cães com suspeita de linfoma, a avaliação diagnóstica deve incluir exame físico minucioso, hemograma, perfil bioquímico sérico e exame de urina. O ideal é mensurar a concentração de cálcio ionizado, em vez de cálcio total. Por fim, é fundamental a obtenção de amostras de tecidos e/ou para exame citológico a fim de definir o diagnóstico.

Exame físico

Em cães, o exame físico minucioso deve incluir palpação de todos os linfonodos passíveis de avaliação, bem como exame retal digital (ver Capítulo 2). As membranas mucosas devem ser inspecionadas em busca de palidez ou petéquias indicativas de anemia, de trombocitopenia secundária à mieloftise e de evidências de insuficiência importante de órgãos, inclusive a presença de icterícia ou úlceras urêmicas. A palpação abdominal pode revelar organomegalia, espessamento da parede intestinal

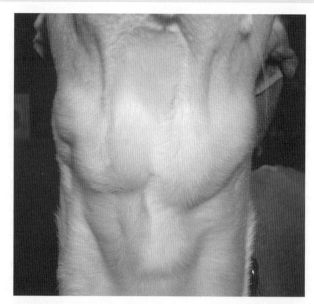

Figura 344.1 Linfadenopatia generalizada em um cão da raça Greyhound Italiano com linfoma (note os linfonodos mandibulares).

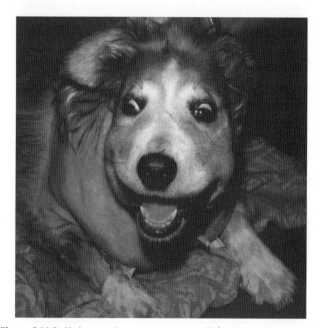

Figura 344.2 Síndrome pré-cava em um cão com linfoma no mediastino. Note o edema, com sinal de Godet na cabeça e no pescoço.

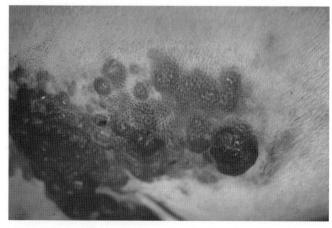

Figura 344.3 Linfoma cutâneo de células T (micose fungoide) em um cão.

ou linfadenopatia mesentérica. A presença de uma massa tumoral no mediastino e/ou de efusão pleural pode ser suspeita, com base nos achados à compressão torácica, em gatos, e à auscultação, em cães e gatos. O exame oftalmológico (ver Capítulo 11) revela anormalidades (p. ex., uveíte, hemorragia de retina e infiltração ocular) em aproximadamente um terço à metade dos cães e gatos com linfoma.[96,97]

Anormalidades hematológicas

Na maioria dos casos, ocorrem anormalidades hematológicas. A anemia, quando presente, geralmente é normocítica normocrômica não regenerativa, refletindo a anemia comum à doença crônica. Anemia regenerativa pode indicar perda de sangue ou hemólise concomitante. Gatos com doença associada ao FeLV podem ter anemia macrocítica. Se houver mieloftise significativa, a anemia pode ser acompanhada de trombocitopenia e leucopenia. Linfócitos atípicos circulantes podem ser indicativos de envolvimento da medula óssea e leucemia. A hipoproteinemia é mais comumente observada em animais com linfoma alimentar.

Recomenda-se o exame citológico de aspirado da medula óssea para o estadiamento devido ao significado prognóstico do envolvimento marcante da medula (ver Capítulo 92); também é recomendado no caso de suspeita de linfoma, mas não é indicado para avaliação dos linfonodos periféricos.

Anormalidades no perfil bioquímico sérico

Aproximadamente 15% dos cães com linfoma (40% dos cães com tumor no mediastino) apresentam hipercalcemia (ver Capítulo 297), quase sempre devido à produção ectópica do peptídio relacionado ao paratormônio (ver Capítulo 352).[95,98] Em caso de hipercalcemia de origem desconhecida, o linfoma deve sempre ser considerado uma das principais hipóteses na lista de diagnósticos diferenciais. Além disso, a presença de hipercalcemia pode servir como indicador da resposta à terapia. Pode ocorrer aumento na concentração de nitrogênio ureico sanguíneo e na concentração sérica de creatinina, secundárias à infiltração neoplásica nos rins, à nefrose hipercalcêmica ou à desidratação. Elevações nas atividades de enzimas específicas do fígado ou na concentração de bilirrubina podem ser causadas por infiltração tumoral no parênquima hepático. O aumento da concentração sérica de globulinas, geralmente monoclonal, é uma ocorrência rara em casos de linfoma de células B.

Condição de infecção por retrovírus

Em gatos, os testes para retrovírus (i. e., FeLV [ver Capítulo 223] e FIV [ver Capítulo 222]) são importantes para o diagnóstico, o prognóstico e o manejo dos animais. A frequência relativa de associações com o FeLV é apresentada na Tabela 344.2.

Exames de imagem

Os exames de imagem (radiografia, ultrassonografia [US], tomografia computadorizada [TC], tomografia por emissão de pósitrons [PET]) podem ser importantes no diagnóstico (especialmente na ausência de linfadenopatia periférica) e na avaliação da resposta ao tratamento, além de serem igualmente importantes para o estadiamento clínico (i. e., a determinação da extensão da doença), já que os resultados podem influenciar de forma significativa o prognóstico geral e o interesse do proprietário pelo tratamento. As anormalidades constatadas em radiografias do tórax podem incluir evidências de infiltrados pulmonares e linfadenomegalia torácica (Figura 344.4). Radiografia ou US do abdome pode revelar evidências de linfadenopatia abdominal e/ou envolvimento esplênico e/ou hepático. A US de abdome (ver Capítulo 88) é mais importante quando há suspeita de linfoma intestinal na ausência de linfadenopatia periférica. Outros exames de imagem, incluindo exames contrastados do trato gastrintestinal, TC, PET/TC, ressonância magnética (RM) ou exames mielográficos do SNC e radiográficos/cintilográficos esqueléticos são reservados para os casos com suspeita de envolvimento da localização anatômica apropriada. A PET/TC representa o padrão de cuidado para o estadiamento e a resposta do monitoramento em pessoas com linfoma; entretanto, a pouca disponibilidade desse procedimento impede o uso rotineiro em oncologia veterinária.[99-102] Na experiência do autor, a menos que haja sinais clínicos atribuíveis à anormalidade abdominal, os exames de imagem se limitam às radiografias de tórax para casos típicos de linfoma multicêntrico canino, já que não há diferença no prognóstico de cães em estágio III ou IV da doença (i. e., envolvimento hepático/esplênico); entretanto, a presença de linfadenopatia no mediastino cranial é de significado prognóstico.

Diagnóstico citológico e histopatológico

Na opinião do autor, uma combinação de exame histopatológico (Tru-Cut, biopsia em cunha, todo o linfonodo) e citometria de fluxo de aspirado com agulha devem ser o padrão para o diagnóstico de linfoma multicêntrico (ver Capítulo 95).[68,103-105] Isso possibilita uma subtipagem acurada, fornece informações prognósticas adicionais e, por fim, pode resultar em protocolos terapêuticos desenvolvidos exclusivamente para o subtipo detectado. Embora o exame citológico do aspirado com agulha fina (AAF) por um patologista clínico geralmente seja adequado para confirmar o diagnóstico de linfoma em cães, não é possível realizar a subtipagem clinicamente importante apenas pela citologia. A predominância de uma população homogênea de células linfoides imaturas é sugestiva de linfoma (Figura 344.5), embora haja diversas variantes de células pequenas nodulares indolentes, e recomenda-se o exame histológico/imunofenotípico dessas formas menos comuns de neoplasia.

Exames citológicos ou histológicos adicionais específicos para algumas localizações de neoplasias podem ser justificáveis quando há suspeita de tumores não localizados em linfonodos. A toracocentese (ver Capítulo 102), seguida de exame citológico ou citometria de fluxo do líquido pleural, geralmente tem valor diagnóstico em gatos com linfoma no mediastino, mas é menos provável que seja útil em cães com efusão secundária ao envolvimento do mediastino. Por outro lado, o exame do liquor (ver Capítulo 115) é normalmente mais útil em cães do que em gatos com linfoma no SNC, pois a forma medular mais comum em gatos geralmente é extradural.[106-108] Em gatos com suspeita de linfoma no SNC, em geral há envolvimento da medula óssea (ver Capítulo 92) e dos rins (ver Capítulo 321), e o exame citológico desses órgãos quase sempre é mais fácil do que da neoplasia localizada no SNC.

Nos casos de linfoma gastrintestinal, ainda há controvérsia quanto à sensibilidade diagnóstica de amostras obtidas por

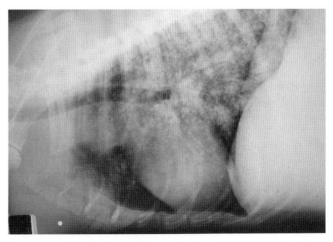

Figura 344.4 Imagem radiográfica lateral do tórax de um cão com linfoma, mostrando intenso infiltrado intersticial e linfadenopatia intratorácica (p. ex., hilar e esternal).

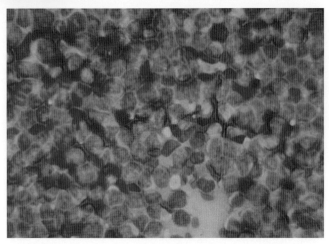

Figura 344.5 Citologia de aspirado por agulha fina (AAF; coloração Wright-Giemsa, ×1.000) de um linfonodo periférico de um cão com linfoma de alto grau. A característica tecidual do linfonodo é ofuscada por uma população homogênea de células linfoides imaturas. (*Esta figura se encontra reproduzida em cores no Encarte.*)

biopsia guiada por endoscopia em relação às amostras de espessura total obtidas por biopsia cirúrgica; o primeiro procedimento (ver Capítulo 113) ainda é considerado padrão-ouro, porém o último está ganhando espaço com o avanço das técnicas.[70-74,109,110] Isso é particularmente relevante para casos de linfoma gastrintestinal indolente, que representam a forma mais comum de linfoma em gatos, porém rara em cães. Nessas situações, podem ser necessárias técnicas de diagnóstico avançadas (p. ex., citometria de fluxo ou reação em cadeia da polimerase [PCR] para rearranjo de receptor do antígeno [PARR]). Para gatos e cães com linfoma gastrintestinal de grau intermediário ou alto, geralmente a constatação de linfadenopatia abdominal, tumores intestinais/gástricos mensuráveis ou qualquer outro envolvimento de órgãos abdominais possibilita uma abordagem diagnóstica definitiva menos invasiva, em que o exame citológico de amostras de aspirado ou obtidas por biopsia central guiadas por US pode ter valor diagnóstico, sem necessidade de biopsia intestinal por meio de laparotomia/laparoscopia.

Técnicas avançadas de diagnóstico

Além de sua importância na confirmação do diagnóstico de linfoma, as amostras destinadas a exames histológicos e citológicos podem ser analisadas por diversas técnicas histoquímicas, imuno-histoquímicas e por citometria de fluxo, a fim de determinar o imunofenótipo (p. ex., células B, células T, célula nula, expressão do complexo principal de histocompatibilidade [MHC]), o tamanho da célula, a taxa de proliferação tumoral (p. ex., Ki-67, o antígeno nuclear celular em proliferação [PCNA], as regiões organizadoras nucleolares argirófilas [AgNOR]) e o subtipo da neoplasia (tumores de alto grau, de grau intermediário ou de baixo grau/indolentes), bem como a presença ou ausência de quantidade crescente de marcadores moleculares sob investigação, com potencial prognóstico, preditivo e terapêutico.[68,103-105,111-113] Atualmente, vários laboratórios disponibilizam na rotina análise imunofenotípica de amostras com um painel cada vez maior de marcadores imunofenotípicos (p. ex., células B, células T, classe de MHC), que fornecem ao clínico e ao tutor informações mais confiáveis quanto ao prognóstico; esse autor atualmente utiliza o Colorado State University's Clinical Immunology Laboratory para tais análises (*http://csu-cvmbs.colostate.edu/academics/mip/ci-lab/Pages/default.aspx*). À medida que mais amostras são analisadas e correlacionadas com os resultados após o tratamento, as recomendações terapêuticas direcionadas para subtipos de linfoma específicos e para cada paciente de fato se tornam disponíveis para pacientes veterinários, como acontece com pacientes humanos.

Em raras condições, as avaliações citológicas e histológicas de rotina dos tecidos ou líquidos celulares não são apropriadas para confirmar sequer um diagnóstico inespecífico de linfoma. Quando tecidos sólidos suspeitos, linfócitos circulantes e amostras de efusão apresentam uma população de células mista ou não possibilita a diferenciação confiável de populações de células malignas das proliferações reativas benignas, a realização de ensaios de clonalidade celular pode ser útil, além da análise por citometria de fluxo.[103,114,115] A clonalidade é a característica da malignidade, ou seja, a população de células malignas teoricamente deve ser oriunda da expansão de um único clone maligno caracterizado por uma região particular do DNA para aquele tumor. Por exemplo, em um cão com linfoma de células T, todas as células malignas devem conter a mesma sequência de DNA na região variável do gene de receptor de células T. Da mesma forma, um cão com linfoma de células B deve ter células malignas com sequências de DNA idênticas na região variável do gene de receptor de imunoglobulina. Diferentemente, na linfocitose reativa benigna, as células são policlonais para seus receptores de antígeno. A técnica da reação em cadeia da polimerase é utilizada para amplificar as regiões variáveis da célula T e dos genes de receptores de imunoglobulina, a fim de detectar a clonalidade. Em cães, a sensibilidade desses testes é de aproximadamente 70 a 90%, com percentuais menores nos gatos. Podem ocorrer taxas de falso-negativos (p. ex., populações de células nulas e primers inapropriado para o DNA) e de falso-positivos (erliquiose e doença de Lyme) de, aproximadamente, 5%. Nesses casos, o diagnóstico deve ser confirmado somente após considerar os resultados de todas as avaliações diagnósticas, inclusive exame histológico/citológico, imunofenotipagem e testes de clonalidade, juntamente a informações epidemiológicas e achados do exame físico. Em geral, para amostras suspeitas, mas não diagnósticas para linfoma, o desempenho da citometria de fluxo é superior ao da análise de PARR; entretanto, pode-se preferir a realização de ambas.

Atualmente, as análises moleculares e proteômicas do DNA e de biomarcadores séricos estão sendo pesquisadas quanto a sua utilidade como testes de diagnóstico e prognóstico, respectivamente.[116-123] Essas técnicas moleculares, ao mesmo tempo que são úteis para o diagnóstico, poderiam também ser úteis para a definição mais confiável do estágio clínico, indicando a resposta terapêutica e a ocorrência de recidiva, bem como a taxa de remissão molecular e os níveis de doença residuais mínimos.

Diagnóstico diferencial

Os diagnósticos diferenciais para linfoma, que variam de acordo com a forma anatômica da doença, estão apresentados na Tabela 344.3.

Tratamento

A sobrevida média de cães e gatos não tratados varia de 4 a 6 semanas após o estabelecimento do diagnóstico de linfoma de grau intermediário ou alto, embora variações significativas dependam da localização e subtipo da neoplasia. Em geral, o linfoma é uma doença sistêmica e requer uma abordagem terapêutica sistêmica (*i. e.*, quimioterapia ou imunoterapia). No caso de linfoma solitário em linfonodo ou fora dele, pode-se indicar tratamento local, mediante extirpação cirúrgica ou radioterapia.

Quimioterapia sistêmica em cães com linfoma de grau intermediário e alto

Inicialmente, o tratamento de linfoma é bastante gratificante em ambas as espécies, já que as taxas de recuperação chegam a 90% em cães e 70% em gatos submetidos à quimioterapia com múltiplos agentes. É importante ressaltar que a percepção do tutor sobre as experiências do animal durante a quimioterapia geralmente

Tabela 344.3	Diagnósticos diferenciais comuns para linfoma.
FORMA ANATÔMICA	**LISTA DE DIAGNÓSTICOS DIFERENCIAIS**
Generalizado	Linfadenopatia disseminada causada por infecções (p. ex., bacterianas, virais, riquetsioses, parasitárias e fúngicas)
	Distúrbios imunomediados (p. ex., lúpus, poliartrite, vasculite, dermatopatia)
	Outras neoplasias hematopoéticas (p. ex., leucemia, mieloma múltiplo, histiocitose maligna ou sistêmica)
	Tumores metastáticos em linfonodos
	Diversas síndromes hiperplásicas reativas benignas, em gatos (ver texto)
Alimentar	Enterite infiltrativa (p. ex., enterite plasmocítica linfocítica)
	Neoplasias intestinais não linfoides
	Enterite granulomatosa
	Tumor de célula redonda granular, em gatos
	Tumor de mastócito gastrintestinal, em gatos
Cutâneo	Dermatite infecciosa (p. ex., piodermite avançada)
	Dermatite imunomediada (p. ex., pênfigo)
	Outras neoplasias cutâneas
Mediastinal	Timoma
	Tumor na base cardíaca (quemodectoma)
	Tumor de tireoide ectópico
	Granulomatose linfomatoide pulmonar
	Doença granulomatosa (p. ex., linfadenopatia hilar)

é positiva, e a vasta maioria dos clientes percebe que o tratamento é válido e resulta em melhora do bem-estar e da qualidade de vida geral.[124-126] Infelizmente, a maioria dos animais sucumbe, no final, à recidiva de doença disseminada resistente à quimioterapia. Foram publicados e previamente revisados vários protocolos quimioterápicos para cães com linfoma,[127,128] refletindo nossa incapacidade em alcançar a cura na maioria dos casos. Diversos fatores devem ser considerados e discutidos com os proprietários ao escolher um protocolo para uma situação particular, incluindo o custo, o comprometimento de tempo, a eficácia, a toxicidade e a experiência do clínico com o protocolo em questão. De forma geral, os protocolos que combinam quimioterápicos, mais complexos, são mais caros, consomem mais tempo (*i. e.*, necessitam de repetidas visitas ao consultório e monitoramento mais próximo), e mais provavelmente resultam em eventos adversos do que os protocolos mais simples com um único quimioterápico. Entretanto, em gral, os protocolos que combinam quimioterápicos, mais complexos, inicialmente resultam em duração da remissão e sobrevida mais longas do que os protocolos com um único antineoplásico. Protocolos que empregam combinação, mais complexos, são modificações do protocolo "CHOP", inicialmente desenvolvido para uso em oncologia humana. O protocolo CHOP consiste na combinação de ciclofosfamida (C), doxorrubicina (hidroxidaunorrubicina [H]), vincristina (Oncovin® [O]) e prednisona (P). Na década de 1990, amplos estudos clínicos aleatórios em pessoas com linfomas de grau intermediário e alto, envolvendo várias instituições, estabeleceram que protocolos mais complexos ou protocolos que *não* resultam em melhora da eficácia, na verdade, resultaram em maior frequência de eventos adversos.[129] Por essa razão, CHOP continua sendo o protocolo quimioterápico padrão para a maioria dos linfomas de grau intermediário e alto em pessoas. Embora ainda não tenham sido realizados amplos estudos clínicos aleatórios em cães, parece que, independentemente de qual protocolo à base do CHOP for utilizado, os tempos medianos gerais de remissão e sobrevida são de aproximadamente 8 e 12 meses, respectivamente.[127,128] Aproximadamente 20 a 25% dos cães

tratados permanecem vivos 2 anos após o início desses protocolos. As taxas de resposta e a duração da resposta variam, dependendo da presença ou ausência de fatores prognósticos, discutidos na sequência. Historicamente, os protocolos terapêuticos do linfoma começam com uma fase de indução intensiva, durante a qual os fármacos são administrados semanalmente; isso é acompanhado de uma fase de manutenção, durante a qual os intervalos terapêuticos são lentamente espaçados e os fármacos, administrados com menor frequência. Protocolos terapêuticos mais recentes abandonaram o uso da fase de manutenção, já que a maioria dos dados atuais demonstra que não há benefício algum com a sua inclusão.[130-137] De forma geral, os protocolos quimioterápicos de menor duração estão associados a taxas de recuperação e duração da primeira remissão semelhantes às obtidas em protocolos de duração mais longa e têm a vantagem de menor tempo de quimioterapia, bem como de menor custo e menor ocorrência de eventos adversos associados. Ademais, o tempo de sobrevida geral não é diferente, desde que realizados protocolos de reindução ou resgate. Para linfomas multicêntricos, por convenção, a condição de remissão é avaliada de acordo com os critérios de avaliação da recuperação do Veterinary Cooperative Oncology Group (VCOG).[138] Essa avaliação, simples e facilmente aplicável, leva em consideração nossa incapacidade de atingir remissão molecular completa verdadeira ou cura e possibilita uma comparação mais confiável da resposta a diferentes protocolos. O protocolo de indução de combinação de quimioterápicos baseada no protocolo CHOP mais frequentemente utilizado pelo autor é apresentado na Tabela 344.4.

A administração de doxorrubicina (30 mg/m^2, intravenoso [IV], a cada 3 semanas, por cinco sessões), junto à administração oral de prednisona, ainda é o protocolo quimioterápico citotóxico com um único agente mais efetivo e comumente utilizado em cães com linfoma.[139-142] Por volta de 70% dos casos respondem ao tratamento, com tempos medianos de remissão e de sobrevida de aproximadamente 5 e 7 meses, respectivamente. Esse protocolo com um único quimioterápico consome menos tempo, é menos caro e requer menos visitas hospitalares. Se os tutores optarem pela administração apenas de medicamentos de uso oral, é possível utilizar lomustina (CCNU; 70 mg/m^2 por via oral [VO], a cada 3 semanas) ou ciclofosfamida (250 a 300 mg/m^2 VO ou IV, a cada 2 a 3 semanas) e terapia com prednisona, embora a taxa e a duração da resposta sejam menores do que aquelas obtidas com a doxorrubicina.[143]

Se questões dos tutores relacionadas ao custo do tratamento ou a outro problema impedirem o uso de quimioterapia sistêmica mais agressiva, a terapia alternativa com prednisona (2 mg/kg, VO, a cada 24 h) quase sempre resulta em período de remissão curto de, aproximadamente, 1 a 2 meses. É aconselhável informar aos tutores que, se posteriormente decidirem tentar tratamento mais agressivo, os cães submetidos à terapia prévia com prednisona mais provavelmente desenvolverão a forma da doença resistente a medicamentos e apresentarão tempo de remissão e sobrevida mais curtos quando optarem por protocolos quimioterápicos subsequentes.[144-146] No caso de eventos adversos (EA) excessivos (ver Capítulo 343), pode ser necessário o ajuste de dose e/ou da frequência do quimioterápico. Na ausência de EA clinicamente relevantes, em particular quando não se constata a contagem mínima de neutrófilos esperada, incrementos da dose também são justificados, já que isso poderia indicar dose inadequada, com base na farmacogenética individual do paciente. Raças de cães (p. ex., Collie, Shetland Sheepdog e outras raças de pastoreio) com risco de anormalidades na glicoproteína-P transportadora de fármacos, que prediz o risco de EA induzidos pela quimioterapia, devem ser avaliados quanto à mutação no gene MDR1 antes da administração de medicamentos que atuam como substrato para MDR1.[147]

Quando ocorre hipercalcemia, se o cão estiver no subestágio a da doença e se alimentando e ingerindo água, geralmente não há necessidade de terapia auxiliar para hipercalcemia, pois a quimioterapia resulta em normalização da concentração

Tabela 344.4 Protocolo quimioterápico Wisconsin-Madison, com combinação de medicamentos, para cães com linfoma.

SEMANA DE TRATAMENTO	MEDICAMENTO, DOSE, VIA DE ADMINISTRAÇÃO	SEMANA DE TRATAMENTO	MEDICAMENTO, DOSE, VIA DE ADMINISTRAÇÃO
1	Vincristina: 0,5 a 0,7 mg/m² IV Prednisona: 2 mg/kg VO, a cada 24 h, durante 7 dias	11	Vincristina: 0,5 a 0,7 mg/m² IV
2	Ciclofosfamida: 250 mg/m² IV/VO Furosemida: 1 mg/kg IV* Prednisona: 1,5 mg/kg VO, a cada 24 h, durante 7 dias	12	Ciclofosfamida: 250 mg/m² IV/VO Furosemida: 1 mg/kg IV
3	Vincristina: 0,5 a 0,7 mg/m² IV Prednisona: 1 mg/kg VO, a cada 24 h, durante 7 dias	13	Vincristina: 0,5 a 0,7 mg/m² IV
4	Doxorrubicina: 30 mg/m² IV/VO Prednisona: 0,5 mg/kg VO, a cada 24 h, durante 7 dias	14	Doxorrubicina: 30 mg/m² IV
6	Vincristina: 0,5 a 0,7 mg/m² IV	16	Vincristina: 0,5 a 0,7 mg/m² IV
7	Ciclofosfamida: 250 mg/m² IV/VO Furosemida: 1 mg/kg IV	17	Ciclofosfamida: 250 mg/m² IV/VO Furosemida: 1 mg/kg IV
8	Vincristina: 0,5 a 0,7 mg/m² IV	18	Vincristina: 0,5 a 0,7 mg/m² IV
9[†]	Doxorrubicina: 30 mg/m² IV	19[‡]	Doxorrubicina: 30 mg/m² IV

*Furosemida é administrada concomitantemente à ciclofosfamida, com intuito de diminuir a incidência de cistite hemorrágica estéril. [†]Se o paciente apresentar remissão total na semana 9, o tratamento deve continuar até a semana 11. [‡]Se o paciente apresentar remissão total na semana 19, a terapia é descontinuada e o cão é reavaliado mensalmente por conta de recidivas. Nota: Antes de cada sessão de quimioterapia, deve-se realizar hemograma. Se a contagem de neutrófilos estiver abaixo de 2.000 células/μℓ, o clínico deve esperar 5 a 7 dias e então repetir o hemograma; administra-se o fármaco assim que a contagem de neutrófilos atingir valor acima do limiar de 2.000 células/μℓ.

sérica de cálcio dentro de alguns dias. Se o animal estiver doente, com azotemia ou sinais clínicos relevantes atribuíveis à hipercalcemia, justifica-se o tratamento específico da hipercalcemia (ver Capítulos 69 e 297), concomitante no início da quimioterapia sistêmica.

Quimioterapia sistêmica em gatos com linfoma de grau intermediário e alto

Diversos protocolos quimioterápicos com combinação de medicamentos para gatos foram relatados e revisados previamente.[148-150] A adição de doxorrubicina ao protocolo COP (Ciclofosfamida; Oncovin® [vincristina]; Prednisolona) parece superior ao uso exclusivo do COP, em gatos. Entretanto, alguns estudos constataram que os gatos submetidos a esse protocolo apresentam tempo de remissão e sobrevida comparáveis aos gatos tratados com o protocolo CHOP.[151,152] Diferentemente do que acontece em cães, a doxorrubicina não parece tão efetiva quanto a terapia com um único antineoplásico em caso de linfoma felino. De forma geral, os gatos com linfoma de grau intermediário ou alto não apresentam taxa de resposta alta, tampouco longo período de remissão e sobrevida, como ocorre em cães com linfoma de mesmo grau. A taxa de resposta total varia de 50 a 80%, e o tempo mediano geral da remissão e a sobrevida são de aproximadamente 4 a 6 meses e 6 a 8 meses, respectivamente. Entretanto, um percentual significante de gatos (30 a 40%) que apresentam resposta total à quimioterapia com combinação de medicamentos tem tempo de remissão total e sobrevida mais longos (ou seja, de 2 anos) do que aqueles observados em cães. O protocolo CHOP modificado preferido do autor, para gatos, é apresentado na Tabela 344.5.

Terapia de reindução ou resgate

Por fim, a maioria dos cães e gatos com linfoma de grau intermediário ou alto tratada com sucesso mediante quimioterapia de indução apresenta recidiva com a forma mais resistente aos medicamentos. Na primeira recidiva, se mais de 2 meses se passaram após o fim da quimioterapia, recomenda-se tentar a reindução mediante a repetição do protocolo de indução, inicialmente efetivo. Embora a probabilidade de resposta seja alta após a reindução, sua duração geralmente é mais curta do que a

observada na terapia inicial.[153] Se a reindução falhar, se o paciente não responder à indução inicial ou se ocorrer recidiva durante a indução inicial, então são utilizados medicamentos denominados fármacos de resgate ou protocolos de resgate. Esses fármacos ou a combinações deles tipicamente não constam do protocolo CHOP padrão, e o seu uso é reservado aos casos resistentes aos medicamentos. Uma série de protocolos de resgate, com uso de um único agente ou de múltiplos, foi relatada e revisada na literatura veterinária.[138,148,154,155] Relatam-se taxas de resposta de resgate total de 40 a 90%; entretanto, quase nunca as respostas são duráveis, com resposta mediana típica de 1,5 a 2,5 meses, independentemente da complexidade do protocolo. A administração sequencial de diversos protocolos de resgate diferentes pode resultar em vários meses adicionais de sobrevida com qualidade de vida aceitável.

Imunoterapia para linfoma (ver Capítulo 341)

O avanço mais significativo no tratamento do LNH em pessoas nas últimas duas décadas foi o desenvolvimento de terapias com anticorpos monoclonais combinadas com o protocolo CHOP padrão (p. ex., rituximabe-CHOP [R-CHOP]). Esse anticorpo monoclonal anti-CD20 humano aumentou de forma significativa o tempo livre da doença e a sobrevida em pessoas com LNH, comparativamente ao uso do protocolo CHOP.[156] A terapia com anticorpos monoclonais se tornou padrão (em combinação com a quimioterapia) para diversos tumores hematopoéticos em pessoas (p. ex., LNH, leucemia linfocítica crônica (LLC), linfoma cutâneo, linfoma de células T gama delta). Quanto à oncologia veterinária, em vários centros estão sendo realizados estudos aleatórios nacionais para determinar a eficácia das terapias com anticorpos monoclonais contra linfoma de células B (anti-CD20 canino; Aratana AT-004®) e células T (anti-CD52 canino; Aratana AT-005®) de cães, que foram totalmente aprovados pelo USDA. Embora tenha sido estabelecida a segurança para esses dois agentes, por ocasião da elaboração desse texto somente havia disponibilidade de dados preliminares (resumos) sobre sua eficácia, que representam uma expectativa razoável, mas não completa, da atividade antitumoral. Assim que esses testes (combinando quimioterapia monoclonal e quimioterapia padrão) forem finalizados e os resultados sujeitos à rigorosa revisão por seus pares, a verdadeira eficácia desses

Tabela 344.5	Protocolo quimioterápico Wisconsin-Madison, com combinação de medicamentos, para gatos com linfoma.		
SEMANA DE TRATAMENTO	MEDICAMENTO, DOSE, VIA DE ADMINISTRAÇÃO	SEMANA DE TRATAMENTO	MEDICAMENTO, DOSE, VIA DE ADMINISTRAÇÃO
1	Vincristina: 0,5 a 0,7 mg/m² IV L-asparaginase: 400 UI/kg SC Prednisolona: 2 mg/kg VO, a cada 24 h, durante 14 dias	11	Vincristina: 0,5 a 0,7 mg/m² IV
2	Ciclofosfamida: 200 mg/m² IV/VO Prednisolona: 2 mg/kg VO, a cada 24 h (contínua)	13[†]	Ciclofosfamida: 200 mg/m² IV/VO
3	Vincristina: 0,5 a 0,7 mg/m² IV Prednisolona: 1 mg/kg VO, a cada 24 h, durante 7 dias	15	Vincristina: 0,5 a 0,7 mg/m² IV
4	Doxorrubicina: 25 mg/m² IV Prednisolona: 1 mg/kg VO, a cada 48 h*	17	Doxorrubicina: 25 mg/m² IV
6	Vincristina: 0,5 a 0,7 mg/m² IV	19	Vincristina: 0,5 a 0,7 mg/m² IV
7[†]	Ciclofosfamida: 200 mg/m² IV/VO	21[†]	Ciclofosfamida: 200 mg/m² IV/VO
8	Vincristina: 0,5 a 0,7 mg/m² IV	23	Vincristina: 0,5 a 0,7 mg/m² IV
9[‡]	Doxorrubicina: 25 mg/m² IV	25[§]	Doxorrubicina: 25 mg/m² IV

*A partir desse momento, administra-se prednisolona (1 mg/kg, VO) em dias alternados. [†]No caso de linfoma renal ou de SNC, substitua por citosina-arabinosídeo (600 mg/m² SC, a cada 12 h, durante 2 dias) nessas sessões. [‡]Se o paciente apresenta remissão total na semana 9, o tratamento continua até a semana 11. [§]Se o paciente apresenta remissão total na semana 25, a terapia é descontinuada e o gato é reavaliado mensalmente por conta de recidivas. Nota: Antes de cada sessão de quimioterapia deve-se realizar hemograma. Se a contagem de neutrófilos estiver abaixo de 1.500 células/$\mu\ell$, o clínico deve esperar 5 a 7 dias e então repetir o hemograma; administra-se o medicamento quando a contagem de neutrófilos for superior ao limiar de 1.500 células/$\mu\ell$.

produtos será conhecida. É esperado que essas e outras potenciais terapias[157] com anticorpos monoclonais em desenvolvimento revolucionem de forma semelhante o tratamento de LNH em cães.

Também estão sendo realizadas pesquisas sobre o desenvolvimento de outras terapias imunológicas, incluindo vacinas antilinfoma e técnicas de transplante de medula óssea ou células-tronco após terapias ablativas da medula óssea.[158,159] Atualmente, elas possuem escopo investigacional.

Radioterapia para linfoma

A radioterapia para linfoma geralmente se limita a casos nos quais há localização anatômica solitária, sem envolvimento sistêmico ou a testes de investigação que utilizam protocolos de radiação de corpo inteiro ou de metade dele, em combinação com quimioterapia (ver Capítulo 340).[160-168]

Tratamento de linfoma indolente (de baixo grau)

Linfomas indolentes incluem um grupo variado de tumores incomuns em cães,[63-69] mas representam a forma de neoplasia mais comum em gatos (linfoma gastrointestinal felino indolente).[70-79] Cães com linfoma indolente (p. ex., linfoma da zona marginal, linfoma do manto, linfoma da zona T) quase sempre apresentam sobrevida longa, geralmente sem quimioterapia. Esses pacientes podem não manifestar sinais clínicos além do aumento de linfonodos ou do baço e, apesar de seus tumores serem menos responsivos à quimioterapia, apresentam sobrevida longa. Devido à natureza menos comum dos linfomas indolentes em cães, as recomendações terapêuticas ainda não estão bem estabelecidas. Inicialmente, uma decisão sobre o tratamento consiste na presença de sinais clínicos que comprometem a qualidade de vida, presença de organomegalia ou de citopenias clinicamente relevantes secundárias à mieloftise. Em tais casos, quase sempre se inicia o tratamento exclusivo com clorambucila (20 mg/m² VO, a cada 2 semanas) ou ciclofosfamida (250 mg/m² VO, a cada 2 a 3 semanas) combinada com prednisona. Em cães com linfomas indolentes confinados ao baço ou a um linfonodo solitário, a esplenectomia ou a extirpação do linfonodo, sem quimioterapia adjuvante, geralmente propicia controle a longo prazo, e vários pacientes apresentam vida normal e morrem em decorrência de outras doenças, não de linfoma indolente.

Gatos com linfoma alimentar de *pequenas células* de baixo grau (*i. e.*, gastrintestinal ou hepático) são mais bem tratados com um protocolo quimioterápico menos agressivo, como o uso oral de clorambucila (20 mg/m² VO, a cada 2 semanas) e prednisolona. Pode-se esperar sobrevida mediana de aproximadamente 2 a 3 anos.

Tratamento de linfoma extralinfonodal

Se há envolvimento extralinfonodal (ou extranodal) como parte de um processo mórbido mais generalizado ou multicêntrico, devem ser instituídas as terapias sistêmicas previamente discutidas. Caso contrário, se a localização extranodal for solitária, pode-se tentar terapia local sem necessidade de quimioterapia sistêmica. Nesses casos, justifica-se a adesão estrita aos exames de estadiamento (*i. e.*, exame da medula óssea, exames radiográficos, US, TC ou PET/TC), a fim de assegurar que a doença seja localizada. A cirurgia local e/ou radioterapia quase sempre é efetiva, e, embora o linfoma sistêmico possa por fim ocorrer meses a anos depois, a opinião do autor é que a terapia sistêmica pode ser resguardada até a constatação de doença sistêmica.

Em casos nos quais o envolvimento do SNC é parte de uma doença mais generalizada, a penetração de fármacos quimioterápicos através da barreira hematencefálica (BHE) pode ser um problema. No protocolo CHOP padrão, somente a prednisona penetra consistentemente a BHE. Tem-se recomendado a adição de citosina-arabinosídeo, que atinge concentração terapêutica no liquor, a um protocolo CHOP; entretanto, são escassas as evidências de sua atividade nessa situação. Embora a L-asparaginase não atravesse a BHE, ela atua no liquor (por causar depleção de asparagina). A radioterapia direcionada a todo o eixo neural (linfoma multifocal do SNC) ou a localização específica do SNC (linfoma solitário central ou espinal) também pode ser efetiva. Tentou-se a cirurgia de citorredução em um pequeno número de casos de linfoma extradural, com resultados diversos.

O linfoma cutâneo solitário pode ser efetivamente tratado por meio de radioterapia ou cirurgia local, mas a probabilidade de envolvimento sistêmico final é alta. São mais comumente encontradas lesões cutâneas múltiplas (ver Figura 344.3), sendo necessária terapia sistêmica. Em geral, o linfoma cutâneo é menos responsivo à quimioterapia do que o linfoma multicêntrico, porém com o passar do tempo podem ocorrer recidivas consideráveis dos sinais clínicos e recuperação a longo prazo. Atualmente, a terapia de primeira linha para cães com linfoma cutâneo consiste em lomustina (CCNU, 50 a 70 mg/m^2 VO, a cada 3 semanas) e prednisona, com taxa de resposta de aproximadamente 80% e duração da resposta mediana de 3 meses.[169,170] Outros quimioterápicos com atividade relatada são Doxil (uma forma de doxorrubicina encapsulada em lipossomos), L-asparaginase, dacarbazina, mostarda nitrogenada de uso tópico e protocolo CHOP padrão. A terapia com anticorpos monoclonais (anti-CD52) é efetiva em pessoas com linfoma cutâneo de célula T, e atualmente estão sendo coletados dados sobre casos tratados com anticorpo monoclonal canino (Aratana, AT-005®) para determinar sua eficácia em cães.

Gatos com linfoma nasal sem terapia sistêmica concomitante podem também ser tratados com radioterapia local e geralmente são beneficiados por sobrevida mais longa.[171-173]

Prognóstico

Fatores prognósticos em cães

Uma lista de fatores que influenciam a taxa de remissão e/ou o período de remissão e a sobrevida de cães com linfoma, conhecidos ou suspeitos, é mostrada na Tabela 344.6.[63-79,122,123,174-186]

Os três fatores que mais consistentemente se relacionam com o prognóstico em cães são as caraterísticas imunofenotípicas e as observadas na citometria de fluxo, o subtipo histológico e o subestágio da OMS. Em cães com linfoma de célula T, quase sempre o período de remissão e a sobrevida são significativamente mais curtos; entretanto, os pacientes com linfoma de zona T indolente apresentam sobrevida mais longa.

Fatores prognósticos em gatos

Os fatores mais fortemente associados a um prognóstico mais favorável em gatos parecem ser a presença de linfoma indolente, a resposta completa à terapia (que infelizmente não pode ser determinada antes do tratamento), a condição de negatividade aos retrovírus, o estágio clínico inicial, a localização anatômica e, talvez, a adição de doxorrubicina ao protocolo terapêutico.[71,75,81-83,87,88,90] Em geral, os gatos negativos ao FeLV que respondem completamente ao protocolo CHOP apresentam alta probabilidade de sobrevida a longo prazo (aproximadamente 35% deles permanecem vivos 1,5 ano após o diagnóstico). Em geral, gatos com linfoma alimentar de pequenas células apresentam melhor prognóstico, com sobrevida mediana de 2 anos ou mais após a terapia. Em gatos com linfoma nasal, o prognóstico é reservado, já que a radioterapia (ou quimioterapia, se a

Tabela 344.6 Fatores prognósticos para linfoma em cães.[63-79,122,123,174-186]			
FATOR	**ASSOCIAÇÃO FORTE**	**ASSOCIAÇÃO MODESTA QUE NECESSITA MAIS PESQUISAS**	**COMENTÁRIOS**
Estágio clínico da OMS		X	Estágio I/II: favorável Estágio V com envolvimento significativo da medula óssea: desfavorável
Subestágio clínico da OMS	X		Subestágio b (doença clínica): associado à diminuição da sobrevida
Histopatologia	X		Alto grau/grau médio: associado a alta taxa de resposta, mas com redução da sobrevida. Quase sempre, a sobrevida de pacientes com linfomas indolentes é mais longa, geralmente na ausência de terapia sistêmica
Características do imunofenótipo e da citometria de fluxo	X		Fenótipo de células T associado à redução da sobrevida. Baixa expressão de MHCII em células B associada à redução da sobrevida
Características do sangue periférico na citometria de fluxo	X		Inclui a análise combinada do tamanho e do imunofenótipo
Sexo		X	Alguns estudos sugerem que fêmeas apresentam melhor prognóstico
Anemia	X		
Avaliação molecular de doença residual mínima (p. ex., PARR)		X	Provavelmente se tornará muito mais importante quando mais abordagens terapêuticas "curativas" forem desenvolvidas e instituídas
Medidas de proliferação		X	Há relatos contraditórios
Pré-tratamento prolongado com esteroide	X		A maioria dos relatos sugere que o uso prévio de esteroide reduz a duração da resposta; entretanto, o tempo de exposição necessário é desconhecido
Expressão da glicoproteína-P (fatores de resistência ao medicamento)		X	Pode estar associada à baixa taxa de resposta e período de remissão mais curto
Linfadenopatia no mediastino cranial	X		Grande compilação de casos relata período de remissão e sobrevida mais curtos
Localização anatômica	X		Formas leucêmica, cutânea difusa, alimentar e hepatoesplênica associadas a prognóstico desfavorável
Toxicidade hematológica induzida por quimioterapia		X	Cães que apresentam neutropenia de grau III/IV têm período da primeira remissão longo

MHC, complexo principal de histocompatibilidade; *PARR*, reação em cadeia de polimerase (PCR) para rearranjo do receptor de antígeno.

radioterapia não estiver disponível) resulta em sobrevida mediana de 1,5 ano. Pouco se sabe sobre a progressão clínica do linfoma de Hodgkin em gatos; após a extirpação cirúrgica do linfonodo acometido, a ocorrência de recidiva pode demorar meses, e a resposta à quimioterapia é variável. Em gatos, os linfomas granulares grandes parecem ter evolução mais agressiva e respondem menos à terapia.

LEUCEMIA LINFOIDE

Leucemia é definida como a proliferação de células neoplásicas na medula óssea. As células malignas podem ou não estar presentes na circulação sanguínea periférica. A classificação de leucemia linfoide em leucemia linfoblástica aguda (LLA) e LLC é importante do ponto de vista diagnóstico, prognóstico e terapêutico (Figura 344.6).[103,186-193] A análise de marcadores imunofenotípicos por meio de citometria de fluxo (ver seções anteriores) é particularmente útil.

Leucemia linfoblástica aguda

A LLA é caracterizada por proliferações de linfoblastos morfologicamente imaturos na medula óssea e pode ser confundida com linfoma multicêntrico em estágio V (i. e., infiltração secundária da medula óssea). O curso clínico da LLA é rápido, progressivo e com resposta ruim à terapia, embora algumas subclassificações imunofenotípicas estejam associadas a melhor prognóstico geral. Gatos com LLA são mais jovens e frequentemente possuem antígenos de FeLV no sangue. As manifestações clínicas são inespecíficas e podem incluir letargia, perda de peso, pirexia intermitente, hepatoesplenomegalia, dor abdominal inespecífica e sintomas neurológicos. A maioria dos animais apresenta anemia e graus variados de trombocitopenia e leucopenia. O diagnóstico é sugerido pela proliferação marcante de linfoblastos na medula óssea ou no sangue periférico. Amostras de aspirado ou de biopsia de medula óssea (ver Capítulo 92) e hemograma geralmente são todo o necessário para o diagnóstico de leucemia aguda; entretanto, pode ser difícil classificar as formas imaturas, exceto uma forma blástica, e realiza-se citometria de fluxo para obter o imunofenótipo, para a confirmação. O exame citológico de aspirado do linfonodo (ver Capítulo 95) e de órgãos envolvidos (ver Capítulo 89) e a confirmação da condição de infecção por retrovírus em gatos podem ser procedimentos auxiliares úteis. Aproximadamente 10% dos casos são classificados como leucemia "aleucêmica", porque há infiltrado na medula óssea, mas não há linfoblastos na circulação periférica. A LLA pode ainda ser diferenciada clinicamente do linfoma multicêntrico em estágio V por sua progressão mais rápida, ausência de linfadenopatia significante, baixa resposta à quimioterapia e imunofenótipo CD34+. O prognóstico de cães e gatos com LLA é ruim. O período de remissão é curto e a sobrevida além de alguns meses é rara. Ainda não se sabe qual a importância, se houver, das novas terapias com anticorpos monoclonais no tratamento de leucemia linfoide.

Leucemia linfocítica crônica

A LLC é caracterizada pela proliferação de linfócitos fenotipicamente maduros, e não de linfoblastos. A maioria dos casos de LLC em cães e gatos é de linhagem de células T, sendo que os cães acometidos apresentam principalmente células T CD8+, várias das quais com morfologia linfocítica granular.[147] A LLC ocorre em cães e gatos idosos atendidos com sintomas inespecíficos, incluindo letargia, organomegalia, pirexia, poliúria/polidipsia, hemorragia (devido à trombocitopenia), claudicação intermitente e colapso. Entretanto, em alguns animais, é possível detectar linfocitose assintomática em exames de triagem pré-anestésicos ou de pacientes geriátricos. A linfocitose periférica pode variar de 10.000 a 300.000 ou mais células/$\mu\ell$. Anemia, trombocitopenia e neutropenia podem ser secundárias à mieloftise. Em gatos, não há comprovação de sua associação com a infecção causada por FeLV. Diferentemente da LLA, a LLC quase sempre apresenta progressão perene e, no início, é altamente responsiva à quimioterapia. O tratamento não é iniciado a menos que haja sinais clínicos, organomegalia ou citopenias periféricas relevantes (anemia, neutropenia, trombocitopenia) que comprometam a qualidade de vida do animal. Foram acompanhados casos de LLC por vários meses, sem necessidade de terapia. Caso haja recomendação de tratamento, administra-se clorambucila (cães: 0,2 mg/kg VO, a cada 24 h, durante 10 dias e então 0,1 mg/kg, por dia; gatos: 2 mg/gato VO, a cada 48 h ou, como alternativa, 20 mg/m^2 VO, a cada 2 semanas), juntamente a prednisona, diariamente ou em dias alternados. A maioria dos animais responde bem e apresenta boa qualidade de vida, com tempo de sobrevida mediano de aproximadamente 1 a 1,5 ano. Embora o prognóstico a curto prazo seja bom, eventualmente a LLC se torna resistente à terapia ou progride para LLA. Embora o anticorpo monoclonal anti-CD52 seja aprovado para uso em pessoas com LLC, as novas terapias com anticorpos monoclonais ainda não foram avaliadas em cães com LLC.

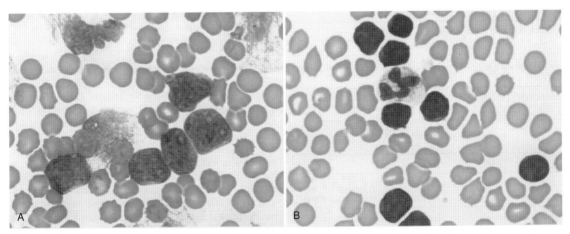

Figura 344.6 A. Esfregaço de sangue periférico (coloração de Wright-Giemsa, ×1.000) de um cão com leucemia linfoblástica aguda (LLA). Note os linfoblastos imaturos morfologicamente característicos de LLA. **B.** Esfregaço de sangue periférico (coloração de Wright-Giemsa, ×1.000) de um cão com leucemia linfocítica crônica (LLC). Note os linfócitos morfologicamente maduros de LLC. (Cortesia de Dr. Karen Young, da Universidade de Wisconsin-Madison.) (*Esta figura se encontra reproduzida em cores no Encarte.*)

LEUCEMIA LINFOIDE E DISTÚRBIOS MIELOPROLIFERATIVOS

Distúrbios mieloproliferativos (DMP) são definidos como um grupo de anormalidades de células da medula óssea não linfoides, nas quais ocorre proliferação de uma, várias ou todas as linhagens celulares da medula. As anormalidades podem ser condições pré-neoplásicas ou neoplásicas, que teriam progressão benigna ou maligna. Com poucas exceções (p. ex., ver policitemia vera [PV], Capítulo 200), a literatura veterinária sobre DMP é escassa, na melhor das hipóteses, sendo composta quase inteiramente de relatos de caso. Os DMP são inicialmente classificados com base na origem da célula em questão e, em seguida, no grau de diferenciação celular. Se a população celular em proliferação for fenotipicamente bem diferenciada, a anormalidade é classificada como crônica; se imatura ou pouco diferenciada, a doença é classificada como aguda. Na Tabela 344.7, há uma lista de possíveis variantes de DMP relatadas em espécies de animais de companhia. Como há envolvimento de células-tronco pluripotentes da medula óssea, um tipo de DMP pode progredir para outro, e há envolvimento de mais de uma linhagem celular no mesmo distúrbio.

Animais com DMP crônico podem não manifestar sinais clínicos até que o envolvimento do órgão ou mieloftise da medula óssea resulte em sinais clínicos, que quase sempre são inespecíficos e podem incluir organomegalia, palidez, sepse e hemorragia causada por trombocitopenia. Em gatos, a maioria dos DMP está associada à infecção por FeLV.

O diagnóstico de DMP é baseado na demonstração da linhagem celular em proliferação, na ausência de doenças não neoplásicas associadas à hiperplasia ou hipoplasia da medula óssea. Portanto, os diagnósticos diferenciais incluem doenças inflamatórias crônicas (p. ex., erliquiose), linfoma multicêntrico, toxicidade por estrógeno, intoxicação por chumbo e, no caso de trombocitose essencial ou primária, deficiência de ferro. Como vários desses DMP agudos são pouco diferenciados e/ou representam combinações de linhagens celulares, a morfologia verificada em microscopia óptica frequentemente é insuficiente, e, por fim, é necessária citometria de fluxo e exame histoquímico para o diagnóstico preciso. Uma lista completa dos testes disponíveis está além do escopo deste capítulo, mas eles foram revisados em outras publicações.[191,193,194]

Os DMP agudos respondem mal aos protocolos quimioterápicos de um único medicamento ou de combinação de quimioterápicos, e o prognóstico é ruim. Caso se tente quimioterapia, são necessários tratamento de suporte agressivo e terapia para citopenias secundárias à mieloftise. Os DMP crônicos apresentam prognóstico reservado; entretanto, são mais prováveis respostas iniciais duradouras à terapia. Não há necessidade de tratamento até que ocorram sinais clínicos ou citopenia periférica relevante. Relata-se que a hidroxiureia ocasionalmente resulta em remissão parcial de vários tipos de DPM crônico, principalmente PV, trombocitopenia essencial, leucemia basofílica e leucemia mieloide crônica (LMC). Em cães com LMC, a hidroxiureia é administrada em dose inicial de 20 a 25 mg/kg, VO, a cada 12 h. Essa dose é mantida até que a contagem de leucócitos diminua para menos de 20.000 células/$\mu\ell$, ocasião em que a dose é reduzida para 10 a 15 mg/kg, a cada 24 h, ou para 50 mg/kg VO, uma vez a cada 2 ou 3 semanas. Um efeito colateral comum da terapia com hidroxiureia em cães é a onicomadese (descamação das unhas). Por fim, vários dos DMP crônicos progridem para uma fase terminal ou crise blástica, na qual ocorre uma fase leucêmica aguda fatal. Inibidores do receptor de tirosinoquinase (p. ex., toceranib ou masitinib) ainda não foram minuciosamente avaliados para os casos de DMP, mas podem ser considerados.

A PV (ver Capítulos 57 e 200) é definida como uma proliferação anormal de precursores eritroides na medula óssea; isso ocorre independentemente da eritropoetina (EP), e as células seguem um padrão de maturação ordenado normal.[150,151] O resultado é uma elevação anormal do hematócrito, da contagem de eritrócitos e da concentração sanguínea de hemoglobina. A PV deve ser diferenciada da policitemia relativa ou policitemia secundária. Cães e gatos de meia-idade são tipicamente afetados, apresentando sintomas variados que incluem emia de membranas mucosas, tortuosidade de vasos da esclera e da retina, fraqueza, intolerância ao exercício, hemorragia franca (epistaxe, hematúria, melena), sintomas neurológicos (demência, convulsões, paralisia, ataxia) e esplenomegalia ocasional. Também pode haver comprometimento cardíaco ou renal. A maioria dos sintomas relatados é secundária à síndrome da hiperviscosidade, discutida no item sobre tumor de plasmócitos, neste capítulo. O diagnóstico é confirmado pela constatação de eritrocitose relevante (hematócrito: 60 a 75%), com concentração sérica de EP normal ou diminuída, e ausência de condições associadas à policitemia relativa ou secundária. Radiografia e US de tórax e abdome, hemogasometria, exames de aspirado da medula óssea e concentração sérica de EP devem ser avaliados para excluir a possibilidade de diagnósticos diferenciais. No exame citológico da medula óssea, nota-se hiperplasia eritroide com padrões relativamente normais de maturação. O tratamento consiste na redução da quantidade de hemácias (flebotomia; 15 a 20 mℓ de sangue/kg de peso corporal e reinfusão do plasma do paciente) e supressão da produção eritroide na medula óssea.[150,151] Para suprimir a produção de eritrócitos, utiliza-se fósforo radiativo (^{32}P) ou, mais comumente disponível, quimioterapia (p. ex., hidroxiureia, melfalana, ciclofosfamida, busulfan), com resultados controversos.

DISTÚRBIOS RELACIONADOS AO MIELOMA

Distúrbios relacionados ao mieloma (DRM) surgem quando uma célula da linhagem de precursores de plasmócitos ou linfócitos B produtores de imunoglobulina se transforma e prolifera até originar uma população de células neoplásicas semelhantes. Na maioria das vezes, essa população é monoclonal, produzindo uma imunoglobulina homogênea; todavia, há neoplasias biclonais e policlonais. Os DRM incluem mieloma múltiplo (MM), macroglobulinemia por IgM (macroglobulinemia de Waldenstrom), plasmocitoma solitário (inclusive plasmocitoma ósseo solitário e plasmocitoma extramedular [PEM]) e linfomas e leucemias que secretam imunoglobulinas (inclusive leucemia de plasmócitos). O mieloma múltiplo é o DRM mais importante, em razão de sua incidência e gravidade. Em gatos, há algumas discordâncias e controvérsias sobre a distinção entre MM e PEM multicêntrico.

Tabela 344.7 Distúrbios mieloproliferativos possíveis em cães e gatos.

CLASSIFICAÇÃO	LINHAGEM CELULAR
Distúrbios mieloproliferativos agudos	
Leucemia mieloide aguda (LMA)	Mieloblastos
Leucemia mielomonocítica aguda (LMMA)	Mieloblastos/monoblastos
Leucemia monocítica aguda (LmoIA)	Monoblastos
Leucemia megacarioblástica aguda	Megacarioblastos
Eritroleucemia	Eritroblastos
Distúrbios mieloproliferativos crônicos	
Leucemia mieloide crônica (LMC)	Neutrófilos, precursores tardios
Trombocitopenia primária	Plaquetas
Leucemia basofílica	Basófilos e precursores
Leucemia eosinofílica	Eosinófilos e precursores
Policitemia vera	Eritrócitos

Mieloma múltiplo

O MM representa 8% de todos os tumores hematopoéticos de cães, mas é relativamente raro em gatos.[195-202] No MM, o componente M pode ser qualquer classe de imunoglobulina ou apenas uma parte da molécula, como a sua cadeia leve (proteína de Bence-Jones) ou pesada (doença da cadeia pesada). Embora na maioria dos casos o mieloma felino/DRM envolva a medula óssea, ele parece envolver locais extramedulares (p. ex., pele e vísceras abdominais) mais comumente do que em cães.[198,200-202,204] Em sua maior parte, a etiologia do MM é desconhecida. Predisposições genéticas, alterações moleculares (p. ex., anormalidades no receptor TKI), infecções virais, estímulo imune crônico e exposição a carcinógenos foram sugeridas como fatores contribuintes. O MM não foi associado às infecções causadas por FeLV e FIV.

Fisiopatologia

Uma ampla gama de anormalidades patológicas e síndromes clínicas relacionadas pode ocorrer como resultado da infiltração tumoral em vários sistemas orgânicos, da presença de alta concentração do componente M circulante ou de uma combinação destas. A síndrome da hiperviscosidade (SHV) é uma das anormalidades clinicopatológicas decorrentes do aumento da viscosidade sérica. A magnitude da SHV está relacionada ao tipo, tamanho, morfologia e concentração do componente M no sangue. É mais comum em casos de macroglobulinemia por IgM, devido ao seu alto peso molecular.[203] A SHV pode resultar em diátese hemorrágica, sintomas neurológicos (p. ex., demência, depressão, atividade convulsiva ou coma; ver Capítulo 260), anormalidades oftalmológicas (p. ex., dilatação/tortuosidade de vasos da retina, hemorragia na retina ou descolamento de retina; ver Capítulo 11) e aumento da pós-carga cardíaca com subsequente cardiomiopatia ou insuficiência cardíaca congestiva. Essas consequências supostamente são resultado do aumento da viscosidade do sangue em pequenos vasos, fornecimento insuficiente de oxigênio e de nutrientes e anormalidades de coagulação. A SHV é menos comum em gatos.[204] Nota-se doença renal em 30 a 50% dos cães com MM, como resultado da proteinúria de Bence-Jones (cadeia leve), infiltração tumoral no tecido renal, hipercalcemia, amiloidose, diminuição da perfusão devido à SHV, desidratação ou infecção do trato urinário ascendente. Nota-se hipercalcemia em 15 a 20% dos cães com MM, devido principalmente à produção do fator ativador de osteoclastos, outras citocinas ou da proteína relacionada ao paratormônio N-terminal pelas células neoplásicas (ver Capítulo 352). A hipercalcemia é rara em gatos com MM.

A suscetibilidade a infecções e imunodeficiência são frequentemente as causas finais de morte em animais com MM. A concentração de imunoglobulina pode estar severamente reduzida, e pode haver leucopenia secundária à infiltração medular (mieloftise). Aproximadamente dois terços dos cães apresentam anemia normocítica normocrômica não regenerativa, o que pode ser decorrência de mieloftise, perda de sangue por distúrbios da coagulação, anemia que acompanha doença crônica ou maior destruição eritrocitária secundária à alta viscosidade sérica. Fatores semelhantes podem levar à trombocitopenia e leucopenia em 25 a 30% dos cães afetados. A diátese hemorrágica pode resultar de um ou da combinação de eventos. O componente M pode interferir na coagulação, inclusive inibindo a agregação plaquetária e a liberação do fator plaquetário-3, adsorção de proteínas da coagulação pequenas, polimerização anormal da fibrina, produção de anticoagulantes semelhantes à heparina e redução na função do cálcio.

Manifestação clínica

Nota-se MM em cães e gatos idosos, sem predileção racial ou sexual. Os sinais clínicos são variáveis devido a uma ampla gama de efeitos patológicos possíveis e podem estar presentes até 1 ano antes do diagnóstico. No cão, os sinais clínicos mais comuns,

em ordem decrescente de frequência, são letargia e fraqueza, claudicação como resultado da osteólise, hemorragia (ver Capítulo 135), poliúria/polidipsia (ver Capítulo 45) e déficits neurológicos (ver Capítulos 259 e 260). Em geral, a diátese hemorrágica é caracterizada por epistaxe e hemorragia de gengiva (ver Capítulo 29). Os sintomas relativos ao SNC podem incluir demência, atividade convulsiva e deficiências em reflexos oriundos do mesencéfalo ou do tronco encefálico secundárias à SHV ou à hipercalcemia extrema. Também pode ocorrer sintomas que refletem mielopatias transversas secundárias à infiltração da coluna vertebral, fraturas patológicas ou compressão por massa tumoral extradural (ver Capítulo 267). Nos gatos, anorexia e perda de peso são os sinais clínicos mais comuns,[198,200-202,204] e pode ocorrer claudicação devido a lesões ósseas e hepatoesplenomegalia, mais comumente do que em cães. Há relato de epistaxe, efusões hemorrágicas pleural (ver Capítulo 244) e peritoneal (ver Capítulo 17), hemorragia na retina e sintomas neurológicos centrais. Polidipsia e poliúria podem ser secundárias à doença renal; e desidratação é possível.

Diagnóstico

Em geral, o diagnóstico de MM baseia-se na detecção de plasmocitose de medula óssea e de proteínas do mieloma no soro ou na urina (componente M), bem como na constatação de lesões osteolíticas e/ou outros locais de envolvimento visceral. Na ausência de lesões osteolíticas ou de envolvimento evidente de vísceras, o diagnóstico pode ser confirmado quando a plasmocitose da medula está associada a um aumento progressivo no componente M. Todos os animais com suspeita de tumor de plasmócito devem ser avaliados com base no hemograma, contagem de plaquetas, perfil bioquímico sérico e exame de urina. Eletroforese de proteínas do soro sanguíneo e imunoeletroforese são realizadas para detectar gamopatia monoclonal (Figura 344.7) e classificar o isótipo da imunoglobulina envolvida. Em publicações anteriores, o componente M quase sempre era da classe de IgG ou IgA, em incidência quase igual em cães;[195] entretanto, na experiência do autor, a vasta maioria dos cães apresenta doença com a forma IgA.[205] No gato, o MM em geral está associado a elevação de IgG; somente alguns poucos casos de gamopatia de IgA ou IgM foram relatados.[198,200-202,204] Raramente nota-se crioglobulinemia em cães e gatos com MM. Crioglobulinas são paraproteínas insolúveis em temperatura inferior a 37°C e necessitam coleta e coagulação do sangue em temperatura de 37°C, antes da separação do soro. Se houver suspeita de proteinúria de Bence-Jones, há necessidade de precipitação por calor e eletroforese das proteínas da urina, pois as fitas reagentes disponíveis no comércio não possibilitam essa determinação. Em cães, há raros relatos de tipos de MM "não secretores".

O diagnóstico definitivo quase sempre requer aspirado de medula óssea ou biopsia. A medula normal contém menos que 5% de plasmócitos, enquanto a medula com mieloma geralmente excede em muito esse percentual. Os plasmócitos malignos podem apresentar aparência microscópica variável, desde aquela de plasmócitos normais até de plasmócitos em estágios iniciais de diferenciação.

Para determinar a presença e extensão de lesões osteolíticas, recomendam-se radiografias simples de ossos, o que pode ter implicações diagnósticas, prognósticas e terapêuticas. Raramente é necessária biopsia de lesões osteolíticas (i. e., biopsia com agulha Jamshidi) para o diagnóstico. As lesões ósseas podem ser lesões discretas isoladas (inclusive fraturas patológicas; Figura 344.8) ou osteopenia difusa.

Aproximadamente 25 a 75% dos cães com MM apresentam evidências de osteólise ou osteoporose difusa. Os ossos envolvidos na hematopoese ativa são mais comumente afetados (p. ex., vértebras, costelas, pelve, crânio e ossos longos proximais). Notam-se lesões ósseas em 8 a 68% dos gatos acometidos.[198,200-202,204] Na macroglobulinemia, frequentemente há infiltração de células malignas no baço, fígado e tecido linfoide, mas não no osso, embora ocasionalmente nota-se envolvimento ósseo.

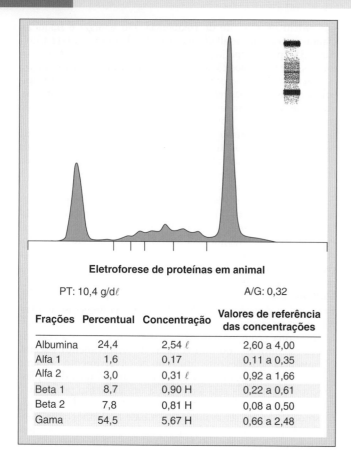

Figura 344.7 Eletroforese de proteínas séricas de um gato com anormalidade relacionada ao mieloma. Fita de acetato de celulose corada (canto superior direito) e respectivo traçado densitométrico. Note o grande pico do componente M (representando a gamopatia monoclonal de IgG) na região gama. (Cortesia de Dr. Frances Moore, Marshfield Laboratories, Marshfield, WI.)

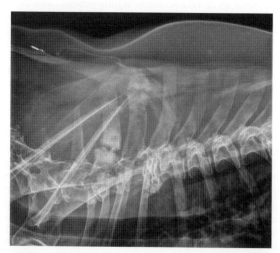

Figura 344.8 Radiografia lateral da vértebra torácica de um cão com mieloma múltiplo, mostrando múltiplas lesões líticas expansíveis e fraturas patológicas no esqueleto axial, mais evidentes nos processos espinhosos das vértebras e em uma fratura por colapso do corpo vertebral de T3.

No caso de evidências clínicas de hemorragia, devem ser realizados testes para avaliação da coagulação (p. ex., contagem de plaquetas, tempo de protrombina [TP] e tempo de tromboplastina parcial [TTP]), bem como a mensuração da viscosidade sérica. Quase metade desses pacientes apresentam valores anormais de TP e TTP. Todos os animais devem ser submetidos à avaliação minuciosa do fundo do olho: possíveis anormalidades incluem hemorragia na retina, dilatação venosa com saculações e tortuosidade, descolamento da retina e cegueira.

Diagnósticos diferenciais

Outras síndromes mórbidas podem estar associadas a gamopatia monoclonais, inclusive tumores linfoides (linfoma, LLC e LLA), infecções crônicas (p. ex., erliquiose, leishmaniose e peritonite infecciosa felina [PIF]) e gamopatia monoclonal de importância desconhecida (GMID). A GMID (benigna, essencial ou idiopática) é uma gamopatia monoclonal benigna não associada à osteólise, infiltrado em medula óssea ou proteinúria de Bence-Jones.

Tratamento

Tratamento inicial do mieloma múltiplo. A terapia tem como alvo a massa de células tumorais e os efeitos sistêmicos secundários. A quimioterapia é altamente efetiva na redução da população de células do mieloma, no alívio da dor óssea, no início da cicatrização dos ossos e na redução das concentrações séricas de imunoglobulinas. O tratamento melhora significativamente a qualidade de vida e a sobrevida da maioria dos pacientes. Contudo, a eliminação total das células neoplásicas do mieloma é rara; ademais, eventualmente deve-se esperar a ocorrência de recidivas.

O melfalana, em combinação com a prednisona, é o tratamento preferido. No cão, administra-se 0,1 mg de melfalana/kg, VO, a cada 24 h, durante 10 dias e, em seguida, reduz-se a dose para 0,05 mg/kg, a cada 24 h, mantendo indefinidamente. A dose de prednisona é de 0,5 mg/kg VO, a cada 24 h, durante 10 dias, e então reduzida para 0,5 mg/kg VO, em dias alternados. Mantém-se o tratamento até que ocorra recidiva clínica ou quando a mielossupressão requerer a redução da dose. A toxicidade do melfalana clinicamente mais significativa é a mielossupressão, sobretudo a trombocitopenia. Hemogramas devem ser realizados quinzenalmente durante 2 meses após o início da terapia e, em seguida, mensalmente. Se ocorrer mielossupressão significativa, pode ser necessária redução da dose ou da frequência de tratamento. Um protocolo terapêutico em pulsos alternados para o melfalana (7 mg/m^2, VO, a cada 24 h, durante 5 dias consecutivos, a cada 21 dias) tem sido utilizado com sucesso na Universidade de Wisconsin, em um pequeno número de casos nos quais a mielossupressão limitou a terapia com baixa dose contínua, mais convencional. O tratamento com melfalana e prednisona também tem sido utilizado em gatos com DRM, embora com resultados menos efetivos. Também tem sido utilizada em gatos uma combinação de ciclofosfamida, vincristina e prednisona.

A ciclofosfamida pode ser utilizada como um quimioterápico alquilante alternativo, às vezes em combinação com o melfalana; entretanto, não há evidência sugestiva de superioridade. Na prática do autor, a administração de ciclofosfamida (250 mg/m^2) é limitada aos pacientes que apresentam hipercalcemia grave ou envolvimento sistêmico disseminado, nos quais o uso de um medicamento alquilante de ação mais rápida pode ser benéfico. A ciclofosfamida é administrada por via IV, no momento do início da terapia oral com melfalana. Em cães com macroglobulinemia por IgM, tem-se utilizado clorambucila (0,2 mg/kg, VO, a cada 24 h).

Avaliação da resposta ao tratamento. A resposta terapêutica é baseada na melhora dos sinais clínicos, dos parâmetros clinicopatológicos e das lesões ósseas mostradas nas radiografias. O alívio da dor óssea, da claudicação, da letargia e da anorexia deve ser evidente dentro de 3 a 4 semanas. Em geral, a melhora das anormalidades laboratoriais objetivas, inclusive redução da concentração sérica de imunoglobulina ou da proteinúria de Bence-Jones, é notada dentro de 3 a 8 semanas.[205] A melhora radiográfica de lesões osteolíticas pode demorar meses, e a resolução pode ser apenas parcial. Conforme previamente discutido, a resolução completa do MM é rara; uma boa resposta terapêutica é definida como redução do componente M mensurado em até, pelo menos, 50% do valor verificado antes do tratamento. Para o acompanhamento de rotina, obtém-se, mensalmente, a concentração sérica da imunoglobulina ou a mensuração da proteína de Bence-Jones na urina, até que haja uma boa resposta e, então, a cada 2 a 3 meses. Realiza-se novamente o aspirado de medula óssea, se justificado, e é possível avaliar PARR para confirmar remissões moleculares.[205]

Tratamento cujos alvos são as complicações do mieloma múltiplo. O controle a longo prazo de complicações, inclusive de hipercalcemia, SHV, diátese hemorrágica, doença renal, imunossupressão e fraturas ósseas patológicas, depende do controle da massa tumoral. Entretanto, a terapia direcionada mais especificamente a essas complicações pode ser indicada a curto prazo. Se a hipercalcemia for acentuada e existirem sinais clínicos significativos, indicam-se tratamentos padrões (ver Capítulo 69). A hipercalcemia moderada tipicamente regride em 2 a 3 dias após o início da quimioterapia.

A SHV é mais bem tratada a curto prazo por meio de plasmaférese. A diátese hemorrágica em geral é resolvida com a SHV; entretanto, nos casos de trombocitopenia, podem ser necessárias transfusões com plasma rico em plaquetas.

Doenças renais podem necessitar terapia hídrica agressiva. Recomendam-se atenção cuidadosa e terapia antimicrobiana apropriada às infecções secundárias do trato urinário. Fraturas patológicas de ossos longos que sustentam o peso corporal e de vértebras podem necessitar intervenção imediata, juntamente a quimioterapia sistêmica. Realiza-se a estabilização ortopédica de fraturas, podendo ser seguida de radioterapia. A inibição da atividade osteoclástica por fármacos bifosfonatos tem sido utilizada, com resultados conflitantes, cujo intuito é reduzir a incidência/gravidade de complicações ósseas.[206,207]

Tratamento de resgate. Em recidivas ou em casos inicialmente resistentes ao melfalana, é possível tentar o tratamento de resgate. Esse autor tem utilizado uma combinação de doxorrubicina (30 mg/m^2, IV, a cada 21 dias), vincristina (0,7 mg/m^2, IV, nos dias 8 e 15 do ciclo de quimioterapia) e fosfato sódico de dexametasona (0,5 mg/kg, IV, nos dias 1, 8 e 15 do ciclo), administrada em ciclos de 21 dias. A maioria dos cães inicialmente responde ao tratamento de resgate; entretanto, a duração da resposta tende a ser curta. A ciclofosfamida em altas doses e a doxorrubicina encapsulada em lipossomos também têm sido utilizadas na terapia de resgate.[208] São utilizados o tratamento ablativo da medula óssea e o resgate da medula ou de células-tronco, a talidomida (e outros medicamentos antiangiogênicos), o bortezomibe (um inibidor do proteassomo), o trióxido de arsênio, os bisfosfonatos, o VDC-1011 e outras terapias moleculares direcionadas; entretanto, atualmente, o seu uso em espécies veterinárias é limitado ou completamente ausente.[205] Em um cão com MM resistente a melfalana, obteve-se resposta parcial ao tratamento com inibidor da tirosinoquinase (toceranib), mantido por 6 meses.[209]

Prognóstico

Em cães com MM o prognóstico é bom, em termos de controle inicial da neoplasia e um retorno à boa qualidade de vida. Em 60 cães com MM, constatou-se que mais de 90% tiveram remissão total ou parcial do tumor com o uso de melfalana ou prednisona.[195] A sobrevida a longo prazo é o normal, com uma média relatada de 540 dias. Hipercalcemia, proteinúria de Bence-Jones e lise óssea extensa são fatores prognósticos negativos, em cães. O prognóstico a longo prazo é ruim, devido à doença recidivante resistente aos medicamentos.

O prognóstico para DRM de gatos não é tão favorável como o de cães, porque, em geral, o período de remissão é de 2 a 4 meses; entretanto, há relatos ocasionais de sobrevida a longo prazo.[198,200-202,204]

Plasmocitoma solitário

Coleções de tumores plasmocíticos monoclonais solitários podem ser originadas em ossos ou tecidos moles e são denominadas plasmocitomas ósseos solitários (POS) e plasmocitoma extramedular (PEM), respectivamente. Por fim, a maioria dos POS progride para MM sistêmico.[172,173] O PEM cutâneo solitário, inclusive PEM em cavidade bucal, é tipicamente uma anormalidade benigna em cães.[174-180] Diferentemente, o comportamento natural do PEM não cutâneo parece mais agressivo. Relata-se que os PEM gastrintestinais envolvem esôfago, estômago, intestino delgado e intestino grosso ou cólon.[181-185] Metástases aos linfonodos associados são normais, embora o envolvimento da medula óssea e a gamopatia monoclonal seja menos comum. As formas colorretais progridem lentamente e podem ser curadas após extirpação.[185] Há poucos relatos em gatos; embora alguns sejam controlados mediante extirpação cirúrgica, é mais provável que ocorra envolvimento sistêmico disseminado.[155-158,186-191]

Sinais clínicos

Os sinais clínicos associados ao plasmocitoma solitário estão relacionados à sua localização. Em geral, o POS está associado a dor e claudicação, quando há comprometimento do esqueleto apendicular, ou a sintomas neurológicos, quando há envolvimento dos corpos vertebrais. O PEM cutâneo em geral tem um curso benigno, enquanto o PEM gastrintestinal ocasiona sintomas inespecíficos que sugerem envolvimento do trato digestório.

Diagnóstico

O diagnóstico de POS e PEM requer exame citológico ou biopsia tecidual. O estadiamento minucioso de POS e PEM não cutâneo por meio de exame de aspirado de medula óssea, eletroforese de proteínas séricas e radiografias simples de ossos é importante para assegurar que a doença esteja confinada antes do início da terapia. Em tumores plasmocíticos solitários pouco diferenciados, o exame imuno-histoquímico (p. ex., MUM1) pode ser útil para confirmar o diagnóstico.[190,192-194] Técnicas de PCR podem também ser utilizadas para determinar a clonalidade.

Tratamento

Na indisponibilidade de quimioterapia sistêmica, os animais com tumores de plasmócitos solitários podem ser submetidos a tratamento local (p. ex., cirurgia e/ou radioterapia), desde que o estadiamento clínico minucioso não revele envolvimento sistêmico. Cães com POS não cutâneo e PEM podem, por fim, desenvolver DRM sistêmico. Em humanos, a disseminação sistêmica pode não ocorrer por vários meses a anos após o diagnóstico, e não se constata benefício algum com o início da quimioterapia sistêmica antes da comprovação do envolvimento sistêmico subsequente. Recomenda-se o acompanhamento a longo prazo de pacientes com plasmocitoma solitário, a fim de detectar recidiva da doença e disseminação sistêmica.

REFERÊNCIAS BIBLIOGRÁFICAS

As referências bibliográficas deste capítulo se encontram online no Ambiente de Aprendizagem.

CAPÍTULO 345

Tumores Cutâneos

Kenneth M. Rassnick

A pele é o local mais comum de ocorrência de neoplasias em cães e o segundo local mais comum em gatos. Tumores subcutâneos (SC) e cutâneos, juntos, correspondem a mais de 1/3 de todos os tumores em cães. Aproximadamente 20 a 30% são histologicamente malignos.[1] Mastocitomas, adenomas perianais (sebáceos), lipomas, adenomas de glândulas sebáceas, histiocitomas, tricoblastomas (anteriormente classificados como tumores de células basais), carcinomas de célula escamosa, melanomas, fibrossarcomas, hemangiopericitomas e papilomas são os tipos histológicos mais comuns de neoplasias em cães.[1-4] Tumores cutâneos e SC correspondem a ≈ 1/4 de todos os tumores em gatos, e 50 a 65% são histologicamente malignos.[1,2,5] A aparência histológica de malignidade não necessariamente está relacionada à tendência de metástase. Os tumores cutâneos mais comuns em gatos incluem tumores de células basais, mastocitomas, carcinomas de célula escamosa, fibrossarcomas, melanomas e hemangiomas.[2,5,6]

Neoplasias de tecidos cutâneo e subcutâneo podem ser amplamente classificados, histologicamente, de acordo com o tecido de origem: epitelial, mesenquimal, de células redondas ou melanocíticos (Boxe 345.1). Eles ainda podem ser classificados de acordo com a célula de origem, quando sua diferenciação é suficiente para tal. Este capítulo tem como foco tumores de origem epitelial, tumores melanocíticos e alguns tumores de células redondas.

Boxe 345.1 Tumores cutâneos e subcutâneos comuns

Tumores epiteliais
Papiloma
Epitelioma cornificante intracutâneo
Carcinoma de célula escamosa
Tumores de células basais (epitelioma de células basais)
Tricoepitelioma
Carcinoma de células-tronco foliculares
Pilomatricoma
Tricoblastoma
Tumores de glândulas sebáceas
Tumores de glândula hepatoide (tumores de glândula perianal)
Tumores de glândulas sudoríparas (tumores de glândulas apócrinas)
Tumores de glândulas ceruminosas
Tumores de glândula apócrina de saco anal

Tumores mesenquimais
Sarcomas de tecidos moles (ver Capítulo 346)

Tumores de células redondas
Plasmocitoma
Mastocitoma (ver Capítulo 349)
Linfoma (ver Capítulo 344)
Histiocitoma (ver Capítulo 350)
Tumor venéreo transmissível (ver Capítulo 351)

Tumores melanocíticos
Melanoma

CONSIDERAÇÕES GERAIS

Histórico e exame físico

Como as lesões e massas teciduais que envolvem a pele são facilmente observadas, elas são razões comuns para tutores buscarem atendimento veterinário. A obtenção do histórico geral deve incluir a duração e a velocidade de crescimento do tumor, alteração na aparência com o passar do tempo, resposta a tratamentos prévios e anormalidades clínicas relacionadas. Tumores benignos mais provavelmente apresentam histórico de crescimento lento durante meses a anos. Diferentemente, os tumores malignos tendem a ter rápido crescimento e alteração na aparência. Todas as neoplasias devem ser minuciosamente relatadas no registro clínico (localização, diagramas/fotografias, mensurações do diâmetro). O registro também deve incluir a aparência macroscópica (cor, alopecia, ulceração), consistência (firme, mole), margens (circunscritas, infiltrativas) e aderências aos tecidos subjacentes (fixos, móveis). A maioria das neoplasias cutâneas benignas é bem circunscrita e móvel. Diferentemente, os tumores cutâneos malignos quase sempre são fixos, aderidos a estruturas subjacentes, e suas margens são mal definidas. Como parte do exame físico completo do paciente, os linfonodos que drenam um tumor cutâneo sempre devem ser examinados minuciosamente.

Diagnóstico

Geral

A chave para o tratamento apropriado dos tumores cutâneos é um diagnóstico específico. Frequentemente, o diagnóstico e a caracterização de uma massa tumoral cutânea devem ser definidos antes da excisão cirúrgica, de forma que o clínico possa planejar o procedimento cirúrgico; decidir quanto à necessidade de radioterapia, quimioterapia ou imunoterapia adjuvante; e discutir as respostas terapêuticas realistas e o prognóstico com os tutores. A Figura 346.2, no Capítulo 346, mostra uma abordagem geral para o diagnóstico de tumores superficiais com base nos resultados dos exames de amostras de aspirado por agulha fina (AAF) e de biopsia.

Análises hematológicas e bioquímicas rotineiras raramente são úteis no diagnóstico de neoplasias cutâneas; entretanto, alguns tumores cutâneos podem estar associados a complicações paraneoplásicas (ver Capítulo 352). Recomendam-se exames de sangue para triagem antes do planejamento de um procedimento definitivo.

Para o estadiamento dos tumores cutâneos malignos, são necessárias radiografias do tórax; a ultrassonografia do abdome pode ser útil para avaliar locais potenciais de metástases de algumas neoplasias. No caso de tumores aderidos aos tecidos subjacentes, o exame radiográfico, a tomografia computadorizada (TC) ou a ressonância magnética (RM) pode ajudar a delinear as margens do tumor antes da excisão cirúrgica.

Os linfonodos com aumento de volume sempre devem ser avaliados por meio de exames citológicos ou histológicos (ver Capítulo 95). No caso de alguns tumores (mastocitomas, melanomas), pode ocorrer metástase em linfonodos que parecem normais à palpação; portanto, o exame de linfonodos deve ser parte rotineira da avaliação de um animal com tumor cutâneo.

Aspirado por agulha fina

O aspirado por agulha fina (ver Capítulo 86) para obtenção de amostra para exame citológico (ver Capítulo 87) é um procedimento fácil e rápido, que quase sempre fornece informações sobre o tipo de célula neoplásica.[7] É mais útil no diagnóstico de neoplasias de células redondas (mastocitomas, linfoma cutâneo, histiocitoma) e na identificação de tumores cutâneos benignos ou pápulas, nódulos e massas teciduais não neoplásicas. Quando o resultado do exame citológico não define o diagnóstico, o paciente deve ser submetido à biopsia. Da mesma forma, quando se obtém o diagnóstico citológico de neoplasia, deve-se realizar biopsia sempre para confirmar o diagnóstico e avaliar informações prognósticas importantes, como o grau de diferenciação ou grau do tumor, a descrição da invasão vascular e a avaliação das margens teciduais,[8] quando se faz biopsia excisional.

Biopsia

Pode-se utilizar uma série de técnicas de biopsia (ver Capítulo 86). Biopsia incisional, com agulha ou com *punch* são indicadas para massas tumorais grandes e infiltrativas ou para tumores em uma área de difícil reconstrução, como membros e região perineal ou periocular. Para lesões exofíticas superficiais, a biopsia por meio de raspagem com uma lâmina de bisturi pode ser adequada. Para massas dérmicas pequenas e móveis, a biopsia excisional pode ser útil tanto para o diagnóstico quanto para nortear o tratamento. Mesmo quando o diagnóstico é definido antes da biopsia, o exame histopatológico da amostra final é essencial, pois pode fornecer informações para o planejamento terapêutico.

Para a realização de biopsia não excisional, o local deve estar em uma área que possa ser facilmente incluída em um campo de ressecção ou radiação definitiva. Como regra geral, nos membros, todas as incisões de biopsia devem ser longitudinais, ao longo do eixo do membro. Deve-se evitar a aplicação de anestésicos locais em tumores cutâneos e subcutâneos em razão da deformidade tecidual. A biopsia deve ser profunda o suficiente para evitar a presença de tecido necrosado superficial e inflamação circundante. O procedimento de biopsia nunca deve prejudicar os planos teciduais. Deve-se evitar a colocação de dreno porque possibilita que as células neoplásicas do líquido drenado tenham contato com todos os tecidos nos quais o dreno é posicionado.

Uma amostra ideal para exame histológico deve incluir a junção entre o tumor e o tecido normal adjacente. Em geral, amostras com menos de 1×1 mm são inapropriadas, mas amostras de 1×5 mm coletadas com agulha podem ser adequadas. Amostras que se desintegram na solução de formalina são oriundas de material sanguinolento, mucoso ou necrótico e em geral não têm valor diagnóstico. Grandes amostras obtidas por múltiplas amostras obtidas de diferentes locais do tumor, coletadas da mesma incisão, podem aumentar a probabilidade de um diagnóstico acurado. Instrumentos de cauterização não devem ser utilizados durante o procedimento de biopsia; a cauterização para hemostasia pode ser utilizada assim que a amostra for removida. Com aparelho de *laser* de diodo cirúrgico, frequentemente obtêm-se amostras inapropriadas; *laser* de dióxido de carbono causa menor lesão térmica, mas as amostras obtidas podem ser pequenas e sem valor diagnóstico.[9] Por fim, a fixação em formalina pode causar acentuada contração tecidual.[10] Antes da fixação em formalina, a aplicação de tinta nanquim ou outros corantes em todas as superfícies de corte do tumor ajuda o patologista a distinguir margens cirúrgicas de artefatos de preparação.

TUMORES EPITELIAIS

Papiloma

Papilomas cutâneos são proliferações benignas da epiderme, comuns em cães, mas relativamente raras em gatos. Macroscopicamente, elas são massas teciduais esbranquiçadas ou acinzentadas, com aparência pedunculada ou de couve-flor, frequentemente denominadas de *verrugas*. Há ambas as formas, viral e não viral.[11,12] Papilomavírus são vírus DNA espécie-específicos; a causalidade não foi comprovada em um relato de caso de papiloma cutâneo em um gato, a partir do qual um papilomavírus humano foi amplificado.[13] Os papilomavírus podem sobreviver por mais de 2 meses em temperatura de 4 a 8°C e por 6 horas em 37°C.[14] Podem ser transmitidos por contato direto ou indireto (p. ex., fômites). De forma geral, a infecção por papilomavírus se instala na pele lesionada, e o período de incubação varia de 1 a 2 meses.[14]

Papilomas cutâneos se desenvolvem em cães idosos, e podem ser observadas lesões solitárias ou múltiplas. Mais comumente elas ocorrem na cabeça, nas pálpebras e nas patas, e não estão associadas ao papilomavírus. Em cães, a papilomatose bucal é uma doença viral contagiosa que quase sempre acomete cães jovens ou com imunossupressão (ver Capítulos 228 e 272).[15] Papilomas invertidos cutâneos, lesões em formato de cálice observadas em cães jovens, também são causadas por infecção pelo papilomavírus. Desenvolvem-se no abdome ventral e na região inguinal.[16] Casos raros de múltiplas placas pigmentadas, ou papilomas papulares, foram relatados em cães.[17] Cães da raça Pug parecem predispostos a desenvolver essas placas pigmentadas, e a doença é causada por um novo papilomavírus.[18] Por fim, em alguns cães raramente o papiloma viral progride para carcinoma.[11,12]

Em gatos, a maioria dos papilomas cutâneos solitários não é causada por papilomavírus. Diferentemente, em gatos os papilomas que ocorrem na parte ventral da língua geralmente são de origem viral, bem como os papilomas cutâneos múltiplos. Esses papilomas virais podem ser precursores do carcinoma de célula escamosa multicêntrico felino, ou doença de Bowen (ver Carcinoma de célula escamosa felino, adiante).[19]

A extirpação cirúrgica dos papilomas cutâneos solitários é curativa. Em cães, a papilomatose bucal em geral sofre regressão espontânea dentro de 3 meses; o cão é imune à reinfecção.[14] Animais com imunossupressão ou submetidos à terapia imunossupressora, como corticosteroides, podem apresentar lesões e infecção persistente por papilomavírus.[15,20] Foram utilizadas vacinas autógenas (para induzir regressão); tentativas recentes almejam a produção de vacinas recombinantes, profiláticas e terapêuticas.[21] Relata-se que a administração oral de retinoides foi efetiva em casos de papiloma invertido canino.[22] Interferona ou azitromicina podem ser efetivos no tratamento da papilomatose viral grave, bucal ou cutâneo.[23,24]

Epitelioma intracutâneo cornificante (acantoma infundibular queratinizante)

Epiteliomas intracutâneos cornificantes (queratoacantomas) surgem da parte externa do folículo piloso. Quase sempre se desenvolvem em cães de raças puras relativamente jovens. A maioria dos tumores é solitária, mas há formas generalizadas. Cães das raças Norwegian Elkhound e Keeshonden são predispostos à forma generalizada da neoplasia.[25] Esses tumores frequentemente apresentam um poro central preenchido por material queratinoso condensado. A leve pressão digital aplicada à neoplasia resulta na expulsão de um material queratinoso branco-acinzentado. O diagnóstico entre os patologistas que avaliam essas lesões é geralmente controverso; o diagnóstico variante mais comum para queratoacantoma é o carcinoma de célula escamosa bem diferenciado.[26]

Epiteliomas intracutâneos cornificantes são benignos e não ocasionam recidiva após sua remoção cirúrgica adequada. Na forma generalizada, novos tumores podem se desenvolver durante toda a vida do cão. A administração oral de retinoides pode ser útil no tratamento de epiteliomas intracutâneos cornificantes múltiplos (em um estudo constatou-se remissão total em 5 de 7 pacientes, e remissão parcial em 2 desses 7 animais).[23] A regressão espontânea foi também relatada em um cão com a forma generalizada da neoplasia.[27]

Carcinoma de célula escamosa em cães

O carcinoma de célula escamosa (CCE) é uma neoplasia maligna comum em cães. Quase sempre a etiologia é desconhecida. Tumores que se desenvolvem em pele não pigmentada ou pouco pigmentada, como no abdome ou na região inguinal, supostamente são causados por radiação ultravioleta (dano solar).[28] Ocasionalmente, o CCE pode ser causado por queimadura, infecção crônica ou doença imunomediada, ou é uma progressão de papilomas virais.[11,12,24] Em um estudo imuno-histoquímico de 40 cães com CCE, constatou-se que 100% das lesões expressaram ciclo-oxigenase-2 (COX-2).[29] A COX-2 foi incriminada como oncogênica para várias neoplasias humanas, mas os mecanismos que levam à suprarregulação da COX-2 não são conhecidos. Em cães, o CCE pode ser proliferativo, ulcerativo ou erosivo. As características clínicas e o tratamento de CCE em cães dependem muito de sua localização anatômica.

Carcinoma de célula escamosa cutâneo em cães

Inicialmente, o CCE cutâneo pode ser diagnosticado como uma lesão pré-neoplásica, mas ele, por fim, progride para um tumor invasivo. Metástase aos linfonodos regionais e pulmões é rara.[30] O CCE cutâneo de cães é mais bem tratado com excisão cirúrgica adequada. Lesões pré-neoplásicas podem responder ao tratamento oral com retinoides,[28] e a terapia intralesional, com cisplatina de liberação contínua, 5-fluoruracila, ou carboplatina pode ser efetiva no tratamento de alguns cães com CCE superficial.[31] A excisão cirúrgica abrangente é o tratamento de escolha para CCE cutâneo invasivo. Em casos de neoplasias metastáticas, pode-se utilizar radioterapia para tumores que foram parcialmente extirpados; quimioterapia à base de platinas, doxorrubicina ou gencitabina; ou, às vezes, tratamento com inibidores de COX-2, mas sua eficácia ainda não foi comprovada.

Carcinoma de célula escamosa no plano nasal de cães

O CCE no plano nasal pode ser tratado por excisão cirúrgica abrangente do plano nasal e pré-maxila, mas o prognóstico é extremamente reservado. A seleção de casos é importante: em um estudo de 6 cães tratados cirurgicamente constatou-se que 2 apresentaram recidiva da lesão em menos de 2 meses, provavelmente por conta de ressecções incompletas.[32] A radioterapia tem sido amplamente insatisfatória, pois todos os 7 cães submetidos à radioterapia para tumores parcialmente extirpados manifestaram recidivas 8 a 12 semanas depois do tratamento.[32]

Carcinoma de célula escamosa digital em cães

O CCE se origina do epitélio subungueal ou, às vezes, de outros tecidos do digito; é o tumor digital mais comum em cães. Há relato de predisposição em cães de raças de grande porte e de pelame preto – inclusive Schnauzer Gigante, Poodle Standard, Labrador Retriever, Rottweiler e Flat Coated Retriever.[33] Cães da raça Teckel de pelame preto podem ser mais predispostos.[33] Aproximadamente 80% dos CCE digitais invadem o tecido ósseo da terceira falange. Inicialmente, a ocorrência de metástases é incomum, mas podem ser diagnosticadas após o tratamento em até 30% dos casos.[33-35] Raramente, os cães podem desenvolver CCE em múltiplos dígitos, simultaneamente ou com o passar do tempo.[33,34] A amputação ampla, com desarticulação da primeira falange e do osso metacarpo/metatarso, é o tratamento de escolha. De forma geral, menos de 50% dos cães com CCE digital morrem em consequência da doença, de forma que a sobrevida mediana não pode ser determinada.[34] Em um estudo, as taxas de sobrevida em 1 e 2 anos foram de 95 e 74%, respectivamente, para CCE epitelial subungueal, e 60 e 40%, respectivamente, para CCE que surgiram de outras partes do dígito.[34] Para tumores metastáticos, pode-se utilizar quimioterapia à base de platinas, doxorrubicina ou gencitabina, ou, às vezes, o tratamento com inibidores da COX-2; contudo, a eficácia não foi comprovada.

Carcinoma de célula escamosa em gatos

Assim como acontece em cães, o CCE em gatos se desenvolve mais frequentemente na pele lesionada pelo sol e em geral é precedida de queratose actínica (solar).[24] Em gatos, os vírus também podem ser causas primárias de CCE. Em um estudo, constatou-se que 24% dos gatos infectados pelo vírus da imunodeficiência felina (FIV) desenvolveram CCE.[36] Nesses gatos, é incerto se há uma relação causal direta ou se a neoplasia ocorre devido à exposição à luz solar. Papilomavírus foi identificado em lesões de CCE multicêntrico *in situ* (doença de Bowen).[24,37] Assim como acontece no CCE canino, notou-se imunorreatividade de COX-2 em todos os casos de CCE cutâneo de gatos,[38] embora os mecanismos sejam desconhecidos. Assim como ocorre em cães, o CCE é a neoplasia digital mais comum em gatos.[39] Em gatos, pode ser difícil a diferenciação histológica entre o CCE digital primário e o adenocarcinoma pulmonar metastático nos dígitos, de forma que se recomenda a radiografia do tórax quando ocorre recidiva de CCE.[39,40]

Carcinoma de célula escamosa cutâneo em gatos

O CCE cutâneo em gatos quase sempre começa como uma área crostosa que progride para uma lesão erosiva ou ulcerativa. Os locais mais comumente envolvidos são áreas despigmentadas expostas à luz solar, inclusive narinas, pavilhão auricular, pálpebras e lábios. Lesões múltiplas ocorrem em ≈ 45% dos gatos afetados.[41] Metástases são raras.

Há diversas opções terapêuticas para CCE cutâneo de gatos, incluindo excisão cirúrgica abrangente (pinectomia, nosectomia), crioterapia, radiação por feixe externo, plesioterapia com estrôncio-90, terapia fotodinâmica, imunoterapia tópica (creme de imiquimode), eletroquimioterapia e quimioterapia intralesional. Esses tratamentos são mais efetivos em lesões pequenas (< 5 cm) e superficiais; portanto, o diagnóstico precoce e o tratamento imediato são essenciais. Na maioria dos gatos, as lesões pequenas e minimamente invasivas de CCE podem ser controladas por mais de 1 ano, sendo possível o controle a longo prazo (2 a 7 anos) em 10 a 60% delas. O tratamento de tumores maiores (> 5 cm) ou invasivos é decepcionante, com período de controle geralmente menor que 2 anos.[41-48] Em todos os gatos, é importante evitar a luz solar para prevenir lesões adicionais.

Carcinoma de célula escamosa multicêntrico in situ em gatos (doença de Bowen)

A doença de Bowen é uma condição caracterizada por pequenas lesões de CCE com aparência de placas crostosas que histologicamente não invadem a membrana basal. Diferentemente do CCE causado por luz solar, o CCE multicêntrico *in situ* se desenvolve em áreas pigmentadas e com pelos, e pode ser causado por infecção por papilomavírus.[37]

As lesões são multifocais, na cabeça, no pescoço, no tórax, no abdome e nos membros. Ocasionalmente, notam-se áreas focais de CCE invasivo ou lesões por CCE invasivo concomitantes.[49,50] Quando possível, a excisão cirúrgica é o tratamento preferido. A plesioterapia com estrôncio-90 pode ser efetiva em pequenas lesões (< 8,5 mm de diâmetro); para lesões maiores, são necessários campos sobrejacentes múltiplos.[46] Pela natureza multicêntrica da doença, alguns gatos podem necessitar de tratamento alternativo. O imiquimode é um modulador da resposta imune, e há relato de regressão das lesões da doença de Bowen tratadas com creme à base desse medicamento.[50] A eficácia do tratamento oral com retinoides é variável.[12]

Tumores de células basais (epitelioma de células basais)

Tumores de células basais (epiteliomas de células basais) são neoplasias benignas que surgem a partir de células basais da epiderme. São os tumores cutâneos mais comuns em gatos.[51] Em cães, a neoplasia previamente classificada como tumor de células basais foi reclassificada como tricoblastoma. Em geral, os tumores de células basais são solitários, firmes, redondos e bem circunscritos. Às vezes, podem ser císticos. Quase sempre os tumores de células basais são pigmentados, o que pode levar a um diagnóstico errôneo de melanoma. A excisão cirúrgica adequada é o tratamento de escolha.

Carcinoma de células basais

Em geral, os carcinomas de células basais são solitários e semelhantes a tumores de células basais; quase sempre são pigmentados, de cor marrom ou preta. Esse tumor é invasor local; portanto, o tratamento deve incluir ampla excisão cirúrgica. Na maioria dos casos, a excisão local é curativa. Há raros relatos de animais com recidiva local[52] e/ou metástases.[53] Quando não é possível obter margens cirúrgicas apropriadas, pode-se utilizar radioterapia adjuvante.

Tricoepitelioma

Tricoepiteliomas são neoplasias benignas que se desenvolvem na bainha do folículo piloso. São relativamente comuns no cão e incomuns no gato. A excisão cirúrgica é o tratamento de escolha. O tricoepitelioma maligno com metástase a linfonodos e pulmões foi raramente relatado.

Carcinoma de célula-tronco folicular

O carcinoma de célula-tronco folicular é um tumor epitelial incomum no cão, ainda não relatado em outras espécies.[54] Neoplasias anteriormente denominadas como *carcinomas sebáceos* agora são nomeados como *carcinomas de célula-tronco foliculares*.[54] Apresentam áreas de diferenciação apócrina ou tricoepiteliomatosa (folículo piloso), ou de ambas. O comportamento biológico ainda não foi bem descrito, mas em alguns tumores nota-se invasão linfática; há relato de metástases.[54]

Pilomatricoma

Pilomatricomas são tumores benignos incomuns que surgem do folículo piloso. Em geral, são solitários e bem circunscritos. Na área de corte, o tumor consiste em várias camadas de tecido arenoso branco-acinzentado. A excisão cirúrgica é o tratamento de escolha. Pilomatricomas malignos foram relatados raramente; a invasão linfática é observada histologicamente, e podem ocorrer metástases aos ossos, linfonodos, pulmões, pele e sistema nervoso.[55]

Tricoblastoma

Os tricoblastomas são tumores benignos comuns predominantemente oriundos do epitélio germinativo de pelos primários. Essa neoplasia foi anteriormente classificada como tumor de célula basal. Tricoblastomas geralmente são solitários e podem ser pigmentados. A excisão cirúrgica é curativa.

Outros tumores foliculares

Outros tumores foliculares incomuns (tricolemoma, tricofoliculoma, poro dilatado de Winer e disqueratoma verrucoso) são lesões benignas, e a excisão cirúrgica adequada deve ser curativa.

Tumores de glândulas sebáceas

Tumores de glândulas sebáceas são oriundos de sebócitos, produzem sebo (um líquido branco oleoso) e estão entre os tumores de pele mais comuns em cães. Raças predispostas incluem English Cocker Spaniel, Cocker Spaniel, Samoyeda, Husky Siberiano, Cockapoo, Malamute do Alasca, West Highland White Terrier, Cairn Terrier, Teckel, Poodle Miniatura e Toy e Shih-tzu. Esses tumores são incomuns em gatos.

Histologicamente, os tumores de glândulas sebáceas são classificados como hiperplasia sebácea, epiteliomas, adenomas ou, raramente, carcinomas. As lesões têm aspecto de verruga ou couve-flor e podem surgir em todo o corpo, inclusive nas pálpebras. Quase sempre são solitários, mas podem ocorrer

múltiplos tumores de glândula sebácea. Neoplasias anteriormente denominadas *carcinomas sebáceos* na literatura agora são definidas como *carcinomas de célula-tronco foliculares*.[54]

A excisão cirúrgica é o tratamento de escolha para todos os tipos de tumores de glândula sebácea. Recidiva local é rara, mas até 10% dos cães podem desenvolver lesões em outros locais.[56] Cães com hiperplasia sebácea podem responder ao tratamento oral com retinoides.[23] Parece que os carcinomas sebáceos apresentam baixo potencial para metástase.[56]

Tumores de glândula hepatoide (tumores de glândula perianal)

Os tumores de glândula perianal são oriundos de glândulas que circundam o ânus, que são glândulas sebáceas modificadas, não secretoras.[57-60] Esses tumores são discutidos no Capítulo 278.

Tumores de glândula sudorípara (tumores de glândula apócrina)

Em cães e gatos, os tumores de glândula sudorípara comumente se desenvolvem na região inguinal ou axilar. Clinicamente, essas neoplasias se manifestam de diversas maneiras, inclusive como massas nodulares solitárias ou de crescimento difuso, inflamatório e ulcerativo, semelhante a uma placa. Gatos com diagnóstico histológico de carcinoma de glândula apócrina no dígito podem ter metástases digitais oriundas de carcinoma pulmonar.

Histologicamente, a maioria das neoplasias de glândula sudorípara é carcinoma maligno, e mais de 20% podem ter evidência de invasão linfática ou vascular.[61-63] Ampla excisão cirúrgica é o tratamento de escolha. Em duas séries de casos em cães, constatou-se que menos de 2% dos carcinomas de glândula sudorípara desenvolveram metástases distantes, possivelmente em associação à invasão vascular.[61,62]

Tumores de glândulas ceruminosas

Tumores de glândulas ceruminosas são oriundos de glândulas sudoríparas apócrinas modificadas no canal auditivo externo. Otite externa crônica pode ser um fator predisponente (ver Capítulo 237).[64] Sinais clínicos comuns associados a tumores de canal auditivo incluem a presença de uma massa tecidual, secreção auricular, odor prurido e dor. Também pode haver sintomas neurológicos, inclusive síndrome de Horner e doença vestibular. Radiografias e/ou TC do crânio são importantes exames de imagem que devem preceder a cirurgia. O exame cuidadoso dos linfonodos mandibulares e periauriculares é fundamental.

Adenomas de glândulas ceruminosas podem ser tratados por meio de ressecção cirúrgica conservadora. Entretanto, para casos de carcinoma de glândula ceruminosa, o tratamento preferido é a excisão cirúrgica abrangente, inclusive com ablação do canal auditivo e osteotomia lateral da bula. Esse procedimento terapêutico propicia remissão mediana de 42 meses, taxa de recidiva de 25% e taxa de sobrevida em 1 ano de 75%, comparado a uma remissão mediana de 10 meses, taxa de recorrência de 40% e taxa de sobrevida em 1 ano de 33%, quando se faz apenas ressecção lateral da orelha.[65] A ablação completa do canal auditivo, com osteotomia lateral da bula, em 7 cães, resultou em ausência de recidiva durante um período de acompanhamento de 36 meses, comparativamente à taxa de recidiva dentro de 4 meses em 75% dos cães submetidos à ressecção lateral do canal auditivo mais conservadora.[66] Pode-se utilizar radioterapia como adjuvante à ressecção parcial. Obteve-se intervalo mediano livre de progressão de 40 meses e taxa de sobrevida em 1 ano de 56%, em 6 gatos e 5 cães submetidos à radioterapia após ressecção parcial de adenocarcinomas de glândula ceruminosa.[67]

Adenocarcinoma de saco anal

Adenocarcinoma de saco anal é oriundo de glândulas apócrinas localizadas na região ventrolateral do ânus. Sua ocorrência é semelhante em cadelas e cães machos, mas é rara em gatos.[68] Até 30% dos adenocarcinomas de saco anal são detectados incidentalmente no exame físico de rotina, destacando a importância do exame retal cuidadoso na avaliação de rotina. Cerca de 25 a 50% dos adenocarcinomas de saco anal produzem a proteína relacionada ao paratormônio (PTHrP), levando à hipercalcemia maligna[68,69] (ver Capítulos 297 e 352); quase sempre a hipercalcemia se resolve rapidamente após a ressecção do tumor primário, mas em alguns casos pode ser necessário tratamento de suporte (p. ex., soluções de uso intravenoso, corticosteroides e/ou bifosfonatos), até que a cirurgia possa ser realizada ou quando não é possível controlar a hipercalcemia apenas com a cirurgia. Quase sempre as metástases surgem nos linfonodos ilíacos, embora também possam ocorrer metástases distantes no fígado, baço, pulmões, ossos e outros locais. Ocasionalmente, pode ocorrer extensão da lesão a partir de linfonodos ilíacos para as vértebras lombares.[69] O diagnóstico e o tratamento desses tumores[70,71] são discutidos com mais detalhes no Capítulo 278.

O tamanho do tumor geralmente é um importante indicador preditivo da sobrevida de cães com adenocarcinoma de saco anal. Após excisão cirúrgica, o prognóstico em cães com pequenos tumores (< 2,5 cm de diâmetro) e sem metástase é excelente (sobrevida mediana ≈ 3,5 anos[73]). No caso de tumores com mais de 2,5 cm de diâmetro, a sobrevida após excisão cirúrgica é de apenas ≈ 1,5 ano.[73] Em um estudo de 24 cães com tumores de saco anal com ≥ 10 cm de tamanho, constatou-se sobrevida inferior a 1 ano.[74] A taxa de recidiva local após excisão cirúrgica de adenocarcinoma de saco anal é de aproximadamente 50%. É incerto se isso está relacionado às margens histológicas inapropriadas;[69,70] contudo, em cães com tumores submetidos à ressecção parcial, a radioterapia adjuvante pode aumentar a sobrevida.[75]

Por ocasião do diagnóstico inicial, em 40%[69] a 80%[70] dos cães com adenocarcinoma de saco anal há metástases aos linfonodos ilíacos, mas a saculectomia anal e linfadenectomia sublombar conferem uma sobrevida mediana de ≈ 2 anos.[76]

É incerto se a hipercalcemia paraneoplásica maligna ou a E-caderina (uma proteína transmembrana mediadora de adesões entre células epiteliais e a matriz extracelular) influencia a recuperação de cães com adenocarcinoma de saco anal.[67,73,74,77]

Os medicamentos antineoplásicos mais amplamente avaliados são cisplatina, carboplatina, doxorrubicina, mitoxantrona, actinomicina e melfalan,[70,73-75] mas a exata importância da quimioterapia nessa doença não é conhecida. Evidências biológicas sugerem que o fosfato de toceranibe é efetivo no tratamento de adenocarcinoma de saco anal em cães (ver adiante e Capítulo 341).[78] Como indicações para o uso de quimioterapia e/ou inibidores de receptores da tirosinoquinase, podem-se incluir tumores sem possibilidade de ressecção, doença metastática, ou até mesmo evidências de invasão linfática; são necessários estudos adicionais para tal avaliação.

TUMORES DE CÉLULAS REDONDAS

Tumores de células redondas também podem ser denominados *tumores de células distintas*. Citologicamente, eles surgem como células redondas individuais, sem ligações óbvias entre elas. Tumores de células redondas incluem linfomas, mastocitomas, plasmocitomas, histiocitomas e tumor venéreo transmissível. Ocasionalmente, melanomas e tumores de células basais podem mimetizar padrões de células redondas. Em alguns casos, o tipo de tumor não é prontamente distinguível citologicamente; uma amostra da lesão obtida por biopsia deve ser enviada para exame histopatológico. Se mesmo assim a linhagem celular não for determinada, pode-se realizar exame imuno-histoquímico ou colorações especiais. Exemplos incluem CD3/CD4/CD8 (linfoma de célula T), CD21/CD79a (linfoma de célula B), CD-117/azul de toluidina/Giemsa (mastocitoma), MUM1/RF4 (plasmocitoma), CD 18 (histiocitoma) e Melan A/PNL2/S100 (melanoma).

Linfomas, mastocitomas, histiocitomas e tumor venéreo transmissível

Esses tipos de neoplasias são discutidos nos Capítulos 344, 349, 350 e 351, respectivamente.

Plasmocitoma

Tumores de plasmócitos cutâneos (plasmocitomas extramedulares cutâneos) em geral são solitários, e os locais comuns de ocorrência são dígitos, lábios, pavilhão auricular, cavidade bucal e reto.[78,79] Em cães, a maioria dos plasmocitomas cutâneos é benigna e não está relacionada ao mieloma múltiplo (ver Capítulo 344). Em cães, o comportamento dos plasmocitomas não parece ter qualquer relação com o grau de atipia histológica ou pleomorfismo.[79,80] Informações adicionais estão disponíveis na seção Distúrbios relacionados ao mieloma (ver Capítulo 344).

O tratamento de escolha para plasmocitoma cutâneo é a excisão cirúrgica. A ocorrência de recidiva local pode ser decorrência de margens cirúrgicas incompletas.[79] No caso de tumor sem possibilidade de ressecção, pode-se realizar radioterapia (ver Capítulo 340), mas as informações a respeito são limitadas.[81,82]

A maioria dos tumores de plasmócitos relatados em gatos é sistêmica (doença relacionada ao mieloma), de forma que é indicada a avaliação conforme mencionada para os casos de mieloma múltiplo (ver Capítulo 344).[83] Em gatos, os plasmocitomas cutâneos solitários devem ser extirpados. No caso de doença multicêntrica, recomenda-se quimioterapia adjuvante com predniso(lo)na e medicamentos alquilantes (*i. e.*, melfalana, clorambucila ou ciclofosfamida). Assim como acontece em cães, para tratamento de lesão cutânea sem possibilidade de ressecção, pode-se realizar radioterapia.

TUMORES MELANOCÍTICOS

Melanoma

A etiologia de melanomas cutâneos em cães e gatos é desconhecida, mas predisposições raciais em cães sugerem uma causa genética. Raças de maior risco incluem Scottish Terrier, Airedale, Boston Terrier, Cocker e Springer Spaniel, Boxer, Golden Retriever, Schnauzer Padrão e Miniatura, Irish e Gordon Setter, e Dobermann Pinscher.[24] Em cães, as lesões quase sempre são solitárias, marrons a pretas. Locais comuns incluem pálpebra, focinho, tronco, pele interdigital e epitélio subungueal (leito da unha). Melanomas digitais são o segundo tumor digital mais comum em cães após o CCE.[33] Em gatos, o tumor cutâneo pigmentado mais comum é o tumor de célula basal. Entretanto, melanomas também são pretos. Locais comuns em gatos incluem pavilhão auricular, nariz e pescoço.

O comportamento biológico de melanomas cutâneos pode ser benigno ou maligno. A localização do tumor é de fundamental importância. Como regra geral, tumores oriundos de pele com pelos são benignos. Aqueles que surgem em junções mucocutâneas são malignos, sendo as únicas exceções aqueles que surgem nas pálpebras. Melanomas de dígitos podem ser altamente malignos; melanomas malignos comumente se disseminam pelos vasos linfáticos aos linfonodos que drenam o local e aos pulmões. Às vezes ocorrem metástases em locais distantes, como fígado, baço, cérebro, coração e medula óssea.

Em cães, os critérios histológicos tradicionais de malignidade parecem ser apropriados para o diagnóstico de neoplasias de origem melanocítica, mas nenhuma característica ou nenhum padrão particular se relaciona à recuperação.[84-86] O índice mitótico histológico geralmente parece ser preditivo do comportamento biológico.[84,87-89] Índice mitótico inferior a 3 em 10 campos de visão parece estar associado a comportamento benigno.[87,93] Em gatos, é difícil prever o comportamento biológico de melanomas cutâneos com base no índice mitótico, porque 25% dos tumores malignos podem não apresentar figuras de mitose.[90]

Em cães e gatos, o tratamento de escolha de melanoma cutâneo é a excisão cirúrgica. Em 59 cães nos quais o índice mitótico era < 3 constatou-se sobrevida mediana de 26 meses e taxa de mortalidade relacionada ao tumor, em 2 anos, de 10%, comparativamente à sobrevida mediana de 7,5 meses e taxa de mortalidade relacionada ao tumor, em 2 anos, de 73%, em 26 cães nos quais o índice mitótico era ≥ 3.[87] Mais de 50% dos cães com melanoma digital apresentaram metástases.[33,35] Há relato de sobrevida mediana de 12 meses em cães tratados mediante a amputação do dígito acometido.[33,34,85] Outros estudos relataram sobrevida mediana de 18 a 24 meses.[87,88]

Em gatos com melanoma cutâneo o prognóstico é reservado. Em um estudo de 57 gatos com esses tumores, por ocasião do diagnóstico inicial foram constatadas metástases em 11 (19%). Quarenta e cinco gatos foram submetidos à excisão cirúrgica, dos quais 22 desenvolveram recidiva local ou metástases.[91]

A radioterapia fracionada é útil no tratamento de cães com melanoma bucal e pode ser benéfica no controle local de melanoma cutâneo sem possibilidade de ressecção em cães e gatos.[92]

Além disso, é possível obter resposta clínica ao tratamento com carboplatina em cães com melanoma bucal. Portanto, esse pode ser considerado um tratamento adjuvante em cães com melanoma digital ou em cães e gatos com tumores malignos ou sem possibilidade de ressecção, ou com doença metastática.[93,94] Por fim, no mercado há disponibilidade de uma vacina de DNA xenogênica para melanoma canino (Canine Melanoma Vaccine®, Merial) (ver Capítulo 341). O produto imuniza com DNA

humano que codifica tirosinase, a enzima essencial para a síntese de melanina. Há relato de sobrevida longa em cães em estágio clínico II (tumor com 2 a 4 cm de diâmetro) ou em estágio III (tumor > 4 cm de diâmetro ou com metástases aos linfonodos locais) do melanoma bucal, com controle local adequado (*i. e.*, com cirurgia e/ou radioterapia), que receberam a vacina. Entretanto, a confiabilidade dos dados de eficácia da vacina é muito prejudicada pela carência de testes clínicos randomizados.[95-97]

Uma vacina xenogênica com DNA de tirosinase mostrou-se segura quando utilizada juntamente com controle local e regional da doença, em um grupo de 58 cães com melanoma digital maligno. A sobrevida mediana geral foi de 476 dias, com taxa de sobrevivência, em 1 ano, de 63%. A vacina xenogênica utilizada no estudo era à base de DNA murino, diferentemente da vacina disponível no mercado, que contém DNA humano. Entretanto, os autores acreditam que a resposta imune e, portanto, a resposta ao tratamento vacinal devem ser as mesmas.[98] A vacina para o melanoma de cães pode ser importante no tratamento de melanoma cutâneo maligno, mas isso ainda precisa ser comprovado.

REFERÊNCIAS BIBLIOGRÁFICAS

As referências bibliográficas deste capítulo se encontram online no Ambiente de Aprendizagem.

CAPÍTULO 346

Sarcomas de Tecidos Moles[a]

Margaret C. McEntee

INTRODUÇÃO

Definições

Os sarcomas de tecidos moles (STM) possuem diversas subcategorias histológicas derivadas de neoplasias de origem mesenquimal (Boxe 346.1). Foram descritos comportamentos biológicos distintos para os tumores de cada uma das subcategorias, mas a experiência de patologistas e especialistas em tratamento de sarcomas em cães possibilitou a elaboração de um esquema de graduação histológica que descreve o comportamento previsto do tumor pelo grau de diferenciação, e não pelo tipo histológico específico (Tabela 346.1). O grau histológico de um tumor pode sugerir a escolha entre cirurgia radical e funcional ou ser utilizado na tomada de decisão quanto ao uso de radioterapia (RT) ou quimioterapia. O tamanho e a localização da neoplasia também influenciam as opções cirúrgicas para o controle local.

Apesar do consenso de que o grau pode influenciar a eficácia da remoção total do tumor, ainda há controvérsia sobre a aplicabilidade universal do grau histológico dos STM como indicador preditivo clinicamente relevante da resposta ao tratamento em cães. Até o momento, não há qualquer evidência convincente para comparação do grau com a recuperação de STM em

Boxe 346.1 Categorias histológicas de sarcomas de tecidos moles em cães e gatos
Fibrossarcoma
Tumor de bainha de nervo periférico (schwanoma maligno, neurofibrossarcoma, hemangiopericitoma)
Mixossarcoma
Histiocitoma fibroso maligno
Sarcoma de célula sinovial
Neurofibrossarcoma
Rabdomiossarcoma
Leiomiossarcoma
Lipossarcoma
Schwanoma
Sarcoma não diferenciado

gatos. Em cães com STM, foram pesquisadas a proliferação celular mensurada pelo grau de argirofilia nas regiões organizadoras nucleolares e a densidade intratumoral de microvasos com a utilização do antígeno relacionado ao fator VII como marcador endotelial, as quais podem suplementar a informação prognóstica baseada no grau da neoplasia.[1,2] Os tipos histopatológicos específicos de tumores relatados em gatos com sarcomas associados ao local de injeção (SAI; anteriormente denominados *sarcomas associados a vacinas [SAV]*) incluem fibrossarcoma,

---

[a]O material original deste capítulo foi financiado por Vaccine Sarcoma Task Force.

SEÇÃO 25 • Câncer

Tabela 346.1	Critérios de estadiamento propostos para sarcomas de tecidos moles em cães.

ESCORE	GRAU DE DIFERENCIAÇÃO	ÍNDICE MITÓTICO*	NECROSE
1	Aparência normal	0 a 9	Nenhuma
2	Tipo histológico específico	10 a 19	< 50%
3	Não diferenciado	≥ 20	> 50%
Grau (escore cumulativo)			
1	3 ou 4		
2	5 ou 6		
3	7, 8 ou 9		

*Quantidade de figuras mitóticas/10 campos de visão (40×). (Adaptada de Kuntz CA, Dernell WS, Powers BE *et al.*: Prognostic factors for surgical treatment of soft-tissue sarcomas in dogs: 75 cases (1986-1996). *J Am Vet Med Assoc* 211:1147-1151, 1997.)

sarcoma não diferenciado, osteossarcoma, rabdomiossarcoma, lipossarcoma, histiocitoma fibroso maligno (ou miofibrossarcoma) e leiomiossarcoma. Hemangiossarcomas (ver Capítulo 347), sarcomas de célula sinovial (ver Capítulo 348) e mastocitomas (ver Capítulo 349) são discutidos separadamente. Outros sarcomas menos comuns não estão incluídos por causa de informações insuficientes para considerá-los na terminologia coletiva (p. ex., rabdomiossarcoma).

Descrições

Os STM são nódulos focais, solitários, palpáveis, macios ou firmes, que se desenvolvem na derme, no tecido subcutâneo (SC) ou em compartimentos musculares e musculofasciais mais profundos. As massas tumorais que cresceram rapidamente ou as que estão grandes porque se instalaram há muito tempo podem apresentar superfície ulcerada e ser dolorosas. Por ocasião do exame clínico inicial, a maioria dos STM possui de 2 a 4 cm de diâmetro. O tamanho do tumor pode variar por causa de uma série de fatores, inclusive a localização; especificamente, a massa tumoral localiza-se na derme ou em músculo profundo? Outros fatores incluem o quão rapidamente o tutor detecta um novo nódulo e a condição corporal geral, pois as neoplasias são mais facilmente observadas em um animal magro ou naqueles com pelos mais curtos.

Os STM podem se desenvolver em qualquer local do corpo, mas são mais comuns nos membros ou na cabeça. Dependendo da localização do tumor, podem ocorrer outros sinais clínicos, inclusive êmese, diarreia e/ou perda de peso, em casos de tumores gastrintestinais; dor e/ou claudicação, se houver tumores de raiz de nervo periférico; halitose, dificuldade de preensão de alimentos e outros sintomas, em casos de tumores na boca. Em gatos, quase sempre os STM se desenvolvem em locais de vacinação/injeção e, portanto, são mais comumente localizados no tronco, seja na região interescapular, dorsolombar, ou no flanco, em diferentes locais, dependendo das recomendações quanto aos melhores locais para vacinar gatos (ver Capítulo 208).

Fatores aplicados ao diagnóstico e tratamento

Em geral, os STM são tumores SC indolores semelhantes a outros nódulos benignos ou malignos. Portanto, o diagnóstico acurado é crítico para o planejamento terapêutico apropriado. Antes do planejamento cirúrgico definitivo, recomenda-se biopsia incisional de todos os nódulos, com exceção dos menores, a fim de prevenir alterações do tecido normal circundante. Deve-se evitar biopsia excisional, a menos que o tumor seja pequeno (< 1 a 2 cm, proporcional ao tamanho do cão ou gato) e circundado por tecido normal abundante. Além disso, no caso

de nódulos SC os procedimentos de biopsia devem ser cuidadosamente planejados a fim de evitar contaminação acidental dos tecidos circundantes. A cirurgia definitiva requer extirpação do trajeto da biopsia e, embora seja esperado o controle local após remoção cirúrgica total da neoplasia, quase sempre ocorre recidiva local após a realização de procedimentos cirúrgicos abaixo do ideal. É necessário tratamento inicial agressivo para a terapia bem-sucedida dos STM. O desafio do planejamento cirúrgico, a melhora do prognóstico pelo uso de terapia multimodal em várias situações e o risco de metástases apesar do controle local de sarcomas de alto grau (44% de taxa de metástases, em um relato[3]) tornam complexo o processo de tomada de decisões. É particularmente importante atender a esses desafios para o tratamento efetivo de SAI em gatos.

ETIOLOGIA

Fatores genéticos, bioquímicos e exposição à radiação

Os mecanismos genéticos ou bioquímicos específicos responsáveis pelo desenvolvimento de STM em cães e gatos permanecem amplamente desconhecidos.[4,5] A maioria dos STM em cães ocorre esporadicamente, embora haja evidências de que os cães da raça Golden Retriever sejam, em geral, mais predispostos a tumores, inclusive STM.[6] Em pessoas foram confirmadas mutações em linhagens germinativas ou formas familiares de sarcomas. Evidências epidemiológicas empíricas provocadas sugerem que mecanismos semelhantes podem ocorrer em cães. Entretanto, ainda não há pesquisas detalhadas sobre a caracterização genética ou a linhagem/raça de cães que desenvolvem STM em idade jovem (< 2 anos), ou nos quais parece provável a predisposição racial.

Está bem estabelecido que a exposição à radiação, infecções virais (vírus do sarcoma felino), traumatismo ou doenças inflamatórias crônicas podem estar associadas ao desenvolvimento de sarcomas em cães e gatos. Os protocolos de radiação convencionais para o tratamento de um câncer primário apresentam o risco de desenvolvimento de um segundo câncer em < 5% dos casos. Tumores induzidos por radiação surgem 3 anos ou mais após a RT.[7] Os benefícios do controle do tumor primário superam o risco de desenvolvimento de tumor secundário induzido por radiação. Uma única dose alta intraoperatória de RT mais provavelmente causa sarcoma (20 a 25%) em cães, após um período de latência mediano de 4 anos.[8]

Sarcomas associados à injeção (SAI)

Fatores de risco

Em um amplo estudo sobre fatores de risco associados ao desenvolvimento de SAI em gatos, nenhuma marca específica de medicamento, nenhuma classe de antígenos vacinais e nenhuma prática vacinal alteraram o risco de desenvolvimento de SAI.[9] Ademais, alguns medicamentos injetáveis de ação prolongada (penicilina, acetato de metilprednisolona) também podem estar associados à ocorrência de sarcoma, daí o termo sarcoma associado à injeção (SAI).[9,10] Também em gatos há relatos de STM nos locais de administração de cisplatina, de fio de sutura não absorvível profundo, esponjas cirúrgicas retidas, microchip ou acesso para administração subcutânea de líquido.[11-15] Provavelmente, há envolvimento de uma combinação de reação inflamatória local e fatores genéticos.[16] De modo semelhante, o desenvolvimento de sarcoma ocular em gatos está frequentemente associado a histórico de traumatismo ocular.[17]

Anormalidades moleculares e celulares

O desenvolvimento molecular de SAI em gatos ainda não está completamente definido. Há diversos relatos que excluem as infecções virais felinas mais comuns (oncornavírus, papilomavírus, poliomavírus) como etiologias.[18-20] Foram identificadas características moleculares particulares de SAI. As expressões do fator/receptor de crescimento epidérmico (EGFR), do fator/receptor de crescimento derivado de plaquetas (PDGF) e do fator de transformação do crescimento beta são marcantes em células tumorais e linfócitos infiltrados em SAI. Tais alterações não são expressas em células de sarcomas felinos fora de locais de injeção.[21] Uma expressão excessiva de C-Jun, um proto-oncogene, foi também identificada em SAI felino e pode ser decorrência da estimulação persistente do fator de crescimento.[21] Fibrossarcomas em locais presumidos de injeção foram relatados em cães, assim como em locais de implante de microchip em dois cães, mas não foram documentados como uma entidade distinta.[22-24]

Anormalidades de *p53* foram relatadas em SAI felino. Em um relato, aproximadamente 43% das amostras obtidas de sarcomas expressaram fortemente a proteína *p53* e, em outro, 5 de 8 amostras tumorais que expressavam excessivamente a proteína *p53* continham genes que haviam sofrido mutação.[25,26] Nenhum gato de um grupo controle de 13 animais com SAI, sem expressão excessiva da proteína *p53*, apresentavam mutações gênicas.[26] Nesse último estudo, nenhum tecido circundante tinha mutações em *p53*, sugerindo que não havia anormalidades na função de *p53* antes do desenvolvimento do tumor. Um estudo mostrou uma associação de polimorfismos de linhagem germinativa no gene *p53* com a predisposição genética para SAI felino.[27] Esses dados indicam que anormalidades moleculares e celulares existem e sugerem diversas hipóteses, mas nenhuma causa específica foi associada ao desenvolvimento de SAI felino.

Anormalidades em *p53* e *MDM2*, um gene cujo produto suprime a expressão de *p53*, foram relatadas em STM canino.[28] Em 20% dos sarcomas, ocorreram substituições de bases, resultando em aminoácidos particulares lidos erroneamente no gene *p53*. Três de 6 tumores com mutações eram tumores malignos de bainha nervosa. A amplificação genética do *MDM2* canino (3 vezes ou mais) foi identificada em 5 de 30 sarcomas. Em todas, com exceção de uma dessas amostras combinadas, houve coordenação dessas anormalidades, resultando em alteração do *p53* (mutações) ou supressão secundária de *p53* devido à expressão excessiva de *MDM2*. Assim, direta ou indiretamente, quase 1/3 dos sarcomas caninos parece ter alteração da função de *p53* e 5 de 7 tumores malignos de bainha nervosa periférica tinham anormalidades funcionais de *p53*.

AVALIAÇÃO CLÍNICA INICIAL

Histórico, exame físico e avaliações iniciais

A avaliação de cães e gatos deve iniciar com minucioso histórico clínico (ver Capítulo 1) e exame físico (ver Capítulo 2). O estadiamento tumoral inclui a avaliação da extensão da doença local e a detecção de qualquer evidência de metástase regional e/ou distante. Ademais, comorbidades e tumores primários concomitantes devem ser identificados por meio de exames laboratoriais, radiografia de tórax e ultrassom (US) abdominal.[29] A descrição minuciosa e a mensuração tridimensional das neoplasias podem ser valiosas para a documentação do crescimento subsequente, se houver atraso no início do tratamento e/ou documentação da resposta à terapia. STM, de forma geral, possuem taxa de metástase relativamente baixa, mas ela aumenta com o aumento do grau do tumor. A maior preocupação com metástase por via hematógena acontece nos casos de sarcomas de alto grau. Os locais de propagação tumoral mais comuns são os pulmões e o fígado. Os linfonodos regionais devem ser avaliados por meio de aspiração e/ou biopsia, particularmente se aumentados ou se o STM for um tumor de alto grau, mesmo que esse não seja o local mais provável de disseminação. Nos casos de diagnóstico precoce de sarcomas, a ocorrência de metástases é considerada baixa;

contudo, sem a avaliação específica dos linfonodos regionais ou o acompanhamento cuidadoso, a real ocorrência é desconhecida. Em gatos com fibrossarcomas associados à vacina, os locais de metástases incluem pulmões, pele, tecido subcutâneo, linfonodos regionais, mediastino, fígado e pelve.

Diagnóstico por imagem

Caso seja confirmada a malignidade, devem-se realizar exames de imagem apropriados para a avaliação do tumor primário, bem como radiografias do tórax e US do abdome (ver Capítulos 88 e 89), durante o processo de estadiamento da neoplasia. Exames de imagem também podem auxiliar no planejamento da biopsia e de opções terapêuticas. A avaliação US do tumor primário pode auxiliar na determinação do melhor local para biopsia. A coleta de amostras guiada por ultrassom pode ser necessária para tumores profundos. Exames de imagem de STM cada vez mais envolvem estudos transversais, como tomografia computadorizada (TC) ou ressonância magnética (RM).[30] A TC com uso de contraste IV pode auxiliar a delinear a extensão de lesões locais, assim como a invasão de tecidos circundantes. É altamente recomendado que os exames de imagem precedam a intervenção terapêutica. Particularmente para SAI em gatos, a extensão da invasão de tecidos circundantes pode ser fundamental e uma biopsia por meio de excisão inicial pode prejudicar a capacidade de atingir o controle do tumor local. O volume do tumor, mensurado a partir de estudos de TC contrastada de sarcomas felinos, pode exceder as mensurações físicas em 2 a 5 vezes. Ademais, a ligação do tumor aos músculos e tecidos circundantes pode ser mais extensa do que o esperado (Figura 346.1).[31]

Em casos de sarcomas felinos associados à injeção, não se recomenda cirurgia sem conhecimento prévio acurado da extensão do tumor. Ademais, em cães, os STM frequentemente ocorrem em membros, locais de difícil ressecção com margens de segurança adequadas. Uma biopsia inicial e exames de imagem podem fornecer tanto um diagnóstico como o conhecimento da extensão da doença, com possível planejamento prévio, de tal forma que o tutor possa ser informado se há indicação de combinação de terapia, considerando a possibilidade de maior duração do tratamento clínico e o custo. É interessante o relato de resultados da cirurgia em 350 cães com STM tratados em clínicas veterinárias. Esse estudo revelou diferenças na extensão do estadiamento antes da cirurgia e tendência aparente de tratamento de tumores de menor grau em clínicas gerais, e não em centros especializados.[32]

DIAGNÓSTICO

Aspirado por agulha fina e citologia

Para determinar a melhor estratégia terapêutica, é necessário o diagnóstico definitivo. A citologia de aspirado pode fornecer informações iniciais sobre um nódulo cutâneo ou subcutâneo que podem sustentar o diagnóstico de uma lesão não neoplásica (ver Capítulos 87, 89, 93 e 95). A citologia de aspirado pode ser diagnóstica para neoplasias e pode sugerir que mais provavelmente o tumor tenha origem em células redondas, epiteliais ou mesenquimais. Todavia, o exame citológico não costuma ser definitivo para a classificação histológica específica. Provavelmente, os tumores mesenquimais são menos esfoliativos durante a aspiração. Nos casos de STM, a citologia de aspirado é realizada principalmente para excluir outras doenças, embora possa ter valor diagnóstico para alguns sarcomas.

Biopsia

Uma biopsia por meio de incisão é recomendada para obter um diagnóstico definitivo e determinar o tipo histopatológico específico e o grau do tumor (ver Capítulo 86). O procedimento de biopsia para sarcomas deve ser cuidadosamente planejado para

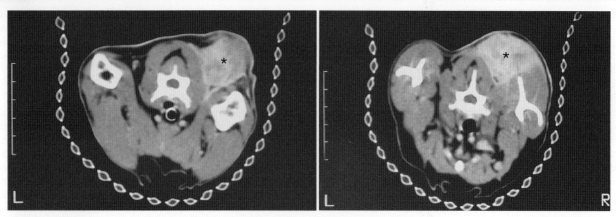

Figura 346.1 Imagem de tomografia computadorizada contrastada de sarcoma felino associado à vacina (*asteriscos*), no espaço pré-escapular. É evidente a extensa infiltração de tecidos moles envolvendo diversos músculos adjacentes ao tecido tumoral.

obter uma amostra representativa do tumor e prevenir quaisquer complicações desnecessárias ou contaminação do tecido circundante ao tumor. Caso utilize uma agulha cortante, é preciso ter cuidado para não penetrar além do perímetro conhecido do tumor, a fim de evitar a propagação de células neoplásicas. Quase sempre os sarcomas se aderem aos tecidos adjacentes, e pode ser difícil verificar a extensão ao longo de planos fasciais durante o exame físico. Portanto, preferem-se amostras de biopsia obtidas por meio de incisão limitada, de *punch* ou de agulhas cortantes, em detrimento de biopsias excisionais, a fim de minimizar o dano tecidual. A obtenção de uma amostra por biopsia possibilita o estadiamento do tumor com base na avaliação de uma série de características histopatológicas, embora possa haver discordâncias entre a biopsia pré-tratamento e os resultados de biopsia excisional, subestimando ou superestimando o grau do tumor.[33]

Histologia

As características histológicas de STM avaliadas para definir o grau do tumor incluem o grau de diferenciação, a porcentagem de necrose e o índice mitótico (ver Tabela 346.1, ver Capítulos 87 e 93). Em cães, o grau do tumor em casos de STM pode ser indicador do prognóstico; tumores de alto grau apresentam um curso mais progressivo e maior probabilidade de metástases. A verificação de margens completas no exame histopatológico é preditiva de não ocorrência de recidiva. Em cães, o grau histológico mostrou ser um forte indicador preditivo de recidiva de STM subcutâneo submetido à extirpação marginal; quanto maior o grau, maior a probabilidade de recidiva local.[34,35] Em gatos, um relato sobre o prognóstico após extirpação cirúrgica de fibrossarcomas mostrou correlação entre o índice mitótico (quantidade de figuras mitóticas em 10 campos de visão [em aumento de 400×]) e a sobrevida.[36] Em gatos com índice mitótico menor que 6, a sobrevida mediana foi de 32 meses; com índice mitótico ≥ 6, a sobrevida foi de 4 meses. A maioria dos estudos não demonstrou correlação entre o grau do tumor e a sobrevida de gatos com sarcomas em locais de injeção, o que, de forma geral, pode ser um tumor mais agressivo.

CONSIDERAÇÕES GERAIS SOBRE O TRATAMENTO

Tratamento cirúrgico *versus* multimodal

A extirpação cirúrgica de qualquer tumor sem planejamento prévio pode resultar na remoção incompleta e necessidade de um segundo procedimento cirúrgico mais extenso, RT e maior taxa de complicação e/ou falha. STM, em particular, provavelmente são removidos de modo incompleto com extirpação marginal próximo ao tumor por causa da extensão da lesão além do tecido tumoral visível ou porque eles podem parecer bem encapsulados. Entretanto, essas estruturas, em geral, são pseudocápsulas: tecido tumoral comprimido e tecido fibrovascular reativo. A maior taxa de morbidade e o maior custo associados à ressecção incompleta justificam o encaminhamento dos animais com STM, com neoplasias grandes ou de alto grau, para avaliação multidisciplinar e possivelmente terapia multimodal. A Figura 346.2 representa um algoritmo de tomada de decisões para sarcomas de tecidos moles, ou qualquer nódulo superficial, com base na estimativa inicial do sucesso cirúrgico. Nesse algoritmo, pontos de decisão primordiais incluem a determinação se a cirurgia curativa é possível; o sucesso da cirurgia com base na avaliação minuciosa das margens cirúrgicas; e a necessidade de quimioterapia adjuvante com base no grau e estadiamento da neoplasia.

A decisão quanto à ressecção cirúrgica de STM talvez seja o ponto mais crítico do algoritmo. A decisão de tentar a ressecção deve ser tomada a partir da mensuração acurada da massa tumoral, da avaliação de infiltrações aos tecidos profundos, da localização do tumor, das limitações de tecidos normais circundantes para a ressecção profunda e da habilidade do cirurgião. Um estudo retrospectivo de 100 cães com mastocitoma ou STM mostrou que o nível de treinamento cirúrgico influenciou o sucesso da extirpação completa da neoplasia.[37] O procedimento cirúrgico deve ser bem planejado, de modo a obter a ressecção completa e reduzir ou prevenir o risco de propagação acidental do tumor, do local ou de tecidos circundantes. Novas e agressivas técnicas cirúrgicas oncológicas estão sendo avaliadas e implementadas.[38-41] Em um estudo piloto de um novo sistema de imagem, cães com sarcomas receberam uma sonda fluorescente por via IV para auxiliar na detecção de tumor residual após ampla ressecção cirúrgica; em 9 de 10 casos, notou-se correlação entre o exame histopatológico das margens cirúrgicas e a imagem transcirúrgica.[42] A ressecção planejada com uma borda tecidual vascularizada, para fechar o defeito, facilita o início oportuno da RT pós-cirúrgica, com alta taxa de sucesso associada a bordas teciduais irradiadas.[43]

Consideração da ocorrência de contaminação do campo cirúrgico com células tumorais

Após um procedimento cirúrgico, deve-se considerar que todo o campo cirúrgico, inclusive a cicatriz, está potencialmente contaminado. O uso de técnica apropriada é essencial, incluindo o planejamento da incisão, a manipulação desnecessária do próprio tumor, ou a colocação de drenos com dissecção tecidual distante. Durante o procedimento podem ser utilizadas pinças hemostáticas para definir a extensão profunda e lateral do tumor e o plano cirúrgico. Isso é útil para determinar a área de uma nova ressecção ou RT, se necessário.[44,45]

A avaliação das margens laterais e profundas para a conclusão da ressecção é fundamental para determinar o controle do tumor local. Isso explica a importância primordial do envio da

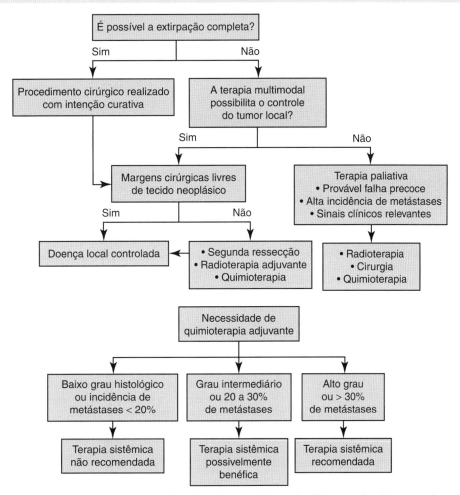

Figura 346.2 Algoritmo para tratamento de tumor sólido periférico (estadiamentos clínico e histológico completos). *Mets*, metástases; *Rad Tx*, radioterapia.

lesão extirpada completa, e não apenas de parte dela. O exame histopatológico das margens tumorais é facilitado pela marcação das margens cirúrgicas com um corante permanente e pela descrição minuciosa da amostra.[46-48] Em um estudo, os pesquisadores utilizaram uma técnica histológica tridimensional para avaliar as margens cirúrgicas laterais e profundas de 48 SAI extirpados de gatos; esse procedimento tem o potencial de aumentar a acurácia do exame da margem cirúrgica.[49] Quando o tecido foi submetido à fixação para o exame microscópico, pode ser difícil avaliar se as margens ao redor do tecido tumoral são adequadas. Na literatura, as definições das margens cirúrgicas são variáveis e incluem, mas não se limitam, à classificação: incompletas (extirpação com presença de células neoplásicas em até 1 mm de margem cirúrgica), estreitas ou próximas (extirpação sem a presença de células tumorais na margem cirúrgica, mas com tecido histologicamente normal que se estende por menos de 1 cm além das margens histológicas, ou menos que 3 mm), e amplas ou completas (extirpação com tecido histologicamente normal com mais de 1 cm além da margem cirúrgica, ou um mínimo de 3 a 5 mm).[35] Para a classificação de uma massa tumoral como completamente extirpada, recomenda-se um mínimo de diâmetro de 10 células entre o tumor e a superfície profunda. Esse procedimento arbitrário deve ser cuidadosamente avaliado com medidas de distância mais bem definidas que podem estar correlacionadas com a margem necessária para prevenção de recidiva de sarcomas de diferentes graus.

Tratamento paliativo

Para neoplasias não passíveis de abordagens definitivas, como cirurgia agressiva ou terapia multimodal, pode ser necessário tratamento paliativo. A terapia paliativa deve ser ativamente realizada; foram desenvolvidas diversas opções terapêuticas especificamente para pacientes com tumores incuráveis ou aqueles com morbidade significativa associada à presença do tumor.

TRATAMENTO DE SARCOMAS DE TECIDOS MOLES EM CÃES

Detecção

Não há fatores de risco conhecidos, de uso clínico, que possibilitam a detecção precoce ou predição de STM em cães. Portanto, as recomendações gerais de triagem e detecção do câncer (exames físicos frequentes, radiografias, outros exames de imagem) são as únicas formas de diagnóstico precoce de STM. Qualquer massa tumoral deve ser caracterizada por meio de mensurações, imagens apropriadas e biopsia o mais cedo possível. No caso de detecção de STM, devem ser implementados os procedimentos mencionados anteriormente para definição do protocolo terapêutico.

Protocolo terapêutico e grau de agressividade da cirurgia (ver Figura 346.2)

O ideal é que as decisões quanto ao tratamento do tumor primário e à necessidade de quimioterapia como terapia adjuvante após o controle do tumor local sejam tomadas, juntamente, pela equipe veterinária e pelo tutor. A ressecção cirúrgica deve ser o primeiro procedimento para qualquer STM. A conclusão de que um tumor é potencialmente curável após cirurgia deve ser minuciosamente analisada, pois a recidiva local é uma séria complicação de uma cirurgia inadequada e influencia as futuras opções terapêuticas.[50] A importância da escolha do tipo de cirurgia foi demonstrada em um relato de 56 cães com lipossarcoma, no qual se constatou sobrevida mediana de 1.188, 649 e 183 dias, respectivamente, após realização de extirpação ampla, extirpação marginal ou biopsia por meio de incisão.[51]

Um relato sobre os resultados da extirpação marginal de sarcomas de célula fusiforme de baixo grau localizado em membros de cães documentou baixa taxa de recidiva local (10,8%), com sobrevida média de 703,5 dias (mediana ainda não foi alcançada).[52] A ampla extirpação local (2 cm de margem lateral, e 1 plano fascial profundo) de STM em 31 cães (extirpação primária em 21 cães; revisão da cicatriz após ressecção incompleta em 10 cães) com tumores localizados na parte distal do membro mostrou excelente controle local a longo prazo; a maioria das feridas cicatrizou completamente por segunda intenção (tempo mediano de 53 dias, com variação de 25 a 179 dias).[53] A maioria dos STM de dígito, o terceiro tumor digital mais comum, é tratada pela amputação do dígito.[54] Nos casos de STM em regiões anatômicas musculofasciais complexas, recomendam-se o encaminhamento para avaliação mais abrangente e o tratamento agressivo do tumor, pois a remoção adequada de tecido normal ao redor do sarcoma melhora o controle local.[55] A terapia multimodal é um procedimento apropriado para tumores cuja ressecção não é tão fácil, sendo de fundamental importância o planejamento prévio.

Radioterapia

A RT mostrou-se muito benéfica para o controle local de STM que não foram completamente removidos (ver Capítulo 340). Pode-se recomendar o uso de RT definitiva, pré-cirúrgica ou pós-cirúrgica, embora o ideal seja um esquema de aplicação de RT definido antes do início do tratamento.[56] Ademais, existem considerações específicas para ter em mente ao combinar cirurgia e RT, como a influência da radiação pré-cirúrgica na cicatrização da ferida.[57] Diversos estudos mostraram que a RT resulta em controle a longo prazo de STM em cães.[58,59] A taxa de sobrevida livre de recidiva local foi estimada em 75 a 85%, em acompanhamento por 3 anos ou mais, e essa combinação deve ser recomendada para todos os STM de cães não removidos completamente. Protocolos de radiação hipofracionada foram utilizados em casos de doença microscópica e propiciam controle a longo prazo na maioria dos cães.[60,61] A extirpação marginal intencional de STM em um membro do cão, seguida de RT hipofracionada (8 a 9 Gy/fração, semanalmente; dose total de 32 a 36 Gy) reduz potencialmente as complicações cirúrgicas, mas pode estar associada a maior ocorrência de efeitos colaterais tardios da radiação por utilizar uma alta dose por fração.[60] Esquemas terapêuticos e tecnologias atuais tornam menos prováveis a ocorrência de efeitos colaterais que limitam o uso de RT em tumores locais.[62] Entretanto, STM pode surgir em qualquer tecido e pode ser difícil preservar as estruturas adjacentes normais sem o comprometimento do tratamento do tumor.

Quimioterapia

Há várias indicações para quimioterapia em casos de STM (ver Capítulo 339): quando o paciente apresenta um STM inoperável, mas uma redução mensurável do tumor pode possibilitar a ressecção com preservação da função; para pacientes com STM recidivante não passíveis a novos procedimentos cirúrgicos; em cães com STM de alto grau, a fim de reduzir ou retardar o desenvolvimento de nódulos metastáticos; e em cães com STM que apresentem maior probabilidade inerente de metástases.[63,64] A doxorrubicina tem sido utilizada como o agente único mais ativo em casos de STM canino; todavia, com base em um estudo não foi efetiva no tratamento de sarcomas de alto grau em cães.[3] Outras opções incluem antineoplásicos que contêm platina e ifosfamida. Durante a cirurgia tem-se utilizado cisplatina no tratamento de STM canino, com intuito de aumentar a concentração local do medicamento, ao mesmo tempo que reduz a toxicidade sistêmica; entretanto, um número inaceitável de 16 entre 19 cães apresentaram complicações locais.[65] A quimioterapia metronômica pode ser útil no tratamento de STM de alto grau ou de STM cuja remoção foi incompleta, com o objetivo de inibir a angiogênese, diferentemente da citotoxicidade direta associada à quimioterapia com dose total, bem como da modulação do sistema imune.[64,66-68] A quimioterapia metronômica com ciclofosfamida e piroxicam retardou significativamente a ocorrência de recidiva do tumor em 30 cães com STM cuja remoção foi incompleta, em comparação com 55 cães do grupo controle; porém, 40% dos cães desenvolveram efeitos adversos discretos relacionados ao tratamento.[67] Embora não haja evidência definitiva para recomendação geral de quimioterapia adjuvante para cães com STM de alto grau, vários especialistas mencionam que o risco (≈ 40%) de metástases distantes, mesmo após tratamento local, justifica a recomendação do tratamento quimioterápico.[3,55]

Tratamento paliativo

Há disponibilidade de tratamento paliativo para cães com anormalidades funcionais relevantes diretamente relacionadas à massa tumoral. Os protocolos de radiação para tratamento paliativo são desenvolvidos para administrar uma dose significativa de radiação no tumor, sem efeitos colaterais debilitantes e com tempo mínimo de hospitalização; tal procedimento pode ser efetivo a curto prazo.[69] Tumores que causam dor, disfagia, dispneia, disquezia ou disúria, e aqueles que sabidamente são incuráveis pela cirurgia, devem ser submetidos a RT paliativa. A quimioterapia paliativa também pode ser utilizada na tentativa de reduzir a massa tumoral que causa sinais clínicos debilitantes. Os procedimentos cirúrgicos paliativos desenvolvidos especificamente para melhorar a qualidade de vida dos pacientes com doença extensa incluem o tratamento de úlcera e de infecção secundária.

SARCOMAS DE TECIDOS MOLES COM CARACTERÍSTICAS CLÍNICAS PARTICULARES EM CÃES

Considerações gerais

A maioria dos STM (ver Boxe 346.1) pode ser tratada de acordo com os princípios descritos anteriormente, após definição do grau histológico e da possibilidade de controle local. Deve-se dar atenção especial à seleção de sarcomas devido às apresentações ou biologia particulares do tumor como, por exemplo, a localização retroperitoneal de sarcomas de tecidos moles, embora rara, está associada à alta taxa de recidiva local e de metástases, com sobrevida curta (mediana de 37,5 dias).[70] O sarcoma de célula sinovial (ver Capítulo 348) e o hemangiossarcoma (ver Capítulo 347) são discutidos em seus respectivos capítulos.

Leiomiossarcoma/tumor estromal gastrintestinal (GI)

Sarcoma de músculo liso se desenvolve mais frequentemente no trato GI e requer procedimentos terapêuticos especiais de acordo com o seu local de origem. Após reclassificação dos tumores de músculo liso GI de cães, os tumores de estroma gastrintestinal (TEGI) são considerados diferentes de leiomiomas e leiomiossarcomas.[71-74] TEGI expressam o gene c-kit, detectado por meio de imuno-histoquímica (IHQ), e vários apresentam mutações ativadoras que supostamente levam à oncogênese.[75] TEGI podem ser responsivos aos inibidores do receptor de tirosinoquinase direcionados ao KIT.[76-78] Mais recentemente, o DOG1 (presente na proteína 1 de tumor de estroma GI) mostrou ser um marcador diagnóstico sensível e específico de tumor estromal gastrintestinal em cães.[79] Foi recomendado que tanto o DOG1 quanto o IHQ do KIT sejam incluídos nos painéis diagnósticos, a fim de melhorar a acurácia diagnóstica de TEGI em cães.

Como é improvável uma segunda cirurgia, recomenda-se a ampla remoção de tumores GI, e quaisquer linfonodos ou outros locais abdominais que causam preocupação também devem ser removidos para auxiliar no estadiamento. Diversas revisões relataram a recuperação clínica em aproximadamente 100 cães com leiomiossarcoma intestinal.[80-82] Além disso, foram resumidos os dados que descrevem o local ou a origem da neoplasia, bem como metástases, em 158 cães e 22 gatos com leiomiossarcomas.[83] Leiomiossarcomas estão mais frequentemente localizados no estômago, intestino delgado, baço ou trato urogenital. Parece que TEGI se desenvolvem mais frequentemente no intestino grosso, principalmente no ceco, embora em um estudo seja relatada sua ocorrência principalmente no intestino delgado.[71,84] Em gatos, os leiomiossarcomas são incomuns, mas são mais frequentes no trato GI do que em outros locais. Caso seja possível a ressecção cirúrgica completa, a sobrevida mediana é de cerca de 18 a 37 meses. Vários cães morrem por outras causas que não sejam recidivas ou metástases tumorais. Há relatos controversos quanto à diferença na sobrevida dependendo se for TEGI ou leiomiossarcoma; um relato menciona sobrevida mediana mais curta em casos de leiomiossarcomas.[71] Lesões metastáticas são relatadas em 15 a 30% dos cães com leiomiossarcomas e mais provavelmente são verificadas no mesentério, baço ou fígado. Metástases podem ter desenvolvimento lento (1 a 2 anos) e progressão relativamente longa. As informações sobre a resposta à quimioterapia são limitadas.[71]

TRATAMENTO DE SARCOMAS EM GATOS

Estão sendo realizadas pesquisas para determinar o melhor protocolo terapêutico para SAI. As melhores taxas de eficácia envolvem diagnóstico precoce e tratamento agressivo. O ideal é impedir o desenvolvimento de SAI.[110] A análise de alterações de $p53$ pode ser útil para nortear o tratamento de alguns gatos com maior risco de recidiva e, no futuro, para uso como alvo molecular de $p53$ mutante.[96,111]

Cirurgia

Necessidade para amplas margens

Em gatos, a extirpação cirúrgica de sarcomas de tecidos moles representa a melhor chance de controle efetivo de tumor local.[31,85-88] Na suspeita de STM em um gato, uma biopsia inicial, juntamente com exames de imagem transversais (TC ou RM) propicia avaliação mais acurada da extensão do tumor e ajuda no planejamento terapêutico.[89,90] Uma biopsia por meio de excisão de um SAI raramente é completa, provavelmente resultará em recidiva local, e será necessária uma segunda cirurgia mais difícil. A recidiva tumoral foi documentada em até 2 semanas após a cirurgia, mas tipicamente ocorre dentro de 6 meses após ressecção incompleta.[91] Uma resseção cirúrgica agressiva é necessária para o tratamento local efetivo, e isso pode implicar ressecção do tumor com margens de 3 a 5 cm, remoção do osso associado (p. ex., processos espinhosos dorsais, escapulectomia parcial), e pelo menos um plano fascial profundo aos tecidos envolvidos.

Não há concordância entre os estudos em termos de fatores prognósticos identificados para gatos com sarcomas de tecidos moles. Em um grupo de 42 gatos com uma série de STM tratados somente com cirurgia, a sobrevida mediana foi mais longa em gatos com tumores com menos de 2 cm de diâmetro e em gatos com fibrossarcomas ou tumores de bainha nervosa, comparativamente aos gatos com histiocitoma fibroso maligno; a sobrevida mediana para todos os gatos foi de 608 dias.[92] Em um relato de 91 gatos tratados por meio de extirpação radical com margens de 5 cm ao redor do tumor palpável e margens profundas, incluindo 2 planos musculares ou ossos profundos em relação ao tumor, sem tratamento adjuvante, constatou-se que a sobrevida mediana geral foi de 901 dias, apesar da não realização de imagens transversas pré-cirúrgicas.[93] A cirurgia radical foi completa em 88 de 91 gatos e a taxa de recidiva local de 14% é menor do que previamente relatada em animais submetidos apenas à cirurgia ou à combinação com terapia adjuvante. Complicações importantes ocorreram em 10 gatos (7 com deiscência na ferida cirúrgica).[93]

Recidiva e metástase

Recidiva e metástase do tumor foram significativamente associadas à sobrevida. A sobrevida mediana de gatos com (n = 13; 14%) e sem recidiva foi de 499 e 1.461 dias, respectivamente. A sobrevida mediana de gatos com (n = 18; 20%) e sem metástase foi de 388 e 1.528 dias, respectivamente. Em um estudo retrospectivo de 49 gatos submetidos à ampla extirpação (3 cm de margem, com base em imagens de TC contrastadas) de SAI no tronco, a duração da cirurgia foi relacionada à complexidade do procedimento.

A duração da cirurgia foi identificada como o melhor preditor de complicações de cicatrização da ferida cirúrgica; 19 gatos (importantes em 8 gatos; menores em 11 gatos).[94] Embora alguns patologistas considerem todos os SAI como de alto grau, com base em seu comportamento biológico, em um estudo os gatos com SAI de alto grau mais provavelmente desenvolveram metástases (SAI foram graduados como de baixo, médio e alto graus), condição que foi associada à sobrevida mediana significativamente menor (165 *versus* 929 dias).[95] Parece haver uma forte associação da deleção somática na região conservada do gene $p53$ e a recidiva pós-cirúrgica e menor sobrevida.[96]

Localização do tumor e uso de terapias multimodais

Quase sempre os SAI se desenvolvem no espaço interescapular, um local de difícil acesso para cirurgia; portanto, há necessidade de remoção dos processos espinhosos dorsais e da musculatura circundante. Por essa razão, a Vaccine-Associated Feline Sarcoma Task Force (VAFSTF) recomenda a vacinação contra os vírus da raiva e da leucemia felina (FeLV) na parte distal do membro pélvico (membro direito e esquerdo, respectivamente), de tal forma que a amputação seja possível, caso desenvolva SAI (ver Capítulo 208). Mesmo após amputação ou hemipelvectomia, pode não ser possível a extirpação completa do SAI.

Geralmente é necessário utilizar uma abordagem multimodal, combinando radioterapia (RT) e cirurgia. Em algumas situações, pode ser necessária a radiação pré-cirúrgica de um sarcoma situado na parte proximal do membro, antes da amputação. O uso de RT no pré-operatório geralmente reduz o tamanho do tumor e, teoricamente, esteriliza os componentes tumorais periféricos que poderiam, de outra forma, resultar em ressecção incompleta e risco para um novo crescimento tumoral rápido (ver Capítulo 240).[56,97] Um estudo com radioterapia corporal estereotática (24 a 32,5 Gy administrada em 3 a 5 frações) empregada para tratar 11 gatos com SAI constatou uma resposta parcial em 5 gatos e resposta total em 3 gatos. O intervalo mediano livre de progressão tumoral foi de 242 dias, e a sobrevida geral foi de 301 dias.[98] Essa abordagem é uma opção de terapia paliativa de tumores, mas requer estudos adicionais para determinar sua importância na terapia de combinação. Em um estudo retrospectivo de 79 gatos com STM submetidos ao tratamento com RT pré-cirúrgica (n = 24) ou pós-cirúrgica (n = 55), verificou-se sobrevida mediana geral de 520 dias.[99] A sobrevida mediana de gatos tratados com RT pré-cirúrgica (310 dias) foi significativamente mais curta do que a de gatos irradiados no período pós-operatório (705 dias), mas isso pode ter ocorrido devido à seleção tendenciosa, pois os gatos com tumores maiores foram irradiados no período pré-cirúrgico. É importante ressaltar que a anemia foi considerada um indicador de prognóstico ruim, com sobrevida mediana de 308 dias para os gatos com volume globular (VG) < 25%, e 760 dias para gatos com VG ≥ 25%.[99]

Quimioterapia

A quimioterapia pode ser utilizada no tratamento de SAI, como terapia adjuvante, em casos de doenças potencialmente metas-táticas; como terapia neoadjuvante para reduzir o tamanho do tumor antes da ressecção cirúrgica; ou como terapia paliativa para tumores sem possibilidade de ressecção. Relata-se que a combinação de doxorrubicina e ciclofosfamida utilizada em 12 gatos com tumores sem possibilidade de ressecção teve uma taxa de resposta total de 50%.[100] A sobrevida mediana foi significativamente maior nos gatos que responderam (242 dias) do que naqueles que não responderam (83 dias). Em um estudo de 69 gatos, não se constatou diferença significativa na sobrevida ou no intervalo livre de doença em gatos submetidos apenas à cirurgia em comparação com aqueles submetidos a cirurgia e tratamento com doxorrubicina.[101] Vinte e um gatos com SAI receberam 3 ciclos de quimioterapia neoadjuvante com epirru-bicina antes da ressecção cirúrgica, seguidos de 3 ciclos adicionais como terapia adjuvante.[102] A quimioterapia foi bem tolerada e a sobrevida média foi de 2.014 dias. Gatos com doença macroscópica tratados com ifosfamida tiveram uma duração mediana de resposta de 70 dias.[103] Gatos com SAI tratados com doses de carboplatina baseadas na taxa de filtração glomerular podem apresentar melhor resposta.[104,105] Em um estudo prospectivo de fase I/II de 28 gatos com SAI tratados com lomustina, a taxa de resposta total foi de 25%, com duração de resposta mediana de 82,5 dias.[106]

Combinação de cirurgia, radioterapia e quimioterapia

Uma combinação de cirurgia, radioterapia e quimioterapia pode resultar em maior eficácia do tratamento tumoral a longo prazo. Em 92 gatos submetidos à RT pré-cirúrgica para SAI, o tempo mediano entre o início do tratamento e a ocorrência de recidiva local, metástase ou data de morte ou eutanásia foi significativamente mais longo (986 dias, n = 59 gatos) quando submetidos à ressecção completa do tumor, em comparação com aqueles submetidos à ressecção parcial (292 dias, n = 28 gatos).[97] Houve tendência de aumento da sobrevida após a adição de quimioterapia (carboplatina ou outro antineoplásico), com intervalo mediano para o primeiro evento de 1.059 dias (n = 33 gatos) em gatos que receberam quimioterapia, contra 584 dias (n = 59 gatos) em gatos tratados apenas com RT e cirurgia. A taxa geral de metástase foi de cerca de 20%, embora o acompanhamento completo não tenha sido possível para todos os gatos. Em 71 gatos, a administração concomitante de doxorru-bicina estendeu o intervalo livre da doença em gatos submetidos à RT pós-cirúrgica (intervalo mediano livre da doença de 15,4 *versus* 5,7 meses), mas não influenciou significativamente a sobrevida.[107] Dez gatos com STM avançado foram tratados com doxorrubicina lipossomal e 5 a 7 frações diárias paliativas concomitantes de RT com dose total mediana de 20 Gy (com variação de 20 a 31,5 Gy).[108] Uma dose de doxorrubicina lipos-somal foi administrada no início da RT e 7 gatos receberam, adicionalmente, doxorrubicina livre ou lipossomal após a conclusão do protocolo doxorrubicina lipossomal/RT. Cinco dos 10 gatos apresentaram uma resposta parcial e 2 tiveram uma resposta total; a duração de resposta mediana foi de 237 dias.

O intervalo mediano livre de progressão (ILP) foi de 117 dias e a sobrevida geral mediana foi de 324 dias. Em geral, a radio-quimioterapia lipossomal concomitante foi bem tolerada.

Um estudo retrospectivo de 73 gatos tratados com RT definitiva (n = 46, maioria com margens limpas; 1 gato também recebeu quimioterapia), ou RT fracionada (n = 27, a maioria com doença macroscópica ou margens incompletas) demonstrou que ambas as abordagens são opções para o tratamento de SAI.[109] Gatos tratados com RT definitiva pós-cirúrgica tiveram sobrevida mediana de 43 meses e ILP mediano de 37 meses. No grupo tratado com RT fracionada, a sobrevida mediana foi de 24 meses, e o ILP, de 10 meses. Nesse último grupo, os preditores de melhor resultado foram ausência de massa tumoral visível (n = 10), diferentemente da doença macroscópica (n = 17, sobrevida de 30 meses *versus* 7 meses); quimioterapia adjuvante para doença macroscópica (n = 5/17, sobrevida de 29 meses *versus* 5 meses) e um pequeno número de cirurgias antes da RT.

PREVENÇÃO

Em cães, a etiologia da maioria dos STM é desconhecida; portanto, não é possível implementar estratégias para sua prevenção. Entretanto, em gatos é possível diminuir o risco de desenvolvimento de STM. As razões incluem a limitação do número de vacinas administradas aos gatos para somente aquelas necessárias para manter a saúde (ver Capítulo 208). Ademais, o clínico deve seguir as recomendações da VAFSTF: limitar uma vacina por local e documentar o local de aplicação de cada vacina (membro pélvico direito, para raiva; membro pélvico esquerdo, para FeLV, e região escapular lateral direita para vacina contra rinotraqueíte viral felina, calicivírus e vírus da panleucopenia felina). Essas recomendações foram aperfeiçoadas pela American Association of Feline Practitioners, de modo a vacinar gatos na região distal ao cotovelo ou abaixo do joelho, especificando cada vacina e seu local de aplicação apropriado.[112] Dessa forma, mesmo que ocorra um tumor, os tutores podem ser informados onde e o que procurar ao avaliar um possível tumor.

Um estudo piloto demonstrou que a vacinação na cauda é bem tolerada, com respostas sorológicas semelhantes àquelas da aplicação da vacina na parte distal dos membros.[113] Foram produzidas vacinas que parecem não resultar em resposta inflamatória local e podem, portanto, causar menor risco de desenvolvimento de tumor naquele local. Entretanto, um estudo de prevalência de envio de SAI de gatos no período de 1992 a 2010 não indicou diminuição na prevalência ou aumento na idade dos gatos acometidos, apesar de alterações instituídas na formulação da vacina ou de alterações recomendadas nos protocolos vacinais.[114] Ademais, embora um estudo de 392 gatos com SAI tenha demonstrado que veterinários cumprem parcialmente as recomendações, mais atenção precisa ser dada à vacinação em locais mais distais possíveis do membro.[115] Há relatos isolados de tumores que ocorrem em gatos em locais não associados à vacinação, mas sim devido a outros eventos que resultaram em resposta inflamatória local. O aumento do conhecimento das várias causas incitantes de sarcomas felinos provavelmente auxilia na detecção precoce e impede a exposição a esses produtos, quando possível.

REFERÊNCIAS BIBLIOGRÁFICAS

As referências bibliográficas deste capítulo se encontram online no Ambiente de Aprendizagem.

CAPÍTULO 347

Hemangiossarcoma

Craig A. Clifford e Louis-Philippe de Lorimier

CARACTERÍSTICAS GERAIS, PATOLOGIA E COMPORTAMENTO BIOLÓGICO

Hemangiossarcoma (HSA; angiossarcoma, hemangioendotelioma maligno) é um tumor altamente maligno, com um comportamento biológico agressivo.[1-5] Foi suposto que essa doença tinha uma ontogenia endotelial; entretanto, dados recentes sugerem que esses tumores surgem a partir de células progenitoras da medula óssea, com parada de diferenciação no estágio de angioblasto ou hemangioblasto e transferência subsequente para os locais vasculares periféricos.[6,7] HSA é diagnosticado mais frequentemente em cães do que em qualquer outra espécie de animal doméstico e corresponde a ≈ 2 % de todos os tumores de cães.[1-5,8,9] HSA tende a afetar cães idosos de ambos os sexos (embora diversos relatos tenham sugerido uma predominância em machos), com idade mediana de 10 anos por ocasião do diagnóstico.[1-5,9,10] Embora cães de qualquer raça podem desenvolver HSA, aqueles das raças Pastor-Alemão, Golden Retriever e de outras raças grandes ou gigantes parecem ser predispostos.[1-5,9,10]

Em cães, há relato de HSA primário em vários locais. Entretanto, o baço, o coração (átrio ou aurícula direita), tecidos cutâneos ou subcutâneos e fígado são os quatro locais primários mais comuns (Figura 347.1). Outras localizações primárias relatadas incluem rins, espaço retroperitoneal, músculo, osso, cavidade bucal/nasal, bexiga e pulmões.[2-5,9,11-15] O comportamento biológico varia dependendo da localização do tumor primário; em alguns locais, como a pele, o prognóstico é mais favorável em comparação a outros. Geralmente, a infiltração local e disseminação metastática ocorrem precocemente no curso da doença, seja por via hematógena seja por propagação local após ruptura do tumor e subsequente implantação intra-abdominal (Figura 347.2). Metástases podem ocorrer em qualquer local; fígado, omento e pulmões são os locais mais frequentes de disseminação da neoplasia.[1-5] Às vezes, é difícil discernir o verdadeiro local de origem por conta da natureza multifocal da doença. De forma interessante, é o sarcoma que mais comumente causa metástase ao sistema nervoso central (SNC).[16,17]

O baço é o órgão primário mais comumente acometido em cães, e com base em uma série de estudos patológicos, estabeleceu-se informalmente a "regra dos dois terços". O resumo desses achados sugeriu que aproximadamente dois terços dos cães com tumor esplênico possuem neoplasia maligna e, portanto, um terço são benignos. Dos dois terços de tumores esplênicos malignos, aproximadamente dois terços são HSA.[8,10] Dois outros grandes estudos patológicos que avaliaram o baço de cães constataram que quase 50% dos animais tinham doença maligna, sendo que 50 a 74% das neoplasias eram HSA.[18,19] Estudos retrospectivos mais recentes que avaliaram pacientes atendidos com hemoabdômen não traumático constataram que 68 a 80% dos casos eram secundários à neoplasia visceral, sendo que 63 a 70% de todos os cães apresentavam, comprovadamente, HSA.[20-22] Embora haja certa discrepância na prevalência exata do HSA esplênico, sem dúvida é a neoplasia esplênica primária mais comum em cães. Entretanto, na lista de diagnósticos diferenciais de tumor esplênico devem ser incluídas outras neoplasias, como histiocitoma fibroso maligno, leiomiossarcoma, fibrossarcoma, sarcomas anaplásicos/indiferenciados e linfoma. Enfermidades não neoplásicas comuns incluem hiperplasia nodular, hematopoese extramedular e hematoma

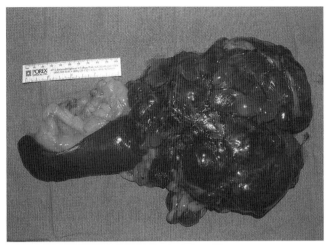

Figura 347.1 Hemangiossarcoma esplênico. Note a natureza multilobulada do tumor. (Cortesia de Julius Liptak, BVSc, MVetLinStud, FACVSc, DACVS, DECVS.)

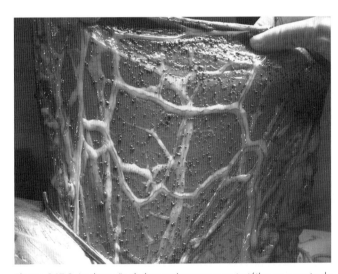

Figura 347.2 Implantação de hemangiossarcoma metastático no omento de um cão da raça Labrador Retriever de 7 anos. (Cortesia de Julius Liptak, BVSc, MVetLinStud, FACVSc, DACVS, DECVS.)

esplênico.[8,18,19] Macroscopicamente, o HSA intra-abdominal pode se apresentar como uma massa tecidual solitária ou pode ser caracterizado por lesões multifocais que parecem macias, com aparência vermelho-escura, que podem ser hemocomponentes oriundos de exsudação.

O coração é outro local primário comum de HSA em cães, sendo o tumor primário mais comum do coração de cães. Especificamente, a neoplasia mais comumente se origina no átrio/aurícula direita; entretanto, há relatos de desenvolvimento do tumor em outros locais do coração (ver Capítulos 254).[5,23-27] Foi previamente relatado que ≈ 25% dos cães com HSA esplênico também possuem um segundo HSA primário no coração, compatível com doença concomitante ou metacrônica.[28] Dados mais recentes sugerem que essa ocorrência é menos comum (8,7%).[29] Os rins, embora um local incomum de HSA primário, podem estar associados a um histórico clínico mais longo, geralmente com lesões menores, doença menos avançada no momento do diagnóstico, e prognóstico mais favorável, comparado a outras apresentações internas de HSA.[12] O HSA é o de tumor mais comum que se instala no espaço retroperitoneal, e está associado a altas taxas de metástases e de recidivas, com sobrevida muito curta (< 40 dias), quando se desenvolve nesses locais.[13]

Há dados escassos quanto à real incidência de HSA em gatos. Entretanto, parece ocorrer muito menos comumente do que em cães, e provavelmente representa < 0.5% de todos os diagnosticados em gatos. Geralmente, o HSA acomete gatos idosos, sem constatação de predisposição quanto ao sexo. Baço, fígado, trato gastrintestinal, tecido cutâneo/subcutâneo e mesentério são os locais primários mais comuns. Hemangiossarcoma incomumente tem sido relatado como uma variante do sarcoma secundário à aplicação de injeção, em gatos (ver Capítulo 346). Embora o HSA ocorra menos comumente em gatos do que em cães, o seu comportamento biológico parece ser semelhante, com locais de metástases comuns, incluindo pulmões, fígado e omento.[30-37] Um estudo que avaliou a ocorrência de hemoperitônio espontâneo em 65 gatos mencionou que 30/65 (46%) tinham neoplasia abdominal, e 54% apresentavam doenças não neoplásicas. Constatou-se que 60% (18/30) dos gatos com doença neoplásica tinham HAS, e o baço foi o local mais comum de origem dessas neoplasias (11/30; 37%).[38] Outro estudo que avaliou 26 gatos com hemangiossarcoma visceral relatou metástase pulmonar e doença multifocal em 33 e 77% dos gatos, respectivamente.[34]

Etiologia e biopatologia

A etiologia definitiva do HSA canino permanece incerta; entretanto, diversos fatores de risco associados foram relatados, incluindo exposição à luz UV e radioterapia.[39-41] Em raças de cães de pelo curto pouco pigmentados, como Saluki, Whippet, Italian Greyhound e Greyhound, em caso de HSA superficial (dérmico) localizada na parte ventral do abdome e na conjuntiva ocorre exposição crônica à luz UV.[40] Há relato de desenvolvimento de lesões de HSA em locais submetidos à radioterapia, mas o risco real é considerado bastante baixo. A exposição a toxinas, como cloreto de vinila, dióxido, radiação e arsênico foi associada às ocorrências de angiossarcoma e HSA em humanos,[42-44] mas não há dados dessas ocorrências em animais de companhia.

Alguns estudos sugeriram uma associação hormonal com o HSA relacionado à castração (ver Capítulo 313). Especificamente, em um estudo que avaliou tumores de origem cardíaca, o HSA cardíaco em fêmeas castradas foi quatro vezes mais comum do que em fêmeas não castradas.[23] De modo semelhante, um estudo que avaliou o HSA esplênico constatou que a prevalência de HSA em fêmeas castradas foi duas vezes maior, comparativamente às fêmeas não castradas.[1] Mais recentemente, um estudo que avaliou os efeitos da castração precoce em cadelas da raça Golden Retriever verificou que a porcentagem de HSA em fêmeas "castradas tardiamente" foi quatro vezes maior do que em naquelas não castradas ou castradas precocemente.[45] É importante ressaltar que o número de cães afetados nesses estudo foi baixo; entretanto, essa é uma área ativa de interesse tanto no contexto veterinário quanto de saúde pública.

Com o advento de plataformas que possibilitam avaliar a expressão gênica de amplo genoma, nós estamos começando a elucidar genes específicos associados ao HSA. Um estudo recente que utilizou tais técnicas identificou três subtipos tumorais distintos em cães com hemangiossarcoma primário. Especificamente, eles estavam associados à angiogênese, inflamação e adipogênese.[46] Esses achados sugerem que tumores podem surgir tanto de células progenitoras multipotentes únicas, que se diferenciam em várias linhagens como parte de um processo de adaptação, ou que linhagens progenitoras múltiplas podem contribuir para a formação do tumor, com uma célula progenitora originando células semelhantes a células endoteliais e semelhantes a células adipogênicas, e outra célula progenitora originando células semelhantes a células mieloides. Outras pesquisas que utilizaram citometria de fluxo multiparamétrica mostraram que em cães o HSA s se origina de precursor hematopoético, com comprometimento da linhagem endotelial.[7,47] Esses dados semelhantemente refutam a crença por muito tempo mantida de que o HSA é uma transformação maligna de células endoteliais maduras nos vasos sanguíneos periféricos. Ademais, é concebível que essa modalidade, que pode avaliar os padrões de expressão dos marcadores de superfície celular observados naquelas células-tronco derivadas da medula óssea multipotenciais, pode auxiliar na confirmação do diagnóstico precoce de HSA e possivelmente ser útil no monitoramento de doença residual mínima.[7,47,48]

Diferenças entre células endoteliais malignas e não malignas foram documentadas com relação ao aumento da expressão de genes envolvidos na inflamação, angiogênese, adesão, invasão, metabolismo, ciclo celular, sinalização e padronização em células neoplásicas. De forma interessante, essa "assinatura" refletiu não somente um fenótipo angiogênico associado ao câncer, mas distinguiu o HSA de outras neoplasias.[49] Ademais, anormalidades específicas em oncogenes e em genes supressores tumorais foram identificados em casos de HSA, ambos os quais podem ser importantes na formação do tumor.[50,51] Essa explosão de pesquisas identificou vários genes que "acionam" o desenvolvimento de câncer associado a vias de sinalização celular aberrantes. É interessante ressaltar que várias dessas vias estão associadas à angiogênese,[46,49] um mecanismo que frequentemente está desregulado nas neoplasias. No HSA nota-se expressão excessiva de múltiplos fatores angiogênicos e seus receptores associados, bem como aumento da quantidade de fatores angiogênicos no sangue de cães com HSA (ver também Capítulo 338).[52-57]

HISTÓRICO E SINAIS CLÍNICOS

A manifestação clínica, o histórico clínicos e os sintomas associados dependem da localização do tumor; entretanto, a maioria dos pacientes com HSA de origens esplênica, hepática e cardíaca é atendida em instituições de atendimento veterinário de emergência devido à ruptura do tumor e hemorragia interna (ver Capítulos 135 e 143). Em alguns casos, isso pode levar ao colapso (ver Capítulo 127) e morte súbita. Pacientes com HSA intra-abdominal ou intratorácico comumente tem um histórico de fraqueza aguda, colapso e palidez de membranas mucosas secundária à anemia por perda de sangue. Frequentemente, na consulta emergencial pode não ser a primeira vez que sintomas semelhantes, embora menos graves, tenham ocorrido; a obtenção de um histórico clínico minucioso pode revelar episódios anteriores. Nos casos de HSA esplênico ou hepático, é provável que após a cessação da hemorragia aguda e a reabsorção do sangue da cavidade acometida os pacientes se recuperam e assumem aparência clinicamente normal, até que ocorra nova crise hemorrágica. Outros achados do histórico incluem anorexia, perda de peso, letargia, distensão abdominal, êmese, dispneia e vocalização.[4,5,20-22,26,27] Sinais clínicos semelhantes são notados em casos de HSA renal, às vezes com hematúria.[12] Pacientes com HSA cardíaco podem necessitar de atenção ainda mais urgente devido ao desenvolvimento de tamponamento cardíaco com risco de morte (ver Capítulo 254). Ao exame físico, os sinais clínicos em tais pacientes, semelhantes àqueles de insuficiência cardíaca direita, são secundários à efusão pericárdica. Especificamente, o abafamento de bulhas cardíacas e as arritmias secundárias são comumente notadas em pacientes com efusão pericárdica.[25-27] Embora a condição clínica interfira no prognóstico, pode ser necessário um retardo no estadiamento clínico completo, de modo a possibilitar a intervenção emergencial, com subsequente estadiamento realizado somente após a estabilização do quadro clínico do paciente. A manifestação clínica de casos de HSA do sistema nervoso central (SNC) pode variar amplamente, dependendo da localização do tumor, sendo as convulsões e as alterações de comportamento os sinais mais comuns (ver Capítulo 260).[16,17]

As manifestações cutâneas do HSA variam dependendo se a lesão é primariamente dérmica ou subcutânea (ver Capítulos 10 e 345). No HSA dérmico essas lesões são tipicamente pequenas, discretas e semelhantes a bolhas de sangue, enquanto no HSA subcutâneo são mais profundas, geralmente maiores e mais parecidas com tumores, com hematomas associados. O HSA intramuscular tipicamente se apresenta como uma grande massa tumoral ou com "efeito de massa", com edema distal associado e claudicação, quando ocorrem em um membro ou próximo a ele.[39,40,58-62] Metástases em locais externos e/ou internos são muito mais comuns nos casos de HSA subcutâneo e intramuscular do que HSA dérmico.[59-62]

DIAGNÓSTICO E ESTADIAMENTO

Embora o exame histopatológico da neoplasia seja o padrão-ouro para o diagnóstico desse tumor, geralmente obtém-se um diagnóstico presuntivo de HSA com base nos dados do histórico clínico, da resenha e do exame físico. Portanto, muitas vezes o estadiamento clínico completo é realizado antes mesmo da obtenção do diagnóstico histológico, quando a manifestação clínica é sugestiva de HSA. O estadiamento completo consiste em exames laboratoriais de rotina (hemograma, perfil bioquímico sérico, exame de urina e perfil de coagulação), radiografias do tórax em três projeções, ultrassonografia abdominal (ver Capítulo 88) e, se aplicável e disponível, ecocardiograma em vários planos de imagem (ver Capítulo 104). No diagnóstico e estadiamento dessa neoplasia também pode ser importante a realização de exames de imagem avançados e testes com novos biomarcadores. Os resultados do estadiamento clínico possibilitam a avaliação acurada do estágio da doença do paciente (Boxe 347.1), informação que ajudam a nortear o prognóstico e o protocolo terapêutico.

Exame histopatológico

Dependendo da lesão específica e da manifestação clínica, pode-se realizar exame histológico, enviando todo o órgão acometido, após remoção cirúrgica; massa tecidual de local externo (i. e., dérmica/subcutânea/intramuscular) obtida por meio de extirpação, ou mediante biopsia diagnóstica simples (i. e., por meio de incisão em cunha, ou de agulha/*tru-cut*) de lesões internas ou externas, se o procedimento é considerado clinicamente seguro. Histologicamente, o HSA é composto por canais vasculares irregulares que apresentam anastomose, delimitados por células fusiformes pleomórficas, com grandes cavidades multifocais preenchidas por sangue. Anisocariose e anisocitose acentuadas são comuns, e frequentemente nota-se um alto índice mitótico[1,2,9,18,19,26,39,40,58] (Figura 347.3). Uma causa clássica de frustação do clínico e do tutor está relacionada aos resultados clínicos e histopatológicos discordantes. Geralmente, essa situação pode estar associada ao envio de amostras pequenas ou em cunha, a partir de uma grande massa esplênica, para reduzir o gasto devido ao alto custo do envio de grande quantidade de formalina ou quando não há disponibilidade de um grande recipiente de formalina. Em tais casos, a amostra pode ser cortada em série ("fatias de pão"), de modo a possibilitar a fixação completa por formalina durante a noite, com remoção da formalina e envio do material envolvido por toalhas umedecidas com formalina, no dia seguinte. Ademais, embora o exame citológico seja um procedimento clinicamente valioso e não invasivo para o diagnóstico de câncer em geral, a sua importância no diagnóstico de HSA é relatada como baixa.[5,63,64] Entretanto, em alguns casos de tumor subcutâneo ou intramuscular, o exame citológico de esfregaços pode fornecer o diagnóstico, em vez do exame histopatológico (Figura 347.4).

Além dos achados histopatológicos, há diversos fatores cirúrgicos que devem ser ressaltados. Dada a natureza altamente metastática do HSA visceral e a influência do estágio da doença no prognóstico, quaisquer lesões suspeitas notadas no momento da cirurgia devem ser coletadas e submetidas a exame histológico. Um recente estudo retrospectivo de 79 cães avaliou a associação entre a aparência macroscópica de lesões hepáticas e os achados histológicos correspondentes em cães com HSA esplênico submetidos à laparotomia. Todas as amostras positivas para HSA foram obtidas de fígados macroscopicamente anormais; entretanto, 59% das lesões histologicamente benignas também foram obtidas de fígados histologicamente anormais. Ademais, somente 50% dos fígados macroscopicamente anormais apresentavam metástases de HSA; os diagnósticos relatados nos outros 50% dos casos incluíram hiperplasia nodular,

> **Boxe 347.1** Sistema de estadiamento clínico TNM de hemangiossarcoma em cães
>
> **T = Tumor (tumor primário)**
> T0 = Sem evidência de tumor
> T1 = Tumor restrito ao local primário e/ou à derme, com menos de 5 cm de diâmetro
> T2 = Tumor que invade o tecido SC e/ou com ≥ 5 cm de diâmetro
> T3 = Qualquer neoplasia T1 ou T2, com invasão tumoral de estruturas adjacentes e/ou músculo
>
> **N = Linfonodos (linfonodos regionais)**
> N0 = Sem evidência de envolvimento de linfonodos regionais
> N1 = Envolvimento de linfonodos regionais
> N2 = Envolvimento de linfonodos distantes
>
> **M = Metástases (distantes)**
> M0 = Sem evidência de metástase distante
> M1 = Metástases distantes
>
> **Estágios TNM**
> I = T0 ou T1, N0, M0
> II = T1 ou T2, N0 ou N1
> III = T2 ou T3, N0 ou N1 ou N2, M1

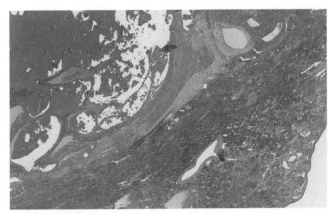

Figura 347.3 Amostra tecidual para exame histopatológico de um cão da raça Pastor-Alemão de 9 anos com hemangiossarcoma esplênico. Note que a arquitetura esplênica normal é substituída por massa tecidual com canais vasculares que formam anastomoses irregulares delimitadas por células fusiformes pleomórficas, com grandes cavidades multifocais preenchidas com sangue. As células fusiformes possuem margens celulares indistintas, pouco citoplasma eosinofílico e núcleos grandes, irregulares, ovais, hipercromáticos ou pontilhados, com nucléolos imperceptíveis. Anisocariose e anisocitose são moderadas a acentuadas, e são comuns figuras mitóticas atípicas. (Cortesia de Danielle Reel, DVM, DACVP, Eastern VetPath.)

degeneração hepática vacuolar, lipogranulomas, hematopoese extramedular e hemossiderose.[65] Fígados que tinham múltiplos nódulos e/ou lesões vermelho-escuras ou pretas mais provavelmente apresentavam HSA (Figura 347.5). Portanto, a presença de anormalidades hepáticas macroscópicas foi associada à alta sensibilidade (100%), porém com baixa especificidade e baixo valor preditivo positivo (VPP) (41 e 48%, respectivamente) para HSA, reafirmando a importância da confirmação histológica da neoplasia antes da tomada de decisão clínica. Ademais, embora não se deva superenfatizar que o diagnóstico definitivo de HSA pode ser confirmado apenas por exame histológico, um estudo recente que avaliou 65 cães submetidos à esplenectomia, incluindo 30 cães (46%) com HSA, constatou que tumores esplênicos maiores e baços mais pesados (como porcentagem do peso corporal), eram mais provavelmente benignos e menos provavelmente HSA.[66] Embora esses resultados sugiram que um tumores esplênicos maiores, com base em maior proporção volume do tumor:volume do baço, e baço mais pesado (em porcentagem do peso molecular) podem ser úteis para diferenciação entre hemangiossarcoma e lesões benignas em cães que apresentam neoplasias esplênicas, sem realização de tentativas de determinar a sensibilidade ou especificidade dessas variáveis ou de identificar os melhores pontos de corte (valores limiares) no estudo referenciado.

Avaliação laboratorial

Em pacientes com HSA podem ser verificadas diversas anormalidades no hemograma, sendo a anemia a mais comum. Geralmente a anemia é regenerativa e com presença de esquisócitos, acantócitos e hemácias nucleadas, compatíveis com dano relacionado à microangiopatia secundária à vasculite, insuficiência hepática, deficiência do sistema reticuloendotelial e hemorragia aguda.[67-71] Leucocitose por neutrofilia é outra anormalidade hematológica comum e foi postulada como resultado de uma síndrome paraneoplásica e/ou necrose que ocorre em grandes neoplasias e em tumores de rápido crescimento.[27,72] Pesquisas mais recentes sugerem que essa neutrofilia (e geralmente monocitose) associada ao tumor pode ser parcialmente compostas de células supressoras de linhagem mieloide (CSLM), um subgrupo de granulócitos responsáveis pela supressão da imunidade antitumoral inata e associado a um mal prognóstico, em algumas neoplasias.[73-76] Em até 75% dos cães com HSA nota-se trombocitopenia, que pode ser decorrência de hemorragia tumoral, destruição via ligações cruzadas de fibrina nos vasos sanguíneos da neoplasia, ou coagulopatias por consumo de plaquetas secundárias, como acontece na coagulação intravascular disseminada (CID; ver Capítulo 197), relatada em até 50% dos cães com hemangiossarcoma.[27,70,71] Como consequência da CID pode haver anormalidades no perfil de coagulação (tempo de protrombina, tempo de tromboplastina parcial, produtos de degradação de fibrina[ogênio], fibrinogênio, D-Dímero; ver Capítulo 196). O perfil bioquímico sérico e o exame de urina raramente auxiliam no diagnóstico de HSA por terem baixa especificidade, embora em um estudo, constatou-se que 53% dos gatos com HSA visceral apresentavam aumento da atividade de aspartato aminotransferase (AST).[38]

Outros testes diagnósticos auxiliares mais recentes podem auxiliar no diagnóstico precoce de HSA, já que a maioria dos pacientes provavelmente terá disseminação metastática microscópica no momento do diagnóstico histológico. Trabalhos iniciais com citometria de fluxo demonstraram capacidade de identificar células de linhagem específica que se expressam simultaneamente com alguns marcadores de superfície celular detectados em grande quantidade no sangue periférico de cães com HSA, comparativamente àqueles de cães saudáveis do grupo controle ou cães que livres de HSA mensurável após extirpação cirúrgica.[6]

Diagnóstico por imagem

Tipicamente, para detecção de doença metastática, são realizadas radiografias do tórax em três projeções – laterais direita e esquerda, e ventrodorsal. A aparência radiográfica típica da doença pulmonar metastática mensurável é a de um padrão miliar coalescente; entretanto, também pode-se observar padrão intersticial miliar nodular ou generalizado (Figura 347.6). Em um estudo comparativo entre radiografia torácica e achados pós-morte em cães com HSA comprovado por exame histológico constatou-se que a sensibilidade radiográfica foi de 78% e o valor preditivo negativo foi de 74%, para casos de HSA pulmonar metastático.[77]

A ultrassonografia abdominal é uma das modalidades de imagem mais comumente utilizada em medicina veterinária, sendo prontamente capaz de detectar efusões, lesões hepáticas

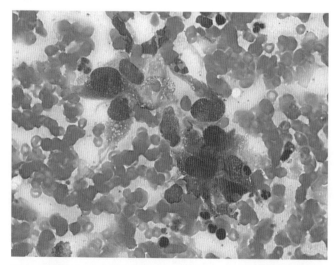

Figura 347.4 Preparação citológica de aspirado por agulha fina do baço de um cão da raça Golden Retriever, macho castrado, de 6 anos, com hemangiossarcoma esplênico e metástase pulmonar. Note o agregado de células fusiformes ou de formato irregular, com citoplasma ligeiramente basofílico, com alguns vacúolos pontilhados. Os núcleos são ovais ou de formato irregular e exibem anisocariose moderada. Objetiva de 50×/aumento de 500×. (Cortesia de Casey J. LeBlanc, DVM, PhD, DACVP, Eastern VetPath.) (*Esta figura se encontra reproduzida em cores no Encarte.*)

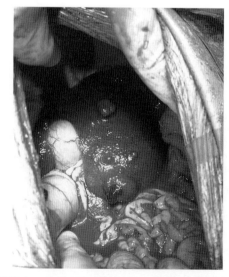

Figura 347.5 Imagem intraoperatória da cavidade peritoneal em Golden Retriever de 10 anos apresentando hemangiossarcoma secundário no abdome. Notam-se lesões múltiplas, elevadas e vermelho-escuras ao longo do fígado, algumas das quais estavam sangrando ativamente. (Cortesia de Julius Liptak, BVSc, MVetLinStud, FACVSc, DACVS, DECVS.) (*Esta figura se encontra reproduzida em cores no Encarte.*)

e esplênicas, assim como lesões metastáticas no omento, dependendo da habilidade do operador. O hemangiossarcoma pode ter várias diferentes características ecogênicas (anecoicas a hipoecoicas, ou mistas) e frequentemente possui áreas de cavitação (Figura 347.7).[78] Técnicas mais avançadas, como ultrassonografia harmônica contrastada, que pode avaliar a dinâmica da perfusão tecidual, podem ser promissoras.[79,80] Um estudo demonstrou melhora do valor diagnóstico de casos de HSA hepático por detectar nódulos não observados no exame ultrassonográfica tradicional, em escala de cinza.[80] Diversos estudos que avaliaram lesões esplênicas demonstraram que a hipoecogenicidade da lesão esplênica durante as fases vasculares precoce e tardia está altamente associada à malignidade.[81-83]

Sem dúvidas, a presença de hemoabdômen agudo (ver Capítulo 143), juntamente com achados ultrassonográficos de tumor esplênico, é altamente sugestivo de HSA. Em um estudo que avaliou 39 cães com hemoabdômen não traumático agudo, verificou-se que 80% deles eram secundários a neoplasias viscerais, dos quais 70% foram confirmados como HSA.[20] Em um segundo estudo que avaliou uma população semelhante de 60 cães, o HSA foi confirmado em 63% dos cães.[22] Embora esses dados possam ser considerados convincentes, o autor acredita que nenhum paciente com hemoabdômen deve ser submetido à eutanásia com base em lesões esplênicas ou hepáticas "compatíveis com HSA", pois várias lesões esplênicas não malignas, como hematomas, parecem semelhantes no exame ultrassonográfico e apresentam prognóstico muito bom a excelente, apenas com a realização de esplenectomia.[8,18,19] Como mencionado anteriormente, um estudo recente que avaliou anormalidades hepáticas presentes no momento da esplenectomia, em casos de HSA esplênico, constatou que apenas 50% dos cães que apresentavam fígados macroscopicamente anormais tinham evidências histológicas de metástase hepática.[65]

Alguns grupos de pesquisadores estão investigando combinações de parâmetros clínicos e laboratoriais, juntamente com achados ultrassonográficos, na tentativa de aumentar a confiança no diagnóstico de HSA, antes da cirurgia. Um estudo desse porte avaliou a prevalência de HSA esplênico em 71 cães anêmicos que apresentavam neoplasia esplênica e hemoperitônio, a fim de identificar fatores que possibilitassem diferenciar cães com HSA e com outros tumores esplênicos no momento da admissão hospitalar. Em 76% dos cães foram identificadas neoplasias esplênicas malignas, dos quais 92,6% tinham HSA; notou-se correlação significativa entre o diagnóstico de HSA e baixa concentração sérica de proteína total e trombocitopenia.[21]

O ecocardiograma ainda é o procedimento preferido para a detecção de tumores cardíacos (átrio/aurícula direita); a presença de efusão pericárdica facilita a detecção desses tumores (ver Capítulo 254 e Vídeo 347.1).[84,85] Seu uso para o estadiamento de rotina de HSA inicialmente detectado em outros locais é considerado controverso, já que de forma geral a detecção de lesões concomitantes é baixa.[29] Entretanto, o ecocardiograma também pode ser utilizado como procedimento de triagem antes do início da quimioterapia com doxorrubicina, a fim de avaliar a função cardíaca em raças sujeitas à cardiomiopatia dilatada; portanto, seu valor para tais pacientes com HSA pode ser duplo.[86] Ademais, do ponto de vista cardíaco, arritmias ventriculares perioperatórias foram documentadas em até 44% dos cães submetidos à esplenectomia, em casos de HSA.[25,87-89] É possível que as arritmias ventriculares em cães com neoplasia esplênica se devam ao comprometido do retorno venoso ao coração, micrometástases no coração e/ou CID, e foram associadas de forma significativa à ruptura do tumor e anemia. Vários cães que desenvolvem arritmias cardíacas nos períodos pré-operatório e pós-cirúrgico poderiam não ser clinicamente afetados diretamente por essas anormalidades, e geralmente seu tratamento pode consistir no controle de fatores desencadeadores de arritmias (p. ex., tratamento de anemia com transfusões sanguíneas, ou correção de desequilíbrios de eletrólitos do soro sanguíneo), em vez da terapia antiarrítmica (ver Capítulo 248). Em um estudo, verificou-se que os cães que desenvolveram arritmias intraoperatórias tiveram uma razão de probabilidade de morte maior que o dobro daquela de cães que não apresentavam arritmias intraoperatórias.[89] A resolução de arritmias perioperatórias deve ser confirmada antes da liberação do paciente e subsequentes tratamentos adjuvantes, já que em um pequeno número de casos elas podem representar disfunção cardíaca primária, uma importante contraindicação para quimioterapia com doxorrubicina.[90]

Com o maior acesso a técnicas de imagem mais avançadas, tanto a tomografia computadorizada (TC) quanto a ressonância magnética (RM) podem ser utilizadas para avaliação de HSA subcutâneo, intramuscular, cardíaco, esplênico e hepático. TC e RM podem auxiliar na determinação da exata origem anatômica, bem como a extensão e disseminação da doença, auxiliando, assim, no planejamento da ressecção cirúrgica e/ou de radioterapia.[91] Ademais, tanto RM quanto TC possuem alta

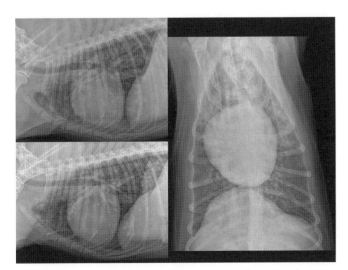

Figura 347.6 Radiografias do tórax em três projeções de uma cadela da raça Labrador Retriever castrada, de 12 anos. Notam-se diversos nódulos de tecidos moles pequenos, pouco a bem delimitados, disseminados por todo o pulmão, condição compatível com hemangiossarcoma metastático. (Cortesia de Chris Ryan, VMD, DABVP, DACVR.)

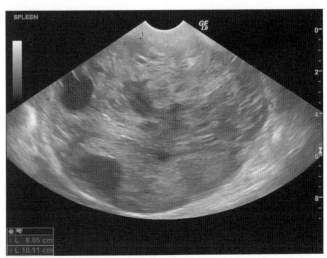

Figura 347.7 Imagem ultrassonográfica do abdome de um cão, macho, sem raça definida, castrado, atendido por apresentar colapso agudo secundário ao hemoabdome. Note uma grande massa tecidual de ecogenicidade mista, com múltiplas cavitações centrais que se sobrepõem à arquitetura esplênica normal e ocupa a maior parte da imagem. (Cortesia de Chris Ryan, VMD, DABVP, DACVR.)

sensibilidade e especificidade para diferenciar lesões esplênicas e hepáticas benignas e malignas (Figura 347.8).[92,93] Também, foi documentado alta sensibilidade da TC do tórax para detecção precoce de metástases pulmonares.[94,95] Com a redução dos custos para realização desses procedimentos, eles logo devem se tornar comuns no estadiamento de rotina de cães com HSA.

Biomarcadores

O uso de biomarcadores específicos para HSA pode ser clinicamente útil não somente para possibilitar a detecção e intervenção precoces, mas também para monitorar a condição da doença do paciente durante e após o tratamento. Diversos estudos recentes avaliaram tais marcadores no sangue e efusões de cães com HSA. A troponina I cardíaca (xcRnI) provou ser um marcador altamente específico e sensível para dano de cardiomiócitos (ver Capítulo 246).[96,97] Uma pesquisa recente mostrou que a concentração plasmática mediana de cTnI em cães com HSA cardíaco foi significativamente maior do que em cães com hemangiossarcomas em outros locais, em cães com outras neoplasias, e em cães com efusão pericárdica não causada por hemangiossarcoma (ver Capítulo 254). Especificamente, o aumento da concentração de cTnI pode detectar o envolvimento cardíaco em cães com HSA em qualquer local (sensibilidade: 78%; especificidade: 71%), bem como detectar HSA cardíaco em cães com efusão pericárdica (sensibilidade: 81%; especificidade: 100%).[96] De forma semelhante, a concentração sérica de peptídio colágeno XXVII foi mensurada no soro de cães com hemangiossarcoma e constatou-se que a concentração em cães com grandes cargas tumorais foi 9,5 vezes maior do que aquela de cães saudáveis.[97] Foi proposto que a elevação pode estar relacionadas à clivagem ou degradação da proteína no tecido circundante, ou estar associada ao comportamento invasivo ou a processos angiogênicos. De forma interessante, a concentração do peptídio do colágeno XXVII em cães com outras formas de neoplasias (osteossarcoma, linfoma, carcinoma) e com doenças inflamatórias também estava aumentada, mas os valores eram consistentemente menores do que aqueles verificados em casos de HSA. A redução da concentração do peptídio do colágeno XXVII após ressecção cirúrgica de HSA e subsequente aumento após recidiva do tumor mostram que esse peptídio pode ser um biomarcador útil de HSA.[97] Outro marcador avaliado em cães com HSA é a enzima citosólica timidina quinase (TK1), cuja atividade está intimamente relacionada à síntese e expressão de DNA restrita às células em proliferação.[99] Um estudo recente demonstrou que a atividade sérica de TK1 foi significativamente maior no soro sanguíneo de cães com HSA quando comparados àquele de cães saudáveis. A TK1 sérica foi então avaliada prospectivamente em 62 cães com hemoabdômen secundário a um tumor esplênico benigno ou a HSA. Estatisticamente, não se constatou diferença na atividade média de TK1, mas foi possível notar diferença entre os dois grupos quando se utilizou um sistema de corte em camada específico.[99]

TRATAMENTO E PROGNÓSTICO

Tratamento local

Cirurgia

A cirurgia ainda é a base do tratamento de HSA; também foram relatadas esplenectomia, lobectomia hepática, nefrectomia, extirpação de tumores dérmicos, subcutâneos, intramusculares ou retroperitoneais, e auriculectomia direita. Tais cirurgias são realizadas para remover os tumores macroscópicos e prevenir maior risco de hemorragia aguda, CID e morte. O prognóstico pós-cirúrgico de HSA depende muito da localização do tumor, do estadiamento, da extirpação completa e do uso de terapias adjuvantes.

Especificamente, o HSA cutâneo, limitado à derme sem invasão hipodérmica (diferentemente de lesões subcutâneas/intramusculares), possui taxa metastática inferior e geralmente pode ser submetido apenas ao tratamento cirúrgico. Após extirpação de HSA dérmico em cães constatou-se sobrevida mediana (SM) de 780 a 987 dias.[58,59] Em um estudo de 94 cães verificou-se que raças predispostas, com tumoral ventral localizado e alterações histológicas solares tiveram sobrevida ainda mais longa. O desenvolvimento de metástases de tumores com invasão subcutânea é mais provável. Fato interessante nesse estudo é que mesmo com o relato de sobrevida a longo prazo, notou-se recidiva local regional em 77% dos cães.[59] Esses dados de sobrevida estão em contraste brutal àqueles relatados para tumores com envolvimento subcutâneo ou intramuscular, nos quais foram relatadas SM de 172 e 307 dias, respectivamente.[58] Em casos de HSA subcutâneo ou intramuscular, a extirpação cirúrgica deve ser a mais minuciosa possível, de modo a obter amplas margens cirúrgicas. Às vezes, a extirpação parcial ou com margens estreitas requer amputação do membro ou uso de radioterapia adjuvante, pois a taxa de recidiva local de HSA inadequadamente extirpados é substancial.[59,60,62] Ademais, por conta do alto risco associada à sobrevida a longo prazo relacionado ao HSA subcutâneo/intramuscular, para essa particular apresentação do tumor também se justifica terapia sistêmica adjuvante. Relata-se que gatos com HSA cutâneo tratados com excisão cirúrgica apresentam SM de ≈ 9 meses a 4 anos.[35,36] Semelhante à situação em cães, o HSA felino com envolvimento subcutâneo foi associado à extirpação incompleta, maior taxa de metástases e eutanásia devido ao tumor.[35,36]

Por conta do alto risco de metástase, os casos de HSA visceral (mais comumente esplênico primário) considera-se a cirurgia como paliativa, e associada à sobrevida mediana de apenas 19 a 86 dias, para cães submetidos apenas à esplenectomia, e 77 dias para gatos submetidos à laparotomia.[1-5,34,100] Portanto, a quimioterapia adjuvante, discutida anteriormente, é recomendada após a cirurgia para praticamente todas as formas de HAS visceral.

Para cães com HSA cardíaco, tipicamente a extirpação cirúrgica do tumor é impossível devido à localização de difícil acesso, ou não é indicada devido aos riscos e/ou ao prognóstico mal a grave. Entretanto, há alguns relatos de caso e de séries de casos que mencionam sobrevida longa após a excisão do tumor.[101-106] Pericardectomia por meio de toracotomia ou toracoscopia é realizada mais comumente e pode aliviar o tamponamento cardíaco com risco à vida, mas é improvável que prolongue significativamente a sobrevida quando utilizada isoladamente (ver Capítulo 254).[107]

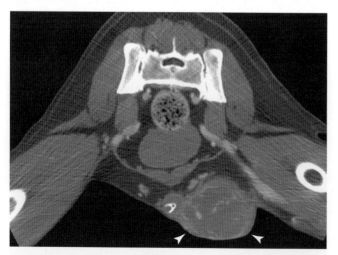

Figura 347.8 Imagens obtidas em tomografia computadorizada de um hemangiossarcoma subcutâneo em um cão da raça Boxer, macho, de 9 anos. A imagem transversa na altura da pelve mostra uma grande massa tecidual subcutânea na região inguinal esquerda (*pontas de seta*). Em sua periferia a massa é exacerbada de modo heterogêneo pelo contraste, sem que isso ocorra na região central; ademais, há exacerbação de diversos septos irregulares e espessos pelo contraste. (Cortesia de Chris Ryan VMD, DABVP, DACVR.)

CAPÍTULO 347 • Hemangiossarcoma

Embora sendo uma variante incomum, o HSA renal primário sem evidência de hemoperitônio ou metástase pode ter prognóstico mais favorável quando tratada apenas com cirurgia. Em um estudo de 14 cães com HSA renal constatou-se que por ocasião da consulta, a maioria dos pacientes apresentava doença localizada e 10 foram tratados somente com a cirurgia. Verificou-se SM de 286 dias em cães submetidos apenas ao tratamento cirúrgico (n = 10); mesmo assim, 10 de 14 cães morreram em decorrência do HSA.[12] O HSA é o diagnóstico histológico mais comum em casos de sarcomas retroperitoneais em cães e é extremamente agressivo localmente, possui alta taxa de invasão local e metástases, e dessa forma, está associado à sobrevida baixa, mesmo quando submetido à terapia multimodal.[13]

Radioterapia

Devido à predileção do HSA por locais anatômicos inacessíveis, sua manifestação frequentemente aguda e sua alta taxa metastática, o uso de radioterapia para HSA tem sido limitado. Um estudo de 20 cães com HSA não esplênico mensurável confirmado no exame histológico, tratados com RT paliativa, demonstrou redução subjetiva do tamanho do tumor em 14 cães (70%), com quatro respostas completas e SM de 95 dias.[108] Esses resultados são encorajadores, sendo necessária uma maior validação com protocolos de combinação terapias consistindo em RT e quimioterapia sistêmica. Ademais, embora não ainda formalmente avaliada ou relatada, também pode ser importante na aplicação de plesioterapia com estrôncio-90 em HSA dérmico pequeno e superficial, pois demonstrou propiciar alta taxa de resposta completa e controle tumoral a longo prazo em outros tipos de neoplasias superficiais.[109]

Terapias sistêmicas

Quimioterapia convencional

A doxorrubicina (DOX) parece ser o antineoplásico mais efetivo e até o momento foi o medicamento que propiciou a melhor extensão da sobrevida pós-esplenectomia. Protocolos comuns consistem no uso de DOX como agente único; da combinação de DOX e ciclofosfamida (protocolo AC); da combinação de vincristina, DOX e ciclofosfamida (protocolo VAC); e da combinação de DOX e ifosfamida.[110-114] A sobrevida mediana depende do estágio da doença e tipicamente estão na faixa de 5 a 7 meses, com os protocolos já mencionados à base de DOX. Em um estudo prospectivo recente comparando os protocolos AC e DOX/DTIC em 27 cães com HSA em diversos locais (20/27 esplênicos), relatou-se SM geral de 142 dias para 18 cães tratados com protocolo AC; a SM de nove cães tratados com DOX/DTIC foi maior que 550 dias.[115] Entretanto, o pequeno número de cães do grupo DOX/DTIC levanta a questão sobre a real significado desses resultados. Um estudo mais antigo que avaliou o uso de muramil tripeptídio fosfatidiletanolamina (L-MTP-PE), um imunomodulador oriundo da parede de célula micobacteriana que aumenta a ação tumoricida dos monócitos, juntamente com a DOX, relatou as maiores sobrevidas até hoje; todos os cães que receberam DOX/L-MTP-PE apresentaram sobrevida mediana de 277 dias, sendo que a SM de cães em estágio clínico I que receberam a combinação foi de 425 dias.[116] Infelizmente, o L-MTP-PE não está mais disponível para uso clínico. Portanto, na ausência de L-MTP-PE, é incerto se qualquer dos protocolos remanescentes à base de DOX é realmente superior aos demais (Tabela 347.1).

Tentou-se aumentar a SM relatada com o uso de protocolo com a DOX como agente único, com dose maior,, juntamente com a administração intravenosa (IV) e intraperitoneal (IP) da forma de DOX encapsulada em lipossomo (Doxil®), mas essa tentativa não resultou em benefício significativo no aumento da sobrevida.[117-119] Entretanto, de forma interessante, os cães submetidos à administração IP tiveram menores taxas de metástases em membranas serosas, mesentério e omento do que os animais dos grupos controles históricos tratados com doxorrubicina sistêmica.[119]

A epirrubicina, um esteroisômero da doxorrubicina, foi desenvolvida na tentativa de minimizar a cardiotoxicidade em pessoas, e foi avaliada em cães. Em um estudo de 18 cães que receberam epirrubicina após esplenectomia constatou-se SM de 144 dias.[120] A epirrubicina foi associada à maior taxa de efeitos colaterais gastrintestinais, geralmente necessitando de hospitalização, do que a taxa de tais efeitos colaterais comumente observados com a monoterapia com DOX. Independentemente disso, esse medicamento pode ser uma boa alternativa aos pacientes que apresentam cardiomiopatia preexistente. Ademais, em um pequeno estudo, administrou-se ifosfamida a seis cães com HSA, após esplenectomia, resultando em SM comparável de 147 dias.[121]

Para cães com HSA subcutâneo ou intramuscular, a quimioterapia geralmente é utilizada no pós-operatório, a fim de evitar taxa metastática considerável. De acordo com diversos estudos, o prognóstico de cães com doença em estágios menos avançados e com tumores menos sujeitos à propagação local parece ser melhor.[58,60,62] De forma interessante, os resultados de dois estudos retrospectivos recentes que avaliaram cães submetidos à terapia local seguida de terapia adjuvante com doxorrubicina foram bastante diferentes. No primeiro estudo, relata-se sobrevida mediana de 1.189 dias para cães submetidos à cirurgia e doxorrubicina adjuvante, com ou sem radioterapia, para HSA subcutâneo não metastático (n = 17) e 272,5 dias para cães que receberam tratamento semelhante para HSA intramuscular não metastático (n = 4).[60] O segundo estudo, que avaliou 71 cães (HSA subcutâneo n = 55, HSA intramuscular n = 16) relatou sobrevida geral de 246 dias para aqueles que foram submetidos a controle local adequado de tumores menores (< 4 cm), sem metástase.[62] As possíveis causas dessa discrepância pode envolver a terminologia utilizada para HSA cutâneo e subcutâneo (no primeiro estudo, cães com HSA cutâneo primário com extensão subcutânea podem ter sido incluídos, enquanto o segundo estudo incluiu somente aqueles cães com tumores que surgiam do espaço subcutâneo e excluíram aqueles com HSA cutâneo primário) e o pequeno número de cães em cada grupo.

A SM de cães com HSA cardíaco (ver Capítulo 254) permanece notadamente inferior aquela verificada nos casos de manifestação esplênica, provavelmente devido à dificuldade em obter controle local do tumor cardíaco, comparativamente ao HSA originado em outros locais anatômicos. Entretanto, quando a extirpação cirúrgica é viável e combinada com quimioterapia adjuvante, pode ser possível sobrevida comparável àquela alcançada após esplenectomia e quimioterapia. Especificamente, um estudo recente que avaliou 23 cães com HSA cardíaco constatou SM de 42 dias em cães tratados somente com cirurgia *versus* 175 dias em cães que receberam quimioterapia adjuvante.[122] Quando a biopsia cirúrgica não é possível, o diagnóstico de HSA cardíaco se torna apenas presuntivo. Somente recentemente foram disponibilizados alguns dados sobre os resultados obtidos em pacientes submetidos à quimioterapia para HSA macroscópico presumivelmente cardíaco. Um pequeno estudo de 16 cães com neoplasia de átrio direito tratados com DOX como agente único ou em combinação com ciclofosfamida, ifosfamida ou dacarbazina, documentou SM de 140 dias.[123] Um segundo estudo retrospectivo mais amplo avaliou 64 cães tratados com protocolo padronizado de DOX como agente único. A taxa de resposta objetiva foi de 41% e a taxa de resposta biológica (respostas mensuráveis mais doença estável), ou "benefício clínico", foi de 68%. A SM de cães tratados foi de 116 dias e foi significativamente maior, comparada à SM de 12 dias de 76 cães do grupo controle atual não tratados.[124]

Pacientes atendidos com HSA sem possibilidade de ressecção ou em estágios avançados da neoplasia representam um desafio terapêutico e há poucas informações sobre o tratamento desses pacientes em grande escala. Devido à possibilidade de mal

Tabela 347.1 Sobrevida mediana selecionada relativa a diversos tratamentos de cães com hemangiossarcoma.

LOCALIZAÇÃO DO TUMOR	TRATAMENTO	SM* (DIAS)	REFERÊNCIAS
Baço	Esplenectomia	19 a 86	1, 2, 10, 100
	Esplenectomia + VAC	140 a 145	10, 113, 126
	Esplenectomia + AC	140[‡] a 180	112, 115, 116
	Esplenectomia + AC + L-MTP-PE	277	116
	Esplenectomia + LDC	178	127
	Esplenectomia + EPI	144	120
	Esplenectomia + A	172 a 210[†]	117, 118
	Esplenectomia + A + VAX	182	145
	Esplenectomia + A/DER	150	111
	Esplenectomia + DOXIL (IV)	166	118
	Esplenectomia + DOXIL (IP)	131	119
	Esplenectomia + IFOS	147	121
	Esplenectomia + A/IFOS	123	114
	Esplenectomia + A/DTIC	> 550[§]	115
	Esplenectomia + A + TOC	172	151
	Esplenectomia + PSP	117 a 199	154
Coração	Pericardectomia + ressecção do tumor	42 a 120	25, 122
	Pericardectomia + ressecção do tumor + A	175	122
	A[ǁ]	139,5	123
	A	116	124
Rim	Nefrectomia, com ou sem quimioterapia	278	12
Retroperitoneal	Diversos	37,5[¶]	13
Cutâneo	Ressecção do tumor	780 a 987	58, 59
Subcutâneo (SC)	Cirurgia	172	58
	Cirurgia + A, com ou sem RT	1189	60
	A	140,5	61
Intramuscular (IM)	Ressecção do tumor	302	58
	Ressecção do tumor + A, com ou sem RT	272,5	60
Miscelânea Misto SC/IM	Variável	172	62
	Ressecção do tumor + quimio, com ou sem RT	246	62
Diversos (não esplênicos)	RT	89	108
Diversos (incluindo esplênicos)	Ressecção do tumor + A	60 a 172	110
	Ressecção do tumor + AC	202	112
	Ressecção do tumor + AC + MINO	170	134
Diversos em estágio avançado (metastático e/ou inoperável)	VAC, com ou sem ressecção do tumor	195	126
	DAV	125	125

*Não separado por estágio da doença. [†]Apenas dados do estágio II esplênico. [‡]Somente 15 de 18 cães tinham HSA esplênico. [§]Somente 5 de 9 cães tinham HSA esplênico. [ǁ]Vários protocolos à base de DOX. [¶]Somente 9 de 14 cães tinham HSA. *A*, adriamicina; *C*, ciclofosfamida; *DER*, deracoxibe; *doxil*, doxorrubicina pegilada encapsulada em lipossomo; *DTIC*, dacarbazina; *epi*, epirrubicina; *HSA*, hemangiossarcoma; *IFOS*, ifosfamida; *LDC*, quimioterapia em baixa dose (ciclofosfamida, etoposida, piroxicam); *L-MTP-PE*, muramil tripeptídio fosfatidiletanolamina lipossômico; *PSP*, polissacaropeptídio (*Coriolus versicolor*); *ref*, referências; *RT*, radioterapia; *SM*, sobrevida mediana; *TOC*, fosfato de toceranib; *V*, vincristina; *VAX*, vacina de lisado tumoral.

prognóstico, os pacientes frequentemente não são tratados; entretanto, há dados que sugerem que um subgrupo pode responder à terapia. Um estudo de 18 cães que receberam quimioterapia à base de DOX para HSA subcutâneo sem possibilidade de ressecção relatou taxa de resposta de 38% para uma duração mediana de apenas 53 dias.[66] Assim, esse procedimento pode ser um tratamento mais paliativo ou uma possível terapia neoadjuvante, para diminuir o tamanho do tumor, a fim de facilitar possível ressecção. Um protocolo terapêutico mais intensivo combinando dacarbazina, DOX e vincristina (protocolo DAV) foi avaliado em 24 cães com HSA inoperável em estágio avançado, relatando-se taxa de resposta de 47,4%, incluindo cinco respostas completas e quatro parciais.[125] Nesse estudo, o tempo mediano de progressão do tumor foi de 101 dias. Outro estudo retrospectivo avaliou 67 cães em estágio III (n = 25) ou estágio I/II (n= 42) submetidos a protocolo quimioterápico.[126] Dos 25 cães em estágio III, a localização do tumor primário variou,

mas notou-se predileção pelo baço (n = 11), tecido subcutâneo (n = 5), e átrio direito (n = 4). A SM geral para os 67 cães foi de 189 dias; fato interessante foi que não houve diferença significativa entre a SM entre o estágio III (195 dias) e estágio I/II (189 dias). Os dados de resposta relativos a 28 cães e a taxa de resposta objetiva geral para esses pacientes foi de 86%.[126]

Quimioterapia metronômica

Está ocorrendo uma modificação no paradigma da administração de quimioterapia. Especificamente, o uso de quimioterapia metronômica (baixa dose, contínua) está se tornando mais comum e foi avaliado em cães com HSA.[127] A quimioterapia convencional tipicamente envolve o uso de ciclos ("pulsos" ou "picos" de quimioterapia administrada na dose máxima tolerada (DMT), com longos intervalos, a fim de possibilitar que as células normais se recuperem do dano causado pelo quimioterápico. Diferentemente, a quimioterapia metronômica consiste na administração contínua (tipicamente 1 vez/dia) de quimioterápicos em dose bem abaixo da DMT, sem intervalos longos sem o uso do medicamento.[127-131] Uma característica-chave da quimioterapia metronômica é a redução do protocolo de administração do antineoplásico, com dose cumulativa significativamente menor do que a utilizada na quimioterapia à base de DMT, o que deve resultar em um perfil de toxicidade mais favorável e a possibilidade de administração a longo prazo, sem interrupção. Diferentemente da quimioterapia com DMT, na qual as células tumorais são os principais alvos do tratamento, a terapia metronômica parece almejar as células que sustentam e nutrem o tumor. Nesse contexto, os quimioterápicos podem atuar como agentes antiangiogênicos.[127-131] Os mecanismos de ação incluem apoptose direta de células endoteliais em fase de multiplicação, supressão da mobilização das células progenitoras endoteliais circulantes (PEC) oriundas da medula óssea, e maior produção de inibidores naturais da angiogênese pelo próprio organismo.[127-131] Ademais, a quimioterapia metronômica demonstrou inibir seletivamente e causar depleção de linfócitos T reguladores (Treg), diminuindo desta forma a tolerância imune.[127-131] Um estudo piloto avaliou um protocolo metronômico que consistia em ciclofosfamida, etoposida e piroxicam em nove cães com HSA em estágio II submetidos à esplenectomia. Constatou-se SM de 178 dias, comparado favoravelmente à SM de 133 dias de 24 cães com HSA em estágio II submetidos à esplenectomia e cinco doses de DOX adjuvante.[127] Não foram notados efeitos adversos graves nos cães tratados com o protocolo de quimioterapia metronômica. Além disso, cães com hemangiossarcoma primário macroscópico e metastático tratados com lomustina (CCNU) metronômica tiveram sobrevida mediana de 120 dias, sem respostas mensuráveis, de fato, documentadas.[132] Em outro estudo, a administração de baixas doses de clorambucila resultou em doença estável em três de cinco cães com HSA macroscópico.[133] Por fim, a minociclina é um antibiótico com discreta ação antiangiogênica que mostrou ser seguro em combinação com quimioterapia AC adjuvante, em cães com HSA. Entretanto, não se verificou aumento da sobrevida, em comparação aos animais do grupo controle.[134]

Inibidores da ciclo-oxigenase

As ciclo-oxigenases (COX) catalisam as etapas iniciais que limitam a velocidade da conversão do ácido araquidônico em prostaglandinas e tromboxanos. Foram identificadas duas isoformas dessa enzima: COX-1 e COX-2. Pesquisas mostraram que a COX-2 tem importância relevante no desenvolvimento e progressão do câncer e, dessa forma, representa um novo alvo à terapia antineoplásica.[135-139] Inibidores da COX-2 são comumente utilizados como parte de protocolos metronômicos e possuem atividade documentada como medicamentos únicos para alguns tipos de câncer, especificamente carcinomas.[138-142] Diferentemente da maioria dos carcinomas de cães pesquisados até o momento, parece que em cães o HSA tipicamente não expressam excessivamente COX-2.[143] Entretanto, como anti-inflamatórios não esteroides inibidores da COX-2 apresentam eficácia clínica contra outros tumores que não expressam excessivamente COX-2 é razoável utilizá-los, ambos, como parte da quimioterapia metronômica[127] e em combinação com a quimioterapia convencional para HSA. De fato, a adição de um inibidor seletivo de COX-2, o deracoxibe, foi avaliado como parte de um protocolo para cães com HSA tratados com protocolo padrão com DOX.[111] Notou-se sobrevida mediana geral de 150 dias e os cães com doença em estágio III tiveram sobrevida mediana de 149 dias, que é mais longa do que a previamente relatada para cães com manifestação mais avançada da doença.[111]

Tratamentos recentes

Imunoterapia

A imunoterapia tem sido por muito tempo um campo de pesquisa ativa na medicina oncológica humana e mais recentemente está cada vez mais empregada em oncologia veterinária (ver Capítulo 341). Os protocolos de imunoterapia incluem modificadores da resposta biológica, citocinas recombinantes e vacinas tumorais.[144] Foi publicado um pequeno número de estudos sobre imunoterapia em cães com HSA. Por exemplo, avaliou-se o uso de uma vacina tumoral recente, juntamente com DOX, em 28 cães com diversas manifestações de HSA. A vacina consistia em lisados oriundos da linhagem celular do HSA canino alogênico misturados com um adjuvante composto de complexo DNA/lipossomo. Os cães vacinados apresentaram alta resposta de anticorpos contra células do HSA canino, mas essa resposta não aumentou a sobrevida, com sobrevida mediana de 182 dias, em 13 cães com HSA esplênico em estágio II que receberam a vacina tumoral, juntamente com quimioterapia com DOX.[145] A combinação do protocolo AC com o imunomodulador L-MTP-PE resultou em um aumento significativo na sobrevida livre da doença e na sobrevida geral (277 dias), comparativamente aos cães que receberam quimioterapia com lipossomos placebos.[116] Essa melhora foi mais evidente em cães que por ocasião da consulta apresentavam HSA em estágio I, enquanto cães com HSA em estágio II não pareceram ter benefício adicional significativo da sobrevida, além daquela obtida somente com quimioterapia à base de DOX.[116] Como mencionado anteriormente, no momento não há disponibilidade de L-MTP-PE no mercado, fato que limita o seu uso clínico.

Terapia molecular direcionada

Compreensivelmente, dada a incapacidade de protocolos quimioterápicos e imunoterapêuticos melhorarem a recuperação de cães com HSA visceral, o potencial para o uso de terapias mais direcionadas propicia uma nova área de pesquisa para essa doença (ver Capítulo 342). A exploração da natureza angiogênica desse tipo de câncer é um dos caminhos, e a análise das linhagens celulares do HSA canino, de amostras tumorais, e de amostras de sangue/efusão de cães com a doença são vias angiogênicas ativas.[6,7,46,48] Ademais, foi documentada a expressão de receptores de tirosinoquinase, inclusive do receptor do fator de células-tronco (KIT), receptor do fator de crescimento derivado de plaquetas (PDGFR), e membros da família do receptor de fator de crescimento endotelial vascular (VEGFR).[52-57] Inibidores direcionados a pequenas moléculas, como o masitinib, que bloqueia as funções de KIT e PDGFR, inibiram o crescimento e a capacidade de induzir apoptose em linhagens celulares do HSA canino, in vitro.[146,147] O desafio, assim como acontece com vários medicamentos inicialmente avaliados em condição in vitro, é que é improvável que as concentrações de fármacos necessárias para esse efeito sejam alcançadas in vivo, sem toxicidade relevante. Dois outros inibidores de pequenas moléculas – imatinibe, que bloqueia KIT e PDGFR, e dasatinibe, que bloqueia KIT, PDGFR e SRC– também são efetivos contra linhagens celulares de HSA, in vitro.[54] Ademais, relata-se que o imatinibe inibe o crescimento significativo de xenotransplantes de HSA canino, em ratos. O fosfato de toceranib (Palladia®) é outro inibidor de pequenas moléculas que bloqueia a sinalização dos membros da família KIT, PDGFR e VEGFR. O toceranib mostrou-se efetivo contra vários tipos de tumores, inclusive mastocitoma, adenocarcinoma de saco anal, osteossarcoma metastático, carcinoma nasal, carcinoma de tireoide e carcinoma de célula escamosa bucal.[148-150] Um estudo prospectivo recente avaliou o impacto da administração de toceranib na sobrevida livre de progressão tumoral em 31 cães com HSA em estágio I ou II após esplenectomia e tratamento com DOX como agente único. De forma desapontante, não houve aumento significativo no intervalo mediano livre de doença (ILD = 161 dias) ou da sobrevida geral (SM = 172 dias) em cães que receberam toceranib como tratamento de manutenção.[151]

Produtos naturais

Terapias alternativas utilizando produtos naturais se tornaram a mais nova área de pesquisa de HSA. A Yunnan Baiyao é uma erva medicinal chinesa que, de forma anedótica, foi utilizada para controlar hemorragia em cães com HSA. Um estudo *in vitro* avaliou os efeitos da Yunnan Baiyao em três linhagens celulares de HSA e constatou morte celular dose-dependente e tempo-dependente mediante apoptose mediada por enzimas caspases.[152] O polissacaropeptídio (PSP), agente bioativo oriundo do cogumelo *Coriolus versicolor*, apresenta possíveis efeitos antitumorais *in vitro* e *in vivo*.[153] Em um recente estudo-piloto duplo-cego aleatório com uso de múltiplas doses, o PSP em alta dose retardou de forma significativa a progressão de metástases e aumentou o tempo de sobrevida de cães com HSA, quando comparado aos dados de controle histórico de cães submetidos somente à cirurgia.[154] Embora os resultados desse estudo tenham sido promissores, é importante salientar que cada grupo continha apenas cinco cães.

RESUMO

Conforme discutido anteriormente, há variação na manifestação e no prognóstico associados aos diferentes tipos anatômicos de HSA. Independentemente, o HAS permanece como uma das neoplasias mais agressivas e letais em animais de companhia. Certamente, a remoção cirúrgica do tumor seguida de quimioterapia adjuvante com DOX, assim como é o tratamento atual de escolha para HSA esplênico, continua sendo o procedimento que mais provavelmente propicia o benefício de aumentar a sobrevida em qualquer apresentação anatômica dessa neoplasia. Entretanto, o surgimento de terapias recentes pode ser promissor para melhoras potenciais na sobrevida historicamente estagnada, associada a esse tipo de câncer.

REFERÊNCIAS BIBLIOGRÁFICAS

As referências bibliográficas deste capítulo se encontram online no Ambiente de Aprendizagem.

CAPÍTULO 348

Tumores Ósseos e Articulares

Julius M. Liptak

OSTEOSSARCOMA APENDICULAR EM CÃES

Os quatro tumores ósseos primários são osteossarcoma (OSA), condrossarcoma (CSA), fibrossarcoma (FSA) e hemangiossarcoma (HSA).[1] Lipossarcoma, rabdomiossarcoma, tumores de plasmócitos (plasmocitoma solitário e mieloma múltiplo) e linfoma também podem envolver os ossos, porém mais tipicamente como um processo secundário.[1] O OSA é o tumor ósseo primário mais comum, correspondendo a mais de 85 a 98% de todos os tumores ósseos apendiculares.[1,2] Ele também pode acometer primariamente o esqueleto axial e tecidos extraesqueléticos, inclusive vísceras, pele e glândula mamária.

A causa de OSA é desconhecida. A lesão repetida à fise foi proposta como causa devido à alta incidência desse tumor na região metafisária de cães de raças de grande porte com fechamento tardio das fises, mas evidências publicadas não sustentam essa teoria.[1,3] Outras causas potenciais incluem infecção viral e predisposição genética.[1,4] O OSA foi relatado em associação a fraturas e/ou implantes prévios, principalmente na diáfise femoral, e em outras doenças ósseas, como infarto e cisto ósseo.[4] Também propôs-se uma associação entre osteotomia para nivelamento do platô tibial (ONPT) e OSA na região proximal da tíbia, porém é mais provável ser decorrência de mecanismos associados aos sarcomas relacionados a fraturas do que especificamente ao procedimento de ONPT.[5,6] Foi igualmente documentado OSA induzido por radiação, que pode estar associado a protocolos envolvendo doses de radiação maiores que 3,5 Gy por sessão (ver Capítulo 340).[1]

Etiologia

O OSA apendicular em geral é uma doença de cães de raças grandes a gigantes,[1] mas também acomete raças menores, ainda que a probabilidade seja 20 vezes menor.[7] Foram relatadas predisposições raciais, entretanto o tamanho e particularmente a altura são fatores de risco mais importantes do que a raça.[1,8] Cães castrados, independentemente do sexo, possuem risco 2 vezes maior de desenvolverem OSA em comparação aos cães não castrados.[8] A distribuição etária no momento do diagnóstico é bimodal: a maioria dos cães tem entre 7 e 9 anos e uma menor população tem 1 a 2 anos.[1,8]

Diagnóstico

Claudicação e edema localizado no membro são os sintomas mais comuns.[1] Dor e claudicação são causadas por microfraturas, alteração do periósteo após extensão do tumor e fraturas patológicas.[1] O OSA apendicular se desenvolve na região metafisária de ossos longos. O membro torácico está envolvido 1,7 vezes mais frequentemente do que o membro pélvico.[1,9] A região distal do rádio (23,1% dos casos) e a proximal do úmero (18,5%) são os dois locais mais comuns.[1,9] No membro pélvico, o OSA se desenvolve na tíbia e no fêmur, com igual frequência. O fêmur é o local mais comum em cães que pesam menos que 15 kg.[7]

É necessário exame ortopédico (ver Capítulo 353) para localizar a origem da claudicação e diferenciar dor metafisária de outras doenças comuns (p. ex., osteoartrite, ruptura do ligamento cruzado cranial, displasia do quadril). O exame físico e uma base de dados mínima consistindo em hemograma, perfil bioquímico sérico e exame de urina são importantes para avaliar o estado geral de saúde e a capacidade de tolerar cirurgia e quimioterapia.

Recomendam-se radiografias regionais para estabelecer um diagnóstico presuntivo e diferenciar tumores ósseos primários de outras doenças ortopédicas. Há três tipos básicos de OSA: endosteal, periosteal e parosteal.[1,10] O periosteal e parosteal são raros e se originam na superfície de ossos longos,[1,10] enquanto o endosteal é muito mais comum.[1] A aparência radiográfica do OSA endosteal pode variar de lítica a blástica e, em geral, é uma mistura de ambos os padrões.[1,10] Outros sinais radiográficos característicos de tumores ósseos primários incluem lise cortical, proliferação periosteal, neoformação óssea em paliçada perpendicular ao eixo do osso cortical (efeito de queimadura solar), elevação periosteal devido à hemorragia subperiosteal (triângulo de Codman), perda do padrão trabecular delgado no osso metafisário e fratura patológica com colapso da metáfise.[1,10] FSA e CSA apendiculares possuem aparência radiográfica semelhante ao OSA e não podem ser diferenciados radiograficamente. Entretanto, a epidemiologia clássica e os achados radiográficos são em geral suficientes para o diagnóstico de um tumor ósseo primário.[1,10]

Diagnósticos diferenciais para tumores ósseos primários incluem osteomielite fúngica, especialmente aquelas causadas por *Coccidioides immitis* (ver Capítulo 232) e *Blastomyces dermatitidis* (ver Capítulo 233).[1,10] É necessário um histórico clínico minucioso para determinar se o cão vive ou visitou uma região onde a doença fúngica é endêmica. Cães com osteomielite fúngica frequentemente apresentam doença sistêmica e doença óssea poliostótica.[1,10] Por outro lado, cães com tumores ósseos primários raramente manifestam sintomas de doença sistêmica, e o envolvimento ósseo em geral é confinado a um local.[1,10] Osteomielite bacteriana, cistos ósseos atípicos e neoplasia metastática são outros potenciais diagnósticos diferenciais.

Pode-se realizar biopsia óssea para confirmar o diagnóstico, utilizando-se técnicas fechadas (ver Capítulo 92) ou abertas.[11-16] A aspiração com agulha fina (AAF; ver Capítulo 93), guiada ou não por ultrassom, é uma técnica útil e minimamente invasiva para diagnosticar sarcomas e diferenciar tumores ósseos primários de doenças metastáticas e osteomielite fúngica.[11-14] O exame citológico de aspirado central utilizando uma agulha de biopsia de medula óssea apresenta uma melhor taxa de sucesso de 95% no diagnóstico de OSA em cães, comparada à taxa de 85% do exame citológico de AAF.[13] O uso de coloração por fosfatase alcalina (ALP) após citologia de AAF ou aspirado central apresentou sensibilidade de 100% para o diagnóstico de OSA.[12,13] A biopsia central com agulha fechada, utilizando uma agulha Jamshidi ou trépano trefina Michele, é invasiva e requer anestesia geral.[1] As biopsias devem ser planejadas e realizadas com muito cuidado, de preferência pelo cirurgião principal, de forma a não comprometer as opções cirúrgicas[1] e assegurar que o trajeto da agulha possa ser extirpado em bloco, junto ao tumor, e que os tecidos não afetados não sejam contaminados durante o procedimento ou pelo hematoma pós-biopsia.[1] Podem ser obtidas grandes amostras centrais com auxílio de um trépano trefina Michele, resultando em uma taxa de acurácia diagnóstica de 94%, mas o aumento do risco de fratura patológica é proporcional ao tamanho do defeito ósseo.[1,15] A taxa de acurácia de biopsias ósseas obtidas com agulha Jamshidi é de 82%; o uso de agulhas de menor diâmetro diminui o risco de complicações e cria um trajeto muito menor.[16] Duas a quatro amostras devem ser coletadas do centro e da periferia da lesão por meio de uma incisão única na pele. O risco de fratura patológica aumenta quando a agulha penetra ambas as partes do córtex, próxima e distante.[1] Amostras múltiplas aumentam a acurácia diagnóstica, pois pequenas amostras podem levar ao diagnóstico errado, devido à heterogeneidade do OSA.[1] Recomendam-se biopsias ósseas centrais, pois as partes periféricas dos tumores ósseos frequentemente contêm osso reativo.[1] Após a cirurgia definitiva, todo o tumor deve ser enviado para exame histológico, a fim de confirmar o diagnóstico.

O OSA apendicular é um tumor altamente agressivo. Mais de 60% dos cães acometidos morrem por conta de doenças metastáticas; entretanto, menos de 15% apresentam metástases clinicamente detectáveis no momento do diagnóstico inicial.[1] A metástase ocorre sobretudo pela via hematógena, particularmente aos pulmões e ossos, embora haja relatos de metástase aos linfonodos regionais em 4,4% dos casos.[17,18] Palpação de linfonodos regionais, radiografias do tórax e cintilografia nuclear são procedimentos essenciais para o estadiamento minucioso de cães com suspeita de tumor ósseo primário (Figura 348.1). A presença de doença metastática detectável influencia sobremaneira as opções de tratamento para cães com OSA.[1,19-21] Para o diagnóstico de metástases pulmonares, são necessárias radiografias do tórax durante a inspiração em três projeções, com altos níveis de detalhamento, incluindo projeções laterais direita e esquerda e ventrodorsal ou dorsoventral.[1,10] Lesões de 7 mm ou mais de diâmetro podem ser detectadas em radiografias de boa qualidade.[1,22] A tomografia computadorizada (TC) possui maior sensibilidade para detectar lesões metastáticas, mas tem sido associada a diagnósticos falso-positivos de metástases.[1,19,22-24] Lesões pulmonares metastáticas são detectadas significativamente com mais frequência na TC do tórax (28 a 64%), comparativamente a radiografias do torácicas em três projeções (5 a 52%).[23,24] Entretanto, embora o número de nódulos metastáticos influencie significativamente a sobrevida, a constatação de lesões pulmonares metastáticas na TC não foi associada de forma significativa à sobrevida.[23] A cintilografia óssea de corpo inteiro, utilizando tecnécio na forma de pertecnetato radioativo, é altamente sensível para detecção de anormalidades ósseas concomitantes, incluindo tumores primários e metastáticos, mas não é específica para o diagnóstico de neoplasias.[1,20,21] Em um estudo, foi identificada uma segunda lesão óssea assintomática, compatível com doença metastática, em 7,8% de 399 cães com OSA.[21] Se uma lesão suspeita for identificada, devem ser obtidas radiografias com alto nível de detalhes da região. É possível realizar biopsia óssea para confirmar os resultados radiográficos caso sejam incertos. Como alternativa à indisponibilidade da cintilografia, as radiografias ósseas simples, consistindo em radiografias laterais de ossos longos e ventrodorsais da pelve, podem detectar metástases ósseas.[25] Quando presente, a doença óssea metastática é um indicador prognóstico negativo. Isso é extremamente importante quando se planeja a amputação do membro, pois metástases ósseas ocultas podem se tornar clinicamente sintomáticas após a cirurgia, fazendo o cão parar de andar.

Tratamento

Tratamento paliativo: geral

As opções terapêuticas para cães com OSA apendicular podem ser classificadas em: intenção paliativa e intenção curativa. A terapia paliativa é indicada para cães com doença metastática ou quando os tutores não pretendem optar por terapias mais intensivas. Essa terapia é direcionada ao controle da dor e da claudicação associada ao tumor ósseo primário, mas ela não aumenta a sobrevida. A analgesia é o ponto-chave desse tratamento (Tabela 348.1).[26] Anti-inflamatórios não esteroides (AINEs) podem inicialmente ser suficientes para tratar a dor e melhorar a qualidade de vida (ver Capítulo 164). Preferem-se AINE que não inibem a ciclo-oxigenase-1, já que os efeitos adversos são minimizados.[26] Para o alívio efetivo da dor, quase sempre são necessários analgésicos mais potentes ou uma combinação de medicamentos (ver Tabela 348.1 e Capítulo 356).[26] Fármacos bifosfonatos, como o pamidronato, quando combinados com AINE, mostraram ser seguros e com efeito analgésico que durava mais de 4 meses em 28% dos cães, com duração média de analgesia de 231 dias.[27,28] Combinações de múltiplos fármacos são mais efetivas no controle de dor refratária, induzindo ação analgésica aditiva ou sinérgica. Não há relato da sobrevida mediana (SM) de cães com OSA apendicular tratados apenas com analgésicos, embora evidências anedóticas sugiram que 1 a 3 meses é uma expectativa razoável.

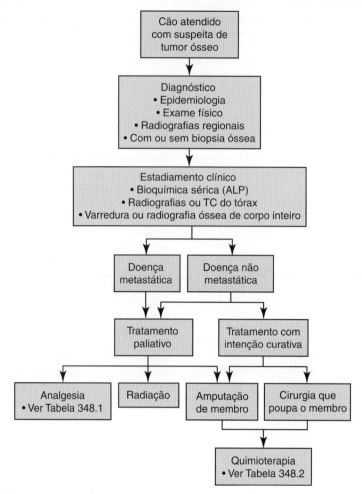

Figura 348.1 Algoritmo para diagnóstico e tratamento de osteossarcoma (OSA) apendicular em cães. Esse algoritmo pode não ser o mais correto para tumores de ossos longos não OSA. *ALP*, fosfatase alcalina; *TC*, tomografia computadorizada.

Radioterapia paliativa

A radioterapia (ver Capítulo 240) é efetiva como tratamento paliativo de cães com tumores ósseos primários. Vários protocolos diferentes foram descritos, e o mais comum é a administração de 4 a 10 Gy, em um protocolo de 0, 7 e 21 dias ou mensal.[29-36] Esses protocolos são relativamente baratos e não necessitam hospitalização prolongada. A radiação reduz a inflamação local, minimiza a dor, retarda a progressão de lesões metastáticas e melhora a qualidade de vida de cães com lesões primárias e metastáticas.[29-36] Relata-se resposta de 50 a 92%, com início mediano da resposta em 11 a 14 dias após o início da radioterapia e duração mediana de 53 a 130 dias.[29-36] A duração da resposta é significativamente maior quando o comprimento do osso acometido pelo tumor é menor que 50%. Foi relatado que tumores ósseos primários localizados no úmero proximal[32,33] e rádio distal[35] apresentaram melhores respostas. Doses cumulativas mais altas, maior intensidade do tratamento e adição de quimioterapia aos protocolos de radiação paliativa melhoram a taxa e a duração da resposta.[31-33,36] A radioterapia paliativa não está associada a efeitos agudos e não influencia negativamente a qualidade de vida.[29-36] A SM de cães com OSA apendicular submetidos à radiação paliativa é de 122 a 313 dias.[29-36] Radiofármacos, como o samário, têm sido utilizados como terapia paliativa de lesões ósseas primárias e metastáticas, mas são caros e não estão amplamente disponíveis na medicina veterinária.[37-39] A combinação de radiação paliativa e pamidronato foi recomendada, mas um estudo demonstrou SM significativamente menor em cães que receberam esse tratamento (122 dias), comparada ao uso exclusivo de radioterapia paliativa ou quando combinada à quimioterapia (307 dias).[36]

Amputação de membro

A amputação de membro pode ser utilizada como terapia paliativa e como parte do tratamento com intenção curativa em cães com tumor ósseo primário.[1,17,40,41] A amputação é um meio efetivo de controle da dor, particularmente em cães com fratura patológica e claudicação não responsiva aos medicamentos analgésicos ou à radioterapia. Osteoartrite, doença neurológica, obesidade e tamanho corporal grande foram citados como contraindicações relativas.[1,40,41] Entretanto, experiência mostra que osteoartrite, peso e tamanho corporal raramente representam problemas para a amputação (ver Capítulo 355).[41] A maioria dos cães com OSA é de grande porte, meia-idade a idosos, com moderada osteoartrite preexistente. Cães com doença neurológica ou sintomas de osteoartrite grave são exceções; nesses pacientes, devem ser empregados tratamentos paliativos ou procedimentos que poupam o membro.

Quando o membro torácico é amputado, deve-se remover a escápula, pois assim é obtido melhor controle do tumor, principalmente em cães com OSA da parte proximal do úmero, além de melhora da aparência estética.[1] No membro pélvico, deve-se realizar a desarticulação coxofemoral em cães com OSA distal ao fêmur proximal, enquanto cães com OSA femoral proximal devem ser submetidos à acetabulectomia em bloco ou hemipelvectomia parcial para obter controle adequado do tumor e minimizar o risco de recidiva local.

Tabela 348.1	Medicamentos analgésicos de uso oral e transdérmico utilizados no tratamento paliativo de cães com osteossarcoma apendicular.[26-28]		

MEDICAMENTO ANALGÉSICO	DOSE	INTERVALO ENTRE DOSES	COMENTÁRIOS
AINE			
Carprofeno	2,2 mg/kg	12 h	Insuficiência hepática idiossincrática, úlcera gástrica, lesão renal e letargia
Deracoxibe	1 a 2 mg/kg	24 h	Úlcera gástrica, lesão renal
Etodolaco	10 a 15 mg/kg	24 h	Úlcera gástrica, lesão renal
Meloxicam	0,05 a 0,1 mg/kg	24 h	Úlcera gástrica, lesão renal
Cetoprofeno	0,5 a 1 mg/kg	24 h	Úlcera gástrica, lesão renal e inibição da agregação plaquetária
Piroxicam	0,3 mg/kg	48 h	Úlcera gástrica e lesão renal
Agonistas parciais			
Butorfanol	0,55 mg/kg	1 a 2 h	Medicamento controlado; ação de curta duração, efeito teto de analgesia, sedação e depressão respiratória
Opioides			
Morfina	0,5 a 1 mg/kg	8 a 12 h	Medicamento controlado; sedação, euforia, bradicardia, êmese, retenção urinária e constipação intestinal
Adesivo de fentanila	50 µg/h (10 a 20 kg) 75 µg/h (20 a 30 kg) 100 µg/h (> 30 kg)	72 h 72 h 72 h	Medicamento controlado; concentração sérica variável devido ao local de aplicação, temperatura e fluxo sanguíneo cutâneo, e hidratação; é necessário descarte correto, pois a dose residual pode ser letal para humanos
Miscelânea			
Pamidronato	1 a 2 mg/kg	28 dias	Fármaco bifosfonato com ação antiosteoclástica e, possivelmente, antineoplásica; melhor efeito analgésico quando combinado com AINE; contraindicado em caso de doença renal
Tramadol	2 a 5 mg/kg	8 a 12 h	Constipação intestinal pelo uso crônico; letargia em altas doses
Codeína-paracetamol	0,5 a 2 mg/kg	6 a 8 h	Medicamento controlado; anemia
Amantadina	3 mg/kg	24 h	Antagonista de NMDA
Prednisona	0,5 a 1 mg/kg	12 a 24 h	Anti-inflamatório, ação sinérgica com opioides, contraindicado com AINE
Amitriptilina	1 a 2 mg/kg	12 a 24 h	Antidepressivo tricíclico; altera efeitos da serotonina e norepinefrina

AINE, anti-inflamatórios não esteroides; *NMDA*, N-metil-D-aspartato.

A maioria dos cães não é capaz de andar sem auxílio 12 a 24 horas após a amputação do membro. Os animais submetidos à amputação devem ser encorajados pelos tutores a andar em casa após alta hospitalar para acelerar a recuperação. Estudos demonstraram que a maioria dos cães se adapta completamente à amputação em 4 semanas após a cirurgia. Se o cão apresentava claudicação relevante causada pelo tumor antes da cirurgia, a recuperação completa em geral é mais rápida, antes das 4 semanas. Além disso, uma atitude positiva dos tutores abrevia o tempo de adaptação.[41] O peso corporal e a amputação de membro, tanto o torácico quanto o pélvico, não influencia significativamente o tempo para adaptação após a amputação; entretanto, no período pós-cirúrgico inicial, cães submetidos à amputação de membro torácico têm maior dificuldade para se equilibrar.[41] Também foram observadas alterações comportamentais, como aumento da ansiedade e perda de dominância, mas são relativamente incomuns.[41] As complicações associadas à amputação do membro são raras, enquanto as intraoperatórias podem incluir hemorragia, embolia gasosa e toracotomia acidental (durante amputação do membro torácico), e as pós-cirúrgicas incluem infecções, formação de seromas e recidiva no coto. A sobrevida de cães tratados apenas com amputação é significativamente maior com o uso de medicamentos analgésicos ou radioterapia paliativa.[14] A SM de cães com OSA tratados apenas

com amputação de membro é de 103 a 175 dias, com taxa de sobrevida em 6 meses de 47 a 52%, em 12 meses de 11 a 21% e em 24 meses de 0 a 4%.[17,42-45] A SM maior (257 dias) é verificada em animais de raça de pequeno porte com OSA apendicular, tratados apenas com amputação.[46]

Cirurgia com preservação do membro

As técnicas que poupam o membro são mais comuns, apesar do sucesso da amputação em cães com tumor ósseo primário.[1,40,47-61] A razão mais frequente para poupar o membro em cães com OSA é a relutância do tutor em realizar a amputação. Indicações clínicas para preservar o membro incluem amputação prévia de outro membro, osteoartrite concomitante grave ou doença neurológica.[1,40]

A cirurgia que preserva o membro é mais efetiva em cães com tumor ósseo primário na parte distal do rádio e na ulna.[40,47-58] A cirurgia que poupa membro em casos de neoplasia em outros locais anatômicos frequentemente está associada a alta taxa de complicações e pouca função do membro no período pós-cirúrgico.[55-58] Candidatos para essa cirurgia são os cães com tumor restrito ao osso, com disseminação mínima aos tecidos moles adjacentes e envolvimento inferior a 50% do comprimento do osso.[1,40] A extensão do envolvimento ósseo é mais acuradamente determinada utilizando TC,[62] pois ela é sobrestimada por radiografias, cintilografia nuclear e ressonância magnética (RM).[62-64] Fraturas patológicas são contraindicações relativas devido à contaminação local oriunda de hemorragia e hematoma, embora o risco de recidiva local do tumor possa ser reduzido mediante quimioterapia ou radioterapia pré-cirúrgica.[40]

Há relatos de várias técnicas cirúrgicas que preservam a função do membro.[1,40,47-58] Após a ressecção marginal do componente de tecido mole do tumor ósseo, o defeito ósseo é preenchido com aloenxerto cortical massivo, endoprótese, enxerto ulnar vascularizado, autoenxerto pasteurizado ou irradiado ou osteogênese por transporte de osso segmentar.[1,40,47-58] Geralmente, é necessária artrodese da articulação adjacente;[1,40] a artrodese pancarpal é bem tolerada pelos cães, mas a artrodese de ombro, joelho ou articulação do tarso resulta em mau funcionamento do membro. A preservação da articulação é possível em casos de OSA na ulna ou na diáfise de qualquer osso longo,[65] e as opções que preservam o membro e a articulação podem ser mais utilizadas à medida que artroplastias articulares totais são adaptadas para os casos oncológicos.[66] Exercícios com sustentação de peso e amplitude de movimentação podem ser iniciados imediatamente no período pós-cirúrgico, mas durante as primeiras 4 semanas a atividade deve ser restrita ao acesso à rua controlado.[1,40] O exercício é importante para prevenir contraturas e flexão dos dígitos e para minimizar o edema dos coxins e dígitos (ver Capítulo 355). O uso bom a excelente do membro é obtido em mais de 75% dos cães.[1,40,47-49]

Falha do implante, recidiva do tumor e infecção no local são as complicações mais comumente relatadas em procedimentos cirúrgicos que preservam o membro.[1,40,47-59] A falha do implante ocorre em até 40% dos casos, mas há técnicas que reduzem esse risco.[49] A recidiva local do tumor é causada por ressecção incompleta ou, mais comumente, por células neoplásicas residuais que permanecem no tecido mole adjacente à cápsula tumoral.[1,40] A recidiva local não influencia[49] ou tem efeito negativo na sobrevida,[57] dependendo do estudo citado. Infecção é a complicação pós-cirúrgica mais relevante em casos de cirurgia que preserva o membro, ocorrendo em até 70% dos casos em que a reconstrução é realizada com o emprego de técnicas não autógenas.[1,40,47-61,68] Foram isoladas diversas bactérias.[61] Inicialmente, as infecções são tratadas com antibióticos apropriados, selecionados com base nos resultados do antibiograma, lavagem com solução salina isotônica e bandagens úmidas-secas.[1,61] Outras opções incluem implante de esferas de metilmetacrilato embebidas em antibióticos, no caso de infecção persistente, ou amputação do membro, quando a infecção é incontrolável.[1,59,61]

Uma variação na técnica cirúrgica que preserva o membro é a fixação interna ou externa de fraturas patológicas. Em um estudo com 16 cães, o uso do membro imediatamente após a cirurgia foi bom a muito bom, com exceção de 2 cães.[69]

Radioterapia

A radioterapia (ver Capítulo 340) é um procedimento mais comumente utilizado como tratamento paliativo, mas também pode ser usado para controle do tumor ósseo primário em casos cujas outras opções não são indicadas ou são rejeitadas.[70-72] A radiação estereotática tem sido utilizada com sucesso em cães com OSA apendicular em diversas localizações anatômicas.[70] Um gradiente de doses de radiação decrescentes é administrado no local, e o centro da lesão recebe 45 a 60 Gy e a periferia 30 a 35 Gy.[70] Há pesquisas com radioterapia com feixe externo, em ciclo completo,[71,72] que usam dose total de 24 a 54 Gy.[71,72] As complicações após radiação estereotática de curso completo incluem descamação cutânea úmida, alopecia, despigmentação, mielossupressão e fraturas patológicas.[70-72] A SM de cães com OSA tratados com radioterapia com intenção curativa e quimioterapia adjuvante é de 363 dias e de 7 meses, respectivamente.[70-72] Fraturas após radiação estereotática são complicações relativamente comuns e podem ser tratadas por meio de fixação interna da fratura.[73]

Quimioterapia

O controle definitivo de cães com OSA apendicular requer o tratamento tanto do tumor ósseo local quanto da doença micrometastática. A eficácia da quimioterapia em outros tipos de tumores ósseos primários é menos clara. A cirurgia, a menos que combinada à quimioterapia, é considerada paliativa.[42-45] Já a quimioterapia sem cirurgia não propicia benefício quanto à sobrevida, se comparada a outros procedimentos paliativos, embora tenha sido constatada maior SM com a combinação de quimioterapia e radioterapia paliativa.[74,75] Na maioria das clínicas especializadas em oncologia, a quimioterapia é iniciada no momento da remoção da sutura, mas é algo variável, podendo ocorrer antes da cirurgia, no perioperatório ou até 21 dias após a cirurgia.[76] Os protocolos de quimioterapia atuais incluem o uso de cisplatina, carboplatina, doxorrubicina e gencitabina, como agentes únicos ou combinados (Tabela 348.2).[1,42-45,76-88] Estudos não demonstraram diferença na sobrevida entre os diferentes protocolos, utilizando agentes únicos ou múltiplos;[86,87] entretanto, com o uso exclusivo de carboplatina, obteve-se um intervalo livre de doença (ILD) significativamente mais longo do que o de protocolos que alternavam carboplatina e doxorrubicina, de acordo com um estudo,[86] e foi associado a efeitos adversos significativamente inferiores, em outro estudo.[87] Na prática, a escolha do protocolo geralmente depende do custo do medicamento, dos efeitos adversos e da intensidade do tratamento. Embora esses agentes quimioterápicos sejam administrados por via intravenosa, relata-se que uma única dose SC de carboplatina em 17 cães com OSA apendicular, após amputação do membro, obteve SM de 365 dias.[89] Se a cisplatina for utilizada, é necessário induzir diurese salina, a fim de minimizar o

| **Tabela 348.2** | Protocolos quimioterápicos utilizados no tratamento de cães com osteossarcoma apendicular.[42-45,76-88] |

AGENTE(S)	DOSE	INTERVALO ENTRE DOSES	NÚMERO DE DOSES	COMENTÁRIOS
Cisplatina	70 mg/m²	3 semanas	5	Êmese durante a administração, nefrotoxicidade, toxicidade gastrintestinal, discreta mielossupressão; concentração mínima aos 10 dias; SM de 262 a 413 dias
Carboplatina	300 mg/m²	3 semanas	4	Mielossupressão, toxicidade gastrintestinal; concentração mínima aos 11 a 14 dias; SM de 321 a 366 dias
Doxorrubicina	30 mg/m²	2 a 3 semanas	5	Anafilaxia durante a administração, toxicidade gastrintestinal, toxicidade ao miocárdio, mielossupressão, concentração mínima aos 10 dias; SM de 366 dias
Cisplatina Doxorrubicina	50 mg/m² 15 mg/m²	3 semanas	4	Administração de cisplatina no dia 1 e de doxorrubicina no dia 2; SM de 300 a 540 dias
Carboplatina Doxorrubicina	300 mg/m² 30 mg/m²	3 semanas	6	Administração alternada de carboplatina e doxorrubicina a cada 3 semanas, três doses cada (no total, seis doses); SM de 388 dias

SM, sobrevida mediana.

| Tabela 348.3 | Protocolos de diurese salina utilizados para minimizar a nefrotoxicidade associada à cisplatina.[1] |

PROTOCOLO	FASE I	FASE II	FASE III
6 h	Solução salina: 18,3 mℓ/kg/h, 4 h	Cisplatina durante 20 min	Solução salina: 18,3 mℓ/kg/h, 2 h
24 h	Solução salina: 3,75 mℓ/kg/h, 16 h	Cisplatina durante 16 h	Solução salina: 3,75 mℓ/kg/h, 6 h

risco de nefrotoxicidade (Tabela 348.3).[1] A nefrotoxicidade pode ser igualmente minimizada pela utilização de carboplatina ou pela administração simultânea de amifostina.[1,81-83,90] A doxorrubicina foi associada à toxicidade ao miocárdio, particularmente em doses cumulativas maiores que 180 mg/m². Portanto, recomenda-se a avaliação cardíaca (ecocardiograma e/ou mensuração da concentração sérica de troponina cardíaca-I) antes do início da quimioterapia, especialmente em raças de alto risco.[1,90a,90b]

Após a administração da quimioterapia, especialmente a primeira dose, os cães devem ser liberados com recomendação de uso domiciliar de antibiótico e antiemético para abrandar a doença gastrintestinal e a náuseas, se necessário (ver Capítulo 343). Deve-se obter o hemograma quando ocorre a contagem mínima de leucócitos, geralmente 7 a 10 dias após a quimioterapia, e imediatamente antes das doses subsequentes da quimioterapia, a fim de verificar possível mielossupressão. Se a contagem de neutrófilos for inferior a 2.000/μℓ ou a contagem de plaquetas for inferior a 100.000/μℓ, deve-se postergar a administração do quimioterápico ou diminuir sua dose.[1] Em cães submetidos à cirurgia e quimioterapia, a SM varia de 235 a 366 dias (sobrevida em 12 meses: 33 a 65%; sobrevida em 24 meses: 16 a 28%).[42-45,76-88] Em cães de raças pequenas com OSA apendicular tratados com intenção curativa, a SM é de 415 dias.[46]

A combinação de terapia em ciclo completo e quimioterapia metronômica foi avaliada, porque a quimioterapia metronômica pode melhorar os resultados terapêuticos em cães com OSA. Em 30 cães com OSA apendicular, notou-se que a quimioterapia metronômica (piroxicam e ciclofosfamida em baixa dose) foi bem tolerada quando combinada apenas com carboplatina ou com administração alternada de carboplatina e doxorrubicina, porém ocorreram mais casos de toxicidade de graus 3 e 4 relevantes quando combinada apenas com carboplatina.[91]

A importância da imunoterapia (ver Capítulo 341) não está definida. Há relatos de ILD e sobrevida significativamente mais longos em cães tratados com um imunoestimulante inespecífico, o muramil tripeptídio fosfatidiletanolamina.[92,93] O uso do medicamento antimicrobiano suramina, juntamente a doxorrubicina, em 47 cães com OSA apendicular após amputação foi bem tolerado, com SM de 369 dias.[88] Também suspeita-se de maior estimulação imune em cães com sobrevida longa após cirurgia infectada que preservou o membro e em 4 cães com regressão espontânea de lesões de OSA.[49,68,94,95]

Metástase

A doença metastática é a causa mais comum de morte ou eutanásia em cães com OSA apendicular após tratamento definitivo.[1] As metástases pulmonares (Figura 348.2) e ósseas são as mais frequentemente envolvidas; outros locais incluem tecido subcutâneo, mediastino, miocárdio, diafragma, rins, baço, intestino delgado, medula espinal, cérebro e linfonodos.[1,14,17] Curiosamente, são raros os casos de doença metastática em cães submetidos a tratamento paliativo não cirúrgico, mas é a principal causa de morte em cães tratados apenas com cirurgia, apesar da mínima diferença na sobrevida. Um estudo recente,

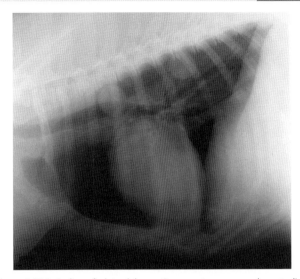

Figura 348.2 Radiografia lateral de um cão com osteossarcoma da parte distal do rádio 8 meses após cirurgia que preservou o membro. Note duas lesões metastáticas nos campos pulmonares dorsais.

utilizando um modelo de OSA em ratos, demonstrou que a ressecção do tumor primário aumentou a angiogênese sistêmica, resultando na progressão de lesões metastáticas distantes.[96] A distribuição de lesões metastáticas depende do tipo de tratamento. Metástases pulmonares são mais comuns quando é feita ablação somente do tumor local, enquanto metástases ósseas são mais prevalentes quando a quimioterapia é incluída no protocolo terapêutico. A metástase pulmonar representa 61% de todas as lesões metastáticas em cães tratados apenas com amputação e 26% quando submetidos à amputação e à administração de cisplatina.[17,78] Em comparação, ocorrem metástases ósseas em até 47% dos cães após cirurgia e tratamento com cisplatina no período pós-cirúrgico.[97]

Indisposição generalizada é o sinal mais comum em cães com metástase pulmonar. Sintomas respiratórios normalmente se manifestam em um estágio mais tardio. A osteopatia hipertrófica pode ser a primeira indicação de metástase pulmonar em algumas ocasiões. A quimioterapia com platina e o uso de antibiótico não são efetivos para prolongar a sobrevida de cães com metástase pulmonar mensurável.[97,98] Em alguns casos, a ressecção cirúrgica de lesões metastáticas, por meio de ressecção subpleural ou lobectomia pulmonar parcial, pode aumentar de forma significativa a sobrevida (Figura 348.3).[99,100] Os candidatos à metastatectomia pulmonar são os cães que desenvolvem metástases pulmonares mais de 300 dias após o diagnóstico inicial de OSA apendicular, possuem 3 ou menos lesões metastáticas radiograficamente evidentes, apresentam lesões que não tenham dobrado de tamanho e não desenvolvem novas lesões em um período de 4 semanas.[99] A SM de cães com metástases pulmonares varia de 61 a 95 dias quando submetidos à quimioterapia[97,98] e 176 dias após metastatectomia.[99] A metastatectomia pulmonar é também recomendada para cães com osteopatia hipertrófica, independentemente do tempo após o diagnóstico, já que a extirpação cirúrgica de uma lesão metastática pode resultar em resolução imediata dos sinais clínicos.[100]

As opções terapêuticas para cães com metástases ósseas incluem controle da dor com medicamentos analgésicos, bifosfonatos e radioterapia paliativa. Os bifosfonatos bloqueiam a atividade osteoclástica, minimizando o risco de fraturas patológicas.[27,28,101,102] Cães com metástases ósseas tratados com radioterapia paliativa e quimioterapia apresentam SM significativamente maior (130 dias), em comparação a outras modalidades terapêuticas paliativas e de combinações.[103] A combinação de pamidronato e AINE também pode ter efeito paliativo em cães com dor óssea relacionada ao tumor, com até 28% dos pacientes sob ação

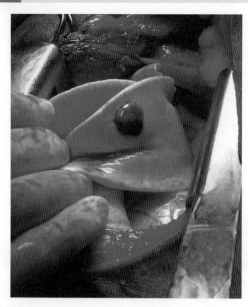

Figura 348.3 Imagem transcirúrgica de lesão metastática oriunda de osteossarcoma apendicular. Realizou-se lobectomia pulmonar parcial, mas o cão morreu de causas não relacionadas à neoplasia 294 dias após a metastatectomia.

analgésica que dura mais de 4 meses (mediana de 231 dias).[28] Em alguns casos, tem-se utilizado cirurgia que preserva o membro e radioterapia com intenção curativa no tratamento de lesões metastáticas ósseas, mas não são rotineiramente recomendadas.[103]

Fatores e indicadores de prognóstico

Em cães com OSA, os fatores de prognóstico ruim incluem idade abaixo de 7 anos ou acima de 10 anos, peso corporal acima de 40 kg, tumor de grande volume, localização da neoplasia no úmero proximal, aumento de atividades séricas pré-cirúrgicas de fosfatase alcalina (ALP) total e de ALP específica de ossos que não se normalizam dentro de 40 dias após a remoção cirúrgica do tumor, tumor de alto grau e presença de metástases.[1,77,84,86,104-107] Em cães com OSA no úmero proximal, o ILD e a SM são significativamente mais curtos daqueles observados em outras localizações de OSA apendicular; entretanto, isso pode ser decorrência do volume do tumor, não de sua localização.[77,86,106,107] Em cães com ALT sérica total normal e elevada, a SM é de 12,5 e 5,5 meses, respectivamente;[105] em cães com ALT sérica específica de ossos normal e elevada, a SM é de 16,6 e 9,5 meses, respectivamente.[105] No caso das atividades de ALP sérica específica de ossos e de ALP total, a cada aumento de 100 UI/ℓ, cresce em 25% o risco de morte decorrente do OSA.[104,105] Cães com infecções relacionadas ao membro preservado durante o tratamento apresentam SM significativamente maior (685 dias), comparada à de cães sem infecção cirúrgica (289 dias).[49,68,94] O OSA pode ser histologicamente subclassificado como osteoblástico, condroblástico, fibroblástico, telangiectásico e indiferenciado, mas o subtipo histológico não foi considerado indicador de prognóstico em cães e humanos.[1]

CONDROSSARCOMA APENDICULAR EM CÃES

O condrossarcoma (CSA) apendicular é o segundo tumor ósseo primário mais comum em cães.[1] Ele corresponde a 9 a 17% de todos os casos de CSA em cães.[108-111] A causa é desconhecida, embora haja relato de que o CSA seja oriundo de osteocondroma ou de locais de traumatismos prévios. Cães das raças Golden Retriever, Pastor-Alemão e Boxer são mais predispostos à neoplasia. A idade mediana no momento da consulta é de 6 a 8,7 anos.[108-115] Os achados clínicos são semelhantes aos de OSA apendicular, sendo necessária biopsia para diferenciar os tipos de tumores. O fêmur é mais comumente envolvido, e o CSA pode ter uma aparência radiográfica de lise maior do que a de OSA.[110,111] Amputação e procedimentos de salvamento do membro podem ser utilizados no tratamento de tumor local. Relata-se doença metastática em até 31% dos cães com CSA, o que depende do grau histológico, com relato de metástases distantes em 0, 31 e 50% dos cães com CSA graus I, II e III, respectivamente.[108-112,115] A quimioterapia não propicia benefícios à sobrevida de pessoas com CSA; provavelmente ocorre o mesmo com cães.[112,113]

Em cães com CSA não tratado, a SM é de 46 dias, enquanto para cães tratados exclusivamente com amputação do membro a SM varia de 540 dias até mais de 2.618 dias.[111,112,115] Os critérios prognósticos incluem localização do tumor e o seu grau histológico.[110,112,114,115] Em cães com CSA apendicular de graus I, II e III tratados apenas com amputação do membro, as SM são de 6, 2,7 e 0,9 anos, respectivamente.[115]

FIBROSSARCOMA APENDICULAR EM CÃES

O fibrossarcoma (FSA) apendicular é a terceira neoplasia óssea mais comum em cães e ocorre mais comumente em locais axiais, não apendiculares.[109] Há dois FSA apendiculares distintos: central e parosteal.[116] Uma massa palpável frequentemente é notada no FSA parosteal, mas não no central. O FSA parosteal pode ser um tumor de origem em tecidos moles, com invasão óssea secundária.[109,116] As características radiográficas do FSA apendicular são semelhantes àquelas do OSA, embora sejam relatadas lesões líticas e fraturas patológicas em até 50% dos cães com FSA.[116] A amputação e a preservação do membro são as principais opções terapêuticas cirúrgicas. A importância da quimioterapia é desconhecida. O FSA apendicular causa metástase tardia durante o curso da doença, com frequência em locais para além dos pulmões, como miocárdio, pericárdio, pele e ossos.[116] É difícil avaliar a sobrevida, pois mais de 50% dos casos de OSA fibroblástico são diagnosticados erroneamente como FSA.[1,116] Em cães com FSA apendicular tratados somente com a amputação do membro, a SM em 12 meses é de 66%.[116]

HEMANGIOSSARCOMA APENDICULAR EM CÃES

O hemangiossarcoma (HAS) apendicular ósseo é raro, correspondendo a 3,6% de todos os tumores ósseos primários (ver Capítulo 347). Cães das raças Pastor-Alemão, Dogue Alemão e Boxer são as mais predispostas, com idade média ao atendimento de 6,2 a 8,2 anos. Essa é uma idade mais jovem ao atendimento do que a relatada na maioria dos outros tumores ósseos primários.[109] A distribuição entre localizações apendiculares e axiais é semelhante, com 43% dos casos se desenvolvem no esqueleto apendicular.[109,117] O úmero proximal é a localização apendicular mais comum.[117] O HSA ósseo apresenta comportamento biológico diferente de outros tumores ósseos primários: a maioria dos HSA apendiculares possui aparência radiográfica lítica, e as alterações corticais e periosteais podem ser mínimas.[109,117] A doença poliostótica, a extensão aos tecidos moles e as fraturas patológicas são comuns.[109,117] Em cães com HSA apendicular, recomendam-se ultrassonografia abdominal e ecocardiograma, além de outros testes-padrão de estadiamento, pois relata-se que 82% dos pacientes apresentam doença extraóssea ou metástases.[117] O benefício do tratamento local e sistêmico é incerto, pois a maioria dos cães desenvolve metástases antes dos 6 meses, e a taxa de sobrevida em 12 meses é menor que 10%.[109,117] Entretanto, pode-se indicar amputação do membro e protocolo quimioterápico com doxorrubicina para cães com HSA apendicular monostótico não metastático.[118] A radioterapia paliativa pode ser utilizada em cães com doença poliostótica.

TUMORES ÓSSEOS AXIAIS EM CÃES

O OSA do esqueleto axial corresponde a 25% de todos os casos de OSA e 59% dos casos de OSA em cães que pesam menos que 15 kg.[7,119] Entretanto, cães de raças de médio e grande porte são comumente afetados.[118,120] A raça Boxer pode ser mais predisposta, e a propensão de fêmeas é relatada em todas as localizações axiais, com exceção de costelas e vértebras.[119,120] As localizações mais comuns de OSA axial são mandíbula (27% dos OSA axiais), maxila (16 a 22%), vértebras (7 a 15%), escápula (13%), crânio (11 a 12%), costelas (10 a 11%), seios nasais e paranasais (9%) e pelve (4 a 5%).[119,120] Também foram relatados OSA de palato duro e patela.[121,122]

Técnicas de imagem avançadas, particularmente TC, são úteis para o estadiamento e planejamento cirúrgico. Recomenda-se ressecção cirúrgica, embora a radioterapia também possa ser utilizada para controle local do tumor.[119,120,123] A recidiva local é relatada em até 80% dos cães, sendo a causa mais comum de morte. A taxa de metástase é de 11 a 46%.[119,120,123-125] A importância da quimioterapia é incerta.[119,120,123-130]

Em cães com OSA axial, a SM é de 120 a 154 dias, com taxas de sobrevida em 12 meses e 24 meses de 26,3 e 18,4%, respectivamente.[119,120,123] Fatores ou indicadores de prognóstico incluem localização anatômica, tamanho corporal, raça, aumento da atividade sérica de ALP total e margens cirúrgicas.[120,123-130] Raças menores apresentam sobrevida significativamente mais longa do que as de grande porte.[120] Em cães da raça Golden Retriever com OSA axial, a SM é de 100 dias, enquanto em cães de raça pura é de 182 dias e em cães sem raça definida é 264 dias.[123] O prognóstico do OSA mandibular é melhor do que o de costela, escápula e crânio;[120] em outro estudo, constatou-se que o OSA escapular foi associado a um aumento de 2,8 vezes do risco de morte relacionada ao tumor, comparativamente a outras localizações do OSA axial não calvarial.[131] Em cães com OSA de mandíbula, maxila ou crânio, a SM após extirpação cirúrgica (329 dias) foi significativamente maior do que a da radioterapia (132 dias).[125] A ressecção cirúrgica incompleta aumenta significativamente o risco de recidiva local e de metástase.[125-130] Após radioterapia com intenção paliativa e curativa do OSA axial em cães de grande porte, notou-se SM de 79 e 265 dias, respectivamente,[123] enquanto o samário-153 propiciou melhora subjetiva em 4 de 25 cães com tumores de crânio.[39]

Tumores de crânio

O OSA de crânio pode envolver o calvário, os seios nasais e paranasais, a maxila e a mandíbula. O OSA de calvário corresponde a 11 a 12% dos casos de OSA axial.[119,120] Os sintomas consistem em uma massa externa visível e sinais neurológicos devido à compressão extradural do cérebro; a invasão direta do cérebro é rara.[1] Recomenda-se ressecção cirúrgica após realização de TC. Complicações perioperatórias podem incluir edema cerebral, herniação cerebral, pneumomeningocele, pneumonia aspirativa e morte.

O OSA axial pode envolver a maxila e a mandíbula, mas é menos comum do que outros tumores que acometem esses ossos. Em cães, os tumores bucais mais comuns são melanoma, carcinoma de célula escamosa, FSA, OSA e epúlide benigna, que são discutidos no Capítulo 272.[126-130]

A causa mais comum de morte em cães com OSA axial é a recidiva local do tumor, não a metástase. Relata-se metástase em até 30% dos casos de OSA craniano. A SM do OSA mandibular tratado com mandibulectomia é de 7 a 18 meses, com sobrevida em 12 meses de até 71%.[124,126-128] A quimioterapia pós-cirúrgica aumenta de forma significativa a sobrevida em cães com OSA mandibular.[124] O escore e o grau histológico são preditivos da sobrevida em cães com OSA mandibular.[124,128] Já a SM de OSA maxilar tratado mediante maxilectomia é de 4,5 a 10 meses, com taxa de sobrevida em 12 meses de 17 a 27%.[129,130] A extirpação cirúrgica radical, com margens histológicas amplas, melhora de forma significativa as taxas de recidiva local e de sobrevida.[125] Radioterapia e quimioterapia pós-cirúrgica não prolongam a sobrevida, mesmo em cães com ressecção incompleta do tumor.[123,125] De forma semelhante, o samário-153, como terapia única, propicia benefício mínimo para os casos de AS de calvário ou osteocondrossarcoma multilobular em cães.[39]

Tumores de escápula

O OSA escapular corresponde a até 13% de todos os casos de OSA axial.[109,120,121,123] Também há relatos de CSA, FSA, HSA, sarcoma histiocítico e sarcoma de tecidos moles na escápula.[110,132-136] Claudicação é o sinal clínico mais comum.[136] Alterações radiográficas são compatíveis com OSA apendicular, tipicamente com padrão misto de alterações líticas e produtivas.[132] Entretanto, devido às dificuldades de posicionamento e sobreposição da parede corporal, pode ser difícil determinar a extensão da doença por meio de radiografias simples. A TC é útil para determinar o local e a extensão da lesão (Figura 348.4). Recomenda-se escapulectomia parcial ou total, com manutenção boa a excelente da função do membro após ressecção de até 90% da escápula.[132-136] Uma alta taxa de metástases foi relatada em cães com OSA escapular, e quimioterapia pós-cirúrgica é recomendada.[120,121,136]

Tumores de pelve

O OSA de ossos pélvicos corresponde a 4 a 6% dos casos de OSA axial.[109,119,120] FSA, CSA e OSA de pelve ocorrem em frequências semelhantes.[109,110,111,137,138] Cães da raça Boxer podem ser predispostos a CSA pélvico.[108] Claudicação é comum, embora também tenham sido observados tenesmo, devido à compressão do reto, e déficits neurológicos, como resultado da compressão de nervos periféricos.[138] Anormalidades radiográficas são semelhantes àquelas do OSA apendicular (Figura 348.5). A TC é útil para o estadiamento local e o planejamento cirúrgico.[138] A hemipelvectomia subtotal ou total é o tratamento recomendado para cães com tumores de pelve.[137-139] Se necessário, pode-se fazer a ressecção em bloco do terço lateral do sacro, lateral ao forame sacral dorsal, com a pelve acometida.[138,139] É possível salvar o membro se o eixo de apoio do peso for preservado, por meio de hemipelvectomia interna.[139] Cães com OSA pélvico devem ser submetidos à quimioterapia, pois o comportamento biológico da neoplasia pode ser semelhante àquele do OSA apendicular.[137,138] Em um estudo, constatou-se

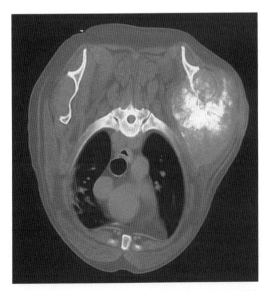

Figura 348.4 Imagem sagital de osteossarcoma da escápula obtida em TC. Esse exame é recomendado para obtenção de imagem de tumores escapulares, para planejamento cirúrgico e pesquisa de metástases pulmonares, por conta do detalhamento superior e da melhor capacidade de determinar a localização e a extensão do tumor em comparação a radiografias.

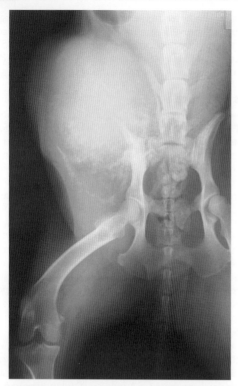

Figura 348.5 Radiografia ventrodorsal de condrossarcoma de grau I no íleo direito. Note o grande volume tumoral e a compressão, e não invasão, do processo transverso da sexta e sétima vértebra lombar. Realizou-se hemipelvectomia, e o cão estava vivo e livre da doença na última consulta de acompanhamento, 640 dias depois.

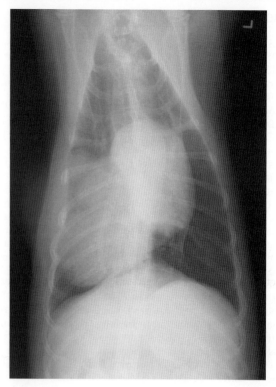

Figura 348.6 Radiografia ventrodorsal de osteossarcoma na sétima costela, deslocando o coração e os lobos pulmonares caudais para o lado esquerdo, o que ocasiona deslocamento medial da pleura parietal e resulta em sintoma extrapleural.

que 11 de 28 cães com OSA pélvico tratados mediante hemipelvectomia desenvolveram metástases, e 15 cães morreram por complicações relacionadas ao tumor.[138] A SM desses cães foi de 533 dias, com taxas de sobrevida em 1 e 2 anos de 51 e 35%, respectivamente.[138] A SM de cães com CSA pélvico foi de 1.232 dias, com taxa de sobrevida em 1 ano de 87%, enquanto a SM de cães com sarcoma de tecidos moles pélvicos e parapélvicos foi de 373 dias, com taxas de sobrevida em 1 e 2 anos de 47 e 38%, respectivamente.[138]

Tumores de costelas

Tumores de costela são incomuns, e os tipos relatados são OSA, CSA, FSA, HSA, osteocondrossarcoma multilobular (OML; ver adiante), e mastocitoma (ver Capítulo 349).[1,119,120,123,140-143] OSA é o mais comum, correspondendo a 73% dos tumores de costela e 11% dos casos de OSA axial.[119,120,140-143] Não há relato de predisposição racial ou sexual, mas podem ocorrer em cães de raças de grande porte mais jovens, com idade média de 4,5 a 6 anos.[119,120,123,140-143]

Tumores de costela em geral se desenvolvem no terço distal da costela, próximo a articulação costocondral.[140-142] Uma massa palpável, firme e fixa é o sinal clínico mais comum, embora dor e dispneia sejam também relatadas.[143] Alterações radiográficas incluem lise, esclerose ou uma mistura de padrões líticos e blásticos, com deslocamento das costelas adjacentes e estruturas intratorácicas, como o coração e os pulmões, e deslocamento medial da pleura parietal, resultando em sintoma extrapleural (Figura 348.6).[140-143] Disseminação intratorácica e invasão do pericárdio e lobos pulmonares são relativamente comuns.[143] A TC é recomenda para determinar a localização e extensão do tumor, a invasão potencial para estruturas adjacentes e a presença de metástases. Metástases pulmonares são comuns (especialmente em casos de OSA telangiectásico), e até 45% dos cães com OSA de costela apresentam metástases no momento do diagnóstico.[140,141] Na necropsia, metástases foram detectadas em 100% dos cães com OSA de costela, 53 a 57% com CSA, 67% com HSA e 100% com FSA de costela.[140,141] Devido aos comportamentos biológicos semelhantes dos OSA de costela e apendicular, o OSA de costela deve ser tratado por meio de ressecção e quimioterapia pós-cirúrgica.[141,143] A importância da quimioterapia em outros tipos de neoplasias não foi definida, mas sua realização é justificada devido à alta taxa de metástases.

Em animais com OSA submetidos apenas à ressecção da costela, a SM foi de 90 dias; em cães com CSA, ela varia de 1.080 dias até mais de 3.820 dias.[112,140-143] A maioria dos cães com CSA de costela primário pode ser curada somente com cirurgia.[112,143] Para cães com OSA de costela primário, os fatores ou indicadores de prognóstico são atividade sérica de ALP total no período pré-cirúrgico e administração de quimioterapia após a cirurgia. Em pacientes com alta atividade sérica de ALP total, ocorre redução significativa da SM de 675 para 210 dias.[143] A quimioterapia pós-cirúrgica prolonga de forma significativa a SM de cães com OSA de costela primário, para 240 a 290 dias.[141,143] Cães submetidos à extirpação cirúrgica incompleta possuem até 6,7 vezes mais chance de desenvolver recidiva local e, possivelmente, doença metastática.[141,143]

Tumores vertebrais

O OSA é o tumor extradural mais comum do sistema nervoso e corresponde a até 16% dos casos de OSA axiais.[119,120,144,145] Outros tumores vertebrais são CSA, FSA, HSA, exostoses cartilaginosas múltiplas, linfoma, lipossarcoma, tumor de célula gigante, tumores de plasmócitos (plasmocitoma solitário ou mieloma múltiplo) e carcinomas e sarcomas metastáticos.[144,145] Não há relato de predisposição racial, embora um estudo constatou que os cães das raças Pastor-Alemão, Labrador Retriever e Poodle Standard são mais predispostos.[144] Raças de grande porte são comumente acometidas; somente 5% dos cães com tumores vertebrais pesam menos que 20 kg.[144,145]

Tumores vertebrais primários tendem a ocorrer em um grupo de cães mais jovens do que os tumores de vértebras metastáticos.

A idade mediana de cães com tumores vertebrais primários é de 6 a 8 anos; para tumores secundários, é de 8 a 9 anos.[145] Deve ser realizado um exame físico minucioso (ver Capítulo 2) para detectar possíveis tumores primários ocultos. Carcinomas de glândula mamária, tireoide, bexiga e próstata e HSA viscerais sabidamente causam metástases em vértebras. Vértebras torácicas e lombares são mais comumente envolvidas.[144] Tumores de tecidos moles, particularmente sarcomas histiocíticos (ver Capítulo 350), podem envolver secundariamente as vértebras.

Dor e déficits neurológicos (ver Capítulo 259) são os sintomas mais comuns em cães com tumores vertebrais.[144,145] Déficits neurológicos são causados por compressão das raízes nervosas ou da medula espinal (ver Capítulo 267).[144,145] Os sintomas neurológicos apresentam progressão tipicamente lenta, mas fraturas patológicas podem causar deterioração aguda. Foi desenvolvido um sistema de graduação neurológica, o que indica prognóstico quanto à recuperação e à sobrevida do paciente.[145]

Um espectro de alterações radiográficas é observado em cães com tumores vertebrais. Essas alterações podem ser difíceis de detectar devido ao formato vertebral inconsistente e a sobreposição de costelas sobrejacentes e de tecidos moles.[144] A lise cortical por colapso do corpo vertebral é um achado característico em tumores vertebrais primários, mas um evento tardio em tumores metastáticos.[144,145] Metástases salteadas (skip) e tumores múltiplos são relatados em até 25% dos cães com OSA vertebral e podem ser difíceis de diferenciar de tumores metastáticos.[144] Osteocondromas são lesões benignas bem circunscritas que frequentemente envolvem a lâmina dorsal e o processo espinhoso, mas não o corpo vertebral.[146]

Exames de imagem incluem mielografia, TC, RM e cintilografia nuclear.[147] Esta pode detectar o local de lesões únicas ou múltiplas, mas não é capaz de diferenciar OSA multifocal de lesões metastáticas múltiplas. Ademais, a maioria dos tumores de plasmócitos são fotopênicos devido à osteólise marcante e à mínima produção de novo osso. Alterações mielográficas incluem colapso do espaço subaracnoide e deslocamento unilateral ou assimétrico da medula (Figura 348.7).[144] Exames de imagem avançados são melhores para a avaliação do envolvimento vertebral (Figura 348.8), mas a diferenciação entre envolvimento intradural e extradural pode ser difícil.[147] A ressecção cirúrgica por meio de vertebrectomia é raramente viável, embora a descompressão dorsal possa ser um procedimento paliativo relevante em cães com tumor dorsal localizado.[145,148] A radioterapia, seja com intenção paliativa, seja com intenção curativa, pode ser benéfica para cães com tumores vertebrais.[145] A importância da quimioterapia é desconhecida, mesmo em cães com OSA vertebral, pois a maioria dos pacientes é submetida à eutanásia devido ao tumor local, não à doença metastática.[145]

Em cães com tumores vertebrais malignos, a SM é de 135 dias.[145] A sobrevida não é influenciada de forma significativa pelo escore neurológico pré-cirúrgico, pelo tipo de tumor (OSA ou FSA), pela doença primária ou metastática, pela localização anatômica (cervical, torácica ou lombar), por quimioterapia ou por radioterapia.[145] Embora não seja relevante, o escore neurológico pode fornecer informações úteis, pois cães com escore pré-cirúrgico de 1 tiveram sobrevida de 330 dias, comparado a 10 dias do escore neurológico maior que 1.[145] Ademais, cães com escore neurológico pós-tratamento de 1 ou 2 tinham 12 vezes mais chance de sobreviver do que os com escore de 3 ou 4.[145] A radioterapia com intenção curativa propicia aumento significativo da sobrevida, comparativamente à radioterapia paliativa, com sobrevidas de 150 e 15 dias, respectivamente.[145]

Osteocondrossarcoma multilobular

O osteocondrossarcoma multilobular (OML) é um tumor incomum que surge do periósteo dos ossos formados por ossificação intramembranosa.[149,150] O crânio é mais comumente envolvido, incluindo calcário, órbita, arco zigomático, mandíbula e maxila.[149,150] Outros locais incluem pelve, costelas e palato duro. Também há relatos de OML em gatos.

Em geral, o OML é uma doença de cães de meia-idade, de raças de grande porte.[149,150] Não há predisposição sexual nem racial conhecida. Os sinais clínicos dependem da localização do tumor e incluem massa palpável firme e fixa, sintomas neurológicos em casos de OML do calvário, dor ao abrir a mandíbula em casos de OML mandibular ou do arco zigomático, exoftalmia em casos de OML orbital e dispneia em casos de OML da bula timpânica.[149,150] Em exames de imagem (radiografias e TC), as alterações associadas à OML são características, descrevendo o tumor com aparência de "pipoca", com margens bem definidas e um padrão lobulado.[149,152] Exames de imagem avançados são indicados para o planejamento cirúrgico de OML de calvário, pois a extensão do envolvimento intracraniano pode ser grande (Figura 348.9).[149,150]

Opções terapêuticas incluem ressecção cirúrgica e radioterapia.[149,150] Há relato de cranioplastia após ressecção do calvário, mas pode não ser necessária. A recuperação neurológica, particularmente em casos de envolvimento intracraniano marcante, pode ser demorada, embora a maioria dos cães retorne à função normal dentro de 2 semanas. Os OML crescem lentamente, quase sempre se encaminhando para resistência relativa e pouca resposta à radioterapia. Foram demonstradas recuperações preliminares variáveis, utilizando radioterapia com feixe externo e radiofármacos.[39,150]

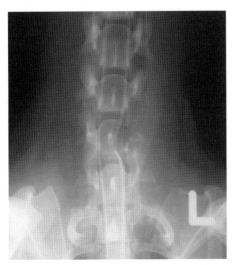

Figura 348.7 Mielograma ventrodorsal de cão com osteossarcoma na sexta vértebra cervical. Note que o tumor desloca e comprime a medula espinal em direção ao lado direito do canal espinal.

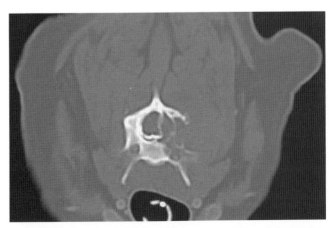

Figura 348.8 Imagem sagital de tomografia computadorizada (TC) do cão da Figura 348.7. Exames de imagem avançados, como TC ou ressonância magnética (RM), fornecem maiores informações sobre a extensão do tumor e a possibilidade de ressecção cirúrgica, para o planejamento cirúrgico e/ou radioterápico.

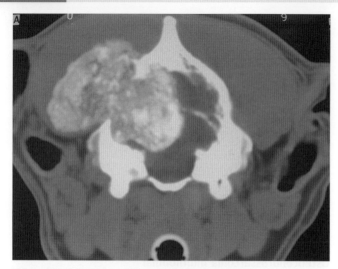

Figura 348.9 Imagem sagital de tomografia computadorizada (TC) de osteocondrossarcoma multilobular de grau I. Note a aparência de "pipoca", característica do tumor, e o extenso envolvimento intracraniano.

Um esquema de graduação histológico para OML tem valor prognóstico para recidivas locais e metástases.[120] Outros fatores prognósticos incluem o local e a ressecção cirúrgica completa.[149,150] A taxa de recidiva local é de 47 a 58%, com ILD mediano de 426 a 797 dias, dependendo do grau histológico.[149,150] A taxa de recidiva local de OML é de 30% para grau I, 47% para grau II e 78% para grau III.[149,150] Recomenda-se uma abordagem cirúrgica abrangente, pois a ressecção incompleta aumenta de forma significativa o risco de recidiva local. O ILD mediano após ressecção incompleta é de 330 dias, mas foi maior que 1.332 dias em casos de ressecção completa do OML.[149,150]

Para casos não tratados de OML, a SM é de 24 dias, comparada a 669 a 797 dias para OML tratados por meio de ressecção cirúrgica.[149,150] A localização do tumor tem valor prognóstico, com animais com OML mandibular apresentando SM significativamente mais longa do que aqueles com tumor em outros locais: 1.487 dias para casos de OML mandibular e 528 dias para casos de OML não mandibular.[150] A SM para OML de grau I é maior que 897 dias, enquanto a SM para OML de graus II e III é de 520 e 405 dias, respectivamente.[150]

OSTEOSSARCOMA APENDICULAR EM GATOS

Tumores ósseos primários são incomuns em gatos.[153-158] Diferentemente de cães, 10 a 33% dos tumores ósseos primários de gatos são benignos.[154] O OSA corresponde a 70 a 80% de todos os tumores ósseos felinos, mas também foram relatados FSA, CSA, HSA e rabdomiossarcoma.[153-155,159] A idade média ao diagnóstico de OSA apendiculares é de 10 a 11 anos; os machos são mais predispostos, com proporção macho:fêmea de 1,5 a 1,7:1.[154,157] Há várias diferenças na manifestação clínica e no comportamento biológico do OSA em gatos, comparativamente aos cães.[157] Em casos de OSA felino, os ossos do membro pélvico estão envolvidos 1,6 vezes mais frequentemente do que aqueles dos membros torácicos.[154] Os dígitos e o úmero proximal são os locais mais comuns, seguidos de perto pelo fêmur distal e pela tíbia proximal.[153-158] As características radiográficas são semelhantes em gatos e cães, embora lesões líticas e justacorticais sejam mais comuns.[153-157] Metástases são incomuns (menos que 10% dos gatos com OSA).[153-158] Os locais de metástases incluem pulmões, cérebro, fígado, rins e baço. Devido à infrequência da doença metastática, recomenda-se a amputação do membro, sem quimioterapia, para o tratamento de gatos com OSA apendicular. Relata-se SM após a amputação do membro de 11,8 a 49,2 meses.[153-158]

OUTROS TUMORES APENDICULARES EM GATOS

O FSA e o CSA apresentam comportamento biológico semelhante ao do OSA. A amputação do membro pode ser curativa, embora haja relato de doença metastática em ambos os tumores.[153,154]

TUMORES AXIAIS EM GATOS

O OSA é o tumor do esqueleto axial mais comum em gatos.[153,157] Também há relatos de FSA e CSA envolvendo o esqueleto axial.[153,154] No momento da consulta, a idade média dos gatos com OSA axial é de 10,4 anos, que é significativamente maior do que a de gatos com OSA apendicular.[157] O crânio e a pelve frequentemente são acometidos; outros locais incluem costelas, vértebras e escápula.[153-157] Os sintomas apresentados, as características radiográficas e as recomendações terapêuticas são semelhantes aos de tumores axiais malignos em cães. A neoformação óssea periosteal e de tumores justacorticais são mais comuns em gatos acometidos por OSA axial.[153,157] A ressecção cirúrgica completa é dificultada pela localização do tumor, resultando em ressecção incompleta e mal controle tumoral. Em gatos com OSA axial, a SM é de 5,5 a 6,1 meses, com a maioria deles submetida à eutanásia devido à recidiva local, não à doença metastática.[156,157]

TUMORES ÓSSEOS METASTÁTICOS

Tumores ósseos metastáticos são infrequentemente diagnosticados em gatos e cães. Quase sempre as metástases se instalam por via hematógena. Em cães, carcinomas urogenitais, principalmente de bexiga e próstata, são os tumores primários que mais originam metástases nos ossos.[7,160] A metástase óssea também é relatada em cães com OSA, carcinoma mamário, carcinoma de tireoide, carcinoma pulmonar, carcinoma nasal, adenocarcinoma de saco anal apócrino e neoplasias renais.[1,7,160-163] Lesões metastáticas representam 24% de todos os tumores ósseos em cães que pesam menos de 15 kg e somente 5% em cães de grande porte.[1,7,162] As localizações metastáticas mais comuns são o esqueleto axial e apendicular proximal, com menos de 11% dos cães desenvolvendo lesões metastáticas distais ao cotovelo ou joelho.[160] Já a acrometástase envolvendo um ou mais dígitos é a manifestação mais comum em gatos com carcinoma pulmonar metastático ("síndrome "pulmão-dígito").[161-164]

Recomenda-se cintilografia nuclear para detectar lesões ósseas múltiplas. As opções terapêuticas para metástases ósseas incluem cirurgia, radioterapia e medicamentos.[28,61] A curetagem cirúrgica e a estabilização de lesões metastáticas são incomumente realizadas na medicina veterinária, mas podem propiciar recuperação relevante em alguns casos. É indicada radioterapia para tratamento de dor e inflamação.[33]

TUMORES ARTICULARES EM CÃES

Quase sempre os tumores articulares são primários e malignos.[165-169] Previamente, o sarcoma de células sinoviais foi considerado o tumor de articulação mais comum em cães.[165,166] Entretanto, evidências recentes sugerem que outros sarcomas de tecidos moles periarticulares são mais prevalentes. É necessário exame imuno-histoquímico (IHQ) para diferenciar esses tipos de neoplasias.[167,168] Outros tumores articulares relatados são sarcoma histiocítico e histiocitoma fibroso maligno, mixoma sinovial e mixossarcoma, OSA, FSA, CSA, HSA, lipossarcoma, rabdomiossarcoma e sarcoma indiferenciado.[1,167-171] Foi detectada uma associação entre sarcoma histiocítico e artropatia preexistente em cães da raça Bernese Mountain (ver Capítulo 350).[170]

Os sarcomas de células sinoviais são tumores malignos que surgem de células mesenquimais do tecido tenossinovial de articulações, bursas e bainhas tendíneas.[165] Joelho, cotovelo, ombro, carpo, tarso e quadril são mais comumente envolvidos, em ordem decrescente de frequência.[1,165] A idade média no momento da consulta é de 6 a 8 anos.[165-169] Machos são mais predispostos, principalmente da raça Flat Coated Retriever.[165-169] Metástases aos linfonodos regionais e aos pulmões se desenvolvem em até 32% dos cães no momento do diagnóstico e em 41 a 54% dos cães durante o curso da doença.[165-169]

Tipicamente, os cães acometidos apresentam claudicação, sinais de dor articular e efusão sinovial. Cães com suspeita de tumor articular devem ser submetidos ao estadiamento por meio de palpação de linfonodos regionais e de radiografias regionais do tórax em três projeções. Quase sempre as radiografias regionais revelam opacidade de tecidos moles adjacentes à articulação acometida. Ocasionalmente, nota-se mineralização da massa de tecidos moles em humanos, mas raramente em cães. Ocorre envolvimento ósseo em 11 a 100% dos casos; pode ser macio ou bem delimitado, devido à necrose por pressão secundária à massa tumoral em expansão, ou permeado a lítico pontilhado, como resultado da invasão óssea.[165-169]

Para o diagnóstico definitivo é necessário biopsia. O exame do líquido sinovial quase sempre é compatível com inflamação crônica de baixo grau, e raramente são identificadas células neoplásicas. Biopsias de fragmentos centrais grandes, obtidos com agulha Jamshidi ou biopsia em cunha, podem definir o diagnóstico e o grau histológico.

Sarcomas de células sinoviais possuem duas populações distintas de células: epitelioides e fusiformes.[1,165] Com base nas características histológicas, os sarcomas de células sinoviais são subclassificados como monofásicos, com um tipo celular, ou bifásicos, com ambos os tipos celulares.[165] Entretanto, essa aparência histológica não é adequada para diferenciar sarcomas de células sinoviais de outros sarcomas de tecidos moles. Colorações imuno-histoquímicas têm sido utilizadas para diferenciar tumores articulares: sarcomas de células sinoviais são corados positivamente com anticorpo citoqueratina AE1/AE3, sarcomas histiocíticos são corados positivamente com anticorpo CD18 e histiocitomas fibrosos malignos são corados positivamente com actina de músculo liso.[168]

A amputação do membro é o tratamento recomendado para cães com tumor articular confirmado em exame histológico.[165-169] Recidiva local é comum após extirpação conservadora e foi relatada com frequência relativa no coto do membro amputado.[165] A importância da radioterapia e quimioterapia é desconhecida, mas relata-se que a quimioterapia não prolonga a sobrevida em pessoas com sarcomas de células sinoviais.[172]

Entretanto, recomenda-se um protocolo quimioterápico à base de doxorrubicina para sarcomas de células sinoviais de alto grau, devido ao seu alto potencial metastático.

Diversos fatores ou indicadores de prognóstico foram identificados em cães com sarcoma de células sinoviais, incluindo estadiamento clínico, tratamento, grau histológico e coloração imuno-histoquímica.[165-169] O estadiamento de sarcoma de células sinoviais local pode ser bem delimitado, sem evidências de invasão de estruturas regionais (T1), com invasão de tecidos moles (T2) ou de ossos e articulações (T3).[165] O estadiamento local não é prognóstico; entretanto, cães com metástases em linfonodos regionais ou pulmões apresentam SM inferior a 6 meses. A ressecção cirúrgica abrangente é importante para o prolongamento do ILD e da sobrevida. O controle do tumor é ruim após extirpação local conservadora, com ILD mediano de 4,5 meses, comparado aos 30 meses após a amputação do membro.[165,169] Ademais, a sobrevida é significativamente mais longa quando são utilizados protocolos terapêuticos locais mais extensos: 93 dias sem tratamento, 455 dias com ressecção conservadora e 840 dias com amputação de membro.[169] O grau histológico também tem valor prognóstico, pois a SM de cães com sarcoma de células sinoviais de grau I é maior que 48 meses; com grau II, 36 meses; e com grau III, 7 meses.[165]

O estadiamento clínico e as recomendações cirúrgicas (amputação do membro) são os mesmos para cães com sarcoma histiocítico (ver Capítulo 350). Cães com sarcoma histiocítico periarticular possuem melhor prognóstico do que cães com localizações não periarticulares, com SM de 391 dias e 128 dias, respectivamente.[169] Entretanto, apesar do melhor prognóstico, 68% dos cães com sarcoma histiocítico periarticular apresentam metástases. Cães sem metástases no momento do diagnóstico tiveram SM significativamente mais longa (980 dias) do que cães com metástases (253 dias).[169] Em cães com sarcoma histiocítico periarticular, recomenda-se o CCNU no período pós-cirúrgico, por conta do alto risco de metástase.[173]

TUMORES ARTICULARES EM GATOS

Sarcoma de células sinoviais é raramente diagnosticado em gatos. Com base em relatos de casos individuais, o comportamento biológico pode ser mais benigno do que em cães.[174,175] Entretanto, foram relatados dois casos de gatos com sarcoma de célula sinovial metastático (em ambos, metástase em linfonodos regionais, e, em um, metástase pulmonar 12 meses após a cirurgia).[176] Recomenda-se amputação do membro para o controle local, porque, como acontece em cães, há relato de recidiva local após extirpação conservadora.[174,175]

REFERÊNCIAS BIBLIOGRÁFICAS

As referências bibliográficas deste capítulo se encontram online no Ambiente de Aprendizagem.

CAPÍTULO 349

Mastocitose

Douglas H. Thamm

TUMORES DE MASTÓCITOS EM CÃES

Introdução

Prevalência

Mastocitomas (MCT) é a neoplasia cutânea mais comum em cães, oscilando entre 16 e 21% de todos os tumores cutâneos (ver Capítulos 10 e 345).[1] Diversas raças são predispostas a MCT, incluindo braquicefálicas (Boxer, Boston Terrier, Buldogue Inglês, Pug), Retriever, Cocker Spaniel, Schnauzer, Staffordshire Terrier, Beagle, Rhodesian Ridgeback, Weimaraner e Shar-pei.[1-3] Embora as raças braquicefálicas sejam mais predispostas ao desenvolvimento de MCT, os mastocitomas são mais provavelmente de baixo grau nesses cães.[1,4] Já as evidências anedóticas sugerem que cães da raça Shar-pei possam desenvolver MCT biologicamente mais agressivos.

Fisiopatologia

É provável que a anormalidade molecular mais bem descrita no MCT de cães envolva o receptor KIT da tirosinoquinase (RTK). O KIT é expresso normalmente em uma série de células, inclusive em células-tronco hematopoéticas, melanócitos e mastócitos.[5,6] O ligante do KIT, o fator de células-tronco (SCF), induz dimerização do KIT, fosforilação e geração de sinalização intracelular, que promove proliferação, diferenciação e maturação de mastócitos normais.[5,6] A expressão do KIT foi demonstrada em MCT de cães, e a localização citoplasmática aberrante do KIT no MCT pode estar associada à sua função desregulada.[7-9] Ademais, 25 a 30% dos MCT em cães de graus intermediário e alto possuem mutações no gene *c-kit*, o que resulta em ativação constitutiva independente de SCF do KIT.[10-13] A presença de mutação ativadora em *c-kit* está associada a maior risco de recidiva local, metástase e pior prognóstico.[10,12,14-16]

Histórico e sinais clínicos

Em cães, a maioria dos MCT se desenvolve nos tecidos dérmico e subcutâneo e é uma lesão solitária, embora 11 a 14% dos cães apresentem lesões múltiplas.[17-21] Uma forma visceral de MCT também foi descrita.[22,23] MCT cutâneos apresentam uma gama extremamente variada de manifestações clínicas e, às vezes, são inadvertidamente confundidos com lesões não neoplásicas. Em cães, o histórico e os sinais clínicos de MCT podem ocasionalmente ser complicados por sintomas atribuíveis à liberação de histamina, heparina e outras aminas vasoativas pelos grânulos de mastócitos, como eritema e edema nos tecidos circundantes, pelo prurido ou pelas alterações no tamanho do tumor. Cães com cargas tumorais substanciais (*i. e.*, tumores grandes, doença metastática) mais provavelmente manifestam sinais sistêmicos relacionados à liberação de mediadores de mastócitos. Esses podem incluir êmese, diarreia, febre, melena e edema periférico. Colapso é um evento raro. A histamina liberada por grânulos de MCT supostamente atua em células parietais gástricas através de receptores H2, resultando em aumento da secreção de ácido clorídrico.

Diagnóstico, estadiamento, prognóstico

Aspiração com agulha fina

A maioria dos MCT é prontamente diagnosticada com base no exame citológico de amostra de aspirado com agulha fina (AAF; ver Capítulos 86 e 87). Os mastócitos se assemelham a células redondas de tamanho pequeno a médio, com abundantes grânulos citoplasmáticos pequenos e uniformes que em geral são corados de vermelho-arroxeado (metacromático), mas um pequeno número deles não cora prontamente.[1,24] Nesses casos, quase sempre a coloração de Wright-Giemsa ou de azul de toluidina mostra os grânulos; entretanto, pode ser necessário exame histológico de uma amostra obtida por biopsia. O diagnóstico de MCT agranulares altamente anaplásicos por meio de microscopia óptica de rotina pode ser um desafio. A imuno-histoquímica para CD117 (KIT) frequentemente é utilizada para diferenciar MCT anaplásico de outros tumores de célula redonda.[7]

Avaliação do paciente

O estadiamento completo inclui uma base de dados mínima (hemograma, perfil bioquímico sérico), exame citológico de linfonodo(s) regional(is) (ver Capítulo 95), ultrassonografia de abdome (US; ver Capítulo 88), exame citológico do baço ou do fígado, se justificada (ver Capítulos 89 e 93), e radiografias do tórax. É provável que não seja necessário estadiamento extenso em cães com MCT, exame de linfonodos negativo, nem indicadores de prognóstico negativo (ver adiante; Figura 349.1). Se a localização do MCT é passível de ampla extirpação cirúrgica e não há indicadores de prognóstico negativo, então não são necessários outros exames além daqueles dados mínimos e do exame citológico dos linfonodos regionais (mesmo se apresentarem tamanho normal). Se a localização do tumor não possibilita ampla extirpação cirúrgica ou se há indicadores de prognóstico negativo, são recomendados exames adicionais antes da terapia definitiva, incluindo US de abdome, exame citológico de amostra de AAF de órgãos anormais e radiografias do tórax.[25,26] Se necessário, pode ser realizada uma biopsia por meio de incisão da lesão para determinar seu grau histológico, a fim auxiliar o tutor na tomada de decisão quanto ao tratamento.

Com relação ao exame citológico de linfonodos, um mastócito solitário ocasional não necessariamente indica metástase; já agrupamentos e agregados de mastócitos são mais preocupantes.[27] A doença no linfonodo regional (mas não além) não deve ser considerada uma razão para evitar a cirurgia; em vez disso, o linfonodo deve ser extirpado e enviado para exame histopatológico no momento da ressecção do tumor primário. Pode ser necessário exame histológico para determinar com acurácia se os mastócitos em um linfonodo representam doença metastática. Foi proposto um esquema de graduação para quantificar melhor o grau de infiltração do linfonodo para MCT em cães.[28] Com exceção da leucemia mastocítica primária, extremamente rara, é improvável o envolvimento da medula ou do sangue periférico na ausência de doença em linfonodos regionais ou de vísceras abdominais.[29] Portanto, raramente são necessários esfregaços da papa leucocitária e exame citológico de amostra obtida por aspiração da medula óssea.

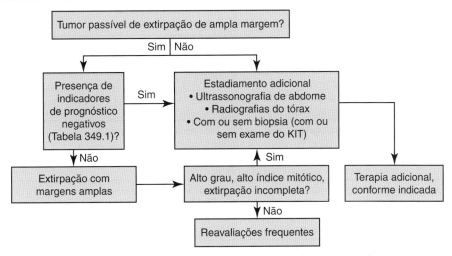

Figura 349.1 Algoritmo sugerido para o diagnóstico de tumores de mastócito cutâneos em cães.

Fatores ou indicadores de prognóstico

Em cães com MCT, devem ser avaliados os principais fatores ou indicadores de prognóstico (Tabela 349.1). É importante ressaltar que nenhum fator é inteiramente preditivo do comportamento biológico do tumor, e, desta forma, todos os indicadores de prognóstico devem ser considerados ao avaliar o paciente.

Tratamento

Mastocitoma de "baixo risco"

Cirurgia Decisões terapêuticas são baseadas na presença ou ausência de fatores prognósticos negativos e no estágio clínico da doença. Para tumores cutâneos localizados em áreas passíveis de ampla extirpação, a cirurgia é o tratamento de escolha. A excisão cirúrgica deve incluir uma margem de 3 cm de tecido normal circundante. Entretanto, algumas evidências sugerem que margens laterais de 1 a 2 cm e um plano fascial profundo não envolvido pela lesão podem ser suficientes para a extirpação total de vários MCT, principalmente dos pequenos e de menor grau.[30-33] Deve-se submeter as margens cirúrgicas ao exame histológico para confirmar a remoção total da neoplasia. Não se recomenda o uso rotineiro de corticosteroides neoadjuvantes com intuito de facilitar a ressecção cirúrgica, com exceção dos casos em que a excisão marginal não é possível devido à localização ou extensão da doença.

Remoção cirúrgica incompleta. Nos casos de obtenção de margens cirúrgicas incompletas ou parciais, justifica-se o uso de terapia local adicional para prevenir a ocorrência de recidiva;[34-36] entretanto, nem todos os MCT com margens cirurgicamente incompletas causam recidiva.[37,38] Se possível, deve-se repetir a extirpação da cicatriz cirúrgica com margens mais amplas. Se a cirurgia adicional não for possível, a radioterapia (RT) adjuvante pode ser bastante efetiva (ver Capítulo 240). É possível esperar uma taxa de controle em 2 anos de 85 a 95% após RT de tumores de grau baixo a intermediário submetidos à ressecção incompleta.[39-41] Uma alternativa menos recomendada é a combinação de cirurgia e quimioterapia (discutida adiante).[42,43] Para os tumores em que não seja possível a extirpação com margem segura, pode-se realizar exclusivamente RT,[41,44,45] RT junto a toceranib[46] ou apenas terapia medicamentosa (ver adiante).

Monitoramento. Independentemente da terapia local escolhida, cães com tumores de grau baixo a intermediário devem ser reavaliados com regularidade em busca de recidiva local, com ou sem metástase. Deve ser realizada uma avaliação local e uma de linfonodos regionais, um exame físico completo e uma aspiração de toda a massa tecidual cutânea nova ou de linfonodos com aumento de tamanho. Se o cão apresentar MCT com alto risco de metástase, deve-se obter um estadiamento mais completo, inclusive US de abdome.

Mastocitoma de "alto risco"

Considerações gerais. O tratamento de MCT de "alto risco" continua sendo um desafio. Essa categoria de pacientes inclui cães com tumores de alto grau, tumores de grau intermediário com metástases regionais ou distantes e tumores de alta atividade proliferativa, indicada pelo índice mitótico ou por colorações especiais. Também estão inclusos os MCT oriundos de membrana mucosa ou de junção mucocutânea. Alguns estudos sugerem que o prognóstico de tumores de grau baixo/intermediário é melhor quando há apenas envolvimento de linfonodos regionais, em comparação ao tumor de alto grau. Entretanto, este autor recomenda que tais tumores sejam tratados como se tivessem alta capacidade de causar metástase.[47-50] Além da terapia local apropriada, como discutido anteriormente, deve ser administrado tratamento medicamentoso adjuvante aos cães com MCT de alto risco, na tentativa de retardar ou prevenir metástases adicionais. Relata-se que os corticosteroides apresentam algum efeito benéfico,[45,51,52] mas a maioria das respostas é incompleta e transitória. A redução do edema/inflamação peritumoral induzida por corticosteroides pode interferir na avaliação da resposta.

Uso da quimioterapia. Diversos estudos avaliaram as taxas de resposta do MCT mensurável em cães a vários protocolos quimioterápicos citotóxicos.[36,53-59] Foram relatadas taxas de resposta de até 64%; protocolos com vários antineoplásicos podem conferir maior taxa de recuperação do que a terapia com um único agente.[36,53,55,57,58] Os medicamentos de primeira linha mais comumente empregados, vimblastina (VBL) e lomustina, são com frequência administrados junto aos corticosteroides.[36,54,57,59] É importante ressaltar que, na maioria das situações, a resposta de um grande MCT a qualquer protocolo quimioterápico tende a ser de curta duração, reforçando a necessidade do controle local da doença, se possível, antes de iniciar o tratamento medicamentoso. Alguns poucos estudos retrospectivos de um único segmento avaliaram a eficácia da quimioterapia pós-cirúrgica com vimblastina ou lomustina no tratamento de MCT de "alto risco". Cães submetidos à quimioterapia tendem a apresentar sobrevida média (SM) e intervalo livre da doença (ILD) mais longos, quando comparados àqueles submetidos apenas à cirurgia, com SM superior a 2 anos, na maioria dos estudos.[15,48,55,57,60]

Toceranib. Foram desenvolvidos inibidores da tirosinoquinase (TKI) de uso oral para inibir a sinalização através da KIT. Os dois KIT dessa classe aprovados para uso veterinário são

Tabela 349.1 Fatores ou indicadores de prognóstico para tumores de mastócito em cães.

FATOR/INDICADOR	COMENTÁRIO	REFERÊNCIAS
Grau histológico	Tumores de alto grau apresentam maior risco de recidiva local e metástases	2, 35, 91 a 93
Estágio clínico	Alguns estudos sugerem que o envolvimento de linfonodos regionais é um indicador de prognóstico negativo. A influência de tumores múltiplos na recuperação do paciente é questionável	17, 18, 20, 21, 27, 36, 41, 48, 50, 53, 55, 92, 94, 95
Localização	A localização subungueal, bucal ou em outras membranas mucosas está associada a tumores de maior grau e pior prognóstico. O prognóstico de tumores viscerais é muito ruim. Tumores subcutâneos geralmente estão associados a um melhor prognóstico	22, 23, 47, 96 a 98
Taxa de proliferação celular	Índice mitótico, frequência relativa de regiões argirofílicas organizadoras de nucléolos (AgNOR) e percentual de antígeno nuclear celular em proliferação (PCNA) ou imunopositividade para Ki-67 são preditivos da recuperação pós-cirúrgica	15, 37, 91, 93, 94, 98 a 107
Recidiva	Recidiva local após extirpação cirúrgica pode indicar um prognóstico mais reservado	36
Sintomas sistêmicos	A presença de sintomas sistêmicos (p. ex., anorexia, êmese, melena, úlcera gastrintestinal) pode estar associada a um estágio mais avançado da doença	18, 23
Raça	Mastocitomas (MCT) em cães da raça Boxer (e potencialmente outras raças braquicefálicas) tendem a ser de grau baixo a intermediário e estão associados a melhor prognóstico. MCT em cães Shar-pei pode ser de maior grau	1, 4
Mutação no *c-kit*	A presença de mutação ativadora no gene *c-kit* está associada a pior prognóstico	10, 14, 15
Localização da proteína KIT	A localização predominantemente aberrante (citoplasmática) de KIT está associada a pior prognóstico	108

toceranib (Palladia®, Zoetis) e masitinib (Masivet/Kinavet®, AB Science). Em algumas pesquisas, também se utilizou o inibidor de KIT humano, o imatinibe (Gleevec®, Novartis).[61] Após estudos clínicos de fase inicial encorajadores, realizou-se um estudo aleatório duplo cego controlado com placebo em cães com MCT de grau intermediário ou alto recidivante ou metastático em diversos centros.[13,62] A taxa de resposta objetiva nos cães tratados com toceranib foi de 37,2% (7 completas, 25 parciais) *versus* 7,9% (todas parciais) de cães do grupo placebo. A duração mediana da resposta e o tempo de progressão tumoral foi de 12 e 18,1 semanas, respectivamente. Cães cujo MCT apresentava mutações ativadoras do *c-kit* tiveram taxas de resposta objetiva mais alta do que aqueles que apresentavam *c-kit* do tipo selvagem (69% *versus* 37%). A toxicidade gastrintestinal (inapetência, perda de peso, diarreia e ocasionalmente êmese ou melena) foi o efeito adverso mais comum e em geral controlado com tratamento sintomático, maior intervalo entre as doses e redução da dose. Outros efeitos adversos incluem leucopenia discreta à moderada e dor muscular ocasional.[62] A experiência clínica com toceranib sugere que é possível obter atividade antitumoral equivalente e menor taxa de efeitos adversos com doses menores do que as recomendadas na bula. Atualmente, muitos clínicos utilizam dose de 2,4 a 2,75 mg/kg, em dias alternados ou 3 dias por semana (segunda-feira, quarta-feira e sexta-feira).[46,63]

Masitinib. Foi realizado um estudo clínico com delineamento semelhante utilizando o masitinib em cães com MCT recidivante ou sem possibilidade de ressecção; constatou-se melhora do tempo de progressão da doença em cães tratados com masitinib, comparativamente aos animais do grupo que recebeu placebo, e, novamente, o resultado foi melhor em cães que apresentavam mutações ativadoras no gene *c-kit* e nos submetidos a tratamento de primeira linha.[64] O acompanhamento subsequente por longo tempo de cães tratados com masitinib constatou um número maior de animais com controle da doença a longo prazo, comparativamente àqueles tratados com placebo (40% *versus* 15% vivos em 2 anos).[65] Efeitos gastrintestinais adversos (êmese ou diarreia) foram mais comuns, porém normalmente eram discretos e autolimitantes. Mielossupressão discreta também foi observada. Uma pequena porcentagem de cães desenvolveu nefropatia com perda de proteína e edema. Em alguns cães, notou-se aumento das concentrações de nitrogênio ureico sanguíneo (NUS) e de creatinina sérica. Anemia hemolítica foi uma ocorrência rara.[64]

Combinação de TKI e outras terapias. Há poucos estudos que avaliam a combinação de inibidores da KIT e protocolos-padrão de terapia, como RT ou quimioterapia citotóxica, mas ainda não foram demonstradas evidências de benefícios quando utilizadas no período pós-cirúrgico. Um estudo clínico recente avaliou a combinação de toceranib e vimblastina em cães com MCT mensurável. Foram necessárias reduções significativas na dose e na frequência de administração da vimblastina, devido à mielossupressão aditiva.[66] Entretanto, constatou-se atividade clínica animadora (taxa de resposta objetiva de 71%), mesmo com as reduções da dose necessária. Outro estudo avaliou a combinação de toceranib, prednisona e RT hipofracionada em cães com MCT sem possibilidade de ressecção e/ou metastática.[46] A taxa de resposta geral foi de cerca de 76%, com quase 60% dos cães apresentando remissão completa e outros 17% tendo remissão parcial. O ILD foi de 10,5 meses.

Terapia paliativa. Às vezes, o uso de terapia paliativa auxiliar é justificado com a minimização dos efeitos sistêmicos dos mediadores de mastócitos, utilizando bloqueadores de H1 e H2 (p. ex., difenidramina, famotidina). O omeprazol, um inibidor da bomba de prótons, pode ser mais efetivo na redução da secreção de ácido gástrico, principalmente quando há mastocitoma grande. Esses medicamentos são particularmente úteis em casos em que: (1) há sintomas sistêmicos; (2) o tumor provavelmente será extensamente manipulado durante a cirurgia (i. e., cirurgia para citorredução, biopsia por meio de incisão); ou (3) o tratamento é realizado no contexto de doença macroscópica (p. ex., RT ou terapia medicamentosa para tumores não submetidos à citorredução). Não há evidência clínica de que bloqueadores H1 e H2 ou omeprazol tenham qualquer ação antineoplásica.

MASTOCITOMAS EM GATOS

Diferentemente dos MCT de cães, que são primariamente cutâneos ou SC, as manifestações típicas dos MCT de gatos aparecem na forma de três síndromes distintas: cutânea, esplênica/visceral e intestinal. Em um estudo, constatou-se que 67% dos MCT cutâneos e esplênicos/viscerais apresentam mutações ativadoras do gene *c-kit*.[67]

Mastocitomas cutâneos em gatos

Definições

Os MCT são o segundo tumor cutâneo mais comum em gatos, correspondendo a cerca de 20% dos casos.[68,69] É um nódulo solitário, elevado, firme, bem circunscrito, alopécico e com 0,5 e 3 cm de diâmetro. Aproximadamente 20% são múltiplos, embora uma série de relatos tenha constatado múltiplas lesões na maioria dos casos.[1] Há relatos de dois tipos distintos de MCT cutâneo em gatos: o MCT mastocítico mais típico, histologicamente semelhante ao MCT de cães, e o MCT histiocítico, menos comum. O MCT histiocítico possui características morfológicas dos mastócitos histiocíticos, e pode regredir espontaneamente após 4 a 24 meses.[70,71] Gatos Siameses parecem ser predispostos a ambos os tipos de lesão.[68-72] A forma mastocítica pode ser subdividida em duas categorias, com base na aparência histológica: compacta (50 a 90% de todos os casos) e difusa (anaplásica).[68,70,73] Tumores compactos bem diferenciados tendem a ser benignos, e a ocorrência de metástase é incomum, enquanto tumores anaplásicos podem apresentar alto índice mitótico, pleomorfismo celular e nuclear marcantes e infiltração SC. Segundo a literatura, o comportamento clínico desses tumores anaplásicos é variável.[71,72,74-76]

Diagnóstico

A maioria dos MCT de gatos é facilmente diagnosticada mediante o exame citológico de AAF (ver Capítulos 86 e 87). Gatos com MCT cutâneo devem ser avaliados em busca de evidências de tumores adicionais, bem como a partir do potencial envolvimento esplênico, por meio de US de abdome (ver Capítulo 88). Um estudo sugeriu que alguns gatos com MCT cutâneos múltiplos também apresentam doença esplênica.[74] É recomendada uma base de dados mínima, juntamente à avaliação cuidadosa de linfonodos locais. O sistema de graduação histológica descrito para MCT de cães não propiciou informações prognósticas para os gatos e, portanto, não é utilizado. Parece que tumores com alto índice mitótico apresentam maior risco de recidiva local e metástases.[71,72,76,77]

Tratamento

O tratamento recomendado para a maioria dos MCT de gatos é a extirpação cirúrgica. Relatos mencionaram taxas de recidiva local após extirpação de 0 a 24%[68,71,72,74-76] e taxas de metástases de 0 a 22%.[71,72,74-76] Tumores histologicamente anaplásicos ou com alto índice mitótico podem ser melhor controlados com tratamento sistêmico, como recomendado para MCT de cães, embora estatísticas relacionadas à eficácia sejam escassas.[76,78] Após confirmação da forma histiocítica em amostra obtida por biopsia, pode-se realizar ressecção conservadora ou monitoramento ativo do paciente. Alguns neoplasias podem regredir espontaneamente.[68-70] A RT pode ser utilizada em tumores submetidos a extirpação completa (ver Capítulo 240).[79] Há informações limitadas sobre a importância de quimioterapia em gatos com MCT. Respostas objetivas à lomustina (CCNU) foram relatadas em gatos.[80,81] Com base em informações anedóticas, o uso de prednisona/vimblastina em alguns gatos, como

mencionado para cães, parece ter atividade antitumoral. A administração de imatinibe foi associada à recuperação parcial em gatos com MCT que expressam mutações ativadoras do gene *c-kit*.[67,82,83] O masitinib e o toceranib não foram formalmente avaliados em gatos com MCT.

Mastocitomas esplênicos/viscerais em gatos

Prevalência e sintomas

MCT é o diagnóstico diferencial mais comum para doença esplênica em gatos e representa 15% dos diagnósticos em uma série de casos.[84] A maioria dos gatos com MCT esplênico não tem histórico de MCT cutâneo, embora evidências recentes sugiram que alguns animais com MCT cutâneos múltiplos podem também ter envolvimento esplênico.[74] Embora o baço seja o principal local de ocorrência dessa doença, outros órgãos podem estar igualmente envolvidos.[68,85] Há relato de mastocitose de sangue periférico na maioria dos casos, com contagens de mastócitos no sangue periférico de 32.000 células/$\mu\ell$.[68,86] Gatos com MCT esplênico podem apresentar sinais de doença sistêmica, inclusive êmese, inapetência e perda de peso.[68,85] Também é possível verificar sinais clínicos associados à degranulação de mastócitos, como úlcera gastrintestinal, hemorragia, choque hipotensivo e respiração laboriosa. A palpação abdominal quase sempre revela organomegalia cranial marcante. Gatos com suspeita de MCT esplênico devem ser submetidos a exames padrões, que incluem uma base de dados mínima, US de abdome (ver Capítulo 88) e radiografias do tórax. Em geral, o exame citológico de AAF guiada por US (ver Capítulos 89 e 93) ou de efusões fornece diagnóstico para MCT esplênico.

Tratamento

Esplenectomia é o tratamento preferido para gatos com MCT esplênico, mesmo se houver envolvimento de outros órgãos. A sobrevida a longo prazo com boa qualidade de vida é comum. Mesmo em gatos com envolvimento relevante da medula óssea e do sangue periférico, a SM é de 12 a 19 meses.[68,85,87] Assim como em casos de MCT cutâneo de alto risco, a utilidade do tratamento medicamentoso adjuvante é desconhecida.

Mastocitomas intestinais em gatos

O MCT intestinal é o terceiro tumor intestinal primário mais comum em gatos, após o linfoma e o adenocarcinoma.[68] A maioria dos gatos tem histórico de êmese, diarreia e inapetência. Uma massa abdominal palpável é frequentemente evidente.[68,88] Linfonodos mesentéricos aumentados e/ou hepatomegalia podem ser notados ao exame físico. Efusão peritoneal contendo mastócitos e eosinófilos é possível. Quase sempre o diagnóstico é baseado em amostras de AAF da massa tecidual ou de órgãos envolvidos. Gatos com MCT intestinal devem ser submetidos ao estadiamento com uma base de dados mínima, radiografias do tórax e US do abdome. O prognóstico de MCT intestinal em gatos é o pior, já que é comum detectar metástase no momento do diagnóstico.[68,88-90] O tratamento de escolha é a cirurgia, com necessidade de amplas margens cirúrgicas (5 a 10 cm), pois a neoplasia em geral se estende histologicamente bem além da doença macroscópica evidente.[68,88] Há informações limitadas quanto ao uso de tratamento medicamentosa para MCT intestinal de gatos.

REFERÊNCIAS BIBLIOGRÁFICAS

As referências bibliográficas deste capítulo se encontram online no Ambiente de Aprendizagem.

CAPÍTULO 350

Doenças Histiocíticas em Cães e Gatos

Laurel E. Williams

Doenças histiocíticas representam um espectro diverso e potencialmente confuso de síndromes que variam desde lesões solitárias que regridem espontaneamente (histiocitoma) até tumores altamente malignos que envolvem várias regiões corporais (sarcoma histiocítico disseminado). Estão inclusos nessa categoria condições reativas associadas à desregulação imune subjacente (histiocitose cutânea, histiocitose sistêmica). O objetivo deste capítulo é caracterizar a origem, o comportamento, a manifestação clínica e o tratamento dessas diversas doenças.

ORIGEM CELULAR E DESENVOLVIMENTO

Os histiócitos se desenvolvem a partir de células-tronco CD34+ da medula óssea, migram para o sangue como monócitos e adentram vários tecidos, onde sofrem diferenciação em macrófagos e células dendríticas (CD). Sob a influência do fator estimulante de colônia de monócitos/macrófagos, os monócitos do sangue se diferenciam em macrófagos, enquanto o fator estimulante de colônias de granulócitos-macrófagos, a interleucina-4 e o fator de necrose tumoral-alfa levam a diversas linhagens de CD, inclusive CD intersticial e células de Langerhans (CL), sendo esta criticamente dependente da estimulação do fator transformador de crescimento beta-1.[1-3] CD intersticiais se desenvolvem em localizações perivasculares de vários órgãos, enquanto CL predominam na epiderme, com populações mais recentemente definidas em linfonodos e outros locais.[4,5]

Histiócitos têm importância fundamental no sistema imune, por meio de fagocitose (macrófagos) e processamento e apresentação de antígenos (CD, CL). As CD são as células apresentadoras de antígenos (APC) mais potentes na indução de respostas imunes pelos linfócitos T (ou células T) que ainda não tiveram contato com determinado antígeno (ou seja, linfócitos T *"naïve"*). As células são definidas com base em sua expressão de moléculas essenciais para sua função, como APC (Tabela 350.1). Anticorpos monoclonais específicos de cães e gatos para essas moléculas funcionalmente importantes auxiliam na identificação de macrófagos, CD e CL nos tecidos e podem ser úteis na distinção de doenças histiocíticas. Por essa razão, além da coleta de amostras de rotina para exames citológicos e histopatológicos, com frequência é recomendada a coleta de tecido fresco que é rapidamente congelado.

DOENÇAS HISTIOCÍTICAS

Histiocitoma em cães

Em cães, o histiocitoma é um tumor cutâneo benigno comum que se origina das CL. Normalmente acomete cães jovens, mas a incidência diminui após os 3 anos. Em um estudo retrospectivo de diagnósticos histológicos de tumores em cães com menos de 1 ano de idade no Reino Unido, o histiocitoma cutâneo foi o diagnóstico mais comum, representando 89% dos casos.[6]

Tipicamente, as lesões são solitárias e se apresentam como massas teciduais alopécicas em formato de domo ou de botão na superfície cutânea. A cabeça é um local frequentemente acometido, embora as lesões possam ocorrer em qualquer parte do corpo. O diagnóstico requer exame citológico. As características citológicas são variáveis, mas tipicamente consistem em uma população de células redondas com características nucleares benignas, citoplasma abundante e quase sempre alto índice mitótico.

Os histiocitomas em geral apresentam regressão espontânea dentro de 3 meses, e a ocorrência de recidiva é incomum. A regressão é mediada por células T CD8+, e, com o passar do tempo, a infiltração linfocítica progressiva é evidente nos tumores.[7] Geralmente, não é necessário tratamento cirúrgico ou medicamentoso, mas pode ser recomendado em casos de lesões persistentes, recorrentes ou problemáticas para o animal.

Histiocitose de células de Langerhans cutânea em cães

A presença de múltiplos histiocitomas em cães é incomum e pode ser mais bem considerada no espectro de histiocitose de células de Langerhans (HCL) cutânea, já que a pele está consistentemente envolvida e é considerada o local de origem.[8] As lesões podem ser limitadas à pele ou se estender até envolver linfonodos regionais e, raramente, órgãos internos. O diagnóstico requer exame citológica, com realização de exame histopatológico e imunofenotipagem

---

Tabela 350.1 Caracterização das doenças histiocíticas de cães e gatos.[8]

DOENÇA	ESPÉCIE	CÉLULA DE ORIGEM	IMUNOFENÓTIPO
Histiocitoma	Cão	CL	CD1a, CD11c/CD18, E-caderina
Histiocitose de CL cutânea	Cão	CL	CD1a, CD11c/CD18, E-caderina
Histiocitose de CL pulmonar	Gato	CL	CD1a,* CD18, E-caderina
Histiocitose cutânea	Cão	CD	CD1a, CD4, CD11c/CD18, CD90
Histiocitose sistêmica	Cão	CD	CD1a, CD4, CD11c/CD18, CD90
Sarcoma histiocítico	Cão, gato	CD	CD1a, CD11c/CD18
Sarcoma histiocítico hemofagocítico	Cão, gato	Macrófago	CD1a (baixo), CD11c/CD18 (cão)
Histiocitose progressiva felina	Gato	CD	CD1a, CD11†/CD18, CD5 (50%)

*CD1a esperado; ainda não avaliado. †CD11c esperado, ainda não foi avaliado em gatos. *CD*, célula dendrítica; *CL*, célula de Langerhans.

CAPÍTULO 350 • Doenças Histiocíticas em Cães e Gatos 2145

para o diagnóstico definitivo. O exame dos linfonodos, as radiografias do tórax e a ultrassonografia (US) do abdome são úteis para determinar a extensão da doença.

Pode ocorrer regressão espontânea das lesões e, às vezes, é demorada, com persistência de lesões por vários meses antes da regressão. Infelizmente, a ausência de regressão e o difícil tratamento de extensas lesões ulceradas quase sempre levam à eutanásia. Há informações limitadas sobre tratamentos efetivos, embora um relato de caso tenha descrito melhora transitória após administração de quimioterapia com lomustina.[9]

Histiocitose de células de Langerhans pulmonar em gatos

Anormalidades proliferativas de CL são raras em gatos. Um relato mencionou doença proliferativa primariamente pulmonar oriunda de CL em três gatos.[10] Esses animais eram de idade avançada (10 a 15 anos) e apresentavam sinais de doença respiratória, inclusive angústia respiratória há 5 dias a 7 meses. Radiografias do tórax detectaram um padrão bronco-intersticial difuso grave nos três gatos, com opacidades miliares a nodulares difusas em dois deles. Em dois gatos, o tratamento com glicocorticoide não melhorou os sinais clínicos. Em ambos, optou-se por eutanásia devido aos sintomas respiratórios progressivos. O diagnóstico de HCL foi confirmado no exame pós-morte, por meio de exames histopatológicos, imuno-histoquímicos e microscopia eletrônica. Também foram detectadas metástases em outros locais, inclusive pâncreas, fígado, rins e linfonodos viscerais.

Histiocitose reativa em cães (cutânea, sistêmica)

A histiocitose reativa consiste em um grupo de doenças não neoplásicas oriundas de CD. Em cães acometidos, as lesões podem ser restritas a pele, tecido subcutâneo e linfonodos regionais (histiocitose cutânea) ou podem envolver pele e diversos outros locais, que incluem linfonodos, fígado, baço, pulmões, medula óssea, olhos e membranas mucosas (histiocitose sistêmica). Em ambas as formas da doença, as lesões cutâneas são semelhantes, sendo possível a progressão de histiocitose cutânea para a forma sistêmica. A etiologia e a patogenia exatas são desconhecidas, mas propôs-se a desregulação dos mecanismos de resposta imune como causa.

Histiocitose cutânea

A histiocitose cutânea tende a ocorrer em cães mais jovens. Em um estudo retrospectivo de 32 cães, constatou-se idade mediana de 4 anos (variando de 1 a 8 anos).[11] O tempo de manifestação dos sintomas antes do diagnóstico é variável, com média de 1,75 mês e variação de 0 a 30 meses, dados relatados no mesmo estudo.[11] As lesões se apresentam como nódulos multifocais, placas e crostas na pele e no tecido subcutâneo. Ulceração da pele sobrejacente é comum.

O diagnóstico requer exame histopatológico e, se possível, imunofenotipagem. As lesões são caracterizadas por infiltrado histiocítico, com angiocentricidade variável, na derme e no tecido subcutâneo. Infiltrado linfoide é comum, compreendendo até 50% dos infiltrados dérmicos.[11,12] Os padrões de expressão dos antígenos dos histiócitos são compatíveis com origem em CD.[12] Exame de linfonodos (ver Capítulo 95), radiografias do tórax e US do abdome (ver Capítulo 88) são úteis para distinção entre as formas cutânea e sistêmica da doença.

A progressão da doença pode ser pontuada por remissões e recidivas, especialmente no início da enfermidade. Dada a natureza difusa, em geral o tratamento cirúrgico tem uso limitado. Em vez disso, o tratamento típico consiste na administração de medicamentos imunomoduladores (ver Capítulo 165). Em um estudo, foram observadas respostas variáveis após o tratamento sistêmico em sete cães.[12] Em outra série de casos, relatou-se cura completa das lesões cutâneas em cães que receberam uma variedade de fármacos imunomoduladores dentro de um período mediano de 45 dias (com variação de 14 a 162 dias).[11]

Medicamentos imunomoduladores incluíam o uso de prednisona como agente único ou em combinação com tetraciclina/niacinamida ou azatioprina, de tetraciclina/niacinamida (exclusivo) e de ciclosporina.

Pode ser necessária terapia de manutenção a longo prazo ou cursos repetidos de tratamento. No relato que descreve a resolução completa das lesões, é mencionado que 30% dos cães apresentaram recidivas, e todos os cães responderam ao tratamento adicional.[11] No final do estudo, após acompanhamento por um período mediano de 25 meses, 26 dos 32 cães (81%) estavam vivos, sem lesões. Os outros 6 cães haviam falecido sem sintomas de histiocitose cutânea.

Histiocitose sistêmica

A histiocitose sistêmica foi incialmente relatada em um grupo de cães Bernese Montanhês com parentesco próximo, sugerindo uma predisposição genética nessa raça.[13] Também foi sugerida predisposição das raças Rottweiler, Golden Retriever e Labrador Retriever.[12] A histiocitose sistêmica acomete predominantemente cães de meia-idade (mediana de 5 anos; com variação de 1 a 9 anos).[12,13]

Em geral, os sintomas apresentados são inespecíficos e incluem depressão, anorexia e perda de peso, variando de acordo com a distribuição e a extensão das lesões. Lesões cutâneas e subcutâneas são semelhantes, embora possivelmente mais disseminadas, em comparação àquelas verificadas na histiocitose cutânea. O envolvimento de linfonodos, fígado, baço, pulmão, medula óssea, olhos (conjuntiva, esclera, órbita, terceira pálpebra) e membranas mucosas (gengival, nasal) é variável.[12,14]

O diagnóstico requer exame histopatológico e, se possível, imunofenotipagem. As lesões são idênticas àquelas descritas em casos de histiocitose cutânea; infiltração angiocêntrica com invasão vascular pode ser mais consistentemente observada na forma sistêmica da doença.[12] Exame de linfonodos (ver Capítulo 95), radiografias do tórax e US de abdome (ver Capítulo 88) são úteis para determinar a extensão da doença. Essas características coletivas também são úteis para distinguir histiocitose sistêmica das doenças histiocíticas malignas e não histiocíticas.

Assim como acontece na histiocitose cutânea, a progressão da doença pode ser pontuada por remissões e recidivas. Medicamentos de uso sistêmico que mostraram certa eficácia incluem prednisona, ciclosporina, leflunomida, fração 5 da timosina bovina experimental e o quimioterápico doxorrubicina.[12,13] A progressão clínica pode ser lenta; recidivas frequentemente estão associadas a sintomas mais graves e resposta menos efetiva ao tratamento.

A progressão oscilante da doença e a remissão espontânea ocasional complicam a avaliação da eficácia terapêutica. Entretanto, repetidas respostas à terapia com agentes imunomoduladores capazes de inibir a ativação de linfócitos T sustentam a teoria de que a histiocitose reativa se deve à regulação imune desordenada que surge a partir de interações anormais entre CD/linfócito T, e não de um processo neoplásico.

Histiocitose progressiva em gatos

As doenças histiocíticas proliferativas são incomuns em gatos. A histiocitose progressiva felina é uma síndrome oriunda de CD. Tipicamente, os gatos acometidos apresentam idade mais avançada, com média de 10 anos (com variação de 2 a 17 anos).[15] Os animais apresentam pápulas intradérmicas e nódulos cutâneos que são ocasionalmente solitários, porém com muita frequência são múltiplos. À semelhança da histiocitose reativa em cães, as lesões apresentam tamanhos variáveis, mas, diferentemente da histiocitose canina, em uma série de 30 gatos não se constatou regressão espontânea total.[15]

O diagnóstico requer exame histopatológico e, se possível, imunofenotipagem. As lesões microscópicas consistem em infiltrados histiocíticos dérmicos difusos que podem se estender ao tecido subcutâneo. Algumas lesões apresentam epiteliotropismo. A atipia celular e a extensão profunda em direção ao subcutâneo são mais notáveis em lesões em estágio avançado.[8,15] Os padrões de expressão dos antígenos de histiócitos são compatíveis com origem de CD.[8,15]

Com o passar do tempo, o tamanho dos nódulos aumenta; alguns deles se unem e formam placas maiores que podem se tornar ulceradas e dolorosas. Na maioria dos gatos, as lesões são restritas à pele por um longo período. Ocasionalmente, nota-se envolvimento interno no momento do diagnóstico, como foi o caso em 4 de 22 gatos (18%) da série anteriormente mencionada.[15] Exame de linfonodos, radiografias do tórax e US do abdome são úteis para determinar a existência de lesões internas. Quase sempre a doença é progressiva ao longo de meses a anos (tempo mediano de 13,4 meses); no cenário da doença avançada, a disseminação para locais internos se torna mais comum, como relatado em 4 de 18 gatos (22%).[15]

Dada sua natureza difusa, a cirurgia tem benefícios limitados e deve ser reservada para lesões que são particularmente incômodas ou que causem morbidade. No estudo citado anteriormente, 8 gatos foram submetidos à cirurgia.[15]

Recidiva tumoral local foi observada em 4 gatos; todos os 8 animais examinados desenvolveram lesões adicionais distantes do local da cirurgia. Foram desapontadores os resultados do tratamento medicamentoso incluindo corticosteroides, quimioterápicos (L-asparaginase, vincristina, vimblastina, ciclofosfamida, mostarda nitrogenada) e agentes imunomoduladores (corticosteroides, ciclosporina, leflunomida, interferona gama, retinoides).

A histiocitose progressiva felina é caracterizada por múltiplos nódulos cutâneos e progressão clínica lenta. As lesões podem ser variáveis, e a doença pode ser restrita à pele por longos períodos. A etiologia é desconhecida. Embora algumas características sejam semelhantes à histiocitose reativa canina, a ausência de remissão espontânea e a carência de resposta aos fármacos imunomoduladores tornam improvável uma etiologia ligada à desregulação imune. Em vez disso, parece que a histiocitose progressiva felina representa um processo neoplásico inicialmente indolor e, por fim, mais agressivo.

Complexo sarcoma histiocítico

É uma doença maligna de origem histiocítica inicialmente relatada em cães no final da década de 1970.[16] Um relato inicial descreveu o sarcoma histiocítico (SH) em 11 cães Bernese Montanhês, 9 dos quais possuíam parentesco próximo, sugerindo uma predisposição genética dessa raça.[17] Cães das raças Flat-Coated Retriever, Rottweiler, Golden Retriever e Labrador Retriever também parecem mais predispostos.[18,19] Embora não seja considerada uma raça predisposta à SH em outras regiões corporais, os cães da raça Pembroke Welsh Corgi tem mais predisposição a casos da doença oriundos do sistema nervoso central (SNC), correspondendo a 47% da população de um estudo.[20,21] Os cães acometidos tipicamente são de meia-idade.

Embora a classificação continue sendo atualizada, o *sarcoma histiocítico* se tornou o termo preferido para esse grupo de neoplasias, descrevendo duas formas da doença: SH localizado e SH disseminado (anteriormente denominado histiocitose maligna). Ambas são oriundas de CD, com coloração positiva característica para anticorpos contra CD11 c e CD18. Embora análises de microarranjos tenham detectadas variações na expressão do gene entre o SH localizado e o SH disseminado,[22] eles são morfológica e imunofenotipicamente idênticos e distinguidos com base na manifestação clínica. O SH localizado é oriundo de um único órgão, enquanto o SH disseminado é uma doença multissistêmica. O SH histiocítico hemofagocítico é outro subtipo, singular em sua origem macrofágica e caracterizado por coloração positiva para anticorpos contra CD11 d e CD18.

Sarcoma histiocítico localizado

O SH localizado acomete mais comumente a pele e o subcutâneo, com mais frequência de membros e tecidos periarticulares, embora possa se desenvolver em outros locais, como baço, pulmão, cérebro, medula espinal, cavidade nasal, ossos e medula óssea.[18-21,23-26] Formas periarticulares e de SNC da doença foram descritas como subgrupos singulares de SH localizado.[20,21,23,26] O SH periarticular pode ser mais comum em cães da raça Rottweiler.[23] Claudicação e/ou edema de tecidos moles periarticulares são os sinais clínicos mais comuns, relatados em 79 e 68% dos cães, respectivamente, em um estudo.[26] O joelho parece ser o local mais frequente, relatado em 37 a 61% dos cães.[23,26] Um fato interessante mencionado em um estudo foi que 55% dos cães tinham histórico de ruptura de ligamento cruzado cranial (LCC) na mesma articulação, após o desenvolvimento de HS.[23] Em cães com ruptura do LCC, a sinóvia inflamada contém diversas CD, embora não tenha sido bem definida uma relação entre a inflamação e o subsequente desenvolvimento tumoral.[27] Radiografias são indicadas para cães com suspeita de HS periarticular. Em um estudo, constatou-se que 60% dos cães tinham evidências radiográficas de osteólise ou proliferação no local do tumor.[26] O SH do SNC pode estar restrito a um único local no cérebro ou na medula espinal ou ser multifocal (ver Capítulos 260 e 267). Os sinais refletem a localização neuroanatômica (ver Capítulo 259) e incluem convulsões, alterações do estado mental ou do comportamento, déficits de reações posturais e paresia.[20,21] Ocorre metástase em 15 a 70% dos cães com HS localizado no momento do diagnóstico, e 50 a 90% dos cães, por fim, desenvolvem doença metastática em linfonodos, pulmão e vísceras abdominais.[18,21,23,24,26]

Sarcoma histiocítico disseminado

O SH disseminado envolve diversos sistemas orgânicos, sugerindo progressão e metástase a partir da forma localizada da doença ou uma doença multicêntrica primária oriunda de tumores simultâneos em diversos locais. Pulmões, baço, fígado, linfonodos e/ou medula óssea são mais comumente afetados.[18] O diagnóstico de SH requer exame citológico (ver Capítulo 93) ou exame histopatológico, além de, se possível, imunofenotipagem. Após o diagnóstico de SH, recomenda-se o estadiamento da doença, incluindo aspirado de linfonodos para exame citológico (ver Capítulo 95), exame histopatológico de amostra obtida por biopsia, radiografias do tórax, US do abdome (ver Capítulo 88) com ou sem exame citológico da medula óssea (ou biopsia de medula óssea; ver Capítulo 92) para caracterizar a extensão da doença.

Tratamento do sarcoma histiocítico

Relatos limitados documentam o resultado após extirpação cirúrgica do SH localizado. Um estudo mencionou sobrevida mediana (SM) de 6 meses em 5 cães com SH sinovial tratado apenas com amputação.[23] Sempre deve-se utilizar quimioterapia, seja como tratamento adjuvante para SH localizado, seja para tratamento de SH metastático ou disseminado. A lomustina parece ser o quimioterápico mais efetivo no tratamento de SH em cães. Foram relatadas taxas de resposta gerais de 29 a 46% quando utilizada lomustina para o tratamento da doença macroscopicamente mensurável, com duração de resposta mediana de 90 dias (com variação de 29 a 805 dias).[28,29] Um melhor resultado pode ser alcançado em casos de SH localizado quando a terapia local é combinada à quimioterapia adjuvante com lomustina. Um grupo de 16 cães com SH localizado e sem evidência de doença metastática distante foi submetido à tratamento local intensivo (cirurgia e/ou radioterapia) e quimioterapia com lomustina.[30] Linfonodos regionais metastáticos, detectados em 4 de 16 (25%) cães no momento do diagnóstico, foram removidos no momento da extirpação do tumor primário. Nesse estudo, constatou-se intervalo livre da doença mediano de 8 meses e SM geral de 18,6 meses.[30]

Um resultado mais favorável foi sugerido para cães com SH periarticular. Um estudo relatou SM de 391 dias (com variação de 48 a 980 dias) em cães submetidos a diferentes tratamentos, incluindo tratamento local combinado com quimioterapia (47%), quimioterapia exclusiva (42%) ou apenas tratamento local (11%). Obteve-se esse resultado apesar de uma taxa geral de metástase de 68% no momento do diagnóstico.[26]

A quimioterapia combinada pode ser superior à terapia com um único antineoplásico, embora ainda seja preciso determinar os quimioterápicos e as combinações ideais. Há informações limitadas relativas a outros medicamentos quimioterápicos efetivos, embora a doxorrubicina, o paclitaxel e a vinorelbina tenham mostrado resultados promissores.[26,31-33] Um estudo relatando o uso de doxorrubicina e lomustina de forma alternada mencionou taxa de resposta geral de 58% e tempo de progressão mediano de 185 dias (com variação de 59 a 268) em cães com doença macroscópica mensurável.[34]

Outra área de estudo visa determinar a importância potencial do bifosfonato clodronato, que destrói osteoclastos e outros macrófagos por indução de apoptose. Quando o clodronato é incorporado a lipossomos, a captação de células fagocíticas é amplamente aumentada, resultando em direcionamento seletivo de macrófagos. A suscetibilidade de células do SH a esse medicamento foi demonstrada *in vitro*.[35] Um estudo-piloto mostrou regressão de lesões em 2 de 5 cães (40%) com SH.[35] A combinação de bifosfonatos com quimioterápicos pode ser benéfica. Resultados de pesquisas *in vitro* sugerem aumento da citotoxicidade do SH quando bifosfonatos selecionados são combinados com vincristina ou doxorrubicina.[36]

Sarcoma histiocítico hemofagocítico

Embora a origem de CD seja um elemento comum a outras doenças histiocíticas, os histiócitos neoplásicos são oriundos de macrófagos no SH hemofagocítico. As células expressam um perfil de antígenos de superfície distinto, compatível com sua origem, na polpa vermelha esplênica e medula óssea. O SH hemofagocítico parece ser mais comum em algumas raças de cães, como Bernese Montanhês, Golden Retriever e Rottweiler.[37]

Suas características clinicopatológicas são singulares, e talvez a mais marcante seja a eritrofagocitose acentuada por histiócitos neoplásicos, resultando em anemia hemolítica regenerativa moderada à marcante. Em um estudo, constatou-se que 94% dos cães apresentavam anemia regenerativa (hematócrito [HT] mediano de 22,6%, com variação de 10,1 a 37%).[37] Outros achados comuns incluem trombocitopenia (88%), hipoalbuminemia (94%) e hipocolesterolemia (69%).[37] Nota-se, consistentemente, esplenomegalia com alteração nodular difusa e mal definida. Fígado, medula óssea e pulmões quase sempre apresentam infiltrado difuso, e a disseminação ocorre via invasão intravascular insidiosa, com mínima formação de tumores.

O diagnóstico é baseado no exame citológico ou histopatológico e, se possível, imunofenotipagem. Parece haver variação marcante nas características citológicas de histiócitos neoplásicos, embora a eritrofagocitose intensa acompanhada de focos de hematopoese extramedular seja uma característica consistente.[37] Diferentemente de anemia hemolítica e trombocitopenia imunomediada (síndrome de Evans; ver Capítulo 198 e 201), os cães com SH hemofagocítico apresentam teste de Coombs negativo. O estadiamento da neoplasia é recomendado, que inclui exame de linfonodos (ver Capítulo 95), radiografias do tórax, US do abdome (ver Capítulo 88) e aspirado da medula óssea (ver Capítulo 92) para exame citológico (ou biopsia), para caracterizar a extensão da doença.

O SH hemofagocítico carreia o pior prognóstico, e relatos de tratamentos efetivos duradouros são escassos. Em um estudo com 17 cães, constatou-se que todos morreram ou foram submetidos à eutanásia, com tempo mediano de 4 semanas (com variação de 2 a 32 semanas), desde o início dos sinais clínicos até a morte ou eutanásia;[37] não foram fornecidas informações sobre os tratamentos tentados. Dada a atividade relatada contra outras formas de SH, a lomustina pode ser uma opção terapêutica razoável. Infelizmente, em um estudo que relatou o uso de lomustina, embora não especificamente caracterizado como portadores de SH hemofagocítico, os cães com anemia, trombocitopenia, hipoalbuminemia e envolvimento esplênico pareciam menos propensos a responder ao tratamento. Ademais, trombocitopenia e hipoalbuminemia foram associadas à menor SM, de 28 dias ou menos, comparada a 163 dias ou mais de ausência desses sintomas.[28]

O SH raramente foi relatado em gatos. Em um grupo de 3 gatos, a doença lembrou muito o SH hemofagocítico em cães.[38] A idade de manifestação foi variável (1, 4 e 9 anos). Anemia (hematócrito: 9 a 15%) e trombocitopenia (31.000 a 94.000 plaquetas/$\mu\ell$) foram detectadas nos três animais. Todos foram submetidos à eutanásia logo após o diagnóstico e apresentaram células histiocíticas malignas que exibiam eritrofagocitose no fígado, baço e medula óssea no exame pós-morte. Outros locais da doença incluíram linfonodos, pulmões, rins, cérebro e bexiga.

REFERÊNCIAS BIBLIOGRÁFICAS

As referências bibliográficas deste capítulo se encontram online no Ambiente de Aprendizagem.

CAPÍTULO 351

Tumores do Trato Urogenital e da Glândula Mamária

Juan F. Borrego

BEXIGA E URETRA

Prevalência e fatores de risco

Tumores de bexiga são incomuns em cães e raros em gatos, mas sua prevalência parece estar aumentando nos últimos 30 anos.[14] A maioria dos tumores vesicais e uretrais é epitelial e maligna. O carcinoma de célula de transição (CCT) invasivo e de grau intermediário a alto é, de longe, o mais diagnosticado em ambas as espécies.[1] Outros diagnósticos diferenciais incluem carcinoma de célula escamosa, adenocarcinoma, rabdomiossarcoma, linfoma e outros tumores mesenquimais.[15] Nesse tipo de tumor, é frequente sua localização no trígono, com envolvimento da uretra e da próstata, quase sempre causando obstrução do trato urinário (Figura 351.1; ver Capítulo 335).[15] A ocorrência de doença metastática é detectada em 10 a 20% dos cães no momento do diagnóstico e em até 58% por ocasião da necropsia.[16] Localizações comuns de metástases de CCT de cães incluem linfonodos, pulmões, ossos e pele.[1,17,18] O CCT felino é incomum, acomete gatos idosos, raramente causa metástase, e a maioria não envolve o trígono vesical.[19,20]

Diversos fatores de risco para CCT foram descritos em cães. Cadelas de idade avançada (9 a 11 anos) parecem predispostas; raças de pequeno porte, como Scottish Terrier, têm risco 21 vezes maior de desenvolver CCT. Cães das raças West Highland White Terrier, Shetland Sheepdog e Beagle têm risco 3 a 5 maior de apresentar CCT do que cães sem raça definida.[14,17,21] Outros fatores de risco potenciais incluem obesidade, estado reprodutivo e terapia com ciclofosfamida. A exposição a produtos mais antigos para controle de ectoparasitas e herbicidas foi associada ao CCT, enquanto produtos para controle de

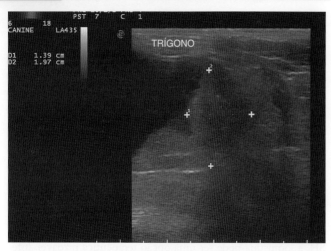

Figura 351.1 Carcinoma de célula de transição na bexiga. Imagem sagital da bexiga com um tumor lobulado no trígono.

ectoparasitas *spot-on* mais recentes, como o fipronil, parecem seguros.[21-23] Relata-se que o consumo de vegetais reduz o risco de CCT em cães Scottish Terrier.[24]

Sintomas e diagnóstico

Sinais clínicos comuns causados por neoplasias de bexiga ou de uretra mimetizam cistite bacteriana ou urolitíase e são típicos de infecção ou inflamação do trato urinário (ITU): estrangúria, polaquiúria (ver Capítulo 46), hematúria (ver Capítulo 47), disúria, incontinência urinária (ver Capítulo 46) ou qualquer combinação desses. Temporariamente, a terapia antimicrobiana pode resolver os sintomas, já que infecções concomitantes são documentadas em cerca de 25% dos casos no momento do diagnóstico.[25] Se não há resolução total dos sinais clínicos após a terapia antimicrobiana ou se ocorre recidiva, deve-se pesquisar a presença de cálculos ou de câncer, especialmente em raças predispostas (Figura 351.2). Em casos avançados, uma massa tumoral é palpável na parte caudal do abdome; anormalidades, como espessamento da uretra ou aumento de linfonodos sublombares ou intrapélvicos, podem ser detectadas no exame retal. É menos comum os cães apresentarem claudicação causada pela dor decorrente de metástase óssea. Metástases cutâneas podem surgir como lesões eritematosas, ulceradas ou proliferativas.[18]

Após exame físico minucioso (ver Capítulo 2), deve-se obter hemograma e perfil bioquímico sérico e realizar exame de urina. Devido à alta taxa de ITU, a urocultura e o antibiograma são incluídos na avaliação inicial e periodicamente durante o tratamento.[25] A urina desses pacientes deve ser obtida durante micção espontânea ou por meio de cateterismo. Se houver necessidade de cistocentese, é realizada uma coleta guiada por ultrassom, de modo a evitar a penetração da massa tumoral pelo cateter ou pela sonda. A presença de células epiteliais anormais no sedimento urinário de animais com tumor ou espessamento da parede da bexiga é sugestiva de CCT; entretanto, em outras doenças inflamatórias, há células epiteliais "reativas" (Figura 351.3). A radiografia torácica deve ser realizada para avaliar possíveis metástases pulmonares. A ultrassonografia (US) do abdome é o exame preferido para verificar a localização e a extensão da doença, porém não pode ser o único método de avaliação, devido à variabilidade inter e intraoperador.[26,27] O exame histológico de amostras de tecido ou daquelas obtidas para citologia coletadas por meio de cateterismo traumático (Vídeos 351.1 e 351.2), cirurgia ou biopsia cistoscópica frequentemente propicia o diagnóstico definitivo (ver Capítulo 93). A aspiração ou biopsia guiada por ultrassom não é recomendada, pois a disseminação de células tumorais viáveis no trajeto da biopsia é uma possível complicação.[28,29] A biopsia cistoscópica é um método efetivo para obter amostras em cães com CCT de bexiga e uretra. É mais provável que a cistoscopia (ver Capítulo 108) propicie uma amostra, por biopsia, de melhor qualidade diagnóstica em fêmeas com CCT (96%) do que em machos com essa neoplasia (65%).[30]

Tratamento

A maioria dos cães com CCT é submetida a tratamento medicamentoso e, menos comumente, radioterapia ou cirurgia. A cirurgia deve ser realizada quando o tumor se localiza na parte cranial da bexiga; entretanto, como a região do trígono está normalmente envolvida, a ressecção completa com preservação de função pós-cirúrgica aceitável é raramente viável. O CCT também foi relatado na parede abdominal, mais provavelmente devido à sua natureza altamente esfoliativa. É provável que o CCT da parede abdominal seja implantado durante procedimentos como coleta de amostra por meio de biopsia, remoção do tumor inteiro ou de parte dele, implantação de sonda de cistotomia ou aspirado com agulha fina (AAF) do CCT de bexiga, uretra e próstata.[31] O CCT de parede abdominal apresenta o pior prognóstico, de forma que seja necessária precaução para evitar a disseminação do tumor no abdome ou no local da cirurgia durante esses procedimentos, sobretudo cirurgia (Figura 351.4).[31] Após manusear o tumor, devem ser utilizados novos instrumentos e luvas esterilizados para a sutura de fechamento do abdome.

Quimioterapia, uso de inibidores da ciclo-oxigenase (COX) e suas combinações representam a base do tratamento de CCT em cães. As taxas de remissão são tipicamente menores que 20% após terapia com um único agente (anti-inflamatório não esteroide [AINE] ou quimioterapia) e 35 a 50% com quimioterapia combinada, incluindo um inibidor da COX.[15,16] Medicamentos à base de platina parecem mais efetivos em casos de CCT, especialmente quando combinados com um inibidor da COX,[32] embora deva-se evitar a combinação de cisplatina e piroxicam devido às altas taxas de nefrotoxicidade e insuficiência renal.[33,34] Alguns outros fármacos quimioterápicos mais frequentemente utilizados como agentes únicos são mitoxantrona, doxorrubicina, vimblastina e gencitabina.[14] A sobrevida mediana (SM) de cães com CCT tipicamente varia de 130 a 195 dias após o tratamento com um único medicamento, sendo superior a 250 dias após o tratamento com uma combinação de fármacos.[16] As recomendações atuais para o tratamento com único agente consistem no uso de um inibidor de COX não seletivo, como piroxicam (0,3 mg/kg VO, a cada 24 h),[16] ou um inibidor mais seletivo de COX, como deracoxibe ou firocoxib.[33,35] Em caso de terapia combinada, deve-se usar um inibidor da COX e um quimioterápico com atividade antitumoral conhecido, utilizando a resposta à terapia a cada 4 a 8 semanas como diretriz para a continuidade do tratamento.[16] Uma estratégia terapêutica emergente envolve a quimioterapia metronômica com clorambucil, via oral, que mostrou bons resultados, inclusive em 67% dos pacientes com doença estável e 3% com remissões parciais.[36]

Em gatos, como o CCT está frequentemente localizado na parte cranial da bexiga, a cirurgia é uma opção a ser considerada. Inibidores da COX (piroxicam e meloxicam) utilizados como agentes terapêuticos únicos ou em protocolos de combinação podem ser importantes no tratamento paliativo de CCT da bexiga de gatos, com sobrevida relatada de 261 a 311 dias.[19,20]

Equipamentos de radioterapia de última geração, que possibilitam a administração de uma dose altamente ajustada de radiação a um alvo selecionado, tornaram possível tratar CCT como parte de um protocolo de combinação com tratamento medicamentoso, com risco muito menor de dano aos tecidos circundantes.[37,38] Essa técnica tem a vantagem de não ser invasiva, manter a continência urinária e controlar local da neoplasia. As desvantagens estão relacionadas ao custo e à disponibilidade de tais equipamentos de radiação.

CAPÍTULO 351 • Tumores do Trato Urogenital e da Glândula Mamária

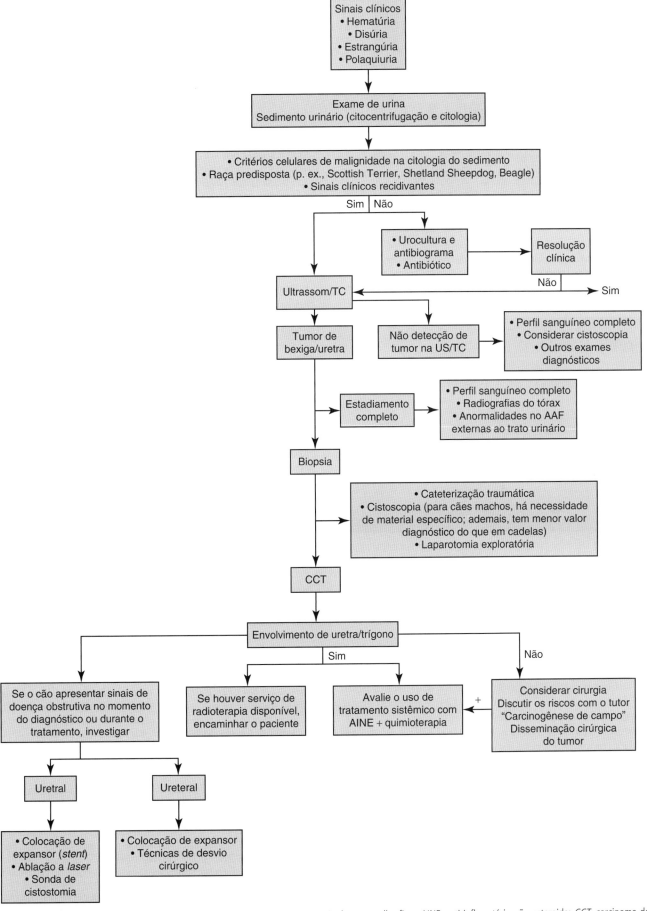

Figura 351.2 Algoritmo para avaliação de tumores de bexiga e uretra. *AAF*, aspirado por agulha fina; *AINE*, anti-inflamatório não esteroide; *CCT*, carcinoma de célula de transição; *TC*, tomografia computadorizada; *US*, ultrassonografia.

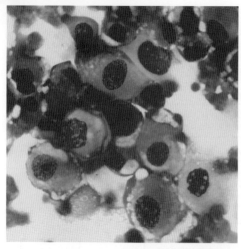

Figura 351.3 Citologia de amostra obtida com a técnica de cateterização traumática. A amostra contém densos agregados de células redondas a poligonais. Note diversos critérios de malignidade, inclusive anisocitose e anisocariose moderadas, proporção núcleo:citoplasma variável e nucléolos proeminentes.

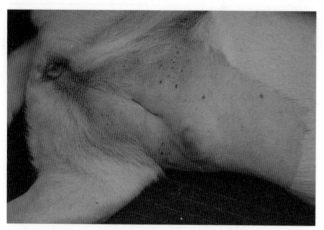

Figura 351.4 Disseminação tumoral de carcinoma de célula de transição na parede abdominal após cistectomia parcial para remoção de tumor de bexiga primário. CCT na parede abdominal apresenta pior prognóstico do que aqueles localizados no trato urinário. (*Esta figura se encontra reproduzida em cores no Encarte.*)

Procedimentos paliativos e prognóstico

A maioria dos cães com CCT morre por complicações secundárias à obstrução do trato urinário, antes do desenvolvimento de doença metastática relevante. Foram descritas diversas técnicas cirúrgicas destinadas a propiciar efeitos paliativos da obstrução da uretra pelo CCT (ver Capítulo 124); entretanto, elas não são comumente realizadas devido à morbidade e ao custo. A anastomose ureterocolônica não é recomendada, pois está associada a complicações neurológicas e gastrintestinais secundárias à hiperamonemia, acidose metabólica, uremia e pielonefrite crônica. Outras técnicas com melhores resultados incluem cistectomia total e remoção do colo e do trígono vesical.[39,40] Para casos de neoplasias restritas à uretra, foram descritas vaginouretroplastia e ressecção transuretral.[16,41,42]

Foram utilizadas sondas de cistotomia como um procedimento muito mais simples e mais bem tolerado para desviar a obstrução urinária, que permitem que animais sobrevivam por, em média, 3 meses adicionais.[43,44] Técnicas para implantação de sonda de cistostomia incluem abordagens abertas no abdome caudal, procedimentos minimamente invasivos no abdome, laparoscopia ou fluoroscopia e um cateter "rabo de porco" autossustentável. Complicações são frequentes, mas facilmente tratadas, sendo a mais comum a remoção acidental da sonda e de ITU.

Outra opção paliativa é a implantação de um extensor ("*stent*") uretral por meio de radiografia intervencionista (ver Capítulo 124).[45,46] Com a ressalva da ocorrência de incontinência urinária em 26 a 39% dos cães, os extensores uretrais são bem tolerados e resolvem as obstruções do trato urinário em 97% dos casos.[45,46] Apesar da boa taxa de resolução a curto prazo da obstrução do trato urinário, essa técnica é paliativa, com SM curta.[45-47] Outra opção paliativa envolve ablação a *laser* endoscópica guiada por US e uso de *laser* de dióxido de carbono para remover porções teciduais e lesões de TCC obstrutivas ou potencialmente obstrutivas. O principal risco desse procedimento é a perfuração da bexiga.[48]

TUMORES DE PRÓSTATA

Prevalência, fatores de risco e sintomas

Tumores de próstata são raros em cães, com prevalência inferior a 1% (ver Capítulo 337). A idade mediana no momento do diagnóstico é de 10 anos. Cães castrados, das raças Shetland Sheepdog e Scottish Terrier, são mais predispostos.[49-51] A maioria consiste em carcinoma que pode surgir do epitélio glandular, dos ductos prostáticos ou da uretra prostática. Outras condições a serem incluídas nos diagnósticos diferenciais de prostatomegalia, especialmente em cães machos não castrados, são prostatite crônica, abscesso de próstata, hiperplasia prostática benigna (HPB) e cisto de próstata.[52] Devido ao rápido crescimento e alto risco de metástase (até 80% em exames durante a necropsia),[53] os cães podem ser atendidos no estágio final da doença, quando os sinais clínicos são representativos de doença metastática (perda de peso, claudicação de membros pélvicos, dor ou sintomas neurológicos), em vez de doença urogenital primária (estrangúria, hematúria, polaquiúria). Metástases ósseas são documentadas em até 40% dos cães no momento do diagnóstico, causando dor, anormalidades de marcha ou claudicação. Outros sinais clínicos causados pelo aumento de tamanho da próstata ou metástases aos linfonodos incluem disquesia, tenesmo, constipação intestinal ou bolo fecal em formato de fita.

Diagnóstico

No exame retal, geralmente nota-se próstata assimétrica, fixa e firme à palpação. Ao continuar a palpação retal cuidadosa, o clínico também pode detectar aumento de linfonodos intrapélvicos. Hemograma e perfil bioquímico sérico podem revelar anemia não regenerativa, leucocitose, azotemia devido à doença obstrutiva e/ou hipercalcemia paraneoplásica (ver Capítulo 352). No exame de urina, quase sempre se verifica bacteriúria, porque, nesses cães, é comum a ocorrência de ITU. Células neoplásicas podem ser observadas no sedimento urinário, embora possa não ser possível a diferenciação entre células epiteliais reativas e neoplásicas.[53] Devido à alta porcentagem de doença metastática distante no momento do diagnóstico, recomendam-se radiografias do tórax em três projeções. Prefere-se US de abdome (ver Capítulo 88) em relação à radiografia abdominal para detectar metástases em linfonodos regionais, envolvimento da bexiga/ureter e outros órgãos intra-abdominais potencialmente acometidos. A mineralização da próstata em radiografias ou US do abdome não é patognomônica de carcinoma de próstata, pois outros tumores benignos também causam mineralização; entretanto, esse achado é altamente sugestivo de neoplasia.[54] Embora possam ocorrer metástases ósseas na forma de lesões líticas, proliferativas ou mistas em qualquer local, as vértebras lombares são as localizações mais comuns, seguidas de pelve e fêmur (Figura 351.5).

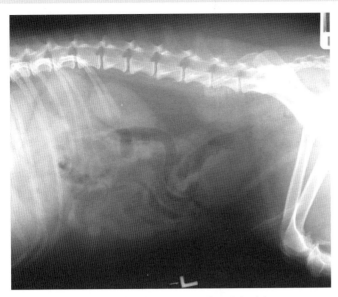

Figura 351.5 Carcinoma de próstata. Imagem lateral do abdome com tumor sublombar que se estende da vértebra L6 até o sacro. Note a reação periosteal irregular e lise mal definida em L6.

O exame histológico ainda é o padrão-ouro para o diagnóstico de câncer de próstata. Apesar de infecção e inflamação secundárias serem comuns, no carcinoma de próstata a concordância entre os achados citológicos e histológicos é alta.[52,55] As amostras para o exame citológico (ver Capítulo 93) podem ser coletadas por meio de cateterização traumática (ver Capítulo 111), lavado de próstata (ver Capítulo 111) ou aspiração com agulha guiada por US (ver Capítulo 89). A citologia ou histologia de qualquer outra lesão suspeita de metástase (p. ex., linfonodos, ossos) pode auxiliar no diagnóstico e no estadiamento. Aspiração e biopsia guiada por US devem ser realizadas cuidadosamente devido à possibilidade de disseminação do tumor. Entretanto, foi publicado apenas um caso de disseminação de tumor de próstata.[28] O adenocarcinoma de próstata é o tumor mais comum, seguido de CCT.[53] Pode-se realizar exame imuno-histoquímico para definir melhor a célula de origem; entretanto, o carcinoma de próstata em cães expressa marcador de origem urotelial e ductal, dificultando a diferenciação entre adenocarcinoma e CCT.

Tratamento e prognóstico

Há relatos de diversos subtipos histológicos, sem diferença no prognóstico.[53,56,57] Como a maioria dos cães com câncer de próstata é diagnosticada em estágio avançado, o prognóstico geral é reservado. O tratamento é considerado amplamente paliativo, focando no controle da doença local e de metástase distante. Diversas técnicas cirúrgicas foram descritas para obter o controle local da neoplasia; entretanto, tipicamente estão associadas a alta morbidade e piores resultados (menos de 3 a 4 meses). A prostatectomia intracapsular subtotal pode ser realizada em cães no estágio inicial da doença, já que pode ter efeito paliativo imediato nos sinais clínicos locais e está associada à menor taxa de complicações pós-cirúrgicas do que a prostatectomia total.[58]

Obstruções uretrais podem ser tratadas por meio de cistostomia ou colocação de expansor da uretra (ver Capítulo 124). A implantação paliativa do extensor pode aliviar imediatamente a obstrução na maioria dos cães, com baixa taxa de complicações. Incontinência urinária e deslocamento do expansor são as complicações comuns.[47] Não há consenso sobre o tratamento sistêmico padrão para carcinoma de próstata, e a importância da quimioterapia ainda está sendo pesquisada. Entretanto, a maioria das opções terapêuticas inclui um inibidor da COX-2. O uso de piroxicam ou carprofeno foi associado a maior taxa de sobrevida em pacientes tratados, comparado a um grupo não tratado. A radioterapia de intensidade modulada (RTIM) guiada por exame de imagem mostrou resultados promissores no tratamento de doença local, com poucos efeitos colaterais, e deve ser realizada quando houver evidência de doença metastática distante.[37]

TUMORES DE TESTÍCULO

Prevalência, diagnóstico e estadiamento

O segundo tumor mais comum em cães machos não castrados (de meia-idade a idosos) é a neoplasia do testículo, com três tipos histológicos comuns: tumor de célula intersticial (célula de Leydig), seminoma, e tumor de célula de Sertoli. Estudos recentes sugerem menor prevalência de sertolioma (8 a 16%) e maior incidência de tumor de célula de Leydig e seminoma.[64,65] Cães criptorquídicos são mais sujeitos ao desenvolvimento de sertolioma do lado direito ou de seminoma, mais comumente em testículos situadas na região inguinal do que na região abdominal, e em idade mais jovem do que em machos não castrados.[65] A maioria dos tumores testiculares não causa metástase. Caso ocorra disseminação de sertolioma ou seminoma (menos de 15%), quase sempre ocorre em linfonodos regionais. Embora a maioria dos tumores testiculares seja um achado incidental notado no exame físico, os sinais clínicos podem incluir diminuição da libido, sinais de prostatomegalia (estrangúria, tenesmo) e inapetência e/ou fraqueza secundária à anemia. Testículos assimétricos, edema escrotal ou inguinal e prostatomegalia secundária à metaplasia escamosa induzida por estrógenos podem ser notados durante os exames físico e retal. Sintomas de hiperestrogenismo, que incluem alopecia, ginecomastia, prepúcio pendular e pelame de má qualidade, podem ser observados em até 50% dos cães com sertolioma. Os sinais de feminilização são raros em cães com seminoma e tumor de célula de Leydig. Cerca de 20% dos cães diagnosticados com tumor em um dos testículos na verdade possuem nos dois. Portanto, é essencial sempre palpar ambos os testículos para comparar tamanho, formato e consistência.[66]

O estadiamento completo desses tumores deve incluir hemograma, US do abdome – para avaliar o tamanho de linfonodos regionais e auxiliar na detecção de testículos criptorquídicos – e radiografias do tórax em três projeções. A US do testículo pode auxiliar a excluir a possibilidade de doenças não neoplásicas, como orquite e torção testicular. O exame histológico possibilita a definição do diagnóstico; entretanto, o diagnóstico também pode ser obtido em exame citológico de AAF (ver Capítulo 93).[67] A supressão da medula óssea é uma complicação rara, porém bem documentada, do hiperestrogenismo, caracterizada inicialmente por leucocitose neutrofílica, que, por fim, progride para pancitopenia (ver Capítulos 57, 92 e 199).

Tratamento e prognóstico

A orquiectomia bilateral com ablação escrotal é a cirurgia preferida e curativa na maioria dos casos (Figura 351.6). Se houver metástase aos linfonodos, deve-se realizar biopsia por meio de excisão. A importância da radioterapia, da quimioterapia adjuvante ou de novas terapias destinadas aos cães com doença metastática é desconhecida, com apenas alguns poucos relatos demonstrando certo grau de eficácia.[68,69] Caso ocorra mielossupressão induzida por estrógeno, o prognóstico é reservado a grave, necessitando de meses de suporte hematológico e de antibióticos.

NEOPLASIA DE ÚTERO

Tumores do útero, inclusive de corno, corpo e cérvice, são relativamente raros em cães e gatos, sendo os leiomiomas (85 a 90%) e os leiomiossarcomas (10%) a vasta maioria. Outros tumores

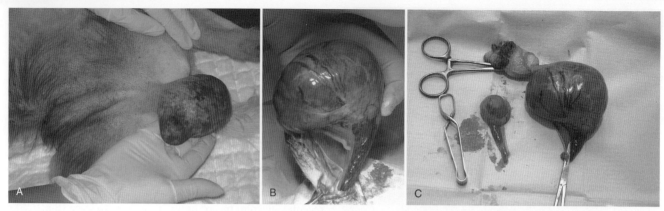

Figura 351.6 A. Grande tumor de células de Leydig à *esquerda*, com atrofia discreta do testículo direito livre de neoplasia, detectado como um achado incidental durante o exame físico. **B** e **C.** Realizou-se orquiectomia bilateral, com ablação do escroto. (*Esta figura se encontra reproduzida em cores no Encarte.*)

mesenquimais (fibroadenomas, adenocarcinomas, lipomas, linfomas e mastocitomas) são menos frequentes. Fêmeas castradas podem desenvolver tumores oriundos do coto uterino.[75] Adenocarcinoma é o tumor uterino mais comum em gatas de meia-idade a idosas, com relatos ocasionais em animais com menos de 1 ano de idade.[76-78] Algumas cadelas da raça Pastor-Alemão manifestam uma síndrome hereditária caracterizada por cistoadenocarcinoma renal, dermatofibrose nodular e leiomioma uterino.[79] Em cadelas, a maioria dos tumores de útero apresenta crescimento não invasivo e lento e não causa metástase. Em gatas, quase sempre os tumores uterinos são agressivos, e as pacientes apresentam metástases disseminadas no momento do diagnóstico.[76]

Em cadelas, os tumores de útero raramente estão associados a sinais clínicos, embora haja relato de aumento uterino, distensão abdominal, secreção vaginal e sintomas relativos ao trato urinário. Gatas também podem manifestar sintomas relacionados à doença metastática. Exames laboratoriais e radiografias do tórax devem ser incluídos na avaliação da paciente, mesmo que as anormalidades não sejam frequentemente detectadas. Radiografias do abdome podem confirmar a presença de um tumor de tecido mole na parte caudal. A US pode ser mais efetiva na detecção do tumor e na determinação do tecido provavelmente envolvido (tumor de corpo uterino ou de cérvice). Em cadelas, a aparência ultrassonográfica de tumores uterinos é variável. O diagnóstico definitivo é confirmado pelo exame histológico de amostras obtidas durante a cirurgia (Figura 351.7).[80] Geralmente, a ovário-histerectomia (OH) é um procedimento curativo para cadelas. Em gatas, entretanto, o comportamento biológico agressivo de tumores uterinos impede que a OH seja curativa, e o prognóstico é reservado. A eficácia da quimioterapia em cadelas e gatas é amplamente desconhecida.

TUMORES DE GLÂNDULA MAMÁRIA

Prevalência e fatores de risco

Tumores de glândula mamária (TGM) são as neoplasias mais comuns em cadelas não castradas e o terceiro tumor mais comum, de forma geral, em gatas.[88] A incidência de tumores mamários varia amplamente entre os países, provavelmente devido a diferentes atitudes com relação à castração. Fêmeas idosas de ambas as espécies são mais prováveis de desenvolver tumor mamário, e aquelas com tumores benignos são pouco mais jovens do que as cadelas que desenvolvem neoplasia maligna. Tumores mamários malignos em cadelas com menos de 5 anos são raros.[89] Raças de cães mais predispostas incluem Poodle, Cocker Spaniel Inglês, Bretão Spaniel, Setter Inglês e Pastor-Alemão. Gatas da raça Siamês também são predispostas. A exposição a hormônios ovarianos durante os primeiros 2 anos de vida é um fator de risco bem reconhecido para o desenvolvimento de tumores, e a OH diminui sobremaneira o risco de TGM em ambas as espécies.[90,91] Cadelas castradas antes do primeiro cio apresentam risco de 0,5%; após o primeiro cio, o risco é de cerca de 8%; e, após o segundo, ele sobe para 26%. Após o terceiro ciclo estral ou ao redor dos 4 anos, a OH propicia apenas proteção modesta. Há risco menor de desenvolvimento de tumores mamários adicionais quando a OH é realizada por ocasião da remoção do primeiro tumor, o que sugere um efeito contínuo dos hormônios.[92]

Em gatas, a castração antes do primeiro cio reduz o risco em 91%; antes do segundo, em 86%; e, antes do terceiro, a redução do risco é apenas 11%.[93] Em gatas com mais de 2 anos, a OH não propicia benefício. A exposição a hormônios exógenos também aumenta o risco de desenvolvimento de tumores benignos. Em TGM de cadelas e gatas foram detectados receptores de estrógeno e progesterona, embora haja uma expressão menor em tumores pouco diferenciados. Embora a associação hormonal seja aceita, cães e gatos machos podem desenvolver TGM. Em cães, eles são em geral benignos, mas em gatos são altamente malignos.[94-96] A obesidade em idade jovem e dieta com alto teor de gordura foram relacionados a maior risco de TGM em cães, e seus tumores são normalmente de maior grau e diagnosticados em idade mais jovem.[97-99]

Exame físico e diagnóstico

Ao exame físico, os animais podem apresentar nódulos mamários únicos ou múltiplos (mais de 50% dos casos). Tumores benignos tendem a ser pequenos, bem circunscritos e firmes à

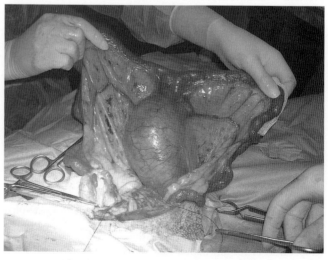

Figura 351.7 Grande leiomiossarcoma no útero.

palpação. Em cadelas, as glândulas mamárias caudais são as mais frequentemente envolvidas (Figura 351.8), enquanto em gatas os tumores ocorrem com igual frequência em todas as glândulas mamárias.[89] Os TGM podem ser móveis ou aderidos à pele ou à parede abdominal, estar ulcerados, inflamados e edemaciados ou apresentar secreção no mamilo. Carcinomas mamários inflamatórios (CMI) são tumores de rápido crescimento, acompanhados de dor, inflamação e, ocasionalmente, edema de extremidades (Figura 351.9). A lista de diagnósticos diferenciais para TGM em gatas incluem neoplasias cutâneas, mastite, hiperplasia lobular e hiperplasia fibroepitelial.

A avaliação diagnóstica de animais com neoplasia mamária deve incluir hemograma, perfil bioquímico sérico e exame de urina. O exame histológico do tumor extirpado é considerado padrão-ouro para o diagnóstico de neoplasias mamárias em cadelas. Quase sempre realiza-se o exame citológico do tumor (ver Capítulo 87), procedimento que pode ajudar a distinguir lesões benignas e malignas; entretanto, o exame histopatológico ainda é necessário, devido à possível subestimativa do potencial maligno do tumor. A citologia é mais útil para excluir outros diagnósticos diferenciais, detectando metástases de linfonodos regionais, e casos em que há suspeita de disseminação dérmica (TGM ou CMI agressivo; Figura 351.10). A disseminação metastática de TGM malignos ocorre através de vasos linfáticos para os linfonodos regionais ou via hematógena para os pulmões.[97] O exame histológico de linfonodos é necessário para diagnosticar definitivamente a presença de metástases/micrometástases.[100] Radiografias do tórax são importantes para avaliar a possibilidade de doença metastática pulmonar ou efusão pleural (comum em gatas). A US do abdome deve ser um componente do estadiamento minucioso, a fim de avaliar linfadenopatia metastática regional (linfonodos inguinais superficiais e axilares) ou intra-abdominal, especialmente nos casos em que os tumores mamários estão localizados nas glândulas mamárias caudais. A suspeita de metástase baseada em US deve ser confirmada pelo exame citológico de AAF. Há relato de tumor mamário detectado pela US; entretanto, a correlação com o exame histológico e a detecção de malignidade entre as pesquisas é variável.[101,102]

Tumores mamários em cadelas

Em cadelas, quase 60% dos TGM são benignos e frequentemente fibroadenomas (tumores mistos benignos).[103] Os tipos mais comuns de neoplasias são carcinomas sólidos ou adenocarcinomas tubulares. Somente cerca de 3 a 5% são sarcomas e 1% são CMI. Entre os tumores malignos, 50% desenvolvem recidivas ou metástase após a primeira ressecção cirúrgica.[104] Fatores

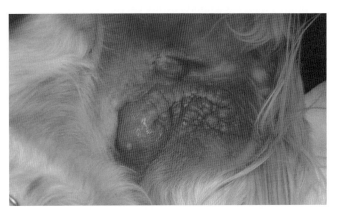

Figura 351.9 Cadela mestiça da raça Pastor-Alemão de 12 anos com carcinoma mamário inflamatório. Esse tumor quase sempre apresenta crescimento rápido e é doloroso.

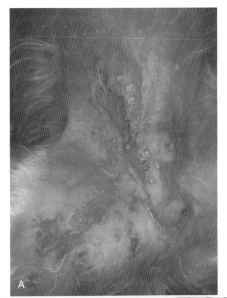

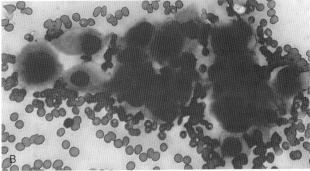

Figura 351.10 A. Disseminação dérmica de adenocarcinoma mamário de grau III submetido a extirpação incompleta. **B.** O exame citológico de lesões cutâneas indicou agregados de células epiteliais glandulares pleomórficas com diversos critérios de malignidade (anisocariose, anisocitose, macrocariose e macronucléolos). (*Esta figura se encontra reproduzida em cores no Encarte.*)

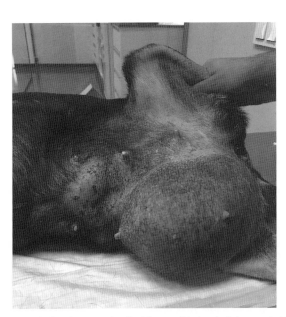

Figura 351.8 Grande tumor de glândula mamária inguinal. As características da manifestação clínica são úteis no prognóstico, inclusive o padrão de crescimento, fixação e ulceração.

associados à sobrevida mais curta incluem o tipo histológico (tumores pouco diferenciados, sarcomas e carcinomas inflamatórios apresentam o pior prognóstico), o grau histológico, o estágio, o tamanho do tumor (maior que 3 cm), o envolvimento de linfonodos, as evidências histológicas de invasão linfática ou vascular, a condição reprodutiva, a intensidade do infiltrado linfocítico, a expressão de receptores hormonais (RE e RP), a expressão de COX-2, a densidade de microvasos, os marcadores de proliferação, o comportamento clínico (padrão de crescimento, fixação, ulceração) e as metástases distantes.[105-108]

Tumores mamários em gatas

A maioria (80 a 90%) dos TGM de gatas é adenocarcinoma maligno.[109] Os CMI também foram relatados como biologicamente agressivos, com alta taxa de metástase. A sobrevida varia significativamente. Relata-se que o tamanho do tumor, o estágio da doença, a graduação histológica e a extensão de intervenção cirúrgica influenciam o prognóstico.[110-112] Tumores com mais de 3 cm estão associados à sobrevida de apenas 4 a 12 meses.[113,114] O tipo de cirurgia e a ressecção completa mostraram ter valor prognóstico para o intervalo livre da doença, mas não para a sobrevida.[109] A graduação histológica baseada no sistema de Elston e Ellis e em um sistema de graduação recente revisado mostrou correlação significativa com a sobrevida.[115]

Tratamento

Cirurgia

Em cadelas e gatas, a cirurgia permanece sendo o tratamento padrão-ouro para tumores mamários. Uma importante contraindicação para a cirurgia envolve CMI associados a altas taxas de metástases regionais e distantes precoces e à alta incidência de recidiva regional. O CMI deve ser considerado uma doença sistêmica, mesmo se não forem detectadas metástases.[116] Em cães com outros tipos de TGM, o objetivo da cirurgia é remover todo o tumor pelo procedimento mais simples possível. Por exemplo, a lumpectomia é aceitável para nódulos mamários superficiais pequenos (por volta de 1 cm), já que eles são, em sua maioria, benignos. Tumores de 1 a 2 cm de diâmetro podem necessitar mastectomia. Se houver massas tumorais em várias glândulas, elas podem ser submetidas à ressecção individual ou em cadeia. Novamente, a cirurgia escolhida deve ser a mais fácil para remover todo o tecido anormal. Deve-se considerar a drenagem linfática das glândulas acometidas.

Recomenda-se OH no momento da mastectomia para prevenir futuras doenças de ovário ou de útero e para reduzir o risco de desenvolvimento de neoplasia mamária.[90,92,105] Pode-se realizar mastectomia profilática de tecido mamário normal, especialmente quando o tumor localiza-se em uma glândula caudal, a fim de prevenir o desenvolvimento de novos tumores mamários. Até 60% dos cães submetidos à remoção de um único tumor mamário desenvolvem novos tumores ipsilaterais.[104] A maioria dos TGM se cura somente com a cirurgia. Em gatas, por conta de possíveis conexões linfáticas entre glândulas individuais e laterais, recomenda-se mastectomia unilateral ou bilateral completa, incluindo a fáscia subjacente "em bloco" (Figura 351.11). Para mastectomia bilateral em etapas, recomenda-se um intervalo mínimo de 2 semanas. Os linfonodos inguinais devem sempre ser removidos com a glândula mamária caudal, enquanto o linfonodo axilar deve ser removido apenas quando o seu tamanho estiver aumentado.

Radioterapia e tratamento medicamentoso

A radioterapia não é rotineiramente utilizada no tratamento dessa doença em cães ou gatos. Apesar de tumores mamários serem comuns, há poucas informações disponíveis quanto à

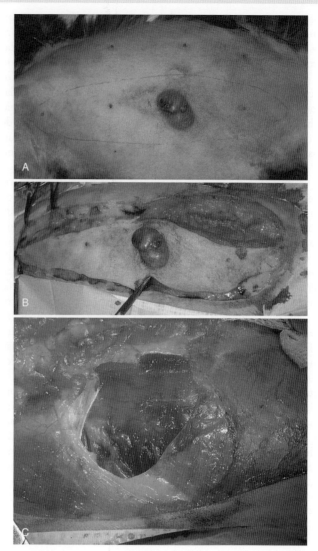

Figura 351.11 Em gatas com tumores mamários, tipicamente recomenda-se mastectomia unilateral completa com remoção da fáscia abdominal em bloco.

eficácia da quimioterapia para TGM canino ou felino. Os tratamentos clínicos, em sua maioria, são considerados experimentais, sobretudo aqueles utilizados como adjuvantes, após a cirurgia. Em cadelas com tumores mamários malignos e indicadores de prognóstico ruins adicionais, doença local avançada ou metastática ou um tipo histológico biologicamente agressivo, pode ser benéfico o tratamento adjuvante com quimioterapia ou terapia antiangiogênica. Diversos fármacos foram utilizados como agentes únicos ou em protocolos de combinação na doença macroscópica com resultados modestos e taxas de resposta ao redor de 20%, sendo o protocolo mais comum constituído por doxorrubicina, carboplatina, mitoxantrona, 5-fluoruracila e ciclofosfamida.[108] As novas formulações de paclitaxel, um fármaco efetivo contra neoplasias mamárias, causam menos reações alérgicas e taxas de resposta moderadas.[117]

Há poucas informações disponíveis quanto à importância da quimioterapia como tratamento adjuvante após a cirurgia. A expressão de COX-2 é maior em TGM maligno, comparada à de TGM benigno ou de tecido mamário normal, e está associada a um pior prognóstico.[118,119] Inibidores da COX-2 foram somente descritos em casos de CMI como parte de tratamento multiterapêutico para melhorar a qualidade de vida e aumentar a taxa de sobrevida, comparativamente à quimioterapia exclusiva.[120] São necessários outros estudos com tumores mamários distintos de cadelas, antes que o uso de inibidores da COX-2 possa ser rotineiramente recomendado como terapia adjuvante.

Apesar do prognóstico reservado em animais com CMI (1 a 2 meses), o tratamento medicamentoso pode melhorar o resultado.[116,120] A administração de 1 mg de desmopressina/kg IV, 30 min antes da cirurgia e 24 horas após, aumentou a sobrevida livre da doença e a sobrevida geral em um grupo de cadelas com TGM.[121] Terapias antiangiogênicas com fosfato de toceranib foram efetivas contra TGM de cadelas e gatas com neoplasia macroscópica, encorajando mais pesquisas sobre sua importância no tratamento adjuvante de TGM.[122,123] A quimioterapia pós-cirúrgica é em geral recomendada às gatas, assim como doxorrubicina, embora haja relatos conflitantes quanto a sua

importância em prolongar a sobrevida.[113,114,124] Recentemente, realizou-se quimioterapia adjuvante com carboplatina e mitoxantrona; entretanto, esses estudos incluíram poucos casos, e a importância da quimioterapia adjuvante permanece amplamente desconhecida nesse tipo de tumor em gatas.[125,126]

REFERÊNCIAS BIBLIOGRÁFICAS

As referências bibliográficas deste capítulo se encontram online no Ambiente de Aprendizagem.

CAPÍTULO 352

Síndromes Paraneoplásicas

Timothy J. Stein

Síndromes paraneoplásicas (SPN) são sintomas que surgem a partir dos efeitos indiretos da produção e liberação de substâncias biologicamente ativas pela neoplasia. Embora alguns oncologistas atribuem o termo "síndrome paraneoplásica" somente para situações em que o composto liberado pelo tumor não é normalmente produzido pela célula tumoral de origem, essa definição restritiva excluiria várias SPN comumente citadas, inclusive hipoglicemia secundária ao insulinoma pancreático. Os sinais de SPN tipicamente surgem em locais distantes do tumor e podem ser a primeira evidência de doença neoplásica. Frequentemente são resolvidos com o tratamento efetivo do processo neoplásico primário. Pode ocorrer recrudescência desses sinais antes da recidiva macroscopicamente detectável ou da recidiva da neoplasia incitante; portanto, é importante o monitoramento permanente.

SÍNDROMES PARANEOPLÁSICAS RELACIONADAS AO SISTEMA ENDÓCRINO

Hipercalcemia maligna

Câncer é a causa mais comum de hipercalcemia em cães, enquanto condições não neoplásicas predominam em gatos.[1-3] Anormalidades na regulação do cálcio podem ser causadas por uma ampla variedade de doenças não neoplásicas; a abordagem diagnóstica da hipercalcemia é discutida com detalhes no Capítulo 69. A hipercalcemia maligna (HM) responde por até dois terços dos casos em cães e um terço dos casos em gatos.[2,3] O mecanismo primário da ocorrência de HM é a promoção de reabsorção óssea pelos osteoclastos e a subsequente liberação de cálcio na corrente sanguínea. Compostos liberados por células neoplásicas podem também influenciar a capacidade do rim e do sistema digestivo de modular a concentração de cálcio. O mais comum desses compostos é o peptídio relacionado ao paratormônio (PTHrP).[4,5] Outros fatores produzidos e liberados por células neoplásicas que demonstram contribuir para a ocorrência de HM incluem o receptor do ativador do fator nuclear kappa-B (RAN-kappa-L), o fator de transformação do crescimento-beta, a interleucina-6 (IL-6) e o fator de necrose tumoral.[6]

Linfoma, adenocarcinoma da glândula do saco anal e mieloma múltiplo são as neoplasias mais comumente associadas à HM em cães.[7] Embora essa lista não seja amplas, outros tipos de neoplasias incluem tumor de glândula mamária, melanoma,

leucemia linfocítica crônica e timoma.[8-11] No adenocarcinoma de glândula de saco anal, há correlação linear entre as concentrações séricas de cálcio e de PTHrP; tal correção não foi verificada no linfoma canino,[12] o que sugere contribuição de outros fatores para a ocorrência de HM no linfoma canino.

Em gatos, a HM é mais frequentemente relatada em casos de carcinoma de célula escamosa e linfoma, embora seja relatada com mieloma múltiplo, osteossarcoma e adenocarcinoma broncogênico.[3,13,14] Semelhante ao mencionado para cães, o PTHrP é considerado o principal responsável pela ocorrência de HM felina.

A concentração sérica de cálcio ionizado deve normalizar rapidamente após o tratamento efetivo do tumor incitante. A mensuração da concentração sérica de cálcio ionizado deve ser incluída e monitorada continuamente em todos os pacientes com HM. No caso de pacientes em que o tumor incitante não é passível de remoção completa ou é refratário ao tratamento, deve-se tentar outras medidas de suporte para o tratamento de hipercalcemia (ver Capítulos 69 e 297), embora o sucesso dessas medidas tenha geralmente curta duração.

Hipoglicemia

A hipoglicemia paraneoplásica deve constar da lista de diagnósticos diferenciais para animais hipoglicêmicos (ver Capítulo 61). Essa SPN está mais comumente associada a neoplasia de célula beta das ilhotas pancreáticas (insulinomas).[15] Com exceção do insulinoma, outros tumores associados à hipoglicemia são carcinoma hepatocelular, hemangiossarcoma, tumor mamário, melanoma bucal, mieloma múltiplo, plasmocitoma, neoplasia renal, tumor de glândula salivar e neoplasias de músculos lisos (leiomioma e leiomiossarcoma).[16-20]

A hipoglicemia associada a insulinoma se deve à produção excessiva de insulina pelo tumor primário. Já a hipoglicemia verificada em casos de tumores extrapancreáticos foi associada a baixa concentração de insulina, causada pelos fatores de crescimento semelhantes à insulina I e II e por somatomedinas.[16] Outras causas potenciais de hipoglicemia paraneoplásica incluem o aumento da expressão de receptores de insulina ou do uso de glicose por células neoplásicas, a diminuição da gliconeogênese ou glicogenólise hepática e a ligação da insulina à proteína M no mieloma múltiplo.

O tratamento ideal de hipoglicemia paraneoplásica consiste na remoção cirúrgica da neoplasia. Entretanto, pode ser necessário o tratamento sintomático da hipoglicemia antes da cirurgia ou controle da hipoglicemia com medicamento (ver Capítulos 61 e 303) se a cirurgia não for viável.

Síndrome do hormônio adrenocorticotrófico ectópico

Em animais, a produção ectópica do hormônio adrenocorticotrófico (ACTH) ou de substâncias semelhantes por neoplasias é extremamente rara. Há relatos de casos que descrevem essa síndrome em cães com neoplasia pulmonar primária, tumor neuroendócrino abdominal e carcinoide hepático.[21-23]

Hiperestrogenismo

A causa neoplásica mais comum de hiperestrogenismo é o tumor de célula de Sertoli.[24] É mais provável que os sertoliomas oriundos de testículo criptorquídico induzam à maior produção excessiva de estrógeno, comparativamente ao tumor de célula de Sertoli que se desenvolve em testículos na bolsa escrotal.[25,26] De forma geral, 30 a 50% dos cães com sertolioma manifestam sintomas de hiperestrogenemia.[25,26] Nem todos os cães com sinais clínicos de hiperestrogenemia apresentam concentração de estrógeno altamente detectável. O aumento da produção de alfainibinas reduz a produção de testosterona e, por fim, reduz a proporção testosterona:estrógeno, condição que provavelmente contribui para a ocorrência dos sinais clínicos.[27]

Os sinais clínicos de hiperestrogenismo incluem alopecia bilateral simétrica, hiperpigmentação cutânea, adelgaçamento epidérmico, ginecomastia, galactorreia, atração de outros machos, atrofia prepucial e atrofia do testículo não neoplásico.[27] No hemograma de animais acometidos, pode-se observar pancitopenia, e o exame da medula óssea (ver Capítulo 92) revela medula hipocelular.[24] Animais com pancitopenia grave podem manifestar letargia, hemorragia secundária à trombocitopenia, petéquias e palidez de membranas mucosas.[24]

O tratamento efetivo de hiperestrogenismo paraneoplásico depende da extirpação cirúrgica do sertolioma. A recorrência de sinais de feminilização foi documentada em um cão com doença metastática de início retardado.[28] Animais com pancitopenia podem necessitar de cuidados pré-cirúrgicos, inclusive administração de antibióticos de amplo espectro e transfusão de sangue total ou de concentrado de hemácias. A recuperação da medula óssea pode demorar semanas a meses após a remoção do tumor.

SÍNDROMES PARANEOPLÁSICAS HEMATOLÓGICAS

Anemia

Anemia é uma das SPN mais comuns em cães e gatos, e o câncer é uma das causas mais frequentes de anemia em cães.[29] A maioria das anemias paraneoplásicas provavelmente é secundária à anemia causada por doença crônica (ADC), anemia hemolítica imunomediada, anemia hemolítica microangiopática e anemia decorrente de hemorragia. Para que esta última seja considerada uma SPN, a perda de sangue deve ocorrer em um local distante do tumor primário. Exemplos disso são a hemorragia devido à ulceração gastrintestinal secundária à secreção excessiva de histamina pelos mastocitomas (MCT) ou a produção excessiva de gastrina em caso de gastrinoma.

ADC é a forma mais comum em pacientes com câncer. Ela surge secundariamente a anormalidades de armazenamento e metabolização do ferro, resultando em supressão da diferenciação celular de eritroides progenitores, redução da produção de eritropoetina e diminuição da meia-vida dos eritrócitos. Em geral, a ADC é caracterizada por anemia normocítica e normocrômica não regenerativa discreta/moderada. Esse tipo de anemia apresenta progressão lenta e raramente requer tratamento de suporte.

A anemia hemolítica imunomediada (AHIM) paraneoplásica está mais comumente associada a neoplasias hematopoéticas, mas foi relatada em associação a tumores sólidos. A SPN é considerada uma AHIM secundária, pois os anticorpos contra os antígenos da membrana celular do tumor apresentam reação cruzada com eritrócitos, resultando em sua destruição. Os sinais clínicos comumente associados à AHIM são letargia, fraqueza,

taquicardia, palidez, icterícia, hepatoesplenomegalia, hemoglobinúria e anorexia. Os testes para diagnóstico de AHIM secundária são discutidos com mais detalhes no Capítulo 198.

Assim como mencionado para a maioria dos casos de SPN, o tratamento preferido para a AHIM paraneoplásica é a remoção do tumor primário; entretanto, isso pode não ser imediatamente viável. Portanto, com frequência utilizam-se doses imunossupressoras de prednisona no tratamento de AHIM secundária. Para casos de AHIM refratários à prednisona, pode ser necessário o uso de outros medicamentos imunossupressores, que incluem azatioprina, ciclosporina e ciclofosfamida, embora a eficácia não esteja bem definida.[30,31]

A anemia hemolítica microangiopática está mais frequentemente associada a tumores microvasculares sólidos, como hemangiossarcoma (HSA; ver Capítulo 34), embora possa ocorrer em outras neoplasias, inclusive tumores hematopoéticos, associadas à coagulação intravascular disseminada (CID; ver Capítulo 197).[32] Pode ocorrer fragmentação de eritrócitos à medida que essas células passam através da fibrina intravascular formada na CID ou secundariamente à anormalidade vascular anormal no tumor, aos êmbolos tumorais pulmonares intraluminais ou ao estreitamento de arteríolas pulmonares.[32] O tratamento efetivo da neoplasia primária é considerado a única terapia efetiva para anemia hemolítica microangiopática paraneoplásica.

Eritrocitose

A eritrocitose, ou policitemia, é uma SPN incomum em animais, mais frequentemente associada a neoplasia renal primária ou secundária.[33-38] Outras neoplasias que foram relatadas como causa de eritrocitose são linfoma, Schwannoma, fibrossarcoma nasal, tumor venéreo transmissível, carcinoma bronquioalveolar e leiomiossarcoma de ceco.[38-43]

A eritrocitose paraneoplásica é uma forma de eritrocitose secundária (ver Capítulo 200), já que o mecanismo primário envolve aumento da concentração de eritropoetina. Em casos de policitemia, os achados clínicos podem incluir eritema de membranas mucosas, polidipsia e sintomas neurológicos, como desorientação, ataxia e convulsões secundárias à hiperviscosidade ou à hipervolemia.

Leucocitose neutrofílica e eosinofílica

A presença de um grande número de neutrófilos maduros na ausência de infecção ou de leucemia caracteriza a leucocitose neutrofílica paraneoplásica. Carcinomas renais (de célula de transição e de célula tubular), linfoma, fibrossarcoma metastático, carcinoma pulmonar e pólipos adenomatosos no reto foram associados à essa síndrome.[44-50] A leucocitose neutrofílica é também comum em cães com osteopatia hipertrófica paraneoplásica.[51] É ocasionada pela produção tumoral de fatores estimulantes de colônia de granulócitos (G-CSF) em gatos e de G-CSF e fatores estimulantes de colônia de granulócito-monócito (GM-CSF) em cães.[47,49,52] Essa SPN é mais comumente um achado incidental e regride com o tratamento efetivo do tumor primário.

A eosinofilia paraneoplásica é rara em cães e gatos. Há relatos dessa condição em cães com leiomiossarcoma de pericárdio, linfoma célula-T intestinal, pólipo retal, carcinoma mamário e fibrossarcoma bucal.[48,53-56] Eosinofilia paraneoplásica foi relatada em gatos com MCT, linfoma células-T intestinal, leucemia aguda e carcinoma de célula de transição da bexiga.[57-61] Como uma SPN, a eosinofilia quase sempre é um achado incidental.

Trombocitopenia

A trombocitopenia paraneoplásica (ver Capítulo 201) foi associada a casos de linfoma, melanoma, HSA, osteossarcoma (OSA), MCT, neoplasia histiocítica e diversos carcinomas.[62-64] Em um estudo, constatou-se que até 36% dos cães com neoplasias não tratadas apresentavam trombocitopenia.[30] Os mecanismos primários dessa SPN são comuns a quaisquer causas de trombocitopenia. A diminuição da produção de plaquetas pode ser secundária à mieloftise induzida por neoplasias infiltrativas na medula ou decorrer de neoplasias de testículos ou de ovários que secretam estrógeno.[65-67] Em neoplasias esplênicas, pode ocorrer trombocitopenia secundária ao sequestro de plaquetas.[67] O aumento da destruição plaquetária é uma possível decorrência de mecanismos imunomediados e foi associado a linfoma ou mieloma múltiplo. Pode ocorrer trombocitopenia secundária ao consumo de plaquetas em casos de neoplasias que causam hemorragia (HSA ou MCT) ou coagulopatia, como CID (tumores metastáticos múltiplos e HSA).[62,68]

Sinais clínicos de trombocitopenia, inclusive a existência de petéquias, não são tipicamente evidentes até que a contagem plaquetária diminua para menos que $30 \times 10^9/\ell$. O tratamento de trombocitopenia, enquanto SPN, depende do mecanismo incitante da trombocitopenia, embora a resolução do tumor primário seja o melhor tratamento. Pode-se recomendar a administração de sangue total fresco antes da ressecção do tumor (ver Capítulo 201).

Trombocitose

A trombocitose como uma SPN é reconhecida menos frequentemente do que a trombocitopenia. Em estudos retrospectivos que avaliaram gatos e cães com trombocitose, verificou-se que a neoplasia foi o diagnóstico mais comum.[70,71] Trombocitose foi descrita em animais com OSA, carcinoma de gengiva, leucemia mieloide crônica, carcinoma broncoalveolar e carcinoma de célula escamosa metastático, além dos animais submetidos à quimioterapia.[70-74]

A trombocitose paraneoplásica é um diagnóstico de exclusão. As causas de trombocitose incluem administração de alcaloides da vinca, esplenectomia, deficiência de ferro e anormalidades mieloproliferativas. A resolução ocorre após tratamento efetivo da neoplasia primária.

Hiperagregação plaquetária, hipercoagulação e coagulação intravascular disseminada

Alterações na função plaquetária foram demonstradas em cães com câncer.[75-78] Tanto a hiperagregação de plaquetas quanto à hipercoagulação foram constatadas como anormalidades hemostáticas comuns em cães com câncer.[75,78] A avaliação e o tratamento de anormalidades hemorrágicas são discutidos no Capítulo 197.

A CID é uma síndrome complexa caracterizada pela ativação excessiva da cascata de coagulação, resultando em microtrombose disseminada e falência múltipla de órgãos. Como uma SPN, a CID foi associada a neoplasias vasculares e tumores sólidos, com incidência relatada de 9,6%.[79] Ela pode estar presente em até 50% dos casos de HSA, na avaliação inicial.[79,80] Juntamente aos mecanismos comuns a outras doenças, o fator tecidual (FT) é expresso em células cancerígenas e forma complexos com o fator VIIa para estimular a formação de trombina e ativação dos fatores de coagulação IX e X. O prognóstico de pacientes com CID paraneoplásica quase sempre é ruim.

Hiperglobulinemia

A hiperglobulinemia é uma SPN mais comumente associada ao mieloma múltiplo, embora também tenha sido notada em casos de linfoma, leucemia linfocítica crônica e plasmocitoma.[81-83] A hiperglobulinemia se deve à produção excessiva de imunoglobulinas pelos plasmócitos ou linfócitos.[83,84] A maioria dos animais com mieloma múltiplo apresenta gamopatia monoclonal de IgG ou IgA. Os sinais clínicos estão relacionados à hiperviscosidade sanguínea secundária ao excesso de globulinas na circulação. Além de hipertensão e hipoxia tecidual, a diminuição da produção normal de imunoglobulinas pode levar a infecções. A hiperviscosidade consegue resultar em cardiomegalia, insuficiência renal, anormalidades neurológicas e doenças oculares, inclusive retinopatia.[85-88] Tendências hemorrágicas são comuns em casos de hiperglobulinemia e estão relacionadas à diminuição da adesão

de plaquetas às superfícies endoteliais lesadas, ao revestimento de plaquetas com imunoglobulinas e à liberação de fator plaquetário III. A confirmação de hiperglobulinemia é feita por eletroforese do soro sanguíneo.[104] O tratamento de animais com hiperglobulinemia paraneoplásica depende do tratamento efetivo do tumor incitante, quase sempre com quimioterapia. Casos em que a neoplasia incitante não é passível de rápida resolução podem necessitar de plasmaférese.[88]

SÍNDROMES PARANEOPLÁSICAS CUTÂNEAS

Alopecia paraneoplásica em gatos

Uma SPN singular de alopecia é verificada em alguns gatos com carcinoma pancreático e biliar (ver Capítulos 10 e 280).[89-93] Ocorre alopecia aguda simétrica progressiva não pruriginosa, com lesões caracterizadas pela facilidade de desprendimento de pelos, abaixo das quais nota-se pele lisa e brilhosa.[89-93] A ressecção do tumor primário pode ser um procedimento paliativo.

Dermatite necrolítica superficial

A dermatite necrolítica superficial (ver Capítulo 285) é uma SPN rara mais comumente associada a neoplasias secretoras de glucagon em cães. Assim como uma SPN, foi relatada em um gato com carcinoma neuroendócrino produtor de glucagon (carcinoide hepático).[94] A hipoaminoacidemia é um achado característico e pode ser fundamental à etiologia dessa síndrome. Histologicamente, ritema, formação de crostas, exsudação, ulceração e alopecia não pruriginosa são caracterizadas por paraqueratose epidérmica com degeneração hidrópica laminar do estrato espinhoso, hiperbasofilia na epiderme profunda e hiperplasia do estrato basal.[95] Notou-se resolução da dermatite necrolítica superficial após remoção cirúrgica de tumor pancreático e tratamento com somatostatina.[96,97]

Dermatofibrose nodular

A dermatofibrose nodular está associada ao cistoadenocarcinoma ou cistoadenoma renal e, raramente, ao leiomioma uterino e adenoma ovariano.[97-101] Essa SPN é comum em cães da raça Pastor-Alemão e relacionada a mutações na região cromossômica sobreposta ao *locus* Birt-Hogg-Dubé.[97-100]

SÍNDROMES PARANEOPLÁSICAS GASTRINTESTINAIS

Caquexia do câncer

A perda de peso e as anormalidades metabólicas observadas em pacientes oncológicos, mesmo com consumo de dieta adequada, são denominadas *caquexia do câncer*. Em pessoas, essa condição tem sido associada a efeitos negativos na força física, na função imune, na cicatrização de feridas e na sobrevida.[102] De forma semelhante, a má condição corporal foi associada à sobrevida mais curta em pacientes oncológicos felinos.[103] A caquexia é revisada com mais detalhes no Capítulo 177.

Ulceração gastrintestinal

A ulceração gastrintestinal (GI) paraneoplásica é mais comumente secundária à liberação excessiva de histamina pelos mastocitomas. A histamina em excesso estimula os receptores H2 gástricos, ocasionando aumento da secreção de ácido gástrico. Estudos demonstraram que até 75% dos cães com MCT macroscópico apresentam aumento da concentração plasmática de histamina, manifestando sinais clínicos de hiperacidez GI em aproximadamente 30% dos casos.[104,105] As terapias de suporte inespecíficas, como inibidores da bomba de prótons, bloqueadores H2, misoprostol e sucralfato, podem beneficiar pacientes que apresentam úlcera GI; entretanto, a cura da ulceração GI paraneoplásica é esperada apenas para tumores primários adequadamente tratados. Além dos MCT, os gastrinomas também foram associados à ulceração GI enquanto SNP.[106,107]

SÍNDROMES PARANEOPLÁSICAS NEUROLÓGICAS

Miastenia *gravis*

A miastenia gravis (MG), como uma SPN, ocorre com mais frequência em casos de timoma, mas foi descrita em associação a colangiossarcoma, linfoma, OSA e sarcoma bucal.[11,108-110] O tumor produz anticorpos contra receptores nicotínicos da acetilcolina, resultando em falha na transmissão sináptica. Sinais clínicos de MG incluem fraqueza, disfagia, regurgitação e pneumonia aspirativa secundária ao megaesôfago. Recomenda-se a remoção do tumor primário; entretanto, a MG pode não ser resolvida, mesmo com a remoção da causa incitante. Informações adicionais sobre testes diagnósticos e tratamento de MG são fornecidas nos Capítulos 117 e 269.

Neuropatia periférica

Há relato de neuropatia periférica paraneoplásica (ver Capítulo 268) em cães e gatos com HSA, tumor pulmonar primário, leiomiossarcoma, tumor mamário, mieloma múltiplo, linfoma, insulinoma e sarcoma não diferenciado.[111-114] A neuropatia periférica paraneoplásica provavelmente se deve à produção de anticorpos contra antígenos compartilhados entre o tumor primário e os nervos periféricos. A remoção do tumor é o único tratamento efetivo para essa SPN.

SÍNDROMES PARANEOPLÁSICAS RENAIS

Glomerulonefrite e nefropatia

A deposição de imunocomplexos relacionados ao tumor nos glomérulos renais pode resultar em anormalidades glomerulares em pacientes com câncer. Embora a prevalência de glomerulonefrite paraneoplásica seja desconhecida na medicina veterinária, há um relato de glomerulonefrite por imunocomplexos em um cão com leucemia linfocítica.[115] A nefropatia em cães e gatos com neoplasias pode ser secundária à hipercalcemia paraneoplásica, resultando em mineralização da membrana basal. O tratamento de nefropatia e glomerulonefrite paraneoplásica deve ser direcionado à remoção do tumor incitante (ver Capítulo 325).

SÍNDROMES PARANEOPLÁSICAS DIVERSAS

Osteopatia hipertrófica

A osteopatia hipertrófica (OH) é uma SPN bem caracterizada, mais frequentemente associada a tumor intratorácico primário. Neoplasias renais, adrenais, sertolioma metastático e tumor de bexiga também foram associados a essa SPN.[51,116-121] A osteopatia hipertrófica é caracterizada por proliferação periosteal ao longo dos eixos de ossos longos, tipicamente nas extremidades distais, associada a edema de tecidos moles dos membros. A síndrome muitas vezes acomete os quatro membros, começando distalmente e se estendendo em direção proximal. Embora esteja mais comumente associada a doenças neoplásicas, a OH também foi associada a doenças pulmonares infecciosas/inflamatórias, granuloma esofágico causado por *Spirocerca lupi* e endocardite bacteriana.[51,122-124] Cães e gatos com OH frequentemente apresentam claudicação ao apoiar o membro e/ou relutância em deambular. Em geral, nota-se hipertermia nasextremidades distais à palpação, além de edema. Um diagnóstico de OH é auxiliado por radiografias dos ossos afetados e subsequente exame radiográfico do tórax. Se as radiografias do tórax forem negativas para doenças intratorácicas, devem ser realizados outros exames para avaliar causas infecciosas/inflamatórias.

A estimulação dos nervos aferentes supostamente está envolvida na ocorrência de OH, resultando em aumento do fluxo sanguíneo aos membros e proliferação periosteal. A resolução dos sintomas em alguns pacientes submetidos a vagotomia sustenta essa possibilidade. O tratamento efetivo do tumor primário resulta em resolução da OH.[51] Deve-se tentar o controle da dor utilizando doses anti-inflamatórios não esteroides (AINE) ou de esteroides.

Febre

A febre paraneoplásica deve-se à produção de citocinas pirogênicas pelo tumor ou à resposta imune do hospedeiro à neoplasia. Esses pirógenos incluem IL-1, IL-6, interferons e fator de necrose tumoral-alfa, que atuam no centro termorregulador do hipotálamo anterior. Além dos pirógenos, a infiltração neoplásica no hipotálamo é outro fator determinante de febre. O tratamento depende da causa primária, embora a terapia sintomática com AINE possa propiciar algum efeito paliativo, caso a neoplasia primária não possa ser removida.

REFERÊNCIAS BIBLIOGRÁFICAS

As referências bibliográficas deste capítulo se encontram online no Ambiente de Aprendizagem.

SEÇÃO 26
Doenças Musculoesqueléticas

CAPÍTULO 353

Anormalidades Esqueléticas em Animais de Companhia

Denis J. Marcellin-Little

Anormalidades esqueléticas em cães e gatos interferem na movimentação e mobilidade livres de dor e na qualidade de vida; ademais, podem necessitar cirurgia ou levar à eutanásia. Problemas ortopédicos resultam de lesões ortopédicas ou de anormalidades esqueléticas. As lesões ortopédicas afetam todos os tecidos musculoesqueléticos: ossos, ligamentos, músculos e tendões. Como cães e gatos são sujeitos a uma ampla gama de traumatismos, o início e a gravidade das lesões ortopédicas é imprevisível. O diagnóstico e tratamento de traumatismos ortopédicos é descrito em outra parte.[1,2] Comparativamente, as anormalidades esqueléticas apresentam início e progressão muito mais previsíveis e são mais frequentemente desencadeadas pela presença de genes anormais, por dieta inapropriada, por infecções, por distúrbios metabólicos ou por anormalidades de desenvolvimento que afetam ossos ou articulações. Apesar dessas causas e da fisiopatologia amplamente variadas, as anormalidades esqueléticas têm consequências comuns na saúde e na mobilidade esquelética. O propósito deste capítulo é revisar as causas e a fisiopatologia de anormalidades esqueléticas em cães e gatos, bem como a sua relevância clínica, o diagnóstico e as opções terapêuticas com foco no tratamento medicamentoso.

CAUSAS DE ANORMALIDADES ESQUELÉTICAS

Em animais de companhia, as anormalidades esqueléticas frequentemente apresentam uma base genética.[3] Problemas ortopédicos podem resultar de um único gene defeituoso ou de vários genes anormais (doenças multigênicas). Em geral, suspeita-se de uma causa genética com base em dados da população, mas não foram detectadas relações genéticas específicas.[4-6] Por exemplo, a condrodistrofia em cães pode resultar de um de vários distúrbios genéticos, mas pouco se sabe sobre as mutações genéticas específicas que causam esses distúrbios.[7] Em humanos, o nanismo (acondroplasia) é uma doença autossômica dominante que resulta da mutação do gene do receptor 3 do fator de crescimento do fibroblasto (FGFR3). Em cães, várias formas de nanismo (ver Capítulo 295) encurtam ou deformam ossos longos e acometem os membros (raças Basset Hound ou Teckel) ou o crânio (braquicefalia em cães da raça Boxer).[8-10] Também relata-se nanismo em gatos (ver Capítulo 294),[10] quase sempre relacionado a doenças metabólicas,

inclusive hipotireoidismo congênito (ver Capítulo 300), mucopolissacaridose (ver Capítulo 260) e hipossomatotropismo congênito (ver Capítulo 294).[11-13] Gatos podem ter uma morfologia condrodistrófica clássica (gatos Munchkin) na ausência de anormalidades metabólicas.

Testes genéticos e genômicos para detectar marcadores de doença ortopédica estão em fase inicial.[14] A identificação de genes específicos responsáveis por doenças ortopédicas do desenvolvimento é um desafio, e apenas alguns poucos marcadores genéticos são utilizados em ortopedia. Por exemplo, a mutação SERPINH1/HSP47 é responsável pela ocorrência de osteogênese imperfeita em cães da raça Teckel.[15] Foi sugerida a seleção genômica, e não a seleção baseada em marcadores, como estratégia para redução da prevalência de displasia coxofemoral em cães[16] e outras doenças ortopédicas.[17]

A dieta pode influenciar a ocorrência dessas anormalidades esqueléticas, diretamente ou indiretamente, pela promoção da expressão de genes defeituosos ou pela aceleração da progressão de doenças ortopédicas. O desequilíbrio nutricional pode causar anormalidades esqueléticas (ver Capítulo 192).[18] O desequilíbrio nutricional mais comum é o hiperparatireoidismo secundário nutricional (ver Capítulos 171, 172, 174, 187 e 297). Cães e gatos que recebem dieta à base de carne consomem baixo conteúdo de cálcio e alto de fósforo (ver Capítulo 192), condição que desencadeia o aumento da concentração de paratormônio. Esse aumento promove a perda de cálcio dos ossos. Pacientes afetados manifestam perda da rigidez óssea, que ocasiona aumento da elasticidade do osso (*mandíbula de borracha*; ver Capítulo 324) ou fraturas. A cicatrização óssea não é influenciada negativamente. Outros distúrbios nutricionais que afetam ossos e articulações incluem hipervitaminose A e osteopetrose (densidade óssea excessiva).[19-21] A dieta influencia diretamente o crescimento ósseo[22] e as taxas de aumento do conteúdo mineral ósseo, de gordura e de tecido magro.[23] As concentrações de cálcio e de fósforo na dieta fornecidas aos filhotes refletem em seus ossos até os 5 e 6 meses de idade.[23] O excesso de energia (ver Capítulos 171 e 187) na dieta e a ingestão excessiva de cálcio influenciam negativamente o crescimento ósseo (pela sua aceleração) e parecem promover a expressão de genes ligados a doenças ortopédicas de desenvolvimento.[22,24]

Pode ocorrer infecção de articulações e ossos.[25] Doenças transmitidas por carrapatos, particularmente a doença de Lyme (*Borrelia burgdorferi*; ver Capítulo 211), podem causar artrite fibrinopurulenta após vários meses de incubação.[26] A erliquiose (ver Capítulo 218) pode causar poliartrite (ver Capítulo 203).[27] Em neonatos, a onfaloflebite pode levar à embolia bacteriana em placas de crescimento (fisite séptica), articulações (artrite séptica) ou ossos (osteomielite). A fisite séptica ocasiona anormalidades do crescimento fisário e frequentemente resulta em grave deformidade óssea, porque ocorre em idade muito precoce. A artrite séptica, se não for diagnosticada ou tratada, causa danos às cartilagens e osteoartrite. Há relato de bacteriemia por *Escherichia coli* associada à osteodistrofia hipertrófica.[28] Em humanos, a artrite pode decorrer de inflamação associada a infecção bacteriana, uma síndrome descrita como espondiloartrite, que inclui artrite reativa, artrite psoriática e espondilite anquilosante (ver Capítulos 15 e 203).[29] Infecções ósseas causadas por fungos são incomuns e geralmente secundárias: histoplasmose (ver Capítulo 233) em geral envolve uma lesão intestinal primária; aspergilose (ver Capítulos 234 e 235) quase sempre envolve uma lesão sinonasal; e blastomicose (ver Capítulo 233) e coccidioidomicose (ver Capítulo 232) normalmente envolvem uma lesão pulmonar primária.[30-32] Lesões ósseas ou articulares associadas à doença fúngica não são incomuns. Há relato de inoculações focais de blastomicose e coccidioidomicose.[33] Paecilomicose (ver Capítulo 336) da epífise distal do osso rádio foi relatada em um cão.[34] Há relato deosteomielite viral em cães.[35] O vírus da cinomose (ver Capítulo 228) foi incriminado na patogênese de várias doenças ósseas proliferativas: osteodistrofia hipertrófica e panosteíte, em cães, e doença de Paget, uma doença óssea proliferativa do crânio, em humanos.[36-38] Vários parasitas podem causar problemas ortopédicos. A leishmaniose (ver Capítulo 221) foi associada à poliartrite.[39-41] A artrite em cães com leishmaniose pode estar relacionada à presença de infecção por *Bartonella* (ver Capítulo 215).[42] Larvas de *Dirofilaria immitis* foram encontradas no líquido sinovial (ver Capítulo 255).[43,44] Em regiões com alta prevalência de *Toxocara canis*, a soroprevalência foi associada à artrite reumatoide em cães.[45]

Mesmo que a literatura científica relevante seja escassa,[46] diversos problemas ortopédicos parecem relacionados a anormalidades metabólicas, entre eles: hiperadrenocorticismo (ver Capítulo 306), hipotireoidismo (ver Capítulo 299), diabetes (ver Capítulos 304 e 305) e altas concentrações de estrógeno e progesterona (em cadelas, durante o parto; ver Capítulo 315). Os problemas ortopédicos em cães com doenças metabólicas são ruptura de ligamento cruzado cranial, do tendão calcâneo comum, da fibrocartilagem palmar e hiperextensão carpal secundária, da fáscia plantar e do tendão de inserção do músculo tríceps braquial. Eles parecem resultar do enfraquecimento do colágeno associado ao *balanço de nitrogênio negativo*. O excesso de hormônio de crescimento (acromegalia; ver Capítulos 294 e 295) ou seu déficit (nanismo proporcional; ver Capítulos 294 e 295) influencia o desenvolvimento do osso.

Doenças ortopédicas do desenvolvimento são multifatoriais, sendo influenciadas por fatores genéticos e nutricionais, bem como por crescimento e condição mecânica das articulações A base genética das doenças ortopédicas do desenvolvimento quase sempre é uma suspeita, com base na predisposição racial. Um estudo avaliou o risco de ocorrência de 10 doenças ortopédicas comuns do desenvolvimento.[47] As mais frequentes são displasia coxofemoral, displasia do cotovelo, luxação da patela e osteocondrite dissecante, enquanto as menos comuns são panosteíte, osteodistrofia hipertrófica, osteopatia craniomandibular, doença de Legg-Perthes e ossificação incompleta do côndilo umeral.

Em cães, a **displasia coxofemoral** é uma doença onipresente que acomete a maioria, se não todas as raças de cães, considerada a doença ortopédica do desenvolvimento mais comum; em um amplo estudo de cães tratados em hospitais-escola, os pacientes com displasia coxofemoral representaram 10% dos pacientes ortopédicos[48] Em dois relatos científicos, menciona-se que a displasia coxofemoral estava presente em mais de 40% dos cães das raças Golden Retriever, Labrador Retriever e Rottweiler.[49,50] A displasia coxofemoral é uma doença do desenvolvimento hereditária que envolve frouxidão articular e ausência de encaixe da cabeça do fêmur ao acetábulo, condição que provoca osteoartrite.[51] Quando presente, a displasia coxofemoral é mais frequentemente bilateral. O crescimento acelerado resultante de alta ingestão calórica aumenta a gravidade da displasia coxofemoral (ver Capítulo 187).[52] Gatos apresentam displasia coxofemoral, mas pouco se sabe sobre a doença nessa espécie. Em um estudo envolvendo 78 gatos, notou-se baixa associação entre displasia coxofemoral e luxação de patela: os gatos tiveram probabilidade 3 vezes maior de ter displasia coxofemoral com luxação de patela do que ter cada doença isoladamente.[53]

A **displasia do cotovelo** é comum em cães. De acordo com estatísticas fornecidas pela Orthopedic Foundation for Animals para as 50 raças mais acometidas, havia displasia do cotovelo em 16% de 180 mil cães examinados. Entre os veterinários, criadores e tutores, há uma clara ausência de percepção de displasia do cotovelo. É de longe a origem mais comum de dor em cães em fase de crescimento, com claudicação de membro torácico, e de osteoartrite na articulação do cotovelo. Foram propostos diversos mecanismos fisiopatológicos para explicar a displasia do cotovelo. A maioria dos patologistas concorda que a doença tem origem mecânica e que é uma consequência do crescimento anormal do rádio com relação à ulna ou ao côndilo umeral; outros pesquisadores acreditam que há um desequilíbrio entre o côndilo umeral e a incisura troclear da ulna (curvatura umeroulnar). Anormalidades do crescimento longitudinal do rádio, em relação à ulna, podem ocasionar subluxação umerorradial transitória ou permanente, que causa lesão à cartilagem do cotovelo dentro de semanas.[54] De forma semelhante, os cães com condrodistrofia geralmente apresentam osteoartrite precoce do cotovelo como resultado de anormalidades do crescimento do antebraço. Uma razão-chave para a falta de diagnóstico precoce de displasia do cotovelo no cão jovem e de subluxação do cotovelo secundária ao nanismo é sua visualização difícil em radiografias. Vários pacientes com displasia do cotovelo não apresentam um problema que possa ser previsivelmente observado em radiografias da articulação do cotovelo. Embora a não união do processo ancôneo e a osteocondrite dissecante do côndilo umeral possam ser previsivelmente observadas em radiografias, essas anormalidades afetam uma minoria de pacientes com displasia do cotovelo.[55] Entretanto, uma discreta incongruidade articular (subluxação umeroulnar distal ou umerorradial distal) ou a presença de processo coronoide medial anormal é verificada na grande maioria de animais com displasia do cotovelo. Essas anormalidades não podem ser prontamente observadas em radiografias.[56] Exames de imagem avançados (tomografia computadorizada [TC], ressonância magnética [RM]) e artroscopia (ver Capítulo 94) aumentam amplamente a chance de detectar esses problemas, mas possuem disponibilidade limitada e são dispendiosos, comparados à radiografia.

A **luxação de patela** é um dos problemas ortopédicos mais comuns em cães, sobretudo de pequeno porte, sendo a causa de 6% dos encaminhamentos ortopédicos.[48] A luxação da patela é definida como o deslocamento completo da patela medial ou lateral à fissura troclear.[48] As luxações são classificadas como: luxação de grau 1, quando pode ser manualmente percebida por meio de pressão digital e reduzida assim que a pressão é liberada; luxação de grau 2, quando é percebida mediante pressão digital, mas não ocorre redução quando a pressão é liberada; luxação de grau 3, quando a articulação apresenta luxação na maior parte do tempo, mas pode ser reduzida por pressão digital; e luxação de grau 4, quando a luxação articular permanece e não é possível reduzi-la por meio de pressão digital. A luxação medial é mais comum do que a lateral. Alguns cães podem apresentar ambas, mais provavelmente como resultado da frouxidão de tecidos moles (p. ex., cães da raça Basset Hound). Pode ocorrer luxação traumáticas da patela, mas são raras. Na maioria das vezes, a luxação da patelar é um sintoma secundário de um problema ortopédico primário. Em termos gerais, há anormalidade no eixo *mecânico* do membro pélvico (uma linha virtual que une o centro da cabeça do fêmur ao coxim metatársico). O centro da articulação do joelho pode estar deslocado medial ou lateralmente, quando comparado ao eixo mecânico do membro. Em termos mais específicos, quase sempre a luxação da patela é consequência de uma gama de problemas geométricos que afetam o fêmur e a tíbia, inclusive angulação anormal ou torção da parte proximal ou distal do fêmur, angulação anormal ou torção da tíbia, patela anormalmente alta (em geral, descrita como *patela alta*) ou baixa (*patela baixa*) e torção por frouxidão anormal da articulação do joelho (Figura 353.1). Essas anormalidades frequentemente coexistem. Elas podem estar presentes em cães com problemas de conformação, como postura com membros arqueados e postura valga.

Se uma luxação de patela ocorre no início da vida do animal, quando os ossos e as articulações estão em desenvolvimento, provavelmente outras anormalidades se desenvolvem, inclusive uma fenda troclear rasa ou ausente e deslocamento medial da crista tibial. Geralmente, um padrão que inclui a posição varus e a rotação interna da parte distal do fêmur é a causa inicial da luxação medial da patela. Às vezes, o subdesenvolvimento do côndilo femoral lateral, resultando em orientação valga da tíbia, é a principal causa da luxação lateral da patela.[57,58] Em pacientes com grave deslocamento medial e caudal da patela, a ausência de extensão da articulação do joelho pode resultar do fato de que o quadríceps femoral deixa de atuar como músculo extensor do joelho quando a tensão gerada por contrações musculares é direcionada ao longo de uma linha que não é mais cranial ao fêmur (Figura 353.2). Com o passar do tempo, à medida que o fêmur cresce, o quadríceps deslocado em posição caudomedial não cresce em comprimento e atua como fixador, limitando a extensão do joelho. Nesses cães, a extensão do joelho é dolorosa, complicando a implementação de programas de alongamento manual ou baseado em exercícios (ver Capítulo 355). Ao examinar cães com luxação de patela, deve-se avaliar os formatos do fêmur e da tíbia, a torção por frouxidão e a extensão do joelho. A avaliação inicial é realizada com o cão em estação e caminhando lentamente. O clínico deve avaliar a conformação do membro, questionando se os membros pélvicos estão retos, arqueados ou em posição varus. Os coxins estão apontados para frente ou rotacionados interna ou externamente? As articulações dos joelhos estão apropriadas ou estão excessivamente flexionadas ou estendidas? Também são avaliados os membros com o cão em decúbito lateral. A luxação é graduada de 1 a 4, e a posição próximo-distal da patela é anotada (patela alta ou patela baixa). A presença de angulação (varus ou valgo) e torção do membro (interna ou externa) é avaliada com a articulação coxofemoral relaxada (nem estendida, nem flexionada), e o joelho é mantido em extensão. O formato do osso é confirmado por radiografias ortogonais do fêmur e da tíbia. Se o cão é suficientemente pequeno, obtém-se uma única radiografia craniocaudal que inclua o fêmur, a tíbia e as patas, utilizada para avaliar o eixo mecânico do membro. Em cães de grande porte, isso pode ser feito com duas radiografias craniocaudais, em feixes horizontais, das partes proximal e distal do membro, respectivamente, por meio da mudança de posição da fonte de raios X, sem alterar a posição do membro. Reconstruções tridimensionais baseadas em imagens do membro obtidas em TC possibilitam uma avaliação mais rápida e acurada do formato do osso do que as radiografias (ver Figura 353.1). A frouxidão rotacional da articulação do joelho é avaliada com o joelho posicionado em ângulo neutro (90°). A rotação tibiofemoral normal é de aproximadamente 20°. Alguns pacientes apresentam rotação tibiofemoral de 60 a 90°, potencialmente como resultado do torque aplicado na tíbia pelo quadríceps femoral. Na palpação da articulação do joelho, devem sempre ser observados sinais de efusão articular, crepitação, gaveta cranial e resposta à dor após a palpação. A efusão articular, palpável em local imediatamente caudal ao ligamento patelar, no aspecto medial do joelho, é incomum em cães com luxação de patela. A presença de efusão deve fazer os clínicos suspeitarem de um problema além da luxação de patela – mais comumente de ruptura do ligamento cruzado cranial. Em caso de luxação traumática da patela, a efusão na articulação do joelho pode resultar de laceração da fibrocartilagem parapatelar medial ou lateral. Crepitação é incomum em cães com luxação

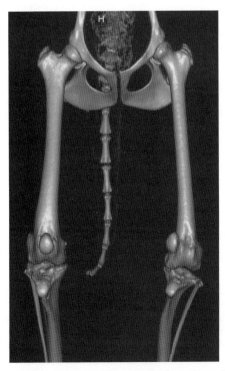

Figura 353.1 Essa reconstrução tridimensional é baseada em imagens dos membros pélvicos de um cão com luxação medial da patela do joelho esquerdo obtidas em tomografia computadorizada (TC). A angulação e torção do fêmur e da tíbia, o formato da tróclea e do côndilo femoral e a posição da patela são avaliados em ambos os membros pélvicos por meio de sua manipulação.

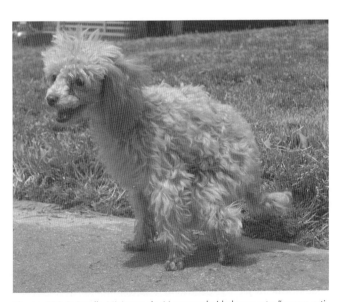

Figura 353.2 Poodle Miniatura de 11 meses de idade em estação, com articulações dos joelhos flexionadas. O cão apresenta luxação de patela de grau 4 em ambos os membros pélvicos. São perdidos aproximadamente 60° de extensão em ambas as articulações do joelho, porque a rotação interna da tíbia é tão grave que o quadríceps não funciona mais como um músculo extensor da articulação do joelho.

de patela. A crepitação pode resultar com mais frequência em dano de toda a cartilagem da patela e da crista da tróclea onde há luxação da patela. Pode haver gaveta cranial se o cão apresentar luxação de patela e lesão do ligamento cruzado cranial simultâneas. Aparentemente, a presença de luxação de patela predispõe os cães a lesões do ligamento cruzado cranial, por conta de potenciais alterações nas forças mantidas pelo ligamento, devido ao deslocamento do músculo quadríceps femoral ou da tíbia em relação ao fêmur. De forma geral, a resposta à dor após a palpação do joelho ou a redução da luxação de patela em cães é incomum. Entretanto, quando há dor, pode ser muito intensa. A resposta à dor após a palpação é mais frequentemente notada em cães com dificuldades para estender a articulação do joelho (por conta da contratura do quadríceps, como mencionado anteriormente), com ruptura do ligamento cruzado (por conta da intensa inflamação articular resultante da ruptura do ligamento cruzado), com patela *justa* que requer esforço significante para reduzi-la, com patela alta e reabsorção óssea no aspecto proximal da tróclea ou com osteoartrite.

Osteocondrose é o desenvolvimento anormal da superfície articular com retardo na ossificação focal do osso subcondral, potencialmente levando à formação de uma aba de cartilagem articular, uma condição denominada **osteocondrite dissecante** (OCD). Em cães, a OCD se desenvolve no aspecto caudal da cabeça do úmero, no aspecto medial do côndilo do úmero, na parte distal dos côndilos femorais medial e lateral e na parte proximal das cristas medial e lateral da tróclea do tálus. A patogenia da osteocondrose envolve duas teorias concorrentes (mecânica e vascular), ambas plausíveis. A teoria mecânica da OCD é baseada no fato de que em cães o osso subcondral de rápido crescimento é grosseiro e mecanicamente fraco, predispondo a fraturas em locais que sustentam a altas cargas.[22] A teoria vascular da OCD é baseada na perda de suprimento sanguíneo à epífise como resultado da degeneração dos vasos de canais da cartilagem.[59] A partir de uma perspectiva genética da população, a OCD do côndilo umeral e a fragmentação do processo medial parecem ser doenças genéticas distintas.[4] A OCD do côndilo umeral, dos côndilos femorais e da tróclea do tálus é acompanhada de inflamação intensa das articulações acometidas (com efusão articular intensa e palpável) e frequentemente desencadeia o rápido desenvolvimento de alterações osteoartríticas. Por outro lado, parece improvável que a OCD da cabeça do úmero desencadeie rápidas alterações osteoartríticas na articulação do joelho.

Várias doenças ósseas inflamatórias acometem cães em crescimento. Elas podem comprometer o eixo de ossos longos (panosteíte), as regiões metafisárias de ossos longos (osteodistrofia hipertrófica) ou o crânio (osteopatia craniomandibular). Mais frequentemente, a panosteíte afeta ossos longos (rádio, ulna, úmero, fêmur) de cães de grande porte e, em geral, se desenvolve em uma única localização, mas pode acometer vários locais em sucessão, recebendo o nome de *claudicação de diferentes membros*. A aparência radiográfica da panosteíte é variável em cada fase de desenvolvimento. Na fase aguda, ocorre perda do padrão trabecular no local acometido (o osso parece borrado). Após algumas semanas, a área afetada se torna radiopaca, potencialmente porque o novo osso está justaposto durante o remodelamento do osso trabecular anormal. Em casos graves, é possível notar discreta reação periosteal focal no centro da lesão. A causa de **panosteíte** não é conhecida, mas alguns pesquisadores sugerem uma causa infecciosa. O genoma do vírus da cinomose canina foi associado a lesões ósseas parecidas com panosteíte, semelhante à osteodistrofia hipertrófica (descrita posteriormente).[38,60] A panosteíte é autolimitante; as lesões são abrandadas após algumas semanas.

A **osteodistrofia hipertrófica**, também denominada osteopatia metafisária, é uma doença óssea inflamatória que se desenvolve nas regiões metafisárias dos ossos longos. A causa de osteodistrofia hipertrófica não é conhecida; o RNA viral (cinomose) foi detectado em osteoblastos da região metafisária de ossos longos em cães acometidos, e lesões metafisárias foram detectadas em cães com cinomose.[37,38] A vacinação com vírus vivo modificado foi relatada como um fator desencadeante de osteodistrofia hipertrófica.[61] Há relato de bacteriemia por *E. coli* em um filhote com osteodistrofia hipertrófica,[28] mas é incerto se a bacteriemia é resultado ou consequência. O rápido crescimento do animal em decorrência do aumento do consumo alimentar foi sugerido como causa de maior risco de osteodistrofia hipertrófica.[62,63] Em casos de osteodistrofia hipertrófica discreta, quase sempre as lesões são restritas à porção distal do rádio, ulna e tíbia. Em casos graves, as lesões frequentemente podem se desenvolver nas metáfises proximais e distais de todos os ossos longos. A osteodistrofia hipertrófica grave desencadeia uma reação periosteal espessa ao redor da região metafisária da porção distal do rádio e da ulna. Essa reação periosteal quase sempre está associada a grave angulação caudal (arqueamento cranial) do rádio.[64] A osteodistrofia hipertrófica é uma doença autolimitante que é abrandada na maioria dos pacientes (85% em um estudo)[65] no momento do fechamento fisário. Entretanto, a angulação resultante de formas graves de osteodistrofia hipertrófica persiste. Há relato de osteodistrofia hipertrófica em gatos.[66]

Núcleos cartilaginosos retidos são lesões radiograficamente visíveis que se desenvolvem nas regiões metafisárias de ossos longos, em especial na ulna distal.[67] Esses núcleos foram relatados em combinação com a osteodistrofia hipertrófica.[68] Embora os núcleos cartilaginosos retidos na ulna e, em menor extensão, no rádio sejam frequentemente associados à anormalidade do crescimento longitudinal, à ocorrência de valgo multiapical bilateral e à deformidade angular causal do rádio, a sua etiologia é incerta. Em outras palavras, os núcleos cartilaginosos retidos e as deformidades angulares podem ser consequências da mesma anormalidade do crescimento, ao contrário do distúrbio de crescimento, que não seria a consequência dos núcleos cartilaginosos retidos. Filhotes de raças de grande porte às vezes apresentam deformidades bilaterais valgas do rádio e ainda podem ter um núcleo cartilaginoso retido visível em um único membro, sugestivo de consequência da anormalidade do crescimento longitudinal, não sua causa.

Osteopatia craniomandibular é uma doença óssea proliferativa que acomete a mandíbula e a maxila de cães imaturos do ponto de vista esquelético.[69,70] A doença ocorre mais frequentemente na raça West Highland White Terrier, mas foi relatada em outras, inclusive Boxer, Dogue Alemão e Doberman Pinscher. A osteopatia craniomandibular também é autolimitante.

A doença de **Legg-Perthes** é uma doença degenerativa da cabeça e do colo do fêmur que ocorre em cães de raças de pequeno porte em fase de crescimento. A doença geralmente é unilateral, mas pode afetar ambas as articulações coxofemorais. Pouco se sabe sobre a fisiopatologia da doença de Legg-Perthes. Acredita-se que o colapso e remodelamento da cabeça do fêmur seja resultado do colapso de vasos sanguíneos que nutrem a cabeça do fêmur.[71] Fraturas na fise femoral proximal (também denominadas fraturas fisárias capitais, fises capitais separadas, fraturas de cabeça do fêmur e epifisiólise) que ocorrem na ausência de traumatismos conhecidos foram relatadas em cães e gatos.[72,73] Em 2 gatos, essas fraturas fisárias femorais proximais foram decorrências de displasia epifisária multicêntrica.[74] Osteonecrose do osso carporradial, semelhante à doença de Legg-Perthes, foi relatada em um cão.[75]

Ossificação incompleta ocorre em ossos de cães geralmente nas regiões subcondrais de pequenos ossos (próximo a superfícies articulares). Ela pode ocorrer devido a pressões anormais aplicadas aos ossos em crescimento, como resultado de condrodistrofia ou outra anormalidade do crescimento (Figura 353.3).[76-78] Predisposição racial foi relatada em algumas formas de ossificação incompleta, sugerindo a participação de fatores genéticos desencantes. Por exemplo, nota-se não união do processo ancôneo em cães da raça Pastor-Alemão, ossificação incompleta

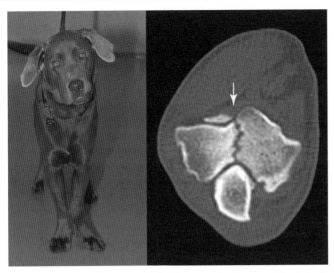

Figura 353.3 Cão da raça Labrador Retriever de 11 meses de idade (*à esquerda*) com desvio do peso do corpo para o lado direito, pois há deformação do rádio esquerdo. Realizou-se tomografia computadorizada (TC) dos membros torácicos para avaliar a geometria da deformação. O cão apresentava ossificação incompleta dos côndilos umerais esquerdo e direito. A região não ossificada do côndilo direito era completa (*seta*), e a região não ossificada do côndilo esquerdo era parcial. Os côndilos foram estabilizados com a colocação de parafusos ósseos transcondilares.

do côndilo umeral em cães de raças Spaniel e ossificação incompleta do osso carporradial em cães da raça Boxer.[76,79-81] A superfície articular sobrejacente ao osso com ossificação incompleta pode ser descontínua, possibilitando a troca de líquido entre a articulação e o osso subcondral. A ossificação incompleta potencialmente leva à osteoartrite por conta de desnível na superfície articular, instabilidade articular ou troca de líquido entre a articulação e osso subcondral.[76] Além disso, a ossificação incompleta consegue atuar como ativador de estresse, desencadeando a incapacidade mecânica catastrófica de um osso longo, como mencionado para o côndilo umeral.[76] Além da ossificação incompleta do processo ancôneo, côndilo umeral e osso carporradial, há relato de ossificação incompleta do aspecto caudal do glenoide e do atlas.[82,83] Ossificação retardada da parte proximal da tíbia foi relatada em cães Greyhound e outros cães de grande porte.[84,85]

Anormalidades ósseas também incluem **cistos** ósseos. Grandes cistos em ossos são raros. Os cistos podem predispor a fraturas[86,87] e surgir como resultado de fístulas arteriovenosas (ver Capítulos 250 e 257).[88] Pequenos cistos ósseos subcondrais são comuns, consequentes de osteoartrite crônica.[89] Há relato de cisto subcondral na incisura ulnar em um cão.[90]

Osteoartropatia hipertrófica, conhecida como doença de Marie em humanos, é uma doença óssea proliferativa na qual ocorre proliferação periosteal difusa ligeiramente irregular nas partes distais dos membros. A doença é causada pela presença de um tumor ou uma lesão com efeito de massa no tórax ou no abdome, mais comumente por tumores pulmonares.[91] A osteoartropatia hipertrófica também foi relatada em cães e gatos como consequência de pneumonia, bronquite, megaesôfago, endocardite, neoplasias intra-abdominais (renal, hepática, de bexiga) e espirocercose.[92-95] Em éguas[96] e em mulheres, a osteoartropatia hipertrófica foi associada à gravidez. A proliferação periosteal é considerada a consequência mais provável do aumento de fluxo sanguíneo resultante do reflexo vagal aferente parafisiológico, mas outras teorias foram propostas.[94,97]

Lesões do **ligamento cruzado cranial** (LCC) estão entre os problemas ortopédicos mais comuns em cães. Em um amplo estudo, verificou-se que 8% dos pacientes apresentavam lesões do LCC.[48] Embora uma minoria resulte de traumatismo direto, a maioria das lesões se deve a anormalidades esqueléticas. Frequentemente, as lesões do LCC são diagnosticadas quando o veterinário examina um cão de grande porte de meia-idade, sem histórico de traumatismo, com claudicação crônica por apoio de peso em um membro pélvico. Em um estudo envolvendo mais de 1,2 milhões de cães tratados ao longo de 40 anos, constatou-se que 9 raças eram mais predispostas a lesão do LCC; as raças com maior risco foram Terranova e Rottweiler.[98] Não há consenso entre os pesquisadores quanto à cadeia de eventos que ocasiona lesão do LCC; claramente, são multifatoriais, e a luxação da patela é um fator predisponente.[99] Alguns pesquisadores acreditam que uma série de eventos mecânicos seria o gatilho para lesão do LCC, como inclinação do platô tibial, ângulo de anteversão femoral, largura da incisura troclear e momento da extensão da articulação do calcâneo.[100,101] Outros acreditam na participação de uma cadeia de eventos biológicos, que inclui doença imunomediada, metaplasia fibrocartilaginosa e degradação da matriz, como fatores desencadeantes.[102,103] Detectou-se DNA bacteriano em articulações do joelho com osteoartrite.[104] A obesidade (ver Capítulo 176) predispõe os cães à lesão do LCC.[105] Castração e ovariosterectomia também estão associadas a maior risco,[106,107] mas ainda não foi demonstrada uma relação causal. Após lesão do LCC, é comum ocorrer ruptura do LCC oposto, cuja sobrevida mediana é relatada em 947 dias.[108] Lesões de menisco são consequências comuns, principalmente quando ocorre ruptura total do LCC, quando os cães são de grande porte e quando o tratamento é postergado.[109,110]

Neoplasias afetam ossos e articulações. O tumor ósseo mais comum é o osteossarcoma (ver Capítulo 348). Outras neoplasias se desenvolvem em ossos e articulações, inclusive condrossarcoma, fibrossarcoma e melanoma maligno. Múltiplas exostoses cartilaginosas foram relatadas em cães[111] e observadas em filhotes da mesma ninhada e por várias gerações.[112,113] Além de osteossarcoma, melanoma e hemangiopericitoma, vários tipos de tumores se desenvolvem especificamente nos dígitos de cães, inclusive carcinoma de célula escamosa em cães de pelame escuro, carcinoma pulmonar metastático e papiloma.[114-118] Neoplasias de ossos longos foram relatadas em associação com infarto medular ósseo multifocal, como acontece em cães da raça Schnauzer com hiperlipidemia, e em associação com infartos medulares focais secundários à substituição total da articulação coxofemoral.[119-121]

Problemas ortopédicos incluem fraturas patológicas em ossos enfraquecidos por doenças preexistentes. As fraturas patológicas mais comuns são as fraturas por fadiga, também conhecidas como fraturas por estresse, ocasionadas por forças normais aplicadas ao osso anormal – diferentemente das fraturas convencionais, que são ocasionadas por forças anormais em um osso normal.[122]

Fraturas por fadiga foram relatadas apenas em cães de corrida da raça Greyhound, que podem fraturar o osso central do tarso, os ossos metacarpianos e metatarsianos e o acetábulo.[122-125] Fraturas patológicas também ocorrem como resultado da perda óssea secundária à doença periodontal,[126] osteossarcoma,[127,128] ou cistos ósseos.[86,87] Ademais, elas ocorrem em cães e gatos com osteogênese imperfeita (ver Capítulo 187).[129,130]

CONSEQUÊNCIAS GERAIS DAS ANORMALIDADES ESQUELÉTICAS

Dor

Os sinais clínicos de problemas ortopédicos com muita frequência resultam da *dor* oriunda de articulações, ossos ou outros tecidos musculoesqueléticos (ver Capítulo 126). Subjetivamente, as dores articulares e ósseas são têm mais relevância clínica do que a dor oriunda de ligamentos, músculos ou tendões. Em cães com ruptura muscular, o uso do membro não parece ser particularmente comprometido. Por exemplo, espera-se que um cão de corrida Greyhound, cujo músculo grácil se rompe durante uma corrida, reduza sua velocidade em alguns segundos, um retardo de aproximadamente 3% (1 segundo durante uma corrida de 35 segundos). De forma semelhante, a tendinite é raramente diagnosticada como causa de claudicação em cães (presumivelmente porque a tendinite não ocasiona claudicação), mas, quando um tendão cruza a articulação, se inflama e causa sinovite nessa articulação, os sinais clínicos podem ser muito intensos. Por exemplo, quando ocorre inflamação do tendão oriundo do músculo bíceps braquial, um tendão que passa pela articulação do ombro, os sintomas geralmente são muito graves.[131]

A principal causa de dor articular é a osteoartrite. A dor articular pode também ser decorrência de artropatia imunomediada, artrite séptica, neoplasia articular (sarcoma de célula sinovial), ossificação incompleta, presença de fragmentos ou abas osteocondrais e de outras causas. Subjetivamente, alguém poderia estimar a dor articular secundária à osteoartrite como causa de 99% da dor relacionada à articulação, pois a osteoartrite é comum em cães e outras causas de dor articular são raras. Artropatias podem ser agudas ou crônicas, inflamatórias ou degenerativas. A dor articular aguda quase sempre é causada por sinovite. A claudicação causada pela sinovite é tão previsível que a sinovite induzida por cristais de urato é utilizada como modelo experimental de claudicação transitória.[132-134] A sinovite pode resultar da presença de um fragmento osteocondral na articulação (p. ex., aba de OCD, fragmentação do processo coronoide medial), de dano em toda a cartilagem (displasia coxofemoral, displasia do cotovelo), em razão da troca de líquido entre a articulação e o osso subcondral (aba de OCD, ossificação incompleta) ou da presença de fibras de colágeno rompidas na articulação (lesão do LCC, lesão do tendão do bíceps braquial). A hemorragia intra-articular induz à sinovite[135] e danifica a cartilagem, particularmente a imatura.[136] Ademais, ocorre inflamação do osso subcondral exposto ao líquido articular.[137] A doença inflamatória aguda resulta em dor, mas não está associada a alterações estruturais da articulação. Nessa situação, a claudicação está presente, mas a amplitude do movimento está dentro dos limites normais. A resposta de dor aos problemas articulares inflamatórios agudos é tratada como dor aguda induzida por lesão ou cirurgia (ver Capítulos 126 e 166). Se a inflamação articular persistir, com o passar do tempo a artropatia se torna crônica: a cápsula articular se torna espessa e a movimentação articular diminui. É provável que ocorra exacerbação da dor local (sensibilização primária periférica) e sensibilização espinal (central). A perda do movimento articular é imprevisível e varia entre as articulações e com os diferentes movimentos articulares. Por exemplo, na displasia coxofemoral crônica, o cão da raça Labrador Retriever perde a capacidade de extensão, mas não a de flexão da articulação.[138] A artropatia crônica é tratada como mencionado adiante para dor crônica.

Os sinais clínicos também podem ser causados por dor óssea, que, de forma geral, é muito menos comum em cães do que a dor articular. Nos EUA, pode-se estimar que milhões de cães apresentem dor articular, enquanto milhares sofrem de dor óssea.[48,98,139] As duas causas mais comuns de dor óssea são iatrogênicas: falha de fixação após procedimento ortopédico e osteomielite. Outras causas de dor óssea, em ordem decrescente de frequência, incluem doenças ósseas inflamatórias juvenis (panosteíte, osteodistrofia hipertrófica e osteopatia craniomandibular), neoplasias (osteossarcoma, condrossarcoma, carcinoma metastático), osteoartropatia hipertrófica e fraturas patológicas. A falha de fixação é uma fonte de dor óssea, porque o primeiro estágio da cicatrização da fratura é inflamatório, que persiste e aumenta de intensidade em fraturas tratadas sem cirurgia e após falha de fixação. Inflamação intensa crônica é o provável mecanismo que causa dor associada à osteomielite.[140] O edema intramedular foi incriminado como fator indutor de dor em cães com doenças ósseas inflamatórias.[141] A atividade osteoclástica excessiva é um fator crítico na dor resultante de osteossarcoma.[142]

Marcha anormal

O surgimento de marcha ou andar anormal é uma consequência comum dos problemas ortopédicos, pois os ossos podem apresentar angulação anormal ou ser curtos, ou da instabilidade articular, resultante de enfermidades sistêmicos ou focais do tecido conjuntivo, que incluem hiperextensão do carpo ou tarso. A hiperextensão do carpo é mais frequentemente relatada em cães de grande porte em fase de crescimento, principalmente na raça Pastor-Alemão (Figura 353.4), em cães com doenças metabólicas, particularmente hiperadrenocorticismo, e em cães com doença articular imunomediada (Figura 353.5; ver Capítulo 203). A marcha anormal também se deve à claudicação, que pode ser definida como uma alteração voluntária da marcha de modo a minimizar a dor percebida durante a locomoção. Em cães, a claudicação varia dependendo da natureza, da gravidade e da cronicidade de problemas ortopédicos, tamanho e comportamento ("personalidade") do paciente, além de outros fatores.

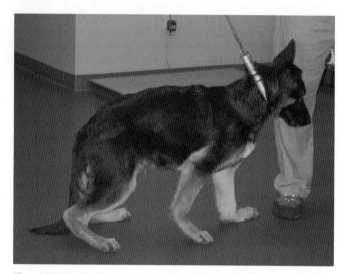

Figura 353.4 Cão da raça Pastor-Alemão de 4 meses de idade com hipertensão das articulações do carpo. O cão está em posição palmígrada. Também se nota frouxidão entre o calcâneo e o quarto osso társico.

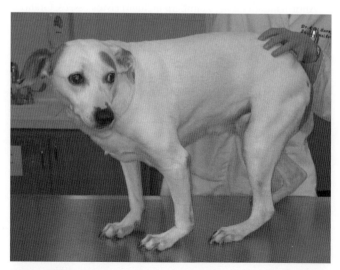

Figura 353.5 Cão sem raça definida com hiperextensão do carpo por conta de poliartrite não erosiva de baixo grau. Em cães com poliartrite imunomediada, embora os carpos e tarsos sejam frequentemente acometidos, em geral a hiperextensão do carpo é notada mais precocemente e é mais grave do que a hiperextensão do tarso.

Sinais clínicos

As consequências de anormalidades esqueléticas variam amplamente, desde claudicações não detectáveis até claudicação sem apoio de peso corporal no membro, mantido em posição flexionada sem ser utilizado. Tutores, clínicos e pesquisadores utilizam diferentes parâmetros para julgar a gravidade dos problemas ortopédicos e a resposta ao tratamento. Tutores quase sempre monitoram se seus animais estão "felizes" (uma avaliação moderadamente subjetiva), se são capazes de realizar suas atividades rotineiras diárias (caminhar para dentro e fora de casa, subir degraus, entrar e sair de um veículo), se vocalizam em resposta à dor e se estão brincando normalmente. Os tutores rotineiramente acompanham a claudicação, por exemplo para avaliar a progressão da doença ou a resposta ao tratamento. Pouco se sabe sobre a acurácia da avaliação da claudicação pelo tutor. Com o passar do tempo, os tutores tendem a subestimar a gravidade da claudicação.[143] Os clínicos julgam a gravidade dos distúrbios ortopédicos com base na gravidade da claudicação, normalmente pelo uso de escalas qualitativas simples, como claudicação com ou sem apoio de peso no membro discreta, moderada ou severa.[144-146] Às vezes, os clínicos tentam documentar problemas ortopédicos com mais especificidade do que a simples utilização de escores de claudicação qualitativos, como a avaliação da reabilitação física (ver Capítulo 355).[147] Avaliações ortopédicas específicas podem incluir presença de efusão articular e de crepitação, resposta à dor após palpação e movimentação da articulação avaliada subjetivamente ou mensurada objetivamente utilizando um goniômetro plástico (Figura 353.6).[148,149]

Desuso de membro

O desuso de membro é uma consequência comum de anormalidades ortopédicas graves responsáveis pela dor crônica sustentada (Figura 353.7). Com o desuso, os cães tocam no solo com as pontas dos dedos ou não apoiam o peso corporal sobre o membro (Figura 353.8) quando em estação ou caminhando. O cão com desuso de um único membro desvia o seu peso para o membro contralateral (Figura 353.9 e Vídeo 353.1). O cão com desuso de dois membros desvia o peso para frente, se os membros afetados são os pélvicos (Figura 353.10), ou para trás, se os membros acometidos são os torácicos. Com isso, o cão modifica os ângulos da coluna e das articulações dos membros (Figura 353.11). Essas alterações de postura se tornam intensamente consolidadas com o passar do tempo, tornando difícil sua recuperação, mesmo quando o problema ortopédico original é tratado com sucesso. Fisiologicamente, o desuso do membro ocasiona perda de massa óssea, de massa muscular, de espessura e rigidez da cartilagem e da força do ligamento. Entretanto, a maioria dessas alterações é lentamente reversível, após o tratamento da causa do desuso do membro.

A aparência radiográfica ou a progressão da osteoartrite é frequentemente utilizada como mensuração da progressão dos problemas ortopédicos. Entretanto, informações sobre a relação entre anormalidades funcionais, dor e alterações radiográficas são escassas. Essa relação foi avaliada em gatos com osteoartrite, e os achados verificados na palpação da articulação e nas alterações radiográficas foram pouco correlacionados.[150,151] No joelho do cão, foram relatadas progressão da osteoartrite após cirurgia para tratar lesão do LCC[152-155] e estabilização cirúrgica da luxação da patela;[156] na articulação do cotovelo do cão, progressão da osteoartrite após cirurgia para remover processos coronoides mediais fragmentados,[157,158] como consequência do sobrepeso;[159] na articulação coxofemoral do cão, progressão da osteoartrite devido ao sobrepeso (ver Capítulo 176).[50,159] Em um estudo não relacionado, a gravidade da osteoartrite em cães da raça Labrador Retriever com displasia coxofemoral não pareceu estar associada à gravidade da claudicação.[138] Exames de imagem avançados, inclusive TC, RM ou cintilografia óssea, às vezes são realizados como procedimento de avaliação. A TC é amplamente utilizada para avaliar a articulação do cotovelo, e há correlação de seus achados com aqueles verificados na artroscopia.[160] Pesquisadores também julgam a gravidade dos problemas ortopédicos com base em mensurações cinéticas objetivas (mensurações da placa de força ou sensibilidade à pressão durante a caminhada), em medidas cinemáticas objetivas (análise cinemática em 2D ou 3D), em biomarcadores séricos ou em exame histológico.

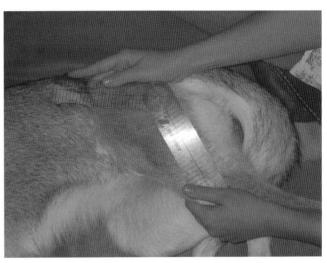

Figura 353.6 Mensuração da extensão da articulação coxofemoral com um goniômetro plástico, cujos "braços" estão alinhados ao longo de uma linha que une a tuberosidade sacral à tuberosidade isquiática e de uma linha que une o trocânter maior ao ponto médio craniocaudal entre a patela e a fabela lateral, respectivamente. Em cães, a extensão normal da articulação coxofemoral é de aproximadamente 160°. Nesse cão submetido à ostectomia da cabeça do fêmur, a extensão era de 123°.

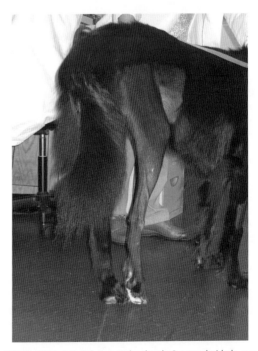

Figura 353.7 Cão mestiço da raça Labrador de 3 anos de idade com desuso do membro pélvico direito, devido a infecção da articulação do joelho após remoção cirúrgica do menisco medial rompido. Problemas biológicos iatrogênicos (infecção) ou mecânicos (falha de fixação do reparo cirúrgico) são causas comuns de desuso do membro.

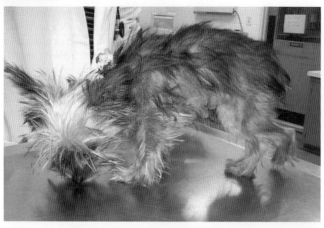

Figura 353.8 Cão da raça Yorkshire Terrier de 4 meses que não apoia o peso corporal no membro pélvico esquerdo, por conta de luxação de patela medial de grau 4. A tíbia está rotacionada internamente em relação ao fêmur. A luxação da patela é a causa mais comum de desuso de membro em cães em fase de crescimento.

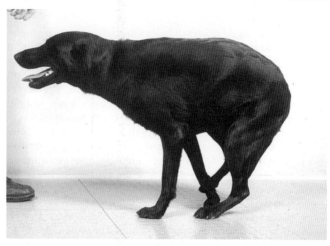

Figura 353.10 Cão da raça Labrador Retriever com ruptura parcial do ligamento cruzado cranial em ambas as articulações do joelho. Embora o cão desvie a maior parte do seu peso aos membros torácicos, esse desvio de peso geralmente é mais discreto.

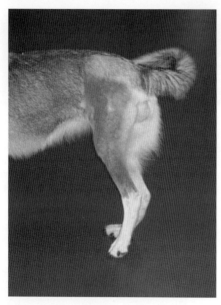

Figura 353.9 Cão da raça Husky Siberiano de 11 meses com sinais de desuso do membro pélvico esquerdo. O desuso se deve a duas cirurgias – a primeira para tratar luxação de patela, a segunda para realizar ostectomia da cabeça do fêmur e tratar displasia coxofemoral. À palpação, detectou-se resposta de dor intensa à extensão da articulação coxofemoral de 123°, uma perda de aproximadamente 40° (ver Figura 353.6).

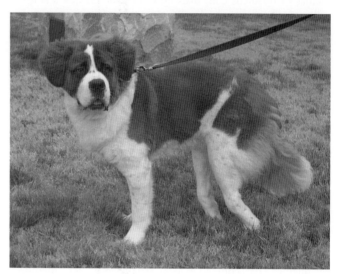

Figura 353.11 Cão São Bernardo macho de 11 meses com desvio de peso corporal para a frente e hiperextensão de articulações talocrurais. A hiperextensão do tarso resultante do desvio do peso é mais frequentemente observada em cães jovens de raças de grande porte e gigantes, que desviam o peso corporal para a frente devido à dor na articulação coxofemoral causada pela subluxação da articulação. Esses cães relutam em estender a articulação coxofemoral quando permanecem em estação e caminham e, de outra maneira, estendem as articulações talocrurais com hiperextensão.

Os sinais clínicos em cães e gatos com distúrbios ortopédicos específicos são raramente descritos com precisão e pesquisados. Logicamente, a maioria das informações disponíveis na literatura está relacionada aos problemas ortopédicos mais comuns: displasia da articulação coxofemoral, displasia do cotovelo e lesões do LCC. Os sintomas de displasia coxofemoral são mais frequentemente descritos como agudos em cães imaturos do ponto de vista esquelético ou em adultos jovens e crônicos em cães idosos. Sinais clínicos agudos refletem dor aguda: geralmente claudicação grave e quase sempre unilateral. Os sintomas agudos em geral surgem durante a fase de rápido crescimento ósseo, dos 4 aos 8 meses de idade. Os cães acometidos podem ser relutantes em realizar atividades propulsivas, inclusive pular, subir degraus, galopar ou caminhar por longo tempo, ou podem manifestar alterações comportamentais, inclusive relutância em brincar, introversão ou comportamento agressivo. Os sintomas crônicos de displasia coxofemoral refletem dor crônica e, como consequência, perda de força. Esses sintomas incluem intolerância ao exercício, relutância em pular e subir degraus e marcha anômala caracterizada por "pulos de lebre" durante o galope. De forma surpreendente, na literatura há poucas informações sobre as alterações fisiológicas em cães com displasia coxofemoral crônica.[138,161-164] Cães com esse tipo de displasia manifestam dor oriunda de superfícies do fêmur e do acetábulo articulares e da cápsula da articulação coxofemoral, principalmente ao se movimentar em maior velocidade e durante extensão dessa articulação. Com o passar do tempo, os cães com displasia podem perder a capacidade de extensão da articulação coxofemoral, mas não parecem perder sua flexão. Em um estudo que avaliou uma coorte de 60 cães da raça Labrador Retriever com displasia coxofemoral, um modelo estatístico indicou perda de 1° de extensão da articulação por ano.[138] A articulação coxofemoral com displasia pode perder a capacidade de extensão por conta da fibrose da cápsula articular ou do desenvolvimento de grandes osteófitos ou entesiófitos nas faces caudal e ventral do acetábulo e do colo do fêmur e na face caudal do trocânter maior ou por conta de alterações nos tecidos periarticulares ou em músculos regionais. A resposta à dor durante a flexão da articulação coxofemoral, subjetivamente, é muito incomum e pode ser consequência de outros problemas, como artrite séptica ou tumor ósseo. A maioria dos cães com displasia perde massa muscular de membros pélvicos. Alguns podem desviar seu centro de gravidade para frente mediante a flexão da coluna e das articulações do ombro e do cotovelo. Os sinais clínicos de displasia coxofemoral variam amplamente entre as raças afetadas. Vários cães manifestam sintomas muito discretos, que podem surgir após longo período de atividade física ou após exercício extenuante;[138] outros são severamente incapacitados de se movimentar em trote ou galope ou de pular. Pouco se sabe sobre a relação entre os aspectos específicos da doença da articulação coxofemoral (subluxação dorsal, luxação dorsal, desgaste da cartilagem, desgaste do rim dorsal, espessamento da cápsula articular, produção de osteófitos, presença de fragmentos na articulação) e o tipo e gravidade dos sinais clínicos. No coorte de cães da raça Labrador Retriever mencionado anteriormente, 94% dos cães não manifestavam claudicação ou apresentavam claudicação discreta ou moderada e 6% tinham claudicação grave.[138] Dois fatores exacerbam a gravidade da claudicação: a presença de luxação coxofemoral (comparada à subluxação e à ausência de luxação ou subluxação dessa articulação) e menos de 20 minutos de exercícios diários (comparado a mais de 60 minutos de exercícios por dia). Nesse estudo, notou-se pouca correlação entre o tamanho e a localização de osteófitos com os sinais clínicos da displasia coxofemoral.

Os sintomas parecem relacionados ao tamanho do cão, mas há escassos dados científicos que confirmam a associação entre tamanho e claudicação ou que avaliam fatores que influenciam os sinais clínicos (comportamento, treinamento, relação entre pessoa e animal).

Subjetivamente, os clínicos frequentemente afirmam que é menos provável que cães de grande porte não apoiem o peso corporal ou apresentem desuso de membro grave, em comparação aos cães menores. Essa tendência aparentemente é aplicada a todas as anormalidades esqueléticas. É menos provável que cães de maior porte apresentem claudicação com toque da ponta do dedo no solo ou sem apoiar o peso corporal do que cães menores, possivelmente porque é mais difícil para os cães grandes permanecer em estação ou deambular com três membros.

A displasia coxofemoral também é comum em gatos,[150,165] mas pouco se sabe sobre os sintomas dessa displasia nesses animais. A baixa correlação entre sinais radiográficos de osteoartrite, lesão de cartilagem e achados anormais durante a avaliação ortopédica dificulta a detecção de doença articular em gatos.[151]

Os sinais clínicos da displasia de cotovelo foram descritos,[79] mas a relação das características dessa displasia e dos sinais clínicos foi relatada apenas em um estudo que envolveu 55 filhotes de cães da raça Rottweiler.[166] Esses sintomas podem incluir claudicação intermitente ou contínua de membros torácicos, efusão articular, perda da amplitude da movimentação durante a flexão e (em menor grau) a extensão e postura anormal ao repousar em posição esternal (flexão do carpo e antebraço em posição supina; Figura 353.12).[77]

Foram relatados sinais clínicos de lesões do LCC,[167] mas a relação entre as características de lesões do LCC e a claudicação ainda não foi avaliada. A palpação do ligamento patelar parece ser o sintoma de maior sensibilidade para a detecção de lesão do LCC.[167] Em cães com lesão do LCC, a constatação de um "clique" do menisco é fortemente sugestiva de laceração dessa estrutura.[109,168] As consequências clínicas da luxação da patela variam amplamente, desde ausência de sintomas até a incapacidade de deambulação. Pouco se sabe sobre os fatores que influenciam esses sinais clínicos. Subjetivamente, cães com

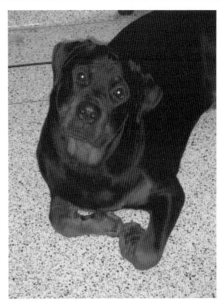

Figura 353.12 Cão da raça Rottweiler repousando em uma sala de exame com os dois antebraços em posição supina e carpos flexionados. Essa posição incomum do membro mais provavelmente resulta da dor oriunda das articulações do cotovelo. A resposta à dor após manipulação das articulações dos cotovelos foi detectada durante a palpação. O cão apresenta displasia bilateral dos cotovelos.

patela *frouxa* toleram bem a luxação. Cães com patela *justa* manifestam sinais de claudicação. A claudicação está também presente em cães com patela alta (eles podem manifestar sinais de reabsorção óssea proximal à tróclea femoral) e com perda da capacidade de extensão da articulação do joelho, como resultado de deslocamento grave da patela.

Avaliação do paciente

A avaliação das anormalidades ortopédicas inclui a obtenção do histórico clínico, a inspeção do paciente e a palpação do membro, bem como exames de imagem.

Histórico clínico

A maioria dos tutores reconhece o início e o impacto dos problemas ortopédicos nas atividades diárias dos seus animais, mas esses pensamentos raramente são organizados. O objetivo do histórico clínico é discutir e registrar de forma acurada informações que identificam distúrbios ortopédicos e mensuram sua gravidade e progressão (ver Capítulo 1). O histórico clínico também almeja detectar a presença de sinais clínicos relativos a outros sistemas orgânicos, principalmente sintomas neurológicos, pois as manifestações de problemas ortopédicos e neurológicos são semelhantes. Ademais, o histórico clínico é igualmente valioso para discriminar entre lesões ortopédicas e distúrbios ortopédicos não traumáticos e para avaliar a cronicidade e a progressão da doença. Questões relacionadas às atividades diárias (o cão consegue urinar, subir degraus e sair para caminhar sozinho?) e à atividade lúdica fornecem informações sobre o impacto de uma anormalidade ortopédica na qualidade de vida. A intolerância ao exercício relatado por tutores pode ser consequência da incapacidade ou falta de vontade. A incapacidade pode resultar da perda de força, perda de movimentação articular, carência de preparo físico (raramente) ou de comprometimento neurológico. A falta de vontade geralmente se deve à dor. A duração de um problema ortopédico é mais frequentemente subestimada, porque os tutores tendem a pensar que a claudicação começou quando eles a descobriram, o que raramente é verdadeiro. Além disso, as anormalidades ortopédicas quase sempre são crônicas e é difícil lembrar a data de início de um evento que ocorreu meses ou anos atrás. Pode ser útil questionar os tutores se o paciente já estava claudicando no momento de um feriado ou evento específico (p. ex., "Seu cão já estava claudicando no 7 de setembro?").

Inspeção do paciente

A inspeção do paciente fornece informações valiosas para os clínicos (ver Capítulo 2). Cães reagem à dor ortopédica de forma previsível, e as informações que seguem referem-se aos cães avaliados. A inspeção do paciente começa com o animal em posição de repouso. Os cães estão mais relaxados antes da palpação dos membros; portanto, a avaliação de sua postura em repouso e ao levantar, permanecer em pé, andar e caminhar em trote deve ocorrer antes da palpação. O cão pode ser inspecionado durante o repouso na sala de espera e ao levantar para caminhar em uma sala de exame. Se a claudicação for difícil de determinar, o tutor pode levar o cão para fora, como se estivessem deixando a clínica, e o clínico acompanha para observar. O cão pode estar mais relaxado, e a claudicação pode se tornar óbvia. É importante assegurar que qualquer claudicação observada corresponda à claudicação percebida pelo tutor. Embora a maioria dos tutores seja objetiva, alguns sobrestimam ou subestimam a gravidade da claudicação. Cães utilizados em apresentação de conformação (cães de eventos) às vezes são levados à consulta porque mais correm do que trotam, quando a corrida é inaceitável durante esses eventos. Alguns cães correm por conta de problemas ortopédicos; outros correm na ausência de qualquer problema ortopédico. Um conhecimento sólido dos padrões de marcha é útil para diferenciar marcha normal de anormal. Uma câmera digital, particularmente uma que possa registrar ou demonstrar a marcha em câmera lenta, é útil para observar e registrar a claudicação.

Cães adotam a posição que propicia o melhor resultado entre a dor percebida e a energia gasta. Ao se manter em pé, os cães com claudicação geralmente desviam o peso corporal sustentado pelos membros doloridos. Se um único membro está comprometido, os cães desviam o peso para o lado oposto. Desvios de peso de um lado para o outro não requerem grande esforço. Se ambos os membros pélvicos estiverem doloridos, os cães desviam o peso para frente mediante a flexão da coluna torácica, do ombro e dos cotovelos, e alargamento da posição dos membros torácicos. Diferentemente, se ambos os membros torácicos estiverem doloridos, os cães desviam o peso para trás, flexionando a coluna lombar, a articulação coxofemoral e os joelhos e alargando a posição dos membros pélvicos. O desvio de peso corporal mais clássico é para a frente, em resposta à grave displasia bilateral das articulações coxofemorais ou lesões bilaterais do LCC. Cães com desvio de peso crônico para frente apresentam ampla caixa torácica, abdução de cotovelos e antebraços com rotação interna (como acontece em cães da raça Buldogue). Desvios de peso para frente ou para trás requerem um grande esforço. Enquanto o cão ainda estiver em pé, os desvios de peso podem ser apreciados quando as patas são tiradas do solo. Cães que desviam o peso sustentado pelo membro podem manifestar respiração ofegante ou ter tremores de membros por conta do esforço e da dor percebida. A hiperextensão do tarso pode ser decorrência de desvio de peso para frente (ver Figura 353.11). O desvio de peso para frente em anormalidades de conformação dos membros pélvicos (geno valgo ou joelho valgo) pode ocasionar torção devido à frouxidão das articulações intertársicas.[169]

Cães levantam o membro dolorido do chão apenas quando a dor percebida diminui ao elevar o membro e quando o esforço para se levantar é compensado pela diminuição da dor percebida. Como o esforço para levantar os membros é menor em pequenos cães do que em grandes e gigantes, os animais pequenos mais frequentemente não apoiam o peso. Quando vários membros estão envolvidos (p. ex., após traumatismo veicular, poliartrite imunomediada ou doença óssea inflamatória multifocal), os cães permanecem em decúbito.

Quando sentados, os cães precisam hiperflexionar as articulações do joelho e do tarso. Cães com articulações do joelho doloridas, mais frequentemente após lesão do LCC, relutam em sentar retos e preferem estender o(s) membro(s) dolorido(s) para o lado. Quando eles levantam, desviam o peso para a frente do corpo para não precisar empurrá-lo com os membros pélvicos (ver Figura 353.10).

Claudicação

A claudicação é geralmente avaliada em uma caminhada e durante o trote. É importante diferenciar a claudicação de uma anormalidade da marcha que possa ser secundária a um problema que interfira na locomoção, mas que não é um problema ortopédico ativo – por exemplo, nanismo condrodistrófico, deformidade de crescimento secundária à lesão fisária, má consolidação de fratura ou doença neurológica. Cães com anormalidades de marcha podem ou não ter membros doloridos. Em casos de claudicação de membros torácicos, o animal balança a cabeça para cima quando o membro dolorido alcança o chão e para baixo quando o membro sadio toca o solo. De forma semelhante, em casos de claudicação do membro pélvico, a base da cauda se move para cima e para baixo. No caso de dor no quadril, o cão pode evitar a flexão da articulação coxofemoral ao movimentar o membro para frente; em vez disso, desvia a pelve de um lado para o outro. Isso ocasiona um movimento oscilante da base da cauda quando o cão é observado por trás. Alguns problemas ortopédicos podem ser mais facilmente detectados com o paciente em pé, enquanto outros são durante caminhada, trote ou galope. O animal deve ser examinado em pé em busca de movimentação articular ausente ou excessiva. Algumas anormalidades ortopédicas são mais visíveis em marcha mais rápida. Por exemplo, problemas associados à subluxação articular, como displasia coxofemoral, ocasionam a característica de "pulo de lebre" durante o galope. Se a claudicação for incerta quando o cão estiver andando, geralmente é útil observar o cão durante o trote ou galope. Inclinação da cabeça ("head tilt") é mais frequentemente evidente durante o trote e menos durante a caminhada. A maioria dos filhotes com displasia coxofemoral apresenta "pulo de lebre" característico ao galopar. Pode ser útil observar um cão pular ou subir escadas. Por exemplo, cães com contratura de músculo semimembranoso apresentam marcha anormal durante o trote, enquanto cães (de caça) com contratura fibrosante do músculo infraespinhoso apresentam circundução característica do membro torácico ao subir escada. Em geral, é mais difícil inspecionar gatos do que cães. Embora seja fácil examinar alguns gatos enquanto andam em uma sala de exame, vários outros relutam em caminhar durante a consulta (ver Vídeo 2.24). Eles podem preferir permanecer na caixa de transporte, agachar no local ou fugir para se esconder.

Palpação

A palpação deve incluir o pescoço, os ombros, o tronco e todos os membros. O ideal é iniciar a palpação com o cão em pé, posição que facilita a comparação entre os lados esquerdo e direito do corpo. A atrofia muscular de um membro torácico frequentemente torna a espinha da escápula mais proeminente, por conta da atrofia dos músculos supraespinhoso e infraespinhoso. No membro pélvico, a atrofia muscular é mais prontamente detectada devido à atrofia do músculo bíceps femoral. Essa diferença pode ser vista comparando as circunferências de ambas as coxas, utilizando uma fita métrica. Deve-se avaliar a propriocepção consciente dos quatro membros. Se estiver diminuída, deve-se realizar um exame neurológico completo do cão. Em pacientes traumatizados, especialmente aqueles que não conseguem andar, o exame neurológico deve incluir a avalição do tônus anal, o reflexo do panículo, o reflexo de retirada e a sensibilidade à dor profunda.

A palpação do membro é mais bem realizada enquanto o cão está deitado com a pata na direção do examinador. Se o cão for

CAPÍTULO 353 • Anormalidades Esqueléticas em Animais de Companhia

pouco colaborativo ou nervoso, pode ser preferível iniciar o exame com o membro no qual a claudicação se origina. De outra forma, pode ser preferível a coleta de informações sobre os membros não doloridos (presumivelmente) antes da palpação dos membros doloridos. A informação obtida durante a palpação deve ser comparada entre os lados esquerdo e direito do corpo. É melhor realizar a palpação utilizando um método consistente, de modo a evitar omissões e maximizar a eficácia (ver Capítulo 2). A palpação do membro torácico inclui dígitos, ossos metacarpianos, carpo, rádio, ulna, cotovelo, côndilos umerais, tubérculo maior e articulação do ombro. A palpação do membro pélvico inclui dígitos, ossos metatarsianos, tarso, tíbia, joelho, côndilos femorais, trocânter maior e articulação coxofemoral. Ao palpar articulações, devem ser avaliadas a crepitação, a amplitude de movimentação, a efusão (ou edema), a resposta à dor após palpação e a instabilidade. As primeiras letras desses parâmetros formam o acrônimo CREPI (do inglês *crepitus, range of motion, effusion, pain reponse to palpation* e *instability*), as primeiras letras da palavra "crepitação". Esses parâmetros são avaliados simultaneamente: enquanto uma mão move a articulação por toda sua amplitude de movimentação, a outra mão verifica se há crepitação, efusão ou instabilidade, e o examinador observa a resposta à dor. A avaliação da amplitude de movimentação é a parte mais crítica da palpação, porque em muitas situações a inflamação ou fibrose periarticular limita o movimento articular, especialmente em articulações menores mais complexas. *Ao palpar ossos, avaliam-se crepitação (quando há fratura), formato anormal e resposta à dor.* Algumas articulações necessitam exames específicos. Por exemplo, pode-se avaliar o sinal ou manobra de Ortolani na articulação do joelho em cães jovens, sendo reflexo do grau de subluxação da articulação. Outros sinais específicos da articulação coxofemoral incluem o sinal de Barlow e o sinal de Bardens (descritos posteriormente), bem como a palpação do triângulo formado pela tuberosidade sacral, tuberosidade isquiática e trocânter maior. O formato desse triângulo se altera quando o cão apresenta luxação coxofemoral. No joelho, o sinal de gaveta cranial indica instabilidade translacional craniocaudal que ocorre após ruptura do ligamento cruzado cranial. No final da palpação ortopédica, o clínico deve reconhecer quais membros estão acometidos e quais as alterações nas articulações afetadas.

Tomada de decisão quanto ao tratamento de anormalidades ortopédicas

Anormalidades ortopédicas podem ser submetidas a tratamento conservador (*i. e.*, não cirúrgico) ou a tratamento cirúrgico. Sem dúvida, o tratamento cirúrgico é o preferido para estabilização de fraturas, principalmente aquelas que envolvem superfícies articulares e placas de crescimento. Poucas fraturas são tratadas de modo conservador: algumas fraturas pélvicas com deslocamento mínimo ou colapso do canal pélvico, algumas fraturas de ossos longos com deslocamento mínimo, entre outras.[84,170,171] Como tão poucas publicações se referem ao tratamento conservador, a recuperação de fraturas tratadas de forma conservadora em geral não é cientificamente conhecida; em dados de experiências clínicas e poucas publicações, parece que o resultado é ruim. Ao tratar distúrbios ortopédicos, os benefícios da cirurgia geralmente são menos óbvios.[138,172] Vários problemas ortopédicos são submetidos a tratamento conservador, inclusive displasia coxofemoral, displasia do cotovelo, deformidades de membros, luxação de patela e lesões do ligamento cruzado cranial.[173-175]

TRATAMENTO CIRÚRGICO DE ANORMALIDADES ORTOPÉDICAS

Embora a descrição técnica do tratamento cirúrgico dos problemas ortopédicos esteja além do escopo deste capítulo, os princípios do tratamento cirúrgico são relevantes, descritos a seguir.

Diversos procedimentos cirúrgicos são realizados com a intenção de **alterar o crescimento ósseo**. A sinfisiodese púbica juvenil é um procedimento cirúrgico no qual as placas de crescimento púbicas parassagitais são aquecidas (ou mecanicamente removidas) em uma idade jovem, a fim de minimizar o crescimento longitudinal do púbis. A diminuição do comprimento do púbis propicia uma posição mais horizontal do acetábulo e maior tolerância da subluxação coxofemoral.[176,177] A sinfisiodese púbica juvenil geralmente é realizada com 16 semanas de idade, após a mensuração da frouxidão coxofemoral. Essa frouxidão pode ser mensurada objetivamente utilizando o método PennHIP.[178] Em cães com fechamento prematuro da fise ulnar distal, podem ser realizar ostectomias ulnares segmentares para evitar a interferência da ulna no crescimento do rádio.[179] O crescimento ósseo da parte proximal da tíbia pode ser alterado com a intenção de diminuir a inclinação do platô tibial. Essa cirurgia foi proposta aos cães jovens com lesões do ligamento cruzado cranial.[180] Procedimentos cirúrgicos também são realizados para **alterar o formato dos ossos** – por exemplo, para tratar deformidades dos membros. A correção de deformidades pode ser feita mediante correção intraoperatória aguda ou progressiva, baseada na formação do osso dentro de uma fenda de desvio, um procedimento denominado distração osteogênica.[181]

Procedimentos cirúrgicos são realizados para **alterar as posições relativas dos ossos no interior de articulações** e, assim, melhorar a saúde articular. Ostectomias ulnares segmentares são também realizadas com o intuito de melhorar as distribuições de carga na articulação do cotovelo.[182] Procedimentos cirúrgicos são realizados para **aumentar a estabilidade de articulações** e influenciar positivamente a mecânica da articulação. O aumento da estabilidade articular pode ser obtido por meio de artrodese, a fusão dos ossos que se articulam. As artrodeses de articulações distais (particularmente intercarpianas, carpo-metacarpianas intertársicas e tarso-metatársicas) são realizadas mais rotineiramente e propiciam melhor resultado funcional do que artrodeses das articulações proximais.

TRATAMENTO NÃO CIRÚRGICO DAS ANORMALIDADES ORTOPÉDICAS

Vários distúrbios ortopédicos são tratados sem necessidade de cirurgia. Ademais, vários problemas ortopédicos tratados cirurgicamente necessitam de tratamento não cirúrgico, além da cirurgia. O tratamento não cirúrgico de anormalidades ortopédicas inclui avaliação ortopédica, otimização do desenvolvimento musculoesquelético, alívio da dor, controle do peso e otimização das atividades e exercícios. O tratamento não cirúrgico pode incluir objetivos mais específicos, como fortalecimento (em pacientes fracos), alongamento (em pacientes desprovidos de movimentação articular) ou assistência para deambulação (em pacientes com distúrbios de mobilidade). Esses objetivos específicos são frequentemente parte de um programa de reabilitação física (*i. e.*, terapia física, fisioterapia). Embora não seja necessário um ambiente de reabilitação física para tratar problemas ortopédicos (e geralmente não está disponível), o fato de existir uma sobreposição tão grande entre a reabilitação física e o tratamento de problemas ortopédicos a longo prazo torna a reabilitação uma condição muito lógica para desenvolver, implementar e monitorar o tratamento de distúrbios ortopédicos (ver Capítulo 355). Também podem ser utilizadas órteses para tratar problemas ósseos específicos (Figura 353.13). A utilização de órteses é um campo em expansão que potencialmente pode ser parte do tratamento de várias anormalidades ortopédicas. O uso efetivo de órteses se baseia em uma avaliação ortopédica específica, modelo da órtese, fabricação, encaixes, ajustes e treinamento do paciente e do tutor. O uso de órteses é descrito em outra publicação.[183]

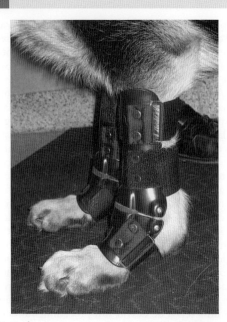

Figura 353.13 Órteses de carpo podem ser utilizadas para limitar ou propiciar a movimentação articular. Essas órteses foram desenvolvidas para limitar a extensão do carpo em um cão da raça Pastor-Alemão jovem palmígrado. As órteses são articuladas para possibilitar a flexão do carpo. A espessura da borracha na parte cranial do carpo pode ser modificada para ajustar o ponto final de extensão do carpo.

Avaliação inicial

Como vários cães com distúrbios ortopédicos manifestam sintomas discretos que frequentemente não são detectados pelos tutores ou são tidos como imperícia ou como marcha ou postura "estranha" ou "engraçada", a avaliação ortopédica deve ser iniciada pelos clínicos, e não pelos tutores. A avaliação ortopédica pode ser feita em qualquer momento da vida, mas é particularmente relevante nos primeiros meses, quando ocorrem doenças ortopédicas do desenvolvimento, e antes que ocorram danos às articulações ou alterações de postura. A articulação coxofemoral, por exemplo, pode ser avaliada pelo uso dos métodos PennHIP ou Orthopedic Foundation for Animals, depois dos 4 meses de idade. A avaliação inicia pelo questionamento do tutor com perguntas específicas relacionadas a postura, marcha e capacidade do animal em realizar atividades diárias. A avaliação deve incluir a observação da posição do filhote em repouso, a mudança na posição do corpo (p. ex., levantar, agachar), de caminhar e de andar em trote. A avaliação deve também incluir o exame ortopédico. Na maioria das situações, esse exame é realizado sem sedação. A palpação de pacientes imaturos do ponto de vista esquelético requer paciência e atitude gentil. Mesmo que os filhotes tenham treinamento limitado e pouca atenção, o clínico deve ser capaz de detectar uma resposta repetida à dor após palpação das principais articulações, particularmente durante flexão e extensão das articulações do cotovelo, extensão do joelho e extensão da articulação coxo femoral.

Por conta da alta prevalência de displasia coxofemoral em várias raças, particularmente de grande porte com tecido subcutâneo espesso e desenvolvimento muscular relativamente modesto (São Bernardo, Bernese Mountain, Mastiff, Welsh Corgis), é comum realizar o exame do quadril. A subluxação coxofemoral é a manifestação precoce da displasia coxofemoral, e as articulações do quadril devem ser avaliadas à procura de subluxação coxofemoral em idade jovem. A subluxação coxofemoral pode ser detectada aproximadamente aos 4 meses de idade (16 semanas) utilizando a palpação com o animal acordado ou sob sedação. Na palpação, geralmente realizada com o paciente em decúbito lateral com a articulação coxofemoral mantida em posição semelhante à posição em estação, pode-se colocar uma mão espalmada nos aspectos proximal e medial da coxa e com pressão abaxial (elevação da coxa em relação à pelve), palpa-se a translação abaxial do fêmur em relação à pelve, sentindo a posição relativa do trocânter maior e da tuberosidade isquiática (Figura 353.14 e Vídeo 353.2). Essa translação é denominada *sinal de Bardens*. Pode-se realizar a palpação da redução da cabeça do fêmur previamente com subluxação no acetábulo devido à abdução do fêmur (Figura 353.15 e Vídeo 353.3). Essa palpação é mais facilmente realizada com o cão em decúbito dorsal, segurando as articulações do quadril em uma posição semelhante à posição em estação, com a articulação do joelho flexionada e lentamente submetida à abdução. O fêmur mantido verticalmente corresponde a um ângulo de 0°. Ângulos positivos correspondem à abdução, enquanto ângulos negativos correspondem à adução que passou a linha média. Também se pode realizar a manobra de Ortolani, com o cão em decúbito lateral, mas, subjetivamente, a pelve é mais móvel, e é mais difícil controlar a direção da pelve ao mensurar os ângulos de redução e subluxação. Se ocorrer inicialmente a subluxação da articulação coxofemoral, pode-se sentir ou ouvir um ruído de estalo, denominado *sinal de Ortolani*, à medida que a cabeça do fêmur se realoca em direção ao acetábulo. O ângulo no qual o sinal de Ortolani ocorre é um reflexo do desgaste potencial do rim acetabular dorsal: ângulos maiores correspondem a desgastes mais graves. A *sensação* de Ortolani também importa: um sinal de Ortolani sutil e nítido sugere que o rim acetabular dorsal está normal ou próximo do normal, mas um sinal de Ortolani sutil ou com crepitação indica perda significativa da cartilagem articular e dano ao rim acetabular dorsal e à cabeça do fêmur. Quando o fêmur é lentamente aduzido em direção à posição em estação, percebe-se discreta translação, à medida que a cabeça do fêmur novamente sofre subluxação. Essa subluxação é conhecida como "sinal de Barlow". Assim como para os ângulos de redução, os ângulos de subluxação maiores indicam dano mais grave ao rim acetabular dorsal. A diferença entre os ângulos de redução e subluxação frequentemente varia entre 20 e 40°. Cães com frouxidão de articulação coxofemoral sem danos ao rim acetabular dorsal geralmente possuem ângulos de redução de 10 a 20° e ângulos de subluxação de aproximadamente −10 a −20°. Cães com dano grave ao rim dorsal geralmente possuem ângulos de redução ao redor de 45° e ângulos de subluxação ao redor de 20°. Subjetivamente, parece que maiores ângulos de redução e subluxação resultam de desgaste do rim dorsal, e não de pura frouxidão da articulação. Cães com pequenos ângulos de redução e ângulos de subluxação negativos podem ser capazes de manter a articulação coxofemoral reduzida ou reduzir intermitentemente essa articulação durante a locomoção mediante abdução discreta do fêmur, assim como os cães com luxação de patela podem relocar sua patela pela extensão da articulação do joelho, perceptível durante caminhada ou trote. Com o passar do tempo, a maioria dos cães com subluxação coxofemoral desenvolve desgaste do rim dorsal, e o sinal de Ortolani positivo desaparece por conta da subluxação permanente dorsal da articulação coxofemoral. A frequência e a idade na qual o sinal de Ortolani desaparece em cães com displasia ainda não foram cientificamente avaliadas, até nosso conhecimento. Clinicamente, a maioria dos sinais de Ortolani desaparece até aos 18 meses de idade. A maioria dos cães com sinais de Ortolani positivos desenvolve displasia coxofemoral nos primeiros anos de vida da fase adulta.

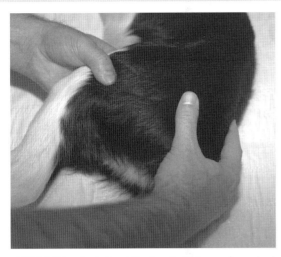

Figura 353.14 Palpação de frouxidão da articulação coxofemoral colocando uma mão na parte medial da coxa com os dedos posicionados ao longo do eixo do fêmur, estabilizando o fêmur com o polegar e lateralizando o fêmur em relação à pelve, enquanto o outro polegar detecta a translação do trocânter maior em relação à tuberosidade isquiática. Essa manobra é conhecida como *sinal de Bardens*. A manobra de Bardens causa desconforto, de forma que é realizada sob sedação.

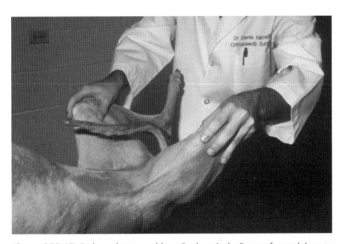

Figura 353.15 Pode-se detectar subluxação da articulação coxofemoral durante a palpação. Com o cão mantido em decúbito dorsal, faz-se a abdução de um membro pélvico. A abdução aumenta a cobertura dorsal da cabeça do fêmur e pode propiciar a redução de uma articulação com subluxação. A redução da articulação coxofemoral resultante da abdução é denominada *sinal de Ortolani*. O ângulo de redução pode ser mensurado.

A avaliação radiográfica de articulações em cães jovens com frequência não é recompensadora, particularmente se o clínico basear o diagnóstico de uma doença articular do desenvolvimento apenas na presença de osteófitos, pois pode demorar semanas, meses ou anos para ter osteófitos detectáveis na articulação. Projeções radiográficas especializadas são utilizadas para detecção precoce da doença articular. Elas incluem o método PennHIP, bem estabelecido para a avaliação de subluxação coxofemoral e realizado sob sedação. Embora haja métodos de avaliação radiográfica, o método PennHIP é o mais acurado para avaliar a presença de frouxidão da articulação coxofemoral. Consiste em uma projeção em distração que quantifica o grau de deslocamento abaxial da cabeça do fêmur em relação ao acetábulo durante uma manobra que lembra o sinal de Barden. Obtém-se distração confiável da articulação coxofemoral utilizando tubos de acrílico ajustáveis recobertos com espuma. O índice de distração (ID) é a distância que separa os centros do acetábulo e da cabeça do fêmur durante a distração, dividida pelo raio da cabeça do fêmur. É muito improvável que os cães com baixo ID (menos de 0,30) desenvolvam displasia coxofemoral. Cães com ID maior (acima de 0,70) muito provavelmente desenvolvem displasia coxofemoral. Algumas raças de cães são mais tolerantes à frouxidão do que outras. Por exemplo, em um estudo envolvendo 3.729 cães da raça Pastor-Alemão e 6.278 cães da raça Labrador Retriever com mais de 24 meses, a probabilidade de ocorrer osteoartrite (OA) da articulação coxofemoral em cães com índice de distração de 0,6 foi de aproximadamente 58% para Pastor-Alemão, comparado a aproximadamente 16% para cães Labrador Retriever. Isso demonstra que a frouxidão articular não é o único fator que causa artrite na articulação coxofemoral e sugere que diferenças na anatomia e na mecânica da articulação são importantes na ocorrência de displasia nessa articulação.[184] Em um relato que avaliou 459 cães clinicamente normais, a palpação mostrou, na melhor das hipóteses, correlação moderada com as mensurações radiográficas de frouxidão articular, indicando a necessidade de combinar a palpação com o exame radiográfico por estresse ao avaliar cães com suspeita de frouxidão articular.[185] Uma projeção oblíqua denominada projeção oblíqua distomedial-proximolateral demonstrou melhorar a detecção do processo coronoide medial fragmentado na articulação do cotovelo de cães.[56]

Otimização do desenvolvimento musculoesquelético

A otimização do desenvolvimento musculoesquelético é um aspecto crítico do tratamento de anormalidades ortopédicas, porque várias delas interferem no crescimento dos pacientes e a expressão de genes anômalos é maior quando o crescimento é acelerado. Em cães, a aceleração do crescimento se deve à excessiva ingestão calórica (consumo exagerado de carboidratos) ou à suplementação com cálcio (ver Capítulo 189).

Cães que se alimentam à vontade crescem muito rapidamente. Uma restrição modesta do consumo alimentar em 25% comparada ao fornecimento à vontade (*ad libitum*) retarda sobremaneira o crescimento. Por exemplo, em cães machos da raça Dogue Alemão em crescimento, uma restrição de 25% ocasiona um peso médio de 26 kg aos 6 meses, comparado à média de 52 kg de cães alimentados à vontade com a mesma idade.[22] Cães com restrição de ingestão alimentar atingem o mesmo tamanho adulto daqueles alimentados à vontade, mas apresentam menos problemas ortopédicos. Tutores devem ser instruídos a restringir a ingestão alimentar de cães em crescimento, particularmente de raças grandes e predispostas a doenças ortopédicas do desenvolvimento. O conteúdo proteico da dieta não influencia a taxa de crescimento; portanto, cães em crescimento devem consumir dieta com teor apropriadamente alto de proteínas. Cães em fase de crescimento não devem receber cálcio suplementar, além do cálcio incluído na ração balanceada.

Controle da dor

A dor é frequentemente a consequência principal das anormalidades ortopédicas e, portanto, sua minimização é o aspecto primordial do controle conservador dos distúrbios ortopédicos, alcançada pela otimização das condições de vida dos pacientes, adequando-o às atividades, encorajando a perda de peso (ver Capítulo 176) e administrando analgésicos (ver Capítulos 126, 164 e 166) e suplementação alimentar.

Embora pouco se saiba sobre a influência das condições de vida nos sinais clínicos de anormalidades ortopédicas em cães, parece lógico adaptar as condições dos cães, de modo a minimizar os desafios associados à vida domiciliar e propiciar exercícios regulares. Foi relatado que alterações na temperatura (onda de frio), na umidade ambiente e na pressão barométrica (diminuição da pressão) influenciam a dor em articulações com artrite em humanos. Para minimizar a influência potencial das condições climáticas em cães com artrite, pode ser benéfico mantê-los dentro de casa, em ambiente controlado. A redução do risco de escorregões e quedas pode igualmente beneficiá-los, propiciando melhor superfície de caminhada que pode melhorar a tração e evitando atividades que necessitem de alterações súbitas de direção ou velocidade.

Em pessoas, os sintomas de doença articular (p. ex., osteoartrite) se alteram com o passar do tempo. Há períodos de relativo conforto e de exacerbação súbita dos sintomas, denominados surtos. Com o passar do tempo, os surtos se tornam mais frequentes, mais graves, mais longos e com controle mais difícil. De forma semelhante, os surtos podem resultar de atividade excessiva de cães com doença articular com baixa condição física ("*weekend warrior syndrome*") ou de eventos que causam estresse excessivo em articulações anormais, como pular ou pisar em buracos. Os surtos podem durar algumas horas ou várias semanas. A determinação se uma articulação anormal está ou não em surto é uma parte importante da avaliação inicial, porque os métodos terapêuticos e os objetivos de manejo são diferentes. Os surtos são prováveis em cães cujos sinais clínicos estão significativamente mais graves do que estavam em semanas anteriores. Pacientes com doença articular estão frequentemente no meio de um surto no momento da primeira avaliação, pois os tutores buscam cuidados veterinários devido ao aumento súbito dos sinais clínicos. A perda repentina do desempenho (incapacidade de subir degraus ou em um veículo, intolerância ao exercício) geralmente se deve a um surto, mas pode ser resultado de perda progressiva de força e de físico secundária à OA, combinada com envelhecimento, ou pode ser decorrência de alteração na condição de uma articulação com artrite (p. ex., uma articulação coxofemoral com subluxação se torna com luxação). Decisões irreversíveis, como cirurgia ou eutanásia, não devem ser tomadas durante surtos, porque os pacientes podem parecer excessivamente acometidos e ter uma perda dramática da mobilidade ou da independência, condição que melhora após o surto. Em vez disso, o foco deve ser no amplo controle da dor e em repouso. Entre os surtos, os tutores devem evitar atividades extenuantes que desencadeiam os surtos e, em consequência, o agravamento dos sinais clínicos. As atividades extenuantes incluem pular, perseguir, buscar algo e brincar com outros cães. Infelizmente, os tutores em geral preferem essas atividades, porque os cães gostam muito, são fáceis de realizar e requerem mínima participação do tutor.

Em cães com anormalidades ortopédicas graves, pode-se auxiliar a deambulação com o uso de tala ou tipoia de apoio. As tipoias de neoprene com faixa fixadora de velcro são populares, porque são ergonômicas, relativamente macias, duráveis e laváveis. Para cães grandes, pesados ou independentes com dificuldade de locomoção, um carrinho de deambulação pode propiciar auxílio efetivo à deambulação. Na maioria das situações, quando a dor e a fraqueza se limitam à região pélvica, utiliza-se um carrinho de duas rodas. Quando os cães apresentam problemas nos quatro membros, pode-se utilizar um carrinho de quatro rodas (quadriciclo). O carrinho sustenta a região pélvica durante a atividade externa. Carrinhos são muito mais convenientes para cães pequenos do que para os grandes. Alguns cães aprendem a passar por portinholas e podem utilizar o carrinho dentro de casa, enquanto outros não. Subjetivamente, as tipoias de neoprene podem funcionar melhor do que um aparato rígido (anéis de metal recobertos por espuma) em carrinhos de pacientes com problemas ortopédicos, pois eles apresentam função motora normal durante a atividade, comparativamente aos cães com paralisia, que podem se dar melhor ao utilizar carrinhos com plataformas rígidas.

Sem o alívio apropriado da dor, a manutenção da mobilidade articular ou a recuperação da força perdida raramente é alcançada. O alívio da dor é obtido pela interferência com os mecanismos periféricos (inflamação e dano tecidual) e centrais (neuropáticos, que envolvem o sistema nervoso central) da dor. Anti-inflamatórios não esteroides (AINE) consistem na base do controle farmacológico da dor musculoesquelética periférica (ver Capítulos 126, 164 e 166).[186] A administração de AINE aos cães com doença articular pode ocasionar melhora dramática do uso do membro e da função geral. Diversos relatos científicos, frequentemente utilizados como estudos de suporte para a aprovação de um fármaco, demonstraram que a administração de AINE ocasiona aumento no pico de força vertical e impulso vertical nos membros pélvicos de cães com arritmia.[186] Não há estudos revisados por pares que comparam AINE disponíveis no mercado, utilizando delineamentos cegos, prospectivos, randomizados e cruzados. Além disso, a ocorrência relativa e a gravidade dos efeitos colaterais após a administração de diversos AINE em cães ainda não foram cientificamente avaliadas. Todos os AINE induzem efeitos colaterais infrequentes, mas potencialmente graves (ver Capítulo 169) e devem ser utilizados com precaução, particularmente em pacientes com comprometimento da função hepática ou renal, com hipovolemia e com doença gastrintestinal. Isso é particularmente relevante, já que vários cães com artrite manifestam agravamento dos sinais clínicos posteriormente, quando é mais provável a ocorrência de problemas hepáticos, renais e gastrintestinais. Em cães que recebem AINE, recomenda-se a avaliação periódica da função hepática, inclusive a avaliação de enzimas. Embora não haja consenso sobre a frequência dessas avaliações, parece razoável realizá-las antes da administração de AINE, algumas semanas após a administração e quando ocorrem sinais clínicos de seus efeitos colaterais. O risco de efeitos colaterais dos AINE não parece aumentar quando são administrados por longo tempo.[187]

Como acontece em todas as formas de dor crônica, no caso de displasia coxofemoral crônica ocorre sensibilização periférica e maior sensibilização da medula espinal (ver Capítulo 356). Para controle de dor crônica, tem-se recomendado tratamento medicamentoso e não medicamentoso multimodais. Isso inclui o uso "extralabel" (ou seja, não indicado na bula) de medicamentos analgésicos que são adjuvantes ou alternativos aos AINE. Os medicamentos adjuvantes podem ser indicados para cães intolerantes a AINE ou cujos sinais clínicos apenas melhoram parcialmente durante o tratamento com AINE. As informações científicas que sustentam o uso desses medicamentos alternativos são escassas, mas pesquisas clínicas nessa área estão ativas. O tramadol, um análogo sintético da morfina, aparentemente é o fármaco adjuvante mais utilizado para dor coxofemoral crônica. Outros medicamentos emergentes utilizados no controle farmacológico multimodal de OA incluem o medicamento análogo ao ácido gama-aminobutírico, a gabapentina, e o fármaco antiviral amantadina.[188] Subjetivamente, os cães com surtos de artrite graves podem ser beneficiados pela infusão intravenosa contínua de uma combinação de agonista alfa2-adrenérgico (medetomidina), de um bloqueador de canais de sódio (lidocaína) e de um antagonista de receptor N-metil-D-aspartato (cetamina). Em um estudo prospectivo, verificou-se que injeções de glicosaminoglicanos polissulfatados 2 vezes/semana, entre 6 semanas e 8 meses de idade, propiciaram menor taxa de subluxação e indicaram tendência de menor dano à cartilagem em filhotes predispostos à displasia coxofemoral.[189]

Em humanos, a suplementação nutricional foi por muito tempo utilizada para diminuir potencialmente a dor causada por artrite, com mais frequência pelo uso de ervas e vegetais manipulados, como acontece na medicina tradicional chinesa e medicina ayurvédica indígena. Em estudos randomizados prospectivos em humanos com OA, mais de 30 ervas ou compostos mostraram algum grau de analgesia. Na medicina ocidental, a atenção focou principalmente no uso de glucosamina, sulfato de condroitina e ácidos graxos poli-insaturados (ômega-3) para o controle de dor articular causada por artrite, com diversos estudos bem estruturados documentando seus benefícios. Já em cães com artrite, pouco se sabe sobre os benefícios dos suplementos nutricionais. Entretanto, diversos estudos clínicos documentaram os benefícios de uma dieta contendo glucosamina, condroitina e ácido eicosapentaenoico (EPA), um ácido graxo ômega-3, em cães com sintomas de displasia coxofemoral. Vários relatos documentaram os efeitos anti-inflamatórios ou anticatabólicos dos ácidos graxos ômega-3, glucosamina, ou condroitina em condrócitos de humanos e de cães, in vitro. O aumento do consumo dietético de EPA demonstrou diminuir a dor osteoartrítica, provavelmente por diminuir a concentração de ácido araquidônico e aumentar a concentração de EPA nas membranas celulares dos condrócitos de cães. Suplementos à base de mexilhão verde também parecem aliviar os sintomas de osteoartrite em cães.[190] O conhecimento atual sugere que os protocolos nutricionais e o tratamento medicamentoso mais razoáveis para cães com artrite seria mantê-los livres de sintomas pelo uso de AINE, ácidos graxos ômega-3, glucosamina e sulfato de condroitina e pela adição potencial de fármacos adjuvantes, se necessário, com base nos sinais clínicos, ou como alternativa aos AINE, caso surjam sintomas de intolerância.

Há diversas opções medicamentosas que não seja o uso de anti-inflamatórios para o controle da dor periférica, inclusive massagem e terapia pelo frio, também conhecida como crioterapia, que propicia alívio direto da dor por diminuir a velocidade da condução nervosa e alívio secundário por reduzir o edema (por si só uma fonte de dor) e diminuir a hiperatividade de enzimas catabólicas na cartilagem osteoartrítica por algumas poucas horas após sua aplicação. Deve-se considerar o uso de crioterapia em animais com episódio de osteoartrite ou após um período de exercício ou antes de dormir. Cubos de gelo ou vegetais congelados não são recomendados, porque possuem bolsões de ar que diminuem a condução do frio. Sacos de gelo preenchidos com pedaços de gelo ou com gelo esmagado ou bolsas frias são mais efetivos na indução de frio. A maioria das bolsas de gelo atinge temperatura terapêutica depois de duas horas mantidas em freezer. Para pacientes com pelo longo, uma possibilidade é a colocação e manutenção de uma bolsa de gelo diretamente na articulação com artrite, prendendo com uma faixa autoadesiva. Algumas bolsas de gelo já possuem uma faixa autoadesiva. Uma fita de neoprene pode também ser utilizada para fixar a bolsa ou o saco de gelo. Em pacientes com pelo curto ou alopécicos, pode-se colocar uma fronha de travesseiro entre a bolsa e a pele. A aplicação de crioterapia pode durar 10 a 15 minutos. A maioria dos pacientes tolera o tratamento. A pessoa que aplica a crioterapia deve ter certeza de que o paciente não está desconfortável e que a superfície da pele se apresenta fria ao toque após a conclusão do procedimento.

Os efeitos a curto e longo prazo da massagem em animais de companhia não são conhecidos. A massagem pode diminuir a dor miofascial e a tensão muscular. As opções não farmacológicas de controle da dor de origem central incluem aquecimento em baixo nível, massagem e, possivelmente, acupuntura, acupressão e eletroacupuntura. Esses métodos primariamente estimulam fibras sensoriais A-beta, que apresentam velocidade de condução mais rápida (30 a 70 m/s) do que as fibras A-delta (12 a 30 m/s) e fibras C (0,5 a 3 m/s). O calor é amplamente considerado como um fator benéfico aos pacientes com osteoartrite dolorosa. O uso do calor é duplo. O calor em baixo nível (elevação da temperatura tecidual em 1 a 2°C) alivia a dor mediante a estimulação de fibras sensoriais A-beta não nociceptivas, bem como por causar vasodilatação e normalização do fluxo sanguíneo. O relaxamento tecidual pode ser obtido mantendo o paciente com osteoartrite em temperatura relativamente quente e umidade ambiente baixa durante todo o dia (dormir em ambientes internos aquecidos ou fornecer camas aquecidas). O calor mais intenso (elevação da temperatura tecidual em 3 a 4°C) é utilizado para aumentar a efetividade do alongamento ao minimizar o dano tecidual. O calor intenso é mais frequentemente aplicado por um profissional da saúde utilizando uma bolsa quente, que é aquecida por uma almofada térmica ou forno micro-ondas. Quatro camadas de toalhas secas geralmente são colocadas entre uma bolsa quente e a pele, e o calor é aplicado durante 15 a 20 minutos. É preciso ter cuidado ao colocar uma bolsa quente sobre um cão, pois pode ocorrer queimadura. De início, as bolsas podem não parecer excessivamente quentes ao toque, mas elas podem induzir dano térmico após vários minutos de contato. Portanto, é importante verificar se há hiperemia excessiva, edema cutâneo ou formação de bolhas, em intervalos de poucos minutos, durante a terapia com calor intenso.

Manutenção da condição física e da força do membro

Os benefícios vitalícios de ter um menor peso corporal para osteoartrite e longevidade foram claramente documentados em um estudo com cães da raça Labrador Retriever, que foram acompanhados durante toda a vida.[50] Nesse estudo, comparativamente aos seus parceiros com sobrepeso, os cães mais leves viveram 1,8 ano a mais. Entretanto, em ambos os grupos, a falta de mobilidade no final da vida devido à OA foi a principal causa de eutanásia.[191] Esse estudo provou que a OA teve uma progressão mais lenta e foi mais facilmente controlada em cães de menor peso. Pacientes adultos com anormalidades musculoesqueléticas rotineiramente apresentam excesso de peso corporal, que interfere clara e negativamente no paciente com problemas ósseos, diferentemente do que acontece quando há perda do excesso de peso.[192,193] Em um estudo, notou-se diminuição subjetiva na claudicação detectada, utilizando uma escala de classificação numérica, quando a perda de peso foi maior que 6,1%; ademais, verificou-se diminuição objetiva na claudicação detectada mediante o uso de uma placa de força, quando a perda de peso foi maior que 8,5%.[194] Aos cães com sobrepeso, recomenda-se taxa de perda de peso semanal de 1 a 2% do peso corporal. Essa perda pode ser obtida pelo fornecimento de uma quantidade próxima a 60% das calorias necessárias para manter o peso corporal. A perda de peso em cães com osteoartrite não parece estar associada a um aumento de atividade física espontânea.[195]

Foi demonstrado que a força muscular diminui em pessoas com OA e que a perda de força é tanto quantitativa (devido à perda de massa muscular) quanto qualitativa (devido à perda do desempenho muscular), potencialmente como resultado de desuso do membro e inibição do reflexo de contração dos músculos adjacentes às articulações com artrite. A perda de massa muscular é comumente observada em cães com enfermidade óssea crônica. Entretanto, a extensão da perda de força não foi avaliada em cães com diversos distúrbios esqueléticos crônicos e poucas pesquisas focaram em estratégias específicas para proteger contra a perda ou recuperação de força. Com poucas exceções, a manutenção da força muscular é obtida com a prática ativa de atividade física. Essas exceções incluem estimulação elétrica neuromuscular e amplitude ativa mediante fisioterapia. A estimulação elétrica neuromuscular pode ser realizada em cães com artrite e com grave perda de força muscular, nos quais não é possível uma atividade física efetiva por conta da dor ou desuso grave do membro. Como regra geral, é mais simples e efetivo utilizar exercícios terapêuticos do que estratégias para fortalecer os pacientes (Tabela 353.1).

| Tabela 353.1 | Atividades físicas potencialmente terapêuticas incluídas no controle de displasia coxofemoral em cães. |

FINALIDADES	ATIVIDADES FÍSICAS TERAPÊUTICAS
Aumentar a força do membro	Caminhada ou trote diário por mais de 10 min; repetições dentro de túnel; repetições de sentar e levantar
Aumentar a força central	Caminhada ou trote diário por mais de 10 min; natação
Melhorar a função cardiovascular	Caminhada ou trote diário por mais de 10 min
Alongar os membros pélvicos	Subir rampas, colinas e escadas; pulos de baixa altura
Melhorar a propriocepção	Caminhada ou trote diário por mais de 10 min; caminhar em superfícies macias: areia, palha, folhas, grama; gangorra; zigue-zague.

A condição física cardiovascular e a resistência muscular foram pouco descritas em cães. Como as anormalidades ósseas crônicas provavelmente têm influência negativa na mobilidade, na resistência muscular e na condição física cardiovascular, faz sentido promover atividades físicas aeróbicas regulares aos cães com anormalidades esqueléticas (ver Capítulo 359).

O aumento da resistência muscular requer movimentos repetidos durante vários minutos. É improvável que a obtenção dessa resistência seja alcançada mediante prática de atividades autônomas em áreas com espaço limitado, como manter o cão sem acompanhamento em um quintal de tamanho médio cercado. Em vez disso, os cães devem ser exercitados regularmente, com um propósito. Em humanos, as enfermidades ósseas e o envelhecimento contribuem para perda da propriocepção. Pouco se sabe sobre o impacto negativo da osteoartrite de ocorrência natural na propriocepção de cães. Entretanto, há evidências claras de que a osteoartrite progride rapidamente em pacientes com lesões articulares que apresentam déficits sensoriais. Em pessoas idosas com diminuição da propriocepção, os exercícios de equilíbrio prontamente melhoram a propriocepção. Em cães com osteoartrite, uma etapa do programa de atividades físicas deve focar em exercícios que estimulam a propriocepção, como aqueles que necessitam de desvios de peso corporal de um lado para outro, rápidos e imprevisíveis, e, em menor extensão, desvios de peso da frente para trás e vice-versa. Esses exercícios incluem caminhada sobre superfícies macias ou irregulares e exercícios suaves de agilidade, incluindo caminhada em zigue-zague e em uma gangorra, caminhada simples ou sobre traves (ver Capítulo 355).

Pouco se sabe sobre o impacto da artrite de articulação coxofemoral na movimentação da articulação. Como mencionado anteriormente, a articulação coxofemoral com displasia aparentemente perdem a extensão, mas não a flexão. Uma perda de extensão de 30° ou mais provavelmente leva o cão à incapacidade de galopar, trotar, pular ou subir degraus. Portanto, parece benéfico avaliar a movimentação articular em cães com displasia coxofemoral crônica. Já que é muito mais fácil manter a movimentação articular do que recuperá-la após sua perda, parece razoável recomendar atividades físicas intermitentes que aumentam a extensão da articulação coxofemoral sem ocasionar sintomas relevantes. Essas atividades podem incluir caminhadas ladeira acima ou dançar para trás. Se a recuperação da movimentação articular é considerada importante, pode-se implementar um programa de alongamento. O alongamento é mais efetivo quando os tecidos são aquecidos imediatamente antes e durante a sessão de alongamento. Empiricamente e baseado em técnicas utilizadas em humanos, pode-se considerar a realização de 10 a 20 alongamentos, mantidos por 20 a 40 segundos, em cada sessão. As sessões podem ser realizadas 2 a 3 vezes/dia. Com a perda crônica da movimentação, é previsto um ganho de 3 a 5° de movimentação articular por semana como resultado de um protocolo de alongamento sustentado.

Cães portadores de enfermidades ósseas e com problemas discretos de locomoção são submetidos a um programa de manejo focado no alívio da dor, na manutenção da força do membro e de origem central, no alongamento das articulações acometidas e no estímulo da propriocepção. O controle da dor geralmente é obtido com simples etapas de procedimentos farmacológicos, repouso e atividades físicas. Os métodos farmacológicos e outros de alívio da dor podem ser intermitentes, contanto que os cães colaborem na prática de um programa de exercícios a longo prazo. Para cães com anormalidades ósseas e problemas de locomoção importantes, é criticamente importante implementar diversas estratégias de suporte para diminuir o impacto da doença no bem-estar e na mobilidade desses animais. Essas estratégias podem incluir repouso, controle farmacológico multimodal, crioterapia, uso de calor, massagem, acupuntura, acupressão, eletroacupuntura ou estimulação nervosa elétrica transcutânea. Assim que é obtido o controle da dor, é importante iniciar um programa de exercícios progressivos. Pacientes com osteoartrite grave podem necessitar auxílio temporário ou permanente para caminhar. Tipoias são os aparatos de auxílio para caminhar mais utilizados e com melhor custo-benefício. Cães com anormalidades graves podem ser beneficiados pelo uso de um carrinho. De forma geral, um programa de controle para animais de companhia com osteoartrite deve ser simples e racional: o controle da dor é a principal prioridade. O programa deve então abordar os aspectos mais críticos de cada situação particular de cada paciente e, com o passar do tempo, melhorar a mobilidade, a força, a propriocepção e, acima de tudo, a qualidade de vida.

REFERÊNCIAS BIBLIOGRÁFICAS

As referências bibliográficas deste capítulo se encontram online no Ambiente de Aprendizagem.

CAPÍTULO 354

Doenças Musculares

G. Diane Shelton

CONSIDERAÇÕES CLÍNICAS GERAIS

O diagnóstico de doenças musculares (miopatias) pode ser um desafio, pois há diversas doenças diferentes (Figura 354.1) que compartilham relativamente poucos sinais clínicos. O reconhecimento do fenótipo miopático é o primeiro passo importante (ver Capítulos 2, 31 a 35 e 259). Os sinais clínicos de doença muscular incluem graus variados de fraqueza muscular, rigidez, mialgia e atrofia ou hipertrofia muscular. Os sintomas podem envolver apenas os músculos dos membros ou podem afetar grupos musculares especiais, como os músculos da laringe e da faringe, os músculos mastigatórios, a língua e o coração. A raça, idade de início e progressão clínica da doença devem auxiliar nos diagnósticos diferenciais.

Os exames laboratoriais de rotina, hemograma, perfil bioquímico sérico e exame de urina, podem detectar algumas das anormalidades sistêmicas que mais comumente causam fraqueza muscular e mialgia (ver Capítulos 12 e 21).[1] A atividade da enzima creatinoquinase ou creatinoquinase (CK) (ver Capítulo 66) e a avaliação da função de tireoide (ver Capítulo 299) devem ser incluídas em todas as bases de dados mínimas para a avaliação da função neuromuscular. Mesmo se apenas discretamente elevada, a constatação de atividade de CH persistentemente elevada pode ser uma indicação para investigação de doença muscular. Em pessoas, no momento do diagnóstico inicial de hipotireoidismo, até 80% relatam problemas atribuídos à disfunção do músculo esquelético, e quase 40% apresentam evidências clínicas de fraqueza muscular.[2] De forma semelhante, rigidez muscular e mialgia podem ser indicadores precoces de hipotireoidismo em cães sem sinais clínicos clássicos óbvios. A detecção de miopatia hipotireoidiana pode evitar gastos com testes diagnósticos desnecessários, se confirmada em exames diagnósticos de rotina.

Como a miastenia gravis autoimune (ver Capítulo 269) pode mimetizar qualquer doença neuromuscular, deve-se incluir a mensuração de anticorpos antirreceptores de acetilcolina (AChR) na base de dados mínima para cães ou gatos com sinais clínicos adquiridos de fraqueza e, em particular, em cães com megaesôfago adquirido. O teste de anticorpos contra AChR permanece como o padrão-ouro para o diagnóstico de miastenia gravis adquirida e confirma uma resposta autoimune contra AChR nicotínicos.[1,3]

O único teste mais importante para o diagnóstico de doença muscular é a biopsia muscular (ver Capítulo 116). Esse procedimento é minimamente invasivo e não requer amplo treinamento cirúrgico. As biopsias musculares devem ser avaliadas em cortes congelados por um laboratório com experiência no exame de amostras de músculo. A menos que a miopatia tenha natureza inflamatória ou neoplásica, os cortes histológicos de amostra obtida por biopsia fixada em formalina e parafina têm valor diagnóstico limitado; ademais, várias miopatias não são diagnosticadas. Amostras de músculo fixadas são úteis para a avaliação ultraestrutural de miopatias congênitas, após diagnóstico presuntivo em cortes histológicos de amostras de biopsia congeladas. Em razão do surgimento de testes genéticos para doenças musculares hereditárias e o desenvolvimento de novos testes com base na análise do DNA, um diagnóstico acurado é fundamental.

As pesquisas na área de doença muscular estão em rápida expansão, tanto na medicina humana quanto na veterinária.[4] Esse tópico não pode ser totalmente abordado no espaço limitado dedicado a este capítulo. Assim, os distúrbios clínicos mais comuns serão abordados com referências citadas às miopatias menos frequentemente observadas.

MIOPATIAS INFLAMATÓRIAS

Miosite dos músculos mastigatórios

A miosite dos músculos mastigatórios (MMM) é uma doença muscular focal, autoimune, relativamente comum, que acomete principalmente cães[5] e raramente gatos. Todas as raças, em qualquer idade, podem ser afetadas. Uma forma particularmente grave de MMM acomete filhotes com 2 a 3 meses de idade, principalmente da raça Cavalier King Charles Spaniel.[6] Os sinais clínicos se limitam aos músculos mastigatórios e podem variar desde um início agudo de edema desses músculos, com restrição da mobilidade mandibular e dor na mandíbula, até atrofia lentamente progressiva dos músculos mastigatórios, com ou sem dor mandibular ou restrição da mobilidade da mandíbula. Deve-se excluir a possibilidade de abscesso retrobulbar e doença da articulação temporomandibular (ver Capítulo 272). O teste sérico para detecção de autoanticorpos contra fibras de músculos mastigatórios do tipo 2 M é útil para o diagnóstico de MMM.[5,7-9] Para resultados mais acurados, a amostra de soro deve ser coletada antes da administração de corticosteroides. A biopsia do músculo temporal também é útil para o diagnóstico e prognóstico de MMM (ver Capítulo 116). É importante não realizar biopsia do músculo frontal que recobre o músculo temporal, pois a amostra dele obtida indicará resultado falso negativo.[5]

A resposta ao tratamento deve ser boa, desde que a MMM seja tratada de modo precoce e apropriado.[5] Devem ser utilizadas doses imunossupressoras de corticosteroides até que a mobilidade da mandíbula retorne ao normal e não haja sinal evidente de dor mandibular. A dose deve ser gradualmente diminuída até se obter a menor dose efetiva, em dias alternados, a qual mantém o cão livre dos sintomas. A terapia com baixa dose deve ser mantida durante 6 a 8 meses, acompanhada por monitoramento

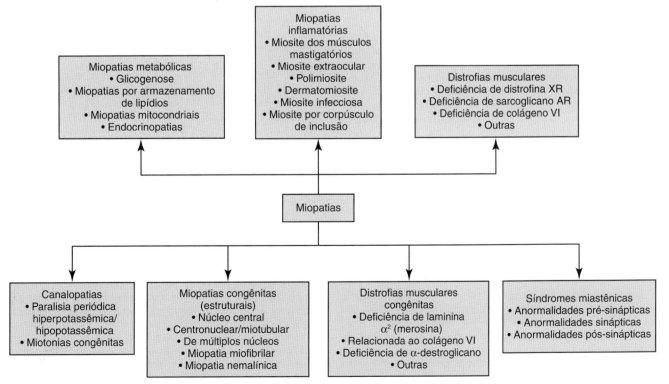

Figura 354.1 O diagrama mostra o amplo espectro clínico das miopatias.

da mobilidade mandibular. Se o tratamento for interrompido muito precocemente, é comum a ocorrência de recidiva. Para MMM grave ou em estágio terminal, a resposta ao tratamento pode ser apenas parcial. Nesse caso, a biopsia muscular é particularmente útil.

Miosite do músculo extraocular

A miosite do músculo extraocular (MEO) é uma miopatia inflamatória focal que acomete seletivamente os músculos extraoculares, poupando os músculos mastigatórios e dos membros. A manifestação clínica consiste em exoftalmia aguda; no estágio crônico, podem ocorrer endoftalmia e estrabismo restritivo.[10,11] A atividade sérica de CK em geral está normal. O título de anticorpos séricos contra 2 M é negativo. O diagnóstico de MEO é mais confiavelmente confirmado por meio de exame ultrassonográfico ou de imagem da órbita, como tomografia computadorizada (TC) ou ressonância magnética (RM). A resposta à corticoideterapia é em geral boa no estágio agudo, e o tratamento é semelhante ao mencionado para MMM (ver anteriormente).

Polimiosite imunomediada

A polimiosite (PM) imunomediada é uma miopatia inflamatória generalizada na qual há invasão de vários grupos de músculos esqueléticos por infiltrados mistos de células mononucleares não supurativos.[12,13] A manifestação clínica pode variar de acordo com os grupos musculares afetados; pode incluir fraqueza generalizada (ver Capítulo 21) com marcha rígida e hipermétrica, megaesôfago (ver Capítulo 273), disfagia (ver Capítulo 38), miocardite (ver Capítulos 252 e 253) e glossite.[14-18] Embora a PM possa ocorrer em todas as raças, foram detectadas predisposições genéticas em cães das raças Terranova[14] e Vizsla.[19,20] A PM também pode ocorrer como parte de uma síndrome poliartrite/PM[21] ou como uma doença paraneoplásica (ver Capítulo 352).[22] A PM é incomum em gatos e pode estar associada a timoma, miastenia gravis, linfoma ou neurite concomitantes.[23]

Na PM, a atividade sérica da CK pode ser variável, com elevações discretas a moderadas (2.000 a 20.000 UI/ℓ), dependendo da gravidade do dano à miofibra.[1] Uma atividade de CK normal ou minimamente elevada não deve excluir a possibilidade de PM, assim como uma atividade de CK acentuadamente elevada não deve confirmar o diagnóstico de PM. Atividades de CK acentuadamente elevadas (> 20.000 UI/ℓ) em geral são observadas nas miopatias necrosantes[24,25] e nas distrofias musculares.[26-28] O exame de amostra muscular obtida por biopsia é a forma mais direta de distinguir miopatias inflamatórias, necrosantes ou distróficas (Figura 354.2). A constatação de anticorpos contra proteínas do sarcolema não identificadas é útil no diagnóstico de PM em cães das raças Boxer e Terranova.[29] Causas infecciosas de miosite (ver adiante) devem ser excluídas antes do início do tratamento com corticosteroide ou com outro imunossupressor. A terapia com corticosteroides é comumente utilizada, como mencionado para MMM e MEU. A expressão de antígenos do complexo de histocompatibilidade principal (MHC) I e II provou ser diagnosticamente útil em amostras obtidas de locais distantes da inflamação.[30-32] O tratamento deve ser iniciado precoce e apropriadamente, de modo a prevenir a perda irreversível de fibras musculares, a ocorrência de fibrose e contraturas.

Dermatomiosite

A dermatomiosite (ver Capítulo 10) é uma doença inflamatória imunomediada que envolve músculo estriado, pele e vaso sanguíneo. Em cães, as lesões cutâneas predominam com características miopáticas menos óbvias. Uma forma familiar de dermatomiosite foi descrita em cães das raças Collie,[33] Shetland Sheepdog[34] e, ocasionalmente, em outras raças.[35] O tratamento consiste na administração de prednisona, pentoxifilina e vitamina E.

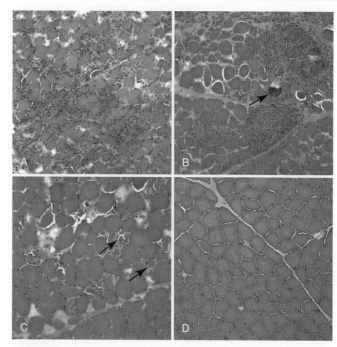

Figura 354.2 Cortes histológicos congelados corados por hematoxilina e eosina (H&E) de amostras obtidas por biopsia muscular em cães com miopatia inflamatória (**A**), distrofia muscular (**B**, a *seta* aponta para fibra muscular calcificada), miopatia necrosante (**C**, as *setas* apontam para fibras musculares necrosadas), comparativamente com o músculo normal em cães (**D**). Aumento de 20× para todas as imagens. (*Esta figura se encontra reproduzida em cores no Encarte.*)

Miosite por corpúsculo de inclusão

A miosite por corpúsculo de inclusão esporádica é a miopatia mais comum em pessoas com mais de 50 anos de idade; também pode ocorrer em cães idosos.[36] A manifestação clínica consiste em fraqueza e atrofia muscular crônica progressiva. O diagnóstico é confirmado pelo exame de amostra de músculo obtida por biopsia e constatação de alterações degenerativas, como vacúolos e depósitos amiloides positivos para a coloração com vermelho-Congo e inflamação. Embora não haja tratamento específico disponível, os suplementos que incluem L-carnitina e antioxidantes podem propiciar algum benefício.

Miosite infecciosa

A miosite de origem protozoária é causada pelos microrganismos *Toxoplasma gondii*, *Neospora caninum*, *Hepatozoon canis*, *Babesia canis*, *Leishmania* ou *Trypanosoma* (ver Capítulo 221).[37] Embora supostamente seja um achado incidental verificado em amostra de músculo obtida por biopsia, recentemente foram detectados casos graves de miosite causados pela infecção por *Sarcocystis* spp. em dois cães.[38] De forma geral a miosite é rara em gatos; contudo, o vírus da imunodeficiência felina foi relatado como a causa de miopatia subclínica.[39]

Miopatia necrosante

Miopatias necrosantes são caracterizadas histologicamente por necrose e fagocitose, sem infiltração linfocítica.[24,25] Deve-se considerar a possibilidade de miopatia necrosante em todos os casos de início agudo e atividade sérica acentuadamente elevada de CK, rabdomiólise e mioglobinúria, ou em casos com elevações periódicas de CK e mioglobinúria esporádica. Etiologias incluem reações a fármacos e exposição a toxinas, picadas de insetos venenosos, anormalidades eletrolíticas e doenças infecciosas. Infelizmente, a causa desses distúrbios é raramente identificada.[25] Suporte respiratório e terapia hídrica intensiva devem resultar em recuperação do paciente. O tratamento com corticosteroide pode agravar os sinais clínicos.[40,41] Em casos recorrentes, deve-se considerar a possibilidade de anormalidades metabólicas relativas ao glicogênio e aos lipídios. Biopsia muscular é útil para identificar produtos de armazenamento e para outros testes diagnósticos diretos.

MIOPATIAS CONGÊNITAS (ESTRUTURAIS)

Miopatias congênitas consistem em um grupo de anormalidades musculares genéticas caracterizadas clinicamente por fraqueza, hiporreflexia e hipotonia, em geral desde o nascimento.[42] As miopatias congênitas são classificadas histopatologicamente com base nas características morfológicas particulares observadas em amostra de músculo obtida por biopsia (Figura 354.3) e incluem bastões (miopatia nemalínica),[43,44] núcleos (doença de núcleo central e doença de múltiplos núcleos),[45] núcleos centralizados (centronuclear[46-49] e miopatia miotubular),[50-52] hipotrofia seletiva de fibras musculares tipo 1 (desproporção congênita de miofibras)[53] e miopatia miofibrilar.[54] Biopsia muscular (ver Capítulo 116) e exames histológicos, histoquímicos, imuno-histoquímicos e ultraestruturais do músculo por meio de microscopia óptica e eletrônica são necessários para obter o diagnóstico de miopatia congênita.[42]

Após detecção de anormalidade estrutural, pode-se iniciar a busca direcionada à mutação genética. Atualmente há disponibilidade de teste de DNA para um número crescente de doenças neurológicas[55] e a lista de testes disponíveis para miopatias hereditárias também está aumentando. Nas miopatias congênitas pode-se verificar heterogeneidade genética, com mutações em mais de um gene, causando uma miopatia específica. Por exemplo, há pelo menos oito diferentes *locus* genéticos que podem resultar em miopatia nemalínica.[42] Diferentes raças de cães acometidas por miopatia miotubular ligada ao cromossomo X podem apresentar mutações em diferentes *locus* do gene

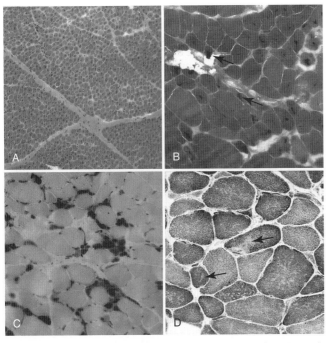

Figura 354.3 Miopatias congênitas detectadas em exame de amostra de músculo obtida por biopsia, incluindo: **A.** Miopatia miotubular ligada ao cromossomo X (coloração H&E). **B.** Miopatia nemalínica (coloração com tricrômio de Gomori modificada; as *setas* mostram agregados de corpúsculos de bastonetes). **C.** Desproporção congênita do tipo de fibra (reação miofibrilar da ATPase em pH 4,3; fibras tipo 1 são escuras). **D.** Doença de múltiplos núcleos (reação NADH-TR; as *setas* apontam para locais desprovidos de atividade enzimática oxidativa compatíveis com núcleos ou mininúcleos). Aumento de 20× para todas as imagens. (*Esta figura se encontra reproduzida em cores no Encarte.*)

MTM1, como foi demonstrado nas raças de cães Labrador Retriever,[50] Rottweiller[52] e Husky Siberiano (Shelton, não publicado). Para essas anormalidades não há disponibilidade de tratamento clínico específico, mas a prevenção da doença com alteração das estratégias de acasalamento deve ser efetiva porque a maior parte dessas miopatias ocorre no início da vida.

As miopatias centronucleares (MCN) persistiram na população de cães das raças Labrador Retriever e Dogue Alemão por vários anos, mas eram conhecidas por diversos nomes. Em cães Labrador Retriever a miopatia centronuclear era denominada deficiência de fibras do tipo 2,[56] distrofia muscular autossômica recessiva[57] e miopatia hereditária do cão Labrador Retriever.[58] Em cães Dogue Alemão, a MCN era denominada miopatia de núcleo central.[59] Com a identificação de mutações específicas nos genes associados às MCN, essas miopatias agora podem ser corretamente definidas, alinhadas com classificações utilizadas em medicina humana.

DISTROFIAS MUSCULARES

As distrofias musculares (DM) consistem em um grupo heterogêneo de mais de 40 diferentes doenças genéticas que resultam em degeneração muscular progressiva, ciclos repetidos de regeneração e fraqueza muscular progressiva. As DM mais comuns envolvem mutações no gene que codifica a proteína citoesquelética distrofina[60] e no complexo associado à distrofina (CAD),[61] que liga a matriz extracelular ao citoesqueleto de actina, estabilizando a membrana da célula muscular durante a contração. Mutações no gene da distrofina resultam em distrofias musculares de Duchenne ligada ao cromossomo X e do tipo Becker em humanos.[62] Mutações em outros genes do CAD, como de sarcoglicanos, resultam em um grupo de distrofias denominadas DM da cintura pélvica, que apresentam modo de hereditariedade autossômica dominante ou autossômica recessiva.[63] Biopsia muscular (ver Capítulo 116) é um importante componente do diagnóstico de DM (ver Figura 354.1) e o exame imuno-histoquímico é um teste essencial para detectar uma forma específica de DM.[64]

DISTROFIA MUSCULAR LIGADA AO CROMOSSOMO X (DEFICIÊNCIA DE DISTROFINA)

A DM por deficiência de distrofina é a forma mais comum de DM em cães;[65] foram identificadas mutações no gene da distrofina em várias raças de cães, incluindo Golden Retriever,[66] Rottweiler,[67] Pointer Alemão de Pelo Curto,[68] Cavalier King Charles Spaniel,[69] Welsh Corgi,[70] Cocker Spaniel, Terrier Tibetano e Labrador Retriever.[71] Os cães acometidos apresentam fenótipo miopático grave progressivo, inclusive perda gradual de massa muscular e desenvolvimento de contraturas. Hipertrofia da língua e disfunção de faringe e esôfago resultam em sialorreia, disfagia e regurgitação. Nota-se elevação marcante e persistente da atividade sérica de CK, que pode ser detectada com poucas semanas de idade. Atualmente não há disponibilidade de tratamento específico. Pode ocorrer morte precoce em decorrência de cardiomiopatia, complicações de disfagia e disfunção esofágica, ou distúrbios respiratórios por espessamento importante do diafragma. Foi detectada uma família de cães Labrador Retriever deficientes em distrofina, com nenhum ou muito poucos sinais clínicos de distrofia muscular, porém com elevação acentuada e persistente da atividade sérica de CK.[72] Em gatos, os sinais clínicos de deficiência de distrofina podem variar desde hipertrofia à atrofia muscular, espessamento diafragmático, megaesôfago e aumento de tamanho da língua, com placas esbranquiçadas.[73,74] Ocorre elevação acentuada e persistente da atividade sérica de CK. O prognóstico quanto à recuperação é ruim. Em gatos, foram identificadas mutações no gene da distrofina.[74]

Distrofia muscular autossômica por deficiência de sarcoglicanos

Sarcoglicanos são componentes do CAD e, no músculo estriado, são compostos de subunidades alfa, beta, gama e delta. Mutações nos genes que codificam os sarcoglicanos resultam no grupo diverso classificado em humanos com DM da cintura pélvica.[63] DM por deficiência de sarcoglicanos foram descritas em cães das raças Boston Terrier,[75] Cocker Spaniel,[76] além de uma cadela Dobermann[77] e um Gato Doméstico de Pelo Curto.[78] Em cães da raça Boston Terrier detectou-se deficiência de sarcoglicanos com mutação no gene que codifica o sarcoglicano delta (Shelton, não publicado). A manifestação clínica de sarcoglicanopatia é semelhante àquela da distrofinopatia, e o exame de amostra de músculo obtida por biopsia mostra o fenótipo distrófico degenerativo e regenerativo. É necessário realizar imunocoloração para proteínas sarcoglicanos a fim de distinguir essa forma de DM daquela da deficiência de distrofina.

Distrofia muscular congênita por deficiência de laminina alfa-2

Lamininas são grandes glicoproteínas que contribuem para a membrana basal no músculo e estão conectadas ao sarcolema pelo CAD.[79] A DM por deficiência de laminina alfa-2 foi relatada em gatos[80,81] e em um cão mestiço da raça Springer Spaniel.[82] Os sinais clínicos variaram de fraqueza muscular generalizada e atrofia até rigidez progressiva com limitação da amplitude de movimentação das articulações dos membros e abertura limitada da mandíbula. A laminina alfa-2 também está presente na membrana basal de células de Schwann.[83,84] Há relato de neuropatia desmielinizante evidente em um dos gatos com distrofia, no qual o nervo periférico foi examinado.[80] Ainda não foi identificada mutação no gene da laminina alfa-2.

Distrofia muscular por deficiência de colágeno VI

A anormalidade progressiva da marcha e múltiplas deformidades articulares foram descritas em um cão jovem da raça Labrador Retriever com deficiência de colágeno VI.[85] Identificou-se mutação no gene do colágeno VI (Shelton, não publicado). Esse caso mostra a importância de considerar uma forma de DM congênita em animais jovens atendidos primariamente por apresentar contraturas de membro.

SÍNDROMES MIASTÊNICAS CONGÊNITAS

Síndromes miastênicas congênitas (SMCs) são anormalidades heterogêneas nas quais a margem de segurança para transmissão neuromuscular é comprometida por defeitos em proteínas presentes nas regiões pré-sinápticas, sinápticas e pós-sinápticas da junção neuromuscular (JNM) (ver Capítulo 269).[86] SMCs em geral acometem animais com 6 a 12 semanas de vida aparentados; são caracterizadas por fraqueza muscular intensa e generalizada. Os animais afetados nunca foram clinicamente normais. Até o momento, há relatos de SMC em cães das raças Jack Russell Terrier,[87,88] Fox Terrier de Pelo Liso,[89] Springer Spaniel,[90] Teckel de Pelo Liso[91] e Braco Dinamarquês.[92] Em cães Braco Dinamarquês com SMC detectou-se mutação no gene da colina acetiltransferase (CHAT).[93] Recentemente, detectou-se deficiência de acetilcolinesterase (AChE) na placa nervosa terminal causada por uma mutação no COLQ, o gene que codifica a extremidade colagenosa da AChE, em uma família de cães jovens Labrador Retriever.[94] Recentemente detectou-se uma mutação no CHRNE, o gene que codifica a subunidade épsilon do AChR nicotínico do músculo, em cães Jack Russell Terrier (Shelton, não publicado). SMC também ocorre em filhotes de cães Golden Retriever, embora o defeito molecular ainda não tenha sido identificado.

De forma geral, o prognóstico de SMC em cães é ruim, já que os sinais clínicos em geral são graves e pode ocorrer dessensibilização aos medicamentos, como a piridostigmina. Medicamentos efetivos em um tipo de SMC podem não ser efetivos ou podem ser danosos em outro tipo.[95] Em cães Labrador Retriever com mutação no COLQ, um inibidor da AChE resultou em agravamento da fraqueza muscular. Em contrapartida, inibidores da AChE em cães Jack Russell Terrier com mutação no CHRNE resultaram em aumento da força muscular. Em pessoas, os agonistas adrenérgicos salbutamol e efedrina foram empiricamente efetivos na SMC causada por mutação no COLQ.[95]

DOENÇAS ENDÓCRINAS E METABÓLICAS

Comparativamente à frequência de miopatias inflamatórias e congênitas na população de cães e gatos de companhia, as doenças metabólicas que envolvem o metabolismo de glicogênio, lipídios ou mitocôndrias são relativamente incomuns.

Doenças de armazenamento de glicogênio

Doenças de armazenamento de glicogênio (DAG) representam um grupo de anormalidades autossômicas recessivas do metabolismo de glicogênio que resultam no acúmulo de glicogênio no tecido e na alteração da homeostase da glicose (ver Capítulo 260). O fenótipo clínico se manifesta precocemente na vida e pode variar dependendo da gravidade do defeito da enzima e tecidos específicos nos quais a enzima é normalmente expressa. Um fenótipo miopático pode estar presente na DAG tipo II (deficiência da enzima α-glicosidase ácida lisossomal, doença de Pompe) em cães das raças Finnish Lapphund e Swedish Lapphund,[96] na DAG III (deficiência de enzima desramificadora do glicogênio) em cães Pastor-Alemão[97,98] e Retriever de Pelo Crespo,[99] e na DAG tipo VII (deficiência de fosfofrutoquinase, PFK) em cães English Springer Spaniel,[100] American Cocker Spaniel,[101] Whippets[102] e Wachtelhund.[103] Diferentemente de humanos, nos quais a miopatia por esforço é a manifestação mais comum da deficiência de PFK, a crise hemolítica é a manifestação clínica predominante em cães. A doença de armazenamento do glicogênio tipo IV foi identificada em gatos da raça Norwegian Forest.[104]

Miopatias mitocondriais e anormalidades de armazenamento de lipídios

O diagnóstico clínico da doença mitocondrial geralmente é um desafio. Além da manifestação predominantemente miopática ou neuropática, podem ocorrer manifestações sistêmicas em vários órgãos, nas quais o envolvimento muscular é apenas uma parte do quadro clínico. Anormalidades mitocondriais podem ocorrer em qualquer idade. Órgãos com alta demanda energética geralmente são acometidos, incluindo músculos esqueléticos, miocárdio, órgãos endócrinos, rins, componentes não mucosos do trato intestinal, retina e sistema nervoso central.[105]

Uma mutação no gene da piruvato desidrogenase fosfatase 1 (PDP1) foi detectada em cães das raças Clumber e Sussex Spaniel, com capacidade muito limitada para realizar atividades físicas já no primeiro ano de vida.[106] A constatação de concentrações plasmáticas de lactato e de piruvato acentuadamente elevadas em repouso e após atividade física, com proporção lactato: piruvato < 10, sustenta o diagnóstico de anormalidade mitocondrial. O fornecimento de dieta com alto teor de gordura e baixo conteúdo de carboidratos, além de suplementação com L-carnitina, coenzima Q10 e vitaminas do complexo B, resulta em maior tolerância a exercícios, embora reduza a expectativa de vida. Há relato de miopatia mitocondrial associada à alteração da atividade de citocromo C oxidase em ninhadas de cães da raça Old English Sheepdog.[107]

Miopatias por armazenamento de lipídios estão associadas a anormalidades primárias ou secundárias do metabolismo da carnitina ou da betaoxidação de ácidos graxos.[108,109] Os sinais clínicos incluem fraqueza generalizada progressiva e mialgia intensa. O diagnóstico pode ser realizado apenas pela constatação de grandes gotículas lipídicas em excesso no interior das miofibras de fibras musculares tipo 1, utilizando um corante para triglicerídeos neutro. A acidemia láctica pode ser um achado concomitante. Em geral, o tratamento é efetivo, utiliza-se uma combinação de L-carnitina, antioxidantes e vitaminas do complexo B.

Miopatias associadas a doenças endócrinas

Mialgia, rigidez e atrofia ou hipertrofia muscular são achados comuns em cães adultos com distúrbios endócrinos, principalmente hipotireoidismo (ver Capítulo 299) e síndrome de Cushing (ver Capítulo 306). Podem ocorrer sintomas neuromusculares sem os sinais clínicos clássicos de endocrinopatia.[110] Alterações patológicas em músculos, como atrofia de fibras tipo 2 e predominância de fibras do tipo 1, podem ser a primeira indicação de miopatia associada a anormalidades endócrinas.[111] No hipotireoidismo, a resposta à suplementação com hormônios da tireoide é excelente. Em gatos com hipertireoidismo, a fraqueza muscular responde bem ao tratamento (ver Capítulo 301). Na síndrome de Cushing crônica, não tratada, pode ocorrer pseudomiotonia (ver Vídeo 306.2), que pouco responde à terapia específica para hiperadrenocorticismo. Há relato de cãibras musculares em cães com hipoadrenocorticismo (ver Capítulo 309).[112]

CANALOPATIAS

Miotonia congênita e paralisia periódica

Miotonias congênitas são causadas por disfunção de canais iônicos do sarcolema, o que resulta em excitabilidade anormal das miofibras. Os sinais clínicos ocorrem antes dos 6 meses de idade e incluem hipertonicidade muscular marcante, hipertrofia e formação de uma depressão tecidual visível após a percussão dos músculos acometidos com martelo. A hipertrofia da língua é proeminente em gatos. O exame eletromiográfico (ver Capítulo 117), com constatação de potenciais de ação *dive bomber*, é diagnóstico. Mutações específicas foram identificadas em cães Schnauzer Miniatura,[113] Australian Cattle Dogs[114] e gatos domésticos;[115] há disponibilidade de testes de DNA para triagem. Agentes estabilizadores de membrana, como procainamida e mexiletina, são considerados os medicamentos mais efetivos.

Paralisia periódica raramente é descrita em medicina veterinária. Fraqueza episódica resultante de hipopotassemia foi descrita em filhotes de gatos Birmaneses.[116] A suplementação oral com potássio previne episódios de paralisia. Uma mutação foi identificada e um teste genético para sua detecção está disponível.[117] A paralisia periódica hiperpotassêmica responsiva à acetazolamida foi relatada em um único cão da raça American Pit Bull Terrier.[118]

REFERÊNCIAS BIBLIOGRÁFICAS

As referências bibliográficas deste capítulo se encontram online no Ambiente de Aprendizagem.

CAPÍTULO 355

Fisioterapia e Reabilitação

David Levine e Darryl L. Millis

A fisioterapia é uma atividade profissional com base científica estabelecida em humanos e animais de companhia. Ela possui inúmeras aplicações clínicas no restabelecimento, na manutenção e na promoção de uma condição física ótima.

Ao optar por fisioterapia e reabilitação, o objetivo é restabelecer, manter e promover melhor função, condição física, bem-estar e qualidade de vida, comprometidos por anormalidades de movimentação e estado geral de saúde.[1-7] Em cães, isso pode incluir o tratamento de pacientes durante a recuperação de procedimentos cirúrgicos ortopédicos, como reparo de fraturas e cirurgias de ligamento cruzado, programas de monitoramento de perda de peso (ver Capítulo 176), fornecimento de reabilitação geral após lesões neurológicas, como em casos de doença do disco intervertebral (ver Capítulo 266), e auxílio ao tratamento de doenças crônicas, como osteoartrite (ver Capítulo 353), ou enfermidades progressivas, como a mielopatia degenerativa (ver Capítulo 266).[8-14] A principal ênfase envolve a prevenção ou o retardo do início de sinais clínicos e da progressão dos transtornos, das limitações funcionais e das incapacidades que podem resultar de doenças, distúrbios, condições e lesões.

A fisioterapia e a reabilitação na clínica de pequenos animais está se tornando cada vez mais comum e provavelmente continuará a emergir como uma atividade essencial da medicina veterinária, à medida que a literatura científica se expande. Em várias condições ortopédicas e neurológicas, a reabilitação física está se tornando rotineira como forma de abreviar o tempo de recuperação, como acontece em medicina humana. Bem-estar e medicina preventiva (p. ex., redução de peso, manutenção da força e função muscular, melhora da capacidade física cardiorrespiratória e condicionamento esportivo específico) também são tendências crescentes na reabilitação e na medicina esportiva. Na literatura relativa a humanos e aos cães, a terapia de reabilitação mostrou-se efetiva em numerosas áreas relacionadas à medicina interna, inclusive controle da dor, função cardiorrespiratória, recuperação e função musculoesquelética e neurológica, bem como oncologia, para citar algumas.[15-24]

Em 2012, o American College of Veterinary Sports Medicine and Rehabilitation (ACVSMR) foi aprovado como uma especialidade certificada por um conselho, sob tutela da American Veterinary Medical Association's American Board of Veterinary Specialties (ABVS). Esse colegiado recém-formado almeja a especialização de médicos-veterinários que possuam excelência em medicina esportiva e reabilitação. Programas certificados em reabilitação de cães também estão disponíveis e requerem atividades *on-line* e presenciais, estágios e processos de avaliação.

A reabilitação é uma especialidade que demanda tempo e envolve uma abordagem colaborativa multiprofissional para maximizar os resultados, incluindo veterinários, técnicos veterinários, fisioterapeutas, ortotistas e prostéticos, etologistas, treinadores e, sem dúvida, os tutores.

AVALIAÇÃO DA FISIOTERAPIA/REABILITAÇÃO

O processo de fisioterapia/reabilitação começa com o diagnóstico pelo veterinário e uma cuidadosa avaliação do fisioterapeuta. A avaliação do fisioterapeuta difere da avaliação clínica pelo fato de que a função é o componente primordial. Amplitude da movimentação, força, marcha, dor, equilíbrio, resistência e outros fatores funcionais são todos documentados, e elabora-se um plano de reabilitação juntamente com o tutor (Apêndice ao fim do capítulo). O protocolo terapêutico deve ser apropriado ao paciente e deve levar em consideração todos os achados anormais e outros fatores, inclusive a gravidade da doença, a idade e a disposição do cão, as expectativas para a função e o desempenho futuros, a urgência da recuperação, o equipamento disponível e as habilidades técnicas do fisioterapeuta, e as limitações financeiras do tutor. O plano de tratamento é então continuamente modificado conforme necessário com base em avaliações frequentes. Um profissional de reabilitação qualificado pode estar ou não presente no local, de forma que às vezes são necessários programas domiciliares.

Durante a avaliação, é importante saber quais são as expectativas do tutor para ajudar a determinar o tipo e a duração do programa necessário para atender aos objetivos. Na maioria dos casos, os tutores são realistas quanto às expectativas, especialmente para animais com doenças crônicas graves em que se deseja a melhora da mobilidade e o controle da dor. Ocasionalmente, um tutor terá objetivos fora da realidade, e é importante discutir a realidade da(s) doença(s) primárias(s) e se os objetivos serão provavelmente atingidos ou não.

Técnicas de avaliação

A avaliação do resultado da fisioterapia e da reabilitação é essencial para determinar como o animal está progredindo e avaliar a efetividade do tratamento. Essas técnicas devem consistir em dados objetivos, sempre que possível, porque geralmente tutores e veterinários subjetivamente acreditam que um paciente está se saindo melhor do que os dados sugerem. Além disso, a documentação do progresso é importante para incentivar os tutores a continuar a reabilitação e justificar o tratamento continuado. Diversas mensurações são úteis para a avaliação dos resultados, incluindo a capacidade de realizar atividades funcionais diárias, análise da marcha, movimentação e função articular (Figura 355.1), massa e força muscular, condição corporal e alteração de peso, avaliação da dor, níveis de atividade física e escalas funcionais.[25-37]

INTERVENÇÕES COMUNS NA FISIOTERAPIA/REABILITAÇÃO

Termoterapia e crioterapia

A aplicação de calor (termoterapia) e frio (crioterapia) na superfície é utilizada terapeuticamente em tecidos moles e articulações há séculos. A crioterapia é comumente utilizada após traumatismo tecidual acidental (torções, estiramentos etc.) ou intencional (cirurgia, exercício intenso), com o objetivo de reduzir a inflamação, o edema e a dor, bem como melhorar a função.[38] O aquecimento de tecidos conjuntivos pela utilização de calor superficial, como bolsas e compressas de calor, geralmente é utilizado em doenças crônicas, como artrite e outras anormalidades que causam rigidez; isso ajuda a aumentar a

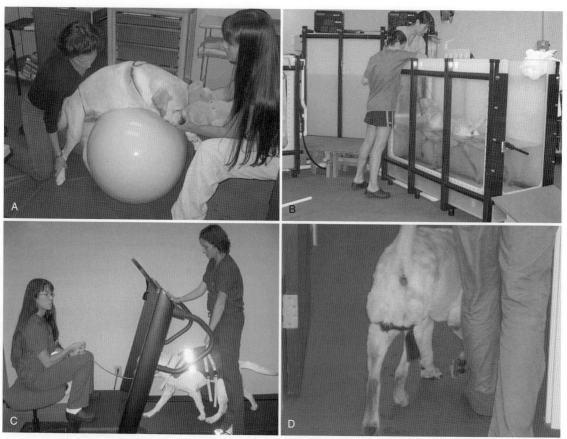

Figura 355.1 Cão da raça Labrador Retriever de 6 meses de idade em recuperação para estabilização extracapsular da articulação do joelho esquerdo após avulsão do ligamento cruzado cranial. O cão está sendo submetido a exercícios de troca de peso corporal estático entre os membros (**A**), caminhada em esteira subaquática (**B**), trote em esteira (**C**), caminhada com uma faixa elástica que impede a rotação externa que havia no membro pélvico direito durante o período de recuperação (**D**). (De Millis DL, Levine D: *Canine rehabilitation and physical therapy*, 2 ed., St. Louis, 2014, Saunders.)

capacidade de extensão do tecido conjuntivo. A termoterapia também pode ser utilizada para aliviar a dor e facilitar a cicatrização.[39] Ambos os tratamentos são facilmente ensinados aos tutores e podem ser realizados no domicílio.

Ultrassom terapêutico

O ultrassom terapêutico (UST) é utilizado principalmente como um agente de aquecimento profundo (até 5 centímetros), utilizado na clínica de pequenos animais para aquecimento de articulações, músculos e tendões, comumente antes do alongamento. Também é utilizado para auxiliar na cicatrização e reparo tecidual, bem como para melhorar a absorção transdérmica de medicamentos (fonoforese). Somente duas frequências são utilizadas na UST (em comparação ao ultrassom diagnóstico), 1 MHz para o tratamento de tecidos situados a 3 a 5 cm de profundidade e 3 MHz para o tratamento de tecidos com 1 a 2 cm de profundidade.[40-42]

Estimulação elétrica

A estimulação elétrica (EE) é uma modalidade comumente utilizada em fisioterapia e pode ser efetiva para vários propósitos, inclusive aumento da força muscular e alívio da dor.[14,43-47] Esse procedimento estimula nervos motores, até causar contração muscular, e nervos sensoriais ou sensitivos, para aliviar a dor. Vários cães toleram bem a EE, mas alguns podem não gostar da sensação; portanto, deve ser utilizada com cuidado.

Laser terapêutico

LASER é um acrônimo de *light amplification by stimulated emission of radiation* (amplificação de luz por emissão estimulada de radiação). O conceito do uso de luz para fins terapêuticos, denominado fototerapia, foi originado da crença de que o sol e outras fontes de luz propiciam benefícios terapêuticos. O *laser* terapêutico tem se tornado cada vez mais popular na reabilitação veterinária para uma série de condições. O *laser* utilizado na reabilitação supostamente ajuda a modular as funções celulares, um processo conhecido como fotobiomodulação (FBM). Relata-se que a FBM atua como moduladora de vários mecanismos biológicos, como a respiração mitocondrial e a síntese da adenosina trifosfato (ATP), de modo a acelerar a cicatrização da lesão e da articulação e promover a regeneração muscular.[48-58] Também é comumente utilizado para alívio da dor; em alguns estudos, verificou-se que foi um adjuvante efetivo no tratamento de dor musculoesquelética. Geralmente, há *laser* terapêutico da classe IIIb (5 a 500 mW) ou da classe IV (> 500 mW), que apresentam comprimentos de onda infravermelhos apropriados para penetrar em tecidos situados em várias profundidades (Figura 355.2).

Amplitude da movimentação e alongamento

A amplitude da movimentação (ADM) e exercícios de alongamento são extremamente importantes para obter a melhor movimentação de articulações após traumatismo agudo ou cirurgia (fraturas articulares) ou para o tratamento de pacientes com doenças crônicas (osteoartrite). Também são procedimentos importantes para aumentar a flexibilidade, prevenir aderências entre tecidos moles e ossos, remodelar a fibrose periarticular e melhorar a capacidade de extensão muscular e de outros tecidos moles de modo a evitar novas lesões.[59] A movimentação articular pode ser mensurada por goniometria, que foi validada para cães e gatos (Figura 355.3).[60,61] Esses exercícios também podem ser realizados no domicílio, desde que o tutor seja cuidadosamente instruído.

Massagem

Há várias formas de massagem, empregada por vários profissionais, em diversos contextos. A massagem é definida como a manipulação científica e sistemática dos tecidos moles do corpo. Em pessoas, o uso de massagem é comum para relaxamento, alívio da dor, recuperação da lesão e melhora da flexibilidade,[62-66] e está se tornando cada vez mais aceita e comum na clínica veterinária. Em alguns estados (mas não em todos), os massoterapeutas são licenciados e regulados, mas isso não é comum na clínica de pequenos animais. Há disponibilidade de cursos de educação continuada e escolas que ensinam as técnicas de massagem.

Exercício terapêutico

O exercício terapêutico (Vídeos 355.1 a 355.19) é muito provavelmente a modalidade mais comum e valiosa utilizada na fisioterapia e reabilitação. O exercício terapêutico é um importante método para retorno do animal ao melhor nível funcional e de independência.[13,14,67,68] Alguns dos objetivos comuns dos exercícios são melhorar a amplitude ativa da movimentação, a flexibilidade, a massa e força muscular, o equilíbrio, a resistência e o desempenho de atividades diárias de rotina.[11,59,68-74] Programas de exercício terapêutico desenvolvidos para o ambiente doméstico também propiciam a oportunidade de os tutores se envolverem ativamente na reabilitação de seus animais (Figuras 355.4 a 355.8).

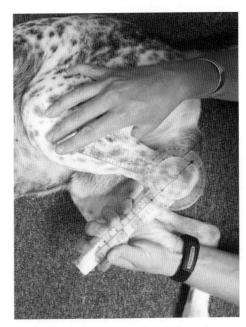

Figura 355.3 Ângulos de flexão e extensão articulares são mensurados com um goniômetro.

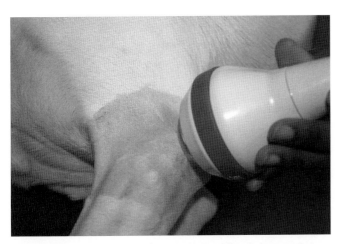

Figura 355.2 Tratamento de articulação com artrite utilizando *laser* terapêutico.

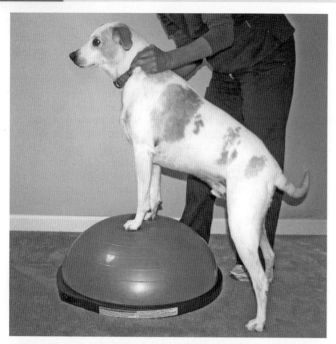

Figura 355.4 Para o posicionamento do animal a fim de realizar exercícios de fortalecimento de músculos profundos, pode-se utilizar uma cúpula de equilíbrio (metade da superfície redonda e metade plana) ou uma bola BOSU.

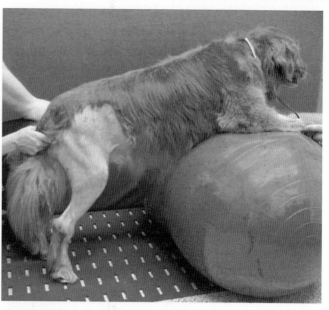

Figura 355.5 Atividades de dança podem ser obtidas com o auxílio de rolo de fisioterapia ou de uma bola oval. O paciente posiciona os membros torácicos no rolo ou na bola e o terapeuta rola lentamente a bola na direção do paciente e para longe dele, forçando-o a movimentar os membros pélvicos para trás e para a frente.

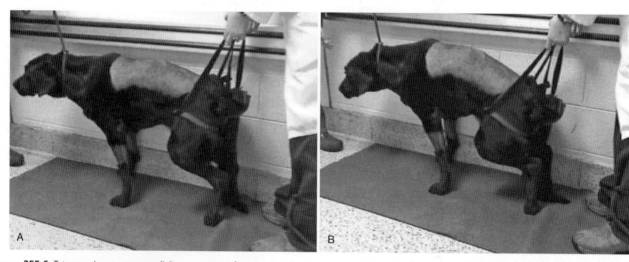

Figura 355.6 Tetraparesia ou outras condições que causam fraqueza em vários membros. **A.** Utilização de um aparato de apoio para auxiliar na sustentação do peso quando o paciente está em pé. **B.** À medida que o paciente começa a cansar e tenta sentar, o terapeuta levanta o cão novamente em posição de estação.

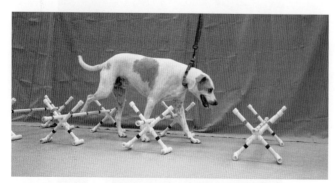

Figura 355.7 Caminhada sobre uma trilha de cavaletes ajuda os cães a aprender como desviar de obstáculos e sobrepô-los pela elevação dos membros até uma altura apropriada.

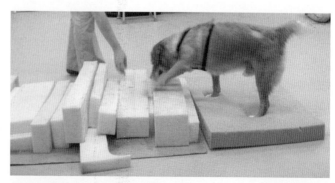

Figura 355.8 Posição de estação ou caminhada em espuma, colchão, colchão de ar ou trampolim altera a textura do solo e estimula o equilíbrio funcional e a capacidade proprioceptiva do animal.

Hidroterapia

A hidroterapia se tornou um componente muito útil na fisioterapia e reabilitação veterinária. Esteiras subaquáticas (ESA) e piscinas se tornaram comuns em instalações de reabilitação veterinária (Figuras 355.1 B e 355.9). Um benefício importante da utilização de ESA é a flutuabilidade, que reduz a carga nas articulações durante o exercício.[12,14,75,76]

Em um estudo realizado com cães, constatou-se que o peso corporal suportado quando o cão está imerso na água (como porcentagem de peso corporal em piso seco) foi de aproximadamente 91%, quando a água estava na altura do maléolo lateral da tíbia, 85% na altura do côndilo lateral do fêmur, e 38% quando na altura do trocânter maior do fêmur.[75] Essa informação pode ser particularmente útil ao tratar pacientes com doenças articulares, como artrite, pois as articulações podem não receber carga por causa da flutuação na água (Figura 355.10). A utilização de ESA é a preferida para melhorar algumas funções, como a marcha. Ela também estimula a movimentação articular em um padrão de marcha mais normal, comparada à natação. A natação tende a aumentar a flexão e a amplitude geral da movimentação dos membros, mas a extensão articular é menor comparada à caminhada na ESA. No entanto, a natação é uma atividade muito mais difícil da perspectiva de resistência e função cardiovascular, e apenas um a dois minutos de natação podem ser exaustivos, especialmente em cães que apresentam má condição física. Dispositivos de flutuação também são úteis para possibilitar melhor flutuabilidade e facilidade do exercício.

A hidroterapia, tal como ESA e natação, é realizada naturalmente por vários pacientes, o que é especialmente benéfico porque exercícios em animais devem ser de forma que eles realizem naturalmente ou possam ser facilmente treinados para fazê-los. Ademais, é um exercício que os tutores podem realizar com o seu cão no próprio domicílio, caso possua as instalações necessárias.

DISPOSITIVOS PARA AUXÍLIO DA REABILITAÇÃO (CARRINHOS, TALAS, CINTOS, SUPORTES, ÓRTESES E PRÓTESES)

Diversos dispositivos auxiliares são utilizados na reabilitação, de modo a auxiliar a marcha e a atividade dos animais (Figuras 355.11 e 355.12). Esses dispositivos vão desde equipamentos

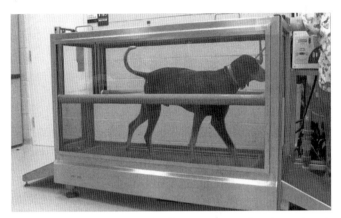

Figura 355.9 Protetores laterais de plástico em uma esteira rolante subaquática para impedir que o animal se posicione em seus lados sem movimentação. (De Levine D, Millis DL, Flocker J et al.: Aquatic therapy. In Millis DL, Levine D, Taylor RA, editors: *Canine rehabilitation and physical therapy*, St. Louis, 2014, Saunders, p 532; com permissão.)

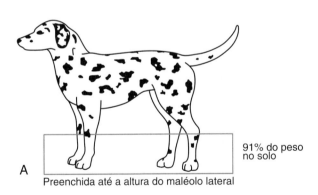

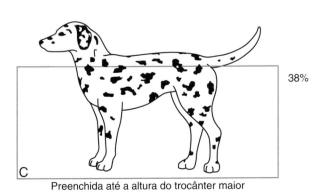

Figura 355.10 A. Cão na água até a altura do maléolo lateral. **B.** Cão na água até a altura do epicôndilo lateral. **C.** Cão na água até a altura do trocânter maior. (Dados de Levine D, Marcellin DJ, Millis DL et al.: Effects of partial immersion in water on vertical ground reaction forces and weight distribution in dogs. *Am J Vet Res* 71:1413-1416, 2010.)

de adaptação, cintas e suportes de baixo custo, até carrinhos e cadeiras de rodas que podem ser customizados ao paciente (Figura 355.13). Vários desses suportes ajudam a propiciar benefícios ergonômicos para o tutor e fornecem conforto e segurança para o cão.[77,78] Órteses envolvem avaliação, fabricação e customização de suspensórios. Próteses envolvem avaliação, fabricação e customização de membros artificiais (Figura 355.14). Profissionais que oferecem serviços de reabilitação possuem equipe capacitada para a obtenção desse equipamento, bem como para treinamento de tutores sobre sua utilização.

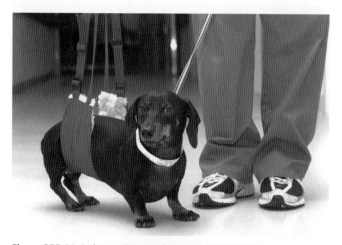

Figura 355.11 Pode-se utilizar um dispositivo de assistência, como uma faixa abdominal, para ajudar um paciente com lesão toracolombar a se manter em pé e caminhar. (De Millis DL, Levine D: *Canine Rehabilitation and Physical therapy*, 2 ed., St. Louis, 2014, Saunders.)

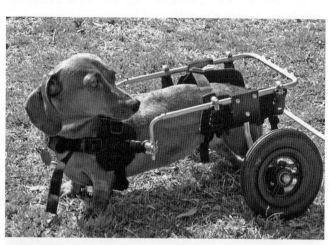

Figura 355.13 Pode-se utilizar um dispositivo de assistência, como um carrinho, para ajudar um paciente com lesão toracolombar a se manter em pé e caminhar. (De Millis DL, Levine D: *Canine Rehabilitation and Physical therapy*, 2 ed., St. Louis, 2014, Saunders.)

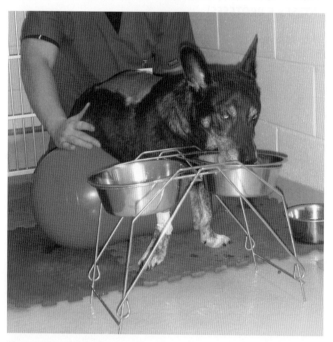

Figura 355.12 Exercício em pé assistido sobre um rolo de fisioterapia, realizado no momento da alimentação, a fim de encorajar o posicionamento em estação e estimular reforço positivo. (De Millis DL, Levine D: *Canine Rehabilitation and Physical therapy*, 2 ed., St. Louis, 2014, Saunders.)

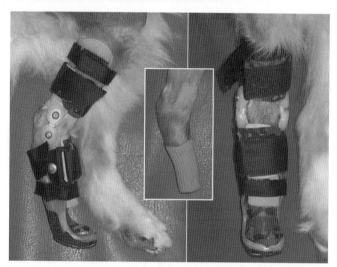

Figura 355.14 Cão da raça Sheltie que perdeu os dígitos após ressecção cirúrgica de sarcoma de tecido mole na coxa. A porção distal do coto é sensível ao toque. Seu coto foi colocado em um dedo de luva revestido com silicone e encaixado em uma prótese articulada mantida no local por meio de quatro fixadores com gancho e velcro.

APÊNDICE

AVALIAÇÃO INICIAL DE FISIOTERAPIA

Nome do paciente:	
Data:	

EXAME FÍSICO:

Pele/incisões:		Cor/temperatura:	
Frequência cardíaca:		Respiração:	

POSTURA/MARCHA:

Observação geral:			
Lesão/claudicação pré-operatória:	Caminhada:		Trote:
Lesão/claudicação pós-operatória:	Caminhada:		Trote:
Posição do membro em pé:		Posição do membro sentado:	

Circunferência (cm):	70% fêmur	80% úmero	Linha da articulação	Outro
Afetado:				
Não afetado:				
Outro:				

AMPLITUDE DE MOVIMENTO:

Articulação(s): alinhada/desalinhada	Flexão	Extensão	Abdução/adução	Varo/Valgo	Outro
Quadril:					
Articulação do joelho:					
Jarrete:					
Ombro:					
Cotovelo:					
Carpo:					
Outro:					

PALPAÇÃO:

Membro anterior	
Membro posterior	
Coluna vertebral	
Outro	

TESTES ESPECIAIS:

Neurológico:	
Ortopédico:	
Funcional:	
Outro:	

Millis and Levine: Canine Rehabilitation and Physical Therapy, 2nd edition.
Copyright© 2014 by Saunders Inc., an affiliate of Elsevier Inc.

TRATAMENTO:

Modalidades:		Manual:		Treino de marcha:	
Interferencial atual	☐	Massagem	☐	Treino de marcha	☐
Estimulação elétrica neuromuscular	☐	Imobilização	☐	Aquático	☐
		Faixa passiva de movimento	☐	Funcional	☐
				Bola suíça	☐
Outros estímulos	☐			Rolo de espuma	☐
Ultrassom	☐	Outro:		Educação do proprietário	☐
Gelo	☐			Revisão do protocolo	☐
Aquecimento	☐			Outro:	
Outro	☐				

AVALIAÇÃO/METAS:

Diminuir a dor	
Diminuir o edema	
Aumentar o suporte de peso	
Realizar programa de exercícios independente em casa	
Retornar à função anterior	
Outras	

PLANO:

Visita de retorno	
Ligar para fazer acompanhamento	
Ligar para DVM	
Outro	

Assinatura DVM _____

Millis and Levine: Canine Rehabilitation and Physical Therapy, 2nd edition.
Copyright© 2014 by Saunders Inc., an affiliate of Elsevier Inc.

REFERÊNCIAS BIBLIOGRÁFICAS

As referências bibliográficas deste capítulo se encontram online no Ambiente de Aprendizagem.

CAPÍTULO 356

Dor Crônica: Fisiopatologia, Identificação e Procedimentos Gerais de Controle

Lisa Moses

A dor crônica é um problema enigmático e complexo em medicina veterinária. A natureza mal adaptativa da dor crônica e incapacidade de autocomunicação do animal são fatores adicionais à complexidade de seu controle. As preocupações dos tutores dos animais quanto à dor crônica não são surpreendentes, dada a prevalência desse problema em pessoas. Em adultos, a dor crônica é considerada uma crise global de saúde pública, que afeta 1 em 5 adultos, por um período mediano de 7 anos.[1] Síndromes de dor crônica suficientemente significativas para impactar a qualidade de vida são quase sempre consequências do controle sustentado de doenças crônicas e de animais de companhia que vivem por mais tempo. A importância do desafio clínico da dor crônica aumenta à medida que aumenta a longevidade de cães e gatos. A inclusão desse novo capítulo é o reconhecimento de que o controle da dor crônica é uma parte integrante da medicina veterinária interna.

O diagnóstico e tratamento efetivo da dor crônica em pacientes que não podem buscar atendimento por vontade própria é feito por um representante. Isso pode parecer desconfortável, comparado à prática geral da medicina na qual um diagnóstico é confirmado com base em dados objetivos e o progresso é aferido em mensurações de resultados aparentemente concretas. Consequentemente, em animais de companhia a dor crônica ainda é muito subdiagnosticada e subtratada, apesar da evidência de sua frequente ocorrência.[2,3]

Todos os tipos de dor são experiências subjetivas, definidas em termos sensoriais e emocionais. Embora veterinários e tutores assumam que a dor seria relativamente fácil de avaliar em pacientes que verbalizam, comparados a animais, uma mensuração "objetiva" da dor em pessoas atualmente é matéria de intensa pesquisa. Até mesmo médicos possuem dúvidas sobre a confiabilidade do relato do paciente como padrão-ouro.[4] Por enquanto, o diagnóstico da dor crônica depende de alterações comportamentais funcionais e resposta ao tratamento. Os estados de dor crônica podem ser inferidos a partir de dados do histórico clínico e do exame físico, tratados da mesma forma, sem causar risco substancial ao paciente. Embora o problema do subdiagnóstico possa ser reduzido pela alteração da abordagem dos pacientes com provável dor crônica, dados sobre estratégias terapêuticas efetivas para animais ainda são escassos, e a prática depende da extrapolação a partir da clínica da dor crônica em adultos e crianças.

DOR CRÔNICA: FISIOPATOLOGIA

Há uma clara distinção entre a fisiologia da dor e a fisiopatologia da dor crônica. A dor pode ser um processo fisiológico destinado a proteger tecidos de danos potenciais ou lesão adicional (dor nociceptiva e aguda, respectivamente; ver Capítulo 126) ou pode ser uma síndrome mórbida mal adaptativa sem função conhecida (dor crônica).[5,6] Na literatura há várias "definições" de dor crônica, mas nenhuma transmite a complexidade ou totalidade dessa doença. Mesmo a definição concisa e precisa de Greene, "[...] processamento somatossensorial aberrante no sistema nervoso periférico ou central (SNC) que é sustentado

além do tempo esperado normal com relação ao estímulo", é tida como parcial.[6] Do ponto de vista fisiopatológico e clínico, a dor crônica é um estado mórbido do SNC, e não um sinal clínico de lesão tecidual de longa ação.[7] Os sinais clínicos da dor crônica são respostas alteradas à estimulação nociceptiva por alodinia (dor provocada por estímulos normalmente não nocivos), hiperalgesia (aumento da sensibilidade a um estímulo nocivo) e sensibilização (aumento da responsividade de neurônios a estímulos nocivos).[8] A dor crônica também pode ser gerada espontaneamente a partir de atividade do SNC, sem lesão aos tecidos, ou pode persistir após a cicatrização tecidual.[8] Essas características são clinicamente muito confusas já que uma lesão estrutural que possa explicar a dor pode ser discreta, pode ter sido resolvida ou pode ser inexistente. Em estados de dor crônica, a percepção e experiência de dor são desconectadas da lesão periférica.[9]

A dor crônica é causada por alterações estruturais e funcionais em vias fisiológicas da dor. Os mecanismos neuronais incluem desinibição, facilitação da via descendente e potencialização a longo prazo na medula espinal e no córtex.[10] Um importante contribuinte para a geração de dor crônica é a sensibilização do sistema de sinalização de dor. A sensibilização central é um tipo de plasticidade do SNC que tem sido mais bem caracterizada como um processo no corno dorsal da medula espinal, envolvendo de forma importante o recrutamento do receptor N-metil-D-aspartato (NMDA).[7] Pesquisas recentes sugerem que um processo semelhante de sensibilização provavelmente ocorre em outros locais do SNC.[11] Fatores desencadeantes neuronais, imunes e gliais da sensibilização central parecem todos importantes, além dos mecanismos do receptor NMDA já mencionados.[8] Tanto a sensibilização quanto a ativação tônica (outro elemento importante) são estimuladas por mediadores liberados em todos os níveis do sistema nervoso relacionado à dor.[11]

Elementos não neuronais, como células da glia e imunes, são fundamentais para a transição da dor aguda para dor crônica.[8] De fato, pesquisas recentes postularam que a dor crônica é uma "gliopatia", ou desregulação da função das células da glia no sistema nervoso.[10] A ativação da interação entre células da glia e neuroglia envolvendo três tipos de células gliais (astrócitos, micróglia e glia satélite) é considerada como um mecanismo fundamental na transição para dor crônica e sua manutenção.[10-12]

Na dor persistente ocorre alteração significativa na expressão gênica em nociceptores (alteração epigenética), assim como na atividade cortical mensurada por exames de imagem funcionais por ressonância magnética.[11] Outros fatores que contribuem para a ocorrência de dor crônica são diferenças genéticas e de gênero, bem como bactérias que causam infecção crônica (que podem estimular diretamente os nociceptores).[8]

A dor crônica não é inevitável após dor aguda ou até mesmo persistente. A suscetibilidade à dor crônica é uma equação completa que envolve predisposição genética e fatores ambientais. Pesquisas recentes tentaram associar técnicas de imagem cerebrais com fenótipos genéticos ou biomarcadores, a fim de caracterizar melhor a base biológica da dor crônica.[13,14]

Um aspecto funcional importante da fisiologia da dor é a existência de um sistema inibidor endógeno (analgésico) da dor.[15] A capacidade de o sistema nervoso reduzir a dor parece envolver a inibição em rede a partir de múltiplos e integrados circuitos sensíveis a opioides, em todos os níveis do sistema nervoso, os quais ocasionam modulação descendente dos sinais de dor.[7,15] Esse sistema é responsável pelas ações da maioria dos medicamentos analgésicos e de vários métodos não farmacológicos indutores de analgesia, inclusive efeito placebo, acupuntura e exercícios.[7,14-16] Vários medicamentos analgésicos utilizam esse circuito mimetizando o efeito de opiáceos endógenos.[15]

IDENTIFICAÇÃO DA DOR CRÔNICA E AVALIAÇÃO DA RESPOSTA AO TRATAMENTO

Diferentemente do que ocorre na espécie humana, há pouca informação sobre a incidência de dor crônica em espécies veterinárias.[17,18] O reconhecimento da dor crônica em condição clínica seguramente é mais difícil do que a da dor aguda. Pesquisas de veterinários em várias culturas relataram o desafio da detecção da dor como um obstáculo para o tratamento de dor crônica.[19-21] Embora haja amplo conhecimento sobre o significado da dor crônica nessas pesquisas, também há uma grande variação na frequência, na duração e no tipo de tratamento utilizado.

O conhecimento dos sinais da dor crônica é fundamental para sua detecção. É importante ter em mente que alguns pacientes *não* demonstram sinais óbvios de dor crônica e alguns ocultam ativamente os sinais. Sinais importantes de dor crônica em cães incluem posturas e movimentos anormais, menor interesse em adotar comportamentos sociais, desvios da conduta usual, tremores, respiração ofegante, vocalizações diferentes, alterações no nível geral de atividade, mordida ou lambedura de áreas doloridas ou de membros torácicos e diminuição do apetite.[22-24] Em gatos, os sinais importantes de dor crônica incluem alterações do ato de saltar ou pular, alterações no comportamento de defecação, menores níveis de atividade, diminuição do *grooming* e autoisolamento social.[25,26]

Esforços têm sido feitos para identificar mensurações objetivas de alterações devido à dor (principalmente) musculoesquelética. O exame físico e exames de imagem podem fornecer informações auxiliares para o diagnóstico da dor crônica, mas sua importância é incerta na ausência de um contexto de alterações funcionais e/ou comportamentais. Os métodos de mensuração do escore de claudicação e os achados do exame físico (p. ex., amplitude de movimentação da articulação) apresentam pouca variabilidade interobservadora e ainda não foram validados.[22,27] Assim como para avaliação da dor aguda, mensurações da homeostase e respostas fisiológicas à dor não são específicas para dor crônica. Nem sempre há correlação entre os índices radiográficos de osteoartrite e os níveis de dor, principalmente em gatos.[28-30] Métodos que avaliam forças de reação do solo, como análise da força da placa, são considerados como padrão-ouro para avaliação da claudicação, mesmo que haja limitações substanciais na utilidade clínica dessa técnica.[27,31] A utilização da análise da força da placa como mensuração da dor é baseada na suposição de que a claudicação é equiparada à dor, mas a relação entre dor e claudicação é inconsistente e variável individualmente. Monitores de atividade física demonstraram ser promissores em alguns estudos, mas não em outros, como indicadores do alívio da dor e têm sido utilizados clinicamente em cães e gatos.[26,32-34]

A dor crônica em humanos é reconhecida como uma experiência complexa e individual que não pode ser descrita completamente pela utilização de escalas simples que apenas avaliam a gravidade (unidimensional).[35] A dor crônica em animais supostamente é semelhante, dado que o "mecanismo" que envolve a experiência de dor é o mesmo entre as espécies.[22] A maioria dos autores concorda que a dor crônica pode ser

identificada por meio de alterações do comportamento, da conduta e da função, conforme observado por veterinários e cuidadores.[26,36,37] Entretanto, a situação pode ser mais complicada em gatos. A claudicação não é o sinal mais consistente ou relatado de dor musculoesquelética em gatos, e os tutores podem ser menos capazes de reconhecer os comportamentos de dor em gatos do que em cães.[28,38] Evidências sugerem que veterinários podem não verificar muitas dessas alterações durante uma visita de rotina ao consultório ou até mesmo durante um exame físico minucioso. A limitação mais óbvia é a falta de relatos pelo paciente, mas há contribuição de outros fatores. Estes incluem sinais de dor atenuados pela liberação de hormônios de estresse durante a avaliação, a natureza inconstante da dor crônica e o fato de que a dor neuropática ou visceral crônica frequentemente não é estimulada durante a palpação da lesão. Felizmente, cuidadores podem relatar de modo acurado alterações na locomoção, no comportamento e na conduta, mesmo que eles não percebam que a dor é a causa das alterações.[39-41] Portanto, a orientação de cuidadores quanto aos comportamentos de dor é crucial para sua compreensão sobre a dor que o animal sente. Por exemplo, vários tutores atribuem os sinais de dor ao envelhecimento normal.

Foram desenvolvidas e validadas mensurações de escore multidimensionais para avaliar a dor crônica causada por osteoartrite, em cães e gatos, e por neoplasias ósseas, em cães, bem como para mensurar os efeitos da dor crônica e câncer na qualidade de vida relacionada à saúde em cães.[26,42-44] Os instrumentos de mensuração da qualidade de vida relacionada à saúde são utilizados em medicina humana para avaliar o impacto adverso da dor (ou outros problemas de saúde) na saúde e no bem-estar de modo mais global do que as escalas unidimensionais.[35] Essa abordagem pode descrever melhor como os pacientes manifestam a dor crônica e pode ser utilizada para a tomada de decisões terapêuticas.

Também têm sido utilizados procedimentos veterinários para avaliar a resposta à cirurgia e ao tratamento clínico da dor crônica, bem como para comparar os resultados submetidos ou não à cirurgia.[25,26,37,40,43,45] Exemplos de alguns desses procedimentos podem ser obtidos em: *www.vetmed.helsinki.fi/english/animalpain/hcpi* e *www.CanineBPI.com*.

A resposta à terapia analgésica e remoção da analgesia é um método válido para avaliação da dor crônica, principalmente em pacientes que ocultam sinais ou cujos tutores têm dificuldade para aferir os níveis de dor crônica nos animais.[39] Para serem úteis, os testes com e sem analgésico devem ser realizados juntamente com mensurações de respostas específicas dos pacientes.

Na avaliação da dor crônica ou da resposta ao tratamento, o efeito "placebo" do cuidador é uma fonte frequente de tendência e deve ser considerado ao avaliar os resultados de avaliações.[33,46] A tendência pode-se originar de qualquer avaliador (veterinário ou tutor). Embora esse não seja um verdadeiro efeito placebo (i. e., o paciente não tem um efeito terapêutico a partir de falso tratamento), ele influencia a tomada de decisão terapêutica e deve ser considerado ao avaliar um paciente.

ABORDAGEM GERAL DO PACIENTE COM DOR CRÔNICA

O tratamento da dor crônica é frequentemente frustrante ao veterinário e ao tutor (e provavelmente ao paciente). Algumas das frustações se devem aos limites da abordagem desse problema clínico complexo como uma sucessão de eventos agudos e não de uma verdadeira doença crônica. Muito da frustração pode ser gerada por expectativas irreais dos tutores, que assim como os pacientes com dor crônica, frequentemente buscam uma simples intervenção médica que resolve o problema e os impactos negativos concomitantes em sua qualidade de vida. Embora veterinários e médicos saibam que isso é raramente provável, eles podem ser sido incompetentes ou negligentes quando não conseguem um alívio imediato da dor. Como a dor crônica geralmente é incurável e progressiva, a orientação do tutor e a elaboração de objetivos e expectativas compartilhados são fundamentais para o sucesso do procedimento. A alteração do paradigma de pacientes que buscam o simples alívio do sintoma comparativamente àquele do cenário de objetivos e responsabilidade compartilhados em direção a soluções a longo prazo é descrita como "cuidado de saúde direcionado ao objetivo".[47] Essa abordagem está sendo utilizada para tratar melhor a dor crônica em pessoas e também pode ser útil aos pacientes veterinários. Os objetivos são identificados pela avaliação do impacto da dor crônica na vida diária no paciente e no cuidador, sua relação, e a perda de funções fundamentais para o bem-estar do paciente. A contextualização da dor crônica como parte da vida diária pode ajudar a apontar o que é mais importante, tentar e restaurar. Questionários de tutores simplificam o processo de avaliação diária e o reconhecimento de objetivos realísticos. Um exemplo de pesquisa com o tutor, do autor, pode ser obtido para utilização e adaptação em: *www.angell.org/painsurvey* e *www.angell.org/catpainsurvey* (adaptado de Taylor *et al.*[48]). Aos animais com suspeita de dor crônica, aqueles com doenças crônicas que podem causar dor crônica, ou pacientes geriátricos, o preenchimento prévio de questionários descrevendo o comportamento funcional e social pode melhorar a eficiência da consulta e facilitar a identificação de pacientes com dor mais crônica.

ABORDAGEM GERAL PARA O CONTROLE DE DOR CRÔNICA

Em razão de diferenças entre tipos distintos de dor crônica e a importância do fenótipo genético individual e da epigenética no processamento da dor, não é possível elaborar uma fórmula padronizada para o tratamento. O controle efetivo da dor depende da investigação minuciosa de todas as fontes de dor, já que várias comorbidades impactam as condições dolorosas.

A identificação de mensurações específicas de resultados para o tutor e o paciente, oriundas de pesquisas e consultas iniciais, é fundamental para aferir o progresso ou a falha do procedimento. O aconselhamento de tutores a manter um "diário da dor" ou "diário do conforto", com quatro ou cinco questões simples e personalizadas, pode ser útil, principalmente para aqueles clientes que têm dificuldade em identificar as alterações. Pode ser especialmente útil a inclusão de mensurações personalizadas dos resultados no diário (p. ex., "hoje o seu animal subiu em sua cadeira favorita sem auxílio?"), de modo a instruir os clientes a responder às questões 1 vez/dia, aproximadamente no mesmo horário, e dizer a eles para não revisar o diário de várias semanas de uma só vez, de modo que seja mais útil.

Nas reavaliações presenciais, e não por telefone ou *e-mail*, é possível detectar alterações sutis e permitir ajustes mais acurados do plano terapêutico. A avaliação acurada da dor é melhor quando há reavaliações frequentes pelo mesmo observador. Visitas de reavaliação também ajudam a solidificar a parceria entre o cuidador e o veterinário na abordagem dos cuidados de saúde direcionados aos objetivos.

Planos terapêuticos multimodais e uso de analgésicos não tradicionais e terapias não farmacológicas geralmente são necessárias para o tratamento efetivo de dor crônica significativa.[5,41,49] A detecção do(s) tipo(s) e/ou fonte de dor pode possibilitar uma comparação mais precisa entre as estratégias terapêuticas apropriadas.[50] O clínico deve reconhecer que as condições de dor crônica frequentemente envolvem vários tipos de dor e, à medida que a doença progride, a origem da dor pode se modificar.

A fisiopatologia e o controle apropriado de doença articular degenerativa receberam grande atenção, já que provavelmente é a causa mais comum de dor crônica em pacientes veterinários.[30,41,51] Recomenda-se ao leitor consultar os Capítulos 353 e 355 para informações adicionais sobre esse importante tema.

A dor crônica pode ser classificada como dor somática inflamatória, dor visceral e dor neuropática.[52] Embora as dores somáticas inflamatórias, como dor associada à doença articular degenerativa e otite externa crônica, sejam familiares e frequentemente de fácil detecção, a percepção de dor visceral e neuropática pode ser mais difícil. A dor visceral ou neuropática é frequentemente episódica e espontânea, e seus sinais podem não ser estimulados pela palpação.[52] A dor visceral parece difusa, difícil de ser localizada mesmo quando relatada pelo próprio paciente.[53] A dor referida é a dor visceral sentida em uma estrutura somática próxima ou distante da fonte de dor. A dor visceral, referida ou não, pode se correlacionar pobremente à lesão visceral.[53] O diagnóstico e tratamento de dor visceral e neuropática crônica podem ser um desafio, mas a atenção a elas pode melhorar a resposta terapêutica em doenças crônicas que não respondem a tratamento que apenas almeja a cura da causa incitante.

A etiologia da dor do câncer é diferente e frequentemente mais complexa do que a de outros tipos de dor. As fontes e os mecanismos específicos de geração de dor se modificam durante a progressão proliferativa do câncer, da invasão tecidual e de metástases; da mesma forma, o tratamento da dor deve ser ajustado ao longo da progressão da doença.[54] No microambiente do câncer, são liberados os mediadores que estimulam diretamente nociceptores primários e causam, indiretamente, maior liberação de mediadores nociceptivos. Algumas dessas substâncias algogênicas (indutoras de dor) afetam as células cancerígenas e nociceptoras. Isso leva a alterações marcantes no sistema nervoso periférico e no SNC devido à sensibilização periférica e central. Além das alterações no microambiente do câncer, ocorrem alterações teciduais e sistêmicas durante a invasão tecidual e metástase.[54,55] Portanto, a dor do câncer pode ser inflamatória, neuropática e pode ocorrer no nível central. Para serem efetivos, os protocolos terapêuticos para dor devem considerar todas as fontes de dor.

REFERÊNCIAS BIBLIOGRÁFICAS

As referências bibliográficas deste capítulo se encontram online no Ambiente de Aprendizagem.

SEÇÃO 27
Comorbidades

CAPÍTULO 357

Cardiopatia e Nefropatia

Mark A. Oyama, Shelly L. Vaden e Clarke Atkins

VISÃO GERAL

Doenças cardiovasculares e renais são altamente prevalentes em cães e gatos geriatras. Ambos os sistemas estão envolvidos na regulação do tônus vasomotor e no balanço hídrico. Tanto na saúde quanto na doença, a interação entre os sistemas é fundamental para determinação da pressão sanguínea e volemia. Graças a essa interdependência, o diagnóstico, a terapia e o monitoramento de animais que sofrem de doenças cardiovasculares e renais concomitantes podem ser desafiadores. Em humanos, o termo *síndrome cardiorrenal* é usado para descrever condições nas quais a disfunção de um sistema leva à lesão e à disfunção do outro.[1] Uma importante faceta da síndrome cardiorrenal é o "se e como": se a íntima relação entre os dois sistemas, por meio de mecanismos fisiopatológicos comuns, impacta o resultado. Em pessoas, há evidências crescentes de que o "eixo cardiorrenal" contribui para a morbidade e a mortalidade em vários tipos de doenças cardiovasculares e renais primárias.[2-4] Em 2014, o Cardiorenal Consensus Study Group agrupou especialistas veterinários em cardiologia e nefrologia para desenvolverem uma nota de resumo com relação à definição, à epidemiologia, à fisiopatologia, ao diagnóstico e ao manejo de distúrbios cardiovasculares-renais (DCvRs) em pacientes veterinários. O conteúdo deste capítulo é baseado amplamente em deliberações e conclusões daquele grupo.[5]

EPIDEMIOLOGIA

DCvRs são definidos como danos estruturais e/ou funcionais relacionados com doenças, toxinas ou fármacos ao sistema cardiovascular e/ou renal, levando a distúrbios das interações normais entre os sistemas, até o detrimento contínuo de um ou ambos. Os DCvRs incluem situações nas quais a doença primária de um dos sistemas supostamente leva ao outro – por exemplo, hipertensão sistêmica com lesão do glomérulo –, assim como situações nas quais a doença primária coexiste em ambos os sistemas – por exemplo, um gato com cardiomiopatia hipertrófica e fibrose tubulointersticial –, complicando o tratamento das condições. O clínico não deve considerar só a doença em ambos os órgãos, mas também a direcionalidade da lesão, partindo do órgão primário e indo até o "espectador" (Boxe 357.1).

Boxe 357.1 Etiologias potenciais de distúrbios cardiovasculares renais em cães e gatos

Doença cardiovascular primária causando lesão renal
- Hipertensão sistêmica causando glomerulopatia
- Tromboembolismo arterial sistêmico causando infarto das artérias renais
- Dirofilariose ou doença caval causando glomerulonefrite
- Congestão passiva da veia renal durante insuficiência cardíaca congestiva causando piora da função renal.

Doença renal primária causando lesão cardíaca
- Hipertensão sistêmica mediada pelo rim levando a aumento da pós-carga, hipertrofia ventricular esquerda, piora da insuficiência mitral ou aórtica, arritmias, vasculopatia ou retinopatia
- Sobrecarga volêmica levando à congestão ou à hipertensão sistêmica
- Hipopotassemia ou hiperpotassemia levando a arritmias cardíacas
- Redução da depuração renal de fármacos (p. ex., digoxina) levando à toxicidade

- Oligodipsia, anorexia ou êmese urêmica levando à depleção volêmica e à redução do débito cardíaco e perfusão
- Pericardite urêmica
- Ativação do eixo renina-angiotensina-aldosterona levando à retenção de sódio e água, ao remodelamento cardíaco e vascular ou à congestão
- Anemia secundária a doença renal crônica levando à sobrecarga volêmica e à redução da oxigenação do tecido cardíaco.

Condições sistêmicas causando lesão cardiovascular e renal
- Êmbolos sépticos ou neoplásicos levando a infarto renal e cardíaco
- Dilatação gástrica e vólvulo levando a arritmias cardíacas e azotemia
- Doença infecciosa (p. ex., *Trypanosoma cruzi*)
- Armazenamento de glicogênio levando ao depósito de glicogênio nos rins e no coração
- Amiloidose levando à deposição amiloide nos tecidos renais e cardíacos.

Adaptado de Pouchelon JL, Atkins CE, Bussadori C *et al.*: Cardiovascular-renal axis disorders in the domestic dog and cat: a veterinary consensus statement. *J Small Anim Pract, 56*(9):537-552, 2015.

Mecanismos fisiopatológicos provavelmente importantes em DCvRs incluem alterações hemodinâmicas, ativação neuro-hormonal e espécies reativas de oxigênio (Figura 357.1). Entretanto, a natureza exata e a existência de DCvRs em pacientes veterinários é amplamente teórica e subestudada. Um objetivo fundamental para cardiologistas e nefrologistas no Cardiorenal Study Group foi fomentar a pesquisa colaborativa, baseada na homeostase hemodinâmica dependente de ações cooperativas dos sistemas cardiovascular e renal.

FISIOPATOLOGIA

Existem efeitos adversos conhecidos e suspeitos da doença renal sobre o sistema cardiovascular, os quais envolvem anormalidades eletrolíticas – por exemplo, hiperpotassemia (hiperK) –, intoxicações envolvendo fármacos primariamente depurados pelos rins – por exemplo, digoxina ou enalapril –, depleção volêmica, sobrecarga volêmica e hipertensão sistêmica. Da mesma forma, efeitos adversos conhecidos e suspeitos da doença cardiovascular sobre a função renal incluem diminuição da perfusão renal, ativação de sistemas neuro-hormonais – como os sistemas renina-angiotensina-aldosterona (SRAA) e nervoso simpático –, geração de espécies reativas de oxigênio por tecido endotelial lesado e congestão venosa passiva dos rins. Alguns desses efeitos podem ser ainda piorados pela administração de diuréticos usados para tratar insuficiência cardíaca congestiva (ICC; ver Capítulo 247). Por exemplo, a insuficiência renal aguda discreta (IRA; ver Capítulo 322), definida como uma concentração de creatinina > 1,6 g/dℓ (> 1,7 a 2,5 [> 141 mcmol/ℓ; 142 a 220]), é frequente em cães ou gatos tratados para ICC.[6] Vários clínicos, ao tratarem a ICC, negligenciam essas elevações como insignificantes, independentemente de serem transitórias ou permanentes, o que pode fazer com que a IRA discreta leve a danos estruturais permanentes aos rins e piora do resultado. Além da doença primária do coração ou dos rins, DCvRs também compreendem condições fora desses sistemas.

Exemplos de problemas que podem causar arritmias e/ou comprometimento da perfusão renal incluem sepse, doenças infecciosas e dilatação vólvulo-gástrica.

MANEJO DA CARDIOPATIA E DA NEFROPATIA

Coração

O diagnóstico, o estadiamento e o tratamento clínico de ICC, IRA e doença renal crônica (DRC), como entidades separadas, foram extensivamente descritos.[7-9] Em resumo, a insuficiência cardíaca é a condição na qual o coração doente não consegue fornecer débito adequado ou o faz somente na presença de pressões de preenchimento venosas adequadas e risco de congestão (ver Capítulo 246). O tratamento envolve o uso de diuréticos, como a furosemida; vasodilatadores, incluindo inibidores da enzima conversora de angiotensina (iECA), como o enalapril ou benazepril, e agentes como amlodipino, nitroglicerina e nitroprussiato; agentes bloqueadores neuro-hormonais, como iECAs, espironolactona e bloqueadores beta-adrenérgicos; e inotrópicos positivos, como digoxina, dobutamina e pimobendana.

Rins

A IRA (ver Capítulo 322) e a DRC (ver Capítulo 324) são condições nas quais os rins doentes falham em excretar adequadamente produtos do catabolismo ou em manter o volume hídrico e o balanço eletrolítico adequados. Azotemia, alterações volêmicas, anormalidades eletrolíticas e sinais clínicos resultantes da uremia ocorrem conforme a insuficiência progride. O tratamento pode envolver o uso de fluidos parenterais, vasodilatadores arteriais, iECAs, protetores gastrintestinais, agentes alcalinizantes e estimulantes da eritropoese, quelantes de fosfato e modificação dietética. Diuréticos podem ser indicados quando houver oligúria, sobrecarga volêmica ou hiperK. Com relação a essa discussão, assim que a doença for identificada e se iniciar a terapia, a avaliação da função do órgão pode ser complicada pela

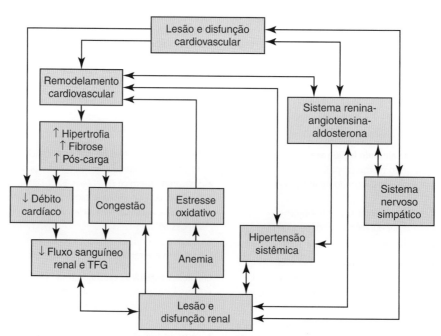

Figura 357.1 Esquema fisiopatológico proposto que liga a lesão e a disfunção cardiovascular e renal em cães e gatos. Lesões nos sistemas cardiovascular, renal ou ambos podem causar ativação de sistemas neuro-hormonais, remodelamento cardíaco patológico, diminuição da função e do débito cardíacos, congestão, baixo fluxo sanguíneo renal, estresse oxidativo e desregulação do tônus vascular. Por fim, há a deterioração progressiva de um ou ambos os sistemas. Essa série de eventos interconectada e complexa requer consideração cuidadosa ao tratar a doença de cada sistema. *TFG*, taxa de filtração glomerular. (Adaptada de Pouchelon JL, Atkins CE, Bussadori C *et al.*: Cardiovascular-renal axis disorders in the domestic dog and cat: a veterinary consensus statement. *J Small Anim Pract*, 56(9):537-552, 2015.)

azotemia, que pode ocorrer em animais submetidos ao tratamento com diuréticos ou iECA, assim como aqueles com cardiopatia e ICC, ao serem tratados com fluidos.

TRATAMENTO DE CONDIÇÕES CONCOMITANTES

Visão geral
Um aspecto crítico do tratamento da doença cardiovascular ou renal é a necessidade de restaurar e manter a homeostase hídrica normal. A IRA e a DRC necessitam de volume e pressão intravascular adequados para suficiente perfusão renal, ao mesmo tempo que se evitam sobrecarga hídrica e desequilíbrios eletrolíticos. A ICC requer redução do volume intravascular e pressão hidrostática por meio de diuréticos e outras terapias redutoras da pré-carga. O tratamento de DCvRs é bastante desafiador, uma vez que cães ou gatos com doença renal avançada costumam necessitar de terapia de reposição hídrica para restaurar a perfusão, enquanto animais com ICC muitas vezes exigem terapia diurética para aliviar a congestão – isto é, edema pulmonar ou efusões em terceiro espaço. A redução do volume vascular em casos de ICC ou aumento no volume vascular em casos de doença renal oligúrica pode levar a efeitos adversos no outro sistema. Diretrizes baseadas em evidências para o reconhecimento e o tratamento de DCvRs são escassas. As recomendações de tratamento do grupo de estudo são baseadas, primariamente, na teoria e na opinião de especialistas.

Manejo da doença cardiovascular em consideração ao rim
Em pacientes com ICC, o alívio da congestão deve se dar com a menor dose necessária de diuréticos, em particular após a fase aguda de resgate. A diurese excessivamente zelosa pode levar à depleção volêmica e a efeitos adversos sobre a perfusão e a função renal. Estratégias para diminuir a incidência de lesão renal incluem a redução da dose diária de diuréticos e o aumento concomitante do débito cardíaco com fármacos inotrópicos, como pimobendana ou dobutamina. Uma minoria de clínicos elege retardar a administração de iECAs na ICC aguda, em razão do risco percebido de lesão renal mediada por iECA na presença de um parenteral agressivo de diuréticos. Uma estratégia potencial, considerada pelo grupo de estudo, é introduzir o iECA no limite inferior da faixa recomendada da dose e ajustá-la conforme a função renal e o estado de hidratação permitirem. A maioria dos clínicos recomenda disponibilidade *ad libitum* de água durante a diurese para ICC, já que a restrição pode levar à contração volêmica excessivamente grave. Em situações de depleção volêmica grave após terapia diurética, a reidratação cuidadosa com atenção às concentrações de sódio (Na) e potássio (K) utilizando fluidos IV SC ou orogástrico é considerada. Sondas de alimentação (ver Capítulo 82) devem ser consideradas em animais anoréxicos para fornecer nutrição e hidratação com níveis reduzidos de Na (ver Capítulos 177 e 189).

Manejo da doença renal em consideração ao coração
A IRA, a DRC ou uma combinação costuma requerer correção do equilíbrio hidreletrolítico anormal para melhorar a função renal, mas aumenta o risco de insuficiência cardíaca em animais com cardiopatia preexistente. Fluidoterapia, diuréticos e agentes anti-hipertensivos devem ser administrados com base no estado de hidratação e pressão sanguínea sistêmica. Os objetivos são restaurar e manter o equilíbrio hídrico normal e a pressão sanguínea, ao mesmo tempo que se evita a sobrecarga de Na ou de fluidos. Em animais com significativa depleção volêmica e sem evidências de ICC, a reposição hídrica parenteral muitas vezes é realizada para restaurar a homeostase hídrica e eletrolítica, bem como para aumentar a produção de urina. Pacientes com IRA e oligoanúria costumam ser submetidos a tratamento com diuréticos, apesar de não haver evidência de qualquer redução na morbidade ou na mortalidade. Uma abordagem cautelosa e passo a passo para reposição hídrica e fluidoterapia de manutenção é recomendada para cães ou gatos com ou sem risco de congestão. Fluidos com baixas concentrações de Na, como o Normosol M ou NaCl 0,18%, em 1,5 ou 4% de dextrose, são administrados ao mesmo tempo que são monitorados peso corporal, frequência e esforço respiratório, além de pressão sanguínea arterial e distensão venosa jugular e/ou ascite.

Necessidades hídricas e de fármacos devem ser continuamente avaliadas, a fim de evitar a congestão. Mesmo sem sinais clínicos de ICC, a suplementação hídrica deve ser intimamente monitorada e descontinuada, caso o ganho de peso seja excessivo. Em situações nas quais ocorrerem sinais de hiperidratação e congestão, a administração de fluidos deve ser descontinuada e a terapia com diuréticos, considerada. As frequências respiratórias em repouso ou dormindo – ou seja, não ofegantes – superiores a 40 movimentos por minuto são um indicador sensível de edema pulmonar inicial. Em pacientes com cardiopatia preexistente ou naqueles que estão recebendo grandes doses de fluidos, a expansão volêmica coloca estresse adicional sobre o sistema cardiovascular e aumenta o risco de congestão. Com exceção de casos de hipotensão sistêmica, a dopamina não é indicada para manejo de pacientes com doença renal, em razão da ausência de eficácia comprovada e de potencial para efeitos colaterais cardíacos adversos, como arritmias e taquicardia sinusal. Terapias de reposição renal, como hemodiálise (ver Capítulo 110), permitem o melhor controle da volemia. Seu papel no tratamento de pacientes com DCvRs necessita de estudos.

Considerações gerais para o tratamento de DCvRs

Hipertensão sistêmica
A hipertensão sistêmica, em razão de sua capacidade de causar lesão cardíaca e renal, é uma causa importante de distúrbios cardiorrenais em humanos e um problema importante, provavelmente subdiagnosticada em cães e gatos. A detecção e o tratamento da hipertensão sistêmica são objetos de várias revisões minuciosas,[10-12] assim como capítulos neste livro-texto (ver Capítulos 99, 157 e 158). Em suma, a mensuração precisa da pressão sanguínea sistólica requer especial atenção ao equipamento e à técnica. O tratamento crônico envolve bloqueadores dos canais de cálcio (amlodipino) e iECA (benazepril ou enalapril) como agentes de primeira escolha em gatos e cães, respectivamente. Outros fármacos anti-hipertensivos, como diuréticos e bloqueadores beta-adrenérgicos, são usados conforme necessários. Os autores costumam recomendar que gatos com hipertensão sistêmica recebam a terapia de combinação com anlodipino e iECA. Em cães e gatos com DCvRs, o objetivo é manter a pressão sanguínea sistólica normal, entre 120 e 160 mmHg, prevenindo ou minimizando o dano hipertensivo aos órgãos-alvo, os quais incluem olhos, cérebro, vasculatura, coração e rins. Conforme a pressão sanguínea aumenta acima de 160 mmHg, o potencial para dano aos órgãos-alvo aumenta e o tratamento anti-hipertensivo é recomendado, a despeito de evidências de danos. Em cães e gatos, a restrição dietética moderada de Na é recomendada em conjunto com a terapia farmacológica concorrente (ver Capítulos 183 e 184).

Fluidos, diuréticos, cardíacos e outros fármacos
Ao que parece, animais com DCvRs são menos tolerantes a alterações extremas do estado volêmico (ver Capítulo 129). Dessa forma, as doses de diuréticos, iECA, inotrópicos e/ou fluidos devem ser cuidadosamente delineadas para as necessidades do paciente, considerando em especial o peso corporal, cada método de eliminação de fármacos e a gravidade relativa das

funções renal e cardíaca. A alteração em diuréticos ou fluidos (tipo e dose) é feita de forma gradual, com monitoramento concorrente do estado de hidratação, do peso corporal, da função renal, da pressão sanguínea e das frequências cardíaca e respiratória em repouso. Quando animais com IRA ou DRC necessitam de expansão volêmica, a administração de fluidos deve ser realizada com precaução. Fluidos parenterais com baixas concentrações de Na ou hidratação enteral com redução de Na por meio de sondas de alimentação devem ser utilizados. Entretanto, qualquer tipo de fluido pode precipitar a ICC ou uma crise hipertensiva se o conteúdo de sal for alto, se os fluidos forem administrados muito rapidamente ou se houver volumes excessivos.

Durante o tratamento, os membros da equipe veterinária e/ou tutores devem monitorar função renal, frequência e esforço respiratório, ingestão hídrica e alimentar, peso corporal e débito urinário do animal. De forma ideal, nos primeiros 3 a 5 dias depois de qualquer ajuste de dose, função renal, peso corporal, hidratação, estado eletrolítico e pressão sanguínea sistólica devem ser reavaliados. Alterações em qualquer parâmetro podem sinalizar mudanças no estado da doença, mas também uma mudança no estado de hidratação e a necessidade de ajuste de medicações. Em situações de DCvRs graves, nos quais o equilíbrio terapêutico é difícil de alcançar, o encaminhamento a um hospital de atendimento secundário ou terciário deve ser considerado. De forma ideal, um cardiologista e um intensivista/nefrologista poderiam formular conjuntamente planos diagnósticos e terapêuticos em pacientes com DCvRs.

Farmacocinética e farmacodinâmica dos medicamentos

Propriedades farmacocinéticas e farmacodinâmicas de medicamentos podem ser alteradas em pacientes com distúrbios da função cardíaca ou renal. Por exemplo, a diminuição da perfusão renal e/ou lesão tubular diminuem a secreção ativa de furosemida por meio de células tubulares renais proximais, ligação aos cotransportadores Na/Cl e resposta esperada frente ao diurético. Vários fármacos cardiovasculares prescritos, como digoxina, enalapril e atenolol, são primariamente excretados pelos rins e podem necessitar de redução de dose em animais com IRA ou DRC. Pacientes com DCvRs podem ter acidose metabólica ou hipoalbuminemia. Doses de fármacos com alta ligação a proteínas (pimobendana ou digoxina) ou alterados por diminuição do pH podem exigir ajustes. Em animais com persistentes efusões em terceiro espaço, ascite ou efusão pleural alterará o volume de distribuição do fármaco, e a dose deve ser realizada por estimativas de peso corporal magro, a fim de evitar a superdosagem.

Suporte nutricional

A garantia de nutrição apropriada é um importante componente do tratamento de DCvRs (ver Capítulos 183 e 184). O apetite e as necessidades nutricionais do paciente devem ser monitorados, com consideração dada ao fornecimento de uma dieta com redução de Na e fosfato (PO_4), ao mesmo tempo que se fornece a ingestão apropriada de proteínas e calorias. A restrição proteica grave, ocasionalmente prescrita em animais com doença renal grave, pode contribuir para caquexia cardíaca em pacientes com cardiopatia coexistente (ver Capítulo 177). O desenvolvimento da caquexia cardíaca muitas vezes necessita de redução da dose, já que o volume de distribuição ou ligação a proteínas podem estar alterados. Dietas com restrição moderada de Na são apropriadas para animais com doença renal ou cardiovascular. A restrição grave de Na pode levar à má ingestão calórica, em razão da diminuição da palatabilidade, ou contribuir para a hiponatremia dilucional em animais com insuficiência cardíaca grave. Animais com doença renal podem ser beneficiados por alterações adicionais no conteúdo de nutrientes, incluindo (mas não limitadas a) alterações do conteúdo de PO_4 e ácidos graxos. Como mencionado, cães com cardiopatia em estágio terminal muitas vezes perdem massa muscular e condição corporal. Portanto, a manutenção da ingestão adequada de proteínas e calorias é um importante objetivo nutricional. Em animais com DCvRs, essas necessidades devem ser balanceadas em relação à ingestão de proteínas e PO_4 para azotemia, lesão renal progressiva e sinais clínicos de uremia. O planejamento cuidadoso dietético, potencialmente em conjunto com um nutricionista veterinário, é recomendado.

REFERÊNCIAS BIBLIOGRÁFICAS

As referências bibliográficas deste capítulo se encontram online no Ambiente de Aprendizagem.

CAPÍTULO 358

Diabetes Melito e Doenças Responsivas a Corticosteroides

Lucy J. Davison

O DILEMA

Corticosteroides têm uma ampla gama de indicações para uso em veterinária (Tabela 358.1). Cães (ver Capítulo 304) e gatos (ver Capítulo 305) afetados por diabetes melito (DM) muitas vezes sofrem de doenças concorrentes, que poderiam se beneficiar do tratamento com corticosteroides. Entretanto, essa situação deixa o clínico com um dilema. Benefícios antecipados da corticoidoterapia devem ser cuidadosamente pesados contra seus efeitos potenciais prejudiciais ao controle glicêmico, como profunda resistência insulínica. Além disso, um animal pré-diabético assintomático pode desenvolver DM evidente assim que

tratado com corticosteroides. Este capítulo revisa o tópico da corticoidoterapia em pacientes pré-diabéticos e diabéticos, incluindo discussão de riscos associados e efeitos colaterais, tomada de decisão clínica e opções alternativas potenciais para indicações específicas.

MEDICAÇÕES CORTICOSTEROIDES

Ações

Corticosteroides são análogos sintéticos dos hormônios adrenocorticais naturais, como cortisol, e podem ter atividades

CAPÍTULO 358 • Diabetes Melito e Doenças Responsivas a Corticosteroides 2195

Tabela 358.1 Indicações comuns para terapia esteroide e possíveis tratamentos alternativos ou que reduzem a necessidade de esteroides que podem ser considerados.

ESPECIALIDADE	CONDIÇÃO	DOSE INICIAL USUAL	CRONICIDADE	POTENCIAIS ALTERNATIVAS AOS ESTEROIDES ORAIS OU POSSÍVEIS MEDICAÇÕES ADICIONAIS QUE POUPAM OS ESTEROIDES
Dermatologia	Urticária (G,C)	Anti-inflamatória	Dias	Anti-histamínicos, esteroide tópico, se localizado
	Dermatite atópica (G,C)	Anti-inflamatória	Semanas a meses, possivelmente permanente	Ciclosporina,[70] ácidos graxos essenciais,[71] oclacitinibe,[70,72] imunoterapia
	Doenças autoimunes (p. ex., pênfigo) (G,C)	Imunossupressora	Semanas a meses, possivelmente permanente	Ciclosporina[73] ± azatioprina[74] (C somente), tacrolimus tópico (C)[75]
Endocrinologia	Hipoadrenocorticismo primário (G,C)	Fisiológica	Permanente	Nenhum, mas use a menor dose possível diariamente. Considere desoxicorticosterona mais um glicocorticoide,[76] se a fludrocortisona estiver impactando o controle glicêmico pela ação glicocorticoide
	Hipoadrenocorticismo atípico (deficiência de cortisol) (G,C)	Fisiológica	Permanente	Nenhum, mas use a menor dose diária possível
	Hipoadrenocorticismo secundário à cirurgia hipofisária (G,C)	Fisiológica	Permanente	Nenhum, mas use a menor dose diária possível
Gastrenterologia	Doença intestinal inflamatória (G,C)	Anti-inflamatória	Semanas a meses, possivelmente permanente	Ciclosporina,[77] manejo dietético, azatioprina (C somente), clorambucila,[78,79] budesonida,[7] metronidazol
	Colangite imunomediada, colângio-hepatite ou hepatite (G,C)	Imunossupressora	Semanas a meses, possivelmente permanente	Ciclosporina, clorambucila, budesonida, metronidazol
	Pancreatite crônica (G)	Anti-inflamatórioa	Dias	Manejo dietético, cuidado de suporte, antieméticos, antibióticos e analgesia[64]
Hematologia	Anemia hemolítica imunomediada (G,C)	Imunossupressora	Semanas a meses, possivelmente permanente	Gamaglobulina intravenosa e leflunomida[80] (C somente), ciclosporina, micofenolato mofetila,[81] esplenectomia[82]
	Trombocitopenia imunomediada (sobretudo C)	Imunossupressora	Semanas a meses, possivelmente permanente	Gamaglobulina intravenosa e leflunomida[80] (C somente), ciclosporina
Doença ortopédica	Poliartrite imunomediada (sobretudo C)	Imunossupressora	Semanas a meses, possivelmente permanente	Ciclosporina (± anti-inflamatórios não esteroidais) ou uso de um segundo imunossupressor para minimizar a dose do esteroide ou leflunomida[83]
Sistema cardiovascular	Vasculite (G,C)	Imunossupressora	Semanas a meses, possivelmente permanente	Fármacos imunossupressores alternativos ou que poupem esteroides[84] (p. ex., ciclosporina[85])
Sistema nervoso	Meningite e arterite responsiva a esteroides (sobretudo C)	Imunossupressora	Semanas a meses, possivelmente permanente	Anti-inflamatório não esteroide em baixa dose pode ser apropriado em casos discretos[86]
	Neoplasia cerebral (G,C)	Anti-inflamatória	Potencialmente permanente, se tolerado	Esteroide em baixa dose pode ser preferível em relação à cirurgia ou eutanásia
Sistema respiratório	Asma (G)	Anti-inflamatória	Semanas a meses, possivelmente permanente	Esteroides inalados (p. ex., budesonida[9] e flucatisona), broncodilatadores, ciclosporina[87]
	Broncopneumopatia eosinofílica (C)	Anti-inflamatória	Semanas a meses, possivelmente permanente	Terapia esteroide inalada[8] (p. ex., flucatisona)
	Complicações secundárias de doenças parasitárias (sobretudo C)	Anti-inflamatória	Dias a semanas	Esteroide em dose baixa pode ser preferível para a inflamação associada a doença parasitária grave
	Rinite alérgica (sobretudo C)	Anti-inflamatória	Semanas a meses, possivelmente permanente	Esteroides inalados, nebulizados ou em gotas nasais, ou anti-inflamatórios não esteroidais com doxiciclina[88] (C)
	Bronquite crônica (sobretudo C)	Anti-inflamatória	Semanas a meses, possivelmente permanente	Esteroides inalados,[8] broncodilatadores

Continua

SEÇÃO 27 • Comorbidades

| Tabela 358.1 | Indicações comuns para terapia esteroide e possíveis tratamentos alternativos ou que reduzem a necessidade de esteroides que podem ser considerados. (*Continuação*) |

ESPECIALIDADE	CONDIÇÃO	DOSE INICIAL USUAL	CRONICIDADE	POTENCIAIS ALTERNATIVAS AOS ESTEROIDES ORAIS OU POSSÍVEIS MEDICAÇÕES ADICIONAIS QUE POUPAM OS ESTEROIDES
Oftalmologia	Uveíte (G,C)	Anti-inflamatória	Dias a semanas	Gotas de esteroides tópicos, ou considere imunossupressão sistêmica, se apropriado
Renal	Glomerulonefrite (G,C)	Imunossupressora	Semanas a meses, possivelmente permanente	Micofenolato mofetila,[89] ciclosporina
Imunologia	Anafilaxia (G,C)	Anti-inflamatória	Dias	Tratamento esteroide pode ser necessário como uma medida que salva vidas ± epinefrina
	Alergia a fármacos (G,C)	Anti-inflamatória	Dias	Dependendo do fármaco que desencadeou a reação, um anti-inflamatório não esteroide ou um anti-histamínico pode ser apropriado em casos mais leves
	Síndrome gengivite-estomatite crônica (G)	Anti-inflamatória ou imunossupressor	Meses	Interferona ômega recombinante[90]
Oncologia	Protocolos quimioterápicos (G,C)	Anti-inflamatória	Permanente, se tolerado em alguns casos	Protocolos que poupam esteroides ou livres deles (p. ex., doxorrubicina como agente único para linfoma[91] [C]), Lomustina[92] ou exclusão da prednisolona do protocolo

C, cão; G, gato.

glicocorticoides e mineralocorticoides.[1] *Ações glicocorticoides* incluem efeitos sobre o metabolismo de carboidratos, proteínas e gordura; antagonismo à insulina; e propriedades anti-inflamatórias dose-dependentes, imunossupressoras, vasoconstritoras e antineoplásicas (ver Capítulo 164 e 165). A *atividade mineralocorticoide* mimetiza a ação da aldosterona de ocorrência natural e impacta o equilíbrio hidreletrolítico nos túbulos renais, primariamente levando à retenção de sódio e água, bem como à perda de potássio (ver Capítulo 67 e 68).

Ao tratar o DM, o antagonismo insulínico associado aos glicocorticoides costuma ser o mais difícil de vencer, por causa de seu impacto sobre o controle glicêmico e o apetite. Receptores de glicocorticoides são amplamente expressos no citoplasma, e a terapia esteroide afeta vários sistemas corporais.[2] Glicocorticoides alteram a expressão de vários genes anti-inflamatórios e pró-inflamatórios. Seu efeito geral é reduzir as respostas inflamatórias e imunes, tornando-os o tratamento de escolha em várias condições imunomediadas e inflamatórias (ver Capítulos 198 e 201 a 204).[3] Além dos efeitos sobre o sistema imune, corticosteroides também afetam o metabolismo com um efeito final de elevação da glicemia.[4,5] Glicocorticoides estimulam a gliconeogênese no fígado pelo aumento da expressão de enzimas envolvidas na geração de glicose a partir de aminoácidos e glicerol.[4,6] Eles promovem lipólise, estimulam a mobilização de aminoácidos pelos tecidos e antagonizam os efeitos da insulina, inibindo a captação de glicose pelas células. Em um animal saudável, a redução da sensibilidade periférica à insulina induzida por corticosteroides é balanceada pelo aumento da função das células beta. A hiperglicemia ocorre se essa compensação não for completamente efetiva, mas isso pode ser problemático em pacientes diabéticos ou pré-diabéticos.[2]

Formulações

Formulações de corticosteroides têm relação de atividade glicocorticoide e mineralocorticoide, efeitos colaterais, potências e durações de ação variáveis (Tabela 358.2). Alguns são predominantemente glicocorticoides; outros, mineralocorticoides.[6]

Tópico e inalado

Além das formulações parenterais, algumas medicações tópicas (olhos, orelhas, pele) e inalantes contêm doses anti-inflamatórias de glicocorticoides. Como os corticosteroides quase sempre são metabolizados pelo sistema p450 hepático, a aplicação tópica desvia do fígado e de seu efeito de primeira passagem hepática, minimizando as doses necessárias e os efeitos colaterais associados.[6] Outras preparações esteroides incluem budesonida, um glicocorticoide designado a humanos com doença de Crohn, que sofre extenso metabolismo hepático de primeira passagem, resultando em efeitos intestinais locais e, teoricamente, evitando efeitos sistêmicos.[7] A flucatisona e a budesonida podem ser usadas como formas inaladas para algumas doenças respiratórias, mas os efeitos sistêmicos foram demonstrados em gatos e pessoas, potencialmente com impactos negativos sobre o controle glicêmico (ver Capítulo 241).[8-11]

Orais e injetáveis

A prednisona costuma ser utilizada graças à alta relação de atividade glicocorticoide e mineralocorticoide. Ela é semelhante à prednisolona, mas bem menos absorvida por via oral em gatos.[12] A dexametasona tem uma relação glicocorticoide/mineralocorticoide semelhante à prednisolona, porém é mais potente, pode ser administrada por via oral ou parenteral e apresenta uma duração mais longa de atividade. A cortisona e a hidrocortisona são glicocorticoides menos potentes, embora sua atividade mineralocorticoide relativamente alta possa ser benéfica

CAPÍTULO 358 • Diabetes Melito e Doenças Responsivas a Corticosteroides

Tabela 358.2 Comparação das atividades glicocorticoide e mineralocorticoide de diferentes fármacos corticosteroides.

FÁRMACO	PROPRIEDADES GLICOCORTICOIDES	PROPRIEDADES MINERALOCORTICOIDES	INDICAÇÃO TERAPÊUTICA GERAL
Glicocorticoides			
Hidrocortisona (C)	1	1	A atividade mineralocorticoide relativamente alta torna seu uso a longo prazo incompatível
Cortisona (C)	0,8	0,8	Semelhante à hidrocortisona
Prednisolona (I)	4	0,8	A alta atividade glicocorticoide a torna útil para tratamento a longo prazo e como anti-inflamatório e imunossupressor
Metilprednisolona (I)	5	Mínima	Anti-inflamatório e imunossupressor
Dexametasona (L)	30	Mínima	Anti-inflamatório e imunossupressor, utilizada especialmente quando a retenção hídrica é indesejável, já que tem atividade mineralocorticoide insignificante. A longa duração de ação a torna útil em algumas condições
Betametasona (L)	30	Negligenciável	Anti-inflamatório e imunossupressor, utilizada em especial quando a retenção hídrica é indesejável, já que tem atividade mineralocorticoide insignificante. A longa duração de ação a torna útil em algumas condições
Mineralocorticoides			
Aldosterona	Nenhuma	500	Útil na deficiência mineralocorticoide. Sem atividade glicocorticoide, então não é útil como anti-inflamatório ou imunossupressor
Fludrocortisona	15	150	Útil na deficiência mineralocorticoide. Atividade glicocorticoide muito baixa, então não é útil como anti-inflamatório ou imunossupressor

C, ação curta, meia-vida biológica 8 a 12 horas; I, ação intermediária, meia-vida biológica 18 a 36 horas; L, ação longa, meia-vida biológica 36 a 54 horas. (Adaptada de http://cks.nice.org.uk/corticosteroids-oral#!scenario.)

no tratamento do hipoadrenocorticismo. O fármaco mineralo-corticoide oral mais usado é a fludrocortisona, prescrita para casos de hipoadrenocorticismo. Ainda que altas doses possam resultar em sinais de excesso de glicocorticoides, a hiperglicemia é rara. Outro efeito colateral importante dos fármacos minera-locorticoides, incluindo o pivalato de desoxicorticosterona, é a perda de potássio. Portanto, é importante que os eletrólitos sejam monitorados, em especial no DM, quando a insulina pode também reduzir o potássio sérico.

EFEITOS COLATERAIS E RISCOS DA TERAPIA ESTEROIDE NO DIABETES MELITO

Antes de qualquer recomendação com relação ao tratamento com corticosteroides em cães e gatos diabéticos, é necessário revisar a patogenia do diabetes nessas espécies e os efeitos cola-terais da terapia esteroide (ver Capítulos 304 e 305).

Diabetes canino e seu tratamento

Em cães, o DM (ver Capítulo 304) é quase sempre uma doença relacionada com deficiência insulínica total e, dessa forma, uma condição insulinodependente, que guarda algumas seme-lhanças no tratamento com o DM tipo 1 humano.[13] O DM é diagnosticado com mais frequência em cães com mais de 7 anos, e a maioria dos pacientes responde melhor às adminis-trações de insulina a cada 12 h, combinadas com alimentação cuidadosa e exercício rotineiro para alcançar o controle glicê-mico.[14] Ao contrário de gatos, cães diabéticos não tendem a ter períodos de remissão diabética, nem existem evidências con-vincentes de que a obesidade contribua para o risco de DM, embora possa contribuir para a resistência insulínica.[15-17] As causas subjacentes da deficiência insulínica são heterogêneas em cães, incluindo inflamação pancreática exócrina – pancre-atite aguda ou crônica –, exaustão das ilhotas como resultado da resistência insulínica crônica – por exemplo, hiperadreno-corticismo, diestro em fêmeas – e possível autoimunidade.[18,19]

O DM reversível canino pode ocorrer em situações específicas nas quais uma síndrome de resistência insulínica, como a pio-metra, pode ser tratada por ovário-histerectomia de forma rápida.[20] De modo geral, entretanto, o DM em cães é irrever-sível. Fatores de risco para DM em cães incluem causas gené-ticas, demonstrados pelo aumento da prevalência em determinadas raças – como Samoyeda, Terrier Tibetano e Poodle Miniatura –, assim como maior risco em cães com histórico de pancreatite, fêmeas inteiras, prenhes e com hipe-radrenocorticismo.[14,21-24] Pode ser prudente evitar a terapia corticosteroide em cães com fatores de risco conhecidos para o DM, pois eles podem já ser pré-diabéticos.

Diabetes felino e seu tratamento

O DM felino (ver Capítulo 305) compartilha várias caracterís-ticas com o DM humano tipo 2, caracterizado por resistência insulínica, e não por deficiência.[13] Além dos fatores de risco relativos à raça (p. ex., gatos Birmaneses), obesidade e inativi-dade aumentam o risco de DM felino.[25] A maioria dos gatos com acromegalia[26] – excesso de secreção de hormônio de cres-cimento por um macroadenoma hipofisário – e a maioria com hiperadrenocorticismo[27] têm DM. Gatos com pancreatite aguda ou crônica apresentam risco maior de desenvolver DM. Ao contrário de cães, não há evidências para DM autoimune em gatos. Felinos diabéticos também costumam ter certa função das células betapancreáticas no momento do diagnóstico.[25] A escolha da terapia depende da glicemia, dos sinais clínicos e da causa subjacente da resistência insulínica. Em alguns casos, a doença discreta pode ser tratada com perda de peso, redução dos carboidratos da dieta e/ou medicamentos hipoglicêmicos. De forma crescente, a insulinoterapia é empregada no início do curso da doença para tentar alcançar um período de remissão do DM,[28,29] que é possível em vários gatos, mesmo naqueles com histórico de cetoacidose diabética ou pancreatite no momento do diagnóstico, porém menos provável naqueles com acrome-galia ou hiperadrenocorticismo, particularmente sem trata-mento específico da condição subjacente.[30] Clínicos devem evitar esteroides em gatos normoglicêmicos com histórico de DM, que provavelmente apresentam redução da sensibilidade à insulina. De forma semelhante, é prudente evitar a terapia corticosteroide, quando possível, em gatos não diabéticos com conhecidos fatores de risco, em especial obesidade e/ou inatividade, pois eles podem já ser pré-diabéticos.[31]

Efeitos colaterais gerais da terapia esteroide

A terapia corticosteroide está associada a uma série de efeitos colaterais potenciais, mesmo em animais saudáveis. O risco de efeitos colaterais aumenta com a dose e a duração do tratamento, e eles são muito variáveis entre determinados indivíduos que recebem doses semelhantes, talvez em razão da variabilidade no número de receptores glicocorticoides.[3] Cães parecem sofrer mais efeitos colaterais esteroides do que gatos, os quais podem ser mais tolerantes a doses maiores, embora o risco de DM ser induzido por corticosteroides seja maior em gatos. É também provável que pacientes muito jovens ou velhos sejam mais suscetíveis aos efeitos colaterais dos esteroides. Determinadas medicações podem interagir com glicocorticoides, como cetoconazol, que pode diminuir o metabolismo de glicocorticoide; e digoxina, que pode resultar em hipopotassemia, se administrada com prednisolona. Assim, tratamentos concorrentes podem aumentar o risco de efeitos prejudiciais pela terapia corticosteroide.

Com o uso a longo prazo de glicocorticoides, sobretudo em altas doses, cães e gatos podem desenvolver os sinais clínicos clássicos de hiperadrenocorticismo: aumento abdominal, perda de massa muscular, polifagia, alopecia bilateral simétrica, poliuria e polidipsia. Outros potenciais efeitos colaterais, além da hiperglicemia induzida pela resistência insulínica, incluem osteoporose, desestabilização da doença cardiovascular, hipertensão, hiperlipidemia, caquexia muscular, proteinúria, estado de hipercoagulabilidade e aumento da suscetibilidade a infecções oportunistas, em especial infecções bacterianas, fúngicas e por leveduras.[32]

Efeitos colaterais da terapia esteroide em pacientes com diabetes melito

Todos os efeitos colaterais de esteroides discutidos previamente são indesejáveis no DM, em particular a resistência insulínica. De fato, há potencial para determinados efeitos colaterais esteroides serem mais comuns ou graves, por diversas razões. Em primeiro lugar, a maioria dos cães com DM[22] e dos gatos[33] é de meia-idade ou idosa, de forma que provavelmente terão condições preexistentes, como nefropatias ou cardiopatias, que podem ser exacerbadas por terapia esteroide. Em segundo lugar, existe uma considerável sobreposição nos sinais clínicos do DM e nos efeitos colaterais da terapia esteroide – poliúria, polidipsia, polifagia, hepatomegalia, ofegação ou fraqueza –, alguns dos quais podem ser exacerbados. Além disso, como animais diabéticos têm maior risco de infecções[22,34] por causa da hiperglicemia persistente, o emprego de esteroides exacerbará esse risco pela imunossupressão. A resistência insulínica como consequência de uma infecção pode complicar as coisas. Se bem que alguns efeitos do início da corticoidoterapia possam ser previsíveis e dose-dependentes, a resposta do paciente com DM depende de uma gama de fatores individuais, incluindo síndromes preexistentes de resistência insulínica – por exemplo, acromegalia em gatos e diestro em cães –, infecções ou doença inflamatória e o grau atual de controle glicêmico.[3] A resistência insulínica induzida por corticosteroides, sem os ajustes adequados na insulinoterapia, pode ter consequências catastróficas, como desenvolvimento de cetoacidose diabética ou síndrome hiperosmolar não cetótica (ver Capítulo 142). De maneira controversa, incrementos na dose de insulina que antecipam a resistência insulínica graças à corticoidoterapia podem levar a episódios hipoglicêmicos perigosos e devem ser evitados.

Tomada de decisão no tratamento de doenças responsivas a corticosteroides em pacientes diabéticos

Visão geral

A decisão de usar medicações à base de corticosteroides em pacientes com DM é desafiadora. Os riscos devem ser pesados em relação aos benefícios (Figura 358.1). Corticosteroides são preferidos em detrimentos de outros medicamentos em diversas condições alérgicas, inflamatórias e autoimunes, por conta de sua efetividade, sua rápida ação e a familiaridade clínica com esses fármacos.[3] Entretanto, o DM é uma doença complexa para tratar, e se qualquer alternativa estiver disponível, deve ser considerada. Em algumas situações, não existe alternativa à terapia esteroide, como na deficiência de cortisol associada ao hipoadrenocorticismo (ver Capítulo 309), em que uma dose fisiológica diária de corticosteroide é vital. A terapia tópica ou local (inalada) pode ser preferível, se apropriada, pois isso pode limitar os efeitos colaterais sistêmicos (ver Tabela 358.1).

Tratamento esteroide de humanos diabéticos

Para pacientes humanos com DM tipo 1 e 2, as diretrizes foram desenvolvidas com relação ao tratamento para doenças responsivas a esteroides concorrentes comuns – asma, doença inflamatória intestinal ou doenças autoimunes.[35] As declarações mais recentes da American Diabetes Association e da European Association for the Study of Diabetes enfatizam a necessidade de monitoramento íntimo e de objetivos terapêuticos individualizados para cada paciente.[36] Diversos tratamentos preventivos podem ser usados para estabilizar a glicemia, desenvolvidos para a farmacodinâmica do glicocorticoide empregado.[37,38] Não há consenso sobre a "melhor prática", destacando a dificuldade em tratar o DM e uma condição "responsiva a esteroides" concorrente.[39] Embora provavelmente haja diferenças espécie-específicas entre cães, gatos e humanos, ainda é benéfico revisar os amplos princípios por trás das diretrizes humanas.

Os efeitos da dexametasona sobre a glicemia em humanos ocorre poucas horas após a administração e são dose-dependentes, de modo que a terapia com altas doses aumenta a resistência insulínica, caracterizada por diminuição da utilização periférica de glicose e distúrbios do transporte de glicose em casos de DM preexistente e recém-diagnosticado.[40,41] Pessoas com DM que recebem terapia esteroide mais de 1 vez/dia tendem a ser hiperglicêmicas durante todo o dia. Aquelas que recebem prednisolona somente 1 vez/dia, pela manhã, costumam passar por hiperglicemia durante a tarde e a noite. Os níveis plasmáticos de prednisolona atingem o pico 2 a 3 horas depois e retornam aos níveis basais em 12 horas.[35,42] A adaptação na função da célula beta frente à resistência insulínica induzida pela dexametasona não ocorre em humanos com baixa sensibilidade insulínica inerente.[43,44] Ainda que a hiperinsulinemia induzida pela dexametasona quase sempre seja acompanhada por normoglicemia em repouso, a desregulação dinâmica da homeostase da glicose por esteroides é enfatizada pela hiperglicemia pós-prandial em alguns indivíduos.[45] Esse efeito de má compensação pode ser observado também em modelos de roedores obesos e relevante para o uso de corticosteroides em gatos obesos,[46] os quais provavelmente apresentam diminuição da sensibilidade insulínica e podem, portanto, ter maior risco de hiperglicemia induzida por esteroides e diabetes.[13]

A colite ulcerativa serve como exemplo de abordagem individualizada recomendada com relação ao tratamento esteroide de pessoas diabéticas. Isso envolve inicialmente a avaliação do DM e a análise dos riscos e dos benefícios da terapia esteroide para a doença concorrente. Na colite ulcerativa, decisões com relação ao tratamento são baseadas na atividade e na localização da doença.[47,48] Em casos de doença grave, o paciente com DM *bem controlado* deve ser tratado com corticosteroides. Entretanto, o início da corticoidoterapia requer monitoramento intenso da

CAPÍTULO 358 • Diabetes Melito e Doenças Responsivas a Corticosteroides 2199

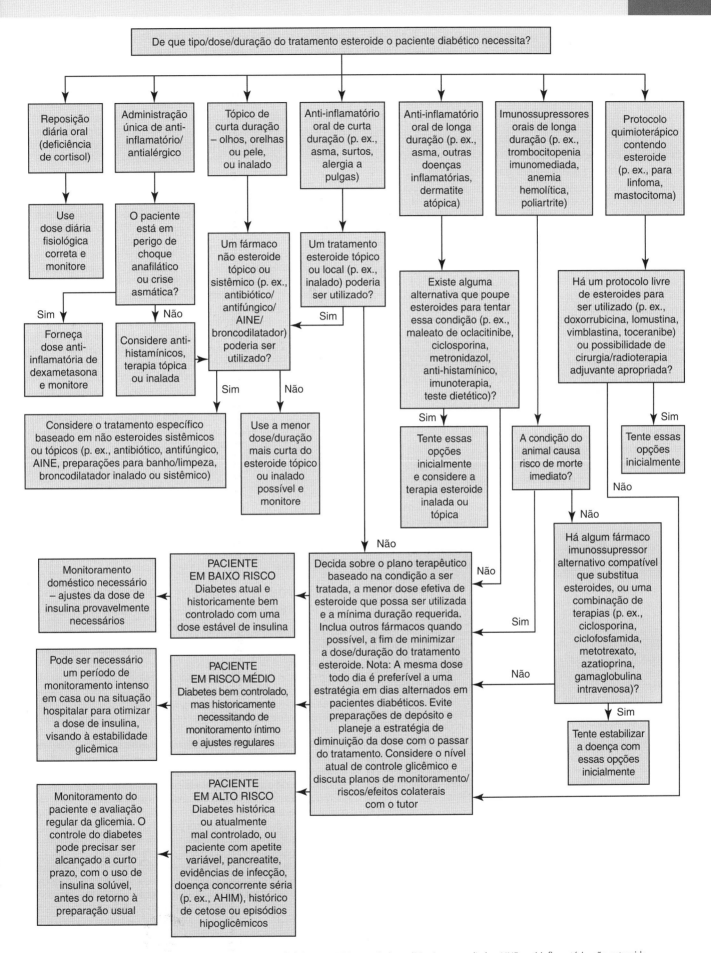

Figura 358.1 Uso de corticosteroides em pacientes diabéticos. *AHIM*, anemia hemolítica imunomediada; *AINE*, anti-inflamatório não esteroide.

glicemia, avaliação para possíveis sepse e cetoacidose, bem como cuidadoso controle eletrolítico. Se o paciente com colite ulcerativa tiver DM *instável*, o risco da terapia esteroide é considerado muito alto e fármacos alternativos são utilizados – ciclosporina, terapia com anticorpos monoclonal.[49] Em casos mais moderados de colite ulcerativa com DM concorrente, para evitar esteroides sistêmicos, a mesalazina tópica ou oral e esteroides tópicos, como a beclametasona, são recomendados.

Evidências do impacto do corticosteroide sobre o controle glicêmico em gatos

O tratamento com esteroides imunossupressores administrados a gatos saudáveis resultou em aumentos significativos de albumina sérica, glicose, triglicerídeos e colesterol após 56 dias.[50] Em um estudo semelhante, na investigação do potencial diabetogênico da prednisolona e da dexametasona, 14 gatos saudáveis receberam prednisolona (4,4 mg/kg) ou dexametasona (0,55 mg/kg) diariamente, por 56 dias, seguida pela avaliação da glicosúria e da frutosamina sérica, além da tolerância à glicose. Na conclusão do estudo, diversos gatos estavam glicosúricos, e os níveis de frutosamina estavam elevados. Também houve uma tendência a maior impacto da dexametasona sobre a glicemia do que a prednisolona em doses "equipotentes".[5] Em uma pesquisa separada, gatos saudáveis foram tratados com metilprednisolona por injeção, resultando em aumento substancial na concentração sérica de glicose 3 a 6 dias depois. Variáveis só retornaram aos níveis basais 16 a 24 dias após o tratamento, com a cinética da resposta variando entre indivíduos.[51,52]

Evidências do impacto do corticosteroide sobre o controle glicêmico em cães

O potencial para a corticoidoterapia impactar a glicemia é ilustrado clinicamente por dois relatos de caso de cães com DM transitório pela terapia com prednisolona.[53,54] De modo experimental, em cães saudáveis, a metilprednisolona aumentou bastante a gliconeogênese e a hiperglicemia induzida por norepinefrina. Esse efeito foi mais marcante quando o glicocorticoide foi administrado por pelo menos 2 dias consecutivos antes do desafio com a epinefrina, sugerindo uma *nova* síntese de enzimas gliconeogênicas e efeitos mais imediatos.[4] O tratamento tópico com glicocorticoides também demonstrou impactar a glicemia em cães. Duas aplicações de dexametasona (dérmica e otológica) foram associadas a um aumento exagerado nos níveis da insulina em Beagles, apesar da manutenção de níveis normais séricos de glicose.[55] Após a remoção do fármaco, levou 1 semana para que a secreção de insulina retornasse aos níveis basais. De forma semelhante, em cães atópicos tratados com prednisolona, as concentrações séricas de frutosamina e glicose não foram afetadas, mas as de insulina aumentaram, enfatizando a necessidade de as células betafuncionais e responsivas manterem a euglicemia.[56] Efeitos do cortisol endógeno sobre o metabolismo de glicose foram examinados em um modelo canino de DM utilizando um desafio IV por glicose, demonstrando uma tendência à tolerância à glicose e que a sensibilidade insulínica diminui após 60 minutos.[57] Isso enfatiza o impacto relativamente imediato do tratamento esteroide sobre o controle glicêmico.

Uso de corticosteroides em cães e gatos diabéticos

Ao tratar comorbidades, o melhor para o tratamento de distúrbios combinados nem sempre é igual à soma dos melhores tratamentos para os dois distúrbios separadamente.[38] Existe também uma diferença importante entre o DM canino e felino a ser considerada: a questão da sensibilidade e da secreção de insulina. Cães diabéticos costumam não ter células betafuncionais. Gatos diabéticos podem ter um número significativo mantido dessas células, sendo importante preservar ou melhorar sua sobrevida e função.[13] Em algumas situações, como anafilaxia com risco de

morte, o uso imediato e a curto prazo de esteroides é prioritário sobre o impacto potencial no manejo do DM.[3] Entretanto, em doenças imunomediadas crônicas ou neoplásicas, pode-se analisar o uso de fármacos imunossupressores ou quimioterápicos alternativos (ver Tabela 358.1).[3] Os últimos podem ser usados sozinhos ou em combinação com doses menores de esteroides, a fim de minimizar o impacto sobre o controle glicêmico. Preparações de esteroides de longa ação podem controlar algumas condições inflamatórias com menores efeitos colaterais, como doenças respiratória e inflamatória intestinal.[7,8]

Uso de alternativas aos corticosteroides

De forma importante, alguns fármacos imunossupressores alternativos também impactam negativamente o controle glicêmico ou a função pancreática. Por exemplo, a ciclosporina, um imunossupressor muito usado na doença atópica, pode aumentar as concentrações de glicose e frutosamina em cães por conta de seu efeito negativo sobre a secreção insulínica.[58] Ao que parece, a ciclosporina precipita o DM em cães com distúrbios da tolerância à glicose.[59-61] É improvável, entretanto, que impacte de forma significativa o controle glicêmico de cães que já sofrem de DM, pois não tem ilhotas funcionais. De forma semelhante, o imunossupressor azatioprina[62] – não recomendado para gatos – foi associado ao desenvolvimento de pancreatite em cães, uma doença que, ao que tudo indica, complica o controle glicêmico.

De fato, a relação entre tratamento corticosteroide e pancreatite é completa e não é bem caracterizada em cães ou gatos, embora a doença seja associada ao DM em ambas as espécies (ver Capítulo 290).[63] Alguns clínicos têm utilizado, com sucesso, doses anti-inflamatórias de prednisolona para o tratamento de pancreatite crônica em gatos (ver Capítulo 291), enquanto evidências experimentais *ex vivo* sugerem que corticosteroides podem ter um efeito prejudicial sobre a função pancreática em cães.[65] Outra opção ao utilizar corticosteroides em casos de DM, sobretudo em gatos, podem ser fármacos hipoglicemiantes orais ou sensibilizadores da insulina como a pioglitazona, que parece ser promissora em gatos obesos.[66,67] Há também benefícios potenciais na suplementação pelo crômio em gatos com distúrbios da tolerância à glicose.[68]

RESUMO: PONTOS IMPORTANTES AO CONSIDERAR CORTICOSTEROIDES PARA CÃES OU GATOS DIABÉTICOS

Assim que a decisão de tratar um cão ou um gato diabético com corticosteroides for tomada, é recomendado seguir as seguintes diretrizes:

1. Corticosteroides orais ou parenterais só devem ser usados quando um diagnóstico certo for alcançado e sob cuidadosa supervisão. Deve-se valer da menor dose efetiva, pelo mínimo período possível, evitando preparações de depósito de longa ação.

2. Cada paciente deve ser avaliado quanto ao risco de exacerbação da doença pelo tratamento esteroide. Os clínicos devem considerar a idade, outras comorbidades – em especial, infecção e síndromes de resistência insulínica –, outros tratamentos – com anti-inflamatórios não esteroidais – e a condição a ser tratada.

3. O tipo e a dose do glicocorticoide deve ser selecionado e utilizado para definir ajustes iniciais no regime da insulina. Preparações de curta ação são preferíveis.[37]

4. Embora a variação diurna do cortisol varie em cães e haja poucos artigos publicados sobre o assunto, muitos veterinários recomendam administrar esteroides em gatos durante a noite e, em cães, durante o dia, a fim de minimizar a supressão adrenal.[69] A despeito do tempo e da frequência escolhidos, é importante que esses momentos de administração sejam respeitados em pacientes diabéticos. Isso minimizará a ampla flutuação nas concentrações de esteroides e a grande

flutuação no controle glicêmico. Aplicações em um momento no dia podem ser preferíveis a protocolos em dias alternados, de modo a tornar mais fácil a manutenção do controle glicêmico – ainda que isso possa levar à maior supressão adrenal. Em pacientes que recebem insulina 2 vezes/dia, alguns clínicos elegem fornecer o esteroide com a dose noturna da insulina, minimizando questões de hiperglicemia pós-prandial, pois uma menor quantidade de alimento é consumida à noite. De forma alternativa, alguns clínicos podem escolher dividir a dose diária do esteroide em duas, para que, em cada período de 12 horas, o paciente receba o mesmo alimento, a mesma dose de esteroide e a mesma dose de insulina.

5. O clínico deve reconhecer que, para o uso de esteroides a longo prazo, a dose de insulina provavelmente necessitará de ajustes para ser compatível com as necessidades do paciente. Ao contrário, assim que a terapia com esteroide for sendo desmamada, o ajuste cuidadoso na dose de insulina deve ser feito, a fim de evitar hipoglicemia.

6. O monitoramento íntimo do paciente é necessário. Para a terapia esteroide em baixas doses em um animal diabético estável, o acompanhamento da glicemia ou da urina em casa, de modo a evitar hiperglicemia profunda ou cetose, pode ser apropriado. Mas, para doenças mais graves ou pacientes diabéticos previamente instáveis, o acompanhamento em ambiente hospitalar pode ser necessário. Atenção rigorosa a glicemia, eletrólitos, pancreatite, infecção ou desestabilização de outras doenças é necessária.

7. Quando doses muito altas de esteroides são necessárias e o paciente apresentar hiporexia, pancreatite ou infecção, deve ser considerada a troca para uma preparação de insulina solúvel de ação curta durante a fase inicial de terapia esteroide, a qual pode ser ajustada mais precisamente, de acordo com a glicemia e o apetite.

8. É útil fornecer ao tutor do animal que estiver recebendo tratamento com corticosteroide um folheto informativo (um exemplo acompanha esse capítulo) para avisá-lo sobre os efeitos adversos e garantir que o tratamento seja ajustado aos poucos, sem interrompê-lo abruptamente.

REFERÊNCIAS BIBLIOGRÁFICAS

As referências bibliográficas deste capítulo se encontram online no Ambiente de Aprendizagem.

CAPÍTULO 359

Comorbidades Associadas à Obesidade

Angela L. Witzel

Taxas de obesidade entre seres humanos subiram muito nos últimos 30 anos e, hoje, têm proporções epidêmicas.[1] Enquanto o tecido adiposo, no passado, era considerado um depósito de armazenamento de energia inativo metabolicamente, hoje sabemos que uma série de hormônios, citocinas e mediadores inflamatórios são produzidos e disseminados por ele.[2] As combinações do excesso de massa exercendo pressão e força sobre o corpo, inflamação em baixo grau causando dano oxidativo e alterações hormonais levando a transtornos metabólicos resultam na associação com a progressão da obesidade para uma série de doenças. Este capítulo revisa a literatura veterinária e humana aplicável para discutir as condições nas quais a obesidade desempenha um papel proeminente no desenvolvimento ou na progressão da doença.

O sobrepeso pode indiretamente contribuir para o desenvolvimento de algumas enfermidades, pois avaliações de saúde geral são mais difíceis em pacientes obesos. Por exemplo, palpação abdominal, auscultação torácica, coleta de sangue, cistocentese, palpação de linfonodos periféricos e exames de imagem são todos mais desafiadores quando camadas espessas de gordura estão presentes.[3] Como resultado, o diagnóstico de doenças sérias, como câncer, doença renal crônica e distúrbios cardíacos valvares pode ser retardado ou perdido. A obesidade (ver Capítulo 176) também pode aumentar riscos e complicações associados a procedimentos anestésicos. O excesso de tecido adiposo pode levar à redução das reservas cardiovasculares, aumentando o risco de comprometimento respiratório e retardando a recuperação após anestesia inalatória em razão da maior deposição do fármaco no tecido adiposo.[4] Consequentemente, as chances de morte anestésica em gatos com mais de 6 kg são quase três vezes maiores do que naqueles que pesam entre 2 e 6 kg.[5]

IMPACTO DA OBESIDADE SOBRE A DOENÇA RESPIRATÓRIA

Foi bem documentado em humanos que a obesidade impacta negativamente a função respiratória. A frequência respiratória média de pacientes obesos (índice de massa corporal ≥ 40 kg/m^2) é de 15 a 21, comparada com 10 a 12 movimentos por minuto em indivíduos de peso normal.[6] Pacientes obesos também tendem a ter volumes corrente e pulmonar reduzidos. Possíveis mecanismos para a redução no volume pulmonar são que a gordura abdominal desloca o diafragma no abdome ou que o excesso de gordura na parede torácica comprime a cadeia torácica.[7] A complacência do sistema respiratório é também reduzida em humanos obesos graças a uma combinação de limitada complacência da parede torácica e pulmonar. A hipoxemia discreta é uma ocorrência comum e pode resultar da microatelectasia nos pulmões. A redução do peso costuma reverter essas alterações respiratórias.[6]

Existe somente um grupo de estudos que avaliam a contribuição da obesidade para a doença respiratória em pacientes veterinários. Uma pesquisa documentou que gatos obesos têm reduções no volume corrente e volume-minuto, além de diminuições dos picos de fluxo inspiratório e expiratório, quando comparados com felinos de peso normal.[8] O volume corrente respiratório também é reduzido em cães obesos.[9] Uma notável diferença entre cães e gatos é o efeito da obesidade sobre a frequência respiratória em repouso. Cães obesos tiveram sua frequência respiratória média aumentada em três vezes ($11,41 \pm 0,94$ *vs.* $33,80 \pm 7,89$).[9] Ao contrário, as frequências respiratórias em repouso de gatos obesos não diferiram daquelas em felinos magros.[8] Outra alteração respiratória característica em cães obesos é o aumento da broncorreatividade.[9] Isso pode contribuir para o broncospasmo e está intimamente associado à asma e à doença pulmonar obstrutiva crônica em humanos.[10]

Relatos anedóticos sugerem que a obesidade contribui para a gravidade de determinadas doenças de vias respiratórias superiores, como a paralisia laríngea e o colapso traqueal em cães, bem como a asma em gatos (ver Capítulo 241).[11] Em humanos, a obesidade é um fator de risco para apneia obstrutiva do sono (AOS), que é resultado do relaxamento do músculo dilatador faríngeo e do colapso das vias respiratórias superiores durante a inspiração (ver Capítulo 238).[12] O Buldogue Inglês é considerado o modelo potencial para AOS.[13] Ao mesmo tempo que a AOS pode levar à hipoventilação e à hipercapnia em humanos dormindo ou conscientes,[14] alterações na Pa_{CO_2} não foram detectadas em cães obesos sob sedação pesada antes ou após a perda de peso.[15] Enquanto somente alguns poucos estudos avaliaram a conexão entre obesidade e doença respiratória em veterinária, uma relação forte foi estabelecida em humanos, e cães e gatos obesos provavelmente têm consequências respiratórias semelhantes. Mais pesquisas são necessárias para explorar o impacto da obesidade sobre as doenças respiratórias como asma, AOS, paralisia laríngea e colapso traqueal em pacientes veterinários (ver Capítulos 176, 238, 239 e 241).

IMPACTO DA OBESIDADE SOBRE A DOENÇA CARDIOVASCULAR

A ligação entre obesidade e doença cardiovascular em humanos é bem estabelecida e foca primariamente no desenvolvimento de cardiopatia isquêmica e hipertensão.[16,17] A obesidade parece ter certa influência sobre o desenvolvimento da hipertensão em cães, mas as alterações atribuídas ao ganho de peso são discretas (5 a 20 mmHg) e, ao que parece, não apresentam consequências patológicas.[18-20] Uma afirmação em consenso pelo American College of Veterinary Internal Medicine concluiu que a obesidade tem impacto mínimo sobre a patogênese da hipertensão canina e felina.[21]

A aterosclerose é rara em cães, gatos, e parece não estar conectada à obesidade.[20] Ao mesmo tempo que cães obesos terão elevações nas concentrações séricas de colesterol total e triglicerídeos, os níveis permanecem abaixo dos esperados como aterogênicos.[20,22,23] Em um estudo comparando gatos cronicamente obesos e magros, o acúmulo de colesterol total não foi diferente, mas o de triglicerídeos dobrou (21 vs. 48 mg/dℓ).[24] Cães e gatos apresentam diferenças importantes de humanos que podem protegê-los do desenvolvimento de aterosclerose e infartos miocárdicos. Primeiro, eles têm elevadas concentrações de colesterol da fração da lipoproteína de alta densidade (HDL). O colesterol HDL é importante para o transporte do colesterol reverso, que o movimenta por artérias e tecidos periféricos até as moléculas do HDL, para o descarte no fígado.[25] Cães e gatos também parecem ter deficiência na enzima proteína de transferência de colesterol esterificado (CETP), que auxilia no transporte do colesterol reverso.[26] A CETP tem o potencial de ser aterogênico pelo aumento do número de moléculas de colesterol de fração de lipoproteína de muito baixa e baixa densidade (VLDL e LDL).[25]

Embora cães obesos possam não ter riscos clinicamente significativos de cardiopatia isquêmica ou hipertensão, há alterações estruturais documentadas no coração. A hipertrofia ventricular esquerda (VE) ocorre em cães obesos e pode ser corrigida com a perda de peso.[27-29] Em humanos, a hipertrofia VE associada à obesidade supostamente é resultado de elevações discretas na pressão sanguínea ou secundárias à hipoxemia crônica pela AOS.[30]

Em humanos, o sobrepeso ou a obesidade moderada está associado ao aumento das sobrevidas em pacientes com insuficiência cardíaca (o "paradoxo da obesidade"; ver Capítulo 177).[31] Entretanto, essa relação é menos evidente em cães e gatos. Em um estudo com 101 felinos com insuficiência cardíaca secundária à cardiomiopatia, houve uma associação em formato U entre o peso corporal e o tempo de sobrevida, na qual os mais leves e mais pesados tiveram sobrevidas mais curtas, quando comparados com gatos no centro da curva.[32] Ao mesmo tempo que não houve relação significativa entre o escore de condição corporal (ECC; ver Capítulos 2, 170 e 177) e a sobrevida, os achados do peso corporal poderiam sugerir que gatos em sobrepeso discreto a moderado poderiam ser beneficiados por um fator protetor.[32] Em um estudo semelhante que avalia cães com insuficiência cardíaca, o tempo de sobrevida também não foi correlacionado ao ECC.[33] Enquanto existem diversas teorias que explicam o motivo pelo qual humanos em sobrepeso mais provavelmente viverão por mais tempo com insuficiência cardíaca do que indivíduos magros, o fato de infartos miocárdicos e cardiopatia isquêmica serem as causas mais comuns de insuficiência cardíaca em humanos significa que extrapolações para cães e gatos não são confiáveis.[31] Em resumo, as consequências cardiovasculares da obesidade em cães e gatos não são tão aparentes quanto em humanos.

IMPACTO DA OBESIDADE SOBRE DOENÇAS MUSCULOESQUELÉTICAS E DO DISCO INTERVERTEBRAL

Em humanos, a obesidade é um fator de risco bem reconhecido para o desenvolvimento de osteoartrite (OA) do joelho.[34] A combinação do aumento da carga sobre a articulação e alterações na direção das forças articulares secundárias à instabilidades explicam a elevação do risco de desenvolvimento de OA com a obesidade.[35] Enquanto alterações nas forças biomecânicas contribuem para a OA no joelho, há também mudanças entre obesidade e OA em articulações que não suportam peso, como a mão.[36] É bem estabelecido que a obesidade leva a um estado de inflamação crônica de baixo grau. Aumentos nas espécies reativas de oxigênio, mediadores inflamatórios, produtos finais avançados de glicosilação e hormônios como a leptina também podem contribuir para o desenvolvimento e/ou a progressão da OA.[37]

Resultados de uma série de projetos que utilizam dados de um estudo sobre a obesidade canina demonstraram um impacto negativo do sobrepeso no desenvolvimento e na gravidade da osteoartrite (ver Capítulos 187 e 353).[38-40] Quarenta e oito filhotes de Labrador foram avaliados por evidências radiográficas de osteoartrite em vários pontos de tempo durante toda a vida. Metade deles foi alimentada ad libitum pelos primeiros 3 anos de vida (grupo-controle), ao passo que a outra metade foi alimentada com 75% da quantidade de alimento dada aos controles (grupo restrito). Os cães do grupo-controle tiveram ECCs maiores durante toda a vida (6,7/9 vs. 4,6/9 aos 12 anos).[41] Os cães com restrição na ingestão calórica apresentaram redução da prevalência e início mais tardio da osteoartrite de quadril quando comparados com os controles (12 vs. 6 anos).[40] Cães em sobrepeso no estudo também tiveram aumento da gravidade radiográfica da artrite do cotovelo e do ombro.[38,39] Enquanto os resultados desses estudos fornecem claras evidências de que o sobrepeso impacta o desenvolvimento e a progressão da OA, os cães nesses estudos estavam somente em discreto sobrepeso, com escores de condição corporal médios de 6,7/9 aos 12 anos. Os resultados provavelmente seriam mais dramáticos em uma população de cães obesos ou obesos mórbidos. Além dos estudos demonstrando que o sobrepeso contribui para a OA em cães, há também evidências de que a redução de peso pode melhorar os sinais clínicos de artrite. A redução de peso em somente 6% resultou em diminuição da claudicação em um estudo de 14 cães obesos com OA, oriundos de tutores.[42]

A obesidade não afeta só o desenvolvimento da OA; é também um contribuinte importante para outras doenças ortopédicas em cães. Os obesos têm quatro vezes mais chances de ter ruptura de ligamento cruzado cranial, enquanto aqueles em sobrepeso apresentam quase o dobro de chances de ter lacerações bilaterais.[43,44] A displasia de quadril é também menos provável em Labradores Retrievers magros, quando comparados com cães em sobrepeso.[45] O risco de desenvolvimento de extrusão de disco intervertebral (EDIV; ver Capítulo 266) é maior em cães obesos de várias raças e tamanhos.[46] Por exemplo, Teckels Miniatura com escores de condição corporal de 9/9 têm quatro vezes mais chances de ter EDIV, quando comparados com Teckels magros.[46]

Comparados com cães, a pesquisa que conecta obesidade à doença musculoesquelética em gatos é esparsa. Em um estudo epidemiológico de quase 1.500 felinos, aqueles em sobrepeso tiveram quase cinco vezes mais chances de necessitar de cuidado veterinário por conta de claudicação, quando comparados com gatos em peso ideal.[47] Em um estudo separado de cerca de 8 mil gatos, animais em sobrepeso tiveram taxas discretamente maiores de artrite (0,4 vs. 0,3%) e obesos tiveram taxas maiores de doença musculoesquelética (0,8 vs. 0,7%), quando comparados com aqueles em peso ideal.[48] Um estudo prospectivo sobre a avaliação da taxa de osteoartrite em 100 gatos com mais de 6 anos não observou correlações entre OA e ECC. Entretanto, somente 14 gatos no estudo tinham ECC maior que 6 em uma escala de 9 pontos, e nenhum deles estava em escore 9.[49] Está claro que mais pesquisas são necessárias para compreender o impacto do sobrepeso ou da obesidade na doença musculoesquelética em gatos.

DOENÇA URINÁRIA

A obesidade é uma doença sistêmica com mediadores inflamatórios, citocinas e hormônios que afetam quase todos os órgãos, incluindo os rins. Em humanos, a obesidade tem sigo ligada a maiores taxas de proteinúria, insuficiência renal, insuficiência renal crônica e mortalidade entre pacientes em diálise.[50] Pacientes obesos apresentam maiores taxas de fluxo plasmático renal, frações de filtração e filtração glomerular, quando comparados com indivíduos não obesos.[51,52] Além disso, a massa renal e o diâmetro dos glomérulos também aumentam com o ganho de peso.[53] A elevação do tamanho glomerular sem expansão concorrente dos podócitos suportando a membrana basal glomerular poderia levar a fendas e perda na seletividade da filtração de proteínas.[50] Se os podócitos se desprenderem ou forem incapazes de cobrir a membrana basal, essas áreas se tornam desnudas, com subsequente glomeruloesclerose.[54] A obesidade também estimula o sistema renina-angiotensina-aldosterona (SRAA), levando à hipertensão glomerular.[50]

Em um estudo avaliando a incidência de proteinúria em cães em sobrepeso e obesos, não houve diferença significativa entre aqueles com escores de condição corporal maiores ou menores que 6 em uma escala de 9 pontos.[55] Em humanos, a obesidade provavelmente resultará mais em alterações renais do que o sobrepeso, e, ao mesmo tempo que os dados foram sugestivos, o estudo não contou com cães obesos suficientes (n = 6 de um total de n = 44) para detectar diferenças significativas em um subgrupo de obesos.[55,56] Quando cães obesos foram admitidos em um programa de perda de peso, múltiplos marcadores de doença renal precoce melhoraram, incluindo relação proteína-creatinina urinária, albumina urinária corrigida pela creatinina, densidade urinária específica, homocisteína, cistatina C e clusterina.[57] Com as altas taxas de obesidade e doença renal em cães e gatos, a caracterização da relação entre essas doenças pode levar ao melhor tratamento e à prevenção da doença renal crônica.

Em humanos, é bem estabelecido que a obesidade aumenta o risco de desenvolvimento de cálculos renais.[58] Cálculos de cálcio correspondem à maioria dos cálculos renais em humanos, e a obesidade pode aumentar o oxalato e reduzir os inibidores dos cálculos de oxalato, como o magnésio e o citrato na urina.[59]

Associações entre cálculos vesicais e obesidade em humanos ainda não foram determinadas, e poucos dados estão disponíveis para cães ou gatos. Um estudo recente avaliando os fatores de risco para o desenvolvimento de cálculos vesicais de oxalato de cálcio não encontrou cães com ECCs maiores em risco aumentado.[60] Uma pesquisa epidemiológica mais antiga observou que cerca de 29% dos cães com urolitíase também estavam em sobrepeso.[61] Entretanto, a taxa de obesidade na população geral do estudo não foi fornecida. Enquanto existem certas evidências de que a obesidade poderia contribuir para o desenvolvimento de cálculos no trato urinário em cães, mais dados são necessários para determinar se ela é um fator significativo no desenvolvimento da doença.

Ao mesmo tempo que a doença urinária é abundante em felídeos, quase não existem dados que avaliem o papel da obesidade na doença renal ou do trato urinário inferior em gatos. A obesidade parece aumentar o risco de cistite idiopática felina (CIF) (ver Capítulo 334).[62] Todavia, alguns fatores de risco para CIF parecem predispor à obesidade. Por exemplo, gatos mantidos confinados têm mais chances de serem inativos, e o ganho de peso e a falta de enriquecimento ambiental também contribuem para a cistite induzida pelo estresse.[62] Um estudo buscando fatores de risco associados ao diagnóstico da doença renal crônica (DRC) em gatos observou uma relação inversa entre ECC e desenvolvimento da doença.[63] Esse estudo avaliou gatos que já tinham sido diagnosticados com DRC, sendo a perda de peso geralmente uma manifestação da doença. Portanto, é difícil determinar se sobrepeso ou obesidade diminui o risco de desenvolvimento da doença, ou se estar mais magro é apenas uma sequela da doença. Em um estudo separado, a prevalência da doença urinária foi aproximadamente 1,5 vez maior em gatos obesos e em sobrepeso, em comparação com animais normais ou abaixo do peso.[64] Dadas as claras associações entre obesidade e doença urinária em humanos, mais trabalhos são necessários em cães e gatos para determinar se as associações epidemiológicas são traduzidas em fatores causadores.

CÂNCER

É estimado que o aumento da adiposidade cause entre 20 e 35% de todos os casos de câncer em humanos.[65] Em 2007, o World Cancer Research Fund observou que a obesidade esteve associada ao aumento das taxas de carcinomas renais, neoplasias colorretais e câncer de mama pós-menopausa.[66] Outras metanálises também demonstraram relações entre obesidade e câncer de próstata, endometrial e esofágico; neoplasias hematológicas; melanoma maligno; e linfomas de células B grandes.[67-74] Conforme o tecido adiposo se expande, os adipócitos se movem além da vasculatura, causando hipoxia local tecidual,[74] que resulta em inflamação crônica de baixo grau, conforme são liberadas citocinas pró-inflamatórias, como TNF-alfa, interleucina 6, proteína quimiotática de monócitos, leptina e inibidor do ativador de plasminogênio tipo 1.[75,76] Além das citocinas inflamatórias, as células estromais/tronco adiposas (CTAs) podem aumentar a proliferação e metástases de células cancerígenas. As CTAs podem se diferenciar em tecido mesenquimal e são privilegiadas do ponto de vista imunológico, já que não expressam moléculas MHC de classe II. Elas podem também ser recrutadas para locais de tumores e, como no caso do câncer de mama, aumentam a liberação de fatores promotores tumorais.[74] Os mecanismos por trás da obesidade e o desenvolvimento do câncer também são específicos de tumores. Por exemplo, alterações em hormônios reprodutivos são importantes fatores para neoplasias de mama e endometriais, enquanto o aumento da produção de insulina provavelmente afetará neoplasias de cólon e próstata.[65,77] Vários outros tipos de câncer podem ocorrer de maneira secundária a condições inflamatórias.[65]

Outra área de preocupação com relação à obesidade e ao câncer é o efeito do excesso de peso corporal sobre a dose dos quimioterápicos. Questões relacionadas com a superdosagem de pacientes obesos que utilizam seu peso atual, em vez de um peso mais próximo do ideal, geralmente são consideradas infundadas na medicina humana. Um artigo de consenso da American

Society of Clinical Oncology recomenda o cálculo da dose de quimioterápicos com base no peso corporal atual ou pela utilização de uma dose fixa, a despeito do índice de massa corpórea.[78]

Enquanto existem claras evidências de que a obesidade contribui para o desenvolvimento e a progressão de vários tipos de câncer em humanos, há muito menos evidências sobre cães e gatos. Cães em sobrepeso ou obesos parecem ter maior risco de neoplasias vesicais e mamárias.[79-81] Existem conexões prováveis entre adiposidade e outros tipos tumorais em cães e gatos, mas são necessárias mais pesquisas para determinar se tais relações existem.

ENDOCRINOPATIA

Desde a descoberta do hormônio adiposo leptina, em 1996, milhares de investigadores confirmaram que o tecido adiposo é um órgão endócrino ativo. Entretanto, o objetivo desta seção é discutir o papel da obesidade no desenvolvimento ou no manejo de endocrinopatias clínicas. A doença endócrina quintessencial relacionada com a obesidade é o diabetes melito tipo 2 (ver Capítulos 304 e 305). Está bem estabelecido que indivíduos obesos são menos sensíveis aos efeitos da insulina em tecidos periféricos, como músculo, fígado e tecido adiposo. Conforme excessos de ácidos graxos livres são depositados nos tecidos, eles alteram a sinalização da insulina, a captação de glicose mediada pela insulina e a síntese de glicogênio.[82,83] Como resultado, a glicose acumula na corrente sanguínea. A hiperglicemia prolongada lesa as células betapancreáticas que secretam insulina. Esse dano provavelmente é resultado de uma combinação da produção sempre crescente da insulina e do acúmulo de espécies reativas de oxigênio. Às vezes, as células beta se tornam "exaustas" e ocorre hipoinsulinemia.[84] Assim que a produção de insulina se torna incapaz de manter os níveis circulantes de glicose normais, ocorre diabetes melito.

Diversos estudos confirmaram uma associação direta entre obesidade e diabetes melito tipo 2 em gatos (ver Capítulo 305).[85-89] Appleton et al. demonstraram que o ganho de peso de apenas 2 kg reduziu a sensibilidade à insulina em cerca de 50%.[85] Gatos obesos também apresentam quase quatro vezes mais chances de desenvolver diabetes melito do que aqueles com o peso ideal.[47]

A associação entre obesidade e diabetes é menos clara em cães (ver Capítulo 304). Enquanto a obesidade demonstrou induzir resistência insulínica em cães,[23] isso não parece progredir para diabetes tipo 2, sendo o tipo 1 é muito mais comum.[90] Há notáveis diferenças entre espécies que desenvolvem diabetes tipo 2 (humanos e gatos) e cães. Primeiro, cães não formam espontaneamente agregados de amiloide nas ilhotas nos pâncreas. O polipeptídio amiloide da ilhota (IAPP), também conhecido como amilina, é cossecretado com a insulina. Conforme a produção de insulina e IAPP aumentam para combater a hiperglicemia, oligômeros intracelulares tóxicos de IAPP e amiloide extracelular são depositados no pâncreas de humanos e gatos, mas não em cães.[90] Outra diferença potencialmente fundamental entre humanos, gatos e cães é a resposta da insulina de primeira fase. Apesar de anos de obesidade e resistência insulínica documentada, os cães ainda conseguem secretar quantidades adequadas de insulina logo após um desafio de glicose.[91] A diminuição da resposta inicial da insulina à glicose em humanos é considerada um importante marcador de danos de células beta.[92]

Enquanto distúrbios da sensibilidade insulínica que acompanham cães obesos podem potencialmente tornar a regulação do diabetes tipo 1 mais difícil, a obesidade provavelmente não é um fator crítico no desenvolvimento da doença. Com isso, cães obesos têm risco discretamente mais alto de desenvolver pancreatite e uma prevalência maior de diabetes melito, em comparação com cães magros (0,7 vs. 0,3%).[48,93]

A relação entre obesidade e outros distúrbios endócrinos comuns além do diabetes melito em cães ainda é incerta. Enquanto a obesidade pode ser um efeito colateral do hipotireoidismo (ver Capítulo 299) e do hiperadrenocorticismo (ver Capítulo 306), parece não ser um fator causador. Em humanos, o hormônio tireoestimulante se correlaciona negativamente com as necessidades energéticas em repouso, mesmo quando as concentrações séricas de hormônio tireoestimulante (TSH) estão nos limites normais.[94] Em um estudo que avalia a função hormonal de cães obesos sem sinais clínicos de doenças endócrinas, os níveis de TSH estavam elevados (> 0,5 ng/mℓ) em 15 de 31 cães. Onze dos 15 cães com TSH elevado também tinham valores baixos de T4 livre. Dos 20 cães obesos que não tinham um padrão clássico de hipotireoidismo nos resultados dos exames, somente 13 apresentavam concentrações normais de T4 livre e TSH.[95] As implicações desse estudo são que a obesidade pode interferir na função tireoideana, mas também seria possível que níveis baixos de hormônios tireoideanos contribuíssem para o desenvolvimento de obesidade (ver Capítulos 299 e 300).

A adiposidade central é uma característica importantíssima do hiperadrenocorticismo ou da doença de Cushing em humanos e cães.[96] O tratamento da doença costuma resultar em perda de gordura abdominal. Existem poucas informações com relação ao papel da obesidade no desenvolvimento da doença de Cushing em cães, e o excesso de adiposidade é visto mais como um efeito colateral do que como uma comorbidade.

DISTÚRBIOS QUE LIMITAM EXERCÍCIOS

Os benefícios dos exercícios para manutenção da saúde física e mental em humanos são bem estabelecidos.[97] Ansiedade, depressão, força muscular e flexibilidade, câncer, saúde cardiovascular e condições crônicas de saúde melhoram todas com atividade física regular.[97-100] Além disso, exercícios moderados e condicionamento físico reduzem taxas de mortalidade. Por exemplo, um estudou demonstrou que corredores com hábitos de corrida de baixa à moderada intensidade tiveram um risco 30% menor de mortalidade por todas as causas e 45% menor de mortalidade cardiovascular, com aumento da expectativa de vida de 3 anos.[101] O Centers for Disease Control and Prevention recomenda que os adultos recebam cerca de duas horas e meia de atividade aeróbica moderada, combinada a 2 dias de treinamento com peso, por semana.[102]

Poucos trabalhos foram realizados em veterinária para estabelecer os benefícios da saúde e níveis ótimos de exercícios em cães e gatos. Entretanto, estudos em cães sugerem que o exercício pode reduzir a sensibilidade a ruídos e comportamentos de ansiedade por separação, melhoram a qualidade de vida para pacientes com doença valvar mitral crônica e diminuem peso corporal e ECC.[103-106] A maioria dos trabalhos relacionados com gatos e exercício focou na relação negativa entre atividade física – estilo de vida confinado vs. fora de casa – e ECC.[107,108]

A capacidade de um indivíduo de se exercitar consistentemente pode ser afetada por várias doenças, incluindo obesidade, cardiopatia, pneumopatia, dor ortopédica, anormalidades neurológicas e doenças sistêmicas, que resultam em letargia e apatia. Os benefícios do exercício vão além do controle do peso, e a atividade física deve ser encorajada em todos os pacientes veterinários. Além disso, os veterinários devem estar cientes das barreiras aos exercícios em nossos pacientes e ajudar a facilitar um maior nível de atividade. Exemplos incluem controle da dor para pacientes com doença ortopédica e redução do peso para animais obesos. Dados os resultados em humanos, mesmo exercícios de baixa intensidade provavelmente fornecerão melhoras de saúde em cães e gatos.[109,110]

RESUMO

A obesidade é a forma mais comum de desnutrição em cães e gatos, com taxas de prevalência maiores que 35%. É uma das doenças mais comuns observadas em animais de companhia.[48,64,111-113] As consequências fisiológicas da obesidade são numerosas e oriundas das combinações de alterações inflamatórias, hormonais e mecânicas no corpo. O impacto da obesidade sobre a saúde geral pode ser demonstrado por seus efeitos sobre a mortalidade. Em um estudo que acompanhou toda a vida de animais em sobrepeso em comparação com cães magros, os segundos viveram quase 2 anos a mais, em média.[114] O controle da obesidade é crítico para a prevenção ou o tratamento de condições referentes aos sistemas respiratório, cardíaco, urinário, musculoesquelético e endócrino. A obesidade também parece influenciar os resultados de vários tipos de câncer. Além disso, a atividade física melhora a saúde mental e física de cães e gatos. A incapacidade de se exercitar deve ser considerada uma comorbidade a condições que impedem a atividade física regular, como obesidade, artrite e doenças cardíacas e respiratórias.

REFERÊNCIAS BIBLIOGRÁFICAS

As referências bibliográficas deste capítulo se encontram online no Ambiente de Aprendizagem.

CAPÍTULO 360

Infecções e Imunossupressão Simultâneas

Nathaniel T. Whitley

Um sistema imune funcional protege contra patógenos e surgimento de neoplasias, evitando respostas adversas a autoantígenos e antígenos inofensivos comensais, ambientais e alimentares. Sempre que o sistema imune for comprometido, há risco de infecção. O comprometimento imune ocorre em razão do uso de fármacos imunossupressores (FI), de imunodeficiência congênita ou de estados adquiridos de imunodeficiência, que incluem dano de patógenos aos tecidos do hospedeiro e subversão do sistema imune ao patógeno. Assim, é necessário que os clínicos previnam, diagnostiquem e tratem infecções em face de imunossupressão. Essa comorbidade apresenta diversos desafios. Algumas infecções só são observadas em pacientes imunocomprometidos, como pneumonia por *Pneumocystis jirovecii*, e o conhecimento de tais patógenos incomuns poderia ser baixo. Alguns sinais clínicos atribuídos a infecções comuns em indivíduos imunocompetentes são resultado de ativação imune e respostas inflamatórias associadas, que podem estar alteradas ou ausentes em indivíduos imunossuprimidos. Maior vigilância é necessária em tais pacientes, algumas vezes exigindo a supervisão e o monitoramento ativos por testes laboratoriais em busca de infecções. Testes comerciais para pesquisar vários componentes da resposta imune não estão disponíveis. Portanto, alguns estados de imunodeficiência podem ser suspeitos ou inferidos com base em padrões ou infecções, mas são difíceis de diagnosticar definitivamente sem acesso a um laboratório de pesquisa.

INFECÇÃO E USO DE FÁRMACO IMUNOSSUPRESSOR

Infecção e tratamento de doença imunomediada

A autoimunidade na ausência de um gatilho identificável é denominada de autoimunidade primária (idiopática). Quando uma infecção provoca uma resposta imune contra tecidos do hospedeiro, trata-se da autoimunidade secundária. Entretanto, algumas infecções mimetizam autoimunidade, e é provável que algumas condições hoje tidas como autoimunidade primária possam ser reconhecidas como distúrbios infecciosos no futuro. Um notável exemplo recente desse desvio é a colite ulcerativa histiocítica em Boxers, que por muito tempo foi considerada uma doença imunomediada idiopática, porém estudos recentes demonstraram ser causada por *E. coli* aderente e invasiva, respondendo a antibióticos apropriados (ver Capítulo 277).[1] Infecções que desencadeiam autoimunidade secundária ou mimetizam algumas vezes autoimunidade primária podem somente ser desmascaradas após semanas ou meses de terapia com FI, como a endocardite bacteriana, de modo que a vigilância e o monitoramento constantes são apropriados. A terapia imunossupressora muitas vezes precisa ser iniciada a curto prazo. No entanto, antes de prescrevê-la, o veterinário deve apreciar os estados mórbidos prévios e atuais que possam conferir maior risco de infecções, a fim de informar aos tutores, abordar comorbidades tratáveis e planejar qualquer terapia suplementar e monitoramento. Exemplos de tais considerações estão listados na Tabela 360.1.

Várias doenças autoimunes causam risco de morte e tendem a recidivar; portanto, a terapia imunossupressora de altas doses, longa duração e generalizada (não direcionada) tem sido a norma. Existe escopo considerável para o refinamento e a redução do uso de FI atuais pela escolha cuidadosa deles, bem como da dose, da duração e do monitoramento, o que deve reduzir todas as complicações, incluindo infecções (Boxe 360.1; ver Capítulo 165 para mais informações).

Tratamento de infecções em pacientes em uso de imunossupressores para doença imunomediada

As permutações incontáveis dessa comorbidade tornam impossível desenvolver um algoritmo universal para guiar o clínico por todos os cenários. Em alguns casos, a tomada de decisão é direta. Os seguintes cenários de casos são exemplos típicos:

- Infecção assintomática do trato urinário com uma bactéria sensível a uma ampla gama de antibióticos é documentada no monitoramento de rotina em um cão que estava sendo desmamado da terapia glicocorticoide. Em primeira instância, 7 a 10 dias de antibióticos bactericidas são prescritos, seguidos por urocultura 7 dias após a conclusão do tratamento com antibiótico
- Sinais discretos de trato respiratório superior com reativação de herpes-vírus latente em um gato tratado com glicocorticoides e ciclosporina para anemia hemolítica imunomediada idiopática, que acabou de entrar em remissão. Como os sinais respiratórios superiores permanecem discretos e não debilitantes, não são necessários ajustes terapêuticos. Se os sinais se

tornarem debilitantes, o clínico necessitará fornecer um maior nível de cuidado de suporte e considerar a redução da dose de um dos FIs antes do planejado. A terapia antiviral também poderia ser instituída.

Em outros casos, em especial aqueles nos quais ocorre infecção com risco de morte em um paciente com autoimunidade que, por si só, seja debilitante ou que cause risco de morte, a tomada de decisão será consideravelmente mais desafiadora. Aqui, respostas muitas vezes são baseadas na opinião profissional oriunda de experiência, anedóticas ou níveis fracos de evidências publicadas. Isso não deve desvalorizar a importância dessas questões, tomando decisões imediatas e procedendo a observações frequentes para determinar o efeito da decisão sobre o estado do paciente. A Tabela 360.2 lista as decisões que precisam ser feitas e questões que devem ser realizadas para tomar as melhores decisões em tais casos. O seguinte exemplo detalhado demonstra a aplicação de diversos desses amplos princípios para dificultar os pontos de decisão durante o tratamento de doenças imunomediadas concorrentes e uma complicação infecciosa.

Tabela 360.1 Diretrizes sobre a prescrição de fármacos imunossupressores – considerações pré-tratamento que influenciam o risco de complicações infecciosas.

FATOR PREEXISTENTE OU COMORBIDADE E EXEMPLOS	COMPLICAÇÃO INFECCIOSA QUE PODERIA SER PRECIPITADA OU PIORADA PELO USO DE FÁRMACOS IMUNOSSUPRESSORES	COMENTÁRIO
Infecção latente Calicivírus felino (ver Capítulo 229) Herpes-vírus felino (ver Capítulo 229) Herpes-vírus canino (ver Capítulo 228) *Toxoplasma gondii* (ver Capítulo 221)	Reativação da infecção latente e eliminação do vírus	A maioria dos casos de reativação de *Toxoplasma* foi associada à terapia com ciclosporina
Implantes cirúrgicos Ortopédicos – prótese de quadril Cardíacos – marca-passo (ver Capítulo 249) Trato urinário – *stents* uretrais e ureterais, dispositivos de desvio ureteral (ver Capítulo 124)	Implante infectado/osteomielite Marca-passo infectado/endocardite Infecção do trato urinário	Implantes de trato urinário ainda são relativamente novos em veterinária. Consequentemente, recomendações de melhores práticas para vigilância de infecções e tratamento ainda estão evoluindo
Cateteres intravenosos Cateter jugular (ver Capítulo 76)	Flebite local, trombo infectado	Potencial para embolização de material infectado a partir do cateter
Sondas de alimentação Esofagostomia (ver Capítulo 82) Gastrotomia endoscópica percutânea (ver Capítulo 82)	Infecções bacterianas ou fúngicas da pele ou cavidade oral, abscesso local	Vários imunossupressores impedem a cicatrização da ferida, comprometendo a formação de aderências estáveis entre a pele e o lúmen esofágicos ou gástricos
Inflamação/infecção de superfície corporal Gengivite/doença periodontal (ver Capítulo 272) Piodermite Otite externa (ver Capítulo 237)	Bacteriemia	
Osteoartrite grave Herança de osteocondrite de cotovelo em Labrador Retriever idoso (ver Capítulo 353)	Artrite séptica	Fluxo sanguíneo e drenagem linfática estão comprometidos ao redor de articulações severamente artríticas
Decúbito prolongado Úlceras de pressão Depuração das vias respiratórias reduzida	Piodermite local, abscesso, bacteriemia, pneumonia, rinite	
Comprometimento de vias respiratórias Paralisia laríngea (PL) (ver Capítulo 239)	Pneumonia por aspiração	Risco ainda se aplica após a correção cirúrgica. A PL costuma ser a primeira manifestação de uma neuropatia mais generalizada
Disfagia Megaesôfago (ver Capítulo 273)	Pneumonia por aspiração	Cuidado particular é necessário quando glicocorticoides são prescritos, já que podem exacerbar a fraqueza muscular
Defeito cardíaco congênito Estenose subaórtica grave (ver Capítulo 250)	Endocardite bacteriana	Associação de doenças foi descrita principalmente com estenose subaórtica, mas também pode se aplicar para outros defeitos congênitos

CAPÍTULO 360 • Infecções e Imunossupressão Simultâneas

Boxe 360.1 Diretrizes sobre refinamento e redução sobre o uso de fármacos imunossupressores para reduzir o risco de infecções

1. **A doença precisa do uso de FI?** Nem todas as doenças autoimunes precisam. Por exemplo, a miastenia *gravis* adquirida canina tem potencial para remissão espontânea com cuidado de suporte apropriado e terapia anticolinesterásica.[2]

2. **Consulte a última literatura sobre a doença em questão.** Alguns estudos de boa qualidade, prospectivos e frequentemente controlados com placebo, estão surgindo, melhorando o nível de evidências disponíveis para guiar as práticas de prescrição. Por exemplo, estudos sequenciais sobre a trombocitopenia imunomediada canina demonstraram que a vincristina, em combinação com a terapia glicocorticoide, reduziu o tempo para o aumento da contagem plaquetária, resultando em tempos de hospitalização mais curta, e que a vincristina foi tão efetiva quanto a imunoglobulina humana IV nesse papel.[3-5]

3. **Faça o melhor uso das opções de monitoramento disponíveis.** Em cães com poliartropatia imunomediada idiopática, mensurações seriadas da proteína C reativa (PCR) e interleucina-6 se correlacionam bem com os níveis de atividade da doença e inflamação sinovial, fornecendo informações objetivas para direcionar o desmame de fármacos imunossupressores, ao mesmo tempo que reduzem a necessidade de artrocenteses seriadas,[6] reduzindo o risco de morbidade. Testes comerciais de PCR estão amplamente disponíveis.

4. **Use glicocorticoides de curta ação orais, injetáveis ou tópicos,** em vez de preparações de longa ação ou de depósito, de forma que a imunossupressão provavelmente ceda logo após descontinuação do agente. Considere o cálculo da dose de prednisolona com base na área de superfície corporal (ASC) para cães maiores, e não com base no peso corporal. Dose máxima imunossupressora sugerida: 50 mg/m²/24 h (Trepanier L, comunicação pessoal, 8 de abril de 2015).

5. **Farmacogenômica.** Tenha ciência do potencial de variações individuais ou relativas às raças na capacidade de metabolizar ou transportar fármacos para dentro ou fora das células. Exemplos incluem variações nos níveis de tiopurina metiltransferase – a enzima que metaboliza azatioprina – e mutações que influenciam a expressão da molécula glicoproteína-p transportadora de efluxo do fármaco. Alguns agentes quimioterápicos, como doxorrubicina, vincristina e vimblastina, são substratos de glicoproteína-p.[8]

6. **Interações farmacológicas.** Por exemplo, a ciclosporina tem inúmeras interações farmacológicas potenciais em razão do seu metabolismo por citocromo P450.[9]

7. **Considere monitorar os níveis sanguíneos do fármaco** – por exemplo, existem testes comerciais para ciclosporina e leflunomida –, a fim de garantir níveis sanguíneos adequados atingidos o mais rapidamente possível, ao mesmo tempo que se evita a superdosagem com o aumento associado do risco de infecções. Para a ciclosporina, o monitoramento farmacodinâmico está também disponível – mensuração de mRNA de células T ativadas para interleucina-2 e interferona-gama – para maior refinamento da dose do fármaco em cães individuais.[10] É provável que novos testes para níveis e efeito de fármacos se tornem disponíveis no futuro.

8. **Examine o horizonte.** Novos agentes permitirão melhor direcionamento de vias específicas de resposta imune em condições mórbidas específicas, para as quais fármacos mais potentes que causam maior imunossupressão generalizada teriam sido utilizados no passado. Exemplos incluem o inibidor de Janus quinase oclacitinibe, aprovado para uso na dermatite atópica canina,[11] e terapia emergente com anticorpos monoclonais "caninizados".[12]

Tabela 360.2 Auxílio à tomada de decisões quando infecções com risco de morte ocorrem em um paciente submetido a tratamento imunossupressor por autoimunidade.

TIPO DE DECISÃO E OPÇÕES	QUESTÕES RELEVANTES ANTES DA TOMADA DE DECISÃO	COMENTÁRIOS
Decisões sobre a infecção		
Tratar a infecção Sim/Não	• A infecção pode ser tratada? • Existem relatos de sucesso terapêutico desse tipo de infecção em pacientes que recebem FIs? • Existe apenas uma infecção? • Quaisquer implicações zoonóticas?	Bem-estar do paciente, desejos do tutor, finanças e prognóstico são fundamentais. Algumas infecções – por exemplo, endocardite de valva aórtica – carreiam um prognóstico ruim mesmo na ausência de terapia com fármaco imunossupressor.
Quando tratar a infecção Imediatamente ou depois	*O que matará primeiro o paciente: infecção ou autoimunidade?*	Em geral, a terapia antimicrobiana é iniciada logo, mas o tratamento cirúrgico da infecção poderia necessitar de ajuste de dose do FI.
Como tratar a infecção Tratamento clínico, cirúrgico ou ambos?	• A infecção é localizada ou generalizada? • Se a cirurgia puder oferecer um melhor prognóstico, o paciente pode estar estável para a cirurgia?	Autoimunidade mal controlada pode impedir anestesia (doença neuromuscular, anemia grave) ou cirurgia (trombocitopenia grave).
Decisões sobre os fármacos imunossupressores		
Alterar a dose/posologia do FI Sim/Não	• A doença autoimune está controlada? • Essa infecção está exacerbando a autoimunidade? • A infecção surgiu por conta de imunossupressão induzida por fármacos? • Existem mielossupressão ou qualquer toxicidade por outro fármaco? • As interações serão prováveis quando os antimicrobianos forem iniciados?	Infecções graves muitas vezes exacerbam a autoimunidade – diversos mecanismos, predominantemente associados ao aumento de citocinas inflamatórias –, mas também podem suprimir as respostas imunes. Portanto, a dose do FI pode precisar ser aumentada ou diminuída. Isso deve ser avaliado com base em cada paciente.
Quando alterar a dose/posologia do FI Imediatamente ou depois	*O que matará primeiro o paciente: infecção ou autoimunidade?*	
Como alterar a dose/posologia do FI • Aumentar a dose • Iniciar outro fármaco • Sem alteração • Redução a curto prazo • Desmame acelerado • Interrupção completa	Veja questões relacionadas com a troca de dose do FI. Também considere: esse é o primeiro episódio, autoimunidade ou uma recidiva?	Autoimunidade recidivante requer desmame mais gradativo dos imunossupressores ou terapia por toda a vida, comparada com o primeiro surto de autoimunidade.

FI, fármaco imunossupressor.

Exemplo: tratamento de miastenia *gravis* e pneumonite/pneumonia por aspiração concomitantes. A miastenia *gravis* adquirida (MGA) é uma doença imunomediada com apresentações clínicas variadas (ver Capítulo 269). Cerca de 85% dos casos têm megaesôfago, sendo a pneumonia por aspiração (ver Capítulo 242) a principal causa de morte em pacientes com MGA. O uso de FIs está destinado a permanecer controverso para o futuro próximo, pois é difícil realizar estudos controlados significativos de uma doença de baixa prevalência com o potencial para remissão espontânea. Quando a pneumonia por aspiração ocorre, uma camada adicional de complexidade é adicionada para o processo de tomada de decisão. O manejo exitoso dessas duas comorbidades e de pares semelhantes de comorbidades requer uma boa compreensão dos mecanismos das comorbidades e das complicações associadas a suas interações, a seleção apropriada de FIs, a escolha correta de antibióticos e outras medidas de suporte essenciais, bem como o monitoramento e a modificação do tratamento.

1. Razões para que pacientes com MGA desenvolvam e sucumbam à pneumonia por aspiração:
   - Ataque mediado autoimune associado à MGA dos receptores nicotínicos de acetilcolina (AChRs) pode causar disfunção esofágica e megaesôfago
   - Risco de aspiração aumenta com a fraqueza dos músculos faríngeos e laríngeos
   - Pacientes com MGA muitas vezes estão em repouso e alguns têm fraqueza de músculos respiratórios, prejudicando os mecanismos normais de limpeza das vias respiratórias
   - Outras doenças imunomediadas que podem afetar a função neuromuscular algumas vezes acompanham a MGA, que, se não forem reconhecidas e tratadas prontamente, podem exacerbar a disfagia. Elas incluem hipoadrenocorticismo, hipotireoidismo e polimiosite. A MGA também ocorre como um fenômeno paraneoplásico, em especial secundário ao timoma
   - Os fármacos anticolinesterásicos – piridostigmina e, algumas vezes, neostigmina – que constituem a terapia-padrão para a MGA apresentam um estreito índice terapêutico e podem causar sialorreia e êmese, aumentando o risco de aspiração maior. Os efeitos colaterais colinérgicos podem ser reduzidos por administração concorrente de atropina ou fornecimento do fármaco com alimento.

2. Indicações e escolha dos fármacos imunossupressores na MGA
   Indicações:
   - Cães com títulos de anticorpos AChR repetidamente aumentados que persistem, apesar da passagem de tempo e da provisão de cuidado de suporte
   - Cães que não respondem bem à terapia anticolinesterásica ou nos quais tais fármacos estejam causando efeitos colaterais inaceitáveis. Cães com títulos positivos para anticorpos AChR, mas em que desafios terapêuticos com edrofônio negativos poderiam em tese responder mal a outros fármacos anticolinesterásicos e, assim, serem candidatos ao tratamento precoce com FI
   - Remoção cirúrgica do tecido neoplásico, se possível, é indicada na MGA paraneoplásica, em detrimento da terapia com FIs – isto é, eliminação da causa de base
   - Dogmas com relação à MGA afirmam que FIs não devem ser iniciados até que a infecção esteja controlada. Entretanto, se um paciente estiver passando por uma pneumonia com risco de morte resultante de frequentes e contínuos eventos de aspiração e a terapia anticolinesterásica não estiver melhorando a transmissão neuromuscular a ponto de cessar esses eventos, a terapia imunossupressora de rápido início para controlar a disfunção neuromuscular imunomediada poderia ser a única esperança para prevenir mais eventos de aspiração. O clínico pragmático perceberá que, em tais situações extremas, há pouco a perder pelo início da terapia com FIs em face da infecção.

Escolha do fármaco:
- Glicocorticoides, se utilizados, podem ser iniciados em uma baixa dose – por exemplo, prednisolona 0,5 mg/kg a cada 24 a 48 h PO ou via tubo de alimentação, ou uso de dose equipotente de um glicocorticoide injetável – e aumentados a cada 2 a 4 dias. Ao mesmo tempo que isso pode ser benéfico e que glicocorticoides injetáveis são fáceis de administrar, razões muitas vezes citadas para evitar glicocorticoides incluem:
- Exacerbação da fraqueza muscular (efeitos sobre a excitação-acoplamento e alteração do canal iônico de AChR)
- Aumento da sede e do apetite, tornando a regurgitação mais provável
- Aumento da ofegância
- Imunossupressão global, incluindo a resposta imune inata (função neutrofílica e macrofágica), piorando a pneumonia
- O succinato sódico de metilprednisolona IV em alta dose foi sugerido para casos de MGA fulminante, já que não exacerba a fraqueza muscular
- Opções que não sejam glicocorticoides ou que os substituam incluem azatioprina, micofenolato mofetila e ciclosporina, que são mais seletivos aos linfócitos com menores efeitos sobre as respostas imunes inatas (ver Capítulo 165)
- Azatioprina atua lentamente, mas em pacientes muito doentes, uma resposta rápida é desejável – mielossupressora e, algumas vezes, hepatotóxica
- Ciclosporina – existem formulações aprovadas para uso veterinário. Há formulações injetáveis. Atua em dias. Monitoramento farmacocinético e farmacodinâmico disponível. Uma proporção significativa (cerca de 25%) de casos com transtornos gastrintestinais nos primeiros dias de terapia
- Micofenolato mofetila – rápida ação. Existem comprimidos, suspensão oral e preparações intravenosas. Menos imunossupressora que a azatioprina, mas doses altas cumulativas podem causar gastrenterite hemorrágica. Benefício a longo prazo não foi comprovado, mas pode ser útil como terapia de resgate na forma grave generalizada de MGA.

3. Escolha do antibiótico e outras medidas de suporte
   - O material aspirado nos pulmões na MGA pode ser uma combinação de conteúdos orofaríngeos, esofágicos e gástricos, provavelmente com substancial contaminação bacteriana
   - De forma ideal, a antibioticoterapia é guiada por resultados de amostras de trato respiratório inferior (ver Capítulo 101), em especial se a terapia prévia falhar ou se fatores de risco estiverem presentes para resistência a vários fármacos. Entretanto, a morbidade associada à sedação ou à anestesia para tais procedimentos de coleta e estudos que demonstram que a maioria dos pacientes com pneumonia por aspiração apresenta resultados de isolados múltiplos bacterianos obrigam o uso de antibioticoterapia de espectro de ação muito amplo para o tratamento empírico inicial
   - Diversos antibióticos têm o potencial de piorar o bloqueio neuromuscular – aminoglicosídeos, ampicilina, ciprofloxacino, eritromicina, imipeném – e devem ser evitados
   - Assim como para outros pacientes com megaesôfago, o oferecimento de alimento e água em uma posição elevada é essencial (ver Capítulo 273). Se não obtiver sucesso, medicações orais provavelmente serão ineficazes, e as administradas por via parenteral devem ser prescritas, ou coloca-se um tubo de gastrotomia endoscópico percutâneo (GEP) (ver Capítulo 82). Como um tubo GEP necessita de anestesia geral, a oportunidade para coleta concorrente das vias respiratórias inferiores deve ser explorada se o estado do paciente permitir. Nota: A terapia glicocorticoide impedirá a formação de aderência estável entre um tubo recém-colocado e a parede corporal, provavelmente mais do que outros fármacos imunossupressores

- Oxigenoterapia e nebulização com solução salina também podem ser benéficos, se tolerados (ver Capítulos 97 e 131)
- Tapotagem deve ser utilizada com cuidado em pacientes com megaesôfago.

4. Monitoramento
- Melhora do estado respiratório e infiltrados pulmonares nas radiografias indicam progresso na pneumonia por aspiração. A antibioticoterapia deve ser mantida por pelo menos 1 semana além do período de resolução clínica
- Títulos seriados de anticorpos AChR costumam estar bem correlacionados com a atividade da doença na MGA. Enquanto uma diminuição do título em resposta a fármacos imunossupressores é encorajadora, não deve ser interpretada como remissão completa da doença até que os FIs tenham sido completamente desmamados com títulos de anticorpos AChR, permanecendo abaixo do nível normal de 0,6 nmol/ℓ
- Se o título de AChR permanecer aumentado, a terapia deve ser continuada mesmo se os sinais clínicos forem resolvidos.

Infecção e quimioterapia antineoplásica (ver Capítulo 343)

FIs citotóxicos (mielossupressores) formam o pilar de vários regimes quimioterápicos antineoplásicos. Assim que a carga tumoral for reduzida de um nível macroscópico para um microscópico, uma diminuição na contagem sanguínea de neutrófilos para menos que 3 mil células/$\mu\ell$ tem sido utilizada como um marcador substituto de provável eficácia do fármaco. Foi sugerido que a intensidade ótima da dose é definida pela administração de doses de fármacos imunossupressores que fornecem um nadir de neutrófilos entre mil e 1,5 mil células/$\mu\ell$, devendo-se considerar o aumento da dose do fármaco para o próximo ciclo, se isso não for alcançado.[13] Se esse objetivo for adotado, é essencial que a lógica por trás dessa prática seja compreendida pelo tutor do paciente e todos os clínicos envolvidos, bem como que o monitoramento hematológico estabeleça o nadir de neutrófilos para cada fármaco mielossupressor. Entretanto, sendo a grave neutropenia a toxicidade dose-limitante mais comum desses medicamentos, poucos oncologistas veterinários estão preparados para agir no limite da legalidade, com muitos considerando um nadir de 3 mil células/$\mu\ell$ ou logo abaixo. Contagens de neutrófilos e plaquetas devem sempre ser verificadas antes da administração de qualquer outro agente mielossupressor, com adiamento até que a contagem de neutrófilos exceda 3 mil células/$\mu\ell$. Uma contagem de neutrófilos menor que mil células/$\mu\ell$, ou longa duração da neutropenia independentemente da gravidade, deve levar à redução imediata de todas as doses subsequentes daquele fármaco mielossupressor, geralmente em 20 a 30%. A maioria dos oncologistas veterinários acredita que uma contagem de neutrófilos maior que mil células/$\mu\ell$ seja adequada para lutar contra a infecção e que esse nível confere ainda um baixo risco de infecções.[14] O risco de sepse aumenta muito com contagens de neutrófilos menores que 500 células/$\mu\ell$. Fatores de risco para neutropenia grave induzida por quimioterapia incluem baixo peso corporal, tumores hematológicos, medicamento utilizado e estar na fase de indução.[15] Portanto, é necessária vigilância do tutor e do veterinário com relação a quaisquer sinais clínicos que poderiam sugerir uma infecção relacionada com a neutropenia e uma compreensão de que infecções ainda ocorrem em pacientes não neutropênicos em quimioterapia. A necessidade para uso profilático ou terapêutico de antibióticos em pacientes em quimioterapia depende da presença ou da ausência de sinais clínicos, em especial febre, e da contagem sanguínea absoluta de neutrófilos. Deve ser notado que a neutropenia, por si só, não causa sinais clínicos.

Tratamento de pacientes neutropênicos assintomáticos

Se a contagem de neutrófilos estiver entre mil e 3 mil células/$\mu\ell$, antibióticos não são necessários, a menos que outros fatores de risco independentes para infecções estejam presentes (ver Tabela 360.1). Quando a contagem de neutrófilos estiver abaixo de mil células/$\mu\ell$, antibióticos orais profiláticos são indicados e a contagem de neutrófilos deve ser reavaliada em 3 a 7 dias. A escolha do antibiótico pode ser restrita às diretrizes de prescrição institucionais. Como se acredita que a sepse em pacientes neutropênicos supostamente resulta de translocação gastrintestinal de bactérias aeróbicas gram-negativas e que bactérias anaeróbicas previnem o crescimento excessivo de aeróbicos no intestino, deve ser dada consideração à prescrição de agentes com mínimo espectro anaeróbico.[15] Embora a hospitalização, em geral, não seja necessária, a observação íntima é essencial, e qualquer alteração nos sinais vitais ou na atitude, redução do apetite ou sinais gastrintestinais em casa devem desencadear reavaliação urgente pelo veterinário em busca de evidências de infecções/sepse.

Tratamento de pacientes neutropênicos sintomáticos

A deterioração do estado físico de um paciente neutropênico deve levar à imediata intervenção para prevenir ou abordar a septicemia. Enquanto o início da febre é de preocupação particular, sua presença não deve ser tida como um marcador obrigatório da sepse, sobretudo em gatos, já que alguns pacientes sépticos têm disfunção imune tão grave que não podem liberar quantidades suficientes de citocinas para gerar uma febre.[16] Após medidas padronizadas apropriadas para qualquer paciente com doença séria – exame físico meticuloso, hemograma, perfil bioquímico e urinálise –, o clínico não deve permitir tentativas exaustivas de identificar a fonte da infecção que tenham prioridade sobre o estabelecimento de acesso IV, utilizando técnica asséptica meticulosa, e instituição de antibioticoterapia parenteral em conjunto com apropriada fluidoterapia IV e monitoramento hemodinâmico. Qualquer medida de suporte adicional necessária – por exemplo, antieméticos, analgesia ou hemocomponentes – pode ser iniciada. Em geral, cobertura antibiótica de muito amplo espectro (quatro quadrantes) é apropriada inicialmente, a menos que haja evidências fortes que impliquem um sistema específico de órgãos e classe de bactérias na doença. Antibióticos podem precisar ser utilizados no limite superior das doses recomendadas para compensar a redução da perfusão de órgãos na sepse.[17] A antibioticoterapia pode ser refinada quando os resultados de cultura estiverem disponíveis e em luz da progressão do caso, levando em conta o problema crescente da resistência antibiótica nas medicinas humana e veterinária. A maioria dos pacientes neutropênicos sintomáticos em quimioterapia responde ao cuidado de suporte apropriado nas primeiras 24 horas. O fator de estimulação da colônia de granulócitos (G-CSF) recombinante poderia ser considerado em pacientes que receberam uma superdosagem inadvertida por fármaco mielossupressor ou quando persistir a neutropenia profunda por mais de 1 semana. Todavia, o uso rotineiro de G-CSF deve ser desencorajado, haja vista que cães neutropênicos devem ter altas concentrações endógenas de G-CSF e que a terapia com o produto recombinante humano carreia o risco de reação cruzada para formação de anticorpos.[18]

Em comparação, o tratamento de pacientes humanos com febre e neutropenia é direcionado pelas avaliações do risco estratificado, baseadas em evidências maiores e opinião de corpo de especialistas, comparadas com o que está disponível em veterinária. Algoritmos estão sendo desenvolvidos para compreender o uso empírico ou preventivo de terapia antifúngica e antiviral além dos antibióticos em alguns grupos de pacientes. Aqueles em alto risco são os com neutropenia antecipada prolongada (> 7 dias) e profunda (< 100 células/$\mu\ell$) e/ou com comorbidades significativas, como hipotensão, pneumonia, novos episódios deflagrados de dor abdominal ou alterações neurológicas. Pacientes em baixo risco são aqueles com uma neutropenia antecipada como breve (< 7 dias), com nenhuma ou poucas comorbidades, os quais são tratados com antibióticos orais profiláticos.[19]

Infecções no transplante de órgãos (ver Capítulo 323)

O transplante renal está disponível para gatos que sofrem de doença renal irreversível em alguns poucos centros na América do Norte e em um na Austrália. Os receptores recebem terapia imunossupressora por toda a vida, incluindo glicocorticoides e ciclosporina. As infecções pós-transplante são uma causa comum de deterioração do enxerto, morbidade e mortalidade. Também podem ser responsáveis por alta hospitalar adiada e admissões múltiplas e, muitas vezes, prolongadas. No maior estudo publicado sobre infecções em gatos após transplante renal, a infecção correspondeu à morte de 14% dos receptores, ficando atrás somente após da rejeição ao enxerto.[20] Metade das infecções ocorreu dentro de 2,5 meses do transplante, quando a imunossupressão foi maior. Gatos com diabetes melito têm risco significativamente maior de infecção. Infecções bacterianas foram as mais comuns, incluindo aquelas associadas a trato urinário, tubos de alimentação, *Mycobacterium* spp. e *Nocardia* spp. Infecções virais – afetando sobretudo o trato respiratório superior – foram as segundas mais comuns, seguidas por fúngicas e protozoáricas.[20]

A avaliação pré-cirúrgica do doador e do receptor é minuciosa (ver Capítulo 32). Infecções do trato urinário devem ter sido tratadas com sucesso, com duas culturas negativas pós-tratamento. Um desafio com ciclosporina pode ser realizado se houver suspeita de pielonefrite, com urina ressubmetida para cultura após 7 dias da administração de ciclosporina. Uma instituição aceitou gatos com doença do trato respiratório superior viral crônica para transplante se a doença estivesse bem controlada no momento da avaliação e os sinais clínicos não piorassem após teste com ciclosporina.[21] A toxoplasmose disseminada foi diagnosticada em receptores felinos e caninos de transplante renal.[22] Como resultado, algumas instituições colocam gatos soropositivos para *T. gondii* em um tratamento com clindamicina por toda a vida, a fim de evitar recrudescência. É importante notar que, em um pequeno estudo a curto prazo realizado como parte da aplicação de licenciamento da ciclosporina, gatos saudáveis soronegativos para *T. gondii* e que receberam ciclosporina sofreram com uma forma mais grave da doença do que soropositivos quando a terapia com ciclosporina foi iniciada.[23]

Quando ocorre infecção em um receptor de transplante renal, em conjunto com a terapia antimicrobiana apropriada, é imperativo que o clínico verifique que a imunossupressão esteja em seu maior nível. Acúmulos sanguíneos de ciclosporina não devem estar anormalmente altos, o que sugeriria imunossupressão excessiva, nem anormalmente baixos, o que poderia comprometer o enxerto. Assim como em outros pacientes imunocomprometidos, a terapia antimicrobiana pode precisar ser administrada por um período mais prolongado e em maiores doses do que o ideal.

O transplante renal em cães é minado por desafios que costumam expor taxas intransponíveis muito altas de morbidade e mortalidade por infecções associadas aos regimes terapêuticos imunossupressores substancialmente mais agressivos, necessários para prevenir rejeições do enxerto.[24-26]

Uso de glicocorticoides no tratamento de doenças infecciosas

Contrário ao dogma, não existe contraindicação absoluta ao uso de fármacos imunossupressores na presença de infecções. Há situações clínicas selecionadas nas quais o uso a curto prazo de agentes anti-inflamatórios ou imunossupressores, predominantemente glicocorticoides, é de grande benefício ao paciente. Entretanto, como existem poucos estudos veterinários que avaliam a segurança e a eficácia da terapia combinada imunossupressora e antimicrobiana, os clínicos devem avaliar riscos e benefícios dessa prática em cada indivíduo. O uso empírico de glicocorticoides em todos os pacientes com certa infecção não é apropriado, porém não é proibido na presença de infecções.

Infecções que causam autoimunidade secundária

Várias infecções podem desencadear processos imunomediados secundários com um efeito adverso sobre o hospedeiro, incluindo formação de anticorpos contra eritrócitos, plaquetas, megacariócitos e neutrófilos, bem como formação de imunocomplexos.[27] Ao mesmo tempo que diversas infecções virais, bacterianas, protozoáricas e helmínticas podem estar envolvidas, as transmitidas por vetores são cada vez mais incriminadas. A crescente literatura sobre doenças transmitidas por vetores (DTV), alterações na taxonomia, identificação de novos agentes e coinfecções –[28] e, algumas vezes, testes demorados e caros necessários para o diagnóstico de DTV – contribui para o desafio significativo que o clínico encontra para identificar e tratar essa comorbidade particular, na qual os limites entre autoimunidade primária e secundária podem ser difíceis de definir. Se os resultados de testes para infecções estiverem pendentes, todavia o estado do paciente ditar que o tratamento seja iniciado, a terapia antimicrobiana empírica apropriada para o agente suspeito deve ser iniciada antes ou junto com a terapia com glicocorticoide. A terapia glicocorticoide não será necessária para todos os casos, e a antimicrobiana imediata aumenta as chances de resolução espontânea da autoimunidade secundária sem o uso de glicocorticoides. Se a suspeita de infecção perdurar, apesar de resultados negativos de exames, o clínico deve permanecer cético sobre a longevidade de qualquer melhora clínica que segue a terapia glicocorticoide inicial e vigilante a sinais sutis que poderiam refletir a piora da infecção. A repetição do teste deve ser considerada, em especial para condições nas quais a cultura é apropriada, já que a terapia glicocorticoide pode aumentar a probabilidade de identificação da infecção. Um dos poucos estudos publicados relacionados com a autoimunidade secundária descreve a febre das Montanhas Rochosas experimentalmente induzida. Cães tratados com doxiciclina e doses imunossupressoras de glicocorticoides não tiveram doença mais grave do que aqueles tratados somente com doxiciclina[29]. No entanto, outros relatam recidiva da parasitemia quando cães que tinham se recuperado de infecções por riquétsias, após tratamento com doxiciclina, foram tratados com doses imunossupressoras de glicocorticoides.[30] Também foi sugerido que a terapia glicocorticoide poderia ser benéfica em citopenias cíclicas associadas a leucemia felina (FeLV), anemias associadas à FeLV nas quais um componente autodestrutivo está envolvido ou coinfecção com micoplasma hemotrópicos existe, e para uso a curto prazo na babesiose. Foi sugerido que a aplasia pura de células vermelhas em gatos com infecção por FeLV seria beneficiada pela terapia com glicocorticoide e ciclosporina.[30]

Infecções que causam inflamação debilitante ou com risco de morte

Em algumas infecções, a inflamação secundária ao dano celular, resposta imune adversa aos antígenos do patógeno, e uma liberação maior de mediadores inflamatórios durante a morte/lise do patógeno durante o tratamento se tornam mais perigosas do que a destruição tecidual pelo próprio patógeno. Isso é especialmente pertinente em infecções que envolvem pulmões, olhos ou sistema nervoso central. Uma recente metanálise oferece visões fascinantes sobre os potenciais benefícios e malefícios da administração de glicocorticoides sistêmicos em combinação com antimicrobianos apropriados para a doença no tratamento de infecções em humanos.[31] Infecções foram categorizadas em grupos de acordo com a possibilidade de melhora da sobrevida com glicocorticoides (p. ex., meningite bacteriana ou tuberculose, tétano grave, pneumonia por *Pneumocystis*), redução da incapacidade a longo prazo (artrite bacteriana), alívio significativo dos sintomas – efusão crônica de orelha média, laringotraqueobronquite aguda, celulite – ou benefício ou malefício incerto (hepatite viral).[31] A duração da terapia geralmente foi a curto prazo (< 14 dias), e a dose do glicocorticoide variou muito entre os estudos.

Em veterinária, o uso de glicocorticoides anti-inflamatórios foi sugerido como benéfico ao manejar a pneumonite com risco de morte induzida pelo tratamento de micoses sistêmicas, dirofilariose ou leptospirose grave; para tosse prolongada em cães com traqueobronquite infecciosa; para redução da inflamação na peritonite infecciosa felina; e para estomatite ulceroproliferativa associada ao calicivírus felino – algumas vezes com ciclosporina.[30,32] Doses imunossupressoras de glicocorticoides são consideradas apropriadas para a celulite juvenil ("garrotilho de filhotes").[32]

Um estudo retrospectivo sobre uso concorrente de antifúngicos e glicocorticoides sistêmicos (prednisolona 0,7 mg/kg/dia PO por uma duração média de 3 meses) para o tratamento de blastomicose ocular em 12 cães concluiu que esteroides não afetaram a taxa de sobrevida de forma adversa.[33] Um breve relato comparando a terapia glicocorticoide com a anti-inflamatória não esteroide para casos de blastomicose pulmonar grave em cães não observou diferença no resultado.[34] Outro estudo sobre o uso de prednisolona ou prednisona (2 a 4 mg/kg/dia PO), com ou sem antifúngicos sistêmicos, levou a uma resolução mais rápida da linfadenopatia hilar causada por histoplasmose crônica do que a terapia antifúngica solo, novamente sem disseminação da doença. Os casos foram cuidadosamente triados, a fim de descartar histoplasmose aguda.[35]

Glicocorticoides no choque séptico

Alguns veterinários utilizam a terapia de reposição de glicocorticoide (hidrocortisona) em baixa dose na hipotensão refratária a vasopressores com sobrecarga volêmica associada a choque séptico e condições relacionadas (ver Capítulo 132). Controvérsias com relação às melhores estratégias diagnósticas e terapêuticas para esse fenômeno, chamado de insuficiência corticosteroide relacionada com doença crítica, foram recentemente revisadas[36] e são discutidas no Capítulo 133.

ESTADOS DE IMUNODEFICIÊNCIA NÃO INDUZIDOS POR FÁRMACOS IMUNOSSUPRESSORES

Estados de imunodeficiência de ocorrência natural podem ser divididos em imunodeficiências primárias (congênitas, em geral hereditárias) e secundárias (adquiridas). Características principais consistentes com a imunodeficiência incluem:
- Infecções recorrentes ou crônicas (especialmente respiratórias, cutâneas, gastrintestinais ou urinárias), em geral com resposta incompleta a antimicrobianos
- Infecções oportunistas por organismos normalmente inofensivos ou incomuns, em geral com manifestações graves de doença
- Resposta adversa a vacinas vivas modificadas
- Neonatos doentes desnutridos/fracos.

Imunodeficiências primárias são incomuns em cães e raras em gatos. O conhecimento dos distúrbios mais prevalentes e raças afetadas, ou previsão para consultar uma lista de tais distúrbios quando apresentados por um paciente com características clínicas sugestivas, é fundamental para a confirmação do diagnóstico. Distúrbios específicos foram revisados em outros capítulos.[37] O prognóstico varia de acordo com a natureza do déficit, sendo que várias das imunodeficiências graves são fatais.[38]

Estados de imunodeficiência secundária são comuns em cães e gatos, compreendendo um grande grupo heterogêneo de distúrbios que afetam animais nascidos com todos os componentes do sistema imune intactos, mas que desenvolvem distúrbios imunes transitórios ou permanentes graças ao estágio de vida, a um estado mórbido ou à exposição a fármacos específicos, infecções ou toxinas. Amplas categorias de imunodeficiência secundária estão relacionadas com idade (p. ex., privação do colostro), disfunção de órgãos (em especial endocrinopatias), dano de barreiras (p. ex., queimaduras e cateteres), distúrbios nutricionais e coinfecções imunossupressoras. Em várias imunodeficiências secundárias, o distúrbio de base é transitório ou pode ser corrigido ou controlado, maximizando o potencial para controle de qualquer infecção resultante. Por exemplo, infecções bacterianas do trato urinário são comuns em pacientes que sofrem de diabetes melito ou hiperadrenocorticismo. O controle rígido da endocrinopatia deve reduzir a frequência e a gravidade de infecções urinárias, mas não remove a necessidade de vigilância rotineira (uroculturas) em diabéticos.

Imunossupressão causada por infecção

Patógenos de sucesso, por definição, devem romper barreiras físicas e suprimir ou subverter as respostas imunes do hospedeiro para facilitar a própria sobrevida e propagação. Assim, a infecção gera imunossupressão, que, por sua vez, gera outras infecções. Mecanismos de imunossupressão induzida pelo patógeno são tão numerosos e variados quanto os próprios patógenos, com o braço comprometido do sistema imune influenciando diretamente o tipo de infecções secundárias. O dano a barreiras físicas e os distúrbios da função de granulócitos facilitam a invasão bacteriana e, algumas vezes, fúngica. A imunidade celular alterada pode permitir que patógenos oportunistas (p. ex., *Nocardia* spp., *Toxoplasma gondii*) se estabeleçam,[39] e a imunidade humoral comprometida favorece bactérias piogênicas. A infecção imunossupressora é arquetípica pelo vírus da imunodeficiência felina, o qual tem efeitos complexos sobre o sistema imune,[40] com depleção de células T CD4$^+$ (células T-helper) e ativação de células T-reguladoras como principais eventos.[40,41] Vários outros patógenos importantes infectam células do sistema imune (FeLV, cinomose canina, *Ehrlichia canis*, *Anaplasma phagocytophilum* e *Leishmania*). Parvovírus canino e felino têm tropismo por células em rápida divisão, causando a combinação devastadora de dano massivo à barreira – perda de células da cripta epitelial intestinal –, com sequestro associado de neutrófilos, e mielossupressão. Outros patógenos apresentam efeitos em cascata sobre células imunes – a cápsula de polissacarídeos glicuronil-xilomannan do *Cryptococcus* sp. inibe fagocitose, migração leucocitária, respostas do complemento e Th1 – ou efeitos diretos sobre a função de barreira – *Bordetella bronchiseptica* paralisa os cílios respiratórios.[39]

Tamanha é a diversidade dos efeitos de patógenos sobre o sistema imune e outros tecidos-alvo que coinfecções e infecções secundárias são inevitáveis. O reconhecimento, o tratamento e a prevenção dessas infecções secundárias necessitam de capacidade de diagnosticar a infecção primária e de compreensão detalhada sobre os efeitos do patógeno e da estratégia de sobrevida.

REFERÊNCIAS BIBLIOGRÁFICAS

As referências bibliográficas deste capítulo se encontram online no Ambiente de Aprendizagem.

Índice Alfabético

A

Abdome
- agudo, 593
- médio, 345
Abdominocentese, 348, 598
- de grande volume, 349
- de quatro quadrantes às cegas, 349
- simples
-- às cegas, 349
-- guiada por ultrassom, 349
Aberrações cromossômicas, 1887
Abertura da boca, 1480
Ablação
- a *laser* guiada por cistoscopia de ureteres
  ectópicos intramurais em cães, 498
- endoscópica a *laser*
-- de vestígios vestibulovaginais, 496
-- guiada por ultrassom de carcinomas de células de
  transição do trato urinário inferior, 493
- pelo calor percutânea guiada por ultrassom, 1740
- percutânea com etanol guiada por ultrassom, 1739
- total de canal auditivo, 1064
Abordagem
- ao paciente com estupor ou coma, 139
- ao proprietário do animal, 1
- clínica e avaliação laboratorial da doença renal, 1925
- da febre, 195
- da questão do odor corporal, 105
- diagnóstica de manifestações ortopédicas de
  doenças sistêmicas, 70
- geral do paciente
-- com dor crônica, 2188, 2189
-- com trauma, 612
-- mecanicista da anemia, 228
- nutricional
-- de afecções dermatológicas, 781
-- do câncer, 788
-- do hipertireoidismo em gatos, 761
- para avaliação de leucocitose e leucopenia, 233
- revisada da fluidoterapia, 1947
Aborto medicamentoso, 1885
Abscesso(s)
- do saco anal, 1612
- hepáticos e esplênicos, 605
- prostático, 2059
- pulmonar, 1139
Absorção, 677
- e secreção de água e eletrólitos, 1527, 1577
Acantócitos, 229
Acantoma infundibular queratinizante, 2107
Ação diurética, 1949
Acepromazina, 628, 2040
Acesso
- perineal percutâneo para uretrocistoscopia rígida
  em cães machos, 496
- vascular, 424
Acetato de megestrol, 1876
Acidente vascular encefálico, 1435
Ácido(s)
- 5-amino salicílico, 1589
- acetilsalicílico, 1309, 1335, 1355
- alfalipoico, 633, 642
- biliares, 1627, 1817
-- não conjugados séricos, 1559

- docosa-hexaenoico, 753
- graxos, 750
-- de cadeia curta, 751
-- essenciais, 727
-- poli-insaturados, 817
--- ômega-3, 747, 753, 1973
- linoleico conjugado, 741
- tióctico, 642
- ursodeoxicólico, 1633, 1634
Acidose, 593
- láctica, 277
- metabólica, 528, 1953, 1966, 1976
-- por ácidos minerais, 1952
- respiratória, 528
- tubular renal, 1997
Acidúrias orgânicas, 1394
Aconselhamento genético, 30
Acrodermatite letal, 52
Acromegalia, 54, 1721, 1809
ACTH endógeno, 1820
Actinomicose, 922, 926
Actinomyces spp, 926
Açúcares, 731
Acúmulo de líquido no abdome, 79
Adenite sebácea, 874
Adenocarcinoma, 1524
- colorretal, 1595
- de saco anal, 2109
- intestinal, 1571
- prostático, 1918
Adenoma(s)
- de paratireoide, 1739
- hepatocelulares, 1685
- intestinal, 1571
Adenovírus canino
- tipo 1, 1015
- tipo 2, 1009, 1017
Adequação nutricional das dietas caseiras, 807, 808
Adiamento do estro
- com acetato
-- de medroxiprogesterona, 1877
-- de megestrol, 1876
- com andrógenos, 1877
- com proligestona, 1877
Adipocinas, 736, 737
Adipsia, 3
Aditivos, 536
Administração
- da transfusão, 544
- de corticosteroides, 1800
- de doses pequenas de glargina e detemir, 1806
- de medicamentos por meio de inaladores com
  dosímetro, 369
- de nutrição parenteral, 795
- de soluções de uso intravenoso, 581
- de vacinação, 906
- intramuscular ou subcutânea de insulina, 592
- oral de cálcio, 1745
Adrenal, 345
Adrenalectomia, 1826
Adrenomedulina, 1169
Adsorção, 422
Adsorventes, 627
Adubo composto, 633

Aelurostrongylus abstrusus, 1121
Aerossolização, 1005
Aflatoxinas, 1682
Afogamento, 1137
Agalaxia, 1897
Agenesia
- da bexiga, 2054
- renal, 2004
Agentes
- alquilantes, 704, 2067
- anestésicos, 1895
- bloqueadores, 1332
- de contraste, 462
- embólicos, 461
- estimuladores de eritropoese, 847
- estimulantes de eritrócitos, 1978
- infecciosos e lúpus eritematoso sistêmico, 878
- modificadores da motilidade e da secreção, 1547
- procinéticos do cólon, 1602
Aglepristone, 1901
Aglutinação, 229
- espermática, 1913
Agonistas
- da dopamina, 1902
- de hormônio liberador de gonadotrofina, 1878
- do adrenorreceptor alfa-2, 707
- do receptor
-- alfa-2 adrenérgico, 520
-- de dopamina, 1875
-- kappa, 706
- dopaminérgicos, 1878
- e antagonistas opioides, 569
- GNRH, 1884
- parciais do receptor mu, 706
Ajuste
- de Bonferroni, 38
- de comparações múltiplas, 38
Alanina aminotransferase, 255, 256, 1624, 1817
Albumina, 537, 1845
Albuterol, 642, 1952
Alcalose
- metabólica, 529
- respiratória, 528
Aldosterona sérica, 1839
Alelo, 25, 28
Alendronato, 1776
Alergia(s), 801
- alimentar, 802, 1555
Alfaxalona, 570, 573
Algas, 1593
- verde-azuladas, 1683
Algoritmo do eletrocardiograma, 579
Alimentação
- assistida, 722
- com dieta crua, 810
- do paciente com doença cardíaca, 774
- do recém-nascido, 724
- dos gatos e cães com câncer, 788
- e apetite, 2
- por esofagostomia, 1975
Alimentos
- comerciais não convencionais, 806
- de origem vegetal e fertilizantes, 633
- tóxicos, 651

Índice Alfabético

Aloenxerto, 1958
Aloimunização de plaquetas, 545
Alongamento do palato mole, 1080
Alopecia, 2087
- areata, 874
- associada às doenças sistêmicas, 50
- paraneoplásica felina, 52, 2157
Alopurinol, 2027
Alquilantes, 2067
Alterações
- cíclicas durante o ciclo estral, 452
- da capacidade de concentração urinária, 1963
- da síntese de hormônios renais, 1962
- de pulso, 221
- do peso corporal, 3
- do tipo de gordura, 767
- geriátricas no sono e ritmo circadiano, 1420
- na biologia do miócito, 1171
- na cor da urina, 189
- na pigmentação, 2087
- na prática de vacinação, 902
- neuro-hormonais, 1164
-- da função renal, 1167
-- dos vasos sanguíneos periféricos, 1168
- no padrão respiratório, 141
- nos miócitos e não miócitos, 1169
- relacionadas com nutrientes e com animais de
   estimação em envelhecimento, 733
Alucinógenos, 646
Alvos moleculares, 2084
Amantadina, 707, 708
Amarílis, 651
Ameloblastomas, 1485
Amidos, 731
Amilase, 253
Amilina, 1798, 1808
Amiloide, 1677
Amiloidose, 1677, 1988, 2004
- canina, 1678
- familiar, 2004
- hepática felina, 1677
Aminoácidos, 726
Aminoacidúria, 1933
Aminoglicosídeos, 688, 1945
Aminotransferases, 255
Amiodarona, 1681
Amitraz, 633
Amônia, 278, 1627
Amostra(s)
- de biopsia com *punch*, 339
- de tamanho pequeno, 38
- do líquido articular, 360
Amplitude
- da movimentação e alongamento, 2181
- do pulso, 1213
Amputação de membro, 2130
Anaerobiospirillum, 1591
Anafilaxia, 566
Analgesia, 1700
- farmacológica sistêmica, 519
- locorregional, 519
- multimodal, 519
- preemptiva, 519
- preventiva, 519
Analgésicos, 1514
- adjuntos para a dor crônica e direções futuras, 709
- anti-inflamatórios não esteroides, 698
Análise
- da composição do cálculo, 2031
- da efusão, 1147
- de hormônios séricos, 1866
- do(s) líquido(s)
-- abdominal livre, 601
-- cefalorraquidiano, 993, 1392, 1402
-- corporais, 289
-- da efusão, 992
- dos gases sanguíneos, 525
- química, 281
Análogos da insulina, 591, 1789
Anaplasma
- *phagocytophilum*, 953
- *platys*, 954
Anaplasmose, 953
Anatomia
- da cartilagem, 1085

- do pericárdio, 1312
- do peritônio, 1615
- dos ureteres, 2009
- funcional
-- do intestino delgado, 1526
-- do sistema imune de mucosa, 1529
Ancilostomídeos, 1553
Ancylostoma caninum, 1553
Anemia(s), 94, 225, 539, 593, 1964, 2156
- caracterização da, 843
- causas da, 225
- da doença renal crônica, 1978
- hemofagocíticas, 838
- hemolítica
-- hereditárias, 838
-- imunomediada, 821, 828, 833, 838
--- canina, 839
--- felina, 841
-- não imunes adquiridas, 837
- não regenerativa, 227, 842, 845
- regenerativa, 122, 833, 834
Anestesia, 302
- e cesariana, 610
Anestésicos locais, 708
Anestro, 452, 1864, 1868, 1883
- primário, 1885
- secundário, 1885
Anfetaminas, 643
Anfotericina B, 689, 691
- lipossomal, 691
Angiodisplasia, 1598
Angiogênese, 2065
Angiografia, 1358
- por ressonância magnética, 1658
- por tomografia computadorizada, 1658
Angiostrongylus vasorum, 1122
Angiotensinogênio, 737
Angústia respiratória, 116, 573
- aguda, 1087, 1116
Animal cianótico, 209
Animal-alvo e formulação, 694
Anlodipino, 1180, 1776
Anomalia(s)
- arteriais, 1254
- cerebrais, 1393
- da bexiga, 2054
- da junção ureterovesical, 2053
- da uretra, 2055
- de câmara, 402
- de Pelger-Huët, 860
- de úraco, 2055
- do cérebro, 1419
- vasculares, 1253, 1457
-- hepáticas, 1651
- venosas, 1254
Anorexia, 98, 1962
- induzida pela quimioterapia, 2089
Anormalidade(s)
- clínicas potenciais em cães, 49
- clinicopatológicas, 225
-- diagnóstico diferencial de, 225
- com destruição e consumo de plaquetas, 238
- com sequestro de plaquetas, 238
- congênitas
-- do intestino delgado, 1533
-- do pericárdio, 1313
- da cavidade pleural, 574
- da condução, 1201
- da córnea, 57
- da excitabilidade, 1189
-- atrial, 1192
-- ventricular, 1197
- da medula óssea, 985
- da micção, 2050
- da mielinização, 134
- da multiplicação celular, 71
- de armazenamento, 2036
- de consumo e ativação plaquetária, 238
- de esvaziamento, 2039
- de movimento tipo tremor, 132
- de ureter congênitas, 2014
- detectadas no exame físico, 193
- do anel vascular, 1496
- do ciclo estral, 1885
- do ritmo cardíaco, 1188

- e alterações da excitabilidade sinusal, 1190
- eletrolíticas, 62, 93
- eritrocitárias, 229
- esqueléticas em animais de companhia, 2159,
   2163
- hematológicas, 2095
- na produção de plaquetas, 236
- no neurônio motor
-- inferior da bexiga, 2039
-- superior da bexiga, 2040
- no ritmo cardíaco, 1189
- ortopédicas
-- tratamento cirúrgico de, 2169
-- tratamento não cirúrgico das, 2169
- por diluição da quantidade de plaquetas, 238
- radiográficas dos pulmões, 1096
- relacionadas
-- ao potássio, 288
-- ao sódio, 286
- relativas ao hormônio de crescimento
-- em cães, 1720
-- em gatos, 1715
- vasculares, 71, 215
Anovulação, 1886
Ansiedade, 46
Antagonistas
- alfa-2, 570
- da N-metil-D-aspartato (NMDA), 708
- de canais de cálcio, 1949
- do receptor
-- da neuroquinina-1, 708
-- de progesterona, 1875
Anti-inflamatórios, 1700
- não esteroides, 200, 640, 1945
Antibacterianos, 1560
Antibióticos, 1514, 1647, 1700, 1945
- antineoplásicos, 2067, 2068
- betalactâmicos, 688
- derivados de lactonas macrocíclicas, 1330
Anticoagulação, 424
Anticoagulantes, 631, 829, 1951
- adquiridos, 831
- mais recentes, 1356
Anticolinérgicos, 570, 581
Anticorpo(s)
- anti-histona, 880
- anti-insulina, 1795
- antifosfolipídios, 880
- antinucleares, 880
- contra vírus da imunodeficiência felina
   maternos, 982
- em líquidos corporais, 899
- induzidos por agentes estimulantes de
   eritrócitos, 1978
- monoclonais, 2081
- para DNA, 880
- patogênicos, 877
- séricos, 898
Antidepressivos tricíclicos, 639
Antídotos para etilenoglicol, 636
Antieméticos, 1513, 1700
Antifúngicos, 689
- azóis, 1680
Antígenos
- das hemácias
-- de gatos, 540
-- dos cães, 543
- de coronavírus felino em macrófagos, 993
- nucleares extraíveis, 880
Antimetabólitos, 2069
Antimicrobianos, 1951
- betalactâmicos, 906
Antioxidantes, 709, 710, 753, 773, 1973
Antiplaquetário, 829
Antitoxina, 935
Antitrombina, 1932
Antivirais, 692
Anúria, 1948
Aparatos de iscas para insetos, 633
Aparência, 1815
- radiográfica dos urólitos, 2023
Apatita de CaP, 2022
Apelina, 737
Apetite, 1815

Índice Alfabético

Aplasia
- da faceta articular, 1449
- uretral, 2046, 2055
Apneia do sono, 1421
Aprovação de vacinas, 901
Aquecimento
- ativo, 202
- passivo, 202
- por ar forçado, 202
- por resistência, 202
Aquisição de potencial de replicação ilimitado, 2064
Aranha viúva-negra, 656
Área sob a curva, 683
Arginina vasopressina, 1168
Armazenamento
- da insulina, 1806
- do endoscópio, 331
Arritmia, 126, 584
- cardíacas, 1186, 1515
- sinusal
-- respiratória, 1190
-- ventriculofásica, 1190
- ventricular, 1281
Artefatos, 399
Artérias, 298
Arteriograma mesentérico cranial, 1659
Articulações sinoviais, 359
Artrite
- bacteriana associada à forma l, 866
- de Lyme, 918
-- em cães, 920
- proliferativa periosteal felina, 870
- reumatoide, 75, 870
- séptica, 73, 866
Artrocentese, 75, 359
Artroscopia, 359
Ascarídeos, 1552
Ascite, 1623, 1638
Aspartato aminotransferase, 255, 256, 1624
Aspergilose
- do trato respiratório superior, 1046
- em cães, 1042
- em gatos, 1046
- invasiva disseminada, 1050
- nasossinusal, 1042
- sinonasal, 1078
- sistêmica, 1045
Aspiração
- com agulha fina, 1630, 1687, 2140
- de linfonodos, 361
- de medula óssea, 353, 354
- por agulha fina, 338, 886
- pulmonar de conteúdo da sonda, 327
- testicular por agulha fina e biopsia, 1909
- transbronquial com agulha fina, 382
Aspirado
- por agulha fina, 2107, 2113
-- renal e biopsia, 1943
- transtorácico com agulha e biopsia, 1101
Astenia, 92
- cutânea, 54
Astenozoospermia, 1913
Astrocitoma, 1399
Astrovírus, 1025
Ataxia, 135, 136, 1375
- cerebelar, 136, 1376
- espinocerebelar, 130
- proprioceptiva, 136
-- generalizada, 1375
- vestibular, 136, 1375, 1430
Atelectasia, 1138
Atenção, 1373
Atenolol, 1310, 1776
Atipamezol, 628
Atitudes bucais repetitivas, 49
Ativação
- dependente do comprimento, 1165
- do sistema
-- nervoso simpático, 1165
-- renina-angiotensina-aldosterona, 1166
-- inadequada da imunidade no intestino delgado, 1531
- neuro-hormonal, 745
Ativador do plasminogênio tecidual, 1354

Atividade(s), 728
- de enzimas hepáticas, 589
- espontânea na eletromiografia, 444
- insercional, 444
- plasmática da renina, 1839
- sérica
-- da amilase, 253, 254, 1698
-- da lipase, 253, 254
--- total, 1698
Ato
- de caçar mosca, 49
- de lamber o ar, 49
Atonia do músculo detrusor, 2039
Atresia
- de coana, 1075
- valvar, 1251
Atrofia
- das vilosidades, 1532
- tubular, 1958
Atropina, 570, 572, 628
Aumento
- da concentração de nitrogênio ureico sanguíneo, 248
- da perda de cálcio, 275
- do enchimento cardíaco, 1183
- do fluxo sanguíneo, 1353
- lento de P4, 1870
- no gasto energético, 741
Auscultação, 221
- cardíaca, 1294
Ausência de alterações histológicas na biopsia intestinal, 1559
Autoanticorpos, 880
- antitireoglobulina, 1754
Automutilação, 49
Autotransfusão, 543
Avaliação
- acidobásica e do pH urinário, 1933
- clínica
-- das doenças do estômago, 1507
-- do trato respiratório, 1091
- da ação diurética, 1949
- da adequação nutricional de dietas caseiras, 808
- da estrutura e da função cardíaca, 401
- da fisioterapia/reabilitação, 2180
- da função
-- cardíaca global, 405
-- renal, 1927
- da hipercoagulabilidade na doença glomerular, 1932
- da libido, 1906
- da pressão arterial, 373
- da proteinúria, 1929
- da resposta terapêutica, 2071
- diagnóstica
-- da função hepática, 1621
-- de doença do parênquima pulmonar, 1118
- do animal cianótico, 209
- do eletrocardiograma, 579
- do espécime de biopsia renal, 1984
- do esvaziamento gástrico, 1509
- do paciente, 721
- do padrão respiratório, 574
- e cuidado com os neonatos, 1922
- geral da saúde, 2066
- indireta da motilidade intestinal, 1542
- inicial de emergências respiratórias, 573
- laboratorial
-- de doenças hepatobiliares, 1624
-- do trato gastrintestinal, 1475
- mineralocorticoide, 1846
- nutricional, 721, 791
-- do animal sênior, 734
- prostática adicional, 1909
- ultrassonográfica do abdome e das glândulas adrenais, 1822
Aves, 917
Avulsão de ureter, 625
Azatioprina, 702, 820, 848, 1635, 1680
Azoospermia, 1911
Azotemia, 247, 1760, 1966
- hemodinâmica, 1940
- pós-renal, 248, 1927
- pré-renal, 247, 1927

- renal intrínseca, 247, 1927
- responsiva ao volume, 1940
- *versus* uremia, 1969

B

Babesiose, 837, 976
Bacilo de Calmette e Guérin, 2080
Baclofeno, 642, 2040
Baço, 345, 348, 2119
Bactérias, 284, 451
- associadas à piometra, 1898
Bacteriemia, 549
Bacteriúria, 1935
- assintomática, 2016
- relevante, 2018
Bainha introdutora, 458
Baixa libido, 1910
Balanço
- de nitrogênio negativo, 2160
- hídrico, 1948
Balantidium coli, 1593
Balões de oclusão, 458
Balsalazida, 1590
Banco de dados emergenciais mínimo, 598
Barreira(s)
- mucosa gástrica, 1505
- teciduais, 687
Bartonelose
- em cães, 935
- em gatos, 940
Baterias, 633
Benazepril, 1180, 1309, 1776
Benefícios
- da febre, 193
- da nebulização, 367
Benzodiazepínicos, 565, 570, 639
Betabloqueadores, 638, 1183, 1310
Betalactamase de espectro estendido, 906
Betanecol, 2040
Betapolissacarídeos, 751
Bexiga, 2147
- pélvica, 2054
Bicarbonato, 1849, 1952
Bifosfonatos, 1738
Biguanidas, 1807
Bile, 82, 1688
Bilirrubina, 211, 282, 1625
Biliverdina, 211
Bioequivalência, 683
Biologia tumoral na quimioterapia, 2066
Biomarcadores, 1306, 1944, 2124
- cardíacos, 938, 1278
- urinários, 1999
Biopsia, 382, 2107, 2113
- assistida por laparoscopia, 1646
- cerebral, 1392
-- e histopatologia, 1403
- cirúrgica em cunha, 1646
- com *punch*, 339
- de linfonodos, 361
- de medula óssea, 353
- de músculos e nervos, 442, 1490
- de nervos, 443
- de próstata, 429
- em cunha/elipse, 339
- esplênicas, 887
- excisional/incisional, 339
- hepática, 1631
-- guiada por laparoscopia, 351
- intestinal, 1543, 1562, 1563, 1571
- muscular, 442
- nasal, 116, 364, 365, 1099
- pancreática, 1705
- para obtenção de fragmento (biopsia core) de medula óssea, 355
- por aspiração percutânea com agulha fina, 1859
- por endoscopia, 1587
- por raspado, 339
- pulmonar por meio de cirurgia e toracoscopia, 1101
- renal, 1930, 1971, 1984
-- e diagnósticos histológicos, 1984
Bioquímica sérica, 1743, 1765, 1832

Bisfosfonatos, 708
Blastomicose, 1034
Blastomyces dermatitidis, 896
Bleflarite, 56
Bleomicina, 2068
Bloqueador(es)
- de canais de cálcio, 637, 1180, 1310
- de receptores de progesterona, 1901, 1902
Bloqueio(s), 1189
- atrioventricular, 1201, 1209
-- de primeiro grau, 1202
-- de segundo grau, 1202
-- de terceiro grau, 1203
- de ramos do feixe, 1204
- de receptores de progesterona, 1885
Bócio nodular tóxico, 1762
Bolhas pulmonar, 1139
Borborigmos, 1534
Bordetella bronchiseptica, 1010, 1125
Bornavírus, 1019
Borrelia burgdorferi, 1951
Bosentana, 1182
Botulismo, 930, 934, 1466
Bougienagem, 482
Brachyspira pilosicoli, 1592
Bradiarritmias, 585
Bradicardia sinusal, 1190
Braquicefalia, 1078
Braquiterapia, 2073
Brometalina, 630
Brometo, 146
3-bromotirosina, 1541
Broncolitíase, 1111
Broncomalacia, 1113
Broncopneumopatia eosinofílica em cães, 1108
Broncoscopia, 379, 381, 1114
Bronquiectasia, 1111
Brônquios, 152
Bronquite crônica em cães, 1107
Brucella, 927
- *canis*, 915
Brucelose, 927, 1889
Brushita (fosfato de cálcio), 2022
Budesonida, 1565
Bulbos relacionados, 651
Buprenorfina, 570, 571, 706
Butirato, 751
Butorfanol, 570, 571, 706, 1311

C

Cabergolina, 1885, 1902
Cães como onívoros, 726
Cafeína, 642
Câimbra em cães da raça Scottish Terrier, 130
Calcinose cutânea, 53, 1816
Cálcio, 272, 1740, 1817, 1953
- ionizado, 1736
- total, 1736
Calcipotrieno, 642
Calcitonina, 1731, 1739
Calcitriol, 642, 1731, 1744, 1776
Cálculo(s)
- de requisitos nutricionais, 792
- de urato, 2028
Calicivírus felino, 897, 1650
Calprotectina fecal, 1541
Câmara(s)
- cardíacas do lado
-- direito, 1262
-- esquerdo, 1261
- olfatória, 1068
- respiratória, 1068
Campylobacter
- *jejuni*, 1905
- spp, 965, 967, 1550, 1592
-- patogênico, 1475
Camundongos, 917
Canais iônicos, 1369
Canalopatias, 2179
Câncer, 740, 2063, 2203
- características/origem do, 2063
- pulmonar, 1130
-- metastático e especial, 1131
-- primário, 1133
- tireoidiano de ocorrência natural, 1772

Candidíase, 1052
Canetas de aplicação de insulina, 1790
Canine Inherited Disorders Database, 29
Canulação arterial, 375
Cânulas nasais, 547
Capacidade de concentração urinária, 1932
Captação e apresentação de antígeno, 1530
Caquexia, 742, 744
- cardíaca, 742, 768
- do câncer, 742, 788, 2157
- renal, 742
Características dos tecidos, 344
Carbamatos, 632
Carboidratos, 729, 731, 760
- /fibras na ração, 751
Carbonato de fosfato de cálcio, 2022
Carboplatina, 2068
Carcinoides, 1855
Carcinoma(s), 294
- biliar, 1692
- de(s) célula(s)
-- basais, 2109
-- escamosas, 1485
--- cutâneo
---- em cães, 2108
---- em gatos, 2108
--- digital em cães, 2108
--- em cães, 2108
--- em gatos, 2108
--- multicêntrico *in situ* em gatos, 2108
--- no plano nasal de cães, 2108
- de célula-tronco foliculares, 2109
- hepatocelular, 1684
-- nodular ou difuso, 1687
-- solitário, 1687
- nodulares ou difusos de ductos biliares, 1687
- sebáceos, 2109
Cardíacos, 2193
Cardiomegalia, 1301
Cardiomiopatia(s)
- arritmogênica do ventrículo direito, 1299
- cães, 1276
- dilatada, 1281, 1282, 1297
-- e insuficiência cardíaca congestiva, 1281
-- em cães, 1276
-- específica da raça
--- Cão d'Água Português, 1280
--- Cocker Spaniel, 1278
--- Dálmata, 1279
--- Doberman Pinscher, 1279
--- Dogue Alemão (Grande Dinamarquês), 1280
--- Manchester Terrier Toy, 1280
--- Newfoundland, 1280
--- Schnauzer Padrão, 1280
--- Wolfhound Irlandês, 1280
-- subclínica (oculta), 1281
- do ventrículo direito arritmogênica em cães da
  raça Boxer, 1282
- gatos, 1285
- hipertrófica, 829, 1284, 1288
-- de gatos, 1306
--- da raça Maine Coon, 1292
- hipertrófica
-- em outras raças de gatos, 1292
-- no homem, 1292
-- não classificadas, 1301
- nutricional, 1280
- primárias em gatos, 1301
- relacionada à taurina, 1280
- restritiva, 1295
-- em gatos, 1295
-- no homem, 1295
- secundária(s), 1301
-- nutricional, 1298
Cardiopatia(s), 2191, 2192
- congênitas, 1215
-- cianótica, 1251
- manejo nutricional das, 768
- primárias de gatos, 1306
Cardiotoxicidade, 2090
Cariotipagem, 28
Cariótipo, 1909
Carnitina, 773, 1995
Carnitinúria, 1995
Carprofeno, 1682

Carrapato, 917
Carreadores de oxigênio à base de
  hemoglobina, 532
Carrinho(s), 2183
- de mão, 1376
Casos
- graves, 44
- não graves, 44
Castração, 732, 1884, 1885
Catarata, 1796
Catárticos, 629
Catecolaminas urinárias, 1859
Cateter(es)
- arterial, 298
- de drenagem, 459
- de oxigênio nasal, 547
- de uso intraósseo, 302, 303
- em escova, 381
- seletivos, 458
- urinário
-- de demora, 409, 2050
-- transuretral, 406
- venoso(s)
-- centrais de inserção periférica, 300
-- periférico, 297
Cateterismo
- cardíaco, 1220
- cardiovascular, 469
Cateterização
- da veia jugular, 299
- traumática, 428
- uretral anterógrada percutânea, 489
Causas
- endócrinas do déficit de crescimento, 89
- femininas de falha na introdução, 1911
- infecciosas de infertilidade e subfertilidade em
  cães e gatos, 1903
- não endócrinas de déficit de crescimento, 90
Cavidade nasal, 1068, 1079
- média, 1069
- rostral, 1069
Cebolas, 652
Ceco, 1575
Célula(s)
- de túbulos renais, 283
- dendríticas, 1529
- do metaestro, 451
- do sistema imune, 1529
- e moléculas do sistema imune de mucosa, 1529
- epiteliais, 283, 450, 1935
-- de transição, 284
-- escamosas, 284
- espumosas, 451
- neoplásicas, 284
- neoplásticas, 452
- T autorreativas, 877
Células-tronco cancerosas, 2065
Centro cirúrgico, 456
Ceratoconjuntivite seca, 56
Cerebelo, 1384, 1388
Cérebro, 94, 1388
Cervos, 917
Cesariana, 1894
Cetamina, 644, 707, 708
Cetoacidose diabética, 587, 590, 1799
Cetoconazol, 690, 691
Cetonas, 281, 589
Cetose diabética, 1799
Choque, 522
- distributivo, 523
- espinal, 1384
- hipovolêmico, 523, 1947
- hipoxêmico, 523
- metabólico, 523
- neurogênico, 523
- obstrutivo, 523
- séptico, 549
Cianose, 208
- central, 208, 211
- periférica, 208, 211
Cicádeos, 650
Ciclo
- de vida (meia-vida) das plaquetas, 234
- estral, 1882
- reprodutivo, 1863

Ciclo-oxigenases, 2127
Ciclobenzaprina, 642
Ciclofosfamida, 704, 847, 2067, 2104
Ciclosporina, 701, 820, 1590, 1635
Cilindro(s)
- bacterianos, 285
- céreos, 1936
- de células epiteliais, 284
- de hemácias, 285
- epiteliais, 1936
- eritrocitários, 1936
- gordurosos, 284, 1936
- granulosos, 284, 1936
- hialinos, 284, 1936
- largos, 285
- leucocitários, 284, 1936
- pigmentados, 285
- serosos, 284
Cilindrúria, 284, 1936
Cimetidina, 1954
Cinacalcete, 1739
Cinomose, 52, 1012
- canina, 1012, 1073
Cintilografia, 1657
- da tireoide, 1760
- portal
-- por via retal, 1630
-- transesplênica, 1630
-- utilizando tecnécio (99mtc)-enxofre coloidal, 1630
- tireoidiana, 1767
Cintos, 2183
Cio, 1863
- permanente, 1863
Cipionato de testosterona, 2038
Cipro-heptadina, 628
Circovírus, 1019
Circuito simples no sistema nervoso, 1372
Cirurgia
- com preservação do membro, 2131
- de ureter, 2013
- laparoscópica, 352
- /ovário-histerectomia, 1895
Cisaprida, 1954, 2040
Cisplatina, 2068
Cistadenoma biliar, 1692
Cistatina C, 1929
Cistina, 780, 2022, 2029
Cistinúria, 285, 1995
Cistite
- hemorrágica estéril, 2091
- idiopática felina, 780, 2041
Cistocentese, 408
Cistolitotomia percutânea transvesical, 491
Cisto(s)
- de laringe benignos, 1090
- em seios paranasais, 1078
- no mediastino, 1156
- ósseos, 2163
- paraprostáticos, 2060
- pericárdicos, 1314
- sinoviais extradurais, 1439
Cistoscopia, 415
Citauxzoonose, 977
Citocinas, 1169, 1530, 2081
- inflamatórias, 744
Citocromo P450, 31
Citogenética, 28
Citologia, 894, 961, 1545, 1582
- da próstata, 359
- de baço, 358
- de coração, 358
- de diferentes órgãos internos, 357
- de fígado, 358
- de linfonodos, 358
- de órgãos internos, 356
- de pele e tecidos subcutâneos, 340
- de pulmões, 357
- de rins, 358
- de timo, 358
- de tireoide, 357
- durante o diestro, 452
- durante o proestro, 452
- fecal, 602
- retal, 1540

- vaginal, 453, 1865, 1866, 1872
-- comportamento, 1866
- *versus* biopsia às cegas, 356
Citrato
- de potássio, 2027
- de tamoxifeno, 1876
Classes de medicamentos, 2067
Claudicação, 2168
- de diferentes membros, 2162
Clearance
- de água positivo *versus* negativo, 287
- urinário de água livre, 286
Cliques sistólicos, 218
Clopidogrel, 1309, 1355
Clorambucil, 704, 2067
Cloridrato
- de apomorfina, 627
- de xilazina, 627
Cloro, 262
Clorpromazina, 1954
Clostridium
- *botulinum*, 1466
- *difficile*, 964, 967, 1476, 1592
- *perfringens*, 963, 967, 1476, 1592
- spp, 1551
- *tetani*, 930
Club drugs, 646
Coagulação, 202, 1817
- intravascular disseminada, 830, 2157
Coagulopatias hereditárias tratamento de, 833
Coana, 1068
Cobalamina, 1477
Cobertura
- e ovulação, 1884
- vegetal com palha de cacau, 634
Cobra-coral, 654
Cobras venenosas, 653
Cobre, 815, 1676
Cocaína, 645
Coccidioides immitis, 896
Coccidioidomicose, 1031
Coccídios, 971
Coenzima q10, 774
Cogumelos amanita, 1683
Colangiocarcinoma, 1692
Colangiografia endoscópica retrógrada, 486
Colangite
- /colângio-hepatite neutrofilica, 1645
- linfocítica, 1649
Colapso, 124
- de laringe, 1088
- de traqueia, 1102
- induzido pelo exercício do Labrador Retriever, 1468
- não associado à síncope, 126
- traqueal, 462
Colar elisabetano, 547
1,25-[OH]2-colecalciferol), 1731
Colecalciferol, 630, 642
Colecistite, 1690
- enfisematosa, 1691
Colecistocinina, 738, 1852
Coledocolitíase, 1689
Colelitíase, 1689
Colesterol, 248, 1625, 1817, 1845
Coleta
- de amostras
-- da próstata, 428
-- de fígado, 1630
-- para citologia por meio de escovação transtraqueal e uso de agulha, 1101
-- para o diagnóstico de doenças do trato respiratório, 1099
- de líquido cefalorraquidiano, 439
-- complicações da, 441
-- da cisterna cerebelomedular, 439
-- da região lombar, 440
- de sêmen, 1888
-- e avaliação, 1906
- de urina, 406
- do ejaculado, 1906
- do histórico nutricional, 721
- e armazenamento de amostras de fezes, 311
- e cuidados com as amostras de urina, 280

Colite
- aguda, 1585
- crônica idiopática, 1585
- granulomatosa, 1590
- linfoplasmocitária, 1587
Colocação
- de cateter
-- arterial, 298
-- venoso periférico, 297
- de esfíncter uretral artificial, 494
- de *stent*, 482
-- biliar, 486
-- esofágico, 483
-- gastrintestinal, 485
-- intracardíaco para obstrução venosa central, 474
-- uretral, 492
- de tubo torácico, 377
- do cateter, 299
- paliativa de um *stent* para obstruções malignas, 508
- percutânea de tubo de cistostomia, 490
Coloides, 532
- sintéticos, 537
Cólon
- distal, 1576
- proximal, 1575
Colonoscopia, 1583
Coma, 139
Combinação de quimioterápicos, 2067
Comorbidades, 2191
- associadas à obesidade, 2201
Compartimentos dos fluidos, 530
Complementação do exame físico, 24
Complexo(s)
- atriais prematuros, 1192
- granuloma eosinofilico, 1482
- sarcoma histiocítico, 2146
- trombina-antitrombina, 822
- ventriculares prematuros, 1197
Complicações
- após oclusão do desvio postossistêmico, 1666
- associadas ao reaquecimento, 203
- da coleta de líquido cefalorraquidiano, 441
- da doença glomerular, 1993
- da mielografia, 441
- da nutrição enteral, 326
- da otoendoscopia, 337
- da terapia antineoplásica, 2085
- decorrentes do uso de marca-passo, 1214
- dermatológicas, 2087
- em longo prazo do diabetes melito, 1796
- gastrintestinais, 2088
- oculares, 1796
- urêmicas, 1952
Componentes do sangue, 538
Comportamento maternal inapropriado, 1896
Composição
- da microbiota em animais saudáveis, 1501
- da ração, 749
Compostos
- 2,4-D, 636
- de platina, 2067
- dietéticos não nutritivos, 817
- semelhantes à anfetamina, 643
Compressões torácicas, 576
Comunicação(ões)
- neuronal, 1371
- oronasais adquiridas, 1072
- uterovesical, 2055
Conceito de PICR, 33
Concentração(ões)
- basais de cortisol, 1846
- da fosfatase alcalina seminal, 1908
- de eletrólitos na urina, 286
- de folato sérico, 1476
- de oxigênio no sangue, 613
- de T3T, 1753
- de T4L, 1754
- de T4T, 1754
- de TSHC, 1754
- de ureia nitrogenada sanguínea, 1968
- fecal do inibidor da alfa1-antitripsina, 1477
- hormonais, 1760
- plasmática máxima, 682
- sanguínea de gordura, 762

Índice Alfabético

- sérica
-- de cobalamina, 1477
-- de creatinina, 1968
-- de folato e cobalamina, 1541, 1559
-- de fosfato e magnésio, 592
-- de glicose e insulina, 1779
-- de proteína c reativa, 1477
-- de vitaminas, 1562
-- ou fecais de marcadores de inflamação, 1478
-- ou plasmáticas de GH e IGF-1, 1718
Concentrado
- de granulócitos, 539
- de hemácias, 538
- de plaquetas, 539
Concha
- etmoidal, 1068
- ventral, 1068
Condição(ões)
- autoimunes orais, 1482
- comumente associadas à hipertensão, 660
- corporal e exercício, 728
- da glândula salivar, 1484
- de escore muscular, 743
- inflamatórias, 94
- mental, 139
Condrossarcoma apendicular em cães, 2134
Condução, 201
- nervosa
-- motora e sensitiva, 444
-- sensitiva, 445
Configuração
- da concha, 1080
- da gestação, 1873
- do diagnóstico de doença renal crônica, 1968
Confundimento por indicação, 37
Congestão, 889
Conjuntiva, 56
Consciência, 139
Conscientização do tutor, 732
Consistência, frequência e quantidade da
    refeição, 748
Constipação intestinal, 171, 172, 1600
Constrição
- da uretra, 2052
- e hipoplasia da uretra, 2048
- uretral, 2056
Contagem de plaquetas, 235, 824
Contaminação do ejaculado, 1913
Contaminantes, 451
Contenção química, 302
Conteúdo gastrintestinal, 82
Controle
- da concentração sérica de cálcio, 1730
- da resistência antimicrobiana, 907
- de carrapatos, 921
- de rigidez e espasmo, 933
- estratégico *versus* preventivo dos parasitas, 694
- glicêmico estrito, 1800
- medicamentoso da hiperlipidemia, 767
- motor, 1373
- nutricional da doença do trato urinário
    inferior, 778
- permanente e temporário de reprodução, 1884
- pré-terapêutico de hipercalcemia, 1738
Contusão(ões)
- da bexiga, 625
- pulmonar(es), 620
-- traumáticas, 124
Convecção, 201, 421
Conversões de pressão, 331
Convulsões, 143
- classificação das, 143
- epilépticas, 1404
Coprocultura de rotina, 1540
Coração, 1764, 2192
Córnea, 57
Cornetos aberrantes
- caudais, 1080
- rostrais, 1080
Coroide, 58
Coronavírus
- entérico canino, 989
- pantrópico, 989
- respiratório canino, 990, 1009

Corpo(s) estranho(s), 1066
- esofágicos, 1495
- intestinal, 1600
- na traqueia, 1105
- na uretra, 2052
- nasais, 1072
- oral, 1483
Corpúsculos de Heinz, 229
Corrimento vaginal, 1864
Córtex adrenal, 1812
Corticosteroides, 521, 1335, 1453, 1634, 2194
- em cães e gatos diabéticos, 2200
Cortisol, 1825
- do pelo, 1819
Coxiella burnetii, 915, 916
Creatinina, 246, 1928, 1966
- e nitrogênio ureico sanguíneo, 246
- sérica, 1943
Creatinoquinase, 260
Crenosoma vulpis, 1121
Crescimento esquelético, 1880
Criação de filhotes órfãos, 724
Crioprecipitados, 538
Criosobrenadantes, 538
Crioterapia, 2180
Criptococose, 1026
Criptorquidismo, 1887
Crise
- aguda de hipoadrenocorticismo, 1848
- de hipertensão tratamento da, 670
Cristais
- de ácido úrico, 285
- de bilirrubina, 285
- de colesterol, 285
- de fosfato
-- de amônio magnesiano, 285
-- de cálcio, 285
- de tirosina, 285
- de urato, 285
Cristalino, 58
Cristaloides, 531
Cristalúria, 187, 285, 1935
Cronobiologia, 1419
Cronologia da sequência de eventos, 3
Cryptococcus
- *gattii*, 1026
- *neoformans*, 896, 1026
Cryptosporidium spp, 1554
Cuidados
- com o equipamento de endoscopia, 328
- de suporte em animais submetidos a
    quimioterapia, 2071
- dos neonatos durante o período pós-parto, 1921
- intensivos, 513
Cultura
- de fezes, 964, 966
-- para parasitas, 317
- e secreção vaginal, 1904
- microbiológica, 893, 1043, 1647
- vaginal
-- durante proestro e estro, 1904
-- pré-cobertura, 1903
Cúpula vaginal, 608
Cura, 2066
Curta duração de ação da insulina, 1795
Curvas glicêmicas e ajustes da dose de
    insulina, 1792
Cyniclomyces guttulatus, 1552
Cytauxzoon felis, 977

D

D-penicilamina, 1635
Dacarbazina, 2067
Dactinomicina, 2068
Dados de identificação do animal, 43
Dano oxidativo, 1798
Dantroleno, 2040
Darbepoietina, 1979
Débito cardíaco, 403
Débito urinário, 536, 1946
Defecação, 1604
Defeito(s)
- adquiridos do palato mole, 1077
- cardíacos variados, 1252

- congênitos do palato, 1077
- de septo, 1227
-- atrial, 220, 1226, 1228, 1229
-- atrioventricular, 1232
-- ventricular, 220, 1226, 1228, 1230
- do pericárdio, 1314
Deficiência(s)
- de adesão de leucócitos, 860
- de alfa1-antitripsina, 1677
- de crescimento, 1534
- de distrofina, 2177
- de fator hereditárias, 832
- de ferro, 1979
- de hormônio do crescimento
-- adquirida, 1724
-- e do fator de crescimento semelhante à insulina
    tipo 1, 89
- de insulina, 90
- de piruvatoquinase, 860
- de pró-coagulante plaquetário, 858
- de taurina em gatos, 1298
- de tiamina, 62, 1436
- de vitamina
-- D, 275
-- K, 830
- do fator de coagulação herdadas, 833
- nutricionais, 782
-- decorrentes de doença do trato
    gastrintestinal, 752
Déficit(s)
- de crescimento, 89
- do nervo craniano, 1431
Deformidade(s)
- congênitas, 1072
- flexural do carpo, 786
Degeneração, 70
Deglutição, 1486
Deiscência incisional, 1480
Densidade urinária, 1932
- e osmolalidade, 280
- específica, 1969
Depleção de volume, 1178
Depósitos teciduais, 72
Depuração, 682
- plasmática, 1927
- renal ou urinária, 1927
Dermatite
- acral, 52
- esfoliativa felina associada ao timoma, 51
- necrolítica superficial, 52, 1675, 2157
-- em gatos, 1676
- responsiva ao zinco, 52
Dermatofibromas nodulares, 53
Dermatofibrose nodular, 2157
Dermatomiosite, 51, 2176
Dermátomo, 1386
Dermatoparaxia, 54
Derrame, 1435
- abdominal, 1656
- hemorrágico, 1408
- peritoneal, 625
1-desamino-8-d-arginina-vasopressina, 184
Descargas
- miotônicas, 444
- repetitivas complexas, 444
Descompensação
- gástrica, 1515
- precoce, 534
- tardia, 534
Desconforto, 97
Descontaminação, 627
Descrição do ambiente doméstico, 3
Desequilíbrio(s)
- anatômico da via respiratória superior, 1080
- microbianos e doença entérica, 1502
- na relação ventilação-perfusão, 208
- nutricionais, 95
Desidratação, 533
- e fluidoterapia, 1975
Desinfecção
- de alto nível, 330
- manual, 330
Deslizamento, 391
Deslocamento da sonda de alimentação, 327
Desmame à idade adulta, 725

Desmopressina, 857
Desnutrição associada ao câncer
- caquexia do câncer, 788
- obesidade, 788
Desobstipação, 436
Desobstrução
- anterógrada
-- por compressão da bexiga, 413
-- por meio de relaxamento farmacológico da
      uretra, 413
- da uretra, 411
-- de cães, 414
-- em gatos, 412
Desordens
- de pênis, 1887
- urogenitais não neoplásicas, 1880
Destruição imunomediada, 238
Desuso de membro, 2165
Desvios (shunts) portossistêmicos, 1621
- em gatos, 1667
- extra-hepáticos, 1664
- intra-hepáticos, 1665
Detecção
- de ácido nucleico, 943
- de anticorpos, 898
- de bacteriúria, 2017
- de complexo antígeno-anticorpo específico para
      coronavírus, 993
- de coronavírus felino ou vírus mutante por reação
      em cadeia da polimerase via transcriptase
      reversa, 994
- do microorganismos, 893
Detemir, 1804
Detergentes, 632
Determinação da dieta felina, 731
Dexametasona, 1875
Dexmedetodimina, 570, 571, 707
Dexmetilfenidato, 642
Dextrometorfano, 708
Diabetes
- canino tratamento, 2197
- dieta
-- na prevenção do, 1806
-- no tratamento do, 1807
- felino tratamento, 2197
- gatos diabéticos mal controlados, 1809
- insípido, 181, 1724, 1725
-- central, 1725, 1728
--- e nefrogênico versus polidipsia primária, 1726
-- nefrogênico, 1726, 1729, 1998
- melito, 63, 152, 587, 759, 1461, 1719, 1828,
      1881, 2194
-- canino, 1783
-- complicações em longo prazo do, 1796
-- efeitos colaterais
--- da terapia esteroide em pacientes com, 2198
--- e riscos da terapia esteroide no, 2197
-- em gatos, 760, 1797
-- em longo prazo sem remissão, 1801
-- hipertensão sistêmica e, 661
-- juvenil, 90
-- manejo nutricional do, 758
-- tipo(s)- , 1797
--- 2, 739, 1797
- objetivos da terapia e remissão do, 1800
Diacilgliceróis, 741
Diafragma, 1159, 1160
Diagnóstico
- das lesões de medula espinal, 1451
- de doença do intestino delgado, 1535
- de infecção do trato urinário, 2017
- de parada cardiopulmonar, 576
- de trombocitose, 238
- diferencial(is)
-- da febre, 195
-- das queixas principais, 43
-- de anormalidades clinicopatológicas, 225
- e tratamento
-- de doenças edematosas, 84
-- de reações transfusionais, 545
- laboratorial de doenças infecciosas, 893
- neuroanatômico, 1374, 1381
- por imagem, 938
-- do sistema respiratório, 1095

Diálise peritoneal, 418, 1950
Diâmetro uretral, 1880
Diarreia, 164, 328, 1533, 1535
- aguda induzida por dieta medicamentos ou
      toxinas, 1548
- idiopática antibiótico-responsiva, 1557, 1558
- responsiva a antibióticos, 1503
-- idiopática, 1558, 1560
- riquetsial, 1552
- secretora, 1533
Diazepam, 570, 571, 1682, 2040
Diazóxido, 1782
Dicamba, 636
Diencéfalo, 1388
Diestro, 1863, 1866
- sem gestação, 1883
Dieta(s)
- caseiras, 806, 810
- com restrição de cobre, 756
- comercial, 732
- de eliminação
-- caseiras, 804
-- comerciais, 804
- de exclusão, 781
- irradiada, 62
- na prevenção do diabetes, 1806
- não convencionais, 730, 806
- no tratamento do diabetes, 1807
- ricas em
-- fibra, 740
-- proteínas, 740
- utilizadas em doenças do trato gastrintestinal, 748
Dietilenoglicol, 633
Dietilestilbestrol, 2038
Diferenciação entre
- alterações de comportamento e doenças
      clínicas, 46
-- intoxicações e doenças não tóxicas agudas, 64
Difusão, 421
Digestão e assimilação de nutrientes, 1506
Digestibilidade, 799
Digoxina, 1308
- imune Fab, 628
Dilatação
- da câmara, 401
- esofágica com balão, 482
- volvulogástrica, 1514
Diltiazem, 1181, 1310
Diluição, 627
Dímero-D, 822, 826
Dimetilarginina simétrica, 246, 1929
- na doença renal crônica, 1969
Dimetilsulfóxido, 1989
Diminuição
- da concentração de creatinina, 248
- da produção de glicose, 242
- da secreção de paratormônio, 275
- na concentração de nitrogênio ureico
      sanguíneo, 248
- na ingestão de energia, 744
Dióxido de carbono, 526
Dipylidium caninum, 1553
Diretrizes para a administração de oxigênio, 549
Dirofilaria immitis, 1122, 1323
Dirofilariose, 124, 829
- assintomática, 1337
- canina, 1323
- felina, 1342
- prevenção de, 1330
Disautonomia, 2041
Discinesia
- ciliar primária, 1110
- induzida por medicamento, 130
- paroxística, 129
-- em cães da raça Chinook, 129
-- em outras raças, 130
Discopondilite, 1450
Disfagia, 155, 1428, 1486, 1963
- cricofaríngea, 1492
Disfunção
- cognitiva em cães e gatos idosos, 1422
- crônica do aloenxerto, 1958
- do nodo sinusal, 1208, 1209
- gonadal

-- adquirida, 1911
-- congênita, 1912
-- no enterócitos, 1531
- plaquetária
-- adquirida, 859
-- hereditária, 858
Dislipidemias, 739
Dismetria, 1384
Dismielopoese secundária, 863
Dismorfogênese tireoidiana, 1758
Disormonogênese tireoidiana, 1758
Displasia
- coxofemoral, 786, 2160
- de valva atrioventricular, 1233
- do cotovelo, 2160
- renal, 2004
- valvar, 1232
Dispneia, 116
Dispositivo(s)
- de aquecimento externos, 202
- de derivação (bypass) ureteral subcutânea, 2013
- para auxílio da reabilitação, 2183
- SUB, 504
Disquesia, 171, 173
Dissinergia
- detrusor-uretral, 2039
- reflexa, 2051
- uretral do detrusor, 2051
Dissociação
- atrial, 1197
- atrioventricular isorrítmica, 1201
- eletromecânica, 1205
Distensão abdominal, 79
- grave, 574
Distocia, 607, 608, 1892
- causas de, 1893
Distribuição, 678
- de fluidos e barreira microvascular, 530
- e farmacocinética de medicamentos, 677
Distrofia(s) muscular(es), 2177
- autossômica por deficiência de sarcoglicanos, 2178
- congênita por deficiência de laminina alfa-2, 2178
- ligada ao cromossomo X, 2177
- por deficiência de colágeno VI, 2178
Distúrbio(s)
- acidobásico, 94, 525, 526
- cerebrais inflamatórios e não infecciosos, 1412
- com perda de proteína, 829
- complexos que envolvem anormalidades da
      excitabilidade e da condução, 1205
- concomitantes causadores de resistência à
      insulina, 1795
- da junção neuromuscular, 1465
- de células sanguíneas secundárias/adquiridas, 862
- de comportamento do sono rem, 1420
- de função de plaqueta, 858
- de reprodução em cães machos, 1906
- de tremor focais, 135
- degenerativos, 1419, 1460
- do movimento, 128
- do potássio, 1976
- do receptor P2Y12, 858
- do sistema nervoso central de origem
      desconhecida, 1471
- do sono, 1419
- esqueléticos relacionados com a nutrição, 783
- gastrintestinais e pancreatite, 1954
- hematológicos, 1953
- hemostáticos primários, 852
- imunomediados e não neoplásicos em
      leucócitos, 860
- infecciosos e inflamatórios, 1462
- intestinais cirúrgicos, 1573
- metabólicos, 63, 1461
- mieloproliferativos, 2102
- na motilidade, 1532
- não neoplásicos dos ossos da mandíbula, 1484
- orais e das glândulas salivares, 1479
- paroxísticos específicos de origem
      desconhecida, 1473
- plaquetários, 851
- primários/congênitos de células sanguíneas, 860
- que limitam exercícios, 2204
- relacionados ao mieloma, 2102

Índice Alfabético

- reprodutivos em cães ou cadelas castrados, 1913
- respiratórios do sono, 1421
- secundários do sono, 1420
- tóxicos, 1464
- traumáticos, 1464
- tubulares, 2006
- vasculares, 72
Disúria, 3, 184
Diurese
- do frio, 202
- osmótica, 181
- pós-obstrução, 2050
Diuréticos, 1177, 1310, 2193
- de alça, 1949
- tiazídicos, 1178
Divertículo(s)
- aracnoide espinal, 1440
- do trígono vesical (parauretérico), 2055
- esofágico, 1497
- uretral, 2047
DL-metionina, 2027
DNA em proteína, 25
Dobutamina, 1182, 1311
Doença(s)
- adquiridas do pericárdio, 1315
- aguda do intestino delgado, 1546
- anatômica congênita da uretra, 2045
- anorretais, 1603, 1604
- arterial tromboembólica, 1351
- articular, 72
-- inflamatória, 295
-- não inflamatória, 295
- autoimunes/imunomediadas e terapia
    imunossupressora, 819
- bacterianas, 917
- biliar extra-hepática, 605
- brônquica(s)
-- inflamatória felina, 1114
-- primárias, 1107
-- secundárias, 1111
- cardíaca, 829
- cardiovascular(es), 94, 1163
-- e dieta, hipertensão sistêmica e, 661
-- no início da idade adulta, 1256
- causadas por protozoários, 968
- cerebrais inflamatórias, infecciosas e
    multifocais, 1411
- congênita(s), 1085
-- do trato urinário inferior, 2053
- crônica do intestino delgado, 1549
- da cripta, 1569
- da faringe, 1486, 1491
- da laringe, 1085
- da medula espinal, 94, 1437, 1451
- da nasofaringe, 1067, 1074
- da órbita, 59
- da parede torácica, 1153
- da próstata, 2057
- da traqueia, 1102
- da uretra, 2045
- da vesícula biliar e do sistema biliar extra-
    hepático, 1688
- de armazenamento
-- de glicogênio, 2178
-- lisossomal, 1395
- de Bowen, 2108
- de costelas, 1159
- de desenvolvimento, 2004
- de disco
-- cervical, 1443
-- toracolombar, 1444
- de Graves, 1762
- de Legg-Perthes, 2162
- de Lyme, 917
-- comparação entre pessoas e cães, 918
-- em cães prevenção da, 921
-- sintomas da em cães no campo, 918
- de Plummer, 1762
- de pseudoaddison, 1846
- de traqueia obstrutivas e/ou traumáticas, 1105
- de ureter, 2009
- de vasos linfáticos, 1357
-- periféricos, 1364
- de veias, 1357, 1360

- de via respiratória inferior em gatos, 1113
- de von Willebrand, 215, 825, 851
-- em felinos, 857
-- hereditária, 855
- degenerativas, 1436
-- cerebrais primárias, 1393
- dermatológicas imunomediadas, 871
- do armazenamento lisossomal, 861
-- e o fígado, 1678
- do cão Dobermann dançarino, 131
- do cérebro, 1387
- do diafragma, 1153
- do disco intervertebral, 1443
- do esôfago, 1486, 1492
- do espaço pleural, 1146, 1152
- do esterno, 1159
- do estômago, 1504, 1507
- do gato cambaleante, 1023
- do intestino
-- delgado, 1526, 1572
--- aspectos clínicos da, 1533
--- diagnóstico de, 1535
--- grosso, 1575
- do mediastino, 1153, 1154
- do nariz, 1067, 1071
- do ouvido, 1059
- do pâncreas exócrino manejo nutricional da, 752
- do parênquima pulmonar, 574, 1117, 1118
-- manifestações de, 1117
- do pericárdio, 1312
- do reto, 1605
- do saco anal, 1612
- do sistema
-- nervoso central, 1469
-- neuromuscular, 1472
- do timo, 1158
- do trato
-- gastrintestinal, manejo nutricional das, 747
-- urinário inferior, 778, 2009
- dos nervos, 72
- dos seios paranasais, 1067, 1078
- edematosas diagnóstico e tratamento de, 84
- endócrinas, 94, 237, 1715
-- e metabólicas, 2178
-- manejo nutricional de, 758
- entéricas causadas por protozoários, 968
- específicas do cérebro, 1393
- esplênica, 891
- fúngicas, 1026
- gastrintestinal, 1475
- glomerular(es), 1985, 2004
-- complicações da, 1993
- hematológicas e imunológicas, 819
- hepática crônica energia metabólica e necessidade
    de proteínas na, 754
- hepatobiliares, 1621, 1624
-- infecciosas, 1649
-- manejo nutricional das, 754
- hepatocutânea, 52
- hepatotóxicas, 1678
- histiocíticas, 2144
- imunomediadas, 94
- infecciosas, 94, 893, 1434
-- diagnóstico laboratorial de, 893
-- do cérebro, 1414
- infiltrativas, 236
- inflamatórias, 1434, 1585
-- da laringe, 1090
-- de vasos linfáticos, 1365
-- do sistema nervoso central
--- infecciosas e não infecciosas, 1469
--- que podem se manifestar com tremor, 134
-- intestinal, 1560
--- idiopática, 1502
--- raça-específicas, 1567
-- não infecciosas do cérebro, 1434
- intestinal(is)
-- bacterianas, 963
-- inflamatória, 748
- intracranianas primárias, 98
- intranasais, 122
- mamárias, 1897
- metabólicas, 93
-- hepáticas, 1671

- metastática, 2133
- mieloproliferativa, 863
- mixomatosa da valva mitral, 1256
- musculares, 72, 2174
- musculoesqueléticas, 2159
- não neoplásicas do baço, 881
- nasofaríngea, 1074
- neurológicas, 94, 1369
- neuromusculares
-- adquiridas, 1472
-- hereditárias, 1472
- ortopédica do desenvolvimento, 786
- ósseas, 70
- pancreáticas, 1695
- parasitárias do sistema
-- biliar, 1692
-- nervoso central, 1471
- pericárdica, 1149
- periodontal, 151
- polissistêmicas causadas por protozoários, 971
- por lesão mínima, 1990
- pós-sinápticas da junção neuromuscular, 1467
- pré-sinápticas da junção neuromuscular, 1465
- prion, 1469
- pulmonar(es)
-- eosinofílica granulomatosa, 1325
-- específicas, 1120
-- intersticial, 1134
-- obstrutivas e restritivas, 1093
-- parasitária, 1120
-- restritiva, 1093
- que causam
-- obstrução, 1599
-- sintomas relacionados com o sistema nervoso
--- central, 60
--- periférico, 63
- relacionadas com a micção anormal, 2035
- renal(is), 64, 739, 1925
-- aguda, 247
-- idiopática identificação de, 1559
--- versus crônica, 1970
-- crônica, 1810, 1959, 247, 273, 775, 776
--- causas de, 1960
--- como minimizar a progressão da, 1980
--- consequências clínicas da, 1961
--- dimetilarginina simétrica na, 1969
--- estadiamento da, 1970
--- hipopotassemia como causa de, 1967
--- prognóstico, 1960
---- de cães com, 1961
---- de gatos com, 1961
--- tratamento da, 1972
-- familiares e congênitas de gatos e cães, 2003
-- hipertensão sistêmica e, 660
-- indicadores na urinálise, 1934
-- manejo nutricional das, 775
-- policística, 2006
- reprodutivas, 1863
- respiratória(s), 94, 740, 1091
-- infecciosa canina, 1009
- responsivas a corticosteroides, 2194
-- em pacientes diabéticos, 2198
- riquetisial transmitida por carrapatos, 866
- sistêmica(s)
-- acompanhadas de
--- alopecia e pele brilhante na região periocular,
     região ventral de pescoço, abdome e patas,
     52
--- alopecia, eritema, descamação e crostas na face
     nos membros e na cauda, 51
--- eritema, alopecia, descamação e formação de
     crostas faciais e dorsais, 51
--- eritema cutâneo, alopecia, descamação e crostas
     na junção mucocutânea e nos coxins
     plantares, 52
--- espessamento cutâneo, 54
--- fragilidade cutânea, 54
--- nódulos cutâneos, 53
--- placas cutâneas, 53
-- associada a hemorragia e trombose na medula
     espinal, 1457
-- com hipotricose difusa descamação e crostas, 51
-- manifestações
--- dermatológicas de, 50

--- neurológicas de, 60
--- oftálmicas da, 54
--- ortopédicas de, 70
- superfície apical da membrana, 1531
- tireoidiana uni e bilateral e histologia, 1763
- traumáticas, 1453
- tubulares renais, 1994
- uretral
-- idiopática, 2051
-- inflamatória/infecciosa, 2052
-- metabólica, 2048
-- neoplásica, 2050
-- traumática, 2052
- urinária, 2203
- uterinas, 1896
- vascular(es), 1455
-- cerebral, 1408
- vestibular(es), 1383, 1429
-- centrais, 1434
-- idiopática, 1433
-- periféricas, 1432
-- unilateral congênita, 1434
-- tratamento de suporte e compensação em, 1432
- virais, 977
- do sistema nervoso central, 1469
Dolasetrona, 1954
Dopamina, 1869, 1949
Doppler
- com esfigmomanômetro, 376
- com fluxo colorido, 398, 1303, 1305
- de ondas
-- contínuas, 398, 1303, 1305
-- pulsadas, 396, 1303, 1304
- espectral, 393
- IDT 2D colorido dos movimentos radial e
   longitudinal do miocárdio, 1305
- PW, 397
- tecidual, 400
Dor, 95, 97, 2163
- aguda, 516, 518
- clínica, 516
-- patológica, 516
- crônica, 516, 2187
-- fisiopatologia, 2187
-- identificação da, 2188
- e tumefação articulares, 73
- em um ambiente de cuidados intensivos
   identificação da, 516
- fisiológica, 516
- funcional, 516
- grave a excruciante, 518
- indicadores comportamentais e fisiológicos da, 517
- inflamatória, 516
- leve a moderada, 518
- moderada a grave, 518
- musculoesquelética que impede a introdução, 1910
- neuropática, 516
- nociceptiva, 516
- suave a leve, 518
Dose, 2073
- da quimioterapia, 2069
- de sêmen/inseminação artificial, 446
Doxiciclina, 1336, 1952
Doxorrubicina, 2068, 2125
Drenagem transcervical, 1902
Drogas
- comuns ("de rua"), 645
- utilizadas para fins recreativos, 643
Ducto nasolacrimal, 1068
Ductus diverticulum, 1220
Duodeno/lobo pancreático, 345
Dupla via de saída do ventrículo direito, 1252
Duplicação
- da uretra, 2047, 2056
- de bexiga, 2055
Duração
- curta de ação da insulina, 1809
- do ciclo estral, 1884
- e progressão, 44
- prolongada do efeito da insulina, 1795

E
Eclâmpsia, 611, 1891
Ecocardiografia, 388, 1219, 1277, 1304, 1318, 1329

- 2D, 390
- bidimensional, 1303
- com contraste, 400
- com Doppler, 392
- tecidual, 400
- em modo M, 391, 1303
- transesofágica, 399
- tridimensional, 399
Ecocardiograma normal, 389
Ectasia
- ureteral, 2053
- vascular colônica, 1598
Edema
- cerebral, 139, 591, 1388
- extracelular, 531
- gestacional, 1889
- periférico, 82
- pulmonar, 124, 1129
-- secundário a insuficiência cardíaca esquerda, 124
Educação do tutor, 1787
Efeito(s)
- a longo prazo da esterilização e da castração na
   saúde de cães e gatos, 1879
- adversos
-- do tratamento da dor aguda, 521
-- dos opioides, 707
-- e contraindicações ao uso de AINEs, 700
-- e contraindicações para o uso de
   glicocorticoides, 697
-- relacionados à eritropoetina, 1978
-- tardios, 2075
- cardíacos de anormalidades sistêmicas do potássio
   e do cálcio, 1205
- cardiovasculares, 201
- colaterais
-- da terapia esteroide em pacientes com diabetes
   melito, 2198
-- e riscos da terapia esteroide no diabetes
   melito, 2197
-- gerais da terapia esteroide, 2198
- de fármacos, 96
- do sistema imune, 801
- neuromusculares, 202
- prejudiciais da febre, 194
- renais e metabólicos, 202
- respiratórios, 202
- Somogyi, 1795, 1811
- tróficos, 1501
Eficácia, 710
- dos parasiticidas, 694
Efusão(ões)
- classificação das, 290
- crônicas, 1150
- exsudativas, 292
- hemorrágicas, 80, 294
- neoplásicas, 294
- pericárdica, 1315
-- em gatos, 1323
- pleural, 1097, 1151
- quilosa, 81, 290, 1150
Ehrlichia
- *canis*, 950
- *ewingii*, 953
Eixo(s)
- hipotálamo-hipófise-adrenal, 555, 1812
- hipotálamo-pituitária-tireoide, 556
- somatotrópico, gonadal e lactotrópico, 557
Ejaculação
- do líquido prostático, 428
- incompleta, 1911, 1912
- retrógrada, 1911, 1912
Ejaculado, 1907
Elementos do histórico clínico, 2
Eletrocardiografia, 385, 937, 1186, 1277, 1318,
   1328
Eletrocardiograma, 1743
Eletrocauterização gastrintestinal, 483
Eletroencefalograma, 1393
Eletrólitos, 202, 730
Eletromiografia, 443, 444
- de fibra única, 444
Eliminação, 680
Eliptócitos, 229
ELISA, 965

- de trombina-antitrombina, 826
- para *Giardia lamblia*, 1476
Embalagem com gel de sílica, 633
Embolia
- fibrocartilaginosa, 1455
- paradoxal, 1351
- pulmonar, 1338
Embolização/quimioembolização transarterial, 511
Emergências
- cardíacas, 582
- gastrintestinais, 599
- hepáticas e esplênicas, 603
- reprodutivas, 606
-- em fêmeas, 606
-- em machos, 611
- respiratórias, 573
Êmese, 1962
Emulsão intralipídica, 628
Enalapril, 1180, 1309, 1776
Encefalite necrosante, 1413
Encefalomielite, 130
Encefalopatia
- espongiforme felina, 1469
- hepática, 60, 1623, 1638, 1653
- metabólica, 98, 1393
- mitocondrial, 1394
- urêmica, 61
Encurtamento do crânio, 1080
Endocardite infecciosa, 829, 1272
Endocrinologia
- gastrintestinal, 1479, 1851
- reprodutiva, 1863
Endocrinopatias, 829, 2204
Endopróteses expansivas (*stents*) de ureter, 2012
Endoscopia, 328, 456, 1043, 1074, 1509, 1512,
   1543, 1864, 1865
- desinfecção de alto nível, 330
- documentação, 331
- gastrintestinal, 432
-- baixa, 435
- instrumentação, 329
- intervencionista, 455, 457
- limpeza manual, 329
- manuseio, 329
- nomenclatura, 328
Endoscópios, 328
Endotelina, 1169
Enemas, 436, 1601
- contraindicados, 438
- e extração manual
-- como executar, 437
-- quando usar, 436
Energia, 728
Enfisema
- pulmonar, 1139
- subcutâneo ou submucoso, 1480
Engasgamento, 152
Enostose, 785
Ensaio(s)
- de fator de von Willebrand qualitativos, 856
- de imunoabsorção enzimática, 948
- de penetração, 1908
- quantitativo de doença de von Willebrand, 856
Entamoeba histolytica, 1594
Enterite(s)
- bacterianas, 1550
- eosinofílica, 1566
- granulomatosa, 1567
- linfocítico-plasmocítica, 1566
- linfoplasmocítica e deficiência de cobalamina em
   cão da raça Shar-pei, 1568
- neutrofílica, 1567
- proliferativa, 1567
- virais, 1550
Enterócitos, 1529
Enterocolite urêmica, 1963
Enteropatia com perda de proteína, 748
- familiar e nefropatia com perda de proteína em
   cães Wheaten Terrier de Pelo Liso, 1567
- com perda de proteínas, 1534, 1536
- do cão Basenji, 1567
- sensível ao glúten, 1557
Enterotoxina de *C. perfringens*, 964
Entrada nasal, 1068, 1069

Envenenamento
- por cobras elapídeas, 1466
- por salmão, 1552
Enzima(s)
- colestáticas, 256
- hepáticas, 254, 1624, 1845
- histona desacetilase, 2084
- urinárias, 1934
Enzimologia
- clínica, 254
- hepática, 254
Ependimoma, 1399
Epidemiologia da vacinação, 901
Epidermólise bolhosa adquirida, 872, 876
Epilepsia, 143
- idiopática, 1404
- primária, 1404
- refratária, 1407
Episódios vestibulares, 1436
Epispadia, 2046, 2056
Epistaxe, 120, 665
Epitelioma
- de células basais, 2108
- intracutâneo cornificante, 2107
Eprinomectina, 1332
Equilíbrio acidobásico, 589
Equimoses, 214
Equipamento de imagem auxiliar, 457
Ergocalciferol, 642, 1745
Eritema
- migratório necrolítico, 52
- multiforme, 1482
Eritrocitose, 210, 225, 230, 848, 2156
- causas de, 231
Eritrodisestesia palmoplantar, 2087
Eritropoese
- diminuída e ineficaz, 843
- na policitemia, 849
- normal, 848
Erliquiose, 950
Erosão gástrica, 1511
Erros inatos do metabolismo, 1393, 1469
Escalas de dor, 517
Escape imune, 2079
Escherichia coli, 967, 1551, 1592
- associada à colite granulomatosa, 967
Escleroterapia, 506
Escolha
- da dieta, 735
- da insulina, 1806
Escore
- clínico de otite em cães, 1061
- de condição corporal, 722, 723
Escova nasal, 1099
Escroto, 1906
Esferas de polietileno impregnadas com bário, 1543
Esferócitos, 229, 835
Esfíncter
- anal, 171
- ileocólico, 1575
Esfregaço(s)
- de sangue, 835
- direto, 1540
- fecal, 311, 1476
Esmolol, 1308
Esofagite, 1493
Esofagogastroduodenoscopia, 434
Esofagoscopia, 1490
Espaço pleural, 119
Espasticidade, 128, 1378
Especificidade
- analítica, 893
- diagnóstica, 893
Espectro de atividade, 694
Espermatozoides, 1907
Espessamento do palato mole, 1080
Espironolactona, 1177, 1308
Espirro, 112, 1070, 1091
- reverso, 112, 1070, 1091
Esplenectomia, 887
Esplenomegalia em cães e gatos
- doenças não neoplásicas, 889
- doenças neoplásicas, 887
Esplenomegalia inflamatória, 890

Espondilomielopatia cervical, 1437
Espondilose deformante, 1441
Esporotricose, 1051
Esqueleto laríngeo, 1082
Esquisócitos, 229
Estabilidade hemodinâmica, 552
Estabilização do paciente, 65
Estadiamento, 2066
- da doença renal crônica, 1970
- da lesão renal aguda, 1939
Estado(s)
- de imunodeficiência não induzidos por fármacos
  imunossupressores, 2211
- de sono REM e não REM, 1419
- epiléptico, 563
- hereditários hipocoaguláveis, 832
- hipercoaguláveis adquiridos, 827, 828
- hipocoaguláveis adquiridos, 827, 830
- reprodutivo do hospedeiro, 695
Estafilococos resistentes à meticilina, 906
Estalidos de abertura, 218
Estatinas, 767
Estatística biomédica, 34
Esteatose, 1671
- hepática, 1672
Estenose, 1600
- aórtica, 219, 1242
- da cavidade nasal, 1071, 1079
- da entrada nasal, 1071
- da laringe, 1089
- da saída nasal, 1072, 1079
- da uretra, 2052
- de narinas, 1078
- e obstrução
-- da nasofaringe, 1075
-- das vias nasais, 1071
-- do meato nasofaríngeo, 1074
- esofágica, 1493
- lombossacral degenerativa, 1438
- mitral, 221
- nasofaríngea, 466, 1075
- pulmonar, 220, 1237
- retal e anal, 1608
Estertores, 112
Estimativa da composição mineral, 2021
Estimulação
- com hormônio
-- liberador de tireotrofina, 1755
-- tireoestimulante, 1754
- elétrica, 2181
Estímulo(s)
- da diurese, 778
- para secreção, 1725
Estomatite, 1481
Estrabismo, 1431
Estrangulamento intestinal, 1573
Estrangúria, 3, 184
Estratégias para quimioterapia, 2066
Estreptoquinase, 1353
Estreptozocina, 1782
Estresse, 1887
- fetal via monitoramento, 1894
- físico e psicológico, 95
Estriol, 2038
Estro, 1863, 1864, 1882
- persistente, 1871
- prolongado, 1869, 1885
- silencioso, 1886
Estrógeno(s), 1876, 1885
- conjugado, 2038
Estruturas da laringe internas, 1082
Estruvita, 285, 779, 2022, 2027
Estudo(s)
- experimentais, 35
- videofluoroscópico da deglutição, 1489
Estupor, 139
Esvaziamento gástrico, 1509
- retardado, 1521
Etanol, 628, 636, 1952
Etilenoglicol, 635
Etomidato, 570, 573
Eucoleus aerophilus, 1121
Eutanásia, 38
Evaporação, 201

Evento(s)
- adversos após a vacinação, 901
- medicamentoso adverso, 716, 717
-- alérgicas e de hipersensibilidade, 718
-- em humanos associadas a medicamentos
   veterinários, 719
-- prevenção e tratamento de, 719
-- relacionadas à espécie, raça e interação
   medicamentosa, 717
-- sobre sistemas orgânicos, 718
- normais na eletromiografia, 444
Eversão dos ventrículos laterais, 1082
Exame(s)
- adequado da lamínula, 317
- citológico, 1043, 1061
-- tipos celulares observados no, 450
- complementares que auxiliam no diagnóstico, 44
- da genitália externa e interna, 1906
- da nasofaringe, 1074
- das biopsias, 1545
- de animais braquicefálicos, 1083
- de espéculo vaginal, 1872
- de fezes, 311, 897, 965, 1114
- de imagem, 602
-- avançados, 599
-- da próstata, 426
-- do fígado, 1628
-- nuclear, 1859
- de sangue iniciais, 601
- de saúde reprodutiva, 1906
- de urina, 183, 280, 589, 1628, 1743, 2023
- do cerume, 1061
- do esfregaço sanguíneo, 235
- do LBA, 1114
- do líquido
-- pericárdico, 1320
-- sinovial, 75
- do nariz, 1071
- do sistema respiratório, 1094
- dos seios paranasais, 1078
- e biopsia endoscópicos, 435
- ecocardiográfico e doppler, 1303
- fecais, 1540, 1562, 1582
- físico, 4, 8, 44, 70, 77
-- do paciente com problema respiratório, 1092
-- e abdominal, 597
- macroscópico da amostra de fezes, 311
- microscópico do sedimento, 283
- neurológico, 1374
- oftálmico, 55
- oral tradicional da laringe, 1086
- otoendoscópico, 335
- otoscópico, 1061
- retal, 21
- sorológicos, 1043, 1095
- ultrassonográfico
-- abdominal completo, 344
-- do trato reprodutivo, 1908
- virológico, 1541
- visual (cor, turbidez e odor), 280
Excentrócitos, 229
Excesso
- de base, 526
- de esteroides gonadais, 90
- de glicocorticoides, 90
Excisão de massas aurais, 336
Excreção
- alterada de eletrólitos e água, 1962
- de hidrogênio respiratório, 1559
- espontânea de ureterólitos, 2011
- fracionada de sódio, 1944
- reduzida de solutos orgânicos, 1962
Exercício(s), 1788
- físicos, 747
- terapêutico, 2181
Exposição, ambiente e hábitos, 44
Expressão, 28
Expressividade genética, 30
Exsudação, 292
Exsudato, 79, 1149
Extração
- de dirofilárias, 473
- manual, 1602
Extrassístoles ventriculares, 1197

Índice Alfabético

Extravasamento(s)
- do medicamento, 2087
- gastrintestinal, 294
- pelo local de ostomia, 327
- subcutâneo de urina, 625
- viscerais ou vasculares, 294
Extrofia, 2055
Extrusão traumática de disco, 1454

F
Falha(s)
- da medula óssea como causa da anemia não regenerativa, 845
- de concepção com estro e cobertura aparentemente normal, 1886
- em atingir ereção ou introdução, 1910
- na distribuição de nutrientes, 1533
- na ejaculação, 1911
- na emissão do ejaculado, 1911, 1912
- no desenvolvimento não relacionada com a doença, 45
- no fechamento da nasofaringe, 1077
- ovulatória, 1869
Falta de eficácia como reação, 716
Famotidina, 1954
Faringe, 1096
Faringite, 1491
Faringoscopia, 1490
Farmacocinética de medicamentos, 677, 2194
Farmacodinâmica dos medicamentos, 2194
Farmacogenética, 31
Farmacologia, 696
Farmacologia e indicações clínicas para anti-inflamatórios não esteroides, 698
Fármacos
- anestésicos, 1086
- ansiolíticos, 521
- anti-inflamatórios/imunossupressores, 1634
- anticoagulantes, 1355
- antifúngicos azóis, 691
- antiplaquetários, 1309, 1355
- antitireoidianos tioureilenos, 1769
- antitrombóticos, 1355
- citoprotetores, 1632
-- hepáticos, 1633
- comumente utilizados no tratamento de hepatopatias, 1632
- de reversão, 579
- e lúpus eritematoso sistêmico, 878
- e toxinas, 95
- que diminuem o volume
-- pós-carga, 1179
-- pré-carga, 1176
- que facilitam a função inotrópica, 1182
- que inibem a função inotrópica, 1183
- sedativos/ analgésicos, 1311
- tempo-dependentes, 688
- usados
-- no tratamento de insuficiência cardíaca, 1176
-- para sedação e anestesia, 569
Fascículo anterior esquerdo, 1205
Fase(s)
- da deglutição, 1487
- esofágica, 1488
- faríngea, 1487
- folicular, 1882
- oral, 1487
- preparatória oral, 1487
Fator(es)
- ambientais e lúpus eritematoso sistêmico, 878
- de conversão felino, 1932
- de crescimento
-- de fibroblastos básico, 2065
-- derivado de plaquetas, 2065
-- do endotélio vascular, 2065
- de segurança dos tecidos, 531
- de von Willebrand, 825
- locais que afetam a eficácia do antibiótico, 687
- nuclear kappa-b, 744
Febre, 193, 2158
- abordagem da, 195
- benefícios da, 193
- de origem desconhecida, 193
- diagnósticos diferenciais da, 195

- efeitos prejudiciais da, 194
- maculosa das Montanhas Rochosas, 955, 1434
- patogênese da, 193
- tratamento da, 197
Fechamento da mandíbula ou qualquer pressão na região ventral de cabeça e pescoço, 1082
Feijão-castor, 650
Feijão precário, 650
Fendas de lábio e palato, 1072
Fenilpropanolamina, 640, 2038
Fenobarbital, 146, 565, 1680
Fenoldopam, 1949
Fenômeno
- de ricochete, 1384
- de Wenckebach, 1202
Fenótipo, 25, 28
Fenoxibenzamina, 2040
Fentanil, 706
Fentanila, 570, 571
Feo-hifomicose, 1056
Feocromocitoma, 1856
Fermentabilidade, 798
Ferramentas laboratoriais para avaliação da função e da doença intestinal, 1476
Ferro, 815
Fertilidade, 1910
Fertilizantes orgânicos, 633
Fibra(s), 727, 731
- alimentar(es)
-- em alimentos para animais de estimação, 797
-- tipos de, 796
-- uso terapêutico da, 797
-- usos nutricionais da, 796
- na dieta, 759
Fibratos, 767
Fibrilação
- atrial, 1194
- ventricular, 1200
Fibrinogênio, 825
Fibroelastose endocárdica, 1253
Fibromas odontogênicos periféricos, 1484
Fibroplasia esclerosante eosinofílica felina, 1567
Fibrose
- hepática, 1638
- intersticial, 1958
- peritoneal, 1958
- pulmonar idiopática, 1136
Fibrossarcoma, 1485
- apendicular em cães, 2134
Fígado, 344, 347, 1621, 1671, 1676
Filaroides, 1121
Filhotes com tremedeira, 134
Fimose, 1910
Fios-guia, 457
FISH para *Escherichia coli* aderente e invasiva, 1476
Física
- da eletrocardiografia, 385
- do ultrassom, 343
Fisiologia
- acidobásica, 525
- da defecação, 1604
- da dor, 513
- da flatulência, 175
- da micção, 2035
- do intestino grosso, 171
- do pericárdio, 1312
- do peritônio, 1615
- dos ureteres, 2009
- e metabolismo do lactato, 276
- nutricional única do gato adulto saudável, 730
Fisioterapia/reabilitação, 2179, 2180
Fissura palpebral e simetria de terceira pálpebra, 1379
Fístula(s)
- broncoesofágica, 1105, 1111
- colovesical, 2055
- esofágica, 1497
- perianal, 1611
- traqueoesofágica, 1105
- ureterovaginal, 2016, 2047, 2056
- ureteroperineal, 2047, 2056
- uretrorretal, 2016, 2047, 2056
Fita reagente de urina bioquímica colorimétrica, 1930

Fixação dos tecidos, 339
Flagelados, 974
Flatulência, 175, 1534
- fisiopatologia da, 175
Flebotomia, 850
Flotação fecal, 1476
Fluconazol, 690, 692
Fluidos, 531, 2193
- de manutenção, 531
- de reposição, 531
- tipo de, 1948
Fluidoterapia, 198, 533, 1510, 1513
- com cristaloides e coloides, 530
- de manutenção, 1948
- tradicional, 1947
Flumazenil, 628
Fluorescência indireta para pesquisa de anticorpos, 898
Fluoroquinolonas, 688
Fluoroscopia, 1098
5-fluoruracila, 641
Flutter
- atrial, 1193
- ventricular, 1200
Flutuação fecal, 312
Fluxo(s)
- arterial, 1353
- da veia pulmonar, 404
- linfático e venoso sistêmicos, 1357
- retrógrado
-- com oclusão do orifício uretral distal, 413
-- sem cistocentese descompressiva, 413
-- transmitral, 404
Foetor hepaticus, 152
Folato, 1476
Fomepizol, 628, 636, 1952
Força(s)
- de Starling tradicionais, 530
- muscular, 1815
Forma do coração, 1301
Formação
- de cálculos nos rins e no trato urinário, 1736
- de cilindros, 1936
- de edema, 1993
- de Rouleaux, 229
Formados dos sopros cardíacos, 219
Formulações lipossomais, 689
Fornecimento de proteção da mucosa, 1513
Fosfatase alcalina, 256, 1624
- sérica, 1817
Fosfato, 275, 1817
- de cálcio, 780, 2029
- de toceranib, 2082
Fosfetos, 630
Fósforo, 272, 275, 1736, 1737, 1953
- dietético, 1973
Fração, 2073
- de ejeção, 402, 403
- de encurtamento, 402
- de excreção de eletrólitos, 1933
Fracionamento, 2073
Fragilidade cutânea felina, 54
Fraqueza, 92
- faríngea, 1491
Fratura(s)
- de costelas, 621
- de pênis, 1910
Frênulo persistente do pênis, 1910
Frequência
- cardíaca, 536
- de inseminação, 1873
- dos sopros cardíacos, 219
Frutosamina, 1800, 1802
- sérica, 1791
Função
- cardíaca, 401
-- global, 405
- cognitiva, 1373
- da laringe, 1085
- diastólica, 404
- do cálcio, 1729
- hepática, 1621
- metabólicas, 1501
- renal, 1927

Índice Alfabético

- retardada do enxerto, 1957
- sistólica, 402
- vestibular, 1381
- vitais, 44
Fundamentos básicos da medicina veterinária, 1
Fungos, 1593
Furosemida, 1177, 1310

G

Gabapentina, 146, 520, 707, 708
Gaiola de oxigênio, 546
Galactostasia, 1897
Galope pré-sistólico, 218
Gamaglutamiltransferase, 256, 259
Gamaglutamiltranspeptidase, 1625
Ganho de peso, 77
Gás(es), 82
- sanguíneos, 525
Gasto energético
- de manutenção, 748
- de repouso, 748
Gastrenterite
- hemorrágica, 1548
- infecciosa, 1503
Gastrina, 1852
- sérica, 1512
Gastrinoma, 1853
Gastrite
- aguda, 1510
- associada a *Helicobacter*, 1520
- crônica, 1516
-- de causa desconhecida, 1521
- parasitária, 1519
Gastropatia urêmica, 1963
Gastroscópios, 328
Genética
- básica, 25
- clínica, 28
- do lúpus eritematoso sistêmico, 877
Gengivite, 151
- hiperplásica juvenil, 1481
Genitália externa, 1880
Genoma
- canino, 25
- felino, 25
Genômica clínica, 27
Genótipo, 25, 28
Gestação, 1868, 1892
- e parto, 1884
Giardia
- *intestinalis*, 1594
- sp., 1554
Glândula
- nasal lateral, 1070
- tireoide, 1745
Glargina, 1803
Glicemia, 1799, 1802, 1817
- única, 1791
Glicocálice endotelial, 531
Glicocorticoides, 200, 696, 701, 847, 1565, 1590, 1738, 1844, 1849, 1885
- no choque séptico, 2211
- no tratamento de doenças infecciosas, 2210
Glicopirrolato, 570, 572
Glicose, 281, 1625, 1845, 1849, 1949, 1952
Glicosímetros portáteis, 1791
Glicosúria, 1791, 1933
- renal, 1997
Glifosato, 636
Gliomatose cerebral, 1399
Glomeruloesclerose, 1991, 2006
Glomerulonefrite, 1337, 2158
- membranoproliferativa, 1985
- mesângio-capilar, 1985
- proliferativa, 1987
Glomerulopatia, 1981
- tratamento imunossupressor de cães com, 1992
Glucagon, 1852
Glucagonoma, 1810, 1854
Gonadectomia cirúrgica, 1879
Gordura, 729, 750, 772
- dietética, 754
Gotejamento de antígenos e biopsia, 1519

Gradiente(s)
- de pressão instantânea, 394
- transtubular de potássio, 288
Granulomas
- parasitários, 1106
- piogênico, 1481
- traqueais, 1106
Granulomatose
- eosinofílica, 1337
- linfomatoide pulmonar, 1131
Grelina, 738, 1852, 1853
Griseofulvina, 690
Gurltia paralisante, 1471

H

Halitose, 147, 150
- bucal, 151
- causas da, 151
- com odor de urina ou amoniacal, 151
- com odor doce, 151
- fisiológica, 150
- frutado, 151
- patológica, 150
- sulfurosa, 150
- verdadeira, 150
Hantavírus, 1026
Helicobacter spp., 1517
- entero-hepáticos, 1592
Helmintos, 1552, 1594
Hemácias, 451
Hemangiossarcoma, 887, 2119
- apendicular em cães, 2134
- esplênico felino, 889
Hematimetria, 1114
Hematócrito, 964, 1946
Hematologia e testes de coagulação, 1686
Hematoma extradural, 1456
Hematopoese
- cíclica em Grey Collies, 861
- extramedular, 890
Hematoquezia, 167, 170, 1595
Hematúria, 189, 282, 283, 1934
- renal idiopática, 505
Hemilocomoção, 1376
Hemivértebras, 1448
Hemocomponentes, 537
Hemocromatose, 1676
Hemocultura, 929, 1274
Hemodiálise, 421
- intermitente, 422
Hemofilias A e B, 122, 832
Hemogasometria, 525
- arterial, 210
Hemoglobinúria, 282
Hemograma, 839, 1562, 1743, 1750, 1765, 1817, 1832, 1845, 2001
- completo, 183, 589
Hemólise, 226, 835, 837
- aloimune felina, 841
- pré-transfusão, 545
Hemoperitônio, 604
Hemoplasmose canina, 838
Hemoptise, 120, 123
Hemorragia, 225, 561, 835, 1149
- arterial causada por lesão invasiva, 124
- no mediastino, 1155
- no timo, 1158
Hemospermia, 1911
Hemostase *in vivo*, 826
Hemostasia primária, 851
Hemotórax, 621, 1149
Heparina(s)
- de baixo peso molecular, 1353, 1356
- não fracionada, 1353
Hepatite
- aguda, 1639
-- causada por toxinas, 1642
- crônica, 1636, 1640
Hepatomas, 1685
Hepatopatias, 1622
- causadas por armazenamento anormal ou normal excessivo de metal ou metabólito, 1676
- esteroide, 1672
- inflamatórias/infecciosas

-- em cães, 1639
-- em gatos, 1645
- metabólica, 1671
- princípios gerais do tratamento de, 1632
- vacuolar semelhante àquela causada por glicogênio em cães Scottish Terrier, 1672
- vacuolares, 1671
Hepatotoxicidade, 1678, 2090
- idiossincrática, 1679
-- induzidas por fármacos, 1681
- induzidas por fármacos dose-dependentes, 1679
Hepatotoxinas presentes no domicílio e no ambiente, 1682
Hepatozoonoses, 971
Herança(s)
- autossômica
-- dominante, 26
-- recessiva, 26
- ligada ao cromossomo X, 27
- poligênica, 27
Herbicidas, 635
Hérnia
- da bexiga, 625
- de hiato, 1161, 1498
- diafragmática, 622, 1152, 1160
-- peritônio-pericárdica, 1161, 1313
- perineal, 1605
Herniação
- do forame magno, 139
- transtentorial, 139
Heroína, 646
Herpes-vírus
- canino, 1009, 1014, 1890
- felino-1, 693
Heterobilharzia americana, 166, 1594
Heterozigoto, 25, 28
Hialo-hifomicose, 1056
Hidratação, 1922
Hidrocarbonetos, 634
Hidroclorotiazida, 1310, 2027
Hidromorfina, 706
Hidromorfona, 570, 571
Hidropulsão salina, 1099
Hidroterapia, 2183
Hidroxiureia, 848
Hiper-reflexia do músculo detrusor/bexiga hiperativa, 2039
Hiperadrenocorticismo, 50, 62, 63, 1760, 1810, 1827
- adrenal-dependente, 1835
- canino, 1812
- felino, 1828
- hipertensão sistêmica, 661
- hipófise-dependente, 1812, 1813, 1818, 1820, 1822, 1825, 1835
Hiperagregação plaquetária, 2157
Hiperaldosteronismo primário em gatos como causa de doença renal crônica, 1967
Hiperalgesia, 515
Hipercalcemia, 62, 1207, 1953, 1967
- em cães, 272
- em gatos, 273
- maligna, 2155
Hipercapnia, 528
Hipercloremia, 266
Hipercoagulabilidade na doença glomerular, 1932
Hipercoagulação, 2157
Hiperemese *gravidarum*, 1889
Hiperemia, 206
Hiperestrogenismo, 50, 2156
Hiperfosfatemia, 275, 1966
Hiperglicemia, 242, 244, 587
- induzida por estresse, 244
- pós-prandial em cães e gatos com diabetes, 759
Hiperglobulinemia, 2157
Hiperlipidemia, 762, 763, 1671, 1994
- canina, 1675
- em cães, 249
- felina, 251
- manejo nutricional de, 765
- primárias, 249, 765
- secundárias, 249, 765
Hipermagnesemia, 271, 1967
Hipernatremia, 63, 262, 263, 288, 629
- isovolêmica, 262
- secundária à perda de líquido hipotônico, 262

Índice Alfabético

Hiperostose
- calvariana, 1484
- esquelética idiopática disseminada, 1441
Hiperparatireoidismo
- primário, 273, 1729
-- em cães, 1732
-- em gatos, 1741
-- humano, 1732
- secundário
-- nutricional, 784
-- renal, 1965
Hiperplasia
- de vagina, 610
- endometrial cística, 1898, 1899
- esplênica, 890
- linfoide, 1910
- mamária, 1886
- nodular, 890, 1684, 1813
- prostática benigna, 2057
Hiperpotassemia, 268, 288, 1206, 1952, 1976
Hiperproteinemia, 239
- causas de, 241
Hipersensibilidade, 1214, 1482, 1532, 1555
- alimentar, 781
-- manejo a longo prazo da, 782
-- prognóstico da, 782
Hipersomatotropismo felino, 1716
Hiperstenúria, 1932
Hipertensão, 1828, 1953
- arterial, 1963, 1977
- de consultório, 661
- do jaleco branco, 661
- idiopática, 661
- manifestações
-- cardíacas da, 662
-- clínicas da, 661
-- do sistema nervoso, 664
-- oculares da, 662
-- renais da, 663
-- vasculares da, 662
- pulmonar, 1141
- sistêmica, 59, 60, 1993, 2193
-- em cães, tratamento de, 668
-- em gatos, tratamento da, 669
-- fisiopatologia da, 659
-- tratamento da, 666
Hipertermia, 63, 193, 1480
Hipertireoidismo, 62, 63, 1810
- canino, 1772
- felino, 1762, 1763
- hipertensão sistêmica e, 661
- humano, 1762
- iatrogênico, 1772
Hipertonia, 1378
Hipertrigliceridemia, 1695
Hipertrofia de tonsilas palatinas, 1082
Hiperuricosúria, 1996
Hipervitaminose A, 787
Hipervolemia, 288
Hiperxantinúria, 1996
Hipnóticos não benzodiazepínicos, 639
Hipoadrenocorticismo, 63, 273, 1842
- felino, 1851
- primário, 1843
- secundário, 1843, 1846
Hipoalbuminemia, 275, 1932
Hipoaldosteronismo isolado, 1846
Hipocalcemia, 62, 274, 611, 1206, 1891, 1953, 1967
Hipocloremia, 265
Hipocoagulabilidade adquirida, 831
Hipocolesterolemia, 252
Hipocortisolismo, 1825
Hipófise, 1812
- anterior, 1812
- posterior, 1812
Hipofosfatemia, 276, 837, 1719, 1825
- felina, 838
Hipofunções endócrinas, 90
Hipoglicemia, 62, 242, 1625, 1796, 1810, 1923, 2155
- aguda, 1781
- induzida pela insulina com hiperglicemia de rebote, 1811
Hipoglicemiante orais, 1807
Hipoluteísmo em cães e gatos, 1890

Hipoluteoidismo, 1870
Hipomagnesemia, 270
Hiponatremia, 63, 263, 287
- hipertônica, 264
- hipotônica, 265
- hipovolêmica, 265
- por diluição, 265
Hipoparatireoidismo, 1742
Hipoplasia
- da bexiga, 2054
- da uretra, 2046, 2055
- de traqueia, 1083
- do centro, 1448
Hipopotassemia, 64, 267, 288, 1205, 1952, 1976
- e doença renal crônica primária, 1967
Hipoproteinemia, 239
- causas de, 240
Hipospadia, 2046, 2056
Hipossensibilidade, 1214
Hipossomatotropismo felino, 1715
- adquirido, 1716
- congênito, 1715
Hipostenúria, 1932
Hipotálamo, 1812
Hipotalamotecto-tegumentar, 1384
Hipotensão, 374
- sistêmica, 671
Hipotermia, 201, 202, 1480, 1922
- como tratamento, 203
Hipótese da célula-tronco cancerosa, 2065
Hipotireoidismo, 50, 61, 63, 1285, 1434, 1461, 1746, 1754, 1760
- adquirido, 1747
- congênito, 1747, 1750, 1758, 1759
- em cães, 1745
- em gatos, 1758
- em idade adulta, 1758
- espontâneo, 1760
- iatrogênico, 1758, 1759
- juvenil, 90
Hipotonia dos músculos abdominais, 82
Hipotrigliceridemia, 252
Hipoventilação, 208
Hipovolemia, 287, 288, 533
Hipoxemia, 371, 529
- secundária a doença sistêmica, 60
Hipoxia, 63
Histiocitoma(s), 2110
- em cães, 2144
Histiócitos, 2144
Histiocitose
- cutânea, 2145
- de células de Langerhans
-- cutânea em cães, 2144
-- pulmonar em gatos, 2145
- maligna, 1132
- progressiva em gatos, 2145
- reativa em cães, 2145
- sistêmica, 2145
Histologia, 2114
Histopatologia, 894
Histoplasma capsulatum, 896, 1593
Histoplasmose, 1034, 1039
História das vacinas e vacinação, 900
Histórico clínico, 44, 70, 77
Homeostase do cálcio em cães e gatos, 1729
Homing dos linfócitos no tecido linfoide associado ao intestino, 1530
Homozigoto, 25, 28
Hormônio(s)
- antidiurético, 1168, 1932
- associados à hiperplasia endometrial cística e à piometra, 1898
- da fome, 738
- do crescimento, 1715, 1720
- liberador
-- de corticotrofina, 1812
-- de gonadotrofina, 1869
- livre (não ligado), 1752
- pancreáticos e intestinais, 1851
- séricos, 1866
- tireoestimulante, 1765
-- no desenvolvimento tumoral, 1773
- tireoidianos, 1745

I

Icterícia, 211, 1622
Idade de início dos sinais de transtornos de comportamento, 47
Identificação dos ingredientes dietéticos agressores, 782
Ifosfamida, 2067
Íleo adinâmico, 1572
Imagem
- cerebral, 1389
- de Doppler tecidual
-- com onda pulsada do anel mitral, 1305
-- para avaliação dos movimentos do miocárdio, 1303
- por ressonância magnética, 1391, 1490
-- do coração, 1303
Imatinib, 2084
Imidapril, 1180, 1309
Imidazolinona, 636
Impactação, 1612
Impedância esofágica, 1490
Implantação
- de marca-passo, 1209
-- permanente, 1213
-- transvenoso, 1213
- de *stent* biliar, 1690
Imunocomplexos patogênicos, 877
Imunodeficiência
- combinada
-- autossômica recessiva grave, 861
-- grave ligada ao X, 861
- comum variável, 861
Imunoedição, 2079
Imunofluorescência, 1540
- para *Giardia* e *Cryptosporidium*, 1476
Imunoglobulina intravenosa, 538
Imunologia
- da vacinação, 900
- e nutrição, 813
- tumoral, 2079
Imunomodulação, 854
- relacionada com a transfusão, 545
Imunorreatividade
- da lipase pancreática, 1698
- semelhante à tripsina, 1698
Imunossupressão, 854, 986, 1957
- causada por infecção, 2211
Imunoterapia, 2127
- no tratamento de câncer, 2079
- para linfoma, 2098
- tumoral
-- específica, 2081
-- inespecífica, 2079
Inalação de fumaça, 1138
Inaladores
- com dosímetro, 369
- de aspersão, 369
Inanição, 815
Incapacidade
- de abrir a boca, 150
- de fechar a boca, 150
Incidentalomas, 1836
Inclinação, 391
Incompatibilidades de células não vermelhas, 543
Incompetência
- congênita do esfíncter uretral, 2056
- do mecanismo do esfíncter uretral, 2036, 2045
Incontinência, 1880
- de urgência, 184
- fecal, 171, 174, 1614
- urinária, 184
-- congênita, 2048
-- na cadela ovariectomizada, 1913
Incretinas, 1808
Índice(s)
- cardíaco, 403
- de atividade da doença inflamatória intestinal, 1563
- de desempenho do miocárdio, 405
- TEI, 405
Indução
- da ovulação, 1884
- do estro, 1869, 1878, 1886
Inervação para o cólon, 1576

Infarto
- do miocárdio, 1285
- esplênico, 605, 890
- isquêmico, 1408
Infecção(ões), 453
- abortiva, 985
- após implantação de marca-passo, 1215
- bacteriana, 864, 1649
- causadas por coronavírus, 989
- de glóbulos vermelhos, 837
- do trato
-- respiratório superior de gatos, 1020
-- urinário, 686, 1810
--- causada por cateter, 410
--- complicada, 2018
--- diagnóstico de, 2017
--- inferior, 2016
--- não complicada, 2018
--- tratamento de, 2018
- e imunossupressão simultâneas, 2205
- e quimioterapia antineoplásica, 2209
- e uso de fármaco imunossupressor, 2205
- fúngicas, 864, 865, 1552, 1651
-- diversas, 1051
-- oportunistas, 1056
- gastrintestinais, 1591
- hemotrópicas por *Mycoplasma*, 837
- intestinais causadas por *Escherichia coli*, 967
- micobacterianas, 865
- no transplante de órgãos, 2210
- nosocomiais, 906
- pelo vírus
-- da cinomose canina, 896
-- da imunodeficiência felina, 864, 977
-- da leucemia felina, 864, 984
- persistentes, 2018
- por *Ancylostoma* spp, 1553
- por astrovírus, 1025
- por *Bartonella* em cães e gatos, 864
- por cianobactérias e algas, 1552
- por cinomose, 864
- por coronavírus felino, 990
- por dermatófitos, 689
- por hantavírus, 1026
- por kobuvírus, 1026
- por morbilivírus, 1026
- por paramixovírus, 864
- por parvovírus, 864
-- em cães e gatos, 997
- por poxvírus, 1024
- por protozoários, 864, 865, 968
- por reovírus felino, 1025
- por retrovírus, 2095
- por rotavírus, 1025
- por torovírus, 1026
- por vírus espumoso felino, 1025
- progressiva, 985
- que causam
-- autoimunidade secundária, 2210
-- inflamação debilitante ou com risco de
   morte, 2210
- regressiva, 985
- riquetsiais, 864
- sistêmicas, 689
- virais, 1650
-- em cães, 864, 1012
-- em gatos, 864, 1023
Infertilidade no gato macho, 1887
Inflamação, 70, 356, 829
- da mucosa, 1532
- oral, 1481
- séptica *versus* asséptica, 341
Influenza em gatos, 1023
Ingestão de alimentos, 800
Inherited Diseases in Dogs, 29
Inibição da absorção de colesterol, 768
Inibidor(es)
- da absorção de gordura, 768
- da alfaglicosidase, 1808
- da ciclo-oxigenase, 2127
- da ECA, 1309
- da enzima conversora de angiotensina, 1180
- da mitose, 2067
- da proteinase, 1700
- da recaptação de serotonina e norepinefrina, 520

- de alpha1-protease, 1541
- de lipase, 741
- de mitose, 2068
- de proteína microssômica de transferência de
   triglicerídeos, 741
- do receptor, 520
- seletivos da recaptação de serotonina e outros, 638
Inibina sérica, 1860
Início
- da reanimação cardiopulmonar, 576
- de sinais anormais e sua progressão, 3
Inotrópicos, 1311
Inquietação, 95
Inseminação
- artificial, 1888
-- em cadelas, 445
-- vaginal ou intrauterina, 445
- intrauterina
-- cirúrgica, 449
-- com visualização endoscópica da cérvice, 448
-- por meio de laparoscopia, 449
-- usando cateter escandinavo, 447
- vaginal, 447
Inseticidas, 632
Insolação, 557
Instabilidade atlantoaxial, 1446
Instrumentação na radiologia intervencionista, 457
Insuficiência(s)
- anterógrada, 1163
- aórtica, 220
- cardíaca, 582, 1174
-- congestiva, 1149, 1163, 1338
--- direita devido à hipertensão pulmonar, 1270
-- de alto débito, 1164
-- de baixo débito, 1163
-- diastólica, 1163
-- fisiopatologia da, 1163
-- tratamento clínico, 1173
- do miocárdio induzida por deficiência de
   taurina, 1298
- do pâncreas exócrino, 753
- hepática, 152, 830
-- aguda, 605, 1636
- mitral, 219
- pancreática exócrina, 1708
- pulmonar, 221
- renal, 152
-- intrínseca, 1941, 2050
-- pós-tratamento, 1771
-- retrógrada, 1163
- tricúspide, 219
Insuflação do manguito do tubo endotraqueal, 1480
Insulina, 591, 1789, 1849, 1952
- inteligente, 1808
- lenta, 1802
- protamina zíncica, 1803
Insulinoma, 1853
Insulinoterapia, 1787, 1802
Integrinas, 1169
Intenção de tratar, 36
Intensidade (sonoridade) dos sopros cardíacos, 219
Interação(ões)
- bactéria-mucosa, 1528
- entre microrganismo e hospedeiro na superfície
   mucosa, 1502
- entre plaquetas e fator de von Willebrand, 852
- fisiológicas microrganismo-hospedeiro, 1501
- hospedeiro-microbiota na saúde e doença
   gastrintestinal, 1500
Interestro, 1883
Interleucinas, 738
Interpretação
- da leitura do oxímetro de pulso, 371
- das lesões no fundo de olho, 55
- dos resultados do exame citológico do
   linfonodo, 364
- dos testes de suscetibilidade, 686
Interrupção da gestação, 1885
Intervalo(s)
- de acoplamento, 1189
- interestrais, 1863
-- curtos, 1871
Intervenção(ões)
- híbridas, 481

- no coração
-- direito, 470
-- esquerdo, 474
- nutricional na encefalopatia hepática, 757
Intolerância(s), 801
- alimentar, 801, 1557
- ao exercício, 1078
- farmacológicas, 1557
Intoxicação, 96
- alimentar, 1557
- causadas por produtos químicos, 629
- por aminoglicosídeos, 1952
- por drogas utilizadas para fins recreativos, 643
- por etilenoglicol, 275, 1952
- por fármacos, 236
- por medicamentos que necessitam de receita e
   por medicamentos de venda livre, 637
- por oxigênio, 549
- por plantas, 647
- tremorgênicas, 133
Introdução
- do cateter intraósseo, 303
- gradual da suplementação com T4, 1757
Intubação gástrica, 430
Intussuscepção, 1573, 1599
- cecocólica, 1598
Inversão cecal, 1598
Iodo radioativo, 1770
Ioimbina, 628
Íris, 57, 651
Isospora spp, 1554
Isquemia global, 1409
Itraconazol, 690, 692
Ivabradina, 1308
Ivermectina, 1330

J
Janela paraesternal direita, 390

K
Kobuvírus, 1026

L
Lactato, 276, 536
Lactonas macrocíclicas como adulticidas, 1334
Lactulose, 1661
Lagenidiose, 1054
Lambedura de superfície, 49
Lantus®, 1803
Laparoscopia, 350
- indicações para, 351
Laringe, 1082, 1096
Laringectomia parcial e ventriculocordectomia
   bilateral, 1087
Laringofaringe, 1381
Laringoscopia, 1490
Laser, 461
- terapêutico, 2181
Lateralização unilateral da cartilagem
   aritenoide, 1087
Lavado
- broncoalveolar, 1099
-- guiado por endoscopia, 382
-- técnica às cegas, 380
- endotraqueal, 380, 1100
- nasal, 364, 366
- peritoneal diagnóstico, 598
- transtraqueal, 379, 1100
- traqueal, 1100
Lavagem
- aural, 336
- da orelha, 334
- gástrica, 431, 627
- peritoneal diagnóstica, 348, 349
Laxantes, 1601
- emolientes, 1601
- estimulantes, 1601
- hiperosmóticos, 1601
- lubrificantes, 1601
Leflunomida, 703, 820
Lei de Laplace, 1170
Leiomiossarcoma, 1525, 2116
Leishmania spp, 974
Leishmaniose, 51, 866, 974

Leptina, 736, 737
Leptospira
- *interrogans*, 1640, 1941
- *kirschneri*, 1941
- spp., 915, 916
Leptospirose, 945, 1640, 1905, 1941
- em gatos, 949
- prevenção de, 949
Lesão(ões)
- cardíaca, 623
- de medula espinal diagnóstico das, 1451
- da membrana de microvilosidades (apical), 1531
- de vasos sanguíneos renais, 625
- do ligamento cruzado cranial, 2163
- hepática aguda, 1636
- melanocíticas primárias, 1398
- neoplásicas, 342, 1457
-- *versus* não neoplásicas, 342
- por reperfusão, 1353
- pulmonar(es)
-- aguda relacionada com a transfusão, 545
-- cavitárias, 1138
-- física, 1136
- renal aguda, 1939
-- adquirida no hospital, 1944
-- estadiamento da, 1939
-- pós-renal, 1942
-- quatro fases da, 1942
- tecidual, 70
- tubular aguda, 1999
- tubulointersticiais associadas à doença
    glomerular, 1991
Letargia, 2089
Leucemia
- granulocítica crônica, 863
- linfoblástica aguda, 2101
- linfocítica crônica, 2101
- linfoide, 2101, 2102
- mieloide aguda, 2065
Leucócitos, 283, 451
Leucocitose, 231, 232
- eosinofílica, 2156
- por neutrofilia, 971, 2156
Leucopenia, 231, 233
Levemir®, 1804
Levetiracetam, 146
Levotiroxina, 1776
Liberação
- de tampões uretrais de matriz cristalina em
    gatos, 2049
- de urólitos, 2049
Libido, 1906
Lidocaína, 707, 1308
Ligação espermatozoide-oócito, 1908
Limiar pruriginoso, 804
Limitações do sistema de registros, 716
Limpadores domésticos, 632
Limpeza
- auricular profunda, 336
- e armazenamento de endoscópios, 436
Linfadenite, 1365
Linfadenopatia, 361
- no mediastino, 1157
Linfangiectasia, 1568
Linfangioma, 1368
Linfangiossarcoma, 1368
Linfangite, 1365
Linfedema, 1366
- primário, 1366
- secundário, 1366
Linfocintilografia, 1359
Linfócitos, 1529
- T, 1529
Linfoma, 294, 1075, 1524, 2092, 2110
- alimentar, 1597
- canino em outras localizações, 2094
- cutâneo
-- em forma de placa, 53
-- /epiteliotrófico de células T, 51
- e neoplasias hematopoéticas, 1398, 1400
- extralinfonodal, 2099
- felino, 2094
- indolente (de baixo grau), 2099
- intestinal, 1570

- multicêntrico canino, 2093
- pulmonar, 1131
Linfonodos, 348
- internos, 362
- periféricos, 362
- sublombares, 345
Língua, 1381
Linhagens tumorais, 1685
Lipase, 253
Lipidose hepática
- em gatos manejo nutricional da, 757
- felina, 1671, 1673
Lipofuscinose ceroide neuronal, 1395
Líquido(s), 79
- abdominal livre, 601
- articular, 295
- cefalorraquidiano, 993, 1392, 1402
- cerebroespinal, 899
- corporais, 289
- da efusão, 992
- das cavidades torácica e abdominal, 289
- para limpador de para-brisa, 634
- sinovial, 76
Litotripsia
- intracorpórea do trato urinário inferior, 491
- por ondas de choque
-- em casos de ureterólitos, 2013
-- extracorpóreas, 499
Lobo
- intermediário, 1812
- pancreático esquerdo, 345
Localização
- e irradiação dos sopros cardíacos, 219
- multifocal e difusa no sistema nervoso central, 1386
Lomustina, 1681, 2067
Lúpus
- cutâneo vesicular eritematoso, 873
- eritematoso, 51
-- cutâneo, 876
--- esfoliativo, 51, 873
-- discoide
--- forma clássica, 873
--- forma generalizada, 873
-- sistêmico, 867, 877
--- fatores ambientais e, 878
- mucocutâneo eritematoso, 873
Luteinização pré-ovulatória, 1864
Luxação de patela, 2160, 2161

M
Má absorção, 1534
Maconha (*Cannabis sativa*), 645, 649
- sintética, 645
Macroglossia, 1082
Macronutrientes, 726
Magnésio, 267, 270, 536, 773, 1953
Malformações
- anorretais, 1609
- arteriovenosas hepáticas, 1668
- atriais, 1252
- congênitas, 1469
- congênitas da medula espinal, 1447
- uretrogenitais, 2047, 2056
- ventriculares, 1253
Malnutrição na imunidade, 815
Manejo
- alimentar dos gatos, 732
- da dor
-- como um padrão na prática, 517
-- em procedimentos diagnósticos, 521
- de condições estressantes, não dolorosas, 521
- nutricional
-- da doença do pâncreas exócrino, 752
-- da lipidose hepática em gatos, 757
-- das cardiopatias, 768
-- das doenças
--- do trato gastrintestinal, 747
--- endócrinas e metabólicas, 758
--- hepatobiliares, 754
--- renais, 775
-- de hiperlipidemia, 765
-- do cão atleta, 728
-- do diabetes melito, 758
- reprodutivo da cadela, 1863

Manifestação clínica das doenças familiares, 30
Manipulação
- do ciclo reprodutivo canino, 1876
- oral e de estruturas adjacentes, 1480
- pelo médico-veterinário e pelo farmacêutico, 714
Manitol, 1949
Manobra vagal, 1188
Manometria esofágica, 1490
Manuseio
- de cateteres urinários, 409
- seguro do medicamento quimioterápico, 2072
Manutenção
- do maquinário, 1372
- do peso ideal, 768
Marca-passo
- atrial
-- inibido, 1212
-- sincrônico, 1212
- cardíaco, 470, 1209
- complicações decorrentes do uso de, 1214
- de câmara
-- dupla, 1212
--- e sensibilidade com inibição e rastreamento, 1213
-- única, 1211
- e hemodinâmica, 1211
- errante, 1186, 1190
- transvenoso temporário, 1213
- ventricular inibido, 1211
Marcadores
- de disfunção/dano tubular, 1933
- de hipoxia, 1934
- de lesão tubular, 1934
- fluorescentes, 1928
- inflamatórios, 1934
- plasmáticos/séricos substitutos da taxa de
    filtração glomerular, 1928
- pró-fibróticos, 1934
- radioisótopos, 1928
Marcha, 1375
- anormal, 2164
Maropitant, 1954
Máscara de oxigênio, 547
Masitinib, 2084, 2142
Massa(s)
- mediastínicas, 1155
- muscular, 1378
- orais, 1485
- teciduais
-- múltiplas, 356
-- na laringe, 1089
Massagem, 2181
- prostática, 428
Mastite, 1897
Mastocitomas, 294, 2110
- cutâneos em gatos, 2143
- de "alto risco", 2141
- de "baixo risco", 2141
- em gatos, 2143
- esplênicos/viscerais em gatos, 2143
- intestinais em gatos, 2143
Mastocitose, 2140
Matéria seca, 748
Meato nasofaríngeo, 1068
Mecanismo(s)
- da tosse, 108
- de disfunção espinal, 1451
- de escape, 1187
- de formação do edema, 83
- e causas de síncope, 125
- fisiopatológicos na doença intestinal, 1531
- neurológicos, 739
- patogênicos da leptospirose, 946
- pseudoalérgicos, 1557
Mecloretamina, 2067
Mediastinite, 1155
Mediastino, 1153
Medicações, 3
Medicamentos
- antibacterianos, 684
- antifúngicos, 1044
- ativo contra o microrganismo, 684
- citotóxicos, 1565
- cuja aquisição requer receita médica, 643
- de liberação transdérmica, 714
- de venda livre, 637

- eméticos, 627
- fornecidos por meio de inalador com dosímetro, 369
- genéricos, 683
- imunossupressores, 1565
- manipulados, 683, 712
- nebulizados, 368
- que necessitam de receita, 637
- quimioterápicos, 2069
- utilizados no tratamento de acúmulo de cobre no fígado, 1635
Medicina
- hiperbárica, 331
-- complicações, 333
-- contraindicações, 333
-- equipamentos de segurança, 333
-- fisiologia, 331
-- indicações, 332
-- protocolo de tratamento, 334
- intervencionista, 455
- nuclear, 1098
- veterinária baseada em evidências, 32
Medula espinal, 1384
Meduloblastoma, 1399
Megacólon idiopático felino, 1602
Megaesôfago, 152, 1428
- congênito, 1495
- secundário adquirido, 1495
Meglitinidas, 1807
Meia-vida, 681
Melanoma, 2110
- maligno, 1485
Melarsomina, 1332
Melatonina, 1885
Melena, 167, 1534, 1536
Melfalana, 2067, 2104
Membranas excitáveis, 1369
Membros torácicos e pélvicos, 1378
Meningioma, 1399, 1400
Meningite-artrite responsiva a esteroides, 1449
Meningoencefalite
- bacteriana, 1414
- eosinofílica, 1414
- fúngica, 1415
- não supurativa do galgo, 1414
- viral, 1416
Meningoencefalomielite
- granulomatosa, 1412
- linfo-histiocítica vagarosa progressiva, 1472
Meningomielite, 1449
Mensuração
- da concentração de lactato, 277
- da pressão
-- arterial para um diagnóstico imediato, 374
-- pleural, 1150
-- sanguínea, 372, 674
-- venosa central, 299, 301
- da temperatura corporal, 194
- das proteínas do soro e do plasma, 239
- de eletrólitos, 183
- de eritropoetina, 850
- do cálcio e sua regulação no soro sanguíneo, 1729
Mesencéfalo, 1388
Mesilato de masitinib, 2084
Mesocestódios spp, 1553
Mesotelioma, 295
Metabolismo, 679
- da glicose, 799
- de proteínas/nitrogênio, 800
- do cálcio, 783
- lipídico, 800
Metabolização da gordura (lipídios), 762
Metadona, 570, 571, 706, 708
Metaestro, 1863
Metaldeído, 633
Metanol, 634
Metaplasia escamosa prostática, 1919
Metástase, 356, 2064, 2133
Metemoglobina, 208
Metimazol, 1682, 1769, 1776
Metocarbamol, 628, 2040
Metoclopramida, 1954
Método(s)
- de alimentação, 734
- de Baermann, 317

- de concentração fecal, 1540
- de cultura, 939
- de diagnóstico molecular, 938
- de remoção de urólitos em animais
-- assintomáticos, 2023
-- sintomáticos, 2025
- estatísticos, 38
- não farmacológicos de analgesia, 521
- sorológicos, 939
Metrite, 1897
Metronidazol, 1589
Miastenia gravis, 1475, 2158
- adquirida, 1467
- congênita, 1468
- formas fulminantes e focais de, 1467
- generalizada, 1467
Micção espontânea, 406
Micetoma, 1057
Micobactérias
- de crescimento lento, 923
- de crescimento rápido, 924
Micobacteriose, 922
- saprofítica, 923
- tuberculosa, 922
Micofenolato de mofetil, 703, 820
Micoplasma, 866
- hemotrópicos, 957
Micotoxicose, 133
Microalbuminúria, 1930
Microambiente tumoral, 2065
Microbioma, 798
- colônico, 1578
- do intestino delgado, 1527
- intestinal, 1500
Microbiota
- gástrica, 1506
- intestinal, 1500
Microrganismo(s), 917
- do tipo *Helicobacter*, 1475
Microscopia, 939
Midazolam, 570, 571
Mielofibrose primária, 863
Mieloftise, 864
Mielografia, 439, 441
- complicações da, 441
Mieloma múltiplo, 2103, 2104
Mielopatia degenerativa, 1442
Mielossupressão, 864, 2085
Mielotoxicose, 864
Migração errática, 1341
Milbemicina oxima, 1331
Minerais, 727, 730, 754, 772
Mineralização brônquica, 1111
Mineralocorticoides, 1844, 1849
Miocardiopatia hipertrófica obstrutiva, 1211
Miocardite, 1284
- atrial, 1284
Mioclonia, 130
Mioglobinúria, 282
Miopatia(s), 94
- associadas a doenças endócrinas, 2179
- congênitas (estruturais), 2177
- inflamatórias, 2175
- mitocondriais e anormalidades de armazenamento de lipídios, 2178
- necrosante, 2176
- visceral e impactação cecal, 1598
Mioquimia, 130
Miosite
- de músculo(s)
--- extraocular, 2176
--- mastigatórios, 1483, 2175
- infecciosa, 2176
- por corpúsculo de inclusão, 2176
Miostatina, 745
Miotonia, 128, 1815
- congênita, 2179
Miringotomia, 334, 337
Mirtazapina, 1954
Miscelânea de líquidos, 633
Misoprostol, 1513, 1954
Mitotano, 1827
Mitoxantrona, 2068
Mitramicina, 1739
Mixedema, 1757

Modelo(s)
- de gato feral, 731
- experimentais de asma felina, 1117
- "meat-in-the-box", 1080
Modificação da dieta, 1563
Modo(s)
- de herança, 26
- de movimento, 391
Modulação
- de nutrientes específicos, 769
- dos sinais de dor, 515
- nutritiva da imunidade, 816
Momento
- da inseminação, 445
- da ovulação e manejo do sêmen, 1872
- dos sopros cardíacos, 219
Monitoramento
- ambulatorial, 387
- cardíaco, 1946
- contínuo da pressão arterial
-- pacientes anestesiados, 374
-- pacientes conscientes, 374
- da frequência respiratória em repouso, 1185
- da glicemia em amostra de sangue obtida da veia auricular, 306
- da progesterona, 1873
- das intervenções nutricionais, 723
- de "entradas e saídas", 410
- do diabetes melito, 1791
- do hormônio luteinizante, 1873
- doméstico, 1793
- e ajuste da terapia para insuficiência cardíaca, 1183
- fetal e uterino, 1894
- glicêmico contínuo, 1793
Monitores de útero e fetos, 609
Monoartropatias, 75
Morbilivírus, 1026
Mordida ou picada
- de cobra, 653
- por animais peçonhentos, 653
Morfina, 570, 571, 706
Morfologia espermática, 1907
Morte
- associada ao uso de medicamentos, 718
- tecidual, 70
Motilidade, 1527, 1578
- espermática, 1907
- gástrica, 1505
- intestinal, 1542
Motilina, 1852, 1853
Motivação, 1373
Movimentos
- anormais, 131
- oculares, 140
Moxidectina, 1331
Mucinose, 54
Muco
- das vias respiratórias, ou respiratórias, 1070
- do cólon, 1577
Mucocele
- biliar, 1692
- de vesícula biliar, 1675
Mucosas, 536, 799, 1576
Mudança(s)
- na composição da dieta, 740
- no apetite, 746
- no nível de consciência, 1431
Multiplicação anormal e neoplasia, 71
Mutação
- *missense*, 28
- *nonsense*, 28
Mycoplasma, 1125, 1905
- *cynos*, 1010
- *haemofelis*, 958

N

N-acetilcisteína, 628, 1633
N-metil histamina, 1541
Nadir, 2085
Nalbufina, 570, 571, 706
Naloxona, 570, 571, 628
Nanismo hipofisário, 51, 1722
Nanophyetus salmonicola, 1552

Narcolepsia, 1421
- canina primária, 1421
Narcolepsia-cataplexia, 1421
Narinas, 1068
Nariz, 152, 1067
Nasofaringe, 1068, 1073
Nasofaringoscopia, 116
Náuseas e vômito, 1431
Nebulização, 367
- indicações para a, 367
- limitações da, 368
Nebulizadores, 367
Necessidades
- de manutenção, 732
- proteicas para cães atletas, 729
Necrólise epidérmica tóxica, 1482
Necrose
- adrenocortical induzida pelo trilostano, 1825
- epidérmica metabólica, 52
- felina hipocampal, 1471
- gástrica por pressão, 326
Nefrite
- de Lyme, 919
-- em cães, 920
- hereditária, 1990, 2006
Nefrolitíases, 499
Nefrolitotomia endoscópica, 499
Nefropatia, 2158, 2191, 2192
- crônica do aloenxerto, 1958
- diabética, 1796
- membranosa, 1986
- por imunoglobulina A, 1987
Nefrotoxicidade, 2090
Nefrotoxinas, 1941, 1942
Neoplasia(s), 63, 95, 356, 829
- auricular, 1067
- biliares, 1691
- comumente surgem do plexo braquial, 1461
- de base do coração, 1316
- de células da ilhota secretoras de insulina
    no gato, 1783
- de intestino grosso, 1595
- de mediastino, 1157
- de próstata, 2060
- de útero, 2151
- do intestino delgado, 1533, 1569
- do pâncreas exócrino, 1712
- do saco anal, 1613
- do tronco encefálico e cerebelo, 1435
- e tumores nasofaríngeos não malignos, 1075
- esofágicas, 1496
- gástrica, 1523
- gastrintestinais, 1572
- hepáticas, 1684
- intracraniana, 1398
-- primárias, 1398
- malignas, 272
- metastáticas, 59
- mieloproliferativa, 863
- peniana, 1910
- perianal, 1613
- relacionadas às meninges, 1398
- retal, 1607
- vesical primária, 2055
Neorickettsia
- *elokominica*, 1552
- *helminthoeca*, 954, 1552
- *risticii*, 955
Neorriquetsioses, 954
Neospora caninum, 972
Neosporose, 972
Nervo(s)
- abducente, 1427
- acessórios, 1428
- cranianos, 1379, 1426
- facial, 1381, 1428
- glossofaríngeo, 1428
- oculomotor, 1427
- óptico, 1426
- periféricos sensoriais, 1386
- peroneal comum, 443
- trigêmeo, 1381, 1427
- troclear, 1427
- vago, 1428
- vestibulococlear, 1428

Neurite
- do plexo braquial, 1463
- óptica, 1426
Neuroanatomia funcional, 1429
Neurofisiologia, 1369
Neurolocalização, 1431
Neurônio(s)
- entéricos, 1529
- motor inferior/sistema neuromuscular, 1386
Neuropatia(s), 94
- autonômicas, 1464
- cranianas, 1426
- diabética, 1796
- facial, 1428
- idiopáticas diversas, 1464
- paraneoplásica, 1462
- periférica, 1460, 1801, 2158
- trigeminal, 1427
Neuroplasticidade, 515
Neurotoxicidade, 2090
Neurotransmissores, 131
Neutralização da toxina não ligada, 932
Neutropenia imunomediada, 862
Niacina, 768
Niacinamida, 704
Nistagmo, 1430
Nitrogênio ureico sanguíneo, 246, 1625, 1817
Nitroprussiato, 1180
Nível de consciência, 139
Nocardia, 926
Nocardiose, 922, 926
Nocicepção, 1379
Noctúria, 1963
Nódulo(s)
- esplênico, 890
- piogranulomatosos/infecciosos, 54
Nomenclatura dos marca-passos, 1211
Normospermia, 1913
Normovolemia, 287, 288
Novas terapias para doença inflamatória
    intestinal, 1565
Núcleos cartilaginosos retidos, 2162
Nutracêuticos, 709
- na doença hepática, 755
Nutrição, 746
- de cães e gatos geriátricos saudáveis, 733
- e imunidade, 813
- em cuidados intensivos, 791
- enteral complicações da, 326
- neonatal e pediátrica, 724
- para cães adultos saudáveis, 725
- para o gato adulto saudável, 730
- parenteral, 793

O

Obesidade, 732, 736, 769, 788, 816, 1082,
    1695, 1880
- como inflamação crônica de baixo grau, 738
- comorbidades associadas à, 2201
- e hipertensão arterial sistêmica 660
- e hormônios reprodutivos, 738
- impacto sobre a(s) doença(s)
-- cardiovascular, 2202
-- musculoesqueléticas e do disco
    intervertebral, 2202
-- respiratória, 2201
Observação
- da alimentação e ingestão de líquidos, 1488
- do animal de estimação e encontro com seu
    cuidador, 4
Obstrução
- da faringe, 1080
- da sonda, 327
- de via(s) respiratória(s), 1093
-- inferiores, 574
-- intranasal em braquicefálicos, 1079
-- superiores, 573
- do fluxo
-- de ar, 1071
-- ventricular, 1237
- funcional da uretra, 2051
- intestinal, 1573
- tubular, 1911
- ureterais, 1951, 2013

- benignas, 500
-- em gatos, 2048
-- malignas, 504
Obtenção
- da amostra de sangue capilar com lanceta
-- a vácuo, 307
-- convencional, 306
- de acesso vascular, 579
- do máximo de uma biopsia de pele, 338
- dos fatos, 2
- e processamento do espécime de biopsia
    renal, 1984
Obturação do lúmen, 1075
Oclusão
- da uretra distal, 413
- de defeito de septo, 479
- do desvio postossistêmico complicações após, 1666
- periventricular de defeito de septo ventricular, 481
Octreotida, 1782
Odontomas, 1485
Odor(es)
- corporais, 105
- desagradável no animal, 106
- normais, 106
Óleo de melaleuca, 633
Oligodendroglioma, 1399
Oligoelementos, 1808
Oligozoospermia, 1912
Oligúria, 1948
Ollulanus tricuspis, 1519
Olsalazina, 1589
Omeprazol, 1954
Ondansetrona, 1954
Ondas F, 1195
Onicodistrofia lupoide simétrica, 874
Online Mendelian Inheritance in Animals
    (OMIA), 29
Opiáceos, 644
Opioides, 520, 569, 644, 705
Opistótono
- descerebelado de rigidez, 1375
- descerebrado, 1375
Organofosforados, 632
Órteses, 2183
Oslerus osleri, 1121
Osmolalidade, 262, 281, 590
- urinária, 1932
Osmolaridade, 262
Ossificação incompleta, 2162
Osteoartrite, 738, 787
Osteoartropatia hipertrófica, 2163
Osteocondrite dissecante, 2162
Osteocondrose, 786
Osteocondrossarcoma
    multilobular, 2137
Osteodistrofia
- fibrosa, 1484
- hipertrófica, 2162
Osteopatia
- craniomandibular, 1484, 2162
- hipertrófica, 2158
Osteossarcoma, 1485
- apendicular
-- em cães, 2128
-- em gatos, 2138
Osteotomia bular lateral, 1064
Otimização
- da frequência e do ritmo cardíacos, 1183
- do desenvolvimento musculoesquelético, 2171
- dos regimes de administração com princípios
    PK-PD, 687
Otite(s)
- eritematosa, 1059
-- ceruminosa, 1059
-- estenosante, 1059
-- externa, 1059
-- crônica eritematosa ceruminosa, 1062
-- supurativa, 1063
- interna/média, 1432
- pegajosa, 1059
Oto-hematoma, 1066
Otocaríase, 1066
Otoendoscopia complicações da, 337

Índice Alfabético

Otoscopia, 334
Ototoxicose, 1067, 1434
Ovariectomia prévia, 1886
Ovário-histerectomia, 1885, 1895, 1902
Oxalato de cálcio, 779, 2025
- di-hidratado, 2022
- monoidratado, 2022
Óxido nítrico, 1169
Oxigenação, 529, 1118
- *versus* ventilação, 371
Oxigênio transtraqueal, 548
Oxigenoterapia, 546
- nasal de alto fluxo, 548
Oximetria, 525
- de pulso, 210, 370
Oximorfina, 706
Oximorfona, 570, 571

P

P-glicoproteína, 32
Pacotes de oxidação de alimentos, 633
Padrão(ões)
- de absorção de luz, 370
- de ingestão de água, micção e defecação, 3
- de referência, 44
- irregulares da ciclicidade ovariana, 1869
- pulmonares
-- alveolares, 1097
-- brônquicos, 1097
- respiratório(s), 1093
-- paradoxal, 1093
Painéis entéricos fecais, 963
Paintball, 633
Palidez, 203
Palpação
- da tireoide, 1763
- de feto na cúpula vaginal, 609
- do colo uterino (cérvice) em cadelas, 446
Pálpebra, 56
Pamidronato, 628, 707, 1776
Pan-hipoproteinemia, 123
Pâncreas, 1704, 1817
- exócrino, 1709
Pancreatite, 1695, 1810
- aguda, 752, 1695
- aguda grave, 1699
- crônica, 1696
-- branda, 1701
- em cães, diagnóstico e tratamento, 1697
- em gatos, diagnóstico e tratamento, 1702
Paniculite nodular estéril, 54
Panleucopenia felina, 1469
Panosteíte, 785, 2162
- esosinofílica, 785
Pantoprazol, 1954
Papilomas, 1484, 2107
Papilomavírus canino, 1017
Paracetamol, 641, 1679
Parada
- atrial, 1205, 1209
- cardiopulmonar diagnóstico de, 576
- e reanimação cardiopulmonares, 576
Paradoxo da obesidade, 742
Parafimose, 611
Paragonimus kellicotti, 1120
Paralagenidiose, 1054
Paralisia, 135, 137
- da laringe em gatos, 1088
- de laringe em cães, 1085
- do carrapato, 1465
- facial, 1428
- laríngea, 1428
- periódica, 2179
Parâmetros
- e testes de função hepática, 1625
- farmacocinéticos, 681
Parasitas
- de parênquima pulmonar, 1120
- de vias respiratórias, 1121
Parasiticidas compostos, 695
Parassístole ventricular, 1201
Paratireoidectomia cirúrgica, 1739
Paratormônio, 1730, 1736, 1737, 1744
Parede torácica, 120, 1159

Parênquima pulmonar, 119
Paresia, 135, 137, 1375
Parte cervical da traqueia, 1096
Parto, 1868
- normal, 1892
- prematuro, 1890
Parvovirose, 1475
Patela
- alta, 2161
- baixa, 2161
Patogênese da febre, 193
Patógenos
- bacterianos que causam pneumonia bacteriana, 1125
- protozoários, 1905
PCR
- em tempo real, 898
- fluorogênico, 898
- para heterobilharzia americana, 1476
- para *Tritrichomonas foetus*, 1476
Pectus excavatum, 1159
Penetração
- do medicamento em outros tecidos, 686
- tecidual dos antibióticos, 686
Penetrância, 28, 30
Pênfigo
- foliáceo, 871
- paraneoplásico, 52, 872
- vulgar, 871
Penfigoide
- bolhoso, 872
- de membrana mucosa, 872, 875
Pênis, 1906, 1910
Pentatrichomonas hominis, 1594
Peptídio(s)
- inibitório gástrico, 1852
- natriuréticos, 1119, 1167
- semelhante ao glucagon-1, 738, 1852
Percepção
- da dor, 1379
-- visceral, 516
- dos sinais da dor, 515
Perda
- de peso, 86, 1534
- gestacional, 1889
-- tardia, 1890
Perfil
- bioquímico
-- clínico, 183
-- sérico, 1562, 1751, 1817, 1845, 2001
- de coagulação, 1655
- hormonal, 1864, 1865
- molecular (*molecular fingerprinting*), 1541
Perfuração
- colônica, 1598
- intestinal, 1574
Perfusão sanguínea aos tecidos, 614
Perguntas para o caso de queixa clínica vaga, 3
Pericardiocentese, 382, 383
Pericardite
- constritiva, 1322
- idiopática, 1317
- infecciosa, 1317
Período(s)
- pós-parto imediato, 1895, 1921
- refratário, 1214
- singulares de vulnerabilidade, 2064
Peritônio, 1615
Peritonite, 1615
- biliar, 294
- infecciosa felina, 864, 989, 990, 1469, 1650
- pelo sêmen, 1888
Permeabilidade intestinal, 1541, 1559
Peróxido de hidrogênio, 627
Persistência de ducto arterioso, 474, 1220
- com hipertensão pulmonar e *shunt* da direita para a esquerda, 1224
- com *shunt* da esquerda para a direita, 1222
Perturbação luminal, 1531
Peso corporal, 536
Pesquisa de vírus, 1909
Peste bubônica, 1126
Petéquias, 214
Petiscos, 741
pH, 281, 526

- gástrico, 1512
- urinário, 1933
Physaloptera spp, 1519
Pica, 49
Picada de aranha-marrom, 655
Picos da placa terminal, 444
Pielonefrite, 2000
Pigmentação, 72
Pilomatricoma, 2109
Pimobendana, 1180, 1181, 1182, 1311
Piometra, 606, 1898, 1899
- de coto uterino, 1902
Piretrinas, 632
Piretroides, 632
Piridínicos, 636
Pirógenos, 193
Piroplasmida, 976
Pitiose, 1053
- gástrica, 1519
Piúria, 283, 1934
Pivalato de desoxicorticosterona, 1849
Placas
- eosinofílicas, 53
- virais hiperpigmentadas, 53
Plano nutricional, 791
Plantas que contêm oxalato, 649
Plasma, 538
- fresco congelado, 538, 1700
- rico em plaquetas, 539
Plasmaférese terapêutica, 423
Plasmocitoma, 2110
- extramedular, 1571
- solitário, 2105
Platinas, 2068
Platinossomose, 1650
Plesioterapia, 2073
Plicamicina, 1739
Pneumocystis carinii, 1127
Pneumomediastino, 1154
Pneumonia
- bacteriana, 1122
- causada por
-- micobactérias, 1125
-- protozoário, 1127
-- *Yersinia pestis*, 1126
- eosinofílica, 1134, 1337
- lipídica, 1135
- micótica, 1127
- por aspiração, 1127
-- e outras complicações, 1088
- viral, 1126
Pneumotórax, 621, 1097, 1150, 1151
- espontâneo, 1152
- iatrogênico, 1152
- por tensão, 1151
- traumático, 1151
Pneumovírus canino, 1010
Podocitopatia, 2006
Poiquilócitos, 229
Polaciúria, 184
Poliadiculoneurite por protozoários, 1462
Poliartrite, 865
- erosiva, 74
- imunomediada, 74, 865
-- idiopática, 865, 868
- não erosiva, 75
- periosteal proliferativa felina, 75
Poliartropatias, 75
- imunomediada(s)
-- erosivas, 870
-- primárias, 867
--- não erosiva, 867
- infecciosas, 866
- secundárias a estímulo imunogênico distante ("reativo"), 867
Policitemia, 225, 849
- primária, 848
- vera (rubra), 863
Policondrite, 874
Polidipsia, 3, 181, 1735, 1963
- primária, 1726
Polifagia, 101
Poligangliorradiculoneurite sensorial, 1463
Poligênico, 25

Polimiosite imunomediada, 2176
Polimorfismo, 28
Polineuropatia
- inflamatória desmielinizante crônica, 1463
- motora de origem desconhecida em gatos
    jovens, 1472
Polioencefalomielite felina, 1472
Polipectomia, 483
Polipeptídio amiloide da ilhota, 1798
Polipeptidoma pancreático, 1855
Pólipo(s)
- colorretal adenomatoso, 1597
- inflamatórios nasofaríngeos, 1075
- nasofaríngeos, 1433
Polirradiculoneurite aguda, 1462
Poliúria, 3, 181, 1735, 1963
Pontos de contato com a mucosa intranasal, 1080
Pool de soro de adultos, 539
Portovenografia, 1658
Posaconazol, 690, 692
Posição e movimento dos olhos, 1381
Postura, 1094, 1375
Potássio, 267, 589, 591, 773, 1849
Potência estatística, 35
Potencial(is)
- de ação, 1370
-- da unidade motora, 444
- de equilíbrio para potássio, 1369
- de fibrilação e ondas agudas positivas, 444
- de placa terminal em miniatura, 444
- de repouso de membrana, 1369
- hemostático global, 826
Poxvírus, 1024
Pralidoxima, 628
Prazosina, 2040
Pré-anestésicos, 1895
Pré-parto, 1921
Pré-síncope, 124
Prebióticos, 1503, 1548, 1565
- fruto-oligossacarídeos, 748
Precipitação do cálcio, 275
Predição da fertilidade, 1908
Prednisolona, 840, 1565
Prednisona, 1565
Pregabalina, 146, 520
Pregas vocais, 1082
Prepúcio, 1910
Prescrição da radiação, 2073
Pressão
- arterial, 373, 536
- hidrostática, 530
- intracraniana aumentada, 1387
- parcial de oxigênio, 530
- sanguínea, 94, 659, 1764, 1946
-- sistêmica, 1858
- venosa central, 1946
Priapismo, 1919
Primeira bulha cardíaca, 217
Princípio(s)
- da distribuição e farmacocinética de
    medicamentos, 677
- da física do ultrassom, 388
- da intenção de tratar, 36
- da oximetria de pulso, 370
- e práticas
-- da quimioterapia, 2066
-- de radiologia oncológica, 2073
- farmacocinético-farmacodinâmicos, 687
Probióticos, 709, 711, 753, 1503, 1548, 1549,
    1565, 1588
Problemas
- da medicina veterinária baseada em evidências, 34
- na cobertura, 1886
- na gestação, no parto e no periparto em cães e
    gatos, 1888
Procarbazina, 2067
Procedimento
- de Bougienagem, 483
- de dilatação por balão, 482
- e análise de amostras de líquido
    cefalorraquidiano, 441
- guiados por ultrassom, 347
- para biopsia nervosa, 443
Processo sensorial, 1373

Proclorperazina, 1954
Proctite, 1605
Produtos
- de degradação de fibrina[ogênio], 822, 825
- de uso doméstico, 632
- domésticos comuns prejudiciais a cães e
    gatos, 633
- tóxicos utilizados em oficinas, 634
Proestro, 1863, 1869, 1882
Progestágenos, 1884
Progesterona, 1868
Programação
- da amplitude do pulso e da amplitude da
    voltagem, 1213
- da frequência, 1214
- do marca-passo, 1213
Programas de controle antimicrobiano, 908
Progressão
- de doença cardíaca para insuficiência cardíaca, 1164
- tumoral, 2064
Projeção dos sinais de dor, 515
Prolactina, 1868
Prolapso
- da uretra, 2048
- retal, 1608
- uterino, 1896
Prolongamento do tempo de sangramento na
    mucosa bucal, 310
Propentofilina, 1425
Propilenoglicol, 635
Propofol, 570, 572
Proporção albumina/globulina, 1625
Propranolol, 1776
Propulsão extensora, 1376
Prosencéfalo, 1381
Prostaglandinas, 1874, 1885, 1900, 1902
Próstata, 345, 406, 1906, 1909
Prostatite bacteriana
- aguda, 2058
- crônica, 2059
Proteína, 726, 749, 769, 815, 1973
- C reativa, 738, 1477
- de baixo peso molecular, 1934
- de coagulação, 1628
- de fase aguda positivas e negativas, 239
- e aminoácidos, 730
- relacionada com o paratormônio, 1731, 1736, 1737
- tubulares, 1934
Proteinúria, 281, 1929
Próteses, 2183
Protetores
- /adsorventes, 1510
- ao epitélio, 1501
Protocolo(s)
- de radioterapia, 2074
- imunossupressor, 820
- terapêuticos paliativos versus definitivos, 2075
Prototheca spp, 1593
Protozoários, 1553, 1593
Pseudo-obstrução intestinal, 1572
Pseudoefedrina, 642
Pseudogestação, 1868, 1883
Ptialismo, 147
Puberdade, 1882, 1910
Pulmões, 152
Pulso
- paradoxal, 1316
- venoso, 224
Punção
- arterial, 298, 375
- aspirativa com agulha fina, 428
- venosa e arterial, 297
Purificação do sangue, 421
Púrpura pós-transfusão, 545
Pythium insidiosum, 1053, 1593

Q
Quadro tóxico versus não tóxico, 65
Qualidade
- de sêmen ruim, 1911
- do produto, 710
- seminal pobre, 1887
Queda episódica em cães da raça Cavalier King
    Charles Spaniel, 129

Queimaduras orais, 1483
Queixa inespecífica de falha no
    desenvolvimento, 43
Quelação do cálcio, 275
Quelantes intestinais, 1974
Queratócitos, 229
Quilo, 81
Quilotórax, 1150
Quimioproteção, 2071
Quimiorradioterapia, 2067
Quimioterapia, 1404, 2066
- combinada com outras modalidades
    terapêuticas, 2067
- e imunoterapia inalatória, 370
- e radioterapia, 2078
- estratégias para, 2066
- intra-arterial, 510
- metronômica, 2070, 2126
- neoadjuvante, 2067
- sistêmica
-- em cães com linfoma de grau intermediário e
    alto, 2096
-- em gatos com linfoma de grau intermediário e
    alto, 2098

R
Radiação, 201
- com feixe externo, 1776, 2073
Radiocirurgia
- estereotática, 1826
- estereotáxica, 2073
Radiografia, 1277
- abdominal, 598, 882, 1509, 1628, 1818
- cervical e torácica, 1489
- de contraste, 1542
- do crânio, 114
- do tórax, 1096
- do trato respiratório superior, 1096
- simples, 1542
- torácica, 1301, 1818
Radiologia
- intervencionista, 455
- oncológica, 2073
Radioterapia, 1403, 2125
- adjuvante, 2077
- clínica, 2074
- conformacional 3D, 2073
- de intensidade modulada, 2073
- estereotáxica, 2073
- guiada por imagem, 2073
- hipofisária, 1835
- paliativa, 2075, 2130
- para hiperadrenocorticismo hipófise-
    dependente, 1826
- para linfoma, 2099
- pré-cirúrgica, 2078
Raiva, 1002
Ramipril, 1180, 1309
Ramo do circuito de reentrada, 1207
Ranitidina, 1954
Raquitismo, 784
Raspados de pele, 337
- profundos, 338
- superficiais, 337
Razões para a interrupção da gestação, 1874
RC:CU/TSADD combinados, 1820
RC:CU/TSBDD combinados, 1820
Reabilitação, 2179
Reação(ões)
- à vacina, asma e pele, 1881
- adversas
-- a medicamentos, 716
-- ao trilostano, 1825
-- aos alimentos, 801, 1555
- alérgicas à transfusão, 545
- de hipersensibilidade, 2091
- de imunocomplexo, 545
- em cadeia da polimerase, 929, 964
-- de material fecal, 1541
-- para provírus do vírus da leucemia felina, 988
- imunológicas, 545
- metabólicas, 1557
- posturais, 1376
- transfusionais, 544

-- agudas não imunológicas, 545
-- diagnóstico e tratamento de, 545
-- imunológicas agudas, 544
-- tardias, 545
Reanimação
- cardiopulmonar com tórax aberto, 581
- inicial, 552, 553
- volêmica, 535
Reaquecimento complicações associadas ao, 203
Reavaliação uma avaliação nutricional, 725
Recesso maxilar, 1078
Recomendações gerais de alimentação, 727
Reconhecimento das bactérias na mucosa, 1502
Redução
- da formação de trombos, 1353
- da ingestão de calorias, 740
- da secreção de ácido, 1513
- da vida útil do eritrócito, 843
- do débito cardíaco, 1178
- do volume pré-carga, 1176
- na produção de eritrócitos, 227
Reflexo(s)
- bicipital e tricipital, 1378
- de aspiração mecanossensitivo, 1070
- de Bezold-Jarisch, 126
- de retirada/flexor, 1378
- de tosse, 108
- de vômito, 1381
- espinais, 1378
- extensor cruzado, 1379
- musculocutâneo, 1379
- patelar, 1378
- perineal, 1379
Refluxo gastresofágico, 1499
Região(ões)
- geográfica, 3
- nasal e facial, 1096
Registro do eletrocardiograma, 386
Regulação
- da secreção de ácido, 1505
- térmica por meio de respiração ofegante, 1073
Regulamento dos alimentos para animais de
    estimação, 811
Regurgitação, 157, 159
- aórtica, 1233
- da tricúspide causada por doença mixomatosa da
    valva, 1259
- das valvas pulmonar e aórtica, 1232
- mitral, 1266
- mitral causada por doença mixomatosa da valva
    mitral, 1258
- pulmonar, 1232
- tricúspide, 1266
Reidratação, 1947
Reincidência, 356
Rejeição crônica, 1958
Relação
- corticoide:creatinina urinária, 1819, 1834
- cortisol:ACTH endógeno, 1846
- proteína:creatinina urinária, 1930
Remifentanil, 706
Remoção
- da fonte de infecção, 932
- de fezes impactadas, 1601
- de sondas de esofagostomia gastrostomia e
    GEP-J, 325
- de urólito, 2023
Remodelamento cardíaco, 1169
Reovírus felino, 1025
Repelentes inseticidas, 1332
Repetibilidade e reprodutibilidade na
    ecocardiografia veterinária, 399
Repetição do tratamento, 695
Reprocessador automático para endoscópio, 330
Reprodução felina clínica, 1882
Requerimentos nutricionais para imunidade, 814
Requisitos
- de energia, 726
- para a obtenção de um histórico detalhado, 2
Resfriamento físico, 198
Resinas de trocas, 1952
Resistência
- à insulina, 739
- antimicrobiana, 906, 907

-- em pequenos animais, 906
- aos fármacos quimioterápicos, 2072
- aos medicamentos antiparasitários, 695
- insulínica, 1797
- tumoral, 2069
Resistina, 737
Resolução, 46
Respiração, 1815
- com a boca aberta/postural, 1092
Resposta(s)
- cerebral à lesão, 1387
- de linfócitos T e B, 1530
- de posicionamento da pata e de colocação
    tátil, 1376
- dermatológicas
-- em cães, 802
-- em gatos, 803
- empírica aos antibióticos, 1559
- endócrina às enfermidades graves, 555
- gastrintestinais em cães e gatos, 804
- imunes
-- adquiridas do tecido linfoide associado ao
    intestino, 1530
-- na nutrição, 816
- imunológicas inatas do intestino delgado, 1530
- motoras esqueléticas, 141
- pupilares, 140
- terapêutica, 2071
Ressecção da parede lateral do canal auditivo
    vertical, 1064
Ressonância magnética, 116, 1098
Restrição
- antimicrobiana, 908
- dietética de PO4, 1974
- e modificação da dieta, 1510
Resultados
- de triagem da glicemia, 1799
- do teste genético, 30
-- heterozigoto positivo, 30
-- homozigoto positivo, 31
-- negativo, 30
Retenção de fósforo, hiperfosfatemia e
    hiperparatireoidismo secundário renal, 1973
Retina, 58
Retirada de cálculos do trato urinário inferior com
    cesto endoscópico, 490
Reto, 1576
Retropulsão de urólitos em cães machos com
    obstrução, 2049
Rhuepo® versus darbepoietina, 1979
Rim(ns), 345, 348, 406, 2192
- hipoplásicos, 2004
Rinite, 1073
- alérgica, 1073
- bacteriana, 1073
- linfoplasmocitária, 1073
- viral, 1073
Rinoscopia, 116, 123, 364
Riquetsioses
- em gatos, 957
- transmitidas por carrapatos, 955
Riscos aos tutores de animais, 2072
Ritmo(s)
- de escape, 1187
- juncional, 1187
- de parada
-- chocáveis, 579
-- não chocáveis, 581
- idioventricular acelerado, 1199
- sinoventricular, 1206
Rodenticidas, 630
Rododendros, 650
Ronco, 1082
Rotação, 391
Rotavírus, 1025
- canino, 1018
Ruídos (knocks) pericárdicos, 218
Ruptura(s)
- da barreira epitelial, 1532
- da bexiga, 625
- da pelve renal, 625
- de uretra, 625
- do átrio esquerdo e, 1272
- do vaso sanguíneo/ hematomielia, 1456
- gastrintestinal, 294

- uterina, 1896
- viscerais ou vasculares, 294

S
S-adenosilmetionina, 1632, 1633
S. aureus resistente à meticilina, 906
S. pseudintermedius resistente à meticilina, 906
Saculite, 1612
Sagu-de-jardim, 1683
Saída nasal, 1068, 1070
Sais
- biliares não conjugados, 1542
- de degelo, 634
- de urato, 2022
Sala para angiografia, 456
Salmonella spp., 966, 967, 1475, 1551, 1593
Saltitar, 1376
Sangramento oral e hemostasia, 1480
Sangue, 80, 282
- oculto, 1541
- total
-- armazenado, 538
-- fresco, 538
Sarcoma(s)
- associados
-- à injeção, 2112
-- a vacinas, 2111
- de tecidos moles, 2111
-- com características clínicas particulares em
    cães, 2116
-- em cães, 2115
-- em gatos, 2117
- histiocítico, 888, 1400
-- disseminado, 2146
-- hemofagocítico, 2147
-- localizado, 2146
- não angiomatosos não linfoides do baço, 888
Sarcopenia, 742, 744
Saturação de oxigênio da hemoglobina, 530
Sazonalidade, 1882
Sazonalidade dos ciclos estrais, 1863
Secreção
- de insulina reduzida, 1798
- ectópica de hormônio adrenocorticotrófico, 1813
- nasal, 112, 1070, 1091
- prepucial, 178, 180
- vaginal, 178
-- mucopurulenta em cadelas e gatas
--- não castradas, 178
--- submetidas a ovariectomia, 180
-- serossanguinolenta em cadelas e gatas
--- após ovariectomia, 178
--- não castradas, 178
-- vulvar, 178
-- hemorrágica, 453
Secretina, 1851, 1852
Sedação e anestesia em pacientes em unidade de
    tratamento intensivo, 569
Sedativos/hipnóticos, 644
Sedimentação fecal, 317
Segunda bulha cardíaca, 217
Segurança, 710
- alimentar
-- de animais de estimação, 812
-- e aspectos regulatórios de alimentos, 811
Seio(s)
- esfenoide, 1078
- nasais, 152
- paranasais, 1077
Selamectina, 1332
Seleção empírica de medicamentos
    antibacterianos, 684
Selênio, 815
Sensação de Ortolani, 2170
Sensibilidade, 1214
- analítica, 893
- cutânea, 1378
- diagnóstica, 893
Sensibilização, 514
- periférica, 515
Separação septal do ponto, 403
Sepse, 523, 549, 550, 829, 1944
- grave, 549
- nasal, 1068

Serotonina, 1853
Sevoflurano, 571
Shunt da direita para a esquerda, 1218
Sialadenite, 1484
Sialadenose, 1484
Sialocele, 1484
Sialometaplasia necrosante, 1484
Siderócitos, 229
Sildenafila, 1181
Silêncio atrial, 1205
Sílica, 2022, 2029
Silimarina, 1633
Simbióticos, 1503, 1504, 1548
Sinal(is)
- anabólicos reduzidos, 745
- clínicos de insuficiência cardíaca, 1172
- de insuficiência cardíaca congestiva, 1302
- de Ortolani, 2170
- gastrintestinais da uremia, 1975
- ortopédicos, 72
Sinapse, 1371
Síncope, 124
- cardiogênica, 125
- neurocardiogênica, 126
- vasovagal, 126, 1209
Síndrome(s)
- braquicefálica, 1078
- da angústia respiratória aguda, 549
- da câimbra epileptoide em cães da raça Border
  Terrier, 129
- da degeneração retiniana adquirida súbita, 1816
- da disfunção múltipla de órgãos, 549
- da dor orofacial felina, 1473
- da negligência, 1383
- da resposta
-- anti-inflamatória compensatória, 551
-- inflamatória sistêmica, 523, 549, 753
- da serotonina, 639
- da veia cava, 1339
- de Chédiak-Higashi, 860
- de disfunção cognitiva, 1422
- de Ehlers-Danlos, 54
- de Fanconi, 1997, 2007
- de fragmentação de hemácias, 838
- de Horner, 1426, 1429, 1461
- de imunoendocrinopatias, 1750
- de neutrófilos aprisionados, 860
- de pré-excitação e macrorreentrada, 1207
- de Schiff-sherrington, 1384
- de Scott, 832, 858
- de tremor generalizado de início
-- agudo, 133
-- crônico, 134
- de tremor, 132
- de von Willebrand adquirida, 857
- de Wolff-Parkinson-White, 1208
- do definhamento neonatal, 1924
- do hormônio adrenocorticotrófico ectópico, 2156
- do intestino
-- curto, 1574
-- irritável, 1574, 1600
- do macrotumor, 1818
- do ovário remanescente, 1902, 1916
- do seio
-- doente, 1189, 1209
-- sinusal doente, 1208
- do tremor generalizado idiopático, 134
- epiléptica, 1404
- hepatocutânea, 1622
- hiperglicêmica hiperosmolar, 587, 590
- leproides, 925
- miastênicas congênitas, 2178
- mielodisplásica(s)
-- primária, 862
-- secundárias, 863
- mielodisplásica-blastos em excesso, 862
- mielodisplásica-citopenia refratária, 862
-- com displasia multilinhagem, 862
- nefrítica, 1983
- paradoxal, 1431
- paraneoplásicas, 64, 2155
-- cutâneas, 2157
-- diversas, 2158
-- gastrintestinais, 2157

-- hematológicas, 2156
-- neurológicas, 2158
-- relacionadas ao sistema endócrino, 2155
-- renais, 2158
-- serotoninérgica, 97
- uveodermatológica, 873
- vestibular pós-anestésica em gatos, 1436
Sintomas
- neuro-oftálmicos, 140
- neurológicos, 591
Sistema(s)
- cardiovascular, 1764
- de avaliação da condição corporal
-- do cão, 12
-- do gato, 13
- de condução cardíaca, 1186
- de monitoramento contínuo da glicose, 1802
- de termorregulação, 1070
- gastrintestinal, 430, 737, 1765
- imune gastrintestinal, 1528
- nervoso
-- central, 899, 1815
--- e trato urinário, 614
-- periférico, 1386
- porta hipotálamo-hipofisário, 1812
- reprodutor, 445
- sensitivo e comportamental, 1375
- urinário, 1764
Sobrecarga
- de ferro, 1676
- de fluidos, 537
Sobredose de insulina e contrarregulação da
  glicose, 1795
Sobrepeso, 1880
Sódio, 262, 589, 772, 1849, 1952
- corporal *versus* quantidade de água, 262
Sólidos totais, 1946
Solução
- carreadoras de oxigênio, 537
- de albumina, 538
- de flutuação, 313
- de problemas de produção contínua de ar, 379
Somatostatina, 1852, 1853
Sondas
- colocadas por meio de esofagostomia, 320
- de alimentação enteral e dispositivos de
  acesso, 319
- de gastrostomia, 322
- de jejunostomia, 323
- nasoesofágicas, 319
Soníferos, 639
Sono normal, 1419
Sons
- cardíacos
-- anormais, 217
-- transitórios, 217
- de ejeção, 218
- pulmonares, 18
- respiratórios, 1094
-- audíveis, 1092
Sopros cardíacos, 217, 218
- contínuos, 221
- diastólicos, 220
- fisiológicos e inocentes, 220
- sistólicos, 219
Sorologia, 962
Sotalol, 1309
Split heat, 1870
SPO$_2$ *versus* SAO$_2$, 370
Sporothrix schenckii, 896, 1051
SRIS, 549
Stents, 460
- intraluminais, 1494
- metálicos, 460
-- autoexpansíveis, 460
-- expansíveis por balão, 460
-- não metálicos, 460
-- ureterais, 461, 500
Streptococcus equi subespécie
  zooepidemicus, 1010, 1125
Strongyloides
- spp., 1553
- *tumefaciens*, 1553, 1595
Suabe, 1099
Subdose de insulina, 1795

Subinvolução de sítios da placenta, 1896
Substâncias tremolíticas, 131
Substituição
- de tubos de gastrostomia e esofagostomia, 325
- molar, 532
Sucção
- contínua, 378
- de flanco, 49
- intermitente, 378
Suco duodenal, 1543
Sucralfato, 1954
Sulfassalazina, 1589
Sulfonamidas potencializadas, 1681
Sulfonilureias, 1807
Supercrescimento bacteriano do intestino
  delgado, 1557
- secundário, 1558, 1559, 1560
Suplementação
- com T4, 1756
- de ferro, 847
- de potássio, 536
- de taurina, 1298
- de vitaminas
-- B, 536
-- e minerais, 756
- nutricional para o manejo de doenças de pele, 782
Suplementos
- de L-carnitina, 741
- nutricionais, 709
Suporte(s), 2183
- avançado à vida, 578
- básico à vida, 576
- de fluidos, 1515
- de nutrição enteral com baixo teor de
  gordura, 765
- nutricional, 791, 792, 1954, 2194
Suposição de distribuição normal, 38
Supositórios retais, 1601
Supressão do estro, 1876
Suprimentos alimentares, 710
Surdez, 1066
- neurossensorial
-- adquirida, 1067
-- congênita, 1066
- pós-inflamatória, 1067
Suspeitas de quadro tóxico *versus* não tóxico, 65
Swabs nasais, 123

T
T4
- livre, 1766
- total e livre, 1766
Tabaco, 652
Talas, 2183
Tamanho
- da amostra, 35
- do coração, 401
Tampões, 526
- uretrais de matriz cristalina, 2048
Tamponamento cardíaco, 586, 1272
Tansulosina, 2040
Taquiarritmias, 585, 1209
Taquicardia(s)
- atriais, 1192
- sinusal, 1191
- ventricular, 1199
Taquipneia, 116
Taurina, 769, 1298, 1311
Taxa
- de filtração glomerular, 1927, 1928, 1943
- de infusão contínua, 304
Tecido(s)
- adiposo, 736
- linfoide associado a mucosa, 1529
- mole no abdome, 79
Técnica(s)
- com Doppler ultrassônico, 376
- com pinça curva De Carmalt, Mixter ou
  Schnidt, 320
- de amplificação de ácido nucleico, 897
- de citologia de linfonodos, 362
- de diagnóstico
-- de anormalidades da próstata, 426
-- laboratorial, 1095

- de *flow-by*, 547
- de flutuação fecal, 312
- de inseminação artificial em cadelas, 446
- de mensuração da pressão arterial, 374, 375
- de oscilometria de alta definição, 376
- de Seldinger, 299
- e complicações da gastrostomia
-- endoscópica percutânea, 322
-- percutânea às cegas, 323
- ecocardiográficas especiais, 399
- imunológicas, 897
-- e moleculares, 318
- oscilométrica, 375
- para a colocação de *stent* uretral, 508
- para TAE/TACE hepática, 511
- percutânea(s)
-- guiadas por ultrassom e complicações, 1646
-- utilizando cateter com agulha, 321
-- utilizando aplicador percutâneo de sonda de
   alimentação, 321
Telomerase, 2064
Temperatura normal, 194
Tempo
- de coagulação ativado, 825
- de preenchimento capilar, 536
- de protrombina, 825
- de relaxamento isovolumétrico, 405
- de sangramento
-- da cutícula, 824
-- da mucosa bucal, 309, 824
- de trombina, 825
- de tromboplastina parcial ativada, 825
- para concentração plasmática máxima, 682
Tenesmo, 171, 173
Tênias, 1553
Terapia(s)
- adjuvante para choque endotóxico e lesão por
   reperfusão, 1515
- analgésica, 705
- anti-inflamatória, 696
- antibacteriana, 198, 1565
- antiemética, 1975
- antifúngica e antiviral, 689
- antimicrobiana, 1547
- antineoplásica complicações da, 2085
- antiparasitária, 693
- baseadas em incretinas, 1808
- com calcitriol, 1979
- com hemocomponentes, 537
- com heparina, 1336
- de alcalinização, 581
- de hemocomponentes, 857
- de reindução ou resgate, 2098
- de reposição renal, 1950
-- extracorpórea, 1951
- de suporte avançado à vida, 579, 581
- dietética, 1972
- para pancreatite aguda, 752
- fracionada, 2074
- gênica, 2081
- glicocorticoide, 1849
- hídrica, 590
- imunossupressora, 701
-- para anemia hemolítica imunomediada, 821
- intervencionistas
-- gastrintestinais, 482
-- minimamente invasivas, 455
-- neoplásicas, 507
-- no sistema
--- cardiovascular, 469
---- respiratório, 462
-- urológicas, 489
- médica para distocia, 1894
- medicamentosa, 819
- microfilaricida, 1336
- mielossupressora, 851
- molecular
-- direcionada, 2127
-- dirigida, 2082
- orexígena, 1975
- por radionuclídeo, 1776
- precoce alvo-direcionada, 535
- renal substitutiva contínua, 421, 422
- respiratória e inalatória, 367

- transfusional, 854
- trombolítica, 829
Terapia-padrão da doença glomerular, 1991
Teratozoospermia, 1913
Terbinafina, 691
Terceira e a quarta bulhas cardíacas, 217
Terminologia
- genética importante, 25, 28
- PK-PD, 687
- radiológica comum, 2073
Termorregulação no cão, 1070
Termoterapia, 2180
Teste(s)
- bioquímicos, 1859
- da função da tireoide, 1751
- de "cabeceira" e limpeza, 329
- de absorção intestinal, 1541
- de aglutinação
-- direta, 836
-- em tubo, 929
-- microscópica, 947
-- rápida em lâmina, anticorpo e imunodifusão em
   gel de ágar, 929
- de antígenos, 1540
- de audição, 1066
- de Brucella, 1871
- de células de lúpus eritematoso, 880
- de citotoxicidade em cultura celular, 965
- de coagulação, 822, 825, 839
- de compatibilidade, 540
- de diagnóstico, 907
- de dieta de exclusão, 1556
- de discriminação em cães com
   hiperadrenocorticismo, 1820
- de DNA, 27, 856
- de eletrodiagnóstico, 1490
- de estimulação
-- por ACTH, 1819, 1846
-- por hormônio
--- adrenocorticotrófico, 1672, 1834
--- liberador de tireotrofina, 1767
- de fibrinogênio e fibrinólise, 825
- de flutuação
-- direta, 314
-- pós-centrifugação, 314
- de fragilidade osmótica, 835
- de função
-- hepática, 1655, 1686
-- plaquetária, 215, 824
-- pulmonar, 1115
-- renal, 589
-- tireoidiana, 1817
--- dinâmicos, 1760
- de hipótese, 34
- de imunofluorescência, 948
-- para pesquisa de antígeno do vírus da leucemia
   felina, 987
- de linha basal, 1401
- de permeabilidade gastrintestinal, 1477
- de pH, 1490
- de plaquetas e da parede vascular, 824
- de privação
-- de água modificado, 184
-- hídrica, 1933
--- modificado, 1727
- de provocação, 782
- de reação
-- em cadeia da polimerase, 948, 962
-- postural, 1376
- de respiração, 1542
- de resposta à atropina, 1188
- de rotina, 1086
- de secreção gástrica, 1510
- de supressão
-- com baixa dose de dexametasona, 1820
-- por alta dose de dexametasona, 1820
-- por dexametasona, 1834
-- por T3, 1767
- de suscetibilidade, 685
- de tiroxina total e livre, 1765
- de vazamento, 329
- diagnósticos para detecção de exposição à doença
   de lyme, 919
- diversos de atividade bacteriana, 1542
- do acetato de desmopressina, 184

- do ácido sulfossalicílico, 1930
- do eixo adrenal, 1846
- endócrinos, 1819, 1833
- específicos da função renal, 1943
- genéticos, 1306
-- na doença renal, 1932
-- para hiperparatireoidismo primário em cães da
   raça Keeshond, 1738
-- tipos de, 31
- hemostático, 827
- hormonais basais no contexto de informação
   clínica, 1754
- imunodiagnósticos para pesquisa de antígenos, 1326
- indiretos
- especiais, 1541
-- para SBID/DRA, 1559
- para autoanticorpo antitireoglobulina, 1752
- para distinguir hiperadrenocorticismo hipófise-
   dependente de hiperadrenocorticismo
   adrenal-dependente, 1834
- para doenças
-- específicas, 1944
-- infecciosas, 602
- para enteropatia com perda de proteínas, 1542
- para hormônio tireoestimulante, 1752
- para mensuração
-- de hormônios tireoidianos totais, 1751
-- de paratormônio, 1730
- para o vírus da leucemia felina, 986
- para pesquisa de anticorpos contra o vírus da
   leucemia felina, 988
- provocativos, 1854
- rápido
-- de fragilidade osmótica, 835
-- para pesquisa de antígeno do vírus da leucemia
   felina, 987
- sorológicos, 1556
- terapêutico com desmopressina, 1728
- úmido hiposmótico, 1908
Testículos, 1906
Tetania, 129
Tétano, 129, 930
Tetraciclina, 704, 1681
Tetralogia de Fallot, 1248
TFG estimada, 1928
Tiazolidinediona, 1808
Timoma, 1159
Tiopronina, 2027
Tiopurina metiltransferase, 31
Tipo selvagem, 28
Tireoidectomia cirúrgica, 1770
Tireotrofina endógena, 1760
Tiroxina
- livre, 1760
- total, 1760, 1765
Títulos de anticorpos, 993
TNF-α, 738
Toceranib, 2082
- na doença metastática microscópica, 2083
Tolerância, 710
- à glicose, 1799
- da mucosa, 1530
- prejudicada à glicose e pré-diabetes melito, 1799
Tolypocladium inflatum, 701
Tomografia computadorizada, 115, 1097, 1928
- abdominal, 886
- do crânio, 1389
- do tórax, 1097
Tonsilas, 152
Tônus muscular, 1378
Toracocentese, 382, 1147
Torção, 391
- de lobo esplênico e hepático, 605
- de lobo pulmonar, 1139
- de testículo, 612
- e ruptura do útero, 610
Torovírus, 1026
Torsade de pointes, 1201
Torsemida, 1178
Tosse, 108, 1092
- devido à compressão do brônquio principal
   esquerdo, 1270
Toxascaris leonina, 1552
Toxemia da gestação, 1891

Toxicidade(s)
- aguda da radiação, 2075
- ao trato urinário, 2090
- como reação, 717
- do metronidazol, 1436
- teciduais, 2074
- urotelial, 2091
Toxicologia, 627
Toxicose, 1436
- de estrógeno na cadela ovariectomizada, 1916
Toxinas de células vermelhas, 837
Toxocara
- *canis*, 1552
- *cati*, 1552
Toxoplasma gondii, 973
Toxoplasmose, 973
Tradução, 25
Tramadol, 706, 707
Transcrição, 25
Transdução, 513, 514
Transfusão(ões), 846
- consequências adversas das, 544
- de grandes volume, 545
- de hemácias, 562
- de plaquetas, 540
- indicações para, 539
- massivas, 545
- sanguíneas, 537
Trânsito intestinal, 799
Translação, 391
Transmissão
- de estimulação, 1370
- e processamento no corno dorsal, 515
- natural e condição de vacinação, 1004
- por contato, 1004
Transpeptidase, 256, 259
Transplante
- de microbiota fecal, 1504
- fecal microbiano, 1588
- renal, 1956, 1958
-- em gatos, 1956
Transporte axonal, 1372
Transposição das grandes artérias, 1252
Transtornos
- de comportamento, 46
- de motilidade, 1521
- neurológicos exclusivos de felinos, 1469
Transudação, 290
Transudato
- com alto teor proteico, 290
- com baixo teor proteico, 290
- modificado, 79, 1149
- puro, 79, 1149
Traqueia, 1083
Traqueíte/traqueobronquite infecciosa, 1106
Tratamento
- com agentes de volume uretral em casos de
    insuficiência do mecanismo do esfíncter, 494
- com antídoto, 628
- com intuito curativo, 2066
- com medicamentos antibacterianos, 684
- de exposição a toxinas, 627
- medicamentoso expulsivo, 2011
- paliativo, 2066
Trato(s)
- gastrintestinal, 1500
- internodais, 1186
- respiratório, 1091
Trauma
- de microchip, 1454
- iatrogênico, 1434
- torácico, 618
Traumatismo
- craniano, 1436
- cranioencefálico, 615
- do trato urinário, 624
- do ureter, 2014
- torácico, 1137
Tremor(es), 131
- associado a neuropatia periférica, 135
- cerebelar, 134
- cinético
-- de tarefa específica, 132
-- intencional, 132
-- simples, 132

- de ação postural, 132
- de cabeça episódico, 130
- de intenção, 1384
- de repouso, 132
- fisiológico, 133
-- exacerbado, 133
- fisiopatologia do, 131
- isométrico, 132
-- de membros, 134
- ortostático primário, 134
- paroxístico da cabeça idiopático, 135
Trepanação temporária e infusão, 1044
Triancinolona transendoscópica, 1494
Trichuris spp, 1595
Tricoblastoma, 2109
Tricoepitelioma, 2109
Trientina (2,2,2-tetramina), 1635
Triglicerídeos, 248, 1817
- de cadeia média, 754
Trilostano, 1823, 1825, 1835
Tripanossomíase, 975
Tripeptídio muramil encapsulado em lipossomo, 2080
Tritrichomonas foetus, 1594
Troglostrongylus spp, 1121
Trombocitemia
- essencial, 863
- primária, 238
Trombocitopatia, 122
- adquiridas, 310
- hereditárias, 310
Trombocitopenia(s), 214, 234, 2156
- classificação da, 236
- hereditárias, 237
- imunomediada, 851, 852
-- e anemia hemolítica imunomediada simultâneas
    em cães, 855
-- felina, 855
-- primária, 852
-- secundária, 852
- infecciosas, 236
Trombocitose, 234, 2157
- classificação da, 238
- diagnóstico de, 238
- secundária, 238
Tromboelastografia, 822, 826, 1932
Tromboelastometria, 822, 826
Tromboembolismo, 1993
- aórtico em gatos, 586
- arterial, 1351
- pulmonar, 1140, 1141, 1145
Trombografia automatizada calibrada, 822
Tromboprama calibrado automatizado, 826
Trombopatias, 215
Tromboprofilaxia, 840
Trombose na gestação, 1889
Tronco encefálico, 1383, 1388
Trypanosoma cruzi, 975
TSH sérico, 1766
Tuberculose, 1552
Tubos de toracostomia, 377, 1147
Túbulos renais, 1995
Tumor(es)
- adrenal(is), 1818
-- descoberto ao acaso, 1859
-- secretores
--- de aldosterona, 1838
--- de hormônios sexuais, 1841
- adrenocorticais, 1827
-- funcionais, 1813, 1818, 1820
--- concomitantes, 1813
-- não secretores de cortisol, 1836
-- secretores de hormônios sexuais
--- em cães, 1842
--- em felinos, 1841
- apendiculares em gatos, 2138
- articulares
-- em cães, 2138
-- em gatos, 2139
- astrocíticos, 1398
- axiais em gatos, 2138
- benignos
-- do baço
--- canino, 889
--- felino, 889

-- do estômago, 1523
-- *versus* malignos, 342
- cerebrais
-- primários, 1398, 1402
-- secundários, 1401
- cutâneos, 2106
- da bainha
-- de nervo periférico, 1485
-- nervosa, 1461
- da região
-- pineal, 1398
-- selar, 1398, 1400
- das meninges, 1398
- de adrenal e hipertensão arterial sistêmica, 661
- de captação e descarboxilação de precursores da
    amina, 1572
- de células
-- basais, 2108
-- distintas, 2110
-- germinativas, 1398
-- granulares, 1400
-- meningoteliais, 1398
-- musculares lisas do estroma, 1572
-- redondas, 2110
- de costelas, 2136
- de crânio, 2135
- de ductos biliares, 1685
- de escápula, 2135
- de glândula(s)
-- apócrina, 2109
-- ceruminosas, 2109
-- hepatoide, 2109
-- mamária, 2152
-- perianal, 2109
-- sebáceas, 2109
-- sudorípara, 2109
- de mastócitos, 889, 1513
-- em cães, 2140
- de meninges, 1399
- de origem neuroepitelial, 1399
- de pelve, 2135
- de próstata, 2150
- de tecido neuroepitelial, 1398
- de testículo, 2151
- do canal auditivo ou orelha média, 1434
- do plexo coroide, 1398, 1399
- do trato urogenital e da glândula mamária, 2147
- embrionários, 1398
- ependimários, 1398
- epiteliais, 2107
- estromal gastrintestinal, 2116
- extradurais, 1458
- hematopoéticos, 2092
- hepático, 1684
- hepatocelulares, 1684
- hipofisários grandes, 1827
- intradurais/extramedulares, 1458
- intramedulares, 1459
- intratraqueais, 1106
- malignos, 1524
-- do baço canino, 887
-- do baço felino, 889
- mamários
-- em cadelas, 2153
-- em gatas, 2154
- melanocíticos, 2110
- mensenquimais, 1398
-- e outros, 1686
-- maciços solitários e outros, 1687
-- metastático(s), 1400
-- do baço
--- canino, 889
--- felino, 889
-- na ressonância magnética, 1402
- nasais, 1073
-- benignos, 1073
- nasofaríngeos, 1073
- neuroendócrinos, 1685, 1855
- neuroectodérmico primitivo, 1399
- neuronais e neuronais-gliais mistos, 1398
- oligoastrocíticos, 1398
- oligodendrogliais, 1398
- orais
-- benignos, 1484
-- malignos, 1485

- ósseos
-- axiais em cães, 2135
-- e articulares, 2128
-- metastáticos, 2138
- secretores
-- de aldosterona
--- em cães, 1840
--- em felinos, 1838
-- de insulina, 1777
-- de mineralocorticoides que não a
    aldosterona, 1841
- sinonasais, 1073
- venéreo transmissível, 2110
- vertebrais, 2136
Turgor cutâneo, 536

U

Ulceração, 1511
- gastrintestinal, 2157
- neurogênica do cólon, 1598
Úlceras de contato, 1481
Ultrassom
- de emergência, 598
- terapêutico, 2181
Ultrassonografia, 1098
- abdominal, 343, 346, 426, 883, 1509, 1543, 1583, 1656, 1686, 1832, 1858
-- total, 598
- com avaliação focalizada no trauma, 620
- contrastada, 1818
- da tireoide, 1755
- e aspirado com agulha fina guiado por ultrassom, 1645
- escrotal, 1908
- hepática, 1628
Umidificação, 548
Urato, 780, 2031
Ureaplasma, 1905
Ureia, 246, 1928
- nitrogenada sanguínea, 1966
Uremia, 1961
Ureteres, 2009
- ectópicos, 2014, 2045, 2053
-- extramurais, 2053
-- extravesiculares, 2053
-- intramurais, 498, 2053
-- intravesiculares, 2053
Ureterocele, 2015, 2054
Ureterólitos, 2010
- de estruvita em cães tratamento de, 2011
Ureteroscopia com eletrocauterização, 506
Uretra, 2147
- ectópica, 2047, 2056
Uretrite, 2052
Uretrolitíase, 2048
Uretroscopia, 415
Urina, 81, 188
- amarelo-clara, 189
- de aspecto branco-leitoso, 192
- normal, 189
- vermelha, marrom ou preta, 189
Urinálise, 1765, 1817, 1832, 1845, 1932
Uroabdômen, 294
Urografia
- excretora, 1937
- intravenosa, 1937
Urolitíase, 778
- causada por cálculo
-- de cistina, 2032
-- de purinas, 2031
-- de urato, 2031
-- de xantina, 2032
- no trato urinário inferior
-- de cães, 2021
-- de gatos, 2030
Urólito(s)
- aparência radiográfica dos, 2023
- compostos, 2029
- de estruvita, 2032
- de oxalato de cálcio, 2033
- de sílica e compostos mistos, 2032
- de xantina, 2029
- prevalência de, 2021
- prevenção de formação de, 2025

Uroperitônio, 624
Uroquinase, 1353
Urospermia, 1911
Uso racional de antimicrobianos, 1480
USP, 715
Útero, 345
- em anestro, 1869
Uvas, 652

V

Vacina tipos de, 901
Vacinação, 3
- de animais de companhia, 900
- prévia com FEL-O-VAX vírus da imunodeficiência felina, 982
Vacina(s)
- contra câncer, 2081
- contra doença de Lyme, 922
- essenciais, 902
-- para cães, 902
-- para gatos, 904
- não essenciais, 902
-- para cães, 903
-- para gatos, 905
- não recomendadas para cães, 904
Vaginite em cadela madura, 180
Vaginoscopia
- durante o proestro, 452
- e citologia
-- durante o estro, 452
-- vaginal em cadelas, 449
Validade, 35
Valor
- preditivo de um teste
-- negativo, 893
-- positivo, 893
- mitral e câmaras cardíacas do lado esquerdo, 1262
- tricúspide e câmaras cardíacas do lado direito, 1265
Valvuloplastia
- aórtica por balão, 477
- pulmonar por balão, 470
Varfarina, 1355
Variabilidade, 35
Variante(s)
- de DNA, 29
- da paniculite pancreática, 54
Varredura(s)
- com tecnécio-99m, 1756
- de tomografia computadorizada, 1490
Vasculite, 1889
Vasodilatadores pulmonares, 1181
Vasopressina, 1724
- arginina, 1725
Vasopressores, 581
Vasos linfáticos do cólon, 1576
Velocidade de condução nervosa, 443, 445
Venodilatadores, 1179
Venopunção, 297
Ventilação, 578
- com pressão positiva, 623
- por pressão inspiratória positiva, 548
Ventrículos, 1082
Vértebra(s)
- bloqueadas, 1449
- de borboleta, 1448
- transicional, 1449
Vesícula
- biliar, 1688
- pulmonar, 1139
- urinária, 345
Vestíbulo nasal, 1068
Vestibulovaginite crônica, 1914
Vestígios vestibulovaginais, 496
Vetsulin Caninsulin®, 1802
Via(s)
- acessória, 1207
- ascendentes da dor, 515
- de administração de quimioterápicos, 2070
- de nutrição, 816
- endócrinas, 739
- inflamatórias, 739
- internodais, 1186

- respiratórias, 152
-- de pequeno calibre, 119
-- nasofaríngea, 1067
-- superiores, 119, 620
- urinárias, 406
Vigilância, 906
- imune, 2079
- imunológica, 1578
Vimblastina, 2068
Vincristina, 2068, 2089
Vinorelbina, 2068
Víru(s)
- da cinomose canina, 1009
- da doença
-- de Aujeszky, 1018
-- de Borna, 1023
--- felina, 1471
- da imunodeficiência felina, 693, 897, 1471, 1650
-- gatos doentes infectados por, 983
-- gatos saudáveis infectados por, 983
- da influenza canina, 1009
- da leucemia felina, 693, 1471, 1650
- da parainfluenza canina, 1009
- do Nilo ocidental, 1019
- espumoso felino, 1025
- influenza, 1126
- sincicial felino, 1025
Visão e respostas pupilares à luz, 1379
Visfatina, 737
Vitamina, 727, 731, 730, 754, 773
- A, 787, 815
- B$_6$, 2027
- B$_{12}$, 1477
- D, 1731, 1740
- D$_2$, 642
- D$_3$, 642, 1731
- do complexo B, 773
- E, 815, 1633, 1634
- K$_1$, 628
Vitiligo, 873
Volume(s)
- de distribuição, 682
- e taxas de administração, 533
- globular, 964
- sistólico, 402, 403
- ventricular esquerdo, 403
Vólvulo intestinal, 1574
Vômito, 159, 160
- crônico e alimentação parenteral, 753
- do conteúdo gástrico e intestinal, 1509
Voriconazol, 690, 692

W

Wolbachia pipientis, 1336

X

Xantinas, 285, 780, 2022, 2031
Xantomas, 53
Xilitol, 634, 1683

Y

Yersinia enterocolitica, 1593
Yersinia
- *pestis*, 1126
- *pseudotuberculosis*, 1552

Z

Zidovudina, 693
Zigomicose, 1055
Zinco, 815, 1635
Zonisamida, 146
Zoonoses, 909, 929
- causadas por
-- mordida ou arranhão, 913
-- vetores compartilhados, 916
- de ambiente compartilhado, 917
- do trato urogenital, 915
- entéricas, 909
- oculares e de trato respiratório, 914
- por exposição e exsudatos, 912
Zootoxicoses, 653